EMERGENCY AND TRAUMA CARE FOR NURSES AND PARAMEDICS

FOURTH EDITION

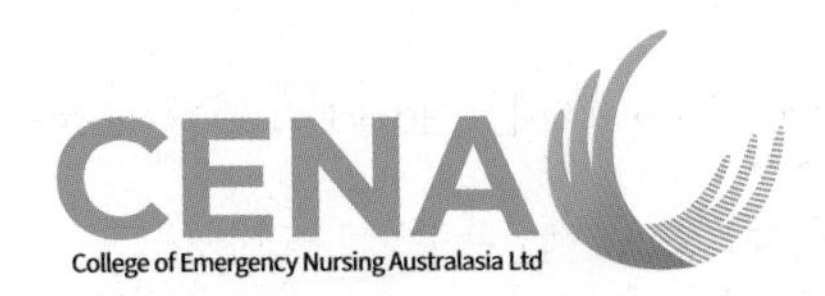

Endorsed by the College of Emergency Nursing Australasia (CENA)

CENA is the peak professional association representing emergency nurses across Australasia.

EMERGENCY AND TRAUMA CARE FOR NURSES AND PARAMEDICS

FOURTH EDITION

Kate Curtis RN, GradDipCritCare, MNurs(Hons), PhD, FCENA

Professor Emergency and Trauma Care, University of Sydney, NSW, Australia

Director Emergency and Critical Care Research, Illawarra Shoalhaven Local Health District, Warrawong, NSW, Australia

Registered Nurse, Wollongong Hospital Emergency Department, Wollongong, NSW, Australia

Honorary Professorial Fellow, The George Institute for Global Health, Sydney, NSW, Australia

Margaret Fry RN, NP, BSc(Nurs), MEd, PhD, FCENA

Professor Emergency and Critical Care, University of Technology Sydney, Sydney, NSW, Australia

Northern Sydney Local Health District Nursing and Midwifery Directorate, Sydney, NSW, Australia

Adjunct Professor, University of Sydney, Sydney, NSW, Australia

Senior Editor, Australasian Emergency Care, College of Emergency Nursing Australia, Sydney, NSW, Australia

Bill Lord AM, BHlthSc(Pre-HospCare), GradDipCBL, MEd, PhD, FACPara

Adjunct Associate Professor, Department of Paramedicine, Monash University, Frankston, Victoria, Australia

Adjunct Professor, Australian Catholic University, Faculty of Health Sciences, North Sydney, NSW, Australia

Director, Australasian College of Paramedicine, Sydney, NSW, Australia

Co-Deputy Chair, Paramedicine Accreditation Committee, AHPRA

Clair Ramsden RN, GradCertCardiol, MHCE, MHServMgt

Executive Director Clinical Services, Opal HealthCare, Australia

Ramon Z. Shaban BSc(Med), BN, GradCertInfCon, PGDipPH&TM, MEd, MCommHealthPrac(Hons1), PhD, RN, FCENA, FACN, FACIPC, CICP-E

Clinical Chair of Communicable Diseases Control and Infection Prevention, Sydney Institute for Infectious Diseases and Susan Wakil School of Nursing and Midwifery, Faculty of Medicine and Health, University of Sydney, Sydney, NSW, Australia

Clinical Chair of Communicable Disease Control and Prevention and Infection Prevention, Public Health Unit, Centre for Population Health, Western Sydney Local Health District, North Parramatta, NSW, Australia

Director and Chief Infection Control Practitioner, Western Sydney Local Health District, Westmead, NSW, Australia

Associate Director, New South Wales Specialist Service for High Consequence Infectious Diseases, Westmead, NSW, Australia

Editor-in-Chief, Australasian Emergency Care, College of Emergency Nursing Australia, Sydney, NSW, Australia

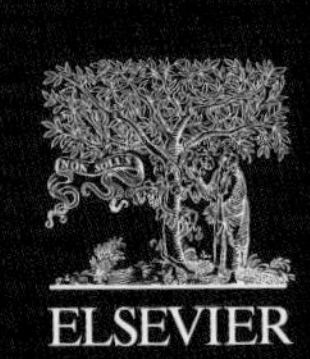

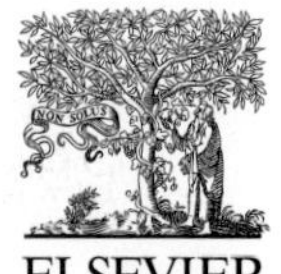

Elsevier Australia. ACN 001 002 357
(a division of Reed International Books Australia Pty Ltd)
Tower 1, 475 Victoria Avenue, Chatswood, NSW 2067

ISBN: 978-0-7295-4441-2

Notice

Practitioners and researchers must always rely on their own experience and knowledge in evaluating and using any information, methods, compounds or experiments described herein. Because of rapid advances in the medical sciences, in particular, independent verification of diagnoses and drug dosages should be made. To the fullest extent of the law, no responsibility is assumed by Elsevier, authors, editors or contributors for any injury and/or damage to persons or property as a matter of products liability, negligence or otherwise, or from any use or operation of any methods, products, instructions or ideas contained in the material herein.

National Library of Australia Cataloguing-in-Publication Data

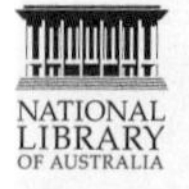

A catalogue record for this book is available from the National Library of Australia

Content Strategist: Melinda McEvoy
Content Project Manager: Fariha Nadeem
Edited by Margaret Trudgeon
Proofread by Annabel Adair
Cover and Internal Design by Natalie Bowra
Index by Innodata Indexing

Typeset by GW Tech

Printed in China by 1010 Printing International Ltd

Last digit is the print number: 9 8 7 6 5 4 3 2 1

CONTENTS

PREFACE

Emergency and Trauma Care for Nurses and Paramedics 4e is a comprehensive, contemporary, practical and evidence-based resource for emergency and trauma nurses, paramedics and other healthcare workers, and students working in urban, rural and remote settings. It provides everyday clinicians with invaluable information relevant to their local practice environment that is informed by best-available global evidence. Our 93 contributing authors are recognised practitioners of standing in Australia or Aotearoa New Zealand, and were chosen for their expertise to ensure relevant, practical information.

Emergency and Trauma Care for Nurses and Paramedics 4e is organised into four sections. Section 1 comprehensively documents the foundations and development of paramedic and emergency and trauma nursing practice, as well as the fundamentals of emergency care, including quality and safety, ethics, leadership and patient education. Section 2 addresses the clinical and health service system concepts of scene assessment, patient assessment, triage and the physiology of emergency care, and contains a chapter featuring essential clinical skills, which are cross-referenced throughout this edition. Section 3 then explores contemporary recognition and management of specific body system emergencies, including cardiovascular, respiratory, neurological and endocrine. Other areas of emergency are also covered in depth, including toxicology, envenomation and ocular and environmental emergencies, as well as end-of-life care. Emergency care for unique population groups, including older adults, disabled people, obstetric and paediatric patients, is also presented. Section 4 provides a detailed review on major trauma assessment and management, examining trauma systems, trauma assessment and trauma to specific body regions.

Throughout the 49 chapters, cross-references are made to other areas of the text that are of relevance. The 547 figures and 264 tables actively support the hands-on clinical approach of the text. Clinical assessment, physiology, decision-making and rationale for interventions of common and not-so-common emergency presentations are provided. Case studies are provided at the end of each chapter to enable consolidation of knowledge for practice.

Emergency and Trauma Care for Nurses and Paramedics 4e reflects expert knowledge, published research and literature available at the time of production. It is important that readers continue to search for the most recent sources of appropriate information to guide their practice. To assist the reader in this, useful websites are also provided at the end of each chapter. Feedback from readers is welcome to facilitate the growth and development of the disciplines of emergency and trauma care and the professions who practise it.

We commend *Emergency and Trauma Care for Nurses and Paramedics 4e* to you in support of our shared efforts to provide high-quality, safe, effective and timely emergency care for patients and their families.

Kate Curtis
Margaret Fry
Bill Lord
Clair Ramsden
Ramon Z. Shaban
July 2023

ACKNOWLEDGEMENTS

A textbook of this size requires the professional dedication and personal support of many clinical and organisational leaders. An incredible amount of expert knowledge, clinical expertise and academic work is necessary to ensure the content is comprehensive and correct, and that the book is completed within specified timeframes. The editors would like to thank:

- the chapter contributors, some of whom have written for the first time. Their patience, persistence, expertise and knowledge are greatly valued. This book has been written by an extremely skilled expert group of clinicians and academics.
- the team at Elsevier, in particular, Fariha Nadeem and Margaret Trudgeon.

On a more personal note, we would particularly like to thank our partners (George, Jason, Sally and Judy), children (Sarah, Beatrix, Edward, Grace and Lewis, Aimee and Aaron), family and friends who have endured the many months of hard work and have been tremendously patient and encouraging. You have our sincere appreciation and gratitude.

CONTRIBUTORS

David Anderson MBChB, FCICM
Medical Director, Medical Directorate, Ambulance Victoria, Melbourne, Victoria, Australia
Intensivist, Department of Intensive Care and Hyperbaric Medicine, The Alfred Hospital, Melbourne, Victoria, Australia
Adjunct Senior Lecturer, Department of Paramedicine, Monash University, Melbourne, Victoria, Australia

Natalie Anderson RN, BHSc, BA, MSc(Hons), PhD
Senior Lecturer, School of Nursing, Faculty of Medical and Health Sciences, Auckland, Aotearoa New Zealand
Registered Nurse, Auckland Emergency Department, Te Whatu Ora Te Toka Tumai, Auckland, Aotearoa New Zealand

Glenn Arendts MBBS, MMed, PhD, FACEM
Senior Honorary Research Fellow, Medical School, University of Western Australia, WA, Australia

Ann Bonner RN, BAppSc(Nurs), MA, PhD, MACN, MAICD
Professor and Head of School of Nursing and Midwifery, Griffith University, Brisbane, Queensland, Australia
Honorary Research Fellow, Kidney Health Service, Metro North Health, Brisbane, Queensland, Australia
Honorary Skou Professor, Aarhus University, Aarhus, Denmark
Adjunct Professor, School of Nursing and Midwifery, Queens University Belfast, Belfast, United Kingdom

Leanne Brown RN, NP, MNSc(NP), GradDipAppSc(Nephrology), Grad DipAppSc(Nsg), GradCertHMgt, PhD
Nurse Practitioner, Cape York Kidney Care, Torres and Cape Hospital and Health Service, Cape York, Queensland, Australia
Adjunct Assoc Professor, James Cook University (School of Rural and Remote); Griffith University (School of Nursing and Midwifery), Queensland, Australia
Sessional Academic, Queensland University of Technology, Brisbane, Queensland, Australia

Mary Chiarella AM, RN, RM, LLB(Hons), PhD, FACN, FRSM, HFACNP
Professor Emerita, Susan Wakil School of Nursing and Midwifery, The University of Sydney, Sydney, NSW, Australia
Adjunct Professor, University of South Australia, Adelaide, South Australia, Australia

Lisa Clegg RP, MHlthSc(Ed), PhD, SFHEA
Senior Lecturer, Paramedicine, Head of Discipline (Undergraduate), Charles Sturt University, Port Macquarie, NSW, Australia

Julie Considine RN, RM, CertAcuteCareNurs(Emerg), GDipNurs(AcuteCare), GCertHigherEd, MNurs, PhD, FACN, LFCENA, SFHEA
Professor of Nursing, Deakin University – Eastern Health, Burwood, Victoria, Australia
Director, Centre for Quality and Patient Safety Research – Eastern Health, Box Hill, Victoria, Australia
Senior Editor, Australian Emergency Care, College of Emergency Nursing Australasia, Beaumaris, Victoria, Australia

Dianne Crellin RN, NP, CertEmerg, GradDip(Paeds), MN(Res), PhD, FCENA
Senior Lecturer Nursing, Melbourne School of Health Sciences, The University of Melbourne, Melbourne, Victoria, Australia
Nurse Practitioner, Emergency Medicine Royal Children's Hospital, Melbourne, Victoria, Australia
Research Fellow, Murdoch Children's Research Institute, Melbourne, Victoria, Australia

Benjamin Crook RN, MEd
Clinical Nurse Educator, Sutherland Hospital Emergency Department, Carinbah, NSW, Australia

Kate Curtis RN, GradDipCritCare, MNurs(Hons), PhD, FCENA
Professor Emergency and Trauma Care, University of Sydney, Sydney, NSW, Australia
Director Emergency and Critical Care Research, Illawarra Shoalhaven Local Health District, Warrawong, NSW, Australia
Registered Nurse, Wollongong Hospital Emergency Department, Wollongong, NSW, Australia
Honorary Professorial Fellow, The George Institute for Global Health, Sydney, NSW, Australia

Natalie Cutler RN, GradCertForenMHlth, MNurs(MHlth), MPubHlth, PhD
Senior Lecturer, Assistant Course Director, University of Technology Sydney, Sydney, NSW, Australia
Specialty Performance Assessor, NSW Nursing and Midwifery Council, Sydney, NSW, Australia

Justin Dunlop ASM, CStJ, DipLead&Mgt, AssDipHlthSc, BSc(Hons), GradDipEmergMgt
Director, Emergency Management, Ambulance Victoria, Melbourne, Victoria, Australia

Alan Eade RN, RP, ASM FACPara
Adjunct Associate Professor, Department of Paramedicine, Monash University, Frankston, Victoria, Australia
Chief Paramedic Officer, Safer Care Victoria, Victoria, Australia

Kate Emond RN, PGDipMHlth, MNurs, ACP
Academic Mental Health Nursing and Paramedicine, La Trobe University, Bendigo, Victoria, Australia

Benjamin Fisk BArts, BHSc, GradCertRemHlth, GradCertAeromedRetriev, GradDipEmergHlth(MICA), MPH, PhD
Intensive Care Flight Paramedic, Air Ambulance Victoria, Melbourne, Victoria, Australia

Lesley Fitzpatrick RN, GradDipCritCare, MN(Hons)
Clinical Nurse Consultant, Royal North Shore Hospital Emergency Department, St Leonards, NSW, Australia

Belinda Flanagan PhD, MPH, MMid, GradCertProfLearning, BAppSci(Nurs), AssDipSci (Ambulance), SFHEA
Associate Professor, Head of School, Paramedicine, University of Tasmania, Hobart, Tasmania, Australia

Associate Professor Tracy Flenady RN, BN(Dist), PhD
Deputy Dean (Research), Research Ready Grant Program (RRGP) Program Coordinator, School of Nursing, Midwifery and Social Sciences, CQUniversity Australia, North Rockhampton, Queensland, Australia

David Foley RN, BSc, CertEmergNurs, GradDipAcCare, MNurs, PhD
Program Director Pre-Registration, Course Coordinator and Lecturer, Adelaide Nursing School, University of Adelaide, Adelaide, South Australia, Australia

Margaret Fry RN, NP, BSc(Nurs), MEd, PhD, FCENA
Professor Emergency and Critical Care, University of Technology Sydney, Sydney, NSW, Australia
Northern Sydney Local Health District Nursing and Midwifery Directorate, Sydney, NSW, Australia
Adjunct Professor, University of Sydney, Sydney, NSW, Australia
Senior Editor, Australasian Emergency Care, College of Emergency Nursing Australia, Sydney, NSW, Australia

Mark Goodhew MNurs(MHlth), GradDipPsych, GradDipCouns, PhD
Senior Lecturer, Faculty of Medicine, Nursing & Midwifery and Health Sciences, The University of Notre Dame, Sydney Campus, Darlinghurst, NSW, Australia

Anna Grant RN, GradCertNurs(IntCareN)
Clinical Nurse Consultant Trauma Service, Townsville University Hospital, Townsville, Queensland, Australia

Rachael Elizabeth Grist RN, RM, CNC, BN, GDipMidwifery
Flight Nurse NSW Ambulance, Nurse Immuniser, Clinical Nurse Consultant Communicable Diseases, Hunter New England Health, Newcastle, NSW, Australia

Kellie Gumm CNC, GradCertITU, GradDipHlthProm, MEd
Trauma Program Manager, The Royal Melbourne Hospital, Parkville, Melbourne, Victoria, Australia

Karel Habig MBBS, BSc(Med), FACEM, DipRTM, DipPHR
Prehospital and Retrieval Staff Specialist and Medical Manager, NSW Ambulance Aeromedical Operations, Bankstown, NSW, Australia
Emergency Physician, Northern Beaches Emergency Department, NSW, Australia

Bernie Hiess RN, GradCert(EmergNurs), MN(AdvPrac)
Clinical Nurse Specialist 2, Wollongong Hospital Emergency Department, Wollongong, NSW, Australia

Andrew J. A. Holland BSc(Hons), MB, BS, GradCertEdSt (HEd), PhD, FRCS(Eng), FRACS(Paed), FACS
Professor of Paediatric Surgery, The Children's Hospital at Westmead Clinical School, Sydney Medical School, Faculty of Medicine and Health, The University of Sydney, NSW, Australia
Consultant Paediatric Surgeon, The Children's Hospital at Westmead and Royal North Shore Hospital, Westmead, NSW, Australia
Director, The Children's Hospital at Westmead, Burns Research Institute, Westmead, NSW, Australia

Claire Hutchinson RN, MCN (Emerg), PhD
Nurse Lecturer, Southern Cross University, Coffs Harbour Campus, Coffs Harbour, NSW, Australia
Registered Nurse, Coffs Harbour Emergency Department, Coffs Harbour, NSW, Australia

Kelli Innes RN, BN, GCertEmergNurs, GCertHlthProfEd, MN, PhD, FCENA
Associate Professor, School of Nursing and Midwifery, Monash University, Clayton, Victoria, Australia

Natasha Jennings RN, NP, GradDipAdvNurs, MNurs, PhD, FACN
Nurse Practitioner, Emergency and Trauma Centre, Alfred Health, Melbourne, Victoria, Australia
Director, Nurse Practitioner Locum Solutions, Melbourne, Victoria, Australia

Paul Jennings BN, GradCertBiostats, MClinEpi, AdvDipMICAParaStud, GCHPE, PhD, FACPara
Intensive Care Paramedic and Improvement Lead, Ambulance Victoria, Melbourne, Victoria, Australia
Adjunct Associate Professor, Monash University, Clayton, Victoria, Australia

Tamsin Jones RN, BN(Hons), BHealth Promotion, GradDipCritCareHlth, MHPE, PhD, FCENA
Senior Lecturer, Nursing and Midwifery, Monash University, Clayton, Victoria, Australia

Jessica Keady RN, GradCertHlthMgt, MNurs
Clinical Nurse Consultant Emergency and Critical Care, Western NSW Local Health District, NSW, Australia

Toby Keene PSM, MPH, GradCertAeroMed, GradCertAppMgt, GradDipAppPsych, BSc, BA, MACPara
Registered Paramedic, Research School of Psychology, School of Medicine and Psychology, The Australian National University, Canberra, ACT, Australia

Jeff Kenneally ASM, Reg ICP, BBus, AssDipAppSci (Paramedic), GradCertMICA
Lecturer Paramedicine, Victoria University, Melbourne, Victoria, Australia

Belinda Kennedy RN, BN, GradCertEmerg, MPhil
Project Manager, Susan Wakil School of Nursing and Midwifery, Faculty of Medicine and Health, The University of Sydney, Sydney, NSW, Australia

Kate King RN, BN, MNurs
Clinical Nurse Consultant – Trauma, John Hunter Trauma Service, John Hunter & John Hunter Children's Hospitals, Newcastle, NSW, Australia
Conjoint Senior Lecturer, College of Health, Medicine and Wellbeing, University of Newcastle, NSW, Australia
Senior EMST Coordinator, Royal Australian College of Surgeons, East Melbourne, Victoria, Australia
Trauma Verifier – trauma verification program, Royal Australian College of Surgeons, East Melbourne, Victoria, Australia

Robert John William Knight MBBCh, MRCS, MD, FRACS (Plast)
Consultant Specialist Plastic and Reconstructive Surgeon, Consultant Specialist Craniomaxillofacial and Paediatric Plastic Surgeon, Supervisor of Training, Plastic and Reconstructive Surgery, The Wollongong Hospital, Wollongong, NSW, Australia
Senior Clinical Lecturer, Faculty of Medicine, University of Wollongong, Wollongong, NSW, Australia

Sarah Kourouche RN, BSN, MNurs, PhD
Lecturer Acute Care Nursing, Implementation Science Research Fellow, Susan Wakil School of Nursing and Midwifery, Faculty of Medicine and Health, The University of Sydney, Sydney, NSW, Australia

Russell Krieger GradCertPublichealth, MBChB(Bristol,UK), FACEM
Emergency Staff Specialist, Deputy Director, Royal North Shore Hospital Emergency Department, St Leonards, NSW, Australia

Kelly Lambert BSc(Nutr), MSc(NutrDiet), Grad CertMgt, GradeCertHlthEcon, PhD
Associate Professor, Advanced Accredited Practising Dietitian
Academic Program Director Nutrition and Dietetics
Councillor (elected), International Society of Renal Nutrition and Metabolism
Co-Director, Kidney Lifestyle Research Group, School of Medical, Indigenous and Health Sciences, Faculty of Science, Medicine and Health, University of Wollongong, NSW, Australia

Bill Lord AM, BHlthSc(Pre-HospCare), GDipCBL, MEd, PhD, FACPara
Adjunct Associate Professor, Department of Paramedicine, Monash University, Frankston, Victoria, Australia
Adjunct Professor, Australian Catholic University, Faculty of Health Sciences, North Sydney, NSW, Australia
Director, Australasian College of Paramedicine, Sydney, NSW, Australia
Co-Deputy Chair, Paramedicine Accreditation Committee, AHPRA

Matthew Lutze RN, NP, BN, MN (Critical Care), MN (NP)
Clinical Senior Lecturer, Sydney Nursing School, Faculty of Medicine and Health, University of Sydney, NSW, Australia
Nurse Practitioner, Hornsby Ku-Ring-Gai Hospital Emergency Department, Northern Sydney Local Health District, NSW, Australia
Principal Advisor Nursing Practice, NSW Ministry of Health, St Leonards, NSW, Australia

Sam Maalouf Qualified Ambulance Paramedic, BA(HlthSci)
A/Area Manager 1, Metropolitan Region – Clinical Operations, Ambulance Victoria, Melbourne, Victoria, Australia

Deborough Macbeth BN, MA AppEthics, PhD, CICP-E, PSM
Assistant Director of Nursing, Infection Control, Gold Coast Hospital and Health Service, Gold Coast, Queensland, Australia

James Marshall Dip AmbParaStud, BA (Hons), GradCertClinEd, MPH, MPA
Specialist Paramedic Educator – Ambulance Victoria, Melbourne, Victoria, Australia

Daniel Martin RN, BN, GradCertEmerg, BNursPracEmerg, GradCertNursSciRet, PostGradCertAeromedRet
Director of Nursing, South Australia Ambulance Service MedSTAR Emergency Medical Retrieval, SA, Australia
Adjunct Associate Professor, School of Public Health and Tropical Medicine, James Cook University, Queensland, Australia
Wing Commander, Health Operational Conversion Unit, Royal Australian Air Force

Michelle McCarthy NP, PGradAdvClinNurs(Emerg), MNSc(NP)
Nurse Practitioner, Royal Children's Hospital, Emergency Department, Melbourne, Victoria, Australia

Joanna McCulloch RN, BHlthSci, MANurs(NursePrac), CertOphthalNurs ENB 346, BA(Psych) (RehabCounsel), Cert IV TAE
Clinical Nurse Consultant, Opthalmology, Sydney Eye Hospital, Sydney, NSW, Australia

Debra McDougall RN, BN, GradCertEd, MNurs
Clinical Nurse Consultant – Trauma, John Hunter Trauma Service, Newcastle, NSW, Australia

Leigh McKay RN, BAS (Nursing), GradCertICU, MPH
Education Coordinator, NSW Organ and Tissue Donation Service, Kogarah, NSW, Australia

Tegwyn McManamny ICP, GradDipEmergHlth (ICP), BEmergHlth(Hons), PhD, MACPara
Intensive Care Paramedic, Ambulance Victoria, Melbourne, Victoria, Australia
Teaching Associate, Department of Paramedicine, Monash University, Melbourne, Victoria, Australia

Ben Meadley BAppSc, GradDipICP, GradDipEmergHlth, GradCertAeromed, PhD, FACPara
Adjunct Senior Lecturer, Department of Paramedicine, Monash University, Victoria, Australia
Intensive Care Flight Paramedic, Ambulance Victoria, Victoria, Australia
Improvement Lead, Ambulance Victoria, Melbourne, Victoria, Australia

Eleanor Milligan BSc, BA(Hons), GradDipEd, PhD, FCHSM, GAICD
Professor of Ethics and Professional Practice, School of Medicine and Dentistry, Griffith University, Brisbane, Queensland, Australia
Board Member and Deputy Chair, North West Hospital and Health Board, Queensland, Australia
Board Member and Deputy Chair, Voluntary Assisted Dying Review Board, Queensland, Australia

Brett Mitchell RN, BN, MAdvPrac, DTN, PhD, FACN, FACIPC
Professor of Nursing and Health Services Research, Avondale University, Lake Macquarie, NSW, Australia
Conjoint Scholar, Central Coast Local Health District, Gosford Hospital, Gosford, NSW, Australia
Adjunct Professor of Nursing, School of Nursing and Midwifery, Monash University, Clayton, Victoria, Australia

Julia Morphet RN, GradDipEmerg, GradCertHlthProfEd, MNurs(Ed), GradDipHlthEcon, PhD, FCENA
Professor, Monash University, Clayton, Victoria, Australia
Head of School, Monash Nursing and Midwifery, Clayton, Victoria, Australia

Peter Moules RN, GradCertCritCare, GradCertHlthLeadMgt
Emergency Services Lead, Illawarra Shoalhaven Local Health District, NSW, Australia

Judy Mullan BA, BPharm, PhD, FSHPA
Associate Head of School: Research; Academic Lead: Research and Critical Analysis, Graduate School of Medicine, Science, Medicine and Health Faculty, University of Wollongong, Wollongong, NSW, Australia

Belinda Munroe RN, BN, MNurs(AdvPrac), PhD, FCENA
Emergency Clinical Nurse Consultant, Illawarra Shoalhaven Local Health District, NSW, Australia
Honorary Lecturer, Faculty of Science, Medicine and Health, University of Wollongong, Wollongong

Margaret Murphy RN, GradDipCritCare, GradDipChangeMgt, MHscEd, PhD
Clinical Nurse Consultant, Westmead Hospital Emergency Department, Westmead, NSW, Australia
Co-Director Emergency Research Unit, Westmead Hospital, Westmead, NSW, Australia
Senior Lecturer, University of Sydney, Sydney, NSW, Australia

Ziad Nehme ASM BEmergHlth(Paramedic)(Hons), PhD, FACPara
Director Centre for Research and Evaluation, Ambulance Victoria, Melbourne, Victoria, Australia
Senior Research Fellow and Adjunct Senior Lecturer, Monash University, Clayton, Victoria, Australia
Registered Paramedic, Ambulance Victoria, Melbourne, Victoria, Australia

Meredith Oatley RN, NP GradcertOncology, MNurs(Nurse Practitioner)
Nurse Practitioner Medical Oncology, Northern Sydney Cancer Centre, Royal North Shore Hospital, St Leonards, Sydney, NSW, Australia

Cameron Palmer BOrth(Hons), GradDip(ClinEpi), PhD, CAISS
Trauma Data Manager, Royal Children's Hospital, Melbourne, Victoria, Australia
Adjunct Research Fellow – Clinical Registries, Monash University, Clayton, Victoria, Australia

Alison Partyka RN, MNurs, GradDipCritCare
Acting Clinical Nurse Consultant, Royal North Shore Hospital, Emergency Department, St Leonards, NSW, Australia

James Pearce BHSc(Para), BN, GradCertInfPrevCtrl, MAdvPrac, GradCertHEd, FACPara, FHEA
Senior Lecturer in Paramedicine, College of Medicine and Public Health, Flinders University, SA, Australia
Paramedic, South Australian Ambulance Service, SA, Australia

Amber Preece BSW, MPS
Senior Social Worker, Coffs Harbour Health Campus, Coffs Harbour, NSW, Australia

Linda Quinn RN, GradDipBurns, CertPaed
Burns Advanced Nurse Consultant, Women's and Children's Hospital, Adelaide, SA, Australia

Clair Ramsden RN, GradCertCardiol, MHCE, MHServMgt
Executive Director Clinical Services, Opal HealthCare, Sydney, NSW, Australia

Dr Jamie Ranse RN, PhD, FACN, FCENA
Associate Professor, School of Nursing and Midwifery, Griffith University, Griffith, Queensland, Australia
Disaster Health Lead, Disaster Management Network, Griffith University, Queensland, Australia
Founder, Mass Gathering Collaboration, Griffith University, Griffith, Queensland, Australia
Visiting Research Fellow, Department of Emergency Medicine, Gold Coast Health, Gold Coast, Queensland, Australia

Helen Rawson RN, MSc, BSc(Hons), PhD, MACN, FHEA
Associate Professor, Deputy Head of School, Monash University Nursing and Midwifery, Clayton, Victoria, Australia

Dwight Robinson RN, BN, MAdvN(ClinPracCritCare), GradCertEmergNurs, Cert III Public Safety (SES Rescue), Cert II Public Safety (SES), MACCCN, MAIES
Senior Project and Policy Officer, State Preparedness and Response Unit, NSW Ministry of Health, St Leonards, NSW, Australia
Registered Nurse, Nepean Hospital Intensive Care Unit, Nepean Blue Mountains Local Health District, NSW, Australia

Michael Anthony Roche RN, MHCert, DipAppSc(Nursing), BHlthSc(Nurs), MHlthSc(Nurs), PhD, FACN
Professor of Mental Health Nursing, Clinical Chair, University of Canberra and ACT Health, Canberra, ACT, Australia
Adjunct Professor, University of Technology Sydney, Sydney, NSW, Australia

Bernadine Romero RN, BN, GradCert(EmergNurs)
Lecturer, Faculty of Health, Discipline of Nursing, Southern Cross University, Gold Coast, Queensland, Australia

Philip Russo BN, MClinEpid, PhD
Associate Professor
Director Nursing Research, Monash Nursing and Midwifery, Clayton, Victoria, Australia
Director, Cabrini Monash University Department of Nursing Research, Malvern, Victoria, Australia
Adjunct Associate Professor, Avondale University, Cooranbong, NSW, Australia

Jacqueline Ryan NP, RN, GradCertCritCare, MN(NP)
Nurse Practitioner, The Injury Clinic Blacktown/Narellan, NSW, Australia
Nurse Practitioner, Emergency Department, The Sutherland Hospital, Caringbah, NSW, Australia

Dr Simon Sawyer RP, BPara, BPsychMan/Mar, GCHPE, PhD
Director of Education, Australian Paramedical College, Burleigh Heads, Queensland, Australia
Adjunct Senior Lecturer, Griffith University – Paramedicine, Gold Coast, Queensland, Australia

Myra Serrano RN, GradCertIntCare, GradCertRes, GradCertHlthMgt, MNurs(Hons)
Policy Manager, Sydney Local Health District, Sydney, NSW, Australia

Ramon Z. Shaban BSc(Med), BN, GradCertInfCon, PGDipPH&TM, MEd, MCommHealthPrac(Hons), PhD, RN, FCENA, FACN, FACIPC, CICP-E
Clinical Chair of Communicable Diseases Control and Infection Prevention, Sydney Institute for Infectious Diseases and Susan Wakil School of Nursing and Midwifery, Faculty of Medicine and Health, University of Sydney, Sydney, NSW, Australia
Clinical Chair of Communicable Disease Control and Prevention and Infection Prevention, Public Health Unit, Centre for Population Health, Western Sydney Local Health District, North Parramatta, NSW, Australia
Director and Chief Infection Control Practitioner, Western Sydney Local Health District, Westmead, NSW, Australia
Associate Director, New South Wales Specialist Service for High Consequence Infectious Diseases, Westmead, NSW, Australia
Editor-in-Chief, Australasian Emergency Care, College of Emergency Nursing Australia, Sydney, NSW, Australia

Dr Paul Simpson AdvDipParamedScience(ICP), BEd, BHSc(PrehospCare), GradCertPaedEmerg, GradCertClinEd, MScM(ClinEpi), PhD
Associate Professor in Paramedicine, Western Sydney University, Western Sydney, NSW, Australia
Intensive Care Paramedic, NSW Ambulance, Sydney, NSW, Australia

Julija Sipavicius BSc, MN(Lead), MN(NP)
Nurse Practitioner: Blood and Marrow Transplantation, Royal North Shore Hospital, Sydney, NSW, Australia
Clinical Senior Lecturer, Faculty of Medicine and Health, The University of Sydney, Sydney, NSW, Australia

Tony Skapetis BDS, MEd, PhD, FIADT
Clinical Director Education – Oral Health, Western Sydney Local Health District, NSW, Australia
Clinical Professor, University of Sydney School of Dentistry, NSW, Australia

Audette Smith BA(Psych), GradDipLegPrac, GradDipArts, LLB
Senior Lecturer Medical Education (Law & Ethics), School of Medicine and Dentistry, Griffith University, Gold Coast, Queensland, Australia
Research Ethics Advisor, Griffith University Human Research Ethics Committee (GUHREC), Gold Coast, Queensland, Australia

Toby St. Clair DipEmergHlth(Paramedic), GradDipEmergHlth(MICA), GradCert(Aeromed Retrieval), MSpecPara(AR), MACPara
Intensive Care Flight Paramedic, Air Ambulance Victoria, Ambulance Victoria, Australia
Teaching Associate – Faculty of Medicine, Nursing and Health Sciences, Monash University, Clayton, Victoria, Australia
Honorary Prehospital Trauma Affiliate, Trauma Service, Royal Children's Hospital, Parkville, Victoria, Australia

Jane Treloggen RN, MHlthSc(Nurs)
Clinical Stream Manager, South Eastern Sydney Local Health District, Sydney, NSW, Australia

Wayne Varndell RN, MN, BSc(Hons), PGDip(AP), DipHE(Nurs), FCENA
Clinical Nurse Consultant, Prince of Wales Hospital, Emergency Department, Randwick, NSW, Australia
Visiting Scholar, Faculty of Health, University of Technology Sydney, Sydney, NSW, Australia
National President, College of Emergency Nursing Australasia, Hobart, Tasmania

Catherine Viengkham BPsych(Hons), PhD
Research Fellow, Susan Wakil School of Nursing and Midwifery, Faculty of Medicine and Health, University of Sydney, Sydney, NSW, Australia

James Vine RN, Dip HE Nursing, BSc Paramedic Science
Critical Care Paramedic, RAC Rescue Helicopter, Perth, WA, Australia
Critical Care Paramedic, St John WA, Perth, WA, Australia

Ioana Vlad MD, FACEM DipClinTox
Emergency Medicine Physician and Clinical Toxicologist, Sir Charles Gairdner Hospital, Nedlands, WA, Australia

Timothy Wand RN, NP, MN(Hons), PhD
Associate Professor and Nurse Practitioner in Mental Health, University of Sydney and Sydney Local Health District, Sydney, NSW, Australia

Nicole Watts RN, RM, MMid
Undergraduate Midwifery Academic Lead, College of Nursing and Midwifery, CDU Sydney Campus, Sydney, NSW, Australia

Diana Williamson RN, MN(ClinPrac-Emerg), GradCertEmerg, DipHlthScNurs, Cert IV TAA
Conjoint Lecturer, University of Newcastle, Newcastle, NSW, Australia
Senior Consultant – Safety & Quality, HNE Clinical Governance, New Lambton, NSW, Australia

Taneal Wiseman RN, GradDipCritCare, PhD
Acute Care Lecturer, Sydney Nursing School, University of Sydney, NSW, Australia
Registered Nurse, Sutherland Hospital Emergency Department, Sutherland, NSW, Australia

Jessica Wood RN, RM, MMid, PhD, GCCE
Lecturer in Midwifery, The University of Newcastle, Newcastle, NSW, Australia

SECTION ONE

OVERVIEW OF EMERGENCY CARE

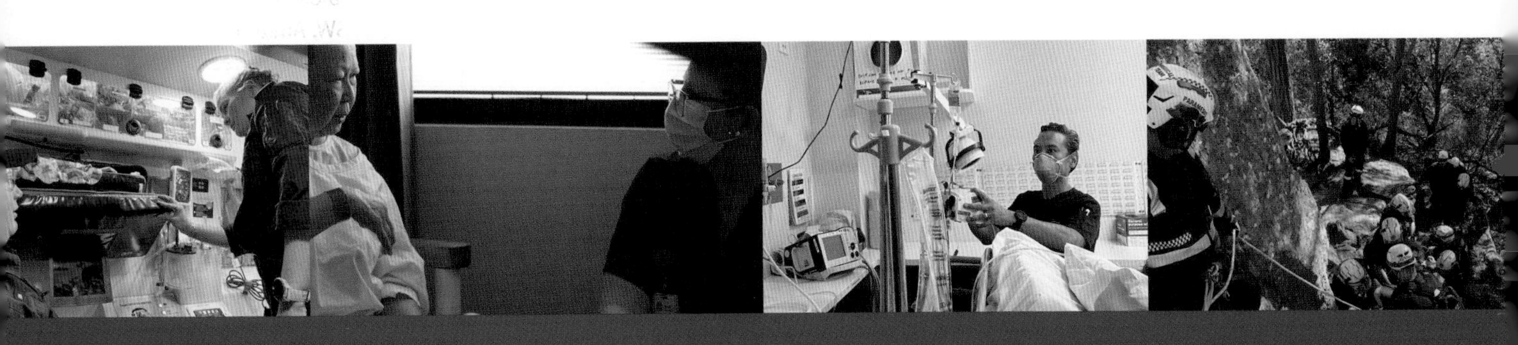

CHAPTER 1
EMERGENCY NURSING IN AUSTRALIA AND AOTEAROA NEW ZEALAND

MARGARET FRY, RAMON Z. SHABAN, JULIA MORPHET AND JULIE CONSIDINE

ESSENTIALS

- Emergency departments (EDs) are a key entry point for patients entering the acute hospital system.
- Clinical care demands mean that EDs share similar characteristics.
- To meet service demand and optimise workforce supply and retention, staff roles and new models of care need further consideration and evaluative research.
- Clinical performance indicators provide an opportunity to compare services and quality and to strive for consistency.
- The cultural context of care has embedded beliefs and values, which drive behaviour, activities and interactions.
- Emergency nurses are responsible for direct patient care and management, policy, education and research within the specialty of emergency nursing.
- Professional development is an ongoing process by which an emergency nurse identifies learning needs and addresses them to maintain safety of practice.
- Self-direction and reflection on practice and learning needs are essential to focusing professional development activities.
- Continual professional development has a positive impact on healthcare outcomes and relies upon a strong partnership and a shared responsibility between individual practitioners and their employers.
- Professional development can take many forms; both formal and informal activities can be effective in their own right.
- All emergency nurses need to champion the translation of research and thereby anchor practice in best evidence.

INTRODUCTION

This chapter provides an overview of the specialty of emergency nursing and the function of emergency departments (EDs) across Australasia. The key challenges, research and professional and management issues confronting emergency nurses are explored. A brief overview of Australasian ED role delineation is provided. Given

that emergency nursing is practised within a specific context of care, embedded cultural beliefs which drive and motivate behaviour and interaction are discussed. The development of the different nursing clinical roles and specialist education and industrial awards are described.

The challenge for emergency nurses is in (re-)designing the Australasian healthcare system to better ensure patient safety, while accommodating an ageing population, population growth, communicable diseases, increased chronic disease rates and workforce shortages. To reform the landscape of healthcare provision requires new ways of thinking that will reshape and define roles, models of care, activities and clinical expertise, and thereby reduce the fragmentation of care that exists within and between sectors, while leading to greater consistency of practice and healthcare accessibilities and equity for patients.

EMERGENCY NURSING

Designated emergency departments (EDs) were first established in Australia in the early 1970s and functioned mainly as an after-hours patient entry point where a nurse from the wards came to monitor the patient's condition until the arrival of a doctor. However, the increasing number of patients presenting to EDs, demand for more emergency care, advances in technology and improvements in resuscitation procedures, led to the need to expand services and create a specialty area for the delivery of emergency care. By 1985, these changes raised the expectation that both nursing and medical staff needed to become highly trained, specialised in emergency care and permanently based in EDs.[1]

The formation of formally designated EDs led to the establishment of emergency nursing as a discrete area of practice, evolving into a specialty practice over the ensuing 45 years. Emergency nurses deliver care to a diverse population experiencing episodic, abrupt, potentially life-threatening health or psychosocial conditions. Emergency care may require minimal intervention or advanced life-support practices. Emergency nurses require in-depth and specialised knowledge, skills and clinical expertise to provide care and to manage situations, such as patient overcrowding and the use of complex technology.[2]

Emergency nurses make risk assessment clinical decisions and deliver complex care under conditions of uncertainty in a stressful and time-pressured environment. Emergency nurses are adaptive and responsive professionals who systematically engage and develop rapport with individuals from a diverse range of cultural and socioeconomic backgrounds.[3] Emergency nurses blend theoretical knowledge systems, past experiences, collated patterns of knowing and ways of doing, with a patient's physiological, interpersonal and communicative signs.[4] Convergences of these knowledge systems with cognitive domains that include assessment, diagnosis, treatment and evaluation skills, enable greater accuracy and speed in the decision-making, troubleshooting, prioritisation and delivery of emergency care.[5,6]

The practice environment of emergency nursing is as diverse as the nursing profession itself. Box 1.1 identifies some of the practice environments of Australasian emergency nurses. In keeping with the nursing profession as a whole, emergency nursing roles include assessment, diagnosis, patient care and management, referral, education, consultation, advocacy and research.[7,8]

BOX 1.1 EMERGENCY CARE PRACTICE ENVIRONMENTS[9]

Emergency departments
Emergency treatment areas
Minor injury units
Urgent Care Centres
Military services
Community health clinics
Remote and very remote health clinics
Industrial areas
Multipurpose centres
Māori health providers
Medical centres
Pre-hospital/retrieval services
Disaster response teams

In Australasia, emergency nursing practice is guided by various professional and government bodies, which include the Nursing Council of New Zealand (NCNZ), New Zealand Nurses Organisation (NZNO), the Nursing and Midwifery Board of Australia (NMBA), Australian Health Practitioner Regulation Agency (Ahpra), the Australian Nursing and Midwifery Accreditation Council (ANMAC), the Australian Nursing and Midwifery Federation (ANMF), the College of Emergency Nursing Australasia (CENA), the College of Emergency Nurses New Zealand (CENNZ), the Council of Remote Area Nurses of Australia (CRANAplus), and local, state, territory and federal governments. However, the demands of the clinical environment also determine the scope of practice roles in emergency nursing. Consequently, role function may vary between and within service providers.

EMERGENCY DEPARTMENTS

The geographical landmass of Australasia (Australia and Aotearoa New Zealand) is vast—(Australia 7,741,220 square kilometres; Aotearoa New Zealand 268,838 square kilometres)—with a combined population in 2020 of over 30.5 million.[10,11] Throughout Australia, the roles of EDs differ depending on the type of hospital, geographical location and position within the healthcare system network (Table 1.1). Within each designated level, physical design, function, staffing and resources are similar.[12] Aotearoa New Zealand's ED role delineation structure is similar to Australia's (Box 1.2).[13]

In the urban setting, most metropolitan and regional areas have a designated ED. However, rural, remote and very remote health centres have designated treatment areas/rooms that provide limited resuscitation practices. To be designated as an ED or service the facility must provide 24-hour specialist medical officer and nurse cover, on-site diagnostic services, and intensive care and surgical operating services.[14] In rural, remote and very remote locations, urgent care centres (multi-purpose centres) are more common. Urgent care centres share attributes with EDs, but do not provide the same level of emergency care, and may not be open 24 hours a day. Urgent care centres are typically staffed by nurses and nurse practitioners, who assess

TABLE 1.1 AUSTRALIAN EMERGENCY DEPARTMENTS BY PEER GROUP[12]

TYPE OF HOSPITAL	DESCRIPTION	NUMBER
Principal referral and specialist women's and children's	Provides broad range of specialist services such as cardiac or neurosurgery, infectious diseases. Located in major cities. 24-hour ED.	40
Public Acute Group A	Provides wide range of services including intensive care, coronary care, and oncology. Located in major cities and regional areas, and one remote hospital. 24-hour ED.	60
Public Acute Group B	Specialist services may include obstetrics, paediatrics, mental health, oncology. Located in major cities and inner and outer regional areas. 24-hour ED.	42
Public Acute Group C	Services may include obstetric and surgical services. Will have either an ED or urgent care centre, that may not be staffed by a doctor 24 hours per day.	64
Other hospitals with emergency departments or urgent care centres	These services are not grouped elsewhere. Services vary.	85
Total		291

BOX 1.2 **NEW ZEALAND EMERGENCY DEPARTMENT DISTRIBUTION[13]**

T1 Higher-level tertiary
T2 Lower-level tertiary
S1 Secondary
S2 Subacute
Health centre/Rural and remote

and manage patients, with general practitioners (GPs) available on call.[15]

The Aotearoa New Zealand healthcare system has historically had 20 District Health Boards (DHBs) across 16 regions. However, at the time of writing, in 2022 the DHBs will be disestablished and a single entity, Te Whatu Ora – Health New Zealand, will manage all health services, including hospital and specialist services, primary and community care.[16] Similarly, Australian state and territory governments are responsible for health services, although service models vary. Australia has 291 and Aotearoa New Zealand 42 designated public hospital EDs.[13,17] Australia and Aotearoa New Zealand each has a national healthcare system that provides universal free access to emergency services, free public hospital care, subsidised pharmaceuticals and out-of-hospital care. A reciprocal healthcare agreement exists between Australia and Aotearoa New Zealand.

Emergency care throughout Australasia is a right of citizens as universal healthcare, and this care must be of an appropriate standard and quality. The challenge for emergency care clinicians is the increasing complexity of the emergency environments, and of the care being delivered, in a context of rising patient presentation rates, an ageing population and increasing comorbidities.

The ED is one of the key entry points for patients entering the hospital system and provides an interface between the primary health and acute care sectors. Throughout Australasia, the increased patient attendance rate is largely due to an ageing population, decreased availability of GP services, increased chronic disease rates and the availability of new technologies and procedures.[12] The need to deliver care for all age groups and respond to patients with minor injuries and illnesses through to critical or life-threatening conditions, requires EDs to be responsive by having specifically designated clinical areas. EDs are largely configured in the same way, although size and bed capacity differ between departments.

CLINICAL ENVIRONMENT

The clinical environment must be designed and allocated appropriate resources to meet the demands of a range of patient conditions and injuries across the life span, and so all EDs share similar architectural commonalities between sites that make them recognisable and consistent with each other. The organisation of emergency care work, purpose and function is shaped and ordered by patient case-mix and architecture. Emergency care is usually provided to patients in a range of specifically designated geographical areas, which are further configured into waiting and ambulance arrival areas, triage, resuscitation, acute, sub-acute and/or fast-track/consultation areas. For mixed adult and paediatric EDs, best practice requires children to be allocated to a separate waiting, clinical and resuscitation area, away from adult patients. There are also increasing calls to have elder-specific models of care within EDs to meet the specific needs of older ED users.[18] Increasingly, assessment or 24-hour short-stay units are being co-located within or near EDs; for example, short-stay mental health or medical aged assessment units.

Patients with critical and/or life-threatening conditions are best managed in resuscitation areas with appropriate lifesaving and continuous-monitoring equipment, and enough to allow a range of skilled staff to provide care. Designated resuscitation areas are often resourced to provide care for both paediatric and adult patients.[18] Urgent patient conditions, with the potential for deterioration, need close monitoring for a period of time and are often located in an acute area where there is provision for continuous vital signs, and invasive and cardiac monitoring. In contrast, patients who self-present with minor injuries and illnesses can be managed in a fast-track and/or consultation-type area with equipment targeting minor procedure and/or illness management. Some patient groups might require isolation, privacy and/or reduced stimulation, and may be more appropriately managed in a single room, with or without continuous-monitoring capabilities. The diverse clinical environment of the ED is challenging, given the requirement for clinicians to provide care for patients across the life span, and with diverse clinical presentations and comorbidities.[18]

The primary distinguishing feature of emergency nursing is the need to care for diverse patients with undifferentiated diagnoses in a time-pressured environment, so the process of patient assessment is vital. Emergency nurses require in-depth knowledge and clinical expertise to provide care and manage situational events, such as patient overcrowding, infectious diseases and complex technology.

Emergency nurses have a broad scope of practice and independently make complex clinical decisions. For example, in a resuscitation context, emergency nurses are responsible for decisions such as setting mechanical ventilation parameters; titrating medications such as sedation and analgesia; and managing advanced respiratory and haemodynamic monitoring, all of which carry high levels of clinical risk and are vital to patient safety.[19–21]

EMERGENCY DEPARTMENT WORKFORCE

The ED workforce is largely driven by patient case-mix, local demand and presentation rates. Therefore, workforce planning, staff ratios and skill-mix, and development and work practice (re-)design should be focused on the challenge of making the patient's journey through the ED as efficient, safe and satisfying as possible.

The most appropriate staff ratio and skill-mix profile for an ED is unclear, and development of staffing models remains an urgent priority.[22,23] Some, but not all, Australian states have legislated nurse-to-patient ratios in EDs, but they are blunt workforce tools and are not flexible to ED workload patterns or specific patient needs,[24,25] and do not recognise the varied skill-set required. Greater clarity is required to understand and define the appropriate workforce model for EDs, which would also give shape to possible advanced practice emergency nursing roles.[24,26–29] Refer to Chapter 6 for further discussion on nursing ratios.

Nevertheless, roles within EDs are diverse, and staff include nursing, medical, allied health, transport and administrative support and communication staff members.[12,13] The workforce profile of an ED is usually individually responsive to local demands and needs, and to patient presentation rates and acuity.

A diverse range of staff is needed to sustain the delivery of emergency care. The emergency doctor's primary role is to assess, stabilise, manage and refer patients. They also oversee/supervise other junior medical staff providing care, including emergency medicine and other specialty trainees, career medical officers, locum practitioners, GPs and junior medical officers.[30] Emergency nurses undertake patient assessment, prioritise nursing care, initiate diagnostics and care interventions, and provide ongoing nursing management for the range of patients. EDs now offer a range of nursing roles that require varying levels of advanced knowledge, expertise and skills.[31] For example, the nurse practitioner[32–34] and clinical initiative nurse (CIN).[35]

Emergency nurses are the largest emergency care workforce.[36] Their scope of practice and ways of work are fundamental considerations for the redesign of ED and emergency care in the future. Reforms must focus on increasing interdisciplinary teamwork and promotion of collaboration between disciplines, staff development to enable the acquisition of advanced skills and experience required for alternative models of care, building staff capacity and expertise of staff in allocating innovative tasks and roles while recognising experience, knowledge, skills, competencies and qualifications, and using technologies, if proven to enhance efficiency and ensure there is adequate support for implementation.

Across Australasia, various EDs are developing innovative approaches to the deployment of emergency care clinicians, including extended practice for experienced nurses, and nurse practitioners and allied health professionals being employed to provide autonomous assessment and treatment.[5,37,38] The delivery of effective emergency care in out-of-hospital, EDs and acute care settings, requires innovative, flexible and collaborative systems that support creative thinking and research about the range and roles of staff working in the area.[39,40]

SUPPORT STAFF

The complexity of the ED environment requires dedicated support staff who can assist directly or indirectly with patient management, admission, disposition and/or discharge processes. The range of dedicated support staff essential to improve ED services and efficiency include clerical staff, clinical and communication support staff, volunteers, orderlies, transport/transfer staff, security personnel and cleaners.[30] Support staff require appropriate education and development and are essential for the efficient provision of ED services. Support staff are necessary to release healthcare workers from non-clinical tasks, enabling their focus to remain on patient safety, care and management.

OPTIMISING WORK PRACTICES

Optimising patient service, flow and management has led to diverse, extended practice roles being undertaken by nursing and allied health staff; roles and/or activities that were traditionally undertaken by medical staff. Emergency nurses have been able to undertake a range of extended patient-management activities through the establishment of reference tools such as clinical practice guidelines, clinical pathways and standing orders.[41,42] Medically endorsed patient-management guidelines have enabled emergency nurses to undertake an extended range of activities, including assessment, pharmacological and investigative interventions, and targeted management activities, such as the commencement of intravenous fluids.[4143,44] By initiating interventions for a range of patients, the experienced emergency nurse optimises work practices. Significant improvements in ED services' flow and costs have been demonstrated in many EDs that have established such reference tools.[45,46] Reference tools, such as clinical guidelines, go some way to securing consistency within practice, and offer clinicians and managers the opportunity to make comparisons with other like services.

COMMUNICATION SUPPORT

Communication, both non-clinical and clinical, consumes a significant proportion of ED staff time.[40,47] The need to better coordinate and centralise non-medical communication is growing. Within many EDs, the coordination of patient and staff communications requires a dedicated communications support role.[48,49]

In addition, communication processes concerning patient care and management are also growing in complexity as increasing numbers of healthcare clinicians and hospital managers become involved.[50,51] Shared decision-making about high-quality patient treatment, care and disposition has led to complex and multilayered communication processes. The communication support role provides a pivotal conduit to better facilitate the patient's journey and provide a consistent link between local, hospital and community engagement. Greater integration of communication processes between primary care and the acute care sector is needed. Refer to Chapter 8 for more discussion on decision-making.

A secondary advantage to having a centralised ED communication role is the ability for patients' carers and family to have access to a consistent communication portal. Providing high-quality patient care is challenged by the pressures of communication in an emergency setting. Communication processes need to be considered within pre-hospital and emergency settings to ensure safety and alleviate patient, family and/or carer stress and anxiety. Clear information about emergency processing and care while in the ED should be provided systematically and consistently to patients, families and/or carers. Refer to Chapters 6 and 8 respectively for further discussion on communication and safety.

PERFORMANCE IMPROVEMENT

With an increasing demand and expectation on service delivery, EDs are challenged to provide consistent, safe and timely high-quality care. EDs have been proactively examining ways to provide a more satisfying and appropriate service. Hence, much has been done through examination of various practice models, at federal, state and local levels, to improve service delivery. However, consistency in ED practice remains elusive, as organisational comparisons are often difficult, given the (often significant) variation in local demand, population mix, geographical location, workforce characteristics and resource availability between sites.

Across Australasia, national accreditation organisations have sought to champion high-quality improvement programs for healthcare. These national accreditation bodies have provided various quality frameworks for healthcare evaluation, which are focused on demonstrating appropriate and consistent patient care practices, staff development and education practices and patient safety review processes. For example, the Australian Commission on Safety and Quality in Health Care National Safety and Quality Health Service (NSQHS) Standards aim to protect the public from harm, improve the quality of health service provision, and provide a quality assurance mechanism that tests whether relevant systems are in place to ensure that expected standards of safety and quality are met.[52]

Traditionally, throughout Australasia, ED comparisons relating to service delivery have largely focused on triage code allocation and the associated 'seen by doctor' times, patient case-mix and mortality and presentation rates. However, ED staff have been concerned that service comparisons have often failed to accommodate the different levels of service providers. For example, rural EDs may not have a doctor on-site and so triage code benchmarks can be an unreliable indicator for service comparison between metropolitan/urban and rural EDs.

Clinical performance indicators, often referred to now as Emergency Treatment Performance (ETP) targets, are important and enable services to make comparisons between each other throughout Australasia.[53] However, it is timely that consideration be given to the development of other system indicators. Examples may include time to analgesia and time to first antibiotic.[54–57] Additional performance indicators need to be identified that will maximise equitable comparisons, while focusing on the patient's journey and drivers of quality and satisfaction for staff and patients. In addition, many external services (e.g. radiology, surgery and pathology) contribute directly or indirectly towards the patient flow. These external services are often outside the control of ED staff, but may limit, impede or reduce the capacity for patient flow. Many external services are critical to ED patient management and decision-making, and so future external service benchmarking is needed to enhance patient flow broadly.

EMERGENCY SERVICE (RE-)DESIGN OF MODELS OF CARE

While there has been a significant increase in ED demand, there has been little debate about patient flow and the use and appropriateness of current and future emergency staff roles, including the contribution of allied health and paramedicine staff within the ED.[18,30] Workload demands and workforce issues continue to dominate the healthcare debate. For example, governments have sought to drive service change through national emergency performance targets.[58]

Optimising ED workforce models to better meet service need is important, given workforce projections concerning supply, distribution and skill-mix needed to meet future demands for services.[12,24] In Australasia, 10–39% of ED presentations have been estimated to be non-urgent and could be managed in a primary healthcare setting.[12] A proportion of this group, both nationally and internationally, is considered to be able to be redirected to new models of care or other healthcare agencies.[59] Extensive research was undertaken of new models of care in many countries, particularly in the United Kingdom, United States, Ireland, Canada, Denmark and Sweden, and to a lesser degree in Australasia. A literature review[60] identified six practice-based new models of care:

1. Minor injuries units
2. Urgent care/walk-in centres
3. Telephone triage and advice services
4. GP cooperatives services
5. Primary care health centres
6. Paramedical services ('see and treat' and 'treat and refer').

Models were not mutually exclusive from each other, EDs or GP clinics. The outcomes of these models of care demonstrated a positive impact on acute service-use patterns.

While there was a wide range of care models beyond traditional GPs and EDs, telephone triage advice centres, minor injury unit walk-in centres were the most effective due to ease of access, convenience and prompt service delivery. The evidence of impact was stronger for services co-located or streamed with EDs. In 2010, Australia opened its first walk-in centre in Canberra, ACT.[61] The widespread implementation of fast-track areas aimed at rapid assessment and care of patients with minor illnesses and injuries has been a successful strategy in facilitating timely emergency care for this patient group.[5,27,62]

A collaborative and integrative relationship between emergency staff, paramedics, GPs, nurse practitioners and other primary healthcare clinicians would enhance the timely delivery of emergency services. Importantly, greater integrative care would also enhance the delivery of discharge interventions by emergency clinicians and result in improved safety and greater adherence.[62–64]

For those in geographically isolated areas throughout Australasia, concerns remain about healthcare equity and access, and limited healthcare options.[16,65,66] The application or impact that re-design models may have in rural, remote and regional areas is unclear. While the different models of care may benefit those living in more-isolated regions, it is difficult to extrapolate the findings of research to these areas. While a portion of these new models could be considered, others would be difficult and/or impractical to implement in geographically isolated areas. Implementation barriers and enablers have been identified within the literature.[60,67,68]

In Australia, the professionalisation of paramedics as a registered health profession is seen as a significant step in the (re-) designing of emergency services.[69] The registration of paramedics enables significant expansion of the scope of paramedics and better position, them to continue to advance their contributions to the quality of the patient experience and the quality of their care. This is particularly relevant as it relates to paramedic clinical judgement and decision-making, which is a hallmark of professionalism.[70,71] In the UK, evidence has identified that extended paramedicine activities, including 'see and treat' and 'treat and refer' protocols, may reduce ED activity.[72–75] A paramedicine pilot 'see and treat' protocol for assessing and treating minor injury or illness in the community was evaluated.[76] This cluster-randomised controlled trial involved 56 UK urban ambulance stations and 3018 patients. The patients treated by a paramedic were less likely to be transported to an ED or need hospital admission within 28 days. The 'see and treat' paramedicine model had a positive impact on healthcare agencies, and paramedics reported high levels of satisfaction. Extended paramedicine roles have been shown to redirect activity away from acute care services.[76,77]

Similarly, Snooks and colleagues[78] evaluated a 'treat and refer' paramedicine protocol. Patients could be assessed, managed and left at the scene with either a referral plan or self-care advice. The evaluation identified that there was no difference in the proportion of patients left at the scene in the intervention or control groups, although job time was longer for the 'treat and refer' group. Paramedicine 'treat and refer' protocols were found to be used appropriately. Further testing and validation of protocols, decision support systems and training was required.

Another paramedicine re-design model included a minor injuries unit (MIU) referral protocol.[79] This 12-month UK study introduced a protocol aimed at reducing ED activity by enabling paramedic crews to directly refer patients to an MIU. In the randomised-cluster control group, 37 people attended an MIU, 327 attended an ED and 61 were not transported. For the intervention group, 41 people attended an MIU, 303 attended an ED and 65 patients were not transported. Ambulance service case times were shorter for those attending an MIU compared with an ED. The MIU patients were 7.2 times as likely to rate care as excellent. The results suggest that paramedics make appropriate referrals to alternative healthcare agencies and thereby reduce ED activity. Extending the role of paramedics could build service capacity and job satisfaction, while redirecting activity away from acute care services.[69,73,77] The shift of paramedic education into the tertiary sector will potentially facilitate the extended-care practitioner (ECP) role. Postgraduate courses are now becoming available, as well as industry-based ECP training. However, it is unclear exactly how the role of the ECP will develop in Australasia. This is discussed further in Chapter 2.

AUSTRALASIAN EMERGENCY NURSE PRACTICE STANDARDS

Emergency nurses require capabilities and skills, specialist knowledge and expertise to meet the challenge of delivering safe emergency care. Various iterations of Australasian competency standards, which detail the combination of skills, knowledge, attitudes, values and abilities that underpin effective performance within a profession/occupational area, have attempted to define these care dimensions. Practice standards have therefore been defined as a set of core standards that describe the current practice of nurses. Such standards can be developed to the professional levels expected of both the beginning nurse and the advanced nurse practitioner.

The Nursing and Midwifery Board of Australia (NMBA), in collaboration with Ahpra, is responsible for the regulation of nurses and midwives. Within Australasia, nursing and midwifery regulating authorities have established standards of practice that apply to the registration of nurses, nurse practitioners and midwives, with a focus on safety of practice.[80–83] These practice standards accommodate the diverse roles that nurses and midwives undertake, provide a framework for undergraduate and postgraduate curricula, define behaviour and are a means of ensuring high-quality care through safe and effective work practices. In Australia and Aotearoa New Zealand, the developed and endorsed enrolled nurse, registered nurse, nurse practitioner and midwife practice standards provide a framework for ongoing professional development. Many peak nursing and midwifery bodies have given support for these practice standards.

In addition, the College of Emergency Nursing Australasia (CENA) and College of Emergency Nurses New Zealand (CENNZ) have developed practice standards for the specialist emergency nurse. These build on the registered nurse practice standards to provide broad practice and performance guidelines in line with national legislation.[8,84] The emergency nursing specialist standards cover nine domains: clinical expertise, communication, teamwork, resources and environment, professional development, leadership, lawful practice, professional ethics and research, and quality improvement.[8] The standards represent the unique characteristics that give shape to the specialty of emergency practice.

Recent Australian research has established evidence-based minimum practice standards for Australian graduate emergency nursing programs. These standards detail the professional practice expectations of graduates. The practice standards present a guide for higher education to anchor their graduate emergency nursing curricula. Consistent and transparent expectations inform clinical practice, which ultimately leads to safer delivery of informed patient care, and improves workforce planning.[7,85,86]

DEVELOPMENT OF EMERGENCY NURSING PROFESSIONAL BODIES

To support nurses in emergency nursing, professional organisations such as the Emergency Nurses Association (ENA) were formally established in the United States (1970), UK (1972), Australia (1983) and Aotearoa New Zealand (1990).[87,88] These associations promote clinical, educational and professional development of emergency nurses by producing policy statements on levels of role performance and by fostering specialty recognition. The associations publish professional journals, newsletters and provide financial sponsorship for emergency nurses to attend conferences and conduct research. Many also provide introductory specialty education courses to update knowledge and skills. In Australia, the Emergency Nursing Association (ENA) from each state and territory merged to form the College of Emergency Nursing Australasia (CENA), the peak professional body for emergency nurses throughout Australia, with professional links to Aotearoa New Zealand and Singapore emergency nursing groups.[8] The *Australasian Emergency Nursing Journal*, first published in 1996 by the New South Wales ENA, became Australasia's first international, peer-reviewed emergency nursing journal. In light of the collaborative nature of emergency care, diversity of its workforce and variety of settings, the journal is known today as *Australasian Emergency Care*. In Aotearoa New Zealand, the College of Emergency Nursing New Zealand aims to promote excellence in emergency nursing within Aotearoa New Zealand, through the development of frameworks for clinical practice, education and research.[84]

EMERGENCY NURSE SPECIALISATION

Nursing specialisation was necessary because of the recognition that nurses could no longer master the volume of knowledge and skills required to work in all clinical areas.[72,89] To assist emergency nurses in gaining in-depth knowledge and clinical expertise, specialty postgraduate courses were developed, with the first established in Victoria in 1974. In the 1970s and 1980s, these were hospital-based vocational specialty courses in emergency nursing. By 1979, professional bodies, such as the New South Wales College of Nursing, had extended their nursing education profile to include advanced emergency nursing programs. By 1995, university-based Emergency Nursing Graduate Certificate courses had been established in Australia.[85]

In 1985, Australian hospital-based pre-registration nurse education began to transfer to the tertiary sector, with completion for all states and territories by 1994. With the shift to tertiary education there was a corresponding demand for postgraduate tertiary qualifications.[85,90] To meet this demand, tertiary programs were developed to articulate with specialist certificate courses and extend nursing knowledge, attributes and clinical skills beyond mere technical competence. Today, Australasian universities provide postgraduate courses in specialty areas such as emergency nursing.[85] Registered nurses can now pursue graduate certificate, graduate diploma, master and/or doctoral degrees in their area of specialisation.[85]

Today nurses are recognised and defined by their area of specialty practice, such as emergency. As a result, each specialty area has its own cultural context. While all types of nursing have similar characteristics, in each specialty there is a unique collection of individuals who share knowledge systems, including values, beliefs and ways of being that make them and their work distinct from other communities of practice.[40,91,92] Emergency nurses share common knowledge sets that provide understanding and bring meaning to activities, shape the boundary of emergency work and make them recognisable to each other.[4,5] This creates systems of meaning which allow people to build conceptual maps and orientate activity and behaviour during interaction. Thus, shared information contributes towards a level of stability and coherence. Within an ED, notions of efficiency, timeliness and equity shape meaning through which expectations of patient behaviour are conveyed and a culture of ED care sustained.[4] Through these knowledge sets of meaning, emergency staff come to learn, communicate and understand how practice is viewed and conducted, and how the notion of care is perceived.[4,92]

A cultural context of ED care is reflected in a standard geography of care that is orientated towards the notions of efficiency and timeliness that are shared and understood through patient movement. Patient movement is normalised by architecture, embedded expectations, urgency codes and bed allocations, and creates a spatial web recognisable to all emergency staff.[40] These embedded cultural mores make explicit a particular cadence of care from which a culture of ED care emanates and within which emergency nursing is enacted.

CLINICAL ROLES

To keep pace with nursing specialisation across Australasia, local, state, territory and regional governments and nurse associations introduced industrial nursing awards to recognise, support and financially reward advanced clinical nurses. For example, the industrial award classification of Clinical Nurse Specialist (CNS) was introduced in New South Wales in 1986 and in Victoria in 1987 and Clinical Nurse Specialist 2 in 2015.[93] Inherent in this classification is the recognition that advanced level practitioners deliver and coordinate care appropriate to the needs of the patient, act as clinical resource people, provide leadership, and support less-experienced staff. However, CNS award classifications did not mandate an academic qualification for the position, preferring instead to maintain the focus on clinical experience and knowledge, and professional leadership.[82] By the 1990s, other award classifications, such as Clinical Nurse Consultant (CNC) and Nurse Practitioner (NP), had been introduced and have added to the clinical career pathways available to registered nurses.[85,94]

These industrial award classifications meant that experienced nurses no longer had to move away from direct patient care to gain career advancement and financial incentives.[95,96] However, specialty definition, qualifications, levels of competency, accreditation processes and extended practice roles have developed without consistency or national unification throughout Australasia,[97] with variations in role title and description between states and territories. In addition, emergency nurses in

Australasia can expand their area of chosen professional development and can develop extended clinical nurse roles, such as a Clinical Initiatives Nurse (CIN)[41] or an Advanced Practice Nurse (APN), Clinical Nurse Specialist (CNS), Clinical Nurse Educator (CNE), Clinical Nurse Consultant (CNC) and Nursing Unit Manager (NUM).[95,97] Extended nursing practice roles require organisational support and governance, and are commonly supported by protocols or standing orders.[96]

Across Australia and Aotearoa New Zealand, emergency nurses have implemented innovative extended clinical practice roles to meet service demands. Hence, a wider range of patient diagnoses are being managed by nurses with specialist education to optimise patient safety.[96] Emergency nurses rely on delegated responsibility to enable the commencement of episodic care for extended practice roles.[45,98] A significant example of episodic care includes pain management interventions.[20,99] Given the range of extended practice roles within Australasian EDs, there is little doubt regarding the positive impact on patient and system services.

EMERGENCY NURSE PRACTITIONERS

Nationally and internationally, Nurse Practitioners (NPs) are recognised as undertaking advanced practice roles.[38,100–102] NPs provide leadership, expertise, support and direction within clinical settings; they undertake assessments, make diagnoses and initiate treatment within their scope of practice, and provide monitoring and care coordination for particular patient groups. Emergency NPs are expert clinicians with advanced skills and theoretical knowledge that enable them to autonomously treat, manage, refer and discharge a range of patient conditions in partnership with medical and other allied health workers.[24,68,103] NP authorisation requires the nurse or midwife to hold general registration, demonstrate extensive advanced clinical expertise and recency of practice, hold a master's degree and demonstrate capability in the NP practice standards.[81,83]

The NP role is well established in the United States (1960s), UK (1980s), Canada (2000) and, to a lesser extent, Australia (1995) and Aotearoa New Zealand (2000). In a US census survey, there were 325,000 authorised NPs with 363,000 being educated annually.[68,104,105] Within the role, 42.5% hold hospital privileges, 12.8% have long-term care privileges, and 96.2% prescribe medications. Within Australia (2020), there were 337,000 registered nurses[106] and approximately 1556 authorised NPs.[107] In Aotearoea New Zealand (2017), there were 51,700 practising registered nurses and 365 authorised NPs.[105]

There is national and international evidence of NP impact in relation to contribution to workload,[32,34,38,100] appropriate care,[33,38,100] patient satisfaction,[108] documentation and guideline adherence,[109] and efficiency and timeliness.[110,111] No clinical difference was found between NPs and doctors in patient health outcomes.[24,112–114] Nurse practitioners were found to be more reliable in following practice guidelines and completing medical record documentation. Of note has been the positive economic impact of NP models compared with 'routine medical care'.[114–116] Cost reductions related specifically to resource use, shorter hospital length of stay and reduced patient complication and re-admission rates.

In Australia, regulation of NP authorisation is promoted and maintained by Ahpra, the Australian statutory authority which implements the National Registration and Accreditation Scheme (NRAS), and in Aotearoa New Zealand, the NCNZ have established practice standards that apply to the authorisation of NPs.[105] Practice areas include metropolitan, district, regional and rural and remote centres with minimal or no medical coverage. In 2010, Australasian NPs gained prescribing and investigation privileges which should be co-endorsed by their scope of practice and organisation. Embedded into authorisation processes are the nurse practitioner standards for practice.[81,83] Within Australasian universities, NP curricula embed the standards and cover care practices for acute and non-acute patient conditions and situations, physical assessment, pharmacology, procedures, leadership, and ethics and the law (see Chapters 3, 4 and 12).

A lack of clarity, internationally, surrounds the NP name. The term 'Nurse Practitioner' was often used interchangeably with 'Clinical Nurse Specialist' (United States), 'Clinical Nurse Consultant' (UK) and 'Advanced Practice Nurse'.[95,97,103] Consequently, for consistency, greater clarity is needed to define, understand and measure advanced practitioners. Nonetheless, emergency NPs are caring for patients, from preterm to aged care, and managing acute and chronic conditions in a variety of different models of care and services. The volume, breadth, depth and consistency of research findings provide strong support for the expansion of NP roles and numbers.

LEADERSHIP AND MANAGEMENT

Emergency leaders create opportunities to redefine nursing roles to create innovative solutions that reshape service and meet service demands.[117,118] The quality and safety of emergency care delivery has been largely shaped and defined by nursing leadership.[117–119] Across Australasia, evidence of emergency nursing leadership and management has led to new models of care, enhanced workforce capability and intellectual capacity.[120,121] Refer to Chapter 6 for more information on leadership.

However, those in leadership and management positions face increasing challenges in meeting service provision demand and consumer expectations. Current challenges include: the COVID-19 pandemic; workforce sustainability; equitable access planning; overcrowding; staff recruitment and retention; and the agility of models of care to reshape emergency roles, referrals and care options. While there are innovative strategies being explored to meet the challenge of service provision, success is often dependent on the ability of clinical leaders and managers to motivate, enthuse and engage with staff to drive new visions of practice.[122,123]

In Australasia, sustainable access planning remains a major ED management issue.[32,124–126] Part of sustainable access planning is resolving access block issues. An 'access block' is defined as a patient who is ready to go to a ward bed, but remains in the ED for longer than 8 hours because of the lack of an inpatient bed.[126] This leads to overcrowding. There is an association between overcrowding, increased hospital length of stay and mortality in Australian hospitals.[126,127] Known effects of overcrowding include delays in patient management, poor hospital processes, poor infection control, patients not being placed on the appropriate ward, and so forth.[128,129]

Hospital strategies and new models of care which aim to improve inpatient bed access include medical admission units, reforming bed management practices, discharge planning and patient processing.[124] Other complementary strategies include the development of new models of care that include: rapid assessment teams, emergency medical units and the use of CINs, APNs, NPs, aged-care assessment teams and community and chronic disease initiative programs.[18,46,130,131]

The delivery of emergency care is dependent on sustaining a sufficient and appropriately skilled workforce. It is essential that the complexities of patient safety, staff recruitment, retention and the development of emergency nursing roles be made explicit to enable strategic planning to sustain and/or enhance nursing workforce density. To this end, transactional leadership can provide a basis for responding creatively to workforce issues and the reshaping of emergency nursing roles (see Chapter 6). Further continuing professional development is central for an innovative, safe and responsive workforce. Emergency managers and clinical leaders everywhere are continually finding new and innovative ways to sustain a responsive workforce to provide timely and equitable emergency care, and meet the challenging demands of contemporary service provision.

PROFESSIONAL DEVELOPMENT

Professional development is synonymous with terms such as 'in-service' education, continuing education, self-directed learning, competencies, etc. The NMBA suggests that continuing professional development (CPD) is the means to maintain, improve and broaden practice knowledge, expertise and competence, and develop attributes and skills to maintain professional practice and improve patient safety and outcomes.[132] CPD should be undertaken to promote more capable practitioners able to provide demonstrable improvements in patient care.[19]

CPD and lifelong learning skills are essential to providing good quality care to patients and communities by emergency clinicians.[19,133] Research suggests that better-educated nurses are associated with better patient outcomes, with many authors espousing that CPD is crucial to patient safety and quality standards of patient care.[134,135] However, fewer studies acknowledge the impact that advanced education within the paramedic profession has had on patient outcomes. One area that has been extensively researched is the relationship between the practice of endotracheal intubation and adverse patient outcomes.[136,137]

Nonetheless, there is good evidence that inadequacy of professional education is associated with adverse patient outcomes. Education can be delivered correctly and effectively, and can be linked to improved patient outcomes.[135] It is clearly advantageous to be able to target CPD in areas of clinical need, with learning outcomes that are desired and measurable to be able to demonstrate benefit. Failure to undertake professional development can affect patient morbidity and mortality and may also affect other important measures, such as ED length of stay and cost of care.[19,134]

PRACTICE TIP

Improved patient care is the objective of any educational strategy undertaken as a clinician. It is often difficult to measure the impact this education has on patient health outcomes, but evaluation of educational strategies should demonstrate patient benefit.

Australian and Aotearoa New Zealand nurses on the national register are required to participate in, and keep written documentation of, at least 20 hours of CPD per year,[132] although there are no quality requirements for CPD offerings, nor stipulation regarding the frequency of engagement.[138] A crucial component of developing a unique body of knowledge is ongoing or lifelong learning, both of which are central to CPD, and indeed are considered important professional traits.[139,140] Professional development activities include such things as undertaking policy work, involvement in quality improvement activities, research, attending conferences and subscription to refereed journals, or in the workplace, such as the transition to specialty practice programs that support the transition of novice emergency nurses into the specialty,[19] to name but a few. In addition, formalised professional development can be undertaken in the tertiary sector in the form of postgraduate certificates, diplomas and degrees in chosen specialties, as described above. While education course structure and content can vary within the different awards, undertaking professional development tertiary qualifications in a specialist area of practice is valuable, and needs to be encouraged as it expands knowledge and skill bases required for nurses to better care for patients of increased complexity and acuity.[85,141] From personal perspectives, advanced or higher-level education also tends to be associated with added self-confidence, and workplace opportunity and mobility.[85]

PRACTICE TIP

Innovative strategies are required to ensure learning needs are met for practitioners working in fluid clinical environments. Similarly, educators, clinical leaders, instructors and mentors are required to be creative and flexible in educational facilitation.

Emergency nurses require advanced assessment skills to be creative and effective in problem-solving, have well-developed communication and teaching skills, as well as emotional intelligence, caring and management expertise. As a result, emergency nurses need to be constantly critiquing the care being provided and the outcome of that care. Therefore, professional development should include the support, translation or undertaking of research and dissemination of evidence-based practice (EBP).[142,143] Research findings can provide insight into and understanding of the complexity of emergency practice and the challenges experienced by emergency care staff.[143,144] By researching everyday nursing practice, insight can be gained into the experiences of emergency nurses and how they make sense of reality. From this insight, new ways to practice, and to educate and support health professionals, can be developed.

SUMMARY

Emergency care and nursing practice have been shaped by many factors. These include advances in resuscitation and technology, recognition of emergency as a specialty practice, increased patient presentation rates, population demands, increased rates of chronic conditions and changing case-mix. These factors and the growing demand on the healthcare system have increased the complexity and demands experienced in emergency nursing. The increasing focus on emergency care provides an opportunity for clinicians to collectively drive the healthcare agenda, policy direction and research agenda. In this way, emergency care services can be strategically directed and reformed. There remains great capacity to reshape and redesign emergency care service delivery within Australasia. Better use of the skills, expertise and qualifications of all healthcare clinicians would go some way towards meeting the challenge for more timely and appropriate healthcare delivery throughout Australasia.

USEFUL WEBSITES

Australian Health Practitioner Regulation Agency (Ahpra). Provides information for regulation of health professionals, www.ahpra.gov.au.

Australian Institute for Health and Welfare. Australia's national agency for health and welfare statistics and information, www.aihw.gov.au/.

Australian Nursing and Midwifery Federation. Provides information and resources for health professional, www.anmf.org.au/education.

College of Emergency Nursing Australasia. Provides policy, guidelines and educational resources relating to emergency nurses, www.cena.org.au.

Council of Remote Area Nurses of Australia Plus. Provides policy, guidelines and educational resources relating to rural and remote nursing and midwifery, www.crana.org.au.

Emergency Care Institute NSW. Provides policy, guidelines and educational resources relating to emergency care, aci.health.nsw.gov.au/networks/eci.

NSW Agency for Clinical Innovation (ACI). Provides policy, guidelines and educational resources relating to healthcare delivery, www.aci.health.nsw.gov.au/.

New Zealand Guidelines Group and Evidence Based Healthcare. Provides evidence-based guidance, tools and implementation frameworks for clinicians, www.health.govt.nz/about-ministry/ministry-health-websites/new-zealand-guidelines-group.

New Zealand Ministry of Health. Provides information for regulation of health professionals, www.health.govt.nz/.

New Zealand Ministry of Health websites, www.health.govt.nz/about-ministry/ministry-health-websites.

New Zealand Nurses Organisation. Provides information for regulation of nurses and midwives, www.nursingcouncil.org.nz/

Nursing and Midwifery Board of Australia. Provides information for regulation of nurse professional, www.nursingmidwiferyboard.gov.au.

Nursing Council of New Zealand. Provides information for regulation, standards and policies for nurses and midwives, www.nursingcouncil.org.nz/Public/Nursing/NCNZ/Nursing.aspx?hkey=4c7f36f6-42c3-40fa-b35c-88875eb2dcd5.

REFERENCES

1. Fry M, Shaban R, Considine J. Emergency nursing in Australia and New Zealand. In: Curtis K, Ramsden C, editors. Emergency and trauma care. Sydney: Elsevier; 2019.
2. Considine J, Curtis K, Shaban RZ, Fry M. Consensus-based clinical research priorities for emergency nursing in Australia. Australas Emerg Care 2018;21(2):43–50.
3. Kennedy B, Curtis K, Waters D. The personality of emergency nurses: is it unique? Australas Emerg Nurs J 2014;17(4):139–45.
4. Fry M. An ethnography: understanding emergency nursing practice belief systems. Int Emerg Nurs 2012;20(3):120–5.
5. Wise S, Duffield C, Fry M, Roche M. A team mental model approach to understanding team effectiveness in an emergency department: a qualitative study. J Health Serv Res Policy 2022;27(1):14–21.
6. Wise S, Duffield C, Fry M, Roche M. Nurses' role in accomplishing interprofessional coordination: lessons in 'almost managing' an emergency department team. J Nurs Manag 2022;30(1):198–204.
7. Jones T, Curtis K, Shaban RZ. Practice expectations for Australian graduate emergency nursing programs: a Delphi study. Nurse Educ Today 2021;99:104811.
8. College of Emergency Nursing Australasia (CENA). Practice standards for the Specialist Emergency Nurse. 2020. Online. Available from: www.cena.org.au/news-item/6021/practice-standards-for-the-specialist-emergency-nurse.
9. NSW Ministry of Health. Role delineation of clinical services. Emerg Med Australas. 2021. Online. Available from: www.health.nsw.gov.au/services/publications/role-delineation-of-clinical-services.PDF.

10. New Zealand Government. National population estimates. 2021. Online. Available from: www.stats.govt.nz/topics/population-estimates-and-projections.
11. Australian Bureau of Statistics (ABS). Population clock. Commonwealth of Australia; 2021. Online. Available from: www.abs.gov.au/ausstats/abs@.nsf/0/1647509ef7e25faaca2568a900154b63?OpenDocument.
12. Australian Institute of Health and Welfare (AIHW). Emergency department care 2020–2021. 2021. Online. Available from: www.aihw.gov.au/reports-data/myhospitals/sectors/emergency-department-care.
13. New Zealand Ministry of Health. Emergency departments. 2021. Online. Available from: www.health.govt.nz/our-work/hospitals-and-specialist-care/emergency-departments.
14. ACEM. Hospital data and accreditation 2012 survey—Part 1: report findings 2013. Online. Available from: acem.org.au/getmedia/27f56ecc-183b-4a57-a9d0-cb44afa0d865/Hosp_Data__Accreditation-_Part_1_Report.aspx.
15. Health.vic. Urgent care in regional and rural areas. 2021. Online. Available from: www.health.vic.gov.au/rural-health/urgent-care-in-regional-and-rural-areas.
16. Department of the Prime Minister and Cabinet (NZ). Future of Health/Te Anamata O Te Oranga. 2021. Online. Available from: www.futureofhealth.govt.nz.
17. Australian Institute of Health and Welfare (AIHW). Admitted patients 2019–2020. 2021. Online. Available from: www.aihw.gov.au/reports-data/myhospitals/sectors/admitted-patients.
18. NSW Ministry of Health. Models of care. 2021. Online. Available from: aci.health.nsw.gov.au/resources/models-of-care.
19. Morphet J, Kent B, Plummer V, Considine J. Transition to specialty practice program characteristics and professional development outcomes. Nurse Educ Today 2016;44:109–15.
20. Varndell W, Fry M, Elliott D. Pain assessment and interventions by nurses in the emergency department: a national survey. J Clin Nurs 2020;29(13–14):2352–62.
21. Varndell W, Fry M, Elliott D. Emergency nurses' perceptions of sedation management practices for critically ill intubated patients: a qualitative study. J Clin Nurs 2015;24(21–22):3286–95.
22. Wise S, Fry M, Duffield C, Roche M, Buchanan J. Ratios and nurse staffing: the vexed case of emergency departments. Australas Emerg Nurs J 2015;18(1):49–55.
23. Weichenthal L, Hendey G. The effect of mandatory nurse ratios on patient care in an emergency department. J Emerg Med 2011;40(1):76–81.
24. Gardner G, Gardner A, Middleton S, Considine J, Fitzgerald G, Christofis L, et al. Mapping workforce configuration and operational models in Australian emergency departments: a national survey. Aust Health Rev 2018;42(3):340–7.
25. Health.vic, Department of Health and Human Services. Safe patient care (nurse to patient and midwife to patient ratios) act 2015. 2015. Online. Available from: www.health.vic.gov.au/nursing-and-midwifery/safe-patient-care-nurse-to-patient-and-midwife-to-patient-ratios-act-2015.
26. Ministry of Health (NZ). A quality framework and suite of quality measures for the emergency department phase of acute patient care in New Zealand. Wellington: Ministry of Health; 2014.
27. Wise S, Duffield C, Fry M, Roche M. Clarifying workforce flexibility from a division of labor perspective: a mixed methods study of an emergency department team. Hum Resour Health 2020;18(1):17.
28. Ang BY, Lam SWS, Pasupathy Y, Ong MEH. Nurse workforce scheduling in the emergency department: a sequential decision support system considering multiple objectives. J Nurs Manag 2018;26(4):432–41.
29. NSW Ministry of Health. Emergency department workforce analysis tool (EDWAT) Edition 2. 2011. Online. Available from: www.health.nsw.gov.au/workforce/Pages/edwat-ed2.aspx.
30. Australian Government. Emergency medicine – Australia's future health workforce report. 2017. Online. Available from: www.health.gov.au/resources/publications/emergency-medicine-australias-future-health-workforce-report.
31. Morphet J, Kent B, Plummer V, Considine J. Profiling nursing resources in Australian emergency departments. Australas Emerg Nurs J 2016;19(1):1–10.
32. Jennings N, Lowe G, Tori K. Nurse practitioner locums: a plausible solution for augmenting health care access for rural communities. Aust J Prim Health 2021;27(1):1–5.
33. Jennings N, Gardner G, O'Reilly G, Mitra B. Evaluating emergency nurse practitioner service effectiveness on achieving timely analgesia: a pragmatic randomized controlled trial. Acad Emerg Med 2015;22(6):676–84.
34. Lutze M, Fry M, Mullen G, Connell JO, Coates D. Highlighting the invisible work of emergency nurse practitioners. J Nurse Pract 2018;14(1):26–32.e1.
35. Innes K, Jackson D, Plummer V, Elliott D. A profile of the waiting room nurse in emergency departments: an online survey of Australian nurses exploring implementation and perceptions. Int Emerg Nurs 2019;43:67–73.
36. Williams G, Crilly J, Souter J, Veach K, Good N. A state wide validation and utilisation study of the Queensland emergency nursing workforce tool. J Nurs Manag 2014;22(8):1076–88.
37. Innes K, Jackson D, Plummer V, Elliott D. Exploration and model development for emergency department waiting room nurse role: synthesis of a three-phase sequential mixed methods study. Int Emerg Nurs 2021;59:101075.
38. Wilson E, Hanson LC, Tori KE, Perrin BM. Nurse practitioner led model of after-hours emergency care in an Australian rural urgent care centre: health service stakeholder perceptions. BMC Health Serv Res 2021;21(1):819.

39. Wise S, Duffield C, Fry M, Roche M. Workforce flexibility – in defence of professional healthcare work. J Health Organ Manag 2017;31(4):503–16.
40. Nugus P, McCarthy S, Holdgate A, Braithwaite J, Schoenmakers A, Wagner C. Packaging patients and handing them over: communication context and persuasion in the emergency department. Ann Emerg Med 2017;69(2):210–7.e2.
41. Fry M, Ruperto K, Jarrett K, Wheeler J, Fong J, Fetchet W. Managing the wait: clinical initiative nurses' perceptions of an extended practice role. Australas Emerg Nurs J 2012;15(4):202–10.
42. Fry M, Jones K. The clinical initiative nurse: extending the role of the emergency nurse, who benefits? Australas Emerg Nurs J 2005;8(1):9–12.
43. Innes K, Jackson D, Plummer V, Elliott D. Emergency department waiting room nurse role: a key informant perspective. Australas Emerg Nurs J 2017;20(1):6–11.
44. Sobolewski KA, Koo S, Deutsch RJ. Improving the flow: optimization of available triage standing medication orders in the pediatric emergency department. Pediatr Emerg Care 2022;38(4):157–61.
45. Considine J, Lucas E, Martin R, Stergiou HE, Kropman M, Chiu H. Rapid intervention and treatment zone: redesigning nursing services to meet increasing emergency department demand. Int J Nurs Pract 2012;18(1):60–7.
46. Crawford K, Morphet J, Jones T, Innes K, Griffiths D, Williams A. Initiatives to reduce overcrowding and access block in Australian emergency departments: a literature review. Collegian 2014;21(4):359–66.
47. Nugus P, Forero R, McCarthy S, McDonnell G, Travaglia J, Hilman K, et al. The emergency department 'carousel': an ethnographically-derived model of the dynamics of patient flow. Int Emerg Nurs 2014;22(1):3–9.
48. Nugus P, Holdgate A, Fry M, Forero R, McCarthy S, Braithwaite J. Work pressure and patient flow management in the emergency department: findings from an ethnographic study. Acad Emerg Med 2011;18(10):1045–52.
49. Kilner E, Sheppard LA. The role of teamwork and communication in the emergency department: a systematic review. Int Emerg Nurs 2010;18(3):127–37.
50. Nugus P, Greenfield D, Travaglia J, Westbrook J, Braithwaite J. How and where clinicians exercise power: interprofessional relations in health care. Soc Sci Med 2010;71(5):898–909.
51. Nugus P, Braithwaite J. The dynamic interaction of quality and efficiency in the emergency department: squaring the circle? Soc Sci Med 2010;70(4):511–17.
52. Australian Commission on Safety and Quality in Health Care (ACSQHC). National safety and quality health service standards. ACSQHC; 2022. Online. Available from: www.safetyandquality.gov.au/wp-content/uploads/2017/12/National-Safety-and-Quality-Health-Service-Standards-second-edition.pdf.
53. ACEM. Quality Standards for emergency departments and other hospital-based emergency care services. 2015. Online. Available from: acem.org.au/getmedia/cbe80f1c-a64e-40ab-998f-ad57325a206f/Quality-Standards-1st-Edition-2015.aspx.
54. Romero B, Fry M, Roche M. The impact of evidence-based sepsis guidelines on emergency department clinical practice: a pre-post medical record audit. J Clin Nurs 2017;26(21–22):3588–96.
55. Northcott KMT, Gibson K, Peters MDJ. Nurse-initiated protocols in the emergency department management of pediatric oncology patients with fever and suspected neutropenia: a scoping review protocol. JBI Evid Synth 2021;19(5):1243–50.
56. Kabil G, Hatcher D, Alexandrou E, McNally S. Emergency nurses' experiences of the implementation of early goal directed fluid resuscitation therapy in the management of sepsis: a qualitative study. Australas Emerg Care 2021;24(1):67–72.
57. Hatozaki C, Sakuramoto H, Okamoto M, Nakajima H, Shimojo N, Inoue Y. Improving antibiotic administration rate for patients with sepsis in the emergency department. J Nurs Care Qual 2021;36(4):322–6.
58. The Australian Council on Healthcare Standards. Assessment to the national safety and quality health service standards. 2nd ed. Sydney: ACSQHC; 2021.
59. Ismail SA, Gibbons DC, Gnani S. Reducing inappropriate accident and emergency department attendances: a systematic review of primary care service interventions. Br J Gen Pract 2013;63(617):e813–20.
60. Fry M. Barriers and facilitators for successful after hours care model implementation: reducing emergency department utilisation. Australas Emerg Care J 2009;12:137–44.
61. Parker RLF, McRae I, Boyland T. Independent evaluation of the nurse-led ACT health walk in centre. Australian National University; 2011.
62. Stevens L, Fry M, Browne M, Barnes A. Fast track patients' satisfaction, compliance and confidence with emergency department discharge planning. Australas Emerg Care 2019;22(2):87–91.
63. Elliott R, Mei J, Wormleaton N, Fry M. Interventions for the discharge of older people to their home from the emergency department: a systematic review. Australas Emerg Care 2022;25(1):1–12.
64. Fry M, Elliott R, Curtis K, Mei J, Fitzpatrick L, Groth R, et al. Family members' perceptions of older person discharge from emergency departments. Int J Older People Nurs 2021;16(3):e12365.
65. Curtis E, Paine SJ, Jiang Y, Jones P, Tomash I, Raumati I, et al. Examining emergency department inequities: descriptive analysis of national data (2006–2012). Emerg Med Australas 2020;32(6):953–9.
66. Curtis E, Paine S, Jiang Y, Jones P, Raumati I, Tomash I, et al. Examining emergency department inequities between Māori and non-Māori: do they exist? Eur J Public Health 2020;30(Suppl. 5). doi:10.1093/eurpub/ckaa166.734.
67. Fry M, Elliott R, Fitzpatrick L, Warton J, Curtis K. Measuring nurses' perceptions of their work environment and linking with behaviour change theories and implementation strategies to support evidence based practice change. Appl Nurs Res 2020;56:151374.

68. Adams S, Carryer J. Establishing the nurse practitioner workforce in rural New Zealand: barriers and facilitators. J Prim Health Care 2019;11(2):152–8.
69. Flynn D, Francis R, Robalino S, Lally J, Snooks H, Rodgers H, et al. A review of enhanced paramedic roles during and after hospital handover of stroke, myocardial infarction and trauma patients. BMC Emerg Med 2017;17(1):5.
70. Shaban R. Paramedic clinical judgement and decision-making of mental illness in emergency contexts: research: practice and tools of the trade. Australas J Paramed 2006;4(2):1–13.
71. Woollard M. Professionalism in UK paramedic practice. Article 990391. J Emerg Prim Health Care 2009;7(4). doi:10.33151/ajp.7.4.181.
72. Stenner K, van Even S, Collen A. Paramedic independent prescribing: a qualitative study of early adopters in the UK. Br Paramed J 2021;6(1):30–7.
73. Abetz JW, Olaussen A, Jennings PA, Smit V, Mitra B. Review article: pre-hospital provider clinical judgement upon arrival to the emergency department: a systematic review and meta-analysis. Emerg Med Australas 2020;32(6):917–23.
74. Power B, Bury G, Ryan J. Stakeholder opinion on the proposal to introduce 'treat and referral' into the Irish emergency medical service. BMC Emerg Med 2019;19(1):81.
75. McQueen C, Crombie N, Hulme J, Cormack S, Hussain N, Ludwig F, et al. Prehospital anaesthesia performed by physician/critical care paramedic teams in a major trauma network in the UK: a 12 month review of practice. Emerg Med J 2015;32(1):65–9.
76. Mason S, Knowles E, Colwell B, Dixon S, Wardrope J, Gorringe R, et al. Effectiveness of paramedic practitioners in attending 999 calls from elderly people in the community: cluster randomised controlled trial. BMJ 2007;335(7626):919.
77. Woollard M. The role of the paramedic practitioner in the UK. J Paramedicine 2015;4(1):1–9.
78. Snooks H, Kearsley N, Dale J, Halter M, Redhead J, Cheung WY. Towards primary care for non-serious 999 callers: results of a controlled study of 'treat and refer' protocols for ambulance crews. Qual Saf Health Care 2004;13(6):435.
79. Snooks H, Foster T, Nicholl J. Results of an evaluation of the effectiveness of triage and direct transportation to minor injuries units by ambulance crews. Emerg Med J 2004;21(1):105–11.
80. Nursing Council of New Zealand. Competencies for registered nurses. Nursing Council of New Zealand; 2017. Online. Available from: www.nursingcouncil.org.nz/NCNZ/nursing-section/Continuing_Competence.aspx.
81. Nursing Council of New Zealand. Nurse practitioner required qualifications and competencies. 2017. Online. Available from: www.nursingcouncil.org.nz/Public/Nursing/Scopes_of_practice/Nurse_practitioner/NCNZ/nursing-section/Nurse_practitioner.aspx?hkey=1493d86e-e4a5-45a5-8104-64607cf103c6.
82. Nursing and Midwifery Board of Australia (NMBA). Registered nurse standards for practice. 2017. Online. Available from: www.nursingmidwiferyboard.gov.au/codes-guidelines-statements/professional-standards/registered-nurse-standards-for-practice.aspx.
83. Nursing and Midwifery Board of Australia (NMBA). Nurse practitioner standards for practice. 2021. Online. Available from: www.nursingmidwiferyboard.gov.au/codes-guidelines-statements/professional-standards/nurse-practitioner-standards-of-practice.aspx.
84. College of Emergency Nursing New Zealand. Knowledge and skills framework. 2016. Online. Available from: www.voced.edu.au/content/ngv%3A89475.
85. Jones T, Curtis K, Shaban RZ. Academic and professional characteristics of Australian graduate emergency nursing programs: a national study. Australas Emerg Care 2020;23(3):173–80.
86. Jones T, Shaban RZ, Creedy DK. Practice standards for emergency nursing: an international review. Australas Emerg Nurs J 2015;18(4):190–203.
87. Royal College of Nursing (RCN). Our history: the Royal College of Nursing from 1916 to the present. 2021. Online. Available from: www.rcn.org.uk/About-us/our-history.
88. Emergency Nurses Association. Organizational and systems leadership in nursing. Emergency Nurses Association. Online. Available from: nursinganswers.net/essays/emergency-nurses-association-organizational-and-systems-leadership-in-nursing.php?vref=1.
89. Russell L, Gething L, Convery P. National review of specialist nurse education. Sydney: University of Sydney; 1997.
90. Whyte S. The specialist nurse: a classification system. Contemp Nurse 2000;9(1):6–15.
91. Kirk K, Cohen L, Edgley A, Timmons S. 'I don't have any emotions': an ethnography of emotional labour and feeling rules in the emergency department. J Adv Nurs 2021;77(4):1956–67.
92. Pavedahl V, Holmström IK, Summer Meranius M, von Thiele Schwarz U, Muntlin Å. Fundamentals of care in the emergency room—an ethnographic observational study. Int Emerg Nurs 2021;58:101050.
93. Duffield C, Forbes J, Fallon A, Roche M, Wise W, Merrick ET. Nursing skill mix and nursing time: the roles of registered nurses and clinical nurse specialists. Aust J Adv Nurs 2005;23(2):14–21.
94. Whyte S. Specialist nurses in Australia: the ICN and international regulation. J Prof Nurs 2000;16(4):210–18.
95. Gardner G, Duffield C, Doubrovsky A, Bui UT, Adams M. The structure of nursing: a national examination of titles and practice profiles. Int Nurs Rev 2017;64(2):233–41.
96. Whitehead L, Twigg DE, Carman R, Glass C, Halton H, Duffield C. Factors influencing the development and implementation of nurse practitioner candidacy programs: a scoping review. Int J Nurs Stud 2022;125:104133.
97. Gardner G, Duffield C, Doubrovsky A, Adams M. Identifying advanced practice: a national survey of a nursing workforce. Int J Nurs Stud 2016;55:60–70.
98. Fry M, MacGregor C, Ruperto K, Jarrett K, Wheeler J, Fong J, et al. Nursing praxis, compassionate caring and interpersonal relations: an observational study. Australas Emerg Nurs J 2013;16(2):37–44.

99. Fry M, Holdgate A. Nurse-initiated intravenous morphine in the emergency department: efficacy, rate of adverse events and impact on time to analgesia. Emerg Med (Fremantle) 2002;14(3):249–54.
100. Ryder M, Jacob E, Hendricks J. An integrative review to identify evidence of nurse practitioner-led changes to health-care delivery and the outcomes of such changes. Int J Nurs Pract 2020;26(6):e12901.
101. Oatley M, Fry M. A nurse practitioner-led model of care improves access, early assessment and integration of oncology services: an evaluation study. Support Care Cancer 2020;28(10):5023–9.
102. Gardner G, Gardner A, Middleton S, Della P, Kain V, Doubrovsky A. The work of nurse practitioners. J Adv Nurs 2010;66(10):2160–9.
103. Carryer J, Wilkinson J, Towers A, Gardner G. Delineating advanced practice nursing in New Zealand: a national survey. Int Nurs Rev 2018; 65(1):24–32.
104. American Association of Nurse Practitioners. NP fact sheet. 2021. Online. Available from: www.aanp.org/about/all-about-nps/np-fact-sheet.
105. Te Kaunihera Tapuhi o Aotearoa/Nursing Council of New Zealand. The New Zealand nursing workforce: a profile of nurse practitioners, registered nurses and enrolled nurses 2018–2019. 2019. Online. Available from: www.nursingcouncil.org.nz/NCNZ/News-section/news-item/2020/2/Council_publishes_Workforce_Report_2018-2019.aspx.
106. Australian Government. Nurses and midwives in Australia. 2021. Online. Available from: www.health.gov.au/health-topics/nurses-and-midwives/in-australia.
107. Australian Government. Nurse practitioner 2017 fact sheet. 2018. Online. Available from: hwd.health.gov.au/resources/publications/factsheet-nrpr-2017.pdf.
108. Roche TE, Gardner G, Jack L. The effectiveness of emergency nurse practitioner service in the management of patients presenting to rural hospitals with chest pain: a multisite prospective longitudinal nested cohort study. BMC Health Serv Res 2017;17(1):445.
109. Rogers T, Ross N, Spooner D. Evaluation of a 'See and Treat' pilot study introduced to an emergency department. Accid Emerg Nurs 2004;12(1):24–7.
110. Fry M, Rogers T. The transitional emergency nurse practitioner role: implementation study and preliminary evaluation. Australas Emerg Nurs J 2009;12(2):32–7.
111. Considine J, Martin R, Smit D, Winter C, Jenkins J. Emergency nurse practitioner care and emergency department patient flow: case-control study. Emerg Med Australas 2006;18(4):385–90.
112. Bunn F, Byrne G, Kendall S. Telephone consultation and triage: effects on health care use and patient satisfaction. Cochrane Database Syst Rev 2004;(4):CD004180.
113. Laurant M, Reeves D, Hermens R, Braspenning J, Grol R, Sibbald B. Substitution of doctors by nurses in primary care. Cochrane Database Syst Rev 2005;(2):CD001271.
114. Martin-Misener R, Downe-Wamboldt B, Cain E, Girouard M. Cost effectiveness and outcomes of a nurse practitioner–paramedic–family physician model of care: the Long and Brier Islands study. Prim Health Care Res Dev 2009;10(1):14–25.
115. Chenoweth D, Martin N, Pankowski J, Raymond LW. Nurse practitioner services: three-year impact on health care costs. J Occup Environ Med 2008;50(11):1293–8.
116. Sylvia ML, Griswold M, Dunbar L, Boyd CM, Park M, Boult C. Guided care: cost and utilization outcomes in a pilot study. Dis Manag 2008;11(1): 29–36.
117. Soco C, Simonovich SD, Dillon D, Bishop-Royse J, Lattner C. Communication, leadership and organizational support facilitate successful transition into practice for nurse practitioners in the emergency department. J Am Assoc Nurse Pract 2020;33(12):1156–65.
118. Duignan M, Drennan J, McCarthy VJC. Impact of clinical leadership in advanced practice roles on outcomes in health care: a scoping review. J Nurs Manag 2021;29(4):613–22.
119. Singhal S, Hosking I, Ward J, Boyle AA. A qualitative study: what do nurses in charge in emergency departments do? Cureus 2021;13(9):e17912.
120. Grover E, Porter JE, Morphet J. An exploration of emergency nurses' perceptions, attitudes and experience of teamwork in the emergency department. Australas Emerg Nurs J 2017;20(2):92–7.
121. Carryer J, Gardner G, Dunn S, Gardner A. The core role of the nurse practitioner: practice, professionalism and clinical leadership. J Clin Nurs 2007;16(10):1818–25.
122. Adams A, Hollingsworth A, Osman A. The implementation of a cultural change toolkit to reduce nursing burnout and mitigate nurse turnover in the emergency department. J Emerg Nurs 2019;45(4):452–6.
123. Kane-Urrabazo C. Management's role in shaping organizational culture. J Nurs Manag 2006;14(3):188–94.
124. Chan SS, Cheung NK, Graham CA, Rainer TH. Strategies and solutions to alleviate access block and overcrowding in emergency departments. Hong Kong Med J 2015;21(4):345–52.
125. Forero R, Hillman KM, McCarthy S, Fatovich DM, Joseph AP, Richardson DB. Access block and ED overcrowding. Emerg Med Australas 2010;22(2):119–35.
126. Fatovich DM, Hughes G, McCarthy SM. Access block: it's all about available beds. Med J Aust 2009;190(7):362–3.
127. Sprivulis PC, Da Silva JA, Jacobs IG, Frazer AR, Jelinek GA. The association between hospital overcrowding and mortality among patients admitted via Western Australian emergency departments. Med J Aust 2006;184(5):208–12.
128. Nouri Y, Gholipour C, Aghazadeh J, Khanahmadi S, Beygzadeh T, Nouri D, et al. Evaluation of the risk factors associated with emergency department boarding: a retrospective cross-sectional study. Chin J Traumatol 2020;23(6):346–50.

129. O'Dowd A. Emergency departments must not return to pre-COVID days of overcrowding and lack of safety, says college. BMJ 2020;369:m1848.
130. McKenna P, Heslin SM, Viccellio P, Mallon WK, Hernandez C, Morley EJ. Emergency department and hospital crowding: causes, consequences, and cures. Clin Exp Emerg Med 2019;6(3):189–95.
131. Wachtel G, Elalouf A. Addressing overcrowding in an emergency department: an approach for identifying and treating influential factors and a real-life application. Isr J Health Policy Res 2020;9(1):37.
132. Nursing and Midwifery Board of Australia and Ahpra. Continuing professional development. 2021. Online. Available from: www.nursingmidwiferyboard.gov.au/registration-standards/continuing-professional-development.aspx.
133. Martin J. The challenge of introducing continuous professional development for paramedics. Aust J Paramedicine 2006;4(2). doi:10.33151/ajp.4.2.368.
134. Sloane DM, Smith HL, McHugh MD, Aiken LH. Effect of changes in hospital nursing resources on improvements in patient safety and quality of care: a panel study. Med Care 2018;56(12):1001–8.
135. Harrison JM, Aiken LH, Sloane DM, Brooks Carthon JM, Merchant RM, Berg RA, et al. In hospitals with more nurses who have baccalaureate degrees, better outcomes for patients after cardiac arrest. Health Aff (Millwood) 2019;38(7):1087–94.
136. Lossius HM, Røislien J, Lockey DJ. Patient safety in pre-hospital emergency tracheal intubation: a comprehensive meta-analysis of the intubation success rates of EMS providers. Crit Care 2012;16(1):R24.
137. von Goedecke A, Herff H, Paal P, Dörges V, Wenzel V. Field airway management disasters. Anesth Analg 2007;104(3):481–3.
138. Ross K, Barr J, Stevens J. Mandatory continuing professional development requirements: what does this mean for Australian nurses. BMC Nurs 2013;12:9. doi:10.1186/1472-6955-12-9.
139. Halfer D. Supporting nursing professional development: a magnet hospital's story. J Nurses Staff Dev 2009;25(3):135–40.
140. Cooper E. Creating a culture of professional development: a milestone pathway tool for registered nurses. J Contin Educ Nurs 2009;40(11):501–8.
141. Theobald KA, Coyer FM, Henderson AJ, Fox R, Thomson BF, McCarthy AL. Developing a postgraduate professional education framework for emergency nursing: a co-design approach. BMC Nurs 2021;20(1):43.
142. Curtis K, Fry M, Shaban RZ, Considine J. Translating research findings to clinical nursing practice. J Clin Nurs 2017;26(5–6):862–72.
143. Considine J, Shaban RZ, Fry M, Curtis K. Evidence-based emergency nursing: designing a research question and searching the literature. Int Emerg Nurs 2017;32:78–82.
144. Shaban RZ, Considine J, Fry M, Curtis K. Case study and case-based research in emergency nursing and care: theoretical foundations and practical application in paramedic pre-hospital clinical judgment and decision-making of patients with mental illness. Australas Emerg Nurs J 2017;20(1):17–24.

CHAPTER 2
PARAMEDICINE IN AUSTRALIA AND AOTEAROA NEW ZEALAND

PAUL JENNINGS

ESSENTIALS

- The history of organised ambulance services in Australia and Aotearoa New Zealand can be traced back to the late 1800s. These services provided basic care, consistent with community expectations of the times.
- There were a number of influences that were common in the development of the ambulance services. First-aiders, trained by St John Ambulance, were often the providers of ambulance services, but—depending upon their location—ambulance services were also provided by hospitals, police, industry groups, government entities, and, in some cases, commercial operators.
- Early ambulance services often focused on the means of transport from the scene, rather than treatment at the scene. Over time, the mode of transport changed from human-powered Ashford litters to horse-drawn wagons, then progressed to mechanical means of transport on the land and through the air.
- In the late 1960s and early 1970s, a change in the focus of ambulance services occurred as a result of parallel developments in the way the sick and injured were treated before they arrived at hospital.
- Advances in the care of cardiac and road-trauma patients led to the development of contemporary paramedicine practices and systems.
- Paramedics are the interface between the community and emergency department and acute hospital care, so play a vital role in improving patient outcomes from illness and injury.

INTRODUCTION

History of Paramedicine

Most of the ambulance services that exist today have long and varied histories. Many have their foundations in the late 1800s and were set up by enthusiastic groups of community-minded people with an interest in first aid. St John Ambulance was an influential factor in their formation, as they were the providers of first aid training for many of the members of these newly created ambulance services.

The increasing number of people with first aid qualifications who were looking for an opportunity to maintain and utilise their newly acquired skills led to the formation of St John Ambulance brigades, which catered for the treatment and sometimes transport of the sick and injured on a voluntary basis. However, not all ambulance services in Australia owe their origins to St John Ambulance; there were also several community-based groups, government bodies, hospitals and private individuals who initially provided this important function.

In their earliest days, the main role of ambulance services was to facilitate the transport of the sick and injured to hospital. The standard of care for the treatment of these patients was at the level of basic first aid and the provision of comfort measures. Medical care was solely within the domain of doctors, who, ably assisted by nurses, provided much of the care for the sick or injured following their arrival at hospital.

Many of the advances that occurred during the early history of ambulance services related to the modes of transport that were available to facilitate the safe arrival of a patient to a hospital. The earliest mode of transport used in Australia and Aotearoa New Zealand was the Ashford litter, which could be best described as a stretcher on detachable cart wheels with retractable supporting legs. This litter owes its origin to Sir John Furley, one of the founders of St John Ambulance. His design was patented in 1875 and was known as 'St John ambulance'. However, the concept of having a system that involved the quick retrieval and transport of the injured can be traced back to Dr Dominique Jean Larrey, a military surgeon in Napoleon's army. In 1792, he developed a system that facilitated initial treatment and retrieval of injured soldiers from the battlefield to field hospitals, where they were treated by military surgeons. The system required the use of lightweight horse-drawn carriages that entered the battlefield and swiftly removed the wounded, taking them to a designated location set up to treat the injured, often situated behind the battle front. These carts were called flying volantes and later became known as flying ambulances.[1] Larrey's approach was, in essence, the principle upon which modern-day trauma systems are founded.

Over time, the Ashford litter was replaced by horse-drawn vans, wagons or carts, but not before the litter was adapted to enable it to become bicycle-powered. The Ashford litter was certainly an improvement on a stretcher carried by two stretcher-bearers, although ultimately its successful utilisation was determined by the patient's proximity to the hospital and by the state of the roads and pathways upon which it was to be deployed.

As motor vehicles became increasingly popular and more affordable, their potential for use by ambulance services was obvious. They were able to transport patients to hospital more quickly and cover greater distances. Initially, trucks, upon whose flat tray the sick and injured were placed, were used by some services, while other services utilised fitted out, motorised vans equipped with stretchers (Fig. 2.1). Eventually, special vehicles were commissioned by ambulance services and built by coach and body builders on a truck chassis. Much later, passenger vehicles and station wagons were modified to satisfy the unique requirements of ambulance vehicles, thus significantly reducing the cost of new purchases (only modifications were required instead of the need for completely new designs) as demands for service increased and old-model ambulances in fleets that had become outdated were replaced.

Over time, ambulances became more specialised, and bespoke vehicles were developed by some ambulance services to meet the specific needs of the communities that they served. During the 1918–19 Spanish flu epidemic and during wartime, tram carriages[2] were transformed into multi-patient modes of transport to move patients to either infectious disease centres or military hospitals. In the Australian outback, motorised rail trikes have been used to transport patients between outlying towns and regional centres.[3] Boats have been adapted to be used in aquatic environments. Planes and helicopters have made a significant contribution to the ability to quickly transport critically ill or seriously injured patients, and are covered in more detail later in this chapter.

FIGURE 2.1
AN EARLY-MODEL MOTORISED AMBULANCE
C. 1910–1920

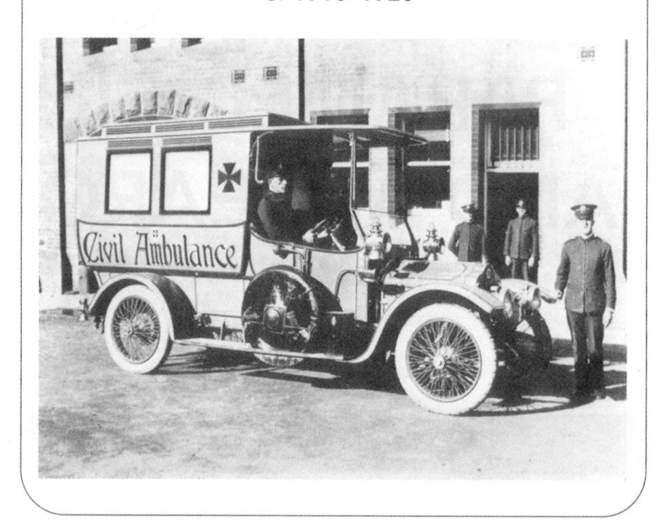

Courtesy of NSW Ambulance.

It is easy to see why the modern-day paramedic was once often referred to as an ambulance driver. Staff, either employed or volunteers, who had mechanical ability were highly regarded by ambulance service managers. A first aid certificate was often the only qualification that was required to become an ambulance driver, the precursor of the modern-day paramedic.[4]

HISTORICAL OVERVIEW OF PARAMEDICINE BY JURISDICTION

NEW SOUTH WALES

New South Wales has the earliest documented ambulance service in Australia, dating back to 1881, when the Board of Health, in response to a smallpox epidemic, organised a transport service to a hospital for infectious diseases for patients located on the outskirts of the Sydney urban area.[4] While a number of hospitals developed their own ambulance services, there were also localised, community-based and industrially orientated groups that provided ambulance transport services.[4] One of the largest and best organised of these groups was the Civil Ambulance and Transport Brigade (CATB). It was established in 1895 and is generally regarded as the original ambulance group from which the present-day Ambulance Service of New South Wales developed.

St John Ambulance also played a part in the original development of ambulance services in the state. While its main role at this time was to provide first aid instruction, it did fund the provision of an Ashford litter that could be used to transport the sick and injured. By 1900 St John Ambulance had provided 14 such litters, which were strategically positioned around the city of Sydney. It was not until 1912 that the CATB took delivery of its first motorised ambulance.

In the early part of the 20th century, CATB became the Civil Ambulance and Transport Corps (CATC) under the auspices of St John Ambulance. A number of other ambulance services also existed during these times, and rivalry between

CATC and other suburban services led to the government of the day enacting legislation to create the Ambulance Transport Service Board via the *Ambulance Transport Service Act 1919*. In 1925 the Central District Ambulance Service (CDAS) was formed, based in the Sydney region. In the years that followed, ambulance services in regional areas replicated the service delivery initiated by CDAS. In 1972 all these services were united together when the *Ambulance Service Act 1972* came into being. This Act created a statewide ambulance service with a common administrative framework, known as the New South Wales Ambulance Service. Later its name was changed to the Ambulance Service of New South Wales. To this day, it remains under the control of the state's Department of Health.

VICTORIA

The first ambulance service in Victoria commenced in 1896 when St John Ambulance placed an Ashford litter at the Eastern Hill Fire Station, Melbourne's main fire station, staffed by trained assistants.[4] It is from this single event that Victoria's state ambulance service grew. Initially the fire brigade provided the service for free, but as demand increased their board sought recompense for the service. Government grants initially assisted the financing of this vital service, but in 1902 the Chief Secretary refused requests for further grants, declaring that police would provide the service using Hansom cabs (horse-drawn taxis) and Ashford litters.[4]

Ambulance services continued, but became increasingly expensive as the method of transport changed from human- and horse-powered transportation to that provided by automobiles. In 1916, the Victorian Civil Ambulance Service (VCAS) was formed. Although legally separate from St John Ambulance, there was a high degree of cross-membership between the two organisations. Over time, VCAS became the main provider of ambulance services in Melbourne and its surrounds. In 1922 a country division was formed to service and support the development of ambulance services in rural and regional areas. This was a loose amalgamation of rural and regional ambulance services and continued until the Victorian Hospital and Charities Commission established regional ambulance boards in 1955, making the country division redundant. VCAS continued until 1973, when the state government restructured ambulance services and created an entity called Ambulance Service Victoria. In 1986, the *Ambulance Services Act 1986* established the Metropolitan Ambulance Service (MAS) and Rural Ambulance Victoria (RAV); RAV was divided into further administrative and operational regions. In July 2008, MAS, RAV and the Alexandra and District Ambulance Service were amalgamated to form Ambulance Victoria, thus creating a single ambulance service for the entire state.[4]

QUEENSLAND

The Queensland Ambulance Transport Brigade (QATB) came into existence in 1902.[4] This organisation has its origins in the City Ambulance Transport Brigade, established in 1892. Many of the members of this Brisbane-based group had a strong affiliation with St John Ambulance, having gained their first aid qualification from them. Over time, QATB prospered and enjoyed a great deal of community support, allowing it to extend its operations to other metropolitan locations and regional centres.

In 1916, QATB took over the St John Ambulance Queensland Centre and became the agent for the Order of St John in Queensland. Ambulance services continued to develop as a result of community endeavour and these brigades were very parochial in nature, with the fund-raising activities that supported their services forming part of the social fabric of many communities.[4]

From the time QATB was established until 1967, ambulance services came under the *Hospitals Acts* of 1923 and 1944. The *Ambulance Services Act 1967* provided a separate legislative framework for ambulance services, and specified that local area committees were to be formed and a State Council established as the regulatory body of QATB.[4]

QATB, which had a large number of single brigades operating within it, became the Queensland Ambulance Service, as we know it today, in 1991, when the brigades amalgamated.[3] The level of training and equipment available to each brigade differed according to each local committee's fund-raising effectiveness and the economic conditions of the time. It was once said that 'when there were 96 brigades the only thing in common was the colour of the shirts'.[4]

WESTERN AUSTRALIA

In 1903 the Perth metropolitan fire brigade began an ambulance service using a horse-drawn van. In the same year, the police acquired an Ashford litter. In the following years, ambulance services spread to industrial workplaces as Ashford litters were located at wharves, railway workshops and railway stations. By 1910 all the major railway stations in Perth had an Ashford litter located in their vicinity. Four Perth municipalities also had their own horse-drawn ambulance services.

As a result of the increasing workload associated with providing ambulance services, the fire brigade decided to concentrate on activities associated with fire-fighting and reduce their involvement in the provision of non-core business. In 1922 St John Ambulance took over formal control of the Perth metropolitan ambulance service, later expanding its activities throughout the state. A second metropolitan ambulance centre was established in Fremantle in 1929. During the 1930s approximately 50 ambulance centres were established throughout the state, and by 1970, the number of ambulance locations had risen to 96. By the late 1980s there were 17 metropolitan ambulance depots and 105 locations outside the metropolitan area. Some ambulance services in remote locations chose to remain outside the St John umbrella, but these were few in number.[4]

SOUTH AUSTRALIA

The early history of ambulance services in South Australia is not well documented.[4] Up until the early 1950s there was no unified system as in the other Australian states; rather, there was a 'haphazard series of small, independent and uncoordinated services in the capital city, Adelaide, as well as in the State's other cities and regional centres'.[4]

In 1951, the state government outsourced ambulance services to the St John Council for South Australia Inc. Prior to this government initiative, metropolitan Adelaide was serviced by a collection of organisations. These included the South Australia Ambulance Transport Inc (previously Hindmarsh Volunteer Ambulance), Northern Suburbs Ambulance Association, the Civil Ambulance run by the police department and Joe Myren's Private Ambulance. St John Ambulance amalgamated these services, and over the next few decades developed regional and rural services to such a degree that by the 1970s South Australia had a statewide service similar to those existing in most other states of Australia.[4]

The *Ambulance Service Act 1992* legislated responsibility for ambulance services to a joint venture between the Minister of Health and the Priory in Australia of the Grand Priory of the Most Venerable Order of the Hospital of St John of Jerusalem. In 2005 it became known as the South Australian Ambulance Service (SAAS), and in 2008 SAAS officially became part of South Australia Health.[4]

TASMANIA

Tasmania's first ambulance service began in Launceston in 1915 when the proprietor of the local livery stable had a horse-drawn ambulance van built.[4] In 1922 the responsibility for this service was transferred to the local municipal authority, which engaged the fire brigade to operate the service. During this time, Hobart City Council also established an ambulance service to serve that city.

By the 1950s there were 13 regional and local boards operating a total of 33 ambulance vehicles. Each board acted independently of the others with little or no coordination between any of the providers. This lack of coordination, along with differing standards of training and equipment and widespread community dissatisfaction, finally led to the state government establishing an Ambulance Commission, whose role was to oversee all these services.

The state's Minister for Health persuaded the St John Council for Tasmania, based in Hobart, to take control of ambulance services. Within two years, St John provided ambulance coverage to about two-thirds of the state's area, along with services to most cities and main towns. A number of issues affected the ability of St John to provide their planned service, and in 1965 they announced they would withdraw from the provision of ambulance services. An external consultation reviewed the state's ambulance service and it was recommended that the government take direct control. Thus, the Tasmanian Ambulance Service came into being, changing its name to Ambulance Tasmania in 2013.

AUSTRALIAN CAPITAL TERRITORY (ACT)

Canberra has had an ambulance service since about 1915 when construction on the nation's capital began.[4] In 1925 the Federal Capital Commission (FCC) was established, with one of its roles being to commission an ambulance service.

By 1930 the FCC had been abolished and the local fire brigade organised the service that was to become known as the Canberra Fire and Ambulance Service. In 1955 the Canberra Ambulance Service came into existence under the control of the Commonwealth's Department of Interior. It soon changed its name to the ACT Ambulance Service. In the next year, control of the service was handed to the board of the Canberra Community Hospital. In 1989 the ACT became self-governing and the service was brought under the control of the ACT Emergency Services Authority.[4]

NORTHERN TERRITORY

Ambulance services in the Northern Territory were initially provided and run by the local hospitals in its two main towns, Darwin and Alice Springs.[4] The first motorised ambulance commenced in 1929. In the early 1950s, St John Ambulance provided after-hours ambulance services.

The outstanding assistance that St John Ambulance service was able to provide during Cyclone Tracy (in 1974) and its aftermath became a catalyst to draw together the various Public Health Department ambulance services in an effort to provide a unified service throughout the territory. In 1977 the Northern Territory government passed control of the ambulance services to the St John Ambulance Council of the Northern Territory, which proceeded to develop a territory-wide service encompassing all the main cities and towns of the territory.[4]

AOTEAROA NEW ZEALAND

There were predominantly four providers of ambulance services in Aotearoa New Zealand—St John Ambulance, Wellington Free Ambulance, and the Taranaki and Wairarapa District Health Boards. St John Ambulance is responsible for ambulance services that cover just over 85% of the nation's land mass. The establishment of St John in Aotearoa New Zealand was first mooted during a public meeting in Christchurch in 1885. By 1889 Christchurch had four Ashford litters based at police and fire stations. They were more fortunate than the people of Auckland—in 1892 St John reported that the equipment there consisted of a stretcher and a set of bandages, but fortunately by 1903 their fleet had expanded to nine litters. In the same year, the city of Dunedin formed the first division of the St John Ambulance Brigade and began to provide first aid services.[4]

St John rapidly established itself throughout Aotearoa New Zealand, proving especially popular in localities where medical services were scarce and where the local industry was labour-intensive. In 1975 the government of the day revamped the Ambulance Transport Advisory Board, resulting in St John reviewing their ambulance service activities. Staff were encouraged to obtain and eventually required to hold formal qualifications. The days of patients being tended to by ambulance personnel who held a basic first aid certificate were over.[4]

Since 1927, the people of Wellington and its surrounds have been the beneficiaries of free ambulance transport from the Wellington Free Ambulance, an organisation that claims to be the only free ambulance service operating in the Southern Hemisphere.

EVOLUTIONS IN OUT-OF-HOSPITAL CARE

Peter J Safar MD[5] made a significant contribution to the development of out-of-hospital emergency care throughout the world. He is known as the father of CPR (cardiopulmonary resuscitation), and is credited with identifying the Airway and Breathing elements of the ABC of resuscitation. Some of his notable achievements were the establishment of the first intensive-care unit in a hospital in the United States; assisting in the development of the first advanced life support (ALS) ambulances; and assisting in the development of the 'Resusci Anne' manikin. Most important, however, was his role in the modern history of emergency medical services—he organised one of the first, if not *the* first, out-of-hospital emergency medical service in the United States.

In 1967, Freedom House Enterprises commenced a paramedic service in Pittsburgh, Pennsylvania. It was a welfare project with a two-fold purpose: to provide an ambulance service to an impoverished area, and also provide employment and training to unemployed members of a minority group. This project led to a partnership between Dr Safar and Freedom House Enterprises, an outreach of the United Negro Protest Committee. The Freedom House Ambulance Service trainee paramedics were African-American men and women drawn from the ranks of Pittsburgh's unemployed.[6,7] The resultant ambulance service provided the most sophisticated emergency care to one of the most disadvantaged groups of people in the United States.

In 1974 Dr Safar appointed Nancy Caroline[8] as medical director of Freedom House Ambulance Service. She was to become a prominent author of textbooks for paramedics. For many years her first textbook, now in its eighth edition, was the only one specifically written for paramedics. The 1975 report she prepared for the US government played a significant role in the development of the first national paramedic training course. To many she is affectionately known as the 'mother of paramedics'.[9]

In early 1966, in Belfast, Northern Ireland, Frank Pantridge, who has sometimes been called the 'grandfather of out-of-hospital ALS', set up a mobile intensive care unit to assist in the management of patients with myocardial infarction. He recognised that in cases of cardiac arrest due to ventricular fibrillation, the defibrillator needed to be brought to the patient rather than the patient being brought to the defibrillator.[10] No portable defibrillators existed at this time, but Pantridge utilised some technology developed by the NASA space program to develop a lightweight, portable defibrillator capable of being carried to the scene of a cardiac arrest by paramedics.[11] His ground-breaking program confirmed that it was possible to treat cardiac arrests that occurred outside hospitals. As a result of this work, similar programs in many centres were set up throughout the developed world over the next decade.

In 1971, the Mobile Intensive Care Ambulance (MICA) program was set up in Victoria. This was the first MICA system in Australia and the third in the world after Belfast, Northern Ireland, and Seattle, Washington. Initially, a paramedic and a medical registrar staffed the MICA vehicle, but by 1973 the medical officer was replaced by another suitably trained paramedic, making it a 'paramedic-only' response (Fig. 2.2).

By the late 1960s and early 1970s, paramedic programs had either begun planning for their implementation or had commenced in a number of locations. Most notably were the centres of Miami, Florida, under the guidance of Eugene Nagel; Seattle, Washington, overseen by Leonard Cobb; Los Angeles, California, with medical director Ron Stewart; Portland, Oregon, and Nassau County, New York. There were two major influences on the development of such paramedic programs. The work of Pantridge in Northern Ireland inspired a number of cardiologists to become advocates for the advanced

FIGURE 2.2
AN INJURED WORKER IN A RURAL SETTING BEING TREATED BY FIRST RESPONDERS AND PARAMEDICS

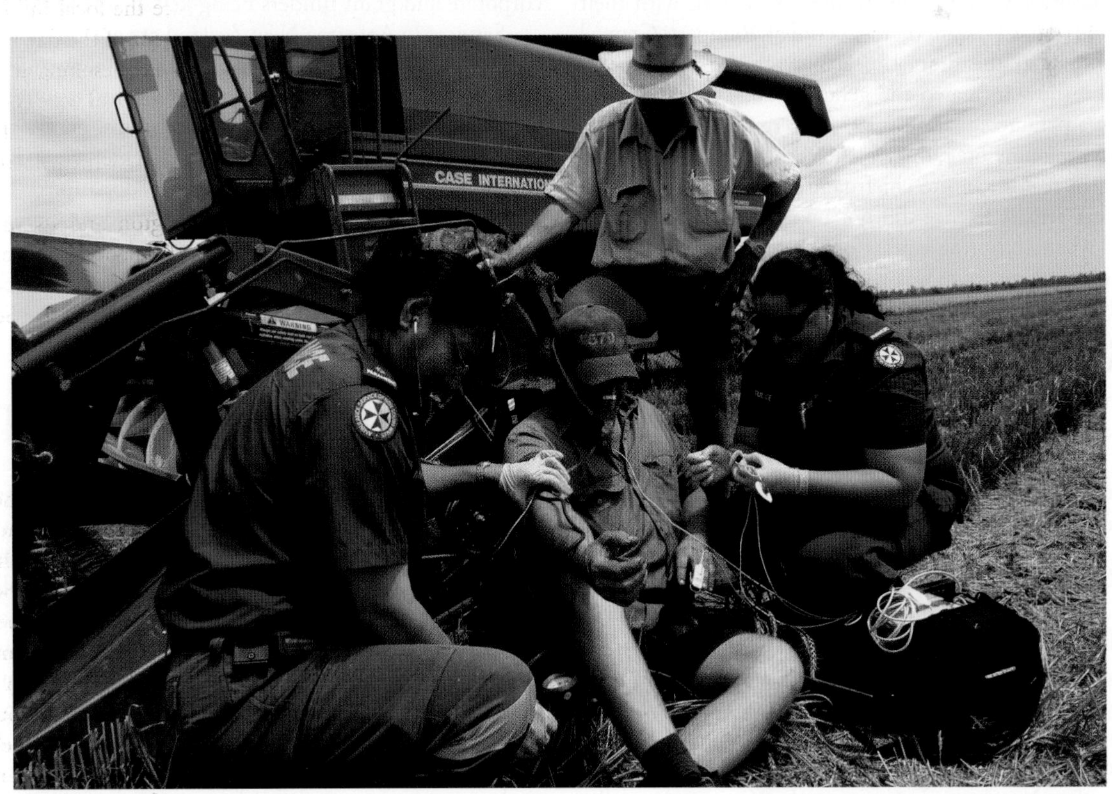

Courtesy of NSW Ambulance.

treatment of myocardial infarction and cardiac arrest outside the hospital setting. This was to occur in multiple locations throughout the world in the decade following Pantridge's initial research and successful implementation of a coronary care program.

Similarly, another quiet revolution occurring in out-of-hospital treatment related to the care of the trauma patient. At about the same time Pantridge was implementing out-of-hospital coronary care in Belfast, US legislators were enacting laws to improve patient outcomes from automobile trauma. The *National Highway and Safety and Traffic Act 1966* funded the development of a national curriculum for out-of-hospital personnel, as well as distributing funds to improve emergency medical services in the United States.[12] Importantly, the national curriculum that was developed included CPR instruction. This, along with the observation that US servicemen injured in Vietnam could be evacuated, on average, in 35 minutes from time of injury and be in surgery within 1–2 hours with an overall mortality rate of just 2.3%,[13] added impetus to the call for improvements in out-of-hospital trauma care. The stage was now set. The treatment of both trauma and coronary care patients was to become the domain of the modern-day paramedic.

The ALS program that had begun in Los Angeles became the basis for the TV series *Emergency!* The series ran from 1972 to 1977 in the United States and was subsequently syndicated throughout the world. It was inspired by a TV producer who, while scouting a location for a new TV show, heard firefighters who spoke like doctors on a visit to a hospital's emergency department (ED). These firefighters were in fact paramedics in the new ALS program. A seed was planted for a new TV show centred on the exploits of two fictitious firefighters, Roy de Soto and John Gage, who worked out of Squad 51 in the Los Angeles County Fire Department. The interactions with their patients and the ED staff of the fictional Rampart General Hospital provided the dramatic setting for the new weekly show.[14] The show increased the general public's awareness of the role of a paramedic, and by 1975, 46 out of 50 states had paramedic programs operating.[12] The technical adviser to the series was, in real life, a fire chief named James O Page.[15] He ensured that artistic licence did not take precedence over authenticity when technical aspects of the paramedic role were part of the storyline. Page was later to become the founder of the widely read *Journal of Emergency Medical Services*.

AIR AMBULANCE SERVICES

In nations that are either as sparsely populated as Australia or as challenged by its unique topography and weather as Aotearoa New Zealand, it is easy to see why air ambulance services have become a key component in the day-to-day functions of ambulance services.

AUSTRALIA

Australia owes its rich tradition of air ambulance services to the Reverend John Flynn OBE. In 1928, he oversaw an air ambulance service as a year-long trial, based at Cloncurry in Central Queensland. The service proved so successful that it was adopted throughout rural and remote Australia. Within the next decade, operations had extended to Victoria, NSW, South Australia, the Northern Territory and Western Australia. Currently, the Royal Flying Doctor Service (RFDS) provides aircraft, pilots and engineering resources to the ambulance services of NSW, Victoria and Tasmania.[16]

Originally called the Australian Inland Mission Aerial Medical Service, Flynn's concept was to provide a 'mantle of safety' to the residents of the outback where your next-door neighbour might be 100 kilometres away. True to its original charter, the RFDS remains a not-for-profit organisation that provides both emergency assistance and primary healthcare for patients unable to readily gain access either to hospitals or to a general practice.

Australia has embraced the use of helicopters as an adjunct for providing quick transport for the trauma patient to the most appropriate hospital, as well as for providing an efficient retrieval service for patients already in hospital but requiring more specialised care at a major referral hospital. A number of public and private enterprises conduct these services throughout Australia and Aotearoa New Zealand. In Australia, some are heavily sponsored by business enterprises, such as large banks and insurance companies, as a community service; others are 'for profit' enterprises contracted by state governments or state ambulance authorities to provide commercial helicopter operations.

AOTEAROA NEW ZEALAND

Aotearoa New Zealand's air ambulance services began later than those in Australia; it is only since the 1980s that there has been a significant increase in the use of aircraft to complement the largely road-based ambulance sector. The clinical crews operating many of these services are provided primarily by the road-based ambulance services. The driving factor in forming many of these services often occurred as a response to a significant local incident. This led to a high degree of community ownership of the services, with local community donors and corporate and grant funders being key stakeholders.

Services in Aotearoa New Zealand are operated by a combination of charitable trusts and private companies located throughout the country. Almost 60% of the revenue for emergency helicopters comes from sponsorships, grants and donations. Funding for the operation of emergency helicopters comes from sponsorships, grants and donations. Te Whatu Ora – Health New Zealand and the Accident Compensation Corporation (ACC) also fund this service.

ROLE OF VOLUNTEERS IN OUT-OF-HOSPITAL CARE

Australia is a large country in terms of landmass, yet has a population density of just under three people per square kilometre—one of the lowest concentrations of people to landmass globally. Its topography is among the lowest, flattest and driest of the continents with its population highly concentrated on the south-eastern sea border. Aotearoa New Zealand, a nation consisting of two main islands, has a much smaller landmass and a population density of approximately 16 people per square kilometre. Its topography is different from Australia's, in that mountainous regions dominate, along with some large coastal plains. Due to the large proportion of sparsely populated areas of Australia and Aotearoa New Zealand, both countries have had a rich tradition of volunteerism from their earliest days to the present time, and this has extended to the provision of ambulance services. The Council of Ambulance Authorities (CAA; collectively Papua New Guinea, and all Aotearoa New Zealand and Australian ambulance services) estimates that there are 18,670 volunteers working in Aotearoa New Zealand and Australian ambulance services, which accounts for approximately 42% of the entire workforce.[17]

Volunteers are engaged in both urban and rural areas. In urban and metropolitan areas, up until the last few decades, volunteers served their communities alongside their salaried counterparts by assisting in the staffing of after-hours services and making themselves available at times of peak demand. In rural and remote areas, the only cost-effective ambulance service that was available was one staffed either predominantly or entirely by volunteers. In these communities, the role of the volunteer paramedic varied. In some locations, it was a community responder role (Fig. 2.3), providing care to the patient prior to the arrival of an ambulance from a location further away, while in other communities there were volunteers who had both treatment and transport capability.

In the metropolitan and regional areas until recently, volunteers had largely been phased out; however, they proved critical to ensuring service delivery during the COVID-19 pandemic, where they stepped up to bolster shortfalls in paramedic rosters and provide surge response.

In regional and rural areas, volunteer paramedics continue to provide a vital first link in the provision of emergency care for many of the residents of Australian and Aotearoa New Zealand rural communities. Given that these areas are sparsely populated and have a low workload, it is easy to understand why a full-time service with salaried staff is not justified. The goal for ambulance services will always be to recruit, retain and train volunteers to serve these communities.

The ambulance volunteer is similar to other Australian volunteers in terms of age and gender. In research conducted as part of a study of volunteer ambulance officers in Australia and

FIGURE 2.3
INTENSIVE-CARE PARAMEDICS TREATING A PATIENT IN THE LATE 1970S

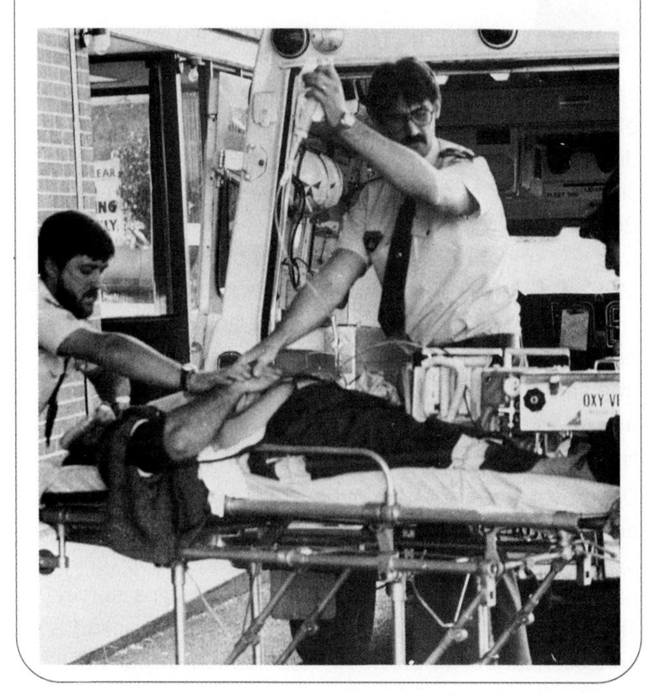

Courtesy of NSW Ambulance.

Aotearoa New Zealand, volunteers stated they enjoy both the training and the opportunity to maintain their skills, sustained by an enjoyment of helping people and making friendships within the group.[18] The difficulties facing ambulance volunteers are lack of time and the inadequate provision of resources.[18] Ongoing training and skills maintenance are critical to maintaining volunteer competence and currency. Most volunteer services now use part of the Australian Qualification Training Framework, associated with the National Training Framework, in a structured approach to ensure that consistent standards and assessments occur in line with vocational education.

When delivered well, training can be a powerful motivator. Conversely, if done poorly it can be a great deterrent to the process of recruiting, engaging and retaining volunteers. The challenge for ambulance service managers is to provide the resources that allow just the right amount of training in just the right amount of time, to keep the volunteer committed to the role of providing ambulance services in their local community.

CURRENT STATUS OF PARAMEDICINE

The primary goal of any discipline in health and medicine, whether emergency medicine, general practice, nursing, allied health or paramedicine, is to reduce pain and suffering and restore health. This goal is supported by most ambulance service mission statements, which identify that the health and wellbeing of the community is achieved through the efficient delivery of high-quality out-of-hospital patient care and specialised patient transport services. Today most ambulance services have a long history of modernisation and adapting services provided to the community.

An emergency medical system (EMS) is identified as a comprehensive network that delivers prompt health services to victims of sudden illness or injury, with their aim being to deliver the patient to the most appropriate facility in the most appropriate time.

Globally, healthcare providers are striving to deliver the best emergency medical systems. While each country has its own systems, protocols and guidelines, most can be categorised by role title or scope of practice, Basic Life Support (BLS) or Advanced Life Support (ALS).

The title given to a member of an ambulance service has varied across Australia compared with Aotearoa New Zealand. Prior to the late 1980s, paramedics were commonly referred to as ambulance officers in most states and territories of Australia. Historically, the term paramedic has not been enshrined in legislation, so virtually anyone can call themselves a paramedic. In December 2018 this changed in Australia and in March 2021 in Aotearoa New Zealand, with the introduction of national registration, which included the protection of the title paramedic. Only those registered as a paramedic are now entitled to call themselves a paramedic. The primary role of paramedics is to treat trauma and medical emergencies outside the hospital setting and during transport to the most appropriate medical facility. They also transfer patients between various healthcare facilities. A number of services have programs in place that allow paramedics to provide primary health as well as emergency care. Each ambulance authority has titles for their staff based upon the level of care that they can provide, but there is no common nomenclature used across Australia or

Aotearoa New Zealand. Many terms are used, but there is, in most cases, a degree of similarity between terms for ambulance operatives with similar skill sets. These are outlined below.

FIRST RESPONDER

An individual who is trained in advanced first aid and responds to emergencies to provide initial management in the out-of-hospital setting.

PATIENT TRANSPORT ATTENDANT

An individual who has completed training in first aid and patient transport and who provides care and transport to patients with lower acuity conditions, often between health facilities.

PARAMEDIC

A health professional who provides rapid assessment, treatment and transport in the out-of-hospital setting. In Australia and Aotearoa New Zealand paramedics are usually degree qualified and must be registered to use the protected title paramedic. They are competent in ALS, with enhanced skills that include defibrillation, advanced airway management, intravenous cannulation, administration of analgesia, antiemetics and hypoglycaemic agents, cardiac and respiratory drug therapies and intravenous fluids. They are capable of maintaining intravenous infusions, patient assessment, including pulse oximetry, vital sign assessment and cardiac monitoring (ECG).

INTENSIVE CARE PARAMEDIC

A paramedic with advanced training, usually at the postgraduate level, who provides advanced assessment, treatment and transport of patients with higher acuity injuries or illnesses. They possess advanced airway skills, and are credentialled to administer a wider range of medications and interventions than paramedics. They practise under either clinical practice guidelines or approved protocols, depending on their jurisdiction.

FLIGHT PARAMEDIC/RETRIEVAL PARAMEDIC/CRITICAL CARE PARAMEDIC

These paramedics work on either fixed-wing or rotary-powered aircraft. They perform emergency, retrieval and routine transports. Most are trained to the level of an intensive care paramedic, but have additional training in rescue techniques and aviation medicine. Registered nurses with postgraduate qualifications staff some fixed-wing air ambulances, completing mostly retrieval operations. In some states, the rotary-powered aircraft are staffed by a combination of a doctor and a flight paramedic.

EXTENDED CARE PARAMEDIC/GENERAL CARE PARAMEDIC

The extended care paramedic (ECP) is a relatively new type of paramedic, who is able to attend emergency cases and provide advanced care and can also attend patients with subacute and non-acute healthcare needs. The ECP has additional training at a postgraduate level in the application of a range of clinical pathways, assessment and management that may not result in the patient being transported to an ED. Working together as a team, ambulance services, and emergency health models more broadly, work best when each component contributes to a system of care. Working as part of a team in the out-of-hospital setting is not only critical to better patient health outcomes, but also to connecting patients to the right care, in the right time-frame.

The following case study illustrates the important role each level of care within the out-of-hospital setting has to play in ensuring optimal health outcomes for people sustaining serious injuries or illness.

CASE STUDY

A is a 12-year-old and a keen equestrian, who lives in rural Victoria. At a weekend gymkhana she was competing in a cross-country race with her gelding, Sinbad. As A and Sinbad were about to leap over a large fallen tree trunk, Sinbad was spooked, and inadvertently tossed A over the tree trunk, where she landed heavily on the ground. A was unconscious and despite several people (including her mother) attending to her quickly, she was unarousable.

A gymkhana official immediately called 000 (Australia's emergency number) and requested an ambulance. While the ambulance call-taker was collecting additional information and providing first aid advice, they alerted the ambulance dispatch area of a potentially time-critical case. The ambulance dispatcher immediately notified their duty manager and clinician (intensive care paramedic working with an operations centre with responsibility for clinical oversight and advice) of the case, given the acuity of the patient and the remoteness of the incident. The ambulance dispatcher also dispatched the closest first responder and paramedic crews. The first responders were approximately 20 minutes from the incident and the paramedic crew was 30 minutes. The nearest Helicopter Emergency Medical Service (HEMS) was also dispatched, with their crew consisting of an intensive care flight paramedic, a paramedic and a pilot. The HEMS crew were 40 minutes away from the incident. Police were also dispatched to assist with scene control and to communicate with HEMS regarding appropriate landing sites.

On arrival, the first responders were able to provide advanced first aid measures, take a full history (from the bystanders and the patient's mother), and undertake a patient assessment, including a full vital signs survey. They immediately positioned A on her side, applied a soft cervical collar, provided stabilisation of her neck, spine and airway, and commenced oxygen therapy. Their secondary survey assessment revealed no obvious injuries, apart from some abrasions around her head and face. They provided a situation report (sitrep) to the communications centre, updating the centre and crews of the patient's condition, vital signs and management initiated.

Following arrival of the paramedic crew, the first responders were able to provide a detailed handover. The paramedic crew undertook a further secondary survey and reassessed all vital signs. The paramedic crew provided a second sitrep, updating the communications centre and the HEMS crew. Given the mechanism, and that the patient was tachycardic (HR 140) and hypotensive (BP 70/40), they decided to apply a pelvic splint. A formal assessment of conscious state revealed A remained unconscious and did not respond to pain. Her Glasgow Coma Scale score was 7 (eye opening = 1, verbal response = 2, motor response = 4). The paramedics carefully repositioned the patient into a supine position, inserted a supraglottic airway without incident and connected a bag–valve–mask resuscitator to the airway. A continued to breathe spontaneously with good tidal volume and oxygen saturation remained greater than 98%. The paramedics commenced transfer of the patient onto a vacuum mattress at the same time as they could hear the helicopter circling overhead.

After the helicopter had landed and shut down, the intensive care flight paramedic arrived and received a handover from the paramedic crew. She requested another set of vital signs, quickly reassessed A's conscious state, and assessed the abdomen. Given there was no improvement in blood pressure and heart rate, the flight paramedic inserted an intravenous cannula, commenced the administration of intravenous fluids, and asked the helicopter crew member to set up for a rapid sequence induction (RSI). RSI is an emergency airway management technique using medications to induce immediate unresponsiveness and muscular relaxation. The flight paramedic decided that RSI was required to protect the child's airway in flight (and prior to getting airborne), and to control oxygenation and ventilation in this child with a closed head injury. With the aid of the paramedic crew, the flight paramedic intubated the child using a RSI technique, and the child was loaded into the aircraft. The child was transported to the nearest paediatric major trauma service.

Answers to Case Study Questions can be found on evolve http://evolve.elsevier.com/AU/Curtis/emergency/

These type of cases occur daily in ambulance organisations that service large populations. Optimal outcomes for patients are reliant on a system that allows teams of care providers to work harmoniously together. Each care provider knows and is proficient at their role and understands the roles of others who are critical to the system.

CAREER STRUCTURE

The career structure for paramedics can be broadly divided into three streams—clinical, management and education/research. The Australian Qualifications Framework provides very broad discipline-free nomenclature,[19] which is associated with many roles within each of the three streams commonly encountered within paramedicine (Table 2.1).

REGULATION OF PARAMEDICINE

Registration of paramedics in Australia and Aotearoa New Zealand has been actively pursued by the profession, ambulance associations and paramedic colleges since the early 2000s. Regulation schemes have been established to ensure the safety of consumers who receive care from registered health practitioners. In Australia, the *Health Practitioner Regulation National Law and Other Legislation Bill 2017*[20] was passed by the Queensland Parliament in September 2017, paving the way for the inaugural Paramedicine Board of Australia to be established under the auspices of the Australian Health Practitioner Regulation Agency (Ahpra).[21] The Paramedicine Board of Australia is one of 15 national boards, one each for the 15 health professions that form part of the National Registration and Accreditation Scheme (National Scheme), and paramedic registration commenced in December 2018. Paramedic services in Aotearoa New Zealand were designated as a health profession in January 2020 and paramedic registration in Aotearoa New Zealand commenced in March 2021, administered by the Te Kaunihera Manapou Paramedic Council, under the *Health Practitioners Competence Assurance Act 2003*.

Broadly, the regulation is responsible for protecting the public, and registering students and practitioners. Regulation of paramedicine has a number of benefits, including the protection of the title paramedic, national mobility for registered paramedics, recognition of international qualified paramedics, development of registration standards and approval of paramedic qualifications and programs of study.[22]

Continuing professional development (CPD) is important for healthcare professionals from all disciplines, and is one of the standards the Paramedicine Board of Australia and the Te Kaunihera Manapou Paramedic Council consider prior to renewal of registration annually. Paramedics need to complete at least 30 hours of CPD each year, and maintain a portfolio that documents learning goals and completed CPD activities.[23]

THE FUTURE OF PARAMEDICINE

The range and complexity of clinical interventions utilised by paramedics has expanded considerably over the last few decades. Furthermore, we have seen paramedic education shift largely from in-service and vocational training to the university sector. Focus will continue to be on paramedic-driven research, contributing to the out-of-hospital evidence base for clinical practice. The role of

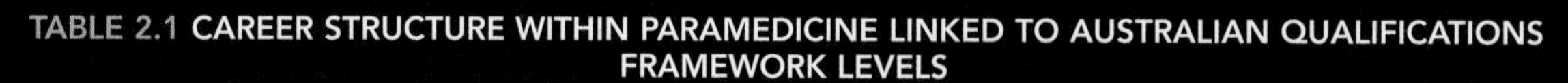

TABLE 2.1 CAREER STRUCTURE WITHIN PARAMEDICINE LINKED TO AUSTRALIAN QUALIFICATIONS FRAMEWORK LEVELS

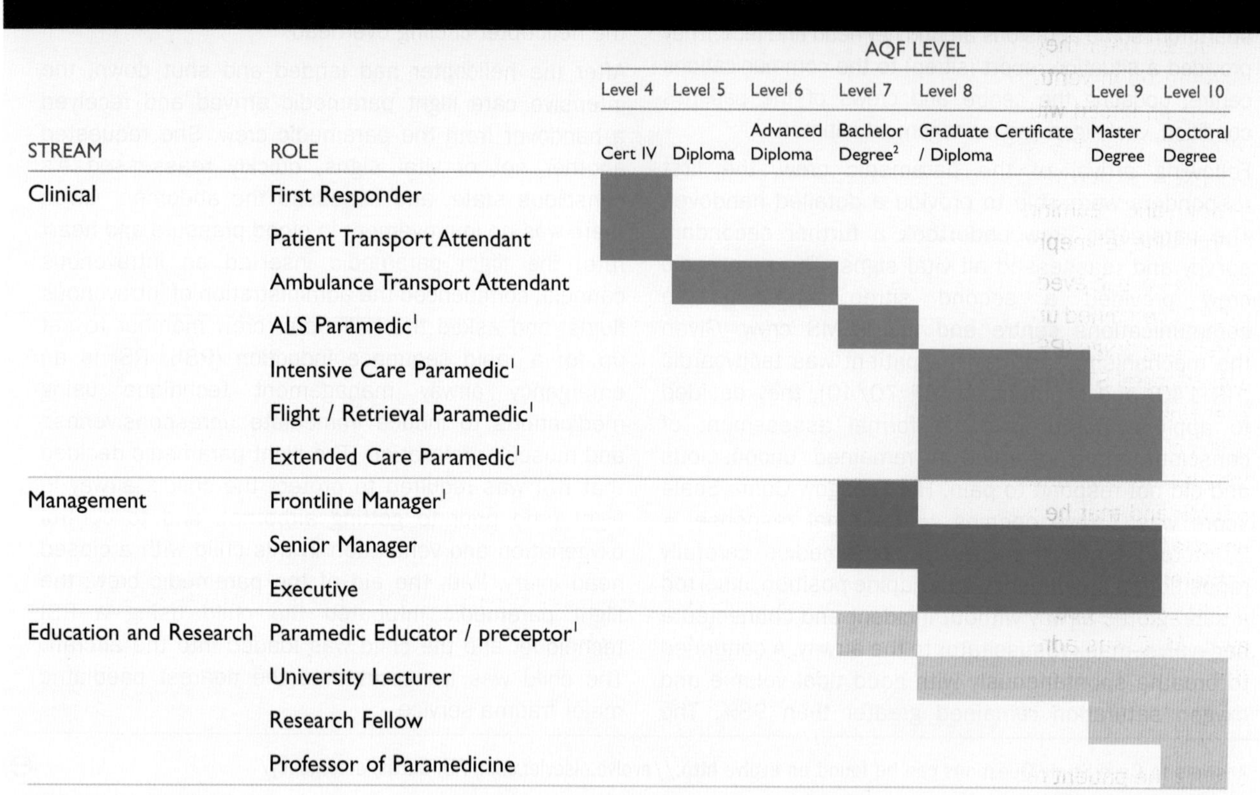

		AQF LEVEL						
		Level 4	Level 5	Level 6	Level 7	Level 8	Level 9	Level 10
STREAM	ROLE	Cert IV	Diploma	Advanced Diploma	Bachelor Degree[2]	Graduate Certificate / Diploma	Master Degree	Doctoral Degree
Clinical	First Responder							
	Patient Transport Attendant							
	Ambulance Transport Attendant							
	ALS Paramedic[1]							
	Intensive Care Paramedic[1]							
	Flight / Retrieval Paramedic[1]							
	Extended Care Paramedic[1]							
Management	Frontline Manager[1]							
	Senior Manager							
	Executive							
Education and Research	Paramedic Educator / preceptor[1]							
	University Lecturer							
	Research Fellow							
	Professor of Paramedicine							

[1] With the introduction of Paramedic Registration in Australia and New Zealand, each of these roles require professional registration.

[2] Some universities offer double degrees in paramedicine and nursing or paramedicine and public health.

the paramedic is currently expanding beyond emergency response, into areas such as primary healthcare and population health. A patient-centred approach, which takes into account the needs and values of patients and consumers, is being embraced by many ambulance services. All healthcare must be patient-centred, and informing and involving patients in decisions about their care and disposition (GP, ED, other healthcare professional) not only results in an improved patient experience, but has been associated with improved health outcomes.[24] Out-of-hospital advancements in technology and availability of point-of-care testing will dramatically change the way paramedics assess, manage and refer patients. Telemedicine will have a great impact on the way paramedics practise, increasing the capability of consulting with other specialties and participating in shared decision-making in terms of appropriate management and choice of patient destination. Some advancements in practice are already acheiving positive outcomes. These include the introduction of focused assessment with sonography in trauma (FAST) into out-of-hospital trauma models, pre-hospital thrombolysis and mobile stroke units. There is certainly scope for further improvement of current processes and expansion of practice, including:

- direct referral of first-time seizure patients to neurology departments
- improved accuracy of call-taking and dispatch systems
- increased health system integration, including referral to alternative healthcare providers
- stroke and neuroprotective drug pilot programs
- diagnosis and early treatment of sepsis.

CASE STUDY

Mr C is a 72-year-old male who lives at home with his wife and dogs in a regional centre in Australia. Mr C was walking his dogs at approximately 9 am one morning with his wife when he suddenly felt pain in both his hips. He sat down and shortly became unresponsive. A young male bystander realised he was in cardiac arrest and called the ambulance emergency phone number. The ambulance call-taker provided the bystander with real-time CPR instruction via his mobile phone. The patient was attended by the local mobile intensive care ambulance (MICA) unit and MICA single responder and the first paramedic crew arrived 4 minutes after they were dispatched. The patient was found to be in ventricular fibrillation, and resuscitation was commenced with the assistance of the bystander. Over the following 9 minutes, paramedics continued CPR, defibrillated Mr C five times, inserted a supraglottic airway and administered intravenous medications (adrenaline (epinephrine) and amiodarone).

Mr C then achieved return of spontaneous circulation (ROSC), remained unconscious and was intubated using paralysing drugs (RSI). A 12-lead ECG revealed an acute anterolateral ST elevation myocardial infarction (STEMI). The Helicopter Emergency Medicine Service (HEMS) was activated because the attending crew identified that his cardiac arrest was probably secondary to his STEMI, and that he would benefit from going to a large hospital with interventional cardiologists and a cardiac catheterisation laboratory; the closest interventional cardiology service was approximately 200 kilometres away. Mr C was administered pre-hospital thrombolysis (PHT) and stabilised while awaiting the HEMS, with the use of intravenous adrenaline (epinephrine) to achieve an adequate blood pressure and sedative agents to ensure the patient remained comfortable and pain-free.

The HEMS arrived within 20 minutes, landing on a football oval nearby, and received a handover from the attending paramedics before loading the patient into the helicopter. The receiving hospital was notified of the impending arrival of Mr C. On arrival, he was immediately transferred to the cardiac catheterisation laboratory and angiography showed moderate-to-severe occlusion of several coronary vessels (50% occlusion of mid left anterior descending artery (mLAD), 65% occlusion of his dominant left circumflex artery LCx). He had normal functioning of his left ventricle. Mr C had coronary bypass graft surgery (×3 vessels) on day 8 following his cardiac arrest. He was transferred back to his local base hospital for rehabilitation 21 days following his cardiac arrest. Mr C was discharged from rehabilitation without any serious deficit following his cardiac arrest.

QUESTIONS

1. Which component of the system of care was the most important for Mr C in the case study described above?
2. What were the different levels of paramedic involved in Mr C's care, and what were the differences in their scope of practice?

Answers to Case Study Questions can be found on evolve **http://evolve.elsevier.com/AU/Curtis/emergency/**

SUMMARY

Out-of-hospital care has evolved considerably over time, with perhaps the most substantial change occurring over the last three decades. No longer is the paramedic considered a 'stretcher bearer', but rather an integral link in the healthcare system. The scope of first responders and paramedics in the out-of-hospital setting is continually expanding in order to address the changing needs of our communities and the healthcare system. In addition, paramedics now work in an ever-expanding range of settings and roles, but are most commonly associated with emergency ambulance systems. With professional regulation and registration fast approaching, the future role of paramedics and their contribution to the broader health system is exciting. Paramedics are now commonly engaged in driving the healthcare agenda through consultation on policy, regulation, education and research.

USEFUL WEBSITES

Australasian College of Paramedicine, the peak professional association representing practitioners who provide paramedic services to the community, www.paramedics.org/.

Paramedicine Board of Australia, regulating Australia's paramedics, supported by the Australian Health Practitioner Regulation Agency (Ahpra), www.paramedicineboard.gov.au/.

St John New Zealand, the largest emergency ambulance service in New Zealand, www.stjohn.org.nz/.

Te Kaunihera Manapou Paramedic Council, regulating New Zealand's paramedics, paramediccouncil.org.nz/.

Wellington Free Ambulance, provides a free paramedic service for the Greater Wellington and Wairarapa region in New Zealand, www.wfa.org.nz/.

REFERENCES

1. St. John Ambulance Australia. The commandery in Western Australia. 113th Annual report. 2005. Online. Available from: www.stjohnambulance.com.au/docs/corporate-publications/2004-05-annual-report.pdf?sfvrsn=0.
2. State Records NSW. Photographic collection, Ambulance tram, c.1915. 2007.
3. Queensland Ambulance Service. Queensland Ambulance Service history and heritage. Online. Available from: www.ambulance.qld.gov.au/history.html.
4. O'Meara P, Grbich C. Paramedics in Australia—contemporary challenges of practice. Sydney: Pearson Education; 2009.
5. Mitka M. Peter J. Safar, 'Father of CPR', innovator, teacher, humanist. JAMA 2003;289(19):2485–6.
6. Freedom House. Street saviours: the documentary. n.d. Online. Available from: www.freedomhousedoc.com.
7. Corbett-Bell R. The next page—Freedom House ambulances: 'We were the best'. 2009. Online. Available from: www.post-gazette.com/news/portfolio/2009/10/25/The-Next-Page-Freedom-House-Ambulance-We-were-the-best/stories/200910250176.
8. Baskett P, Safar P. The resuscitation greats. Nancy Caroline—from mobile intensive care to hospice. Resuscitation 2003;57(2):119–22.
9. Pollak AN. Nancy Caroline's emergency care in the streets. Sudbury MA: Jones and Bartlett; 2008.
10. Pantridge JF, Geddes JS. A mobile intensive care unit in the management of myocardial infarction. Lancet 1967;2(7510):271–3.
11. National EMS Museum Foundation. The virtual EMS Museum. 2010. Online. Available from: emsmuseum.org/virtual_museum/.
12. Déziel J. Past medical history. Paramedics in the United States. 2006. Online. Available from: docplayer.net/8824980-Past-medical-history-paramedics-in-the-united-states-jackson-deziel-spring-2006.html.
13. Neel S. Medical Support of the U.S. Army in Vietnam 1965-1970. Chapter IV: Hospitalization and evacuation. 1991. Online. Available from: https://history.army.mil/html/books/090/90-16/index.html.
14. Emergencyfans.com. Biography of Robert A. Cinander. 2017. Online. Available from: www.emergencyfans.com/people/robert_cinader.htm.
15. Emergencyfans.com. Biography of James O Page; Researcher, Technical Advisor, Writer. 2004. Online. Available from: www.emergencyfans.com/people/jim_page.htm.
16. Royal Flying Doctor Service. Our bases. 2017 Online. Available from: www.flyingdoctor.org.au/about-the-rfds/our-bases/.
17. Council of Ambulance Authorities. Home. Online. Available from: www.caa.net.au/.
18. Fahey C, Walker J, Lennox G. Flexible, focused training: keeps volunteer ambulance officers. Aust J Paramed 2003;1(1). doi:10.33151/ajp.1.1.74.
19. Australian Qualifications Framework. AQF qualifications. 2022. Online. Available from: www.aqf.edu.au/framework/aqf-qualifications.
20. Queensland Government. Health Practitioner Regulation National Law and Other Legislation Amendment Act 2017. Online. Available from: www.legislation.qld.gov.au/view/pdf/asmade/act-2017-032.
21. Paramedicine Board of Australia 2018. Regulating Australia's paramedics. Online. Available from: www.paramedicineboard.gov.au/.
22. Paramedicine Board of Australia. Registration standards. 2022. Online. Available from: www.paramedicineboard.gov.au/Professional-standards/Registration-standards.aspx.
23. Kaunihera Manapou Paramedic Council. Standards. 2022. Online. Available from: paramediccouncil.org.nz/PCNZ/Standards/PCNZ/Standards.
24. National Ageing Research Institute. What is person-centred health care? A literature review. 2006. Online. Available from: www2.health.vic.gov.au/about/publications/researchandreports/What-is-person-centred-health-care-A-literature-review.

CHAPTER 3
CLINICAL ETHICS FOR EMERGENCY HEALTHCARE

ELEANOR MILLIGAN, AUDETTE SMITH AND SARAH WINCH

ESSENTIALS

- Remember the values that inform your practice. Why are you in healthcare?
- Slow down ... where possible.
- Ethically sensitive care happens in every interaction you have with your patients and colleagues, and is not limited to resolving the big dilemmas.
- There are many ways to harm a patient—patients may remember the 'moral harms' (of feeling excluded, ignored, uncared for, or misunderstood) long after their physical illness subsides. Act to minimise all harms.
- Every action in an organisation either contributes to or undermines its ethical culture; choose your actions carefully.
- Treat yourself, your colleagues and your patients with kindness and respect.
- Seek help if you are struggling with the ethical aspects of your professional role.

INTRODUCTION

> We are discussing no small matter, but how we ought to live. *Socrates, in Plato's Republic.*
>
> Medicine being simultaneously the scientific and humanistic study of man cannot escape being based in an explicit or implicit philosophy of human nature. *ED Pellegrino, in 'From medical ethics to a moral philosophy of the professions'.*[1]

Most societies recognise healthcare as a fundamental 'good'—something of great value that is collectively nurtured, protected and preserved. Human communities, even ancient ones, developed traditions of healthcare, ranging from the diagnoses and treatments offered by medicine men and shamans within indigenous communities to the healing traditions provided within Chinese medicine, Islamic traditions and the early Western tradition of medicine derived from the ancient Greeks. These formalised systems of healthcare delivery, and the collective desire to improve and progress medical knowledge, flow from the recognition that the preservation of life and good health are integral to every person's ability to flourish.

While life is valued and we collectively (through the provision of collective funding of healthcare systems) and individually (through personal choices) seek to maintain health, the human body is fragile, subject to illness, disease and trauma. In the context of medical emergency, healthcare professionals are called upon to respond to the needs of patients at times of unexpected trauma, in addition to expected and unexpected illness. Often, patients are in distress, possibly confronting their own (or a loved one's) mortality. They enter the healthcare system seeking skilled and competent treatment, and, importantly, reassurance, understanding and 'care' in the true sense of the word. The families and loved ones of patients similarly look to emergency healthcare professionals for reassurance that the trust placed in them to provide care is deserved and will not be misused. Hence, for healthcare to be effective, health professionals, and the organisations in which they operate, must be worthy of the trust placed in them; that is, they must be trustworthy.

At such times when the fragility of life is a stark reality for patients and their families, the ethical response of emergency healthcare professionals is triggered by the personal vulnerability that comes hand-in-hand with illness and trauma. Illness is not simply a matter of physical threat to the body; it is equally a threat to a person's sense of identity and wellbeing—who they are, and how others see them, their future possibilities and present capabilities. It is this vulnerability of the ill person that invites a caring response from healthcare professionals. Barry Hoffmaster writes that: 'vulnerability is an even more basic feature of our human constitution than rationality, because while all human beings are vulnerable, not all are rational or even possess the potential to become rational ... it is our very vulnerability that creates the need for morality'.[2] Thus, healthcare, including the provision of emergency healthcare, occurs within a moral relationship between the carer and the cared for. It is 'ethically laden practice'[3] because it requires healthcare professionals to respond to the needs of others at times of personal fragility and disempowerment, and to care for patients and families, both in the physical and in the human sense.

While emergency healthcare shares this ethical foundation of providing care and relieving suffering with other healthcare disciplines, it also raises particular and unique ethical challenges. The physical landscape of emergency and trauma care is one in which a pre-existing relationship with the patient often does not exist, potentially impeding critical understandings on both sides. Frequently, organisational resources are limited, creating ethically confronting situations such as 'ramping', where patients are unable to be handed over from ambulance staff to be triaged in hospital emergency departments (EDs), or poor response times where the best care possible is unable to be given. The inherent unpredictability of emergency, the need to make time-pressured treatment decisions, and the professional isolation of emergencies in rural practice can create ethical tension. Similarly, community expectations that emergency healthcare staff will respond to the needs of others and even compromise their own safety in times of pandemic or natural disaster can breed fear and resentment in practitioners. Confusion over what to do when a patient lacks capacity or does not appear to have given appropriate informed consent can generate anxiety and unease in healthcare professionals. Decisions concerning the instigation of futile treatment can also generate moral distress. Added to this mix are the hierarchical structures within healthcare organisations that can negatively shape interprofessional communication, sometimes to the detriment of patient care. All of these considerations define the unique and complex environment of emergency and trauma care; all can lead to moral anguish in the individual practitioner; and all can contribute to stress, burnout and even poor retention in the workforce.[4] However, when clinical staff develop the skills and tools to work through, understand and engage with the ethical and human dimensions of their practice, they can become more effective, both personally and professionally.

ETHICS: AN ANCIENT AND EVOLVING FIELD

A working knowledge of the approaches available to understand ethical issues is important because it clarifies the emergency healthcare professional's role in ethical situations and the associated decision-making. There are many different ethical perspectives, and considering a clinical scenario through these different lenses can lead to different outcomes.

Ethical concepts drawn from the classical, modern and post-modern centuries of thought are useful tools for understanding, explaining and deciding how to resolve contemporary ethical issues. In this brief review, we consider four of the more well-known approaches to understanding ethics: virtue ethics, deontology, utilitarianism and narrative ethics. For a more detailed discussion on ethical theory, a number of good texts are available, such as *Ethics in nursing: the caring relationship*[5] and *Ethics and law for the health professions*.[6]

This chapter begins with a brief review of the ethical theory from which the principles for ethical practice and decision-making are drawn, then considers the role of professional codes of ethics and codes of conduct in guiding practice. All approaches have strengths and weaknesses; hence, in a given clinical situation the ability to recognise and use these various ways of thinking can help you navigate the ethical aspects of care. It concludes with an example of one model of ethical decision-making that may assist health carers in developing their skills of ethical analysis.

VIRTUE ETHICS

Ideas from the ancient Greek philosopher Aristotle (384–322 BC) underpin *virtue ethics*, an approach that has seen resurgence in popularity since the publication of *Modern moral philosophy* in 1958.[7] Virtue ethics, in common with Aristotle's thinking, focuses on inner character and/or motives rather than rules or consequences of actions. Virtues are qualities that make their possessor good; a virtuous person is a morally excellent or admirable person who acts and feels well. Virtues are not innate in a person, but can be cultivated. Thus, moral education and the development of a virtuous character are central to virtue ethics.[8] The ethical or moral character of an individual develops over a long period of time, and can be encouraged by family, teachers and the peer group. Professional education plays an important role in developing moral character. For example, it is a requirement of a variety of undergraduate health degree programs to teach ethics as part of the core curriculum. The inclusion of ethics tutoring creates an educational space in which healthcare providers can extend and consolidate understanding of how their existing values and beliefs can be actualised in the professional context. Such education can also be an opportunity for personal transformation and growth. Moral training can also be provided by role models, such as senior staff in healthcare organisations, who are expected to model ethical behaviour.

DUTY-BASED ETHICS AND UTILITARIANISM

The age of modernity, commonly understood to have begun with the Enlightenment in the 18th century, promoted *rationalism* (the capacity for human reason), *universalism* (truths that can be applied to all) and *individualism* (valuing the individual). These ideas have influenced contemporary approaches to ethical decision-making. Deontology, drawn from the work of Immanuel Kant (1724–1804), takes its name from *deon*, the Greek word for 'duty'. Deontological, or duty-based ethics, examines the nature of actions and the will of agents, rather than goals achieved. That is, a person has a duty to perform particular actions and to do the right action for its own sake. We see this in the well-accepted notion that health carers have a duty to care for patients, no matter what the outcome.

Utilitarianism, conceptualised initially by Jeremy Bentham (1748–1832) and developed further by John Stuart Mill (1806–1873), refers broadly to the greatest happiness (or good) for the greatest number. It is known as a consequentialist theory, in that it judges an act as morally right or wrong depending on the consequences of that act. This argument is frequently applied to modern resource allocation in the notion of getting the best value out of scarce resources.[9] The ethics of triage can be understood as a form of utilitarianism. If our ultimate goal is to give the best care possible for all patients in the ED, then the sickest patients need to be seen first. If we used an alternative method to prioritise patient care, such as when the patient actually arrived in the ED, as opposed to their clinical need, then some patients would suffer significantly poorer outcomes. Resources in the ED are finite and the system of seeing patients according to their clinical urgency actually provides the greatest good for the greatest number, in terms of patient outcomes. An enduring criticism of taking a purely utilitarian approach is that needs and perspectives of marginalised or minority groups become discounted or silenced when the majority rule. This can have particularly devastating impacts on already vulnerable groups.

NARRATIVE ETHICS

Narrative ethics acknowledges the *subjective* nature of ethical and moral aspects of any situation. It differs from other philosophical approaches that seek to uncover universal truths through the systematic and objective application of rational thought to ethically challenging circumstances. The narrative approach seeks to uncover each individual stakeholder's personal story as a rich way of understanding their individual perspective and life. Taking a narrative approach, moral rules and principles can be best understood in the context of each person's circumstances, and the subjective meaning each individual places on particular aspects of their situation.[10,11] Narrative ethics draws its concepts and methodologies from literary criticism and phenomenology and is a postmodern approach to understanding ethics.

An example of a clinical situation in which a narrative approach may be useful is in considering the ethical issues surrounding domestic violence that emergency care workers face in their practice.[12] In such cases, the emergency care worker needs to hear the patient's story to make sense of the situation, and the moral rules that may influence the patient's life, which may be significantly different from the care worker's values, beliefs and expectations. For example, the emergency care worker might be concerned about a young adult patient who presents regularly to the department with injuries that indicate they may be experiencing domestic violence. The care worker feels that it is their moral duty to counsel the patient to leave this situation and seek a safer place to live. Using a narrative approach, the care worker listens to the patient's story and is told that the patient is staying in the situation in order to protect younger siblings. The care worker can now gain an appreciation of the complexity involved. The patient feels they have a moral duty to stay and protect their siblings; the care worker is concerned for the patient. In this case, the care worker may decide to support the patient to stay in their situation and put into place actions that help protect them and their siblings.

THE ETHICAL FRAMEWORK OF EMERGENCY HEALTHCARE: OUR MORAL COMMITMENTS AND OBLIGATIONS

> Our practices … are the visible manifestations of invisible values.
> *G Hofstede*[13]

A useful starting point for all healthcare workers when confronting ethical decision-making is to examine the values that they hold as individuals. Values are embedded deeply in our psyche, developing from our family, schooling and cultural background. Further education and experience will shape and sharpen these values considerably, particularly through the enculturation into the professional norms and values of healthcare practice. These are then expressed consciously or unconsciously in the work environment. Values have three components: emotional, cognitive and behavioural. This means that when our values clash with what we see or hear, we are likely to feel upset or worried about what we see happening. This feeling can be made worse if we feel we have little control over the situation, which may be the case in many emergency presentations. A simple example that may challenge us is the case of the 30-year-old alcoholic single mother who is admitted with liver failure following a wild drinking binge the night before. Her two children are with her and look malnourished and dishevelled. This case challenges values that we hold regarding self-care and monitoring, as well as care of children.

In cases such as these, it is timely to remind ourselves of the professional values that we hold. These are often articulated in professional codes of ethics, and are a good reference point to guide our attitudes and subsequent clinical practice. The International Council of Nurses first developed a Code of Ethics in 1953, and most recently updated it in 2021, now in effect for all nurses in Australia.[14] The Nursing and Midwifery Board of Australia now work from the joint Code of Conduct for Nurses and Code of Conduct for Midwives.[15] This code is founded firmly in the values of nursing, which promote person-centred care, culturally safe and respectful care of all patients, integrity, compassion and honesty. Since the inclusion of paramedics under the National Scheme and registration with AHPRA, the Paramedicine Board of Australia has adopted a shared Code of Conduct to guide practitioners.[16]

These codes encompass the ethical aspects of everyday care. Importantly, they also communicate a shared professional standard to the community. They can provide a framework for determining whether certain behaviours have breached the expected professional standard of care. Codes are often criticised for their broad aspirational statements, for being self-generated and self-monitored within professions, and for lacking independent critique. Professional codes of ethics and conduct are not legally binding. They do not provide a means of sanctioning individual professionals who do not abide by them. Legislative pathways to deal with negligent actions or poor professional standards are discussed in Chapter 4. Despite their limitations, however, codes of ethics play a critical role in expressing the underlying values of healthcare practice, while assisting clinicians to develop a shared understanding of their collective moral obligations and to develop a strong professional culture. They can also act as a touchstone to anchor clinical practice and practitioners back to their purpose.

In addition to considering aspects of clinical ethical decision-making, healthcare professionals also need to be aware of the research ethics codes that govern the conduct of research involving patients, colleagues and others. In Australia, the *National statement on ethical conduct in human research*, issued by the National Health and Medical Research Council (NHMRC),[17] provides ethical guidance for conducting research. The NHMRC outlines four fundamental principles that must be considered in determining whether any research proposal meets the ethical standards expected by the community. The four principles are: 1) that the research must have *merit and integrity*; 2) it must be done *justly* (without unfairly burdening or including/excluding particular groups); 3) it should be carried out with *beneficence* (designed to minimise the risks, harms or discomfort to participants); and 4) it should *respect* participants as having intrinsic value, not as a means to a research agenda. Similarly, the Health Research Council of New Zealand has published *HRC Research ethics guidelines*.[18] Box 3.1 discusses some of the ethical issues which arose during the COVID-19 pandemic and the guidelines produced to try to deal with them.

ETHICAL DECISION-MAKING

While codes provide general guidance for healthcare professionals, specific guides to moral decision-making and problem-solving also exist. The 'four principles' approach developed by Tom Beauchamp and James Childress[21] (see Box 3.2)—also known as 'principlism'—is popular in the healthcare field because of its accessibility and ease of application.

BOX 3.1 PROVIDING CARE IN A PANDEMIC

The COVID-19 Pandemic, which is still active across the globe at the time of writing in 2022, has raised many ethical issues for practitioners. In the emergency setting, issues have included decision-making on how limited resources can be fairly and compassionately allocated, the scarcity of PPE, which has impacted practitioner health, and in some cases resulted in loss of life, the exposing of practitioners' loved ones to harm, and challenges to the assumption that there is a duty to treat—that the 'social contract' requires health practitioners to place themselves in harm's way to care for others. Each of these issues is complex with no straight forward answer; however, each can cause moral distress as personal, professional and organisational values collide when trying to navigate an ethical solution to these pressing realties in emergency care. The recently published NHMRC *Ethical issues arising from the COVID-19 pandemic*[19] and NHMRC *Decision-making for pandemics: an ethics framework*[20] provide guidance and case examples based on the values of respect, justice, solidarity and common good, resting on the procedural principles of transparency, accountability, inclusiveness, verifiability, responsiveness and proportionality.

BOX 3.2 THE FOUR PRINCIPLES TO GUIDE ETHICAL DECISION-MAKING[21]

- **Respect for autonomy—respect people's decisions and values.**
- **Beneficence—help people.**
- **Non-maleficence—don't harm people.**
- **Justice—treat like cases alike; distribute benefits and burdens fairly.**

Based on a combination of common moral theory, virtue ethics and utilitarianism, the four principles seek to guide reflection and decision-making within the context of the specific duties that healthcare professionals owe to patients. These duties are seen to be *prima facie*. This means they are always considered to be in effect, in all situations. While Beauchamp and Childress[21] made it clear that all of the principles should be considered equally, in practice many clinicians tend to place the principle of patient autonomy above the others.

A simple example of how these principles may be applied is to consider a patient who needs a blood transfusion, but refuses it because it violates her religious beliefs. Using the principlist approach, there are two ethical principles in conflict—the right of the patient to decide her own treatment (autonomy) and the duty of the healthcare professional to provide the best assistance possible (beneficence). If the patient is deemed competent to make the decision (that is, she is an adult with capacity), the patient's right to refuse the treatment because of her religious beliefs would be absolute, and to treat her without consent, in the name of beneficence, could result in a charge of assault or battery. If the patient in this scenario is a child, the situation would be considered differently. Children are not automatically considered to have the legal capacity to make autonomous decisions. If a parent requests the withholding of a life-sustaining treatment from their child, this poses a very serious situation that emergency staff need to report immediately to senior staff; it may require legal intervention, particularly if the child's life is at risk.

While this approach to ethical decision-making appears straightforward, it has been widely criticised for oversimplifying what are inevitably complex and multifaceted deliberations and viewing the 'problem' primarily from the clinician's perspective.[22,23] The attributes that make this model so accessible, such as the temptation to simplify and reduce the complexity, and to decontextualise difficult ethical decisions, are also its greatest weakness. Pullman[24] suggests that principlism may be better thought of as a sort of 'first aid' response, which may be helpful in the immediate term, but cannot fulfil the role of thorough exploration.

AUTONOMY AND INFORMED CONSENT

Seeking informed consent from a patient demonstrates respect for the patient as a person and for their ability to act autonomously when participating in healthcare. For informed consent to occur, the patient (or the patient's representatives, if they are a minor or lack capacity) needs to understand:

- the health intervention that is being proposed
- what alternatives are available
- the risks attached to any course of action.

In addition, a patient should be able to act freely in choosing or rejecting proposed health interventions without undue influence or control by others.[25,26] Consent may be implied, such as when a patient rolls up their sleeve to receive an injection, or can be assumed in a true emergency situation where delaying care may cause serious or permanent harm.[27] The legal aspects of the Doctrine of Necessity (Emergency) are discussed more fully in Chapter 4.

Australian law recognises that individuals aged 18 years and over have full legal capacity, such that they are capable of making decisions relating to their own healthcare. In South Australia and Aotearoa New Zealand, the law allows persons 16 years and over to make decisions about their own medical treatment. Prior to 18 years (or 16 years in SA and Aotearoa New Zealand), parents (or legal guardians) are entitled to consent to their child's medical and dental treatment. A parent's authority in this respect is not, however, absolute, as the law in Australia recognises that children become increasingly competent as they move towards adulthood. Parents and healthcare professionals should consider the parents' and guardians' responses carefully. Childress[28] provides the following guidance for clinicians to evaluate this response: Do they have adequate knowledge and information to make the decision? Are they emotionally stable and able to make reasoned judgements? Is the decision in the best interests of the child? In this complex area of ethical decision-making, junior staff need to alert senior clinicians and managers who can assist them. In turn, senior staff may have to seek legal opinion for the correct course of action. Competent minors may be able to give consent if they demonstrate understanding of the decision and its consequences; however, this must be decided on a case-by-case basis, as there is no prescribed age below 18 at which a child may be considered a 'mature minor' in Australia; similarly, those aged below 16 years in Aotearoa New Zealand and South Australia can give or refuse consent if considered competent to do so. If children are not considered competent to make a decision, their views should still be considered.

MODEL FOR ETHICAL DECISION-MAKING

When healthcare professionals experience competing ethical considerations, or a choice between two competing good outcomes, and are not able to resolve them, they are often left feeling burdened.[29] Box 3.3 details a general model of ethical decision-making that clinicians in Australia have found useful in such cases. This model draws upon a number of the ethical approaches discussed earlier in this chapter and provides a useful framework for health carers to use in their practice. For a more detailed discussion of this method, see Kerridge, Lowe and Stewart.[6]

BOX 3.3 A MODEL FOR ETHICAL DECISION-MAKING[6]

- **Identify the ethical problem.**
- **What facts are available?**
- **Consider the ethical principles.**
- **Consider how the problem would look from another perspective or using another theory.**
- **Identify ethical conflicts.**
- **Consider the law.**
- **Make the decision.**

In emergency and trauma care, clinical ethics questions arise urgently and often without any prior established relationship with the patient or family. It is sometimes difficult to ascertain the patient's preferences for treatment when they are unaccompanied and unable to speak for themselves. This may hinder the application of ethical decision-making frameworks that are of use in other healthcare settings. One key aspect is to try to slow the decision-making process to allow all the options to be considered for the patient and, if necessary, to secure additional information about the patient's preferences and wishes. In end-of-life situations, where the patient may or may not be able to consent to or refuse treatment, the emergency care worker needs to be aware of the laws guiding end-of-life intervention in the geographical area where they practise. Chapter 4 considers these issues in more detail.

ETHICAL DECISION-MAKING IN PRACTICE

The following discussion applies the ethical decision-making framework outlined in Kerridge et al[6] to a particular case.

CASE SCENARIO

You are called to a 48-year-old male, Lincoln, who has widely disseminated kidney cancer, including multiple abdominal and cerebral secondary tumours. He is experiencing widespread malignant abdominal ascites and pleural effusion, making breathing and communication difficult. He is clearly approaching the end of life, but has no advance care planning documentation. He is also in pain. His wife Sarah, who informs you that she holds his enduring power of attorney (Lincoln confirms this), requests that you treat and transport Lincoln to the ED for a palliative admission.

Following assessment, ED medical staff are clear that the ascites and pleural effusion should be drained to enable respiration and reduce the pain Lincoln is feeling. He can then be admitted to the palliative care unit for appropriate end-of-life care. Sarah is adamant that Lincoln wants to end his life, and requests increased morphine to make her husband comfortable. She is anxious, sarcastic and angry.

Meanwhile, Lincoln's pain is increasing. Despite his brain tumours, he appears to have the capacity to make decisions regarding his healthcare and he is also requesting the morphine for his pain. He clearly states that he does not want any more tubes stuck in him. He does not consent to the drainage procedures. The doctors argue that this is an emergency case and consent is not required. You are aware that patients with capacity can refuse treatment, and feel that the wishes of the patient and his wife should be upheld, so a morphine infusion started as requested. You communicate these views to the others, who counter that Lincoln cannot really have capacity because of his cerebral metastasis and that if he was fully cognisant he would consent to treatment. Further, his lung capacity is now so compromised that his oxygen saturation levels are dropping. Meanwhile, Sarah is getting more and more angry and threatening to call a friend who is a health lawyer to 'sort things out' and 'witness and document' this lack of care and compassion towards her husband. The relationship between Lincoln and Sarah and the treating team is becoming fraught. What should happen next?

Answers to Case Study Questions can be found on evolve http://evolve.elsevier.com/AU/Curtis/emergency/

IDENTIFY THE ETHICAL PROBLEM

Ethical problems may be considered as those arising from an imbalance or misuse of power, or from a clash of underlying values. In this case, we might consider the following points:

- The patient has refused consent to the proposed medical treatment and this may hasten his death. The aim of the treating team is to preserve life.
- The patient's wishes not to receive any more active treatment are in conflict with the preferred action of the treating team, which is to relieve physical symptoms by draining fluid.
- Can staff override his autonomy, and use their power in this situation to impose the drainage procedure?
- The patient's cognitive capacity, and thus his ability to make healthcare decisions, has been questioned due to the unconfirmed possibility of brain metastasis and low oxygenation.
- Ask yourself whose interests are served by questioning the patient's capacity? The patient's or the treating clinician's?
- The patient and his wife are in a very vulnerable position: Lincoln is dying. They sense there may be an imposition of an unwanted treatment and may be feeling increasingly helpless due to the power imbalance in this context.

The initial question that must be resolved in this scenario is whether Lincoln has capacity. While this is largely a clinical determination, the answer to this question influences all subsequent deliberations. *It is important to remember that adults are presumed to have capacity.* If he has capacity, his refusal to consent to treatment must be respected. If he doesn't, he has a clearly appointed substitute decision-maker in Sarah, who is affirming his stated position of refusal of the procedure and request for pain relief only.

What facts are available?

- Lincoln is the patient.
- Lincoln is in the end-stage of a terminal illness.
- He is dying; he appears to know and accept this.
- He has not consented to the drainage procedure.
- He appears to have capacity, but this is being questioned.
- The presence of brain metastasis is not confirmed.
- His wife is his substitute decision-maker.
- He is in pain.
- He has requested sedation.
- There is some disagreement among the treating team.

Consider the ethical principles

If a patient's autonomy is being respected, they will participate in shared decision-making with clinical staff at all times. This means that all efforts should be made to determine whether the patient is capable of engaging in decisions about their care. If Lincoln has capacity, his wishes and refusal to consent must be respected. If he doesn't, we must look for ways to ascertain what his wishes are likely to have been. He has clearly appointed a substitute decision-maker in his wife, Sarah, to act in his best interests, in the way he would have wanted, and clinical staff must trust that he made this appointment in good faith. However, if Sarah appears to be making requests on his behalf that appear not to be in his best interests, her status as substitute decision-maker can be legally challenged. In this case, both Sarah and Lincoln are making the same request for pain relief, and refusal of drainage procedure, even if this shortens his life.

Acting with beneficence means seeking to do good for the patient. What 'good' means to the patient can only be ascertained by communicating with the patient and his wife, in seeking to understand what aspects of the proposed intervention they perceive as harmful. Occasionally, what the patient perceives as 'good' and what the clinical staff regard as 'good' conflict. Disagreement over what is the best course of action should not be a trigger to question a patient's capacity.

Non-maleficence, or not causing harm, can also only be determined by taking into account what the patient perceives as harmful. Would the drainage procedure inflict additional pain and suffering on a person who has already endured enough? To what end is this procedure being performed? Are we really acting in Lincoln's best interests by imposing an unwanted procedure, even if this procedure may relieve some of his physical symptoms? Does lengthening the patient's life, perhaps by only a few days, warrant the imposition of this procedure when the extreme discomfort he is feeling can be managed another way?

Consideration of justice usually refers to issues of resource allocation and the costs associated with patient care.[6] In a case like this, where the patient is at the end of life, the difference in life span as a consequence of this intervention may not represent a significant cost of care. In our healthcare system, considerations of cost are not usually the primary driving factor in determining what treatments are made available to patients.

Consider how the problem would look from another perspective or using another theory

- The key stakeholders in this case are the patient, his wife and the treating clinicians.
- The patient has stated he is tired of being treated, saying he *does not want any more tubes stuck in him.*
- His wife is *anxious, sarcastic and angry*, possibly already in a phase of anticipatory grief.
- Members of the team may feel that their professional relevance and credibility is being undermined by a non-compliant patient.
- Healthcare staff may feel that the patient is under-equipped to make a good decision in such circumstances, and their desire to achieve the best health outcome for the patient may encourage them to act in a paternalistic way—to look for ways to override his stated wishes.
- Paramedical staff may feel guilty that the patient is now in a situation where his options are becoming more limited, and question their role in bringing a palliative patient to the ED.
- Consider what outcome delivers the best outcome for most people. Answering this question depends upon subjective interpretations of what 'best' means in this circumstance. It also depends on whose perspective is privileged when deciding who among the 'most' count. As Verkerk and collegues[30] note, 'Man has almost limitless ability to convince him/herself that what s/he wants to do is morally justifiable'. The skill of ethical decision-making is the ability to see the problem from perspectives other than your own, to understand, then respectfully accept and negotiate difference.

Identify ethical conflicts

- There are a number of ethical conflicts—between the patient, his wife and the treating team. There are also interprofessional conflicts within the treating team, who disagree over the best course of action.
- The powerful voices within the team have a desire to intervene and relieve pain and suffering.
- The patient and his wife are rejecting the intervention.
- The different type of psychological pain and suffering being experienced by the patient and his wife demand equal consideration, but appear not to have been heard by all members of the clinical team.
- In this case, the conflict could be represented as existing between preservation of the autonomy of the patient and the desire of the treating team to do good for the patient.
- Interprofessional disagreement within the clinical team has not yet been resolved constructively.

Consider the law

- Adults are presumed to have capacity and Lincoln's wishes should automatically be respected.
- If there is doubt about Lincoln's capacity, you must be able to identify the reasons why.
- If it is decided that he doesn't have capacity, his wife, who is his nominated substitute decision-maker, can make healthcare decisions on his behalf, within the law, and in accordance with his values and beliefs. Lincoln doesn't have an advance care plan, but this would only come into effect if he lacked capacity.
- Sarah has the legal authority to make decisions for him, as though he were making them.
- Although Lincoln has arrived in hospital through the ED, this situation may not be a medical emergency negating the need for consent. Treatment in an emergency can only be undertaken to the point that averts the emergency; additional treatment without consent should not be initiated. Sarah has requested sedation for her husband. This is not illegal in Australia: sedation can be given for the purpose of relieving pain. If an unintended consequence of such pain relief is that an imminent death occurs more quickly, this is legally acceptable, provided that the primary purpose of administering the drug is for pain relief only.

Make the decision

- Lincoln appears to have capacity and you cannot impose the procedure on him. To do so would constitute an assault or battery. If this is unclear, you may request an independent assessment. In some situations, due to time pressures or lack of appropriate personnel, this might not be possible.
- In general terms, if the patient has made a decision, appears to understand it, has not been coerced, and can communicate the decision, they are regarded as having capacity.
- You cannot override Lincoln's request, even in the ED, as he is in a position to make his wishes known. In an emergency, you can only act to the extent that the emergency is averted. You cannot intervene beyond this without consent from the patient or substitute decision-maker.
- A clinician cannot administer morphine for the sole purpose of hastening death. However, pain relief that has the unintended consequence of hastening an imminent death may be administered, but only with the primary intent of relieving pain.
- You should reassure Lincoln that even though he has rejected the treatment advice of the treating team, he will not be abandoned; he will receive appropriate and ongoing care, including pain relief in the last days of his life.
- Document your decision and conversations with the patient and his wife.
- Reflect on this decision and consider what you can learn for future care of patients in similar situations. You may reflect upon constructive ways to resolve disagreement within the treating team when the immediate pressure has subsided, to equip yourselves as a professional community to better cope in the future.

Initially, this process may seem onerous and overly complex; however, as you become more experienced you will learn to undertake this level of analysis as second nature in your clinical practice. It is also a good idea to debrief with colleagues when there is a particularly challenging case, as you will learn from each other, and build a supportive and collegial community.

SEQUELAE—ANOTHER KEY VALUE: TAKING CARE OF YOURSELF

Clashing professional and personal values, differences in cultural background and expectations and the ongoing pressures of working in frequently under-resourced EDs can increase the personal burden on clinical staff.[31] Frequently when we talk about ethics and morals we have the patient in mind as the focus of our attention. This absolute focus on the patient is important, but sometimes the caregiver can get lost in this process. As we conclude this chapter, we invite you to add another very important value and ethical obligation to the many we have discussed thus far. This is the value of taking care of *you*, of treating yourself well and kindly. Having friends and interests outside of work is important. Making time for exercise and family will not only keep you physically robust, but will also help you be mentally able to face the many moral challenges that come your way. This is not entirely selfish, as work stress and overload for health carers has been associated with poor patient outcomes in the clinic.[32–34]

Moral distress is described as painful feelings and associated emotional and mental anguish as a result of being conscious of a morally appropriate action that despite all effort cannot be performed due to organisational or other obstacles.[35] Examples of such obstacles may include onerous policies, hierarchical power structures that inhibit action, inadequate numbers of staff, time limitations or legal constraints; all of which can undermine the provision of the best patient care.

GETTING SUPPORT

Empathy and support from colleagues can be most beneficial in times of moral distress and conflict. Ethical dilemmas can be difficult to resolve, and often emerge not from determining what is good or bad, but from having to choose between competing 'goods' or competing 'bads'.[36] In Australia and Aotearoa New Zealand, there are only a few facilities which have access to a hospital-based ethicist or a facility-based clinical ethics committee, although this is becoming increasingly more common and is recognised as adding value to organisations in the NHMRC Consensus Statement and *Clinical ethics capacity building resource manual*.[37] If you work in an area without specialist ethics services, you may wish to discuss any ethical concerns with a team leader, director, nursing manager or trusted senior colleague. Often organisations have pastoral care or staff counselling services, the staff of which often have some ethics training. However, all healthcare staff should strengthen their competence in the area of ethical decision-making by regularly attending education sessions and seminars, or by seeking professional development through organisations such as the Australasian Association of Bioethics and Health Law (see aabhl.org for more information).

SUMMARY

In most cases, shared moral values, such as mutual respect, honesty, trustworthiness, compassion and a commitment to pursue shared goals, make the provision of healthcare in emergencies ethically straightforward between the carer and the patient. However, as the healthcare system grows more complex, ethical decision-making will also become more complex. In the context of emergency, anchoring practice to the underlying purpose of healthcare—which is to preserve life and relieve suffering—and considering this goal within the guiding ethical principles and processes for resolving ethical dilemmas, form an essential part of practice knowledge. As with any clinical skill, regular training and updates ensure that, when required, emergency healthcare practitioners can act competently in what is likely to be a complex and urgent situation, in a way that does not add a moral burden to the patient or to themselves.

REFERENCES

1. Pellegrino ED. From medical ethics to a moral philosophy of the professions. In: Walter JK, Klein EP, editors. The story of bioethics. Washington: Georgetown University Press; 2003.
2. Hoffmaster B. What does vulnerability mean? Hastings Cent Rep 2006;36(2):38.
3. Gastmans C. A fundamental ethical approach to nursing: some proposals for ethics education. Nurs Ethics 2002;9(5):494-507.
4. Schluter J, Winch S, Holzhauser K, Henderson A. Nurses' moral sensitivity and hospital ethical climate: a literature review. Nurs Ethics 2008;15(3):304-21.
5. Tschudin V. Ethics in nursing: the caring relationship. 3rd ed. London: Elsevier; 2003.
6. Kerridge I, Lowe M, Stewart C. Ethics and law for the health professions. 4th ed. Sydney: Federation Press; 2009.
7. Anscombe G. Modern moral philosophy. Philosophy 1958;33:1-19.
8. Aristotle. Nicomachean ethics. Grinnell: Peripatetic Press; 1984.
9. Fry ST, Johnstone MJ. Ethics in nursing practice. 2nd ed. Oxford: Blackwell; 2002.
10. Charon R, Montello M. Stories matter: the role of narrative in medical ethics. London: Routledge; 2002.

11. Charon R. Narrative medicine: honouring the stories of illness. New York: Oxford University Press; 2006.
12. Mayer B. Dilemmas in mandatory reporting of domestic violence: carative ethics in emergency rooms. Nurs Connect 1998;11(4):5–21.
13. Hofstede G. Culture's consequences: international differences in work-related values. London: Sage Publications; 1984.
14. International Council of Nurses (ICN). The ICN code of ethics for nurses. Geneva. Revised 2021. Online. Available from: www.icn.ch/system/files/2021-10/ICN_Code-of-Ethics_EN_Web_0.pdf.
15. Nursing and Midwifery Board of Australia (NMBA). Code of conduct for nurses. 2018. Online. Available from: www.nursingmidwiferyboard.gov.au/Codes-Guidelines-Statements/FAQ/Fact-sheet-Code-of-conduct-for-nurses-and-Code-of-conduct-for-midwives.aspx.
16. Paramedicine Board of Australia. Code of conduct. 2022. Online. Available from: www.ahpra.gov.au/Publications/Code-of-conduct/Shared-Code-of-conduct.aspx.
17. National Health and Medical Research Council (NHMRC). Statement on ethical conduct in research involving humans. 2007 (updated 2018). Online. Available from: www.nhmrc.gov.au/about-us/publications/national-statement-ethical-conduct-human-research-2007-updated-2018.
18. Health Research Council of New Zealand (HRC). HRC Research ethics guidelines. 2017. Online. Available from: www.hrc.govt.nz/sites/default/files/2019-10/HRC%20Research%20Ethics%20Guidelines-%20December%202017.pdf.
19. National Health and Medical Research Council (NHMRC). Ethical issues arising from the COVID-19 pandemic. 2020. Online. Available from: www.nhmrc.gov.au/sites/default/files/2020-06/nchrac-report-Ethical-issues-arising-from-the-COVID-19-pandemic0620.pdf.
20. National Health and Medical Research Council (NHMRC). Ethics frameworks for pandemics. Online. Available from: www.nhmrc.gov.au/file/17452/download?token=a363M_PE.
21. Beauchamp T, Childress J. Principles of biomedical ethics. 5th ed. New York: Oxford University Press; 2001.
22. Dodds S. Choice and control in feminist bioethics. In: Mackenzie C, Stoljar N, editors. Relational autonomy. New York: Oxford University Press; 2000.
23. Donchin A. Understanding autonomy relationally: toward a reconfiguration of bioethical principles. J Med Philos 2001;26(4):365–86.
24. Pullman D. Ethics first aid: reframing the role of 'principlism' in clinical ethics education and practice. J Clin Ethics 2005;16(3):223–9.
25. Zawistowski C, Frader J. Ethical problems in paediatric critical care: consent. Crit Care Med 2003;31(5):407–10.
26. Manson NC, O'Neill O. Rethinking informed consent in bioethics. Cambridge: Cambridge University Press; 2007.
27. Luce J. Ethical principles in critical care. J Am Med Assoc 1990;263:696–700.
28. Childress J. Protecting handicapped newborns. In: Milunsky A, Annas G, editors. Genetics and the law III. New York: Plenum Press; 1985.
29. Lützén K, Dahlqvist V, Eriksson S, et al. Developing the concept of moral sensitivity in health care practice. Nurs Ethics 2006;13(2):187–96.
30. Verkerk M, Lindemann H, Maeckelberghe E, et al. Enhancing reflection: an interpersonal exercise in ethics education. Hastings Cent Rep 2004;34:31–8.
31. Corley MC, Minick P, Elswick RK, et al. Nurse moral distress and ethical work environment. Nurs Ethics 2005;12(4):381–90.
32. Aitken LH. Hospital nurse staffing and patient mortality, nurse burnout, and job dissatisfaction. J Am Med Assoc 2002;288(16):1987–93.
33. Cameron ME. Legal and ethical issues: ethical distress in nursing. J Prof Nurs 1997;13(5):280.
34. Sundin-Huard D, Fahy K. Moral distress, advocacy and burnout: theorising the relationships. Int J Nurs Pract 1999;5(1):8–13.
35. Jameton A. Nursing practice: the ethical issues. New Jersey: Prentice-Hall; 1984.
36. Taylor C. Sources of the self. Cambridge: Harvard University Press; 1989.
37. National Health and Medical Research Council (NHMRC). Clinical ethics capacity building resource manual. Online. Available from: www.nhmrc.gov.au/about-us/publications/clinical-ethics-capacity-building-resource-manual.

CHAPTER 4
EMERGENCY CARE AND THE LAW

MARY CHIARELLA

ESSENTIALS

- It is important to understand the relationship between law, ethics and professionalism to ensure optimum patient care is able to be provided.
- All nurses and midwives and paramedics need to understand the legal framework in which they practise.
- There is a range of processes and procedures that health practitioners need to know in relation to the Australian court system; in particular, the aspects of the court system in which they might become involved.

Disclaimer: The law referred to in this chapter is predominantly NSW and Commonwealth law, but reference is made to general principles. Where possible, reference is made to corresponding law in other states and it is advisable that practitioners in those states refer directly to that law.

INTRODUCTION

Emergency nurses and paramedics frequently find themselves faced with legal issues within the workplace. These include issues relating to maintenance of privacy, obtaining consent, fulfilling a duty of care and maintaining professional standards, to name but a few. It is important that health practitioners understand the law that governs their practice. Our society is structured around a legal system that was adopted from an English system of rules that were essentially designed to govern a community's behaviour and, more specifically, an individual's behaviour and rights within that community. Laws are shaped by societal values and are designed to reflect those. The law provides a range of remedies, depending on the type and focus of the law. For example, health professional regulation is about protecting the public, whereas criminal law is designed to punish offenders and deter potential offenders. Civil law is about disputes between individuals and is often about compensatory redress. The system derives from two main sources of law: common law or judge-made law and statutory or parliamentary-made law.

This chapter will explore the responsibilities of health professionals to comply with the law and the particular pieces of law that most commonly apply to them, and why it is important to do so. We will start with a brief explanation of what the law is.

WHAT IS THE LAW?[1]

The law is a system of rules and regulations that are designed to ensure that individual human rights, such as our rights to liberty, justice and equality, are able to be upheld. A law is a rule that comes from a legitimate authority, for example, a democratically elected parliament, and applies to everyone equally. Laws are created to make sure that everyone in a society understands what is expected of them as a member of that society (obligations and duties), and what they can expect from others, including the government (their rights). An example of a law made by the parliament that sets out the rules of behaviour is the *Crimes Act 1900 (NSW)*.[2]

In addition to setting out the rules by which we live, another function of the legal system is to resolve disputes. The resolution of disputes commonly occurs in civil law matters. For example, contract law is an example of civil law. A contract is an agreement made between two or more parties on the basis of some form of transaction between the parties. Sometimes disputes arise as to the terms of the contract. These disputes can be resolved by the court.

DIFFERENT TYPES OF LAWS

COMMON LAW

Common law is based on principles that have arisen in previous decisions made in cases relating to certain facts and the reapplication of those principles to new cases. This form of law allows for expansion and development of the law, as each case contributes to the body of law in that area. This is also known as case law or precedent.

PARLIAMENTARY LAW

Parliamentary (or statute) law is also known as legislation, and a piece of legislation is referred to as an Act. This law is made by the people we elect to Parliament as our representatives. This law is often written to accommodate the social and technological changes that occur within our society. There are various pieces of statute law that apply to nurses, midwives and paramedics; for example, most states have legislation that controls the use of drugs and poisons. There is also subordinate legislation, usually referred to as regulations or by-laws. Regulations have the force of the law and usually contain a lot of details that are not present in the Act, thus allowing the law to be updated and amended to change with time, without having to go through the extended process of putting new legislation through Parliament.[3] This allows the law to be more flexible.

BRANCHES OF LAW

The law is divided into many branches, but for the purposes of this chapter we will briefly outline the difference between criminal law and civil law. A criminal case deals with a crime which is an offence against the Crown and punishable by fine or imprisonment, whereas a civil case generally involves disputes between citizens involving liability for damages (such as in a motor vehicle collision) or breach of contract.

LEGAL JURISDICTIONS

Both criminal and civil cases are dealt with in the general courts (in NSW the Local Court, the District Court and the Supreme Court), but there are other courts and tribunals which deal with legal issues outside the general courts. Matters relating to unexpected or unexplained deaths are heard by the Coroner in the Coroner's Court; whereas other criminal or civil matters, such as assault or negligence, will be heard by the Supreme Court. There are many others. One legal jurisdiction that is particularly relevant to healthcare staff is the professional regulatory jurisdiction that hears matters pertaining to professional competency and patient safety. We will examine that area first.

PROFESSIONAL REGULATION AND PATIENT SAFETY

In July 2010 the Australian Health Practitioner Regulation Agency (Ahpra) became the organisation underpinning the national registering Boards for regulated health practitioners in Australia, including medical and nursing professionals. The legislation regulating the National Registration and Accreditation Scheme (the Scheme) for health practitioners is the *Health Practitioner Regulation National Law* of each state and territory.

Paramedics were not originally included in the Scheme. However, in late 2017, paramedics became the fifteenth health profession to be regulated by the National Law.[4] The passing of this law authorised the establishment of a Paramedicine Board of Australia, which was tasked with establishing the governance of paramedics under the Scheme. Paramedics commenced being regulated under the National Registration and Accreditation Scheme (NRAS) in 2018.

The traditional purpose of a professional regulatory scheme is to protect the public; it has been said that those presiding over disciplinary tribunals and committees for the purpose of professional regulation exercise a 'protective jurisdiction'.[5] However, NRAS also has a number of other objectives relating to workforce mobility and flexibility. The system now works in the same way as an Australian drivers' licensing system—a person may register in one state, but their licence enables them to drive anywhere in Australia. Similarly, now, although a person might register, say, with the Northern Territory State Board of the Nursing and Midwifery Board of Australia, they will be able to practise nursing and/or midwifery in any jurisdiction in Australia. The state Boards for Nursing and Midwifery have their authority delegated from the Nursing and Midwifery Board of Australia, and this is because of the sheer scale of numbers of nurses and midwives that require registration each year (479,526 registrants as at December 2021).[6] By contrast, the Paramedicine Board of Australia has a much smaller cohort of registrants (22,563 as at December 2021),[7] and so is able to operate more centrally.

The model for professional regulation in most countries is one of co-regulation, most usually with government, through a range of government agencies. This is the case in Australia.

Within the domain of professional self-regulation are four key elements:

- who should enter the profession (registration)
- how they might properly conduct themselves as members of that profession (codes and guidelines)
- what criteria would need to be breached for them to be excluded from the profession (complaints and notifications)
- what those who enter might look like (accreditation).[8]

THE NATIONAL REGISTER

There are national registers for each profession that the public can access online by entering a practitioner's name into a search engine and viewing the results.[9] The search will confirm that the person is registered and identify whether there are any specific regulatory requirements on their registration. If a health practitioner has the word 'registered' in the column 'registration status' they are registered and legally able to practise.

STUDENT REGISTRATION

Under the National Law, students undertaking courses leading to qualification as registered health practitioners have been registered from 2011. The only student group not to be registered are psychology students. (The Psychology Board of Australia has determined to register these students through provisional registration.) There are no fees for student registration.

Any student who is currently enrolled in an approved program of study is required to be registered. Students do not need to apply for registration personally, as Ahpra works directly with education providers to do this.

REGISTRATION AS A HEALTH PRACTITIONER

All health professionals who have been off the register and wish to renew, and those who are applying for the first time, either because they have just completed an approved course of study in Australia or because they are applying from overseas, are required to meet the national registration eligibility criteria, including certain registration standards, some of which are mandatory across all health professions.

The National Law states that an individual is *qualified* for general registration in a health profession if:

a. the individual holds an approved qualification for the health profession; or
b. the individual holds a qualification the National Board established for the health profession considers to be substantially equivalent, or based on similar competencies, to an approved qualification; or
c. the individual holds a qualification, not referred to in paragraph (a) or (b), relevant to the health profession and has successfully completed an examination or other assessment required by the National Board for the purpose of general registration in the health profession; or
d. the individual:
    i. holds a qualification, not referred to in paragraph (a) or (b), that under this Law or a corresponding prior Act qualified the individual for general registration (however described) in the health profession; and
    ii. was previously registered under this Law or the corresponding prior Act on the basis of holding that qualification.[10]

Each Board may set its own standards, but whenever possible, the National Boards prefer to develop common or similar standards across professions. Certainly the criminal history registration standard is common to all National Boards and the English language skills registration standard is common to all, except the Nursing and Midwifery Board of Australia and the Aboriginal and Torres Strait Islander Board of Australia. However, the recency of practice, continuing professional development and professional indemnity insurance registration standards are specific to the individual National Boards.[11]

There are also codes and guidelines in place for each profession, the NMBA having published new Codes of Conduct for Nursing and Midwifery in 2018,[12] and having adopted the International Council of Nurses' Code of Ethics[12] and the International Confederation of Midwives' Code of Ethics[12] in the same year. The Paramedicine Board has a new Code of Conduct that came into effect on 29 June 2022.[13]

COMPLAINTS HANDLING

The third element of professional self-regulation is the management of complaints and notifications, which includes expressions of concern about the health, performance or conduct of a registered health professional.[14] The general public, including other health professionals, has a right (and in some instances a duty) to notify the relevant registration authority of a concern about a health practitioner's:

- conduct, if it appears in some way to be putting the public at risk;
- health, insomuch as it affects their ability to practise safely;
- clinical competence or performance.

Ahpra explains in simple terms what a notification can be about. These are set out in Box 4.1.

The notification process is quite complex and also differs between certain states, such as NSW and Queensland, which have co-regulatory processes with the NRAS.[16] A notification can be made electronically, by mail, by telephone or in person. There are forms that need to be completed, but Ahpra staff can assist the public where necessary.

When a notification is received, Ahpra will assess it to determine whether a Board must consider taking immediate action to

BOX 4.1 WHAT CAN A NOTIFICATION BE ABOUT?[15]

Concerns that a practitioner is working or providing patient care in an unsafe way, such as:

- serious or repeated mistakes in carrying out procedures, in diagnosis or in prescribing medications for a patient
- a failure to examine a patient properly or to respond reasonably to a patient's needs
- serious concerns about the way in which a practitioner managed someone's personal information
- serious concerns about the way a practitioner is prescribing medication
- serious concerns about the practitioner's ability to understand and communicate in English, or
- serious concerns about the practitioner's skills, knowledge or judgement in their profession.

Concerns about the way a practitioner behaves, including:

- a practitioner abusing their professional position; for example, by engaging in an sexual or personal relationship with a patient or someone close to a patient
- inappropriate examinations of a patient
- acts of violence, sexual assault or indecency
- acts of fraud or dishonesty
- any serious criminal acts, or
- any other behaviour that is inconsistent with the practitioner being fit and proper to be a registered health practitioner.

Concerns that a practitioner has a health issue or impairment that might cause harm to a member of the public if it is not appropriately managed, including that a practitioner might have a problem with alcohol or drugs.

protect public health or safety. This may result in suspending or imposing conditions on the registration status of a student or practitioner. If immediate action is not required, Ahpra will assess the notification thoroughly to enable the relevant Board to make an informed decision about it. Each investigation is tailored to the notification received, and complex matters take more time. Notwithstanding the differences mentioned in NSW and Queensland, there is a nationally consistent process across the NRAS for managing notifications, which can include the following stages:

- lodgement
- assessment
- health complaints entity (HCE) consultation
- investigation
- health or performance assessment
- immediate action
- panel hearings
- tribunal hearings.[16–19]

New guidelines came into force on 1 March 2020 regarding mandatory notifications.[18] These guidelines mean that health practitioners are able to seek help for mental health problems without fearing a mandatory notification. The new guidelines are applicable to registered health practitioners and their employers. Four possible concerns might lead a practitioner to necessitate a mandatory notification and these concerns must be based on a reasonable belief and a substantial risk of harm. The concerns are: impairment, intoxication while practising, significant departure from professional standards, and sexual misconduct. There are different thresholds for notifications, depending on your relationship with the practitioner about whom you are making the notification. These are set out clearly in the documentation on the webpage.[20] However, regardless of your relationship, there is always the requirement for a reasonable belief that the risk exists. For example, there is a need to 'have direct knowledge, or a report from a reliable source about their experience or observations. A mandatory notification should not be made based on rumors or gossip.'[21]

The Ahpra website provides useful information in relation to notifications, but it is important to remember that the advice on the NMBA website, and also on the Paramedicine Board website in relation to professional standards, is there specifically to protect the public. Practitioners who practise within their professional practice framework, while not being immune from public dissatisfaction or concern, would be less likely to attract disapprobation.

THE CORONER'S COURT

The role of the Coroner's Court is an ancient one. The role of the Coroner is to determine the manner and cause of a person's death, or to determine the identity of a deceased person where the identity is not known. In general, the Coroner investigates deaths that are violent or unnatural; sudden and of unknown cause; deaths in suspicious or unusual circumstances; deaths during or following surgery or other invasive procedures; or deaths that occur in custody. The role of the Coroner is not to make a finding of guilt or innocence in a case, but to instead establish the way in which a death has occurred and recommend actions that may prevent such a death from occurring in the future. For example, the Coroner has recently made the recommendation 'to ensure that no patient proceeds to surgery without first having obtained all necessary medical consultation and clearances'.[22] Many recommendations are made by the Coroner that have led to the development of protocols and procedures, which may help to reduce the risk of a recurrence of an incident that has previously come before the Coroner.

PREPARATION OF BODY FOR THE CORONER

After a patient's death, provided this death falls under the jurisdiction of the Coroner, it is necessary for paramedics or hospital staff to contact the police. The police may wish to take statements from staff and gather evidence. The body should be left exactly as it was at the time death was declared. All interventions should remain in situ, including IV lines, drainage bags, catheters, endotracheal tubes, defibrillation pads, dressings and the like. These should obviously be capped or sealed as necessary. The body can then be transported to the morgue per local protocol or hospital procedure and, if necessary, arrangements can be made for a post-mortem. The requirements and circumstances in which this must occur vary across jurisdictions and should be set out in procedure manuals.

APPEARANCE AT CORONER'S COURT

If a health practitioner is called to appear before the Coroner, they can expect that the following processes will occur. Note the points about record-keeping and the stages at which the practitioner is advised to seek advice.

1. They will be approached by police to give a statement pertaining to an event in which they have been a witness or directly involved. The role of the police in Coroner's Court proceedings is to work to assist the Coroner by gathering information that will assist the court to identify the circumstances surrounding an event. A practitioner has the right to refuse to give evidence until they have received legal advice. Each person has a right to refuse to give evidence if they feel they might incriminate themselves. However, this protection was altered by a change in the law in 2000 (s 61 of the NSW Act) which enables the Coroner to require a person objecting to giving evidence on the grounds of self-incrimination to give evidence, but they are given a certificate which prevents that evidence being given against the witness in other court proceedings. If a practitioner does not cooperate with the police, a subpoena may be issued by the court that will compel this witness to attend. If that person does not attend they may be arrested. Note that it is advisable to give evidence or make statements as close to the time of the incident as possible. Contemporaneous evidence is most reliable and is most highly sought. It is advisable to keep a copy of the statement made. If a request for a statement comes sometime after the event it may be necessary to access a copy of the patient's notes from records storage and review them. This is where good documentation serves an important purpose.
2. Prior to making a statement, it may be necessary to seek legal advice from your employer's legal representatives, or, if there is a conflict, contact your own solicitor or union solicitor.
3. A subpoena will be issued stating the date, time and location to appear.
4. When the practitioner arrives at court, they should check that the case has been listed and in which court it will be heard.
5. The practitioner should notify the court officer they have arrived.
6. The practitioner waits outside the court until called.

7. They are called to the stand to give evidence, at which time they will be asked to take an oath or an affirmation.
8. The practitioner will be asked to give their account of events, which may involve revisiting the content of their statement.
9. The rules of evidence do not apply in the Coroner's Court as they do in other courts, so the way in which evidence is presented is different. For example, the practitioner may be called upon to give hearsay evidence—evidence of what they have heard someone else say. This is not normally permitted in court, but there are provisions within the Coroner's Act that authorise a Coroner holding an inquest or inquiry to not be bound to observe the rules of procedure and evidence applicable to proceedings before a court of law. This is because the purpose of the Coroner is not to make a determination as to a person's guilt, but rather to establish the truth of a matter.
10. The practitioner may be cross-examined, but the purpose of the Coroner's inquest is not to put the healthcare practitioner on trial. Instead, its purpose is to ascertain the circumstances surrounding an incident in the hope that such information will lead to a satisfactory explanation of the events that have led to the inquest.
11. Only if the Coroner determines there is enough evidence to suggest that a witness is guilty of a criminal offence will the matter be referred to the Director of Public Prosecutions (DPP) for further examination. There are very few instances of practitioners being pursued by the DPP in this regard.[22] It is more likely that if the Coroner finds the healthcare staff negligent they will refer the matter to the relevant disciplinary body for investigation and possible disciplinary action. Ahpra publishes regular updates on cases referred to the National Boards from the jurisdictional Coroners.[23]

INVESTIGATIONS AND COURT

MAKING A STATEMENT

The healthcare system is complex. Mistakes are made and oversights and omissions occur. From time to time this may result in an internal or external investigation being undertaken. The most common way in which an investigator will engage those staff who might be able to help them with their investigation is via an interview. This interview may form part of or remain separate from a formal oral statement that you may also give. You may also be asked to provide a written statement of your experience, knowledge and understanding of a certain event or series of events. An affidavit is a written statement sworn as to the truth of its contents before a legal representative or justice of the peace. This statement can be used in court. It is always advisable to seek legal advice before providing a statement, even to your employer, so as to avoid self-incrimination.[24] You may prepare a statement yourself or have your lawyer or other person draft it for you. It is an offence to give a false or misleading statement.[24]

However, although each individual has the right to refuse to give a statement, there may be occasions where remaining silent is not in the healthcare practitioner's best interest. For example, if there is an innocent explanation for a sequence of events that occurred or if the practitioner has a sound alibi, then offering the explanation or alibi may relieve the practitioner of having to engage in any further discussion regarding the events, and they should be forthcoming with this information.

If a practitioner is required to give a statement of events, the statement should be precise and factual. It should be written in numbered paragraphs and should commence with the practitioner's name and, if relevant to the inquiry, place of work and role. A chronological recitation of events leading up to and including the event being examined is almost always what is required. Statements may include conversations that the writer has engaged in directly. For example, 'The patient said "I have some pain in my chest". I [the practitioner] asked, "How long have you had it for?"' Avoid attempting to interpret or explain this direct evidence. Simply recite exactly what happened without embellishment. Where possible, avoid the use of hearsay in statements as hearsay is only admissible as evidence in certain circumstances or in certain jurisdictions, for example, the Coroner's Court in NSW. An example of hearsay is, 'When I went to the nurses' station, Jill B said that the patient's wife had told her yesterday that the patient was complaining of chest pain.' This is hearsay because the patient's complaint was not heard directly by the nurse making the statement. Just as with any evidence, it is advisable to recite only what *you* heard, saw, did, and when and where you heard, saw or did it.

LEGAL PRIVILEGE

In some circumstances the issue of privilege arises between professionals and their clients. For healthcare professionals in all states, with the exception of Tasmania,[25] this is not the case. Nurses in these states are compellable, and thus required, if asked, to disclose patient information in court. The sharing of confidential patient information with the court is an authorised disclosure of personal information. If the witness has any doubt as to whether it is lawful to share private patient information in court, the witness can ask the judge hearing the matter, or their lawyer, for clarification as to whether the information can or should be disclosed. The exception to this rule is in sexual assault communications. In these cases any counselling communication that is made by, to or about a victim or alleged victim of sexual assault, may not be compellable as evidence in court.[26]

VICTIM IMPACT STATEMENTS

If the practitioner is the victim of a crime (for example, is assaulted in the workplace) and the crime is prosecuted, the practitioner will be required to make a statement to police regarding the matter. Once the case has been heard and the offence found to be proved, the victim (practitioner) may have the opportunity to write a victim impact statement, which can be taken into account by the judge when considering the appropriate sentence.[27] This statement is presented to the court and explains how the crime has harmed the victim. A practitioner may not have been directly injured as a result of the crime, but instead have been a witness to it and suffered some loss as a result of witnessing the event. A victim impact statement may also be written in this instance.[27] If someone is physically unable to write the statement themselves, then they may have someone else do it for them.

THE PRESERVATION AND COLLECTION OF EVIDENCE

Often patients will present to an emergency department (ED) as a result of being involved in a criminal offence, such as an assault. In this instance it is a healthcare practitioner's first priority and duty to provide care to the patient. However, there may be moments during the care and treatment of the patient when it is possible for healthcare staff to gather and preserve evidence for the police to use at a future time for the purposes of investigating the incident.

Police are generally interested in any object or item left either with a victim, offender or witness at a scene of inquiry, no matter how insignificant it may appear to be. Advances in forensic science, specifically in the area of DNA testing, mean that a wide range of evidence is now suitable for analysis by police, to assist them in determining the events surrounding an offence.

The general rule with the gathering of evidence is simply, 'Don't touch'. However, it is unlikely that in all circumstances this will be possible. The rule then is that if a piece of evidence is handled, the handling is minimised. Staff should wear fresh gloves when handling evidence so as not to contaminate it with DNA from themselves or elsewhere. It should be noted, however, that even gloves can smear fingerprints.

It is important that staff note the placement of certain objects and note who has touched what, where and why. This documentation is important so that the *chain of evidence* remains intact. The chain of evidence is necessary for police to demonstrate that evidence has not been tainted or tampered with. This maintains the integrity of the exhibit, so that it may be used in court proceedings. These rules apply equally to all medical professionals, including doctors, nurses and paramedics. It is also important for staff to be aware of the evidence they may inadvertently discard. For example, the gloves worn by healthcare workers handling materials may come into contact with items of interest, so the gloves themselves can also be gathered as evidence. Other materials used by or taken from a patient suspected of being involved in an event that may be of interest to the police should be placed in a contaminated waste bag assigned to that patient only and passed on to the police at a later time. Almost any item has the potential to hold incriminating evidence, so, as a general rule, everything that is used on the patient should be preserved. To wilfully destroy evidence is an offence.[28]

If emergency staff, including paramedics, have reason to believe that their patient has been involved in an event that might be of interest to the police, then they should do all they can to assist the police. For example, a patient presents to emergency with a knife impaled in their body. It is important that someone notes the position of the knife prior to its removal. This position should be documented with the names of all persons who come into contact with the knife and the reasons why it was removed. This procedure should be followed for any piece of evidence removed from a person.

Paper bags are the preferred vessel for storage. Paper preserves evidence for a longer period of time than plastic. Plastic sweats and therefore is more likely to destroy or affect the quality of the evidence. Once clothing, weaponry, drugs, personal items or the like are gathered by the emergency staff, the items should be placed in a paper bag or box and stored in a secure area. This area could be a safe; alternatively, security staff could be required to supervise the items until police arrive. Refer to local hospital policy in these cases.

It should be noted that police do have the power to seize exhibits if they suspect that an indictable (serious) offence has been committed.[29] Relatives may ask to hold on to a patient's possessions, but police do have the authority to seize such items for the purpose of ascertaining information regarding the offence. The only item police are not authorised to seize is the Sexual Assault Investigation Kit.[30] Police are only entitled to seize this item if the patient has signed the relevant documentation permitting them to do so. Police can seize any clothing or other items belonging to the patient.

PARAMEDICS: PRE-HOSPITAL TEAMS AND EVIDENCE

Health and emergency service workers in the pre-hospital environment should also be aware that their actions can directly affect the ability of police to gather and preserve evidence. While it is understood that the priority for health workers in this setting is the health and wellbeing of the patient, workers should be mindful of the way in which they enter and work in the environment. If, for example, paramedics are called to a 'concern for welfare' case or are called to attend a scene by the police, they should be aware of the way in which their presence at the scene may disturb it. For example, if an intruder has accessed premises unlawfully and is known to have walked across the middle of the room, leaving behind evidence of their presence, and a paramedic, called to that scene, also proceeds across the middle of the room, evidence of this movement will be left as well. Where practicable, pre-hospital care teams should try to preserve as much evidence as possible. This includes items such as the gloves they wear. DNA evidence from the patient may also become embedded in the officers' uniforms. They should be mindful of evidence such as blood splatter and make all attempts to ensure that it remains untouched. Pre-hospital care teams may also take note of anything touched, moved, noticed or smelt at the scene. This may be called upon at a later date as evidence in court.

In the case of *Jackson v Lithgow City Council* [2010] NSW CA 136, the court considered the question of whether the records made by ambulance officers attending the scene of a man who had allegedly fallen 1.5 metres were admissible as evidence of that fact which the man was attempting to prove in his case of negligence against the council. The records showed that the recording officer had written next to Patient History: *"? Fall from 1.5 metres on to concrete."* The question mark appearing in the record suggested that the height and indeed the fall was not confirmed. Neither of the officers were called to give evidence and so the court was asked to consider if the documentation provided any admissible evidence that could contribute to the case. The court accepted that the document added a legitimate opinion (an inference) that from all that he or they could see there was a question whether the plaintiff had fallen off the wall. The inference (and thus the opinion) was based upon what the ambulance officers perceived. This case demonstrates the importance of taking and recording accurate notes of events and findings at the scene, as they can later be used and relied upon in court for a variety of reasons.

BLOOD ALCOHOL TESTING

If a person over the age of 15 years presents to the ED for examination or treatment as a result of a motor vehicle collision, and has been a pedestrian, cyclist, horse rider, motorboat or train driver, then it is the duty of the medical officer to take a sample of the patient's blood for analysis, whether or not the patient consents, and within 12 hours of the patient presenting.[31] If no medical officer is present, the blood or urine sample is to be taken by the registered nurse attending the patient. It is an offence to fail to take a sample. The penalty for failing to take a sample is $2200. The defences to the offence include believing that the patient was younger than 15 years, that they had not been involved in a motor vehicle collision or that to take the sample would in some way impair the patient's care and treatment.[31] It is an offence for a person to prevent a health professional from obtaining a sample for the purposes of the Act.[31]

CHILD VICTIMS

In dealing with a child suspected of being the victim of an offence, medical personnel should first treat the child's injuries. However, at no time should medical personnel attempt to elicit evidence from the child about the circumstances surrounding the child's injuries. For example, medical staff should not ask, 'Who did this to you?' To do so could compromise future court proceedings against any offender. It is the responsibility of teams such as the Joint Investigative Response Team (NSW) to gather evidence from the child. This team, made up of Child Protection Unit police officers and Department of Family and Community Services (FACS) staff, are specially trained for this purpose. The medical staff should notify police that they believe such an investigation is required.[32] All staff have a mandatory duty to report any cases where they believe a child is the victim of abuse.[32]

CHILD PROTECTION LEGISLATION AND MANDATORY REPORTING[33]

Law

Child protection laws fall under the 'protective' jurisdiction of the court. This jurisdiction also covers mental health patients and those under guardianship. Every parent or guardian has responsibility to ensure the care and protection of their child until that child turns 18 years of age. The definition of maltreatment of a child varies in each state and territory, but broadly the term encompasses neglect and sexual, physical or emotional abuse. That is, omitting to provide care is considered maltreatment, just as assaulting a child is considered maltreatment. The scope of the area is too large to be effectively covered in this chapter, but each healthcare provider should have a policy in place to assist staff to take action if they suspect that a child is a victim of neglect or abuse.

Mandatory reporting

It is an offence in every state and territory for nominated health professionals to fail to report suspected child abuse or neglect to the authorities. Under the revised, shared Code of Conduct that came into force in June 2022, paramedics are now expected to comply with mandatory notification relating to children, aged care residents and other vulnerable groups.[13]

A person who reports a suspected case of abuse, in good faith, cannot be considered to have breached privacy laws and cannot be sued for defamation. On the contrary, it is more likely there could be ramifications for a healthcare professional if they fail to report.

Prenatal reporting

In some states and territories, a person who reasonably believes that a child, once born, may be at risk of harm and in need of care and protection, may make a report to the Director-General of Family and Community Services. This will trigger an investigation into the child's future home environment. This provision only allows for care and protection to be given once the child has been born alive.[34]

DOCUMENTATION

In nursing and paramedicine, there exists a culture of verbal handover of information regarding a patient and their condition.[35] While the verbal exchange of this information has its place in the healthcare setting, this information should also be recorded in the patient's healthcare record. Records can be used in a variety of ways. For example, they can allow for the exchange of information between different parties, they can be used as evidence that something has or has not been done and they can be used to record incidents that occurred, for the purposes of implementing effective risk management measures. The guide to effective record-keeping is:

1. Records should be accurate. Pre-printed fourth-hourly observation charts can cause problems with accuracy. For example, it is not accurate to say the patient's temperature was 38°C at 1800 hrs when the temperature was taken at 1825 hrs.
2. They should be written contemporaneously, that is, at the time of the event.
3. They should be brief and objective. They should not be embellished with interpretation.
4. They should be legible.
5. They should avoid the use of abbreviations and jargon, unless this is widely used and accepted in the healthcare community. This avoidance limits misunderstanding among the allied health workforce who all contribute to the patient's integrated record.
6. Errors should be left in the report with a simple line drawn through them.
7. The report should be written for the correct patient. Just as with medication, the notes should be checked to ensure that the notes refer to the patient being written about.
8. Patients should be referred to by name, not number alone.
9. Do not write notes on behalf of someone else. Write only what *you* saw, heard or did.
10. Read the patient's notes. Do not just rely on a verbal handover.

The more information recorded in the patient's health record, the better able the healthcare practitioner is to accurately recall issues surrounding the event. Courts will rely on not only oral evidence, but also written evidence. A case may not get to court until sometime after the incident that led to the proceedings, and a witness's recollection of events over time can become clouded and unreliable. This can lead the court to question the witness's credibility and the evidence they give may not be able to be relied upon. This highlights the importance of keeping good written records.[36]

PRACTICE TIP

Complete documentation during and immediately after treating your patient to ensure that it is contemporaneous. This will also help with accuracy and completeness.

PERSONALLY CONTROLLED ELECTRONIC HEALTH CARE RECORD (PCEHR)

A Personally Controlled Electronic Health Care Record (PCEHR) is an electronic form of medical records which, as the name suggests, is able to be controlled by the patient to some extent. Where previously medical records were only able to be owned, at law, by the creator of that record, under the laws governing the PCEHR, patients are able to legally own and make notes in their own healthcare record. With regards to patient control over the record, there will be a section of the record for personal information that the patient can control and change as they wish. There will also be a clinical component of the record. Within the clinical component of the record, blood test results may be listed on the record. These results cannot be altered by the patient, but the patient can control who sees that part of the record. The record will include the patient's prescribed medication, test results, care plans, immunisations and health alerts, such as allergies. The electronic nature of the record means that, with the patient's permission, the record is able to be accessed by the patient or their doctor anywhere in Australia at any time and would be likely to prove invaluable in an emergency.

There are a number of reasons for implementing the e-health system, including to assist in the reduction of the high rate of medical errors that occur from inadequate patient information, reduce unnecessary hospital admissions and save doctors from collecting a full medical history each time they see a new patient.

There have been some difficulties in implementing the national opt-in program, which has meant the e-health record is not able to be utilised in all health facilities, including paramedic services where a localised form of electronic record-taking is used.

Confidentiality

In order to ascertain the information needed to treat patients safely and effectively, healthcare workers rely on their patients to disclose personal details to them which they would not necessarily disclose to others. Healthcare practitioners encourage their patients to disclose this information on the basis that the information disclosed will remain confidential and will not be discussed with others without the patient's permission. A breach of confidentiality is *any* disclosure of a person's healthcare record without permission. This disclosure may include verbal, written or electronic communication of any sort with respect to the patient and/or the institution's records.[37]

Healthcare workers and public or private health organisations owe a common law duty of confidentiality to their patients. Confidentiality extends to all patients within that facility, whether the healthcare practitioner directly cares for them or not. If confidentiality is breached the healthcare worker can be prosecuted by the patient and/or institution and may be required to pay the injured party damages. They may also face a disciplinary charge by their respective health board.

There are several exceptions to the rule with respect to the disclosure of confidential personal information. Along with the patient agreeing to the disclosure, they also include the mandatory reporting of child abuse, the mandatory reporting of infectious diseases (although this may be de-identified information), and there is also a duty to the public to disclose, by the order of a court for the assistance of police in the investigation of an offence, by subpoena for a civil action or by a government minister.

Privacy

All public or private sector health service providers are subject to the provisions of the Privacy Act in each state and territory,[38] which aims to regulate the way in which private institutions collect and use personal information. In NSW, the *Health Records and Information Privacy Regulation 2022* is intended to promote the fair and responsible handling of health information by health service providers and to protect the privacy of an individual's health information, whether it is held by the public or private sector. There is equivalent legislation in Victoria. The Act was designed to enhance and promote the individual's ability to be informed about their healthcare and to assist individuals to access their healthcare information. It is designed to allow individuals access to a dispute resolution process regarding the handling of their health information should such a process be required.

Another important consideration for practitioners with regards to the protection of patient privacy is the impact of advances in technology, which has increased risks associated with the use of patient information. There have been recent examples of paramedics and ambulance services sharing patient cases on social media like Twitter without the patient's permission. The sharing of this information by those involved has been justified on the basis that the information does not identify the patient, and that the sharing of the detailed work of what paramedics do is in the public interest and therefore excusable. This is a false understanding of the 'public interest' test for the sharing of patient information and it demonstrates a lack of confidence in the way in which even de-identified information can be triangulated with other pieces of data to make a patient identifiable. The action also demonstrates a lack of understanding in the way in which assurance in the trustworthiness of healthcare staff to keep patient information private is absolutely essential to maintaining confidence in the healthcare system, particularly the ambulance system, where people have suggested they are less likely to call for help if they believe their private information will be shared with others without their permission.[39] In Australia, Ahpra has a strong policy about the sharing of patient information by health professionals. This policy now applies to paramedics as they are now a registered health profession.[40]

INCIDENT REPORTS

Most health services have an incident management system that is used to improve patient safety and support improvements and maintenance of quality clinical practice. Incident reports allow for the identification of work practices, equipment or environments that could lead to a lower quality of service being provided to a consumer, or that may pose a risk to staff or visitors of a facility. Any accident or near-miss is able to be reported anonymously and able to be investigated by the administration to allow it to put in place policy, procedures and resources to limit the possibility of an accident recurring. Once a service becomes aware of an incident or accident, they have an obligation to take 'reasonable' measures to address the matter.

Incident reports should contain information on the date, time and place of the incident, the names and details of the parties concerned, a brief but factual and accurate account of the incident with no hearsay or personal interpretation of the events, the harm that the incident caused, any action taken and by whom, including, for example, that faulty equipment has been decommissioned and labelled in compliance with Workplace Safety requirements.

Incident management systems are designed to encourage staff to feel that they will not be punished if they admit they have made an error. It stipulates that the obligation of reporting such incidents rests with the individual healthcare worker. It is an attempt when an error is made to move the focus of blame from the individual to the system.[41]

OPEN DISCLOSURE

If an adverse event occurs and the practitioner believes that they have contributed to it, there is provision at law for health practitioners to make an honest expression of regret to a patient and/or their loved ones and to give an explanation of what has happened.[42]

ASSAULT AND CONSENT

ASSAULT

There is a legal requirement that healthcare practitioners obtain the consent of their patient prior to performing any form of intervention upon them. Without this consent, any attempt to treat the patient could be considered unlawful and amount to a tort of assault or battery upon that person. Today there are typically few instances where a distinction is made between assault and battery. Assault is the threat of harm one may feel from another. This may not involve any actual physical contact. It is sufficient that a patient simply feels that they will be subjected to a form of treatment to which they have not consented for it to constitute an assault. Battery is the actual physical action of touching someone without consent. The patient does not have to have sustained any injury for it to be a battery. It is the physical contact without consent that constitutes the battery. An assault may fall within the criminal or the civil jurisdiction. Even if a healthcare practitioner states that they contacted the patient with all good intentions, it may not amount to a defence for assault or battery.[43]

There are exceptions to the law of assault. Accidentally making contact with someone in public is an example. Another is 'reasonable force' used by police officers in performing their duty.[44] However, this provision is limited, as in NSW, s 230 of the *Law Enforcement (Powers and Responsibilities) Act 2002* ('the LEPRA') states that police can only use force that 'is reasonably necessary to exercise the[ir] function'. Section 231 makes it clear that such force cannot go beyond what is required 'to make the arrest or to prevent the escape of the person after arrest'. In EDs healthcare staff often deal with patients in a 'time critical' environment where the patient is unable to give consent to contact, and, in these instances, staff must be able to explain their interference with the patient in a legally justifiable way or risk being charged with assault. This legal justification exists in the form of the 'doctrine of necessity'.

PRACTICE TIP

To avoid issues of assault and as a matter of professional courtesy, it is best, wherever possible, to ask your patient's permission to do something to them before doing it.

DOCTRINE OF NECESSITY

Time-critical life-and-death decisions are made on an almost daily basis in any ED and by paramedics. Often patients who present to emergency are unconscious or incompetent and therefore unable to give or refuse consent to treatment. In these circumstances, under the doctrine of necessity, staff are able to treat patients who are unable to give consent to or refuse treatment, without the risk of litigation for assault.[45] That is, where it is not possible to communicate with the patient and treatment is needed to preserve life or reduce the risk of further harm and where treatment is given in the best interests of the patient, it can be given without the patient's consent (see also below, 'When consent is not required').

CONSENT

In the medical context, consent is the permission given by one person to another to lawfully touch them. Consent is arguably the strongest representation of patient autonomy and the principle of self-determination is necessary to avoid a claim of battery or charge of assault. Failure to obtain informed consent may also lead to claims of negligence, but informed consent is different from consent per se (see below). Consent from a patient is required for direct or indirect touching and both major and minor treatment. Consent can be given in writing, verbally or implied. When a patient sees you approaching with a sphygmomanometer and holds out their arm, this constitutes implied consent to perform the blood pressure reading. As a matter of good practice, you should tell your patient what you are doing and explain that they may feel a tightness in their upper arm for a minute while you take the pressure reading.[46]

THREE ELEMENTS OF VALID CONSENT

There are three components that need to be met in order for a consent (or refusal of consent) to be considered valid. The first is that the consent must be given freely by the patient with no coercion, the patient must be informed of the broad nature and effect of the treatment and the risks and benefits associated with it; and the patient must be competent to consent to the treatment.[46]

Competence (capacity)

Any person over the age of 18 years is presumed to be competent to give or refuse consent for medical treatment. If a health professional believes that a patient is not competent to give or refuse consent for treatment, the onus rests on the health professional to show that the patient is not competent. The test for competence has three steps. The patient should be able to take in, retain and understand the treatment information. The patient should believe the information they have been given (for example, some patients with anorexia may not believe that they are unwell at all and therefore not be able to demonstrate competence). Finally, the patient should be able to weigh up the risks and benefits of the treatment and communicate a decision.

REFUSAL OF TREATMENT

The right to consent to or refuse treatment is conferred on all patients by common law.[46] The law acknowledges an individual's right to determine whether they wish to undergo medical treatment or not even if the refusal of treatment results in the patient's death. Professional issues may arise when a health practitioner is confronted by a patient's decision that conflicts with their own. It is a requirement of all health practitioners that they reflect upon and consider carefully their professional position when confronted by such dilemmas. The issue goes beyond just the legal considerations and becomes an ethical and professional concern.

PROVIDING INFORMATION TO PATIENTS—INFORMED CONSENT

Prior to commencing a procedure or treatment a clinician is required, as part of their duty of care, to inform the patient about the broad nature and effects of the treatment and has a duty to inform the patient about material risks involved in the treatment so that the patient can give or refuse consent for that proposed treatment/procedure. A material risk is a risk that a reasonable person in the patient's position would, if placed in the patient's position, be likely to attach significance to or that the medical practitioner is or ought reasonably to be aware that the patient would, if warned of the risk, attach significance to. This is distinct from informing the patient of ALL risks. The principle of 'material risk' obviously values the patient's view of what is material over those of the doctor who may think the risk is immaterial and therefore encourages patient autonomy over medical paternalism. These duties developed from the case of *Rogers v Whitaker*.[47]

This case turned largely on the fact that Dr Rogers failed to inform Mrs Whitaker of the material risks involved in an ophthalmic surgical procedure he recommended to her. The causative relationship between the duty of care between the doctor and his patient and the damage that was ultimately done was also examined. This will be discussed later with respect to negligence. Mrs Whitaker had lost sight in her right eye when she was young. She retained normal vision in her left eye and led a normal life. In her mid-40s she consulted Dr Rogers, an ophthalmic surgeon, to see if he could do anything to help her right eye, even if the improvement was just cosmetic. Dr Rogers told Mrs Whitaker that he could operate on her right eye and remove scar tissue from it, thus improving its appearance and possibly restoring some sight. Mrs Whitaker asked Dr Rogers about the risks associated with the operation. None were mentioned, despite Mrs Whitaker repeatedly asking and making comments of concern that she had regarding the risk of loss of sight (this was later recognised as a material risk). Mrs Whitaker agreed to the operation. Just after the operation she developed complications, not only with her right eye but also with her left, in a rare condition called 'sympathetic ophthalmia'. This condition can result in sympathetic inflammation of the untreated eye, which can result in loss of sight, and this occurred with Mrs Whitaker. Mrs Whitaker brought an action against Dr Rogers for not warning her of the risk of this complication developing. Mrs Whitaker stated that if she had known that the risk existed, she would not have consented to the operation. The causative link between Dr Rogers' negligence and the blindness was provided by Mrs Whitaker relying upon Dr Rogers' advice that there would be no risk. 'But for' this negligent advice, Mrs Whitaker would not have had the surgery and would not have suffered the damage.[48]

CHILDREN AND CONSENT

Unlike with adults, there is a presumption that a person under the age of 18 DOES NOT have capacity to consent or refuse consent for treatment (excluding South Australia and New Zealand where it is 16 years). A parent or guardian can also consent for medical or dental treatment for a child, but they must justify their decisions as being in the child's best interest. If there is some doubt from healthcare staff as to whether healthcare decisions are being made in the child's best interest and that decision is not immediately life threatening, then the matter can be referred to the Supreme Court or Guardianship Division of the Administrative Tribunal for determination. If a parent or guardian of a child under the age of 14 refuses treatment for a child where that treatment is necessary to prevent death or serious injury, treatment may be instituted under s 174 of the *Children and Young Persons (Care and Protection) Act 1998* (NSW), and under similar provisions in other states, or the common law doctrine of necessity.

There is also a limit to the type of treatment that a parent or guardian can consent to. For example, a parent or guardian does not have the authority to refuse life-sustaining treatment to a person under 18. That is a matter that would have to be determined by a court. A parent or guardian is also not able to consent to gender reassignment surgery. Again, that is a matter for the court operating under its *parens patriae* (protective) jurisdiction. A minor (a person under 18) can consent to minor medical treatment, provided they can demonstrate competency. There is a presumption against competency in children and rather than healthcare professionals having the onus to challenge competency, as they do with adults, in the case of children, the onus is on the child to demonstrate that they are competent to make a healthcare decision. This type of competence is referred to as Gillick competency, after the case where the issue of competency in children was first established. Gillick competency is most commonly assumed in a minor who is over the age of 14 and is consenting to minor medical treatment. There is no reason why Gillick competency could not be established in children under 14, but no child under the age of 18 is able to refuse consent for life-sustaining treatment, even if they demonstrate competence.[48]

WHEN CONSENT IS NOT REQUIRED

As an example of a statutory provision that allows treatment without consent, under the *Guardianship Act 1987* (NSW), medical or dental treatment may be carried out without consent if the treatment is considered necessary, as a matter of urgency, to save a patient's life or to prevent serious damage to the patient's health.[5,49] The purpose of this part of the Act is to ensure that patients are treated even when they lack the capacity to consent to treatment and that the treatment that is undertaken without their consent is done so for the purposes of promoting and maintaining their health and wellbeing.

Minor treatment, that is, treatment which is not major or special, may be carried out without any consent if there is no person responsible for the patient or that person cannot be contacted or they do not wish to make a decision regarding treatment. However, the clinician carrying out the treatment must certify in writing in the patient's clinical record that the treatment was required to promote the patient's health and wellbeing, and that the patient has not made known their objection to the carrying out of the treatment.[50] In short, this means that the clinician must be clear that the patient does not object to the treatment prior to it being initiated.

WHO MAY GIVE CONSENT WHEN THE PATIENT CANNOT

For patients aged 16 years and above where substitute consent is required, because the patient is incapable of giving consent to the carrying out of medical or dental treatment, the 'person responsible' under legislation such as the *Guardianship Act 1987* (NSW) is able to consent on the patient's behalf. If a young person is under 16 and without parents, in NSW the Director-General of the Department of Family and Community Services (FACS) is the guardian. In this instance, the child is effectively a ward of the state. If a person responsible is unable to be contacted to give consent, then the Guardianship Division of the Administrative Tribunal is able to act as the substitute decision-maker. If a patient presents who falls within the jurisdiction of the Mental Health Act, then the provisions of that Act will prevail.

Any person may request a person responsible for a patient to give consent for the carrying out of medical or dental treatment on the patient.[51] This request should specify the following:

1. The condition of the patient and why they require treatment.
2. The alternative courses of treatment available in relation to the condition.
3. The nature and effect of those courses of treatment.
4. The nature and degree of risk associated with those courses of treatment.
5. The reason why a course of treatment should be carried out.[51]

THE INCOMPETENT PATIENT, GUARDIANSHIP AND THE 'BEST INTERESTS' TEST

Guardianship laws in all states and territories were written for the purposes of providing protection to those within our community who would otherwise be vulnerable to neglect, abuse and exploitation from others. The law essentially applies to patients over the age of 18 who are incapable of consenting to medical treatment and who meet the criteria set out in the law. Under s 3(2) of the *Guardianship Act 1987* (NSW) a reference to a person who has a disability is a reference to a person:

> (a) who is intellectually, physically, psychologically or sensorily disabled,
>
> (b) who is of advanced age,
>
> (c) who is a mentally ill person within the meaning of the *Mental Health Act 2007*, or
>
> (d) who is otherwise disabled,
>
> and who, by virtue of that fact, is restricted in one or more major life activities to such an extent that he or she requires supervision or social habilitation.[52]

The purpose of the statute (and indeed all jurisdictional legislation) is to ensure that a surrogate decision-maker is appointed to make those decisions in the person's best interest.

The laws broadly aim to apply a set of principles that serve to ensure that the welfare and interests of people with a disability are observed. Those principles include that the decision-making freedom of those with a disability is restricted as little as possible, that they are encouraged to share in decisions that affect their lives and be as independent in this process as possible, that their cultural and family ties are recognised and preserved, and that the community is encouraged to apply and promote these principles. Similar legislation exists in other states and under the Act that law is recognised as corresponding law in NSW.

Guardians have much of the authority of the individual they advocate for, including consent to medical and dental treatment, provided those treatments do not fall into the category of 'special treatments'. An example of a 'special treatment' includes the sterilisation of a person with a disability. This is to limit the infringement on the human right of those with a disability to have a family.

Guardians can be appointed via an enduring power of attorney document or via the Guardianship Board. The process of appointment varies in each state, but the obligations and powers of the guardian are broadly the same.

The fundamental principle to be applied by guardians making healthcare decisions on behalf of their charge is to act in the best interests of that person. If healthcare staff form a reasonable belief that the guardian is not acting in the best interests of the patient, staff can take the matter to the Supreme Court or Guardianship Tribunal for review.[53]

OFFENCES UNDER THE GUARDIANSHIP ACT

It is an offence under the Guardianship Act to perform a medical or dental treatment on a patient without consent. A penalty of imprisonment may be imposed for a special treatment (experimental, including clinical trials) or, with respect to minor or major treatment, imprisonment or a fine or both.

PERSON RESPONSIBLE/STATUTORY HEALTH ATTORNEY

In NSW, Queensland, Victoria, Tasmania and Western Australia, there is a hierarchical system whereby a person responsible is authorised to consent to treatment. Under s 33A(4) of the *Guardianship Act* (NSW), a list of the hierarchy of persons who may be considered 'persons responsible' is listed. In descending order of authority, the list is:

> 1. the person's guardian. 'Guardian' means a person who is, whether under this Act or any other Act or law, a guardian of

the person of some other person (other than a child who is under the age of 16 years) and includes an enduring guardian. However, this only applies if there is an order or instrument that appoints a guardian for the purpose of giving consent to the carrying out of medical or dental treatment on the person or, if not applicable then

2. the spouse of the person if the relationship is close and continuing. 'Spouse' means a husband or wife, or de facto or, if not applicable, then
3. a person who has the care of the person. A person is deemed to fit this description for the purposes of the Act if on a regular basis they provide domestic services and support to that person or arrange for that person to be provided with that support. This does not apply to those carers who are paid for their services. It also does not include those who care for a person at an institution. The person who has care of the person is that person who cared for the patient prior to them being admitted to that institution, then
4. a close friend or relative of the person. Under the Act a close friend or relative is defined as a person who maintains both a close personal relationship with the other person through frequent personal contact and a personal interest in the other person's welfare. However, a person is not to be regarded as a close friend or relative if that person has any financial interest in any service that is related to the care of that person.[54]

The person responsible should always have regard to the views of the patient (if they are known) when considering any medical or dental treatment of a patient. The information supplied to them from the medical or dental practitioner with respect to the details of the treatment, any alternatives, the nature of the treatment and any risks associated with the treatment must also be considered.

In South Australia, powers of consent are able to be given to the closest relative in the absence of a guardian. A relative is a spouse, a parent, a person who acts *in loco parentis* in relation to the person, a brother or sister over 18, a son or daughter over 18.[55] The NT and the ACT do not have person responsible legislation. This means that family, friends and carers have no immediate legal right to consent to the treatment of incompetent patients and a guardian is required to be appointed if there is no formal instrument doing so. Decisions concerning patients are made by medical practitioners for emergencies, but otherwise require the consent of an administrative tribunal or the Supreme Court. There is a useful guide outlining who can do what at the ACT Public Trustee and Guardian website.[56]

ENDURING GUARDIAN

In NSW there exists in the legislation a provision for the enduring guardian to act as the person responsible for a patient who is incapable of consenting to medical or dental treatment. In Schedule 1 of the *Guardianship Regulation 2016* there is a proforma for an enduring guardian appointment form.[57]

ADVANCE CARE DIRECTIVE

An advance care directive (ACD), or living will, is a document drafted by a patient which contains instructions from the patient outlining their wishes with respect to any medical intervention they may consent to or refuse to consent to, in the event that they are incapable of giving consent directly. ACDs act as the patient's consent. (See Chapter 20 for ACDs in relation to end of life.) The Victorian, WA, NT, Qld, SA and ACT laws[58] allow refusal of any treatment. A failure to comply with an ACD acts in the same way as ignoring a patient's refusal of consent in any other instance. It leaves the healthcare practitioner open to an action of civil or criminal liability. It should be noted that these documents can serve as protection to medical and nursing staff when dealing with issues surrounding withholding and withdrawing of treatment and end-of-life decision-making. They can act as evidence that staff were, for example, complying with the patient's decision by upholding the patient's refusal of treatment. It should be noted that a lack of formal documentation does not in any way negate the validity of the patient's right to refuse treatment and if they have made their decision known in any form, provided the patient is competent, staff have an obligation to comply.

In some instances there may be doubt surrounding the validity of an ACD; for example, whether it applies in the circumstances that exist at the time or if the patient was competent at the time the ACD was made. If there is doubt about the validity or existence of an ACD and the situation is time critical—that is, a life-or-death decision must be made immediately—then healthcare staff should actively treat the patient. In this instance they will be protected by the doctrine of necessity. Once the patient has been stabilised, there will be an opportunity for staff to meet with the patient or their person responsible in order to determine the patient's wishes. If healthcare practitioners suspect that the patient has been subjected to undue influence with respect to this decision-making process, they should seek legal advice and continue to treat the patient according to the patient's best interests. The healthcare practitioner must bear in mind that their primary focus of responsibility is in caring for their patient, not their family. Family involvement in treatment discussions is permissible only when the patient gives permission for such involvement or, if they are incapable, with their person responsible or equivalent. All decisions should be documented.

WITHHOLDING AND WITHDRAWING TREATMENT[59]

When a patient refuses treatment, it can be withheld. Health practitioners are lawfully able to withhold treatment at the patient's request provided the patient is competent to refuse consent, and that the healthcare staff do so in good faith and without negligence.

Healthcare staff are also able to withdraw life-sustaining treatment like artificial ventilation. Protections for health practitioners who withdraw treatment that results in the patient's death are provided under a variety of laws.[60]

There are other instances where treatment of the patient is futile and, in this instance, treatment may also be withheld.[61] There is no obligation on staff to provide treatment that is futile because this treatment would not be in the patient's best interest. There are two situations in which the futility of treatment can be easily determined. The first is when the patient is obviously dead. In NSW a definition of death is contained within s 33 of the *Human Tissue Act 1983*:

> For the purposes of the law of New South Wales, a person has died when there has occurred–
>
> (a) irreversible cessation of all function of the person's brain, or
>
> (b) irreversible cessation of circulation of blood in the person's body.[62]

The second is when the patient is known to be at the end-stage of a terminal illness, all available avenues for treatment have been exhausted and there is no prospect of a better outcome for the patient. This circumstance may arise when a patient with a known terminal illness suffers a cardiac arrest and for whom resuscitation may be futile. If it is not known that the patient is suffering from a terminal illness and it is not known to the healthcare staff that the patient wishes to refuse treatment, then treatment should be given. If a dispute arises between the parties involved, the matter can be referred to a guardianship authority in an administrative tribunal or application can be made to the Supreme Court.

PALLIATIVE CARE

The legal and ethical basis for treatment of palliative care patients is that the treatment should neither intentionally hasten nor hinder the patient's death.

VOLUNTARY ASSISTED DYING LEGISLATION

As of May 2022, when the NSW Parliament passed its *Voluntary Assisted Dying Act*, legislation has been passed to enable voluntary assisted dying (VAD) in every state in Australia. The NSW legislation will not be in force for 18 months, and the legislation in Tasmania, South Australia and Queensland is also not yet in force, but will be soon. Victoria passed its legislation in 2019, followed by Western Australia in 2021. The NSW legislation is similar to the legislation in the other states.

The legislation makes VAD available to an adult (with decision-making capacity) who has an advanced and progressive illness that will cause death, likely within 6 months (or 12 months for neurodegenerative conditions). In addition, the patient must be suffering, and their choice must be voluntary and enduring. Two senior doctors, who have completed mandatory training, will each conduct a rigorous eligibility assessment. A VAD board will be established to ensure the system is operating safely.

Each state has slight variations in its VAD laws. One of note in NSW is that a person is able to choose between self-medication or having a health practitioner administer the medication to them. Similarly, in the other states, although both methods are allowed, self-administration is the default method. Victoria's processes arc operable now and more medical practitioners are currently being educated in the mandatory training.[63]

MEDICINES

There are strict laws that govern the manufacture, importing, testing, registration, dispensing, storage, supply, possession and prescription of drugs in every jurisdiction in Australia. It is essential that healthcare providers are familiar with these laws and are knowledgeable about their employer's policy and procedures about handling medicines.

There are criminal sanctions for the unauthorised possession, supply, administration and self-administration of restricted drugs. In addition to criminal sanction, the most common cause for redress by disciplinary tribunals is the wrongful use of drugs by healthcare staff.[64]

MENTAL HEALTH AND INVOLUNTARY DETENTION

Paramedics and ED staff will encounter patients with mental health issues on a regular basis. Each state and territory in Australia has its own legislation with respect to the care and treatment of the mentally ill.[65] It is worthwhile noting that not all mental health legislation is confined to legislation that is labelled as such. For example, there are additional provisions for dealing with a person with a 'major disturbance in mental capacity' in Chapter 4A of the *Public Health Act 2005* (Qld). This chapter of the Act makes reference to the power of an 'ambulance officer' (now called paramedics) and provides them with the power to take a patient who may be at risk of harming themselves (e.g. suicidal) to a place for treatment and care (s 157B). Ambulance officers have a statutory obligation, that is, a requirement beyond the common law, to tell the person they are being detained for treatment and how that may affect that person (s 157C). This approach is consistent with that provided for in the Queensland *Mental Health Act 2016*, and indeed in all Mental Health Acts throughout the country to ensure that mentally ill persons receive the best possible care and treatment in the least restrictive environment. This includes limiting any restriction or interference with their civil liberties, rights, dignity and self-respect to the minimum necessary to effectively provide care and treatment.

DEFINITION OF MENTAL ILLNESS, MENTALLY ILL PERSON AND MENTALLY DISORDERED

Each state and territory have a different definition of mental illness, but they all have similarities and the principles underpinning the legislation are essentially the same. The definition of what constitutes a mental illness in the ACT, NSW, Tasmania and the NT is essentially:

> a condition that seriously impairs, either temporarily or permanently, the mental functioning of a person and is characterised by the presence in the person of any one or more of the following symptoms:
>
> (a) delusions,
>
> (b) hallucinations,
>
> (c) serious disorder of thought form,
>
> (d) a severe disturbance of mood,
>
> (e) sustained or repeated irrational behaviour indicating the presence of any one or more of the symptoms referred to in paragraphs (a)–(d).[66]

A mentally ill person is defined as a person:

> (1) suffering from mental illness and, owing to that illness, there are reasonable grounds for believing that care, treatment or control of the person is necessary:
>
> (a) for the person's own protection from serious harm, or
>
> (b) for the protection of others from serious harm.
>
> (2) In considering whether a person is a mentally ill person, the continuing condition of the person, including any likely deterioration in the person's condition and the likely effects of any such deterioration, are to be taken into account.[67]

In Victoria and Queensland, a person is considered mentally ill if he or she has a 'medical condition that is characterised by a significant disturbance of thought, mood, perception or memory'. There is then a long list of conditions and behaviours that do not constitute being mentally ill; for example, engaging in particular political activities or sexual promiscuity. But the serious temporary or permanent physiological, biochemical or psychological effects of using drugs or consuming alcohol may be regarded as an indication that a person has mental illness.[68] In SA 'mental illness' means any illness or disorder of the mind,[69] and in WA a person has a mental illness if they have a condition that: 'a) is characterised by a disturbance of thought, mood, volition, perception, orientation or memory; and b) significantly impairs (temporarily or permanently) the person's judgement or behaviour'.[70]

Mentally disordered

Some of the statutes also provide a definition for a person who is not mentally ill, but may be mentally disordered or disturbed. That is, this section of the Act may apply to a person who is experiencing a crisis which results in behaviour that may be dangerous to themselves or others, but which exists only temporarily. The NSW legislation defines them as:

> A person (whether or not the person is suffering from mental illness) is a mentally disordered person if the person's behaviour for the time being is so irrational as to justify a conclusion on reasonable grounds that temporary care, treatment or control of the person is necessary—
>
> (a) for the person's own protection from serious physical harm, or
>
> (b) for the protection of others from serious physical harm.[71]

THE PRINCIPLES OF CARE AND TREATMENT OF THE MENTALLY ILL OR DISORDERED

In NSW, as in other states, the principles underpinning the care and treatment of people with a mental illness or mental disorder include the following:

> (a) people with a mental illness or mental disorder should receive the best possible care and treatment in the least restrictive environment enabling the care and treatment to be effectively given,
>
> (b) people with a mental illness or mental disorder should be provided with timely and high quality treatment and care in accordance with professionally accepted standards,
>
> (c) the provision of care and treatment should be designed to assist people with a mental illness or mental disorder, wherever possible, to live, work and participate in the community,
>
> (d) the prescription of medicine to a person with a mental illness or mental disorder should meet the health needs of the person and should be given only for therapeutic or diagnostic needs and not as a punishment or for the convenience of others,
>
> (e) people with a mental illness or mental disorder should be provided with appropriate information about treatment, treatment alternatives and the effects of treatment and be supported to pursue their own recovery,
>
> (f) any restriction on the liberty of patients and other people with a mental illness or mental disorder and any interference with their rights, dignity and self-respect is to be kept to the minimum necessary in the circumstances,
>
> (g) any special needs of people with a mental illness or mental disorder should be recognised, including needs related to age, gender, religion, culture, language, disability or sexuality,
>
> (g1) people under the age of 18 years with a mental illness or mental disorder should receive developmentally appropriate services,
>
> (g2) the cultural and spiritual beliefs and practices of people with a mental illness or mental disorder who are Aboriginal persons or Torres Strait Islanders should be recognised,
>
> (h) every effort that is reasonably practicable should be made to involve persons with a mental illness or mental disorder in the development of treatment plans and recovery plans and to consider their views and expressed wishes in that development,
>
> (h1) every effort that is reasonably practicable should be made to obtain the consent of people with a mental illness or mental disorder when developing treatment plans and recovery plans for their care, to monitor their capacity to consent and to support people who lack that capacity to understand treatment plans and recovery plans,
>
> (i) people with a mental illness or mental disorder should be informed of their legal rights and other entitlements under this Act and all reasonable efforts should be made to ensure the information is given in the language, mode of communication or terms that they are most likely to understand,
>
> (j) the role of carers for people with a mental illness or mental disorder and their rights under this Act to be kept informed, to be involved and to have information provided by them considered, should be given effect.[72]

DETENTION

There are strict provisions made under the Act for the involuntary detention of a person in a mental health facility. A person may only be detained or continued to be detained involuntarily in a hospital or other place if they meet the criteria of a mentally ill person or mentally disordered person as it is defined under the Act. They may only be detained for the purposes of care and treatment or determining whether the person should be the subject of a community treatment order. This course of action can only be undertaken if there is no other less restrictive course available.[73]

Admission of an involuntary patient to hospital

A doctor or accredited person is able to schedule a mentally ill or mentally disordered patient to a hospital provided that the patient is admitted within a short statutorily defined time from when the admission certificate is issued. The certificate must be in the statutory form. The doctor must have personally examined or observed the patient shortly before completing the certificate and be satisfied that there is no more appropriate way of dealing with the patient. The doctor must not be a near relative of the patient.[6,74]

Paramedics and involuntary patients

If a paramedic has reasonable grounds to believe that a person appears to be mentally ill or mentally disordered and that it would be beneficial to the person's welfare for them to be treated in accordance with the Mental Health Act, then the paramedic may transport the person to a declared mental health facility. Police may be requested if there are serious concerns about safety of the person or other persons.[75]

Who else can request a patient get help

A relative or friend may submit a written request to the medical superintendent of a hospital to detain a person because it would not be feasible to expect that a medical practitioner should travel a great distance to examine the patient and the matter is urgent.[76]

The police may apprehend a person if they believe that person may harm themselves or others or is committing an offence or has recently committed an offence and police believe it would benefit the welfare of the person to be dealt with under the Mental Health Act. They may take the person to a hospital.[77]

A magistrate, who is of the opinion that a person who appears before them is mentally ill, may order that police take that person to hospital for assessment.[78]

What happens at the hospital?

Once the involuntary patient arrives at the ED, an examination must be undertaken as soon as practicable, but no later than 12 hours after admission, to determine if the patient is suffering from a mental illness or mental disorder. Medication prescribed must be the minimum that is able to be given and still preserve the patient's ability to communicate adequately. Before a person is certified they must be informed of their rights both orally and in a written statement. A psychiatrist must perform a second examination. If there is a dispute between the first and second examiners, a third examination must take place. The medical practitioner who wrote the schedule must not perform any of these examinations. If the person is found not to have a mental illness or disorder they must be released.[79]

DURATION OF DETENTION

A mentally disordered person should not be detained for a continuous period in excess of 3 days (this excludes long weekends). A medical officer must examine the person once every 24 hours and the person must not be detained on more than three occasions in 1 month.[80] A mentally ill person must present before a magistrate as soon as practicable after detention so that the court may determine if the person is in fact mentally ill and to confirm, inquire into or overrule the decision made with respect to the period of detention and the care to be given to the patient.[81] Voluntary or involuntary patients retain their right to give or withhold consent for treatment unless they fall under a specific section of the Act that presumes they would be incapable of giving informed consent. In addition, a person is presumed to be incapable of giving informed consent if at the time consent was sought the patient received medication that would impair the patient's ability to give consent. However, it must be remembered that all patients have the right to be informed, the right to the least restrictive environment that is reasonable and the right to an independent review of any decision made regarding their treatment and detention.[82] Under no circumstances is it permissible for health staff to wilfully abuse, neglect or assault a patient. Penalties for this behaviour include imprisonment.[83]

Use of medications

The appropriate use of medications is laid out in the Act.[84] A patient with a mental illness must not be prevented from communicating with any person that may be engaged to represent the person or an authority making enquiries with respect to that person, for example, the Mental Health Review Tribunal. The patient is also able to request details of their medications.

RESTRAINT

There are often times in the healthcare setting when a patient becomes dangerous to themselves or to others. In these instances, it may be appropriate for staff to restrain the patient to protect them from harming themselves or harming others, including staff. Every workplace should have a policy related to these issues. It is suggested that restraints be used as a last resort and only when the benefits of their use outweigh the potential harm they can cause. There have been cases where the restraint of a patient has contributed to their death. If a person is wrongfully and intentionally restrained it may constitute false imprisonment and this is relevant particularly to paramedics who may transport a patient to hospital against that patient's wishes. Being confined in the back of the ambulance may constitute a form of imprisonment. In order to find for a case of false imprisonment two elements must be met: that the restraint was intentional and that it was a total restraint of the liberty of another person against their will.

In the case of *Sayers v Harlow Urban District Council*,[85] Mrs Sayers was inadvertently trapped in a toilet operated by the council when the inside door handle fell off. In an attempt to get out of the toilet cubicle, Mrs Sayers stood on the toilet roll dispenser. Under her weight, the toilet roll dispenser broke from the wall and Mrs Sayers was injured. Mrs Sayers sued the council for false imprisonment and negligence. In hearing her case, the court determined that Mrs Sayers had not been falsely imprisoned because there was no intention on the part of the council to restrain her. However, if a person is threatened and consequently believes that their movement is restricted, that may be sufficient to constitute false imprisonment.

If restraint must be used with a patient it should be the minimum restraint required to prevent the patient from harming themselves or others. For example, if a patient with dementia or confusion was pulling out tubes and intravenous lines, then the least restrictive option for a means of restraint would be gloves or bandages of slippery material like 'boxing gloves' to prevent the patient being able to grip and pull at the tubes and lines. This method is preferable to using arm restraints that tie the patient's arms to the bed, or chemical restraints which also limit an individual's freedom when a less restrictive option may be available.

NEGLIGENCE

Negligence is difficult to define succinctly, but in essence it occurs when person/party A (the defendant) has a duty of care to person/party B (the plaintiff) and person/party B suffers damage as a direct result of a breach of duty by person/party A.[86] Four elements contribute to an act of negligence. The plaintiff must establish on the balance of probabilities that all four elements exist to be successful in their claim. The four elements are:

a) duty of care—the plaintiff must demonstrate a duty was owed to them by the health practitioner
b) breach—the health practitioner breached their duty of care by providing treatment that was below the standard expected
c) damage—that damage was suffered as a result of the breach and the damage suffered by the plaintiff was reasonably

foreseeable.[87] That is, any reasonable healthcare professional would have been able to foresee that the breach of duty would result in an injury being suffered

d) causation—a clear relationship exists between the act or omission that caused the action or omission to act. That is, 'but for' the breach of duty the injury would not have been suffered.

DUTY OF CARE

Wherever there is a health practitioner–patient relationship there will exist a duty of care. In *Donoghue v Stevenson*,[88] Lord Atkin stated that it is necessary to give thought to those who 'are so closely and directly affected by my acts that I ought reasonably to have them in contemplation as being so affected when I am directing my mind to the acts or omissions which are called in question'. The duty can also apply to people who are not your patients. The law imposes a duty on a health practitioner to take all reasonable care and skill in the provision of advice and treatment. This extends 'to the examination, diagnosis and treatment of the patient and the provision of information in an appropriate case'.[89]

DUTY TO RESCUE

There is no common law duty to attend an emergency when a health practitioner is off-duty. If a health practitioner attends a person in need in good faith and without expectation of a reward—as a 'good Samaritan'—then they are unable to be sued in negligence unless they are under the influence of alcohol, drugs or where they caused the emergency.[90]

Paramedics in NSW and Queensland are offered specific protections under s 67I of the *Health Services Act* (NSW) and ss 38 and 39 of the *Ambulance Services Act 1991* (Qld), where they are carrying out duties in relation to ambulance service or protecting people from injury or death.

BREACH OF DUTY

Once a duty of care is established, the person bringing the action to court (the plaintiff) must provide evidence that the defendant breached their duty of care by failing to provide the requisite standard of care. An example of the standard of care is determined in s 50 of the *Civil Liability Act NSW* (2002). Similar legislation was introduced into most states in or around 2002–03. It states that:

> (1) A person practising a profession ('a professional') does not incur a liability in negligence arising from the provision of a professional service if it is established that the professional acted in a manner that (at the time the service was provided) was widely accepted in Australia by peer professional opinion as competent professional practice.
>
> (2) However, peer professional opinion cannot be relied on for the purposes of this section if the court considers that the opinion is irrational.
>
> (3) The fact that there are differing peer professional opinions widely accepted in Australia concerning a matter does not prevent any one or more (or all) of those opinions being relied on for the purposes of this section.
>
> (4) Peer professional opinion does not have to be universally accepted to be considered widely accepted.[91]

To put this into a clinical perspective, the standard of reasonableness for a paramedic would be to act in accordance with the standard of their peers in the same area. This would apply equally to nurses. In determining what a reasonable standard of care might be for a nurse, the court would have regard to what the 'reasonable' or 'average' nurse might do in a particular situation.

Healthcare workers will also be held to peer group standards of practice, departmental guidelines, policy and procedure directives and responsibilities and obligations as they are set out in other relevant laws, such as the relevant poisons legislation in the various jurisdictions. If a nurse, for example, were to practise below the reasonable standard of practice for a nurse with an equivalent level of training in an equivalent area and it was reasonably foreseeable that a person would be harmed as a result, and the patient was harmed as a direct result of that breach of the standard of care, then the nurse would be at high risk of being found negligent in the performance of their duty.

DAMAGE AND CAUSATION

In any action for negligence, there must be not only a breach of the duty of care, but also damage sustained as a result of that breach. For example, a nurse may put a prescribed medication in the wrong ear of the patient and this could be considered a breach of his or her duty because a reasonable nurse would not make such a mistake. However, if no damage has been suffered by the patient because of this breach then there can be no action taken for negligence. Additionally, in order to make a finding of negligence, there must be a link between the breach of the duty owed to the patient and the harm caused to the patient. For example, an elderly patient presents to the ED with a heavily bleeding leg, but she is triaged as a low priority and then has a stroke while waiting for medical attention. Clearly the triage nurse is in breach of their duty to the patient for prioritising the patient incorrectly with respect to the bleeding leg. However, it is unlikely that the delay in treatment of the leg resulted in the stroke. If it could be established, on the balance of probabilities, that a causal relationship did in fact exist between the two events, then the patient would be entitled to rely on the delay in treatment as a basis for a claim.[92]

REASONABLE FORESEEABILITY

To recap, to be successful in a negligence claim the plaintiff must establish that a duty of care existed between the parties, that there was a breach in the duty of care, that damage occurred as a result of that breach and that the damage should be compensated only to the extent that it was reasonably foreseeable. In the High Court case of *Annetts v Australian Stations Pty Ltd*[93] the court heard that James Annetts, the 16-year-old son of the applicants, left home in August 1986 and went to work as a jackaroo on a WA sheep station. Mrs Annetts (James' mother) was assured by the station manager that James would be constantly supervised. After 7 weeks of work James was assigned to work as a caretaker on a station under the same management about 100 kilometres from the main station. About 8 weeks after that Mr and Mrs Annetts learned that James had gone missing. An intensive search was begun, but it was not until April 1987 that Mrs Annetts was telephoned and told that a car had been found with two sets of human remains nearby. Mr and Mrs Annetts were told that James had most likely died not long after moving to the second station as a result of dehydration, exhaustion and hypothermia. James' parents claimed that he had died as a result of the station manager's negligence. The Annetts argued that the station manager owed not only James a duty of care, but that he also owed them a duty of care because he had said that he would constantly supervise James. The Annetts claimed that they had been psychologically damaged as a result of the station manager's breach of his duty of care and that they should be compensated. The issue was not only whether the defendant owed the parents a duty of care (proximity), but also whether the psychological damage sustained by the Annetts was reasonably foreseeable. Could they say, 'but for' the breach of duty of the station manager, the Annetts would not have suffered the harm? The High Court found that the defendant did owe the Annetts a duty of care and it was reasonably foreseeable that a breach of the station manager's duty would lead to a psychological harm to the Annetts.

VICARIOUS LIABILITY

Vicarious liability exists when one person is held legally responsible for the acts or omissions of another. In the healthcare setting, an example of vicarious liability is the employer, for example, the state health department, being responsible for the negligence of its employee—a nurse or paramedic.[94] Although the health department may be completely blameless with respect to its direct involvement with the act or omission to act that has led to the cause of the action, it is vicariously liable for the acts or omissions of those who work for it.

However, where an employee engages in serious or wilful misconduct, or where the act does not arise out of the course of the individual's employment, then an employer does have the right to take action to recover any compensation it has paid out to a claimant from the employee.[95] Essentially this means that if employees fail to comply with guidelines and protocols set down by their employer with respect to the way in which they should conduct their work and as a consequence the employee is found to have been negligent and is required to pay compensation to the injured party, the employer may have a cause of action against them. Paramedics are exempt from personal liability in NSW under s 67I of the *Health Services Act 1997*. Similar protection for paramedics is found in other jurisdictions.

TRIAGE AND NEGLIGENCE

Triage is the system used to sort the order in which patients should be treated. The order in which a patient is treated is determined by need. That is, the patient most in need of treatment will be treated first. As per the Australasian Triage Scale, those most in need will be labelled category 1 patients and should be seen immediately for treatment. These people have life-threatening conditions. Those with a less urgent condition may be classified as category 5 patients and should be seen within 2 hours of presenting. In rural and remote areas where a doctor is not available to see the patient within the timeframe recommended by the guidelines, staff should refer to the health department policy or guidelines on triaging at a location with no on-site doctors. A legal risk associated with triage includes failing to appropriately assess a patient's treatment priority. This could raise the issue of negligence. The policy documents for each jurisdiction in relation to triage need to be read with great care.[15]

NURSE PRACTITIONER RESPONSIBILITIES

Nurse practitioners (NPs) were first recognised in Australia in 2000. Since then, many nurses have undertaken further education at Masters level to become eligible to apply for positions as nurse practitioners throughout Australia. They are endorsed as NPs under s 95 of the *Health Practitioner Regulation National Law Act (2009)* (The National Law). The National Law was originally passed through the Queensland Parliament (which is unicameral) and then adopted by each of the jurisdictions. Section 95 states that:

> (1) the National Board for the nursing profession may endorse the registration of a registered health practitioner whose name is included in the Register of Nurses as being qualified to practise as a nurse practitioner if the practitioner—
> (a) holds either of the following qualifications relevant to the endorsement–
> (i) an approved qualification;
> (ii) another qualification that, in the Board's opinion, is substantially equivalent to, or based on similar competencies to, an approved qualification; and
> (b) complies with any approved registration standard relevant to the endorsement.[96]

NPs are now legally authorised to prescribe medications and order diagnostic tests relative to their scope of practice—activities that were previously permitted to be done only by medical practitioners. The scope of practice of an NP is usually established via state health department guidelines and/or employer policies and procedures. There are no statutory restrictions on the scope of NP practice, except in pieces of legislation that specifically make mention of the responsibilities and obligations of medical practitioners. For example, the *ACT Health Act 1993* (Part 6) makes provision for abortion to be performed, but it must be undertaken by a suitably qualified medical practitioner.

The scope of practice of NPs is limited by the qualifications and experience that each individual NP holds. For example, if an NP has a qualification in mental healthcare, then their scope of practice in the role of the NP extends only to mental health, but they would be expected to perform to the level of a NP exercising and professing to have skills in mental health. In contrast, if an emergency situation arises which falls outside the NP's usual scope of practice, the standard that the practitioner is likely to be held to by a court is that of the registered nurse—not of the nurse practitioner. That is, the NP in this example will only be expected to perform the same interventions and provide the same level of care as a registered nurse.

PRESCRIBING MEDICATION

In prescribing drugs for a patient, the NP is expected to inform the patient of everything that is associated with the administration of the medication. This includes the drug's action, its side-effects, its interaction with other substances, the importance of compliance, how long the patient can expect to have to take the medication and any specific precautions. The practitioner is also expected to undertake regular monitoring of the drug and its effectiveness.[64]

It should be noted that, although over-the-counter (OTC) drugs do not require a prescription, if the NP prescribes an OTC drug to a patient, the same responsibilities and accountability apply as if the drug were a prescription-only medication. This also applies to complementary therapies. NP prescribing is governed by the same laws as those that govern the prescribing of drugs by medical practitioners.

SUMMARY

Whole texts have been written on the subject of health law because of its complexities. This chapter has set out to provide only an introduction to the fundamentals of health law. A basic understanding of the law is critical for all professionals, including nurses and paramedics, because it establishes boundaries on behaviours. The emergency setting provides some exceptions to rules that would apply in other environments and it is critical that practitioners have an understanding of when and to whom those exceptions apply, so as not to breach the rights of another person and thus do no harm. The law serves to protect both patients and practitioners and thus a working understanding of it and how it applies to healthcare practice is required of all practitioners.

CASE STUDY

You are called to assess and assist 54-year-old Karen, who has kidney disease and is a renal dialysis patient. She has to travel to hospital from her home in the country to undertake dialysis in a regional centre three times a week. The trip takes 3 hours each way. Karen has been making this trip for the past 5 years and is now telling her family that she has had enough and doesn't want to continue this treatment. She says she just wants to stay at home with her family and let nature take its course. Knowing that you are the only health practitioner in town, the family have asked you to come and speak with Karen about her decision.

QUESTIONS

Identify the legal issues that arise from this case. Consider the following:

1. What are the issues with respect to consent?
   a. What are the legal obligations of the care team when it comes to upholding Karen's decision or not?
   b. Is there the potential for assault to be committed? If so, how?
2. What is the final outcome? Does Karen go home or not? Why or why not?

Answers to Case Study Questions can be found on evolve http://evolve.elsevier.com/AU/Curtis/emergency/ 

REFERENCES

1. For a more in-depth account of the Australian legal system see Chapter 1 of Staunton P, Chiarella M. Law for nurses and midwives. 9th ed. Sydney: Elsevier; 2020.
2. Crimes Act 1900 No. 40 (NSW). Available from: legislation.nsw.gov.au/view/html/inforce/current/act-1900-040.
3. For a succinct explanation of the parliamentary process see Parliamentary Education Office. How Parliament works. 2022. Online. Available from: https://peo.gov.au/understand-our-parliament/how-parliament-works/bills-and-laws/making-a-law-in-the-australian-parliament/#:~:text=A%20bill%20can%20only%20become,as%20an%20Act%20of%20Parliament.
4. Paramedicine Board of Australia. About. 2019. Online. Available from: www.paramedicineboard.gov.au/About.aspx.
5. Great Britain Department of Health. Trust, assurance and safety: the regulation of health professionals in the 21st century. Norwich: HMSO; 2007. p. 16.
6. Nursing and Midwifery Board of Australia and Ahpra. Statistics. 2022. Online. Available from: www.nursingmidwiferyboard.gov.au/about/statistics.aspx.
7. Paramedicine Board of Australia and Ahpra. Statistics. 2022. Online. Available from: www.paramedicineboard.gov.au/News/Statistics.aspx.
8. Chiarella M, White J. Which tail wags which dog? Exploring the interface between professional regulation and professional education. Nurse Educ Today 2013;33(11):1274–8.
9. Ahpra and National Boards. Register of practitioners. 2022. Online. Available from: www.ahpra.gov.au/Registration/Registers-of-Practitioners.aspx?m=Search.

10. Health Practitioner Regulation National Law Act 2009 (Qld), Schedule, Part 7, s 53.
11. Ahpra and National Boards. Registration Standards. 2019. Online. Available from: www.ahpra.gov.au/Registration/Registration-Standards.aspx.
12. Nursing and Midwifery Board of Australia and Ahpra. Professional Standards. 2021. Online. Available from: www.nursingmidwiferyboard.gov.au/Codes-Guidelines-Statements/Professional-standards.aspx.
13. Ahpra and National Boards. Shared code of conduct. 2022. Online. Available from: www.ahpra.gov.au/Resources/Code-of-conduct/Shared-Code-of-conduct.aspx.
14. Health Practitioner Regulation National Law Act 2009 (Qld), Schedule, Part 8.
15. Ahpra. Concerns about practictioners: How to submit a concern. 2022. Online. Available from: www.ahpra.gov.au/Notifications/How-to-submit-a-concern.aspx.
16. Ahpra and National Boards. Concerns about practitioners. How we manage concerns. 2021. Online. Available from: www.ahpra.gov.au/Notifications/Find-out-about-the-complaints-process.aspx.
17. Satchell C, Walton M, Kelly P, et al. Approaches to management of complaints and notifications about health practitioners in Australia. Aust Health Rev 2016;40(3):311–18.
18. Forrester K. Notifications and mandatory reporting: two years on. J Law Med 2012;20(2):273–9.
19. Bismarck MM, Spittal MJ, Plueckhahn TM, et al. Mandatory reports of concerns about the health, performance and conduct of health practitioners. Med J Aust 2014;201(7):399–403.
20. Australian Health Practitioner Regulations Agency (Ahpra). Mandatory notifications: what you need to know. 2020. Online. Available from: www.ahpra.gov.au/Notifications/mandatorynotifications.aspx.
21. Coroners Court NSW. Inquest into the death of Anthony Barrett. 2020. S.12.8, p. 23. Online. Available from: coroners.nsw.gov.au/coroners-court/download.html/documents/findings/2022/Inquest_into_the_death_of_Anthony_Barrett.pdf.
22. See, for example, Coroners Court NSW. When a death is reported to the coroner. Investigation. 2020. Online. Available from: www.coroners.nsw.gov.au/coroners-court/the-coronial-process/investigation.html.
23. Ahpra and National Boards. Recommendations from the coroner. 2022. Online. Available from: www.ahpra.gov.au/News/Recommendations-from-the-Coroner.aspx.
24. NSW Government Communities and Justice. Affidavits. 2020. Online. Available from: www.lawaccess.nsw.gov.au/Pages/representing/lawassist_readingwritinghome_wysk/lawassist_affidavits_wysk/lawassist_affidavits.aspx#.
25. Evidence Act 1910 (Tas).
26. Criminal Procedure Amendment (Sexual Assault Communications Privilege) Act 1999 No 48.
27. See for example: Victims of Crime. How Victim Impact Statements are used at court. 2022. Online. Available from: www.victimsofcrime.vic.gov.au/going-to-court/how-victim-impact-statements-are-used-at-court.
28. Crimes Act 1914 (Cth) s 39.
29. Law Enforcement (Powers and Responsibilities) Act 2002 s 49.
30. Women's Legal Service NSW. Your rights after a sexual assault. 2022. Online. Available from: www.wlsnsw.org.au/resources/sexual-assault/your-rights-after-a-sexual-assault/.
31. NSW Consolidated Acts. Road Transport Act 2013 Schedule 3. Online. Available from: www5.austlii.edu.au/au/legis/nsw/consol_act/rta2013187/sch3.html.
32. NSW Health. Child protection units. 2018. Online. Available from: www.health.nsw.gov.au/parvan/childprotect/Pages/cp-units.aspx.
33. For an overview of all the child protection legislation see the Australian Institute of Health and Welfare. Child Protection. 2019. Online. Available from: www.aihw.gov.au/reports-data/health-welfare-services/child-protection/child-protection-legislation-by-jurisdiction.
34. Legal Aid Queensland. Child protection legal information. 2021. Online. Available from: www.legalaid.qld.gov.au/Find-legal-information/Relationships-and-children/Child-protection-overview/Child-protection-legal-information#toc-reporting-child-abuse–2.
35. Barnard A. Technology and professional empowerment in nursing. In: Daly J, Speedy S, Jackson D, editors. Contexts of nursing an introduction. 5th ed. Sydney: Elsevier; 2017. p. 236.
36. For a detailed account of how to document see Staunton P, Chiarella M. Law for nurses and midwives. 9th ed. Sydney: Elsevier; 2020, p. 215.
37. Australian Digital Health Agency. My Health Record. Health professionals: recognise your privacy and security obligations. 2022. Online. Available from: www.myhealthrecord.gov.au/for-healthcare-professionals/howtos/recognise-your-privacy-and-security-obligations.
38. Privacy Act 1988 (Cth); Privacy and Personal Information Protection Act 1998 (NSW); Privacy and Data Protection Act 2014 (Vic); Information Privacy Act 2009 (Qld); Freedom of Information Act 1992 (WA); Personal Information Protection Act 2004 (Tas); Information Act 2002 (NT). NB: South Australia operates the principles from the Privacy Act 1988 (Cth).
39. Baron A, Townsend R. Live tweeting by ambulance services: a growing concern. J Paramedic Pract 2017;9(7):282–6.
40. Ahpra and National Boards 2019. New social media guide. 2019. Online. Available from: www.ahpra.gov.au/News/2019-11-11-Social-media-guide.aspx.
41. For a useful account of incident management systems, see the Australian Commission on Safety and Quality in Health Care (ACSQHC). Incident management and sentinel events. 2022. Online. Available from: www.safetyandquality.gov.au/our-work/indicators-measurement-and-reporting/incident-management-and-sentinel-events.

42. ACSQHC. Australian open disclosure framework: better communication, a better way to care. 2014. Online. Available from: www.safetyandquality.gov.au/sites/default/files/migrated/Australian-Open-Disclosure-Framework-Feb-2014.pdf.
43. Canada. Ontario. Supreme Court, Court of Appeal. Malette v. Shulman. Dom Law Rep 1990;67:321–39. Online. Available from: pubmed.ncbi.nlm.nih.gov/12041075/.
44. R v Turner (1962) VR 30.
45. See also Eburn M. Australian Emergency Law. The doctrine of necessity – explained. In re F (1990) 2 AC 1. January 31, 2017. Online. Available from: australianemergencylaw.com/2017/01/31/4203/.
46. For an in-depth explanation of consent see Staunton P, Chiarella M. Law for nurses and midwives. 9th ed. Sydney: Elsevier; 2020. p. 119.
47. Rogers v Whitaker (1992) 109 ALR 625.
48. Gillick v West Norfolk and Wisbech Area Health Authority [1986] AC 112.
49. Guardianship Act 1987 (NSW) s 37(1).
50. Guardianship Act 1987 (NSW) s 37 (2) and (3).
51. Guardianship Act 1987 (NSW) s 40.
52. Guardianship Act 1987 (NSW) s 3(2).
53. For an in-depth discussion of guardianship and ethical principles, see Lamont S, Stewart C, Chiarella M. Decision making capacity and its relationship to a legally valid consent: ethical, legal and professional context. J Law Med 2016;24(2):371–86.
54. Guardianship Act 1987 (NSW) s 33A.
55. Consent to Medical Treatment and Palliative Care Act 1995 (SA) s 14.
56. Office of the Public Trustee and Guardian. Guardianship. 2022. Online. Available from: www.ptg.act.gov.au/guardianship.
57. Guardianship Regulation 2016 (NSW) Schedule 1. Available from: classic.austlii.edu.au/au/legis/nsw/consol_reg/gr2016227/sch1.html.
58. Guardianship and Administration Act 1990 (WA) s 110S; Medical Treatment Planning and Decisions Act 2016 (Vic) s 3(1); Medical Treatment (Health Directions) Act 2006 (ACT) s 7; Advance Personal Plan (NT Government). Online. Available from: nt.gov.au/law/rights/advance-personal-plan; Powers of Attorney Act 1998 (Qld). Online. Available from: www.qld.gov.au/law/legal-mediation-and-justice-of-the-peace/power-of-attorney-and-making-decisions-for-others/advance-health-directive; Advance Care Directives Act 2013 (SA). Online. Available from: www.sahealth.sa.gov.au/wps/wcm/connect/public+content/sa+health+internet/about+us/legislation/advance+care+directives+act+2013.
59. For a more in-depth discussion of the right to refuse treatment, see Staunton P, Chiarella M. Law for nurses and midwives. 9th ed. Sydney: Elsevier; 2020. p. 154–8.
60. Medical Treatment (Health Directions) Act 2006 (ACT); Advance Personal Planning Act 2013 (NT); Powers of Attorney Act 1998 (Qld); Consent to Medical Treatment and Palliative Care Act 1995 (SA); Guardianship and Administration Act 1995 (Tas); Medical Treatment Planning and Decisions Act 2016 (Vic); Guardianship and Administration Act 1990 (WA).
61. Airedale NHS Trust v Bland (1993) AC 789.
62. Human Tissue Act 1983 (NSW) s 33.
63. For a helpful discussion on the latest NSW developments and links to other articles, see White B & Willmott L. Voluntary assisted dying will soon be legal in all states. Here's what's just happened in NSW and what it means for you. The Conversation; 2022. Online. Available from: theconversation.com/voluntary-assisted-dying-will-soon-be-legal-in-all-states-heres-whats-just-happened-in-nsw-and-what-it-means-for-you-183355.
64. For an extensive discussion on medication administration, see Staunton P, Chiarella M. Law for nurses and midwives. 9th ed. Sydney: Elsevier; 2020. Chapter 6.
65. Mental Health Act 2015 (ACT); Mental Health Act 2007 (NSW); Mental Health and Related Services Act 1998 (NT); Mental Health Act 2016 (Qld); Mental Health Act 2009 (SA); Mental Health Act 2013 (Tas); Mental Health Act 2014 (Vic); Mental Health Act 2014 (WA).
66. Mental Health Act 2007 (NSW) s 4.
67. Mental Health Act 2007 (NSW) s 14.
68. Mental Health Act 2014 (Vic) s 4; Mental Health Act 2016 (Qld) s 10.
69. Mental Health Act 2009 (SA) s 3.
70. Mental Health Act 2014 (WA) s 6.
71. Mental Health Act 2007 (NSW) s 15.
72. Mental Health Act 2007 (NSW) s 68.
73. Mental Health Act 2007 (NSW) s 18.
74. Mental Health Act 2007 (NSW) s 19, s 20.
75. Mental Health Act 2007 (NSW) s 20.
76. Mental Health Act 2007 (NSW) s 26.
77. Mental Health Act 2007 (NSW) s 22.
78. Mental Health (Criminal Procedure) Act 1990 (NSW) s 33.
79. Mental Health Act 2007 (NSW) s 27.

80. Mental Health Act 2007 (NSW) s 31.
81. Mental Health Act 2007 (NSW) s 34.
82. Mental Health Act 2007 (NSW) s 68.
83. Mental Health Act 2007 (NSW) s 69.
84. Mental Health Act 2007 (NSW) ss 81–86.
85. Sayers v Harlow Urban District Council [1958] 1 WLR 623.
86. Donoghue v Stevenson (1932) AC 562 at 580.
87. Jaensch v Coffey (1984) 155 CLR 549 at 579.
88. Donoghue v Stevenson (1932) AC 562.
89. Rogers v Whitaker (1992) 109 ALR 625.
90. Civil Law (Wrongs) Act 2002 (ACT) s 5; Civil Liability Act 2002 (NSW) Part 8; Personal Injuries (Liabilities and Damages) Act 2005 (NT) s 8; Civil Liability Act 2003 (Qld) s 26; Civil Liability Act 1936 (SA) s 74; Civil Liability Act 2002 (Tas) Part 8A; Wrongs Act 1958 (Vic) Part VIA; Civil Liability Act 2002 (WA) Part 1D.
91. Civil Liability Act 2002 (NSW) s 50.
92. See Staunton P, Chiarella M. Law for nurses and midwives. 9th ed. Sydney: Elsevier; 2020. Chapter 3 for an extensive discussion.
93. Annetts v Australian Stations Pty Ltd. Torts Law Journal, 11(1):11–19.
94. Employees Liability Act 1991 (NSW) s 3.
95. Employees Liability Act 1991 (NSW) s 5.
96. Health Practitioner Regulation National Law Act (2009) s 95.

CHAPTER 5
CULTURAL CONSIDERATIONS IN EMERGENCY CARE

NATALIE CUTLER AND MARK GOODHEW

ESSENTIALS

- To meet the needs of diverse populations, healthcare workers must have a deep understanding of culture and cultural considerations.
- The worldviews, personal beliefs and traditions embraced by an individual, their family and carers, and their community, will influence how healthcare is experienced.
- Misunderstandings about culture can present barriers to the provision and receipt of effective healthcare. Healthcare workers must be aware that cultural differences can impact their communication and interaction with individuals receiving healthcare, their family and carers, and their community.
- Cultural misunderstandings can cause discomfort or distress, leading to suboptimal or even adverse health outcomes.
- By being culturally sensitive, healthcare workers in Australasia can enhance their interactions with people who receive healthcare.
- To be effective, healthcare workers and the systems they work in must be sensitive to the worldviews, personal beliefs and traditions embraced by an individual, their family and carers, and their community.

INTRODUCTION

This chapter orients healthcare workers to the importance of culture as a factor that can influence individuals' experience, and the outcomes, of healthcare. The chapter aims to assist healthcare workers gain an insight into, and appreciation of, some of the issues, concerns and needs of people who belong to the cultural (often) minority groups in Australia and Aotearoa New Zealand. Healthcare workers meet and work with people from diverse cultural and social groups that may be different from the healthcare worker's own. As a result, healthcare workers must develop and continually build their knowledge and skills in working with cultural differences to provide safe, effective and culturally sensitive care. In this chapter, 'healthcare workers' refers to pre-hospital workers, paramedical and ambulance personnel, assistive caregivers, and nurses who work with and care for people and their families in the community, and in the hospital emergency and acute care setting.

Healthcare workers need to develop an appreciation of the ways in which cultural difference impacts their interactions and communications with individuals, their family, carers and community. Cultural beliefs affect attitudes and comprehension and therefore influence the tone and quality of all pre-hospital care and acute care encounters. Cultural differences can result in misunderstanding, distress and even

conflict, especially during times of stress related to illness, trauma and personal crisis, of the type that will be encountered by pre-hospital healthcare workers and those working in an emergency department (ED) or acute care service.

Lack of cultural sensitivity by a healthcare worker may also lead to suboptimal, or even harmful, outcomes by increasing the possibility of non-engagement with care and treatment, and increasing the likelihood of adverse events. This chapter aims to inspire healthcare workers to reflect on the importance of understanding diverse cultures to deliver high-quality, person-centred care that is culturally safe and effective.

WHAT DOES 'CULTURE' MEAN?

In Australia and Aotearoa New Zealand, a frequent interpretation of 'culture' is where social 'difference' is manifested through nationality and ethnicity. Therefore, in healthcare settings the perception of culture may only be associated with people who are different from the healthcare worker in an obvious way. Typically, difference is correlated or linked to physical appearance or different country of origin from the healthcare worker. While defining culture primarily by ethnicity or nationality might seem the easiest way to understand culture, it can also lead to an oversimplistic way of understanding culture, cultural difference and diversity.[1,2] This view of culture does not acknowledge the diversity between members of the same cultural group, nor does it consider the contributions of sociopolitical and historical events that can create, shape and change cultures. An alternate way of understanding culture is that it is dynamic, and involves the sharing of knowledge, meaning and experiences between individuals who are similarly influenced by social and political structures. This broader view of culture is not limited to ethnicity or nationality, and incorporates cultures that are associated with attributes such as disability/ability, sexuality, gender, religion, lifestyle, socio-economic status and age.[3] Cultural diversity can and should include any individuals or groups/communities that might differ from the healthcare worker in terms of worldview or beliefs. This will also necessarily include minority social groups or subcultures that are represented in contemporary society.[1,2,4] Cultural identity infers belonging to, or identifying with, a particular social group; however, it is important to recognise that diversity also occurs within and between social groups.

In Aotearoa New Zealand, it is important that people self-identify with a particular culture, for example, as Māori, rather than the healthcare worker making assumptions about a person's cultural identity or worldview.[4] While it is important for healthcare workers to understand the shared beliefs associated with different cultures, making assumptions about culturally specific beliefs and practices can lead to a stereotypical view of that cultural group, which then makes it more challenging to respond to individual diversity. For healthcare workers, it is important not to treat people according to cultural stereotypes, but to treat each person as an individual. Culturally sensitive care is best understood as care that is individualised, through the healthcare worker seeing each person as unique and different. The term *cross-cultural difference* should be applied to 'any people who might differ from the healthcare provider because of such things as socioeconomic status, age, gender, sexual orientation, ethnic origin, migrant/refugee status, religious belief or disability'.[5] Any social, worldview or lifestyle-related issue that might have an impact on a person's capacity to receive safe, high-quality, effective and equitable healthcare should be considered as having a cultural origin. If this understanding is applied when providing care, then any aspect of diversity or difference must be considered by the healthcare worker.[1–6]

Culturally sensitive healthcare can be supported by cultural competence training of the healthcare workforce,[7–9] with culturally competent practice linked to improved health outcomes in patients.[7,8,10] Cultural competence refers to the range of skills, attitudes and knowledge demonstrated by healthcare workers, and the strategies implemented by healthcare services to ensure that culturally appropriate healthcare is provided.[8,9] The need for cultural competence is not only confined to healthcare in hospitals, community and pre-hospital settings, but also applies to the conduct of research in healthcare.[11]

CULTURE AND WHAT IT MEANS FOR HEALTHCARE WORKERS

For people in need of emergency or acute care, interacting with healthcare workers in a crisis situation, or in the ED and acute care settings of a hospital, will generally be associated with stress and distress. An individual's first encounter with the healthcare system has the potential to affect not only that interaction and its outcomes, but may also have a long-term impact on an individual's health status and health-seeking behaviours. Healthcare workers will meet individuals from a variety of cultural groups and subgroups, and they are required to interact professionally and appropriately across a wide range of values–belief systems, and behavioural norms to support positive health outcomes.

Illness or injury are not just physical events; they are experienced and understood in a variety of ways by different individuals. It is important for healthcare workers to have a fundamental understanding of the impact of the cultural world of individuals and their interpretations of what takes place in a healthcare encounter. It is also important for healthcare workers to be cognisant of the impact of their own interactions on individuals, their families, carers and community. Culturally-based beliefs, worldviews, lifestyles and social traditions affect both the course and the outcome of the health–illness encounter, and significantly shape the lived experience of healthcare. In a therapeutic encounter, both the individual and the healthcare worker will hold points of view, beliefs and practices that might be unfamiliar and very different from each other. While this is an opportunity for growth and enrichment, it also has the potential to cause discomfort, isolation and distress, especially for the person receiving care.

Many individuals and their families will have had a range of different experiences of healthcare in their home country, and may have previously encountered healthcare workers who behave very differently from those in Australia and Aotearoa New Zealand. Particularly in the case of refugees or asylum seekers, these previous encounters may have been negative or unpleasant. For some, previous experiences can be 'reawakened' by the hospital environment. For example, when receiving healthcare, individuals or their families who are survivors of torture and trauma might be reminded of previously distressing or disturbing experiences. Common responses by people to the unknown or unfamiliar can include anxiety, fear and anger, which healthcare workers must understand and acknowledge in order to facilitate positive health outcomes.

PRACTICE TIP

Make sure you become familiar with the information available about professional standards in relation to culturally competent healthcare provision. All healthcare providers should become familiar with the relevant standards and codes of conduct that apply to their professional group. For nurses, these can be accessed on the websites of the Australian Nursing and Midwifery Board (available via the Ahpra website), the Nursing Council of New Zealand (NCNZ) and the College of Emergency Nursing Australasia (CENA). Paramedics should ensure that they consult their own regulatory standards (see Chapter 3). All such standards are updated regularly, and each healthcare worker group should have a knowledge of and clear understanding about relevant professional mandates. It is also important to understand your professional responsibility in terms of equity and diversity legislation, which changes from time to time.[5,12,13]

Cultural differences can present barriers to the delivery of appropriate treatment and care. Factors that contribute to the quality of healthcare include the degree of respect afforded to cultural traditions and beliefs, and the quality of the interpersonal relationship and communications between professionals, people receiving care and their families, carers and community.[10] Healthcare workers must develop and possess effective skills in therapeutic communication and remain empathetic and respectful towards people receiving care.

The rights of the healthcare consumer have been protected in terms of equity, diversity and anti-discrimination legislation. These rights are also enshrined in the professional practice standards that must be embodied in the practice of all professional healthcare workers in both Australia and Aotearoa New Zealand. One of the fundamental rights accorded to individuals is access to healthcare services that allow freedoms related to cultural, religious, spiritual and social needs, and that recognise the values and beliefs of the individual. Resources outlining these rights and responsibilities should be freely available and easily accessible in all healthcare facilities.[5,12,13]

UNDERSTANDING THE HEALTH–ILLNESS EXPERIENCE FROM THE HEALTHCARE CONSUMERS' PERSPECTIVE

There is a difference in the patterns of various diseases and responses to illness among the diverse social and cultural groups of Australia and Aotearoa New Zealand. It is important that healthcare workers understand how individuals, including themselves, are shaped by their social world, as well as the way in which healthcare workers shape the environment and context of healthcare through their actions and interactions with others.

The particular form of Western-based scientific knowledge and the allopathic medical model currently used in healthcare in Australasia is influential and authoritative. Healthcare knowledge and its associated practices are usually considered by healthcare workers in Australasia to be based on unquestionable 'truths' and supported by sound reasoning and seemingly logical beliefs. When providing care to people from diverse cultural groups, especially those who may be unfamiliar with Western ideology, it is important to realise that there can be any number of ways to view the world and that there are many forms of legitimately held ideas about health and healthcare. All understanding is appropriate in its context and environment, but some ideas might be unfamiliar to healthcare workers in Australasia and perhaps very different to the views held by individual healthcare workers.

Holding particular ideas about health and illness that are considered socially legitimate in our own country can dominate healthcare workers' thinking about what is right or correct for others. Understanding that the 'facts' relied upon in Western healthcare institutions might sometimes be seen very differently by people belonging to other cultural groups is important if healthcare workers are to work effectively with those who hold alternative ways of thinking and understanding. Commonly, healthcare providers in Western society will consider their own beliefs to be 'common sense' or 'straightforward and unbiased'. Recognising that there are many and varied ways to view health and healthcare will assist healthcare professionals to see the world from the point of view of the person receiving care, and may make healthcare workers more sensitive to the perspectives of others.

MATTERS SPECIFIC TO AUSTRALIA

On 10 June 2022, the Australian population was estimated to be 25,906,397 persons.[14] The original population of Australia are Aboriginal and Torres Strait Islander peoples. There were 812,728 people who identified as Aboriginal and Torres Strait Islander people in the 2021 Census, and they spoke more than 150 Australian Indigenous languages at home. This represented about 3.2% of the total Australian population and was an increase of 25.2% from the 2016 Census.[15] Historically, Australia has been characterised by successive waves of immigration, and since World War II there have been waves of immigrants from the United Kingdom, Europe, South-East Asia, and, more recently, the Pacific nations, India and Africa, arriving here in growing numbers. Australia is now one of the most multicultural countries in the world, with people from approximately 200 countries calling it home.

For some years immigration has exceeded natural population increase, and under current immigration policy this will continue to be the main contributor to Australia's population growth. The 2021 Census showed that 28% of the Australian population, or 7.3 million people currently in Australia, were born overseas; this percentage has risen from 25% in 2011.[16] After Australia, the top five countries of birth are England (3.5%), India (2.6%), China (2.1), New Zealand (2%) and the Philippines (1.1%).[17]

The cultural diversity of Australia is considered to be one of its great social and economic resources. Australian unity in diversity is based on moral values, such as respect for difference, tolerance, a common commitment to freedom and an overriding commitment to Australia's national interests. These values are based on the following principles:[18]

- *Civic duty*—obliges all Australians to support those basic structures and principles of Australian society, which guarantee freedom and equality, and enable diversity in the society to flourish.
- *Mutual respect*—subject to the law, this gives all Australians the right to express their own culture and beliefs and obliges them to accept the right of others to do the same.
- *Social equity*—entitles all Australians to equality of treatment and opportunity, so that they are able to contribute to the social, political and economic life of Australia, free from discrimination on the grounds of race, culture, religion, language, location, gender, sexuality or place of birth.
- *Productive diversity*—maximises for all Australians the significant cultural, social, and economic dividends arising from the diversity of the population.

ABORIGINAL AND TORRES STRAIT ISLANDER HEALTH

The poor health of the Aboriginal and Torres Strait Islander peoples of Australia is one of the more pressing issues facing this country. Indigenous Australians do not enjoy the same level of health and wellbeing as other Australians, and levels of chronic disease, mental illness, neonatal and child morbidity and mortality, and harmful poly-substance use and addiction are significantly higher than in the general population. At all ages and stages, the quality of life for Aboriginal and Torres Strait Islander peoples is not as good as that of non-Indigenous Australians. As early as 2005, the Australian National Health and Medical Research Council (NHMRC) urged Australian healthcare providers to recognise the unique position in this country of Aboriginal and Torres Strait Islander people, because the Indigenous population was disadvantaged by Australia's current healthcare system.[8] The Australian Productivity Commission's Biennial Review, in 2009, found that the gap between Indigenous and other Australians, in terms of disadvantage, was actually growing, not diminishing.[19] This disadvantage has been well documented and is widely recognised as the worst experienced by any population cohort in the country.[20,21]

The life expectancy of an Indigenous person a decade ago was approximately 11 years lower than for the rest of the population. Life expectancy at birth for Indigenous males was 69 years, compared to 80 years for non-Indigenous males. For Indigenous females, life expectancy at birth was 74 years, compared to 83 years for non-Indigenous females. The mortality rate for Indigenous people is 1.6 times that of non-Indigenous people, with almost two-thirds of deaths of Indigenous people occurring in those younger than 65 years of age. The three most common causes of death are cardiovascular-related; cancers, particularly lung cancer; and external injury and poisoning, with the death rate from cardiovascular disease 1.5 times that of non-Indigenous people.[22,23]

Since 2008, Australian federal, state and territorial governments, in partnership with Aboriginal and Torres Strait Islander peoples and Indigenous and non-Indigenous healthcare organisations, have sought to achieve equality in health outcomes and life expectancy for Indigenous people by 2030. Known as *Closing the Gap* of disadvantage between Indigenous and non-Indigenous Australians, seven targets, including health, education and employment, have guided the redress of these inequalities. The health targets focus on reducing child mortality rates, addressing chronic health conditions that contribute to a reduced life expectancy, and improving mental health and emotional and social wellbeing, including reducing rates of suicide and substance use.[24] Underpinning *The National Aboriginal and Torres Strait Islander Health Plan*, a framework for policy development to close the gap, is a rights- and strengths-based approach to accessible, culturally appropriate healthcare and services for Aboriginal and Torres Strait Islander people.[20]

Much of the negative epidemiology associated with indigeneity is related to economic and social disadvantage. The Indigenous population has had a different life experience as a result of Australia's colonial history, with a values system, language, religion, lifestyle, as well as educational, legal, health and social institutions, imposed on their communities.[25,26] Colonisation has left an enduring legacy into the 21st century, which has been recognised in recent public policy. The long-term effects of colonisation have been characterised by a continued lack of access to health, education, economic power, and the resources needed for Indigenous peoples to have the same quality of life as the rest of Australian society.

Despite an increased level of expenditure and a commitment to improving Indigenous health, data regarding health outcomes over the last 15 years demonstrates that progress is slow. Outcomes have not been encouraging and there is only a minimal improvement in the health status of this specific demographic group. This lack of improvement is directly related to the domination of the Western worldview in healthcare research, policy and praxis, the pre-eminence of the biomedical model, and personal and institutional racism, which although 'unwitting and systemic', occurs when cultural assumptions become embodied in a society's established institutions and processes. Racism or negative discrimination occurs when a practice or policy appears to be fair because it treats everyone the same, but it actually disadvantages people from one racial or ethnic group.[27] Today, in Australia, Indigenous people appear to have access to the same healthcare services as the rest of the community; however, the impact of the history and issues outlined above must be considered carefully when caring for Indigenous peoples. Healthcare workers need to make this a priority and support the Indigenous effort, recognise the need to develop a deeper understanding of Indigenous lifeways and experience, and build trust to genuinely address these healthcare inequalities. Collaborative ventures and increased concern for, and consideration of, how to work with the Indigenous population can assist pre-hospital carers and healthcare professionals in this process.

In 2016, only 2.6% of Aboriginal or Torres Strait Islander people over the age of 15 years were employed in health-related fields, compared to 4.1% of non-Indigenous people. The most substantial gap in the rates of employment between Indigenous and non-Indigenous health workers was in nursing, medicine and allied health.[28,29] In the main, Australian healthcare workers are predominantly of European background and are likely to have had little contact with Indigenous people. There is significant evidence confirming that Indigenous health will continue to be a major challenge to healthcare professionals, and in the face of this there is an urgent need for healthcare professionals to be better prepared to work with Indigenous people and communities. This requires adequate educational preparation of all students of health professions about the factors related to the health outcomes of Aboriginal and Torres Strait Islander peoples. Until there is a change on the part of healthcare workers, this inequity will remain a reality. This comment is not intended to engender feelings of guilt or anger in non-Indigenous healthcare workers, although it will sound challenging to some; rather it is about healthcare workers developing a concern for and a commitment to social justice.

MATTERS SPECIFIC TO AOTEAROA NEW ZEALAND

Aotearoa New Zealand has a smaller population than Australia, with some 4,699,755 people residing in that country in the 2018 Census.[30] The country remains legislatively a bicultural rather than a multicultural nation and is distinguished principally by its Indigenous Māori peoples (comprising 16.5% of the population) and the descendants of British settlers—identified as Pakeha. Just under three-quarters of the Aotearoa New Zealand population in the 2018 Census identified as European (70.2%).[30] Aotearoa New Zealand, like Australia, is a former British colony and was recognised as a legally constituted territory during British settlement with the full rights of citizenship being accorded to the Indigenous Māori inhabitants. Similar to the experience of the Indigenous population of Australia, however, it became clear that Māori had disproportionately high levels of mortality and morbidity in their population compared with the non-Māori people of that country. Over the last several decades a more inclusive concept of health has been encouraged, and healthcare professionals have been urged to rethink their attitudes to culture as it pertains to health and healthcare.

The Treaty of Waitangi (1848) is now commonly considered to be the founding document of Aotearoa New Zealand, and today, after much negotiation, it guides all governmental and governing policy and standards in that country relating to healthcare. From this original document, principles were developed by the 1987 Royal Commission on Social Policy, which were, and continue to be, applied across the healthcare sector, and are believed to be integral to future development.[31]

They are the principles of:

- partnership—working together with iwi, hāpu, whānau and Māori communities to develop strategies for Māori health gain and appropriate health and disability services.
- participation—involving Māori at all levels of the sector, in decision-making, planning, development and delivery of health and disability services.
- protection—working to ensure Māori have at least the same level of health as non-Māori, and safeguarding Māori cultural concepts, values and practices.

These concepts have been mandated across the healthcare sector in Aotearoa New Zealand, and in the last few years have become foundational and integral to the delivery of high-quality and appropriate healthcare services in that country. These concepts are the drivers behind Māori health development and underpin healthcare-based initiatives with a positive correlation to some improvements in mortality and morbidity within this population. Healthcare workers in Aotearoa New Zealand have specific and collective responsibilities to respond to and address Māori health issues, and considerable value is attached to achieving the goal of offering culturally safe healthcare services.

Nurses in Aotearoa New Zealand were the forerunners in developing cultural care guidelines in the form of cultural safety, a construct unique to that country, which constitutes a mandatory framework for ensuring quality in nursing and healthcare service.[1,2,5,12,32] The formal definition of cultural safety is: the effective nursing practice of a person or a family from another culture as determined by that person or family, while unsafe nursing practice is: any action which diminishes, demeans or disempowers the cultural identity and wellbeing of an individual.[5] The philosophy of cultural safety, while developed within a nursing framework, nonetheless has much to offer all professional healthcare workers.[1,2,4,12,32]

Much remains to be done into the future, as Māori remain over-represented in relation to most types of diseases. Higher levels of mental ill health, asthma, diabetes mellitus, drug and alcohol dependency, rheumatic fever, involvement in road injury and rates of sudden infant death syndrome in this population will ensure that this group will be seen commonly in presentations to EDs.

LGBTIQA+ CULTURE

The LGBTIQA+ culture is complex, comprising a diverse group of people. LGBTIQA+ refers to lesbian, gay, bisexual, transgender, intersex, queer, questioning, asexual, and the + sign refers to other sexual and gender orientations that don't fit within the letters.[33,34] Australia's First Nations people add S and B to the acronym, and S stands for sistergirl and B for brotherboy.[35]

In Australia, Aotearoa New Zealand and the United Kingdom, homosexuality has gradually been decriminalised, and LGBTIQA+ people have gained more equal rights, such as having legal protection from discrimination and being able to adopt children, marry and serve in the military.[34] Despite these advances, LGBTIQA+ people do not possess the same rights and levels of safety as heterosexual and cisgender people.[34] Cisgender people identify with their corresponding sex at birth. LGBTIQA+ people are more likely to be discriminated against,[36,37] bullied at school,[38] victims of violent crimes,[39] and experience poor mental health,[36] and these factors are much worse for transgender people.[37] In Australia, 73% of LGBTIQA+ people over 18 experience a mental health diagnosis within their lifetime, and young people aged between 16–27 are five times more likely to attempt suicide.[40] Suicide attempt rates among transgender people aged 14–25 are even more alarming, as they are 15 times more likely to make attempts.[40] As a result of these significant health challenges, healthcare workers in prehospital and hospital emergency and acute care settings must understand the needs of people who identify as part of LGBTIQA+ culture.

Despite being a high-need group for healthcare, LGBTIQA+ people often experience homophobia, biphobia or transphobia, abuse, discrimination, misgendering, and incorrect assumptions about their gender or sexuality by healthcare workers.[41] It is common for LGBTIQA+ people not to be acknowledged within health services' mission statements, admission forms, databases, posters, pamphlets and toilets.[42] Not being recognised by health systems pressures LGBTIQA+ to disclose their sexuality/gender identity and determine their own healthcare needs.[42] Failure to disclose sexuality/gender identity may result in LGBTIQA+ people receiving inappropriate healthcare, including misdiagnosis, under-diagnosis, and delays in seeking treatment.[43]

The following are tips to enable you to provide culturally appropriate and humanising care to LGBTIQA+ people:

- Learn about LGBTIQA+ culture—many health services offer education.
- When learning about LGBTIQA+, be aware that it is a two-way process. Rather than just learning about the culture, also learn from LGBTIQA+ people by asking questions and carefully listening.[42]
- Don't assume a person is heterosexual or cisgender. If you are unsure about someone's sexuality/gender identity, respectfully ask.
- Ask transgender people their preferred pronouns, e.g. he/him, she/her or they/them.
- If you get a person's pronouns wrong, apologise. Many gender-diverse people are thankful, as they can see that you are trying and acknowledging who they are.
- Don't ignore it if you witness an LGBTIQA+ person being mistreated by healthcare staff or other people. Either intervene or report the incident and ensure the person is okay.

ISSUES AND CONCERNS

The concerns most commonly articulated by recipients of healthcare relate to issues around communication style, variation in beliefs, attitudes and social custom, and differences regarding healthcare knowledge and self-care practices.[2,44,45] In an Australian study of healthcare providers, including health professionals and health services managers, and culturally and linguistically diverse (CALD) consumer groups, Johnstone and Kanitsaki found that the majority of participants were unfamiliar with the terms 'cultural competence' and 'cultural safety'.[46] The knowledge they had was informally acquired; however, participants recognised that culturally inappropriate care resulted in poorer health outcomes, including sentinel events.[45] In an Aotearoa New Zealand study of senior acute care nurses, stereotypical views of healthcare recipients' culture were often used, and the comprehensive assessment of individuals' cultural needs was often poorly addressed.[12]

In another Australasian study,[47] nurses attested to feeling greater uncertainty when caring for individuals from other cultures, as a result of being more aware of cultural differences. The participants in this study expressed feelings of inadequacy in establishing relationships with people who were culturally different from themselves. As a result, participants' perception of their ability to provide individualised and appropriate care was compromised. The inability of the participants to form effective relationships meant that healthcare recipients failed to divulge crucial information to the nurse. Because of this, the needs of the individual were often not clearly understood or utilised in the planning and delivery of care, which adversely affected the individual's healthcare experiences. This demonstrates that apprehension and uncertainty about interacting with people from different cultures affects the ability of nurses to gain a deeper understanding of healthcare needs.

It is likely that this cause-and-effect dynamic is relevant to other healthcare provider groups. In an Australian study of experienced medical registrars and consultants who were the clinical supervisors of junior doctors,[45] few of the participants had knowledge of cultural differences, nor of the effects of culture on health outcomes. The concept of cultural competence was poorly understood, along with strategies such as the specific communication skills necessary for the development of culturally competent practice. The participants mostly underestimated the number of people on the wards from culturally diverse backgrounds, rarely sought out professional interpreters for interactions between the junior doctors and their patients, and Aboriginal and Torres Strait Islander peoples were not identified as requiring any specific support. To develop a culturally competent healthcare workforce, cultural competence training of those health professionals responsible for the clinical education of less experienced staff is paramount.[46,48,49]

PRACTICE TIPS

While most healthcare workers acknowledge the importance of issues around culture and appreciate the need for competent and culturally safe nursing care, quite how to achieve this is less certain. In the fast-moving environment of a busy ED and acute care services, it is easy to become focused on 'what to do' and rather less on 'how to do it'. The 'how' can become eclipsed into the background in the face of multiple presentations, busy triage stations and many demands for attention. Culturally competent care is fundamentally good care that is person-centred and involves using well-developed communication skills. Working effectively in cultural care encounters will become easier if some time is taken to consider the following points.

COME TO UNDERSTAND 'YOURSELF'

Know what your own thoughts and ideas are; these are always apparent to healthcare recipients as you work alongside and with them. If time is taken in coming to recognise and challenge your assumptions, by 'seeing yourself' as others might see you, you will have a fuller understanding of what you bring to each healthcare encounter. Through self-reflection, explore your beliefs and attitudes because you will draw on these to form and shape your reactions and responses to healthcare recipients. Ramsden[1] identifies the crucial importance of the healthcare worker exploring and understanding their own attitudes and beliefs, and this work (available online) makes it worthwhile reading if you want to further develop your skills in this area.[5,13,49]

TREAT EVERYONE AS AN INDIVIDUAL

Treat each person as an individual and do not make assumptions about their beliefs and customs based on their outward appearance. Healthcare workers should regard each individual and their family, carers and community as unique, and develop the skills to better understand the impact of their culture on any situation. The individual and their family and carers might appreciate being asked about their cultural or religious beliefs, sexuality or gender identity, or they might not. Most people are cooperative and helpful when they can see that an effort is being made to understand their culture or belief systems to better understand and meet their needs.

Some individuals may adhere closely to the traditional beliefs and practices of a birthplace, while others, born in the same location or country, may be fully acculturated into the way of life of their adopted country.

COMMUNICATION SKILLS

Develop your therapeutic communication skills, both spoken and non-verbal, and actively and intentionally listen to the people you are providing care for. In a crisis, healthcare recipients are actively seeking out someone in whom they can place trust, find reassurance, depend on for security and gain help and support to enable them to cope in what might be an unfamiliar, anxiety-provoking or frightening emergency experience. You, as the healthcare professional, will unwittingly be constantly in communication with your patients through your body language and facial expressions, which convey your attitude and expectations every time you meet people.[1,2,47]

Different cultural groups will communicate with you in different ways; there are many variations in the way that requests can be put to others, the physical or personal space that is comfortable for different people, or the extent to which personal information is shared with strangers. Healthcare recipients will remain cautious and apprehensive if they feel they are in an environment that might potentially be unsafe or 'hostile' towards them.

Signage in all health services should, where possible, be written in several different and relevant languages to make things as easy as possible for those who are not native English speakers. While it would be impossible to accommodate all the languages used in Australia or Aotearoa New Zealand, if you know your local population's needs well, then a careful and helpful selection used in pamphlets and available resources will assist patients.

HOW HELPFUL ARE CULTURAL PROFILES AND CHECKLISTS?

Using a specific profile or a 'checklist' of how other cultures might be expected to behave, what beliefs they hold or how they are likely to 'think' is not very efficient, as it is 'best guess' only and is, in a real sense, just a series of generalisations. Such aids are secondary to making yourself open to the 'real' messages that are being conveyed by healthcare recipients about what 'works for them as individuals'. There is as much variation within cultural groups as there is between them.

Caution is advised about assuming what is 'normal' for those with different cultural values and beliefs to you. Everyone has their own idiosyncrasies and considers that they know the way to go about things; for example, food choices, bathing preferences and what constitutes an uncomfortable topic of conversation, will vary within and across different groups of people. Providing intimate care and touching people during caregiving is always an activity that must be approached with sensitivity and respect. Take the time to observe what makes healthcare recipients comfortable or uncomfortable, and always ask for their preference as a way of showing respect in how you provide care.

INFORMATION SHARING AND TEACHING

Be prepared to negotiate knowledge; much of the information that healthcare workers provide to individuals receiving care is often complex and can be confusing to those unfamiliar with the terminology and concepts you are talking about. Try to establish the information needs of the individual and their family. Information will be culturally 'filtered' by the recipient to gain comprehension, and at times of stress language difficulties are magnified and any inability to understand the healthcare worker only leads to greater stress, which further reduces understanding.

Try to give people 'thinking' time—to translate, ascertain meaning, evaluate what words mean and determine what response they need to provide to the healthcare worker. If you cannot establish a shared meaning, you can attempt the sentence again and vary your word choice. Be patient and provide positive feedback to the recipient and avoid displays of impatience or irritation. Remember to avoid medical jargon, and to utilise professional healthcare interpreters as necessary, allow the person time to think and to ask questions, and remember to check the person's understanding of what was said.[45]

WORKING IN A REAL PARTNERSHIP

Value the importance of working in a real partnership with the healthcare recipient, as an equal. Developing a partnership starts with openness, involves remaining receptive to others, and relies upon the establishment of trust. Undertake your work as a healthcare provider in the knowledge that you have a great deal of 'role power'—use that wisely. It is unreasonable to assume that healthcare recipients will have the knowledge and understanding of healthcare in the same way as you, the healthcare worker.

CULTURALLY COMPETENT CARE INTO THE FUTURE

Goold, an Indigenous Australian nurse, and Ramsden, from Aotearoa New Zealand, have both voiced concern that nurses and indeed all healthcare workers have, to an extent, currently failed to ensure that they have a significant impact on healthcare encounters or have been part of effecting any significant improvement on the quality of healthcare service delivery and its related outcomes.[1,25] Australian Indigenous nurse Renee Blackman contends that to develop a culturally competent workforce, healthcare professionals must regularly and critically engage in self-reflection and reflect on their practice before they can begin to understand and assist healthcare consumers.[50]

To move forwards, healthcare workers in Australasia need to reflect upon the way that they, as a body of professionals, interact with people who are from culturally marginalised and disempowered groups accessing the healthcare system.[47] A person-centred, rather than a task-centred, approach has been advocated for effective care to take place. Healthcare workers must individualise care for each person and consider their personal and unique circumstances more deeply when responding to and caring for people. Healthcare workers themselves have traditionally articulated this as an important part of their role and must continue to prioritise a person-centred approach; one that values the individualisation of each person's illness experience.[51]

Good health outcomes are 'a product of reciprocal interactions between individuals and the environments that shape their lives'.[5,6,13,26] The need for considerations of 'culture' to become a specific focus in the delivery of emergency healthcare and a priority for the healthcare worker is now undeniable. Healthcare workers in Australasia have traditionally been accustomed to working within a predominantly monocultural, historically European workforce. This is changing as the demographic of the healthcare workforce begins to mirror that of the wider community. Culturally competent interaction must be one of the issues considered important into the future because of the growing heterogeneity in the population and in the healthcare provider workforce. Healthcare providers must assume responsibility for becoming more engaged with ideas around culture and culture's place in contemporary society.[48]

SUMMARY

In terms of health, it is well established that cultural beliefs shape human understanding of and responses to health and illness; that is, the 'culture' of an individual will affect their perceptions and experience of healthcare. Ideas and beliefs about health and illness generally will have a significant impact on individuals, their families, carers and communities, in fashioning their understanding of illness, the treatment of disease and the prevention of ill-health. When individuals seek assistance in times of sickness, their conceptualisation and understanding of social roles and their own personal beliefs and expectations will have an impact on healthcare encounters. Any healthcare encounter will be influenced by the attitudes and understandings of both the healthcare recipient and the healthcare worker. For people from marginalised or disadvantaged cultural groups, there is a risk of a mismatch between their values and belief systems and those of the healthcare system or individual healthcare providers they encounter. All of these might constitute barriers to service appropriateness and quality, and if cultural needs are not addressed, this might lead to negative outcomes and adverse events.

Healthcare workers have an obligation to ensure that individuals are cared for in the best manner possible. It is imperative that healthcare workers remain open to the idea that there are many different ways of 'thinking, doing and being' in the world. If the healthcare worker is unsure of an individual's beliefs and practices, the best place to start is to seek advice from the individual, their family, carer or their social support system. It is also wise to avoid guessing, by seeking advice from other healthcare professionals or consulting a textbook, 'expert' or pamphlet. The best way forward is to ensure that as a healthcare professional, you try to provide the most respectful care possible for individuals and their families.

CASE STUDY

It is a busy night, and a young pregnant female arrives at the ED accompanied by two paramedics; the male paramedic states that this patient's family made a telephone call for help saying the patient was in pain, bleeding and distressed, but her baby is not due yet.

The history is very vague, as are the details of this patient's situation; the accompanying paramedics state that they could not understand what was or is actually happening as English is not the first language of the patient or her family. Everyone at the home was quite upset, and when the paramedics tried to examine the patient, she became even more distressed and resisted their intervention.

You and the paramedics take the patient inside the ED. You need to establish what is happening here and determine what to do next.

QUESTIONS

1. What issues do you need to consider, in order of priority, in light of the cultural background that might be having a significant impact on this situation?
2. How can you develop an open and supportive relationship with this patient and her family group?
3. Describe how you might modify the way in which you undertake your physical assessment and history-taking.
4. What information will you decide to relay to other staff that will ensure culturally appropriate care is provided to this patient into the future?
5. How would you engage with the patient if you suspect they identify as LGBTIQA+?

Answers to Case Study Questions can be found on evolve **http://evolve.elsevier.com/AU/Curtis/emergency/**

USEFUL WEBSITES

Australian Bureau of Statistics, www.abs.gov.au.

Australian Indigenous Health InfoNet, www.healthinfonet.ecu.edu.au.

Australian Institute of Aboriginal and Torres Strait Islander Studies (AIATSIS), www.aiatsis.gov.au.

Australian Institute of Health and Welfare (AIHW), www.aihw.gov.au.

Central Australian Aboriginal Congress, www.caac.org.au.

College of Emergency Nursing Australasia (CENA), www.cena.org.au.

Congress of Aboriginal and Torres Strait Islander Nurses and Midwives (CATSINaM), www.catsinam.org.au.

LGBTIQ+ Health Australia, www.lgbtiqhealth.org.au/

New Zealand Ministry of Health/Manatu Hauora for the health of Pacific peoples, Asian peoples and Māori, disability strategy and the health of New Zealanders, www.health.govt.nz.

Nganampa Health Council, www.nganampahealth.com.au.

Nursing and Midwifery Board of Australia (Australian Health Practitioners Regulatory Authority), www.nursingmidwiferyboard.gov.au/.

Nursing Council of New Zealand/Te Kaunihera Tapuhi o Aotearoa, www.nursingcouncil.org.nz.

Public Health Association of New Zealand Inc./Kāhui Hauora Tumatanui, www.pha.org.nz.

Rainbow Organisations Te Ngākau Kahukura, www.tengakaukahukura.nz/rainbow-organisations

Statistics New Zealand/Tatauranga Aotearoa, www.stats.govt.nz.

The Rainbow Network, www.rainbownetwork.com.au/.

REFERENCES

1. Ramsden I. Cultural safety and nursing education in Aotearoa and Te Waipounamu. Unpublished PhD thesis. Wellington: Victoria University of Wellington; 2002.
2. DeSouza R. Wellness for all: the possibilities of cultural safety and cultural competence in New Zealand. J Res N Z 2008;13(2):125–35.
3. Blanchet Garneau A, Pepin J. Cultural competence: a constructivist definition. J Transcult Nurs 2015;26(1):9–15.
4. Durie M. Cultural competence and medical practice in New Zealand. Presented at the Australian and New Zealand Boards and Council Conference; Wellington, New Zealand on 22 November 2001.
5. Nursing Council of New Zealand. Guidelines for cultural safety, the Treaty of Waitangi and Māori health in nursing education and practice. Wellington, New Zealand: NCNZ Whanau Kawa Whakaruruhau; 2011. Online. Available from: ngamanukura.nz/sites/default/files/basic_page_pdfs/Guidelines%20for%20cultural%20safety%2C%20the%20Treaty%20of%20Waitangi%2C%20and%20Maori%20health%20in%20nursing%20education%20and%20practice%282%29_0.pdf.
6. Phiri J, Dietsch E, Bonner A. Cultural safety and its importance for Australian midwifery practice. Collegian 2010;17(3):105–11.
7. National Health and Medical Research Council (NHMRC). Road map II: a strategic framework for improving the health of Aboriginal and Torres Strait Islanders through the support of health research and its translation 2010. Online. Available from: www.nhmrc.gov.au/guidelines-publications/r47.
8. National Health and Medical Research Council (NHMRC). Cultural competency in health: a guide for policy, partnership and participation 2006. Online. Available from: www.nhmrc.gov.au/about-us/publications/cultural-competency-health#block-views-block-file-attachments-content-block-.
9. Jongen C, McCalman J, Bainbridge R. Health workforce cultural competency interventions: a systematic scoping review. BMC Health Serv Res 2018;18(1):232.
10. Olaussen SJ, Renzaho AMN. Establishing components of cultural competence healthcare models to better cater for the needs of migrants with disability: a systematic review. Aust J Prim Health 2016;22(2):100–12.

11. Woodland L, Blignault I, O'Callaghan C, Harris-Roxas B. A framework for preferred practices in conducting culturally competent health research in a multicultural society. Health Res Policy Syst 2021;19(1):24.
12. Richardson S, Williams T, Finlay A, Farrell M. Senior nurses' perceptions of cultural safety in an acute clinical practice area. Nurs Prax N Z 2009;25(3):27–36.
13. Nursing and Midwifery Board of Australia and Ahpra. Professional standards, standards for practice, codes of ethics and codes of conduct 2018. Online. Available from: www.nursingmidwiferyboard.gov.au/codes-guidelines-statements/professional-standards.aspx
14. Australian Bureau of Statistics (ABS). National, state and territory population. 2022. Online. Available from: www.abs.gov.au/statistics/people/population/national-state-and-territory-population/sep-2021.
15. Australian Bureau of Statistics (ABS). Snapshot of Australia: national data summary 2021. Online. Available from: www.abs.gov.au/statistics/people/people-and-communities/snapshot-australia/2021.
16. Australian Bureau of Statistics (ABS). 2016 Census: multicultural. Media release. 2017. Online. Available from: www.abs.gov.au/ausstats/abs@.nsf/lookup/media%20release3.
17. Australian Bureau of Statistics (ABS). Cultural diversity: Census 2021. Online. Available from: www.abs.gov.au/statistics/people/people-and-communities/cultural-diversity-census/2021.
18. Australian Government, Department of Social Services. Beginning a life in Australia. Online. Avaiable from:immi.homeaffairs.gov.au/settling-in-australia/settle-in-australia/beginning-a-life-in-australia. Canberra, ACT 2020.
19. Australian Government, Australian Institute of Health & Welfare and the Institute of Family Studies. Closing the Gap: what works to overcome Indigenous disadvantage—key learnings and gaps in the evidence. 2011–12. 2013. Online. Available from: www.aihw.gov.au/getmedia/47bcb156-74a2-4f6e-bb3f-4698c54026d2/15161.pdf.aspx?inline=true.
20. Australian Government. National Aboriginal and Torres Strait Islander health plan 2013–2023. 2013. Online. Available from:www.health.gov.au/resources/publications/national-aboriginal-and-torres-strait-islander-health-plan-2013-2023.
21. Australian Medical Association (AMA). Indigenous health report card 2012–2013. The healthy early years—getting the right start in life. 10th series 2013. Online. Available from:ama.com.au/article/best-practice-and-good-news-stories-2012-13-ama-indigenous-health-report-card-healthy-early.
22. Australian Institute of Health and Welfare (AIHW). The health and welfare of Australia's Aboriginal and Torres Strait Islander peoples: 2015. Online. Available from: www.aihw.gov.au/reports/indigenous-health-welfare/indigenous-health-welfare-2015/contents/life-expectancy-and-mortality-key-points.
23. Council of Australian Governments (COAG). 2020–25 National Health Reform Agreement (NHRA). 2022. Online. Available: www.health.gov.au/initiatives-and-programs/2020-25-national-health-reform-agreement-nhra.
24. Aboriginal and Torres Strait Islander Social Justice Commissioner and the Steering Committee for Indigenous Health Equality. Close the Gap: national Indigenous health equality target 2008. Human Rights and Equal Opportunity Commission. Online. Available from: humanrights.gov.au/our-work/aboriginal-and-torres-strait-islander-social-justice/projects/close-gap-indigenous-health.
25. Goold S. Transcultural nursing: can we meet the challenge of caring for the Australian Indigenous person? J Transcult Nurs 2001;12(2):94–9.
26. McMurray A, Clendon J. Community health and wellness: primary health care in practice. 4th ed. Sydney: Churchill Livingstone Elsevier; 2011.
27. Levey G. The political theories of Australian multiculturalism. University of New South Wales Law Journal. Online. Available from: www.unswlawjournal.unsw.edu.au/article/thepolitical-theories-of-autralian-multiculturalism.
28. Australian Institute of Health and Welfare (AIHW). Nursing and midwifery workforce, 2015. 2015. Online. Available from: www.aihw.gov.au/reports/workforce/nursing-and-midwifery-workforce-2015/contents/who-are-nurses-and-midwives.
29. Australian Institute of Health and Welfare (AIHW). Health workforce, 2022. 2022. Online. Available from: www.aihw.gov.au/reports/australias-health/health-workforce.
30. Statistics New Zealand. 2018 Census. 2018. Online. Available from: www.stats.govt.nz/census.aspx.
31. The Royal Australian and New Zealand College of Psychiatrists. Recognising the significance of Te Tiriti o Waitangi. Position statement 107. 2022. Online. Available from: www.ranzcp.org/news-policy/policy-and-advocacy/position-statements/te-tiriti-o-waitangi.
32. Mackay B, Harding T, Jurlina L, et al. Utilising the Hand Model to promote a culturally safe environment for international nursing students. Nurs Prax N Z 2011;27(1):13–24.
33. La Trobe University. What does LGBTIQA+ mean? 2022. Online. Available from: www.latrobe.edu.au/students/support/wellbeing/resource-hub/lgbtiqa/what-lgbtiqa-means#:~:text='LGBTIQA%2B'%20is%20an%20evolving,sexuality%20and%20physiological%20sex%20characteristics.
34. Grundy-Bowers M, Read M. Developing cultural competence in caring for LGBTQI+ patients. Nurs Stand 2019;35(2):29–34.
35. Spurway K, Sullivan C, Leha J, et al. 'I felt invisible': First Nations LGBTIQSB+ young people's experiences with health service provision in Australia. J Gay Lesbian Soc Serv 2022:1–24.
36. Balakrishnan K, Haregu T, Hill AO, et al. Discrimination experienced by sexual minority males in Australia: associations with suicidal ideation and depressive symptoms. J Affect Disord 2022;305:173–8.
37. Bretherton I, Thrower E, Zwickl S, et al. The health and well-being of transgender Australians: a national community survey. LGBT Health 2021;8(1):42–9.
38. Chan ASW, Wu D, Lo IPY, et al. Diversity and inclusion: impacts on psychological wellbeing among lesbian, gay, bisexual, transgender, and queer communities. Front Psychol 2022;13:726343.

39. Flores AR, Langton L, Meyer IH, et al. Victimization rates and traits of sexual and gender minorities in the United States: results from the National Crime Victimization Survey, 2017. Sci Adv 2020;6:eaba6910.
40. LGBTIQ+ Health Australia. Snapshot of mental health and suicide prevention statistics for LGBTIQ+ people. 2021. Online. Available from: assets.nationbuilder.com/lgbtihealth/pages/549/attachments/original/1648014801/24.10.21_Snapshot_of_MHSP_Statistics_for_LGBTIQ__People_-_Revised.pdf?1648014801.
41. Carman M, Rosenberg S, Bourne A, et al. Research matters: why do we need LGBTQ-inclusive services? A fact sheet by Rainbow Health Victoria. Melbourne: La Trobe University; 2020.
42. Baker K, Beagan B. Making assumptions, making space: an anthropological critique of cultural competency and its relevance to queer patients. Med Anthropol Q 2014;28(4):578–98.
43. Polonijo AN, Hollister BA. Normalcy, boundaries, and heterosexism: an exploration of online lesbian health queries. J Gay Lesbian Soc Serv 2011;23(2):165–87.
44. Spence D. Nursing people from cultures other than one's own: a perspective from New Zealand. Contemporary Nurse 2003;15(3):222–31.
45. Berger G, Conroy S, Peerson A, Brazil V. Clinical supervisors and cultural competence. The Clinical Teacher 2014;11(5):370–4.
46. Johnstone MJ, Kanitsaki O. Culture, language, and patient safety: making the link. Int J Qual Health Care 2006;18(5):383–8.
47. Health Navigator New Zealand. Patient and patient-centred care. 2022. Online. Available from: www.healthnavigator.org.nz/clinicians/p/patient-centred-care/.
48. Health Quality and Safety Commission New Zealand. Health literacy, equity, cultural safety and competence. 2022. Online. Available from: www.hqsc.govt.nz/our-work/leadership-and-capability/kaiawhina-workforce/health-literacy-equity-cultural-safety-and-competence/.
49. Stewart S. Ringing in the changes for a culturally competent workforce. 3rd ed. Parramatta, Multicultural Mental Health Australia; 2006.
50. Blackman R. Understanding culture in practice: reflections of an Australian Indigenous nurse. Contemporary Nurse 2010;37(1):31–4.
51. Johnstone MJ, Kanitsaki O. Health care provider and consumer understandings of cultural safety and cultural competency in health care: an Australian study. J Cult Divers 2007;14(2):96–105.

CHAPTER 6

PATIENT SAFETY AND QUALITY IN EMERGENCY CARE

JULIE CONSIDINE, RAMON Z. SHABAN, MARGARET FRY, KATE CURTIS, CLAIR RAMSDEN AND PAUL A. JENNINGS

ESSENTIALS

- Key performance indicators and performance targets in emergency care must be grounded in safety and quality.
- It is not possible to improve the quality and safety of emergency care without measurement.
- Patients are safer when emergency clinicians have appropriate workloads and are well educated.
- Patient safety is dependent on a sustainable and engaged emergency care workforce.
- Emergency clinicians are inextricably linked to patient wellbeing, and thus are poised to help bridge the gap between equity, safety and access for patients.
- There is clear evidence that patient (and family) experience, engagement and participation in care increases patient safety.
- Emergency care information systems should support care delivery, the management of patient information, and enable reporting and monitoring.
- Effective communication is fundamental to patient safety and quality of care and directly impacts on interprofessional relationships, staff morale, care delivery, evidence-based practice and safe transitions in care.
- The scope of practice of emergency clinicians continues to evolve to meet the needs of patients, including advanced and extended practice roles for both nurses and paramedics.
- Leadership is fundamental to a safety culture that enables emergency clinicians to practise to their fullest scope of practice in a safe and supportive environment.
- Emergency clinicians have a professional responsibility to ensure the care they deliver is evidence-based and patient-centred.

INTRODUCTION

Emergency nurses and paramedics comprise the largest component of the emergency health workforce in Australia and Aotearoa New Zealand. They are vital to the safety of emergency care and effective health service delivery and fulfil a critical role in the development of the socioeconomic framework for these countries. Patient safety is defined as 'reducing the risk of unnecessary harm to an acceptable minimum level', and quality in healthcare is defined as 'the degree to which health services for individuals and populations increase the likelihood of desired health outcomes and are consistent with current professional knowledge'.[1]

Safety and quality are important tenets of healthcare, including emergency care. Emergency clinicians care for patients of all ages, with varying degrees of clinical urgency and care requirements, and who are undifferentiated and undiagnosed. In addition, emergency clinicians make complex decisions in an unpredictable, busy environment under conditions of uncertainty and time pressure. The patient safety imperatives in emergency care are important as many patients are solely in the care of emergency nurses and paramedics prior to medical assessment. Systems of care ensure that the right patient is being delivered to and treated in the right place in the right time and improve clinical outcomes for a range of patients, including those with major trauma, stroke, cardiac arrest, acute coronary syndrome and sepsis.[2-5] Nurses and paramedics contribute substantially to such systems of care, which aim to improve both quality and safety in these settings.

Australasian emergency nurses make complex clinical decisions, such as setting mechanical ventilation parameters; titrating vasoactive medications, sedation and analgesia; and managing advanced respiratory and haemodynamic monitoring; all of which carry a high level of clinical risk.[6,7] Australian paramedics provide rapid response, emergency medical assessment and apply advanced life support (ALS) and critical care interventions in the pre-hospital setting. They make decisions on appropriate destinations, commence cardiac and haemodynamic monitoring, administer a range of analgesic, vasoactive, antiarrhythmic and sedative medications, and intervene with a range of invasive emergency procedures in order to stabilise patients prior to hospital handover.[8]

The Australian Commission on Safety and Quality in Health Care (ACSQHC) is Australia's peak safety and quality authority. ACSQHC was established in 2006 by the Council of Australian Governments (COAG) to coordinate national improvements in the safety and quality of healthcare based on the best available evidence. The Commission works in partnership with patients, clinicians, policy-makers and healthcare organisations to achieve safe, high-quality and high-performance healthcare and protect patients from preventable harm. One of the key safety and quality initiatives from the Commission was the development and implementation of the National Safety and Quality Health Service (NSQHS) Standards in 2011.[9] From 2013, the NSQHS Standards were used as the basis to accredit all publicly funded Australian hospitals. The second edition of the NSQHS Standards was released in 2017,[10] and revised in 2021.[11] The 2021 version of the NSQHS Standards (2nd edn) includes the Preventing and Controlling Infections Standard, which supersedes the NSQHS Preventing and Controlling Healthcare-Associated Infection Standard (2nd edn) and incorporates lessons learnt from the COVID-19 pandemic to better support health service organisations to prevent, control and respond to infections that cause outbreaks, epidemics or pandemics, including novel and emerging infections.[11] There are now eight NSQHS Standards focused on high-prevalence high-risk adverse events: clinical governance, partnering with consumers, preventing and controlling infections, medication safety, comprehensive care, communicating for safety and recognising and responding to acute deterioration.[11]

In Aotearoa New Zealand, the Health Quality and Safety Commission New Zealand fulfils a similar function to the ACSQHC. The Health Quality and Safety Commission works with clinicians and consumers to improve health and disability support services, reduce harm, improve healthcare experience and decrease ineffective spending and healthcare costs.[12] The Health Quality and Safety Commission program areas include medication safety, infection prevention and control, adverse events, reducing harm from falls, health quality evaluation, consumer engagement, reducing perioperative harm and mortality review.[12]

SAFETY AND QUALITY FRAMEWORKS

One of the most well-known quality frameworks is that created by Avedis Donabedian,[13,14] which has three broad principles: Structure–Process–Outcome. This framework will be used to organise the chapter. Donabedian's framework recognises that the structure of, and processes within, an organisation or an emergency department (ED) are interrelated: structure influences process, and both structure and process influence outcomes.[15] Therefore, emergency care outcomes are dependent on both the structure (setting) and processes of care. In the context of this chapter and safety and quality of care in pre-hospital and ED settings, structure refers to physical and human resources in the setting where care is delivered, while process refers to how care is delivered (practices and interventions), and outcomes are the end-result of care delivery.

Another important quality framework is the 'Six Domains of Health Care Quality' from the Institute of Medicine:[16]

1. Safe: Avoiding harm to patients from the care that is intended to help them.
2. Effective: Providing services based on scientific knowledge to all who could benefit and refraining from providing services to those not likely to benefit (avoiding underuse and misuse, respectively).
3. Patient-centred: Providing care that is respectful of and responsive to individual patient preferences, needs and values, and ensuring that patient values guide all clinical decisions.
4. Timely: Reducing waits and sometimes harmful delays for both those who receive and those who give care.
5. Efficient: Avoiding waste, including waste of equipment, supplies, ideas and energy.
6. Equitable: Providing care that does not vary in quality because of personal characteristics such as gender, ethnicity, geographic location and socioeconomic status.

SAFETY AND QUALITY FRAMEWORKS FOR EMERGENCY CARE

Quality Standards for Emergency Departments and Other Hospital-Based Emergency Care, published by the Australasian College for Emergency Medicine (ACEM), 'aim to provide guidance and set expectations for the provision of equitable, safe and high quality emergency care in EDs and other hospital-based emergency care services' in Australia and New Zealand (see Useful websites).[17] These Standards are organised into five domains: clinical care, administration, professionalism, education and training, and research. Within each domain there are standards which articulate the overall goal and expected objective or outcome; objectives that are measurable elements of service provision and usually related to the desired outcome or performance of team members or services within the ED; and criteria which are components of service provision that are required to be in place in order to achieve the objective.[17] Ambulance services have historically developed their own safety and quality frameworks. In addition, some Australian ambulance services have commenced preparing for accreditation against the NSQHS Standards, in a similar way to other traditional health services.[18]

OUTCOMES

Australian and Aotearoa New Zealand emergency care providers and the acute hospital sector have experienced significant changes in patient demographics, demand for services, patient complexity, changing patient expectations, ambulance transports and referral patterns, and use of emergency services by aged care facilities.[19,20] EDs are experiencing increased usage by the older patient population and there are increasing numbers of patients with chronic disease requiring emergency care.[21] Demand for emergency ambulance services also continues to grow, exceeding population growth.[22] Increased emergency ambulance demand has been associated with delayed response times, which in turn may negatively impact on survival and patient outcomes for time-critical conditions.[22] Patients with mental health issues, alcohol and other drug abuse, and those with multiple or severe comorbidities tend to account for the greatest growth.[22] Emergency clinicians make critical decisions every day to ensure safe, high-quality care for sicker, older, frailer patients, and are increasingly integrating advanced technology into emergency care provision. The care provided by emergency clinicians is inextricably linked to patient wellbeing, and thus emergency clinicians are fundamental to the equity, safety, access and coordination of increasingly complex care for the wide range of ED patients.[7,8]

SYSTEM OUTCOMES AND PERFORMANCE MONITORING

The demand for safety and quality of healthcare is a global priority for hospitals, healthcare workers and patients.[23,24] Evidence-based practice underpins the increasing obligations for, and expectations of, safer and higher quality healthcare. At the core of the evidence-based practice movement is the patient or consumer voice garnished by systematic programs capturing their experience. The demand for safe and quality healthcare is also being aided and abetted by an increasingly litigious society, where individuals, community and society as a whole demand better. The vision for quality care championed by luminaries such as Florence Nightingale,[25] Avedis Donabedian,[13,14] and many others over the last centuries has been realised in ways not imagined. Their efforts gave rise to the importance of systems and measures to determine the quality and safety of healthcare.

Today, the most successful and comprehensive medical systems are those centred on universal healthcare that is enabled by a range of free and subsidised public enterprises and supported by private enterprise, all of which operates as a system. These systems are, however, complex. Emergency healthcare systems in particular are extraordinarily complex, as they have high-pressured, high-risk environments laden with uncertain, finite resources where demand for healthcare often exceeds supply and predispose the emergency care setting to error. The actions and omissions of individuals and the system overall directly influence the safety and quality of healthcare patients receive. When the many moving parts in the emergency healthcare systems do not operate optimally, or they fail, error arises. In the contemporary context these are referred to as hospital-acquired complications. Hospital-acquired complications and their consequences can be catastrophic for patients, particularly in emergency care situations.

The ACSQHC defines hospital-acquired complications as 'a complication for which clinical risk mitigation strategies may reduce, but not necessarily eliminate, the risk of that complication occurring'.[24] The ACSQHC has established and published a list of 16 hospital-acquired complications following reviews of the literature, clinical engagement and testing of the concept with public and private hospitals (Table 6.1).[24] The Grattan Institute suggests that one in every nine hospital patients in Australia suffers a hospital-acquired complication, or more than 900,000 patients every year.[26] The costs of these hospital-acquired complications, in human and financial terms, and other ways, are well documented.[27] At the core of contemporary clinical quality frameworks in hospital and other healthcare settings are efforts to prevent these and other forms of hospital-acquired complications. As such, hospitals across the country are required to focus their efforts on reducing the rate of, and ultimately preventing, these hospital-acquired complications. Measures aimed at emboldening efforts to prevent hospital-acquired complications include restricting public funding for serious hospital-acquired complications, by way of a financial penalty.[24] Financial penalties for preventable hospital-acquired infections already exist and operate in Australia, such as for preventable bloodstream infections.[28] There are reports of health insurance companies requiring hospitals to provide warranties on surgical procedures and imposing financial penalties on hospitals where patient outcomes result in a hospital-acquired complication.[24] What is clear is that there are firm efforts to reduce healthcare-associated complications and associated financial penalties for such events, and equally firm efforts to make every complication count.[27,29]

A range of specific performance measures is used to determine how well emergency care systems are functioning, for example, ambulance response times, ambulance off-load time, time to treatment, ED length of stay, and National Emergency Access Target (NEAT) (also called Emergency Treatment Performance (ETP) in some jurisdictions) standards. There are a range of injury- or disease-based measures that have been used to measure emergency care performance for conditions such as stroke, trauma and acute coronary syndrome. The sensitivity and specificity of these measures varies, and each has strengths and limitations. For example, time-based measures may not reflect emergency nursing quality and safety, given emergency care clinicians' limited capacity to influence overall patient time in the ED. Such measures are used systematically to determine and demonstrate effectiveness and efficiency of emergency care within healthcare more broadly, and to communicate care outcomes to policy-makers, organisational leaders and the community. If emergency care systems manage patients appropriately, with minimal duplication and referral, then the impact is likely to be a significant improvement in patient safety.

TABLE 6.1 IDENTIFIED HOSPITAL-ACQUIRED COMPLICATIONS IN AUSTRALIA[24]

HOSPITAL-ACQUIRED COMPLICATION	DIAGNOSIS
Pressure injury	• Stage III ulcer • Stage IV ulcer • Unspecified decubitus ulcer and pressure area • Unstageable pressure injury • Suspected deep tissue injury
Falls resulting in fracture or intracranial injury	• Intracranial injury • Fractured neck of femur • Other fractures
Healthcare-associated infection	• Urinary tract infection • Surgical site infection • Pneumonia • Bloodstream infection • Infections or inflammatory complications associated with peripheral/central venous catheters • Multi-resistant organism • Infection associated with prosthetics/implantable devices • Gastrointestinal infections • Other high-impact infections
Surgical complications requiring unplanned return to theatre	• Postoperative haemorrhage/haematoma requiring transfusion and/or return to theatre • Surgical wound dehiscence • Anastomotic leak • Vascular graft failure • Other surgical complications requiring unplanned return to theatre
Unplanned intensive care unit admission	• Unplanned admission to intensive care unit
Respiratory complications	• Respiratory failure including acute respiratory distress syndrome requiring ventilation • Aspiration pneumonia • Pulmonary oedema
Venous thromboembolism	• Pulmonary embolism • Deep vein thrombosis
Renal failure	• Renal failure requiring haemodialysis or continuous veno-venous haemodialysis
Gastrointestinal bleeding	• Gastrointestinal bleeding
Medication complications	• Drug-related respiratory complications/depression • Haemorrhagic disorder due to circulating anticoagulants • Movement disorders due to psychotropic medication • Serious alteration to conscious state due to psychotropic medication
Delirium	• Delirium
Persistent incontinence	• Urinary incontinence • Faecal incontinence
Malnutrition	• Malnutrition
Cardiac complications	• Heart failure and pulmonary oedema • Arrhythmias • Cardiac arrest • Acute coronary syndrome, including unstable angina, STEMI and NSTEMI • Infective endocarditis
Third- and fourth-degree perineal laceration during delivery	• Third- and fourth-degree perineal laceration during delivery
Neonatal birth trauma	• Neonatal birth trauma • Hypoxic ischaemic encephalopathy

Clinical quality registries are useful in improving the quality of care and reduce health costs.[30] Clinical quality registries collect minimum data about patients undergoing a specific procedure, who have a specific diagnosis, or are using a healthcare resources.[31] Data is captured from administrative systems, medical records or directly from clinicians or patients.[31] There is evidence that the longer duration of clinical quality registries, the better data quality.[31]

STRUCTURE OF EMERGENCY CARE

Emergency care provision involves complex care systems that encompass the physical environment; patients with increasingly complex care needs and significant comorbidities and their families; inter- and intra-professional relationships, communication and collaborations to achieve a systems-based approach to care; use of technology to manage information and enhance treatment options; and a support services workforce. All of these factors influence safety and quality of care.

THE EMERGENCY CARE WORKFORCE

Emergency clinicians have many patient safety responsibilities, including surveillance, prevention of complications and adverse events and symptom management. Emergency clinicians have a right to be well supported by organisational management and administration and work within teams with the skill-mix, expertise and competency to provide high-quality emergency care.[17] There is a substantial body of evidence on the importance of nurses in patient safety. Nurses make up the largest component of the health workforce and have more direct patient contact than any other healthcare professional. Paramedics also are responsible for the safety of patients, themselves and bystanders. Often working in uncontrolled, emergent and austere environments, paramedics often contend with the added complexity of a different work environment for every case. This increases the risk to patient (and personal) safety. Paramedics utilise a range of guidelines, checklists and standard practices to reduce the likelihood of adverse events and errors.

Staffing and skill-mix

A sustainable and agile health workforce is needed to manage the ongoing challenges of emergency care. There is clear evidence from ward settings that patients are safer when nurses have appropriate workloads. When nurses have six or fewer patients each (compared to 10 or more), there is a 20% decrease in risk of death in medical wards and a 17% decrease in risk of death in surgical wards.[32] For each additional patient added to nursing workloads, there is a 7% increase in the risk of inpatient death within 30 days of admission[33] and substituting one nurse assistant for a professional nurse for every 25 patients is associated with a 21% increase in the odds of 30-day mortality.[34] Modelling by Aiken and colleagues shows that when compared to a 1:8 nurse-to-patient ratio, a 1:4 nurse-to-patient ratio with 90% registered nurses (RNs) would improve mortality rates from 25.1 to 15.6 per 1000 hospital admissions and failure-to-rescue rates from 105.9 to 68.2 per 1000 hospital admissions.[35] Australian data show that each additional patient per nurse is associated with 12% higher odds of 30-day mortality and poorer nurse outcomes (15% higher odds of emotional exhaustion, 14% higher odds of job dissatisfaction, 12% higher odds of concerns about quality of care and 32% higher odds of concerns about patient safety).[36] The optimum number and skill-mix for emergency nurses in terms of patient safety in EDs is unknown. Nurse-to-patient ratios have been adopted in many parts of the world to ensure that nurse staffing is appropriate for the delivery of safe, high-quality care. Appropriate nurse staffing has several benefits, including better patient outcomes,[32,35,36] decreased nurse burnout,[37,38] increased nurse recruitment and retention and reduced nurse turnover.[39] Nurse burnout has been clearly linked to adverse patient safety outcomes and poor quality of care.[40,41]

Australia has been a world leader in nurse staffing and the legislation of nurse-to-patient ratios which are now in place in a number of states, beginning in Victoria in 2000 and introduced in Queensland in 2016.[42,43] On acute care hospital wards, Victoria has legislated that nurses care for gazetted 4:1 nursing ratio;[44] however, at the time of writing, much of Australia and Aotearoa New Zealand do not have nurse-to-patient ratios.[45] For example, in Victoria and Queensland nurse-to-patient ratios are one nurse to four patients on morning and afternoon shifts and one nurse for seven to eight patients overnight,[42,43] and in Victoria, no more than 20% of nurses on acute wards can be enrolled nurses.[43] Data from Queensland showed that following implementation of nurse-to-patient ratios, there were significant reductions in 30-day mortality (OR = 0·89, 95% CI 0·84–0·95, p = 0·0003), 7-day re-admissions (OR = 1·06, 95% CI 1·01–1·12, p = 0·015), and hospital length of stay (incident rate ratio (IRR) = 0·95, 95% CI 0·92–0·99, p = 0·010).[46] Staffing improvements by one patient per nurse reduced 30-day mortality (OR 0·93, 95% CI 0·86–0·99, p = 0·045), 7-day re-admissions (OR = 0·93, 95% CI 0·89–0·97, p <0·0001), and hospital length of stay (IRR 0·97, 0·94–0·99, p = 0·035).[46] Further, the costs savings from reduced re-admissions and shorter hospital stay were more than double the cost associated with additional nurse staffing.[46]

In Australia, 95.2% of nurses working in EDs are RNs;[47] however, the optimum ED nursing staff ratios are unknown. To date, ED nurse-to-patient ratios in Victoria are 1:3 plus the nurse in-charge of the shift[43] and triage nurse(s), and since 2021 there are 1:1 nurse-to-patient ratios in ED resuscitation cubicles.[48] In Queensland, ED nurse-to-patient ratios are 1:3 plus team leader plus triage and 1:1 in ED resuscitation cubicles.[49] In addition, Queensland has a requirement for minimum 90% RNs rostered on every shift in EDs and that Assistants in Nursing (AINs) (however described) will not be included in the direct care hours.[49] Further, when there is an appropriate skill-mix (i.e. an increased proportion of RNs), hospital length of stay decreases, pain management is improved, and adverse events, such as infections, gastrointestinal bleeding events, falls and medication errors, are decreased.[50]

Different paramedic agencies have different models of paramedic skill-mix and many paramedic services employ other staff, such as volunteers or community first responders, to support out-of-hospital care.[51] Paramedic scope of practice in Australia and Aotearoa New Zealand typically ranges from advanced life support (ALS) paramedics to extended care paramedics, intensive care paramedics and intensive care flight paramedics.[52] The most common model of emergency paramedicine in Australia and Aotearoa New Zealand is two ambulance paramedics. Ambulance crewing may consist of two advanced life support (ALS) paramedics, two intensive care paramedics, or one ALS and one intensive care paramedic. Many services also employ 'single responder' models consisting of an ALS or intensive care paramedic responding in a non-stretcher bearing vehicle. In addition, ALS paramedics may also have specific training to become flight paramedics.[8] There has been little research to investigate the safest or clinically optimal paramedic skill-mix to date.

Educational preparation of emergency clinicians

Patients are also safer when nurses are well educated, with numerous studies over the last two decades showing that as the number of degree-prepared nurses increases, mortality decreases.[34,53] For every 10% increase in nurses with bachelor degrees, there was a 7% decrease in the risk of inpatient death within 30 days of admission.[33] A ten-year longitudinal study published in 2021 showed that between 2006 and 2016, patients in hospitals that increased their proportion of bachelor-prepared nurses over time had significantly reduced odds of risk-adjusted mortality (OR 0.95, 95% CI 0.92–0.98, p = 0.002), 7-day re-admissions (OR 0.96, 95% CI 0.94–0.99), p = 0.01) and 30-day re-admissions (OR 0.98, 95% CI 0.95–1.00, p = 0.03), and shorter length of hospital stay (IRR 0.98, 95% CI: 0.97–0.99, 0.003).[54] In real terms, if a hospital where 30% of nurses are degree-prepared and caring for an average of eight patients changed to ensure that nurses cared for an average of six patients and 60% of the nursing workforce had bachelor degrees, mortality would decrease by 30%.[53] In Australia, 30% of emergency nurses have a postgraduate qualification.[47] Improving nurse-to-patient ratios, nurses' educational preparation and clinical education support could prevent as many as 40,000 patient deaths per year.[55]

Educational preparation for ambulance officers (as they were then known) commenced in the early 1960s and comprised on-the-job first aid training. Since this time, Australasian paramedic education has moved through the vocational educational training sector to where it sits today, in the university sector, the first paramedic (conversion) degree being offered in New South Wales.[56] Since the late 1990s, entry-level paramedic preparation has occurred predominantly within the university sector at the bachelor degree level.[56]

Patient engagement, experience, satisfaction and relationship with safety and quality

Although the terms patient (and family) experience, engagement and participation are used interchangeably, they are conceptually different. Refer to Chapter 8 for more details about patient and family engagement. Specifically, patient engagement is different to patient satisfaction. Patient satisfaction is a momentary emotional judgement made by the patient about how positive they feel about an encounter.[57,58] Patient experience encompasses more than satisfaction and is a lasting phenomenon of perceptions, understanding and memories. Patient experience is not about making patients and families happy, but about ensuring the best in quality, safety and service outcomes. A systematic review of 55 studies showed clear links between patient experience (self-rated and objectively measured) and clinical effectiveness and patient safety outcomes across a wide range of clinical conditions, practice settings and outcome measures.[59] Patient engagement had positive associations with health outcomes, adherence to recommended management plans and medications, preventive care (health-promoting behaviours, use of screening services and immunisation) and resource use (hospitalisation, length of stay and primary-care visits).[59]

There is evidence that patient (and family) experience, engagement and participation in care increases patient safety.[60] Engagement between emergency clinicians and patients and their families is an important aspect of the service delivery and a measure of quality of care.[61] Indeed, carers and relatives can play an important role in providing information about the presenting person's medical history and condition to emergency clinicians.[60] This has been shown to be the case particularly in the care of the older person.[62] Greater engagement with families and carers can also ensure safer discharge and potentially reduce ED representation and/or hospital re-admission.[62,63]

Burnout of emergency clinicians

Caring for emergency clinicians is important not only for the clinician, but also the patients they care for. The emergency care workforce is experiencing greater workloads, resulting from increased demand, increased patient acuity and care needs, access block resulting in ambulance ramping and prolonged ED length of stay, and national workforce shortages. Professional burnout is characterised by emotional exhaustion; increasing mental distance from one's job or feelings of cynicism or negativity; and decreased professional efficacy.[40,64] Burnout in healthcare providers is associated with mental health disorders such as depression and anxiety; poor physical health; absenteeism, poor retention and increased turnover that further exacerbate job dissatisfaction related to staff shortages and increased workloads.[64] A systematic review and meta-analysis of 82 studies involving over 200,000 healthcare providers showed that clinician burnout is consistently associated with poorer quality of healthcare and reduced patient safety.[40] Emotional exhaustion is the burnout element that has the strongest relationship with poor quality of care and the impact of burnout seems to be greater for nurses than for doctors or mixed groups of healthcare professionals.[40] A systematic review of 17 studies of the determinants and prevalence of burnout in emergency nurses highlights that on average 26% of the emergency nurses suffer from burnout.[65] A systematic review of five studies reported the prevalence of burnout in paramedics ranged between 16% and 56%.[64]

Individual factors associated with increased risk of burnout are younger age, flexibility, stubbornness, judgemental behaviour and difficulty in adaptation, and avoidance behaviour following a traumatic event.[64,65] The work-related factors associated with burnout are exposure to traumatic events, psychological demands (work/time pressure) and low levels of social support from managers and peers.[64,65] The organisational characteristics that were determinants of burnout are poor interprofessional collaboration, understaffing, lack of material resources, outdated organisational culture and lack of quality assurance initiatives.[64,65]

THE EMERGENCY CARE ENVIRONMENT

The emergency care environment should cater to the needs of different patient groups and their families, and to the needs of emergency clinicians.[17] Patients and families have a right to expect that the emergency care environment is safe, has the requisite amenities, enables access for people of all abilities, supports privacy and dignity, and enables the delivery of high-quality emergency care.[17] Emergency clinicians have a right to expect that their working environments are safe, functional, have the requisite equipment, and enable care delivery to meet the needs of patients and their families.[17]

Communication

ED information systems should support care delivery, the management of patient information, and enable reporting and monitoring.[17] Communication is fundamental to patient safety and quality of care. This is because communication directly impacts on interprofessional relationships, staff morale, streamlined care, implementation and sustained uptake of evidence-based practice and accurate handover; all of which are crucial to patient safety. The complex, high-stress, unpredictable and dynamic work of emergency care poses particular challenges for effective communication,[66] and has a direct impact on patient outcomes. There is clear evidence that patients are safer when interprofessional relationships are effective and productive.[67,68] Rudeness lowers diagnostic and procedural performance scores; however, deficits in diagnostic performance are mediated by information-sharing behaviours and help-seeking behaviours mediate the negative effect of rudeness on procedural performance.[69–71]

The key elements of communicating for safety are recognised in the ACSQHC National Safety and Quality Health Service Standards:[11]

- Clinical governance and quality improvement to support effective communication
- Correct patient identification and procedure matching
- Communication at clinical handover
- Communication of critical information
- Documentation of information.

The ACSQHC has developed a National Clinical Handover Initiative that has generated practical tools and solutions for improving handover. Use of these tools, in particular ISBAR (see Chapter 14), is known to improve the accuracy and consistency in clinical handover.[11] However, tools and guides on how to communicate are not useful unless they are implemented, and implemented sustainably.[72] Examples of how to achieve effective communication are through regular and repeated high-fidelity simulation training programs that focus on non-technical skills,[73] or embedding the specific communication tools in clinical practice by incorporating them into mandatory clinical information systems or clinical assessment techniques.[74] Patient advocacy is a key aspect of emergency clinician practice, particularly in the deteriorating patient. Techniques such as graded assertiveness (discussed in detail in Chapter 13) should also be embedded in clinical education programs and modelled by senior clinicians.

Technology in the form of uniformly introduced and mandated information systems are another form of communication that we are reliant on in our day-to-day practice, and is a huge infrastructure investment.[20] System functionality varies greatly and affects clinician decision-making, workflow, communication, and ultimately the overall quality of care and patient safety.[17] Following wide face-to-face consultation at the frontline of care, any information system that is to be used by clinicians should be tested extensively by all those who are potentially impacted, for example, clerical, medical, nursing, pharmacy and allied health across the span of patient care. The system should support care delivery, the management of patient information, and enable reporting and monitoring.[17]

EMERGENCY CARE PROCESSES

Processes of emergency care include the models of care delivery; the degree to which emergency care is grounded in a quality and safety culture; resource management strategies, such as leadership and governance; capabilities for decision support and evidence-based practice and the use of technology.

MODELS OF EMERGENCY CARE

To improve patient safety and timely access to emergency care, innovative models have been developed to meet increasing emergency care demand. All the models of emergency care operate based on the principle that care needs to be delivered to the right patient at the right time and that staff have the capacity and capability to make the right decisions to inform and meet patient care needs. Many models of care are pragmatically allocated to a geographical location within the ED. For example, patients with minor conditions and injuries may be allocated to a specific area such as fast track.[75] 'Streaming' models of care have been introduced in many EDs, whereby patients with similar care needs are co-located and care is delivered by a team of clinicians.[75] Streaming aims to reduce ED crowding and improve ED efficiency and is often based on the anticipated discharge destination (admission vs discharge), patient demographics (children, adults and elders), diagnostic groups or care requirements (simple vs complex).[75] Other models of ED care are based on staffing and specific roles within the ED, such as the clinical initiatives nurse.[76,77] However, the different models of ED care lack standardisation across Australia and Aotearoa New Zealand, have had varied implementation strategies, and have not been subject to rigorous evaluation.[77]

New models of ED care have often resulted in concurrent development of new nursing roles, which have enabled emergency nurses to broaden their scope of practice and achieve greater recognition of their expertise and skills. However, across Australia and Aotearoa New Zealand the titles for advanced and extended nursing roles, such as nurse practitioner, advanced practice nurses, and clinical initiative nurses[77–79] have varied, creating confusion and inconsistency in nomeclature.[80,81] Examples of increased scope of practice for emergency nurses include independent initiation of investigations and interventions to reduce service delays, nurse-initiated medications (analgesics, antiemetics, intravenous fluids), and ordering x-rays and pathology testing.[82–84] Many of these advanced and extended nursing roles are formalised locally and often allocated to specific patient areas and/or diagnostic groups.

Many emergency nurses practise at an advanced level; however, nurse practitioners (NP) are the pinnacle of autonomous nursing practice. NPs have the capability to provide high levels of clinically focused nursing care in a variety of contexts in Australia and independently manage whole episodes of care.[85] In contrast to the registered nurse, NPs are legislated to autonomously diagnose, prescribe and refer when treating and managing patients within their scope of practice.[85] Across Australasian EDs, it is common for a NP to be the leader of the ED's fast-track service, which is aimed at the timely management of patients with single-system illness or injury.[86,87] The introduction of emergency NPs has significantly improved the safety and timeliness of care for patients.[86–89] Further details about different emergency nursing roles and nurse practitioners can be found in Chapter 1. Nurses and paramedics continue to respond to demand by reviewing their roles in healthcare systems. However, role implementation and impact measurements need to be considered to ensure patient safety.

Paramedics within Australia, Aotearoa New Zealand and internationally are increasingly taking on advanced care roles. Known as extended care paramedics, advanced care paramedics or paramedic practitioners, these clinicians specialise in managing patients with low or medium acuity injuries or illnesses within the community.[8,52,90,91] The aim of the role is to manage the patient in their home, and avoid unnecessary transportation to already overburdened EDs. Like the roles of NPs and physicians' assistants, the utility of advanced care paramedics has undergone much evaluation. Advanced care paramedics have proved themselves in many jurisdictions by offering a clinically effective alternative to ED treatment.[52]

QUALITY AND SAFETY CULTURE/ LEADERSHIP

Safety culture is defined as a culture:[1]

i) where all workers (including frontline staff, doctors and administrators) accept responsibility for the safety of themselves, their co-workers, patients and visitors
ii) that prioritises safety above financial and operational goals
iii) that encourages and rewards the identification, communication and resolution of safety issues

iv) that provides for organisational learning from accidents, and
v) that provides appropriate resources, structure and accountability to maintain effective safety systems.

The ED should foster a safe and supportive culture with the intent of improving patient and emergency clinician experience.[17]

Leadership styles

For the past decade, research has shown the relationship between various leadership styles of healthcare leaders and outcomes for clinicians, work environments and patients. Through a series of systematic reviews of the nursing research literature, a clear relationship has been shown to exist between nursing leaders in healthcare management roles and outcomes for nurses, including job satisfaction, health and wellbeing, motivation to perform, intent to remain, and their work environments.[92–94] Outcomes for nurses are highly important, as they are the largest group of healthcare professionals in the health system, and therefore represent a substantial investment, cost and quality driver into achieving patient outcomes, and providing safe quality care.

The influence that nurses in leadership roles can have on the health system and nurse outcomes can be profound, both positively and negatively.[92–94]

Four elements characterise transformational leadership: 1) idealised influence, which occurs when leaders are perceived as having high ideals and a strong sense of ethics; 2) inspirational motivation, which describes leaders who communicate high expectations and inspire commitment to a shared vision; 3) intellectual stimulation, which describes leader behaviours that promote innovation and new ways of approaching problems; and 4) individualised consideration, which includes creating a supportive environment and attending to the needs and concerns of followers.[95] The current evidence to date suggests there is a clear relationship between relational leadership styles and lower patient mortality and reduced errors, including medication errors, restraint use and hospital-acquired infections. Strategies that leaders and managers use in practice build positive work environments that optimise patient safety and outcomes.[96]

Safety culture

Developing a culture of safety is a core element of many efforts to improve patient safety and care quality in acute settings. Several studies show that safety culture and the related concept of safety climate are related to clinician behaviour, such as error reporting, reduction in adverse events and reduced mortality.[97] Safety culture refers specifically to shared perceptions or attitudes about norms, policy and procedures related to patient safety among groups such as care teams or departments.

Promotion of patient safety culture can best be described as a collection of interventions entrenched in principles of leadership, teamwork and behavioural change, rather than a specific process, team or technology. Strategies to promote a culture of patient safety may include a single intervention or several interventions combined into a multifaceted approach or sequences. They may also include system level change, such as those in governance or reporting structures. For example, team training, interdisciplinary rounding or executive walk-arounds and department-based strategies that include a series of interventions, have all been characterised as interventions that promote a culture of safety.[97]

Leadership walkarounds are an interventional strategy that engage the leadership team in an organisation directly with frontline care providers. Executive or senior leaders visit frontline care providers of all levels, with the goal of observing and discussing current or potential threats to patient safety, as well as supporting frontline staff in addressing challenges such as workforce and equipment resources. Leadership rounding aims to show commitment to safety, foster trust and psychological safety and provide support, which includes motivational feedback and celebration of achievements, and for frontline providers to proactively address concerns around patient safety.

DECISION SUPPORT AND EVIDENCE-BASED PRACTICE

Evidence-based care is safer care. Early studies showed that 30–40% of patients do not receive the recommended care, and as many as 20% receive diagnostic tests or medications that are not evidence-based, are unnecessary and potentially harmful.[98,99] In Australia, it is estimated that appropriate care is provided in only 57% of healthcare encounters and compliance with indicators of appropriate care ranged from 32% to 86%.[99] There are a number of decision support tools available to emergency clinicians to help improve patient safety and the key features are summarised below. Refer to Chapter 7 for more detail about evidence-based practice and evidence implementation and Chapter 11 for more detail about clinical decision-making and clinical reasoning.

Consistency of care and decreasing unwarranted variation

Emergency care delivery requires balancing best available evidence with available resources and patient and family preferences. Therefore, some variation in emergency care delivery is warranted and desirable if it is beneficial to patients. However, unwarranted variation is variation in care delivery that is not explained by patient needs or preferences and is a source of potential harm in healthcare, as patients either do not receive care they should have or receive care they do not need and unwarranted variation increases healthcare costs.[100–102]

There are many examples of unwarranted variation in emergency care practices. The 2021 *Australian Atlas of Healthcare Variation*[103] showed that 43–56% of the planned caesarean sections performed at less than 39 weeks' gestation did not have a documented obstetric or medical indication. Of more than 330,000 preventable hospitalisations, the greatest variations in hospital admissions were for COPD (18 times higher than the lowest), cellulitis (about 16 times higher than the lowest) and diabetes complications (about 12 times higher than the lowest).[103] National Stroke Foundation Audit data show that across Australian states and territories, the percentage of patients who receive a validated stroke screen in the ED varies from 31% to 83%, thrombolysis in ischaemic stroke varied from 4% to 18% and median time from stroke onset to thrombolysis varied from 2 hours 41 minutes to 3 hours 17 minutes.[104]

Clinical practice guidelines

The National Health and Medical Research Council (NHMRC) defines clinical practice guidelines as 'evidence-based statements that include recommendations intended to optimise patient care and assist healthcare practitioners to make decisions about appropriate health care for specific clinical circumstances. Clinical practice guidelines should assist clinicians and patients in shared decision making'.[105]

Checklists

The use of safety checklists in healthcare has increased since World Health Organization (WHO) Surgical Safety Checklist trials showed that the use of checklists dramatically decreased postoperative mortality.[106] Safety checklists differ from protocols, algorithms and guidelines that provide detailed recommendations and are additional tools designed to ensure that an operation, procedure or task is performed as planned. A 2018 systematic review and meta-analysis involving 11 studies of 453,292 patients, showed that for patients where a surgical safety checklist was used, there were lower mortality rates and fewer complications.[106]

Care bundles

A care bundle is a set of evidence-based interventions for a defined patient group and context of care, which, when implemented together, give significantly better outcomes than when implemented individually.[107] Care bundles have improved care and outcomes for patients with blunt chest injury, hip fracture and sepsis and have reduced complications such as ventilator-acquired pneumonia and central-line infection.[107–109]

Patient decision aids

Patient decision aids are tools that enable patients and family participation in shared decision-making with health professionals by providing evidence-based information about care options, risks and benefits, and assist patients in considering what is most important to them in terms of outcomes.[110] Patient decision aids can be delivered using many formats (videos, booklets, websites) that can be tailored to the patient population and context of care.[110]

DIGITAL HEALTH

Digital health is described as 'using digital information data and communication technologies to collect, share, and analyse health information for purposes of improving patient health and health care delivery'.[111] Digital health aims to increase access to, and equity of, healthcare; improve communication between clinicians and patients and between clinicians; provide easier access to critical information; monitor variation; deliver clinical decision-making support at the point of care; facilitate delivery of evidence-informed healthcare; and reduce errors and near-miss adverse events through alerts and forcing functions. It is now increasingly clear that healthcare is unlikely to see transformation without successful implementation of advanced technologies and the presence of a culture that accepts information technology as part of providing care.[112]

Initiatives such as telehealth enable patients to receive quality care closer to home, thus improving access to specialist healthcare for people in regional communities and reducing the need to travel for specialist advice. In the emergency care context, technology has enabled a systems approach to care across the emergency care continuum via initiatives such as transmission of pre-hospital electrocardiography to emergency departments for patients with acute coronary syndrome, mobile stroke units enabling pre-hospital CT scan or telehealth support for emergency care clinicians practising in rural or remote areas.

Healthcare informatics is a specialty area that integrates science with multiple information management and analytical sciences to identify, define, manage and communicate data, information, knowledge and wisdom in practice.[112] Healthcare informatics supports clinicians, consumers, patients and other stakeholders in their decision-making in all roles and settings to achieve desired outcomes.[112]

SUMMARY

The safety and quality of emergency care relies on complex interactions between patients and families and emergency clinicians in both out-of-hospital and ED environments that have unique characteristics and within a system that is under increasing pressure. Emergency care performance indicators and performance targets must be grounded in safety and quality rather than time-based measures. There is clear evidence that patient safety is enhanced when emergency clinicians are engaged and have reasonable workloads, good interprofessional relationships, effective systems for communication and information management and whose wellbeing is an organisational priority. In addition, patient (and family) experience, engagement and participation in care further increases patient safety. Emergency clinicians have a professional responsibility to deliver evidence-based and patient-centred care and are vital to ensuring that emergency care is accessible, equitable and safe.

USEFUL WEBSITES

Australian Commission on Safety and Quality in Health Care (ACSQHC), body established by Australian, state and territory governments to lead and coordinate national improvements in safety and quality in health care, www.safetyandquality.gov.au/.

Australian Institute for Health and Welfare (AIHW), Australia's national agency for information and statistics on Australia's health and welfare used to inform discussion and policy decisions on health, community services, www.aihw.gov.au/.

Australian Resuscitation Outcomes Consortium (AUS-ROC), aims to increase research capacity in the area of out-of-hospital cardiac arrest, with specific focus on improving rates of survival and outcomes for survivors, www.ausroc.org.au/.

Australasian College of Emergency Medicine (ACEM), the organisation responsible for training emergency doctors and advancement of professional standards in emergency medicine in Australia and Aotearoa New Zealand, acem.org.au/.

Australasian College of Emergency Medicine (ACEM), Quality Standards for Emergency Departments and Hospital-based Emergency Care Services, https://acem.org.au/getmedia/f4832c56-2b59-4654-815b-cdd1a66b27a8/ACEM_QualityStandardsEDs_Report

College of Emergency Nursing Australasia (CENA), peak professional association representing emergency nurses, www.cena.org.au/.

Emergency Care Clinical Network, brings together emergency clinicians, health organisations and patients to improve the quality of care and patient experience in Victorian emergency departments, www2.health.vic.gov.au/hospitals-and-health-services/quality-safety-service/clinical-networks/clinical-network-emergency.

Emergency Care Institute, is a subsidiary of the Agency for Clinical Innovation (ACI) with a primary role to improve outcomes for patients presenting at hospital emergency departments (EDs) across NSW through coordination, networking and research, www.aci.health.nsw.gov.au/networks/eci/about.

Institute for Healthcare Improvement (IHI), leading innovator, convener, partner and driver of results in health and healthcare improvement worldwide with five key areas of focus: improvement capability; person- and family-centred care; patient safety; quality, cost and value; and applying integrated approaches to simultaneously improve care, improve population health and reduce costs, www.ihi.org/.

Institute of Medicine, non-profit organisation devoted to providing leadership on healthcare. It serves as an excellent source for leaders and managers to gain access to current research and publications devoted to healthcare, www.ihi.org/resources/Pages/OtherWebsites/TheInstituteofMedicine.aspx.

National Health and Medical Research Council (NHMRC), Australian Clinical Practice Guidelines, this portal provides links to high-quality, NHMRC approved guidelines; evidence-based guidelines not approved by NHMRC and guidelines developed by Australian guideline developers, www.clinicalguidelines.gov.au/portal.

REFERENCES

1. World Health Organization (WHO) and WHO Patient Safety. Conceptual framework for the international classification for patient safety: final technical report. Geneva: World Health Organization; 2009. Online. Available from: apps.who.int/iris/handle/10665/70882.
2. Moore L, Champion H, Tardif P-A, Kuimi B-L, O'Reilly G, Leppaniemi A, et al. Impact of trauma system structure on injury outcomes: a systematic review and meta-analysis. World J Surgery 2018;42(5):1327–39.
3. Fatima N, Saqqur M, Hussain MS, Shuaib A. Mobile stroke unit versus standard medical care in the management of patients with acute stroke: a systematic review and meta-analysis. Int J Stroke 2020;15(6):595–608.
4. Hyun K, Redfern J, Woodward M, D'Souza M, Shetty P, Chew D, et al. Socioeconomic equity in the receipt of in-hospital care and outcomes in Australian acute coronary syndrome patients: the CONCORDANCE registry. Heart Lung Circ 2018;27(12):1398–405.
5. Aliprandi-Costa B, Morgan L, Snell L-C, Kritharides L, French J, et al. ST-elevation acute myocardial infarction in Australia—temporal trends in patient management and outcomes 1999–2016. Heart Lung Circ 2019;28(7):1000–8.
6. Fry M, Shaban RZ, Considine J. Clinical reasoning, problem solving and triage. In: Curtis K, Ramsden C, Shaban RZ, et al. (eds). Emergency and trauma care for nurses and paramedics. 3rd ed. Chatswood NSW: Elsevier Australia; 2019.
7. Fry M, Shaban RZ, Considine J. Emergency nursing in Australia and New Zealand. In: Curtis K, Ramsden C, Shaban RZ, et al. (eds). Emergency and trauma care for nurses and paramedics. 3rd ed. Chatswood NSW: Elsevier Australia; 2019.
8. Jennings PA. Paramedicine in Australia and New Zealand. In: Curtis K, Ramsden C, Shaban RZ, et al. (eds). Emergency and trauma care for nurses and paramedics. 3rd ed. Chatswood NSW: Elsevier Australia; 2019.
9. Australian Commission on Safety and Quality in Health Care (ACSQHC). National Safety and Quality Health Service Standards. Sydney: Australian Commission on Safety and Quality in Health Care; 2011. Online: Available from: www.safetyandquality.gov.au/standards/nsqhs-standards.
10. Australian Commission on Safety and Quality in Health Care (ACSQHC). National Safety and Quality Health Service Standards. 2nd ed. Sydney: Australian Commission on Safety and Quality in Health Care; 2017. Online: Available from: www.safetyandquality.gov.au/wp-content/uploads/2017/12/National-Safety-and-Quality-Health-Service-Standards-second-edition.pdf.
11. Australian Commission on Safety and Quality in Health Care (ACSQHC). National Safety and Quality Health Service Standards. 2nd ed. Updated May 2021. Sydney: Australian Commission on Safety and Quality in Health Care; 2021. Online: Available from: www.safetyandquality.gov.au/publications-and-resources/resource-library/national-safety-and-quality-health-service-standards-second-edition.
12. Health Quality and Safety Commission New Zealand. Health Quality and Safety Commission Annual Report 2019–20. Wellington: Health Quality and Safety Commission New Zealand; 2021. Online: Available from: www.hqsc.govt.nz/assets/Core-pages/About-us/Annual-reports/AnnualReport2019-20.pdf.

13. Donabedian A. Evaluating the quality of medical care. Milbank Mem Fund Q 1966;44(3):166–206.
14. Donabedian A. The quality of care: how can it be assessed? J Am Med Assoc 1988;260(12):1743–8.
15. Donabedian A. Quality of care: problems of measurement. II. Some issues in evaluating the quality of nursing care. Am J Public Health Nations Health 1969;59(10):1833–6.
16. Institute of Medicine and Committee on Quality and Health Care in America. Crossing the quality chasm: a new health system for the 21st century. Washington DC: National Academy Press; 2001.
17. Australasian College for Emergency Medicine (ACEM). Quality standards for emergency departments and other hospital-based emergency care services. 2nd ed. West Melbourne: ACEM; 2021. Online: Available from: https://acem.org.au/getmedia/f4832c56-2b59-4654-815b-cdd1a66b27a8/ACEM_QualityStandardsEDs_Report.
18. SA Ambulance Service. NSQHS standards accreditation. Australas Ambulance 2018;Winter:33.
19. Lowthian JA, Curtis AJ, Jolley DJ, Stoelwinder JU, McNeil JJ, Cameron PA. Demand at the emergency department front door: 10-year trends in presentations. Med J Aust 2012;196(2):128–32.
20. Australian Institute of Health and Welfare (AIHW). Emergency department care 2020–2021. Canberra: AIHW; 2021. Online: Available from: www.aihw.gov.au/reports-data/myhospitals/sectors/emergency-department-care.
21. Fry M, Fitzpatrick L, Considine J, Shaban RZ, Curtis K. Emergency department utilisation among older people with acute and/or chronic conditions: a multi-centre retrospective study. Int Emerg Nurs 2018;37:39–43.
22. Andrew E, Nehme Z, Cameron P, Smith K. Drivers of increasing emergency ambulance demand. Prehosp Emerg Care 2020;24(3):385–93.
23. Institute of Medicine. To err is human: building a safer health system. Washington DC: The National Academies Press; 2000.
24. Australian Commission on Safety and Quality in Health Care. Hospital-acquired complications. 2019. Online: Available from: www.safetyandquality.gov.au/our-work/indicators/hospital-acquired-complications.
25. Nightingale F. Notes on nursing: what it is, and what it is not. New York: D Appleton and Company; 1860.
26. Duckett S, Jorm C, Danks L, Moran G. All complications should count: using our data to make hospitals safer. Melbourne: Grattan Institute; 2018.
27. Shaban RZ, Mitchell B, Russo P, Macbeth D. Epidemiology of healthcare-associated infections in Australia. Sydney: Elsevier Health Sciences; 2021.
28. Russo P, Mitchell B, Allen CC, Hall L. Healthcare-associated infection in Australia: tackling the 'known unknowns'. Aust Health Rev 2018;42(2): 178–80.
29. Shaban RZ. Tackling errors in healthcare: the rise of financial penalties for preventable hospital-acquired complications. Aust Hosp Healthcare Bull 2018;Autumn:22–3.
30. Ahern S, Evans S, Hopper I, Zalcberg J. Towards a strategy for clinical quality registries in Australia. Aust Health Rev 2019;43(3):284.
31. Hoque DME, Ruseckaite R, Lorgelly P, Mcneil JJ, Evans SM. Cross-sectional study of characteristics of clinical registries in Australia: a resource for clinicians and policy makers. Int J Qual Health Care 2018;30(3):192–9.
32. Griffiths P, Ball J, Murrells T, Jones S, Rafferty AM. Registered nurse, healthcare support worker, medical staffing levels and mortality in English hospital trusts: a cross-sectional study. BMJ Open 2016;6(2):e008751.
33. Aiken LH, Sloane DM, Bruyneel L, Van den Heede K, Griffiths P, Busse R, et al. Nurse staffing and education and hospital mortality in nine European countries: a retrospective observational study. Lancet 2014;383(9931):1824–30.
34. Aiken LH, Sloane D, Griffiths P, Bruyneel L, McHugh M, et al. Nursing skill mix in European hospitals: cross-sectional study of the association with mortality, patient ratings, and quality of care. BMJ Qual Saf 2017;26(7):559–68.
35. Aiken LH, Clarke SP, Sloane DM, Lake ET, Cheney T. Effects of hospital care environment on patient mortality and nurse outcomes. J Nurs Adm 2008;38(5):223–9.
36. McHugh MD, Aiken LH, Windsor C, Douglas C, Yates P. Case for hospital nurse-to-patient ratio legislation in Queensland, Australia, hospitals: an observational study. BMJ Open 2020;10(9):e036264.
37. Gomez-Urquiza JL, De la Fuente-Solana EI, Albendin-Garcia L, Vargas-Pecino C, Ortega-Campos EM, Canadas-De la Fuente GA. Prevalence of burnout syndrome in emergency nurses: a meta-analysis. Crit Care Nurse 2017;37(5):e1–9.
38. Vahedian-Azimi A, Hajiesmaeili M, Kangasniemi M, Fornes-Vives J, Hunsucker RL, Rahimibashar F, et al. Effects of stress on critical care nurses: a national cross-sectional study. J Intensive Care Med 2019;34(4):311–22.
39. Van Osch M, Scarborough K, Crowe S, Wolff AC, Reimer-Kirkham S. Understanding the factors which promote registered nurses' intent to stay in emergency and critical care areas. J Clin Nurs 2018;27(5–6):1209–15.
40. Salyers MP, Bonfils KA, Luther L, Firmin RL, White DA, Adams EL, et al. The relationship between professional burnout and quality and safety in healthcare: a meta-analysis. J Gen Inter Med 2017;32(4):475–82.
41. Garcia C, Abreu L, Ramos J, Castro C, Smiderle F, Santos J, Influence of burnout on patient safety: systematic review and meta-analysis. Medicina 2019;55(9):553.
42. Queensland Health. Nurse-to-patient ratios – frequently asked questions. 2016. Online. Available from: www.health.qld.gov.au/ocnmo/nursing/nurse-to-patient-ratios/nurse-patient-ratios-faqs.
43. State Government of Victoria. Safe Patient Care (Nurse to Patient and Midwife to Patient Ratios) Act 2015. Melbourne: Department of Health and Human Services, State Government of Victoria, Australia; 2015. Online. Available from: www.legislation.vic.gov.au/in-force/acts/safe-patient-care-nurse-patient-and-midwife-patient-ratios-act-2015/005.

44. Victorian Hospitals' Industrial Association. Nurses and Midwives (Victorian Public Sector) (Single Interest Employers) Enterprise Agreement 2020–2024. Melbourne: 2022. Online. Available from: www.anmfvic.asn.au/~/media/files/anmf/eba%202020/campaign%20updates/200120-NandM-EBA-master-clean.pdf.
45. New Zealand Nurses Organisation (NZNO). District Health Boards/NZNO Nursing and Midwifery Multi-Employer Collective Agreement (2 August 2020–21 October 2022). Wellington. Online. Available from: www.bopdhb.health.nz/media/2ydajwiy/nzno-meca-2-aug-2020-31-oct-2022-final-signed.pdf.
46. McHugh MD, Aiken LH, Sloane DM, Windsor C, Douglas C, Yates P. Effects of nurse-to-patient ratio legislation on nurse staffing and patient mortality, readmissions, and length of stay: a prospective study in a panel of hospitals. Lancet 2021;397(10288):1905–13.
47. Morphet J, Kent B, Plummer V, Plummer V, Considine J. Profiling nursing resources in Australian emergency departments. Australas Emerg Nurs J 2016;19(1):1–10.
48. State of Victoria DoHaHS. Guide to implementation of amendments to the Safe Patient Care (Nurse to Patient and Midwife to Patient Ratios) Act 2015. Melbourne: Department of Health & Human Services, State Government of Victoria, Australia; 2020. Online: Available from: www.health.vic.gov.au/sites/default/files/migrated/files/collections/policies-and-guidelines/g/guide-to-implementation-of-amendments-to-the-safe-patient-care-112020.pdf.
49. Queensland Nurses and Midwives Union. Ratios save lives phase 2: extending the guarantee. Brisbane: Queensland Nurses & Midwives Union; 2018. Online: Available from: www.qnmu.org.au/DocumentsFolder/Ratios%20website/Phase%202/Ratios%20Save%20Lives%20Phase%202%201017%20FINAL.pdf.
50. Needleman J. Nursing skill mix and patient outcomes. BMJ Qual Saf 2016;26(7):525–8.
51. O'Meara P, Duthie S. Paramedicine in Australia and New Zealand: a comparative overview. Aust J Rural Health 2018;26(5):363–8.
52. Wilkinson-Stokes M. A taxonomy of Australian and New Zealand paramedic clinical roles. Australas J Paramed 2021;18:1–20.
53. Aiken LH, Clarke SP, Cheung RB, et al. Educational levels of hospital nurses and surgical patient mortality. JAMA 2003;290(12):1617–23.
54. Lasater KB, Sloane DM, Mchugh MD, et al. Changes in proportion of bachelor's nurses associated with improvements in patient outcomes. Res Nurs Health 2021;44(5):787–95.
55. Aiken LH, Cimiotti JP, Cheung RB, Sloane DM, Silber JH. The effects of nurse staffing and nurse education on patient deaths in hospitals with different nurse work environments. Med Care 2011;49(12):1047–53.
56. Brooks IA, Grantham H, Spencer C, Archer F. A review of the literature: the transition of entry-level paramedic education in Australia from vocational to higher education (1961–2017). Australas J Paramed 2018;15(2). doi:10.33151/ajp.15.2.584.
57. Hefner JL, McAlearney AS, Spatafora N, Moffatt-Bruce SD. Beyond patient satisfaction: optimizing the patient experience. structural approaches to address issues in patient safety. In: Advances in health care management. Emerald Publishing; 2019.
58. LaVela SL, Gallan A. Evaluation and measurement of patient experience. Patient Exp J 2014;1(1):28–36.
59. Doyle C, Lennox L, Bell D. A systematic review of evidence on the links between patient experience and clinical safety and effectiveness. BMJ Open 2013;3(1):e001570.
60. Fry M, Chenoweth L, MacGregor C, Arendts G. Emergency nurses' perceptions of the role of families and carers in the care of cognitively impaired older person in pain: a qualitative study. Int J Nurs Stud 2015;52(8):1323–31.
61. Stein-Parbury J, Gallagher R, Fry M, Chenoweth L, Gallagher P. Expectations and experiences of older people and their carers in relation to emergency department arrival and care. Nurs Health Sci 2015;17(4):476–82.
62. Fry M, Elliott R, Murphy S, Curtis K. The role and contribution of family carers accompanying community-living older people with cognitive impairment to the emergency department: an interview study. J Clin Nurs 2021;31(7–8):975–84.
63. Fry M, Elliott R, Curtis K, Mei J, Fitzpatrick L, Groth R, et al. Family members' perceptions of older person discharge from emergency departments. Int J Older People Nurs 2021;16(3):e12365.
64. Reardon M, Abrahams R, Thyer L, Simpson P. Review article: prevalence of burnout in paramedics: a systematic review of prevalence studies. Emerg Med Australas 2020;32(2):182–9.
65. Adriaenssens J, De Gucht V, Maes S. Determinants and prevalence of burnout in emergency nurses: a systematic review of 25 years of research. Int J Nurs Stud 2015;52(2):649–61.
66. Slade D, Manidis M, McGregor J, Scheeres H, Chandler E, Stein-Parbury J, et al. The role of communication in safe and effective health care. In: Communicating in hospital emergency departments. Berlin, Heidelberg: Springer; 2015.
67. Wise S, Duffield C, Fry M, Roche M. A team mental model approach to understanding team effectiveness in an emergency department: a qualitative study. J Health Serv Res Policy 2022;27(1):14–21.
68. Wise S, Duffield C, Fry M, Roche M. Nurses' role in accomplishing interprofessional coordination: lessons in 'almost managing' an emergency department team. J Nurs Manag 2022;30(1):198–204.
69. Katz D, Blasius K, Isaak R, Lipps J, Kushelev M, Goldberg A, et al. Exposure to incivility hinders clinical performance in a simulated operative crisis. BMJ Qual Saf 2019;28(9):750–7.
70. Riskin A, Erez A, Foulk TA, Kugelman A, Gover A, Shoris I, et al. The impact of rudeness on medical team performance: a randomized trial. Pediatrics 2015;136(3):487–95.
71. Guo L, Ryan B, Leditschke IA, Haines KJ, Cook K, Eriksson L, et al. Impact of unacceptable behaviour between healthcare workers on clinical performance and patient outcomes: a systematic review. BMJ Qual Saf 31(9):679–87.

72. Eggins S, Slade D. Communication in clinical handover: improving the safety and quality of the patient experience. J Public Health Res 2015;4(3):666.
73. Murphy M, Curtis K, Lam MK, Palmer CS, Hsu J, McCloughen A. Simulation-based multidisciplinary team training decreases time to critical operations for trauma patients. Injury 2018;49(5):952–8.
74. Munroe B, Curtis K, Murphy M, Strachan L, Hardy J, Considine J, et al. A structured framework improves clinical patient assessment and non-technical skills of early career emergency nurses: a pre-post study using full immersion simulation. J Clin Nurs 2016;25(15–16):2262–74.
75. Grant KL, Bayley CJ, Premji Z, Lang E, Innes G. Throughput interventions to reduce emergency department crowding: a systematic review. CJEM 2020;22(6):864–74.
76. Austin EE, Blakely B, Tufanaru C, Selwood A, Braithwaite J, Clay-Williams R. Strategies to measure and improve emergency department performance: a scoping review. Scandinavian J Trauma Resusc Emerg Med 2020;28(1):55.
77. Pryce A, Unwin M, Kinsman L, McCann D. Delayed flow is a risk to patient safety: a mixed method analysis of emergency department patient flow. Int Emerg Nurs 2021;54:100956.
78. Cashin A, Waters CD, O'Connell J, Christofis L, Lentakis A, Rossi M, Clinical initiative nurses and nurse practitioners in the emergency department: what's in a name? Australas Emerg Nurs J 2007;10(2):73–9.
79. Putri AF, Tocher J, Chandler C. Emergency department nurses' role transition towards emergency nurse practitioner: a realist-informed review. Int Emerg Nurs 2022;60:101081.
80. Gardner G, Gardner A, Middleton S, Considine J, Fitzgerald G, Christofis L, et al. Mapping workforce configuration and operational models in Australian emergency departments: a national survey. Aust Health Rev 2018:42(3):340–7.
81. Duffield C, Gardner G, Chang AM, Fry M, Stasa H. National regulation in Australia: a time for standardisation in roles and titles. Collegian 2011;18(2):45–9.
82. Considine J, Shaban RZ, Curtis K, Fry M. Effectiveness of nurse-initiated X-ray for emergency department patients with distal limb injuries: a systematic review. Eur J Emerg Med 2019;26(5):314–22.
83. Varndell W, Fry M, Elliott D. Quality and impact of nurse-initiated analgesia in the emergency department: a systematic review. Int Emerg Nurs 2018;40:46–53.
84. Burgess L, Kynoch K, Theobald K, Keogh S. The effectiveness of nurse-initiated interventions in the emergency department: a systematic review. Australas Emerg Care 2021;24(4):248–54.
85. Nursing and Midwifery Board of Australia. Nurse practitioner standards for practice. 4th ed. Dickson, ACT: NMBA; 2021. Online: Available from: www.nursingmidwiferyboard.gov.au/Codes-Guidelines-Statements/Professional-standards/nurse-practitioner-standards-of-practice.aspx.
86. Lutze M, Fry M, Gallagher R. Minor injuries in older adults have different characteristics, injury patterns, and outcomes when compared with younger adults: an emergency department correlation study. Int Emerg Nurs 2015;23(2):168–73.
87. Lutze M, Fry M, Mullen G, O'Connell J, Coates D. Highlighting the invisible work of emergency nurse practitioners. J Nurs Pract 2018;14(1): 26-32.
88. Fox A, Gardner G, Osborne S. Nursing service innovation: a case study examining emergency nurse practitioner service sustainability. J Adv Nurs 2018;74(2):454–64.
89. Jennings N, Gardner G, O'Reilly G, Mitra B. Evaluating emergency nurse practitioner service effectiveness on achieving timely analgesia: a pragmatic randomized controlled trial. Acad Emerg Med 2015;22(6):676–84.
90. O'Meara P, Wingrove G, Nolan M. Frontier and remote paramedicine practitioner models. Rural Remote Health 2018;18(3):255–62.
91. Acker JJ, Johnston T. The demographic and clinical practice profile of Australian remote and industrial paramedics: findings from a workforce survey. Australas J Paramed 2021;18. doi:10.33151/ajp.18.959.
92. McCay R, Lyles AA, Larkey L. Nurse leadership style, nurse satisfaction, and patient satisfaction: a systematic review. J Nurs Care Quality 2018;33(4):361–7.
93. Agyeman-Prempeh C, Ndaago AI, Setordzi M, Abu P, Tia MB, Aboba TA, et al. Challenges to effective nursing leadership: a systematic review. 2021. doi:10.21203/rs.3.rs-948602/v1.
94. Yodang Y, Nuridah N. Nursing leadership models in promoting and improving patient's safety culture in healthcare facilities: a systematic review. Evid Based Health Policy, Manage Econ 2020.
95. Daly J, Speedy S, Jackson D. Leadership and nursing: contemporary perspective. Sydney: Elsevier; 2015.
96. Fry M, Elliott R, Fitzpatrick L, Warton J, Curtis K. Measuring nurses' perceptions of their work environment and linking with behaviour change theories and implementation strategies to support evidence based practice change. App Nurs Res 2020;56:151374.
97. Alshyyab MA, FitzGerald G, Dingle K, Ting J, Bowman P, Kinnear FB, et al. Developing a conceptual framework for patient safety culture in emergency department: a review of the literature. Int J Health Plann Manage 2019;34(1):42–55.
98. Grimshaw JM, Eccles MP, Lavis JN, Hill SJ, Squires JE. Knowledge translation of research findings. Implement Sci 2012;7(1):50.
99. Runciman WB, Hunt TD, Hannaford NA, Hibbert PD, Westbrook JI, Coiera EW, et al. CareTrack: assessing the appropriateness of health care delivery in Australia. Med J Aust 2012;197(2):100–5.
100. Harrison R, Hinchcliff RA, Manias E, Mears S, Heslop D, Walton V, et al. Can feedback approaches reduce unwarranted clinical variation? A systematic rapid evidence synthesis. BMC Health Serv Res 2020;20(1). doi:10.1186/s12913-019-4860-0.

101. Nouhi M, Hadian M, Jahangiri R, Hakimzadeh M, Gray S, Olyaeemanesh A. The economic consequences of practice style variation in providing medical interventions: a systematic review of the literature. J Educ Health Promot 2019;8(1):119.

102. Sutherland K, Levesque JF. Unwarranted clinical variation in health care: definitions and proposal of an analytic framework. J Eval Clin Prac 2020;26(3):687–96.

103. Australian Commission on Safety and Quality in Health Care, Welfare (AIHW). The fourth Australian Atlas of healthcare variation. Sydney, NSW: ACSQHC & AIHA; 2021. Online: Available from: www.safetyandquality.gov.au/publications-and-resources/australian-atlas-healthcare-variation-series.

104. National Stroke Foundation. National Stroke Audit. Acute Services Report 2021. Melbourne: National Stroke Foundation; 2021. Online: Available from: informme.org.au/stroke-data/Acute-audits.

105. National Health and Medical Research Council (NHMRC). Guidelines for guidelines handbook. n.d. Online. Available from: www.nhmrc.gov.au/guidelinesforguidelines.

106. Abbott TEF, Ahmad T, Phull MK, Fowler AJ, Hewson R, Biccard BM, et al. The surgical safety checklist and patient outcomes after surgery: a prospective observational cohort study, systematic review and meta-analysis. Br J Anaesth 2018;120(1):146–55.

107. Gilhooly D, Green SA, McCann C, Black N, Moonesinghe SR. Barriers and facilitators to the successful development, implementation and evaluation of care bundles in acute care in hospital: a scoping review. Implement Sci 2019;14(1). doi:10.1186/s13012-019-0894-2.

108. Curtis K, Kourouche S, Asha S, Considine J, Fry M, Middleton S, et al. Impact of a care bundle for patients with blunt chest injury (ChIP): a multicentre controlled implementation evaluation. PLOS ONE 2021;16(10):e0256027.

109. Kourouche S, Curtis K, Munroe B, Asha S, Carey I, Considine J, et al. Implementation of a hospital-wide multidisciplinary blunt chest injury care bundle (ChIP): fidelity of delivery evaluation. Aust Crit Care 2022;35(2):113–22.

110. Joseph-Williams N, Abhyankar P, Boland L, Bravo P, Brenner AT, Brodney S, et al. What works in implementing patient decision aids in routine clinical settings? A rapid realist review and update from the international patient decision aid standards collaboration. Med Decis Making 2021;41(7):907–37.

111. Sharma A, Harrington RA, McClellan MB, Turakhia MP, Eapen ZJ, Steinhubl S, et al. Using digital health technology to better generate evidence and deliver evidence-based care. J Am Coll Cardiol 2018;71(23):2680–90.

112. Sittig DF, Wright A, Coiera E, Magrabi F, Ratwani R, Bates DW, et al. Current challenges in health information technology–related patient safety. Health Informatics J 2020;26(1):181–9.

CHAPTER 7
RESEARCH FOR EMERGENCY CARE

JULIE CONSIDINE, RAMON Z. SHABAN, MARGARET FRY, PAUL SIMPSON AND KATE CURTIS

ESSENTIALS

- Emergency clinicians require capability (knowledge and skills), opportunity and motivation to evaluate research studies and determine that they have sufficient rigour to provide findings that are reliable, useful and safe for practice.
- When formulating a research question, always ask yourself about the significance of the research for knowledge, practice, education, workforce or policy. Your research should answer the following questions: What do we know? What don't we know? What should we know? Why should we know it? In answering these questions, you will be able to discern a research question from the problem statement.
- Research questions should always be clear and concise. Research may not be viable if:
  - it is expensive to undertake and there is little or no funding
  - it is poorly or incorrectly designed
  - there are barriers to accessing data or sufficient data relative to the methodology
  - data collection procedures are overly complex or onerous.
- Make sure before you attempt even a pilot project that you have sufficient funding or resources to undertake the project.
- Engage a mentor or a supervisor to guide you with your research from the beginning, especially if you are an inexperienced researcher. Seek out opportunities to join and contribute actively to an established research team or group and begin to establish your own research track record.
- All researchers must act ethically, with honesty and integrity, throughout the research process, including publication of the findings, irrespective of whether the findings were positive or negative, significant or not.
- When planning your research, be sure to consider how you will disseminate the findings through publications, presentations, social media and professional events.

INTRODUCTION

Research, the systematic search for new knowledge, is essential for the continuing evolution of professional emergency nursing and paramedicine practice. It is the foundation to evidence-based decision-making and the provision of quality emergency

care. Importantly, it provides the necessary basis to challenge our practice and goes beyond intuition, traditional behavioural norms and opinion. Evidence gained from scholarly research informs practice decisions and enables practice change and improvement. Evidence-based care is reliant on the best available research findings, patient preferences and available resources, and is essential to safe, effective and efficient healthcare that meets the expectations of patients, families and colleagues. Where the evidence for practice is strong, protocols based on the research findings should guide clinical practice. This chapter provides an overview of the basics of the research process and assists you to read and understand research literature. In this chapter, emergency clinicians are encouraged to support and engage in collaborative research as part of research teams to identify new knowledge and/or evaluate the outcomes of practice change.

EVIDENCE-BASED PRACTICE

Evidence-based practice started with Professor Archie Cochrane, who, in the late 1970s, made the statement:

> It is a great criticism of our profession that we have not organised a critical summary, by speciality or subspeciality, adapted periodically, of all relevant randomised controlled trials.[1]

More contemporary definitions of evidence-based practice include the 'conscientious, explicit and judicious use of current best evidence in making decisions about the care of individual patients'[2] and the 'integration of best research evidence with clinical expertise and patient values'.[3] Evidence-based practice has changed the way nurses and paramedics make clinical decisions and how they behave in practice.[4] Rather than make decisions about practice actions based on routine or how one was taught, there are professional and consumer expectations that nurses and paramedics will translate the best available evidence as a basis for all clinical decisions and behaviours. Other considerations in the application, evaluation and translation of research evidence include the clinical expertise of the healthcare professional, the acceptability of evidence to specific patients, the context of practice and the availability of resources. Consequently, evidence-based healthcare requires a whole-of-organisation approach to the translation of evidence, whereby clinicians are engaged across all disciplines, and includes support staff, managers and policy-makers.[4,5]

LEVELS OF EVIDENCE

Evidence generated from research is classified according to the research design. These classifications are called 'levels of evidence' and organise evidence in a hierarchical structure according to quality. The levels of evidence reflect the degree of confidence in the research findings. The most commonly used system of rating the quality of evidence and strength of recommendations is GRADE: Grading of Recommendations, Assessment, Development and Evaluation.[6] The GRADE system classifies the certainty of evidence as high, moderate, low or very low (Table 7.1).[7] A high recommendation means that further research is unlikely to change our confidence in the estimate of effect, while very low means that any estimate of effect is very uncertain.[6,7] The GRADE system also has two classifications of recommendation: strong and weak. Strong recommendations are made when the desirable effects of an intervention clearly outweigh the undesirable effects.[7] Weak recommendations are made when there is less certainty, either because the quality of evidence is low or because there are both desirable and undesirable effects. The factors that influence the strength of recommendation are the quality of evidence, uncertainty about the balance between desirable and undesirable effects, uncertainty or variability in values and references and uncertainty about whether an intervention is a sound use of resources.[7] The National Health and Medical Research Council (NHMRC) has also moved to using the GRADE system and considers GRADE to be the international standard for guideline development.[8]

TABLE 7.1 GRADE QUALITY OF EVIDENCE AND DEFINITIONS[7]

High quality	Further research is very unlikely to change our confidence in the estimate of effect
Moderate quality	Further research is likely to have an important impact on our confidence in the estimate of effect and may change the estimate
Low quality	Further research is very likely to have an important impact on our confidence in the estimate of effect and is likely to change the estimate
Very low quality	Any estimate of effect is very uncertain

Reproduced from BMJ, Guyatt et al, vol. 7650, pp. 924–6, © 2008 with permission from BMJ Publishing Group.

While GRADE was traditionally used to appraise evidence from quantitative studies,[6] there are many important research questions that can only be answered using qualitative methods. In 2018, GRADE-CERQual (Confidence in the Evidence from Reviews of Qualitative Research) was published[9] to provide guidance for assessing confidence in the findings from systematic reviews of qualitative research or qualitative evidence syntheses. Assessment of confidence using CERQual is based on four key considerations: i) methodological limitations, ii) coherence, iii) adequacy of data, and iv) relevance.[9]

PRACTICE TIP

To source evidence and enhance your research knowledge and skills:

- enrol in a postgraduate degree that includes coursework in research methods
- subscribe to emergency care journals, such as *Australasian Emergency Care*
- attend seminars and conferences relevant to emergency practice.

RESEARCH AND THE PROCESS

Research is a process used to generate knowledge about a problem or reality using a systematic and logical series of steps.[10] Research is frequently classified as taking one of two approaches: quantitative (numerical), moving from more general concepts to specific observations or hypothesis testing or qualitative (narrative), in which specific subjective observations move to general concepts or theories.[10,11] Many studies in emergency care use a combination of both approaches, to gain a deeper and richer understanding of phenomena, and are referred to as 'mixed methods'. There are many different mixed-methods research design, and all are suitable for the complexity of emergency settings. Further detail on mixed-methods research can be found in textbooks by authors such as Creswell[12] or Field and Morse.[13] Field and Morse wrote that while the steps in qualitative research are less encapsulated than those in quantitative research, they are seen to flow in the same directions and together offer a richer understanding of the phenomena under interest.[13]

Within these two classifications there is a variety of methods available to researchers to answer research questions or problems. Clinicians reading journal articles to inform their practice require a basic knowledge of research elements or steps, because these elements are reflected in the way journal articles are traditionally structured and presented. New researchers obviously require a more comprehensive understanding of research processes. It is advisable for new researchers to seek support in selecting an appropriate approach and method from more experienced colleagues or from supervisors, prior to proposal submission to a human research ethics committee and prior to the collection of any data even for a pilot study. Larger research projects are usually undertaken by a research team involving a group of clinicians from one discipline, or members from various disciplinary groups. The term 'collaborative' is used to refer to research groups formed through a varied membership. For example, a research team may include doctors, pharmacists, nurses and paramedics, as well as a psychologist, a communication expert and a statistician.

The following section provides an overview of the elements of the research process as a beginning point. There are many excellent research texts written by experienced researchers which you are encouraged to read for detailed explanations of research concepts.[10–12,14]

IDENTIFICATION OF A RESEARCH PROBLEM OR PHENOMENON

Clinical research starts with a question, a problem or a phenomenon of interest. An identified problem may concern patient care or a clinical problem, nurses, systems of administration or any issue of nursing or paramedical interest. Research problems generally address practice differences or discrepancies, and what clinicians consider is ideal or desirable for the patient. At this stage the question needs to be asked if the problem or difference is something that really matters, is able to be researched and whether it relates to more general conceptual issues. However, deciding on and formulating a specific research question is often difficult for the beginning researcher. One starting point is for nurses and paramedics to reflect on their personal and clinical experiences as an initial source of potentially researchable problems. An observation and reflection can be turned into a question, which can start a research plan.

For example: I wonder …

- if administration of intravenous adrenaline (epinephrine) during cardiac arrest increases survival to hospital discharge with favourable neurological outcome?
- if the early management with humidified high-flow nasal oxygen, physiotherapy and multi-modal analgesia in patients with blunt chest trauma decreases complications?
- if the use of cervical spinal immobilisation in trauma patients is beneficial or harmful?
- how emergency nurses and paramedics feel when resuscitation is terminated?
- how emergency nurses and paramedics interact with each other during patient handover?

At this early stage of the research process it is usually necessary to 'refine' the problem area or phenomenon to form a question that enables a search of the literature by the use of key terms. It is usually possible to discuss ideas with a colleague who has some research experience, or if you have a mentor from your own or other disciplinary areas, seek their advice. The PICO format: **P**atient (or population), **I**ntervention (drug, diagnostic test, model of care), **C**omparison (other drug, test or intervention) and **O**utcome, is commonly used to refine a research idea into an answerable question.[15] The PICO format can be used to clarify and refine a research idea about the effectiveness of an intervention or process of care into an answerable research question (Table 7.2). For questions that are qualitative in nature, the SPIDER format is an alternative to PICO: Sample, Phenomenon

TABLE 7.2 PICO QUESTIONS: PATIENT (OR POPULATION), INTERVENTION (DRUG, DIAGNOSTIC TEST, MODEL OF CARE), COMPARISON (OTHER DRUG, TEST OR INTERVENTION) AND OUTCOME

	EXAMPLE 1	EXAMPLE 2	EXAMPLE 3
P	In adult patients in cardiac arrest	In adult patients with blunt chest trauma	In patients with suspected spinal injury
I	Does the use of intravenous adrenaline (epinepherine)...	Does the use of humidified high-flow nasal oxygen, physiotherapy and multi-modal analgesia as a bundle of care...	Does the use of spinal immobilisation (hard collars, back boards, sand bags, head blocks)...
C	compared with no adrenaline...	compared with usual practice...	compared with no immobilisation...
O	improve survival to hospital discharge with favourable neurological function?	decrease complications – in-hospital death – the need for and duration of non-invasive ventilation – pneumonia?	affect outcomes – neurological outcome – prevention of movement – complications – pain?

of Interest, Design, Evaluation, Research type.[16] As you can see, the PICO and SPIDER formats force you to clearly define your population, the intervention and the outcomes.

The refinement process continues until each term (variable) within the research question is defined. Even at this early point it is important to be very clear about each term or variable, and it can be useful to define your use of a term to ensure you are clear about the meaning you are trying to communicate to others.[15] Other sources of potential research questions are the recommendations for further research in many published research reports. When reviewing research articles, a nurse or paramedic may identify research questions based on the state of the science about a given area or clinical problem. The same research question answered in a publication can be asked again in a different country to verify the findings of the primary study (replication), or for a different sample of patients or clients. When an aspect of practice is changed, based on the available evidence, it is useful to evaluate the impact of that change by measuring the outcomes of the change in a specific location, institution or service. The evaluation of outcomes could be a measure of cost changes or staff time, as well as the impact on patients or clients.

SEARCHING AND REVIEWING THE LITERATURE

The purpose of the literature search is to identify published research work conducted previously in the particular area of interest to assist the researcher to clarify and specify the research problem and to identify whether similar studies have already been published. The statement of the problem or research question is used to guide the literature search question. For example, in a systematic review of the effectiveness of nurse-initiated x-ray for emergency department (ED) patients with distal limb injury, search terms included:[17]

- 'emergency' OR 'emergency department*' OR 'emergency room*' OR 'accident and emergency' OR 'A&E' OR 'emergency medicine' OR 'emergency nursing' OR 'ED' OR 'ER' OR 'emergency care' OR 'emergency service' OR 'trauma centres' OR 'accident and emergency department' OR 'emergency departments' OR 'emergency ward' OR 'hospital emergency service'
- 'nurs*' OR 'nurs*?initiated' OR 'triage' OR 'triage nurs*' OR 'registered nurse' OR 'nursing staff' OR 'registered nurses' OR 'nursing personnel'
- 'x-ray*' OR 'radiograph*' OR 'imaging' OR 'diagnostic imaging' OR 'radiological' OR 'x-ray therapy' OR 'roentgenography' OR 'diagnostic x-ray' OR 'diagnostic x-ray radiology' OR 'roentgen rays'.

Electronic searches of databases, such as the Cumulative Index for Nursing and Allied Health Literature (CINAHL), Medline, PubMed or EMBASE, normally start with broad terms and then the search is narrowed. It is often worthwhile to ask a librarian to check that you have identified all the appropriate databases, if you are unsure. Once you start the search with specific terms, keywords can be combined to narrow the search output; for example, 'spinal injuries' and 'spinal immobilisation' as a combined search term will provide references containing both terms. MeSH is the Medical Index of Subject Headings and was established in 1960 as a comprehensive vocabulary that is maintained for the purpose of indexing journal articles and books in the life sciences.[18] It is a useful resource when developing keywords for database searches. You can also limit your search by checking specifications such as the language the article is written in and the year of publication. Depending on the nature of the question, it may be appropriate to explore 'grey' literature in addition to published literature. 'Grey' literature refers to reports relating to research published outside the traditional commercial or academic publishing process. OpenDOAR and BASE are examples of search portals used to search for and identify grey literature. Once you have a listing of the articles, you move to the next stage of the review process.[15]

It takes practice to read each section of a research article and understand exactly what is meant. If this process is new to you, re-reading articles will enable better comprehension of the meaning of the text. Many ways to achieve an informed read have been suggested. For example, some people skim over the article first before focusing on any particular sections. Others read the abstract several times. You will choose your preferred method, which might include making notes in the margins or using a bibliographic software package. When you understand each section, you then need to judge if the sections are consistent in answering the research question. For example, you would consider whether the research design can answer the question asked, whether the sample was selected appropriately and is of a sufficient size, whether data were analysed according to the design and whether the results answered the question/s asked.

After reading and critiquing previous research in a specific area, the reviewer summarises what has been previously studied. This summary of previous research findings is helpful in making decisions about the usefulness or significance of the evidence to inform practice decisions. If the reviewer is interested in undertaking new research, how this new study will contribute to the state of the science can be delineated. A thorough review reinforces the need for the study in light of previous research findings, and what is accepted as truth from other studies is the groundwork on which new studies or replication studies are based. A written literature review will include summaries of articles in which the conclusions may differ from or agree with the proposed point of view.

Sources of information for literature reviews can include both primary and secondary sources. A primary source of information is the description of an investigation written by the person who conducted it. A secondary source is a description of a study written by someone other than the original researcher. Both sources can be helpful, but written literature reviews should be based on primary sources whenever it is possible to locate those primary sources. A secondary source is useful when the primary source is unavailable, or when the secondary source is providing a different perspective or emphasis to the primary source. At times, grey literature is useful and includes sources such as government reports, professional associations and blogs summarising evidence; however, the cited references and authority of the sources should always be considered. If the topic is a general practice issue, such as the emergency management of patients with abdominal pain, it is important to check whether a systematic review (scientific summary) has been undertaken. Librarians at your local hospital are generally more than willing to assist with the sourcing of literature. If you are enrolled in tertiary education, your college or university faculty librarians can be consulted for assistance.

PRACTICE TIP

Check the literature for a systematic review on the chosen topic before looking for single articles. The review will identify the 'strongest' articles and provide a summary of the evidence for you to read.

Comprehensive literature searches and reviews should be systematic and detail the critical review of scholarly papers, government reports, unpublished works and even personal communications. Emergency clinicians need to be able to critically review to deliver evidence-based care. The critical review process can be assisted by using a series of appraisal questions that are based on the elements of the research process.[15] When the literature review process is complete, the reviewer summarises and synthesises all information on the topic into a written summary. If a research study is subsequently conducted, ongoing updates of the literature need to be undertaken to ensure the literature review remains current.

THEORETICAL AND CONCEPTUAL FRAMEWORKS

Theoretical and conceptual frameworks provide a structure to guide the study of clinical problems. A *theoretical framework* defines the concepts and proposes relationships among those concepts. It enables the findings of the researcher's study to be linked to existing knowledge. A framework consists of definitions of concepts and propositions about the relationships of those concepts to each other. It helps to interpret beliefs about what is observed, and provides a systematic way to organise information about a particular aspect of interest in a research study.[19]

Two components of a theory are *concepts* and a statement of *propositions*. *Concepts*, the building blocks of a theory, are abstract characteristics, categories or labels of things, persons or events. Examples of concepts employed by nurses and paramedics are health, stress, adaptation, caring and pain. *Propositions* are statements that define the relationships among concepts. A set of propositions may state that one concept is associated with another or is contingent upon another. Examples of theories are critical social theory, systems and adaptation theory. The power of theories lies in the ability to explain the relationship of variables and the nature of this relationship. Theories also help stimulate research by giving direction.[19] *Conceptual frameworks* represent a less-well-developed system for organising phenomena. Frameworks contain concepts that represent a common theme, but lack the deductive system of propositions which gives the relationship among concepts. Research grounded in clinical practice often uses conceptual frameworks rather than theories because they tend to be more flexible and descriptive and often draw on one or more theories.[20] These conceptual frameworks can lay the groundwork for more formal theories.[19]

Each methodology in qualitative research has a basic belief system that is manifest in the particular conventions of sampling, data collection, data management and auditing, analyses and conceptualisation that the researcher is required to follow. If no existing theory or conceptual framework has been applied to the phenomenon of interest, the researcher chooses a methodological approach that will enable the research question to be explored. For example, Fry used an exploratory descriptive qualitative methodology to explore and describe the role of family carers accompanying the older person with a cognitive impairment to the ED, and of their support by family during emergency care and in preparation for discharge home in the community (see Research Highlight 7.1).[21] A different qualitative method, the Delphi technique, was used by Considine, Curtis, Shaban and Fry[15] to establish the clinical research priorities for Australian emergency nursing. Using this method, the researchers sent the results of the research questions back to the respondents for further refinement. The number of times this process occurs varies for each situation, but the process usually continues until a predetermined consensus rate is reached by all respondents. In this project, 48 research themes were identified by emergency nurses and then ranked according to priority. The end-result of this process was 17 research themes organised into four research priority areas.

Exploratory or explanatory studies may use 'mixed methods'. That is, qualitative data are collected as well as quantitative data, with the intent of integrating data to achieve a richer understanding of a situation or the phenomena under study. In mixed-methods studies, the numerical results (quantitative data) are further explored and understood through the collection of qualitative data obtained from what participants say or write. For example, in a study of patient participation in nursing handover, data from observations of nursing handovers were combined

RESEARCH HIGHLIGHT 7.1

Study using a quantitative design[21]

Title—The role and contribution of family carers accompanying community-living older people with cognitive impairment to the emergency department: An interview study

Aim—To explore and describe the role and contribution of family carers accompanying the older person with cognitive impairment to the ED

Method—Exploratory descriptive qualitative study in three metropolitan emergency departments in Sydney, Australia. Telephone interviews were conducted with 28 family carers: five interviews were conducted with the family carer and older person together.

Results—Reflexive thematic analysis resulted in three themes: i) 'communicating knowledge of the older person's health status and usual behaviour'; ii) 'providing advocacy, translation, surrogacy and care co-ordination'; and iii) 'ensuring safe transition from the emergency department to home'.

Conclusions—Family carers created an important safety net while the older person was in the ED, through advocacy and the communication of vital health information. Family carers' knowledge influenced the older person's healthcare management and was a key factor in safe discharge and care coordination in the community.

RESEARCH HIGHLIGHT 7.2

Study using mixed methods[22]

Title—Enhancing active patient participation in nursing handover: A mixed-methods study

Aim—To explore: i) the frequency and nature of patient participation in nursing handover and ii) patients' and nurses' perceived strategies to enhance patient involvement in nursing handover.

Method—A multi-site prospective mixed-methods study design; 117 nursing handovers were observed on ten randomly selected wards followed by semi-structured interviews with 33 patients and 20 nurses.

Results—Patients were active participants in 33.3% and passive participants in 46.7% of handovers; in 20% of handovers the patient had no input at all. Active participation was more likely in women (vs men), surgical patients (vs medical patients) and when nurses displayed engagement behaviours (eye contact, opportunity to ask questions, explanations). Three major themes were identified from the interviews: 'Being involved', 'Layers of influence' and 'Information exchange'.

Conclusion—There was a low level of patient participation in nursing handover, even when conducted at the bedside. Patients' preferences to participate in nursing handover were variable. Both patients and nurses considered accurate and consistent communication delivered in an open, honest and clear format to be important. There was conflict between patients' views who did not want information withheld, and nurses' concern to protect sensitive information.

with data from semi-structured interviews with patients and nurses[22] (see Research Highlight 7.2). The other two common mixed-methods designs are the sequential exploratory model, in which qualitative data are collected first followed by the quantitative, and the convergent design in which the quantitative and qualitative data are collected concurrently.[12]

RESEARCH QUESTIONS OR HYPOTHESES

As previously stated, before a problem can be researched it must be focused and refined, so that it is possible to develop a research design (plan) that can potentially answer the problem or question of interest. The research interest can be stated as a research question or as a hypothesis. The term 'research question' is used in qualitative approaches where findings are presented as narrative themes or theories. A research question also directs the processes of numerical descriptive studies. Quantitative research questions that are used in descriptive studies should be specific and not attempt to describe too much, because data analysis may be complex and confusing to interpret. A research project can (and frequently does) answer more than one question or hypothesis in the same study. As previously mentioned, research questions and hypotheses should define key variables or terms.

Questions formulated about what will occur in specific situations in quantitative approaches are called *hypotheses*. Hypotheses are tested to identify significant associations between variables or significant differences between groups and to determine how results fit existing theory. A hypothesis expands on a research question because it is a tentative prediction or explanation of the relationship between two or more variables,[23] which the researcher postulates before the initiation of the research study. For example, one hypothesis might be that adults (20–50 years of age) with severe abdominal pain who are managed with a nurse-led pain protocol soon after arrival in the ED will report a perception of better management (satisfaction) than will adults with similar presentations who wait longer to see a doctor and have delayed analgesia. In this example, the researcher is postulating not only a relationship between the time of treating pain and adults' perception of better management (satisfaction), but is also predicting an outcome from this relationship. The null (or 'no effect') hypothesis indicates that the two populations (the sample of adults treated quickly for pain and the sample of adults with delayed pain treatment) have the same perceptions of hospital management (satisfaction) score. Therefore, the *null* hypothesis, stated as 'there is no relationship between the length of time waiting for analgesia and satisfaction' or 'there will be no difference in the satisfaction scores between the two groups', is generated as a position of non-bias towards finding the result the researcher seeks, as well as guiding the statistical analyses and discussion.[10,11]

There are different kinds of variables for hypotheses. An independent variable is what is assumed to cause or thought to be associated with the dependent or outcome variable. Changes in the dependent variable are presumed to depend on the independent variable's effects. The dependent variable is explained through its relationship with the independent variable, and it is what the researcher wants to explain or understand. The dependent variable in the example above is 'adults' perceptions of better management (satisfaction score)'. The independent variable is 'the time taken to provide the adult in pain with analgesia'. It is known that while many factors affect an adult's perception of good hospital management (satisfaction), only one independent variable (time to analgesia) is intended to be measured in the proposed research question to keep the variables under consideration specific and clear.[10,11]

Often the dependent (outcome) variable can be the result of several influences (factors), such as (in our example) age of the participant, gender or pain level. A study might be designed to examine several factors and their impact on a phenomenon or dependent variable. For example, you may want to know whether experience with triage or an educational program concerning triage influences the ability to perform triage adequately. Both independent variables (education and experience) can influence triage performance ability (dependent variable). Another research design could have several dependent or outcome variables designated as measures of treatment effectiveness. An example of multiple dependent variables identified in a research question is, 'Does a comprehensive triage system influence length of stay in the ED, patient satisfaction and patient outcome?' In this question it is proposed that the length of stay in ED, patient satisfaction and patient outcome are all dependent on the system of triage.[10,11]

METHOD

The method section of a research study identifies how the researcher plans to implement the research study to answer the research questions or test the hypotheses. The components of the method section include:

- the study design
- participants or subjects in the study, commonly labelled the sample
- the study procedure, which describes how data will be collected and analysed
- the measures used to collect data, including any instruments (tools), such as a questionnaire or an apparatus such as a thermometer.

It is essential that the validity of an instrument (basically, testing what it purports to be testing) and its reliability (consistency of results over repeated use) are established prior to data collection. In some cases, a questionnaire will require testing in a pilot study to establish validity and reliability prior to the main study being conducted. Then these results are reported in the section discussing the instrument. A description of how data will be analysed is also required. Box 7.1 identifies some commonly used quantitative approaches.

DESIGN

The study design tells a reader how the research is planned. Each different approach/method incorporates a way of structuring the study, selecting participants and collecting and analysing data. There are several literature review designs: systematic review, scoping review and integrative review: each are a study in their own right, but they serve different purposes. A systematic review is used when the researchers have a precise and clearly defined question and their aim is to identify, evaluate and summarise the available research evidence.[24] A scoping review is a useful method when the research question is less well developed and researchers wish to undertake a 'horizon scan' or map the research related to a specific topic.[24] In a scoping review, the outcome is the characteristics, concepts, methods or outcomes of studies to date rather than clinical outcomes derived from a systematic review.[24] If the topic to be explored requires use of a diverse range of data sources and the aim is to understand the current state of research evidence and synthesise different theoretical or philosophical positions, then an integrative review is an appropriate study design.[25,26]

In quantitative research, the design statement includes information on the variables: whether the variable (also called a factor) has different levels or classes, such as high and low, the number of groups participating in the research, and the occasions on which data will be collected. For example, in a design that is called a pre-test/post-test design, an experimental or treatment group and a control group (two randomly selected or matched groups) will be tested for the variable (e.g. physical fitness) before the experimental group is given a treatment or intervention that

BOX 7.1 RESEARCH USING QUANTITATIVE RESEARCH APPROACHES[10,11]

- Descriptive research is a means of discovering new meanings by describing what exists, or the frequency at which something occurs, or the categorising of information. Descriptive studies provide the knowledge base and potential hypotheses to direct correlational or experimental studies subsequently. Descriptive data can be obtained by auditing records, observations of events or by questionnaires. Descriptive studies undertaken over a long time period (months and years) are called longitudinal.
- Correlational research involves the investigation of relationships between two or more variables. The strength or degree of a relationship between variables can be measured and a numerical coefficient provided that identifies the strength of the relationship. Where two variables are strongly related, by knowing the value of one variable, it is possible to predict the likely value of the other. It is important to note that a significant relationship between two variables does not imply that one variable caused the other.
- Experimental research is defined as an objective, systematic, controlled investigation for the purpose of examining causality. That is, the intervention and nothing else is responsible for the result. Experimental or comparative studies have three main characteristics: controlled manipulation of the treatment or independent variable (one group gets the treatment and the other group doesn't), treatment and control groups, and each subject has an equal chance of random selection for either the treatment or the control group (randomisation). This design is considered to provide the highest level of research evidence for an individual study, when the researcher does not know what intervention the subject received. That is, the researcher is 'blind' to knowing what group the subject is in or whether the subject received the treatment or not. It is often difficult in nursing for an investigator to be 'blind' to an intervention, because the treatment or intervention can be identified, even when the researcher is not informed. An example is a study to compare patient outcomes from the use of peripherally inserted central lines and midline lines for low irritant antibiotic administration. Even when patients are randomly assigned to type, the investigator monitoring the outcomes will know what has been inserted from expert knowledge of the different vascular access devices.
- Quasi-experimental research is used to explain relationships and/or clarify why certain events occur. This design is not considered to be as 'controlled' as experimental studies, because there is a lack of control over the setting or the intervention or the subjects have not been assigned randomly. This design is useful in some clinical situations where the population receiving the intervention is very small, or where random assignment of subjects to a control group is not possible because of ethical considerations (see Research Highlight 7.5).
- Mixed methods: some studies combine both qualitative and quantitative methods. An investigator may choose to do this because of small populations or difficulty sampling from a large population because of access restrictions. In a research study, the method of data collection may include narrative data about a phenomenon provided by a sufferer of an illness combined with physiological measures of the illness. Mixed methods are often used in case study research.

RESEARCH HIGHLIGHT 7.3

Study using a randomised crossover trial design[27]

Title—Impact of hand dominance on effectiveness of chest compressions in a simulated setting: a randomised, crossover trial

Aim—To investigate the impact of hand dominance on effectiveness of ECC.

Method—This was a single-blinded, prospective randomised crossover trial design. Using a simulation manikin and health science students, Group 1 ($n = 37$) performed 3 minutes of chest compressions with their dominant hand on the chest and non-dominant hand supporting, followed by a 'rest and recovery' period and then a second 3-minute period of chest compressions with the hand reversed such that the non-dominant hand was on the chest. Group 2 ($n = 38$) performed the same series of chest compressions in the reverse order.

Results—There was no significant difference in CPR scores between groups (69.9% (SD = 29.9) vs 69.1% (SD = 34.1) ($p = 0.92$)). There were also no differences in compression rate and depth, though compression release was improved when the dominant hand was on the chest (53% vs 42%) ($p = 0.02$).

Conclusion—In a simulation context there was no difference in chest compression effectiveness according to placement of the dominant or non-dominant hand on the chest during compressions. A modest improvement in chest compression release was seen in the dominant hand on chest group.

the control group will not receive. Following the treatment or intervention, both groups are re-tested within a similar timeframe for physical fitness. The pre-test/post-test design seeks to determine if a treatment or intervention had any effect on physical fitness while controlling for extraneous or outside events the researcher has no control over. The pre-test results from both groups should be similar, or at least not statistically different, indicating that both groups started with a similar level of fitness. Following the intervention, if fitness is statistically different in the two groups (called significantly different), then the researcher can conclude that the treatment or intervention had some effect that changed the level of fitness of the group receiving it. A randomised crossover design has been used in Research Highlight 7.3, where Cross and colleagues examined the impact of hand dominance on chest compression effectiveness.[27]

In qualitative research, the design statement reflects the research approach and method, for example, the constructivist-interpretive, feminist or critical approaches.[28]

RECRUITMENT AND SAMPLING

Robust sampling methods in quantitative studies ensure that the research results are accurate, representative of the population and generalisable to other populations.[29] It is usually not feasible, practical or necessary to study everyone from the population of interest, therefore sampling is used to derive a group of participants from a population to conduct the study.[29] When designing quantitative studies and the sampling methods, researchers are trying to minimise the risk of sampling error and bias. Sampling error occurs when the sampling method results in random imprecision, for example, a study shows a difference between the sample and the population due to chance.[29] Sampling bias occurs when the sampling methods result in study participants not being representative of the population, for example, if participants are self-selected or if there is non-response or non-participation bias.[29]

There is a range of different sampling methods for designing studies. *Probability sampling* relies on random selection (e.g. a table of random numbers) to choose the subjects or units to be sampled; any member of the defined population has an equal chance of being selected. A number of inclusion criteria will be identified by the researcher. These might be the participant's (subject's) age, gender, illness diagnosis or language spoken. Potential participants who do not meet the inclusion criteria are excluded from the study. A statistical technique, known as 'power analysis', is used by researchers to estimate the sample size required to get an accurate result when data are analysed.[10,11]

Non-probability sampling is used in both qualitative and quantitative methods. There are different types of non-probability sampling, including accidental or convenience, quota, purposive and snowballing. Accidental samples are based on convenience of gathering subjects, such as surveying the first 100 patients in the ED on a particular day. Quota samples are used when a researcher knows an element of the population and bases sampling on the known representativeness within the population. For example, if a researcher knows that 25% of emergency nurses are males, the researcher attempts to ensure that 25% of the sample of emergency nurses selected for a study of emergency nurses are male. This technique improves the representativeness of the population within the sample.

Purposive sampling occurs when a researcher 'hand-picks' cases to be included in the sample that represent the typical subjects within a given population based on predetermined criteria or characteristics. A study may use purposive sampling to ensure a variety of responses or because the choices are judged to be typical of a specific population or matching samples (see Research Highlight 7.4). Purposive sampling is said to provide information-rich cases for in-depth study in qualitative research.

Snowball sampling is used in qualitative or quantitative research to locate participants who might be difficult for the researcher to identify. Researchers access the networks of participants who meet the inclusion criteria to locate other participants. Qualitative methods require a direct relationship between the researcher and the research participants because data are collected through in-depth interviews or direct encounters in focus groups. This level of direct relationship may not be required in quantitative research; for example, the use of questionnaires or surveys where the respondent may be anonymous. Participants may not benefit directly from participating in a research study, but give informed consent to be involved because they want to progress the development of knowledge for the benefit of others. Some researchers provide a financial or material incentive, such as a small amount of money or a movie ticket, as a token of appreciation for the participant's time. The use of incentives for recruitment and sampling must be approved by the governing human research ethics committee, which is explored later in this chapter.

RESEARCH HIGHLIGHT 7.4

Study using a retrospective cohort design[30]

Title—COVID-19 in Australia: Our national response to the first cases of SARS-CoV-2 infection during the early biocontainment phase

Aim—To report the clinical and epidemiological features, laboratory data and outcomes of the first group of 11 returned travellers with COVID-19 in Australia.

Method—Retrospective, multi-centre case series. All patients with confirmed COVID-19 infection were admitted to tertiary referral hospitals in New South Wales, Queensland, Victoria and South Australia.

Results—The median patient age was 42 years: six were men and five were women. Nine patients had returned from China (Wuhan $n = 8$ and Shenzhen $n = 1$), one from Japan and one from Europe. In two cases, there was possible human-to-human transmission from close family contacts in gatherings overseas. Symptoms on admission were fever, cough and sore throat ($n = 9\%$). No patients required intensive care unit admission or mechanical ventilation. All patients were discharged from hospital and the median hospital stay was 14.5 days.

Conclusion—This study documents a historical record of the first COVID-19 cases in Australia and the national early biocontainment phase.

DATA COLLECTION AND DATA MEASUREMENT

Data collection refers to a description of the processes used or proposed to be used to implement the study and gather data. Different research designs require different methods of data collection. An example of the types and characteristics of data are summarised in Table 7.3.

INSTRUMENTS: DATA MEASUREMENT, VALIDITY AND RELIABILITY

When instruments are used for measuring data about subjects, the validity and reliability of the instrument needs to be determined by the researcher. Instruments, or tools as they are more commonly called, used for research measurement refer not only to physiological and psychometric measures, but also to questionnaires and surveys used in studies. Validity is the degree to which an instrument measures what it is intended to measure.[10,11] There are three main types of validity: content-related, construct-related or criterion-related. Although an instrument may appear to measure some aspect of a concept or construct, it must be evaluated to determine whether it really does provide such measurement. Face validity is the subjective assessment of the relevance and presentation of research instruments.[29] Content validity is the degree to which an instrument measures the total content of the construct that it is said to represent or measure. Content validity is often determined by a panel of experts in the field in which the research is being conducted. If a researcher wanted to measure bereavement behaviours in the ED, for example, a variety of knowledgeable opinions from social workers, members of the clergy and emergency nurses could be sought out to review the instrument that will be used to measure bereavement behaviour. Construct validity is the degree to which an instrument measures the construct that is being studied.[29] Construct validity has two major components: convergent construct validity, whereby similar measures or constructs are identified, and discriminant construct validity, whereby differing constructs are identified. For example, a survey of emergency clinicians' perceptions of the key elements of pain management in patients with chest injuries, may ask emergency clinicians to rate their responses to 20 items using a 5-point scale, giving a score out of 100. Convergent construct validity enables the identification of an expected relationship between pain management and the patient's ability to deep breathe and cough.

Discriminant construct validity is assessed by comparing the score with a variable that is not expected to be related, such as pain management and type of footwear worn by the patient.[29] *Criterion validity* relates to the agreement between two or more measures and has two major components: concurrent and predictive validity. Concurrent validity is the independent validation that the instrument is measuring what it is designed to measure.[29] For example, a survey of emergency clinicians' preferences for pain management in patients with chest injuries may be compared with objective measures, such as patient medication charts. Predictive validity determines if

TABLE 7.3 TYPES OF DATA, FEATURES OF DATA AND EXAMPLES OF EACH TYPE

TYPE OF DATA	FEATURE	EXAMPLE
Biophysical measures	Sensitive and precise	Electronic thermometer to measure temperature
Direct observation	Entities difficult to measure by instruments or interview	Interactions between patients, nurses and doctors are observable
Interview–unstructured or structured; think-aloud technique	Participants can report data about themselves or what they are thinking	People with illicit drug use and pain management following injury. Nurses' decision-making
Questionnaire/scales	Participants can report the degree to which they possess an attitude or trait	Questionnaire about state and trait anxiety. Visual analogue scale for pain
Records or existing databases	Convenient and can provide insight	Information on a patient's chart to identify variance in the clinical pathway

the instrument can predict future changes in key variables.[29] For example, high levels of knowledge of the evidence-based management of patients with chest injuries may be related to the time to analgesia and quality of pain relief provided by an emergency clinician.

The *reliability* of an instrument is a measure of the extent to which it produces the same results when it is used to measure a specific criterion or behaviour repeatedly. In other words, whether the instrument produces the same measurement when a measurement is repeated several times. The less an instrument varies in repeated measurements, the greater the reliability of the instrument.[10,11] An example for a physiological measurement might be a thermometer that records two different oral temperatures, 37.2°C one moment and 39°C shortly after, in a person with no obvious febrile illness. You would suspect that the instrument (the thermometer) is not giving reliable readings. Problems with reliability can also arise when more than one data collector is used for the same study. When more than one data collector is required to administer the same instrument to measure participants' responses, it is essential that they administer the instrument in the same way. The process, called inter-rater reliability, is the degree of agreement (consistency) between the scores of two or more data collectors for the same observation. Inter-rater reliability should be tested by the researcher prior to formal data collection and throughout data collection for members of the research team collecting data.

PRACTICE TIP

Always check the literature to find if there is an existing instrument with established validity and reliability that measures the construct of your research before you try to develop a new instrument.

The accuracy and quality of data are just as important in qualitative research as they are in quantitative research. In qualitative approaches, such as grounded theory, information spoken to the researcher by a participant is summarised by the researcher and provided as narrative for the participant to check that it was an accurate reflection of what was said.[31] Similarly, a researcher can write an account of the observed behaviours of participants using fieldnotes for observational studies and ask participants at a later stage, or another observer of the event, to comment on the accuracy of the account of the observations and/or fieldnotes.[32] Given the complexity of emergency settings, observation data collection can provide greater insight into practice, social processes, interactions and context. Specifically, observation as a method of data collection can generate new knowledge and answer clinical and system questions that can improve the quality, safety and consistency of care.[32] Criteria used in narrative methods to ensure the 'truthfulness' of data, credibility, auditability and fittingness, are discussed in the section below on data analysis.

DATA ANALYSIS

After completing data collection, the researcher summarises, with the support of a statistician if necessary, quantitative data through statistical procedures to answer the study questions or hypotheses. Researchers who use quantitative methods for data collection should plan the analysis before the research data are collected to ensure there are sufficient participants in the sample to provide an accurate result. Statistical tests give meaning to quantitative data because they reduce, summarise, organise, evaluate, interpret and communicate numerical data. One does not need to know all the statistical tests to understand the common principle that the statistical test will reveal whether the findings are statistically significant. This means the findings are probably valid and replicable with a new sample of subjects. The level of statistical significance is an index of the probability of reliability of the findings, and is reported as the 'p value'. If findings are reported as significant at the 0.05 level, this means that five times out of 100 there is a risk that the result would be different from the reported finding; in other words, 95 out of 100 times the findings would be the same.[10,11] A researcher can set a higher level of significance: 0.01 means that only one time out of 100 is there a risk that the result has occurred by chance. Researchers should also consider clinical significance and what their findings mean in terms of world costs and benefits.[33]

Many papers are reporting odds ratios or relative risks and 95% confidence intervals in preference to, or in conjunction with, p values. Relative risk (RR) is the likelihood of an event or outcome after exposure to a risk factor compared with the likelihood of that event or outcome in a control or reference group.[34] A RR of 1.00 indicates that the event or outcome is equally likely in the exposed and the control groups.[34] A RR is considered clinically significant if it is less than 0.5 (i.e. the risk is at least halved) or more than 2.0 (i.e. the risk is doubled).[34] An odds ratio (OR) compares the odds of an event or an outcome after exposure to a risk factor with the odds of that event or outcome in a control or reference group.[34] An OR of 1.00 indicates equal risk in both groups. An OR < 1.00 means that exposure to the risk factor reduces the likelihood of the event or outcome and an OR that is > 1.00 indicates the risk of the event or outcome is increased.[34] OR are often reported with 95% confidence intervals (95% CI), which indicate that researchers can be 95% sure that values presented are true for 95% of the population. If the 95% CI for the OR crosses 1.00, the OR is not statistically significant.[34]

Statistical tests are referred to as either descriptive or inferential. *Descriptive statistics* describe and summarise data. Examples are the mode, median, mean, average, percentage and frequency. *Inferential statistics* are used to draw conclusions, to make judgements and to generalise information about a large population based on a sample from a study. Inferential statistics are used to test hypotheses to determine if they are correct. Two categories of inferential statistics are non-parametric and parametric. Most statistical tests undertaken by researchers are parametric tests, which focus on populations, require measurements on at least one interval or ratio scale and make assumptions about the distribution of the variables. The distribution of the scores of a variable should be close to the shape of a bell curve, called a 'normal' distribution, before they are statistically tested. Alternatively, non-parametric tests are used when measured variables are nominal or ordinal (ranked). These tests do not require the assumption that the variables in the research are distributed normally. An example of a study finding a statistical significance is provided in Research Highlight 7.5, in which the incidence of

RESEARCH HIGHLIGHT 7.5

Study using a descriptive design[35]

Title— Impact of a care bundle for patients with blunt chest injury (ChIP): A multicentre controlled implementation evaluation.

Aim—To identify the effects of this multidisciplinary chest injury care bundle (ChIP) on patient and health service outcomes in two centres in regional New South Wales (NSW), Australia.

Method—Controlled pre- and post- test study with two intervention and two non-intervention sites.

Results—Following implementation of ChIP, the intervention sites had a 58% decrease in non-invasive ventilation (OR = 0.42; 95% CI 0.18–0.96, $p < 0.05$) and 69% decrease in unplanned ICU admissions (OR = 0.31, 95% CI 0.12–0.78, $p < 0.05$). In the post-test period, the ChIP sites had 90% decreased odds of unplanned ICU admissions (95% CI 0.04–0.29, $p < 0.05$) compared to the control sites. There was no significant change in mortality.

Conclusion—The implementation of a chest injury care bundle using behaviour change theory was associated with a sustained improvement in evidence-based practice, resulting in reduced unplanned ICU admissions and need for non-invasive ventilation.

non-invasive ventilation and unplanned ICU admission reduced significantly in patients with blunt chest injury following implementation of a bundle of care protocol when compared to usual care.[35]

Qualitative research provides narrative data that are often referred to as 'rich' data. The challenge for researchers collecting qualitative data is to subject what is usually a large amount of observation or narrative to a rigorous and systematic analysis that is not distorted from the initial representation when it is summarised as overarching themes. Researchers undertaking observational studies can make the choice to collect structured or unstructured observations. These can take the form of field notes, surveys or audits.[32] As a result, the process of analysing narrative data usually starts with a transcription of the verbal or observational encounters into a textual account. Then the researcher undertakes an interpretative analysis that is an iterative process, whereby data is clustered and re-conceptualised into a higher level of abstraction (interpretation) that will be presented as overarching themes. The focus of the analysis and the formulation of themes is guided by the theoretical basis of the study—for example, grounded theory that is trying to distil participants' meanings accurately and without researcher bias.[28,36]

Whereas in quantitative research, validity and reliability are markers of the quality and rigour of data collection and analysis, in qualitative research, *trustworthiness* and *credibility* are important measures.[37] The scientific rigour of qualitative analysis is evaluated by four criteria. The findings should reflect participants' experience of the phenomenon when their feedback is sought.[37] This process is called *credibility*. *Credibility*, or truth-value, depends further on transferability, dependability, and confirmability. It is established when the descriptions and interpretations made by the researcher are recognised by the participants as their own. *Dependability* is achieved when the reader is clearly able to identify and follow the steps taken by the researcher throughout the research. Confirmability is achieved when credibility, transferability and dependability are established.[37] *Auditability* is used to gauge the adequacy of information leading from the question and raw data through the analysis and interpretation of findings that is logical and consistent. *Fittingness* is the match between the research findings and other published research, and can indicate the accuracy of interpretation; while *confirmability* is the process of scrutinising the accuracy of data using various ways of checking. Confirmability demonstrates the rigour of the analytical process used.[37] Ultimately, the measure of *trustworthiness* and *credibility* of qualitative research is a measure of the extent to which the researcher and the study have come to understand the problem, issue or phenomenon of interest. Various techniques were employed in qualitative research to afford trustworthiness and credibility, including triangulation, prolonged engagements, member checks, and leaving an audit trail. Box 7.2 identifies some commonly used quantitative approaches.

ETHICAL CONSIDERATIONS IN RESEARCH

Healthcare research raises questions about what is acceptable and 'right' or unacceptable and 'bad'. In 1964, the World Medical Association developed the Declaration of Helsinki as a statement of ethical principles in research.[38] The Declaration of Helsinki is grounded in the best interests and safety of research participants, and principles of privacy, confidentiality, dignity, autonomy to choose (to participate, not participate or withdraw) and consent, and protection of vulnerable populations.[38] The practices of all those involved in human research are guided by the National Statement on Ethical Conduct in Human Research, a document that has been compiled by the NHMRC, the Australian Research Council and the Australian Vice-Chancellors' Committee.[39] The statement is intended for use by any researcher conducting research with human participants, members of an ethical review body, those involved in research governance and potential research participants. The five sections of the review document are presented in Box 7.3. Further reading on critiquing ethical issues in published research is available in textbooks[10,11] or on the NHMRC website.

Before research on humans can be undertaken, it must be evaluated and approved by members of an institutional human research ethics committee (HREC) that manages research proposals in that area or institution. In 2022, there were more than 200 HRECs in institutions and organisations across Australia.[39,40] The constitution of an HREC is determined in Australia by policies and standards of the NHMRC. Members of an HREC make decisions about each research project and give approval for specified periods for the research to be conducted. Any person undertaking health-related research on humans is required to submit an ethics application to an HREC. An interactive web-based tool for researchers of all disciplines has been developed to assist researchers to submit well-formulated ethics proposals to HRECs. The Human Research Ethics Application (HREA) is now the standard way to submit an ethics application (see Useful websites).

BOX 7.2 RESEARCH USING QUALITATIVE RESEARCH APPROACHES[10,11]

- *Qualitative research* approaches provide data (information) in a non-numerical form, most commonly as writing (stories) or spoken language obtained during an interview. These methods are used to investigate phenomena that are difficult to categorise or where there has been little previous research conducted. Specific observations and/or interviews are analysed to develop themes and, in some instances, theories to explain a phenomenon.
- *Phenomenological interpretative research* is an inductive, descriptive approach developed from phenomenological philosophy. The aim of the research is to describe experience as it is lived by the person. The focus of the research is an attempt to understand the whole human being rather than specific behaviours or parts, and the numerous ways human beings experience the complexity of their world.
- *Grounded theory research* seeks to identify social problems and the processes people use to manage these problems. Through observations and interviews, the researcher develops an understanding of the relations between variables and formulates propositions that are tested with participants and redeveloped until 'saturation' (no new information arises). The grounded new theory that emerges from data has its basis in data and it evolves from these propositions.
- *Ethnographic research* seeks to understand the behaviours of people within the context of their culture. It is considered naturalistic research, in that the social milieu is observed without control or manipulation to gain insights into the subjective experiences and actions of people. Analysis of the observations enables the researcher to develop a theory about the culture.
- *Critical social research* seeks to understand how people communicate and how they develop symbolic meanings in a social group. Symbolic meanings may take on factual status and they are not disputed or challenged, but taken for granted. In the method of critical social research, the researcher seeks to identify the constraints that impede autonomous and uncoerced participation in the society. Action research, in which the researcher works with a group to effect technical or emancipatory change, is a major method of critical social research. An action research method can be used in practice development projects.

BOX 7.3 SECTIONS OF THE AUSTRALIAN NATIONAL STATEMENT ON ETHICAL CONDUCT IN HUMAN RESEARCH DOCUMENT[39]

- *Section 1* sets out the values and principles of ethical conduct that apply to all human research, and stipulates that researchers and review bodies consider these values and principles and be satisfied that the research proposal addresses and reflects them. For example, research confidentiality means that any data provided by a participant will not be reported in a way that could identify that person, or be accessible to anyone outside the research team.
- *Section 2* identifies the themes in research ethics: risk, benefit and consent. Research users need to identify the level of risk involved in the planned research, and how to minimise, justify and manage that risk. Researchers must identify the information that needs to be disclosed to participants. The statement will help researchers to draft information for participants and plan the consent process (or develop a proposal for waiver of consent). It will help reviewers to assess the suitability of the proposed consent process and help participants understand what information they are entitled to receive, and what their participation in research will characteristically involve.
- *Section 3* provides ethical considerations specific to research methods or fields to assist researchers and reviewers to identify ethical matters specific to the research methods proposed.
- *Section 4* identifies ethical considerations specific to participants to help researchers and reviewers identify ethical matters relating to specific categories of research participants.
- *Section 5* identifies the processes of research governance and ethical review to help those involved in research governance to understand their responsibilities for research ethics, ethical review and monitoring of human research, as well as criteria for accountability.

Over the last decade, a much greater appreciation of the ethical and moral dilemmas in conducting clinically-based research with colleagues has been discussed. A good example is the ethical considerations of the Paramedic-2 trial, which was a randomised controlled trial comparing adrenaline (epinephrine) and placebo in out-of-hospital cardiac arrest.[41] A study of paramedics' experiences of participation highlighted differing viewpoints and moral conflict. For example, some viewed the study as an opportunity to improve patient outcomes, while others felt the study was unethical and led to withholding of care and reported feelings of guilt and regret.[42]

RESULTS, CONCLUSIONS AND RECOMMENDATIONS

Results of quantitative studies are usually organised using the research hypotheses or questions of the study. The research question may be re-stated and the results reported in tables and/or graphs because they can be more easily interpreted. Based on the findings of the study, the research draws conclusions and then uses these conclusions as the foundation for the discussion section of the research report or manuscript. The researcher should attempt to give meaning to 'why' the findings occurred by interweaving the findings of previous related studies.

Recommendations can stem from changes the researcher plans in sample, design or analysis if the study is repeated. Other explanations for results should be discussed so that progress can be made with the research problem in future studies. The implications of research, such as how findings can be used to improve clinical practice and patients' outcomes, or how to advance knowledge through additional research, should be provided.[10,11]

The findings from qualitative research are written up in a carefully categorised and organised way. Data presented as themes can be interpreted at different levels of abstraction.[43] The 'writing up' of results is considered a crucial part of the research process because the act of writing explicates patterns, linkages and themes as the writer reflects within the process. In the grounded theory method, the categorisation continues until a core category emerges from data that provide the basis for a new theory.[44] The objective tone of quantitative research reporting is often replaced by a more personable account that frequently uses the first person in reporting the meaning and interpretation of data. Examples of participants' active speech may be used to demonstrate authenticity and confirmability. While the findings of qualitative research are not considered to be generalisable, they can provide emergency care clinicians with new insights into phenomena that are potentially transferrable and important to clinical practice.[43,45,46]

DISSEMINATION AND TRANSLATION OF RESEARCH FINDINGS

Disseminating and applying the results of a research project to clinical practice can be as difficult, or more difficult, than doing the research. However, doing the study, getting a result and drawing conclusions is only part of a researcher's role. Researchers have a professional and ethical responsibility to ensure that the research findings are made known to others and, where possible, used to research findings to improve clinical practice.

PUBLICATION AND PRESENTATION OF THE FINDINGS

A researcher's job is not completed until the findings of a study have been written up and attempts made to present the results at a conference or published in a peer-reviewed journal. It is no longer acceptable for research to be undertaken with no attempt made to publish the findings. Research is a costly process that involves the thinking and time commitment of a lot of people, including that of the participants. Consequently, researchers have a moral obligation to share the findings of their project with others. The World Health Organization (WHO), in its position on Interventional Clinical Trial Results, states that it is unethical to conduct human research without publication and dissemination of the results of that research, as withholding results may subject future volunteers to unnecessary risk,[47] and, that clinical trial results be submitted for publication in a peer-reviewed journal within 12 months of study completion.[48] Fortunately, there are many opportunities for sharing new knowledge, not only by writing for journals or books, but also by speaking at conferences and other events about the research outcomes, or disseminating research findings using social media platforms. Within any clinical area there will be opportunities for you to assist in maintaining published protocols and practice guidelines with the most recent evidence. Involvement in guideline development or revision is an excellent way to become familiar with new knowledge and publication requirements. Many organisations managing population healthcare have established organisational structures and processes, such as clinical governance committees that support the revision of protocols by clinicians working in specific clinical areas across an institution.

There is support available for clinicians to get assistance in writing for publication if they initially lack confidence. It is very likely there will be at least one colleague in the clinical area or nearby who has published successfully in a journal. If not, then try contacting an academic supervisor or member of staff from a local university to critique a draft of the article. It is important to carefully select several journals that are more likely to be interested in the topic or the research approach prior to writing up the findings, because different journals have specific publication requirements that you need to follow when writing the draft. It is also important to be aware of bogus or predatory journals and ensure that the journal you are submitting to is legitimate.

PRACTICE TIP

Predatory publishing is on the rise globally. There are many ways to identify a predatory journal:

- Predatory or suspicious journals aggressively solicit scholars to submit papers. These offers come in the form of unsolicited emails that are usually individually flattering. Legitimate journals usually do not solicit authors, but instead usually have the authors contact them.
- Predatory journals agree to publish your article for a fee before reviewing it. Don't let a claim that a journal is peer reviewed sway you. Almost all predatory journals claim to be peer reviewed. In predatory journals, the time for peer review is extremely short.
- The members of the predatory journal's editorial board lack qualifications or expertise in the field. Different journals by the same publisher have the same editorial board. Predatory journals will sometimes solicit well-known scholars to join their boards to lend credibility to their journal, but then don't let them make decisions. Academics are often listed as members of editorial boards without their permission and are not allowed to resign or be removed from editorial boards.
- Predatory journals are not typically indexed in the major indexes in the field or general indexes, even though they might claim to be. Some journals falsely claim to be indexed by Thomson Reuters. Be wary of journals that cite bogus impact factors, such as the GIF (Global Impact Factor), Index Copernicus Value, Citefactor, or the UIF (Universal Impact Factor). Some may falsify legitimate impact factors. Other things to look out for are if the journal is difficult to locate in established library catalogues; the journal is listed on Beall's List of Predatory Journals; the website contains spelling and grammatical errors, images that are distorted/fuzzy, intended to look like something they are not, or which are unauthorised.

- Check that the scope of a predatory journal is not overly broad and/or that it fits well with your research. Predatory journals may be published infrequently or irregularly or it might not be stated. They may have the same or similar name to a legitimate journal. The former is characteristic of hijacked journals. The email address is often non-professional (@yahoo.com, ao.com or @gmail.com) rather than being associated with a journal or publisher.

If you are unsure, always check first. Contact a librarian at a local university or within your health service and seek assistance.

When a local review and critique of the draft article from colleagues has been completed (it may take several drafts when you are new to this process), you are ready to submit your article to a journal. Review the author guidelines of the selected journal prior to submission. When submitting an article for publication to a peer-reviewed journal, the article will be reviewed by professionals who are familiar with writing for publication and possibly expert in the area or topic. The most common review process is a double-blinded peer review, whereby the reviewers do not know who the author is and vice versa. Some journals engage in single-blind peer review, typically where the reviewers know who the author is, but the author doesn't know the identity of the reviewer, while other journals use an open review process where all parties are known to each other. The journal editor will send the reviewers' feedback on your article back to you, and you will have an opportunity to make corrections to the manuscript if the editor decides to accept the article for publication. If not successful initially, then persevere. Writing for publication is a skill that needs to be developed and it is important not to be discouraged if one journal sends a rejection letter. Select a journal with a lower impact rating and try again.

KNOWLEDGE TRANSLATION

While sourcing sufficient evidence to base practice on is an ongoing challenge, so too is identifying established evidence and translating it into practice.[5]The time lapse between the publication of evidence and its implementation into practice is referred to as an *evidence–practice gap*. Addressing this gap requires *knowledge translation*. Synonymous terms are used by researchers around the world. For example, similar processes are called *research utilisation* in the UK and Europe, *research dissemination, diffusion* or *knowledge uptake* in the United States, and *knowledge translation* and *knowledge-to-action* in Australia and Canada.[49]

Knowledge translation (KT) is defined as:

> [a] dynamic and iterative process that includes synthesis, dissemination, exchange and ethically sound application of knowledge to improve the health …, provide more effective health services and products and strengthen the health care system. This process takes place within a complex system of interactions between researchers and knowledge users which may vary in intensity, complexity and level of engagement depending on the nature of the research and the findings as well as the needs of the particular knowledge user.[49]

Multiple factors influence the uptake of research into practice.[4] The increasing volume of research evidence being produced, access to new evidence, the skills to appraise the quality of the evidence, time to locate and read evidence and the capacity to apply evidence, are some of the major factors identified.[5] Strategies to promote the use of research in practice by healthcare workers continue to be devised as the complexity of the application of evidence into practice has been recognised. One strategy now commonly used is *knowledge distillation*, which is the synthesis of findings from the most rigorously conducted research available on a specific topic into systematic reviews.[5] The synthesis can then be presented to clinicians as practice guidelines,[50] clinical care standards,[51] or fact sheets for clinicians and consumers.[52]

The leading global organisation is The Cochrane Collaboration. The Australasian Cochrane Centre in Melbourne is one of many global Cochrane centres. The Cochrane Collaboration coordinates the Cochrane Library, the production and dissemination of systematic reviews, randomised controlled trials and other information for an international audience. Guidelines provided by the NHMRC grade the strength of the evidence, as outlined earlier. JBI coordinates the conduct and dissemination of systematic reviews of clinical nursing and midwifery research, and publishes best practice information sheets based on the findings from systematic reviews, and evaluates the impact these have on clinical care. Emergency nurses and paramedics are increasingly publishing systematic reviews and reviews of current guidelines.

Research utilisation implies not only the implementation of new knowledge into practice, but also the evaluation of consequent changes in practice.[5] It is no longer acceptable to implement a change in practice and not evaluate the impact of that change. That is, if the research evidence is applied in a given context, the resulting change should be evaluated in terms of the outcomes, for example for patients, consumers, clinicians and the organisation. Outcome research assesses the effectiveness of healthcare services and workforce.[10] There are eight Australian National Safety and Quality Health Service Standards that seek to improve the quality of health service provision and minimise risk to patients.[53]

Barriers to translation of research into practice

Any attempt to improve the quality of care for patients must incorporate a clear understanding of the associated barriers and facilitators. It is challenging to apply evidence and evidence-based protocols in the context of competing priorities in the challenging pre-hospital and ED environments. Despite high-level recommendations to improve implementation of evidence-based practice, implementation remains variable, with numerous organisational and individual factors influencing healthcare workers' behaviour. These factors include a lack of time, difficulties in developing evidence-based guidelines, a lack of continuing education and an unsupportive organisational culture,[54] the availability of evidence, its relevance to practice, the dissemination of evidence and guidelines, individual motivation, the ability to keep up with current changes, clarity of roles and practice and the culture of specific healthcare practices.

Research and evidence-based practice is taught in Australian and New Zealand nursing and paramedic bachelor degrees and there are a number of postgraduate research training options including honours, masters and doctoral degrees. The Nursing and Midwifery Board of Australia (NMBA) sets clear expectations of registered nurses that they will think critically and analyse nursing practice and use best available evidence in making decisions and providing nursing care.[55] Similarly, the Paramedicine Board of Australia also sets clear expectations that registered paramedics will be evidence-based practitioners.[56]

Ways to improve clinicians' research use—implementation science

Closing the gap between high-standard health-research evidence and everyday clinical practice is an international healthcare priority and implementation science is a key strategy by which to do this.[57] Implementation science is the study of methods to promote the integration of research findings and evidence into healthcare policy and practice.[58] It seeks to understand the behaviour of healthcare professionals and other stakeholders as a key variable in the sustainable uptake, adoption and implementation of evidence-based interventions. Implementation science addresses the major barriers (e.g. social, behavioural, economic, management) that impede effective implementations.[5]

Behaviour change is key to improving healthcare and health outcomes, particularly the implementation of evidence-based practice.[59] Improving the implementation of evidence-based practice by healthcare workers depends on changing multiple behaviours of multiple types of people (e.g. health professionals, managers, administrators).[60] Changing behaviour is not easy, but is more effective if interventions are based on evidence-based principles of behaviour change. The validated theoretical domains framework[61] is a well-accepted tool on which to structure implementation strategies to introduce new policies and practice. It provides comprehensive coverage of possible influences on behaviour in 14 domains: 'Knowledge', 'Skills', 'Social/professional role and identity', 'Beliefs about capabilities', 'Optimism', 'Beliefs about consequences', 'Reinforcement', 'Intentions', 'Goals', 'Memory, attention and decision processes', 'Environmental context and resources', 'Social influences', 'Emotions' and 'Behavioural regulation'. The intent of implementation science and related research is to investigate and address major bottlenecks (e.g. social, behavioural, economic, management) that impede effective implementation, test new approaches to improve health programming, as well as determine a causal relationship between the intervention and its impact.[58] Australian and New Zealand nursing, midwifery and paramedicine joint clinical–academic appointments are increasing and are a key strategy to enable research evidence to be filtered, disseminated and introduced into the clinical arena using implementation approaches supported by science.

The Canadian Institutes of Health Research promote knowledge translation by the use of the model of knowledge-to-action cycle as the preferred approach (Fig. 7.1).[62] The knowledge-to-action cycle is based on the combination of a knowledge creation process and more than 31 planned-action

FIGURE 7.1 KNOWLEDGE-TO-ACTION PROCESS[62]

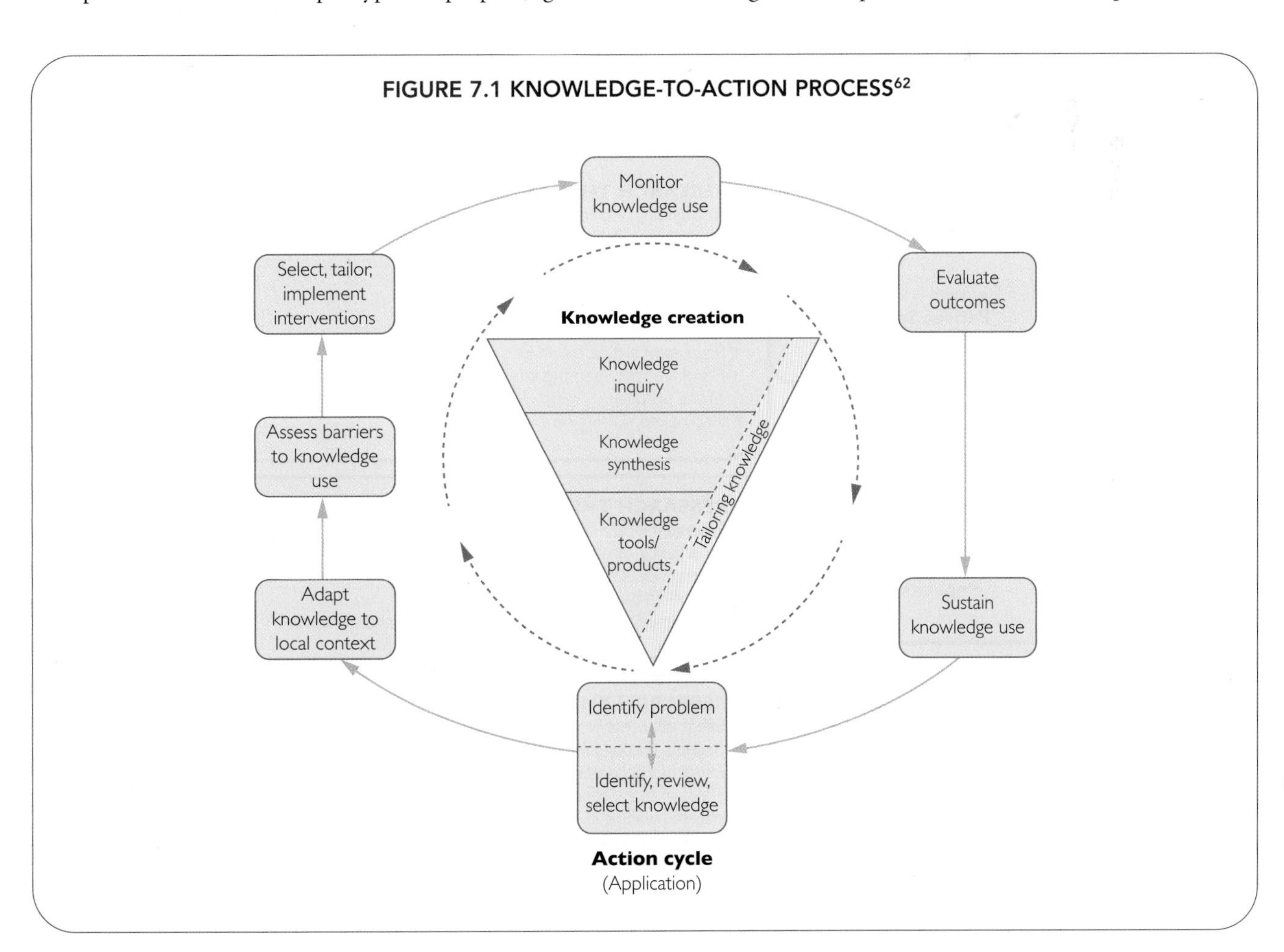

theories. The knowledge-to-action framework has two major concepts: knowledge creation and the action cycle.[62] Knowledge creation consists of: knowledge inquiry, knowledge synthesis, and knowledge instruments or product creation, and is surrounded by the action cycle. Knowledge creation and the action cycle are considered iterative with dynamic boundaries.

The action cycle describes the dynamic process of knowledge application in practice through seven phases that can occur sequentially or simultaneously:

1. Identify a problem and select knowledge
2. Adapt knowledge to local context
3. Assess barriers to knowledge use
4. Select, tailor and implement interventions
5. Monitor knowledge use
6. Evaluate outcomes
7. Sustain knowledge use.

The seven action phases of the action cycle can occur sequentially or simultaneously.[62]

RESEARCH PRIORITIES FOR EMERGENCY CARE

Research and the generation of new knowledge is key to providing consistent, high-quality and safe emergency care. A number of professions have, to a varying extent, established research priorities to guide and support the professional practice needs of emergency doctors, emergency nurses and emergency paramedics. How the research priorities of these disciplines is presented varies with priority research themes, research objectives and formal research questions reported for emergency care in general,[63–66] emergency medicine specifically,[67–70] and emergency nursing in the United States.[71] In Australia, a study of the research priorities for emergency nursing conducted in 2017 identified four research priority areas based on 27 research themes (Fig. 7.2).[72] The five research themes with a content validity index ≥ 0.90, so therefore ranked as most important by participants, were:

1. Recognising and responding to deteriorating ED patients

FIGURE 7.2 EMERGENCY NURSING RESEARCH PRIORITIES[72]

Research Priority 1
Professional Issues

- **RESEARCH THEMES**
- Scope of practice of specialist emergency nurses
- Emergency nursing education
- Emergency department leadership
- Patient flow through the ED
- Effect of nurse-initiated investigations (e.g. pathology and imaging)
- Burnout in emergency nursing
- Nursing skill-mix: optimum mix of RNs, ENs and AINs in EDs
- Occupational violence
- Methods of implementing evidence into practice
- Barriers and facilitators to implementing evidence into practice

Research Priority 2
Patient Safety

- **RESEARCH THEMES**
- Recognising and responding to deteriorating ED patients
- Medication safety in EDs
- Nursing skill-mix: optimum % postgraduate prepared registered nurses in EDs
- Nurse:patient ratios in EDs
- Patient assessment approaches and frameworks
- Sources of clinical risk in EDs
- Handover between the emergency department and other areas of the hospital
- Incomplete nursing care in EDs

Research Priority 3
Care of Vulnerable Populations

- **RESEARCH THEMES**
- Emergency care of children
- Emergency care of mental health patients
- Emergency care of older patients
- End-of-life care in the ED
- Emergency care of patients with behavioural disturbance

Research Priority 3
Healthcare System Issues

- **RESEARCH THEMES**
- Effect of access block on the clinical care of admitted ICU patients waiting in ED for a bed
- Effect of ED overcrowding on clinical care
- Effect of block effects on the clinical care of admitted ward patients waiting in ED for a bed
- Effect of ED overcrowding on patient (+/- carer) experience of emergency care

2. The effect of access block on clinical care of admitted ICU patients
3. Effects of ED overcrowding on clinical care
4. Scope of practice of specialist emergency nurses
5. The effect of access block on clinical care of admitted ward patients.

These are reflected in four broad research priority areas: professional issues, patient safety, emergency care of vulnerable populations, and healthcare system issues.[72]

SUMMARY

Research is critical for paramedic and emergency nursing practice. This chapter has provided a basic overview of the steps of the research process and the language used to describe this process for clinicians in the earlier stages of this continuum. The steps in research, guided by either a research question or a hypothesis, collecting narrative or numerical data, have been represented. Well-defined systems, such as evidence-based practice and implementation science, exist to support clinicians engaging in research and research application in practice. The outcome that most clinicians want from research activity is knowledge to improve patient care. It is imperative for all healthcare professionals to understand their professional responsibility to support, use and engage in research to ensure that new, useful knowledge is continuously generated, implemented and evaluated for the benefit of the people for whom they care.

CASE STUDY

You are a registered nurse or paramedic enrolled in a postgraduate course at the local university. While undertaking a literature review for an assignment you identify that there are new guidelines for the management of adults presenting to the ED with acute coronary syndrome. When you read the new guideline and the practice recommendations by the National Heart Foundation of Australia/Cardiac Society of Australia and New Zealand Guidelines for the Management of Acute Coronary Syndromes (ACS), you realise that the existing practice protocol at your organisation is out of date and there are some changes in practice that need to occur to ensure patients receive evidence-based care.

After careful consideration of the issues, and engaging the support of colleagues who are experienced researchers, you decide to lead a project as part of your master's degree. After gaining some knowledge of the action research method and implementation science at university, you agree to facilitate the process in your organisation with the help of your supervisors. You develop a proposal and attach a copy of the new guideline from the National Heart Foundation website.

Once you have gained the necessary permissions, including HREC approval for the project to be conducted, you start to talk to your colleagues about the new guidelines, because their engagement in the process is central to effective change. Also, you are fully aware that your colleagues are busy and the pre-hospital and ED environments are chaotic and unpredictable, and that some colleagues are concerned about the amount of time required to participate in the project. The first meetings are held, and the majority of your colleagues are prepared to discuss the new guideline and decide how practice needs to change to accommodate the new evidence.

QUESTIONS

1. Using the steps of the research process, make a list of the information you would include in the proposal.
2. Identify the stakeholders you need to speak with about your proposal to implement a new guideline using the knowledge-to-action framework as a guide.
3. Identify some ways to schedule the first meetings to involve as many of your colleagues as possible in the implementation. How will staff on evening and night-duty shifts be involved if the meetings are conducted during the day?
4. What suggestions would you give your colleagues about maintaining records of the processes and outcomes of meetings, particularly as you may not be able to attend every meeting?
5. You are required to write an assignment for your course, evaluating the project. How will you determine the 'success' of your project? How will you know whether clinicians are implementing the new guideline correctly and completely?

Answers to Case Study Questions can be found on evolve http://evolve.elsevier.com/AU/Curtis/emergency/ 

USEFUL WEBSITES

Australasian Cochrane Centre, acc.cochrane.org.

Human Research Ethics Application (HREA), www.nhmrc.gov.au and hrea.gov.au/.

JBI, www.joannabriggs.org.

REFERENCES

1. Cochrane AL. Effectiveness and efficiency: random reflections on health services. Nuffield Trust; 1972.
2. Sackett DL, Rosenberg WM, Gray JA, Haynes RB, Richardson WS. Evidence based medicine: what it is and what it isn't. Br Med J 1996;312(7023): 71–2.
3. Sackett D. Evidence-based medicine: how to practice and teach EBM. 2nd ed. Edinburgh: Churchill Livingstone; 2000.
4. Fry M, Attawet J. Nursing and midwifery use, perceptions and barriers to evidence-based practice: a cross-sectional survey. Int J Evid-based Healthc 2017;16(1):47–54.
5. Curtis K, Fry M, Shaban RZ, Considine J. Translating research findings to clinical nursing practice. J Clin Nurs 2017;26(5–6):862–72.
6. GRADE Working Group. Online. Available from: www.gradeworkinggroup.org.
7. Guyatt GH, Oxman AD, Vist GE, et al. GRADE: an emerging consensus on rating quality of evidence and strength of recommendations. Br Med J 2008;336(7650):924–6.
8. National Health and Medical Research Council (NHMRC). Assessing certainty of evidence. September, 2019. Online. Available from: www.nhmrc.gov.au/guidelinesforguidelines/develop/assessing-certainty-evidence.
9. Lewin S, Booth A, Glenton C, Munthe-Kaas H, Rashidian A, Wainwright M, et al. Applying GRADE-CERQual to qualitative evidence synthesis findings: introduction to the series. Implement Sci 2018;13:2.
10. Polit D, Beck C. Essentials of nursing research: appraising evidence for nursing practice. Lippincott Williams & Wilkins; 2020.
11. Whitehead D, Ferguson C, LoBiondo-Wood G, Haber J. Nursing and midwifery research: methods and appraisal for evidence based practice. 6th ed. Chatswood NSW: Elsevier Australia; 2020.
12. Creswell JW, Creswell JD. Research design: qualitative, quantitative, and mixed methods approaches. 5th ed. Thousand Oaks, California: Sage Publishing; 2017.
13. Morse JM, Field P-A. Nursing research: the application of qualitative approaches. 2nd ed. Netherlands: Springer Science+Business Media B.V.; 2013.
14. Whitley G, Siriwardena AN, editors. Prehospital research methods and practice. Somerset: Class Publishing; 2022.
15. Considine J, Shaban RZ, Fry M, Curtis K. Evidence-based emergency nursing: designing a research question and searching the literature. Int Emerg Nurs 2017;32(Supp C):78–82.
16. Cooke A, Smith D, Booth A. Beyond PICO. Qual Health Res 2012;22(10):1435–43.
17. Considine J, Shaban R, Curtis K, Fry M. Effectiveness of nurse-initiated X-ray for emergency department patients with distal limb injuries: a systematic review. Eur J Emerg Med 2019;26(5):314–22.
18. U.S. National Library of Medicine. Medical subject headings. 2021. Online. Available from: www.nlm.nih.gov/mesh/.
19. Ravitch SM, Riggan M. Reason and rigor: how conceptual frameworks guide research. 2nd ed. Thousand Oaks: Sage Publications; 2017.
20. Passey D. Theories, theoretical and conceptual frameworks, models and constructs: limiting research outcomes through misconceptions and misunderstandings. Stud Technol Enhanc Learn 2020;1(1). doi:10.21428/8c225f6e.56810a1a.
21. Fry M, Elliott R, Murphy S, Curtis K. The role and contribution of family carers accompanying community-living older people with cognitive impairment to the emergency department: an interview study. J Clin Nurs 2022;31(7):1016–29.
22. Street M, Dempster J, Berry D, Gray E, Mapes J, Liskaser R, et al. Enhancing active patient participation in nursing handover: a mixed methods study. J Clin Nurs 2022;31(7–8):975–84.
23. Crookes P, Davies S. Research into practice: essential skills for reading and applying research in nursing and health care. Edinburgh: Bailliere Tindall; 2004.
24. Munn Z, Peters MDJ, Stern C, Tufanaru C, McArthur A, Aromataris E. Systematic review or scoping review? Guidance for authors when choosing between a systematic or scoping review approach. BMC Med Res Methodol 2018;18(1):143.
25. Da Silva RN, Brandão MAG, Ferreira MDA. Integrative review as a method to generate or to test nursing theory. Nurs Sci Q 2020;33(3): 258–63.
26. Cronin MA, George E. The why and how of the integrative review. Organ Res Methods 2020:168–92.
27. Cross J, Lam T, Arndell J, Quach J, Reed B, Thyer L, et al. Impact of hand dominance on effectiveness of chest compressions in a simulated setting: a randomised, crossover trial. Australas J Paramed 2019;16.
28. Denzin NK, Lincoln YS. The handbook of qualitative research. 5th ed. Thousand Oaks, CA: Sage Publications; 2017.
29. Bruce N, Pope D, Stanistreet D. Quantitative methods for health research: a practical interactive guide to epidemiology and statistics. Oxford: John Wiley; 2018.

30. Shaban RZ, Li C, O'Sullivan MVN, Gerrard J, Stuart RL, Teh J, et al. COVID-19 in Australia: our national response to the first cases of SARS-CoV-2 infection during the early biocontainment phase. Intern Med J 2021;51(1):42–51.
31. Glaser BG, Strauss A. The discovery of grounded theory: strategies for qualitative research. New York: Aldine; 1967.
32. Fry M, Chenoweth L, Arendts G. Can an observational pain assessment tool improve time to analgesia for cognitively impaired older persons? A cluster randomised controlled trial. Emerg Med J 2018;35(1):33–8.
33. McShane BB, Gal D, Gelman A, Robert C, Tackett JL. Abandon statistical significance. Am Stat 2019;73(1):235–45.
34. Andrade C. Understanding relative risk, odds ratio, and related terms: as simple as it can get. J Clin Psych 2015;76(7):e857–61.
35. Curtis K, Kourouche S, Asha S, et al. Impact of a care bundle for patients with blunt chest injury (ChIP): a multicentre controlled implementation evaluation. PLOS ONE 2021;16(10):e0256027.
36. Silverman D. Qualitative research. 5th ed. Los Angeles: Sage; 2020.
37. Guba EG, Lincoln YS. Epistemological and methodological bases of naturalistic inquiry. ECTJ 1982;30(4):233–52.
38. Rickham PP. Human experimentation. Code of ethics of the World Medical Association. Declaration of Helsinki. Br Med J 1964;2(5402):177.
39. National Health and Medical Research Council (NHMRC). National Statement on ethical conduct in research involving humans. Canberra: NHMRC; 2018.
40. National Health and Medical Research Council (NHMRC). Human Research Ethics Committees (HRECs). n.d. Online. Available from: www.nhmrc.gov.au/research-policy/ethics/human-research-ethics-committees#.
41. Perkins GD, Ji C, Deakin CD, Nolan JP, Scomparin C, et al. A randomized trial of epinephrine in out-of-hospital cardiac arrest. NEJM 2018;379(8):711–21.
42. Charlton K, Franklin J, McNaughton R. Phenomenological study exploring ethics in prehospital research from the paramedic's perspective: experiences from the Paramedic-2 trial in a UK ambulance service. Emerg Med J 2019;36(9):535–40.
43. Neville S, Whitehead D. Analysing data in qualitative research. In: Whitehead D, Ferguson C, LoBiondo-Wood G, Haber J, editors. Nursing and midwifery research methods and appraisal for evidence based practice. Chatswood: Elsevier; 2020.
44. Glaser B, Strauss A. Grounded theory: the discovery of grounded theory. Sociology 1967;12:27–49.
45. Whitehead D, Disler R. Common qualitative methods. In: Whitehead D, Ferguson C, LoBiondo-Wood G, Haber J, editors. Nursing and midwifery research methods and appraisal for evidence based practice. Chatswood, NSW: Elsevier; 2020.
46. Whitehead D, Whitehead L. Data collection and sampling in qualitative research. In: Whitehead D, Ferguson C, LoBiondo-Wood G, Haber J, editors. Nursing and midwifery research methods and appraisal for evidence based practice. Chatswood: Elsevier; 2020.
47. Matosin N, Frank E, Engel M, Lum JS, Newell KA. Negativity towards negative results: a discussion of the disconnect between scientific worth and scientific culture. Dis Model Mech 2014;7(2):PMC3917235.
48. Moorthy VS, Karam G, Vannice KS, et al. Rationale for WHO's new position calling for prompt reporting and public disclosure of interventional clinical trial results. PLoS Med 2015;12(4):e1001819.
49. Canadian Institutes of Health Research. About us: knowledge translation and commercialization. 2016. Online. Available from: www.cihr-irsc.gc.ca/e/29418.html.
50. National Stroke Foundation. Clinical guidelines for stroke management. Early assessment and diagnosis. 2021. Melbourne. Online. Available from: informme.org.au/guidelines/clinical-guidelines-for-stroke-management#.
51. Banks G. Australian Council on Healthcare Standards. ACHS 30 years. Ultimo: ACHS; 2004.
52. Australian Commission on Safety and Quality in Health Care (ACSQHC). Osteoarthritis of the knee clinical care standard – consumer fact sheet. Darlinghurst: ACSQHC; 2007. Online. Available from: www.safetyandquality.gov.au/publications-and-resources/resource-library/osteoarthritis-knee-clinical-care-standard-consumer-fact-sheet.
53. Australian Commission on Safety and Quality in Health Care (ACSQHC). National safety and quality health service standards. 2nd ed. Sydney: Australian Commission on Safety and Quality in Health Care; 2021. Online. Available from: www.safetyandquality.gov.au/publications-and-resources/resource-library/national-safety-and-quality-health-service-standards-second-edition.
54. Wallis L. Barriers to implementing evidence-based practice remain high for US nurses: getting past 'we've always done it this way' is crucial. Am J Nurs 2012;112(12):15.
55. Nursing and Midwifery Board of Australia (NMBA). Registered Nurse standards for practice. 4th ed. Dickson, ACT: NMBA; 2016. Online. Available: www.nursingmidwiferyboard.gov.au/Codes-Guidelines-Statements/Professional-standards.aspx.
56. Paramedicine Board of Australia. Professional capabilities for registered paramedics. Dickson: Paramedicine Board of Australia; 2021. Online. Available from: www.paramedicineboard.gov.au/Professional-standards/Professional-capabilities-for-registered-paramedics.aspx.
57. McKee G, Codd M, Dempsey O, Gallagher P, Comiskey C. Describing the implementation of an innovative intervention and evaluating its effectiveness in increasing research capacity of advanced clinical nurses: using the consolidated framework for implementation research. BMC Nurs 2017;16(1):21.
58. Bauer MS, Damschroder L, Hagedorn H, Smith J, Kilbourne AM. An introduction to implementation science for the non-specialist. BMC Psychol 2015;3(1). doi:10.1186/s40359-015-0089-9.
59. Fry M, Elliott R, Fitzpatrick L, Warton J, Curtis K. Measuring nurses' perceptions of their work environment and linking with behaviour change theories and implementation strategies to support evidence based practice change. App Nurs Res 2020;56:151374.

60. Grol R, Grimshaw J. From best evidence to best practice: effective implementation of change in patients' care. Lancet 2003;362(9391):1225–30.
61. Cane J, O'Connor D, Michie S. Validation of the theoretical domains framework for use in behaviour change and implementation research. Implement Sci 2012;7:37.
62. Graham ID, Logan J, Harrison MB, Theodosis C, Totten VY, Radeous MS, et al. Lost in knowledge translation: time for a map? J Contin Educ Health Prof 2006;26(1):13–24.
63. Calvello EJB, Broccoli M, Risko N, Theodosis C, Totten VY, Radeous MS, et al. Emergency care and health systems: consensus-based recommendation and future research priorities. Acad Emerg Med 2013;20(12):1278–88.
64. Gazmuri RJ, Nadkarni VM, Nolan JP, Arntz H, Billi JE, Bossaert L, et al. ILCOR Consensus Statement: scientific knowledge gaps and clinical research priorities for cardiopulmonary resuscitation and emergency cardiovascular care identified during the 2005 International Consensus Conference on E and CPR science with treatment recommendations. Circulation 2007;116:2501–12.
65. Plint AC, Stang AS, Calder LA. Priorities in Patient Safety Research in Emergency Medicine Consensus Panel. Establishing research priorities for patient safety in emergency medicine: a multidisciplinary consensus panel. Int J Emerg Med 2015;8(1):5.
66. Thom O, Keijzers G, Davies S, McD Taylor D, Knott J, Middleton PM. Clinical research priorities in emergency medicine: results of a consensus meeting and development of a weighting method for assessment of clinical research priorities. Emerg Med Australas 2014;26(1):28–33.
67. Deane HC, Wilson CL, Babl FE, Dalziel SR, Cheek JA, Craig SS, et al. PREDICT prioritisation: establishing the research priorities of paediatric emergency medicine physicians in Australia and New Zealand. Emerg Med J 2018;35(1):39–45.
68. Keijzers G, Thom O, Taylor D, Knott J, McD Taylor D. Clinical research priorities in emergency medicine. Emerg Med Australas 2014;26(1):19–27.
69. Lecky F, Benger J, Mason S, Cameron P, Walsh C. The International Federation for Emergency Medicine framework for quality and safety in the emergency department. Emerg Med J 2014;31(11):926–9.
70. Smith J, Keating L, Flowerdew L, O'Brien R, McIntyre S, Morley R, et al. An emergency medicine research priority setting partnership to establish the top 10 research priorities in emergency medicine. Emerg Med J 2017;34(7):454–6.
71. Bayley EW, MacLean SL, Desy P, McMahon M. ENA's Delphi study on national research priorities for emergency nurses in the United States. J Emerg Nurs 2004;30:12–21.
72. Considine J, Curtis K, Shaban RZ, Fry M. Consensus-based clinical research priorities for emergency nursing in Australia. Australas Emerg Care 2018;21(2):43–50.

CHAPTER 8

PATIENT AND CARER ENGAGEMENT AND COMMUNICATION

JUDY MULLAN AND KELLY LAMBERT

ESSENTIALS

- Simple strategies can be used to help improve healthcare professional–patient engagement and communication.
- It is important to target patient education interventions for all patients, especially for those with poor health literacy skills.
- A range of instruments and tools can be used to assess the readability, presentation, quality and suitability of written patient information resources.
- Medication adherence and health promotion needs to be encouraged to further improve patient health outcomes.

INTRODUCTION

The notion of person-centred care, with patient engagement and communication as a central focus, has been increasingly incorporated into healthcare models worldwide.[1–4] There are many different definitions of person-centred care, but essentially it is about treating the patient with dignity and respect and involving them in all decisions about their health.[5] This involves developing a collaborative and respectful partnership between the healthcare professional and the patient.[5]

It is understandable, and professionally responsible, that today's healthcare professionals and many healthcare organisations have been seeking to improve the quality of their patient education by supporting the use of person-centred communication standards.[1,3,4] These person-centred communication standards recommend strategies which encourage patients, and, where appropriate, their family member/carer to become active participants in the decision-making process about their care.[3–5] The standards are a result of evidence indicating that active patient/family engagement and partnerships with healthcare professionals can result in reductions in mortality and healthcare utilisation, as well as improved patient outcomes, patient satisfaction and patient self-management skills.[6–13]

The move towards person-centred care promotes the provision of high-quality care based on an individual's needs and expectations.[10,11] Healthcare professionals, including nurses and paramedics, are in a good position to foster and promote patient education and engagement from a person-centred viewpoint. This is an important consideration because healthcare professionals play a pivotal role in providing patient education and information in a wide range of healthcare environments, which

includes busy hospital emergency departments (EDs). Despite the challenges,[14] it is important to acknowledge that ED presentations may be the most regular contact many patients suffering from chronic diseases, such as asthma, diabetes, cardiovascular disease and mental illness, may have with a health service.[15–17]

Effective patient education requires good communication between the healthcare professional and the patient, in order to develop a mutual understanding.[18] However, having a mutual understanding is reliant upon establishing good rapport, as well as respectful and trusting relationships.[18] This, in turn, promotes collaborative partnerships and effective communications, which are key factors to consider when providing patient education. Other key factors include the provision of clear verbal communication and simple, easy-to-read written patient information (where appropriate), as well as the use of the teach-back technique[19] to promote good therapeutic and medication adherence and the provision of patient follow-up.

The process of effective patient education begins with the provision of information, but also includes interpretation and integration of information to bring about attitudinal or behavioural change(s) that benefit the patient's health status.[20] Since effective patient education helps patients actively participate in their healthcare and to make informed choices,[20,21] healthcare professionals need to focus upon providing information based on the needs of the patient, and, where appropriate, their family members and carers.[2–4] These include, but are not limited to, their reading and literacy skills, their learning preferences, as well as their religious and cultural beliefs.[1,2] It is also important to consider the needs of patient populations most at risk of poor health outcomes, such as those who are older (> 65 years of age);[22–25] those with poor health literacy skills;[26–29] and those from ethnically diverse backgrounds.[30–32] These patient populations are considered most at risk because they are often overwhelmed and may not realise they have misunderstood or seldom voluntarily admit that they have not understood the information they receive during patient education sessions.

HEALTH LITERACY

Poor health literacy, a pervasive and under-recognised problem worldwide, is a concern because these patients are more likely to experience challenges with adherence to treatment, poorer health outcomes and increased healthcare costs.[27,33–39] Patients with poor health literacy may struggle to find, read or understand written information, fill out consent forms and comply with treatment recommendations.[27,40–42] They may also struggle with knowing when to seek appropriate healthcare.[36,43,44] It is important for all healthcare professionals to be aware that many of their patients will have poor health literacy.

For effective patient education, when using both verbal and written communication methods, health literacy is an important concept to consider. It is essential, however, to recognise that there are two aspects to health literacy: the health literacy of the environment and individual health literacy.[45] The health literacy of the environment includes the systems, processes, people, information and practices involved in the provision of healthcare.[46] There are strategies that organisations and healthcare professionals can adopt to support people with low health literacy, for example, provision of well-designed patient information, educational strategies, support groups for people with chronic illnesses and the use of shared decision-making processes.

MEASURING INDIVIDUAL HEALTH LITERACY

It is not essential to measure a person's health literacy. However, there are a number of tests available to assess the literacy and/or health literacy levels of individual patients. These include simple word recognition tests such as the Wide Range Achievement Test-Revised (WRAT-R)[47] and the Rapid Estimate of Adult Literacy in Medicine (REALM).[48] In addition, the Test of Functional Health Literacy in Adults (TOFHLA)[49] is considered useful because it has good content validity and uses text from real healthcare settings, measuring a patient's comprehension and numeracy skills. More recently, the Health Literacy Questionnaire (HLQ) has been added to this health literacy assessment toolbox.[50] The HLQ was designed to identify health literacy strengths and limitations of both individuals and groups. The questionnaire contains 44 items across nine scales with each scale examining a different domain of health literacy:[50]

- Scale 1: Feeling understood and supported by healthcare providers
- Scale 2: Having sufficient information to manage my health
- Scale 3: Actively managing my health
- Scale 4: Social support for health
- Scale 5: Appraisal of health information
- Scale 6: Ability to actively engage with healthcare providers
- Scale 7: Navigating the healthcare system
- Scale 8: Ability to find good health information
- Scale 9: Understanding health information well enough to know what to do.

The Newest Vital Sign (NVS),[51] accessible in English and Spanish, provides a quick screening test for limited literacy in primary healthcare settings. The NVS consists of a nutrition label with six questions which investigate the participant's ability to read and apply the information from the label. Unlike the other health literacy assessment tests, which tend to be time-consuming to administer, the NVS is quick (1–3 minutes) and convenient, which makes it more appealing for busy healthcare professionals. In addition to the quick and easy-to-administer NVS tool, Chew and colleagues[52] developed the following three questions to screen for limited health literacy:

1. How often do you have someone help you read hospital materials?
2. How often do you have problems learning about your medical condition because of difficulty understanding written information?
3. How confident are you filling out forms by yourself?

Further research has shown that a modified version of the Chew's 'confident with forms'[52] question, 'How often do you need to have someone help you when you read instructions, pamphlets, or other written material from your doctor or pharmacy?' can be used alone to detect patients who will have difficulty reading health-related information.[53]

Given the busy nature of EDs, it is recommended that all healthcare professionals and the organisations they work for adopt the universal precautions approach to health literacy.[54,55] In brief, this means that every patient is treated as though they have low health literacy, especially in terms of difficulty accessing and understanding health information. By taking this approach, everyone benefits from the provision of clear information in plain language and not just those who most need it.

EFFECTIVE PATIENT COMMUNICATION

Effective communication involves two-way communication between the patient and the healthcare professional,[56–58] which often involves more than just the spoken word. To be effective, communication needs to be tailored to the individual, allowing patients the opportunity for clarification and feedback and tailored to the person's health literacy and needs.

WAYS TO IMPROVE HEALTHCARE PROFESSIONAL–PATIENT COMMUNICATIONS

Healthcare professionals can help foster and facilitate effective communication with patients by using the following guiding principles:[58–60]

- plan and think about the needs and desired outcomes for each session
- clarify the needs and desired outcomes for each session with the patient and carer/family member
- consider providing information in meaningful blocks, spread over multiple sessions
- make the sessions interactive and use the teach-back technique[61] to gauge understanding
- engage the patient and their carer/family members during each session.

Effective communication between healthcare professionals and patients can be further encouraged by providing patient education and information in a timely manner, and by offering encouragement, reinforcement, reassurance and feedback.[58,62,63] Encouragement can be given to patients by developing rapport, establishing trust, asking questions, inviting patients to make comments,[64] and by respecting the patient's opinions, assumptions and attitudes.[65] Verbal reinforcement can be offered by reiteration and repetition of important points.[59] Reassurance can be promoted by addressing patients in a positive, caring and motivating manner, while ensuring that they are as comfortable as possible and confident enough to ask questions.[66]

The teach-back technique is an effective method of gauging patient understanding of the concepts prior to them being discussed.[61] Teach-back is not about testing the patient, but rather asking the patient to explain in their own words what they have understood based on the information they have been provided.[19] Other useful strategies for providing effective communication include providing feedback regarding responses to open-ended questions, rather than questions that require 'yes' or 'no' answers.[67] This feedback allows the healthcare professionals to correct any misunderstandings. In the event that patients have misunderstood or misinterpreted information, healthcare professionals can use this opportunity to revise the explanation and correct misunderstanding in a positive manner. Further reinforcement can be offered through the provision of written information with key points highlighted.[68]

ACTIVE LISTENING

Active listening is a core component of effective communication and can positively impact patient health outcomes.[18,59,69] Healthcare professionals who actively listen to their patients make them feel valued and confident,[18] thereby fostering a collaborative and supportive partnership. When culturally appropriate, it is also important to use non-verbal cues to demonstrate active listening. This includes maintaining appropriate eye contact and direction of gaze, sitting slightly forward, facing the patient, displaying positive facial expressions and nodding when appropriate.[59,67] Similarly, verbal cues, such as asking questions associated with the patient's last comment, as well as using appropriate tone, rate and volume of speech can be used to further demonstrate active listening.[59,67]

The physical proximity of the healthcare professional to the patient and/or their carer/family member can have an impact upon the effectiveness of the communication during the education session. A close but comfortable position is important[70] because sitting too close may make the patient feel threatened, while sitting too far away may suggest disinterest.[67] When communicating with patients in both hospital and community settings, it is also important to be sitting at the same level as the patient, rather than speaking to them from a standing position, which could make them feel vulnerable or intimidated.[67]

LEARNING ENVIRONMENTS

Learning environments play an important role in patient education. To be effective, learning environments should encourage patients and their carers/family members to listen, feel confident enough to ask questions, access information and seek reassurance about their knowledge and understanding.[71,72] Positive learning environments occur in three key phases: (i) before learning (i.e. logistics about where learning will take place, preparation of information based on learning goals and providing a welcoming environment); (ii) during learning (i.e. making introductions, ensuring a balance of power, encouraging open communication and providing a safe and supportive environment); (iii) after learning (i.e. recapping key points, giving and getting feedback, and providing contact information for future questions).[72] In busy environments such as EDs, it is not always possible to find a quiet area in which to offer education to patients and their carer/family members. However, it is important to try to ensure that the surroundings are as private and comfortable as possible, thereby facilitating communication between all parties.[16,73]

PRIVACY

Privacy is another important consideration required for effective communication. For example, a patient in a hospital bed in a shared room may not wish to discuss personal health-related matters or may be distracted by what is happening around them.[74] Education/information sessions should, where possible, take place in a quiet setting with appropriate lighting, seating and temperature arrangements.[18,67] For healthcare professionals working in the community environment, educating patients in their home environment provides an excellent opportunity to educate them in a comfortable and familiar environment with fewer distractions, and the possibility of having important carer/family members present.

TEACHABLE MOMENTS

Despite the challenges of providing patient education in busy healthcare settings such as EDs, these settings often present opportunities described as 'teachable moments'.[15,75] Teachable moments are unplanned opportunities, often created by a unique situation, that allow for the discussion of a specific topic, such as a health issue, and may lead to positive behaviour change which helps to improve the patient's health status.[76] For healthcare professionals to effectively use these 'teachable moments' they could engage in a number of strategies, which include the provision of verbal instruction; the use of problem-solving techniques; the provision of up-to-date written information; and, where possible, participation in role-playing or simulations.[16,73] These 'teachable moments' may also involve the use of health information websites and multimedia education programs.[77–79] Such opportunities would be particularly important in promoting and reinforcing positive health behaviours and therapeutic management strategies that help to optimise patient health outcomes.[63,80,81] In addition, emerging research has identified that patient educational interventions in the ED, using a variety of teaching methods, have been effective at improving health outcomes.[15,16,82]

INVOLVEMENT OF FAMILY MEMBERS AND CARERS

Perhaps one of the more valuable interventions to help improve healthcare professional–patient communication is to urge family members and/or significant others to attend patient education sessions.[1,3,4,40,83] The active participation of patients and their carers/family members in the learning process helps to ensure that the patient understands the information given to them, which should build on what they already know to improve their health outcomes.[80,84] This is particularly beneficial for patients with cognitive impairment, poor health literacy skills and those living with intellectual disabilities.

PATIENT FOLLOW-UP

Patient follow-up is another important intervention which can be used to improve patient engagement and communication with their healthcare professionals.[85,86] Patient follow-up, which can occur individually, as part of a group, over the telephone, by letter or via electronic means, is useful to reinforce and clarify important information, provide reassurance and suggest changes to health behaviours when appropriate.[55,87,88] Patient follow-up, especially after discharge from hospital or the ED, significantly reduces the incidence of hospital readmission.[84,87–89] Healthcare professionals working in both hospital and community healthcare settings are ideally placed to provide patient follow-up.

TARGETING PATIENT EDUCATION ABOUT MEDICATION ADHERENCE

Estimates of poor medication adherence among patients who have been prescribed medications range from 20% to 70% for all medications,[90,91] and 50% to 65% for long-term medications for chronic disease.[92] This is of concern because poor medication adherence has been found to be associated with poorer health outcomes and increased healthcare costs.[93,94] For patients who are taking medications as part of their therapeutic regimen, healthcare professionals can promote medication adherence by addressing the following when delivering their patient education:[92,94–96]

- inform the patients and their carer/family members about the importance of regular adherence to prescribed medications
- tailor the information to the patient's needs
- suggest appropriate dosing schedules in plain language
- inform the patient about potential medication-related side-effects
- identify possible drug-to-drug interactions and/or contraindications
- explain the implications of poor medication adherence
- when appropriate, recommend medication adherence aids and dosage reminders, such as blister packs, dosette boxes, medication alarms or medication cards, especially for patients with physical (e.g. poor eyesight) and/or cognitive impairments (e.g. dementia).

HEALTH PROMOTION ACTIVITIES AND DISEASE PREVENTION STRATEGIES

In addition to the provision of patient education, healthcare professionals working both within and outside of the hospital environment have the opportunity to promote positive health behaviours that will help lead to better health outcomes.[20,97] Health promotion activities enable people to increase their control and management of their own health behaviours, with a view to improving their health.[98,99] Such activities often target diet, physical activity, smoking, alcohol use, recreational drug-taking and sun safety, and may also include community education and education about disease prevention strategies. Community education strategies can encompass a broad range of activities, depending on the needs of the community, which include education about road safety, marine safety, injury prevention, harm minimisation and first aid training.[100,101] Disease prevention strategies occur at three levels: primary disease prevention strategies are designed to eradicate health risks (e.g. vaccination); secondary disease prevention strategies can lead to an early diagnosis of disease (e.g. screening); and tertiary disease prevention strategies refer to rehabilitation activities that assist with the recovery process following ill-health (e.g. referral to a cardiac rehabilitation clinic after a heart attack).[102] The choice of health promotion activities, and uptake of disease prevention strategies, can be influenced by many factors, including government health policies and priorities, available programs and societal influences.[103] At an individual level, there can also be the impact of factors such as age, gender, socioeconomic status, education level and cultural issues.[103] It is important for healthcare professionals to be aware of the influences of these factors when promoting and encouraging the uptake of these health promotion activities and disease prevention strategies.

When educating patients and their carer/family members, healthcare professionals should take every opportunity to encourage or 'nudge' patients to change unhealthy behaviours. These behaviours should include: undertaking regular exercise, eating nutritious foods, minimising alcohol intake, smoking cessation (when and if appropriate), stress management and the development and maintenance of social support networks. When appropriate, healthcare professionals should also recommend disease prevention strategies such as: immunisation programs, identification of age-appropriate screening examinations (e.g.

breast screening, cervical screening, prostate screening); and the clarification of safety issues (e.g. child safety, safe sex behaviours, occupational health). Although healthcare professionals working in busy environments may not necessarily view their role as supporting disease prevention strategies, it is important they recognise that many patients would benefit from receiving reinforcement regarding the value of these strategies.[16,104] Emerging evidence suggests that ED staff are often involved in assessing modifiable risk factors for acute and chronic illness and are therefore well placed to offer health promotion interventions and advice.[104,105] For example, on a patient level ED staff can be involved in assessing vaccination status and providing advice, as well as providing health information for a wide variety of health issues. They may also be involved in referring patients for screening for different issues (e.g. mental health, substance abuse or domestic violence screening).[106] ED staff can also play an important role in promoting the health of the community by addressing sustainability initiatives (e.g. infection control, disposal of hospital waste and limiting the use of plastic cups).[106]

VERBAL PATIENT EDUCATION AND COMMUNICATION

GUIDELINES FOR EFFECTIVE VERBAL PATIENT EDUCATION AND COMMUNICATION SESSIONS

Verbal communication is the most frequently used patient education strategy and a key component of effective patient education. Healthcare professionals use verbal communication during both formal and informal patient education sessions, with the added bonus of being able to readily tailor their education session(s) based on the patient's needs and their current understanding of their health status. Simple and useful tips to assist in achieving effective verbal patient education sessions include:[4,18,27,59,67,84,107,108]

- use plain language which is clear, simple and direct (e.g. 'eat' rather than 'consume')
- avoid medical jargon, where possible (e.g. heart rather than cardiac; kidney rather than renal)
- avoid giving vague advice (e.g. 'take this every day at 10 am' rather than 'take this regularly')
- speak slowly in a clear, active voice
- confirm the patient's understanding of the information provided by asking them to repeat what they have heard and what it means to them (e.g. use the teach-back technique)
- avoid giving too many directives at once, which may overwhelm the patient
- ask the patient to repeat the key points before they leave the session
- provide simple, easy-to-read and actionable written information (when available)
- encourage patients to ask questions through the use of open-ended questions (e.g. 'What questions do you have?' rather than 'Do you have any questions?')

When speaking with older patients, as well as those with low literacy skills, it may also be necessary to:[27,40]

- ensure enough time is spent with the patient
- allow for frequent short appointments, rather than one long appointment (when possible)
- provide pictures and visual images (when available)
- encourage patients to bring along a family member
- demonstrate respect and empathy.

Healthcare professionals should be aware of the following potential issues, which can have a negative impact on effective communication during patient education sessions:[59,67]

- failing to recognise both verbal and non-verbal cues
- not giving patients and/or families enough time to have their say or consider options presented
- asking too many questions
- using slang, medical jargon or vague terms that could be misinterpreted
- experiencing unnecessary disruptions
- rushing through information without assessing patient understanding.

Box 8.1 provides some practical guidelines, based on communication principles, which can be used by healthcare professionals during patient education sessions.[59] The generic nature of these guidelines makes them suitable for both formal and informal patient education sessions in any healthcare setting.

BOX 8.1 PRACTICE GUIDELINES FOR EFFECTIVE PATIENT COMMUNICATION[59,109]

- Assess the patient's knowledge prior to providing information.
- Address underlying concerns that the patient and/or family member express.
- Ensure that the information provided relates to the patient's perspectives and/or concerns.
- Provide information and explanations in an organised, logical sequence.
- Engage the patient in an interactive conversation through the use of open-ended questions.
- Use simple language and examples to teach-back to ensure important concepts are understood.
- Encourage patients to be involved in the learning process by contributing their ideas and suggestions.
- Elicit the patient's responses, reactions and attitudes regarding information provided and/or therapeutic management plans suggested.
- When tailoring a therapeutic management plan, negotiate a mutually acceptable plan which takes into consideration the patient's lifestyle, beliefs, cultural background and abilities.
- Encourage patients to be involved in implementing their therapeutic management plans and taking responsibility for self-management of their health conditions.
- Use suitable non-verbal encouragement when appropriate (e.g. a pat on the shoulder, nodding, smiling) and verbal encouragement when appropriate.

PATIENT ENGAGEMENT AND COMMUNICATION WITH ETHNICALLY DIVERSE PATIENTS

Healthcare professionals need to recognise that language and communication barriers can be major contributors to poor health outcomes and adverse events for many ethnically diverse patients.[110–112] For example, ethnically diverse patients with limited English experience are at greater risk of infections, falls, hospital re-admissions, extended length of hospital stays and surgical delays, compared to their English-speaking counterparts.[113–116]

Cultural competence is often used to describe the knowledge, skills and attitudes that healthcare professionals require when providing effective patient education to patients from diverse ethnic and cultural backgrounds.[59,117] This may involve sensitivity towards issues, such as gender, family relationships, religion, spiritual and cultural beliefs,[107,117,118] as well as support and a mutual respect for these patients.[67,119] Healthcare professionals should be mindful that patients from ethnically diverse backgrounds may have certain expectations and beliefs about their healthcare needs. It is important for healthcare professionals to be aware of these needs and expectations prior to the patient education sessions.[67,118,120]

Cultural differences might also affect the patient's therapeutic management. As such, healthcare professionals should try to ask open-ended questions, allowing the patient to contribute to the session, thereby gaining a better understanding of the cultural differences without compromising the quality of care.[18,59,67] Healthcare professionals also benefit from recognising possible cultural differences in non-verbal behaviours such as touching, proximity and eye contact, which may make the patient feel uncomfortable. In addition, awareness and knowledge about cultural competency issues when communicating with vulnerable groups, such as refugees and asylum seekers, is important.[121] For example, when communicating with refugees, healthcare professionals need to appreciate that in addition to the language and cultural barriers experienced by these patients,[122] refugees often experience higher rates of psychological and physical health problems, resulting from a lack of access to appropriate healthcare services and possible exposure to trauma.[123,124] These experiences may negatively impact on their attitudes and health-seeking behaviours, which is why good listening skills are essential when communicating with and caring for this vulnerable patient population.[122]

PATIENT ENGAGEMENT AND COMMUNICATION WITH ABORIGINAL AND TORRES STRAIT ISLANDER PEOPLE

When providing patient education to Aboriginal and Torres Strait Islander people, it is particularly important to acknowledge that there are different languages, communication needs and cultural preferences across the country.[125] It is suggested that patient education is most successful when the healthcare professional takes a respectful, non-judgemental approach.[126] Further, asking local Indigenous staff to provide support and mentorship is recommended.[126,127] Such partnerships can provide guidance around the local meaning of words, traditional practices such as men's and women's business and non-verbal communication.[125,127] For example, avoiding eye contact is often seen as a mark of respect, as is the use of extended silences.[127] It is also important to understand how European colonisation has affected the lives of Aboriginal and Torres Strait Islander people, including access to healthcare and health services.[126]

THE USE OF INTERPRETERS

Healthcare professionals have legal and ethical obligations to ensure effective communication with their patients from ethnically diverse backgrounds, including Aboriginal and Torres Strait Islander people. Qualified professional healthcare interpreters should always be used, in preference to family members, friends or bilingual staff, as they have received specific training in interpreting medical terminology.[128–130] This is important because the use of informal interpreters has been reported to contribute to adverse events[131] and longer hospital stays.[132,133] Moreover, the use of professional interpreters has been found to improve the quality and safety of care and promotes access to healthcare.[134,135]

In situations where access to and use of qualified professional healthcare interpreters may be problematic and logistically difficult, telephone interpreter services are a suitable alternative.[54] However, when an interpreter is able to attend, it is preferable for both the interpreter and the healthcare professional to face and speak directly to the patient.[136] The following tips should be considered when communicating with ethnically diverse patients via an interpreter:[18]

- If possible, liaise with the interpreter prior to the patient education session to introduce yourself and to clarify any areas of uncertainty.
- At the beginning of the patient education session, introduce everyone and describe their role.
- Always speak to the patient and their family members rather than the interpreter.
- Use plain language and short sentences.
- Avoid medical jargon.
- Observe non-verbal cues.
- Encourage patient engagement by asking open-ended questions and using the teach-back technique.
- Summarise and reinforce key issues.

WRITTEN PATIENT INFORMATION

PROVIDING SIMPLE, EASY-TO-READ WRITTEN PATIENT INFORMATION

Written information resources are a convenient, economical and useful way of providing information to patients.[137,138] Evidence suggests that use of good quality written information, in addition to verbal information, increases patients' knowledge, understanding, adherence and satisfaction with therapeutic regimens.[108,139,140] Healthcare professionals should therefore always try to provide additional written information where possible, especially since patients remember approximately 25% of what they hear, but more than 50% of what they hear and read.[141] Another important reason for providing written information is that patient recall is an essential component for improving treatment adherence and health outcomes.[142]

THE READABILITY OF WRITTEN PATIENT INFORMATION

The goal of written patient information is to increase patient knowledge and understanding by providing a cheap, portable, reusable and self-paced learning resource.[63,137,143] It is important, therefore, that the written information can be read and understood by the patients and/or their carer/family member(s). To ensure that appropriate written information resources are provided or recommended it is important to assess the readability level of the written patient information and to ensure that the information is suitable and of good quality.

ASSESSING THE READING GRADE LEVEL OF WRITTEN PATIENT INFORMATION

It is important to consider the educational reading grade required to read and understand written patient information. There are many different tools available to assess written information; these include the Simple Measure of Gobbledygook (SMOG) index;[144] the Fry Readability Formula (FRY);[145] the Gunning FOG formula;[146] and the Flesch Reading Ease (FRE) formula.[147] Several of these tools can be accessed online. See Useful websites section.

The Flesch Reading Ease test and Flesch-Kincaid Grade Level tests are also included in Microsoft Word. These functions can be readily accessed by enabling 'show readability statistics', under 'File', 'Options'. Once this feature is enabled, MS Word will check the document for spelling, grammar and readability when a spell check is performed.[148]

Perhaps the major limitation for each of these tools, as far as written patient information is concerned, is that they are not healthcare-specific, and, as such, inclusion of medical terms often results in higher readability scores.

It is worth checking readability with more than one tool, as research shows there is concern about inconsistency between scores from different readability tools.[149–151] This problem is caused by the different tools using different formulas which consider syllables, word length and sentence length,[152] as well as font size, font type and the inclusion of pictures and illustrations.[153,154]

PRESENTATION OF WRITTEN PATIENT INFORMATION

Written patient information should be presented clearly and in a format suitable for patient needs. The validated Suitability Assessment of Materials (SAM) instrument[155] provides a thorough assessment of written patient information because it reviews the content, as well as the graphics, layout and cultural appropriateness of the information. In addition, the SAM[155] instrument can be used to evaluate the learning stimulation, motivation and cultural appropriateness of the written information for different patient populations, including those with low literacy. The Bernier Instructional Design Scale (BIDS)[156] is another instrument designed to identify and measure the presence (or absence) of learning principles within written patient information.

The Baker Able Leaflet Design (BALD)[157] was developed to assess the standardised Australian consumer medicine information leaflets,[158] and contributed to the development of the Medicine Information Design Assessment Scale (MIDAS),[159] which assesses the layout, design and quality of written medication information. Healthcare professionals can use any of these instruments to evaluate existing resources and/or to help guide the development of new written patient information resources.

QUALITY OF WRITTEN PATIENT INFORMATION

The quality of the written information being presented and/or developed for patients and their carer/family members is another important element to consider. The Patient Education Materials Assessment Tool (PEMAT) is a 26-item tool that evaluates the understandability and actionability of written health information.[160] This tool is a validated tool and helps to determine whether patients will be able to understand and act on the information provided.[160] Other tools which can be used by both health professionals and patients to assess the quality of written health information include the DISCERN instrument[161,162] and the Brief DISCERN instrument,[163] which can be used to identify good information on the internet. The CDC Clear Communication Index is a 20-item tool that allows health professionals to develop and assess the quality of patient education materials against criteria that enhance clarity and aid understanding by ensuring that the materials are written in plain language.[164] The Ensuring Quality Information for Patients (EQIP) scale[165] and the EQIP36[166] are two additional instruments that can be used to assess the quality of written information, in terms of language, tone and text organisation. EQIP36 also assesses the quality of information in terms of risk and consequences for medical procedures, procedural steps and other background information.[166]

PATIENT COMPREHENSION AND SATISFACTION WITH WRITTEN INFORMATION

Ultimately patients and their carer/family members need to be able to understand and be satisfied with the written information they receive. Apart from asking the patients themselves about whether or not they are satisfied and can understand the written information received, there are some tools that can be used to assess their comprehension and satisfaction. For example, in addition to the aforementioned PEMAT instrument,[160] the Cloze test[155,167] can be used to assess patients' understanding of the written information, as well as the reading difficulty of the written information. The Satisfaction with Information about Medicines Scale (SIMS)[168] and the Consumer Information Rating Form (CIRF)[169] can be used to specifically target written information about medication. SIMS is a 17-item tool designed to assess patient satisfaction with the written information they receive about their prescribed medicines.[170] The CIRF measures patients' perception about the comprehensibility, design quality and utility of the written medicine information[169] and has been translated for use into different languages.[170]

DEVELOPING WRITTEN PATIENT INFORMATION

There are legal, moral, ethical and financial incentives that warrant the time needed to develop good-quality written patient information resources. It is known that good-quality written information helps to improve patient health outcomes by supporting informed decision-making and reducing healthcare co sts.[46,86,119,152,171] Consequently, it is important for healthcare professionals who are developing new written information resources for their patients to ensure that the information can be easily read, understood and acted upon.[51,54,137,160]

The development of health information materials is a highly skilled activity.[55,172,173] Written information should ideally be created using plain English, an active voice and be personalised (using the pronouns we and you).[55,140,173] The information should be targeted at Grade 6–8 levels (ages 11–13 years),[155,174] and complex information should be conveyed via the use of bullet points.[144,152,174] Other factors, such as the font used, the font size, the contrast between text and background, and the use of pictures, infographics, illustrations and white space, also need to be considered.[140,175] These can enhance patients' knowledge, understanding, satisfaction and engagement with the written information.[63,176–180]

Visual aids and graphic illustrations provide quick and effective ways of disseminating information to patients and their cares/family members.[108,175,181] The use of appropriate visual aids and illustrations (including cartoons, pictographs and infographics), in combination with verbal/written information, has been found to improve patient understanding, recall and retention of medical information.[177,180,182] It follows that when creating patient education materials for specific patient groups (e.g. older people and/or ethnically diverse people) that relevant and appropriate images are used. Furthermore, for patient education materials developed for use with patients from Indigenous backgrounds (e.g. Aboriginal and Torres Strait Islander people), it is important to try and include photos of local people and places and use Indigenous-specific graphics.[125] When using visual aids and graphic illustrations it is also important to be aware of colour combinations that may be appropriate for people who are colourblind.[175]

Box 8.2 contains a summary of tips to assist healthcare professionals in the development of good-quality written patient information.

The following online resources can be used to ensure that written information complies with these design guidelines:

- Guidelines for Creating Materials: resources for assessing and developing materials[137]
  - cdn1.sph.harvard.edu/wp-content/uploads/sites/135/2012/09/resources_for_creating_materials.pdf.
  - www.hsph.harvard.edu/healthliteracy/
- Simply Put: A Guide for Creating Easy-to-Understand Materials
  - www.cdc.gov/healthliteracy/
  - www.cdc.gov/ccindex/index.htm
- Toolkit for making written material clear and effective
  - www.cms.gov/outreach-and-education/outreach/writtenmaterialstoolkit
- The United Kingdom Department of Health 'Toolkit for Producing Patient Information'
  - ppitoolkit.org.uk/PDF/toolkit/patient_info_toolkit.pdf
- The Agency for Healthcare Research and Quality (AHRQ) Health Literacy Universal Precautions Toolkit, 2nd edition
  - www.ahrq.gov/health-literacy/improve/precautions/index.html

WRITTEN INFORMATION FOR ETHNICALLY DIVERSE PATIENTS

When selecting and/or developing written information for ethnically diverse patients and their family members, it is important to include information and illustrations that are culturally sensitive.[27] Seeking the advice of members from the cultural group should ideally occur prior to and during the development of these written patient resources.

For ethnically diverse patients and carers/family members who are literate in their native language, information that has been translated into their first language would be the preferred option.[54] Notably, however, limited health literacy and poor English-speaking proficiency often co-exist in this patient population.[183–186] This suggests that many ethnically diverse patients will require additional education sessions, supplemented with materials with low-health literacy demand, including resources in the form of visual aids and/or, where possible, multimedia tools.[108,177,187,188]

ONLINE HEALTH INFORMATION RESOURCES

Online health information resources can be used by healthcare professionals to reinforce important information and improve patients' knowledge and understanding about the information provided. Like written patient education, online health information is useful for patients as they can access the information

BOX 8.2 TIPS TO ASSIST WITH DEVELOPING EASY-TO-READ WRITTEN INFORMATION[108,137,173]

ORGANISATION

- Information needs to be presented in a logical order
- Include necessary background information or context
- Provide small blocks of text with clear headings
- Emphasise and summarise main points
- Help patients make decisions by giving them facts about risks, side-effects and benefits—link information to other reputable and reliable sources

STYLE

- Use everyday plain language—avoid jargon and acronyms
- Write at or below Grade 6–8 reading levels
- Use short sentences—approximately 15–20 words long
- Use lower-case letters where possible
- Use present and active tenses
- Use a question and answer format to help engage readers

LAYOUT AND DESIGN

- Use sans serif type with a minimum font size of 12 point
- Ensure a good amount of white space on the page
- Bullet points are preferable to blocks of text
- Use appropriate space between lines (e.g. 1.2 to 1.5 spacing between lines)
- Use a large bold font to emphasise text. Avoid uppercase letters, italics and underlining
- If appropriate, provide clearly labelled, simple and instructive visual aids/illustrations.

whenever and wherever they need to. From an organisational point of view, online health information is relatively cheap to produce and update. These online resources can be created to be interactive and allow the information provided to be tailored specifically to the patients' needs.

RELIABLE AND REPUTABLE SOURCES OF ONLINE HEALTH INFORMATION

Healthcare professionals should be aware of the many sources of online information available to patients and their carers/family members. It is important, however, to consider the quality and the accuracy of this information, as well as the needs of the patients and their carer/family members. Many non-profit organisations provide online patient education and support resources, such as Asthma Australia and Kidney Health Australia. While global information is readily available, often country-specific, or even state-specific, resources are preferable as they refer to the treatment regimens and healthcare structures that the patients are familiar with. Other useful sites for patient information resources include department of health websites, national prescribing websites, university websites and other sources listed at the end of this chapter. Healthcare professionals should provide guidance to patients about trustworthy sites to visit to avoid patients aimlessly searching the internet for information that may not always be useful or trustworthy.[189–192] Health professionals should also be conscious of the fact that older people are increasingly accessing web-based information sources to help make better-informed decisions about their health.[193] In addition to providing guidance about trustworthy sites, healthcare professionals could also recommend that patients use tools such as the PEMAT,[160] DISCERN,[161] the CDC Clear Communication Index,[164] or ensure that the sites are HON-code certified.[194]

MOBILE APPLICATIONS

Applications relating to health and health information are readily available on smartphones and tablet devices. Data indicates that health and fitness apps are the leading category of apps downloaded, and that 64% of US adults regularly use a health app to manage their health and lifestyle behaviours, and to share health information with their doctors.[195] While apps have enormous potential to influence how patients and carers engage in the management of their health, there are also numerous non-evidence-based apps available that do not provide good-quality information and can create confusion.[196–198] In addition, there is evidence that people prefer apps as an adjunct to, rather than a replacement for, in-person consultations with healthcare professionals.[199,200] This may be because the use of health apps requires a high level of digital literacy,[201] and patients prefer not to have to actively input data.[200] Health professionals who recommend the use of health apps should be aware that this may potentially worsen health inequalities, given that mobile technologies are typically adopted by affluent, well-educated consumers with the technical skills needed to operate apps.[201]

If health professionals wish to suggest mobile apps for the management of health to their patients, there are a number of recommendations that can help to ensure the most appropriate app is recommended:[202]

- Search the literature and app clearing house websites for reviews of apps.
- Search app stores to ensure that the apps suggested are evidence-based and user-friendly.
- Review app descriptions, their user ratings and read their reviews.
- Pilot potentially suitable apps to evaluate functionality, usability and content accuracy.
- Obtain feedback from patients about the apps used to better understand which apps may be more useful for different patient groups.

TELEHEALTH

Telehealth is a broad term, which refers to the provision of healthcare over distance using telecommunications technologies, such as video, phone, text messaging, web-based services and remote patient monitoring.[203] The delivery of healthcare via telehealth has been touted to improve access to healthcare and patient health outcomes, as well as contribute to a reduction in healthcare costs.[204] However, many of the telehealth initiatives used prior to, and during, the COVID-19 pandemic were supported by weak evidence of their effectiveness.[204,205] The Cochrane Library has collated the available evidence from systematic reviews,[206] suggesting that the benefits of telehealth are limited and that patient outcomes appear similar to in-person care.[207]

Prior to the pandemic, there were three discernible telehealth trends, which included greater access and convenience to healthcare, greater focus on the management of chronic conditions, and a shift of telehealth from hospitals and clinics to the home and the use of mobile devices.[208] In theory, these initiatives are achievable; however, the evidence suggests that healthcare providers using telehealth often experience issues with usability, implementation issues, bandwidth and connectivity.[205]

The need to protect healthcare professionals and patients during the rapid spread of COVID-19, between 2020 and 2021, led to the rapid expansion of telehealth.[209,210] During the pandemic, telehealth has been used to expand access to a wide range of healthcare services, such as primary care, chronic disease management, mental health, mild-to-moderate COVID-19 support, contact tracing and staff training.[211,212] It is anticipated that at least some of these changes in healthcare delivery will continue beyond the pandemic,[213] even though others feel that telehealth could exacerbate health inequalities and poor health outcomes.[210]

If telehealth is to be adopted more broadly, then it is important to ensure that patients, carers and healthcare professionals have the necessary skills to optimise its utilisation. Patients and carers need instructions on how to use telehealth and directions on how to handle patient–healthcare professional interactions. Healthcare professionals need training on how to set up joint agendas remotely, handle effective telehealth engagement and communication, and assess patient comprehension. They also need to be aware of the challenges that telehealth can present when trying to build rapport and establish therapeutic relations, especially with new patients.[214] At a systems level, successful telehealth requires convenient, fast and secure internet connections, user-friendly telehealth platforms and affordable cost structures.[215–217] Attention should be paid to adequately resource technological infrastructure and to promote positive attitudes towards the technology, with plenty of time for capacity building and sharing best practice.[218]

SUMMARY

In this chapter it has been established that healthcare professionals, including nurses and paramedics, play a pivotal role in helping patients to understand how to achieve optimal health and therapeutic outcomes by providing them with effective patient education. In order to do this successfully, healthcare professionals need to:

- promote good healthcare professional–patient communication and partnerships
- provide good-quality, easy-to-understand verbal and written information in an effective manner
- promote medication and treatment adherence (where appropriate), via well timed and appropriate health promotion and disease prevention activities.

It is also important for healthcare professionals to recognise that they may need to spend more time educating patients who are older, those with poor health literacy and patients from ethnically diverse backgrounds, to ensure that they have understood the information provided. Qualified health interpreters should also be used when communicating with patients from ethnically diverse backgrounds, especially if they have limited English proficiency. Furthermore, all patients should be provided with high-quality, easy-to-understand information. In this chapter, a number of simple tests and instruments have been suggested for use in assessing the readability, quality and suitability of information that is already available and/or being developed for patients and their family members.

CASE STUDY

Paramedics are called out to the home of Miss PG, a 5-year-old child, who is distressed and experiencing breathing problems, that is, rapid and shallow breathing. Her mother is extremely agitated and informs the paramedics that her child used to suffer bronchiolitis as a baby, but has never had an experience as bad as this one before. Clinical examination of the child by the paramedics confirms evidence of hypoxaemia associated with impaired ventilation and expiratory wheeze. Following the administration of oxygen, and nebulised salbutamol, Miss PG's condition only improves slightly and she is transported by the paramedics via ambulance to the local hospital emergency department (ED). En route to the hospital, the paramedics gently but firmly reassure the mother about the child's safety to allay her fears and they also ensure that the child is comfortable, relaxed and continues to receive appropriate care.

On arrival at the hospital, the paramedics inform the triage nurse about the child's condition and as a result she is immediately seen by a paediatric registrar, who diagnoses her with an acute exacerbation of asthma. The paediatric registrar prescribes a salbutamol inhaler (reliever) and a steroid inhaler (preventer) for the child to use and writes a discharge letter for the mother to take to their local doctor.

The nurse is then asked to educate the mother and child about asthma medications, correct inhaler technique, the importance of medication adherence and the importance of follow-up consultations with their local doctor. The nurse is also asked to provide the mother with information resources on asthma and asthma medication.

QUESTIONS

1. In this scenario, what strategies could the paramedic and the ED nurse use to communicate most effectively with the child and her mother?
2. Describe the most appropriate location for the nurse to educate both the mother and the child about the new asthma medications and correct inhaler technique.
3. What barriers to effective communication might the nurse encounter?
4. Where would the nurse search to find reliable, valid and appropriate information about asthma, asthma medications and correct inhaler technique?
5. What advice should the nurse provide to the mother for the ongoing management for her daughter's asthma following her discharge from the hospital emergency department?

Answers to Case Study Questions can be found on evolve **http://evolve.elsevier.com/AU/Curtis/emergency/** 

USEFUL WEBSITES

Advisory Committee on Medicine (AM), www.tga.gov.au/committee/advisory-committee-medicines-acm.

Alcohol and Drug Foundation, adf.org.au/.

Arthritis Australia, arthritisaustralia.com.au/.

Asthma Australia, asthma.org.au/.

Australian Commission on Safety and Quality in Health Care (ACSQHC), www.safetyandquality.gov.au/.

Australian Government Department of Health and Ageing, www.health.gov.au/.

Australian Institute of Health and Welfare (AIHW), www.aihw.gov.au/.

Beyond Blue, www.beyondblue.org.au/.

Cancer Council, www.cancer.org.au/.

Clinical Excellence Commission, www.cec.health.nsw.gov.au/.

Dementia Australia, www.dementia.org.au/.

Diabetes Australia, www.diabetesaustralia.com.au/.

Heart Foundation, www.heartfoundation.org.au/.

Kidney Health Australia, kidney.org.au/.

National Institutes of Health, www.nih.gov/.

National Prescribing Service (NPS), www.nps.org.au/.

National Tobacco Campaign, www.health.gov.au/initiatives-and-programs/national-tobacco-campaign/.

Plain language in health care, www.plainlanguage.gov/resources/content-types/healthcare/.

Pregnancy, Birth and Baby, www.pregnancybirthbaby.org.au/.

Readability checkers, www.readabilityformulas.com/free-readability-formula-tests.php or Hemingway readability app: hemingwayapp.com/.

Sport Australia, www.sportaus.gov.au/.

Teach-back, teachback.org/.

The Australian Immunisation Handbook, immunisationhandbook.health.gov.au/.

World Health Organization (WHO), www.who.int/.

REFERENCES

1. Joint Commission International. International Patient Safety Goals (IPSGs). Oakbrook Terrace, Illinois: 2021. Online. Available from: www.jointcommission.org/standards/national-patient-safety-goals/.
2. Euromed Info. Patient Teaching into Practice. Online. Available from: www.euromedinfo.eu/.
3. NSW Government Clinical Excellence Commission. Partnering with patients, carers and families. Online. Available from: www.cec.health.nsw.gov.au/improve-quality/teamwork-culture-pcc/partnering-with-people/partnering-with-patients.
4. Australian Commission on Safety and Quality in Health Care (ACSQHC). Partnering with patients in their own care. Online. Available from: www.safetyandquality.gov.au/standards/nsqhs-standards/partnering-consumers-standard/partnering-patients-their-own-care.
5. National Ageing Research Institute. What is person-centred health care? A literature review. Melbourne: Victorian Government Department of Health; 2006/2011. Online. Available from: www.health.vic.gov.au/publications/what-is-person-centred-health-care-a-literature-review.
6. Bertakis KD, Azari R. Patient-centered care is associated with decreased health care utilization. J Am Board Fam Med 2011;24(3):229–39.
7. Saha S, Beach MC. The impact of patient-centred communication on patients' decision making and evaluations of physicians: a randomized study using video vignettes. Patient Educ Couns 2011;84(3):386–92.
8. Meterko M, Wright S, Lin H, Lowy E, Cleary PD. Mortality among patients with acute myocardial infarction: the influences of patient-centered care and evidence-based medicine. Health Serv Res 2010;45(5 Pt 1):1188–204.
9. NHS Health Improvement Scotland (ihub). How is person-centred care understood and implemented in practice? 2021. Online. Available from: strathprints.strath.ac.uk/76933/1/Miller_HIS2021_person_centred_care_review.pdf.
10. Bergeson SC, Dean JD. A systems approach to patient-centered care. JAMA 2006;296(23):2848–51.
11. Sidani S. Effects of patient-centered care on patient outcomes: an evaluation. Res Theory Nurs Pract 2008;22(1):24–37.
12. Bauman A, Fardy J, Harris P. Getting it right: why bother with patient-centred care? Med J Aust 2003;179:253–6.
13. Robinson JH, Callister LC, Berry JA, Dearing KA. centred care and adherence: definitions and applications to improve outcomes. J Am Acad Nurse Pract 2008;20(12):600–7.
14. Jenkins J, Calabria E, Edelheim J, Hodges J, Markwell K, Walo M, et al. Service quality and communication in emergency department waiting rooms: case studies at four New South Wales hospitals. Southern Cross University; 2011.
15. Wei HG, Camargo Jr CA. Patient education in the emergency department. Acad Emerg Med 2000;7(6):710–7.
16. Szpiro AK, Harrison BM, Van Den Kerkhof GE, Lougheed DM. Patient education in the emergency department: a systematic review of interventions and outcomes. Adv Emerg Nurs J 2008;30(1):34–49.
17. Australian Institute of Health and Welfare (AIHW). Emergency department mental health services. 2022. Online. Available from: www.aihw.gov.au/reports/mental-health-services/mental-health-services-in-australia/report-contents/emergency-department-mental-health-services.

18. O'Toole G. Communication: core interpersonal skills for health professionals. 4th ed. Elsevier; 2020.
19. Shersher V, Haines TP, Sturgiss L, Weller C, Williams C. Definitions and use of the teach-back method in healthcare consultations with patients: a systematic review and thematic synthesis. Patient Educ Counsel 2021;194(1):118–29.
20. Rankin SH, Duffy Stallings K. Patient education: principles and practice. 4th ed. Philadelphia: Lippincott, Williams & Wilkins; 2001.
21. Redman Klug B. The practice of patient education. 10th ed. Detroit, Michigan: Mosby; 2006.
22. Hastings S, Oddone EZ, Fillenbaum G, Sloane RJ, Schmader KE. Frequency and predictors of adverse health outcomes in older Medicare beneficiaries discharged from the emergency department. Med Care 2008;46(8):771–7.
23. Hesselink G, Sir O, Koster N, Munsterman M, Olde Rikkert M, Schoon Y. Teach-back of discharge instructions in the emergency department: a pre-post pilot evaluation. Emerg Med J 2022;39(2):139–46.
24. Forster AJ, Murff HJ, Peterson JF, Gandhi TK, Bates DW. The incidence and severity of adverse events affecting patients after discharge from the hospital. Ann Intern Med 2003;138(3):161–7.
25. Lowthian J, Straney LD, Brand CA, Barker AL, De Villiers Smit P, Newnham H, et al. Unplanned early return to the emergency department by older patients: The Safe Elderly Emergency Department Discharge (SEED) project. Age Ageing 2016;45(2):255–61.
26. Feifer R. How a few simple words improve patients' health. Manag Care Q 2003;11(2):29–31.
27. Scudder L. Words and well-being: how literacy affects patient health. J Nurse Pract 2006;2(1):28–35.
28. Sudore RL, Landefeld CS, Pérez-Stable EJ, Bibbins-Domingo K, Williams BA, Schillinger D. Unraveling the relationship between literacy, language proficiency, and patient-physician communication. Patient Educ Couns 2009;75(3):398–402.
29. Sagi D, Spitzer-Shohat S, Schuster M, Daudi L, Rudolf MCJ. Teaching plain language to medical students: improving communication with disadvantaged patients. BMC Med Educ 2021;21(1):407.
30. Phillips TM, Moloney C, Sneath E, Beccaria G, Issac H, Mullens AB, et al. Associated factors, assessment, management, and outcomes of patients who present to the emergency department for acute exacerbation of chronic obstructive pulmonary disease: a scoping review. Respirat Med 2022;193:106747.
31. Williams A, Manias E, Liew D, Gock H, Gorelik A. Working with CALD groups: testing the feasibility of an intervention to improve medication self-management in people with kidney disease, diabetes, and cardiovascular disease. (Report). Renal Soc Australas J 2012;8(2):62.
32. Wechkunanukul K, Grantham H, Damarell R, Clark RA. The association between ethnicity and delay in seeking medical care for chest pain: a systematic review. JBI Database System Rev Implement Rep 2016;14(7):208–35.
33. Nutbeam D. Health literacy as a public health goal: a challenge for contemporary health education and communication strategies into the 21st century. Health Promot Int 2000;15(3):259–67.
34. Nutbeam D. The evolving concept of health literacy. Soc Sci Med 2008;67(12):2072–8.
35. Kickbusch I, Pelikan JM, Apfel F, Tsouros AD, editors. Health literacy: the solid facts. Geneva: WHO; 2013. p. 4.
36. Baker DW, Wolf MS, Feinglass J, Thompson JA. Health literacy, cognitive abilities, and mortality among elderly persons. J Gen Intern Med 2008;23(6):723–6.
37. Baker DW, Wolf MS, Feinglass J, Thompson JA, Gazmararian JA, Huang J. Health literacy and mortality among elderly persons. Arch Intern Med 2007;167(14):1503–9.
38. Adams RJ, Stocks NP, Wilson DH, Gravier S, Kickbusch I, et al. Health literacy: a new concept for general practice? Austral Fam Phys 2009;38(3):144–7.
39. Choudhry FR, Ming LC, Munawar K, Zaidi STR, Patel RP, Khan TM, et al. Health literacy studies conducted in Australia: a scoping review. Int J Environ Res Public Health 2019;16(7):1112.
40. Rajda C, George NM. The effect of education and literacy levels on health outcomes of the elderly. J Nurse Prac 2009;5(2):115–9.
41. Cameron KA, Ross EL, Clayman ML, Bergeron AR, Federman AD, Bailey SC, et al. Measuring patients' self-efficacy in understanding and using prescription medication. Patient Educ Couns 2010;80(3):372–6.
42. Singh S, Acharya SD, Kamath A, Ullal SD, Urval RP. Health literacy status and understanding of the prescription instructions in diabetic patients. J Diabetes Res 2018;2018:4517243.
43. Jordan JE, Buchbinder R, Osborne RH. Conceptualising health literacy from the patient perspective. Patient Educ Couns 2010;79(1):36–42.
44. McCaffery KJ, Dodd RH, Cvejic E, Ayre J, Batcup C, Isautier JMJ, et al. Health literacy and disparities in COVID-19-related knowledge, attitudes, beliefs and behaviours in Australia. Public Health Res Prac 2020;30(4):30342012.
45. Australian Commission on Safety and Quality in Health Care (ACSQHC). Health literacy. 2018. Online. Available: www.safetyandquality.gov.au/our-work/patient-and-consumer-centred-care/health-literacy/.
46. Australian Commission on Safety and Quality in Health Care (ACSQHC). Health literacy: taking action to improve safety and quality. Sydney; 2014.
47. Wilkinson G, Robertson G, editors. The Wide Range Achievement test revised: Administration manual (WRAT-3). Delaware: Wide Range Inc; 1993.
48. Murphy PW, Long SW, Jackson RH, et al. Rapid estimate of adult literacy in medicine (REALM): a quick reading test for patients. J Read 1993;37(2):124–30.
49. Nurrs JR, Parker RM, Williams MV, Baker DW. Test of functional health literacy in adults. Atlanta: Centre for the Study of Adult Literacy; 1995.
50. Osborne RH, Batterham RW, Elsworth GR, Hawkins M, Buchbinder R. The grounded psychometric development and initial validation of the Health Literacy Questionnaire (HLQ). BMC Public Health 2013;13(1):658.
51. Weiss BD, Mays MZ, Martz W, Castro KM, DeWalt DA, Pignone MP, et al. Quick assessment of literacy in primary care: the Newest Vital Sign. Annals Fam Med 2005;3(6):514–22.

52. Chew LD, Bradley KA, Boyko EJ. Brief questions to identify patients with inadequate health literacy. Fam Med 2004;36(8):588–94.

53. Chew LD, Griffin JM, Partin MR, Noorbaloochi S, Grill JP, Snyder A, et al. Validation of screening questions for limited health literacy in a large VA outpatient population. J Gen Internal Med 2008;23(5):561–6.

54. Dewalt DA, Callahan LF, Hawk VH, et al. Health literacy universal precautions toolkit. Chapel Hill: North Carolina Network Consortium Agency for Healthcare Research and Quality; 2010.

55. AHRQ. Health literacy universal precautions toolkit. 2nd ed. Rockville: Agency for Healthcare Research and Quality. Online. Available from: www.ahrq.gov/health-literacy/improve/precautions/index.html.

56. Kwame A, Petrucka PM. A literature-based study of patient-centered care and communication in nurse-patient interactions: barriers, facilitators, and the way forward. BMC Nurs 2021;20(1):158.

57. Ratna H. The importance of effective communication in healthcare practice. Harvard Public Health Rev 2019;23.

58. Paterick TE, Patel N, Tajik AJ, Chandrasekaran K. Improving health outcomes through patient education and partnerships with patients. Proc (Bayl Univ Med Cent) 2017;30(1):112–13.

59. Silverman J, Kurtz S, Draper J. Skills for communicating with patients. 3rd ed. London: Radcliffe Publishing; 2013.

60. Talevski J, Shee AW, Rasmussen B, Kemp G, Beauchamp A. Teach-back: a systematic review of implementation and impacts. PLoS One 2020;15(4):e0231350.

61. Ha Dinh TT, Bonner A, Clark R, Ramsbotham J, Hines S. The effectiveness of the teach-back method on adherence and self-management in health education for people with chronic disease: a systematic review. JBI Database System Rev Implement Rep 2016;14(1):210–47.

62. Ross L. Facilitating rapport through real patient encounters in health care professional education. Australas J Paramed 2013;10(4): Online. Available from: doi.org/10.33151/ajp.10.4.50.

63. Hoffmann T, McKenna K. Analysis of stroke patients' and carers' reading ability and the content and design of written materials: recommendations for improving written stroke information. Patient Educ Couns 2006;60(3):286–93.

64. Price B. Developing patient rapport, trust and therapeutic relationships. Nurs Stand 2017;31(50):52–61.

65. Epstein RM, Street Jr RL. The values and value of patient-centered care. Ann Fam Med 2011;9(2):100–2.

66. Finset A. Patient participation, engagement and activation: increased emphasis on the role of patients in healthcare. Patient Educ Couns 2017;100(7):1245–6.

67. Lloyd M, Bor R. Communication skills for medicine. 3rd ed. London: Churchill Livingstone Elsevier; 2009.

68. Doak CC, Doak LG, Lorig K. Selecting, preparing, and using materials. 2nd ed. Thousand Oaks: SAGE; 1996.

69. Bramhall E. Effective communication skills in nursing practice. Nurs Stand 2014;29(14):53.

70. Tamparo CT, Lindh WQ. Therapeutic communications for health professionals. 2nd ed. Delmar Thomson Learning; 2000.

71. van Schaik SM, Reeves SA, Headrick LA. Exemplary learning environments for the health professions: a vision. Acad Med 2019;94(7):975–82.

72. Bannister SL, Hanson JL, Maloney CG, Dudas RA. Practical framework for fostering a positive learning environment. Pediatrics 2015;136(1):6–9.

73. Szpiro KA. Providing asthma self-management education in the emergency department: a systematic review and feasibility study. ProQuest: UMI Dissertations Publishing; 2007.

74. Anderson WG, Winters K, Arnold RM, Puntillo KA, White DB, Auerbach AD. Studying physician–patient communication in the acute care setting: the hospitalist rapport study. Patient Educ Couns 2011;82(2):275–9.

75. Rasler F. Letter to the Editor: ED patients and teachable moments. Emerg Med News 2021;43(8):4.

76. Lawson PJ, Flocke SA. Teachable moments for health behavior change: a concept analysis. Patient Educ Counsel 2009;76(1):25–30.

77. Fox MP. A systematic review of the literature reporting on studies that examined the impact of interactive, computer-based patient education programs. Patient Educ Couns 2009;77(1):6–13.

78. Kandula NR, Nsiah-Kumi PA, Makoul G, Sager J, Zei CP, Glass S, et al. The relationship between health literacy and knowledge improvement after a multimedia type 2 diabetes education program. Patient Educ Couns 2009;75(3):321–7.

79. White JV, Pitman S, Denny SC. Tool kits for teachable moments. J Am Dietetic Assoc 2003;103(11):1454, 1456.

80. Gruman J, Rovner MH, French ME, Jeffress D, Sofaer S, Shaller D, et al. From patient education to patient engagement: implications for the field of patient education. Patient Educ Couns 2010;78(3):350–6.

81. Johnson SB, Bradshaw CP, Wright JL, Haynie DL, Simons-Morton BG, Cheng TL. Characterizing the teachable moment: is an emergency department visit a teachable moment for intervention among assault-injured youth and their parents? Pediatr Emerg Care 2007;23(8):553–9.

82. Harrison R. News: 'Sick or not sick' isn't the only question to ask. Emerg Med News 2021;43(5):29.

83. Smith SK, Dixon A, Trevena L, Nutbeam D, McCaffery KJ. Exploring patient involvement in healthcare decision making across different education and functional health literacy groups. Soc Sci Med 2009;69(12):1805–12.

84. Ross J. Health literacy and its influence on patient safety. J Perianesth Nurs 2007;22(3):220–2.

85. Dudas V, Bookwalter T, Kerr KM, Pantilat SZ. The impact of follow-up telephone calls to patients after hospitalization. Am J Med 2001;111(9B):26s–30s.

86. Bombard Y, Baker GR, Orlando E, Fancott C, Bhatia P, Casalino S, et al. Engaging patients to improve quality of care: a systematic review. Implement Sci 2018;13(1):98.

87. Hendricks LE, Hendricks RT. The effect of diabetes self-management education with frequent follow-up on the health outcomes of African American men. Diabetes Educ 2000;26(6):995–1002.

88. Waterman AD, Milligan PE, Banet GA, Gatchel SK, Gage BF. Establishing and running an effective telephone-based anticoagulation service. J Vasc Nurs 2001;19(4):126–32.
89. Health Quality Ontario. Effect of early follow-up after hospital discharge on outcomes in patients with heart failure or chronic obstructive pulmonary disease: a systematic review. Ont Health Technol Assess Ser 2017;17(8):1–37.
90. Barat I, Andreasen F, Damsgaard EM. Drug therapy in the elderly: what doctors believe and patients actually do. Br J Clin Pharmacol 2001;51(6):615–22.
91. Heneghan C, Glasziou P, Perera R. Reminder packaging for improving adherence to self-administered long-term medications (Review). The Cochrane Collaboration; 2007.
92. Haynes RB, Ackloo E, Sahota N, McDonald HP, Yao X. Interventions for enhancing medication adherence. Cochrane Database Syst Rev 2008;(2):CD000011.
93. Walsh CA, Cahir C, Tecklenborg S, Byrne C, Culbertson MA, Bennett KE. The association between medication non-adherence and adverse health outcomes in ageing populations: a systematic review and meta-analysis. Br J Clin Pharmacol 2019;85(11):2464–78.
94. Yang C, Zhu S, Lee DTF, Chair SY. Interventions for improving medication adherence in community-dwelling older people with multimorbidity: a systematic review and meta-analysis. Int J Nurs Stud 2022;126:104154.
95. Kröger E, Tatar O, Vedel I, Giguère AMC, Voyer P, Guillaumie L, et al. Improving medication adherence among community-dwelling seniors with cognitive impairment: a systematic review of interventions. Int J Clin Pharm 2017;39(4):641–56.
96. Usherwood T. Encouraging adherence to longterm medication. Aust Prescr 2017;40:147–50.
97. Kumar S, Preetha G. Health promotion: an effective tool for global health. Indian J Community Med 2012;37(1):5–12.
98. World Health Organization (WHO). Health promotion. 2018. Online. Available from: www.who.int/topics/health_promotion/en/.
99. Brydges M, Denton M, Agarwal G. The CHAP-EMS health promotion program: a qualitative study on participants' views of the role of paramedics. BMC Health Serv Res 2016;16(1):435.
100. McManamny T, Jennings PA, Boyd L, Sheen J, Lowthian JA. Paramedic involvement in health education within metropolitan, rural and remote Australia: a narrative review of the literature. Aust Health Rev 2019;44(1):114–20.
101. Reeve C, Pashen D, Mumme H, De La Rue S, Cheffins T. Expanding the role of paramedics in northern Queensland: an evaluation of population health training. Aust J Rural Health 2008;16(6):370–5.
102. Celentano DD, Szklo M. Gordis epidemiology. 6th ed. Philadelphia: Elsevier; 2020.
103. Corcoran N, editor. Communicating health: strategies for health promotion. Thousand Oaks, CA; Sage; 2007.
104. Phillips A, Laslett S. Health promotion in emergency care: rationale, strategies and activities. Emerge Nurse 2022;30(1):32–40.
105. Robson S, Stephenson A, McCarthy C, et al. Identifying opportunities for health promotion and intervention in the ED. Emerg Med J 2021;38(12):927.
106. Phillips A, Laslett S. Health promotion in emergency care: rationale, strategies and activities. Emerg Nurse 2022;30(1):32–40.
107. Kripalani S, Weiss BD. Teaching about health literacy and clear communication. J Gen Intern Med 2006;21(8):888–90.
108. Weiss BD. Health literacy and patient safety: help patients understand: manual for clinicians. Chicago: AMAF and AMA; 2007.
109. Clark NM, Gong M, Schork MA, Evans D, Roloff D, Hurwitz M, et al. Impact of education for physicians on patient outcomes. Pediatrics 1998;101(5):831–6.
110. Divi C, Koss RG, Schmaltz SP, Loeb JM. Language proficiency and adverse events in US hospitals: a pilot study. Int J Qual Health Care 2007;19(2):60–7.
111. Egede LE. Race, ethnicity, culture, and disparities in health care. J Gen Internal Med 2006;21(6):667–9.
112. Krishnan A, Rabinowitz M, Ziminsky A, Scott SM, Chretien KC. Addressing race, culture, and structural inequality in medical education: a guide for revising teaching cases. Acad Med 2019;94(4):550–5.
113. John-Baptiste A, Naglie G, Tomlinson G, Alibhai SM, Etchells E, Cheung, et al. The effect of English language proficiency on length of stay and in-hospital mortality. J Gen Intern Med 2004;19(3):221–8.
114. Graham CL, Ivey SL, Neuhauser L. From hospital to home: assessing the transitional care needs of vulnerable seniors. Gerontologist 2009;49(1):23–33.
115. Ash M, Brandt S. Disparities in asthma hospitalization in Massachusetts. Am J Public Health 2006;96(2):358–62.
116. Jiang HJ, Andrews R, Stryer D, Friedman B. Racial/ethnic disparities in potentially preventable readmissions: the case of diabetes. Am J Public Health 2005;95(9):1561–7.
117. The Joint Commission. Advancing effective communication, cultural competence, and patient- and family-centred care: a roadmap for hospitals. Oakbrook Terrace, IL: The Joint Commission; 2010.
118. Seeleman C, Suurmond J, Stronks K. Cultural competence: a conceptual framework for teaching and learning. Med Educ 2009;43:229–37.
119. The Joint Commission. 'What did the doctor say?' Improving health literacy to protect patient safety. Oakbrook Terrace IL: The Joint Commission; 2007.
120. Diamond L, Jacobs E. Let's not contribute to disparities: the best methods for teaching clinicians how to overcome language barriers to health care. J Gen Intern Med 2010;25(Suppl. 2):189–93.
121. Lau LS, Rodgers G. Cultural competence in refugee service settings: a scoping review. Health Equity 2021;5(1):124–34.

122. Rowe J, Paterson J. Culturally competent communication with refugees. Home Health Care Manag Prac 2010;22(5):334–8.
123. Farley R, Askew D, Kay M. Caring for refugees in general practice: perspectives from the coalface. Aust J Prim Health 2014;20(1):85–91.
124. World Health Organization (WHO). Report on the health of refugees and migrants in the WHO European Region: no public health without refugee and migrant health. Geneva: WHO; 2018.
125. Australian Government. Communicating with Aboriginal and Torres Strait Islander audiences. Canberra, Australia: Cabinet DotPMa; 2016.
126. Abbott P, Dave D, Gordon E, Reath J. What do GPs need to work more effectively with Aboriginal patients? Views of Aboriginal cultural mentors and health workers. Aust Fam Phys 2014;43(1–2):58–63.
127. Queensland Health. Communicating effectively with Aboriginal and Torres Strait Islander people 2015. Online. Available from: www.health.qld.gov.au/__data/assets/pdf_file/0021/151923/communicating.pdf.
128. Jacobs EA, Diamond LC, Stevak L. The importance of teaching clinicians when and how to work with interpreters. Patient Educ Couns 2010;78(2):149–53.
129. Kale E, Syed HR. Language barriers and the use of interpreters in the public health services. A questionnaire-based survey. Patient Educ Couns 2010;81(2):187–91.
130. NSW Government Health. Interpreters – standard procedures for working with health care interpreters directive PD2017_044. 2017. Online. Available from: www1.health.nsw.gov.au/pds/ActivePDSDocuments/PD2017_044.pdf.
131. AHRQ. Improving patient safety systems for patients with limited English proficiency: a guide for hospitals. Rockville: Agency for Healthcare Research and Quality; 2012.
132. Lindholm M, Hargraves JL, Ferguson WJ, Reed G. Professional language interpretation and inpatient length of stay and readmission rates. J Gen Intern Med 2012;27(10):1294–9.
133. Flores G, Abreu M, Barone CP, Bachur R, Lin H. Errors of medical interpretation and their potential clinical consequences: a comparison of professional versus ad hoc versus no interpreters. Ann Emerg Med 2012;60(5):545–53.
134. Flores G. The impact of medical interpreter services on the quality of health care: a systematic review. Med Care Res Rev 2005;62(3):255–99.
135. Johnstone MJ, Kanitsaki O. Culture, language, and patient safety: making the link. Int J Qual Health Care 2006;18(5):383–8.
136. Illawarra Forum. Fact Sheet. Working with interpreters. 2018. Online. Available from: communityindustrygroup.org.au/wp-content/uploads/Working-with-Interpreters.pdf.
137. Rudd RE. Guidelines for creating materials. Harvard T.H. Chan School of Public Health. Online. Available from: cdn1.sph.harvard.edu/wp-content/uploads/sites/135/2012/09/resources_for_creating_materials.pdf.
138. Harvard T.H. Chan School of Public Health. Health literacy studies. Online. Available from: www.hsph.harvard.edu/healthliteracy.
139. Baker DW. The meaning and the measure of health literacy. J Gen Intern Med 2006;21(8):878–83.
140. Karnieli-Miller O, Adler A, Merdler L, Rosenfeld L, Eidelman S. Written notification of test results: meanings, comprehension and implication on patients' health behavior. Patient Educ Couns 2009;76(3):341–7.
141. Bateman WB, Glassman KS, Kramer EJ. Patient and family education in managed care and beyond: seizing the teachable moment. New York: Springer; 1999.
142. Richard C, Glaser E, Lussier MT. Communication and patient participation influencing patient recall of treatment discussions. Health Expect 2017;20(4):760–70.
143. Washington KT, Meadows SE, Elliott SG, et al. Information needs of informal caregivers of older adults with chronic health conditions. Patient Educ Couns 2011;83(1):37–44.
144. McLaughlin GH. SMOG Grading–a new readability formula. J Read 1969;12(8):639–46.
145. Fry E. A readability formula that saves time. J Read 1968;11(7):513–78.
146. Gunning R. The technique for clear writing. New York: McGraw-Hill; 1952.
147. Flesch R. A new readability yardstick. J App Psych 1948;32(3):221–33.
148. Microsoft. Get your document's readability and level statistics–Microsoft Support. Online. Available from: support.microsoft.com/en-us/office/get-your-document-s-readability-and-level-statistics-85b4969e-e80a-4777-8dd3-f7fc3c8b3fd2.
149. Sabharwal S, Badarudeen S, Unes Kunju S. Readability of online patient education materials from the AAOS web site. Clin Orthop Relat Res 2008;466(5):1245–50.
150. Shedlosky-Shoemaker R, Sturm AC, Saleem M, Kelly KM. Tools for assessing readability and quality of health-related web sites. J Genet Counsel 2009;18:49–59.
151. Fitzsimmons PR, Michael BD, Hulley JL, Scott GO. A readability assessment of online Parkinson's disease information. J R Coll Physicians Edinb 2010;40:292–6.
152. Tasmanian Government Department of Health. Assessing readability. 2021. Online. Available from: www.health.tas.gov.au/professionals/health-literacy/health-literacy-workplace-toolkit.
153. Walsh TM, Volsko Ta. Readability assessment of internet-based consumer health information. Respiratory Care 2008;53:1310–5.
154. Weih M, Reinhold A, Klein H, Kornhuber J. Unsuitable readability levels of patient information pertaining to dementia and related diseases: a comparative analysis. Int Psychogeriatr 2008;20(6):1116–23.

155. Doak CC, Doak LG, Root JH. Teaching patients with low literacy skills. 2nd ed. Philadelphia: Lippincott; 1995.
156. Bernier MJ. Establishing the psychometric properties of a scale for evaluating quality in printed education materials. Patient Educ Couns 1996;29(3):283–99.
157. Baker SJ. Who can read consumer product information? Aust J Hosp Pharm 1997;27(2):126–31.
158. Luk A, Aslani P. Tools used to evaluate written medicine and health information: document and user perspectives. Health Ed Behav 2011;38(4):389–403.
159. Krass I, Svarstad BL, Bultman D. Using alternative methodologies for evaluating patient medication leaflets. Patient Educ Couns 2002;47(1):29–35.
160. Shoemaker SJ, Wolf MS, Brach C. Development of the Patient Education Materials Assessment Tool (PEMAT): a new measure of understandability and actionability for print and audiovisual patient information. Patient Educ Couns 2014;96(3):395–403.
161. Charnock D, Shepperd S, Needham G, Gann R. DISCERN: an instrument for judging the quality of written consumer health information on treatment choices. J Epidemiol Community Health 1999;53(2):105–11.
162. Charnock D. The DISCERN Handbook: quality criteria for consumer health information on treatment choices. 1998. Report No: 1 85775 310 0.
163. Khazaal Y, Chatton A, Cochand S, Coquard O, Fernandez S, Khan R, et al. Brief DISCERN, six questions for the evaluation of evidence-based content of health-related websites. Patient Educ Couns 2009;77(1):33–7.
164. Centers for Disease Control and Prevention. The CDC clear communication index. Online. Available from: www.cdc.gov/ccindex/index.html.
165. Moult B, Franck LS, Brady H. Ensuring quality information for patients: development and preliminary validation of a new instrument to improve the quality of written health care information. Health Expect 2004;7(2):165–75.
166. Charvet-Berard AI, Chopard P, Perneger TV. Measuring quality of patient information documents with an expanded EQIP scale. Patient Educ Couns 2008;70(3):407–11.
167. Taylor WL. 'Cloze Procedure': a new tool for measuring readability. JMCQ 1953;30(4):415–33.
168. Horne R, Hankins M, Jenkins R. The Satisfaction with Information about Medicines Scale (SIMS): a new measurement tool for audit and research. QHC 2001;10(3):135–40.
169. Koo MM, Krass I, Aslani P. Evaluation of written medicine information: validation of the Consumer Information Rating Form. Ann Pharmacother 2007;41(6):951–6.
170. Wongtaweepkij K, Krska J, Pongwecharak J, Pongpunna S, Jarernsiripornkul N. Development and psychometric validation for evaluating written medicine information in Thailand: The Consumer Information Rating Form. BMJ Open 2021;11(10):e053740.
171. Murray TS, Hagey J, Wilms D, et al. Health literacy in Canada: a healthy understanding. Ottawa: Canadian Council on Learning; 2008. Online. Available from: https://escholarship.org/uc/item/890661nm.
172. Buchbinder R, Hall S, Grant G, Mylvaganam A, Patrick MR. Readability and content of supplementary written drug information for patients used by Australian rheumatologists. Med J Aust 2001;174(11):575–8.
173. National Health Service (NHS) UK. Toolkit for producing patient information. v. 2. London: Dept of Health Crown Print; 2003. Online. Available from: www.uea.ac.uk/documents/746480/2855738/Toolkit_for_producing_patient_information.pdf.
174. Leonard K. Evaluating patient education materials for grade level. J Consum Health Internet 2017;21:87–94.
175. Nersesian S, Vitkin N, Grantham S, Bourgaize S. Illustrating your research: design basics for junior clinicians and scientists. BMJ 2020;370:m2254.
176. Houts PS, Doak CC, Doak LG, Loscalzo MJ. The role of pictures in improving health communication: a review of research on attention, comprehension, recall, and adherence. Patient Educ Couns 2006;61(2):173–90.
177. Clark KL, AbuSabha R, von Eye A, Achterberg C. Text and graphics: manipulating nutrition brochures to maximize recall. Health Educ Res 1999;14(4):555–64.
178. Koo MM, Krass I, Aslani P. Factors influencing consumer use of written drug information. Ann Pharmacother 2003;37(2):259–67.
179. Ngoh LN, Shepherd MD. Design, development, and evaluation of visual aids for communicating prescription drug instructions to nonliterate patients in rural Cameroon. Patient Educ Couns 1997;31(3):245–61.
180. Choi J. Pictograph-based discharge instructions for low-literate older adults after hip replacement surgery: development and validation. J Geron Nursing 2011;37(11):47–56.
181. Green MJ, Myers KR. Graphic medicine: use of comics in medical education and patient care. BMJ Online 2010;340:c863.
182. Roberts NJ, Partridge MR. Evaluation of a paper and electronic pictorial COPD action plan. Chron Respir Dis 2011;8(1):31–40.
183. Yiu AW, Bajorek BV. Health literacy and knowledge in a cohort of Australian patients taking warfarin. Pharm Prac 2018;16(1):1080.
184. Nadar S, Begum N, Kaur B, Sandhu S, Lip GYH. Patients' understanding of anticoagulant therapy in a multiethnic population. J R Soc Med 2003;96(4):175.
185. Sentell T, Braun KL, Davis J, Davis T. Colorectal cancer screening: low health literacy and limited English proficiency among Asians and whites in California. J Health Commun 2013;18(Suppl. 1):242–55.
186. Mohammad A, Saini B, Chaar BB. Exploring culturally and linguistically diverse consumer needs in relation to medicines use and health information within the pharmacy setting. Res Soc Admin Pharm 2015;11(4):545–59.
187. Sobel RM, Paasche-Orlow MK, Waite KR, Rittner SS, Wilson EA, Wolf MS. Asthma 1-2-3: a low literacy multimedia tool to educate African American adults about asthma. J Commun Health 2009;34(4):321–7.

188. Ngo-Metzger Q, Hayes GR, Chen Y, Cygan R, Garfield CF. Improving communication between patients and providers using health information technology and other quality improvement strategies: focus on low-income children. Med Care Res Rev 2010;67(Suppl. 5):246s–67s.

189. Wu JT, McCormick JB. Why health professionals should speak out against false beliefs on the internet. AMA J Ethics 2018;20(11):1052–8.

190. Burns P, Jones SC, Iverson D, Caputi P. Where do older Australians receive their health information? Health information sources and their perceived reliability. J Nurs Educ Pract 2013;3:60–9.

191. Diviani N, Fredriksen EH, Meppelink CS, Mullan J, Rich W, Sudmann TT. Where else would I look for it? A five-country qualitative study on purposes, strategies, and consequences of online health information seeking. J Public Health Res 2019;8(1):33–9.

192. Daraz L, Morrow AS, Ponce OJ, Beuschel B, Farah MH, Katabi A, et al. Can patients trust online health information? A meta-narrative systematic review addressing the quality of health information on the internet. J Gen Int Med 2019;34(9):1884–91.

193. Zhao YC, Zhao M, Song S. Online health information seeking behaviors among older adults: systematic scoping review. J Med Internet Res 2022;24(2):e34790.

194. The Health on the Net Foundation. HONcode. Online. Available from: hon.ch/en/tools.html.

195. McCarthy J. Survey: 64 percent of patients use a digital device to manage health. mobihealthnews.com; 2017. Online. Available from: www.mobihealthnews.com/content/survey-64-percent-patients-use-digital-device-manage-health.

196. Lambert K, Mullan J, Mansfield K, Owen P. Should we recommend renal diet-related apps to our patients? An evaluation of the quality and health literacy demand of renal diet-related mobile applications. J Renal Nutr 2017;27(6):430–8.

197. Thornton L, Quinn C, Birrell L, Guillaumier A, Shaw B, Forbes E, et al. Free smoking cessation mobile apps available in Australia: a quality review and content analysis. Aust N Z J Public Health 2017;41(6):625–30.

198. Pagoto S, Schneider K, Jojic M, DeBiasse M, Mann D. Evidence-based strategies in weight-loss mobile apps. Am J Prev Med 2013;45(5):576–82.

199. Shen H, van der Kleij R, van der Boog PJM, Chang X, Chavannes NH. Electronic health self-management interventions for patients with chronic kidney disease: systematic review of quantitative and qualitative evidence. J Med Internet Res 2019;21(11):e12384.

200. Dawson J, Campbell KL, Craig JC, Tong A, Teixeira-Pinto A, Brown MA, et al. A text messaging intervention for dietary behaviors for people receiving maintenance hemodialysis: a feasibility study of KIDNEYTEXT. Am J Kidney Dis 2021;78(1):85–95.e1.

201. Norman CD, Skinner HA. eHEALS: the eHealth literacy scale. J Med Internet Res 2006;8(4):e27.

202. Boudreaux ED, Waring ME, Hayes RB, Sadasivam RS, Mullen S, Pagoto S. Evaluating and selecting mobile health apps: strategies for healthcare providers and healthcare organizations. Transl Behav Med 2014;4(4):363–71.

203. Cochrane Library. Special Collection-Coronavius (COVID-19): remote care through telehealth. 2020. Online. Available from: www.cochrane.org/news/special-collection-coronavirus-covid-19-remote-care-through-telehealth.

204. Flodgren G, Rachas A, Farmer AJ, Inzitari M, Shepperd S. Interactive telemedicine: effects on professional practice and health care outcomes. Cochrane Database Syst Rev 2015;(9):CD002098.

205. World Health Organization (WHO). WHO guideline: recommendations on digital interventions for health system strengthening. Geneva: WHO; 2019.

206. Cochrane Library. Remote care through telehealth 2020. Online. Available from: www.cochranelibrary.com/collections/doi/SC000043/full.

207. Shigekawa E, Fix M, Corbett G, Coffman J, Roby DH. The current state of telehealth evidence: a rapid review. Health Affairs 2018;37(12):1975–82.

208. Ray DE, Topol EJ. State of telehealth. N Engl J Med 2016;375(2):154–61.

209. Greenhalgh T, Wherton J, Shaw S, Morrison C. Video consultations for COVID-19. BMJ 2020;368:m998.

210. Totten AM, McDonagh MS, Wagner JH. The evidence base for telehealth: reassurance in the face of rapid expansion during the COVID-19 pandemic. Rockville, MD: Agency for Healthcare Research and Quality; 2020.

211. Ministers Department of Health and Aged Care. COVID-19: whole of population telehealth for patients, general practice, primary care and other medical services. 2020. Online. Available from: www.health.gov.au/ministers/the-hon-greg-hunt-mp/media/covid-19-whole-of-population-telehealth-for-patients-general-practice-primary-care-and-other-medical-services/.

212. Mahmood S, Hasan K, Colder Carras M, Labrique A. Global preparedness against COVID-19: we must leverage the power of digital health. JMIR Public Health Surveill 2020;6(2):e18980.

213. Duckett S. What should primary care look like after the COVID-19 pandemic? Aust J Prim Health 2020;26(3):207–11.

214. Reay RE, Looi JCL, Keightley P. Telehealth mental health services during COVID-19: summary of evidence and clinical practice. Australas Psychiatry 2020;28(5):514–6.

215. Dinesen B, Nonnecke B, Lindeman D, Toft E, Kidholm K, Jethwani K, et al. Personalized telehealth in the future: a global research agenda. J Med Internet Res 2016;18(3):e53.

216. Olson CA, McSwain SD, Curfman AL, Chuo J. The current pediatric telehealth landscape. Pediatrics 2018;141(3):e20172334.

217. Association AM. Telehealth implementation playbook. 2022. Online. Available from: www.ama-assn.org/system/files/ama-telehealth-playbook.pdf.

218. Wherton J, Shaw S, Papoutsi C, Seuren L, Greenhalgh T. Guidance on the introduction and use of video consultations during COVID-19: important lessons from qualitative research. BMJ Leader 2020;4(3):120.

SECTION TWO

CLINICAL CONCEPTS AND SYSTEMS

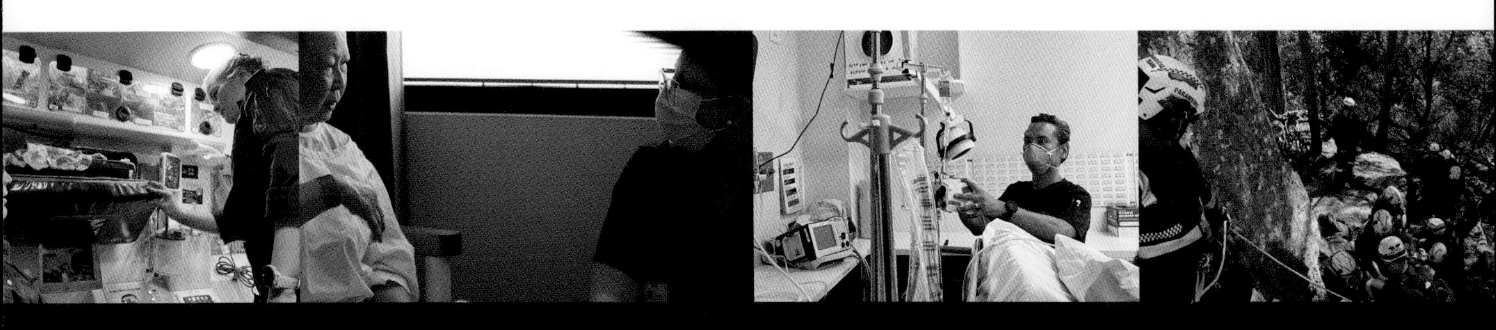

CHAPTER 9
SCENE ASSESSMENT, MANAGEMENT AND RESCUE

KAREL HABIG

ESSENTIALS

- Safety comes first in all emergency responses and is fundamental from the time of the emergency call to the conclusion of scene management.
- Accurate and comprehensive information gathered from the emergency caller is essential, as it determines not only the urgency but also the composition, skill set and degree of the response.
- Personal protective equipment (PPE) should be used routinely as it protects against common hazards such as water, body fluids, chemicals and some variation in temperature, but also has high-visibility characteristics to enable the wearer to be seen easily in traumatic or confused scenes. It should always be worn and donned prior to approaching or entering a scene.
- Good planning, leadership, command and teamwork, both within the organisation and by the scene responders, should be a priority to ensure the safety and health of personnel and patients.
- Adapting the environment is essential in ensuring safety. Response vehicles should be used, where possible, to enhance safety for rescuers, such as parking in the 'fend-off' position.
- An essential prerequisite to moving in to treat patients is to take control of the scene, then assess, communicate and triage, treat and transport.
- Emergency healthcare providers must maintain a high level of situational awareness of the overall scene and consider all potential hazards as they approach the patient and while on-scene.
- Crowds present a unique challenge to emergency service providers and a cautious approach using 'lights' but not sirens to move slowly through mass gatherings is recommended.
- The principles of vehicle extrication include protection of the scene, stabilisation of the vehicle, patient assessment, triage and treatment, creation of space and physical extrication of the patient.
- During an extrication the aim is to focus on limiting clinical procedures to 'meaningful interventions' to minimise unnecessary delays on-scene.

SAFETY FIRST—KEEPING YOU AND THE PATIENT SAFE

Safety in emergency responses, whether by an ambulance service or by the police or fire services, starts as soon as the emergency call is received, and includes appropriate dispatch prioritisation, well-planned procedures and equipment for scene care and clear protocols for high-risk situations.

DISPATCH AND PRE-ARRIVAL INFORMATION

In Australia, a call to 000 (111 in New Zealand) elicits the help of a call-taker who directs the caller to the appropriate emergency service to deal with the call.[1] At this stage of the operation of an emergency paramedic response, the caller is asked a structured set of important questions that are intended to identify and prioritise life-threatening emergencies, elicit essential information to allow dispatch of appropriate resources and give a clear picture of the speed of response necessary by clinicians. In a typical computer-aided dispatch system, like the Medical Priority Dispatch System,[2] software prompts call-takers to ask 'case-entry' questions, a process which has been likened to the primary survey: the location and a call-back number for the incident are verified, and the patient's age, status of consciousness, status of breathing and 'chief complaint' are determined. If information is given that the patient is unconscious and not breathing (for any reason), a maximal response is dispatched before any further interrogation or instructions continue. In this way, ambulance services can implement a degree of triage, ensuring that most rapid responses are made to only the most urgent cases that need this, rather than sending an urgent response to all cases, a common occurrence before the implementation of these sorts of triage and decision-support systems.

After these case-entry questions, 'key questions' are asked from the appropriate protocol, which is determined from the chief complaint. These key questions have been described as being equivalent to the secondary survey, and provide an ordered view of the patient complaint, to ensure that the pre-hospital care provided is appropriate and in keeping with the severity of the injury or illness. Finally, the structured elicitation of key facts from a 000 (or 111) caller also allows the delivery of pre-arrival instructions to the caller, including coaching on cardiopulmonary resuscitation, even allowing coaching in non-standard resuscitation.[3] Early research has shown that the proportion of inappropriate advance life support (ALS) responses was able to be reduced significantly by the use of emergency medical dispatch software.[4]

Dispatch information is also essential in ensuring that the paramedic is able to appropriately prepare to manage the scene. Data, such as the type of vehicle and number of patients, can prompt rescuers to consider situations very differently; very different procedures may be needed in a school bus incident compared with a single motorcyclist trauma. The following items of data are extremely useful in ensuring safety en route to an incident:

- traffic congestion, preferred routes and potential delays
- other delays, such as raised bridges or blocked railway crossings
- pertinent weather information
- the fastest, safest route to follow
- identified alternative routes
- pre-arrival instructions regarding care for the patient.

Essential dispatch information also includes as complete a description of the scene as possible, and enables the paramedic to determine whether the call:

- is a call to a trauma or to a potential medical case
- includes any life-threatening conditions
- involves multiple vehicles, if trauma, or multiple victims, which may indicate the need for more personnel
- involves fire or unstable building hazards
- involves other hazards, such as downed power lines, broken gas lines, chemical spills or dangerous animals
- requires special rescue equipment, personnel, or the possibility of helicopter evacuation
- involves very hot or cold conditions that may aggravate the patient's condition
- involves any type of reported violence—paramedics are taught never to enter a scene in these circumstances until it is secured by law enforcement officers
- includes pre-arrival instructions, such as CPR coaching, that have been given to the caller to provide care to the patient until paramedics arrive.

The location and type of call help to determine if a need for more than one response unit is required, such as in a cardiac arrest situation, where two crews may potentially be needed to transport the patient while continuing effective CPR. They may also help to determine if an immediate need for specialised resources exists, such as Hazmat teams.[5] In Australia, fire services assume the responsibility for managing hazardous materials and have specially trained personnel to handle these types of calls.[5]

Notification of an incident can also come through other sources, such as police or fire services, and it is essential that data can be shared between systems to ensure rapid dispatch of ambulance resources. A shared computer-aided dispatch platform, as exists in most states of Australia, is the ideal model.

Jurisdictions around the world are now exploring how to best use the added functionality of near ubiquitous smartphone penetration to geo-locate callers, utilise video and image acquisition and to provide visual aids to first aid.

TRAVELLING TO THE SCENE

Collisions involving emergency vehicles are rare, but have resulted in serious injury or death.[6] Most data on this phenomenon comes from the United States in incidents that occur when primary responders[7] are using 'lights and sirens'.[8] One study showed that there were 67 ground-transportation-related fatalities in the United States from 1992 to 1997;[7] another study revealed that the collision rate for emergency medical service (EMS) road transportation was 5 in 10,000 responses.[8]

It has been identified that situations where emergency vehicles are responding to emergencies under lights and sirens are particularly dangerous because they may be performing manoeuvres, such as entering intersections against red lights and using lanes not commonly employed. Most drivers, however, if obeying the road rules, stop at red lights and keep to the appropriate lanes. A contradiction is apparent where emergency vehicle drivers believe they are following the road rules that apply to them in an emergency, believing that other drivers will

BOX 9.1 EMERGENCY VEHICLE RESPONSE AND TRAVEL GUIDELINES

1. The first arriving ambulance should be responsible for determining the response status for any additional ambulance vehicles going to the scene of the call.
2. Ambulance service vehicles should not exceed posted speed limits by more than 15 kph.
3. Ambulance service vehicles should not exceed posted speed limits when proceeding through intersections with a green light.
4. Ambulance service vehicles approaching a red light, stop sign or railway crossing must come to a complete stop before proceeding with caution.
5. When traffic conditions require ambulance service vehicles to travel in the oncoming traffic lanes, the maximum speed should be 30 kph.
6. When ambulance service vehicles use the turning lane or oncoming traffic lane to approach intersections, they must come to a complete stop before proceeding through the intersection with caution.

FIGURE 9.1 HIGH-VISIBILITY VEST AND PERSONAL PROTECTIVE EQUIPMENT

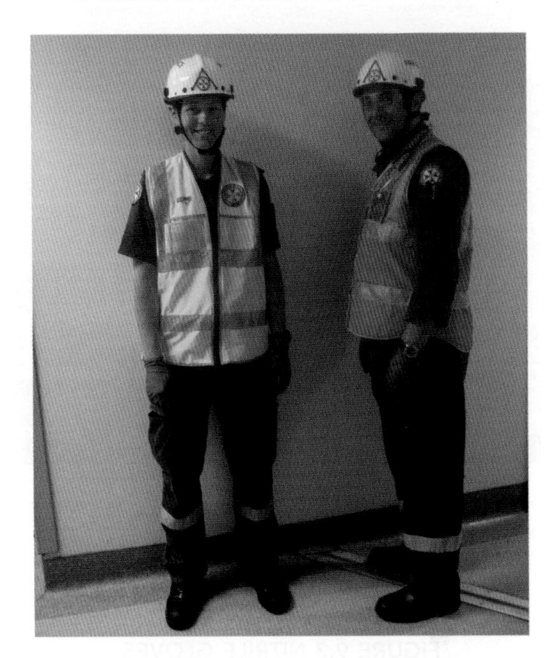

Courtesy of NSW Ambulance and Kate Curtis.

always yield, whereas a 'civilian' driver is conditioned to believe that other vehicles will give way when they have the right of way.[9] One report into an incident involving a fire engine and a train in the United States described the phenomenon of 'sirencide', 'used to describe the emotional reaction of emergency vehicle drivers when they begin to feel a sense of power and urgency that blocks out reason and prudence, leading to the reckless operation of the emergency vehicle'.[10]

It has been suggested that there should be a set of strict criteria defined for the response to any emergency situation, as paraphrased in Box 9.1.[11]

It has been pointed out that driver training for emergency vehicles is now widely available and should be part of every paramedic's training.[12] The purpose and intent of any well-regarded program is to minimise injury, death and damage to expensive equipment, with a parallel decrease in risk of liability likely to occur for agencies that provide driver training. It is recommended that instruction should include all aspects of both non-emergency and emergency vehicle operation, including the use of the emergency warning systems, communications system, vehicle locating system, on-board computer system, location-of-area emergency facilities, proper parking and backing procedures, and safe driving practices. It was also proposed that a new driver should have the assistance of a trained driving instructor for a certain number of initial kilometres of driving, in both emergency and non-emergency modes.

PERSONAL PROTECTIVE EQUIPMENT

Personal protective equipment (PPE) refers to protective clothing, helmets, goggles and other garments designed to protect the body from injury by blunt impacts, infection, electrical hazards, traffic, caustic substances, extremes of temperature, and assault by patients, relatives or bystanders, for job-related occupational safety and health purposes. PPE therefore comprises garments with specific protective properties, and equipment that may contribute to maximising personal protection for paramedics working in uncontrolled pre-hospital scenes. Although unpredictability is part of pre-hospital care, the potential harmful effects of factors, such as those described above, need to be minimised to ensure the safety of clinicians. The ability of these articles of protective clothing and equipment to perform their function appropriately is usually mandated through national quality agencies, which are often members of the International Organization for Standardization (www.iso.org) or organisations such as Standards Australia (www.standards.org.au) or the American National Standards Institute (www.ansi.org).

Routinely worn PPE protects against common hazards, such as water, body fluids and some variation in temperature, but also has high-visibility characteristics to enable the wearer to be easily seen in traumatic or confused scenes. There are often strips or patches of reflective material that form distinctive patterns seen easily in car headlights, for example (Figs 9.1 to 9.3). Added PPE for the purposes of physical safety are safety glasses and helmets. In traumatic incidents, these items of protective equipment should always be worn and donned prior to approaching or entering the scene.

Protection against infection is an essential prerequisite to arrival at any incident, and standard PPE of this nature includes gloves and the safety glasses mentioned above, which provide a barrier to protect the healthcare worker from contamination. Medical examination gloves, which may be latex or a latex substitute, are worn in situations where there is direct contact anticipated with blood, body fluids, mucous membranes or non-intact skin. Facial protection, such as glasses and/or fluid-resistant face masks with transparent eye shields, should be worn if there is a likelihood of splashing or splattering of body substances or blood.

FIGURE 9.2 SAFETY GLASSES AND HELMET

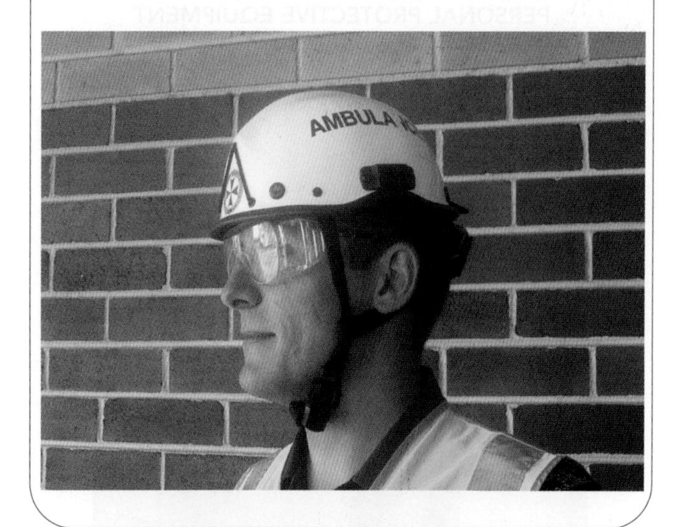

Courtesy NSW Ambulance.

FIGURE 9.3 NITRILE GLOVES

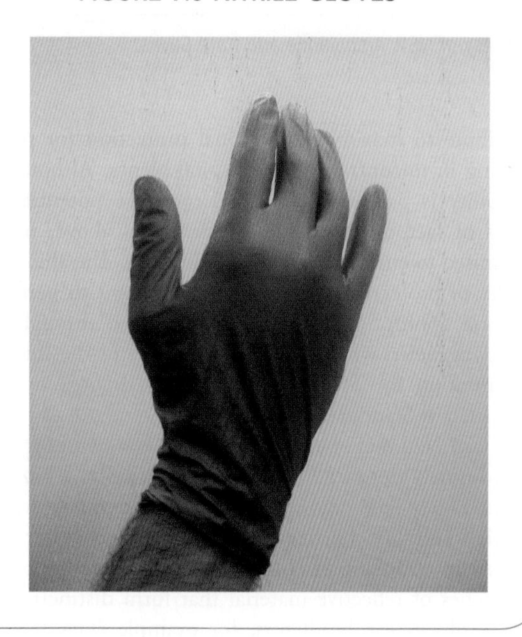

Courtesy NSW Ambulance.

The performance of hand hygiene has been seen to be essential in the prevention of cross-infection,[13] and has also been shown to be achievable and effective with simple measures.[14]

PRACTICE TIP

Alcohol-based hand rubs are the best way to clean hands and should be available in all vehicles, as well as on-scene before and after all patient contacts.

Specific PPE may also be used in higher-risk situations where there are defined hazards; these may often be termed Hazmat suits (for hazardous materials) and are discussed in relation to mass-casualty incidents in Chapter 12. The US Department of Homeland Security defines a Hazmat suit as 'an overall garment worn to protect people from hazardous materials or substances, including chemicals, biological agents or radioactive materials'.[15] These may provide protection from:

- chemical agents—through the use of appropriate barrier materials like Teflon, heavy PVC or rubber
- nuclear agents—possibly through radiation shielding in the lining, but more importantly by preventing direct contact with or inhalation of radioactive particles or gas
- biological agents—through fully sealed systems (often at overpressure to prevent contamination even if the suit is damaged)
- fire/high temperatures—usually by a combination of insulating and reflective materials which reduce or retard the effects.[15]

The most common classification of Hazmat protective clothing uses the US system,[16] which classifies garments as Level A, B, C or D, based on the degree of protection the clothing provides; these are outlined in Box 9.2 and discussed in detail in Chapter 12.

WORKING WITH OTHER AGENCIES AT A SCENE

Teamwork, whether on a scale involving inter-agency interactions with colleagues on-scene or most commonly between individual paramedics forming the two-person treating team, is a fundamental component of pre-hospital care. Although it

BOX 9.2 CLASSIFICATIONS OF HAZMAT PROTECTIVE CLOTHING[16]

LEVEL A

The highest level of protection against vapours, gases, mists and particles is Level A, which consists of a fully encapsulating chemical-entry suit with a full-facepiece, self-contained breathing apparatus (SCBA) or a supplied air respirator (SAR) with an SCBA escape cylinder.

LEVEL B

Level B protection requires a garment (including SCBA) which provides protection against splashes from a hazardous chemical. Since the breathing apparatus is worn on the outside of the garment, Level B protection is not vapour-protective.

LEVEL C

The same type of garment used for Level B protection is worn for Level C, but there are differences in the equipment needed for respiratory protection, allowing any of the various types of air-purifying respirators. Level C equipment does not offer the protection needed in an oxygen-deficient atmosphere.

LEVEL D

Level D protection does not protect from chemical exposure and, therefore, this level of protection can only be used in situations where a crew member has no possibility of contact with chemicals. Most firefighter gear is considered to be Level D.

might be obvious that partners within an ambulance need to work together, good teamwork is also an essential component of successful organisations at every administrative and corporate level. On a small scale, and particularly in longer-term partnerships, teamwork contributes to safety on multiple levels, including improved vigilance for environmental hazards, coordination of patient care and manual handling, dealing with and defusing intense emotional scenes, negotiating traffic safety and recognising stress and burnout. On a multi-agency level, teamwork becomes particularly important as the specialised activities and talents of individual organisations directly affect, and need to be closely coordinated with, each other.

Although ambulance personnel may be an early arrival at the scene of an incident, there are defined responsibilities attributable to and expected of other emergency service personnel. These may be summarised as police being in control of an incident scene, fire services being in control of hazardous materials and situations and ambulances/paramedics being in control of patient management. The discrete responsibilities of each service mean that as the scene evolves different priorities will emerge requiring a high level of communication between agencies. One team may continue a high level of control, such as in a dangerous situation involving weapons, where the police will assume extended control even in the presence of wounded patients (discussed in the section below on scene safety), or one agency may temporarily default to another, such as in the management of violent patients where paramedics may need police assistance to manage them. Some agency interactions may have local variations, such as rescue operations, which may be managed primarily by a range of services including ambulance, fire/rescue services or volunteer agencies such as the State Emergency Service (SES) in rural Australia.[17]

In disaster situations, either a natural calamity or a human-made catastrophe, and defined in health terms, as when affected patient load overwhelms the available resources, similar but more formalised arrangements apply: police maintain a defined perimeter around the incident, the fire service takes responsibility for direct rescue operations and healthcare services, including ambulance services, manage immediate trauma scenes, of which there may be several, and the triage, stabilisation and orderly evacuation of casualties. The Major Incident Medical Management and Support (MIMMS)[18] course manual describes this in terms of a major incident, defined as causing so many live casualties that special arrangements are necessary to deal with them, an incident that disrupts the health service or an incident that presents a serious threat to the health of the community.

SCENE MANAGEMENT PRIORITIES—WHY AN ORGANISED SCENE IS PRICELESS

A summary of the priorities at an incident scene can be remembered as CONTROL and ACT. An essential prerequisite to moving in to treat patients is to take control of the scene, and then to assess, communicate and triage, treat and transport (Box 9.3). The following sections elaborate on this theme.

TEAM FUNCTION

Leadership, command and control are important. In emergency incident terms, a scene without adequate leadership may deteriorate quickly. One approach, which is being adapted to the paramedical environment, is the Incident Management System (IMS), an outgrowth of the US Incident Command System (ICS).[12] The US National Fire Protection Association states that 'the purpose of an incident management system is to provide structure and coordination to the management of emergency incident operations in order to provide for the safety and health of ... persons involved in those activities'.[20] It is described[12] as a process for creating order from disorder through a comprehensive approach to leadership and task delegation. Versions of IMS have been used for handling wildland fires, urban fire scenes, Hazmat situations and everyday emergency medical service (EMS) scenes.

BOX 9.3 SCENE MANAGEMENT PRIORITIES—THE ACT MNEMONIC[19]

A Assess
C Communicate
T Triage, treat and transport

Effective, consistent scene leadership is a vital issue in pre-hospital safety, and no matter how a system is organised or functions on a day-to-day basis, this leadership may be routinely achieved through use of the primary principle of defining one leader who makes all scene management decisions. There is no doubt that the presence of this one leader at a pre-hospital scene, no matter how large or small, ensures that the scene is both more orderly and more organised. This has parallels with other team decision-making, such as in the trauma team setting where decisions are based on the big picture rather than piecemeal as new information becomes known, or subsumed in a mass of hands-on detail that prevents perception of the greater picture.

Even when a two-person crew is handling a routine emergency call, this may improve incident coordination. The clinician assuming the leadership role should prepare to take on certain functions, delegating them as needed depending on circumstances; for example, an available first responder might be asked to scout out the best path from the scene to the ambulance vehicle. The incident commander, even in a single-paramedic response, should be the individual with the best ability to assemble the resources necessary and the experience to take an overview of the scene while allowing the other clinician to attend directly to the patient. Roles should be clearly delineated in standard operating procedures, although allowing for training, mentoring and guidance of more junior staff.

Scene management begins prior to the actual arrival of the paramedical crew at the patient. The NSW Ambulance Service (NSWAS) scene management skill training manual[21] states: 'Scene assessment is commenced as soon as visual contact is made with the scene and is as equally important at medical situations as at trauma scenes'. Communications are also of great value at this point—the NSWAS protocol also directs paramedics arriving at the scene of a motor vehicle collision to provide a brief preliminary report once visual contact is made with the scene. It suggests a script such as 'Car approaching scene. I observe a single motor vehicle collision. Car into a tree.'

VEHICLE PLACEMENT

Pre-hospital scenes, particularly roadside trauma, can be extremely hazardous; many paramedics' lives have been lost in this environment. In an ideal world, police maintain scene control in this sort of incident, but to rely on this would be naive, as they are not always in a position to provide traffic control. This is particularly true when pre-hospital clinicians are first on the scene, and in many areas assistance is patchy, slow to arrive or unavailable. Paramedics and other pre-hospital clinicians need to know how to provide the safest environment to assure their own protection.

Vehicles should be positioned in a lane that is already blocked or on the same side of the carriageway as the incident, unless there are some specific reasons not to do so. There are several advantages to this apart from being efficient for patient care. First, it prevents clinicians from crossing busy roads to gain access to the patients and possibly being injured themselves; second, as the lane is already blocked, the ambulances and other emergency vehicles occupy little further space. Third, leaving other lanes open ensures that other traffic can move past, albeit at a slower pace, which may in itself prevent further accidents. Passers-by in other vehicles are often a source of further accidents as they drive with their attention on what is happening in the more interesting accident scene. Finally, and related to the last point, if ambulances and other rescue vehicles, such as fire engines and police rescue, are parked across other lanes, bringing equipment and hydraulic lines across the carriageways would not only block these lanes to other traffic, but would effectively stop the egress of emergency vehicles themselves.

Vehicles should be parked in such a way as to create a barrier to oncoming traffic that might cause injury to rescuers, in the 'fend-off' position (Fig. 9.4). The steering wheel should be turned so that any vehicle that is struck by another would move away from the scene, entrapped patients and rescuers. Even this is not that simple, however; there is a belief that it is safest if the ambulance is placed between oncoming traffic and the involved vehicles, providing emergency warning beacons at that end of the crash site, illuminating the scene with the ambulance headlights, and providing a physical barrier from approaching traffic. However, once the patient(s) and paramedics are actually in the ambulance, they are endangered by being closest to oncoming traffic during preparations for leaving the scene. Therefore, although it makes sense to position an emergency vehicle at the end of the crash site, using the ambulance for this is probably not the best choice if another emergency vehicle is available. It is probably better for the ambulance to be moved ahead of the crash site when another vehicle arrives to create a barrier against traffic.

FIGURE 9.4 PARKING AT A MOTOR VEHICLE COLLISION SCENE

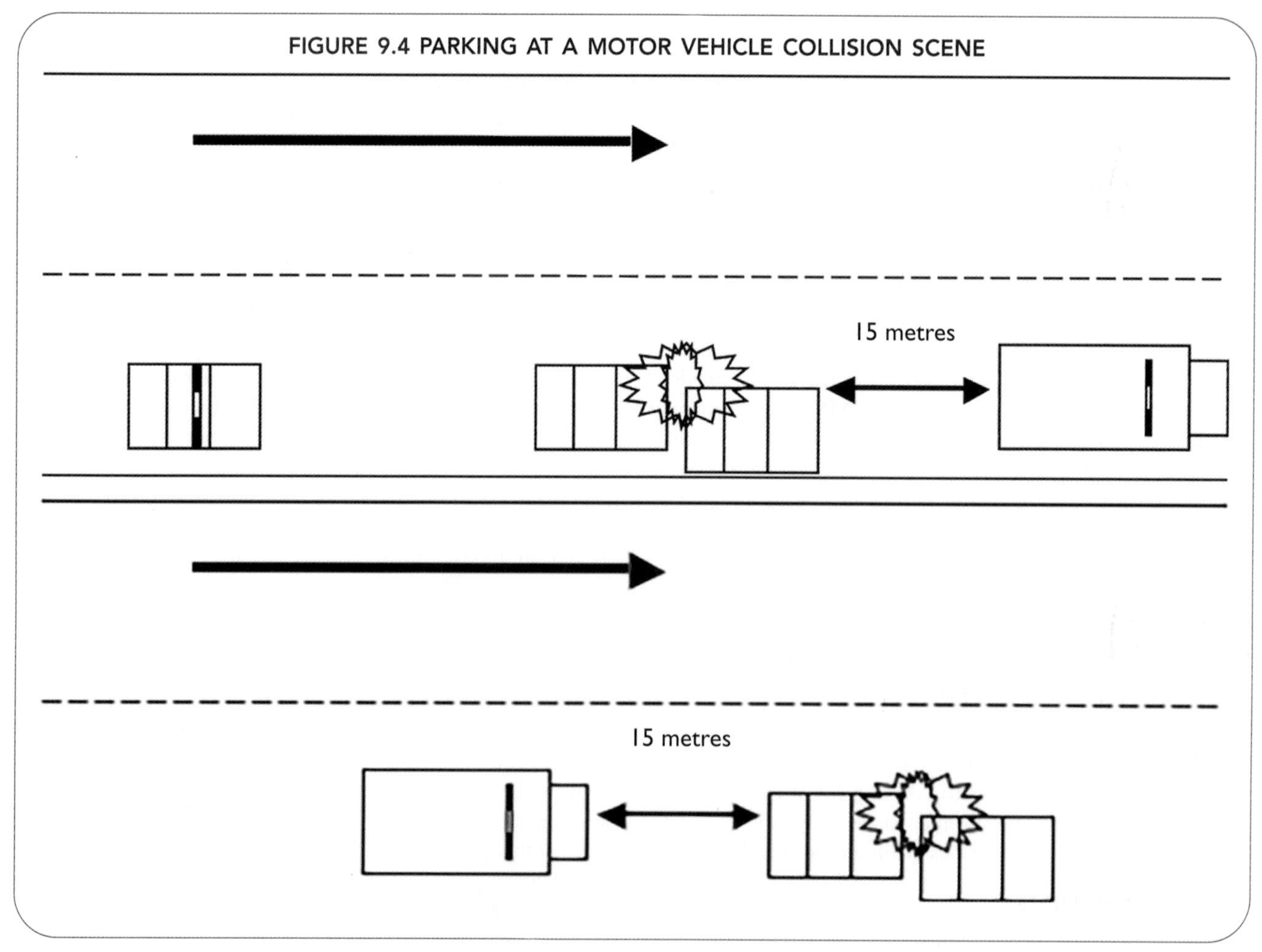

Courtesy PM Middleton.

BOX 9.4 **THE PROTECTION MNEMONIC**[20]

P Proceed slowly, using your vehicle as a safety shield for personnel.
R Remember: passing motorists are watching you, not where they are going.
O Observe types of vehicles, placards, condition of containers and fire hazards.
T Take the time to stabilise all vehicles before beginning operations.
E Evacuate as necessary to ensure the safety of public and EMS personnel.
C Call for additional assistance early. Overtaxed personnel become a safety liability.
T Treat the incident scene with great caution. Wear full protective clothing and use all warning devices.
I In the interests of safety, appoint a safety officer and dedicate adequate resources.
O Once assessment is complete, close the road when necessary to protect personnel.
N Never let your guard down.

It has been suggested that when parking on the side of a road, one front and one rear wheel should be left on the solid surface of the road, to ensure that there is sufficient traction to move the vehicle when it attempts to leave the scene. It is often safer, even when there are urgent interventions that need to be performed, to briefly move the vehicle and patient to a location away from passing traffic. Considerations when parking the ambulance may include:

- which spot is safest
- which is most convenient for patient care
- which will best facilitate traffic flow around the scene
- which allows the best outlet for departure
- whether other emergency personnel are already on the scene or will arrive later.

Headlights should be kept on low beam, and, if needed to illuminate the scene, should be pointed specifically in that direction to avoid blinding other drivers. Exhaust fumes should be considered, and vehicles parked in such a way as to minimise the possibility of these affecting both patients and rescuers.

The following aide memoire for securing safety at the scene is a version of that in the publication *EMS Safety: Techniques and Applications*,[20] a guide for firefighters which is also very appropriate for all EMS and ambulance personnel. It describes the mnemonic PROTECTION, which is outlined in Box 9.4.

SCENE ASSESSMENT

RISK AND HAZARD ASSESSMENT

One of the first decisions that needs to be made by paramedics arriving at the scene of any sort of incident, whether trauma scene or medical case, is whether it is actually safe to get out of the vehicle or not. There are many factors that make a scene unsafe or potentially hazardous, and in a substantial proportion of these not actually approaching or entering the area without further information or back-up may be recommended. Although it can be seen by some to be contrary to the priorities of routine clinical intervention and behaviour, the priorities for safety are paramedic, scene and patient, in that order (Fig. 9.5).

FIGURE 9.5 SAFETY PRIORITIES

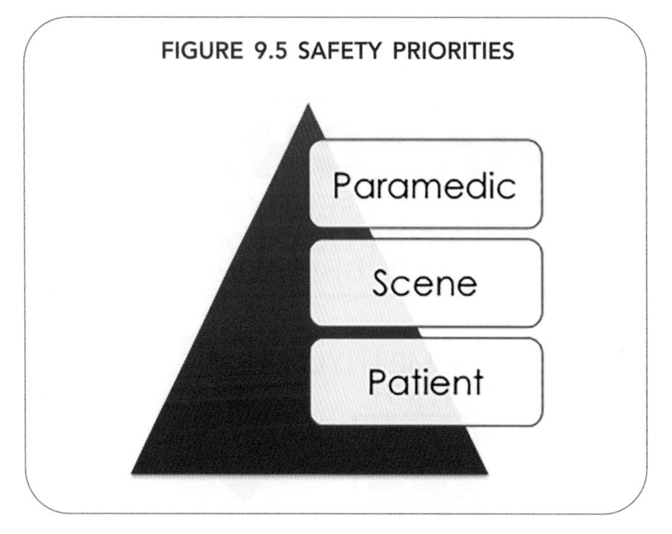

Courtesy PM Middleton.

Scene assessment (otherwise known as 'scene size-up'[20] or 'reading the scene'[22]) is a quick analysis of the scene on arrival, and is vital for safe and efficient operations in order to enforce a rapid and accurate evaluation, particularly of obvious hazards. This initial reading of the scene comprises a scan for immediate hazards—fire, power lines and potential assailants with weapons—which need to be mitigated prior to operating at the scene. EMS personnel in the United States are taught that the driver of the rescue vehicle should stay behind the wheel to facilitate rapidly leaving the scene if attacked, and treating clinicians are taught to approach a vehicle from behind, close any opened car boot to prevent attack by a hidden assailant, not to move forward of the B pillar of a car (the rear frame of the front door) and always to keep the hands of the driver or passenger in sight. These precautions are less often required in Australia and other similar regions, although may still be valid and life-saving in particular areas. The 1994 US Department of Transport EMT-Basic National Standard Curriculum[23] lists five key components of the scene size-up process:

1. Number of patients.
2. Mechanism of injury/nature of illness.
3. Resource determination (heavy rescue, Hazmat, etc).
4. Standard precautions before leaving the ambulance.
5. Scene safety.

ENVIRONMENTAL FACTORS

Another important aspect of reading the scene is evaluation of environmental hazards, such as rain, snow, ice, bright sunlight, extreme temperatures and humidity. The environment may provide significant physical and mental stress, which can decrease resistance to disease, and decrease emotional tolerance and responsiveness to others. The environment obviously may have a profound impact on the patient's physical condition and ability to maintain core body functions, and heat stress or cold exposure may have increasingly significant effects on both patient and clinician during prolonged incidents.

FIGURE 9.6 SAFETY SIGNS USED IN AUSTRALIA

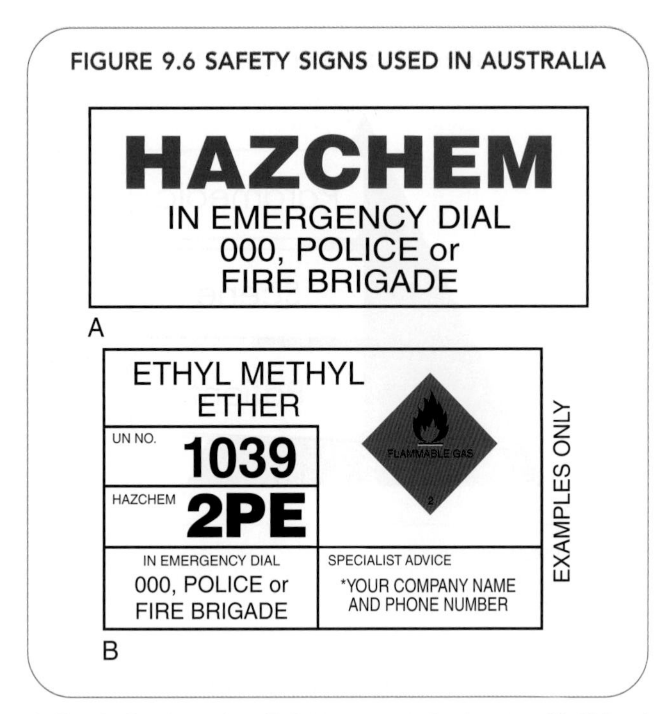

A Simple Hazchem sign. **B** Dangerous goods signage, with UN and Hazchem substance identification numbers in the middle left panels, emergency number in the bottom left panel, warning symbol indicating the danger represented by the hazard in the top right panel, and telephone number for specialist advice in the bottom right panel. *Courtesy Signs of Safety www.signsofsafety.net.au.*

Hazardous materials have been discussed above in relation to PPE, but their potential or actual presence at a scene may have great importance as they are indiscriminate in causing harm to patients and rescuers alike. Paramedics and other pre-hospital staff need to have a substantial index of suspicion, particularly in motor vehicle collisions involving large vehicles or industrial transport, and also in industrial or rural areas. Hazardous materials are subject to clear labelling, which may be common between countries. In the United States the Department of Transport and the Environmental Protection Agency regulate transport of hazardous goods[24] as well as their labelling, whereas Australia and the UK follow the Hazchem labelling system which uses standard United Nations codes.[25] Plates that use the Hazchem system are displayed on vehicles and storage facilities, and give coded information describing the hazard, the level of protection needed and the actions required (Figs 9.6 and 9.7).

Correct and adequate illumination of a night-time trauma scene is vital to operations that are safe and efficient for paramedic and patient. Vehicle-mounted or portable lights powered by a generator or 12-volt vehicle supply are in common use, and portable fluorescent or LED lights provide ample light with minimal heat output. Special care should be taken to avoid the use of lights or other appliances that produce heat near either patients or flammable materials.

USING YOUR SENSES

Less speed, more haste

Pre-hospital work is often intense and stimulates the release of endogenous catecholamines, which often clouds the judgement of inexperienced practitioners. The sense of urgency when another's life is potentially at stake, and the perception that resolution of the situation is in the hands of the clinician, is often a trigger for rushing, which diminishes the chance of carrying out a well thought out and coordinated plan.[20] Although there exists a degree of urgency to any emergency, running to the patient does not allow time to 'absorb' the scene.

Looking

While walking briskly to the patient, time can be spent not only scanning for hazards, as already described, but also assessing the incident scene for clues to causation, including mechanism of injury pointers, such as skid marks, airbag deployment, 'bullseye' fractures of windscreens, deformation of vehicles and distance of patients from vehicles. A rapid global overview of the patients, both in numbers and in appearance, potentially prompts the call for increased resources and back-up, and contributes to the clinician's expectation of the likelihood of significant illness or injury.

Other key visual cues, particularly when responding to a potential crime scene or calls to an assault, may be vital for the safety of clinicians and others. Importantly, when approaching on-scene civilians and bystanders, attempt to 'read' their body language on three levels:[20] their overall body language, their facial expressions and their eyes. Although the most dominant emotion is usually demonstrated, there may be conflict between facial expression, body language and eyes. A typical example might be in the responsibility felt by the parent of an injured child, where potential guilt at contributing or causing an event may conflict with anger, often displaced onto paramedics, and fear for the potential outcome. Weapons of any kind, as well as signs of intoxication with alcohol or drugs, should be actively looked for by paramedics, as should the presence of other emergency service vehicles, particularly police and fire service; and signs of fire, smoke and downed power lines are other essential visual cues to the potential harm in any situation.

Listening

Listening on approach to a scene may give important insights into the potential number of victims, the type of incident and the immediate situation that may be encountered at the scene. Typical auditory cues may be human, animal or environmental, and may obviously include calls for help and cries of pain, crowd noise and voices associated with attempts to help, rescue or organise the scene. Sounds of conflict—loud, argumentative voices or screams—are especially important. Animal noises are less common, but may include dogs barking; this may represent a potentially severe injury risk to clinicians, particularly when attempting to access private or industrial premises where dogs will have a real or perceived guard function. The family dog, however harmless-looking, always has the potential to attack; always summon trained assistance where there is a perceived risk of this. Environmental noise is potentially very significant, and includes traffic noise—or the lack of it, as an unusual silence may have important connotations.

Feeling

Feeling has less of a role in the assessment of a scene, but a great role in the assessment of a patient, as palpation and appropriate movement are two of the key methods to identify injury and some illnesses. Even on approach to an accident scene or into a

FIGURE 9.7 STANDARD SYMBOLS USED IN HAZARD WARNING SIGNS

CLASS	LABEL	DESCRIPTION
1	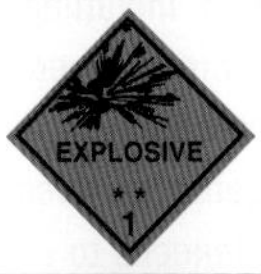 EXPLOSIVE * * 1	EXPLOSIVE Orange Background Black Text & Symbol
2.1	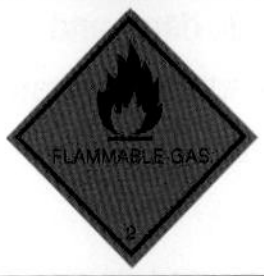 FLAMMABLE GAS 2	FLAMMABLE GAS Red Background Black Text & Symbol
2.2	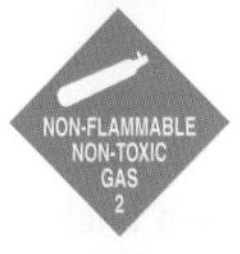 NON-FLAMMABLE NON-TOXIC GAS 2	NON-FLAMMABLE NON-TOXIC GAS Green Background White Text & Symbol
2.2	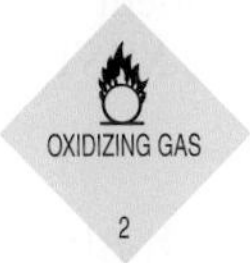 OXIDIZING GAS 2	OXIDIZING GAS Yellow Background Black Text & Symbol Subsidiary Risk 5.1
2.3	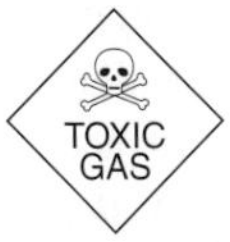 TOXIC GAS	TOXIC GAS White Background Black Text & Symbol
3	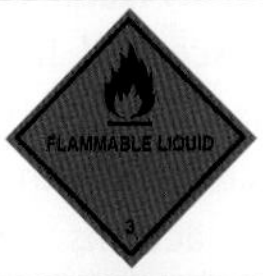 FLAMMABLE LIQUID 3	FLAMMABLE LIQUID Red Background Black Text & Symbol
4.1	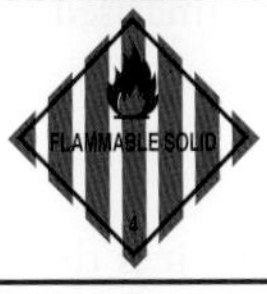 FLAMMABLE SOLID 4	FLAMMABLE SOLID Red/White Vertical Striped Background Black Text & Symbol
4.2	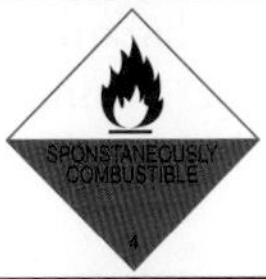 SPONTANEOUSLY COMBUSTIBLE 4	SPONTANEOUSLY COMBUSTIBLE White Upper Background Red Lower Background Black Text & Symbol
4.3	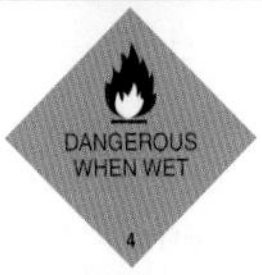 DANGEROUS WHEN WET 4	DANGEROUS WHEN WET Blue Background Black Text & Symbol

CLASS	LABEL	DESCRIPTION
5.1	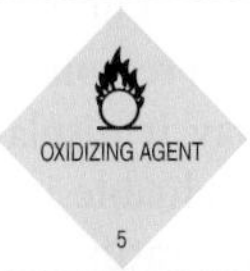 OXIDIZING AGENT 5	OXIDIZING AGENT Yellow Background Black Text & Symbol
5.2	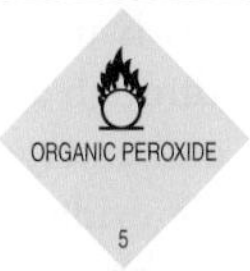 ORGANIC PEROXIDE 5	ORGANIC PEROXIDE Yellow Background Black Text & Symbol
6.1(A)	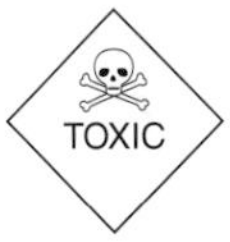 TOXIC	TOXIC White Background Black Text & Symbol
6.1(B)	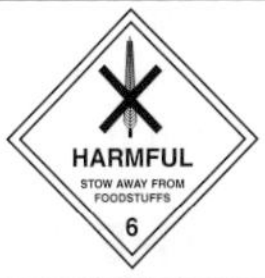 HARMFUL STOW AWAY FROM FOODSTUFFS 6	HARMFUL White Background Black Text & Symbol
6.2	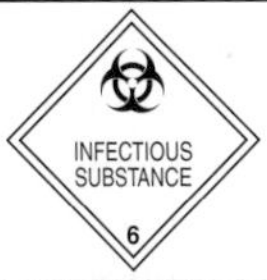 INFECTIOUS SUBSTANCE 6	INFECTIOUS SUBSTANCE White Background Black Text & Symbol
7	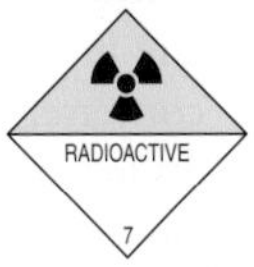 RADIOACTIVE 7	RADIOACTIVE Yellow Upper Background White Lower Background Black Text & Symbol
8	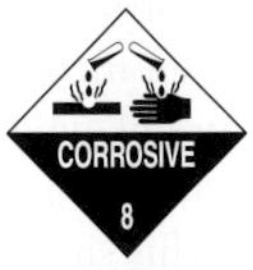 CORROSIVE 8	CORROSIVE White Upper Background Black Lower Background White Text & Symbol
9	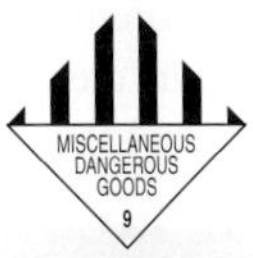 MISCELLANEOUS DANGEROUS GOODS 9	MISCELLANEOUS White & Black Vertical Striped Upper Background Black Text
10	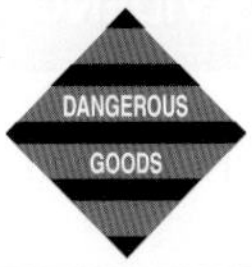 DANGEROUS GOODS	DANGEROUS GOODS Orange & Black Horizontal Striped Background White Text

Courtesy Signs of Safety www.signsofsafety.net.au.

dwelling, there is a need to use all the senses. Feeling for heat, or cold, is particularly important if there is a possibility of burn injury or hypothermia. The presence of a cold draught has been seen to signify everything from an open window to a gas jet from a leaking propane cylinder.

Smelling

Smelling has a vital role in the scene size-up, as there are many things that could give a clue to mechanism of injury, potential harm to rescuers or need for intervention. Some of these are the smell of gas in a house and the smell of caustic chemicals in road traffic incidents and particularly in tanker accidents; remember to look for the Hazchem sign. Smells of smoke and sulfur from discharged firearms, and even the smell of body fluids such as blood, urine or sweat, all may be a pointer to possible hazards, patients or pathologies about to be encountered. The smell of a cigarette or a match being struck where there is a potential fuel spill or gas leak may certainly prove to be a warning of the possibility of harm for all concerned, and prompts urgent action to ensure protection.

PROTECTING THE SCENE

Protection of the integrity of a scene of an incident or accident is exceptionally important for several reasons. First, in the short term the environment and the way it displays the habitat or habits of an individual may give valuable information, which can assist in the diagnosis and risk stratification of a newly encountered patient. Ensuring that this is undisturbed until the clinician has had a chance to work through a process of clinical reasoning, structured examination and emergency intervention may prevent vital pieces of diagnostic evidence being found or used. All the senses of a seasoned pre-hospital clinician should be routinely alert to notice factors relevant to safety, medical intervention priorities and interpersonal communication (the 1-2-3 of pre-hospital care). In a similar way, when there is a suspicion of a crime being committed, it is essential to avoid inadvertent disruption or destruction of potential evidence. Preservation of evidence can be promoted by observing some simple rules and principles, as outlined in Box 9.5.

COMMUNICATION FROM THE SCENE

Communication is important in many aspects of scene and patient management: between clinician and patients, relatives and bystanders; between clinical colleagues; and between emergency services—but it is absolutely vital to have clear and structured communication from ambulance to control or operations centre. It has been shown that lack of structure in information transfer leads to information loss,[26,27] and conversely that applying a structure to the handover process results in a decrease in information loss and an improvement in handover quality.[28]

There are three situations where a structured set of information has great value. It has already been mentioned that a situation report ('sitrep') is extremely useful when arriving at the scene of an incident or accident, in order to give a brief overview of the appearance as a crew arrives. This sitrep enables the control centre to gain some sense of the potential scale of the problems encountered by the first clinician crew, and to put other resources on standby. Following an accurate, complete but rapid scene size-up as described above, it is often essential to transmit another set of structured information back to the control centre; this is the result of the systematic patient assessment. Worldwide this is most commonly given in the MIST format:

M Mechanism of injury
I Injuries identified
S Signs. Vital signs including PR, BP, RR, SaO_2, GCS
T Treatment. Interventions and medications administered.

Early notification of the severity of illness or injury of the patients assessed by paramedics enables actions to be carried out, including prewarning of emergency departments and activation of medical teams or retrieval services, not only to increase the level of care available at the scene if necessary but also to shorten the time to definitive care. Finally, in the situation of a major incident or disaster scenario, an accurate picture of the scale of the incident, the actions taken and the need for extra resources may be summarised by the mnemonic ETHANE (Box 9.6).[29]

BOX 9.5 PRESERVATION OF EVIDENCE PROMOTION

- Avoid moving furniture or other articles apart from to provide vital medical care.
- Take a photograph of the scene prior to moving a body if this is possible in the context of the ambulance system. Many paramedics carry mobile phones that are able to take high-quality digital images, although patient privacy and confidentiality hampers the use of these in many jurisdictions.
- Do not cut through bullet holes or stab holes in clothing when attempting to expose the patient in trauma. Investigators often use minute evidence from these areas in forensic examination relevant to the pursuit of a criminal prosecution.
- Be careful with clothing, and place in a paper bag if possible.
- Try to avoid tracking through blood and other items of evidence; this is a damaging mistake to make at a crime scene.
- Clean up and carry away any debris that is generated from treating the patient, such as wrappings from cannulae, dressings, etc.

BOX 9.6 THE ETHANE MNEMONIC[29]

E Exact location—the precise location of the incident.
T Type—the nature of the incident, including how many vehicles, buildings and so on are involved.
H Hazards—both actual and potential.
A Access—best route for emergency services to access the site, or obstructions and bottlenecks to avoid.
N Numbers—numbers of casualties, dead and uninjured on-scene.
E Emergency services—which services are already on-scene, and which others are required.

SCENE ACCESS

Following assessment of the scene, it is then time to access the patient; specific considerations and hazards will vary depending on the type of scene and incident. Planning scene access is a critical element of the overall successful management of pre-hospital incidents.[30]

PLANNING

Emergency healthcare providers must have a high level of situational awareness of the overall scene and consider all potential hazards as they approach the patient.[31] Special circumstances will be dealt with later in the chapter; for most incidents, patient access is straightforward and readily achievable.

Where possible, following the call for an ambulance, the operations centre dispatchers should advise callers to assist EMS staff finding the scene. This may be done by sending a bystander, friend or family member to wait by the road or entrance to escort the team. At night, switching on external lights can be of great assistance; however, patients on their own or incapacitated by their illness or injury may not be able to help in this way.

HOUSES

Most patients are easily accessed via the front door or main entrance. As the team approaches, it is imperative to remain vigilant to hazards, and assess and plan an egress route, should this be required urgently. When approaching at night, look for lights and listen for voices, which may indicate the number of people inside; knock firmly or ring the door bell, announcing yourself as an emergency healthcare provider. Standing to the side of the door and leaving screen or security doors closed, if present, is a sensible safety measure if there is any concern about personal security. Establish rapport as soon as possible and identify the whereabouts of the patient; it is best to follow the person who met you rather than have them follow you.[31] At night, turn illumination on as you proceed through the house; this will assist with planning the egress of the patient and identification of hazards. Always be aware of your closest egress point as well as an alternative.

UNITS

Identification of, and gaining access to, units or apartment blocks is often much more challenging for EMS providers than are single dwellings. Locating the correct block of units can be difficult in high-density residential areas, as numbering is often inadequate or absent or insufficient information has been provided by the caller. Security buildings have intercom systems, which require the resident to activate to enable access, and if this is not possible due to injury, illness or incapacity then neighbouring residences will need to be tried. As always, it is imperative to clearly identify yourself and your organisation. If an elevator is available, this is usually the quickest way to access the patient, but take careful note of the internal dimensions in relation to your stretcher as many elevators will not accommodate a stretcher in a standard configuration, necessitating an alternative route of egress where patients must be moved using a stretcher. Some units do not have elevators and the team will be required to ascend stairs while carrying their equipment. It is vital that packs and equipment for all likely eventualities are carried by the team to the first contact, as it is rarely easy to rapidly undo an error of omission upon assessing the patient. As one moves through the building it is essential to consider how egress might be accomplished once the patient is loaded, as it is always easier to get equipment to a patient than to extricate the patient once loaded on a stretcher or extrication board. On arrival outside the unit, it is important not to block egress with equipment, should you need to retreat quickly. Once on-scene, seeking local knowledge of alternative routes for egress can be invaluable.

OUTDOORS

A large proportion of situations requiring emergency medical care occur outdoors. These include simple falls, vehicle collisions, environmental emergencies (such as heat-related illness or envenomation) and sporting injuries or medical illnesses occurring outside. The general principles of access for such scenes include getting the ambulance as close as possible to the patient, and then using the vehicle to protect you and the patient, both in physical terms ('fending off' at motor vehicle collisions on roadways) and as a privacy screen (where crowds of onlookers are present).[31] Experienced EMS providers always consider how they will load the ambulance and egress the scene when choosing a place to park. Where practical and safe to do so, parking with the ambulance facing downhill generally makes loading the patient easier.

CROWDS

Crowds present unique challenges, and vary from the quiet and courteous to the angry and anti-social. Individuals within a crowd commonly have a reduced awareness of the approach of EMS, even when they arrive in a vehicle the size of an ambulance. Use of sirens is typically unhelpful and can increase the unpredictability of the crowd; therefore their use is discouraged in close proximity.[2] Judicious use of 'lights' is generally a satisfactory way to move slowly through a crowd. Emergency healthcare providers need to be particularly mindful of children, patrons affected by drugs or alcohol and individuals who seem unaware of your presence and intent. Windows should be closed and doors locked to avoid interference and delay. If proceeding on foot, the notification of your response to your control centre is imperative; move purposefully through the crowd, announcing your approach to indicate the urgent medical nature of your response. A key barrier to moving within crowds is your equipment, which generally significantly increases your width and can cause harm or injury to others; backpacks are helpful, if available, to assist in moving through densely packed people. It may be very challenging to locate a patient requiring assistance among large crowds, and it requires careful observation on the part of the responders and accurate directions by dispatchers. Always have access to a radio and stay together with a partner, keeping a close eye on each other. Inadvertently coming across another person who is ill or injured is not uncommon, and this needs to be managed in accordance with the urgency of your task; priorities should be reconciled with the assistance of the control centre.

EQUIPMENT

Choice and carriage of equipment is very important when accessing scenes and will vary greatly depending on the skills of the provider. Typically, a minimum of oxygen, suction, medication kit with approved medications and a monitor/defibrillator would be carried to all scenes. Emergency healthcare professionals will need to consider whether other specialised equipment that is not routinely carried may be required (such as maternity packs, pelvic sheeting, burns dressings, etc). Emergency healthcare responders need to keep a close eye on their equipment, as it is not uncommon for equipment to be left behind or even taken by bystanders. Equipment taken to the side of the patient and opened also requires time to repack, and in certain circumstances it may be prudent to expeditiously load the patient and commence treatment in the ambulance rather than take all equipment to the patient.

PATIENT EXTRICATION

THEORY OF EXTRICATION

Vehicle extrication is the process of removing or deforming parts of a vehicle from around a person following a motor vehicle collision, where conventional means of exit are impossible or hazardous. There are several steps to all extrications, as outlined in Box 9.7.

A practical approach to extrication is to seek to perform the least effort for the greatest gain. Typically, effort is associated with increased time on-scene and often unnecessary delay. For example, if a patient could be safely extricated from a crashed vehicle by simply removing a single door, then this is likely to be more appropriate than removing the roof and the entire side of the vehicle. Extrication must be tailored to meet the specific needs of the patient, the severity of illness or injury, the environment and the available resources (Figs 9.8 to 9.12).

BOX 9.7 EXTRICATION PROCESS/STEPS[32]

1. Protection of the scene—avoid further collisions by marking the scene and fending off with vehicles, and mitigate obvious risks such as downed power lines, fire or leaking fuel.
2. Stabilisation of the vehicle by blocks or cribbing to prevent unintended movement.
3. Patient assessment, triage and first aid.
4. Creation of space by cutting or opening the structure with tools.
5. Removal of the patient(s) (physical extrication) from the vehicle with the least amount of movement consistent with urgency of their clinical needs. Where patients are physically compressed, this is called disentanglement.

FIGURE 9.8 SCENE SAFETY IS A PRIORITY FOR ANY EXTRICATION

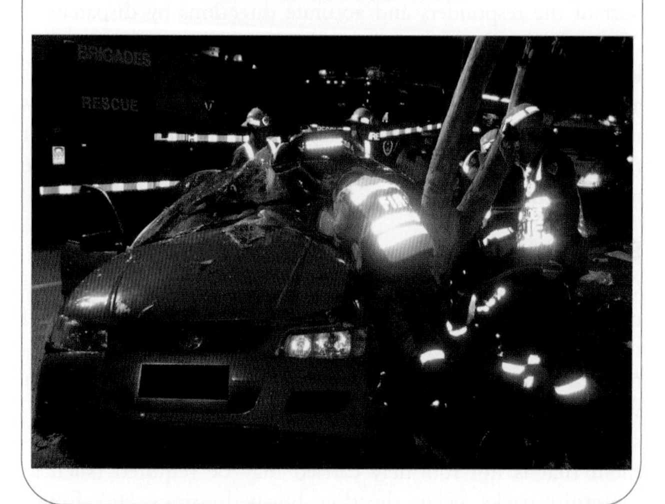

Courtesy NSW Ambulance.

FIGURE 9.9 EFFECTIVE ANALGESIA AND SEDATION CAN FACILITATE EXTRICATION

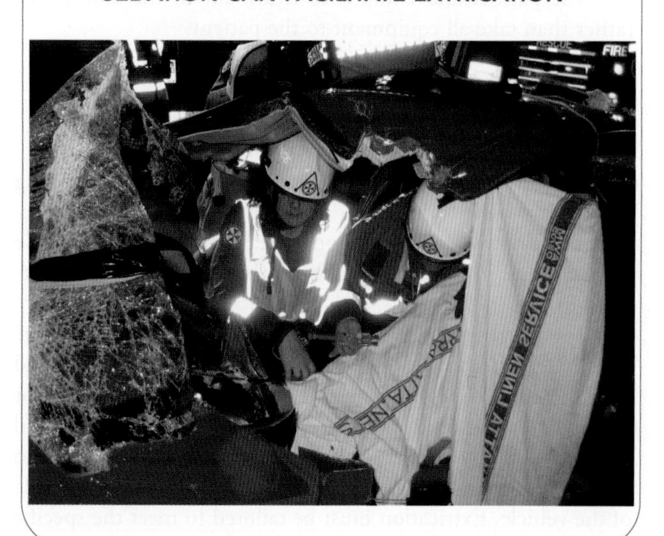

Courtesy NSW Ambulance.

FIGURE 9.10 LONG EXTRICATION BOARD READY FOR THE PATIENT

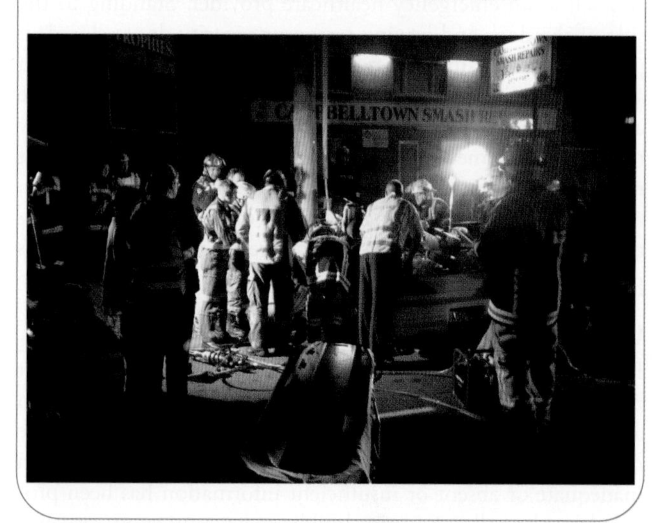

Courtesy NSW Ambulance.

FIGURE 9.11 A DIFFICULT EXTRICATION REQUIRES THE WHOLE TEAM TO WORK TOGETHER

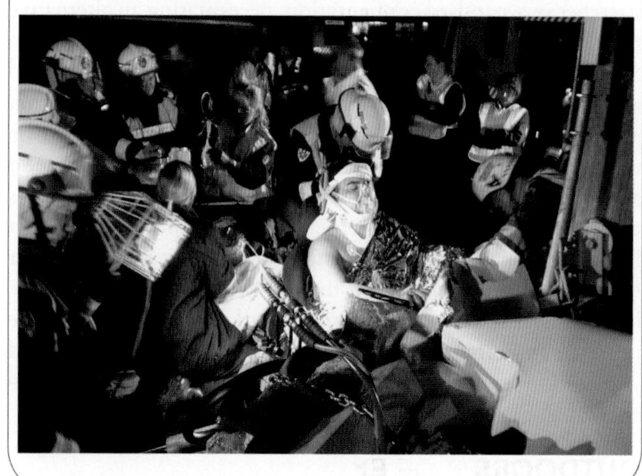

Courtesy NSW Ambulance.

INDICATIONS FOR RAPID EXTRICATION[32]

Rapid extrication is indicated when the clinical condition of the patient mandates urgent clinical interventions which cannot be delivered in situ. Rapid extrication is indicated for the following situations:

1. Deteriorating level of consciousness or haemodynamic parameters
2. Penetrating trauma to the torso
3. Threatened airway unable to be managed on the scene
4. Uncontrolled haemorrhage
5. Potentially reversible life-threatening medical conditions, such as myocardial infarction or cardiac arrhythmia.

FIGURE 9.12 HYDRAULIC CUTTING TOOLS BEING USED BY RESCUERS

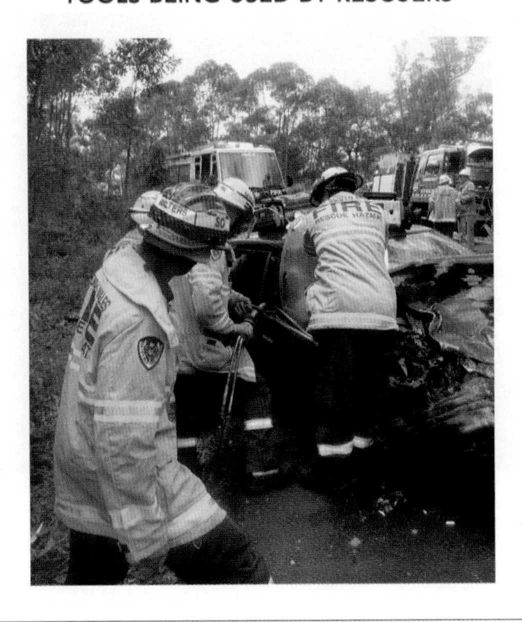

Courtesy NSW Ambulance.

Following extrication, the patient should be reassessed and immediately life-threatening conditions treated, followed by rapid transport to a centre able to provide definitive care.

PRACTICE TIP

Decisions about the speed of extrication are inevitably a compromise between reducing patient movement (especially of the spinal column) and enabling life-threatening injuries to be managed effectively. Discussion with the designated rescue agency should ALWAYS include an estimate of time required for standard extrication, but with a plan B briefed in case of patient deterioration.

TECHNIQUES OF EXTRICATION

There are many techniques and types of specialised rescue equipment used for extrication of patients, and it is beyond the scope of this book to describe the more technical aspects. The key role of emergency healthcare providers is to access the patients (where safe to do so), and control and coordinate their clinical management. It is vital to liaise closely with rescue services regarding the extrication plan and have a plan B to expedite in case of sudden clinical deterioration. Emergency medical care providers must have a good understanding of commonly used extrication equipment such as stretchers and spinal boards, and extrication aids, such as the Kendrick Extrication Device (KED) or Neann Immobilisation and Extrication Jacket (NEIJ).

SCENE EGRESS

Planning egress from the scene is a key component in the overall management of ill or injured patients, and this planning should begin at the initial scene assessment. The route taken to access the patient may not be the best way of leaving the scene, particularly if the patient is immobile or stretcher-bound.[31] Emergency healthcare providers must carefully plan the egress route considering terrain (surface, gradient, stairs), patient condition, ongoing treatment (oxygen, intravenous fluids, etc) and the need for, and manipulation of, a stretcher or carry-chair. Ambulance vehicle egress becomes another important factor, especially in urban environments, and nowhere is this more important than when multiple units respond to an incident, where subsequently arriving vehicles can interfere with egress routes.

MANAGEMENT OF SPECIFIC HAZARDS

REMOTE CLINICAL ACCESS

Remote areas are defined as inaccessible or difficult-to-access places due to their terrain (dense bush, mountains, coastlines, water, etc) or extreme distances from transport infrastructure (Fig. 9.13). Remote clinical access refers to the ability to attend, triage, treat and evacuate[33] patients who are ill or injured in areas inaccessible to usual EMS resources such as road ambulances.

The skills and procedures required for remote access overlap significantly with other aspects of 'difficult' access missions, such as confined space, safety at heights and helicopter operations; details of these will be considered within their respective sections. The defining nature of remote clinical access missions is that they all require a team approach and thoughtful systematic planning.

The basic principles[33] of such missions are:

1. plan
2. brief
3. execute
4. review.

FIGURE 9.13 RESCUE OF AN INJURED BASE JUMPER IN THE BLUE MOUNTAINS, NSW

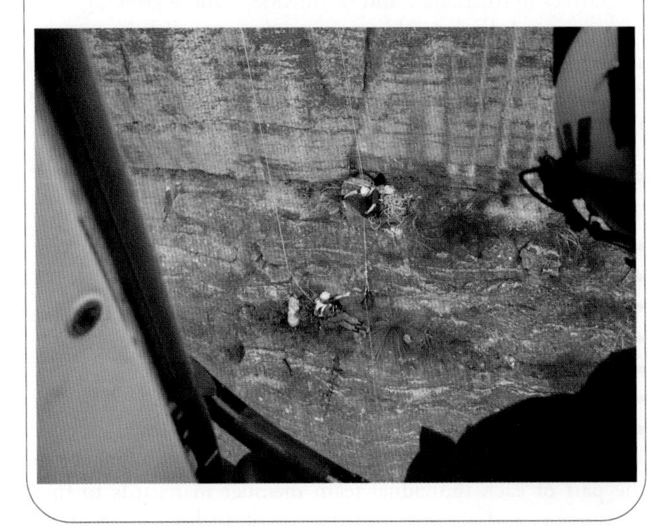

Courtesy NSW Ambulance.

Mission planning

Planning may be considered on a strategic or operational level, but both levels involve the process of gathering relevant information, determining the key priorities, assessing alternatives and coming to a final decision about the plan which must be executed. Relevant considerations include:

- logistics—requirements for food, water, equipment and additional personnel
- communication methods—direct, radio, mobile phone, satellite phone
- back-up—are there any other resources coming and do they know the 'plan'?
- helicopter resources—are these available?
- alternative/contingency plan—is there another way to do this mission?

Team briefing

The mnemonic SMEACS is a useful one; it has been adapted from the Australian armed forces guide[34] to assist in organising the briefing of a mission:

S	Situation—brief statement of the current situation
M	Mission—clear explanation of the goal of the operation
E	Execution—step-by-step list of how the mission will be performed
A	Administration and logistics—description of the stores, job delegations and contingency plans
C	Communications and signals—chain of command, communications and timings
S	Safety—all identified hazards and abatements

Execution

Carry out the plan as briefed.

Review

Constant evaluation and review should take place. A timeframe for completion of the mission and an interim set of goals to work towards can assist in this process.

SAFETY AT HEIGHTS

Falls from heights are the most common cause of fatal injury to employees in Australia[35] and worldwide,[36] and a growing cause of injury and death in domestic settings as well.[37] Emergency medical service staff must understand the risks of accessing patients at height and ensure that these risks are minimised (see Fig. 9.14).

FIGURE 9.14 EDGE SAFETY

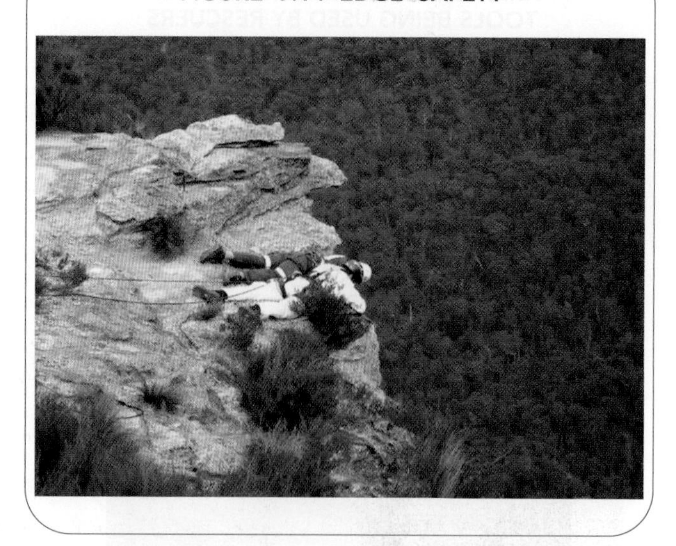

Courtesy NSW Ambulance.

Settings in which to consider safety at heights

There are a broad range of relevant settings, including:

- roof structures
- building sites
- industrial sites
- ladders
- trees
- cliff edges/mountains
- truck or other large vehicle extrications.

The keys to working safely at heights are constant vigilance on the part of each individual team member in regards to their movements and actions, and the use of anchors to secure all personnel and equipment at risk of falling.[33,38]

Casualties that have fallen from a height require particular safety considerations; consequently there is always the risk that an unstable structure (or debris that is about to fall) is directly above the casualty; this must be considered and anticipated on approaching the scene. Wherever possible, the patient should be removed from a dangerous position as early as possible during their treatment. This 'rule' applies to all pre-hospital situations and settings, but vigilance is even more vital where risk of falling from a height exists.

As well as individual awareness of the dangers, it is important to appoint a 'safety officer' who is not involved in any other activities to supervise the safety of the team. All staff should remain 2 metres or more from hazardous edges at all times, unless secured to an anchor. If there is a need to look over an edge before an anchor is set up, then the safest way is to lie prone and inch slowly up to the edge. Remember that edges that are unstable or undermined may give way when weight is applied from above.

In any situation where there will be prolonged exposure to the risk of falling from a height, it is essential that anchors are secured, and all staff and equipment are tied to an anchor in such a way as to avoid or minimise injury should they fall. Anchors should be set up by appropriately trained rescue staff and must be capable of sustaining the intended load of personnel or equipment, including 'shock-loading' due to sudden falls where there is slack in attachment lines. Attachment lines must be kept as short as possible and always shorter than the distance to the edge.

In some cases, it is necessary for rescue teams to descend to the casualty by way of roping equipment such as belay systems. This must only be undertaken by appropriately credentialled rescue operators who undertake regular training in the use of ropes, anchors and climbing equipment.[1] Such technical aspects are beyond the scope of this book to describe.

CAVES AND CONFINED SPACES

Caves and other confined spaces pose significant dangers to those who must work within them and those who choose to

FIGURE 9.15 CONFINED SPACE RESCUE

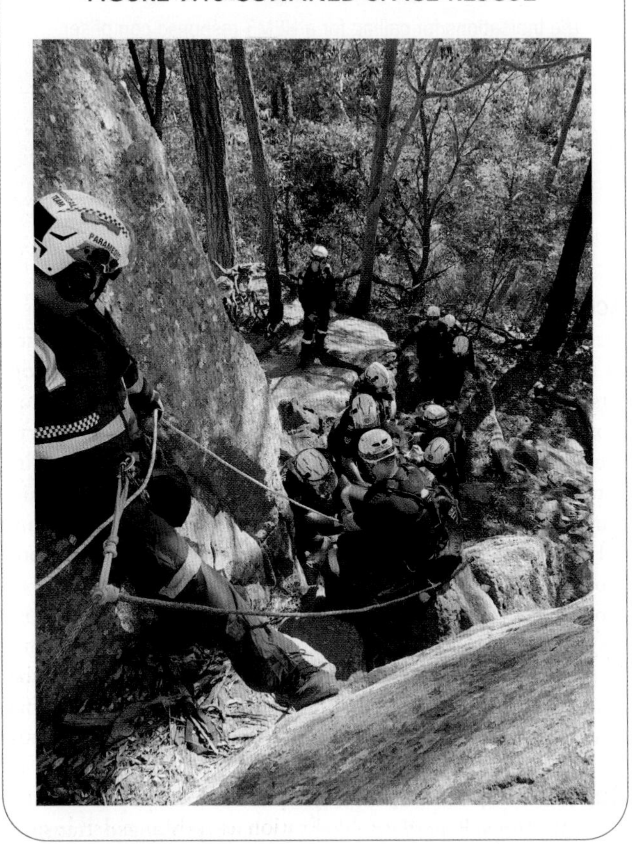

Courtesy K. Habig, NSW Ambulance.

recreate within them. Access and rescue of patients suffering illness or injury from confined spaces presents many hazards to rescuers and clinical teams and should only be undertaken by staff with appropriate training and a thorough understanding of the risks (Fig. 9.15).

A confined space is any space of an enclosed nature where there is risk to human health from dangerous conditions or hazardous substances. Some examples of enclosed spaces include:

- mine shafts
- caves
- collapsed buildings
- machinery rooms
- silos
- storage tanks
- drains or sewers
- small, poorly ventilated rooms or compartments.

Possible hazards of enclosed spaces

A range of dangers may exist within enclosed spaces, as listed below,[38,39] and the mnemonic 3TVIPS should be followed (Box 9.8).

- irrespirable atmospheres
- toxic substances or residues
- fires/explosions
- physical injury due to falls, moving equipment, unstable structures, etc
- environmental exposure—hypothermia, hyperthermia

BOX 9.8 **CONFINED SPACE OPERATIONS MNEMONIC—3TVIPS[33]**

T Test (oxygen)
T Test (flammable)
T Test (toxic)
V Ventilate (prior and after)
I Isolate (lock out/tag out)
P Personal protective equipment
S Safety and standby teams

- electrical hazards
- concentrations of dust
- psychological responses
- confined space operations.

Confined space entry

Prior to entering confined spaces it is essential to assess the risks involved and be prepared for potential hazards. The following vital elements should be considered.

- *Risk assessment*—the safety of the entry teams must be the prime consideration.
- *Safety officer*—a single individual should be appointed to this role, and they must remain outside the dangerous environment to oversee the operation.
- *Communications*—confirm communication systems and back-up communication plan. Such a plan must also include a specific determination of when to send a back-up team if contact is lost.
- *Team assembly*—ensure that all staff entering the hazardous area have had the relevant training to be competent in confined space access. Such training usually includes hazard identification and mitigation, escape and rescue procedures and confidence with PPE, lighting, communications and environmental monitoring equipment. Record all staff in and out (tag in/out).
- *PPE*—check all staff have appropriate PPE. This must include adequate means of illumination, with back-up in case of failure.
- *Safe atmosphere*—set up atmospheric monitoring and maximise ventilation. Atmospheric monitoring using multi-gas detection systems must be undertaken prior to rescuer access.

Specific hazards of enclosed spaces/caves

Hazardous/irrespirable atmospheres

High concentrations of gases can displace oxygen from the atmosphere in enclosed spaces. This is particularly common in underground settings, where gas may naturally vent from surrounding rocks and where heavier-than-air gases such as carbon dioxide collect in particular areas. Where concentrations of such gases rise sufficiently to displace a significant proportion of the atmospheric oxygen, there is a risk of hypoxic asphyxia. In addition, any inhaled gases may have their own toxic effects. The most common three such gases are carbon dioxide, carbon monoxide and 'sewer gas'.[39]

- 'Foul air' refers to an atmosphere with a high level of carbon dioxide. Carbon dioxide is a colourless and odourless gas that causes physiological effects in proportion to its concentration. Symptoms begin at concentrations as low as 1%,[39] with initial headache, increased respiratory rate and 'panting' respirations. Death is possible at concentrations as low as 10%. Treatment is removal from the toxic atmosphere and administration of 100% oxygen.

- Carbon monoxide is produced by the incomplete combustion of carbon fuels, and is also odourless and colourless. It may build up due to emissions from internal-combustion engines or from poorly ventilated gas or charcoal fires. Once inhaled, it binds preferentially to circulating haemoglobin and displaces oxygen from red blood cells. Early symptoms include headache, nausea and confusion, followed by coma. Treatment is removal from the source and administration of 100% oxygen.
- Sewer gas[38] comprises a variable combination of hydrogen sulfide, methane, sulfur dioxide and trichloroethylene. These gases are poisonous and highly explosive, making them a particular risk when naked flames or cutting tools are used. Treatment is removal from the source and administration of 100% oxygen.

Fires/explosions

Flammable gases (such as methane) or vapours (such as petroleum vapour) and dusts (such as coal dust or grain dust) are a threat to rescuers in many environments, but particularly in mines and industry. Naked flames pose a high risk in such environments and should never be used unless continuous atmospheric monitoring can be undertaken.

Physical injury

Enclosed spaces present a multitude of ways in which the rescuer can become a victim. These range from rock falls, trip hazards and slippery surfaces in caves to unstable structures and falling debris in damaged buildings. Enclosed spaces with tight passages present a real risk of entrapment due to rescuers becoming physically jammed within tight passages or spaces and unable to extricate themselves. The entrapped person then may succumb to physical restriction on chest excursion, hypothermia or dehydration.

Psychological responses

It is easy for inexperienced staff to become disoriented and lost in enclosed spaces, and particularly in cave systems. Fear and panic can threaten the safety of rescuers unused to these environments.

HELICOPTER EMS OPERATIONS

Helicopters are a vital part of EMS responses around the world. There is a large variety of aircraft types, capabilities and crew mix, but in general the utility of helicopters in pre-hospital responses relates to their ability to gain access to difficult scenes, extricate the patient and rapidly transport them 'as the crow flies' to definitive treatment, usually with an enhanced level of clinical care over typical ground EMS responses. The ability to call for helicopter EMS (HEMS) support can provide a vital link in the chain of survival for patients suffering major trauma[40] or medical illness remote from major hospital resources. An understanding by each EMS provider of the capabilities of their local HEMS response is vital in decision-making about utilising these resources.

PRACTICE TIP

The indications for calling for a HEMS response comprise:

- Patient access issues (need for winching, etc)
- Rapid transport requirements (critically ill remote from suitable hospital, etc)
- Provision of enhanced clinical resources (medical teams, etc)

Access problems requiring helicopters

Helicopters are able to take off and land vertically, and can land in unprepared sites distant from road infrastructure. Helicopters equipped with a winch or 'long-line' provide even more flexibility, and allow clinical and/or rescue teams to directly access ill or injured parties where no suitable helicopter landing zone exists near the scene, such as with wilderness areas, mountains, coastal zones, oceans, boats or waterways (Figs 9.16 and 9.17). Access issues requiring helicopter response most commonly involve a patient who is ill or injured in a location remote from roads and therefore remote from a standard road EMS response. Other scenarios where access by helicopter may be preferable include extreme road conditions that inhibit usual road responses, such as following an earthquake, flood, rock fall or extreme road traffic congestion.

Rapid transport capability

Critically unwell patients likely to have prolonged transport times to definitive care may benefit from aeromedical helicopter transport.[41] In general, helicopters are able to provide faster transfer times (from emergency call to arrival in hospital) where

FIGURE 9.16 HELICOPTER WINCHING OPERATIONS

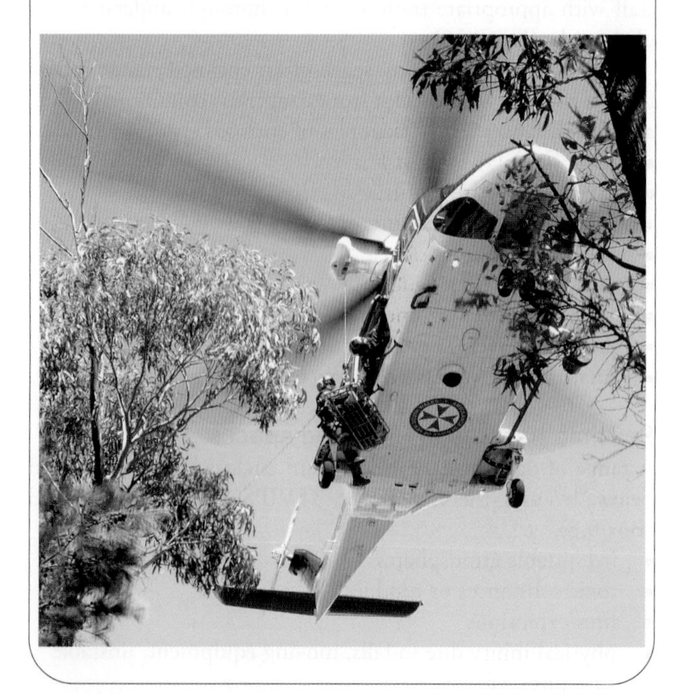

Courtesy NSW Ambulance.

FIGURE 9.17 COASTAL ACCESS BY WINCH-CAPABLE HELICOPTER

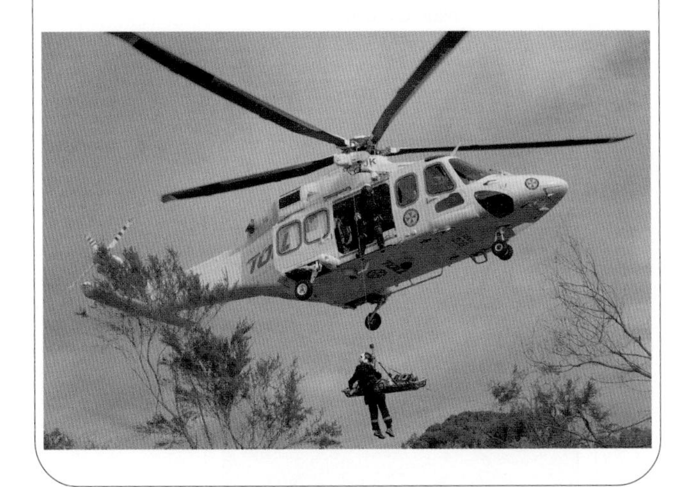

Courtesy K. Habig, NSW Ambulance.

FIGURE 9.18 SPECIAL CASUALTY ACCESS TRAINING (SCAT) PARAMEDICS

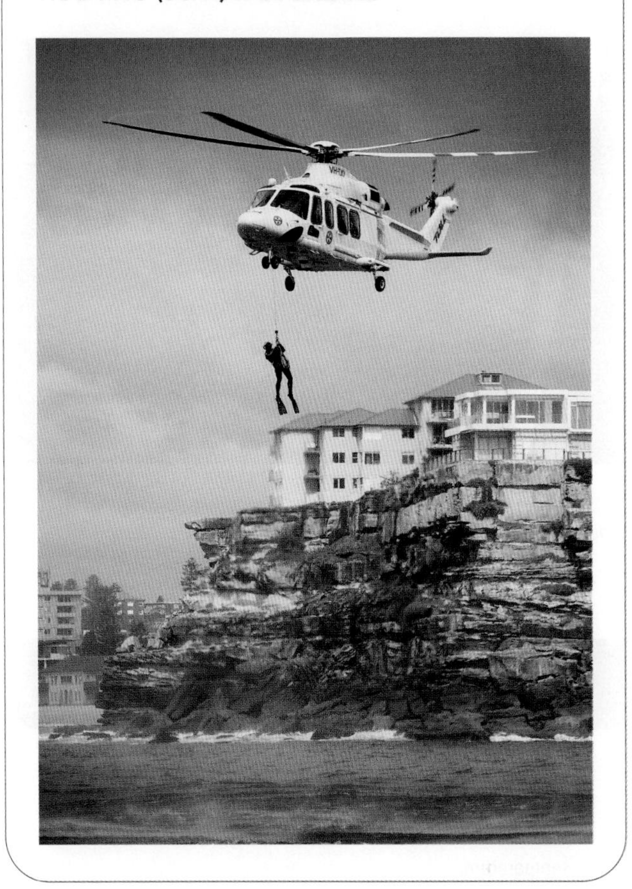

Courtesy K. Habig, NSW Ambulance.

anticipated road transport times exceed 20 minutes or approximately 16 km when tasked simultaneously, and approximately 60 km where helicopter dispatch occurs after road ambulance arrival and report.[42] Transport times must always factor in the time for engine start-up and spool-down, as well as loading and unloading at each end of the transfer. Helicopters have the advantage of travelling 'as the crow flies' at speeds between 220 and 350 kph,[42] and are not subject to issues of road traffic congestion or limited by terrain. They can also take the patient from the scene directly to the most appropriate hospital, bypassing smaller hospitals if necessary.

Enhanced clinical resources

Worldwide, HEMS typically provides enhanced clinical resources and crewing over standard road-based paramedical systems. In Australia, Europe and the UK, HEMS crew mix is most commonly a doctor and a paramedic or flight nurse team. In the United States, most HEMS utilise a paramedic or flight nurse team only, though usually these teams have significantly higher levels of training and skills than the road-based EMS systems where they operate (Fig. 9.18). Critical interventions available to HEMS include emergency pre-hospital anaesthesia, procedural sedation and more-advanced pharmacological interventions, advanced surgical interventions, such as thoracostomy or amputation and advanced imaging such as Point-of-Care Ultrasound (POCUS).

Helicopter landing zones

Once the decision has been made to call for HEMS support the next important step, where possible, is to identify and prepare a suitable helicopter landing zone (LZ). The largest flat, open and unobstructed area close to the accident scene should be chosen for the LZ. Consider carefully hazards to helicopter flight or landing, such as buildings, towers, wires, animals, loose objects or debris. Helicopters will always try to land 'into wind' (towards the wind direction), and so wind direction is a crucial factor in the approach path. The LZ must be a minimum of 25 m × 25 m, and preferably 40 m × 40 m in size.

By day, a ground-marshalling officer wearing appropriate PPE (including ear, eye and head protection and safety vest), standing at the upwind end of the area with their back to the wind, should indicate the area. If a smoke flare is available, it should be activated when the aircraft approaches overhead to show position, wind direction and wind speed (Fig. 9.19). If the area is large enough (40 m × 40 m), and there are sufficient responsible ground personnel, then four people standing one at each corner should indicate the area. At night, the four corners of the area should be indicated using vehicles, lights or 'Cyalume' (glow) sticks. Information helpful to the HEMS team is outlined in Box 9.9 and a landing plan is given in Fig. 9.20.

Helicopter safety

Working around helicopters poses risks to EMS providers. Apart from the obvious risk of injury or death due to contact with moving main or tail rotors, hazards also include injury due to 'downwash' (which is proportional to the size of the helicopter), and dust or debris being blown around, particularly into the eyes causing temporary blindness. The same rules of safety around helicopters should apply whether the helicopter's

FIGURE 9.19 LANDING ZONE MARKED BY SMOKE FLARE

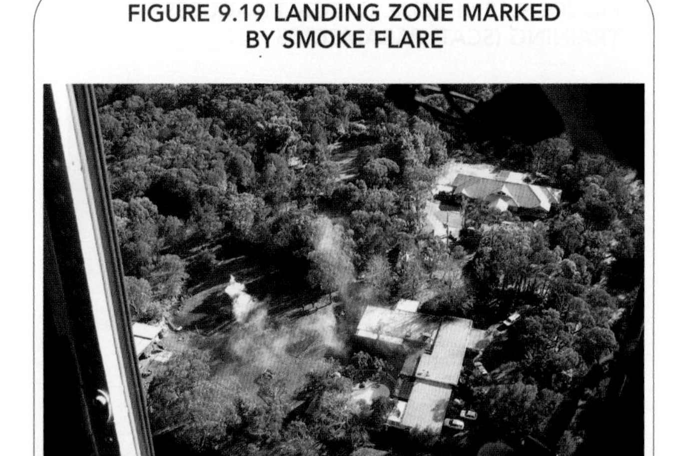

Courtesy NSW Ambulance.

FIGURE 9.20 HELICOPTER LANDING PLAN

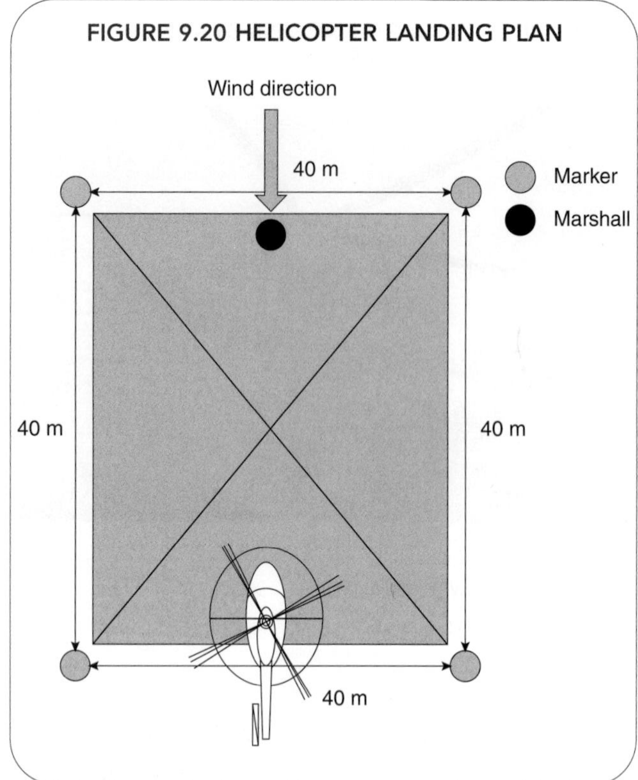

Courtesy Jason Bendall.

BOX 9.9 INFORMATION HELPFUL TO THE HEMS TEAM

- Location–GPS coordinates (latitude and longitude) if possible or street-grid map reference.
- Weather–wind speed and direction, fog, rain, clouds, temperature.
- Obstacles on approach–wires, towers, buildings, trees, bystanders, animals.
- Supporting resources on-scene–ambulance service commander, police, rescue, etc.
- Patient details–e.g. MIST-formatted report (Mechanism, Injuries, Signs and Treatment).
- Landing site–terrain, slope, surface, dust conditions.

engines and rotors are running or shut down, and are outlined in Box 9.10 and shown in Figs 9.21 to 9.26.

BOX 9.10 HELICOPTER SAFETY[33]

- Remain clear of the helicopter at all times unless accompanied by a helicopter crewperson.
- Follow all instructions (verbal or hand signal) given by the helicopter pilot and flight crew.
- During engine shut-down in gusty winds, the helicopter blades may dip below head height ('blade-sailing'). Do not approach the helicopter until the rotor blades have ceased rotating.
- If blinded by helicopter downwash or dust, sit down and await assistance.
- When approaching the helicopter always approach from the front–in the 'ten-to-two-o'clock' safe area of the helicopter–and depart in the same direction.
- Never walk around or approach a helicopter from the tail-rotor area.
- When approaching a helicopter on a slope, always approach from the downhill side.
- Never reach for, especially above head height, or chase after articles which have blown away.
- Intravenous drips or other objects must be carried below shoulder level at all times, and long objects carried parallel to the ground between two officers.

RAILWAY INCIDENTS

Railway incidents present a multitude of dangers to rescuers, and working close to railway lines requires a great deal of common sense, understanding of the components of railway systems and careful coordination of operations. The most common reason for EMS to need to access railway lines is a person falling or jumping onto tracks. Patients injured or trapped beneath trains represent a great challenge to rescuers and require a coordinated multidisciplinary approach.

POSSIBLE HAZARDS AT RAILWAY INCIDENTS

Such hazards include:

- contact with moving trains/rolling stock
- electrical injury from overhead systems, the 'third rail', pylons and signalling systems
- mechanical track-switching equipment
- trip/slip hazards
- falling from platforms.

In Australia, the majority of railway lines operate with overhead power systems that supply electricity to the engine units

FIGURE 9.21 NEVER APPROACH OR DEPART WITHOUT PERMISSION[33]

PERMISSION TO APPROACH OR DEPART HELICOPTER ROTOR DISC ZONE — Hand signal

Do not enter or depart rotor disc zone UNTIL PERMISSION IS GIVEN BY THE PILOT

– THUMBS UP returned or FLASHED LANDING-LIGHT

Edgar C. SCAT (Special Casualty Access Training) reference text. NSW Ambulance 2006.

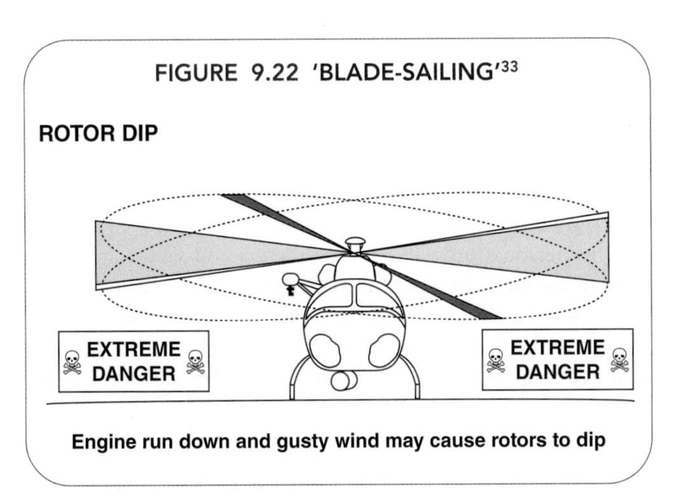

FIGURE 9.22 'BLADE-SAILING'[33]

Edgar C. SCAT (Special Casualty Access Training) reference text. NSW Ambulance 2006.

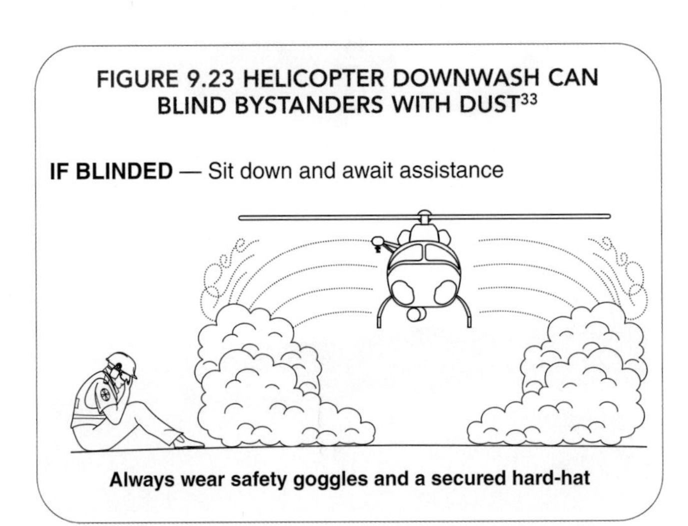

IF BLINDED — Sit down and await assistance
Always wear safety goggles and a secured hard-hat

FIGURE 9.23 HELICOPTER DOWNWASH CAN BLIND BYSTANDERS WITH DUST[33]

Edgar C. SCAT (Special Casualty Access Training) reference text. NSW Ambulance 2006.

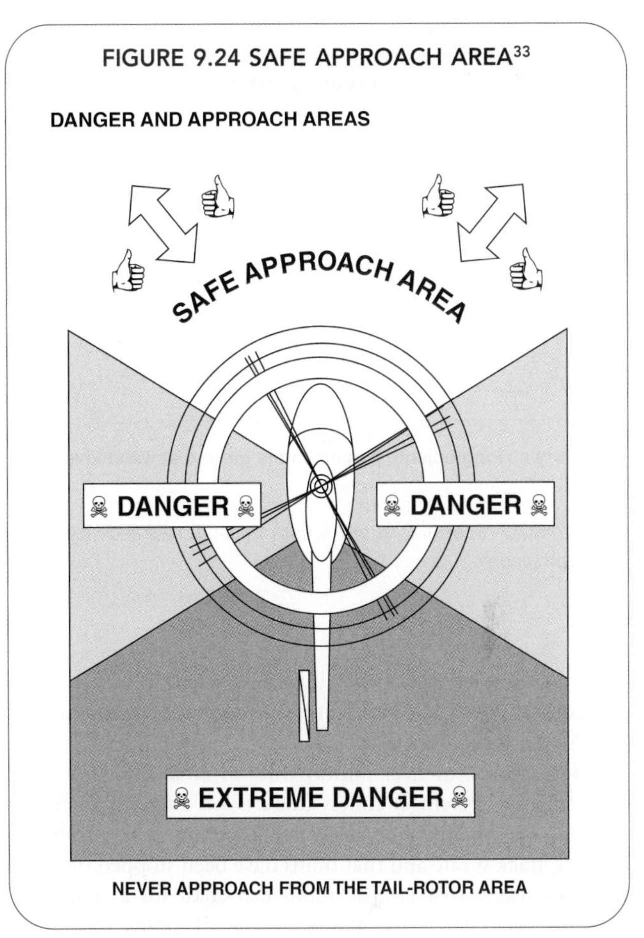

FIGURE 9.24 SAFE APPROACH AREA[33]

Edgar C. SCAT (Special Casualty Access Training) reference text. NSW Ambulance 2006.

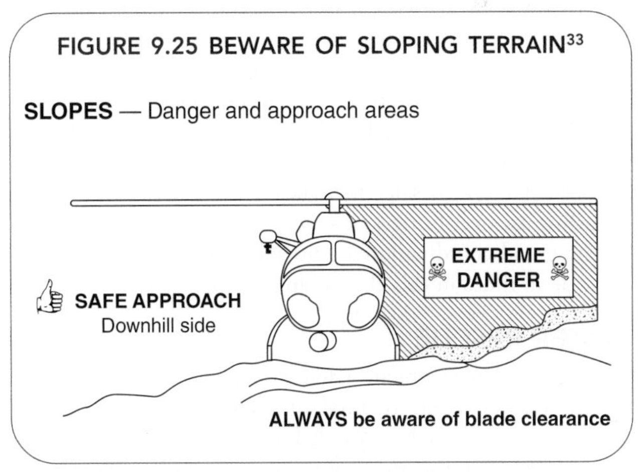

FIGURE 9.25 BEWARE OF SLOPING TERRAIN[33]

Edgar C. SCAT (Special Casualty Access Training) reference text. NSW Ambulance 2006.

through lines at up to 25,000 volts. While the supporting pylons are not electrified, all lines or wires suspended from them should be considered so. Electrical injury can result from contact or even close proximity to overhead power transmission lines due to arcing, and so all personnel, clothing and equipment must be kept back at least 3 m from overhead lines. If

FIGURE 9.26 TAKE CARE WHEN LOADING AND UNLOADING[33]

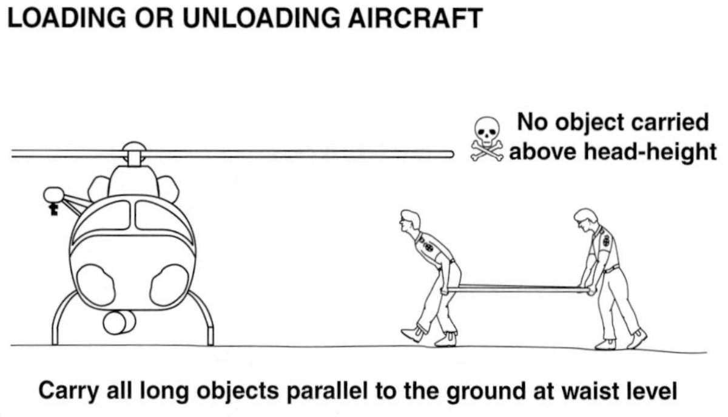

LOADING OR UNLOADING AIRCRAFT

No object carried above head-height

Carry all long objects parallel to the ground at waist level

Edgar C. SCAT (Special Casualty Access Training) reference text. NSW Ambulance 2006.

there are powered rails—the 'third rail'—then it must be confirmed that power has been cut to all lines prior to anyone accessing the track area.

Never go on or near railway lines or cross rails (except at marked level crossings) unless there is no alternative. Before entering the vicinity of railway tracks, it must be confirmed that the track is safe and that trains have been stopped on those lines. Be aware that electric trains can coast for a significant distance even when the power is cut. If trains cannot be stopped on all lines in the vicinity, then ensure that everyone has a clear understanding of the direction trains will move in, and have a lookout stationed for protection. It is worth assuming that trains can come from either direction at any time. High-visibility vests with reflective markings should be worn whenever accessing the track area.

Besides the obvious dangers of electricity and fast-moving vehicles, working close to or on railway tracks poses serious risks from falls or trips. Rail lines are a tripping hazard and become slippery, particularly in wet weather, as can timber sleepers. It is much safer to walk on the ballast (stone chippings) or use over-bridges or other safer routes where possible. Training and coordination are no substitute for constant vigilance at all times in this challenging environment.

WATER RESCUE

The aquatic environment refers to open ocean/sea, coastal zones, beaches, dams (natural or man-made), lakes, creeks/rivers, swimming pools or flooded urban environments (stormwater drains, flooded streets or buildings). These environments pose a wide variety of hazards to rescuers. Possible hazards of water rescue include:

- drowning/immersion
- hypothermia
- ocean waves, tides, rips
- hidden sandbars or rocks
- slip hazards on rocks/rock pools
- whitewater/rapids
- boats—collision, propellers
- debris in running water
- underwater snags
- disease due to contaminated water
- sea creatures—sharks, venomous stingers, etc.

Access to patients in open water or on boats requires very specialised rescue skills and equipment, but rescuers and EMS staff may be called to a casualty requiring rescue in an inland or inshore waterway without immediate access to additional resources.

Inshore/inland waterway rescue

The principle of inshore and inland waterway water rescue is to Reach, Throw, Wade, Row and only finally consider Swim and Tow.[38]

This means that where possible it is much better to reach out to a person using a pole or branch than to enter the water to effect a rescue. If this is not possible, the next best option is to throw a rope, life-preserver or other buoyant object to the person. If you can wade out to the person safely, then this is the next option, but rescuers must beware of fast-flowing water in rivers or streams and unseen underwater hazards. If a boat is available, then this may be utilised in the rescue. There is always the risk of capsize, particularly in a small dinghy if a panicked casualty tries to clamber aboard unsafely. In inshore rescues, such as at a beach, a boat such as a powered inflatable or water bike may be the only safe way of accessing the patient. Only if all other options are exhausted should one ever consider swimming to the victim and attempting to tow them back to shore. This should only be contemplated with appropriate equipment such as personal inflatable life-preservers and safety lines with enough assistants to pull both the victim and the rescuer out of the water. Finally, a winch-equipped helicopter may be able to access the patient most safely; however, such specialised resources require time to reach the scene (Fig. 9.27).

FIGURE 9.27 WATER RESCUE OPERATIONS

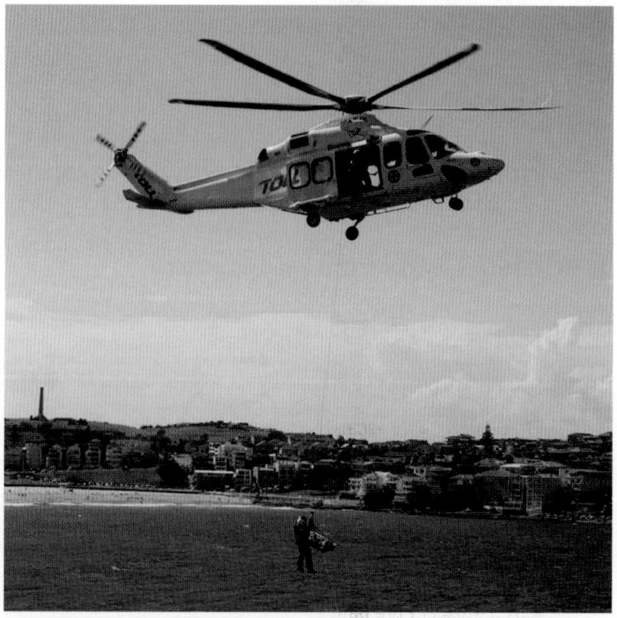

Courtesy K. Habig, NSW Ambulance.

VIOLENT PRESENTATIONS

Apart from dangers posed by the pre-hospital environment, patients themselves can pose a risk to emergency medical crews. There is evidence that violent attacks on paramedics are common and increasing in frequency.[43] Patients or bystanders may be violent for a variety of reasons, including alcohol intoxication, use of drugs such as methamphetamines and cocaine, psychiatric conditions, such as schizophrenia, psychosis or personality disorder, dementia, head injury or medical illness, such as hypoglycaemia or epilepsy. The risk of violence to EMS staff increases in cases of domestic dispute, where the patient has been the subject of a violent act, such as stabbing or shooting, in large crowds or in episodes of civil disturbance.[43]

Violent behaviour may come after clear warning signs with a period of escalation, but may occasionally come without warning. When approaching a scene it is essential to learn to look beyond the usual physical and environmental threats to safety, and consider risks from patients, family or bystanders. Where a risk of violence is perceived or anticipated, police should be called as early as possible. This should be a routine policy for any incident where a person has been injured by someone else (especially where firearms or knives are suspected), or where there is a previous history of violent or criminal behaviour. Most ambulance service dispatch systems enable flagging of such individuals and incidents, so that police are dispatched simultaneously. Never enter such an incident until police are present and have confirmed that the scene is safe. Ask whether the alleged assailant has been secured.

On occasion, EMS providers find themselves arriving at a scene where a domestic or other dispute is occurring or recurs on their arrival. In such cases it is important to have training and knowledge of how to de-escalate an aggressive situation (Chapter 39).

De-escalation

Where possible, always position yourself close to an exit and keep yourself and your partner between the aggressor and the exit.[38,44] Lower the tone and volume of speech, to convey calmness. Be polite, and address the person by name, if possible. Maintain eye contact in a non-threatening manner. Stand at least 1 m from the person and ask permission before taking any action which may be seen as an invasion of personal space. People involved in a heated argument are usually highly emotional and not thinking logically. Asking questions relevant to the patient's condition can help the person revert to logical behaviour. Remove distractions from the scene, such as bystanders, and do not allow others to interact with the person.

Mental health considerations

The legislative framework for management of patients with a mental illness or mental disorder differs between states of Australia and throughout the world.[45–47] EMS providers must ensure that they understand the particular rights and obligations of themselves and their patients in the jurisdiction where they work. In all states of Australia and many places in the world, EMS providers have the power under legislation to detain a person against their will for the purposes of transportation to a mental health facility for further evaluation and treatment, where that person refuses voluntary transport and where that patient's behaviour is such that it presents a risk of serious harm to themselves or others. Police will often be involved in assisting with this process. Police generally have similar powers to enact involuntary transport of patients to a mental health service or facility for the purposes of further assessment or treatment. Physical restraint by EMS providers may be allowed under local standard operating procedures, and police have further powers of restraint. Chemical restraint, or administration of psychoactive medications for behavioural control, is generally only permitted under the direction of a medical practitioner (Chapter 36).

SUMMARY

Assessment and management begins long before any arrival at the scene of an injury or an illness. The key principles of safety, including dispatch and pre-arrival information, planned and cautious travel to scene, personal protective equipment (PPE), planning an approach to the scene and careful and meticulous scene assessment, pave the way for the next stage of systematic patient assessment and structured intervention. Much of this may be summarised in the first stage of Caroline's Six Rs of Paramedic Practice—read the scene (Box 9.11).

BOX 9.11 CAROLINE'S SIX R's OF PARAMEDIC PRACTICE[22]

1. **READ THE SCENE**—scan the environment, review the surroundings, gather information regarding mechanisms of injury, identify and resolve dangers or threats to safety.
2. **READ THE PATIENT**—observe the patient, talk with the patient and others, take vital signs, identify life-threatening conditions, obtain complete vital signs through primary and secondary survey.
3. **REACT**—discern the patient's problems, determine provisional diagnosis, provide treatment, develop and implement plan for outcome.
4. **RE-EVALUATE**—obtain revised patient data, examine response to treatment, discern secondary problems and their significance, provide treatment, suitability of outcome.
5. **REVISE THE PLAN**—reconsider the plan and goal for achieving the outcome in light of emerging changes identified during ongoing data collection and analysis.
6. **REVIEW YOUR PERFORMANCE**—reflect on the case using continuous quality improvement. Integrate review outcomes into future practice.

CASE STUDY

You have responded to a three-car motor vehicle collision on the highway approximately 30 minutes south of the regional town where you work. There have been multiple calls and regular updates arriving via the mobile data terminal, indicating the severity of the incident. There is a report of one car on fire, multiple patients and one vehicle over a 5-metre steep embankment, with both the driver and a passenger trapped. As you approach the scene, you find that the traffic is not moving in either direction and there is a significant amount of smoke in the area. You are the first emergency service to arrive at the scene; however, the police, fire rescue and other emergency service resources are on the way. You find many bystanders already on the scene. The control centre has launched the helicopter emergency medical service (HEMS) from the closest facility, which will be overhead in approximately 45 minutes.

QUESTIONS

1. Describe the key principles of your initial scene assessment.
2. Describe key considerations regarding scene access and egress.
3. Describe the principles of patient extrication following vehicular collisions.
4. Describe key considerations when dealing with bystanders and other emergency services.
5. Describe the principles for establishing a landing site for the helicopter.

Answers to Case Study Questions can be found on evolve **http://evolve.elsevier.com/AU/Curtis/emergency/** 

USEFUL WEBSITES

Robert Simpson@AmboFOAM, ambofoam.wordpress.com—an interesting and insightful Twitter feed by a Victorian ICP.

REFERENCES

1. NSW Health. Calling an ambulance. Online. Available from: www.ambulance.nsw.gov.au/our-services/emergency-services.
2. National Academies of Emergency Dispatch. What is MPDS? Online. Available from: www.emergencydispatch.org/what-we-do/emergency-priority-dispatch-system/medical-protocol.
3. Roppolo LP, Pepe PE, Cimon N, et al. Modified cardiopulmonary resuscitation (CPR) instruction protocols for emergency medical dispatchers: rationale and recommendations. Resuscitation 2005;65(2):203–10.
4. Bailey ED, O'Connor RE, Ross RW. The use of emergency medical dispatch protocols to reduce the number of inappropriate scene responses made by advanced life support personnel. Prehosp Emerg Care 2000;4(2):186–9.
5. Fire Brigades Act 192 of 1989, Part 3. Fighting and preventing fires and dealing with hazardous material incidents. Online. Available from: legislation.nsw.gov.au/view/whole/html/inforce/2009-11-09/act-1989-192.
6. Lutman D, Montgomery M, Ramnarayan P, et al. Ambulance and aeromedical accident rates during emergency retrieval in Great Britain. EMJ 2008;25(5):301–2.
7. Maguire BJ, Hunting KL, Smith GS, et al. Occupational fatalities in emergency medical services: a hidden crisis. Annals Emerg Med 2002;40(6):625–32.
8. Biggers Jr WA, Zachariah BS, Pepe PE. Emergency medical vehicle collisions in an urban system. Prehosp Disaster Med 1996;11(3):195–201.
9. Solomon SS. Emergency response and vehicle operation. In: Solomon SS, Hill PF, editors. Emergency vehicle accidents: prevention, reconstruction and survey of state law. Tucson, AZ: Lawyers and Judges; 2002.
10. National Transportation Safety Board report by Chairman James L. Kolstad, January 4, 1991 regarding the incident in Catlett, Virginia on 28 September 1989. Firefighter's News 1990; Aug–Sep:36–7.
11. Elling R. Dispelling myths on ambulance accidents. JEMS 1989;14(7):60–4.
12. Federal Emergency Management Agency (FEMA), United States Fire Administration. EMS safety practices. 2022. Online. Available from: www.usfa.fema.gov/downloads/pdf/publications/ems-safety-practices.pdf.
13. Pittet D, Allegranzi B, Boyce J. World Health Organization, World Alliance for Patient Safety First: Global Patient Safety Challenge Core Group of Experts. The World Health Organization guidelines on hand hygiene in health care and their consensus recommendations. Infect Control Hosp Epidemiol 2009;30(7):611–22.
14. McLaws ML, Pantle AC, Fitzpatrick KR, et al. Improvements in hand hygiene across New South Wales public hospitals: clean hands save lives, part III. Med J Aust 2009;191(Suppl. 8):S18–24.
15. O'Leary MR, editor. Dictionary of Homeland Security and Defense. iUniverse; 2006. Online. Available from: en.wikipedia.org/wiki/Splash_suit#cite_note-0.

16. Naval Sea Systems Command. Protective clothing–hazmat gear online. Online. Available from: www.dcfpnavymil.org/Personnel%20Protection/HMUG/OPNAVINST_5100.28_(Previous_HMUG).pdf.
17. Australasian Fire and Emergency Service Authorities Council (AFAC). How we operate. Online. Available from: www.afac.com.au/insight/operations.
18. Advanced Life Support Group. MIMMS: the practical approach at the scene. Online. Available from: onlinelibrary.wiley.com/book/10.1002/9781444398236.
19. Greaves I, Hodgetts T, Porter K. Emergency care. A textbook for paramedics. London: WB Saunders; 1997.
20. Federal Emergency Management Agency. United States Fire Administration. EMS safety: techniques and applications. Scotts Valley CA: Createspace Independent Publishing Platform; 2013.
21. Ambulance Service of New South Wales 2003. Skills Manual Index Section 4, Patient Assessment.104.12 Scene management procedure.
22. Caroline N. Nancy Caroline's emergency care in the streets. 6th ed. Sudbury, MA: Jones and Bartlett; 2008.
23. National Highway Traffic Safety Administration. Emergency medical technician: basic refresher curriculum instructor course guide. US Department of Transport EMT–Basic National Standard Curriculum, 1994.
24. Dangerous goods. Online. Available from: en.wikipedia.org/wiki/Dangerous_goods#Classification_and_labeling_summary_tables.
25. National Chemical Emergency Centre. Dangerous goods emergency actions codes list 2017. Norwich: AEA Group; 2018. Online. Available from: the-ncec.com/en/resources/the-dangerous-goods-emergency-action-code-list-201.
26. Wong K, Levy RD. Interhospital transfers of patients with surgical emergencies: areas for improvement. Aust J Rural Health 2005;13(5):290–4.
27. Mikos K. Monitoring handoffs for standardization. Nurs Manage 2007;38(12):16–20.
28. Alem L, Joseph M, Kethers S, et al. Information environments for supporting consistent registrar medical handover. Health Inf Manag 2008;37(1):9–25.
29. Hodgetts TJ, Abraham K, Homer T, editors. Major incident medical management and support. The practical approach (Australian supplement). Sydney: SWSAHS Staff Development Unit; 1995.
30. Eaton CJ. Essentials of immediate medical care. 2nd ed. Edinburgh: Churchill Livingstone; 2006.
31. Calland V. Safety at scene: manual for paramedics and emergency care doctors. London: Elsevier Health Sciences; 2001.
32. Moore R. Vehicle rescue life cycle. In: Moore R, editor. Vehicle rescue and extrication. 2nd ed. St Louis: Mosby: JEMS; 2002.
33. Edgar C. SCAT (Special Casualty Access Training) reference text. NSW Ambulance Special Operations Unit Student Manual V2.0 2017.
34. Casey S. Challenges in converting training needs analysis (TNA) findings into a comprehensive language for defence purposes (LDP) course. In: de Silver Joyce H, Thomson EA, editors. Language in uniform: language analysis and training for defence and policing. Cambridge: Cambridge Scholars Publishing; 2015.
35. Australian Bureau of Statistics (ABS). Australian social trends 2007–work-related injuries. Online. Available from: www.abs.gov.au/ausstats/abs@.nsf/0/63ED457234C2F22DCA25732C002080A7?opendocument.
36. Health and Safety Commission, UK. Statistics of workplace fatalities and injuries–falls from a height. National statistics. Online. Available from: www.hse.gov.uk/statistics/pdf/fatalinjuries.pdf.
37. Australian Bureau of Statistics (ABS). 3303.0 Causes of death, Australia, 2011. Online. Available from: www.abs.gov.au/AUSSTATS/abs@.nsf/Lookup/3303.0Main+Features12007?OpenDocument.
38. Calland V. Safety at scene: safety at scene manual for pre-hospital emergency care providers and police officers. Rev. 1st ed. aLL2easyIT; 2008.
39. WorkSafe, Queensland Government. Workplace Hazards: Dangers in your workplace: confined spaces. 2023. Online. Available: from: www.worksafe.qld.gov.au/safety-and-prevention/hazards/workplace-hazards/dangers-in-your-workplace/confined-spaces. 2003.
40. Thomas SH, Harrison TH, Buras WR, et al. Helicopter transport and blunt trauma mortality: a multicentre trial. J Trauma 2002;52(1):136–45.
41. Frankema SP, Ringburg AN, Steyerberg EW, et al. Beneficial effect of helicopter emergency medical services on survival of severely injured patients. Br J Surg 2004;91(11):1520–6.
42. Diaz MA, Hendey GW, Bivins HG. When is the helicopter faster? A comparison of helicopter and ground ambulance transport times. J Trauma 2005;58(1):148–53.
43. Pozzi C. Exposure of prehospital providers to violence and abuse. J Emerg Nurs 1998;24(4):320–3.
44. Ambulance Service of NSW. Standard operating procedure SOP2007-075. ASNSW safety and security information for ambulance officers 28 Sept 2007.
45. Mental Health Act 2016. Queensland. Online. Available from: www.legislation.qld.gov.au/view/pdf/asmade/act-2016-005.
46. NSW Mental Health Act 2007 no. 8. Online. Available from: www.austlii.edu.au/au/legis/nsw/consol_act/mha2007128/.
47. Victorian Mental Health Act 1986. Online. Available from: www.legislation.vic.gov.au/repealed-revoked/acts/mental-health-act-1986/101.

CHAPTER 10

PHYSIOLOGY AND PATHOPHYSIOLOGY FOR EMERGENCY CARE

PETER MOULES

ESSENTIALS

- The early assessment and identification of abnormal physiology is central to the work of emergency clinicians. Early sets of vital signs can provide an indication of the existence of clinical deterioration and provide clinical cues to guide interventions.
- Physiological responses form the basis for signs and symptoms observed in emergency patients.
- The sympathetic nervous system is activated and the parasympathetic nervous system is slowed in most stressful situations.
- Shock is the process resulting from inadequate cellular perfusion.
- The 'diamond of death' (acidosis, hypothermia, hypocalcaemia and coagulopathy) is linked to death following blood loss.

INTRODUCTION

Physiology in emergency care forms the basis of the many signs and symptoms displayed in patients who use emergency health services. Many research articles and textbooks have been published on the physiological phenomena of the stress response, or 'general adaptation syndrome' (GAS), first introduced and popularised by Hans Selye.[1,2] Selye's research identified three very distinct phases within the GAS: alarm, resistance and exhaustion. These phases are triggered after the body's exposure to injury or illness, resulting in the disruption of homeostasis. This chapter examines the physiological principles that apply to patients seen in the pre-hospital and hospital emergency department (ED) setting.

HOMEOSTASIS

Homeostasis may be defined as the body's maintenance of a relatively constant internal environment in the face of an ever-changing external environment. The factors that are being kept relatively constant are called *regulated variables*. Examples include the concentration of virtually all blood chemicals, core temperature, partial pressure of carbon dioxide, vertical posture, withdrawal reflexes, blood pressure, blood glucose, energy usage, metabolic rate—even weight.

In general, these variables are regulated by negative feedback loops (Fig. 10.1). For any variable to be kept relatively constant there must be a feedback loop which corrects (or negates) any deviation of that variable from the set point. This is the healthy range for every variable.

In principle, every feedback loop must contain the following elements:

- Set point—the level at which the regulated variable should be maintained, as determined by a process that is connected to the control centre, i.e. the control centre has to have some knowledge of what the set point should be.
- Receptors—sensitive cells or tissues that measure or monitor the regulated variable; this together with the neural or hormonal signalling mechanism is the *afferent* component.
- Control centre—compares the regulated variable with the set point and initiates the 'error signal'.
- Error signal—a signal (electrical or chemical) initiated by the control centre in proportion to the difference between the regulated variable and the set point. The error signal brings about a response from the effector organ(s). This is the *efferent* component.
- Effector organ(s)—the organ(s) that respond to the error signal and shift the regulated variable up or down towards the set point.

FIGURE 10.1 A NEGATIVE FEEDBACK LOOP

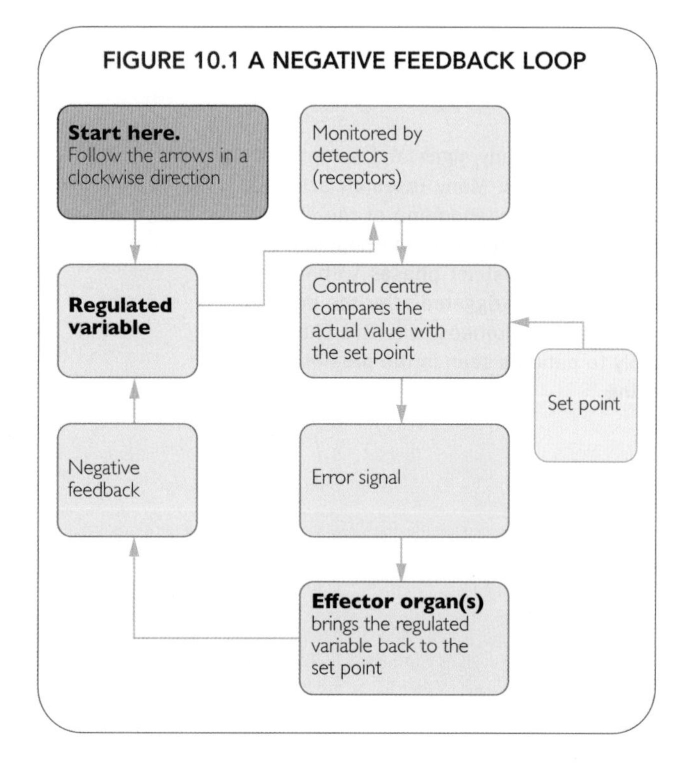

FIGURE 10.2 A REGULATED VARIABLE OSCILLATING AROUND ITS SET POINT

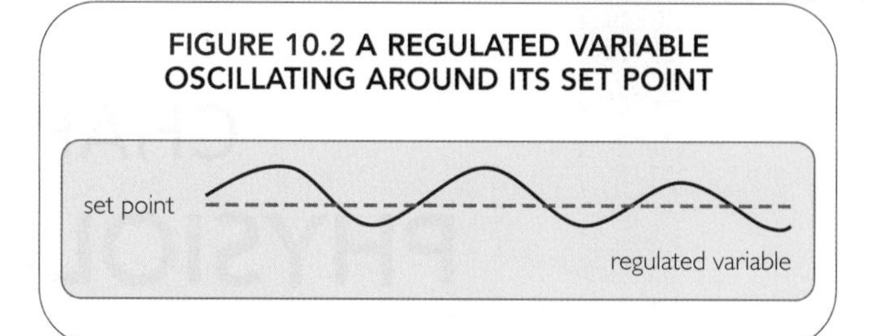

As a consequence, regulated variables are always oscillating around a set point, as shown in Fig. 10.2.

PRACTICE TIP

The principle of regulated variables oscillating around a set point explains why 'normal' vital signs are given as a range, rather than a value. For example, a normal temperature may be between 36°C and 37.2°C in most people.

If the regulated variable rises above the set point, this is monitored by receptors and the control centre compares this high value with the set point. The control centre sends an error signal to the effector organs to bring the regulated variable back towards the set point. The regulated variable then, generally, overshoots the set point; the lower value is detected by receptors and the control centre sends an error signal that causes the regulated variable to trend upwards, back to and over the set point, and so on.

A simple example is the control of core temperature when moving from a cool temperature to a slightly warmer one. The thermoreceptors in the hypothalamus constantly monitor the temperature of the blood. As it starts to warm, the control centre senses the difference between the temperature of the blood and the set point. The control centre then generates an error signal through the vascular portion of the sympathetic nervous system that controls the dilation and constriction of the small arterioles in the skin vascular beds. Dilation of these vessels allows the blood's heat to radiate into the environment. If too much heat is lost, constriction of the same vessels helps to conserve heat. At more extreme changes of temperature, other mechanisms such as perspiration, and shivering are recruited to assist cooling and warming.

If any part of a feedback loop is damaged or missing, a loss of homeostasis may result. Feedback loops can become pathological when, rather than taking the regulated variable back to the set point, it moves it *further* from the set point. Instead of *negating* the difference between the regulated variable and the set point, a pathological feedback loop will increase and amplify the difference. This is called *positive feedback* and is a central principle in the pathophysiology of emergency care.

An example will help to make the point. Consider a panic attack. A patient becomes aware of their own heart beating (normally this cannot be felt). The anxiety caused by these palpitations increases the release of adrenaline, which causes the heart to beat faster and with increased force, which causes more anxiety, more adrenaline release, and yet more rapid and forceful palpitations: even though the patient is not in danger, the 'fight or flight' feedback mechanism has entered a vicious cycle.

Examples of some relevant regulated variables, receptors, control centres, error signals, effector organs and outcomes are shown in Table 10.1.

TABLE 10.1 RECEPTOR PATHWAYS FOR HOMEOSTASIS

REGULATED VARIABLE	RECEPTOR	CONTROL CENTRE	SET POINT	ERROR SIGNAL	EFFECTOR ORGAN(S)	RESULT
Arterial partial pressure of carbon dioxide, $PaCO_2$	Central chemoreceptors—neurons in the medulla that are sensitive to CO_2 and hydrogen ions	Respiratory neurons in the pons and medulla	40 mmHg, determined by automatic neurons associated with the respiratory centres	Modulation of the medullary respiratory neurons that project down the spine	Intercostal and diaphragm muscles	Modulation of the rate and depth of respiration and maintenance of $PaCO_2$ at the set point
Plasma osmolarity	Hypothalamic osmoreceptors—neurons that shrink or swell depending on the particle content of the hypothalamic interstitial fluid. This changes their firing patterns depending on their degree of hydration	Paraventricular hypothalamic neurons whose axons project to the posterior pituitary	Approx. 300 Osm. Determined by automatic neurons associated with the hypothalamic control centre	Modulation of the secretion of ADH	Primarily the cells of the collecting ducts in the kidney	ADH binds to V-2 receptors in the kidney collecting-duct cell membranes, initiating an intracellular second messenger cAMP which promotes the manufacture and installation of aquaporins (water channels) in the apical and basolateral cell membranes. This increases their permeability to water and, providing the kidney medulla is of a higher osmolarity than the collecting ducts, water is reabsorbed, and a more concentrated urine is produced.
Core temperature	Hypothalamic temperature receptors which change their discharge patterns depending on the temperature of the perfusing blood	Hypothalamic neurons whose axons connect to the vascular component of the sympathetic nervous system	37°C, determined by automatic neurons associated with the hypothalamic control centre	Modulation of discharge down the sympathetic nerves which control flow in the cutaneous circulation	The arterioles in the dermis of the skin	An increase in core temperature results in cutaneous vasodilation; a decrease in core temperature results in cutaneous vasoconstriction
Sodium and potassium—short route	Low plasma sodium or high plasma potassium stimulate the glomerulosa cells of the adrenal gland	Glomerulosa cells of the adrenal gland	Na^+ approx. 140 mmol/L; K^+ approx 4–5 mmol/L. Determined by the glomerulosa cells of the adrenal gland	Aldosterone secretion	Tubular cells of the distal convoluted tubule of the kidney	Aldosterone binds to nuclear receptors and stimulates the transcription of more Na^+-K^+-ATPase pumps. These retrieve more Na^+ from the filtrate and allow K^+ loss
Sodium and potassium—*long route*	A drop in blood pressure or volume or a lowering of plasma sodium stimulates the cells of the JGA in the kidney	Cells of the JGA	Na^+ approx. 140 mmol/L; K^+ approx. 4–5 mmol/L. Determined by cells of the JGA	Renin secretion ⟶ angiotensin I formation ⟶ angiotensin II formation ⟶ stimulates aldosterone secretion from glomerulosa cells of adrenal gland	Tubular cells of the distal convoluted tubule of the kidney	Aldosterone binds to nuclear receptors and stimulates the transcription of more Na^+-K^+-ATPase pumps. These retrieve more Na^+ from the filtrate and allow K^+ loss

Continued

TABLE 10.1 RECEPTOR PATHWAYS FOR HOMEOSTASIS—cont'd

REGULATED VARIABLE	RECEPTOR	CONTROL CENTRE	SET POINT	ERROR SIGNAL	EFFECTOR ORGAN(S)	RESULT
Calcium (Ca^{2+})	Low calcium detected by cells of the parathyroid gland	Cells of the parathyroid gland	Approx 5 mEq. Determined by cells of the parathyroid gland	Secretion of parathyroid hormone	(i) Bone, releases some Ca^{2+} from bone (ii) Gut, enhances Ca^{2+} absorption from the gut (iii) Kidney tubule cells, enhance Ca^{2+} reabsorption from kidney filtrate	Raises plasma calcium levels
	High plasma calcium stimulates interstitial cells in the thyroid gland	Interstitial cells of the thyroid gland	Approx. 5 mm. Determined by interstitial cells of the thyroid	Secretion of calcitonin	Opposes reabsorption of Ca^{2+} from bone	Lowers plasma calcium levels
Hydrogen ions and bicarbonate ions	The respiratory system controls hydrogen ions and bicarbonate ions (see above). The tubule cells of the kidney are sensitive to hydrogen ions	Kidney tubule cells	pH approx 7.4; 40 nM. Bicarbonate approx. 24 mmol/L. Determined by the kidney tubule cells	Activation of proton pumps when plasma is too acidic, inhibition if the plasma is too alkaline	Protons are pumped from the plasma into the tubular fluid and bicarbonate is retrieved. In alkalosis this is inhibited so acid accumulates and bicarbonate is lost	Plasma pH and bicarbonate concentrations are maintained within homeostatic limits
Mean arterial pressure (MAP)	Stretch receptors called baroreceptors in the carotid bifurcation and the aortic arch	Medulla cardiac and vasomotor centres	Approx. 100 mmHg (13.25 kPa). Determined by neurons associated with the cardiac and vasomotor centres in the medulla	Activation of sympathetic nerves to heart and blood vessels	Increases heart rate, stroke volume and constriction of arterioles in response to a drop in MAP	MAP is kept within homeostatic limits

ADH: antidiuretic hormone; cAMP: cyclic adenosine monophosphate; JGA: juxtaglomerular apparatus; K^+: potassium ions; Na^+: sodium ions.

CELLULAR METABOLISM

The internal environment of cells is quite different from the tissue fluid that surrounds them. Forty per cent of the energy we extract from our diet is expended in maintaining the difference between the intracellular and extracellular environments.

Just about all cellular machinery use energy stored in the form of adenosine triphosphate (ATP). The whole process of carbohydrate metabolism is directed towards the extraction of energy from sugars and the manufacture of ATP, in which the extracted energy is temporarily stored, then used for virtually all cellular processes. Primary among these is the operation of the ion pumps that actively pump sodium ions out of cells and potassium ions into cells, both up a concentration gradient. Not only does this generate an ion imbalance across the cell membrane (low sodium inside, high sodium outside), but it also creates a negative electrical potential of nearly one-tenth of a volt between the inside and the outside of the cell. The rest of the energy is used in the manufacture of all the other molecular structures inside the cell. Many proteins are biological catalysts, or enzymes, which foster the conversion of ATP into adenosine diphosphate (ADP). The reconversion of ADP into ATP requires energy input. This is achieved by other enzymes that work in a series of steps to break down some form of metabolic fuel, such as simple carbohydrates (sugars), fatty acids, proteins or ketone bodies. Thus, ATP can be thought of as the 'universal energy currency' of the body.

There are generally two processes inside cells which harvest the energy contained in the chemical bonds of sugars. The first is the anaerobic process. Cells lacking mitochondria, or *sufficient oxygen* for normal metabolic processes, use *glycolysis*. This involves a series of reactions to convert glucose to pyruvate, with a net gain of 2 ATP molecules for every glucose molecule. Without sufficient oxygen, pyruvate is converted to lactic acid. If left untethered (as in shock or cardiac arrest), lactic acid increases and is detectable in large quantities in the blood as lactate. If this process only occurs for a short period, as in strenuous exercise, lactic acid is reconverted to pyruvate, and used by the liver to create glucose in *gluconeogenesis*.

PRACTICE TIP

In the pre-hospital or emergency setting, lactate is used as a measure of severity of illness. As lactate is produced in anaerobic metabolism, it can be viewed as a measure of failure to supply adequate oxygen to the cells—due to inadequate perfusion or hypoxaemia.

The second process is aerobic. Aerobic metabolism occurs in the cells' mitochondria. This process converts glucose to ATP with the use of oxygen. The end-result of this process is between 36 and 38 ATP molecules. The by-products of this are CO_2 and H_2O, which are generally harmless and easily eliminated from the body.[3]

OXYGEN/CARBON DIOXIDE

Oxygen/carbon dioxide homeostasis

As explained above, oxygen is crucial for aerobic cellular metabolism. When mitochondria produce ATP through the conversion of glucose and oxygen (aerobic metabolism) the by-products of water, heat and carbon dioxide are produced. Due to the crucial role of CO_2 in the maintenance of acid–base balance via carbonic anhydrase, the respiratory system controls $PaCO_2$ very tightly (Fig. 10.3 and Table 10.1).

FIGURE 10.3 THE RESPIRATORY SYSTEM'S HOMEOSTATIC CONTROL OF BLOOD CARBON DIOXIDE

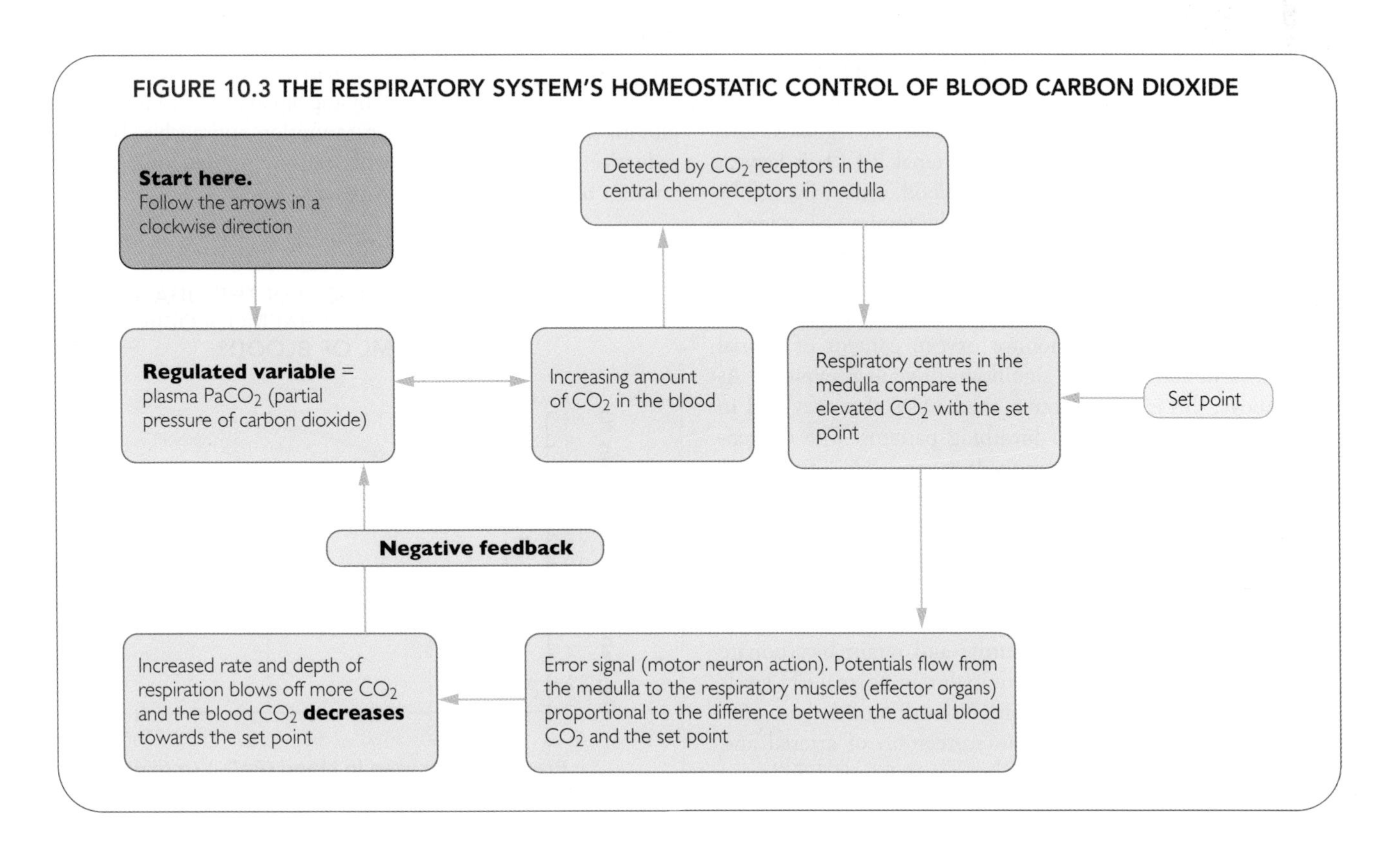

When the $PaCO_2$ gets above 40 mmHg (5.3 kPa), there is a reflex increase in the rate and depth of respiration, so more carbon dioxide diffuses from the blood into the alveoli and is 'blown off'. When the $PaCO_2$ drops below 40 mmHg (5.3 kPa), there is a reflex decrease in the rate and depth of respiration, so more carbon dioxide is retained. The respiratory muscles, the diaphragm and the intercostals, are the effector organs. They are driven by motor neurons in the spinal cord, which are in turn driven by descending motor neurons that originate in the medulla oblongata. In the medulla and pons are respiratory centres; they consist of pacemaker cells which determine the rate of respiration, and amplifier circuits which determine the depth of respiration. These respiratory centres are influenced by central chemoreceptors that are sensitive to $PaCO_2$ and hydrogen–ion concentration ($[H^+]$), and by peripheral chemoreceptors situated in the aortic arch and carotid bodies that are sensitive to arterial $PaCO_2$, $[H^+]$ and also PaO_2, but only if oxygen drops to dangerously low levels. This hypoxic sensitivity and the associated respiratory drive are, essentially, emergency devices. Hyperventilation (may be voluntary or caused by anxiety or fever) blows off carbon dioxide. $PaCO_2$ may be reduced to as low as 20 mmHg (2.6 kPa; normally 40 mmHg, 5.3 kPa), thus reducing the respiratory drive. Hyperventilation cannot, however, increase the amount of oxygen carried in arterial blood if all the haemoglobin is already fully saturated and has no further carrying capacity. Consider the effects of hyperventilation on the equation:

$$CO_2 \quad H_2O \leftrightarrow H_2CO_3 \leftrightarrow HCO_3 \quad H \qquad \text{(a)}$$

As carbon dioxide is 'blown off', the equation will be *pulled* from right to left reducing the concentration of HCO_3^- and H^+ (i.e. the pH will increase—respiratory alkalosis).

Consider the effects of breath-holding or hypoventilation on the same equation: carbon dioxide will accumulate and *push* the equation from left to right, thus *increasing* the concentration of HCO_3^- and H^+ (i.e. the pH will decrease—respiratory acidosis). Therefore, in the ordinary daily moment-to-moment control of the blood gases oxygen and carbon dioxide, the regulated variable is, largely, carbon dioxide. If the arterial $PaCO_2$ is kept at around 40 mmHg (5.3 kPa), then the blood, ordinarily, will be close to fully saturated with oxygen. If the respiratory system is compromised, for example, by brain injury, and respiration is reduced, the brain becomes relatively insensitive to the rising carbon dioxide levels and at a certain point the peripheral chemoreceptors, which alone monitor oxygen content of arterial blood, kick in and provide a significant drive to respiration. As noted above, this is an emergency mechanism that may lead to intermittent (Cheyne-Stokes) breathing patterns. The oxygen-sensitive peripheral chemoreceptors do not provide a significant amount of drive to the respiratory centres until the arterial blood is approaching the PaO_2 of venous blood (PaO_2 40–50 mmHg, 5.3–6.6 kPa), by which time cyanosis may well be evident.

In chronic respiratory acidosis (lasting more than an hour or so), the kidney tubule cells progressively increase their expulsion of hydrogen ions into the urine and retain bicarbonate ions in the plasma in an attempt to maintain normal pH levels in the blood. A more comprehensive discussion of the measurement of acid–base balance and interpretation of arterial and venous blood gases is provided in Chapter 16 Clinical skills and Chapter 21 Respiratory emergencies.

Oxygen transport

The atmosphere at sea level has a pressure of 760 mmHg. Twenty-one per cent of this is oxygen, which has a proportionate, or partial, pressure of $0.21 \times 760 = 160$ mmHg. If this atmosphere is in contact with a body of fluid, the partial pressure of that particular gas dissolved in the fluid will equilibrate. The partial pressure can be thought of as the 'driving force' that causes the gas to dissolve in the fluid. The amount of gas in the fluid depends on other factors as well, in particular, the solubility.

Unlike carbon dioxide, oxygen is not very soluble in water or plasma. At 37°C, only 1.5% of the oxygen carried by 100 mL of blood is dissolved in plasma. The only reason that blood can carry a significant amount of oxygen is the presence of approximately 15 g of haemoglobin per 100 mL of blood. The haemoglobin is contained in the red blood cells. Haemoglobin is a globular protein with four subunits, each of which has a central iron atom capable of binding reversibly with one oxygen molecule, with an S-shaped affinity curve (Fig. 10.4).

Under experimental conditions it is possible to vary the partial pressure of oxygen in blood, and measure the resulting amount of bound *oxyhaemoglobin* as a percentage of total haemoglobin. This is termed the oxygen *saturation*. A gradient exists between alveolar air, across the alveolar wall, into the blood. At sea level, breathing room air, the typical partial pressure of oxygen in the arterial blood (PaO_2) in a healthy person is about 100 mmHg (Fig. 10.5).

The oxygen–haemoglobin dissociation curve turns out to be S-shaped rather than linear. The shape of this curve (with a flat top) is primarily due to the fact that when all the haemoglobin molecules are carrying four oxygen molecules, no more oxygen can be carried by blood, except if dissolved in the plasma. This dissolved amount is very small (0.3 mL O_2/100 mL plasma at 100 mmHg PaO_2). Each gram of haemoglobin can combine with a maximum of about 1.34 mL of oxygen, so an individual with 15 g of haemoglobin per 100 mL of blood can carry about 20 mL of oxygen per 100 mL of blood.[4] It can be seen that the vast majority of oxygen carried by the blood is bound to haemoglobin, thus even if the oxygen saturation approaches 100% a reduction in haemoglobin will lead to a reduction in the amount of oxygen delivered to tissues.

FIGURE 10.4 EFFECT OF PaO_2 ON THE QUANTITY OF OXYGEN BOUND WITH HAEMOGLOBIN IN EACH 100 ML OF BLOOD[4]

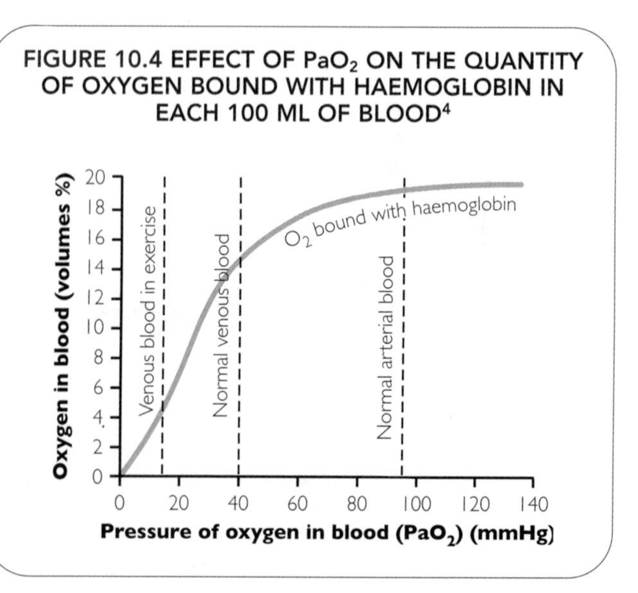

FIGURE 10.5 EXCHANGE OF GASES AT THE ALVEOLUS AND THE BODY TISSUES WITH BLOOD AND TRANSPORT OF OXYGEN AND CARBON DIOXIDE[5]

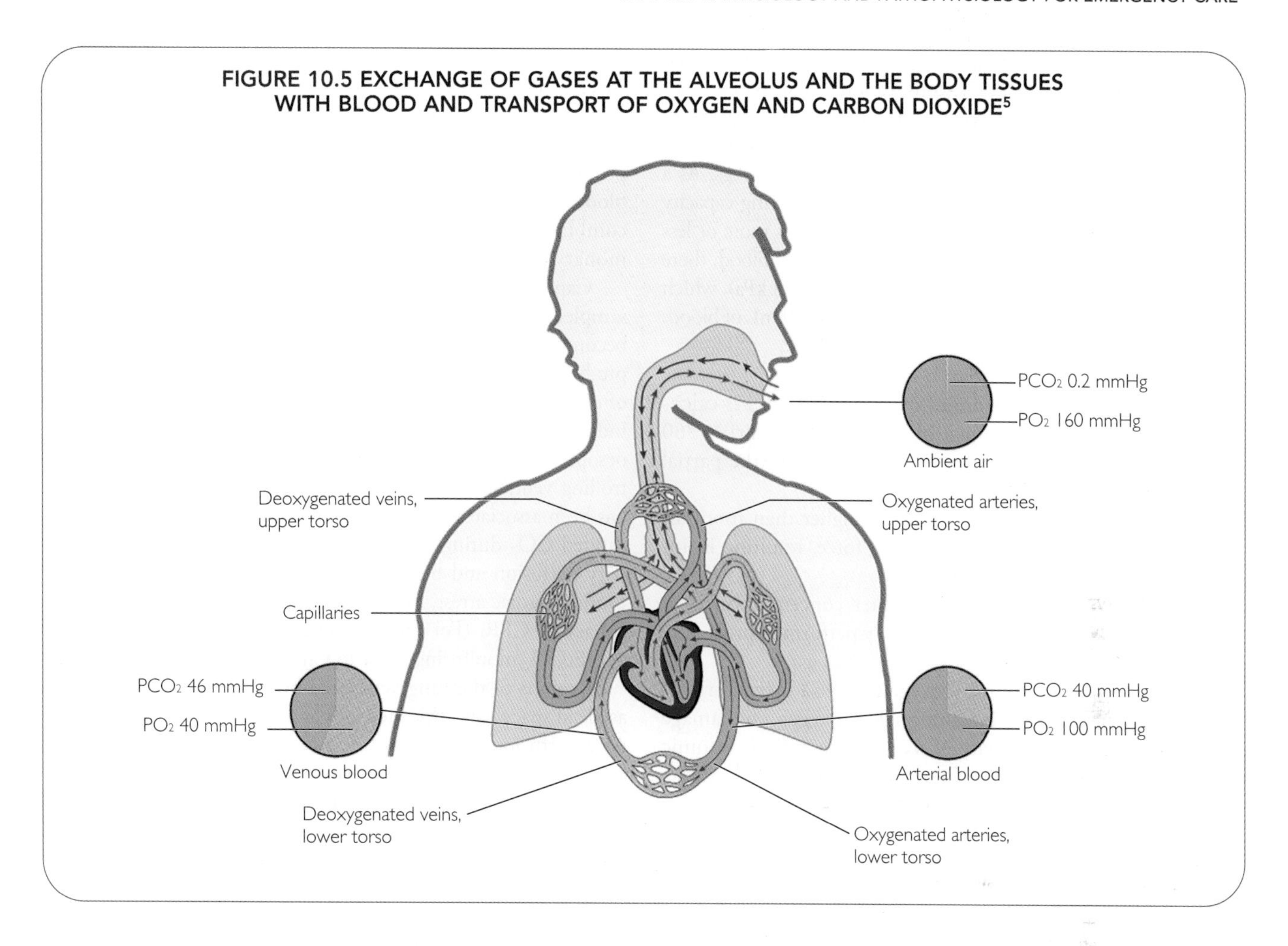

Symptoms of cardiac ischaemia may result from severe anaemia. No amount of supplemental oxygen will compensate for the reduced oxygen carriage in such a patient. As foreshadowed above, another trick that haemoglobin has up its molecular sleeve is that its affinity for oxygen changes depending on the environment in which it is operating. Most of the time it flows from the lungs saturated with oxygen and is then pumped through working vascular beds, the tissue of which has relatively low metabolic rates. On average, each haemoglobin molecule delivers only one oxygen molecule to the tissue and goes back to the heart and lungs still three-quarters saturated.

But in hardworking tissue like exercising muscle, the tissue is hot and acidic. This environment twists the haemoglobin molecule a touch and reduces the affinity between oxygen and haemoglobin, so that more than one oxygen molecule is liberated from each haemoglobin molecule (Fig. 10.6). In extremely hot acidic working muscle, all the oxygen is stripped off the haemoglobin. In this way, the oxygen supply to tissue can be increased four-fold without an increase in blood supply.

FIGURE 10.6 SHIFT OF THE OXYHAEMOGLOBIN DISSOCIATION CURVE TO THE RIGHT CAUSED BY AN INCREASE IN HYDROGEN-ION CONCENTRATION (DECREASE IN PH)[4]

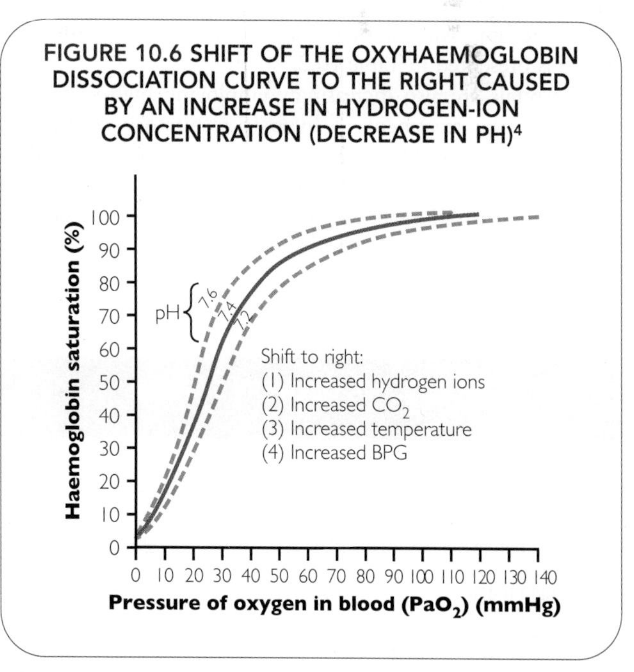

BPG: 2,3-bisphosphoglycerate.

Carbon dioxide transport

Carbon dioxide does not bind to haemoglobin at the same sites as oxygen. It is carried as carbamino (N–COO$^-$) compounds on all the blood protein molecules, including haemoglobin, but this only accounts for 18% of carbon dioxide carriage. Five per cent of carbon dioxide is carried dissolved in the plasma. Approximately 77% of carbon dioxide is carried as bicarbonate ions that result from the chemical reaction between carbon dioxide and water. Carbon dioxide easily diffuses into red cells and is hydrated by the enzyme carbonic anhydrase, producing carbonic acid which ionises into bicarbonate ions and hydrogen ions:

$$CO_2 \quad H_2O \leftrightarrow H_2CO_3 \leftrightarrow HCO_3 \quad H \qquad \text{(a)}$$

The bicarbonate ions produced in this way diffuse out of the red cells and are replaced by chloride ions. In lung capillaries, the opposite of this happens: bicarbonate ions are converted back into carbon dioxide and carbon dioxide flows down a concentration gradient out of the blood and into the alveoli of the lungs. As a result of this increased solubility and chemical buffering capacity in plasma and red blood cells, the carriage of CO_2 is more or less linearly proportional to its partial pressure. In arterial blood, there is a partial pressure ($PaCO_2$) of about 40 mmHg (5.3 kPa), which represents around 400 mL of carbon dioxide per 100 mL of blood.

Oxygen therapy

Remember the partial pressure of oxygen at sea level is calculated as follows, 0.21 (percentage of oxygen in room air) × 760 (atmospheric pressure at sea level) = 160 mmHg (the partial pressure of oxygen at sea level).

Delivering oxygen at concentrations higher than room air increases the partial pressure, or driving force, resulting in increased oxygen dissolved in fluid.

The provision of oxygen at a greater concentration than room air (i.e. above 21%) is a commonly performed procedure in emergency situations.

Very high concentrations of oxygen are also toxic. Particularly in premature infants, breathing 100% oxygen can damage lung tissue due to the activity of oxygen-free radicals (atomic oxygen) that occur in the gas. The unpaired electrons of atomic oxygen damage structural and functional proteins in the lung. However, in the first 24 hours it is important to titrate oxygen delivery according to oxygen saturation measurements, but oxygen should not be withheld for fear of toxicity in adults.[6]

The most common delivery devices used in emergency environments are nasal cannula, masks or masks with reservoir bags. The approximate percentage oxygen delivery for each device is presented in Table 10.2.[6]

Hospitals are also increasingly employing high-flow nasal prongs in the treatment of hypoxic respiratory conditions. These devices provide warmth and humidification to the flow supplied. They can supply between 1 and 60 L of flow, with oxygen concentrations between 0.21 and 1. These devices can provide PEEP of up to 7.4 cmH_2O.[7]

TABLE 10.2 O_2 DELIVERY SYSTEMS[6]

APPARATUS	OXYGEN FLOW (L/MIN)	OXYGEN CONCENTRATION (%)
Nasal catheters	1-4	24-40
Semi-rigid mask	6-15	35-60
Semi-rigid mask with double O_2 supply	15-30	Up to 80
Semi-rigid mask with reservoir bag	12-15	60-90
High-flow nasal catheter	1-70	21-100

Capnography

Arterial $PaCO_2$ can be estimated by infrared assay of end-expiratory air samples. This air, essentially alveolar air, in normal haemodynamic and pulmonary states has a PCO_2 approximately 1–5 mmHg (0.14–0.68 kPa) below that of arterial blood. End-expiratory, or end-tidal, CO_2 ($EtCO_2$) reflects a combination of the arterial CO_2 level and the amount of pulmonary perfusion.

Capnography is the real-time graphical representation of sampled CO_2 in air inspired and expired by the patient. It has become a standard monitoring tool for intubated patients in the pre-hospital setting and ED for several reasons. First, the presence of expired CO_2 confirmed by the monitor waveform (Fig. 10.7) indicates that the endotracheal tube is in the trachea and not the oesophagus.[8] Second, in brain-injured patients, for example, controlling ventilation to maintain arterial PCO_2 in normal ranges has been associated with improved outcomes. Lastly, the level of expired CO_2 during steady ventilation is a reflection of pulmonary perfusion and hence a useful indicator of cardiac output.[9] During cardiac arrest, for example, the $EtCO_2$ can reflect the adequacy of CPR. (For more information regarding capnography and $EtCO_2$ monitoring, refer to Chapter 14.)

Regions of the lung ventilated but not perfused are known as 'dead space', and this increases as a result of decreased pulmonary perfusion. These areas do not contribute to gas exchange between the blood and the atmosphere and thus decrease the efficiency of the lung as a functional unit. An increase in dead space results in an increased gradient between arterial CO_2 and end-expiratory CO_2 (increased $PaCO_2$ in relation to $EtCO_2$). As the gradient between $EtCO_2$ and $PaCO_2$ may be significant in ill or injured patients, it is good practice to obtain a measure of arterial PCO_2 and correlate this with the $EtCO_2$. Some examples of the clinical scenarios that affect $PaCO_2$:$EtCO_2$ gradient include: decreased pulmonary blood flow (low cardiac output states); pulmonary embolism; cardiac arrest; PEEP; hypovolaemia; and lateral decubitus positioning.[9]

PRACTICE TIP

Capnography is used in EDs in a variety of scenarios, including sedation monitoring (especially in procedural sedation), ventilation monitoring and endotracheal tube confirmation, assessing adequacy of CPR, diagnosis through waveform interpretation (such as bronchospasm), and detection of respiratory dead space.

HOMEOSTATIC TEMPERATURE CONTROL

In normal health, core body temperature is a regulated variable. The normal body temperature (recorded via a tympanic thermometer) is in the range of 35.4–37.8°C, and has a slight diurnal variation.[10] The detectors and control centre are temperature-sensitive receptors in the skin, and specialised neurons in the hypothalamus. In other species, and in human infants, metabolically active 'brown' adipose tissue plays a role in temperature homeostasis. In adults, the principal effector organs are the blood vessels and sweat glands in the skin. In temperate climates, the skin serves as an adjustable radiator for heat loss and heat retention and, depending on the requirement to either eliminate or retain heat, blood is redistributed either to or from the peripheral

FIGURE 10.7 NORMAL FINDINGS ON A CAPNOGRAM[9]

A⟶B indicates the baseline;
B⟶C, expiratory upstroke;
C⟶D, alveolar plateau;
D, partial pressure of end-tidal carbon dioxide;
D⟶E, expiratory downstroke.

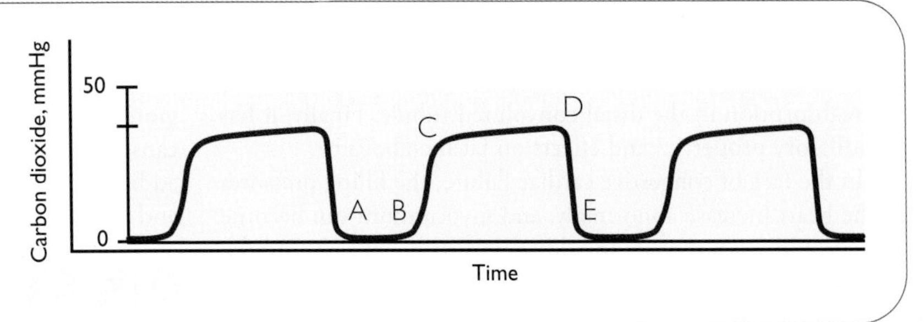

skin circulation. A change in temperature below the 'set point' of the body's thermostat is detected by skin and hypothalamic receptors, and results in vasoconstriction of the skin arterioles, reducing the rate of heat loss. Conversely, if the body core starts to heat up, vasodilation results, increasing skin blood flow and dissipating excess heat into the environment. In low-melanin persons this can be seen as a change in skin colour—pale in cold and pink in warm environments.

In response to more extreme changes in temperature, other mechanisms are used to warm or cool the body. As ambient temperature approaches body temperature, radiant heat loss becomes less effective and is augmented by sweating and evaporative cooling. The sweat glands are also under the control of the sympathetic nervous system. When water evaporates it has to draw heat from the skin to change it from a liquid to a gas. This can provide a cooling effect, even if the ambient temperature is above body temperature. However, the effectiveness is reduced in the presence of humid heat, and excessive sweating also reduces plasma volume, serum sodium and potassium and urinary output (see Chapter 28 on environmental emergencies). Individuals acclimatise to heat over several days to weeks, with an increase in sweat production and a reduction in sweat sodium losses.

When the body is exposed to extreme cold, the drop in core temperature detected in the hypothalamus results in shivering—involuntary contractions of skeletal muscles that produce some waste heat. At the same time, the contraction of the arrector pili muscles at the base of each hair follicle (goose-bumps) is an ancient reflex harking back to our evolutionary heritage when humans were a lot hairier. The generalised erection of body hair improves the skin's insulating properties.

FLUID AND ELECTROLYTE BALANCE IN HOMEOSTASIS

The amount of fluid, water and the concentration of electrolytes are all under the control of homeostatic mechanisms. Ultimately the kidney is the main effector organ. Life processes depend on water and electrolytes being kept within strict limits.

Water

An increase in osmotic pressure (i.e. particle concentration in the blood) is caused, for example, by a loss of water when sweating is detected by osmoreceptors in the hypothalamus. Essentially, the osmoreceptors are neurons that swell or shrink depending on the solute concentration of the perfusing fluid and change their electrical discharge rates as a result. The information is processed by the nearby control centre, also in the hypothalamus. The nerves that emerge from the control centre descend to the posterior pituitary and secrete the peptide antidiuretic hormone (ADH), also known as vasopressin. ADH is secreted into the bloodstream and ultimately binds to V-2 receptors, mainly on the collecting ducts deep in the medulla of the kidney. The ADH-receptor complex initiates the manufacture of the second messenger cyclic adenosine monophosphate (cAMP) in the cytoplasm of cells, which in turn brings about the incorporation of aquaporins—water pores—in the apical and basolateral membranes of the collecting duct tubules. This increases the permeability of the membranes, allowing water to be drawn back into the relatively hyperosmotic (dry) kidney medulla and subsequently back into systemic circulation. A concentrated urine is produced; it has up to four times the osmotic concentration of blood. The hypothalamus also governs the subjective feeling of thirst, leading to increased oral water intake.

Excess water has the opposite effect: in the presence of hypo-osmolar plasma ADH secretion is inhibited, and excess water is allowed to pass through the collecting ducts producing a dilute urine (see Table 10.1).

The osmoreceptors in the hypothalamus are not the only receptors involved in the ADH reflex. Baroreceptors in the aortic arch and at the bifurcation of the carotid arteries detect pressure. If the pressure is lowered due to blood loss or dehydration, the reduced pressure also results in increased ADH release from the posterior pituitary and retention of water. This accounts for about 10–15% of the response.

Importantly, both ADH and the baroreceptor reflex cause vasoconstriction of both the resistance vessels (arterioles) and the capacitance vessels (venules). Sensibly, when faced with loss of blood volume the vasculature contracts, both keeping the pressure up on the arterial side and reducing the capacitance on the venous side. This accommodates the reduced circulating volume and preserves venous return of blood to the heart.

As noted earlier, the constriction of the arterioles generally reduces the capillary blood hydrostatic pressure, and so tissue fluid is drawn into the circulation in capillaries where the osmotic pressure of the blood exceeds the capillary hydrostatic pressure. This bolsters blood volume.

The antidiuretic effect of ADH and the baroreceptors is opposed to some extent by atrial natriuretic peptide (ANP). ANP is secreted by the atria of the heart in response to stretch, and therefore helps regulate intravascular volume. The secretion of ANP is inhibited when blood volumes are reduced and venous return to the heart reduced. When venous return increases, ANP secretion follows suit. ANP antagonises the effects of ADH by inhibiting its release, both from the posterior pituitary and at its site of action in the collecting duct of the kidney. ANP, as the term 'natriuretic' suggests (from the Latin word for sodium, 'natrium'), also antagonises the effects of aldosterone and reduces renin production (see next section) and promotes the loss of sodium, and hence water, from the kidney by reducing reabsorption in the distal convoluted tubule. Finally, it has vasodilatory properties and effects on fat metabolism.

In the face of congestive cardiac failure, the filling pressures of the heart increase abnormally, and myocardium can become hypertrophic in response. In addition to its beneficial modulation of blood volume in this situation, ANP is thought to have a protective effect on cardiac muscle by directly limiting this 'remodelling'.

Electrolytes

Sodium and potassium

The levels of sodium and potassium in the blood are ultimately controlled by action of the steroid hormone aldosterone, mainly on the distal convoluted tubules of the kidney. Essentially, aldosterone binds to nuclear receptors in the nuclei of tubular cells and promotes the transcription of genes for specific proteins that increase the number of sodium channels in the cell membranes and also increase the number of sodium-potassium-ATPase pumps in the basolateral membrane that pump sodium back into the kidney capillaries and allow potassium to be lost in the urine. The relative abundance of aldosterone will determine how much sodium is being retained and potassium is lost, and vice versa.

There are two feedback loops that control the secretion of aldosterone from the adrenal cortex. First, the cells of the adrenal cortex itself sense reductions in plasma sodium levels and secrete aldosterone as a response. Second, some sensitive tissue (the juxtaglomerular apparatus, JGA), lodged between the glomeruli and the distal convoluted tubules of the kidney, senses the loss of sodium, and releases the enzyme renin as a result. Renin, when released into the plasma, converts angiotensinogen into angiotensin I; this is converted in turn by angiotensin-converting enzyme (ACE) into angiotensin II, which causes the release of aldosterone from the adrenal cortex. In addition, angiotensin II causes vasoconstriction of arterioles and venules (Fig. 10.8).

PRACTICE TIP

The Renin-Angiotensin-Aldosterone (RAA) system plays an important role in regulating blood volume and systemic vascular resistance, thus affecting cardiac output and arterial pressure.

In this way, the kidneys play an important role in maintaining homeostatic blood pressure.

Calcium

Ninety-nine per cent of the body's calcium is in the form of calcium phosphate in bone. Calcium in plasma exists in an ionised, or free, form and an electrically neutral form bound to albumin and other plasma proteins. Only the ionised form is biologically active, and is important for many cellular functions, including nerve transmission, blood coagulation and muscle contraction. A reduction in plasma albumin or acidosis tends to favour an increase in the ionised, active form. Conversely, alkalosis tends to decrease ionised calcium. A clinical example is respiratory alkalosis caused by hyperventilation. The profound reduction in ionised calcium causes paraesthesia and tetany of skeletal muscles, which is reversible once normal ventilation is restored.

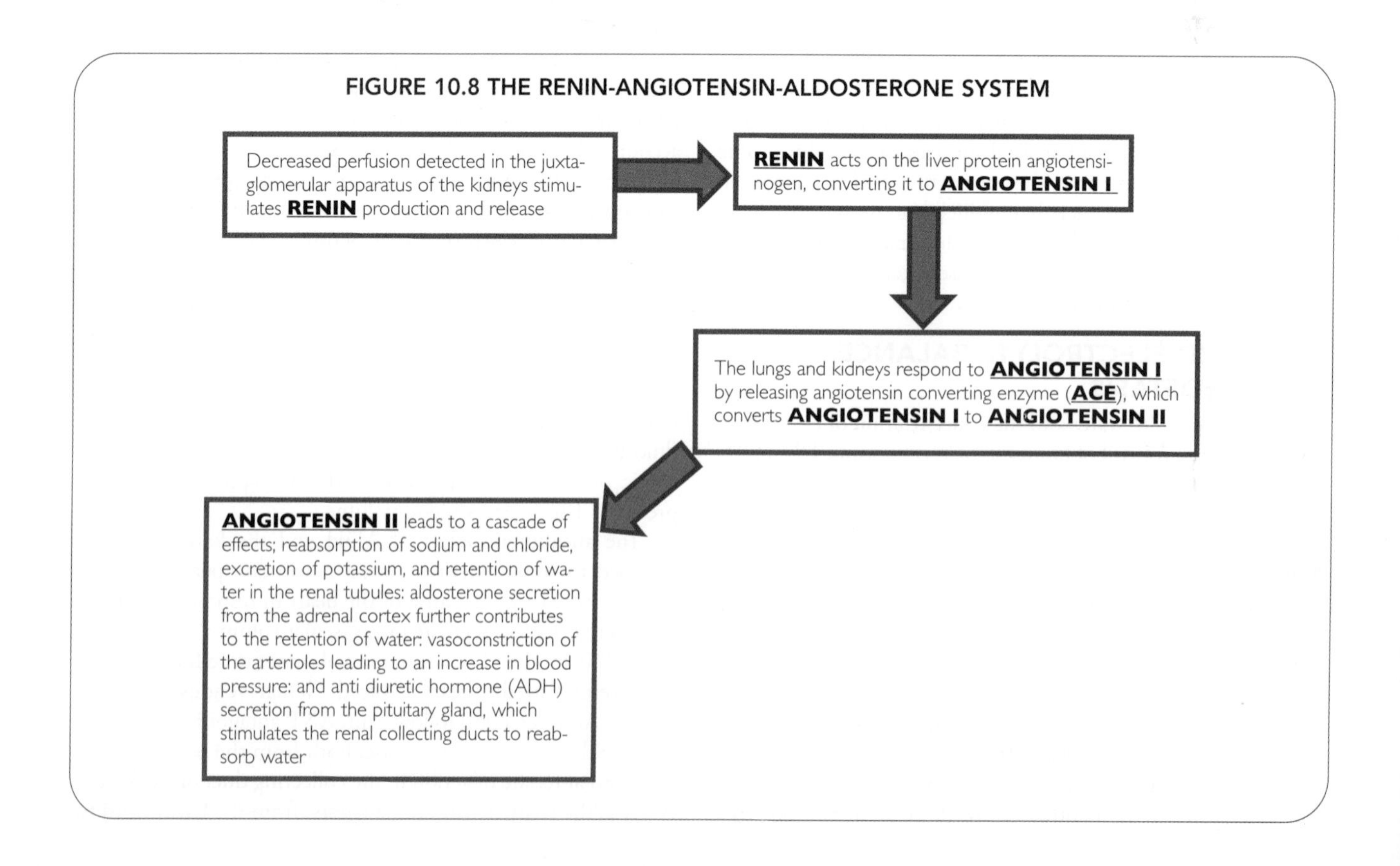
FIGURE 10.8 THE RENIN-ANGIOTENSIN-ALDOSTERONE SYSTEM
Decreased perfusion detected in the juxtaglomerular apparatus of the kidneys stimulates RENIN production and release
RENIN acts on the liver protein angiotensinogen, converting it to ANGIOTENSIN I
The lungs and kidneys respond to ANGIOTENSIN I by releasing angiotensin converting enzyme (ACE), which converts ANGIOTENSIN I to ANGIOTENSIN II
ANGIOTENSIN II leads to a cascade of effects; reabsorption of sodium and chloride, excretion of potassium, and retention of water in the renal tubules: aldosterone secretion from the adrenal cortex further contributes to the retention of water: vasoconstriction of the arterioles leading to an increase in blood pressure: and anti diuretic hormone (ADH) secretion from the pituitary gland, which stimulates the renal collecting ducts to reabsorb water

The total concentration of calcium in plasma is controlled by two hormones—parathyroid hormone (PTH) and calcitonin—secreted, respectively, by the parathyroid gland and the interstitial cells of the thyroid gland. When plasma calcium starts to drop, this is detected by the cells of the parathyroid gland and increased amounts of PTH are released. PTH has three actions:

1. It stimulates the synthesis of calcitriol, which increases the number of calcium pumps in the gut epithelium, thereby increasing the absorption of calcium from the gut.
2. It binds to PTH receptors in the kidney tubules and via a second messenger increases the number of calcium pumps in the tubules, thereby increasing the reabsorption of calcium from the kidney tubules back into the blood.
3. It recruits calcium from bone by stimulating the recruitment of osteoclasts.

As the plasma calcium concentration rises, the release of PTH is progressively inhibited and the release of calcitonin is progressively stimulated.

Calcitonin opposes the effects of PTH. There is some evidence that, paradoxically, pulsatile release of PTH and some PTH fragments have the effect of increasing calcium deposition in bone rather than decreasing it.[11]

Magnesium

The control of plasma magnesium concentration is primarily under the control of the tubular cells of the proximal convoluted tubules of the kidney and the loops of Henle. These tubes convey the glomerular filtrate through the kidney, and the cells of these tubes are sensitive to plasma and tubular levels of magnesium and reabsorb magnesium as required. This may vary from almost total reabsorption during time on a low-magnesium diet to low reabsorption on a high-magnesium diet.

HOMEOSTATIC ACID–BASE REGULATION

All biological enzyme systems are dependent on a very tight control of acid–base balance for optimal function. pH is a mathematical expression of the degree of acidosis or alkalosis in a solution:

$$\mathrm{pH} \quad \log_{10}[\mathrm{H}] \qquad \text{(b)}$$

Hence for each decrease in pH by 1, there is an increase in hydrogen ion concentration by a factor of 10. The physiological range of plasma pH is 7.35 to 7.45. Two interrelated systems, the respiratory system and the renal system, are responsible for maintaining this critical acid–base balance, by contributing hydrogen ions or bicarbonate ions to the various *buffers* present in body fluid. A buffer is a system of molecules that exists in equilibrium in a solution, and which, by gaining or losing a bicarbonate or a hydrogen ion in response to an alkali or acid load, tends to resist changes in pH. An important example was outlined above in the case of carbon dioxide and bicarbonate, catalysed by carbonic anhydrase. By increasing or decreasing ventilation, the respiratory system has the capacity to blow off or retain carbon dioxide and hence can control pH over a course of minutes to hours.

The kidney, by altering the acidity of urine, has an even more profound influence on body pH maintenance, albeit exerted over a longer time-frame of hours to days. The renal tubule has several mechanisms to control H^+ excretion and HCO_3^- reabsorption, in response to pH, sodium and potassium concentration and hormonal influences. Essentially, carbon dioxide is distributed evenly through the kidney, but inside tubular cells the enzyme carbonic anhydrase catalyses a chemical reaction between carbon dioxide and water. This results in the production of bicarbonate ions and hydrogen ions (as in Equation a). The hydrogen ions are pumped by an ATP-powered proton pump into the tubular fluid where they are mostly buffered by phosphate and ammonium ions. The bicarbonate is retrieved into the peritubular capillaries and then into the systemic circulation. The buffered and unbuffered hydrogen ions are voided in the urine.

NERVOUS SYSTEM FUNCTIONS—FRIGHT, FIGHT AND FLIGHT, OR REST AND DIGEST

The nervous system has structural and functional components. Structurally, the central nervous system (CNS) comprises the brain and spinal cord and the peripheral nervous system is comprised of afferent (signalling *towards* the brain, or sensory) and efferent (signalling *from* the brain, or motor) nerves. The 31 spinal nerves serve as both afferent and efferent pathways, or mixed nerves. Functionally, the peripheral nervous system is comprised of the enteric, somatic and autonomic nervous systems. The enteric nervous system controls the gastrointestinal tract, independently, or in coordination with the autonomic nervous system (parasympathetic and sympathetic branches). The somatic nervous system is associated with skeletal muscle and movement. The autonomic nervous system is comprised of the sympathetic and parasympathetic nervous systems.

SYMPATHETIC NERVOUS SYSTEM

Physiologically, emergencies are generally accompanied by the activation of the sympathetic nervous system (SNS). The resulting secretions of noradrenaline from sympathetic nerve endings, adrenaline from the adrenal medulla and cortisol from the adrenal cortex have a profound effect on the functioning of all organ systems. In evolutionary terms, the sympathetic nervous system prepares the body for physical activity—to fight or to run.

The sympathetic nerves flow out of the spinal cord between the first thoracic and second lumbar vertebrae, synapse in the paravertebral ganglia and extend postsynaptic fibres back up to the head and down to the organs of the thorax and abdomen, the arms and the legs. The sympathetic nervous system is also directly wired to the adrenal medulla, which, when stimulated, secretes adrenaline and some noradrenaline directly into the bloodstream. These bind to receptors on cell membranes in addition to the noradrenaline that is secreted by the sympathetic nervous system.

In most physiologically stressful situations, the sympathetic nervous system is activated, and the parasympathetic nervous system slows. The majority of noradrenaline in a stress response is secreted from the sympathetic nerve endings. The adrenal medulla secretes adrenaline:noradrenaline in approximately 4:1 ratio. The noradrenaline and adrenaline then flood into the bloodstream to bind to any available receptors. The effect at a cellular level differs according to the subtype of adrenergic receptor activated by these hormones in various end organs. In the cardiovascular system, alpha-adrenergic receptors respond by causing a constriction of the arterioles of non-essential vascular beds—as in the gut, skin, kidneys and liver—while beta-adrenergic receptors respond by relaxing muscle arterioles and increasing the heart rate and contractile force of myocardium. The background vascular tone of muscle arterioles is simultaneously reduced by centres in the medulla oblongata. The resultant effect is to raise blood pressure, increase cardiac output and divert blood away from the temporarily non-essential organs to skeletal muscle.

In the liver, muscle and adipose tissue, adrenergic receptor stimulation leads to an increase in available levels of glucose and free fatty acids, as an immediate source of energy. In the lungs, beta-2 receptors lead to dilation of bronchial smooth muscle.

In extreme situations, excess adrenaline and noradrenaline can cause evacuation of the contents of the upper and lower digestive tract while the activity of the rest of the intestines is dramatically slowed, as blood is diverted from non-essential vascular beds to working muscle. The circulating adrenaline and noradrenaline also bring about increased alertness, anxiety and, at high levels, cognitive impairment, and sometimes nausea associated with slowing gastric motility.

Sympathetic activation also increases the secretion of adrenocorticotrophic hormone (ACTH) from the anterior pituitary gland, which increases the secretion of steroids from the adrenal cortex. This has the effect of inhibiting inflammation, retaining water and sodium, and breaking down proteins and fats for their energy content.

PARASYMPATHETIC NERVOUS SYSTEM

The sympathetic nervous system is countered by the aptly named parasympathetic nervous system. Nearly every organ system has a dual supply of sympathetic and parasympathetic nerves which have largely opposite effects on the organs in question. A major exception is the vast majority of blood vessels which have, primarily, only sympathetic innervation.

The outflow of parasympathetic nerves from the central nervous system is mainly contained in the cranial nerves which service the head and most of the thorax and abdomen (via the vagus nerve). There is a small outflow in the sacral nerves at the base of the spine which service the bladder, genitals and the distal end of the digestive tract.

The sympathetic nerve endings generally secrete noradrenaline onto their target cells, while the parasympathetic nerve endings secrete acetylcholine.

The target organs have specific adrenergic and cholinergic receptors in their cell membranes to which the noradrenaline and acetylcholine specifically bind. This brings about changes in the target cells' activity by activating 'second messengers' in the cells and/or by opening ion channels in the cell membranes. An example of this is the heart. It has both a sympathetic and a parasympathetic nerve supply. Both the sympathetic and the parasympathetic nerves are continuously secreting small amounts of noradrenaline and acetylcholine onto heart muscle. In cardiac pacemaker cells—for example, the sinoatrial node—an electrical potential difference is maintained across the cell membrane. This is due to the opposing effects of potassium and sodium ion concentrations in the intracellular compared with the extracellular fluid. A membrane protein 'pump' maintains the potential difference, termed polarisation. The resting electrical potential of the inside of the cell membrane compared to the outside is about –70 mV, comparable to other excitable cells. Highly regulated protein 'channels' allow specific ions to flow back down their concentration and/or electrical gradients leading to depolarisation. If a cell depolarises enough and reaches 'threshold', an 'action potential' is propagated by the pacemaker and conducting cells and that initiates contraction of the myocardium. The *rate* of discharge is affected by both the degree of baseline electrical polarisation across the cell membrane and the amount of channel leakage leading the cell to reach its threshold for action potential propagation. The sympathetic nerves thus increase the heart rate by speeding up the depolarisation of the pacemaker cells slightly (a few extra sodium channels are opened) and the parasympathetic nerves slow it down by hyperpolarising the cells slightly (a few extra potassium channels are opened). The resulting heart rate is essentially a net result of opposing sympathetic and parasympathetic activity.

PRACTICE TIP

Atropine is an anticholinergic (muscarinic acetylcholine receptor antagonist). Acetylcholine is the main parasympathetic neurotransmitter. Atropine, therefore, blocks the cardiac actions of the parasympathetic nervous system in the short term, and thus leads to a rise in heart rate.

The gastrointestinal tract also has a dual innervation, but in this instance the parasympathetic nervous system increases peristaltic activity and other aspects of digestion in the gut from the stomach to the colon while noradrenaline secreted by the sympathetic nervous system slows it down. Although the transmitters bind to very similar receptors on the gut cell membranes as on cardiac cells, they are linked to different second messengers and ion channels, and consequently mediate different cellular responses.

The sympathetic nerve terminals may also directly inhibit the output of parasympathetic nerve terminals, through presynaptic inhibition. Put simply, the parasympathetic nervous system plays the major role in our vegetative being—digesting food, for example—while the sympathetic nervous system mediates 'fight or flight'.

For a summary of the anatomical structures and function of the autonomic nervous system, see Table 10.3.

CAPILLARIES AND NUTRITIVE BLOOD FLOW

During activation of the sympathetic nervous system, the blood flow to non-essential organs is dramatically reduced. Normally organs are adequately supplied with oxygen, glucose, amino acids and fats and produce by-products of cellular metabolism, such as carbon dioxide, lactate and other acids. Tissue perfusion through these capillary beds is tightly regulated at both a central and a local level. The sympathetic nervous system generally ensures an adequate flow of blood to organs by controlling the diameter of the feeding arterioles. In the perfused tissues, most of the time, the majority of the capillaries are actually closed off by pre-capillary sphincters, which only open when waste products accumulate in the surrounding tissue. Under increased demand, metabolic by-products accumulate, leading to dilation of these sphincters and hence increased local blood supply.

Oxygen, carbon dioxide, fats and urea are fat-soluble and can diffuse easily through capillary endothelium down their respective concentration gradients. Water-soluble components

TABLE 10.3 THE FUNCTIONS OF THE AUTONOMIC NERVOUS SYSTEM

ORIGIN OF EFFERENT PATHWAY	PARASYMPATHETIC	ORGAN	SYMPATHETIC	ORIGIN OF EFFERENT PATHWAY
Cranial	Constricts pupils	Eyes	Dilates pupils	Thoracic
Cranial	Stimulates salivation	Salivary glands	Inhibits salivation	Thoracic
Cranial	Decreases heart rate	Heart	Increases heart rate	Thoracic
Cranial	Constricts bronchi	Lungs	Dilates bronchi	Thoracic
Cranial	Stimulates digestion	Stomach	Inhibits digestion	Thoracic, lumbar
Cranial	Stimulates bile release	Liver, gall bladder	Stimulates glucose release	Thoracic, lumbar
Cranial		Kidneys	Stimulates adrenaline and noradrenaline release	Thoracic, lumbar
Cranial, sacral	Stimulates peristalsis and secretion	Intestines	Inhibits peristalsis and secretion	Thoracic, lumbar
Sacral	Contracts bladder	Bladder	Relaxes bladder	Lumbar
Sacral	Stimulates	Sex organs	Inhibits	Lumbar

have to be filtered through 4-nm clefts in the capillary wall. This allows the flow of water and small molecules (glucose, amino acids, ions, etc), but not proteins, through the capillary walls. The proteins and other large molecules remaining in plasma are an important determinant of fluid equilibrium between the blood and extravascular tissue. By raising 'oncotic pressure' (a form of colloid osmotic pressure exerted by proteins, notably albumin, in the blood that pulls water into the circulatory system) they cause a tendency for fluid to move across the capillary wall into the vascular space. Opposing this is the *capillary hydrostatic pressure*, equal to the difference between capillary blood pressure and tissue pressure. At the arterial end of the capillary beds the hydrostatic pressure is greater than the colloid osmotic pressure and there is net flow of water and solute into the extravascular tissue. At the venous end of the capillary beds the hydrostatic pressure has fallen beneath the colloid osmotic pressure, and now there is a net flow of water and its dissolved components back into the capillaries. Hundreds of litres of fluid are shifted across capillary walls each day, but the process is usually finely balanced. A slight excess, roughly 500 mL per day, flows out into extravascular tissue and is collected and recirculated by the lymphatic system, ultimately draining via the cisterna chyli into the left supraclavicular vein.

If capillary hydrostatic pressure is elevated past a certain point, fluid will filter out through the 4-nm clefts in the capillary walls, accumulate in the extravascular tissues and cause swelling. The disturbance in this balance of oncotic and hydrostatic pressures is known as oedema. Capillary venous pressure might be elevated, as in the case of congestive cardiac failure or venous obstruction from thrombosis. Alternatively, the capillary hydrostatic pressure can be lower than normal; for example, by hepatic failure, malnutrition, protein-losing renal diseases, or blockage, for example, by malignant infiltration. Then the protein in the blood can draw liquid out of the tissues and bolster blood volume. The section below on hypovolaemic shock is a case in point.

Another means of transporting blood molecules into the tissues is *vesicular transport*. This is used for transporting large molecules, especially proteins, out of capillaries and into the extracellular space. Proteins such as insulin, or any of the anterior pituitary hormones, are too large to get out of the 4-nm clefts in the capillary walls. Instead they bind to the surface of the endothelial cells lining the capillaries and are then surrounded by endothelial cell membrane, which forms a tiny vesicle around the protein. The vesicle then travels through the endothelial cell to the outer membrane and the contents are discharged into the tissue surrounding the capillary (the extravascular space). These transport mechanisms are protein-specific and highly regulated.

PATHOPHYSIOLOGY

PHYSIOLOGICAL RESPONSES TO TISSUE HYPOPERFUSION

Tissue hypoperfusion may result from a systemic shock state, such as hypovolaemia, or may result from activation of the sympathetic nervous system in susceptible organs. Mechanisms exist to mitigate against this low flow state, with the dual problems of reduced oxygen and nutrient delivery, and reduced waste product removal. Commonly the blood flow is reduced to 25% of the normal blood flow, potentially reducing the supply of vital nutrients and reducing the removal of toxic wastes. The supply of water, soluble nutrients and those requiring vesicular transport will be reduced in proportion to the reduction in blood flow. The fat-soluble components fare a little better.

As we saw earlier, accumulation of CO_2 and various acids leads to relaxation of precapillary sphincters, allowing access to the perfusing blood. Flow is sluggish, but there *is* flow.

Second, the acidic waste products cause haemoglobin to dissociate from most of the oxygen it is carrying, and consequently the perfusing blood can deliver up to four times as much oxygen to the tissue as it normally would. Similarly, hypoxic and acidic haemoglobin can take up and remove proportionately more carbon dioxide than in normal conditions. So even at a quarter of the normal flow, oxygen supply would remain adequate and carbon dioxide removal would keep pace. For details, see the previous sections on oxygen and carbon dioxide transport.

The reduction in the supply of glucose and amino acids is countered by the effects of the stress hormone *cortisol* (from the adrenal cortex), which promotes the breakdown of cellular glycogen to glucose and also promotes the breakdown of some cellular protein to amino acids, both of which can be used to generate adenosine triphosphate (ATP) through glycolysis and through the Krebs cycle. This can supply some of the metabolic needs of cells in under-perfused tissues, but prolonged under-perfusion leads to cell starvation, cell death and ultimately multiple-organ failure.

CELL DETERIORATION

Under-perfused tissues are on the verge of oxygen starvation and frequently glycolysis alone cannot generate enough ATP to maintain cellular processes. This under-perfusion may result from a global abnormality, such as asphyxia or haemorrhagic shock, or from local disruption of blood supply, such as during a stroke or myocardial infarct. The first thing that happens is that the energy-dependent sodium–potassium exchange pump slows. Then the cell membranes start to lose their voltage and the membrane potential is gradually lost. This depolarisation can lead to catastrophic consequences for the cells in question *and* for the cells in the vicinity of the dying cells. A small number of dying cells can, literally, kill thousands of adjacent cells by inadvertently initiating a massive amplification of the initial disturbance. This amplification is called a 'cascade' effect. The important cascade effects on a cellular level may be electrical or chemical.

Electrical and chemical cascades

Electrical anomalies occur in excitable cells, such as nerve cells and cardiac muscle. As the sodium-potassium-ATPase pumps fail and the cell starts to depolarise, the cell may experience electrical 'death shudders' in the form of abnormally triggered action potentials that stimulate other cells in the vicinity to follow suit. If confined to a small area of myocardium, this abnormal pacemaker is termed an ectopic focus. Spread of the action potential through the heart's conducting system and myocardium would give a mistimed but coordinated contraction called an ectopic beat. Under more critical conditions a greater amount of myocardial tissue may have a reduced threshold for action potential propagation. Abnormal electrical activity might spread in an uncoordinated fashion, causing sustained ventricular fibrillation rather than effective rhythmic contractions.

Pathological depolarisation may precipitate calcium entry into the cell by the uncontrolled opening of voltage-regulated calcium channels in the plasma membrane, the endoplasmic reticulum and the mitochondria. The influx of calcium has a deleterious cascade effect on a number of cellular functions. These include maintaining the integrity of the mitochondrial membrane, cellular metabolism, neurotransmitter release in the nervous system and control of muscle cell contraction and relaxation.

Loss of cell contents

The process of cellular death in an uncontrolled, widespread manner is termed necrosis. This is distinct from the orderly removal of individual senescent cells, termed apoptosis. One of the hallmarks of cellular necrosis is release of intracellular contents, such as potassium, intracellular enzymes and lactate. Clinically, the release of contents from a significant mass of dying cells may be detected by the presence of metabolic acidosis (a low arterial blood pH in the presence of a low bicarbonate level) and hyperkalaemia.

In addition, some of the cellular contents may appear in the blood. Depending on the type of tissue involved, specific intracellular contents might have diagnostic utility. For example, pancreatic cells contain a variety of powerful digestive enzymes that can damage the protein and lipid components of surrounding tissue in an amplifying cascade of necrosis that characterises severe pancreatitis. One of these proteins is lipase, which when detectable in large quantities confirms the diagnosis.

PRACTICE TIP

Pathology results that raise suspicion of cellular necrosis include:

- hyperkalaemia
- lactate
- metabolic acidosis (low blood pH and bicarbonate)
- creatine kinase (muscle cells, especially after crush injury)
- troponin (cardiac muscle)
- lipase (pancreatic cells)

The release of potassium from dying cells will also affect the electrical activity of neighbouring cells. This is because membrane potential is primarily due to the ratio of the intracellular and extracellular potassium concentrations. If cells lose potassium into the extracellular space, the remaining cells will have a reduced ratio of potassium inside and outside the cell membrane, and consequently will have a lower (less-negative) membrane potential. This may tip adjacent cells into cell death, causing the release of even more potassium and hence initiating a potassium cascade.

Nerve cells may become ischaemic during a stroke, or due to systemic hypoxia. Normal cellular function rapidly ceases. Within minutes, ongoing ischaemia causes the neurons to release excess glutamate (an excitatory amino acid neurotransmitter) as their electrical potential fails. This binds to and opens NMDA (*N*-methyl-D-aspartate) receptor-mediated calcium-ion channels in neighbouring cells, initiating a calcium cascade (see above), which causes the release of even more glutamate. This release results in a synergistic calcium and glutamate cascade, which propagates through nervous tissue, damaging cells in addition to those areas deprived of oxygen during the initial insult.

SHOCK

Shock refers to an insufficient circulatory state leading to inadequately perfused body tissues. The lack of oxygen and nutrients and the non-removal of waste products impair normal metabolism. The cells cannot generate enough ATP for their metabolic requirements and are consequently prone to cell death. When cells die, as outlined in the cell deterioration section earlier in the chapter, their membranes allow the cell contents to leak into the extracellular space and generate an even more toxic environment for the adjacent cells—resulting in even more cell death. This is yet another example of a positive (vicious-circle) feedback mechanism (Fig. 10.9). A review of the normal functioning of the cardiovascular system will demonstrate the major reasons for inadequate perfusion. In order to function adequately, the cardiovascular system requires the following components:

- an adequate blood volume with sufficient oxygen-saturated haemoglobin that is circulating through the arteries, arterioles, capillaries, venules and veins
- an adequate pump (i.e. the heart) to provide circulatory force
- sufficient vascular tone (i.e. degree of arteriolar constriction) to resist blood flow and maintain adequate arterial pressure, yet allow adequate tissue perfusion
- sufficient vascular tone in the venules to supply a capacitance that is related to the blood volume, and in the venous system to ensure blood return to the heart.

Finally, the major vessels must be free of any kind of functional obstruction, such as pulmonary emboli or pericardial tamponade. Variations in any of these factors may give rise to inadequate perfusion of the tissues. The process of shock is an example of the positive (or vicious-circle) feedback system causing further physiological derangement if left uninterrupted (Fig. 10.9).[4]

PRACTICE TIP

Timely interventions, such as oxygen therapy early in the shock process, can impede the positive feedback mechanism that leads to cellular death and organ failure. These interventions are generally directed by treatment protocols established to respond to vital signs.

Stages and causes of shock

Varying any of the critical elements in the cardiovascular system beyond homeostatic limits will give rise to inadequate tissue perfusion. These are summarised in Table 10.4. It can be

FIGURE 10.9 DIFFERENT TYPES OF POSITIVE FEEDBACK THAT CAN LEAD TO THE PROGRESSION OF SHOCK[4]

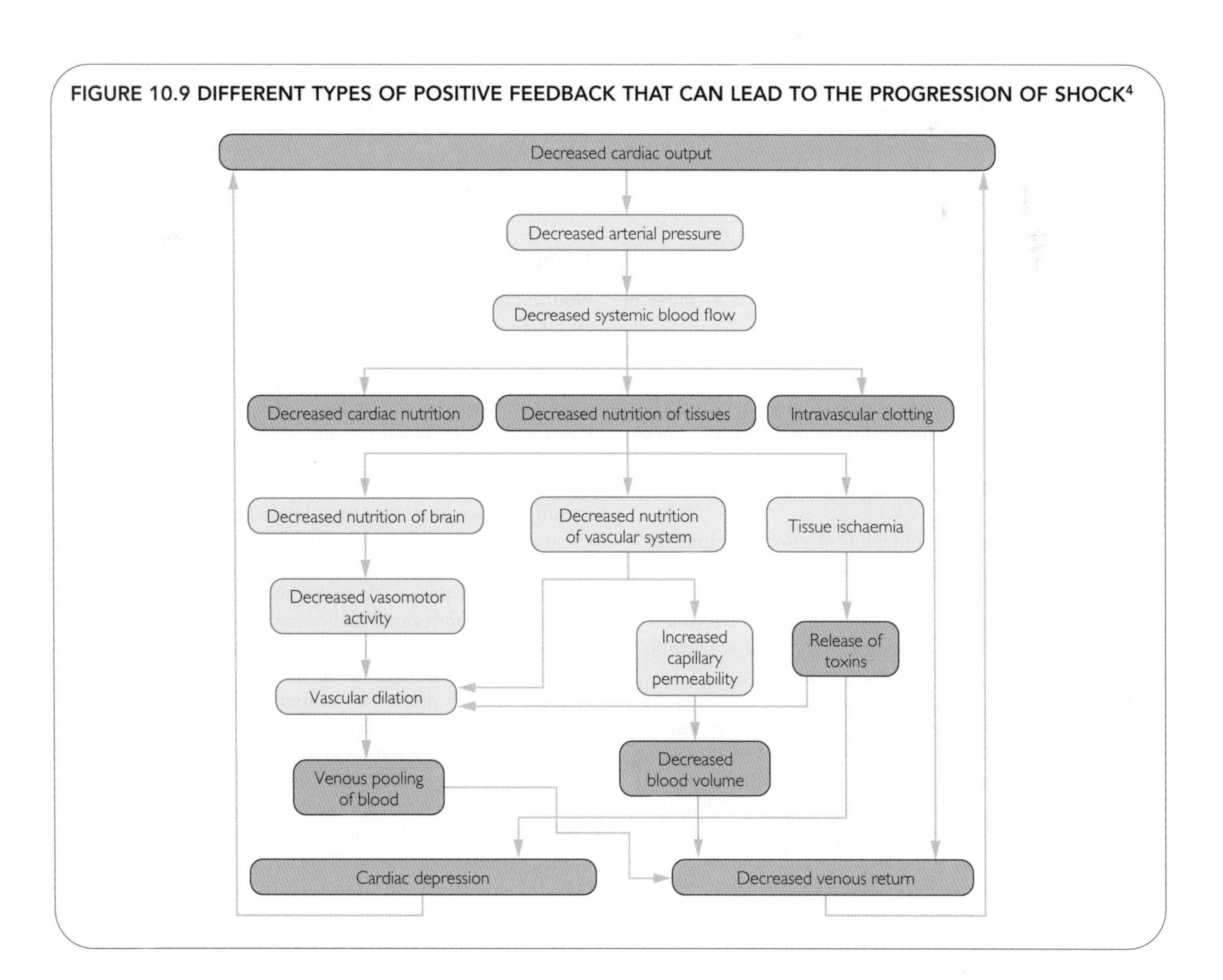

TABLE 10.4 CLASSIFICATION AND PRECIPITATING FACTORS OF SHOCK[12]

CLASSIFICATION	PRECIPITATING FACTORS
Low blood flow	
Cardiogenic shock	• Systolic dysfunction: inability of the heart to pump blood forward (e.g. myocardial infarction, cardiomyopathy) • Diastolic dysfunction: inability of the heart to fill during diastole (e.g. cardiac tamponade) • Dysrhythmias (e.g. bradycardia, tachycardia) • Structural factors: valvular abnormality (e.g. stenosis or regurgitation), papillary muscle dysfunction, acute ventricular septal defect
Hypovolaemic shock	
Absolute hypovolaemia	• Loss of whole blood (e.g. haemorrhage from trauma, surgery, GI bleeding) • Loss of plasma (e.g. burn injuries) • Loss of other body fluids (e.g. vomiting, diarrhoea, excessive diuresis, diaphoresis, diabetes insipidus, diabetes mellitus)
Relative hypovolaemia	• Pooling of blood or fluids (e.g. ascites, peritonitis, bowel obstruction) • Internal bleeding (e.g. fracture of long bones, ruptured spleen, haemothorax, severe pancreatitis) • Massive vasodilation (e.g. sepsis)
Maldistribution of blood flow	
Neurogenic shock	• Haemodynamic consequence of injury and/or disease to the spinal cord at or above T5 • Spinal anaesthesia • Vasomotor centre depression (e.g. severe pain, drugs, hypoglycaemia, injury)
Septic shock	• Infection (e.g. urinary tract, respiratory tract, invasive procedure, indwelling lines and catheters) • At-risk patients: older adults, patients with chronic diseases (e.g. diabetes mellitus, chronic renal failure, congestive heart failure), patients receiving immunosuppressive therapy or who are malnourished or debilitated • Gram-negative bacteria most common; also Gram-positive bacteria, viruses, fungi and parasites
Anaphylactic shock	• Contrast media, blood/blood products, drugs, insect bites, anaesthetic agents, food/food additives, vaccines, environmental agents, latex

GI: gastrointestinal

helpful for the clinician to approach a patient in shock using the following classification, as defining the type of shock can yield clues to the specific diagnosis and suggest a course of treatment:

- *hypovolaemic*—resulting from a loss of intravascular volume
- *cardiogenic*—resulting from pump failure, due to a problem with myocardial contractility, heart rate or rhythm or valvular apparatus
- *obstructive*—resulting from any impedance to flow in the major vessels
- *distributive*—resulting from a loss of vasomotor tone (i.e. resistance) in the arterioles and the venules. Distributive shock results from a drop of pressure due to the drop in arteriole resistance and a reduction in venous return due to the loss of tone in the post-capillary venules. Distributive shock may be further categorised as:
  - *septic shock:* caused by infection; either toxins from the pathogenic organism or an adverse effect of the host's immune response (an excess of the periphery's own antibacterial gas (nitric oxide, a potent vasodilator))
  - *neurogenic shock:* where the descending sympathetic control of vascular tone is disrupted, e.g. in spinal cord injury, again relaxing the arterioles and venules
  - *anaphylactic shock:* a hypersensitivity to a substance leading to an overproduction of vasodilator mediators resulting in a gross relaxation of blood vessels.

Compensatory responses

Neural control of blood pressure and flow

Although the cardiovascular system is primarily concerned with perfusing tissue, thereby providing an adequate supply of oxygen and nutrients, and removing waste products, by and large the regulated variable in the cardiovascular system is systemic pressure (Table 10.1). Blood pressure is maintained by an adequate pump discharging into a vascular resistance that both maintains systemic pressure and allows enough blood through to the downstream tissues to keep those tissues alive. Equally, having perfused the tissues the blood must return through the venules and the veins back to the heart to ensure a continuity of flow.

The arterial pressure is monitored by baroreceptors in the aortic arch and the carotid bifurcation. This pressure information is continually fed, beat by beat, up the vagus and glossopharyngeal nerves to the control centres in the medulla oblongata. If the systemic pressure drops, two centres in the medulla oblongata respond through connections to the autonomic nervous system to increase the heart rate and stroke volume (i.e. increase the cardiac output) and mildly constrict the systemic arterioles and the venules below the heart to increase the pressure and direct flow towards the head. Unless affected by some form of autonomic dysfunction, this happens every time an individual stands up from a lying position. In addition to the sympathetic nervous system providing continuing tonic constriction of the vasculature, some tonic constriction is provided by circulating and local hormones.

Endocrine and paracrine control of blood pressure and flow

Adrenaline and noradrenaline from the adrenal medulla and sympathetic nerve terminals constrict the skin, gut (splanchnic) and kidney circulation through alpha-receptors. The second messenger system involves the inositol triphosphate–calcium–calmodulin pathway. Adrenaline also binds to beta-receptors in muscle blood vessels and activates the cyclic-GMP (guanosine monophosphate) pathway that leads to smooth muscle relaxation and dilation of the muscle blood vessels. Additionally, adrenaline also binds to beta-receptors in the heart and increases both the force of contraction and the heart rate.

As noted above, hormones involved in fluid and electrolyte balance, ADH and angiotensin II, also provide some of the background vasoconstriction. Angiotensin II binds to AT_1 receptors and, again, via the inositol triphosphate–calcium–calmodulin pathway causes the constriction of vascular smooth muscle. This latter effect provides the rationale for using ACE inhibitors and angiotensin II receptor antagonists as drugs to lower blood pressure.

Also contributing at the tissue level are local pressure and flow mediators, notably nitric oxide (a vasodilator) and endothelin (a vasoconstrictor). A number of other local mediators produced by damaged or inflamed tissue affect local vascular tone and the permeability of the capillaries in those vascular beds. Vascular compensation for various types of shock depends on the origin of the problem.

Systemic response to a drop in blood pressure

The body's responses to a drop in arterial pressure are summarised in Fig. 10.10.[11] The drop in pressure is detected by the baroreceptors which cause a reflex increase in heart rate and stroke volume and a generalised vasoconstriction if this is possible. This assists with venous return to the heart and should assist with cardiac output. The sympathetic nervous system also restricts renal blood flow and triggers the release of renin which leads to the production of angiotensin II, causing further vasoconstriction and the release of aldosterone. Aldosterone increases renal sodium reabsorption, which in turn causes more water to be reabsorbed in the kidney tubules. If the drop in pressure is not too severe, these homeostatic mechanisms will maintain blood pressure and reasonably adequate tissue perfusion.

Hypovolaemic shock

Hypovolaemic shock is the loss of circulating volume (see Fig. 10.11).[11] The resulting drop in pressure generally results in a baroreceptor reflex which initiates a massive vasoconstriction that holds up the systemic pressure but may drastically restrict the perfusion of most organs. In extreme shock, blood flow to the peripheries and the splanchnic circulation is sacrificed and diverted to 'vital organs' (brain, heart and lungs). Arteriolar constriction results in a drop in capillary hydrostatic pressure. Unopposed oncotic pressure from plasma proteins in the capillary blood draw tissue fluid out of the interstitial space, bolstering the plasma volume by up to 30% over the ensuing 24 hours. The massive constriction on the venous side ensures that no blood pools in the capacitance vessels. Often the systemic pressure remains within normal limits, even though tissue perfusion, particularly of the skin, gut and kidney, may be reduced.

A clue to the presence of vasoconstriction is the rise in diastolic pressure and hence a reduction in pulse pressure. Peripheral pulses may be reduced in amplitude or entirely absent.

Traditionally, hypovolaemic shock has been classified into four stages according to typical signs expected with increasing degrees of volume loss. Much variation exists between individuals, however, and this classification is often misleading (Table 10.5).

Clinical manifestations are produced according to the degree to which tissue perfusion is compromised and the response of the body's compensatory mechanisms. Physiological responses can be related to the level of fluid loss.[3] Tachypnoea is often present, particularly after haemorrhage; this is a respiratory compensation associated with the reduction of circulating haemoglobin and may also reflect a 'thoracic pump' mechanism to augment venous return. Acute haemorrhage represents one end of a spectrum of hypovolaemia, where fluid is lost from the intravascular space. Circumstances such as diabetic ketoacidosis, diarrhoea or heat stress may also lead to a reduction in interstitial, intracellular and intravascular volume. This is identified by clinical manifestations of shock plus evidence of dehydration such as dry tongue, reduced skin turgor and excessive thirst. General fluid resuscitation is discussed in Chapter 14.

Trauma-induced coagulopathy and the diamond of death

Shock by definition involves the under-perfusion of tissues and thus there is a reduced supply of oxygen. This severely limits cellular oxidative processes. This has three effects:

1. ATP can only be produced by anaerobic glycolysis, resulting in lactic acidosis.
2. The heat produced as a by-product of the use of ATP is dramatically reduced.
3. Tissue damage and associated inflammatory response.

This accounts for the frequently observed acidosis and hypothermia. The microcirculation plays a crucial contributory role. Haemorrhage and resuscitation induce cellular changes that are characteristic of ischaemia–reperfusion injury—for example, production of reactive oxygen species, activation of inflammation and apoptotic cell death. In severe shock, a large range of inflammatory mediators, cytokines and oxidants are almost instantaneously produced and released in large quantities (Fig. 10.12).[13]

Coagulopathy, known as trauma-induced coagulopathy, usually accompanies severe haemorrhage in trauma patients and commences within minutes of injury.[14] It is characterised by systemic anticoagulation and fibrinolysis.[15] As many as 25% of severely injured trauma patients have an established coagulopathy when they arrive in the emergency department.[16] It is driven by severe shock in the presence of some degree of physical tissue trauma,[17] and the protein C feedback system has a central role.[18] Within a normal coagulation cascade, protein C is intended to deactivate clotting factors once they have performed their 'duty' of clotting and ceasing bleeding. However, in the major trauma patient, it appears that protein C is present in elevated levels, and continues to deactivate clotting factors, even though clots have not formed or more clotting is required. Early control of bleeding and haemostatic resuscitation, incorporating correction of coagulopathy and minimal volume replacement, are likely to improve outcomes at least in part by facilitating recovery in the microcirculation. The biggest impact of hypocalcaemia is on those pathways reliant upon calcium such as platelet

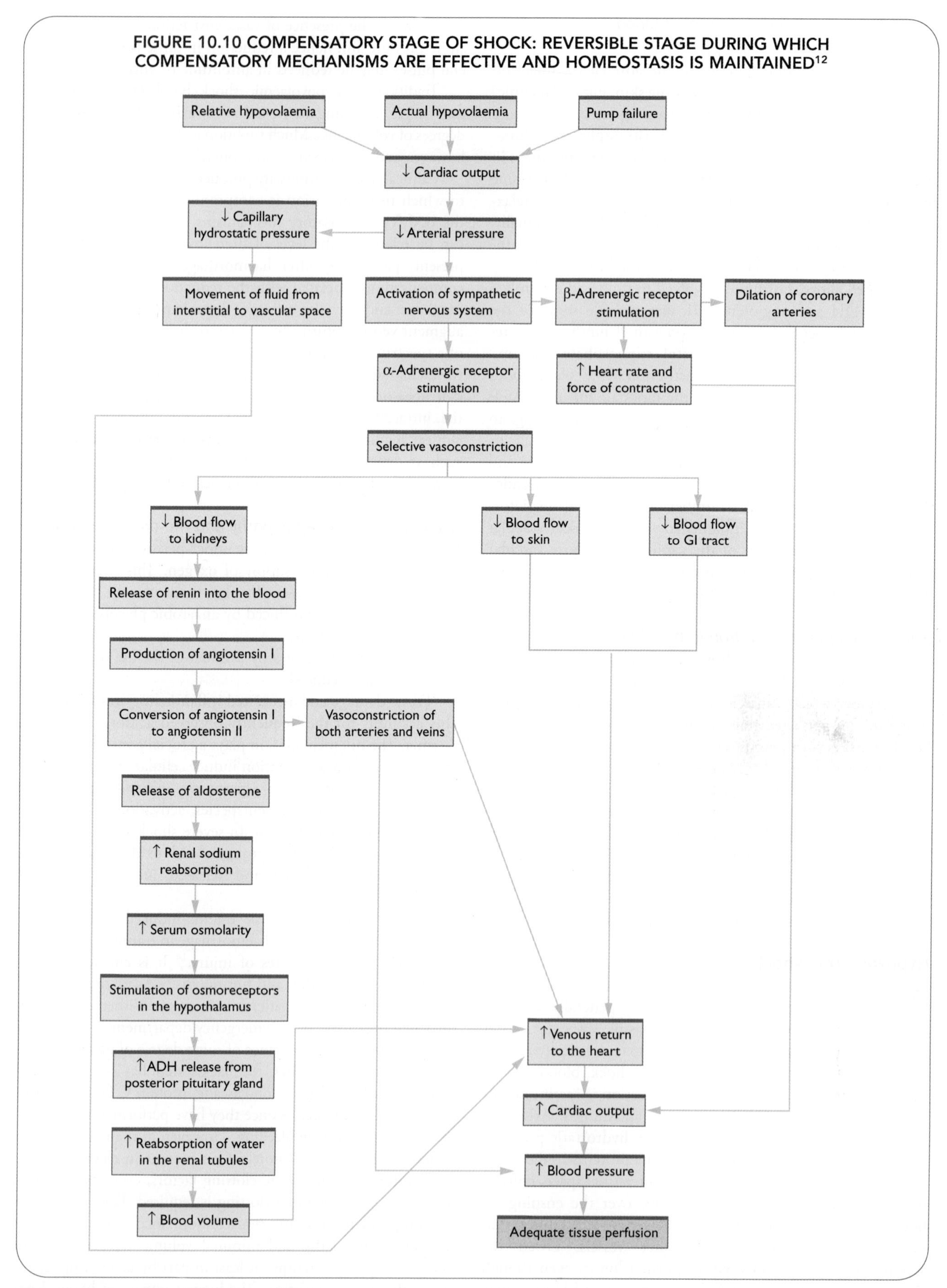

ADH: antidiuretic hormone; GI: gastrointestinal.

FIGURE 10.11 PATHOPHYSIOLOGY OF HYPOVOLAEMIC SHOCK[12]

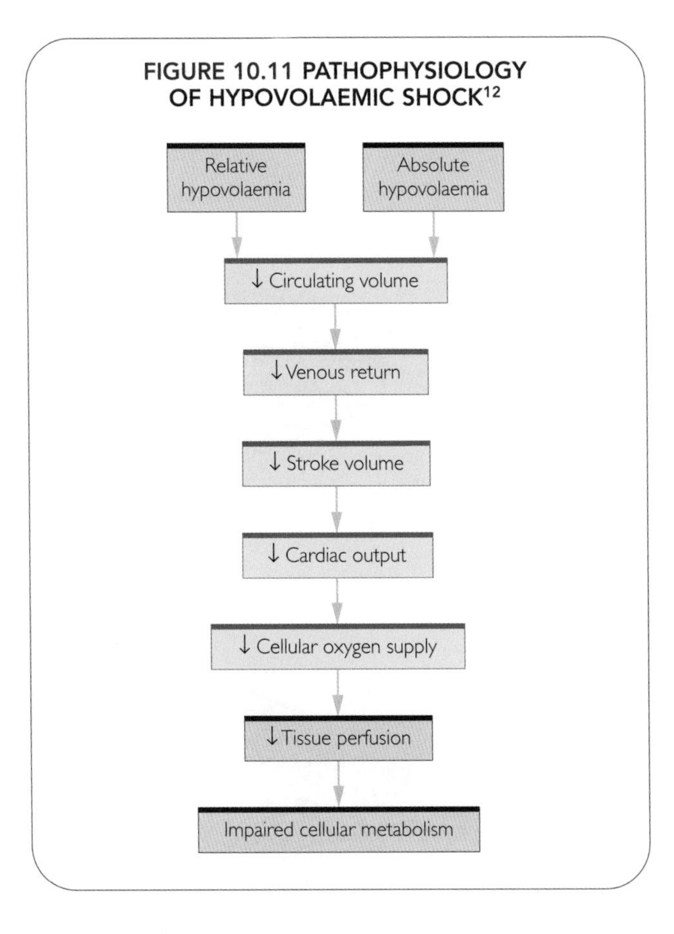

TABLE 10.5 SIGNS FOR EACH CLASS/STAGE OF HYPOVOLAEMIC SHOCK

	HEART RATE	BLOOD PRESSURE	PERIPHERY
Class II	↑	unchanged	Cool, pale
Class III	↑	↓	Cool, pale
Class IV	↓	↓	Cool, cyanosed

function, intrinsic and extrinsic haemostasis and cardiac contractility. Calcium is lost in haemorrhagic shock and this loss is exacerbated by the blood products transfused which contain citrate.

Hypothermia is known to be an indicator and result of severe injury (rather than an independent predictor of mortality), which has its own impacts on coagulopathy and the shock process by impacting on both platelet function and the oxyhaemoglobin dissociation curve. Hypothermia causes sequestration and inhibited release of platelets, thereby diminishing clotting capacity,[19] while shifting the oxyhaemoglobin curve to the left and impairing oxygen availability to cells.[20] Along with hypoperfusion, hypocalcaemia and coagulopathy, hypothermia feeds back into the vicious circle: the 'diamond of death' (see also Chapter 42 and Chapter 48).

Distributive shock

Distributive shock is due to a loss of vascular tone in the systemic arterioles and venules. The three types of distributive shock—septic, anaphylactic and neurogenic—are all associated with hypotension, but differentiated by the cause. With septic and anaphylactic shock, the drop in pressure detected by the baroreceptors is compensated for initially by an increase in force and rate of the heart, but no increase in peripheral resistance as the vasomotor centre and the sympathetic supply to blood vessels and the autonomic nervous system are overridden by peripheral mediators (Fig. 10.13). In contrast to hypovolaemic shock, anaphylactic and septic shock are often characterised by a bounding pulse and warm, pink skin.

Sepsis and septic shock

Sepsis is a systemic response to a severe, usually bacterial, infection, characterised by varying degrees of cardiovascular and other organ system dysfunction. The source of the infection may be anywhere in the body but tends to occur with organisms that produce endotoxins or that incite a disproportionate and destructive immune response. The various inflammatory mediators, including nitric oxide, interleukins, cytokines and prostaglandin, are responsible for many of the features of the 'systemic inflammatory response syndrome', such as tachycardia, fever and leucocytosis, which are the hallmarks of sepsis. The hypotension is the result of a relaxation of the arterioles and venules, due partly to bacterial endotoxins and partly to the nitric oxide gas released by macrophages in an attempt to kill off the pathogens. Nitric oxide is a potent vasodilator.

Septic shock is identified by the presence of hypotension with evidence of infection. The evidence of infection can be fever and an elevated white blood cell count and an identifiable source of infection, such as a wound or chest infection. The high metabolic demands of sepsis result in a high cardiac output, and often the key clinical manifestation is a bounding pulse in the presence of hypotension. Later, circulating cardiac depressants may add to the worsening haemodynamic state.[21]

Treatment of septic shock requires a combination of fluid resuscitation to fill the expanded vascular space, vasopressor drugs (such as noradrenaline) to constrict the vasculature and identification and eradication of the infective process. Management of sepsis is discussed in Chapter 27.

PRACTICE TIP

The ARISE study[22] provides a snapshot of the management of patients presenting to Australian and New Zealand emergency departments (EDs) with septic shock from September 2006 to January 2007 (n = 324; mean age 63.4 [SD 19.2] years).

Most common causes of sepsis:

1. pneumonia (n = 138/324, 42.6%)
2. urinary tract infection (n = 98/324, 30.2%)

Common interventions within 6 hours of presentation to ED:

3. intra-arterial catheter (n = 144/324, 44.4%)
4. central venous catheter (n = 120/324, 37.0%)
5. vasopressor infusion (n = 104/324, 32.1%)
6. mechanical ventilation (n = 60/324, 18.5%)

Admission to ICU rate: 52.4% (n = 170/324)

7. In-hospital mortality rate: 23.1% (n = 75/324)

FIGURE 10.12 MICROCIRCULATORY CHANGES IN HAEMORRHAGIC SHOCK AND RESUSCITATION[13]

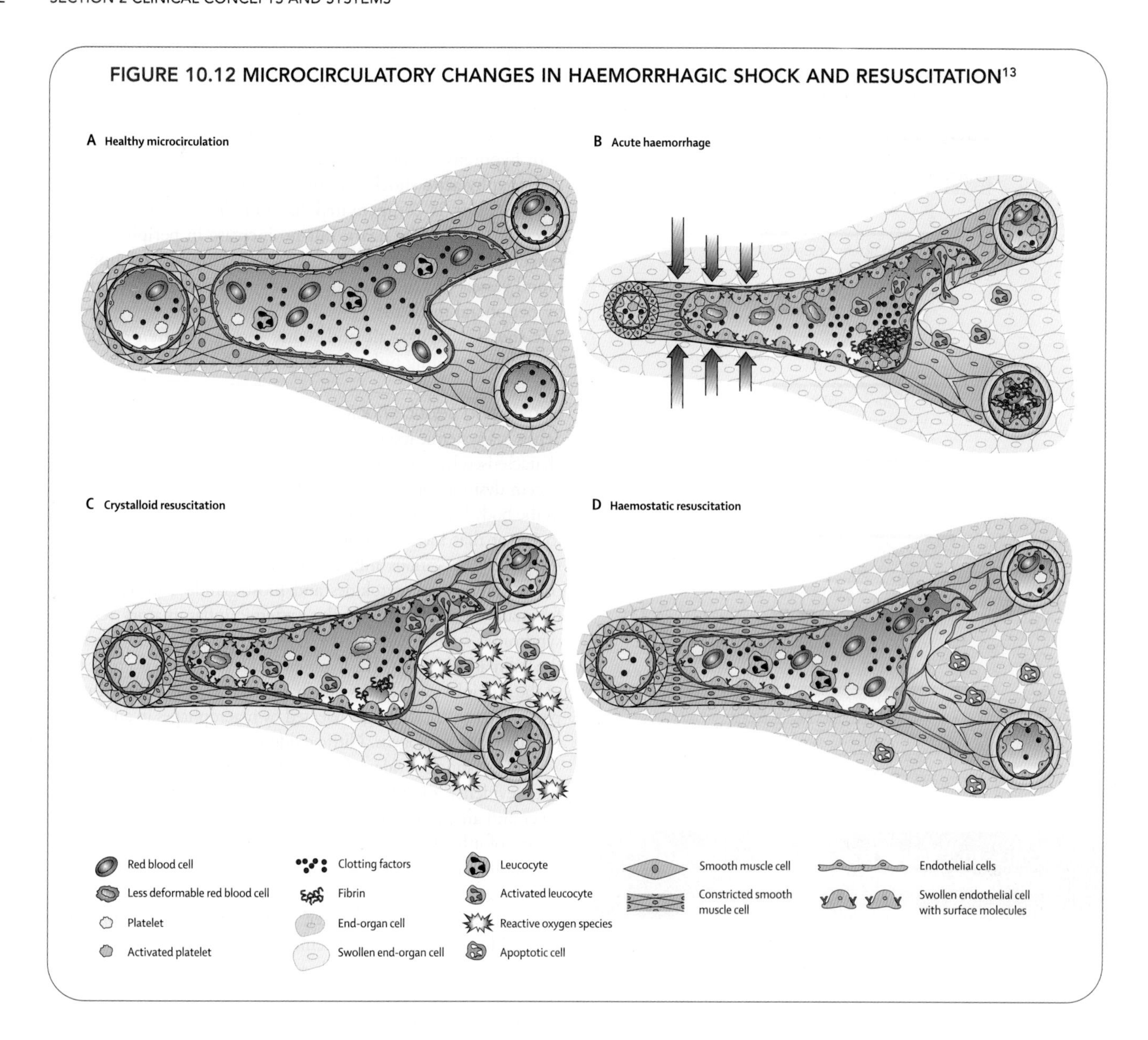

Anaphylactic shock

Anaphylaxis results from an exaggerated antibody–antigen reaction after exposure to an antigen to which the patient is allergic. Prior exposure to the antigen is a prerequisite, and 'primes' mast cells with antibodies. Subsequent exposure to the same antigen causes degranulation of mast cells and a massive release of histamine and other vasodilatory substances. Vascular smooth muscle relaxes, resulting in a drop in the total peripheral resistance and a consequent drop in blood pressure. The smooth muscle on the venous side of the circulation also relaxes, causing blood to pool and reducing venous return to the heart with a consequent reduction in cardiac output. The antigen–antibody reaction also causes bronchoconstriction in the lungs, and increased vascular permeability in the laryngeal mucosa, resulting in oedema. Death can be rapid, particularly when a compromised circulation is combined with the dual threats of upper airway obstruction and bronchospasm. At times, the diagnosis of anaphylaxis may be obvious, for example, urticaria, wheeze and collapse following a bee sting in a patient with a known hypersensitivity. At other times, the manifestations may be subtle or confounded by other causes of hypotension; for example, a severely injured trauma patient who becomes difficult to ventilate and then arrests following induction of general anaesthetic.

Neurogenic shock

Neurogenic shock is produced by a lesion of the spinal cord that disrupts the sympathetic nervous system. Spinal shock is a separate phenomenon describing a complete but usually transient disruption of all spinal cord activity below the level of an acute injury.

Parasympathetic nerves are largely unaffected as these are located in cranial nerves. A complete collapse of the sympathetic nervous system allows all the peripheral vessels to relax, dramatically increasing vascular capacity.[4] If the spinal cord lesion is above the lower cervical segments, then the sympathetic supply to the heart is also disrupted, leading to a paradoxical bradycardia in the face of hypotension. Common

FIGURE 10.13 PATHOPHYSIOLOGY OF SEPTIC SHOCK[12]

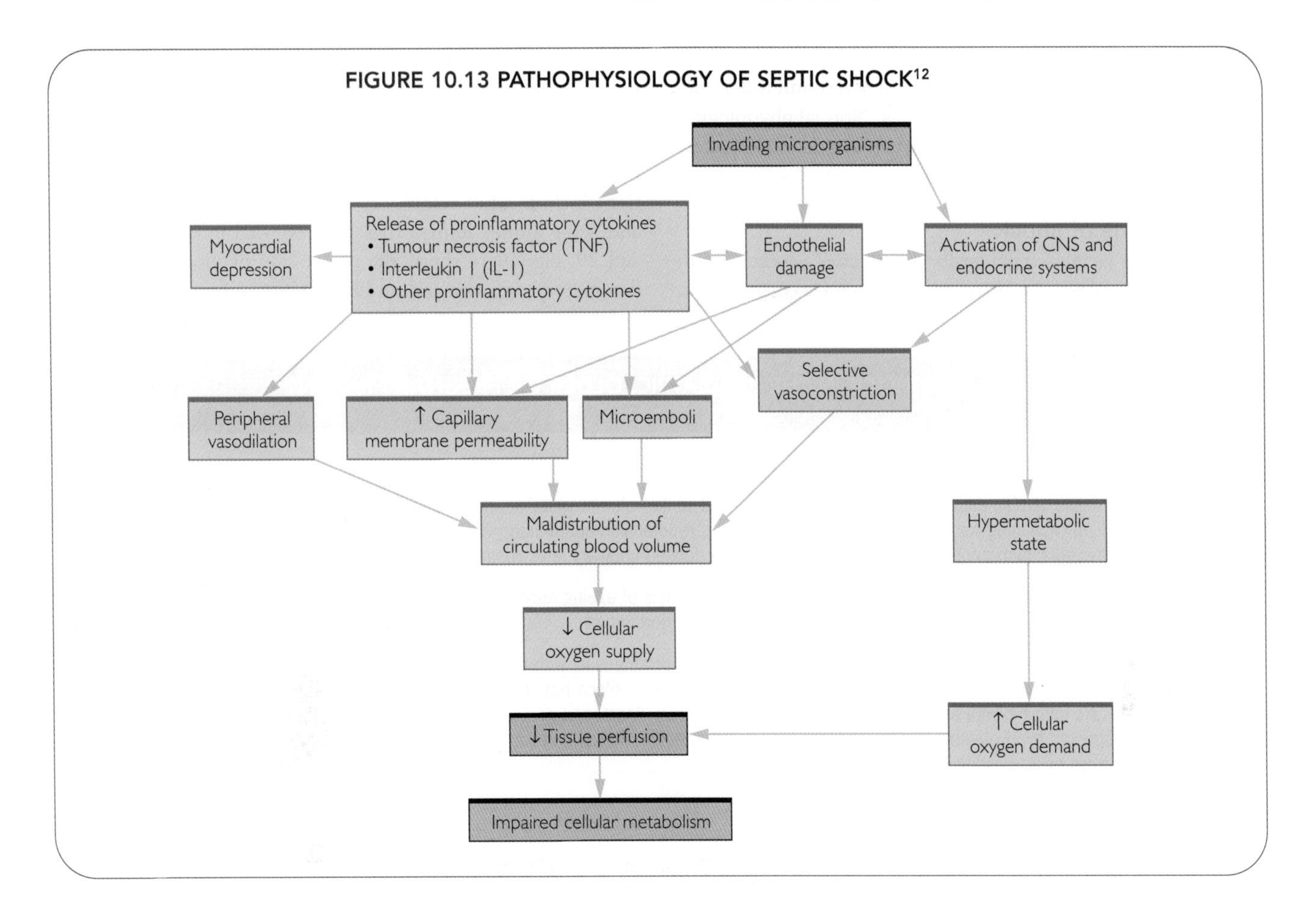

examples of lesions or interventions that may block impulses from spinal nerves include spinal trauma, spinal anaesthetic, and epidural infusion.

Treatment of neurogenic shock comprises support of blood pressure and/or heart rate. If fluid resuscitation alone is ineffective, vasopressor and chronotropic drugs may be required. If possible, the underlying cause needs to be addressed; for example, shock due to spinal or epidural interventions requires reduction or removal of the anaesthetic or infusion. Neurogenic shock as a result of trauma is discussed in Chapter 47.

Cardiogenic shock

Cardiogenic shock is the reduction of cardiac output and a consequent reduction in blood pressure. This precipitates a baroreceptor response to increase the heart rate and stroke volume and initiate a fight or flight response that, through peripheral vasoconstriction, limits flow to the skin, gut and kidneys, favouring flow to the brain, heart and lungs. The reduction in kidney blood flow precipitates water retention by way of ADH and the renin–angiotensin–aldosterone system, further increasing the load on the heart. This is another example of a damaged feedback loop making matters worse rather than returning the system to its set point. It explains the use of diuretics in heart failure.

The clinical manifestations of cardiogenic shock relate to the inadequate cardiac output and evidence of cardiac damage or failure. Hypotension, significant peripheral shutdown, tachycardia, oliguria and extreme lethargy reflect the low cardiac output. The classic presentation of the patient with cardiogenic shock is a person with chest pain or cardiac failure who develops hypotension. The treatments of cardiogenic shock are provided in greater detail in Chapter 22. In principle, the treatment involves minimising cardiac damage due to acute myocardial infarction, maximising oxygen delivery and minimising oxygen consumption. Cardiogenic shock is associated with a high mortality rate. Irreversible cardiogenic shock is reached when other organs fail due to inadequate perfusion.

Obstructive shock

Obstructive shock occurs when, despite a relatively healthy cardiovascular system and operating baroreceptor reflexes, tissue perfusion is compromised by an obstruction in a major vessel; for example, an embolus in a major artery, lung or major vein. The reduction in flow again initiates baroreceptor reflexes that restrict blood flow to non-essential organs.

Clinical manifestations of obstructive shock vary according to the site of the obstruction. There may be signs of reduced blood flow and hypoxaemia, such as a cold periphery and cyanosis, combined with typical signs of shock, including tachycardia, hypotension and oliguria. Identification and management of the cause, such as a pulmonary embolus, tension pneumothorax, cardiac tamponade, or aortic aneurysm, are covered in detail in Chapters 21 and 45.

Unique population groups

Paediatric, older and pregnant patients may respond differently to hypovolaemia and other causes of shock. Normal physiological responses and indicators of shock may be compromised; these are summarised in Table 10.6.[23]

Complications of shock

The positive (or vicious circle) feedback processes associated with shock result in worsening tissue perfusion and oxygen deficit. When the mean systemic pressure drops below 50 mmHg (6.6 kPa), the baroreceptors fail and the cardiovascular system is essentially out of control because a vital part of the feedback loop is missing. If tissues continue to be grossly under-perfused, multiple-organ failure will result followed by death. Typical complications include adult respiratory distress syndrome (ARDS), DIC and acute kidney injury. These are reviewed in Chapters 21, 25 and 29. Fig. 10.14 shows the progression of shock, systemic inflammatory response and multiple-organ dysfunction syndrome.

TABLE 10.6 SHOCK IN THE PAEDIATRIC, OLDER OR PREGNANT PATIENT[24]

PATIENT	DESCRIPTION
Paediatric	Increases cardiac output by increasing heart rate; fixed stroke volume; sustains arterial pressure despite significant volume loss; loses 25% of circulating volume before signs of shock occur; hypotension and lethargy are ominous signs. Early clinical manifestations are tachycardia, tachypnoea, pallor, cool mottled skin and delayed capillary refill; volume replaced with 20 mL/kg bolus of crystalloid
Older adult	Shock progression often rapid; normal physiological changes of ageing reduce compensatory mechanisms; predisposed to hypothermia; pre-existing disease states contribute to comorbidities
Pregnant	Hypervolaemia of pregnancy means patient can remain normotensive with up to a 1500 mL blood loss; compression of inferior vena cava by gravid uterus reduces circulating volume by 30%; place patient on left side, manually displace uterus to the left or elevate right hip with towel; risk for aspiration resulting from decreased gastric motility and decreased gastric emptying; treat suspected hypovolaemia to prevent placental vasoconstriction associated with catecholamine release; potential for fetal distress exists despite maternal stability

FIGURE 10.14 RELATIONSHIP OF SHOCK, SYSTEMIC INFLAMMATORY RESPONSE AND MULTIPLE-ORGAN DYSFUNCTION SYNDROME[12]

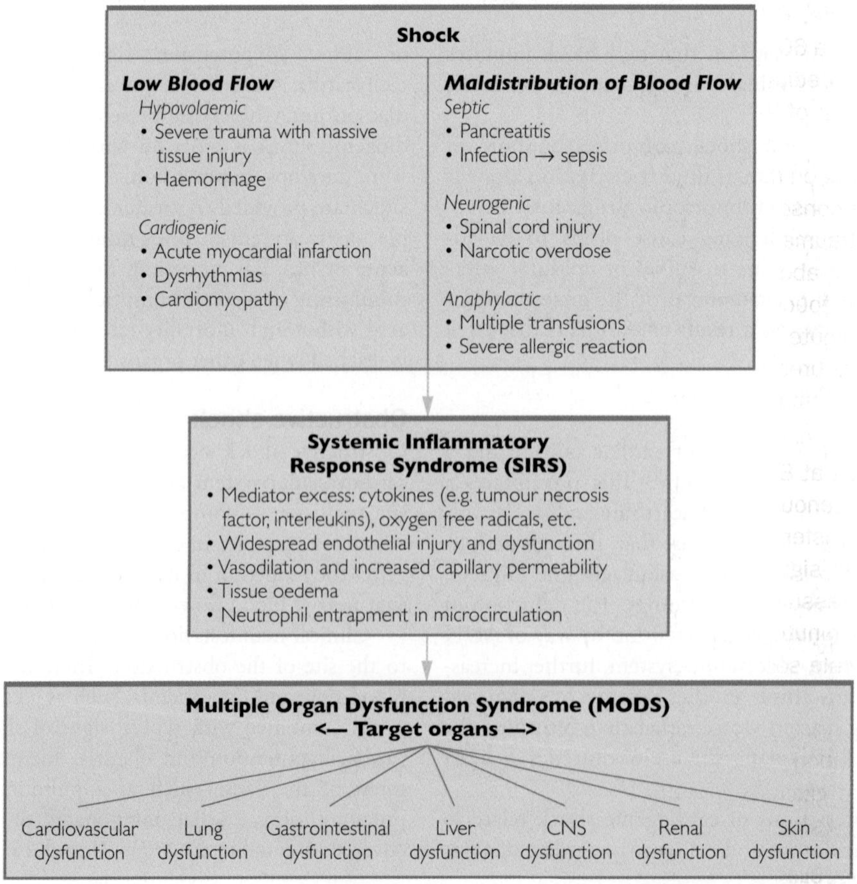

Shock

Low Blood Flow

Hypovolaemic
- Severe trauma with massive tissue injury
- Haemorrhage

Cardiogenic
- Acute myocardial infarction
- Dysrhythmias
- Cardiomyopathy

Maldistribution of Blood Flow

Septic
- Pancreatitis
- Infection → sepsis

Neurogenic
- Spinal cord injury
- Narcotic overdose

Anaphylactic
- Multiple transfusions
- Severe allergic reaction

Systemic Inflammatory Response Syndrome (SIRS)
- Mediator excess: cytokines (e.g. tumour necrosis factor, interleukins), oxygen free radicals, etc.
- Widespread endothelial injury and dysfunction
- Vasodilation and increased capillary permeability
- Tissue oedema
- Neutrophil entrapment in microcirculation

Multiple Organ Dysfunction Syndrome (MODS)
<— Target organs —>

Cardiovascular dysfunction
Lung dysfunction
Gastrointestinal dysfunction
Liver dysfunction
CNS dysfunction
Renal dysfunction
Skin dysfunction

Minimisation of the severity and duration of the dysfunctional microcirculatory response in the first minutes and hours after injury might prevent complications.[12] Early control of bleeding and haemostatic resuscitation, incorporating correction of coagulopathy and minimal volume replacement, are likely to improve outcomes at least in part by facilitating recovery in the microcirculation.[25]

PRACTICE TIP

The assessment and management of abnormal vital signs play a vital role in rectifying feedback loops and mitigating the impact that the shock process has on the patient.

SUMMARY

Physiology is the study of feedback loops, while pathology is the study of failing feedback loops. As a consequence, an understanding of pathology requires an appreciation of the underlying physiology. Failure of any links in the physiological chain will affect the whole mechanism. The feedback loops explored in this chapter include gas carriage, temperature control, fluid and electrolyte balance and the control of tissue perfusion.

Health is adversely affected when negative feedback mechanisms that usually keep the regulated variables close to the set point actually do the reverse—shifting the regulated variables away from the set point and initiating mechanisms that move the regulated variables even further away from the set point; so-called positive feedback. Ideally, clinical interventions are aimed at restoring the damaged physiological link(s), so that the regulated variables return to their set points.

CASE STUDY

Dale is a 24-year-old man who has crashed his car head-on into a power pole. He was the only occupant. The incident occurred in a 60 kph zone, but witnesses report that the car was speeding. The car is quite old and has no airbags; the front of the car is caved in against the pole, but the windscreen is intact. When paramedics arrive, Dale is sitting on the footpath beside the vehicle. He is noted to be conscious and alert, and there is no obvious external trauma or bleeding. He is complaining of pain in his lower abdomen and is pale and sweaty; his skin is cool to touch. Dale's vital signs are: heart rate 126 beats/minute, blood pressure 85/50 mmHg, respiratory rate 28 breaths/minute, oxygen saturation 96% and Glasgow Coma Scale score 15.

Spinal motion restriction practices are applied, oxygen applied via a mask at 8 L/minute, intravenous access obtained and intravenous analgesia administered. Dale is prepared for transfer to the nearest trauma centre. On arrival his vital signs are: heart rate 128 beats/minute, blood pressure 90/60 mmHg, respiratory rate 26 breaths/minute, oxygen saturation 99% and Glasgow Coma Scale score 15. He is receiving oxygen via mask at 8 L/minute, and continues to complain of lower abdominal pain. The following blood tests are ordered: venous blood gas, full blood count, urea and electrolytes, blood glucose and blood cross-matching. A trauma radiology series is also requested, including plain chest and pelvis x-rays. Prior to x-rays being taken, an abdominal ultrasound is performed and a significant amount of intraperitoneal blood is detected.

QUESTIONS

1. Explain the physiological basis for the vital sign findings—the patient has no significant medical history and is not taking any medications that may cause vital sign changes.
2. What determines the affinity between oxygen and haemoglobin, and how does hypothermia impact this affinity?
3. In the presence of hypotension, what changes will occur to heart rate and peripheral perfusion in the following types of shock?
   a. hypovolaemic
   b. septic
   c. neurogenic
   d. anaphylactic
   e. cardiogenic.
4. What mechanism initiates a systemic response to a reduction in blood pressure? Briefly outline the main stages of the body's response to a reduction in blood pressure and describe potential masking agents.

Answers to Case Study Questions can be found on evolve **http://evolve.elsevier.com/AU/Curtis/emergency/**

REFERENCES

1. Selye H. A syndrome produced by diverse nocuous agents. Nature 1936;138:32.
2. Selye H. The stress of life. New York: McGraw-Hill; 1956.
3. Norris TL. Porth's pathophysiology: concepts of altered health states. 10th ed. Philadelphia: Wolters Kluwer; 2018.
4. John E. Hall MEH. Guyton and Hall textbook of medical physiology. 14th ed. Saint Louis: Elsevier Health Sciences; 2020.
5. Clark MA, Choi J. Biology 2e. Gas exchange across respiratory surfaces. OpenStax; 2018. Online. Available from: openstax.org/books/biology-2e/pages/39-2-gas-exchange-across-respiratory-surfaces.
6. Cameron PA, Little M, Mitra B, et al. Textbook of adult emergency medicine. 5th ed. Sydney: Elsevier; 2019.
7. El-Khatib MF. High-flow nasal cannula oxygen therapy during hypoxemic respiratory failure. Respir Care 2012;57(10):1696–8.
8. Urden LD, Stacy KM, Lough ME. Critical care nursing: diagnosis and management. 8th ed. Maryland Heights, Missouri: Elsevier; 2018.
9. Frakes MA. Measuring end-tidal carbon dioxide: clinical applications and usefulness. Crit Care Nurse 2001;21(5):23–6.
10. Sund-Levander M, Forsberg C, Wahren LK. Normal oral, rectal, tympanic and axillary body temperature in adult men and women: a systematic literature review. Scand J Caring Sci 2002;16(2): 122–8.
11. Rang HP, Ritter J, Flower RJ, Henderson G. Rang and Dale's pharmacology. 8th ed. London, England: Elsevier Churchill Livingstone; 2016.
12. Harding MM, Roberts D, Hagler L, Reinisch C. Lewis's medical-surgical nursing: assessment and management of clinical problems. 11th ed. St Louis: Elsevier; 2019.
13. Gruen RLP, Brohi KP, Schreiber MP, Balogh ZJP, Pitt VP, Narayan MMD, et al. Haemorrhage control in severely injured patients. Lancet 2012;380(9847):1099–108.
14. Floccard B, Rugeri L, Faure A, Denis MS, Boyle EM, Peguet O, et al. Early coagulopathy in trauma patients: an on-scene and hospital admission study. Injury 2010;43(1):26–32.
15. Brohi K, Cohen MJ, Ganter MT, et al. Acute coagulopathy of trauma: hypoperfusion induces systemic anticoagulation and hyperfibrinolysis. J Trauma 2008;64(5):1211–17.
16. Brohi K, Singh J, Heron M, Schultz MJ, Levi M, Mackersie RC, et al. Acute traumatic coagulopathy. J Trauma 2003;54(6):1127–30.
17. Frith D, Goslings JC, Gaarder C, Maegele M, Cohen MJ, Allard S, et al. Definition and drivers of acute traumatic coagulopathy: clinical and experimental investigations. J Thromb Haemost 2010;8(9):1919–25.
18. Brohi K, Cohen MJ, Ganter MT, Matthay MA, Mackersie RC, Pittet J-F. Acute traumatic coagulopathy: initiated by hypoperfusion: modulated through the protein C pathway? Ann Surg 2007;245(5):812–18.
19. Boffard KD. Manual of definitive surgical trauma care: incorporating definitive anaesthetic trauma care. 5th ed. Boca Raton: CRC Press; 2019.
20. Bacher A. Effects of body temperature on blood gases. Applied physiology in intensive care medicine. Berlin, Heidelberg: Springer; 2006.
21. Jozwiak M, Persichini R, Monnet X, Teboul JL. Management of myocardial dysfunction in severe sepsis. Semin Respir Crit Care Med 2011;32(2):206–14.
22. Peake SL, Bailey M, Bellomo R, Cameron PA, Cross A, Delaney A et al. Australasian resuscitation of sepsis evaluation (ARISE): a multi-centre, prospective, inception cohort study. Resuscitation 2009;80(7):811–18.
23. Foley A, Sweet V, editors. Shock emergencies. In: Sheehy's emergency nursing: principles and practice. 7th ed. St Louis: Elsevier Health Sciences; 2019.
24. Hammond B, Zimmermann P, editors. Sheehy's manual of emergency care. 7th ed. St Louis: Mosby, Elsevier; 2013.
25. Duchesne J, McSwain NE, Cotton BA, Hunt JP, Dellavolpe JD, Lafaro KJ, et al. Damage control resuscitation: the new face of damage control. J Trauma 2010;69(4):976–90.

CHAPTER 11
CLINICAL REASONING, PROBLEM-SOLVING AND TRIAGE

MARGARET FRY, JULIE CONSIDINE, BERNADINE ROMERO, RAMON Z. SHABAN AND TOBY KEENE

ESSENTIALS

- Clinical reasoning and problem-solving are core elements of professional practice for emergency clinicians.
- Essential to clinical reasoning is the gathering and organising of information, discerning of relevant data from irrelevant data and concept formation of the patient's problem, making comparisons with similar situations and experiences, and maintaining analytical distance.
- In emergency care, clinical reasoning and critical thinking are focused on problem-solving, but there is always the risk of uncertainty, inevitable error and unavoidable injustice.
- Clinical records from pre-hospital and emergency settings are an essential element of continuity of care for ongoing patient assessment, care and transport. They are factual and legal documents, and information that is omitted from formal clinical records is largely treated as not having occurred.
- Triage is the sorting of patients into urgency categories to optimise care delivery within available resources.
- Triage roles require advanced communication and interpersonal skills to optimise clinical handover and the patient's understanding of the ED journey.
- The emergency nurse triage role requires advanced knowledge, experience and skills to discriminate between life-threatening, urgent and non-urgent conditions.
- There are many validated and reliable emergency department triage tools used to determine patient urgency.
- The role and responsibilities of the triage nurse require advanced skills to enable the fast-tracking of patients and management of overcrowding.
- Effective communication is essential to the delivery of high-quality and safe pre-hospital and emergency care.
- Legible, timely, accurate, complete, original, factual and objective documentation is the healthcare professional's best protection from liability action.

INTRODUCTION

This chapter provides an understanding of clinical reasoning, problem-solving and triage practice in the out-of-hospital and emergency department (ED) settings. Essential to the delivery of high-quality and safe triage in emergency care settings are: (i) the science of clinical reasoning; (ii) the application of clinical reasoning science to emergency healthcare practice by way of problem-solving and triage; and (iii) the communication of these within the broader healthcare setting.

With emergency care demand increasing, formalised triage systems have been developed to identify and prioritise those patients presenting with actual or potentially life-threatening conditions. Triage guidelines and protocols have been developed to assist in the discrimination between life-threatening, urgent and non-urgent conditions. However, triage involves more than the application of guidelines. In the ED, triage nurses determine the need for a bed, allocate ED resources, fast-track patient care, deliver first aid and provide a safety net for waiting room patients. In the out-of-hospital environment, triage decisions will influence resources deployed to the scene and transport decisions. To undertake accurate out-of-hospital and ED triage and achieve additional extended roles requires discipline specific knowledge, advanced practice expertise, and clinical reasoning and decision-making skills. All these aspects will be discussed in this chapter.

CLINICAL REASONING FOR QUALITY EMERGENCY CARE

Within Australia, Aotearoa New Zealand and around the world there is an unprecedented demand for quality and safety in healthcare.[1–3] The provision of high-quality healthcare ultimately depends on the services provided by individual healthcare professionals. In recent times, individuals and the organisations they work within have been called to account for the quality of their clinical judgements and decisions, more than ever before.[4,5] The clinical judgement and decision-making of healthcare professionals and their ability to understand, diagnose and respond to clinical problems are fundamental to the delivery of high-quality healthcare and medical care.[6–8]

Critical thinking and clinical reasoning are vital antecedents to high-quality and safe out-of-hospital healthcare and professionalism.[9,10] Making sound clinical judgements is an 'intrinsic and inescapable imperative'[11] for all healthcare professionals if they are to render high-quality and safe healthcare. The ability of healthcare workers to solve clinical problems with clinical judgements and make decisions are skills that are critical features of professionalism.[12,13] Higgs and Jones suggest that professions must build and maintain a formidable store of knowledge and skills. They must learn to absorb information through the various senses and to assess its validity, reliability and relevance, and must acquire the art and culture of their calling. Most importantly, they must learn to use these qualities to solve practical clinical problems.[12]

The terms 'clinical thinking and clinical reasoning' and 'clinical judgement and decision-making' are used interchangeably within the literature. Generally speaking, the *clinical* care that healthcare professionals provide is concerned with the treatment of patients.[14] Their *judgement* is a critical faculty of discernment, good sense or an opinion or estimate;[14] and a *decision* is the act or process of deciding a conclusion or other future action after consideration.[14] Broadly speaking, *clinical judgement and decision-making* may be viewed as 'an assessment of the alternatives in treatment from which decisions or choices between alternatives for optimal treatment are made'.[5] Clinical reasoning is a series of cognitive processes that is informed by evidence to optimise patient safety and outcomes, thereby minimising risk.[15] For brevity, we will refer to these terms collectively as *clinical reasoning*, although we acknowledge that therein exist different philosophical and theoretical perspectives.

THEORETICAL CONSIDERATIONS

The ability to form clinical judgements, to make decisions and to exercise clinical reasoning is fundamental to the delivery of high-quality healthcare.[13,15] The origins of this work are largely connected to the desire to deal with uncertainty and the unknown,[16,17] and are interconnected with the highly contested and controversial study of emotion, cognition and perception. Moreover, there is no single or universal way to arrange or organise the literature on judgement and decision-making.[13,18] All that is known and recorded cannot be considered as 'singularly paradigmatic, but rather as immersed in a number of competing schools of thought that identify issues as interesting and deem different methods as appropriate'. Each of the theoretical positions is contextually bound and has contested philosophical origins. Many of their meanings and understandings are not sharply demarcated—they overlap, often because of shared theoretical and philosophical positions.[13,18] Much of the debate in the literature is focused on how to view, define and categorise judgement and decision-making.[13,19]

The science of decision-making dates back to the early 1950s. The original dominant paradigm of judgement and decision-making was *classical decision-making*. This views the decision-maker as an element in a context of complete certainty.[12] The problems decision-makers face are clearly defined, and they know all the possible alternatives for action, and their consequences. The action they choose provides for an optimum outcome. They are characteristic of laboratory settings, and articulate the correct way to make an optimum decision in an ideal situation, environment or world. Theories derived from this paradigm have been applied to decision-making in many contexts, although Chapman[20] and others note that it does not fit well in chaotic contexts, uncontrolled environments or critical situations.[5,10]

Growing criticism of classical decision-making and its limitations in the 1980s spurred a rethink of judgement and decision-making theory. Instead, *naturalistic* (or *behavioural*) *decision-making* is an alternative position that has attracted recent attention.[19] Within this dichotomy, classical and naturalistic decision-making, lie three models or theoretical positions of clinical judgement and decision-making: descriptive, normative and prescriptive. The relationship between these and a description of them is illustrated in Box 11.1 and Fig. 11.1.

Unlike classic decision-making, naturalistic decision-making acknowledges that individuals exist and function within cognitive limitations in a bounded rationality. According to Lipshitz and colleagues,[24] within this paradigm individuals are presented with ill-structured problems in uncertain, dynamic environments with shifting, ill-defined and competing goals such as emergency settings. Of particular importance here is the significance of time as a constraint, especially when individuals

BOX 11.1 DESCRIPTIVE, NORMATIVE AND PRESCRIPTIVE MODELS[5]

DESCRIPTIVE THEORIES

Naturalistic and behavioural in nature, these theories originate from the philosophies and professions of psychology and behavioural science.[21,22] Specifically, descriptive theories are concerned with understanding how individuals actually make judgements and decisions. Descriptive theories place no restriction on whether the individual is rational and logical or irrational and illogical, and seek to understand how individuals make judgements and decisions in the real world, focusing on the actual conditions, contexts, ecologies and environments in which they are made.[22] Irrationality in this context refers to instances where individuals have not given any thought to the process of judgement or decision-making (JDM), and, even if they have, are unable to implement the desired process.[21] These theories seek to understand the learning and cognitive capabilities of 'ordinary people' and aim to determine if their behaviour is consistent or 'rational'.[22] Context, interactions and ecology are central to the interpretation.

NORMATIVE THEORIES

These are classical and positivist in nature, and are born from the statistical, mathematical and economic philosophies.[22] In this domain, researchers (often referred to as decision theorists) seek to propose rational procedures for decision-making that are logical and may be theorised. The focus of normative theory is to discover how rational people make decisions with the aim of determining how decisions *should be made* in an ideal or optimal world, where decisions are based on logical and known conclusions supported by clear or probable evidence. Normative theories, often based on statistics and probabilities within the positivist domain, propose to evaluate how good judgements should be made and how good outcomes should be achieved.[21,22] Normative theories give little or no consideration to how judgements are made by 'ordinary people' in reality and everyday practice, and place little or no emphasis on the context or ecology of the judgement.[21] They are concerned only with optimal conditions and environments, and assume that decision-makers are 'super-rational',[23] with little or no emphasis on how JDM occurs in the 'real' world.[22]

PRESCRIPTIVE THEORIES

These theories set out to 'improve' the clinical reasoning of individuals by investigating how people make decisions.[21,22] The focus of prescriptive theories is to *help* or *improve* individuals' judgements. In evaluating the application of prescriptive models and theories that attempt to aid in the JDM process, the central question asked is pragmatic—did it make the judgement any better? Prescriptive theories have been applied in multiple settings and contexts. Decision analysis and decision trees (described later in the chapter) are used commonly in prescriptive modelling in medicine to improve clinician reasoning.[21] A recently introduced but now common prescriptive model for assisting JDM in clinical settings is the use of clinical guidelines and clinical policies. Clinical guidelines are prescriptive tools used to assist practitioner and patient decisions about appropriate healthcare for specific circumstances.[21] They are largely guidelines that outline operational information, procedures and guidelines with options, and are often referred to as 'protocols'. Primarily aimed at improving the quality of care or standardising care, guidelines are mechanisms for reducing variations in clinical practice and discouraging practices that are not based on sufficient evidence.[21] While they have been found to provide improvements in the quality of care,[21] the effects of their application are significantly variable and the extent to which they are routinely applied is not clear.[22]

FIGURE 11.1 CRITICAL ELEMENTS TO PARAMEDIC CLINICAL THINKING AND REASONING

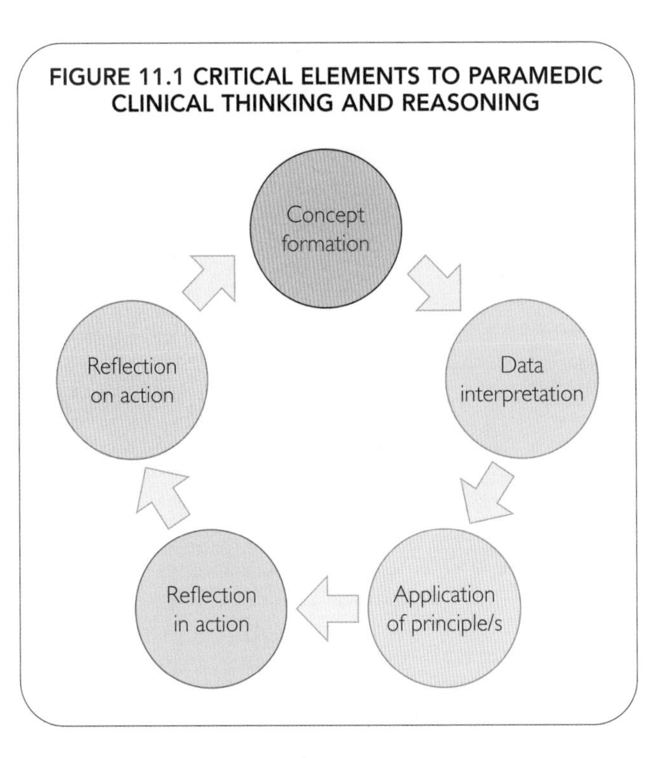

are required to assess, interpret and assimilate multiple data from multiple sources, often in settings where the stakes are high. The problem faced by the naturalistic decision-maker lacks clarity, and can limit knowledge of possible action alternatives and their consequences. The action they undertake is more geared towards achieving a satisfactory outcome rather than the optimal outcome, out of sheer necessity.[25]

Naturalistic decision-making holds particular relevance in chaotic environments where conditions are uncertain, and individuals have limited information. In these situations, such as in the out-of-hospital and emergency setting, individuals most often rely on their experience to resolve patient problems and comprehensively gather and record appropriate relevant information.[5] When it comes to out-of-hospital emergency settings, the clinical reasoning of emergency nurses and paramedics is focused on problem-solving.[17,25]

PRACTICE TIP

A definitive diagnosis is no substitute for comprehensive description and documentation of the patient's presenting problems that require intervention.

CLINICAL GUIDELINES AND PROTOCOLS FOR PROBLEM-SOLVING

Clinical guidelines and protocols and other forms of decision support are fundamental to clinical judgement and decision-making, and evidence-based practice. Research supporting the use of decision support resources exists for many areas of emergency care, including triage and telephone triage,[26] ambulance service telemedicine,[27] COVID-19 ambulance dispatch screening tool,[28] ambulance triage,[29] management of sepsis[30,31] management of hip and chest trauma,[32,33] paediatric recognition of severe injury,[34,35] cardiac arrest and resuscitation,[36] disasters and mass gatherings[37] and determining the need for further treatment and transport.[38,39] The findings of the majority of this research recommend the use of decision-support processes, such as protocols and guidelines, for health professional judgement practice.

Much of this existing research advocates the use of computer-assisted decision support systems,[40,41] which is increasingly being adopted. Computer-assisted decision-making software for accurate ambulance call-taking and the management of emergency health services is an international standard.[41,42] Farrand and colleagues[43] examined the introduction of a computerised dispatch system into an emergency medical system call centre traditionally staffed by nurses. The study found that in attempting to formalise nurse decision processes using artificial intelligence, the complexities of the decision processes therein were revealed. An assessment of the accuracy of the decision process—using an expert panel review of 1006 calls—found almost perfect sensitivity with telephone triage and decision as to whether to send an EMS resource or not. In this instance, the study demonstrated that nurses' clinical judgement and decision-making processes in this setting were sophisticated.[20] Other studies have reported similar findings.[44,45]

Researchers[46–48] have suggested that clinical judgement and decision-making regarding the futility of resuscitation is best supported by the use of an algorithm and doctor-guided clinical guidelines. Dunne and colleagues[49] conducted a study to estimate the proportion of patients transported by paramedics who do not need emergency medical care. They found that paramedics could not reliably identify those patients in need of emergency medical treatment when unaided by protocols or specific training. Although the use of computer-aided decision support is common, recent research reveals a poor uptake of electronic decision support and information systems for evidence-based practice.[50]

Clinical guidelines and other decision support are often presented as decision trees and are a direct application of normative theories of judgement and decision-making. They outline how decisions should be made. Decision trees, such as the one illustrated in Fig. 11.2, work by breaking down problems

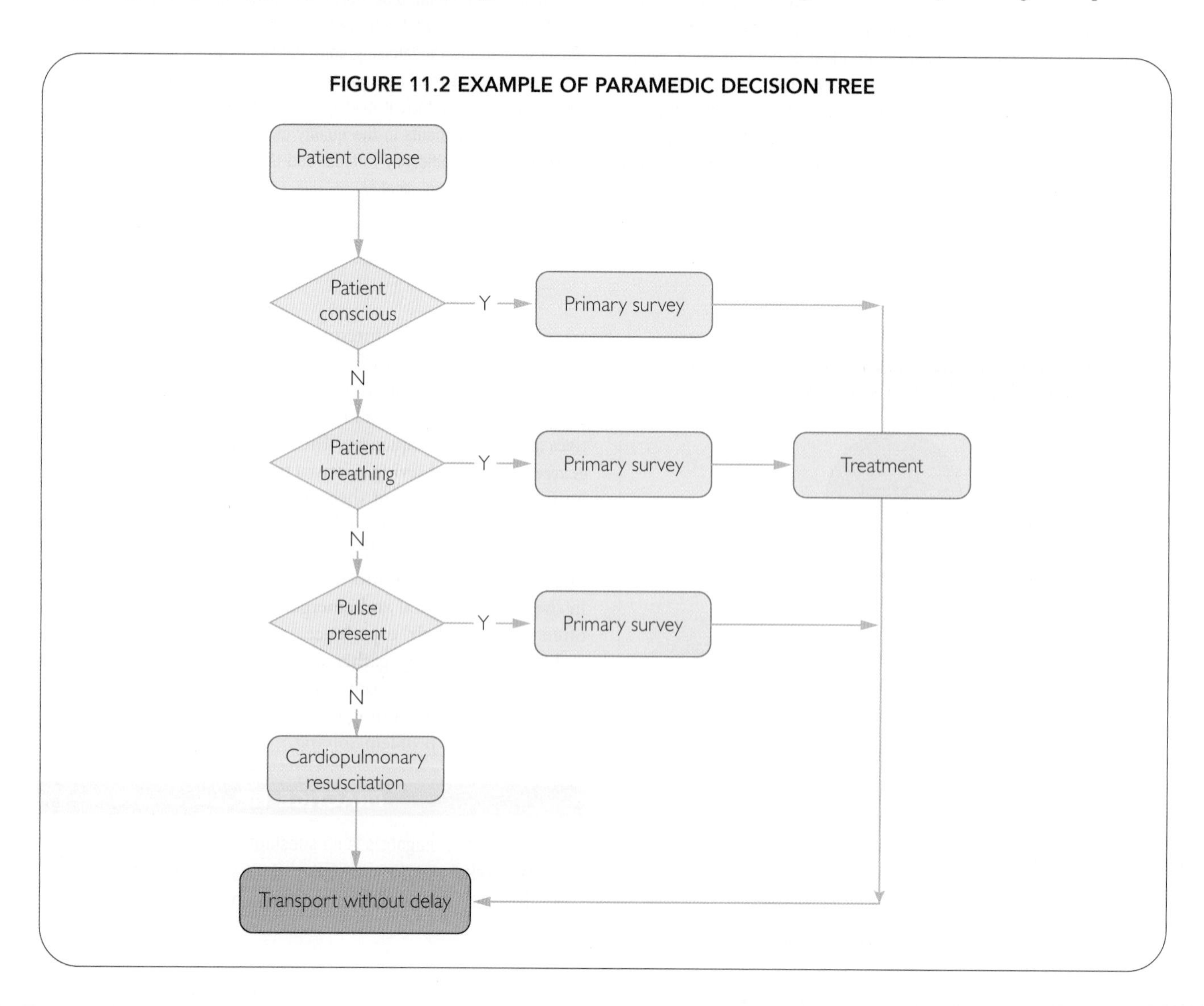

into smaller decisions and choices.[6,40] Traditionally, determining how judgements and decisions should be made by healthcare professionals required comprehensive risk analyses, which were then weighted.[19] The decisions alluded to within the tree are based on the predictability of events using probability and statistical occurrence. Once each choice has been assigned a probability—assuming this is possible—the option with the highest utility for the decision-maker can be calculated.[19] Such models attempt to quantify the probability of the most likely and most desirable event in an attempt to assist the individual or group in making that judgement or decision by making this probability known.

PRACTICE TIP

When developing and reviewing a clinical decision tree, both qualify and quantify the clinical problem that it seeks to solve.

Decision trees also assist emergency clinicians to make decisions about the transportation and transfer of patients.[51,52] There is considerable evidence in the literature demonstrating the improvement that clinical guidelines can have on standards of care.[6] Though intended to guide judgement and decision-making to obtain high-quality outcomes, protocols and procedures, and their implementation, clinical guidelines are far from infallible. Clinical guidelines and protocols are socially constructed—that is, they 'propose regulatory principles of action for adoption by individuals, groups and organisations'.[53] Protocols, policies and procedures are a form of social policy, and the 'uncertainty in the creation of social policy makes error inevitable, and error makes the injustice unavoidable'.[53] Being socially constructed, they provide accounts and representations of people, events and contexts at one point in time and are crafted, communicative objects. Culturally and ideologically, they play an important role.[54] Many factors influence the ways in which individuals interpret and enact these texts and their enactment will inevitably precipitate problems in practice.[6]

Although clinical guidelines are at the heart of quality-improvement strategies, Rycroft-Malone argues that they are not the panacea for professional clinical decision-making or judgement.[55] They are official texts designed to assist individuals in making quality judgements and decisions about patient care. In principle, they are 'systematically developed statements to assist practitioner and patient decisions about appropriate health care for specific circumstances'.[56] Clinical guidelines that are not evidence-based, are not comprehensive, are without context or are applied incorrectly or inconsistently, can have detrimental effects on patient quality and safety. Their use is intended to reduce variability in individual decision-making, to deal with notions of uncertainty and therefore to minimise risk and the generation of error. Recent research illustrates that protocols only provide part of the answer for clinical judgement and decision-making for emergency health professionals. One Australian study explored paramedic clinical judgement and decision-making and determined that decisions were not wholly governed by protocols, legislation, policies, guidelines and other normative and prescriptive instruments. Rather, their practice was highly individualised and influenced by the contextual and mediating elements, as illustrated in Fig. 11.3.[6] Their clinical judgement

FIGURE 11.3 CONCEPTUALISING PARAMEDIC CLINICAL JUDGEMENT AND DECISION-MAKING OF MENTAL ILLNESS IN THE FIELD[6]

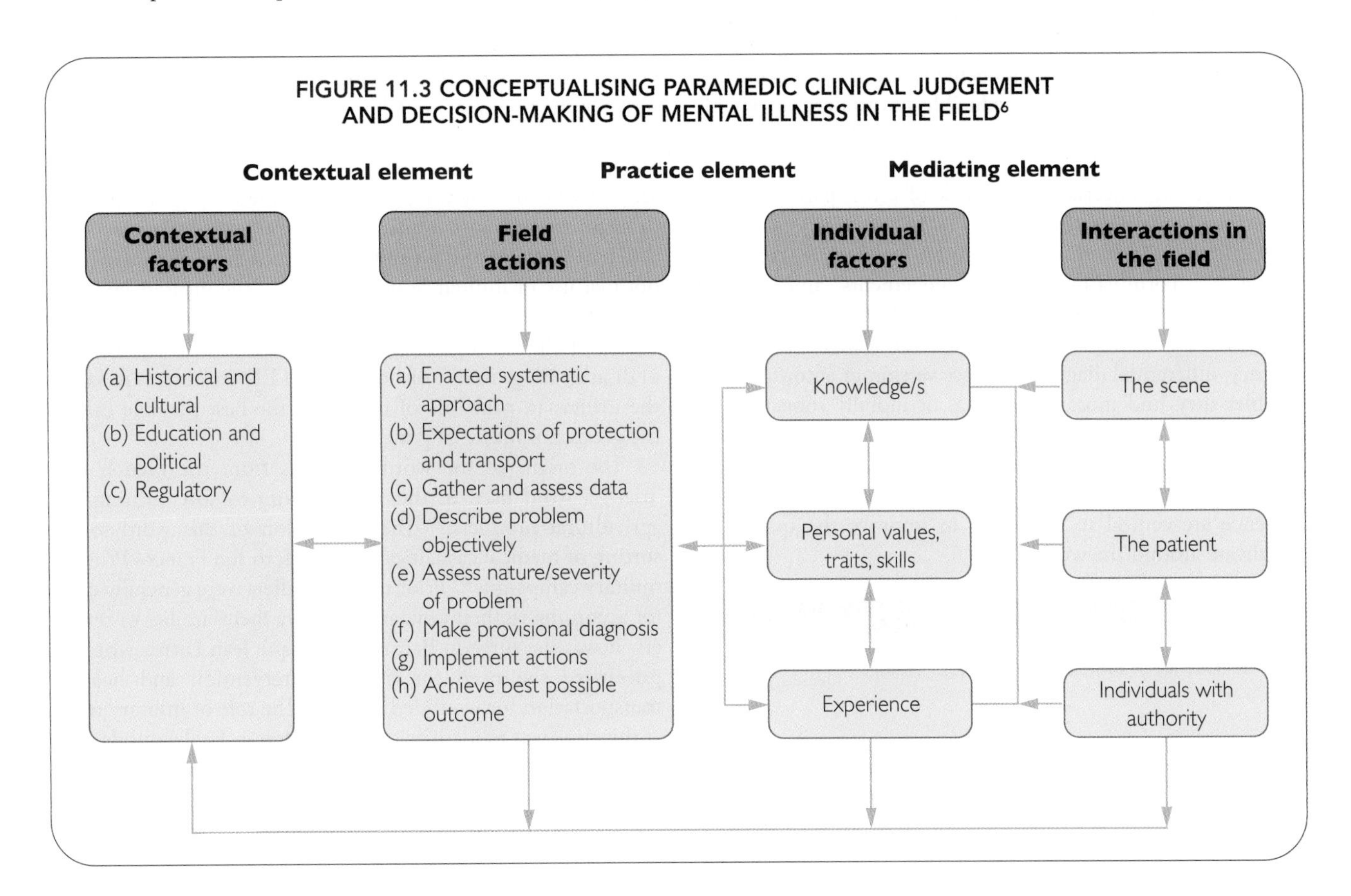

and decision-making comprised three different interconnected elements—contextual, practice and mediating. Fundamental to judgement practice was the *contextual element*, an amalgam of organisational and occupational factors associated with various historical, cultural, educational, political and regulatory dimensions. The *practice element* consisted of field actions for problem-solving and a range of individual-specific factors. The *mediating element* was comprised of social interactions within the scene, with the patient and with individuals in authority. These interactions influenced the success of clinical judgement and decision-making, in particular their interactions with the patient, doctors, relatives, bystanders and other individuals in authority.[6] The use of an interpretive, naturalistic case study that adopted this descriptive theoretical framework unearthed the complex mix of elements that characterised the paramedics' accounts of their own judgement practice. At issue in this study was the preparedness of paramedics to recognise, assess and manage mental illness in everyday practice and the sufficiency of education and training programs, clinical standards, policy and legislation for ensuring safe practice and accountability in the field.[6]

PRACTICE TIP

Clinical reasoning should always feature more than the individual nurse or paramedic, and include the patient and others.

Sometimes the clinical judgements and decisions made by healthcare professionals are insufficient or inaccurate, and sometimes inappropriate.[11] The fallibility of clinical judgement and decision-making has always presented problems for individuals, professions, communities and societies.[53] Broadly speaking, when it comes to judgement and decision-making, there is always the risk of 'irreducible uncertainty, inevitable error and unavoidable injustice'.[53] Because of this, research into judgement and decision-making has for decades focused heavily on reducing uncertainty and risk of error, particularly in professional practice settings.[11]

Clinical judgement and decision-making is far from simple.[57,58] Formulating clinical judgements and making decisions for high-quality and safe healthcare are complex processes.[57,58] Making judgements and decisions about triage urgency, differential diagnoses, whose version or account of the troubles they find most convincing, or morally robust,[40,57] is challenging. One notable priority for healthcare professionals for ensuring quality healthcare is the mandate for evidence-based practice. Production and use of the best available evidence are central to all efforts to improve the quality of healthcare around the world.[59,60]

PRACTICE TIP

The absence of evidence is not always evidence of absence.

Providing evidence-based healthcare may be a contemporary imperative, but there are many challenges to achieving this goal. In emergency care, there are some areas of practice where there is comparatively little evidence on which to base practice and the evidence–practice gap is substantial.[61] Some kinds of evidence—namely randomised controlled trials, systematic reviews and meta-analyses—carry greater weight in the hierarchy of evidence for knowledge generated in this way often limits or undervalues the influence of context in generating the best available evidence. In the context of emergency care, evidence-based healthcare can be particularly challenging. Refer to Chapter 7 for further discussion of levels of evidence.

The demands that the context of emergency healthcare places on doctors, nurses and paramedics to render life-saving care to the sick and injured are complex, time-pressured and often high-stakes.[62,63] Healthcare professionals, or first-contact practitioners,[12] such as paramedics and triage nurses, often have scant evidence to support their clinical practice. Nevertheless, they 'go about their ordinary but complicated business of making sense of the symptoms and troubles of their patients and clients'.[11]

TRIAGE

The role of triage is central to quality and safety in emergency care and paramedic practice. Healthcare workers in emergency care routinely use triage to prioritise patients according to their level of clinical urgency. As a clinical tool, triage is commonly enacted when the resources on hand are inadequate for the number or nature of those injured, such as during a multi-casualty event. In instances where demand exceeds supply, the allocation of resources for care is aimed at achieving the best possible clinical outcome for the greatest number of patients.

The philosophical underpinnings of triage are utilitarian—arguing for the rational use of limited resources to ensure the greatest good for the greatest number; and egalitarian—intended to achieve fair treatment of patients. Under normal circumstances where the number of patients is manageable in terms of the resources available, triage is egalitarian and patients with a high degree of clinical urgency are treated first and are allocated the most resources. In circumstances where resources are overwhelmed by the numbers of patients (e.g. in a disaster or mass casualty situations—see Chapter 12), triage serves a different purpose and a utilitarian approach is taken to ensure optimal use of limited resources; that is, the greatest good for the greatest number. Under disaster triage, patients with a high degree of clinical urgency may be the lowest priority. The aim of disaster triage in out-of-hospital and ED contexts is to satisfy the utilitarian principle of providing the best possible care to the greatest number of patients.

The origin of the word 'triage' is from the French verb 'trier', a word used in the 18th century to sort farming and agricultural products.[64] The application of this word to the sorting of medical casualties dates back to the Franco–Prussian military campaigns.[65] Prior to this, soldiers were generally cared for according to their rank and often by their families or retainers. It was the surgeon Baron Dominique Jean Larrey who first prioritised the need for medical intervention and hospital transportation for wounded soldiers. The role of military triage at this time was to identify soldiers with non-fatal wounds. This meant that soldiers with minor injuries were medically treated while those mortally wounded were left to die. The main benefit of implementing a triage system was to accelerate the return of soldiers to the battlefield.[66]

While triage remained a process confined to military campaigns, it underwent extensive refinement during subsequent wars (World War I and II, and the Korean, Vietnam, Falkland and Gulf wars). Evidence was building of mortality-rate reduction by early assessment, prompt resuscitation and fast patient transfer in military hospital settings and battlefields. Soldier mortality rate reduced from 5% during World War II to 1% by the end of the Vietnam War.[66] By the 1970s, the patient outcome benefits evident in military triage had captured the interest of governments and hospital service providers, resulting in formal triage systems being implemented in some civilian EDs.[67]

In Australia, before the introduction of triage into civilian EDs, medical and non-medical personnel, such as clerks, performed the initial patient assessment. The need to obtain patient and financial details saw the role commonly performed by clerical staff.[66] Generally, patients were processed on a first-come first-served basis. While this was an efficient system when patient presentation numbers were low, it proved unsafe when large numbers of patients arrived at the same time.

The ED nurse triage role was introduced to improve the timely recognition of patients with life-threatening conditions, and to ensure the safety of waiting room patients, the appropriate allocation of resources and the overall efficiency of ED services.[68] By the late 1980s, people presenting to an Australasian ED for care were met by the triage nurse who assessed their clinical urgency. Since this time, decision-making and activity by triage nurses has been shown to significantly influence the patient's experience of emergency care, mortality, morbidity and satisfaction rates.[69,70]

In emergency care settings, triage outcomes are used during clinical audit to assess patient outcome.[71] The quality of triage can influence patient length of stay, rates of admission to intensive care units and morbidity and mortality. The majority of research literature related to triage decision-making has been conducted by expert emergency nurses from a number of perspectives. Studies have also focused on inter-rater and intra-rater reliability of triage decisions;[70,72–74] influences on triage decision-making, including triage nurse characteristics;[72,74–76] ED workload;[77–79] financial incentives;[80] and patient populations.[81,82] Knowledge and experience of triage personnel are two factors that have dominated research related to triage decision-making, although no research has found a significant relationship between experience and triage decision-making.[75,76] In contrast, factual knowledge appears to be more important than years of triage experience in improving the accuracy of triage decisions.[4,76,83]

PRACTICE TIP

Review triage decisions systematically, particularly in light of the deteriorating patient.

TRIAGE DECISION-MAKING TOOLS

There have been many triage tools developed to assist paramedics and emergency nurses to determine medical urgency, treatment priority and location.[28,38,84–86] Globally, EDs in many countries, such as Australia, Aotearoa New Zealand, Canada and the United Kingdom, have adopted a five-level urgency triage system.[87] For example, Australasia has endorsed the Australasian Triage Scale (ATS), the UK has widely adopted the Manchester Triage System (MTS), Canada has adopted the Canadian Triage and Acuity Scale (CTAS), and Germany and the United States commonly use the Emergency Severity Index (ESI).[86,88] There is significant evidence that a five-level triage scale is better than a three-level triage system.[86,88]

Paramedic triage systems have also been developed and implemented to improve recognition of medical urgency and triage assessment. Common paramedical decision tools include: SALT (sort-assess-lifesaving intervention-treatment/transport); jumpSTART (simple triage and rapid transport); and Triage sieve.[38,89–91] Often these decision tools are applied in a mass casualty situation and evidence suggests that the triage tool SALT compared to START, Triage sieve and CareFlight has greater accuracy for patient outcomes.[38,89–91] However, all tools demonstrated a moderate level of under triage.[90] Compared with ED triage systems, there is a lack of evidence to support the effectiveness of paramedical triage tools.[92,93]

THE AUSTRALASIAN TRIAGE SCALE

Across Australia and Aotearoa New Zealand, governments were seeking ways to improve safety, regulate, compare and predict the cost of emergency services. To gain some control over the escalating ED cost of healthcare, financial models started including triage data.[94] Given that triage codes were being examined to predict costs and that many EDs had developed their own guidelines, clinicians were motivated to establish national triage guidelines to secure greater equity of access, potentially within funding models.[95]

Australian triage guidelines were developed to assist triage nurse recognition of patient urgency; to achieve greater safety, consistency and uniformity within practice; and to create equity within ED funding models.[95] In 1994 the National Triage Scale (NTS), which in 2002 became known as the Australasian Triage Scale (ATS), was introduced in Australia.[96] The ATS, implemented across Australia and Aotearoa New Zealand, consisted of five scales that link patient history, signs and symptoms, and diagnosis to clinical urgency,[97] and incorporates a hierarchy of medical and nursing response times for patients (Table 11.1).

To aid the application, veracity and standardisation of ED triage, a number of healthcare information systems integrate triage processes into electronic Medical Record (eMR) systems. The purpose of the eMR information system is to enable clinicians to view an integrated patient record, order and

TABLE 11.1 AUSTRALASIAN TRIAGE SCALE[96]

ATS CODE	RESPONSE TIME
Code 1 (resuscitation)	Requires immediate intervention
Code 2 (emergency)	Requires intervention within 10 minutes
Code 3 (urgent)	Should be seen within 30 minutes
Code 4 (semi-urgent)	Should be seen within 1 hour
Code 5 (non-urgent)	Should be seen within 2 hours

TABLE 11.2 TRIAGE PERFORMANCE BENCHMARKS[96,99]

	ACEM%	NZ%
Triage code 1	100	100
Triage code 2	80	80
Triage code 3	75	75
Triage code 4	70	70
Triage code 5	70	70

ACEM – Australian College of Emergency Medicine

review investigations and track the patient journey. The eMR enables greater standardisation, consistency, safety and auditing of healthcare data, thus enabling greater triage surveillance, regulation and prediction of healthcare costs for EDs. With the implementation of the eMR, governments can calculate, audit and predict current and future ED funding needs.[2]

Throughout Australasia, triage code waiting times are also being used to measure and compare ED performance. Waiting times provide a quality indicator for the efficiency and timeliness of ED services.[98,99] Hence, with the implementation of the ATS there was increasing expectation that EDs would demonstrate timely service by meeting the agreed-upon triage code benchmarks. Triage code benchmarks are determined by the percentage of patients seen by a medical officer or nurse practitioner (NP) or extended practice emergency nurse within the specified triage code time-frame (Table 11.2). By the early 1990s, Australia, Aotearoa New Zealand and Canada had adopted the five-scale triage guideline.[66,100,101]

Jelinek and Little[102] assessed the inter-rater reliability of the ATS by having 115 nurses allocate a triage code to 100 hypothetical patient scenarios. The findings from this study demonstrated that between nurses there was high concordance (95% within one category of the modal response) and that despite triage experience and hospital type, the ATS appropriately and consistently measured clinical urgency. The results are supported by other researchers who found inter-rater reliability at between 80% and 95%.[103,104] While these studies confirmed that the ATS was a reliable measure of patient urgency, they identified that some patients continued to be over- or under-triaged—accounting for inter-rater disagreement rates of between 5% and 20%.[103,105]

As a result, ongoing modification and review of the ATS occurs to ensure that vulnerable groups are not marginalised and/or disadvantaged.[95,98,100] For example, the triage guidelines initially were not sensitive in identifying the urgency of acutely ill children.[106] Browne and colleagues[106] provided evidence that the ATS did not consistently identify children with urgent conditions. Similarly, Durojaiye and O'Meara's[107] study confirmed inconsistent application of the guidelines for seriously ill children. This indicated that the guidelines needed to be revised for specific vulnerable population groups. Consequently, the ATS was revised to accommodate these vulnerable populations.

Researchers were also interested in identifying the reliability of the ATS when measuring a range of patient outcomes, such as admission rates. Hollis and Sprivulis[108] identified that, despite ED activity, admission rates for codes 1, 2 and 3 were consistent with ATS guidelines. Other researchers examined and demonstrated a strong association between triage codes and patient diagnoses, management, admission, morbidity and mortality rate.[98,105,109,110]

Australasian studies convincingly established the inter-rater reliability of the ATS and identified that greater consistency and recognition of clinical urgency were present when triage nurses used these guidelines. There is Level II,[111,112] Level III[100,102,106] and Level IV[75,108] evidence to support the continued use and acceptance of the five-level ATS guidelines. (See Chapter 7 for a more detailed understanding of research evidence levels.)

TRIAGE NURSE DECISION-MAKING

Emergency nurses, when undertaking triage, are required to determine a patient's medical urgency, the allocation of departmental resources (allocation of beds and clinical areas), initiation of interventions and management of incidents and service flow.[113] To this end, the role of triage requires the nurse to undertake primary and secondary triage.

Across Australia and Aotearoa New Zealand, healthcare infrastructure is composed of hospitals that provide different levels of emergency care (see Chapter 1). Designated EDs are located largely in urban settings, while rural, remote and very remote health centres have designated treatment rooms that provide limited resuscitation practices. Rural and remote healthcare providers face significant challenges, specifically relating to access, staff retention, resources and distances between geographically isolated locations.[114]

Work demands on healthcare workers in rural and regional areas would appear to be different compared with metropolitan areas.[115] One Australian study examined general practitioner (GP) income, work hours and dependence on Medicare reimbursement in rural settings. The cross-sectional, retrospective analysis of rural and urban doctors demonstrated that GPs in rural and regional areas provided greater after-hour patient contact episodes, worked longer and earnt less than metropolitan-based GPs.[114] The trend was also evident within the international literature.[116] In addition, non-metropolitan healthcare workers often lacked separation between work and private life.

Across Australia, there are 217 very remote communities and 271 health services, sites or facilities that provide emergency services with limited resuscitation capabilities. Compared with remote, rural or regional communities, Indigenous Australians largely compose the populations that live in remote and very remote communities (18% of the total population). Many of the very remote services ($n = 133$) are staffed by, and for, Indigenous communities.[117] By contrast, Māori healthcare providers are under-represented in Aotearoa New Zealand rural and semi-rural healthcare communities. In Aotearoa New Zealand, a Māori health provider is an organisation that delivers health services largely for Māori and is managed by Māori.[118]

Rural, remote and very remote emergency nurses undertake triage, but then go on to provide first-line emergency care (FLEC) and definitive patient management and/or referral.[119] For emergency services, where medical review is limited, the ATS waiting time benchmark is examined with respect to the 'nurse seen time'. Many rural, remote and very remote communities experience significant healthcare isolation.[101,120,121] To reduce isolation and improve healthcare access throughout Australasia, telephone triage initiatives, such as HealthDirect hotline and the Bush Support Line have been developed.[122–124]

In geographically isolated regions, nurses and paramedical staff have extended their scope of practice through successful completion of educational courses. For example, nurses in rural Aotearoa New Zealand are able to expand their scope of practice through the PRIME (Primary Response in Medical Emergencies) program. To improve Aotearoa New Zealand rural health, the PRIME program was implemented nationally.[125] Equivalent first-line emergency care courses are available throughout Australia.[126] These educational initiatives aim to meet the needs of healthcare providers working in rural, remote and very remote emergency settings, where, as the first responder, they must triage, resuscitate and manage the patient.

PRIMARY TRIAGE DECISIONS

Primary triage decisions are focused on identifying life-threatening conditions and then delivering appropriate interventions and first aid. The initial assessment evaluates the patient's airway, breathing, circulation and infection risk and only if the patient is determined stable should the triage nurse then focus on the patient's primary complaint. Using this primary decision, triage nurses determine the appropriate urgency code. In this way, triage code allocation regulates the timing of medical and nursing care.[66]

The determination of a patient's clinical urgency must be independent of ED activity, patient behaviour, benchmarking practices and incentive funding.[68,100,127] The most urgent clinical patient feature should determine triage code selection and infection risk. This may be identified during the history, physical assessment or when the clinician obtains vital signs. The COVID-19 pandemic experience has impacted on triage processes and heightened vigilance of infection control risk to limit transmissible events within the ED. Refer to Chapter 27 for guidance on infection control management. Selection of the correct triage code will avoid incidences of over- or under-triaging and provide for safer patient outcomes. To minimise over- or under-triaging, triage nurses need to have emergency experience to become skillful in the recognition of a range of conditions and injuries and develop information-gathering skills to be able to determine patient urgency.[128]

Central to achieving this primary outcome is the triage nurse's ability to systematically trawl for information, recognise and discriminate between patterns of clinical urgency, develop a working diagnosis, predict patient care needs and evaluate collected information.[128,129] Triage nurses collect objective and subjective data, which enable clinical urgency to be determined. Mass casualty and trauma triage concepts and guidelines are presented in Chapters 12 and 42 respectively.

PRACTICE TIP

If you are unsure in your decision-making, the best and safest approach is to triage up and/or seek clarification from senior emergency staff.

Objective data

Triage nurses should begin each patient assessment with a primary survey. This information process begins with inspection (visual observation of the patient). It is important 'just to look at the patient'. Initial observations of a patient should include general appearance and the degree of distress and emotional responses. This information provides an opportunity to form working diagnoses or suppositions. Triage nurses should also obtain collateral information from sources such as family.[130,131] For example, a patient may present with pathology, radiological and/or interventional reports. These information sources can help to support triage decision-making. In the ED, a triage working diagnosis frames impressions of a patient's urgency and the need to allocate a bed. A working diagnosis can be confirmed or refuted during the triage interview and on the collection of physiological data.

Physiological data

Triage nurses should regularly choose to collect respiratory and haemodynamic data. Such data should inform triage decision-making and discriminate between more- or less-urgent cases. For example, tachypnoea is a more accurate predictor of serious illness than any other vital sign change.[132–134] Physiological assessment can assist in the identification of red flags. Physiological red flags are suggestive of actual or potential threats to patient safety.[128,129] Yet, assessment of all vital signs may not be required for life-threatening conditions, actual or potential (triage code 1 and 2 patients); only the information required to make a triage decision should be collected. For vital sign values see Chapter 13.

PRACTICE TIP

All triage decisions should be supported by physiological data to ensure patient safety.

Subjective data

The triage nurse concurrently collects and collates subjective data.[129] This involves collecting information that provides an understanding of 'why' the patient is presenting to the ED (primary complaint). Additional patient information to be elicited and collated includes: the precipitating event, onset of symptoms, medical history and medications and allergies. This information enables a more complete clinical picture, early detection of red flags and accurate triage decision-making.

Triage nurses typically gather information using focused questioning.[26] Triage nurse questioning should target the main reason for a patient presenting to an ED (chief complaint). By using open-ended questioning techniques, triage nurses should be able to gather information that 'funnels down' from the broad complaint to specific signs and symptoms. This funnelling process enables triage nurses to determine risk, quickly problem-solve and use critical reasoning to gain insight into the patient's chief complaint.[128,129]

PRACTICE TIP

Questions to consider asking at triage include: What brought you to hospital today? Do you have any medical conditions or injuries? Do you have any allergies? In determining urgency, it is important to explore the duration and potential cause(s) of presenting signs and symptoms to identify red flags and minimise over- or under-triaging.

Patient problems and potential diagnosis

When triage nurses gather patient information, they measure this against clinical templates stored from practical experience and theoretical knowledge. By taking a patient's history, undertaking a focused physical examination, obtaining relevant vital signs and symptoms and then comparing this information with mental models, triage nurses are able to discriminate between the different levels of urgency. Triage nurses rely on pattern recognition when gathering information to refine decision-making processes, direct choice and accelerate decision-making.[4,135]

While pattern recognition enables triage nurses to discriminate between more- or less-urgent cases, the prioritisation of a patient's need for care is accelerated through the development of a working diagnosis based on clinical problems. A working diagnosis is used by triage nurses as a strategy to confirm or refute life-threatening conditions, patient urgency, determine an appropriate clinical area and predict care interventions. A triage working diagnosis helps to make sense of the act of triage, assists decision-making processes, reduces patient and family anxiety, expands professional confidence and adds an element of personal satisfaction to the role.[129,136]

PRACTICE TIP

In some instances, physical examination of a patient at triage can assist with the determination of urgency and differentiation between triage categories. In this way physical examination can alert the triage nurse to more or less urgent conditions and/or minimise over- or under-triaging.

SECONDARY TRIAGE DECISIONS

Secondary triage decisions involve the appropriate allocation of ED resources and the initiation of emergency care. Secondary decisions are based on assessment data and a working diagnosis, which inform decisions about further investigations, or interventions. The aim of secondary triage decisions is to ensure patient safety, promote comfort and expedite timely and appropriate emergency care.

PRACTICE TIP

It is important to obtain sufficient history as synthesis of this information assists with diagnostic determination, investigations and disposition considerations.

Triage extended practices

Triage nurses often initiate extended practices, which modulate a timing of ED care that creates a process of 'timekeeping'. Triage nurses use timekeeping practices to maintain, regulate or restore a normal rhythm of emergency care to the waiting area. Triage timekeeping processes sustain and maintain appropriate patient flow and resource use, while supporting patient assessment and urgency recognition decision-making. The decision to undertake investigational and/or extended activities occurs simultaneously with triage code and clinical area allocation. Evidence suggests that triage nurse pain management[137–139] and radiological investigations[140,141] contribute to improved patient outcomes and more timely, efficient and equitable healthcare services.

Triage gatekeeping processes

Primary and secondary triage decision-making is sustained through a process of gatekeeping. Gatekeeping regulates patient flow, and through this process a patient's clinical need is appropriately matched with a geographical ED workspace 'inside'.[113] For example, a patient requiring urgent medical intervention would be allocated to an appropriate resuscitation workspace where care is optimised and delivered by appropriately qualified nursing and medical staff. Triage nurses know that clinical areas provide different levels of care appropriate for a patient's condition or injury and that this determines a normal pattern of patient movement.

The fragmentation of workspaces into 'place' enables a process of gatekeeping to occur and triage decision-making to be ordered and consistent. Different meanings of time punctuate clinical areas, which hierarchically order practice and staff activities. Consequently, each ED clinical area reflects varying levels of urgency, timeliness, efficiency and control, characterising different workspaces into 'places'. Once nurses have learnt the meanings applied to work 'places' and the different patient groups, they are able to make effective triage choices and predict care needs. Triage nurses use gatekeeping processes to accomplish the appropriate allocation of service resources to a patient's medical need, thereby minimising risk and securing patient flow, consistency and patient safety.[66]

TRIAGE NURSE EDUCATION

The triage role requires the nurse to have advanced cognitive, communication and decision-making skills and the ability to collate knowledge systems, patterns of knowing and ways of doing with a patient's physiological, interpersonal and communicative signs. In addition, the ATS guidelines, well validated and reliable, provide a frame of reference for nurses to determine an appropriate urgency scale for presenting patients.[136]

Triage education programs need to develop strategies, in combination with the Emergency Triage Education Kit (ETEK), that foster advanced skills and provide practical opportunities to develop patterns of 'knowing'.[136] To this end, emergency educators can support triage decision-making by adapting local educational initiatives that target systematically high levels of problem-solving and questioning in order to achieve more thoughtful triage practice responses.[128,129]

PRACTICE TIP

Blended triage educational learning opportunities that comprise mentoring, patient urgency scenario practice, interviewing skills and simulation will better support knowledge translation and build triage skill capacity.

Triage education programs can assist nurses to understand the character of the role. Patients, families and carers and triage nurses have established values and expectations of services that are not often aligned. Greater patient, family and carer engagement can increase awareness of differing expectations and increase tolerance, particularly when experiencing a clash of expectations in the allocation of beds, resources and the management of incidents, such as with patient overcrowding (refer to Chapter 6).[130,142] Triage educational strategies should provide opportunity for novice triage nurses to work beside an experienced clinician to assist the development of these practical aspects of gatekeeping.[66]

When EDs are overcrowded, time pressures increase and can often induce negative experience patterns for both patients and clinicians.[143,144] By making this dimension of triage practice transparent, conflicting interests and knowledge systems that compete to build 'threatening' or 'blame' environments can be avoided. In addition, novice triage nurses may benefit from an introductory period free of extended-role activities. Once adjustment to the role is complete, extended practices can be introduced into the nurse's craft repertoire. This may result in greater consistency in triage practice.[141]

Triage nurses need to be provided with opportunities to reflect on belief systems, biases, assumptions, expectations and ways of thinking, which are embedded within emergency care. Through reflective practices, nursing independence within the context of triage practice can be secured; and more-responsible decision-making, disciplined and compassionate work practices achieved.[145] This educational process should give triage nurses the wherewithal to extract complex meanings from experiences and analyse practice patterns.

Educational forums need to be structured, whereby experienced and novice triage nurses are brought together as a group. These focus groups provide opportunity for triage nurses to share their experiences and practices for information gathering, managing difficult triage situations and resource allocation, thus improving gatekeeping, timekeeping and decision-making skills. This process would assist nurses to understand what makes practice reasonable and would promote ethical and compassionate patterns of knowing and acting.

To reduce the potential influence of an emotionally charged triage response to a particular situation or event, triage nurses must develop emotional intelligence to learn how emotions can hold sway over gatekeeping, timekeeping and decision-making processes.[66,146] The convergence of different expectations (patient and/or nurse) often precipitates emotionally labile situations that escalate troubling or aggressive behaviour. Triage nurses must be prepared to confront and mediate ethical issues, contradictions, conflict and practical dilemmas in order to foster more tolerant and caring triage practices.

PARAMEDIC APPLICATIONS: PATTERNS AND PROTOCOLS AND TRIAGE FOR PROBLEM-SOLVING

In the contemporary context, paramedics encounter a diverse range of problems, for which they are expected to arrive at a single, correct solution. The emphasis is on the early identification of the most serious problems, which in turn enables the paramedic to achieve their core goal of providing the best outcome for the patient.[21,147] In 2013, the Convention of Ambulance Authorities and Paramedics Australasia[148] established professional competency standards for paramedics. These underpin practice standards for paramedic curriculum and practice. Bendall and Morrison[25] describe clinical judgement and decision-making as 'fundamental to the role of a professional paramedic' and 'core business'. In their view, the acquisition of good quality information and its synthesis are essential to clinical judgement and decision-making: 'best information best judgement'. Bendall and Morrison describe how expertise is developed in paramedic decision-making. Citing Billett,[149] they suggest that there are five cognitive decision-making strategies that are common to emergency medical services, these being algorithmic, pattern recognition, worst-case scenario (rule out), event-driven and hypothetico-deductive. They suggest that algorithms are common in ambulance services to support pattern recognition.[25,150] Bendall and Morrison argue that when problem-solving, paramedics make use of five elements,[25] which is consistent with guidelines in popular paramedic textbooks from the United States.[150,151]

A cognitive assessment of paramedics' and triage nurses' problem-solving has been reported in recent studies.[7,152,153] For example, Alexander examined the cognitive processes by which paramedics in the United States undertook clinical reasoning.[153] Verbal protocol analysis and think-aloud methods were used to analyse the current and retrospective clinical reasoning of ten paramedics when solving two vignettes. Alexander argues that paramedic clinical decision-making is derived from the practice of emergency medicine, which renders the cognition literature on medicine and emergency medicine a suitable comparison for research purposes in the absence of paramedic-specific literature.[153] Moreover, Alexander argues that in the United States, emergency doctors are intimately involved with all aspects of paramedic practice, are the primary authors and content editors of paramedic training textbooks, and are required to approve all accredited paramedic training programs and all paramedic provider services.[153] Paramedics in Alexander's study[153] were found to solve problems primarily by pattern recognition without adequate hypothesis testing. According to Alexander, paramedics' patient assessment and illness scripts for both sets of vignettes were 'inadequately developed, disorganised, and, in some ways, faulty'.[153] Moreover, in the absence of adequate illness scripts for pattern recognition and adequate hypothesis testing, paramedics in the study generated pseudo-information and used cognitive biases in their problem-solving. For the vignettes presented, the paramedics had a low threshold for initiating treatment, and provided inappropriate treatment. Alexander has called for additional research and argues that 'changes in paramedic education practice should focus on providing meaningful learning experiences, promoting learner reflection on problem-solving and giving feedback on clinical reasoning processes in order to improve the quality of paramedics' illness scripts and clinical reasoning processes'.[153]

The use of pattern recognition by paramedics is underpinned by clinical guidelines and protocols. Individuals and organisations use clinical guidelines and protocols to limit the occurrence and impact of error. Ambulance services provide paramedics with case-management guidelines and protocols to assist them in achieving the desired outcome in the best interests of the patient. Box 11.2 provides practical tips for minimising error in clinical judgement and decision-making, particularly in emergency healthcare.

PRACTICE TIP

Review guidelines and protocols systematically based on evidence and the extent to which they enable timely, effective problem-solving.

BOX 11.2 TIPS FOR MINIMISING ERROR IN JUDGEMENT PRACTICE[5,6]

- Maintain a systematic assessment and judgement practice.
- Gather and organise data, and form concepts and patterns of injury and illness.
- Focus on specific and multiple elements of data concurrently.
- Identify and deal with uncertainty as much as is possible.
- Differentiate between relevant and irrelevant data.
- Analyse events and situations in light of past experience.
- Recall cases in which judgements and decisions were incorrect or inaccurate.
- Construct and articulate arguments in support of your judgement practice and clinical reasoning.
- Seek the advice and opinion of others, particularly those with different skills and expertise.
- Communicate your assessments and plans to others in a clear and concise manner.
- Test and critically evaluate your assessment and assumptions with your peers and colleagues.

TRIAGE DOCUMENTATION AND LEGAL ASPECTS

The documented triage assessment should constitute the first part of the patient's emergency care notes and may commence in out-of-hospital or ED contexts. Triage clinicians should document every triage episode undertaken within their institution or service. Triage clinicians should also enter treatment contemporaneously, as this avoids reliance on personal memory.

PRACTICE TIP

Triage documentation should include the clinician's name, date and time of assessment, presenting complaint (history), a focused patient assessment, infection risk and red flags, triage code, treatment area and interventions implemented.[129,136,154]

The triage documentation should be sufficient to explain the allocated triage code, clinical area and interventions instigated by the emergency care clinician. The triage clinicians should not make an entry on behalf of someone else. Triage documentation has the potential to be admitted as legal evidence if it is relevant to a matter being dealt with in a court of law or a coronial inquest. While medical records are not legal documents, they can be submitted as legal evidence. In some instances, medical records are used to determine whether a coronial investigation is required to determine the cause of death. High-quality nursing documentation remains part of a nurse's accountability. Good documentation can assist a nurse if called upon to account for their professional actions.

Medical records require explanation of actions.[51] The triage clinician should only document the facts, relevant patient assessment and interventions. Triage clinicians should document treatments/procedures and reasons why. Triage assessments and reassessments must be contemporaneous, and notes and information should never be obliterated (see Chapter 4).

If triage clinicians are using telephone or radio orders from supporting medical officers, it is important to adhere to organisational requirements. This may include another person listening to, and counter-signing, the order on the phone. If this is not possible, make sure the medical officer repeats the order and then, for confirmation, repeat the order back to them. It is also important that telephone or radio orders are accurately recorded in the patient's notes.

The consequences of poor documentation are significant for the patient and emergency care clinicians. Not only does poor documentation present a significant risk to patient safety and the quality of their health experience and outcomes, but it also exposes emergency care clinicians to actions for negligence and breaches in tort. There is perhaps no greater professional risk to emergency care clinicians than failure to adequately document patient refusal of treatment and/or transportation.

There are a variety of systems used by emergency care clinicians for gathering and documenting information for high-quality and safe out-of-hospital and ED care within Australia and Aotearoa New Zealand. The more common of these are described in Table 11.3. Recent research into the practices of Australian paramedics shows that paramedics' gathering and reporting of information follows the requirements of the formal document, particularly with the move to electronic ambulance records. Such systems prompt paramedics for the information required.[6]

Regardless of the individual system or method used, there are critical features of the gathering, documenting and

TABLE 11.3 POPULAR MNEMONICS FOR GATHERING AND DOCUMENTING INFORMATION

ISBAR[155]	SOAP[150]	HIRAID[129]	SAMPLE[150]	CHART[150]	IMIST-AMBO[156]
Identify	**S**ubjective data	**H**istory	**S**igns and symptoms	**C**hief complaint	**I**dentification of the patient
Situation	**O**bjective data	**I**nfection-risk	**A**llergies	**H**istory	**M**echanism/Medical complaint
Background	**A**ssessment data	**R**ed flags	**M**edications	**A**ssessment	**I**njuries/Information relative to the complaint
Assessment/Agreed plan	**P**lan for patient management	**A**ssessment	**P**ast medical history	t**R**eatment	**S**igns/vitals/GCS
Recommendations/Read back		**I**nterventions	**L**ast meal or intake	**T**ransport	**T**reatment and trends/response to treatment–
		Diagnostics	**E**vents pre-emergency		**A**llergies
					Medications
					Background history
					Other (social) information

communicating of information for providing high-quality and safe pre-hospital emergency care. These include:

- accuracy
- timeliness
- completeness
- legibility
- originality
- objectivity.

Attention paid to such measures will ensure that emergency care clinicians augment efforts to provide high-quality and safety in pre-hospital emergency care.

PRACTICE TIP

Ensure records are legible, timely, accurate, complete, original, factual and objective.

SPECIAL CONDITIONS

EMERGENCY DEPARTMENT OVERCROWDING

Emergency department overcrowding is a pandemic whole-of-health-system problem and often results in ambulance patients experiencing prolonged waits for transfer to an appropriate clinical area bed (ramping).[157,158] ED overcrowding jeopardises care practices, patient and staff safety and the overall functioning of the ED.[159–161] Within Australasia, ED overcrowding is commonly attributed to an increase in patients with non-urgent problems seeking ED care; however, this is often not the case. ED overcrowding is largely the result of increasing demand for healthcare services and declining hospital bed numbers.[160,161] This has meant that ambulance patients and/or admitted patients are waiting longer in the ED for a ward bed to become available.[44,157,158,162,163] Overcrowding has specific implications for paramedics and triage nurses, in that their ability to obtain handover and allocate an appropriate clinical area to match the patient's need is significantly reduced.[157,158] Hence, for triage nurses, overcrowding usually results in patients with higher urgency conditions being placed in the waiting room until an appropriate clinical area bed and staff resources become available.

ED overcrowding poses a great challenge to patient safety, as the risk of deterioration for patients in the waiting room escalates. In addition, during periods of overcrowding, aggression and behaviours of concern are a common experience for the triage nurse. To ensure patient safety during episodes of ED overcrowding, strategies need to be in place that enable regular patient reassessment, communication and evaluation to occur.[44,164] Additional nursing resources and/or new models of care may need to be implemented to enable more-frequent patient re-evaluations to take place until an appropriate clinical area becomes available.

Triage nurses need to regularly undertake a risk assessment to maintain or restore a safe triage environment for staff, patients, families and/or carers. During periods of overcrowding, waiting rooms and ambulance corridors can be overflowing with acute patients.[157,158,163,165] In these instances, frequent re-assessment is required to minimise the risk of patient deterioration within the waiting room. To date, while EDs may have dedicated nurse–patient ratios for bed areas, the waiting room and ambulance waiting areas have never been included in workforce planning numbers and hence are unstaffed areas. As a result, triage nurses may need to seek assistance to better ensure the safety and early identification of deterioration for those waiting.[132,166] For ED staff and patient safety, the following hospital resources and equipment should be viewed as standard: security personnel should be located within the ED to ensure a timely and active security presence and the resolution of troubling behaviour; the triage and clerical areas should have access to direct telephone lines to police and security. Other security features to be considered include personal staff mobile duress alarms, metal detectors and camera surveillance equipment. All ED staff should be required to undertake educational courses in aggression minimisation.[167,168]

PRACTICE TIP

Maintaining or restoring a safe environment can often be achieved by the triage nurse's ability to implement aggression minimisation strategies.[169,170]

EMERGENCY TREATMENT PERFORMANCE TARGET

Across Australia and Aotearoa New Zealand, time performance targets have been implemented for EDs.[169] In Australia, this target is known as the Emergency Treatment Performance (ETP) target or National Emergency Access Target (NEAT) depending on the jurisdiction. This performance indicator was introduced to ensure that 81% of patients presenting to ED are managed and discharged within 4 hours.[171] In contrast, Aotearoa New Zealand has a time target of 6 hours.[172] In part, time targets were introduced to drive service delivery and reduce ED overcrowding, commonly the result of ED processing patterns and/or hospital admission delays. A key emergency performance target broadly accepted globally is measured from the time of triage (first clinician assessment) to ED discharge. While emergency performance is also a hospital issue, meeting this performance target should assist to reduce the number of patients within the ED. Triage decisions determine how long a patient can safely wait for emergency care, so have been reported as a key influence on an ED's capability to meet NEAT or ETP targets. This is a false assertion, as it is the responsibility of the whole ED to ensure patients receive emergency care according to their clinical urgency as assessed by the triage nurse, and it is a whole-of-hospital responsibility to support patient flow and the effective function of the ED. Further research is needed to explore the impact of performance targets on the triage role, activities and function.[173]

TELEPHONE OR TELEHEALTH TRIAGE

Telephone triage has evolved alongside ED triage to better manage ED workload.[174,175] During the late 1990s, the strategy was widely implemented to reduce ED patient overcrowding.[176] The purpose of telephone triage is to reduce the burden on GPs and acute services, particularly after-hours, by screening and referring patients to appropriate services.[177] In the UK, a national telephone triage centre independent of EDs was initiated, a model that is increasingly being adopted.[65,178,179]

Internationally, telephone triage and advice services have been highly effective in reducing ED utilisation.[179–181] Within the context of healthcare reform, there was already widespread acceptance of nurses providing autonomous, safe, competent and often more-timely care for a range of patient conditions. There was broad engagement with medical staff in the development of agreed protocols and computer software triage progr ams.[36,177,182] Incentives for those calling included the additional provision of screening, health information, secondary urgency triage and a residential care online care service. Across the UK telephone triage advice centres, including ambulance telephone triage enabled quicker access to health information and advice, reducing the need to attend an ED.[36,177,182] Utilisation was better when one contact number was available, and service was timely, national, free and advertised.

Telephone triage has its own unique difficulties when compared with ED triage.[182] These difficulties include the lack of visual cues for assessment and patient compliance. Given legal and patient safety concerns, many Australasian EDs do not provide telephone triage. As a result, governments have developed triage centres with specific telephone triage guidelines. Throughout Australasia, telephone triage systems are able to refer patients to local practitioners, EDs or community services.

Australasia has adult and paediatric telephone triage systems which include: PlunketLine (1994) and Healthline (2005) in Aotearoa New Zealand; and in Australia Kidsnet (1997), HealthDirect (1999), Health-Connect (2000), Nurse-On-Call and HealthDirect (Victoria, 2006). In Western Australia, HealthDirect commenced with experienced nurses to manage telephone calls and provide a range of services, from screening, health information, secondary-urgency triage and a residential care online care service. In July 2007, HealthDirect became part of the National Health Call Centre Network (NHCCN), a nationwide system operating from a single telephone number.

Aotearoa New Zealand's PlunketLine provides expert telephone advice to healthcare workers, parents and caregivers.[177] PlunketLine is now incorporated into Healthline, the free 24-hour 7-day-a-week national service and receives more than 1000 calls a day.[124] Evaluation of Healthline reported high consumer satisfaction, a good safety record and reduced demand on health services. Despite legal and safety concerns, the implementation of telephone triage systems has provided significant positive outcomes for EDs, ambulance personnel, GPs and consumers.[122,177,181,182]

Telehealth has emerged broadly across the Australasian emergency care system largely in response to COVID-19.[183,184] However, in Australia enhanced government funding to support the COVID-19 pandemic response has led to the more recent implementation of telehealth-enabled programs. Telehealth across Australasia now provides a significant role in improving access and equity, especially for rural and regional areas and for people with disability through consultation and triage.[183,185] Telehealth has been shown to reduce ED waiting times, ambulance presentations and community transfers.[183,185,186] Many emergency telehealth programs have been shown to also improve access, clinical effectiveness and patient safety while reducing the risk of COVID-19 infection.[184] Unlike telephone triage, telehealth is reliant on appropriate and reliable internet services, digital technologies and security.[183] When seeking to establish telehealth-enabled programs, clinicians need to consider how patient consent, physical assessment and treatments will be obtained, provided and/or managed.

COMMUNICATING FOR PATIENT SAFETY

Effective communication is vital to safe and quality healthcare and communication failures are a leading cause of harm.[128,129] Through communication processes, health professionals act as a cultural broker for patients and family, staff and other healthcare professionals.[187] A patient's first encounter with the healthcare system is often with a triage nurse. Professional conduct needs to be conveyed within all communication processes and informed patient consent obtained before undertaking relevant triage activities. Indeed, ineffective or inappropriate communication is often the primary source of patient complaints and dissatisfaction.[128,129]

Advanced communication and interpersonal skills are critical to ensure that information from the patient, primary care sector and/or paramedic is appropriately interpreted and synthesised.[180,182] In this way, triage decision-making can be supported and appropriate. Triage nurses and paramedics need to be expert in timely, efficient and effective communication, which is essential to the high-quality functioning of a contemporary emergency medical system. To provide quality pre-hospital and emergency care, paramedics and emergency nurses rely on communication centre staff, comprising experienced and highly trained telephonists, call-takers, dispatchers and clinicians.[188],[189] The dynamic nature of the pre-hospital emergency care setting makes communications challenging.[189] Communicating in the emergency medical system is typically event- or incident-centred, and occurs in five stages, as illustrated in Fig. 11.4.

One of the most important forums for information transfer during the emergency care process is clinical handover.[52,187] Clinical handover is defined as 'the transfer of professional responsibility and accountability for some or all aspects of care for a patient, or group of patients, to another person or professional group on a temporary or permanent basis'.[190] Clinical handover processes are also referred to as hand-off, shift report and patient transfer.[191] The aim of clinical handover is efficient transfer of high-quality clinical information and transfer of responsibility for patient care.[52,187]

Transition of care and associated clinical handover is a high-risk time for patients.[51,52] During this time there is a risk that communication and documentation will be inadequate or ineffective, resulting in loss of key pieces of information that may negatively impact on patient care. Further, the information handed over and clinician conduct during the handover process can predispose the patient to decision biases, which again have negative impacts on patient care and patient safety implications. Common decision biases arising during the handover process include fundamental attribution error, whereby the patient is blamed for their condition, diagnostic labelling, gender bias and premature closure.[62,192] Many of these cognitive biases result in clinicians being 'closed' to new information and ideas and are a major cause of diagnostic error.

Important elements of communication handover in healthcare include information about the patient's current state and

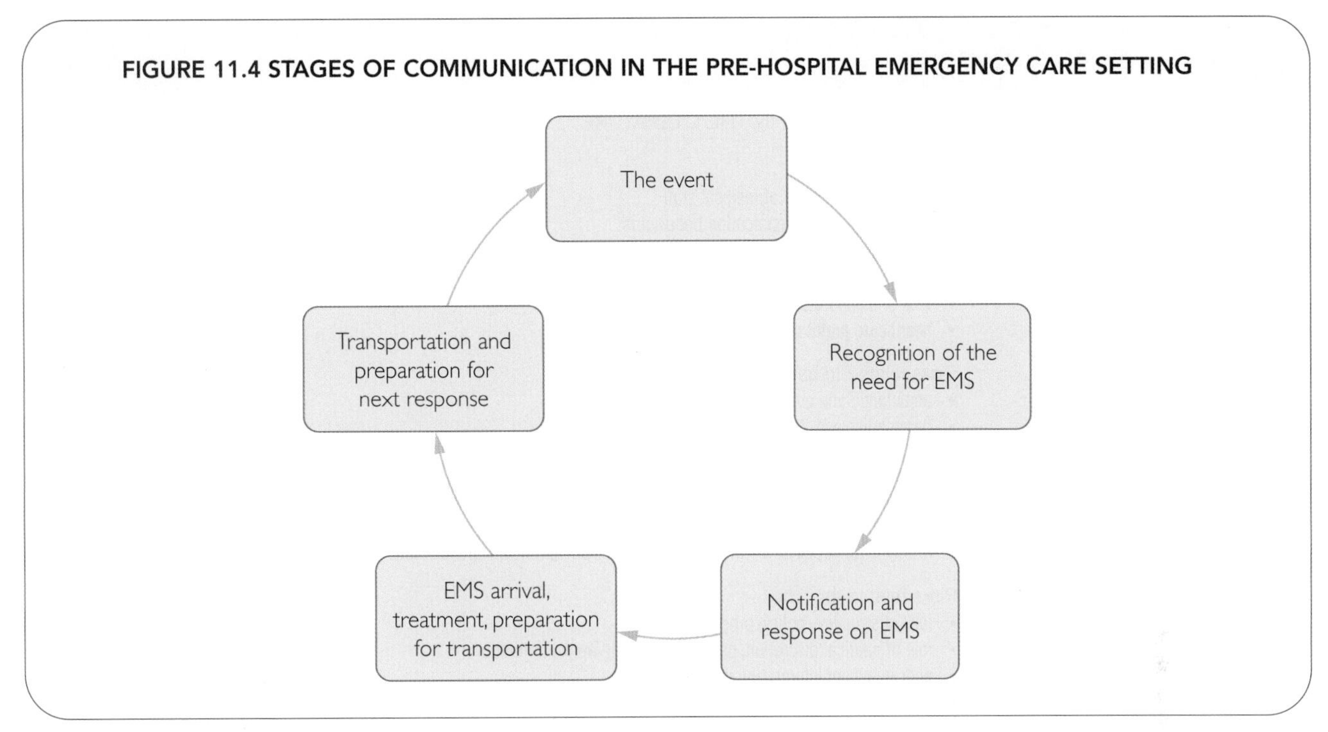

EMS: emergency medical services.

future events or goals.[128,129] A possible strategy for improving information transfer is the use of a standardised framework for clinical handover communication.[51,52] Advantages of such standardised systems and use of a predetermined structure are a decrease in omission of important information and clear expectations about the order in which information will be conveyed.[129] Studies of interprofessional communication comparing standard information transfer with communication using the ISBAR mnemonic (see Table 11.3) showed that the content and clarity of communication was higher when ISBAR was used, and that use of a structured method improved communication.[51,52] For emergency clinical handovers, patients should be involved where clinically appropriate. The Australian Commission on Safety and Quality in Health Care (ACSQHC) has established standards and implementation tool kits for quality clinical handover via the National Safety and Quality Health Service Standard for Clinical Handover, which adopts the ISBAR framework.[193]

The ability to receive, understand and forward information within the out-of-hospital, ED and broader healthcare setting is critical to patient welfare and the quality and safety of the care that paramedics and emergency nurses provide. Communicating information in the emergency medical system requires the use of a variety of methods and equipment, all of which have advantages and limitations. This is also discussed in Chapter 13.

PRACTICE TIP

Role clarification and delineation is critical to timely and effective clinical handover.

A rigorous approach to clinical handover protects both patients and clinicians.[52,129] Benefits of competent handover practices for patients include increased safety, decreased error, decreased morbidity and mortality, increased continuity of care, decreased repetition and increased satisfaction. For clinicians, high quality affords professional protection, makes accountability and responsibility transparent, decreases stress associated with feeling ill-informed, provides opportunities for education and improves job satisfaction by enabling provision of a high standard of care.[194]

Numerous studies clearly show that clinical handover is a high-risk event with potential for fragmentation of care and adverse events.[52,191,194] A review of the literature[191] identified a number of major themes related to high-risk scenarios in clinical handover, summarised in Table 11.4. The elements of handover in the out-of-hospital care setting include a verbal report, the handing over of documented accounts and the physical handover of the patient from ambulance to the hospital, which one study claims is symbolic.[195,196]

PRACTICE TIP

To de-escalate negative emotions, triage nurses should inform patients of the waiting times and comfort family, carers and/or patients by explaining the triage process, the technology that is being used and the potential procedures and care interventions that may take place at the bedside.[130,142]

Providing patient- and family-centred communication

Paramedics and emergency nurses must communicate with a caring and compassionate professional attitude towards patients, families and carers.[130,142,145] Specifically, triage nurses should take the opportunity to explain to patients, families and carers about activities taking place in the triage area and

TABLE 11.4 RISKS DURING HANDOVER[191]

ASPECT OF HANDOVER	RISKS IDENTIFIED IN THE LITERATURE
Handover risks generally	Risks related to: • seniority/experience of medical staff • nature/type of communication behaviours • quality/content of information recorded and/or exchanged • discontinuity in patient care • lack of standardised protocols • healthcare professional fatigue
Interprofession handover	Risks related to handover between: • ambulance and emergency department • paramedics and first responders
Interdepartment handover	Risks related to handover: • between ED and intensive care • between ED and inpatient team in which interdepartmental boundaries/responsibilities are unclear
Shift-to-shift handover	Risks related to: • lack of structure/policy/procedures • role of medical discretion, particularly during weekend handover • poor quality of information in ED handover • uncertainty over responsibility in an intensive care unit • importance of the maintenance of core values/relationships in nursing handover • lack of guidelines for handover of anaesthetised patients • impact of fragmentation of handover among mental health nurses • information overload • dangers of long handovers
Hospital-to-community handover	Risks related to: • poor hospital-to-community discharge processes due to shift-to-shift handover • poor communication and differences in information quantity/quality depending on a patient's community destination • increased incidence of medical errors and re-hospitalisations
Provision of verbal handover only	Risks related to: • limitations of human memory • loss of information across each handover
Use of abbreviations in handover	Risks related to: • use of non-standard abbreviations by specific groups of clinicians (paediatrics) that were not understood by other healthcare professionals
Patient characteristics affecting handover	Risks related to: • varying responses by emergency staff to handover information from paramedics depending on patient condition • complex patient problems receiving poorer quality handover than more-defined patient conditions • failures in communicating patients' mental health status during transfer between hospital and residential aged care
Characteristics of handover	Risks related to: • lack of clarity over the effectiveness of verbal versus tape-recorded versus face-to-face handover • communication failures • handover being complex and cognitively taxing • interruptions

potentially along the patient journey. Triage nurses need to be aware that patients, families and carers typically experience anxiety and fear. [130,131] Being a skillful communicator enables clinicians to elicit appropriate information and to facilitate a patient's understanding of the ED journey.

It is well documented that effective communication with patients and families and between healthcare professionals is a significant factor in the quality and safety of care.[142,193] Communication failures (either between staff and patients or between staff and other staff) are a well-documented factor in adverse events, and as many as 70% of serious incidents in healthcare are related to communication failure.[193] Despite clear evidence of gaps in communication between patients and healthcare professionals, the majority of safety and quality initiatives focus on improving communication between doctors and nurses, and tend to exclude patients.[197]

A recent systematic review of the literature related to nurse–patient communication showed that the terms 'interaction' and 'communication' are often used interchangeably without consideration of the true theoretical definition.[197] In the nurse–patient context, the main intent of communication and interaction is to promote a positive patient health outcome or state of wellbeing.[197,198] Though not a subject of systematic research, similar phenomena apply in the pre-hospital care setting.

Involving patients and families in their care and using language free from medical jargon are both important aspects of effective communication between patients, families and healthcare professionals.[197] There are many challenges to effective communication between healthcare professionals and patients/families. Time constraints, patient stress and poor health literacy may mean that patients often do not understand their care.[198,199] One study found that 78% of ED patients did not understand one or more critical element of their treatment,[200] and a study of surgical patients showed that 40–80% of information covered in a consultation is immediately forgotten.[201] Poor or inappropriate communication between patients and healthcare professionals has significant clinical consequences: patients who do not fully understand their care have longer lengths of hospital stay and higher mortality rates.[202] Further, patients from diverse and particularly minority cultural and language backgrounds, or those who have physical communication problems, are at increased risk of preventable adverse events.[198,203]

Communication and documentation skills enable emergency clinicians to convert patient language into an urgency code and allocate a hospital/clinical area, a useable currency which provides an understanding for emergency clinicians to orientate their practice. In this way the paramedic and/or triage nurse is responsible for ensuring ED staff receive an appropriate and relevant handover to enable the continuity of care to match the patient's need. This ensures patients receive the appropriate care and intervention in the 'right' clinical area. To achieve effective 'cultural brokering', paramedics and triage nurses require advanced communication and interpersonal skills. Further discussion on communication is found in Chapters 8 and 12.

SUMMARY

Paramedics and emergency nurses undertake triage. Emergency care clinicians optimise clinical reasoning and problem-solving skills during triage practice in out-of-hospital and ED settings. When triaging, health professionals must decide within a few minutes the patient's level of clinical urgency, allocate appropriate resources and initiate or direct interventions according to patient need. The development of out-of-hospital triage and the triage nurse role has led to improved patient outcomes and the delivery of safer emergency care. Standardised triage guidelines have assisted health professionals to discriminate between more- and less-urgent conditions. In this way, for example, the ATS has contributed towards safer, consistent and ethical triage nursing practice.

The increasing complexity and acuity of patient presentations requires the emergency nurse to be highly experienced and have advanced knowledge, communication and problem-solving skills. There is overwhelming evidence that triage nurses bring about a quality difference in ED services and patient outcomes. However, it remains unclear how new models of care may impact, change or influence the role of triage nursing or out-of-hospital triage in the future.

CASE STUDY

A 36-year-old First Nations male presents to the emergency department at 8.30 am with fever, cough, dyspnoea and chest pain experienced over 3 days. He is able to walk to the triage desk unassisted. He was on his way to work, but felt too unwell and so decided to come to the ED.

PRACTICE TIP

The aim of the triage assessment is to gain relevant information quickly and efficiently. Your attitude is important and may well govern what type of reply you receive. Always speak with and observe the client yourself.

At triage you begin your assessment and discover:

- he is alert, lucid and well perfused, with no evidence of respiratory distress or cyanosis.
- he has no accessory muscle usage and can comfortably talk in full sentences.
- his chest pain is pleuritic and worse with coughing (pain 4 out of 10); he has a productive cough with green sputum and feels mildly short of breath only on exertion. He has not sought any medical intervention for the presenting condition.
- on auscultation, he has reduced breath sounds at the right lung base with some coarse inspiratory crepitations and bronchial breathing. He has

increased vocal resonance at the right lung base but there is no pleural rub.
- his vital signs are: temperature 38.4°C; heart rate/min 90; BP 125/75; respiratory rate/min 22 and oxygen saturation 98%.

QUESTIONS

1. What information and observations would you obtain?
2. What potential life-threatening risks are there for this patient?
3. What triage category would you allocate to this patient?
4. Where would you allocate this patient within the ED?
5. What fast-track activities or additional interventions could you provide or initiate at triage?
6. What would have to be different in this scenario for you to change your decision-making?
7. What do you think is the likely diagnosis of this patient?
8. How do you ensure the safety of patients in waiting areas?

Answers to Case Study Questions can be found on evolve http://evolve.elsevier.com/AU/Curtis/emergency/ 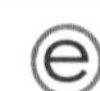

USEFUL WEBSITES

Aotearoa New Zealand Government, information publications relating to policy, education and workforce issues, www.health.govt.nz/publications/health?f0=im_field_category%3A41.

Australasian College for Emergency Medicine, information relating to emergency medicine policy, education and workforce issues, www.acem.org.au.

Australasian College of Paramedicine, Paramedicine online courses and role descriptions, paramedics.org/.

Bush Crisis Line, information relating to healthcare choices and services for consumers in rural and remote areas, crana.org.au/mental-health-wellbeing/call-1800-805-391#:~:text=Bush%20Support%20Line%20%7C%201800%20805%20391%20%7C%20CRANAplus.

Clinical Excellence Commission Clinical Handover, www.cec.health.nsw.gov.au/improve-quality/teamwork-culture-pcc/teamwork/clinical-handover.

College of Emergency Nursing Australasia, information relating to emergency medicine policy, education and workforce issues, www.cena.org.au.

Council of Remote Area Nurses of Australia (CRANA) (including rural triage), policy, education and workforce information relating to nursing and midwifery in rural and remote areas, crana.org.au/.

Council of Remote Area Nurses of Australia Plus (CRANA Plus), Triage Emergency Care, crana.org.au/learning-opportunities/courses/triage-emergency-care.

Department of Health and Aged Care, Australian Government, information publications relating to policy, education and workforce issues, www1.health.gov.au/internet/main/publishing.nsf/Content/publications-all.

Department of Health and Ageing, Emergency Triage Education Kit, acem.org.au/getmedia/c9ba86b7-c2ba-4701-9b4f-86a12ab91152/Triage-Education-Kit.aspx.

Emergency Care Institute, aci.health.nsw.gov.au/networks/eci.

National Emergency Management Agency (Aotearoa New Zealand), government information relating to emergency disaster response at a national level, www.civildefence.govt.nz/.

National Health Call Centre Network, www1.health.gov.au/internet/main/publishing.nsf/Content/national-health-call-centre-network-team-overview.

National Health Emergency Management (Australia), information relating to emergency disaster response at a national policy, education and workforce level, www.health.gov.au/resources/publications/national-health-emergency-response-arrangements?utm_source=health.gov.au&utm_medium=callout-auto-custom&utm_campaign=digital_transformation.

PRIME Programme, information relating to emergency education, www.stjohn.org.nz/What-we-do/Community-programmes/Partnered-programmes/PRIME/.

Reconciliation Action Plan, demonstrating inclusive and respectful language, www.reconciliation.org.au/wp-content/uploads/2018/05/language-guide.pdf.

Te Whatu Ora Health New Zealand, NZ emergency department triage, www.tewhatuora.govt.nz/our-health-system/hospitals-and-specialist-services/emergency-departments/emergency-department-triage.

REFERENCES

1. The Australian Council on Healthcare Standards. Assessment to the National Safety and Quality Health Service Standards. 2nd ed. Sydney: ACHS; 2021.
2. Australian Institute of Health and Welfare (AIHW). Emergency department care 2020–2021. Canberra: AIHW; 2021.
3. Australian Institute of Health and Welfare (AIHW). Australian hospital statistics 2019–2020. Canberra: AIHW; 2021.
4. Considine J, Botti M, Thomas S. Do knowledge and experience have specific roles in triage decision-making? Acad Emerg Med 2007;14(8):722–6.
5. Shaban RZ. Theories of judgment and decision-making: a review of the theoretical literature. J Emerg Prim Health Care 2005;3:1–2.
6. Shaban RZ. Paramedic clinical judgment of mental illness: a case study of accounts of practice. Brisbane: Arts, Education and Law Group, Griffith University; 2011.

7. Clarke DE, Boyce-Gaudreau K, Sanderson A, et al. ED triage decision-making with mental health presentations: a 'think aloud' study. J Emerg Nurs 2015;41(6):496–502.
8. Fernandes M, Vieira SM, Leite F, Palos C, Finkelstein S, Sousa JMC. Clinical decision support systems for triage in the emergency department using intelligent systems: a review. Artif Intell Med 2020;102:101762.
9. Jones CM, Cushman JT, Lerner EB, Fisher SG, Seplaki CL, Veazie PJ, et al. Prehospital trauma triage decision-making: a model of what happens between the 9-1-1 call and the hospital. Prehosp Emerg Care 2016;20(1):6–14.
10. Shaban RZ. Paramedics and the mentally ill. Paramedics in Australia: contemporary challenges of practice. Melbourne: Pearson Education; 2009.
11. White S, Stancombe J. Clinical judgment in the health and welfare professions: extending the evidence base. Philadelphia, USA: Open University Press; 2003.
12. Higgs J, Jones M. Clinical reasoning in the health professions. 3rd ed. Melbourne: Butterworth–Heinemann; 2008.
13. Watkins S. Effective decision-making: applying the theories to nursing practice. Br J Nurs 2020;29(2):98-101.
14. The Australian Oxford Dictionary. The Australian Oxford Dictionary. 5th ed. Melbourne: OUP Australia; 2011.
15. Lehane E, Leahy-Warren P, O'Riordan C, Savage E, Drennan J, O'Tuathaigh C et al. Evidence-based practice education for healthcare professions: an expert view. BMJ Evid Based Med 2019;24(3):103–8.
16. Angie AD, Connelly S, Waples EP, Kligyte V. The influence of discrete emotions on judgement and decision-making: a meta-analytic review. Cogn Emot 2011;25(8):1393–422.
17. Clemett VJ, Raleigh M. The validity and reliability of clinical judgement and decision-making skills assessment in nursing: a systematic literature review. Nurse Educ Today 2021;102:104885.
18. Dowding D, Thompson C. Measuring the quality of judgement and decision-making in nursing. J Adv Nurs 2003;44(1):49–57.
19. Clemen RT. Naturalistic decision making and decision analysis. J Behav Decis Mak 2001;14(5):359–61.
20. Chapman G, Sonnenberg F. Decision making in health care: theory, psychology and applications. Cambridge: CUP; 2000.
21. Thompson C, Dowding D. Clinical decision making and judgment in nursing. London: Churchill Livingstone; 2002.
22. Bell DE, Raiffa H, Tversky A. Descriptive, normative, and prescriptive interactions in decision making. In: Tversky A, Bell DE, Raiffa H, editors. Decision making: descriptive, normative, and prescriptive interactions. Cambridge: CUP; 1988.
23. Pruitt JS, Cannon-Bowers JA, Salas E. Search of naturalistic decisions. Decision making under stress: emerging themes and applications. Aldershot: Ashgate Publishing; 1997.
24. Lipshitz R, Klein G, Orasanu J, Salas E. Taking stock of naturalistic decision making. J Behav Dec Mak 2001;14(5):331–52.
25. Bendall J, Morrison A. Clinical judgement. Paramedics in Australia: contemporary challenges of practice. Frenchs Forest: Pearson Education Australia; 2009.
26. Duke T. New WHO guidelines on emergency triage assessment and treatment. Lancet 2016;387(10020):721–4.
27. Karlsten R, Sjoqvist BA. Telemedicine and decision support in emergency ambulances in Uppsala. J Telemed Telecare 2000;6(1):1–7.
28. Albright A, Gross K, Hunter M, O'Connor L. A dispatch screening tool to identify patients at high risk for COVID-19 in the prehospital setting. West J Emerg Med 2021;22(6):1253–6.
29. Marks P, Daniel T. Emergency ambulance triage. J Royal Soc Med 2002;95(5):270.
30. Burrell AR, McLaws ML, Fullick M, Sullivan RB, Sindhusake D. SEPSIS KILLS: early intervention saves lives. Med J Aust 2016;204(2):73.
31. Romero B, Fry M, Roche M. The impact of evidence-based sepsis guidelines on emergency department clinical practice: a pre-post medical record audit. J Clin Nurs 2017;26(21–22):3588–96.
32. Curtis K, Kourouche S, Asha S, Considine J, Fry M, Middleton S, et al. Impact of a care bundle for patients with blunt chest injury (ChIP): a multicentre controlled implementation evaluation. PLoS One 2021;16(10):e0256027.
33. Curtis K, Moules P, McKenzie J, Weidl L, Selak T, Binks S, et al. Development of an early activation hip fracture care bundle and implementation strategy to improve adherence to the National Hip Fracture Clinical Care Standard. J Multidiscip Healthc 2021;14:2891–903.
34. Jones T, Woollard M. Paramedic accuracy in using a decision support algorithm when recognising adult death: a prospective cohort study. Emerg Med J 2003;20(5):473–5.
35. Figgis K, Slevin O, Cunningham JB. Investigation of paramedics' compliance with clinical practice guidelines for the management of chest pain. Emerg Med J 2010;27(2):151–5.
36. Deakin CD, England S, Diffey D, et al. Can ambulance telephone triage using NHS pathways accurately identify paediatric cardiac arrest? Resuscitation 2017;116:109–12.
37. Neal D. Prehospital patient triage in mass casualty incidents. An engineering management analysis and prototype strategy recommendation. USA: The George Washington University; 2009.
38. Deluhery MR, Lerner EB, Pirrallo RG, Schwartz RB. Paramedic accuracy using SALT triage after a brief initial training. Prehosp Emerg Care 2011;15(4):526–32.
39. Schmidt T, Atcheson R, Federiuk C, et al. Evaluation of protocols allowing emergency medical technicians to determine need for treatment and transport. Acad Emerg Med 2000;7(6):663–9.
40. Zlotnik A, Alfaro MC, Perez MC, et al. Building a decision support system for inpatient admission prediction with the Manchester triage system and administrative check-in variables. Comput Inform Nurs 2016;34(5):224–30.

41. Bennett P, Hardiker N. A quantitative study investigating the effects of computerised clinical decision support in the emergency department. Stud Health Tech Inform 2016;225:53–7.
42. Clawson J, Olola C, Heward A, et al. Ability of the medical priority dispatch system protocol to predict the acuity of 'unknown problem' dispatch response levels. Prehosp Emerg Care 2008;12(3):290–6.
43. Farand L, Leprohon J, Kalina M, et al. The role of protocols and professional judgement in emergency medical dispatching. Euro J Emerg Med 1995;2(3):136–48.
44. Wachtel G, Elalouf A. Addressing overcrowding in an emergency department: an approach for identifying and treating influential factors and a real-life application. Isr J Health Policy Res 2020;9(1):37.
45. Poole SR, Schmitt BD, Carruth T, et al. After-hours telephone coverage: the application of an area-wide telephone triage and advice system for pediatric practices. Pediatrics 1993;92(5):670–9.
46. Donnelly PD, Weston CF. Ambulance staff exercise discretion over resuscitation decision. BMJ 1995;311(7009):877–8.
47. Marsden AK, Ng GA, Dalziel K, et al. When is it futile for ambulance personnel to initiate cardiopulmonary resuscitation? BMJ 1995;311(6996): 49–51.
48. Hick J, Mahoney B, Lappe M. Factors influencing hospital transport of patients in continuing cardiac arrest. Annals Emerg Med 1998;32(1):19–25.
49. Dunne RB, Compton S, Welch RD, et al. Prehospital on-site triaging. Prehosp Emerg Care 2003;7(1):85–8.
50. Westbrook J, Westbrook M, Gosling A. Ambulance officers' use of online clinical evidence. BMC Med Inform Dec Mak 2006;6:31.
51. Kerr D, Klim S, Kelly A-M, et al. Impact of a modified nursing handover model for improving nursing care and documentation in the emergency department: a pre- and post-implementation study. Int J Nurs Prac 2016;22(1):89–97.
52. Shah DY, Alinier PG, Pillay Y. Clinical handover between paramedics and emergency department staff: SBAR and IMIST-AMBO acronyms. Int Paramed Prac 2016;6(2):37–44.
53. Hammond KR. Human judgment and social policy: irreducible uncertainty, inevitable error, unavoidable justice. London: OUP; 1996.
54. Freebody P. Qualitative research in education: interaction and practice. London: SAGE Publications; 2004.
55. Rycroft-Malone J. Clinical guidelines. Clinical decision making and judgement in nursing. London: Churchill Livingstone; 2002.
56. Grimshaw JM, Russell IT. Effect of clinical guidelines on medical practice: a systematic review of rigorous evaluations. Lancet 1993;342(8883):1317–22.
57. Stanfield LM. Clinical decision making in triage: an integrative review. J Emerg Nurs 2015;41(5):396–403.
58. Fry M, MacGregor C. Confidence and impact on clinical decision making and behaviour in the emergency department. Australas Emerg Nurs J 2014;17(3):91–7.
59. Curtis K, Fry M, Shaban RZ, et al. Translating research findings to clinical nursing practice. J Clin Nurs 2017;26(5–6):862–72.
60. National Institute of Clinical Studies. Implementation of a state-wide emergency department mental health triage tool in Victoria. Melbourne: National Institute of Clinical Studies; 2006.
61. Considine J, Shaban RZ, Fry M, et al. Evidence based emergency nursing: designing a research question and searching the literature. Int Emerg Nurs 2017;32:78–82.
62. Croskerry P. To err is human—and let's not forget it. CMAJ 2010;182(5):524.
63. Campbell SG, Croskerry P, Bond WF. Profiles in patient safety: a 'perfect storm' in the emergency department. Acad Emerg Med 2007;14(8):743–9.
64. Mitchell GW. A brief history of triage. Disaster Med Public Health Prep 2008;2(Suppl. 1):S4–7.
65. Hughes G. Giving emergency advice over the telephone: it can be done safely and consistently. N Z Med J 2003;116(1177):U493.
66. Fry M. Triage nursing practice in Australian emergency departments 2002–2004: an ethnography. Sydney: University of Sydney; 2005.
67. McKay JI. The emergency department of the future – 2014: the challenge is in changing how we operate! J Emerg Nurs 1999;25(6):480–8.
68. Lahdet EF, Suserud BO, Jonsson A, et al. Analysis of triage worldwide. Emerg Nurse 2009;17(4):16–19.
69. Vatnoy TK, Fossum M, Smith N, et al. Triage assessment of registered nurses in the emergency department. Int Emerg Nurs 2013;21(2):89–96.
70. Farrohknia N, Castren M, Ehrenberg A, et al. Emergency department triage scales and their components: a systematic review of the scientific evidence. Scand J Trauma Resusc Emerg Med 2011;19:42.
71. Australasian College for Emergency Medicine (ACEM). Policy on the Australasian Triage Scale. Melbourne: ACEM; 2013.
72. LeVasseur SA, Considine J, Charles A, et al. Consistency of triage in Victoria's emergency departments: triage consistency report. Monash Institute of Health Services Research. Report to the Victorian Department of Human Services; Clayton: Monash Institute of Health Services Research; 2001.
73. Fernandes CMB, Wuerz R, Clark S, et al. How reliable is emergency department triage? Ann Emerg Med 1999;34(2):141–7.
74. Dilley SJ, Standen P. Victorian nurses demonstrate concordance in the application of the national triage scale. Emerg Med 1998;10(1):12–18.
75. Considine J, Ung L, Thomas S. Triage nurses' decisions using the national triage scale for Australian emergency departments. Acad Emerg Nurs 2000;8(4):201–9.
76. Considine J, Ung L, Thomas S. Clinical decisions using the national triage scale: how important is postgraduate education? Acad Emerg Nurs 2001;9(2):101–8.
77. Richardson D. No relationship between emergency department activity and triage categorization. Acad Emerg Med 1998;5(2):141–5.

78. Cameron M, Shaw V. Expanding the emergency nurse role to meet demand: nurse and physician perspectives. Emerg Nurse 2020;28(6):26–33.
79. Cameron PA, Joseph A, McCarthy SM. Access block can be managed. Med J Aust 2009;190(7):364–8.
80. Cameron PA, Kennedy M, McNeil JJ. The effects of bonus payments on emergency service performance in Victoria (Australia). Med J Aust 1999;171(5):243.
81. Considine J, LeVasseur SA, Villanueva E. The Australasian Triage Scale: examining emergency department nurses' performance using computer and paper scenarios. Ann Emerg Med 2004;44(5):516–23.
82. Crellin DJ, Johnston L. Poor agreement in application of the Australasian Triage Scale to paediatric emergency department presentations. Contemp Nurse 2003;15(1–2):48–60.
83. Grossmann FF, Bingisser R, Nickel CH. Comment on the validity of emergency department triage tools. Am J Emerg Med 2017;35(9):1376.
84. van Rein EAJ, van der Sluijs R, Voskens FJ, et al. Development and validation of a prediction model for prehospital triage of trauma patients. JAMA Surg 2019;154(5):421–9.
85. Voskens FJ, van Rein EAJ, van der Sluijs R, Houwert RM, Lichtveld RA, Verleisdonk EJ, et al. Accuracy of prehospital triage in selecting severely injured trauma patients. JAMA Surg 2018;153(4):322–7.
86. Weyrich P, Christ M, Celebi N, Riessen R. [Triage systems in the emergency department]. Med Klin Intensivmed Notfmed 2012;107(1):67–78.
87. Kuriyama A, Urushidani S, Nakayama T. Five-level emergency triage systems: variation in assessment of validity. Emerg Med J 2017;34(11):703–10.
88. Christ M, Grossmann F, Winter D, Bingisser R, Platz E. Modern triage in the emergency department. Dtsch Arztebl Int 2010;107(50):892–8.
89. Jones N, White ML, Tofil N, Pickens M, Youngblood A, Zinkan L, et al. Randomized trial comparing two mass casualty triage systems (JumpSTART versus SALT) in a pediatric simulated mass casualty event. Prehosp Emerg Care 2014;18(3):417–23.
90. McKee CH, Heffernan RW, Willenbring BD, Schwartz RB, Liu JM, Colella MR, et al. Comparing the accuracy of mass casualty triage systems when used in an adult population. Prehosp Emerg Care 2020;24(4):515–24.
91. Cuttance G, Dansie K, Rayner T. Paramedic application of a triage sieve: a paper-based exercise. Prehosp Disaster Med 2017;32(1):3–13.
92. Tsai LH, Huang CH, Su YC, et al. Comparison of prehospital triage and five-level triage system at the emergency department. Emerg Med J 2017;34(11):720–5.
93. Follin A, Jacqmin S, Chhor V, et al. Tree-based algorithm for prehospital triage of polytrauma patients. Injury 2016;47(7):1555–61.
94. Hindle D. Health care funding in New South Wales: from health care needs to hospital outputs. Aust Health Rev 2002;25(1):40–71.
95. Holroyd BR, Rosychuk RJ, Jelinski S, et al. Is triage score a valid measure of emergency department case mix? Canad J Emerg Med 2016;18:S99–100.
96. Australasian College for Emergency Medicine (ACEM). The Australasian Triage Scale. Melbourne: ACEM; 2002.
97. Australasian College for Emergency Medicine (ACEM). Guidelines for implementation of the Australasian Triage Scale in emergency departments. Melbourne: ACEM; 2016.
98. Ducharme J, Tanabe P, Homel P, et al. The influence of triage systems and triage scores on timeliness of ED analgesic administration. Am J Emerg Med 2008;26(8):867–73.
99. District Health Board. DHB hospital benchmark information. Wellington: Aotearoa New Zealand Ministry of Health; 2010.
101. Aotearoa New Zealand Ministry of Health. Emergency department triage. Wellington: Aotearoa New Zealand Ministry of Health; 2011.
101. Aotearoa New Zealand Ministry of Health. Māori providers: primary health care delivered by doctors and nurses. Wellington: Aotearoa New Zealand Government; 2004.
102. Jelinek GA, Little M. Inter-rater reliability of the national triage scale over 11,500 simulated occasions of triage. Emerg Med 1996;8(4):226–30.
103. Creaton A, Liew D, Knott J, et al. Interrater reliability of the Australasian Triage Scale for mental health patients. Emerg Med Australas 2008;20(6):468–74.
104. Westman J, Grafstein E. The interrater reliability of triage in an acute care ED setting. J Emerg Nurs 2003;29(5):413.
105. Doherty SR, Hore CT, Curran SW. Inpatient mortality as related to triage category in three New South Wales regional base hospitals. Emerg Med (Fremantle) 2003;15(4):334–40.
106. Browne GJ, Gaudry PL, Lam L. A triage observation scale improves the reliability of the national triage scale in children. Emerg Med 1997;9(4):283–8.
107. Durojaiye L, O'Meara M. A study of triage of paediatric patients in Australia. Emerg Med (Fremantle) 2002;14(1):67–76.
108. Hollis G, Sprivulis P. Reliability of the national triage scale with changes in emergency department activity level. Emerg Med 1996;8(4):231–4.
109. Mould-Millman NK, Dixon JM, Burkholder T, Pigoga JL, Lee M, de Vries S, et al. Validity and reliability of the South African Triage Scale in prehospital providers. BMC Emerg Med 2021;21(1):8.
110. Yamamoto A, Kuriyama A, Ikegami T. Validity of a five-level prehospital triage system in Japan: a cohort study. Am J Emerg Med 2021;45:329–34.
111. Whitby S, Ieraci S, Johnson D, et al. Analysis of the process of triage: the use and outcomes of the national triage scale. Sydney: Commonwealth Ambulatory Care Reform; 1999.
112. Wuerz RC, Travers D, Gilboy N, et al. Implementation and refinement of the emergency severity index. Acad Emerg Med 2001;8(2):170–6.
113. Fry M, Stainton C. An educational framework for triage nursing based on gatekeeping, timekeeping and decision-making processes. Accid Emerg Nurs 2005;13(4):214–19.

114. Weeks WB, Wallace AE. Rural-urban differences in primary care physicians' practice patterns, characteristics, and incomes. J Rural Health 2008;24(2):161–70.

115. Mira M, Cooper C, Maandag A. Contrasts between metropolitan and rural general practice in the delivery of after-hours care. Aust Fam Physician 1995;24(6):1064–7.

116. Scott A, Simoens S, Heaney D, et al. What does GP out of hours care cost? An analysis of different models of out of hours care in Scotland. Scott Med J 2004;49(2):61–6.

117. Australian Institute of Health and Welfare (AIHW). Expenditure on health for Aboriginal and Torres Strait Islander people 2010–11 to 2016–17. Health and welfare expenditure series no. 39. Canberra: AIHW; 2021.

118. Aotearoa New Zealand Ministry of Health. Annual update of key results 2019/20: Aotearoa New Zealand Health Survey. Auckland: Aotearoa New Zealand Government; 2021.

119. Grant AW, Buckley DJ. Nurse experiences and confidence in treating critically ill and injured patients following the completion of the First Line Emergency Care Course. Australas Emerg Care 2019;22(4):236–42.

120. Ministry of Health. Health workforce Aotearoa New Zealand Annual Report to the Minister of Health Wellington. MOH; 2018.

121. Ellison-Loschmann L, Pearce N. Improving access to health care among New Zealand's Māori population. Am J Public Health 2006;96(4): 612–17.

122. HealthDirect Australia. Annual report 2017–2018. Western Australia: HealthDirect Australia; 2012.

123. St. George I, Cullen M, Gardiner L, et al. Universal telenursing triage in Australia and Aotearoa New Zealand – a new primary health service. Aust Fam Phys 2008;37(6):476–9.

124. Aotearoa New Zealand Ministry of Health. More about Healthline. Wellington: Aotearoa New Zealand Government; 2021.

125. Aotearoa New Zealand Rural General Practice Network. Submission on Service Specifications Review: Primary Response in Medical Emergencies (PRIME). Wellington: 2006.

126. CRANAPlus. First Line Emergency Care Northern Territory. Cairns: CRANAPlus; 2013.

127. Varndell W, Hodge A, Fry M. Triage in Australian emergency departments: results of a New South Wales survey. Australas Emerg Care 2019;22(2):81–6.

128. Curtis K, Munroe B, Fry M, Considine J, Tuala E, Watts M, et al. The implementation of an emergency nursing framework (HIRAID) reduces patient deterioration: a multi-centre quasi-experimental study. Inter Emerg Nurs 2021;56:100976.

129. Munroe B, Curtis K, Murphy M, Strachan L, Buckley T. HIRAID: an evidence-informed emergency nursing assessment framework. Australas Emerg Nurs J 2015;18(2):83–97.

130. Fry M, Elliott R, Murphy S, Curtis K. The role and contribution of family carers accompanying community-living older people with cognitive impairment to the emergency department: an interview study. J Clin Nurs 2022;31(7–8):975–84.

131. Fry M, Chenoweth L, MacGregor C, Arendts G. Emergency nurses, perceptions of the role of family/carers in caring for cognitively impaired older persons in pain: a descriptive qualitative study. Int J Nurs Stud 2015;52(8):1323–31.

132. Considine J, Fry M, Curtis K, Shaban RZ. Systems for recognition and response to deteriorating emergency department patients: a scoping review. Scand J Trauma Resusc Emerg Med 2021;29(1):69.

133. Scott BM, Considine J, Botti M. Unreported clinical deterioration in emergency department patients: a point prevalence study. Australas Emerg Nurs J 2015;18(1):33–41.

134. Mochizuki K, Shintani R, Mori K, Sato T, Sakaguchi O, Takeshige K, et al. Importance of respiratory rate for the prediction of clinical deterioration after emergency department discharge: a single-center, case-control study. Acute Med Surg 2016;4(2):172–8.

135. Jeffries D. Should triage nurses trust their intuition? J Emerg Nurs 2008;34(1):86–8.

136. Commonwealth Department of Health and Ageing. Emergency triage education kit. Canberra: Commonwealth of Australia; 2007.

137. Varndell W, Fry M, Elliott D. Pain assessment and interventions by nurses in the emergency department: a national survey. J Clin Nurs 2020;29(13–14):2352–62.

138. Fry M, Hearn J, McLaughlin T. Pre-hospital pain management patterns and triage nurse documentation. Int Emerg Nurs 2012;20(2):83–7.

139. Vuille M, Foerster M, Foucault E, Hugli O. Pain assessment by emergency nurses at triage in the emergency department: a qualitative study. J Clin Nurs 2018;27(3–4):669–76.

140. Fry M. Triage nurses order x-rays for patients with isolated distal limb injuries: a 12-month ED study. J Emerg Nurs 2001;27(1):17–22.

141. Considine J, Payne R, Williamson S, Curtis K. Expanding nurse initiated x-rays in emergency care using team-based learning and decision support. Australas Emerg Nurs J 2013;16(1):10–20.

142. Fry M, Elliott R, Curtis K, Mei J, Fitzpatrick L, Groth R, et al. Family members' perceptions of older person discharge from emergency departments. Int J Older People Nurs 2021;16(3):e12365.

143. Morley C, Unwin M, Peterson GM, Stankovich J, Kinsman L. Emergency department crowding: a systematic review of causes, consequences and solutions. PloS One 2018;13(8):e0203316.

144. Forero R, McCarthy S, Hillman K. Access block and emergency department overcrowding. Crit Care 2011;15(2):216.

145. Fry M, MacGregor C, Ruperto K, et al. Nursing praxis, compassionate caring and interpersonal relations: an observational study. Australas Emerg Nurs J 2013;16(2):37–44.

146. Acorn M. Nurses' triage assessments were affected by patients' behaviours and stories and their perceived credibility. Evid Based Nurs 2009;12(2):61.
147. United States Department of Transportation. Emergency Medical Technician Paramedic (EMT-P) national standards curriculum. National Highway Traffic Safety Administration; 1998.
148. Convention of Ambulance Authorities and Paramedics Australasia. Professional competency standards—paramedics. St. Kilda, Victoria: Convention of Ambulance Authorities and Paramedics Australasia; 2013.
149. Billett S. Learning in the workplace: strategies for effective practice. Crows Nest: Allen & Unwin; 2001.
150. Sanders MJ, editor. Mosby's paramedic textbook. 3rd ed. St. Louis: Mosby Elsevier; 2006.
151. Elling B, Smith MG, Pollack AN, editors. Nancy Caroline's emergency care in the streets. 6th ed. Sudbury, Mass: Jones and Bartlett; 2009.
152. Abetz JW, Olaussen A, Jennings PA, Smit V, Mitra B. Review article: pre-hospital provider clinical judgement upon arrival to the emergency department: a systematic review and meta-analysis. Emerg Med Australas 2020;32(6):917–23.
153. Alexander M. Reasoning processes used by paramedics to solve clinical problems. Columbia: The George Washington University; 2010.
154. NSW Health. Emergency department system. Sydney: NSW Department of Health; 2008.
155. Marshall S, Harrison J, Flanagan B. The teaching of a structured tool improves the clarity and content of interprofessional clinical communication. Qual Safe Health Care 2009;18(2):137–40.
156. Iedema R, Ball C, Daly B, et al. Design and trial of a new ambulance-to-emergency department handover protocol: 'IMIST-AMBO'. BMJ Qual Safety 2012;21(8):627–33.
157. Boyle LM, Mackay M, Stockman K. Ambulance ramping, system pressure, and hospitals in crisis: what do the data tell us? Med J Aust 2021;215(11):526–7.
158. Sedgman R, Aldridge E, Miller J, Fleming D, Buntine P. Pre-triage wait times for non-ambulance arrivals in the emergency department: a retrospective video audit. Australas Emerg Care 2022;25(2):126–31.
159. Crowe S, Grieco L, Vindrola-Padros C, et al. Multidisciplinary embedded research to identify solutions to emergency department overcrowding. Int J Qual Health Care 2017;29(Suppl. 1):55–6.
160. Kenny JF, Chang BC, Hemmert KC. Factors affecting emergency department crowding. Emerg Med Clin North Am 2020;38(3):573–87.
161. McKenna P, Heslin SM, Viccellio P, et al. Emergency department and hospital crowding: causes, consequences, and cures. Clin Exp Emerg Med 2019;6(3):189–95.
162. O'Dowd A. Emergency departments must not return to pre-covid days of overcrowding and lack of safety, says college. BMJ 2020;369:m1848.
163. Lee Y, Shin S, Lee E, et al. Emergency department overcrowding and ambulance turnaround time. PLoS One 2015;10(6):e0130758.
164. Lindner G, Woitok BK. Emergency department overcrowding: analysis and strategies to manage an international phenomenon. Wien Klin Wochenschr 2021;133(5–6):229–33.
165. Cremonesi P, di Bella E, Montefiori M, et al. The robustness and effectiveness of the triage system at times of overcrowding and the extra costs due to inappropriate use of emergency departments. App Health Econ Health Policy 2015;13(5):507–14.
166. Varndell W, McGregor C, Gallagher R, et al. Measuring patient dependency – performance of the Jones dependency tool in an Australian emergency department under review. Australas Emerg Nurs J 2013;16(2):64–72.
167. Gerdtz MF, Daniel C, Dearie V, et al. The outcome of a rapid training program on nurses' attitudes regarding the prevention of aggression in emergency departments: a multi-site evaluation. Int J Nurs Stud 2013;50(11):1434–45.
168. Fry M, Ruperto K, Jarrett K, et al. Managing the wait: clinical initiative nurses' perceptions of an extended practice role. Australas Emerg Nurs J 2012;15(4):202–10.
169. Angland S, Dowling M, Casey D. Nurses' perceptions of the factors which cause violence and aggression in the emergency department: a qualitative study. Int Emerg Nurse 2014;22(3):134–9.
170. Rippon TJ. Aggression and violence in health care professions. J Adv Nurs 2000;31(2):452–60.
171. Perera ML, Gnaneswaran N, Roberts MJ, et al. The 'four-hour target' and the impact on Australian metropolitan acute surgical services. ANZ J Surg 2016;86(1–2):74–8.
172. ACEM. 2020 Annual Site Census – Part Two: Emergency department resources, hospitals and networks. Melbourne: Australasian College for Emergency Medicine; 2020.
173. Jones P, Wells S, Harper A, et al. Impact of a national time target for ED length of stay on patient outcomes. N Z Med J 2017;130(1455):15–34.
174. Gamst-Jensen H, Lippert FK, Egerod I. Under-triage in telephone consultation is related to non-normative symptom description and interpersonal communication: a mixed methods study. Scand J Trauma Resusc Emerg Med 2017;25(1):52.
175. Griffin E, McCarthy JP, Thomas F, et al. New Zealand Healthline call data used to measure the effect of travel time on the use of the emergency department. Soc Sci Med 2017;179:91–6.
176. Breslin E, Dennison J. The development of telephone triage: historical, professional and personal perspectives. J Orthop Nurs 2002;6(4):191–7.
177. Huibers L, Smits M, Renaud V, Giesen P, Wensing M. Safety of telephone triage in out-of-hours care: a systematic review. Scand J Prim Health Care 2011;29(4):198–209.

178. Morreel S, Philips H, Colliers A, Verhoeven V. Performance of a new guideline for telephone triage in out-of-hours services in Belgium: a pilot study using simulated patients. Health Serv Manag Res 2020;33(4):166–71.

179. Dunt D, Wilson R, Day SE, et al. Impact of telephone triage on emergency after hours GP Medicare usage: a time-series analysis. Aust New Zealand Health Policy 2007;4:21.

180. Riley LM, Manton A. ED utilization by uninsured and Medicaid patients after availability of telephone triage. J Emerg Nurs 2017;43(2):98.

181. Eastwood K, Smith K, Morgans A, et al. Appropriateness of cases presenting in the emergency department following ambulance service secondary telephone triage: a retrospective cohort study. BMJ Open 2017;7(10):e016845.

182. Gibson A, Randall D, Tran DT, et al. Emergency department attendance after telephone triage: a population-based data linkage study. Health Serv Res 2018;53(2):1137–62.

183. NZ Telehealth Forums and Resource Centre. Regulations, standards and guidelines. 2022. Online. Available from: www.telehealth.org.nz/regulations-and-policies/regulations-and-standards/.

184. Heslin SM, Nappi M, Kelly G, Crawford J, Morley EJ, Lingam V, et al. Rapid creation of an emergency department telehealth program during the COVID-19 pandemic. J Telemed Telecare 2020;38(3):207–12.

185. Langabeer JR II, Gonzalez M, Alqusairi D, Champagne-Langabeer T, Jackson A, Mikhail J, et al. Telehealth-enabled emergency medical services program reduces ambulance transport to urban emergency departments. West J Emerg Med 2016;17(6):713–20.

186. Williams Jr D, King K, Kruis RD, Ford DW, Sterling SA, Castillo A, Robinson CO, et al. Do hospitals providing telehealth in emergency departments have lower emergency department costs? Telemed J E Health 2021;27(9):1011–20.

187. Odone A, Bossi E, Scardoni A, Orlandi C, Arrigoni C, et al. Physician-to-nurse handover: a systematic review on the effectiveness of different models. J Pat Safe 2022;18(1):e73–84.

188. Gaston C. How an ambulance service can contribute to the health care continuum. Sydney: Centre for Policy Development; 2007. Online. Available from: cpd.org.au/2007/07/how-an-ambulance-service-can-contribute-to-the-health-care-continuum/.

189. Steinkopf B, Reddin RA, Black RA, Van Hasselt VB, Couwels J. Assessment of stress and resiliency in emergency dispatchers. J Police Crim Psych 2018;33(4):398–411.

190. Bergman LM, Pettersson ME, Chaboyer WP, et al. Safety hazards during intrahospital transport: a prospective observational study. Crit Care Med 2017;45(10):e1043–9.

191. Wong MC, Yeek KC, Turner P. A structured evidence-based literature review regarding the effectiveness of improvement interventions in clinical handover. Canberra: ACSQHC; 2008.

192. Croskerry P. Achieving quality in clinical decision making: cognitive strategies and detection of bias. Acad Emerg Med 2002;9(11):1184–204.

193. Australian Commission on Safety and Quality in Health Care (ACSQHC). National Safety and Quality Health Service Standards. 2019. Online. Available from: www.safetyandquality.gov.au/wp-content/uploads/2017/12/National-Safety-and-Quality-Health-Service-Standards-second-edition.pdf.

194. Australian Medical Association. AMA—Safe handover: safe patient: Guidance on clinical handover for clinicans and managers. Kingston, ACT: AMA; 2007.

195. Munroe B, Curtis K, Fry M, Shaban RZ, Moules P, Elphick TL, et al. Increasing accuracy in documentation through the application of a structured emergency nursing framework: A multisite quasi-experimental study. J Clin Nurs 2022;31(19–20):2874–85.

196. Munroe B, Curtis K, Murphy M, Strachan L, Considine J, Hardy J, et al. A structured framework improves clinical patient assessment and nontechnical skills of early career emergency nurses: a pre-post study using full immersion simulation. J Clin Nurs 2016;25(15–16):2262–74.

197. Fleischer S, Berg A, Zimmermann M, et al. Nurse–patient interaction and communication: a systematic literature review. J Public Health 2009;17(5):339–53.

198. Brady AM, Byrne G, Quirke MB, et al. Barriers to effective, safe communication and workflow between nurses and non-consultant hospital doctors during out-of-hours. Int J Qual Health Care 2017;29(7):929–34.

199. Meuter RF, Gallois C, Segalowitz NS, et al. Overcoming language barriers in healthcare: a protocol for investigating safe and effective communication when patients or clinicians use a second language. BMC Health Serv Res 2015;15:371.

200. Engel KG, Heisler M, Smith DM, et al. Patient comprehension of emergency department care and instructions: are patients aware of when they do not understand? Ann Emerg Med 2009;53(4):454–61.

201. Kessels RPC. Patients' memory for medical information. J Royal Soc Med 2003;96(5):219.

202. Curtis K, Elphick T-L, Eyles M, Ruperto K. Identifying facilitators and barriers to develop implementation strategy for an ED to ward handover tool using behaviour change theory (EDWHAT). Implement Sci Comm 2020;1(1):71.

203. van Rosse F, de Bruijne M, Suurmond J, et al. Language barriers and patient safety risks in hospital care. A mixed methods study. Int J Nurs Stud 2016;54:45–53.

CHAPTER 12
MAJOR INCIDENT PREPAREDNESS AND MANAGEMENT

JUSTIN DUNLOP AND JAMIE RANSE

ESSENTIALS

- When planning for a major incident (MI), all facets of the incident must be considered—before, during and after.
- It is essential that all staff involved in an MI response are aware of their roles and the roles of others within their context.
- Communication is key to any effective MI response and planning for increased communications needs to be in place to ensure good information flow.
- Effective MI triage is 'doing the greatest good for the greatest number of survivors'.
- The development of standardised processes assists in streamlining mass casualty incident (MCI) survivor flow by determining what essential tests and investigations are required in an MCI event.
- Triage is a dynamic process and should be repeated regularly at all stages of the MI.
- Understanding the nexus between pre-hospital and hospital MI response, such as pre-hospital and hospital triage, is important for transitioning patient care responsibilities.
- Development of agreed key coordinator positions will assist in prioritising care and assisting flow of MI survivors.
- Ensure robust back-up systems exist that are easily understood and have been tested prior to an MI.
- Keep all documentation simple and relevant.
- Practise MI responses in regular education sessions for all staff.
- Ensure that the emergency department (ED) and organisations have surge capacity strategies ready to be deployed in an MI.
- In a CBRN (chemical, biological, radiological and nuclear) MI, it is essential to ensure that staff and facilities minimise contamination. This can be achieved by controlling access to sites including EDs and ensuring that staff treating patients have the appropriate personal protective equipment (PPE) available.

INTRODUCTION

This chapter describes the broad categories of major incidents (MIs), arising from any hazard. The principles of prevention, preparedness, response and recovery (PPRR) management described in this chapter are applicable to all MIs. The PPRR cycle can be more simply described as the activities and actions that can be undertaken

by health professionals before, during and/or after an MI. Throughout this chapter, Australian and Aotearoa New Zealand government legislation and terminology are outlined with recent MI incidents highlighted as examples. However, it is important that local plans and arrangements are sought out and applied to ensure a contextually relevant, consistent and coordinated approach. Early consideration towards PPRR of MIs goes some way to mitigating risk and therefore lessening the impact of MIs on pre-hospital and hospital health services, and subsequently patient morbidity and mortality. The chapter also includes a section on chemical, biological, radiological and nuclear (CBRN) response, which is designed to enhance the reader's understanding of the important considerations of these types of CBRN MIs.

WHAT IS A MAJOR INCIDENT?

The Australian *Health and Disaster Management* handbook identifies a range of terms used to describe MIs that impact on the health system. These include 'emergency', 'disaster' or 'mass casualty incident'.[1] The *Australian Emergency Management Arrangements* describe an 'emergency' as:

> an event, actual or imminent, which endangers or threatens to endanger life, property or the environment, and which requires a significant and coordinated response.[2]

The World Health Organization (WHO) describes a 'mass casualty incident' (MCI) as:

> An incident which generates more patients at one time than locally available resources can manage using routine procedures. It requires exceptional emergency arrangements and additional or extraordinary assistance.[3]

A more descriptive definition is offered by the Aotearoa New Zealand Ministry of Health:

> [A]ny occurrence that presents a serious threat to the health of the community or disruption to the health services, or causes (or is likely to cause) numbers or types of casualties that require special measures to be implemented by appropriate responding agencies, including ambulance services, District Health Boards (DHBs) e.g. hospitals, primary care and public health and the ministry. This is undertaken in order to maintain an effective, appropriate and sustainable response.[4]

Devastating large-scale MIs continually occur worldwide, resulting in the need to put into action response systems and processes to deal with these incidents. The WHO maintains an online list of current international health emergencies, including disease outbreaks, disasters and humanitarian crises.[5] Additionally, both the Australian and Aotearoa New Zealand governments maintain online registers of historical emergencies which are a good resource for people to gain an understanding of previous MIs of significance.[6,7] Figs 12.1 to 12.5 show examples of natural disasters. A list of major incident categories based on the abovementioned registers is provided in Box 12.1.

BOX 12.1 TYPES OF MAJOR INCIDENTS[6,7]

Biosecurity	Industrial
Criminal	Infrastructure failure
Cyclone	Landslide
Drought	Maritime/Coastal
Earthquake	Pandemic
Environment	Radiation incident
Fire - Bushfire	Storm
Fire - Urban	Terrorism
Flood	Tornado
Food Safety	Transport
Hazardous substances	Tsunami
Health	Volcanic unrest

FIGURE 12.1 6.3 MAGNITUDE EARTHQUAKE STRUCK CHRISTCHURCH, NZ, IN 2011

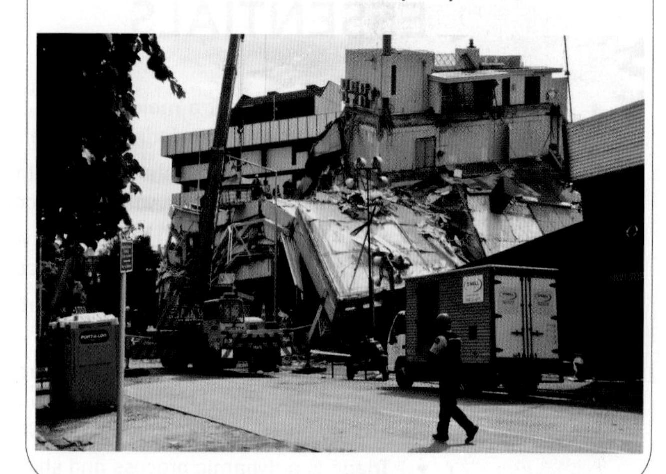

Gabriel/Flickr CC BY 2.0.

FIGURE 12.2 FIRE ON THE HILLS NORTH OF LITHGOW, NSW, DURING BUSHFIRES, OCTOBER 2013

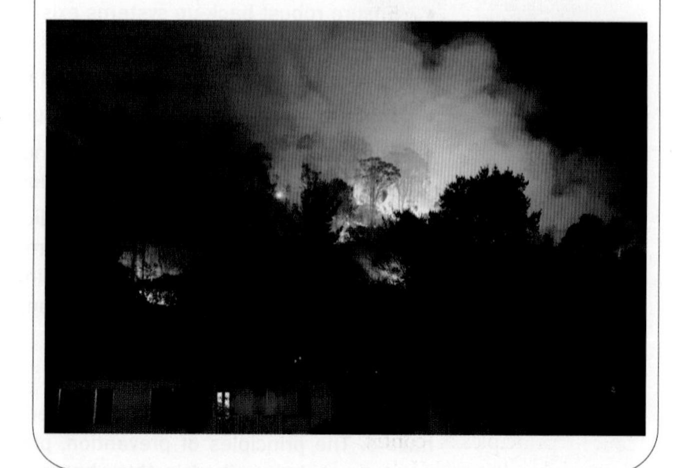

LithgowLights, CC BY 3.0.

MAJOR INCIDENT PRINCIPLES

A comprehensive approach to managing MIs includes actions that occur before, during and after an event. The Australian Emergency Management Arrangements use the PPRR framework, mentioned in the introduction, to further describe this comprehensive approach,[2] while the Aotearoa New Zealand Ministry of Health use the four Rs—Reduction, Readiness, Response and Recovery—to mitigate and manage a risk or

FIGURE 12.3 BUSHFIRE SMOKE OVER NEW SOUTH WALES, 2019

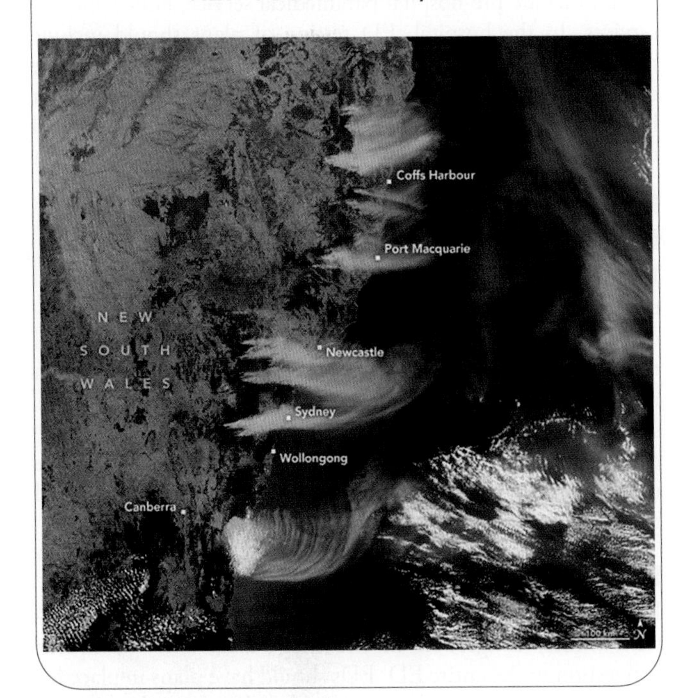

NASA Earth Observatory image by Lauren Dauphin.

FIGURE 12.4 LOCALS AND TOURISTS EVACUATED TO THE BEACH AT MALLACOOTA, VICTORIA, 2020

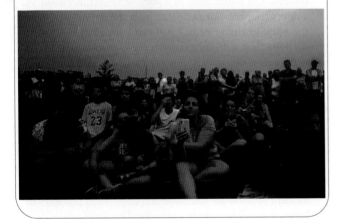

Rachel Mounsey, The Guardian.

consequence.[8] Regardless of the before, during and after MI framework used, a general principle in managing MIs is to apply this comprehensive approach to 'all emergencies', regardless of the nature of the risk or hazard. This should include 'all communities' and provide an integrated response from all organisations, and extensive community and stakeholder engagement.

A multi-agency response is generally managed following the 'Triple C' principles of 'control', which is the overall direction of activities related to an MI: 'command', which relates to the internal direction of an organisation's personnel; and 'coordination' of

FIGURE 12.5 AOTEAROA NEW ZEALAND VOLCANO: WHITE ISLAND'S ERUPTION, 2019

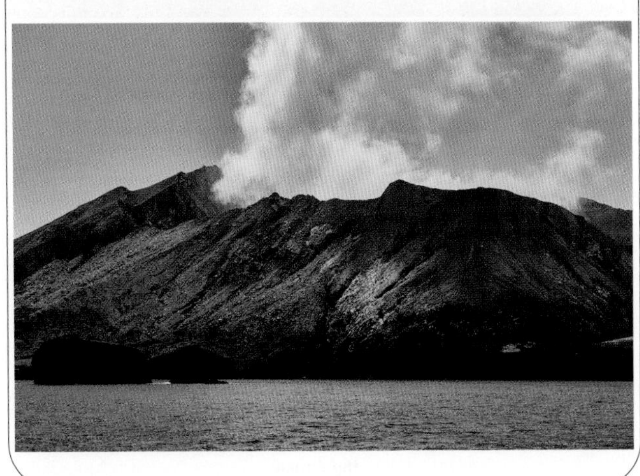

Shutterstock/Peter Gudella.

the various organisations and groups involved in the MI. As a result of experiences, some jurisdictions have added some additional 'C's'. These can include 'consequence', reminding those involved that the impact of the MI may be larger than the hazard alone; 'communication', to ensure that information flow remains a priority; and 'community connection', to ensure that community and stakeholder engagement remain front of mind.[9]

INCIDENT MANAGEMENT SYSTEMS

Internationally, there is a range of incident management systems available. They all have similar principles, including:

- unity of command
- management by objectives
- predetermined delegation of functional management
- span of control
- flexibility.

A popular system used in Australia is the Australasian Inter-Service Incident Management System (AIIMS),[10] while the Aotearoa New Zealand Government uses the Coordinated Incident Management System (CIMS).[11]

PLANNING

In most jurisdictions and organisations there will be pre-existing emergency and/or MI plans. Under the international Sphere humanitarian standards, there is an expectation that existing, local risk assessments and plans will be used to guide activities.[12] It is important to seek out and understand the existing local organisational and jurisdictional emergency plans to inform your preparedness.

Governments in Australia and Aotearoa New Zealand have developed plans to cover the high-level and often strategic considerations for MIs. Both plans aim 'to minimise the health impacts to individuals and the community during an emergency'.[13,14] These high-level, overarching plans are often focused on key national, state or territory MI arrangements. However, these plans do not often provide operational considerations for the PPRR of individual clinicians Instead, they provide guidance for local government areas and organisations to follow to ensure

TABLE 12.1 AUSTRALIA AND AOTEAROA NEW ZEALAND PRINCIPAL KEY PLANS

AUSTRALIAN GOVERNMENT	
Australian Emergency Management Arrangements (AEMA)[2]	The arrangements provide an overview of the Australian federal, state, territory and local governments' collective approach to the management of emergencies, including catastrophic MCI events.
Australian Government Disaster Response Plan (COMDISPLAN)[19]	The aim of COMDISPLAN is to describe the coordination arrangements for the provision of Australian Government physical assistance to states or territories or offshore territories in the event of a disaster. The plan can be activated for any disaster regardless of the cause.
Australian Health Emergency Response Arrangements (NatHealth Arrangements)[20]	The NatHealth Arrangements describe the strategic arrangements and mechanisms for the coordination of the Australian health sector in response to emergencies of national consequence.
Australian Domestic Health Response Plan for All-Hazards Incidents of National Significance (AUSHEALTHRESPLAN)[21]	The AUSHEALTHRESPLAN describes the national health coordination and response arrangements with a particular focus on patient management and transfer, health workforce availability, and the provision of resources.
AOTEAROA NEW ZEALAND GOVERNMENT	
National Civil Defence Emergency Management Plan (National CDEM Plan)[22]	The Aotearoa New Zealand National CDEM Plan identifies core functions for national management of the consequences of emergencies.
National Health Emergency Plan: A framework for the health and disability sector[8]	This plan provides guidance on the effective health emergency management and describes the roles and responsibilities at all levels across the areas of reduction, readiness, response and recovery for Aotearoa New Zealand.
National Health Emergency Plan: Mass Casualty Action Plan[4]	This plan provides an agreed framework, outlines the relationship between local, regional and national plans, and describes mechanisms for effective national coordination arrangements in the event of an MCI in Aotearoa New Zealand.

a consistent approach following the Australia– Aotearoa New Zealand standard for risk management.[15–18]

Table 12.1 describes some of the key plans that are in place.

A key to preparedness of pre-hospital and hospital MI systems is testing of plans on a regular basis. This testing should include focusing on the individual agency or department for which the plan is designed. Additionally, testing should include agencies and departments that have key interactions during an MI. For example, emergency department (ED) testing of plans should include pre-hospital paramedical service, police and fire services. In the hospital, ED testing of plans should include medical imaging service, pathology, operating theatres, intensive care and in-patient wards/units. There is no evidence to suggest how frequently these plans should be tested; however, annual testing seems to be recognised as a benchmark for testing plans.

BUSINESS RESILIENCE PLANNING FOR HEALTH ORGANISATIONS

In addition to planning for external disasters, organisational emergency planning committees need to consider internal incidents, such as power outages, downtime of electronic medical records, flooding, fire damage and chemical spillage, which may disrupt normal operations.[23,24] Business resilience plans should be developed to mitigate internal incidents and help the organisation get back to normal business, or at least to ensure that organisational capability is either partially or fully restored to ensure continued emergency care.[25]

EMERGENCY DEPARTMENT PLANS

Paramedics and ED staff are quite familiar with the peak patient influx, congestion in the triage area, and subsequent congestion in the entire ED. EDs should have plans in place for managing MIs. These plans may be scalable depending on the number of patients expected, the type of MI event and the expected duration of the MI.

- *Small-scale MI:* When small numbers of survivors are expected, with mixed injuries, and it is deemed manageable within currently available resources and operational systems. On notification of a small-scale MI, normally via a direct telephone or radio call from the ambulance service, the nurse in charge of ED puts out a preselected message notifying key staff, for example, surgical and trauma staff, patient flow officer, hospital executive staff and orderlies. A brief meeting should be held to ensure all involved are agreed on the plan of action.
- *Large-scale MI:* When there are large numbers of survivors and injuries of high complexity, requiring a whole-hospital response and the establishment of a Hospital Command Centre and Incident Command Structure. The MI messaging system may be increased to include further critical care areas and other clinical areas for early notification of the incident to allow for discharge and disposition processes to begin; this will be a multi-operational response (Figs 12.6, 12.7).

RISK PREVENTION/REDUCTION

Risk prevention and reduction measures seek to eliminate or reduce the impact of hazards and/or to reduce the susceptibility and increase the resilience of the community subject to the impact of those hazards. Prevention covers a range of activities and strategies by individuals, communities, businesses and governments. State and territory governments have the primary role in prevention within their respective jurisdictions. This role is supported by legislation and policy; however, government agencies at all levels undertake prevention programs as part of their day-to-day functions within their responsibilities.

FIGURE 12.6 MCI MAJOR DOCTOR TASK CARD

Code Brown Major Task Card

DOCTOR IN CHARGE ED

MAJOR MCI CODE BROWN TASK CARD

Responsible for:	Liaising with medical and nursing staff and organising ED to respond to a Major MCI incident		
Report to:	**Hospital disaster controller**	**Direct Report Contact Number:**	**XXXX**

- **CONVENE A BRIEF MEETING IN THE NUMS OFFICE WITH KEY ED STAFF TO OUTLINE THE PLAN.**
- **WEAR THE SILVER "DOCTOR IN CHARGE EMERGENCY" TABARD.**
- **DO NOT ATTEND THE DCC UNTIL REQUESTED TO DO SO VIA THE PAGING SYSTEM.**
- **DELEGATE THE IDENTIFICATION OF PATIENTS FOR IMMEDIATE WARD ADMISSION OR DISCHARGE TO RED AND YELLOW PRE-MCI MEDICAL TEAM LEADERS. THEY WILL THEN LIAISE WITH THE DOCTOR AND NUM IN CHARGE OF THE ED and ED IMAGING COORDINATOR (IF REQUIRED).**
- **ALLOCATE THE FOLLOWING ROLES** (TASK CARDS AND TABARDS KEPT IN TRIAGE CUPBOARD):
  - ED Imaging coordinator (Ideally ED SS with an Intern to assist) Tick when complete ☐
  - Surgical coordinator (Ideally surgical Consultant) ☐
  - Doctor in charge of Red Area (Ideally ED SS) ☐
  - Doctor in charge of Yellow Area (Ideally ED Registrar) ☐
  - Doctor in Charge of Green Area (ACC level 3 or Fast Track, Ideally ED Registrar) ☐
  - Doctor in Charge of TED (Ideally ED Registrar) ☐

  These positions have task cards that outline preparation for MCI and the "Rules of MCI Management"
- **ED LAYOUT**
  - Admitted patients are to be transferred to ward areas.
  - **Resuscitation rooms are not to be used for MCI victims**.
  - North End (Beds 1–12) – Red Label Victims
  - South End (Beds 13–22) +/– Fast Track – Yellow Label victims
  - Clinic 8 ACC level 3 – Green Label victims. If ACC is not operational, Green Victims will go to Fast Track
  - Green label victims will be triaged, given a pre-allocated MCI MRN, have an ID band attached and then will be escorted to ACC via the ambulance corridor and access the brown lifts in the south corridor. If ACC is not operational (outside working hours 7am to 7pm Mon–Fri), green victims will be directed to fast track, at least in the initial phase of the MCI response.
  - Temporary Emergency Department (TED) is in EMU/Resus for non-MCI patients.
  - The moribund are to be nursed in the side rooms in fast track, and if required, there will be two to a room.
  - Mortuary arrangements: 15 deceased MCI victims may be placed in the 2H and 2I tutorial rooms.
- **RULES OF MCI MANAGEMENT**
  - **Disaster trauma forms** will be used for all MCI victim documentation and management plans
  - **Damage control resuscitation** and damage control surgery should be employed if appropriate
  - **Radiology requests** are to be made on the "Radiology and Surgical Request Forms". These are sent to the ED Imaging Coordinator who will prioritise and negotiate time slots in the radiology department and their assistant will enter the order on FirstNet®
  - **Surgical requests** for OT are to be written on the "Radiology and Surgical Request Forms". These are to be sent to the ED Surgical Coordinator who will prioritise and negotiate time slots in theatre
  - **Victim movements** will be recorded by a clerk on the "Code Brown MCI Victim Tracking Form"
  - **Admissions**: victims will be admitted under the Upper GI Surgeon of the day
  - **Antibiotics** are only prescribed from the preselected list (to be found in the pre-packaged victim folders)
  - **Pharmacy** will set up a satellite unit in A.A.A. and A.C.C. for analgesia, ADT and antibiotics
  - **Pathology** will send a "Blood Safety Officer" who is responsible for ensuring all blood specimens meet the zero tolerance labelling policy. **Transfusion requests must be witnessed**
  - **Documentation** for ALL staff is only to be on the papers provided in the pre-registration packs
  - **A management plan** is to be written before the victims leave the ED
  - **Victim flow is one way** i.e. MCI victims do not return to the ED once they leave for radiology
  - **Non-MCI patients in radiology** will return to the ED for review and management prior to disposition
- **KEY ROLES AND RESPONSIBILITES**
  - ED NUM and Doctor in Charge will provide overall coordination of the ED
  - ED Surgical Coordinator will determine the priority for all surgical interventions for MCI Victims and liaise with the Operating Theatres Duty Director
  - ED Imaging Coordinator will determine the priority and suitability for all radiological interventions for all MCI and non-MCI victims and liaise with the Radiology Imaging Coordinator

Sample Task Card Courtesy: Emergency Department, Royal North Shore Hospital, St Leonards NSW 2065 Australia (2014) Page 1 of 2

Continued

FIGURE 12.6 cont'd

- **NURSING POSITIONS TO BE ALLOCATED BY NUM**
  - Nurse in Charge ED
  - Triage all MCI Victims
  - Nurse team leader Yellow Victims
  - Nurse team leader Red Victims
  - Nurse in Charge of Temporary Emergency Department (TED)
  - TED Communication Clerk
  - Triage Clerk assigned to the MCI Triage nurse
- **STAFF TO BE SENT FROM THE DDC**
  - Tracking coordinators Red × 1 Yellow × 2
  - Imaging tracker
  - Surgical tracker
  - Administration assistance to in charge nurse and doctor
  - Tracker in TED
- **TRACKING PAPERWORK**
  The following MCI registration and tracking forms will be used:
  - Triage Code Brown MCI Registration Form
  - Code Brown MCI Victim Tracking Form
  - Radiology and Surgical request Form
  - Surgical Coordinator Tracking Form
  - Radiology Coordinator Tracking Form
  - Green Label Registration and Tracking Form
- **VICTIM PAPERWORK**
  All victims will have a pre-registration MRN and a pre made, pre labelled, paperwork pack containing:

Arm band	Victim ID stickers × 10	Disaster Trauma forms	Adult "BTF" obs charts
Blood request forms	Radiology/Surgical request forms × 4	Antibiotic prescribing guidelines	Victim Admission Summary

- **STAFF CALL-IN**
  - There is a staff call-in book in the triage MCI folder.
  - Telephone numbers are kept with the ED NUMs and department secretary
- **STAND DOWN:**
  - ED will receive notification from the DCC of de-escalation and of final MCI victims being received
- **CONTINUATION OF CORE BUSINESS**
  - **Non-MCI** victims will receive a regular MRN via the FirstNet registration system and be directed to TED, AAU or RR.
  - Paediatric patients will be assessed and triaged to EP or RR.
  - Mental health patients will be kept in the ED waiting room and reviewed by the CNC mental health. Patients requiring close observation and monitoring will be admitted directly to the Cummins Unit.
  - Code Blue Emergencies: the ED will continue its usual responses
- **DEBRIEF**
  - The ED will hold a departmental "hot" debrief for ED staff.
  - An operational debrief will be conducted at which the ED along with other departments will provide a documented report on the operational response.

DCC PHONE NUMBERS:	
HDIC	XXXX
COMMUNICATIONS	XXXX
LOGISTICS	XXXX
DCC FAX NUMBER:	XXXX XXXX

Sample Task Card Courtesy: Emergency Department, Royal North Shore Hospital, St Leonards NSW 2065 Australia (2014) Page 2 of 2

Courtesy: Emergency Department, Royal North Shore Hospital, St Leonards, NSW 2065, Australia, 2014.

FIGURE 12.7 MCI MAJOR NURSE TASK CARD

Code Brown MAJOR Task Card

NURSE IN CHARGE ED

MAJOR MCI CODE BROWN MCI TASK CARD

Responsible for:	Liaising with medical and nursing staff and organising ED to respond to a Major MCI incident		
Report to:	**Hospital disaster controller**	**Direct Report Contact Number:**	**XXXX**

- **IF NOT ALREADY DONE, PUT OUT THE "CODE BROWN MAJOR" PAGE VIA SWITCHBOARD ON XX**
- **ATTEND A BRIEF MEETING IN THE NUMS OFFICE WITH KEY ED STAFF TO OUTLINE THE PLAN**
- **WEAR SILVER "NURSE IN CHARGE EMERGENCY" TABARD**
- **DO NOT ATTEND THE DCC UNTIL REQUESTED TO DO SO VIA THE PAGING SYSTEM**
- **LIAISE WITH NURSE T/LS AND BED MANAGER (LOCATED IN ED) REGARDING PT ADMISSIONS**
- **ALLOCATE THE FOLLOWING ROLES:** (TASK CARDS AND TABARDS KEPT IN TRIAGE CUPBOARD):
  - Triage (all MCI Victims) Tick when complete ☐
  - Triage (non-MCI Patients) ☐
  - Nurse team leader Yellow Victims ☐
  - Nurse team leader Red Victims ☐
  - Nurse in Charge of Temporary Emergency Department (TED) ☐
  - TED Communication Clerk ☐
  - Clerk assigned to the MCI Triage nurse ☐
  - Nurse in Charge Green label victims (ACC or Fast Track) ☐

  The above positions have task cards that outline preparation for MCI and the "Rules of MCI Management"

- **ED LAYOUT**
  - Admitted patients are to be transferred to ward areas.
  - **Resuscitation rooms are not to be used for MCI victims.**
  - North End (Beds 1–12) – Red Label Victims
  - South End (Beds 13–22) +/– Fast Track – Yellow Label victims
  - Clinic 8 ACC level 3 – Green Label victims. If ACC is not operational, Green Victims will go to Fast Track
  - Green label victims will be triaged, given a pre-allocated MCI MRN, have an ID band attached and then will be escorted to ACC via the ambulance corridor and access the brown lifts in the south corridor. If ACC is not operational (outside working hours 7am to 7pm Mon–Fri), green victims will be directed to fast track, at least in the initial phase of the MCI response.
  - Temporary Emergency Department (TED) is in EMU/CDU for non-MCI patients.
  - The moribund are to be nursed in the side rooms in fast track, and if required, there will be two to a room.
  - Mortuary arrangements: 15 deceased MCI victims may be placed in the 2H and 2I tutorial rooms.

- **RULES OF MCI MANAGEMENT**
  - **Disaster trauma forms** will be used for all MCI victim documentation and management plans
  - **Damage control resuscitation** and damage control surgery should be employed if appropriate
  - **Radiology requests** are to be made on the "Radiology and Surgical Request Forms". These are sent to the ED Imaging Coordinator who will prioritise and negotiate time slots in the radiology department and their assistant will enter the order on FirstNet®
  - **Surgical requests** for OT are to be written on the "Radiology and Surgical Request Forms". These are to be sent to the ED Surgical Coordinator who will prioritise and negotiate time slots in theatre
  - **Victim movements** will be recorded by a clerk on the "Code Brown MCI Victim Tracking Form"
  - **Admissions**: victims will be admitted under the Upper GI Surgeon of the day
  - **Antibiotics** are only prescribed from the preselected list (to be found in the pre-packaged victim folders)
  - **Pharmacy** will set up a satellite unit in A.A.A. and A.C.C. for analgesia, ADT and antibiotics
  - **Pathology** will send a "Blood Safety Officer" who is responsible for ensuring all blood specimens meet the zero tolerance labelling policy. **Transfusion requests must be witnessed**
  - **Documentation** for ALL staff is only to be on the papers provided in the pre-registration packs
  - **A management plan** is to be written before the victims leave the ED
  - **Victim flow is one way** i.e. MCI victims do not return to the ED once they leave for radiology
  - **Non-MCI patients** in radiology will return to the ED for review and management prior to disposition

- **KEY ROLES AND RESPONSIBILITES**
  - ED NUM and Doctor in Charge will provide overall coordination of the ED

Sample Task Card Courtesy: Emergency Department, Royal North Shore Hospital, St Leonards NSW 2065 Australia (2014) Page 1 of 2

Continued

FIGURE 12.7 cont'd

- ED Surgical Coordinator will determine the priority for all surgical interventions for MCI Victims and liaise with the Operating Theatres Duty Director
- ED Imaging Coordinator will determine the priority and suitability for all radiological interventions for all MCI and non-MCI victims and liaise with the Radiology Imaging Coordinator

❧ **MEDICAL POSITIONS TO BE ALLOCATED BY DR IN CHARGE ED**

- ED Imaging coordinator and Assistant (Intern)
- Surgical coordinator
- Doctor in charge of Red area
- Doctor in charge of Yellow area
- Doctor in Charge of Green area
- Doctor in Charge of TED

❧ **STAFF TO BE SENT FROM THE DDC**

- Tracking coordinators Red × 1 Yellow × 2
- Imaging tracker
- Surgical tracker
- Administration assistance to in charge nurse and doctor
- Tracker in TED

❧ **TRACKING PAPERWORK**

The following MCI registration and tracking forms will be used:

- Triage Code Brown MCI Registration Form
- Code Brown MCI Victim Tracking Form
- Radiology and Surgical request Form
- Surgical Coordinator Tracking Form
- Radiology Coordinator Tracking Form
- Green Label Registration and Tracking Form

- **VICTIM PAPERWORK**

All victims will have a pre-registration MRN and a pre made, pre labelled, paperwork pack containing:

Arm band	Victim ID stickers × 10	Disaster Trauma forms	Adult "BTF" obs charts
Blood request forms	Radiology/Surgical request forms × 4	Antibiotic prescribing guidelines	Victim Admission Summary

❧ **STAFF CALL-IN**

- ❧ There is a staff call-in book in the triage MCI folder.
- ❧ Telephone numbers are kept with the ED NUM's and department secretary

❧ **STAND DOWN:**

- ED will receive notification from the DCC of de-escalation and of final MCI victims being received

❧ **CONTINUATION OF CORE BUSINESS**

- ❧ **Non-MCI** victims will receive a regular MRN via the FirstNet registration system and be directed to TED, AAU or RR.
- ❧ Paediatric patients will be assessed and triaged to EP or RR.
- ❧ Mental health patients will be kept in the ED waiting room and reviewed by the CNC mental health. Patients requiring close observation and monitoring will be admitted directly to the Cummins Unit.
- ❧ Code Blue Emergencies: the ED will continue its usual responses

❧ **DEBRIEF**

- ❧ The ED will hold a departmental "hot" debrief for ED staff.
- ❧ An operational debrief will be conducted at which the ED along with other departments will provide a documented report on the operational response.

DCC PHONE NUMBERS:	
HDIC	XXXX
COMMUNICATIONS	XXXX
LOGISTICS	XXXX
DCC FAX NUMBER:	XXXX XXXX

Sample Task Card Courtesy: Emergency Department, Royal North Shore Hospital, St Leonards NSW 2065 Australia (2014) Page 2 of 2

Courtesy: Emergency Department, Royal North Shore Hospital, St Leonards NSW 2065, Australia, 2014.

Prevention strategies include:

- hazard-specific control programs, such as building flood levees, bushfire mitigation and installation of fire alarms
- land-use planning and building controls in legislation and regulations
- quarantine and border control measures
- public health strategies
- community education and awareness
- hazardous material safety and security initiatives
- critical infrastructure protection programs
- mass gathering safety and protection programs.

PREPAREDNESS

Planning is a key element of being prepared. However, there are many other aspects associated with being prepared, such as training, identification of appropriate equipment, public education, public communication arrangements and stockpiling of essential items. Australia addresses these issues at several levels, with individuals encouraged to make appropriate provision for their own preparedness, as well as at community and multi-government levels. In addition to stockpiling essential items, such as generators and medicines, there are education and training programs; interoperability across the country, testing of procedures through exercise programs, and warning systems for the public. An example of preparedness is the critical infrastructure protection planning and cooperation by all spheres of government in partnership with the private sector.

AWARENESS TRAINING AND EDUCATION

Education and training for major incidents are provided in a haphazard manner in many undergraduate programs and rely on the interest or expertise of the academic staff within the undergraduate institution.[26] Undergraduate nursing education should include topics such as general disaster knowledge, assessment and triage, critical thinking, technical skills, and most importantly, mental wellbeing and teamwork in stressful environments.[27] As a result of limited undergraduate education and training for MIs, reliance is either on individuals to seek opportunities or on pre-hospital or hospital and health services to provide education and training. If MI education and training are offered by pre-hospital or hospital and health services, they should focus on the realities of what is likely to be seen within the context of the service being provided. For example, perennially, Australia and Aotearoa New Zealand are impacted by floods, fires and cyclone. As such, these should be a focus in education and training, alongside other MIs such as motor vehicle collisions (MVCs).[28] Local training and testing of plans are included in standards and hospital accreditation programs.

Tabletop exercises are a useful tool to help raise awareness of MI plans and to test specific incident management system roles. However, tabletop exercises do not test real timeframes for clinical decision-making and application of treatment. A more realistic test of MI plans is to simulate survivors and events with actors in realistic scenarios. This method requires the use of sophisticated equipment and large numbers of personnel. An alternative method is using simulation exercises that do not require so many resources yet still provide a realistic test of emergency planning procedures and emergency response plans in real time. An example of such a system is the Emergotrain System™ (ETS), which is used across Australian and Aotearoa New Zealand jurisdictions.[29] The ETS is a training system that is modular and may commence at the scene of the incident or anywhere through to the provision of definitive care. It is therefore ideal for pre-hospital paramedical, medical, nursing and support service personnel. The main strength of ETS is that it is interactive and enables decision-making by providing enough clinical information for attending staff to make decisions. Exercise evaluation of clinical judgement, staff allocation, communication systems and how MI plans interlink becomes a powerful tool for future MI organisational planning.[29]

Points to consider

The following points need to be considered when developing training and education programs:

- Recognition of the numbers and types of staff to be trained to enable safe cover during annual leave and sickness.
- Testing of equipment and rotating stock to be encouraged to increase staff awareness of equipment location and content; regular checking and rotation of stock will prevent stock wastage and re-educate staff about equipment available.
- Practising MI responses requires regular exercises.
- Education and training should focus on the realities of being in an MI.
- Education and training should focus on the types of MIs that the pre-hospital and hospital services are likely to encounter.

RESPONSE

Emergency response involves actions taken in anticipation of, during and immediately after an emergency to ensure that its effects are minimised, and that people affected are given immediate response and support. The response to an emergency is managed first at the local level. Assistance from adjacent local areas and districts, elsewhere within the jurisdiction, other jurisdictions or from the national government is provided according to the scale of the emergency and requests for assistance made according to relevant government arrangements.

A response may include:

- development of warning messages and public information
- evacuating people or communities
- firefighting
- containment and neutralisation of hazardous materials
- provision of medical support
- providing food, water and shelter
- searching and rescue
- establishment of control, command, coordination, or evacuation centres
- animal/stock welfare, e.g. fodder drops
- damage assessment.

THE PRE-HOSPITAL PHASE OF RESPONSE

PRE-HOSPITAL MI MANAGEMENT

The pre-hospital health role remains predominantly the responsibility of the local ambulance services. The first crew on-scene play a pivotal role in escalating resources to the area and activating major incident processes. In a protracted MI, a commander will be deployed to the incident site to lead the pre-hospital health response, working in conjunction with all health organisations on-site, and becoming part of the multi-agency incident management team. Based on the information received, the health commander will make a decision as to any additional health resources needed, including whether medical teams are to be deployed to the MI site.

The incident management and supporting agency operations areas will be set up surrounding the incident site, at a safe distance from the hazard and positioned uphill and upwind from possible contamination. The incident site may have no physical boundary, and there may also be a number of incident scenes within the overall MI site—for example, the wreckage of an aircraft, which may have broken up on impact into many pieces over a wide area. The incident site may also be a forensic crime scene for police purposes. If the site is deemed a crime scene, the police will take control of the site and manage access, egress and forensics on scene.

THE FIRST RESPONDERS ON SCENE

The first crew to arrive on scene at an MI normally take on leadership and triage roles, and must act quickly in order to assist the most people. The roles and responsibilities of the first crew on scene vary in different jurisdictions; however, the processes focus on the following five points:

1. Assess the scene visually to determine if a major incident exists.
2. Declare the incident in a timely manner to prepare the systems that will be implicated, for example, other emergency services and receiving hospitals.
3. Maintain high-end communication while on scene and relay information on scene to dispatch.
4. Commence triage and lifesaving care for survivors.
5. Coordinate resources that arrive on scene.

Assessing the scene at an MCI

It is important to undertake an assessment of the scene, including: identifying any risks to patients or emergency workers, the nature of injuries, number of casualties, best access for emergency workers to gain entry to the scene and to set up clearing stations. In situations where the paramedic suspects a chemical, biological or radiological (CBRN) incident, the STEP 1-2-3 approach may contribute to paramedics staying safe (Table 12.2).[30]

TABLE 12.2 STEP 1-2-3[30]

STEP	EXPLANATION
1	1 casualty exists, approach the scene and treat the patient in the usual way
2	2 casualties exist, use caution when approaching the scene. Provide reports to dispatch and consider all options
3	3 or more casualties exist, do not approach the scene. Isolate yourself and send for specialist help

Declaring a major incident

Declaring a major incident should occur as soon as possible. Several mnemonics exist which can assist the practitioners on scene in relaying the necessary information to dispatch, who will then activate the major incident plans (Table 12.3). An acronym that has been widely utilised and adopted in the prehospital setting is METHANE: M: Major incident declared, E: Exact location, T: Type of incident, H: Hazards or potential hazards on scene, A: Access to the scene, N: Number of casualties, E: Emergency service required.[31] The use of METHANE allows the first responder to provide integral information for an MI to allow for a tactical response from emergency services.

Communication during a major incident

Numerous communication challenges exist when managing a complex scene. Understanding the factors that impact upon communication (Table 12.4) may allow the paramedic to consider these when making decisions and problem-solving.

Communication during MIs has been cited as the biggest problem in achieving optimal patient outcomes.[32,33] The paramedic responsible for maintaining high-end communication must be able to not only communicate effectively with everyone on scene, but to identify and select essential information from the scene to feed back to dispatch.

COORDINATING THE RESOURCES THAT ARRIVE ON SCENE (COMMANDER ROLE)

The scene of an MI soon becomes filled with other medical personnel, emergency service workers and volunteers of all categories. The commander must keep meticulous notes of who has arrived on scene, and where they have been deployed to. It is important that staff wear identification so their skills can be used effectively.

TABLE 12.3 METHANE, CHALETS AND SAM MNEMONICS FOR MAJOR INCIDENT DECLARATION

METHANE	CHALETS	SAM
Major incident declared	**C**asualties–**N**umber, type, severity	**S**ituation unfolding–state what you see, including number of casualties, types of hazards, resources needed
Exact location	**H**azards present	**A**ccess–state the best access to the incident
Type of incident	**A**ccess	**M**ajor incident declared
Hazards	**L**ocation	
Access/Egress	**E**mergency services required	
Number and severity of casualties	**T**ype of incident	
Emergency services required	**S**afety issues	

TABLE 12.4 FACTORS IMPACTING ON COMMUNICATION

FACTORS IMPACTING ON COMMUNICATIONS ON SCENE	FACTORS IMPACTING ON COMMUNICATIONS TO AND FROM DISPATCH
• Size and nature of the incident • Skill and experience of the paramedics on scene • Familiarity and experience of the paramedics in practice/training for mass casualty events • Number of paramedics and other services arriving on scene • Speed of additional support arriving on scene • Time of day • Weather conditions	• Procedures that do not support what is occurring on the scene • Technology that cannot cope with the situation • Experience of dispatchers in managing mass casualty incidents • Leadership challenges

FIGURE 12.8 SMART TAG TRIAGE TAGS

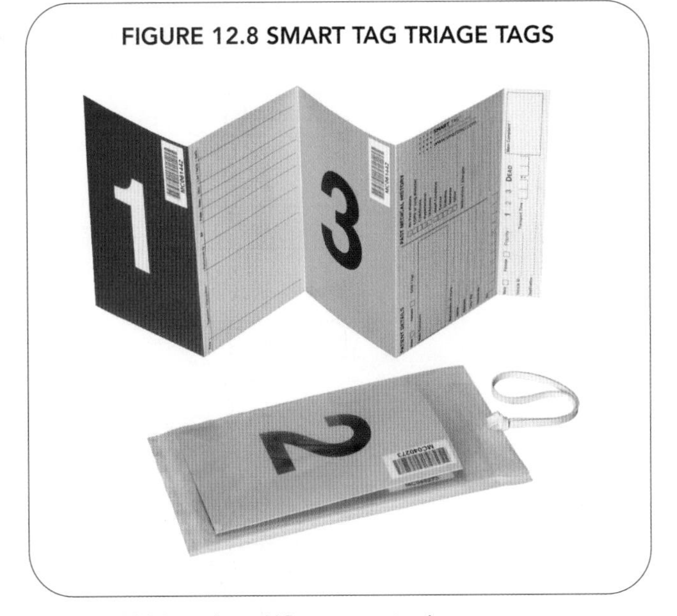

Copyright TSG Associates LLP, www.smartmci.com.

MAJOR INCIDENT TRIAGE

Triage is a fundamental component of MI survivor management and may well determine the outcome for many MI survivors. Triage is performed by trained first responders, paramedics, medical and nursing staff. The principles of MI triage must be applied strictly whenever the number of casualties would overwhelm the available resources.

PRACTICE TIP

It is important to follow all training guidelines and not become emotionally involved in the appearance or age of the survivors. Maintain the MI philosophy of 'do the greatest good for the greatest number'.

Simple pre-hospital MI triage

Simple triage is usually used at a scene of an MI to separate survivors into two distinct groups:

1. Survivors who need immediate attention and rapid transport to hospital.
2. Survivors with less-serious injuries, for whom treatment can be delayed.

To date, however, approaches to triage have become progressively more evidence-based. The triage category of the survivor is frequently the result of an alteration in the survivor's vital (physiological) signs and physical assessment findings.

The Simple Triage and Rapid Treatment (START) model, which has been adopted by Australasian emergency medical services and is taught in the Major Incident Medical Management and Support (MIMMS) training program, as devised by Hodgetts in 1998,[34] is encouraged to be practised and memorised by responders, and an algorithm system is used to assist with this. START is a simple triage system that can be performed by trained first responders, paramedics and emergency clinicians in emergencies. Previous experience, however, reminds us that it is important to undertake simple, immediate lifesaving treatment as part of this initial triage.[35]

Treatment and transport decisions are determined by using the Triage Revised Trauma Score (TRTS), a medically validated scoring system incorporated in some triage cards and discussed later in this chapter.[36] Once a triage decision is made, categorisation and identification of survivors is aided with the use of printed triage tags (Fig. 12.8).

The START triage technique separates MCI survivors into four priority groups:

1. The injured who can be helped by immediate transportation.
2. The injured whose transport can be delayed.
3. Those with minor injuries, who may need help less urgently.
4. The deceased.

It should be noted that the 'expectant' label, issued to survivors who are not dead but are severely injured and might not survive their injuries if treated and transported, does not exist in this triage system. For ethical reasons, a priority 1 label (or an urgent, red, label) is allocated by first responders, paramedics and nursing teams. Ethical decisions are made by senior medical staff either at the site or in a hospital setting. Further discussion of this type of triage is outlined below.

Triage sieve

Triage sieve involves assessment of airway, breathing and circulation (Fig. 12.9) against an established system, as follows:

The system is:

- Immediate (Red)—those survivors who require immediate lifesaving interventions.
- Urgent (Yellow)—those survivors who require urgent and immediate intervention and treatment.
- Delayed (Green)—those survivors who have no serious life-threatening injuries and may wait longer to receive treatment.
- Deceased (White or Black)—individuals who require no further treatment or intervention.[34]

Some authors have debated which physical parameters are the best predictors for those survivors requiring urgent care.[37,38] A decrease in level of consciousness has been shown to be a predictor of those survivors requiring immediate care. The triage tools used most commonly are those devised by Hodgetts and colleagues where the GCS is not formally assessed in the sieve

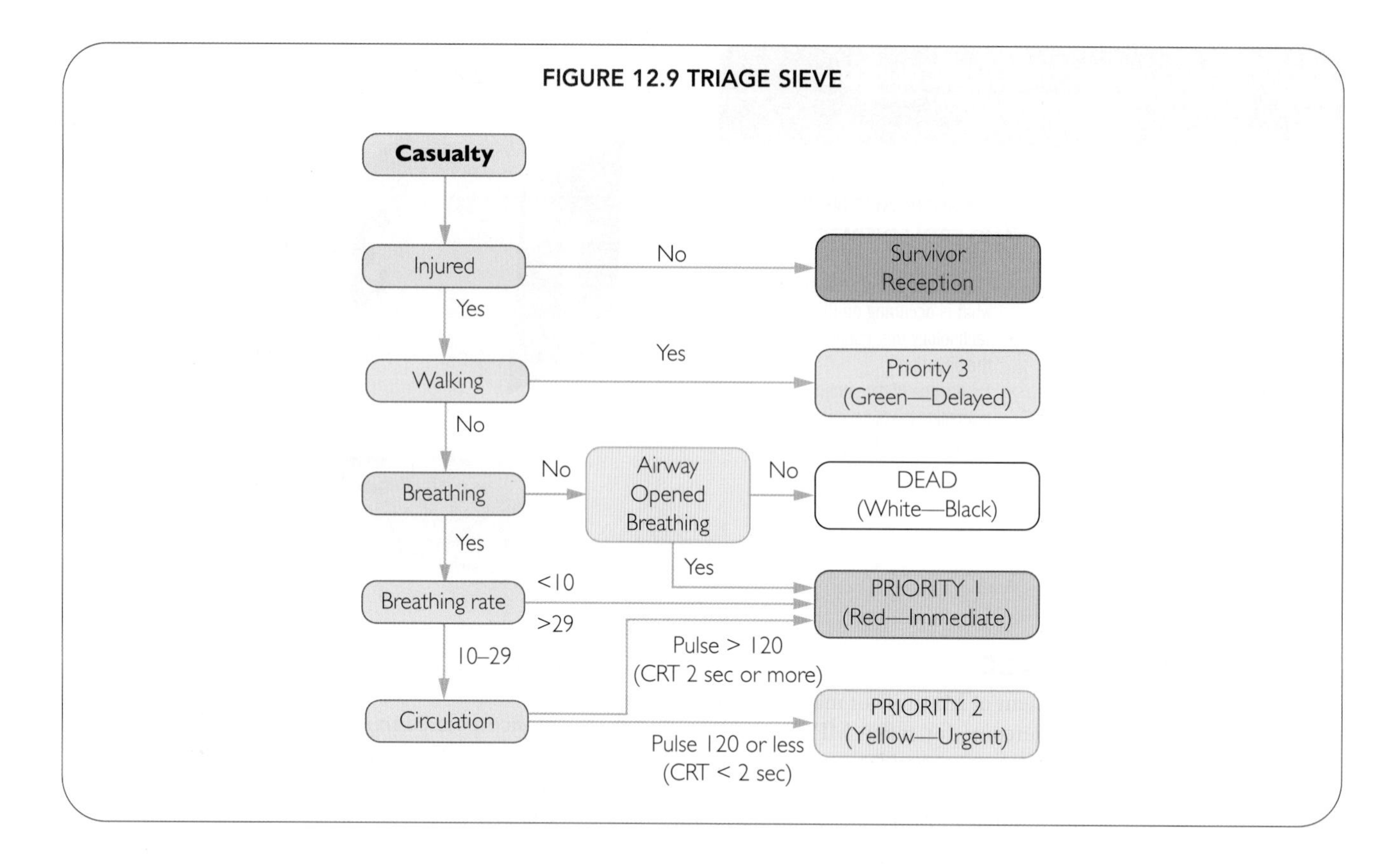

FIGURE 12.9 TRIAGE SIEVE

process, but is used extensively in the sort process.[34] Other key vital signs and characteristics are important. Those survivors able to walk—who therefore must be breathing—are allocated a Priority 3 Delayed category. Survivors who are unable to walk have their airway, breathing and circulation assessed. Survivors unable to breathe despite airway opening are allocated a Dead label. Those survivors able to breathe with a respiratory rate $<$ 10 or $>$ 29 breaths/minute are allocated Priority 1 Immediate, and those survivors with a respiratory rate between 10 and 29 breaths/minute have their capillary refill assessed. A survivor with a capillary refill time below 2 seconds—brisk response—is allocated Priority 2 Urgent. A capillary refill time longer than 2 seconds—sluggish response—is allocated a Priority 1 Immediate. The use of capillary refill time as an assessment of circulation is controversial because the ambient temperature may well affect the speed of the capillary refill. However, the pulse is considered a good circulatory assessment tool.[34] A pulse rate $>$ 120 beats/minute receives a Priority 1 Immediate. A survivor with a pulse rate $<$ 120 beats/minute receives a Priority 2 Urgent. Note that taking the pulse only takes 2 seconds: if the pulse beats twice in 1 second then the rate is 120 beats/minute. If the pulse does not beat twice in 1 second, then it is assumed to be below 120 beats/minute.

Using the SMART triage pack, Delayed (Green) treatment goes to those who can walk; however, it can be difficult to define 'walking'. If a patient is physically able to move and remove themselves to the clearing station, or to a safer location in the absence of an established clearing station, they must do so. This can be achieved by the paramedic shouting to all injured persons and requesting that they move to the clearing station, or a temporary, safe location. Some ambulance services have attempted to clarify this group by defining what constitutes walking. For example, the Australian Capital Territory Ambulance Service defines this group as those who do not have any of the following:

- burns greater than 20%
- airway burns
- respiratory distress
- mental confusion, or
- other conditions of concern.[39]

Such explanations can be useful to paramedics in clarifying which patients should be categorised as walking or non-walking and therefore receive the most appropriate help at the right speed.

'Sort' aspects of MI triage process

Triage sort occurs once the casualties arrive in a casualty clearing post. There are two useful methods of sorting, as described below.

Physiological triage

Physiological triage is a method that uses the TRTS.[34] It is not designed to be descriptive of the casualty's injuries, but is indicative of the physiological consequences of injuries sustained, whether the injuries are overt or covert. In the TRTS, a score from 0 to 4 is given to each of the following clinical parameters:

- GCS
- respiratory rate
- systolic blood pressure.

TRTS combines all three clinical parameters and awards a top score of 12 to indicate that all physiological parameters measured are within acceptable limits. A Green (Delayed) label is allocated to such a survivor. If any one of the clinical parameters scores 1 point lower, giving a total score of 11, a yellow (Urgent) label is allocated to the survivor. If another 1 point or more is lost (a total score of 10 or below), the survivor will be allocated a Red (Immediate) label. A zero score indicates death.

Anatomical triage

Anatomical triage does not require the triage officer to refer to a TRTS; however, an extensive knowledge of the consequences of the mechanism of injuries is used as a good predictor of injury patterns. Some would argue that to perform anatomical triage, a secondary assessment would have to be performed.[34] However, some injuries are so overt that a detailed secondary survey is not required. A well-planned education program would develop fast head-to-toe assessment of MCI survivors. Naturally, a combination of physiological and anatomical triage would complement each other during the sort phase of triage (Fig. 12.10).

Labelling of survivors

In an MI situation, the triage system should facilitate identification of the survivor's medical needs and encompass a documentation system for treatment given, enabling appropriate medical and nursing resource deployment and management. The use of survivor triage labels is part of this process. The issue of multiple triage systems for mass-casualty situations throughout Australasia was resolved by an agreement reached between state and territory governments in Australia and Aotearoa New Zealand's Civil Defence Emergency Management Group (CDEM) in 2011; the resultant changes improved collaborative efforts and uniformity in disaster management within Australasia.

In early 2010, the SMART triage tags were approved as an Australian standard mass casualty triage label by the Council of Ambulance Authorities (CAA) following consultation with jurisdictional health departments.[40] These tags also provide, for the first time, a national consistency for mass casualty triage tags across Australia and allow inter-operability.

The SMART triage tags meet world's best practice and have been tested and evaluated for Australian conditions.

Survivor transport

Different modes of survivor transport are useful to facilitate an even survivor distribution across metropolitan and rural areas. In MIs, ambulance services are the main mode of survivor transport. Large buses may be used to transport large numbers of non-critically ill survivors away from the MI scene to reception centres or definitive care in a non-trauma centre. However, international experience has demonstrated the importance of providing appropriate clinical escort.[41] Air ambulance fixed-wing and rotary-wing craft are used to move critically ill survivors rapidly to trauma centres. An example of an incident site flow process and survivor transfer is illustrated in Fig. 12.11.

In an MI there may be an overwhelming influx of survivors who are not critically injured.[42,43] Therefore, planners need to put in place an effective triage system for Green label survivors and those not requiring medical attention. Triage distribution of Green label survivors to non-trauma centres will enable stretched resources in trauma centres to be concentrated on the Red and Yellow label survivors.[44,45] Those people involved in an MI who do not require medical assistance are triaged to a survivor reception area where social workers and mental health support responders are deployed. The remaining survivors are assessed using sieve and sort.

A well-planned casualty clearing post effectively filters out those who do not require treatment and those with minor injuries who may be best transferred to non-trauma centres. However, experience has proven that despite the intentions of site organisers, a large number of survivors will attend the closest or most familiar hospital and potentially overwhelm the ED. Planning for this should be covered in ED MI plans.

Typical casualty mix of an MI

Several authors have analysed the injuries caused by bombing incidents and note that, apart from those immediately killed, about 10–15% of survivors are severely injured, and the remainder have mild to moderate injuries. For example, in the terrorist attack on a federal building in Oklahoma City in 1995, 88% of people in or near the building were injured and 11% required hospitalisation.[43] In the September 2001 terrorist attack on the World Trade Center, 15% of survivors were admitted to hospital and 85% were walking wounded.[46] It may be possible to extrapolate these figures to non-explosive MCIs where multiple injuries are experienced, for example, bridge collapse, train crash, earthquake and aeroplane crash. The

FIGURE 12.10 TRIAGE SORT

GLASGOW COMA SCALE

Eye opening	Code	Verbal response	Code
Spontaneous	4	Oriented	5
To voice	3	Confused	4
To pain	2	Inappropriate words	3
None	1	Incomprehensible	2
		None	1
Motor response	**Code**		
Obeys commands	6		
Localises to pain	5		
Withdraws to pain	4		
Flexes to pain	3		
Extends to pain	2		
None	1		

REVISED TRAUMA SCORE

Glasgow Coma Scale	AVPU	Code	Respiratory rate	Code
13–15	Awake	4	10–29	4
9–12	Verbal	3	≥ 29	3
6–8	Pain	2	6–9	2
4–5	Unresponsive	1	1–5	1
3		0	0	0
Systolic blood pressure		**Code**		
≥ 90		4		
76–89		3		
50–75		2		
1–49		1		
0		0		

FIGURE 12.11 CASUALTY CLEARING STATION

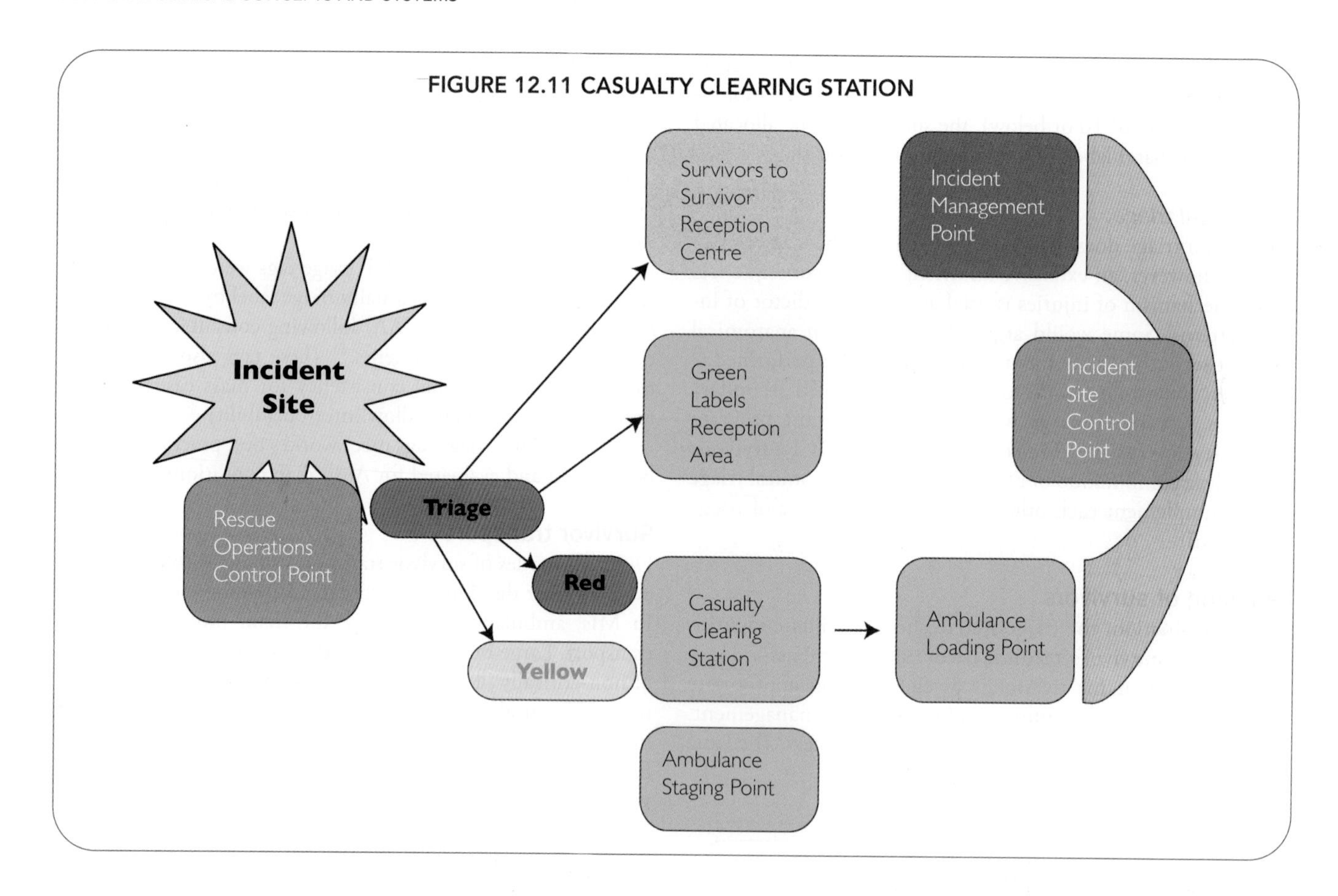

clinical assessment and management of blast injuries is described in Section 4, Major trauma.

Hirshberg, Stein and Walden estimate that if a hospital could assemble seven trauma teams to treat the expected 10–15% patient load of injured survivors following an MCI, then a realistic patient load presentation to an ED would be 7–10 patients who are severely injured (Red labels) and 60–70 patients in the 'Urgent' and 'Delayed' label categories combined.[47]

The principle of doing 'the greatest good for the greatest number' in an MI involving multiple injuries that require surgical intervention hinges on the availability of trauma surgical teams. This availability should determine the hospital's capacity to receive and treat survivors. To accept patient numbers far in excess of available resources might well be detrimental to survivor care and outcome.[46,47]

EMERGENCY DEPARTMENT PHASE OF RESPONSE

This section outlines the key considerations for emergency departments in MIs.

TRIAGE AT RECEIVING HOSPITAL

During business as usual practice, many EDs use a four-or-five point triage scale, such as the Australasian Triage Scale.[48] During an MI, ED triage processes may need to be altered. This alteration may include a more rapid triage process and/or the adoption of triage tags, similar to those tags used in the pre-hospital setting. It is important to note that the MI triage process applied at the ED may differ from that of the pre-hospital paramedical service triage systems. Claudius and colleagues found that introducing a pre-hospital triage model in a hospital setting resulted in inappropriate actions and increased time to perform triage, which is not meeting the ideals of the right patient to the right place in the right time in an MI.[49] To limit confusion among ED staff, usual triage processes should be adhered to as much as possible.

In addition to changes in the triage process, the place where triage occurs may differ. It may be of importance to triage patients outside of the ED; for example, in nearby carparks or in an ambulance bay. This may be important for some MIs, such as chemical, biological, radiological or nuclear events, whereby triage and decontamination should occur prior to patients entering the ED. If triage locations are changed, there are several processes to consider, including reach of information technology, communication to patients, liaison with local ambulance services, relocation of equipment and additional staffing.

PATIENT TRACKING

Depending on the ED, the tracking of patients may differ. Examples of patient tracking include the use of whiteboards or computer systems. Regardless of the MI patient-tracking system in use, the system should be familiar to ED staff and additional human resources may be required to ensure information is updated in a timely manner. In hospitals that have electronic medical records (eMRs), a bank of predetermined MI medical record numbers should be preloaded into the eMR system. Electronic records have a significant advantage over paper records as all users are able to view progress notes and management plans throughout a hospital and inside the hospital command centre. All investigation orders and results are readily available, along with vital sign observations. Planned surgical procedures are able to be booked electronically. Some areas have developed a 'Disaster' section within electronic medical systems to allow for a quick electronic registration of patients and earlier interventions and ordering.

Care considerations

It is important to resist the temptation to order multiple non-urgent radiological investigations, because such investigations may congest survivor flow and jeopardise lives. The development of standing operational procedures (SOPs) involving key stakeholders should be undertaken in the early planning stages to determine which essential tests and investigations are required in an MI event. A senior clinician should be involved in triaging pathology and medical imaging tests that are sent from the ED.

CREATING SURGE CAPACITY

Receiving hospitals are required to have MI plans to deal with an increase in patient presentations and/or increased acuity of patients. Surge capacity 'refers to more than just the maximum survivor load a hospital can handle during a crisis situation'.[47] Hospitals need to be able to respond rapidly to such a surge by creating bed capacity, making operating theatres available, increasing levels of staffing and ensuring supplies and equipment are adequate (Fig. 12.12). Rural and regional facilities, although smaller in size, follow the same concepts, although creating capacity for any number of survivors may exceed the capability of maintaining a standard service level of care. The capacity to rapidly clear patients out of the ED and prepare for the reception of MI survivors is of paramount importance. Individual hospitals and health services will have strategies to manage this differently.

It is worth noting that not all survivors of an MI need to be admitted into hospital or remain in the ED. Following initial triage and/or assessment, it should become apparent that many survivors of MIs can be triaged, treated and discharged from areas outside of the ED. Models of care that exemplify this approach are influenza assessment clinics, which provide rapid assessment and decisions of disposition of those with mild symptoms,[50] or evacuation centres temporarily assessing and managing people due to an MI, such as a bushfire or flood.

Coordination and liaison

The coordination of staff within the ED, and liaison with agencies and services outside of the ED are important for patient outcomes. Best practice in coordination and liaison will ensure that staff roles do not overlap, and that lines of communication are clear and adhered to. There are several strategies to ensure that coordination and liaison is effective. A growing trend is the use of 'role action cards'. Role action cards are small, usually A5 or A6 in size, outlining the roles and responsibilities of each person within the ED. Role action cards should be developed for all roles, not limited to and including individual clinicians,

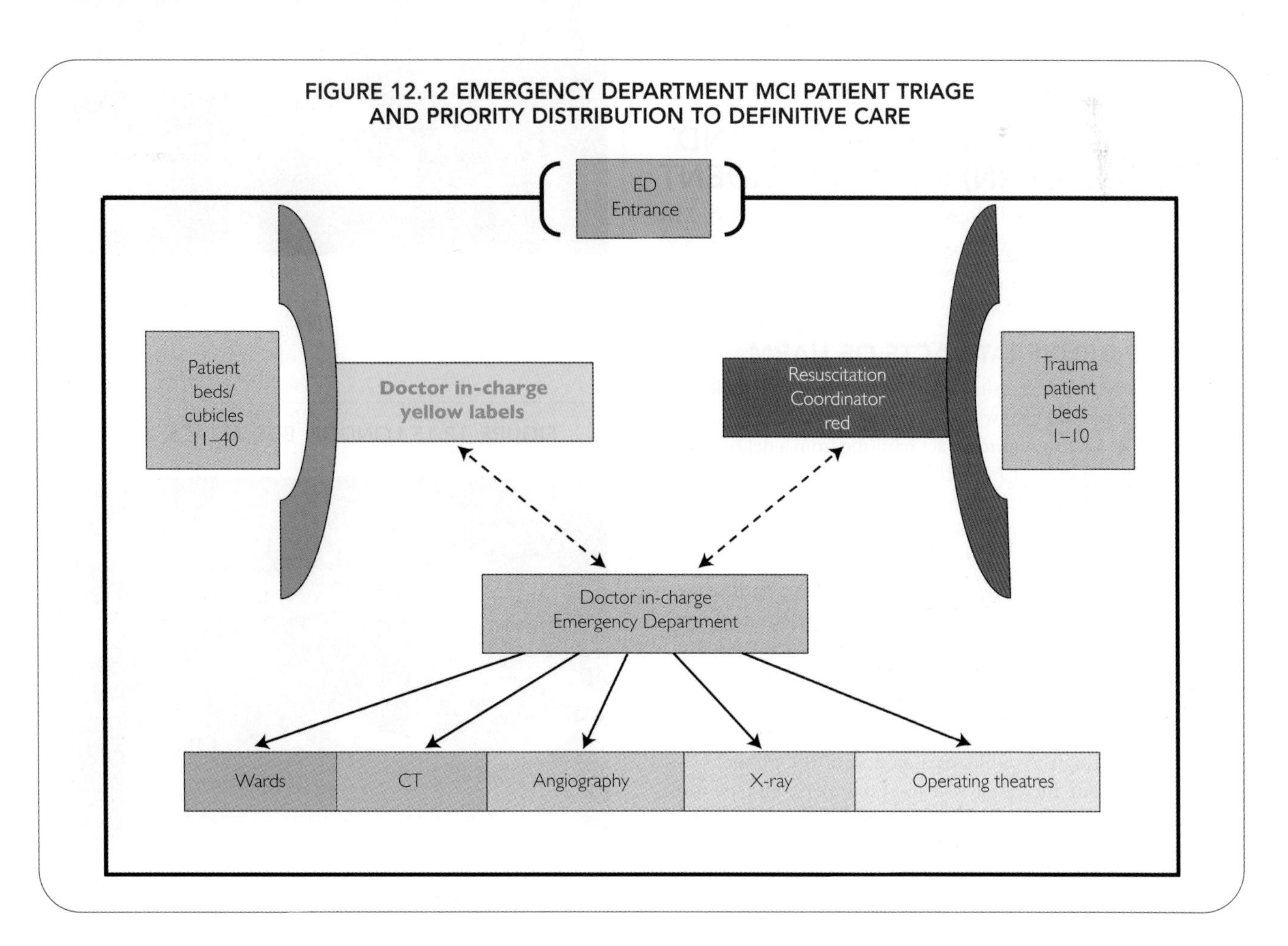
FIGURE 12.12 EMERGENCY DEPARTMENT MCI PATIENT TRIAGE AND PRIORITY DISTRIBUTION TO DEFINITIVE CARE

clinical leads, team leaders, care or flow coordinators, triage staff, managers and administrative staff. Role action cards remain physically with an individual. For example, the clinical team lead of the ED will have their action card visible, usually by attaching it to their name tag. At the end of their shift, they physically hand their action card to the oncoming clinical team lead. This process of handing over role action cards is done for all staff in all positions.

SPECIAL RESPONSE: ACTIVE SHOOTER HOSTILE ENVIRONMENT INCIDENTS

The multi-agency Joint Committee to Create a National Policy to Enhance Survivability from Intentional Mass Casualty and Active Shooter Events have held a series of meetings and developed the Hartford Consensus statements. These include an acronym to describe the priorities in responding to an intentional MI: THREAT.[51] While health personnel may not be equipped to safely undertake some of these actions (for example: suppress a threat), it does indicate the priority actions required for a multi-agency team in order to save the maximum number of patients from such MIs.

THREAT

Threat suppression
Haemorrhage control
Rapid **E**xtrication to safety
Assessment by medical providers
Transport to definitive care

SPECIAL RESPONSE: CHEMICAL, BIOLOGICAL, RADIOLOGICAL AND NUCLEAR (CBRN) MAJOR INCIDENT

Chemical, biological, radiological and nuclear (CBRN) MIs may be the result of unintentional incidents or deliberate acts of harm. The following text outlines MI considerations for CBRN events.

CBRN AS DELIBERATE ACTS OF HARM

There have been an increasing number of large-scale deliberate acts of harm around the world resulting in MIs (Fig. 12.13, Fig. 12.14, Fig. 12.15). A terrorist act resulting from a deliberate act of harm is defined in the *Criminal Code Act 1995* (Australia) as:

an action or threat of action where:

(a) the action falls within subsection (2) and does not fall within subsection (3); and
(b) the action is done, or the threat is made with the intention of advancing a political, religious or ideological cause; and
(c) the action is done, or the threat is made with the intention of:
 (i) coercing, or influencing by intimidation, the government of the Commonwealth or a State, Territory or foreign country, or of part of a State, Territory or foreign country; or
 (ii) intimidating the public or a section of the public.[52]

These MIs present increased risk to responders, and in some cases actually target responders. The following information is presented for awareness only, and additional equipment, training and exercise are required for those who respond to this form of MI.

FIGURE 12.13 FIRST RESPONDERS AT THE WORLD TRADE CENTER 2001

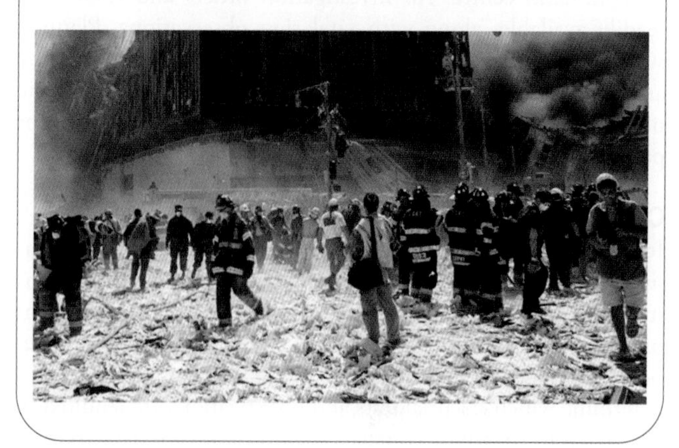

Antony Correia/Shutterstock.

FIGURE 12.14 MEMBERS OF THE PUBLIC ARE GIVEN MEDICAL TREATMENT IN BOURKE ST MELBOURNE FOLLOWING A DRIVER ATTACK 2017

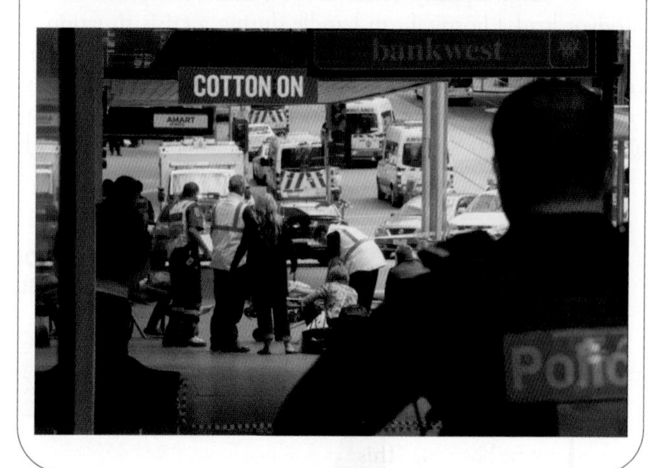

Darrian Traynor/Stringer via Getty Images.

FIGURE 12.15 LONDON BUS ATTACK 2005

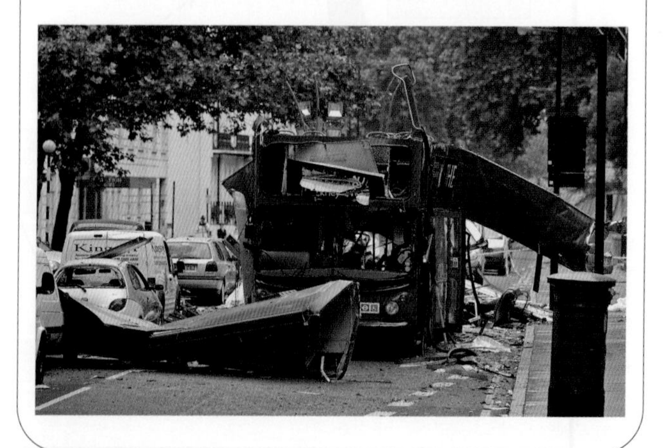

AP/AAP/PA Wire/Peter Macdiarmid.

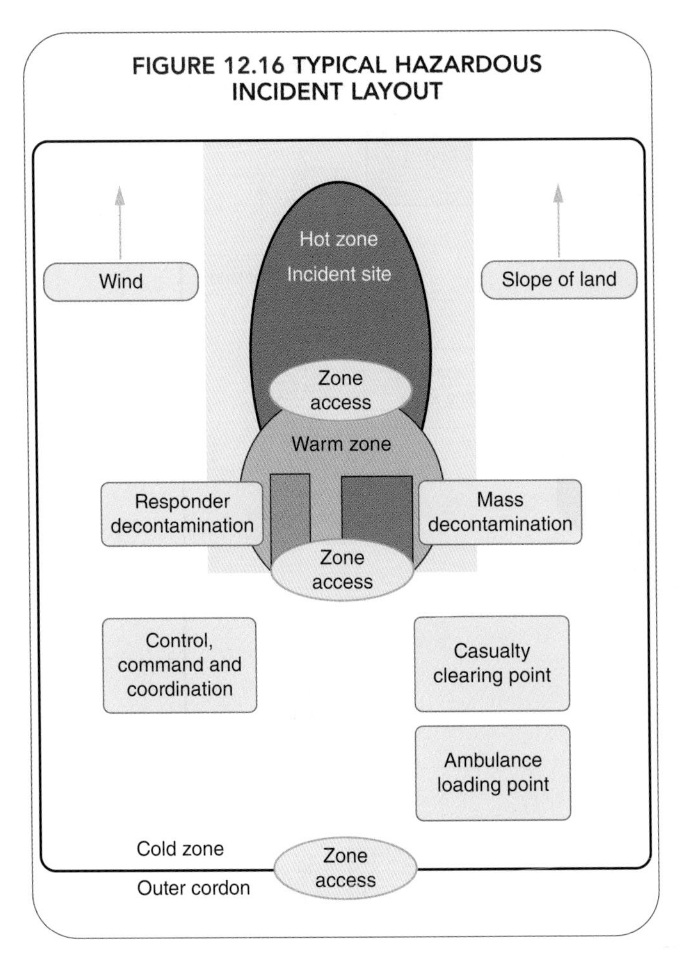

FIGURE 12.16 TYPICAL HAZARDOUS INCIDENT LAYOUT

Due to the high level of risk associated with these hazards, a common language is being used to describe the location of the hazard. The term 'hot zone' is used to describe the area immediately surrounding the hazard where it is dangerous.[6] The term 'warm zone' is used to describe the controlled corridor from the safe area to the hot zone. This is the area where any decontamination will occur. The 'cold zone' is the area that is considered safe and where command posts and other support functions, such as casualty clearing posts, will operate.[6] There may also be an 'outer cordon', which is an area surrounding the entire incident site that has been secured to control access to the site (Fig. 12.16).

Hot zone

In a CBRN MI, the hot zone is the area of known contamination (Fig. 12.17). This zone will be controlled by the nominated lead agency, usually the fire services, and is usually only staffed by specially trained fire, police and paramedical personnel. In the hot zone, the lead agency will determine the level of PPE required. Usually this is the highest level of PPE, Level A. Specially trained paramedics may enter this area if rapid assessment and treatment are required.

Warm zone

The warm zone in a CBRN MI is where decontamination is undertaken. Only minimal response staff are deployed into this area. In the warm zone, the lead agency will determine the level of PPE required. A medium level of PPE is usually worn, for example, Level B or C. All patients presenting to an ED from a hot zone of a CBRN event should be considered contaminated. As such, all patients should undergo decontamination processes. The only exceptions to this are patients who are presenting to the ED from a hot zone via pre-hospital providers, where decontamination has already occurred at the CBRN site.

Cold zone

In this area usually no special PPE is required. Caution must be considered in deployment to a CBRN MI because of the likelihood of hazards such as a secondary explosion or building collapse.

PRE-HOSPITAL MANAGEMENT OF A CBRN MCI

The actions to be considered when responding to a CBRN MCI should include:

- minimising CBRN agent injuries by utilising personal protective equipment (PPE)
- controlling the spread of CBRN contamination by setting up incident management systems
- fast and timely response of appropriate services and rapid establishment of good communication pathways
- timely and accurate information dissemination to enable rapid identification of hazards
- rapid set-up of decontamination facilities on-site and at hospitals
- preventing aggravation of traumatic injuries during first aid and decontamination procedures.

DECONTAMINATION PROCESS AND TREATMENT

Survivor decontamination is essential for the removal of the agent from the survivor and to ensure that the agent does not leave the incident site or enter the hospital facility. The following six steps are an overview of the decontamination process:

1. Wet down the survivor to reduce the likelihood of secondary contamination from materials that may be adhering to clothing and skin.
2. Remove wet contaminated clothing from the survivor.
3. Secure the individual's clothing in a large plastic bag. Jewellery and personal items should be secured in a small clear plastic bag, which is to stay with the survivor. All items are to be taken through the shower process.
4. Shower the survivor with warm water and soap (if available) to remove any remaining contamination from skin and hair. Showering is considered to be effective in removing hazardous substances from the survivor's body (Fig. 12.18).[53]
5. Cover the survivor to maintain modesty and to prevent hypothermia. Return personal items such as jewellery to the survivor.
6. Register and remove survivor from the decontamination area to a safe zone where social and medical services are available if required.

INITIAL PRESENTATIONS TO HEALTHCARE FACILITIES

What we know from previous CBRN MIs is that survivors flee the scene of a CBRN incident before on-scene decontamination facilities are able to be erected,[54] and arrive at EDs via private vehicle or on foot and not by ambulance.[55,56] The ma-

FIGURE 12.17 TYPICAL CBR SITE LAYOUT

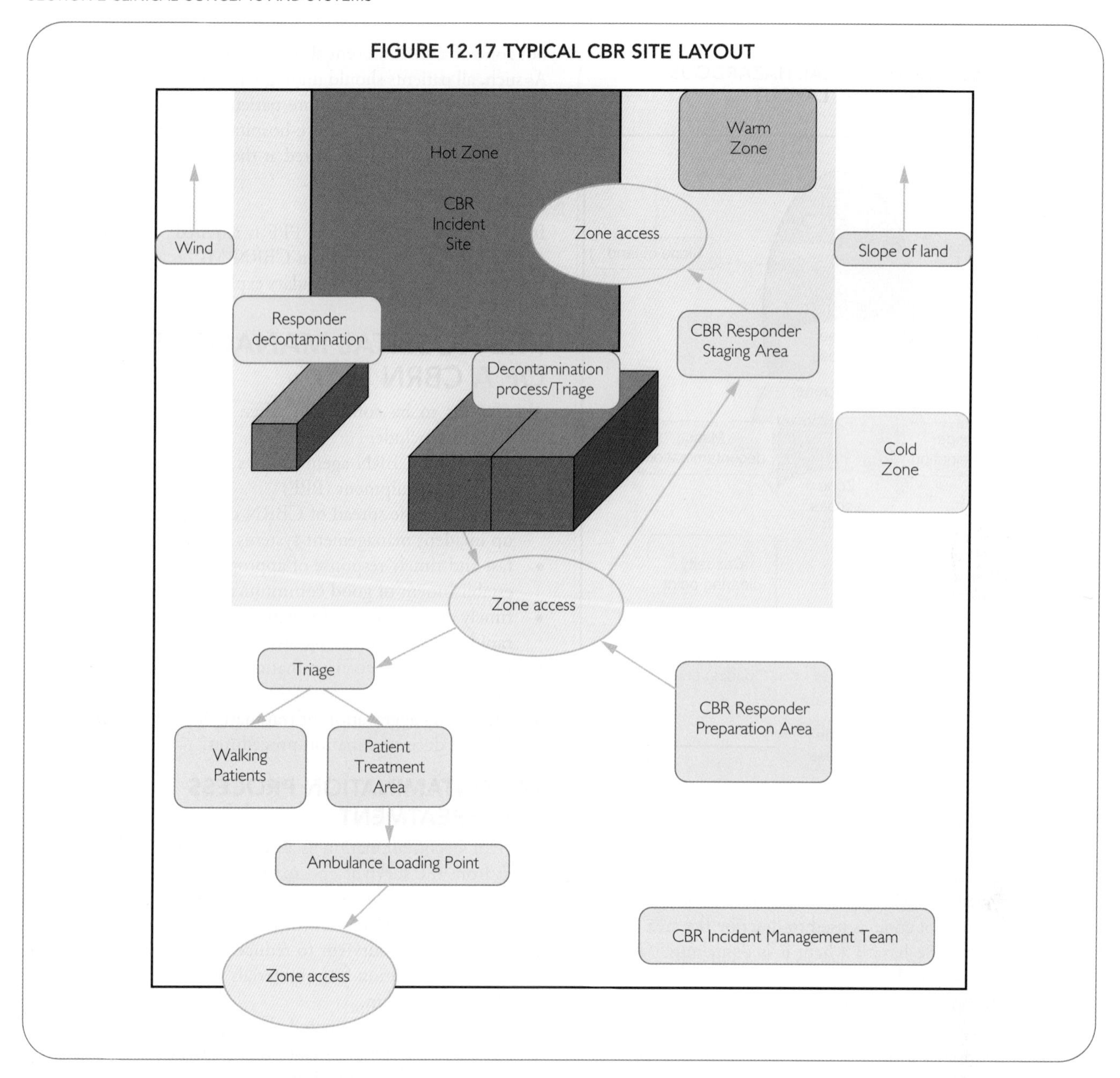

FIGURE 12.18 MASS DECONTAMINATION SHOWER

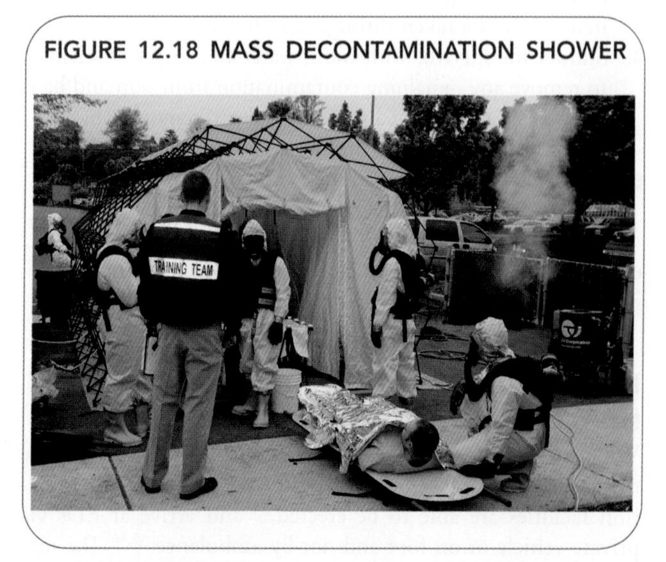

jority of survivors involved in a bomb or chemical attack are seen by EDs,[54,56] and the initial surge will overwhelm hospital resources.[57,58] Most survivors are seen within the first 6 hours following an attack. Hospital emergency procedures should detail how, in the event of a surge of CBRN-contaminated survivors, the facility is quickly locked down to protect it from contamination. The hospital CBRN plan should also detail the corralling of large numbers of survivors to be decontaminated and their movement to a treatment area, or a reception centre for registration and counselling.

CBRN AGENTS

CHEMICAL AGENTS

Chemical agents fall into five major categories: nerve, blister, choking, blood and riot control (Table 12.5). Other chemical agents that affect the nerves are organophosphates. Chemical agents are able to penetrate the body via inhalation, dermal

TABLE 12.5 EXAMPLES OF CHEMICAL AGENTS

CHEMICAL AGENT GROUP	NAME	CODE	ONSET	ENTRY MODE	PHYSICAL STATE AT 20°C	SIGNS AND SYMPTOMS		TREATMENT
Nerve	Tabun	GA	Very rapid	All*	Colourless to brown liquid	*Nicotinic*	*Muscarinic*	Decontamination
	Sarin	GB	Very rapid	All*	Colourless liquid	Mydriasis	Diarrhoea	Pralidoxime
	Soman	GD	Very rapid	All*	Colourless liquid	Tachycardia	Urination	Atropine
	VX	VX	Rapid	All*	Colourless liquid to brown liquid	Weakness	Miosis	Benzodiazepine
						Hypertension	Bradycardia	
						Fasciculations	Emesis	
							Lacrimation	
							Salivation	
Blister	Lewisite	L	Rapid	All*	Dark brown or yellow oily liquid	Immediate pain with blister formation (vesiculations)		Decontamination British antilewisite (BAL) Supportive care
	Distilled mustard	HD	Delayed	All*	Colourless to pale yellow liquid	Blister formation (vesiculations) chemical burns to skin and mucous membranes		Decontamination Supportive care
	Nitrogen mustard	HN3	Delayed	All*	Dark liquid			
	Phosgene oxime	CX	Immediate	All*	Colourless solid	Immediate pain with delayed blister formation (vesiculations)		Decontamination Supportive care
Choking	Phosgene	CG	Rapid	Respiratory	Colourless gas	Short of breath, chest tightness, hypoxaemia, noncardiac pulmonary oedema		Decontamination Supportive care
Blood	Hydrogen cyanide	AC	Very rapid	Respiratory	Colourless gas	Cyanosis, cellular asphyxia, lactic acidosis, seizures and coma		Decontamination Amyl nitrate Sodium nitrate Sodium thiosulfate
	Cyanogen chloride	CK	Rapid	Respiratory	Colourless gas			
	Arsine	SA	Delayed	Respiratory	Colourless gas			
Riot control	Orthochloro-benzylmalonitrile	CS	Instant	Respiratory	White solid	Mucous membrane and skin irritation, lacrimation (tearing)		Decontamination Supportive care
	Chloroacetophenone	CN	Instant	Respiratory	Solid			

absorption, ingestion and injection. It should be noted that clothing is not a protective barrier to these agents, and may well, if not removed, provide a continual source of exposure to the chemical agent.[59] The list of potential chemical agents resulting in injury is long. The average Australian ED chemical injury is more likely to arise from an industrial or a domestic incident. The severity of the injury and the number of people involved will be directly related to the chemical, its concentration, the length of time of exposure and the location of the incident.

BIOLOGICAL AGENTS

Biological agents are broken down into three main types: viruses, bacteria and toxins (Table 12.6). The effectiveness of biological agents is determined by their ability to disseminate disease, to multiply in the object they target and to spread quickly. Signs and symptoms of all types of biological agent poisoning are delayed and can range from 1 day up to 21 days or longer, and usually present as influenza-like symptoms, such as cough, malaise, fever and muscle pains. Specific symptoms, such as rashes, pustules and ulcerations, as noted in cutaneous anthrax, may be visible.

RADIOLOGICAL AGENTS

Many organisations use a variety of radioactive materials as part of normal business: laboratories, universities, the construction industry, hospitals and factories. The risk of radiological incidents occurring and causing industrial contamination from radioactive material release is therefore always present. Radioactive material availability is strictly controlled; however, the probability of unscrupulous people stealing radioactive materials or obtaining 'discarded' radioactive materials is always a threat.

NUCLEAR AGENTS

Similar to radiological material, nuclear material can be found in facilities such as nuclear power plants and medical imaging facilities. Nuclear and radiological incidents can be managed in a similar manner. However, a key difference is the way in which the materials are transmitted. Nuclear events normally involve the detonation of an explosive, resulting in a rapid release of radioactive material, whereas radiological events can result from exposure over time, and a leaking of radioactive material. As a result, nuclear incidents may need special considerations, given the number of severe burns that may be experienced from these events.

RECOVERY

It is not possible to prevent all emergencies. Therefore, recovery activities are needed to address reconstruction, rehabilitation and re-establishment demands across physical, social, emotional,

TABLE 12.6 EXAMPLES OF BIOLOGICAL AGENTS[59]

BIOLOGICAL AGENT GROUP	DISEASE NAME	TIME OF ONSET OF SYMPTOMS	TRANSMISSION (HUMAN TO HUMAN)	MODE OF DISSEMINATION	SIGNS AND SYMPTOMS	TREATMENT
Viruses	Venezuelan equine encephalitis	1–5 days	No	Aerosol/direct	Headaches, pains, fever, malaise, photophobia, myalgia of legs	Supportive
	Smallpox	7–17 days	Yes. High	Aerosol	Severe fever, pox blisters on skin–starts on face and hands	Supportive
Virus (haemorrhagic)	Ebola	2–21 days	Yes. High	Direct	Fever, muscle joint pain, abdominal discomfort, vomiting, bleeding into skin and abdomen	Supportive
	Dengue fever	3–15 days	No	Vector/aerosol		
	Yellow fever	3–6 days	No	Vector/aerosol		
Bacteria	Anthrax (inhalation)	1–7 days	No	Vector/aerosol	Flu-like symptoms, tachycardia, cyanosis and shock	Antibiotics
	Pneumonic plague	2–5 days	Yes. High	Vector/person to person/aerosol	Extreme weakness, glandular swelling, skin haemorrhages	Antibiotics
	Tularaemia	1–10 days	No	Vector/direct/aerosol	Extreme weakness, glandular swelling, skin ulcers	Antibiotics
	Q fever	10–20 days	No	Vector	Headaches, pains, fever, chills, coughs	Antibiotics
Toxins	Botulism	1–12 hours	Non-transmissible	Aerosol	Fevers and cough, weakness, respiratory failure	Supportive
	Ricin	4–8 hours				
	Staphylococcal enterotoxin B	1–12 hours				

psychological, environmental and economic elements. Recovery is, however, more than simply the replacement of what has been destroyed and the rehabilitation of those affected. The aim is to leave the community more resilient than it was before. Planning for recovery is integral to emergency preparation and mitigation actions may often be initiated as part of recovery. Recovery starts with the initial response and may continue for a long period of time, well after the physical damage has been repaired. It requires the collaboration of all spheres of government, the private sector and, most importantly, the community.

RECOVERY ARRANGEMENTS

Australia has in place coordinated recovery arrangements across all levels of government. Recovery agencies are part of each jurisdiction's emergency management committees to ensure continuity and consistency between response and recovery.[16] This includes input from the community and non-government agencies. The arrangements in each state and territory are detailed in stand-alone state-wide plans or as sub-plans of broader emergency management plans. Generally, these plans:

- outline arrangements for managing recovery activities at local and state or territory levels
- identify and provide protocols for establishing and managing local evacuation, relief or recovery centres
- provide processes for disaster relief and assistance measures
- suggest arrangements for establishing and managing public appeals
- recommend approaches for providing continuing information to the affected population
- identify the types of activities which rebuild communities, including the need to capture 'lessons learned' to improve recovery operations in the future.

RECOVERY PRINCIPLES

Successful recovery management in Australia follows six nationally endorsed principles:

1. It is based on an understanding of the community context.
2. It acknowledges the complex and dynamic nature of emergencies and communities.
3. It is responsive and flexible, engaging communities and empowering them to move forward.
4. It requires a planned, coordinated and adaptive approach based on continuing assessment of impacts and needs.
5. It is built on effective communication with affected communities and other stakeholders.
6. It recognises, supports and builds on community, individual and organisational capacity.[60]

ROLES AND RESPONSIBILITIES

The roles and responsibilities during the recovery phase include the following:

- States and territories have primary responsibility for the management of emergencies within their jurisdictions.
- When emergencies occur, the Australian Government provides physical and financial assistance to states and territories when requested to do so, and may also provide financial and other assistance to individuals directly affected by an emergency.
- The Australian Government also has specific responsibilities in relation to national security and defence, border control, aviation and maritime transport, quarantine and the enforcement of Commonwealth legislation and international relations.
- Each jurisdiction is responsible for determining its own internal coordination mechanisms to give effect to these arrangements.[57]

DEBRIEFING AND AFTER-ACTION REVIEW

During an MI or following on from this event, people directly involved, and other members of the community, may exhibit psychological symptoms as a result of the catastrophic nature of the MI.[60] Mental health planning will provide counselling and other ongoing supportive programs. 'Hot' debriefs are usually held immediately after the event to allow for agency and services personnel to voice their thoughts on operational (not emotional) aspects of the MI response. A cautionary note about debriefs is made by Reid,[61] who states: 'The kind of terse questioning often seen in "debriefing" should be avoided.' Carlier and colleagues[62] cite recent studies which indicate that critical incident stress debriefing (CISD) may in fact increase the symptomatology of those airing their emotional reactions to the event. Therefore, debriefing should be offered to, but not be compulsory for, those members of response services involved in the MI.

SUMMARY

MIs can occur at any time, and authorities and professional groups need to be prepared. The development and frequent rehearsal of MI plans are the keys to a controlled and effective response. Risk analysis assists planners in exploring inside and outside their organisations for events that may well have catastrophic effects on their organisations. The triage process has some pitfalls, and the initial reception processes of MI survivors into hospitals should be discussed to assist planners in choosing which members of staff are most suitable to perform the various functions of the MI plan.

Members of staff who may be deployed to the site of a CBRN MI need an overview of the site layout, scene management and knowledge of the CBRN agent effects and antidotes required. Staff responding need to be trained in using the appropriate PPE. This chapter has given an overview of the more common CBRN agents that may be involved in CBRN incidents; note that Tables 12.5 and 12.6 only give examples and are not definitive information documents. Further reading on CBRN is listed below.

The associated response to and the initial surge reception of survivors from an MI can be complex, especially when CBRN agents are involved. The training of as many staff as possible to make them familiar and competent in their response to an MI will assist greatly in any response the institution has to an MI. Such training cannot be emphasised enough. It is important to offer frequent refresher courses and updates.

USEFUL WEBSITES

Australian Institute for Disaster Resilience (AIDR), www.aidr.org.au/.

Australian National Security, www.nationalsecurity.gov.au/.

Australian Radiation Protection and Nuclear Safety Agency, www.arpansa.gov.au.

Centers for Disease Control and Prevention (CDC) (USA), www.cdc.gov.

Department of Health and Ageing (Australia) Emergency Health Management, www.health.gov.au/health-topics/emergency-health-management.

Department of Home Affairs (Australia) Emergency Management, www.homeaffairs.gov.au/about-us/our-portfolios/emergency-management.

Department of Homeland Security (USA), www.dhs.gov.

Federal Emergency Management Agency (FEMA)(USA), www.fema.gov.

International Atomic Energy Agency (IAEA), www.iaea.org.

National Emergency Management Agency (Aotearoa New Zealand), www.civildefence.govt.nz

Ministry of Health (Aotearoa New Zealand) Emergency Management, www.health.govt.nz/our-work/emergency-management.

New Zealand's national security system, dpmc.govt.nz/our-programmes/national-security-and-intelligence/national-security/new-zealands-national-security.

Sphere, spherestandards.org/.

World Health Organization (WHO), www.who.int.

REFERENCES

1. Australian Institute for Disaster Resilience. Health and disaster management. 2nd ed. Melbourne: Australian Institute for Disaster Resilience; 2019.
2. Australian Institute for Disaster Resilience. Australian emergency management arrangements. 3rd ed. Melbourne: Australian Institute for Disaster Resilience; 2019. Available from: https://knowledge.aidr.org.au/resources/handbook-australian-emergency-management-arrangements/.
3. World Health Organization (WHO). Mass casualty management systems: strategies and guidelines for building health sector capacity. Geneva: WHO; 2007.
4. Ministry of Health. National Health Emergency Plan: mass casualty action plan. Wellington: Ministry of Health; 2011.
5. World Health Organization (WHO). Health emergencies list. Online. Available from: www.who.int/emergencies/situations/2022.
6. National Emergency Management Agency. Historical emergencies (NZ). 2022. Online. Available from: www.civildefence.govt.nz/resources/previous-emergencies/historical-emergencies/.
7. Australian Institute for Disaster Resilience. Australian Disaster Resilience Knowledge Hub. Australian Government; 2022. Online. Available from: https://knowledge.aidr.org.au/about/.
8. Ministry of Health. National Health Emergency Plan: A framework for the health and disability sector. Wellington: Ministry of Health; 2015.
9. Emergency Management Victoria. Online. Available from: www.emv.vic.gov.au/about-us/what-we-do/the-six-cs.
10. Australasian Fire and Emergency Service Authorities Council (AFAC). Australasian Inter-service Incident Management System. 2022. Online. Available from: www.afac.com.au/initiative/aiims.
11. Officials' Committee for Domestic and External Security Coordination. Coordinated Incident Management System (CIMS). 3rd ed. Wellington: Department of the Prime Minister and Cabinet; 2019.
12. Sphere Association. The Sphere handbook: Humanitarian charter and minimum standards in humanitarian response. 4th ed. Geneva: Sphere Association; 2018.
13. National Emergency Management Agency. Guide to the National Civil Defence Emergency Management Plan 2015. NEMA. Wellington: National Emergency Management Agency. Online. Available from: www.civildefence.govt.nz/cdem-sector/plans-and-strategies/national-civil-defence-emergency-management-plan-and-guide/.
14. Australian Government. Emergency management. 2022. Online. Available from: www.homeaffairs.gov.au/about-us/our-portfolios/emergency-management/emergency-response-plans.
15. Cocco A, Patel B, Jansen M, Ranse J. Expression of ethical principles in Australia's disaster plans. Emerg Med Australas 2022;34(6): 989–[94]doi:10.1111/1742-6723.14035.
16. Ministry of Health. Response planning in CDEM: Director's Guideline for Civil Defence Emergency Management Groups [DGL 19/15]. Wellington: MOH; 2015.
17. Australian Institute for Disaster Resilience. Emergency planning handbook. 2020. Online. Available from: https://knowledge.aidr.org.au/resources/emergency-planning-handbook/.
18. Standards Australia. Risk management—Risk assessment techniques AS/NZS IEC 31010:2020. Sydney: Standards Australia; 2020.
19. Emergency Management Australia. Australian Government Disaster Response Plan (COMDISPLAN). Canberra: Emergency Management Australia; 2020.

20. Department of Health and Ageing. National Health Emergency Response Arrangements (NatHealth Arrangements). Canberra: Australian Health Protection Committee; 2011.
21. Australian Government Department of Health. Domestic health response plan for all hazards incidents of national significance (AUSHEALTHRESPLAN). Canberra: DOH; 2021.
22. National Emergency Management Agency. National Civil Defence emergency management plan 2015 and guide to the plan. Wellington: National Emergency Management Agency; 2015.
23. Standards Australia. Australian/New Zealand Standard (AS/NZS 4083) infrastructure protection. Sydney: Standards Australia; 2010.
24. Hammad KS, Wake M, Zampatti C, Neumann S, Ranse J. Working in the dark—The impact of a state-wide black systems event on emergency departments: a case study from clinician perspectives. Collegian 2019;26(2):262–6.
25. Standards Australia. Planning for emergencies – Health care facilities AS 4083–2010. Sydney: Standards Australia; 2010.
26. Usher K, Mayner L. Disaster nursing: a descriptive survey of Australian undergraduate nursing curricula. Australas Emerg Nurs J 2011;14(2): 75–80.
27. Ranse J, Ituma OW, Bail K, Hutton A. Disaster education in undergraduate nursing curriculum: a Delphi study to prioritise content for nursing students. Collegian 2022;29(5):590–7.
28. Ranse J, Hammad K, Ranse K. Future considerations for Australian nurses and their disaster educational preparedness: a discussion. Aust J Emerg Manage 2013;28(4):49–53.
29. Lennquist S. The Emergotrain system for training and testing disaster preparedness: 15 years of experience. Int J Disaster Med 2003;1(1):25–34.
30. Kahn C, Koenig K, Boylan M. Emergency preparedness: chemical, biological, radiation and nuclear incidents. In: Nutbeam T, Boylan M, editors. ABC of prehopsital emergency medicine. West Sussex: Wiley Blackwell; 2013.
31. Keene D, Nutbeam T, Scanlon C. Emergency preparedness: major incident management. In: Nutbeam T, Boylan M, editors. ABCs of prehospital emergency medicine. West Sussex: Wiley Blackwell; 2013.
32. Fish JA, Peters MDJ, Ramsey I, Sharplin G, Corsini N, Eckert M. Effectiveness of public health messaging and communication channels during smoke events: a rapid systematic review. J Environ Manage 2017;193:247–56.
33. Palttala P, Boano C, Lund R, Vos M. Communication gaps in disaster management: perceptions by experts from governmental and non-governmental organizations. J Conting Crisis Manage 2012;20(1):2–12.
34. Hodgetts T, Mackaway-Jones K, editors. Major incident medical management and support, the practical approach. Plymouth: BMJ Publishing; 1998.
35. Coroner HM, editor. The Rt Hon Lady Justice Hallett DBE. Coroner's inquests into the London bombings of 7 July 2005. London: UK Government; 2012.
36. European Resuscitation Council. European Trauma course. Online. Available from: www.erc.edu/courses/european-trauma-course.
37. Garner A, Lee A, Harrison K, Schultz CH. Comparative analysis of multiple-casualty incident triage algorithms. Ann Emerg Med 2001;38(5):541–8.
38. Meredith W, Rutledge R, Hansen AR, Oller DW, Thomason M, Cunningham P. Field triage of trauma patients based upon the ability to follow commands: a study in 29,573 injured patients. J Trauma 1995;38(1):129–35.
39. ACT Ambulance Service. Clinical Management Guidelines: Mass casualty triage flow chart. 2022. Online. Available from: https://esa.act.gov.au/sites/default/files/wp-content/uploads/28-MASS-CASUALTY-TRIAGE-FLOW-CHART-right-justified.pdf.
40. NSW Health. Mass casualty triage – SMART triage packs. Document Number PD2017_037. Sydney: NSW Health; 2017.
41. European Court of Human Rights. Case of Finogenov and others v. Russia (Applications nos. 18299/03 and 27311/03). Strasbourg: European Court of Human Rights; 2012.
42. Jacobs Jr LM, Ramp JM, Breay JM. An emergency medical system approach to disaster planning. J Trauma 1979;19(3):157–62.
43. Teague DC. Mass casualties in the Oklahoma City bombing. Clin Orthopaed Related Res 2004;(422):77–81.
44. Ammons MA, Moore EE, Pons PT, Moore FA, McCroskey BL, Cleveland HC. The role of a regional trauma system in the management of a mass disaster: an analysis of the Keystone, Colorado, chairlift accident. J Trauma 1988;28(10):1468–71.
45. Frykberg ER. Medical management of disasters and mass casualties from terrorist bombings: how can we cope? J Trauma 2002;53(2):201–12.
46. Cushman JG, Pachter HL, Beaton HL. Two New York City hospitals' surgical response to the September 11, 2001, terrorist attack in New York City. J Trauma 2003;54(1):147–54; discussion 54–5.
47. Hirshberg A, Stein M, Walden R. Surgical resource utilization in urban terrorist bombing: a computer simulation. J Trauma 1999;47(3):545–50.
48. Australasian College for Emergency Medicine. Policy on the Australasian triage scale. Melbourne: The Australasian College for Emergency Medicine; 2013.
49. Claudius I, Kaji AH, Santillanes G, Cicero MX, Donofrio JJ, Gausche-Hill M, et al. Accuracy, efficiency, and inappropriate actions using JumpSTART Triage in MCI simulations. J Prehosp Disaster Med 2015;30(5):457–60.
50. Ranse J, Lenson S, Luther M, Xiao L. H1N1 2009 influenza (human swine influenza): a descriptive study of the response of an influenza assessment clinic collaborating with an emergency department in Australia. Australas Emerg Nurs J 2010;13(3):46–52.
51. Jacobs LM. The Hartford Consensus IV: a call for increased national resilience. Bull Am Coll Surg 2016;101(3):17–24.
52. Australian Government, Federal Register of Legislation. Criminal Code Act 1995. No 12. Compilation 144. Part 5.3 Terrorism, Division 100—Preliminary. 100.1 Definitions. Australia; 1995 (2 April 2022). Online. Available from: www.legislation.gov.au/Details/C2022C00156.

53. Macintyre AG, Christopher GW, Eitzen Jr E, Gum R, Weir S, DeAtley C, et al. Weapons of mass destruction events with contaminated casualties: effective planning for health care facilities. JAMA 2000;283(2):242–9.
54. Okumura T, Suzuki K, Fukuda A, Kohama A, Takasu N, Ishimatsu S, et al. The Tokyo subway sarin attack: disaster management, Part 1: community emergency response. Acad Emerg Med 1998;5(6):613–7.
55. Okumura T, Suzuki K, Fukuda A, Kohama A, Takasu N, Ishimatsu S, et al. The Tokyo subway sarin attack: disaster management, Part 2: hospital response. Acad Emerg Med 1998;5(6):618–24.
56. Bradt D. Rapid assessment of injuries among survivors of the terrorist attack on the World Trade Center. New York City, September 2001. MMWR Morb Mortal Wkly Rep 2002;51(1):1–5.
57. Okudera H, Morita H, Iwashita T, et al. Unexpected nerve gas exposure in the city of Matsumoto: report of rescue activity in the first sarin gas terrorism. Am J Emerg Med 1997;15(5):527–8.
58. Okumura T, Takasu N, Ishimatsu S, Miyanoki S, Mitsuhashi A, Kumada K, et al. Report on 640 victims of the Tokyo subway sarin attack. Ann Emerg Med 1996;28(2):129-35.
59. Walter FG. Advanced Hazmat Life Support provider manual. 5th ed. Tucson: University of Arizona Emergency Medicine Research Center, American Academy for Clinical Toxicology; 2017.
60. Social Recovery Reference Group Australia. National Principles for Disaster Recovery. 2018. Online. Available from: knowledge.aidr.org.au/resources/national-principles-for-disaster-recovery/.
61. Reid W. Psychological aspects of terrorism. J Psychiatr Pract 2001;7(6):422–5.
62. Carlier IVE, Lamberts RD, Van Uchelen AJ, Gersons BPR. Disaster-related post-traumatic stress in police officers: a field study of the impact of debriefing. Stress Med 1998;14(3):143–8.

CHAPTER 13

PATIENT ASSESSMENT AND ESSENTIALS OF CARE

BELINDA MUNROE, CLAIRE HUTCHINSON AND TAMSIN JONES

ESSENTIALS

- Patient assessment should always begin with DRSABCDE (Danger, Response, Send for help, Airway, Breathing, Circulation, Disability and Exposure). Once life-threatening conditions have been identified and treated, a more comprehensive assessment can be completed, focusing on relevant body regions and systems.
- HIRAID™ is the only evidence-based comprehensive emergency nursing framework, and is applicable to all patient presentations.
- If a patient deteriorates, then reassessment should always start again at DRSABCDE.
- Use an aid such as the SAMPLE mnemonic to ensure that all relevant history data is obtained. Risk of infection and communicable diseases should be considered when collecting a patient history, including appropriate precautions required.
- 'Red flags' may become evident at any stage of the patient assessment and should never be ignored.
- A set of vital signs comprises respiration rate, oxygen saturation, blood pressure, pulse rate temperature, conscious state and new onset confusion or behaviour change.
- When performing a physical assessment, remember to inspect, auscultate, percuss and palpate. Use a structured handover tool, such as IMIST-AMBO or ISBAR; this ensures that no vital information is forgotten. Use a structured approach to and double-check your documentation for errors.
- Patients should be screened to identify risk of falls, pressure injuries, poor nutrition and cognitive impairment, and appropriate strategies put into practice to prevent or minimise complications.

INTRODUCTION

Assessment is the ability to observe and interpret any clinical situation, thereby influencing the decisions of emergency nurses and paramedics. Accurate patient assessment enables the evaluation of actions and practices and lies at the core of both professions. How well patients are cared for has a direct effect on their sense of wellbeing and recovery. This chapter also discusses the essential elements of nursing care.

Assessment enables emergency clinicians to prioritise care. The triage nurse or first-responder paramedic will perform a rapid patient assessment, but, as every patient's condition has the potential to change, there is a need to recognise the importance of a more comprehensive assessment, followed by the ability to determine how often reassessment should take place. Patient reassessment in emergency departments

(EDs) has never been more important, given the prevalence of access block, which results in prolonged length of stay in the ED.[1] Different assessment models exist with their own distinct purpose. The triage assessment is brief with the aim of sorting patients into order of urgency and determining how long they can wait for emergency care.[2] The primary survey ensures life-threatening conditions are identified and treated first.[3] The HIRAID™ emergency nursing framework provides a systematic approach to the comprehensive assessment of patients.[4] Assessment models such as these ensure a structured evidence-based approach to assessment and are imperative to enhance the clinician's performance and optimise patient safety.[5–9]

Emergency clinicians make important clinical decisions every day and these decisions have an effect on the patient's healthcare and the actions of healthcare professionals. As care provision is becoming increasingly complex, emergency clinicians have to rely on sound clinical decision-making skills to maintain up-to-date care and positive outcomes.

THE ASSESSMENT PROCESS

Assessment starts from the first moment you see your patient and begins with a primary survey assessment and collection of details about the patient's history, followed by a systematic assessment of relevant body regions and systems. Assessment findings inform the selection and prioritisation of interventions. Diagnostic tests also contribute to developing a complete picture of the patient's condition.

THE PRIMARY SURVEY

The primary survey, as the first element of patient assessment, ensures a consistent, evidence-informed and sequenced approach promoting patient safety in all clinical settings.[5] The primary survey consists of DRSABCDE (**D**anger, **R**esponse, **S**end for help, **A**irway, **B**reathing, **C**irculation, **D**isability and **E**xposure) (see Box 13.1). There are some slight variations to the primary survey components (e.g. D for Defibrillator in the event of an unconscious collapse, and D for Disability for a primary survey of a conscious patient), but the general principles are the same.[3,10–12] The patient environment should always be checked for danger before commencing patient assessment, to ensure it is safe to approach the patient. Any foreseeable risks should be removed to prevent injury prior to commencing the assessment. A scan of the surroundings will inform you of any danger or hazards that need to be negotiated. These can include a patient who has collapsed in the waiting room bathroom and is lying in a pool of water, or at a motor vehicle collision (MVC), where traffic is still passing at speed. As a paramedic arriving on the scene, assessment can also tell you about the mechanism of injury, how many casualties there are and what resources you may need. You will need to note the position of the casualties and any points of impact, as this is important information to include when handing over your patient. Once the scene has been assessed and any danger removed, an initial patient assessment of ABCDE can take place. See Chapter 9 for a detailed discussion of scene assessment and management.

The Australian Resuscitation Council recommends the primary survey follows DRSABCD (**D**anger, **R**esponse **S**end for help, **A**irway, **B**reathing, **C**PR and **D**efibrillator) to preserve and restore life when resuscitating the unconscious patient.[3] The Advanced Trauma Life Support guidelines also teach the step called 'exposure', which involves the removal of the patient's clothing to expose and identify any immediate life-threatening injuries and ensure adequate temperature control is achieved.[13] Undressing and exposing all patients is necessary to enable a complete physical assessment, particularly once the patient has reached the ED, where privacy may be maintained. Early measurement of temperature is important to identify hypothermia, hyperthermia and febrile illnesses in both trauma- and non-trauma-related presentations such as sepsis, which requires urgent identification and treatment to reduce morbidity and mortality.[14] Exposure is also recommended by the Australian Resuscitation Council when reassessing the patient after the return of spontaneous circulation; targeted temperature control as part of post-resuscitation care has been demonstrated to improve patient outcomes.[3] See Chapter 14 for patient resuscitation and Chapter 42 for a detailed assessment of the major trauma patient.

During this phase, life-threatening problems are identified and interventions commenced if required. The clinician should ensure each step of the primary survey is complete and any identified life-threatening conditions are treated first, before moving on to the next stage of assessment. If nothing imminently life-threatening is detected, a further, more-focused assessment can take place.[3,4] It is important to have a systematic approach to this assessment to ensure that important information is not missed, and prevent further patient deterioration.[15]

BOX 13.1 ASSESSMENT OF DRSABCDE

DR–Danger and Responsiveness	Check for danger and patient responsiveness
S–Send for help	If patient unresponsive send for help
A–Airway	Is the airway patent and protected? Is there any sign of obstruction? Is the cervical spine immobilised (for trauma patients)?
B–Breathing	Is the chest rising and falling? Is breathing adequate?
C–Circulation	Is the circulation sufficient to meet the needs of the patient? Is there ongoing bleeding?
D–Disability	What is the patient's neurological status? Assess using AVCPU. (**A**lert, responding to **V**oice, new onset of **C**onfusion, responding to **P**ain or **U**nresponsive) scale Check pupil response Don't forget the glucose
E–Exposure	Remove clothing and look for immediate threats to life or limb What is the patient's temperature?

HIRAID™: AN EMERGENCY NURSING FRAMEWORK

The emergency nursing framework HIRAID™, by Curtis and colleagues,[16] can ensure that a systematic approach is taken when performing an initial nursing assessment and ongoing patient care.[17] In the ED setting, HIRAID™ has been shown to

FIGURE 13.1 HIRAID™: AN EVIDENCE-INFORMED EMERGENCY NURSING FRAMEWORK[4]

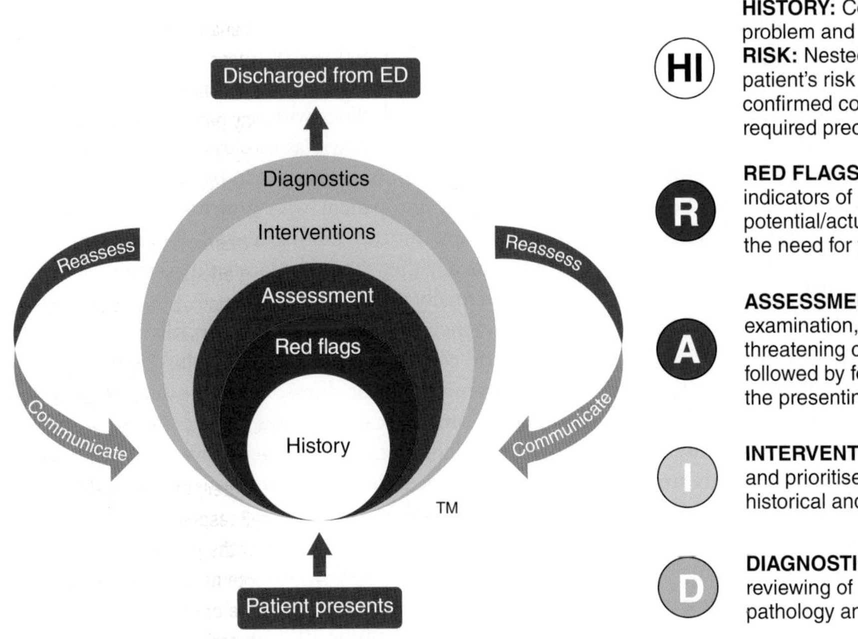

HISTORY: Collection of the presenting problem and health history. **INFECTION RISK:** Nested within history; refers to the patient's risk of infection or suspected/confirmed communicable disease; includes required precautions.

RED FLAGS: Historical or physiological indicators of urgency that identify potential/actual threat to life or limb; highlights the need for timely escalation of care.

ASSESSMENT: Comprehensive physical examination, prioritised to ensure life threatening conditions are identified first, followed by focussed assessments guided by the presenting problem.

INTERVENTIONS: The delivery of appropriate and prioritised interventions based on historical and physical assessment findings.

DIAGNOSTICS: The ordering, performing and reviewing of further investigations, including pathology and diagnostic imaging.

The HIRAID framework encapsulates the cyclical nature of patient assessment, in which more than one element of the framework may be performed simultaneously. It also embraces the importance of **reassessment** and **communication**, which are vital components of emergency nursing.

REASSESSMENT: The evaluation of care and monitoring of patient progress using a structured approached and repeated at appropriate intervals per condition of the patient.

COMMUNICATION: Verbal/non-verbal skills necessary to effectively communicate with patients, families and clinicians, includes using: a structured approach to comunicate clinical handovers; graded assertiveness to escalate if needed; and, accurate and comprehensive clinical documentation.

significantly reduce ward patient deterioration of emergency admissions and associated healthcare costs.[15,18] The HIRAID™ process is comprised of seven critical components:

- **H**istory (including **I**nfection risk)
- Identify **R**ed flags
- **A**ssessment (clinical examination)
- **I**nterventions
- **D**iagnostics
- Reassessment
- Communication.[4]

Fig. 13.1 illustrates the relationship between the steps. They do not necessarily occur in this order, as in reality they often happen simultaneously. The assessment is a cyclic process, supported by ongoing reassessment and communication.

The history is gained from the patient, relative, carer or significant other. It should include details about the chief complaint and the patient's individual health history, such as past medical history, medications and allergies. Infection risk should be considered as part of the patient's history, comprising of infection and/or suspected or confirmed communicable disease, including personal protective equipment (PPE) required. Identification of red flags involves recognition and response to clinical indicators of urgency identified during any stage of the assessment process. The emergency clinician must respond to red flags and escalate care as required in a timely manner to prevent deterioration and optimise patient recovery. Assessment involves the clinical examination of the patient, including skills such as inspection, auscultation, percussion and palpation. Interventions that may be required include giving first aid, applying oxygen and giving analgesia. Once the patient has arrived at an ED and life-threatening conditions are identified and treated, diagnostic and laboratory testing can take place.

On the patient's arrival to hospital, the triage nurse is initially responsible for identifying the chief complaint and the ideal location within the ED. Once the patient is moved to a treatment area, a more thorough and detailed assessment is performed to ensure that any life-threatening illnesses or injuries not found initially are detected and treatment commenced. Emergency clinicians are often responsible for patients for extended periods and required to commence treatment and monitor response to therapies prior to medical review. Therefore, it is vital that every emergency clinician has the ability to perform an accurate clinical assessment with a view to determining the chief complaint and not just record a set of vital signs which, taken in isolation, is often meaningless.

HISTORY (INCLUDING INFECTION RISK)

Taking a history requires collection of subjective data. This is the information that you gather from the patient, relative, carer or significant other. In the pre-hospital setting this may also be a witness to an accident. Developing and maintaining rapport are central to good communication and effective information gathering.[19] It is important to take some time at the beginning of any assessment to explain who you are and what it is you are planning to do. Ask open-ended questions and let the patient speak for a minute or two without interruption, and the main problem and any concerns should become apparent. Examples of open-ended questions are: 'What's troubling you today?', 'Why have you come to hospital?' or 'Why did you call the ambulance?'. Emergency clinicians should then be able to focus the assessment and gather required additional information, and allay any immediate anxieties. Asking open-ended questions of Indigenous people is very important, as they may not respond well to direct questioning (see Chapter 5 for further discussion of cultural considerations). When the patient is acutely unwell, the amount of time spent asking open-ended questions should be limited so that the assessment can move promptly to the area of concern, allowing quick evaluation and management.[20]

It is important to also speak to family, carers or witnesses, as they may be able to add pertinent information that the patient considers insignificant or is unable to give due to an altered mental state. If the patient has an altered level of consciousness, then the nurse or paramedic has to rely more heavily on other assessment skills, and once the patient has arrived in the ED the nurse may need to obtain old hospital records or contact the general practitioner if friends or relatives are not able to help or are uncontactable. However, such searches can be quite time-consuming. The emergency nurse responsible for assessing the patient once they have been allocated to a treatment space should review the ambulance case sheet and triage form to ensure information has not been omitted during the handover process.

When taking a history, it is useful to develop a systematic approach to ensure that all the important questions are asked. The SAMPLE mnemonic (Box 13.2) is a way to structure history-taking in a pre-hospital environment.[21]

It is also important to consider if the patient is at increased risk of acquiring an infection or transmitting an infection to others, and the relevant infection prevention and control requirements. Focused questioning should be used to identify patients who are immunocompromised. For example, patients on immunosuppressive drugs such as corticosteroids or chemotherapy, or with an immune deficiency disorder such as cancer, diabetes mellitus or human immunodeficiency virus (HIV). Infants (< 1 month of age) are also at increased risk of infection as their immune system is underdeveloped, as well as elderly people (> 65 years old) as the immune response declines with age.[22] Knowledge of the patient's increased infection risk will assist clinicians to put in place appropriate infection control measures to prevent infection in these patients. Placing the patient who presents to the ED 5 days post chemotherapy in the waiting room, for example, should be avoided; ideally they should be located in a single room away from other potentially infectious patients.

Emergency clinicians must be especially vigilant in detecting carriers of communicable diseases, who present an increased risk of transmission of disease to healthcare workers and other patients. Communicable diseases may be spread via direct contact (e.g. methicillin-resistant *staphylococcus aureus* (MRSA), vancomycin-resistant enterococcus (VRE), transmission of large droplet particles that travel short distances (e.g. influenza, meningococcal) or smaller airborne particles that can remain in the air for several hours (e.g. SARS-COV-2, measles, tuberculosis and varicella (chickenpox)).[23] Knowledge of the disease and how it spreads can help clinicians determine PPE and isolation requirements. Obtaining a detailed history of potential exposure risk such as contact with carriers of a disease, recent travel, vaccination status and signs and symptoms of diseases is critical to detecting infections early.[24] Appropriate questioning of a child who presents with a pustule rash and fever, for example, will help identify if they are unvaccinated and have recently attended daycare where there is an outbreak of chickenpox. During outbreaks of disease, clinicians may be required by public health to undertake specific screening questions. See Chapter 27 for more information on healthcare-associated infections and infectious diseases.

Once the patient has arrived at an ED, details about the patient's history can be handed over to the accepting nurse. The patient's condition may have changed during transportation, so conducting a thorough assessment on arrival in a more controlled environment is important. See Box 13.3 for the questions that should be asked and the rationale for these.

When assessing a patient's pain, the mnemonic PQRST can be very useful. It helps determine the Provoking factors, Quality, Radiation, Severity and Timing of the pain, and is a useful tool to assist in exploring all realms of the pain. (See Box 13.4 for full explanation of terms, and Chapter 18 for discussion of pain management.) The information gathered while taking the history will guide emergency clinicians as to which body systems need to be examined, as well as the extent of the investigation. However, during history-taking it is important not to make assumptions about the patient's clinical presentation until a comprehensive assessment has been completed.

BOX 13.2 THE SAMPLE MNEMONIC FOR HISTORY-TAKING

S	Signs and symptoms
A	Allergies
M	Medications
P	Pertinent past history
L	Last oral intake
E	Events leading up to the illness/injury

PRACTICE TIP

When taking a history, it is useful to develop a systematic approach to ensure all the important questions are asked.

BOX 13.3 PERTINENT QUESTIONS TO OBTAIN A HISTORY

PRESENTING PROBLEM

Chief complaint

What is the reason the patient has presented to hospital? It is advisable to document this using the patient's own words. It is then very clear what the patient complained of on presentation, as symptoms can change.

Characteristics

It is important to identify the location and characteristics of the chief complaint and any related symptoms (both ones you may expect and ones that are absent). For example, centralised abdominal pain associated with vomiting or diarrhoea.

Pain history

This can be explored using PQRST (see Box 13.4).

Aggravating causes and relieving factors

What exacerbates or relieves the symptoms? This can provide clues as to the cause. For example, cough started after being commenced on new medication.

Timing

You need to explore when the symptoms started, and whether they are continuous or intermittent. How long do they last?

Medications taken to relieve symptoms and effectiveness

Some patients take multiple pain medications when pain is severe. If one type over another is more effective, this can also offer clues.

INDIVIDUAL HEALTH HISTORY

Past medical/surgical history

This is an essential component of your assessment. Patients may not realise the significance of prior problems and may not think them relevant. You should prompt your patient to divulge all past medical history and previous surgeries, however irrelevant it may seem to them.

Current medications (including smoking, alcohol, illicit drugs)

It is important to elicit details of current medications as they may be linked to the problem. Not only prescription medications, but also over-the-counter and herbal or homeopathic ones.

Allergies

Information about allergies is important. However, many patients attribute adverse reactions or intolerance to allergies. Therefore, the reaction to any drug should be noted, e.g. 'Patient states they are allergic to morphine, but the reaction they suffered was nausea and vomiting. This is a common side-effect and not a true allergy.'

Relevant family and social history

The patient's problem may be hereditary or genetic. Important diseases to ask about are cardiovascular, respiratory, cancer, diabetes, renal disease, allergies and mental health problems. Although family history is not diagnostic, it allows risk stratification. The social history should be tailored to the individual, but an understanding of the patient's social habits helps to determine further risk factors. Recognition of social supports at home for an elderly person can assist with early identification of the likelihood of needing admission. It is also important to identify the carer responsible for paediatric patients and any child protection concerns that need to be considered.

Tetanus status; last menstrual period

These are asked about only if relevant to the presenting problem.

BOX 13.4 PAIN ASSESSMENT USING PQRST

P–Provoking factors	What factors precipitated the patient's discomfort? What were they doing at the onset of pain?
Q–Quality	Get the patient to describe the pain/ache/dullness. Ask them to tell you its characteristics: 'Describe the pain and how it feels.'
R–Region/radiation	Ask the patient to show you where the pain is and where it radiates to, if applicable. Ask if there is pain anywhere else.
S–Severity	Get the patient to rate their pain/ache/dullness on a pain scale.
T–Time	How long has the patient had the pain; or, if it has gone, how long did it last? Does anything make it worse or better?

IDENTIFY RED FLAGS

In determining the severity of the patient's illness and how urgent the need for intervention is, the emergency clinician relies on a combination of clinical signs and historical data. These may be actual or potential cues that indicate presence or risk of serious illness or injury, including abnormal vital signs, a history of pre-existing illness or time-sensitive presentations (such as chest pain or the onset of acute neurological signs). These can be referred to as clinical or historical indicators of urgency, also termed 'red flags'. They can be identified when listening to the patient's history or conducting a clinical assessment. See Table 13.1 for examples. Identification of red flags prompts the clinician to initiate appropriate management early on. Early recognition and response to signs of clinical deterioration or issues that increase the risk of deterioration improve the delivery of care and save lives.[25] Each patient should be assessed using the 'worst first' approach, and no assumptions should be made until all high-morbidity and high-mortality conditions have been ruled out.[16]

TABLE 13.1 HISTORICAL AND CLINICAL RED FLAGS

PRESENTING COMPLAINT	HISTORICAL RED FLAG	CLINICAL RED FLAG
Chest pain	History of ischaemic heart disease	Abnormal ECG
	Prolonged chest pain	Pale and diaphoretic
	Diabetes or chronic renal failure	Abnormal vital signs
Abdominal pain	Recent abdominal surgery	Pregnancy
	Vascular disease	Rigid abdomen
	Haematemesis or melaena	Abnormal vital signs
Fever	Prolonged fever	Infected wound
	Recent surgery	Elevated white blood cell count
	Immunosuppressed	Abnormal vital signs
Vomiting	Elderly or paediatrics	Hypo/hyperglycaemia
	History of diabetes	Haematemesis
	Pregnancy	Abnormal vital signs
Shortness of breath	Sudden onset	Abnormal CXR
	History of COPD	Use of accessory muscles
	Productive cough	Abnormal vital signs

ECG: electrocardiogram; COPD: chronic obstructive pulmonary disease; CXR: chest x-ray.

PRACTICE TIP

Red flags can be found at any stage of the assessment process, when listening to the patient's history or conducting a clinical assessment.

ASSESSMENT (CLINICAL EXAMINATION)

The next step of the assessment process is the clinical examination. Once life-threatening problems have been identified and stabilised in the primary survey, the general survey of the patient and collection of vital signs should be performed. It is advisable to use the ABCDE approach and reassess for potential or actual threats to the airway, breathing, circulation, disability (neurological status) and exposure, before moving on to a focused assessment. If any of the ABCs are compromised, then interventions will need to be performed before moving on with the assessment. In airway management, this could be as simple as performing a jaw thrust or chin lift (while maintaining cervical spine precautions), through to intubating the patient and securing the airway for transportation. If at any stage during the assessment the patient appears to deteriorate, you must return to ABCDE and reassess these again, stopping if any interventions are required and only moving forwards once the patient is stable.

A head-to-toe review of the relevant body regions and systems should follow. The examination sequence is then inspection, auscultation, percussion and palpation. The emergency clinician should also consider the patient's ability to perform everyday tasks, such as eating, drinking, mobilising, toileting and personal hygiene.[26] A decline in the ability to perform these tasks can threaten the safety of the patient while in hospital and once discharged.[27–29] It is also important to screen for specific risk of harm. Patients should be screened for pressure injuries, falls, poor nutrition and cognitive impairment to prevent or minimise harm. Preventing complications is discussed in more detail under 'Essentials of care' later in this chapter.

GENERAL SURVEY

Your general survey commences the moment you first see your patient. This may be as you approach them in their house or at the scene of an accident, or as they approach you at the triage window. Posture and gait should be noted. Listening to the patient speak will reveal clues to neurological and respiratory function. The overall appearance of the patient can also give clues to mood, altered level of consciousness and signs of pain and distress.

PRACTICE TIP

The overall appearance of the patient can give clues to mood, altered level of consciousness and signs of pain and distress.

Vital signs

Taking vital signs and identifying clinical deterioration is an essential part of the role of the nurse or paramedic, and they must know the normal limits. Monitoring of vital signs, in addition to other objective data, such as urine output and lactate results, have been shown to assist in the early detection of clinical deterioration and prevents loss of life.[30,31] The initial vital signs performed pre-hospital can be a predictor of adverse hospital outcomes.[32] The majority of patients who suffer an in-hospital cardiac arrest or unplanned ICU admission have abnormal vital signs in the hours prior to the event.[33,34] Failure to recognise and respond to clinical deterioration in a timely manner increases the incidence of high-mortality adverse events such as cardiac arrest[35] and unplanned admissions to the intensive care unit.[34] One Australian study reported that clinical deterioration goes undetected in as many as one in seven ED patients (12.9%).[36] There are times when seriously ill patients are not recognised because of the staff's busy, unpredictable workload.[37,38] This is particularly prevalent in areas of lower staff to patient ratios such as the ED waiting room.[39]

A set of vital signs is considered to consist of:

- respirations (R)
- oxygen saturations (SpO_2)
- blood pressure (BP)
- pulse (P)
- temperature (T)
- level of consciousness
- new onset confusion or behaviour change.[40]

Patients who present to the ED for the first time do not have any baseline observations to compare their condition against. It

TABLE 13.2 NORMAL VALUES FOR BLOOD PRESSURE (BP), PULSE (P) AND RESPIRATIONS (R) IN PAEDIATRICS[43] AND ADULTS[38]

AGE	SYSTOLIC BP*	P?	R‡
< 3 months	60-100	110-160	30-55
3-12 months	70-110	100-160	30-45
1-4 years	90-110	90-140	20-40
5-11 years	90-110	80-120	20-30
12-16 years	90-120	60-100	15-20
Adult (>16 years)	90-120	60-100	12-20

**mmHg*
?beats per minute
‡breaths per minute

can therefore be challenging to determine if the patient's vital signs are within normal limits for them. Repeating vital signs at appropriate intervals helps to determine trends and to detect clinical deterioration.[41] Studies have shown wide variation in the frequency of vital signs performed in the emergency context.[42] The time interval between vital signs should be determined by the clinical situation and local protocols. The clinician may be required to increase or decrease frequency of vital sign measurement if the patient's condition changes.

Normal ranges for vital signs differ in paediatric patients and adults (see Table 13.2 for normal values). Changes that occur in pregnancy also affect vital signs; blood pressure decreases and heart rate increases according to the effects of increased progesterone and increased circulating blood volume.[44] Once the patient has arrived at the hospital, an accurate history and a review of hospital records may assist in determining what is normal for the patient. The Australian Commission of Safety and Quality in Health Care (ACSQHC) recommend the use of observation charts with parameters that indicate when vital signs are abnormal and when escalation should occur.[40] It should be noted that having normal vital signs does not necessarily guarantee a stable physiological status. Examples of this include: failure to detect large blood losses in a fit, healthy person; failure to identify serious illness in infants, and inability to detect an inadequate plasma volume in burn injury patients or a patient taking beta-blockers who cannot mount a tachycardic response to correct hypotension. Therefore, it should be remembered that although the vital signs may appear within normal limits, this may be due to compensatory mechanisms and/or be masked by medications; the patient may in fact be compromised.

PRACTICE TIP

Vital signs may appear within normal limits; however, this may be due to compensatory mechanisms and/or may be masked by medications; the patient may in fact be compromised.

Respirations

The respiratory rate is considered one of the most important vital signs as it is the most accurate in detecting clinical deterioration, as well as predicting the need for admission to the intensive care unit (ICU) and for cardiac arrest.[41,45] Despite this, the respiratory rate, often called the 'forgotten vital sign', is commonly not accurately measured and is poorly documented.[46] Abnormal respiratory rate is a significant predictor of deterioration, cardiac arrest and/or need for admission to the ICU.[47,48] Clinical deterioration can be detected early on by a change in respiratory rate of as few as four breaths per minute either side of the normal range, which would otherwise go undetected through monitoring of other vital signs.[46,49] A rise in respiratory rate from 24 to 28 breaths per minute in an adult has been reported to increase mortality by 5% and a respiratory rate from four to eight by 10%.[50] Respiratory rate is normally more rapid in infants and children.[51] For normal ranges of respiratory rates see Table 13.2.

The rate, depth, rhythm and effort of respiration should be assessed and recorded.[51] To obtain the most accurate respiratory rate it is recommended that respirations be counted for a full 60 seconds and not telling the person you are measuring their respiratory rate as awareness of this can alter their normal breathing patterns.[52] It can often be difficult to count respirations in paediatric patients, particularly if they are crying or moving around. Counting respirations in paediatric patients may be made easier by the use of a stethoscope or by placing a hand on the child's chest. The depth of respiration can be established by watching the person's chest rise and fall, and is best done at a distance, so that the patient is not aware of what you are counting. It can be described as shallow, normal or deep. The chest wall should expand symmetrically. The rhythm of breathing should be regular, without presence of tracheal tug, nasal flaring, accessory muscle use or signs of intercostal, substernal or suprasternal recession. On auscultation, air entry should be clear and equal, with no added breath sounds, such as wheeze or crackles.

PRACTICE TIP

The depth of respiration can be established by watching the person's chest rise and fall, and is best done at a distance, so that the patient is not aware of what you are counting.

Oxygen saturation

Oxygen saturation (SpO_2) is measured using a pulse oximeter, which detects the amount of haemoglobin that is bound to oxygen, and is used as an adjunct to assessing respiratory function. Peripheral probes are commonly used on the fingers, toes or ears; they are easy to apply and non-invasive. However, these probes will not work through nail varnish, dirt or dried blood. Dysrhythmias or poor peripheral circulation may also cause low readings because of inadequate and irregular perfusion.[53] Forehead probes should be used when an accurate reading is not obtainable via peripheral means.[53] Anaemic patients will have a normal SpO_2 reading, but may be hypoxic. The pulse oximeter measures how much haemoglobin is saturated, but the patient may have insufficient haemoglobin to attain tissue perfusion. Following smoke or exhaust inhalation, SpO_2 readings are of no value as carbon monoxide has a greater affinity to haemoglobin than to oxygen, so saturation levels could be 99% while the haemoglobin molecule is saturated with carbon monoxide, not oxygen, placing the patient in a hypoxic state.[53] An arterial blood gas should be performed in these patients to accurately measure the partial pressure of oxygen, partial pressure of carboxyhaemoglobin and saturation levels. The oximetry probe can cause pressure areas on the skin if left in one position for an extended period of time, so it is recommended to change and document probe placement regularly.[54]

PRACTICE TIP

The pulse oximeter tells how much haemoglobin is saturated, but the patient may have insufficient haemoglobin to attain tissue perfusion.

Blood pressure

Blood pressure (BP) is the force of the blood pushing against the blood vessel wall. This measurement of force is determined by: (1) cardiac output (how much blood is pumped by the heart with each contraction); (2) the ability of the vessels to stretch; (3) the volume of the circulating blood; (4) the amount of resistance the heart must overcome when it pumps blood; and (5) blood viscosity (thickness of the blood).[51] The systolic pressure is the pressure within the arterial system when the ventricles contract. The diastolic pressure is the pressure within the arterial system when the ventricles relax and fill with blood. The pulse pressure is the difference between the two; a pulse pressure of between 30 and 50 mmHg is considered a normal range.

There are several factors that can influence BP, which need to be taken into account. These include the patient's age, gender, fitness, emotional state and medications (see Box 13.5). It is important to remember that a fit, healthy person has compensatory mechanisms and may not display signs of depleted circulating volume until late. For normal ranges of systolic blood pressure according to age, see Table 13.2.

BOX 13.5 **FACTORS AFFECTING BLOOD PRESSURE**

AGE

Blood pressure (BP) tends to rise with age—attributed to arteriosclerosis, a process whereby the arteries become rigid and lose elasticity, and atherosclerosis, a narrowing of the arteries caused by cholesterol deposits.

GENDER

Women generally have lower BP than men of a similar age.

FITNESS

Athletes tend to have BP in the lower ranges.

EMOTIONAL STATE

Strong emotions and pain can cause the BP to rise as a result of sympathetic nervous system stimulation.

MEDICATIONS

Consider if the patient is taking antihypertensives. Also drugs such as nicotine, caffeine and cocaine tend to constrict arteries and raise BP.

BP is most commonly measured non-invasively by inflating a cuff on the patient's arm using a manual or automatic sphygmomanometer. However, various factors can affect the accuracy of non-invasive BP measurement, such as the position of the patient, cuff size and cuff placement.[55] If the BP cuff is too large, the result will be a false low reading. If the cuff is too small, the result will be falsely elevated.

To obtain the most accurate BP reading, the patient should ideally be seated, with their back supported and both feet resting on the ground, and remain resting in this position for 5 minutes.[54] The arm should be supported at heart level as the position of the arm affects the pressure observed. If the upper arm is below the level of the heart the BP reading will be too high, and if the arm is above the heart the reading will be too low.[56] It is often not possible to place the patient in a seated position; the emergency clinician should therefore consider the effects that the position of the patient has on the blood pressure reading.

If a patient has poor peripheral circulation or cardiac dysrhythmias, electronic BP machines become inaccurate and may not be able to record a reading at all. In this instance, and with any resuscitation or clinically unwell patient, a manual reading should be obtained. It is also good practice to double-check any high or low reading obtained from an electronic BP machine manually. For the most accurate measurement of blood pressure an arterial catheter should be used; these are very invasive and therefore are usually only used when the patient is critically unwell or when close BP monitoring is required.[55]

While most healthy patients will demonstrate little difference in their lying and standing blood pressure, a significant fall (systolic BP 20 mmHg or diastolic BP 10 mmHg) can occur in older people, patients with diabetes and those with symptoms suggestive of postural hypotension, such as dizziness, syncope and falls on changing position.[57] A lying and standing blood pressure should be recorded for these groups. First, the patient should have been lying down for 5 minutes, and have their arm supported at heart level. Record the blood pressure and then get the patient to stand, keeping the cuff in place. Allow the patient to stand for 3–5 minutes to allow for delayed orthostatic hypotension, which usually occurs in the first 5 minutes of standing. Support the arm at heart level and repeat the reading. If on standing, the patient reports dizziness, faintness or light-headedness, the procedure should be aborted for safety reasons.[57]

For patients with a side affected by stroke, mastectomy or renal fistula, the BP should be taken on the opposite arm. It is important to remove the BP cuff for all patients between readings to prevent injury from prolonged pressure in one area. Significant discrepancies in BP reading between the left and right arm should be escalated to a senior clinician as this can be an indicator of a ruptured abdominal aortic aneurism, which is life-threatening.

PRACTICE TIP

Patients with diabetes and those with symptoms suggestive of postural hypotension, such as dizziness, syncope and falls on changing position, should have a lying and standing blood pressure taken.

Pulse

There is more to a pulse than its rate; pulse rhythm and character should also be noted. The clinician must palpate the pulse to determine its rate, rhythm and aptitude (strength). In healthy adults the normal pulse rate is between 60 and 100 beats/minute,[51] but this is higher for children and babies (see Table 13.2). Tachycardia is defined as a pulse rate greater than 100 beats/minute, while bradycardia is a pulse rate less than 60 beats/minute.[58] Factors which can affect the pulse rate need to be considered when obtaining the patient history. A slow pulse rate may be normal for a fit athlete, but it may also indicate a cardiac dysrhythmia, metabolic disturbance, hypothermia, hypoxia or neurological issue, or be caused by certain medications, such as beta-blockers. A fast pulse rate can be triggered by emotion, exercise, drugs, infection/inflammation, cardiac dysrhythmias, hypovolaemia or haemorrhage and hypoxia.[59] The pulse volume may be described as bounding, normal, weak, thready or absent. A bounding pulse may indicate sepsis, carbon dioxide retention or liver failure, and a thready pulse is indicative of shock. A pulse should be felt for a minimum of 30 seconds to obtain an accurate reading, and a minimum of 60 seconds if the pulse is irregular.[51] In adults, the pulse is generally taken over the radial artery, but in a patient in shock it may be difficult to assess the pulse at this site; the carotid or femoral artery can be used instead. Brachial, carotid and femoral arteries are the preferred sites in children.[3] Palpation or auscultation of the apical heart rate is also recommended in babies[51,60] (see Fig. 13.2). If a patient is found to have an irregular pulse, an ECG should be performed and cardiac monitoring should be considered (see Chapter 16).

PRACTICE TIP

The rate, regularity and characteristic of the pulse should be assessed through palpation.

Temperature

Accurate temperature measurement is essential to identify the presence of illness, as well as enable appropriate and timely treatment to prevent the negative effects of an abnormal temperature. Historically, the focus of temperature management has been on monitoring fever and treating infection; however, there is growing research demonstrating the significance of hypothermia as an indicator of critical illness.[61,62] Temperature measurement is indicated in all patients to identify hypothermia, hyperthermia and other febrile illnesses.

A normal core body temperature is defined as 37°C; however, this may fluctuate by 0.5°C to 1.0°C.[66] The core body temperature is regulated hormonally by the hypothalamus through controlling heat production and conservation.[64] Infants, children and older people are at risk of having difficulty regulating body temperature. Infants have poor heat conservation due to having a greater ratio of body surface area to weight and less subcutaneous fat compared to adults, where it functions as insulation. Elderly people have a poorer response to extreme external temperature variations, resulting from slow circulation and structural and functional changes in the skin.[64]

Maintaining a normal core body temperature is essential to optimise normal cellular function. Hypothermia is defined as a core temperature below 36°C.[65] Hypothermia is commonly caused by prolonged heat loss or exposure to cold environments, but can also be an indicator of critical illness, such as sepsis.[63] Hypothermia has been reported in up to 35% of patients with sepsis,[65] and is associated with higher mortality compared with patients without hypothermia with sepsis.[66,67] Hypothermia causes changes in circulation, coagulation and can cause cellular ischaemia.[64] Clinicians should take care to avoid hypothermia in patients as a result of prolonged exposure to cold environments or to enable assessment and massive intravenous fluid resuscitation, which can result in hypothermia. However, therapeutic hypothermia (32°C to 34°C) has been shown to reduce mortality in patients post-cardiac arrest through preserving ischaemic tissue.[68]

Fever is generally defined as a temperature of 38.3°C or above and is primarily caused by the action of pyrogens on the hypothalamus, such as bacteria or virus.[63] The term fever is often used interchangeably with pyrexia or hyperthermia. An elevated temperature may also result from exposure to extreme environmental temperature, drugs, trauma or autoimmune disease. Fever has been reported to aid the body's response to infection by preventing replication of infective organisms and increasing antimicrobial activity in many classes of antibiotics and improves patient outcomes.[66] A high fever can however be harmful in patients following brain injury or stroke and treatment with antipyretics should be considered to optimise cerebral perfusion.[69,70] Significant cellular changes occur in temperatures above 40°C and are associated with higher mortality, indicating that the harmful effects of fever outweigh the benefits in fighting infection. Temperatures above 41°C are usually drug-related, but can also result from damage to the hypothalamus caused by trauma, prolonged high temperatures (heat stroke) or genetic disorders.[63] Cell death rapidly occurs in adults at 41°C, causing seizures which frequently lead to death.[63,64]

There are a variety of thermometers for use at different sites. The most common types of non-invasive thermometers include tympanic, digital electronic, infrared and single-use chemical-dot thermometers. Both digital electronic and single-use chemical dot thermometers can be used in the oral, tympanic or axillary site. Infrared thermometers may be either contact (touch skin) or non-contact (do not touch skin). Tympanic and infrared thermometers are reported to be more accurate than

FIGURE 13.2 LOCATION OF APICAL PULSE[17]

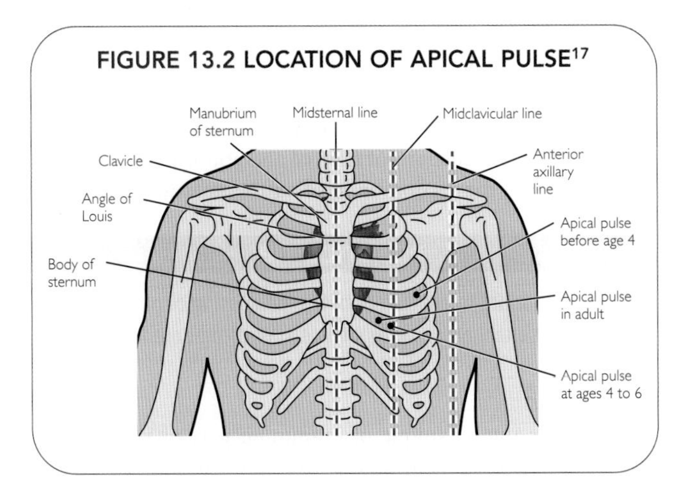

oral or axilla digital thermometers.[71] However, some studies have reported a wide variation of up to 1°C when comparing temperatures in children < 5 years old using non-contact infrared thermometers compared with axillary and tympanic devices.[72] Chemical thermometers have been found to be less precise than digital thermometers.[50,73] The single-use chemical-dot thermometer only has a range between 35.5°C and 40.4°C, so in patients suspected of having a temperature outside this range an alternative thermometer should be used. Temperature strips, which are liquid-crystal strips applied to the forehead, have been found to be inaccurate and can miss fevers in children.

Infrared thermometers measure temperature by measuring the heat emitted from the skin. Temporal artery thermometers measure the heat radiating from the skin when placed flush on the skin and moved from the forehead to behind the earlobe.[74] The non-touch infrared forehead thermometer measures the temperature of the forehead without touching the skin. Simply hold the thermometer 3–15 cm away from the patient's forehead, activate the device and the temperature reading is available within a few seconds.[51] This method is particularly useful when measuring temperatures in children as it does not wake the child.

When taking an oral temperature, it is vital to ensure the thermometer is placed correctly—it needs to sit in the posterior sublingual pocket of the mouth. This method should not be used in children under the age of 5 years due to the difficulty they experience in holding the thermometer in the correct position. A digital electronic thermometer will beep when ready; a single-use chemical-dot thermometer should be left in place for 3 minutes.[75] Factors that can influence the reading are a respiratory rate of greater than 18 breaths/minute and eating, drinking or smoking prior to the reading being taken.[76]

The axillary site is considered similar to the oral site when measuring temperature in adults; however, lack of precision may result in failure to detect low-grade fevers in paediatric patients.[73]

Tympanic thermometers measure the temperature from the tympanic membrane. Historically there was much debate over the accuracy of tympanic thermometers, particularly in the paediatric population. However, there has been significant development of this device in recent years with studies reporting the tympanic thermometer to be superior over other non-invasive methods of temperature measurement in children and adults.[71,77] Tympanic thermometers can be used in patients over 3 months of age. The ear canal must be straightened by pulling the pinna slightly up and back in an adult. Be cautious not to force the probe into the ear so as to avoid risk of perforation. It can be inaccurate in people with a small ear so canal, a build-up of cerumen, otitis media and incorrect placement.[73,76]

Rectal thermometers are considered the gold standard method of temperature measurement and recommended for when an accurate core temperature is required. However, they are invasive and impractical.[71] The rectal temperature probes can be slow to respond to changes in temperature and the probe needs to be accurately placed to a depth of 4 cm to obtain an accurate reading. They are therefore not recommended in children due to the risk of bowel perforation. In critically ill patients requiring continuous monitoring of temperature, urinary thermometers can be inserted easily into the bladder via urinary catheters. Bladder thermometers have been reported to measure core body temperature close to that of rectal thermometers.[78]

It should be carefully noted on the patient's documentation which kind of thermometer and which site was used to record the temperature. It is not possible to accurately convert the temperature taken at one site to compare it with a temperature taken at a different site, with or without using a different kind of thermometer. This is also an important consideration when the paramedic hands over a patient to the accepting emergency nurse.

PRACTICE TIP

In critically ill patients, thermometers can be easily inserted into the bladder via urinary catheters to accurately measure core temperature.

INSPECTION

It is important to look at the patient as a whole before undertaking a more focused assessment. Inspection commences when you first see the patient, either at the scene or when receiving clinical handover in view of the patient. Questions to consider are: Does the patient appear unwell or in pain? Are they unkempt, inappropriately dressed, under- or overweight? Once a general view of the patient has been obtained, observations should become specific, focusing on the chief complaint and affected system. When inspecting as part of your focused assessment you are looking for discharge, skin integrity, swelling, redness and other abnormalities. You should also take note of any diaphoresis and document pallor.

PRACTICE TIP

Inspection commences when you first see the patient, either at the scene or when receiving clinical handover in view of the patient.

Auscultation

Auscultation is the process of listening, usually with a stethoscope, to sounds produced by the movement of gas or liquid within the body. The heart, lungs and abdomen are the areas most often auscultated. The diaphragm of the stethoscope is used to hear high-pitched sounds, such as bronchial sounds, and the bell is used for low-pitched sounds, such as heart sounds. If too much pressure is applied with the bell, it tightens the skin and acts as a diaphragm. It is important to auscultate before percussing or palpating as these techniques may change sounds that are heard. Discussions of normal and abnormal findings are found below in the section on head-to-toe assessment.

PRACTICE TIP

It is important to auscultate before percussing or palpating as these techniques may change sounds that are heard.

Percussion

Percussion is the technique of examining part of the body by tapping it with the fingertips and hearing the resultant vibratory

TABLE 13.3 PERCUSSION SOUNDS

SOUND	INTENSITY	QUALITY	COMMON LOCATION
Flat	Soft	Muted	Muscle, bone
Dull	Medium	Thud-like	Liver, heart, full bladder
Resonant	Loud	Hollow	Normal lung
Tympanic	Loud	Cavernous	Intestine filled with air
Hyperresonant	Very loud	Booming	Emphysematous lung

sounds. The quality of the sound aids in determining the location, size and density of underlying structures. The sound can be described as flat, dull, resonant, tympanic or hyperresonant. See Table 13.3 for sound characteristics and examples of where they can be heard.

Palpation

Palpation is the process of examining parts of the body by careful feeling with the hands and fingertips. Light palpation is used for feeling the surface of the skin, structures that lie just beneath the skin, vibrations in the chest and for the pulsation of peripheral arteries. The examiner uses the fingertips, or the back or palm of one hand. When examining the abdomen, deep palpation may also be used to identify organ structures. This is performed by placing one hand on the other and using the top hand to apply pressure to depress the abdomen by 2.5 cm. The bottom hand remains relaxed. Palpation provides information about the temperature and moisture of the skin, the presence of tenderness, unusual vibrations, distension and the size, shape, consistency and mobility of organs or masses.

Analgesia should be administered if required before palpation is performed to provide comfort during examination. While many patients have concerns that the use of pain relief before seeing a doctor may mask important physical symptoms, the early provision of analgesics has been reported to have no effect on the accuracy of diagnosis,[79] but there is strong evidence to demonstrate it improves comfort[79] and should not be withheld.

PRACTICE TIP

Analgesia should be administered before palpation is performed to provide comfort during physical examination.

HEAD-TO-TOE ASSESSMENT

In the ED and pre-hospital setting, the history taken will assist you in determining which systems you should review. For a more in-depth review of trauma patient assessment using the primary and secondary survey, refer to Chapter 42.

HEENT (HEAD, EARS, EYES, NOSE AND THROAT)

Inspection of the external surfaces of the head will reveal the presence of foreign bodies discharge, redness, abrasions, contusions and bleeding. Palpation can be performed to feel for any unusual lumps or bumps at the same time.

Inspect the face for asymmetry, swelling or involuntary movements, as abnormalities could indicate facial nerve problems or an allergic reaction. Palpation will reveal step-offs, deformity and tenderness (see Chapters 31 and 44 for more detailed HEENT patient assessment).

Ears are inspected for discharge, foreign bodies, deformities and lumps. If infection is suspected, the tympanic membrane (TM) and external auditory canal are viewed with an otoscope (auroscope). The pinna is pulled up and back to straighten the ear canal in an adult, and down and back in a child. The TM should appear pearly-grey; yellow, redness or a bulging TM are signs of infection. In head injury, blood may be seen in the canal or behind the TM.[80]

Common presentations for eyes include foreign bodies, infection and trauma. The standard examination for eyes is to measure visual acuity using a Snellen chart. If the patient wears glasses or contact lenses for distance vision, these should be worn during testing if available; otherwise, the use of a pinhole is advised. The smallest line the patient can read with each eye individually and then together is noted. Acuity is written as a fraction, with the numerator indicating the distance from the chart (usually 6 m, but a 3 m modified chart can also be used) and the denominator describing the distance at which a person with normal vision could read the line. Therefore, 6/6 is a normal finding. It should be noted if glasses or contact lenses are worn during a visual acuity assessment. The eye should be examined for obvious foreign bodies. Inflammation, pain, discharge, tearing and changes in appearance should be noted.[81] Further eye assessment is discussed in Chapter 32.

The mouth can offer several clues as to the wellbeing of the patient. Assess the tongue for dryness and colour: a dry tongue can indicate dehydration. Examine the gums for evidence of bleeding or swelling. If the patient complains of a sore throat, inspect for swelling, redness and ulceration.

Disability (level of consciousness or new confusion)

Assessing a patient's level of consciousness is an essential component of a neurological examination, which is usually performed alongside an assessment of pupil size and reaction, vital signs and focal neurological signs in the limbs.[82] In the pre-hospital setting and at triage, the ACVPU scale is often used when assessing disability to quickly determine a patient's level of consciousness. The ACVPU scale, a superseded version of the AVPU tool, crudely measures response: is the patient Alert, do they have a new onset or worsening Confusion, are they responding to Voice, responding to Pain or Unresponsive? Acute confusion is a significant indicator for clinical risk, thus acute confusion must be assumed new unless proven otherwise.[83,84] The ACVPU should be followed up with a formal assessment of the patient's score on the Glasgow Coma Scale (see below).

Glasgow Coma Scale

When performing a more focused assessment, a neurological observation chart incorporating a Glasgow Coma Scale

(GCS) is used. The GCS was first described in the early 1970s as an objective and reliable measure of conscious state in patients with head injury.[85–88] The GCS is an internationally accepted measure of conscious state in victims with head injury,[87,89,90] and is now used extensively in non-trauma populations.[89,91,92]

The GCS evaluates three key categories of behaviour that most closely reflect activity in the higher centres of the brain: eye opening, verbal response and motor response. These behaviours enable us to determine whether the patient has cerebral dysfunction.[87,93] There are separate scoring criteria for adults, children and babies, and the appropriate chart should be selected. The GCS evaluates each of these parameters by allocating a numerical score (see Tables 13.4 and 13.5). The scores for each parameter are then added up to give a total out of 15.[86] Because the lowest number that can be given for each part of the assessment is 1, the lowest score that can be given is a GCS of 3. 'Coma' is arbitrarily defined as a GCS score of < 8, and a GCS score ≤ 8 has been used to indicate the need for endotracheal intubation.[91,95–97]

Although widely used in emergency care, research has shown variability in the reliability of the GCS,[89,90,93,98] making consistency of its application an important aspect of the nursing management of patients with a neurological emergency.[90] It is best if the same emergency clinician does the assessment each time, so that if there is a change in score it can be attributed to the patient and not the evaluator. At change of shift or transfer of the patient, the nurse escort or paramedic and receiving nurses should perform the evaluation together in order to avoid misinterpretation and to ensure continuity. Sleeping patients must be woken before commencing the evaluation. A deterioration of one point in the 'motor response' or one point in the 'verbal response' or an overall deterioration of two points is clinically significant and must be reported to medical staff.[87,93]

The Paediatric Glasgow Coma Scale (PGCS) is a modification of the GCS. Assessment of conscious state in infants and young children is difficult due to developmental progression and lack of verbal response in young children.[85,89] Well children may have decreased responses because of fear, and crying may be misinterpreted as a normal response in the context of significant neurological pathology.[85,100,101] If using the adult GCS, it is expected that a child will have a reduced score. Refer to Chapter 35 for further details.

GCS assessment

Assessment of eye-opening tests the function of the arousal mechanisms in the brain stem. There are four possible responses when assessing eye opening: spontaneous, to speech, to pressure and none. If the patient is unable to open their eyes due to paralysis, this should be documented as a 'P', and if the patient's eye is closed secondary to swelling, a 'C' should be documented.[102]

TABLE 13.4 GLASGOW COMA SCALE[85,86]

	SCORE
Eye opening	
Spontaneously	4
To speech	3
To pressure	2
None	1
Verbal response	
Orientated	5
Confused	4
Words	3
Sounds	2
None	1
Motor response	
Obeys commands	6
Localising	5
Normal flexion (withdrawal)	4
Abnormal flexion	3
Extension	2
None	1

TABLE 13.5 PAEDIATRIC GLASGOW COMA SCALE[94]

	SCORE
Eye opening	
Spontaneously	4
To speech	3
To pain	2
None	1
Verbal response	
Coos, babbles	5
Irritable, cries	4
Cries to pain	3
Moans to pain	2
None	1
Motor response	
Normal spontaneous movement	6
Withdraws to touch	5
Withdraws to pain	4
Abnormal flexion	3
Abnormal extension	2
None	1

Verbal response may be assessed as: orientated (5), confused (4), inappropriate words (3), incomprehensible sounds (2) and no response (1). To be assessed as orientated, the patient must *correctly* tell the emergency care provider their name, location, day, month and year. Do not assume that a patient is orientated because they are conversing with you in a normal manner; they need to be able to correctly answer the above questions to be assessed as orientated. If verbal response is altered by other processes, for example, dysphasia, aphasia or facial fractures, this should be documented; and if the patient is intubated, a 'T' should be documented.

Motor response may be assessed as: obeys command (6), localises to pressure/pain (5), normal flexion/withdraws from pain (4), abnormal flexion to pain (3), extension to pressure/pain (2) and no response (1). Although responses of all limbs should be documented as part of neurological observations, only the *best* response counts towards GCS.[93] To be assessed as 'obeys commands', the patient needs to squeeze *and let go* of the emergency care provider's hands on command. It is important that the assessor does not place their hands into the patient's hands: this may elicit a reflex response that may be misinterpreted as obeying a command. If the patient is paralysed, a 'P' should be recorded.

There are two types of pressure, often referred to as painful stimuli: central and peripheral painful stimuli. Use caution when applying stimuli and do not cause injury such as bruising. It is recommended that when eliciting a response using pain that supraorbital pressure be used, but this carries a risk of damage to the eye, so should be used with caution and not used if facial fractures are suspected. Other recommended methods include jaw margin pressure (the flat of the thumb is applied to the corner of the maxillary and mandibular junction and pressure is increasingly applied for up to 60 seconds), squeezing the trapezius muscle or applying pressure to the earlobe.[102,103]

Each limb should be assessed. A peripheral painful stimulus needs to be applied if the patient does not appear to be able to voluntarily move the limb. Bilateral responses should be assessed. Assessing pupils is not necessarily effective in the sedated or paralysed patient; however, any changes in pupil reaction, shape or size are a late sign of raised intracranial pressure. Very small pupils may be a result of opiate or barbiturate use. A more detailed assessment of the patient with altered consciousness is discussed in Chapter 23.

Cognitive screening

As part of the neurological assessment, routine cognitive screening in older people is recommended to increase detection and management of cognitive impairment. Studies have reported that cognitive impairment, commonly resulting from dementia or delirium, occurs in up to 40% of older people presenting to the ED; however, it often goes undetected.[104–107] Cognitive impairment in hospitalised patients is associated with higher rates of adverse events, longer length of stay, functional and cognitive decline and increased medical and surgical complaints.[108–111] The presence of delirium has been reported to be an independent predictor for increased mortality in ED patients,[112] and if discharged from the ED with an undetected delirium, 6-month mortality increases by three-fold.[106,113] Patients hospitalised with dementia had a five-times higher length of stay compared to patients without dementia.[114–116]

A range of different tools exist to screen for cognitive impairment in the ED. To exclude delirium and cognitive impairment, the 4AT tool (Abbreviated Mental Test 4) is recommended as it is quick and easy for clinicians to use and no special training is required.[117] The 4AT tool measures four features: alertness, orientation, attention and whether there are any acute changes or fluctuating course. A score out of 12 is calculated: a score of 0 excludes delirium and cognitive impairment, a score of 1 to 3 indicates cognitive impairment and 4 or above is suggestive of delirium.[108,117] The Confusion Assessment Method (CAM) is a validated tool reported to accurately assess for delirium.[110,118] The CAM consists of four clinical features: 1) acute onset and fluctuating course; 2) inattention; 3) disorganised thinking; and 4) altered level of consciousness. The presence of features 1, 2 and either 3 or 4 are required to make a diagnosis of delirium. It is important to note that a poor score on screening is not a diagnosis but a trigger for further assessment.[104,108] The brief CAM (bCAM) was specifically adapted from the CAM algorithm for use in the emergency care environment. It maintains the four clinical features of the CAM; however, it has clear specified limits when determining inattention and disorganised thinking, and should only take 1 to 2 minutes to complete.[119] While the 4AT screens for both cognitive impairment and delirium, the CAM and bCAM do not assess for general cognitive impairment such as dementia. If the presence of delirium or cognitive impairment cannot be excluded, then the patient should be referred to aged care services for further assessment and management. See Chapter 38 for further information on cognitive impairment in older persons.

PRACTICE TIP

When handing over care of your patient, repeat your GCS and pain assessment with the paramedic or nurse receiving the patient to maintain consistency.

CERVICAL SPINE AND NECK

Examine the external neck for swelling and symmetry. Both the front and the back should be inspected for injuries. Look for enlargement of the parotid or submandibular glands and note any visible lymph glands. Palpate for lumps or enlarged lymph nodes.[102] The potential for C-spine injury in trauma patients should be considered as part of 'Airway' in the primary survey (see Box 13.1). All trauma patients should be presumed to have a cervical spine injury until proven otherwise; clearance of the cervical spine is discussed in Chapter 47.

PRACTICE TIP

All trauma patients should be presumed to have a cervical spine injury until proven otherwise.

Thorax

When examining the thorax, both the respiratory and the cardiovascular systems will be assessed. The respiratory assessment focuses on the function of the respiratory system to exchange oxygen and carbon dioxide in the lungs and its role in regulation of the acid–base balance.[120]

Start by looking for signs of respiratory distress, such as tachy/bradypnoea, dyspnoea, nasal flaring, use of accessory muscles and cyanosis. The patient's speech, change in voice and drooling are also important signs. Examine the hands for clubbing, indicative of chronic illness such as bronchiectasis, endocarditis and empyema. Observe for evidence of respiratory failure, for example, hypoxia (central cyanosis), or hypercarbia (drowsiness, confusion, warm hands, bounding pulse, dilated veins and a coarse tremor).[121] Observe the pattern of breathing—see Table 13.6.

Inspect the shape of the chest, and look for deformities or asymmetry. The posterior and anterior surfaces should both be inspected; this is most easily done with the patient sitting on the edge of the bed. Note the position of the trachea and watch for unequal movement of the chest. This is more easily ascertained by placing both hands on the chest wall and feeling for movement. Palpation of the chest should identify any tender areas or crepitus. The clavicles, sternum, ribs, spine and shoulder blades should be palpated for any abnormalities and to determine if there are any factors that will restrict the patient's ability to breathe.[121] Respiratory excursion (thoracic expansion) should be measured. This is best assessed by standing behind the seated patient and placing the thumbs next to each other along the spinal processes at the level of the tenth rib. As the patient breathes in, the thumbs will separate. You should watch for a loss of symmetry, absence or delay in movement. These could indicate complete or partial obstruction of the airway, or underlying lung or diaphragmatic dysfunction on the affected side.[121]

Percuss the chest bilaterally for resonance. Dullness or hyperresonance indicates an abnormality.[54] Hyperresonance occurs when the lungs are hyperinflated with air, such as in chronic obstructive pulmonary disease (COPD), or if identified on one side of the chest it is suggestive of a pneumothorax. Dull sounds indicate underlying dense tissue due to fluid or soft tissue, such as pleural effusion or tumour. Dullness to the anterior lower lung fields is not conclusive, as the heart is on the left side and the liver on the right.[121]

Next, auscultate the chest. It is recommended that the patient cough first to remove sputum that could create adventitious sounds. Use the sequence shown in Fig. 13.3 and always compare one side with the other. Listen for normal breath sounds (summarised in Table 13.7), absent or decreased sounds, and added sounds such as wheeze or crackles. Absent or

TABLE 13.6 PATTERNS OF BREATHING

NAME	PATTERN OF RESPIRATION	AETIOLOGY (examples)
Eupnoea	Normal respiration 12–20 breaths/minute	
Tachypnoea	Rapid respiration > 20 breaths/minute	Fever, pneumonia, pleuritic chest pain
Bradypnoea	Slow and regular < 12 breaths/minute	Drug intoxication, tumour
Cheyne-Stokes	Hyperventilation alternating with apnoea	Left ventricular failure, raised intracranial pressure, high altitude
Biot's or ataxic	Irregular in depth and rate, with periods of apnoea	Neurological disorders/disease
Kussmaul	Deep, rapid respiration	Metabolic acidosis
Pursed-lip breathing	Expiration against partially closed lips	Chronic obstructive pulmonary disease

FIGURE 13.3 RECOMMENDED SEQUENCE TO AUSCULTATE THE CHEST[122]

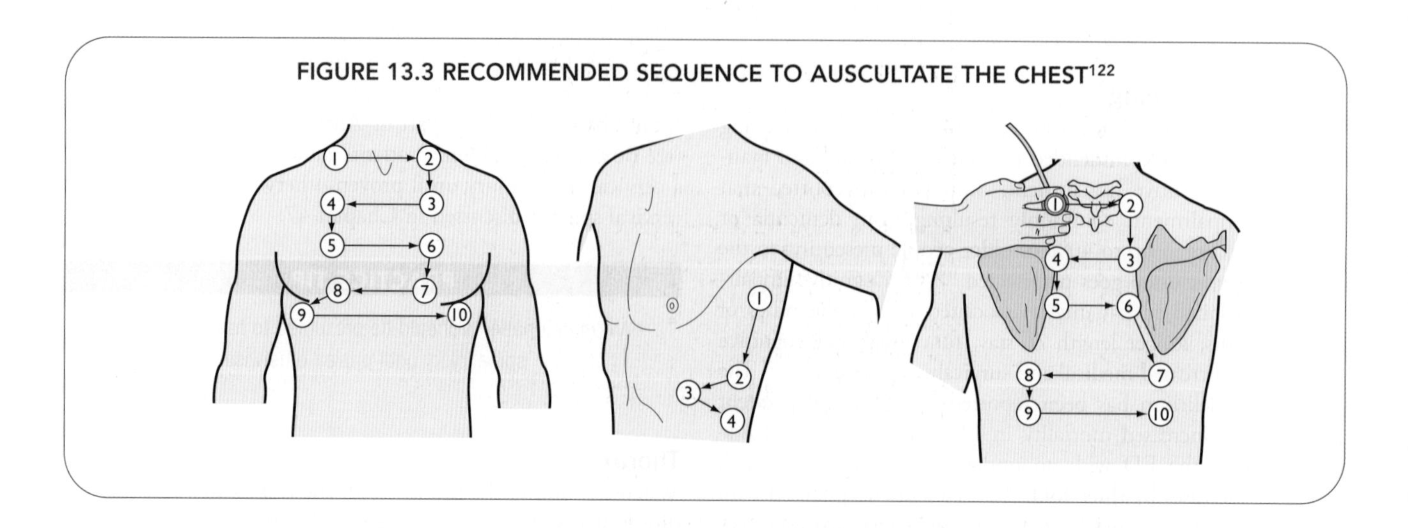

TABLE 13.7 NORMAL BREATH SOUNDS

SOUND	LOCATION
Vesicular	Lung tissue
Bronchovesicular	Near the bronchi
Bronchial	Lower part of trachea
Tracheal	Upper part of trachea

decreased breath sounds may be due to no air movement, caused by an obstructed airway or the presence of air or fluid preventing sound conduction (e.g. pneumothorax or pleural effusion). Wheeze is heard when air rapidly flows through constricted airways, such as in asthma, anaphylaxis or pulmonary oedema. Crackles are caused by either alveoli opening during inspiration or air bubbling through fluid, such as in heart failure, pulmonary oedema or infection. Inspect any sputum produced for colour, consistency, quantity and presence of blood.[121] Fig. 13.4 summarises the clinical findings for certain respiratory pathologies. See Chapter 21 for a more detailed description of respiratory assessment.

PRACTICE TIP

When assessing the patient for chest pain, ask them at rest, then when they take a deep breath and cough.

The purpose of examining the cardiovascular system is to assess the function of the heart as a pump, and of the arteries and veins throughout the body in transporting oxygen and nutrients to the tissues and in transporting waste products and carbon dioxide from the tissues.[124] Refer to Chapter 22 for the anatomy and physiology of these processes.

FIGURE 13.4 CLINICAL FINDINGS OF RESPIRATORY PATHOLOGIES[123]

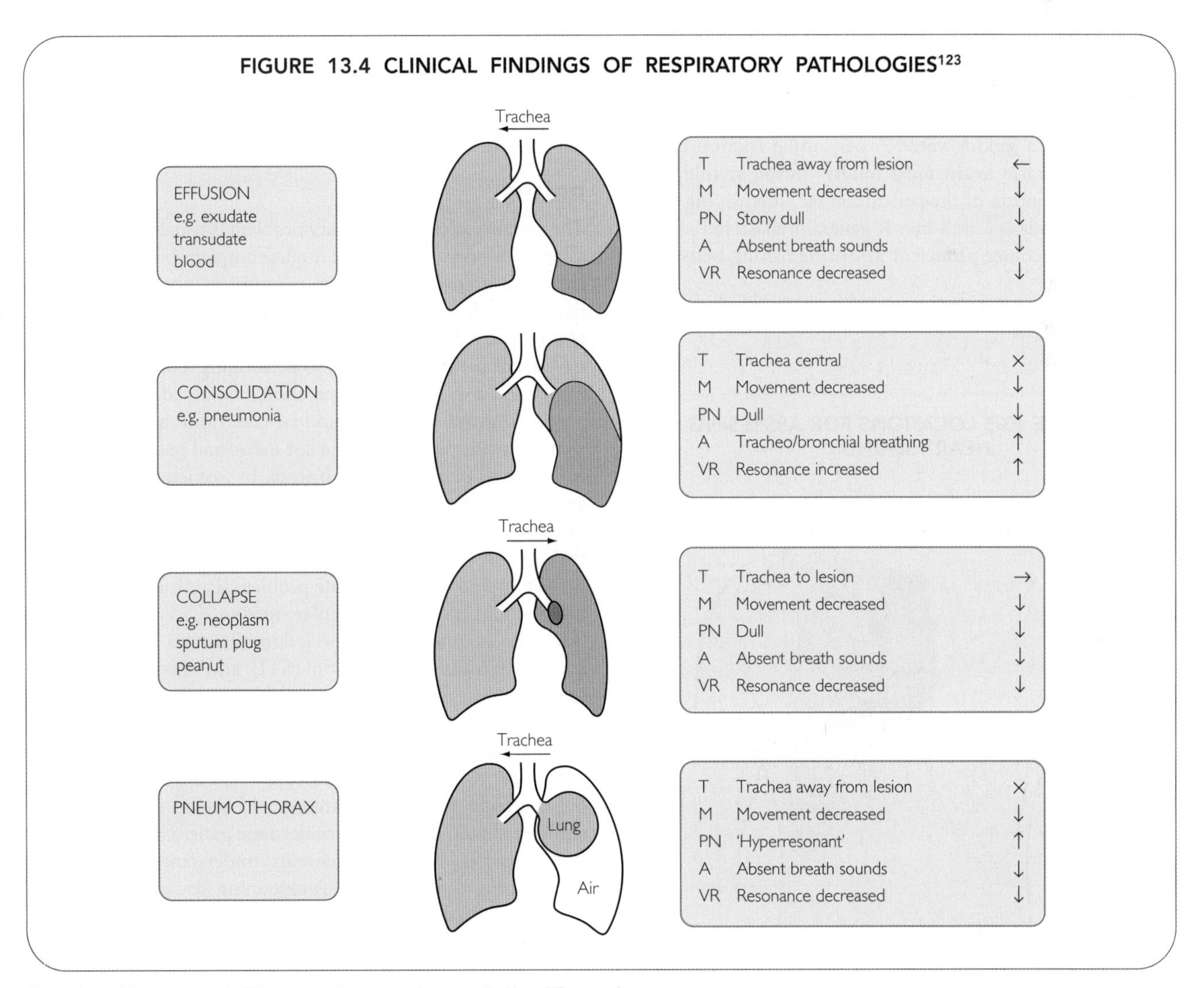

T: trachea; M: movement; PN: percussion note; A: auscultation; VR: vocal resonance.

Sit the patient at 45° and observe the jugular veins. Distension is suggestive of cardiac failure. Auscultate over the main areas of the heart (see Fig. 13.5), listening for normal heart sounds followed by added sounds and then murmurs. Normal heart sounds consist of two distinct parts. The first, named S1, is due to the mitral and tricuspid valves closing at the start of ventricular contraction or systole. It is best heard over the mitral and tricuspid areas (Fig. 13.5). The second sound, S2, is the closing of the aortic and pulmonary valves at the end of systole. It is best heard over the aortic and pulmonary areas[125] (see Fig. 13.5).

Added heart sounds are S3 and S4. S3 is the rapid ventricular filling as soon as the mitral and tricuspid valves open, and is sometimes referred to as a 'ventricular gallop'. It is common in children and young adults, but in the older adult is a sign of failure of the left ventricle, insufficient valves or constrictive pericarditis. S4 occurs from an atrial contraction (also known as atrial kick), which induces ventricular filling towards the end of diastole. This additional heart sound is called an 'atrial gallop'. It may be normal in middle age, but in an older adult it can indicate hypertensive cardiovascular disease, coronary artery disease, aortic stenosis, myocardial ischaemia, infarction and congestive heart failure.[125]

Murmurs are produced by turbulent blood flow. Turbulence occurs when there is high blood flow through a normal valve, or normal blood flow through an abnormal valve or into a dilated chamber. It is also caused by regurgitation of blood through a leaking valve. A pericardial friction rub is a high-pitched noise heard most loudly during systole and is due to inflammation of the pericardial sac. Identifying abnormal heart sounds is a skill that is generally mastered after the practitioner becomes proficient at distinguishing between S1 and S2.[125]

FIGURE 13.5 LOCATIONS FOR ASSESSING HEART SOUNDS[122]

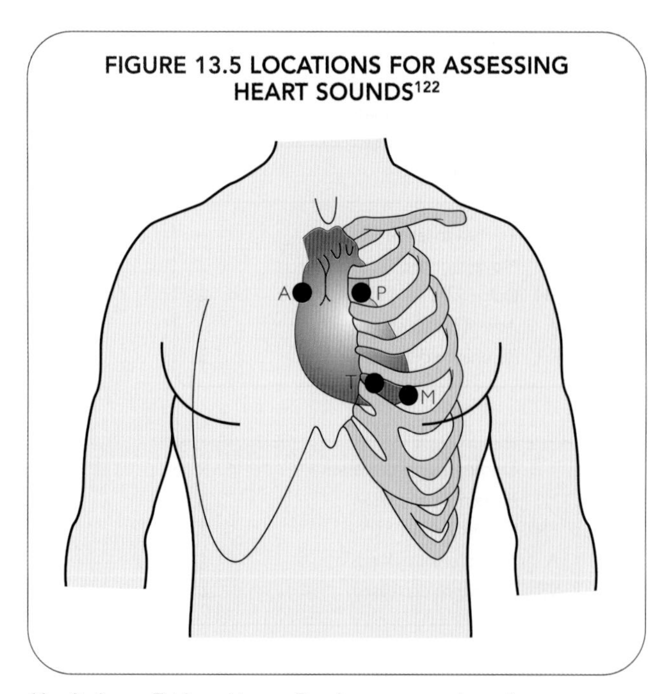

M: mitral area; T: tricuspid area; P: pulmonary area; A: aortic area.

ABDOMEN

The abdomen can be divided into four quadrants (see Fig. 13.6). It is useful to consider this when examining the abdomen, as the area of pain or injury can give clues to the cause and help consider which structures may have been injured in a trauma patient.

The patient is best examined while lying flat with one pillow under the head and knees slightly bent. This allows the abdomen to become as relaxed as possible. Inspect the abdomen for scars, discolouration, distension, symmetry, pulsation and masses. Auscultate over each of the four quadrants. It is important to listen before touching, as palpating can alter the frequency of bowel sounds. Listen for 10–15 seconds, but for up to 4 minutes if bowel sounds are difficult to hear.[122] Normal bowel sounds occur every 5–20 seconds. Hyperactive sounds indicate increased peristalsis. They have a loud tinkling sound and can indicate diarrhoea or an early bowel obstruction. Hypoactive sounds occur infrequently and signify decreased motility of the bowel, and can indicate inflammation or late bowel obstruction. Absent bowel sounds indicate paralytic ileus.[126]

Before palpating the abdomen, allow the patient to empty their bladder, as this makes examination more comfortable. Start away from the pain. Look for tenderness, rebound tenderness, guarding and rigidity (which can indicate peritonism). Rebound tenderness is identified by pressing slowly and deeply over the painful area and then quickly releasing. Sharp pain is felt on release.[126]

PELVIS

The presence of a genitourinary problem is usually elicited when taking a history. The patient might complain of difficulty passing urine, urgency, burning on micturition, altered volume and flank pain. A mid-stream urine sample is obtained for analysis (see Chapter 25 for more detail regarding renal and genitourinary assessment). In addition to performing a urinalysis, colour, clarity and any offensive odour should be noted.[127]

A menstrual history should be taken in female patients. It should include the date of the last menstrual period, contraceptive use and past pregnancy history. In women of childbearing age, a pregnancy test is indicated if pregnancy status is unclear.[128] Males should be assessed for problems specific to their genitourinary anatomy. A slow stream or inability to void may be indicative of a prostate problem. Painful swelling of the testes could mean a testicular torsion.[129] Presence of any discharge (penile/vaginal) or lesions may be indicative of a sexually transmitted infection (STI) and should prompt an inquiry about the patient's sexual history. The patient should be questioned about sexual partners and their health, contraception methods used, previous history of STI or high-risk behaviour.[128,129] It may be difficult to get a full history in the presence of a partner or parents, and so the emergency care clinician should attempt to speak to the patient alone. This may feel awkward, but most patients understand the necessity of acquiring a full history. Ascertaining sexual practices can provide a valuable arena for safe-sex education and referral, if appropriate.

Genitourinary trauma (saddle injuries) in children can be caused by non-accidental injury and the emergency care

FIGURE 13.6 DISTRIBUTION OF COMPONENTS IN THE FOUR IMAGINARY QUADRANTS OF THE ABDOMINAL SYSTEM[123]

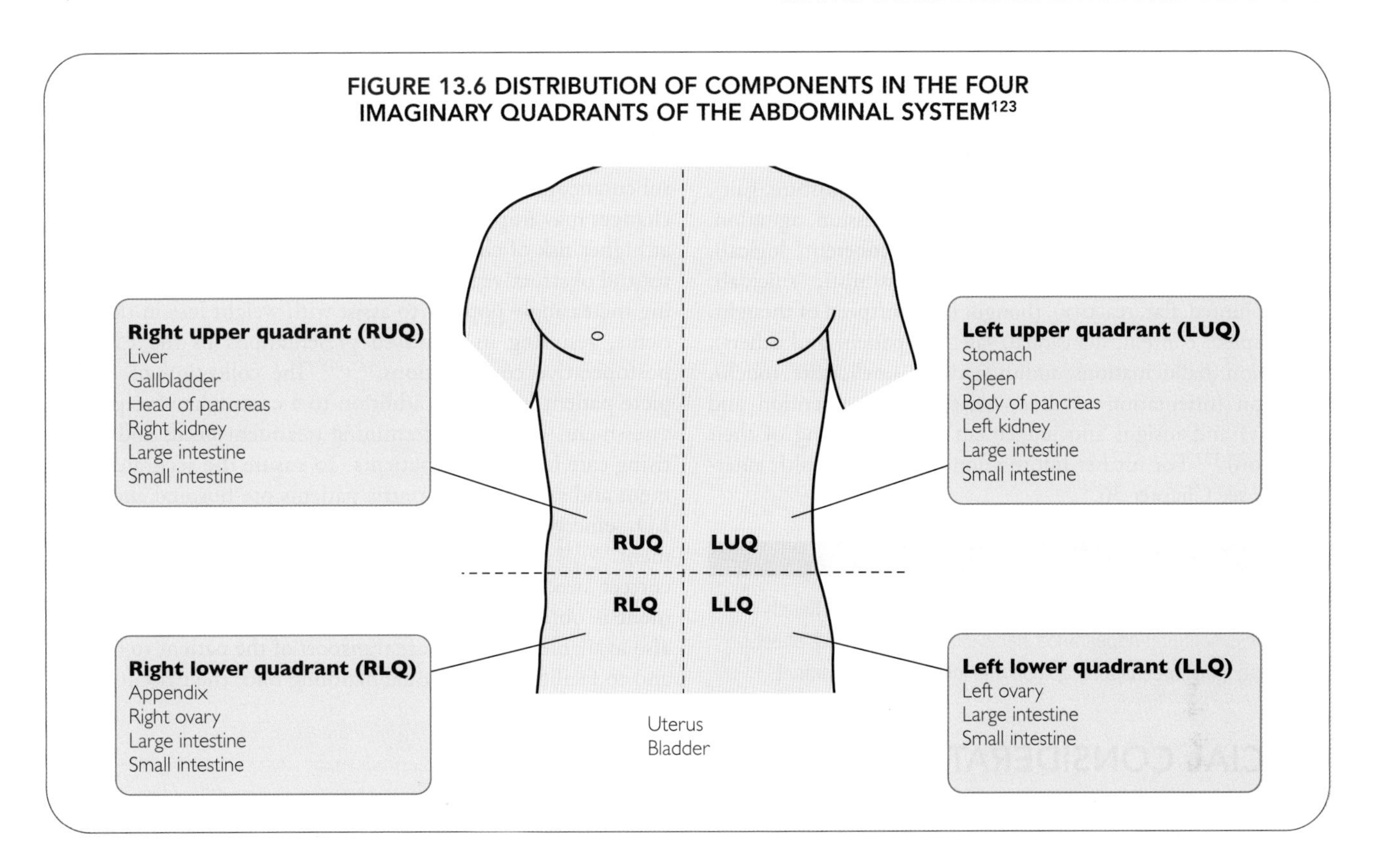

clinician should be alert for this possibility when taking a history (see Chapter 39 for more detail regarding non-accidental injuries).

MUSCULOSKELETAL AND SKIN

Most presentations concerned with the musculoskeletal system are due to pain. This can be caused by trauma, infection and vascular, autoimmune or degenerative disease. Observation and palpation are done simultaneously and should start on the unaffected side to give a base for comparison. Inspect for size, symmetry, deformities, swelling and colour. Palpate for pain, tenderness, swelling and warmth. Compare range of movement to the unaffected side. Assess active range of movement before passive movement. A dislocated limb is considered an emergency if distal circulation and sensation is affected.[130] See Chapter 17 for more information about minor injuries.

Assessment of the skin comprises observation for colour, integrity, rashes, lesions and perspiration and palpation to feel temperature and turgor.[131] Skin colour can also give clues to the underlying pathology; for example, cherry red lips in carbon monoxide poisoning, generalised yellowness in jaundice or the pallor of anaemia.

The hands and feet should also be inspected for colour, warmth, movement and sensation. Adequate peripheral perfusion is established by feeling strong radial and pedal pulses and a capillary refill time of under 3 seconds. Observe the peripheral limbs for pitting oedema, as this can be an indication of heart failure.[125]

PRACTICE TIP

Observation and palpation of both sides/limbs are done simultaneously and should start on the unaffected side to give a base for comparison.

OTHER CONSIDERATIONS

Signs of an endocrine or haematological condition may become obvious during history-taking. Areas to focus on in the clinical examination are discussed in brief here.

Symptoms of an endocrine disorder can include changes in weight, appetite, bowel habits, hair distribution, pigmentation, sweating or alteration in menstruation, as well as lethargy, weakness, polyuria, polydipsia, headaches and impotence.[132] Therefore, it is best to focus on the specific presenting complaint (see Chapter 26 for more information about endocrine emergencies).

A haematological disease can affect red blood cells, white blood cells, platelets and haemostatic mechanisms. Patients may present with anaemia, which is characterised by weakness, tiredness, dyspnoea, fatigue or postural dizziness. Platelet or blood-clotting disorders may present with easy bruising or bleeding problems. Recurrent infections could be an indication of a disorder of the immune system. Laboratory testing of blood confirms the diagnosis. See Chapters 27 and 29 for further discussion.

Mental health assessment

A mental health assessment should consist of gathering general information, then following with more specific questions to clarify ambiguities and confirm or refute initial impressions. The main areas looked at are: appearance (cleanliness, posture, gait), behaviour (facial expression, cooperation, aggression, agitation, activity levels), speech (form and pattern, coherent, logical), mood (apathetic, irritable, optimistic or pessimistic, suicidal), affect (blunted, flat, reactive), thought (stream/speed of thought, preoccupied, content, delusional, safety of patient and others), perception (hallucinations, auditory, visual, smell, taste, touch), cognition (orientation to time, place, person, attention and memory) and insight and judgement (understanding of their condition).[133] For further information on mental health emergencies, see Chapter 36.

PRACTICE TIP

The main areas looked at when performing a mental health assessment are: appearance, behaviour, speech, mood, affect, thought, perception, cognition and insight and judgement.

SPECIAL CONSIDERATIONS

Physiological and anatomical age-specific differences must be taken into account when collecting the patient's history and performing a clinical assessment. Paediatric patients are not just 'small adults', but have physical, cognitive and developmental differences as they progress from infancy and childhood into adulthood. Examination of children can also be challenging as they can often be uncooperative and are often reliant on their carer to provide information about their history.[134] The familiar adage in paediatrics that 'children are not just small adults' could be adapted to the care of geriatric patients. Older people have a higher proportion of chronic diseases, which can make assessment challenging and places them at increased risk of acute illnesses.[135,136] Several age-related structural and physiological changes develop in geriatric patients. See Table 13.8 for a summary of anatomical and physiological differences in paediatric and geriatric patients. For more detail on the assessment and care of paediatric patients and older people, see Chapters 35 and 38 respectively.

PRACTICE TIP

The patient's age must be taken into consideration when performing an assessment.

Changes that occur in pregnancy should also be taken into consideration when assessing the pregnant woman. The development of the baby, as well as hormonal changes, affect the anatomical structure and physiology of the female. See Chapter 34 for further details on the assessment and management of the pregnant patient.

OBESE PATIENTS

The prevalence of obesity is increasing globally and presents several challenges for emergency clinicians, both pre-hospital and in the ED.[137–139] Several physiological changes occur in obese patients which emergency clinicians must be aware of, including chest wall resistance, increased abdominal pressure, decreased lung capacity, increased airway resistance, increased subcutaneous tissue and anatomical distortion.[140–143] These changes may impact on assessment findings and place patients at higher risk of chronic diseases, such as hypertension, diabetes and obstructive sleep apneoa.[144] Bariatric surgery is becoming increasingly popular to assist with weight loss in these patients, resulting in increased presentations to the ED with postoperative complications.[141,145] The collection of a complete patient history, in addition to a comprehensive physical assessment, is key to determining treatment needs and prioritising care for bariatric patients. To ensure the accurate assessment and safe care of bariatric patients pre-hospital and in the ED, emergency services must have the appropriate equipment.[137,144] When measuring blood pressure, for example, the correct sized cuff is essential to ensure an accurate measurement is obtained. A range of manual handling equipment is also available to ensure safe transport of the patient to hospital and to facilitate safe manual handling once the patient has arrived at hospital.[146]

INTERVENTIONS

During the assessment process, a range of interventions may be initiated. This includes simple nursing care, such as repositioning the patient, dressing a wound or the administration of medications such as antibiotics. Some treatments may be nurse-initiated, or carried out in response to a medical order. The delivery of interventions should be prioritised in order of urgency, following the ABCDE approach to ensure all life-threatening conditions are treated first.

Interventions will occur simultaneously with other aspects of the assessment. While helping the patient to get onto the trolley you will already have started to gather historical data, taking note of how the patient moves and signs of pain. You might observe if they have some difficulty breathing, and oxygen therapy may be indicated, or they may appear to have severe pain, so analgesia is given. An intravenous cannula may need to be sited. In the pre-hospital setting this may be used to administer fluid resuscitation or drugs; in the ED setting it could be used to administer analgesia and to collect blood for laboratory testing. It is important to note that isolated pathology is not an indication for the insertion of an IV cannula.

Before delivering care the emergency clinician should question if the care they intend to deliver is best practice. While research knowledge is produced and published at an increasing rate, translation of research into clinical practice remains inconsistent and delayed.[147] Increasing demands for emergency care, and limited support received to change practice, restrict the emergency clinician's capacity to access, critique and adopt research into their clinical practice.[148] As a result, patients who present to the ED frequently do not receive optimal care, with the incidence of preventable adverse errors ranging from 36% to 71%.[149] Clinicians should refer to clinical practice guidelines and pathways available to assist in the delivery of evidence-based care.

TABLE 13.8 AGE-SPECIFIC COMMONALITIES

SYSTEM	PAEDIATRICS		GERIATRICS	
Cardiovascular	S3	Heard in up to a quarter of children	Coronary artery disease	A high incidence over age 60
	Murmurs	Heard in up to 50% of 3- to 7-year-olds		
Respiratory	Inhaled foreign object	At risk of obstruction due to small airway	Lung function	Declines with age
			Pneumonia	Increased risk of death with age
Gastrointestinal	Abdominal pain	Appendicitis, intussusception	Gastric and duodenal ulcers	At greater risk and mortality 4–10 times greater from GI bleeding
	Vomiting and diarrhoea	Caused by viral infection. Give fluids to prevent dehydration	Constipation	Due to decreased mobility and fluid intake or as side-effect of medications
Genitourinary	Scrotal swelling	Generally caused by hernia, but if acutely painful consider torsion	Prostatism	Enlarged prostate causing micturition problems
	UTI	Requires follow-up due to risk of renal scarring	Acute renal failure	Function declines with age, side-effects from medications
			UTI	Due to increased urinary stasis, obstruction or presence of IDC
Neurological	Meningitis	Common in childhood during neonatal period	Dementia	
	Convulsions	Occur in 20% of children under 5 years. Commonly due to fever	Acute confusional state secondary to infection	May be the only sign of infection
			Head injury	Minor trauma can result in significant head injury
Head, ears, eyes, nose and throat	Tonsillitis	If chronic may cause upper airway obstruction, sleep apnoea	Decreased vision	Physiological changes occur in aged eye
	Otitis media	Common until age 7	Ulceration of cornea	Eyelids lose elasticity and turn inwards
			Epistaxis	Due to anticoagulants, hypertension
Integumentary	Jaundice	Common in neonates, but in older children viral hepatitis is the commonest cause	Paper-thin skin	Easily damaged and difficult to heal
	Rashes	Most likely due to measles, chickenpox, with fever	Hypothermia	Increased risk due to fat loss
Musculoskeletal	Painful limb in absence of trauma	Septic arthritis. Present with fever and hot, swollen joint	Osteoporosis	Makes bones more fragile and can sustain fractures from minor trauma
Mental health	Depression and mood swings	Common in adolescence	Depression	Due to social isolation or loss of independence

PRACTICE TIP

Clinicians should refer to clinical practice guidelines and pathways available to assist in the delivery of evidence-based care.

All patients need to be re-evaluated for a response to these interventions and for any deterioration in general condition. Based on the findings of the re-evaluation, more interventions may be required or, in an ED setting, medical review sought earlier.

DIAGNOSTICS/INVESTIGATIONS

Diagnostic tests may commence in the pre-hospital setting, such as the performance of 12-lead ECGs, which, in some settings, are sent to the local hospital during transport to expedite patient transfer to the angiogram suite/catheter lab on arrival to hospital for patients requiring rapid reperfusion. When a patient arrives in the ED there is then an opportunity to obtain more extensive diagnostic and laboratory tests. The availability of this will depend on the facility. Most major metropolitan hospitals will have access to 24-hour facilities; however, in more rural and remote areas access may be restricted, particularly after-hours.[16,150]

While the primary responsibility for determining which diagnostic and laboratory tests are required remains that of the medical practitioner, paramedics and ED nurses need to understand why particular tests might be required and the significance of the results. This will help with the early identification of sick or complex patients, initiating investigations and their subsequent reporting to medical staff. Rather than ordering standard groups of tests for particular sets of presenting symptoms, clinicians need to consider whether the tests they order are relevant to the patient's current condition. For example, ordering thyroid function tests can be fairly common practice for many presentations, yet it is important to think critically about whether this is clinically indicated. If it *is* indicated, findings may not result in clinical intervention in the acute ED setting, for reasons such as time delays in receiving results. However, results can be followed up by the GP if the patient is discharged, or can prevent delay in inpatient treatment; for example, if blood collection did not occur in the inpatient unit until the following day.

There are certain other tests that are performed during an assessment to either confirm or rule out a diagnosis. Electrocardiograms (ECGs) are usually performed on any patient presenting with chest pain, jaw pain, difficulty breathing, nausea and vomiting or collapse. Falls in older persons that are not witnessed could be a result of a cardiac cause, and an ECG should also be recorded.[151] All patients with a suspected cardiac problem should have continuous cardiac monitoring according to department protocol (see Chapters 16 and 22 for more detail on ECGs). Blood glucose levels (BGLs) should be obtained and recorded for all patients with diabetes and in patients who present with collapse, altered consciousness level, multiple abscesses or non-healing wounds, dizziness and nausea and vomiting, and in neonates[84] (see Chapter 16 for more details on BGL).

Nurse-initiated x-rays are also a consideration when a patient presents with pain over a distal limb from trauma. Nurses will have to have completed additional training before being assessed as competent to perform this skill, and it will depend on whether the facility has a policy or procedure in place to support this practice (see Chapter 16).

PRACTICE TIP

Rather than ordering standard groups of tests for particular sets of presenting symptoms, clinicians need to consider whether the tests they order are relevant to the patient's current condition.

REASSESSMENT

Reassessment of the patient is essential to monitor patient progress and to ascertain response to interventions. If at any time the patient's condition deteriorates it is important to return to the DRSABCDEs to ensure life-threatening conditions are identified and treated first. When evaluating care and monitoring patient groups, a structured approach should be employed, focusing on relevant body regions, which is repeated at appropriate intervals according to the condition of the patient.[4] The clinician should also review results from any investigations performed (to gain a complete understanding of the patient's condition) and consider the priorities and ongoing plan for the patient.

COMMUNICATION

Effective communication and respectful human relationships with all those involved in the patient's care impact the delivery of safe patient care, emotional intelligence and job satisfaction, and influence how clinicians feel about themselves.[152–157] As paramedics and nurses, we have a responsibility to provide safe and high-quality care. Throughout the assessment process it is essential that communication occurs on several levels: paramedic to paramedic, paramedic to nurse, paramedic/nurse to patient and family/carers, nurse to nurse, and nurse to medical staff. Although paramedics and ED nurses are extremely busy, a large proportion of their time is spent communicating, so good communication is an essential aspect of care and can either facilitate a relationship or create barriers. On this note, public surveys, practitioner accounts, emerging policy and practice-based research are unanimous: communication determines clinical quality, patient safety, clinicians' wellbeing and public satisfaction.[156–159]

PRINCIPLES OF COMMUNICATION

Communication is a reciprocal process in which messages are sent and received between two or more people. The interaction is often interchangeable, with the speaker receiving messages from the person listening and the listener sending messages while the other is speaking.[160]

In general, there are two parts to communication: the verbal and non-verbal expression of the sender's thoughts and feelings. Verbally, cognitive and affective messages are sent through words, voice inflection and rate of speech; non-verbally, messages are conveyed by eye movements, facial expressions and body language (see Box 13.6). Non-verbal communication can send powerful messages, such as a suspicious glance, a warm smile or eyes widened with fear. However, when telephones or other electronic devices are used to communicate, the effect of gestures and other non-verbal communication is lost.[161] Additionally, mask-wearing creates a physical barrier and reduces the efficiency of non-verbal communication; however, conscious non-verbal communication, particularly use of the eyes, can mitigate some of the challenges experienced.[162] The following basic principles of communication are important to consider:

1. It is impossible not to communicate. All behaviour has a message of some sort. As well as the more obvious carriers of messages like words or gestures, saying or doing nothing is in itself a message. Once a message has been sent it cannot be retracted.
2. Every communication has a context and relationship aspect.
3. A series of communications can be viewed as an uninterrupted series of interchanges. There is no clear beginning or ending to a series of interchanges—communication between two individuals has a history and a future in itself and is affected by the past experiences of each individual.
4. All communication relationships are either symmetrical or complementary, depending on whether they are based on equality or inequality. With a status or power difference between two people, such as between a nurse and a doctor, the complementary relationship will affect any communication between them. In general, how communication is interpreted depends on the relationship the sender has with the receiver.[163]

COMMUNICATION IN THE ED

Effective communication, both among clinicians and between clinicians and patients, is critical in the provision of safe and quality healthcare, yet EDs are becoming increasingly challenging healthcare environments for clinician–patient communication.[158,164] Poor communication practices have consistently been identified as a major cause of adverse events, leading to avoidable patient harm in hospitals around the world.[156,164–166] A number of studies have examined the degree of communication interruptions experienced by clinicians in the ED and the implications for patient safety.[167–170] The ED is well known for being an 'interrupt driven' area,[171] and nurses are interrupted on average once every 6 minutes.[172] Although there have been numerous studies on interruptions in the ED, conclusive strategies to effectively manage these interruptions have not been established.[171,173,174]

One Australian study[164] observed communication across a number of EDs and found two broad areas of communication that affect the quality and safety of the patient journey through the department: how medical knowledge is communicated, and how clinician–patient relationships are established and maintained. Both of these are crucial for effective communication and to deliver care effectively.[164]

BOX 13.6 FACTORS THAT HAVE AN IMPACT ON COMMUNICATION[160]

Type of language used	Jargon, dialect, social linguistics
Paralinguistic features	Pitch, tone, pace, emphasis and volume
Body language	Posture, touch, eye contact, proximity, facial expression, gestures
Social	Age, gender, ethnicity, power, social status, relationship
Psychological	Attitudes and beliefs, prejudices, perceptual distortions, defence mechanisms, frame of mind/mood, stress, trust
Environmental	Privacy, layout of room, odours, lighting, colour

COMMUNICATING WITH OTHER HEALTH PROFESSIONALS

Clinical handover

Paramedics, nurses and doctors undertake segregated and distinct preparation for clinical practice, yet are expected to communicate effectively with each other in the workplace and ensure excellent and accurate clinical handover. There are three distinct transitions of care when handover occurs: the paramedic handing over to the triage nurse or resuscitation team on arrival at the ED; nurse-to-nurse handover at change of shift; and handover by the emergency nurse to the ward nurse. Patients are often critically unwell and may be unstable at the time of handover, while available resources and ED overcrowding may contribute to further constraints.[166,170] The aim of handover in all circumstances is to ensure a seamless exchange of information between care providers.[109] It is acknowledged that without a proper structure to the handover, vital information is likely to be forgotten and this can lead to adverse outcomes.[109,156,165,166,170] Continuing work has been conducted to establish and evaluate structured clinical handovers to reduce communication errors,[156,165] with different tools suited to different practice environments.[175] It is recommended that structured, standardised clinical handovers are implemented, but that flexibility for the context is applied.[109] The mnemonic IMIST-AMBO (**I**dentification of the patient, **M**echanism/Medical complaint, **I**njuries/information relative to the complaint, **S**igns vitals and GCS, **T**reatment and trends/response to treatment—**A**llergies, **M**edications, **B**ackground history and **O**ther (social) information)[176]—is a recommended structure used for handovers from paramedics to emergency staff, and is discussed in detail in Chapter 42. ISBAR (**I**ntroduction, **S**ituation, **B**ackground, **A**ssessment/Agreed plan and **R**ecommendations/**R**ead back) is a demonstrated effective strategy that can be employed to promote good communication with other in-hospital staff (Box 13.7).[177] Variations to ISBAR, such as the use of ISoBAR (**I**dentify, **S**ituation, **O**bservations, **B**ackground, **A**gree to a plan, **R**esponsibility and risk)

BOX 13.7 **THE ISBAR COMMUNICATION TOOL**

I	Introduction: identify yourself and introduce the patient
S	Situation: what is the main problem? What are your observations?
B	Background: pertinent information, including past medical history
A	Assessment/Agreed plan: include the clinical assessment and the plan of care
R	Recommendation/Read back: outline any outstanding items that need attending to and clarify and check for understanding.

and SHARED (**S**ituation, **H**istory, **A**ssessment, **R**isk, **E**xpectation, **D**ocumentation) have been implemented in other clinical settings, highlighting the importance of knowing healthcare guidelines for clinical handover practice. Additionally, it is important to acknowledge that handover is a social, yet stressful time,[156] and that respect and kindness for our colleagues must be maintained.[178]

Using a communication tool allows accurate and relevant information to be shared in a structured format. This leads to a better patient experience, increases the credibility of the handover and allows the person receiving the information to be in possession of all the facts.[109,179] This will lead to them being able to quickly prioritise what they need to do first when taking over the care of the patient.

Escalation of care/graded assertiveness

The ability to escalate care in an assertive manner is a vital skill, particularly in the emergency environment when a patient's condition may be unpredictable. Regardless of how intimidating a situation may be or how senior other staff are, it is important to articulate concerns in order to keep the patient safe. This assertive way of communicating is termed graded assertiveness. Graded assertiveness is a concept adopted from the airline industry where adverse incidents occurred; even though staff knew something wasn't right as they were too afraid to be assertive when communicating.[7] The employment of graded assertiveness aims to assist the staff member in escalating their concerns through a stepped process (Table 13.9).[152]

TABLE 13.9 **LEVELS OF GRADED ASSERTIVENESS AND EXAMPLES**[152]

LEVEL	EXAMPLE
Level one: express concern with an 'I' statement	I am concerned about ...
Level two: make an inquiry and offer a solution	Would you like me to ...
Level three: ask for an explanation	It would help me to understand ...
Level four: a definitive challenge demanding a response	For the safety of the patient you must listen to me

It is important to emphasise that assertiveness is not the same as aggression. Aggression is disrespectful and denies the other person the opportunity to express their opinions, whereas assertiveness is respectful and allows the expression of opinions.[152,180,181]

COMMUNICATION WITH PATIENTS

Dialogue is more than sending and receiving messages verbally and non-verbally, and each patient should be treated as a unique individual.[182] Research has shown that patients who come to the unfamiliar territory of the ED often experience feelings of bewilderment, loss of control, anxiety and frustration, particularly as they are moved through a number of areas, experiencing prolonged and often unexplained waiting times.[159,183] If clinicians are sensitive to the patient's concerns, communication can be improved.[183] Difficulties arise when the patient is unable to communicate clearly due to their clinical condition, cognitive impairment, treatment side-effects or language. This can further aggravate feelings of anxiety, frustration and stress as they lose control over their life and decisions. There is also evidence to support that patients with communication problems are more at risk of preventable adverse events.[164,184]

The AIDET™ (**A**cknowledge the patient, **I**ntroduce yourself, **D**uration of procedures/test/interaction, **E**xplanation of procedure/test/procedure, **T**hank the patient for their cooperation) mnemonic, developed by the Studer Group, encapsulates five principles of communication identified to promote patient satisfaction[185] (see Box 13.8 for an explanation of each principle). These communication strategies assist clinicians in making patients feel safe and calm, and to gather the key pieces of information needed to treat patients safely.[185]

Communication can also occur through physical contact: touch may communicate empathy and demonstrate warmth.[161] Language barriers may necessitate the assistance of an interpreter with knowledge of healthcare terminology to ensure the content is adequately translated.[161,186]

As a result of greater-than-ever access to medical information through superior communication systems and technology, patients and families recognise and may understand the basic definition of many medical terms and jargon. However, there are large variations of comprehension which may be of clinical significance. Healthcare providers should not assume a patient or family member's level of understanding, and an attempt should be made to determine what their level of comprehension is, particularly when new information is given. Using plain language, a range of modalities to provide information and remembering to actively listen to the patient and/or their family member are key strategies.[186,187]

Communication and patient outcomes

It is important to discuss the relationship between communication, suboptimal care and patient outcomes, as there is a direct correlation.[109,188] The most common characteristics of international crisis-prompted healthcare inquiries are: care is not

BOX 13.8 **THE AIDET™ COMMUNICATION PRINCIPLES**[185]

A—ACKNOWLEDGE THE PATIENT

Greet the patient and other visitors with a smile, maintaining appropriate eye contact. Demonstrate a warm, receptive attitude. Address the patient by their name. Ask them what they would like to be called. Acknowledge others present.

I—INTRODUCE YOURSELF AND YOUR ROLE

Introduce yourself by name and role. Indicate your desire to help the patient by providing them with your full attention.

D—DURATION OF THE PROCEDURE/TEST/ INTERACTION

Provide a brief explanation of how long any procedures/tests will take to perform or for results to come back. Let them know who they are waiting for and possible time-frames. Inform them of any delays.

E—EXPLANATION OF PROCEDURE/TEST/ INTERACTION

Keep the patient informed to enable them to make informed decisions and reduce any anxieties they have about the care of their condition. Provide details about tests and procedures, such as why it is being performed, who will perform it, whether there is pain or discomfort associated with the test, and what will happen afterwards. Provide them with an opportunity to ask questions.

T—THANK THE PATIENT FOR THEIR COOPERATION

Thank the patient for their cooperation and patience. Ask if there is anything else you can do.

Courtesy Studer Group.

delivered in multidisciplinary teams; people do not communicate well across the clinical divides; and care is not delivered in a coordinated, organised way. The variety of healthcare areas investigated demonstrates that no one specialty is immune from error if poor communication exists.[109,189,190]

Positive interpersonal relationships between clinicians and patients result in a higher degree of patient involvement, which in turn produces better clinical outcomes.[164] Poor communication can lead to delays in transfer from the ED, and there is a correlation between increased hospital length of stay (LOS) and increased LOS in the ED. This occurs particularly on weekend shifts when patients are not reviewed by specialist teams and are often placed on outlying wards not related to the patient's condition, secondary to insufficient appropriate beds.[191]

Poor communication has been related to staff dissatisfaction, stress and burnout in the nursing profession,[192–194] with stress, wellbeing and burnout linked to patient safety incidents.[195,196] In particular, burnout has been associated with avoidable mistakes, ineffective delivery of care, and nursing shortages.[197] This highlights the need for strategies to be in place to identify and reflect on the causes of stress and burnout, and how it impacts on patient care at both an individual and system level.[198,199]

Patient experience

There is good evidence to suggest that a patient's positive experience is directly associated with safety and clinical effectiveness, across a range of disease areas and population groups.[200] Common public expectations of emergency care include staff communication with patients, appropriate waiting times, the triage process, information management and good quality of care.[157,159,201] Often the healthcare system is portrayed negatively by the media,[199] and while the paramedic and emergency nurse cannot control all of the elements that contribute to this, effective communication is achievable. The way in which communication is conducted is closely related to ED patient satisfaction,[157,159,187,202] and has been linked to the interpersonal skills of staff.[203] Patients and their families need provision of information/explanation on a consistent basis, especially on arrival.[204] Emergency care clinicians need to consider core themes of information sharing during care provision: communication, emotion, waiting, care delivery, physical, and environmental needs.[159] Respectfully communicating the cause of delays, patient management plans and how to get to other locations within the hospital are themes that will improve a patient's satisfaction.[187,205] Regular communication with patients in the waiting room and explaining reasons for any delays improves satisfaction levels, and reduces perceived waiting times.[185,206–209]

OPEN DISCLOSURE

Open disclosure means providing an open, consistent approach to communicating with patients following an adverse event. This includes expressing regret for what has happened, informing the patient about the event and potential consequences, creating a forum for the patient to discuss their experience, and providing feedback on investigations, including the steps taken to prevent an event from recurring.[109] It is also about providing information that will enable systems of care to be changed to improve patient safety. The Australian Open Disclosure Framework provides a nationally consistent basis for open disclosure in Australian healthcare. It was endorsed in 2013 and replaced the former Open Disclosure Standard.[210]

Improving healthcare safety begins with ensuring that communication is open and honest, and immediate. This includes communication between healthcare professionals and patients and their carers. It also includes communication between healthcare professionals, healthcare managers and all staff. It is important that when this framework is put in place people feel supported and are encouraged to identify and report adverse events, so that system improvements can be identified and acted on. This should include the following:

- Providing an environment where patients, their family and carers:
  - receive the information they need to understand what happened
  - can contribute about the adverse event and, where possible and appropriate, participate in the incident review, creating a culture where patients, their family and carers, clinicians and managers all feel supported.
- Integrating open disclosure with investigative processes to identify why adverse events occur.
- Implementing the necessary changes in systems of clinical care based on the lessons learnt.[210]

Disclosure is required where a patient has suffered some harm (physical or psychological) because of treatment. This may be a recognised complication or the result of human or systems error. As soon as an event is noticed, you should ensure patient safety, perform any immediate care interventions required and inform your manager. If the emergency clinician notices harm caused under the care of another clinician, they should always speak first to their manager and the senior clinician of the team involved. If these members of staff are unwilling to initiate the disclosure process, refer the matter to the person responsible for clinical risk or medical administration.

DISCLOSURE WITH THE PATIENT AND FAMILY

The individual making the disclosure should be the most senior healthcare professional involved; for example, the nurse manager, and someone with experience or training in communication and open disclosure. Effective communication is pivotal to the open-disclosure process. Patients, their families and carers, may become upset or angry when they have suffered an adverse event. This is a natural response, so it is important not to become angry or react defensively in this situation. An adverse incident is an emotionally charged event for all parties. Guidelines for communicating with the patient and family can be found on the Australian Commission on Safety and Quality in Health Care (ACSQHC) website,[210] and include the following:

- Arrange a face-to-face meeting that allows adequate time for detailed discussion as soon as possible after an adverse outcome has occurred.
- Listen actively and respectfully to the patient.
- Use plain language and avoid jargon.
- Acknowledge the validity of the emotions the patient and/or carer may feel.
- Where a family member is present, include them in your dialogue where appropriate.
- In all discussions, avoid defensiveness and laying blame. Avoid statements that include terms such as 'fault', 'blame' or 'feel responsible'.[210]

Support for staff involved

If directly involved in an adverse event, staff have the right to seek appropriate legal advice and to disclose information to legal advisers in a manner that ensures it attracts legal professional privilege. The breaking of bad news can be extremely stressful on staff members.[210] They have the right to be treated fairly by the institution and to receive natural justice and procedural fairness, and the right not to be defamed.[210] While an expression of regret and an apology is a part of open disclosure, it is important to avoid speculative statements such as:

- 'I'm sorry—I appear to have made an error in judgement.'
- 'I apologise for this mistake.'
- 'It is my fault that this has happened.'

The best approach is to give an honest and factual account of what happened.

Healthcare professionals who have been involved in an adverse event may be angry with themselves or someone else for what occurred. They may feel that they have let the patient down. It is important to make sure they receive emotional support and advice after the incident, as well as feedback once the investigation has been finalised.[211,212]

Needs of the family

The psychosocial care of family who arrive in the ED with a critically ill relative is stressful for families, as well as complex and challenging for staff.[213,214] Quite often, staff are focused on stabilising a patient and may overlook or ignore anxious family members. Research has shown that communication with family members is the most important need of family members of critically ill patients within the ED.[212,214,219] During such stressful situations, suffering can be exacerbated when there is a lack of information provided.[215] Another important family need is for relatives to be close to their loved one.[213,214,219] Often family members may be left out in the waiting room or be asked to step outside while an assessment or treatment takes place, yet family consider being close to their loved one very important.[214,216] Staff should invite family members to be with the patient whenever possible and engage in family-centred care.[217]

In light of the various definitions of family and the regulations regarding the release of information, how people define themselves has implications for clinicians (see Chapter 4 for further details). It is important to ask the patient who they consider to be family, who they wish to receive information and who should be allowed in the treatment area. When that is not possible, the clinician must be guided by good judgement, policy and regulations and ethics.[218]

Although emergency care clinicians are usually very busy, it can be crucial to conduct a brief family assessment, and determine if social work intervention may be required. There are several ways to develop a dialogue with families and conduct a quick assessment of family strengths and potential resources.

- Introduce yourself to the patient and the family.
- Ask about people at the bedside and determine their relationship to the patient.
- Call patients by name, after having asked how they wish to be addressed.
- Explain procedures and equipment, and be honest about the anticipated length of the wait.
- Repeat information; the anxiety of being in the ED, even in non-urgent situations, decreases the ability to remember what has been said.
- Stop in the patient's doorway or at the foot of the bed to update them and their family whenever the situation in the ED changes.

After any explanation, always ask if anyone has questions. If the answer is not known, say so, then find out the answer. When encountering a family in the initial stages of a life-changing event, paramedics and ED nurses often interact with and provide support for family members who feel despair, fear, anger, guilt or helplessness, or who are in a state of disbelief or denial. Family members present at the scene, or who come to the ED with a loved one nearing the end of a long and debilitating illness, may be fatigued, frustrated or ambivalent. The paramedic or emergency nurse may be the first to recognise a family that is bordering on crisis because of the drain on their emotional and physical resources.

Family needs have been extensively researched, and include the need for information, participation, reassurance, closeness, support and comfort.[213,214] Practical ways to meet these are presented in Box 13.9.

The Australian Institute for Patient and Family-Centred Care (AIPFCC) promotes the relationship between the patient,

BOX 13.9 FAMILY NEEDS[205,211]

Ways to meet families' needs include:

- listen compassionately
- compliment the family on how well members are coping
- involve the family early
- communicate regularly
- praise family strengths
- acknowledge how difficult the experience is
- commend patience
- update them on relative progress and prognosis
- answer questions honestly
- give consistent information
- demonstrate caring (offer a chair and a cup of tea/coffee)
- call them at home to update on patient condition or any change
- inform about transfer plans as they are being made.

their family members and the healthcare professional with the aim to 'ensure safer, more cost effective and satisfying health care experience for all involved'.[219] The core values of patient and family-centred care are:[219]

- compassionate care and communication
- collaboration between patients and carers, both professional and family
- innovation in our practices
- care practices that are sustainable over time
- care that is accessible to both patients and carers
- respectful communication
- ethical behaviour and practice at all times
- openly and honestly sharing information and our experiences.

Documentation

Documentation should occur regularly and be contemporaneous, occurring with each intervention rather than once at the end of a shift. Documentation must also be legible and identify clearly who the author is; this is becoming easier with the implementation of electronic records. Treating clinicians should be able to read the patient notes and determine the patient status (waiting for review, awaiting ward bed), condition, interventions that have been performed and response to those interventions. Up-to-date documentation also allows the patient to be transferred without delay.[109] The use of structured frameworks, such as HIRAID™, have demonstrated improved accuracy of documentation, further evidencing the benefits of structured tools to not only support patient assessment, but communication through documented findings.[220] Documentation is not only a way to communicate the assessment, findings and the plan of care for the patient to other clinicians, it is a legal record of the patient's care (for more details please refer to Chapter 4).

ESSENTIALS OF CARE

Essential care refers to fundamental elements of patient care that have a direct impact on the wellbeing of both patient and healthcare worker.[221] In Australia, NSW Health introduced the Essentials of Care (EOC) program with the intention of improving the experience of everyone involved in patient care (the patient, their families, their carers and staff) by bringing the focus back to caring. Essential care encompasses care that is important to the patient, but is subjective and may be influenced by several factors, such as (but not limited to) culture, age, gender, pain and the patient's previous healthcare experience.[222] Regardless, all patients want to be treated with respect and compassion, particularly when feeling unwell or experiencing pain.[222] Culture and pain are discussed in detail in Chapters 5 and 18 respectively.

While paramedics and ED nurses are expected to work under pressure to many standards, guidelines and protocols related to patient care,[202] it is important that they remain compassionate. Compassionate care is beneficial across a variety of healthcare settings, but it is often reported as lacking among healthcare workers.[223] Recent evidence suggests that healthcare worker empathy declines as clinical experience increases.[223] Therefore, it is important that paramedics and ED nurses regularly consider how the patient and/or their loved ones may be feeling. Paramedics and ED nurses may find it useful to ask themselves: 'How would I want this patient to be cared for if it were me or my mother/grandfather/husband/child?' A similar approach should be taken when interacting with the patient's relatives, but with respect to culture and the wishes of the patient. This question provides an answer that sets a benchmark for nursing practice.[216]

Increasing demands on the health service, increased patient wait times and increased ED length of stay (LOS) impact on both patient and staff experience. Paramedics may need to wait with a patient until a treatment space becomes available, and patients may need to wait extended periods of time for medical review, test results and/or an inpatient bed. This means that paramedics and ED nurses need to consider other essential aspects of patient care such as personal hygiene nutrition and elimination. However, as the roles of the paramedic and ED nurse become more technical, less time is available for direct patient care. Less time for direct patient care has been related to a drecrease in job satisfaction.[224] Paramedics and ED nurses may feel frustrated that they are too busy to provide quality care and may be morally and emotionally torn as they struggle to find the time to meet the basic needs of patients.[225] It is important that paramedics and ED nurses acknowledge these feelings and escalate these issues with management. Care for staff is discussed in more detail later in the chapter.

RISK ASSESSMENT

Increased length of stay in the ED has been associated with adverse events, particularly in elderly patients.[226] While ED length of stay may be outside of our control, performing a risk assessment on each patient will facilitate the identification of potential problems and instigate suitable interventions. Two key areas of care—reducing risk and providing high-quality care—are served by a series of principles (see Table 13.10) and are closely related. Good risk management is an important component of high-quality care; if patients are assessed thoroughly and on a continuing basis then problems may be detected and treated early, thus preventing the development of unnecessary complications.[153] Initial screening and ongoing assessment of patients in line with local and governmental policy will provide information that can help the paramedic and ED nurse plan their care.

TABLE 13.10 PRINCIPLES OF PRACTICE[153]

REDUCING RISKS TO PATIENTS	PROVISION OF HIGH-QUALITY CARE
Recognition of the specific needs of critically ill patients, particularly those who are unconscious, sedated or immobile	Development of knowledge and skills for practice
Recognition of specific complications that may require special observation or treatment	Evidence-based practice
Vigilant monitoring and early recognition of signs of deterioration	Optimal use of protocol-driven therapy
Selection, implementation and evaluation of specific preventive measures	Competent practice
Management of potentially detrimental environmental factors that may affect the patient	Efficient and safe practice
	Selection and application of appropriate nursing interventions
	Monitoring the effects of nursing interventions
	Evaluation of nursing practice

A variety of risk assessment tools are available and include (but are not limited to) falls risk screening in elderly patients, pressure injury risk, non-accidental injury in children and domestic violence screening, to name a few.

CARING

Caring is a core characteristic of healthcare. In emergencies, lifesaving procedures are, of course, the priority, but it is important not to forget to meet the patient's psychological needs as well.[182,211,228] Professional caring consists of three essential elements: competence, caring and connection. *Competence* involves empowering, connecting and educating people, making clinical judgements and being able to do tasks and take action on behalf of people. Aspects of *caring* are outlined below and involve being dedicated and having the courage to be appropriately involved as a professional paramedic and nurse. The *connection* aspects of professional caring involve initiating professional connection, which requires both the patient and the clinician to reach out and respond. A bridge is built when patients realise the connection and feel free to ask for help. Professional intimacy then occurs when patients begin to trust the clinician. As a result of the connection and professional intimacy, emergency clinicians work with patients towards their common goal. Professional boundaries are discussed in more detail in Chapter 3.

An uncaring encounter can consist of incompetence and indifference, lack of trust, mutual avoidance and disconnection between the nurse and the patient. The clinician may be perceived as inconsiderate, insensitive, disrespectful and disinterested.

ASPECTS OF CARING IN EMERGENCIES

- *Being open to and perceptive of others:* patients are often affected by the acute event, as they have abruptly lost control of their own situation and are in a position of dependence. A caring emergency clinician has to be sensitive to such patients and capable of interpreting or predicting their needs. The caring clinician must adopt an open attitude and should communicate openly with the patient.
- *Being genuinely concerned for the patient:* paramedics and nurses with this caring quality display genuine feelings of goodwill towards patients and a holistic view of caring.
- *Being morally responsible:* from the patient's perspective, calling an ambulance and presenting to the ED are not usually planned events. Suddenly, they become dependent on others to help fulfil their basic needs. Clinicians have to act to maintain and strengthen the patient's dignity in this serious situation.
- *Being truly present:* this means that clinicians have to be attentive to the present moment, and be present in dialogue, in listening and responding. They should be present in the situation, physically and emotionally. In order to be truly present in the dialogue, paramedics and nurses require good communication skills.[182]
- *Meeting the patient's psychological needs* could reduce the risk of developing post-traumatic stress syndrome. To create an authentic encounter, paramedics and nurses need to display several aspects of sensitive and effective communication, be dedicated and have the courage to be appropriately involved.[182] It is important to find the balance between being overly involved and too detached.[229]

CARE OF PARAMEDICS

Just as patients require care, so do paramedics. The role of the paramedic has moved away from its focus of giving first aid and transporting patients to hospital, to a more dynamic role that encompasses higher levels of patient care and instigating interventions based on a thorough patient assessment.[230] Paramedics are frequently exposed to highly stressful situations,[229,231] increasing physical and verbal aggression, and there is less down time between calls as the service continues to get busier.[230] There is further concern for the physical and mental wellbeing of not just paramedics, but all healthcare workers as we face the challenges of a global COVID-19 pandemic.[232,233] While formal practices such as debriefing and counselling are advocated to aid resilience, support from colleagues, family and friends, as well as a sense of humour, are reported as methods that assist with resilience.[229] Globally, paramedics have higher rates of post-traumatic stress disorder, anxiety and depression than the general population.[234] Historically it may have been an accepted belief that to do their job well, paramedics should appear 'tough', but by failing to talk about a traumatic incident, the likelihood of suffering stress increases. While it is important that the individual is aware of their own stress and that they act on symptoms,[234] it is just as important that the organisation is responsive to any reports made.[235] Peer support is also imperative,[235] and the value of social support from colleagues cannot be underestimated as it can help to mitigate the impact of traumatic events.[231] Managers in the profession should be empathetic and acknowledge staff reports and, where possible, offer regular debriefing or counselling, and encompass this into the role. Regular debriefing and the promotion of an employee assistance program that offers free, confidential counselling to employees should be encouraged. Even if staff feel it is unnecessary, a regular check-in may be of value, particularly when there has been a significant event.

CARE OF EMERGENCY NURSES

ED nurses also require care. Providing thorough and effective care for emergency patients can be emotionally draining and highly demanding for the busy ED nurse, who often fail to notice or acknowledge their own needs.[236] A certain amount of stress at work can be a motivator, but repeated exposure to stressful events can have adverse outcomes.[237] Nurses have been extensively studied as groups experiencing high levels of stress, burnout and fatigue.[238] Being aware of the signs of stress and developing and implementing coping mechanisms is essential.[239] Nurses depend on colleagues and friends for support and value debriefing sessions, whether it be an opportunity to share feelings or a clinical review of events. The effectiveness of sessions should be evaluated and staff health and welfare monitored by ED managers and colleagues. An awareness of colleagues' needs is key to providing the support they require.[211] Employee assistance programs should also be made available for nursing staff as well as regular debriefings for significant events. Paramedics and ED nurses should also aim to eat a well-balanced diet, exercise regularly and rest when possible. The use of alcohol and/or drugs to alleviate stress should be avoided as this can exacerbate issues. Other strategies such as mindful meditation have proven to improve nurses' stress, anxiety, depression, burnout and wellbeing,[240] with some facilities running weekly mindful meditation programs for staff.[241]

PRIVACY AND DIGNITY

Respect, autonomy, empowerment and communication have been identified within the literature as being the defining attributes of dignity. In the busy ED, maintenance of dignity may be unintentionally overlooked. Patients may be nursed in a corridor, or other patients and relatives may overhear personal information, which does not lend itself to upholding the dignity, privacy and confidentiality of the patient. Discretion should be used if updating relatives in a crowded waiting room; triage assessment should be conducted in a safe and private location, and the patient's dignity should be maintained at all times.[242]

PERSONAL HYGIENE AND PREVENTING COMPLICATIONS

Patients presenting to the ED can be in various states of hygiene as a result of injury, vomiting, incontinence or neglect. Also, despite the 4-hour Emergency Treatment Performance Target (formerly known as National Emergency Access Target),[243] patients may remain in the ED for an extended period of time with the inability to maintain their regular hygiene routine. Personal hygiene is closely related to individual esteem and sense of wellbeing, and is an important sensory determinant by family members that influences their perception of the quality of care the patient is receiving and the confidence they have in the staff. While personal hygiene is a basic right for all patients, it should not be placed above the need for other therapies, forensic requirements and rest.[153]

As with all aspects of care and treatment, the patient has the right to refuse personal hygiene measures. Bathing or washing patients provides opportunities for the emergency nurse to assess the patient's skin and tissue. Often this enables the nurse to identify tissue damage that requires treatment, and to identify dressings or wounds that require attention. Some patients who are sweating, incontinent or bleeding need to be washed and their linen changed more often. Wet, creased sheets alter skin integrity and may cause pressure on dependent areas, increasing the risk of pressure-ulcer development. A bed bath can be a major and painful undertaking, which often requires at least two people to support and move the patient, along with prophylactic pain relief before commencement.[153] The length of time taken to wash a patient, the environmental temperature and the patient's clinical condition are factors that affect cooling. Water on exposed skin causes rapid heat loss and shivering increases metabolism and oxygen consumption, which is detrimental in a compromised patient (see Chapter 28).

It is essential to maintain patient privacy and avoid interruptions that affect the dignity of the patient. All necessary equipment should be prepared prior to performing any procedure with the patient to ensure interruptions are minimised and dignity is maintained. In areas where curtains are used to separate treatment spaces, ensure there are no gaps when they are drawn for procedures. Ensure any necessary discussion remains professional and that the patient is not spoken over. Careful handling of patients to reduce skin friction and shear during repositioning and transfers can prevent skin tears.[153] The management of skin tears is discussed in Chapter 17.

PRACTICE TIP

Consider the length of time a patient has spent, or will spend, in the ED and ensure opportunities are given for attending to their personal hygiene needs. This will differ from person to person and depend on their condition.

EYE CARE

Eye care aims to provide comfort and prevent infection, and is an important aspect of caring for the sedated or unconscious patient.[158] There are a number of physiological processes that protect the eye. The eye is protected from dryness by frequent lubrication, facilitated by blinking. Antimicrobial substances in tears help prevent infection, and the tear ducts provide drainage. When the eye is unable to close properly, tear film evaporates more quickly.[244] If these mechanisms are compromised, the patient is at risk of eye problems. The blink response may be slowed or absent in some patients, such as individuals receiving sedatives and muscle relaxants, which can potentially cause keratopathy, corneal ulceration and viral or bacterial conjunctivitis. Patients who are exposed to high flows of air/oxygen may also be vulnerable to its drying effects.[153] See Chapter 32 for assessment and management of eye injury.

Eye care and the administration of artificial tears should be provided if required, if the patient complains of sore or dry eyes, or if there is visible evidence of encrustation. If a patient is receiving high-flow oxygen therapy via a mask, they may benefit from regular 4-hourly administration of artificial tears to lubricate the eyes and prevent the drying effect of oxygen.[153] Conjunctival oedema is a common problem associated with positive-pressure ventilation with high positive end-expiratory pressure (PEEP) (above 5 cmH_2O), and prone positioning often results in the patient's inability to maintain eye closure.[153] Eye closure may be maintained by applying a wide piece of adhesive tape horizontally to the upper part of the eyelid. This usually anchors the lid in the closed position, but allows the eyelid to be opened for pupil assessment and access for eye care.[153]

PRACTICE TIP

Apply 4-hourly artificial tears to lubricate the eyes to prevent the drying effect of high-flow oxygen therapy.

ORAL HYGIENE

Poor oral hygiene is unpleasant, and causes halitosis and discomfort. Oral care aims to ensure a healthy oral mucosa, maintain a clean and moist oral cavity, prevent pressure ulcers from devices such as endotracheal tubes (ETTs), prevent trauma caused by grinding teeth or biting the tongue and reduce bacterial activity that leads to local and systemic infection.[153] Although mouth care is one of the most basic nursing activities, in some cases lack of oral hygiene can lead to serious complications or increase the risk of complications, such as ventilator-associated pneumonia (VAP) in the ventilated patient.[153,245] Studies have shown that mouth care decreases the risk of VAP and that chlorhexidine mouthwash or gel reduces the risk of developing VAP from 24% to about 18%.[246]

If the ED patient has had an extended stay, a toothbrush, toothpaste and assistance to clean teeth should be provided. The use of mouth swabs only for oral hygiene is ineffective.[247] Many oncology and immunology patients suffer from mouth ulcers and are on oral care regimens at home. The maintenance of such a regimen is essential for patient comfort and may require the emergency nurse to organise and obtain prescribed mouthwashes from the pharmacy department. Regular sips of fluid or mouthwash with water for those patients who are nil by mouth prevents drying, coating and subsequent oral discomfort. If the patient is able to suck and swallow, small pieces of ice can be very refreshing,[153,248] yet it is important to monitor the amount of ice given so as not to give excessive amounts that would equate to numerous glasses of water. The application of lanolin or petroleum jelly will ease the discomfort of dry lips and maintain the integrity of the lips.

For patients with crusty build-up on their teeth (commonly seen in the elderly or dehydrated patient), a single application of warm dilute solution of sodium bicarbonate powder with a toothbrush is effective in removing debris and causes mucus to become less sticky, although its use is sometimes contested as it can cause superficial burns.[153] Its use should be followed immediately by a thorough water rinse of the mouth to return the oral pH to normal.[153,249]

In the sedated, intubated or unconscious patient, absence of mastication leads to a reduction in saliva production. Saliva produces protective enzymes. An endotracheal tube can cause pressure areas in the mouth (which may be exacerbated if the patient is oedematous). Once the patient is in the intensive care unit, an oral care program will be commenced.

PRACTICE TIP

Ensure patients who have an extended stay in ED have access to a toothbrush and toothpaste as using mouth swabs alone is ineffective.

PREVENTION OF DECONDITIONING

Positioning patients correctly and as soon as possible in the ED, while considering cardiovascular stability, respiratory function and cerebral or spinal injury, is important to contribute to the prevention of common short- and long-term complications of immobility.[153] The complications of immobilisation in the critically ill include pressure injuries, venous thromboembolism and pulmonary dysfunction, such as atelectasis, retained secretions, pneumonia and aspiration.[250] Ideally, the immobile patient should be positioned with the head raised by 30° or more, as this prevents the tongue from obstructing the airway, reduces the risk of aspiration from secretions and saliva and aids cerebral venous drainage, helping to reduce intracranial pressure.[8] It is also important to remember that Australian healthcare organisations are required to be accredited for Standard 8: Preventing and Managing Pressure Injuries.[251]

Provided there are no contraindications, function should be stimulated by regular passive movements of all limbs and joints to maintain both flexibility and comfort. One week of bed rest substantially reduces skeletal muscle mass.[252] Movement of the lower legs, ankles and feet can be achieved in conjunction with a gentle massage or application of moisturiser. Family members may wish to undertake this, giving them an opportunity to provide the patient with care and touch. The emergency nurse should encourage the able patient to perform exercises, and conduct an early physiotherapy referral for patients who may have an extended ED stay awaiting a ward bed.

Within the intensive care setting, the standard for body repositioning is 2-hourly, although this may not always happen.[153] Repositioning may be required more frequently, which will be determined by the nurse, based on patient factors and the clinical situation.[251] When planning to reposition the patient, check that there are enough staff available so that all the patient devices (e.g. endotracheal tube, intravenous lines) are managed and to give the patient a feeling of security during the positioning. It is advisable to have a designated leader in such circumstances to avoid injury or dislodgement of any devices.

PRESSURE INJURY PREVENTION

Many ED patients are at risk of pressure injuries due to immobility, lack of sensory protective mechanisms, excessive moisture, suboptimal tissue perfusion and environmental factors that cause pressure and friction: these issues are exacerbated in the critically ill.[110,253] Patients left on ambulance stretchers for prolonged periods due to delays in transfer of care are also at high risk of developing pressure injuries. The most common locations for pressure injuries are the bony prominences, such as the sacrum, the heels and the head.[227,253,254] Significant risk factors include the age of the patient, malnutrition,[253] and delays in the use of pressure-relieving mattresses (see Box 13.10).[255,256] Pressure injury risk-assessment tools, such as the Braden and Waterlow Scales,[257] can help nurses identify at-risk patients early.

Any pressure injuries should be documented and described in relation to size, grade/stage and treatment and monitored closely. Many facilities require pressure injuries to be reported. If a patient develops one pressure injury, there is a good chance they could develop another. While the pressure injury may not

BOX 13.10 RISK FACTORS FOR PRESSURE INJURIES[227]

- Advanced age
- Anaemia
- Contractures
- Diabetes mellitus
- Elevated body temperature
- Immobility
- Impaired circulation
- Incontinence
- Low diastolic blood pressure (< 60 mmHg)
- Mental deterioration
- Neurological disorders
- Obesity
- Pain
- Prolonged surgery
- Vascular disease

be evident in the ED, the initial reddened areas give clues to potential locations for development, and any preventative measures implemented in the ED contribute greatly to prevention.

Simple preventative measures include water-filled gloves under the heels, removing additional bed linen from under the patient which may have been transferred from the ambulance trolley, ensuring the patient is kept clean and dry (particularly patients with spinal precautions and incontinence), the use of foam boots and alternating pressure-relief mattresses and foam mattresses with adequate thickness and stiffness. However, none of these are a substitute for regular repositioning and avoiding pressure on any affected areas.[256] It is also important to document the details of position each time the patient is repositioned and communicate this on handover, as well as to maintain the patient's hydration and nutrition to improve tissue perfusion and integrity.

Patients are also at risk of developing pressure injuries and injury from a number of devices in everyday use, such as endotracheal tubes, backboards and blood-pressure cuffs (Table 13.11).[153] Close attention to detail with frequent observation of the patient, the patient's position and the presence and location of equipment is required to prevent skin damage.[153]

TABLE 13.11 RISK OF PRESSURE INJURIES FROM COMMONLY USED EQUIPMENT[153]

EQUIPMENT	RISKS
Endotracheal (ETT) tubes	Care should be taken when positioning and tying ETT tapes: friction burns may be caused if they are not secure; pressure injuries may be caused if they are too tight (particularly above the ears and in the nape of the neck).
	Moist tapes exacerbate problems and harbour bacteria.
Oxygen saturation probes	Repositioning of oxygen saturation probes 1–2-hourly prevents pressure on potentially poorly perfused skin.
	If using ear probes, these must be positioned on the lobe of the ear and not on the cartilage, as this area is very vulnerable to pressure and heat injury.
Blood-pressure cuffs	Non-invasive blood-pressure cuffs should be regularly reattached and repositioned. If left in position without reattachment for long periods of time, they can cause friction and pressure damage to skin.
	Care should be taken to ensure that tubing is not caught under the patient, especially after repositioning.
Urinary catheters, central lines and wound drainage	The patient should be checked often to ensure that invasive lines are not trapped under the patient. In addition to causing skin injury, they may function ineffectively.
Bed rails	Limbs should not press against bed rails; pillows should be used if the patient's position or size makes this likely.
Oxygen masks	Use the correct-size mask and a hydrocolloid protective dressing on the bridge of the nose to assist with prevention of pressure from non-invasive or CPAP masks, especially when these are in constant or frequent use.
Splints and cervical collars	Devices such as leg/foot splints and cervical collars can all cause direct pressure when in constant use and friction injury if they are not fitted properly.
Hard backboards	Hard backboards or spine-boards used by ambulance personnel for patient extrication cause pressure areas and should be removed on patient arrival to the ED or on initial log roll.

CPAP: continuous positive airway pressure.

NUTRITION

The impact of adequate nutrition on patient outcomes is well documented. The intake of nutrients, such as protein, calories, vitamins, minerals and fluids, provides the energy source required for growth of all body structures and maintenance of body functions, as well as supporting the immune function of the bowel.[258,259] Patients presenting to the ED are often in an altered metabolic state due to the stress response to illness, injury or starvation (when nutrient intake is unable to meet the body's energy demands). Wounds place increased metabolic and hence oxygen and nutritional demands on patients.[260] Patients with poor nutrition, including malnutrition, are at greater risk of complications, including pressure injuries, healthcare-associated infections and mortality, both in hospital and for up to three years following discharge.[110] Malnutrition also increases length of hospital stay and unplanned hospital re-admissions.[261] Critically ill patients are usually in a hypermetabolic state, characterised by rises in oxygen consumption and use of nutritional substitutes such as amino acids. Malnutrition and starvation increases electrolyte imbalances, muscle wasting, morbidity and mortality; delays recovery; impedes healing of acute and chronic wounds; interferes with the body's ability to fight infection; and increases the cost of hospitalisation.[262,264] Understanding the importance of nutrition and its effect on the patient is integral for nurses to predict and promote successful outcomes and is a priority of care.[264]

While it is often inappropriate for the ED patient to have oral intake for a number of reasons (the potential to require emergency surgery, cerebral insult that compromises swallowing and gag reflexes, or altered level of consciousness), it is essential to establish nutritional status as soon as possible. Nutritional status should be assessed early and documented clearly and communicated to all relevant parties. In particular, stroke/TIA patients should have their swallow assessed early as this has been shown to improve patient outcomes.[265] Since the implementation of tools, such as the Acute Screening of Swallow in Stroke/TIA (ASSIST), the assessment can be performed by the emergency nurse.[266] Completion of a swallowing assessment will determine whether the patient can swallow safely and re-establish normal nutritional status or identify the need for further referral. The dietetics department should be notified of special requirements and speech pathology referral and assessment conducted promptly.

Particular consideration should be given to the diabetic patient and the monitoring of their blood glucose levels (BGLs); more so if their condition requires a prolonged fasting status. Alterations to their anti-hyperglycaemic medications may need to be made in consultation with medical staff and careful monitoring implemented.

ED patients who are clinically able to tolerate some form of diet should be encouraged to eat and drink and should be assisted if necessary, enlisting the aid of family members, if they are present and willing. This will help prevent the development of a compromised nutritional state.

ELIMINATION

Effective urine and bowel elimination is a basic human need, and adequate privacy, discretion and dignity is essential. While it can be difficult in a busy ED or in an ambulance, it is important to facilitate prompt toileting and maximise access to toilets while ensuring cardiac monitoring and bedrest are not disrupted.

More than one million people living in Australia and Aotearoa New Zealand suffer from urinary incontinence from causes such as poor pelvic floor tone, central nervous system disorders, spinal cord injury, fistulas and bladder disorders.[267] Also, the normally continent patient may present having been incontinent following a seizure or traumatic event. The paramedic and ED nurse must recognise the physical and emotional problems associated with urinary incontinence and frequency. The patient's dignity, privacy and feelings of self-worth must be maintained. The discreet disposal of soiled pads, patient sponging (wet skin contributes to pressure-injury development), cleansing of the perineum, provision of clean incontinence pads and referral to appropriate continence services, should be done if required. If urinary catheter insertion is needed, thorough cleansing and aseptic techniques are essential to prevent the development of urinary tract infections.

Bowel management

Good bowel care promotes patient comfort and reduces the risks of further associated problems such as nausea, vomiting and abdominal/pelvic discomfort. Maintaining good bowel care can range from promoting defecation to containing diarrhoea, as a result of changing therapies, medications, nutrition, hydration and mobility of the patient.[153] The consequences of constipation are not well defined, but can include increased abdominal distension, impedance of lung function, inability to establish adequate enteral nutrition and increased acquired bacterial infections.[153] Risk factors for constipation include: immobility, medications such as opiates, sedatives, anticonvulsants, diuretics and calcium channel blockers, reduced gut motility, a poor dietary intake, dehydration and older age.[153]

Interventions that can be commenced in the ED include exercise—even in the bed-bound patient—as peristaltic movement of the gut is stimulated. Diet and fluids are also important considerations in maintaining normal bowel function, ensuring, if clinically appropriate, that the patient receives adequate administration of fluid and diet in the ED. Prior to patient transfer to the ward from the ED, if the patient is at risk of constipation, ensure that oral aperients have been charted, if clinically appropriate, so that the risk has been handed over to the ward nursing staff and the patient has been educated on prevention techniques.

Recognising and managing loose stools/diarrhoea is just as important as it may signify a particular condition or medication side-effect. Potential complications, such as fluid and electrolyte imbalance, may occur and skin damage is likely, particularly in the incontinent or immobile patient. Protection for staff providing care, as well as other patients and relatives, should be considered and the requirement for isolation discussed with relevant infection control staff (infection control is discussed in Chapter 27).

Bowel care can be an embarrassing and even quite distressing issue for patients, particularly for those who may have lost control of their bodily functions or perhaps have developed particular routines to maintain regular bowel motions. Coming to the ED can interrupt routines and highlight embarrassing issues with bowel motions for the patient, therefore sensitive nursing care that respects the dignity of the patient is paramount.[153] It can be quite difficult for a patient to relax and open their bowels in the busy ED, particularly if limited to a bed pan behind a curtain that offers very little privacy.

SUMMARY

This chapter has discussed a 'head-to-toe' approach to assessment. The emergency clinician should consider the assessment process as more than just recording a set of vital signs. Although the process appears to be time-consuming, with practice and experience the emergency clinician is able to automatically and quickly proceed through the process. This is made easier by adopting an assessment template such as HIRAID™. Reassessment has been highlighted in monitoring dynamic changes in a patient's condition and comparing them with the baseline. This can help initiate timely and appropriate measures to maximise patient care and outcomes. Effective communication between healthcare providers, the patient and their family, which acknowledges their concerns, is instrumental in patient outcomes and satisfaction. The emergency clinician conducting or commencing the discussed aspects of essential paramedic or nursing care contributes greatly to reducing the risk of the patient developing complications during their hospital stay. Simple measures, such as timely toileting of patients, will assist in maintaining comfort and dignity; documentation of nutritional status will help avoid malnutrition; regular pressure-area and skin care will help to prevent pressure injury development. While it is easy to be distracted by performing advanced procedures, it is vital that these basic but essential elements of patient care are provided and documented for the health, comfort and dignity of the patient and to prevent complications. It is also important to find time to care for ourselves so that we can continue to care for our patients.

CASE STUDY

PART A: PRE-HOSPITAL

You are the treating paramedic of a morbidly obese man in his 40s, who is complaining of shortness of breath. On arrival to his home the patient is sitting upright in a chair talking in short phrases, but complaining primarily of severe left leg pain.

QUESTIONS

1. Where would you start your assessment?
   a. Inspect his leg.
   b. Record a set of vital signs.
   c. Check his BGL.
   d. Assess DRSABCDE.

You assess the scene and identify no immediate dangers to yourself, so you approach the patient. He responds appropriately and you commence taking a history while performing your physical assessment.

2. What mnemonic could you use to structure taking the patient's history?

The patient's wife informs you that she called the emergency number as she is worried that his breathing has become more laboured over the course of the day. You also learn that the patient has a known history of type 1 diabetes and a chronic ulcer on his left leg, which has become malodourous.

3. What 'red flags' have you already identified in this patient?

While undertaking your physical assessment you identify that the patient has a respiratory rate of 28 breaths per minute with some mild accessory muscle use. Oxygen saturations are within normal parameters. On auscultation, air entry is equal. You inspect the left leg ulcer and find a red sloughy, odorous wound. There is decreased sensation to the affected limb, but strong pedal pulses present. You dress the wound to absorb the exudate and transport the patient to hospital.

4. How would you (the paramedic) structure your handover to the receiving emergency nurse on arrival to hospital?

PART B: AT THE ED

You are the emergency nurse receiving care of this patient in the acute treatment area.

QUESTIONS

5. How would you start your assessment?
   a. Collect the patient's history.
   b. Identify red flags.
   c. Perform a set of vital signs.
   d. Apply oxygen.
6. You commence your physical assessment. When attempting to check his blood pressure the cuff keeps popping off. What do you do?
   a. Tape it on with micropore.
   b. Not bother, he only presented with a leg ulcer.
   c. Find an appropriate-size cuff.
   d. Use the manual sphygmomanometer as you can stop inflating before the cuff pops open.

After completing the primary survey you perform a head-to-toe examination, including a focused respiratory assessment. You identify that the patient is still only able to speak in short sentences and has moderate accessory muscle use. The respiratory rate is counted at 32 breaths per minute, oxygen saturations measure 92% on room air and temperature 38.7°C. The patient denies any history of lung disease.

7. What new 'red flags' have been identified and how should you respond to these?
8. What diagnostic test is this patient likely to require?
9. Your patient suddenly becomes very sweaty and disorientated. What do you do next?
10. After medical review and initial treatment the patient is admitted into hospital. There is no access to a bed for several hours. What factors do you need to consider for his ongoing care?

Answers to Case Study Questions can be found on evolve **http://evolve.elsevier.com/AU/Curtis/emergency/**

USEFUL WEBSITES

Australian Institute of Patient and Family Centred Care, www.aipfcc.org.au/about.html.

Australian Resuscitation Council, Australian Resuscitation Council Guidelines, resus.org.au/.

Clinical Excellence Commission, NSW Health Government, www.cec.health.nsw.gov.au/.

College of Emergency Nursing Australasia, Peak professional association representing emergency nurses, www.cena.org.au.

COMPASS ACT Health, provides information on the early recognition of the deteriorating patient and provides a number of learning resources, www.health.act.gov.au/professionals/compass.

HIRAID™: The Emergency Nursing Framework, aci.health.nsw.gov.au/networks/eci/research/current-research-and-quality-activities/hiraid.

New South Wales Emergency Care Institute, set up to provide resources and support to emergency clinicians, www.aci.health.nsw.gov.au/networks/eci.

First2act, interactive online simulation package, first2act.com/.

National Safety and Quality Health Service Standards, www.safetyandquality.gov.au/wp-content/uploads/2011/09/NSQHS-Standards-Sept-2012.pdf.

The 4AT Rapid Clinical Test for Delirium, www.the4at.com/.

REFERENCES

1. Australasian College of Emergency Medicine. Position statement: access block 2021. Online. Available from: acem.org.au/getmedia/c0bf8984-56f3-4b78-8849-442feaca8ca6/S127_v01_Statement_Access_Block_Mar_14.aspx.
2. Australian College of Emergency Medicine. Guidelines on the implementation of the Australasian Triage Scale in Emergency Departments 2016. Online. Available from: acem.org.au/Content-Sources/Advancing-Emergency-Medicine/Better-Outcomes-for-Patients/Triage.
3. Australian Resuscitation Council. Australian Resuscitation Council Guidelines 2021. Online. Available from: resus.org.au/guidelines/.
4. Munroe B, Curtis K, Murphy M, Strachan L, Buckley T. HIRAID™: an evidence-informed emergency nursing assessment framework. Australas Emerg Nurs J 2015;18(2):83–97.
5. Considine J, Currey J. Ensuring a proactive, evidence-based, patient safety approach to patient assessment. J Clin Nurs 2015;24(1–2):300–7.
6. Munroe B, Curtis K, Considine J, Buckley T. The impact structured patient assessment frameworks have on patient care: an integrative review. J Clin Nurs 2013;22(21–22):2991–3005.
7. Munroe B, Buckley T, Curtis K, Murphy M, Strachan L, Hardy J, et al. The impact of HIRAID™ on emergency nurses' self-efficacy, anxiety and perceived control: a simulated study. Int Emerg Nurs 2016;25:53–8.
8. Munroe B, Curtis K, Murphy M, Strachan L, Considine J, Hardy J, et al. A structured framework improves clinical patient assessment and nontechnical skills of early career emergency nurses: a pre-post study using full immersion simulation. J Clin Nurs 2016;25(15–16):2262–74.
9. The HIRAID™ Research Group. The implementation of an emergency nursing framework (HIRAID™) reduces patient deterioration: a multi-centre quasi-experimental study. Int Emerg Nurs 2021;56:100976.
10. Resuscitation Council UK. The ABCDE approach. 2021. Online. Available from: www.resus.org.uk/library/abcde-approach.
11. Whitfield S. The sequence of care – do new methods warrant a shift from the standard ABC to a CABC approach? Australas J Paramed 2019;16.
12. Colbeck MA, Maria S, Eaton G, Campbell C, Batt AM, Caffey M, et al. International examination and synthesis of the primary and secondary surveys in paramedicine. Ontario: Fanshawe College, Faculty and Staff Publications – Public Safety; 2018;21.
13. American College of Surgeons. Advanced Trauma Life Support for doctors (ATLS): student course manual. 10th ed. Chicago: 2018.
14. Society of Critical Care Medicine. Surviving sepsis campaign responds to ProCESS Trial. 2014. Online. Available from: www.icnarc.org/DataServices/Attachments/Download/3d1bc8e1-1ed1-e311-a997-d48564544b14.
15. Curtis K, Munroe B, Fry M, Considine J, Tuala E, Watts M, et al. The implementation of an emergency nursing framework (HIRAID™) reduces patient deterioration: a multi-centre quasi-experimental study. Int Emerg Nurs 2021;56:100976.
16. Curtis K, Murphy M, Hoy S, Lewis MJ. The emergency nursing assessment process—a structured framework for a systematic approach. Australas Emerg Nurs J 2009;12(4):130–6.
17. Berman A, Snyder S, Kozier B, Erb G. Kozier and Erb's techniques in clinical nursing. 5th ed. New Jersey: Prentice Hall; 2003.
18. Curtis K, Sivabalan P, Bedford DS, Considine J, D'Amato A, Shepherd N, et al. Implementation of a structured emergency nursing framework results in significant cost benefit. Durham, NC: Research Square Platform LLC; 2021.
19. Peart P. Clinical history taking. Clin Integr Care 2022;10:100088.
20. Toney-Butler T, Unison-Pace W. Nursing admission assessment and examination. Treasure Island (FL): StatPearls Publishing; 2021.
21. Clinical Quality and Patient Safety Unit—Queensland Ambulance Service. Clinical practice procedures: assessment/primary and secondary survey. 2021. Online. Available from: www.ambulance.qld.gov.au/docs/clinical/cpp/CPP_Primary%20and%20secondary%20survey.pdf.
22. Valiathan R, Ashman M, Asthana D. Effects of ageing on the immune system: infants to elderly. Scand J Immunol 2016;83(4):255–66.
23. Liang SY, Theodoro DL, Schuur JD, Marschall J. Infection prevention in the emergency department. Ann Emerg Med 2014;64(3):299–313.
24. Millán R, Thomas-Paulose D, Egan DJ, Nusbaum J, Gupta N. Recognizing and managing emerging infectious diseases in the emergency department [digest]. Emerg Med Pract 2018;20(Suppl. 5):1–2.

25. Maharaj R, Raffaele I, Wendon J. Rapid response systems: a systematic review and meta-analysis. Crit Care 2015;19(1):254.
26. Roper N, Logan WW, Tierney AJ. The elements of nursing: a model for nursing based on a model of living. Edinburgh: Churchill Livingstone; 2001.
27. Veedfald T, Andersen-Ranberg K, Waldorff F, Anru PL, Masud T, Ryg J. Activities of daily living at hospital admission associated with mortality in geriatric patients with dementia: a Danish nationwide population-based cohort study. Eur Geriatr Med 2021;12(3):627–36.
28. Rondinelli J, Zuniga S, Kipnis P, Kawar LN, Liu V, Escobar GJ. Hospital-acquired pressure injury: risk-adjusted comparisons in an integrated healthcare delivery system. Nurs Res 2018;67(1):16–25.
29. Sharma Y, Miller M, Kaambwa B, Shahi R, Hakendorf P, Horwood C, et al. Malnutrition and its association with readmission and death within 7 days and 8–180 days post discharge in older patients: a prospective observational study. BMJ Open 2017;7(11):e018443.
30. Oedorf A, Day E, Lior R, Novack AT, Shapiro E, Henning S. Lactate as a predictor of deterioration in emergency department patients with and without infection. Critical Care 2014;18(Suppl. 1):P171.
31. Pain C, Green M, Duff C, Hyland D, Pantle A, Fitzpatrick K, et al. Between the flags: implementing a safety-net system at scale to recognise and manage deteriorating patients in the New South Wales Public Health System. Int J Qual Health Care 2016;29(1):130–6.
32. Williams TA, Ho KM, Tohira H, Fatovich DM, Bailey P, Brink D, et al. 14 Initial prehospital vital signs to predict subsequent adverse hospital outcomes. BMJ Open 2017;7(Suppl. 3):A5.
33. Andersen LW, Kim WY, Chase M, Berg KM, Mortensen SJ, Moskowitz A, et al. The prevalence and significance of abnormal vital signs prior to in-hospital cardiac arrest. Resuscitation 2016;98:112–7.
34. van Galen LS, Struik PW, Driesen BE, Merten H, Ludikhuize J, van der Spoel JI, et al. Delayed recognition of deterioration of patients in general wards is mostly caused by human related monitoring failures: a root cause analysis of unplanned ICU admissions. PloS One 2016;11(8):e0161393.
35. Healthcare Safety Investigation Branch. Recognising and responding to critically unwell patients: independent report by the Healthcare Safety Investigation Branch United Kingdom. 2019. Online. Available from: https://hsib-kqcco125-media.s3.amazonaws.com/assets/documents/hsib_report_recognising_responding_critically_unwell_patients.pdf.
36. Considine J, Jones D, Pilcher D, Currey J. Patient physiological status at the emergency department-ward interface and emergency calls for clinical deterioration during early hospital admission. J Adv Nurs 2016;7(2):1287–300.
37. Johnson KD, Winkelman C, Burant CJ, Dolansky M, Totten V. The factors that affect the frequency of vital sign monitoring in the emergency department. J Emerg Nurs 2014;40(1):27–35.
38. Mok WQ, Wang W, Liaw SY. Vital signs monitoring to detect patient deterioration: an integrative literature review. Int J Nurs Pract 2015;21(Suppl. 2): 91–8.
39. Connell CJ, Endacott R, Cooper S. The prevalence and management of deteriorating patients in an Australian emergency department. Australas Emerg Care 2021;24(2):112.
40. Australian Commission on Safety and Quality in Health Care (ACSQHC). National Consensus Statement: essential elements for recognising and responding to acute physiological deterioration. 2021. 3rd ed. Online. Available from: www.safetyandquality.gov.au/sites/default/files/2021-12/essential_elements_for_recognising_and_responding_to_acute_physiological_deterioration.pdf.
41. Churpek MM, Adhikari R, Edelson DP. The value of vital sign trends for detecting clinical deterioration on the wards. Resuscitation 2016;102:1–5.
42. Lambe K, Currey J, Considine J. Frequency of vital sign assessment and clinical deterioration in an Australian emergency department. Australas Emerg Nurs J 2016;19(4):217.
43. Clinical Excellence Commission. NSW Health standardised paediatric observation charts, between the flags. 2018. Online. Available from: www.cec.health.nsw.gov.au/patient-safety-programs/adult-patient-safety/between-the-flags/observation-charts.
44. Costantine MM. Physiologic and pharmacokinetic changes in pregnancy. Front Pharmacol 2014;5:65.
45. Daw W, Kaur R, Delaney M, Elphick H. Respiratory rate is an early predictor of clinical deterioration in children. Pediatr Pulmonol 2020;55(8): 2041–9.
46. Flenady T, Dwyer T, Applegarth J. Accurate respiratory rates count: so should you! Australas Emerg Nurs J 2017;20(1):45–7.
47. Cretikos MA, Bellomo R, Hillman K, Chen J, Finfer S, Flabouris A. Respiratory rate: the neglected vital sign. Med J Aust 2008;188(11):657–9.
48. Barfod C, Lauritzen MM, Danker JK, Sölétormos G, Forberg JL, Berlac PA, et al. Abnormal vital signs are strong predictors for intensive care unit admission and in-hospital mortality in adults triaged in the emergency department – a prospective cohort study. Scand J Trauma Resusc Emerg Med 2012;20:28.
49. Ljunggren M, Castren M, Nordberg M, Kurland L. The association between vital signs and mortality in a retrospective cohort study of an unselected emergency department population. Scand J Trauma Resusc Emerg Med 2016;24:21.
50. Bleyer AJ, Vidya S, Russell GB, Jones CM, Sujata L, Daeihagh P, et al. Longitudinal analysis of one million vital signs in patients in an academic medical center. Resuscitation 2011;82(11):1387–92.
51. Jarvis C, Eckhardt A, Forbes H. General survey and vital signs. In: Jarvis C, editor. Jarvis's Health assessment and physical examination. 3rd ed. Australia: Elsevier; 2021.
52. Kallioinen N, Hill A, Christofidis MJ, Horswill MS, Watson MO. Quantitative systematic review: sources of inaccuracy in manually measured adult respiratory rate data. J Adv Nurs 2021;77(1):98–124.
53. Jubran A. Pulse oximetry. Crit Care 2015;19(1):272.

54. Kim JY, Lee YJ, Korean Association of Wound Ostomy Continence N. Medical device-related pressure ulcer (MDRPU) in acute care hospitals and its perceived importance and prevention performance by clinical nurses. Int Wound J 2019;16(S1):51–61.
55. Kallioinen N, Hill A, Horswill MS, Watson MO, Christofidis MJ. Sources of inaccuracy in the measurement of adult patients' resting blood pressure in clinical settings: a systematic review. J Hypertens 2017;35(3):421–41.
56. Muntner P, Shimbo D, Carey RM, Charleston JB, Gaillard T, Misra S, et al. Measurement of blood pressure in humans: a scientific statement from the American Heart Association. Hypertension 2019;73(5):e35–66.
57. Tzur I, Izhakian S, Gorelik O. Orthostatic hypotension: definition, classification and evaluation. Blood Press 2019;28(3):146–56.
58. Farley H, Zubrow MT, Gies J, Kolm P, Mascioli S, Mahoney DD, et al. Emergency department tachypnea predicts transfer to a higher level of care in the first 24 hours after ED admission. Acad Emerg Med 2010;17(7):718–22.
59. Henning A, Krawiec C. Sinus tachycardia. Treasure Island (FL): StatPearls Publishing; 2022. Online. Available from: www.ncbi.nlm.nih.gov/books/NBK553128/.
60. Sarti A, Savron F, Casotto V, Cuttini M. Heartbeat assessment in infants: a comparison of four clinical methods. Pediatr Crit Care Med 2005;6(2):212–15.
61. Kushimoto S, Abe T, Ogura H, Shiraishi A, Saitoh D, Fujishima S, et al. Impact of body temperature abnormalities on the implementation of sepsis bundles and outcomes in patients with severe sepsis: a retrospective sub-analysis of the focused outcome research on emergency care for acute respiratory distress syndrome, sepsis and trauma study. Crit Care Med 2019;47(5):691–9.
62. Ramgopal S, Noorbakhsh KA, Pruitt CM, Aronson PL, Alpern ER, Hickey RW. Outcomes of young infants with hypothermia evaluated in the emergency department. J Pediatrics 2020;221:132–7.e2.
63. Walter EJ, Hanna-Jumma S, Carraretto M, Forni L. The pathophysiological basis and consequences of fever. Crit Care 2016;20:200.
64. Huether SE, Rodway G. Pain, temperature regulation, sleep and sensory function. In: McCance KL, Huether SE, editors. Pathophysiology: the biological basis for disease in adults and children. 7th ed. St. Louis: Elsevier, Mosby; 2019.
65. Wiewel MA, Harmon MB, van Vught LA, Scicluna BP, Hoogendijk AJ, Horn J, et al. Risk factors, host response and outcome of hypothermic sepsis. Crit Care 2016;20(1):328.
66. Rumbus Z, Matics R, Hegyi P, Zsiboras C, Szabo I, Illes A, et al. Fever is associated with reduced, hypothermia with increased mortality in septic patients: a meta-analysis of clinical trials. PloS One 2017;12(1):e0170152.
67. Thomas-Rüddel DO, Hoffmann P, Schwarzkopf D, Scheer C, Bach F, Komann M, et al. Fever and hypothermia represent two populations of sepsis patients and are associated with outside temperature. Crit Care 2021;25(1):368.
68. Arrich J, Holzer M, Havel C, Müllner M, Herkner H. Hypothermia for neuroprotection in adults after cardiopulmonary resuscitation. Cochrane Database System Rev 2016;2(2):CD004128.
69. Hinson HE, Rowell S, Morris C, Lin AL, Schreiber MA. Early fever after trauma: does it matter? J Trauma Acute Care Surg 2018;84(1):19–24.
70. Ávila-Gómez P, Hervella P, Da Silva-Candal A, Pérez-Mato M, Rodríguez-Yáñez M, López-Dequidt I, et al. Temperature-induced changes in reperfused stroke: inflammatory and thrombolytic biomarkers. J Clin Med 2020;9(7):2108.
71. Pecoraro V, Petri D, Costantino G, Squizzato A, Moja L, Virgili G, et al. The diagnostic accuracy of digital, infrared and mercury-in-glass thermometers in measuring body temperature: a systematic review and network meta-analysis. Intern Emerg Med 2021;16(4):1071–83.
72. Hayward G, Verbakel JY, Ismail FA, Edwards G, Wang K, Fleming S, et al. Non-contact infrared versus axillary and tympanic thermometers in children attending primary care: a mixed-methods study of accuracy and acceptability. Br J Gen Pract 2020;70(693):e236–44.
73. Fadzil FM, Choon D, Arumugam K. A comparative study on the accuracy of noninvasive thermometers. Aust Family Phys 2010;39(4):237–9.
74. Reynolds M, Bonham L, Gueck M, Hammond K, Lowery J, Redel C, et al. Are temporal artery temperatures accurate enough to replace rectal temperature measurement in pediatric ED patients? J Emerg Nurs 2014;40(1):46–50.
75. Rajee M, Sultana RV. NexTemp thermometer can be used interchangeably with tympanic or mercury thermometers for emergency department use. Emerg Med Australas 2006;18(3):245–51.
76. Sund-Levander M, Grodzinsky E. What is the evidence base for the assessment and evaluation of body temperature? Nurs Times 2010;106(1):10–13.
77. Shi D, Zhang L-Y, Li H-X. Diagnostic test accuracy of new generation tympanic thermometry in children under different cutoffs: a systematic review and meta-analysis. BMC Pediatr 2020;20(1):210.
78. Geneva II, Cuzzo B, Fazili T, Javaid W. Normal body temperature: a systematic review. Open Forum Infect Dis 2019;6(4):ofz032.
79. Manterola C, Vial M, Moraga J, Astudillo P. Analgesia in patients with acute abdominal pain. Cochrane Database Syst Rev 2011;(1):CD005660.
80. Jarvis C, Sharrad S. Ear assessment. In: Forbes H, Watt E, editors. Australian and New Zealand Jarvis's health assessment and physical examination. 3rd ed. Sydney: Elsevier; 2021.
81. Jarvis C, Wylie A. Eye assessment. In: Forbes H, Watt E, editors. Australian and New Zealand Jarvis's health assessment and physical examination. 3rd ed. Sydney: Elsevier; 2021.
82. Fairley D, Timothy J, Donaldson-Hugh M, Stone M, Warren D, Cosgrove J. Using a coma scale to assess patient consciousness levels. Nurs Times 2005;101(25):38–41.
83. Williams B. The National Early Warning Score and the acutely confused patient. Clin Med 2019;19(2):190–1.
84. Smith D, Bowden T. Using the ABCDE approach to assess the deteriorating patient. Nurs Stand 2017;32(14):51–63.

85. Teasdale G, Maas A, Lecky F, Manley G, Stocchetti N, Murray G. The Glasgow Coma Scale at 40 years: standing the test of time. Lancet Neurol 2014;13(8):844–54.
86. Teasdale G, Jennett B. Assessment of coma and impaired consciousness. A practical scale. Lancet 1974;2(7872):81–4.
87. Cook N. The Glasgow Coma Scale: a European and global perspective on enhancing practice. Crit Care Nurs Clin North Am 2021;33(1):89–99.
88. Middleton PM. Practical use of the Glasgow Coma Scale: a comprehensive narrative review of GCS methodology. Australas Emerg Nurs J 2012;15(3):170–83.
89. Bodien Y, Barra A, Temkin N, Barber J, Foreman B, Vassar M, et al. Diagnosing level of consciousness: the limits of the Glasgow Coma Scale Total Score. J Neurotrauma 2021;38(23):3295–305.
90. Reith F, Synnot A, van den Brande R, Gruen RL, Maas AI. Factors influencing the reliability of the Glasgow Coma Scale: a systematic review. Neurosurgery 2017;80(6):829–39.
91. Hew R. Altered conscious state. In: Cameron P, Jelinek G, Kelly AM, et al., editors. Adult textbook of emergency medicine. 4th ed. Sydney: Churchill Livingstone; 2015.
92. Gill MR, Reiley DG, Green SM. Interrater reliability of Glasgow Coma Scale scores in the emergency department. Ann Emerg Med 2004;43(2):215–23.
93. Waterhouse C. Practical aspects of performing Glasgow Coma Scale observations. Nurs Stand 2017;31(35):40–6.
94. James HE, Ana NG, Perkins RM. Brain insults in infants and children: pathophysiology and management. Orlando: Grune & Stratton; 1985.
95. Hoffmann M, Czorlich P, Lehmann W, Spiro AS, Rueger JM, Lefering R, et al. The impact of prehospital intubation with and without sedation on outcome in trauma patients with a GCS of 8 or less. J Neurosurg Anesthesiol 2017;29(2):161–7.
96. Hatchimonji J, Dumas R, Kaufman E, Scantling D, Stoecker JB, Holena DN. Questioning dogma: does a GCS of 8 require intubation? Eur J Trauma Emerg Surg 2021;47(6):2073–9.
97. Deasy C. Neurology emergencies. In: Cameron P, Little M, Mitra B, et al., editors. Textbook of adult emergency medicine. 5th ed. Edinburgh: Elsevier; 2019.
98. Verma A, Jaiswal S, Sheikh W, Haldar M. Interrater reliability of four neurological scales for patients presenting to the emergency department. Indian J Crit Care Med 2020;24(12):1198–200.
99. Jevon P, Ewens B, Pooni J. Monitoring the critically ill patient. West Sussex, UK: John Wiley & Sons; 2012.
100. Hoffmann F, Schmalhofer M, Lehner M, Zimatschek S, Grote V, Reiter K. Comparison of the AVPU Scale and the Pediatric GCS in prehospital setting. Prehosp Emerg Care 2016;20(4):493–8.
101. DiBrito S, Cerullo M, Goldstein S, Ziegfeld S, Stewart D, Nasr IW. Reliability of Glasgow Coma Score in pediatric trauma patients. J Pediatr Surg 2018;53(9):1789–94.
102. Jarvis C, Coulton B. Neurological assessment. In: Forbes H, Watt E, editors. Australian and New Zealand Jarvis's health assessment and physical examination. 3rd ed. Sydney: Elsevier; 2021.
103. Jarvis C, Watt E. Physical assessment techniques. In: Forbes H, Watt E, editors. Australian and New Zealand edition: Jarvis's physical examination and health assessment. 2nd ed. Sydney: Elsevier; 2016.
104. Boucher V, Lamontagne M, Nadeau A, Carmichael PH, Yadav K, Voyer P, et al. Unrecognized incident delirium in older emergency department patients. J Emerg Med 2019;57(4):535.
105. Han J, Suyama J. Delirium and dementia. Clin Geriatr Med 2018;34(3):327–54.
106. Oliveira LO, Berning M, Stanich JA, Gerberi DJ, Murad MH, Han JH, et al. Risk factors for delirium in older adults in the emergency department: a systematic review and meta-analysis. Ann Emerg Med 2021;78(4):549.
107. Schofield I, Stott DJ, Tolson D, McFadyen A, Monaghan J, Nelson D. Screening for cognitive impairment in older people attending accident and emergency using the 4-item abbreviated mental test. Eur J Emerg 2010;17(6):340–2.
108. Australian Commission on Safety and Quality in Health Care (ACSQHC). National Safety and Quality Health Service Standards user guide for health service organisations providing care for patients with cognitive impairment or at risk of delirium. Sydney: ACSQHC; 2019.
109. Australian Commission on Safety and Quality in Health Care (ACSQHC). National Safety and Quality Health Service Standards. 2nd ed.—version 2. Sydney: ACSQHC; 2021.
110. Australian Commission on Safety and Quality in Health Care (ACSQHC). Evidence for the safety and quality issues associated with the care of patients with cognitive impairment in acute care settings: a rapid review. 2013. Online. Available from: www.safetyandquality.gov.au/wp-content/uploads/2013/10/Rapid-Review_Evidence-for-the-safety-and-care-of-patients-with-cognitive-impairment-in-acute-care-settings.pdf.
111. Australian Commission on Safety and Quality in Health Care (ACSQHC). National safety and quality health service standards. 2nd ed. Sydney: 2017. Online. Available from: www.safetyandquality.gov.au/wp-content/uploads/2017/12/National-Safety-and-Quality-Health-Service-Standards-second-edition.pdf.
112. Han JH, Shintani A, Eden S, Morandi A, Solberg LM, Schnelle J, et al. Delirium in the emergency department: an independent predictor of death within 6 months. Ann Emerg Med 2010;56(3):244–52.e1.
113. LaMantia MA, Messina FC, Hobgood CD, Miller DK. Screening for delirium in the emergency department: a systematic review. Ann Emerg Med 2014;63(5):551–60.e2.

114. Australian Institute of Health and Welfare (AIHW). Dementia in Australia. Australian Government; 2021. Online. Available from: https://www.aihw.gov.au/reports/dementia/dementia-in-aus/contents/health-services-used-by-people-with-dementia/hospital-care.

115. Draper B, Karmel R, Gibson D, Peut A, Anderson P. The hospital dementia services project: age differences in hospital stays for older people with and without dementia. Int Psychogeriatr 2011;23(10):1649–58.

116. Mukadam N, Sampson EL. A systematic review of the prevalence, associations and outcomes of dementia in older general hospital inpatients. Int Psychogeriatr 2011;23(3):344–55.

117. O'Sullivan D, Brady N, Manning E, O'Shea E, O'Grady S, O'Regan N, et al. Validation of the 6-item cognitive impairment test and the 4AT test for combined delirium and dementia screening in older emergency department attendees. Age Ageing 2018;47(1):61–8.

118. Wei LA, Fearing MA, Sternberg EJ, Inouye SK. The confusion assessment method: a systematic review of current usage. J Am Geriatr Soc 2008; 56(5):823–30.

119. Han J, Suyama J. Delirium and dementia. Clin Geriatr Med 2018;34(3):327–54.

120. Quade BN, Parker MD, Occhipinti R. The therapeutic importance of acid–base balance. Biochem Pharmacol 2021;183:114278.

121. Jarvis C, Allen J. Lower airways assessment. In: Forbes H, Watt E, editors. Australian and New Zealand Jarvis's health assessment and physical examination. 3rd ed. Sydney: Elsevier; 2021.

122. Cox C. Physical assessment for nurses. 2nd ed. West Sussex, UK: Wiley Blackwell; 2010.

123. Timby B. Fundamental skills and concepts in patient care. 7th ed. Philadelphia: Lippincott Williams & Wilkins; 2002.

124. Elder A, Japp A, Verghese A. How valuable is physical examination of the cardiovascular system? BMJ 2016;354:i3309.

125. Jarvis C, Murphy M. Cardiac assessment. In: Forbes H, Watt E, editors. Australian and New Zealand Jarvis's health assessment and physical examination. 3rd ed. Sydney: Elsevier; 2021.

126. Jarvis C, Watt E. Abdominal assessment. In: Forbes H, Watt E, editors. Australian and New Zealand Jarvis's health assessment and physical examination. 3rd ed. Sydney: Elsevier; 2021.

127. Jarvis C, Watt E. Assessment of urinary function. In: Forbes H, Watt E, editors. Australian and New Zealand Jarvis's health assessment and physical examination. 3rd ed. Sydney: Elsevier; 2021.

128. Jarvis C, Lee D. Female sexual and reproductive assessment. In: Forbes H, Watt E, editors. Australian and New Zealand Jarvis's health assessment and physical examination. 3rd ed. Sydney: Elsevier; 2021.

129. Jarvis C, Lee D. Male sexual and reproductive assessment. In: Forbes H, Watt E, editors. Australian and New Zealand Jarvis's health assessment and physical examination. 3rd ed. Sydney: Elsevier; 2021.

130. Jarvis C, Pearce F. Musculoskeletal assessment. In: Forbes H, Watt E, editors. Australian and New Zealand Jarvis's health assessment and physical examination. 3rd ed. Sydney: Elsevier; 2021.

131. Jarvis C, Burton T. Skin, hair and nails assessment. In: Forbes H, Watt E, editors. Australian and New Zealand Jarvis's health assessment and physical examination. 3rd ed. Sydney: Elsevier; 2021.

132. Keithly J, Burton T. Nutritional and metabolic assessment. In: Forbes H, Watt E, editors. Australian and New Zealand Jarvis's health assessment and physical examination. 3rd ed. Sydney: Elsevier; 2021.

133. The Royal Children's Hospital Melbourne. Mental state examination. Melbourne: The Royal Children's Hospital; 2018.

134. Fernández A, Ares MI, Garcia S, Martinez-Indart L, Mintegi S, Benito J. The validity of the pediatric assessment triangle as the first step in the triage process in a pediatric emergency department. Pediatr Emerg Care 2017;33(4):234–8.

135. Malik M, Moore Z, Patton D, O'Connor T, Nugent LE. The impact of geriatric focused nurse assessment and intervention in the emergency department: a systematic review. Int Emerg Nurs 2018;37:52–60.

136. Ellis G, Marshall T, Ritchie C. Comprehensive geriatric assessment in the emergency department. Clin Interv Aging 2014;9:2033–43.

137. Atlantis E, Kormas N, Samaras K, Fahey P, Sumithran P, Glastras S, et al. Clinical obesity services in public hospitals in Australia: a position statement based on expert consensus. Clin Obes 2018;8(3):203–10.

138. Huse O, Hettiarachchi J, Gearon E, Nichols M, Allender S, Peeters A. Obesity in Australia. Obes Res Clin Pract 2018;12(1):29–39.

139. Australian Institute of Health and Welfare (AIHW). Overweight and obesity. Australia: Australian Government; 2020. Online. Available from: www.aihw.gov.au/reports/australias-health/overweight-and-obesity.

140. Roberts K, Gallo AM, Patil C, Vincent C, Binns HJ, Koenig MD. Family management of severe obesity in adolescents. J Pediatr Nurs 2021;60:181.

141. Windish R, Wong J. Review article: postoperative bariatric patients in the emergency department: review of surgical complications for the emergency physician. Emerg Med Australas 2019;31(3):309–13.

142. Sebbane M, Claret P-G, Lefebvre S, Mercier G, Rubenovitch J, Jreige R, et al. Predicting peripheral venous access difficulty in the emergency department using body mass index and a clinical evaluation of venous accessibility. J Emerg Med 2013;44(2):299–305.

143. Rabec C, de Lucas Ramos P, Veale D. Respiratory complications of obesity. Arch Bronconeumol 2011;47(5):252–61.

144. Brown WA, Burton PR, Shaw K, Smith B, Maffescioni S, Comitti B, et al. A pre-hospital patient education program improves outcomes of bariatric surgery. Obes Surg 2016;26(9):2074–81.

145. Hussain A, El-Hasani S. Bariatric emergencies: current evidence and strategies of management. World J Emerg Surg 2013;8(1):58.

146. Australian Safety and Compensation Council. Manual handling risks associated with the care, treatment and transportation of bariatric (severely obese) patients in Australia. 2009. Online. Available from: www.safeworkaustralia.gov.au/system/files/documents/1702/manualhandlingrisks_caretreatmenttransportation_fbariatricseverelyobesepatients_australia_2009_pdf.pdf.

147. Morris Z, Woodings S, Grant J. The answer is 17 years, what is the question: understanding time lags in translational research. J R Soc Med 2011;104(12):510–20.

148. Chan GK, Barnason S, Dakin CL, Gillespie G, Kamienski MC, Stapleton S, et al. Barriers and perceived needs for understanding and using research among emergency nurses. J Emerg Nurs 2011;37(1):24–31.

149. Stang A, Wingert A, Hartling L, Plint AC. Adverse events related to emergency department care: a systematic review. PLoS One 2013;8(9):e74214.

150. Flowerdew L, Brown R, Vincent C, Woloshynowych M. Identifying nontechnical skills associated with safety in the emergency department: a scoping review of the literature. Ann Emerg Med 2012;59(5):386–94.

151. Sampson M. Continuous ECG monitoring in hospital: part 1, indications. Br J Card Nurs 2018;13(2):80.

152. Curtis K, Tzannes A, Rudge T. How to talk to doctors—a guide for effective communication. Int Nurs Rev 2011;58(1):13–20. © 2011 The Authors. International Nursing Review. © International Council of Nurses.

153. Grealy B, Johansson L, Coyer F. Essential nursing care of the critically ill patient. In: Aitken LM, Chaboyer W, editors. ACCCN's critical care nursing. 4th ed. Sydney: Elsevier; 2019.

154. Li X, Chang H, Zhang Q, Yang J, Liu R, Song Y. Relationship between emotional intelligence and job well-being in Chinese clinical nurses: multiple mediating effects of empathy and communication satisfaction. BMC Nurs 2021;20(1):144.

155. Boggs K. Communicating with other health care professionals. In: Arnold E, Boggs K, editors. Interpersonal relationships. 7th ed. Missouri: Elsevier; 2016.

156. Redley B, Botti M, Wood B, Bucknall T. Interprofessional communication supporting clinical handover in emergency departments: an observation study. Australas Emerg Nurs J 2017;20(3):122–30.

157. Graham B, Smith JE. Understanding team, interpersonal and situational factors is essential for routine communication with patients in the emergency department (ED): a scoping literature review and formation of the 'T.IP.S' conceptual framework. J Commun Healthc 2016;9(3): 210–22.

158. Bagnasco A, Tubino B, Piccotti E, Rosa F, Aleo G, Di Pietro P, et al. Identifying and correcting communication failures among health professionals working in the emergency department. Int Emerg Nurs 2013;21(3):168–72.

159. Graham B, Endacott R, Smith JE, Latour JM. 'They do not care how much you know until they know how much you care': a qualitative meta-synthesis of patient experience in the emergency department. Emerg Med 2019;36(6):355–63.

160. Ellis RB, Gates RJ, Kenworthy N, editors. Interpersonal communication. Nursing: theory and practice. 2nd ed. New York: Churchill Livingstone; 2003.

161. Balzer Riley J. Communication in nursing. Missouri: Elsevier; 2017.

162. Marler H, Ditton H. 'I'm smiling back at you': exploring the impact of mask wearing on communication in healthcare. Int J Lang Commun Disord 2021;56(1):205–14.

163. Watzlawick P, Beavin J, Jackson D. Pragmatics of human communication. New York: Norton; 1967.

164. Slade D, Manidis M, McGregor J, Scheeres H, Chandler E, Stein-Parbury J, et al. Communicating in hospital emergency departments. Berlin, Heidelberg: Springer; 2015.

165. Darcy D, Rawson H, Redley B. Nurse-to-nurse communication about multidisciplinary care delivered in the emergency department: an observation study of nurse-to-nurse handover to transfer patient care to general medical wards. Australas Emerg Care 2020;23(1):37.

166. Golling M, Behringer W, Schwarzkopf D. Assessing the quality of patient handovers between ambulance services and emergency department – development and validation of the emergency department human factors in handover tool. BMC Emerg Med J 2022;22(1):10.

167. Kwon YE, Kim M, Choi S. Degree of interruptions experienced by emergency department nurses and interruption related factors. Int Emerg Nurs 2021;58:101036.

168. Schneider A, Williams DJ, Kalynych C, Wehler M, Weigl M. Physicians' and nurses' work time allocation and workflow interruptions in emergency departments: a comparative time-motion study across two countries. Emerg Med J 2021;38(4):263–8.

169. Weigl M, Beck J, Wehler M, Schneider A. Workflow interruptions and stress at work: a mixed-methods study among physicians and nurses of a multidisciplinary emergency department. BMJ Open 2017;7(12):e019074.

170. Flowerdew L, Tipping M. SECUre: a multicentre survey of the safety of emergency care in UK emergency departments. Emerg Med J 2021;38(10):769–75.

171. Werner NE, Holden RJ. Interruptions in the wild: development of a sociotechnical systems model of interruptions in the emergency department through a systematic review. Appl Ergon 2015;51:244–54.

172. Kalisch B, Aebersold M. Interruptions and multitasking in nursing care. Jt Comm J Qual Patient Saf 2010;36(3):126–32.

173. Ratwani RM, Fong A, Puthumana JS, Hettinger AZ. Emergency physician use of cognitive strategies to manage interruptions. Ann Emerg Med 2017;70(5):683–7.

174. Johnson KD, Schumacher D, Lee RC. Identifying strategies for the management of interruptions for novice triage nurses using an online modified Delphi method. J Nurs Scholarsh 2021;53(6):718–26.

175. Cohen M, Hilligoss B. Handoffs in hospitals: a review of the literature on information exchange while transferring patient responsibility or control. Ann Arbor: University of Michigan; 2009.
176. Iedema R, Ball C, Daly B, Young J, Green T, Middleton PM, et al. Design and trial of a new ambulance-to-emergency department handover protocol: 'IMIST-AMBO'. BMJ Qual Saf 2012;21:627–33.
177. Hunter New England NSW Health. ISBAR revisited: Identifying and Solving BARriers to effective clinical handover in inter-hospital transfer. Public report on pilot study for Australian Commission on Safety and Quality in Healthcare as part of the National Clinical Handover Initiative 2009.
178. Brewster DJ, Waxman BP. Adding kindness at handover to improve our collegiality: the K-ISBAR tool. Med J Aust 2018;209(11):482–3.
179. Christie P, Robinson H. Using a communication framework at handover to boost patient outcomes. Nurs Times 2009;105(47):13–5.
180. Geraghty A, Paterson-Brown S. Leadership and working in teams. Surgery 2018;36(9):503–8.
181. Manojlovich M, Harrod M, Hofer T, Lafferty M, McBratnie M, Krein SL. Factors influencing physician responsiveness to nurse-initiated communication: a qualitative study. BMJ Qual Saf 2021;30(9):747–54.
182. Wiman E, Wikblad K. Caring and uncaring encounters in nursing in an emergency department. J Clin Nurs 2004;13(4):422–9.
183. Olthuis G, Prins C, Smits M-J, van de Pas H, Bierens J, Baart A. Matters of concern: a qualitative study of emergency care from the perspective of patients. Ann Emerg Med 2014;63(3):311–9.e2.
184. Bartlett G, Blais R, Tamblyn R, Clermont RJ, MacGibbon B. Impact of patient communication problems on the risk of preventable adverse events in acute care settings. Can Med Assoc J 2008;178(12):1555.
185. Studer Group. AIDET guidelines and keywords. 2013. Online. Available from: https://az414866.vo.msecnd.net/cmsroot/studergroup/media/studergroup/pages/what-we-do/learning-lab/aligned-behavior/must-haves/aidet/aidet_guidelines_and_key_words_aidet1.pdf?ext=.pdf.
186. Parnell T. Health literacy in nursing: providing person-centered care. Secaucus, US: Springer; 2014.
187. Hermann RM, Long E, Trotta RL. Improving patients' experiences communicating with nurses and providers in the emergency department. J Emerg Nurs 2019;45(5):523–30.
188. Alsabri M, Boudi Z, Lauque D, Dias RD, Whelan JS, Östlundh L, et al. Impact of teamwork and communication training interventions on safety culture and patient safety in emergency departments: a systematic review. J Patient Saf 2022;18(1):E351–61.
189. Brummell Z, Vindrola-Padros C, Braun D, Moonesinghe SR. NHS 'Learning from Deaths' reports: a qualitative and quantitative document analysis of the first year of a countrywide patient safety programme. BMJ Open 2021;11(7):e046619.
190. Hindle D, Braithwaite J, Iedema R, Travaglia J. Patient safety: a review of key international enquiries. Sydney: NSW Clinical Excellence Commission; 2005.
191. Sprivulis PC, Da Silva JA, Jacobs IG, Frazer AR, Jelinek GA. The association between hospital overcrowding and mortality among patients admitted via Western Australian emergency departments. Med J Aust 2006;184(5):208–12.
192. Molero Jurado MDM, Herrera-Peco I, Pérez-Fuentes MDC, Oropesa Ruiz NF, Martos Martínez Á, Ayuso-Murillo D, et al. Communication and humanization of care: effects over burnout on nurses. PloS One 2021;16(6):e0251936.
193. Zborowska A, Gurowiec PJ, Młynarska A, Uchmanowicz I. Factors affecting occupational burnout among nurses including job satisfaction, life satisfaction, and life orientation: a cross-sectional study. Psychol Res Behav Manag 2021;14:1761–77.
194. Aitken LH, Clarke S, Sloane D, Lake ET, Cheney T. Effects of hospital care environment on patient mortality and nurse outcomes. J Nurs Admin 2008;38(5):223–9.
195. Park Y-M, Kim SY. Impacts of job stress and cognitive failure on patient safety incidents among hospital nurses. Saf Health Work 2013;4(4):210–5.
196. Hall LH, Johnson J, Watt I, Tsipa A, O'Connor DB. Healthcare staff wellbeing, burnout, and patient safety: a systematic review. PloS One 2016;11(7):e0159015.
197. Balevre PS, Cassells J, Buzaianu J. Professional nursing burnout and irrational thinking: a replication study. J Nurs Staff Dev 2012;28(1):2–8.
198. Grant S, Davidson J, Manges K, Dermenchyan A, Wilson E, Dowdell E. Creating healthful work environments to deliver on the quadruple aim: a call to action. J Nurs Admin 2020;50(6):314–21.
199. Kennedy JF, Trethewy C, Anderson K. Content analysis of Australian newspaper portrayals of emergency medicine. Emerg Med Australas 2006;18(2):118–24.
200. Doyle C, Lennox L, Bell D. A systematic review of evidence on the links between patient experience and clinical safety and effectiveness. BMJ Open 2013;3(1):e001570.
201. de Steenwinkel M, Haagsma JA, van Berkel ECM, Rozema L, Rood PPM, Bouwhuis MG. Patient satisfaction, needs, and preferences concerning information dispensation at the emergency department: a cross-sectional observational study. Int J Emerg Med 2022;15(1):1–8.
202. Curtis K, Wiseman T. Back to basics–essential nursing care in the ED. Australas Emerg Nurs J 2008;11(1):49–53.
203. Toma G, Triner W, McNutt L-A. Patient satisfaction as a function of emergency department previsit expectations. Ann Emerg Med 2009;54(3):360–7.
204. Woloshynowych M, Davis R, Brown R, Vincent C. Communication patterns in a UK emergency department. Ann Emerg Med 2007;50(4):407–13.
205. Saunders K. A creative new approach to patient satisfaction. Top Emerg Med 2005;27(4):256–7.
206. Nyce A, Gandhi S, Freeze B, Bosire J, Ricca T, Kupersmith E, et al. Association of emergency department waiting times with patient experience in admitted and discharged patients. J Patient Exp 2021;8:23743735211011404.

207. Huang YH, Sabljak LA, Puhala ZA. Emergency department patient experience and waiting time. Am J Emerg Med 2018;36(3):510–1.
208. Swancutt D, Joel-Edgar S, Allen M, Thomas D, Brant H, Benger J, et al. Not all waits are equal: an exploratory investigation of emergency care patient pathways. BMC Health Serv Res 2017;17(1):436.
209. Barbarian M, Bishop A, Alfaro P, Biron A, Brody DA, Cunningham-Allard G, et al. Patient-reported experience in the pediatric emergency department: what matters most? J Patient Saf 2021;17(8):e1166–70.
210. Australian Commission on Safety and Quality in Health Care (ACHQHC). Australian Open Disclosure Framework. Better communication, a better way to care. 2013. Online. Available from: www.safetyandquality.gov.au/wp-content/uploads/2013/03/Australian-Open-Disclosure-Framework-Feb-2014.pdf.
211. Mitchell M, Wilson D, Aitken R. Family and cultural care of the critically ill patient. In: Aitken L, Marshall A, Chaboyer W, editors. Critical care nursing. Sydney: Elsevier; 2015.
212. Mahajan RP. Critical incident reporting and learning. Br J Anaesthes 2010;105(1):69–75.
213. Redley B, Phiri LM, Heyns T, Wang W, Han CY. Family needs during critical illness in the emergency department: a retrospective factor analysis of data from three countries. J Clin Nurs 2019;28(15/16):2813–23.
214. Hsiao P-R, Redley B, Hsiao Y-C, Lin CC, Han CY, Lin HR. Family needs of critically ill patients in the emergency department. Int Emerg Nurs 2017;30:3–8.
215. Wong P, Liamputtong P, Koch S, Rawson H. Families' experiences of their interactions with staff in an Australian intensive care unit (ICU): a qualitative study. Intensive Crit Care Nurs 2015;31(1):51–63.
216. Al-Mutair AS, Plummer V, O'Brien A, Clerehan R. Family needs and involvement in the intensive care unit: a literature review. J Clin Nurs 2013; 22(13–14):1805–17.
217. Barretto M, Marcon SS, Garcia-Vivar C. Patterns of behaviour in families of critically ill patients in the emergency room: a focused ethnography. J Adv Nurs 2017;73(3):633–42.
218. Kamienski MC. Emergency: family-centered care in the ED. Am J Nurs 2004;104(1):59–62.
219. Institute for Family and Family-Centred Care. Frequently asked questions. What are the core concepts of family centred care? 2018. Online. Available from: www.aipfcc.org.au/values.html.
220. Munroe B, Curtis K, Fry M, Shaban RZ, Moules P, Elphick TL, et al. Increasing accuracy in documentation through the application of a structured emergency nursing framework: a multisite quasi-experimental study. J Clin Nurs 2022;31(19–20):2874–85.
221. NSW Health. Essentials of care: working with the essentials of care program: a resource of facilitators. North Sydney: 2014. Online. Available from: www.health.nsw.gov.au/nursing/culture/Documents/eoc-facilitation-resources.pdf.
222. Lown BA, Dunne H, Muncer SJ, Chadwick R. How important is compassionate healthcare to you? A comparison of the perceptions of people in the United States and Ireland. J Res Nurs 2017;22(1–2):60–9.
223. Hales C, Deak CK, Popoola T, Harris DL, Rook H. Improving the quality of patient care and healthcare staff well-being through an empathy immersion educational programme in New Zealand: protocol of a feasibility and pilot study. Methods Protoc 2021;4(4):89.
224. Adriaenssens J, De Gucht V, Van Der Doef M, Maes S. Exploring the burden of emergency care: predictors of stress-health outcomes in emergency nurses. J Adv Nurs 2011;67(6):1317–28.
225. Kilcoyne M, Dowling M. Working in an overcrowded accident and emergency department: nurses' narratives. Aust J Adv Nurs 2007;25(2):21–7.
226. Burgess L, Ray-Barruel G, Kynoch K. Association between emergency department length of stay and patient outcomes: a systematic review. Res Nurs Health 2022;45(1):59–93.
227. Lewis S, Finlayson K, Parker C. Inflammation and wound healing. In: Lewis SL, Bucher L, Heitkemper M, editors. Medical surgical nursing assessment and management of clinical problems. 10th ed. Missouri: Elsevier; 2017.
228. NSW Health. NSW health patient study 2008 statewide report. Sydney: NSW Health; 2009.
229. Clompus SR, Albarran JW. Exploring the nature of resilience in paramedic practice: a psycho-social study. Int Emerg Nurs 2016;28:1–7.
230. Ball L. Setting the scene for the paramedic in primary care: a review of the literature. Emerg Med J 2005;22(12):896–900.
231. Lowery K, Stokes M. Role of peer support and emotional expression on posttraumatic stress disorder in student paramedics. J Trauma Stress 2005;18(2):171–9.
232. Heath G, Wankhade P, Murphy P. Exploring the wellbeing of ambulance staff using the 'public value' perspective: opportunities and challenges for research. Public Money Manage 2021.
233. Greenberg N, Docherty M, Gnanapragasam S, Wessely S. Managing mental health challenges faced by healthcare workers during COVID-19 pandemic. BMJ 2020;368:m1211.
234. Petrie K, Milligan-Saville J, Gayed A, Deady M, Phelps A, Dell L, et al. Prevalence of PTSD and common mental disorders amongst ambulance personnel: a systematic review and meta-analysis. Soc Psychiatry Psychiatr Epidemiol 2018;53(9):897–909.
235. Lawn S, Roberts L, Willis E, Couzner L, Mohammadi L, Goble E. The effects of emergency medical service work on the psychological, physical, and social well-being of ambulance personnel: a systematic review of qualitative research. BMC Psychiatry 2020;20(1):1–348.
236. Stockbridge J. Care for the carers. Emerg Nurse 2004;12(7):10–1.
237. Healy S, Tyrrell M. Stress in emergency departments: experiences of nurses and doctors. Emerge Nurse 2011;19(4):31–7.

238. Duffield CM, Roche MA, O'Brien-Pallas L, Diers D, Aisbett C, King MT, et al. Glueing it together: nurses, their work environment and patient safety. Sydney: Centre for Health Services Management, UTS; 2007.
239. Barkway P. Stress and adaptation. In: Brown H, Edwards D, editors. Lewis's medical–surgical nursing. Sydney: Elsevier; 2005.
240. van der Riet P, Levett-Jones T, Aquino-Russell C. The effectiveness of mindfulness meditation for nurses and nursing students: an integrated literature review. Nurse Educ Today 2018;65:201–11.
241. Foureur M, Besley K, Burton G, Yu N, Crisp J. Enhancing the resilience of nurses and midwives: pilot of a mindfulnessbased program for increased health, sense of coherence and decreased depression, anxiety and stress. Contemp Nurse 2013;45:114–25.
242. Griffin-Heslin VL. An analysis of the concept dignity. Accid Emerg Nurs 2005;13(4):251–7.
243. Emergency Care Institute. Emergency Treatment Performance (ETP) – The basics. 2017. Online. Available from: www.aci.health.nsw.gov.au/networks/eci/administration/neat/neat-the-basics.
244. Nair PN, White E. Care of the eye during anaesthesia and intensive care. Anaesth Intensive Care Med 2014;15:40–3.
245. Micik SB, Johnson N, Han M, Hamlyn S, Ball H, Besic M. Reducing risk for ventilator associated pneumonia through nurse sensitive interventions. Intensive Crit Care Nurs 2013;29:261–5.
246. Hua F, Xie H, Worthington HV, Furness S, Zhang Q, Li C. Oral hygiene care for critically ill patients to prevent ventilator-associated pneumonia. Cochrane Database Syst Rev 2016;10(10):CD008367.
247. Berry AM, Davidson PM, Masters J, Rolls K. Systematic literature review of oral hygiene practices for intensive care patients receiving mechanical ventilation. Am J Crit Care 2007;16:552–62.
248. Berry A. A comparison of Listerine® and sodium bicarbonate oral cleansing solutions on dental plaque colonisation and incidence of ventilator associated pneumonia in mechanically ventilated patients: a randomised control trial. Intensive Crit Care Nurs 2013;29(5):275–81.
249. O'Reilly M. Oral care of the critically ill: a review of the literature and guidelines for practice. Aust Crit Care 2003;16(3):101–10.
250. Truong AFE, Brower RG, Needham DM. Bench-to-bedside review: mobilizing patients in the intensive care unit—from pathophysiology to clinical trials. Crit Care Med 2009;13:167.
251. Miles S, Nowicki T, Fulbrook P. Repositioning to prevent pressure injuries: evidence for practice. Aust Nurs Midwifery J 2013;21(6):32–3.
252. Dirks M, Wall BT, van der Valk B, Holloway TM, Holloway GP, Chabowski A, et al. One week of bed rest leads to substantial muscle atrophy and induces whole-body insulin resistance in the absence of skeletal muscle lipid accumulation. Diabetes 2016;65(10):2862–75.
253. Tayyib N, Coyer F, Lewis P. Pressure ulcers in the adult intensive care unit: a literature review of patient risk factors and risk assessment scales. J Nurs Educ Pract 2013;3:28–42.
254. Australian Wound Management Association. Pan Pacific guideline for the prevention and management of pressure injury. Abridged version. WA: Cambridge Publishing; 2012.
255. Weststrate J, Heule F. Prevalence of PU, risk factors and use of pressure-relieving mattresses in ICU patients. Connect Crit Care Nurs Eur 2001;1(3):77–82.
256. Tannen A, Balzer K, Kottner J, Dassen T, Halfens R, Mertens E. Diagnostic accuracy of two pressure ulcer risk scales and a generic nursing assessment tool. A psychometric comparison. J Clin Nurs 2010;19(11–12):1510–8.
257. Lewis SM, Collier IC, Heitkemper MM, Dirksen SR, O'Brien PG, Bucher L., editors. Medical–surgical nursing: assessment and management of clinical problems. 7th ed. St. Louis: Mosby; 2007.
258. Loan T. Determinants and assessment of nutrition and metabolic function. In: Wagner KD, Hardin-Pierce MG, editors. High acuity nursing. 6th ed. Stamford: Pearson; 2014.
259. Brogden BJ. Clinical skills: importance of nutrition for acutely ill hospital patients. Br J Nurs 2004;13(15):914–20.
260. Guo S, Dipietro LA. Factors affecting wound healing. J Dent Res 2010;89(3):219–29.
261. Australian Commission on Safety and Quality in Health Care (ACSQHC). National Consensus Statement: essential elements for recognising and responding to acute physiological deterioration. 2nd ed. Sydney. Online. Available from: www.safetyandquality.gov.au/our-work/recognising-and-responding-to-clinical-deterioration/implementing-r-and-r-systems/the-national-consensus-statement/.
262. Heersink JT, Brown CJ, Dimaria-Ghalili RA, Locher JL. Undernutrition in hospitalized older adults: patterns and correlates, outcomes, and opportunities for intervention with a focus on processes of care. J Nutr Elder 2010;29(1):4–41.
263. Posthauer ME. The role of nutrition in wound care. Adv Skin Wound Care 2006;19(1):43–52.
264. Holmes S. Undernutrition in hospital patients. Nurs Stand 2003;17(19):45–52.
265. Middleton S, McElduff P, Ward J, Grimshaw JM, Dale S, D'Este C, et al. Implementation of evidence-based treatment protocols to manage fever, hyperglycaemia, and swallowing dysfunction in acute stroke (QASC): a cluster randomised controlled trial. Lancet 2011;378(9804):1699–706.
266. National Stroke Foundation. Clinical guidelines for stroke management. 2017. Online. Available from: https://informme.org.au/en/Guidelines/Clinical-Guidelines-for-Stroke-Management-2017.
267. Parsell ST. Renal and urological problems. In: Lewis SB, Heitkemper L, Harding M, editors. Medical surgical nursing assessment and management of clinical problems. 10th ed. Missouri: Elsevier; 2017.

CHAPTER 14
RESUSCITATION

JULIE CONSIDINE, ZIAD NEHME AND RAMON Z. SHABAN

ESSENTIALS

- Prevention of cardiac arrest will save more lives than the best resuscitation. Early recognition and treatment of the deteriorating patient is vital.
- Coronary perfusion pressure has a direct relationship with successful resuscitation. The best way to optimise coronary perfusion pressure, and therefore chance of survival, is to provide effective, uninterrupted chest compressions.
- Attempts at endotracheal intubation should not interrupt chest compressions for more than 5 seconds.
- The time between stopping chest compressions and delivering defibrillation should be as short as possible, and compressions should continue until the time of defibrillation.
- Chest compressions should recommence immediately following defibrillation, irrespective of electrical success.
- Inadequate compression depth, overventilation and excessive interruptions to chest compressions are ongoing problems in resuscitation, even for experienced healthcare professionals.
- Current evidence suggests that vasopressors increase return of spontaneous circulation, survival to hospital discharge and survival at 3 months and antiarrhythmic medications increase return of spontaneous circulation. No benefit or harm in terms of neurological outcomes from medications in cardiac arrest has been demonstrated to date.
- Hypothermic temperature control (32–34° C) is still a core component of post-arrest care in Australia and Aoteroea New Zealand; however, the evidence continues to evolve. At a minimum, the international consensus is for active fever prevention (≤ 37.5° C).

INTRODUCTION

Cardiac arrest is a major focus of the work of emergency clinicians in hospital and out-of-hospital care settings, and there are many different causes of cardiac arrests. Ventricular fibrillation (VF) is the most common primary rhythm in sudden cardiac arrest in adults, and the majority of patients who survive cardiac arrest have had a primary VF arrest.[1] This means that the focus of resuscitation in adults must be on early defibrillation.[1] In infants and children, the primary causes of cardiac arrest are respiratory or circulatory failure (or a combination of both).[2,3] The most common initial cardiac arrest rhythm is asystole or pulseless electrical activity, occurring in 85% of children in cardiac arrest,[2,3] so the focus of advanced life support in paediatric patients is to restore oxygenation and circulating volume. The incidence of VF as the initial rhythm in infants and children in cardiac arrest is between 6% and 8% in out-of-hospital cardiac arrest,[4,5] and 15% overall,[2,3] and is most likely in infants and children with congenital cardiac conditions or as a consequence of poisonings.[2,3]

Basic life support (BLS) is a suite of procedures that preserve or restore life by establishing and maintaining airway, breathing and circulation without the need for adjunctive equipment, although use of an automated external defibrillator (AED) is commonly accepted as part of BLS.[6] Effective BLS may increase the likelihood of successful defibrillation and may enable time to detect and correct reversible causes of cardiac arrest.[7] Advanced life support (ALS) is BLS with the addition of invasive techniques, such as defibrillation, advanced airway management, vascular access and administration of drugs.[7]

Internationally, reviews of resuscitation science are coordinated by the International Liaison Committee on Resuscitation (ILCOR), comprised of regional resuscitation councils from North America, Europe, South Africa, Asia and Australia and New Zealand. Although the Australian Resuscitation Council (ARC) and New Zealand Resuscitation Council (NZRC) are separate organisations, they have high levels of collaboration and in the international arena combine to become the Australian and New Zealand Committee on Resuscitation (ANZCOR). In addition, all resuscitation guidelines pertinent to Australia and New Zealand are now co-badged as ANZCOR guidelines.

This chapter provides an overview of the principles and practice of the resuscitation of adults and children. Please refer to Chapter 34 for details about resuscitation of the newborn infant. It is important to note that the exact age at which paediatric protocols and techniques should be used in preference to neonatal protocols and techniques is unknown.[3] Infants who are newly born or in the first few hours of life should be managed as per neonatal guidelines.[3] Infants aged more than a few hours beyond birth should be managed according to paediatric guidelines.[3]

In this chapter both BLS and ALS are detailed, primarily referenced to the ANZCOR guidelines, which are freely available at www.resus.org.au. In addition, an evidence-based approach to prevention of cardiac arrest, post-arrest care and care of families of patients suffering cardiac arrest is also provided. The importance of effective recognition of, and response to, deteriorating patients is explored, and a summary of the evidence related to predictors of mortality is provided. Non-technical aspects of resuscitation practice, namely communication, teamwork and leadership, which are critical to resuscitation success, are also explored. The anatomy and physiology relevant to cardiac arrest and resuscitation in adults are detailed in Chapter 22. The major anatomical and physiological considerations for resuscitation in children are detailed in Chapter 35, along with discussions on sepsis, respiratory and cardiac illness. Resuscitation of the newly born infant is explored in Chapter 34 and resuscitation of the older person is detailed in Chapter 38.

RECOGNITION AND RESPONSE TO DETERIORATING PATIENTS

It is well documented that preventing cardiac arrest is critical to improving patient outcomes and reducing mortality. Research from both the out-of-hospital and in-hospital context supports the use of physiological criteria as a basis for clinical decisions. There is clear evidence that the majority of out-of-hospital and hospital patients exhibit physiological abnormalities in the hours preceding cardiac arrest,[4,8,9] and that tachypnoea is the most sensitive and specific vital sign predictor of serious illness in adults.[10–12] The primary survey approach is advocated by emergency care personnel as a structured approach to patient assessment, particularly in the critically ill or injured patient.[13,14] The primary survey is defined as the systematic assessment of airway, breathing, circulation and conscious state, and aims to identify and correct life-threatening conditions.[13] A more detailed discussion of patient assessment is presented in Chapter 13.

SYSTEMS APPROACH TO RESUSCITATION

There is clear evidence that early recognition of, and response to, deteriorating patients, preventing cardiac arrest and ensuring critically ill patients have access to expert care saves lives.[15,16] The decisions that paramedics and emergency nurses make when faced with a patient suffering cardiac arrest or critical illness impact on their outcomes. The notion of cardiac arrest centres that specialise in evidence-based post cardiac arrest care is gaining momentum both in Australia and overseas.[17] It is well established that regional systems of care have improved outcomes for patients suffering major trauma, stroke and acute coronary syndrome, and there is clear evidence that hospital factors, such as hospital size and interventional cardiac care capabilities, influence patient outcomes, specifically mortality.[17] The Australian Resuscitation Council recognises that it may be reasonable for patients suffering cardiac arrest or ST elevation myocardial infarction to be transported directly to centres with primary percutaneous coronary intervention capability, even if that means bypassing other hospitals with less cardiac care capability.[18]

In the hospital setting, rapid response systems (RRSs) facilitate early recognition of, and response to, deteriorating ward patients and have reduced in-hospital mortality and in-hospital cardiac arrests.[19,20] In Australia, the most common model of RRS is the Medical Emergency Team (MET), which functions in parallel with the cardiac arrest team and is activated for patients who have not yet suffered cardiac arrest but who have respiratory, cardiovascular or neurological deterioration.[21] Patients who receive a MET review have an in-hospital mortality rate as high as 60%,[22] so waiting for patients to fulfil MET call criteria is possibly too late. Many healthcare organisations have now implemented pre-MET systems with lower thresholds to facilitate earlier calls.[23]

Following decades of research showing positive outcomes of RRSs in general ward areas, the use of RRSs in EDs has increased over time.[24,25] Research related to systems for recognising and responding to deteriorating ED patients to date shows high levels of variability in both recognition and response systems; few studies reported on system use to improve care of patients while in the ED; the systems for recognising clinical deterioration in ED patients were highly variable; and few studies reported on the ED response to patients identified as deteriorating.[24] There are specific features of the ED that increase the risk of unrecognised and unreported deterioration and the ideal response to deteriorating ED patients is unknown. The only Australian study of ED-specific systems for recognition and response to deteriorating patients showed that although most Victorian EDs had a rapid response system in place, there was variability in activation criteria and responding team, both between EDs, and between ED and the ward RRS.[26]

In the out-of-hospital context, the use of systems to identify and respond to clinical deterioration is less well understood and there are currently no standardised definitions for clinical deterioration.[27] Escalation of care in the out-of-hospital environment may involve doctor or paramedic phone consultation or rendezvous with more senior clinical expertise (e.g. intensive or critical care paramedics). In many cases, however, expedited transport to the nearest hospital may be the only timely option for escalation of care. A number of early warning systems exist to identify patients who are at risk of clinical deterioration in the ambulance, although it is unclear if their utility is associated with improved patient outcomes.[28] The most common of these early warning systems include the National Early Warning Score (NEWS) and the simpler Modified Early Warning Score (MEWS) which typically use a combination of physiological parameters (heart rate, respiratory rate, systolic blood pressure, temperature, oxygen saturation, supplemental oxygen, and level of consciousness) to predict the risk of pre-hospital deterioration or short-term death.[28] Although the use of these systems has not been universally adopted in Australasia, they are widely used by emergency medical services in the United Kingdom to systematically identify patients at risk of clinical deterioration and to improve patient safety.[29]

The advantages of a structured and consistent approach to escalation of care include further development of already positive multidisciplinary relationships, enhanced interprofessional communication and increased patient safety. A systematic approach to recognising and responding to deterioration is important as there is clear evidence that clinical deterioration in the ED is associated with an increased risk of in-hospital death, hospital admission and RRS activation on the wards during the first few days of hospital admission.[30–32] An organised approach to recognising and responding to deteriorating patients in both the out-of-hospital and ED environments is a logical progression and builds on other patient safety systems, such as triage and systematic approaches to ED care of critically ill or injured patients.[27,28]

PRACTICE TIP

RECOGNISING AND RESPONDING TO DETERIORATING PATIENTS

One of the key strategies to improving patient outcomes from cardiac arrest is to prevent cardiac arrest by timely recognition of, and response to, clinical deterioration. All clinicians should understand the mechanisms and processes for escalating care of a deteriorating patient related to their specific area of practice and work environment. This is particularly important in the out-of-hospital environment, where efforts to escalate care may be impeded by long travel distances and resourcing of senior paramedics.

SHOCK STATES

In general terms, shock is defined as failure of the circulatory system to adequately perfuse organs and peripheral tissue.[33] It is a condition of severe haemodynamic and metabolic disturbance, resulting in an imbalance between the supply and demand of oxygen at the cellular level.[33] At the cellular level, shock is a secondary physiological response to injury, resulting in an imbalance between the supply and demand of oxygen. It precipitates anaerobic respiration and cellular hypoxia.

There are four broad categories and types of shock:[33]

- Cardiogenic shock is associated with cellular injury of the heart and its related structures, and results in a failure of cardiac function. Common causes of cardiogenic shock include myocardial infarction, cardiomyopathy, valve disease or trauma or anatomical rupture. If unmanaged, the heart progressively decompensates, leading to cardiac failure.
- Hypovolaemic shock, as the name implies, results from a loss of blood or extracellular fluid, typically from haemorrhage, burns, or, in extreme cases, vomiting and diarrhoea.
- Obstructive shock occurs when blockages or disruptions of systemic, pulmonary or coronary circulation interfere with cardiac output, as would occur during cardiac tamponade, pulmonary embolism or dissecting aortic aneurysm.
- The fourth category, distributive shock, occurs because of a shift of fluid into the peripheral vasculature, where an increase in extravascular spaces results in pooling of fluid, resulting in hypotension and poor tissue perfusion. Distributive shock may be anaphylactic, septic or neurogenic in nature.[33]

Collectively, all types of shock result in cellular hypoxia, anaerobic metabolism and respiration, and ultimately irreversible cell injury.[33] For resuscitation to be successful, it is imperative to treat the precipitating injury. Failure to stop uncontrolled haemorrhage in haemorrhagic shock, or untreated anaphylaxis in distributive shock, will render most resuscitative efforts futile. Preventing deterioration of the patient which would otherwise result in aggressive resuscitation is the priority in emergency and trauma care.

EFFECTIVE COMMUNICATION

One of the most important aspects of preventing and responding to clinical deterioration is effectively communicating critical information about the patient, such as their current condition, anticipated clinical course, interventions and response to interventions thus far.[34,35] There is evidence that using standardised tools for communication and handover improves content and clarity of communication between clinicians, patient safety, and clinician satisfaction with communication.[34–38] Advantages of standardised communication systems and using a predetermined structure are reduction in omissions of important information and clear expectations about the order in which information will be conveyed.[34–36] Further detail about communication frameworks is presented in Chapter 11.

PRACTICE TIP

EFFECTIVE COMMUNICATION

An example of a structured approach to communication is the situational briefing tool ISBAR, which stands for:[37,38]

Identify
Situation
Background
Assessment
Recommendation.

Another effective communication strategy for when crises are evolving or when there is a need to rapidly communicate concern is *critical assertiveness*, also known as *graded assertiveness*. Graded assertiveness is assertive communication aimed at preventing adverse events by encouraging a challenge followed by escalation of assertion.[39] A commonly used model is PACE (Probe, Alert, Challenge, Emergency).[39,40] The initial probe may be framed as a question: 'Are you sure we should be …?', and this is a particularly useful strategy when questioning figures of authority. As the levels of assertiveness increase, communication should remain polite and professional, but also draw attention to concern, using phrases such as 'I'm uncomfortable', 'I'm worried', 'I'm concerned'.[39,40] Graded assertiveness focuses on patient wellbeing as a central common interest rather than the merit of individual judgements or actions.

ED and out-of-hospital environments are complex and dynamic working environments prone to crises. A crisis is a situation that engenders a serious threat to patient safety and which is unable to be solved by knowledge alone.[41–43] The need for a standardised approach to communication has been long recognised by other high-risk industries, particularly the aviation industry. Many years of research into airline disasters demonstrated a lack of skills in managing rapidly developing complex situations, so a simulation-based curriculum called Cockpit Resource Management (CRM) was developed to teach teamwork and leadership skills. It is now a standard requirement in the airline industry. In the late 1980s, the principles of CRM were adapted for use in many areas of healthcare and re-termed Crisis Resource Management. These are the principles of CRM:[44]

- Know your team and your environment.
- Anticipate and plan.
- Allocate attention wisely.
- Use all available information and confirm it.
- Use cognitive aids (e.g. checklists).
- Take a leadership role.
- Call for help early.
- Communicate effectively.
- Distribute the workload.
- Mobilise and use all available resources.

TEAMWORK AND LEADERSHIP

Resuscitation in both out-of-hospital and hospital environments may involve a single responder or a large team. The effectiveness of resuscitation is critically dependent on team functioning. An effective team leader is one of the most important determinants of successful resuscitation. Resuscitation team leaders are well established in-hospital, and are also increasingly being used in the out-of-hospital setting.[45–47] The role of the team leader is to ensure that resuscitation priorities are carried out in a structured and efficient manner, therefore minimising delays and errors of omission in critical interventions. All orders/requests coming from other personnel should be directed to the team leader, and staff involved in the resuscitation should only accept orders/requests from the team leader.

It is also important that the team leader communicates effectively with the team. Orders should be stated loudly and clearly and should be directed to the individual expected to carry out the order, not simply announced to the room. As tasks are completed they should be announced loudly and clearly, for example, '1 mg adrenaline given IV', to ensure that all members of the team are aware of what is happening, and duplication of tasks is avoided. If there is a 'scribe' or note-taker, verbalisation of tasks also assists in keeping accurate records.

EPIDEMIOLOGY OF CARDIAC ARREST

In Australia, the Australasian Resuscitation Outcomes Consortium (Aus-ROC) have enabled all Australian and New Zealand ambulance services to contribute data to an Australasian cardiac arrest epistry, which is an epidemiological registry that provides population-based out-of-hospital cardiac arrest (OHCA) data.[48] Using internationally agreed definitions, the epistry records demographics, cardiac arrest features, ambulance response times, treatment and patient outcomes: the primary outcome of interest is 'survival to hospital discharge' and 'return of spontaneous circulation' is a key secondary outcome.[48] Data from 31,778 out-of-hospital cardiac arrests in Australia and New Zealand from 2019 showed that the majority of out-of-hospital cardiac arrests occurred in adults (96%), males (66%), and in private homes (76%). Two-thirds were unwitnessed (63%), 64% had an initial monitored rhythm of asystole, and 12% had an initial rhythm that was shockable. In cardiac arrests not witnessed by paramedics, bystander CPR was initiated in 38% and 2% received public defibrillation.[48]

For patients in whom resuscitation was attempted by paramedics (43%: n = 13,664/31,778), return of spontaneous circulation (ROSC) was achieved in 35% of cases in the pre-hospital environment and in 28% on hospital arrival. Survival to hospital discharge or 30 days occurred in 13% of out-of-hospital cardiac arrests. In bystander-witnessed cardiac arrests with a shockable rhythm (n = 2,285), ROSC on hospital arrival was achieved in 49.5% of cases and 32% survived to hospital discharge or 30 days.[49] Outcome data from Victoria suggests that many survivors of out-of-hospital cardiac arrest have an acceptable quality of life 12 months post their event, particularly when compared to population quality of life norms.[50] In older out-of-hospital cardiac arrest survivors (aged ≥ 65 years), 61% resided at home without additional care and 67% reported a good functional recovery.[51]

Despite detailed and robust national data about out-of-hospital cardiac arrests, the epidemiology and outcomes from in-hospital cardiac arrest remain poorly understood. A systematic review of 30 studies detailing the epidemiology and outcomes of 2345 in-hospital cardiac arrests in Australia and New Zealand shows that the frequency of in-hospital cardiac arrests is 0.58–6.11 per 1000 hospital admissions and cardiac arrests were less frequent in hospitals with RRS (1.32 vs 4.11 per 1000 admissions, $p < 0.001$).[52] ROSC occurred in 46.0% of patients. Overall, 74.6% of patients (range 59.4–77.5%) died in-hospital and survival was higher among patients with monitored cardiac arrest, younger patients, in those with a shockable rhythm, or those whose cardiac arrest occurred during work hours.[52] More recent data from 159 in-hospital cardiac arrests in 152 patients from seven Australian hospitals showed that the median patient age was 71.5 years, most (94%) resided at home and 68% were medical admissions. In two-thirds of in-hospital cardiac arrests (66%), the initial rhythm was non-shockable, the median resuscitation duration was 6.5 minutes and adrenaline was the most common intervention, used in 60% of cases. One-third (30%) of in-hospital cardiac arrests resulted in death on the ward, and 50% were admitted to the intensive care unit. One-quarter (26%) of patients were discharged home and 60.5% died during their hospitalisation (including those in whom ROSC was not achieved).[53]

BASIC LIFE SUPPORT

The purpose of BLS is to maintain myocardial and cerebral oxygenation until advanced life support personnel and equipment are available.[54] Effective BLS may increase the likelihood of successful defibrillation and enable time for reversible causes of cardiac arrest to be diagnosed and/or treated.[54] In all emergency situations, irrespective of whether the event occurs in the out-of-hospital or hospital setting, the priorities in an emergency are to:[55]

- quickly assess the situation
- ensure safety for personnel, patient and bystanders
- send for help
- commence BLS.

PRACTICE TIP

PRIORITIES IN RESUSCITATION

During any resuscitation it is important that:[6,7]

- chest compressions are high-quality (adequate rate and depth) with minimal interruptions
- minimising defibrillation of shockable rhythms occurs as early as possible
- hyperventilation and overventilation are avoided
- attempts to secure the airway should not delay CPR for more than 5 seconds
- vascular access should be obtained.

It is also important to consider reversible causes of cardiac arrest, and if present attempts should be made to correct these causes. To remember these causes, think of the '4 Hs' and '4 Ts' (Box 14.1).[7,54] Patients who are most likely to survive a cardiac arrest with intact neurological function:[54]

- have a witnessed arrest
- receive immediate BLS
- have a shockable cardiac rhythm that is VF or VT (ventricular tachycardia)
- receive early defibrillation.

DANGER

Your safety is paramount. Evidence of danger should prompt first responders to retreat to safety and request support from police, security or other emergency services personnel.

There are many actual and potential sources of danger, both for you and for your patient. Sources of danger can include bystanders, hazardous materials and road traffic. Unfortunately, assault remains one of the leading causes of occupational risk to paramedics.[56,57] It is important to recognise that bystanders respond in different ways to emotionally driven events, and it is common for bystanders to be aggressive or agitated, particularly when there is alcohol and/or illicit drugs involved. In the context of road trauma, both the patient and healthcare personnel should be safe from other vehicles, fire and fuel spills. When working in confined spaces, toxic fumes, exposure to carbon monoxide gas and risk of a low-oxygen environment should be considered. In mass casualty incidents or events with the possibility of terrorism, second-wave attacks should be considered.

BOX 14.1 REVERSIBLE CAUSES OF CARDIAC ARREST—THE '4 Hs' AND THE '4 Ts'[7]

- **Hypoxaemia**
- **Hypovolaemia**
- **Hypo- or hyperthermia**
- **Hypo- or hyperkalaemia**
- **Tamponade: pericardial**
- **Tension pneumothorax**
- **Toxins/poisons/drugs**
- **Thrombosis: pulmonary or coronary**

INFECTION PREVENTION AND CONTROL DURING RESUSCITATION

Resuscitation, like all aspects of emergency care and healthcare in general, is associated with the risk of the transmission of infectious diseases and the acquisition of healthcare-associated infection. As examined in greater detail in Chapter 27, emergency care must be delivered using a combination of Standard and Transmission-based Precautions that follows a comprehensive risk assessment. Infection risk from aerosol or droplet transmission should be considered; however, the risk of disease transmission during CPR in non-pandemic circumstances is very low.[6] Cardiopulmonary resuscitation (CPR) is complex in terms of assessing AGP (aerosol generating procedure) risk. While many procedures undertaken during the course of CPR are considered high-risk AGPs, such as intubation, there is no consensus and a lack of data about whether chest compressions result in aerosol generation or transmission of many infectious diseases, including COVID-19.[58,59] Other aspects of resuscitation, such as defibrillation, are not an AGP, and it is known that early chest compressions and defibrillation may improve survival.

It is uncertain whether chest compressions or defibrillation cause aerosol generation or transmission of COVID-19 to rescuers. A systematic review commissioned by ILCOR in 2020 did not find any direct evidence that chest compressions or defibrillation either are or are not associated with aerosol generation or transmission of infection.[58] A further review in 2021 found very few cases of infection transmission during CPR reported globally and in fact, only 15 isolated cases of infection transmission have been reported from mouth-to-mouth ventilation since its first use in 1744.[60]

Notwithstanding, protecting health workers from infectious diseases is paramount, as is preventing patients from acquiring healthcare-associated infections. There are a range of communicable diseases that are highly infectious and easily spread, such as influenza, tuberculosis and measles. Resuscitation must be performed following Standard and Transmission-based Precautions with a risk assessment for every patient. Patients that are suspected of having, or confirmed with, a respiratory infectious disease must be managed using appropriate contact, droplet and airborne precautions. All participants in resuscitation must have practised and be competent in safe, effective and rapid donning of PPE required for contact, droplet and airborne precautions (see Chapter 27).

RESPONSE

Unconsciousness or unresponsiveness may be caused by lack of cerebral circulation, lack of cerebral oxygenation, metabolic problems (such as hypoglycaemia, diabetic emergencies) or central nervous system problems (such as head injury, stroke or tumour). When assessing response, clinicians should assess for responsiveness and breathing. If the patient is unresponsive and not breathing normally, resuscitation is required.

SEND FOR HELP

Calling for help will be different depending on the context of practice, but examples of common methods of requesting assistance in a hospital context include calling for assistance from colleagues, calling an ambulance, using emergency buzzers, or activation of a Medical Emergency or Cardiac Arrest (Code Blue) team. In the out-of-hospital setting, an early situational report to the communication centre is critical to enable the early mobilisation of specialist ambulance resources for cardiac arrest patients (e.g. intensive/critical care paramedics, manual handling/extrication support, or helicopter retrieval).

AIRWAY

In an unconscious patient, there is a major risk of death from airway obstruction, as the tongue falls against the back of the throat when in a supine position. Airway obstruction may also occur from aspiration of foreign material in the airway, such as blood, vomit or food.[6,61] In unconscious patients, the airway always takes precedence over other injuries, including potential spinal injuries.[62] Risk factors for cervical spine injury and cervical spine immobilisation are detailed in Chapters 12 and 47.

When assessing the airway, there is no need to routinely roll the patient on their side.[61] Loose dentures should be removed, but well-fitting dentures can be left in place.[61] The mouth should be opened and inspected for obvious foreign material:[61] if foreign material is clearly visible, suction should be used to clear the oral cavity and oropharynx. If breathing commences, the patient should be placed on their side and monitored.[61]

Airway management is required when the patient is unconscious, has an obstructed airway or needs rescue breathing. The most common technique to establish and ensure a patent airway in adults is the backward head tilt with chin lift.[61] When using head tilt, do not use excessive force, particularly if neck injury is suspected. Chin lift facilitates airway patency by opening the mouth and pulling the tongue and soft tissues away from the back of the throat.[61]

Children should be managed in a similar manner to adults (as above).[2,61] In infants, the airway is easily obstructed because of the narrow diameters of nasal passages, vocal cords and trachea, and also their soft and pliable trachea may be compressed by excessive backwards head tilt.[2,61] Conversely, given that an infant's head can be disproportionately large in relation to the body, they may require padding under the shoulders to maintain neutral alignment. In infants under 1 year, a neutral head position should be used and the lower jaw should be supported at the chin with the mouth open. If these manoeuvres do not provide a clear airway, a slight backwards tilt to the head may be applied. In patients with suspected cervical spine injury, jaw thrust is a preferable method of opening the airway.[61]

Foreign body airway obstruction (choking)

Foreign body airway obstruction is a life-threatening condition.[63] Signs and symptoms will depend on the cause and severity of obstruction (partial or complete). Table 14.1 shows the signs of partial and complete airway obstruction. Airway obstruction may not be obvious until you attempt rescue breathing or bag–valve–mask ventilation. Assessment of a cough is a useful way to assess severity of foreign body airway obstruction.[61] In mild airway obstruction with an effective cough, the patient should be encouraged to cough and be monitored for recovery or deterioration. If the patient has severe airway obstruction with an ineffective cough, then management will depend on whether the patient is conscious or unconscious. The conscious patient should be given up to five back blows, and if that is not effective, then up to five chest thrusts may be attempted. Abdominal compression (e.g. Heimlich manoeuvre) is not recommended as there have been a number of reports of life-threatening complications from this procedure.[61] BLS should be commenced in the unconscious patient. Fig. 14.1 shows the ANZCOR flow chart for management of foreign body airway obstruction.[61] If scope of practice and organisational guidelines allow, removal of the foreign body under laryngoscopy may be an option.

BREATHING

Breathing may be absent or ineffective due to upper airway obstruction, damage to the respiratory centre in the brain, paralysis of nerves and/or muscles of respiration, lung dysfunction or immersion.[64] Breathing may be assessed by the 'look, listen, feel' approach: look for chest rise and fall, listen for breath sounds and feel for movement of the chest and upper abdomen: chest movement does not necessarily guarantee a patent airway.[64] If there are concerns about infection risk, then breathing should be assessed by looking only.[65] It is important to remember that complete absence of breathing is no longer a prerequisite for cardiac arrest and the need for resuscitation.

Cardiopulmonary resuscitation is indicated in patients who are unresponsive and not breathing normally after the airway has been opened and cleared. Chest compressions should be commenced, followed by rescue breathing or ventilations.[64] If

TABLE 14.1 SIGNS OF AIRWAY OBSTRUCTION[61]

PARTIAL AIRWAY OBSTRUCTION	COMPLETE AIRWAY OBSTRUCTION
Laboured breathing	There may be efforts at breathing
Noisy breathing, e.g. stridor, snoring	There are no sounds associated with breathing
Some escape of air felt at the mouth	There is no escape of air from the nose or mouth

FIGURE 14.1 ANZCOR FLOWCHART FOR MANAGEMENT OF FOREIGN BODY AIRWAY OBSTRUCTION[63]

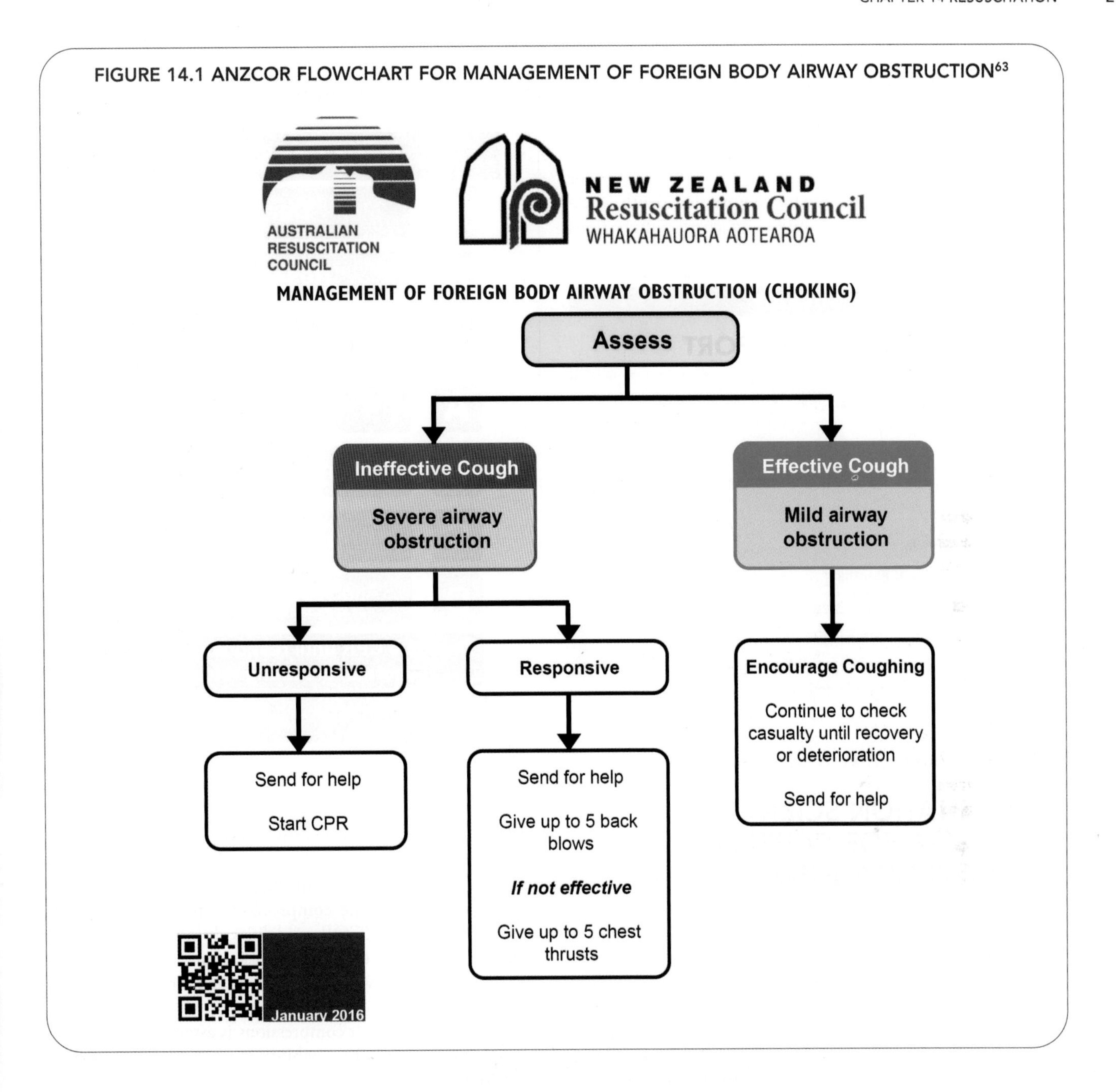

the chest does not rise, consider airway obstruction, insufficient tidal volume, inadequate seal or air leak. It is important to promote to lay rescuers that if they are unwilling or unable to perform rescue breaths, they should do continuous chest compressions.[6,64,66]

COMPRESSIONS

Chest compressions should be commenced if the patient is unresponsive and not breathing normally.[6,66] Palpation of a pulse is unreliable and should not be performed to confirm the need for resuscitation by lay rescuers.[66] Chest compressions in all age groups should be performed on the lower half of the sternum.[66] The chest should be compressed at least 5 cm in adults, approximately 5 cm in children and 4 cm in infants.[66] The compression rate is 100–120 per minute for all ages (almost 2 compressions/second). In adults and children, the heels of both hands should be used; in infants, a two-finger/two-thumb technique is recommended. It is vital that personnel performing chest compressions allow complete recoil of the chest after each compression.[66]

CARDIOPULMONARY RESUSCITATION

The fundamental aim of CPR (chest compressions combined with rescue breathing/ventilation) is to preserve brain function until definitive treatment of cardiac arrest can be provided. CPR should be commenced in patients who are unresponsive and not breathing normally.[6,67] There is no evidence about optimal compression–ventilation ratios from human studies; however, current guidelines recommend a compression-to-ventilation ratio of 30:2 in all age groups and irrespective of the number of rescuers, and that compressions are paused for ventilation.[6,67] The 30:2 compression-to-ventilation ratio was selected to increase the number of compressions, minimise interruptions to compressions, prevent excessive ventilation, simplify teaching, maximise skill retention and maintain consistency with other international guidelines.[6]

Although many healthcare professionals regard themselves as skilled in BLS, research has consistently shown that even for healthcare professionals, inadequate compression depth, overventilation and excessive interruptions to chest compressions are ongoing problems.[54]

PRACTICE TIP

BASIC LIFE SUPPORT

ANZCOR recommend using a DRSABCD sequence for resuscitation:[6]

- check for **D**anger
- assess **R**esponse: is the patient unresponsive?
- **S**end for help
- open the **A**irway
- check for normal **B**reathing
- if unresponsive and not breathing normally, commence 30 chest **C**ompressions followed by 2 breaths
- attach an Automatic External Defibrillator (AED) and provide **D**efibrillation if indicated.

Fig. 14.2 shows the ANZCOR flowchart for BLS.

FIGURE 14.2 ANZCOR BASIC LIFE SUPPORT FLOWCHART[68]

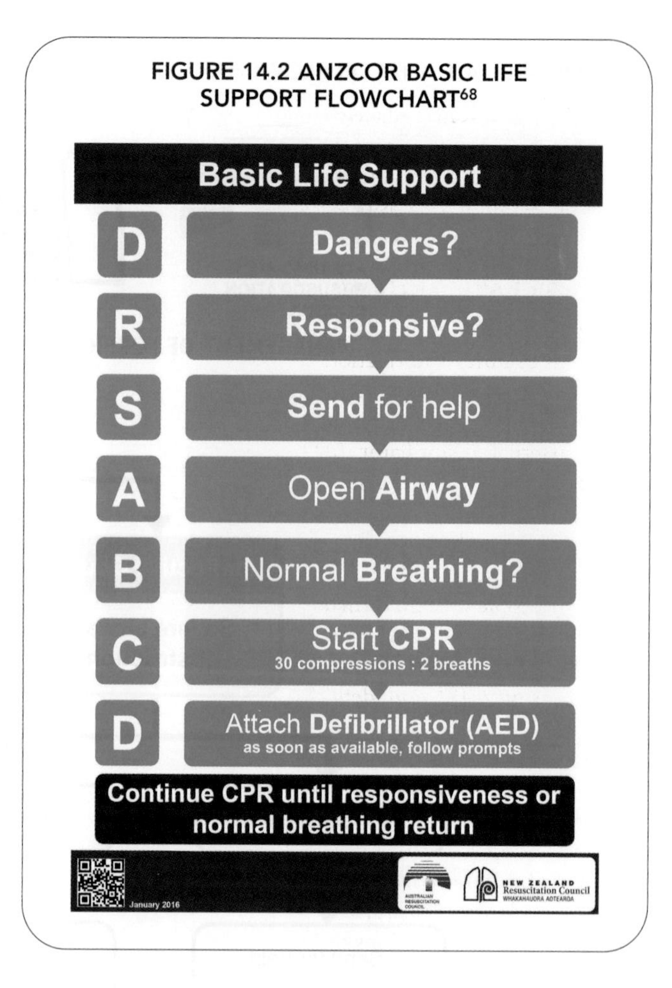

RESUSCITATION SCIENCE: RATIONALE FOR CURRENT RECOMMENDATIONS

In adults with primary cardiac arrest, arterial blood oxygenation is usually satisfactory at the time of cardiac arrest, so the blood flowing through the pulmonary circulation during CPR will have some oxygen content,[69] but as the duration of cardiac arrest progresses, oxygen levels fall and carbon dioxide levels rise.[69] Hyperventilation (excessive rate and/or tidal volume) is detrimental during cardiac arrest.[70] High intrathoracic pressure or prolonged time with positive intrathoracic pressure results in failure to develop negative pressure between chest compressions.[69] Failure to develop negative pressure between chest compressions results in decreased venous return (preload), decreased cardiac output, decreased cerebral and coronary perfusion, and ultimately decreased likelihood of survival.[69] As a result of these physiological processes, there has been a decreased emphasis on ventilation during CPR over the last decade or so.

The de-emphasis of ventilation during CPR has been accompanied by an increased focus on high-quality chest compressions during CPR: adequate rate and depth, complete chest wall recoil between compression and minimal hands-off time.[6,7,67] The optimal rate and depth of chest compressions is unknown; however, at this point in time return of spontaneous circulation and survival to hospital discharge seem to be optimised at a compression rate of 100–120 per minute and a depth of at least 5 cm in adults.[66,67,71] Although there is some evidence suggesting harm with chest compression depths greater than 6 cm, the clinical reality of being able to differentiate between 5 or 6 cm is doubtful.[66] There is a clear association between inadequate compression depth and lower survival, so current ANZCOR guidelines do not have an upper limit on compression depth as the risk of inadequate compression depth likely outweighs the risk of compressions that are too deep.[66]

Interruption of chest compressions is associated with lower survival rates, decreased probability of successful defibrillation and higher incidence of myocardial dysfunction following resuscitation.[7,54] The heart needs a continuous supply of energy (adenosine triphosphate: ATP): increased chest compressions result in increased myocardial blood flow, increased probability that ventricular fibrillation will become more coarse and increased likelihood of successful defibrillation. There is a direct and important relationship between coronary perfusion pressure and survival: a coronary perfusion pressure $\geq$ 15 mmHg is predictive of ROSC.[54] Coronary perfusion pressure increases cumulatively during chest compressions and decreases when compressions are stopped (e.g. for ventilation); therefore interruptions to chest compressions should be minimised.[54] In particular, the time between stopping chest compressions and starting defibrillation should be as short as possible; compressions should continue until the time of defibrillation and compressions should recommence immediately following defibrillation *irrespective of electrical success* (see the following section on defibrillation).[7,54]

In the first minute following defibrillation, the likelihood of developing a rhythm that results in cardiac output is low.[1,7,54] Commencing CPR immediately following defibrillation increases the likelihood of return of spontaneous circulation as cerebral and coronary perfusion are restored. In addition, effective CPR for a period of 1–3 minutes is associated with an increased likelihood of successful subsequent attempts at defibrillation.[1,7,54]

DEFIBRILLATION USING AN AED

Time to defibrillation is a key factor that influences survival. For every minute defibrillation is delayed, there is approximately a 10% reduction in survival if the victim is in cardiac arrest due to VF.[1,72] As a result, defibrillation using an automated external defibrillator (AED) has become a valuable adjunct to BLS.[1,72] Most adults who are salvageable from cardiac arrest are in VF or pulseless VT, making defibrillation the single-most important intervention for these patients. AED use should not be restricted to trained personnel: allowing AED use by lay people with no formal training may be life-saving.[1,72] CPR prior to defibrillation increases the likelihood of successful defibrillation. It is also important to minimise the time between ceasing CPR and defibrillating and to recommence CPR immediately following defibrillation.[1,72] Emergency nurses and paramedics should be familiar with the AED that is available in their clinical environment and the manufacturer's recommendations in terms of its operation. In general, the principles of operation of AED are:

- locate the AED as soon as it is available and turn it on
- apply pads as per manufacturer's recommendations, while minimising interruptions to chest compressions
- follow the verbal prompts.

If shock is advised, ensure safe defibrillation by ensuring the pads are applied correctly and are not touching, following the AED prompts and not touching the patient during shock delivery. If shock is not advised, continue BLS and seek assistance from ALS personnel.[67,72]

ADVANCED LIFE SUPPORT

The techniques and rationales discussed so far in this chapter from a BLS perspective are equally applicable to advanced life support (ALS). Like BLS, ALS should be commenced in patients who are unresponsive and not breathing normally.[6,7]

In adults and children, palpation of a pulse is unreliable and should not be performed to confirm cardiac arrest or the need for resuscitation.[6,7] In the 2010 ILCOR review of resuscitation science, all the studies retrieved showed that pulse check by out-of-hospital and in-hospital health professionals was unreliable in both infants and children, irrespective of whether carotid, femoral and brachial pulses were used.[73] The 2020 ILCOR consensus on science process did not identify any new evidence regarding pulse checks.[67] For healthcare professionals, it is reasonable to check a pulse if an organised rhythm is visible on the monitor at the next rhythm check. Planned pauses in cardiac compressions for rhythm analysis (and/or pulse check) should not take more than 10 seconds.[54]

Given that ALS involves the addition of invasive techniques, such as emergency defibrillation, advanced airway management, vascular access and administration of drugs, it is imperative that these additional therapies do not result in interruptions to chest compressions. Ideally, chest compressions should continue during attempts at intubation and, at worst, interruption to compressions for intubation should be 5 seconds or less. Planned pauses for rhythm analysis and/or pulse check should take no more than 10 seconds.[54] The cardiac rhythm should be checked after 2 minutes of CPR or if the patient becomes responsive and starts breathing; if the rhythm appears compatible with return of spontaneous circulation (ROSC), then the pulse should be checked.[54]

LIFE-THREATENING DYSRHYTHMIAS

Life-threatening dysrhythmias can generally be considered in two categories: shockable and non-shockable rhythms. The shockable rhythms covered in detail in this chapter are ventricular fibrillation (VF) and unconscious, pulseless ventricular tachycardia (VT); as the term suggests, these rhythms are responsive to defibrillation. The non-shockable rhythms covered here are asystole and pulseless electrical activity (PEA), also called electromechanical dissociation (EMD); these rhythms are *not* responsive to defibrillation. In addition, there is a section discussing symptomatic bradycardia.

Shockable rhythms: VF and pulseless VT

The major characteristics of VF and VT are summarised in Table 14.2.

Non-shockable asystole and PEA/EMD

The major characteristics of asystole and PEA are summarised in Table 14.3.

ALS—ADULT

The current ANZCOR protocol for adult ALS is shown in Fig. 14.3.

ALS—PAEDIATRIC

Paediatric ALS presents additional challenges to ED clinicians as the size and weight of children of various ages is different, and almost all paediatric ALS interventions are weight-based (medication doses, endotracheal tube size, defibrillation energy). There are a number of methods which can be used to calculate weight in children and assist with decision-making regarding weight-related interventions (see below). The current ANZCOR protocol for paediatric ALS is shown in Fig. 14.4.

Body length tapes

Body length tapes, such as Broselow tape (Fig. 14.5), were developed to provide a length-based estimate of bodyweight and equipment size during resuscitation. The tape is laid on the trolley with the top end level with the child's head; the coloured section that corresponds with the level of the child's feet is the section to be used for that child.

Weight estimation

All drugs in a paediatric ALS context are given in weight-related doses. There are numerous methods of weight calculation in children, including parental/clinician estimation, body length tapes and a range of formulae based on age (Table 14.4). A systematic review of 58 studies involving 792,209 children showed that the weight-estimation accuracy of the Broselow tape was suboptimal in all populations studied, with weight estimation within 10% of actual weight occurring in just over

TABLE 14.2 CHARACTERISTICS OF VENTRICULAR FIBRILLATION (VF) AND VENTRICULAR TACHYCARDIA (VT)[1,7]

	VENTRICULAR FIBRILLATION	VENTRICULAR TACHYCARDIA
Rate	Rapid, disorganised	150–250 beats/minute
Rhythm	Irregular	Regular most of the time May occasionally be slightly irregular
ECG trace		
Pacemaker	Disorganised electrical activity in the ventricles makes ventricular muscle fibres contract independently. This causes 'quivering' of ventricular myocardium and makes the ventricles incapable of pumping blood	Ventricular pacemaker fires rapidly Impulse spreads through the ventricles via an abnormal pathway
P waves	Not seen	Not seen
QRS complex	Absent Fibrillation waves of various sizes and shapes present	Wide and bizarre Width > 0.12 seconds
P–QRS relationship	–	–
PR interval	–	–
Clinical significance	The cause of VF is still not completely understood. VF is the most common cause of sudden cardiac death and may be preceded by VT Results in no cardiac output Often associated with acute myocardial ischaemia (AMI) and occurs in up to half of cardiac arrest survivors Begins as a coarse, irregular rhythm and then degenerates to a fine irregular rhythm and eventually asystole; the likelihood of successful defibrillation decreases as these changes occur	VT is usually defined as greater than 4 consecutive ventricular beats VT that lasts for longer than 30 seconds is considered sustained Causes significant reduction in cardiac output as ventricular filling time is severely reduced, so cannot be tolerated for long periods of time Can deteriorate into VF then asystole Re-entry (or a single circular pathway of electrical impulse) is the most common mechanism responsible for VT
Intervention	The mainstay of resuscitation for VF is early defibrillation	Pulseless VT → treat as VF → defibrillation VT with pulse → antiarrhythmic drugs

ECG: electrocardiogram.

half the children studied.[77] Further, in low- and middle-income countries there was commonly an overestimation of the child's weight giving rise to potential for harmful medication errors. There are limited data about the value of the Broselow tape as a drug-dosing guide, but data to date shows that the tape is often used incorrectly and contains insufficient information regarding drug therapies.[77] In non-obese paediatric patients, resuscitation medication doses should be based on actual body weight (which closely approximates ideal body weight).[3] If necessary, body weight can be estimated from body length.[3]

DEFIBRILLATION

Early defibrillation provides the best chance of survival for patients (adult and paediatric) with VF or pulseless VT. Defibrillation is the only proven definitive treatment for VF.[1,72] Defibrillation is the application of an electric shock through the chest with the aim of producing simultaneous depolarisation of myocardial cells and restoring organised electrical activity.[1] The discussion in this chapter is focused on emergency defibrillation rather than synchronised cardioversion. Current ALS protocols recommend that defibrillation be indicated for VF and pulseless VT.[1,72] The chance of successful defibrillation decreases as time to defibrillation increases. As time increases, the high-energy phosphate stores in the myocardium decrease, resulting in deterioration of VF amplitude and waveform. Effective CPR will slow the rate of deterioration of VF, but will not stop it from occurring. One of the ongoing debates in ALS is whether CPR should be performed prior to defibrillation. Current recommendations are that for patients with an unmonitored cardiac arrest, a short period of CPR should be provided until the defibrillator is applied and rhythm analysis has occurred. CPR should continue during defibrillator charging and the defibrillation shock should be delivered as soon as the defibrillator is available.[1,67] In a hospital context, if a

TABLE 14.3 CHARACTERISTICS OF ASYSTOLE AND PULSELESS ELECTRICAL ACTIVITY (PEA)[1,7]

	ASYSTOLE	PEA
Rate	None	Variable
Rhythm	None	Variable (remember, can be sinus rhythm)
ECG trace		
Pacemaker	No electrical activity	Variable
P waves	None	Variable
QRS complex	None	Variable
P–QRS relationship	-	Variable
PR interval	-	Variable
Clinical significance	Asystole carries the poorest prognosis of all the ALS-requiring rhythms Asystole has an extremely high mortality rate (> 95%) As asystole is often preceded by VT/VF, the presence of asystole indicates a prolonged state of arrest It is important to confirm the diagnosis of asystole by checking for electrical activity in more than one monitor lead to make sure that it is not a technical problem or fine VF	PEA occurs when there is electrical myocardial activity but no cardiac output. This can occur because of: • no cardiac contractions ('pump failure') • cardiac contractions that are too weak to generate adequate cardiac output • cardiac contractions with no blood flow due to hypovolaemia or obstruction to flow
Intervention	BLS and adrenaline	BLS and adrenaline Correct underlying cause of PEA

ALS: advanced life support; BLS: basic life support; ECG: electrocardiogram; VT: ventricular tachycardia; VF: ventricular fibrillation.

FIGURE 14.3 ANZCOR FLOWCHART FOR ADULT ALS[74]

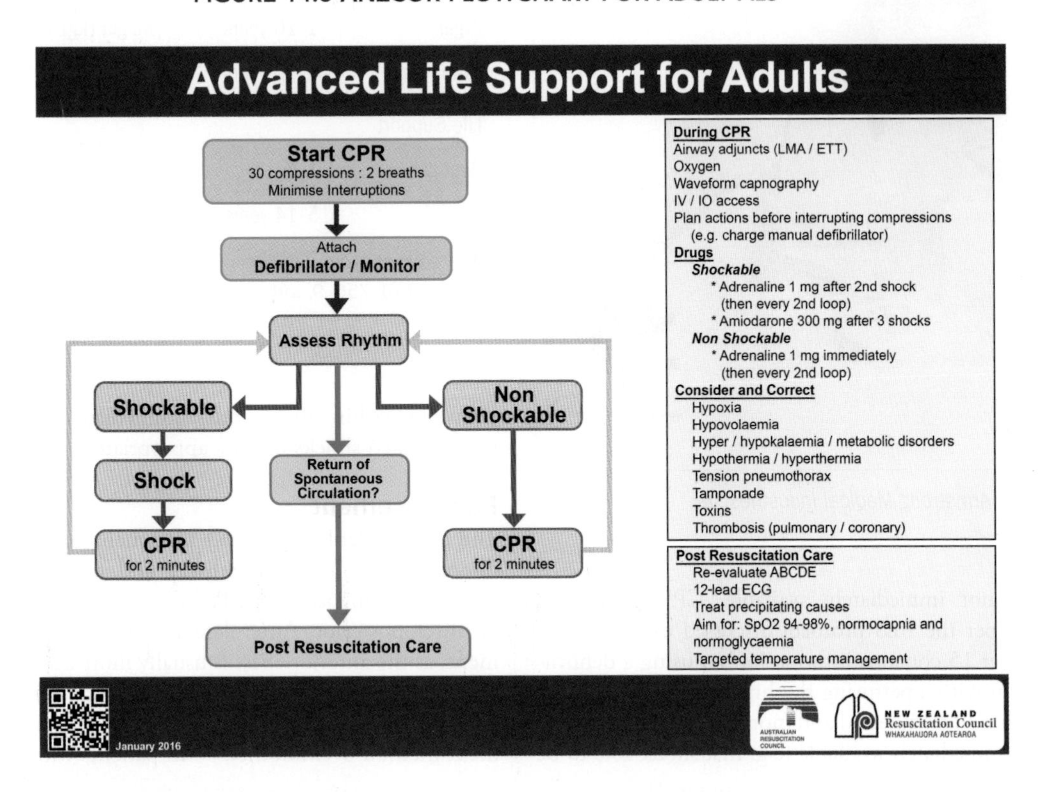

FIGURE 14.4 ANZCOR FLOWCHART FOR PAEDIATRIC ALS[75]

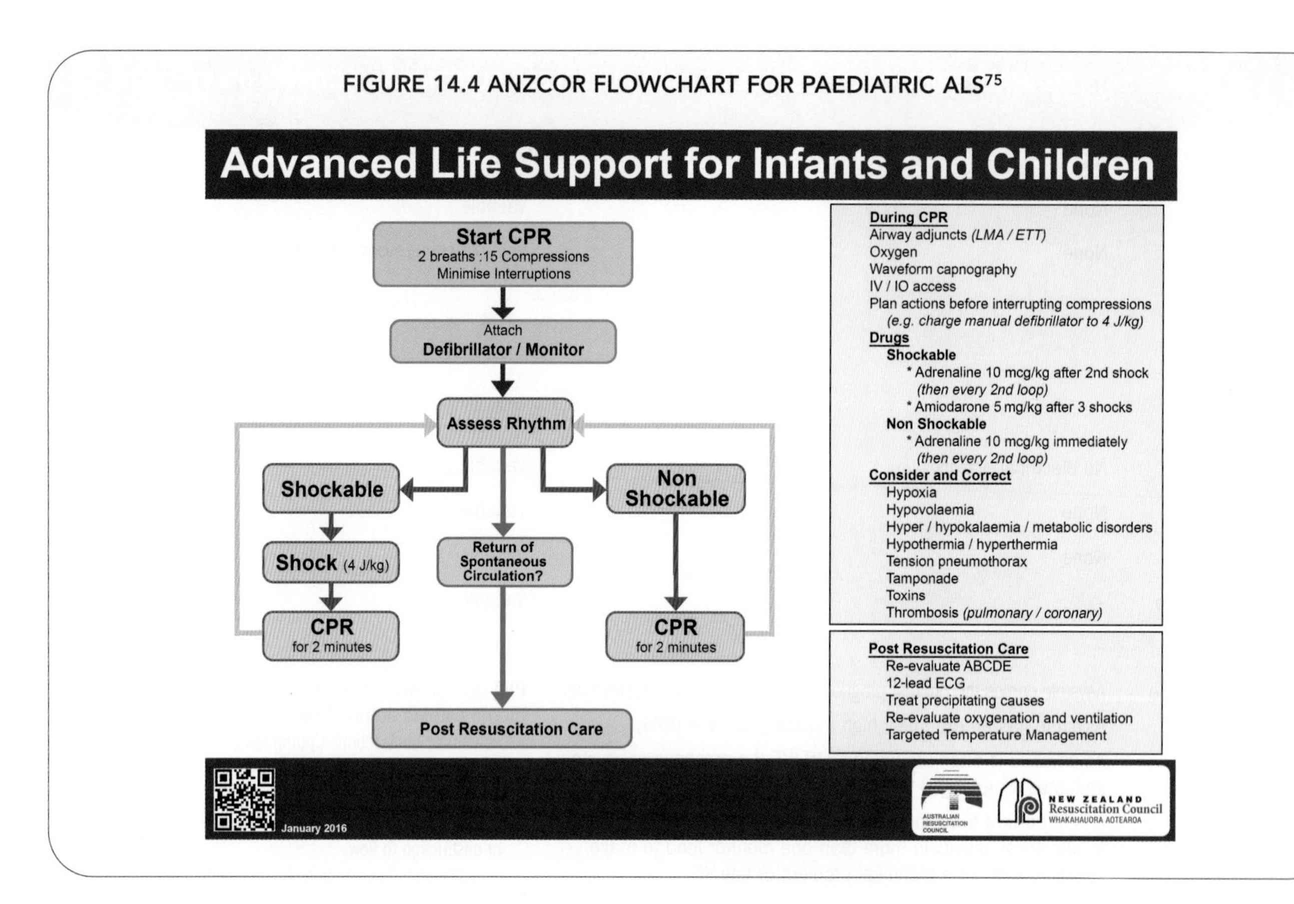

FIGURE 14.5 BROSELOW TAPE

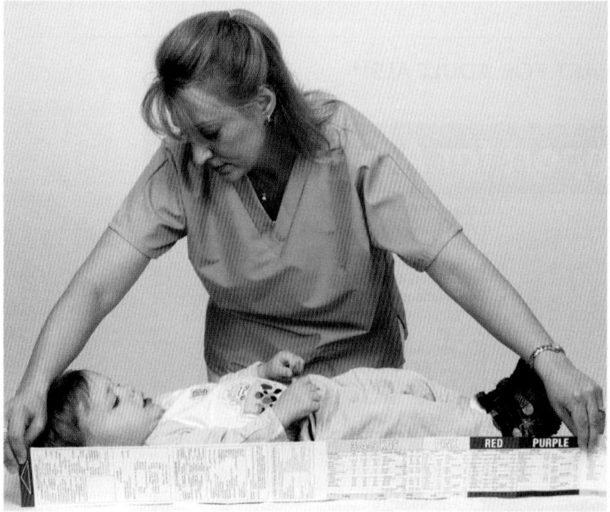

Photo courtesy of Armstrong Medical Industries, Inc.

TABLE 14.4 FORMULAE FOR DETERMINING CHILDREN'S WEIGHT[76]

METHOD	AGE GROUP	FORMULA (AGE IN YEARS)
Argall	1–10 years	Weight (kg) = (age + 2) × 3
Advanced Paediatric Life Support	1–10 years	Weight (kg) = (age + 4) × 2
Best guess	1–4 years	Weight (kg) = (age × 2) + 10
	5–14 years	Weight (kg) = age × 4

Reproduced from Emergency Medicine Journal, Krieser, D. et al. 2007;24(6): 756–9, with permission from BMN Publishing Group Ltd.

defibrillator is not immediately available, CPR should be commenced as per the BLS protocol discussed earlier in this chapter.[6] Chapter 15 contains information on using a defibrillator. If a patient with a perfusing rhythm suddenly develops a shockable rhythm in a witnessed and monitored setting and the defibrillator is immediately available (e.g. first shock able to be delivered within 20 seconds), immediate defibrillation using three stacked shocks may be appropriate.[54]

Pad placement

The aim of defibrillator pad placement is to place the heart directly in the current pathway and maximise current flow through the myocardium. Pad placement may be anterolateral or anteroposterior. Anterolateral is the most common placement, as the anterior chest is usually more accessible. However, both methods are effective as long as pads are positioned correctly; currently there is no evidence to support one pad placement method over another.[1,72] In patients with large breasts, it is acceptable to place the apical pad/paddle lateral to or underneath the breast.[1,72] Irrespective of the pad/paddle placement method chosen, defibrillator pads/paddles should not be placed over electrocardiogram (ECG) electrodes/leads, implanted pacemakers, central venous catheter insertion sites and glyceryl trinitrate (GTN) or other medication patches.[1,72]

Transthoracic impedance

Transthoracic impedance is the resistance to flow of electrical current by the chest wall, lungs and myocardium. Decreased transthoracic impedance results in increased effectiveness of defibrillation. Transthoracic impedance may be minimised by a number of strategies (Box 14.2).[1]

Shock protocols

Current recommendations are that single shocks be used for patients in VF or pulseless VT and that CPR should be commenced immediately following shock delivery.[1,7,54] As discussed earlier, three stacked shocks may be appropriate in a witnessed, monitored arrest when a defibrillator is immediately available.[54] Energy levels in adult patients should be set at 200 J when using a biphasic defibrillator, unless there is clinical data for the specific defibrillator which suggests an alternative energy level that provides greater than 90% shock success.[1] For monophasic defibrillators, energy levels for adult patients should be set at 360 J.[1] In children, the optimal energy dose for VF or pulseless VT is unknown. Current recommendations are that 4 J/kg should be used.[3] A praecordial thump (a single, sharp blow to the patient's mid sternum using the rescuer's fist) may be considered in patients with monitored, pulseless VT if a defibrillator is not immediately available.[54] Praecordial thump is ineffective in VF and is no longer recommended for use in this rhythm.[54]

Defibrillation safety

The operator of the defibrillator is ultimately responsible for defibrillator safety. In terms of patient safety, ensure that the rhythm is a shockable rhythm (VF/pulseless VT), that the patient is not touching any metal objects and that there is proper application of pads to the patient's chest (air pockets increase the risk of burns/arcing). Risk of oxygen-related fire is minimised by correct application of defibrillator pads to prevent arcing and removal of oxygen sources from the patient's chest and immediate bed area. Never place defibrillator pads over transdermal medication patches, such as glyceryl trinitrate (GTN) patches, as there is a risk of burns and/or explosion. To ensure safety of personnel and bystanders, announce loudly and clearly 'CHARGING' as the defibrillator is being charged. Then announce loudly and clearly 'STAND CLEAR' and perform a visual check of the area surrounding the patient before pressing 'SHOCK'.

Troubleshooting

If the defibrillator fails to defibrillate, there are a number of common reasons that need to be excluded. These are shown in Box 14.3.

BOX 14.2 STRATEGIES TO MINIMISE TRANSTHORACIC IMPEDANCE[1]

- **Dry the skin prior to application of pads**
- **Increase pad size. As pad size is increased:**
  - **resistance to current flow decreases**
  - **chance of successful defibrillation increases**
  - **risk of myocardial damage secondary to defibrillation decreases.**
- **Maintain optimal contact between the skin and pad and use conductive pads.**

ADVANCED AIRWAY MANAGEMENT

Decisions about airway management will depend on the availability of devices and the skills and experience of resuscitation team members.[54] Options for advanced airway management during cardiac arrest include:

- manual airway manoeuvres (see BLS section earlier in the chapter)
- oropharyngeal airway
- nasopharyngeal airway
- supraglottic airway
- oesophageal-tracheal combitube
- endotracheal intubation.

A 2019 ILCOR systematic review of 78 observational studies and 11 controlled trials concluded that high risk of bias and heterogeneity across studies precluded any meaningful recommendations.[78] Two adequately powered randomised controlled trials of airway management during out-of-hospital cardiac arrest showed no difference in survival with favourable neurological outcome at 28 days (4.3% for bag–mask ventilation and 4.2% for tracheal intubation, $p = 0.68$)[79] or at hospital discharge or 30 days (6.4% for supraglottic airway and 6.8% for tracheal intubation, $p = 0.24$).[80] The one randomised trial of airway management during out-of-hospital cardiac arrest with a significant difference between groups showed 72-hour survival rates of 18.3% for supraglottic airway and 15.4% for tracheal intubation ($p = 0.04$).[81] Current international recommendations are that if an advanced airway is used, a supraglottic airway for adults with out-of-hospital cardiac arrest in settings with a low tracheal intubation success rate is suggested (weak recommendation, low certainty evidence).[82] For adults with out-of-hospital cardiac arrest in settings with a high tracheal intubation success rate or in-hospital cardiac arrest, supraglottic airway or tracheal intubation is suggested (weak recommendation, very low certainty evidence).[82] Once an advanced airway is inserted (supraglottic airway or endotracheal tube), the ventilation rate should be 6–10 per minute and chest compressions should be continuous without pausing for ventilations.[54] Refer to Chapter 15 for further information on airway management.

Oro- or nasopharyngeal airways

Despite the use of oro- and nasopharyngeal airways in cardiac arrest over many decades, there are no studies examining the use of these medical devices in this clinical context.[70] Current recommendations are that their use is still reasonable when performing bag–valve–mask ventilation.[70] Oropharyngeal airways should be of an appropriate size and not forcibly inserted.[70] To determine the correct-size oropharyngeal airway, the airway should reach

BOX 14.3 TROUBLESHOOTING DEFIBRILLATOR FAILURES

POOR CONTACT BETWEEN DEFIBRILLATOR PADS AND PATIENT

- Defibrillator may have a display prompt or voice alert that indicates pads are ill-applied or missing.
- Check that pads are applied to patient's bare chest.
- If the problem continues, replace defibrillator pads.

PAD CABLE IS NOT CONNECTED TO THE DEFIBRILLATOR

- Defibrillator may have a display prompt or voice alert indicating cable disconnection or pads missing.
- Check cable connection.

DEFIBRILLATOR CHARGE AUTOMATICALLY DISARMS

- Defibrillator may have a prompt that indicates shock cancelled
- After 30 seconds the defibrillator automatically disarms if the 'SHOCK' button is not pressed; if this occurs, recharge defibrillator and deliver shock within 30 seconds.

BATTERY FAILURE

Synchronised mode engaged

- Defibrillator may have a prompt that indicates synchronised mode or 'SYNC' is engaged, and a highlighted R wave on the monitor display.
- Synchronised cardioversion is different to emergency defibrillation, as during emergency defibrillation the shock is delivered at random during the cardiac cycle.
- Synchronised cardioversion is used to treat cardiac dysrhythmias such as conscious VT, SVT, AF or atrial flutter when drugs have failed to revert the dysrhythmia or if the patient becomes haemodynamically unstable.
- During synchronised cardioversion, the shock is delivered during the absolute refractory period after ventricular depolarisation (just after the QRS complex on ECG), thus decreasing the potential for the shock to be delivered during the vulnerable period of repolarisation (upslope of the T wave on ECG).
- 'R on T phenomenon' occurs when a shock is delivered during the vulnerable period—this is dangerous and can result in VF.
- If the 'SYNC' button is activated during emergency defibrillation and the cardiac rhythm is VF, the defibrillator will still attempt to sense an R wave and deliver the shock just after the QRS complex; as there are no R waves in VF, the defibrillator will not discharge.
- If the rhythm is pulseless VT (rapid rate and wide and bizarre QRS complexes), it may be difficult for the defibrillator to sense the R wave or to distinguish the R wave from the T wave; therefore it is recommended that emergency defibrillation is a safer option for pulseless VT.

AF: atrial fibrillation; ECG: electrocardiogram; SVT: supraventricular tachycardia; VT: ventricular tachycardia; VF: ventricular fibrillation.

from the centre of the incisors to the angle of the jaw.[83] To determine the correct-size nasopharyngeal airway, the correct size should reach from tip of the nose to the tragus of the ear.[84] Insertion of an oropharyngeal airway in children is different to that in adults. In adults, the oropharyngeal airway is inserted upside down until it reaches the soft palate, then is rotated 180° so it is 'right way up' and slid over the tongue.[83] In infants and small children, the airway is inserted 'right way up' using a tongue depressor to aid insertion. In large children, the same technique as for adults may be used.[83] An oropharyngeal airway is preferred in the context of head trauma with potential for a fractured base of skull.[70]

Supraglottic airways

Supraglottic airways have the advantage of being easier to insert than endotracheal tubes.[70] Randomised trials comparing supraglottic airways with endotracheal intubation have produced conflicting results and both have been in the out-of-hospital context.[80,81] One trial showed no difference in survival to hospital discharge or 30 days (6.4% for supraglottic airway and 6.8% for tracheal intubation, $p = 0.24$),[80] and the other showed higher 72 hour survival with supraglottic airway use (18.3%) when compared to tracheal intubation (15.4%) ($p = 0.04$).[81] Therefore, there is insufficient evidence to recommend one approach over the other.[70,82] Supraglottic airways should not be used in patients with a gag reflex. See Chapter 16 for details on supraglottic airway insertion.

Endotracheal intubation

Endotracheal intubation has long been considered the gold standard for airway maintenance and protection during CPR; however, there is no high certainty evidence to support endotracheal intubation over other airway management options *during cardiac arrest.*[70] The disadvantages of endotracheal intubation during cardiac arrest include the risk of unrecognised oesophageal intubation (mean 4.3%, range 0–14%) and interruption to chest compressions.[70] Decisions about endotracheal intubation should be informed by assessing the benefit of intubation versus consequences of interrupted chest compressions, and the skills and availability of personnel.[70] In some cases, it may be more appropriate to intubate the patient following return of spontaneous circulation.[70] Attempts at endotracheal intubation should occur with CPR in progress and *should not* interrupt chest compressions for more than 5 seconds.[70] Once the endotracheal tube has been inserted, the cuff should be inflated to prevent air leaks. Endotracheal tube placement should be confirmed by chest inflation, auscultation, direct observation and waveform capnography.[70] Waveform capnography is also recommended to confirm and continuously monitor the endotracheal tube position and to protect against unrecognised oesophageal intubation.[70]

MEDICATIONS/FLUIDS USED IN CARDIAC ARREST

Defibrillation, oxygenation and ventilation always take priority over drug administration.[85]

Methods of administration

It is always preferable in a resuscitation situation to give drugs via the intravenous route using a large-bore peripheral IV cannula inserted into a large peripheral vein; for example, the cubital fossa.[70] Placement of IV cannulae in lower limbs should be avoided because in the arrested patient there is decreased venous return.[70] IV drug administration should always be followed by a normal saline flush of at least 20–30 mL in adults and a full cycle of external chest compressions; in children the flush should be appropriate to the age/size of the child and the length of extension tubing, if present.

Intraosseous (IO) administration is also a good alternative to IV administration. The bone marrow has a rich blood supply and is part of the peripheral circulation, so drugs and fluids administered via the IO route are absorbed and distributed as quickly and in the same concentrations as they would be if they were administered using the IV route. Any drug that can be given via the IV route can also be given using the IO route and the dose is the same as the dose that would be used for IV administration. The most common place for insertion of an IO needle is the anterior surface of the tibia 2–3 cm below the tibial tuberosity.

Bone marrow may also be aspirated for biochemistry and haematology (excluding white cell count). When giving drugs and/or fluids via the IO route, usually they will not run using gravity alone. A common method of fluid administration via the IO route is to place a three-way tap between the IO needle and the fluid line, turn the three-way tap off to the patient, use an appropriate-size syringe to draw up the required amount of fluid from the flask, turn the three-way tap off to the flask and then inject the fluid into the IO needle.

If IV or IO access cannot be established, drugs may be administered via an ETT, although absorption may be variable.[85] The drugs that can be administered via ETT are adrenaline, atropine and lidocaine. Other cardiac arrest drugs should not be given via an ETT as they may cause mucosal and/or alveolar damage. In adults, the ETT dose should be increased (3 to 10 times the IV dose); there is some evidence that dilution with water increases drug absorption.[85]

Pharmacology

Tables 14.5 and 14.6 outline the medications used during resuscitation.

Fluid resuscitation

There is insufficient evidence to recommend for or against routine use of IV fluids during cardiac arrest.[85] If hypovolaemia is suspected as a cause of cardiac arrest, an initial bolus of 20 mL/kg should be given via either the IV or the IO route and additional boluses titrated against response.[85]

e-CPR

Extracorporeal membrane oxygenation (ECMO) during CPR (e-CPR) maintains organ perfusion, while reversible causes of cardiac arrest can be identified and corrected.[87] Given that e-CPR is a relatively new therapy, the benefits in cardiac arrest are not well understood and are an area of emerging research.[87] A 2018 ILCOR systematic review of 25 observational studies (15 adult out-of-hospital cardiac arrest; 7 adult in-hospital cardiac arrest; 3 paediatric in-hospital cardiac arrest) showed inconsistent results from individual studies. A number of studies in adult and paediatric in-hospital cardiac arrest appeared to support e-CPR; however, the overall risk of bias for individual studies was critical, largely due to confounding and the overall certainty of evidence was very low.[87] Current ANZCOR recommendations are that e-CPR as rescue therapy for selected patients with cardiac arrest when initial standard CPR is failing in settings where this can be implemented is suggested (weak recommendation, very low quality of evidence).[70] It is also noted that eCPR is a complex intervention and not available in all settings.[70]

TRAUMATIC CARDIAC ARREST

The three most common causes of preventable early death in trauma are airway obstruction, tension pneumothorax and haemorrhage.[88] Unless there are injuries clearly incompatible with life, resuscitation of patients with cardiac arrest should be attempted. The first priority in shocked trauma patients is to stop any obvious bleeding and restoration of circulating volume may have a higher priority than airway and breathing.[88] To manage hypovolaemia, a fluid bolus of 20 mL/kg should be given as rapidly as possible.[88] Patients in cardiac arrest from chest trauma who are not responding to airway opening and restoration of circulating blood volume should have chest decompression.[88] In cardiac arrest due to trauma, haemorrhage control, restoration of circulating volume, airway patency and decompressing tension pneumothorax take priority over conventional CPR unless a medical cause for cardiac arrest is suspected to have preceded the traumatic event.[88] If there are enough resources available, conventional CPR should occur simultaneously if it does not interfere with resuscitative procedures.[88]

ADDITIONAL PROCEDURES—PERICARDIOCENTESIS AND CHEST DECOMPRESSION

There are a number of procedures that may be undertaken during resuscitation in an attempt to correct reversible causes of cardiac arrest or to increase the effectiveness of resuscitation.

Pericardial tamponade, where impairment of diastolic filling of the right ventricle due to significant amounts of fluid in the sac surrounding the heart results in decreased cardiac output, is a major cause of obstructive shock. It has predicable clinical features that are not dissimilar to other cardiac-related conditions, such as tension pneumothorax. Patients present with Beck's triad (venous pressure elevation, decline in arterial pressure and muffled heart tones), pulsus paradoxus, Kussmaul's sign and ultimately pulseless electrical activity (PEA) (see Table 14.7). The definitive treatment for this form of shock is pericardiocentesis, coupled with hyperoxygenation. Without this intervention, resuscitation is largely futile.

Thoracostomy is a lifesaving procedure used to treat tension pneumothorax. Finger thoracostomy is the preferred method of chest decompression and involves making a 3–4 cm skin incision over the 4th intercostal space just anterior to the mid-axillary line, followed by blunt dissection to the pleura to allow introduction of a finger into the pleural space. Finger thoracostomy should be followed by insertion of an intercostal catheter if available and connection to an underwater seal drain or one-way valve.[88] Further details regarding chest injuries can be found in Chapter 45.

PRONE CPR

While 'proning' has been used to improve oxygenation in critically ill patients for many years, its use has increased dramatically during the COVID-19 pandemic. The increased use of prone positioning and risk of cardiac arrest in these critically ill patients was the impetus for a 2021 ILCOR systematic review on prone CPR and/or defibrillation.[90] The systematic review identified 29 case reports (32 individual cases), two prospective observational studies, and two simulation studies.[90] The two observational studies (17 patients who were declared dead in the supine position) reported higher mean systolic blood pressure from CPR in the prone position (72 mmHg versus 48 mmHg, $p < 0.005$; 79 ± 20 mmHg vs 55 ± 20 mmHg, $p = 0.028$). One simulation study reported prone position was

TABLE 14.5 DRUGS USED IN RESUSCITATION[3,7,85,86]

	ADRENALINE	AMIODARONE	ATROPINE	SODIUM BICARBONATE
Presentation	β	150 mg/3 mL ampoules	600 microg/1 mL ampoules 1 mg/10 mL 'mini-jet'	8.4 g (100 mmol)/100 mL vials (each mL contains 1 mmol each of sodium and bicarbonate)
Actions	Naturally occurring catecholamine with alpha (α) and beta (β) adrenergic effects Causes peripheral vasoconstriction (α effects) directing cardiac output to the brain and myocardium Is thought to facilitate defibrillation by improving myocardial blood flow during CPR	Class III antiarrhythmic drug Has effects on sodium, potassium and calcium channels, as well as alpha (α) and beta (β) adrenergic blocking effects Lowers defibrillation threshold and has antifibrillation effects	Parasympathetic antagonist that blocks the action of the vagus nerve on the heart Increases automaticity and rate of conduction at SA and AV nodes	An alkalising solution which combines with H^+ ions to form carbonic acid (H_2CO_3) which then breaks down to CO_2 and H_2O Theoretically reverses metabolic acidosis that is associated with profound or prolonged ischaemia The need for sodium bicarbonate in cardiac arrest should be avoided by early and effective BLS
Evidence review	Currently there is no evidence that high-dose adrenaline improves long-term outcomes following cardiac arrest or that ETT-administered adrenaline is effective	There is no conclusive evidence that antiarrhythmic medications during cardiac arrest improve survival-to-discharge rates	There is insufficient evidence to support or refute the use of atropine in cardiac arrest to improve survival to hospital discharge	Currently there is no strong evidence that supports the use of alkalinising agents in cardiac arrest Routine use of sodium bicarbonate in cardiac arrest is not recommended
Indications	VF/pulseless VT in conjunction with defibrillation Asystole/PEA as initial treatment	VF/pulseless VT when defibrillation and adrenaline have failed to revert arrhythmia Prophylaxis of recurrent VF/ VT	Asystole Severe symptomatic bradycardia	Hyperkalaemia Documented metabolic acidosis Overdose of tricyclic antidepressants Prolonged arrest (> 15 minutes) as the likelihood of acidosis is increased
Adverse effects	Tachyarrhythmias Increased oxygen requirements Severe hypertension post resuscitation Tissue necrosis if extravasation occurs	Hypotension Bradycardia Heart block	Tachycardia Delirium, hyperthermia in large doses	Alkalosis Hypernatraemia Hyperosmolarity Risk of intracellular acidosis as CO_2 liberated from sodium bicarbonate enters cells If sodium bicarbonate is mixed with adrenaline or calcium, precipitation occurs causing both drugs to be inactivated and block IV lines
Dose	Adult	Adult	Adult	Adult
	IV dose: 1.0 mg repeated at regular intervals (every 2nd cycle)	300 mg IV; an additional dose of 150 mg may be considered May be followed by an infusion once return of spontaneous circulation is achieved	IV dose (asystole): 1 mg repeated to a maximum of 3 mg	IV dose: 1 mmol/kg given over 2–3 minutes; should be guided by arterial blood gases
	Paediatric	Paediatric	Paediatric	Paediatric
	IV or IO: 10 microg/kg	5 mg/kg Amiodarone is incompatible with normal saline, so needs to be diluted in 10–20 mL 5% dextrose	IV or IO dose: 20 microg/kg	IV or IO dose: 1.0 mmol/kg

AV: atrioventricular; CPR: cardiopulmonary resuscitation; ETT: endotracheal tube; H^+: hydrogen ion; IO: intraosseous; IV: intravenous; SA: sinoatrial; VF: ventricular fibrillation; VT: ventricular tachycardia.

TABLE 14.6 ELECTROLYTES USED IN RESUSCITATION[3,85,86]

	POTASSIUM	MAGNESIUM	CALCIUM
Presentation	10 mmol/100 mL bags potassium chloride (KCl)	10 mmol/5 mL ampoules magnesium sulfate ($MgSO_4$)	2.2 mmol/10 mL ampoules calcium gluconate 5 mmol/5 mL ampoules calcium chloride
Actions	An electrolyte essential for membrane stability ↓ K^+ causes ventricular dysrhythmias especially in the presence of ↓ Mg^{2+} and digoxin	An electrolyte essential for membrane stability ↓ Mg^{2+} causes myocardial hyperexcitability, especially in the presence of ↓ K^+ and digoxin	Essential for normal muscle and nerve activity Causes a transient increase in myocardial excitability, contractility and peripheral resistance
Evidence review	Not available	Several studies into the effect of magnesium on cardiac arrest have had contradictory results, so currently there is little evidence to support the routine use of magnesium in cardiac arrest	Routine administration of calcium in cardiac arrest is not recommended Calcium is seldom indicated in the management of cardiac arrest *unless* there is evidence that cardiac arrest is associated with hyperkalaemia, hypocalcaemia or calcium channel blocker toxicity
Indications	Persistent VF Documented hypokalaemia	Torsades de pointes Cardiac arrest associated with digoxin toxicity VF/pulseless VT when defibrillation and adrenaline have failed to revert dysrhythmia Documented hypokalaemia Documented hypomagnesaemia	Hyperkalaemia Hypocalcaemia Overdose of calcium channel blockers
Adverse effects	Inappropriate or excessive use may cause hyperkalaemia which may result in bradycardia, hypotension and asystole Tissue necrosis if extravasation occurs	Hypotension Heart block Muscle weakness and respiratory failure	May mediate cell damage causing possible increase in myocardial and cerebral injury Digoxin causes an increase in intracellular calcium, so calcium should be given with caution in the setting of known or suspected digoxin toxicity Tissue necrosis if extravasation occurs
Dose	Adult	Adult	Adult
	IV dose: 5 mmol KCl	IV dose: 5 mmol $MgSO_4$	IV dose: 5–10 mL calcium chloride IV dose: 10 mL calcium gluconate
	Paediatric	Paediatric	Paediatric
	IV or IO dose: 0.03–0.07 mmol/kg KCl	IV or IO dose: 0.1–0.2 mmol/kg $MgSO_4$	IV or IO dose: 0.2 mL/kg 10% calcium chloride IV or IO dose: 0.7 mL/kg 10% calcium gluconate (20 mg/kg)

IO: intraosseous; IV: intravenous; KCl: potassium chloride; K^+: potassium ions; Mg^{2+}: magnesium ions; $MgSO_4$: magnesium sulfate; VF: ventricular fibrillation.

TABLE 14.7 COMPARISON OF PERICARDIAL TAMPONADE AND TENSION PNEUMOTHORAX[89]

CLINICAL FEATURE	PERICARDIAL TAMPONADE	TENSION PNEUMOTHORAX
Presenting condition	Shock	Respiratory distress
Neck veins	Distended	Distended
Trachea	Midline	Deviated
Breath sounds	Bilaterally equal	Diminished on the side of the injury
Chest percussion	Normal	Hyper-resonant on the side of the injury
Heart sounds	Muffled	Normal

associated with reduced time to defibrillation.[90] ROSC, survival to discharge or 30 days were reported in case reports of both adults and children.[90] Therefore, prone CPR and/or defibrillation may not be plausible if changing the patient to a supine position is not possible or too difficult.[90]

RESUSCITATION QUALITY AND QUALITY IMPROVEMENT

There are a number of modalities that can be used to optimise the quality of resuscitation both in terms of quality of real-time CPR during cardiac arrest or from a systems improvement perspective.

CPR feedback devices

CPR feedback devices during real-time CPR are intended to improve CPR quality and thereby improve the chances of ROSC and ultimately survival.[67] CPR feedback devices can have audio and visual components, such as voice prompts, metronomes, visual dials, numerical displays, waveforms, verbal prompts and visual alarms. Visual displays enable rescuers to see chest compression quality parameters, such as depth, rate and recoil in real time. Audio prompts may guide CPR rate or may give audible prompts to rescuers. There is no high-level evidence that the use of CPR feedback devices during real-time CPR improves survival or return of spontaneous circulation.[67,70] There are some studies that have shown improved CPR quality, none of which are of high quality.[67,70] Current recommendations are that CPR feedback devices may be considered as part of a broader system of care and component of CPR quality improvement initiatives, rather than as an isolated intervention.[67,70]

Waveform capnography (end-tidal carbon dioxide)

Waveform capnography has a number of advantages during CPR in addition to confirming endotracheal tube placement as discussed.[70] Waveform capnography is an objective method of monitoring ventilation rates and assisting clinicians to avoid overventilation. Waveform capnography enables assessment of chest compression quality with higher end-tidal carbon dioxide ($EtCO_2$) values indicative of adequate chest compressions. Further, an increase in $EtCO_2$ is an early indicator of return of spontaneous circulation.[70] $EtCO_2$ of less than 10 mmHg after 20 minutes of CPR has been associated with poor outcomes in observational studies; however, current recommendations are that $EtCO_2$ values should not be used in isolation when making decisions to continue or stop resuscitation.[70] Refer to Chapter 16 for further information on its use.

Arterial blood gases

Current evidence suggests that arterial blood gases (ABGs) are an inaccurate indicator of the degree of tissue acidosis during cardiac arrest.[70] ABGs provide an indication of degree of hypoxaemia and metabolic acidosis and arterial CO_2 is an indicator of adequacy of ventilation during CPR. ABG sampling also enables rapid determination of electrolyte levels, including potassium, calcium and magnesium. ABG sampling should not interfere with provision of effective CPR, nor should it interrupt chest compressions.[70] Refer to Chapter 16 for information on ABG collection and sampling.

POST-EVENT DEBRIEFING

Debriefing is defined as a post-event discussion in which aspects of resuscitation performance are analysed with the intent of improving future resuscitation performance.[91] Although there is no high certainty evidence regarding performance-focused debriefing, the 2020 ILCOR consensus on science and treatment recommendations showed that performance-focused debriefing had no significant effect on survival with favourable neurological outcome, but significantly improved survival to hospital discharge and ROSC when compared to no debriefing.[91] Further, debriefing did appear to significantly improve components of chest compression depth but not chest compression rate or fraction.[91] Therefore, data-driven, performance-focused debriefing of rescuers after out-of-hospital and in-hospital cardiac arrest is suggested for adults and children (weak recommendation, very low-certainty evidence).[91]

EDUCATION, TRAINING AND EXPOSURE

The importance of education and training, and real-life exposure to resuscitation, is receiving considerable interest in the medical literature. A 2020 ILCOR consensus on science and treatment recommendation suggested that emergency medical services should monitor their clinical personnel's exposure to resuscitation and implement strategies to address low exposure or ensure that treating teams have members with recent exposure (weak recommendation, very-low certainty of evidence).[91] The recommendation reflects growing evidence that increasing team exposure to resuscitation is associated with better patient outcomes, including survival to hospital discharge.[92]

In some regions, exposure to resuscitation is declining and may be as low as one attempted resuscitation annually for the average paramedic.[93] There is evidence from randomised controlled trials and observational studies that education and training directed at the mastery of resuscitation skills can help improve skill retention and CPR quality and reduce errors of omission.[94] Similarly, data from observational studies indicate that prior participation in an accredited ALS course by at least one member of the resuscitation team has been shown to improve the likelihood of ROSC and survival to hospital discharge after cardiac arrest.[95]

POST-RESUSCITATION CARE

It is important to recognise that resuscitation is an ongoing process which does not stop when the patient exhibits return of spontaneous circulation.[96,97] The majority of deaths following resuscitation are due to hypoxic brain injury or myocardial injury: the risk of these adverse events can be minimised by the delivery of structured, evidence-based, post-resuscitation care.[96,97] The post-resuscitation care delivered by paramedics and emergency nurses has a profound impact on patient outcomes.[96,97]

Post-cardiac arrest syndrome is a unique and complex combination of the following pathophysiological processes: 1) brain injury, 2) myocardial dysfunction, 3) systemic response to reperfusion and 4) residual issues related to the cause of cardiac arrest.[67,98] There is a growing body of evidence showing that post-cardiac arrest syndrome has a significant impact on mortality and morbidity.[67,98] Protocols for the structured and standardised management of patients who have suffered cardiac arrest have been shown to improve outcomes. The aims of post-resuscitation care are to continue respiratory support, maintain cerebral perfusion, treat and prevent cardiac arrhythmias and determine and treat the cause of the arrest.[98] Factors known to reduce the impact of post-cardiac arrest syndrome include:[67,98]

- active temperature control (or fever prevention at a minimum), blood pressure control, airway protection and ventilation, oxygenation and seizure control to limit brain injury
- blood pressure control, intravenous fluids, inotropic support and in some cases intra-aortic balloon pump (IBP) or extra corporeal membrane oxygenation (ECMO) to minimise myocardial dysfunction
- blood pressure control, vasopressors, active temperature control, glucose control and early administration of antibiotics if evidence of infection to limit the systemic response to reperfusion
- strategies, such as early reperfusion, percutaneous coronary intervention (PCI), fibrinolysis, management of traumatic injury and antidote therapy, to address residual issues related to the cause of cardiac arrest.

PRACTICE TIP

POST-RESUSCITATION CARE

The aims of post-resuscitation care are to:[96-98]

- continue respiratory support and maintain adequate oxygenation
- maintain cerebral perfusion by restoration and maintenance of adequate blood pressure
- prevent and treat cardiac dysrhythmias
- identify and treat the cause of cardiac arrest:
  - hypoxaemia
  - hypovolaemia-hypo- or hyperkalaemia
  - hypo- or hyperthermia
  - pericardial tamponade
  - tension pneumothorax
  - toxins/poisons/drugs
  - thrombosis: pulmonary embolism or acute myocardial infarction.

Ventilation should continue via an endotracheal tube in the immediate post-arrest period. Arterial blood gases should be taken as a guide to pH, PaO_2 and $PaCO_2$. PaO_2 and $PaCO_2$ should be maintained at normal levels. Hypoxaemia, hyperoxia and hypocapnia should be avoided.[96,97] ABGs should be used to monitor ventilation in the immediate post-resuscitation period, rather than $EtCO_2$ levels.[96] Systolic blood pressure should be at least 100 mmHg and hypotension should be treated with inotropes, vasopressors and/or restoration of circulating volume.[96]

Cardiac monitoring should continue and a 12-lead ECG should be performed to determine if any time-critical re-perfusion is warranted: if there is evidence of ST-segment elevation myocardial infarction (STEMI) or new left bundle branch block (LBBB), PCI is the preferred re-perfusion strategy if primary PCI can be achieved in less than 90 minutes.[96] (Refer to Chapter 16 for further information on cardiac monitoring and how to perform ECGs.) Fibrinolytic therapy is an alternative if there is limited access to primary PCI. Thrombolysis may be indicated for pulmonary embolism. Although there are no studies of the prophylactic use of anti-arrhythmics, if anti-arrhythmic drugs have been given during the resuscitation, it is reasonable to continue those drugs as an infusion.[96]

Hyperglycaemia has been associated with poor neurological outcomes following cardiac arrest.[96] Evidence about the optimal blood glucose level following cardiac arrest is lacking; however, blood glucose should be frequently monitored following cardiac arrest, hypoglycaemia should be avoided and hyperglycaemia (blood glucose $>$ 10 mmol/L) should be treated with insulin.[96] Blood should be taken for serum electrolytes; anticonvulsant drugs may be considered if fitting occurs; and analgesia and/or sedation should be given as required. Complications of resuscitation, such as rib fractures or other injuries, should be assessed and treated, and the location of all tubes and lines placed during resuscitation should be confirmed. It may also be necessary to replace IV lines inserted under emergency conditions. If in a rural or remote location, preparation for transfer will also be required.

ACTIVE TEMPERATURE MANAGEMENT FOLLOWING CARDIAC ARREST

Targeted management following ROSC is an area of evolving evidence. The impetus for use of therapeutic hypothermia as part of post-arrest care was two landmark randomised controlled trials, both published in 2002, showing improved neurological outcomes in patients cooled to a target temperature of 33°C.[99,100] In 2013, a randomised trial of targeted temperature management at either 33°C or 36°C for 28 hours showed no significant differences between the two groups in overall mortality or neurological function or death at 180 days.[101] Unfortunately this study has been interpreted by some as supporting the notion that targeted temperature management is unnecessary in patients following resuscitation from cardiac arrest. In 2021, another randomised trial of hypothermia (target temperature of 33°C for 28 hours) versus targeted normothermia and early treatment of fever ($\geq$ 37.8°C) showed no significant difference in 6-month mortality (50% in hyperthermia group and 48% in normothermia group, p = 0.37).[102] A 2021 ILCOR systematic review and meta-analysis of 32 studies of targeted temperature management had a number of key findings that will inform national and international guidelines.[103] Nine trials comparing a target temperature of 32–34°C versus normothermia (which often required active cooling), showed that targeted temperature management did not result in an improvement in survival or favourable neurologic outcome at 90 to 180 days after the cardiac arrest (low certainty of evidence).[103] Three trials examined different hypothermic temperature targets (32°C versus 34°C, 33°C versus 36°C and 32–33°C versus 34°C) and found no difference in outcomes (survival 90 days – 6 months) (low certainty of evidence).[103] The ten trials that compared pre-hospital cooling versus no pre-hospital cooling showed no improvement in survival or favourable neurologic outcome at hospital discharge (moderate certainty of evidence).[103]

At the time of writing, the ILCOR recommendations were that active fever prevention by targeting a temperature $<$ 37.5°C for patients who remain unconscious after ROSC from cardiac arrest is suggested (weak recommendation, low certainty evidence).[104] Unconscious patients with mild hypothermia after ROSC should not be actively warmed to achieve normothermia (good practice statement),[104] and active fever prevention for at least 72 hours is suggested (good practice statement).[104] The routine use of pre-hospital cooling with rapid infusion of large volumes of cold IV fluid immediately after ROSC is not recommended (strong recommendation, moderate certainty evidence).[104] It is uncertain whether sub-populations of cardiac arrest patients may benefit from targeting hypothermia at 32–34°C.[104]

At the time of writing, the current recommendations are that for patients who remain unconscious following return of spontaneous circulation, targeted temperature management is recommended for those who have suffered out-of-hospital cardiac arrest from a shockable rhythm and suggested for patients who have suffered out-of-hospital cardiac arrest from non-shockable rhythms or in-hospital cardiac arrest.[96,105] Current recommendations are that targeted temperature management should maintain temperature between 32°C and 36°C for at least 24 hours and that fever should be avoided; if fever occurs, it is to be actively treated.[96,105]

WITHHOLDING AND CEASING RESUSCITATION

In Australia and New Zealand, almost 60% of cardiac arrest patients have their resuscitation attempts withheld on arrival of paramedics.[49] Emergency medical services have specific criteria for withholding resuscitation in patients with cardiac arrest, and although these differ nationally, most guidelines recommend withholding resuscitation where there are obvious signs of death (e.g. rigor mortis, morbid lividity, injuries incompatible with life) or where an advance care directive, medical power of attorney or medical treatment decision-maker indicates that resuscitation is not desired.[106] In some regions, resuscitation may also be withheld where the initial presenting rhythm is asystole and there is evidence of prolonged downtime before the commencement of CPR.

After a resuscitation attempt has commenced, as many as 65% of out-of-hospital and 55% of in-hospital cardiac arrest patients do not achieve ROSC.[49,52] Most emergency medical service clinical practice guidelines recommend that paramedics consider ceasing resuscitation after 20–30 minutes of resuscitation (depending on the circumstances) if the patient remains in asystole despite ALS techniques.[106] Terminating or ceasing resuscitation may also be guided by evidence-based criteria. The ILCOR conditionally recommends the use of validated Termination of Resuscitation rules to help guide paramedics in making termination of resuscitation decisions.[107] In the in-hospital setting, cessation of resuscitation should be guided by clinical examination, the clinician's experience, and the patient's condition and wishes.[107]

CARE OF FAMILIES AND FAMILY PRESENCE DURING RESUSCITATION

The majority of studies on family presence during resuscitation are surveys of health professionals aimed at investigating their attitude to having families present during CPR. There are few studies comparing actual family or patient outcomes associated with family presence during resuscitation.[108] In the out-of-hospital environment, paramedics often do not have a choice about whether families are present during resuscitation and in the in-hospital context, families of patients who are undergoing active resuscitation were often excluded from the resuscitation room on the premise that invasive procedures and active resuscitative efforts would be distressing to families and distracting to staff. Over recent years, research findings have suggested that, in fact, witnessing resuscitation is beneficial for families, patients and staff, and that the routine exclusion of families by staff is not supported by evidence.[108]

Current guidelines recommend that families should be offered the choice of being present during the resuscitation of their family member.[108] The decision of family members who choose not to witness resuscitation should be respected and these family members supported. Family members who choose to be present during resuscitation should be accompanied at all times by an experienced member of staff, who should:

- prepare the family prior to entering the resuscitation area (this includes the patient's appearance, number of people in the room and their roles, resuscitative efforts in progress)
- make it clear that resuscitation of the patient is the first priority and that the family will be removed from the room if they are disruptive or combative
- explain interventions and the patient's response to those interventions
- interpret medical and nursing jargon
- provide comfort measures such as tissues or chairs
- give the opportunity for the family to ask questions
- facilitate touching and talking to the patient if possible.

SUMMARY

Prevention of cardiac arrest is one of the most important things that emergency care clinicians can do for their patients, as prevention of cardiac arrest will save more lives than even the best resuscitation. Should cardiac arrest occur, the things that save lives are early CPR, good quality chest compressions and early defibrillation if there is a shockable rhythm. Inadequate compression depth, overventilation and excessive interruptions to chest compressions are ongoing problems in resuscitation, even for experienced healthcare professionals. Defibrillation, oxygenation and ventilation always take priority over medication administration as these are the cornerstones of evidence-based resuscitation. Resuscitation does not stop once there is return of spontaneous circulation and evidence-based post-resuscitation care is vital to patient outcomes.

CASE STUDY

Abe is a 3-year-old boy found by his mother floating face-down in a home swimming pool. It is not known how long he was in the water; he was last seen playing with siblings approximately 20 minutes earlier. When his mother pulled him from the water he was pale, floppy, unconscious and did not appear to be breathing. A neighbour heard Abe's mother screaming and called an ambulance.

When paramedics arrive, Abe's mother is performing cardiopulmonary resuscitation with both chest compressions and mouth-to-mouth ventilation. Paramedics suction Abe's airway and continue with bag–valve–mask ventilation and chest compressions. Application of a cardiac monitor shows a sinus tachycardia of 160 beats/minute; however, Abe has no palpable pulse.

Paramedics achieve return of spontaneous circulation and transport Abe to the emergency department (ED). On arrival, Abe has poor blood pressure and poor peripheral perfusion, so an adrenaline infusion is commenced. He is hypothermic at 29°C so is re-warmed to 33°C. Abe then has a ventricular fibrillation arrest. The ED staff achieve return of spontaneous circulation after administration of adrenaline, amiodarone and defibrillation.

QUESTIONS

1. While the ambulance is en route, what is the best thing that Abe's mother can do to improve the chance of her child's survival?
2. What are the priorities for paramedics in this case?
3. How should paramedics treat Abe?
4. How should ED staff treat Abe?
5. What are the management priorities for Abe now he is in a post-arrest state?

Answers to Case Study Questions can be found on evolve http://evolve.elsevier.com/AU/Curtis/emergency/ 

USEFUL WEBSITES

Australian Resuscitation Council (ARC), represents all major groups involved in the teaching and practice of resuscitation and develops resuscitation guidelines for Australia and New Zealand, www.resus.org.au.

European Resuscitation Council, ERC aims to preserve human life by making high-quality resuscitation available to all, www.erc.edu/.

First2Act, interactive video simulation software that allows students and professionals to practise medical emergency scenarios in an engaging but safe environment, https://first2act.com.

ILCOR (International Liaison Committee on Resuscitation), provides a discussion and coordination of all aspects of cardiopulmonary and cerebral resuscitation worldwide, and, reviewing and sharing international scientific data on resuscitation, www.ilcor.org/home.

REFERENCES

1. Australian Resuscitation Council. ANZCOR guideline 11.4: electrical therapy for adult advanced life support. Melbourne: Australian Resuscitation Council; 2016. Online. Available from: www.resus.org.au.
2. Australian Resuscitation Council. ANZCOR guideline 12.1: Paediatric Basic Life Support (PBLS) for health professionals. Melbourne: Australian Resuscitation Council; 2021. Online. Available from: www.resus.org.au.
3. Australian Resuscitation Council. ANZCOR guideline 12.2: Paediatric Advanced Life Support (PALS). Melbourne: Australian Resuscitation Council; 2021. Online. Available from: www.resus.org.au.
4. Inoue M, Tohira H, Williams T, Bailey P, Borland M, McKenzie N, et al. Incidence, characteristics and survival outcomes of out-of-hospital cardiac arrest in children and adolescents between 1997 and 2014 in Perth, Western Australia. Emerg Med Australas 2017;29(1):69–76.
5. Nehme Z, Namachivayam S, Forrest A, Butt W, Bernard S, Smith K. Trends in the incidence and outcome of paediatric out-of-hospital cardiac arrest: a 17-year observational study. Resuscitation 2018;128:43–50.
6. Australian Resuscitation Council. ANZCOR guideline 8: cardiopulmonary resuscitation. Melbourne: Australian Resuscitation Council; 2021. Online. Available from: www.resus.org.au.
7. Australian Resuscitation Council. ANZCOR guideline 11.2: protocols for adult advanced life support. Melbourne: Australian Resuscitation Council; 2018. Online. Available from: www.resus.org.au.
8. Nehme Z, Andrew E, Bray JE, Cameron P, Bernard S, Meredith IT, et al. The significance of pre-arrest factors in out-of-hospital cardiac arrests witnessed by emergency medical services: a report from the Victorian Ambulance Cardiac Arrest Registry. Resuscitation 2015;88:35–42.
9. Nishiyama C, Iwami T, Kawamura T, Kitamura T, Tanigawa K, Sakai T, et al. Prodromal symptoms of out-of-hospital cardiac arrests: a report from a large-scale population-based cohort study. Resuscitation 2013;84(5):558–63.

10. Cretikos M, Chen J, Hillman K, Bellomo R, Finfer S, Flabouris A, et al. The objective medical emergency team activation criteria: a case-control study. Resuscitation 2007;73(1):62–72.
11. Cretikos MA, Bellomo R, Hillman K, Chen J, Finfer S, Flabouris A. Respiratory rate: the neglected vital sign. Med J Aust 2008;188:657–9.
12. Fieselmann J, Hendryx M, Helms C, Wakefield DS. Respiratory rate predicts cardiopulmonary arrest for internal medicine inpatients. J Gen Int Med 1993;8(7):354–60.
13. Considine J, Currey J. Ensuring a proactive, evidence-based, patient safety approach to patient assessment. J Clin Nurs 2015;24(1-2):300–7.
14. Curtis K, Murphy M, Hoy S, Lewis MJ. The emergency nursing assessment process—a structured framework for a systematic approach. Australas Emerg Nurs J 2009;12(4):130–6.
15. Jones D, Bhasale A, Bailey M, Pilcher D, Anstey MH. Effect of a national standard for deteriorating patients on intensive care admissions due to cardiac arrest in Australia. Crit Care Med 2018;46(4):586–93. doi:10.1097/CCM.0000000000002951.
16. Martin C, Jones D, Wolfe R. State-wide reduction in in-hospital cardiac complications in association with the introduction of a national standard for recognising deteriorating patients. Resuscitation 2017;121:172–8.
17. Yeung J, Matsuyama T, Bray J, Reynolds J, Skrifvars MB. Does care at a cardiac arrest centre improve outcome after out-of-hospital cardiac arrest? – A systematic review. Resuscitation 2019;137:102–15.
18. Australian Resuscitation Council. ANZCOR guideline 14.3: acute coronary syndromes: reperfusion strategy. Melbourne: Australian Resuscitation Council; 2016. Online. Available from: www.resus.org.au.
19. Maharaj R, Raffaele I, Wendon J. Rapid response systems: a systematic review and meta-analysis. Crit Care 2015;19(1):254.
20. Rocha HAL, Alcântara ACdC, Rocha SGMO, Toscano CM. Effectiveness of rapid response teams in reducing intrahospital cardiac arrests and deaths: a systematic review and meta-analysis. Rev Bras Ter Intensiva 2018;30(3):366–75.
21. Jones DA, DeVita MA, Bellomo R. Rapid-response teams. New Eng J Med 2011;365(2):139–46.
22. Tirkkonen J, Tamminen T, Skrifvars MB. Outcome of adult patients attended by rapid response teams: a systematic review of the literature. Resuscitation 2017;112:43–52.
23. Sprogis SK, Currey J, Jones D, Considine J. Use of the pre-medical emergency team tier of rapid response systems: a scoping review. Intens Crit Care Nurs 2021;65:103041.
24. Considine J, Fry M, Curtis K, Shaban RZ. Systems for recognition and response to deteriorating emergency department patients: a scoping review. Scan J Trauma Resusc Emerg Med 2021;29(1):69. doi:10.1186/s13049-021-00882-6.
25. Considine J, Jones D. Rapid response systems and the emergency department. In: Cameron P, Little M, Mitra B, Deasy C, editors. Textbook of adult emergency medicine e-book. Edinburgh: Elsevier Health Sciences; 2019.
26. Considine J, Rhodes K, Jones D, Currey J. Systems for recognition and response to clinical deterioration in Victorian emergency departments. Australas Emerg Care 2018;21(1):3–7.
27. Bourke-Matas E, Bosley E, Gowens P, Smith K, Bowles KN. Defining and recognising clinical deterioration in the prehospital setting (PRECLuDE study): a systematic scoping review. Irish J Paramed 2020;5(1). doi:10.32378/ijp.v5i1.245.
28. Patel R, Nugawela MD, Edwards HB, Richards A, Le Roux H, Pullyblank A, et al. Can early warning scores identify deteriorating patients in pre-hospital settings? A systematic review. Resuscitation 2018;132:101–11.
29. Royal College of Physicians. National Early Warning Score (NEWS) 2: standardising the assessment of acute-illness severity in the NHS. London: Royal College of Physicians; 2017. Online. Available from: www.rcplondon.ac.uk/projects/outputs/national-early-warning-score-news-2.
30. Considine J, Jones D, Pilcher D, Currey J. Patient physiological status during emergency care and rapid response team or cardiac arrest team activation during early hospital admission. Euro J Emerg Med 2017;24(5):359–65.
31. Curtis K, Munroe B, Fry M. The implementation of an emergency nursing framework (HIRAID) reduces patient deterioration: a multi-centre quasi-experimental study. Int Emerg Nurs 2021;56:100976.
32. Considine J, Jones D, Pilcher D, Currey J. Patient physiological status at the emergency department - ward interface and emergency calls for clinical deterioration during early hospital admission. J Adv Nurs 2016;72(6):1287–300.
33. McCarthy G. Shock overview. In: Cameron P, Little M, Mitra B, Deasy C, editors. Adult textbook of emergency medicine. 5th ed. Sydney: Elsevier; 2020.
34. Alimenti D, Buydos S, Cunliffe L, Hunt A. Improving perceptions of patient safety through standardizing handoffs from the emergency department to the inpatient setting: a systematic review. J Am Assoc Nurse Pract 2019;31(6):354–63.
35. Müller M, Jürgens J, Redaèlli M, Klingberg K, Hautz WE, Stock S. Impact of the communication and patient hand-off tool SBAR on patient safety: a systematic review. BMJ Open 2018;8(8):e022202.
36. Maddry JK, Simon EM, Reeves LK, Mora AG, Clemons MA, Shults NM, et al. Impact of a standardized patient hand-off tool on communication between emergency medical services personnel and emergency department staff. Prehosp Emerg Care 2020;25(4):530–8.
37. Haig KM, Sutton S, Whittington J. SBAR: a shared mental model for improving communication between clinicians. Jt Comm J Qual Patient Saf 2006;32(3):167–75.
38. Marshall S, Harrison J, Flanagan B. The teaching of a structured tool improves the clarity and content of interprofessional clinical communication. Qual Saf Health Care 2009;18(2):137–40.
39. Sameera V, Bindra A, Rath GP. Human errors and their prevention in healthcare. J Anaesthesiol Clin Pharmacol 2021;37(3):328–35.

40. Stewart-Parker E, Galloway R, Vig S. S-TEAMS: a truly multiprofessional course focusing on nontechnical skills to improve patient safety in the operating theater. J Surg Ed 2017;74(1):137–44.
41. Bishop R, Porges C, Carlisle M, Strickland R. Crisis resource management in medicine: a clarion call for change. Curr Treat Options Pediat 2020;6(4):299–316.
42. Reznek MA, Lei C, Yashar MD. Crisis resource management. In: Strother C, Okuda Y, Wong N, editors. Comprehensive healthcare simulation: emergency medicine. Cham Switzerland: Springer International Publishing; 2021.
43. Rowland M, Adefuye AO, Vincent-Lambert C. The need for purposeful teaching, learning and assessment of crisis resource management principles and practices in the undergraduate pre-hospital emergency care curriculum: a narrative literature review. Australas J Paramed 2021;18: doi.org/10.33151/ajp.18.820.
44. Fanning RM, Goldhaber-Fiebert SN, Udani AD. Crisis resource management. In: Demaria S, Levine A, Sim A, Schwartz A, editors. The comprehensive textbook of healthcare simulation. New York: Springer; 2013.
45. Nehme Z, Ball J, Stephenson M, Walker T, Stub D, Smith K. Effect of a resuscitation quality improvement programme on outcomes from out-of-hospital cardiac arrest. Resuscitation 2021;162:236–44.
46. Hopkins CL, Burk C, Moser S, Meersman J, Baldwin C, Youngquist ST. Implementation of pit crew approach and cardiopulmonary resuscitation metrics for out-of-hospital cardiac arrest improves patient survival and neurological outcome. J Am Heart Assoc 2016;5(1):e002892.
47. Pearson DA, Darrell Nelson R, Monk L, Tyson C, Jollis JG, Granger CB, et al. Comparison of team-focused CPR vs standard CPR in resuscitation from out-of-hospital cardiac arrest: Results from a statewide quality improvement initiative. Resuscitation 2016;105:165–72.
48. Beck B, Bray J, Smith K, Walker T, Grantham H, Hein C, et al. Establishing the Aus-ROC Australian and New Zealand out-of-hospital cardiac arrest Epistry. BMJ Open 2016;6(4):e011027.
49. Bray J, Howell S, Ball S, Lester W, Morton S, Coleman J, et al. The epidemiology of out-of-hospital cardiac arrest in Australia and New Zealand: a binational report from the Australasian Resuscitation Outcomes Consortium (Aus-ROC). Resuscitation 2022;172:74–83.
50. Smith K, Andrew E, Lijovic M, Nehme Z, Bernard S. Quality of life and functional outcomes 12 months after out-of-hospital cardiac arrest. Circulation 2015;131(2):174–81.
51. Andrew E, Mercier E, Nehme Z, Bernard S, Smith K. Long-term functional recovery and health-related quality of life of elderly out-of-hospital cardiac arrest survivors. Resuscitation 2018;126:118–24.
52. Fennessy G, Hilton A, Radford S, Bellomo R, Jones D. The epidemiology of in-hospital cardiac arrests in Australia and New Zealand. Intern Med J 2016;46(10):1172–81.
53. Australia and New Zealand Cardiac Arrest Outcome and Determinants of ECMO (ANZ-CODE) Investigators, Determinants of ECMO (ANZ-CODE) Investigators. The epidemiology of in-hospital cardiac arrests in Australia: a prospective multicentre observational study. Crit Care and Resuscitation 2019;21(3):180–7.
54. Australian Resuscitation Council. ANZCOR guideline 11.1: introduction to and principles of in-hospital resuscitation. Melbourne: Australian Resuscitation Council; 2019. Online. Available from: www.resus.org.au.
55. Australian Resuscitation Council. ANZCOR guideline 2: managing an emergency. Melbourne: Australian Resuscitation Council; 2021. Online. Available from: www.resus.org.au.
56. Maguire B. Violence against ambulance personnel: a retrospective cohort study of national data from Safe Work Australia. Pub Health Res Prac 2018;28(1):e28011805.
57. Maguire BJ, O'Meara PF, Brightwell RF, O'Neill BJ, Fitzgerald GJ. Occupational injury risk among Australian paramedics: an analysis of national data. Med J Aust 2014;200(8):477–80.
58. Couper K, Taylor-Phillips S, Grove A, Freeman K, Osokogu O, Court R, et al. COVID-19 in cardiac arrest and infection risk to rescuers: a systematic review. Resuscitation 2020;151:59–66.
59. Tran K, Cimon K, Severn M, Pessoa-Silva CL, Conly J. Aerosol generating procedures and risk of transmission of acute respiratory infections to healthcare workers: a systematic review. PLoS ONE 2012;7(4):e35797.
60. Fragkou PC, Dimopoulou D, Latsios G, Koudounis P, Synetos A, Dimopoulou A, et al. Transmission of infections during cardiopulmonary resuscitation. Clin Microbiol Rev 2021;34(4):e0001821.
61. Australian Resuscitation Council. ANZCOR guideline 4: airway. Melbourne: Australian Resuscitation Council; 2021. Online. Available from: www.resus.org.au.
62. Australian Resuscitation Council. ANZCOR guideline 3: recognition and first aid management of the unconscious victim. Melbourne: Australian Resuscitation Council; 2021. Online. Available from: www.resus.org.au.
63. Australian Resuscitation Council. ANZCOR choking flowchart (Management of Foreign Body Airway Obstruction). Melbourne: Australian Resuscitation Council; 2016. Online. Available from: www.resus.org.au.
64. Australian Resuscitation Council. ANZCOR guideline 5: breathing. Melbourne: Australian Resuscitation Council; 2021. Online. Available from: www.resus.org.au.
65. National COVID-19 Clinical Evidence Taskforce. Cardiopulmonary resuscitation of adults with COVID-19 in healthcare settings. Melbourne, Australia: National COVID-19 Clinical Evidence Taskforce; 2021. Online. Available from: covid19evidence.net.au/.
66. Australian Resuscitation Council. ANZCOR guideline 6: compressions. Melbourne: Australian Resuscitation Council; 2021. Online. Available from: www.resus.org.au.

67. Olasveengen TM, Mancini ME, Perkins GD, Avis S, Brooks S, Castrén M, et al. Adult basic life support: 2020 international consensus on cardiopulmonary resuscitation and emergency cardiovascular care science with treatment recommendations. Circulation 2020;142 (16 – suppl 1):S41–91.
68. Australian Resuscitation Council. ANZCOR basic life support flowchart. Melbourne: Australian Resuscitation Council; 2021. Online. Available from: www.resus.org.au.
69. Neth MR, Idris A, Mcmullan J, Benoit JL, Daya MR. A review of ventilation in adult out-of-hospital cardiac arrest. J Am Coll Emerg Phys Open 2020;1(3):190–201.
70. Australian Resuscitation Council. ANZCOR guideline 11.6: equipment and techniques in adult advanced life support. Melbourne: Australian Resuscitation Council; 2016. Online. Available from: www.resus.org.au.
71. Considine J, Gazmuri RJ, Perkins GD, Kudenchuk PJ, Olasveengen TM, Vaillancourt C, et al. Chest compression components (rate, depth, chest wall recoil and leaning): a scoping review. Resuscitation 2020;146:188–202.
72. Australian Resuscitation Council. ANZCOR guideline 7: External Automated Defibrillation (AED) in Basic Life Support (BLS). Melbourne: Australian Resuscitation Council; 2021. Online. Available from: www.resus.org.au.
73. Koster RW, Sayre MR, Botha M, Cave DM, Cudnik MT, Handley AJ, et al. Part 5: adult basic life support: 2010 International consensus on cardiopulmonary resuscitation and emergency cardiovascular care science with treatment recommendations. Resuscitation 2010;81(1):e48–70.
74. Australian Resuscitation Council. ANZCOR adult cardiorespiratory arrest flowchart. Melbourne: Australian Resuscitation Council; 2016. Online. Available from: www.resus.org.au.
75. Australian Resuscitation Council. ANZCOR paediatric cardiorespiratory arrest flowchart. Melbourne: Australian Resuscitation Council; 2016. Online. Available from: www.resus.org.au.
76. Krieser D, Nguyen K, Kerr D, Jolley D, Clooney M, Kelly AM. Parental weight estimation of their child's weight is more accurate than other weight estimation methods for determining children's weight in an emergency department? Emerg Med J 2007;24(11):756–9.
77. Wells M, Goldstein LN, Bentley A, Basnett S, Monteith I. The accuracy of the Broselow tape as a weight estimation tool and a drug-dosing guide—a systematic review and meta-analysis. Resuscitation 2017;121:9–33.
78. Granfeldt A, Avis SR, Nicholson TC, Holmberg MJ, Moskowitz A, Coker A, et al. Advanced airway management during adult cardiac arrest: a systematic review. Resuscitation 2019;139:133–43.
79. Jabre P, Penaloza A, Pinero D, Duchateau FX, Borron SW, Javaudin F, et al. Effect of bag-mask ventilation vs endotracheal intubation during cardiopulmonary resuscitation on neurological outcome after out-of-hospital cardiorespiratory arrest. JAMA 2018;319(8):779.
80. Benger JR, Kirby K, Black S, Brett SJ, Clout M, Lazaroo MJ, et al. Effect of a strategy of a supraglottic airway device vs tracheal intubation during out-of-hospital cardiac arrest on functional outcome. JAMA 2018;320(8):779.
81. Wang HE, Schmicker RH, Daya MR, Stephens SW, Idris AH, Carlson JN, et al. Effect of a strategy of initial laryngeal tube insertion vs endotracheal intubation on 72-hour survival in adults with out-of-hospital cardiac arrest. JAMA 2018;320(8):769–78.
82. Soar J, Berg KM, Andersen LW, Böttiger BW, Cacciola S, Callaway CW, et al. Adult Advanced Life Support: 2020 International consensus on cardiopulmonary resuscitation and emergency cardiovascular care science with treatment recommendations. Resuscitation 2020;156:A80–119.
83. Queensland Ambulance Service. Clinical practice guideline: oropharyngeal airway insertion. Brisbane: Queensland Ambulance Service; 2018. Online. Available from: www.ambulance.qld.gov.au/docs/clinical/cpp/CPP_Oropharyngeal%20airway%20insertion.pdf.
84. Johnson M, Miskovic A, Ray S, Chong K, Hickson M, Bingham B, et al. The nasopharyngeal airway: estimation of the nares-to-mandible and nares-to-tragus distance in young children to assess current clinical practice. Resuscitation 2019;140:50–4.
85. Australian Resuscitation Council. ANZCOR guideline 11.5: medications in adult cardiac arrest. Melbourne: Australian Resuscitation Council; 2016. Online. Available from: www.resus.org.au.
86. Australian Resuscitation Council. ANZCOR guideline 12.3: management of other (non-arrerst) arrhythmias in infants and children. Melbourne: Australian Resuscitation Council; 2021. Online. Available from: www.resus.org.au.
87. Holmberg MJ, Geri G, Wiberg S, Guerguerian AM, Donnino MW, Nolan JP, et al. Extracorporeal cardiopulmonary resuscitation for cardiac arrest: a systematic review. Resuscitation 2018;131:91–100.
88. Australian Resuscitation Council. ANZCOR guideline 11.10.1: management of cardiac arrest due to trauma. Melbourne: Australian Resuscitation Council; 2016. Online. Available from: www.resus.org.au.
89. American Academy of Orthopaedic Surgeons, Pollak AN, Elling B, Aehlert B. Nancy Caroline's emergency care in the streets. Burlington MA: Jones and Bartlett Learning; 2018.
90. Hsu CH, Considine J, Pawar RD, Lassen AT, Moskowitz A. Cardiopulmonary resuscitation and defibrillation for cardiac arrest when patients are in the prone position: a systematic review. Resuscitation Plus 2021;8:100186.
91. Greif R, Bhanji F, Bigham BL, Bray J, Breckwoldt J, Cheng A, et al. Education, implementation, and teams. Resuscitation 2020;156:A188–239.
92. Bray J, Nehme Z, Nguyen A, Lockey A, Finn J. A systematic review of the impact of emergency medical service practitioner experience and exposure to out of hospital cardiac arrest on patient outcomes. Resuscitation 2020;155:134–42.
93. Dyson K, Bray J, Smith K, Bernard S, Straney L, Finn J. Paramedic exposure to out-of-hospital cardiac arrest is rare and declining in Victoria, Australia. Resuscitation 2015;89:93–8.
94. Donoghue A, Navarro K, Diederich E, Auerbach M, Cheng A. Deliberate practice and mastery learning in resuscitation education: a scoping review. Resuscitation Plus 2021;6:100137.

95. Lockey A, Lin Y, Cheng A. Impact of adult advanced cardiac life support course participation on patient outcomes—a systematic review and meta-analysis. Resuscitation 2018;129:48–54.

96. Australian Resuscitation Council. ANZCOR guideline 11.7: post-resuscitation therapy in adult advanced life support. Melbourne: Australian Resuscitation Council; 2016. Online. Available from: www.resus.org.au.

97. Australian Resuscitation Council. ANZCOR guideline 12.5: Management after Return of Spontaneous Circulation (ROSC). Melbourne: Australian Resuscitation Council; 2021. Online. Available from: www.resus.org.au.

98. Nolan JP, Sandroni C, Böttiger BW, Cariou A, Cronberg T, Friberg H, et al. European Resuscitation Council and European Society of Intensive Care Medicine Guidelines 2021: post-resuscitation care. Resuscitation 2021;161:220–69.

99. Bernard SA, Gray TW, Buist MD, Jones BM, Silvester W, Gutteridge G, et al. Treatment of comatose survivors of out-of-hospital cardiac arrest with induced hypothermia. New Eng J Med 2002;346(8):557–63.

100. The Hypothermia after Cardiac Arrest Study Group. Mild therapeutic hypothermia to improve the neurologic outcome after cardiac arrest. New Eng J Med 2002;346(8):549–56.

101. Nielsen N, Wetterslev J, Cronberg T, Erlinge D, Gasche Y, Hassager C, et al. Targeted temperature management at 33°C versus 36°C after cardiac arrest. New Eng J Med 2013;369(23):2197–206.

102. Dankiewicz J, Cronberg T, Lilja G, Jakobsen JC, Levin H, Ullén S, et al. Hypothermia versus normothermia after out-of-hospital cardiac arrest. New Eng J Med 2021;384(24):2283–94.

103. Granfeldt A, Holmberg MJ, Nolan JP, Soar J, Andersen LW. Targeted temperature management in adult cardiac arrest: systematic review and meta-analysis. Resuscitation 2021;167:160–72.

104. Soar J, Nolan JP, Andersen LW. Temperature management in adult cardiac arrest consensus on science with treatment recommendations [Internet]. Brussels, Belgium: International Liaison Committee on Resuscitation (ILCOR) Advanced Life Support Task Force; 30 August 2021. Online. Available from: ilcor.org.

105. Australian Resuscitation Council. ANZCOR guideline 11.8 Targeted Temperature Management (TTM) after cardiac arrest. Melbourne: Australian Resuscitation Council; 2016. Online. Available from: www.resus.org.au.

106. Beck B, Bray JE, Smith K, Walker T, Grantham H, Hein C, et al. Description of the ambulance services participating in the Aus-ROC Australian and New Zealand out-of-hospital cardiac arrest Epistry. Emerg Med Australas 2016;28(6):673–83.

107. Nolan JP, Maconochie I, Soar J, Olasveengen TM, Greif R, Wyckoff MH, et al. Executive summary: 2020 International consensus on cardiopulmonary resuscitation and emergency cardiovascular care science with treatment recommendations. Circulation 2020;142(16-suppl 1):S2–27.

108. Australian Resuscitation Council. ANZCOR guideline 10.6: family presence during resuscitation. Melbourne: Australian Resuscitation Council; 2021. Online. Available from: www.resus.org.au.

CHAPTER 15
STABILISATION AND TRANSFER

DANIEL MARTIN AND BEN MEADLEY

ESSENTIALS

- Taking time to appropriately expose and package the patient prior to transport maximises patient comfort and safety, and reduces the risk of missed injury. Wherever possible, all anticipated interventions and procedures must be completed prior to moving the patient.
- High-risk, high-complexity and low occurrence procedures should be trained for and based on robust and contemporary, evidence-based standard operating procedures.
- Using a checklist, talking through the plan for any attempt at intubation, allocating roles and preparing the patient increases the likelihood of a successful first attempt at endotracheal intubation.
- Transport staff must be able to weigh up the risks versus benefits for all patient transport, whether within a hospital or between locations.
- Internationally recognised minimum standards for the transport of the critically ill patient should be adhered to.[1]
- The transport environment places specific stressors on both the patient and the team and must be accounted for.
- The effects and risks of each transport platform must be fully appreciated and understood by all transport staff.
- Centralised clinical coordination provides advice to both metropolitan and rural healthcare teams, and allows for effective and safe movement of teams and asset tracking.
- A formalised handover tool increases the opportunity for a complete and brief handover of all patient details.
- Monitoring equipment must be lightweight, robust and easy to use. All staff must be completely familiar with the workings of all equipment and how to troubleshoot during the transport.
- Each member of the team, and the organisation on the broader scale, facilitates and undertakes regular debriefing, auditing and quality improvements for all retrieval activities.

INTRODUCTION

The critically ill patient will often require transport, both within (intra-facility) and between (inter-facility) facilities. These tasks require critical care clinicians to be highly trained, current in their practice and able to be flexible and adaptive to the environment and the circumstances in which they are placed. The transport environment places specific demands on both the patient and the team caring for them, and these must be keenly understood and appreciated. These may include, but are not limited to, noise, vibration, temperature and barometric pressure changes, and any intervention may need to be undertaken under extreme circumstances where access to the patient is limited or taking place while on the move.

Even the most closely attended transfer can be subjected to delays due to external factors. Ambulances arrive late, weather can ground aircraft, and taxis for team transport may never arrive. Time can be of the essence and treatment may be time-critical; these factors must be considered and accounted for when coordinating the retrieval.

The key to good transport practice is to bring definitive or optimal care to the patient as soon as possible. For example, definitive care can be maximised through cardiovascular support, securing an airway, intubation and mechanical ventilation or lifesaving surgical procedures. Fundamentally, the care that is provided by the transport team should be at least equal to if not exceed that which is offered at the referring facility.[2] Teamwork, leadership and good communication are paramount to successful integration of teams and missions in often austere and stressful circumstances.

Transport teams are staffed with a variety of skill sets and healthcare professionals. The team composition should suit the patient's condition and treatment requirements. Whichever combination of doctor, nurse or paramedic, each has its advantages and disadvantages. In deciding on which team to task, there needs to be a risk–benefit analysis in deciding which skill-mix is the most appropriate. The ultimate goal of the mission is to get the patient to the right place, by the right means, in a timely fashion, at the right cost and—most importantly—safely.

Transport platforms include road ambulances, rotor-wing aircraft, fixed-wing aircraft and, for long-haul missions, commercial and private jet aircraft, and in special circumstances Australian Defence Force (ADF) assets. Selection is dependent on distance travelled, landing options, the patient's clinical status, availability, weather and cost. The focus of this chapter is on team preparation; retrieval/transport types; patient assessment and preparation; stabilisation and transfer of critically ill patients; and the factors that influence the mission.

The following list broadly outlines the types of missions that transport teams are likely to be tasked with in Australasia:

- metropolitan inter-facility transfer of patients
- rural/remote medical centre/hospital transfer to tertiary centres
- ambulance service activation for roadside trauma
- international repatriation of patients back to their country of origin
- major incident (local or international) activation and field medical team response.

INTRA- AND INTER-FACILITY PATIENT TRANSPORT

Incumbent in the treatment of the critically ill patient is a transport phase of care, either intra- or inter-facility. Moving a critically unwell patient takes great consideration, planning and execution. Patients are regularly moved for a variety of reasons. Movement may be as basic as to radiology for simple imaging, or as complex as a decompensating patient being moved rapidly to an operating theatre for definitive surgical intervention. The mode or urgency may differ, but the fundamentals remain the same.

STAFFING AND PREPARATION

The staff transferring the critically ill patient should be senior, experienced clinicians who are familiar with the equipment and travel times, whether between the emergency department (ED) and intensive care unit (ICU) or between a rural hospital and the tertiary facility. Intra-facility transport requires the same level of planning and preparation as does transport over longer distances—the team should be able to provide the equivalent standard of care during the transport as is available in the ED or ICU, and should therefore be ALS (advanced life support) accredited with consummate knowledge of the necessary interventions and equipment. High-level and autonomous clinical decision-making is key, especially given the urgent nature of such cases. The transport team should be self-sufficient during patient transfer, prepared for any eventuality, and able to perform independently. They often do not have at-hand support, so need to be able to respond to any emergency or change in patient condition. However, they are not isolated, as good two-way communication ensures that advice and coordination are available.

Preparation for transfer should be carefully completed for every movement and the risk of movement should be weighed against the potential benefit for the patient. The team should reassess the patient prior to movement, ensure that the receiving facility/unit is aware of the impending arrival, consider the route, agree on plans to address patient deterioration, and ensure that communication devices are working and at hand.[3]

Preparation tips to remember prior to patient transport include, but are not limited to, the following:

- Staff doing the transferring should be experienced and accredited.
- Plans for worst-case scenarios should be discussed and formulated, to ensure mutual understanding.
- Reassess the patient (primary survey) prior to each movement.
- The number and type of infusions should be rationalised; be prepared to discontinue those not deemed necessary.
- Ensure all intravenous, arterial or other (i.e. indwelling urinary catheter) lines are secure, and equipment or monitor cables are accessible to aid in troubleshooting or manipulation.
- Ensure emergency equipment, i.e. bag–valve–mask assembly, medications are close at hand in the event of a mid-transit emergency.
- Ensure the patient is secure and kept warm to minimise hypothermia and actively warm if indicated.
- Check that monitoring is attached correctly, working with sufficient battery life for the duration of the mission, and with maximal visibility around the patient.
- Communicate the plan for movement with the patient and family where possible.
- Communicate with the receiving facility regarding the patient's impending arrival and any pertinent clinical information.
- Ensure all documentation, x-rays, blood results etc, are up to date and available.
- Prepare and rehearse a systematic handover strategy prior to arrival.

Every effort should be made to minimise the effects of hypothermia when travelling through air-conditioned corridors or out in the elements. At a minimum, monitoring should include electrocardiogram, pulse oximetry and non-invasive blood-pressure monitoring. The equipment must be safely secured to either the bed or a stretcher bridge. A capacity to increase the level and complexity of monitoring must be readily available. There must be enough power, whether this be from an internal battery or an ability to plug-in to an external power source to ensure full functionality throughout the transfer, and ideally there should be back-up means, such as spare 'hot swappable' batteries; that is, the monitor continues to function when the battery is removed and replaced, or mains power access in the transport platform. The monitor, and indeed any infusion devices, must be able to withstand accidental damage and be lightweight enough to be carried with ease by any member of the retrieval team. Knowing the capability and limitations of the equipment being used in retrieval medicine ensures that the team does not expect the equipment to perform beyond its limits. All equipment must be rigorously tested prior to the introduction and use on any aircraft, with compliance to electro-magnetic interference limitations required by national aviation regulators.[4]

Inter-facility transfer is necessary when a critically ill patient requires movement from a referring facility to a receiving one. This may be from a regional or country setting to a metropolitan location or between two city-based facilities for specialist therapy. Historically, utilisation of the sending facility staff to effect the transfer removes valuable resources from rural/district facilities, potentially leaving those hospitals with inadequate specialist care. Ideally, the retrieval service should be a stand-alone source so as to not draw valuable staff from the ED or ICU, and these staff should be specifically trained and accredited in retrieval or transport medicine.[5] Transport teams are at times required to move patients who are undergoing very complex and highly sophisticated treatment. Common examples of these include intra-aortic balloon pump (IABP) and extra-corporeal membrane oxygenation (ECMO) therapies. In such circumstances, the coordination and logistical issues are compounded by the size and weight of the equipment and the need for specifically trained personnel to manage them, who are not usually part of the retrieval team. These extra staff may not be familiar with the transport environment, so it is important that they are well briefed and advised throughout the entirety of the transport. Oxygen consumption, calculation and sourcing are paramount when in transit, and this is especially important for intubated and non-invasively ventilated patients. A careful calculation of anticipated oxygen requirements must be carried out prior to the commencement of the mission. Box 15.1 shows a suggested formula for calculating oxygen requirements.[6] Oxygen cylinders are heavy and expensive and on commercial airlines and military aircraft are considered dangerous goods. Knowing if the ventilator is gas or power/turbine-driven, and having a contingency back-up in the form of a bag–valve–mask assembly, is part of the planning and preparation needed prior to commencing the mission. See Table 15.1 for oxygen bottle capacity and approximate life at varying flow rates.

Central coordination and communication are vital to the success of an organised transfer—continual downstream communication to the destination via a centralised clinical coordination centre is a must. Providing the receiving facility with an estimated time of arrival and by which means, and with up-to-date clinical details, will give the receiving facility enough time to have appropriate staff ready to accept the patient, and any infusions or equipment ready to go immediately.

Likewise, distance plays an important factor in the coordination. Transferring a patient over vast distances, over a great period of time, requires careful consideration, communication and execution. Issues such as patient safety, team fatigue and movement between transport platforms must be appreciated. The further away the patient is from their destination facility, the more planning is required.

The Joint Faculty of Intensive Care Medicine, the Australian and New Zealand College of Anaesthetists and the Australasian College for Emergency Medicine have developed minimum standards for the transfer of the critically unwell. They make recommendations as to the basic essential standards for equipment, monitoring capability and minimum training requirements for staff, among other items.[1]

BOX 15.1 SUGGESTED FORMULA FOR CALCULATING IN-TRANSIT OXYGEN REQUIREMENTS[3]

OXYGEN REQUIREMENTS DURING TRANSFER

2 × Transport time in minutes × [(MV × FiO_2) + ventilator driving gas]

where:

MV = minute volume

FiO_2 = inspired oxygen fraction.

Ventilator driving gas is dependent on ventilator make (e.g. an Oxylog 3000 uses 0.5 litres per minute)

Note that transport time is doubled, for safety.

SAMPLE CALCULATION FOR A 1-HOUR TRANSPORT

MV = 6 litres per minute

FiO_2 = 0.6

Ventilator driving gas = 0.5 litres per minute

REQUIREMENTS

$2 \times 60 \times [(6 \times 0.6) + 0.5]$

$= 120 \times 4.1 = 492$ litres of oxygen

EN ROUTE TO TRANSFER

The en route time to the referring facility for an inter-hospital transfer is time that can be well used to plan for the upcoming mission. Detailed plans can be developed by all team members to deal with any potential deterioration in patient condition, or indeed any threats to safety while travelling. Relevant medications can be pre-drawn-up and labelled to facilitate quicker administration and a reduction in workload at the scene or hospital; these must remain the responsibility of the team until they are administered or correctly disposed of. Further, paediatric calculations can be checked by the team to reduce errors, equipment can be identified as priority for attachment to the patient and building team cohesion can also be achieved.

A mental rehearsal and checklist of how to assess, treat and package the patient is a cheap, reproducible and effective

TABLE 15.1 OXYGEN CYLINDER SIZE, CONTENTS AND DURATION AT VARYING FLOW RATES (DURATION IS APPROXIMATE ONLY)[6]

CYLINDER SIZE	400 C	400 CD	400 ND	400 NE	400 NG
CONTENTS (LITRES)	490	630	1600	4000	8075
1 L/min	8:10	10:30	26:40	66:40	134:35
2 L/min	4:05	5:15	13:20	33:20	67:17
3 L/min	2:43	3:30	8:53	22:13	44:51
4 L/min	2:03	2:37	6:40	16:40	33:38
5 L/min	1:38	2:06	5:20	13:20	26:55
6 L/min	1:21	1:45	4:26	11:06	22:25
7 L/min	1:10	1:30	3:48	9:31	19:13
8 L/min	1:01	1:18	3:20	8:20	16:49
10 L/min	0:49	1:03	2:40	6:40	13:27
15 L/min	0:32	0:42	1:46	4:26	8:58

method of preparation. It is useful to try to anticipate any problems before being faced with them, and the time without the patient on the way is the perfect opportunity to do this.

TYPES OF TRANSPORT

The type of transport platform used for each mission will be dependent on a variety of factors. Some are directly patient-focused, and others are environmental or logistical in nature. Transfer generally takes place in two very distinct environments: on the ground or by air via fixed- or rotary-wing aircraft. Each has its advantages and disadvantages, and these must be appreciated when determining the type of transport platform to be used. Table 15.2 highlights the strengths and weaknesses of the various transport platforms.

Regardless of transport platform, all staff require significant training and orientation in terms (where relevant) of flight safety, loading and unloading patients, hazardous materials, emergency exits, fire procedures, seatbelts, life jacket operation and location of emergency oxygen and masks for rapid decompression. All flight teams should receive a pre-flight brief before departure to familiarise themselves with the unique safety aspects of each aircraft, and be briefed on patient oxygen outlets, suction operation, power outlets and advanced life support equipment. Further, a mental rehearsal of Helicopter Underwater Escape Training (HUET) drills is advised whenever the flight path takes the aircraft and team over a body of water.

The Civil Aviation Safety Authority (CASA) has orders in place (specifically 20.11) that stipulate requirements with regards to emergency and lifesaving equipment. These orders apply to all Australian registered aircraft and all team members who board an aircraft must have a current safety brief in place.

For all missions in the aviation environment, the pilot-in-command has ultimate responsibility for the safety of all those on board their aircraft. As such, they have the final say if they perceive an actual or potential risk to the mission; therefore, it is vital that the pilot is aware of the patient's condition and any requirements for the transport phase. It is therefore incumbent on the retrieval team to voice any of these prior to take-off. This should not be confused with trying to rush the pilot for clinical reasons.

GROUND TRANSPORT

Ground transport of patients is the mainstay of ambulance services throughout Australasia. Most patient transports in the metropolitan environment are performed by road and over short distances. Long distances in the rural setting compound the issue of timely patient transport, and here it may be necessary to rendezvous and use rotary- or fixed-wing aircraft.

Adverse weather conditions may influence the decision of the transport medium, and on occasion, ground transport may be the only option. Additionally, aircraft are not always the faster option when factoring in loading and unloading to the aircraft, as well as start-up and lift-off times. Conversely, when traffic is heavy, roads are impassable or the topography contains mountains, winding roads, etc. air transport may be a better option. Other considerations are transport time and the number of casualties/patients requiring transport.

Specialised options, including bariatric transport platforms and teams, are now standard in our society. Obtaining a clear and current weight of the patient is important fact-finding; once over 130 kg, safe transport becomes a complex task. As with the transport of patients undergoing complicated, specialist therapies, the bariatric patient also requires specialised teams and lifting equipment. This further increases the workload of the coordinating team, who need to ensure that the patient destination is aware of any special needs (i.e. bariatric bed and lifting team made available on arrival). This can at times pose delays for the movement of the patient and access to definitive care.

The bariatric patient is subject to all the stressors of flight or transport in the same way as any other patient; however,

TABLE 15.2 COMPARISON OF TRANSPORT PLATFORMS[7]

	FIXED-WING	ROTARY-WING	ROAD
Speed	450 kph approximately	240 kph approximately	140 kph maximum
Landing	Requires landing strip	Versatile landing options	Not required
Altitude	0–35,000 ft, pressurised	5000–6000 ft, non-pressurised	Ground level
Cost	A$3000–$5000 approximately	$5000/h approximately	Dependent on crew wage level
Patient capacity	1–2 only	1 as standard; 4 at maximum	Single patient only
Activation time	40 minutes minimum needed before take-off	Rapid activation possible	Immediate activation possible
Gas laws	Can be pressurised	Nil pressurisation ability	Not affected, aside from alpine services
Range	3300 km	760 km	Limitless, though dependent on resource availability
Weather	Able to fly above weather	Can be affected by poor weather	Unaffected by weather, unless flood or road damage present

consideration must be made for vibration (increased potential for pressure areas), temperature and hypoxia. Time allowed for close attention to patient positioning to maximise chest excursion and ventilation is worthwhile, utilising a low threshold for supplemental oxygen delivery. The utilisation of lifting aids, safe manual handling techniques and teamwork is vital to both patient and team safety.

ROTARY-WING AIRCRAFT

Rotary-wing aircraft provide rapid transport from point-to-point or from incident scene direct to a trauma centre, and can bypass traffic conditions in urban areas or topographical obstacles (i.e. bodies of water or mountain ranges) in the regional setting. In addition to those at major metropolitan hospitals, there are helipads at many rural and regional centres, facilitating quicker delivery of the team. Alternative landing zones can be created quickly at trauma scenes; for example, country sporting fields can be used as temporary helicopter landing zones easily by ground staff (i.e. local ambulance and/or fire services). In discussion with the aircraft pilot-in-command, teams may request an orbit over a pre-hospital scene. This allows the team to get an appreciation of the scene, inform them of the mechanism and identify the most likely and suitable place to land. However, the final decision of where the helicopter will land always sits with the pilot-in-command.

Although in some regions there is a survival benefit for major trauma patients when treated by a helicopter medical retrieval team,[7] helicopter transport is expensive,[8] and can expose the patient and crew to risks. Safety of helicopter aeromedical transport in Australia has been reviewed by Holland and Cooksley,[9] who reported that from 1992 to 2002, the crash rate was 4.38 per 100,000 flying hours, with one patient fatality as a result of a helicopter crash in 50,164 journeys. Other limitations of helicopter transport are excessive noise and vibration, small cabins and limited payload (thus limiting staffing numbers). Further, helicopter operations can be restricted by adverse weather conditions, resulting in delays, cancellations or alternative transport methods needing to be found. The captain has the over-arching authority to base the decision for flight on safe conditions regardless of clinical urgency. Additionally, helicopters are maintenance-intensive and prone to grounding secondary to minor or major faults. As such, coordinating staff must always consider alternative transport means and have them readily available should the team be unable to fly (grounded by potentially unsafe circumstances).

FIXED-WING AIRCRAFT

In 1928 the Royal Flying Doctor Service (RFDS) was the first comprehensive aero-medical organisation in the world and remains unique for the range of primary healthcare and emergency services it provides to the rural population of Australia.[10] With an average cruising speed of 240 knots (450 kph), the fixed-wing aircraft has the ability to cover vast distances in a relatively short time period, but is dependent on runways. The pressurised cabin provides the pilot with flight options regarding cruising altitude, as this can have negative effects on the patient and flight crew (see the section below on stresses of transport). When clinically indicated, the pilot can pressurise the cabin to ground-level pressure, but this can restrict flight options and increases fuel consumption and slows down the journey. However, this must be articulated to the pilot prior to take-off.

Dependent on aircraft and configuration, most aeromedical fixed-wing aircraft in Australasia can carry two patients and up to five crew, giving flight crew the option of allowing family members to accompany the patient (if appropriate). All-weather navigational equipment allows the fixed-wing aircraft to fly in adverse weather conditions, which may not be possible for rotary-wing aircraft. Once again, the fixed-wing captain needs to make an autonomous decision regarding flight safety. The mission is *never* more important than the safety of the crew.

The destination of fixed-wing aircraft is limited to the location of the nearest airstrip, so transport teams still rely on ground transport at both ends of the mission, adding time and potentially increasing the clinical risk to the patient. All equipment must be secured in the aircraft in accordance with CASA regulations. All mounting brackets must comply with CASA regulations. This requirement ensures that flight crew and patients are not subjected to flying objects or missiles in the cabin during turbulence or in the event of a crash.

COMMERCIAL TRANSPORT

For patient transport beyond the range of turbo-prop, fixed-wing aircraft, commercial aircraft can be used in two distinct environments: commercial passenger aircraft and medically configured jet aircraft. With notice, the major commercial airliners can install a stretcher over 9–12 seats of domestic and international passenger aircraft. This would be at an additional cost, in terms of both a dollar value as well as space. This allows transport teams to transfer patients over long distances in relative comfort in a relatively larger working environment. With passengers surrounding the stretcher, interventions should be kept to a minimum and privacy needs to be maintained for the patient. Similar to an in-hospital ward environment, patient care requirements, such as hygiene, toileting and nutrition, must be attended to with discretion. Given the proximity to other passengers on board, issues such as confidentiality and patient privacy are acutely important to consider. There is always a risk of patient deterioration in any patient transport; however, when using commercial national or international aircraft, the risk of diversion or delays due to patient need is ever-present and must be considered.

Oxygen supply should be pre-organised and approved, and must be able to be secured at all times. Patient monitoring can be difficult, as access to onboard power supplies may be difficult due to incompatibility, and few biomedical devices have a battery life that will last the length of a long-haul flight. Backup power supplies, such as spare batteries, must be accounted for during the planning phase for this type of transport.

Using a roster system to manage fatigue in the team is vital in these long-haul missions and sufficient rest periods will go a long way to ensuring the team is able to care for and respond to any patient need. Further, hydration and nutrition will also enable the team members to stay vigilant over long periods. In Australasia, there are a number of medically configured jets that are used for patient transport. Commercial transport costs are expensive, with most funded by the patient's travel insurance company or by outright payment. The jet provides similar challenges in patient management to the fixed-wing aircraft in terms of stressors of transport. These aircraft have ranges of 3300 km or more and can fly at speeds exceeding 800 km/hr, making them a swift option for flight. For example, Adelaide to Darwin (approximately 2600 km flight distance) via propeller fixed-wing aircraft takes approximately 6 hours, while a Lear jet takes approximately 3.5 hours.

Australian Defence Force assets

At times, special needs, such as a natural disaster (e.g. 2019/2020 Victorian bushfires, the Bundaberg floods, the evacuation of Cairns Base Hospital) or patient need (e.g. a bariatric patient who exceeds the size and weight limits for civilian ambulance services), require the assistance of the Australian Defence Force through the Defence Aid to the Civil Community (DACC) system. The Royal Australian Air Force (RAAF) provides the aeromedical evacuation capability Defence-wide, and this mature, responsive system can be provided to the civilian community. The RAAF has highly trained and experienced personnel, as well as airframes with a large patient load capacity.

CLINICAL COORDINATION AND COMMUNICATION

A single point of contact, attended 24 hours a day, 7 days a week, answered by clinically experienced staff, provides invaluable support to rural/regional referring facilities. Medical coordination staff provide clear advice for all types of presentations and for numerous and, at times, simultaneous requests for assistance. Clinical coordinators benefit from a background in aeromedical retrieval, giving them an inherent awareness of tasking, teams, platforms and resources.

The National Clinical Handover Initiative of the Australian Commission on Safety and Quality in Health Care (ACSQHC) has identified a need for a standardised handover checklist.[11,12] The failure of effective communication is a recurring theme in the patient safety literature, specifically as it relates to handover. A review of local clinical incidents confirmed that this pattern was particularly evident for acutely ill, deteriorating patients who require transfer to a higher level of care.[10]

The ISBAR handover tool has been suggested as one appropriate tool for safe and effective handover.[12] Like the primary survey, there is safety in following a process to make it easier to communicate all the relevant detail and information. The handover should be short, concise and practised prior to delivering the patient to the destination facility.

PRACTICE TIP

Rehearsing your pre-written handover to your teammate prior to arrival at the destination hospital allows them to remind you of any missed details, as well as practising a clear and succinct final delivery of information to the receiving team.

Prior to commencing handover, it is useful to advise the receiving team of any immediate concerns. These could be additional medications, further fluid or blood product resuscitation, commencement of a resuscitative surgical procedure or the ordering and preparation of urgent imaging.

I **Identify.** This is the time to introduce both yourself and the patient.
- Who are you and what is your role?
- Patient identifiers (at least three).

S **Situation.** This is where you can provide information regarding where the patient has come from, a presenting complaint or provisional diagnosis and/or the mechanism of injury in the presence of trauma.
- What is going on with the patient?
- Patient stability/level of concern.

B **Background.** Any pertinent treatment and medical history must be relayed to the receiving facility.
- What is the clinical background/context?
- History of presentation.

A **Assessment.** Providing physiological data is a place from which the primary assessment can take place. It is useful to provide the observations at the time of referral, in transit and when you arrive at the receiving facility.
- What do you think the problem is?
- What have you done so far?

R **Recommendation/Response/Rationale.** This may be the most important phase of the handover, as it confirms a shared understanding of patient care priorities. Any questions or concerns can be discussed at this stage.
- What would you recommend or want done?
- What are you most concerned about?
- Risk—patient/occupational health and safety.
- Assign and confirm acceptance of responsibility/accountability.
- What is the plan from here?

This is just a suggested tool for handover; the facility you work in may have a separate process in place. It merely highlights the need for a structured, reproducible handover tool that is easy to remember and use. In the electronic age there are many additional resources, such as the ISBAR smartphone application produced by NSW Health and South Australian Health as a handy guide and prompt when formulating a handover (see Useful websites).

Telemedicine is a useful means of communication between the regional setting and central clinical coordination services. A combination of digital photography, real-time vision and the internet, has made it possible for doctors to provide accurate advice and interpret clinical imaging and monitoring to directly influence patient care. Studies have found that 75% of coordinators felt that telemedicine improved patient care, and, further, that both the referring doctors and the medical coordinators felt that telemedicine improved communication and patient assessment.[13] Time spent organising and utilising telemedicine must not be at the expense of clinical care to the patient, or cause delay. In reality it can occur simultaneously and will influence decisions, such as active resuscitation of the patient, while the team is en route; high-fidelity patient information could dictate the urgency, speed of activation or determine the need for retrieval at all. Most smartphones or other handheld communication devices have face-to-face or video call capabilities. These can be very effective tools in those areas where reception is intact. They do have limitations in rural and remote locations or areas where mobile coverage is poor. Careful consideration about patient confidentiality and call security must be in place when using these devices to avoid third parties from listening in, or receiving unwanted patient details.

TEAM PREPARATION

TRAINING

Team members who are to be involved in the transfer of the critically ill must have appropriate situational awareness, experience and training. Each organisation will have specific training and experience requirements for their own services, but in general terms these should include:
- entry-level nursing or paramedic qualifications, including professional registration
- a critical care specialty:
  - emergency
  - intensive care (neonate, paediatric and adult, specific to service)
  - intensive care paramedicine
- postgraduate aeromedical/retrieval qualifications
- Emergency Management Severe Trauma (EMST) or Emergency Trauma Management
- Advanced Paediatric Life Support (APLS)
- Major Incident Medical Management Support (MIMMS)
- Helicopter Underwater Escape Training (HUET).

Keen patient assessment skills and the ability to diagnose and treat independently are ideal. Teamwork and excellent communication skills are also vital for safe and efficient transport of patients. Service-specific standing operating procedures (SOPs), clinical guidelines and work instructions are site-specific and should be evidence-based.

Accreditation

Continual service accreditation and currency maintenance are prerequisites for the transport environment. The level of skill required to safely practise in these circumstances is high, and team members are expected to be able to think and react very quickly and in difficult scenarios. Each team member has their own specialisation or craft mix, requiring ongoing registration, maintenance of professional standards and continual professional education.

Nationally recognised accreditation systems, such as the ACSQHC's National Safety and Quality Health Service Standards, can form a basis by which services can be assessed to ensure they provide safe and quality assured care to their patients.

Simulation training and mock scenarios are methods for introducing new theoretical and practical skills to those starting in retrieval medicine, and also a way to hone existing skills and maintain currency for the experienced practitioner. Consistent reorientation of all transport modes must be adhered to, to maintain currency and familiarity. Retrieval and transfer of the critically ill is a dynamic and evolving profession. New safety upgrades and technological improvements are continual, so the team must be current and up to date with these issues.

Helicopter Underwater Escape Training (HUET)

Helicopters are noisy, distracting and generate an enormous amount of down-force from rotor wash, with almost invisible tail rotors located at head height in some models. Training and orientation are key to providing the safest working environment and reducing the opportunity for adverse outcomes when involved in rotary-wing aircraft emergencies or ditching over water. HUET has been made mandatory across many rotary-wing services and is at times a service standard for all flight crew. The training involves the demonstration and actual participation in how to exit an underwater rotary-wing aircraft in any orientation; that is, upside down or right way up (Figs 15.1 and 15.2). This training improves the chances of survival for the aircraft passengers, flight crews, patients and passengers.[14]

PRACTICE TIP

On every entry into the rotor-wing aircraft, identify primary and secondary exits and undertake a personal rehearsal of the escape drill.

FIGURE 15.1 HUET CAGE ROLLING ON ENTRY INTO WATER

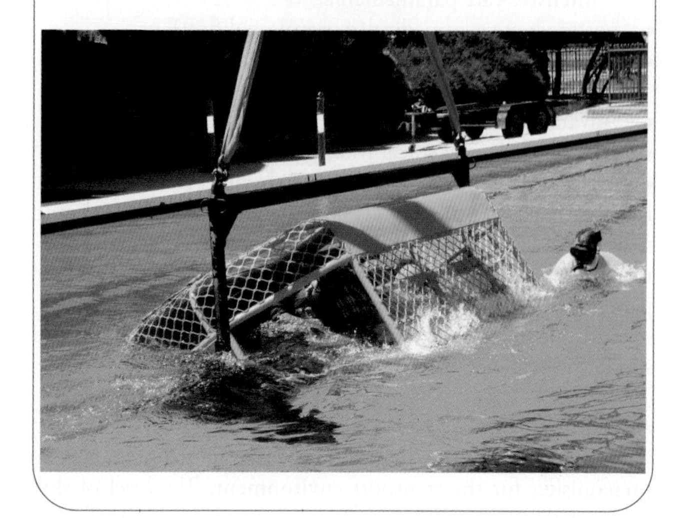

FIGURE 15.2 HUET CAGE UNDERWATER AND UPSIDE DOWN, PERSON EXITING

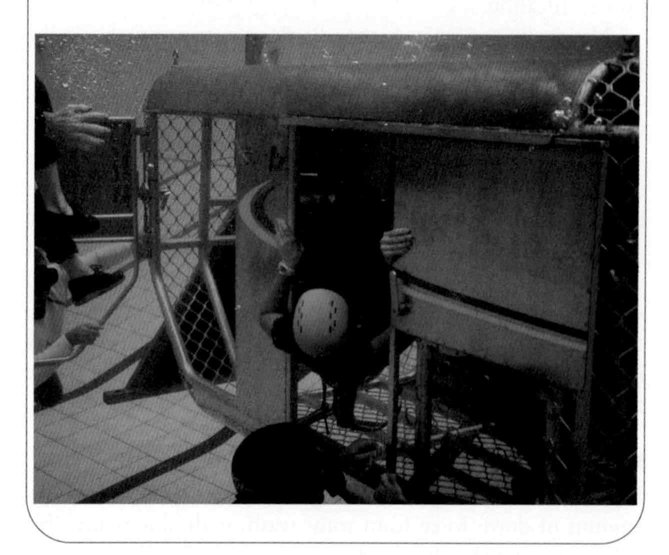

PERSONAL PROTECTIVE EQUIPMENT (PPE) AND UNIFORMS

A properly sized and fitted uniform is essential as PPE, and for identifying team members and roles. It should contain multiple pockets in which items such as gloves, a notebook, pens, food etc. can be carried, and form part of a safety standard. A brightly coloured uniform, complete with reflective tape, offers increased safety and visibility, especially after dark where ambient light will be low and provided by electrical means. A fire-resistant Kevlar fabric is a standard in the aeromedical environment to reduce the effects of fire and the potential for burns to the team members. Helmets, rigger's gloves, eye and ear protection, hard-soled boots and life jackets with specific survival equipment when flying in rotary-wing aircraft are also essential in the out-of-hospital transport environment. When responding to roadside trauma scenes, high visibility tabards and safety helmets provide further safety in this, at times, austere environment. See Chapter 9 for scene assessment and management, and Chapter 12 for information on different types of PPE.

FITNESS

Team members should have a reasonable level of fitness in order to be able to perform clinical duties in the relevant transport platform. A fit-for-task assessment prior to inclusion in the team is a method of identifying areas of need and will reduce the opportunity for adverse events and injury. A combination of aerobic fitness and strength will enable the team to adapt to any circumstances, such as carrying packs over great distances, handling stretchers over uneven surfaces or working in confined spaces. While this area is controversial, there is growing evidence that some of the tasks performed by retrieval teams invoke extreme physiological strain; therefore, staff should be selected for their capacity to perform such work.[15,16]

PRINCIPLES OF TRANSPORT

PRE-DEPARTURE PACK CHECKING

Mission success is dependent on gear that is complete and regularly checked by all team members at the beginning of the shift, in a challenge and response format.[17] Discovering that equipment is missing from the pack while caring for the patient can have catastrophic effects, and therefore all necessary equipment must be available for use on all missions, at all times. It places the responsibility of mission readiness squarely on the team, as well as keeping them familiar with the contents of the pack sets. Resources such as smartphone apps can hold all checklists and provide an easy-to-use method of checking and re-familiarisation. Case cards or patient records can also contain specific areas for documenting or pre-planning the handover in readiness for delivery to the receiving facility.

PATIENT PACKAGING

Taking the time to adequately package the patient is time well spent. The benefits include, but are not limited to:

- thermoregulation
- return of 'as-close-to' anatomically correct alignment of fractures, both obvious and suspected
- pain reduction and patient comfort
- reduction of undue handling
- reduction of unnecessary intervention or replacement of therapy at the receiving facility
- ease of access to points of vascular access during transport or in an emergency
- minimising further negative effects of illness or injury.

The patient should be totally exposed for a thorough examination, after which they must be kept warm to alleviate the effects of hypothermia. A skin-to-sheet or skin-to-device approach wherever possible is an effective way to prepare the patient for transport, and to reduce unnecessary handling on arrival at the destination facility. Undue rough or multiple movements can disrupt any primary haemostatic clots about long bone or pelvic fractures, increase pain, and expose the patient to unnecessary environmental factors.

FIGURE 15.3 EXAMPLE OF PATIENT PACKAGING[22]

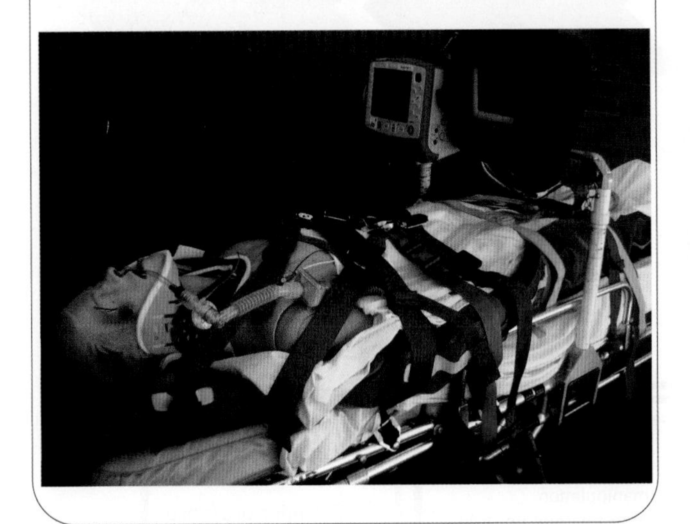

Where the index of suspicion for pelvic fractures is high, the pelvic splint is a device that is wrapped around the pelvic girdle of the traumatically injured patient. When applied correctly and directly to the skin, it can close previously separated or acutely fractured pelvic rings to reduce the haemorrhage and pain experienced by the patient. Likewise, the femoral traction splint can realign femur fractures and thereby reduce pain and the potential for uncontrolled bleeding into the femoral space. The limb extremity must be assessed for perfusion and neurovascular function, both pre- and post-application and during movement. It is useful to mark the site where a pulse is found to ensure the site is accessible during the transport phase for continual reassessment.

Fig. 15.3 shows an example of a patient packaging technique. Note the use of a stretcher bridge for the securing of medical equipment, vacuum mattress, vital signs monitoring and ventilator. Challenges and considerations include reducing hypothermia (in this instance the patient has been kept exposed to show pelvic binder and monitoring leads), securing the ventilator circuit and maintaining stability of the stretcher as the centre of gravity is relatively higher and, as such, poses a tipping risk on uneven surfaces.

PRACTICE TIP

Good patient packaging promotes comfort, can reduce pain and allows for rapid access to the patient in the event of an emergency.

Aeromedical retrieval services have different methods for securing equipment onto the patient stretcher for transport. Often, they will be in the form of stretcher bridges, which are specifically designed to hold all monitoring and ventilation equipment. They are engineered and rated to cope with acceleration and deceleration forces in the event of a sudden deceleration or collision and make the equipment easily viewable and adjustable throughout the mission.

Providing in-transit care is challenging at best. The vehicle or aircraft can be subject to noise, movement and vibration and is a cramped environment. This may hinder any access to the patient and can put the team at risk if they are out of their safety harnesses and moving around in the cabin. Attempts must be made to package the patient in such a way as to optimise access and anticipate any change in clinical state and to remain in a seated position throughout the critical phases of flight (i.e. take-off and landing).

AIRWAY

The protection of any potentially unstable airway is of paramount importance. The airway should be secured prior to departure if there is actual or anticipated airway risk. Plans should be put in place to make sure the first attempt at intubation is successful. A failed attempt at intubating a deteriorating patient in the rear of an aircraft or ambulance adds unnecessary stress to team members and poses a significant risk to the patient's wellbeing.

Methods to improve successful first pass intubation include, but are not limited to:

- *using a checklist* (Fig. 15.4). The successful first pass rapid sequence intubation (RSI)/induction of a critically ill patient is a high complexity/low occurrence procedure and if unsuccessful can have drastic consequences. The use of the pre-formed checklist maximises patient safety and reduces the opportunity for any potential mistakes or omissions to occur.
- *using a 'kit dump' bag* (Fig. 15.5). This is a suggested method for making the first attempt as easy as possible. Essentially, it is a yellow plastic bag (these may differ depending on the service preference) with outlines representing all equipment that is needed to carry out an intubation. It is placed at the right-hand side of the practitioner and is managed by the assistant and allows for easy recognition and access to all equipment including secondary devices.

Once the patient has been successfully intubated, the team must spend time securing the tube, confirming cuff integrity and documenting the intervention. Vital information to be recorded should include: tube position at teeth or lips, size of tube, position of patient, whether in-line immobilisation was utilised, drugs used for induction and doses.

Tying the tube in with tape does not guarantee security. Unexpected extubation, especially in-flight, is a challenging circumstance and all care must be taken to avoid this during any patient movement; a team member must therefore take control of the tube and be responsible for the coordination of the rest of the team.

BREATHING

Assessment of the patient's respiratory state forms part of the continuous assessment and should be carried out throughout the entirety of the patient transport. Subtle pathology has the potential to increase markedly on patient movement, especially at altitude. Close monitoring of arterial oxygen saturation (SaO_2) $\pm$ end-tidal carbon dioxide levels ($EtCO_2$) helps with recognising changes in respiratory state and effectiveness, but these must not be relied on in lieu of clinical assessment. The patient's respiration rate, work of breathing equality and depth

FIGURE 15.4 A PRE- AND POST-RSI CHECKLIST

RSI preparation

- ✓ Optimise patient position & access
- ✓ O_2 cylinder > half full & backup
- ✓ Nasal prongs ApOx
- ✓ Pre-oxygenation
- ✓ OPA & NPA
- ✓ Vascular access
- ✓ Fluids run easily
- ✓ BP set at 2 minute cycles
- ✓ Baseline obs
- ✓ $EtCO_2$ connected to monitor & on

Equipment check

- ✓ BVM with O_2
- ✓ ETT mount & HME
- ✓ Laryngoscopes × 2 tested
- ✓ Blade size
- ✓ Suction tested
- ✓ Bougie or stylet
- ✓ ETT & cuff tested
- ✓ Syringe
- ✓ Tube tie
- ✓ LMA (inc iLMA)
- ✓ Surgical airway kit

Team brief

- ✓ Airway assistant
- ✓ M.I.L.S
- ✓ Drug giver
- ✓ RSI drug doses
- ✓ Consider cricoid pressure

30 second drill options:
1. Release cricoid pressure
2. External laryngeal manipulation
3. Adjust patient position
4. Adjust operator position
5. Change equipment
6. Change operator

JAWS:
- Jaw thrust
- Airways – OPA/NPA
- Work together – 2 person
- Small volumes, easy squeeze

Post-RSI

- ✓ Waveform $EtCO_2$ confirmed
- ✓ Check obs
- ✓ Tube secured & position noted
- ✓ Ventilation
- ✓ Analgesia/Sedation
- ✓ Paralysis
- ✓ Consider oro/naso gastric tube
- ✓ Temperature probe
- ✓ Cuff pressure

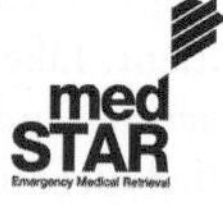

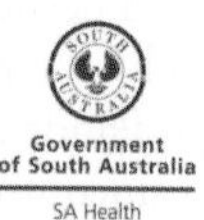

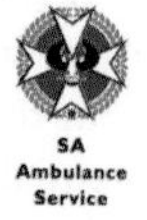

CHALLENGE & RESPONSE

CO_2.B.O.L.T.S

IMMEDIATE/ PERI-ARREST INTUBATION CHECKLIST

CO_2 – $EtCO_2$ connected to monitor and on

B – Bougie/BVM

O – Oxygen

L – Laryngoscope

T – Endotracheal tube

S – Suction/syringe

CHALLENGE & RESPONSE

Confirm ETT placement

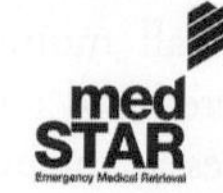

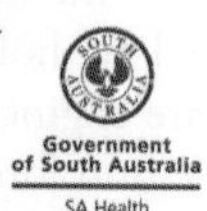

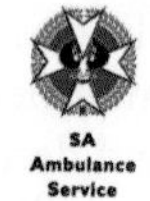

SAAS MedSTAR.

FIGURE 15.5 SUGGESTED KIT DUMP CONFIGURATION[22]

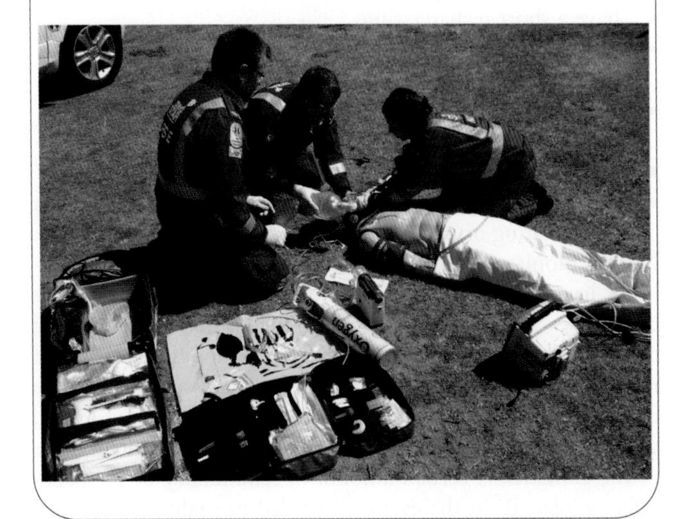

of chest excursion must be continually monitored, all of which can be difficult in different circumstances, such as at night or when the patient's chest is covered by blankets or monitoring equipment leads.

Hypoxia at altitude is of concern; therefore, all patients transferred by aircraft must have supplemental oxygen available to mitigate its effects (see sections below on gas laws and stressors of transport).

The assessment, diagnosis and treatment of a pneumothorax in flight or in the rear of an ambulance is almost impossible due to ambient noise and vibration (see below), and therefore in the presence of trauma, either blunt or penetrating, the transport team should have a low threshold for the insertion of chest drains, and serious consideration should be given to undertaking this prior to departure if clinically appropriate. Ultrasound in the hands of an experienced practitioner can help with diagnosis of intra-thoracic pathology and can be performed prior to, during and post transport.

PRACTICE TIP

Keep basic airway adjunct and bag-valve-mask assemblies close at hand during the transport phase in case of an unexpected airway emergency.

CIRCULATION

Before transporting the patient, at least two peripheral, well-secured and working intravenous (IV) cannula should be present and patent. Having a second line in situ offers redundancy if the first one should be dislodged during transfer. Monitoring should include electrocardiography (ECG), pulse oximetry and non-invasive blood pressure, as a minimum. Refer to Chapter 16 for information on inserting an IV cannula and cardiac monitoring. For patients requiring vasopressor and/or inotropic support, the discussion regarding central access should be considered and discussed by the referring and receiving facilities/units. Medications such as norepinephrine (noradrenaline) should not be infused via peripheral IV access for extended periods of time, although it is safe to do so where no alternative exists.[18]

If the team is having trouble gaining peripheral IV access, intra-osseous access should be the next step. Sites for insertion include the tibial plateau and the humeral head. Both sites are easily accessible and offer quick and effective access to the venous circulation. Any medication and fluid can be infused through these access points; however, they do need supplementary pressure as gravity alone is not strong enough to overcome the intra-osseous tissue. Alternatively, if the team has the equipment and expertise, ultrasound guided vascular access can be achieved quickly and is increasingly used in the retrieval setting.[19]

Blood products are used in transport services across the globe. Adherence to clinical procedure, cold chain management, sound haemovigilance, and product stewardship must be in place to protect and preserve this vital and, at times, scarce resource. Sound working relationships with the transfusion unit or blood bank and a local clinical lead are also useful to monitor usage, wastage and clinical indications for all usage events.

PRACTICE TIP

If done correctly, intra-osseous access is quick, easy and in some cases may be the first choice for intra-vascular access.

Serial observations of the patient's haemodynamic state, including pulse rate and blood pressure, must be taken. The timing of these is determined by the patient's clinical state, but should be documented at least every 30 minutes, with at least 1–2 complete sets being taken during the transport phase (dependent on transport phase length). Once again, reliance on electronic equipment alone to monitor the patient's haemodynamic state can be difficult. At extremes of blood pressure, portable non-invasive blood-pressure (NIBP) monitors are inaccurate, so observe for clinical signs of hypovolaemia and hypoperfusion. Observing skin colour, conscious state and palpating for peripheral pulses are useful techniques to monitor blood pressure. All efforts must be made to halt or reduce the amount of external blood loss, with direct pressure being the most effective method.

Invasive monitoring by arterial lines is a useful tool for continuous haemodynamic monitoring. A decrease or loss of cardiac output can be observed in the sometimes cramped and noisy transport environment. However, lengthy or troublesome insertions should not unduly delay the transport of the patient, especially in a time-critical scenario. However, in secondary transport situations (e.g. hospital to hospital), arterial access for blood pressure monitoring and blood gas analysis is seen as the ideal modality.

DISABILITY

Assessing the patient's neurological state can be done quickly using AVPU (**A**lert, **V**erbalising, responding to **P**ain or **U**nresponsive) or using a formal Glasgow Coma Scale (GCS) (see Chapter 13). AVPU allows a quick assessment, and the GCS allows for a more detailed and thorough examination. Further, pupillary response to light must also be included in any neurological examination, and changes in response acted upon, as well as a baseline blood glucose test.

The agitated patient with an altered conscious state represents a danger to all team members, whether they are flying in an aircraft or travelling by road to the destination. Consideration must be given to sedation techniques, securing devices or elective intubation of the patient, and also the exploration of alternative methods of transport. Likewise, the patient who has a labile conscious state may require intubation to secure the airway and avoid potential intubation in the cramped transport environment.

MONITORING AND EQUIPMENT

The ideal vital signs monitor needs a number of key features to satisfy all the requirements of the transport team. It must:

- be light and easy to carry
- be easily securable and removable throughout the phases of transport
- be 'user-friendly' and intuitive in its operations, both basic and advanced
- have a large, easy-to-read screen that can be read in bright sunlight and backlit when working in the dark or low light
- be robust and able to withstand rough handling and potential dropping
- have a long battery life with all parameters functioning
- have a short recharge time
- be able to measure ECG, SpO_2, NIBP, two invasive pressure lines, $EtCO_2$, temperature
- have consumables and biomedical engineering support readily available
- ideally have an ease of interchangeability between services
- be safe and approved for use in an aircraft, especially when defibrillating or pacing.

Not all monitoring devices are able to provide all of the attributes listed above, and sound understanding of the monitor's capabilities and limitations is imperative. The equipment and consumables carried by the retrieval team should be capable of responding to a variety of patient presentations, such as extremes of age, size and physiology. Care must be given to the overall weight and design of the pack sets, with special consideration as to the contents. A certain amount of redundancy in the packs offers a 'plan B' in the event of a failed procedure attempt or multiple patients. Table 15.3 shows a suggested contents list for a single-team pack set. It is completed by a transport 'suite' of monitor/defibrillator, stretcher bridge and ventilator.

TABLE 15.3 SUGGESTED TRANSPORT PACK CONTENTS LIST

RESUSCITATION PACK	
Outside front pocket	
Bag/mask module – adult	
Adult resuscitation bag with hose	1
Resuscitation mask - size 4 & 5	1 ea
OPA - size 8, 9, 10	1 ea
NPA - size 6, 7, 8	1 ea
PEEP valve	1
Disposable cuff manometer	1
10 mL syringe	1
KY jelly sachet	1
Safety pin	1
Bag/mask module – paediatric	
Paediatric resuscitation bag with hose	1
Resuscitation mask - size 0/1, 2, 3	1 ea
OPA - size 5, 6, 7	1 ea
NPA - size 4, 5	1 ea
PEEP valve	1
Disposable cuff manometer	1
10 mL syringe	1
KY jelly sachet	1
Safety pin	1
Inside top pocket	
Howard Kelly's forceps (L&R)	2 pr
No. 20 scalpel blade	2 ea
Maxiswabs	2 ea
Sterile gloves - size 6, 7, 7.5, 8	1 pr ea
Sterile shears	1 pr
Gigli saw	1
Gigli saw handle	1 pr
Skin stapler 35W	1
Inside middle pocket	
Crepe bandage - 15 cm	2
Combine dressing - 20 × 75 cm	1
Combine dressing - 10 × 20 cm	2
Israeli bandage - 6″	1
1 Mersilk suture	1
Spencer wells forceps	1 pr
Arterial tourniquet	2
Indwelling Foley catheter - 18 fr	1
Inside bottom pocket	
500 mL normal saline	1
IV giving set	1

TABLE 15.3 SUGGESTED TRANSPORT PACK CONTENTS LIST—cont'd

Lever lock cannula	1
Fluid warmer	1
Disposable set	2
100 mL normal saline	1
Velcro support straps	2
Plastic bag	1
Main compartment	
Standard pelvic binder with triangular bandage	1
Flexible splints	2
Hypertonic saline module, complete with:	
• 250 mL 7.5% strong sodium	1
• IV giving set	1
• Lever lock cannula	1
• Dosing guideline	1
Video laryngoscope module - complete with:	
• Video laryngoscope handle/monitor	1
• Laryngoscope blade - size 2, 3, 4 & X 3	1 ea
• Spare battery	1
Airway module	
Panel 1	
Laryngoscope handle	2
Laryngoscope blade, Mackintosh - size 3, 4	1 ea
Laryngoscope blade, Miller - size 1, 2	1 ea
10 mL syringe	1
ETT mount	1
KY lube sachet	2
Panel 2	
Intubating stylet - size S, M, L	1 ea
Cloth tube tie - 1 m	2
Magill forceps, adult & child	1 ea
Dump bag	1
ETT, uncuffed - size 3	1
ETT, cuffed - size 3.5, 4, 4.5, 5, 6, 7, 8	1 ea
Nasogastric tube - 10 g & 14 g	1 ea
Drainage bag	1
Cricothyroidotomy pack	1
Nasal prongs, adult & paediatric	1 pr ea
Panel 3	
Easi-cap	1
Paedi-cap	1
Persist plus swabs	1
No. 20 scalpel blade	1
Tracheal dilator forceps	1 pr
50 mL catheter tip syringe	1
Dental props - adult & child	1 pr ea
Nasal tamponade catheter	2
Tape	1 roll
Panel 4	
LMA - size 2, 3, 4, 5	1 ea
Bougie	2
Suction catheter - size 8, 14	1 ea
Pre/Post-RSI checklist	1
Intra-osseous/vascular access module	
Intra-osseous drill	1
IO needle - adult, paediatric & obese	2 ea
Stabilisers	2
3-way tap	2
10 mL syringe	1
50 mL syringe	1
10 mL normal saline ampoule	2
Persist plus swabs	2
IV cannula - 14 g, 16 g, 18 g, 20 g, 22 g	2 ea
IV bungs	2
Tegaderm	2
25 mm transpore tape	1 roll
Tourniquet	1
PROCEDURE PACK	
Inside top pocket	
Sterile bundle:	
• Sterile gown	
• Sterile drape	
• Surgical mask	
• Surgical cap	
Intercostal catheter 12 fr, 20 fr	1 ea
Intercostal catheter 32 fr	2

Continued

TABLE 15.3 SUGGESTED TRANSPORT PACK CONTENTS LIST—cont'd

Item	Quantity
Main compartment	
Minor surgical module	
Panel 1	
Drainage bag	2
Connector	2
Panel 2	
Tegaderm	2
Gauze swab - 10 cm × 10 cm	4
1.0 Mersilk suture	2
2.0 silk suture	2
Stitch cutter	1
No. 11 scalpel	1
Scissors	1 pr
Spencer Wells forceps	2 pr
Howard Kelly forceps	1 pr
Panel 3	
Sterile plastic drape	1
Sterile regional adhesive drape	1
Maxi-swab	4
Panel 4	
Sterile glove - size 6, 6.5, 7, 7.5, 8, 8.5	1 pr ea
Sterile hypafix dressing - 10 cm × 25 cm	4
Dressing pack	1
Central access module	
7 fr/20 cm triple lumen CVC	1
16 g/20 cm single lumen CVC	1
9 fr Swann sheath/Cook access introducer	1
Spare guide wire	1
18 g spare Cook I.O. needle	1
Arterial line module	
Outside pocket	
Pressure cable	1
Panel 1	
10 mL normal saline ampoule	5
10 mL syringe	2
10 mL springfusor	1
2 mL syringe	1
25G needle	1
Red bungs	4
Steri strip	1 pkt
Gauze swab - 10 cm × 10 cm	1 pkt
Tegaderm	2
2.0 silk suture	1
Stitch cutter	1
Sterile plastic drape	1
Spencer Wells forceps	1
2% lidocaine	1
Panel 2	
Seldinger type radial artery catheter	2
Persist plus swabs	2
Pressure transducer set	2
Side pocket	
Back-up monitor bag:	
• $EtCO_2/SpO_2$ monitor	1
• SpO_2 finger probe	1
• $EtCO_2$ sidestream sampling line	1
• Nasal prong sampling line	1
• AA batteries	4
• $EtCO_2$ nasal sampling line	1
Disposable gowns	2
Safety glasses	2
N95 mask - sml & med	2 pr ea
DRUG PACK	
Panel 1	
Row 1:	
Adrenaline 1 mg / 1 mL	6
Noradrenaline 4 mg / 4 mL	4
Metaraminol 10 mg / 1 mL	1
Amiodarone 150 mg / 3 mL	3
Metoprolol 5 mg / 5 mL	2
Magnesium sulfate 10 mmol / 5 mL	2
Atropine 600 microg / 1 mL	2
Hydralazine 20 mg	2

TABLE 15.3 SUGGESTED TRANSPORT PACK CONTENTS LIST—cont'd

Item	Qty
Row 2:	
Levetiracetam 500 mg / 5 mL	4
Lidocaine 2%	2
Bupivacaine 0.5% 50 mg/10 mL	2
Hydrocortisone 100 mg	2
SNIP 50 mg / 2 mL + shroud (in box)	1
Calcium chloride 1 g / 10 mL	1
Tranexamic acid 1 g / 10 mL	2
Panel 2 (sleeve)	
Paediatric quick reference guide	1
IV medication labels (blank)	6
Ultrasound guided short bevel needle	1
Ziplock rubbish bag	1
Monthly drug and consumables expiry matrix	1
Panel 3	
Row 1:	
Cephazolin 1 g	2
Meropenem 1 g	2
Vancomycin 1 g	2
Aciclovir 500 mg / 20 mL	2
Row 2:	
Salbutamol IV 5 mg / 5 mL	2
Ipratropium 500 microg / 1 mL	2
Salbutamol nebules 5 mg / 2.5 mL	5
Rocuronium 50 mg	4
Suxamethonium 100 mg / 2 mL	2
Thiopentone 500 mg	1
Ondansetron 4 mg / 2 mL	2
Base	
Left-hand side	
Potassium chloride 10 mmol / 10 mL (in red pouch)	2
Sodium bicarbonate 8.4% in 100 mL	1
GTN Spray	1
Left-hand middle compartment:	
MDI tube mount	1
Salbutamol MDI	1
Glucose 50% / 50 mL	1
GTN infusion 50 mg / 10 mL	1
Left-hand bottom compartment:	
Propofol 500 mg / 50 mL	2
Normal saline 10 mL	6
Middle:	
Syringe pump	2
30 mL syringe	2
50 mL syringe	3
Normal saline 100 mL	1
5% Glucose 100 mL	1
Glucometer pouch:	
• Glucometer	1
• Test strips - individual	5
• Lancets	5
Right-hand side (in syringe roll):	
Red bungs	5
Mucosal atomising device	1
Lever lock	2
Minimum volume extension set	4
Lever lock	2
Three-way tap	1
10 mL syringe	5
5 mL syringe	2
5 mL red plunger syringe	2
2 mL syringe	2
1 mL syringe	2
0.5 mL syringe	1
Alcohol swabs	5
18 g drawing up needle	5
Vial access cannula	5
Blunt access cannula	5
21 g needle	5
RSI roll:	
• 30 mL syringe	1
• 10 mL syringe	1
• 10 mL red plunger syringe	1
• Rocuronium 50 mg/5 mL	2
• Suxamethonium 100 mg/2 mL	2
• Vial access cannula	3
• Blunt access cannula	3
• Red bungs	3

Continued

TABLE 15.3 SUGGESTED TRANSPORT PACK CONTENTS LIST—cont'd

MONITOR PACK	
Main compartment	
Monitor/defibrillator - complete with:	
• 4 lead ECG cable	1
• Pulse oximeter lead and reusable finger probe	1 ea
• NIBP tubing and adult cuff	1 ea
• Fully charged battery (installed)	1
Defibrillator pads, adult	2
Defibrillator pads, paediatric	1
Defibrillator cable	1
Portable suction:	
• Suction canister	1 ea
Folder:	
• Patient records	2
• Transfusion record forms	2
• Consent forms	2
• Mass Casualty recording sheet	2
Sharps container	1
Spare suction cannister	1
Inside top flap	
Suction tubing with elbow (attached to suction canister)	1
Yankauer suction catheter	1
Front left pocket	
Pressure infusion bag	1
NIBP cuffs (obese, small adult, child, infant)	1 ea
Front middle pocket	
Tympanic thermometer (with probe covers)	1
SpO_2 probe, disposable, neonatal / adult (< 3 kg > 40 kg)	1
$EtCO_2$ sidestream sampling line	2
$EtCO_2$ nasal sampling line	2
Temperature cable	1
Temperature probe, disposable	1
Front right pocket	
12 lead ECG adaptor cable	1
Spare Zoll battery	1
Adult ECG dots	1 pkt
VENTILATOR PACK	
Main compartment	
Ventilator with high pressure oxygen hose	1
Inside top pocket	
Operational circuit (in ziplock bag):	
• Ventilator circuit (test at start of shift)	1
• ET mount	1
• HME filter (adult)	1
• Cuff manometer	1
• 10 mL syringe	1
Closed suction system	1
Outside pocket	
Spare circuit	1
Spare expiration valve	1
Aide memoire	1
T piece nebuliser set	1
Spare HME filter (adult, child)	1 ea
Spare ETT mount	1
NIV masks (small, medium, large)	1 ea

STRESSORS OF TRANSPORT

The transport environment has specific stressors that must be understood, as they have the potential to have adverse effects on the patient who, in many cases, already has altered physiology, as well as on the team caring for the patient. Once appreciated, the team can anticipate and plan for these. The effects are predictable, and some are specific to the aviation environment (see Table 15.4), but they are also considered of importance in the road-transport platforms.

HYPOXIA

Hypoxia is of concern in the aeromedical environment due to changes of the partial pressure of oxygen at altitude and can be defined as an oxygen deficiency in body tissues, which, when sufficient, will cause impairment, either transient or permanent, of physiological function.[20] Oxygen comprises approximately 21% of inspired gas at sea level (760 mmHg) and its partial pressure is 159 mmHg. As the aircraft ascends in altitude, the atmospheric pressure decreases exponentially, therefore decreasing the partial pressure of oxygen. At 10,000 ft (3000 metres) oxygen is still at 21%; however, the barometric pressure falls to 523 mmHg, resulting in a drop in partial pressure of oxygen to 110 mmHg. All patients transported by air should have supplemental oxygen available to be delivered by the most appropriate device, dependent on clinical state.

TABLE 15.4 BODY CAVITIES, SYMPTOMS AND TREATMENT FOR THE EFFECTS OF ALTITUDE[21]

CAVITY (CONDITION)	SYMPTOMS (CAUSES)	TREATMENT
Middle ear (barotitis media)	Pain on descent due to blocked eustachian tube (viral illness, infection)	Moving jaw, Valsalva manoeuvre, swallowing
Sinuses (barosinusitis)	Pain on descent due to cough/cold, sinus infection	Decongestants, avoiding flying
Teeth (barodontalgia)	Pain on descent in dental decay/abscesses	Avoiding flying when affected, and good dental care
Gastrointestinal tract	Abdominal bloating and pain, respiratory distress Post-operative free gas	Nasogastric tube insertion
Thoracic cage (pneumothorax)	Respiratory distress, chest pain, hypoxia, hypotension	Chest drain insertion, needle thoracocentesis
Cranium (pneumocephalus)	Headache, altered conscious state	Cranial decompression, intraventricular drain, sea-level cabin (or as close as possible)
Endotracheal tube	Gas leak on descent	Cuff check and addition of air to tube, using saline in cuff instead of air

BAROMETRIC PRESSURE

The effects of altitude have direct consequences on the human body and equipment utilised for patient transport missions. Specifically, the effects of Boyle's Law must be understood. Boyle's Law relates to the expansion of gases and states that when temperature remains constant, the volume of a given mass of gas is inversely proportional to its pressure (see Chapter 28). So as an aircraft increases its altitude, the barometric pressure decreases and the volume of gas in an enclosed space will expand. Therefore, any gas trapped in any enclosed space—whether it is a human or equipment space—is subject to this law.

NOISE

Continuous noise has an insidious effect on the retrieval team, and levels vary depending on the type of transport frame utilised. The inability to clearly communicate with your team and hear any audible alarms on monitoring equipment places the patient at risk. Regular visual assessment of the monitor is essential, coupled with noticing any non-verbal cues provided by the patient. Grimacing, agitation, alteration in perfusion and skin colour are some of the signs to watch out for.

In the self-ventilating patient, predetermined hand signals may be useful to alert the team of any increasing symptoms, nausea or anxieties. Patient education of what to expect is important to allay any fears they may have and potentially decrease the workload for the team.

Classic assessment techniques, such as chest auscultation, manual blood pressure measurement and percussion, can be rendered useless in the transport environment; subtle changes or notes will be affected by the ambient noise.

To protect the hearing of both the team and the patient, hearing protection is mandatory in the form of mouldable ear plugs or rigid external muffs. This is still the case for intubated and ventilated patients who are sedated; they are still at risk of hearing damage. The longer the exposure and the more intense the noise, the greater the potential damage.

VIBRATION

Vibration affects the management of the critically ill patient in transit and is present in all forms and all transport platforms. The body's responses to vibration include increased muscle activity, increased metabolic rate, vasoconstriction, disturbed visual acuity and increased respiratory rate.[21] The already compromised patient may be further destabilised by these physiological changes.

It is difficult to minimise the effects of vibration on both the patient and the team alike. Reducing the amount of body contact with the airframe by sitting on cushioned seats for the team and effective packaging of the patient will serve to alleviate the effects. However, it should be relayed to the patient that they will experience vibration and shudder, especially on take-off and landing.

Transport equipment, particularly monitoring, is susceptible to interference. ECG and SpO_2 waveforms can become unrecognisable, even being interpreted as VT/VF. Additionally, NIBP can be subject to artefact and inaccurate data, lowering the threshold arterial line insertion for selected patients. It is therefore required of the team member to visually assess the patient, elicit a response or feel for a pulse. Clear visualisation of all patients at all times is imperative.

TEMPERATURE

During transport, both the team and the patient are exposed to variations in temperature. As the altitude of the aircraft increases, the internal ambient temperature will decrease at a rate of approximately 2°C every 1000 ft (300 metres). In fixed-wing aircraft, temperature is more controlled; however, special consideration must be given to any patient contact with the fuselage of the aircraft, as the walls will be cooler than the ambient temperature. In rotary-wing aircraft, the change in temperature is more important. Depending on the helicopter model, there are varying levels of in-cabin temperature control, ranging from climate control to exhaust-driven piped heating only.

Both hyperthermia and hypothermia create an increase in metabolic rate and subsequent increased oxygen demand and consumption. This additional stress may compound problems for the already compromised patient. Prolonged exposure to extremes of temperature may cause irritability, impaired performance of the team, motion sickness, fatigue, headache and a reduction in any stress-coping mechanisms the patient or team may have.

Strategies to reduce the effect of temperature on the patient include: reducing exposure to the elements when transiting between aircraft, ambulance and hospital and accessing the patient; warm blankets, including space (thermal) blankets; removing any wet clothes from the skin; covering the head; and the use of warmed IV fluids when possible.

FATIGUE

Fatigue is the cumulative end-product of all the stressors combined. The fatigue management of staff must always be considered a high priority for any tasking and coordination. It is important to minimise the effects of fatigue on the team by ensuring appropriate downtime, satisfactory time-off between shifts and the provision of good teamwork in monitoring each other for signs of exhaustion and off-lining those who are fatigued. Additionally, consideration should be given to avoiding the movement of non-time-critical patients overnight, when even the most well-rested clinicians will be working against their circadian rhythms. A culture where team members feel empowered to speak up and advise others of their fatigue is important, and this also must be supported by policy.

DEBRIEF AND POST-MISSION REVIEW

Discussing every mission should be standard procedure for all team members involved in the retrieval of the critically unwell. All attempts should be made to have this discussion as close to the date of the mission as possible. The case details, good and bad, will be fresh in the team members' minds and will offer useful insights for other staff to reflect upon. This can be done in two ways: either a formal audit or an informal debriefing process directly post-mission. Working from a template will offer prompts for detailed conversation. See Table 15.5 for a suggested post-mission debrief form. The audit forum will often take place the next day and provides the opportunity for staff to discuss the case, identify areas for improvement and make innovative suggestions for treatment. It is of value to discuss the case post-mission, when returning to base or to the home unit. Informally debriefing case details while they are fresh in your mind and all team members are available will provide valuable discussion points and an opportunity to acknowledge the team's efforts.

Furthermore, it is just as important to provide the referring hospital with feedback on the patient's treatment and condition post-transfer. Often the sick patient will represent the biggest source of stress and anxiety for these referring staff, and it is important from both a patient safety and a staff morale point of view to provide constructive feedback on the case.

Feedback can be sought from a senior team member, who ensures impartiality and a useful opportunity to discuss the case in full, without any prejudice or preconceived ideas.

PSYCHOLOGICAL CONSIDERATIONS

Open and transparent communication with both the patient and the family cannot be overlooked. The family have been exposed to an increased level of stress already, seeing their loved one acutely ill or injured, and furthermore the patient is to be moved from the local community to a larger, foreign and often city-based receiving facility far away. Clear explanations of procedures (time permitting), plans for movement, destination and expectations during transport will go a long way to reducing anxieties and provide important information that can be disseminated to extended family and friends. Providing phone numbers for the patient's destination is also useful. If the patient survives, they will be returning to the home community and will be cared for by the referring hospital in the future.

The team must demonstrate a cohesive and professional demeanour with the family and patient to instil confidence that the patient will be taken care of to the highest possible standard available to the team. The augmentation of care that the transport team provides will help with this; conversely, a disjointed,

TABLE 15.5 SUGGESTED POST-MISSION TEAM DEBRIEF TEMPLATE

Crew names:	Date and shift:	Mission outline:
Coordination and tasking (involve coordination staff where able)		Action points
En route to scene (including driving, enplaning, in-flight, deplaning etc.)		Action points
Scene safety		Action points
Team organisation and interaction with local team/crew/staff		Action points
Clinical plan		Action points
Interventions, SOP compliance and knowledge		Action points
Communications		Action points
Departing scene, loading into aircraft or vehicle		Action points
En route to destination care		Action points
Handover and documentation		Action points
What if ...?		Action points

disorganised and abrupt approach to the patient will not only put them in jeopardy but will also serve as another source of stress and anxiety. This confidence provided to the patient and family cannot be underestimated.

At times a family member will request that they accompany the patient while in transit. In fixed- and rotary-wing environments this request often cannot be granted due to weight and space limitations. However, the request should not be flatly refused and should be discussed with the team at large, including the pilot and crewperson. The patient's condition should also be factored into the decision-making process, as an unstable patient in transit who may require continual care could represent further opportunities for stress reactions and the family member may in fact cause a hindrance or block to adequate and safe patient access. Alternatively, the family member's presence may alleviate some of the patient's anxiety, especially when the patient is a child. The decision should not be made until the time of the transport, because the patient's condition may change, and promises cannot always be kept. The final decision as to whether the family member accompanies the patient always rests with the aircraft pilot-in-command.

Providing as much information as possible to the family about the receiving facility is also important. The actual destination (ED, ICU or ward number) gives a clear picture of a first port of call for the family, as well as maps and current contact phone numbers. The family should be informed of the estimated length of transport and expected time of arrival at the receiving hospital. Ensuring that the family has time with the patient before departure will prove to be a very valuable part of the transport. This may indeed be the last time they have with their loved one, and the importance of goodbyes and farewells cannot be trivialised. Overestimation of time is always best—if the transport is completed sooner than anticipated, the family will feel relief.

PRACTICE TIP

The stressors of flight and transport are experienced by the team as well. Keep an eye on your teammates and do not be afraid to voice any issues you may identify or are experiencing yourself.

SUMMARY

The successful transfer of the critically unwell patient can have far-reaching consequences for the patient, as there is a large portion of the community that has limited access to an increased scope of care. The transport environment is an emerging specialist role and cannot be considered a part-time job. It is a constantly evolving specialty, with significant improvements and changes occurring on an international scale.

It takes dedicated and motivated retrieval team members to prepare for, respond to and deliver patient care in challenging circumstances, while maintaining perspective on the safety of teams and patients. At times, the team will be expected to work in austere and potentially dangerous environments, so they must be supported by a framework of training, education, teamwork and clinical governance.

CASE STUDY

You are part of a three-person pre-hospital and retrieval team, consisting of a nurse (you), a doctor and a rescue paramedic. You have all been tasked to a primary trauma scene where two cars have collided at high speed on a sweeping turn, resulting in one of the vehicles rolling and stopping on its side approximately 100 metres from the initial collision location. The flying time is approximately 20 minutes from a tertiary major trauma centre, but only one patient can be brought back at a time due to weight and weather considerations.

Police, fire and country emergency service volunteers are in attendance.

You have been advised that there are two patients, in separate vehicles.

PATIENT 1
45-year-old

- Driver of vehicle 1—strong smell of petrol on-scene
- Still in the vehicle, trapped and suspended by the seatbelt
- Oxygen via a non-rebreather mask in situ
- No IV access
- Injuries include:
  - an altered conscious state, only responding to pain
  - obvious deformity to his right forearm
  - multiple abrasions and contusions to face and head

PATIENT 2

12-year-old

- Passenger in vehicle 2
- Out of the vehicle, being cared for by volunteer ambulance officers
- No IV access
- Clothes still on
- Injuries include:
  - swelling and deformity of right ankle and left thigh
  - crying out in pain
  - aware of surroundings

QUESTIONS

1. What are the priorities of the team?
2. How would you allocate the available resources?
3. How would you assess the patients and what would your treatment priorities be?
4. What should the retrieval team expect in terms of patient condition and potential complications in-flight?
5. What configuration of transport teams would you choose?
6. How would you prepare the patients for transport?
7. What methods would you use to integrate with the local paramedic team?
8. What communication needs to occur, and at what time?

Answers to Case Study Questions can be found on evolve **http://evolve.elsevier.com/AU/Curtis/emergency/**

USEFUL WEBSITES

ISBAR Government of South Australia, https://www.sahealth.sa.gov.au/wps/wcm/connect/public+content/sa+health+internet/clinical+resources/clinical+programs+and+practice+guidelines/safety+and+wellbeing/communicating+for+safety/isbar+-+identify+situation+background+assessment+and+recommendation.

REFERENCES

1. Australasian College for Emergency Medicine, Australian and New Zealand College of Anaesthetists, College of Intensive Care Medicine of Australia and New Zealand. Guideline for transport of critically ill patients (PG52(G). 2015. Online. Available from: www.anzca.edu.au/getattachment/bd5938d2-d3ab-4546-a6b0-014b11b99b2f/PG52(G)-Guideline-for-transport-of-critically-ill-patients.
2. Shirley PJ, Hearns S. Retrieval medicine: a review and guide for UK practitioners. Part 1: clinical guidelines and evidence base. Emerg Med J 2006;23(12):937–42.
3. Ellis D, Hooper M. Cases in pre-hospital and retrieval medicine. Sydney: Churchill Livingstone; 2010.
4. Civil Aviation Safety Authority. Advisory Circular – Electromagnetic compatibility (AC 21-53). 2015. Online. Available from: www.casa.gov.au/sites/default/files/2021-08/advisory-circular-21-53-electromagnetic-compatibility.PDF.
5. Australasian College for Emergency Medicine. Pre-hospital and retrieval medicine. 2022. Online. Available from: acem.org.au/Content-Sources/Certificate-and-Diploma-Programs/Pre-Hospital-and-Retrieval-Medicine.
6. BOC Healthcare Australia. Medical gases. Online. Available from: www.boc-healthcare.com.au/en/medical_gases/index.html.
7. Wallace PG, Ridley SA. ABC of intensive care. Transport of critically ill patients. BMJ (Clinical Research Ed.) 1999;319(7206):368–71.
8. Taylor CB, Stevenson M, Jan S, Middleton PM, Fitzharris M, Myburgh JA. A systematic review of the costs and benefits of helicopter emergency medical services. Injury 2010;41(1):10–20.
9. Holland J, Cooksley DG. Safety of helicopter aeromedical transport in Australia: a retrospective study. MJA 2005;182(1):17–9.
10. O'Connor J. The Royal Flying Doctor Service of Australia: the world's first air medical organization. Air Med J 2001;20(2):10–12.
11. Porteous JM, Stewart-Wynne EG, Connolly M, Crommelin PF. iSoBAR—a concept and handover checklist: the national clinical handover initiative. Med J Aust 2009;190(Suppl 11):S152–6.
12. Thompson JE, Collett LW, Langbart MJ, Purcell NJ, Boyd SM, Yuminaga Y, et al. Using the ISBAR handover tool in junior medical officer handover: a study in an Australian tertiary hospital. Postgrad Med J 2011;87(1027):340–4.
13. Mathews KA, Elcock MS, Furyk JS. The use of telemedicine to aid in assessing patients prior to aeromedical retrieval to a tertiary referral centre. J Telemed Telecare 2008;14(6):309–14.
14. CareFlight Safety Services. Helicopter underwater escape training—training manual. CareFlight Safety Services; 2005.
15. Meadley B, Bowles KA, Smith K, Perraton L, Caldwell J. Defining the characteristics of physically demanding winch rescue in helicopter search and rescue operations. Appl Ergon 2021;93:103375.
16. Meadley B, Horton E, Perraton L, Bowles KA, Caldwell J. The physiological demands of helicopter winch rescue in water and over land. Ergonomics 2022;65:828–41.

17. Degani A, Wiener E. Human factors of flight-deck checklists: the normal checklist. National Aeronautics and Space Administration; 1990.
18. Cardenas-Garcia J, Schaub KF, Belchikov YG, Narasimhan M, Koenig SJ, Mayo PH. Safety of peripheral intravenous administration of vasoactive medication. J Hosp Med 2015;10(9):581–5.
19. Schmidt GA, Blaivas M, Conrad SA, Corradi F, Koenig S, Lamperti M, et al. Ultrasound-guided vascular access in critical illness. Intensive Care Med 2019;45(4):434–46.
20. Martin TE. Clinical aspects of aeromedical transport. Curr Anaesth Crit Care 2003;14(3):131–40.
21. Harding J, Goode D. Physical stresses related to the transport of the critically ill: optimal nursing management. Aust Crit Care 2003;16(3):93–100.
22. MedSTAR Emergency Medical Retrieval Services. Agency overview SA Health: SA Ambulance Service. South Australia: Government of South Australia; 2007.

CHAPTER 16
CLINICAL SKILLS

BERNARD HIESS AND BEN MEADLEY

ESSENTIALS

- Clinical skills range from those skills performed frequently on a day-to-day basis to skills that will only be encountered on a very infrequent basis.
- Skills will range from the complex to the simple. It is, of course, beyond the scope of this text to present all the clinical skills that the emergency clinician would require; rather, a broad range of specifically selected skills is presented.
- The skills outlined are presented in association with the relevant anatomy and physiological considerations, and are based upon the latest available evidence.
- The emergency clinician requires the skills outlined, as they are a valuable resource to: (1) refresh previously learnt skills; and (2) acquire knowledge to develop new and more advanced skills to deliver patient care.

INTRODUCTION

The emergency clinician requires a vast repertoire of clinical skills to provide care. This repertoire of skills increases with time and experience. Some skills are used daily, while others may be learnt but rarely used. It is essential that the emergency clinician has a solid theoretical and practical knowledge base to perform these skills competently. Many of these skills may be used outside the hospital emergency department (ED), such as in the pre-hospital setting or in the general ward environment, or by clinicians not normally involved in the provision of emergency care, for example, in outpatient clinics, local doctors' rooms or medical centres.

The goal of this chapter is to introduce the range and type of clinical skills that are important to the safe care of emergency patients.

The procedures outlined in this chapter should only be performed by clinicians who have the necessary knowledge, skill development and demonstrated competency. These skills should be performed in accordance with any professional licensing requirements and in accordance with the employing institutions' policy and procedures.

AIRWAY MANAGEMENT

Assessment of the adequacy of a patient's airway is a priority in any patient's initial assessment and management. Assessment and management of the airway in any critically ill patient is of particular importance, especially for those patients with an altered level of consciousness. Any patient identified as having an inadequate airway will require immediate interventions. Patients will die if there is a failure to recognise and manage airway emergencies.

Interventions used in airway management generally begin simply and move to the more complex and are described here. Even the most basic airway management manoeuvres can have dramatic results.

BASIC AIRWAY MANAGEMENT

Basic airway management involves the assessment of the patient and the implementation of a variety of simple interventions aimed at opening and maintaining the patency of the patient's airway. This often involves suctioning of the airway where required and the administration of oxygen, both of which are described later in this chapter. These simple interventions, while providing a patent airway to assist with ventilation, do not provide airway protection against aspiration into the lungs of vomit and secretions. Airway protection is achieved through the more-complex interventions described below, such as intubation.[1]

Upper airway obstruction can occur by the tongue, substances retained in the mouth, such as saliva, vomitus, blood or foreign bodies, or by laryngospasm, leading to ineffective ventilation. Obstruction may be complete or partial. Complete obstruction results in the absence of air exchange; the patient is unable to breathe. Signs of partial upper airway obstruction include snoring, inspiratory stridor and retractions of the neck and intercostal muscles. The most common cause of upper airway obstruction is from the relaxation of the tongue and jaw, which causes the base of the tongue to fall backwards against the posterior pharyngeal wall in the supine patient.[2] Upper airway obstruction caused by the tongue can be relieved by head tilt/chin lift or jaw thrust manoeuvres and by the insertion of either nasopharyngeal or oropharyngeal airways.[1]

Head tilt/chin lift manoeuvre

To perform the head tilt/chin lift manoeuvre, the palm of one hand is placed on the patient's forehead while the tips of the fingers of the other hand are placed under the patient's chin, avoiding the soft tissues of the submandibular region. The chin is then lifted up and back towards the back of the patient's head and upwards to the ceiling (Fig. 16.1). The upper neck will naturally extend when the head tilts backwards and therefore this manoeuvre is not preferred in the patient with a possible cervical spine injury. An additional step which may be considered with this manoeuvre is to use the thumb to open the patient's mouth.[1,2]

Jaw thrust manoeuvre

To perform the jaw thrust manoeuvre, while at the head of the patient looking down towards their feet, the hands are placed on the patient's face with the middle or index fingers behind the angle of the mandible. The mandible is then lifted vertically towards the ceiling (Fig. 16.2). This manoeuvre may also be performed in combination with a head tilt. The head tilt should not be performed if there is a suspected cervical spine injury.[1,2] The preferred airway manoeuvre in suspected cervical spine injury is the jaw thrust without head tilt, performed with the neck in the neutral position and supported by in-line stabilisation.[1]

FIGURE 16.1 HEAD TILT/CHIN LIFT MANOEUVRE[1]

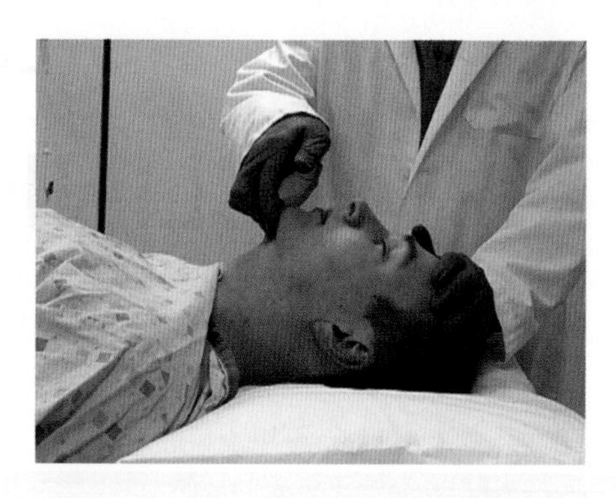

FIGURE 16.2 JAW THRUST MANOEUVRE[1]

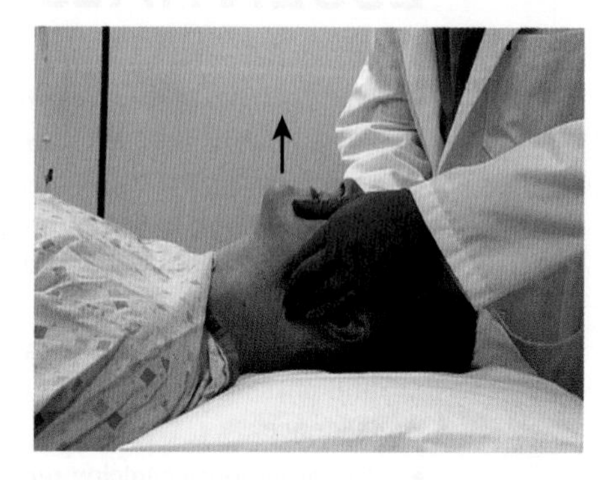

PRACTICE TIP

The preferred airway manoeuvre in suspected cervical spine injury is the jaw thrust without head tilt, performed with the neck in the neutral position and supported by in-line stabilisation.

AIRWAY ADJUNCTS

Airway adjuncts are used in addition to initial airway manoeuvres and suctioning to maintain airway patency, facilitating either spontaneous respirations or assisted bag–mask ventilation. The two most common types of airway adjuncts available are: the *oropharyngeal airway* and the *nasopharyngeal airway*.

Oropharyngeal airway

The oropharyngeal airway (Fig. 16.3) is a semicircular-shaped airway made of hard plastic. Named after the designer, it is commonly called a Guedel airway.

FIGURE 16.3 THE OROPHARYNGEAL AIRWAY[3]

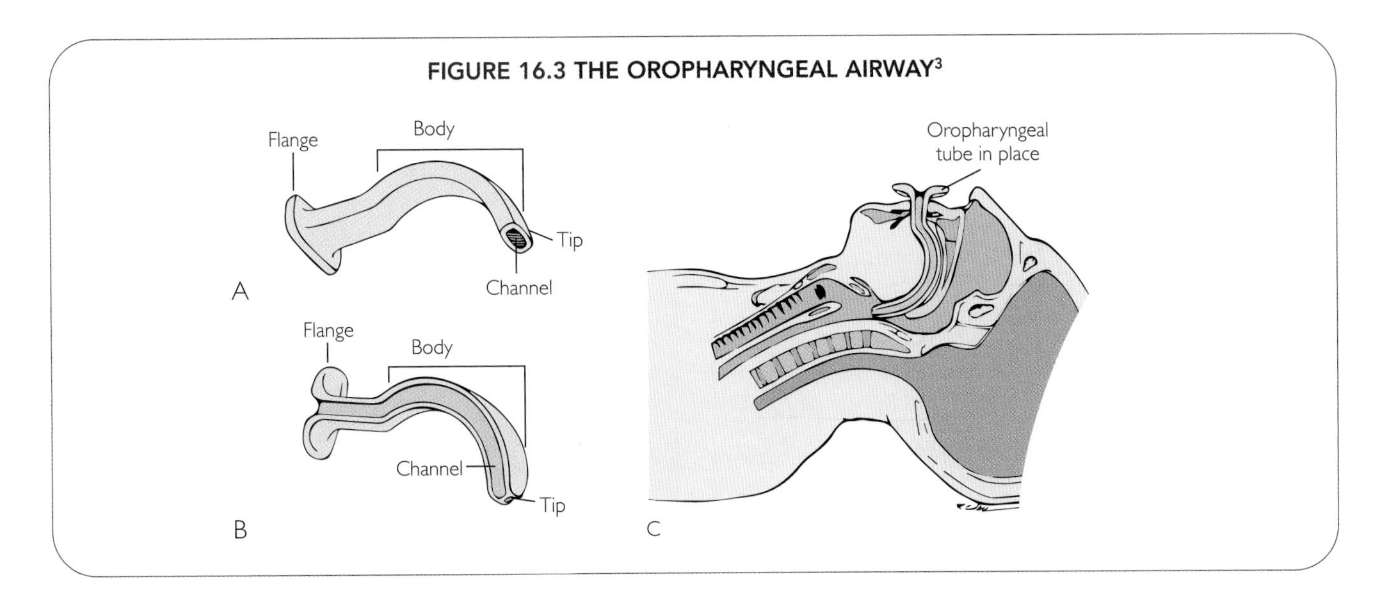

The airway is inserted through the open mouth, over the tongue, with the tip positioned in the patient's pharynx. The airway displaces the tongue forwards off the posterior pharyngeal wall. The airway has four parts: flange, body, tip and channel. The flange protrudes from the patient's mouth, resting against the lips. The body of the airway covers the tongue. The channel allows the passage of a suction catheter.[3]

The oropharyngeal airway is indicated only in unconscious patients; otherwise, it is likely to initiate gagging and vomiting. In patients where the presence of airway tone/gag reflex is not known, and the patient has known or suspected raised intracranial pressure (ICP) (e.g. traumatic brain injury), the oropharyngeal airway may induce a gag, and further raise ICP. Oropharyngeal airways should be used with caution in these patients, and consideration given to bag–valve–mask support alone, or the use of a nasopharyngeal airway.[4] Due to its hard plastic construction, it prevents teeth clenching and is often used in conjunction with an oral endotracheal tube. Care must be taken on insertion not to push the tongue backwards into the posterior pharyngeal wall, causing obstruction.[1,3] Care must also be taken not to cause additional trauma and bleeding to the soft palate when inserting.

Procedure for oropharyngeal airway insertion

1. Wash hands and don personal protective equipment (PPE)—gloves, goggles and a mask.
2. Select the correct-sized airway by selecting an airway measuring the same distance from the central incisors to the angle of the jaw (Fig. 16.4). Commonly the airway flange is coloured to represent different sizes.
3. Suction the mouth and pharynx if required.
4. Open the patient's mouth and remove dentures if present.

5a. Insert the oral airway—method 1 (Fig. 16.5):
- Hold the oral airway with the curve facing upwards.
- Advance the airway towards the hard palate and into the back of the mouth.
- Rotate the airway 180 degrees over the base of the tongue and into the oropharynx.

FIGURE 16.4 OROPHARYNGEAL AIRWAY SIZING[3]

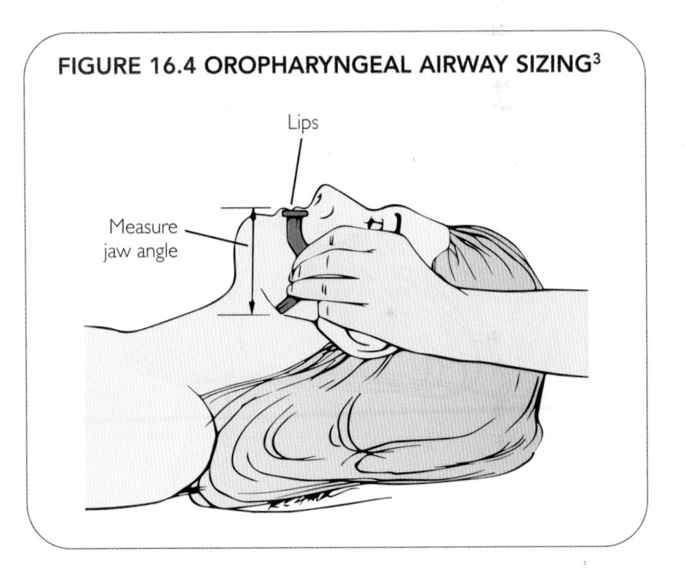

5b. Insert the oral airway—method 2; this method is recommended in paediatric patients due to the size of their tongue and the softness of their hard palate:
- Hold the oral airway with the curve facing downwards.
- With a tongue depressor, displace the tongue down and forwards.
- Insert the airway directly over the tongue into the oropharynx.

6. Recheck the size and position of the airway.
7. Verify patency of the airway: look, listen and feel.

Nasopharyngeal airway

The nasopharyngeal airway (NPA), or nasal trumpet, is a soft, flexible tube consisting of three parts: flange, cannula and bevel or tip. The flange, at the proximal end, is trumpet-shaped to prevent the airway from slipping into the nasal cavity. A hollow cannula allows airflow into the hypopharynx and also facilitates the passage of a suction catheter. The bevelled tip assists with insertion. When inserted correctly, it sits posterior to the base of the tongue (Fig. 16.6).[5]

FIGURE 16.5 OROPHARYNGEAL AIRWAY INSERTION—METHOD 1[3]

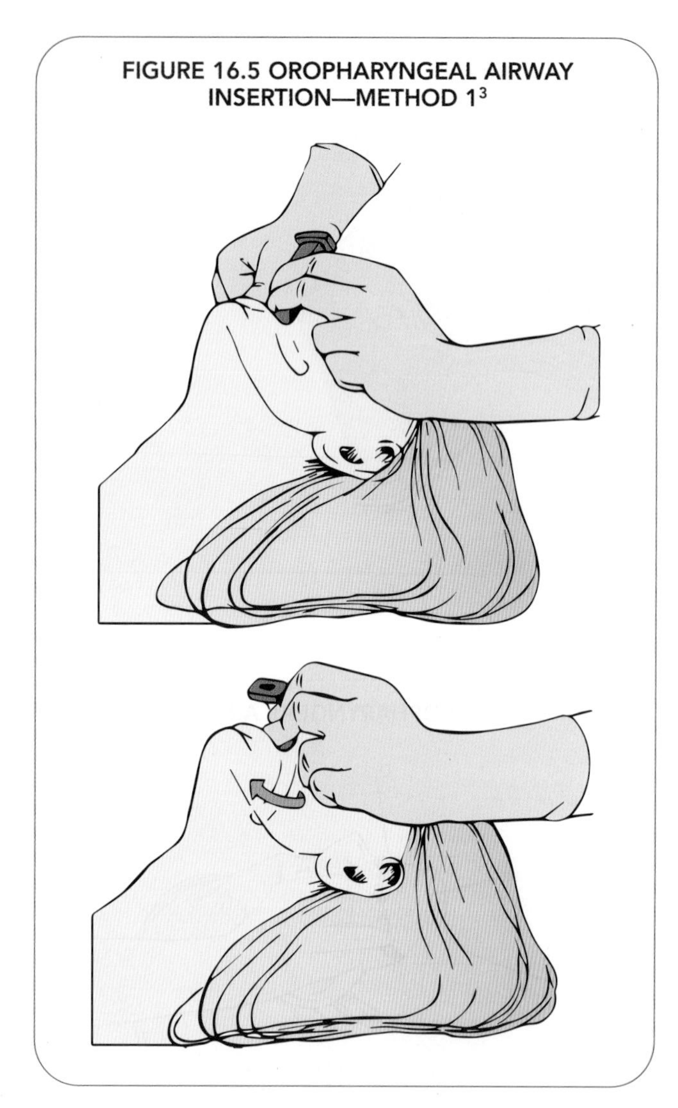

FIGURE 16.6 NASOPHARYNGEAL AIRWAY[5]

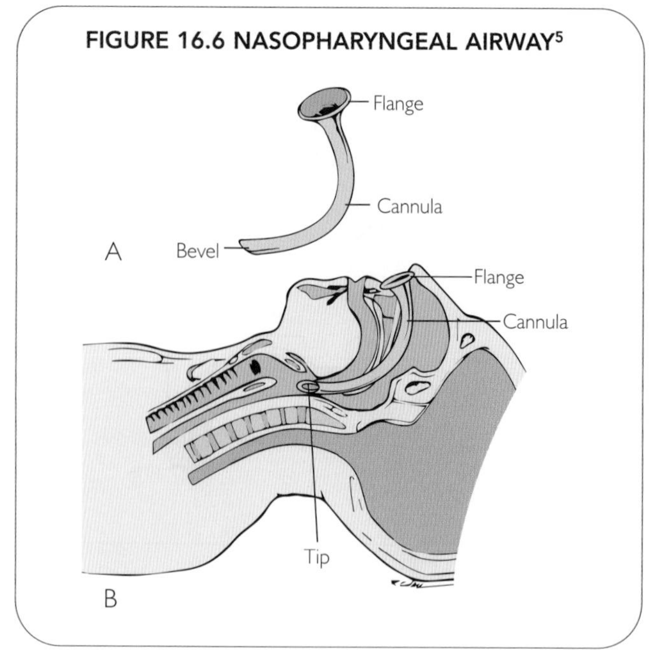

The nasopharyngeal airway has advantages over the oropharyngeal airway as it is better tolerated in semiconscious patients and is less likely to induce vomiting in patients with an intact gag reflex.[1] Other benefits over the oropharyngeal airway include its use in patients with trismus, those with known or suspected raised ICP (e.g. traumatic brain injury) and dental trauma.[6] The nasopharyngeal airway may cause epistaxis and the use of this airway is contraindicated in patients with suspected facial fractures and basilar skull fractures, due to risk of the NPA device entering the cranial vault.[1,2]

Procedure for nasopharyngeal airway insertion

1. Wash hands and don PPE.
2. Select the correct-sized airway by selecting an NPA measuring the same distance from the tip of the patient's nose to the tragus of the ear (Fig. 16.7A).
3. Identify the nasal cannula with the largest diameter. The size of the NPA will be marked on the cannula side or on the flange.
4. Generously lubricate the tip and outer surface of the airway with a water-based lubricant.
5. Gently slide the airway into the nostril and direct the airway medially and downwards along the nasal floor. Care must also be taken not to cause additional trauma and bleeding in the nose when inserting.
6. Advance the airway into the nasal passage until the flanged end sits comfortably at the nostril (Fig. 16.7B).
7. Verify patency of the airway: look, listen and feel.
8. Suction secretions as required.

BAG–MASK VENTILATION

Bag–mask ventilation is the single most important skill in airway management. Although it appears simple, it is one of the more difficult procedures to perform. Performed correctly, bag–mask ventilation provides effective oxygenation and ventilation, allows for adequate pre-oxygenation prior to drug-facilitated intubation, reduces the urgency for intubation and reduces anxiety associated with failed intubation attempts. Proficient use of bag–mask ventilation is a prerequisite for more advanced methods of airway management.[1,7]

Successful bag–mask ventilation is dependent on a patent airway, adequate mask seal and proper ventilation.[7] Bag–mask ventilation may be achieved by one or two operators; however, the two-operator technique is the most effective, and should be used whenever resources allow.[1,7]

With *single-operator bag–mask ventilation*, one hand is used to seal the mask on the face while the other is used to squeeze the bag to ventilate the patient. An E–C clamp technique is often effective in providing a mask seal. The thumb and index finger form a 'C' over the mask and apply pressure anteriorly to form a seal, while the third, fourth and fifth fingers form an 'E' to lift the jaw forwards into the mask (Fig. 16.8). Single-operator success is often dependent on the operator's hand size and on their ability to achieve an adequate seal of the face mask and lift the lower jaw into the mask while providing adequate ventilations with the other hand. Obese patients and men with facial hair pose an additional challenge in obtaining a single-operator mask seal.

The *two-operator technique* has the more experienced person controlling the mask with their thenar eminences and thumbs

FIGURE 16.7 NASOPHARYNGEAL AIRWAY SIZING[5]

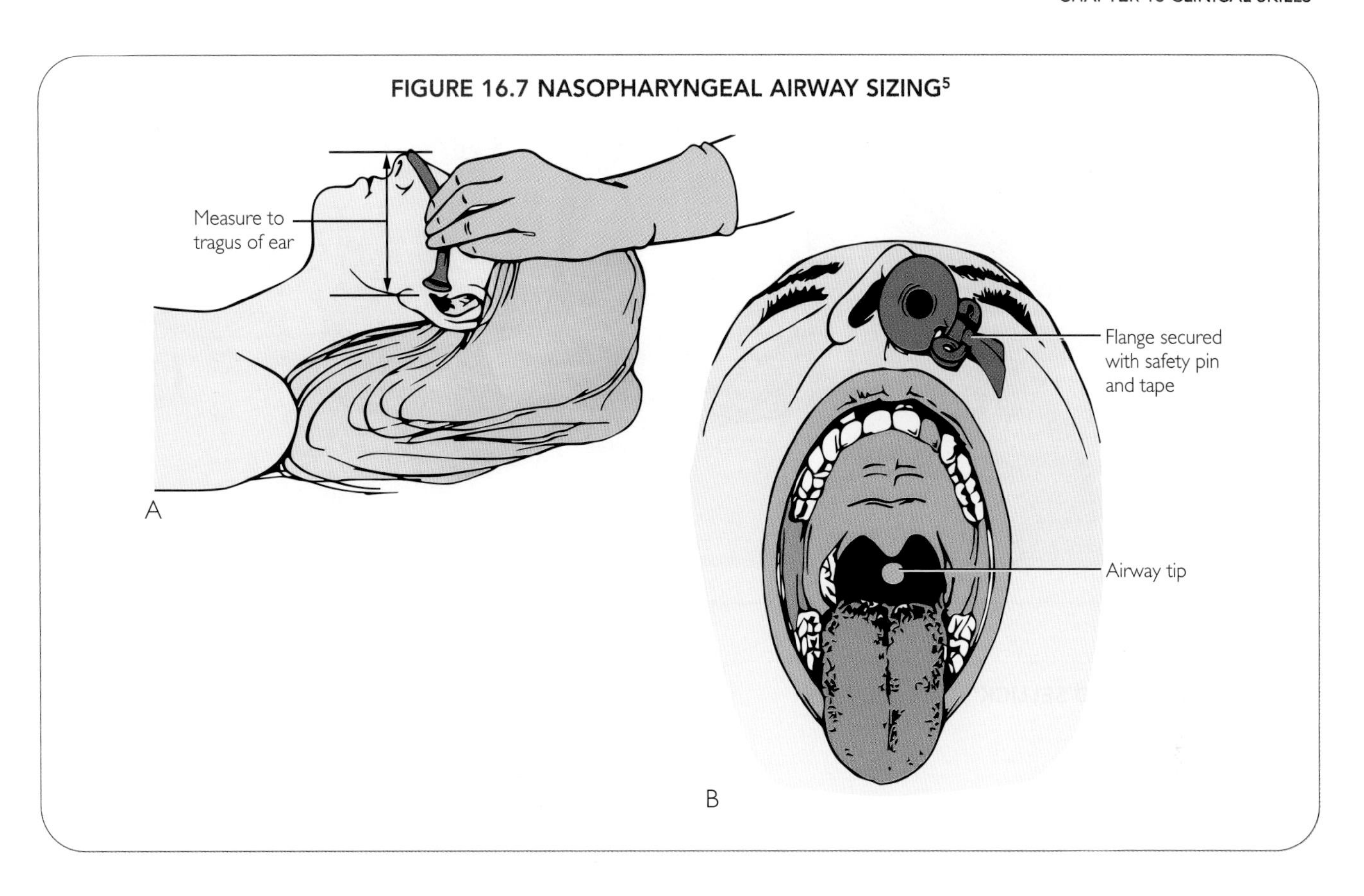

FIGURE 16.8 E–C CLAMP TECHNIQUE FOR SINGLE-OPERATOR BAG–MASK VENTILATION[1]

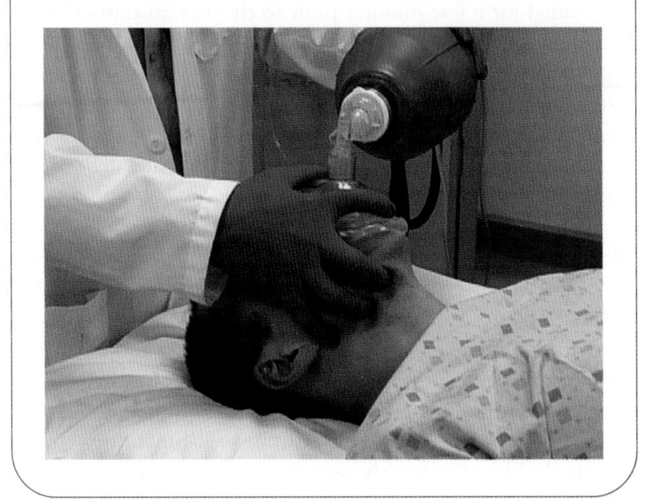

on top of the mask, to maintain an adequate face-mask seal,[7] and their second through to fifth fingers performing a jaw thrust, lifting the mandible up into the mask. The other operator controls the bag, providing ventilations (Fig. 16.9).

To provide ventilation using the bag–mask approach, the ventilation bag must be connected to an oxygen supply with a flow rate of 15 L/min. Ventilations must be delivered in such a way as to provide effective oxygenation while avoiding generating large tidal volumes, high peak airway pressures and gastric inflation. It is recommended that bag–mask ventilations in adults be administered to provide a tidal volume of approximately 500 mL at a rate of 10–12 ventilations/minute, with each ventilation delivered over 1–1.5 seconds. In children and infants, care must be taken to deliver only the volume necessary to achieve effective ventilation. Effectiveness of ventilation can be assessed by the rise of the chest, breath sounds, oxygen saturation and electronic waveform capnography.[1,7]

PRACTICE TIP

It is recommended that bag-mask ventilations in adults be administered to provide a tidal volume of approximately 500 mL at a rate of 10-12 ventilations/minute, with each ventilation delivered over 1-1.5 seconds. The two-operator technique should be used where resources allow.

Cricoid pressure (Sellick's manoeuvre)

Cricoid pressure is no longer considered essential in every instance of rapid sequence induction. Good evidence has not been found to support its efficacy. It is now employed based on clinician preference and case-by-case considerations.[8] Sellick's manoeuvre is performed by placing the thumb and middle finger over the cricoid cartilage and applying downward pressure (see Fig. 16.10). The cricoid cartilage is displaced posteriorly, occluding the oesophagus against the spinal column. The airway is not compressed due to the rigid nature of the cricoid ring.

Cricoid pressure attempts to prevent gastric inflation and passive regurgitation of gastric contents. The manoeuvre should only be used in the unconscious patient.[7] Care should be taken in children whose airways are more pliable, to avoid

FIGURE 16.9 TWO-OPERATOR BAG–MASK VENTILATION[1]

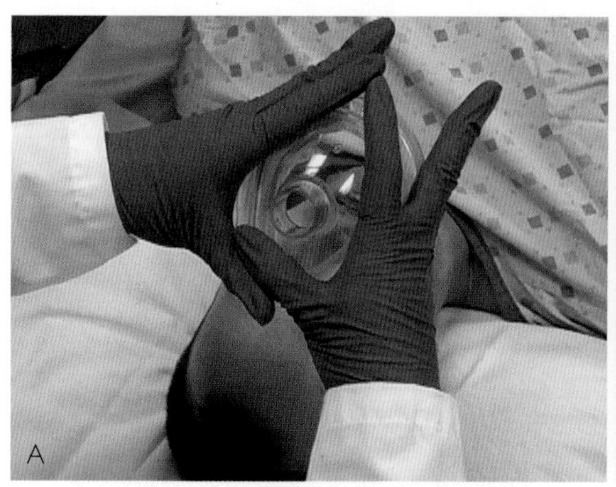

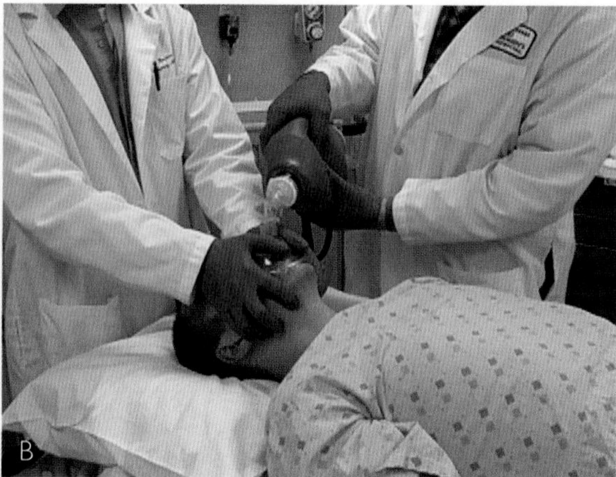

FIGURE 16.10 SELLICK'S MANOEUVRE[9]

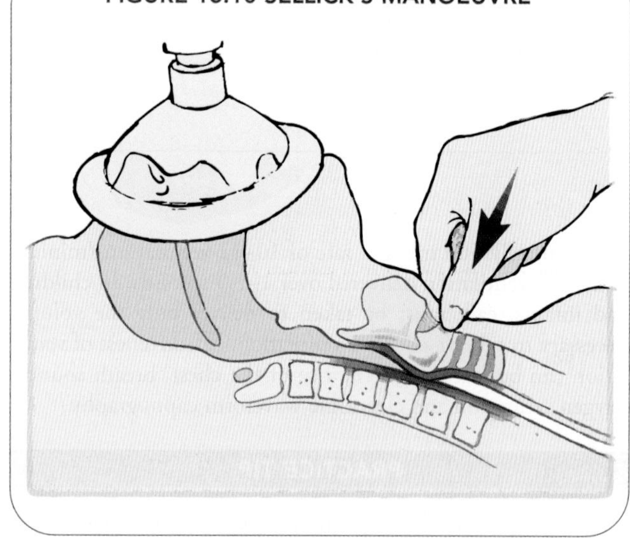

airway obstruction with excessive pressure.[1] Release/removal of cricoid pressure should be considered where the technique may be obscuring either view of the vocal cords or passage of the endotracheal tube. Cricoid pressure can also be adjusted to assist in visualisation of the cords during intubation. This technique, referred to as backwards upwards rightwards pressure (BURP) move, manipulates the cricoid ring.

INTUBATION

Rapid-sequence intubation (RSI) is a technique used for the emergency management of the airway. The basic theory behind RSI is that all pre-hospital patients and those presenting to the ED have a full stomach and therefore pose a significant aspiration risk during intubation.[10] To minimise the risks of aspiration, intubation must be performed in a rapid, safe and controlled manner to stabilise and maintain the airway. RSI is the almost simultaneous administration of an anaesthetic induction agent with a paralysing dose of a neuromuscular blocking agent, followed by the insertion of an endotracheal tube (ETT).[11,12] Pre-oxygenation is provided for a few minutes prior to the administration of the induction agents and paralysing agents. If cricoid pressure is applied during intubation, it should be maintained until the patient is successfully intubated, the ETT cuff is inflated and ETT placement in the trachea has been confirmed.[11,12] If applied, do not release cricoid pressure until instructed. If the patient begins to vomit, it must be released.

RSI can be broken down into a series of seven steps (Box 16.1).[13]

Preparation

Prior to commencing RSI, it is important to spend any available time in preparation. This step should involve preparation of the patient, the team and the necessary equipment.

The patient should have at least one well-functioning intravenous (IV) line (preferably two) and be in an area with readily

CASE STUDY 1

Mr Thomas is a 21-year-old man who was walking and was struck by a fast-moving car. On-scene he is obtunded with traumatic long bone injuries. He has extensive facial injuries from striking the car's windscreen.

QUESTIONS

1. Describe the initial assessment of Mr Thomas.
2. What are your priorities and options for opening his airway?

Answers to Case Study Questions can be found on evolve http://evolve.elsevier.com/AU/Curtis/emergency/

BOX 16.1 THE SEVEN STEPS OF RSI[13]

1. Preparation
2. Pre-oxygenation
3. Pre-treatment
4. Paralysis with induction
5. Positioning
6. Placement with proof
7. Post-intubation management

available resuscitation equipment. The patient should be attached to available monitoring including a cardiac monitor, non-invasive blood pressure and pulse oximetry. Quantitative waveform capnography is mandatory, and confirmation of functionality must occur prior to the procedure.[4]

All equipment should be assembled and checked. An appropriate-size ETT is opened, lubricated and the cuff checked by inflating, squeezing for leaks and deflating. Alternative-sized ETTs must also be readily available. A laryngoscope with appropriate-size blade and the light source is checked. Spare laryngoscopes and blades should be at hand. Video laryngoscopy, specifically with a hyper-angulated blade option, should be considered as an alternative device, depending on operator experience. While there is limited historical evidence that video laryngoscopy is superior to direct laryngoscopy in optimising endotracheal tube 'first-pass' success rates, it is rapidly becoming the preferred first option in the emergency care environment.[14] Suction equipment must be available and functioning. RSI drugs being used should be drawn up into labelled syringes and doses calculated. Additional airway equipment should also be readily available, including intubating stylets, bougies and Magill forceps. Difficult-intubation equipment should also be close at hand. The staff involved should also be adequately prepared in terms of appropriate PPE, and familiarity with the RSI procedure and the equipment being used.[13,15]

The use of a pre-intubation checklist is recommended to improve communication between the resuscitation team and improve outcomes of the emergency procedure (Box 16.2).[17]

BOX 16.2 EXAMPLE OF ITEMS FOR A PRE-INTUBATION CHECKLIST[16]

TEAM

- Is ED staff specialist or anaesthetist aware of proposed RSI? How will you and the team manage a difficult airway when there are fewer staff available, such as out-of-hours?
- Are all members of the resuscitation team aware of their and each other's roles?
- Who is the team leader?
- Plan for difficult intubation?
- Are all team members briefed?
- Difficult airway tray or trolley ready?
- Any team concerns or questions?

PATIENT

- Pre-oxygenation performed—nasal cannula ± NIV?
- Best patient position achieved?
- Haemodynamics optimal? Fluid bolus?
- Will it be difficult—BVM, laryngoscopy, supraglottic airway, cricothyroidotomy?

EQUIPMENT AND DRUGS

- IVC patent, fluids connected and running easily?
- Second IVC?
- Monitoring: ECG, BP, SaO_2 monitoring?
- RSI drugs drawn up? Doses calculated?
- Post-intubation sedation ready?
- Suction working?
- BVM working? Capnography ready?
- X2 laryngoscopes checked, blade sizes, bulbs working?
- ETT sizes checked, cuffs checked?
- Boogie or stylet in ETT?
- Tube ties or tapes ready?
- Ventilator ready?
- LMA sizes and cuffs checked?
- Surgical airway equipment available?

Pre-oxygenation

Wherever possible, the patient should be pre-oxygenated prior to commencing RSI to maximise the period of apnoea while maintaining acceptable oxygen saturations during intubation attempts. To achieve optimum pre-oxygenation, the patient should receive 100% oxygen and breathe at normal tidal volume for 3 minutes or take eight maximal breaths over 60 seconds. In reasonably healthy patients this may maintain acceptable oxygen saturations > 90% for up to 8 minutes of apnoea. However, in the critically ill and a number of specific patient groups; for example, paediatric patients, obese patients and pregnant patients, this time is likely to be considerably less (Fig. 16.11).[13,15]

Pre-oxygenation can be delivered via a non-rebreather mask on maximum oxygen flow rate if the patient is awake and breathing. In a critically ill patient, bag–valve–mask ventilation will be required. This should be delivered with the wall oxygen on the maximum flow rate and using a two-operator technique to obtain a tight face mask seal. Placing a positive end-expiratory pressure (PEEP) valve on the bag–valve–mask should be considered in patients with low oxygen saturation. PEEP should be commenced at 5 cmH_2O,[4] and increased to a maximum of 15 cmH_2O, depending on the patient's haemodynamic status and the effect on oxygenation.

To prevent desaturation during intubation, particularly during the apnoeic period after the administration of sedation and muscle relaxants, apnoeic oxygenation should occur. In the apnoeic patient, high-flow oxygen will cause oxygen to move from the alveoli into the bloodstream, thus preventing significant desaturation.[17] Nasal cannula on 15 L/min oxygen flow rate will deliver near 100% FiO_2 in the apnoeic patient. These can be placed on the patient under any face masks and left in situ until successful tracheal intubation or safe airway has been achieved.

PRACTICE TIP

To achieve optimum pre-oxygenation the healthy patient should receive 100% oxygen and breathe at normal tidal volume for 3 minutes or take eight maximal breaths over 60 seconds.

FIGURE 16.11 TIME TO DESATURATION IN DIFFERENT POPULATIONS[18]

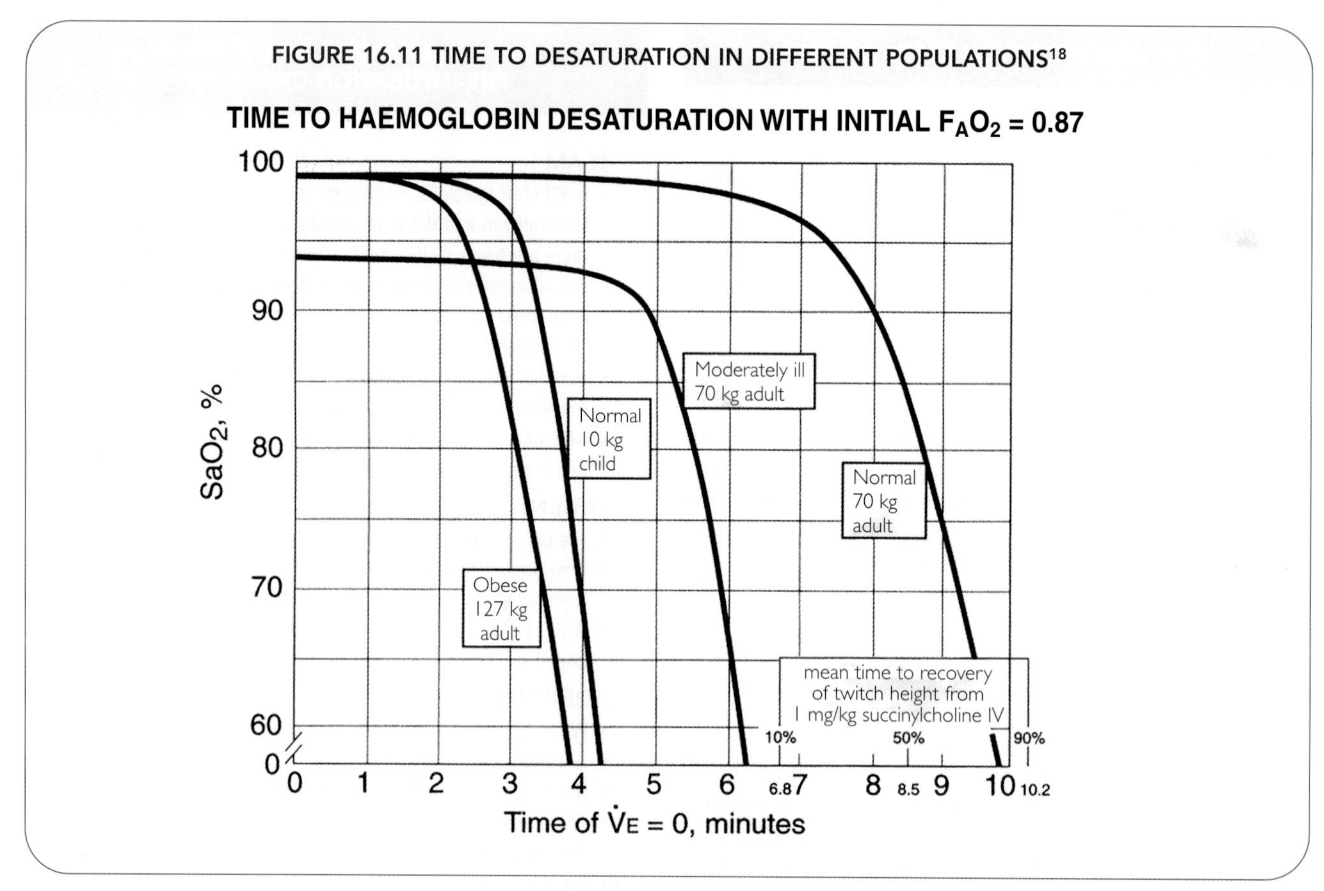

Arterial oxyhaemoglobin saturation (SaO_2) versus time of apnoea in an obese adult, a 10 kg child (low functional residual capacity (FRC) and high oxygen consumption (VO_2)), and a moderately ill adult, compared with a healthy adult. *F_AO_2: fractional alveolar oxygen concentration; VE: expired volume.*

Pre-treatment

This stage involves the administration of drugs to counteract any anticipated adverse effects associated with the intubation or the patient's underlying condition.[13] Pre-treatment medications may be given during pre-oxygenation, but in rapid sequence induction this is uncommon.

Paralysis with induction

This stage involves the administration of a rapid-acting induction agent to produce unconsciousness followed by the administration of a neuromuscular blocking agent leading to paralysis. The induction agents used will often be determined by the clinical situation, the experience and training of the medical staff and the institutional policies.[13,19] Commonly used induction agents include: propofol, ketamine and fentanyl. Neuromuscular blocking agents may be depolarising or non-depolarising. Suxamethonium is a depolarising muscle relaxant that is commonly used during RSI and is characterised by muscle fasciculations at the time of onset. Its duration of action is relatively short, 3–5 minutes, compared with other agents. This is beneficial in failed intubations, providing a return of respiratory function within a short period. Longer-acting non-depolarising agents such as rocuronium, are now increasingly popular as a first-line paralysing agent. They have favourable safety profiles and fewer absolute contraindications than depolarising agents.[20] Cricoid pressure may be applied during this stage at the onset of unconsciousness. Non-depolarising muscle relaxants are generally used following successful intubation if ongoing paralysis is required (see post-intubation management on the following page). These agents include: rocuronium, vecuronium, cisatracurium and pancuronium.

Positioning

The ideal position of the adult patient with normal body habitus is a 'sniffing' position with the head extended and neck flexed slightly. This may be facilitated by placing a small towel under the patient's head, raising it 7–10 cm.[15] Ideal positioning will not be possible in any situation where there is potential for cervical spine injury. Video laryngoscopy should be considered as a first-line intubation procedure. In these circumstances, in-line immobilisation of the neck/cervical spine is provided by a separate staff member, also positioned at the head of the bed. The staff member providing in-line stabilisation is often required to crouch down, allowing the person intubating space to visualise the airway and intubate the patient.

The 'sniffing' position is, however, not ideal for the obese patient. Increased fat in the chest and abdominal wall have a mechanical effect on the thoracic cage, diaphragm and lungs. This decreases functional residual capacity, increases airway resistance and worsens ventilation perfusion mismatch. The recommended position for obese patients is one where the external auditory canal meatus and the sternal notch are aligned, with

FIGURE 16.12 THE RAMP POSITION[21]

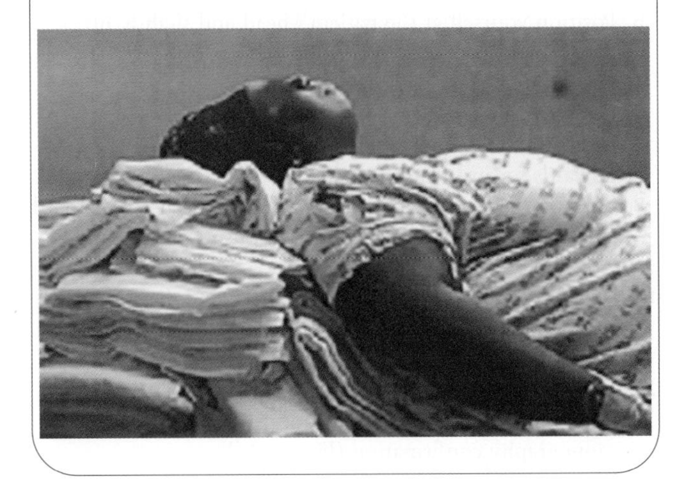

the head up and the head and shoulders supported by pillows or blankets. This is called the 'ramp' position (Fig. 16.12).

Placement

Following intubation, the ETT cuff is inflated using a syringe of air, and placement of the ETT in the trachea must be confirmed. This can be achieved reliably with quantitative waveform capnography (note with caution that during cardiac arrest, due to absence of or low cardiac output, therefore absent or decreased pulmonary blood flow, the capnography trace can be significantly degraded). Supplementary methods to confirm ETT placement include visualisation of the ETT passing through the cords (by the intubator); auscultation of breath sounds; absence of breath sounds over the epigastrium; condensation within the ETT with each breath; rise and fall of the chest with ventilation; and chest x-ray.[15] Quantitative waveform capnography is however the '*gold standard*' for immediate confirmation of endotracheal tube placement in the trachea.

Post-intubation management

Following confirmation of placement, the ETT must be secured in place. Several taping and tying methods and devices are available for securing the ETT. Institutional/departmental policy and procedure should be followed. As a rule, however, patients who have endured a brain injury are better to have their ETT secured with adhesive. This reduces the risk of raised intracranial pressure (through jugular venous outflow obstruction) that may occur from a tightly taped ETT.[22]

Hypotension is common following RSI and the subsequent commencement of positive-pressure ventilation. It may respond to IV fluids in the first instance; however, given the fact that patients requiring RSI are usually critically unwell, the use of a vasoactive agent may also be required. Metaraminol, phenylephrine and adrenaline are examples of such medications. It should be prepared and available for immediate use if required. Persistent hypotension should prompt evaluation for other more ominous causes and guide intervention.[13]

Patients will require ongoing sedation and analgesia while intubated and ventilated. This is often achieved by continuous IV infusion of various agents, which commonly include morphine, midazolam and propofol. In the pre-hospital environment, electronic syringe drivers should be available to ensure controlled delivery of ongoing sedation and/or analgesia.[4] If ongoing paralysis is required, this must always be given in conjunction with sedation. Ongoing paralysis is achieved with intermittent boluses of non-depolarising muscle relaxants, such as rocuronium, vecuronium, cisatracurium and pancuronium. Infusions of paralytics are also possible when extended paralysis is desirable; for example, prolonged pre-hospital or inter-facility transfer.[4]

SUPRAGLOTTIC AIRWAY INSERTION

Supraglottic airways (SGAs) (e.g. the iGel™) may be used in the profoundly unconscious patient who requires artificial ventilation and when a clinician is not credentialled in endotracheal intubation, intubation is not readily available or there has been a failure to establish an airway successfully.[23] SGAs may also be the first-line airway choice in patients with known difficult airways, following cardiac arrest or in severe facial trauma.[1] Historically, a number of devices have been available, but modern SGAs (Fig. 16.13) are a wide-bore tube with an oval cuff or conforming gel head, and when inserted conforms to the contours of the hypopharynx, positioning the opening directly over the laryngeal opening to provide an avenue for ventilation. The seal attained by the SGA provides protection from oral and nasal secretions but does not necessarily protect the airway from aspiration of gastric contents.[1] SGAs are relatively easy to insert and have been successfully used by novice nurses and other healthcare professionals following minimal training.[24] SGAs are also widely used by pre-hospital personnel. Other types of SGAs are available, including SGAs that are specifically designed to facilitate intubation of the trachea, but are beyond the scope of this text.

FIGURE 16.13 SUPRAGLOTTIC AIRWAYS

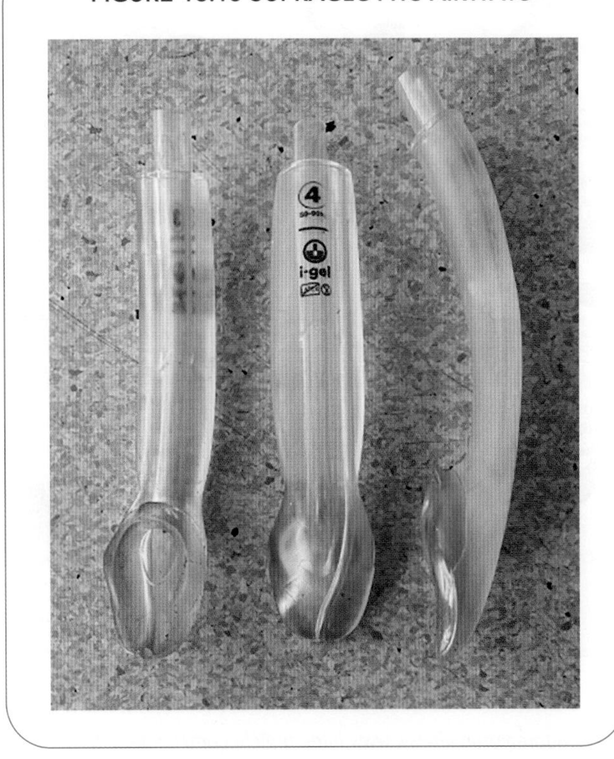

Procedure for supraglottic airway insertion

1. Wash hands and don PPE.
2. Obtain the appropriately sized SGA for the patient (Table 16.1).
3. Lubricate the posterior tip of the cuff with water-based lubricant.
4. Place the patient's head in the sniffing position, unless contraindicated.
5. Position yourself at the patient's head and slightly lift the patient's head with your non-dominant hand.
6. Hold the SGA along the stem with the cuff facing the patient's chin (Fig. 16.14).
7. Insert the SGA into the patient's mouth, directing upwards towards the hard palate (Fig. 16.14).
8. Glide the device downwards and backwards along the hard palate with a continuous but gentle push (Fig. 16.14).
9. Continue to advance until resistance is felt (Fig. 16.14).
10. Remove the non-dominant hand from behind the patient's head and use it to stabilise the SGA and remove the dominant hand index finger from the patient's mouth (Fig. 16.14).
11. Connect a resuscitation bag and gently ventilate, looking for chest rise and fall, breath sounds on auscultation and capnography confirmation (Fig. 16.14).
12. Secure the SGA by taping from maxilla to maxilla (Fig. 16.14).

TABLE 16.1 iGel SUPRAGLOTTIC AIRWAY SIZING CHART[4]

SIZE	PATIENT SELECTION INFORMATION	MAXIMUM SIZE OF GASTRIC TUBE
1	2-5 kg	N/A
1.5	5-12 kg	12
2	10-25 kg	12
2.5	25-35 kg	12
3	30-60 kg	12
4	50-90 kg	12
5	90+ kg	14

CRICOTHYROIDOTOMY

Cricothyroidotomy is the establishment of a surgical opening in the airway through the cricothyroid membrane and the insertion of a cuffed tracheostomy tube or ETT, providing an avenue for ventilation (Fig. 16.15). The indication for cricothyroidotomy occurs in the *'can't intubate, can't oxygenate'* scenario. Where there have been failed attempts at intubation

FIGURE 16.14 SUPRAGLOTTIC AIRWAY INSERTION METHOD

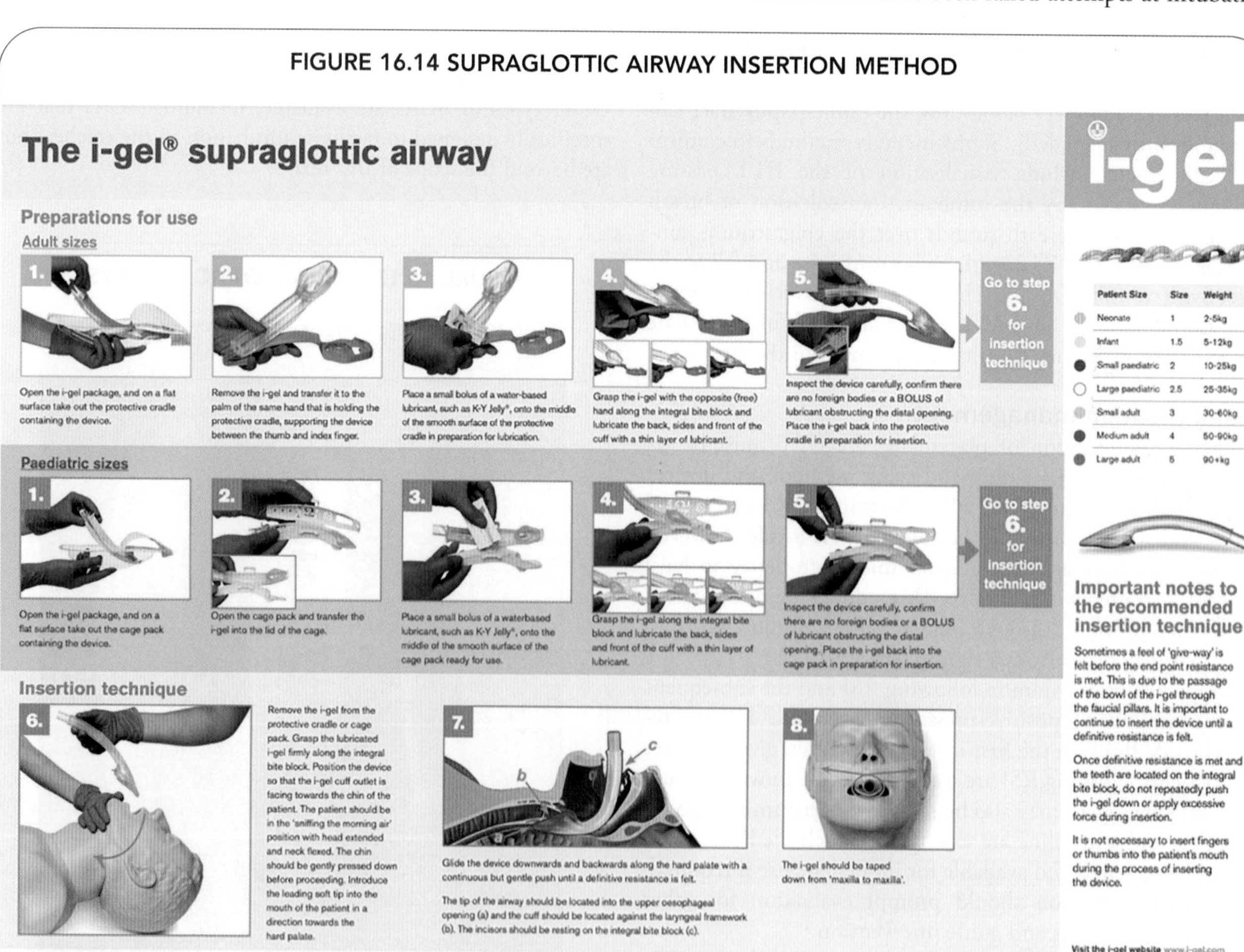

i-gel® Supraglottic Airway. www.intersurgical.com/content/files/62376/-1493058229

FIGURE 16.15

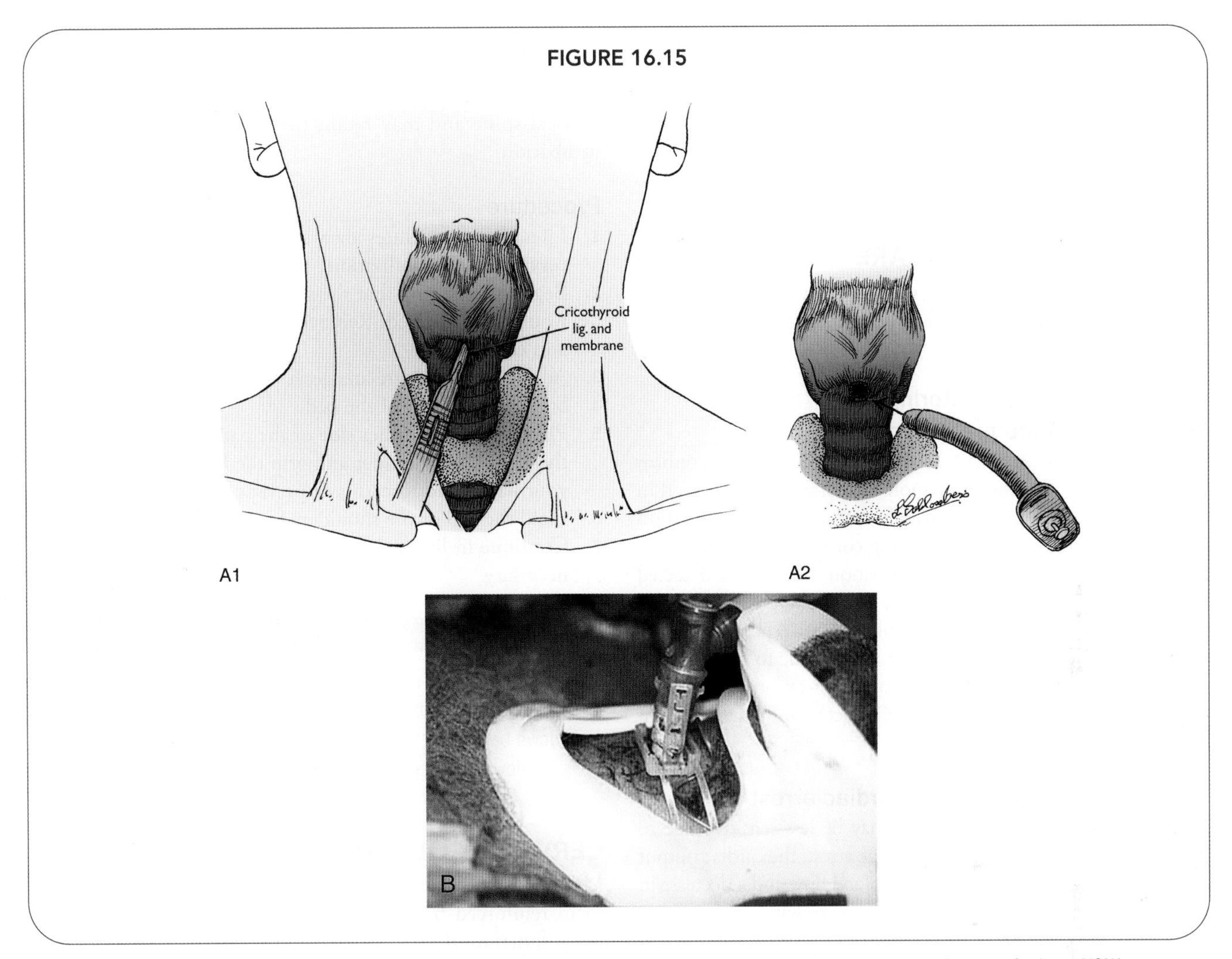

A. Cricothyroidotomy technique.[25] **B.** Completed cricothyroidotomy. B, *Courtesy of Liverpool Hospital Trauma Service, Sydney, NSW.*

and the patient is unable to be ventilated adequately using bag and mask, cricothyroidotomy should be considered. Alternatively, if the patient is unable to be intubated but able to be ventilated, but there is no other device available that is likely to be successful in securing the airway (e.g. SGA/LMA), then cricothyroidotomy should also be considered. Additional and persistent attempts at laryngoscopy and intubation are likely to result in significant hypoxia. The final scenario in which cricothyroidotomy is indicated is in the trauma patient with significant lower facial trauma where airway access through the mouth or nose would be considered too time-consuming or impossible.[26]

Cricothyroidotomy is generally contraindicated in children less than 12 years of age. Children have a small, pliable, mobile larynx and cricoid cartilage, making cricothyroidotomy extremely difficult. Children who require an emergency surgical airway require needle cricothyroidotomy with trans-tracheal jet ventilation. In this technique, a 12- to 14-gauge angiocath or IV cannula is inserted through the cricothyroid cartilage into the trachea. The catheter is left in place, providing an avenue for ventilation. Ventilation is provided by jet ventilation (not described here) or via a ventilation bag attached via a suitable adaptor. Needle cricothyroidotomy should be seen as a rescue technique and is not considered a definitive airway. Needle cricothyroidotomy is a temporary measure to provide oxygenation until a more definitive airway can be secured.[26,27]

The role of the emergency nurse or paramedic in a situation in which cricothyroidotomy is required may be to help the person performing the procedure. In most states and territories of Australia and in Aotearoa New Zealand, intensive care or critical care paramedics can perform emergency cricothyroidotomy. To provide assistance, it is important that the emergency clinician is familiar with the indication for cricothyroidotomy, the equipment, particularly its location within their department or vehicle, and also the techniques for performing this very seldom-occurring procedure. Paramedics credentialled in this skill require ongoing skills maintenance according to local arrangements.

CAPNOGRAPHY/END-TIDAL CARBON DIOXIDE MONITORING

Carbon dioxide (CO_2) is produced as an end-product of cellular metabolism and is transported in the venous blood back to the lungs where it is eliminated during the expiratory phase of breathing. During inspiration minimal amounts of CO_2 are drawn into the lungs, and during alveolar ventilation the high concentrations of CO_2 returning via the pulmonary circulation diffuse down a concentration gradient into the alveoli and are expelled during expiration. In healthy lungs where ventilation matches perfusion, exhaled CO_2 levels closely approximate $PaCO_2$ (arterial partial pressure of CO_2) levels, with expired end-tidal carbon dioxide ($EtCO_2$) levels being approximately 2.5–10 mmHg below the level of arterial CO_2.[28] This gradient may be increased when there is diminished pulmonary perfusion to regions of the lung, resulting in dead-space ventilation.[29]

USES IN EMERGENCY CARE

The assessment and monitoring of $EtCO_2$ has a number of uses in the emergency pre-hospital and in-hospital environments. These include the following:

Confirmation and monitoring of endotracheal tube placement

The measurement of $EtCO_2$ is the 'gold standard' to confirm ETT placement. During intubation, when an ETT is placed in the trachea the CO_2 present is readily detected during expiration by means of capnography, confirming correct ETT positioning. In the event of an oesophageal intubation, no CO_2 is detected and corrective actions can be rapidly undertaken. $EtCO_2$ is also useful in the monitoring of ETT placement, especially during transportation or movement of the patient. Due to the continuous monitoring of CO_2 levels on a breath-by-breath basis by capnography, ETT dislodgement, displacement, disconnection or obstruction is rapidly identifiable.[29,30]

Use of capnography during cardiac arrest

During cardiac arrest, capnography may be less sensitive due to decreased cardiac output. During cardiac arrest, the cardiac output falls resulting in decreased pulmonary blood flow and a decrease in CO_2 elimination. As cardiac output improves with either cardiopulmonary resuscitation (CPR) or return of spontaneous circulation (ROSC), pulmonary blood flow is restored in conjunction with elimination of CO_2. Therefore, capnography is useful in assessing the effectiveness of CPR and in the recognition of the return or loss of spontaneous circulation.[29,30]

CERVICAL SPINE STABILISATION

Cervical spine stabilisation is used for suspected acute cervical injury to prevent potential spinal cord damage. The spine should be always protected during the management of the patient with multiple injuries. There are several different techniques available that can be used to stabilise the cervical spine.

PRACTICE TIP

To maintain neutral spinal alignment in adult patients, place support, such as a folded towel, underneath the patient's head. Patients with spinal kyphosis will require thicker padding, such as a folded blanket or pillow. The best position is one of comfort.

MANUAL IN-LINE CERVICAL SPINE STABILISATION

Manual in-line cervical spine stabilisation involves holding the head and neck in a neutral position and is often used during lifesaving procedures when a hard collar is not indicated or cannot be fitted. Some evidence suggests that manual in-line stabilisation does not effectively immobilise an injured cervical spine and may retard the view of the airway during intubation.[31]

Procedure

1. Lifesaving procedures always take precedence over in-line cervical spine stabilisation.
2. Begin by ensuring that the skin is clean and dry and any wounds are covered. Remove jewellery such as necklaces and earrings.
3. Administer adequate analgesia where possible.
4. Stand at the head of the bed.
5. Place both arms either side of the patient's head down to the top of the shoulder and grip the head and neck with your hands and forearms to prevent movement.
6. Hold the top of the shoulders for additional support.
7. Continue in-line stabilisation until it is no longer deemed necessary.

PRACTICE TIP

When providing manual in-line stabilisation of the cervical spine during intubation, hold the head and neck and crouch down below and to the side of the back of the bed. This will allow the proceduralist a good view during intubation.

CERVICAL COLLARS

Most collars are made from rigid plastic, soft or semi-rigid foam reinforced by plastic struts with Velcro straps. The primary function of these collars is to restrict flexion and extension of the middle and lower cervical spine. The use of hard cervical collars is no longer recommended due to a lack of evidence proving benefit.[32] There is evidence, however, that rigid collars lead to complications, including discomfort, tissue ulceration, increased intracranial pressure (through cerebral venous outflow obstruction), impaired respirations and in some cases compounding spinal injury.[22] Nonetheless, these devices remain in use in some jurisdictions.

A soft collar is a foam collar that does not contain rigid or semi-rigid pieces. The cervical soft (foam) collar is a disposable single-use device made from soft, open-cell foam plastic with a cotton stockinette cover and touch tape closure. Using a cervical soft collar can reduce the complications associated with hard collars while reminding staff that the patient still requires spinal precautions. These devices are preferable, safe and now more commonly used than the cervical hard collar, in both the pre-hospital and emergency department settings.[33]

Fitting a cervical soft collar

1. Lifesaving procedures always take precedence over fitting of a collar.
2. Begin by ensuring that the skin is clean and dry and any wounds are covered. Remove jewellery such as necklaces and earrings.

FIGURE 16.16 APPLICATION OF A SOFTCOLLAR FOR CERVICAL SPINE IMMOBILISATION

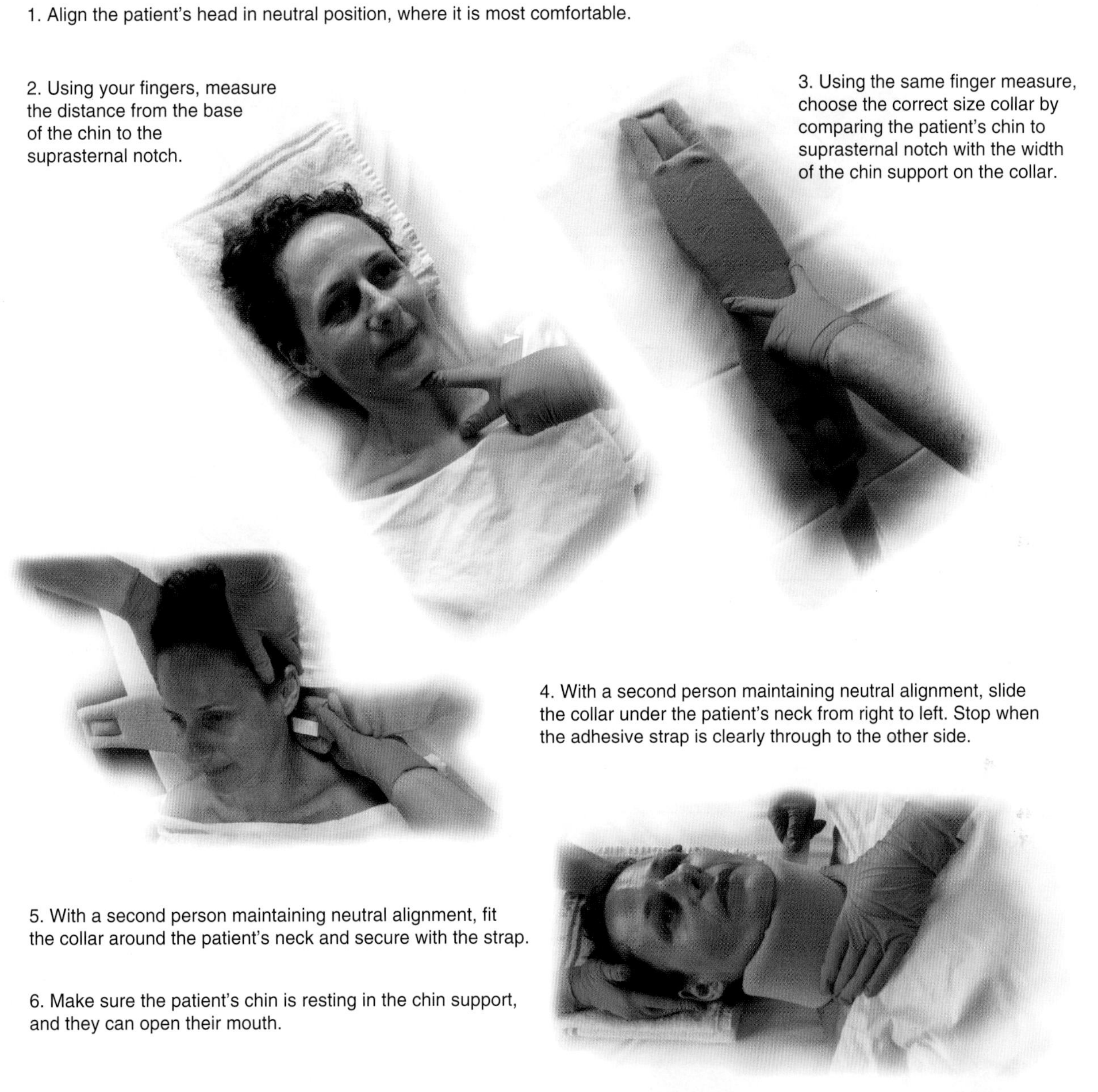

1. Align the patient's head in neutral position, where it is most comfortable.
2. Using your fingers, measure the distance from the base of the chin to the suprasternal notch.
3. Using the same finger measure, choose the correct size collar by comparing the patient's chin to suprasternal notch with the width of the chin support on the collar.
4. With a second person maintaining neutral alignment, slide the collar under the patient's neck from right to left. Stop when the adhesive strap is clearly through to the other side.
5. With a second person maintaining neutral alignment, fit the collar around the patient's neck and secure with the strap.
6. Make sure the patient's chin is resting in the chin support, and they can open their mouth.

Courtesy of James Brinton.

3. Administer adequate analgesia where possible.
4. Align the patient's head to a neutral anatomical position that is most comfortable.
5. Measure between the base of the patient's chin and the suprasternal notch and select a collar with a similar chin support width.
6. Immobilise the patient's head in a neutral position with manual in-line stabilisation.
7. Slide the collar under the neck and secure with the Velcro strap.
8. Check the collar allows the patient to open their mouth and their chin rests on top of the collar (Fig. 16.16).

HELMET REMOVAL

Refer to Fig. 16.17 for in-line removal of various types of motorcycle and sports helmets.

PHILADELPHIA COLLAR

The Philadelphia tracheotomy collar is a semi-rigid foam collar used to support the cervical spine (Fig. 16.18).

Fitting a Philadelphia collar

1. Lifesaving procedures always take precedence over fitting of a collar.

FIGURE 16.17 MOTORCYCLE HELMET REMOVAL[34]

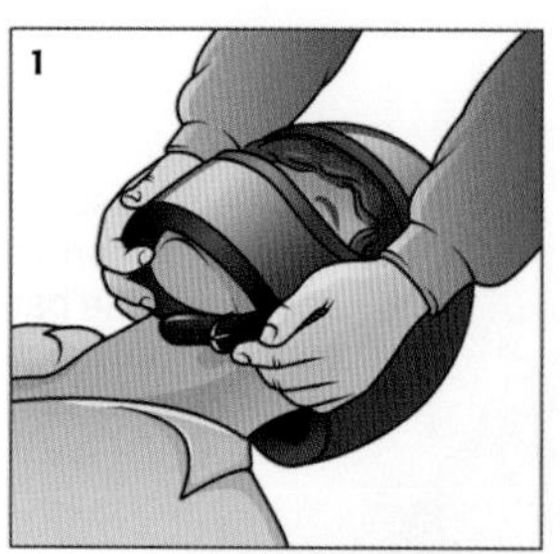

One rescuer maintains in-line immobilisation by placing their hands on each side of the helmet with the fingers on the victim's mandible. This position prevents slippage if the strap is loose.

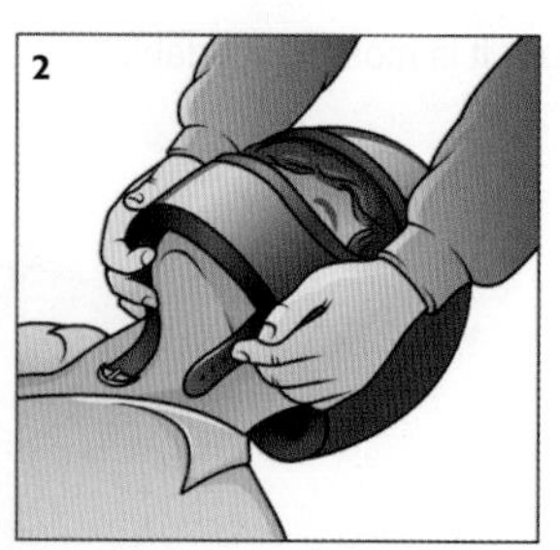

A second rescuer cuts or loosens the strap at the D-ring.

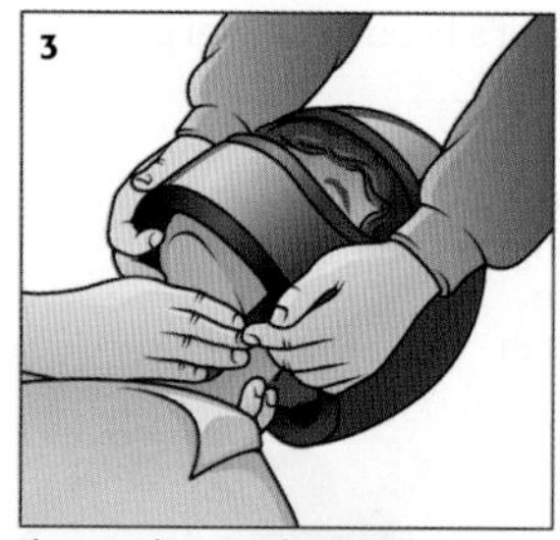

The second rescuer places one hand on the mandible at an angle, the thumb on one side and the long and index fingers on the other. With the other hand, the rescuer applies pressure from the occipital region. This manoeuvre transfers the in-line immobilisation responsibility to the second rescuer.

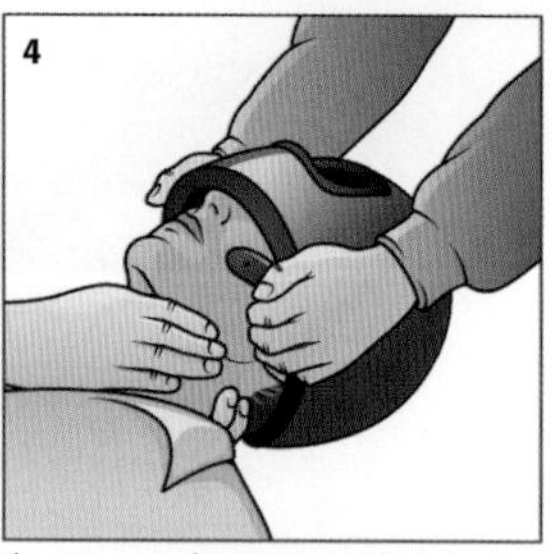

The rescuer at the top moves the helmet. Three factors should be kept in mind:
- The helmet is egg-shaped and therefore must be expanded laterally to clear the ears.
- If the helmet provides full facial coverage, glasses must be removed first.
- If the helmet provides full facial coverage, the nose may impede removal. To clear the nose, the helmet must be tilted backwards and raised over it.

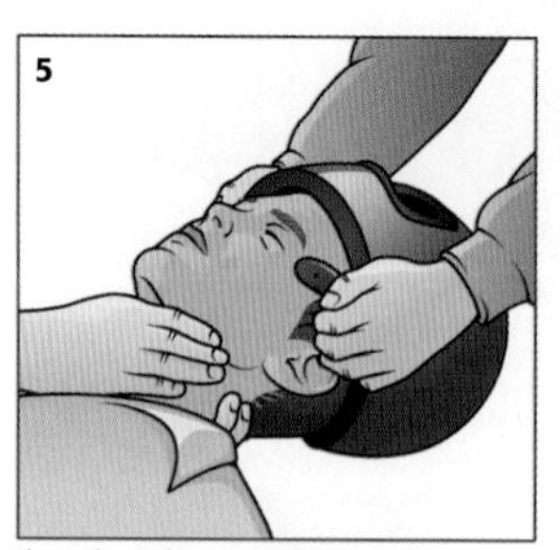

Throughout the removal process the second rescuer maintains in-line immobilisation from below to prevent unnecessary neck motion.

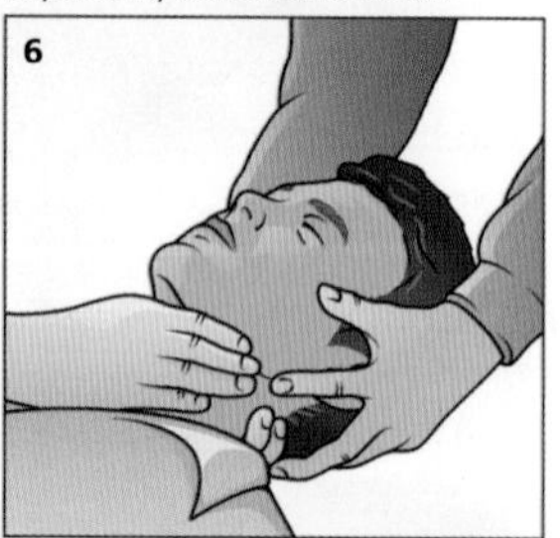

After the helmet has been removed, the rescuer at the top replaces his or her hands on either side of the victim's head with the palms over the ears.

FIGURE 16.18 PHILADELPHIA COLLAR[34]

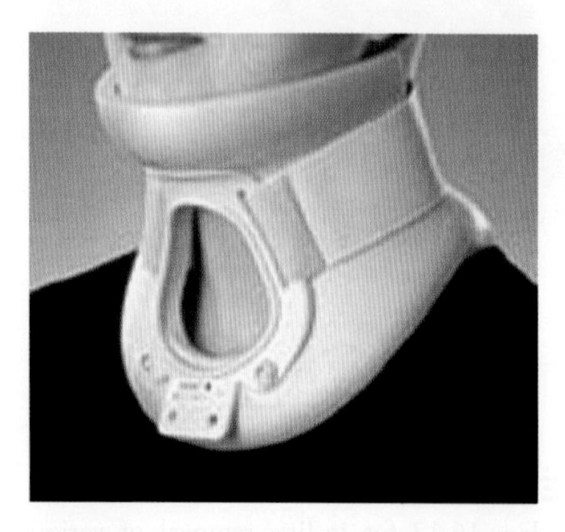

The collar supports the head in a dish-shaped contour formed by the two halves when joined with the Velcro fasteners. When properly sized, it provides excellent support; if too tight, it tends to force the mandible backwards and can cause thyroid compression in some patients.

2. Begin by ensuring that the skin is clean and dry and any wounds are covered. Remove jewellery such as necklaces and earrings.
3. Administer adequate analgesia where possible.
4. Measure the vertical distance from the top of the shoulder to the tip of the chin to give the height of the collar.
5. Measure the circumference of the neck for the second size.
6. Select the correctly sized collar that corresponds with the two measurements. The collar comes in two pieces—do not mix and match sizes.
7. Immobilise the patient's head in a neutral position with manual in-line stabilisation.
8. Fit and centre the back piece of the collar with the black arrow pointing towards the top of the head.
9. Fit the front piece of the collar with the black arrow pointing towards the top of the head.
10. Secure the chin in the cup recess. The front piece of the collar overlaps the back piece and is secured with Velcro straps.

PRACTICE TIP

The Philadelphia collar comes in two pieces and 20 different adult sizes and can remain on for up to 48 hours. To prevent pressure injury, pressure areas should be attended to after 2 hours.

Philadelphia collars are x-ray-lucent and safe to use in magnetic resonance imaging (MRI) scanners.

CASE STUDY 2

Mr Thomas is a 21-year-old man who presents at 0800 hours following a traumatic pedestrian injury. Pre-hospital treatment included rapid sequence intubation.

QUESTIONS

1. Describe how you will initially stabilise his cervical spine.
2. How will this immobilisation change if he requires long-term cervical spine immobilisation?

Answers to Case Study Questions can be found on evolve **http://evolve.elsevier.com/AU/Curtis/emergency/**

Assisting with a spinal collar application

1–6. If providing manual in-line cervical spine stabilisation so that a spinal immobilisation collar can be fitted, proceed as above for the first 6 steps. Then:

7. Maintain in-line stabilisation while the collar is fitted. Usually, the back section of the Philadelphia collar is fitted first.
8. Move hands and forearms up to the patient's ears and grip their head in the palm of the hands as the front section of the collar is applied.
9. Check that the collar is in correct alignment and that the head remains in a neutral position throughout.
10. Release manual in-line stabilisation only when the collar is correctly secured.

SANDBAGS IN HEAD CONTROL

Sandbags can be used to assist with immobilisation of the head and neck following trauma. In the field, rolled towels, full 1-L IV fluid bags, foam blocks or pillows can be substituted.[35] Sandbags or rolled towels may play a role in the stabilisation of children or of patients to whom a collar cannot be adequately fitted. Sandbags can be used with or without a spinal immobilisation collar.

PRACTICE TIP

Pay particular attention to the risk of vomiting and aspiration in any patient who has the cervical spine stabilised. A patient's head should never be taped to a spinal board, sandbags or rolled towels, due to risk of aspiration.

END-TIDAL CARBON DIOXIDE DETECTION DEVICES

The majority of $EtCO_2$ detection devices use infrared radiation technology to calculate CO_2 concentrations in a gas sample. This is achieved through the use of photodetectors that identify the amount of infrared radiation that is absorbed by CO_2 present within a given breath sample. This allows for the calculation of concentration or partial pressure of the CO_2. Depending on the location of the photodetector sensor, this is achieved through either sidestream or mainstream devices.

Mainstream devices have the detector located on the endotracheal tube and directly measure gas from the airway. Mainstream devices are primarily designed for intubated patients as the detector forms part of the ventilation circuit.

Sidestream devices aspirate small samples of gas from within the airway and pump the gas through tubing to a sensor located within the machine. Sidestream devices may be configured to be used in either ventilated or non-ventilated patients. Use in non-ventilated patients is for spontaneously breathing patients where a nasal–oral cannula is used, allowing both the sampling of exhaled CO_2 and the administration of oxygen.[36]

$EtCO_2$ detection devices may be *quantitative* or *qualitative*. Quantitative devices measure and display the exact $EtCO_2$ as either a number (capnometry) or as a number and a waveform (capnography). The capnography devices display a continuous waveform depicting the breath-by-breath rise and fall of the $EtCO_2$; this waveform is known as the *capnogram* (Fig. 16.19). The capnography device has become a standard of care for the ventilated patient and is widely used in several clinical settings, including the ED. Older capnography devices require some form of calibration prior to use to ensure their accuracy. This calibration often involves allowing the sensor to warm to its operating temperature, then zeroing it before calibrating it to a predetermined reference value. In addition to this, the sensor may also need to be calibrated to room air outside the patient circuit and away from any exhaled CO_2.[38] While these calibrations routinely do not take more than a few minutes, this may be difficult to achieve in

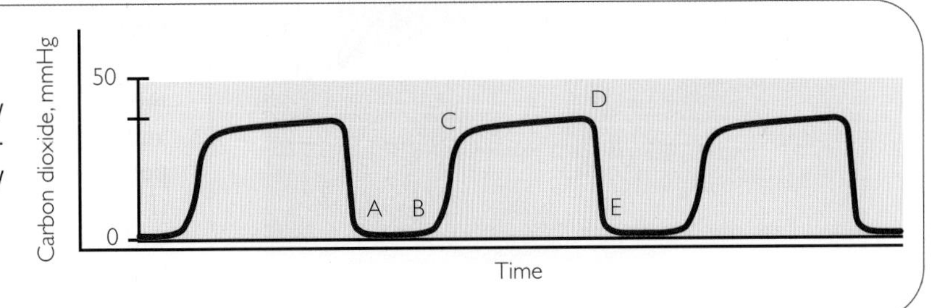

FIGURE 16.19 NORMAL FINDINGS ON A CAPNOGRAM[37]

A → B indicates the baseline; B → C expiratory upstroke; C → D alveolar plateau; D partial pressure of end-tidal carbon dioxide; D → E inspiratory downstroke.

unanticipated emergency situations. In these instances, it would be recommended to use a qualitative $EtCO_2$ detection device (*colourimetric device*—see below) to confirm ETT placement, and, when time permits, calibrate and use the capnograph.

Qualitative devices measure a range in which $EtCO_2$ falls, rather than a precise number. The most used devices are the colourimetric $EtCO_2$ detection devices.

Colourimetric $EtCO_2$ detection devices

Colourimetric devices (Fig. 16.20) change colour in the presence of exhaled CO_2 through the use of a litmus paper. These devices are small, portable and disposable, making them suitable to austere environments where electronic waveform capnography is not practical or available. These devices are primarily used to confirm ETT placement within the trachea. The device is placed between the ETT and the resuscitation bag immediately following intubation; the device is then observed for a change in colour to confirm the presence of CO_2. It is important to allow adequate exhalation time so that the device can change colour. This may require checking the device for a definitive colour change after up to six ventilations.

If there is an oesophageal intubation the device will fail to change colour, indicating the absence of CO_2 and prompting the need for re-intubation. Failure of the device to change colour may also be seen in cardiac arrest (as discussed above); therefore, in these situations the user should confirm correct ETT placement by other acceptable means. A colour change may be subsequently seen with the ROSC or effective CPR.

These devices are available for patients of all ages and sizes. Some devices have a variable colour change and a numerical scale showing the $EtCO_2$. These devices may be accurate for up to 2 hours of continuous use or 24 hours of intermittent use (the exact characteristics of individual devices should be confirmed with the product literature). Those devices that can be used for an extended period provide an additional benefit that they can be used to monitor ETT placement during transport or movement of the patient, assisting in the early identification of ETT dislodgement. Devices which may become contaminated with fluid, such as respiratory secretions, vomitus or blood, should be replaced to ensure their reliability.[30,39] It is important to note that waveform capnography is *vastly* superior to a colourimetric $EtCO_2$ detection device. Ideally, electronic waveform capnography should be the default position in all instances where intubation is being performed, and colourimetric devices reserved for situations where electronic capnography fails, or carriage of such equipment is not practical (e.g. remote area medicine, winch rescue).

FIGURE 16.20 COLOURIMETRIC END-TIDAL CARBON DIOXIDE DETECTION DEVICE[38]

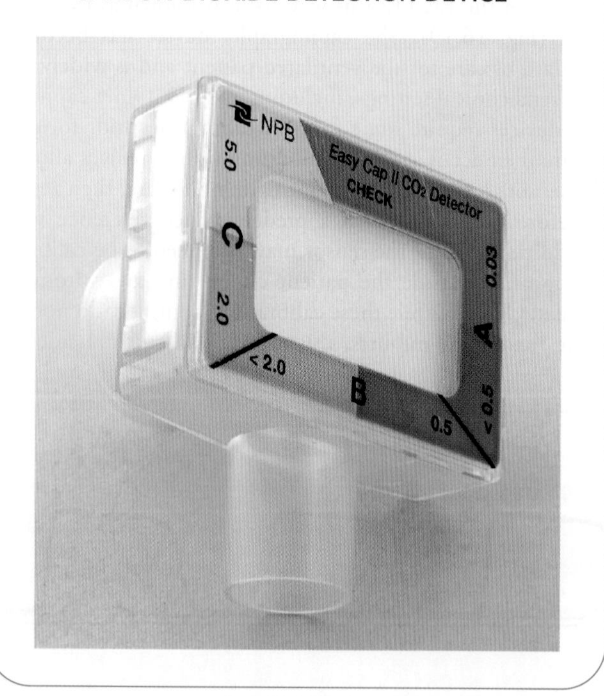

Assessment of respiratory function

Due to the correlation of $EtCO_2$ and $PaCO_2$, the clinician is able to evaluate alterations in pulmonary perfusion, in particular dead-space ventilation.[29]

Monitoring of mechanical ventilation

Capnography is today a standard monitoring tool for the ventilated patient. Capnography allows the caring clinician to readily identify changes in ventilation such as ventilator disconnection, apnoea, patient asynchrony with the ventilator and the depth of neuromuscular blockade.[26] Capnography also assists in identifying hypoventilation and hyperventilation in mechanically ventilated patients. This has been shown to be of significant benefit in patients where the tight control of CO_2 is clinically important, such as the head-injured patient with raised intracranial pressure.[36]

SUCTIONING TECHNIQUES

Many patients who are critically unwell or who have an alteration in their respiratory function may be unable to cough and remove respiratory secretions. These patients require assistance in removing these respiratory secretions by way of suctioning to reduce the risk of consolidation, infection and atelectasis.[40,41]

ROUTES OF SUCTIONING

Suctioning can be performed via various routes. Selection of the most appropriate route will be determined by the requirements of the patient and the clinical setting.

Oral

Oral suctioning involves the removal of secretions in the mouth. These secretions may include sputum, saliva, vomitus and/or blood. Suctioning of the oral cavity is usually performed using a hard plastic Yankauer suction catheter (Fig. 16.21).[40] Solid objects that are not able to be removed with the aid of Yankauer suction device, for example, dislodged teeth or vomitus, may require manual removal with a gloved hand or (Magill) forceps.

FIGURE 16.21 YANKAUER SUCTION DEVICE[42]

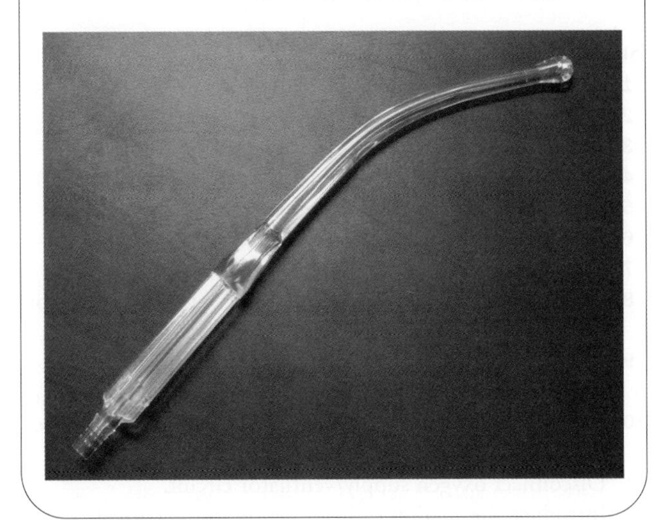

Oropharyngeal

The oropharynx extends from the lips to the pharynx. Oropharyngeal suctioning requires the insertion of a suction catheter through the mouth and into the pharynx and/or trachea to remove respiratory secretions. Patients who need this form of suctioning may often be unable to maintain an open airway and require the insertion of an oropharyngeal airway (see insertion of oropharyngeal airways, p. 316).[40] The oropharyngeal airway may assist in suctioning by allowing a small suction catheter to be passed through the airway to provide suctioning deep in the oropharynx and into the trachea.

Nasopharyngeal

Suctioning of the nasopharynx is performed to remove secretions from within the nasopharynx. This route may also be used for the collection of specific specimen samples such as a nasopharyngeal aspirate. Nasopharyngeal suctioning is commonly performed on patients with an altered level of consciousness and is best performed with the aid of a nasopharyngeal airway. When a nasopharyngeal airway is used, the suction catheter is passed through the airway.

Tracheal

Suctioning of the trachea occurs through an artificial opening in the trachea. Suctioning may be performed directly through a tracheal stoma or via an airway adjunct such as a tracheostomy tube.

Endotracheal

This form of tracheal suctioning occurs through an ETT in either spontaneously breathing or ventilated patients to remove respiratory secretions.

INDICATIONS FOR SUCTIONING

The common indications for suctioning are outlined in Box 16.3.

CONSIDERATIONS FOR SUCTIONING

Frequency of suctioning

Suctioning should be performed only when necessary (see Indications for suctioning, above). In intubated patients it may be advisable to perform suctioning at least every 8 hours to reduce the risk of secretion accumulation and partial tube occlusion.[41]

Catheter size

In general, suction catheters should be as small as possible, yet large enough to facilitate secretion removal. This allows air to enter around the catheter during suctioning, preventing a sudden drop in functional residual capacity and thus reducing the risk of atelectasis. For ETT suctioning, the catheter should occlude less than half of the internal lumen of the ETT (Box 16.4).[41]

Suction pressure

It is recommended to use the lowest possible suction pressure. For ETT suctioning this pressure is usually 80–120 mmHg. A negative pressure of 200 mmHg may be applied, provided that the appropriate suction-catheter size is used.[41]

Insertion depth

For ETT suctioning, a minimally invasive technique should be used where the suction catheter is inserted to the length of the ET tube only. The suction catheter can be inserted to

BOX 16.3 COMMON INDICATIONS FOR SUCTIONING[40]

- Visible or audible secretions—'rattling' or 'bubbling' sounds, audible with or without a stethoscope.
- Sensation of secretions in the chest reported by patient.
- Increased airway pressure in the ventilated patient or pre-set tidal volume not being delivered.
- Deteriorating arterial blood gases.
- Altered chest movement.
- Restlessness.
- Decreased oxygen saturation.
- Altered haemodynamics (increased blood pressure, heart rate).
- Decreased air entry on auscultation.
- Tachypnoea.
- Colour change in patient (e.g. cyanosis, redness, pallor).
- Specimen collection.
- Assessment of airway patency.
- Evaluation of cough reflex.

BOX 16.4 CALCULATION OF SUCTION CATHETER FOR ENDOTRACHEAL TUBE (ETT) SUCTIONING[41]

Suction catheter size [Fr] = (ETT size [mm] - 1) × 2

the carina and withdrawn 1–2 cm before suction is applied, or the catheter length can be estimated against an identical tube.[41]

Suction duration and method

It is recommended that each suction procedure should last no longer than 15 seconds and the suction should be applied continuously rather than intermittently.[41]

Use of saline

The routine instillation of normal saline prior to ETT suctioning is not recommended. There are no reliable positive effects demonstrated in terms of secretion removal, saturation or ventilation.[41]

Pre-oxygenation

It is recommended that pre-oxygenation with 100% oxygen is provided for at least 30 seconds prior to and after ETT suctioning to prevent decreases in oxygen saturation.[41]

CLOSED SUCTION SYSTEMS

The closed suction system consists of a reusable sterile suction catheter protected by a flexible, clear plastic sleeve that prevents contact between the catheter and the environment (Fig. 16.22). The closed suction system attaches to the end of the ETT via an adaptor, becoming an integrated part of the ventilator circuit. The closed suction system allows suctioning of the ETT without disconnecting the ventilator circuit. This maintains PEEP and an uninterrupted oxygen supply, as well as minimising loss of pulmonary volume (in volume-control ventilated patients). These systems often contain an irrigation port for rinsing the catheter or instilling saline. There is little evidence to support closed suction systems over open suction systems and the use of either system is recommended.[40,41]

Suctioning procedure (open)[40–42]

1. Explain the procedure to the patient.
2. Obtain consent (verbal).
3. Calculate correct catheter size.
4. Organise equipment including PPE.
5. Turn on suction to required pressure (80–120 mmHg).
6. If possible, the patient should be sitting upright.
7. Wash hands.
8. Hyperoxygenate for 30 seconds and/or apply hyperinflation before suctioning (if required).
9. Use a sterile, disposable glove on the hand manipulating the catheter and a clean disposable glove on the other.
10. With the clean disposable gloved hand, withdraw catheter from sleeve.
11. Disconnect oxygen supply/ventilator circuit.
12. Introduce the suction catheter gently to the correct length. Do not apply suction on insertion.
13. Apply suction and withdraw catheter slowly (< 15 seconds) in one continuous motion.
14. Reconnect oxygen supply/ventilator circuit.
15. Monitor oxygen saturation levels and heart rate throughout procedure.
16. Wrap the catheter around the sterile-gloved hand and pull the glove back over the soiled catheter and discard.
17. Rinse connection with sterile water and discard other glove.
18. Wash hands.
19. Assess the patient, and if further suctioning is required start the procedure again with another sterile catheter and glove.

FIGURE 16.22 CLOSED SUCTION SYSTEM[43]

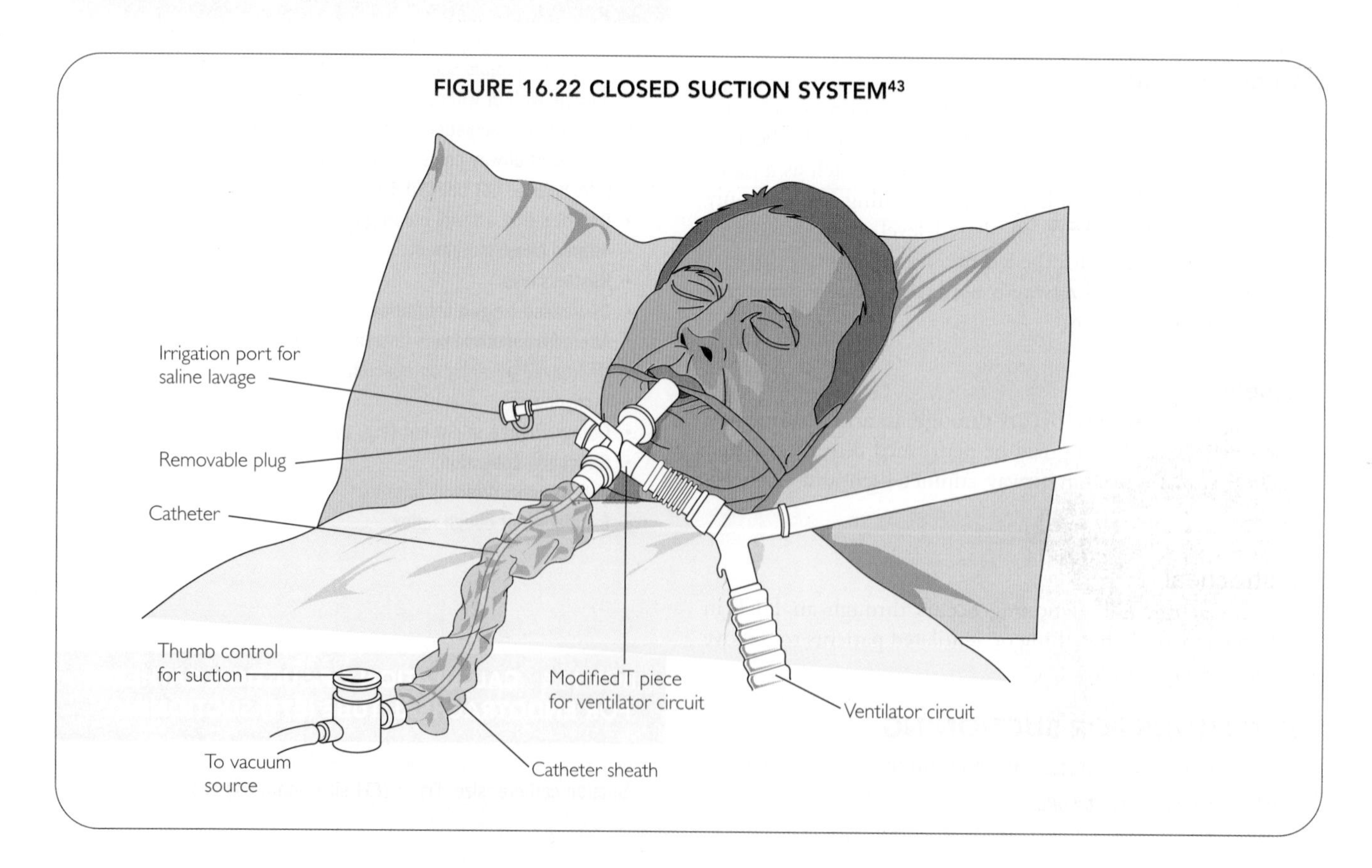

20. Repeat until airway is clear, allowing patient to rest between each suction pass.
21. Clean patient's oral cavity.
22. Wash hands.
23. Document procedure and findings.

ARTERIAL BLOOD GASES

COLLECTION

Arterial blood samples are usually obtained to perform an arterial blood gas (ABG) analysis. There are several possible arterial puncture sites, including the radial, brachial, femoral or dorsalis pedis arteries. Despite these options, the radial artery is the most preferred site for ABG sampling, as the majority of people have collateral circulation supplied by both the radial and the ulnar arteries (Fig. 16.23). This means that there is another supply of circulation should the radial artery become blocked distal to the puncture site due to spasm or thrombosis. Before a radial ABG can be taken, collateral circulation must be assessed, by either using a Doppler or the Allen's test (see opposite).[44] This procedure is common in the hospital environment, but rarely used in emergent pre-hospital patients.

If the patient is receiving oxygen, the oxygen concentration must remain the same for 20 minutes before the ABG is taken; if the test is to be taken without oxygen, the oxygen must be turned off (and any mask removed) for 20 minutes before the test is taken. Blood gas analyser machines measure samples at 37°C. Dissociation of gases is affected by temperature, so it is important to follow hospital policy and either enter the patient's temperature into the analyser or let it default and measure all samples at 37°C.[45]

Samples can be tested at the point-of-care (POC) (in the ward) or in the pathology laboratory. Blood gas analysers require frequent specialised calibration, testing, cleaning and maintenance that is usually performed by pathology laboratory technicians.

FIGURE 16.23 ARTERIAL BLOOD GAS SAMPLING

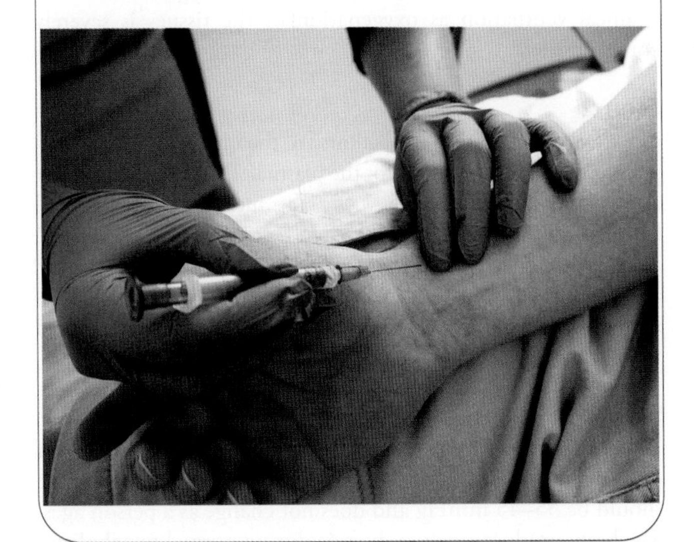

Courtesy Fremantle Hospital and Health Service Pathology Department, WA. OSCE, CC BY 2.0.

Procedure for arterial blood gas sampling

1. Gather all equipment that will be needed:
   - laboratory request form
   - arterial blood gas needle and syringe
   - gloves and PPE
   - alcohol swab
   - patient identification sticker to label blood gas syringe
   - specimen bag with ice (not required if POC testing is available).
2. Position the patient comfortably (lying down if possible).
3. Explain the procedure to the patient and gain verbal consent.
4. Wash hands.
5. Apply gloves and PPE.
6. Position extended arm appropriately on a pillow with wrist extended.
7. Perform Allen's test (see next section).
8. Palpate the pulse and assess the position of the artery.
9. Clean the site with 70% alcohol solution and allow it to dry.
10. Immobilise the artery between your fingers, being careful not to contaminate the puncture site.
11. Insert needle at a 45° to 90° angle perpendicular to the artery, with the needle's bevel up.
12. The syringe will begin to fill spontaneously when inside the artery. (This may not occur if the patient's blood pressure is low or the needle is not fully inside the artery; it may be necessary to reposition the needle slightly and pull back on the plunger to aspirate the blood.)
13. Obtain 0.3 to 0.5 mL of blood. Some blood gas analyser machines are able to perform testing on smaller samples.
14. Remove needle.
15. Apply gauze square and pressure for 5 minutes.
16. Label specimen and immediately send it for sampling
17. Send to laboratory immediately or perform POC testing.
18. Dispose of sharps safely.

It is important after taking the arterial sample to remove any air bubbles inside the syringe, as they can alter PaO_2 (arterial oxygen partial pressure) results. The needle needs to be removed and a cap placed over the end of the syringe to stop leaking and to prevent air from entering the syringe. Label the specimen with a patient identification sticker. If an extended delay to testing is expected, arterial blood gas specimens need to be placed in ice and sent to the lab or tested at the point-of-care immediately. Blood is a living tissue in which oxygen continues to be consumed and carbon dioxide continues to be produced, even after the blood is drawn into the syringe. Placing the blood gas specimen in ice should reduce the specimen temperature to approximately 4°C, which will decrease the metabolic rate to such an extent that the sample may undergo little change over several hours. As a rule, ABG samples should be analysed within 10 minutes. If longer times are expected they must be cooled immediately. Specimens left at room temperature lose 0.01 pH units every 15 minutes.[46]

ALLEN'S TEST

The Allen's test determines the patency of the ulnar and radial artery (Fig. 16.24 and Box 16.5). It involves raising the patient's hand and asking them to make a fist, then occluding the radial and ulnar arteries. Observe the hand for blanching. Then

FIGURE 16.24 ALLEN'S TEST[47]

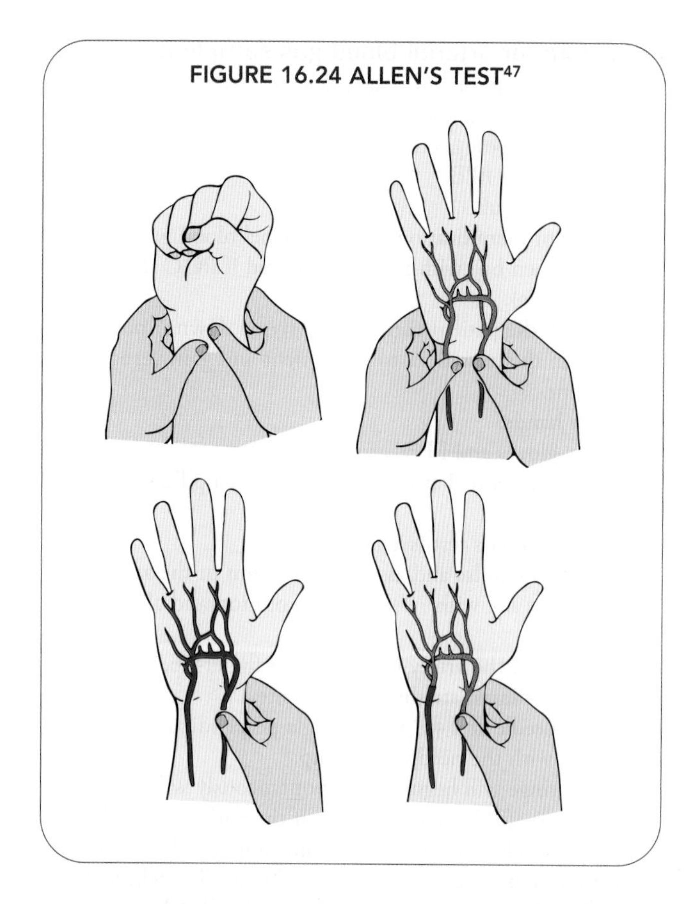

BOX 16.5 **PROCEDURE FOR ALLEN'S TEST**

1. Flex the patient's arm with the hand above the level of the elbow.
2. Have the patient clench their fist to force blood from the hand.
3. Place pressure on both arteries simultaneously, then ask the patient to open their hand. The hand should appear blanched.
4. Remove pressure from the ulnar artery. The blanched area flushes within seconds if collateral circulation is adequate.
5. If the area flushes quickly, this is recorded as a positive Allen's test. The test is negative if the blanched area does not flush quickly.
6. A negative Allen's test means collateral circulation is inadequate to support circulation to the hand; therefore, an alternative site should be selected.

release the pressure from the ulnar artery, lower the arm and ask the patient to unclench their fist. Observe the hand for return of colour (usually within 6 seconds). Return of colour within this time indicates ulnar artery patency. Repeat, testing the radial artery.[15]

ARTERIAL BLOOD GASES INTERPRETATION

ABG sampling and analysis is the gold-standard assessment of the patient's oxygenation and acid–base balance. It is commonly used in EDs and is vital to the management of the patient's condition. Knowledge of normal values for each patient is paramount. Interpretation of these results should follow five simple steps (see Box 16.6).[11,49–51]

BOX 16.6 **STEPS FOR INTERPRETATION OF ABG LEVELS[48]**

STEP 1

Look at the PaO_2 level and answer the question, 'Does the PaO_2 level show hypoxaemia?'

STEP 2

Look at the pH level and answer the question, 'Is the pH level on the acid or alkaline side of 7.40?'

STEP 3

Look at the $PaCO_2$ level and answer the question, 'Does the $PaCO_2$ level show metabolic acidosis, alkalosis or normalcy?'

STEP 4

Look at the HCO_3^- level and answer the question, 'Does the HCO_3^- level show metabolic acidosis, alkalosis or normalcy?'

STEP 5

Look back at the pH level, and answer the question, 'Does the pH show a compensated or an uncompensated condition?'

Step 1

PaO_2 refers to the measurement of the partial pressure of oxygen dissolved in arterial blood. The normal range should be 80–100 mmHg for a person breathing room air at sea level. Normal levels vary in infants and in people over 60 years of age. For older people, normal levels decrease due to ventilation/perfusion (V/Q) mismatch and the normal ageing of the lung.[49–51] A PaO_2 of less than the normal value is indicative of hypoxaemia, which means the amount of oxygen dissolved in the plasma is lower than normal. A PaO_2 level of 40 mmHg or below, at any age, indicates a life-threatening situation. The patient needs immediate administration of oxygen and/or mechanical ventilation as oxygenation of the tissues is severely compromised.[11,46,49–51]

Step 2

pH refers to the acidity or alkalinity of the blood and the hydrogen ion (H^+) concentration of the plasma. The normal values for arterial blood pH are 7.35–7.45. The mean value for arterial blood pH is 7.40. Any result that is below this value is on the acidic side of average, and any result above this value is on the alkaline side of average. An arterial blood pH of less than 7.35 is referred to as acidosis and a result of greater than 7.45 is referred to as alkalosis.[11,46,49–51]

Step 3

$PaCO_2$ refers to the measurement of the partial pressure of carbon dioxide dissolved in arterial blood. The normal range should be 35–45 mmHg and does not change as a person ages. The body produces carbon dioxide during normal metabolism. The $PaCO_2$ values indicate the ability of the patient to effectively ventilate to rid the body of carbon dioxide.

TABLE 16.2 ARTERIAL BLOOD GASES WITH VARIOUS STAGES OF COMPENSATION

STAGE OF COMPENSATION	CAUSE	$PaCO_2$	UNCOMPENSATED pH	UNCOMPENSATED HCO_3^-	PARTIALLY COMPENSATED pH	PARTIALLY COMPENSATED HCO_3^-	FULLY COMPENSATED pH	FULLY COMPENSATED HCO_3^-
Respiratory alkalosis	Hyperventilation	↓	↑	Normal	↑	↓	Normal	↓
Respiratory acidosis	Drug ingestion (hypoventilation)	↑	↓	Normal	↓	↑	Normal	↑
	CAUSE	HCO_3^-	UNCOMPENSATED pH	UNCOMPENSATED $PaCO_2$	PARTIALLY COMPENSATED pH	PARTIALLY COMPENSATED $PaCO_2$	FULLY COMPENSATED pH	FULLY COMPENSATED $PaCO_2$
Metabolic alkalosis	Severe vomiting	↑	↑	Normal	↑	↑	*	↑
Metabolic acidosis	Diabetic ketoacidosis	↓	↓	Normal	↓	↓	*	↓

HCO_3^-: bicarbonate; $PaCO_2$: partial arterial carbon dioxide pressure.
**Metabolic cannot be fully compensated to a normal pH by the respiratory system.*

The definition of respiratory acidosis is a $PaCO_2$ value above 45 mmHg. This is due to hypoventilation and can be the result of a number of conditions including chronic obstructive pulmonary disease (COPD), over-sedation, head trauma or drug overdose. When the levels of $PaCO_2$ are greater than 50 mmHg, ventilatory failure occurs.[11,46,49–51] Acute ventilatory failure will have abnormal pH values of 7.30; this is because the body has not had enough time to compensate by attempting to bring the pH value back towards the normal value. Chronic ventilatory failure has near-normal pH values of greater than 7.30.

The definition of respiratory alkalosis is a $PaCO_2$ value of < 35 mmHg. Respiratory alkalosis is due to hyperventilation and can be the result of a number of conditions including hypoxia, pulmonary embolus, hyperventilation and pregnancy. It can also be the result of a compensatory mechanism to a metabolic acidosis.[11,46,49–51]

Step 4

The bicarbonate (HCO_3^-) result is a reflection of the renal function. The normal range is 22–26 mEq/L. The definition of a metabolic acidosis is a level below 22 mEq/L. This can be a result of renal failure, lactic acidosis, ketoacidosis or diarrhoea. The definition of a metabolic alkalosis is a level above 26 mEq/L and can be the result of loss of fluid and diuretic therapy or long-term compensation.[11,46,49–51]

Step 5

In an *uncompensated* condition (respiratory or metabolic)—if the pH is abnormal, then the $PaCO_2$, HCO_3^-, or both, will also be abnormal, because the body has not had enough time to return the pH value back to the normal range.

In a *compensated* condition (respiratory or metabolic)—if the pH is normal and both the $PaCO_2$ and the HCO_3^- values are abnormal, then the body has had time to return the pH values back to the normal range (Tables 16.2 and 16.3).[46,49,50,52,53]

TABLE 16.3 NORMAL VALUES OF AN ABG SAMPLE[53]

NAME	NORMAL VALUE OR RANGE
pH	7.35-7.45
PaO_2 (mmHg)	85-90
$PaCO_2$ (mmHg)	35-45
HCO_3^- (mEq/L)	22-26

VENOUS BLOOD GASES INTERPRETATION

With the increasing availability of point-of-care (POC) blood-testing devices, it is becoming increasingly common for the emergency clinician to perform venous blood gas (VBG) analysis as a first-line investigation in the initial evaluation of the patient. VBGs have several advantages over ABGs, including ease of collection, less pain for the patient and less significant complications. VBGs will provide results for all the parameters reported on a standard ABG and may also include a number of additional biochemical parameters (depending on the capability of the testing device). These may include potassium (K^+), sodium (Na^+), haemoglobin (Hb) and creatinine. The results for many of the POC devices tend to be quicker than routine pathology testing, providing valuable clinical information in a timely manner. ABG values acceptably compare with the same values collected via venous sampling. Venous values for pH, $PvCO_2$ and bicarbonate have been shown to correlate closely with the values obtained via arterial sampling and are therefore an acceptable alternative to ABG-acquired results.[54,55] There is no acceptable comparison between venous PO_2 and arterial PO_2; therefore, evaluations of oxygenation continue to require ABG analysis.

BLOOD GLUCOSE LEVEL SAMPLING

Blood glucose level (BGL) is the measurable amount of glucose in the blood and is normally between 3 and 8 mmol/L. A bedside BGL is available as quickly as 5 seconds with portable glucose meters. As part of a comprehensive assessment of the emergency patient, a finger-prick blood glucose measure should be collected.[52] Maintaining normal serum glucose levels in critically ill patients improves outcomes by reducing infection rates.[56] BGL should be obtained and recorded for all patients with diabetes and in patients who present with collapse, multiple abscesses or non-healing wounds, dizziness and nausea and vomiting. Paediatric patients and neonates, in most instances, will also require their BGL measured. Hypoglycaemia should be considered a factor in any unresponsive patient until proven otherwise.

PROCEDURE

1. Select a finger of the non-dominant hand.
2. Begin by ensuring the skin is clean and dry.
3. Apply PPE. Ready the glucometer by turning it on and inserting a testing strip.
4. Place the lancet firmly on the side of the distal end of the selected finger and press to trigger the lancet.
5. Gently bleed the wound and wipe away the first drop of blood.[35]
6. Gently bleed the wound to collect sufficient blood by milking the finger from the proximal to the distal end.
7. Touch the testing strip to the blood. Capillary action will draw the sample.
8. Cover the finger wound with a dry dressing and apply momentary pressure.

UNDERWATER-SEAL DRAINS

Trauma to the chest can produce a life-threatening collection of blood or air between the chest wall and the lung. An underwater-seal drain (UWSD) or chest drain is designed to provide a closed system for the one-way removal of air or blood from the pleural space. The water acts to prevent air returning to the pleural space.[57] A pneumothorax with greater than 25% collapse may require the placement of a chest tube or intercostal catheter (ICC). ICCs are inserted in the pleural space to remove air or blood and allow the lung to re-expand under normal negative intrapleural pressures.[48] A UWSD, or a more-simple Heimlich valve, is connected to an intercostal catheter or chest drain, which is inserted between the ribs into the pleural space. For pre-hospital clinicians, the Heimlich valve is more commonly used, but UWSDs may be encountered during inter-facility transfer where a chest tube has been placed at the sending facility.

ASSISTING WITH THE INSERTION OF AN INTERCOSTAL CATHETER

1. Set up a sterile procedure tray containing kidney dishes, clamps, needle holders and bowls. Commonly, a large general sterile procedure set-up is used.
2. Add a large fenestrated or four large sterile drapes if not included in the procedure tray.
3. Open sterile gloves and gowns.
4. Fill a sterile bowl with a skin-cleaning solution such as chlorhexidine with alcohol.
5. Open and place on the tray a 10 mL syringe for local anaesthetic.
6. Open and place a large-bore blunt drawing-up needle to draw up local anaesthetic.
7. Open and place out a 22-gauge injecting needle for the injection of local anaesthetic.
8. Put out a large, long, straight needle with a 2/0 silk suture to secure the drain.
9. Put out a scalpel for cutting the space between the ribs where the catheter will be pushed.
10. Have ready two large clear dressings to cover the drain insertion site.
11. Have ready two rubber-tipped forceps to clamp the catheter. Often these are left at the bedside during the entire time the drain is in place.
12. Open the intercostal catheter.
13. Open and prepare the UWSD. Different products are prepared using different methods, but most have a water reservoir within the drain that needs filling before use.
14. Administer adequate analgesia where possible.
15. Continue cardiorespiratory monitoring throughout the insertion procedure for signs of immediate deterioration or lethal dysrhythmia.
16. When the ICC is inserted, assist with the connection of the UWSD tubing and secure the two with long lengths of Elastoplast tape. Often these are applied in a spiral or trouser-leg fashion.
17. When the catheter is sutured in place, cover the insertion site with occlusive dressings.
18. Check the UWSD is functioning. This will be indicated by bubbling of air through the water within the drain and oscillation or swinging of any blood in the tube on inspiration.
19. Apply low-pressure suction to the UWSD if indicated.
20. Prepare the patient for x-ray to confirm the placement of the ICC.

PRACTICE TIP

The insertion of a chest drain with underwater-seal drain is an immediate priority in chest trauma, as tension pneumothorax can cause life-threatening complications. As the air collects within the pleura, this alters the inter-pleural pressure and can cause the lung to collapse, putting pressure on the heart and affecting stroke volumes.[57]

CARING FOR THE UNDERWATER-SEAL DRAIN AND INTERCOSTAL CATHETER

1. Keep a pair of rubber-tipped artery forceps at the bedside. If there are complications with the drain, these can be used to clamp the ICC close to the insertion site for a short period of time.
2. Keep the UWSD unit at the patient's bedside and below the level of the insertion site. This is to prevent the return of air or fluid to the chest cavity.
3. Maintain the water level within the drain. The drain should bubble gently rather than vigorously, as the latter can increase evaporation.[35]

FIGURE 16.25 UNDERWATER-SEAL DRAINAGE SYSTEM[48]

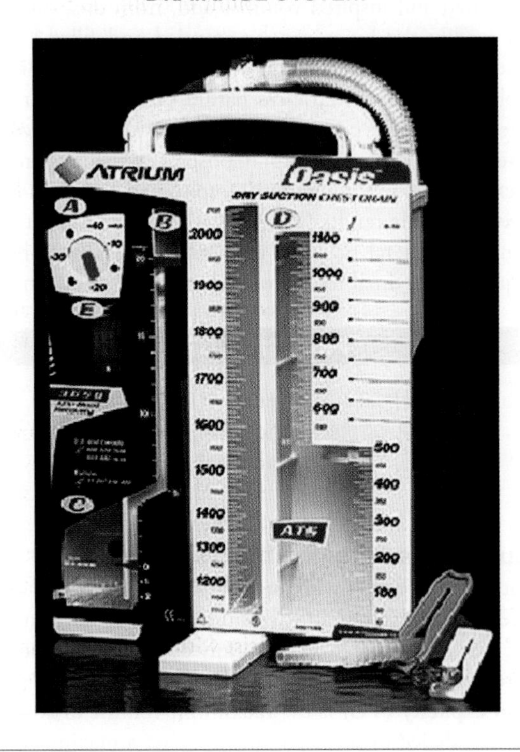

4. Continue the required amount of low-pressure suction if ordered.
5. Check the ICC and UWSD from the point of insertion down to the drain.
6. Check the dressing at the point of insertion. Confirm there is an occlusive dressing covering the whole insertion point.
7. Check for air leaks and check all tubes are well secured with long lengths of spiral or trouser-leg tape.
8. Confirm there are no kinks in the tubing (Fig. 16.25).[42]

HEIMLICH CHEST DRAIN VALVE

The Heimlich chest drain valve or flutter valve (Fig. 16.26) is a simple device used to prevent the return of air into the ICC. The Heimlich valve works without suction, but can only be used to remove air, not blood, from the pleural space. Normal respiration and cough create enough intrathoracic pressure to expel air through the valve.[58] The Heimlich chest drain valve is commonly used to transport patients with ICC as it reduces the need for bulky UWSD. Heimlich is generally used in the pre-hospital setting for suspected pneumothorax, following needle decompression or in patient transport, and less commonly used in the admitted in-hospital patient.

To fit a Heimlich chest drain valve

1. Confirm the ICC is secured in place.
2. Attach the blue end of the Heimlich valve to the distal end of the ICC and tape it in place using lengths of spiral-wrapped tape. There is an arrow on the valve to confirm that it is inserted correctly.

FIGURE 16.26 HEIMLICH VALVE[58]

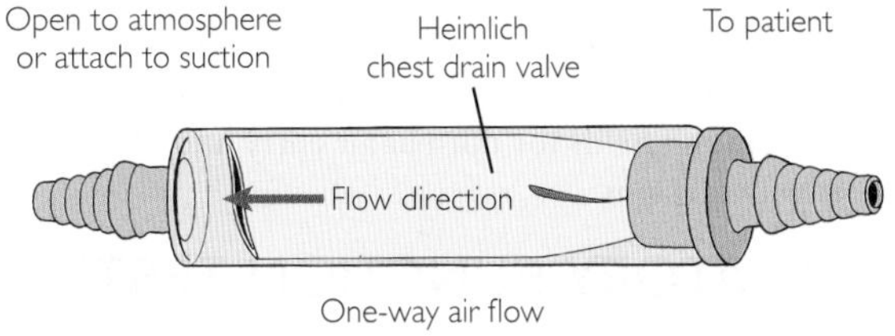

Open to atmosphere or attach to suction
Heimlich chest drain valve
To patient
Flow direction
One-way air flow

A one-way Heimlich valve alone is often sufficient to treat a pneumothorax, but it cannot be used to treat a haemothorax.

3. Attach the clear end of the valve to a drainage bag. There is no need to secure this with lengths of tubing as the one-way valve prevents back-flow of air.
4. Observe fluttering of the valve on cough and respiration. The collection bag may also fill with air and require venting.
5. Low-pressure suction can be applied to the distal end of the Heimlich valve, if required.
6. Beware that the valve will clog with fluids and should be observed closely to ensure it continues to function. To change a blocked valve, clamp the ICC proximally with two rubber-tipped forceps, remove the old valve and replace with a new one.
7. Beware of the weight of the Heimlich valve kinking a smaller bore chest tube (such as cannulae or 'angiocaths') that may be used for needle decompression in the pre-hospital environment. The weight of this equipment can lead to kinking of small-bore intercostal catheters used by pre-hospital services, therefore preventing the drainage of air.

PRACTICE TIP

A modified Heimlich valve can be made by using the fingers of a glove to allow air to escape but prevent its return to the chest cavity. Make a small slit in the glove finger and tape it securely over the end of the ICC.

REMOVAL OF UNDERWATER-SEAL DRAIN AND INTERCOSTAL CATHETER

1. Ensure that the UWSD is no longer bubbling continuously. Confirm on x-ray that the amount of air or blood in the pleural space is adequately reduced and the drain is ready for removal.
2. Have emergency equipment ready for the re-insertion of a new ICC, if urgently required.
3. Administer adequate analgesia where possible.
4. Clamp the ICC proximally above the join of the UWSD with two rubber-tipped clamps.
5. Disconnect the UWSD from the chest tube.
6. Remove the occlusive dressings and cut the sutures at the point of insertion.
7. Instruct the patient to inhale completely and perform a Valsalva manoeuvre and pull the drain out quickly and continuously.[52,58]

8. Apply an occlusive dressing immediately over the insertion site to prevent air from returning to the pleural space. The wound may also be sutured closed, in some cases using a purse-string suture that may have held the drain in place initially.
9. Monitor the patient for signs of pneumothorax by auscultation of lung fields for normal air entry and observing normal vital signs.

RESPIRATORY FUNCTION TESTING

PEAK EXPIRATORY FLOW (PEF) RATE MEASUREMENT

Measurement of peak flow in the ED is performed using a simple assessment device that measures airflow, or peak expiratory flow (PEF). Patients blow into the device quickly and forcefully, and the resulting peak flow reading indicates how open the airways are, or how difficult it is for the patient to breathe.[37] Peak flow meters have limited accuracy and provide only a single-effort-dependent assessment of ventilatory function. They are also dependent on patient technique. PEF is reduced in diseases causing airway obstruction and for asthmatics. The meter is a very useful tool in the home for patients to assess changes in condition and prevent unnecessary attendance at the ED.[11,46,52,59]

SPIROMETRY

Spirometry is a physiological test to measure lung function; it is the broadest non-invasive test of ventilatory function. Spirometry is rarely indicated in the emergency setting. Spirometry is used to detect and assess diseases which limit ventilatory capacity and affect the mechanics of the chest wall and lungs, and it assesses the function of the airways. Spirometry is used to measure timed expired and inspired volumes and, from this, calculation of how readily the lungs can be emptied and filled.[46,59] This assessment provides information on whether the lung disease is of an obstructive or a restrictive nature. Acceptable spirometry measurement requires cooperation by the patient and knowledge of the technique by the operator. Constant verbal reinforcement of patient technique throughout the spirometry test will help to produce favourable results (Fig. 16.27).[11,46,50,52,59] Spirometry is performed in general practice, medical centres and in hospital and requires a maximal respiratory effort from the patient.

PRACTICE TIP

Constant verbal reinforcement of patient technique throughout the spirometry test will help to produce favourable results.

Measurements obtained from spirometry

The data obtained following spirometry is interpreted against predicted normal values and within the clinical context of the patient. The measurements commonly obtained from performing spirometry are outlined below.[60]

- **Vital capacity (VC)** is the maximum volume of air which can be exhaled or inspired during either a maximally forced (FVC) or a slow (SVC) manoeuvre.
- **Forced expired volume in one second (FEV_1)** is the volume expired in the first second of maximal expiration after

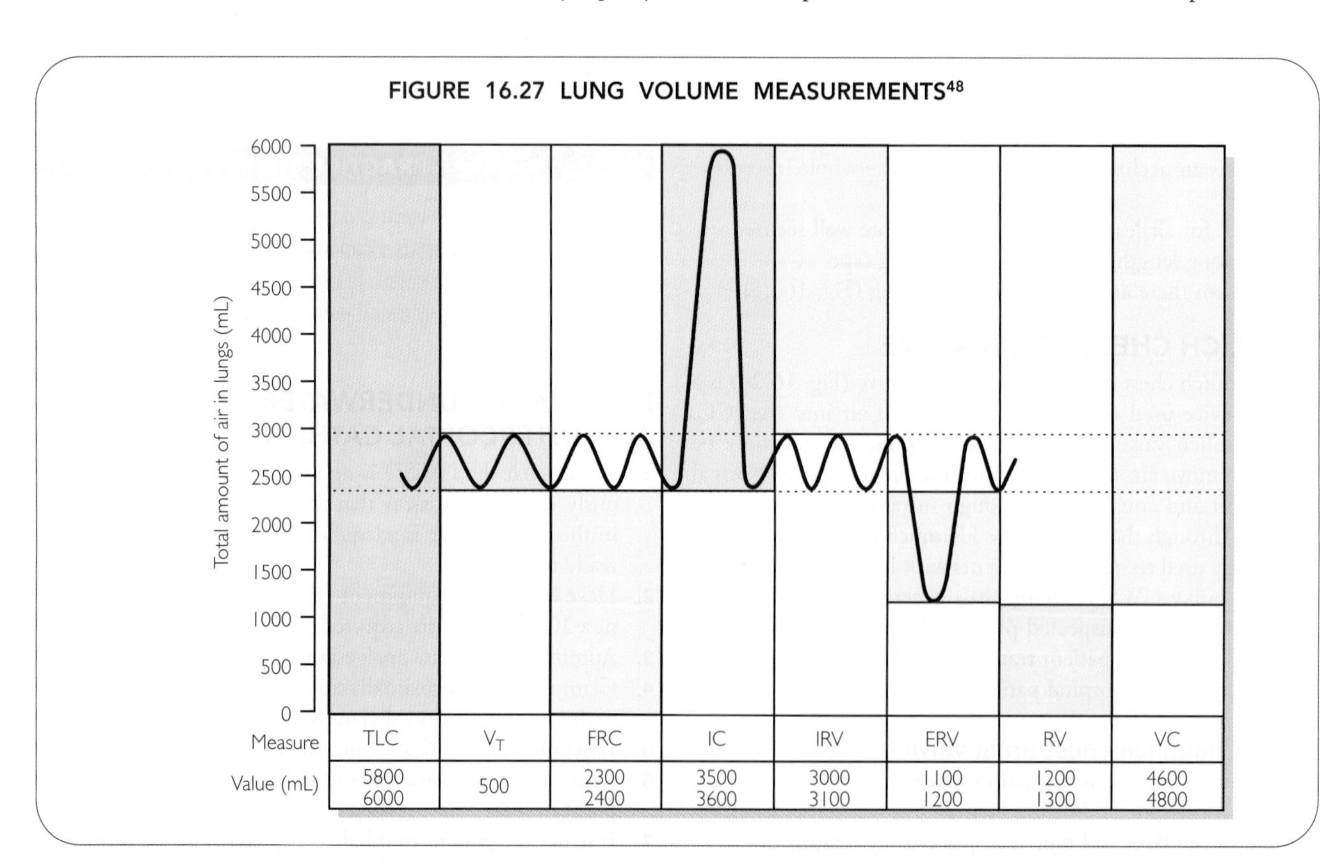

FIGURE 16.27 LUNG VOLUME MEASUREMENTS[48]

All values are approximately 25% less in women. *TLC: total lung capacity; VT: tidal volume; FRC: functional residual capacity; IC: inspiratory capacity; IRV: inspiratory reserve volume; ERV: expiratory reserve volume; RV: residual volume; VC: vital capacity.*

a maximal inspiration and is a useful measure of how quickly full lungs can be emptied.

- **FEV_1/VC (or FEV_1/FVC)** is the FEV_1 expressed as a percentage of the VC or FVC (whichever volume is larger), and gives a clinically useful index of airflow limitation.
- **$FEF_{25-75\%}$** is the average expired flow over the middle half of the FVC manoeuvre and is regarded as a more sensitive measure of small airways narrowing than FEV_1.
- **Peak expiratory flow (PEF)** is the maximal expiratory flow rate achieved; this occurs very early in the forced expiratory manoeuvre.
- **$FEF_{50\%}$ and $FEF_{75\%}$** (forced expiratory flow at 50% or 75% FVC) is the maximal expiratory flow measured at the point where 50% of the FVC has been expired ($FEF_{50\%}$) and after 75% has been expired ($FEF_{75\%}$).
- **FVC_6** is the forced expiratory volume during the first 6 seconds and is a surrogate of the FVC. The FVC_6 (and FEV_1/FVC_6) is gaining popularity because stopping the expiratory manoeuvre after 6 seconds is less demanding and easier to perform for patients with airflow obstruction and the elderly yet is similar to conventional FVC and FEV_1/FVC for diagnosing and grading airflow obstruction.

Performing a spirometry measurement

The procedure for performing a spirometry measurement is given in Box 16.7.

> **BOX 16.7 PROCEDURE FOR PERFORMING A SPIROMETRY MEASUREMENT (FORCED EXPIRATORY MANOEUVRE)[60,61]**
>
> 1. Obtain spirometer and any disposable equipment required (e.g. mouthpiece, filter or nose clip).
> 2. Ensure the spirometer has been calibrated in accordance with the manufacturer's recommendations.
> 3. Measure the patient's weight and height. For patients who are unable to stand, height can be calculated by measuring from the patient's mid-sternum along their outstretched arm to the tip of the middle finger (demispan, in cm) and using the following equations to calculate height:[52]
>   females: height (cm) = (1.35 × demispan) + 60.1
>   males: height (cm) = (1.40 × demispan) + 57.8
> 4. Explain the procedure to the patient, stressing the following points:
>   - Take a full breath in (must be absolutely full).
>   - Place the mouthpiece in your mouth and ensure a good, tight seal.
>   - Immediately blow air out as hard and as fast for as long as possible.
>   - Do not lean forwards during the test.
> 5. Position the patient, preferably in a seated position with feet flat on the floor (adults). Children may stand.
> 6. Turn on the spirometer and enter the required test details. This may include such information as name, age, gender, height, ethnicity, temperature, weight or smoking history.
> 7. Apply the nose clip.
> 8. Instruct the patient to take a full deep breath in and start the test.
> 9. Provide encouragement throughout the test. 'Blow . . . blow . . . good . . . keep going . . . keep going'. The importance of active encouragement cannot be overstated.
> 10. Allow the patient to rest following each forced expiration.
> 11. Repeat the test to ensure that at least three technically acceptable manoeuvres are obtained to ensure reproducibility. Reproducibility is achieved when the best two results are within 5% or 100 mL of each other. The patient should perform no more than eight tests in a single session; however, if reproducibility cannot be achieved within four attempts with proper instruction and active encouragement, it is unlikely that additional testing will be helpful.
> 12. Terminate procedure and dispose of equipment.
> 13. Collect data–generally this is provided in a printed format; however, on older manual-style machines data may have to be obtained from the graphed results.
> 14. Interpret data (see the section 'Measurements obtained from spirometry').

CARDIAC MONITORING

The following section contains information on the skill of performing electrocardiograph (ECG) and continuous cardiac monitoring.

PERFORMING AN ELECTROCARDIOGRAPH

Performing an electrocardiograph (ECG) is an essential skill for all emergency clinicians. An ECG can provide timely and important information about the electrical activity of the heart.

ECG should be performed promptly:

- in patients with chest pain
- following a life-threatening dysrhythmia (ventricular tachycardia, ventricular fibrillation, asystole, atrioventricular blocks or symptomatic bradydysrhythmias)
- in haemodynamically compromised patients
- routinely after cardiac surgery
- following the ingestion of pro-dysrhythmic drugs
- perioperatively
- after a syncopal episode.

Fig. 16.28 overleaf shows placement of the leads on the chest for performing an ECG.

Heavy vertical lines represent the midclavicular, anterior, axillary and midaxillary lines (from left to right). V_1 and V_2 are referenced to the fourth intercostal space and V_4 to the fifth space. V_3 lies on a line between V_2 and V_4. V_5 and V_6 lie on a horizontal line from V_4. Additional praecordial leads can be obtained on the right side (V_3 R, V_4 R), as well as extending further left from V6 (V7).[62]

Procedure

1. Inform the patient of the steps and gain consent.
2. The patient should be supine.
3. Shave the hair at electrode placement if required.
4. Anatomically position the leads.

   Electrode positionss
   - RA (Right arm): Right forearm, proximal to the wrist, or right shoulder between the clavicle and medial deltoid*
   - LA (Left arm): Left forearm, proximal to the wrist, or left shoulder between the clavicle and medial deltoid*

FIGURE 16.28 PLACEMENT OF THE CHEST LEADS FOR ECG[62]

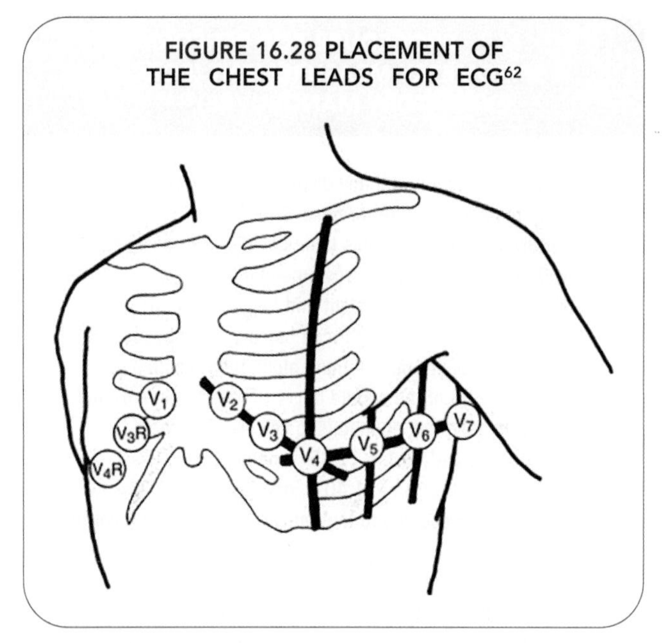

Locations of the precordial leads. Heavy vertical lines represent the midclavicular, anterior, axillary and midaxillary lines (from left to right). V_1 and V_2 are referenced to the fourth intercostal space and V_4 to the fifth space. V_3 lies on a line between V_2 and V_4. V_5 and V_6 lie on a horizontal line from V_4. Additional precordial leads can be obtained on the right side (V_3 R, V_4 R), as well as extending further left from V_6 (V_7).

- LL (Left leg): Left lower leg, proximal to the ankle, or left abdomen at the anterior axillary line, above the iliac crest*
- RL (Right leg): Right lower leg, proximal to the ankle, or right abdomen at the anterior axillary line, above the iliac crest*
- V1: Fourth intercostal space at the right sternal edge
- V2: Fourth intercostal space at the left sternal edge
- V3: Midway between V_2 and V_4
- V4: Fifth intercostal space in the mid-clavicular line
- V5: Left anterior axillary line at same horizontal level as V_4
- V6: Left mid-axillary line at same horizontal level as V_4 and V_5.

  *Pre-hospital monitors are less sensitive than in-hospital devices. Some manufacturers recommend placement of limb leads on the torso. Paramedics should refer to local policy and recommendations from the manufacturer.

5. Ensure the patient is still and relaxed.
6. Record and print a 12-lead ECG at 25 mm/sec with a gain setting of 10 mm/mV.
7. Label the ECG with the patient demographic details, and clinical information such as current and past medical history.
8. Clean the equipment after the procedure.
9. Most emergency services have policies about the interpretation and review of an ECG, but, in general, most ECGs should be reviewed within 10 minutes.

CONTINUOUS CARDIAC MONITORING

Continuous cardiac monitoring should be performed:[62,63]

- in patients with acute coronary syndromes
- post cardiac arrest
- following a life-threatening dysrhythmia (ventricular tachycardia, ventricular fibrillation, asystole, atrioventricular blocks or symptomatic bradydysrhythmias)
- in haemodynamically compromised patients
- for 48 hours after cardiac surgery
- following the ingestion of pro-dysrhythmic drugs.

Patients should be regularly assessed by the medical team for the need for continuous electrocardiogram monitoring.

Procedure

1. Inform the patient of the procedure and gain consent.
2. The patient should initially be supine.
3. Shave the hair at electrode placement, if required.
4. Anatomically position the leads.

   Electrode position for the 5-electrode monitor (Fig. 16.29)
   - RA (Right arm) Right shoulder
   - LA (Left arm) Left shoulder
   - LL (Left leg) Left side torso
   - RL (Right leg) Right side torso
   - V Fourth intercostal space at the right sternal edge

   Electrode position for the 3-electrode monitor (Fig. 16.30)
   - RA (Right arm) Right shoulder
   - LA (Left arm) Left shoulder
   - LL (Left leg) Left side torso
5. Confirm continuous electrocardiogram monitoring.
6. Electronically label the cardiac monitor with the patient demographic details (if required).

TEMPORARY CARDIAC PACING

The following section contains information on the use of temporary cardiac pacing for cardiac dysrhythmia.

TRANSCUTANEOUS (EXTERNAL) PACING

Transcutaneous or external cardiac pacing is the most readily available form of cardiac pacing in the pre-hospital environment

FIGURE 16.29 ELECTRODE POSITION FOR THE 5-ELECTRODE MONITOR

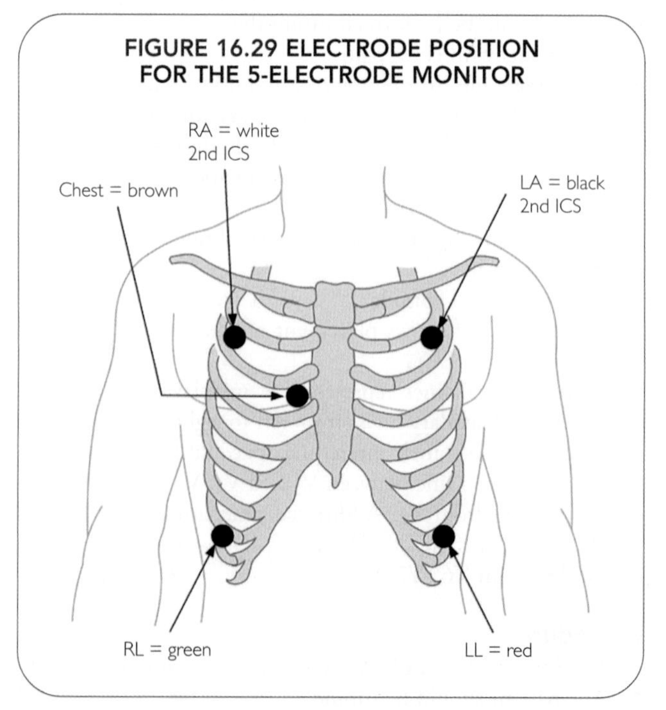

Life in the Fast Lane.

FIGURE 16.30 ELECTRODE POSITION FOR THE 3-ELECTRODE MONITOR

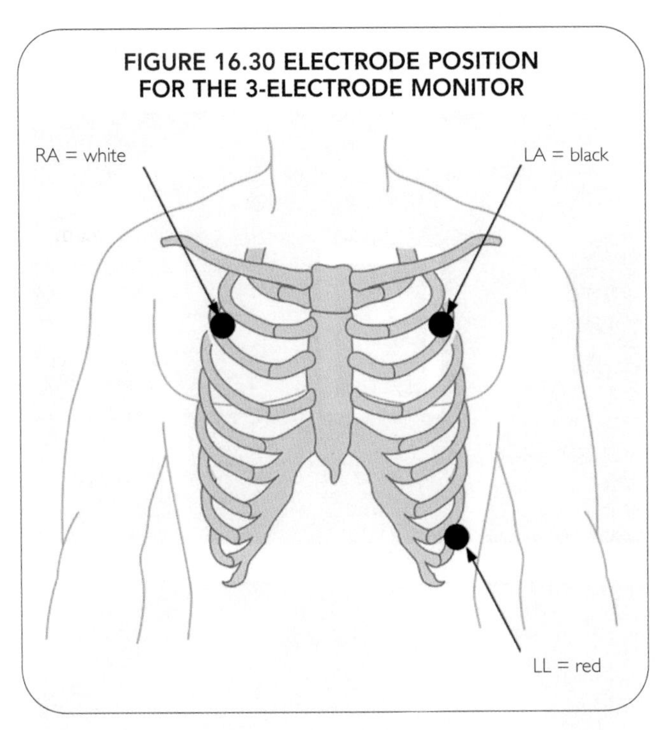

Life in the Fast Lane.

and the ED. Many defibrillators can provide transcutaneous cardiac pacing through self-adhesive multifunctional pads, which are able to defibrillate and pace. This method is non-invasive and relatively fast to initiate and is therefore the preferred method of pacing in an emergency situation. Pads are placed on the chest in either a left anterior/posterior position or an anterior/lateral position. The pacemaker generates an electrical impulse, which is delivered through the pads, causing depolarisation of myocardial tissue as the current travels through the chest wall and heart muscle. External cardiac pacing is generally a temporary measure providing time to make arrangements and decisions regarding transvenous pacing.[64]

External pacing is indicated in haemodynamically compromising bradydysrhythmias (such as complete heart block and second-degree heart block Mobitz type II) if the patient has not responded to medical therapies (e.g. drug therapy, IV fluids).[64] Pacing is not recommended for patients in asystolic cardiac arrest. There is no improvement in the rate of admission to hospital or survival to hospital discharge when pacing is initiated in asystolic patients in the pre-hospital or ED settings.[65]

Procedure

1. Explain the procedure to the patient, where possible.
2. Prepare the patient's skin over which the external pacing pads are to be placed. The skin should be clean and dry to promote good adhesion and contact of pacing electrodes. Any transdermal drug delivery patches should be removed. If time permits, excessive body hair should be removed.[64,66]
3. Apply the electrocardiograph (ECG) electrodes attached to the pacing unit. If using multifunctional pads, an ECG tracing may be obtainable through these; however, if the ECG trace is inadequate the separate ECG electrodes must also be used.
4. Apply the pacing pads in the desired position. Many pads come with an image of the correct position. Avoid positioning the pads over bone as this is likely to increase transthoracic resistance, increasing the amount of energy required. In females, the pad should be placed under the breast.
   - Anterior/posterior positioning—generally the preferred position. The anterior pad is placed on the left anterior chest at the point of maximal impulse (approximately V_3 position) and the posterior pad is placed on the patient's back immediately opposite the anterior pad, to the left of the spinal column and below the scapula (Fig. 16.31A).[67–69]
   - Anterior/lateral positioning—alternative position. One pad is positioned on the right side of the chest at the sternal border and the other pad is placed on the left lateral chest wall (Fig. 16.31B).
5. Provide the patient with analgesia and/or sedation. External pacing can be uncomfortable and wherever possible this should be mitigated. An example of sedation and analgesia combination is fentanyl and midazolam.[4]
6. Select the mode of pacing:
   - *Demand (synchronous) mode*—the pacer senses the patient's own QRS complexes and only generates an impulse to achieve the set rate when the heart does not produce its own intrinsic QRS complex.[68,69] This is the preferred mode of pacing and the most commonly used.
   - *Non-demand (asynchronous) mode*—a fixed-rate mode where impulses are delivered at the set rate regardless of the patient's own intrinsic heart rate. Non-demand or fixed-rate pacing is rarely used as it can have potential complications by delivering an impulse on the T wave and precipitating ventricular fibrillation.[68,69]
7. Select the pacing rate—this is generally set at 60–70 beats/minute to achieve an adequate blood pressure and cerebral perfusion.
8. Slowly increase the energy output level.
9. Observe the ECG tracing for pacing spikes and signs of electrical capture. Electrical capture occurs when every pacing spike is followed by a wide QRS complex.
10. Slightly increase the energy output after the point of electrical capture. Ideally, pacing should be continued at an output level just above the threshold of electrical capture so as to minimise discomfort.[64]
11. Assess the patient for mechanical capture—this is assessed by palpating the pulse. The femoral pulse is preferred, as the muscle contractions associated with external pacing may make the carotid pulse difficult to assess.[64]
12. Assess the patient's haemodynamic response.

Maintain close observation and adequate analgesia/sedation. Patients should be continually observed and assessed. In particular, the patient should be observed for loss of electrical capture which may result from pad dislodgement or patient movement. Patients require ongoing analgesia/sedation as they may become increasingly aware of and distressed by the discomfort associated with external pacing, especially patients who have an improved level of consciousness with external pacing.

FIGURE 16.31 TRANSCUTANEOUS PACING PAD PLACEMENT

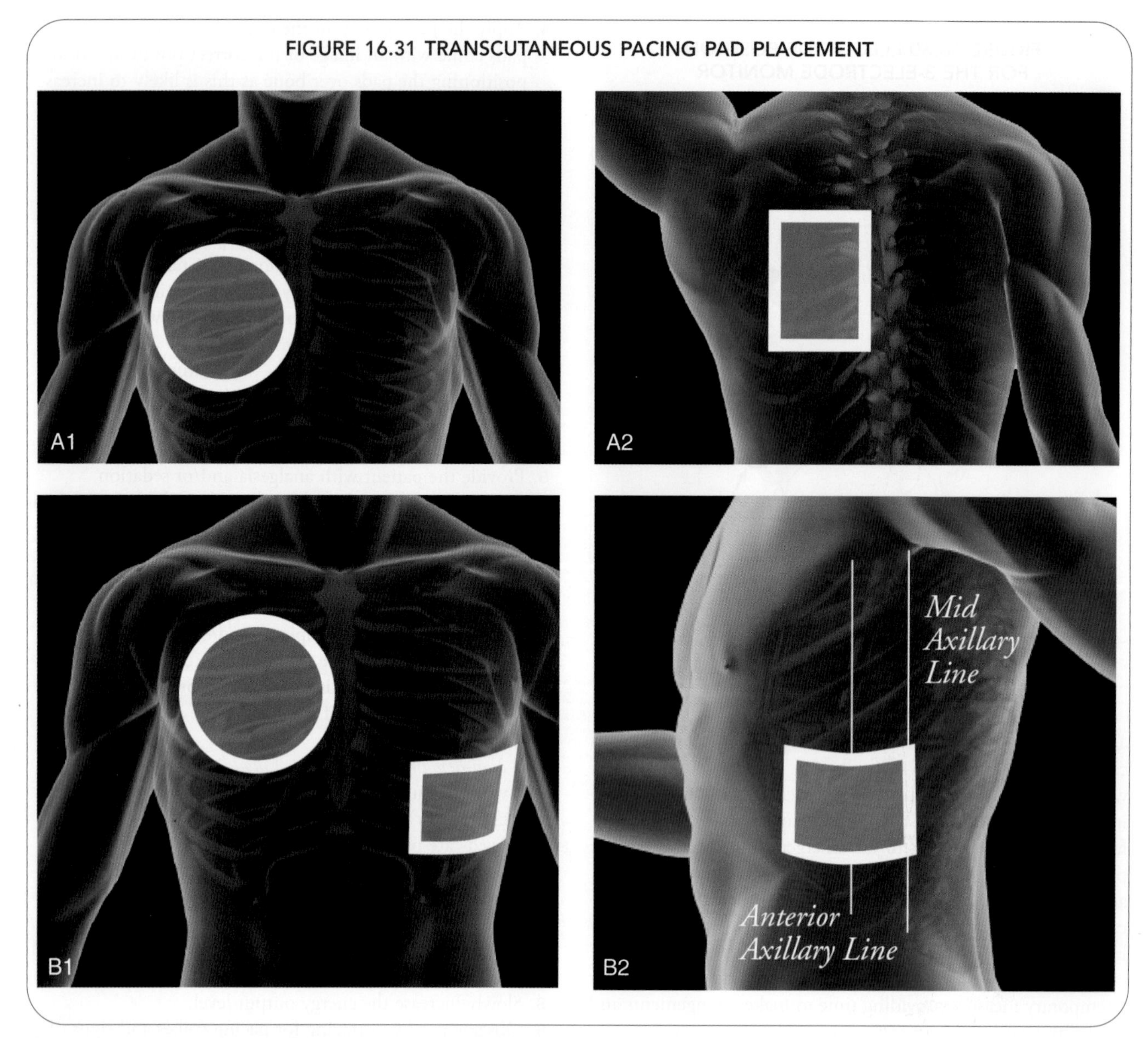

A. Anterior/posterior positioning. **B.** Anterior/lateral positioning. *Courtesy ZOLL Medical Corporation.*

TRANSVENOUS PACING

Transvenous pacing involves the insertion of a pacing electrode into the right ventricle via the subclavian or internal jugular venous route under fluoroscopy or with a flotation-pacing catheter under guidance by the ECG. The electrodes are connected to an external pulse generator where the output can be selected in milliamps along with the rate.[68,69] This type of pacemaker also has a fixed-rate mode or a demand mode.

VASCULAR ACCESS

Inserting peripheral intravenous catheters is an essential core skill for paramedics and emergency nurses. The decision to insert should be made based on clinical need and in consultation with the patient.[70] They should only be inserted if clinically indicated, and not 'just in case'. The traditional sites chosen for peripheral intravenous catheter in both an emergency and an acute situation are the cephalic and basilic veins in the lower arm and veins in the dorsum of the hand. These are large constant and straight, making venous access easy (Figs 16.32 and 16.33).

In some clinical environments the insertion of central catheters may also be required (see pp. 341–342), but this is not a basic skill for most emergency clinicians, and reference to local organisational and departmental policies and procedures is required. Nurses and paramedics have certain responsibilities to use and maintain established vascular access points. Catheters are usually inserted into peripheral veins of the hand and arm. Other sites include veins of the lower extremities, or the external jugular, internal jugular and femoral veins. Cannulation of the lower extremities, such as the foot and leg, are usually avoided due to the risk of complications such as thrombophlebitis and pulmonary embolism.[72]

Vascular access is obtained using aseptic technique. Additionally, many paramedics and nurses may be trained in ultrasound guided peripheral vascular access. While this technique is beyond the scope of this text, note that this procedure may

FIGURE 16.32 VEINS OF THE UPPER ARM[71]

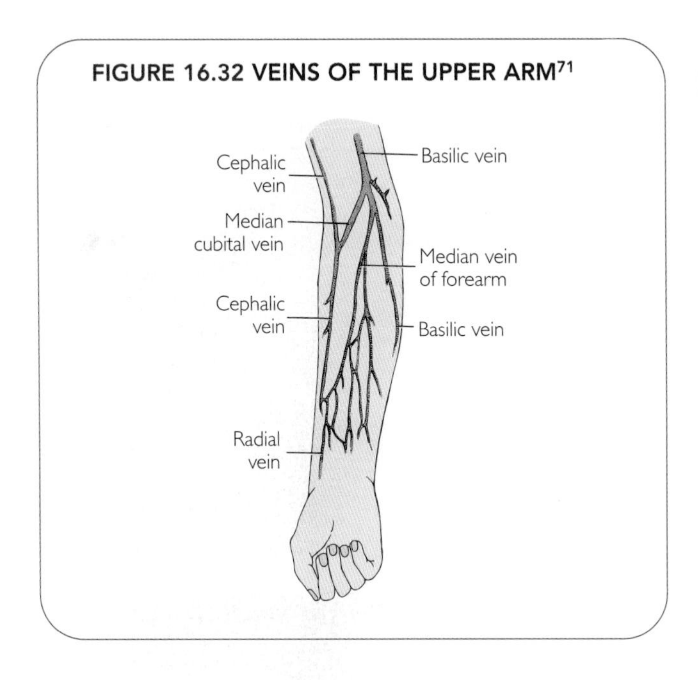

FIGURE 16.33 VEINS OF THE HANDS AND FINGERS[71]

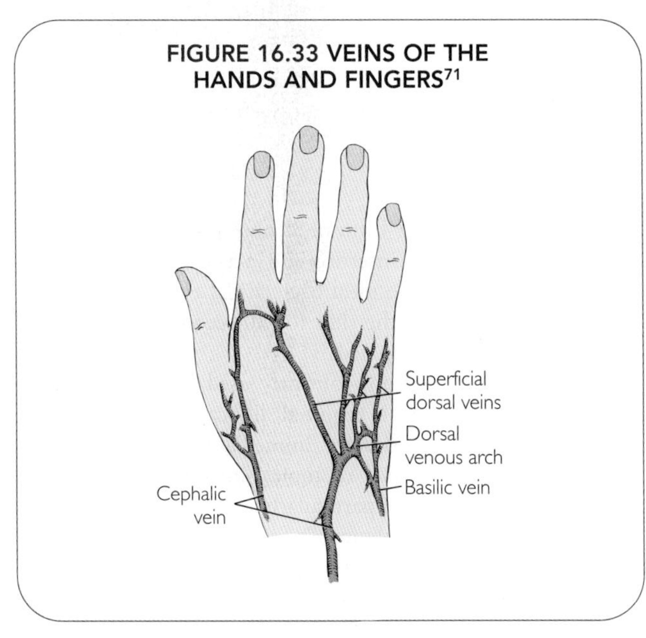

require a full sterile set-up. Initial insertion attempts should begin with distal veins and progress up the extremity. Proximal veins are not routinely used or recommended unless patients need immediate fluid replacement, such as in trauma or hypovolaemic shock. These veins are also used for patients receiving drugs that have an extremely short half-life (e.g. Adenosine). Scalp veins have no valves, so fluid can be infused in either direction; they are also easily visualised, making them an ideal alternative in infants.

Insertion of intravenous catheters is not without risk to the patient and the emergency clinician. Standard precautions must be applied to all patients, especially in emergency care settings, where the risk of blood exposure is increased and the infection status of patients unknown. Potential complications for the patient include infection and haematoma (Box 16.8). Handwashing and aseptic technique remain major prevention strategies for catheter-related infections.[70] The emergency clinician risks exposure to potentially infectious blood through a needle-stick or direct contact with blood or body fluids. Extreme care should be taken to minimise risks through use of standard precautions and appropriate disposal of needles. Intravenous catheters with safety features such as self-capping needles and retracting needles are readily available and should be used.[73]

BOX 16.8 **COMPLICATIONS OF INTRAVENOUS CATHETERS**

- Haematoma at insertion site
- Fluid infiltration
- Phlebitis
- Embolism of blood, air or catheter fragments
- Infection
- Cellulitis

CATHETER SELECTION

The size and type of intravenous catheter are determined by the clinical scenario, urgency of need, patient body habitus, age and vasculature. The general rule when choosing a cannula is the smallest gauge and the shortest length to meet the needs of the patient. Cannula selection is also determined by the purpose of the IV, the type of fluid to be administered, the location of the insertion site, the duration of the IV therapy and the condition of the vein.[74]

The chosen vein should be larger than the cannula, so that blood can flow easily around the catheter after insertion. This allows haemodilution to occur, therefore reducing venous wall trauma and distal oedema.[71] The rate of infusion flow is not determined by the vein itself but by the diameter of the cannula, and is inversely affected by the cannula length.[75] Larger-diameter catheters are used for administering large and rapid volumes, colloid solutions, blood or blood products, whereas smaller-diameter catheters are used for routine vascular access.

A guide for intravenous catheter selection[74]

- 22–24 gauge—children/adults with extremely small and/or fragile veins, e.g. the elderly. Infusion rate will be slow.
- 18–20 gauge—medical and surgical patients (depending on purpose of infusion).
- 16–20 gauge—blood product administration, surgical admissions and trauma.
- 14–16 gauge—life-threatening situations.

All intravenous catheters now use a catheter-over-needle design. Catheters used for peripheral access include a butterfly or winged catheter (Fig. 16.34) and straight catheter-over-needle design (Fig. 16.35). Winged catheters are easily inserted and can be stabilised with minimal effort; however, these catheters are not ideal for rapid fluid replacement. Catheters over needles are ideal for aggressive fluid replacement, but can present problems with stabilisation, particularly in distal veins of the hand.

INSERTION

Aseptic technique is essential to protect the patient from infection during intravenous catheter insertion. Gloves must be

FIGURE 16.34 BUTTERFLY OR WINGED INFUSION SET

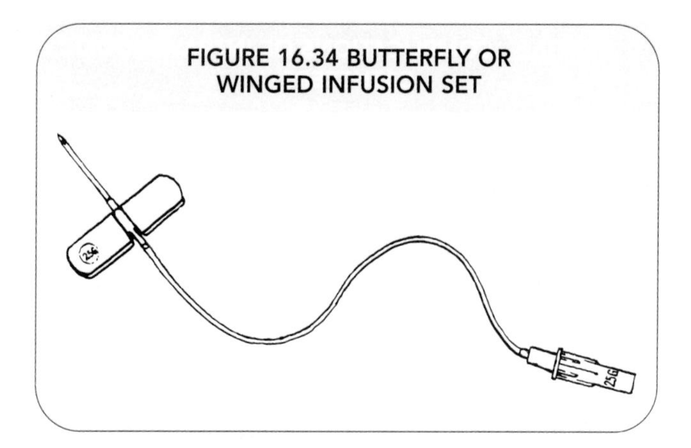

FIGURE 16.35 CATHETER OVER NEEDLE DESIGN OF INTRAVENOUS CATHETER

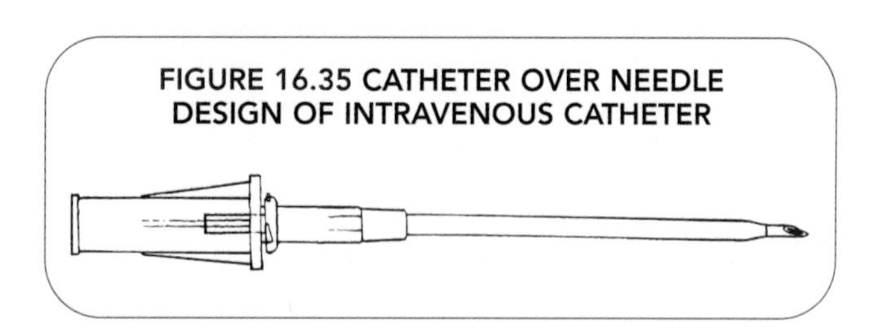

FIGURE 16.36 PREPARING FOR VENEPUNCTURE[71]

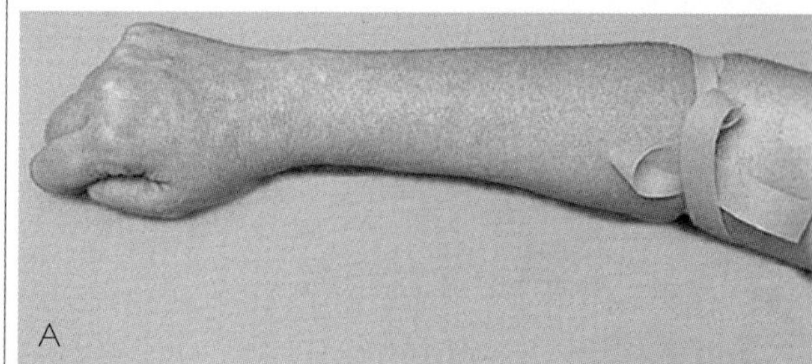

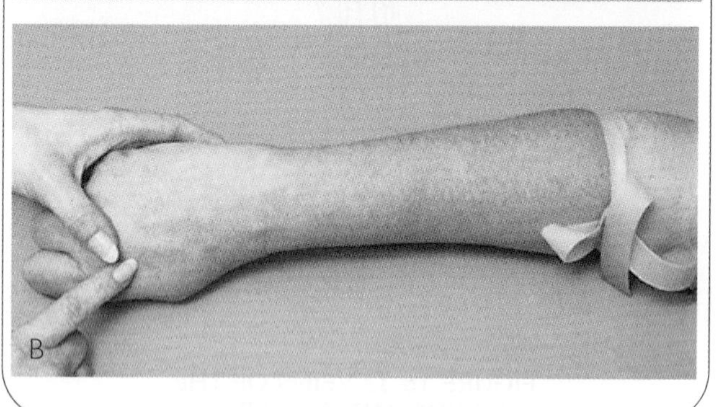

A. Placement of tourniquet. **B.** Technique for increasing vein size by dilation.

worn for site preparation and catheter insertion. The selected insertion site should have adequate circulation and be free of infection. In general, IV cannulation should be performed on the most distal part of the client's arm, but proximal to previous attempts.[74] Peripheral veins in hands and arms are the first choice for intravenous access. The hand veins are appropriate for 22- to 20-gauge IV cannulas. Cephalic, accessory or basilic veins are ideal for larger-bore cannulas. The femoral vein is an excellent choice in cardiac arrest because cardiac compressions can continue. Femoral access also provides an opportunity for haemodynamic pressure monitoring.

Veins should be avoided if they are below previous IV infiltration, close to arteries at points of flexion or show signs of skin inflammation, bruising or infection. If patients have undergone radical mastectomy, avoid the arm on the same side as the surgery because circulation may be impaired, affecting flow, causing oedema and other complications like thrombosis. In renal dialysis patients who have an arteriovenous (AV) fistula in place, this arm should be avoided to prevent damage above and below the fistula. Deep percutaneous antecubital or external jugular vein cannulation are also options in the patient with difficult veins or those who need immediate IV access.[73]

After a site is selected, palpation is the next crucial step in successful cannulation.[73] A tourniquet is placed proximally to distend vessels for easy insertion (Fig. 16.36A). Because veins may be more prominent in older patients, a tourniquet may not be required. Tourniquets may rupture vessels because of increased pressure in fragile veins. Gently tapping or rubbing vessels below the tourniquet increases vessel size by dilation. When vessels are not easily visualised or palpated, applying warm towels over the vein for 5 minutes causes vasodilation and can facilitate catheter insertion (Fig. 16.36B). Be careful not to burn fragile skin.

Skin preparation begins with initial cleansing using an antiseptic solution such as alcohol 75% with chlorhexidine gluconate or some other form of alcohol wipe. The solution is applied directly over the insertion site in a circular pattern moving slowly outwards. The ideal bactericidal effect requires that the solution remain on the skin for 30 seconds. The cleansed area should not be re-palpated.[74]

Local anaesthesia is not routinely used for cannula insertion. If local anaesthetic is required, lidocaine 1% may be injected at the insertion site for immediate anaesthetic effect. Various proprietary brands of topical anaesthetic creams are available for use. They are particularly useful for reducing pain and distress during cannulation.[76]

After the site is prepared, the catheter is inserted by stabilising the vein to prevent movement during puncture. With the needle bevel up, the skin is punctured using the smallest angle possible between the skin and needle (Fig. 16.37). Veins may be entered on the top or side. The catheter is advanced slowly until blood flashes into the catheter, then the catheter is advanced over the needle into the vein and the needle removed. The tourniquet is removed; fingertip pressure is applied at the distal end of the catheter tip to prevent extravasation of blood. The injection port is attached and catheter flushed with 0.9% normal saline or connected to primed IV tubing. The catheter and tubing should be secured with tape according to local policy; however, tape should never be applied directly over the insertion site. The evidence regarding the nature of site dressings is debatable.[70] However, clear, occlusive dressings such as Opsite, Tegaderm or Bioclusive should be applied over the insertion site. Sites should be labelled with the date, time, catheter size and initials of the person inserting to facilitate monitoring and evaluation.[70]

IV lines and the cannula itself should be changed according to local policy, although some hospitals now differentiate

FIGURE 16.37 VENEPUNCTURE[71]

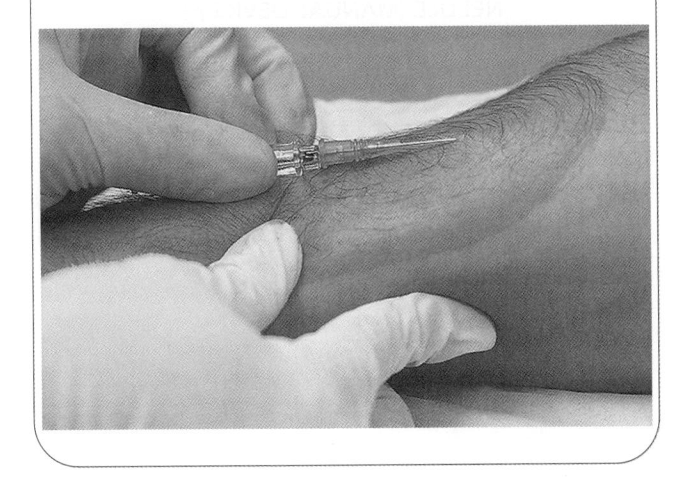

out-of-hospital (paramedic-inserted) and in-hospital-inserted cannulae.

PAEDIATRIC CONSIDERATIONS

Paediatric IV cannulations can be very traumatic for both the child and their parents; therefore, consideration should be given first to the need for the procedure and second to the urgency with which the procedure needs to be performed. Once the need for IV cannulation has been determined, it is important to plan and prepare for the procedure adequately if the clinical situation allows to ensure the best chance at success.

The anxiety and pain associated with cannulation may be limited with the use of topical anaesthetic creams and/or the use of other analgesics such as nitrous oxide during the procedure. Topical anaesthetic creams need to be applied 45–60 minutes prior to performing the procedure for them to successfully anaesthetise the area, an effect which persists for at least 2 hours after removal of the patch.[77] The procedure time therefore needs to be planned in conjunction with the action of the anaesthetic cream. It is also important to apply the patch to a site that has a potentially suitable vein, as the maximum number of patches that can be applied is limited by age. This strategy is generally not applicable to the pre-hospital environment.

The need to provide appropriate psychosocial support to a child cannot be over-emphasised. Anxiety is a significant factor in a child's perception of pain and thereby influences the level of pain experienced during cannulation. Moreover, this may also affect the degree of cooperation by the child. Previous experience may also influence the degree to which the child will cooperate during the cannulation procedure and may even flow on to future procedures and healthcare.[78] It is therefore important to have an adequate understanding of the perception of children of various age groups in terms of how they may react to IV cannulation.

Parental support can also be very beneficial. Most parents prefer to be present during the procedure and almost all children perceive that parental presence 'helps the most'.[79] Parents need to have an active role in the procedure—providing distraction, encouragement and comfort. Caution should be taken with parental involvement where the parents themselves have a needle phobia or show high levels of distress, and this needs to be discussed openly to avoid causing blame or guilt.[79]

Where practical, the procedural steps and what the child may feel should be explained in terms that the child understands. During the procedure, diversional tactics can be beneficial in reducing anxiety and distracting the child from the procedure. Many ambulance services and EDs use a range of distraction equipment. Where possible, it may be of some benefit to develop some more-positive reinforcement for cooperation, for example, a sticker, special toy, smartphone/tablet-based videos, cuddles from a parent, or in-hospital, playing their favourite video after the procedure. This can often assist with cooperation in patients who may be having this procedure on a regular basis, or for future encounters with the procedure.[79]

In some instances, the child may become very objectionable, uncooperative and physically resistant, in an attempt to gain some control over what is happening to them. This may make the procedure very difficult to perform and physical restraint may be required to continue. The restraint should be at the least restrictive level to perform the procedure. The child should be given some reassurance that the pain and restraint they are experiencing is not punishment for any wrongdoings. Parents where possible should not be involved in restraint as their presence is as a resource for the child.[79]

INTRA-OSSEOUS ACCESS

Intra-osseous (IO) access involves the insertion of specifically designed IO devices into the IO space of the bone matrix. The IO space refers to the spongy cancellous bone of the epiphysis and the medullary cavity of the diaphysis. The medullary cavity consists of a vast non-collapsible vascular structure which connects to the central circulation by a series of longitudinal canals which contain an artery and a vein. Volkmann's canals connect the IO vasculature with the major arteries and veins of the central circulation (Fig. 16.38).[80,81] IO access provides a safe, rapid and reliable route for administration of drugs, crystalloids, colloids and blood. A three-way tap can be connected to allow fluid bolus delivery. Medications and fluids administered via the IO route enter the central circulation in comparable concentrations and time as the IV route.[80,82]

IO access is indicated in both children and adults requiring immediate resuscitation and in whom peripheral intravascular access cannot be achieved in a timely or reliable manner.[83] IO

FIGURE 16.38 VASCULAR ANATOMY OF LONG BONES[82]

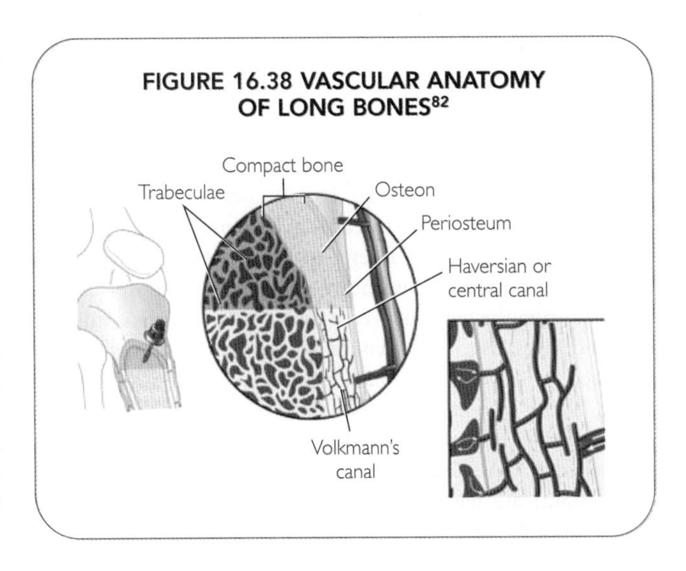

FIGURE 16.39 SCHEMATIC DIAGRAM OF POSSIBLE PROBLEMS ENCOUNTERED WITH INTRA-OSSEOUS INSERTION SITES[82]

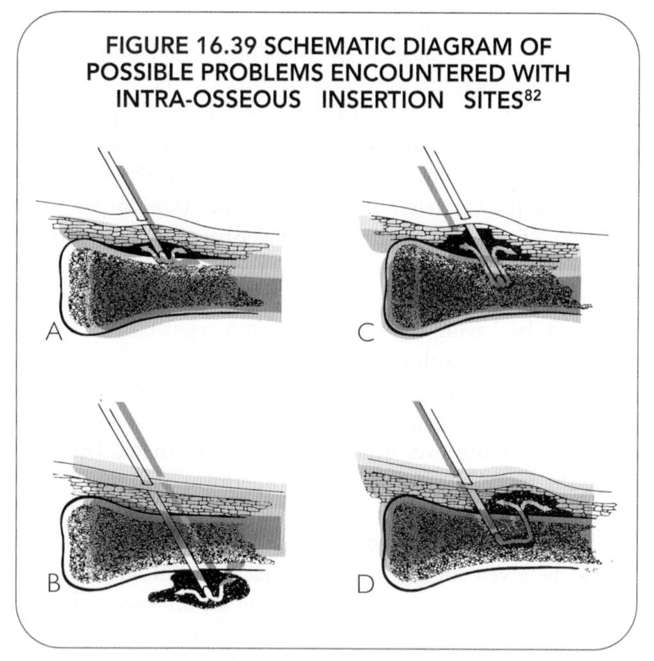

A. Incomplete penetration. **B.** Penetration of posterior cortex. **C.** Fluid escaping around needle. **D.** Fluid leaking through nearby cortical puncture.

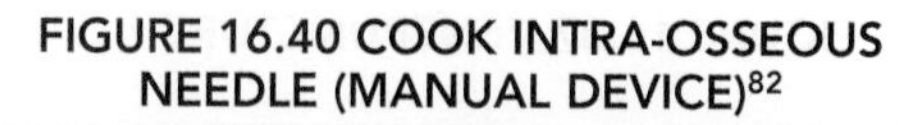

FIGURE 16.40 COOK INTRA-OSSEOUS NEEDLE (MANUAL DEVICE)[82]

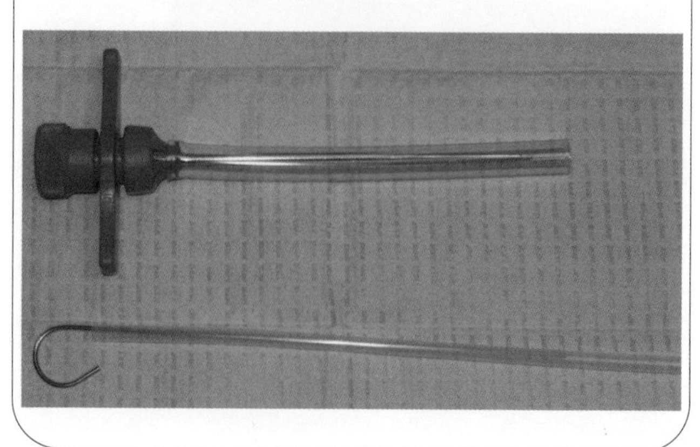

FIGURE 16.41 BONE INJECTION GUN (IMPACT-DRIVEN DEVICE)[82]

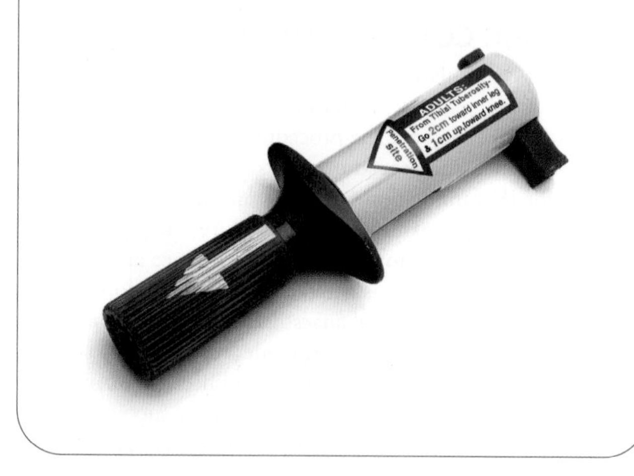

FIGURE 16.42 EZ-IO DEVICE (POWERED DRILL DEVICE)[82]

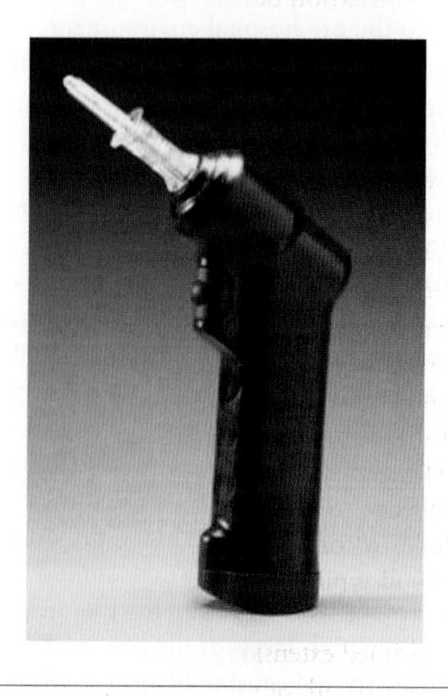

access can be achieved quickly and is as fast as IV access. Successful insertion rates have been shown to be high following failed IV attempts.[82] Contraindications include fracture of the bone, previous IO attempts in the same bone, osteoporosis, osteogenesis imperfecta, infection of the overlying insertion site and inability to identify insertion landmarks.[80,82] Complications related to IO access include extravasation, fat emboli, osteomyelitis and subcutaneous abscess (Fig. 16.39). Epiphyseal damage can occur in children; therefore, careful identification of the appropriate anatomical insertion site is vital.[83]

PRACTICE TIP

IO access is indicated in both children and adults requiring immediate resuscitation and in whom peripheral intravascular access cannot be achieved in a timely or reliable manner.

Various IO devices are available and generally fall into one of three categories: manual, impact-driven or powered drill devices. Manual devices (Fig. 16.40) consist of hollow steel needles with a removable trocar that prevents plugging of the needle with bone during insertion. These are increasingly uncommon in developed healthcare systems. Manual devices are inserted using the hand-delivered force of the clinician. Impact-driven devices (Fig. 16.41) contain a spring-loaded mechanism designed to penetrate through the bone cortex into the IO space. These devices do not use a drill motion, but instead use the force from the spring-loaded mechanism to drive the sharpened IO needle into the IO space. Powered drill devices (Fig. 16.42) are battery powered, handheld drills that insert the IO needle into the IO space with a high-speed rotary

FIGURE 16.43 SCHEMATIC DIAGRAM DEMONSTRATING INTRA-OSSEOUS (IO) INSERTION SITES

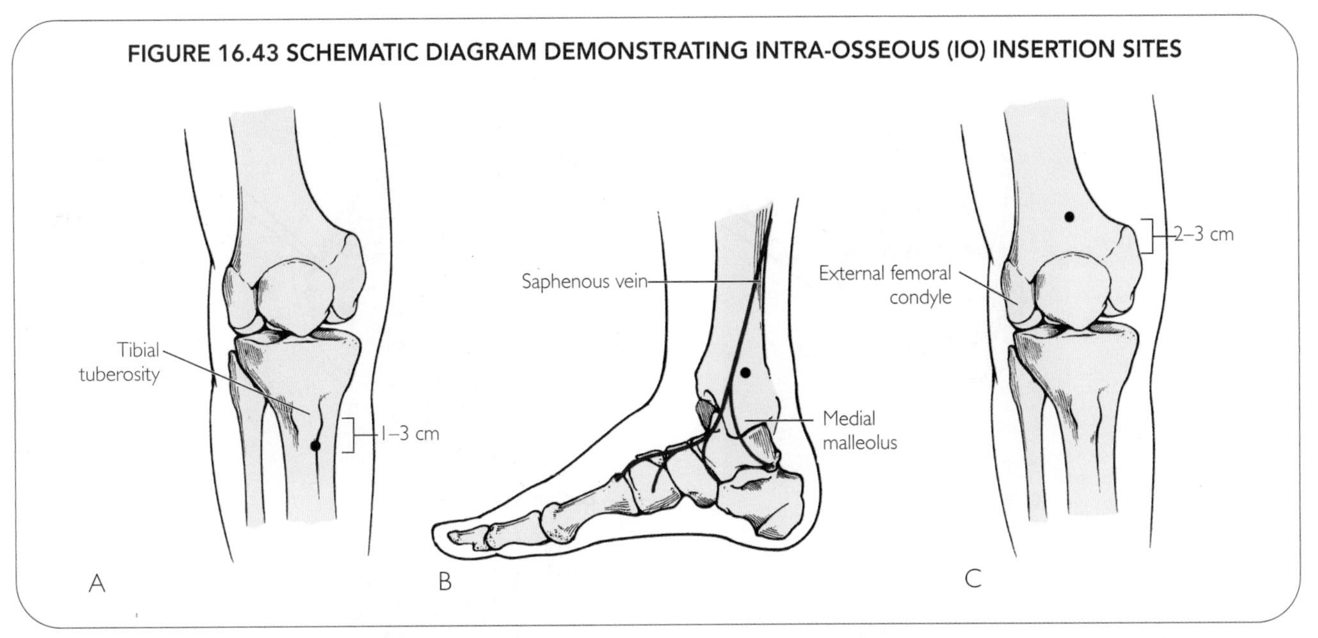

A. The proximal tibia. The IO needle is inserted 1–2 cm distal to the tibial tuberosity and over the medial aspect of the tibia. The bevel of the needle is directed away from the joint space. **B.** The distal tibia. The IO needle is inserted on the medial surface of the distal tibia at the junction of the medial malleolus and the shaft of the tibia, posterior to the greater saphenous vein. The needle is directed cephalad, away from the growth plate. **C.** The distal femur. The IO needle is inserted 2–3 cm above the external condyles in the midline and directed cephalad, away from the growth-plate.

motion.[81] These devices yield the highest success rates, are easy to use, and are readily available to most ambulance services and hospitals.

Sites commonly used for insertion include proximal tibia, distal tibia and distal femur (Fig. 16.43). In infants and children younger than 6 years, the proximal tibia is the preferred site, followed by the distal tibia and distal femur. In adults, the most common site is the distal tibia.[82] The proximal humerus site offers ready access in patients where lower limbs may be inaccessible (e.g. trapped in a vehicle). Other sites include the sternum, calcaneus and clavicle; however, they are rarely employed due to difficult-to-locate landmarks and the requirement for specific insertion devices.[80,82]

Intra-osseous device insertion method

1. Gather equipment.
2. Wash hands and don PPE.
3. Locate insertion site.
4. Prepare insertion site—sterile technique.[81]
5. Prepare IO device.
6. Insert IO device in accordance with manufacturer's instructions.
7. Penetrate the bone cortex. A sudden decrease in resistance is felt, along with a 'pop' or 'crunch' sensation.
8. Remove the stylet from the IO needle. The IO needle should feel secure and stable in position.
9. Attach a syringe to the IO needle and aspirate bone marrow or blood to confirm correct position. Aspirate may be used for blood typing, cross-match and blood chemistry testing.[82]
10. Connect a primed extension set to the hub of the IO needle and flush with 10 mL of normal saline to confirm patency.
11. Apply the stabiliser set to the patient's skin to avoid movement and/or dislodgement of the IO needle. All fluids and medication should be given through the extension set and not directly into the hub of the IO needle as this is likely to cause movement and loss of stability at the insertion site.[84]
12. Dress as appropriate. Avoid covering the insertion site as this may hide evidence of extravasation. Splinting of the limb may also be considered.

VENOUS CUTDOWN

Vascular access may be obtained surgically when a large volume of fluid is required or when peripheral access cannot be obtained. The procedure is used more often in children than in adults but has lost favour with increased use of intra-osseous needles. Venous cutdown involves surgical isolation of the basilic vein or saphenous vein (Fig. 16.44A) followed by insertion of a large-bore catheter, intravenous tubing or feeding tube (5 Fr or 8 Fr), which is sutured in place (Figs 16.44B and C). Disadvantages of this technique include time and skill required to complete the procedure. This implies that cutdown should be resorted to only when percutaneous access has failed or is deemed likely to be unsuccessful.

It is more common, and preferential, to attempt central venous access over venous cutdown. Intra-osseous access is used more often to secure emergent access.

HAEMODYNAMIC MONITORING

Haemodynamic monitoring is used in critically ill patients to allow prompt recognition and accurate assessment of circulatory characteristics and dynamics. Haemodynamic monitoring involves the placement of invasive catheters into the vascular

FIGURE 16.44 VENOUS CUTDOWN

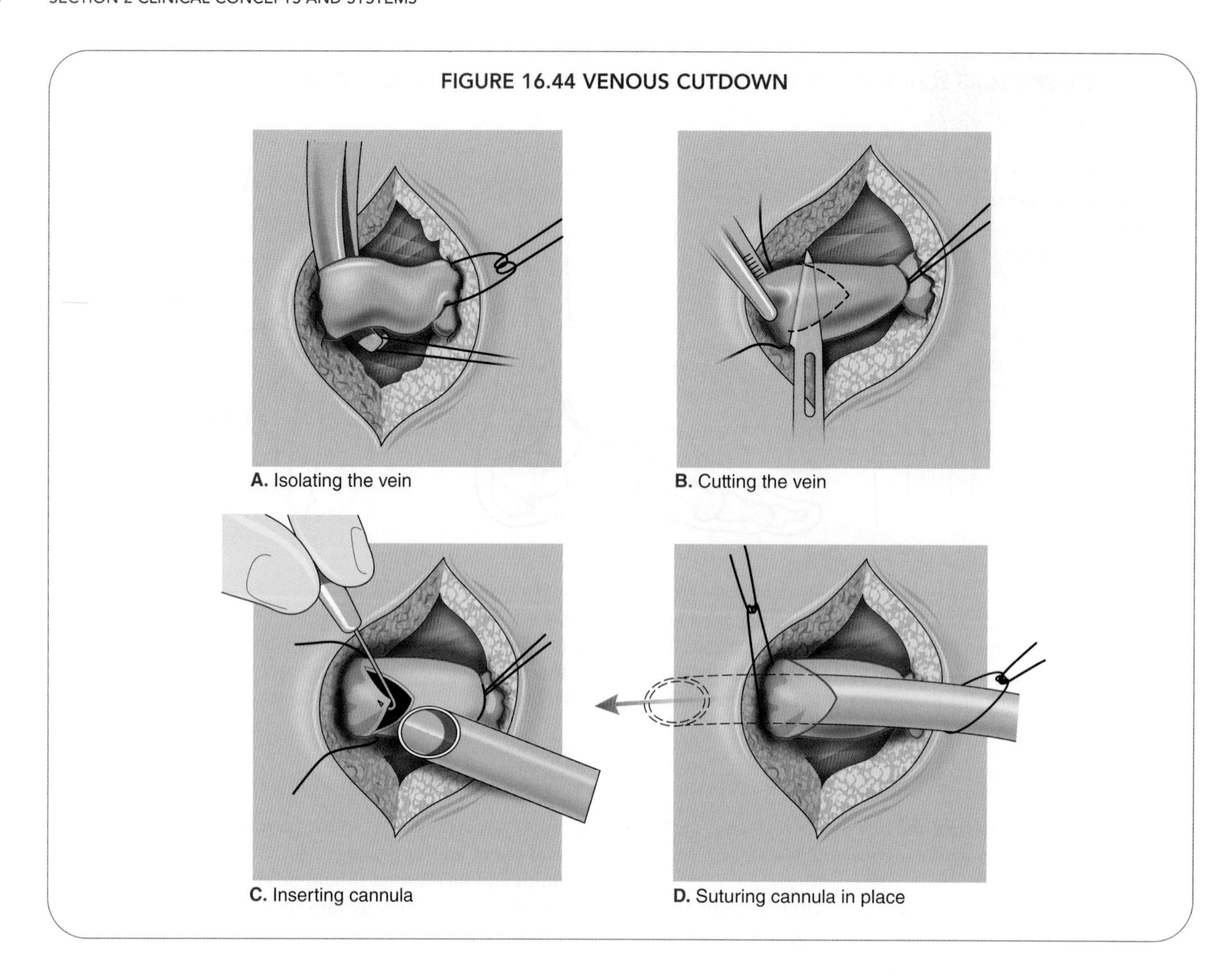

system for the purpose of either continuous or intermittent measurement of haemodynamic parameters. In the emergency environment, these parameters are generally limited to the measurement of arterial blood pressure (ABP) and central venous pressure (CVP), although CVP monitoring is less common nowadays.

For emergency clinicians caring for patients where haemodynamic monitoring is being used, it is important to understand the underlying physiology of arterial and venous pressure and the relationship of these pressures to the production of the waveforms and values which are monitored at the bedside. This knowledge is important when relating and interpreting these waveforms and values to the care and management of these patients.

PRODUCTION OF VISUAL PRESSURE WAVEFORMS

The production of a pressure waveform occurs through the insertion of an intravascular (arterial or venous) catheter, which is connected via fluid-filled rigid plastic tubing to a transducer. The fluid-filled system beyond the transducer is pressurised to 300 mmHg. Changes in pressure are transferred through the tubing to the transducer. These changes in pressure are converted to an electrical signal by the transducer. These signals are then amplified and converted by a monitoring device into graphical and numerical displays.

ARTERIAL LINES

Indications

The indications for ABP monitoring include:

1. conditions requiring continuous arterial pressure monitoring. These may include:
   - uncontrolled hypertension
   - hypovolaemia
   - shock of all aetiology
   - patients receiving vasoactive drugs (e.g. adrenaline, dopamine, dobutamine, metaraminol, sodium nitroprusside).
2. to avoid repeated venepuncture in patients requiring frequent blood samples (e.g. in diabetic ketoacidosis and severe respiratory illnesses).

Sites

The following sites may be used for arterial cannulation and arterial blood pressure monitoring.

- *Radial artery*—this site is the most common site chosen due to the fact that it is easy to access and the site is easy to maintain and manipulate if required. It is important to perform an Allen's test prior to cannulation of the radial artery (Fig. 16.24).
- *Femoral artery*—recommended for use in long-term critically ill patients as it is associated with a lower complication rate.

BOX 16.9 EQUIPMENT FOR ARTERIAL LINE INSERTION[86,87]

- Sterile gloves, eye protection
- Moisture-proof underpad
- Dressing pack/small-procedure pack/sterile field
- Antiseptic solution (e.g. 2% chlorhexidine); refer to hospital policy
- Arterial cannula
- Suture material
- Occlusive and transparent dressing
- Adhesive tape
- Arm board
- 500 mL normal saline
- Pressure transducer set–primed
- Transducer cable
- Infusion pressure bag

- *Axillary artery*—again, this site is also recommended for long-term use.
- *Brachial artery*—not a commonly used site due to concerns regarding lack of effective collateral circulation and the close proximity of the median nerve.
- *Dorsalis pedis artery*—also not commonly used. The anatomy is less predictable and success rates are lower. This site should also be avoided in patients with peripheral vascular disease and diabetes.[85,86]

Equipment

Equipment required for arterial line insertion is given in Box 16.9.

Care of arterial catheter

The care of the arterial catheter and line should include the following:

- The site (e.g. arm) should be immobilised (on an arm board) to prevent movement, which may result in catheter displacement.
- Ensure that lines are secured and connections are tight, to avoid haemorrhage from accidental dislodgement.
- The site and all connections should be always left exposed. An unexposed, disconnected arterial line can result in significant blood loss before being noticed.
- Check distal circulation (colour, warmth, movement and sensation) hourly and report any abnormalities.
- Label the arterial catheter and/or tubing of the arterial line as 'arterial'; labels are generally available in the packaging.
- Never inject anything into the arterial line. Anything injected into the line may cause significant effects distal to the site of the catheter.
- Maintain the pressure bag at 300 mmHg. This ensures that a fluid administration rate of 3 mL/h will be maintained and that no blood will flow back into the tubing.
- Zero the transducer at the beginning of each shift or when the patient has been repositioned (e.g. during inter-facility transfer).

ZEROING

Following insertion and care of the arterial catheter, the arterial line needs to be calibrated to ensure accuracy of the recorded values. Zeroing is the process of eliminating the weight of the air or the atmospheric pressure (usually about 760 mmHg) from the pressure measurements. This is achieved by opening the transducer to air and adjusting the display system (monitor) to read zero. This will eliminate all the pressure contributions from the atmosphere and only the pressure values that exist within the vessel being monitored will be displayed.[88] The procedure is:

1. Prime the transducer giving set and insert into a pressure bag.
2. Pump the pressure bag to 300 mmHg.
3. Connect transducer IV line to arterial cannula and secure.
4. Plug pressure cable into monitor.
5. Connect pressure cable from monitor to transducer set.
6. Adjust transducer to the height of the phlebostatic axis. The phlebostatic axis is found at the intersection of a vertical line from the fourth intercostal space and midway between the anterior and posterior surfaces of the patient's chest, in the supine position. This position correlates to the level of the patient's right atrium.[89]
7. Switch the transducer 'off' to the patient (open to sampling port) by turning the three-way stopcock.
8. Remove the cap from the sampling port, opening the transducer to the atmosphere.
9. Press 'Zero' on the monitoring device.

BLOOD SAMPLING—ARTERIAL LINES

Blood sampling from an arterial line is performed to obtain blood samples for ABG analysis and other pathology testing. Blood sampling from the arterial line may be required frequently, for example, in unstable patients who require frequent ABGs.

The procedure for blood sampling from an arterial line[90,91] is given below.

1. Assemble equipment:
   - clean (non-sterile) gloves
   - goggles/face shield
   - syringe for discarding
   - sampling syringe
   - sterile bung/cap for the access/sampling port
   - sterile gauze.
2. Silence alarm on monitor.
3. Explain the procedure to the patient.
4. Remove the cap from the sampling port and attach the spare syringe.
5. Turn the three-way stopcock off to the transducer and open to the sampling port.
6. Allow sufficient 'dead-space' fluid to enter the syringe until undiluted blood reaches the syringe.
7. Turn the three-way stopcock off to the patient (open to the transducer).
8. Remove the syringe and discard.
9. Attach the sampling syringe.
10. Turn the three-way stopcock off to the transducer and open to the sampling port.
11. Collect sample volume required by allowing blood to flow into the syringe; assist aspiration gently if required.
12. Turn the three-way stopcock off to the patient (open to the transducer).
13. Remove sampling syringe.

14. Flush the sampling port into sterile gauze to remove blood from port.
15. Place a new sterile cap on the sampling port.
16. Turn the three-way stopcock off to the sampling port.
17. Use the fast-flush device to clear the line of blood.
18. Reactivate alarms and ensure arterial waveform is present.
19. Prepare and send collected samples.
20. Discard used supplies.
21. Wash hands.

Some haemodynamic monitoring line systems contain a reservoir into which fluid from between the catheter and the sampling port can be moved, allowing undiluted blood to be accessible without having to discard a sample prior to collection of the true sample. The reservoir is then emptied at the completion of the sample collection to flush the line of blood.

CENTRAL VENOUS CATHETERS

Central venous access plays an important role in the management of critically ill patients, as it affords staff the ability to draw blood samples and instil high doses of multiple medications while simultaneously measuring pressures within the vascular system. Central venous access is commonly used in trauma patients for the restoration of blood volume, and in unwell patients who require vasoactive or inotropic support and multiple antibiotics to stabilise circulation. In patients with vascular compromise or circulatory collapse, central venous access may be the only way to access the venous system.

INDICATIONS

The indications for insertion of a central venous catheter (CVC) include:

- administration of drugs and fluid
- administration of total parenteral nutrition (TPN)
- insertion of a temporary cardiac pacing wire
- to monitor CVP to:
  - assist in the estimation of a patient's hydration status as a guide to fluid replacement
  - assess the extent of right-sided heart failure

SITES

Commonly the following sites are chosen for CVC insertion:

- internal jugular
- subclavian vein
- femoral vein
- brachial vein. The brachial vein is usually used for peripherally inserted central catheters (PICCs).

The advantages and disadvantages of these sites are outlined in Table 16.4.

EQUIPMENT

The equipment commonly used for CVC insertion is outlined in Box 16.10. The nurse needs to be familiar with the equipment required and the main steps in CVC insertion to be able to assist with preparation and insertion. Insertion of CVCs and PICCs by specialised registered nurses is also becoming increasingly common throughout Australasia.

INSERTION

The most common insertion method for CVCs is the use of the Seldinger (guidewire) technique. This technique is performed

TABLE 16.4 ADVANTAGES AND DISADVANTAGES OF COMMONLY USED CVC INSERTION SITES[92,93]

SITE	ADVANTAGES	DISADVANTAGES
Internal jugular	Large vessel Easy to locate, good external landmarks Easy access Short, straight path to vena cava (right side) Low rate of complications	Uncomfortable for patient Hard to maintain dressing Close proximity to carotid artery High infection rate Problematic in patients with tracheostomies
Subclavian	Large vessel with high flow rate Lowest infection rates Easy to dress and maintain Supra to infraclavicular approaches Less restrictive for patient	Lies close to lung apex (pneumothorax risk) Close proximity to subclavian artery Difficult to control bleeding (non-compressible site)
Femoral	Easy access, good external landmarks Large vessel Advantageous during resuscitation	Decreased patient mobility Increased rate of thrombosis and phlebitis High rates of infection Risk of femoral artery puncture Dressing may be problematic
Brachial	Easy access Advantageous during resuscitation	Large incidence of phlebitis Longer time for drugs to access central circulation Catheter tip movement related to arm movement

BOX 16.10 EQUIPMENT COMMONLY USED FOR CVC INSERTION[94]

- CVC–single/triple lumen/size
- Procedure tray
- Moisture-proof underpad
- Personal protective equipment
- Sterile gown/gloves
- Sterile drapes
- Antiseptic solution
- 2 mL, 10 mL syringes
- 10–20 mL normal saline for injection
- 25, 23 and 19 gauge needles
- 1% lidocaine
- Gauze
- Scalpel–11 or 12 gauge
- 2/0 silk suture–straight needle
- Transparent occlusive dressing (sterile)
- Additional equipment may be required based upon local policy/procedures

under sterile conditions and involves the insertion of a small needle into the intended vessel, through which a guidewire is passed into the lumen of the vessel. The needle is then withdrawn, leaving the guidewire within the vessel. The insertion site is often enlarged with a scalpel and a dilator is used over the guidewire to widen the intended path of the catheter. The dilator is then removed and the catheter inserted into the vessel over the guidewire. The guidewire is then removed and the catheter secured in place with a suture, and a transparent dressing is applied. Although this approach has several steps, once mastered, the procedure can be performed quickly.[92,93]

Following insertion involving puncture of the neck or thorax, observe for cardiac dysrhythmias on insertion, as the catheter tip will be inserted to the lower third of the superior vena cava outside the right atrium. A chest x-ray (CXR) should be obtained. The x-ray is assessed to identify any complications associated with insertion, such as haemothorax or pneumothorax, and to confirm the correct position of the catheter tip. Where possible, the CXR should be performed in the upright or semi-upright position as small amounts of air or blood within the intrapleural space may not be seen in the supine patient. The catheter tip should sit in the lower third of the superior vena cava outside the right atrium (Fig. 16.45).[89] Correct position of the catheter tip should be confirmed prior to the commencement of any infusions. A post-procedure CXR is not indicated for CVCs inserted into the femoral vein because, due to the distance away from the heart, there is less risk of misplacement.

The insertion of CVC is beyond the scope of all Australian paramedics at the time of publication, but paramedics in the retrieval environment may assist doctors with the insertion and monitoring of central lines.

CENTRAL VENOUS PRESSURE MEASUREMENT

There are two methods of measuring CVP: these include the water manometer method and, more commonly, the use of a haemodynamic monitoring system. With either system the measurement is taken at the level of the phlebostatic axis. Once the phlebostatic axis point has been determined, a small ink mark may be made on the patient's skin for future reference. It is important that all measurements are taken from the same location to ensure accuracy.

The water manometer measures CVP in centimetres of water (cmH_2O), while haemodynamic monitoring records the CVP in millimetres of mercury (mmHg). This makes it more difficult to compare readings from one system against the other, although conversion formulae are available if required. The water manometer readings are performed intermittently while the haemodynamic monitoring records the CVP continuously, improving its accuracy over the water manometer method.[89,95]

FIGURE 16.45 CHEST X-RAY SHOWING CORRECT PLACEMENT OF CENTRAL VENOUS CATHETER

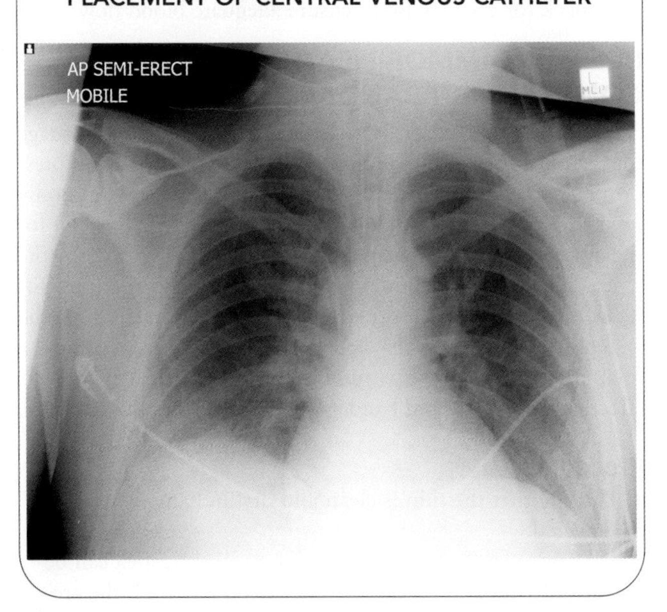

Water manometer method

Box 16.11 shows the recommended procedure for CVP measurement using a water manometer.

SOFT-TISSUE INJURIES

Soft-tissue injures are a common reason for patients to seek help.

An assessment of the affected area should include: noting the colour of the skin and surrounding tissue, feeling the warmth of the area, assessing range of motion and strength, and testing for sensation (colour, warmth, movement, sensation). A measure of the pulses and capillary refill times in the affected area should also be included in the assessment of soft-tissue injuries. It is important to consider the mechanism of injury and potential underlying structures involved. Assessment and management of soft tissue injuries are presented in Chapter 17. Types of bandaging are presented here.

BOX 16.11 PROCEDURE FOR CENTRAL VENOUS PRESSURE (CVP) MEASUREMENT—WATER MANOMETER[95,96]

1. Explain the procedure to the patient.
2. Locate the phlebostatic axis.
3. Position the patient in the supine position (preferred) or semi-recumbent position.
4. Ensure all intravenous fusions running through the manometer line are stopped.
5. Zero the manometer by placing the zero of the water manometer at the level of the phlebostatic axis. To ensure the level is accurate, a spirit or laser level should be used.
6. Close the three-way stopcock off to the patient and allow the manometer to fill with fluid to a level beyond the expected pressure.
7. Close the three-way stopcock off to the fluid supply and open to the patient.
8. Observe the column of water in the manometer. It should fall until gravity pressure equals the CVP. The water level will fluctuate gently with the patient's respiratory cycle.
9. Record the CVP measurement at end expiration.
10. Turn the three-way stopcock open to the flush system and the patient (off to the manometer) and re-establish the IV fluid infusion.

FIGURE OF EIGHT BANDAGE

The figure of eight bandage is used to provide support to joints. The figure of eight bandage encircles below the joint and crosses over to immobilise above the joint like a figure 8. The bandage ascends obliquely in a circular motion in a figure-8 fashion, overlapping, until immobilisation is achieved.[35] To fit:

1. Begin by ensuring that the skin is clean and dry and any wounds are covered.
2. Start by wrapping twice around the limb to stabilise the bandage.[35]
3. Wrap a single layer distally and cross up like a figure 8 over the joint proximally.
4. Continue to wrap proximally and then cross back down over the joint distally, like a figure 8.
5. Continue the figure-8 wrap until immobilisation is attained.
6. Ensure there are no wrinkles or creases which could cause tissue injury.
7. Secure the end of the bandage well with tape.
8. Apply an elasticised tubular compression bandage and ice pack over the figure 8 for additional compression and pain relief.

PRACTICE TIP

Use a figure of 8 dressing in combination with an ice pack and elasticised tubular compression bandage on ankle injuries to provide immobilisation, compression and pain relief.

ELASTICISED TUBULAR COMPRESSION BANDAGES

Elasticised tubular compression bandages, such as Tubigrip™, are strands of cotton-covered elastic and are used to provide support and reduce swelling. The bandage will provide compression but does not immobilise the limb. Acute ankle sprains and strains are a common ED orthopaedic presentation that can be effectively treated with elastic compression bandages.[97] Scarring from burns can be controlled with the use of tubular compression bandaging in the weeks after injury.

Patients can wash and reuse Tubigrip without it losing its effectiveness. Elastic compression bandages can be worn for 2–3 days.

To apply:

1. Begin by ensuring the skin is clean and dry and any wounds are covered.
2. Cut the elasticated tubular bandage to twice the length of the patient's limb.
3. Pull the bandage onto the limb like a sock and then double it over by pulling the second layer up.
4. Ensure the bottom layer is 2–3 cm higher on the limb than the top layer.
5. Ensure there are no wrinkles or creases which can cause tissue injury.
6. Check pulses and capillary refill distally.

PRACTICE TIP

Use elasticised tubular compression bandages (e.g. Tubigrip) to provide compression where immobilisation of the injury is not required, such as soft-tissue ankle injuries. Avoid HARM.

- Patients can wash and reuse tubular compression bandages.

SPICA BANDAGE

The finished spica bandage resembles a spike of wheat with overlapping V-like layers, providing compression, support or retention of wound dressings. The term 'spica cast' is sometimes used to describe a plaster cast that involves the limb and the trunk of the body.

Procedure

1. Begin by ensuring that the skin is clean and dry and any wounds are covered.
2. Start by wrapping twice around the limb, above the joint, to stabilise the bandage.[98]
3. Wrap the first layer down distally across the joint and around, bringing it back up to the beginning point.
4. Repeat the layers, overlapping two-thirds ascending and descending until the final bandaging represents a series of V-like shapes down the limb.
5. Ensure there are no wrinkles or creases that can cause tissue injury.
6. Secure the end of the bandage well with tape.
7. Check for distal pulse to ensure adequate blood flow.

ROBERT-JONES BANDAGE

A Robert-Jones bandage is a heavy, multi-layered application consisting of alternate layers of bandage and padding or wadding. The purpose of the Robert-Jones bandage is to immobilise and support.

Procedure

1. Begin by ensuring that the skin is clean and dry and any wounds are covered.
2. Wrap from distal to proximal with an overlapping layer of wadding or soft, absorbent orthopaedic padding (e.g. Velband).
3. Ensure there are no wrinkles or creases that can cause tissue injury.
4. Wrap an alternate layer of wide elastic compression or crepe bandage firmly enough to allow distal blood flow. Select a bandage that is at least 15 cm wide.
5. Repeat with alternate layers of orthopaedic padding and bandaging for up to six layers in total, with the final layer being bandage.
6. Secure the end of the final bandage well with tape.
7. Check for distal pulse to ensure adequate blood flow.

PRESSURE-IMMOBILISATION OR COMPRESSION BANDAGE

A compression bandage is an elasticised, stretchable bandage that applies pressure to prevent or relieve swelling. Compression or pressure-immobilisation bandaging (PIB) is commonly used to prevent limb swelling but can be used pre-hospital for the management of envenomation. The PIB compresses the lymphatic vessels and inhibits limb muscle movement therefor retarding venom transport and slowing venom entering the systemic circulation.[99] To be effective, a PIB should have a final pressure of 50–75 mmHg.[100] Crepe bandages are less effective than elasticised bandages in maintaining this pressure.

Procedure

1. Ensure that the skin is clean and dry and any wounds are covered.
2. In cases of suspected envenomation, the bite area can be circled with pen for later reference; do not wash the area, to allow easier venom identification.

3. Begin by wrapping at the point of injury down the limb, overlapping the bandage one-third each time. Select an elastic bandage that is at least 15 cm wide.
4. Wrap to the end of the limb, including fingers or toes, and then continue proximally until the entire limb is covered.
5. Use firm pressure to occlude lymphatic flow but preserve blood flow. Check for distal pulse to ensure adequate blood flow.
6. Ensure there are no wrinkles or creases which can cause tissue injury.
7. Secure the end of the bandage well with tape.
8. Splint the limb to further restrict movement. Do not elevate the limb.

PRACTICE TIP

Compression bandaging is an effective first-aid measure in snakebite and where reduction of swelling is desired.

- Compression or pressure-immobilisation bandaging (PIB) must be used in combination with splinting to achieve limb immobilisation.
- A correctly fitted PIB for use in snakebite requires between 50 and 70 mmHg pressure. To determine how tightly to fit a bandage, apply a blood pressure cuff to your own arm and inflate it to this pressure.

Correct bandaging can effectively stabilise injuries and reduce pain. It is important to select the correct type of bandage, as each has different properties. It is also important to select the correct method of bandaging to suit the injury, as each provides different levels of compression and immobilisation.

TOURNIQUET

A tourniquet is a tight cuff, bandage or purpose-made device to control haemorrhage in the pre-hospital or early resuscitation stage of trauma. The use of a tourniquet can prevent exsanguinating haemorrhage that accounts for half of the deaths in the first 24 hours of trauma.[101] In the field the control of life-threatening haemorrhage may even become a priority over the management of airway and breathing assessments, particularly in combat situations,[9] as uncontrolled haemorrhage is a leading cause of battlefield death.[102] Proprietary tourniquets such as the Combat Arterial Tourniquet™ (CAT) can be used in the pre-hospital and in-hospital environments to rapidly arrest life-threatening haemorrhages, particularly in limb trauma. Even though there are some complications of tourniquet application (discussed below), these are not relevant when life-threatening external haemorrhage is evident.

A cuff tourniquet is applied using a sphygmomanometer cuff inflated to 250 mmHg or 300 mmHg or 70–100 mmHg above the systolic pressure, to stop venous and arterial bleeding without crushing underlying tissues (Fig. 16.46).

Direct damage to underlying vessels and nerves and limb ischaemia remain the risks of tourniquet application. Limiting the time a tourniquet is applied and avoiding excessive pressures will reduce the risks.

Tourniquets can be used on arms and legs for haemorrhage control and facilitating a bloodless field for wound care.

FIGURE 16.46 HAEMORRHAGE CONTROL

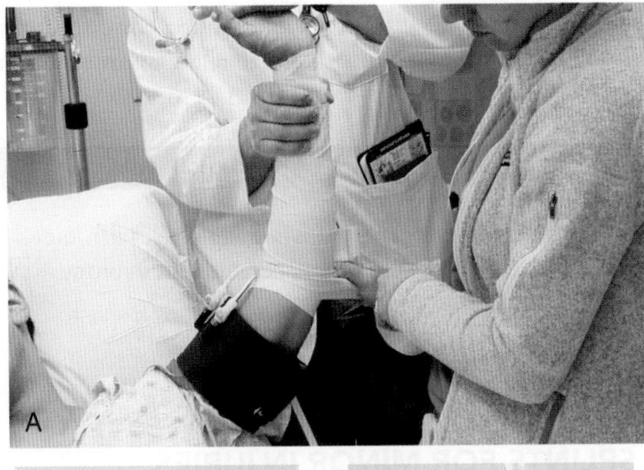

B

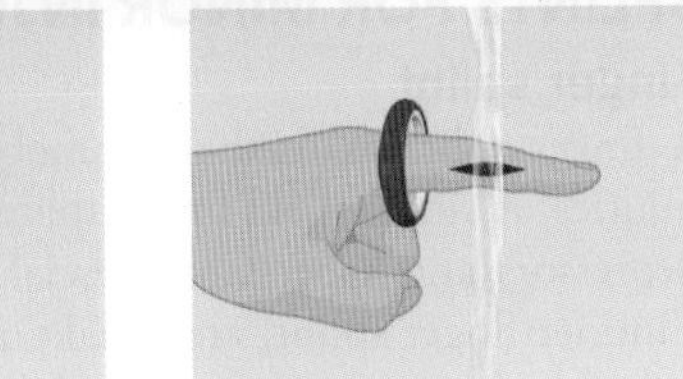

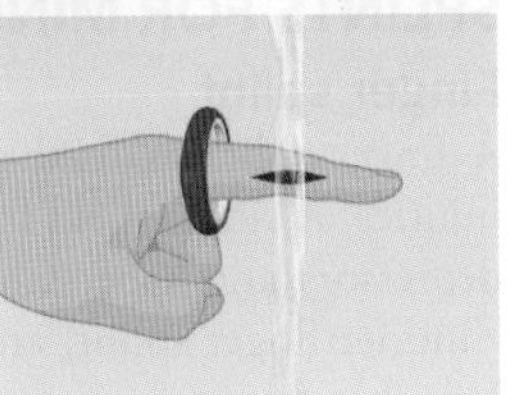

CLEAN
• Rinse thoroughly
• Examine wound
• Dry with gauze

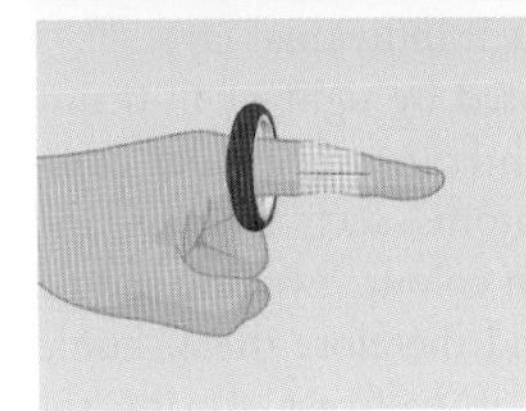

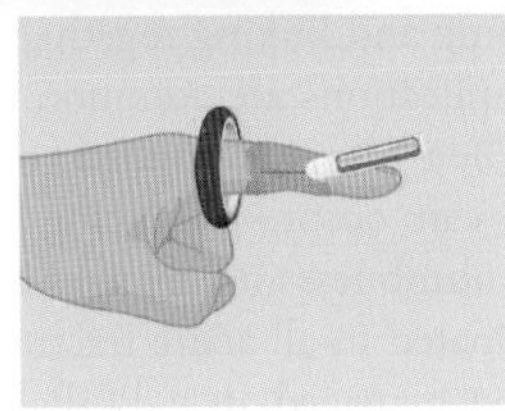

SEAL
• Use a topical skin adhesive to completely coat T-Strip
• REMOVE T-RING
• Apply non-adhesive bandage

A. Haemorrhage control: use of tourniquets.[103] **B, C.** The T-RING™ digit tourniquet immediately stops bleeding on any size digit, and avoids the risks associated with other methods. B, C, *Courtesy of Precision Medical Devices, LLC, www.thetring.com.*

Because of the risk of nerve and vessel injury, tourniquet use should be limited to 1 hour,[104] and conversion to PIB considered.[105] There is no evidence that tourniquet use plays a role in the treatment of envenomation.[99]

Life-threatening haemorrhage will not occur from a finger or toe wound. A simple pressure dressing and elevation will achieve haemostasis. A tourniquet on a digit will then only be needed to create a bloodless field for wound care. Traditional methods of tourniquet application to digits (e.g. surgical glove, Penrose drain tubing, Tourni-Cot™) have all been found to exceed the pressure required for digital haemostasis, and so dramatically increasing the risk of neurovascular injury, These potential injuries can be devastating for the patient. The T-Ring™ tourniquet is now used to replace these other methods. It is a one-size-fits-all tourniquet, which applies even pressure to any digit, creating the required bloodless field with minimal pressure.

PRACTICE TIP

Record the time of application of a torniquet.

CASTS

Plaster of Paris (POP) is still widely used as a splint. Casts are used for three main reasons: to relieve pain, to stabilise a fracture and to immobilise a fracture to promote healing.[106,107] Plaster splinting is performed in the pre-hospital setting by some extended care paramedic services.

Analgesia is essential in the reduction of fractures and the application of a POP cast. Reduction of fractures should only be performed by a trained clinician. A regional block provides good anaesthesia to the limb and can be used safely in the ED and there is some evidence of their utility in pre-hospital care.[107]

When applying POP, first apply wadding from the distal end to the proximal end of the limb, ensuring that padding extends beyond the planned margins of the cast. To prepare the POP roll, water must be added, which causes a chemical reaction that releases heat. Patients should be warned that they might feel heat on application. Place the plaster roll in a bowl of water (the colder the water, the longer the plaster takes to set). Squeeze out excess water by squeezing the ends together. The POP bandage should be rolled in the same direction as the wadding, overlapping at each turn. Each roll should be smoothed by the palms. The strength of the cast relies on the overlapping and linking together of each individual layer.[107]

Complications are commonly caused by tight or ill-fitting casts. When casts are applied too tightly, neurovascular compromise can occur, producing symptoms such as pins and needles, numbness and changes in skin colour. Swelling should be anticipated in all acute fractures and therefore these should always be managed in a POP backslab/half-cast, during the acute phase. These can be reinforced during the sub-acute phase to improve strength of the cast for the long term but should not be removed and changed to a full cast as the reduction will be lost.

Pressure sores can develop from ill-fitting casts; common sites for increased pressure include bony prominences such as the patella, elbow, head of the ulna and the heel. Padding all bony prominences prior to POP application may prevent these pressure sores. Once swelling has subsided the patient may complain that the cast is too loose; in such cases, the cast should be replaced.[106,107]

Advanced practice emergency nurses and, in some Australian states and territories and Aotearoa New Zealand, extended care paramedics should be able to apply backslabs and full casts after education and assessment. The emergency nurse or paramedic must explain to the patient the purpose of the cast, the margins of the cast, the process and equipment used and the need to maintain correct alignment of specific joints during application. Neurovascular observations are essential for at least the first 4 hours after POP application. The clinician must educate the patient regarding warning signs and cast care. The patient should be made aware that the POP cast is not waterproof, and they should be alerted to symptoms of increased pain and swelling, and changes in skin colour and sensation; they should be instructed to seek medical attention immediately as this may indicate ischaemia. Some full POP casts take 24–48 hours to dry completely. The patient should not bear weight on the cast until it is completely dry.[108,109]

The application of a cast may seem a minor procedure; however, if the cast is ill-fitting, the fracture is not aligned or the assessment and care is inadequate, the patient may suffer significant complications, such as lifelong deformity or even amputation of the extremity.[110]

SPLINTING

Splinting plays an important role, in combination with bandaging, to ensure effective limb immobilisation. Early splinting and limb immobilisation can reduce pain and minimise the risk of further injury from bony fragments in fracture or neurovascular injury in sprain. Splinting is important in controlling blood loss and facilitates healing.[35] The basic splints include soft splints, hard splints, inflatable air splints and traction splints.[111]

PRACTICE TIP

- Pad all splints, particularly over the site of injury.
- Immobilise the joints above and below the injury.
- Gentle traction can be applied while fitting a splint.
- Assess neurovascular status before and after splinting.

SPLINTS FOR MINOR INJURIES

Finger splint

A finger splint is used to immobilise carpal and metacarpal injuries. A simple field finger splint can be made using tongue depressors and tape. Commercial finger splints, such as the Zimmer finger splint, are usually made from padded aluminium that can be conformed to the required shape.

To fit an aluminium finger splint

1. Begin by ensuring that the skin is clean and dry and any wounds are covered.
2. Use the corresponding finger on the uninjured hand to measure and mould the splint to the desired shape and size.

CASE STUDY 3

Mr Andrews is an 18-year-old man who presents at 1600 hours following a trip and fall at touch football. He has no medical history. He describes an inversion of the right ankle while running and turning at speed.

He has pain to the right ankle with some localised swelling. His toes are warm with a 2-second capillary return. He has impaired motor function due to moderate pain. He looks unsettled while sitting.

An x-ray reveals a fracture of the right distal tibia and fibula.

QUESTIONS

1. Describe the initial assessment of Mr Andrews.
2. What are the options for initial management of the injury?
3. What are the risks and benefits of different types of immobilisation splints for ankle injuries?

Answers to Case Study Questions can be found on evolve **http://evolve.elsevier.com/AU/Curtis/emergency/**

3. Slide the splint in place on the injured finger.
4. Secure the splint in place with tape.
5. Check for capillary refill to ensure adequate blood flow.
6. Apply ice pack to the hand.

Knee immobiliser

A knee immobiliser (Fig. 16.47) or Zimmer™ knee splint is a three-panelled soft splint with fibreglass or aluminium inserts. They are used in mild to moderate knee injuries that don't require complete knee immobilisation, such as ligament or soft-tissue injuries.[112]

To fit a knee immobiliser

1. Begin by ensuring that the skin is clean and dry and any wounds are covered.
2. Check for distal pulse to ensure adequate blood flow.
3. Administer adequate analgesia where possible.
4. Select the correct size of immobiliser by laying it next to the leg. The proximal end should be just below the buttocks crease and the tapered distal end should be just above the ankle.

FIGURE 16.47 KNEE IMMOBILISER[112]

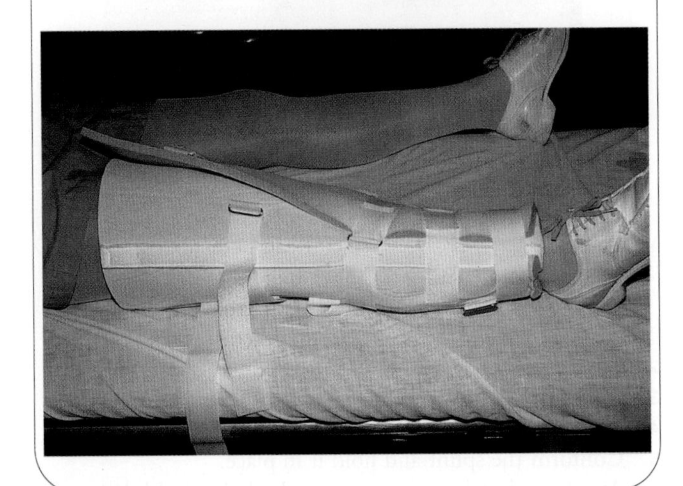

Can be worn over clothes and be easily removed and applied by the patient.

5. Place the splint behind the leg. Align the splint so that when closed, the patella sits within the patella opening.
6. Adjust the two side panels so that when they are closed on the leg, they touch the midline.
7. Close the Velcro straps from bottom to top.
8. Check for distal pulse to ensure adequate blood flow.

SPLINTS FOR MAJOR INJURIES/TRAUMA

Femoral traction splint

Femoral traction splints apply traction to the femur to reduce blood loss and relieve pain.[102] The splints are generally divided into two categories: ring splints, which include Donway, Hare (Fig. 16.48) and Thomas; and non-ring splints, which include Sager, Kendrick Traction Device, Faretec CT-6 (Fig. 16.49) and the Slishman splint.

Instructions on fitting each brand of splint is outside the scope of this chapter and can be accessed from the manufacturer's guiding literature and local health service policies.

Principles of traction splint application

1. Begin by ensuring that the skin is clean and dry and any wounds are covered.
2. Check for distal pulses to ensure adequate blood flow.
3. Administer adequate analgesia.
4. Place the ischial pad against the iliac crest.
5. Adjust the splint so that the bend is in line with the heel and tighten the locking collars.
6. Fit the proximal ring or loop on the splint to the ischial tuberosity on the affected leg. This will apply counter-traction.
7. Apply the pubic strap over the groin and high on the femur.
8. Apply the ankle strap. This will apply longitudinal traction.
9. Apply traction until the legs are approximately the same length.
10. Check for distal pulses and/or perfusion regularly to ensure adequate blood flow.
11. Be aware that regular analgesia will likely be required.

Vacuum splints

Vacuum splints such as the Evac-U-Splint® can be used to splint all limb fractures. They are applied to the affected limb and air is evacuated so the splint conforms around the fracture (Fig. 16.50).

FIGURE 16.48 HARE TRACTION SPLINT[103]

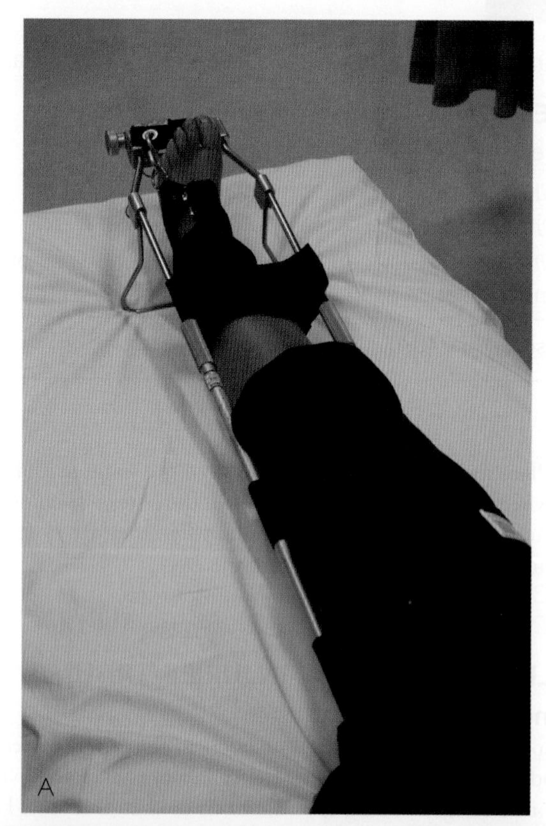

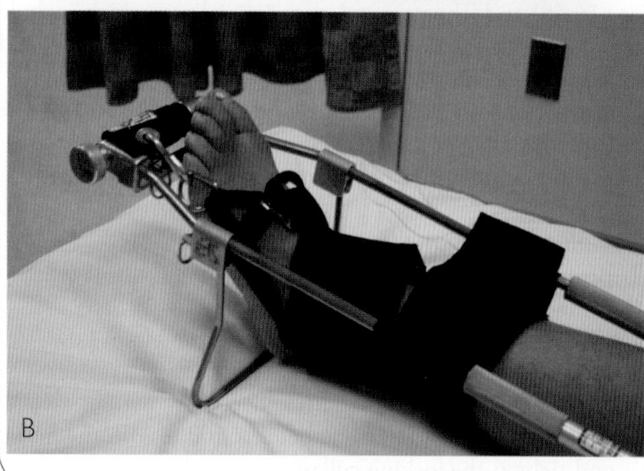

A. Hare traction splint. **B.** Commercial hitch designed to protect the ankle and heel during traction.

FIGURE 16.49 FARETEC CT-6 TRACTION SPLINT

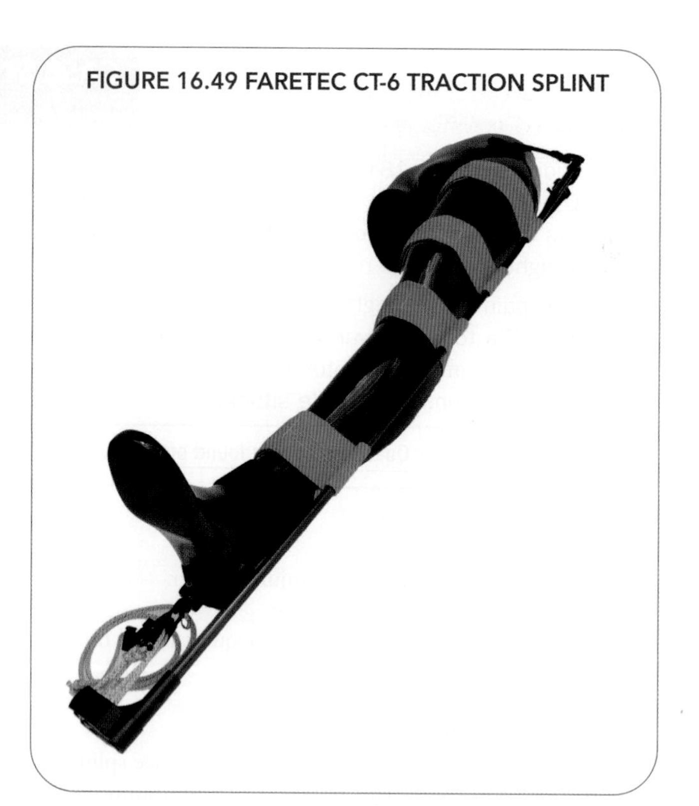

Courtesy of FareTec Inc., www.FareTec.com.

FIGURE 16.50 UPPER EXTREMITY VACUUM SPLINT[103]

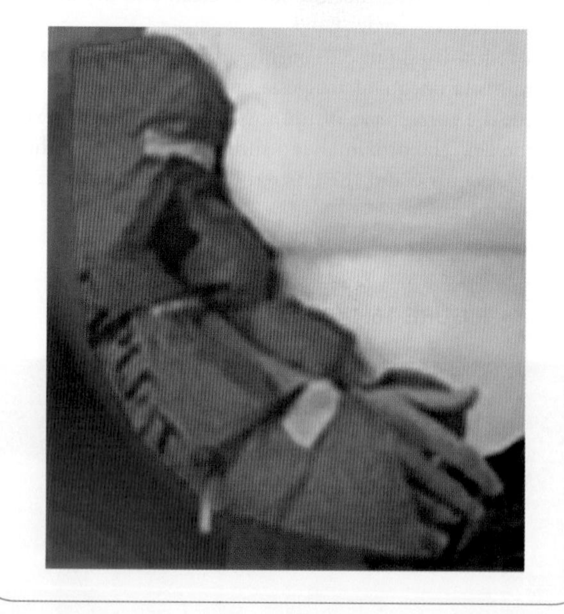

Whole-body vacuum splint mattresses are used to immobilise and transport patients with suspected spinal injuries.

Vacuum splints have the advantage of being able to conform to the exact shape of the wearer. They are much more bulky than other types of splint, require a pump to evacuate air and there may be changes in the conformity in altitude retrieval, requiring adjustment. Vacuum splints are available in multiple sizes and they do not apply any traction to fractures.

Fitting an Evac-U-Splint®

1. Begin by ensuring that the skin is clean and dry and any wounds are covered.
2. Check for distal pulse to ensure adequate blood flow.
3. Administer adequate analgesia where possible.
4. Slide the splint into place.
5. Conform the splint and hold it in place.
6. Attach the hand pump and evacuate the air from the splint.
7. Secure any straps.
8. Check for distal pulse to ensure adequate blood flow.

Pelvic splint

The purpose of a pelvic splint is to reduce the pelvic volume, which in turn reduces potential space for bleeding that may aid in the formation of blood clots. Aligning fracture surfaces may reduce bleeding from bones. Attention is then given to stabilisation of the pelvis by initially using a sheet or a commercially available pelvic binder such as a SAM® Pelvic Sling II or T-POD splint (Fig. 16.51).

PRACTICE TIP

Correct fitting at the level of the greater trochanters is essential. Pelvic splints are commonly misplaced, usually too high, at the level of the iliac crests. Such misplacement is not only ineffective in minimising internal haemorrhage but can cause significant discomfort to the patient.

FIGURE 16.51 APPLICATION OF THE SAM PELVIC SLING[103]

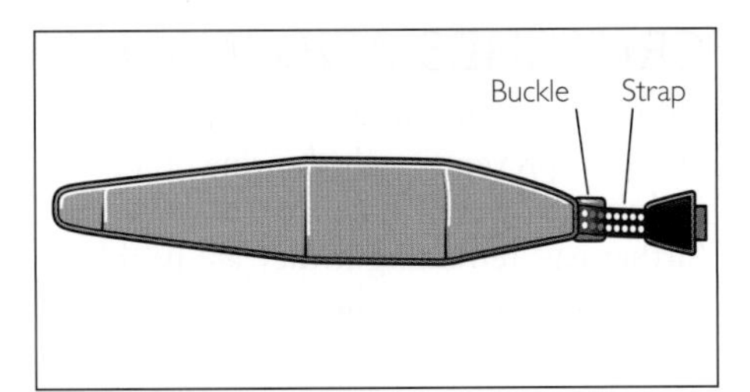

1. Remove objects from patient's pocket or pelvic area. Unfold SAM Pelvic Sling with non-printed side facing up. Keep strap attached to buckle.

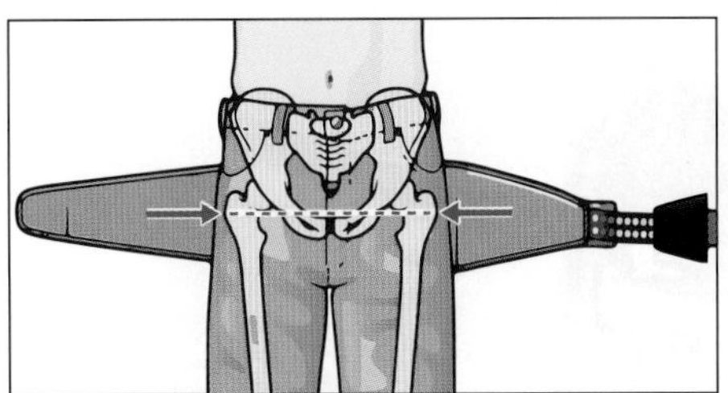

2. Place non-printed side of SAM Pelvic Sling beneath patient at level of buttocks (greater trochanters).
CORRECT PLACEMENT. The correct level of application is at the greater trochanters.

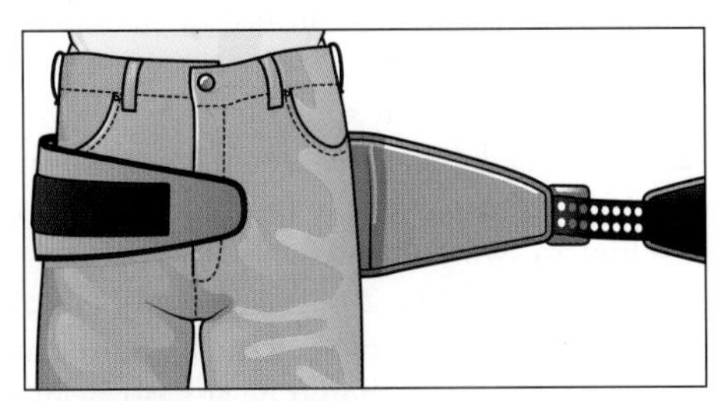

3. Wrap non-buckle side of SAM Pelvic Sling around patient.

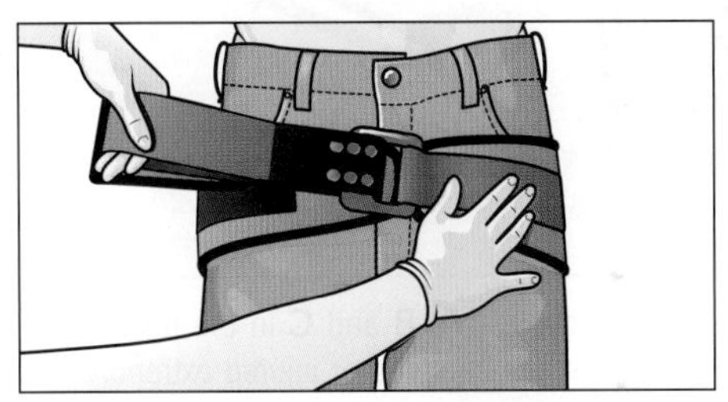

4. FIRMLY WRAP buckle side of sling around patient, positioning buckle in midline. Secure by pressing flap to sling.

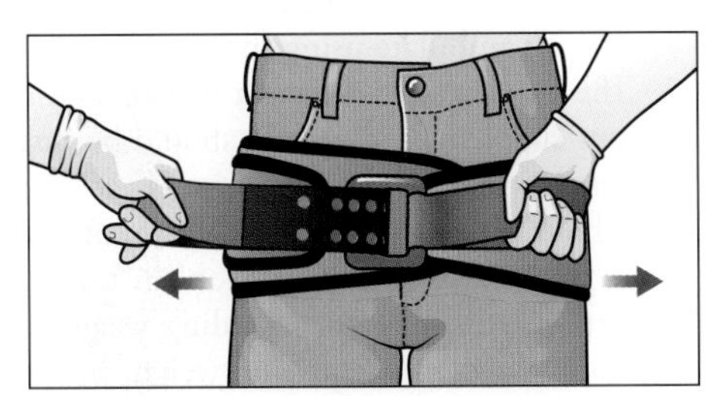

5. Lift the BLACK STRAP away from sling by pulling upwards.

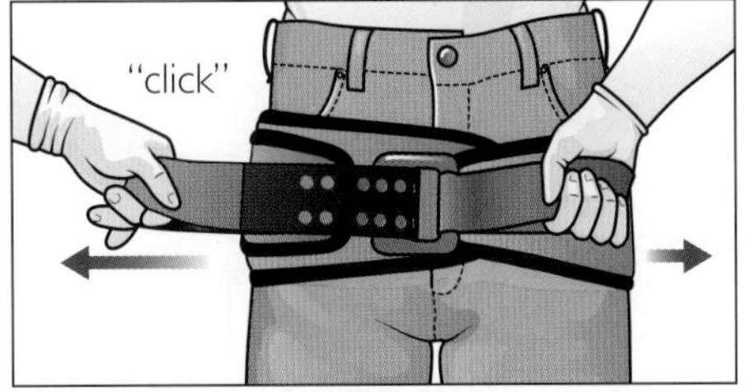

6. With or without assistance, firmly pull orange and black straps in opposite directions until you hear and feel the buckle click.
MAINTAIN TENSION!

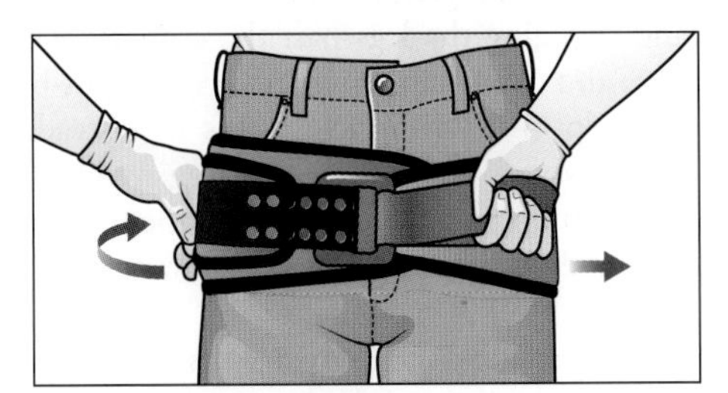

7. IMMEDIATELY press black strap onto surface of SAM Pelvic Sling to secure.
Note: do not be concerned if you hear a second 'click' after sling is secured.

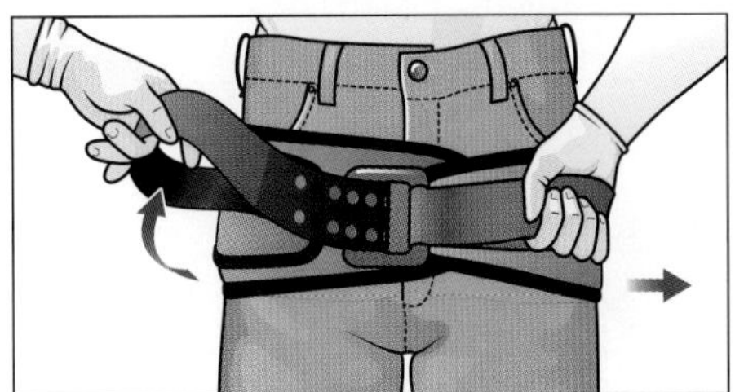

8. To remove, lift black strap by pulling upwards. Maintain tension and slowly allow SAM Pelvic Sling to loosen.

Rigid limb splint

The purpose of a fixed or rigid splint is to prevent the movement of fractured bones, which can cause bleeding and pain. Rigid splints can be made from a variety of materials, including cardboard, aluminium or wood; some come pre-padded (Figs 16.52 and 16.53).

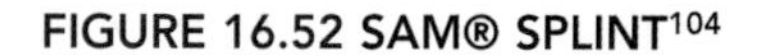

FIGURE 16.52 SAM® SPLINT[104]

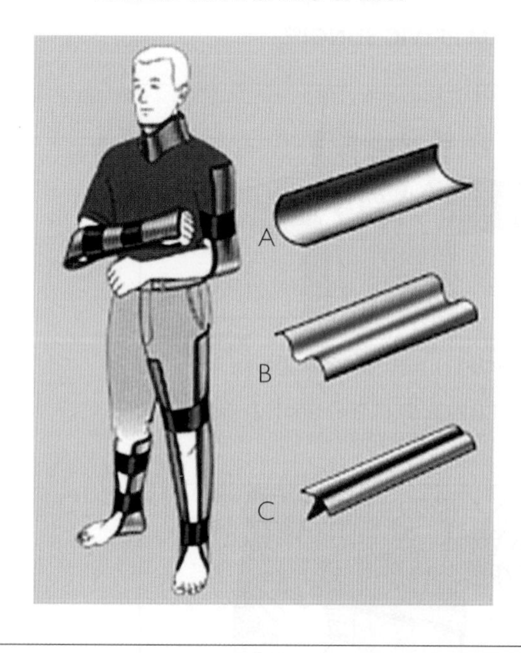

Bent into any of three simple curves (**A**, **B** and **C** in the figure), the SAM splint provides support for any fractured or injured extremity.

FIGURE 16.53 EXAMPLES OF RIGID SPLINTS[103]

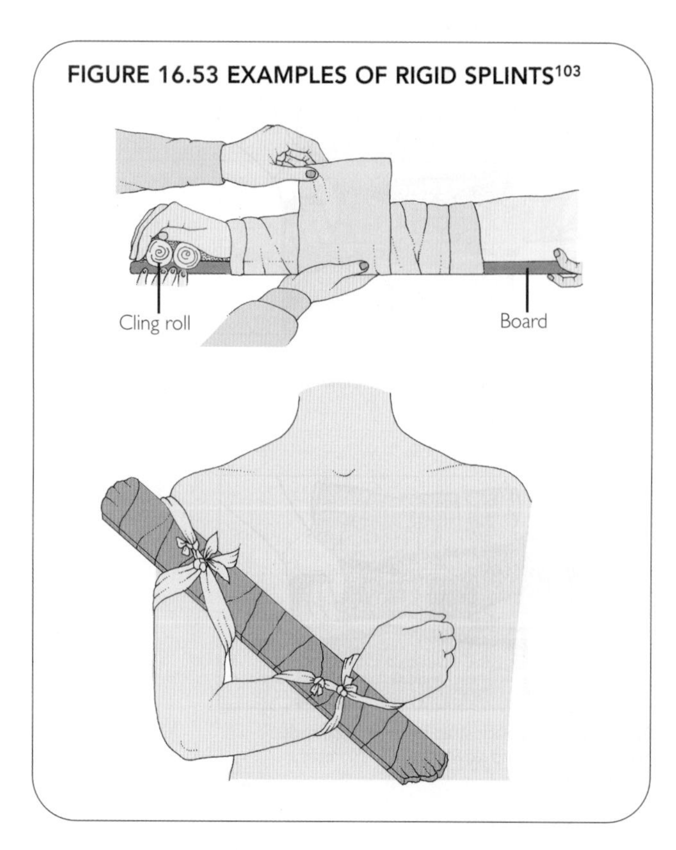

To fit:

1. Begin by ensuring that the skin is clean and dry and any wounds are covered.
2. Check for distal pulse to ensure adequate blood flow.
3. Administer adequate analgesia where possible.
4. Apply gentle traction to deformed and neurovascularly compromised limbs.
5. Apply the rigid splint with additional padding where required.
6. Fix the splint with bandages or tape.
7. Check for distal pulse to ensure adequate blood flow.

CRUTCHES AND WALKING STICKS

Crutches are used to aid walking where there is a lower limb injury, to prevent weight-bearing on the injured leg or to aid in mobility; however, note that patients should be admitted for further gait retraining if they are unable to use them safely or are at risk of falling. The most common type of crutch used in emergency injury is the underarm or axilla crutch.

UNDERARM CRUTCHES

Underarm crutches are the most common type of crutches. They sit under the axilla and are also called axillary crutches.[113] The appropriate height of axillary crutches can be measured with the patient lying supine in bed or standing. To fit (instructions given for standing):

1. Stand the patient straight.
2. Place the base of the crutch 15 cm to the side of and 15 cm in front of the foot. This will allow room for the hips to swing through.
3. There should be 2–3 fingers' width, or about 5 cm, between the top of the crutch and the armpit.
4. The hand piece should be at wrist height allowing the elbow to bend at 30°. This is called the tripod position and provides the most stability.
5. The patient should be provided with information about how to ambulate using the crutches (Fig. 16.54).

The patient should have a pair of well-fitting, flat shoes to prevent slipping. The patient should be instructed not to bear weight through the axilla, as this may cause axillary nerve palsy; they should instead use their hands to support their bodyweight. There should be clear instructions in the medical records from the orthopaedic surgeon regarding weight-bearing status prior to mobilisation, such as non-weight-bearing (NWB), partial weight-bearing (PWB), touch weight-bearing (TWB) or full weight-bearing/weight-bear as tolerated (FWB/WBAT).

The usual gait that is taught to patients who are NWB is the swing-through gait; this involves moving the crutches forwards and swinging the legs past the crutches, before regaining balance and continuing forwards. For weight-bearing patients, use the step-to or swing-to gait, as it is steadier: step up to the crutches with injured leg, putting weight through the hands, and step up to the crutches with the uninjured leg.

Patients should be taught how to go up and down stairs (Fig. 16.55).

When mobilising down stairs, the patient should place the crutches down onto the lower step, followed by the uninjured limb and then the injured limb. This ensures that the patient's stronger limb is used to lower bodyweight onto the lower step and enables the crutches to support the injured limb.

FIGURE 16.54 THREE-POINT GAIT

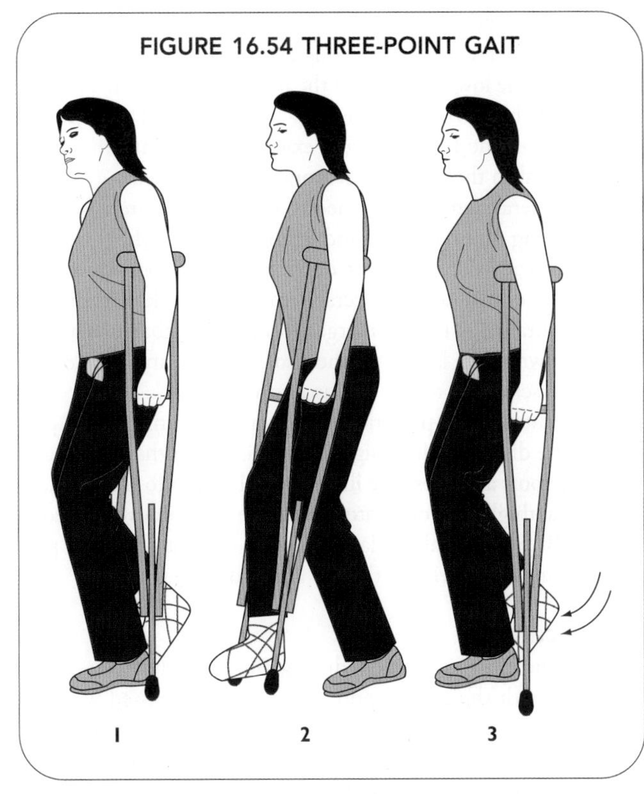

1. Standing with crutches, all weight is on the good leg. **2.** Move crutches and injured leg forward simultaneously. **3.** Bearing weight on the palms of the hands, step forward onto the good leg.

FIGURE 16.55 USING CRUTCHES ON STAIRS

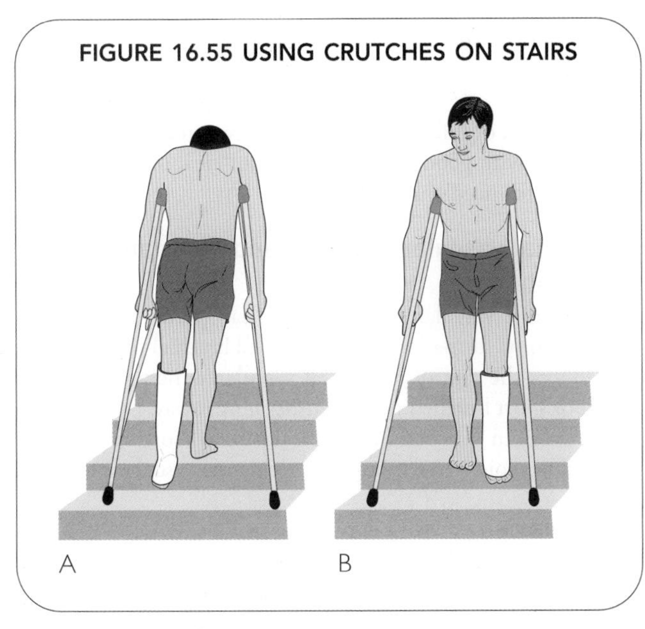

A. Going up stairs. **B.** Going down stairs.

When mobilising up stairs, the patient places the uninjured limb onto the upper step, pushes through the crutches to raise the injured limb up onto the same step, followed by the crutches.

The patient should always have a 'support' person with them in the initial stages when going up and down stairs.

PRACTICE TIP

Crutches are rarely used for older patients because of the risk of brachial plexus injury. There is also an increased risk of falls when used by someone with impaired cognitive function or in patients with insufficient arm and shoulder strength.

FOREARM CRUTCHES

Forearm crutches are used to prevent compressive radial neuropathy caused by excessive underarm pressure rarely caused by axillary crutches. They have a forearm and hand piece but provide less support and require a greater level of skill to use.[113] They are more commonly used in patients requiring long-term crutches or where partial weight-bearing is allowed. To fit:

1. Stand the patient straight.
2. Fit the forearm piece 2.5 cm below the elbow crease. The forearm piece should be firm-fitting enough to prevent the crutch from falling when the wearer opens a door.
3. The hand piece should be at wrist height allowing the elbow to bend at 30°.
4. The patient should be provided with information about how to ambulate using the crutches.

WALKING STICKS

A walking stick is used to assist with balance where weight-bearing on the affected leg is still possible. To fit:

1. Stand the patient straight.
2. Place the base of the walking stick next to the heel.
3. The handpiece of the walking stick should be at wrist height allowing the elbow to bend at 30°.
4. A walking stick should be used on the side opposite to the injury. The patient is provided with information about how to ambulate using a walking stick.

REGIONAL ANAESTHESIA AND NERVE BLOCKS

Regional anaesthesia and regional nerve blocks are simple, convenient and provide effective pain relief for patients in the ED.

Regional nerve blocks may prove superior to local anaesthetic infiltration or systemic delivery of analgesia in providing pain relief in specific scenarios in the emergency care. Emergency clinicians should be aware of the indications for using regional nerve blocks. Advanced practice emergency clinicians, including paramedics, may be able to perform these procedures after appropriate education and assessment.[114] Scenarios in which regional nerve blocks may be appropriate include:

- reduction of pain to digits during procedures, e.g. reduction of dislocations or fractures, repair of wounds
- procedures such as wound repair or foreign body removal in areas where local infiltration is particularly painful, such as the plantar surface of the foot or the palm of the hand
- for manipulation/reduction of fractures, e.g. a Colles' fracture
- to reduce the need for systemic analgesia and improve pain relief in the elderly with a fractured femur.

NERVE BLOCK IN HIP FRACTURE

A particular consideration is analgesia in hip fracture and older patients. Pain management for this vulnerable group of patients is particularly challenging.[115] Multiple comorbidities, polypharmacy and altered pharmacokinetics can limit the range of suitable analgesics. Furthermore, anecdotal evidence from emergency clinicians suggests that time in cannulating, performing frequent observation of blood pressure, drawing-up and administering (in the presence of two nurses) aliquots of intravenous (IV) opioids is a boundary to treatment. An alarming overseas study[116] showed some patients with hip fracture were receiving no analgesia.

A proportion of older hip fracture patients have cognitive impairment from dementia. Some may suffer acute confusion from comorbidities, their injury or because of admission into hospital. This cognitive impairment may prevent them from asking for, or accepting, analgesia.[117]

Older patients often have preconceived ideas about the addictive properties of opioids. Staff may also have misconceptions regarding pain perception and ageing. Together, this can contribute to inadequate prescribing or administration of pain relief in older adults.[118]

Several studies support the use of femoral nerve anaesthesia in emergency situations, for effective pain relief following hip fractures.[114,119,120]

Femoral and fascia iliaca nerve block can provide rapid and effective analgesia for most patients, with a reduction in opioid consumption when compared with controls.[121–123] The result is faster, longer lasting pain relief without the associated side-effects of opioids. Undesirable opioid side-effects can include sedation and respiratory depression. The Australian National Health and Medical Research Council (NHMRC) recommends the use of regional anaesthetics as a standard of care when used in conjunction with oral and parenteral analgesia.

PRACTICE TIP

Femoral and fascia iliaca blocks provide rapid and effective pain relief for patients with hip fractures. A nerve block should be considered in all hip fracture patients.

ANATOMY OF THE FASCIA ILIACA BLOCK

The nerve supply that causes pain as a result of a hip or proximal femur fracture passes through the fascia iliaca compartment. Inserting a local anaesthetic into this space can effectively anaesthetise these nerves and provide up to 12 hours of pain relief.[124] The iliacus muscle is a large, flat, triangular muscle that lines and fills the ilium. It originates from all along the upper portions of the ilium and iliac crest, sacrum and iliolumbar ligaments.[125] The iliacus muscle joins with the lateral side of the psoas major muscle. Together they are referred to as the iliopsoas. The iliopsoas exits the pelvis from beneath the inguinal ligament, wraps around the proximal neck and inserts into the lesser trochanter, acting as a powerful hip flexor.

The fascial covering of the iliopsoas is thin superiorly, becoming significantly thicker as it reaches the level of the inguinal ligament. This thickness provides a great deal of resistance and a large 'pop' as a needle tip is passed through the fascia.

The lumbar plexus is made up of the nerve roots from the T12 through L5 vertebrae. The largest branch of the lumbar plexus is the femoral nerve, arising from the L2, L3 and L4 roots. The femoral nerve descends through the fibres of the psoas major and exits at the lower portion of the psoas's lateral border, passing downwards between the psoas and iliacus muscle, deep to the iliacus fascia. The femoral nerve exits the pelvis into the upper thigh, lateral to the common femoral artery and vein.

The lateral femoral cutaneous nerve is a purely sensory nerve arising from the L2 and L3 nerve roots that provides sensation from the iliac crest down the lateral portion of the thigh to the area of the lateral femoral condyle. The lateral femoral cutaneous nerve emerges from the lumbar plexus and travels downwards lateral to the psoas muscle and crosses the iliacus muscle deep to the iliacus fascia.

The anterior and posterior obturator nerves innervate a portion of the distal, medial thigh. They arise from the L2, L3 and L4 nerve roots and cross the iliacus muscle, deep to the fascia, to the medial thigh. The obturator nerves are sometimes involved in the FICB, but probably play little role in post-operative pain relief for most surgeries of the hip and proximal femur.

Complications

All complications identified during the procedure should be discussed with the patient and their family, discussed with the treating clinicians and documented in the patient record.

Potential complications include inadvertent intravascular injection, haematoma and nerve injury. Complications relating to the local anaesthetic include hypotension and toxicity. Motor block of the affected limb is common.

Block failure

There is a potential that the nerve block will only be partially successful or unsuccessful in relieving pain.

Infection

There is a risk of infection with all invasive procedures that can be reduced with good handwashing, skin-cleaning and a sterile technique for needle insertion.

Accidental vascular puncture and haematoma formation

An accidental vascular (venous or arterial) puncture can result in haematoma formation. A blunt-ended brachial plexus needle set reduces the risk of accidental vascular puncture. A blunt-ended or short bevelled needle pushes fibres away. Needles such as the B Braun Brachial Plexus Plexufix 45° short bevel needle are used to avoid nerve injury and accidental vascular puncture.

Anaphylaxis

Anaphylaxis remains an unavoidable complication of any medication administration. Airway management, oxygenation, ventilation and good basic life support are the necessity of successful resuscitation.

Local anaesthetic systemic toxicity (LAST)

LAST remains an unavoidable complication of regional anaesthesia administration. LAST can result from intravascular injection, absorption from a tissue depot, accumulation of active metabolites, or a combination of these. Attentiveness during the procedure and timely intervention at the earliest signs of toxicity are most important for successful treatment.

The classic description of LAST includes a series of progressively worsening neurological symptoms and signs occurring shortly after the injection of local anaesthetic and mirroring a progressive increase in blood local anaesthetic concentration, climaxing in seizures and coma. In severe cases of LAST, hypotension, bradycardia, confusion, dizziness, agitation, loss of consciousness, followed by seizure, ventricular dysrhythmia or asystole, can occur. Systemic toxic reactions occur in only 0.1% to 0.4% of local anaesthetic administrations. Vagal reactions, anxiety and sensitivity to preservatives have also been incorrectly attributed to LAST.[103]

LAST is usually very rapid, following a single injection by 50 seconds or less, and occurring before 5 minutes in 75% of cases. Peak blood levels are usually within 30 minutes.[103] Rapid onset of symptoms after a single local anaesthetic injection suggests that most systemic toxic reactions are because of inadvertent intravascular injection.

Patients with liver disease may not be able to adequately metabolise local anaesthetics such as bupivacaine for excretion, increasing the risk for toxic plasma concentrations. Additionally, patients with cardiovascular disease may not be able to compensate for the functional changes associated with the prolongation of atrioventricular conduction induced by amide-type local anaesthetics.

Adverse reactions to ropivacaine are rare in the absence of overdosage, exceptionally rapid absorption or inadvertent intravascular injection.

PRACTICE TIP

The rapid injection of a large volume of local anaesthetic solution should be avoided. Always calculate a weight-based dose and consider comorbidities that might lead to systemic toxicity.

MIMS Online[126] states:

> Injection of repeated doses of local anaesthetic may cause significant increase in blood levels with each repeated dose, due to accumulation of the drug or its metabolites, or due to slow metabolic degradation.

Airway management, oxygenation, ventilation and good basic life support are the necessity of successful resuscitation. Seizure suppression is important. Lipid infusion should be considered early, and most EDs have the capability to perform rapid lipid infusion. Literature suggests 'Vigilance, preparedness, and quick action will improve outcomes of this dreaded complication'.[127]

Procedure for femoral and fascia iliaca block

1. Review the x-ray to confirm hip fracture after discussion with the treating clinicians.
2. Consult the relevant medical officer before nerve block to ensure that:
   - a nerve block is required
   - alternatives have been considered
   - the benefits outweigh the risks.
3. Check for allergies to any of the cleaning solutions or anaesthetics used.
4. Identify any transmission-based precautions such as multi-resistant organisms (MRO), so that appropriate precautions can be taken.
5. Identify comorbidities that may pose a problem with the procedure or the anaesthetic, including partial or complete heart block, advanced liver disease or severe renal dysfunction.
6. Discuss the procedure with the patient and their family/carers, outlining the steps involved, the benefits and the potential complications and risks. Treatment and care, and the information patients are given about it, should be culturally appropriate. It should also be accessible to people with additional needs such as physical, sensory or learning disabilities, and to people who do not speak or read English; use an interpreter if required.
7. Obtain verbal or written consent from the patient or their family/carers. Absolute contraindications to the procedure include:
   - infection or haematoma in the vicinity of the puncture site
   - refusal of the procedure by the patient.
8. View the baseline observations.
9. Estimate the patient's weight for drug dose calculation. Calculate the drug dose and volume required. Estimation of weight is required if the patient is unable to provide a recent accurate weight, remembering the patient will not be able to sit or stand to be weighed.
10. Ropivacaine is the anaesthetic of choice due to its reduced cardiac toxicity profile over other local anaesthetic agents.[128] The dose is calculated dependent on the patient's weight. Generally, 0.375% concentration is used to anaesthetise nerves in the fascia iliaca compartment.[129]
    - Ropivacaine preparations come in various concentrations and, as such, should be diluted as per local guidelines.
    - Debilitated or older patients, including those with partial or complete heart block, advanced liver disease or severe renal dysfunction, should be given a reduced dosage commensurate with their physical condition and according to their estimated weight.
11. Collect and open onto a dressing tray all equipment required (Box 16.12).
12. Expose the site without unnecessarily exposing the patient. The patient lies on his or her back with legs spread slightly apart. Clean the skin with neutral soap and water if the insertion site is visibly dirty. Infection in

BOX 16.12 EQUIPMENT COMMONLY USED FOR FASCIA ILIACA AND FEMORAL NERVE BLOCK INSERTION

- Ropivacaine stock solution
- 20 mL 0.9% saline for injection
- 20 mL syringe × 2
- Drawing-up needle
- Blunt-ended needle set
- Alcohol-based chlorhexidine gluconate swabs (0.5% chlorhexidine in 70% isopropyl alcohol) × 2
- Sterile gloves

the vicinity of the puncture site is a contraindication to the procedure.

13. Perform hand hygiene as set out in the Hand Hygiene Policy and identify the landmarks by palpating the anterior superior iliac crest and pubic tubercle. Feel for the femoral artery.
14. Mark the site/side of injury with an arrow denoting the affected hip.
15. Clinicians should wear protective eyewear when performing the procedure due to the low risk of a splash injury occurring.
16. No touch technique
    Touching the insertion site, the shaft or tip of the needle or other sterile equipment breaches aseptic technique. To follow aseptic technique, clinicians should avoid touching:
    - the insertion site after decontamination
    - sterile parts of the brachial plexus set
    - other sterile equipment.
17. Perform hand hygiene (see Chapter 27). Put on sterile gloves.
18. Draw up the calculated dose of anaesthetic agent with the drawing-up needle and attach the brachial plexus set.
19. Decontaminate the skin using a single-use swab. Apply antiseptic to cover an area of approximately 5 × 5 cm in a side-to-side or up-and-down motion with light friction. Repeat with a second swab and allow the skin to air-dry (do not wipe, fan or blot dry the area) for at least 1 minute.
    Alcohol-based chlorhexidine gluconate swabs (> 0.5% chlorhexidine in > 70% isopropyl alcohol) should be used.
    For patients with a history of chlorhexidine sensitivity/allergy, use:
    - 5% alcohol-based povidone-iodine swab
    - ≥ 70% alcohol
    - 10% aqueous povidone-iodine (suitable for patients in whom alcohol is contraindicated).
    Do not use antimicrobial creams/ointment at the insertion site.
    If the site or equipment is contaminated at any stage during the procedure discard it and start again.
20. Identify the landmarks of the anterior superior iliac crest and pubic tubercle. The foot of the leg to be anaesthetised should be turned loosely to the outside, although it may already be rotated due to fracture (Fig. 16.56).
21. The puncture site is located approximately in the region of the inguinal fold, 1.5 cm lateral of the femoral artery, approximately 2–3 cm below the inguinal ligament (IVAN = inner vein artery nerve) (Fig. 16.57).
22. Palpate the femoral artery. Insert the needle at 30 degrees to the skin and advance in a cranial direction. After reaching a depth of around 2–4 cm, the femoral nerve is encountered. Progress the needle downwards.
23. Feel for the 'pop' as the needle passes through the fascia lata and then again as the needle passes into the fascia iliaca.
24. Aspirate intermittently during insertion and injection of anaesthetic to reduce the risk of inadvertent arterial or venous infiltration (Fig. 16.58).

FIGURE 16.56 LANDMARKS FOR FEMORAL AND FASCIA ILIACA BLOCKS[130]

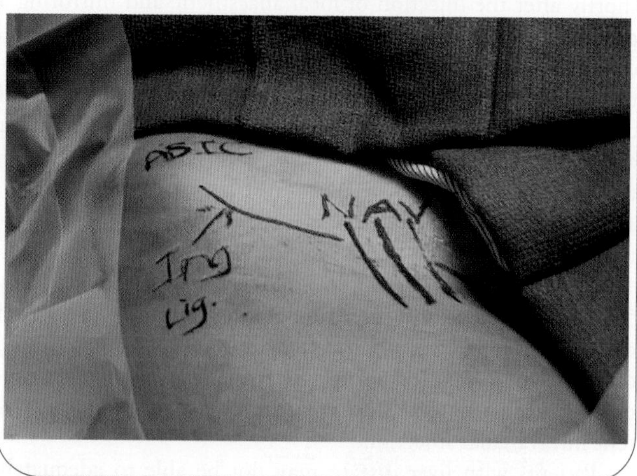

The drawing identifies the anterior superior iliac spine (ASIC), the inguinal ligament ('Ing lig'), and the approximate locations of the femoral nerve (N), femoral artery (A) and femoral vein (V). A good way to remember the relationships is 'NAVEL': going towards the navel, i.e., Nerve, Artery, Vein, Empty, Lymphatics, going from lateral to medial (towards the navel).

25. Slowly inject in 10–15 mL increments, withdrawing regularly to observe for vascular penetration. Advance the needle into the space created by the volume, and inject the anaesthetic slowly. Do not continue to inject if excessive resistance is felt or blood is returned in the needle on withdrawal (Fig. 16.59).
26. Aspirate intermittently during insertion and injection of anaesthetic to reduce the risk of inadvertent arterial or venous infiltration.
27. Remove the needle and dispose of all sharps.
28. Placing pressure over the injection site for 10 seconds after completing the injection may speed up the onset of the block by spreading the local solution with external pressure. This is also a common way of trying to enhance the block's effect. Place pressure below the puncture site to prevent the local anaesthetic from flowing in the distal direction and to promote its dissemination in the cranial direction.
29. Dispose of all sharps. Dispose of all contaminated waste. Cover the patient. Remove gloves and wash hands.
30. Evaluate the occurrence of complete loss of pinprick sensation in the femoral nerve distribution; a sign of nerve block effectiveness.
31. Record a pain score 1 hour after the procedure.
32. Watch for signs of complications. Adverse reactions to bupivacaine are rare in the absence of overdosage, exceptionally rapid absorption or inadvertent intravascular injection.
33. Document the procedure in the clinical record. Record or sign all local anaesthetic doses on the medication chart.
    NB: if this procedure is to be performed in the pre-hospital environment (most likely by advanced paramedics), the guideline of the relevant service/organisation should be followed.

FIGURE 16.57 ANATOMICAL RELATIONSHIPS OF THE INGUINAL LIGAMENT AND FEMORAL NERVE, ARTERY AND VEIN[131]

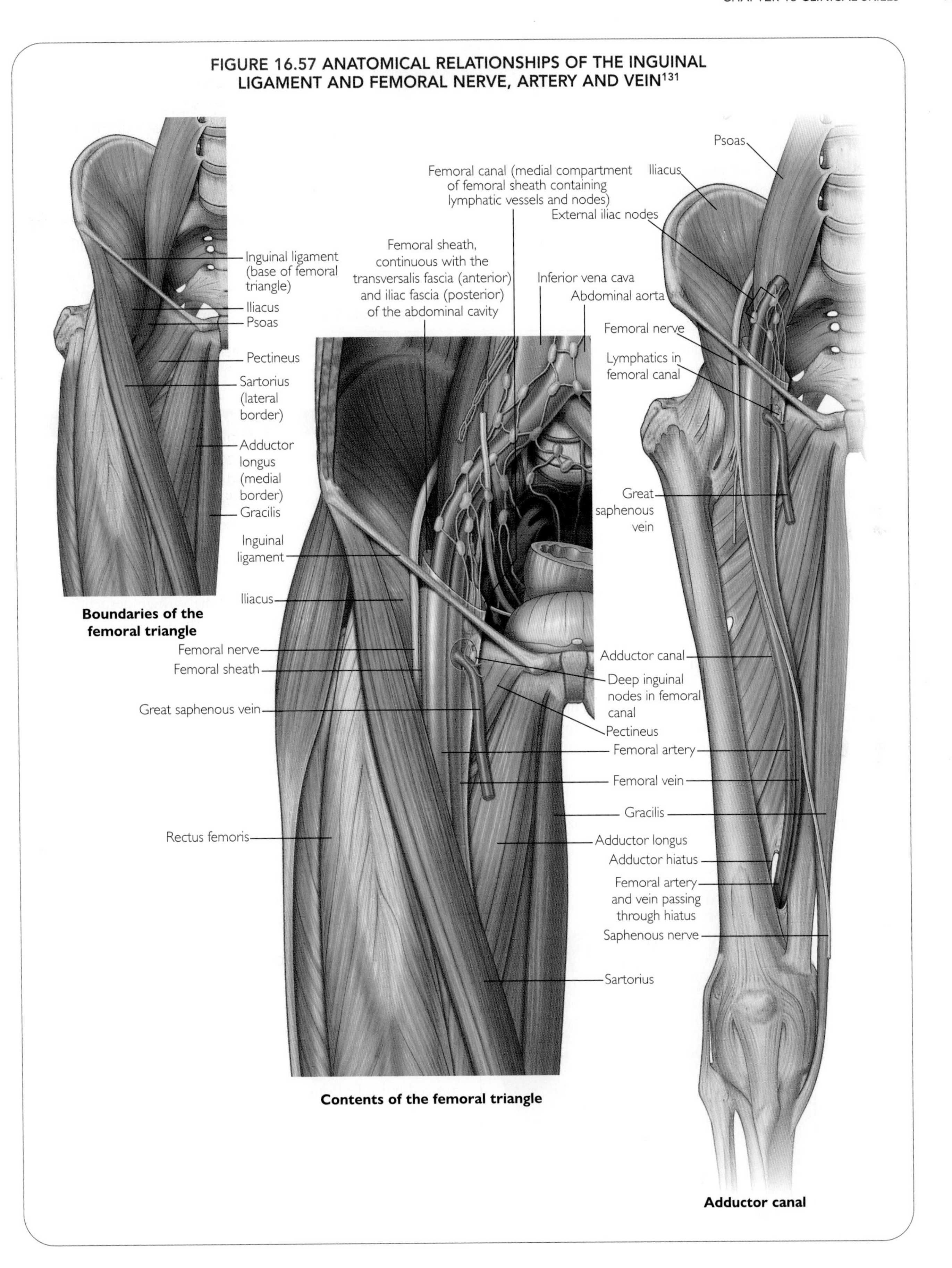

CASE STUDY 4

Mrs Lily is a 91-year-old woman who presents at 0800 hours following a trip and fall. She has an extensive medical history that includes ischaemic heart disease, dementia, osteoporosis and falls.

She has pain to the left hip with shortening of the leg and outward rotation of the foot. Her toes are cool with a 3-second capillary return. She has impaired motor function due to severe pain. She looks unsettled and is agitated in bed.

An x-ray reveals a fracture of the left neck of the femur.

QUESTIONS

1. Describe the initial assessment of Mrs Lily.
2. What are the options for management of Mrs Lily's pain?
3. What are the advantages and disadvantages of using intravenous opioids for pain relief?
4. What are the advantages and disadvantages of using regional anaesthesia for pain relief?

Answers to Case Study Questions can be found on evolve **http://evolve.elsevier.com/AU/Curtis/emergency/** 

DIGITAL NERVE BLOCK

Indications for using a digital nerve block include reduction of dislocations or fractures of phalanges, repair of injuries to nail-beds and nails, assessment and repair of wounds, including lacerations, burns and amputations and drainage of infections.[133]

Each finger is supplied by two sets of nerves—the dorsal and palmar digital nerves—and these run in a 2, 4, 8 and 10 o'clock position around the digit. There are a variety of approaches to blocking these nerves (Fig. 16.60).[134] The most common techniques are the transthecal (flexor tendon sheath) block and the webspace block. For both procedures, aseptic injection technique is used and the skin is prepped with alcohol preparation. The equipment required is minimal: alcohol wipes, examination gloves, local anaesthetic of choice, 5 mL syringe, drawing-up needle, 25 g needle. The onset and duration of anaesthesia to the digit is dependent on the choice of anaesthetic (Table 16.5).[135]

FIGURE 16.58 NEEDLE INSERTION[132]

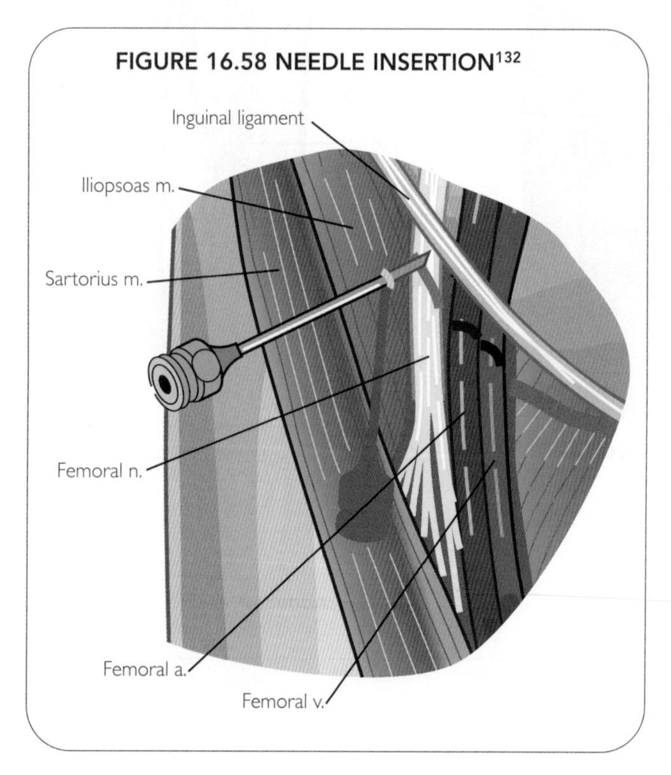

PRACTICE TIP

The clinicians involved in administration of regional nerve blocks must ensure a neurovascular assessment of the digit or limb has been performed prior to administration and regularly post-administration.

The webspace block requires the patient's hand to be palm down on a steady surface. Hold the syringe perpendicular to the digit and insert the needle into the webspace just distal to the metacarpalphalangeal joint. Slowly inject the anaesthetic into the dorsal aspect of the webspace while slowly advancing the needle towards the volar aspect of the hand, injecting 2–3 mL. Repeat on the opposite webspace.

The transthecal approach requires the patient's hand to be palm-up on a steady surface. Palpate just distal to the distal palmar crease over the head of the metacarpal to locate the flexor tendon; gently flex the finger, if required, to help locate the tendon. Insert the needle at a 45-degree angle aimed towards the finger and begin injecting. The anaesthetic should flow freely if the needle is in the potential space—if not, withdraw slightly and try injecting again. You should feel the flow of the local anaesthetic along the flexor surface of the proximal phalanx as you inject. Inject 2–3 mL.

Haematoma block for the reduction of distal radius fractures

A haematoma block is used to anaesthetise the wrist and manipulate deformed distal radius fractures (such as Colles' fracture) in emergency (Box 16.13). Haematoma blocks are a safe method of obtaining analgesia without increased post-procedural infections when compared to other regional blocks (Fig. 16.61).[116]

They are equally effective as conscious intravenous sedation in terms of both quality of fracture reduction and pain control before, during and after the procedure, but without the prolonged recovery time.

There is some evidence that haematoma blocks provide slightly inferior anaesthesia and reductions when compared to intravenous regional anaesthesia such as Bier Block, although they are quicker, easier and less resource intensive.[136] Adequate pain control will assist with adequate fracture reduction (Box 16.14).[137]

FIGURE 16.59 THE FEMORAL NERVE/'THREE-IN-ONE' BLOCK[133]

FEMORAL NERVE/'THREE-IN-ONE' BLOCK

Anatomy

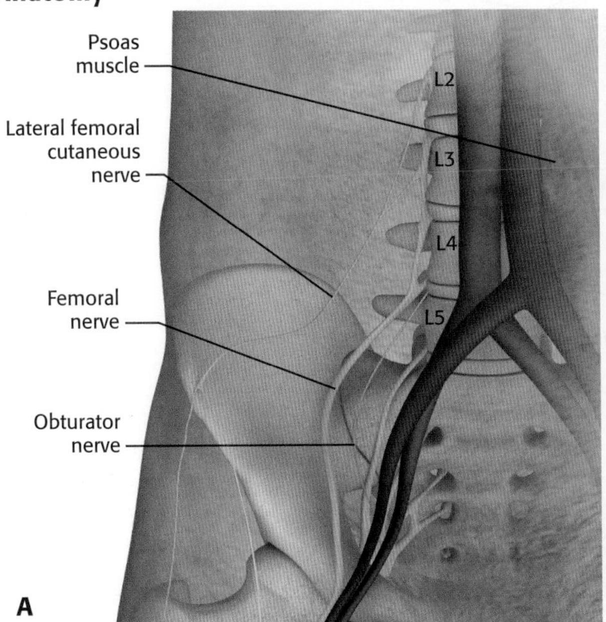

The lumbar plexus lies in the psoas compartment between the psoas major and quadratus lumborum muscles. The femoral nerve is formed from the posterior branches of L2–L4 and is the largest branch of the lumbar plexus. The lateral femoral cutaneous and obturator nerves arise from L2–L3 and L2–L4, respectively.

Technique

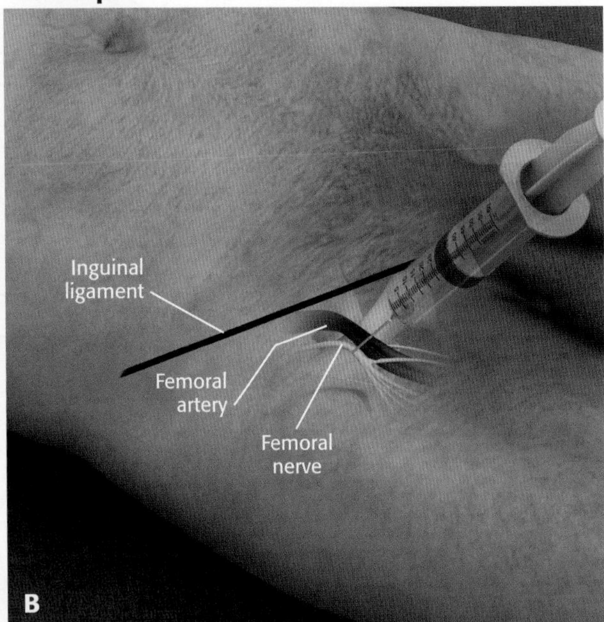

Palpate the femoral artery 2 cm distal to the inguinal ligament. Inject a wheal of lidocaine 1 to 2 cm lateral to this point. Advance the needle at a 45° to 60° angle to the skin until (1) a 'pop' and sudden loss of resistance are felt, (2) paraesthesia is elicited, or (3) the needle pulsates laterally. Inject 25 to 30 mL of anaesthetic. If proximity to the nerve is uncertain, inject in a fanlike distribution lateral to the femoral artery.

PRACTICE TIP

The rapid injection of a large volume of local anaesthetic solution should be avoided. Always calculate a weight-based dose and consider comorbidities that might lead to systemic toxicity.

Procedure for haematoma block for the reduction of distal radius fractures

1. Review the x-ray to confirm the site of the wrist fracture.
2. After explaining the procedure to the patient, family or carer, obtain verbal or written consent for the procedure.
3. Ropivacaine without adrenaline is the anaesthetic of choice. Dose is calculated dependent on the patient's weight, but generally 20 mL is used.
4. Debilitated or older patients, including those with partial or complete heart block, advanced liver disease or severe renal dysfunction, should be given a reduced dosage commensurate with their physical condition.
5. Set up a plaster trolley and prepare appropriate backslab (Box 16.15).
6. Decontaminate the dorsal aspect of the wrist using a single use swab.
7. Identify the deformity by palpating the dorsum of the wrist. Insert the 21-g needle into the fracture site until the needle progresses smoothly into the fracture. Confirmation of the needle location with the fracture haematoma site is obtained by drawing back on the syringe and aspirating blood.
8. Inject local anaesthetic incrementally: 5–7 mL after needle placement. Advance the needle into the space created by the volume and inject the remainder of the anaesthetic.
9. Gently palpate over the injection site for 10–15 seconds after completing the injection as this may help distribute the anaesthetic around the fracture.
10. Wait for the haematoma block to take effect. This may take 10–15 minutes. Evaluate the occurrence of complete loss of pinprick sensation in the forearm nerve distribution, a sign of nerve block effectiveness.
11. Reduce the fracture by pulling the arm and manipulating the displaced portion towards normal alignment (Figs 16.62, 16.63).
12. Apply the under-cast padding 3 cm beyond the extent of the plaster slab with extra layers around bony prominences. Apply the POP backslab and bandage while continuing to manipulate the wrist to normal position. Consider a short arm sandwich POP for unstable fractures.
13. The wrist will need to be held in the desired position until the POP is dry.

FIGURE 16.60 ANATOMY OF DIGITAL NERVES. SCHEMATIC CROSS-SECTION OF THE PHALANX DEMONSTRATING THE RELATIONSHIP OF THE NERVES TO THE BONE[133]

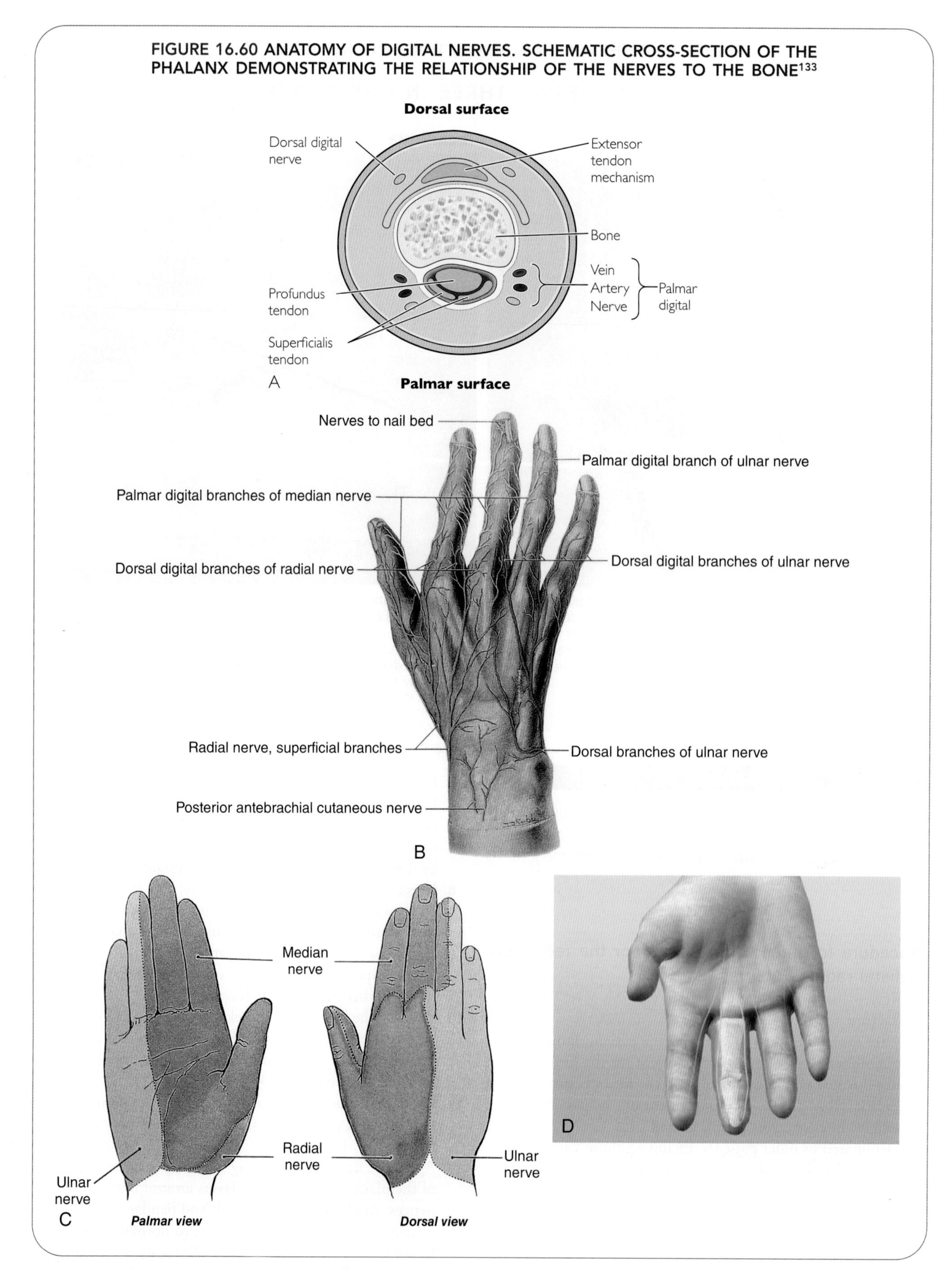

Note that each finger has four digital nerves and that the digital artery and vein run parallel to and near the palmar branches.

TABLE 16.5 COMPARISON OF LOCAL ANAESTHETICS[135]

DRUG	MAXIMUM DOSE[1]		AVERAGE ONSET OF ACTION (MINUTES)		AVERAGE DURATION OF ACTION (HOURS)			
	Without adrenaline[2]	With adrenaline[2]	Topical and/or infiltration	Nerve blockade[3]	Topical	Infiltration	Minor nerve block	Major nerve block
Bupivacaine	2 mg/kg	2 mg/kg	10-15	15-30		3-4	2-6	7-14
Cocaine	1.5 mg/kg		1-5		0.3-0.5			
Levobupivacaine	2 mg/kg		10-15	15-30	0.5-1	3-4	2-6	7-14
Lidocaine	3 mg/kg	7 mg/kg	5-10	5-15	0.5-1	1-2.5	1-2	3-4
Mepivacaine[4]	5-7 mg/kg		5-10	5-15		1-2.5	1-2	
Prilocaine	6 mg/kg	8 mg/kg	5-10	5-15	0.5-1	1-2.5	1-2	3-4
Ropivacaine	3 mg/kg		10-15	15-30	0.5-1	3-4	2-6	7-14
Tetracaine	1 mg/kg		30-60		4-6			

1 When given as a single dose; doses given are guidelines only.

2 Adrenaline is also known as epinephrine.

3 Onset of action of nerve blockade also depends on size of nerve; complete blockade takes longer with larger nerves.

4 Only available as dental cartridge.

BOX 16.13 EQUIPMENT COMMONLY USED FOR HAEMATOMA BLOCK INSERTION

- Bupivacaine (Marcain)
- 10 mL syringe
- Drawing-up needle
- 22 g needle
- Alcohol-based chlorhexidine gluconate swabs (> 0.5% chlorhexidine in > 70% isopropyl alcohol) × 2
- Sterile gloves

14. Watch for signs of complications: adverse reaction to local anaesthetic and neurovascular compromise after manipulation and plaster application.
15. Document the procedure in the clinical record. Record or sign all local anaesthetic doses on the medication record.

PRACTICE TIP

It may take up to 10 minutes to achieve effective anaesthesia following a haematoma block. Waiting until the block has worked will assist with adequate fracture reduction.

CASE STUDY 5

Mrs Lucy is an 86-year-old woman who presents at 0300 hours following a trip and fall onto her outstretched hand. She has pain with an obvious deformity to the right wrist. Her fingers are cool with a 3-second capillary return. The wrist is swollen but a radial pulse is present. She has impaired motor function due to severe pain. An x-ray reveals a transverse fracture of the distal radius with dorsal displacement and angulation. You recognise this as a Colles' fracture that will need reduction.

QUESTIONS

1. Describe the initial assessment of Mrs Lucy.
2. What are the options for management of Mrs Lucy's pain?
3. What are the advantages and disadvantages of using sedation or regional anaesthetic to reduce the fracture?
4. How will you reduce the fracture?
5. What type of splint will you apply?

Answers to Case Study Questions can be found on evolve http://evolve.elsevier.com/AU/Curtis/emergency/

FIGURE 16.61 CONFIRMATION OF NEEDLE LOCATION WITHIN THE FRACTURE HAEMATOMA SITE CAN BE OBTAINED BY DRAWING BACK ON THE SYRINGE PLUNGER AND ASPIRING HAEMATOMA[133]

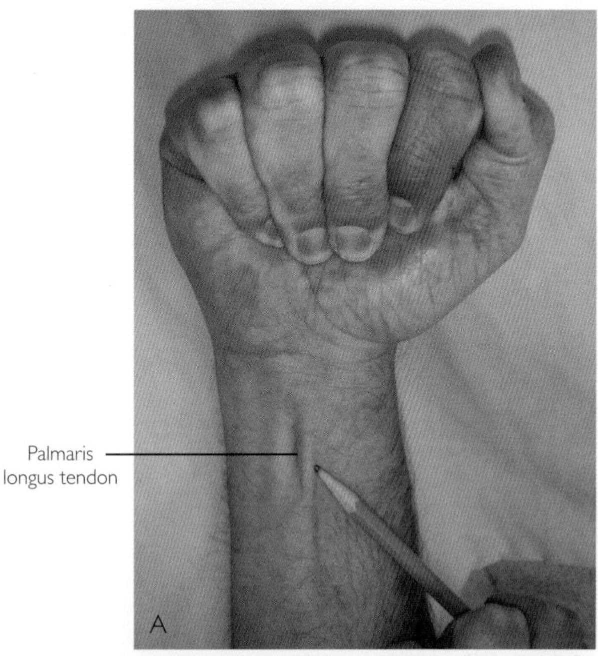

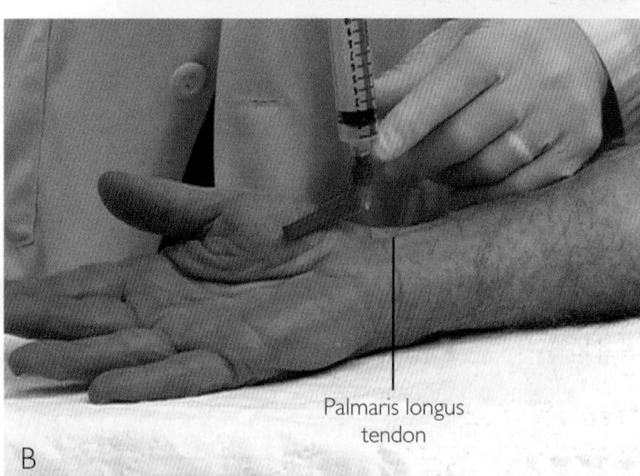

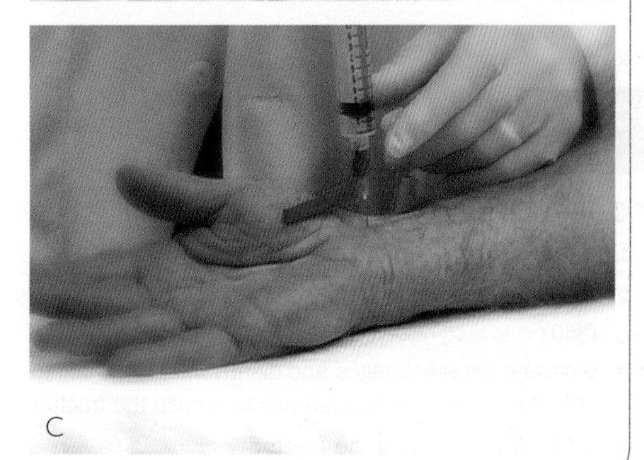

BOX 16.14 POTENTIAL COMPLICATIONS OF HAEMATOMA BLOCK

- All complications identified during the procedure should be discussed with the patient and their family, discussed with the treating clinicians and documented in the patient record.
- Inadvertent intravascular injection
- Nerve injury
- Motor block of the affected limb is common
- Block failure
- Infection
- Accidental vascular puncture
- Anaphylaxis or adverse reactions
- Local anaesthetic systemic toxicity (LAST).

BOX 16.15 EQUIPMENT COMMONLY REQUIRED FOR POP BACKSLAB APPLICATION

- Under cast padding
- Warm water
- Bandages 7.5 cm wide × 3
- Plaster 15–20 cm wide (dependent on the patient size) cut to length with 6–8 layers
- Scissors
- Tape
- Sling

BIER BLOCK: INTRAVENOUS REGIONAL ANAESTHESIA

A Bier Block is a type of intravenous regional anaesthesia most commonly used in the ED for manipulation and reduction of fractures and dislocations below the elbow (Fig. 16.64). A cooperative patient facilitates the procedure, sedation is generally not needed, and minimal haemodynamic monitoring is required, although ready access to resuscitation equipment should be available. Absolute contraindication for the procedure is an allergy to the anaesthetic agent and relative contraindications include Raynaud's disease, Buerger's disease or a vascularly compromised limb.[133]

Equipment includes: 1% lidocaine, sterile saline solution as diluents, 50 mL syringe/drawing-up needle, pneumatic tourniquet, elastic bandage/padding/splinting or plastering materials; the patient should have two IV cannulas, one on the side of injury distal to injury site and one on the other arm for resuscitation. The lidocaine should be prepared as a 0.5% solution (1% lidocaine mixed with equal parts of saline in the 50 mL syringe). The initial dose is 1.5 mg/kg, and usually results in adequate analgesia; the maximum dose is 3 mg/kg.

See Box 16.16 and Fig. 16.65 for procedural steps. Note that the lidocaine is administered in the injured arm in which the circulation has been blocked, not in the IV cannula on the unaffected side. As the lidocaine takes effect, the arm will appear blotchy as a result of the residual blood being displaced from the vascular compartment.[128] Complete anaesthesia

FIGURE 16.62 MANUAL REDUCTION OF A DISTAL RADIUS (COLLES' TYPE) FRACTURE[138]

A. Disimpaction with longitudinal traction and extension of the wrist. **B.** Reduction with flexion of the wrist to restore palmar tilt and ulnar deviation to restore radial inclination. **C, D.** Stabilisation with double-thumb pressure on the distal fracture fragment in neutral forearm rotation, with slight wrist flexion and ulnar deviation. Extreme pronation, flexion and ulnar deviation (Cotton Loder position) should be avoided because of problems encountered with median nerve compression.

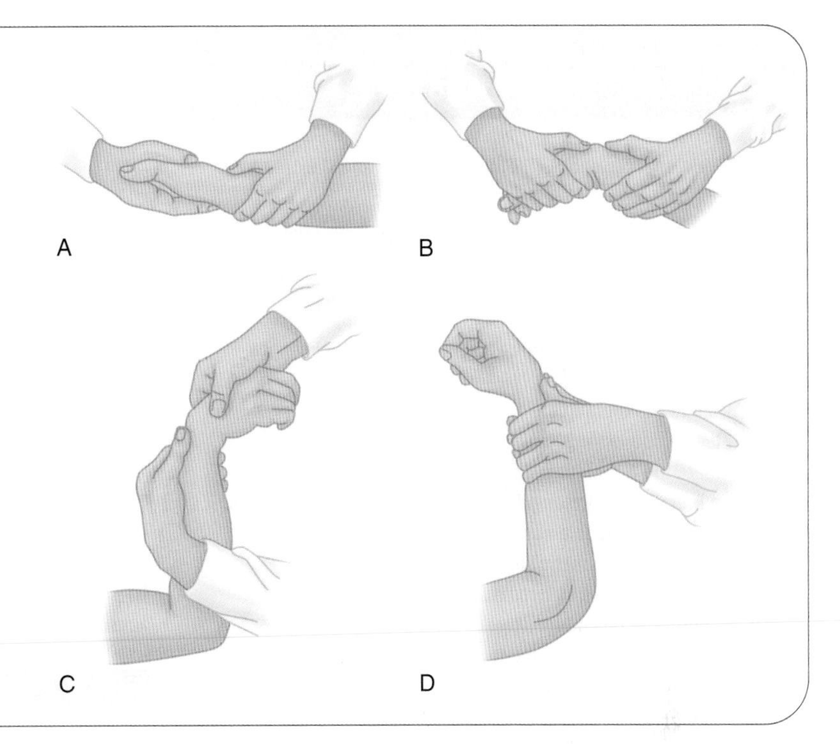

FIGURE 16.63 REDUCTION OF A DISTAL RADIUS (COLLES' TYPE) FRACTURE[137,139]

A
B
C
D

A and **B.** Distal radius (Colles') fracture. **C** and **D.** Recommended reduction of this fracture. After suspending the arm from fingertips and allowing disimpaction of the fracture, pressure is applied with the thumb over the distal fragment.

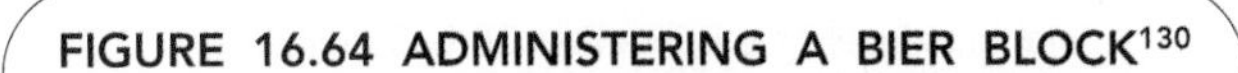

FIGURE 16.64 ADMINISTERING A BIER BLOCK[130]

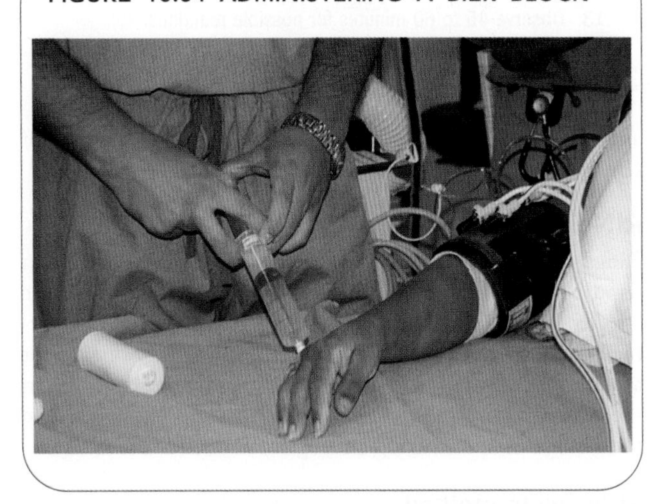

After careful removal of the Esmarch bandage, slowly inject the anesthetic agent in the distal IV cannula.

occurs in 10–20 minutes, although the patient may still sense touch and movement.

REMOVAL OF OBJECTS

Patients with foreign bodies that require removal commonly present for treatment. In general, paramedics are encouraged to leave foreign bodies in situ until arrival at the hospital. This may not be applicable to paramedics in regional and remote areas however, and in these cases consultation with senior clinicians (according to local policy) should occur prior to the removal of a foreign body.

If a foreign body is to be removed, it is important to assess the patient and the affected area, consider the type of object

BOX 16.16 **INTRAVENOUS REGIONAL ANAESTHESIA**[106]

1. Begin an intravenous (IV) line in the uninvolved extremity (optional).
2. Draw up and dilute 1% plain lidocaine (1.5 to 3 mg/kg total lidocaine dose) for a final concentration of 0.5% lidocaine.*
3. Place a padded tourniquet and inflate the upper cuff.
4. Insert a small plastic IV cannula near the pathological lesion and secure it.
5. Deflate the tourniquet.
6. Elevate and exsanguinate the extremity.
7. Inflate the tourniquet (250 mmHg), lower the extremity and remove the exsanguination device. Inflate the proximal cuff only if a double-cuff system is used.
8. Infuse the anaesthetic solution.
9. Remove the infusion needle and tape the site.
10. Perform the procedure.
11. If pain is produced by the tourniquet, inflate the distal cuff first, and then deflate the proximal cuff.
12. After the procedure has been carried out, deflate the cuff for 5 seconds and then reinflate it for 1 to 2 minutes. Repeat this step three times. Do not deflate the cuff if total tourniquet time is less than 20 to 30 minutes.
13. Observe 45 to 60 minutes for possible reactions.

and the risks, such as ischaemia or infection, or benefits of removal.

RINGS

Rings must be removed to prevent vascular compromise in hand and arm injuries.[98] All rings should be removed on the affected limb. Commercial ring cutters, such as the Leatherman™ Raptor Shears, are now available and are very efficient at removing all rings (Fig. 16.66). These shears are common in the pre-hospital environment and are generally more effective than some mechanical ring-cutting tools.

String-wrap method

The string-wrap method of removing a ring is best attempted when there is no finger laceration or underlying fracture. If there is extensive distal swelling or severe pain, a ring cutter may be required.

1. Begin by wrapping the finger distally to proximally with a Penrose drain or compression bandage to reduce oedema. Leave this in place for up to 5 minutes.
2. Unwrap the compression bandage.
3. Using a long piece of tracheostomy tape or thick suture, pull a short section from the distal side under the ring.
4. Wind the long end of the tape from the edge of the ring down to the tip of the finger to provide very firm compression with even rows and no skin bulges.
5. Use the short end that was initially pulled through the ring to pull distally and slowly unwrap it, bringing the ring down the finger over the tightly wrapped area (Fig. 16.67).[140]
6. Apply ice pack to finger once ring is removed.

Ring cutter method

Using a ring cutter is best attempted when there is finger laceration or suspected underlying fracture. Manual ring cutters require patience, as the cutting process is slow. Some EDs use electric or battery-operated ring cutters. Some rings are made of tungsten carbide, stainless steel or titanium and cannot be cut by conventional hospital ring cutters. In these cases, the assistance of the local fire brigade or police rescue using specialised saws will be required.

Procedure

1. Fit the small ring cutter hook under the ring. This acts as a guide for the cutting wheel.
2. Turn the cutting wheel slowly, applying firm but not excessive pressure.
3. Continue cutting until there is a break in the ring.
4. Use two large artery forceps or haemostats on either side of the cut to spread the ring (Fig. 16.68).

In some cases of severe swelling, the ring may need to be cut again into two pieces (Fig. 16.66).

PRACTICE TIP

- The string-wrap method of ring removal can be uncomfortable as a high degree of compression is required. The advantage is that this method can be used for rings that cannot be cut. Because it preserves the integrity of the ring, it also has some psychological benefits to those people reluctant to cut a wedding ring because of the superstition that cutting a wedding ring will result in the end of the marriage.
- Using a ring cutter requires patience and is not always possible with modern ring metals. Cutting a ring may be the only technique possible in the case of laceration, fracture or severe swelling.

BODY PIERCINGS

Body piercings may need to be removed in the case of infection, localised swelling or to permit intubation. Care should be taken when removing any piercing near the mouth or nose, so as to prevent aspiration of the separated pieces. Body piercing can involve the nose, ear, tongue, nipple, genitals, navel and eyebrow, including piercings that involve stretching of the skin of the ears or lips. Extreme piercings include piercing of the uvula or multiple facial piercings. If the patient is conscious, the use of local anaesthetic around the piercing site should be considered as the removal of piercings from infected or injured tissue can be very painful.

Procedure

1. If possible, ask the patient how the piercing comes apart. The types of piercings include clip-on ends, screw-on balls, fixed ends with screw-on balls and balls held on with tension.
2. Ensure that the area is clean and dry.
3. Grip each end of the piercing with artery forceps and unscrew counter-clockwise or pull apart the ring.
4. Remove the piercing and apply ice pack for pain relief if required.

FIGURE 16.65 INTRAVENOUS REGIONAL ANAESTHESIA. A DOUBLE-CUFF TOURNIQUET IS DEPICTED[105]

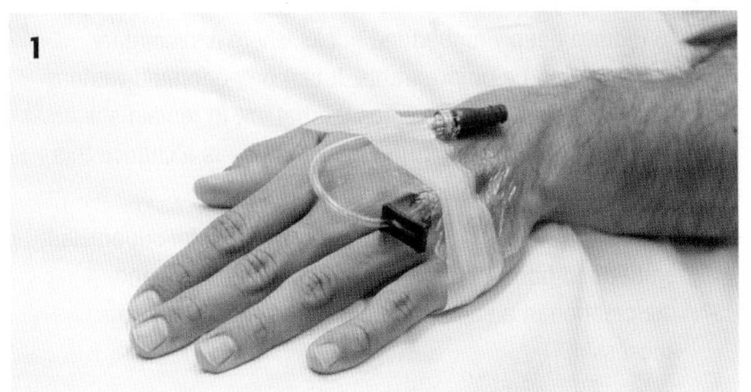

Place an IV catheter or butterfly needle as close to the pathological site as possible. The site should be at least 10 cm distal to the tourniquet. A dorsal hand vein is ideal.

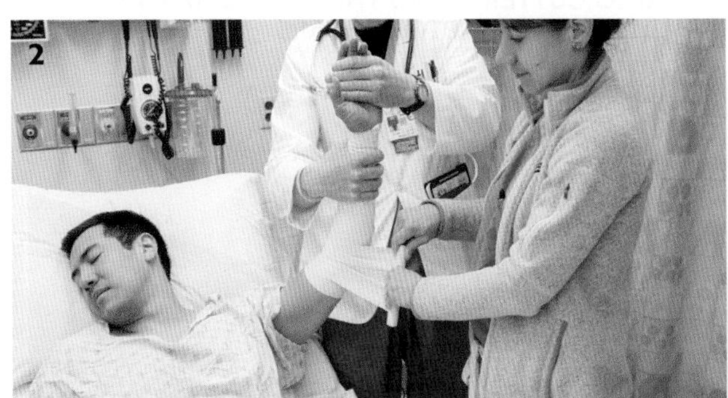

Exsanguinate the extremity by elevating and wrapping it in a distal-to-proximal fashion. Here, an Esmarch bandage is being used.

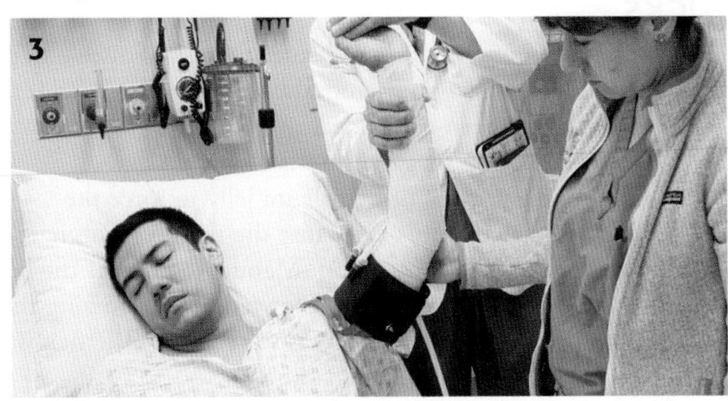

Apply the tourniquet to the patient's arm.

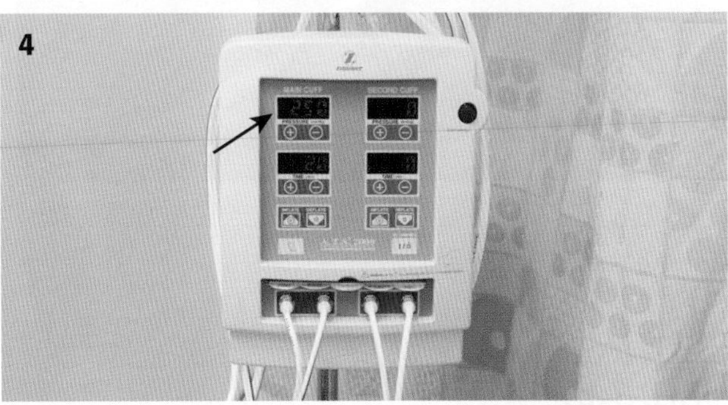

Inflate the tourniquet to 250 mmHg or 100 mmHg above systolic pressure. In the leg, inflate the cuff to 300 mmHg or twice the systolic pressure measured in the arm.

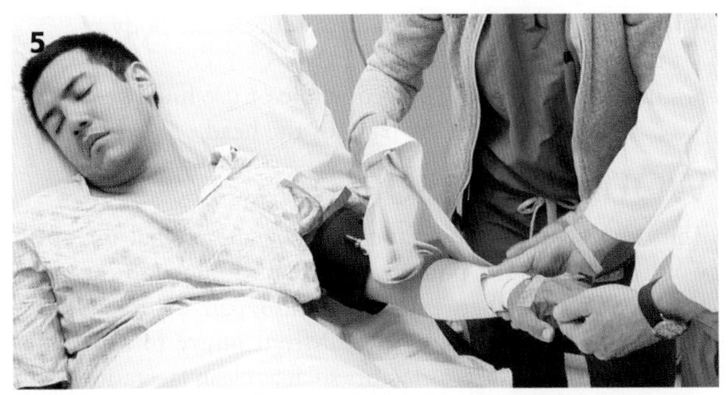

Place the patient's arm by their side and remove the Esmarch bandage. The tourniquet remains inflated.

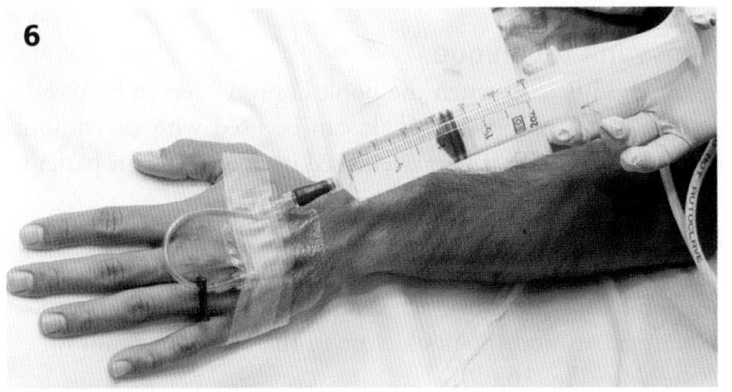

Slowly inject the 0.5% lidocaine solution into the infusion catheter at the calculated dose. See text for details and dosing information.

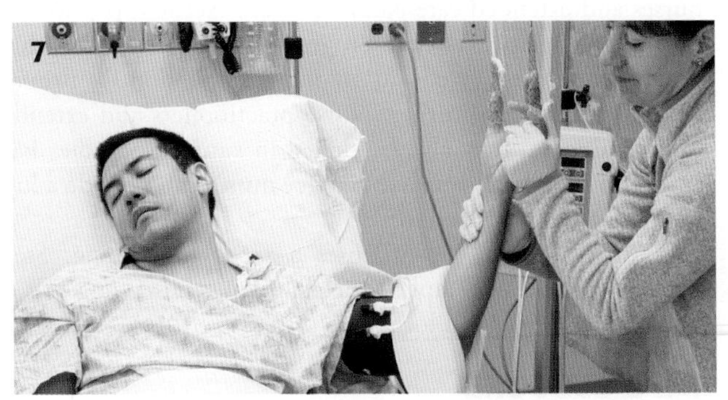

Remove the infusing needle/catheter, and tightly tape the puncture site to prevent extravasation of the anaesthetic agent. Perform the procedure, including post-reduction films and casting.

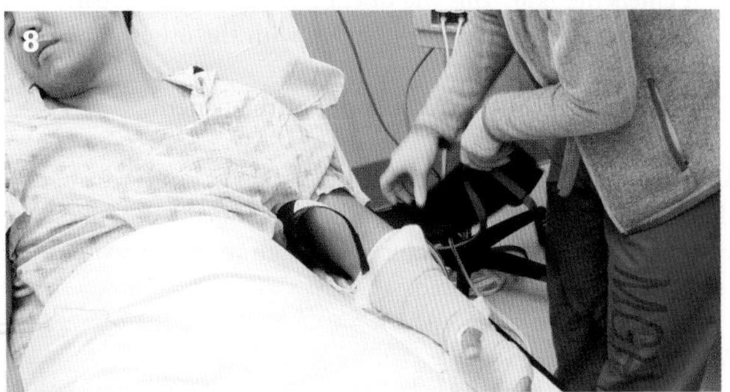

Once the procedure is complete, deflate the tourniquet in a cycling fashion (deflate for 5 seconds, reinflate for 1 to 2 minutes) two or three times. Then remove the tourniquet.

FIGURE 16.66 RING REMOVAL—MANUAL RING CUTTER USING THE LEATHERMAN™ RAPTOR SHEARS

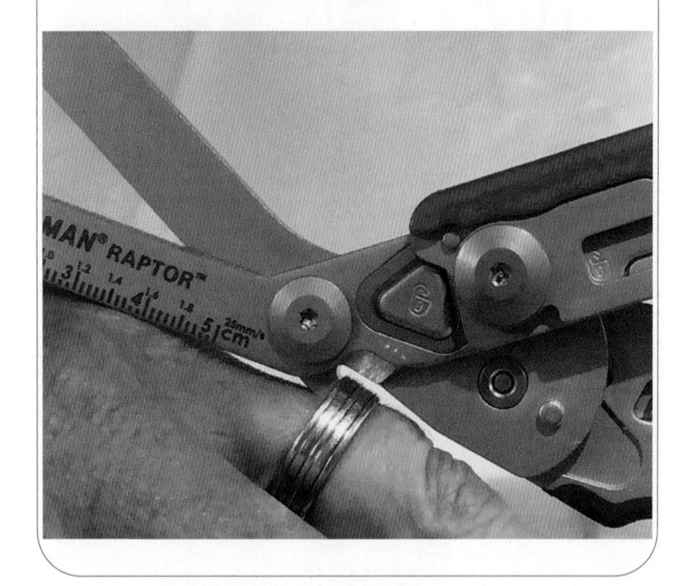

Courtesy of James Brinton and Wendy Fenton.

FISHHOOKS

The method of removing a fishhook depends on the location and the depth of the hook.[140]

String-yank technique

This method is used when the hook lies too deep to be passed out through a second wound. It can be used with or without local anaesthesia and is best attempted in the compliant patient.

Procedure

1. Begin by ensuring that the skin is clean and dry.
2. Loop a long piece of tracheostomy string or thick suture material around the hook close to the insertion point of the skin (Fig. 16.69).
3. Press the long shaft of the hook against the skin while applying downward pressure on the curve of the hook where it enters the skin. This will disengage the embedded barb.
4. Yank or pull sharply on the string with the other hand to remove the hook.
5. Beware of the hook as it flies out of the patient.

Advance and cut technique

This method is best used for superficially embedded hooks as it requires the hook to be advanced through a second wound.[140] Local anaesthesia is required.

Procedure

1. Begin by ensuring that the skin is clean and dry.
2. Inject local anaesthetic into the tissue overlying the barb.
3. Force the barb through the skin.
4. Cut off the barb using pliers.
5. Remove the remaining hook by passing it back through the entry wound.

PRACTICE TIP

- The string-yank technique of fishhook removal can be used to remove deeply embedded hooks where a secondary wound would be unfavourable. It can be performed without local anaesthetic but requires the patient to remain still as the hook is yanked from the skin. There is a chance this technique will be unsuccessful.
- The advance and cut technique can be used for superficially embedded hooks, but requires local anaesthetic and the creation of a second wound. This method is always successful.

TICKS

Ticks should be removed early to reduce the risk of disease transmission and local infection. Removal becomes more difficult the longer the tick has been embedded.

1. Begin by ensuring that the skin is clean and dry.
2. Do not apply alcohol or petroleum jelly to force the tick to disengage as this can cause the tick to regurgitate, increasing the risk of infection. Manual removal is the best method. The preferred method for removal is freezing the tick in situ with an agent such as wart kill.[141] The tick will often fall out after a period of time.
3. If a freezing agent is not available, using a pair of straight tweezers, grasp the tick at the head as close to the skin as possible.
4. Slowly pull, taking care not to squeeze the body of the tick.
5. Ensure the tick is removed whole or use fine tweezers to remove any remaining parts of the head.

WOUND CLOSURE

The time of injury and time to repair are crucial for optimal wound healing. The potential for wound infection increases as the time increases between injury and repair. Six to eight hours is considered a safe time interval from injury to primary closure. This is not exact, as factors such as clean lacerations on the face can extend the time, whereas diabetes and steroid use may place the patient at risk for delayed healing.[142] Emergency nurses and extended care paramedics are excellent providers of wound management. Many programs exist in Australia which provide the necessary education and accreditation for primary wound closure by suturing. Nurse practitioners and extended care paramedics may also be skilled in suturing. Studies have demonstrated that advanced practice nurses can provide a high level of patient satisfaction.[143]

Primary wound closure uses a tape closure (e.g. Steri-Strips™), sutures or staples. The technique chosen depends on wound size, depth and location.

TAPE CLOSURE

Tape closure is used for superficial linear wounds under minimal tension or as an adjunct after suture removal. However, tape closure should not be used for skin tears. Best practice recommendations for the management of skin tears in aged skin are presented in Chapter 17.

FIGURE 16.67

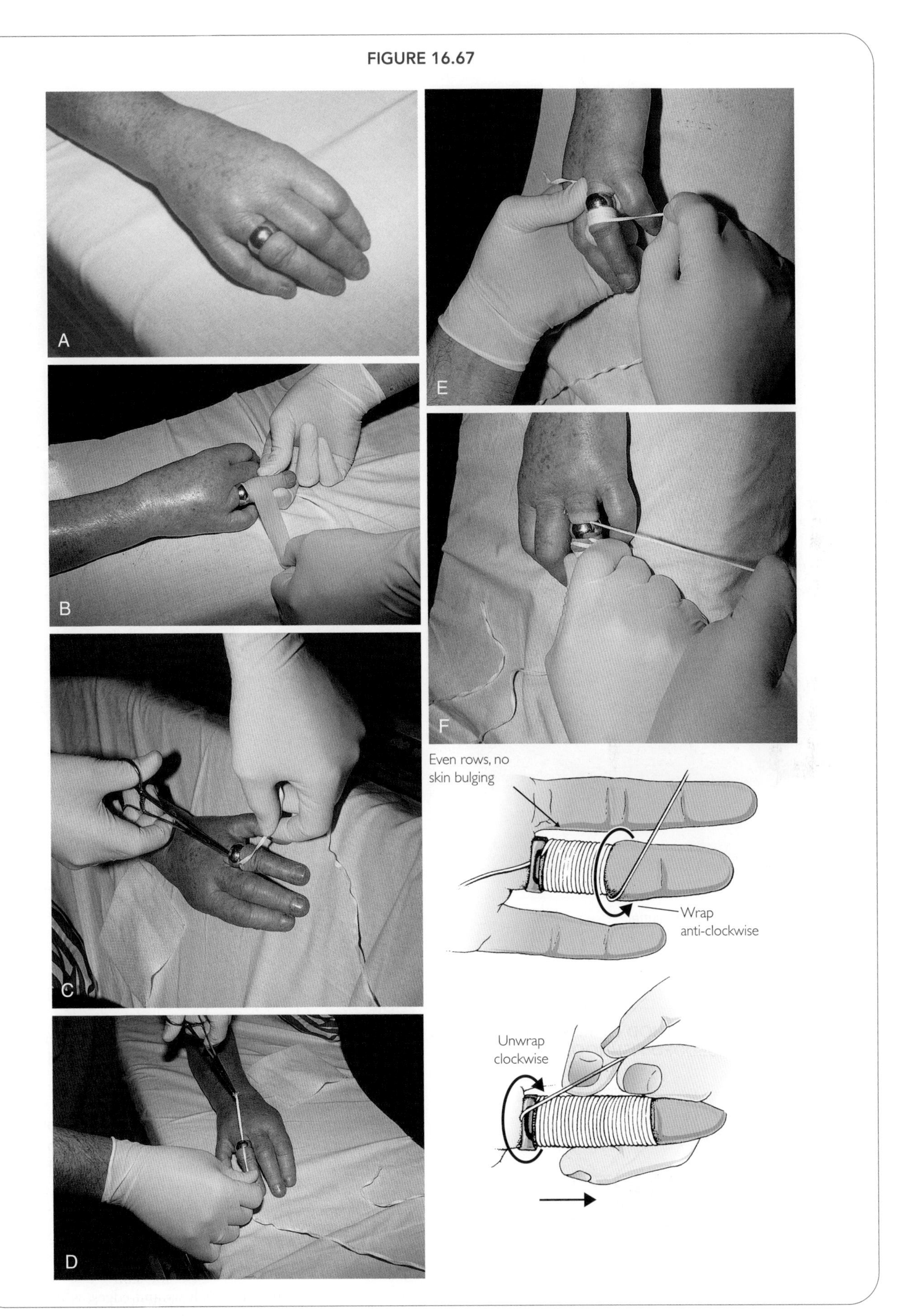

A–G. String removal method for a tight ring.[140]

FIGURE 16.68

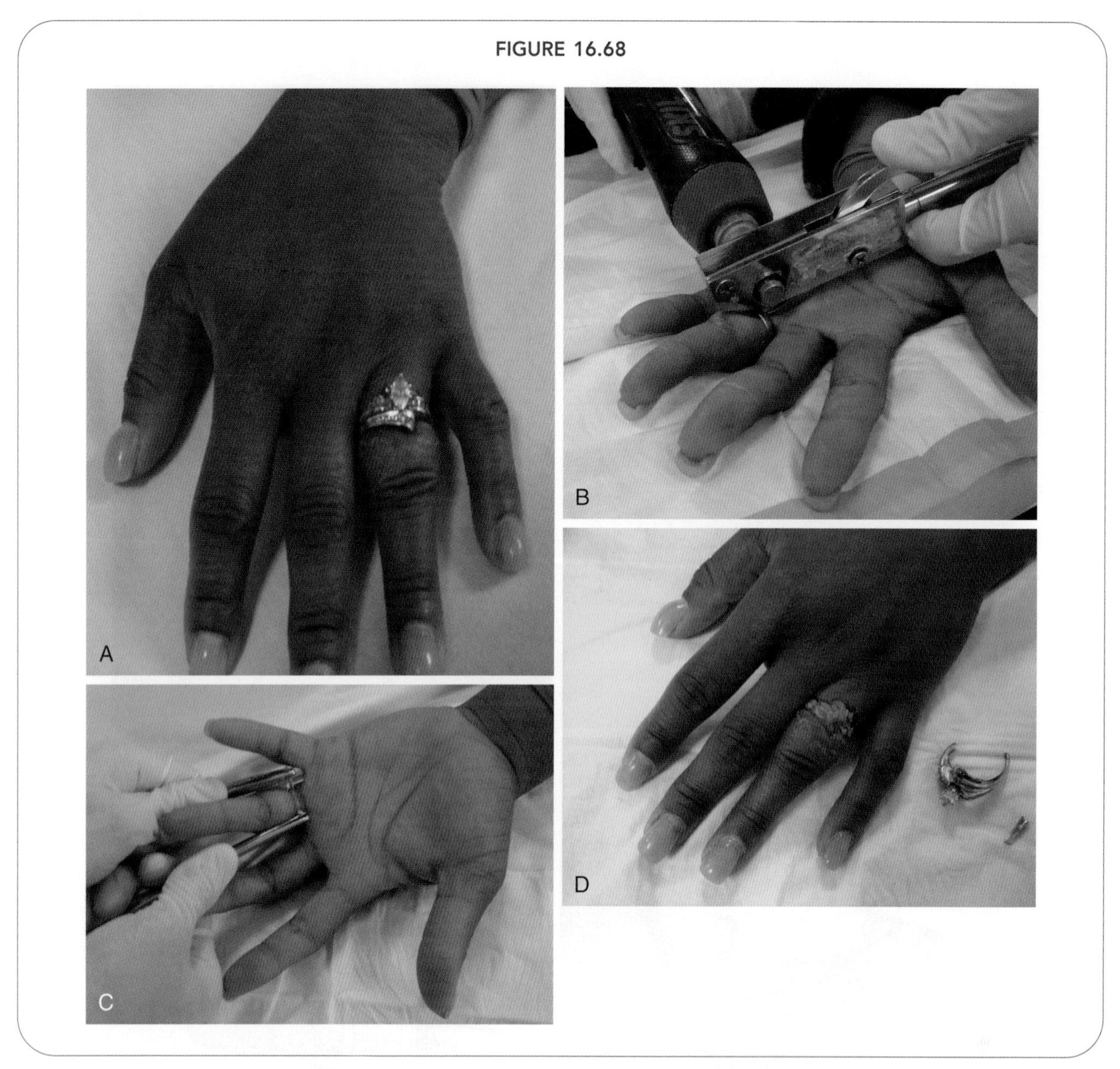

A–D. Ring removal–electric ring cutter.[140]

FIGURE 16.69 METHOD OF REMOVING AN EMBEDDED FISHHOOK[140]

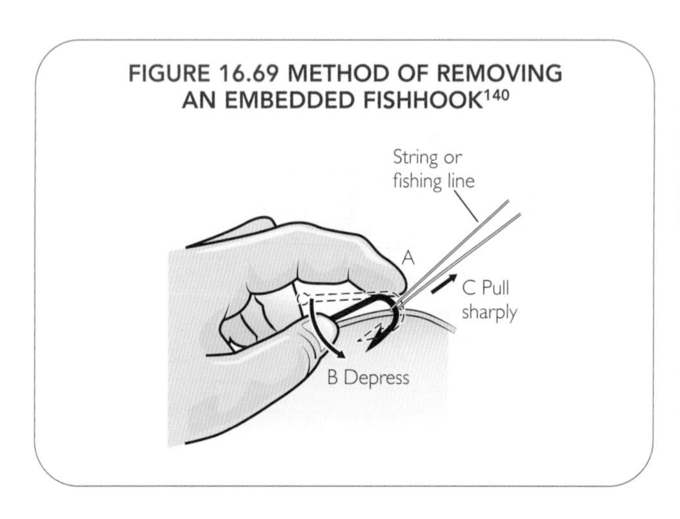

Tincture of benzoin can be applied to the skin before tape application to ensure adherence. Care must be taken to ensure that the tincture does not contact the open wound or injured skin—it will cause pain. A tape closure may also be used after deeper layers are closed with sutures. Dressings may or may not be applied over the tape closure. An anaesthetic is not necessary, and a lower risk of infection and skin necrosis is associated with tape closure.[102] Tape strips remain in place until they fall off. Newer brands of pre-packaged tape closure systems are embedded with wound glue or contain small skin barbs to assist with adherence. Fig. 16.70 illustrates tape closure.

SUTURING

Sutures approximate and attach wound edges, which decreases infection, promotes wound healing and minimises scar formation.

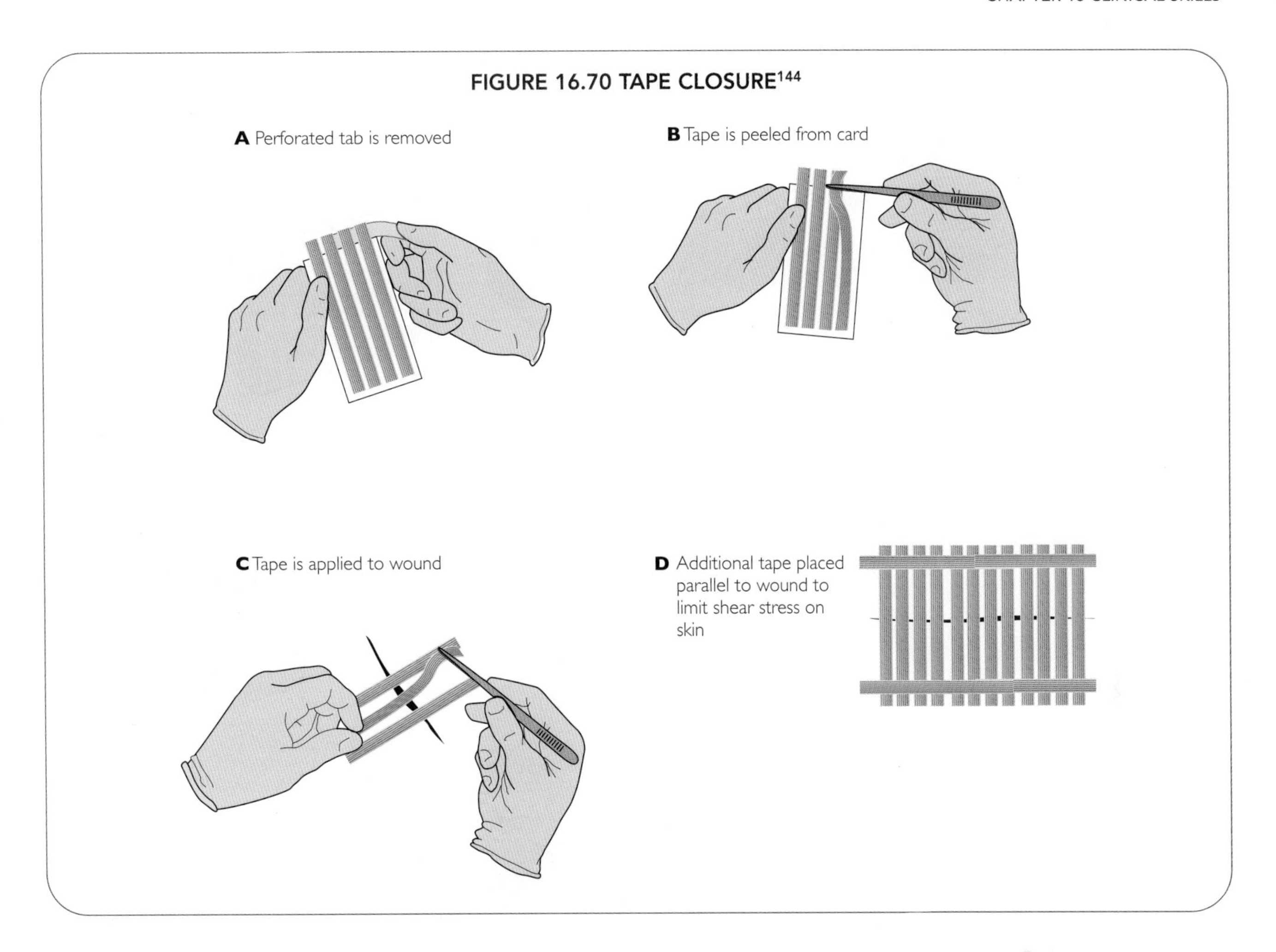
FIGURE 16.70 TAPE CLOSURE144
A Perforated tab is removed
B Tape is peeled from card
C Tape is applied to wound
D Additional tape placed parallel to wound to limit shear stress on skin

A local anaesthetic applied by infiltration or topically is required for suturing. Different suture materials are used to close various wounds depending on depth, location and tension of the wound. Fig. 16.71 shows various stitches and their uses. Sutures may be absorbable or non-absorbable, which means they are generally composed of natural or synthetic material, respectively. Essential qualities of suture material are security, strength, reaction, workability and infection potential. Table 16.6 describes these qualities for various suture materials.[145] Ideal suture materials are strong, easily secured, resistant to infection and cause minimal local reaction.

In suturing, absorbable sutures are for dermal and subcutaneous layers; non-absorbable sutures are used externally. Sutures cause minimal discomfort after insertion; however, they also act as a foreign body and can cause local inflammation. An initial cover with a non-adherent dressing protects the wound and absorbs fluid.

In pre-hospital care, suturing remains the domain of extended care practitioners.

STAPLES

Staples are a fast, economic alternative for closure of linear lacerations of the scalp, trunk and extremities (Fig. 16.72). Wounds closed with staples have a lower incidence of infection and tissue reactivity, but do not provide the same quality of closure as sutures. Scars are more pronounced; therefore, staples are only recommended for areas where a scar is not apparent (i.e. scalp). Staples should not be used in areas of the scalp with permanent hair loss because of poor aesthetic results. Consider the likelihood of the patient attending imaging; for example, head computed tomography (CT) scans, which may be affected by steel staples. If this is a possibility, then suturing using non-absorbable material may be a better option. Local anaesthesia is optional when only one or two staples are required because pain from infiltration of anaesthetic agents may be greater than pain associated with insertion of one or two staples.

Staples usually remain in place for 7–10 days, and they can only be removed using a specialised skin staple remover.

SKIN ADHESIVES

A topical skin adhesive is another method of non-invasive wound management used to close skin edges that are easily approximated. Studies have demonstrated that adhesive is the preferred wound closure method in small and recent facial wounds.[147] This type of wound closure should not be used in areas of high skin tension or across areas of increased skin tension. Wounds should be less than 5 cm long. Application of three thin layers of adhesive is more effective than a single thick layer: the skin adhesive dries within 2.5 minutes.

Discharge education should stress not applying liquid or ointment to the closed wound because these substances can weaken the adhesive, leading to dehiscence. Patients should also be instructed that the adhesive will slough naturally, usually within 5–10 days. If removal of skin adhesive is necessary, use petroleum jelly or acetone.

FIGURE 16.71 STITCHES FOR SUTURING

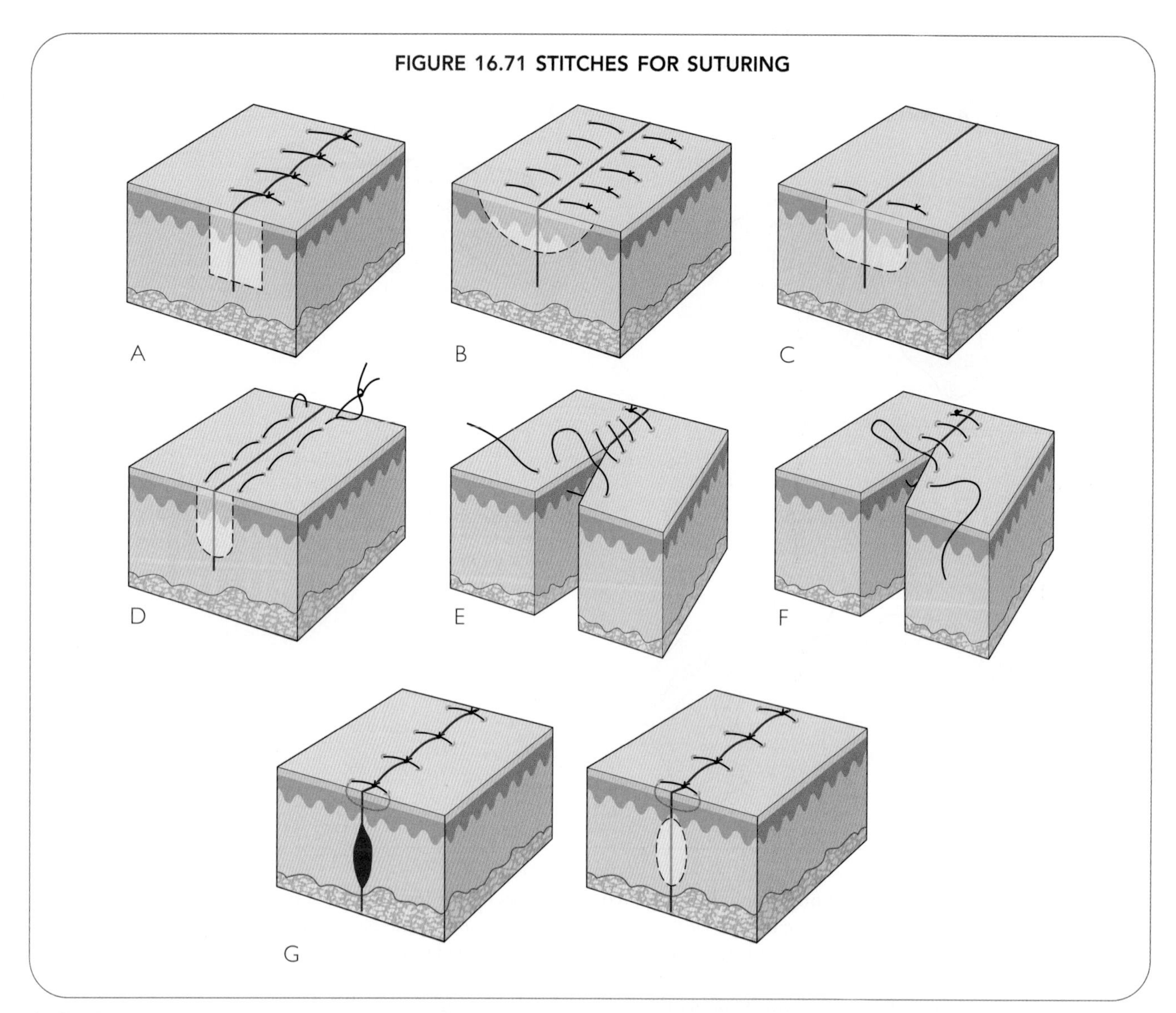

A. Simple interrupted suture: pairing skin edges together evenly; edges are slightly elevated but flatten with healing. **B.** Vertical mattress suture: assures eversion on healing. **C.** Horizontal mattress suture: closely approximates skin edges and has slight amount of eversion, especially in areas under tension. **D.** Half-buried horizontal mattress suture: good with flaps, V-spaced and parallel lacerations. **E.** Subcuticular suture (continuous intradermal suture): good for wounds where sutures should be left in place for longer periods, as in wounds under a great deal of tension. **F.** Continuous suture: good when suture marks will not show, as in scalp. **G.** Buried suture: reduces dead space and reduces surface tension in wound.

Instruct the patient to keep the wound clean and dry. If washing of the wound is required, mild soap and water is all that is required and drying is important. Soaking of the wound and swimming is not advised. Elevation of an affected limb reduces swelling and subsequent pain. Educate about the signs and symptoms of inflammation and early infection. Pain is usually the initial symptom, followed by redness, swelling and discharge. Instruct the patient to seek professional advice from their general practitioner or return to the ED.

REMOVAL OF WOUND CLOSURES

Suture removal

Recommendations for suture removal vary with wound location. For wounds in areas of movement or increased surface tension, sutures should remain longer. Table 16.7 provides guidelines for suture removal. To reduce scarring further, sutures in highly visible areas such as the face may be removed earlier than those in other areas, and surgical skin tape (e.g. Steri-Strips) applied to reinforce the wound.

Suture removal method

1. Begin by ensuring that the skin is clean and dry.
2. Grasp the suture using fine tweezers and lift the suture (Fig. 16.73).
3. Cut the suture as close to the skin as possible using a suture cutter or scissors.
4. Pull the suture out. Never pull a knot through the skin.
5. Apply surgical skin tape to maintain wound repair after suture removal.

Staple removal

Wound staples should be removed after the same interval as sutures and require a specialised staple-removal device (Fig. 16.74).

TABLE 16.6 SUTURE MATERIALS FOR WOUND CLOSURE[145]

<table>
<tr><th>TYPE</th><th>DESCRIPTION</th><th>SECURITY</th><th>STRENGTH</th><th>REACTION</th><th>WORKABILITY</th><th>INFECTION</th><th>COMMENT</th></tr>
<tr><td>Non-absorbables</td><td></td><td></td><td></td><td></td><td></td><td></td><td></td></tr>
<tr><td>Silk</td><td></td><td>||||</td><td>|</td><td>||||</td><td>||||</td><td>||</td><td>Nice around mouth, nose or nipples; too reactive and weak to be used universally</td></tr>
<tr><td>Mersilene</td><td>Braided synthetic</td><td>||||</td><td>||</td><td>|||</td><td>||||</td><td></td><td>Good tensile strength; some prefer for fascia repairs</td></tr>
<tr><td>Nylon</td><td>Monofilament</td><td>||</td><td>|||</td><td>||</td><td>||</td><td>|||</td><td>Good strength; decreased infection rate; knots tend to slip, especially the first throw</td></tr>
<tr><td>Prolene Polypropylene</td><td>Monofilament</td><td></td><td>||||</td><td>|</td><td>|</td><td>||||</td><td>Good resistance to infection; often difficult to work with; requires an extra throw</td></tr>
<tr><td>Ethibond</td><td>Braided coated polyester</td><td>|||</td><td>||||</td><td>||</td><td>|||</td><td>|||</td><td>Costly</td></tr>
<tr><td>Stainless steel wire</td><td>Monofilament</td><td>||||</td><td>||||</td><td>|</td><td>|</td><td>|</td><td>Hard to use; painful to patient; some prefer for tendons</td></tr>
<tr><td>Absorbables</td><td></td><td></td><td></td><td></td><td></td><td></td><td></td></tr>
<tr><td>Gut (plain)</td><td>From sheep intima</td><td>|</td><td>||</td><td>|||</td><td></td><td>|</td><td>Loses strength rapidly and quickly absorbed; rarely used today</td></tr>
<tr><td>Chromic (gut)</td><td>Plain gut treated with chromic salts</td><td>||</td><td>||</td><td>|||</td><td></td><td>|</td><td>Similar to plain gut; often used to close intraoral lacerations</td></tr>
<tr><td>Dexon</td><td>Braided copolymer of glycolic acid</td><td>||||</td><td>||||</td><td>|</td><td></td><td>||||</td><td>Braiding may cause it to ‘hang up’ when tying knots</td></tr>
<tr><td>Vicryl</td><td>Braided polymer of lactide and glycolide</td><td>|||</td><td>||||</td><td>|</td><td></td><td>|||</td><td>Low reactivity with good strength; therefore, nice for subcutaneous healing; good in mucous membranes</td></tr>
<tr><td>Polydioxanone</td><td>Monofilament</td><td>||||</td><td>||||</td><td>|</td><td>Excellent</td><td>Unavailable</td><td>First available monofilament synthetic absorbable sutures; appears to be excellent</td></tr>
</table>

Scale: |||| *, high* → | *, low*

FIGURE 16.72 APPLICATION OF SKIN STAPLES

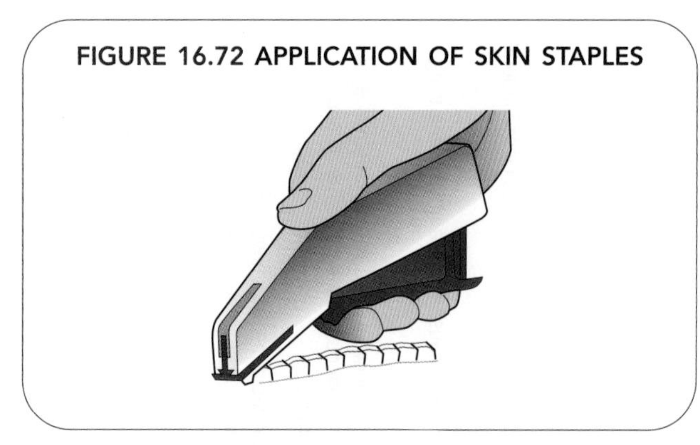

Staples are centred over the incision line using locating arrows or a guideline and placed approximately 10 mm apart.

TABLE 16.7 GUIDELINES FOR SUTURE REMOVAL

LOCATION	REMOVAL DATE
Eyelids	3-5 days
Eyebrows	4-5 days
Ear	4-6 days
Lip	3-5 days
Face	3-5 days
Scalp	7-10 days
Trunk	7-10 days
Hands and feet	7-10 days
Arms and legs	10-14 days
Over joints	14 days

1. Begin by ensuring that the skin is clean and dry.
2. Slide the lower jaw of the staple remover under the staple.
3. Squeeze or close the handle to compress the staple.
4. Ensure the staple is fully compressed to decrease patient discomfort.
5. Lift the staple from the wound.
6. Apply surgical skin tape (e.g. Steri-Strips) to maintain wound repair after staple removal.

Most staple-removal devices are disposable. It is important that the patient has access to a staple-removal device; not all local doctors have them in stock.

EYE EMERGENCIES

Most ocular emergencies do not represent a threat to the patient's life; however, these conditions represent a great threat to the patient's wellbeing. Once lost, vision cannot be replaced. The emergency clinician should assess patients who present with ocular problems and identify those with actual or potential threats to vision. Early recognition of true ocular emergencies and preventing further damage is critical for the patient's optimal visual outcome.

Immediate and copious irrigation of chemical burn injuries is essential, because the area and time of exposure determines the injury and overall outcome.[148] Irrigation can be performed using running tap water, a normal IV giving set or a commercial Morgan lens. The Morgan lens is a moulded plastic lens with tubing that attaches to the end of an IV giving set to run continuous irrigation. It allows hands-free irrigation of unilateral or bilateral eyes. Correct eye irrigation is time-consuming and labour-intensive.

PROCEDURES

Everting an eyelid

1. Ask the patient to look downwards with both eyes gently closed.
2. Use your right hand to hold a cotton bud and left hand to open the lid of the patient's left eye; and the other way round for the right eye.
3. Place the cotton bud horizontally so that the soft tip rests on the top eyelid crease.
4. With the other hand, grip the eyelashes.
5. Apply gentle pressure to the cotton tip and lift the lashes to fold the eyelid over the cotton tip (Fig. 16.75).
6. Hold the lid in place and slide the cotton bud out.
7. Examine, sweep or irrigate under the lid as required.
8. When finished, ask the patient to blink and look up to return the lid to normal.

Double-everting the top eyelid

1. Lifesaving procedures always take precedence over eye emergencies.
2. Apply topical anaesthetic to the eye and wait 3–5 minutes.
3. Ask the patient to look downwards with both eyes gently closed.
4. Use your right hand to hold a cotton bud and left hand to open the lid for the patient's left eye; and the other way round for the right eye.
5. Place the cotton bud horizontally so that the soft tip rests on the top eyelid crease.
6. With the other hand, grip the eyelashes.
7. Apply gentle pressure to the cotton tip and lift the lashes to fold the eyelid over the cotton tip.
8. Hold the lid in place and slide the cotton bud out.
9. Moisten a second sterile cotton tip with anaesthetic or normal saline.
10. Place this on the everted eyelid and apply pressure to view the upper conjunctival fornix deep under the lid.
11. Examine, sweep or irrigate under the lid as required.
12. When finished, ask the patient to blink and look up to return the lid to normal.
13. Hold the lid in place and slide the cotton bud out.

Irrigating an eye using an IV giving set

Lifesaving procedures always take precedence over eye emergencies, but early irrigation can be vital in saving vision.

1. Apply topical anaesthetic to the eye and wait.
2. Begin irrigation with at least 1 litre of normal saline or Hartmann's IV solution via an IV giving line to direct the stream of irrigation, following the steps below.
3. Evert the upper lid and irrigate. Sweep and remove any foreign bodies seen.
4. Open the IV giving set and continue to instil the irrigation into the open eye.

FIGURE 16.73 SUTURE REMOVAL[103]

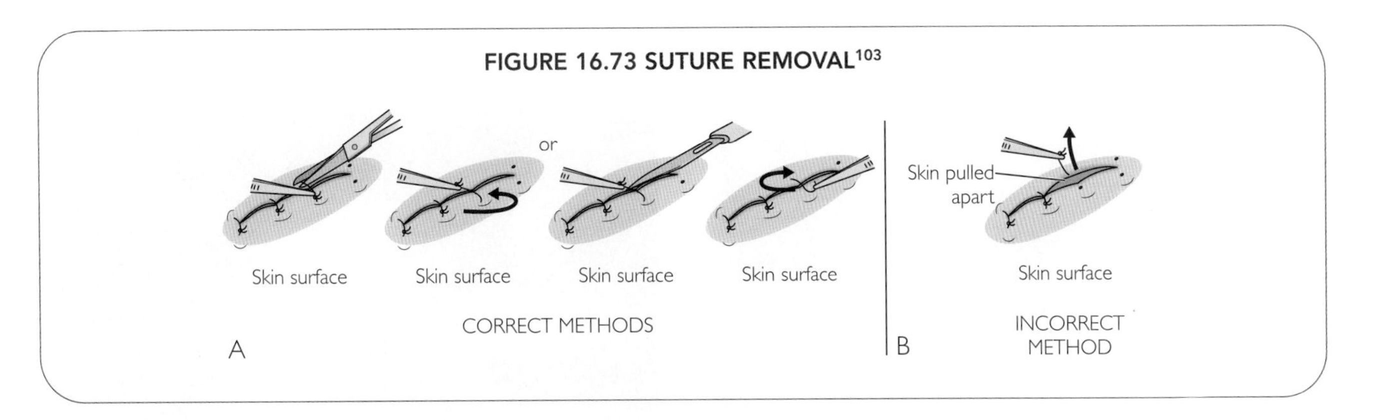

FIGURE 16.74 STAPLE REMOVAL[103]

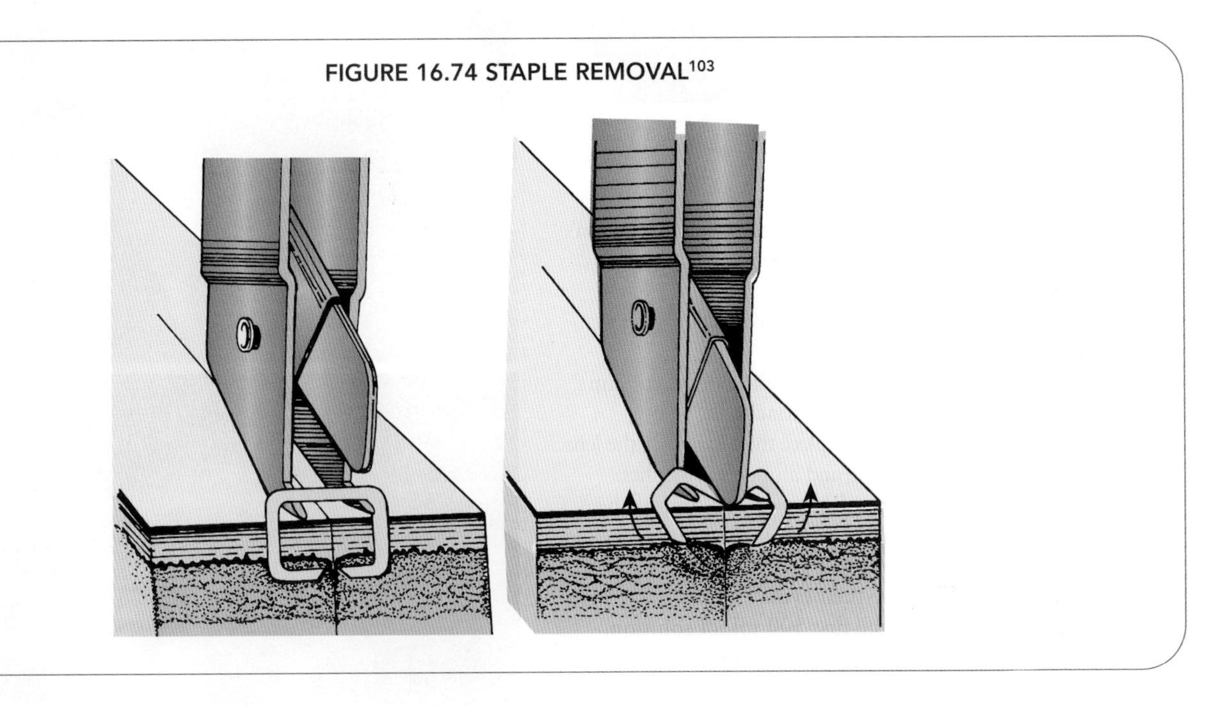

FIGURE 16.75 LID EVERSION[147]

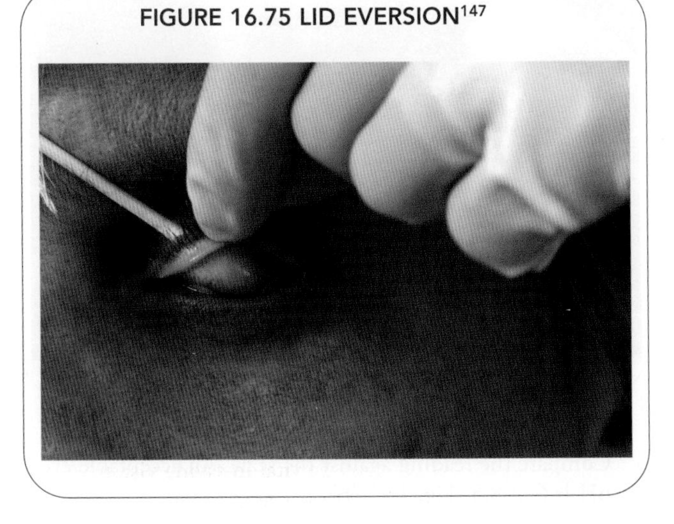

5. Use eyelid retractors or hold the eye open with a gloved hand or gauze.
6. Direct the stream of fluid medially onto the conjunctiva, then across the cornea so that the fluid flows laterally down the side of the head.[149]
7. Begin by rapidly flushing the first 500 mL of solution, then slow the infusion to a continuous trickle.
8. Repeat topical anaesthetic every 10 minutes as required.
9. Infuse at least 1 litre of irrigation. Alkali burns (e.g. caustic soda, lime-plaster/cement and ammonia) penetrate the cornea rapidly because of their ability to lyse with the cell membranes, and prolonged irrigation may be required.
10. Wait 5 minutes after the completion of irrigation before checking the pH at the conjunctival fornices. The average pH of tears is 7.35, but a wide normal variation exists from 5.20 to 8.35.[150]

Irrigating an eye using a Morgan lens

The Morgan lens (Fig. 16.76) allows the medical team to irrigate the eye without the use of eyelid retractors, which can cause abrasions to the eye, or without a dedicated person holding the eyelids open; it is the hands-free option for eye irrigation. The Morgan lens is relatively expensive, and may not adequately irrigate under the lids. Particulate may be trapped under the lens, causing corneal abrasion. New users may find the lens difficult to fit.

1. Lifesaving procedures always take precedence over eye emergencies, but early irrigation can be vital in saving vision.
2. Apply topical anaesthetic to the eye and wait.

FIGURE 16.76 MORGAN LENS[147]

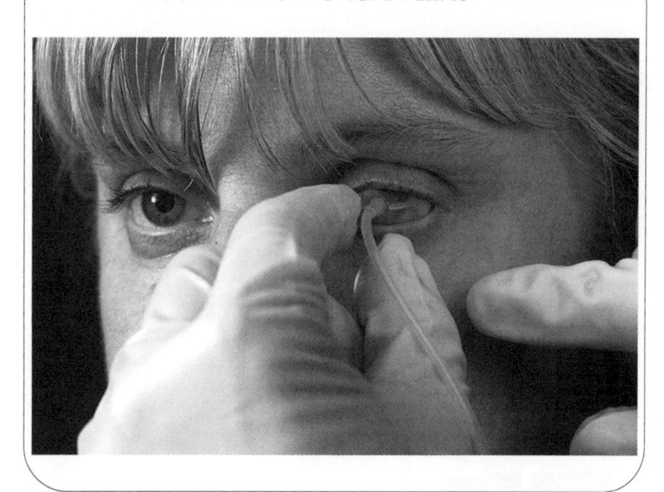

3. Begin irrigation with 1 litre of normal saline or Hartmann's IV solution via an IV giving line before fitting the lens, following the steps below.
4. Evert the upper lid and irrigate. Sweep and remove any foreign bodies seen.
5. Prime an IV giving set with normal saline or Hartmann's IV solution with the Morgan lens attached.
6. Ask the patient to look down and place the top half of the lens under the top eyelid by grasping and lifting the eyelashes.
7. Ask the patient to look up and place the bottom of the lens under the bottom eyelid, so that it sits on the eye like a contact lens.
8. Instruct the patient to close their eyes.
9. Begin by rapidly flushing the first 500 mL of solution, and then slow the infusion to a continuous trickle.
10. Repeat topical anaesthetic every 10 minutes as required.
11. Infuse at least 1 litre of irrigation. Alkali burns (e.g. caustic soda, lime-plaster/cement and ammonia) penetrate the cornea rapidly because of their ability to lyse with the cell membranes, and prolonged irrigation may be required.
12. Wait 5 minutes after the completion of irrigation and remove the Morgan lens before checking the pH at the conjunctival fornices. Do not use the same lens in the other eye and consider changing the lens if the pH is abnormal after prolonged irrigation.

Checking the pH of an eye

1. Do not delay treatment to check the pH of the eye following chemical burns. Irrigation (see above) must start immediately.
2. Wait 5 minutes after the completion of irrigation, and remove the Morgan lens if used, before checking the pH.
3. Use a strip of universal indicator paper. If none is available, the pH section of a urine analysis dipstick may be used but beware of the risk of corneal abrasion from the sharp plastic.
4. Ask the patient to look up, and pull down the bottom lid.
5. Hold the universal indicator paper on the bottom conjunctival fornices until it is wet with tears (Fig. 16.77A).

FIGURE 16.77 CHECKING THE PH OF THE EYE[149]

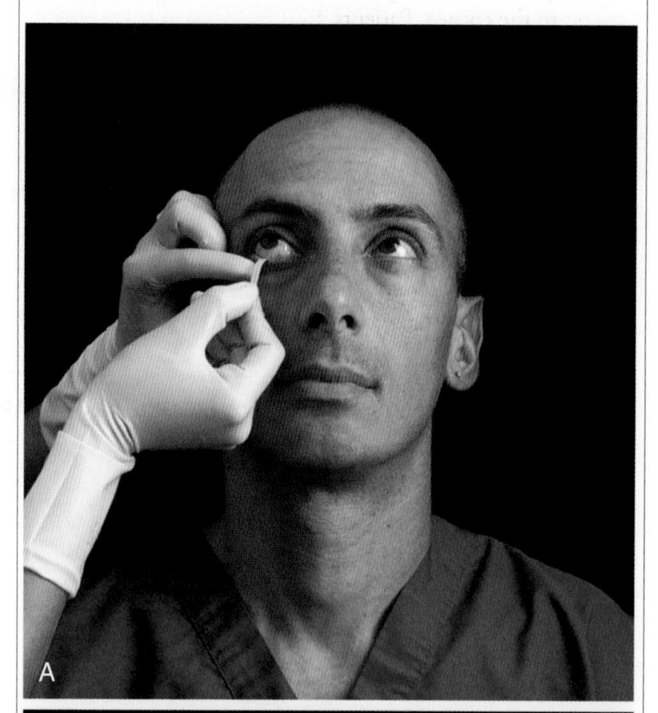

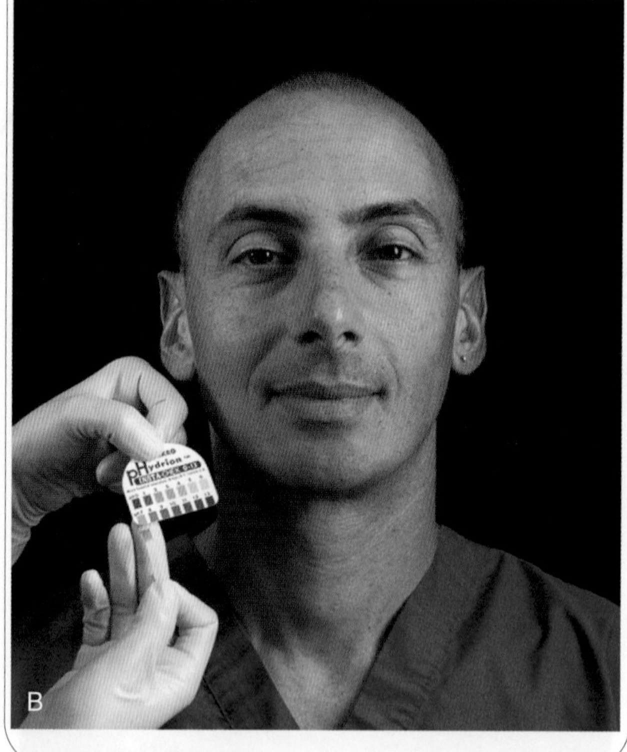

6. Compare the reading against the scale. An acceptable eye pH is 6.5–8.5 (Fig. 16.77B).
7. Recheck the pH after 30 minutes.

Padding an eye

Eye padding is not commonly used, because a padded eye cannot be frequently examined. It is important to leave eye padding on for no longer than 24 hours as there is an increased risk of infection. Correct eye padding must be firm enough not to allow the padded eye to open. Doing so can cause irritation and abrasion to the cornea. Patients must be aware that padding an eye will result in the loss of binocular vision—they must not drive and should take care when walking.

1. Apply topical anaesthetic to the eye and wait.
2. Ask the patient to close both eyes.
3. Apply a generous amount of antibiotic ointment to the conjunctival fornices and the outer lids.
4. Fold an eye pad in half and place it on the closed eye.
5. Secure this with three pieces of tape, taking care not to apply pressure to the centre of the pad.
6. Tape from above the eyebrow medially diagonally down to the cheek.
7. Place a second eye pad on top of the first and tape with three pieces of tape, taking care not to apply pressure to the centre of the pad. The taping should be firm and even, and on completion the patient should not be able to open the padded eye.

Fitting a protective eye shield

A protective eye shield should be used to prevent further compression to an injured eye and where an eye perforation or penetrating eye injury is suspected. A shield prevents secondary injury.[103]

1. Apply topical anaesthetic to the eye if required. Systemic analgesia may also be required for penetrating eye injuries.
2. Ask the awake patient to close both eyes.
3. Apply a generous amount of antibiotic ointment to the conjunctival fornices and the outer lids.
4. Use a commercial eye shield and secure this with three pieces of tape, taking care not to apply pressure to the centre of the shield.
5. Tape from above the eyebrow medially diagonally down to the cheek.
6. A modified eye shield can be made using a polystyrene or paper cup (Fig. 16.78).

FIGURE 16.78 ALTERNATIVE EYE SHIELD[149]

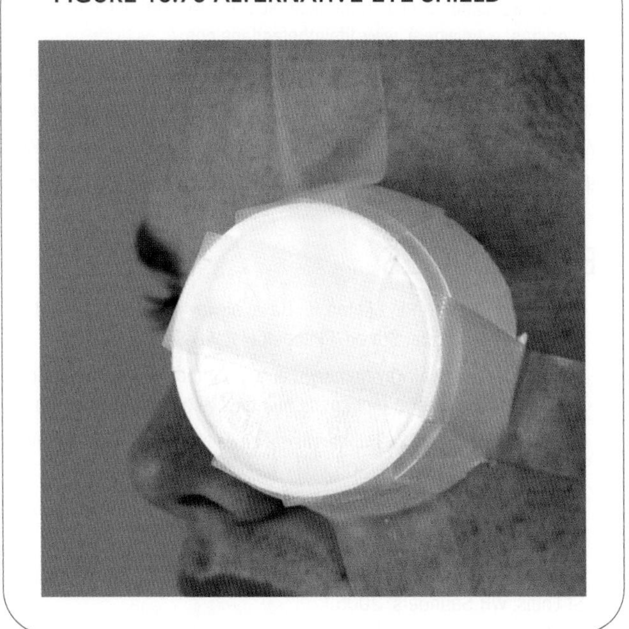

SUMMARY

This chapter has outlined a broad range of clinical skills relevant to the emergency clinician. The relevant theoretical and practical aspects of the procedures have been included in conjunction with the latest available research. The contents of this chapter can be used by the emergency clinician to refresh previously acquired skills and to provide a basis to the attainment of new skills.

ACKNOWLEDGEMENT

The authors acknowledge the work of Mark Wilson, the first edition author.

USEFUL WEBSITES

Australian Commission on Safety and Quality in Health Care. Management of Peripheral Intravenous Catheters (2021) www.safetyandquality.gov.au/publications-and-resources/resource-library/management-peripheral-intravenous-catheters.

Australian Resuscitation Council: useful guidelines for management of emergency presentations, www.resus.org.au.

AO Online: the surgical management of trauma and disorders of the musculoskeletal system, www.aofoundation.org/.

Australian Wound Management Association, www.woundsource.com/resource/australian-wound-management-association-awma.

BestBETs (Best Evidence Topics), www.bestbets.org.

Company resources from Molnlycke, www.molnlycke.com/com/Wound-Care-Products.

Company resources from Smith&Nephew, http://wound.smith-nephew.com/.

Emergency Care Institute Global Airway Registry: a multi-centre database to evaluate what is current practice and to assess future developments in techniques and technology in ED airway management, www.aci.health.nsw.gov.au/networks/eci/research/current-research-and-quality-activities/global-airway-registry.

Emergency Eye Manual (an illustrated guide) written by the Statewide Ophthalmology Service NSW, www.cena.org.au/wp-content/uploads/2014/10/eye_manual.pdf.

Expert in My Pocket is a mobile-enabled repository of learning resources that demonstrate specific skills that nursing and paramedic students must acquire to provide safe and effective healthcare. http://expertinmypocket.com.au/

Intraosseous access devices information (e.g. EZ-IO), www.vidacare.com.

Life In The Fast Lane: LITFL is a medical blog and website dedicated to providing online emergency medicine and critical care insights and education for everyone, everywhere, www.lifeinthefastlane.com/.

MIMS Online: Monthly Index of Medical Specialties pharmaceutical prescribing reference guide, www.mimsonline.com.au.

Neuraxiom: ultrasound guided regional nerve blocks, www.neuraxiom.com/html/ficb.html.

NSW Health Procedural Videos: https://aci.health.nsw.gov.au/networks/eci/clinical/procedures.

Useful information and user guides for fitting Hare traction splints, www.haretractionsplint.com/.

REFERENCES

1. Reardon RF, Mason PE, Clinton JE. Basic airway management and decision-making. In: Roberts JR, Hedges JR, editors. Clinical procedures in emergency medicine. 6th ed. Philadelphia: WB Saunders; 2014.
2. Heard SO, Kaur S. Airway management and endotracheal intubation. In: Irwin RS, Rippe JM, Lisbon A, Heard SO, editors. Procedures, techniques and minimally invasive monitoring in intensive care medicine. 4th ed. Philadelphia: Lippincott Williams & Wilkins; 2008.
3. Skillings KN, Curtis BL. Oropharyngeal airway insertion. In: Wiegand DJ, Carlson KK, editors. AACN procedure manual for critical care. 5th ed. St Louis: WB Saunders; 2005.
4. Ambulance Victoria. Clinical practice guidelines for ambulance and MICA paramedics. Doncaster, Victoria, Australia: Ambulance Victoria; 2022. Available from: cpg.ambulance.vic.gov.au/.
5. Skillings KN, Curtis BL. Nasopharyngeal airway insertion. In: Wiegand DJ, Carlson KK, editors. AACN procedure manual for critical care. 5th ed. St Louis: WB Saunders; 2005.
6. Roberts K, Whalley H, Bleetman A. The nasopharyngeal airway: dispelling myths and establishing the facts. Emerg Med J 2005;22(6):394–6.
7. Barker TD, Schneider RE. Supplemental oxygen and bag-mask ventilation. In: Walls RM, Murphy MF, editors. Manual of emergency airway management. 3rd ed. Philadelphia: Lippincott Williams & Wilkins; 2008.
8. Stewart JC, Bhananker S, Ramaiah R. Rapid-sequence intubation and cricoid pressure. Int J Crit Ill Injury Sci 2014;4(1):42.
9. Auerbach PS. Wilderness medicine. 6th ed. St Louis: Mosby; 2012.
10. Brimacombe JR, Berry AM. Cricoid pressure. Can J Anaesth 1997;44(4):414–25.
11. Wilkins RL, Stoller JK, Scanlan CL. Egan's fundamentals of respiratory care. 8th ed. St Louis: Mosby; 2003.
12. Reynolds SF, Heffner J. Airway management of the critically ill patient: rapid-sequence intubation. Chest 2005;127(4):1397–412.
13. Walls RM. Rapid sequence intubation. In: Walls RM, Murphy MF, editors. Manual of emergency airway management. 3rd ed. Philadelphia: Lippincott Williams & Wilkins; 2008.
14. Guyette FX, Farrell K, Carlson JN, Callaway CW, Phrampus P. Comparison of video laryngoscopy and direct laryngoscopy in a critical care transport service. Prehosp Emerg Care 2013;17(2):149–54.
15. McGill JW, Reardon RF. Tracheal intubation. In: Roberts JR, Hedges JR, editors. Clinical procedures in emergency medicine. 5th ed. Philadelphia: WB Saunders; 2010.
16. RSI Checklist Sunshine 2013 VIC Western Australia. Available from: www.aci.health.nsw.gov.au/__data/assets/word_doc/0008/249083/RSI_Checklist_Sunshine_2013_VIC_Western_Australia.docx.
17. Weingart SD, Levitan RM. Preoxygenation and prevention of desaturation during emergency airway management. Ann Emerg Med 2012;59(3):165–75.
18. Benumof JL, Dagg R, Benumof R. Critical hemoglobin desaturation will occur before return to unparalyzed state from 1 mg/kg succinylcholine. Anesthesiology 1997;87:979–82.
19. Hopson LR, Schwartz RB. Pharmacological adjuncts to intubation. In: Roberts JR, Hedges JR, editors. Clinical procedures in emergency medicine. 5th ed. Philadelphia: WB Saunders; 2010.
20. Joseph J, DiCorpo J, Rice D, Merlin MA, Weber A. Succinylcholine vs. rocuronium: battle of the RSI paralytics. J Emerg Med Serv 2020. Available from: www jems com/2019/05/13/succinylcholine-vs-rocuronium-battle-of-the-rsi-paralytics/.
21. Dargin J, Medzon R. Emergency department management of the airway in obese adults. Ann Emerg Med 2010;56(2):95–104.
22. Mohammed NY, Di Domenico G, Gambaccini M. Cerebral venous drainage through internal jugular vein. Veins Lymphatics 2019;8(3): doi.org/10.4081/vl.2019.8379.

23. Day MW. Laryngeal mask airway. In: Wiegand DJ, Carlson KK, editors. AACN procedure manual for critical care. 5th ed. St Louis: Saunders; 2005.
24. Howes BW, Wharton NM, Gibbison B, Cook TM. LMA Supreme insertion by novices in manikins and patients. Anaesthesia 2010;65(4):343–7.
25. Zuidema GD, Rutherford RB, Ballinger WF. Management of trauma. 4th ed. Philadelphia: WB Saunders; 1996.
26. Vissers RJ, Bair AE. Surgical airway techniques. In: Walls RM, Murphy MF, editors. Manual of emergency airway management. 3rd ed. Philadelphia: Lippincott Williams & Wilkins; 2008.
27. Hebert RB, Bose S, Mace SE. Cricothyrotomy and transtracheal jet ventilation. In: Roberts JR, Hedges JR, editors. Clinical procedures in emergency medicine. 5th ed. Philadelphia: WB Saunders; 2010.
28. Byrne AL, Bennett M, Chatterji R, Symons R, Pace NL, Thomas PS. Peripheral venous and arterial blood gas analysis in adults: are they comparable? A systematic review and meta-analysis. Respirology 2014;19(2):168–75.
29. Zwerneman K. End-tidal carbon dioxide monitoring: a VITAL sign worth watching. Crit Care Nurs Clin N Am 2006;18(2):217–25, xi.
30. DeBoer S, Seaver M, Arndt K. Verification of endotracheal tube placement: a comparison of confirmation techniques and devices. J Emerg Nurs 2003;29(5):444–50.
31. Manoach S, Paladino L. Manual in-line stabilization for acute airway management of suspected cervical spine injury: historical review and current questions. Ann Emerg Med 2007;50(3):236–45.
32. Maschmann C, Jeppesen E, Rubin MA, Barfod C. New clinical guidelines on the spinal stabilisation of adult trauma patients – consensus and evidence based. Scand J Trauma Resusc Emerg Med 2019;27(1):77.
33. Asha SE, Curtis K, Healy G, Neuhaus L, Tzannes A, Wright K. Neurologic outcomes following the introduction of a policy for using soft cervical collars in suspected traumatic cervical spine injury: a retrospective chart review. Emerg Med Australas 2021;33(1):19–24.
34. Klimke A, Furin M. Pre-hospital immobilisation. In: Roberts JR, Hedges JR, editors. Clinical procedures in emergency medicine. 6th ed. Philadelphia: WB Saunders; 2014.
35. Altman GB, Kerestzes P, Wcisel MA. Fundamental and advanced nursing skills. 3rd ed. New York: Delmar; 2010.
36. Nagler J, Krauss B. Devices for assessing oxygenation and ventilation. In: Roberts JR, Hedges JR, editors. Clinical procedures in emergency medicine. 6th ed. Philadelphia: WB Saunders; 2014.
37. Frakes MA. Measuring end-tidal carbon dioxide: clinical applications and usefulness. Crit Care Nurse 2001;21(5):23–6, 8–35.
38. Aehlert BJ. Airway management. Paramedic practice today. Maryland Heights, Miss: Mosby Elsevier; 2010.
39. Kent B, Dowd B. Assessment, monitoring and diagnostics. In: Elliot D, Aitken LM, Chaboyer W, editors. ACCCN's critical care nursing. Sydney: Mosby; 2007.
40. Moore T. Suctioning techniques for the removal of respiratory secretions. Nurs Stand 2003;18(9):47–53.
41. Pedersen CM, Rosendahl-Nielsen M, Hjermind J, Egerod I. Endotracheal suctioning of the adult intubated patient—what is the evidence. Intens Crit Care Nurs 2009;25(1):21–30.
42. Davey AJ. Medical suction apparatus. In: Davey A, Diba A. Ward's anaesthetic equipment. 6th ed. Elsevier; 2012.
43. Chulay M. Suctioning: endotracheal or tracheostomy tube. In: Wiegand DJ, Carlson KK, editors. AACN procedure manual for critical care. 5th ed. St Louis: WB Saunders; 2005.
44. Darovic G. Hemodynamic monitoring: invasive and noninvasive clinical application. 3rd ed. Philadelphia: WB Saunders; 2002.
45. Woodrow P. Arterial blood gas analysis. Nurs Stand 2004;18(21):45–52.
46. Edwards G. Respiratory emergencies. In: Newberry L, editor. Sheehy's manual of emergency care. 6th ed. St Louis: Mosby; 2005.
47. May JL. Emergency medical procedures. New York: John Wiley & Sons; 1984.
48. Urden LD, Stacy KM, Lough ME, editors. Critical care nursing: diagnosis and management. 6th ed. St Louis: Mosby; 2009.
49. Ahern J, Fildes S, Peters R. A guide to blood gases. Nurs Stand 1995;9(49):50–2.
50. Koran Z, Howard PK. Respiratory emergencies. In: Newberry L, editor. Sheehy's emergency nursing: principles and practice. 5th ed. St Louis: Mosby; 2003.
51. Urden LD, Stacy KM, Lough ME, editors. Thelan's critical care nursing: diagnosis and management. 4th ed. St Louis: Mosby; 2003.
52. Urden LD, Stacy KM, Lough ME, editor. Thelan's critical care nursing: diagnosis and management. 5th ed. St Louis: Mosby; 2006.
53. Vincent JL, Abraham E, Moore FA. Textbook of critical care. 6th ed. Philadelphia: WB Saunders; 2011.
54. Kelly AM, McAlpine R, Kyle E. Venous pH can safely replace arterial pH in the initial evaluation of patients in the emergency department. Emerg Med J 2001;18(5):340–2.
55. Malatesha G, Singh NK, Bharija A, Rehani B, Goel A. Comparison of arterial and venous pH, bicarbonate, PCO2 and PO2 in initial emergency department assessment. Emerg Med J 2007;24(8):569–71.
56. Bochicchio GV, Joshi M, Bochicchio KM, Pyle A, Johnson SB, Meyer W, et al. Early hyperglycemic control is important in critically injured trauma patients. J Trauma Nurs 2007;63(6):1353–8.
57. Allen DA, Baranoski S, Barron VE, editors. Lippincott's nursing procedures. 5th ed. Philadelphia: Lippincott Williams & Wilkins; 2008.
58. Kirsch TD, Sax J. Tube thoracostomy. In: Roberts JR, Hedges JR, editors. Clinical procedures in emergency medicine. 6th ed. Philadelphia: WB Saunders; 2014.

59. Johns DP, Pierce R. Pocket guide to spirometry. Sydney: McGraw-Hill; 2005.
60. Johns DP, Pierce R. Spirometry: the measure and interpretation of ventilatory function in clinical practice. The Thoracic Society of Australia and New Zealand; 2008.
61. Booker R. Simple spirometry measurement. Nurs Stand 2008;22(32):35–9.
62. Friedman HH. Diagnostic electrocardiography and vectorcardiography. In: Reich DL, Kaplan J, editors. Essentials of cardiac anesthesia. Elsevier; 2008.
63. Drew BJ, Califf RM, Funk M, Kaufman ES, Krucoff MW, Laks MM, et al. Practice standards for electrocardiographic monitoring in hospital settings: an American Heart Association scientific statement from the Councils on Cardiovascular Nursing, Clinical Cardiology, and Cardiovascular Disease in the Young: endorsed by the International Society of Computerized Electrocardiology and the American Association of Critical-Care Nurses. Circulation 2004;110(17):2721–46.
64. Besseman ES. Emergency cardiac pacing. In: Roberts JR, Hedges JR, editors. Clinical procedures in emergency medicine. 6th ed. Philadelphia: WB Saunders; 2014.
65. Link MS, Atkins DL, Passman RS, Halperin HR, Samson RA, White RD, et al. Part 6: electrical therapies: automated external defibrillators, defibrillation, cardioversion, and pacing: 2010 American Heart Association guidelines for cardiopulmonary resuscitation and emergency cardiovascular care. Circulation 2010;122(18 Suppl. 3):S706–19.
66. Kelly EM. Temporary transcutaneous (external) pacing. 5th ed. Philadelphia: WB Saunders; 2005.
67. Gibson T. A practical guide to external cardiac pacing. Nurs Stand 2008;22(20):45–8.
68. Hatchett R, Thompson D, editors. Cardiac nursing: a comprehensive guide. Edinburgh: Churchill Livingstone; 2002.
69. Woods SL, Sivarajan-Froelicher ES, Halpenny CJ. Cardiac nursing. 4th ed. Philadelphia: Lippincott; 2000.
70. The Joanna Briggs Institute. Best practice: evidence-based practice information sheets for the health professionals. Management of peripheral intravascular devices. 21998. p. 1–6.
71. Potter PA, Perry AG. Fundamentals of nursing. 5th ed. St Louis: Mosby; 2001.
72. Tintinalli JE, Kelen GD, Stapczynski JS, editors. Emergency medicine: a comprehensive study guide. 6th ed. New York: McGraw-Hill; 2004.
73. Liu SW, Zane R. Peripheral intravenous access. In: Roberts JR, Hedges JR, editors. Roberts and Hedges' clinical procedures in emergency medicine. 6th ed. Philadelphia: WB Saunders; 2014.
74. Queensland Health Central Zone. Venepuncture and peripheral intravenous cannulation. Queensland: Queensland Government; 2004.
75. Dolan B, Holt L. Accident and emergency theory into practice. Edinburgh: Baillière Tindall; 2000.
76. Lander JA, Weltman BJ. Topical anaesthetics (EMLA and AMETOP creams) for reduction of pain during needle insertion in children (Protocol). Cochrane Database Syst Rev 2002:4.
77. MIMS Online. [Accessed February 2018].
78. Andreoni C. Paediatric emergencies. In: Sheehy SB, editor. Sheehy's manual of emergency care. 6th ed. St Louis: Mosby; 2005.
79. Duff AJ. Incorporating psychological approaches into routine paediatric venepuncture. Arch Dis Child 2003;88(10):931–7.
80. Fenwick R. Intraosseous approach to vascular access in adult resuscitation. Emerg Nurse 2010;18(4):22–5.
81. Infusion Nurses Society. The role of the registered nurse in the insertion of intraosseous access devices. J Infus Nurs 2009;32(4):187–8.
82. Deitch K. Intraosseous infusion. 6th ed. Philadelphia: WB Saunders; 2014.
83. McCarthy G, O'Donnell C, O'Brien M. Successful intraosseous infusion in the critically ill patient does not require a medullary cavity. Resuscitation 2003;56(2):183–6.
84. Vidacare. EZ-IO needle sets. Directions for use. Available from: www.vidacare.com/.
85. Celinski SA, Seneff MG. Arterial line placement and care. 6th ed. Philadelphia: Lippincott Williams & Wilkins; 2008.
86. Garretson S. Haemodynamic monitoring: arterial catheters. Nurs Stand 2005;19(31):55–64.
87. Becker DE. Arterial catheter insertion (perform). 5th ed. St Louis: WB Saunders; 2005.
88. Daily EK, Schroeder JS, editors. Techniques in bedside hemodynamic monitoring. 5th ed. St Louis: Mosby; 1994.
89. Scales K. Central venous pressure monitoring in clinical practice. Nurs Stand 2010;24(29):49–55.
90. Shaffer RB. Blood sampling from an arterial catheter. 5th ed. St Louis: WB Saunders; 2005.
91. Woodrow P. Arterial catheters: promoting safe clinical practice. Nursing Stand 2009;24(4):35–40.
92. McNeil C, Rezaie S, Adams BD. Central venous catheterization and central venous pressure monitoring. 6th ed. Philadelphia: WB Saunders; 2014.
93. Arrow International. Central venous catheter: nursing care. Guideline. 1996.
94. Munro N. Central venous catheter insertion (assist). In: Wiegand DJ, Carlson KK, editors. AACN procedure manual for critical care. 5th ed. St Louis: WB Saunders; 2005.
95. Woodrow P. Central venous catheters and central venous pressure. Nurs Stand 2002;16(26):45–51.
96. Munro N. Central venous/right atrial pressure monitoring. In: Wiegand DJ, Carlson KK, editors. AACN procedure manual for critical care. 5th ed. St Louis: WB Saunders; 2005.
97. Assal M, Crevoisier X. [Entorse aigue de la cheville: quelle immobilisation?] Acute ankle sprain: which immobilization. Rev Med Suisse 2009;5(212):1551–4.

98. Lewis SM, Heitkemper MM, Dirksen SR. Medical-surgical nursing: assessment and management of clinical problems. 5th ed. St Louis: Mosby; 2000.
99. Australian Resuscitation Council. Envenomation. Pressure immobilisation technique. Revised policy statement: guideline 8912005.
100. Canale E, Isbister GK, Currie BJ. Investigating pressure bandaging for snakebite in a simulated setting: bandage type, training and the effect of transport. Emerg Med Australas 2009;21(3):184–90.
101. Engels PT, Passos E, Beckett AN, Doyle JD, Tien HC. IV access in bleeding trauma patients: a performance review. Injury 2013;45(1):77–82.
102. Marx JA, Hockberger RS, Walls RM. Rosen's emergency medicine. 8th ed. Philadelphia: Saunders; 2014.
103. Roberts JR. Chapter 34, Roberts and Hedges' clinical procedures in emergency medicine. 6th ed. Philadelphia: Saunders; 2014.
104. Geeraedts Jr LM, Kaasjager HA, van Vugt AB, Frölke JP. Exsanguination in trauma: a review of diagnostics and treatment options. Injury 2009;40(1):11–20.
105. Roberts JR. Intravenous regional anesthesia. 6th ed. Philadelphia: WB Saunders; 2014.
106. Solomon L, Warwick D, Nayagam S. Apley's concise system of orthopaedics and fractures. 3rd ed. London: Arnold; 2005.
107. Simon RR, Sherman SC, Koenigsknecht SJ. Emergency orthopedics: the extremities. 5th ed. New York: McGraw-Hill; 2006.
108. Olson SA. An instructional course lecture, the American Academy of Orthopedic Surgeons. J Bone Joint Surg Am 1996;78(9):1428–37.
109. Landry PS, Marino AA, Sadasivan KK, Albright JA. Effect of soft-tissue trauma on the early periosteal response of bone to injury. J Trauma 2000;48(3):479–83.
110. Altizer L. Casting for immobilization. Orthoped Nurs 2004;23(2):136–41.
111. Howard PK, Steinmann RA. Sheehy's emergency nursing: Principles and practice. 6th ed. St Louis: Mosby; 2009.
112. Chudnofsky CR. Splinting techniques. 6th ed. Philadelphia: WB Saunders; 2014.
113. Walsh D, Caraceni AT, Fainsinger R, Foley K. Palliative medicine. Philadelphia: WB Saunders; 2008.
114. McRae PJ, Bendall JC, Madigan V, Middleton PM. Paramedic-performed fascia iliaca compartment block for femoral fractures: a controlled trial. J Emerg Med 2015;48(5):581–9.
115. Cole A. Nurse-administered femoral nerve block after hip fracture. Nurs Times 2005;101(37):34–6.
116. Ardery G, Herr K, Hannon BJ, Titler MG, editors. Lack of opioid administration in older hip fracture patients. Mosby; 2003.
117. Wong J, Wong S, Brooks E. A study of hospital recovery pattern of acutely confused older patients following hip surgery. J Orthopaed Nurs 2002;6:68–78.
118. Willson H. Factors affecting the administration of analgesia to patients following repair of a fractured hip. J Adv Nurs 2000;31(5):1145–54.
119. Finlayson BJ, Underhill TJ. Femoral nerve block for analgesia in fractures of the femoral neck. Arch Emerg Med 1988;5(3):173–6.
120. Stella J, Ellis R, Sprivulis P. Nerve stimulator-assisted femoral nerve block in the emergency department. Emerg Med Australas 2000;12:322–5.
121. Fernandez DL, Palmer AK. Fractures of the distal radius. 5th ed. Philadelphia: Churchill Livingstone; 2005.
122. Fletcher AK, Rigby AS, Heyes FL. Three-in-one femoral nerve block as analgesia for fractured neck of femur in the emergency department: a randomized, controlled trial. Ann Emerg Med 2003;41(2):227–33.
123. Foss NB, Kristensen BB, Bundgaard M, Bak M, Heiring C, Virkelyst C, et al. Fascia iliaca compartment blockade for acute pain control in hip fracture patients: a randomized, placebo-controlled trial. Anesthesiology 2007;106(4):773–8.
124. Agency for Clincial Innovation (ACI). Fascia Iliaca block guide. 2022. Online. Available from: aci.health.nsw.gov.au/__data/assets/pdf_file/0004/285592/ACI-Fascia-iliaca-block-guide.pdf.
125. Neuraxiom. Ultrasound guided regional nerve blocks. 2015. Available from: www.neuraxiom.com/.
126. MIMS. MIMS Online Ropivacaine Medication Information. 2021. Available from: www.mimsonline.com.au.acs.hcn.com.au/Search/QuickSearch.aspx?ModuleName=Product%20Info&searchKeyword=+Ropivacaine+Kabi+Solution+for+injection.
127. Weinberg GL. Treatment of local anesthetic systemic toxicity (LAST). Reg Anesthes Pain Med 2010;35(2):188–93.
128. Australia TG. Dosing local anaesthetics for acute pain management. 2021. Available from: tgldcdp.tg.org.au.acs.hcn.com.au/viewTopic?topicfile=local-anaesthetics-acute-pain-management&guidelineName=Pain%20and%20Analgesia#toc_d1e56.
129. Emergency Care Institute, NSW. Anaesthesia Fascia-iliaca block. Online. Available from: aci.health.nsw.gov.au/networks/eci/clinical/procedures/procedures/554382.
130. Fleisher LA, Gaiser R, editors. Anaesthetic procedures consult. Philadelphia: Elsevier; 2011.
131. Drake R, Vogl AW, Mitchell AWM, Tibbitts R, Richardson P. Gray's atlas of anatomy. Philadelphia: Churchill Livingstone/Elsevier; 2008.
132. Waldman SD. Atlas of interventional pain management. 4th ed. Philadelphia: WB Saunders; 2015.
133. Kelly J, Spektor M. Nerve blocks of the thorax and extremities. In: Roberts JR, Hedges JR, editors. Roberts and Hedges' clinical procedures in emergency medicine. 5th ed. Philadelphia: WB Saunders; 2010.
134. Murphy-Lavoie H, Legros TL. Local and regional anaesthesia. 2nd ed. Philadelphia: Saunders; 2008.
135. Australian Medicines Handbook. Adapted from Table 2-3 Comparison of local anaesthetics. Richmond: Hyde Park Press; 2019:33.
136. Emiley P, Schreier S, Pryor P. Hematoma blocks for reduction of distal radius fractions. Emerg Phys Month 2012;9:16–17.
137. Miller M, Hart J, MacKnight J. Essential orthopaedics, III–III. Philadelphia: Saunders; 2010.

138. Browner B, Fuller R. Musculoskeletal emergencies: Elsevier; 2012.
139. Green DP, Hotchkiss RN, Pederson WC, Kozin SH, Cohen MS. Green's operative hand surgery. 5th ed. Philadelphia: Churchill Livingstone; 2005.
140. Stone DB, Scordino D. Foreign body removal. 6th ed. Philadelphia: WB Saunders; 2014.
141. Allergy ASoCIa. Tick allergy. 2019. Available from: www.allergy.org.au/ticks.
142. Brinker D, Hancox JD, Bernardon SO. Assessment and initial treatment of lacerations, mammalian bites, and insect stings. AACN Clin Issue 2003;14(4):401–10.
143. Cooper MA, Lindsay GM, Kinn S, Swann IJ. Evaluating emergency nurse practitioner services: a randomized controlled trial. J Adv Nurs 2002;40(6):721–30.
144. Meeker MH, Rothrock JC. Alexander's care of the patient in surgery. 11th ed. St Louis: Mosby; 1999.
145. Swanson NA, Tromovitch TA. Suture materials, 1980s: properties, uses, and abuses. Int J Dermatol 1982;21(7):373–8.
146. Feliciano DV, Moore EE, Mattox KL, editors. Trauma. 3rd ed. Stamford: Appleton & Lange; 1996.
147. Carley S. Glue is better than sutures for facial lacerations in children. 2001.
148. Yanoff M, Duker JS, editors. Ophthalmology. 3rd ed. St Louis: Mosby; 2008.
149. Knoop KJ, Dennis WR. Opthalmologic procedures. 6th ed. Philadelphia: WB Saunders; 2014.
150. Riordan-Eva P, Whitcher JP, editors. Vaughan and Asbury's general opthalmology. 17th ed. New York: McGraw-Hill; 2007.

CHAPTER 17
MINOR INJURY AND MANAGEMENT

MATTHEW LUTZE AND NATASHA JENNINGS

ESSENTIALS

- Practising a systematic approach to patient assessment helps to avoid missing injuries. Look, feel and move is the standard approach used to assess all injury presentations.
- Proper wound cleansing is the key to minimising infection.
- Listen to the patient as they describe the mechanism of injury, as this will lead you to the most likely diagnosis.

INTRODUCTION

Although the exact percentage of minor injuries is not well documented in Australia and New Zealand, patients with minor musculoskeletal limb injuries represent a reasonable portion of workload for clinicians in various clinical settings. One in four (25%, or just over 2.0 million) presentations to Australian public hospital emergency departments (EDs) in 2018–19 was due to an injury.[1] Six of the top 20 presentations to EDs were injury related—injury unspecified, open wound head, open wound hand/wrist, fractures at wrist and hand, dislocations/sprains at ankle/foot. The broad term 'minor musculoskeletal limb injury' is also not clearly defined and requires strong history-taking and focused assessment skills to ensure quality patient care. Typically, patients with minor musculoskeletal injuries have traditionally waited the longest time for treatment, when often, with a clear diagnostic pathway, their total treatment time could indeed be very short. Many ambulance services and EDs have recognised this and have implemented additional streaming measures, extended care paramedic roles and nurse practitioners.[2–7] To expedite patient management, these patients are often filtered into a separate queue and area of the ED after triage. Many EDs now use a mixed workforce model specifically trained to manage the care of these patients.[3,8] A growing number of EDs employ nurse practitioners and musculoskeletal physiotherapists and there is good evidence to support higher patient satisfaction levels for people with fast-track conditions.[2–5,8–14]

PRE-HOSPITAL CARE

Initial out-of-hospital care for people with minor injuries follows the same principles of primary and secondary assessment. As for all patients, assessment should be guided by the systematic process of assessing for danger and patient responsiveness, and shouting for assistance where indicated. Assessment begins with DRSABCD—**D**anger (remove patient from danger), **R**esponse (check for response if patient is alert or unconscious), **S**end for help (call 000 in Australia and 111 in New Zealand if needed), **A**irway (check for obstructions to airway), **B**reathing (check if patient is breathing), **C**PR (commence CPR if necessary), **D**efibrillation (source and apply defibrillation if needed).

A systematic approach of examining from 'head to toe' ensures all injuries are identified and need not be time-consuming. Minor injuries can often occur concurrently with other, more significant injuries and risk being overlooked. Patient history should be used to guide assessment; some injuries are clearly isolated; for example, a crush injury to a digit. A mechanical fall onto an outstretched hand may injure any structure of the upper limb and can potentially cause injury elsewhere.

Some patients with an isolated minor injury may not present to a hospital setting, depending on patient preference for care or geographical location. If a suitably qualified and experienced clinician is available (e.g. nurse practitioner, physiotherapist or extended care paramedic), some injuries may be managed in the field and hospital care may not be required.

INITIAL ASSESSMENT

After obtaining a history of the mechanism of injury, approach assessment using the structure of 'look', 'feel' and 'move' for a focused assessment (Box 17.1). Remove clothes, cutting them off if necessary to expose the whole limb. If a fracture is suspected, moving the injured limb may not be appropriate; however, it may be diagnostic to do so; for example, pain on elbow pronation and inability to fully extend the joint helping to diagnose a fracture of the radial head, prior to x-ray.

BOX 17.1 ASSESSMENT OF MUSCULOSKELETAL INJURIES

INSPECT

- Deformity
- Swelling
- Bruising
- Skin perfusion at the site and distal to the injury
- Location and type of any wounds
- Comparison with the other limb

PALPATE

- Crepitus
- Bony tenderness
- Skin temperature
- Distal pulses
- Altered sensation distal to injury

MOVE

- *If appropriate:* gentle active range of movement

This structure can be implemented in any setting; at triage or wherever patient assessment takes place.

PRACTICE TIP

Some patients with multiple minor injuries may be at higher risk for major trauma (e.g. older patients). Consider using a modified assessment approach if major trauma is suspected—see Chapter 42 Major trauma initial assessment and management.

IMMEDIATE PRACTICAL CARE

Immediate interventions for all patients with minor musculoskeletal injuries include the following comfort measures to enhance patient management. Cover all wounds with a clean or ideally sterile dressing and apply pressure if the wound is bleeding. Grossly contaminated wounds can be irrigated with clean tap water, if available and time allows, by simply pouring copious amounts of water onto the wound. In the pre-hospital setting, mechanical irrigation with clean drinking water will aid in the removal of debris and contaminants, reduce microbial contamination and serve to reduce infection risk. Bacteria begin multiplying in as little as 6 hours in contaminated wounds. If the wound is left contaminated, an infection can establish itself within 24 hours.[15]

Consider splinting, particularly if a fracture is suspected (see Chapter 16 for splinting techniques). By minimising movement, the bone ends are less likely to cause further damage to nerves, vessels and other soft tissues and will prevent a closed fracture from becoming compound. Obvious deformity can be gently corrected to as normal anatomical positioning as possible. The distal pulses should be assessed before and after reduction or splinting, and regularly until definitive care is provided.

Elevate the limb to reduce swelling, which may compromise neurovascular status and increase pain. A sling may be useful for upper limb trauma. The acronym RICE (Rest, Ice, Compression, Elevation)[16] is a well-known approach for treating soft-tissue injuries and joint sprains, and may offer some symptomatic relief for the patient. However, a systematic review of RICE therapy for ankle sprains reveals there is limited randomised controlled trial data supporting its use. Applying ice for a period of 20 minutes every 1–2 hours has been demonstrated to reduce pain.[17] An ice pack can be simply made by wrapping a pack of frozen peas or corn kernels in a damp towel; this conforms to the joint shape.

In the field of sports medicine, recent opinions on the management of acute soft tissue injuries suggest that joint protection and encouragement of early, gentle mobilisation may be more beneficial to recovery. The acronym POLICE (**P**rotection, **O**ptimal **L**oading, **I**ce, **C**ompression, **E**levation) is being discussed as a replacement for the acronym of RICE, although more recent commentary suggests soft tissues injuries should be managed using 'PEACE and LOVE' (**P**rotection, **E**levation, **A**void anti-inflammatories, **C**ompression, **E**ducation, and **L**oad, **O**ptimism, **V**ascularisation, **E**xercise).[15,18–20] Provision of oral, inhalational or intravenous analgesia may reduce pain and anxiety.[21]

A SYSTEMATIC APPROACH TO INJURY ASSESSMENT

Minor injury assessment may take place as part of a secondary survey, or in some cases as a focused examination. It is valuable to adopt a methodical examination process, which in due course becomes routine for the clinician.[22] Remember, a clear history and mechanism of injury will often aid in the process. A systematic approach is suggested below.

INSPECTION—'LOOK'

Observe for deformity and asymmetry (comparison to the other limb where possible), local swelling, joint effusion, contusions (bruising), open wounds and their location over underlying structures, likely and actual foreign bodies and contamination of wounds. Assess distal perfusion.

PALPATION—'FEEL'

Is there generalised tenderness or point tenderness indicating a possible underlying structural injury? Assess for bony crepitus, palpable malalignment, soft tissue swelling and joint instability. Assess distal neurovascular sensation status.

MOVEMENT—'MOVE'

Consider testing movement of a limb or joint gently prior to x-ray, if it will help with possible diagnosis.

Be cautious where there is significant swelling, deformity, or where movement exacerbates pain considerably. Assess for normal distal nerve motor function. Range of movement may be best tested after radiological examination results are known and may yield better results, particularly once a fracture has been excluded and pain has been addressed. Anatomical terms of motion are described in Box 17.2.

BOX 17.2 ANATOMICAL TERMS OF MOTION

Flexion: a reduction in angle between two body parts.
Extension: an increase in angle between two body parts.
Internal rotation: rotation of body part towards the midline axis of body.
External rotation: rotation of body part away from the midline axis of body.
Abduction: moving of body part away from midline axis of body, spreading the fingers.
Adduction: moving of body part towards the midline axis of body, or closing the fingers together.
Supination: rotation of forearm or ankle inwards, so that palms of hand/soles of feet turn upwards.
Pronation: rotation of forearm or ankle outwards, so that palms of hand/soles of feet turn downwards.
Inversion: (ankle/foot) tilting of the foot towards the midline of body.
Eversion: (ankle/foot) tilting of the foot away from the midline of body.
Dorsiflexion: where the foot is moved towards the shin.
Plantarflexion: where the foot is moved away from the shin, i.e. standing on tiptoes.
Opposition: touching the tip of the index and thumb together to form a circle shape.

Documenting the patient's range of motion in degrees for a particular body area is a useful way of recording current joint movement. This can be used to judge improvement or deterioration in condition. For example, a knee is considered to be at 0° when it is fully extended and at approximately 135° at full flexion.

INJURIES SURROUNDING THE SHOULDER

ANATOMY AND FUNCTION

The bones of the shoulder, humerus, clavicle, acromion, scapula and sternum form the articulating bony structure of the shoulder complex. It comprises the sternoclavicular, the acromioclavicular and the 'ball and socket' glenohumeral joints, which in combination attach the upper limb to the scapula and sternum. The shoulder has a wide range of movement and is stabilised by many muscles, ligaments and tendons. The humeral head is held into the glenoid by the four rotator cuff muscles. Blood is supplied to the arm via two branches from the axillary artery, the anterior and posterior circumflex arteries. The axillary nerve curls around the humeral neck, clinically important in injuries to this area, and the three main nerves of the arm, the median, radial and ulnar, all pass through the axilla. Anatomy of the shoulder can be found in Fig. 17.1.

PATIENT ASSESSMENT

If any neck movement causes or increases pain in the shoulder, the assessment should be ceased and cervical spine assessment should be undertaken. The shoulder is also predisposed to inflammatory and degenerative changes which may limit a person's range of movement. This needs to be taken into consideration during assessment of the ageing population.

FIGURE 17.1 ANATOMY OF THE SHOULDER[23]

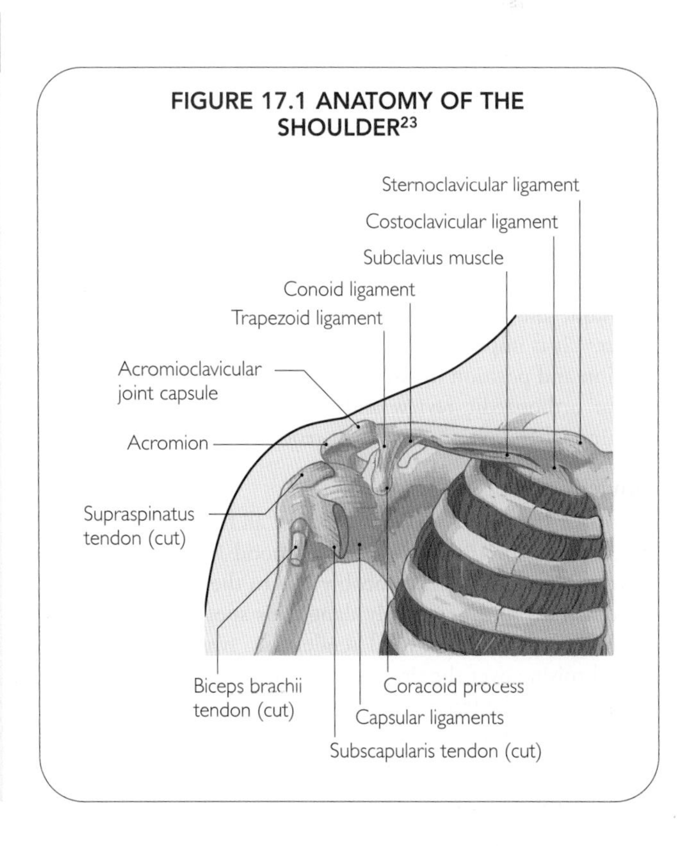

Look. Usually, the injury will be accompanied by swelling, deformity and focal tenderness. Compare the appearance with that of the other shoulder. A patient with an empty glenoid on clinical examination, a slightly externally rotated arm and severe pain is likely to have a shoulder dislocation and should be managed as soon as possible (see Chapter 48). There may be open wounds and/or bruising if the presentation is delayed.

Feel. Palpation should begin with the cervical spine and then include the entire clavicle, acromioclavicular joint, humeral head, neck and shaft to the elbow and wrist. Fractures to the scapula, which usually require a significant mechanism, should be excluded by palpating for bony tenderness. Axillary nerve function is assessed specifically by testing sensation over the deltoid muscle in comparison with the other arm. A palpable radial pulse should also be recorded.

Move. If the patient is able, they can be asked to perform gentle passive shoulder movements to assess range of movement. The drop arm test is used to assess rotator cuff tears and the horizontal flexion test to assess an acromioclavicular sprain.

COMMON INJURIES AROUND THE SHOULDER

Shoulder dislocations

Shoulder dislocations are a common injury from a fall onto an outstretched hand with rotation of the arm. There may have been pull on the arm or a blow to the anterior or posterior aspect of the arm to cause the head of the humerus to be forced anterior or posteriorly. Anterior dislocations are most common with the humerus head displacing forwards, down and medially from the glenoid cavity of the scapula. Previous episodes of dislocation predispose patients to recurrences with the slightest injury.

Patients usually present with their arm held internally rotated against their body and in severe pain. A hollow may be visually observed under the acromion or a palpable gap or asymmetry of the shoulder when comparing both shoulders. It is important to assess the patient's sensations on the lateral deltoid to assess for any injury to the axilla nerve.

X-ray of the shoulder will determine fracture of the humerus or glenoid rim and demonstrated dislocation. There are several methods for reduction dependent on the direction of the dislocation. The most common techniques currently used are either the Cunningham Shoulder technique or the Spaso technique and need to be performed by an experienced practitioner.[24] It is important to assess neurovascular supply after reduction and position in adduction in a broad arm sling. Referral for orthopaedic review and physiotherapy is required for ongoing rehabilitation to prevent reoccurrence.

Clavicle

Clavicular fractures constitute 2–5% of all fractures; they comprise more than 10–15% of all childhood fractures. They are more common in males, probably due to their involvement in more contact and potentially dangerous sports and traffic accidents.[17,25–27] There is focal tenderness, swelling and sometimes bruising over the site and pain on movement of the arm. The skin over the fracture site should be assessed and a referral made to an orthopaedic specialist if skin integrity is at risk, or the fracture is compound. Fractures are generally easily identified on x-ray.

There remains some controversy regarding the indications and value of surgical fixation of displaced mid-clavicular fractures. In Australia, these injuries are increasingly being managed surgically, but most often are treated conservatively in a broad arm sling and mobilised as pain allows (see Chapter 16 for instructions on this technique).[28,29]

Acromioclavicular joint

A sprain of the acromioclavicular joint (ACJ) is common after a blow or fall onto the shoulder, elbow or outstretched hand. A dislocation of the ACJ is rare. There will be focal tenderness and swelling over the ACJ. Try not to confuse a prominent ACJ with a shoulder dislocation, as the deformity seen can occasionally be quite striking. X-rays should be requested specifically of the ACJ, and comparative views of the other shoulder may be provided. The diagnosis is both clinical and radiological. A sprain may damage the ACJ ligaments, but the clavicle remains in contact with the acromion. Treatment consists of a broad arm sling and rest for 4–6 weeks. In more severe injuries, there is separation of the clavicle from the acromion as the trapezoid and coracoid ligaments are torn. These injuries are more likely to be unstable and the patient should be referred for a specialist orthopaedic opinion.

Proximal humerus

Injuries to the proximal humerus are usually as a result of a direct blow or a direct fall onto the shoulder and/or a fall onto the outstretched hand. Some 70% of fractures to the humeral head and neck are seen in the over-60 age group, usually following a fall onto an outstretched hand. Like fractures of the hip, they are a major cause of morbidity in the older person,[30] and osteoporosis may be a contributing factor. As in all falls, particularly in the ageing person, the cause must be established and other injuries excluded. The patient will have pain around the shoulder and restricted range of movement, and often deformity and swelling. If the presentation is delayed, there is often marked bruising around the upper arm and sometimes chest wall. Axillary nerve function should be assessed. Extra-articular fractures that are relatively undisplaced can be treated conservatively in a close-fitting support sling that minimises movement. Fracture or dislocation of the humeral head should be referred on for orthopaedic opinion. Humeral shaft fractures are again often treated conservatively unless they are open or unstable.

INJURIES SURROUNDING THE ELBOW, FOREARM AND WRIST

ANATOMY AND FUNCTION

The synovial hinge joint of the elbow consists of the distal humerus, proximal radius and proximal ulna. They are held in position by ligaments and the associated musculature. The elbow can be flexed and extended, and the forearm pronated and supinated (a rotational movement of the forearm at the radioulnar joint). The elbow has an organised pattern of growth dependent on age and can complicate x-ray interpretation by the unskilled practitioner. The wrist is comprised of a series of joints that are very mobile, particularly between the proximal and distal rows of the carpal bones, allowing a wide range of movement in several planes (Fig. 17.2). The complex ligamentous structure can be easily injured during trauma, particularly in a fall onto the hand.

FIGURE 17.2 ANATOMY OF THE WRIST[23]

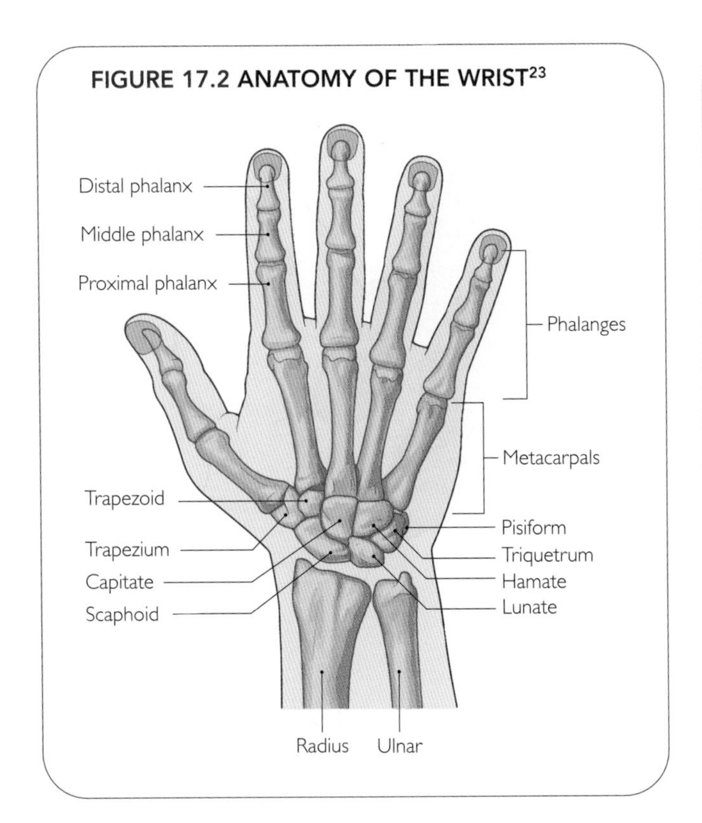

FIGURE 17.3 FAT PAD—A JOINT EFFUSION INDICATING A LIKELY FRACTURE

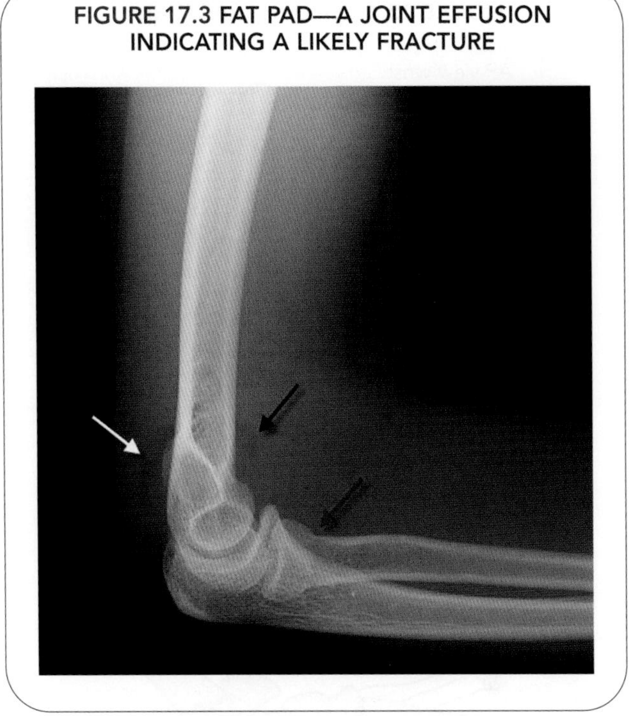

The median, radial and ulnar nerves all travel through the volar wrist (the median nerve passing through the carpal tunnel) and allow the hand and wrist to function and innervate the skin. The radial and ulnar arteries provide the hand with blood and are both palpable on the volar aspect of the wrist.

PATIENT ASSESSMENT

Mechanism of injury is of particular importance and requires a focused examination for injuries surrounding the elbow and wrist. Falls onto the outstretched hand can provide forces that may damage any part of the upper limb. Examination begins by using the acute musculoskeletal approach.

Look. Usually, the injury will be accompanied by likely swelling, deformity and focal tenderness. Compare the appearance with that of the other arm. There may be open wounds and/or bruising if the presentation is delayed.

Feel. Palpation should continue to the wrist and hand. Identify and palpate the distal radius, ulnar styloid and the scaphoid bone (Fig. 17.3). Be alert not to miss a scaphoid fracture in a patient with a swollen wrist after a fall onto the hand with normal x-rays, and take care to differentiate between a scaphoid facture, a Bennett's fracture and a fracture of the distal radius by careful methodical palpation of each. A palpable radial pulse should also be recorded.

Move. Examination should begin with gross movement of the shoulder to exclude injury here. The humerus can then be palpated down to the elbow region, examining for bony tenderness over the medial and lateral epicondyles, the olecranon and the radial head. It is unusual for the elbow or wrist to be swollen without a fracture being present.

In the absence of deformity, and if pain allows, gentle active range of movement at the elbow can be assessed. The 'elbow extension test' can be utilised. The patient is asked to extend both arms with the hands supinated. A UK study found that if patients could fully extend both elbows, the negative prediction for fracture was 98% in adults and 96% for children and is a useful adjunct in the assessment of traumatic elbow injuries.[31] Pain on gentle supination and pronation of the forearm is also a common finding in fractures of the radial head and neck.

X-ray requests depend on the area of tenderness. If there is only elbow tenderness, elbow x-rays alone will suffice. Look carefully for a positive anterior and/or posterior fat pad or 'sail sign' (Fig. 17.4) on the lateral elbow radiograph demonstrating a joint effusion. A posterior fat pad is indicative of a fracture in 90% of elbow injuries radiologically investigated, even if the bony anatomy and cortex appear normal.[33–35] Forearm views include the elbow and forearm, while scaphoid views include the wrist, so this does not need to be requested separately.

COMMON INJURIES AROUND THE ELBOW

Distal humerus

A fracture of the distal third of the humerus or supracondylar fracture is a common injury in childhood and occurs more infrequently in adults, following a fall onto the hand. Significantly displaced fractures pose a risk to neurovascular integrity and should be referred urgently. Excessive swelling may occlude the brachial artery and the radial pulse should be monitored frequently. However, many supracondylar fractures are undisplaced or only identifiable on x-rays by a positive fat pad sign. These are generally treated in a plaster of Paris (POP) above-elbow cast or a 'collar and cuff' sling with hyperflexion of the elbow, depending on local practice.

FIGURE 17.4 COLLES' FRACTURE[32]

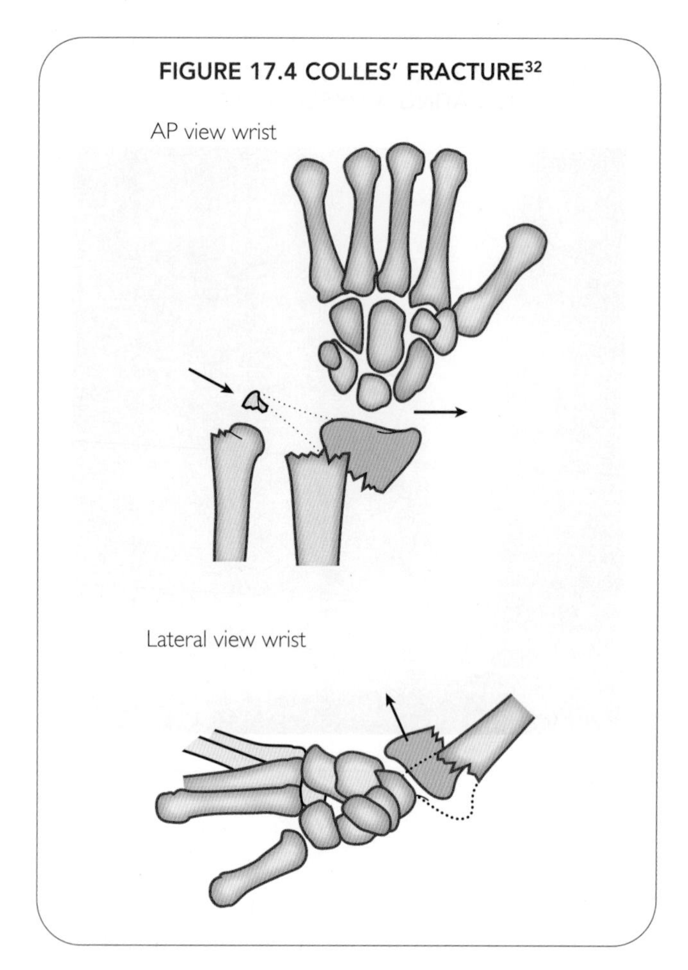

FIGURE 17.5 SCAPHOID TENDERNESS[35]

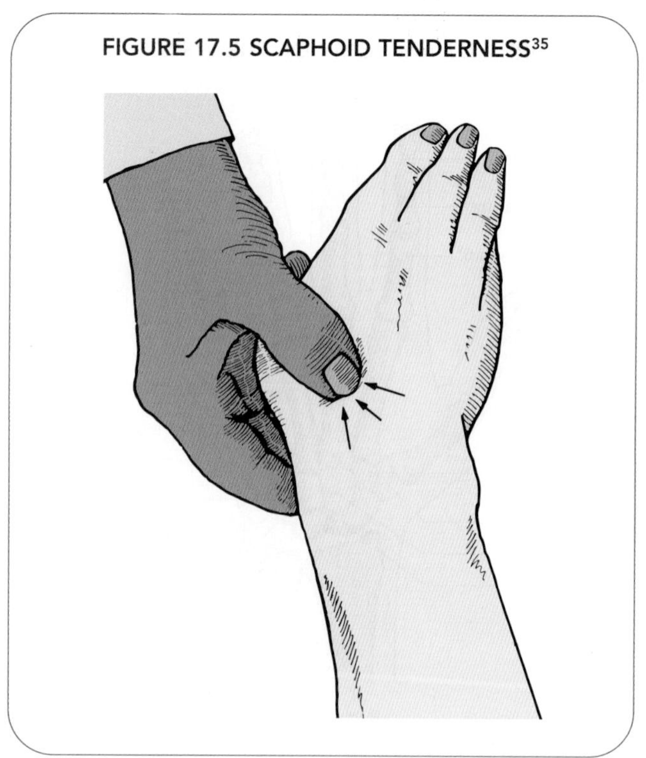

Olecranon

The olecranon can be fractured from a fall directly onto the point of the elbow, and treatment is dependent on the degree of displacement. Undisplaced fractures can be treated again with a broad arm sling, ice and analgesia. Triceps contraction may displace the fracture, which then needs surgical fixation.

Elbow dislocation is seen in both the adult and the paediatric population, and is generally identified clinically by significant pain and deformity at the elbow following a fall onto the hand. Careful neurovascular assessment should be made before and after relocation, which usually requires a general anaesthetic. Post-reduction x-rays should be reviewed to identify associated fractures, such as a medial epicondyle avulsion in a child.

Proximal radius and ulna

The radial head and neck can both be fractured, causing pain and swelling around the elbow. The patient will generally find pronation and supination painful and will have a limited ability to fully extend the elbow. X-rays may show a fracture and/or a positive fat pad sign. Treatment consists of a broad arm sling, ice and analgesia. Some patients may be unable to pronate and supinate, and this may indicate a significant displacement of the radial head fracture fragment and warrant orthopaedic review.

Distal radius and ulna

The ulna and radius can be fractured in isolation, especially if there is a direct blow to the forearm. However, the bones are bound together at both ends by ligaments forming a type of linked parallelogram[35] and therefore it is most common for both bones to break. If there is an angulated fracture of either the radius or the ulna, the bone must become shorter in length, and it is vital to exclude dislocation at one end of the other forearm bone. It is imperative, as previously discussed, for both the joint above and that below an injury to be examined. A Monteggia injury involves a fracture of the ulna with dislocation of the radial head. Conversely, a Galeazzi fracture–dislocation involves a fracture of the radius with dislocation of the radioulnar joint at the wrist. Both require surgical reduction.

One-third of all fractures in older adults will involve the wrist, particularly older osteoporotic women.[36] It is also the most common fracture site in children,[37] with the incidence increasing with age and in boys. A Colles' fracture is a fracture of the distal radius within 2.5 cm of the wrist (Fig. 17.5).[38] With greater force the distal fragment becomes dorsally angulated, leading to the clinical deformity typical of the fracture, which is likened to a dinner fork. There may be an associated fracture of the ulnar styloid. The forearm can be immobilised with a POP splint for comfort while x-rays are taken.

The need for reduction depends on the degree of angulation and the age, frailness and usual activities of the patient. Methods of anaesthesia for reduction of the fracture vary depending on the facilities available, and include general anaesthetic, intravenous regional anaesthesia block, known as a Bier block, and local infiltration of the fracture itself, known as a haematoma block. Bier block, which provides regional anaesthesia, has been well validated for safety and effect;[39] however, resuscitation facilities should be available. Haematoma block effectiveness may vary with individual patients and the technique and expertise of the clinician, but is a technically easy and relatively safe procedure in areas where facilities are limited.[40]

A reverse Colles' fracture, known as a Smith's fracture, is occasionally seen after a fall onto the back of the hand. Here, the distal fragment is displaced anteriorly and usually requires surgical manipulation to correct it.

Scaphoid

The scaphoid bone is the largest carpal bone and a fracture to it is usually the result of a fall onto an outstretched hand.[41] The scaphoid primarily receives blood supply from the distal pole, so a fracture through the scaphoid body could disrupt blood supply to the proximal pole and lead to avascular necrosis. This can cause significant morbidity through hand disability; hence scaphoid injuries should not be overlooked.[41] Clinically the patient will have scaphoid tenderness and often subtle swelling over the anatomical snuffbox when compared with the other hand (see Fig. 17.3). Scaphoid fractures are one of the most commonly missed fractures. It is estimated that 30% or more scaphoid fractures are missed through initial x-ray imaging.[41] This may be partially attributed to clinicians not identifying the exact location of the scaphoid on examination, and also to the difficulty of absolute diagnosis of a fracture at the initial consultation as x-rays are often normal.

For suspected occult scaphoid fractures, further imaging through MRI (magnetic resonance imaging), CT (computed tomography) or bone scan is required, although there is no consensus as to which modality is best.[42] MRI has been shown to be more sensitive for both scaphoid and concurrent occult carpal bone injuries, where CT has been shown to be more useful in monitoring scaphoid bone healing.[41,42] A CT exam is less expensive and more easily accessible than MRI in Australia. Bone scans, completed four or more days after the injury, is a third option for imaging, but require a higher radiation dose and are not able to isolate a specific injury, rather the region of injury, and thus are used less frequently.

Early diagnosis and treatment of scaphoid fractures reducing the risk of non-union result in better patient outcomes through maximising post-injury function. For the patient, early treatment results in less time spent in a cast, less impact on daily activities and, for patients employed, less time off work. Confirmed and suspected scaphoid fractures are placed in a scaphoid cast for immobilisation, which should allow full movement of the finger metacarpophalangeal joints. Displaced fractures may need surgical fixation.

PRACTICE TIP

To locate the scaphoid bone, first locate the base of the radial styloid and the base of the thumb. The anatomical snuff box, which overlies the scaphoid, is between these two points. Palpate over the scaphoid of both hands simultaneously and push the thumb up towards the wrist (telescoping) to identify tenderness.

INJURIES SURROUNDING THE WRIST AND ELBOW IN CHILDREN

Children's fracture patterns vary from those of adults due to increased bone compliance and lower bone density. The bone frequently bends or buckles and a pattern of incomplete fractures is seen. A greenstick fracture involves a break in one bone cortex, while the opposite cortex remains intact. They can vary from obvious clinical deformity and radiological angulation to subtle injuries where the child has few clinical signs of injury and mild pain which restricts use of the arm. Some greenstick fractures are so slight that parents may only seek advice after a few days of subtle symptoms. A torus fracture is also a frequently seen paediatric injury, where x-rays show a compression deformity to the bone surface with the appearance of a bump or ripple to the cortex. Management in a correctly sized wrist splint for 3 weeks is adequate for torus injuries.[43] Both greenstick and torus fractures heal rapidly.

The young skeleton contains many physes, or 'growth plates' at one or both ends of the bone, where proliferation of cartilage cell growth with eventual differentiation into osteocytes occurs. Simply, bone manufacture occurs here and injuries involving the physis can affect subsequent bone growth. These are known as Salter Harris injuries, named by Robert B Salter and W Robert Harris in 1963. Injuries of and around the physis are stratified into five parts of the Salter Harris classification system, with the higher number correlating to poorer outcomes.[44] The management varies and depends on ensuring the epiphyseal surface is restored to promote ongoing cell manufacture.

Pulled elbow

Toddlers may present with a sudden onset of pain and reluctance to move an arm after a traction or pulling type mechanism. The child has no swelling or no bony tenderness, but forearm pronation is painful. In this injury, known as a 'pulled elbow', the radial head becomes subluxed and can be relocated by the simple manoeuvre of either extending the elbow and supinating the forearm or flexing the elbow and pronating the forearm. Either technique can be attempted, as studies to date have not shown either technique to be more effective.[45] If the clinician's thumb is placed over the radial head, a click is usually felt with successful relocation. Relocation is usually painful, but instantly relieving for the child, who quickly starts using the arm again. X-rays are not normally indicated where there is a good history (a clearly understood mechanism of injury) and after successful reduction with clinician-observed return to normal function.

INJURIES SURROUNDING THE HAND AND DIGITS

ANATOMY AND FUNCTION

The hand is an intricate structure with complex motor and sensory functions. An injury to the hand may interrupt any number of structures, which could in turn affect the ability to perform basic functions and potentially affect a patient's livelihood. Many injuries to the hand are associated with open wounds; this will be discussed further in the chapter.

The eight carpal bones, which facilitate movement of the hand and wrist, form two rows that articulate proximally with the distal radius and ulna and distally with the metacarpals. The largest carpal bone is the scaphoid. There are five metacarpals corresponding respectively with each finger and the thumb. The digits should be correctly termed thumb, index, middle, ring and little finger (see Fig. 17.2). Movement of the digits is controlled by four muscle groups, which flex and extend the metacarpal joints and the interphalangeal joints. The back of the hand is known as the dorsal surface and the front as the palmar or volar surface. Sensation is supplied by the median, radial and ulnar nerves leading to the digital nerves in each digit.

PATIENT ASSESSMENT

Determining the mechanism of injury is important to identify potential injuries. A fall onto an outstretched hand will involve a different injury pattern to that of direct trauma, such as a crush or punch injury.

Look. Observe for swelling, deformity and distal perfusion of the digits. Bruising, especially on the palm, often suggests a metacarpal fracture, and bruising over the volar surface of a finger joint is common after an avulsion fracture. Note the location of any wounds and their cause; for example, a bite injury which may be associated with a tendon injury (see the section on Hand and digit wounds later in the chapter).

Feel. Palpate systematically from the clavicle, if indicated, and ending with the digits.

Move. Gently test active movement of the hand by asking the patient to make a fist. Watch for finger rotation, where the nail orientation appears to be different to that of other fingers, as the fingers are gently flexed into a fist. Where possible, comparison with the other hand/digits should be performed as rotation can be subtle. If rotation is noted, this may identify a displaced fracture. A fixed interphalangeal joint with obvious deformity is probably dislocated.

X-ray requests should be specific and based on careful clinical evaluation. Carpal and metacarpal tenderness warrants hand x-rays. For suspected digit fractures and dislocations, ask for views of the specific digit and always obtain a lateral x-ray. Dislocations and, in particular, small avulsion injuries, may be seen on the volar surface of an interphalangeal joint, and can be overlooked if the lateral is not studied carefully.

PRACTICE TIP

If a patient is to be transported to another facility for x-ray or specialist review, the injured hand should be immobilised in a cast in the 'position of safety'. The cast should hold the wrist in extension, the metacarpal joints in flexion at 90° and the fingers extended straight (see Fig. 17.6).

FIGURE 17.6 POSITION OF SAFETY FOR IMMOBILISING AN INJURED HAND (POSI)

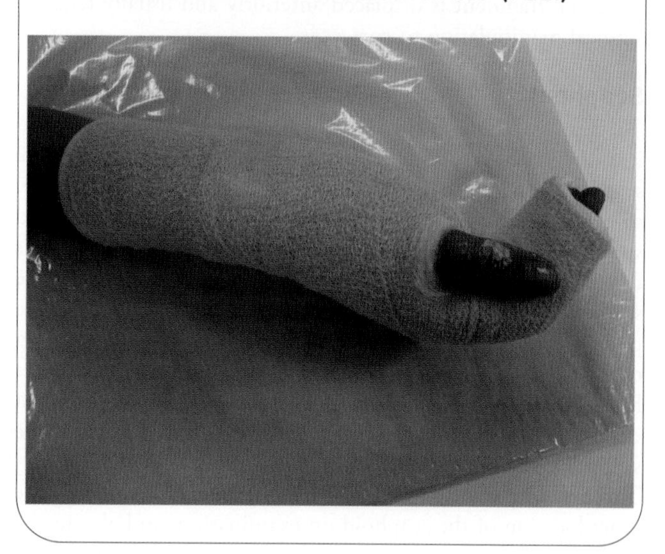

COMMON INJURIES SURROUNDING THE HAND AND DIGITS

All hand injuries should be considered significant; incorrect treatment may cause ongoing pain and limitation of future hand use, which may impact on daily activities and occupational capabilities. For many patients, referral to a hand specialist may be needed, but this will depend on the patient's preference, services available and the experience of the clinician managing the patient.

Metacarpals

Metacarpal fractures are common and may be sustained following a fall onto the hand, crush mechanisms and punch injuries.[46] Check for finger rotation, as this indicates an angulated fracture, which may need reduction and fixation. The clinician should observe for corresponding wounds associated with a fracture and consider any potential damage to nerves and tendons.

A 'boxer's' fracture is one that occurs to the base of the fifth metacarpal, usually following a blow to the knuckles with a clenched fist. Patients may be reluctant to admit the exact mechanism. Unless the fracture is significantly angulated, or there is finger rotation, treatment with a cast or neighbour strapping with soft wrap is satisfactory.[47]

A Bennett's fracture/dislocation occurs at the base of the thumb metacarpal after a fall onto the fist or the hand with the thumb abducted or outstretched, such as a skier falling while holding a ski pole. When the fracture is comminuted, it is referred to as a Rolando fracture and is more difficult to treat.[48] The base of the metacarpal becomes subluxed and needs surgical fixation. The ligaments that secure the thumb metacarpal at the first metacarpal–phalangeal joint can also be damaged by a similar mechanism; specifically, the ulnar collateral ligament on the ulna aspect of the joint can be sprained or torn. There may also be a fracture. Test for instability by passive stressing of the joint with the metacarpophalangeal (MCP) flexed to 30 degrees. Any instability requires plaster immobilisation and a surgical opinion from a hand specialist.

Phalanges

A mallet finger occurs when a straight finger sustains a blow to the end, flexing the distal interphalangeal joint. The extensor tendon is torn from its attachment and the patient presents with a flexion deformity at the distal interphalangeal joint. Patients are usually unable to actively extend or straighten the fingertip and there is sometimes an associated fracture. Treatment involves a mallet splint for 6–8 weeks which holds the finger extended. The patient can remove the splint for washing the finger only if the finger is held strictly in extension by pressing the fingertip against a hard surface.

Digits can be dislocated following a hyperextension type injury, which is usually identified by clinical deformity. If there

FIGURE 17.7 OPEN DISLOCATION IN THE LITTLE FINGER

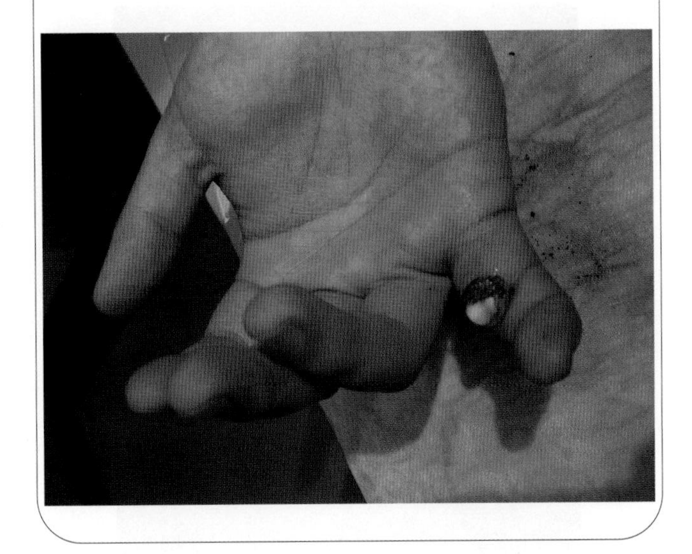

FIGURE 17.8 ANATOMY OF THE KNEE[23]

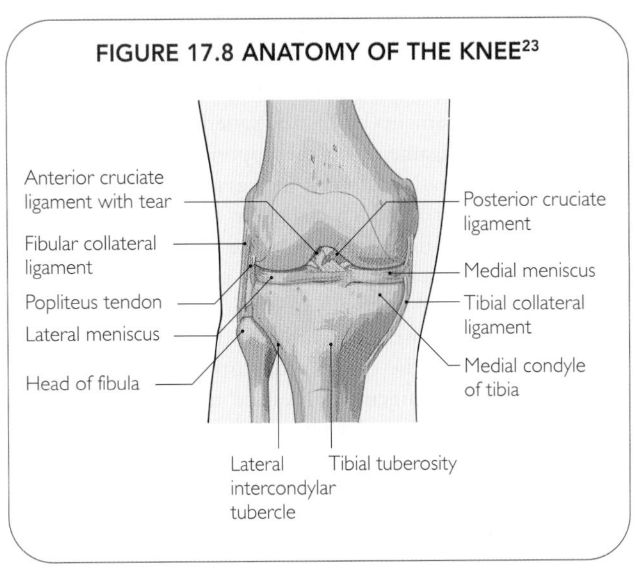

is a wound overlying the dislocation, it is considered an open dislocation (Fig. 17.7). These injuries should be reduced urgently, but will also need to be referred for surgical washout.[49]

Reduction after x-ray can be performed using an inhalational anxiolytic, such as nitrous oxide (e.g. Entonox), or by using a digital nerve block. Care should be taken to identify any fractures, particularly small avulsion fractures, with a post-reduction x-ray. Fingers should be buddy-strapped to the adjacent digit for 2 weeks and the thumb post-dislocation should be splinted.

LOWER LIMB INJURIES

ANATOMY AND FUNCTION

The knee is a large weight-bearing joint where stability of the distal femur, proximal tibia, fibula and the patella are provided by a complex of tendons, ligaments, muscles and the menisci.

The patella is attached proximally to the quadriceps tendon and distally by the patella tendon, which inserts into the tibial tuberosity. The strong medial and lateral collateral ligaments (MCL and LCL) are situated along the inside and outside of the knee and provide stability from lateral stresses. The anterior (ACL) and posterior (PCL) cruciate ligaments provide stability to the knee from rotational forces and run from the femoral condyles to the tibial spines. The menisci lie between the tibial and femoral condyles and function as cushions during articulation (Fig. 17.8). Blood supply to the knee is complex, provided by the popliteal artery, among others.

PATIENT ASSESSMENT

An acutely injured knee is often too painful to fully complete a systematic focused examination. In these cases, careful consideration of the exact mechanism of injury can be of great value in narrowing your differential diagnoses. Try to ascertain the position of their knee at the time of the injury, whether this was sustained through contact or non-contact, if twisting was involved or whether a 'pop' was described. Ask the patient about whether their knee 'gives way' or 'buckles' and whether they have had any previous serious knee injuries (e.g. ruptured cruciate ligament, patella dislocation or meniscal tear). Immediate inability to weight-bear usually signifies a more serious injury.

Look: Observation and the speed of onset of any effusion (swelling over the entire knee joint) may help to distinguish a significant ligamentous or bony injury. Try to distinguish local swelling over a particular structure (e.g. the patella) from a joint effusion (diffuse suprapatellar region swelling). Note any deformity, particularly to the patella as this may indicate a fracture or dislocation. Where possible, always use the other knee for comparison as swelling and deformities can be subtle.

Feel: Palpate all bony landmarks for tenderness including the patella, fibula head and the medial and collateral ligaments. Remember to check the hip and ankle for associated proximal and distal injuries. Remember to check neurovascular status, particularly to the foot and ankle.

Move: The extensor mechanism is tested by asking the patient to lift the leg with a straight knee (straight leg raise) or by having the patient demonstrate they can 'kick'. Examine the patient for active and passive range of movement.

PRACTICE TIP

Consider combining your movement examination and applying the Ottawa rules to determine if the patient requires an x-ray (Box 17.3).

BOX 17.3 THE OTTAWA KNEE RULES[50,51]

- Age 55 years or older
- Tenderness at head of fibula
- Isolated tenderness of patella
- Inability to flex knee to 90°
- Inability to walk four weight-bearing steps immediately after the injury and in the ED.

LIGAMENTOUS INJURIES OF THE KNEE

A force striking the side of the knee while weight-bearing can cause injury to the medial collateral ligament (MCL) or the lateral collateral ligament (LCL). The patient usually experiences an injury to the ligaments on the opposite side to which the force occurred. Rotational forces, such as twisting the knee with a stationary foot or a sudden change in direction can tear the cruciate ligaments, most commonly the anterior cruciate ligament (ACL). A patient may describe a 'pop' at the time of the injury and a haemarthrosis with an effusion may be seen as soon as 2–6 hours, but most often within 48 hours. This pattern of injury usually alerts the clinician to suspect an ACL injury.[52] Posterior cruciate ligament injuries are usually from a direct blow to the proximal anterior tibia.

Look: The patient may have some local swelling or an associated joint effusion or a deformity.

Feel: Lateral and medial collateral ligamentous injuries typically produce focal tenderness over the area of injury. Cruciate ligamentous injuries may be globally tender without a specific area of focal tenderness.

Move: In acute injuries there is usually pain on passive stressing of the joint. There should be an obvious endpoint at full stretch of the ligament (medial collateral or lateral collateral); if not, assume a complete tear. In acute injuries, this may be difficult to determine.

Management: If the patient meets the Ottawa knee rules (see Box 17.3) an x-ray should be obtained to exclude a bony injury. Stable soft tissue injuries are usually treated conservatively, and crutches may be needed. If the knee is unstable on examination, an orthopaedic opinion should be sought as surgical repair may be indicated.

Suspected cruciate ligament injuries can be initially treated with an ice pack to reduce pain and crutches to aid mobilising for short periods. Meniscal tears similarly can occur in patients with twisting of the knee while weight-bearing. Patients with significant meniscal tears often describe a sensation of 'locking' or 'giving way', and they are often worsened by squatting or turning.

Patella dislocation

Patella dislocation may occur following sudden muscle contraction or a blow to the medial side of the knee (Fig. 17.9).[35] Dislocation may be recurrent, and is more common in young teenage girls who have ligamentous laxity.[53] Relocation is usually spontaneous as the patient extends their knee; however, occasionally these will need to be reduced. This can usually be achieved by applying gentle lateral pressure to the patella while the knee is extended. Inhalational analgesia such as nitrous oxide is useful for this procedure. The knee should be splinted post-reduction and the patient referred for orthopaedic follow-up.

FIGURE 17.9 DISLOCATED PATELLA

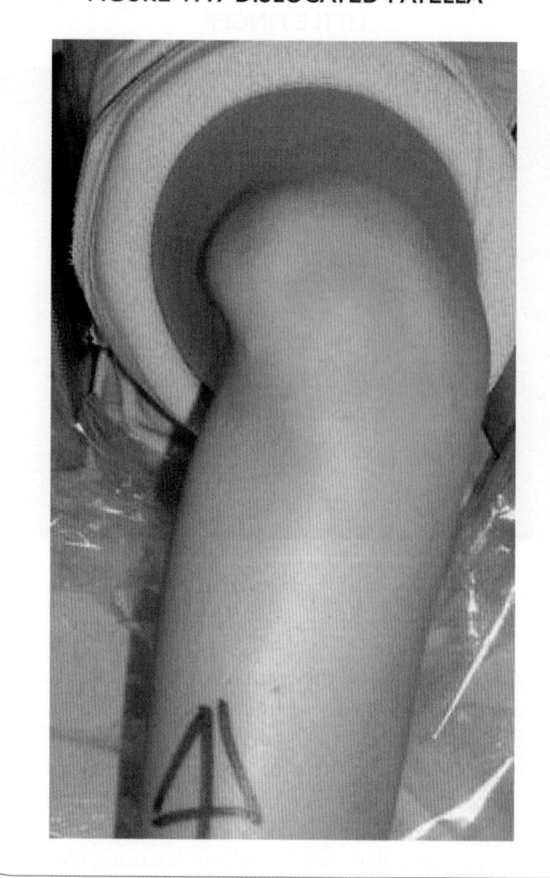

Extensor mechanism injuries

Both the quadriceps and the patella tendons can be ruptured by forcible contraction of the quadriceps; check for a more proximal patella than usual, indicating a quadriceps tendon rupture. These injuries are more common in older patients. There may be a palpable defect to the quadriceps tendon. Patella tendon rupture is common in the young athlete. In both cases, the patient is usually unable to perform a straight leg raise or a kick test, indicating the need for surgical repair and referral to an orthopaedic surgeon.

An avulsion fracture of the tibial tuberosity is commonly seen in male adolescents where a sudden contraction of the quadriceps tendon avulses the insertion site on the anterior tibia. This injury also causes an inability to straighten the knee and requires orthopaedic opinion.

FRACTURES AROUND THE KNEE

The patella may be fractured by a direct fall or blow to the knee. There will be local swelling and tenderness and the patient will find it difficult to mobilise or extend their lower leg. Always check ability to straight-leg raise. Transverse fractures that affect the ability to straight-leg raise will need surgical fixation. Longitudinal or vertical fractures can mostly be treated conservatively.[54]

The tibial plateau may also be fractured by a direct blow or fall onto the knee. The patient will have great difficulty weight-bearing and there will be considerable swelling and localised bony tenderness. Following x-ray, a CT scan is often required to identify the extent of the injury or for surgical planning.[55] The patient should be referred for orthopaedic review as surgery is often required to restore bony alignment of the articulating surface and joint function.

THE LOWER LEG, ANKLE AND FOOT

ANATOMY AND FUNCTION

The tibia and fibula provide the bony structure to the lower leg for movement and weight-bearing. The fibula head can be located just distal to the lateral aspect of the knee joint, ending distally at the lateral malleolus. The tibia extends close to the skin at the shin, ending at the medial malleolus at the medial aspect of the ankle. Here the articulation with the talus forms the mortise of the ankle joint with stability and articulation provided by the medial deltoid ligament and lateral anterior talofibular, calcaneal fibular and posterior talofibular ligaments. The anatomical landmarks provided by the medial and lateral malleoli are important for assessing bony tenderness and deciding on x-ray imaging (e.g. Ottawa foot and ankle rules see Box 17.4, 17.5 and Fig. 17.10).

The foot creates a surface for weight-bearing and is composed of the hind foot, including the calcaneus and talus, the mid foot and its complex ligamentous structure, the metatarsal bones and the toe phalanges, known as the forefoot.

The muscles of the lower leg are contained in individual fascial compartments, along with the tibial and common peroneal nerves, which are susceptible to increasing pressure from swelling and bleeding after injury.

PATIENT ASSESSMENT

Ask the patient to describe how the injury occurred to elicit the likely injury mechanism. The most common ankle injury is usually sustained from an inversion mechanism where the ankle and foot twists inwards towards the midline of their body. A deformity with neurovascular compromise requires immediate

BOX 17.4 THE OTTAWA ANKLE RULES

X-rays are only required if there is any pain in the malleolar zone and *any one* of the following:

- **bone tenderness along the distal 6 cm of the posterior edge of the tibia or the tip of the medial malleolus**
- **bone tenderness along the distal 6 cm of the posterior edge of the fibula or tip of the lateral malleolus**
- **an inability to bear weight both immediately and in the ED for four steps.**

BOX 17.5 THE OTTAWA FOOT RULES

X-rays are only required if there is any pain in the midfoot zone and *any one* of the following:

- **bone tenderness at the base of the fifth metatarsal (for foot injuries)**
- **bone tenderness at the navicular bone (for foot injuries)**
- **an inability to bear weight both immediately and in the ED for four steps.**

FIGURE 17.10 OTTAWA ANKLE AND FOOT LANDMARKS[56]

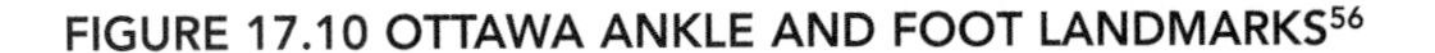
Lateral view
Medial view
Malleolar zone
Mid-foot zone
A Posterior edge or tip of lateral malleolus – 6 cm
B Posterior edge or tip of lateral malleolus – 6 cm
C Base of fifth metatarsal
D Navicular
A series of ankle x-ray films is required only if there is any pain in malleolar zone and any of these findings:
• Bone tenderness at A
• Bone tenderness at B
• Inability to bear weight both immediately and in emergency department
A series of ankle x-ray films is required only if there is any pain in midfoot zone and any of these findings:
• Bone tenderness at C
• Bone tenderness at D
• Inability to bear weight both immediately and in emergency department

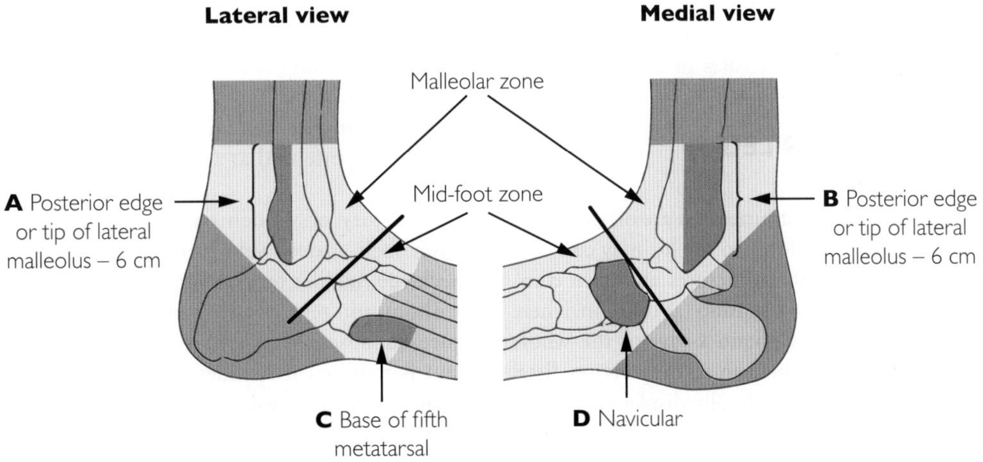

reduction and splintage, often with intravenous pain relief, if available. The primary aim is to restore near normal anatomy and neurovascular status.

Look: Observe for deformity and other signs of injury. Compare the injured site to the opposite limb to appreciate swelling and deformities. Observe the colour of the foot for pallor and vascular supply. Look for wounds and cover suspected compound fractures with a sterile dressing where possible.

Feel: Regularly assess distal circulation by palpation of the dorsalis pedis, palpated over the dorsum of the foot usually just lateral to the base of the first metatarsal and/or the tibialis posterior pulse, which is found just behind the medial malleolus. Systematically palpate the lower leg for bony tenderness, using the mechanism as a guide for potential injury. Also palpate over the ankle ligaments to determine if there is ligamentous injury, not forgetting the calcaneum, mid and forefoot and Achilles, as indicated.

Move: Assess the patient's ability to bear weight. A patient is considered to be weight-bearing if they can take four or more steps on examination. There may be limited range of movement in the acute phase of an ankle or foot injury.

Depending on the site of tenderness and suspected injury, x-ray examination can be undertaken. X-rays of the tibia and fibula will include the ankle; if an isolated ankle fracture is suspected, request an ankle x-ray alone. It is unusual in a simple inversion injury to need to obtain an image of the foot and ankle together, and a systematic, thorough examination should elicit the area of focal tenderness.

In isolated inversion-type ankle injuries in adults, a decision over whether to x-ray the ankle or foot to determine the presence of a fracture may be based on the Ottawa ankle and foot rules.[57]

These rules have an accuracy of nearly 100% for excluding a fracture and have reduced the number of ankle x-rays requested by 30–40%,[56] reducing patient and clinician time and saving hospital resources. Several studies have also positively evaluated the Ottawa ankle and foot rules in children over 6 years of age, with a sensitivity rate of 98.5%.[58]

INJURIES TO THE LOWER LEG

Tibia and fibula fractures

These are commonly encountered injuries and are often sports-related. A blow or rotational-type force to the leg may cause an isolated tibia or fibula fracture. Shaft fractures are often compound, as the bone is near to the skin surface at the shin. There may be clinical deformity. Always obtain x-rays of the whole length of the tibia and fibula to exclude an accompanying distal injury with a proximal fracture.[35] Minimally displaced isolated shaft fractures may be treated in an above-knee plaster back slab or splint. Angulated fractures need referral to the orthopaedic service as these often need to be corrected to avoid longterm complications involving the knee and ankle after they have healed.[30]

Always consider a toddler's fracture (Fig. 17.11) in small children who are reluctant to weight-bear following a relatively minor fall. These children may sustain a subtle undisplaced fracture of the tibia, or a greenstick fracture which can usually be managed in a long leg cast.

Compartment syndrome is a serious potential risk following fractures of the tibia and fibula and should be considered in all patients with increasing pain and a tense, swollen limb; this is discussed further in Chapter 48.

FIGURE 17.11 TODDLER'S FRACTURE

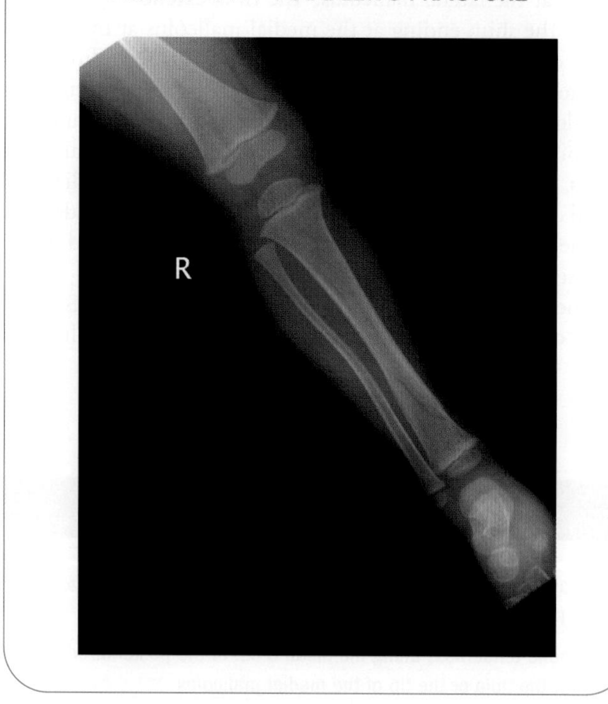

Torn calf muscle

Calf muscle tears mostly occur in the gastrocnemius muscle, primarily the medial head of the calf muscle.[59] Most commonly, this injury occurs during weight-bearing activity where the ankle joint is placed under plantar flexion load and is often sports-related.[60] The patient reports sudden severe pain in the calf, often likening it to being hit or shot in the leg. There is tenderness over the upper calf and walking is very painful. Soleus muscle injuries can also occur but are less common and are normally experienced as a gradual onset from repetitive use or strain.

A history of sudden pain should aid in ruling out other causes such as deep vein thrombosis or a Baker's cyst. Always check the Achilles tendon is intact by performing a Simmonds or Thompson test (presence of plantar flexion when the calf is squeezed, absent if it is ruptured). Referral to an orthopaedic team is required if Achilles tendon rupture is suspected. Calf strain treatment consists of ice, elevation and early mobilisation, where a heeled shoe may be helpful.

Pre-tibial lacerations

Pre-tibial lacerations are common, particularly in older persons. They are often the result of a fall and a thorough assessment should be conducted to exclude other injuries and establish the underlying cause of the fall. The anterior aspect of the tibia has minimal subcutaneous tissue, and as a result pre-tibial lacerations have limited vascular supply and can often expose the surface of the tibia. These wounds are commonly managed conservatively with dressings and referred for skin grafting if the wound fails to heal. Some recent studies have found that early intervention using a split skin graft can significantly reduce healing time of pre-tibial wounds. Regardless of whether these wounds are managed conservatively or surgically, early treatment is key to optimising healing.[61]

Wounds of the lower limb are often slower to heal due to the nature of their vascular supply. For elderly people, the normal physiological changes of ageing, including changes in skin integrity and lower limb vasculature, prolonged healing, comorbidities, polypharmacy and often immobility, further exacerbate poor healing. Pre-tibial lacerations in elderly people are often slow to heal and may not completely heal, often resulting in ulcers and chronic lower limb wounds.

Management includes thorough irrigation. Where possible, the flap of skin should be softened with gauze soaked in normal saline and stretched back over the wound to provide wound coverage. For specific management of pre-tibial wounds, see the wound management and skin tear sections later in the chapter. Integral to optimal healing of lower limb injuries is the application of compression bandaging to the entire lower limb in appropriate patients with no arterial vascular disease to maximise venous return (see Chapter 16 for compression bandaging techniques).

INJURIES AROUND THE ANKLE AND FOOT

Most commonly, the ankle is injured by an inversion mechanism, where the foot is inverted inwards towards the midline. The injury is likely to be on the lateral aspect, injuring the lateral ankle ligaments and sometimes causing a fracture of the distal fibula or the base of the fifth metatarsal of the foot. Ankle injury can also be sustained less frequently by eversion mechanism, where the foot turns outwards. Ligamentous and possible bony injuries can occur on the medial aspect. Greater force often causes more severe ligamentous and bony injuries to both the medial and lateral ankle/foot.

Fractures of the ankle

Ankle fractures may involve one, two or three malleoli. Single, relatively undisplaced fractures of the distal fibula below the level of the ankle mortise may be treated in a non-weight-bearing cast or, increasingly commonly, in a walking cast boot. Distal fibula fractures that extend from the level of the mortise or above the mortise are unstable and may need internal fixation. This is particularly likely if there is tenderness around the medial malleolus, or a medial malleolar fracture is present. Talar tilt or shift, where the normal alignment of the talar mortise is displaced, should be corrected, usually under general anaesthesia, and signifies significant disruption to the ligamentous and bony stability of the ankle.[62]

Ankle dislocation

Where there is obvious deformity to the ankle and a malpositioned foot, relocation is urgently required. The vascular supply to the skin and distal tissues is often compromised and the injury may be open. Patients will require analgesia and/or procedural sedation to facilitate reduction. Obtaining initial x-rays to confirm the joint is dislocated should not delay the reduction and the lower leg should be placed in a below-knee POP backslab for stabilisation. X-rays can then be requested and most (but not all) patients will have evidence of bi-malleolar ankle fractures (the lateral and medial malleoli). All ankle dislocations result in significant ligamentous injuries. Operative management is usually required by the orthopaedic team for definitive treatment.

Ankle sprains

Ankle sprains are one of the most common musculoskeletal injuries sustained through sporting activities with approximately 80% making a full recovery.[17,63]

Localised swelling and focal tenderness over the anterior talofibular ligament and no bony tenderness (see Ottawa ankle rules Box 17.4) is diagnostic of a ligamentous injury, comprising 85% of all ankle injuries.

Treatment for ankle sprains remains varied and dependent on the severity of the sprain, the functional needs of the patient and the resources available. Traditionally, the initial treatment of ankle sprains has been Rest, Ice, Compression and Elevation (RICE). However, a systematic review of RICE therapy for ankle sprains reveals there is limited randomised controlled trial data supporting its use.[17] Despite this, RICE therapy continues to be the initial treatment of choice for most ankle sprains.

Sprains to the ankle can be graded depending on severity and treatment is often based around these gradings.

- *Simple sprain, grade 1*—simple inversion injury, tenderness and swelling over anterior talofibular ligament; patient can weight-bear. Treat with 2 days of rest, with gradual return to mobilisation. Compression can be achieved with elastic soft brace, or ankle tape-strapping, although taping may result in localised skin reaction or breach of the skin on tape removal for some patients.[64]
- *Moderate sprain, grade 2*—inability to weight-bear, marked swelling, tenderness over both the lateral and the medial ligaments. These injuries can be treated as for grade 1; however, several studies have shown benefit of a semi-rigid brace.[65] Patients may also require crutches for a short period of time. A review by a physiotherapist should be recommended.
- *Severe sprain, grade 3*—severe mechanism, inability to weight-bear, marked bimalleolar swelling, clinical or radiological evidence of effusion and signs of ankle instability (although instability is difficult to establish after an acute injury).

These injuries are very painful and there is evidence that a short period of immobilisation, either in a POP below-knee backslab or a more practical air-cast brace, leads to a more rapid recovery at 3 months post-injury. These injuries should be reviewed, depending on the resources available, by the original clinician, an orthopaedic specialist or a physiotherapist to further assess stability. Considering one-third of people will develop some degree of instability after lateral ankle sprain,[66] early referral to a physiotherapist, where available, may be prudent, especially in athletic or older populations.

Achilles tendon rupture

Achilles tendon rupture often occurs during sport when there is a sudden dorsiflexion of the foot. The patient recalls a sudden snapping sensation, pain in the back of the heel and difficulty walking normally. They will be unable to stand on tiptoes. There is a palpable gap on palpation of the tendon. The Simmonds or Thompson test is used to diagnose a complete

Achilles rupture reliably.[67] The patient lies face down with their feet hanging over the edge of the bed and the examiner squeezes the mid-calf region. The test is positive if there is no plantar flexion of the foot.

There is no clear consensus to support surgical versus non-surgical treatment for Achilles tendon rupture, each having its own risk and benefit profiles. Treatment is based on a case-by-case basis, which considers such issues as need/ability to weight-bear quickly, time to full recovery, risk of re-rupture, postoperative wound complications and surgeons' preference.[67] The final decision is one that is made between the consulting orthopaedic surgeon and the patient.

Fractures of the calcaneum

Calcaneus fractures are mostly caused by falling or jumping from a height and is an injury more frequently seen in men than in women.

Fracture of the lumbar spine occurs in 5% of patients with a calcaneal fracture,[68] and should be carefully excluded. There is marked swelling around the heel and it will be tender on palpation. The patient will be unable to walk. Calcaneal x-rays will include an axial view, where the foot is viewed from behind. Operative and non-operative management options depend on the type of fracture and the degree of displacement, and may need to be confirmed with CT scan.

Lisfranc injuries of the midfoot

The Lisfranc ligament provides bony stability to the tarsal–metatarsal area of the midfoot. The midfoot is critical for stabilising the arch and in walking. Any injury to the midfoot that results in a fracture and/or displacement of the tarsometatarsal joints is known as a Lisfranc injury.

A Lisfranc injury can result from a direct crush injury to the foot or from a fall where uneven forces are applied to the midfoot region. The patient usually has significant swelling and tenderness over the midfoot and often is unable to weight-bear. The dorsalis pedis (DP) pulse may be difficult to palpate through swollen tissues; however, other clinical neurovascular findings or a bedside doppler ultrasound can be used to confirm DP pulse.

Lisfranc injuries are easily missed as the abnormality on x-ray can be subtle. Check for normal alignment of the second metatarsal base with the intermediate cuneiform on the anteroposterior foot x-ray and for displacement on the lateral films. There may also be accompanying metatarsal fractures. Beware of the non-weight-bearing patient with significant clinical signs of a midfoot injury and seemingly normal x-rays. Many patients require CT scanning to completely appreciate the injury.[69] Displaced or unstable Lisfranc injuries require an orthopaedic referral for consideration of operative management. Missed or inappropriately managed Lisfranc injuries can result in persistent pain, activity limitations and arthritis in the involved joints.[70]

Metatarsal fractures

An avulsion fracture to the base of the fifth metatarsal commonly follows an inversion injury, as the insertion of the peroneus brevis tendon avulses the bone after sudden contraction. Palpation of the base of the fifth metatarsal is included in the Ottawa foot rules; clinically there will be swelling, tenderness and, later, bruising over the site. Avulsion fractures of the base of the fifth metatarsal are generally treated symptomatically, with supportive bandaging over sturdy closed shoes, weight-bearing as able, along with ice and elevation. However, more recent studies have shown that in instances where the avulsed fragment is displaced more than 3 mm, operative management may be beneficial.[71] When the fracture fragment to the base of the fifth metatarsal is larger, more distal or occurs within the proximal third of the metatarsal, it is at greater risk of healing complications and non-union. These fractures may require immobilising in a walking boot and may also require orthopaedic opinion.[71]

The base of the fifth metatarsal epiphysis in children may mimic a fracture. Generally, single second to fifth metatarsal shaft fractures are treated conservatively. First metatarsal and multiple fractures may be unstable requiring orthopaedic review.

Stress fractures of the foot are sometimes encountered in patients with a history of insidious foot pain, often related to a repetitive impact, such as running, walking or marching. X-ray may demonstrate a calcification at the site of injury, often the second metatarsal. Where x-rays are normal, a bone scan may help identify a fracture.

Most patients make a full recovery after a period of rest from the aggravating activity for 6–8 weeks and then gradually progress to full activity again. A firm, flat-soled shoe may aid comfort.[72]

INJURY TO THE TOES

The toes are frequently damaged by crushing forces or caught against objects such as furniture. Injury to the nail and skin lacerations may be seen. Suspected fractures of the big toe should be x-rayed as the big toe has a role in balance and mobilisation. A stiff-soled shoe or plaster shoe is recommended to limit great toe motion while walking. Alternatively, a walking POP cast with a toe platform or an air-cast boot can be used.[73,74]

Suspected fractures to the lesser toes (2–5), where there is no clinical deformity and the skin is intact, do not require x-ray, as management will be unchanged, even if a fracture is present. Fractures of the lesser toes are generally managed conservatively by strapping the affected toe to the adjacent toe for 3–4 weeks and symptomatic management. Exceptions to this include open fractures and displaced fractures and dislocations that cannot be reduced. Nail and skin wounds involving the toes can be treated similarly to the finger and thumb, covered earlier in the chapter.

WOUNDS

ANATOMY AND FUNCTION OF THE SKIN

The skin is the largest organ of the body, and consists of three distinct layers: the epidermis, the dermis and the subcutaneous layer, often referred to as the hypodermis/subdermis (Fig. 17.12).

The epidermis is the outermost layer of the skin. It is made up of keratinised epithelium consisting of between four and five layers or strata. The thickness of the epithelium varies on the region and on the demands placed upon the skin. The soles of the feet and palms of the hands are the thickest, measuring 1.5 mm thick, compared with the epidermis of the eyelid, which is 0.5 mm thick.[75] The epidermis has pores to allow for release of sweat. Hair follicles protrude through the

FIGURE 17.12 CROSS-SECTION OF THE SKIN, SHOWING STRUCTURE[75]

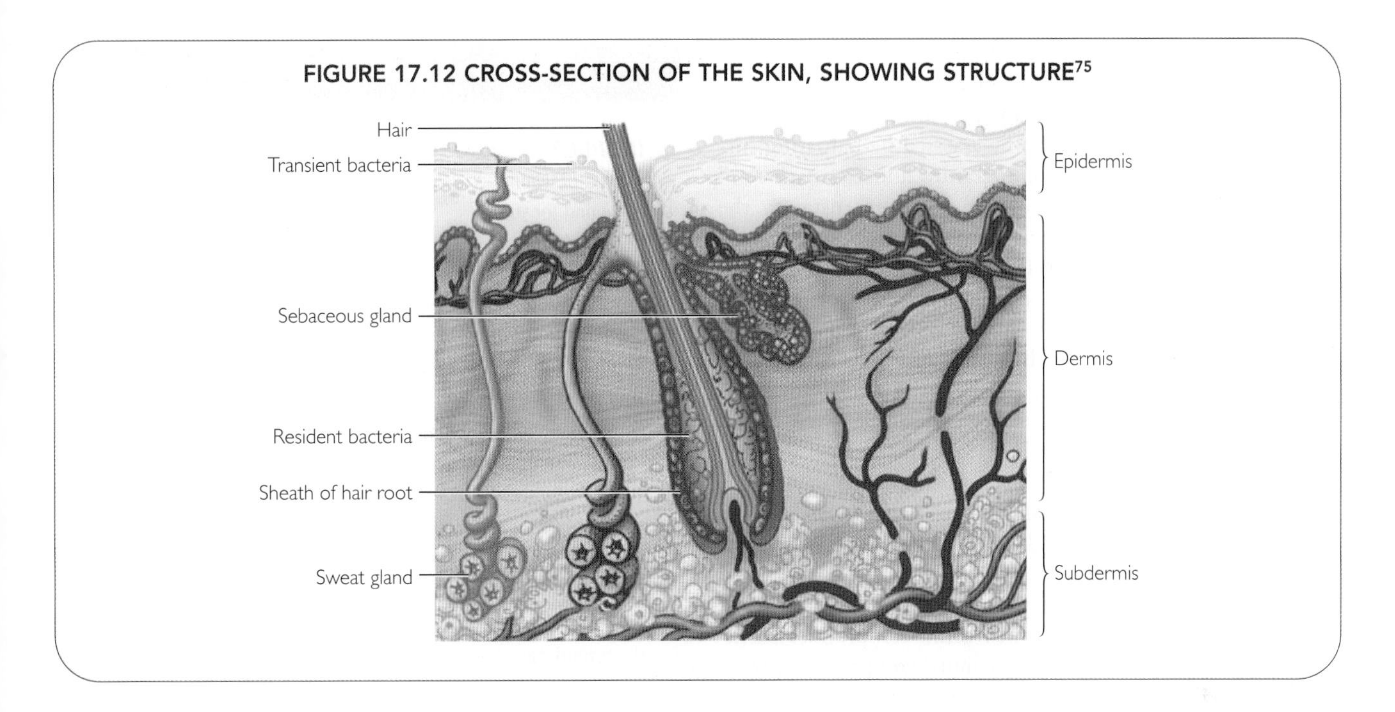

epidermis, depending on the region, and also allow for sebum release from the deeper layers of the skin. The epidermis is avascular, and so receives nourishment via diffusion from the deeper dermis.

The dermis is a strong yet flexible layer of the skin. It contains collagen, reticular and elastin fibres, which provide strength and elasticity and is the thickest of the skin layers. The dermis is highly vascular and is also rich in lymphatic vessels and nerve fibres. Directly beneath the dermis lies the subcutaneous layer.

The subcutaneous layer is loosely arranged connective tissue containing fat, fibrous bands of tissue, blood and lymphatic vessels, nerves and, in the scalp, hair follicles. Subcutaneous tissue anchors the dermis and epidermis to the underlying structures and organs and provides insulation and cushioning.

The appendages of the skin, such as eccrine and apocrine glands secreting sweat, sebaceous glands secreting sebum and the hair follicles and roots, arise from the dermis and subcutaneous layers.

The skin has multiple physiological functions:

- It serves as an anatomical barrier between the internal and external environment, protecting the body from mechanical injury and pathogens.
- It contains an abundance of various nerve endings that respond to heat and cold, touch, pressure, vibration and tissue injury.
- It regulates body temperature through vasodilation and vasoconstriction, convection, conduction and evaporation.
- It synthesises vitamin D, which is an active component of calcium and phosphate metabolism in the body.

The skin plays an integral role in a person's overall emotional and psychological wellbeing. Disruptions to the skin integrity, such as discolourations, wounds or scarring, can affect a person's self-esteem and psychological wellbeing, particularly where they involve cosmetically significant areas such as the face.

WOUND ASSESSMENT

Wound assessment forms part of the systematic primary and secondary physical assessment processes. Life-threatening wounds or wounds resulting in uncontrolled haemorrhage should be identified during the primary survey and steps taken to promote and obtain haemostasis, which may require definitive management of the wound at that time. All other wounds, including those only temporarily managed in the primary assessment, should be reviewed in the secondary survey.

The location of wounds should be considered in relation to the mechanism of injury, particularly those where there may have been substantial impact, such as following a fall or another type of blunt trauma. Once any significant injury has been diagnosed, treated or excluded, wound care will follow the same principles. Before examination of the wound itself, use the mechanism of injury to anticipate associated injuries to the bone, tendon, ligament, muscle or neurovascular structures. When examining a wound, it is important to recall normal anatomy and function of the injured area and the underlying structures to guide the examination and anticipate potential complications.

Wound assessment follows the same systematic approach of inspection, palpation and movement to ensure the examination is thorough.

Look. Note the type of wound: abrasion, laceration, tissue avulsion, puncture, bite or a combination of these. There may be multiple wounds of varying severity, location and depth, as in the case of a trauma or assault.

Note the shape, size and depth of the wound and whether underlying structures are visible at the deepest points of the wound bed. Inspect the colour and condition of the surrounding tissue. Dusky or mottled surrounding tissue may indicate poor circulatory perfusion. Wounds may be contaminated with debris or foreign bodies, which will need to be removed. The depth of the wound can often be concealed beneath a thrombus (clot), which is a normal physiological response to injury. This will require evacuation for further examination. Where wounds involve a limb, inspect the unaffected limb as a comparison, noting oedema and skin colour.

Feel: Palpate the wound and surrounding tissue. Perfusion to surrounding tissues can be assessed by palpating surrounding tissue for colour, temperature and capillary refill time. Assess for changes or loss of sensation distal to the wound as an indication of nerve damage. It is not uncommon to find mild sensation differences due to the physiological response to injury and anxiety. However, there are several techniques that can be used to obtain objective information about sensory changes, including the two-point discrimination technique and assessing the discrimination between sharp and dull sensation. These are conducted distal to the wound. Test the sensation against the same area on the corresponding opposite side, i.e. the other arm, hand or foot. Where possible, assess an unaffected area first to reduce the patient's anxiety and to provide an understanding of what is required.[15]

Palpate arterial pulses distal to the wound. Deep lacerations may sever larger, vital vessels which could compromise perfusion. Where the injury involves a limb, compare quality of pulses between both limbs. Where appropriate, palpate the underlying bony structures, noting crepitus or bony tenderness, which may indicate a fracture. Clear any debris and evacuate any thrombus to assess wound depth. Estimate the depth and size of the wound; if it is difficult to determine, specialist referral may be needed. Note any palpable foreign body beneath the skin surface.

Move: Gently move the adjacent structures surrounding the wound, where appropriate, to establish any actual or potential loss of function. Assess through the full range of motion, noting any loss in power. Deep hand lacerations involving tendons, for example, may affect subsequent function of the hand and/or digits. Where a wound affects a limb, compare motor function to the non-affected limb (Box 17.6). Moving the joints adjacent to the wound will ascertain whether the wound is under tension, such as wounds over joint surfaces. This may prompt specialist referral and affect choice of closure or dressing management.

BOX 17.6 WOUND INSPECTION

INSPECT
- Type of wound
- Wound location
- Wound size
- Wound depth
- Wound contaminants—debris, foreign bodies
- Underlying visible structures
- Surrounding tissue integrity, colour

PALPATE
- Surrounding tissue sensation
- Surrounding tissue perfusion—temperature, capillary refill time
- Pulses distal to the wound
- Underlying bony injury—crepitus, bony tenderness
- Wound tracking beneath skin surface

MOVE

If appropriate:
- Underlying and adjacent structures
- Assess for skin under high tension
- Assess range of motion
- Assess motor power

PATIENT ASSESSMENT

Wounds involving only the skin layers may be cleaned and closed by primary or secondary intention. Care should be taken to ascertain a thorough history of the injury. Wounds sustained on glass or knives, for example, may appear superficial, but may have penetrated deeply.

Lacerations of the hand and digits should be explored through a full range of motion, as the deeper structures move and slide below the laceration. A tendon injury sustained with a clenched fist and flexed digits may not be visible on examination when the digits are extended, as the tendon retracts away from the wound site. Complete lacerations of tendons will result in loss of motor function. The hand can be assessed with the dorsal surface of the hand resting on the examination table. The fingers should normally lie uniformly with a natural curve in slight flexion. An abnormally extended finger in comparison to the other digits has most likely been caused by a complete flexor tendon laceration. Likewise, a drooping finger, when all other fingers are extended, demonstrates a complete extensor tendon laceration. Partial lacerations of tendons controlling flexion or extension of the digit may not affect the motor function of the hand initially but may weaken the tendon and completely rupture at a later stage. Surgery to repair complete tendon rupture can be extensive. Assess for pain at the wound site as the digits are moved against resistance; this is diagnostic of a partial tendon laceration. If a partial or complete laceration is suspected, the patient should be referred for surgical exploration.

Lacerations occurring over a joint may penetrate the joint capsule, risking joint-space infection, or may sever supporting ligaments, leaving the joint unstable. Lacerations resulting in changes or loss of distal sensation may have caused injury to nerve fibres or vasculature and may require surgical repair. Compare the sensation distal to the injury against the same area on the unaffected hand. Remember that different digits are supplied by different nerves, so adjacent digits on the same hand should not be compared with each other. Lacerations with significant blood loss may involve damage to larger vessels.

Where underlying structures are involved and referral is made, the wound should be thoroughly irrigated, under local anaesthesia if needed. A basic moist dressing and non-adherent secondary dressing is normally sufficient, unless an alternative dressing has been advised. If there is to be a delay in review, the injured hand should be splinted in a 'position of safety' and elevated to reduce swelling.

Antibiotic prophylaxis should be considered for high-risk wounds according to mechanism of injury, compound fractures, involvement of underlying structures, contamination and the patient's comorbidities. Primary tetanus vaccination or update may also be required. Tetanus vaccinations are discussed later in the chapter under tetanus immunisation.

WOUND HEALING

The complex process of wound healing can be divided into four distinct, yet overlapping, phases:

1. Initial haemostasis
2. The inflammatory phase
3. The proliferative phase
4. The remodelling phase.

Within these four broad phases is a complex and coordinated series of events.[76] Table 17.1 outlines the overlapping phases and an approximate timeline of the phases of wound healing, excluding complications such as those listed above. Wounds require a number of factors for healing to occur; these include adequate perfusion and temperature of the injured tissue, control of contamination and infection and good general health and nutrition of the patient.

Speed of wound healing varies depending upon the location of the wound. The face and scalp have a greater vascular supply which results in higher baseline skin temperature, better oxygen and nutrient delivery to the skin and therefore more rapid healing. Infection may occur when there is an imbalance between the microbial load at the wound site and the host's immune response. Infection stalls and protracts wound healing and can result in greater scarring.

General health factors of the patient can inhibit healing. Conditions such as diabetes, obesity, haematological, vascular and renal disease, immunocompromised patients, advanced age and many drug therapies, such as corticosteroids, can inhibit the healing process. Other factors such as poor nutrition, smoking, excessive alcohol use or other drug use can also inhibit the healing process. The patient's ability to appropriately care for their wound, or occupational commitments, may restrict adherence to wound care advice, such as rest, elevation and keeping the wound dry. If any of these factors are suboptimal, the wound-healing process will be delayed or protracted.

TABLE 17.1 PHASES OF WOUND HEALING[76]

PHASE	ACTIVITY
Haemostasis (immediate)	Local vasoconstriction
	Clotting to achieve haemostasis
Inflammatory phase (up to 3 days)	Release of vasoactive substances by damaged cells
	Local vasodilation and increased vascular permeability
	Migration of leucocytes and macrophages
	Bacterial balance restored
	Preparation of wound for healing
Proliferative/ reconstruction phase (3 days to 3 weeks)	Reconstruction of tissue
	Granulation tissue–new capillaries, fibroblasts, inflammatory cells, endothelial cells, connective tissue proteins, collagen deposition
	Epithelialisation–epithelial cells migrate across the granular tissue
	Contraction of wound size–myofibroblasts
Maturation phase (3 weeks to 1 year)	Scar development
	Matrix breakdown and reformation
	Continued collagen formation

HAEMOSTASIS

Thorough wound examination is dependent on establishing haemostasis to allow a detailed view of the wound. Haemostasis may have been achieved spontaneously through the normal physiological responses to injury, or in the pre-hospital setting through first-aid measures. Haemostasis may be difficult to achieve in patients with coagulopathies or those on medications affecting normal coagulation. Often, examining a wound will disrupt this process and bleeding will recommence. Haemostasis should be achieved by applying direct pressure and by elevating the wound. Local infiltration of the surrounding tissues with a local anaesthetic containing adrenaline can aid local vasoconstriction and haemostasis, after neurovascular assessment is complete.

In instances where haemostasis cannot be achieved wound assessment is very difficult. Achieving haemostasis is then the main priority and referral may be indicated. Urgent escalation in care and expert advice is needed in these circumstances.

SCARRING

Scarring is an inevitable result of wound healing. Hypertrophic and keloid scarring can be unsightly and, depending upon the location of the wound, can cause problems with tissue and/or joint mobility, as well as causing significant emotional distress to the patient.

Adequate wound cleansing and decontamination, coupled with good primary wound edge apposition are the primary contributors to reducing the size of a scar. Where scarring is considered to be an issue, specialist referral should occur.[77,78]

WOUND MANAGEMENT

The decision to manage or refer a patient with an acute wound is determined after you have completed your focused assessment, including relevant investigations. Wounds that fit into the criteria below may require referral to a specialist surgical team for evaluation. The referral will vary depending on local policy, geographical location and local expertise and patient preference.

- Is there evidence of injury to underlying structures?
- Is there an underlying fracture? Is there neurovascular compromise? Is there motor function compromise?
- Is the wound in a functionally important or cosmetically sensitive area?
- Does the wound involve the vermilion border of the lip, eyelid, nose or ear? Is there tissue avulsion of a sensitive area, inhibiting primary closure?
- Will the wound affect occupational function?
- Will the patient's job be specifically affected by the injury; for example, a professional musician with a hand or digit injury?
- Is closure of the wound technically challenging?
- Is the wound extensive?
- Does the wound require significant debridement or further exploration to retrieve foreign bodies? Are the wound edges jagged or under excessive tension, making alignment difficult?
- Is the patient cooperative?
- Is the patient a young child, particularly anxious, or an elderly patient with dementia? Does the patient have an

intellectual disability, where treatment may cause fear, refusal of or non-compliance with treatment?

Definitions of wounds

A wound is defined as any break in the skin (see below). Wounds can occur from many different mechanisms. There are many different types of wounds and it is important to be able to assess and describe them accurately.

Laceration

- A break in the skin caused by blunt force and the skin is torn or cut.
- Occurs usually where there is little padding between the skin and bone, i.e. top of head or hands.
- Management includes wound irrigation/debridement and closure, if applicable.
- Superficial lacerations involving the epidermis and dermis can be closed with topical adhesive or dressings.
- Lacerations under tension, over moving joints or where the edges are not easily opposed may require closure with sutures.
- Deeper lacerations may require closure in layers, using absorbable sutures at the wound base to oppose muscle facia.

Abrasions

- A wound caused by friction between the skin and a rough or hard surface, causing layers of the epidermis to be removed.
- Management of abrasions includes wound irrigation/debridement and dressings. If debris such as gravel is left in the wound it may be visible through the epidermis after the wound has healed, like a tattoo. Care should be taken, particularly in cosmetically significant areas, to remove debris to avoid tattooing.
- Abrasions should be kept moist to aid healing. This can be achieved with soft white paraffin or dressings, to retain moisture, and a non-adhesive dressing.

Avulsions

- Refers to 'tearing away wound'. An avulsion of tissue results in the loss of both epidermis and dermis. In these instances, approximation of wound edges is not possible.
- Degloving injuries are the result of a circumferential avulsion of skin over a larger surface, such as a digit, hand, foot or limb.
- Management includes wound irrigation and debridement and wound dressings.
- Severe degloving injuries that involve larger areas of tissue loss will require referral to a surgeon for management under general anaesthesia and consideration for skin grafting.

Skin tears

- These are wounds where the skin undergoes a shearing, friction or blunt trauma, which results in separation of skin layers.
- Skin tears can occur in any patient, but those most at risk are the elderly, due to age-related skin changes, and those with chronic illness. Some medications can also predispose skin to becoming friable.
- Management involves thorough wound bed cleansing, ensuring the skin flap is softened. The flap is then approximated as best as possible, and dressing applied.
- Dressing choice must consider the wound characteristics, but should not be highly adhesive products that can result in peri-wound skin stripping or tearing on removal. Wound closure strips, sutures and staples are also not recommended for skin tear closure as they frequently cause further skin tearing.[79,80]

Puncture wounds

- A puncture wound is caused by penetration of the skin by a sharp object, creating a small hole. Minor puncture wounds rarely result in excessive bleeding. Deep wounds can appear relatively minor yet can damage deeper structures.
- Objects causing puncture wounds can deposit foreign matter and infective organisms into the wound itself, leading to an increased risk of infection.
- Management is usually wound cleansing and debridement is necessary.
- Puncture wounds should not be closed, to allow the passage of debris and exudate.
- Dressings should provide wound coverage and manage any potential exudate.

Foreign bodies

- Any wound caused by a foreign object can potentially leave foreign material at the wound site. Certain foreign matter is radio-opaque, including glass > 2 mm long, metal, teeth, pencil graphite, certain plastics, gravel and sand, and may be visible on plain-film x-rays. Other, non-radio-opaque objects, such as wood, will often require ultrasound examination to detect.[81]
- Any foreign matter can be difficult to locate and remove and may require specialist referral. However, small, innocuous material that causes no discomfort or loss of function to the patient can in some instances be left in situ. Attempted removal can often cause more trauma to the local tissue, increase the size of the wound and the risk of scarring or infection or result in cosmetically poor outcomes, frequently without successful retrieval of the foreign material.
- Where an inert foreign body is left in place, a physiological response may occur at the site, where the foreign body is 'walled off' or encased, forming a foreign-body granuloma. Beneath the skin this can be felt as a firm, discreet swelling. Foreign-body granulomas have little clinical significance.

Skin tears

A skin tear is a wound where the skin undergoes a shearing, friction or blunt trauma, which results in separation of skin layers. Skin tears can occur in any patient, but those most at risk are elderly people, due to age-related skin changes, and those with chronic illness. Some medications can also predispose skin to becoming friable. International studies of skin tears occurrence have reported prevalence rates of up to 54% in the long-term care population.[79] Skin tears are classified according to level of epidermal skin loss (Fig. 17.13).

As with all wounds, thorough wound bed cleansing is required, ensuring the skin flap is softened. The flap is then

FIGURE 17.13 SKIN TEAR ASSESSMENT[79]

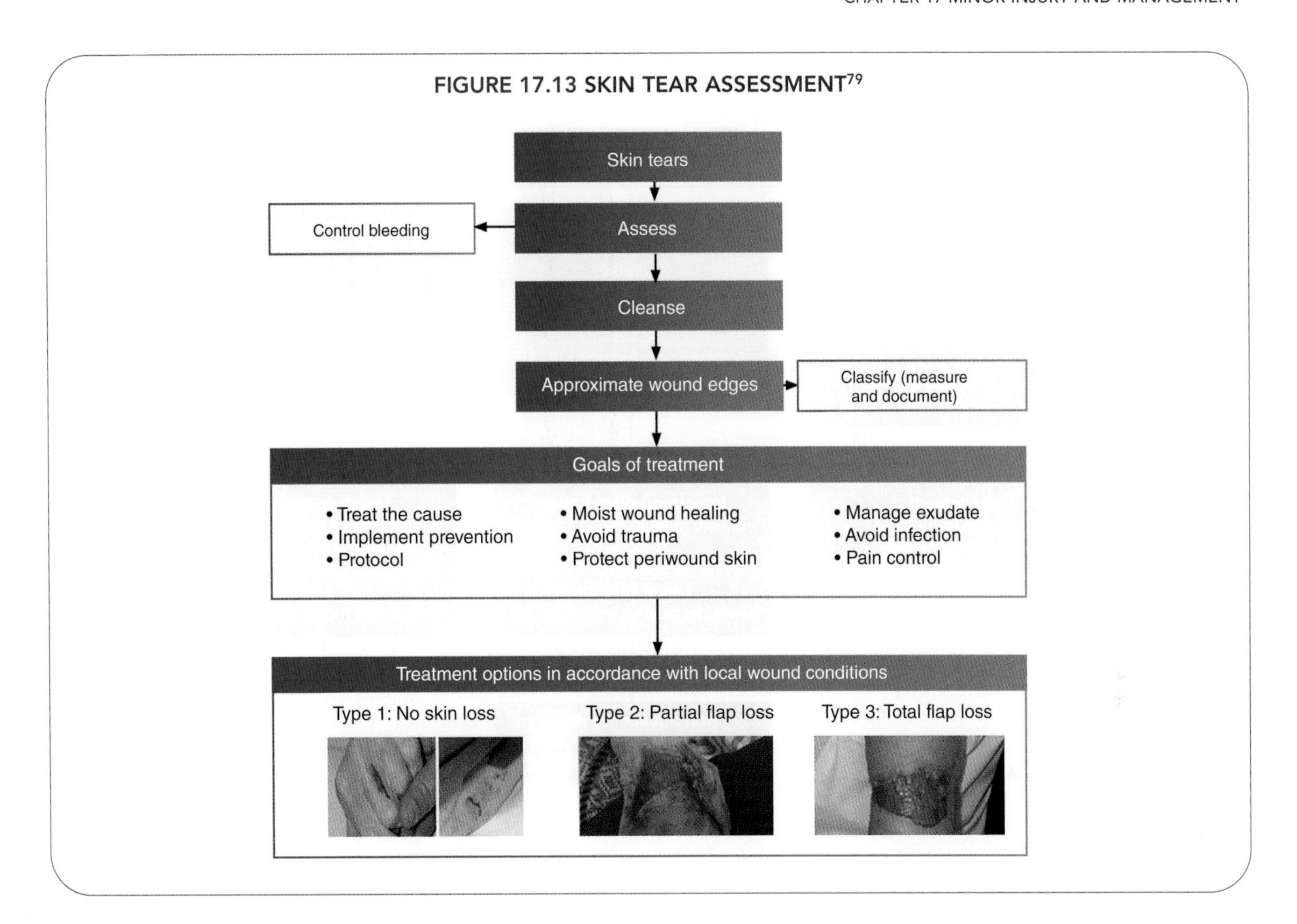

approximated as best as possible and dressing applied. Dressing choice must consider the wound characteristics, but should not be highly adhesive products that can result in peri-wound skin stripping or tearing on removal. Wound closure strips, sutures and staples are also not recommended for skin tear closure as they frequently cause further skin tearing.[79,80] There are several procedures and concerns to be considered when managing a person with a skin tear to prevent further damage (Fig. 17.14).

Contusions and hematomas

A contusion occurs usually due to blunt trauma resulting in rupture of blood vessels and subsequent bleeding into local tissues. A contusion can be superficial, involving the skin, or can involve deeper structures, such as muscles, organs and bones. Most contusions can be managed conservatively.

A more significant blunt trauma can result in a haematoma, a discrete interstitial collection of blood. Where it occurs beneath the surface of the skin it presents initially as a firm swelling. It progresses to a boggy swelling as the collection breaks down. The combination of the collection of blood and the swelling resulting from the local inflammatory process causes an increase in local pressure beneath the skin. This pressure can pose a risk to overlying skin integrity and is detected by local nerve endings causing the sensation of pain. Extravasated blood is an irritant to soft tissues and this also contributes to the pain sensation.

Initial treatment is compression, elevation where appropriate, and ice to promote vasoconstriction and decreased flow from the ruptured vessels. In most instances the hematoma will eventually be reabsorbed. Larger haematomas, or those slow to resolve, may need to be drained or evacuated to promote healing. Infection is a common complication of a haematoma, as the stagnant blood provides an excellent environment for bacteria colonisation. Patients on anticoagulant therapies or with coagulopathies are at increased risk of developing haematomas from a relatively minor injury.

Crush injuries of the digits

A crush injury of a digit is a common injury, resulting from compression between two hard objects. The resulting injury can be any combination of phalangeal fractures, avulsion or laceration of the nail or digit pulp, subungual haematoma, nail bed laceration or partial or complete amputation of the digit. Sudden soft tissue swelling can also result in a burst injury of the pulp, where there is an open wound overlying the pulp and the underlying soft tissue protrudes through the breach.

Hands and fingers have a complex nerve supply, and so when injured can result in significant pain. Examination, debridement and wound preparation often requires analgesia and local or regional anaesthesia. A digital block, using plain lidocaine, is an effective form of anaesthesia to manage digit injuries.

Digit injuries should be managed according to the severity and nature of the injury. An x-ray of the digit may be indicated to exclude a fracture or foreign body. Injuries should be elevated, and ice applied to reduce inflammation and pain. As crush injuries can continue to be painful for several days, advice should be provided about ongoing analgesia, rest and elevation.

FIGURE 17.14 SKIN TEAR MANAGEMENT[79]

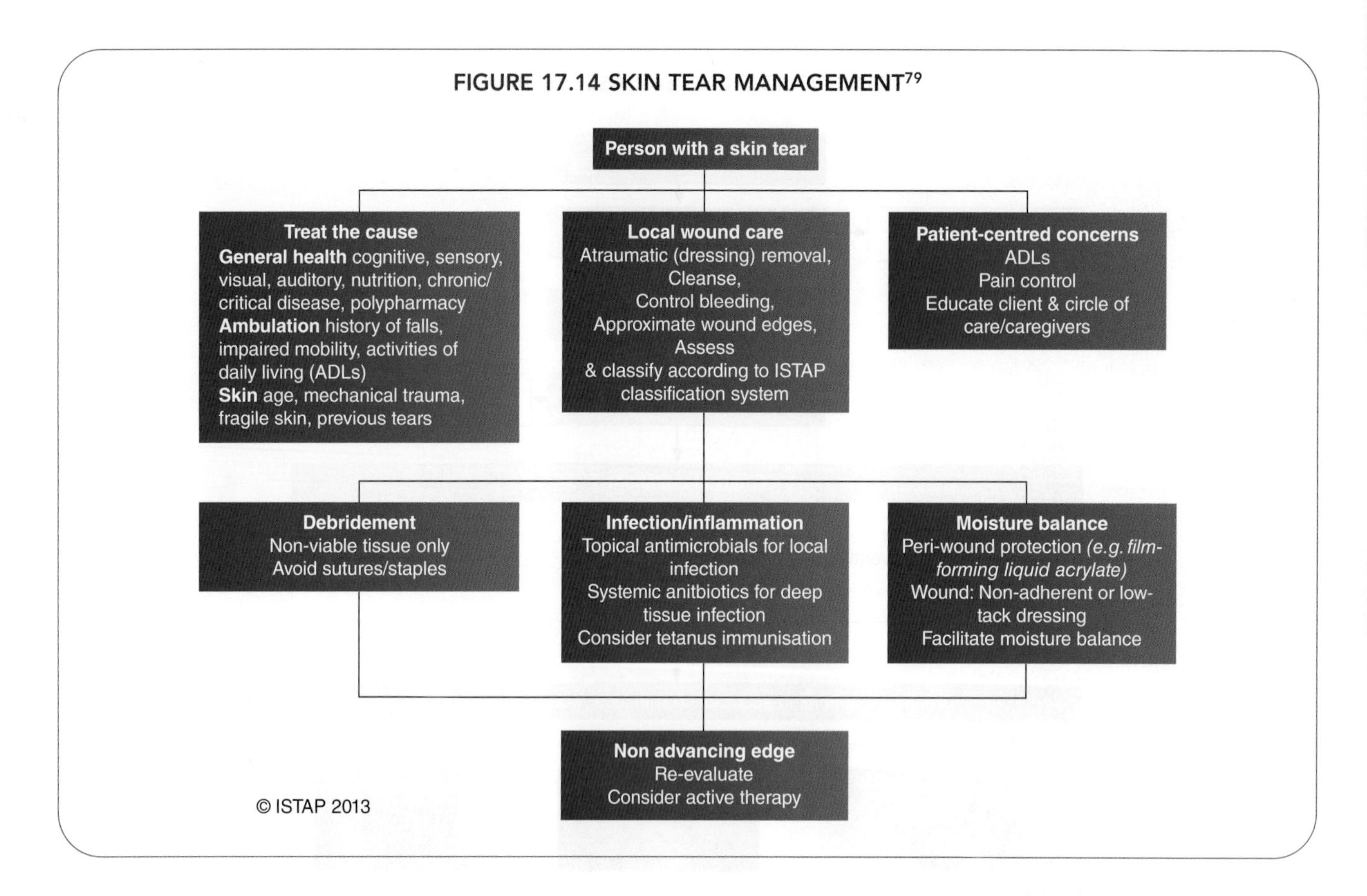

Avulsion of digit pulp

Avulsion of digit pulp can occur as a result of a shearing force applied to the finger or thumb, or by direct laceration from a sharp edge with complete removal of overlying skin (Fig. 17.15 A, B, C).

Haemostasis is difficult to achieve with avulsions of the pulp, as the digit is highly vascular. After thorough irrigation, initial management is elevation and pressure. If this is unsuccessful, a compression dressing can be applied for 1–2 hours, taking care not to apply too much pressure. Excessive pressure will cause a rebound re-bleed when the dressing is removed. Highly compressive digit dressings left in place for an extended period of time can also reduce tissue perfusion at the injury site and potentially result in tissue necrosis. When haemostasis is achieved, a dressing can be applied to encourage healing by secondary intention. These injuries in many circumstances can be successfully healed with ongoing meticulous wound care. For extensive wounds, or wounds that are slow to heal, referral to a surgeon may be required to consider skin grafting.

Nail avulsions and nail bed lacerations

Nail avulsions and partial nail avulsions result from a shearing force applied to the distal digit, tearing the nail away from the nail bed or nail fold. Nail avulsions can often occur as a result of a crush injury, where the nail is avulsed and the nail bed is also lacerated. Nail avulsions rarely occur in isolation of a nail bed laceration. Nail bed lacerations should be repaired to avoid infection and abnormal and problematic subsequent nail growth. This may need referral to a specialist surgeon.

If the original nail is intact but damaged, the patient should be advised of possible nail loss. New nail growth is very slow, taking a period of months, and the new nail is often ridged and not as cosmetically acceptable as the original nail.

Subungual haematoma

A subungual haematoma (Fig. 17.16) is a collection of blood between the nail and nail bed, the result of a crush injury or significant blunt trauma to the distal end of the digit. Such patients usually present with significant throbbing pain secondary to pressure beneath the nail. Associated injuries include nail bed lacerations and distal tuft fractures. More significant subungual haematomas usually indicate an underlying nail bed injury. Studies have shown that if the nail and nail fold remain intact, the haematoma can be drained by trephining the nail. In these instances, the injury does not necessitate nail removal and nail bed repair.[84]

A 22-gauge needle can be rotated against the nail plate at the centre of the haematoma until blood drains and providing immediate relief when the pressure beneath the nail is relieved. This is a relatively painless procedure; however, the patient may feel the sensation of pressure over the nail and nail bed. A battery-powered electric cautery device can be used to aid trephination and is reportedly less discomforting for the patient.[85] Where there is an underlying fracture of the distal phalanx and the nail has been trephined, antibiotics have not shown to be of value in preventing infection.[86]

Digit amputation

In instances where a digit is amputated, the wound should be thoroughly irrigated and a dressing applied. The amputated digit should be wrapped in a sterile gauze moistened in normal saline, placed in a watertight bag and then placed in another

FIGURE 17.15

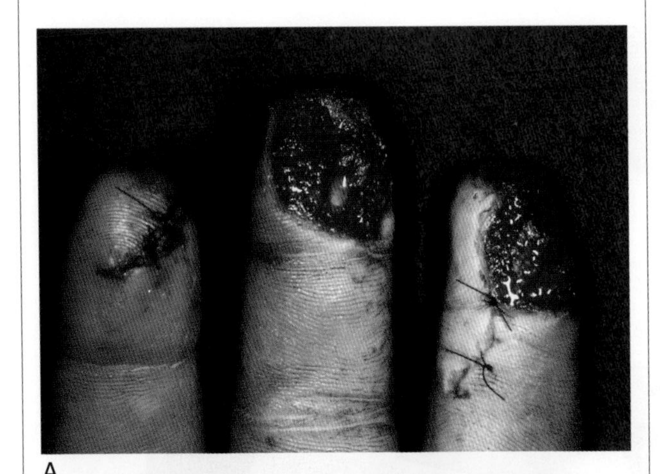

A

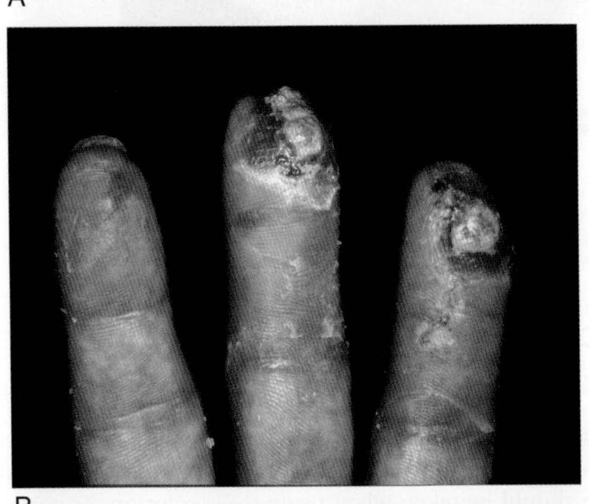

B

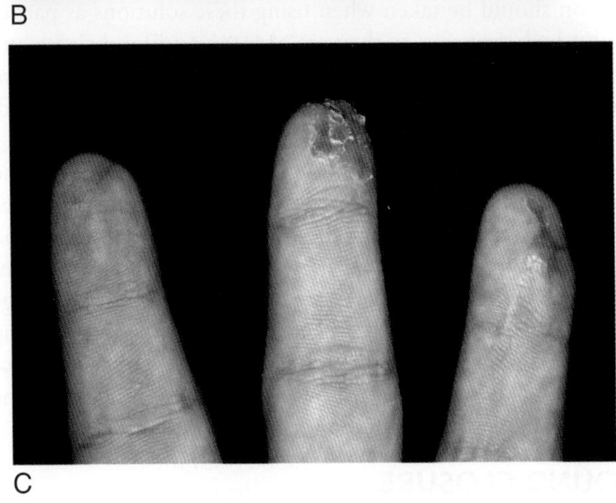

C

Avulsion of the digit pulp before **A** and after **B, C.**[82]

bag filled with ice and water. The patient requires urgent surgical referral for re-implantation.[87] Antibiotic prophylaxis is standard practice for digit amputations.

Interestingly, there are studies indicating that antibiotics can be omitted where the injury is at the tip of the finger, even if there is bone exposed. However, these injuries need to be managed early and surgically. This coincides with evidence recommending thorough irrigation and wound bed decontamination as the mainstay of defence against infection.[88]

Wound investigations

Investigations may be useful to further assess the severity of an injury, prepare a patient for wound repair or aid decisions for antibiotic therapies in high-risk or infected wounds. The recommended wound investigations for common presentations are outlined in Box 17.7.

ANAESTHESIA OF WOUNDS

Examining and preparing a wound for closure or dressing can exacerbate pain and result in increased anxiety for the patient. Providing relief in the form of analgesia and local anaesthesia is essential to maximise wound preparation and compliance to treatment (see Table 17.2). Always assess neurovascular status before administering local anaesthetics. Local anaesthetics work by temporarily inhibiting the influx of sodium through sodium-specific channels of the nerve cells and, subsequently, inhibit both the afferent and efferent conduction of nerve impulses.

For wounds where haemostasis has not been achieved, lidocaine with adrenaline can be used to provide local vasoconstriction and anaesthesia, aiding in haemostasis and examination. Due to its vasoconstrictive quality, historically it has been recommended that anaesthetics with adrenaline are not used on arterial endpoints such as digit tips, ears, nose or penis. There is, however, some evidence of its use in surgery for digital nerve blocks and short procedures.[89] Where local anaesthetic with adrenaline is used expertise is recommended and caution is advised.[90]

Infiltration of local anaesthetic is painful. The pain is caused by a combination of the solution temperature, acidity and the infiltration pressure distorting the surrounding soft tissues. Techniques used to reduce pain include warming the anaesthetic solution to body temperature, using a slow injection rate, buffering the anaesthetic solution to neutralise its pH and using a small-bore needle to infiltrate the wound. The acidity of the anaesthetic can be buffered by adding sodium bicarbonate 8.4% to the solution. Buffering may decrease the time to onset of anaesthesia, but can maintain anaesthesia for longer.[91–93]

Topical application relies on dermal absorption of local anaesthetic. These preparations come in combinations of adrenaline, lidocaine and amethocaine (ALA); tetracaine, adrenaline and cocaine (TAC); or lidocaine, adrenaline and tetracaine (LAT). The combination gives both anaesthesia and local vasoconstriction. It is frequently used for children to alleviate anxiety surrounding the use of needles. Note that emla®, a topical dermal anaesthetic preparation of lidocaine and prilocaine, is not for use on open wounds due to high risk of rapid absorption and lidocaine toxicity.[92,93]

Local anaesthetics are relatively safe to use, but systemic responses can occur due to sensitivity or allergy, or if the recommended maximum dose is exceeded. Signs and symptoms of local anaesthetic toxicity typically include circumoral numbness, tongue paraesthesia dizziness, tinnitus and blurred vision, agitation, nervousness or paranoia, and may progress to muscle twitches and seizures. Early identification is the key with rapid escalation to a senior medical practitioner for consideration of lipid emulsion therapy.

FIGURE 17.16

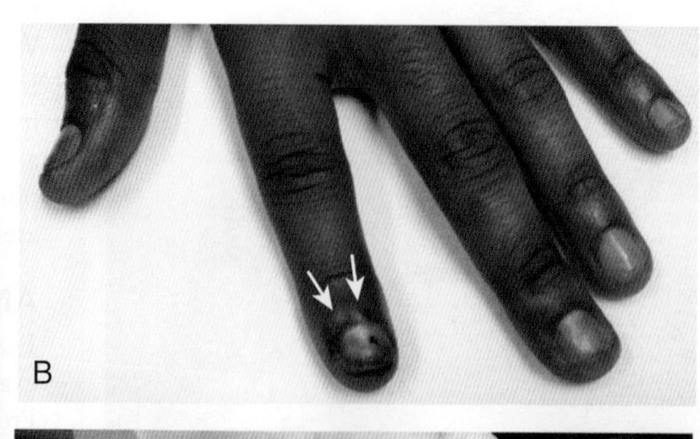

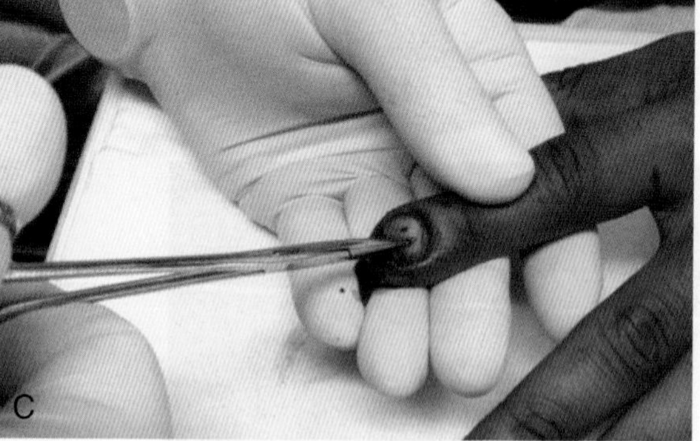

A. Subungual haematoma (with trephine hole). **B.** Position for trephining nail. **C.** Trephining nail.[83]

> **BOX 17.7 WOUND INVESTIGATIONS**
>
> **POINT OF CARE INVESTIGATIONS**
> - Obtain a random blood sugar level for patients with chronic wounds, where there is a history of diabetes or anticipated poor wound healing or signs of localised infections
>
> **PATHOLOGY INVESTIGATIONS**
> - Wound swabs are not usually indicated to diagnose an infection; however, they help identify a pathogen when antibiotic therapy is needed. Seek expert advice for chronic wounds
> - Blood tests are not routinely indicated for wound investigations; however, may be needed where underlying medical conditions (e.g. chronic renal failure, diabetes etc.) is likely to impact the patient's outcome
>
> **RADIOLOGICAL INVESTIGATIONS**
> - X-rays and ultrasounds can be used to identify radio-opaque foreign bodies and underlying fractures
> - Ultrasound is useful to identify organic or non-radio-opaque foreign bodies but is less accessible in the acute setting. Consider clinician-led point-of-care ultrasound if appropriately trained and credentialled

WOUND CLEANSING/PREPARATION

Studies have shown that potable, distilled, cooled boiled or high-quality tap water can be used to irrigate minor acute wounds, demonstrating infection rates to be similar regardless of the solution used.[88,94] It is a relatively common practice to clean wound edges and surrounding tissues with cleansing solutions such as chlorhexidine, povidone–iodine or hydrogen peroxide 3%, to inhibit migration of bacteria into the wound. Caution should be taken when using these solutions as part of wound bed cleansing as they are also toxic to local tissue and may delay wound healing. If these solutions are used to decontaminate the wound they must be well irrigated away with normal saline solution to reduce the risk of tissue death.[87,96]

There are conflicting recommendations on the ideal wound pressure for irrigation and the tools required to provide these pressures. Studies suggest that the ideal pressure for wound irrigation without causing tissue trauma is between 8 psi and 13 psi. Recommendations to achieve this pressure include using a 20 mL syringe and 21-gauge needle.[88,94–97] The key principle for wound cleansing is copious irrigation and removal of foreign debris to reduce infection. Table 17.3 shows the properties and mechanisms of the various wound cleansing solutions currently available.

WOUND CLOSURE

Primary wound healing occurs when wound edges can be approximated and closed with suture material, topical adhesive or wound-closure strip dressings. Healing begins within hours. Wounds closed by primary closure have a better cosmetic appearance and generally have fewer complications, including infection or wound breakdown. Ideally, simple, non-contaminated wounds should be closed as soon as possible after an injury. However, the maximum allowable time between injury and primary wound closure is yet to be clearly defined.[98,99] Various studies recommend that scalp and face wounds can be closed up to 24 hours after the injury with good outcome, while other wounds have a better healing outcome if closed within 12–18 hours of the injury.[95,96,100]

TABLE 17.2 LOCAL ANAESTHETICS COMMONLY USED IN THE ACUTE CARE SETTING[101]

DRUG	DOSE	DURATION	ADVANTAGES/USES	DISADVANTAGES/EXCLUSIONS
Lidocaine 1%	3–5 mg/kg	0.5–2 hours	All locations	
Lidocaine with 1% adrenaline 1 : 100,000	5–7 mg/kg	2–5 hours	Areas likely to bleed Areas already bleeding Easier to see effect and where you are going	Regional blocks Wounds at end arterial points
Bupivacaine	2 mg/kg	2–12 hours	Longer-acting, useful for dental analgesia and situations where long duration is beneficial	Longer onset
Topical anaesthesia				
Lidocaine/adrenaline	Max: 0.1 mg/kg	20–30 minutes	Topical—no infiltration required	Wounds at endpoints
Amethocaine preparation	0.5–1 mL/cm of wound		Areas likely to bleed	Wounds larger than 5 cm Short duration

TABLE 17.3 WOUND-CLEANSING SOLUTIONS[96]

SOLUTION	PROPERTIES	MECHANISM OF ACTION	USES	DISADVANTAGES
Normal saline	Isotonic, non-toxic	Simple washing action	In wound for irrigation	No antiseptic action
Chlorhexidine 0.1 w/v aqueous	Bacteriostatic	Antibacterial and washing action	Cleanse skin surrounding wound	Not for use near eyes (causes keratitis), perforated ear drum or meninges
Chlorhexidine 0.1% w/v + cetrimide 1% w/v	Bacteriostatic	Antibacterial and soap action, removes sebum, 'wetting' the skin	Cleanse skin surrounding wound	Not for use near mucous membranes, eyes (causes keratitis), perforated ear drum or meninges
Hydrogen peroxide (H_2O_2) 3%	Bacteriocidal to anaerobes	Forms superoxide radicals	Severely contaminated wounds with anaerobic-type pathogens	Obstruction of wound surface capillaries and subsequent necrosis
Povidone-iodine 10% w/v	Bacteriocidal, fungicidal, viricidal, sporacidal	Releases free iodine	On surrounding skin, or in severely contaminated wounds (dilute 1% w/v)	Use on/in large wounds, may cause acidosis due to iodine absorption

Secondary wound healing involves no formal wound closure, allowing healing to occur by cellular regeneration from the base and edges of the wound. This form of wound management is used where there has been tissue loss, which inhibits closure by primary intention. Closure by secondary intention has an increased risk of infection due to the lack of epidermis to provide a barrier to the external environment. After cleansing, wounds are dressed to optimise cellular regeneration and healing from the wound bed. Wounds may require ongoing dressing changes and observation. It may take several weeks or even months for a wound to heal by secondary intention.

Wounds that expose vital structures, large wounds over joints or at cosmetically significant sites are not suitable for secondary wound healing. These require early referral to a specialist for consideration.

DRESSINGS

The goal of a wound dressing is to create the optimal environment for wound healing. Some specialised dressings assist in the control of microbial load in infected wounds. For acute wounds, it is best to use a simple dressing moistened with potable tap water or normal saline, as bleeding is likely to recur on removal of a dry dressing that has adhered to the wound. Wound dressing commonly used can be found in Table 17.4, while wound dressing principles can be found in Box 17.8.

Consideration should be given to the nature of the wound and the goal of treatment, whether it is to promote moisture, control exudate or manage contamination. Enzymatic and cellular function is at its optimum when the wound bed is at body temperature.[102] Less-frequent dressing changes supports healing through maintaining wound-bed temperature.

Dressing choice may also be affected by the circumstances of the patient. Issues to consider include whether the patient is to be discharged or admitted to hospital, whether the patient will be able to care for the wound themselves with education and advice, and whether suitable wound care follow-up can be arranged. Consideration should also be given to the ongoing financial costs of dressings. The Therapeutic Guidelines group (TG)

TABLE 17.4 WOUND DRESSINGS COMMONLY USED IN THE ACUTE CARE SETTING[100,102]

PRODUCT	CHARACTERISTICS/PURPOSE	EXAMPLES
Gauze	Provides absorption of exudate Supports debridement if applied and kept moist Maintains wound moisture if applied moistened Filter dressing in sinus tract	Numerous products available
Non-adherent dressings (woven or non-woven)	May be impregnated with saline, petroleum or antimicrobials Minimal absorbency	Adaptic Exu-dry Sofsorb Telfa Vaseline gauze Xeroform
Transparent films	Semipermeable membrane permits gaseous exchange between wound bed and environment For dry, non-infected wounds or wounds with minimal drainage Minimally absorbent—exudate at wound collects beneath dressing Protective barrier to bacteria	Acu-derm Bioclusive Blisterfilm Opsite Polyskin Tegaderm Transeal
Hydrocolloid	Occlusive dressing—no gaseous exchange between wound bed and external environment Occlusion—exudate collects at wound to promote moist wound environment Used for superficial and partial-thickness wounds—light to moderate drainage Not used in infected wounds Supports debridement and prevents secondary infections	Comfeel DuoDerm Intact Intrasite Restore Tegasorb Ultec
Polyurethane foams	Absorptive dressing—moderate to heavy amounts of exudate can be absorbed Can be used on infected wounds Used for partial- or full-thickness wounds with minimal to heavy drainage	Allevyn Epilock Hydrasorb Lyofoam Mitraflex Synthaderm
Absorption dressings	Large volumes of exudate can be absorbed Maintains moist wound surface Supports debridement Can be placed into wounds to obliterate dead space Used for partial- or full-thickness wounds Used for infected wounds	AlgoDERM Bard Absorption Debrisan DuoDerm Paste Hydragan Kaltostat Sorbsan
Hydrogel	Adds moisture to the wound bed Debridement because of moisturising effects—used to hydrate necrosis for debridement Available as a sheet or gel—mostly requires a secondary dressing Limited absorption of exudate (gel sheets) Used for partial- or full-thickness wounds, deep wounds with minimal drainage Used for necrotic wounds	Vigilon Elasto Gel Intrasite Gel Geliperm

BOX 17.8 WOUND DRESSING PRINCIPLES

Dressings have several purposes:

- to apply pressure to control bleeding
- to provide a barrier between the wound and surrounding tissue and the external environment
- to reduce pain
- to eliminate dead space
- to remove non-viable tissue
- to control exudate
- to optimise conditions for wound healing, by providing a moist wound environment and optimal wound-bed temperature.

BOX 17.9 CONSIDERATIONS IN CHOOSING ANTIMICROBIALS

If antimicrobials are indicated, choice is based on:

- knowledge of suspected pathogens involved
- local hospital or other health-setting policy
- national drug prescribing guidelines
- local availability
- patient factors, such as allergy or background medical conditions
- ease of antibiotic dosage regimen and maximisation of compliance.

has published guidelines to aid clinicians in making decisions related to wound dressings and management.[103]

WOUND INFECTIONS

Intact and healthy skin is a poor medium for bacterial growth. It is when the skin is breached, or if it is overly moist and occlusive, that conditions support the growth of bacteria. Thorough wound irrigation and cleansing techniques are the mainstay of antimicrobial treatment. A 'wait and see' approach gives the patient some control over their health, prevents unnecessary antibiotic use and may prevent multiple trips to a healthcare facility for further advice. The approach is, however, reliant on thorough patient education and cooperation, as well as balancing risks and potential benefits.[104]

Antimicrobial prophylaxis should be reserved for high-risk wounds or for those patients who are immunocompromised.[105] High-risk wounds include bite and deep wounds to the hands, feet or face; over joints; grossly contaminated wounds; and wounds involving underlying structures (see Practice Tips: Wounds at higher risk of infection). Contaminated wounds and where there is a delay in treatment, may also be considered high risk. There is debate over the exact time-frame considered to be 'delayed', but many sources suggest 8 hours.[92,106] Patients with comorbidities (such as diabetes)[107] which affect the immune system or wound healing are at greater risk of infection due to their inability to mount an adequate physiological response to infection. For these patients, infection may be the result of both normal skin commensals, such as *Staphylococcus* and *Streptococcus* species, as well as opportunistic Gram-negative bacteria, such as *Pseudomonas* species. Antibiotic prophylaxis should be considered the exception rather than the rule in managing acute wounds (see Box 17.9).

There is well-documented concern regarding increasing resistance to antibiotic therapy.[104,105] This has been attributed to inappropriate antibiotic selection, inappropriate use of antibiotics and over-prescribing. In Australia, the National Prescribing Service (NPS) and TG have published therapeutic guidelines to enhance the appropriate use and choice of antimicrobial therapy and, importantly, when they are not needed.[106,108] The risk of other complications to the patient, such as adverse side-effects and allergy, also need to be considered. Antimicrobial treatment should be tailored to the individual circumstances of each patient.[98,105,109,110]

The most likely contaminants of any wound are normal skin commensals such as Gram-positive *Staphylococcus* and *Streptococcus* species. Generally, penicillins are considered first-line treatment for antibiotic prophylaxis; or, if penicillin allergy exists, first-generation cephalosporins.[106,111] Bite wounds are also likely to be contaminated by a mixture of normal skin commensals and the oral flora of the causative animal (see the section on bite wounds later in the chapter).

Patient education regarding antibiotic use, including appropriate dosing, time intervals and completion of course, is vital to ensure effective results and limit the development of antibiotic resistance.

PRACTICE TIP

WOUNDS AT HIGHER RISK OF INFECTION

Wounds

- Grossly contaminated wounds
- Puncture wounds involving the hand, foot or face
- Cat and human bite wounds, some dog bite wounds
- Contaminated wounds with delay > 8 hours to irrigation treatment
- Wounds involving bone, joints, tendons and ligaments
- Open fractures
- Full-thickness intraoral wounds

Health of host

- Diabetes
- Obesity
- Immunocompromise/autoimmune/haematological disorders, malignancy
- Vascular disease
- Renal disease
- Elderly
- Malnutrition
- Medications–steroids, chemotherapy

Social factors

- Smoker
- Excessive alcohol/illicit drug use

TETANUS IMMUNISATION

Tetanus is a systemic bacterial infection caused by *Clostridium tetani*. The bacterium can be found in the gastrointestinal tract of various animals, and as spores found in soil and dust. It is a hardy bacterium and is resistant to many antiseptics and heat. If a wound is contaminated by the *C. tetani* spore, the bacteria replicate anaerobically, incubating over a period of 2 days to 2 weeks. Once infection is established, the bacteria produce a toxin which acts on the central nervous system causing generalised muscle spasms and rigidity, resulting in trismus, fractures and muscle rupture. If left untreated, it can cause spasm of the ventilatory muscles, seizures, hypertension, cardiac dysrhythmia or arrest, and can be fatal.[112]

In Australia, as in many industrialised countries, most deaths from tetanus occur in people over 70 years of age, with previous vaccination having been a significant number of years prior to the injury; or in those from migrant populations who have had no previous vaccination at all. The case-fatality rate in Australia is about 2%.[112] Widespread immunisation programs, beginning in childhood, have been effective in limiting cases of tetanus. Boosters in adulthood are generally given on presentation to a medical facility to patients with a tetanus-prone wound and are often given prophylactically prior to overseas travel.

Wounds that are considered prone to tetanus infection include:

- wounds contaminated by dirt or soil
- bite wounds
- deep, penetrating wounds
- wounds containing foreign materials
- crush injuries and open fractures.

Care should be taken to establish the immunisation history of any patient presenting with a wound and, where indicated, a tetanus vaccination should be administered (see Table 17.5). Refer to the *Australian Immunisation Handbook* or *New Zealand Immunisation Handbook* for the most current advice.[114]

SPECIAL WOUNDS GROUPS TO CONSIDER

Wounds sustained in fresh, salt or brackish water

Consideration should be given to wounds sustained in or around water. These often result from punctures or lacerations from foreign matter beneath the water's surface, for example, coral cuts, lacerations from boat motor propeller blades and embedded fishhooks. The most common waterborne organisms causing soft-tissue infection include *Aeromonas* species in fresh or brackish water, Vibrio species in salt water or brackish water and *Mycobacterium marinum* in fish tanks.[115] Guidance on use of antibiotics can be obtained through the latest version of the up-to-date reference modality Therapeutic Guidelines.[116]

Bite wounds

A bite wound can be caused by animals or humans. The resulting wound can be a combination of abrasion, laceration or puncture, and may involve underlying muscle, tendons, ligaments, bone, vasculature or organs. Not all animal bites are

TABLE 17.5 AUSTRALIAN TETANUS VACCINATION GUIDELINES[113]

HISTORY OF TETANUS VACCINATION	TIME SINCE LAST DOSE	TYPE OF WOUND	DTPA, DTPA COMBINATION, DT OR DTPA AS APPROPRIATE	TETANUS IMMUNOGLOBULIN (TIG)[1]
3 doses	< 5 years	Clean minor wounds	No	No
		All other wounds[2]	No	No[3]
	5–10 years	Clean minor wounds	No	No
		All other wounds[2]	Yes	No[3]
	> 10 years	Clean minor wounds	Yes	No
		All other wounds	Yes	No[3]
< 3 doses or uncertain[4]		Clean minor wounds	Yes	No
		All other wounds[2]	Yes	Yes

DTPa: infant/child formulation diphtheria–tetanus–acellular pertussis vaccine

dTpa: adult/adolescent formulation diphtheria–tetanus–acellular pertussis vaccine

dT: adult formulation diphtheria–tetanus vaccine

1. The recommended dose for TIG is 250 IU, given by IM injection, as soon as practicable after the injury. If more than 24 hours have elapsed, 500 IU should be given. Because of its viscosity, TIG should be given to adults using a 21-gauge needle. For children, it can be given slowly using a 23-gauge needle.

2. All wounds, other than clean minor wounds, should be considered 'tetanus-prone'.

3. Individuals with a humoral immune deficiency (including HIV-infected persons who have immunodeficiency) should be given TIG if they have received a tetanus-prone injury, regardless of the time since their last dose of tetanus-containing vaccine.

4. Persons who have no documented history of a primary vaccination course (3 doses) with a tetanus toxoid-containing vaccine should receive all missing doses and must receive TIG.

BOX 17.10 BITE WOUNDS CONSIDERED HIGH RISK

Bite wounds considered high risk are:

- all cat bite wounds, complicated dog and human bite wounds
- all bite wounds involving the hand, foot, face and those over a joint
- puncture or crush wounds potentially penetrating underlying structures such as tendons, ligaments, bones or joints
- wounds resulting in vascular or lymphatic compromise
- wounds where there has been a delay of more than 8 hours to cleansing, debridement and treatment
- comorbidities, resulting in immunocompromise.[99,118]

severe enough to prompt a patient to seek medical attention, and the significant risk to public health and safety is potentially underestimated. Animal bites comprise around 2% of emergency presentations each year.[117]

The severity of an injury must be considered in the context of the inflicting animal, the site of the injury and the general health of the patient. Bite wounds considered at high risk of infection are discussed in Box 17.10.

Bite wounds require particular attention due to the high risk of contamination by a combination of the oral flora of the causative animal and the normal skin flora at the bite site. All bite wounds should be considered multimicrobial contaminated wounds. Gram-negative organisms such as Pasteurella and, less commonly, *Capnocytophaga* are particular to dog and cat bites. *Haemophilus* spp., *Eikenella corrodens* and other anaerobes are prevalent in human bites.[118–120]

Copious wound irrigation and debridement for any bite wound is vital to reduce the incidence of infection. Wounds are routinely managed by delayed primary closure. An exception to this is facial bite wounds, extensive lacerations and disfiguring wounds, which require referral to a surgeon for washout and closure by primary intention.[110,121]

If prophylactic antibiotics are indicated, please refer to local guidelines to inform the decision for their use.[106,118] Consider surgical referral for patients with cosmetically significant bites, such as wounds of the face, extensive or disfiguring bite wounds, or bites that involve underlying structures or fractures, particularly of the hand. These may require surgical washout. All bite wounds are considered tetanus-prone wounds and tetanus prophylaxis should be considered.[121]

Dog bites

Dog bites are the most common bite injury, accounting for 80–90% of presentations.[117,119,120] Dog bites can result in abrasions, crush injuries, lacerations and/or avulsion of tissue. Due to the significant pressure exerted by the canine jaw, fractures are common. Studies indicate the infection rate of dog bite wounds is between 4% and 25%.[120]

Cat bites

Cat bite wounds most commonly result in puncture wounds, due to the shape of feline teeth. Bites commonly occur on the arm and hands. The infection rate of cat bites is greater than that of dog bites due to the penetrating nature of the bite. Cat bites press foreign debris and bacteria deep into the tissues, which is difficult to clear with wound cleansing as puncture wounds close over soon after injury. This traps foreign material in the tissues, increasing infection risk. Cat bites are therefore routinely treated prophylactically with antibiotics.[118,119,121]

Human bites

Human bite wounds are often the result of physical fighting and assault. These bite injuries commonly occur on the hand, face and head, including the ear. Mechanical falls can cause accidentally self-inflicted bite wounds to the lip and oral mucosa. Human bite wounds often become infected due to the large load of normal oral flora contaminating the wound site. Human saliva can contain up to 190 different species of organisms.[122] Human bite wounds are associated with a 50% infection rate.[123] This is significantly reduced with the use of antibiotics.[124]

There is a theoretical risk of blood-borne virus transmission from person to person following a human bite injury. Human bites have been shown to transmit hepatitis B, hepatitis C, herpes simplex virus (HSV), syphilis, tuberculosis, actinomycosis and tetanus.[122–124] An attack by an unknown person would raise concern regarding risk. If the patient's immunisation status against hepatitis B is unknown, it is generally recommended that the patient be administered hepatitis B immunoglobulin together with the first vaccination of an accelerated course of hepatitis B immunisation.[123] There is no active or passive vaccination for hepatitis C. Infection with HIV is negligible through a human bite. Many cases of bite injuries from known HIV/AIDS patients have been documented with no viral transmission; therefore, the potential for salivary transmission of HIV is remote—blood-to-blood contact is necessary.[96,125]

COSMETICALLY SIGNIFICANT WOUNDS

Wounds to the face

Wounds to the face can be the cause of significant anxiety due to the potential for scarring or disfigurement.[126] This is particularly so in parents of young children with facial lacerations. Examination should include assessment of underlying facial bones for crepitus or tenderness, and facial sensory and motor function to exclude damage to the branches of the facial and trigeminal nerves. Facial skin is highly vascular, so simple, non-contaminated lacerations generally heal and are rarely complicated by infection.[127] Skin develops along lines of tension (Fig. 17.17). Lacerations following the direction of these lines generally have a better cosmetic outcome. Lacerations perpendicular to these lines often result in the scar widening, as the edges are under constant tension.

Simple, non-contaminated facial wounds can be managed in the acute care setting. Wounds involving underlying fractures or those resulting in motor sensory deficit will require referral. Depending on the skills of the clinician, technically challenging wounds where cosmetic outcome is a concern may also be referred for surgical opinion. Wounds of the face are difficult to dress and are frequently left uncovered and topical paraffin ointment or a microporous paper tape can be applied.[128]

Oral mucosa and lip wounds

Lip and oral lacerations often occur as a result of a blow to the mouth, often the result of a fall or a blow to the face. Lacerations

FIGURE 17.17 SKIN TENSION LINES ON THE FACE[128]

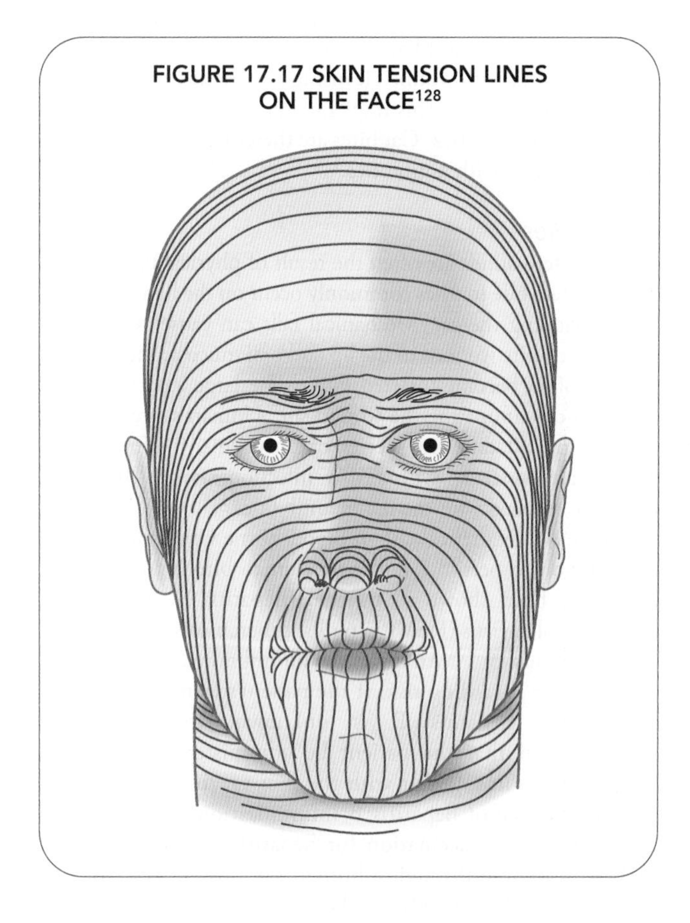

are often caused by the teeth, but can also be from the surface of the causative factor, such as a jewellery ring or the fingernail of an assailant. Oral wounds tend to bleed profusely at the time of injury, often resolving relatively quickly. Minor injuries are often seen in the acute care setting, as the patient equates the blood loss with significant injury.

When examining wounds sustained by a blow to the mouth, it is important to assess for broken or missing teeth, bite malocclusion or trismus (inability to fully open the mouth).[129–131] Patients with crown fractures and misplaced teeth should be referred to a dentist for repair. Care of dental injuries is discussed later in this chapter and in more depth in Chapter 31. Patients with trismus or bite malocclusion may have a mandibular fracture and will require radiological investigation and referral. Consideration should be given to the location and possible involvement of the parotid and submandibular ducts and glands. Involvement of these structures will require referral.

Buccal mucosa and lips heal rapidly due to the nature of mucosal regeneration. Minor wounds not involving muscle or other buccal structures which have ceased bleeding do not require closure. For deeper wounds where a significant gaping or defect exists or the oral musculature is involved, layered closure using absorbable suture material may be required after careful, thorough wound preparation. Where a deep intraoral injury also involves a tooth fracture, the wound should be explored carefully to ensure the tooth fragment is not embedded in the wound.

In full-thickness 'through-and-through' lacerations there is a communication between the internal oral surface and the exterior skin surface. The external surface and intraoral musculature should be closed after careful wound preparation. Minor tongue lacerations will heal with no cosmetic or functional deficit. Large tongue lacerations may need to be referred for closure, to avoid deformity.

Lacerations to the surface of the lip may require closure to prevent cosmetic defect (Fig. 17.18). Lacerations involving the vermilion border require precise approximation of edges. These lacerations are often closed using regional anaesthetic blocks, such as mental nerve blocks, inferior alveolar nerve blocks or infraorbital nerve blocks, so that the wound edges are not distorted by local infiltration.

Meticulous oral hygiene is essential to avoid infection and promote healing. Normal saline mouthwashes, particularly after meals, are advised. The patient should also be advised to avoid hot food and drinks and eat a soft diet. Patients with complex oral lacerations should receive prophylactic antibiotics after repair of oral and perioral laceration. These antibiotics should be targeted to cover for oral flora.[132]

FIGURE 17.18 LIP LACERATION

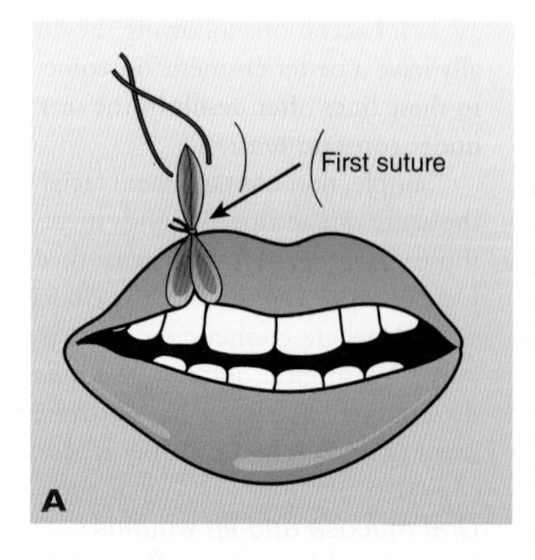

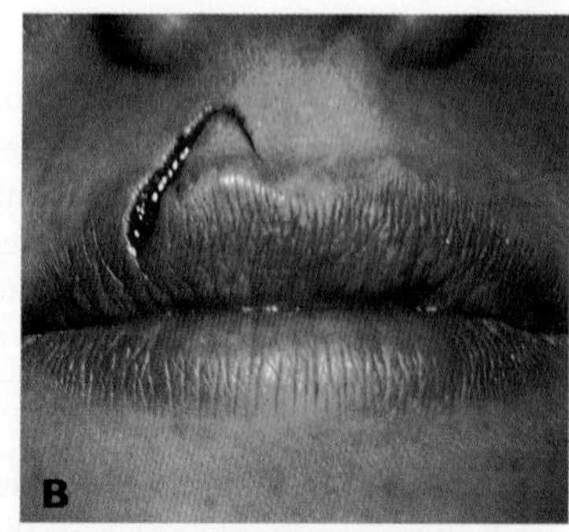

A. Position for first suture. **B.** Lacerated lip alignment.[83]

Wounds of the external ear

The pinna or auricle is the external visible ear. The skin is highly vascular overlying cartilage which provides shape to the ear. Wounds to the ear are cosmetically important. Lacerations of the external ear frequently involve the underlying cartilage. Due to lack of vascular supply, the cartilage is often slower to heal. The goal of repairing auricular lacerations is to cover exposed cartilage. Some literature recommends avoiding using sutures to close auricular cartilage as this causes an increased risk of infection and subsequent delay in healing. Often the closure of the overlying skin laceration will approximate the cartilage edges without the need to suture the cartilage. Where cartilage deformity is significant it can cause distortion of the wound edges, making it difficult to close the overlying tissue. Extensive lacerations or amputations should be referred to specialist surgeons.

Management should include thorough irrigation and removal of debris. Debridement should be done with caution, as even a small loss of tissue may result in wound malunion and cartilage exposure. Haematomas of the auricle should be drained, and a compressive bandage and ice applied to inhibit reformation (Fig. 17.19). Auricular haematomas can result in deterioration of the underlying cartilage and a cosmetic defect known as a 'cauliflower ear'. This is often seen in players of full-contact sport. A compression bandage should be applied to all significant auricular injuries to prevent haematoma development. If injury to the external auditory canal or inner ear is suspected, referral is indicated. Antimicrobial prophylaxis is reserved for contaminated wounds and patients at high risk of infection.

FIGURE 17.19 DRAINED CAULIFLOWER EAR

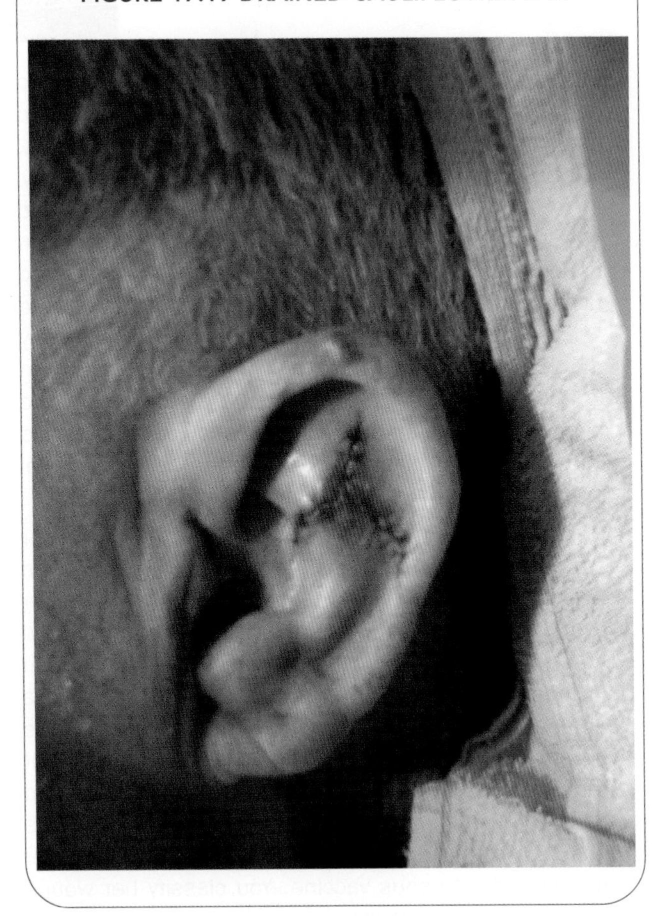

SUMMARY

Minor musculoskeletal injuries comprise a significant proportion of patients presenting to ED care. Timely and appropriate care helps to alleviate patient anxiety, their experience of pain, and, most importantly, result in an overall reduction in severity of the injury. Key points to remember:

1. Use a systematic approach to patient assessment.
2. Look, feel and move is the essential to assess all injury presentations. Always look for a second injury.
3. Thorough and appropriate wound cleansing is the key to minimising infection.
4. Listen to the patient as they describe the mechanism of injury, as this will lead you to the likely diagnosis and clues to avoid missed injuries.

As with all physical assessment, minor injuries should be assessed using a systematic approach. The chapter has addressed the most common upper and lower limb injuries, their assessment and management. It has also covered wound examination, management of general and complex and special areas wounds and adjuncts to care, including dressing choice, appropriate use of antibiotics and scar management.

CASE STUDY

Mrs Chan, a right-handed 54-year-old woman, tripped and fell while walking in a local park. A bystander called an ambulance as she complained of a tender right wrist. She is normally well with no previous medical history. An extended care paramedic (ECP) assessed her and noted a painful right wrist with an associated laceration to her forehead. Although a little shaken, she looks and feels well, her vital signs are within normal limits and she reports no loss of consciousness, and it is noted by the ECP that there are no focal neurological deficits. The ECP was concerned she may have a displaced fracture of her wrist and after administering analgesia, splint and initial wound management, transported her to the local emergency department (ED) for further management.

Mrs Chan was triaged and assessed as safe for assessment in the Fast Track area of the ED. On examination, she has a swollen right wrist and is tender over her distal radius, ulna and scaphoid. An accredited nurse initiated x-rays for Mrs Chan's right wrist, which included scaphoid views as she was tender in the anatomical snuff box. On return from x-ray you manage her facial wound. It is a simple, superficial wound, but requires closure with skin sutures to obtain a good cosmetic result. Mrs Chan recently migrated and is unsure of her tetanus status. She does not recall ever having had a tetanus vaccine. You classify her wound as a clean, minor wound.

You must decide whether to provide antibiotic cover, as Mrs Chan is very concerned about the risk of a wound infection. She has no existing medical conditions and no drug allergies. Her x-ray examination does not demonstrate a fracture.

QUESTIONS

1. In what ways might you attempt to assess and relieve Mrs Chan's pain? Discuss both pharmacological and non-pharmacological measures.
2. Describe how you would systematically exclude other injuries to the right limb. What x-rays would you request? What are the issues with diagnosing scaphoid fractures on a plain x-ray?
3. What would be your choice of cleansing solution for the facial wound? How would you irrigate the wound adequately? Would you use a sterile procedure, as it is a facial wound?
4. What type of prophylaxis against tetanus would you give Mrs Chan now, and what additional injections should she be advised to have, and when, in the future?
5. What is the rationale behind your decision regarding antibiotics? Briefly discuss the explanation you give to your patient.
6. In view of Mrs Chan's scaphoid tenderness, how would you manage her injury? Discuss this comparing the availability of further imaging resources where you presently work and what you would consider to be the gold standard.

Answers to Case Study Questions can be found on evolve http://evolve.elsevier.com/AU/Curtis/emergency/

USEFUL LINKS

New South Wales Emergency Care Institute, clinical conditions and procedure guides (including wounds, splinting and joint reduction techniques)

Clinical tools: https://aci.health.nsw.gov.au/networks/eci/clinical/clinical-tools.

Procedures: https://aci.health.nsw.gov.au/networks/eci/clinical/procedures.

Royal Children's Hospital Melbourne, Clinical Practice Guidelines, www.rch.org.au/clinicalguide/.

Australian and New Zealand Immunisation Handbooks

Australia, https://immunisationhandbook.health.gov.au/contents.

New Zealand, www.health.govt.nz/publication/immunisation-handbook-2020.

Queensland Health, Primary Clinical Care Manual, The principal clinical reference text for health professionals working in rural, remote and isolated health care settings

www.health.qld.gov.au/rrcsu/clinical-manuals/primary-clinical-care-manual-pccm.

REFERENCES

1. Australian Institute of Health and Welfare. Emergency department care. 2022. Online. Available from: www.aihw.gov.au/getmedia/0d0d6cbf-e764-4a89-a71a-b03c5156235d/Emergency-Department-Care-2020-21.xlsx.aspx.
2. O'Brien D, Williams A, Blondell K, Jelinek GA. Impact of streaming 'fast track' emergency department patients. Aust Health Rev 2006;30(4): 525–32.

3. NSW Ministry of Health. Emergency department models of care. Sydney: NSW Government; 2012.
4. Dinh MM, Enright N, Walker A, Parameswaran A, Chu M. Determinants of patient satisfaction in an Australian emergency department fast-track setting. Emerg Med J 2013;30(10):824–7.
5. Gardner G, Gardner A, Middleton S, Considine J, Fitzgerald G, Christofis L, et al. Mapping workforce configuration and operational models in Australian emergency departments: a national survey. Aust Health Rev 2017;42(3):340–7.
6. Hoyle S, Swain AH, Fake P, Larsen PD. Introduction of an extended care paramedic model in New Zealand. Emerg Med Australas 2012;24(6): 652–6.
7. Thompson C, Williams K, Morris D, Lago L, Kobel C, Quinsey K, et al. HWA Expanded scopes of practice program evaluation: extending the role of paramedics sub-project: final report of paramedics sub-project: final report. Wollongong, NSW: University of Wollongong, Australian Health Services Research Institute; 2014.
8. Wallis M, Hooper J, Kerr D, Lind J, Bost N. Effectiveness of an advanced practice emergency nurse role in a minor injuries unit. Aust J Adv Nurs 2009;27(1):21–9.
9. Alkhouri H, Maka K, Wong L, McCarthy S. Impact of the primary contact physiotherapy practitioner role on emergency department care for patients with musculoskeletal injuries in New South Wales. Emerg Med Australas 2020;32(2):202–9.
10. Plath SJ, Bratby JA, Poole L, Forristal CE, Morel DG. Nurse practitioners in the emergency department: establishing a successful service. Collegian 2019;26(4):457–62.
11. Gill SD, Stella J, McManus L. Consumer preferences regarding physiotherapy practitioners and nurse practitioners in emergency departments–a qualitative investigation. J Interprof Care 2019;33(2):209–15.
12. Jennings N, Clifford S, Fox AR, O'Connell J, Gardner G. The impact of nurse practitioner services on cost, quality of care, satisfaction and waiting times in the emergency department: a systematic review. Int J Nurs Stud 2015;52(1):421–35.
13. Lutze M, Ross M, Chu M, Green T, Dinh M. Patient perceptions of emergency department fast track: a prospective pilot study comparing two models of care. Australas Emerg Nurs J 2014;17(3):112–18.
14. Dinh M, Walker A, Parameswaran A, Enright N. Evaluating the quality of care delivered by an emergency department fast track unit with both nurse practitioners and doctors. Australas Emerg Nurs J 2012;15(4):188–94.
15. Tichter A, Carter W, Stone S. Wound preparation. In: Tintinalli J, Mao S, Yearly D, editors. Tintinalli's emergency medicine: a comprehensive study guide. 8th ed. New York: McGraw-Hill Education; 2016.
16. Javorac D, Stajer V, Ratgeber L, Olah A, Betlehem J, Acs P, et al. Hydrotherapy with hydrogen-rich water compared with RICE protocol following acute ankle sprain in professional athletes: a randomized non-inferiority pilot trial. Res Sports Med 2021;29(6):517–25.
17. Van Den Bekerom MP, Struijs PA, Blankevoort L, Welling L, van Dijk CN, Kerkhoffs GM. What is the evidence for rest, ice, compression, and elevation therapy in the treatment of ankle sprains in adults? J Ath Train 2012;47(4):435–43.
18. Bleakley C, Glasgow P, MacAuley D. PRICE needs updating, should we call the POLICE? Br J Sports Med 2012;46(4):220–1.
19. Norton C. How to use PRICE treatment for soft tissue injuries. Nurs Stand 2016;30(52):48–52.
20. Dubois B, Esculier JF. Soft-tissue injuries simply need PEACE and LOVE. Br J Sports Med 2020;54(2):72–3.
21. NPS MedicineWise. Acute pain management. 2022. Online. Available from: www.nps.org.au/pain-management-hub/acute-pain-management.
22. Purcell D. Minor injuries E-book: a clinical guide. 3rd ed. Kindle edition. Sydney: Churchill Livingstone; 2016.
23. Moses KP, Nava PB, Banks JC, Petersen D. Atlas of clinical gross anatomy. St Louis: Mosby Elsevier; 2005.
24. Cunningham NJ. Techniques for reduction of anteroinferior shoulder dislocation. Emerg Med Australas 2005;17(5-6):463–71.
25. Estephan A. Clavicle fracture in emergency medicine treatment and management. New York: Medscape; 2012.
26. Herteleer M, Winckelmans T, Hoekstra H, Nijs S. Epidemiology of clavicle fractures in a level 1 trauma center in Belgium. Eur J Trauma Emerg Surg 2018;44(5):717–26.
27. Kleinhenz B. Clavicle fractures. New York: Medscape; 2017.
28. Devji T, Kleinlugtenbelt Y, Evaniew N, Ristevski B, Khoudigian S, Bhandari M. Operative versus nonoperative interventions for common fractures of the clavicle: a meta-analysis of randomized controlled trials. CMAJ Open 2015;3(4):E396–405.
29. Lenza M, Faloppa F. Conservative interventions for treating middle third clavicle fractures in adolescents and adults. Cochrane Database Syst Rev 2016;12(12):CD007121.
30. Launonen AP, Lepola V, Flinkkilä T, Laitinen M, Paavola M, Malmivaara A. Treatment of proximal humerus fractures in the elderly: a systematic review of 409 patients. Acta Orthopaedica 2015;86(3):280–5.
31. Appelboam A, Reuben A, Benger J, Beech F, Dutson J, Haig S, et al. Elbow extension test to rule out elbow fracture: multicentre, prospective validation and observational study of diagnostic accuracy in adults and children. BMJ 2008;337:a2428.
32. Cameron P, Jelinek G, Kelly A, editors. Textbook of adult emergency medicine. 2nd ed. London UK: Churchill Livingstone: Elsevier; 2005.
33. Chow YC, Lee SW. Elbow and forearm injuries. In: Tintinalli JE, Ma O, Yealy DM, Meckler GD, Stapczynski S, Cline DM, et al., editors. Tintinalli's emergency medicine, a comprehensive study guide. 9th ed. New York: McGraw-Hill Education; 2016.
34. Herring W. Positive fat pad sign – elbow joint effusion. 2015. Online. Available from: http://learningradiology.com/notes/bonenotes/posteriorfatpad.htm.
35. McRae R, Esser M. Practical fracture treatment e-book. Edinburgh: Elsevier Health Sciences; 2008.

36. Nguyen TV, Center JR, Sambrook PN, Eisman JA. Risk factors for proximal humerus, forearm, and wrist fractures in elderly men and women: the dubbo osteoporosis epidemiology study. Am J Epidemiol 2001;153(6):587–95.
37. Upton D, Chorley J. Overview of acute wrist injuries in children and adolescents. UpToDate; 2017. Online. Available from: www.uptodate.com/contents/overview-of-acute-wrist-injuries-in-children-and-adolescents.
38. Jelinek G, Kelly A. Section 4: orthopaedic emergencies. In: Cameron P, Jelinek G, Kelly A, Little M, editors. Textbook of adult emergency medicine. 4th ed. Edinburgh, UK: Churchill Livingstone; 2014.
39. Kraus GP, Rondeau B, Fitzgerald BM. Bier block. In: StatPearls [Internet]. StatPearls Publishing; 2017. Online. Available from: www.ncbi.nlm.nih.gov/books/NBK430760/
40. Tabrizi A, Tolouei FM, Hassani E, Taleb H, Elmi A. Hematoma block versus general anesthesia in distal radius fractures in patients over 60 years in trauma emergency. Anesth Pain Med 2016;7(1):e40619.
41. Rhemrev SJ, Ootes D, Beeres FJ, Meylaerts SA, Schipper IB. Current methods of diagnosis and treatment of scaphoid fractures. Int J Emerg Med 2011;4:4.
42. Mallee WH, Wang J, Poolman RW, Kloen P, Maas M, de Vet HC, et al. Computed tomography versus magnetic resonance imaging versus bone scintigraphy for clinically suspected scaphoid fractures in patients with negative plain radiographs. Cochrane Database Syst Rev 2015;(6):CD010023.
43. Emergency Care Institute. Removeable wrist splints for Buckle fractures. Agency for Clinical innovation NSW; 2022. Online. Available from: https://aci.health.nsw.gov.au/networks/eci/clinical/clinical-tools/orthopaedic-and-musculoskeletal/upper-limb-injuries.
44. Jones C, Wolf M, Herman M. Acute and chronic growth plate injuries. Pediatr Rev 2017;38(3):129–38.
45. Krul M, van der Wouden JC, Kruithof EJ, van Suijlekom-Smit LW, Koes BW. Manipulative interventions for reducing pulled elbow in young children. Cochrane Database Syst Rev 2017;7(7):CD007759.
46. Blomberg J. Metacarpal fractures. OrthoBullets; 2017. Online. Available from: www.orthobullets.com/hand/6037/metacarpal-fractures.
47. Dunn JC, Kusnezov N, Orr JD, Pallis M, Mitchell JS. The boxer's fracture: splint immobilization is not necessary. Orthopedics 2016;39(3):188–92.
48. Krueger C. Base of thumb fractures. Orthobullets; 2017. Online. Available from: www.orthobullets.com/hand/6036/base-of-thumb-fractures.
49. Singer A, Hollander J. Wound closure. In: Tintinallis JE, Ma OJ, Yealy DM, Meckler JD, Cline DM, Thomas SH, editors. Tintinallis emergency medicine: a comprehensive study guide. New York: McGraw-Hill Education; 2015.
50. Yao K, Haque T. The Ottawa knee rules: a useful clinical decision tool. Aust Fam Phys 2012;41(4):223–4.
51. Bulloch B, Neto G, Plint A, Lim R, Lidman P, Reed M, et al. Validation of the Ottawa Knee Rule in children: a multicenter study. Ann Emerg Med 2003;42(1):48–55.
52. Wang JH, Lee JH, Cho Y, Shin JM, Lee BH. Efficacy of knee joint aspiration in patients with acute ACL injury in the emergency department. Injury 2016;47(8):1744–9.
53. Moore B, Bothner J. Recognition and initial management of patellar dislocations. UpToDate; 2022. Online. Available from: www. uptodate.com.acs.hcn.com.au/contents/recognition-and-initial-management-of-patellar-dislocations.
54. Myers D. Patella fracture. OrthoBullets; 2022. Online. Available from: www.orthobullets.com/trauma/1042/patella-fracture.
55. Stiell IG, Greenberg GH, Wells GA, McDowell I, Cwinn AA, Smith NA, et al. Prospective validation of a decision rule for the use of radiography in acute knee injuries. JAMA 1996;275(8):611–15.
56. Bachmann LM, Kolb E, Koller MT, Steurer J, ter Riet G. Accuracy of Ottawa ankle rules to exclude fractures of the ankle and mid-foot: systematic review. BMJ 2003;326(7386):417.
57. Stiell IG, Greenberg GH, McKnight RD, Nair RC, McDowell I, Worthington JR. A study to develop clinical decision rules for the use of radiography in acute ankle injuries. Ann Emerg Med 1992;21(4):384–90.
58. Dowling S, Spooner CH, Liang Y, Dryden DM, Friesen C, Klassen TP, et al. Accuracy of Ottawa Ankle Rules to exclude fractures of the ankle and midfoot in children: a meta-analysis. Acad Emerg Med 2009;16(4):277–87.
59. Bryan Dixon J. Gastrocnemius vs. soleus strain: how to differentiate and deal with calf muscle injuries. Curr Rev Musculoskel Med 2009; 2(2):74–7.
60. Rainbow C. Calf injuries not involving the Achilles tendon. UpToDate; 2017. Online. Available from: www.uptodate.com/contents/calf-injuries-not-involving-the-achilles-tendon.
61. Cahill K, Gilleard O, Weir A, Cubison TCS. The epidemiology and mortality of pretibial lacerations. J Plast Reconst Aesth Surg 2015;68(5):724–8.
62. Yap RY, Babel A, Phoon KM, Ward AE. Functional outcomes following operative and nonoperative management of Weber C ankle fractures: a systematic review. J Foot Ankle Surg 2020;59(1):105–11.
63. Doherty C, Delahunt E, Caulfield B, Hertel J, Ryan J, Bleakley C. The incidence and prevalence of ankle sprain injury: a systematic review and meta-analysis of prospective epidemiological studies. Sp Med 2014;44(1):123–40.
64. Seah R, Mani-Babu S. Managing ankle sprains in primary care: what is best practice? A systematic review of the last 10 years of evidence. Br Med Bull 2011;97(1):105–35.
65. Lardenoye S, Theunissen E, Cleffken B, Brink PR, de Bie RA, Poeze M. The effect of taping versus semi-rigid bracing on patient outcome and satisfaction in ankle sprains: a prospective, randomized controlled trial. BMC Musculoskel Dis 2012;13(1):1–7.
66. Thompson JY, Byrne C, Williams MA, Keene DJ, Schlussel MM, Lamb SE. Prognostic factors for recovery following acute lateral ankle ligament sprain: a systematic review. BMC Musculoskel Dis 2017;18(1):1–14.

67. Gulati V, Jaggard M, Al-Nammari SS, Uzoigwe C, Gulati P, Ismail N, et al. Management of Achilles tendon injury: a current concepts systematic review. World J Orthoped 2015;6(4):380–6.
68. Walters JL, Gangopadhyay P, Malay DS. Association of calcaneal and spinal fractures. J Foot Ankle Surg 2014;53(3):279–81.
69. Gaillard F, Lustosa L. Lisfranc injury. Radiopaedia; 2022. Online. Available from: radiopaedia.org/articles/lisfranc-injury
70. Clare MP. Lisfranc injuries. Curr Rev Musculoskel Med 2017;10(1):81–5.
71. Bowes J, Buckley R. Fifth metatarsal fractures and current treatment. World J Orthoped 2016;7(12):793.
72. Hossain M, Clutton J, Ridgewell M, Lyons K, Perera A. Stress fractures of the foot. Clin Sp Med 2015;34(4):769–90.
73. Watts E. Turf toe. OrthoBullets; 2017. Online. Available from: www.orthobullets.com/foot-and-ankle/7011/turf-toe.
74. Gravlee J. Toe fractures in adults; UpToDate. 2022. Online. Available from: https://www.uptodate.com/contents/toe-fractures-in-adults.
75. Mandell G, Bennett J, Mandell D, editors. Douglas and Bennett's principles and practice of infectious diseases. 7th ed. Philadelphia: Churchill Livingstone; 2010.
76. Doughty D, Sparks-Defriese B. Wound healing physiology. In: Bryant R, Nix D, editors. Acute and chronic wounds. 3rd ed. St Louis: Mosby; 2007.
77. Perez JL, Rohrich RJ. Optimizing postsurgical scars: a systematic review on best practices in preventative scar management. Plastic Reconstruct Surg 2017;140(6):782e–93.
78. Del Toro D, Dedhia R, Tollefson TT. Advances in scar management: prevention and management of hypertrophic scars and keloids. Curr Opin Otolaryngol Head Neck Surg 2016;24(4):322–9.
79. LeBlanc K, Baranoski S, Christensen D, Langemo D, Edwards K, Holloway S, et al. The art of dressing selection: a consensus statement on skin tears and best practice. Adv Skin Wound Care 2016;29(1):32–46.
80. ISTAP. International Skin Tear Advisory Panel (ISTAP): decisions algorithm. 2018. Online. Available from: www.skintears.org/_files/ugd/9d080f_e040fdb2aef5461a831f106d7e4a2178.pdf?index=true.
81. Lewis D, Jivraj A, Atkinson P, Jarman R. My patient is injured: identifying foreign bodies with ultrasound. Ultrasound 2015;23(3):174–80.
82. Canale ST, Beaty JH. Campbell's operative orthopaedics. 11th ed. St Louis: Mosby; 2007.
83. Lammers RL. Methods of wound closure. In: Roberts JR, Hedges JR, editors. Clinical procedures in emergency medicine. 5th ed. Philadelphia: Saunders; 2010. p. 592–633.
84. Patel L. Management of simple nail bed lacerations and subungual hematomas in the emergency department. Pediat Emerg Care 2014;30(10):742–5.
85. Ciocon D, Gowrishankar T, Herndon T, Kimball AB. How low should you go: novel device for nail trephination. Dermatol Surg 2006;32(6):828–33.
86. Metcalfe D, Aquilina A, Hedley H. Prophylactic antibiotics in open distal phalanx fractures: systematic review and meta-analysis. J Hand Surg (European Volume) 2016;41(4):423–30.
87. Ramirez C, Menaker J. Traumatic amputations. Trauma reports website. 2022. Online. Available from: www.reliasmedia.com/articles/140552-traumatic-amputations
88. Queirós P, Santos E, Apóstolo J, Cardoso D, Cunha M, Rodrigues M. The effectiveness of cleansing solutions for wound treatment: a systematic review. JBI Evid Synth 2014;12(10):121–51.
89. Prabhakar H, Rath S, Kalaivani M, Bhanderi N. Adrenaline with lidocaine for digital nerve blocks. Cochrane Database Syst Rev 2015(3):CD010645.
90. Ilicki J. Safety of epinephrine in digital nerve blocks: a literature review. J Emerg Med 2015;49(5):799–809.
91. Newton DJ, McLeod GA, Khan F, Belch JJ. The effect of adjuvant epinephrine concentration on the vasoactivity of the local anesthetics bupivacaine and levobupivacaine in human skin. ASRA Pain Med 2004;29(4):307–11.
92. Dillon D, Gibbs M. Local and regional anesthesia. In: Tintinalli JE, Ma O, Yealy DM, Stapczynski J, Meckler G, editors. Tintinalli's emergency medicine: a comprehensive study guide. 8th ed. New York: McGraw-Hill Education; 2016.
93. Rosenberg PH, Veering BT, Urmey WF. Maximum recommended doses of local anesthetics: a multifactorial concept. ASRA Pain Med 2004;29(6):564–75.
94. Fernandez R, Griffiths R. Water for wound cleansing. Cochrane Database Syst Rev 2008;(1):CD003861.
95. Nicks BA, Ayello EA, Woo K, Nitzki-George D, Sibbald RG. Acute wound management: revisiting the approach to assessment, irrigation, and closure considerations. International J Emerg Med 2010;3(4):399–407.
96. Joanna Briggs Institute JBI. Solutions, techniques and pressure in wound cleansing. Nurs Stand. 2008 Mar 12-18;22(27):35–9.
97. Gabriel A. Wound irrigation. New York: Medscape; 2017.
98. Farion KJ, Russell KF, Osmond MH, Klassen T, Crumley E, Wiebe N, et al. Tissue adhesives for traumatic lacerations in children and adults. Cochrane Database of Syst Rev 2002;2002(3):CD003326.
99. Armstrong D, Meyr A. Basic principles of wound management. UpToDate; 2017. Online. Available from: www.uptodate.com/contents/basic-principles-of-wound-management.
100. Lewis SM, McLean M, Dirksen SR, editors. Medical-surgical nursing: assessment and management of clinical problems. 5th ed. St Louis: Mosby; 2000.
101. Garmon EH, Huecker MR. Topical, Local and regional anaesthesia and anaesthetics. StatPearls - NCBI Bookshelf. 2022. Online. Available from: www.ncbi.nlm.nih.gov/books/NBK430894/

102. Kruse CR, Nuutila K, Lee CC, iwanuka E, Singh M, Caterson EJ, et al. The external microenvironment of healing skin wounds. Wound Rep Regen 2015;23(4):456–64.
103. Therapeutic Guidelines. Fundamentals of ulcer and wound management. In: Therapeutic Guidelines. Melbourne: Therapeutic Guidelines Limited. 2021. Online. Available from: www.tg.org.au
104. Del Mar CB, Scott AM, Glasziou PP, Hoffmann T, van Driel ML, Beller E, et al. Reducing antibiotic prescribing in Australian general practice: time for a national strategy. Med J Aust 2017;207(9):401–6.
105. AAE Group. Principles of prophylactic, empirical and directed antimicrobial therapy. Melbourne: Therapeutic Guidelines Limited; 2017.
106. Turnidge J. Antimicrobial use and resistance in Australia. Aust Prescr 2017;40:2–3.
107. East JM, Yeates CB, Robinson HP. The natural history of pedal puncture wounds in diabetics: a cross-sectional survey. BMC Surg 2011;11(1):1–9.
108. Therapeutic Guidelines. Antibiotics. Melbourne: Therapeutic Guidelines Limited; 2021.
109. Eliya-Masamba MC, Banda GW. Primary closure versus delayed closure for non bite traumatic wounds within 24 hours post injury. Cochrane Database Syst Rev 2013;(10):CD008574.
110. Baddour LM, Brown AM. Infectious complications of puncture wounds; UpToDate; 2023. Online. Available from: www.uptodate.com/contents/infectious-complications-of-puncture-wounds.
111. Leong C, Goulouris T. Skin and soft tissue infections. Medicine 2021;49(11):699–705.
112. Australian Technical Advisory Group on Immunisation (ATAGI). Table. Guide to tetanus prophylaxis in wound management. Australian Immunisation Handbook, Australian Government Department of Health and Aged Care, Canberra. 2018. Online. Available from: immunisationhandbook.health.gov.au/resources/tables/table-guide-to-tetanus-prophylaxis-in-wound-management.
113. Australian Technical Advisory Group on Immunisation (ATAGI). Tetanus. Australian immunisation handbook. 10th ed. Canberra: Australian Government Department of Health and Aged Care; 2022. Online. Available from: https://immunisationhandbook.health.gov.au/contents/vaccine-preventable-diseases/tetanus.
114. Australian Technical Advisory Group on Immunisation (ATAGI). Australian Immunisation Handbook. Canberra: Australian Government Department of Health and Aged Care; 2022. Online. Available from: immunisationhandbook.health.gov.au.
115. Baddour LM. Soft tissue infections following water exposure. UpToDate. 2023. Online. Available from: www.uptodate.com/contents/soft-tissue-infections-following-water exposure#:~:text=For%20most%20soft%20tissue%20infections,until%20signs%20of%20infection%20resolve.
116. Therapeutic Guidelines. Water-immersed wound infections. Melbourne: Therapeutic Guidelines Limited; 2021.
117. Dendle C, Looke D. Management of mammalian bites. Aust Fam Phys 2009;38(11):868–74.
118. ABE Group. Bite wounds and clenched fist injuries. Melbourne: Therapeutic Guidelines Ltd; 2014.
119. Dendle C, Looke D. Animal bites: an update for management with a focus on infections. Emerg Med Australas 2008;20(6):458–67.
120. Broom J, Woods ML. Management of bite injuries. Aust Prescr 2006;29:6–8.
121. Harper M. Clinical manifestations and initial management of animal and human bites. UpToDate. 2023. Online. Available from: www.uptodate.com/contents/animal-bites-dogs-cats-and-other-animals-evaluation-and-management.
122. Revis D. Human bite infections. New York: Medscape; 2009.
123. Therapeutic Guidelines. Fundamentals of antibiotic choice. Melbourne: Therapeutic Guidelines Limited. 2021. Online. Available from: www.tg.org.au.
124. Barrett J. Human bites. New York: Medscape; 2017.
125. Hui AY, Hung LC, Tse PC, Leung WK, Chan PK, Chan HL. Transmission of hepatitis B by human bite—confirmation by detection of virus in saliva and full genome sequencing. J Clin Virol 2005;33(3):254–6.
126. Tebble NJ, Thomas DW, Price P. Anxiety and self-consciousness in patients with minor facial lacerations. J Adv Nurs 2004;47(4):417–26.
127. Hoyt KS, Flarity K, Shea SS. Wound care and laceration repair for nurse practitioners in emergency care: part II. Adv Emerg Nurs J 2011;33(1):84–99.
128. Hollander JE, Stack A, Wolfson AB. Assessment and management of facial lacerations. UpToDate. 2023. Online. Available from: www.uptodate.com/contents/assessment-and-management-of-facial-lacerations?search=assessment%20and%20management%20of%20facial%20lacerations&source=search_result&selectedTitle=1~150&usage_type=default&display_rank=1.
129. Day PF, Duggal M, Nazzal H. Interventions for treating traumatised permanent front teeth: avulsed (knocked out) and replanted. Cochrane Database Syst Rev 2019;2(2):CD006542.
130. Doshi D, Hogg K. Avulsed tooth brought in milk for replantation. Blackburn Royal Infirmary: BestBETs. 2023. Online. Available from: bestbets.org/bets/bet.php?id=187.
131. Skapetis T. Lecture notes: dental trauma. Westmead: Clinical Director of Education, Westmead Centre for Oral Health; 2009.
132. Hollander JE, Conlon LW, Wolfson AB. Assessment and management of lip lacerations. UpToDate; 2022. Online. Available from: www.medilib.ir/uptodate/show/13877.

CHAPTER 18

PAIN MANAGEMENT

BILL LORD AND WAYNE F. VARNDELL

ESSENTIALS

- Pain relief is an important component of the patient care process and is a basic human right.
- Unrelieved acute pain may be associated with morbidities, including the development of persistent pain due to changes in peripheral nerves, the spinal cord, pain pathways in the central nervous systems and sympathetic nerves.
- Pain is a highly personal experience, and the perception and expression of pain are influenced by many factors, which include prior pain experience, culture, gender, coping strategies, expectations of care and the social environment in which the pain occurs. There are no standards of pain expression, and interpersonal comparisons should not be used to set 'norms' for pain-related behaviour.
- Regular assessment of pain should be undertaken to inform pain management decisions and to document the efficacy of care.
- Pain severity should be measured using validated tools. Wherever possible, the patient's self-report should be used to evaluate pain severity.
- Assessment of the presence and severity of pain in patients with communication difficulties or cognitive impairment should involve alternative tools which include assessment of pain-related behaviours.
- The type of pain and severity should inform the choice of analgesic interventions.
- Opioids should be given intravenously and titrated to achieve the desired effect; there are large inter-patient variations in doses required to achieve pain relief and standard doses for adult patients may be ineffective in some cases.
- Intranasal administration of lipid-soluble opioids such as fentanyl produces effective analgesia and may be indicated where intravenous access is not possible.
- Adverse effects, such as respiratory depression, are associated with opioid use, but the risk can be reduced through careful titration and observation of sedation, as sedation is an early and more reliable sign of respiratory depression than a decrease in respiratory rate.
- Non-pharmacological interventions play an important role in the alleviation of pain.
- Although there are contraindications to specific analgesics, there are no contraindications to pain relief.

INTRODUCTION

Pain is a multidimensional phenomenon that results from a complex interaction of physiological and neurochemical effects, with psychosocial and environmental factors, such as culture, context, previous pain experience, personality, coping styles and expectations of cure influencing the individual's perception and expression of pain. Although pain is considered to be an inevitable consequence of tissue injury, and its management is influenced by beliefs that pain in itself is not harmful, evidence shows that unrelieved pain is associated with significant morbidity. Unrelieved pain may increase the risk of delirium in older patients with hip fracture,[1] and may produce significant disability associated with 'emotional, behavioural and social disruption'.[2] Pain has been shown to inhibit immune function,[3] and can have detrimental effects on respiratory, cardiovascular, gastrointestinal and other body systems. Apart from the humane and moral considerations, it is imperative to relieve pain, as the early relief of pain can have a significant effect on the overall health of the individual. Adverse effects of inadequately managed severe acute pain are listed in Box 18.1.

Pain is a common complaint that motivates people to seek emergency care, with evidence showing that over 60% of patients report pain on arrival at an emergency department (ED),[5] with severe pain reported at between 20% and 40% globally.[6] Patients expect their pain to be relieved in the ED, with a significant number expecting complete analgesia.[7] There is, however, evidence that these expectations are not always met, with low rates of analgesia for some painful conditions and evidence that some patients experience long delays between arrival at an ED and analgesic interventions.[8,9] Despite targeted strategies to improve the effectiveness of analgesia in cases of severe pain, research has failed to identify significant change.[10]

Disparities in the relief of pain in the ED setting have been associated with ethnicity[11] and age.[12] The very young and the elderly have been found to be at risk of inadequate analgesia, with these findings attributed to safety concerns associated with opioid administration, as well as difficulties in assessing pain due to communication issues related to age or disease such as dementia.[13,14] However, extremes of age should not result in disparities in the relief of pain. Patient gender has been found to influence pain management practice in the ED,[15] with the gender of the health provider also influencing practice.[16] Gender disparities have been demonstrated in the pre-hospital setting, with females treated by paramedics being less likely to receive morphine, despite having more severe pain than males.[17] Race also appears to influence the odds of receiving analgesia in the pre-hospital setting.[18] Although pain management has been identified as a clinical priority in the pre-hospital setting, there is evidence of inadequate analgesia among patients treated by paramedics,[19] with children less likely to receive paramedic-initiated analgesia for painful injuries.[20] The reasons for the suboptimal management of pain in children include inadequate provider education, inexperience in providing care for children, unfamiliarity with age-specific pain assessment tools, and practice guidelines that are not based on contemporary evidence.[21]

Efforts to reduce disparities in care and to improve the healthcare professional's response to pain require a better understanding of factors that have contributed to inadequate management. Although multiple factors can contribute to ineffective pain management, barriers that have been documented include:

- lack of educational emphasis on pain management practices in nursing and medical school curricula and postgraduate training programs
- inadequate or non-existent clinical quality management programs that evaluate pain management
- a paucity of rigorous studies of populations with special needs that improve pain management in the ED, particularly in elderly and paediatric patients
- clinicians' attitudes towards opioid analgesics that result in inappropriate diagnosis of drug-seeking behaviour and inappropriate concern about addiction, even in patients who have obvious acutely painful conditions and who request pain relief
- inappropriate concerns about the safety of opioids compared with non-steroidal anti-inflammatory drugs (NSAIDs), which result in their under-use (opiophobia)
- unappreciated cultural and sex differences in pain reporting by patients and interpretation of pain reporting by providers
- bias and disbelief of pain reporting according to racial and ethnic stereotyping.[22]

Despite the existence of these barriers, safe, effective and early control of pain is an appropriate and achievable goal for emergency care. Healthcare professionals can achieve these goals by ensuring that a comprehensive pain assessment is performed in the early stage of care, by using a reliable pain scale to measure pain severity and by taking a lead role in the management of the patient's pain. This requires a sound

BOX 18.1 ADVERSE EFFECTS OF UNDERTREATED SEVERE ACUTE PAIN[4]

CARDIOVASCULAR

Tachycardia, hypertension, increased peripheral vascular resistance, increased myocardial oxygen consumption, myocardial ischaemia, altered regional blood flow, deep-vein thrombosis, pulmonary embolism

RESPIRATORY

Reduced lung volumes, atelectasis, decreased cough, sputum retention, infection, hypoxaemia

GASTROINTESTINAL

Decreased gastric and bowel motility, increased risk of bacterial transgression of bowel wall

GENITOURINARY

Urinary retention

NEUROENDOCRINE

- Increased catabolic hormones—glucagon, growth metabolic hormone, vasopressin, aldosterone, renin and angiotensin
- Reduced anabolic hormones—insulin, testosterone
- This catabolic state leads to hyperglycaemia, increased protein breakdown, negative nitrogen balance; leading to impaired wound healing and muscle wasting

MUSCULOSKELETAL

Muscle spasm, immobility (increasing risk of deep-vein thrombosis), muscle wasting leading to prolonged recovery of function

PSYCHOLOGICAL

Anxiety, fear, helplessness, sleep deprivation, leading to increased pain

CENTRAL NERVOUS

Chronic (persistent) pain due to central sensitisation

knowledge of pain and its management, a more active role in the assessment and management of pain, and the development of evidence-based treatment plans to ensure safe and effective pain management. Clinical practice guidelines are available for the assessment and management of pain, and these should inform treatment plans.

DEFINITION OF PAIN

The International Association for the Study of Pain (IASP) defines pain as 'an unpleasant sensory and emotional experience associated with, or resembling that associated with, actual or potential tissue damage'.[23] This definition recognises the emotional interpretation and response to pain that is shaped by gender and cultural, environmental and social factors, as well as prior pain experience. This definition also acknowledges the fact that patients can experience very real pain without evidence of obvious pathology, such as phantom limb pain associated with amputation and some chronic pain syndromes.

It is important to remember that pain is a symptom that cannot be objectively verified in the same way that other clinical findings can. Attempts to judge the patient's pain should be resisted, as this often leads to a devaluing of the patient's experience. Instead, healthcare professionals need to actively seek and accept the patient's self-report of their pain.

Pain can be defined as *acute* if it is of recent onset and probable limited duration (less than 3 months). It usually has an identifiable temporal and causal relationship to injury or disease. In contrast, *chronic*—also known as persistent—pain may not have a clearly identifiable cause, has no obvious biological value, lasts longer than the time taken for injuries to heal (considered to be a duration of greater than 3 months), and may not respond to standard analgesic interventions.

ANATOMY AND PHYSIOLOGY OF PAIN

Several theories of pain exist, but none are complete. One of the first published theories to describe the physiology of pain was developed by the 17th-century French philosopher René Descartes, who proposed a specific pain pathway between pain receptors in the skin and the brain. However, Descartes' purely mechanistic explanation of a stimulus–response model failed to acknowledge the interrelationships between the physical stimulus and the interpretation of the stimulus that is shaped by the individual's characteristics and experience of pain. This theory also assumes that the perception of pain arises from injury and ignores the possibility that pain can have no obvious physical basis. Descartes' theory influenced the study and treatment of pain for the next three centuries, and it was not until the mid-1900s that research into pain began to more correctly describe the complexity of the somatosensory system and multifactorial influences on individual pain perception and expression.

A major breakthrough in the understanding of pain occurred in 1965, when Melzack and Wall described their 'gate theory'.[24] This theory suggested that sensory input from peripheral nerves is transmitted to the dorsal horn of the spinal cord, where it is modulated and then transmitted to the brain for perception. 'Gates' occur at afferent synapses in the spinal cord and brain that are responsible for pain-signal transmission. When sensory stimulation associated with pain reaches the spinal cord, the gates open and uninhibited signals from the periphery ascend via the spinothalamic tract to the brain, where pain is perceived. The pain can be moderated or inhibited if the gates are closed. Other sensory stimuli, such as gently rubbing the injured area, can help to close the gate by stimulating inhibitory neurons, which can reduce the pain an individual is experiencing. This concept forms the basis of transcutaneous electrical nerve stimulation (TENS), which is a therapeutic intervention that can reduce pain through sensory stimulation of the affected area.

Subsequent growth in understanding pain processing recognised that pain had several dimensions other than the obvious sensory dimension. Later work by Melzack proposed that the perception of pain involves:

- a sensory–discriminative system that enables the recognition of the location, intensity and duration of pain
- a motivational–affective component associated with reflexes and strategies designed to avoid or escape from the cause of the pain
- a cognitive–evaluative component that involves the comparison of contextual information about the current pain experience with past experiences in order to evaluate the pain, its significance and consequences, which, when combined with sensory and affective information, helps to inform response strategies.[25]

The ability to perceive and react to threats to our wellbeing is an important protective homeostatic process. In order to detect potential tissue-damaging stimuli, the body needs sensitive somatosensory nerve fibres to relay action potentials to multiple peripheral and central centres. Pain is experienced through pathways in the central, peripheral and autonomic nervous systems. The peripheral sensory organs are known as *nociceptors*. These are widely dispersed throughout the body, and can be identified in skin, periosteum, joints, muscle and viscera.

Two main types of nociceptor—A-delta fibres and C-fibres—give rise to the varied perceptions of pain. The A-delta fibres are myelinated fibres that are stimulated by heat and noxious mechanical injury. Action potentials travel rapidly (2–20 m/s) along these fibres towards the dorsal horn of the spinal cord, where they synapse with second-order neurons to finally convey signals to the brain. Stimulation of A-delta fibres gives rise to pain that is experienced as the initial sharp pain that follows injury. The throbbing, slowly building and sometimes burning pain that follows this initial injury is transmitted along C-fibres. These fibres are unmyelinated and conduct action potentials more slowly (< 2 m/s). C-fibres are activated by heat and by noxious chemical and mechanical stimuli. A C-fibre subclass—the C-fibre polymodal receptor—responds to heat, cold, pressure and chemical stimuli. These pain pathways are illustrated in Fig. 18.1.

Tissue can be damaged by direct mechanical trauma (pressure, extremes of temperature or chemical), or by ischaemia and inflammation. Tissue injury causes the release of chemical mediators such as bradykinins, substance P, histamine and arachidonic acid derivatives, such as leukotrienes and prostaglandins. Several of these mediators are implicated in the stimulation and sensitisation of nociceptors.

Once a nociceptor is stimulated beyond its threshold, a signal is transmitted along the sensory nerve axon to the cell body in the dorsal root ganglion, and then on to a secondary

FIGURE 18.1 POSSIBLE ASCENDING AND DESCENDING PATHWAYS OF A-DELTA FIBRES AND C-FIBRES FROM THE DORSAL HORN IN THE SPINAL CORD TO THE THALAMUS AND OTHER CENTRES. THESE PATHWAYS ARE NOT DEFINITIVE AND MAY CROSS OVER[26]

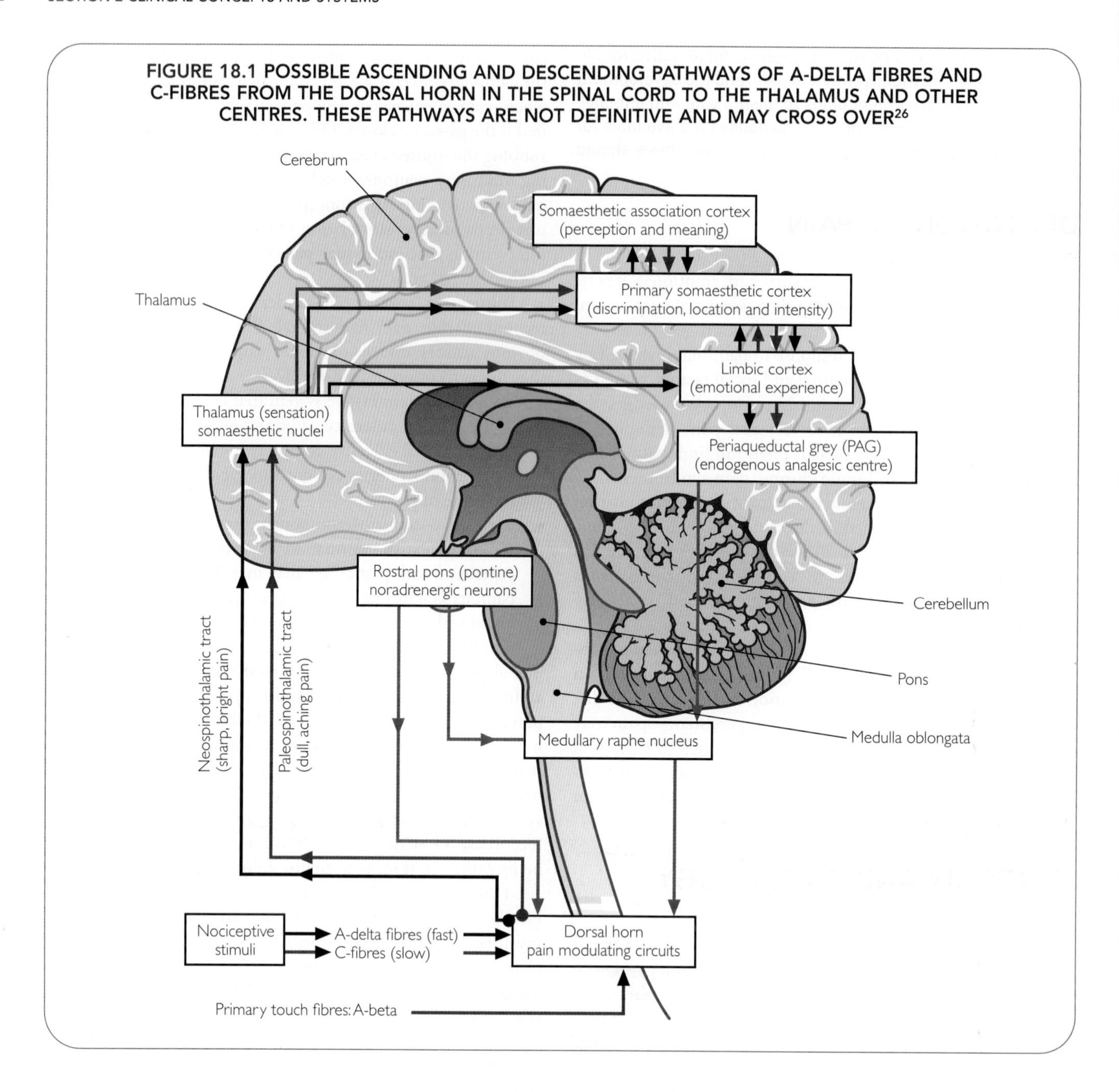

neuron in the dorsal horn of the spinal cord. Nociceptive information can be processed within the spinal cord, as in the case of spinal reflexes, where the nociceptor neuron synapses with an interneuron within the cord. This then synapses with an anterior horn efferent nerve to produce an action such as skeletal muscle contraction to withdraw a hand from a hot surface.

Conscious awareness of pain requires the transmission of the nociceptive signal via the spinothalamic tracts and the dorsal columns. Neurons then transfer information from the thalamus to the sensory cortex of the brain. While this may appear to be a simple connection of neurons, the perception of pain relies on complex interconnections between other areas of the brain, such as the hypothalamus, brainstem nuclei and basal ganglia. Connections to the frontal lobe enable conscious interpretation of the experience and influence our emotional response to pain.[27]

The afferent input from nociceptors is moderated or inhibited by neurons that descend from the cerebral cortex via the periaqueductal grey (PAG) matter to the dorsal horns of the spinal cord. These can facilitate or inhibit the second-order neurons, modifying the sensory input and, consequently, the perception of pain.

Neurotransmitters associated with nociceptive transmission in the spinal cord and brain include substance P, glutamate, monoamines and opioid peptides. Inhibition of pain is a function of endogenous opioid peptides such as the dynorphins, endorphins and encephalins, which inhibit nociceptor transmission and pain perception by binding with specific opioid receptors. Exogenous opioids, such as morphine, also bind to these receptors, which are located in the spinal cord (substantia gelatinosa and primary afferent fibres) and brain (rostroventral medulla and midbrain periaqueductal grey). Receptors have been classified as mu (μ), kappa (κ) and delta (δ). The μ_1

subtype is responsible for the analgesic and euphoric effect of opioids, while activation of the μ_2 subtype produces side-effects of opioid administration, including gastrointestinal slowing, constipation, sedation and respiratory depression. At this time, there is no μ_1-specific analgesic available.

PATHOPHYSIOLOGY

Pain is an important signal that tissue damage is occurring. Without the ability to perceive injury our life would be threatened, as organ ischaemia and inflammation would go undetected until the occurrence of major systemic derangement. However, some pain does not have any obvious pathological basis, and this serves as the basis for the classification of pain. A useful clinical approach involves the classification of pain as *nociceptive* (with subcategories somatic and visceral), and *neuropathic* (with subcategories centrally generated pain or peripherally generated pain). A comparison of the clinical features associated with these major types of pain is outlined in Table 18.1.

NOCICEPTIVE PAIN

Somatic pain occurs following injury to the skin, bone, joints and skeletal muscle. An example of somatic pain is that arising from a laceration to the hand caused by a sharp knife. Pain from cutaneous sites is initially sharp and well localised, although deeper structures such as muscle and joints may be more poorly localised. The initial pain may be followed by a duller, throbbing pain.

Visceral pain arises from stimulation of A-delta fibre and C-fibre nociceptors located near the surface of the organ. Ischaemia, stretching and pressure activate nociceptors, and pain from these structures is usually described as dull, cramp-like, diffuse and poorly localised. There may be associated autonomic stimulation as these afferent nerve fibres are located with sympathetic and sympathetic nerves innervating the same organs. Visceral pain can be referred to other areas of the body, possibly as a result of the fact that afferent fibres from the skin and viscera converge at the same secondary neurons within the spinal cord. This can produce pain that is perceived to be, for example, in the patient's left arm, if afferent signals from an ischaemic myocardium converge at the same level in the cord as cutaneous innervation from the arm. The classic descriptions of visceral pain can be gained from careful questioning, and this information helps to differentiate musculoskeletal and visceral pathologies. However, it should be remembered that patients could have pain arising from several anatomical sites concurrently (Fig. 18.2).

When nociceptors are repeatedly stimulated, their threshold for activation decreases, while the size of the response increases. This is known as *hyperalgesia*: an increased response to a painful stimulus. An associated term, *allodynia*, refers to pain produced by a stimulus that would not normally cause pain, and can be observed as the hypersensitive response to lightly stroking sunburnt skin.

NEUROPATHIC PAIN

Neuropathic pain—which may be acute or chronic—results from injuries or diseases that directly affect the nervous system. Acute neuropathic pain may result from lesions or entrapment of nerves; for example, an entrapped median nerve at the wrist

TABLE 18.1 CLASSIFICATION OF PAIN BY INFERRED PATHOLOGY[28]

TWO MAJOR TYPES OF PAIN	
I. NOCICEPTIVE PAIN	II. NEUROPATHIC PAIN
A. Somatic pain; B. Visceral pain	A. Centrally generated pain; B. Peripherally generated pain
Nociceptive pain: normal processing of stimuli that damages normal tissues or has the potential to do so if prolonged; usually responsive to non-opioids and/or opioids. *Somatic pain:* arises from bone, joint, muscle, skin or connective tissue. It is usually aching and is well localised. *Visceral pain:* arises from visceral organs, such as the gastrointestinal tract and pancreas. This may be subdivided: ◦ Tumour involvement of the organ capsule that causes aching and fairly well-localised pain. ◦ Obstruction of hollow viscus, which causes intermittent cramping and poorly localised pain.	**Neuropathic pain:** abnormal processing of sensory input by the peripheral or central nervous systems; treatment usually involves adjuvant analgesics. **Centrally generated pain** *Deafferentation pain:* injury to either the peripheral or the central nervous system. Examples: phantom pain may reflect injury to the peripheral nervous system; burning pain below the level of a spinal cord lesion reflects injury to the CNS. *Sympathetically maintained pain:* associated with dysregulation of the autonomic nervous system. Examples: may include some of the pain associated with reflex sympathetic dystrophy/causalgia (complex regional pain syndrome, type I, type II). **Peripherally generated pain** *Painful polyneuropathies:* pain is felt along the distribution of many peripheral nerves. Examples: diabetic neuropathy, alcohol-nutritional neuropathy and those associated with Guillain-Barré syndrome. *Painful mononeuropathies:* usually associated with a known peripheral nerve injury, and pain is felt at least partly along the distribution of the damaged nerve. Examples: nerve root compression, nerve entrapment, trigeminal neuralgia.

FIGURE 18.2 TYPICAL AREAS OF REFERRED PAIN[26]

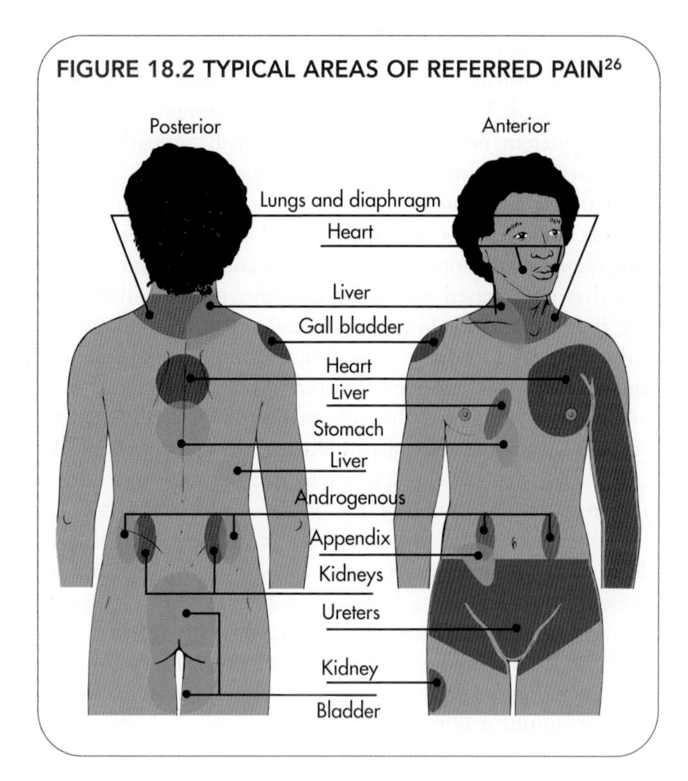

causes burning pain or unpleasant tingling. Sensory neurons in the parasympathetic pathway generate impulses that fire spasmodically at the site of the injury or may be stimulated by movement, causing sharp or burning pain. Neuropathic pain syndromes are complex and difficult to treat.

Hyperalgesia is an exaggerated neuronal response that intensifies the sensory perception of pain, especially in neuropathic pain. It can also be a feature of both somatic and visceral tissue injury and inflammation, occurring not only at the site of injury but also in the surrounding uninjured area (e.g. pharyngitis where swallowing can initiate severe pain).[29]

Chronic neuropathic pain is also referred to as central pain. Central pain is chronic pain that occurs as a result of a lesion or dysfunction in the central nervous system (CNS) rather than from receptor stimulation in the periphery. Diseases such as multiple sclerosis, stroke or traumatic spinal cord injury can produce central pain, and this may be associated with tactile allodynia (peripheral sensitisation). Central pain is usually diffuse and may extend over large areas, such as the whole right or left side or lower half of the body. Many symptoms and effects of central pain are congruent with acute neuropathic pain, and one of the main distinguishing features is the delay in the appearance of central pain after the causative event.[29]

PATIENT ASSESSMENT

APPROACH TO INITIAL EVALUATION

To effectively manage pain, clinicians must recognise that it has both physical and non-physical components. Specific components are the physical stimulus and the patient's cognitive and emotional interpretation of that stimulus. Interpretation of pain is influenced by a diverse range of factors that include the context in which the pain occurs, knowledge of the possible consequences of the injury or disease and trust and fear about interactions with healthcare professionals and health systems. Handling the subjectivity of pain can prove to be challenging, but a knowledgeable, calm, empathetic healthcare professional can do much to minimise the patient's fears and facilitate early pain management.

Pain may be the patient's chief complaint, or one of several symptoms associated with disease or injury. Pain can be an important marker of serious pathology, such as myocardial ischaemia, and a careful assessment of the quality of this symptom can inform clinical judgements regarding the likely cause of the pain and the most appropriate emergency interventions required. However, severe pain associated with significant soft tissue or musculoskeletal injury has the potential to distract the clinician from other clinical management priorities, and, as such, it is important to develop a systematic approach to patient assessment which ensures that, while pain is effectively managed, other priorities, such as airway patency and the patient's ventilation and perfusion status, are assessed and managed before lower-order priorities are addressed.

A comprehensive assessment is essential. A health history should be obtained to identify prior complaints and chronic pain conditions, as well as risk factors that may be associated with the current episode. The assessment of pain includes the measurement of pain severity, and the evaluation of the clinical data to develop a management plan. As the existence of pain cannot be proven or disproven by an independent observer, it is accepted that the patient's self-report is the most reliable indicator of the existence and intensity of pain.

PHYSICAL EXAMINATION

A focused assessment should be conducted to collect data about the patient's pain. The following mnemonic, PQRST, can assist assessment of pain, particularly when the cause of pain is not immediately obvious.

P **Provocation.** What activities were associated with the onset of pain? Did the pain occur during exercise, or did it occur at rest (unprovoked)? What makes the pain worse? Does deep inspiration, movement or palpation of the affected area change the intensity of the pain? When undertaking this assessment, it is important to avoid prompting the patient by asking leading questions and making inferences about the patient's pain.

Q **Quality.** How does the patient describe the pain? Is it dull, sharp, crushing, burning, shooting or cramping? Some of these descriptors are frequently associated with specific pathologies and are therefore useful in identifying possible causes of the pain.

R **Region, radiation and relief.** Ask the patient to describe the region or site of the pain. Patterns of radiation should be elicited using open, non-leading questioning techniques. For example, instead of asking, 'Does the pain radiate to your back?', ask 'Can you tell me about where the pain is located, and whether it can be felt in other areas of your body?' Factors that relieve the pain should be explored. Does a particular body posture, such as lying supine with knees flexed, or sitting forward, help to relieve the pain? Patients should be questioned about prescription or over-the-counter (OTC) medications that they may have taken in an attempt to relieve their pain.

S **Severity and associated symptoms.** Patients should be asked to rate their pain severity using a validated pain scale. Paediatric scales should be used to assess pain in children who cannot understand the instructions used to score pain in adults. Triage decisions in the ED will need to consider the patient's reported level of pain. The Australasian Triage Scale requires assessment and treatment of severe pain from any cause within 10 minutes (triage code/category 2). Patients reporting moderately severe pain from any cause that will require analgesia should be assessed and treated within 30 minutes (ATS category 3).[30] Associated symptoms, such as nausea and paraesthesia, should be sought.

T **Time of onset and duration.** Time of onset is important as this helps to differentiate acute and chronic pain. This information is also important if the patient is to receive thrombolytics for the management of cardiac pain, as the drug must be given within a narrow window of effectiveness (see Chapters 22 and 23 for further discussion of thrombolytics). Information should be sought about whether the pain is constant, or whether there have been periods of remission. Patients may have self-administered analgesics, or received analgesia from paramedics or other healthcare professionals prior to presenting at a healthcare facility. In these cases the drug, dose, time of last administration, analgesic effect and adverse events are important to note as this information informs the continuum of care.

Patients might have difficulty describing key components of their pain. Language barriers, cultural differences, cognitive impairment and other physiological or psychosocial factors may make the assessment more difficult, and require an assessment strategy that addresses these limitations. A general recommendation where self-report is unavailable or unreliable, is to seek evidence of pain-related behaviours, evidence of potential causes of pain, and to use estimates of pain by others such as carers and relatives who can describe changes in a patient's behaviour that may be associated with pain. Pain scales designed for the assessment of acute pain in cognitively impaired adults are available, and these may have utility in emergency health settings.[31] Physiological indicators such as vital signs have been shown to be an unreliable indicator of pain severity, and their use for this purpose is discouraged.[32–34]

PAIN SCALES

Pain-rating scales provide important information regarding the severity and nature of the patient's pain. Measurement of pain helps the clinician to:

- determine pain intensity, quality and duration
- aid in the diagnosis
- help determine the choice of therapy
- evaluate the relative effectiveness of the therapy.[25]

Evidence demonstrates that formal pain measurement reveals unrecognised or under-treated pain, with the consequence that improved recognition of pain can lead to improved pain management practice.[35] Simple pain scales include the adjective rating scale (ARS), numeric rating scale (NRS) and visual analogue scale (VAS). The ARS involves the use of descriptions of pain severity, such as 'none', 'slight', 'moderate', 'severe' or 'agonising', with the patient asked to select the term that best describes their pain. By contrast, the NRS requires the patient to rate their pain between 0 and 10, with 0 representing no pain, and 10 representing the worst pain imaginable. The VAS involves the patient moving a slide on a mechanical scale to a point between two ends of a device that is marked 'no pain' at one end and 'worst pain imaginable' (or similar descriptors) at the other. The result is then read against a 100-point scale on the side that is not visible to the patient. Alternatively, the patient marks a point on a 100 mm line and the result is read as a pain score between 0 and 100. The NRS and VAS have been validated in the emergency health setting, and the resulting scores have good levels of correlation between each scale. However, in non-verbal reporting patient groups, other pain assessment instruments may be more relevant.

PRACTICE TIP

PAINAD is an excellent and validated pain scoring tool for use in the older person with cognitive impairment.

Critically ill adult patients are usually unable to self-report and yet have complex pain management needs. While care of the critically ill patients traditionally occurs in intensive care units, it increasingly happens in the pre-hospital setting and in ED for extended time periods. Adequate pain relief is paramount for optimising comfort in the critically ill patient; however, it has been widely reported that over half of this patient cohort experience moderate-to-severe pain while intubated and mechanically ventilated.[36–42] Pain may be multifactorial in terms of presentation (e.g. trauma), but also iatrogenic during repositioning, physical examination, endotracheal intubation, mechanical ventilation, insertion of central venous catheters and chest drains; which commonly occur during resuscitation and stabilisation in the ED.[42,43] However, pain remains undetected, underestimated and poorly managed, particularly in critically ill intubated patients.[44–46] Critically ill intubated patients require close observation and monitoring during treatment of their underlying condition with titration of analgesia; a role increasingly undertaken by emergency nurses[47] and paramedical services.[48] In the absence of communicating pain levels, observational assessment instruments are preferred to evaluate acute pain in non-verbal, critically ill patients.[49] In a recent systematic review of 26 studies, the CPOT (Critical Care Pain Observation Tool) was identified as the most appropriate instrument in detecting and rating pain intensity in both conscious and unconscious critically ill adult patients, and in critically ill patients with delirium.[50]

PRACTICE TIP

CPOT (Critical Care Pain Observation Tool) is the most appropriate tool for detecting and rating pain intensity in both conscious and unconscious critically ill adult patients.

Pain is a dynamic process, which mandates frequent reassessment. When using a pain-rating scale, it is important to use the same scale consistently with the patient. Using a simple scale is helpful for the patient and clinicians, as it minimises any confusion or misinterpretation that may occur. A review of the pain assessment literature has shown that there is a poor correlation between the patient's pain rating and ratings estimated by the healthcare professional, with the latter tending to underestimate the patient's pain.[51,52] This underestimation may be a result of an individual's values, experience and biases influencing clinical judgements. As these attributes can lead to a devaluing of the patient's pain experience, it is important to recognise the detrimental effect that these attributes can have on the care of patients in pain. Clinicians must also remember that, while there is evidence for a minimally clinically significant change in pain score, the actual score reported by a patient is unique to that person, and interpersonal comparisons are unhelpful.

Assessing pain in children

Assessment tools and strategies for the paediatric patient vary from those used for adults. The ability of a child to accurately self-report pain depends on the stage of their cognitive and emotional development. While children aged eight years or more can generally use a visual analogue scale, those aged between three and eight may require different approaches to assessment of pain due to difficulties in communicating and interpreting instructions regarding the use of pain scales. Parents can contribute to assessing a child's pain by helping to distinguish usual behaviour from the child's current reactions. For further discussion of paediatric assessment refer to Chapter 35.

Observing a child for pain-related facial expressions and body position augments assessment. This is particularly helpful in pre-verbal infants. Pain severity scales suitable for infants and children are described in Table 18.2.

TABLE 18.2 PAIN RATING SCALES FOR CHILDREN[53,54]

DESCRIPTION	INSTRUCTIONS	RECOMMENDED AGE/COMMENTS
FACES pain rating scale, developed by Wong and Baker[53]		
Consists of six cartoon faces ranging from smiling face for 'no pain' to tearful face for 'worst pain'	*Original instructions:* Explain to child that each face is for a person who feels happy because there is no pain (hurt) or sad because there is some or a lot of pain. FACE 0 is very happy because there is no hurt. FACE 1 hurts just a little bit. FACE 2 hurts a little more. FACE 3 hurts even more. FACE 4 hurts a whole lot, but FACE 5 hurts as much as you can imagine, although you don't have to be crying to feel this bad. Ask the child to choose the face that best describes their own pain. Record the number under the chosen face on the pain assessment record.	For children as young as 3 years. Using original instructions without affect words, such as *happy* or *sad*, or brief words resulted in same pain rating, probably reflecting child's rating of pain intensity. For coding purposes, numbers 0, 2, 4, 6, 8, 10 can be substituted for 0–5 system to accommodate 0–10 system.
	Brief word instructions: Point to each face using the words to describe the pain intensity. Ask child to choose the face that best describes their own pain and record the appropriate number.	The FACES provides three scales in one: facial expressions, numbers and words. Use of brief word instructions is recommended.

0 No hurt	1 or 2 Hurts a little bit	2 or 4 Hurts a little more	3 or 6 Hurts even more	4 or 8 Hurts a whole lot	5 or 10 Hurts worst

DESCRIPTION	INSTRUCTIONS	RECOMMENDED AGE/COMMENTS
FLACC scale*, developed by Merkel et al[54]		
The scale consists of descriptors of behaviours that are associated with pain.	The scale was first validated in the postoperative setting, but has subsequently been validated to score pain in infants and children with pain from injury and with procedural pain. The clinician should observe the patient for at least 1 minute with the legs and body uncovered and select the most appropriate score for each of the categories of behaviour listed. It may be necessary to reposition the patient to observe for pain-related behaviour on movement. The numbers for each category are summed to provide a score from 0–10. This scale should be used in conjunction with a self-report if the child is able to do this.	The authors validated this scale in children aged 2 months to 7 years. Further research has validated this scale in older children (up to 16 years) and in neonates. The scale is particularly useful in assessing pain in pre-verbal children or in those with cognitive impairment or communication difficulties.

TABLE 18.2 PAIN RATING SCALES FOR CHILDREN—cont'd

DESCRIPTOR	FLACC SCALE		
Face	0 No particular expression or smile	1 Occasional grimace or frown; withdrawn, disinterested	2 Frequent to constant frown, clenched jaw, quivering chin
Legs	0 Normal position or relaxed	1 Uneasy, restless, tense	2 Kicking or legs drawn up
Activity	0 Lying quietly, normal position, moves easily	1 Squirming, shifting back and forth, tense	2 Arched, rigid or jerking
Cry	0 No cry (awake or asleep)	1 Moans or whimpers, occasional complaint	2 Crying steadily, screams or sobs; frequent complaints
Consolable	0 Content, relaxed	1 Reassured by occasional touching, hugging or being talked to; distractible	2 Difficult to console or comfort

Each of the five categories is scored from 0–2, resulting in a final score of 0–10.

PRACTICE TIP

AN 'A TO G' GUIDE FOR THE ASSESSMENT OF PAIN

(A) Ask about pain regularly, anticipate pain, and assess systematically with appropriate tool[55]—even if unconscious.[56]

(B) Believe the patient and family reports of pain, especially if unresolved.

(C) Choose analgesia that is appropriate for the patient's needs, age, culture[57] and condition; consider ongoing need for analgesia (e.g. stat, regular or continuous administration of analgesia).

(D) Deliver pain relief in a timely manner.

(E) Encourage the patient and family to report the presence of pain, 'If you are in pain, tell us'.

(F) Follow up with non-pharmaceutical pain management such as icepacks, elevation or immobilisation.

(G) Give adjuvant analgesia if appropriate.[27]

MANAGEMENT

Pain is a major human health problem throughout the world. Although relief from pain is considered a basic human right,[58] pain management practices in many healthcare settings have been shown to be deficient, leading to the use of the term 'oligoanalgesia' to describe low levels of analgesic use resulting in unrelieved pain.[59] Patients at particular risk for oligoanalgesia include children and elderly people, and those who are more seriously injured.[60,61] Managing pain is a multifaceted, multidimensional process. Co-existing medical conditions, age, social, cultural and psychological needs, beliefs and experiences, as well as individual variations to pain perception and response to therapy, all influence the process. The endpoint in the management of pain is not a predetermined reduction in pain severity score, as this endpoint varies between individuals. Rather, the aim is to achieve a reduction in pain that corresponds with the patient's assessment of satisfactory relief. This requires an assessment of the risk of dose-dependent adverse effects associated with commonly used analgesics.

There are many barriers to effective pain relief, including fear of addiction among both patients and healthcare professionals. This fear affects decisions regarding the administration of analgesics, but also affects the patient's acceptance of analgesia, particularly when opioids are recommended. This problem arises from a misunderstanding of the action of common analgesics, as well as terminology relating to addiction (see Table 18.3). The actual incidence of addiction in patients receiving opioids for pain management is often overestimated. A systematic review of the literature found a low risk of drug dependence in patients where opioids were used to treat acute pain.[62]

Addiction is defined as a chronic disease that is characterised by 'impaired control over drug use, compulsive use, continued use despite harm, and craving'.[66] It is important to note that patients taking analgesics for pain relief are using drugs for therapeutic reasons. This needs to be contrasted with the use of analgesics, particularly opioids, to satisfy a compulsive desire for the drug's non-analgesic effects such as euphoria. A useful analogy is to consider the therapeutic use of insulin in a patient with insulin-dependent diabetes mellitus. The patient depends on the regular injection of this drug. However, this is a physical dependence, rather than addiction. Physical dependence can occur in patients taking analgesics over time for chronic pain conditions. Withdrawal symptoms can occur by abruptly stopping drug administration, rapid dose reduction or administration of an antagonist that rapidly reverses the analgesic effect.

TABLE 18.3 DEFINITION OF ESSENTIAL TERMS[26]

TERM	DEFINITION
Pharmacokinetics	The movement of drugs throughout the body.[63] The action following the administration of a drug such as an analgesic: its absorption, distribution, metabolism by the cells and elimination from the body, mainly by the kidneys and liver.
Bioavailability	The amount of drug absorbed through the gastrointestinal tract into the bloodstream that determines the subsequent plasma level available from each dose for analgesic effect. Many factors can interfere with drug absorption and bioavailability, such as slower gastric emptying and peristalsis, or a decrease or increase in blood circulating volume and tissue perfusion.
Half-life	The length of time for the concentration of the drug in the bloodstream to be reduced by half.
Pain threshold	The least-intense stimulus that will cause pain or an intensity of stimulation below which pain is not perceived.
Pain tolerance	The level of pain accepted before intervention is requested or required.[64]
Drug tolerance	A decreased response to a drug dose requiring an increase in the dose to provide the original effect experienced.[65]
Physical dependence	Characterised by a tolerance to the drug causing a reduction in effectiveness of analgesia and an increase in dose requirements to relieve the existing pain. Withdrawal symptoms of agitation, anxiety, irritability, nausea and vomiting are likely if the drug is discontinued abruptly.[65]
Psychological dependence	Characterised by craving that influences mood and actions to acquire the drug. This dependence interferes with both the physical and the psychological health of the person concerned.
Minimum effective	The lowest concentration of drug in the blood required to provide a therapeutic effect such as minimum effective concentration (MEC) analgesia.
Titration	The dose adjustment to achieve and maintain the analgesic level within the therapeutic window.

Tolerance is characterised by decreasing effects of a drug at a constant dose of the drug or, conversely, the need for a higher dose of a drug to maintain an effect. Tolerance to opioids is a natural physiological response that should be anticipated with long-term therapy. This response is typically seen in patients suffering chronic pain, particularly those with pain due to cancer, where very large doses of opioids may be required to achieve adequate analgesia. This finding is a reminder that opioids such as morphine have no ceiling effect—the dose of the drug can be continually increased to achieve analgesia, while monitoring for potentially serious adverse effects. The assessment of tolerance is particularly important in managing acute pain in patients with opioid tolerance, whether due to addiction associated with illicit drug use or through long-term use for chronic pain. Patients taking an opioid antagonist such as naltrexone, which is used to manage addiction to alcohol or opioids, may represent a management challenge when they experience acute pain due to injury or disease as their pain may be unresponsive to opioids, requiring consideration of non-opioid alternatives such as ketamine.[67,68] Patients on long-term opioid therapy may also experience opioid-induced hyperalgesia, which is seen as a heightened response to a stimulus that is not normally painful.

Clinicians may occasionally be faced with a patient who they believe may be seeking drugs for non-therapeutic purposes. While this scenario has been found to be uncommon in one ED setting,[69] it can be challenging to determine whether a patient may be displaying drug-seeking behaviour. Drug-seeking behaviour may involve or include: a vague or misleading history; atypical symptoms or absence of expected associated signs or symptoms; requests for injectable rather than oral medicines; unexplained increase in dose of medicines needed; request for multiple opioid prescriptions; refusing or declining alternative medicines; no general practitioner involvement in care; and/or resistant to alternative treatments and advice. Further, people may request additional medicines that historically have been associated with potential abuse and which may be suggestive of drug-seeking behaviour. For example, there is evidence of known abuse potential with medicines such as flunitrazepam and oxycodone (common brands are Hypnodorm and Oxycontin). Research has identified that patient requests for parenteral medication and pain severity reports of greater than 10 out of 10 pain were most predictive evidence of drug-seeking behaviour. However, none of these clues in isolation is completely reliable, and there is a risk that patients may be labelled as 'drug-seekers' when they are actually seeking drugs to relieve a genuine complaint of pain. It is important to be aware of cognitive bias that may occur at a subconscious level when assessing an individual who is reporting pain. Beliefs regarding an individual's motives for reporting pain may compromise the quality of the care provided if incorrect attribution arising from bias is not recognised.[70]

CHOICE OF INTERVENTION

Selection of interventions for the relief of pain is influenced by a host of factors other than fears of addiction. Research has shown that tradition, intuition, stereotypes and ethnicity influence interventions selected for pain management. Burke and Jerrett[71] studied student nurses' perceptions of the best interventions for people of various ages who were in acute pain. Age was identified as a factor that influenced both the number and the type of interventions selected. In this study, student nurses selected more interventions for adolescents and adults, and fewer interventions for infants, toddlers, children and the elderly.

In a study of analgesic administration in the ED, Neighbor, Honner and Kohn[60] found that patients with trauma were less likely to receive opioids if they were young or elderly, intubated or had a lower Revised Trauma Score (RTS). Inadequate analgesia has also been documented in the pre-hospital setting.[72,73]

Alterations in levels of consciousness or cognitive disabilities related to age or illness can complicate the pain assessment and management process. Behavioural cues can be used to judge pain severity in the absence of a self-report. Patients with a decreased level of consciousness can experience severe pain and signs of agitation may be associated with nociception. As such, it is important to attend to these patients' needs once other resuscitation priorities have been established and managed. In cases of altered levels of consciousness due to trauma, the motor component of the Glasgow Coma Scale (GCS) can be used to guide treatment decisions, as a motor score ≥ 3 indicates an intact reaction to painful stimuli. As such, analgesia should be considered in patients suffering trauma which is likely to be painful and where the motor component of the GCS is ≥ 3.[74]

An injury that may result in deterioration of neurological, pulmonary or haemodynamic status is not, in itself, an absolute contraindication for systemic analgesia. While there are contraindications associated with specific analgesics, there is no contraindication to analgesia. However, judicious choice of analgesic agent and careful titration of analgesia is mandatory to prevent complications.

There is strong evidence that early analgesic administration does not affect the diagnosis in cases of acute abdominal pain. Therefore, analgesia should not be withheld until a diagnosis is made in a patient presenting with abdominal pain.[74] Paramedics and nurses have important responsibilities for the provision of early and effective analgesia in patients experiencing pain. This role requires authority to administer a range of analgesics using appropriate clinical judgement that is supported by knowledge of contemporary pain management practices and by evidence-based clinical practice guidelines. Such guidelines should include protocols for nurse-initiated analgesia in the ED, as evidence has shown considerable patient benefits in establishing these programs.[75–80]

Pain management interventions include invasive techniques, such as medication, and non-invasive techniques, such as distraction, cooling burns and splinting fractures. When selecting a technique for a specific patient, the healthcare professional should recognise that each patient is unique and that no single universally superior pain control method exists for all patients. The pathology responsible for the pain will influence the choice of analgesic. For example, in patients with renal colic, NSAIDs have been found to provide effective analgesia with a lower incidence of vomiting than opioids.[74] Patients should be evaluated individually, and interventions tailored to each patient and their situation. The following sections discuss specific aspects of pain management.

PHARMACOLOGICAL PAIN MANAGEMENT

Drugs that act as analgesics are divided into two groups: *non-opioids* and *opioids*. The term opioid includes natural and synthetic compounds that bind to opioid receptors in the nervous system. In 1986 the World Health Organization (WHO) released guidelines for the management of cancer pain, which included a three-step 'analgesic ladder' that advocated the addition of different analgesics to a patient's treatment regimen as pain severity increased.[81] Although this was designed to provide pain relief in patients with chronic pain due to cancer, this strategy can also be applied to the treatment of acute pain.

Non-opioids

Paracetamol and non-steroidal anti-inflammatory drugs (NSAIDs) comprise this group of analgesics. Although the exact mechanism of action of paracetamol is unknown, it is believed to produce analgesia by blocking pain impulses through its prostaglandin inhibitory effect on the CNS. Paracetamol has few adverse effects, but, unlike aspirin, has no significant anti-inflammatory effects. Paracetamol is preferred for patients who are allergic to aspirin or those with platelet or gastrointestinal problems. The usual recommended daily dose of paracetamol should not exceed 4000 mg for adults.[26] Paracetamol has a low therapeutic index, and acute liver failure may occur in overdose due to the hepatocellular necrosis caused by an active metabolite. This metabolite is normally conjugated with glutathione in the liver to form a harmless compound that is excreted by the renal system. However, overdose of paracetamol may deplete glutathione stores, leading to the accumulation of the toxic metabolite and consequent liver damage. This drug should be used with caution in patients with malnutrition or liver disease, who may have low levels of glutathione.

NSAIDs have an anti-inflammatory effect on the peripheral tissues. These drugs act by inhibiting prostaglandin synthesis by blocking cyclo-oxygenase (COX) production. Two forms (COX-1 and COX-2) exist. Many NSAIDs are non-selective. Examples of drugs in this category include aspirin, diclofenac, ibuprofen, indomethacin, ketoprofen, ketorolac, naproxen, piroxicam, sulindac and tiaprofenic acid. Selective (COX-2) inhibitors are less likely to cause the gastrointestinal adverse effects associated with COX-1 agents. Drugs in this class include celecoxib, meloxicam and parecoxib.

NSAIDs may not be effective for the management of severe pain, but can be a useful adjunct when used with opioids. These drugs have significant side-effects, which are more common with long-term use. These include peptic ulceration and effects on renal and platelet function. Aspirin can precipitate bronchospasm in susceptible individuals with a history of asthma.

Paracetamol and NSAIDs are useful for the treatment of mild-to-moderate pain. However, as the common route of administration is oral, these drugs may not be appropriate in an emergency setting where a stress response may affect gastric motility and drug absorption. Readers are advised to consult a specialist pharmacology reference (e.g. MIMS) for advice regarding indications, dose, contraindications, adverse effects and preparation of these analgesics. Table 18.4 provides a summary of common non-opioid analgesics.

Opioids

All classes of analgesics can be used to manage acute pain, but opioids are considered the most effective agents for moderate-to-severe pain control. The effective use of opioids involves

TABLE 18.4 SELECTED NON-OPIOID ANALGESICS AND NSAIDs[82]

ANALGESIC	USUAL ADULT ORAL DOSAGE (mg/day)	DOSES/DAY	CLINICAL CONSIDERATIONS
Aspirin	2400–3600	4–6	Available in effervescent tablet, capsule, enteric coated, sustained-release tablet, suppository Possibility of gastric irritation and bleeding
Paracetamol	2000–4000 (max. 4000)	4–6	Available in tablet, capsule, mixture, suppository Adverse effects rare in normal therapeutic doses Overdose can cause serious damage to liver and kidneys
Ibuprofen	1200–1600 (max. 2400)	3–4	Available in tablet and liquid Possibility of gastric irritation
Indomethacin	50–200 (max. 200)	2–4	Available in capsule, suppository Higher risk for GI effects
Celecoxib	100 (max. 400)	1–2	Does not affect platelet aggregation Long-term effects not established yet
Diclofenac	75–150 (max. 200)	2–3	Available in tablet and suppository Less effect on platelet aggregation
Naproxen	250–500 (max. 1000)	2	Available in tablet, controlled-release tablet and suppository Caution with patients on sodium-restricted diets

GI: gastrointestinal; NSAIDs: non-steroidal anti-inflammatory drugs.

titration of the dose against pain relief while observing the patient for unwanted effects. Both exogenous and endogenous opioids bind to opioid receptors in the brain and spinal cord. These receptors are classified as mu (μ), delta (δ) and kappa (κ), and activation of these different receptors is responsible for the range of effects associated with opioid administration.

The mu agonists (morphine-like) are the largest group and used most often. Examples of drugs in this category include morphine, codeine, fentanyl, hydromorphone, methadone, oxycodone and dextropropoxyphene. The mechanism of action of opioids is complex and not yet fully understood. In the spine, opioids inhibit the release of substance P from dorsal horn neurons. While opioids are considered to act on receptors in the CNS, there is evidence that there is also action of opioids at peripheral sites following tissue injury.

Although little difference is believed to exist among mu agonists and their ability to relieve pain, *morphine* is often the mu agonist of choice and is the standard against which other opioid analgesics are compared. In an emergency setting, morphine should be given intravenously, with adults receiving 2.5–5 mg increments every 5 minutes until pain is relieved. While intramuscular administration is generally discouraged due to variations in absorption in the injured patient, this route of administration should be considered in haemodynamically stable patients where intravenous access is unavailable. If the intramuscular route is chosen, the initial dose of morphine should be based on the patient's weight: 0.1 mg/kg. However, the patient's weight may be poorly correlated with the dose required to achieve clinically significant pain relief, with up to a ten-fold variation in dose required to achieve analgesia between patients of similar age, irrespective of weight.

Immune-mediated reactions to morphine are rare, and the majority of reactions to morphine are classified as side-effects rather than an allergy. When patients report an allergy, they may be referring to an undesirable effect such as nausea, and it may be possible to pre-empt nausea by administering an antiemetic in cases where the patient reports previous episodes of nausea associated with morphine administration. Routine prophylactic use of antiemetics in conjunction with opioid administration is not recommended. Apart from nausea, some more common adverse effects of mu agonists include sedation, euphoria, dysphoria, pruritus, constipation and urinary retention. More serious adverse effects include hypotension and respiratory depression. Monitoring of the patient's respiratory status, perfusion and oxygenation is vital while administering opioids. However, respiratory rate is a poor indicator of respiratory depression. Instead, the level of sedation is a better early indicator of respiratory depression.[74] Common indicators of respiratory depression are listed in Box 18.2. The aim of opioid administration is to achieve satisfactory relief of pain while keeping the sedation score less than 2. It is important to note that respiratory depression in the setting of opioid administration usually results from decreased responsiveness to carbon dioxide within the medullary respiratory centre. Pulse oximetry will not reveal hypercapnia that may be associated with respiratory depression. It is therefore vital that a sedation score is regularly sought in patients receiving opioid therapy.

Tolerance to sedation and respiratory depression occur in patients receiving opioids over a period of several days. If

BOX 18.2 **COMMONLY USED INDICATORS OF RESPIRATORY DEPRESSION**[4]

SEDATION SCORE

1. Wide awake
2. Easy to rouse*
3. Constantly drowsy, easy to rouse but unable to stay awake (e.g. falls asleep during conversation); early respiratory depression
4. Severe; somnolent, difficult to rouse; severe respiratory depression.

RESPIRATORY RATE

- Fewer than 8 breaths/minute is often considered to be a sign of respiratory depression, but this is generally an unreliable indicator.
- Respiratory depression can co-exist with a normal respiratory rate.

OXYGEN SATURATION

- May also be unreliable, especially if the patient is receiving supplemental oxygen.

**Some centres also add '1S', which indicates asleep but easy to rouse.*

clinically significant respiratory depression occurs following the administration of opioids, the patient's ventilations should be assisted. Decisions to reverse the opioid effect using an opioid antagonist such as naloxone should be made cautiously, as this will return the patient to their pre-opioid pain level and may induce withdrawal syndrome in the opioid-dependent patient.

Fentanyl is a short-acting pure opioid agonist that binds to mu-receptors in the brain, spinal cord and other tissues. When administered intravenously, a dose of 100 microgram is equivalent to 10 mg of intravenous morphine. Unlike morphine, fentanyl rarely causes significant histamine release. As such, there is less potential for histamine-mediated hypotension following fentanyl administration. Fentanyl is effective in managing severe pain in the pre-hospital setting, and several emergency medical services allow paramedic administration of fentanyl via the intranasal route using an atomising device attached to a 1 mL syringe. The efficacy of fentanyl delivered via the intranasal and intravenous routes in children has been shown to be similar.[83] However, efficacy of this form of administration depends on delivery technique, as the drug must be atomised and dispersed across a large area of nasal mucosa to be effective. Research has shown that intranasal administration of this drug to children in pain is safe and effective.[84] This is a particularly effective route of administration in children, who may have needle phobias. This study recommended the implementation of nurse-initiated administration of intranasal fentanyl in the ED.

Fentanyl is rapidly absorbed across mucous membranes as it is many times more lipid-soluble than morphine. However, bioavailability via the intranasal route is approximately 70% and a larger morphine-equivalent dose is required when administering the drug via this route. The initial intranasal dose for an adult is 200 microgram. If the patient is aged over 60 years or weighs less than 60 kg, half this dose (100 microgram) should be used. The initial dose for children is 2 microg/kg. If the calculated dose volume exceeds 1 mL a more concentrated preparation must be used to reduce the total volume to be administered via the intranasal route. Onset of action is rapid, with duration of action approximately 30 minutes. A lozenge form for oral transmucosal administration is available and is approved for the treatment of breakthrough pain in palliative-care patients with cancer. While not currently approved for the treatment of acute or postoperative pain, this form of fentanyl has been shown to be effective in treating soldiers injured in combat.[85] Fentanyl has become popular for the initial treatment of pain associated with acute coronary syndrome due to proposed benefits in the setting of haemodynamic instability. However, there is no evidence of significant difference in efficacy or incidence of adverse effects when either morphine or fentanyl is used to treat ischaemic chest pain.[86]

Oxycodone is a semisynthetic thebaine (opium alkaloid) derivative. This drug is a mu receptor agonist which also has affinity for delta and kappa opioid receptors in the brain and spinal cord. The drug is available in oral form for the treatment of moderate-to-severe pain, particularly chronic pain. The use of oxycodone has increased significantly in recent years, with much of this increase attributed to illicit drug use. It is often sought by individuals with opioid dependence who inject the drug, and its use as a substitute for drugs such as heroin (diamorphine) has led to the drug being known as 'hillbilly heroin' in the United States.

Other opioids have significant disadvantages in the emergency setting. *Codeine* is a weak opioid prodrug that is metabolised to morphine to provide an analgesic effect. However, up to 10% of the Caucasian population may lack the enzyme responsible for this conversion process (CYP2D6), rendering the drug ineffective in these individuals. The drug is available in combination with paracetamol or aspirin for oral administration for mild-to-moderate pain, but is no longer available in Australia without prescription due to concerns of abuse.

Pethidine is a synthetic opioid, which was believed to be better than morphine in relieving the pain of renal colic. Research has subsequently shown that it is no more effective than morphine, while producing significant adverse effects due to the accumulation of the active metabolite, norpethidine.[74] This can produce CNS stimulation leading to muscle tremors, myoclonus and seizures. The use of this drug is no longer recommended.[74]

Tramadol is a weak opioid that acts on mu receptors, but also acts as a serotonin and noradrenaline re-uptake inhibitor. The active metabolite is mono-*O*-desmethyltramadol. However, this metabolism depends on the CYP2D6 isoenzyme of cytochrome P450, and patients who are lacking this enzyme may have a reduced analgesic effect (see discussion of codeine, above). The full analgesic action of this drug has not been completely explained. Although it causes less respiratory depression than an equivalent dose of morphine, nausea and vomiting occur at similar rates to other opioids. The interactions of tramadol with other drugs are similar to those of other opioids. However, particular attention should be given to interactions with drugs that increase serotonin by any mechanism, as this can lead to a serotonin syndrome.

Information comparing common opioids is shown in Table 18.5.

TABLE 18.5 OPIOID COMPARATIVE INFORMATION[82]

When changing opioid, start at 50% of the approximate equianalgesic dose; then titrate according to response.

DRUG	APPROXIMATE DOSE EQUIVALENT TO 10 mg IM/SC MORPHINE[a]	APPROXIMATE DURATION OF ACTION (HOURS)[b]	COMMENTS
Agonists			
Codeine[c] (analgesic only)	200 mg oral	3-4	not recommended (contraindicated in children < 12 years)
Fentanyl[d]	100-150 microg SC	1-2	preferred in renal impairment
Hydromorphone[e]	1.5-2 mg SC/IM; 6-7.5 mg oral	2-4; 24 (controlled release)	not for first-line use
Methadone (analgesic only)	complex	8-24 (chronic dosing)	discuss with a pain or palliative care specialist
Morphine[e]	30 mg oral	2-3; 12 or 24 (controlled release)	
Oxycodone	15-20 mg soral	3-4; 12 (controlled release)	preferred in renal impairment (adjust dose)
Pethidine[e]	75-100 mg IM	2-3	not recommended
Tapentadol[f]	75-100 mg oral	4-6; 12 (controlled release)	
Tramadol[e]	100-120 mg IM/IV; 150 mg oral	3-6; 12 or 24 (controlled release)	
Partial agonists			
Buprenorphine (analgesic only)[d]	0.4 mg IM; 0.8 mg sublingual	6-8	not first-line for analgesia

[a]Dose equivalents are a guide only and may be greater than the maximum dose, see relevant monograph

[b]Duration of action depends on dose and route of administration

[c]Inactive; must be metabolised to morphine

[d]See monograph for patch dose equivalence

[e]Has an active metabolite; see monograph

[f]Dose equivalence based on limited data; use caution

Inhalational analgesics

Nitrous oxide (N_2O) is an analgesic and is commonly used to induce anaesthesia. It is a mild analgesic and sedative when given with oxygen in a 50:50 mix; equivalent to 10–15 mg of morphine.[87] This analgesic is used in labour, during painful procedures, such as changing burns dressings, and in dental surgery. This is a safe analgesic with few side-effects. However, if used over prolonged periods (6–8 hours), nitrous oxide can destroy the enzyme methionine synthetase (MS) and deplete vitamin B_{12} stores. Low levels of MS can affect DNA synthesis, resulting in rare but serious bone-marrow and neurological complications.[74] Patients and staff may experience adverse effects after long-term exposure to this gas if effective scavenging systems are not used. Its use in the community-based emergency health setting is becoming uncommon due to the bulk of the gas cylinder and administering apparatus, and safety concerns when the gas is used in confined spaces, including ambulances.

Methoxyflurane is classed as a volatile anaesthetic agent belonging to the fluorinated hydrocarbon group. It is a clear fluid with a distinctive odour that must be vaporised to be administered by inhalation. Unlike other volatile anaesthetics, at low concentrations this agent produces analgesia, which has been found to be effective in relieving acute pain in settings which include the ED.[88] This agent is currently used by several emergency medical services and departments in Australia. The initial dose is 3 mL given via a disposable inhaler. The agent must be self-administered by the patient to avoid sedation. Duration of action is approximately 30 minutes, after which the initial dose may be repeated once. Patients should not be given more than 6 mL of methoxyflurane in 24 hours, and no more than 15 mL in a week. Contraindications include renal failure or impairment, as this agent has been shown to be nephrotoxic with long-term use or when high concentrations are given. Administration of this agent should be done in a well-ventilated environment.

N-methyl-D-aspartate receptor antagonists

Neurotransmitters such as glutamate, glycine and aspartate are involved in central nociceptive modulation, where they bind to

N-methyl-D-aspartate (NMDA) receptors located in the postsynaptic interneurons and ascending neurons in the spinal cord. The action of these neurotransmitters appears to be linked to hyperalgesia and allodynia. Drugs such as ketamine and dextromethorphan block or antagonise these receptors and act as analgesics.

Ketamine has anaesthetic properties without reducing reflexes or muscle tone. At subanaesthetic doses it produces conscious sedation where the patient appears responsive but experiences analgesia while maintaining airway reflexes. The use of ketamine is becoming more common in managing severe pain in the prehospital and ED settings, with evidence supporting its safety and efficacy.[89] Analgesia is usually obtained with an intravenous dose of 0.3 mg/kg.[74] Ketamine stimulates sympathetic activity to increase cardiac output and blood pressure, reducing the risk of hypotension associated with some opioids. However, this may lead to increases in intraocular and intracranial pressure, so its use may be contraindicated in eye injuries and closed head trauma. At analgesic doses ketamine does not depress respiration in the way opioids can. While this drug has been successfully used in procedural sedation in children, its wider use as an analgesic has been constrained by a significant incidence of agitation, vivid dreams and hallucinations in older patients upon emergence from the dissociative state, and it is these properties that have seen an increase in the illegal use of this drug. These effects can, however, be managed by administering a short-acting benzodiazepine such as midazolam.[74]

Given its analgesic and anaesthetic properties, ketamine is particularly useful in disaster, transport and industrial accidents where patient extrication involves the manipulation of fractured limbs, or in cases of entrapment where amputation may be required and where the adverse effects of opioids complicate treatment. It should also be considered when managing severe acute pain in opioid-tolerant patients or in patients with poor response to opioids.

Adjuvants

Adjuvants are medications that are used in combination with opioid or NSAID analgesics to enhance pain relief or to treat symptoms that exacerbate pain. These drugs have analgesic properties but these properties are not their primary function. They are primarily used to treat chronic headaches, back pain and neuropathic pain. Examples of drugs in this group include:

- tricyclic antidepressants and selective serotonin reuptake inhibitors (SSRIs)
- corticosteroids—dexamethasone
- psychotropics—benzodiazepines and phenothiazines
- anticonvulsants—carbamazepine, gabapentin, sodium valproate
- alpha2 agonists—dexmedetomidine, clonidine.

The type of pain determines the drug chosen; for example, patients with chronic continuous neuropathic pain have been shown to benefit from treatment with tricyclic antidepressants, which increase levels of noradrenaline and serotonin by inhibiting their uptake at adrenergic and serotonergic neurons.[74] This action may partly explain the action of tramadol in managing neuropathic pain. The route of administration for drugs in this group varies, but almost all adjuvants are available orally. Although not classified as an analgesic, metoclopramide is recommended as an early treatment for migraine pain.[74]

NON-PHARMACOLOGICAL PAIN MANAGEMENT

Distraction, hypnosis, imagery and relaxation are psychological interventions that may help to relieve pain. Physical adjuvant strategies include massage, application of heat and cold, transcutaneous electrical nerve stimulation (TENS) and acupuncture. These approaches are discussed briefly here.

Distraction

Distraction may facilitate pain management by assisting the patient to focus on a stimulus other than the pain. This technique may be of particular benefit in managing pain in young children. It may minimise, but does not entirely alleviate, pain. For distraction to be effective, the object of that distraction must be of interest to the patient. This can include pleasant images or music. Multiple modes of distraction have been used to reduce pain in children with burns and those undergoing painful procedures. Virtual reality has been shown to alleviate pain in children and adolescents

Hypnosis, imagery and relaxation

Although hypnosis has been found to be useful in reducing procedural pain in children,[74] it is rarely used in emergency health settings because few clinicians have the knowledge, skills or time necessary to undertake this procedure. However, the nurse or paramedic functioning in the capacity of patient advocate can assist the patient in pursuing this method of pain management by referring the patient to available community resources for continued pain management.

Using one's imagination to control pain is a form of distraction that produces relaxation. The imagination is used to develop images that promote pleasant sensations and diminish pain perception. For example, a patient may have decreased pain when imagining lying on the beach listening to the sound of waves washing over sand. By assisting in creating this imaginary setting, the nurse or paramedic can assist the patient with pain management. Effectiveness of imaging depends on familiarity of the image and its pleasantness for the patient and also depends on the environment, with noisy industrial settings or accidents in the middle of busy roads posing special challenges.

Relaxation techniques promote a state free from anxiety. When the patient is relaxed, skeletal muscle tension is minimal. Deep breathing is one way to promote relaxation. The nurse or paramedic can instruct the patient to inhale deeply through the nose and exhale slowly through the mouth. Repeating this sequence several times while concentrating on muscle relaxation may be an effective adjunct to pain management in the ED.

Cutaneous stimulation

This method refers to cutaneous techniques which stimulate the skin for the purpose of pain relief (e.g. vibration, superficial heat and cold, ice application, massage, methanol application to the skin, TENS and acupuncture). These techniques have been shown to be effective in some limited acute pain settings. For example, acupuncture may help to reduce pain associated with childbirth, and there is evidence for the use of TENS in the same clinical context.[74] Acupressure and TENS have been trialled in the paramedic practice setting.[90] However, the evidence for efficacy remains scant.

PRACTICE TIP

AIMS FOR EFFECTIVE PAIN CONTROL

Interventions should be considered to successfully manage pain.

- The goal of pain management is to recognise relief of pain as a clinical priority and to relieve or prevent pain whenever possible. Pain relief may be more effective if initiated soon after onset of pain.
- The underlying cause of pain and the severity of the pain are important considerations in selecting analgesia.
- A calm, quiet patient–or one who is able to sleep despite reporting pain–does not preclude the presence of pain.
- A patient's refusal to accept pain medication may be related to fear of addiction, sedation, loss of control, beliefs about pain or method of administration.
- A patient's request for specific pain medication does not automatically mean he or she is a drug-seeker.
- The endpoint of treatment relies on the patient's assessment of relief rather than achievement of a predetermined reduction in pain score.
- All pain is real. Pain is what a patient says it is.
  - Successful assessment and management of pain is, in part, contingent on establishing a positive relationship between healthcare professionals and patients and their families. Encourage patients and their family to report the presence of pain, and to voice any concerns or preferences they may have to the healthcare team.
  - Unrelieved pain has negative physical and psychological consequences. Systematic assessment and targeted pain management strategies yield both short- and long-term benefits.

Prevention is better than treatment. Pain that is established and severe is difficult to control. Provide analgesia prior to interventions likely to cause pain (e.g. endotracheal suctioning, repositioning).

ANAESTHESIA

LOCAL

Local anaesthesia refers to techniques that reduce or prevent pain without affecting consciousness. Drugs that provide local anaesthesia are often used for minor surgical procedures. These drugs block sodium channels and prevent the influx of sodium through membrane channels involved in depolarisation of the cell. This stops the propagation of action potentials along neurons, including nociceptor afferents. Although the intended site of action is the nerve cells responsible for the transmission of signals that are perceived as pain, all excitable tissue can be affected by sodium-channel blockade, including muscle cells and motor neurons. This action may produce paresis or paralysis. Autonomic neurons are also affected.

Lidocaine is a short-acting local anaesthetic, with a rapid onset and half-life of approximately 90 minutes. Longer-acting local anaesthetics include bupivacaine, ropivacaine and levobupivacaine. Lidocaine/prilocaine cream (Emla®)—a eutectic mixture—is useful as a topical preparation in reducing pain in procedures such as venous ulcer debridement. It is also used in procedural pain relief in children, particularly for venepuncture. However, Emla needs to be applied at least 60 minutes prior to the procedure to be effective.[91] A similar product with the same properties is AnGel®, used topically to reduce pain.

Local anaesthetics may be injected into the epidural space to block transmission of afferent signals along thoracic, lumbar or sacral nerves.

Classification of local anaesthetics

Two groups of local anaesthetics can be described, based on their duration of action. The *amides* include lidocaine, bupivacaine, levobupivacaine and ropivacaine. These are slowly metabolised by the liver and have a long duration of action. In contrast, the *esters* are metabolised more quickly. Examples include procaine, cocaine, benzocaine, tetracaine (amethocaine), oxybuprocaine and proxymetacaine. The ester compounds are metabolised to *p*-aminobenzoic acid metabolites, which may be associated with allergic reactions in some patients. The properties of common local anaesthetics are listed in Table 18.6.

Route of administration

Local anaesthetics can be given via several routes. *Topical* application produces anaesthesia when applied to mucous membranes, conjunctiva and damaged skin. Apart from Emla and AnGel, local anaesthetics do not penetrate unbroken skin. A range of formulations is available for topical administration.

Infiltration involves subdermal and subcutaneous injections to produce an anaesthetic field around the injury or area to be repaired. Nerve blocks involve the injection of a drug such as lidocaine next to a peripheral nerve that may be some distance from the injury or pain-producing lesion. A femoral nerve block provides good analgesia distal to the injection, and is used to treat pain arising from injuries such as a fractured femur. However, ultrasound may be required to facilitate needle placement, and a related technique that does not require technology to guide needle placement, and that has been shown to be effective in the pre-hospital and emergency department setting, is the fascia iliaca compartment block.[94]

Epidural anaesthesia involves injection of a local anaesthetic into the epidural space in the spinal canal where the drug remains localised. This procedure is used to relieve pain associated with labour and surgical procedures such as caesarean section and thoracic and abdominal surgery.

Subarachnoid (intrathecal) anaesthesia involves drug administration into the cerebrospinal fluid (CSF) within the subarachnoid space at a point below the third lumbar vertebra to avoid potential penetration of the spinal cord.

Local anaesthetics, opioids and combinations of both can be administered via the epidural route to provide analgesia while maintaining motor function. Opioids bind to opioid receptors in the substantia gelatinosa of the spinal cord to provide local analgesia without systemic effects. When administered by the epidural route, opioids diffuse into the CSF before reaching the cord. Local anaesthetics act on spinal roots and nerves, as

TABLE 18.6 PROPERTIES OF COMMONLY USED LOCAL ANAESTHETICS[92]

NAME	TYPE/METABOLISM	USES	TOXICITY/NOTES
Short-acting (30–60 minutes)			
Procaine	Ester/plasma	Infiltration, nerve block, spinal	Least toxic LA; low lipid solubility; slow onset; potency 0.5 × lidocaine
Benzocaine	Ester/plasma	Topical: drops, gel, lozenges, paint, suppositories	Relatively non-toxic; very low potency; only active topically
Intermediate duration (1–3 hours)			
Tetracaine (amethocaine) (AnGel®)	Ester/plasma	Topical: IV	Do not apply to broken skin due to increased rate of absorption and risk of adverse effects[93]
Lidocaine	Amide/liver	Infiltration, nerve block, spinal epidural, IV, topical	Prototype LA, potency = 1; more cardiotoxic than prilocaine; rapid onset
Prilocaine	Amide/liver	Infiltration, nerve blocks, caudal, epidural, IV	Lower systemic toxicity than lidocaine; equipotent with lidocaine; products of liver metabolism may cause methaemoglobinaemia
Lidocaine/prilocaine cream (Emla®)	Amides/liver	Topical (venepuncture, cannulation, minor skin surgery)	Local irritation; risk in infants < 6 months old (methaemoglobinaemia); toxic if swallowed by small children
Mepivacaine	Amide/liver	Infiltration, nerve blocks, caudal, epidural	Less toxic than lidocaine; equipotent with lidocaine; avoid use in pregnancy
Articaine	Amide/liver	Dental	Combined with adrenaline 1:100,000 provides 1–3 hours of regional anaesthesia; no significant advantages over lidocaine
Long duration (3–10 hours)			
Bupivacaine, levobupivacaine, ropivacaine	Amides/liver	Infiltration, caudal, epidural, nerve blocks	More cardiotoxic than lidocaine; potency 4 × lidocaine; slow onset; adrenaline not needed; less motor blockade
Tetracaine (amethocaine)	Ester/plasma	Topical anaesthesia	Potency 5 × lidocaine; slow onset; high systemic toxicity; useful for analgesia for venous cannulation

IV: intravenous; LA: local anaesthetic.

well as the spinal cord. As the intrathecal technique provides direct access to the CNS, it is associated with an increased risk of infection and other adverse effects arising from medullary and sympathetic depression.

Intravenous regional anaesthesia of the forearm (Bier block) is used to provide analgesia in procedures such as wound debridement, foreign body removal and reduction of fractures and dislocations. After placing an intravenous cannula in the dorsum of the hand on the affected limb, the limb is exsanguinated by elevation and brachial artery compression, or by winding an Esmarch bandage proximally along the forearm. A blood pressure cuff is placed over the upper arm and inflated to 100 mmHg above systolic blood pressure, and the arm is lowered. A local anaesthetic, such as prilocaine, is injected intravenously slowly via the cannula in the hand, with analgesia achieved within 5–10 minutes. The blood pressure cuff should remain inflated for at least 20 minutes, but no longer than 60 minutes.[26] Continuous monitoring for evidence of systemic toxicity should be undertaken by nursing staff, particularly following release of the tourniquet.

Benefits of local anaesthetics

Local anaesthetics prevent or significantly reduce pain and discomfort associated with injury and medical procedures such as suturing, without affecting the patient's level of consciousness. For example, injecting a local anaesthetic such as lidocaine next to the digital nerve can effectively relieve pain associated with a crush injury to a digit. This technique—known as a nerve block—avoids the potential complications associated with administering a centrally acting opioid, while providing an excellent level of analgesia. Although the use of digital and femoral nerve blocks has had limited use by nurses and paramedics, the wider use of these procedures offers a broader range of pain-control options, and their use could be extended with additional training.

Disadvantages and limitations of local anaesthetics

The interference with sodium-ion transport across cell membranes that results in anaesthesia when this transport is inhibited in afferent nociceptors can also influence the propagation of action potentials in other parts of the body, including the

CNS and heart. This can lead to cardiac dysrhythmias and CNS stimulation if local anaesthetics such as lidocaine are injected intravenously, or if significant systemic absorption occurs following topical administration or infiltration in highly vascular areas. The addition of adrenaline (epinephrine) can produce local vasoconstriction and restrict systemic absorption from the injection site. However, adrenaline (epinephrine) may cause ischaemia in poorly perfused tissue and, as such, it must not be used on the digits, penis, ears or nose because of its vasoconstrictive effects.

Nursing and paramedicine implications for procedures involving local anaesthetics

Local anaesthetics are usually considered to be safe when administered in small doses prior to surgical procedures such as wound debridement. However, the patient's blood pressure, pulse rate and respiratory rate should be monitored during treatment with injectable agents because systemic toxicity may occur when the dose is too high, or the drug is accidentally injected intravenously. Systemic toxicity can result in CNS stimulation and dysrhythmias, such as ventricular fibrillation, heart block and asystole. Resuscitation equipment should be readily available and staff trained in resuscitation procedures.

In explaining the procedure, the nurse or paramedic informs the patient that pain will be blocked, but touch and pressure should remain intact during topical and infiltration administration. Pain management is facilitated if the patient is assisted into a comfortable position before initiating the procedure. As with all drug administration, contraindications to use should be assessed, such as known allergy or hypersensitivity to the drug. Local anaesthetics containing adrenaline (epinephrine) should not be used in poorly perfused areas such as those previously described.

The maximum safe dose of a local anaesthetic should be calculated to avoid systemic side-effects. Doses may need to be modified in children, pregnant patients, elderly patients or patients with liver disease. Solutions containing adrenaline (epinephrine) should be used with caution in hypertensive patients or those taking tricyclic and monoamine oxidase inhibitor antidepressants.

OTHER TYPES AND USES OF ANAESTHESIA

Procedural sedation refers to a technique of administering sedatives or dissociative agents with or without analgesics to induce a state that allows the patient to tolerate unpleasant procedures while maintaining cardiorespiratory function. This technique produces a reduced level of consciousness while maintaining airway reflexes. The continuum of sedation ranges from a state where the patient can respond purposefully to stimuli, to deep sedation where patients cannot be easily roused. Sedation that produces a drug-induced depression of consciousness to the point where patients do not respond to any stimuli is classified as *general anaesthesia*. This stage of sedation requires airway control and cardiorespiratory support, and requires considerable expertise in managing the patient and any complications that may arise. Procedural sedation requires that personnel providing procedural sedation and analgesia have an understanding of the drugs administered, have the ability to adequately monitor the patient's response to medications given and have the skills necessary to manage all potential complications.

Informed consent should be obtained before initiation of analgesia. Patients should be given information regarding the nature of the procedure, risks and benefits and any potential complications. Contraindications for procedural sedation are clinical instability and refusal by a competent patient.

Although there are risks with procedural sedation, these can be minimised if the appropriate agent, dosage and route of administration are considered. Monitoring is mandatory, and should include level of consciousness, heart rate, blood pressure, ECG and respiratory rate and effort. Additionally, pulse oximetry and capnography to measure end-tidal carbon dioxide ($EtCO_2$) should be considered (see Chapter 14). Pulse oximetry may not be as sensitive as $EtCO_2$ in identifying respiratory depression. As patients with respiratory depression will usually have an $EtCO_2$ of > 50 mmHg, this finding may allow more-rapid identification of hypoventilation than pulse oximetry alone.

PRACTICE TIP

ACTIONS FOR EFFECTIVE PAIN CONTROL

Establish an effective, supportive relationship with the patient.

- Believe, collaborate with and respect the patient's response to pain and its management.
- Use a validated pain scale to measure pain severity; the scale used must be appropriate for age.
- Use an appropriate behavioural pain scale to assess preverbal children and patients with cognitive impairment, including patients with dementia.
- Tailor the treatment to suit the individual to accommodate interpersonal differences in response to analgesics.
- Ensure patient safety at all times. Monitoring the patient facilitates assessment of treatment effectiveness and minimises potential adverse occurrences. An opioid antagonist must be available for the management of serious adverse effects associated with opioids such as respiratory depression.
- Monitor the patient's response and effectiveness of treatment.
- Sedation is an early indicator of respiratory depression associated with opioid administration. Sedation should be routinely monitored in this setting.
- Consider other interventions when pain fails to respond to treatment; opioid-tolerant patients may require higher doses or non-opioid therapy such as ketamine to relieve severe pain.
- Inform the patient what they are likely to experience while in the ED to minimise fear of the unknown.
- Communicate effectively with the patient and healthcare professionals responsible for ongoing care regarding the treatment plan and its effectiveness. This may include a pain assessment with the clinician taking over care from you.
- Maintain a calm, empathetic manner.
- Educate the patient about the occurrence, onset and duration of pain; methods of pain relief; and preventive measures.
- Research the multidimensional nature of pain, its assessment and subsequent management. Use this research in practice.
- Maintain current knowledge and competencies.

Opioids are the drug of choice for moderate-to-severe pain, with the titrated IV route preferred. This is considered the safest approach to rapid analgesia. Opioids may be used alone or in combination with other analgesics and sedatives. A combination of fentanyl and midazolam has been found to be safe and effective when used in the ED with appropriate monitoring of the patient.[95] Propofol and ketamine are also recommended for procedural sedation. Before administering a drug, it is important to determine the patient's history of drug use. Patients who have developed drug tolerance may require higher dosages; the elderly and the very young may require lower doses.

If respiratory depression occurs from induction with an opioid, it can be reversed with naloxone. For adults, naloxone can be slowly administered 0.4–2 mg IV, repeated every 2 minutes until the respiratory depression is reversed. However, this can be avoided by careful monitoring for sedation and ventilation support where required.

Patient assessment, patient monitoring and documentation are important before, during and after the procedure. Emergency nurses and doctors should be cognisant of their institution's policies on procedural sedation and accept responsibility for ensuring safe standards of practice.

SUMMARY

Pain is a common complaint in many healthcare settings. Paramedics, nurses and other healthcare professionals have an important role in assessing, evaluating and managing a patient's pain. This requires a knowledge of contemporary principles of pain management practice, which includes the actions and indications of pharmacological agents used to manage pain. In addition, an understanding of non-pharmacological interventions is essential. However, the effectiveness of any care plan depends on the quality of the clinical decision-making process and awareness of the effect of bias on decisions. These include assumptions about pain-related behaviours based on gender, race and age. Being aware of these influences will help to ensure that equitable and effective analgesia is provided to relieve pain and improve the patient's quality of life.

CASE STUDY 1

A 40-year-old cyclist has collided with a car that turned into the path of the rider from a side street in a residential area. On examination, the patient is conscious, orientated and is complaining of severe pain over the right lateral chest wall. The patient tells you that he was wearing a helmet and denies any loss of consciousness. He estimates that he was travelling at 20 km/h when he hit the side of the car. The patient's blood pressure is 110/80 mmHg, pulse is 120 beats/minute and skin is pale and sweaty. He is complaining of exacerbation of pain on inspiration (10/10 severity), but denies any other pain. Auscultation of the chest reveals decreased air entry in right lung fields, but no adventitious sounds. However, the patient refuses to take a deep breath due to the pain. Examination of the chest wall reveals bruising over several ribs over the right anterior axillary line. This area is exquisitely painful on palpation. There is no obvious deformity, flail segment or paradoxical chest wall movement. A comprehensive examination does not reveal any other abnormalities other than abrasions over all extremities, consistent with contact with the road surface. Further observations reveal a saturation of 88% on air by pulse oximetry. The patient's respiratory rate is 24 breaths/minute and shallow.

QUESTIONS

1. Propose causes for the observed decrease in oxygen saturation.
2. Are there any contraindications to analgesia in this case?
3. If you decide to use a pharmacological intervention to manage the patient's pain, what agent/s will you elect to use? Summarise the risks and benefits associated with each agent.
4. What is the endpoint in analgesic administration in this case?

Answers to Case Study Questions can be found on evolve http://evolve.elsevier.com/AU/Curtis/emergency/ 

CASE STUDY 2

A 32-year-old man is complaining of a sudden onset of severe abdominal pain. On examination, the patient appears distressed and is restless. He occasionally paces the room before returning to a sitting position where he sits with knees drawn up. The patient describes the pain as 'agonising' and constant, starting abruptly approximately 20 minutes previously while he was at home. He tells you the pain is in his right flank and that the pain radiates to the umbilical region and groin. The pain is associated with nausea. On palpation the abdomen is soft, with tenderness reported over all quadrants. The patient denies any constipation or other gastrointestinal tract symptoms. He denies any gross haematuria or recent trauma that may be associated with the pain. Vital signs show a pulse of 80 beats/minute, blood pressure of 130/85 mmHg, respiratory rate of 16 breaths/minute, and temperature of 37.2°C. The patient states that he is hepatitis C positive, and denies any current medications or drug use.

QUESTIONS

1. Are there any contraindications to analgesia in this case?
2. You note an absence of signs of sympathetic activity despite a report of severe pain. Describe the utility of vital signs in verifying pain in patients where a self-report is available.
3. Your colleague considers delaying analgesia until further diagnostic tests can be undertaken to rule out the possibility of drug-seeking behaviour. Discuss the clinical and ethical implications of this course of action.
4. If you decide to use a pharmacological intervention to manage the patient's pain, what agent/s will you elect to use? Summarise the risks and benefits associated with each agent.

Answers to Case Study Questions can be found on evolve **http://evolve.elsevier.com/AU/Curtis/emergency/** 

USEFUL WEBSITES

Better Pain Management, online education program developed by the Faculty of Pain Medicine (FPM) of the Australian and New Zealand College of Anaesthetists (ANZCA). Designed for specialist and general medical practitioners, medical students, nurses and allied health practitioners engaged in the care of patients with persistent pain. www.betterpainmanagement.com/.

International Degree Program in Pain Management, provides comprehensive and advanced education on the basic and applied sciences, concepts and approaches underpinning our current understanding of pain, its assessment and management. http://sydney.edu.au/medicine/pmri/education/index.php.

Pain management network. Enables patients to develop skills and knowledge in the self-management of their pain in partnership with your healthcare providers. www.aci.health.nsw.gov.au/chronic-pain.

REFERENCES

1. Morrison RS, Magaziner J, Gilbert M, Koval KJ, McLaughlin MA, Orosz G, et al. Relationship between pain and opioid analgesics on the development of delirium following hip fracture. J Gerontol Series A Biol Sci Med Sci 2003;58(1):76–81.
2. Craig K. Emotions and psychobiology. In: McMahon S, Koltzenburg M, editors. Wall and Melzack's textbook of pain. Philadelphia: Churchill Livingstone; 2006.
3. Liebeskind JC. Pain can kill. Pain 1991;44(1):3–4.
4. Macintyre P, Schug S. Acute pain management: a practical guide. 4th ed. Boca Raton: CRC Press; 2015.
5. Cordell WH, Keene KK, Giles BK, Jones JB, Jones JH, Brizendine EJ. The high prevalence of pain in emergency medical care. Am J Emerg Med 2002;20(3):165–9.
6. Chang HY, Daubresse M, Kruszewski SP, Alexander GC. Prevalence and treatment of pain in EDs in the United States, 2000 to 2010. Am J Emerg Med 2014;32(5):421–31.
7. Fosnocht D, Heaps N, Swanson E. Patient expectations for pain relief in the ED. Am J Emerg Med 2004;22(4):286–8.
8. Forero R, Mohsin M, McCarthy S, Young L, Ieraci S, Hillman K, et al. Prevalence of morphine use and time to initial analgesia in an Australian emergency department. Emerg Med Australas 2008;20(2):136–43.
9. Yeoh M, Huckson S. Audit of pain management in Australian emergency departments. Emerg Med Australas 2008;20:A26–36.
10. Doherty S, Knott J, Bennetts S, Jazayeri M, Huckson S. National project seeking to improve pain management in the emergency department setting: findings from the NHMRC-NICS National Pain Management Initiative. Emerg Med Australas 2013;25(2):120–6.
11. Anderson KO, Green CR, Payne R. Racial and ethnic disparities in pain: causes and consequences of unequal care. Pain 2009;10(12):1187–204.

12. Jones JS, Johnson K, McNinch M. Age as a risk factor for inadequate emergency department analgesia. Am J Emerg Med 1996;14(2):157–60.
13. Fry M, Elliott R. Pragmatic evaluation of an observational pain assessment scale in the emergency department: the Pain Assessment in Advanced Dementia (PAINAD) scale. Australas Emerg Care 2018;21(4):131–6.
14. Fry M, Arendts G, Chenoweth L. Emergency nurses' evaluation of observational pain assessment tools for older people with cognitive impairment. J Clin Nurs 2017;26(9–10):1281–90.
15. Chen EH, Shofer FS, Dean AJ, Hollander JE, Baxt WG, Robey JL, et al. Gender disparity in analgesic treatment of emergency department patients with acute abdominal pain. Acad Emerg Med 2008;15(5):414–18.
16. Safdar B, Heins A, Homel P, Miner J, Neighbor M, DeSandre P, et al. Impact of physician and patient gender on pain management in the emergency department–a multicenter study. Pain Med 2009;10(2):364–72.
17. Lord B, Cui J, Kelly AM. The impact of patient sex on paramedic pain management in the prehospital setting. Am J Emerg Med 2009;27(5):525–9.
18. Lord B, Khalsa S. Influence of patient race on administration of analgesia by student paramedics. BMC Emerg Med 2019;19(1):32.
19. White LJ, Cooper JD, Chambers RM, Gradisek RE. Prehospital use of analgesia for suspected extremity fractures. Prehosp Emerg Care 2000;4(3):205–8.
20. Samuel N, Steiner IP, Shavit I. Prehospital pain management of injured children: a systematic review of current evidence. Am J Emerg Med 2015;33(3):451–4.
21. Murphy A, McCoy S, O'Reilly K, Fogarty E, Dietz J, Crispino G, et al. A prevalence and management study of acute pain in children attending emergency departments by ambulance. Prehosp Emerg Care 2016;20(1):52–8.
22. Rupp T, Delaney KA. Inadequate analgesia in emergency medicine. Ann Emerg Med 2004;43(4):494–503.
23. Carr D, Cohen M, Finnerup N, Finnerup NB, Flor H, Gibson S, et al. The revised International Association for the Study of Pain definition of pain: concepts, challenges and compromises. Pain 2020;161(9):1976–82.
24. Melzack R, Wall PD. Pain mechanisms: a new theory. Science 1965;150(3699):971–9.
25. Melzack R, Katz J. Pain assessment in adult patients. In: McMahon S, Koltzenburg M, editors. Wall and Melzack's textbook of pain. Philadelphia: Churchill Livingstone; 2006.
26. Brown D, Edwards H, editors. Lewis's medical-surgical nursing. 4th ed. Sydney: Elsevier; 2014.
27. Lui F, Ng KF. Adjuvant analgesics in acute pain. Expert Opin Pharmacother 2011;12(3):363–85.
28. McCaffery M, Pasero C. Pain: clinical manual. St Louis: Mosby; 1999.
29. Devor M. Response of nerves to injury in relation to neuropathic pain. In: McMahon S, Koltzenburg M, editors. Wall and Melzack's textbook of pain. Philadelphia: Churchill Livingstone; 2006.
30. Australasian College for Emergency Medicine. Guidelines for implementation of the Australasian Triage Scale in emergency departments. 2016.
31. Lord B. Paramedic assessment of pain in the cognitively impaired adult patient. BMC Emerg Med 2009;9:20.
32. Daoust R, Paquet J, Bailey B, Piette É, Sanogo K, Chauny JM. Vital signs are not associated with self-reported acute pain intensity in the emergency department. Can J Emerg Med 2016;18(1):19–27.
33. Lord B, Woollard M. The reliability of vital signs in estimating pain severity among adult patients treated by paramedics. Emerg Med J 2011;28(2):147–50.
34. Marco CA, Plewa MC, Buderer N, Hymel G, Cooper J. Self-reported pain scores in the emergency department: lack of association with vital signs. Acad Emerg Med 2006;13(9):974–9.
35. Lee JS. Pain measurement: understanding existing tools and their application in the emergency department. Emerg Med (Fremantle) 2001;13(3):279–87.
36. Desbiens NA, Wu AW, Broste SK, Wenger NS, Connors Jr AF, Lynn J, et al. Pain and satisfaction with pain control in seriously ill hospitalized adults: findings from the SUPPORT research investigations. For the SUPPORT investigators. Study to Understand Prognoses and Preferences for Outcomes and Risks of Treatment. Crit Care Med 1996;24(12):1953–61.
37. Li DT, Puntillo K. A pilot study on coexisting symptoms in intensive care patients. App Nurs Res 2006;19(4):216–9.
38. Ma P, Liu J, Xi X, Du B, Yuan X, Lin H, et al. Practice of sedation and the perception of discomfort during mechanical ventilation in Chinese intensive care units. J Crit Care 2010;25(3):451–7.
39. Nelson JE, Meier DE, Litke A, Natale DA, Siegel RE, Morrison RS. The symptom burden of chronic critical illness. Crit Care Med 2004;32(7):1527–34.
40. Nelson JE, Meier DE, Oei EJ, Nierman DM, Senzel RS, Manfredi PL, et al. Self-reported symptom experience of critically ill cancer patients receiving intensive care. Crit Care Med 2001;29(2):277–82.
41. Puntillo KA, White C, Morris AB, Perdue ST, Stanik-Hutt J, Thompson CL, et al. Patients' perceptions and responses to procedural pain: results from Thunder Project II. Am J Crit Care 2001;10(4):238–51.
42. Varndell W, Elliott D, Fry M. Emergency nurses practices in assessing and administering continuous intravenous sedation for critically ill adult patients: a retrospective record review. Int Emerg Nurs 2015;23(2):81–8.
43. Weir S, O'Neill A. Experiences of intensive care nurses assessing sedation/agitation in critically ill patients. Nurs Crit Care 2008;13(4):185–94.
44. Batiha A. Pain management barriers in critical care units: a qualitative study. Int J Adv Nurs Stud 2014;3(1):1–5.
45. Clukey L, Weyant RA, Roberts M, Henderson A. Discovery of unexpected pain in intubated and sedated patients. Am J Crit Care 2014;23(3):216–20.

46. Thomas S. Management of pain in the emergency department. Int Scholarly Res Notice Emerg Med 2013:1–19.
47. Varndell W, Fry M, Elliott D. Emergency nurses' perceptions of sedation management practices for critically ill intubated patients: a qualitative study. J Clin Nurs 2015;24(21–22):3286–95.
48. Delorenzo AJ, Abetz JW, Andrew E, de Wit A, Williams B, Smith K. Characteristics of fixed wing air ambulance transports in Victoria, Australia. Air Med J 2017;36(4):173–8.
49. Herr K, Coyne PJ, Ely E, Gélinas C, Manworren RCB. Pain assessment in the patient unable to self-report: clinical practice recommendations in support of the ASPMN 2019 Position Statement. Pain Man Nurs 2019;20(5):404–17.
50. Varndell W, Elliott D, Fry M. The validity, reliability, responsiveness and applicability of observation sedation-scoring instruments for use with adult patients in the emergency department: a systematic literature review. Australas Emerg Nurs J 2015;18(1):1–23.
51. Solomon P. Congruence between health professionals' and patients' pain ratings: a review of the literature. Scand J Car Sci 2001;15(2):174–80.
52. Varndell W, Fry M, Elliott D. Pain assessment and interventions by nurses in the emergency department: a national survey. J Clin Nurs 2020;29(13–14):2352–62.
53. Hockenberry M, Wilson D, editors. Wong's essentials of pediatric nursing. 8th ed. St Louis: Mosby; 2009.
54. Merkel SI, Voepel-Lewis T, Malviya S. The FLACC: a behavioral scale for scoring postoperative pain in young children. Pediat Nurs 1997;23(3): 293–7.
55. Varndell W, Fry M, Elliott D. A systematic review of observational pain assessment instruments for use with nonverbal intubated critically ill adult patients in the emergency department: an assessment of their suitability and psychometric properties. J Clin Nurs 2017;26(1–2):7–32.
56. Varndell W, Elliott D, Fry M. Assessing, monitoring and managing continuous intravenous sedation for critically ill adult patients and implications for emergency nursing practice: a systematic literature review. Australas Emerg Nurs J 2015;18(2):59–67.
57. Varndell W. Nursing within a diverse cultural environment, and death and dying. In: Hodge A, Varndell W, editors. Professional transitions in nursing: a guide to practice in the Australian healthcare system. Sydney: Allen and Unwin; 2018.
58. International Pain Summit Of The International Association For The Study Of Pain Declaration of Montréal: declaration that access to pain management is a fundamental human right. J Pain Pall Care Pharmacother 2011;25(1):29–31.
59. Todd KH, Sloan EP, Chen C, Eder S, Wamstad K. Survey of pain etiology, management practices and patient satisfaction in two urban emergency departments. Can J Emerg Med 2002;4(4):252–6.
60. Neighbor ML, Honner S, Kohn MA. Factors affecting emergency department opioid administration to severely injured patients. Acad Emerg Med 2004;11(12):1290–6.
61. Silka PA, Roth MM, Geiderman JM. Patterns of analgesic use in trauma patients in the ED. Am J Emerg Med 2002;20(4):298–302.
62. Minozzi S, Amato L, Davoli M. Development of dependence following treatment with opioid analgesics for pain relief: a systematic review. Addiction 2013;108(4):688–98.
63. Galbraith A, Bullok S, Manias E. Fundamentals of pharmacology: a text for nurses and allied health professionals. Sydney: Prentice Hall; 2004.
64. Bowsher D. Mechanisms of pain in man. London: TCI Publications; 1987.
65. Savage SR, Joranson DE, Covington EC, Schnoll SH, Heit HA, Gilson AM. Definitions related to the medical use of opioids: evolution towards universal agreement. J Pain Sympt Manage 2003;26(1):655–67.
66. Heit HA. Addiction, physical dependence, and tolerance: precise definitions to help clinicians evaluate and treat chronic pain patients. J Pain Pall Care Pharmacother 2003;17(1):15–29.
67. Huxtable CA, Roberts LJ, Somogyi AA, MacIntyre PE. Acute pain management in opioid-tolerant patients: a growing challenge. Anaesth Intensive Care 2011;39(5):804–23.
68. Vickers AP, Jolly A. Naltrexone and problems in pain management. BMJ 2006;332(7534):132–3.
69. McNabb C, Foot C, Ting J, Breeze K, Stickley M. Profiling patients suspected of drug seeking in an adult emergency department. Emerg Med Australas 2006;18(2):131–7.
70. Saposnik G, Redelmeier D, Ruff C, Tobler PN. Cognitive biases associated with medical decisions: a systematic review. BMC Med Inform Decis Mak 2016;16(1):138.
71. Burke SO, Jerrett M. Pain management across age groups. West J Nurs Res 1989;11(2):164–78; discussion 178–80.
72. McEachin C, McDermott J, Swor R. Few emergency medical services patients with lower-extremity fractures receive prehospital analgesia. Prehosp Emerg Care 2002;6:406–10.
73. Wisborg T, Flaatten H. Pain management in the pre-hospital/emergency medical service environment: on-site and transport. In: Rosenberg A, Grande C, Bernstein R, editors. Pain management and regional anesthesia in trauma. London: WB Saunders; 1999.
74. Schug S, Palmer G, Scott D, Alcock M, Halliwell R, Mott JF, editors. Acute pain management: scientific evidence. 5th ed. Melbourne: Australian and New Zealand College of Anaesthetists and Faculty of Pain Medicine; 2020.
75. Coman M, Kelly A. Safety of a nurse-managed, titrated intravenous analgesia policy on the management of severe pain in the emergency department. Emerg Med (Fremantle) 1999;11:128–31.
76. Fry M, Holdgate A. Nurse-initiated intravenous morphine in the emergency department: efficacy, rate of adverse events and impact on time to analgesia. Emerg Mede (Fremantle) 2002;14(3):249–54.

77. World Health Organization (WHO). Cancer pain relief. Geneva: WHO; 1986.
78. Barksdale AN, Hackman JL, Williams K, Gratton MC. ED triage pain protocol reduces time to receiving analgesics in patients with painful conditions. Am J Emerg Med 2016;34(12):2362–6.
79. Pierik JG, Berben SA, Ijzerman MJ, Gaakeer MI, van Eenennaam FL, van Vugt AB, et al. A nurse-initiated pain protocol in the ED improves pain treatment in patients with acute musculoskeletal pain. Int Emerg Nurs 2016;27:3–10.
80. Varndell W, Fry M, Elliott D. Quality and impact of nurse-initiated analgesia in the emergency department: a systematic review. Int Emerg Nurs 2018;40:46–53.
81. Carlson CL. Effectiveness of the World Health Organization cancer pain relief guidelines: an integrative review. J Pain Res 2016;9:515–34.
82. AMH. Australian medicines handbook. Adelaide: Australian Medicines Handbook; 2022.
83. Murphy A, O'Sullivan R, Wakai A, Grant TS, Barrett MJ, Cronin J, et al. Intranasal fentanyl for the management of acute pain in children. Cochrane Database Syst Rev 2014;2014(10):Cd009942.
84. Lord B, Jennings PA, Smith K. Effects of the introduction of intranasal fentanyl on reduction of pain severity score in children: an interrupted time-series analysis. Pediatr Emerg Care 2019;35(11):749–54.
85. Kotwal RS, O'Connor KC, Johnson TR, Mosely DS, Meyer DE, Holcomb JB. A novel pain management strategy for combat casualty care. Ann Emerg Med 2004;44(2):121–7.
86. Weldon ER, Ariano RE, Grierson RA. Comparison of fentanyl and morphine in the prehospital treatment of ischemic type chest pain. Prehosp Emerg Care 2016;20(1):45–51.
87. Young A, Ismail M, Papatsoris AG, Barua JM, Calleary JG, Masood J. Entonox® inhalation to reduce pain in common diagnostic and therapeutic outpatient urological procedures: a review of the evidence. Ann Roy Coll Surg Eng 2012;94(1):8–11.
88. Brichko L, Gaddam R, Roman C, O'Reilly G, Luckhoff C, Jennings P, et al. Rapid Administration of Methoxyflurane to Patients in the Emergency Department (RAMPED) Study: a randomized controlled trial of methoxyflurane versus standard care. Acad Emerg Med 2021;28(2):164–71.
89. Bronsky ES, Koola C, Orlando A, Redmond D, D'Huyvetter C, Sieracki H, et al. Intravenous low-dose ketamine provides greater pain control compared to fentanyl in a civilian prehospital trauma system: a propensity matched analysis. Prehosp Emerg Care 2019;23(1):1–8.
90. Simpson PM, Fouche PF, Thomas RE, Bendall JC. Transcutaneous electrical nerve stimulation for relieving acute pain in the prehospital setting: a systematic review and meta-analysis of randomized-controlled trials. Euro J Emerg Med 2014;21(1):10–17.
91. Arendts G, Stevens M, Fry M. Topical anaesthesia and intravenous cannulation success in paediatric patients: a randomized double-blind trial. Br J Anaesth 2008;100(4):521–4.
92. Bryant B, Knights K, Salerno E. Pharmacology for health professionals. Sydney: Mosby; 2014.
93. Warren L, Pak A. Local anaesthetic systemic toxicity. UpToDate; 2022. Available from: www.uptodate.com.acs.hcn.com.au/contents/local-anesthetic-systemic-toxicity.
94. Hards M, Brewer A, Bessant G, Lahiri S. Efficacy of prehospital analgesia with fascia iliaca compartment block for femoral bone fractures: a systematic review. Prehosp Disast Med 2018;33(3):299–307.
95. Deitch K, Chudnofsky CR, Dominici P. The utility of supplemental oxygen during emergency department procedural sedation and analgesia with midazolam and fentanyl: a randomized, controlled trial. Ann Emerg Med 2007;49(1):1–8.

CHAPTER 19

ORGAN AND TISSUE DONATION

MYRA SERRANO, LEIGH McKAY AND JANE TRELOGGEN

ESSENTIALS

- It is important to stay up to date with changing donation practices to maintain high standards of care within the required legal, procedural and ethical frameworks.
- Rapid and early referral of patients meeting the clinical trigger allows staff to explore their wishes and suitability to donate, and provides an opportunity to plan the family donation conversation.
- Medical suitability of potential donors should be determined by the respective tissue banks and organ and tissue donation agency.
- Proactive donor management optimises solid-organ and tissue function following consent to donation.
- Consistent and appropriate bereavement support for families of organ and tissue donors enables them to find comfort and meaning in their loss.
- Collaborative efforts between clinicians in the emergency department, intensive care, operating theatre and hospital administrators develop mutual accountability and responsibility that leads to improved bereavement and end-of-life care, as well as transplant recipient outcomes.
- Maintaining open channels of communication between hospital clinicians, tissue banks and the organ and tissue donation agency will build strong partnerships for success.

INTRODUCTION

Australian medical specialists indicated a few decades ago that human organ and tissue transplantation had become a very effective treatment option for irrevocable failure of vital organs.[1,2] Retrieval and transplantation of organs and tissues from the deceased has been occurring in Australia since 1911, when a portion of pancreas was transplanted unsuccessfully at the Launceston General Hospital in Tasmania.[3] This was followed by the first reported corneal transplant in 1941, kidneys in 1956 and liver and heart in 1968.[3,4] Transplantation began in Aotearoa New Zealand with the first corneal grafting in the 1940s and the first organ to be transplanted was the kidney in 1965.[5] Bone tissue and hearts were first successfully transplanted in the 1980s and the 1990s saw the commencement of skin, lung, liver and pancreas transplantations.[5,6] In 2019 the NSW Organ and Tissue Donation Service commenced an Amnion Donor Program, matching a New Zealand program and addressing a gap left when a similar program in Victoria, Australia, was ceased. The amniotic membrane is turned into tissue graft, known as a biological bandage, and is an effective treatment option for serious wounds, eye injuries and burns.

Long-term graft survival became possible with the discovery and use of immunosuppressive agents in the 1960s,[7,8] and the current era of organ and tissue transplantation in Australia (1982) and Aotearoa New Zealand (1964) began with the enactment of legislation that defined death and addressed the retrieval and use of tissue from living and deceased persons.[3] Since then, programs have commenced for solid-organ and tissue transplantation—heart, lung, liver, kidney, pancreas, islet cell and intestinal, corneal, cardiac, skin, amnion and musculoskeletal tissues.

Organ and tissue donation is a component of end-of-life care, and the variables of how, when and where the person dies will influence which organs and tissues they can donate. With a focus on paramedics, emergency care clinicians and nurses, this chapter will describe in detail the process and clinical implications of deceased organ and tissue donation in Australia and Aotearoa New Zealand with reference to best-practice evidence from the literature. Useful websites are listed at the end of the chapter.

DONATION AND TRANSPLANTATION IN AUSTRALIA AND AOTEAROA NEW ZEALAND

Legislation governing organ and tissue donation in Australia is state- and territory-based. The Australian Organ and Tissue Authority (OTA) was established in 2009 to implement A World's Best Practice Approach to Organ and Tissue Donation for Transplantation.[9] OTA is the peak body that works with all sectors to maximise the potential for organ and tissue donation in Australia. Organ and tissue donation (OTD) agencies are based in each Australian state and two territories, and are known as the DonateLife network. State-based tissue banks facilitate tissue retrieval in partnership with their local OTD agency. National legislation on organ and tissue donation is enforced in Aotearoa New Zealand. Organ Donation New Zealand (ODNZ) is the national organisation with primary responsibility for coordinating the donation of organs and tissues from deceased donors in Aotearoa New Zealand.

Quality and safety processes involved in tissue retrieval, manufacture and transplantation are governed by the Australian Therapeutic Goods Administration (Australian Code of Good Manufacturing Practice—Human Blood and Tissues) and the New Zealand Medicines and Medical Devices Safety Authority (New Zealand Code of Good Manufacturing Practice for Manufacture and Distribution of Therapeutic Goods). The process of potential organ and tissue donor identification and management in the critical care environment is guided by the Australian and New Zealand Intensive Care Society (ANZICS) *Statement on Death and Organ Donation Edition 4* (2021). Donor selection, eligibility and allocation criteria were developed by the Transplantation Society of Australia and New Zealand (TSANZ) and the National Health and Medical Research Council (NHMRC) to ensure that there are equitable and transparent processes in place.

The Australia and New Zealand Organ Donation Registry (ANZOD) records and reports on a wide range of statistics that relate to organ and tissue donation following death, and the Australia and New Zealand Dialysis and Transplant Registry (ANZDATA) collects a wide range of statistics that relate to the outcomes of treatment of those with end-stage kidney failure (Table 19.1).[10]

Following the emergence and spread of the novel coronavirus (SARS-CoV-2) across the world since 2020, precautionary steps were undertaken by the donation and transplant sectors that affected the organ and tissue donation rates in Australia and Aotearoa New Zealand. The National Transplantation and Donation Rapid Response Taskforce was established, which resulted in the temporary suspension of the kidney and pancreas transplant programs, and restriction of liver, heart, lung, paediatric and multi-organ transplant programs. There were also limitations on transport of organs between states and territories due to border closures, as well as freight and COVID-19 restrictions.[10]

TABLE 19.1 SUMMARY OF SOLID-ORGAN DONATIONS 2012–2021[10]

YEAR	AUSTRALIA	NEW ZEALAND
2012	354 (15.6)	38 (9)
2013	391 (16.9)	36 (8)
2014	378 (16.1)	46 (10.2)
2015	435 (18.3)	53 (11.5)
2016	503 (20.8)	61 (11.7)
2017	510 (20.7)	73 (15.2)
2018	554 (22.2)	62 (12.7)
2019	548 (21.6)	74 (15.0)
2020	463 (18.0)	64 (12.6)
2021	421 (16.4)	66 (13.0)

Donors per million population reported in brackets.

A professional education package has been developed for Australian health professionals working within critical care areas and includes IDAT (Introductory Donation Awareness Training) and the Family Donation Conversation (Core and Practical) workshops. This package is funded by OTA and endorsed by the Australian College of Critical Care Nurses (ACCCN), the College of Intensive Care Medicine (CICM) and ANZICS. Donation and transplantation training for health professionals is also offered in Aotearoa New Zealand. Professional associations in organ and tissue donation and transplantation include the Australasian Transplant Coordinators Association (ATCA), Transplant Nurses' Association (TNA), Transplantation Society of Australia and New Zealand (TSANZ), Biotherapeutics Association of Australasia (BAA) and the Eye Bank Association of Australia and New Zealand (EBAANZ).

'OPT-IN' SYSTEM OF DONATION

There are two general systems of approach to consent for deceased organ and tissue donation around the world. Some countries have an 'opt-out' or presumed consent system (e.g. Spain, Belgium, Austria, Singapore, England, Wales, Scotland, Northern Ireland and Crown dependencies—Guernsey, Jersey and Isle of Man), where eligible persons are considered for organ and tissue donation at the time of their death if they have not indicated their explicit objection.[11,12] In Australia, Aotearoa New Zealand, the United States and other common-law countries, the approach is to 'opt in', with specific consent required from the potential donor or their next of kin.[13] In Australia, a person may indicate their consent for organ and tissue donation on the Australian Organ Donor Register and on their driver's licence (South Australia only). Aotearoa New Zealand is the only nation where indicating one's donation decision is compulsory in order to obtain a driver's licence. In Australia and Aotearoa New Zealand, the focus remains on providing compassionate communication, information about donation for transplantation and quality care so that every family can make an informed, proactive and enduring donation decision.[9] In parts of Asia, the informed-consent legislation of Japan and Korea came into force in 1997 and 2000 respectively and is still practised.[14,15]

LEGISLATION

Legislation governing organ and tissue donation in Australia and Aotearoa New Zealand takes the form of an Act that addresses the retrieval and use of human tissue before and after death. The legislation enables a person to choose to be a donor, and organ and tissue donation can proceed unless revoked or objected to by the family. If the deceased's wishes are not known, consent for donation rests with the next of kin. The *New Zealand Human Tissue Act 2008* governs the practice in Aotearoa New Zealand; however, this does not include a statutory definition of death, but rather uses the words 'satisfied … that the individual concerned is dead'.[16] Death is defined in the New Zealand Ministry of Health national strategy to increase deceased organ donation and transplantation.[16] Each Australian state and territory enacts its own legislation or Human Tissue Act and these can be found on state government websites. Australian legislation defines death as the:

- irreversible cessation of all function of the brain of the person, or
- irreversible cessation of circulation of blood in the body of the person.[17]

PATHWAYS OF DONATION

Organs and tissue may be donated by a living or deceased person. Organ and tissue donation from a living person is divided into the categories of *regenerative* and *non-regenerative* tissue. Regenerative tissue includes blood and bone marrow, while non-regenerative tissue includes cord blood, kidneys, liver (lobe/s), lungs (lobe/s), amnion, skin and femoral heads. The implications of consent differ for each type of tissue. For example, the collection of bone marrow or the retrieval of a kidney, the lobe of a liver or a lung are invasive procedures that could potentially put the health and wellbeing of the donor at risk.[18] In contrast, the donation of a femoral head could be the end-product of a total hip replacement where the bone is otherwise discarded. Similarly, cord blood from the umbilical cord and amnion from the amniotic sac would be discarded if not retrieved immediately after birth.

After death, organ and tissue donation are clinically dependent on the variables of medical, surgical and social history, and how, when and where the person died. Legally and ethically, organ and tissue donation is dependent on informed decision-making and consent by the donor and their family. The most common form of donation after death in Australia and Aotearoa New Zealand is tissue donation.

TISSUE-ONLY DONATION

Many people can be tissue donors after their death. Eyes (whole or corneal button) are retrieved for corneal and scleral transplantation. Musculoskeletal tissue is used for bone grafting (long bones of upper and lower limbs and hemipelvis), urology procedures and treatment of sports injuries (ligaments, tendons, fascia and meniscus). Heart tissue (bicuspid and tricuspid valves, aortic and pulmonary tissue) is used for heart valve replacement and cardiac reconstruction. Skin is used as a temporary covering for the treatment of burns. Amnion is an effective treatment option and is used as a biological bandage for non-healing wounds, eye injuries and burns.[19]

The potential tissue-only donor

The most influential component of the tissue-only donation process is the early notification of the potential donor's death to the relevant tissue bank or OTD agency, ideally within hours of circulatory standstill. All deceased persons can be considered potential donors, with assessment for clinical suitability completed on a case-by-case basis.

The process of tissue-only donation

In general, local health, palliative and aged-care facilities notify the tissue bank or OTD agency of any death. People who die in their home are not routinely notified, due to logistical issues and the length of time elapsed since circulatory standstill. However, the family may raise donation and this may be facilitated directly through the funeral home with the tissue bank and OTD agency. The determining factors are age, cause of death, serology results, presence of infection, risk assessment of social and medical history, and time elapsed since circulatory standstill.[20] The legal requirements of obtaining consent mirror those of the multi-organ donor and are discussed later in the chapter.

Following medical suitability assessment and relevant donor registry checks, the tissue bank coordinator or other trained personnel will approach the next of kin with the possibility of tissue donation. Eyes can be retrieved from 12 to 24 hours after circulatory standstill, depending on the techniques used when processing the tissue after retrieval. Heart tissue, skin and musculoskeletal tissue can be retrieved up to 24 hours after circulatory standstill. Of note, eye donors can be up to 99 years of age, heart tissue donors up to 60 years and musculoskeletal donors up to 90 years of age in Australia and Aotearoa New Zealand.

Following tissue retrieval, every effort is made to restore anatomical appearance. Incisions are sutured, closed and covered with surgical dressings as appropriate, limbs given back their form and the eye shape is restored with the lids kept closed with eye caps.

Support requirements for the families of tissue-only donors share many of the aspects of programs provided for the families involved in donation after circulatory and neurological determination of death, as discussed later in the chapter. A sensitive approach, provision of adequate information to assist informed and enduring decision-making, offers of formal bereavement support and follow-up information of recipient outcomes are proven aspects of successful programs.[21,22] A possibility for some potential donor families is solid-organ donation, as confirmation of death using circulatory criteria does not necessarily preclude solid-organ retrieval. See the section on donation after circulatory determination of death.

Clinical trigger

The use of clinical triggers in the emergency department (ED) and the intensive care unit (ICU) facilitate the early identification and referral of potential donors to enable early involvement of the donation specialist.[23] A clinical trigger is a tool used as part of a systematic approach to organ and tissue donation and is based on established international best practice.[24] Australia's OTA developed clinical triggers to optimise the identification and referral of all potential organ, eye and tissue donors.

PRACTICE TIP

Early notification about a potential donor should take place, as it allows for medical suitability assessment by donation and transplant experts, check of the registration status on the Australian Organ Donor Register (AODR) and the involvement of a Donation Specialist to support and plan the family donation conversation.[23,25] ED and ICU staff are asked to contact the hospital-based donation team (where available), OTD agency or tissue bank when a patient meets the trigger criteria, whereby no further treatment options are available or appropriate, and a family discussion regarding end-of-life care has been or is to be conducted.

DONATION AFTER CIRCULATORY DETERMINATION OF DEATH (DCDD)

Donation after circulatory determination of death (DCDD), previously known as non-heart-beating donation and donation after cardiac or circulatory death, is now an established pathway to multi-organ donation in patients with irreversible neurological conditions who do not fulfil the neurological determination of death criteria, or in patients with a catastrophic and irreversible cardio-respiratory condition where withdrawal of cardio-respiratory support (WCRS) is considered appropriate. Prior to legislation in the determination and certification of neurological death in the late 1960s and early 1970s, DCDD was the source of cadaveric kidneys for transplantation.[26,27]

Initially, long-term success of transplantation from organs procured from DCDD donors was limited due to prolonged warm ischaemic time, ineffective immunosuppression, unrefined surgical technique and underdeveloped organ preservation methods.[26] However, DCDD programs around the world were re-established following evidence to suggest that organs from DCDD provide relatively equivalent outcomes when compared with organs from donation after neurological determination of death (DNDD) donors.[28]

The renewed focus on DCDD in Australia and Aotearoa New Zealand has been driven, in part, by stagnant donation rates and greater indications for transplantation. DCDD forms part of a broad approach to expand the donor pool and the availability of organs for transplantation. There have been significant increases in the number of DCDD donors over the last decade in both Australia and Aotearoa New Zealand, 25% and 10% respectively.[17] This has been partly due to families and community acceptance, evolving technologies and excellent transplantation outcomes. In 2021, Australia's OTA released a revised national best practice guideline for DCDD, ensuring clinical consistency, and appropriate and ethical practice to optimise outcomes for both the donor and the recipient.[29] In Aotearoa New Zealand, the ODNZ developed a national protocol for DCDD in consultation with intensive care and transplant professionals that was released in 2007.[30] DCDD allows the families of patients who do not meet the neurological determination of death criteria the opportunity to donate solid organs and tissue after death.

The potential DCDD donor

With consideration of the lessons learnt from the DNDD program, a successful DCDD program is founded on evidence-based ethical and clinical grounds that aim to maintain the dignity of the donor at all times and provide the donor family with support and information to ensure informed decision-making.[31] Five categories of potential DCDD donors have been identified, and are known as the Maastricht Classification of DCDD (see Table 19.2).[17,32]

Uncontrolled categories 1, 2, 4 and 5 are unpredictable and present logistical difficulties in limiting the length of warm ischaemic time; present legal and ethical restrictions in the management of the potential donor; and do not allow enough time for informed decision-making by the potential donor's family.

Category 3 and controlled category 4 are options that are able to be controlled. The category 3 potential DCDD donor is a person ventilated and monitored in ED or ICU who has suffered an irrecoverable condition that is not likely to deteriorate to neurological death, and the decision has been made that further treatment is no longer of benefit to the person and current interventions are to be withdrawn. A controlled

TABLE 19.2 MAASTRICHT CLASSIFICATION OF DCDD[32]

Category 1 (Uncontrolled)	Out-of-hospital cardiac arrest with unsuccessful resuscitation—dead on arrival at hospital	Sudden unexpected cardiac arrest without resuscitation or unknown warm ischaemic time
Category 2 (Uncontrolled)	In-hospital cardiac arrest in ED or ICU	Sudden unexpected irreversible circulatory arrest with unsuccessful resuscitation
Category 3 (Controlled)	Withdrawal of treatment in ICU or OT	Expected cardiac arrest following planned withdrawal of cardiorespiratory support
Category 4 (Controlled / Uncontrolled)	Cardiac arrest in a neurological dead patient in ICU or OT	Sudden circulatory arrest following neurological determination of death prior to planned organ recovery
Category 5 (Uncontrolled)	Cardiac arrest in ICU	Unexpected cardiac arrest in ICU

category 4 potential DCDD donor is a person in ICU who is determined to be neurologically dead and the family wish to be present at the time of WCRS.[17]

Transplant outcomes from this form of donation are influenced by the length of warm ischaemia, which is the time taken from cessation of ventilation and treatment to the certification of death, and then to the commencement of infusion of cold perfusion fluid and/or organ retrieval and/or machine perfusion. The cold perfusion fluid is an electrolyte-specific solution that is used to flush the organs and temporarily reduce their metabolic rate by decreasing temperature and minimising cellular oedema and ischaemic damage.[33] Machine perfusion has a similar effect in organ preservation, except that it enables normothermic and oxygenated perfusion of organs following retrieval, which then leads to adequate graft function.[33]

PRACTICE TIP

The decision to withdraw cardiorespiratory support must be made independently of any decision to donate organs and tissue for transplantation and must be agreed to by the family and the treating healthcare team.[17,34]

The process of donation after circulatory determination of death

The clinical suitability assessment for solid-organ retrieval replicates that of a multi-organ DNDD donor (discussed later in the chapter), with medical, surgical and social history, serology and organ function information collected prior to WCRS. The legal requirements for obtaining consent are the same as in DNDD. Families will be informed that retrieval may not take place due to a number of variables, including the length of time from WCRS to circulatory standstill.[31]

DCDD is deemed not appropriate if, in the judgement of the treating medical practitioner, it is anticipated that the patient is likely to survive after WCRS for significantly longer than the allocated time limit. The time limit ensures a respectful approach to managing the patient's death where the possibility of DCDD might complicate an unexpectedly prolonged dying process.[35] Furthermore, the longer the warm ischaemic time, the greater the risk of irreparable damage to the organ due to hypotension and hypoxaemia.[33] Transplant units determine the specific time limits for the warm ischaemic period, for example: no more than 30 minutes from WCRS for liver, pancreas and heart, 60 minutes for kidneys; and 90 minutes for lungs.[29]

It should be noted that the ability to accurately predict the timing of death is difficult and the use of predictive algorithms to assess the likelihood of the patient dying within the time limit should be at the discretion of the treating medical practitioner. The University of Wisconsin criteria for predicting asystole following WCRS assigns a numerical value to clinical parameters to generate a score predicting the likelihood of death occurring within 90 minutes.[26] The UNOS tool (United Network for Organ Sharing) also uses a set of criteria for identifying potential DCDD patients.[35] While these tools are commonly used within the United States, widespread validation of their effectiveness has not yet occurred in Australia or Aotearoa New Zealand. Clinical indicators such as ventilator support, use of inotropes and sedation, body mass index and Glasgow Coma Scale (GCS) score can be used as an 'informal' guide for predicting death; however, the decision to proceed with DCDD is generally at the discretion of the patient's treating medical practitioner. If the time-frames are not met following WCRS in a potential DCDD donor, the organ retrieval process is abandoned, usual end-of-life care continues and tissue donation pursued following death if indicated.

DCDD retrieval process alternatives

WCRS in a potential DCDD donor most commonly occurs in the ICU, but may also take place in the operating theatre. The location of WCRS is generally dependent upon family requests and hospital policy. Consideration should also be given to logistical constraints, which may have an impact on organ viability. Rapid transfer of the patient to theatre must occur following the certification of death to ensure that warm ischaemic time is kept to a minimum. The operating room is prepared well ahead of the scheduled WCRS and the procurement team and other operating room staff are kept updated until death is certified.

If the patient is donating lungs, an anaesthetist will re-intubate prior to moving the patient on to the operating table to prevent aspiration. The patient will not be attached to a ventilator. For multi-organ procurement (involving both abdominal and thoracic organs), a super-rapid laparotomy is performed in tandem with a sternotomy. The aim is to cannulate the aorta and, if necessary, the pulmonary artery, to initiate the rapid infusion of cold preservation solutions. The thoracic aorta is cross-clamped and the right atrium vented. Topical cooling of the thoracic and abdominal viscera with icy saline slush is also performed. Once organ flushing with preservation solution has occurred, the surgical procedure continues as for a standard multi-organ procurement, or as a renal-only procurement depending on the circumstances.

If WCRS occurs in the operating theatre and circulatory standstill does not occur, the patient is transferred back to the ED or ICU or another appropriate area. The priority at all times is the provision of high-quality end-of-life care, and the donation process should not compromise this aim.

DONATION AFTER NEUROLOGICAL DETERMINATION OF DEATH (DNDD)

In Australia and Aotearoa New Zealand, the term 'neurological determination of death' is now used in preference to 'brain death' as it avoids the implication of two different types of death. However, the term brain death is likely to persist as it is short and convenient.[17]

The most common pathway to deceased donation is DNDD, which is more likely to occur in the ICU than in the ED. There are four main factors that directly influence the number of donors after neurological determination of death:

- the incidence of neurological death
- identification of potential donors
- confirmation of death and informed consent for donation
- clinical management after confirmation of death.

Neurological determination of death (brain death)

The diagnosis of neurological death is now widely accepted, and most developed countries have legislation governing the definition of death and the retrieval of organs and tissues for

BOX 19.1 CONDITIONS ASSOCIATED WITH NEUROLOGICAL DEATH[38]

Hypotension
Diabetes insipidus
Disseminated intravascular coagulation
Dysrhythmias
Cardiac arrest
Pulmonary oedema
Hypoxia
Acidosis

transplantation. In Australia and Aotearoa New Zealand, the most common cause of neurological death is spontaneous intracranial haemorrhage, which has implications for the organs and tissues retrieved as the donors may be older and often have cardiovascular and other comorbidities.[36] There is no legal requirement to formally confirm neurological death if organs and tissues are not going to be retrieved for transplantation.[17]

Neurological death is only observed clinically when the patient is supported with mechanical ventilation, as the respiratory reflex that is lost due to cerebral ischaemia will result in respiratory and cardiac arrest. Mechanical ventilation maintains the oxygen supply to the natural pacemaker of the heart, which functions independently of the central nervous system. Neurological death results in hypotension due to loss of vasomotor control of the autonomic nervous system, loss of temperature regulation, reduction in hormone activity and loss of all cranial nerve reflexes.[37,38] Box 19.1 lists the common conditions associated with neurological death. Irrespective of the degree of external support, circulatory standstill will mostly occur in a matter of hours to days once neurological death has occurred.[38]

Neurological determination of death testing methods

The aim of testing for neurological death is to determine irreversible cessation of brain function. Testing does not demonstrate that every brain cell has died, but that a point of irreversible ischaemic damage involving cessation of the vital functions of the brain has been reached. Two senior medical practitioners with relevant and recent experience and no involvement with transplant recipient selection participate in this process. In Australia, one of the medical practitioners must be a designated specialist appointed by the governing body of their health institution.[17]

There are a number of steps in the process, the first being the observation period. ANZICS recommends that the observation period is a minimum of 4 hours from onset of no response observed until formal testing commences (with the patient being mechanically ventilated, a GCS score of 3, nonreacting pupils, absent cough and gag reflexes and no spontaneous respiratory effort). In cases of acute hypoxic-ischaemic encephalopathy, post cardiac arrest or prolonged hypothermia (<35°C), there should be a waiting period of 24 hours before using clinical testing alone.[17]

The second step is to consider the preconditions (see Box 19.2). Once the observation period has passed, during which time the patient receives ongoing treatment, and the preconditions have been met, formal testing can occur. Formal testing for neurological death in Australia and Aotearoa New Zealand is undertaken using either clinical testing of brainstem function or cerebral blood flow studies.[17] The most common form of testing is clinical testing of the brainstem, involving assessment of the cranial nerves and the respiratory centre (see Table 19.3). Brain death is confirmed if there is no response to stimulation of all of these reflexes, with the respiratory centre tested last and only if the other reflexes prove to be absent. If the patient demonstrates no response to the first set of tests, the testing is replicated to demonstrate irreversibility. It is recommended that the two sets of tests be performed separately and independently by the medical practitioners.[17]

BOX 19.2 PRECONDITIONS OF NEUROLOGICAL DETERMINATION OF DEATH TESTING[17]

- Definite clinical or neuro-imaging evidence of acute brain pathology consistent with irreversible loss of neurological function
- Normothermia (core temperature ≥ 35°C)
- Normotension (systolic blood pressure ≥ 90 mmHg, mean arterial pressure ≥ 60 mmHg in an adult)
- Exclusion of effects of sedative medications (self-administered or otherwise)
- Absence of severe electrolyte, metabolic or endocrine disturbances
- Absence of acute liver failure or decompensated chronic liver disease
- Intact neuromuscular function
- Ability to adequately examine the brainstem reflexes (at least one ear and one eye)
- Ability to perform apnoea testing

PRACTICE TIP

When testing for corneal reflex, take care not to cause corneal abrasion which might prevent the cornea being transplanted if the patient is an eye donor.

The opportunity to observe the second set of clinical tests should be offered to the family with appropriate explanation and support to assist their comprehension of neurological death.[17,39]

If the preconditions listed in Box 19.2 cannot be met, neurological death can be confirmed using cerebral blood flow imaging to demonstrate absent blood flow to the brain, either by intra-arterial catheter angiography, radionuclide imaging or computed tomography angiography (CTA). However, it must be preceded by performance of those parts of the clinical examination that are possible.

A four-vessel angiography is performed by direct injection of contrast medium into both carotid arteries and both vertebral arteries.[40] Neurological death is confirmed if there is no

TABLE 19.3 CLINICAL NEUROLOGICAL DEATH TESTING[17]

		CRANIAL NERVES	TEST TECHNIQUE	OUTCOME
1	Response to noxious stimuli	Trigeminal V (sensory), facial VII (motor)	Stimulus within the cranial nerve distribution and all four limbs and trunk, e.g. firm pressure over supraorbital region, sternal rub and deep nail pressure	If reflex is absent the patient will not grimace or react
2	Pupillary response to light	Optic II, oculomotor III	Use torch to shine bright light into eye	If reflex is absent the pupils are fixed; may or may not be dilated but must be at least midsize in diameter
3	Corneal reflex	Trigeminal V (sensory), facial VII (motor)	Use wisp of sterile cotton wool or gauze to touch the cornea	If the reflex is absent the eyes will not react or blink
4	Gag reflex	Glossopharyngeal IX, vagus X	Use a tongue depressor on the oropharynx or move ETT	If reflex is absent there is no gag or pharyngeal response
5	Cough reflex	Vagus X	Use soft suction catheter down ETT to deliberately stimulate the carina	If reflex is absent there is no cough response
6	Oculovestibular reflex	Vestibulocochlear VIII, oculomotor III, IV, abducens VI	Check first that both tympanic membranes are intact or not obstructed. Then slowly irrigate both ears with 50 mL of iced water while eyes are held open	When the reflex is absent the eyes remain midline rather than deviating towards the stimulus
7	Apnoea test	Medulla respiratory centre	The last test to be performed when all other reflexes have proven to be absent. The patient is pre-oxygenated on 100% oxygen for at least 5 minutes, an ABG analysis is performed to ascertain the baseline carbon dioxide, and then the patient is disconnected from mechanical ventilation but supplied with oxygen via catheter or self-inflating bag and PEEP valve. The patient is observed for signs of respiratory effort.	The period of time disconnected from the ventilator must be long enough for the arterial carbon dioxide level to rise to a threshold high enough to normally stimulate respiration; i.e. an arterial carbon dioxide pressure greater than 60 mmHg and an arterial pH of less than 7.30. For pre-existing hypercapnia wait for $PaCO_2$ rise $>$ 20 mmHg above chronic level. Expose chest and abdomen to observe for spontaneous breathing. No breathing effort is seen.

ABG: arterial blood gas; ETT: endotracheal tube.

blood flow above the level of the carotid siphon or above the foramen magnum (Fig. 19.1).[17,40]

The radionuclide imaging is performed by administering a bolus of short-acting radionuclide isotope intravenously while imaging the head using a gamma camera. No intracranial uptake of the radionuclide isotope confirms absent blood flow to the brain (Fig. 19.2).[17,40]

Computed tomography angiography (CTA) is acceptable if recommended radiological guidelines are followed and the above methods are not readily available.[17]

The time of death is recorded as the time the second medical practitioner determines that neurological death has occurred, whether this is by clinical examination or imaging to confirm the absence of intracranial blood flow, and this should be documented accordingly.[17]

The potential donor after neurological determination of death

A potential DNDD donor is someone who is suspected of or has been confirmed as being deceased by neurological criteria. The inclusion and exclusion criteria for organ and tissue donation are constantly reviewed and amended.[41] Advice regarding medical suitability for organ and tissue donation is available 24 hours a day, 7 days a week from the OTD agency. This advice can be sought at any stage of the process and there is no expectation that the treating clinician and nursing staff at the bedside would make this decision.

Obtaining consent

An important factor that influences the number of donors is the consent process. Historically in Australia and Aotearoa New Zealand, the treating medical practitioner would either initiate or be involved in approaching the next of kin after death has been confirmed or anticipated. Current evidence suggests that the best practice approach is for the senior treating doctor (ideally someone who has completed OTA's core Family Donation Conversation workshop) and Donation Specialist Nurse to discuss donation with the family in a collaborative way.[42] Approaching the next of kin to discuss organ and tissue donation is part of the duty of care to that patient, who may

FIGURE 19.1 NEUROLOGICAL DETERMINATION OF DEATH STUDY—FOUR-VESSEL CEREBRAL ANGIOGRAPHY

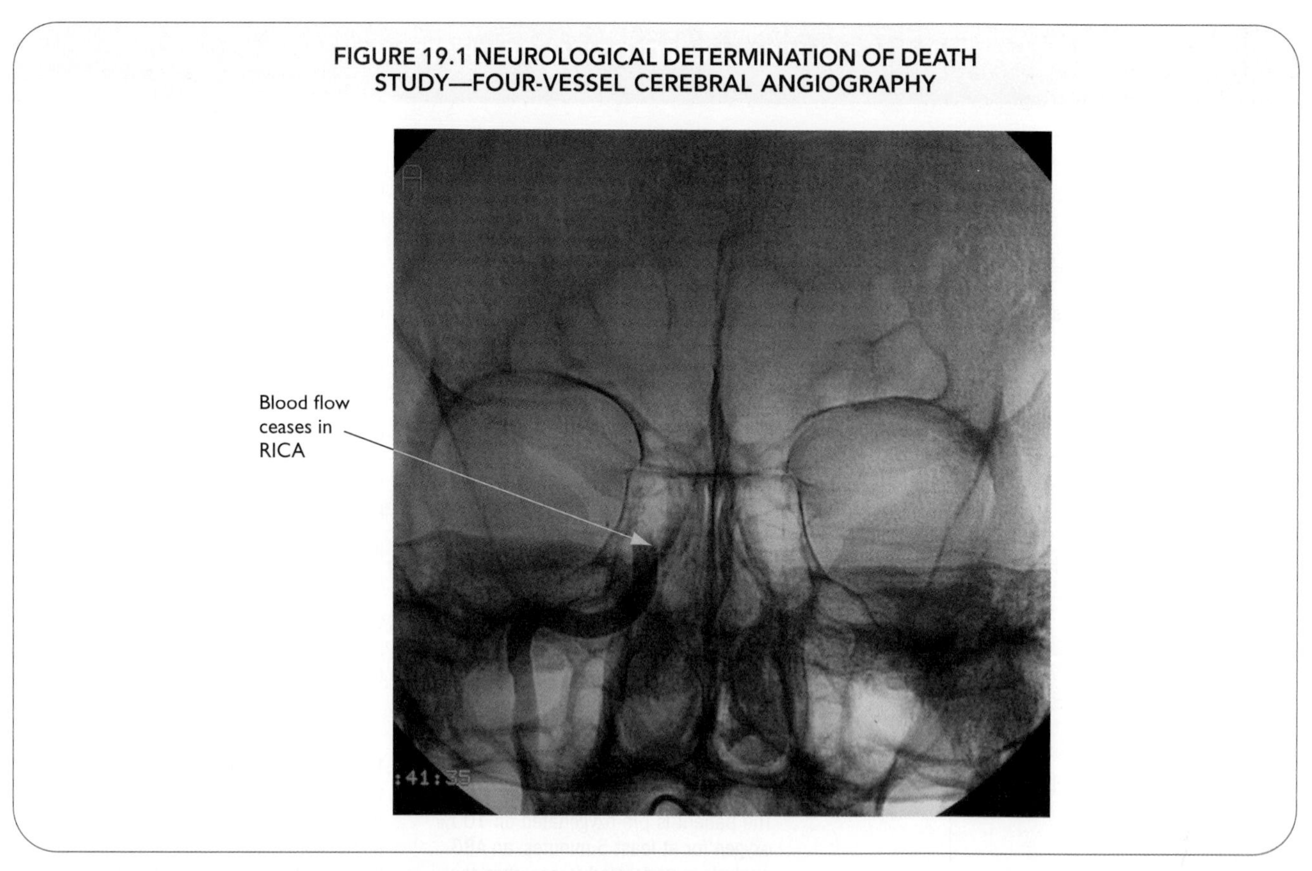

Frontal cranial view of contrast flow in right internal carotid artery (RICA). Blood flow ceases at the carotid siphon (arrow). Conclusion: if blood flow is shown to have ceased in all the vessels there is no functioning cerebrum/cerebellum. *Courtesy Radiology Department, St George Hospital, Sydney.*

FIGURE 19.2 NEUROLOGICAL DETERMINATION OF DEATH STUDY—CEREBRAL PERFUSION HEXAMETHYLPROPYLENE-AMINE OXIME (HMPAO) SCAN

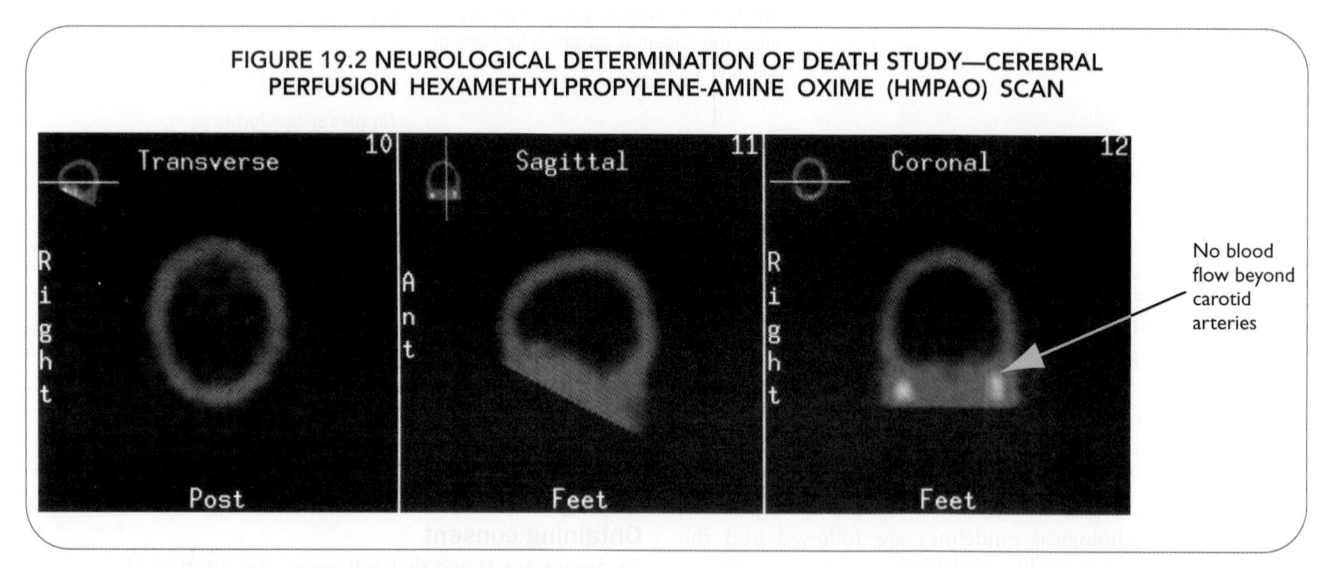

Transverse, sagittal and coronal views. No uptake is seen in the cranial vault within the cerebrum or cerebellum. Blood flow is present in the sagittal and coronal views only to the carotid siphon (arrow). Conclusion: there is no functioning cerebrum/cerebellum within the cranial vault. *Courtesy Nuclear Medicine Department, St George Hospital, Sydney.*

have indicated their wish to be a donor at the time of their death.[17,43] The act of offering information about donation could also be considered part of the duty of care to the family. This view is supported by a survey of donor families who have indicated that donation has brought some long-term meaning to their loss, knowing that their loved one helped others through transplantation.[22] Similarly, a study of Australian donor families revealed that 81% of the respondents felt that organ and tissue donation was an opportunity for something positive to come out of a tragedy therefore helping them to cope with their loss; 96% of respondents were comfortable with their donation decision.[44]

There are three elements involved when discussing organ and tissue donation with the family:[45,46]

- the knowledge, beliefs and attitudes they bring to the situation
- the in-hospital experience they have received
- the biases and beliefs of the health professional/s conducting the conversation.

The outcome of the conversation should not be predicted or anticipated, as it may affect the 'spirit' in which the approach is made. Evidence to support this statement can be found in the results of a large study undertaken in the United States. Evanisko and colleagues[47] endorsed a non-presumptive approach because they found that clinical staff asked to predict the response of the next of kin were incorrect 50% of the time.

Influence of knowledge, beliefs and attitudes

Attitudes towards organ and tissue donation are influenced by spiritual beliefs, cultural background, prior knowledge about donation, views on altruism, and prior healthcare experiences.[22] The next of kin need to consider two aspects associated with existing attitudes and knowledge:[47]

- the thoughts and feelings of the decision-maker(s), and
- the previous wishes and beliefs of the person on whose behalf they are making the decision.

There is evidence of a link between consent rates and prior knowledge of the positive outcomes of organ and tissue donation.[22,44,45,48]

Delivery of relevant information

An important detail to be considered by all health professionals is that families may have a diminished ability to receive and understand information because they are often emotionally and physically overwhelmed at this time of family crisis.[22] It has been suggested in the literature that interviews held with the family are the foundation of the entire organ and tissue donation process.[46] The discussion about death or impending death must be clear and emphatic, using language that is free of medical terminology, and includes an explanation of the physical implications.[49] The use of diagrams, analogies, scans and written materials have been suggested as useful aids for enhancing understanding by next of kin.[39,49] For example, Haddow[49] relates the effective use of the analogy of neurological death being described as a jigsaw puzzle with a piece missing to illustrate the relationship of the brain to the rest of the body. The opportunity to provide intensive training to health professionals in sensitive communication with accredited education programs improves the likelihood of meeting the needs of the family.[42,46,50]

As the time of confirmation of neurological death is the person's legal time of death, a discussion would then be held with the family to discuss the subsequent plan and implications. As death has been confirmed, ventilation will be ceased to allow circulatory standstill to occur. However, if donation is to occur, ventilation and haemodynamic support will be provided to facilitate organ and tissue donation. The donation process must be fully explained, in an open and sensitive manner, to ensure an informed and enduring decision, while not overburdening the next of kin.[39,42] The family should be given information on the benefits of donation, the right of the family to decline, the donation process and the inability to guarantee that the organs and tissues will be transplanted.[42] Of note, a best-practice approach to this discussion aims to assist the family to make the decision that is 'right' for them and not necessarily to result in obtaining consent.[50]

Meetings with the family

Common to all pathways of donation after death, the timing, location, content and process of discussions with the family are all important considerations. An effective protocol for communicating with the family of the potential donor must include:[42,44,46,47,51]

- frequent and honest updates on the patient's prognosis
- clear explanation of cause of death
- the possibility of organ and tissue donation not to be raised until the family accepts that the patient is likely to die or has already been confirmed as dead
- conversations held in a private and quiet setting
- involvement of organ and tissue donation specialists with clearly defined roles.

There is compelling evidence that the meeting confirming the diagnosis of neurological determination of death should be held separately or de-coupled from the conversation about organ and tissue donation.[42,46] In reality, the pace of the discussions should be assessed on a case-by-case basis, as there may be circumstances when the discussion about donation is appropriately held prior to the confirmation of death.[17,47]

Other influential components of this process have been identified from insightful surveys completed with donor and non-donor families. The first is the use of inappropriate terms such as 'harvest' to describe the organ retrieval surgery and 'life support' to describe the ventilator. The first term is considered extremely harsh and undignified, while the second term could perpetuate the hope of a chance of survival or recovery.[43,44,49,51] The health professionals attending the family donation conversation must be mindful of their attire; for example, surgical scrubs or plastic aprons can distract families who may wonder why such a garment is necessary. Another component is the timing or use of the information sourced from organ donor registers and the driver's licence. Careful consideration must be taken when introducing this information in the family donation conversation.[42,49]

Staff roles, delineation and involvement

The process of organ and tissue donation within the emergency and critical care environments is significant for all concerned. When death is confirmed, it marks the end of an episode that has been catastrophic for the patient and their family and a potentially stressful and draining experience for the staff.[47,52,53]

Supporting a potential donor family is very much a multidisciplinary team effort. As noted earlier, the ANZICS guidelines[17] encourage the treating medical staff to continue their involvement with the patient and their family after death is confirmed for continuity of care. Nursing staff involvement in the process of organ and tissue donation is intrinsic. This includes the practicalities of the process and care of the potential donor and their family during the decision-making process.[47,52] Donor families have identified nurses as being the most helpful health professionals in providing information and emotional support.[43,44,51,52]

A holistic approach for supporting families includes the involvement of social workers, pastoral-care workers, as well as interpreters and Aboriginal Liaison Officers where relevant.

Often these health professionals have been working with the family for a number of days, and act as confidants and a resource for information on matters such as the implications of a coronial enquiry and the stance a religious denomination has on organ and tissue donation. It is timely to note that the majority of primary religions are supportive of organ and tissue donation for transplantation, and most would instruct the family to make the decision that they felt was right for them (see Community resources in Useful websites).[44,45]

The organ and tissue donation specialist acts as a resource and is notified and invited into the emergency or critical care area when end-of-life discussions are planned.[41,42] A health professional who is an expert in donation, has had training in sensitive communication and has the time to spend with the family is the best person to conduct a family donation conversation.[17,41,50] Studies have found that the combination of separating the conversations about death and donation, holding the conversations in a private setting and the involvement of an organ and tissue donation specialist improved consent rates.[41,44,46,50]

PRACTICE TIP

All clinical, administrative and management staff must be aware of the possibility of experiencing grief reactions when involved in the organ and tissue donation process and the personal drain it can cause when trying to maintain professional boundaries. Compassion fatigue is a well-recognised phenomenon and staff must be sensitive to their own limitations.[52,53]

Role of designated officers

Under Australian law, a designated officer is appointed by the governing body of the institution to authorise non-coronial post-mortems and the removal of tissue from a deceased person for transplantation or other therapeutic, medical or scientific purposes.[17] The designated officer must be satisfied that all the necessary enquiries have been made and that the necessary consent has been obtained before granting authority. Medical, nursing and administrative staff can be appointed to the role; however, they must not act in a case in which they have a clinical or personal involvement.

The term designated officer is not used in New Zealand legislation. The person with equivalent authority under the *Human Tissue Act 1964* is the person lawfully in possession of the body.[54] In the case of a hospital, this person is specified as the medical officer in charge and in practice the treating clinician undertakes this consultation with the family.

Consent-indicator databases

The most influential contribution that an individual can make to the decision-making process of their family is the existence of an advance care directive or prior indication of consent. Some authors have reported that the existence of such information has made the decision-making 'easier';[44,55] it preserves patient autonomy[49] and could mean that the wishes of the patient are followed even when family decision-makers would have made the opposite decision.[43] Table 19.4 lists prospective donation databases available in Australia and Aotearoa New Zealand.[56]

Documentation of consent

Consent is sought for the individual organs and tissues, rather than a 'global' approach. Once consent is granted, the individual organs and tissues are indicated on the consent form, or named if the consent is being recorded over the phone, and only those organs and tissues will be retrieved. The donation specialist staff might also seek permission to retrieve organs and tissues for approved research projects.

Definition of next of kin

In Australia, the definition of next of kin for adults and children is listed in strict order (see Table 19.5). In Aotearoa New Zealand, there is no stated hierarchy of next of kin, with a surviving spouse or relative able to act in this role.[17,54] In both countries, the next of kin can object on ethical grounds to grant consent, but experience shows that the family rarely disagrees if the wishes of the deceased are known.[17,44]

Role of coroner and forensic pathologist

Due to the nature of their death, many donors are subject to coronial inquiry. If this is the case, permission to undertake organ and tissue retrieval is sought from the respective forensic pathologist and Coroner according to local policy and procedure as part of the authorisation process. The coronial system is very supportive of donation for transplantation and in Australia,

TABLE 19.4 CONSENT-INDICATOR DATABASES IN AUSTRALIA AND AOTEAROA NEW ZEALAND[57]

DATABASE NAME	HOST	ACCESS TO DATABASE INFORMATION	AVAILABILITY TO JOIN
Australia			
Australian Organ Donor Register	Medicare Australia	Limited to coordinators nominated by state donation agencies and tissue banks	Via Medicare offices, online or phone 1800 777 203
Driver's licence	SA Department of Planning, Transport and Infrastructure	Limited to coordinators nominated by state donation agencies and tissue banks	Driver's licence application and renewal form
Aotearoa New Zealand			
Driver's licence	Land Transport Safety Authority	Limited to coordinators nominated by the National Transplant Donor Coordination Office	Driver's licence application and renewal form

TABLE 19.5 DEFINITION OF NEXT OF KIN FOR CHILDREN AND ADULTS IN AUSTRALIAN LEGISLATION[17]

DONOR	ORDER OF SENIORITY	RELATIONSHIP
Child	1	Parent
	2	Adult sibling (over 18 years of age)
	3	Guardian (immediately before death)
Adult	1	Spouse or de facto (at time of death)
	2	Adult offspring (over 18 years of age)
	3	Parent
	4	Adult sibling (over 18 years of age)

54% of donors in 2020 were subject to Coronial inquiry. In Aotearoa New Zealand it was 47% in 2020.[36]

Referral of potential donor after neurological determination of death

If consent is obtained, the referral process usually commences immediately. To ensure organ viability for transplantation, the time from neurological determination of death confirmation to retrieval of the organs is kept to a minimum. The longer the time delay, the more likely organ-failure-related complications will occur.[37]

The referral process starts with the donation specialist collating the past and present medical, surgical, behavioural, social and travel history of the potential donor, and relaying this information to the relevant local transplant units (see Table 19.6). Using this information, local transplant teams allocate the organs to the most suitable and appropriate recipient/s. If the local transplant team does not have a suitable recipient, the offer is extended to another team within Australia or Aotearoa New Zealand on rotation using TSANZ guidelines.[41]

Tissue typing and cross-matching

A vital component of the assessment and referral process is the tissue typing, cross-matching and serology testing of the potential donor's blood. Blood is drawn from the potential donor and sent to the relevant accredited laboratory for testing (see Table 19.7). Tissue typing identifies the human leucocyte antigen (HLA) phenotype from the genes on chromosome 6.[57] The HLA molecules control the action of the immune system to differentiate between 'self' and 'foreign' tissue, and initiate an immune response to foreign matter. A transplanted organ will always be identified as foreign tissue by the recipient's body, hence the use of immunosuppressive drugs to suppress the immune response. A test routinely used to predict the level of this response is the cross-match. Lymphocytes from the potential donor are added to the potential recipient's serum to test if the recipient has an antibody that is specific to the HLA antigens of the donor.[58] A reaction where the recipient's serum destroys the donor's cells is a positive cross-match, and is a contraindication for transplantation.[58,59]

TABLE 19.6 DONOR REFERRAL INFORMATION[60]

SECTION	DETAILS
Personal details	Address, phone number, gender, age, date of birth, height, weight, ethnicity, religion, build
Cause of death	Date and time of hospital admission, intubation, critical care admission, other trauma
Neurological death confirmation	Date, time, method
Consent details	Specific organs and tissues, Designated Officer details, forensic pathologist and Coroner details, police details, next of kin and databases accessed
Donor history	Family history, medical, surgical, travel, social and sexual history
Blood results	Blood group, biochemistry and haematology on admission and within last 12 hours, microbiology, gas exchange
Test results	Chest x-ray, including lung field measurements, electrocardiogram, echocardiogram, bronchoscopy and sputum
Haemodynamics	Blood pressure, mean arterial pressure, heart rate, central venous pressure, urine output and temperature
Admission history	Cardiac arrest, temperature, renal and hepatic function, nutrition, drug and fluid administration
Physical examination	Overall appearance, body habitus, abnormalities or deformities, scars, trauma, lesions, needle marks, tattoos, medical devices etc

Pre-hospital care

Before organ and tissue donation can be considered, paramedics have a duty of care to act in the immediate best interest of their patient. Therefore, paramedics should aim to provide optimal physiological support for the patient to enable the establishment of a diagnosis and assessment of prognosis upon arrival in the ED. Immediate and effective physiological support also preserves the opportunity for organ donation. It allows for the determination of neurological death, ensures best possible organ function for potential recipients and, most importantly, it allows time for the family to make a decision about organ and tissue donation.

Donor management

Another important factor that influences the number of actual donors is the clinical management the donor receives after confirmation of death according to neurological criteria. The ANZICS guidelines recommend maintaining physiological support that provides the opportunity to explain the prognosis to the family and to preserve the possibility of organ donation.[17] If consent for organ and tissue retrieval is given, the aim of donor management is to support and optimise organ function until the retrieval commences, while maintaining the dignity and respect for the donor and support for the family (see Table 19.7). Ideal parameters for biochemistry, vital signs, urine output and clinical management are detailed in Table 19.8.

TABLE 19.7 DONOR MANAGEMENT CARE PLAN[17,37]

MANAGEMENT AIMS	VARIATION IN BRAIN DEATH	CAUSES AND CONSIDERATION	TREATMENT
pH 7.35–7.45 PaO_2 > 300 mmHg on FiO_2 100% and PEEP 5 (if lungs for Tx) $PaCO_2$ 35–45 mmHg	No cough or respiratory drive Hypoxaemia Orthostatic pneumonia Neurogenic pulmonary oedema	Optimise tissue oxygenation Prevent lung injury including over-expansion Aim to reduce atelectasis	Ventilate to normocarbia Lowest FiO_2 PEEP 5 cmH_2O ± bronchodilators Regular suctioning and repositioning 2–3 times in 24 hours Regular ABGs + when treatment or ventilation changed Regular physiotherapy Strict asepsis Broad-spectrum antibiotics (if necessary) CXR within last 12 hours
MAP > 60 mmHg HR < 120 bpm CVP 6–12 mmHg	Decrease in MAP Decrease in CVP Dysrhythmias Hypertension	Blood loss Deliberate dehydration to decrease cerebral oedema Polyuria–diabetes insipidus (DI), diuretics Electrolyte and acid–base disturbance, hypotension, hypothermia Common during herniation Dysrhythmias are usually self-limiting	Optimise intravascular volume as guided by CVP Physical assessment and FBC Choice of replacement fluid depends on fluid loss Consider ceasing contributing medications (diuretics, mannitol and barbiturates) Use of inotropes if not hypertensive, consider using agent with a short half-life Hormone resuscitation for persistent instability
Temperature > 35°C	Decrease in temperature Increase in temperature	Non-functioning hypothalamus Depressed metabolism Inability to shiver or vasoconstrict Cold IV fluid/blood administration Sepsis/infection	Avoid long exposure Active warming Warmed IV fluids Cooling blanket
Electrolytes within normal range	Increase in Na Decrease in K Decrease in Mg Decrease in Ca	Commonly encountered secondary to urinary losses in uncontrolled DI Increase in Na: DI Decrease in K: dysrhythmias Decrease in Mg: dysrhythmias	Frequent serum electrolytes Electrolyte replacement Correct hypernatraemia ECG within last 12 hours Control urine output, i.e. DI
Urine output 1 mL/kg/hr	Decrease in U/O Increase in U/O (> 300–400 mL/hr)	Hypovolaemia DI (lack of ADH leads to an inappropriate and large U/O)	Restore circulating volume Consider correcting 'free water' deficit and replace electrolytes Consider the use of DDAVP in small amounts to decrease urine output
Blood glucose level	Increase in BGL	Insulin resistance–stress response + circulation of catecholamines IV fluids containing dextrose	Insulin infusion Avoid dextrose
Good general nursing care and infection control Maintain patient's dignity and respect	Some may consider unnecessary as patient has been confirmed dead	Demonstrate continuum of care Act as a patient advocate Optimise success of donation and transplantation	2-hourly eye care (for eye retrieval) 2-hourly repositioning 2-hourly mouth care General hygiene

ABG: arterial blood gas; ADH: antidiuretic hormone; BGL: blood glucose level; BP: blood pressure; Ca: calcium; CVP: central venous pressure; CXR: chest x-ray; DDAVP: desmopressin; DI: diabetes insipidus; ECG: electrocardiogram; FBC: full blood count; FiO_2: fraction of inspired oxygen; Hb: haemoglobin; HR: heart rate; IV: intravenous; K: potassium; MAP: mean arterial pressure; Mg: magnesium; Na: sodium; $PaCO_2$: arterial pressure of carbon dioxide; PaO_2: arterial pressure of oxygen; PEEP: positive end-expiratory pressure; Tx: transplant; U/O: urine output.

TABLE 19.8 BLOOD TESTS REQUIRED FOR ORGAN DONATION[41,58,59]

	TEST	RESPONSE TIME FOR RESULTS
Serology	HBsAg, HBsAb, Anti-HBcAb, HBcAb IgM	2-3 hours
	Anti-HIV-1/2	
	Anti-HCV	
	Anti HTLV-I/II	
	CMV IgG, CMV IgM	
	EBV IgG, EBV IgM	
	EBNA	
	Toxo Ab IgG, Toxo AB IgM	
	Chagas	
	WNV	
	Syphilis (next day)	
	Nucleic acid testing (NAT)	High-risk donor–done prior to referral and 4 hours
	NAT HIV	Low-risk donor–next day
	NAT HCV	
	NAT HBV	
Tissue typing	Cross-matching with the blood of potential recipients for relevant ABO blood groups	8 hours

HBsAg: hepatitis B surface antigen; HBsAb: hepatitis B surface antibody; Anti-HBcAb/HBcAb: hepatitis B core antibody; HIV: human immunodeficiency virus; HCV: hepatitis C virus; HTLV: human T-cell lymphotrophic virus; CMV: cytomegalovirus; IgM: immunoglobulin M; IgG: immunoglobulin G; EBV: Epstein-Barr virus; EBNA: EBV nuclear antigen, Toxo: toxoplasmosis; WNV: West Nile virus.

PRACTICE TIP

When managing a potential multi-organ donor after confirmation of neurological determination of death, continuation of eye care, chest physiotherapy, suctioning and positioning is vitally important, and can influence which organs and tissues are able to be retrieved.

THE RETRIEVAL PROCESS

The retrieval surgery occurs in the hospital where the donor is located and the local operating theatre staff are involved in this process. The donor is transferred to theatre after routine pre-operative checks and documentation are completed, including death confirmation and consent for organ and tissue retrieval. Depending on which organs are to be retrieved, the retrieval teams will be tasked to abdominal organs and thoracic organs, and will bring most of their specialised equipment with them. An anaesthetist will be present in DNDD cases to monitor haemodynamics, ventilation and administer medications, but will not deliver anaesthetic agents. In DCDD cases, an anaesthetist from the thoracic retrieval team will reintubate the donor after death if lung donation is to occur. The local operating theatre staff will work with the visiting surgical teams and a donation specialist will be present to document the procedure and its outcomes, and act as a resource for everyone present.

The surgery takes 5–7 hours, depending on the extent of the retrieval. In DNDD, once the surgeons have identified all the various anatomical points, the aorta is cross-clamped with vascular clamps below the diaphragm and at the aortic arch, the heart is stopped and ventilation is ceased. Before the organs are removed, the retrieval teams administer a cold perfusion fluid with an electrolyte-specific mix to the organs. Upon removal, the organs are bagged with sterile slush and perfusion fluid, and transported in ice by the retrieval teams to the transplanting hospitals. Some retrieval teams use machine perfusion technology that allows normothermic preservation of organs such as lungs and hearts. This portable technology pumps warm, oxygenated, nutrient-rich blood through the organ, thus allowing more time between donation and transplant; hence the ability to assess the organ before transplant for better overall outcomes.[60,61]

The incision that extends from the sternal notch to the pubic symphysis is closed by the surgeons in a routine manner and covered with a surgical dressing. If the donor is not a Coroner's case, the remaining lines, catheter and drains are removed according to local policy, the donor is washed and arrangements made to transfer to a specified location for a viewing with the family or to the mortuary. The musculoskeletal tissue, skin and eye retrieval can occur at the end of the solid-organ retrieval in theatre or later in the mortuary.[34,62]

DONOR FAMILY CARE

Family support begins from the time their loved one is admitted to hospital and continues well beyond organ and tissue retrieval. In addition to individual considerations that may influence the grieving process, such as religion, culture, family dynamics, coping skills and prior experiences with loss, the family of an organ and tissue donor will be dealing with a number of unique factors (see Community resources in Useful websites). The death of their family member is likely to have been sudden and unexpected; death by neurological criteria can be difficult to understand when their loved one looks like they are asleep rather than dead; the opportunity of donation might mean having to make a decision on behalf of their loved one if their wishes are not known; in DCDD, the decision to withdraw cardiorespiratory support might set off feelings of guilt and thoughts of prematurely withdrawing treatment; and in DNDD, the process might mean they may not be able to be with their loved one when their heart stops.[45,51]

Donor families benefit from emotional and physical support throughout and following the donation process. In the critical care area, support can take the form of open visiting times, privacy for meetings, clear and precise information, and regular contact with the treating clinical team and the donation specialist.[46] After retrieval, the ongoing care of a donor family can include contact with a bereavement specialist, written resource material, telephone support, counselling and correspondence from recipients.[21,63] ODNZ and the Australian DonateLife network have cost-free, structured aftercare and follow-up programs that offer these features.[42] Holtkamp states that trained personnel involved with a donor family through this process have the unique opportunity to positively influence the family's grief journey.[51]

SUMMARY

In summary, organ and tissue donation is a routine component of end-of-life care. Along with age, medical, surgical and social history, the location, cause and mechanism of the death are determining factors of which donation pathway is possible. Every potential donor is assessed on a case-by-case basis to determine medical suitability for organ and tissue retrieval for transplantation. In Australia and Aotearoa New Zealand, consent for organ and tissue donation is required in writing, which can be indicated by the person themselves before their death or by their next of kin after their death. In some instances, verbal consent can be recorded over the phone. Only the organs and tissues with specific consent will be retrieved.

Notification of the person's impending or confirmed death and participation in the assessment and referral process is seen as a component of end-of-life care by the treating clinical staff. Support and guidance in the process of organ and tissue donation is available 24 hours a day from the tissue banks and OTD agencies in both countries. There is no expectation that the treating clinicians and nursing staff would have to make decisions about medical suitability and are therefore encouraged to contact the relevant tissue bank or OTD agency at any stage of the process. The organ and tissue donation referral and retrieval process has legal, practical and ethical components that must be observed, but the overriding aim is to treat the donor and their family with the care, respect and dignity they deserve.

CASE STUDY

It is 10.15 am and Tony, a 19-year-old electrician, has collapsed on a building site. On arrival, the paramedics find him lying unconscious and surrounded by his workmates, who have placed him in the recovery position. On examination, Tony has a Glasgow Coma Scale (GCS) score of 5 and is spontaneously breathing. He reportedly complained of a severe headache and vomited just prior to collapsing. Tony is intubated and transferred to hospital.

QUESTIONS

1. At the scene and during the transfer, the aim of treatment is to:
   a. resuscitate and optimise oxygenation and organ function for potential organ and/or tissue donation
   b. resuscitate and optimise oxygenation and organ function for assessment of cause of injury and prognosis
   c. limit resuscitation as Tony is likely to have suffered a life-ending event.
2. On arrival at the emergency department, Tony's GCS is 3, his pupils are fixed and dilated, and he has stopped spontaneously breathing. The next intervention should be:
   a. neurological determination of death testing
   b. wait for family to arrive before withdrawing treatment
   c. cerebral computed tomography.
3. Transferred to the intensive care unit (ICU), Tony is kept intubated and ventilated, sedated and inotropes are titrated to maintain blood pressure and cerebral perfusion pressure. After 3 days, the sedation is weaned and ceased. Tony is triggering spontaneous breaths, but only scoring a GCS of 5. After a further 3 days, Tony's condition has not changed. The neurosurgical and ICU team meet with his parents to explain that he is unlikely to survive this incident, and that death is inevitable. After ensuring the family understand that information, the conversation moves to the plan for end-of-life care, including withdrawal of treatment. After consideration, Tony's parents agree to withdrawal of treatment and ask if organ and tissue donation would be possible. Is this possible?
   a. No, Tony has not died with death determined by neurological criteria.
   b. Only tissue donation is possible after determination of circulatory death.
   c. Donation of both solid organs and tissues is possible via the donation after circulatory determination of death pathway (DCDD).
4. If organ and tissue donation is possible, does Tony have to be transferred to a tertiary referral centre?
   a. Yes, smaller hospitals will not have the specialised equipment necessary for the donation coordination and retrieval.
   b. No, the donation coordination staff and retrieval team can travel to regional and metropolitan sites.

Answers to Case Study Questions can be found on evolve http://evolve.elsevier.com/AU/Curtis/emergency/ 

USEFUL WEBSITES

Australasian Transplant Coordinators Association (ATCA), www.atca.org.au.

Australian Code of Good Manufacturing Practice (GMP) for Blood and Blood Components, Human Tissues and Human Cellular Therapy Products, www.tga.gov.au.

Australian Government Organ and Tissue Authority, www.donatelife.gov.au.

Australian and New Zealand Intensive Care Society, www.anzics.com.au.

Australian Organ Donor Register, www.servicesaustralia.gov.au.

Biotherapeutics Association of Australasia, www.bioaa.org.au.

Eye Bank Association of Australia and New Zealand, www.ebaanz.org.

Introductory Donation Awareness Training, www.donatelife.gov.au/resources/professional-education/introductory-donation-awareness-training-idat-workshop.

New Zealand Medicines and Medical Devices Safety Authority, www.medsafe.govt.nz.

Organ Donation New Zealand, www.donor.co.nz.

Transplantation Society of Australia and New Zealand, www.tsanz.com.au.

Transplant Nurses' Association, www.transplantnurses.org.au.

Community resources

Australian Government Organ and Tissue Authority, Multicultural and faith resources, www.donatelife.gov.au/resources/multicultural-and-faith-communities/multicultural-and-faith-resources.

REFERENCES

1. Chapman JR, Deierhoi M, Wight C, editors. Organ and tissue donation for transplantation. London: Arnold; 1997.
2. Mathew TH, Chapman JR. Organ donation: a chance for Australia to do better. Med J Aust 2006;185(5):245–6.
3. Chapman JR. Transplantation in Australia—50 years in progress. Thomas E. Mandel, ed. Transplantation: an effective therapy. MJA 1993;3:3–6.
4. McBride M, Chapman JR. An overview of transplantation in Australia. Anaesth Intens Care 1995;23(1):60–4.
5. George CR. Caring for kidneys in the antipodes: how Australia and New Zealand have addressed the challenge of end-stage renal failure. Am J Kidney Dis 2009;53(3):536–45.
6. Roake J. Editorial: liver transplantation in Australia and New Zealand. ANZ J Surg 2008;78:628–9.
7. Thomas E. Mandel, editor. Transplantation: an effective therapy. Kingsgrove: Australasian Medical Publishing; 1991.
8. Nozohoor S, Stehlik J, Lund L, Ansari D, Andersson B, Nilsson J. Induction immunosuppression strategies and long-term outcomes after heart transplantation. Clin Transplant 2020;34(7):e13871.
9. Australian Government Organ and Tissue Authority. A world's best practice approach to organ and tissue donation for transplantation. 2008. Available from: www.donatelife.gov.au.
10. Australia and New Zealand Dialysis and Transplant Registry. 44th Annual report. Adelaide: 2021. Available from: www.anzdata.org.au/report/anzdata-44th-annual-report-2021-data-to-2020/.
11. Rithalia A, McDaid C, Suekarran S, Myers L, Sowden A. Impact of presumed consent for organ donation on donation rates: a systematic review. BMJ (Clinical Research Ed.) 2009;338:a3162.
12. Abadie A, Gay S. The impact of presumed consent legislation on cadaveric organ donation: a cross-country study. J Heal Econ 2006;25(4): 599–620.
13. Rosenblum AM, Li AH, Roels L, Stewart B, Prakash V, Beitel J, et al. Worldwide variability in deceased organ donation registries. Transplant Int 2012;25(8):801–11.
14. Kim JR, Elliott D, Hyde C. Korean nurses' perspectives of organ donation and transplantation: a review. Transplant Nurses J 2002;11:20–4.
15. Kim JR, Elliott D, Hyde C. The influence of sociocultural factors on organ donation and transplantation in Korea: findings from key informant interviews. J Transcult Nurs 2004;15(2):147–54.
16. New Zealand Ministry of Health. Increasing deceased organ donation and transplantation: a national strategy. Wellington: Ministry of Health; 2017.
17. Australian and New Zealand Intensive Care Society. The ANZICS statement on death and organ donation. 4.1 ed. Melbourne: ANZICS; 2021.
18. Gleeson G. Organ transplantation from living donors. Plunkett centre for ethics in health care. Bioeth Outlook 2000;11(1):5–8.
19. Memmi B, Leveziel L, Knoeri J, Leclère A, Ribes O, Despiaux MC, et al. Freeze-dried versus cryopreserved amniotic membranes in corneal ulcers treated by overlay transplantation: a case-control study. Cornea 2022;41(3):280–5.
20. Cordner S, Ireland L, editors. Tissue banking. London: Arnold; 1997.
21. Beard J, Ireland L, Davis N, Barr J. Tissue donation: what does it mean to families? Prog Transplant (Aliso Viejo, Calif.) 2002;12(1):42–8.
22. Rodrigue JR, Cornell DL, Howard RJ. Organ donation decision: comparison of donor and nondonor families. Am J Transplant 2006;6(1):190–8.

23. Zavotsky KE, Tamburri LM. A case in successful organ donation: emergency department nurses do make a difference. J Emerg Nurs 2007;33(3):235–41.
24. Graham JM, Sabeta ME, Cooke JT, Berg ER, Osten WM. A system's approach to improve organ donation. Prog Transplant (Aliso Viejo, Calif.) 2009;19(3):216–20.
25. Murphy PG, Logan L. Clinical leads for organ donation: making it happen in hospitals. J Intens Care Soc 2009;10(3):174–8.
26. Lewis J, Peltier J, Nelson H, Snyder W, Schneider K, Steinberger D, et al. Development of the University of Wisconsin donation after cardiac death evaluation tool. Prog Transplant (Aliso Viejo, Calif.) 2003;13(4):265–73.
27. Levvey B, Griffiths A, Snell G. Non-heart beating organ donors: a realistic opportunity to expand the donor pool. Transplant Nurse J 2004;13(3): 8–12.
28. Bell MDD, Bodenham AR. Non-heart beating organ donation: can we balance duty of care, the law and recipient need? Care Critically Ill 2004;20:1–2.
29. Australian Government Organ and Tissue Authority. Best Practice Guideline for Donation after Circulatory Determination of Death (DCDD) in Australia 1.0 ed. 2021. Available from: www.donatelife.gov.au.
30. Organ Donation New Zealand. Deceased organ donation and transplantation in New Zealand. 2016. Available from: www.health.govt.nz.
31. American College of Critical Care Medicine SoCCM, Ethics Committee. Recommendations for nonheartbeating organ donation. A position paper by the ethics committee, American College of Critical Care Medicine, Society of Critical Care Medicine. Crit Care Med 2001;29(9):1826–31.
32. Thuong M, Ruiz A, Evrard P, Kuiper M, Boffa C, Akhtar MZ, et al. New classification of donation after circulatory death donors definitions and terminology. Transpl Int 2016;29:749–59.
33. Hameed AM, Hawthorne WJ, Pleass HC. Advances in organ preservation for transplantation. ANZ J Surg 2017;87(12):976–80.
34. Steinbrook R. Organ donation after cardiac death. NEJM 2007;357:209–13.
35. Brieva J, Coleman N, Lacey J, Harrigan P, Lewin TJ, Carter GL. Prediction of death in less than 60 minutes after withdrawal of cardiorespiratory support in potential organ donors after circulatory death. Transplantation 2014:98(10):1112–18.
36. Australia and New Zealand Organ Donation Registry. ANZOD annual report. Adelaide: ANZOD; 2021.
37. Kutsogiannis D, Pagliarello G, Doig C, Ross H, Shemie SD. Medical management to optimise donor organ potential: review of the literature. Can J Anaesthes 2006;53(8):820–30.
38. Power BM, Van Heerden PV. The physiological changes associated with brain death–current concepts and implications for treatment of the brain dead organ donor. Anaesthes Intens Care 1995;23(1):26–36.
39. Siminoff LA, Mercer MB, Arnold R. Families' understanding of brain death. Prog Transplant (Aliso Viejo, Calif.) 2003;13(3):218–24.
40. Welschehold S, Kerz T, Boor S. Computed tomographic angiography as a useful adjunct in the diagnosis of brain death. J Trauma Acute Care Surg 2013;74(5):1279–85.
41. Transplantation Society of Australia and New Zealand. Clinical guidelines for organ transplantation from deceased donors. Version1.7. Canberra: TSANZ; 2021. Available from: www.tsanz.com.au/guidelinesethics-documents/organallocationguidelines.htm.
42. Australian Organ and Tissue Authority. Best practice guideline for offering organ and tissue donation in Australia. Edition 2. Canberra: OTA; 2021. Available from: www.donatelife.gov.au/resources/clinical-guidelines-and-protocols/best-practice-guideline-offering-organ-and-tissue.
43. Streat S. Clinical review: moral assumptions and the process of organ donation in the intensive care unit. Crit Care 2004;8:382–8.
44. Australian Organ and Tissue Authority. National study of family experiences of organ and tissue donation: wave 4 research report. Canberra: OTA; 2020. Available from: www.donatelife.gov.au/resources/donor-families/national-donor-family-study.
45. Siminoff L, Mercer M, Graham G, Burant C. The reasons families donate organs for transplantation: implications for policy and practice. J Trauma 2007;62:969–78.
46. Griffith J, Verble MS, Falvey S, Bell S, Logan L, Morgan K, et al. Culture change initiatives in the procurement of organs in the United Kingdom. Transplant Proc 2009;41(5):1459–62.
47. Evanisko MJ, Beasley CL, Brigham LE, Capossela C, Cosgrove GR, Light J, et al. Readiness of critical care physicians and nurses to handle requests for organ donation. Am J Crit Care 1998;7(1):4–12.
48. Rodrigue JR, Scott MP, Oppenheim AR. The tissue donation experience: a comparison of donor and nondonor families. Prog Transplant 2003;13(4):258–64.
49. Haddow G. Donor and nondonor families' accounts of communication and relations with healthcare professionals. Prog Transplant 2004;14(1):41–8.
50. Potter JE, Gatward JJ, Kelly MA, McKay L, McCann E, Elliott RM, et al. Simulation-based communication skills training for experienced clinicians to improve family conversations about organ and tissue donation. Prog Transplant 2017;27(4):339–45.
51. Holtkamp S. Wrapped in mourning: the gift of life and organ donor family trauma. New York: Brunner-Routledge; 2002.
52. Cohen J, Ben Ami S, Ashkenazi T, Singer P. Attitude of healthcare professionals to brain death: influence on the organ donation process. Clin Transplant 2008;22(2):211–15.
53. Ainsworth K, Sgorbini M. Compassion fatigue: who cares for the carers? Transplant J Australa 2010;19(2):21–25.
54. New Zealand Government. Human Tissue Act 2008. Part 2.

55. Thompson TL, Robinson JD, Kenny RW. Family conversations about organ donation. Prog Transplant (Aliso Viejo, Calif.) 2004;14(1):49–55.
56. Australian Government. Services Australia. Australian organ donor register. 2022. Available from: www.servicesaustralia.gov.au/australian-organ-donor-register?utm_id=9.
57. Tait BD, Süsal C, Gebel HM, Nickerson PW, Zachary AA, Claas FH, et al. Consensus guidelines on the testing and clinical management issues associated with HLA and non-HLA antibodies in transplantation. Transplantation 2013;95:19–47.
58. Australian Red Cross Blood Service. Blood testing: safety and testing. 2021. Available from: www.lifeblood.com.au/blood/learn-about-blood/blood-testing-and-safety.
59. Electronic Donor Record. Standard operating procedure and user guide. Version 6.6. Canberra: Australian Organ and Tissue Authority; 2021.
60. Warnecke G, Moradiellos J, Tudorache I, Kühn C, Avsar M, Wiegmann B, et al. Normothermic perfusion of donor lungs for preservation and assessment with the organ care system lung before bilateral transplantation: a pilot study of 12 patients. Lancet 2012;380(9856):1851–8.
61. Prastein D, Poston R, Gu J, Gage F. Viability markers to assess nonheartbeating donor hearts during ex vivo perfusion. Transplantation 2004;78(2):642.
62. Regehr C, Kjerulf M, Popova SR, Baker AJ. Trauma and tribulation: the experiences and attitudes of operating room nurses working with organ donors. J Clin Nurs 2004;13(4):430–7.
63. Verble M, Worth J. Cultural sensitivity in the donation discussion. Prog Transplant 2003;13(1):33–7.

CHAPTER 20
END OF LIFE

NATALIE ANDERSON, DWIGHT ROBINSON, AND JAMES MARSHALL

ESSENTIALS

- Appreciate the impact of culture on the patient and their family's experience through trauma, death and grief; and the impact of emergency organisational culture on the experience of the individual and their family.
- Understand the skills and processes that are required to facilitate appropriate care of the patient and family in both expected and sudden or unexpected death situations.
- Ensure that emergency clinicians understand their role in the advance care planning process, to respect and safeguard the patient's wishes for care at the end of life.
- Palliative care involves a full and active approach to comfort, and is the collective responsibility of all clinicians involved in a patient's care.
- Ensure emergency clinicians understand the legislation and guidelines in relation to management of death and dying in the country, state or territory in which they work.

INTRODUCTION

The primary focus of emergency departments (EDs) and paramedic services is to minimise morbidity and mortality.[1] Despite this, life and death sit firmly alongside one another in the ED.[2] Providing care for a person who is dying or who has died, and supporting the person's family (both biological and non-biological significant others) during this difficult time are core components of the emergency clinician's role. Managing the practical and emotional aspects of a person's death in the ED and paramedical settings can be confronting for even the most experienced emergency clinician.

There are two broad categories of death in the emergency setting that will be referred to in this chapter: the death of a person from a known chronic life-limiting illness, categorised as an *expected* death. The other category is a *sudden* or *unexpected* death, which can be traumatic or violent in nature. Irrespective of the nature or cause of the death, the emergency clinician's ability to communicate compassion and provide individualised care for the patient and their grieving family can have a lasting impact on the lives of all concerned.

PRACTICE TIP

Emergency clinicians are in a privileged position to be at the front line of care for people who are dying, either from an expected illness or from a sudden or traumatic death. Clinicians must never underestimate the impact of their care on people at this time, memories of which will remain with the survivors for life.

CULTURAL CONSIDERATIONS

When members of the pre-hospital or emergency clinical team are faced with a death, irrespective of the cause, self-awareness and cultural awareness are driving factors in how clinicians respond to the situation. Hence, cognisance of one's personal beliefs and culture in relation to death and dying is crucial. Australia is defined as a multicultural society, with over 29.8% of Australians born in countries outside Australia.[3] Similarly, in New Zealand, just over one-quarter of the population is born overseas.[4]

Culture permeates all aspects of the human experience, and while people from culturally and linguistically diverse (CALD) backgrounds may have particular needs, no individual can or should be reduced to a simplistic set of expected cultural norms, values or practices. The emergency clinician must ensure they are culturally competent to meet the needs of CALD patients and families, acknowledging that EDs and paramedic services have their own organisational culture, expectations and practices. Furthermore, culturally safe service delivery[5] relies on the emergency clinician's ability to encourage empowerment, share respect and foster a safe environment for Indigenous communities of Australia and New Zealand, in order to promote meaningful pathways to self-determination. It is essential that clinicians have the ability to understand and respond to the unique cultural needs of both their workplace and a diversity of people facing death and grief in the emergency care setting.

There are several models to guide clinicians on how to deliver culturally competent and culturally safe care,[5,6] and more information on cultural considerations in emergency care can be found in Chapter 5. The following steps provide some guidance on how to begin to provide cultural support in the context of death and dying:

- Have an awareness of one's own attitudes, beliefs and values about death and dying and how this can impact on the patient and family.
- Ask clear and concise questions about patient and family culture, beliefs and rituals around death and dying.
- Show respect for nationality, culture, age, sex, political and religious beliefs.
- Establish trust and open, non-threatening relationships, often within a short period of time.
- Use effective communication skills to elicit family members' understanding about what is happening to the patient in the situation at hand.
- Provide practical support for CALD families, such as offering to assist with arranging interpreters, spiritual or community leader support.
- Communicate with the family to ascertain if there are any specific cultural needs and/or if particular rituals need to be observed when the patient has died.

Different cultures may require specific management of the deceased. A resource such as an outline of different cultural beliefs at the time of death can be helpful as a general guide for clinicians.[6]

PRACTICE TIP

Each individual clinician, patient or family member will manage death and dying based on his or her own situation, emotion, culture and experience.

Of the 158,500 people who die each year in Australia, the majority are clinically expected deaths from known chronic life-limiting conditions.[3] Furthermore, older people are the fastest growing demographic in developed countries and with this comes increased prevalence of life-limiting chronic conditions, such as cardiovascular, cerebrovascular and respiratory disease and dementia.[7] While many emergency clinicians feel comfortable managing a dying patient and report they find the experience rewarding, an Australian study highlighted that approximately 70% of clinicians felt that the ED was 'not the right place to die'.[1] This is largely due to the busy nature of the ED environment and poor structural design that does not allow for adequate privacy or time to provide appropriate end-of-life care.[8] In addition, emergency clinicians can have significant issues communicating with patients' usual care teams, particularly out-of-hours.[2] Nonetheless, patients who present to the ED with complex psychosocial and medical needs require adequate and appropriate care and such patients are known to use inpatient and ED services extensively in the last year of life.[9] However, while many presentations are warranted, EDs should not be expected to substitute for a lack of appropriate in- and out-of-hours community-based services.

Patients living with life-limiting illness will often present to an ED for management of symptoms, such as gastrointestinal problems, breathing difficulties and pain.[10] The skills that palliative care specialist teams use to effectively communicate and engage with patients and families, and palliate such symptoms, are (and ought to be) transferable to emergency clinicians. However, it has been recognised that more needs to be done to increase the skill capacity of emergency clinicians by fostering partnerships between specialties, and ensuring palliative care is integrated into emergency training and education.[11]

While the main role of paramedics in Australia and New Zealand is perceived to be responding to emergency calls to provide life-sustaining treatment, these emergency clinicians in particular have a key role in supporting palliative care patients who require optimal symptom management and end-of-life care at home, in order to avoid unnecessary ED presentation.[12] Palliative care is commonly associated with patients with cancer in the dying phase; however, educational efforts for paramedics should be focused more broadly on ethical issues, end-of-life communication, increasing understanding of the common causes of death, and understanding of non-malignant illnesses where a palliative approach might be beneficial.[13] Recently, progress has been made in some jurisdictions to empower paramedics to effectively care for people who are dying from expected deaths, and this will be discussed later in this chapter in the section on advance care planning.

PALLIATIVE CARE

At times, emergency clinicians confront a major dilemma relating to whether an accurate prediction of appropriate active treatment is possible and whether decisions about a transition to palliation can or should be made.[14] When goals of care shift from life-sustaining or 'active measures' to 'comfort measures', emergency clinicians have an opportunity to provide not 'just comfort' measures. Rather, *not* escalating treatment means a full, active approach can be taken to reduce suffering and promote comfort. As the goals of care are established through good communication and advance care planning, where possible, it becomes the responsibility of all generalist and specialist clinicians to provide comfort to those who are dying and their families.

PRACTICE TIP

A 'goals of care' discussion with the patient and their family is the appropriate way to begin the advance care planning process.

End-of-life care does not necessarily involve emergency clinicians. Many patients with life-limiting conditions have care pathways established to allow them to remain in their home. Palliative care teams may be involved, who can monitor the patient's condition at home and change medications if increased symptom control is required. In many cases it will not be necessary for a palliative care patient to attend hospital.

While the best efforts may be made to keep palliative care patients at home, paramedics and emergency clinicians stand at the 'front door' of hospital services where patients can receive high-level care when it is needed. This may be for many different reasons, including family discomfort with home care, difficulty in managing symptoms, or a request from the palliative care team.

Although it is acknowledged that the ED is not the ideal place to provide end-of-life care, due to lack of space, privacy and specialist palliative care trained staff, emergency clinicians have the opportunity to provide skilled and attentive care to patients in the last hours of life to enable a 'good death', with a focus on patient dignity, relief of symptoms, relief of physical and emotional suffering and support for grieving families.[8,15] To help achieve this goal, emergency clinicians can benefit from training in basic symptom management to effectively address common end-of-life symptoms such as pain, terminal delirium, restlessness, anxiety and respiratory distress.[16] It is acknowledged that these are a distinct skill set, different from those needed to stabilise non-palliative patients in ED. For particularly complex or challenging symptoms, early palliative care consultation in the ED is recommended.[17]

ADVANCE CARE PLANNING

Advance care planning recognises the importance of integrating a patient's wishes into the holistic management of their chronic, life-limiting illness treatment.[18–20] The process of advance care planning is fluid and begins with a conversation to establish the goals of care, whereby the patient is supported to discuss their life goals, values and choices about their preferred outcomes of care with a trained professional, family and friends, including the patient's substitute decision-maker. This conversation should be ongoing as preferences may change over time.[1] A discussion on goals of care[14] can often result in the creation of an advance care planning document or directive. There is variation between jurisdictions regarding the document title and legislation to enforce it, and advance care directives can be verbal, as well as written.[18,21] When the patient cannot communicate their wishes for themselves, their advance care plan must be respected and should guide family and health professionals in making treatment decisions.

The following elements can strengthen an advance care plan's validity:[18,21]

- It is a written document.
- There is evidence that, when signed, the person was competent and not unduly influenced. Witnessing may provide further support, as may the witness's qualifications (e.g. doctor). Witnessing requirements are specified for statutory documents.
- A more recent advance care plan may be regarded as more valid because it provides more certainty about its currency.
- It relates to a current condition. An advance care plan that clearly contemplates the current clinical circumstances will reduce doubt about its applicability.
- It is appropriately worded. An advance care plan will be stronger if it avoids vague or imprecise language.
- It is recommended that advance care planning documents be incorporated in all electronic health records.[22]

Delays in the communication of appropriate end-of-life care planning can result in:[23]

- continued aggressive, unwanted or unwarranted life-sustaining measures instigated for those approaching end of life, including even those who are imminently dying
- poor experiences for families where distraught family members are called on at a time of grieving to engage in end-of-life decisions, and who often experience distress observing life-sustaining measures in their dying loved one
- potentially avoidable conflicts between families and the healthcare team, or within the healthcare team, about the best course of treatment and care for the dying patient
- care being delivered in acute settings when better patient outcomes could be delivered in supported community or home environments
- stress for health professionals balancing their obligation to act in the best interests of dying patients, sometimes differing views among treating clinicians and families about what that entails, and good stewardship of health resources.

Advance care plans may involve direction around the person's choices regarding resuscitation, but should not be confused with 'Resuscitation plans'. A 'Not for resuscitation' order is just one step in the process of clarifying quality end-of-life care planning. Given the time-sensitive environment of the ED, it is important to diligently clarify the patient's goals of care beyond resuscitation status alone. This includes understanding the patient's functional baseline, how the presenting illness fits into the natural history of their disease and what would constitute a meaningful recovery.[24]

A substitute decision-maker (SDM) is appointed or identified by law to make substitute decisions on behalf of a person whose decision-making capacity is impaired. An SDM may be appointed by the person, appointed for (on behalf of) the person, or identified as the default decision-maker by guardianship legislation. More than one SDM can be appointed.

There are three categories of SDM:[22]

1. Chosen by the person (e.g. one or more enduring guardians appointed under a statutory advance care/health directive or a nominated SDM in a common law directive).
2. Assigned to the person by the law in the absence of an appointed SDM (e.g. family member, carer or 'person responsible').
3. Appointed for the person (e.g. a guardian appointed by a guardianship tribunal).

In Australia and New Zealand, national framework documents[19,22] and advance care planning websites (see 'Useful websites') can be accessed to guide clinicians, as well as local policy between states and territories.

The Australian national framework recognises:[22]

- that under common law the terms of an advance care directive must be respected whether or not the person was medically informed of the consequences when the directive was written
- that a person (or the SDM) can consent to treatment options that are offered, and refuse such treatment, but cannot demand treatment that is not medically indicated
- the need to protect health and aged care professionals from civil and criminal liability if they abide by the terms of an advance care directive that they believe, in good faith, to be valid.

Some Australian ambulance services now have advance care planning tools, such as the NSW Ambulance Authorised Adult Palliative Care Plan.[25] This document outlines the patient's medical history, current medications and preferences for place of death. Doctors can indicate the appropriate medical treatment orders for paramedics to follow, such as a not-for-CPR order in the event the patient is in cardiac arrest or if death has occurred. An Authorised Paediatric Palliative Care Plan[18] is also available in NSW.

This model empowers paramedics to provide treatment to the patient in line with the patient's preferences and established end-of-life care plan, and potentially avoid unnecessary hospital admission.

The culture of EDs and paramedic services can be at odds with the palliative approach and non-escalation of treatment for many reasons previously already discussed in this chapter. Furthermore, emergency clinicians may feel it is not their duty to initiate goals-of-care discussions with patients who are not known to them. However, developing mastery of palliative care core competencies is recommended for all emergency clinicians irrespective of clinical experience.[24]

At the same time, it is acknowledged that palliative care teams are under pressure to ensure their often-limited resources are used for appropriate patients with high-level, complex physical, psychological and/or social needs.

Therefore, it is the collective responsibility of all clinicians involved in the patient's health management to ensure that the treatment and care that is given is guided by the person's wishes and preferences.[26]

SUDDEN AND UNEXPECTED DEATH

A *sudden* death implies the death occurs usually within 24 hours of the first symptoms. Sudden death may also refer to those resuscitated from cardiac arrest who die during the same hospital admission. Most sudden deaths occur over a few seconds or minutes. *Unexpected* death acknowledges a patient's pre-existing medical condition, such as someone who was believed to have been in good health or who had a stable chronic condition (e.g. cardiomyopathy, epilepsy or a respiratory condition such as asthma), in which sudden death was not expected. A person's death may be considered unexpected if it occurs in the presence of an illness that would not be expected to cause death.[27]

The responsibility of notifying the family of a death may fall to the emergency clinician. How, when and where the family is notified can have a significant impact on their bereavement outcomes.[28,29] An optimal outcome may not be achievable; for example, if the family member or friend has witnessed the death of their loved one in the pre-hospital setting, or been the first one to find their body. For emergency clinicians, the emotional toll of communicating death notification and providing emotional support to the family cannot be underestimated. Emergency clinicians report feeling uncomfortable communicating death notifications and these experiences can be very stressful, particularly for inexperienced clinicians.[29–31] Formal training on how to notify someone of a death varies and many learn through experience.[28] The following is a brief outline of the 'steps' in the death notification process:[28]

1. *Preparation:* choose the appropriate individual to attend the notification who is fully aware of the situation.
2. *Initiating contact:* confirm identity of the person to be notified; do not delay notification; allow for privacy in a safe and comfortable environment.
3. *Delivering bad news:* give a chronology of events; avoid euphemisms such as 'passed away'; be compassionate and humanistic.
4. *Responding to the survivor's reaction and providing support:* constantly monitor for emotional and physical support needs; allow time for expression of emotions; offer the person the opportunity to spend time with the deceased; allow customs and rituals; provide anticipatory guidance.
5. *Provision of ongoing support:* provide written information and information about resources; attend/arrange follow-up contact.
6. *Dealing with notifier's response:* provide adequate information and education about death notification; provide opportunities for supportive discussion for those staff involved.

The sudden or unexpected death of a person leaves family members unprepared and, most often, emotionally distraught. Emergency clinicians have an important role to play in supporting grieving family members, even if notification of death falls to other health team members such as medical staff or chaplains.[28] Genuineness, warmth, empathy, active listening and openness[32] are central qualities and skills that are required to provide essential bereavement support to families at a very difficult time.

PRACTICE TIP

Genuineness, warmth, empathy, active listening and openness are central qualities and skills that are required by emergency clinicians to provide support to dying people and their families.

SUDDEN DEATH OF A CHILD

As with adult deaths, good bereavement care provided after the death of a child can have positive long-term effects on the bereavement outcomes of parents and siblings. For emergency clinicians, the death of a child in the emergency setting or in the community may be one of the most distressing and stressful events that can occur.[33] Adequate training and education to prepare staff for how to manage these events is essential. The following are key practice points from Lawrence's[33] guidelines for best practice in supporting parents after the death of their child:

- An emergency-trained clinician or appropriately trained staff member should immediately be allocated to support the parents, particularly through the resuscitation process. The allocated staff member should learn the names and roles of family members present and the child should always be referred to by their name.
- Allow time for parents to hold the child and offer the opportunity for them to assist with washing or dressing the child if permitted by the Coroner.
- Understand that siblings should be told of the death by their parent or a person they know and trust, and offer some supportive literature to parents to help siblings make sense of their loss.
- Reassure parents that their child will continue to receive care and attention after they have left the ED.
- Be aware of agencies that may need to be notified after a child's death and give advice to parents regarding who they may be required to speak to.
- Ensure appropriate after-care, possibly including a condolence card from the ED staff.
- Ensure debriefing for staff, both formal and informal, to allow reflection on this highly emotional, demanding aspect of the emergency clinician's role.
- In many cases, the cause of death will be clear; however, consideration should be given to death from non-accidental injury, and such cases should be referred to the police. Some deaths in childhood remain unexplained, even after autopsy. These are referred to as Sudden Infant Death Syndrome (SIDS), or Sudden Unexplained Death in Childhood (SUDC) for children aged over one year.[34]

FAMILY PRESENCE DURING RESUSCITATION

The presence of family during resuscitation was first explored in the United States in the 1980s, after a landmark study showed that relatives would have preferred to have been present.[35] Since then, a significant amount of research has been published,[36] providing clinical practice guidelines[37,38] that support relatives' presence during resuscitation. Reasons given to support family presence include:

- better communication between family and staff, which can also reduce the risk of liability
- family can realise the seriousness of the situation and that everything was done to try to save their loved one
- family are better able to cope with the outcome of the resuscitation and have a sense of closure, knowing the death was real.

Some limitations to presence of family during resuscitation are recognised in the literature:[36,39]

- witnessing resuscitation could be more traumatic for the family
- stress or distraction for staff is increased
- it could increase litigation and breach patient confidentiality
- the family may interfere during the resuscitation.

Both the Australian and New Zealand Resuscitation Council[37] and the Emergency Nursing Association (ENA) recommend family members be offered the opportunity to be present during resuscitation. The following practical recommendations are given by the ENA[38] for organisations that are considering implementing the practice of relatives' presence during resuscitation:

- Provide an environment that is suitable for the implementation of the program.
- Provide chairs for family to sit on, to ensure that there is less potential for injury of family members while they are witnessing the resuscitation.
- Educate staff on how to work with grieving families.
- Prepare the family with a clear explanation of what to expect when they are in the resuscitation room.
- Provide a support person to accompany the relatives during their presence in the resuscitation room.

Some of these recommendations may not be achievable if the death has occurred in the community, and clinicians may not have the resources to manage family members during the process of resuscitation. Allowing for these limitations, an effort should be made to keep the family updated on progress and to provide support afterwards.

Evidence for a designated emergency clinician to support the family looking on in a resuscitation situation is highly recommended in the literature.[39] However, a designated family support person is not always evident in practice due to staff shortage, and was considered in one study to be 'low on the priority list'.[39] The decision to allow family to be present during resuscitation remains controversial and, ultimately, culturally defined.[35,38–44] Evidence generally suggests that while family presence at resuscitation is recommended, and can reduce the risk of post-traumatic stress disorder (PTSD) in family members[41,42] it is not widely observed in practice, therefore more research is needed.[44]

CARE OF A DECEASED PATIENT

In the pre-hospital setting where resuscitation has been withheld or withdrawn, it may be appropriate to move the deceased patient to a more suitable location.[45] For example, a general practitioner (GP) may certify a patient who has died on a property outside their home. The patient could then be moved inside and placed on a bed until they can be transferred to a funeral director. Movement of the deceased patient should not be carried out if there is a suspicious death or if preservation of evidence is important. Clinicians should refer to the local police service or the jurisdictional Coroner regarding appropriate procedure.

The ED is not an ideal environment for end-of-life care and caring for a deceased patient.[1,46] However, within an ED setting, when there is no requirement for a review of a death by a Coroner, caring for a deceased patient can include core nursing tasks, such as washing the body, replacing dentures and dressing the patient in clean clothes or a hospital gown. Additional tasks that may facilitate interaction for the loved ones with the deceased include slightly elevating the head of the deceased patient, placing hands above the sheet for ease of access and provision of a quiet place for time with the deceased patient. While these undertakings may be challenging to achieve within an ED environment, such tasks can facilitate a therapeutic commencement of the grieving process and a completion of formal patient identification.[47]

Each jurisdiction across Australia and New Zealand will have different specific requirements for the identification of a deceased person. However, in the case of a reportable death, the Coroner will usually require identification of the body by a family member or close friend to be attended in the presence of a police officer. On rare occasions, particularly in rural or remote settings, identification may take place in the presence of an intermediary; such as in the presence of an emergency clinician. The emergency clinician acts as a witness to the identification by the family, then signs a specific identification form to hand over to a police officer once the family has left the hospital. Such a process may assist the family or friends in reducing the time that they are required to remain at the hospital following the death of the patient.

It is implicit that staff caring for deceased patients should follow standard precautions. Consideration should be given to additional precautions in situations where the infection risk is higher. Further consideration should be given to providing infection control education and equipment to the deceased's loved ones.

Note that in the event of a reportable death to the Coroner, many of the above patient care tasks are not permitted. There are a number of legal aspects that pre-hospital and emergency clinicians need to take into consideration. In many jurisdictions clinicians can document that life is extinct, without making a determination of cause, in order to allow funeral procedures to commence. The related legislation will vary across Australia and New Zealand; issues relating to pre-hospital, emergency care and the law is explored in Chapter 4.

REPORTABLE DEATHS

A reportable death is a death that must be referred to the relevant state or territory Coroner.[48] The specific processes and criterion for referral to the Coroner will vary across jurisdictions, so pre-hospital and emergency clinicians should familiarise themselves with the relevant local procedures and legislation. However, as a general guide, the types of death that meet the requirement for a reportable death are sudden, violent and/or accidental in nature. Other criteria include (but are not limited to) the following:

- if the deceased person's identity is unknown or in question
- if the person died under suspicious or unusual circumstances
- if the person was held at, or temporarily absent from, a care facility, mental health facility or was in custody (police or corrective services)
- where the death occurred unexpectedly after a medical procedure
- if the person has not seen a health professional within the 6 months before the death.

Not all reported deaths will result in a post-mortem examination; however, the Coroner may order such an examination to assist with determining identity of the patient, circumstances and cause of death.

POST-MORTEM EXAMINATION

Discussing a post-mortem examination (PME) with a deceased person's family can be awkward and challenging for the pre-hospital or emergency clinician.[48] The main context for discussing a PME would be as part of referring a death to the state or territory Coroner; however, on occasion the deceased's family may also request a full, limited or partial PME.[49] For example, a family may request a limited PME to investigate an insidious lung disease and request a lung tissue sample be collected, but may not want to proceed to a full PME.

A full PME involves a procedure (autopsy) where a detailed examination of the body's external surfaces and internal organs is undertaken to establish a cause of death.[48] A limited or partial PME focuses on specific sections or organs of the body.[49] Additionally, whole organs, tissue, blood and body fluids may be taken from the body for further examination and/or retention for investigative or research purposes.[49]

Family members often have questions about the PME, including how it may affect the body of the deceased and if it will delay funeral arrangements. A PME may seem insensitive at an extremely difficult time; however, due to the circumstances of a patient death, it may be a legal requirement. The pre-hospital and emergency clinician is well placed to provide accurate, compassionate information on the procedure and processes for a PME.[48] A PME may cause additional distress for family, particularly when religious and cultural views place a strong emphasis on the inviolability of the deceased physical body, requirements for ritual cleaning of the body, or stringent time limits for burial.[50] The pre-hospital and emergency clinician should be prepared to address the family's queries on a full or limited PME. PME and coronial information in multiple languages for family members can be sourced through the local state or territory Coroner's office.

DEATHS FOR REVIEW BY THE CORONER AND MANAGEMENT OF EVIDENCE

When a person dies and a death certificate cannot be completed, the death will be referred to the relevant Coroner (state or territory) for further investigation. As previously identified, some variance exists between specific coronial requirements between the different states and territories across Australia and New Zealand. Pre-hospital and emergency clinicians should be familiar with the general principles and any specific local requirements outlined below. Links to relevant resources are provided for further review at the end of this chapter. Additionally, local health, paramedical and ambulance organisations should have specific local procedures to guide clinicians in recognising and managing potential cases for referral to the Coroner.

Within the pre-hospital and emergency setting, it is unlikely that a clinician will interact directly with the Coroner. Instead, the clinician is likely to interact with the local police acting on behalf of the Coroner. Police will prepare a brief or report for the Coroner that may include statements from the clinician and other items of evidence, such as the deceased's clothing and clinical notes. All of the collected evidence, in addition to the PME, will help the Coroner answer a set of key questions.[51]

When there are questions about the deceased's identity, or if the death is suspicious or unexpected, the Coroner will seek to provide answers specifically addressing the following key questions:

- The identity of the deceased.
- The cause of death.
- The circumstances in which the death occurred.

The investigations by the Coroner to answer the key questions can proceed along a continuum from a simple review of patient medical records and a discussion with the local investigating police, which may be completed in days, to a full judicial investigation through the coronial court, which could take several years.[51] It is beyond the scope of the pre-hospital and emergency clinician to determine the likely breadth and depth of the Coroner's investigation. Therefore, all deaths where a death certificate is not going to be completed at the time of death must be treated as a 'Coroner's case'. It is prudent for clinicians to assume they may be called as a witness in the coronial investigative process. Hence it is essential that medical records are accurate and the chain of evidence protocols are adhered to.

The Coroner may be satisfied that there is enough evidence to answer the key questions without having to order a PME. However, if a PME is undertaken and the above questions are still not resolved, the coronial process will be extended into the form of a coronial hearing. The coronial process then extends into further investigations and is generally explored through a formal court proceeding.

If applicable, at the conclusion of the coronial process, the Coroner may go on to make recommendations, which may include:

- suggesting criminal or professional misconduct proceedings be commenced by the relevant authorities
- mitigation or correctional steps to reduce the likelihood of a similar occurrence in the future
- returning an 'open' finding, where there is not enough evidence to answer the three key questions above (note the Coroner may re-examine the case in the future if further information is unearthed).

For all deaths that are being referred to the coronial process, the principles of 'chain of possession' (chain of evidence, chain of custody) and evidence preservation must be maintained.[52]

The chain of possession ensures that there is a record of all people who have contact with a particular item of evidence.[52,53] For example, a piece of clothing that was cut off the deceased patient during a resuscitation attempt would have a recorded chain of possession, including the paramedic or nurse who cut the clothing. This record would then be continued to include the police officer who took custody of the item, the lab technician who received the item and the other lab technician who examined the item.[53]

Evidence preservation refers to the specific methods of handling and treating different pieces of evidence with the aim of preserving physical macro and micro evidence, such as DNA, hair, chemical, blood and gunshot residue. Recommendations for handling and treating evidence include the following:

- Once the person has been confirmed as deceased, nothing should be removed from the patient.
- Leaving any medical devices or equipment that were in situ at the time of death—including endotracheal tubes, venous access devices and gastric tubes.
- The body should not be washed or otherwise tampered with.
- Any bodily fluids should be preserved and stored in clearly marked and sealed containers.
- All items removed from the patient, including clothing, jewellery and the like, should be placed into separate paper bags, allowing preservation of DNA and other trace materials (plastic bags should be avoided due to the build-up of condensation which may degrade any evidence).
- Any sharps related to the above points should be stored or secured in a way that maintains evidence integrity, but also safety for all staff involved in the evidence chain process.
- All medical records, including pre-hospital and hospital records, must be up to date.
- Any other personal items of the deceased, particularly electronic devices, should be secured by the clinician until such time as they can be handed over to police.

CERTIFICATION OF DEATH

New Zealand and states and territories in Australia have resources available to guide clinicians on the legislative requirements on the process for 'certification as to the cause of death'. This certification is a medical form completed by a registered medical officer at the time of a person's death. The certification is only completed when deaths are not to be referred to the Coroner.

The certification form details the medical cause of death. The doctor who certifies a patient's death is also required to separately notify the Registrar of Births, Deaths and Marriages within a designated period after the death.

Establishing that a person is deceased—also referred to as 'verification of death' or 'extinction of life assessment'—can be attended to by a medical officer; it can also be a registered nurse or a paramedic in some jurisdictions in New Zealand and Australia. This process involves a clinical assessment of the body only to establish that death has occurred. For example, relevant policies exist in New Zealand and some states of Australia outlining that a registered nurse or a paramedic can attend an extinction-of-life assessment on a patient known to palliative care services who has died an expected death at home, in the case where a medical officer cannot immediately attend. The medical officer is contacted at the time of death and is then required to complete the certification as to the cause of death within 48 hours.

CARE OF THE DECEASED BARIATRIC PATIENT

In Australia and New Zealand, between 25% and 33% of the general population are considered obese.[54,55] Increasing numbers of morbidly obese patients are interacting with pre-hospital and emergency clinicians, the wider hospital service and the funeral services industry. All staff face potential manual handling challenges during treatment, collection, transport, preparation, funeral service and burial of the deceased bariatric patient. Manual handling of bariatric patients in the pre-hospital setting can be particularly challenging, as resources and equipment are limited.

To aid in management and transport of the deceased bariatric patient, the approximate weight and girth of the patient should be calculated, as this will need to be communicated to hospital and funeral services staff. Pre-hospital and ED environments should have access to bariatric equipment, including beds and trolleys. At times, the facility's mortuary refrigerator may not be large enough to accommodate the deceased bariatric patient. In this case, pre-hospital clinicians or hospital staff should contact relevant funeral services, or state coronial contractors, to collect the bariatric patient directly from the pre-hospital scene or facility.

ORGAN DONATION

Organ donation is the process of transplanting one or more organs or tissues from a donor to a recipient. The live and deceased donation process is covered in detail in Chapter 19. Both New Zealand and Australian federal authorities provide guidelines and clinical triggers that outline when to initiate discussions with family members about organ and tissue donation in patients where ongoing treatment is futile or patient prognosis is poor.[56] When organ donation is to occur, the dying person receives care that is aimed at preserving organ function. This care may include artificial ventilation, inotropic support and strict temperature and blood glucose control.

STAFF SUPPORT

Pre-hospital and emergency clinicians are routinely confronted with human suffering, trauma and death, often in the midst of a hectic work environment. In addition, they are expected to assess, manage, treat and transport critically ill patients and manage both their own emotions and the emotions of others who are potentially in distress.[57,58] It is therefore not surprising that pre-hospital and emergency clinicians are highly vulnerable to post-traumatic stress disorder (PTSD) symptoms, including anxiety, depression, nightmares, intrusive thoughts and loss of concentration.[59] Clearly, this can have a significant impact on the clinician, but also can impact on the quality of patient care. Regehr and LeBlanc[60] conducted research into emergency service personnel, including paramedics. They found that while day-to-day 'core function' decision-making was not affected, situations where professional judgement and risk assessment was required were significantly impacted by the presence of PTSD symptoms.

Critical incident stress debriefing (CISD) allows those involved in an incident to reflect on and process the event; sessions should be led by adequately trained staff.[61] Although most emergency workers believe that CISD is important, many organisations have no formal structures, such as guidelines or policies, in place to ensure this practice is followed. Ongoing debriefing programs, such as clinical supervision, as well as CISD, have been found to reduce occupation stress in emergency settings.[62]

Organisations should take preventive measures to ensure staff have the means to foster and maintain professional resilience.[62] In addition, individuals in the pre-hospital and ED setting are responsible for developing their personal resilience by taking active measures to participate in self-care strategies to 're-fuel' physically, socially, psychologically and spiritually. Such activities could include enjoyable exercise; going out with friends and family; keeping a reflective journal; or participating in meaningful rituals. Collectively, these professional and personal strategies can assist emergency clinicians to ensure their physical and emotional wellbeing, and enable them to provide the best-quality patient care.

SUMMARY

Emergency clinicians have the privilege of being at the frontline of emergency care settings and are involved with people's lives at significant times of trauma, loss and grief. These highly skilled clinicians must provide end-of-life care across a continuum that ranges from patients who have made their wishes clear as they come to the end of a struggle with illness, to those for whom death was entirely unforeseen. Emergency clinicians are tasked with providing the highest quality care to critically ill patients in a highly demanding clinical environment and ensuring the requirements of law in their relevant country, state or territory are met. In addition, emergency clinicians are required to meet the needs of families that often can be in a state of distress and emotional suffering. The ongoing impact of a compassionate and individualised approach to care for families who have suffered a loss cannot and should not be underestimated.

CASE STUDY 1

Peter is a 70-year-old male who has collapsed during a routine appointment with his general practitioner (GP). Clinic staff are doing CPR when paramedics arrive. The attending paramedics continue CPR, as well as initiating protocols for airway management and a shockable cardiac rhythm. Peter's family attend the scene during the resuscitation and are visibly distressed. After an extended period of resuscitation, Peter is found to be in prolonged asystole and resuscitation is ceased. The paramedics verify that all signs of life are extinct at the scene.

QUESTIONS

1. Peter's GP assumes that the cause of death was a sudden cardiac arrest of unknown origin, presumed to be cardiac. Which of the following is true?
   a. A medical certificate of cause of death can be written because cause of death is known.
   b. All tubes, lines and the like can be removed because the cause of death is known.
   c. The police must be informed because the death will be referred to the Coroner.

d. The family will not be able to see Peter because the death will be referred to the Coroner.

2. In providing psychosocial support to Peter's family members, what might be helpful?
   a. Provide the family with information about death, dying and the coronial process.
   b. Discuss organ donation because Peter had an organ donor card in his wallet.
   c. Organise a minister of religion because you heard one of Peter's family praying.
   d. Provide the family with information about screening for cardiac risk factors now they have a family history of cardiac arrest.
3. Which of the following is true in relation to Peter and the coronial process?
   a. Family members are not to be left alone with Peter's body; they must be supervised by police at all times.
   b. All lines, tubes and the like must be left in place to assist in the coronial investigation.
   c. An autopsy will be carried out only if the Coroner requires it to be completed or the family requests it.
   d. All of the above.
4. The manager of the ambulance service has suggested that the resuscitation team, including the GP and clinic staff, meet for debriefing. The purpose of this debrief would best be described as an opportunity to:
   a. Review the treatment of Peter and comment on the performance of individual team members so they can improve next time.
   b. Screen all team members for symptoms of post-traumatic stress response and organise referral to a counsellor.
   c. Allow team members to reflect on and discuss what happened during the resuscitation and ask questions that may arise.
   d. Comply with legislative requirements around unexpected deaths in the community.

Answers to Case Study Questions can be found on evolve http://evolve.elsevier.com/AU/Curtis/emergency/ 

CASE STUDY 2

Sara is a 24-year-old woman who has been in and out of remission of leukaemia since she was 15. Over the last 6 weeks she has transitioned to palliative care with the goal of maximising her quality of life. Sara called the ambulance due to increased, uncontrolled pain. When she arrived in the ED, Sara deteriorated quickly, became unconscious and died a short time later.

QUESTIONS

1. A large number of Sara's family, including her 18-month-old daughter and friends, arrived at the hospital and were understandably very upset. Which of the following strategies do you think would work best for this situation?
   a. Limiting bedside visitors to two at a time in line with your ED visitor policy.
   b. Restricting bedside visitors to immediate family and Sara's closest friends.
   c. Providing an area where the family and friends can gather, separate to the ED waiting room.
   d. Appointing a family spokesperson who can be a point of contact for both ED staff and other family and friends.
2. The ED medical officer is not willing to write a death certificate because they have not seen Sara before. Which of the following actions are indicated in this situation?
   a. Try to contact the relevant haematologist or palliative care doctor to provide further information on Sara's medical history.
   b. Consult any available previous medical records to provide further information on Sara's medical history.
   c. Treat this death as a Coroner's case until a death certificate is completed.
   d. Inform Sara's next of kin that a death certificate will not be written at this stage.
3. Sara's parents have requested that no males be left alone with her as it is in line with their cultural practices. On reflection, this is:
   a. A reasonable request for the parents to make in line with their cultural belief.
   b. An unreasonable request because this cannot be guaranteed by hospital staff.

4. A staff member is upset by Sara's death. An empathic response would include:
   a. Encouraging the staff member to 'move on' as it was an expected death.
   b. Expressing understanding about how sad Sara's death is and how 'only the good die young'.
   c. Discouraging the staff member to express their feelings because it is unprofessional for emergency clinicians.
   d. Allowing the staff member to express their thoughts and feelings without judgement and letting them know about the local Employee Assistance Program.

Answers to Case Study Questions can be found on evolve **http://evolve.elsevier.com/AU/Curtis/emergency/** 

USEFUL WEBSITES

Advance Care Planning

Advance Care Planning Australia, advancecareplanning.org.au/.

Advance Care Planning New Zealand, www.hqsc.govt.nz/our-work/advance-care-planning/.

Department of Birth Deaths and Marriages

Australia

NSW: www.nsw.gov.au/births-deaths-marriages.

Northern Territory: nt.gov.au/law/bdm.

Queensland: www.qld.gov.au/law/births-deaths-marriages-and-divorces.

South Australia: www.cbs.sa.gov.au/births-deaths-marriages.

Tasmania: www.justice.tas.gov.au/bdm/home.

Victoria: www.bdm.vic.gov.au.

WA: www.wa.gov.au/organisation/department-of-justice/the-registry-of-births-deaths-and-marriages.

New Zealand

New Zealand Government, www.govt.nz/organisations/births-deaths-and-marriages/.

Organ donation

Australian Government Organ and Tissue Authority, www.donatelife.gov.au/.

Organ Donation New Zealand, www.donor.co.nz/.

Palliative care

Palliative Care Australia, www.palliativecare.org.au.

Palliative Care New Zealand, www.hospice.org.nz.

REFERENCES

1. Marck CH, Weil J, Lane H, Weiland TJ, Philip J, Boughey M, et al. Care of the dying cancer patient in the emergency department: findings from a national survey of Australian emergency department clinicians. Int Med J 2014;44(4):362–8.
2. Ieraci S. Palliative care in the emergency department. Emerg Med Australas 2013;25:112–13.
3. Australian Bureau of Statistics (ABS). Migration, Australia, 2019-20 financial year. Commonwealth of Australia; 2021. Available from: www.abs.gov.au/statistics/people/population/migration-australia/latest-release.
4. Statistics New Zealand. Census quickstats about national highlights: cultural diversity. New Zealand Government; 2021. Available from: www.stats.govt.nz/topics/ethnicity.
5. Human Rights Commission. Cultural safety and security: tools to address lateral violence: Social Justice Report 2007. Available from: www.humanrights.gov.au/our-work/aboriginal-and-torres-strait-islander-social-justice/publications/social-justice-report-3.
6. Loddon Mallee Regional Palliative Care Consortium. An outline of different cultural beliefs at the time of death; 2011. Available from: http://lmrpcc.org.au/wp-content/uploads/2011/07/Customs-Beliefs-Death-Dying.pdf.
7. Mathers CD, Stevens GA, Boerma T, White RA, Tobias MI. Causes of international increases in older age life expectancy. Lancet 2015;385(9967):540–8.

8. Granero-Molina J, Díaz-Cortés Mdel M, Hernández-Padilla JM, García-Caro MP, Fernández-Sola C. Loss of dignity in end-of-life care in the emergency department: a phenomenological study with health professionals. J Emerg Nurs 2016;42(3):233–9.
9. Goldsbury DE, O'Connell DL, Girgis A, Wilkinson A, Phillips JL, Davidson PM, et al. Acute hospital-based services used by adults during the last year of life in New South Wales, Australia: a population-based retrospective cohort study. BMC Health Serv Res 2015;15(1):537.
10. Spilsbury K, Rosenwax L, Arendts G, Semmens JB. The association of community-based palliative care with reduced emergency department visits in the last year of life varies by patient factors. Ann Emerg Med 2017;69(4):416–25.
11. Kraus CK, Greenberg MR, Ray DE, Dy SM. Palliative care education in emergency medicine residency training: a survey of program directors, associate program directors, and assistant program directors. J Pain Sym Man 2016;51(5):898–906.
12. Swetenham K, Grantham H, Glaetzer K. Breaking down the silos: collaboration delivering an efficient and effective response to palliative care emergencies. Prog Pall Care 2014;22(4):212–8.
13. Rogers I, Shearer F, Rogers J, Ross-Adjie G, Monterosso L, Finn J. Paramedics' perceptions and educational needs with respect to palliative care. Australas J Paramed 2015;12(5):1–8.
14. Mierendorf SM, Gidvani V. Palliative care in the emergency department. Permanente J 2014;18(2):77–85.
15. Meier EA, Gallegos JV, Thomas LPM, Depp CA, Irwin SA, Jeste DV. Defining a good death (successful dying): literature review and a call for research and public dialogue. Am J Geriat Psych 2016;24(4):261–71.
16. Basol N. The integration of palliative care into the emergency department. Turk J Emerg Med 2015;15(2):100–7.
17. Lamba S, Quest TE, Weissman DE. Palliative care consultation in the emergency department #298. J Pall Med 2015;19(1):108–9.
18. Ambulance Service of NSW. Authorised paediatric palliative care plan. Available from: www.slhd.nsw.gov.au/btf/pdfs/Amb/Paediatric_Palliative_Care_Plan.pdf.
19. Ministry of Health New Zealand. Advance care planning: a guide for the New Zealand health workforce. Available from: www.health.govt.nz/system/files/documents/publications/advance-care-planning-aug11.pdf.
20. Alliance NR. Advance care planning New Zealand. 2017. Available from: www.advancecareplanning.org.nz/.
21. Bird S. Advance care planning. Aust Fam Phys 2014;43(8):526–8.
22. Australian Health Ministers Advisory Council. A national framework for advance care directives. 2011. Available from: www.dementia.org.au/sites/default/files/start2talk/5.0.4.1%20AHMAC%20framework.pdf.
23. Ministry of Health NSW. Advance planning for quality care at end of life: action plan 2013–2018. Available from: www.health.nsw.gov.au/patients/acp/Publications/acp-plan-2013-2018.pdf.
24. Wang DH. Beyond code status: palliative care begins in the emergency department. Ann Emerg Med 2016;69(4):437–43.
25. Ambulance Service of NSW. Authorised adult palliative care plan. 2017. Available from: www.slhd.nsw.gov.au/btf/pdfs/Amb/Adult_Palliative_Care_Plan.pdf.
26. Palliative Care Australia. Position statement: workforce for quality care at the end of life. 2015. Online. Available from: palliativecare.org.au/wp-content/uploads/2015/08/PCA-Workforce-position-statement.pdf.
27. Trans-Tasman Response Against Sudden Death in the Young. Post-mortem in sudden unexpected death in the young: guidelines on autopsy practice. Available from: www.cidg.org.
28. Roe E. Practical strategies for death notification in the emergency department. J Emerg Nurs 2012;38(2):130–4.
29. Ombres R, Montemorano L, Becker D. Death notification: someone needs to call the family. J Pall Med 2017;20(6):672–5.
30. Douglas L, Cheskes S, Feldman M, Ratnapalan S. Paramedics' experiences with death notification: a qualitative study. J Paramed Prac 2012;4(9):533–9.
31. Brady M. Mortality face to face: death anxiety in paramedics. J Paramed Prac 2013;5(3):130–1.
32. Scott T. Sudden death in emergency care: responding to bereaved relatives. Emerg Nurse 2013;21(8):36–9.
33. Lawrence N. Care of bereaved parents after sudden infant death. Emerg Nurse 2010;18(3):22–5.
34. Goldstein R, Kinney H, Willinger M. Sudden unexpected death in fetal life through early childhood. Paediatrics 2016;137(6):e20154661.
35. Doyle CJ, Post H, Burney RE, Maino J, Keefe M, Rhee KJ. Family participation during resuscitation: an option. Ann Emerg Med 1987;16(6):673–5.
36. Powers KA. Educational interventions to improve support for family presence during resuscitation: a systematic review of the literature. Dimens Crit Care Nurs 2017;36(2):125–38.
37. Australian Resuscitation Council & New Zealand Resuscitation Council. Guideline 10.6 family presence during resuscitation. Available from: resus.org.au/wpfb-file/anzcor-guideline-10-6-family-presence-during-resuscitation-aug-2016-pdf/.
38. 2017 ENA Clinical Practice Guideline Committee; Vanhoy MA, Horigan A, Stapleton SJ, Valdez AM, Bradford JY, et al. Clincial practice guideline: family presence. J Emerg Nurs 2019;45(1):76.e1–e29.
39. Porter JE, Cooper SJ, Taylor B. Emergency resuscitation team roles: what constitutes a team and who's looking after the family? J Nurs Ed Prac 2014;4(3):124–32.
40. Norton CK, Hobson G, Kulm E. Palliative and end-of-life care in the emergency department: guidelines for nurses. J Emerg Nurs 2011;37(3):240–5.
41. Jabre P, Belpomme V, Azoulay E, Jacob L, Bertrand L, Lapostolle F, et al. Family presence during cardiopulmonary resuscitation. New Eng J Med 2013;368(11):1008–18.

42. Jaques H. Family presence at resuscitation attempts. Nurs Times 2014;110(10):20–1.
43. Fernandes AP, de Souza Carnerio C, Goecze L, Santos B, Guizilini S. Experiences and opinions of health professionals in relation to the presence of the family during in-hospital cardiopulmonary resuscitation: an integrative review. J Nurs Ed Prac 2014;4(5):85–94.
44. Sak-Dankosky N, Andruszkiewicz P, Sherwood PR. Integrative review: nurses' and physicians' experiences and attitudes towards inpatient-witnessed resuscitation of an adult patient. J Adv Nurs 2014;70(5):957–74.
45. Queensland Ambulance Service. Clinical practice guidelines: other/recording of life extinct (ROLE)/management of a deceased person. Queensland Ambulance Service; 2021. Available from: www.ambulance.qld.gov.au/docs/clinical/cpg/CPG_ROLE_Management%20of%20 deceased.pdf.
46. Hogan KA, Fothergill-Bourbonnais F, Brajtman S. When someone dies in the emergency department: perspectives of emergency nurses. J Emerg Nurs 2016;42(3):207–12.
47. Walker W, Deacon K. Nurses' experiences of caring for the suddenly bereaved in adult acute and critical care settings, and the provision of person-centred care: a qualitative study. Intens Crit Care Nurs 2016;33:39–47.
48. Charles A, Cross W, Griffiths D. What do clinicians understand about deaths reportable to the coroner? J Foren Legal Med 2017;51:76–80.
49. Queensland Department of Justice and Attorney-General. Autopsies. In: Queensland Courts, editor. 2017. Available from: www.courts.qld.gov.au/ courts/coroners-court/coroners-process/autopsies.
50. Arnold BB, Bonython W. Autopsies, scans and cultural exceptionalism. Alt Law J 2016;41(1):27–9.
51. NSW Government Justice and Attorney General Department. NSW Coroners Court: a guide to services. Available from: www.coroners.justice.nsw. gov.au/Documents/coroners%20ct%20brochure_guide%20to%20services.pdf.
52. Byrne-Dugan CJ, Cederroth TA, Deshpande A, Remick DG. The processing of surgical specimens with forensic evidence. Arch Path Lab Med 2015;139(8):1024–7.
53. Peel M. Opportunities to preserve forensic evidence in emergency departments. Emerg Nurse 2016;24(7):20–6.
54. Ministry of Health – Manatū Hauora. Annual update of key results 2020/21: New Zealand Health Survey. 2021. Online. Available from: www. health.govt.nz/publication/annual-update-key-results-2020-21-new-zealand-health-survey.
55. Australian Institute of Health and Welfare (AIHW). Overweight and obesity. 2022. Online. Available from: www.aihw.gov.au/reports/australias-health/overweight-and-obesity.
56. Donate Life. Best practice guideline for offering organ and tissue donation in Australia. Commonwealth of Australia: ACT; 2021. Available from: donatelife.gov.au/resources/clinical-guidelines-and-protocols/best-practice-guideline-offering-organ-and-tissue.
57. Shakespeare-Finch J, Rees A, Armstrong D. Social support, self-efficacy, trauma and well-being in emergency medical dispatchers. Soc Indicat Res 2015;123(2):549–65.
58. Waldrop DP, Clemency B, Lindstrom HA, Clemency Cordes C. 'We are strangers walking into their life-changing event': how prehospital providers manage emergency calls at the end of life. J Pain Symptom Manage 2015;50(3):328–34.
59. Skeffington PM, Rees CS, Mazzucchelli T. Trauma exposure and post-traumatic stress disorder within fire and emergency services in Western Australia. Aust J Psychol 2017;69(1):20–8.
60. Regehr C, LeBlanc VR. PTSD, acute stress, performance and decision-making in emergency service workers. J Am Acad Psychiatry Law 2017;45(2):184–92.
61. Dentry SJ, Joannou M, Besemann M, Kriellaars D. Project trauma support: addressing moral injury in first responders. Ment Health Fam Med 2017; 13:418–422.
62. Brucia E, Cordova MJ, Ruzek JI. Critical incident interventions: crisis response and debriefing. In: Khosrow-Pour M., Information Resources Management Association. Police science: breakthroughs in research and practice. Hershey, PA: IGI Publishing; 2019.

SECTION THREE
EMERGENCIES

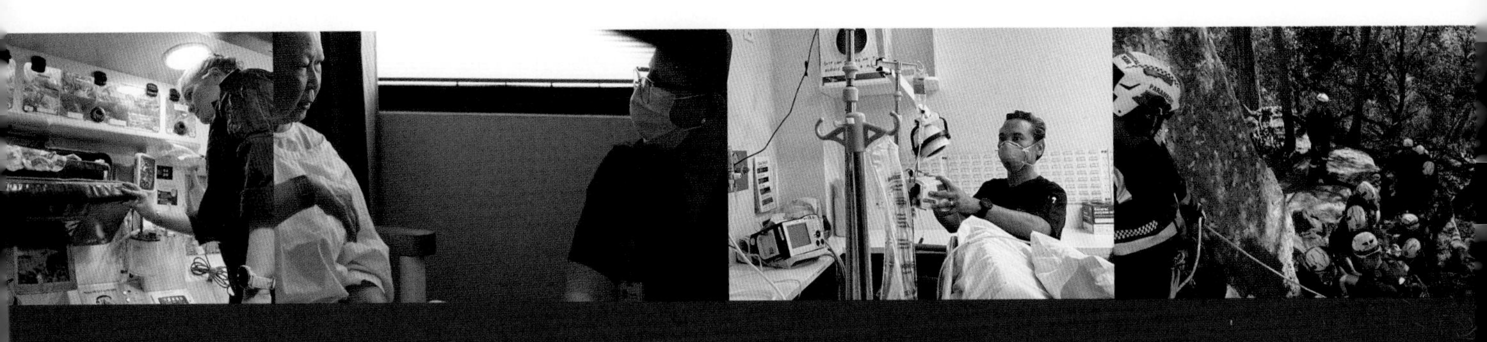

CHAPTER 21
RESPIRATORY EMERGENCIES

JEFF KENNEALLY AND TRACY FLENADY

ESSENTIALS

- Respiratory compromise is a common reason for seeking assistance from healthcare providers, with frequent clinical presentations including chronic obstructive pulmonary disease (COPD), asthma, pneumonia, pulmonary oedema and pulmonary emboli.
- Respiratory dysfunction is a recognised precursor of serious adverse events, including cardiac and respiratory arrest and unplanned intensive care unit admission.
- A comprehensive respiratory assessment should include a patient history and physical assessment incorporating inspection, percussion, palpation and auscultation.
- Pre-hospital decisions are based on comparatively little information with an emphasis on identifying key assessment findings to prompt initial management options.
- Physical assessment can be further informed by appropriate use of investigations, such as pulse oximetry, capnography, arterial or venous blood gases, radiography, peak flows and spirometry.
- The level of respiratory support required will vary according to presentations. Non-invasive ventilation or invasive mechanical ventilation may be required to support optimal gas exchange in some patients.
- Accurate respiratory assessment should inform investigations and plan of care, as well as resource and environment allocation to maintain patient safety.

INTRODUCTION

Respiratory complaints account for a significant proportion of emergency presentations. Symptoms experienced by the patient may range from mild to immediately life threatening. It is essential that emergency clinicians can identify patients at immediate risk of respiratory compromise. Subsequent to assessment, emergency clinicians must be able to implement appropriate interventions to maintain patient safety, provide adequate respiratory support and prevent further deterioration. This chapter will discuss the physiological changes that occur in respiratory failure and will present a methodical approach for assessing respiratory function, explore respiratory support strategies and detail five common adult respiratory emergencies.

RESPIRATORY FAILURE

Almost 7.5 million Australians (31% of population) have one or more chronic respiratory conditions, with 4.7 million (19% population) having hay fever, 2.7 million (11%) with asthma and 599,000 (2.5%) with COPD.[1] The upward trend of respiratory illness since 2007 has seen an increase from 9.9% to 11% of the population with asthma and a relative stability of COPD incidence.[1] Cause of death from respiratory diseases remained slightly higher during 2021 than for the same time in 2020, with the addition of two internationl standards (albeit conservative), the introduction of pulmonary disease and death from COVID-19 (recorded separate to established respiratory disease categories).[2] Three of the top ten causes of death, accounting for as many as one in seven deaths each year in Australia, are attributable to respiratory conditions, such as chronic lower respiratory diseases, pulmonary malignancy and influenza and pneumonia.[3] Respiratory compromise is a common clinical presentation that can be linked to an extensive range of causes (Table 21.1).[4] Common presentations, including asthma, COPD, pneumonia, pulmonary oedema and pulmonary emboli, will be specifically covered in this chapter, although it is acknowledged that there are many other clinical presentations which emergency clinicians may encounter in their practice.

TABLE 21.1 CAUSES OF RESPIRATORY COMPROMISE[4]

CATEGORY	DISEASE
Chest wall disorders	Chest wall restriction such as severe kyphosis or scoliosis Flail chest
Pleural abnormalities	Pneumothorax Haemothorax Pleural effusion Empyema
Restrictive lung disorders	Aspiration Atelectasis Bronchiectasis Bronchiolitis Pulmonary fibrosis Pulmonary oedema Acute respiratory distress syndrome COVID-related ARDS[5]
Obstructive pulmonary disease	Asthma Chronic obstructive pulmonary disease
Respiratory tract infections	Pneumonia Tuberculosis Abscess formation and cavitation Acute bronchitis
Pulmonary vascular disease	Pulmonary embolism Pulmonary artery hypertension

In New Zealand, the story is little different. Respiratory hospitalisations have been climbing since 2000 with the current rate of almost 1800 per 100,000 people in 2019, highest among those < 15 or > 65 years of age.[6] In particular, Pacific peoples and Māori rates of respiratory hospitalisation are both over twice the rate of the non-Indigenous population. The most common disease presentations include asthma, bronchiectasis, bronchiolitis, pneumonia and COPD. Asthma and COPD make up the greatest respiratory illness burden, with over 600,000 people taking medication for asthma alone. Childhood respiratory illnesses were significantly more prevalent (three to four times) among Māori and Pacific peoples. Respiratory disease was New Zealand's third most common cause of death at 3243 in 2017.

Regardless of the cause of respiratory failure, it is important to understand how physiological changes associated with respiratory failure contribute to alterations in gas exchange and increased work of breathing. Respiratory failure occurs when the exchange of oxygen and of carbon dioxide between the lungs and the atmosphere fails. Respiratory failure is defined as a partial pressure of arterial oxygen (PaO_2) that falls below 60 mmHg (hypoxaemia) or pressure of arterial carbon dioxide ($PaCO_2$) above 50 mmHg (hypercapnia).[4] This definition may be accurate yet not sufficient for paramedics where access to arterial blood gas (ABG) analysis may be inconsistent or entirely absent. The differentiation between respiratory distress and failure will be informed by the patient's history and physical signs that the patient has been overwhelmed by hypoxaemia or hypercapnia. Arguably, a critical finding will be a failure of respiration to maintain sufficient gas levels to allow for maintenance of normal consciousness.

Respiratory failure may be acute or chronic in nature, and can occur in patients with a normal respiratory system, as well as in those with existing chronic pulmonary disease. Acute respiratory failure is characterised by life-threatening derangements in PaO_2, $PaCO_2$ and acid–base balance. Those with chronic respiratory failure may have alterations in their arterial blood gas values that impact their activities of daily living (ADL) but are not usually life threatening. Patients with chronic respiratory issues may have very different normal vital signs and presentations which must be appreciated when establishing any baseline with which to make comparisons.

Respiratory failure is an important complication that may be associated with both respiratory and non-respiratory causes. Patients with pre-existing lung disease and those who smoke are at particular risk. A number of clinical conditions may also increase the chance of patients developing respiratory failure, including cardiac failure, renal failure and hepatic disease.[4]

MECHANISMS OF GAS EXCHANGE

For gas exchange to occur effectively there must be balance between alveolar ventilation and pulmonary capillary blood flow. During normal respiration the lungs are in balance and every litre of alveolar ventilation is matched (approximately)

FIGURE 21.1 VENTILATION AND PERFUSION MATCHING[7]

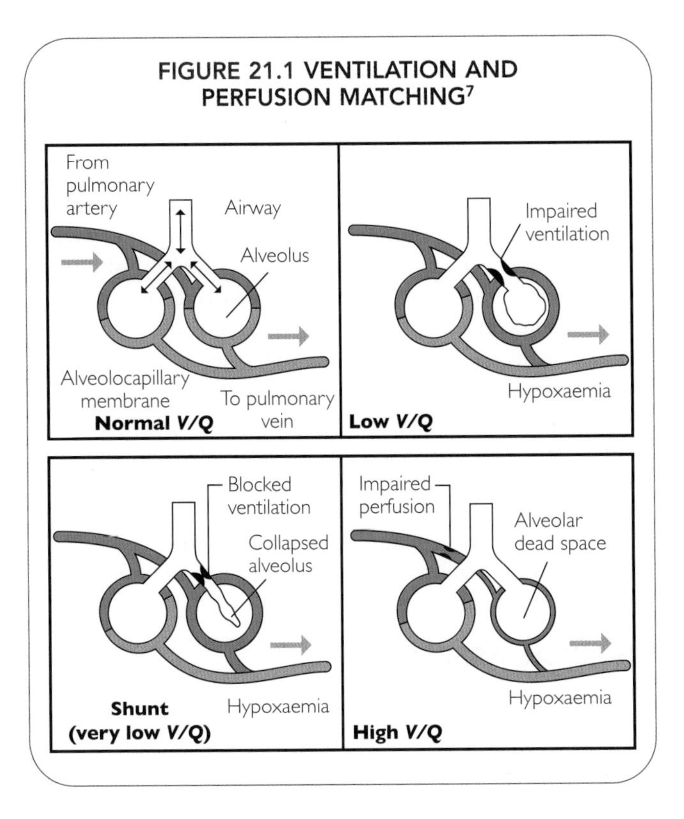

by a litre of pulmonary capillary blood flow. Changes in this balance are expressed as a ratio, called the ventilation–perfusion (V/Q) ratio. A high V/Q ratio is indicative of greater than normal ventilation or lower than normal perfusion, or both. A low V/Q ratio is indicative of lower than normal ventilation or greater than normal perfusion, or both (Fig. 21.1).[4] Alterations in V/Q matching can contribute to both hypercapnia and hypoxaemia. Hypercapnia, the increase in $PaCO_2$, occurs because of a decrease in tidal volume and/or respiratory rate (minute ventilation), in turn decreasing alveolar ventilation and CO_2 removal and can contribute to alterations in acid–base balance. A significant range of physiological effects result from hypercapnia, including decreasing pulmonary vascular permeability and lung oedema, altered airway resistance, and pulmonary vasoconstriction and intrapulmonary shunting.[8] Determinable through ABG analysis or capnography, hypercapnia is difficult to identify through physical assessment alone, since the rate and depth of breathing may appear normal in many hypercapnic patients. For paramedics where blood gas analysis is not available, suspicion of hypercapnia is based on capnography, patient history and patient assessment data.

Hypoxaemia occurs when oxygenation in the arterial blood is decreased. It can occur from the same mechanisms that lead to hypercapnia; however, hypoxia (reduced cellular oxygenation) may occur without alterations in pulmonary function and may be attributed to systemic abnormalities such as cardiac failure. Mechanisms that contribute to hypoxaemia include decreased alveolar oxygenation; decreased diffusion of oxygen from the alveoli into the pulmonary capillary; and decreased pulmonary capillary perfusion.[9] Clinical causes associated with these mechanisms are detailed in Table 21.2.[4]

TABLE 21.2 CAUSES OF HYPOXIA[4]

MECHANISM	COMMON CLINICAL CAUSES
Decrease in FiO_2	High altitude
	Low oxygen concentration of gas mixture
	Suffocation
Hypoventilation of the alveoli	Lack of neurological stimulation of the respiratory centre
	Defects in chest wall mechanics
	Large airway obstruction
	Fatigue/exhaustions in conditions causing prolonged increased work of breathing
Ventilation–perfusion mismatch	Asthma
	Chronic obstructive pulmonary disease
	Pneumonia
	Atelectasis
	Pulmonary embolism
	Acute respiratory distress syndrome
Alveolocapillary diffusion abnormality	Oedema
	Fibrosis
	Emphysema
Reduced oxygen carrying capacity of blood	Anaemia
	Methaemoglobinaemia
	Carbon monoxide poisoning
Inability of cells to utilise oxygen	Carbon monoxide and cyanide poisoning
Decreased pulmonary capillary perfusion (shunting of de-oxygenated venous blood to the systemic arterial circulation)	Intracardiac defects (e.g. atrial and ventricular septal defects)
	Intrapulmonary arteriovenous malformations

RESPIRATORY ASSESSMENT

PRIMARY SURVEY

As with any emergency presentation, patient assessment of a respiratory complaint begins with a primary survey assessment of airway, breathing, circulation, disability, exposure and a set of vital signs. The purpose of the primary survey is to identify life-threatening conditions and manage them immediately.[10–12] Comprehensive descriptions of a primary survey are detailed in Chapters 13 and 42. Gross signs of respiratory compromise that require immediate intervention may be identified during the primary survey. These signs include evidence of airway obstruction evidenced by stridor (an audible high-pitched inspiratory and/or expiratory noise suggestive of glottis/tracheal obstruction)[13] or stertor (audible, low-pitched snoring sound indicating pharyngeal/supraglottic obstruction).[14] Further signs that the patient requires immediate intervention include increased respiratory effort, marked accessory muscle use and work of breathing exhibited by: tachypnoea; decreased speech tolerance; pallor or cyanosis; hypoxia despite oxygen therapy; paradoxical chest wall movement; decreased air entry; and altered level of consciousness.[15,16] With very limited access to past history and without more complex assessment tools, these findings will be critical for paramedics when conducting a respiratory assessment.

At the completion of the primary survey and before proceeding further, clinicians must first reflect on their assessment findings and consider the following questions:

- Are immediate interventions required?
- Does the patient's condition warrant escalation, re-triage to higher category or transfer to an area of higher acuity within the emergency department (ED)?
- Particularly in the out-of-hospital setting, is there a requirement for other resources, including people and devices, to help extricate and move the patient and intensive care support to assist with advanced airway and ventilation management?

If the answer is 'yes' to any question, it may be necessary to immediately commence treatment or summon further assistance before taking a history and progressing to the comprehensive physical examination.[16,17] If no immediate interventions are required, continue on with the respiratory assessment.

CLINICAL HISTORY

The aim of respiratory assessment is to identify the adequacy of gas exchange, tissue oxygenation and the excretion of carbon dioxide.[18] During a comprehensive respiratory assessment, it is vital to review the patient's clinical history (Table 21.3), as this will guide the remainder of the examination and aid interpretation of clinical findings.[19,20]

Detailed patient history is a relative luxury for pre-hospital responders and important information about the patient's previous illnesses can commonly come from sources other than the patient, including family, general practitioner letters, hospital discharge records, nursing notes or residential aged care facility records. The patient themselves may be confused, unclear about their past history, or simply unable to speak. Other past history findings include medications, hospital patient information books, including old electrocardiographs and medical devices in the vicinity of the patient, such as nebulisers, CPAP therapy devices and oxygen cylinders.

The other element of patient history is the description of current events, including defining why help has been requested at this time, duration of the current illness episode and what therapies may have been employed already. The pattern of previous similar episodes, including significant deteriorations and hospital admissions, can be critical in predicting the likely course of events on this occasion.

The medical history will generally provide most of the information vital for determining the aetiology of the patient's respiratory distress. The first step is to determine the presence and duration of current symptoms, such as chest pain, breathlessness or cough. However, as many respiratory and cardiac conditions share similar symptoms, it is vital to question the patient for disease-specific symptoms (e.g. haemoptysis and risk factors for pulmonary embolism; fever and cough for pneumonia; nocturnal dyspnoea; peripheral oedema and a history of cardiac disease for congestive cardiac failure).

It is important to appreciate the distinction between detectable signs of respiratory difficulty and the symptoms of the problem the patient reveals through questioning. In some cases, patients may complain of feeling breathlessness that may be associated with a significant underlying illness. The level of complaint may not always be matched by the level of respiratory difficulty that can be clinically observed and assessed. On occasion, problematic breathlessness can be a significant problem in its own right and not supported by other clinical findings of respiratory difficulty or illness.[23,24]

The patient's medical history is the next important aspect of history-taking. In a patient with a known chronic respiratory illness, the cause of their current respiratory symptoms will most commonly be due to an exacerbation of this chronic respiratory disease or a complication related to it. Likewise, a history of cardiac failure should heighten suspicion for a cardiac cause of the patient's respiration distress.

PHYSICAL ASSESSMENT

Physical assessment includes inspection, palpation, percussion and auscultation. Using a systematic format during physical assessment ensures that clinicians avoid missing subtle signs while practising in the chaotic emergency environment. All patient assessment should start with a primary survey assessment.[10–12] A head-to-toe format may be useful with inspection, palpation, percussion and auscultation; however, another method may be used to identify relevant elements from each domain while assessing a body section before moving on to the next. Although a comprehensive respiratory physical assessment is detailed, clinical judgement should be used to identify the relevant aspects of respiratory assessment in relation to the particular patient presentation; for example, seeking evidence of inhalation injury in a patient with possible airway burns. Once signs of respiratory compromise are identified, escalation of care and implementation of appropriate interventions should take priority.

Elements of respiratory assessment can pose particular difficulties for emergency clinicians. Removal of clothing can increase patient exposure to bystanders or to the environment. It may be difficult to control the ambient noise or light. The paramedic in particular must find balance and compromise between these difficulties to allow proper and full assessment to take place.

PRACTICE TIP

The aim of respiratory assessment is to determine respiratory status, identify deterioration in patients at risk of life-threatening deterioration, and guide and evaluate the effectiveness of management.

Inspection

Inspection involves critical, purposeful direct observation using vision and hearing. The aim of inspection is to identify abnormalities, paying attention to both subtle and obvious changes.[18] Inspection begins with a general inspection, followed by an inspection of the head, neck and thorax.

TABLE 21.3 CLINICAL HISTORY OF A PATIENT WITH RESPIRATORY COMPROMISE[18–20]

AREA OF FOCUS	RATIONALE
Presenting complaint	A statement as to why the patient has attended the ED or called for pre-hospital assistance, e.g. 'increased shortness of breath'. This provides a starting point to guide specific areas of questioning relevant to the problem.
Allergies	Identify whether an allergic reaction is a factor in the current presentation, and avoidance of future exposure to known drug allergies during the hospital stay.
Medications	Identify what medications the patient is currently taking. Take notice of drug classes that may inform interpretation of physical assessment findings; e.g. beta-blocker drugs can inhibit sympathetic compensatory mechanisms such as increased heart rate. Medications may also give an indication of medical conditions that the patient forgets/doesn't understand, or may allude to severity of disease process and potential for future deterioration.
Past medical/surgical history	Identify conditions the patient has been diagnosed with and treated for in the past. Identify chronic illnesses such as chronic obstructive pulmonary disease, recent influenza, COVID, asthma, cystic fibrosis, heart failure, hypertension and cancer. Enquire if the patient is on a specific management plan and whether they adhere to it. Past surgical procedures and historical risk features that may be relevant to the current presentation should be identified; e.g. previous admission to ICU/HDU, previous deterioration requiring intubation or invasive interventions.[21]
Last menstrual period/ last meal	Possible pregnancy should be identified prior to radiation exposure, e.g. chest x-ray, computed tomography pulmonary angiogram (CTPA). Identify last meal if surgery and elective intubation are a possibility.
Familial history	Identify family history of pulmonary and cardiac disease.
Social history	Explore tobacco use (number of pack-years); inhaled drugs, e.g. marijuana. Identify recent overseas travel and exposure to environmental hazards such as chemicals, allergens, extreme heat/cold, animals within the home or worksite.
Events leading to presentation and associated signs and symptoms	Identify the sequence of events that led to the patient coming to hospital, and any associated symptoms. The sequence of events, mechanism of injury and associated symptoms provide clues to the underlying pathophysiology of the complaint, and may indicate particular investigations and interventions.
Dyspnoea	Questions regarding dyspnoea include: Does anything make it worse? Does it occur with exercise? Does it relate to position, e.g. worse when lying down/better when sitting up, or time of day? Does anything help improve the presentation?
Chest pain	Identify the presence of any pain/pressure/tightness in the chest, or radiation of pain to jaw/shoulder/arm. If the patient has had a complaint of chest pain, further questioning aims to help differentiate cardiac ischaemia, pleuritic or musculoskeletal origin. Also identify pain that is exacerbated by breathing with possibility of pleural involvement and adverse impact on inspiratory volume. A useful mnemonic to assess chest pain is PQRST: P—precipitating and palliating factors; Q—quality; R—region and radiation; S—severity, pain scale 1–10; T—time of onset and duration.
Sputum	Questions regarding sputum include changes in amount and colour. Yellow, green and brown sputum typically represent bacterial infection.[21] Clear or white may notify the absence of bacteria. Mucoid, viscid or blood-streaked may be a sign of viral infection. Frothy white or pink-tinged sputum can be a clinical symptom of pulmonary oedema.[22]
Cough	Coughs have various precipitants, such as inflammation to the respiratory mucosa, smoking, allergies, asthma and certain medications. Relevant questions involve identifying onset, precipitant factors, timing, frequency and whether or not it is productive.

HDU: high-dependency unit; ICU: intensive care unit.

General inspection

Note skin and mucous membrane colour as an indication of haemoglobin oxygen saturation.[25,26] Skin colour should be noted, with particular attention to whether the patient's skin is normal for them, pale, mottled or cyanotic. Peripheral cyanosis is noted in the extremities, including lips, earlobes and fingers; central cyanosis is a late sign and is noted in the oral mucous membranes, face and trunk as a bluish colour.[27,28] Where the patient's skin pigmentation is darker, cyanosis may be more difficult to discern. Favour sclera, tongue, fingernails and mucous membrane examination and make use of those who know the patient to comment on any perceived variation in skin appearance.[29] Cyanosis may become visible when arterial saturation drops below 85% and there is increased reduced haemoglobin;[18,27] however, it may not be visible during severe anaemia as there is insufficient haemoglobin present.[18,27] Any form of respiratory disease including pneumonia, COPD, adult respiratory distress syndrome (ARDS) and pulmonary oedema, can lead to cyanosis.[27,28] Peripheral cyanosis secondary to vasoconstriction, decreased cardiac output or vascular occlusion can occur in the presence of normal systemic oxygen saturation.[18,28] A mottled appearance to the skin can indicate poor tissue perfusion, as may occur with shock states. Cyanosis is subjective and should be accompanied by other forms of respiratory assessment, including pulse oximetry and ideally blood gas analysis.[28]

During general inspection, the patient's level of consciousness should be assessed. A baseline Glasgow Coma Scale (GCS) score is critical to note deterioration or improvement. Even minor changes in GCS are highly significant in respiratory distress. Confusion, drowsiness or GCS scores less than 15 can indicate severe distress or even respiratory failure.[30–32] More common are subtle changes in consciousness, which are often dismissed as difficult patient behaviours. An increase in agitation or anxiety or an altered consciousness level may be an indication of cerebral hypoxia or inadequate ventilation and resultant hypercapnia.[18] The patient's speech pattern should be assessed, while noting if they are speaking in sentences, phrases or words, or unable to talk. Moderate-to-severe respiratory distress is often reflected in a decreasing tolerance for speech.[18] This should be reflected during patient assessment by using short-answer questioning or having the patient nod where possible to minimise speech demands.

Identify the posture and activity of the patient and how much exercise the patient can tolerate prior to experiencing dyspnoea. This is particularly applicable for patients with chronic respiratory illness. Patients experiencing respiratory distress may sit or stand leaning forwards in a position known as 'tripoding', with their hands on their knees or a table. This helps to elevate the clavicles, giving a slightly greater ability to expand the chest on inspiration.[18] Alternatively, the patient who is slumped and unable to support themselves may indicate a state of respiratory failure.

Evidence of peripheral vasodilation may indicate hypercapnia. High levels of CO_2 result in dilation of vasculature,[7] and may be apparent in surface capillaries. Hypercapnia may also produce a flapping tremor noticeable in the hands.[7,18]

Clubbing of the fingertips is an abnormal enlargement, thinning and change in the angle of the fingernail bases, or, less commonly, those of the toes, is associated with chronic hypoxia[7,18] and is a good predictor for significant underlying respiratory illness, such as cancer or pulmonary fibrosis.[24]

Head

Pursed-lip breathing and nasal flaring may be seen in patients with respiratory distress;[33] mouth breathing versus via the nose, cyanosis of mucous membranes, decreased speech tolerance and alterations to level of consciousness may also be noted.[18] Pursed-lip breathing, in particular, is a technique often performed spontaneously, but can be taught to patients to use as a self-management strategy. Pursed-lip breathing involves providing resistance to expiration prolonging time for gas exchange and combating airway collapse and is particularly useful in COPD.[34]

Clinicians should listen for sounds of upper airway obstruction, evidenced by a snoring, stridor or gurgling noise on inspiration.[13] When there is a sudden onset of severe respiratory distress in a previously well person, particularly those at risk, including children and older people, the patient should be assessed for foreign body airway obstruction (FBAO).[35] If FBAO is suspected, the ANZCOR flowchart for management of FBAO should be followed and back blows and chest thrusts used as indicated.[35] Further information and the ANZCOR flowchart can be found in Chapter 14.

The oropharynx should be inspected for foreign bodies.[18] Where the patient is conscious, this may include looking for signs of choking, such as clutching the throat, sudden onset of coughing, wheezing from partly obstructed airways or unequal lung sounds. The unconscious patient may require visualisation under laryngoscopy or bronchoscopy to dislodge the foreign body. Signs of vomitus may be evident on the mouth, clothing or near the patient, suggestive of foreign body or aspiration occurrence. If inhalation burns are suspected, search for relevant evidence, including facial and nasal hair singeing, soot particles in mouth or nose, carbonaceous sputum, intraoral oedema or stridor or hoarse voice.[36] The head should also be inspected for signs of trauma, deformity or bruising that may affect the airway.[13]

Neck

Clinicians should inspect the neck for signs of trauma, bruising or swelling. Identify if the trachea is midline or deviated to the left or right.[18] A deviated trachea can indicate mediastinal shift, as may occur with tension pneumothorax, haemothorax or pleural effusion, which pushes the trachea away from the affected side, although it can be difficult to visualise and is a very late sign (see Chapter 45).[18] The trachea can also be pulled towards the affected side with atelectasis, fibrosis, tumours or phrenic nerve palsy.[19] Neck vein distension may be observed as jugular venous pressure rises and may be associated with increased intrathoracic pressure or ventricular dysfunction; this may be useful in assessing patients with cardiac disease and breathing difficulty.[37]

Chest

The chest should be fully exposed to facilitate examination. Out-of-hospital examination of the chest can be very different to the in-hospital examination and care must be taken when exposing any patient where public view is possible. This may be the case even if only other family members or friends are present or where particular observances are encountered, such as religious or cultural norms. Physical exposure of patients can also increase the risk of environmental hazard, if the temperature is low or it is windy. Paramedics may have to consider moving a patient to a more protected location to allow a thorough chest examination. Similarly, the presence of an appropriate chaperone may be sought where the patient is a child, female or has specific religious or cultural observances.

Observe for symmetrical movement of the chest wall during breathing. Asymmetry may indicate bronchial obstruction, pneumothorax, fibrosis or collapse of lobes.[18] Paradoxical movement is seen when some of or the entire chest wall moves inwards during inspiration and outwards on expiration. This may be seen in the presence of a flail segment of ribs, or severe respiratory distress in a young child.[18] Paradoxical breathing can also be seen where there is spinal cord injury and altered nervous control of the normal respiratory muscles.[38] There is more information about specific breathing patterns in chest and spinal injured patients in Chapters 45 and 47.

Observe for accessory muscle use. During breathing at rest, the diaphragm contracts and the intercostal muscles contract, pulling the ribs upwards and outwards.[7,26] This causes an increase in intrathoracic volume and negative pressure compared to the external atmosphere, causing net movement of air into the lungs.[7,26] A patient who is in respiratory distress may use additional muscles to aid the respiratory effort.[26] These include the sternocleidomastoid, scalene and trapezii muscles, which all contract to marginally pull the sternum upwards and increase the anteroposterior (AP) and transverse diameters of the thorax,[7,18,26] aiding in increasing inspiratory volume. Conversely, expiratory effort is typically more passive and largely reliant on natural chest elastic recoil. Internal intercostal muscles can add to this during forced exhalation. The abdominal muscles can be used to compress the abdominal compartment and force the diaphragm upwards, offering further assistance with expiration. This can be particularly prominent in smaller children, where a more upright and soft chest wall gives the diaphragm greater prominence.

The respiratory rate and rhythm should be carefully assessed. A normal rate is between 10 and 20 breaths/minute, with an inspiratory:expiratory ratio of 1:2.[18,26] Alterations to rate or rhythm of this ratio may indicate underlying conditions. Hypoventilation (rate < 10) can suggest a number of conditions, including respiratory centre depression, or increased intracranial pressure.[18] Tachypnoea is a respiratory rate > 20 and is often the first sign of respiratory distress,[18] and the most sensitive predictor of serious illness and risk of clinical deterioration.[39] Kussmaul respirations—breaths that are rapid, deep and caused by stimulation of the respiratory centre secondary to metabolic acidosis—may be observed if there is an attempt to increase removal of CO_2.[14] Prolongation of the expiratory phase of respiration may be noted in some respiratory disease, including COPD and asthma.

The chest wall should be examined for signs of trauma, bruising, deformity and scars from previous injury or surgery.[19,40] The shape of the thorax should also be inspected. The chest wall should be symmetrical, with the transverse diameter larger than the AP diameter. Barrel-shaped chests (where transverse and AP diameter are equal) are commonly associated with chronic obstructive respiratory disorders such as emphysema.[7,18] Other irregular anatomical features affecting the thorax and function include: pectus excavatum, where the sternum is depressed inwards; pectus carinatum, where the sternum and costal cartilages project outwards; kyphosis, a forward curvature of the spine; and scoliosis, a lateral curvature of the spine.[7,18]

Intercostal muscle recession may be commonly seen in children who have underdeveloped intercostal muscles, or thin or elderly patients.[19] Intercostal recession occurs during inspiration, where the intercostal muscles are sucked backwards between the ribs by intrathoracic negative pressure.[19]

PRACTICE TIP

COMPONENTS OF INSPECTION DURING RESPIRATORY ASSESSMENT

General

Level of consciousness

- Agitation/anxiety
- Speech
  - sentences/phrases/words/unable to speak
  - quality (hoarseness)

Skin colour

- Pallor/cyanosis
- Exercise tolerance/body position

Head and neck

- Nasal flaring
- Pursed-lip breathing
- Mouth vs nose breathing
- Evidence of trauma: deformity, bruising, wounds, swelling, burns
- Tracheal position
- Tracheal tug

Thorax

- Symmetry of chest wall movement
- Accessory muscle use, recession
- Rate, rhythm, pattern of breathing
- Evidence of trauma, wounds, deformity, flail, bruising, scars
- Anteroposterior vs transverse diameter of chest
- Alignment of spine: presence of kyphosis, scoliosis

Extremities

- Clubbing
- Oedema
- Peripheral cyanosis

Palpation

Structures in the neck and thorax should be palpated to locate abnormalities.

Neck

Palpate the position of the trachea; the trachea should be midline above the suprasternal notch.[18,19] Palpate for subcutaneous emphysema, which is a condition caused by a disruption to the alveoli, allowing air into the subcutaneous tissue.[19] The cause may be mechanical trauma, barotrauma from a high peak inspiratory pressure (PIP) or use of positive end-expiratory pressure (PEEP). Palpation of subcutaneous emphysema is likened to the sensation of rice paper under the skin.

Chest

The thorax should be palpated systematically, comparing left with right.[18] Commence above each clavicle and progress down the anterior wall, followed by palpation of each axilla and posterior chest wall.[18] Identify areas of bony or soft tissue tenderness, crepitus, depressions, bulges, pulsations, paradoxical movement and subcutaneous emphysema.[18] Respiratory excursion (expansion) is checked by standing behind the patient, placing the palmar surface of the hands on the patient's back with thumbs next to one another along the spinal processes at the approximate level of the 10th rib.[18] The thumbs should separate symmetrically on inspiration. An absence of symmetry indicates a problem with respiratory excursion on one or both sides of the chest.[18] The final stage of palpation is to identify tactile fremitus. This is the palpable vibration of the chest wall during speech. Assessment of tactile fremitus is completed by placing the ulnar aspect of one hand on the chest wall and requesting the patient to say 'ninety-nine'.[18] Vibration is better transmitted through solid than air-filled structures. A decrease in vibration transmission to the hand may be felt when air is present between lung and chest wall, such as with a pneumothorax; or when there is an increase of air per unit of lung tissue; for example, with emphysema.[19] An increase in vibration may be present with lung consolidation.[18]

Auscultation

Auscultation of the chest involves listening and interpreting the sounds transmitted through the thorax with a stethoscope.[18] A structured approach should be taken: auscultating the anterior, posterior and lateral aspects of the chest, comparing the left and right sides and listening throughout inspiration and expiration.[19,41] Auscultation can present difficulties for pre-hospital responders when patients are mechanically trapped, heavily dressed or postured to manage altered consciousness. Nonetheless, compromises in auscultation can deprive the assessor of valuable information and should not be readily accepted.

Breath sounds in the normal chest are created by airflow in the airways.[18] These are described as vesicular (normal) or bronchial (abnormal).[19,41]

- Vesicular sounds are heard in normal lung parenchyma where air flows through smaller bronchioles; the inspiratory phase is longer than the expiratory phase and the sound is soft and low-pitched.[17,18]
- Bronchial breath sounds are heard over areas of lung where the alveoli are filled with fluid (most commonly caused by pneumonia). The sounds of airflow through bronchi are efficiently transmitted through the abnormal fluid to the chest wall. The sound is high-pitched, harsh and loud.[18,19]

Adventitious noises are abnormal sounds created by fluid or sputum accumulation, obstruction, bronchoconstriction, inflammation or pleural lining pathology.[18,19] Common adventitious noises are crackles, wheezes, rhonchi and pleural rubs.[18,19]

- Crackles are caused by the opening of either collapsed alveoli or smaller airways.[18] The sound is a soft, high-pitched, brief clicking or popping sound, heard more commonly during inspiration.[18,19] They are often described as fine or coarse. Coarse crackles occur with fluid accumulations, as may occur if the patient has pneumonia and are typically the smaller airways being forced to reopen. They are heard in late inspiration. Crackles also occur with congestive cardiac failure, atelectasis of lung tissue and sometimes in an acute exacerbation of asthma. Typically, these are the finer crackle sounds and are produced at very end inspiration as alveoli are forced to reopen. Differentiating between these sounds can pose a particular difficulty for paramedics during examination due to noisy environments and where history may be partly unclear and there is no access to detailed medical records or more complex assessment methods, including x-ray. A focus on past and current history may offer further clues in assessment. Management options selected may have to be mindful of an uncertain diagnosis where the different possible options may conflict with each other.
- Wheezes are caused by air movement through narrowed or partially obstructed airways due to bronchoconstriction, increased sputum, mucosal oedema or foreign bodies.[18] Wheezes have a continuous musical sound.[18,19] The degree of airway narrowing may be indicated by the pitch of the wheeze, higher pitches being associated with greater obstruction.[18] During assessment, keep in mind that severely reduced airflow may be insufficient to produce enough wheeze to be audible.
- Rhonchi are a different type of continuous sound typified by a low-pitched rumbling noise.[18,19] They are caused by secretions in the larger airways and sometimes may be cleared by coughing.[18,19]
- A pleural rub, or friction rub, is more commonly heard on inspiration and is a grating or crackling sound.[18] It is caused by the rubbing together of inflamed parietal and visceral pleura.[18,19]

Whispered pectoriloquy refers to being able to hear clear, loud sounds through the stethoscope when the patient whispers.[18,19] Normally the whispered voice is heard only faintly and indirectly while auscultating.[18,19] An increase in sound transmission indicates the presence of consolidation or fluid, such as in pneumonia, pulmonary oedema or haemothorax.[18,19]

Absent air sounds over lung tissue indicate absence of air movement. This may be due to consolidation or obstruction. The absence of sound, or a quiet chest in a patient displaying increased respiratory effort, is an emergent sign requiring immediate escalation and intervention.[18,19]

As with exposing the chest to allow examination to occur, auscultation may also pose some difficulties for emergency clinicians. ED presentation is often sudden and allows the patient little or no time to prepare; therefore patients may be wearing clothes not intended to allow chest auscultation. Often many items of clothing have to be removed to allow access to the posterior and anterior chest. The temptation to leave out auscultation, perform only a partial assessment or listen over clothing is not an adequate assessment technique. Similarly, attempting to auscultate the chest by pushing the stethoscope upwards or downwards beneath clothing removes clues as to correct anatomical locations for performance.

Percussion

Percussion is challenging in the noisy pre-hospital and ED environments, and not often required. However, it does remain part of the formal, comprehensive, respiratory assessment. During percussion, one hand is placed flat to the chest wall with fingers separated. The other hand is used as a hammer, swinging from the wrist, the fingers striking the middle-finger distal inter-phalangeal joint (DIPJ) of the hand on the chest.[18] Percussion should be performed systematically starting from above the clavicles, comparing left and right of the chest, at 3–4 cm intervals.[18] The quality of the sound heard indicates the nature of the structures beneath the hand.[18] A dense structure such as consolidated tissue or liquid will give a dull sound, whereas air-filled structures will give a louder, hollow sound called tympany.[18,19]

EMERGENCY CARE CONSIDERATIONS FOR RESPIRATORY ISSUES

Respiratory issues are a common reason to seek emergency care. The assessment and management priorities remain the same for a respiratory issue (primary survey approach), whether or not the patient is in the pre-hospital or ED environment. Use of the appropriate protocol and related interventions must be dictated by the patient's clinical history and physical assessment. Severe airway and respiratory compromise must be identified early and used to determine the need for escalation of care or additional support for interventions. Respiratory difficulty may be the primary issue or it may be associated with other problems such as chest pain, trauma, infection or metabolic disorders. When respiratory issues are associated with another disorder, emergency clinicians must manage both the respiratory distress and the associated problem. All patients with respiratory difficulty must be treated as unstable with potential for deterioration.

DIAGNOSTICS AND MONITORING

Pulse oximetry

Pulse oximetry non-invasively monitors the saturation of haemoglobin in tissue capillaries by transmitting a beam of light through tissue to a receiver.[18,42] The amount of saturated haemoglobin alters the wavelengths of the transmitted light, which is then translated by the receiver into a percentage of haemoglobin saturation.[18,42] The oxygen saturation as measured by pulse oximetry (SpO_2) has a normal range of 95–99% at sea level when breathing room air.[18,19] The displayed value is an average of multiple readings over a 3–10 second window, reducing the effect of waveform variation caused by patient movement.[18,19] Limitations of SpO_2 monitoring should be taken into consideration when using this technology:

- Nail polish should be removed from the digit used,[18] although the effects of different colours is variable with some less problematic.[43,44]
- Poor peripheral perfusion due to shock or peripheral vasoconstriction will contribute to an inaccurate reading.[18]
- SpO_2 in an anaemic patient is an unreliable indication of oxygen transport to tissues. SpO_2 is only an indication of available haemoglobin saturation, rather than oxygen-carrying capability.[18,19] For example, a patient with haemoglobin of 60 g/L and SpO_2 of 99% will still have reduced capacity for oxygen transport to the tissues.
- During carbon monoxide (CO) poisoning, CO binds preferentially to haemoglobin. Pulse oximetry cannot differentiate between carboxyhaemoglobin and oxyhaemoglobin, and consequently in such cases pulse oximetry will not accurately indicate oxygen saturation of available haemoglobin.[18,19]
- Movement can affect the ability of emitted light to travel between the diode and receiver, affecting the accuracy of the results.[18]
- The SpO_2 value only reflects a part of the ventilation equation. Carbon dioxide is also important and any oxygen saturation must be considered within an overall patient context. Asthma, in particular, can cause a significant rise in CO_2 capable of causing altered consciousness and respiratory failure, but with the patient erstwhile maintaining tolerable oxygen saturation levels.[45,46]
  This can be worsened in the presence of cigarette smoking where pulse oximetry is unable to differentiate oxyhaemoglobin from carboxyhaemoglobin. Relying on pulse oximetry alone as a guide to severity of illness can be deceiving. Similarly, patients with COPD may have lower oxygen and higher carbon dioxide values than other patients as a normal finding for them. In such instances, the value of trend monitoring can be more important than any one finding alone.

PRACTICE TIP

Pulse oximetry is only an indication of saturation of available haemoglobin. Values should be interpreted in conjunction with clinical conditions such as low haemoglobin, poor peripheral perfusion and clinical history, such as exposure to carbon monoxide.

Capnography

End-tidal carbon dioxide ($EtCO_2$) monitoring, known as capnography, quantifies the amount of CO_2 at the end of expiration. It can be used to monitor a patient's level of arterial CO_2 when alveolar carbon dioxide ($PaCO_2$) closely approximates the carbon dioxide dissolved in the arterial blood ($PaCO_2$).[18,19] The $EtCO_2$ is usually 2–5 mmHg lower than the patient's $PaCO_2$. Normal values for $PaCO_2$ range between 35 and 45 mmHg.[18,19] See Chapter 16 for an explanation on applying capnography and end-tidal monitoring.

$EtCO_2$ monitoring is indicated immediately post-intubation as a gold-standard initial confirmation of endotracheal tube placement in the trachea. Thereafter, $EtCO_2$ monitoring can be used to gauge adequacy of mechanical ventilation and guide adjustment of minute volume.[14,47] Correlation between $EtCO_2$ and $PaCO_2$ should be confirmed by ABG measurement at the commencement of invasive ventilation.

Pre-hospital use of $EtCO_2$ can be important, given that point-of-care blood gas analysis is not routinely available, with use of $EtCO_2$ extending beyond confirming endotracheal intubation placement. $EtCO_2$ use is increasing with the recognition that pulse oximetry only reflects one part of the patient's respiratory status. In contrast, $EtCO_2$ has been demonstrated to more sensitively reflect changes in ventilation.[14,48] Use of $EtCO_2$ in non-intubated patients with the device attached to bag/valve/mask circuits or supraglottic airway devices is also increasing. There are other clinical problems for which $EtCO_2$ provides useful information. For patients with diabetic ketoacidosis, who develop a progressive metabolic acidosis, $EtCO_2$ may be useful in assessment and ongoing maintenance of any compensatory respiratory alkalosis.[14,48,49] Similarly, it may be useful to monitor $EtCO_2$ values in patients being intentionally hyperventilated to create a therapeutic respiratory alkalosis following tricyclic acid medication overdose.[19] Reduction in perfusion will cause reduction in alveolar perfusion and CO_2 expiration. Conversely, improvements will enhance this situation. This allows for use of $EtCO_2$ in monitoring cardiac arrest and shocked states.[14,48]

Arterial blood gases

The arterial blood gas (ABG) is an investigation that provides information regarding respiratory function in areas of acid–base balance, oxygenation, ventilation, tissue perfusion and compensation.[8,18,19] This information can be used to guide the respiratory management plan and interventions. Chapter 16 contains information on ABGs and blood glucose level sampling.

PRACTICE TIP

ARTERIAL BLOOD GAS (ABG)

The normal ranges for components of an ABG are as follows:[19]

pH	7.35-7.45
PaO_2	80-100 mmHg
SaO_2	95-99%
$PaCO_2$	35-45 mmHg
HCO_3^-	22-26 mmol/L

pH is a measurement of hydrogen-ion concentration within the blood and indicates acidity or alkalinity. A pH of < 7.35 indicates acidosis; a pH of > 7.45 indicates alkalosis.[18,19]

An ABG measures two factors that alter pH: $PaCO_2$ and bicarbonate (HCO_3^-).[19,50]

- $PaCO_2$ is the respiratory component of pH, and measures CO_2 dissolved in the blood.[18,19] High $PaCO_2$ will contribute to acidosis and low levels will result in alkalosis. CO_2 is a by-product of cellular metabolism and diffuses across the alveolar–capillary membrane for removal during alveolar ventilation.[4]
- HCO_3^- is a buffer produced by the kidneys, and the metabolic component of the pH.[19] If the body produces more acid than the kidneys can buffer ($HCO_3^- < 22$ mmol/L), acidosis will result; if too much HCO_3^- is produced ($HCO_3^- > 26$ mmol/L), alkalosis will result.[19]
- PaO_2 assesses the amount of oxygen dissolved in the blood.[19] After oxygen dissolves, it binds to haemoglobin to form oxyhaemoglobin.[4] The SaO_2 refers to the percentage of haemoglobin saturated with oxygen in arterial blood.

Six-step process to ABG analysis[19]

1. Analyse the pH
   - Determine if the pH is normal (7.35–7.45), acidotic (< 7.35) or alkalotic (> 7.45).
   - If the pH is within normal limits, establish if it is on the acidotic side of normal (7.35–7.39) or on the alkalotic side of normal (7.41–7.45).
2. Analyse the $PaCO_2$ changes (respiratory component of blood gas).
   - A low $PaCO_2$ of < 35 mmHg can be caused by hyperventilation and will result in respiratory alkalosis by removal of high amounts of CO_2.
   - Conversely, hypoventilation causes less CO_2 removal and causes the $PaCO_2$ to increase, resulting in respiratory acidosis (> 45 mmHg).
3. Analyse the HCO_3^- (metabolic component).
   - A value of < 22 mmol/L indicates acidosis; a value of > 26 mmol/L indicates alkalosis.
4. Match either $PaCO_2$ or HCO_3^- with the pH.
   - If $PaCO_2$ is high (acidosis) and pH low (acidosis), there is respiratory acidosis.
   - If $PaCO_2$ is low (alkalosis) and pH high (alkalosis), there is respiratory alkalosis.
   - If HCO_3^- is low (acidosis) and pH is low (acidosis), there is metabolic acidosis.
   - If HCO_3^- is high (alkalosis) and pH is high (alkalosis), there is metabolic alkalosis.
5. Determine if $PaCO_2$ or HCO_3^- move in the opposite direction to the pH.
   - If this occurs, compensation is present. Compensation aims to return the pH to normal parameters and can happen via respiratory (CO_2) or metabolic (HCO_3^-) compensation. The respiratory system can begin compensation immediately; however, metabolic compensation can take many hours.
   - If there is no change in the $PaCO_2$ or HCO_3^-, then compensation is not occurring.
   - If compensation is occurring (as seen by a change in the $PaCO_2$ or HCO_3^-), but the pH has not returned to within normal limits, this is termed a partial compensation. Full compensation is reflected by a pH within normal limits.
6. Analyse the PaO_2 and SaO_2 for hypoxaemia. This must be interpreted in the context of the inspired oxygen concentration. For example, the normal range for PaO_2 is usually between 80 and 100 mmHg when breathing room air, but a patient who has a PaO_2 in this range when receiving high-flow supplemental oxygen is most likely to have serious pulmonary pathology impairing gas exchange.

Examples of ABG results

1. pH 7.20
   $PaCO_2$ 50 mmHg
   HCO_3^- 25 mmol/L
   PaO_2 70 mmHg
   SaO_2 90%
   The pH is acidotic, and this corresponds with a high $PaCO_2$, which is also acidotic. The HCO_3^- is normal, so does not reflect an attempt at compensation. The PaO_2 is low and suggests hypoxaemia. Therefore, this ABG reflects a patient with an uncompensated respiratory acidosis with hypoxaemia.
2. pH 7.50
   $PaCO_2$ 30 mmHg
   HCO_3^- 24 mmol/L
   PaO_2 80 mmHg
   SaO_2 95%
   The pH is alkalotic, and this corresponds with a low $PaCO_2$ that also reflects alkalosis. The HCO_3^- is normal and therefore there are no attempts at compensation. The PaO_2 and SaO_2 are normal. Therefore, this ABG reflects a patient with an uncompensated respiratory alkalosis.

3. pH 7.20
   $PaCO_2$ 38 mmHg
   HCO_3^- 19 mmol/L
   PaO_2 85 mmHg
   SaO_2 96%
   The pH is acidotic which corresponds with a low HCO_3^- (acidosis). The $PaCO_2$ is within the normal range, suggesting no attempts at compensation; the PaO_2 and SaO_2 are also normal. This ABG reflects a patient with an uncompensated metabolic acidosis and normal arterial oxygenation.
4. pH 7.50
   $PaCO_2$ 38 mmHg
   HCO_3^- 29 mmol/L
   PaO_2 85 mmHg
   SaO_2 96%
   The pH is alkalotic which corresponds with a high HCO_3^- (alkalosis). The $PaCO_2$, PaO_2 and SaO_2 are normal. This ABG reflects a patient with an uncompensated metabolic alkalosis and normal arterial oxygenation.
5. pH 7.34
   $PaCO_2$ 50 mmHg
   HCO_3^- 30 mmol/L
   PaO_2 85 mmHg
   SaO_2 96%
   The pH is acidotic which corresponds with a high $PaCO_2$ (acidosis). The HCO_3^- is high (alkalosis). The acidotic pH and acidotic $PaCO_2$ suggest a respiratory acidosis. Because the HCO_3^- is alkalotic (opposite to the pH), this suggests an attempt at compensation. As the pH has not returned to normal limits, the compensation is not complete. This ABG reflects a patient with a partially compensated respiratory acidosis with normal PaO_2 and SaO_2 levels, suggesting adequate arterial oxygenation.
6. pH 7.44
   $PaCO_2$ 50 mmHg
   HCO_3^- 31 mmol/L
   PaO_2 70 mmHg
   SaO_2 92%
   The pH is normal and on the alkalotic side of normal, which corresponds with the HCO_3^- (alkalosis). The $PaCO_2$ is acidotic which is opposite to the pH, indicating that compensation is occurring; because the pH is in normal limits, there is full compensation. The PaO_2 and SaO_2 are low. Therefore, this is a fully compensated metabolic alkalosis with hypoxaemia.

Venous or arterial blood gas? When is a venous blood gas enough?

Arterial puncture for the purpose of obtaining ABGs carries elements of risk to the patient, is often a painful procedure, and presents another potential exposure to a sharp for the emergency care clinician.[51,52] Due to these considerations—and like any investigation—there should be a clear clinical necessity to obtain an arterial blood sample. Venous blood gases are an alternative to ABGs, able to provide clinical information that will influence diagnosis, management and interventions or referral and exposes the patient to less risk and pain. There are a number of elements traditionally acquired from an ABG which can be inferred from a venous blood gas (VBG).

PRACTICE TIP

VENOUS BLOOD GAS (VBG)

Normal VBG values are as follows:

pH	7.35–7.38
$PvCO_2$	44–48 mmHg
PvO_2	40 mmHg
HCO_3^-	21–22 mmol/L

The VBG cannot replace an ABG in all circumstances. While a VBG does give reliable data about arterial pH and HCO_3^- values and can be used to evaluate acid–base balance, it is not a reliable source of information about oxygenation. Measurement of pH on a VBG will be 0.04 less than for an arterial sample, and a venous HCO_3^- value is on average 0.52 mmol/L less than that of an arterial sample.[51] However, in acute illness there is a non-linear relationship between venous and arterial oxygen content. This means that PvO_2 cannot reliably be used as an indicator of PaO_2 in acutely or critically ill patients.

A study comparing VBG and ABG samples of 53 patients in acute respiratory illness or respiratory compromise found arteriovenous agreement for pH was close with narrow limits of agreement making venous pH clinically interchangeable with arterial pH; however, agreement for PCO_2 was poor, with unacceptably wide limits of agreement.[53] A meta-analysis considering this question also found insufficient correlation to allow for VBG to be used as a reliable substitute for ABG.[50]

If frequent ABG sampling is necessary; for example, with an unstable invasively ventilated patient, consider whether the insertion of an arterial line may be more appropriate to minimise trauma associated with frequent arterial puncture.

PRACTICE TIP

The risks and benefits of measuring ABGs should be considered in relation to information that may be more easily obtained through VBGs or non-invasive means such as $EtCO_2$ monitoring and pulse oximetry.

Peak flow and spirometry

Two methods of assessing airflow limitations and obstruction have been commonly available in the ED environment: peak flow and spirometry.

Peak flow testing may also be used in the community, and paramedics should seek information about peak flow if the patient routinely records this information as part of their management plan. The peak flow test measures 'peak expiratory flow rate' (PEFR), which is the maximum flow achievable from a forced expiration starting at full inspiration.[53,54] It only reflects resistance through the larger conducting airways and the reading is reached within the first tenth of a second on expiration.[55] Peak flow is most commonly used for home monitoring of asthma.[55]

More-sensitive information can be gained from *spirometry* although this is rarely used in the ED context. Spirometry measures two main values: forced vital capacity (FVC), which is the maximum volume of air expired from the point of maximal inspiration,[18,19] and forced expiratory volume (FEV_1), which is the volume of air exhaled during the first second of the exercise.[56] The ratio of these two measurements is then calculated (FEV_1 : FVC).[55] A value of < 80% of the predicted norm is indicative of an airflow limitation.[55] The predicted norm is calculated based on sex, height, age and race, and graphs depicting normal values across a range of parameters are commonly available.[7,56] In obstructive diseases, such as COPD or exacerbation of asthma, airflow is reduced and this will be reflected by a decreased FEV_1, and greater time taken to expire the full breath.[55]

For instructions on how to conduct a spirometry reading, see Chapter 16. For emergency clinicians, the additional information from PEFR does not make a major difference to management during acute exacerbations. Further, it can be quite difficult for patients to perform the PEFR during respiratory difficulty or when receiving nebulised therapy.

Chest x-ray

The chest x-ray is an extremely common and informative diagnostic tool for pulmonary and thoracic assessment within the ED. The image is used to assess lung fields, disease processes, the presence of trauma sequelae such as fractures, haemo- or pneumothorax, as well as the position of invasive lines and tubes. For a guide to systematic chest x-ray interpretation, see Box 21.1.[57]

BOX 21.1 A GUIDE TO SYSTEMATIC CHEST X-RAY INTERPRETATION[57]

CHEST X-RAY REVIEW

A. Appearance—chest view (AP, lateral, PA), airway, additional apparatus (ETT/tracheostomy, ECG leads, NGT), lung fields captured
B. Bones—fractures
C. Cardiac shadow—cardiac and costophrenic angles, aortic arch and width of mediastinum
D. Diaphragm—shape, breadth, depth (8th rib viewed) in lung field
E. Exposure—are the posterior spinous processes visible?
F. Fine lines (normal lung markings out to edge of lung field); fat lines (congested fluid volume); fuzzy lines (infection)
G. Gastric bubble
H. Hylus markings
I. Identification (MRN, name), position of patient

AP: anteroposterior; PA: posterior-anterior; ECG: electrocardiogram; ETT: endotracheal tube; MRN: Medical Records Number; NGT: naso-gastric tube.

SUPPORT OF RESPIRATORY FUNCTION

OXYGEN THERAPY

The administration of supplemental oxygen therapy has long been considered one of the most fundamental components of emergency medical and trauma management. Even colloquially referred to as 'the good gas', it was long thought to be unable to do any harm. In recent years the indiscriminate use of oxygen administration has come into question. Already widely criticised when used for managing exacerbations of COPD,[58,59] emergency clinicians now recognise that oxygen is not an inert and harmless therapy and hyperoxia may in fact result in significant patient harm. There is a growing body of evidence reporting that routine oxygen administration for non-hypoxaemic patients with acute coronary syndrome shows little clinical benefit and is in fact associated with increased infarct size and mortality.[60–62] There is also evidence that hyperoxia causes constriction of coronary vessels and worsening ischaemia.[63–65] Similarly, hyperoxia-induced vasoconstriction has been shown to cause reduction in cerebral blood flow and worsen outcomes in some acute neurological emergencies, including stroke severity and one-year survival.[60,66,67] Increasingly, emergency care clinicians are being guided by pulse oximetry to guide oxygen administration rather than indiscriminantly applied therapy. There is no evidence that patients who are normoxaemic with or without the complaint of shortness of breath benefit from oxygen therapy.[63,68] Patients with no history of COPD should have an oxygen saturation target of 94–98%, and in patients with COPD a target of 88–92% is appropriate.[63,68]

Oxygen therapy devices are categorised as low-flow or high-flow devices that provide either a fixed or a variable concentration of oxygen. *Low-flow devices*, such as standard nasal cannula, deliver flows of gas, usually between 1–3 L/min, and no more than about 6 L/min, as rates higher than this are poorly tolerated due to discomfort caused by drying of the nasal mucosa. This rate of flow is well below the normal inspiratory flow demand of 30 L/min, and consequently the remainder of airflow is obtained from room air. The entrainment of room air that occurs with low-flow devices means that the fraction of inspired oxygen (FiO_2) varies from breath to breath and is dependent on the patient's minute ventilation. By contrast, *high-flow devices* are able to accommodate a patient's inspiratory demand and maintain a fixed FiO_2, irrespective of the patient's respiratory rate and tidal volume. A choice regarding appropriate oxygen therapy and delivery device should be dictated by the patient's support requirements, whether in the pre-hospital or the emergency setting. The most commonly used oxygen therapy devices are described in Table 21.4.[18,68] See Chapter 16 for an explanation of inserting a range of airway management devices.

Home oxygen therapy is provided in some cases for the chronically hypoxemic patient, typically with relatively stable COPD or other chronic illnesses such as pulmonary fibrosis. Patients most often make use of oxygen concentrators capable of utilising available room air with nitrogen removed to increase FiO_2. Commonly these are used to provide long-term oxygen therapy for periods of the day or night, usually delivered through nasal cannula at less than 4 L/min. Limited improved quality of life and reduced mortality outcomes have been shown. Similarly, home oxygen therapy can be used to minimally reduce dyspnoea during palliative care.[69]

TABLE 21.4 COMMON OXYGEN THERAPY DEVICES[19,68]

DEVICE	TYPE	DESCRIPTION AND DELIVERY RATES
Nasal cannula	Low flow	Delivers flow rates of 6 L/min or less
		Delivers FiO_2 of 0.24 (at 1 L/min) to 0.40 (at 5-6 L/min)*
Simple mask	Low flow	Design acts as an oxygen reservoir. Holes in the mask allow entrainment of room air
		CO_2 accumulates in the mask, so oxygen flow rates of at least 5 L/min are required to flush CO_2 out of the mask
		Delivers FiO_2 of 0.3-0.6 at flow rates of 5-10 L/min*
Partial-rebreathing mask	Low flow	Simple facemask with the addition of a 300–600 mL reservoir bag
		Oxygen flow should be set so that the bag remains inflated on inspiration (usually 8-15 L is sufficient)
		Delivers FiO_2 of 0.3-0.6 at flow rates of 5-10 L/min*
Non-rebreathing mask	Low flow	Design similar to partial-rebreathing mask, but with a one-way valve between the mask and the reservoir bag. During exhalation the reservoir fills with 100% oxygen. Mask port valves close on inspiration, preventing entrainment of room air
		Oxygen flow rate should be set so that the bag remains inflated on inspiration
		Delivers FiO_2 of 0.6-0.8 at flow rates of 10-15 L/min
Air-entrainment mask (e.g. Venturi mask or multi-vent mask)	High flow	Consists of a facemask, jet nozzle and entrainment ports
		Oxygen is delivered through the jet nozzle which increases velocity. Entrainment of ambient air occurs because of viscous shearing forces between the gas travelling through the nozzle and the ambient air
		FiO_2 is dependent on the size of the nozzle and the entrainment ports, and can vary from 0.24 to 0.70
		Flow to the mask must exceed the patient's peak inspiratory flow in order to deliver a fixed FiO_2
High-flow nasal cannula	High flow	Usual flow rates 30-60 L/min.
		Delivers FiO_2 of 1.0 at flow rates of 60 L/min
		Increasing level of PEEP flow dependent

**Assuming a constant tidal volume, inspiratory–expiratory ratio, inspiratory time and respiratory rate.*

In addition to commonly used oxygen therapy devices, the use of humidified high-flow nasal cannulae (HHFNC) is now a favoured method of delivering oxygen to spontaneously breathing patients who may have high oxygen requirements. Conventional oxygen therapy via nasal cannula or facemask is limited in maximum delivery flow and will not always prove sufficient in relieving hypoxemia. Non-invasive ventilation alternatives are not always well tolerated. HHFNC can provide high oxygen flows greater than 30 L/min allowing for inspired oxygen fraction (FiO_2) to vary from 60 to 100%.[70] The aim of HHFNC use is to exceed the patient's inspiratory flow demands, so that dilution of delivered oxygen does not occur. With the delivery of high flows directly into the nares, a flushing effect occurs in the pharynx.[70–72] The anatomical dead space of the upper airway is flushed by the high incoming gas flows. This creates a reservoir of fresh oxygen available for each and every breath, minimising rebreathing of carbon dioxide (CO_2).[70–72] When using HHFNCs, the mean airway pressure may increase,[19] although this could be influenced by a number of factors, including the flow rate, structure of the upper airway, cannula size, and whether the patient breathes through the nose or the mouth.[71,72] The increasing body of evidence regarding the effectiveness of HHFNCs as an oxygen-delivery method in adults suggests they are effective in improving oxygenation in patients with hypoxic respiratory failure, such as ARDS or pulmonary oedema,[70,73] with some limited improvement shown in COPD exacerbations.[70] HHFNCs are also increasingly used for patients with blunt chest trauma[63,74] and are reasonably well tolerated by patients. HHFNCs may also contribute to a decrease in work of breathing and provide a minimal level of end-expiratory pressure.[70]

The administration of supplemental oxygen is indicated when hypoxaemia is present and should be titrated so that the minimum amount of oxygen required to overcome the hypoxaemia is delivered to the patient. Some patients with chronic respiratory disease will exhibit both hypoxaemia and hypercarbia. The notion of a hypoxic drive theory, which proposed that oxygen administration to this group of patients could result in apnoea, cardiorespiratory arrest and death because administration of oxygen removed the patient's stimulus to breathe, has long been associated with acute COPD exacerbation management, but has been called into question.[69,75] There is no evidence to suggest that patients with hypoxaemia and hypercarbia should not receive oxygen therapy sufficient to address severe hypoxaemia, and failure to do so may result in further clinical deterioration.[68,69]

When supplemental oxygen is administered, elevations in $PaCO_2$ may be observed in some patients. This increase in $PaCO_2$ appears to be related to changes in ventilation–perfusion matching in the lung where the compensatory diversion of circulation away from hypoxic, non-ventilating lung units is overridden by oxygen delivery. This compensatory diversion might improve oxygen delivery, but does little to increase CO_2 removal, which remains in the circulation despite increased oxygenation. Further, the Haldane effect causes a further increase in $PaCO_2$. The better-oxygenated haemoglobin molecules are less able to attach the increasing carbon dioxide molecules and the ability to buffer the excess, causing acidosis.[76] In contrast to previous theory, it is not the consequence of changes in the patient's respiratory drive, respiratory rate or tidal volume. In short, when oxygen is administered $PaCO_2$ will increase, but not because the patient stops breathing.

The clear message for patients who exhibit both hypercarbia and hypoxaemia is that sufficient oxygen needs to be administered to ensure an adequate PaO_2 for the patient, being mindful that excessive amounts of oxygen will needlessly worsen V/Q matching and gas exchange. The critical determinant is what constitutes hypoxaemia in the patient with COPD. While a normal SpO_2 target may be 94% or greater, the desired target range in a patient with COPD may in fact be as low as 88–92%, with supplemental oxygen only required below that.[59,68,76–79] There is good evidence that paramedics administer greater oxygen therapy concentrations than are required without providing sufficient ongoing patient assessment.[80,81]

PRACTICE TIP

Patients, including those with COPD, require sufficient supplemental oxygen to reverse hypoxaemia. Oxygen should be titrated to individual patient requirements. Hypoxaemia in the COPD patient may be defined differently to other clinical problems with intentionally lower targets used to guide management.

NON-INVASIVE VENTILATION

In the absence of an endotracheal tube, non-invasive ventilation (NIV), delivered through the application of positive pressure, can be used as a respiratory support strategy. Compared with invasive mechanical ventilation, the use of NIV has benefits that include improved survival, fewer complications, increased comfort and decreased cost.[77,82–84] NIV can be used in acute, chronic, hypoxaemic and hypercapnic conditions. NIV efficacy is well established in hospitals, and now similarly well supported in pre-hospital application. Prospective and retrospective studies of pre-hospital CPAP looking typically at APO, and less commonly COPD, asthma and pneumonia, have all been able to demonstrate clinical patient vital sign improvement, decreased intubation rates and in some cases decreased mortality.[85–88]

More recently, similar advantages have been demonstrated in the management of respiratory failure associated with COVID-19. Such patients pose particular challenges, including the airborne infectious risk of aerosol formation. NIV, including CPAP, has been demonstrated to achieve desired respiratory support as with other pulmonary pathologies, particularly ARDS, which COVID-19 can be considered a variation of.[5] Somewhat uniquely, this has commonly been in conjunction with prone posturing.[89–91]

Appropriately-applied NIV is usually adequate to support the work of breathing required for adequate ventilation. While reduced ventilator effort is particularly important in the patient with respiratory failure, NIV may also alter cardiac load and therefore contribute to a decrease in cardiac oxygen demands and adrenergic stimulation. With application of NIV, a decrease in respiratory work occurs, which improves the balance between oxygen delivery and demand, and results in increased mixed venous PO_2 and PaO_2.[85] Improvements in oxygenation may also be attributed to the increase in mean airway pressure.

In the setting of acute respiratory failure, the goal of NIV is to rest the respiratory muscles and increase alveolar ventilation. Importantly, alveolar collapse is reduced, leading to substantially reduced work of breathing in reopening them. Through these processes, gas exchange is enhanced. In the ED, NIV is most commonly used as a respiratory support strategy for patients presenting with respiratory failure caused by cardiogenic pulmonary oedema, acute exacerbation of COPD, asthma and hypoxaemic respiratory failure and community-acquired pneumonia.[85,92,93] Despite this, evidence remains less conclusive for pneumonia presentations, with NIV failure rates as high as 50% of patients despite some noteworthy success.[94,95] Current research supports the effectiveness of NIV for exacerbations of both COPD and acute cardiogenic pulmonary oedema.[68]

Evidence supporting the use of NIV in asthma and hypoxaemic respiratory failure is not as abundant and may be conflicting.[96–100] With pulmonary oedema, alveolar collapse arises from surfactant washout. Positive end-expiratory pressure (PEEP) helps to maintain alveoli from this collapse and provide rest from subsequent effort to reopen them. Where the disease is in the lower airways, this same pressure helps to keep those airways from collapsing during expiration, maintaining time available for expiratory airflow.

For NIV to be effective as a respiratory support strategy, there must be careful consideration of patient suitability and selection of appropriate equipment, such as the ventilator and the patient interface.

Patient selection

Success rates with NIV are dependent on its use in appropriate patient populations. NIV is being increasingly used to treat patients with respiratory failure who otherwise meet criteria for intubation and ICU admission, but where underlying poor

BOX 21.2 SELECTION CRITERIA FOR USE OF NON-INVASIVE VENTILATION IN ACUTE RESPIRATORY FAILURE[55,99]

1. Acute respiratory failure with potential to reverse over hours to days.
2. Evidence of need for respiratory support:
   - moderate to severe respiratory distress
   - increased respiratory rate (> 24 breaths/minute for chronic obstructive pulmonary disease, > 30 breaths/minute for hypoxaemia)
   - use of accessory muscles evident
   - arterial blood gases showing respiratory acidosis or PaO_2/FiO_2 of < 200

BOX 21.3 CONTRAINDICATIONS FOR NON-INVASIVE VENTILATION[55,99,103]

- Haemodynamic instability
- Myocardial ischaemia, unstable angina
- Unable to protect airway, including impaired cough or swallowing
- Copious respiratory secretions
- Uncooperative, agitated or depressed level of consciousness
- Difficulty fitting mask (facial burns, trauma)
- Head injury with unstable respiratory drive
- Recent upper airway or gastrointestinal surgery
- Severe vomiting or haematemesis
- Severe haemoptysis

health prognosis makes this undesirable.[101,102] This can include elderly patients and those with chronic or even palliative illnesses. This group can include end-stage COPD, upper airway obstructions, neuromuscular diseases and malignancy, all provided respiratory failure is central and patient suffering and distress is to be minimised. In some instances, use of the high-flow nasal cannula can also offer some palliative benefits.[102] Knowledge of factors that are indicative of success or failure can assist with determining for which patients NIV might be suitable. Patient selection is detailed in Box 21.2.[55,99]

It must be remembered that non-invasive ventilation is only capable of supporting spontaneous ventilation and not substituting for absent or inadequate respiratory effort. Impaired consciousness is a key contraindication to NIV.[100,103] An important general consideration is that NIV is not suitable for patients with advanced respiratory failure, as evidenced by significant CO_2 retention and acidaemia.[99] Further, if a trial period of therapy fails to provide desired improvement, or the patient deteriorates, therapy should be discontinued and an alternative strategy implemented.[103] Additional contraindications for NIV are listed in Box 21.3.

Equipment selection

There are many different ventilators through which NIV can be delivered, including those designed specifically for NIV; critical care ventilators designed for invasive mechanical ventilation; and portable positive-pressure ventilators designed for use in the home. The choice of ventilator will be dependent on availability and suitability for patient need.[55]

For pre-hospital use, any NIV device must ideally be lightweight and compact, easy to use and not excessively expensive. A critical determinant is the need to be sparing in oxygen consumption, given the limited capacity for gas storage in most ambulances.

In the ED, bi-level pressure-limited ventilators are the most common, although critical care ventilators can also be used, some of which may have a specific NIV setting. Bi-level pressure-limited ventilators deliver pressure-assist or pressure-support ventilation. Bi-level ventilators deliver a pre-set inspiratory positive airway pressure (often referred to as IPAP) and positive end-expiratory pressure (PEEP or EPAP). Support of ventilation is provided by the difference between these two set pressure levels. Most ventilators provide a maximum pressure of 20–35 cmH_2O and have the capacity to deliver supplemental oxygen. These ventilators are particularly useful for NIV (where it may be difficult to achieve a leakproof seal with the mask), as there is the ability to increase inspiratory flow and provide leak compensation. Some bi-level pressure-limited ventilators have limited capability to delivery an FiO_2 above 0.50, and therefore may not be suitable for patients with hypoxaemic respiratory failure.

Bi-level pressure-limited ventilators differ from critical-care ventilators in that they usually have a single ventilator tube. This design may contribute to rebreathing and increased $PaCO_2$.[55,105] Rebreathing can be minimised by using masks with in-mask exhalation ports or non-rebreathing valves.[99] Ensuring the EPAP is greater than 4 cmH_2O provides higher flow during exhalation, which assists with removal of CO_2 from the mask and tubing.[55,104]

There are a variety of interfaces available and in an acute care setting it is useful to have a selection at hand, so that the most appropriate mask can be rapidly applied. The oronasal mask is the most commonly used mask in the ED setting, although it limits the patient's ability to communicate verbally, eat and expectorate.[104] The advantages and disadvantages of patient interfaces used in NIV are listed in Table 21.5. The most common challenge with the patient interface is leak minimisation. Using a mask that is too large will often contribute to an increase in leaks.[104] As a general guide, the smallest mask should be selected. When assessing best fit of nasal masks, the landmarks that should come closest to the interface are the nasal bridge, the skin on the side of the nares and just above the upper lip. For oronasal masks, the landmarks should be just outside the sides of the mouth, the area just below the lower lip and the nasal bridge.[55,104] More recently, full-facemasks have been developed that provide better patient comfort and tolerance and often fewer problems with air leaks.

Initiation and management of NIV

Commonly, the initiation of NIV will be pre-hospital or in the ED. The most important step in initiating NIV is patient education and emotional support from the emergency clinician, as patients are often anxious and combative as a result of

TABLE 21.5 ADVANTAGES AND DISADVANTAGES OF PATIENT INTERFACES USED IN NON-INVASIVE VENTILATION[55,105]

INTERFACE	ADVANTAGES	DISADVANTAGES
Nasal mask	Easy to fit	Mouth leaks
	Less feeling of claustrophobia	Eye irritation
	Low risk of aspiration	Facial skin irritation
	Allows patient to cough and clear secretions	Nasal bridge ulceration
	Maintains ability to speak and eat	Oral dryness
	Minimal dead space	Nasal congestion
		Increased resistance through nasal passage
Facemask (oronasal mask)	Reduces air leakage through the mouth	Increased risk of aspiration
	Less airway resistance	Increased risk of asphyxia
		Increased dead space
		Claustrophobia
		Difficult to secure and fit
		Facial skin irritation
		Nasal bridge ulceration
		Patient must remove mask to eat, drink, expectorate
Total facemask	Reduced risk of pressure sores	Increased risk of aspiration
	Less claustrophobic	Increased risk of asphyxia
		Increased dead space

TABLE 21.6 COMPLICATIONS OF NON-INVASIVE VENTILATION AND POSSIBLE SOLUTIONS[55,105]

COMPLICATIONS	SOLUTION
Mask-related problems	
Discomfort	Decrease strap tension
Nasal redness, ulceration	Check mask fit
Poor fit	Try new mask
Air-pressure- and airflow-related problems	
Sinus and ear pain	Lower mask pressure
Nasal dryness	Humidification
Nasal congestion	Decongestants, nasal steroids
Gastrointestinal insufflations	Lower pressures
Air leaks	
Under mask	Re-seat mask, tighten straps
Through mouth	Use chin strap to close mouth
Into eyes	Tighten straps, use new mask
Asynchrony	
Failure to trigger	New ventilator
Failure to cycle	Shorten inspiratory time
Failure to ventilate	Use leak-compensating ventilator

hypoxaemia. It is often useful to allow the patient, if they are able, to hold the mask in place in the initial stages of commencing NIV. To enhance patient comfort, it is best to begin with lower pressure levels; inspiratory pressures of 8–12 cmH_2O and expiratory pressures of 4–5 cmH_2O may provide a useful starting point. Upward titration of these levels (by 1–2 cmH_2O with each adjustment) can occur as the patient begins to tolerate NIV.[103,105] NIV can be used with continuous positive airway pressure (CPAP), where only an expiratory pressure is applied, or with bi-level ventilation, which has both an inspiratory pressure and an expiratory pressure.[55]

Patient tolerance and comfort are key to successful use of NIV. Patient tolerance is identified through a decrease in the respiratory rate, and a reduction in inspiratory muscle activity and compliance with NIV itself. If these clinical signs are not evident, steps should be made to improve tolerance. This may include refitting the mask, adjusting the ventilator settings and, most importantly, providing ongoing patient support. Ongoing patient monitoring should include heart rate, respiratory rate and pulse oximetry. After the patient has had an opportunity to adjust to NIV, an ABG may be taken to assess gas exchange. An improvement in PaO_2, $PaCO_2$ and pH should be evident. If the patient has chronic hypercapnia, an improvement in $PaCO_2$ may occur over a longer period of time.[55]

Common problems encountered with NIV include mask-related problems, air-pressure and airflow-related problems, air leaking and asynchrony.[103] Suggested remedies are provided in Table 21.6. Occasionally patients may become restless during therapy. Some pre-hospital guidelines allow for mild sedation to facilitate providing respiratory support. If sedation is to be considered, then caution must be taken to ensure that consciousness and respiratory effort are not compromised. Sedation may also be used in hospital with the intention of allowing for application of therapy while maintaining the patient sufficiently awake;[103,106,107] however, the safety and efficacy of this practice remains in question due to its association with failure of NIV and increased mortality.[103,108]

Adjuncts to NIV include humidification of the gas. Excessive drying of the mucosa may occur during NIV and may contribute to patient discomfort and non-compliance.[103] Humidification of inspired gases is generally recommended, except for patients with acute cardiogenic pulmonary oedema. Humidification should be achieved through the use of a passover-type heated humidifier, as heated bubble humidifiers and heat–moisture exchangers (HME) can increase airway resistance and the work of breathing.[55] The initial stages of NIV may require considerable nursing time and expertise. Consequently, appropriate patient allocation should occur with, whenever possible, the emergency clinician providing care to the one patient only.[34]

When to initiate therapy in pre-hospital practice can require careful consideration. The usual intention of pre-hospital care is to safely convey a patient from the community to a higher level of care and patient transport to the ED requires a balance between critical at-scene management and in-transit therapies. Preferred posturing of the patient can be challenging as can the logistics of concurrent movement of equipment while maintaining ongoing therapies and avoiding undesirable interruptions. The patient with respiratory distress, in particular, can deteriorate with even mild exertion or if left briefly without sufficient respiratory support. It is sometimes more advantageous to settle the patient with initial therapies, including NIV, and then undertake careful and consider movement of the patient. For patients with NIV, oxygen cylinders and ongoing vital sign monitoring, movement typically requires suitable equipment and sufficient personnel to maintain safety for everyone involved in the move.

PRACTICE TIP

Emergency care management and patient support is critical to the success of non-invasive ventilation. Movement of patients with respiratory distress requires careful planning, appropriate equipment and sufficient personnel to ensure safety and effectiveness.

INVASIVE MECHANICAL VENTILATION

The objectives of mechanical ventilation are to reduce respiratory distress and reverse acute respiratory failure. Patients who require respiratory support, but for whom NIV may not be appropriate, will require endotracheal intubation and mechanical ventilation (see Chapter 16 for information about intubation and airway management). Once intubated, a decision must be made regarding the most appropriate ventilation strategy for the patient. With full ventilator support, the ventilator maintains effective alveolar ventilation irrespective of patient effort. Partial ventilator support is provided when the patient is capable of participating in the work of breathing and contributes to maintaining alveolar ventilation. In the ED, the degree of respiratory distress may mean that full ventilator support is required. However, it is important that patient assessment occurs to avoid inappropriate use of full ventilator support, which may contribute to muscle wasting and atrophy.

PRINCIPLES OF MECHANICAL VENTILATION

There are numerous mechanical ventilators in use across Australia and worldwide. Many EDs and EMS providers use critical-care ventilators, which are commonly seen in the intensive care setting, while others may use ventilators that have less versatility.[55] It is critical to appreciate the capabilities and limitations of the ventilator being used, as key features, such as spontaneous breathing and pressure support, may not be possible with the simpler devices.

Understanding the principles of mechanical ventilation enables healthcare providers to effectively and safely use a wide variety of devices. The four variables that are controlled during inspiration are pressure, flow, volume and time. The primary variable that the ventilator adjusts during inspiration is referred to as the control variable. When volume is controlled, the inspiratory pressure varies. Conversely, when pressure is controlled, volume and flow are variable. Because ventilators are microprocessor-controlled, the ventilator can change, breath by breath, which variable is controlled on inspiration.

There are four phases to the delivery of a single breath: the change from expiration to inspiration (commonly referred to as triggering); the inspiratory phase; the change from inspiration to expiration (commonly referred to as cycling); and exhalation. Table 21.7 provides a description of each phase of the respiratory cycle, and Table 21.8 provides a description of common breath-delivery strategies used in the ED.

Consideration also needs to be given to setting delivery parameters on the ventilator. The respiratory rate, tidal volume (or inspiratory pressure), FiO_2, PEEP and inspiratory: expiratory ratio all need to be set. A general guide to setting ventilation parameters is provided in Table 21.9; however, clinicians are reminded that these settings will need to be modified with consideration for the patient's clinical condition, age and respiratory function. Healthcare practitioners who commonly work with ventilated patients and who make clinical decisions about ventilation strategies are encouraged to read more widely in this area.

Management of the ventilated patient

While the ED is not designed to provide ongoing care to critically ill patients who require invasive mechanical ventilation, resource allocation at times prevents timely admission to the intensive care unit. For this reason, it is imperative that a nurse working in the ED has a sound foundational knowledge of mechanical ventilation.[55,108] Patients who are receiving mechanical ventilation in the pre-hospital setting or ED are likely to have received sedation, analgesia and neuromuscular blockade. The effect of these drugs means that ventilated patients will require frequent and diligent fundamental care, including, but not limited to, mouth care, eye care, pressure-area care, positioning and psychological support (see Chapter 13).[55] Specific issues that relate to the care of the ventilated patient include patient assessment, troubleshooting ventilation and transportation of the intubated and ventilated patient.

PRACTICE TIP

The importance of fundamental care for the mechanically ventilated patient, such as mouth care, eye care, pressure-area care and psychological support, should not be underestimated and is vital to preventing complications.

PATIENT ASSESSMENT

The use of positive pressure ventilation has a direct effect on the pulmonary system and affects the cardiovascular, renal and other organ systems. The pulmonary system is designed to allow increased blood flow simultaneous with lowering of intrathoracic pressure and alveolar filling during inspiration. This allows for maximum pulmonary capillary flow just as alveoli are fully inflating. Positive pressure ventilation produces the opposite of this: intrathoracic pressure increases with alveoli filling meaning reduced capillary blood flow at this optimal time. Ongoing assessment of heart rate, temperature, blood pressure

TABLE 21.7 PHASES OF THE RESPIRATORY CYCLE[4]

PHASE	DESCRIPTION
Beginning of inspiration–triggering	*Time-triggered* when the ventilator delivers a breath after a set time.
	Pressure-triggered when patient effort is sufficient to decrease circuit pressure to the pre-set pressure sensitivity level.
	Flow-triggered when the patient effort is sufficient to drop the flow in the circuit to the pre-set flow trigger level.
Inspiration	Inspiration occurs from the beginning of inspiratory flow until the beginning of expiratory flow.
	Pressure, flow, volume or time can be limited during inspiration. The variable is limited but this does not end inspiration.
	Pressure limiting allows pressure to rise but not to exceed the specified pressure. Pressure-limited breaths may be used where lung compliance is poor.
	Volume limiting establishes the maximum volume to be delivered. If patient lung compliance is poor, volume-limited breaths may be terminated before all volume has been delivered (to avoid generation of excessive airway pressures).
	Flow limiting is not in the interests of the patient, as this limits the flow of gas that can be received. Some older ventilators can limit flow (such as when a specified flow rate is set). More-modern ventilators allow patients to access increased flow to accommodate any increase in demand.
Beginning of expiration–cycling	Pressure, flow, volume or time can be the variable which cycles the breath out of inspiration, but only one can function for each individual breath.
	Volume and time cycling are not influenced by changes in lung compliance and may result in increased airway pressures.
	Pressure cycling is greatly influenced by lung compliance, and the volume delivered is dependent on the flow delivered, the length of inspiration, lung characteristics and the set pressure.
	Flow cycling functions on a pressure-supported breath in that the exhalation valve opens when a predetermined flow rate is reached.
Exhalation	Exhalation is passive. The baseline pressure can be altered and is usually positive.
	Positive end-expiratory pressure (PEEP) is usually applied as this helps to prevent early airway closure and alveolar collapse at end of expiration. The increase in functional residual capacity assists in improving oxygenation.

TABLE 21.8 BREATH-DELIVERY STRATEGIES IN MECHANICAL VENTILATION[4]

BREATH-DELIVERY STRATEGY	CLINICAL APPLICATION	NURSING IMPLICATIONS
Continuous mandatory ventilation (CMV): can be pressure- or volume-controlled. Breaths are time-triggered.	Only appropriate if the patient cannot make the effort to breathe. This mode should not be used unless the patient is sedated and paralysed.	Patients on CMV may not be able to breathe spontaneously. If spontaneous drive is intact, distress may occur.
Assist-control (A/C) ventilation: can be pressure- or volume-controlled. Breaths are patient- or time-triggered. A minimum rate is set and the patient can trigger additional breaths if required.	A minimum breath rate is set and these mandatory breaths, plus any additional breaths, are delivered at the set volume or pressure (whichever is the control variable).	High rates in A/C ventilation may lead to hyperventilation and respiratory alkalosis.
Synchronised intermittent mandatory ventilation (SIMV): delivers a set rate and allows the patient to breathe spontaneously.	Mandatory breaths are time-triggered and deliver the set pressure or volume. Assisted breaths may be initiated by the patient and deliver the set pressure or volume. Patient effort and the level of pressure support determine the volume of spontaneous breaths.	Volume-control SIMV may result in increased airway pressures. If these exceed the pressure-alarm limits, pre-set volume may not be delivered. Pressure-control SIMV results in variable tidal volume. High tidal volume can contribute to volutrauma and hypocapnia. Low tidal volumes may contribute to hypercapnia and respiratory acidosis.

TABLE 21.8 BREATH-DELIVERY STRATEGIES IN MECHANICAL VENTILATION—cont'd

BREATH-DELIVERY STRATEGY	CLINICAL APPLICATION	NURSING IMPLICATIONS
Pressure-support ventilation: a pre-set positive pressure is used to augment the patient's inspiratory effort. The patient controls the rate, inspiratory flow and tidal volume.	Pressure-support ventilation requires a stable respiratory drive and sufficient respiratory muscle strength to overcome airway and equipment resistance. May be used in conjunction with SIMV.	Patients must have an intact respiratory drive and sufficient respiratory muscle strength to generate a tidal volume sufficient for CO_2 clearance. With low rates or tidal volumes, hypoventilation may occur.
Continuous positive airway pressure (CPAP): on most ventilators, CPAP refers to spontaneous breathing with positive end-expiratory pressure.	As with pressure-support ventilation, CPAP requires a stable respiratory drive and sufficient respiratory muscle strength to achieve an acceptable tidal volume.	Hypoventilation may occur with low respiratory rates and low tidal volumes (or both). Patients will need to overcome circuit resistance and this increases work of breathing.

TABLE 21.9 SETTING THE VENTILATOR[55]

VENTILATOR PARAMETER	SETTING	RATIONALE
Tidal volume	6–10 mL/kg (6–7 mL/kg usual)	The injured lung has reduced inspiratory capacity and is more susceptible to further damage as a result of increased volumes and pressures to the lung during mechanical ventilation. Lower tidal volumes can prove lung protective. For patients with acute respiratory distress syndrome or similar bilateral alveolar processes, the lower end of this range (e.g. 6 mL/kg) should be used.
Respiratory rate	Hypoxic respiratory failure, 20–30 breaths/minute	In hypoxic respiratory failure, respiratory rates < 20 breaths/minute are usually poorly tolerated because of existing rapid shallow breathing.
	Hypercapnic respiratory failure, 8–15 breaths/minute	Ventilator respiratory rates should be closely set to the patient's requirements. Clinicians should be mindful of the contribution of respiratory rate to the overall minute ventilation and CO_2 removal.
	Asthma, 12–14 breaths/minute	High respiratory rates should be avoided as these contribute to the development of intrinsic PEEP. With a tidal volume of 8–9 mL/kg, respiratory rates below 12 breaths/minute have not demonstrated significant impact on gas trapping. Lower rates (5–8 breaths/minute) may be indicated when hyperinflation is marked or when small reductions in hyperinflation have significant clinical impact.
Inspiratory pressure	< 30 cmH_2O	Lung inflation beyond total lung capacity increases the chance of barotraumas (extra-alveolar air). At total lung capacity the transpulmonary pressure is 25 cmH_2O and the alveolar pressures are 35 cmH_2O. Consensus regarding the safety of pressures < 30 cmH_2O is lacking.
Inspiratory ratio	1:2 to 1:3	Longer inspiratory times will bring the I:E closer to 1:1 and may improve alveolar recruitment. However, this can be associated with adverse haemodynamic effects and is generally poorly tolerated by the patient (in the absence of sedation and paralysis).
Flow rate	40–90 L/min	Higher flow rates may be required for some patients and may improve comfort, decrease work of breathing and help slow the respiratory rate. Higher flow rates will increase the peak airway pressure, although most of this is dissipated along the length of the endotracheal tube. Flow waveforms can be selected on some ventilators. Selection of decelerating flow waveforms in volume ventilation will extend the inspiratory time.
Positive end-expiratory pressure (PEEP)	5–20 cmH_2O	There is general agreement that a PEEP > 5 cmH_2O should be used in patients with injured lungs, and in this group of patients a starting point of 10 cmH_2O should be considered. However, there is little consensus about target endpoints for PEEP. Adjustments to PEEP should be made during evaluation of ventilator graphics and evidence of lung recruitment.
Trigger sensitivity	Pressure trigger: 0.5–2.0 cmH_2O Flow trigger: 1–3 L/min	Triggering that is too sensitive to the patient's inspiratory effort will result in excessive breaths being delivered, or self-cycling of the ventilator. Insensitive triggering will result in increased work of breathing and patient anxiety or discomfort.
FiO_2	0.21–1.0	The FiO_2 should be adjusted to achieve the desired PaO_2 and SaO_2. Prolonged high levels of oxygen should be avoided if possible. Manipulation of PEEP increases mean alveolar pressure, and may also improve the PaO_2 and SaO_2.

I:E: inspiratory:expiratory ratio; FiO_2: fraction of inspired oxygen; PaO_2: arterial partial pressure of oxygen; SaO_2: arterial oxygen saturation.

TABLE 21.10 PHYSIOLOGICAL EFFECT OF POSITIVE PRESSURE VENTILATION

SYSTEM	PHYSIOLOGICAL EFFECT	ASSESSMENT
Cardiovascular	Increased pressure reduces venous return to the right heart, reducing right ventricular preload. Increased intrathoracic pressures and PEEP also reduce venous return to the left heart and reduce cardiac output.	Close monitoring of blood pressure, especially when ventilation is commenced or when inspiratory pressures are changed.
	Increased pulmonary vascular resistance, making the right ventricle work harder.	Closely monitor patients with known or suspected right ventricular compromise.
	Increased intrathoracic pressure may decrease coronary perfusion.	Monitor patients for signs of myocardial ischaemia.
Neurological	The decrease in cardiac output may result in a decrease in cerebral perfusion pressure (CPP). CPP may also be reduced because of an increase in CVP.	Patients at greatest risk are those with increased intracranial pressure and who may develop cerebral oedema.
Renal	Decreased cardiac output can lead to a decrease in renal blood flow and glomerular filtration rates.	Monitor urine output.
	Redistribution of blood flow within the kidneys so that flow to the outer cortex decreases and flow to the inner cortex and outer medullary tissue increases.	Monitor urine output and creatinine levels.
Liver and gastrointestinal	Decreased cardiac output, downward movement of the diaphragm against the liver, a decrease in portal blood flow and/or increase in splanchnic resistance may contribute to liver ischaemia.	Monitor liver function through blood chemistry.
	Increases in splanchnic resistance may contribute to gastric mucosal ischaemia.	Assess for clinically important gastric bleeding. Treat with histamine-2 receptor antagonists or proton pump inhibitors.
	Gastric distension may occur from swallowing air that leaks around the ETT cuff.	Assess gastric distension and insert a nasogastric tube as required.
Pulmonary	Barotrauma (subcutaneous emphysema, pneumothorax, pneumomediastinum, etc) can occur secondary to increased positive pressure.	Monitor peak airway pressure.
	Volutrauma occurs with overdistension of the alveoli.	Monitor tidal volumes. Tidal volumes of 4–10 mL/kg ideal bodyweight can be used for adults, and of 5–10 mL/kg ideal bodyweight for children. The lower range of tidal volume should be used when lung pathology is present.
	Hospital-acquired infections, such as ventilator-associated pneumonia, may occur secondary to aspiration of subglottic secretions.	Respiratory assessment including chest x-ray is important. Prevention measures include mouth care, head-of-bed elevation 45°, suctioning subglottic secretions.

CVP: central venous pressure; ETT: endotracheal tube; PEEP: positive end-expiratory pressure.

and physical examination of the chest are required in any patient receiving mechanical ventilation. Table 21.10 provides a summary of the physiological effects of positive pressure ventilation and related nursing assessment and management. Comprehensive information about assessment of the mechanically ventilated patient is discussed elsewhere.[109]

ASSESSMENT OF RESPIRATORY SUPPORT EQUIPMENT

Assessment of equipment, including the ventilator, is a fundamental aspect of caring for the mechanically ventilated patient.[109] A self-inflating manual resuscitation bag with appropriate-sized facemask should be readily available and able to be quickly attached to supplemental oxygen. High-flow suction with a Yankauer suction tip and endotracheal suction catheters need to be checked for availability and functioning. Checks should be made to ensure that the ventilator is connected to an uninterrupted power supply and that appropriate ventilator alarm limits have been set. Specific assessment of the endotracheal tube and humidification equipment should also be made.

Assessment of the endotracheal tube

Following intubation, the position of the endotracheal tube (ETT) should be assessed by chest radiograph. The tip of the ETT should be positioned approximately 5 cm above the carina. If the carina is not visible, the tip of the ETT should be positioned at the level of T3 or T4. Once confirmed, the emergency clinician should check markers on the ETT to determine the level at which the tube is inserted. This is measured as the distance from the tip of the ETT to the teeth, using the 1 cm gradated markings on the tube.

Pre-hospital assessment of endotracheal tube placement is more difficult but just as critical. Radiograph assessment is not available, but use of ultrasonography has been shown to be reliable. End-tidal carbon dioxide confirmation is 'gold standard' and should always be available wherever intubation occurs. Though useful in identifying right main bronchus tube placement, secondary assessment tools, including chest and epigastric auscultation and pulse oximetry, should be considered as adjuncts only. End-tidal colourimetric devices are available as a fallback alternative to capnography where device failure occurs.

The ETT must be adequately secured to prevent accidental extubation or tube migration. Methods for securing the ETT vary and there is no evidence to suggest the best way to do so. Options range from cloth and adhesive tape to purpose-produced clamp devices. Whatever method is used to secure the tube, careful consideration must be given to the potential for this to produce pressure areas or cause skin damage. Almost invariably, patients will be moved in the pre-hospital setting. This makes securing the endotracheal tube a critical factor, along with appropriate continuous supervision. Even minor patient head movements or inattentive pulling on equipment can cause tube displacement and continued vigilance is required. Each patient movement must be carefully coordinated by the airway supervisor. Following each movement, correct tube placement should be reconfirmed. This should be finally affirmed on transfer of patient to the destination facility with agreed confirmation provided by the airway attendant taking over responsibility. Patient tolerance of the ETT (and of ventilation itself) may vary, and often sedation is required to blunt CNS activity and achieve patient comfort and tolerance of the tube and ventilator. Depending on the clinical problem and patient level of underlying consciousness, a muscle relaxant may also be necessary. Patient paralysis further heightens the need for constant supervision and vigilance during care.

The high-volume, low-pressure cuff on the ETT is designed to prevent oropharyngeal secretions from entering the airway. Cuff pressures should be kept between 20 and 30 cmH_2O (ideally below 25 cmH_2O) to avoid mucosal circulation impairment and damage.[110] The ETT cuff should be inflated using a minimal occlusion technique that adjusts cuff inflation volume so that during inspiration a leak around the ETT cuff cannot be heard. Enough air should be removed from the cuff to first identify the leak, and then volume slowly added until the leak just disappears. Cuff pressure should be assessed once per shift. Best practice for cuff measurement involves the use of a manometer attached to the ETT cuff balloon, to achieve cuff pressures of not more than 25 cmH_2O—the aim being to maintain the pressure below tracheal mucosal perfusion pressure (34 cmH_2O).[104] Historically, smaller children were typically intubated using non-cuffed tubes; these were intended to neatly fit into the funnel-shaped upper airway, narrowing at the cricoid area and reducing the seal's absoluteness. However, better understanding of the shape of the airway of small children and the effectiveness of cuffed endotracheal tubes has prompted debate and reconsideration of this approach. Cuffed paediatric endotracheal tubes are now considered normal, consistent with adult patients.[111]

Humidification equipment

During mechanical ventilation, the upper airway is bypassed, and consequently inspired gases should be warmed and humidified.[99] This can be achieved using either a heat–moisture exchanger (Fig. 21.2) or a heated humidifier (Fig. 21.3). As the duration of mechanical ventilation increases, humidification becomes particularly important to prevent retention of secretions and maximise mucociliary function. Humidification systems have limitations to consider in use. They can contribute to dead space and increase airway resistance when used, adversely affecting patients by increasing the work of breathing, particularly where low tidal volumes are being used for lung protection.[99]

FIGURE 21.2 HEAT–MOISTURE EXCHANGER

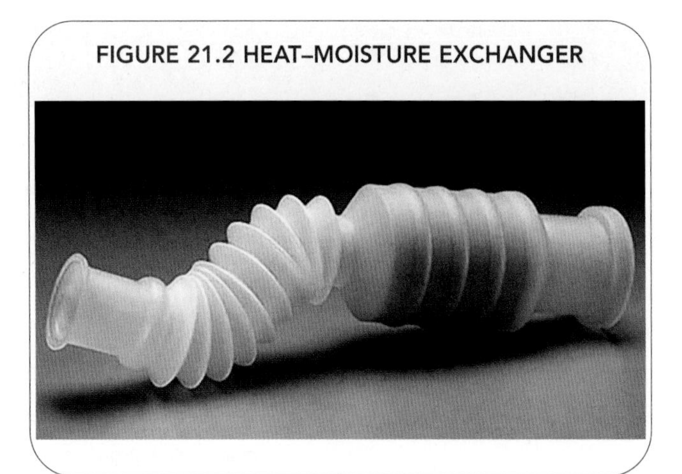

FIGURE 21.3 HEATED WATER CIRCUIT USED TO HUMIDIFY INSPIRED GASES IN MECHANICAL VENTILATION[112]

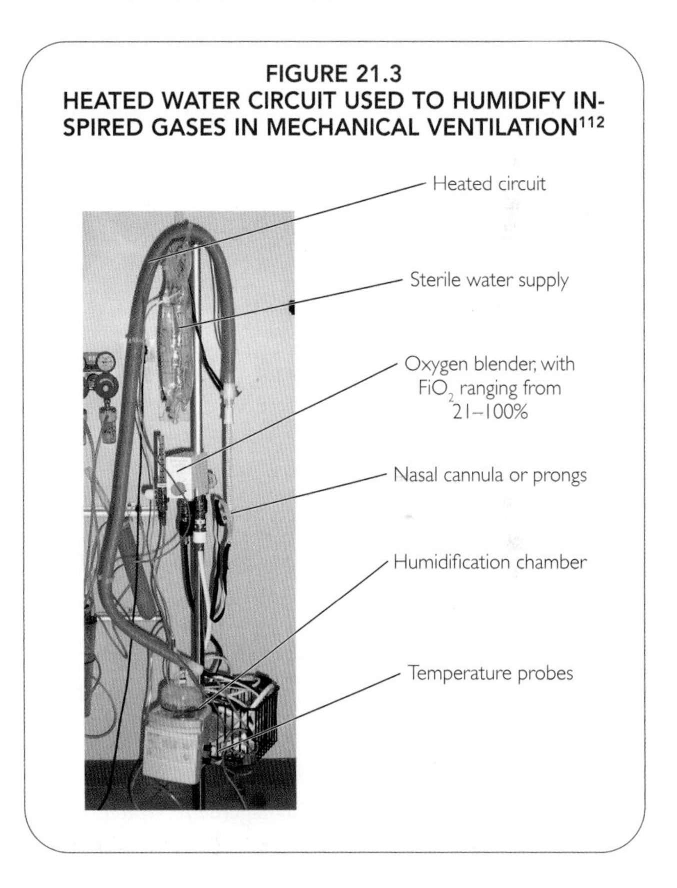

TROUBLESHOOTING AND PROBLEM-SOLVING MECHANICAL VENTILATION

Ventilators, like other complex equipment, can contribute to and help identify problems. Alarm systems on ventilators are designed to identify when there might be a problem with the ventilator or the patient. The two most common alarms are the high and low pressure alarms. Possible reasons for the triggering

TABLE 21.11 VENTILATOR ALARMS—CAUSES AND SOLUTIONS

CAUSE	SOLUTION
Low-pressure alarm: should be set 5–10 cmH_2O below peak inspiratory pressure	
Patient disconnection	Reconnect patient to the ventilator
Circuit leaks	Check all connections are secure
	Assess ventilator tubing for cracks or holes
	Check exhalation valves are correctly seated
Cuff leak	Use minimum occlusion technique for inflating the ETT cuff
	Check pilot balloon
	Check position of ETT as migration into the upper airway (above the vocal cords) can cause leaking
Chest tube leaks	Assess degree of leak. Consider readjusting the low pressure alarm
High-pressure alarm: should be set about 10 cmH_2O above peak inspiratory pressure	
Coughing	Usually self-limiting and does not require treatment. Secretions loosened during coughing may need to be cleared by suctioning
Increased secretions	Suction as required
Patient is biting on the endotracheal tube (ETT)	Consider sedation or use of a bite block. Depending on patient condition, consider neuromuscular blockade
ETT is kinked	Check ETT through visual inspection, and check on x-ray
ETT migration	Check position of ETT on x-ray
ETT cuff herniation	Attempt to pass a suction catheter. If unable to do so, deflate the ETT cuff and reposition the tube before reinflating
Heat-moisture exchanger (HME) blocked	Check and replace HME if indicated
Inspiratory circuit kinked	Assess ventilator tubing
Accumulation of water in the circuit	Drain circuit
Increased airway resistance	Auscultate the chest. Consider bronchodilators
Decreased compliance	Re-evaluate the ventilation strategy

of these alarms, and suggested management strategies, are presented in Table 21.11.

Ventilators can also be the source of problems for the patient. The delivery of gas under positive pressure and imposition of mandatory breaths may be uncomfortable for some patients. Patient–ventilator dyssynchrony results when the delivery of ventilator breaths is no longer in synchronisation with the patient's spontaneous respiratory effort and may result in signs of respiratory distress or increased patient anxiety. Patient–ventilator dyssynchrony can result from patient- or ventilator-related problems.

Patient-related problems

There are many different patient-related problems that may contribute to the development of patient–ventilator dyssynchrony. One of the most common problems is the retention of secretions which increase the work of breathing, and this is usually easily rectified by suctioning the endotracheal tube. Bronchospasm, normally managed with common bronchodilators, can result in increased work of breathing and the generation of high-peak inspiratory airway pressures and/or difficulty in delivering the set tidal volume.

General anxiety associated with endotracheal tube placement and the imposition of mechanical ventilation is usually well managed with low levels of sedation. It is important to determine the cause of patient–ventilator dyssynchrony in order to implement appropriate strategies to alleviate the problem. Increasing sedation is only appropriate when all other physical and mechanical problems have been investigated and corrected. For a more detailed discussion of patient-related problems, readers are encouraged to access publications that specifically focus on this topic.[99,109]

Ventilator-related problems

Ventilator-related problems include leaks, inadequate ventilator support, trigger sensitivity and inadequate flow. Leaks can occur within the ventilator circuitry, especially at the junctions where connections exist, or around the ETT cuff. Less commonly, the presence of a pleural drainage system can contribute to system leak. Before connecting the patient to a ventilator, a leak check should be performed to assess the system.[113]

Inadequate ventilator support may occur when the prescribed minute ventilation cannot be delivered. This can occur as a result of circuit leaks or may be attributed to failure to deliver the prescribed tidal volume because peak inspiratory pressures have been reached.

Trigger sensitivity can be set too low or too high. When the trigger sensitivity is too low, autotriggering will result. Setting the trigger sensitivity too high means that, despite patient respiratory effort, the ventilator will not deliver a spontaneous or assisted breath. This can lead to a considerable increase in work of breathing, patient discomfort and patient–ventilator dyssynchrony.

Inadequate flow can be identified by patient–ventilator dyssynchrony, increased respiratory effort and high negative pressures generated on inspiration. Increasing the flow rate or shortening the inspiratory time can rectify this. If a volume-control ventilation strategy is used, consideration should be given to changing to a pressure-control strategy.

TRANSPORTING THE PATIENT ON MECHANICAL VENTILATION

Patients who require mechanical ventilation in the ED are also likely to be transferred to the intensive care unit (ICU) or to other departments in the hospital for diagnostic tests or therapeutic procedures. When planning to transport a mechanically ventilated patient, it is important that time is taken to stabilise haemodynamics, oxygenation and ventilation. The team transporting the patient will be dependent on local policies, but should take into consideration the severity of illness and the degree of support required. Transport equipment should be lightweight, small, portable and rugged.[114]

Many hospitals have a common ventilator for use in the ICU and the ED. This simplifies transport somewhat, as the patient can remain on the one ventilator from initiation of mechanical ventilation to discontinuation. Additionally, the ventilator used for transport will not be limited in its capabilities. When selecting a ventilator for transport, the power source is an important consideration. Pneumatically powered and operated ventilators are preferable for transport, but they consume gas to function which depletes the gas supply quickly. If the ventilator is an electronically controlled device, consideration should be given to battery longevity.

In addition to the ventilator, a cardiac monitor, pulse oximeter, waveform capnography, bag–valve–mask ventilation device and supply of pharmacology agents and intravenous fluids should be available. During transportation, airway management is of utmost concern and should be a responsibility dedicated to one member of the healthcare team. The person responsible for airway management should be skilled in emergency intubation. Transport of patients receiving mechanical ventilation therapy by paramedics varies considerably between primary and secondary transport and jurisdictions. Mechanical ventilation, and usually intubation, is often restricted in primary roles to intensive care paramedics. Devices used often either lack complexity or only a few of their capabilities are used. Most commonly, the purpose of ventilation for paramedics is to care for paralysed and intubated patients. The key is to provide the patient with adequate respiratory rate and tidal volume sufficient to maintain suitable oxygen saturation and end-tidal capnography. Management of PEEP, as indicated in support of positive pressure ventilation, may also be required.

Ventilators may also be used in secondary hospital transfers and patient retrievals. These transport teams may vary in discipline, including mixtures of paramedics, nurses and doctors. The complexity of the ventilator used may vary depending on the purpose.

The most common ventilator setting used is synchronised intermittent mandatory ventilation (SIMV). The value of this setting is that a predetermined baseline of ventilation will be provided, yet spontaneous breathing by the patient can be detected and allowed for by the device. Where this spontaneous breathing proves ineffective and problematic, the patient may be paralysed to allow for better operator control. Paralysing patients, common in initial patient management by intensive care paramedics, reduces, but does not negate, the value of SIMV. As these patients are intubated, the intrinsic auto PEEP formed by the glottis closing is lost. Typically, a small amount of PEEP, usually 5 cmH_2O, is added to compensate for this. Another variable to be considered by paramedics is the fraction of inspired oxygen. Given the usual emergency nature of most calls, the fraction is usually high and typically 1.0.

The device chosen will be restricted by the same problems that confront all pre-hospital equipment. It must be lightweight and compact. Even in a larger ambulance, space is at a premium, so placing the device near to the patient for immediate use can be challenging. In sedans, helicopters and fixed-wing aircraft, size and weight of appliances becomes even more of an issue. Before embarking on any patient response, a suitable oxygen supply must be ascertained. Typically, this will include at least one and probably two 1500 mL cylinders with regulator attached. Similarly, battery life will have to be assured. Ideally, battery life will be long and beyond the anticipated duration of transfer. Spare batteries should be present and, when practicable, it should be possible to run the ventilator on external power while in the vehicle.

Transferring intubated patients incurs some risk. The endotracheal tube can become dislodged with relatively small amounts of movement shifting from the trachea to the oropharynx or even oesophagus without being noticed. All movements should be coordinated by a team leader who has a secure hold of the endotracheal tube. The patient's head and body should be moved as one each time. It is frequently easier to disconnect the endotracheal tube briefly during movement to reduce any pressure that may be placed on it by hoses. If it is not disconnected the length of hose available must be inspected first to ensure it is sufficient to accommodate the move. At the completion of each move, the tube placement should be reconfirmed with capnography and chest auscultation. Monitoring devices must be kept close to the patient at all times during transfer, including pulse oximetry and end-tidal capnography. The most appropriately qualified paramedic must constantly remain close to the patient's airway to maintain constant scrutiny of the endotracheal tube and ongoing ventilation. Concurrent management of the main presenting problems will usually continue whether it is primary response or secondary retrieval.

ACUTE PULMONARY OEDEMA

Acute pulmonary oedema (APO) is a pathophysiological state typified by fluid in the alveolar space, resulting in gas-exchange problems and decreased lung compliance.[115] APO is a sign of a disease rather than a disease itself and can be linked to a range of cardiogenic and non-cardiogenic causes. The latter are most commonly initiated through changes in pulmonary capillary permeability and include ARDS (the most recognised form), anaphylaxis, neurogenic pulmonary oedema, high altitude pulmonary oedema and problems related to transfusion lung injury.[116] Though there are numerous causes of APO, each on their own is comparatively uncommon.[117] By far, the most commonly encountered APO is cardiogenic in origin as a result of heart failure, discussed herein.[4]

ASSESSMENT

On presentation, most patients are normotensive or hypertensive; the presence of hypotension indicates a concurrent cardiogenic shock.[115,118] Patients demonstrating a thready pulse, pale or cyanosed skin and delayed capillary refill may be systemically hypoperfused despite an adequate systolic blood pressure that is maintained by severe vasoconstriction.[118] Patients are commonly diaphoretic due to sympathetic activation.[118] Orthopnoea is commonly noted at night, particularly in reclined or supine posturing.[117] Cardiac failure can be considered acute or chronic. Clinical findings include breathlessness, even with minimal exertion and particularly nocturnal.

Left ventricular failure typically results in a decreased ventricular ejection fraction ($< 40\%$) and a decrease in cardiac output,[119,120] although in some cases this ejection may be preserved or right heart function might be disturbed.[117,120] Problems with ventricular emptying result in increased left-side heart-filling pressures and a back-up of pressure into the pulmonary vasculature.[4] The increase in pressure within the pulmonary capillaries manifests itself as increased hydrostatic pressure (the mechanical force exerted by a fluid against the walls of a vessel). When the hydrostatic pressure exceeds the oncotic pressure (the osmotic pull of a fluid into a compartment), the fluid will begin to move out of the capillary into the interstitial space between the vessel and the alveolus.[4,37] At first, the fluid in the interstitium is removed via lymphatic drainage; however, when the movement out of the capillary exceeds the ability of the lymphatic system to remove it, the fluid then starts to move into the alveolar space.[4,37] When the alveolus is filled with fluid, it is no longer able to participate in gas exchange.[4] Alterations in gas exchange are reflected in reduced SpO_2, indicating hypoxaemia[119] and increased $PaCO_2$. Hypoxaemia and hypercarbia, in conjunction, may be reflected in the patient being agitated, anxious, restless or having a decreased consciousness level.[115,119] The fluid within the alveolus and interstitium results in reduced pulmonary compliance and reduced functional residual capacity, and is reflected in clinical findings of dyspnoea and diffuse moist crackles on auscultation. Progression to peri-bronchial oedema may cause wheezing or rhonchi. These sounds can complicate diagnosis and suggest bronchospastic disease; patient history and consideration of all assessment signs can assist, but ultimately differentiation may take chest x-ray to confirm. Pulmonary oedema may cause the patient to have a productive cough, producing white- or pink-tinged frothy sputum. The chest may be dull to percussion, especially over the bases. The patient strives to remain in an upright position,[115] and there is marked accessory muscle use with tachypnoea.[119] The left and right sides of the heart do not function in isolation from each other, so that failure of the left side of the heart will lead to eventual deterioration in function of the right side, manifesting as lower limb oedema and raised jugular venous pressure.[115,119]

DIAGNOSTICS AND MONITORING

Consider including the following blood tests: full blood count to identify anaemia; electrolytes, urea and creatinine to identify electrolyte disturbances and renal function; consider troponin for evidence of myocardial injury.[119] An upright chest x-ray will aid differentiation of pulmonary oedema from other causes of dyspnoea. An early ECG is essential for recognition of dysrhythmia and for identification of acute coronary syndrome. Particularly for chronic failure, echocardiography is used to establish left ventricular function.[120] Pulse oximetry allows a non-invasive indication of oxygenation.[117,119] More recently, point-of-care lung ultrasound has proven useful in both differentiating between normal lungs and that of acute pulmonary oedema or ARDS. Further, it has proven to be effective in differentiating between the latter two pathologies.[117,120,121] If myocardial structural abnormality is suspected, echocardiography is indicated.[117,120]

Pre-hospital recognition of the patient in acute pulmonary oedema must be made on rudimentary clinical examination findings. A past history of cardiac disease and previous episodes of pulmonary oedema can be helpful. Clinical findings of breathing difficulty when supine may be noted or be more prevalent at night. These presenting signs and symptoms may not be specific to acute pulmonary oedema.[120] Jugular venous distension may be observed as left ventricular end diastolic pressure rises. Audible crackles on chest auscultation may be heard, but these may be difficult to differentiate from infective crackles or overshadowed by other sounds such as wheezing. Early acute exacerbations may be caused by interstitial oedema without yet progressing to causing alveolar collapse and crackle sounds.

TREATMENT

- *Oxygen therapy*—all patients presenting with APO should be given supplemental oxygen to match their needs and correct hypoxaemia.[119,120] Oxygen use should be guided by pulse oximetry with patients only requiring oxygen when their oxygen saturation is less than 92% on room air.[115,117,120]
- *Nitrates*—nitrates initially cause venous dilation and reduction in preload.[37,115,119] At higher doses, nitrates precipitate arterial dilation, leading to a concurrent decrease in afterload and a resultant drop in systolic blood pressure.[120] The combined effect can allow for increased stroke volume.[117] Coronary artery dilation results in greater myocardial blood flow and oxygen delivery.[99,120] Overall, nitrates achieve decreased demand on the myocardium while increasing oxygen delivery.[115] Nitrate therapy can be provided easily and rapidly using sublingual, buccal or transdermal routes or, if necessary, intravenously.[117,120] Particularly useful in the presence of hypertension, they should be avoided where hypotension is encountered.[117,120]

- *Ventilation support*—patients who have a severe decrease in consciousness level, agonal breaths or respiratory arrest require assisted positive pressure ventilation, intubation and mechanical ventilation.[99,120] For patients not fitting the above exclusion criteria, NIV has allowed many to avoid intubation and its associated risks. The application of CPAP works by aiding the redistribution of intra-alveolar fluid and splinting the alveoli open, resulting in an increased area for gas exchange, increased lung compliance and a decrease in the work of breathing.[99] In terms of APO management using NIV (both CPAP and BiPAP), there is no significant clinical benefit for either method; therefore, the modality should be directed by availability of equipment.[117,122] CPAP has become the mainstay of pre-hospital management of acute episodes of APO, with all other therapies taking on the role of adjunct therapies.[85–88,90,91,117,120]
- *Diuretics (furosemide)*—this is thought to decrease preload by initially causing venous dilation, and then increasing diuresis and a further reduction in preload.[99] Diuretics are recommended in patients with evidence of significant fluid overload;[115,120] however, caution is advised to avoid unnecessary diuresis in patients that are normovolaemic.[115,117] Loop diuretics have the potential to reduce glomular filtration rate and produce electrolyte disturbances; hence, although diuretics may aid in symptom relief, caution must be taken to ensure their use does not trigger overvigorous diuresis.[123] Patients who have not had diuretics before are commonly provided a 20–40 mg intravenous dose. Those who receive ongoing oral therapy should receive a greater intravenous dose, in the vicinity of equivalent to that taken daily.[117,120]
- *Opioids* are no longer a mainstay of treatment for acute pulmonary oedema.[117] Morphine is primarily used to relieve chest pain resistant to nitrates. Morphine also acts upon the sympathetic response and has anxiolytic properties. Resultant decreased heart rate, blood pressure, contractility and vasodilation cause a decrease in myocardial oxygen demand and workload.[115] Negative aspects of morphine that must be taken into consideration include respiratory and central nervous system depression; therefore, the administration of morphine to patients with decreased consciousness levels, hypotension or respiratory depression is not recommended.[115,118]

Chronic heart failure is typically managed pharmacologically including: angiotension converting enzyme (ACE) inhibitors to reduce left ventricular afterload, beta-blockers to maintain heart rate, mineralocorticoid receptor antagonists (MRA) to regulate aldosterone activity, sodium-glucose co-transporter (SGLT2) inhibitors and loop diuretics.[120]

Disposition

In the majority of patients who respond to standard therapy, consider admission to a coronary care unit if there are ongoing cardiac issues such as pain and/or dysrhythmias, and close monitoring is still required. In other cases, such as elderly patients who have had a brief decompensation of chronic heart failure, admission to a non-monitored medical bed may be appropriate.[118]

ASTHMA

ASSESSMENT

Asthma is a common respiratory presentation characterised by bronchial hyper-responsiveness and inflammation that cause episodic reversible bronchospasm and increased mucus production and oedema.[4] This leads to widespread but variable airway obstruction that is often reversible, either spontaneously or with treatment.[124] Inflammation resulting in hyperreactivity of the airways is the hallmark pathological feature of asthma.[4,124] Asthmatics face a variety of trigger factors, severity of presentations and responsiveness to therapies for episode reversal. Ideally, asthmatics should have a tailored asthma action plan that they follow, including clear instructions to guide their responses to presentation and for seeking help.[125] Common asthma trigger factors include viral respiratory infections, cigarette smoke irritation, allergy triggers and some medications such as aspirin. Emotional stress and exercise can also be implicated in triggering or worsening episodes.[125] Individuals should learn to recognise their triggers, where possible, and avoid them if possible.

Allergen- or irritant-induced mast cell degranulation releases a large number of inflammatory mediators such as histamine, and chemotactic factors that cause bronchial infiltration by white cells.[4] These inflammatory mediators produce bronchial smooth muscle spasm, increased permeability, oedema formation, vascular congestion, mucus production and impaired mucociliary function.[4] The resultant airway obstruction causes resistance to airflow (particularly expiratory given the comparatively passive nature of this respiratory phase), increased physiological dead space, hyperventilation, air trapping and impaired gas exchange. This manifests as dyspnoea, wheeze, a feeling of chest tightness, cough, prolonged expiration,[124,125] hypoxaemia and hypercapnia and respiratory muscle fatigue.[4]

Patients with long-term asthma have the potential to develop lung function impairment that becomes irreversible. In some cases, differentiation between asthma and COPD can be difficult with identifiable commonalities, including inflammatory profile and common trigger factors. This condition is effectively the co-existence of both pathologies, called asthma-COPD overlap syndrome, or ACOS, and affects as many as 15% of people diagnosed with COPD or asthma.[126] Persistent and chronic airway inflammation leads to airway remodelling, characterised by loss of the elasticity necessary to accommodate lung expansion during breathing and permanent narrowing. The higher yet less effective treatment requirements and persistence of symptoms is a feature of severe asthma.[127]

High-risk features in a clinical history include a previous serious episode of asthma requiring ventilatory support, or having taken a course of steroids within the last 6 months.[20] Physical assessment findings that highlight a potentially life-threatening episode include an inability to talk normally, a quiet or silent chest on auscultation, agitation or decreased level of consciousness (Table 21.12).[20,125] Other life-threatening risk factors include poorly controlled asthma, inappropriate medical management and social or behavioural factors that can prove adverse to a correct response to avoiding or managing precipitating a dyspnoea episode.[128,129] While peak expiratory flow rate (PEFR) or a $FEV_1 < 80\%$ of that expected is also recognised as an indication of severity, it is an impractical tool for use in the ED in patients who are markedly short of breath and in distress, and are

TABLE 21.12 INITIAL ASSESSMENT OF ACUTE ASTHMA IN ADULTS[125]

	MILD/MODERATE	SEVERE	LIFE THREATENING
Speech	Can finish a sentence in one breath	Can only speak a few words in one breath	Can't speak
Posture	Can walk	Unable to lie flat due to dyspnoea	Collapsed or exhausted
Breathing	Respiratory distress is not severe	Paradoxical chest wall movement: inward movement on inspiration and outward movement on expiration (chest sucks in when person breathes in) Use of accessory muscles of neck or intercostal muscles or 'tracheal tug' during inspiration Subcostal recession	Severe respiratory distress Poor respiratory effort (indicates respiratory exhaustion and impending respiratory arrest)
Consciousness	Alert	Alert, agitated or drowsy	Drowsy or unconscious
Skin colour	Normal	Normal	Cyanosis
Respiratory rate	< 25 breaths/min	25 breaths/min	> 25 breaths/min Bradypnoea (indicates respiratory exhaustion and impending respiratory arrest)
Heart rate	< 110 beats/min	110 beats/min	110 beats/min Bradycardia (indicates impending cardio-respiratory arrest)
Chest auscultation	Wheeze or Normal lung sounds	Wheeze and reduced breath sounds	Markedly reduced breath sounds with few wheezes Silent chest
Oxygen saturation	> 94%	90–94%	< 90% Cyanosis
Blood gas analysis	Not indicated	Not indicated	PaO_2 < 60 mmHg $PaCO_2$ > 50 mmHg $PaCO_2$ within normal range despite increased work of breathing may indicate the patient is tiring and may need respiratory support pH < 7.35

simply unable to complete this test. Life-threatening asthma may be marked by PEFR < 50% less than baseline normal.[129] Severity of a patient's asthma condition (as opposed to a specific episode or attack) is defined by the ability for it to be controlled, particularly by the medications required to do so, and is divided into untreated, difficult to treat and treatment-resistant severe asthma.[124] Severe asthma is also considered in terms of non-medication features of presentation, including symptom frequency, the ability to become life threatening and the severity of symptoms.[128] Severe asthma should have alternative diagnoses excluded, trigger factors removed and the patient should be compliant with medication. Where this has all occurred, yet the asthma remains poorly controlled or there are more than two severe exacerbations per year, or there is dependency on corticosteroids to avoid exacerbations, this is also considered severe asthma.[124]

A phenomenon referred to as thunderstorm asthma, while uncommon, has the potential to trigger fatal episodes of asthma in people who have no previous history of asthma, or those who have previously experienced well-controlled asthma.[125,130] Thunderstorm asthma is effectively asthma whereby the episode is triggered as a result of particular weather conditions. Seasonally, high concentrations of airborne pollens are caught in winds and lifted into clouds where they swell, burst and release copious smaller allergens. Though relatively uncommon and able to be reasonably predicted with weather events and time of year, thunderstorm asthma can result in much larger than normal asthma and hay-fever events, including manifestations in people who normally have minimal respiratory problems. If a thunderstorm event does occur, affected patients are managed using the same protocols as those employed for a severe asthma attack.[130]

DIAGNOSTICS AND MONITORING

In the pre-hospital setting, protocol-driven therapy is primarily in response to physical assessment findings. The level of assessment for paramedics is largely based on clinical observations.

Audible wheeze and prolonged expiratory phase are important clues, keeping in mind that severe asthma might lead to such poor airflow that auscultation may produce little sound at all. Past history is useful in diagnosis, as is perusal of current medications. Of particular interest are previous hospital and intensive care admissions to act as a guide to underlying severity and possible course of acute illness. Pulse oximetry is an adjunct to severity, although it is often not a reliable clue until the episode is severe. By this point other clinical findings, such as consciousness, ability to speak freely and involvement of accessory respiratory muscles, will inform further management decisions.

In the emergency setting, further investigations should be considered. In asthma of mild and moderate severity, investigations should be limited to spirometry or peak flow to compare lung volumes or flow rates with the predicted norm.[20] A chest x-ray is indicated if physical examination suggests possible pneumonia or pneumothorax.[20] In severe asthma, a chest x-ray is necessary. ABGs are not considered routine, but may be useful to gain a full respiratory picture in the following cases: $SpO_2 < 92\%$; if the patient is not responding to treatment; if the patient is tiring; and if intubation is being considered.[20,124] In severe asthma, an ABG may initially show a respiratory alkalosis with hypoxaemia as the patient raises their respiratory rate to maintain oxygenation; as deterioration occurs, a respiratory acidosis will develop as airway obstruction worsens and the patient tires.[20]

TREATMENT

The management of asthma is determined by episode severity. Presentations of asthma are assessed against objective criteria into three classes of severity—mild, moderate and severe—as articulated by the National Asthma Council of Australia.[125] When managing asthmatic episodes, consider the shift from severe to life threatening and potentially catastrophic presentation.[129] Asthma can be classified as mild, moderate or severe in regards to how difficult it is to manage long term. By this measure, mild worsening can include a slight increase in symptoms or the number of episodes each week. Moderate worsening may include symptoms that disturb sleep and the requirement for repeated use of relieving medication. Severe is where there is repeated use of relievers and difficulty with normal daily activities.[125]

The mainstay of asthma management involves the administration of beta-2 agonists, such as salbutamol for bronchodilation, a possible addition of ipratropium bromide and systemic corticosteroids.[20,125] Ipratropium bromide may relieve cholinergic bronchomotor tone and lessen mucosal oedema and secretions, resulting in bronchodilation, and can be delivered via metered-dose inhaler or nebulised.[125] Ipratropium is generally only recommended for severe exacerbations of asthma. Salbutamol can be delivered via metered-dose inhaler with a spacer, or nebulised. Both methods of delivery are equally efficacious, but for most situations delivery by metered-dose inhaler with a spacer has advantages over the nebuliser: droplets are smaller and therefore penetrate quicker and more easily target receptor sites in the distal airways; it is faster to deliver the dose; it is cheaper; it can be taken home with the patient for continued treatment without the need to hire/buy expensive and cumbersome equipment, as required for home nebulisation; it is safer for infection control as respiratory viruses can be transmitted by the nebulised aerosol to nearby patients or staff.[131] However, in severe exacerbations of asthma and when patients find it challenging to coordinate the spacer with inhalation, the nebuliser is generally used as it is more practical for the delivery of continuous aerosolised salbutamol.

Where air entry to the lower airways is significantly reduced through airway narrowing, it may prove too difficult to deliver sufficient bronchodilator therapy for effective result. As such, beta-agonist therapy must be administered via an alternative route. Intramuscular adrenaline is an effective choice for severe asthma episodes when patients are unresponsive to inhaled therapy or they are in respiratory failure (such as attested by altered consciousness).[132] Intravenous adrenaline has become more popular in emergency use instead of salbutamol when a rapid acting intravenous beta agonist is required.[131] Salbutamol can be administered as an intravenous infusion in extreme cases, although it is unclear if this offers a benefit over continuous nebulised salbutamol.

Corticosteroids can be given orally, inhaled or intravenously and act upon the inflammatory cascade.[125,128,133] Other therapies include magnesium sulfate.[133] Magnesium is a smooth muscle relaxant that has been shown to provide effective bronchodilation in severe asthma. Typically, it is provided by intravenous injection and follows unsuccessful beta agonist and steroid therapy,[129,134,135] although there is evidence that it can be effective when administered via nebuliser.[134] All offer some bronchial smooth muscle benefit, but evidence is limited as to whether there is any advantage over nebulised or aerosol therapy. The most likely role is where the patient remains unresponsive or deteriorates following initial therapies.[133]

Oxygen therapy should be employed targeting SaO_2 92–95% for adults or, at a minimum, 95% for children.[124] High-concentration oxygen therapy has been shown to increase transcutaneous partial pressure of carbon dioxide during severe asthma exacerbation. Delivered concentration should be titrated to provide the minimal oxygen therapy to maintain adequate pulse oximetry.[124] As with other respiratory presentations, there is growing evidence of a role for NIV in the management of acute, severe asthma, with observed benefits including decreased drug therapy requirement and shortened hospital stays.[96] Heliox is a blend of helium and oxygen, and is thought to provide advantages in acute asthma due to better gas-flow dynamics.[20]

Critically, when spontaneous ventilation diminishes with the patient in respiratory failure, supportive positive ventilation is required in support. Ventilation of the asthmatic patient can be challenging given the higher pulmonary airway pressures involved and the resistance to airflow. Higher pressures of inspiration are required to encourage air entry with sufficient expiratory flow time allowed to ensure subsequent air escape. Such ventilation rates are typically slower than for many other patients as a result. Potential complications of asthmatic positive pressure ventilation include increased intra-alveolar and intrathoracic pressure leading to barotrauma or compromised venous return and hypotension.[136]

Management of adults with acute asthma is detailed in Table 21.13.

Disposition

Moderate and severe cases of asthma will require admission to hospital; severe cases responding poorly to therapy will require ICU admission. Mild cases of asthma, and moderate exacerbation

TABLE 21.13 INITIAL MANAGEMENT OF ADULTS WITH ACUTE ASTHMA[125]

	MILD/MODERATE	SEVERE	LIFE THREATENING
Immediately	Give 12 puffs salbutamol via MDI and spacer (100 microg/puff)	Give 12 puffs salbutamol via MDI and spacer (100 microg/puff) Use intermittent nebulised salbutamol (5 mg) if patient cannot breathe through spacer Drive nebuliser with air unless oxygen needed Provide oxygen if oxygen saturation less than 95% (titrate to target oxygen saturation of 92–95%)	Give continuous nebulised salbutamol (commence with 2 × 5 mg nebules. Keep the nebuliser chamber approximately half-full by 'topping-up' with nebuliser solution) Start oxygen (if oxygen saturation less than 95%) and titrate to target oxygen saturation of 92–95% Ventilatory assistance if required (non-invasive ventilation; intubation/ventilation)
Reassess response to treatment			
Over 1 hour	Repeat dose every 20 mins in the first hour (or sooner if needed)	Repeat dose every 20 mins in the first hour (or sooner if needed)	Continuous nebulisation until dyspnoea improves. Then change to intermittent bronchodilator therapy via MDI plus spacer or intermittent nebuliser
	If poor response, add ipratropium bromide 8 puffs via MDI and spacer (21 microg/puff) Repeat every 4–6 hours as needed	Give ipratropium bromide 8 puffs via MDI and spacer (21 microg/puff) or 500 microg nebule via nebuliser added to nebulised salbutamol every 20 minutes for the first hour	Give ipratropium bromide 8 puffs via MDI and spacer (21 microg/puff) or 500 microg nebule via nebuliser added to nebulised salbutamol every 20 minutes for the first hour
	Give steroids Oral prednisolone 37.5–50 mg, then continue 5–10 days OR If oral route not possible hydrocortisone 100 mg IV every 6 hours		
Reassess response to treatment			
Consider add-on treatments for persisting severe or life-threatening asthma		IV magnesium sulphate 2 g (20 mmol) infused over 20 minutes IV salbutamol Loading dose 5 microg/kg/min over 1 hour, then 1–2 microg/kg/min IM adrenaline 300–500 microg for adults 10 microg/kg paediatric patients Smaller bolus IV adrenaline or infusion if unresponsive or as an alternative to IV salbutamol Non-invasive positive pressure ventilation Consider if starting to tire or signs of respiratory failure If no improvement, intubate and start mechanical ventilation	

MDI: metered dose inhaler.

responding promptly to therapy, typified by absence of physical exhaustion or decreased speech tolerance, pulse rate less than 100, normal oxygen saturation, variable wheeze intensity and $FEV_1 >$ 75% of predicted,[137] can usually be discharged home after treatment in the ED and at least 1 hour of observation, and the formulation of a treatment plan.[20]

CHRONIC OBSTRUCTIVE PULMONARY DISEASE

Chronic obstructive pulmonary disease (COPD) is a general term for diseases that are not fully reversible and limit airflow due to airway or alveolar abnormalities.[2,138,139] COPD has a strong association with cigarette smoking, progressively limiting airflow. The condition develops over many years, therefore predominantly affects the ageing population. COPD incorporates conditions previously referred to as emphysema and chronic bronchitis.[2] Despite considerable commonality between the two diseases, there are significant differences that should be appreciated. A valuable resource for clinicians to access when providing care for patients with COPD is the *Australian and New Zealand Guidelines for the Management of Chronic Obstructive Pulmonary Disease*, accessible on the Lung Foundation Australia website,[138] or the Global Initiative for Chronic Obstructive Lung Disease strategy.[139]

ASSESSMENT

The continued division of patients with COPD into chronic obstructive bronchitis 'blue bloaters' and emphysema 'pink puffers' is outdated, as many patients do not fit these stereotypes. However, discussion of these two variants is not without benefit in that it discusses the two major pathologies from which COPD is drawn from.[139] Bronchitis is classically characterised by lower airway inflammation, collapsing on expiration, reducing airflow escape and trapping air within the alveoli. Hypoxia predominates, hence blue bloater. Emphysema is classically characterised by alveolar and supportive elastic tissue destruction, leading to reduction in chest recoil on expiration, increased forced, rapid breathing and alveolar gas trapping. Hypoxaemia is less of a problem; hypercapnia is a problem in both conditions.

Most patients with COPD have a varying prominence of these two main pathologies of COPD.[139] Obstruction to airflow and decrease in FEV_1 is primarily caused by inflammation, which is evident from the trachea down to the smallest peripheral airways that become progressively more scarred and narrow. It predominates in the smallest airways. Severity of disease can be graded based on the reduction in FEV_1 predicted. Obstruction to airflow is further impeded by an increased number and size of mucus-secreting goblet cells that create mucus plugs.[139] Ability to clear bacteria and mucus is impeded by damage to the epithelium, which impairs mucociliary function. Lung parenchyma is damaged over time, most commonly in a pattern of centrilobular emphysema.[139] This is typified by a destruction of alveoli, loss of lung elasticity and collapse of small airways that require the support of surrounding connective tissues for patency during expiration. The decrease in lung elasticity and parenchymal destruction further contributes to airflow obstruction,[140] and causes problems with gas exchange.[139] Gas-exchange abnormalities produce hypoxaemia and hypercapnia.[140] Pulmonary hypertension may develop late in the progression of the disease, and this is attributed to hypoxic vasoconstriction of small pulmonary arteries.[140]

In patients where chronic obstructive bronchitis is the predominant pathology, coughing is more prominent due to increased mucus production.[139] When coughing is vigorous, it results in expectoration of sputum. The presence of severe bronchopulmonary secretions is evidenced on auscultation by scattered crackles and wheeze, especially at the lung bases.[139] The primary symptom of airflow obstruction/limitation is chronic and progressive dyspnoea.[139] Gas exchange abnormality is often present with carbon dioxide retention, and hypoxaemia contributes to a cyanotic appearance, and, when hypoxaemia is severe, may lead to a decrease in consciousness level. If emphysema is a minor component, the anterior posterior diameter of the chest will be normal.[139]

When emphysema characteristics predominate, the patient is commonly thin, alert and orientated, dyspnoeic, tachypnoeic and using accessory muscles to ventilate.[139] They often assume a 'tripod' position, hunched forward to aid chest expansion, and create PEEP through pursed-lip breathing during exhalation. The additional PEEP provides increased intraluminal bronchial pressure and internal support for bronchial walls that have decreased support due to destruction of surrounding connective tissues.[139] Parenchymal destruction and loss of elasticity results in gross overinflation of the lungs, increased antero-posterior thorax diameter and a low diaphragm. Percussion of the chest demonstrates hyper-resonance, while decreased breath sounds are heard during auscultation. The patient experiences dyspnoea due to extensive lung parenchyma destruction; however, near-normal ABG values are maintained, while increased mucus production contributes to clinical features of productive cough.[140]

One critical point of patient assessment is to identify the severity of exacerbation. With some patients, chronic respiratory difficulty re-establishes a new normal baseline for the patient. This impacts on normal living function and activities, so must be appreciated for a number of reasons. It is also linked to frequency of exacerbations and mortality. The COPD assessment test (CAT) is one means of assessing a patient's baseline and considers a score for eight items, including cough, phlegm, chest tightness, dyspnoea, daily activities, patient confidence, sleep patterns and energy.[141] Interpretation of this patient 'normal' is important, along with determining any acute changes. In emergency situations, this can be challenging, but subjective questioning on patient appearance, exercise tolerance and levels of breathlessness can assist.[141]

DIAGNOSTICS AND MONITORING

Pulse oximetry is used to evaluate the oxygenation status,[140] and spirometry can be used to confirm the degree of obstruction.[140] An ECG should be taken to identify concurrent dysrhythmias, ischaemic changes and right-side heart hypertrophy.[140] A chest x-ray helps to rule out alternative diagnoses that can mimic an exacerbation and to identify the presence of co-existing diseases requiring specific interventions; for example, pneumonia, pneumothorax or pleural effusion.[140] An ABG is not universally indicated; however, in a severe exacerbation, one may provide information regarding acute versus chronic gas-exchange problems and monitor improvement or deterioration against interventions.[140] Other tests that may be useful, but will have little effect on initial management in the acute setting, include full blood count to identify polycythaemia and raised white cells, and assessing serum electrolyte levels for abnormalities.

MANAGEMENT

- *Oxygen therapy*—not without controversy, this remains the cornerstone of acute treatment of COPD. Supplemental oxygen therapy can improve quality of life and prove to be lifesaving in emergencies. However, its provision must be controlled with targeted administration.[63,68,125,138,139] For the hypoxaemic patient, it is critical that sufficient oxygen is administered to correct oxygen deficits. This oxygen therapy should be titrated to the minimum delivery to maintain tolerable pulse oximetry between 88% and 92%.[63] This has been shown to significantly reduce the risk of respiratory failure and mortality when compared with high-flow oxygen therapy and is particularly applicable to paramedics in acute emergencies.[59] Uncontrolled oxygen administration can lead to hypercapnia.[76] In non-emergency situations, supplemental oxygen therapy to assist with normal ADLs is considered differently and plays an important role in maintaining activity and quality of life.[139,140,142,143] There are various forms this can take place including both short-term use during exacerbations and longer term use. For most patients, this targeted oxygen therapy will not produce clinically significant CO_2 retention.[140]

- *Ventilation*—the use of NIV, both CPAP and BiPAP, has provided consistent positive results in acute respiratory failure.[122,139] NIV improves respiratory acidosis, decreases the work of breathing, decreases respiratory rate and dyspnoea, and also, importantly, decreases rates of intubation.[125,138] For some patients, the use of invasive ventilation may be more appropriate. If volume ventilation is used, it is recommended that the tidal volume not exceed 7–9 mL/kg. An inspiratory to expiratory (I:E) ratio of 1 : 3 should also be used to avoid the development of cumulative air-trapping.[55] This phenomenon (also known as breath stacking) is due to the collapse of small airways during expiration trapping air in the distal lung airspaces. If the expiratory time is too short to allow this gas to escape, more air becomes trapped with each breath, leading to progressive hyperinflation of the lungs. The increased intrathoracic pressure can impair venous return to the heart and, in extreme cases, cardiac arrest. If air-trapping is such that haemodynamic compromise results, then fluid resuscitation may be indicated to maintain adequate preload and cardiac output.[55] However, measures to reverse the air-trapping need to be addressed. This may include reducing ventilator PEEP to zero, reducing the respiratory rate and increasing the expiratory phase of the respiratory cycle. In extreme situations, external manual thoracic compression in time with expiration can be attempted, although the effectiveness of this technique has not been well studied. Air-trapping may develop more readily in the patient with COPD because of changes in pulmonary flow resistance, expiratory flow limitation and decreased respiratory system compliance.[139]
- *Bronchodilators*—these are used because of a possibility of a small reversible component of the airway obstruction.[138,139] Beta-2 agonists, such as salbutamol, and an anticholinergic agent, such as ipratropium bromide, are the most commonly used agents.[139] Just as with asthma management, these agents can be either short-acting, long-acting or both. Variation in responsiveness to bronchodilators appears to be inversely related to the severity of the COPD and not all patients will benefit from bronchodilator therapy[138] though reversibility in some can be as effective as with asthmatics.[144] Bronchodilator therapy is an appropriate starting point for therapy; however, alternative therapy options such as NIV should be considered where necessary.
- *Glucocorticosteroids* are recommended as an addition to other therapies in an acute exacerbation.[3,139]
- *Antibiotics* may be indicated if specific symptoms exist of increased sputum production and increased purulence of sputum, and for patients who require mechanical ventilation for the exacerbation.[138,139]

Exertion should be kept to an absolute minimum during acute exacerbations. This is particularly so for paramedics, where movement of the patient will be imposed. Transfer should involve the use of lifting devices, wheelchairs and mobile stretchers. Patient sliding or standing self-transfers or standing, ambulation or positioning the patient in any way other than their own preference are all capable of worsening breathing difficulty and causing patient deterioration.

Disposition

Decisions regarding hospital admission are based on the severity of exacerbation; how well the patient responds to therapy, and the degree of reversibility of the cause of the exacerbation.[138] For discharge home, the emergency care provider must ensure appropriate social support, including a check that home conditions are suitable, and that follow-up care, such as community nursing or a respiratory chronic care program, has been organised.

PNEUMONIA

Pneumonia is an infection of the lower respiratory tract caused by bacteria, viruses and other organisms. Many individuals in the community are susceptible to the development of pneumonia, particularly the elderly. Other factors that increase the risk of pneumonia include immune system compromise, alcoholism, smoking, malnutrition and immobilisation.[4] Table 21.14

TABLE 21.14 PRECIPITATING CONDITIONS OF PNEUMONIA[145]

CONDITION	AETIOLOGIES
Depressed epiglottal and cough reflexes	Unconsciousness, neurological disease, endotracheal or tracheal tubes, anaesthesia, ageing
Decreased ciliary activity	Smoke inhalation, smoking history, oxygen toxicity, hypoventilation, intubation, viral infections, ageing, COPD
Increased secretions	COPD, viral infections, bronchiectasis, general anaesthesia, endotracheal intubation, smoking
Atelectasis	Trauma, foreign-body obstruction, tumour, splinting, shallow ventilations, general anaesthesia
Decreased lymphatic flow	Heart failure, tumour
Fluid in alveoli	Heart failure, aspiration, trauma
Abnormal phagocytosis and humoral activity	Neutropenia, immunocompetent disorders, patients receiving chemotherapy
Impaired alveolar macrophages	Hypoxaemia, metabolic acidosis, cigarette smoking history, hypoxia, alcohol use, viral infections, ageing

COPD: chronic obstructive pulmonary disease.

lists conditions that may predispose the patient to pneumonia. Community-acquired pneumonia is likely to be the most common type of pneumonia seen in the ED. Causative organisms include *Streptococcus pneumoniae*, *Mycoplasma pneumoniae* and viral pathogens such as influenza.[146]

In the context of community-acquired pneumonia, airborne pathogens released through coughing and sneezing can be inhaled and enter the respiratory system. Airborne pathogens can also be released from aerosolised water. An example of this is when cooling towers are implicated in an outbreak of *Legionella* infection.

The first line of defence is the protective mechanisms of coughing and mucociliary clearance. If organisms are able to bypass these, alveolar macrophages are the next line of defence—but this will only be effective if the virulence and load of the bacteria or virus is low. If this defence is not effective, then the immune system will be activated. Release of inflammatory mediators and immune complexes damage bronchial mucous membranes and alveolocapillary membranes, causing the terminal bronchioles to fill with debris and exudates and results in patients experiencing dyspnoea, pleuritic chest pain, cough with expectoration of purulent sputum, crackles or wheezing and bronchial breath sound on auscultation. Changes in ventilation–perfusion matching contribute to hypoxia. CO_2 levels may remain normal, as it diffuses more easily than oxygen. Pre-existing respiratory compromise may further compromise and complicate the patient's clinical presentation. It is important to remember that elderly people and those with weaker immune systems may have fewer and less-severe symptoms, or non-specific symptoms, such as acute confusion/delirium or deterioration of baseline function.

In 2019, the SARS coronavirus SARS-CoV-2, better known as COVID-19, embedded itself as a global pandemic. This is a highly contagious respiratory disease responsible for an array of symptoms, including fatigue, chills, headache, sore throat, rhinitis, loss of smell and even nausea, vomiting and diarrhoea. Most people recover without major issue, although the aged and those with some comorbidities are at risk of more complex sequalae, including life-threatening viral pneumonia. This has similarities to other infective pneumonia, such as diffuse alveolar injury and pulmonary thrombosis, with some differences noted, such as maintained respiratory compliance despite severe hypoxemia and appearance on x-ray.[147–149] As many as 40% of COVID-19 viral pneumonia cases can progress to develop ARDS, with most requiring intensive care admission.[148]

DIAGNOSTICS AND MONITORING

Pulse oximetry is used to evaluate the oxygenation status where severely low oxygen levels can commonly be encountered.[19] A chest x-ray will demonstrate one or more areas of airspace opacification and helps to rule out alternative diagnoses. Patients with a pleural effusion greater than 5 cm on an upright posterior–anterior chest x-ray may be considered for a diagnostic thoracocentesis with fluid sent for cell count, pH, culture and Gram stain.[145,149] Less specific signs include respiratory rate > 30 breaths/minute, poor pulse oximetry, confusion, alterations in body temperature and hypotension.[150]

A full blood count may demonstrate an elevated white count; however, this information rarely alters diagnostic or management decisions. Creatinine and electrolytes are useful in elderly patients to determine renal function, which may alter dosing of drugs that are eliminated by the kidneys. Sputum cultures, which take 24–48 hours for results, rarely change the choice of antibiotics already made, and are not routinely required. They may be useful in patients at risk of unusual pathogens, such as those with pre-existing chronic lung disease (e.g. bronchiectasis, cystic fibrosis) and immunocompromised patients. Blood cultures are not routinely required although may be considered for higher-risk patients admitted with community-acquired pneumonia.[19] For young patients who are otherwise healthy and have an uncomplicated case of pneumonia, testing can be limited to a chest x-ray and pulse oximetry.

Pre-hospital differentiation of pulmonary infection from acute pulmonary oedema can prove difficult. In many cases increased capillary permeability with infection might produce oedema concurrently compounding this problem. The point is comparatively moot since, drug therapy aside, the patient management may not substantially differ outside the hospital environment.

MANAGEMENT

The vast majority of patients with community-acquired pneumonia can be treated successfully with narrow-spectrum beta-lactam treatment, such as penicillin combined with doxycycline or a macrolide.[146,150] Pneumonia of a viral origin may be treated with antivirals. Patients who are severely affected may require supportive therapy, such as NIV or invasive ventilation.

While the majority of patients presenting with pneumonia are able to be managed outside the hospital environment, pneumonia is one of the top three principal diagnoses for hospital admissions in Australia.[151] An assessment of pneumonia severity is essential to inform decisions regarding the need for admission. Refer to the Practice Tip (Red flags indicating severe CAP requiring hospital admission) for 'red flags' in clinical features and investigations that should prompt hospital admission.

PRACTICE TIP

'RED FLAGS' INDICATING SEVERE COMMUNITY-ACQUIRED PNEUMONIA REQUIRING HOSPITAL ADMISSION

Clinical

- Respiratory rate greater than 30 breaths/min
- Systolic blood pressure less than 90 mmHg
- Pulse rate > 125 beats/min
- Oxygen saturation less than 92%
- Acute onset confusion

Investigations

- Arterial (or venous) pH less than 7.35
- Partial pressure of oxygen (PaO_2) less than 60 mmHg
- Multilobar involvement on chest x-ray

Hospital admissions for pneumonia are based not only on severity of illness, but also underlying comorbid illness and psychosocial reasons, the latter including ability for self-care or any cognitive impairment.[150] Australian studies have developed two severity scoring systems—CORB and SMART-COP—to aid disposition and management decisions of community-acquired pneumonia in adults. These scales are based on predictors of likely requirement of intensive respiratory or vasopressor support, and direct attention to clinical features that predict clinical deterioration; these are now the preferred tools for assessing pneumonia severity.[152] Patients considered for treatment outside the hospital environment should not display high-risk features and should score mild severity or mild–moderate severity on one of the scoring systems.

Severe pneumonia that progresses to include ARDS may require NIV or even intubation and mechanical ventilation to support pulmonary function. In some cases, particularly COVID-19, prone positioning has proven advantageous during ventilated periods.[147] The maintained lung compliance in COVID-19 has also led to variations in ventilation strategy, including the use of lower PEEP levels.[149]

PULMONARY EMBOLI

Pulmonary emboli (PE) cause occlusion of the pulmonary vascular bed. Thrombi, tissue fragments, lipids, foreign bodies and air bubbles can all cause emboli, although the vast majority of emboli occur as a result of deep vein thrombosis (DVT).[4] Risk factors for the development of pulmonary emboli are therefore linked to DVT formation and also include hypercoagulability, venous stasis and injuries to the endothelial lining of blood vessels.

PATHOPHYSIOLOGY

The impact of the embolism is dependent on the size of the emboli and how much blood flow is obstructed. Emboli can cause massive occlusion, such as to the pulmonary artery, and can contribute to infarction of lung tissue. Some patients may develop multiple emboli and experience recurrent pulmonary emboli.

Occlusion of the pulmonary circulation results in ventilation–perfusion mismatch. Hypoxic vasoconstriction, decreased surfactant, atelectasis and the development of pulmonary oedema all contribute to the alterations in ventilation–perfusion matching.

Approximately 90% of patients with non-infarcting PE experience dyspnoea. This is most likely the clinical manifestation caused by ventilation–perfusion mismatch, where alveoli are ventilated but not perfused. This same V/Q mismatch is also the likely primary cause of hypoxaemia in a patient with PE, although not all patients experiencing a PE will actually be hypoxaemic.[153]

If the PE is large enough to result in occlusion of an artery leading to tissue necrosis, the patient can experience a sharp, pleuritic, focal chest pain. In later days after infarction, the infarcted section of lung tissue will become consolidated on chest x-ray and develop a pleural effusion due to the accompanying inflammatory process.[153]

When a PE obstructs $>$ 50% of vasculature, it can result in increased right ventricular pressure, and in the most severe cases arterial hypotension can eventuate. This is associated with a four-fold increase in risk of death.[153]

DIAGNOSTICS AND MONITORING

Diagnosis of PE starts with an estimation of probability. Patient history is important, and questioning should focus on risk factors for pulmonary emboli and DVT. The most commonly used tool to aid decision-making is the 'Wells criteria/scoring for PE' (Table 21.15).[154]

A second very useful clinical decision aid that works in concert with the Wells scoring system is the pulmonary embolism rule-out criteria (PERC) rule. In patients who are considered unlikely to have a pulmonary embolism, the PERC rule can be applied to rule out a PE based on clinical criteria alone, avoiding the problems associated with the frequent false positive D-dimer test. The PERC rule consists of eight items, all of which must be answered 'No' to rule out a PE. The items are: age $\geq$ 50; pulse rate $\geq$ 100; oxygen saturation $<$ 95%; previous history of DVT or PE; recent trauma or surgery; haemoptysis; drug therapy containing oestrogens; and unilateral leg swelling.[155,156]

Chest x-rays rarely show diagnostic features for PE, but are useful for detecting alternative causes for the patient's symptoms, such as pneumothorax, pneumonia and cardiac failure. ABGs may be taken and may show hypoxaemia and hypocarbia. Patients who are considered unlikely to have a PE on Wells risk criteria, but who cannot have PE ruled out using the PERC rule, should have a D-dimer test. If positive, further testing is required to make the diagnosis. A ventilation–perfusion lung scan is a useful modality in young patients with no pre-existing lung disease. A clear CXR may be the preferred test in this population due to the lower radiation exposure. For other patients, spiral computed tomography (CT) is more useful in making the diagnosis of pulmonary emboli and has the added benefit of identifying alternative diagnoses such as pneumonia and aortic dissection. Echocardiography may be used for rapid and accurate risk-stratification of patients with pulmonary embolism.[155]

TABLE 21.15 WELLS CRITERIA AND SCORING FOR PULMONARY EMBOLISM[154]

PRESENT	SCORE
Clinical signs and symptoms of DVT	+3
PE is No. 1 diagnosis or equally likely diagnosis	+3
Heart rate $>$ 100	+1.5
Immobilisation at least 3 days, or surgery in the previous 4 weeks	+1.5
PREVIOUS	
Objectively diagnosed PE or EVT?	+1.5
Haemoptysis?	+1
Malignancy with treatment within 6 months, or palliative?	+1

Pre-test clinical probability of a PE:

Wells score $>$ 4: PE likely, consider diagnostic imaging

Wells score $\leq$ 4: PE unlikely, consider D-dimer to rule out PE

MANAGEMENT

Prevention is the best strategy for managing pulmonary emboli. If PE is diagnosed, anticoagulant therapy (heparin, warfarin, or both) will usually be prescribed. Patients are increasingly being treated with new oral anticoagulants (e.g. dabigatran, rivaroxaban, apixaban), which have the benefit of a rapid onset of action and no need for blood-testing to monitor the level of anti-coagulation. If the pulmonary emboli are life threatening, pulmonary angiography may be used to locate and extract the emboli or inject thrombolytic agents to dissolve the clot. If thrombolysis is contraindicated, surgical embolectomy may be required.[156] There is limited evidence on the efficacy of using vena caval filters to trap emboli from deep veins, although recent evidence success rates continue to rise.[157]

Disposition

Haemodynamically unstable patients, or those with significant hypoxaemia, should be admitted to ICU. The majority of patients diagnosed with a PE can be admitted to a ward; however, early discharge home with low-molecular-weight heparin can be considered with small pulmonary emboli.[158]

RESPIRATORY OUTPATIENT CARE PROGRAMS

Various models of outpatient respiratory care programs have been developed in different locations. The aim of these programs may incorporate some or all of the following areas: to facilitate early discharge from hospital with follow-up care in the home; development of action plans to guide management of future exacerbations, thereby reducing admission rate; provide pulmonary rehabilitation services, and specialist review services within the home or hospital for acute exacerbations.[159] Successful respiratory care programs have been instrumental in decreasing hospital presentation and admission rates for chronic respiratory patients, and decreasing hospital length of stay for some patients by continuing therapy post-discharge in the home.[159]

If a patient is involved with a respiratory outpatient program, early contact should be made with the program to enable input towards management, and determine what supports are available in the home environment. Early liaison with the respiratory outpatient program may present options for management other than admission to an acute-care hospital bed.

INHALATION INJURIES

Three factors to consider when evaluating a patient with an inhalation injury are exposure to asphyxiants (carbon monoxide, cyanide), thermal or heat injury of the airways (see Chapter 28) and inhalation of pulmonary irritants (smoke particles and other gases produced by a fire). Exposure to asphyxiants is the most frequent cause of early mortality, with carbon monoxide (CO) the most frequent asphyxiant from a fire.

CARBON MONOXIDE

Carbon monoxide is extremely common, being produced by the incomplete combustion of carbon-containing fuels, including petrol, coal, wood and gas. It is produced in domestic heating, motor vehicles, industry and cigarette-smoking. Carbon monoxide is also produced naturally within the body as a by-product of haemoglobin breakdown. It has no colour, no smell and cannot be detected by human senses, making it sometimes difficult to identify as the clinical problem. Carbon monoxide diffuses into the lungs in a similar way to oxygen, but has an affinity for attaching to haemoglobin over 200–250 times greater, forming carboxyhaemoglobin.[160] Carbon monoxide also binds to key proteins within the mitochondria of cells that use oxygen for the production of cellular energy (ATP).[160] Cellular respiration is impaired by the failure to deliver expected quantities of oxygen attached to haemoglobin, and the inability of cells to use the oxygen that is delivered. Oxygen that diffuses into the blood remains highly reactive and is more available to form unwanted radical substances. The resultant cellular changes and dysfunction include inflammation, capillary changes and oedema. These are most notable in the brain where susceptible oxygen-demanding tissue can be found, including white matter, cerebral cortex and basal ganglia.[161,162]

Significant exposure, such as from a suicide attempt or exposure to smoke from a house or building fire, will typically raise suspicions of carbon monoxide exposure.[160] In other instances, such as a malfunctioning gas heater, it may be completely unrecognised or overlooked. There may be clues that help, such as other people or animals being unwell or being wintertime with obvious heater usage increase. Patients who may also appear to improve and then have a return of symptoms in certain locations can assist with identifying the cause.[161]

Exhaust fumes containing carbon monoxide was once a well-recognised method of committing suicide; however, changes to vehicle emission laws have produced a steady reduction in available gas and resultant fatalities.[163]

Carboxyhaemoglobin (COHb) levels greater than 10% may indicate smoke inhalation; however, smokers or individuals exposed to vehicle exhaust fumes can have baseline COHb levels of up to 10%, rising to greater than 20% for heavy smokers. The rise in e-cigarette use has only partly offset this with significant, although lesser, levels of COHb still detectable.[164]

The signs and symptoms of acute CO poisoning can be related to the concentration at the time of exposure. Acute exposure to CO usually causes central nervous system and cardiovascular toxicity and injury. Tissues in these regions have high blood flow and oxygen demand. Table 21.16 summarises the

TABLE 21.16 SIGNS AND SYMPTOMS RELATED TO CARBOXYHAEMOGLOBIN (COHb) LEVEL AT TIME OF EXPOSURE TO CARBON MONOXIDE[161]

COHb LEVEL (%)	SIGNS AND SYMPTOMS
0	None
10	Frontal headache
20	Throbbing headache, shortness of breath on exertion
30	Impaired judgement, nausea, fatigue, visual disturbances, dizziness
40	Confusion, loss of consciousness
50	Seizures, coma
60	Hypotension, respiratory failure
70	Death

TABLE 21.17 CLINICAL FEATURES OF CARBON MONOXIDE POISONING[161]

SYSTEM	SYMPTOMS	PATHOLOGY	DIAGNOSTIC
Central nervous system	Early—confusion, coma, seizures	Brain oedema, encephalopathy	EEG
	Late—psychoses, dementia, parkinsonism, ataxia, peripheral neuropathy, gait disturbance	Cerebral atrophy, basal ganglia lesions	CT scan
Cardiac	Dysrhythmias, hypotension angina, tachycardia	Myocardial ischaemia	ECG, CK, CK-MB, troponin
Pulmonary	Shortness of breath	Pulmonary oedema	Chest x-ray
Ophthalmological	Visual disturbances	Flame-shaped retinal haemorrhages, cerebral lesions, retrobulbar neuritis, papillo-oedema	Fundoscopy
Renal	Acute failure	Myoglobinuria	Renal function tests, serum myoglobin, urine myoglobin
Muscular	Ischaemia	Compartment syndrome, rhabdomyolysis	
Auditory and vestibular	Hearing loss, nystagmus, tinnitus		

CK: creatine kinase; CK-MB: creatine kinase-MB enzyme (primarily produced by the heart muscle); CT: computed tomography; ECG: electrocardiogram.

signs and symptoms and Table 21.17 summarises the clinical features of CO poisoning.

Diagnosis of CO poisoning

The presenting signs and symptoms of carbon monoxide poisoning are often vague and non-specific. They can be easily confused with or dismissed as other problems. Even severe illness can be mistaken for another diagnosis, including stroke and seizure.[161] The most common initial complaints are fatigue, nausea, headache and dizziness.

Neurological signs include confusion and anxiety. Ataxia and vision impairment can develop. Reduced consciousness with decreasing GCS score and convulsions occur at higher levels of exposure. Even after recovery some of these complaints can persist for several weeks with reports of symptoms persisting beyond 1 year.[160,165] The onset of Parkinsonism following exposure has been described.[166] Even in patients who present with only mild acute exposure to carbon monoxide, symptoms of headache and dizziness can continue for more than 4 weeks.[161]

Early cardiovascular signs of tachycardia and hypertension are frequently noted.[161] Myoglobin has an even stronger affinity for carbon monoxide. This increases the likelihood of cardiovascular problems.[167,168] Angina, hypotension and myocardial infarction can be caused by significant carbon monoxide exposure. Acute pulmonary oedema can occur.[167]

Cardiovascular signs and symptoms commonly suggest higher exposure levels in acute incidents. Death from carbon monoxide that occurs very quickly is likely to be due to lethal dysrhythmia following myocardial ischaemia.[168]

Carboxyhaemoglobin is a redder colour than oxyhaemoglobin and this has led to the belief that redness in skin colour can be useful in diagnosis. This is not, however, of any use in assessment as the redness only becomes apparent when concentrations are close to lethal levels.[169]

The diagnosis of carbon monoxide poisoning is based on a history of the patient's exposure to the gas, the presence of symptoms of exposure and a finding of elevated carboxyhaemoglobin level in the blood. Venous and arterial blood will have the same reading.[169] Patient presentations may be varied when there is exposure to other gases, such as cyanides that can occur in house fires. The diagnosis of CO poisoning should be considered whenever multiple members of the same family or from the same workplace present with non-specific symptoms, especially headache within 24 hours of each other.

Carboxyhaemoglobin levels in non-smokers are normally close to zero of total haemoglobin. CO levels in light smokers may be 1% and heavy smokers could be as much as 15% as a normal finding. After 3%, high-risk groups, including elderly people, those with cardiovascular disease and children, will begin to show effects.[168] Infant haemoglobin has greater affinity for CO leading to slightly higher natural levels in the circulation than adults. Children may recover more quickly, most likely due to increased minute ventilation, though this can also be a factor in the greater uptake of CO in the first place.[71,170] Pregnant women, and subsequently the unborn child, are at an increased risk with the fetus having even greater affinity than adults.[170,171] In non-smokers, 10% carboxyhaemoglobin in the blood will usually produce symptoms, including nausea, fatigue and confusion; by 20–40%, these symptoms will worsen, including angina presentation, muscular weakness and visual impairment. By 40%, loss of consciousness is encountered; 50% seizures, and coma with fatality by 60%.[170]

Evaluation of blood levels of carboxyhaemoglobin is an accurate way to determine levels. Devices that can measure exhaled levels of carbon monoxide are also accurate.[18] However, the correlation between levels found in the blood and presentation is unreliable. This is because as soon as exposure ceases, carbon monoxide begins to disassociate from haemoglobin and is exhaled. This process is faster if the patient is given oxygen; for example, while being transported by ambulance to hospital. By the time a blood sample is taken in hospital, the carboxyhaemoglobin level may have decreased substantially. Severe presentations can therefore have comparatively low measured levels of carbon monoxide and clinical improvements in presentation do not always correlate with clearance.[160]

Pulse oximeters are unable to differentiate between oxyhaemoglobin and carboxyhaemoglobin. This makes them less reliable for determining severity of exposure and unreliable at providing oxygenation information.[19,160,169] Commercially available carbon monoxide pulse oximeters (SpCO) are available, but while they are potentially useful, their reliability remains in question.[160,169] Where these are used and readings are obtained, their use as a guide to exposure should be supported by clinical examination and detailed history.

MANAGEMENT

Pre-hospital management of the patient exposed to carbon monoxide is comparatively simple and straightforward. The first key is to remove the patient from further exposure after confirming that the scene is safe to enter. Increasing the partial pressure of oxygen available will displace carbon monoxide bound to haemoglobin. High-concentration oxygen therapy should be utilised with either a non-rebreathing mask or bag–valve–mask with high-flow oxygen therapy attached.[160,170]

Hyperbaric oxygen therapy involving high concentrations of oxygen delivered under greater than atmospheric air pressure is supported but controversial. Numerous studies have demonstrated a variety of patient improvements in both short- and long-term evaluations.[160,172,173] While oxygen therapy hastens removal of CO from the haemoglobin, hyperbaric therapy has been shown to hasten its elimination.[172] Hyperbaric oxygen administration has been shown to reduce the half-life of carboxyhaemoglobin from 320 minutes to 80 minutes with 100% oxygen therapy then reduced again to only 22 minutes with hyperbaric therapy.[174] The benefit of this therapy must be provided within 6 hours of exposure. Overall, patient benefit and improvement is not as reliable and predictable.

Cardiac monitoring for dysrhythmias and 12-lead ECG should be performed. Intravenous cannulation and blood testing for full blood count, electrolyte imbalance, urea and creatinine, COHb, blood sugar level and cardiac enzymes should be performed. Measurement of an elevated COHb concentration confirms the diagnosis; ABG analysis may demonstrate an acidosis, with an elevated lactate level. Where lactate levels are measured above 10 mmol/L, concomitant cyanide poisoning should be considered. Blood gas machines calculate the oxygen saturation from measured partial pressure and give a falsely elevated result in CO poisoning.

Other acute presenting problems associated with exposure, including cardiac chest pain, dysrhythmias, acute pulmonary oedema, hypotension, dehydration, external and airway burn injuries, pain and bronchospasm, may have to be managed concurrently depending on the nature of the exposure and examination findings.

An additional consideration with CO poisoning in the setting of fires and smoke in enclosed spaces is the potential for exposure to cyanide. Cyanide can be produced during the combustion of wool, silk, plastics, paper products, rubber and polyurethane (see Chapter 30).[159]

SUMMARY

This chapter has discussed the physiological changes that occur in respiratory failure and presented a methodical approach for assessing respiratory function. Subsequent to assessment, emergency clinicians must be able to implement appropriate interventions to maintain patient safety, provide adequate respiratory support and prevent further deterioration. This chapter explored respiratory support strategies that emergency clinicians may employ to achieve these goals. Respiratory complaints account for a significant proportion of emergency presentations with symptoms experienced by the patient ranging from mild to immediately life threatening. It is therefore essential that emergency clinicians have the ability to identify early signs of respiratory compromise or the patient at immediate risk.

CASE STUDY

A 72-year-old woman reports increased shortness of breath. Her husband reports recent chest infection, and worsening shortness of breath over the past 2 days. Physical examination reveals that the patient is leaning forwards with hands on knees, she is speaking in short phrases, and is tachypnoeic with a respiratory rate of 38 breaths/minute. She is using pursed-lip breathing, is pale and her nails reveal clubbing and are dusky coloured. On palpation, the radial pulse is rapid and thready. The patient has a Glasgow Coma Scale (GCS) score of 15, although she is becoming increasingly irritable and agitated.

QUESTIONS

1. Which of the following is the least paramedic consideration in pre-hospital management?
   a. Expeditious patient movement and transport without causing exertion
   b. Early and continuous monitoring of pulse oximetry and capnography
   c. Provision of sedation to control increasing patient agitation
   d. Preparing non-invasive ventilation options in case of patient deterioration
2. Within which area of the ED could this patient be adequately managed?
   a. Waiting room
   b. Subacute
   c. Acute
   d. Resuscitation bay
3. Which physical assessment findings would indicate acute deterioration?
   a. Recent chest infection with increased shortness of breath
   b. Tripoding, short phrases, peripheral cyanosis, tachypnoea, pursed-lip breathing
   c. Clubbing of fingernails
   d. Being elderly
4. The patient is moved into a resuscitation bay for prompt assessment and management. The first priority of the resuscitation nurse is to complete:
   a. Introduction
   b. Primary survey of ABCD
   c. Intravenous access
   d. Humidified oxygen
5. A decision is made to commence non-invasive ventilation. The initial settings utilised are IPAP 10 cmH_2O, EPAP 6 cmH_2O, FiO2 0.50. Thirty minutes later the patient is reviewed and the nurse finds the following information:
   - Observations: respiratory rate 34 breaths/minute, blood pressure 110/65 mmHg, heart rate 120 beats/minute, GCS 15
   - ABG: pH 7.30, $PaCO_2$ 55 mmHg, HCO_3^- 29 mmol/L, PaO_2 70 mmHg

   Interpret the blood gas results:
   a. Partially compensated respiratory acidosis with hypoxaemia
   b. Uncompensated respiratory acidosis with hypoxaemia
   c. Uncompensated metabolic acidosis with hypoxaemia
   d. Partially compensated respiratory alkalosis with hypoxaemia
6. To decrease the $PaCO_2$ and correct the pH, the ventilation strategy should increase which of the following?
   a. FiO_2
   b. Minute volume
   c. Respiratory rate
   d. Positive end-expiratory pressure
7. Using non-invasive ventilation, what strategies can you use to alter the minute volume?
   a. Increase the respiratory rate
   b. Increase the pressure support, and therefore the IPAP value
   c. Increase the EPAP
   d. Minute volume cannot be altered in non-invasive ventilation
8. Following a significant change to the ventilator settings to EPAP 10 cmH_2O and IPAP 20 cmH_2O, the next set of observations post-ventilation reflect a deterioration in haemodynamic status: blood pressure 90/45 mmHg, heart rate 125 beats/min. What is a probable cause for this sudden change in the scenario?
   a. Dehydration
   b. High settings of positive-pressure ventilation contributing to obstructive shock by raising intrathoracic pressure
   c. Hypoxia resulting in a haemodynamic decompensation
   d. Acute myocardial infarction

Answers to Case Study Questions can be found on evolve http://evolve.elsevier.com/AU/Curtis/emergency/ 

ACKNOWLEDGEMENT

The contributors would like to acknowledge and thank Diane Inglis for her assistance on this chapter.

USEFUL WEBSITES

Australian Institute of Health and Welfare (AIHW) is Australia's leading health and welfare statistics agency, www.aihw.gov.au/.

Australian Resuscitation Council represents all major groups involved in the teaching and practice of resuscitation and produces guidelines to meet its objectives in fostering uniformity and simplicity in resuscitation techniques and terminology, resus.org.au/.

Clinical procedures, NSW Emergency Care Institute. A series of short informative videos including NIV aci.health.nsw.gov.au/networks/eci/clinical/procedures.

COPD Guidelines: The COPD-X plan, COPD-X Plan is the Australian and New Zealand online management guidelines for chronic obstructive pulmonary disease. It has been developed jointly by The Thoracic Society of Australia and New Zealand and the Lung Foundation, copdx.org.au/.

Lung Foundation Australia provides information on lung disease for patients, their families, carers, health professionals and the general community, lungfoundation.com.au/.

National Asthma Council Australia, Australian Asthma Handbook, www.asthmahandbook.org.au.

REFERENCES

1. Australian Bureau of Statistics (ABS). National Health Survey: first results 2017–18. ABS. Online. Available from: www.abs.gov.au/statistics/health/health-conditions-and-risks/national-health-survey-first-results/latest-release.
2. Australian Bureau of Statistics (ABS). Provisional mortality statistics, Jan 2020–Aug 2021. ABS. Online. Available from: www.abs.gov.au/statistics/health/causes-death/provisional-mortality-statistics/jan-2020-aug-2021.
3. Australian Bureau of Statistics (ABS). Causes of death; 2019. ABS. Online. Available from: www.abs.gov.au/statistics/health/causes-death/causes-death-australia/2019.
4. Huether S, McCance SE. Alterations of pulmonary function. In: Understanding pathophysiology. Sydney: Elsevier Health Sciences; 2015.
5. Li X, Ma X. Acute respiratory failure in COVID-19: is it 'typical' ARDS? Crit Care 2020;24(1):1–5.
6. Barnard LT, Zhang J. The impact of respiratory disease in New Zealand: 2020 updates. 2021. Respiratory-Impact-report-final-2021Aug11.pdf (asthmafoundation.org.nz).
7. Morales-Quinteros L, Camprubi-Rimblas M, Bringue J, Bos LD, Schultz MJ, Artigas A. The role of hypercapnia in acute respiratory failure. Intensive Care Med Exp 2019;7(1):39.
8. McCance KL, Huether SE. Pathophysiology: the biologic basis for disease in adults and children. Chatswood: Elsevier Health Sciences; 2018.
9. Creagh-Brown B. Respiratory failure. Medicine 2016;44(6):342–5.
10. Considine J, Currey J. Ensuring a proactive, evidence-based, patient safety approach to patient assessment. J Clin Nurs 2015;24(1–2):300–7.
11. Munroe B, Curtis K, Considine J, Buckley T. The impact structured patient assessment frameworks have on patient care: an integrative review. J Clin Nurs 2013;22(21–22):2991–3005.
12. Curtis K, Hoy S, Murphy M, Hoy S, Lewis MJ. The emergency nursing assessment process: a structured framework for a systematic approach. Australas Emerg Nurs J 2009;12(4):130–6.
13. Macken L, Manning R. Facial trauma. 4th ed. Sydney: Churchill Livingstone; 2014.
14. Aminiahidashti H, Shafiee S, Kiasari AZ, Sazgar M. Applications of end-tidal carbon dioxide ($ETCO_2$) monitoring in emergency department; a narrative review. Emerg (Tehran) 2018;6(1):e5
15. Obe R, Charters A, Dawood M, Bennett P. Oxford handbook of emergency nursing. Oxford: Oxford University Press; 2016.
16. DeVita MA, Hillman K, Bellomo R, Odell M, Jones DA, Winters BD, et al. Textbook of rapid response systems: concept and implementation. New York: Springer; 2017.
17. Smith J, Rushton M. How to perform respiratory assessment. Nurs Stand 2015;30(7):34–6.
18. Forbes H, Watt E, editors. Jarvis's health assessment and physical examination–E-book: Australian and New Zealand. Sydney: Elsevier Health Sciences; 2020.
19. Ringdal M, Gullick J. Respiratory assessment and monitoring. In: Aitken L, Marshall A, Chaboyer W, editors. ACCN's critical care nursing. 3rd ed. Sydney: Elsevier Health Sciences; 2016.
20. Kelly A. Asthma. 4th ed. Sydney: Churchill Livingstone; 2014.
21. Gupta D, Nath A, Agarwal R, Behera D. A prospective randomized controlled trial on the efficacy of noninvasive ventilation in severe acute asthma. Respir Care 2010;55(5):536–43.
22. Gumm K. Emergency department trauma management. Sydney: Mosby; 2006.
23. Simon ST, Higginson IJ, Benalia J, Gysels M, Murtagh FE, Spicer J, et al. Episiodic and continuous breathlessness, a new categorization of breathlessness. J Pain Symptom Manage 2013;45(6):1019–29.
24. Sarkar M, Maheshe DM, Madabhavi I. Digital clubbing. Lung India 2012;29(4):354–62.
25. Wilson S, Giddens J. Health assessment for nursing practice—e-book. St Louis: Elsevier Health Sciences; 2016.
26. Jevon P, Ewens B. Monitoring the critically ill patient. London: John Wiley; 2012.

27. Wang K, Zeng R. Cyanosis. Handbook of clinical diagnostics. Singapore: Springer; 2020.
28. Mukherjee SE. Clinical approach to cyanosis. In: Pal J, Sarkar S, Chakraborty S, editors. Clinical methods in respiratory medicine. New Delhi: Jaypee Brothers Medical Publishers; 2018.
29. Cohen PR. The color of skin: blue diseases of the skin, nails, and mucosa. Clin Derm 2019;37(5):468–86.
30. Jiang-Nan Z, Yao L, Huai-Chen L. Aspiration-related acute respiratory distress syndrome in acute stroke patient. PLoS One 2015;10(3):e0118682.
31. Afshar M, Smith G, Cooper R, Murthi S, Netzer G. Trauma indices for prediction of acute respiratory distress syndrome. J Surg Res 2016;201(2):394–401.
32. Barbas CSV, Lopes GC, Vieira DF, Couto LP, Dourado LK, Caser E. Respiratory evaluation of patients requiring ventilator support due to acute respiratory failure. Open J Nurs 2012;2:336–40.
33. Rambaud-Althaus C, Althaus F, Genton B, D'Acremont V. Clinical features for diagnosis of pneumonia in children younger than 5 years: a systematic review and meta-analysis. Lancet Infect Dis 2015;15(4):439–50.
34. Kaufman J, Kent B. Nursing management: obstructive pulmonary diseases. In: Brown D, Edwards H, Lewis S, editors. Lewis's medical surgical nursing. 2nd ed. Marrickville: Mosby Elsevier Health Sciences; 2016.
35. Australian Resuscitation Council. ANZCOR guideline 4: airway. Melbourne: Australian Resuscitation Council; 2016. Available from: www.resus.org.au.
36. Knighton J, Fong J. Nursing management: burns. In: Brown D, Edwards H, Lewis S, et al. editors. Lewis's medical surgical nursing. 2nd ed. Marrickville: Mosby Elsevier Health Sciences; 2016.
37. Gallagher R, Driscoll A. Cardiovascular alterations and management. In: Aitken L, Marshall A, Chaboyer W, editors. ACCN's critical care nursing. 3rd ed. Sydney: Elsevier Health Sciences; 2016.
38. Berlowitz DJ, Wadsworth B, Ross J. Respiratory problems and management in people with spinal cord injury. Breathe 2016;12(4):328–40.
39. Cretikos M, Chen J, Hillman K, Bellomo R, Finfer S, Flabouris A, et al. The objective medical emergency team activation criteria: a case-control study. Resuscitation 2007;73(1):62–72.
40. Morton P, Fontaine D, Hudak C, Gallo BM. Critical care nursing: a holistic approach. Philadelphia: Lippincott Williams & Wilkins; 2017.
41. Inglis D, Kenneally J, editors. Chapter 2.8 in Clinical skills for paramedic practice ANZ 1e. Sydney: Elsevier Australia; 2020.
42. Inglis D, Kenneally J, editors. Chapter 2.10 in Clinical skills for paramedic practice ANZ 1e. Sydney: Elsevier Australia; 2020.
43. Yont GH, Korhan EA, Dizer B. The effect of nail polish on pulse oximetry readings. Intens Crit Care Nurs 2014;4(30):111–5.
44. Doğan SD, Yikar SK, Arslan S, Nazik E. The effect of nail polish and henna on the measures of pulse oximeters in healthy persons. J Perianesth Nurs 2021;36(5):532–5.
45. Nagurka R, Bechmann S, Gluckman W, Scott SR, Compton S, Lamba S. Utility of initial pre-hospital end tidal carbon dioxide measurements to predict poor outcomes in adult asthmatic patients. Prehospital Emerg Care 2014;18(2):180–4.
46. Agnihotri NT, Saltoun C. Acute severe asthma (status asthmaticus). Allergy Asthma Proc 2019;40(6):406–9.
47. Bernard S. Advanced airway management. 4th ed. Sydney: Churchill Livingstone; 2014.
48. Long B, Kpyfman A, Vivirito MA. Capnography in the emergency department; a review of uses, waveforms and limitations. J Emerg Med 2017;53(6):829–42.
49. Soleimanpour H, Taghizadieh A, Niafar M, Rahmani F, Golzari SE, Esfanjani RM. Predictive value of capnography for suspected diabetic ketoacidosis in the emergency department. West J Emerg Med 2013;14(6):590–4.
50. Byrne AL, Bennett M, Chatterji R, Symons R, Pace NL, Thomas PS. Peripheral venous and arterial blood gas analysis in adults: are they comparable? A systematic review and meta-analysis. Respirology (Carlton, Vic.) 2014;19(2):168–75.
51. Kelly AM. Can VBG analysis replace ABG analysis in emergency care? Emerg Med J 2016;33(2):152–4.
52. Brooks N. Venepuncture and cannulation: a practical guide. United Kingdom: M&K Update Ltd; 2014.
53. Kelly AM, Klim S. Agreement between arterial and venous pH and pCO_2 in patients undergoing non-invasive ventilation in the emergency department. Emerg Med Australas 2013;25(3):203–6.
54. Inglis D, Kenneally J, editors. Chapter 2.11 in Clinical skills for paramedic practice ANZ 1e. Sydney: Elsevier Australia; 2020.
55. Rose L, Butcher R. Ventilation and oxygenation management. In: Aitken L, Marshall A, Chaboyer W, editors. ACCN's critical care nursing. 3rd ed. Sydney: Elsevier Health Sciences; 2016.
56. Graham BL, Steenbruggen I, Miller MR, Barjaktarevic IZ, Cooper BG, Hall GL, et al. Standardisation of spirometry 2019 update. An official American Thoracic Society and European Respiratory Society technical statement. Am J Respir Crit Care Med 2019;200(8):e70–88.
57. Johns D, Pierce R. Spirometry: the measurement and interpretation of ventilatory function in clinical practice. Rev ed. Melbourne: Australia: The Thoracic Society of Australia and New Zealand; 2008.
58. Wijesinghe M, Perrin K, Healy B, Hart K, Clay J, Weatherall M, et al. Pre-hospital oxygen therapy in acute exacerbations of chronic obstructive pulmonary disease. Intern Med J 2011;41(8):618–22.
59. Echevarria C, Steer J, Watson J, Bourke S. Oxygen therapy and inpatient mortality in COPD exacerbation. Emerg Med J 2021;38(3):170–7.
60. Grensemann J, Fuhrmann V, Kluge S. Oxygen treatment in intensive care and emergency medicine. Dtsch Arztebl Int 2018;115(27–28):455–62.
61. Gibbs, LM, Pham K, Langston S, Stigleman S. Supplemental oxygen therapy for nonhypoxemic patients with acute coronary syndrome. Amn Fam Phys 2020;101(11):687–8.

62. Stub D, Smith K, Bernard S, Nehme Z, Stephenson M, Bray JE, et al. Air versus oxygen in ST-segment elevation myocardial infarction. Circulation 2015;131(24):2143–50.
63. O'Driscoll BR, Howard LS, Earis J, Mak V. British Thoracic Guideline for oxygen use in adults in healthcare and emergency settings. BMJ Open Respir Res 2017;4(1):e000170.
64. Kones R. Oxygen therapy for acute myocardial infarction–then and now. A century of uncertainty. Am J Med 2011;124(11):1000–5.
65. Burls A, Cabello JB, Emparanza JI, Bayliss S, Quinn T. Oxygen therapy for acute myocardial infarction: a systematic review and meta-analysis. Emerg Med J 2011;28(11):917–23.
66. Stroke Foundation. Clinical guidelines for stroke management. Melbourne: Australia; 2021.
67. Girardis M, Alhazzani W, Rasmussen BS. What's new in oxygen therapy? Intensive Care Med 2019;45:1009–11.
68. Boatright J, Ward J. Therapeutic gases: management and administration. In: Hess D, Macintyre NR, Galvin W, editors. Respiratory care. 3rd ed. USA: Jones & Bartlett Learning; 2016.
69. Melani AS, Sestini P, Rottoli P. Home oxygen therapy: rethinking the role of devices. Exp Rev Clin Pharmacol 2018;11(3):279–89.
70. Spicuzza L, Schisano M. High flow nasal cannula oxygen therapy as an emerging option for respiratory failure: the present and the future. Ther Adv Chronic Dis 2020;11:2040622320920106.
71. Curtis K, Kouraouche K, Asha S, Considine J, Fry M, Middleton S, et al. Impact of a care bundle for patients with blunt chest Injury (CHiP): a multicentre controlled implementation evauation. PLoS One 2021;16(10):e0256027.
72. Parke RL, McGuinness SP, Eccleston ML. A preliminary randomized controlled trial to assess effectiveness of nasal high-flow oxygen in intensive care patients. Respir Care 2011;56(3):265–70.
73. Nishimura M. High flow nasal cannula oxygen therapy devices. Respir Care 2019;64(6):735–42.
74. Maggiore SM, Idone FA, Vaschetto R, Festa R, Cataldo A, Antonicelli F, et al. Nasal high-flow versus venturi mask oxygen therapy after extubation. Effects on oxygenation, comfort, and clinical outcome. Am J Respir Crit Care Med 2014;190(3):282–8.
75. Li J, Jing G, Scott JB. Year in review 2019: high-flow nasal cannula oxygen therapy for adult subjects. Respir Care 2020;65(4):545–57.
76. Abdo WF, Heunks LM. Oxygen induced hypercapnia in COPD: myths and facts. Crit Care 2012;16(5):323.
77. Cornet AD, Kooter AJ, Peters MJ, Smulders YM. The potential harm of oxygen therapy in medical emergencies. Crit Care (London, England) 2013;17(2):313.
78. Cameron L, Pilcher J, Weatherall M, Beasley R, Perrin K. The risk of serious adverse outcomes associated with hypoxaemia and hyperoxaemia in acute exacerbations of COPD. Postgrad Med J 2012;88(1046):684–9.
79. Pilcher J, Perrin K, Beasley R. The effect of high concentration oxygen therapy on $PaCO_2$ in acute and chronic respiratory disorders. Trans Respir Med 2013;1(1):8.
80. Kopsaftis Z, Carson-Chahhoud KV, Austin MA, Wood-Baker R. Oxygen therapy in the pre-hospital setting for acute exacerbations of chronic obstructive pulmonary disease. Cochrane Database Syst Rev 2020;(1):CD005534.
81. Bentsen LP, Lassen AT, Titlestad IL, Brabrand M. A change from high-flow to titrated oxygen therapy in the prehospital setting is associated with lower mortality in COPD patients with acute exacerbations: an observational cohort study. Acute Med 2020;19(2):76–82.
82. Carron M, Freo U, BaHamman AS, Dellweg D, Guarracino F, Cosentini R, et al. Complications of non invasive ventilation techniques: a comprehensive qualitative review of rendomized trials. Br J Anaesthes 2013;110(6):896–914.
83. Ergan B, Oczkowski S, Rochwerg B, Carlucci A, Chatwin M, Clini E, et al. European Respiratory Society guidelines on long-term home non-invasive ventilation for management of COPD. Euro Respir J 2019;54(3):1901003.
84. Masip J, Peacock WF, Price S, Carlucci A, Chatwin M, Clini E, et al. Indications and practical approach to non-invasive ventilation in acute heart failure. Eur Heart J 2018;39(1):17–25.
85. Ducros L, Logeart D, Vicaut E, Henry P, Plaisance P, Collet JP, et al. CPAP for acute cardiogenic pulmonary oedema from out-of-hospital to cardiac intensive care unit: a randomised multicentre study. Intensive Care Med 2011;37(9):1501–9.
86. Bledsoe BE, Anderson E, Hodnick R, Johnson L, Johnson S, Dievendorf E. Low-fractional oxygen concentration continuous positive airway pressure is effective in the prehospital setting. Prehosp Emerg Care 2012;16(2):217–21.
87. Hensel M, Strunden MS, Tank S, Gagelmann N, Wirtz S, Kerner T. Prehospital non-invasive ventilation in acute respiratory failure is justified even if the distance to hospital is short. Am J Emerg Med 2019;37(4):651–6.
88. Abubacker AP, Ndakotsu A, Chawla HV, Iqbal A, Grewal A, Myneni R, et al. Non-invasive positive pressure ventilation for acute cardiogenic pulmonary edema and chronic obstructive pulmonary disease in prehospital and emergency settings. Cureus 2021;13(6):e15624.
89. Windisch W, Weber-Carstens S, Kluge S, Rossaint R, Welte T, Karagiannidis C. Invasive and non-invasive ventilation in patients with COVID-19. Deutsches Ärzteblatt Int 2020;117(31-32):528–33.
90. Sivaloganathan AA, Nasim-Mohi M, Brown MM, Abdul N, Jackson A, Fletcher SV, et al. Noninvasive ventilation for COVID-19-associated acute hypoxaemic respiratory failure: experience from a single centre. Br J Anaesthes 2020;125(4):e368–71.
91. Mæhlen JO, Mikalsen R, Heimdal HJ, Rehn M, Hagemo JS, Ottestad W. Pre-hospital critical care management of severe hypoxemia in victims of Covid-19: a case series. Scandinavian J Trauma, Resusc Emerg Med 2021;29(1):16.
92. Shah NM, D'Cruz RF, Murphy PB. Update: non-invasive ventilation in chronic obstructive pulmonary disease. J Thoracic Dis 2018;10(Suppl. 1): S71–9.
93. Coleman III JM, Wolfe LF, Kalhan R. Noninvasive ventilation in chronic obstructive pulmonary disease. Ann Am Thoracic Soc 2019;16(9):1091–8.

94. Stefan MS, Priya A, Pekow PS, Lagu T, Steingrub JS, Hill NS, et al. The comparative effectiveness of noninvasive and invasive ventilation in patients with pneumonia. J Crit Care 2018;43:190–6.
95. Al-Rajhi A, Murad A, Li PZ, Shahin J. Outcomes and predictors of failure of non-invasive ventilation in patients with community acquired pneumonia in the ED. Am J Emerg Med 2018;36(3):347–51.
96. Althoff MD, Holguin F, Yang F, Grunwald GK, Moss M, Vandivier RW, et al. Noninvasive ventilation use in critically ill patients with acute asthma exacerbations. Am J Respir Crit Care Med 2020;202(11):1520–30.
97. Althoff M, Holguin F, Moss M, Yang F, Grunwald GK, Kiser TH, et al. Noninvasive ventilation use in critically ill patients with acute asthma exacerbations. Critical care: all's well that ends well—translating practice to outcomes for our patients with critical illness 2019 May. Conference paper. American Thoracic Society; 2019.
98. Landaeta M, Troya Maldonado M, Hoge G, Manglani R, Kasubhai M, Menon V, et al. Outcomes and predictor of the use of non-invasive ventilation in asthma exacerbation. Factors in adherence and control of asthma 2020 May. Conference paper. Philadelphia PA: American Thoracic Society; 2020.
99. Cairo JM. Pilbeam's mechanical ventilation–e-book: physiological and clinical applications. St. Louis, Missouri: Elsevier Health Sciences; 2015.
100. Bond KR, Horsley CA, Williams AB. Non-invasive ventilation use in status asthmaticus: 16 years of experience in a tertiary intensive care. Emerg Med Australas 2018;30(2):187–92.
101. Diaz de Teran T, Barbagelata E, Cilloniz C, Nicolini A, Perazzo T, Perren A, et al. Non-invasive ventilation in palliative care: a systematic review. Minerva Medica 2019;110(6):555–63.
102. Davies JD. Noninvasive respiratory support at the end of life. Respir Care 2019;64(6):701–11.
103. Chawla R, Dixit SB, Zirpe KG, Chaudhry D, Khilnani GC, Mehta Y, et al. ISCCM guidelines for the use of non-invasive ventilation in acute respiratory failure in adult ICUs. Ind J Crit Care Med 2020;24(Suppl. 1):S61–S81.
104. Hare A, Chatwin M. Basic principles of ventilators. In: Simonds AD, editor. ERS Practical handbook of noninvasive ventilation. London: The European Respiratory Society; 2015.
105. Hare A. Problem-solving: case studies of NIV problems and their management. In: Simonds AK, editor. ERS Practical handbook of noninvasive ventilation. London: The European Respiratory Society; 2015.
106. Hilbert G, Clouzeau B, Nam Bui H, Vargas F. Sedation during non-invasive ventilation. Minerva Anestesiol 2012;78(7):842–846.
107. Arroliga AC, Frutos-Vivar F, Anzueto A, Penuelas O, Ferguson ND, Rios F, et al. The use of sedatives and analgesics in patients receiving non-invasive positive pressure mechanical ventilation. American Thoracic Society international conference abstracts, 2012.
108. Jansson M, Ala-Kokko T, Ylipalosaari P, Syrjälä H, Kyngäs H. Critical care nurses' knowledge of, adherence to and barriers towards evidence-based guidelines for the prevention of ventilator-associated pneumonia–a survey study. Intensive Crit Care Nurs 2013;29(4):216–27.
109. Rose L, Ramagnano S. Emergency nurse responsibilities for mechanical ventilation: a national survey. J Emerg Nurs 2013;39(3):226.
110. Mpasa F, van Rooyen DR, Venter D, Jordan P, Ten Ham-Baloyi W. Improving nurses' knowledge of managing endotracheal tube cuff pressure in intensive care units: a quasi-experimental study. Health SA Gesondheid 2020;25:1479.
111. De Orange FA, Andrade RG, Lemos A, Borges PS, Figueiroa JN, Kovatsis PG. Cuffed versus uncuffed endotracheal tubes for general anaesthesia in children aged eight years and under? Cochrane Database Syst Rev 2017;11:CD011954.
112. Sztrymf B, Messika J, Mayot T, Lenglet H, Dreyfuss D, Ricard JD. Impact of high-flow nasal cannula oxygen therapy on intensive care unit patients with acute respiratory failure: a prospective observational study. J Crit Care 2012;27(3):324.e9–13.
113. Al Ashry HS, Modrykamien AM. Humidification during mechanical ventilation in the adult patient. BioMed Res Int 2014;2014:715434.
114. Dellavolpe JD, Lovett J, Martin-Gill C, Guyette FX. Transport of mechanically ventilated patients in the prone position. Prehosp Emerg Care 2016;20(5):643–7.
115. Purvey M, Allen G. Managing acute pulmonary oedema. Aust Prescrib 2017;40(2):59–63.
116. Givertz MM. Noncardiogenic pulmonary edema. Waltham, MA: UpToDate; 2020.
117. Čerlinskaitĉ K, Javanainen T, Cinotti R, Mebazaa A. Acute heart failure management. Kor Circ J 2018;48(6):463–80.
118. O'Brien J, Hunter C, editors. Heart failure. 8th ed. Philadelphia: Elsevier Saunders; 2014.
119. Lightfoot D, editor. Assessment and management of acute pulmonary oedema. 4th ed. Sydney: Churchill Livingstone; 2014.
120. McDonagh TA, Metra M, Adamo M, Gardner RS, Baumbach A, Burri H, et al. 2021 ESC Guidelines for the diagnosis and treatment of acute and chronic heart failure: Developed by the Task Force for the diagnosis and treatment of acute and chronic heart failure of the European Society of Cardiology (ESC) With the special contribution of the Heart Failure Association (HFA) of the ESC. Eur Heart J 2021;42(36):3599–726.
121. Brusasco C, Santori G, Tavazzi G, Via G, Robba C, Gargani L, et al. Second-order grey-scale texture analysis of pleural ultrasound images to differentiate acute respiratory distress syndrome and cardiogenic pulmonary edema. J Clin Monit Comput 2020;36(1):131–40.
122. Masip J. Noninvasive ventilation in acute heart failure. Curr Heart Fail Rep 2019;16(4):89–97.
123. Opie LH, Victor RG, Kaplan NM. Differing effects of diuretics in congestive heart failure and hypertension. In: Opie LH, Gersch BJ. Drugs for the heart. South Asian edition. New Delhi: Elsevier India; 2018.
124. Myers T, Holt T. Asthma. D. In: Hess D, Macintyre NR, Galvin W, editors. Respiratory care. 3rd ed. USA: Jones & Bartlett Learning; 2016.
125. Cosío BG, Dacal D, Pérez de Llano L. Asthma–COPD overlap: identification and optimal treatment. Ther Adv Respir Dis 2018;12:1753466618805662.

126. Table adapted from the Australian asthma handbook, quick reference guide, version 1.1. Melbourne: National Asthma Council Australia; 2020. Available from: www.asthmahandbook.org.au.
127. King GG, James A, Harkness L, Wark PA. Pathophysiology of severe asthma: we've only just started. Respirology 2018;23(3):262–71.
128. Pike KC, Levy ML, Moreiras J, Fleming L. Managing problematic severe asthma: beyond the guidelines. Arch Dis Child 2018;103(4):392–7.
129. Carlsson JA, Bayes HK. Acute severe asthma in adults. Medicine 2020;48(5):297–302.
130. Thien F, Beggs PJ, Csutoros D, Darvall J, Hew M, Davies JM, et al. The Melbourne epidemic thunderstorm asthma event 2016: an investigation of environmental triggers, effect on health services, and patient risk factors. Lancet Planet Health 2018;2(6):e255–63.
131. Inglis D, Kenneally J, editors. Chapter 4.3 in Clinical skills for paramedic practice ANZ 1e. Sydney: Elsevier Australia; 2020.
132. Baggott C, Hardy JK, Sparks J, Sabbagh D, Beasley R, Weatherall M, et al. Epinephrine (adrenaline) compared to selective beta-2-agonist in adults or children with acute asthma: a systematic review and meta-analysis. Thorax 2022;77:563–72.
133. Sellers WF. Inhaled and intravenous treatment in acute severe and life-threatening asthma. Br J Anaesthes 2013;110(2):183–90.
134. Qureshi IS, Fatima U, Akram A. The benefit of nebulized magnesium sulphate therapy in patients with acute severe asthma: a scoping review. South Asian J Emerg Med 2016;4(1):27–32.
135. Stojak BJ, Halajian E, Guthmann RA, Nashelsky J. FPIN's Clinical inquiries: intravenous magnesium sulfate for acute asthma exacerbations. Am Fam Phys 2019;99(2):127.
136. Laher AE, Buchanan SK. Mechanically ventilating the severe asthmatic. J Intens Care Med 2018;33(9):491–501.
137. Lange P. Persistent airway obstruction in asthma. Am J Respir Crit Care Med 2013;187(1):1–2.
138. Yang IA, Brown JL, George J, Jenkins S, McDonald CF, et al. COPD-X Australian and New Zealand guidelines for the diagnosis and management of chronic obstructive pulmonary disease: 2017 update. Med J Aust. 2017 Nov 20;207(10):436–442.
139. Global Initiative for Chronic Obstructive Lung Disease. Global strategy for the diagnosis, management, and prevention of chronic obstructive pulmonary disease. 2019. Available from: https://goldcopd.org/wp-content/uploads/2018/11/GOLD-2019-v1.7-FINAL-14Nov2018-WMS.pdf.
140. Kohli P. Chronic obstructive pulmonary disease. In: Hess D, Macintyre NR, Galvin W, Mishoe SC, editors. Respiratory care. 3rd ed. USA: Jones & Bartlett Learning; 2016.
141. Gulart AA, Munari AB, Queiroz AP, Cani KC, Matte DL, Mayer AF. Does the COPD assessment test reflect functional status in patients with COPD? Chron Respir Dis 2017;14(1):37–44.
142. Wetzig SM, Blackwood B, Currey J. Respiratory alterations and management. In: Aitken L, Marshall A, Chaboyer W, editors. ACCN's critical care nursing. 3rd ed. Sydney: Elsevier Health Sciences; 2016.
143. Lacasse Y, Tan AY, Maltais F, Krishnan JA. Home oxygen in chronic obstructive pulmonary disease. Am J Respir Crit Care Med 2018;197(10):1254–64.
144. Janson C, Malinovschi A, Amaral AF, Accordini S, Bousquet J, Buist AS, et al. Bronchodilator reversibility in asthma and COPD: findings from three large population studies. Euro Respir J 2019;54(3):1900561.
145. Urden LD, Stacy KM, Lough ME. Thelan's critical care nursing: diagnosis and management. 5th ed. St Louis: Mosby; 2006.
146. Johnson D, Crilly J. Emergency presentations. In: Aitken L, Marshall A, Chaboyer W, editors. ACCN's critical care nursing. 3rd ed. Sydney: Elsevier Health Sciences; 2016.
147. Gattinoni L, Chiumello D, Rossi S. COVID-19 pneumonia: ARDS or not? Crit Care 2020;24(1):154.
148. Gibson PG, Qin L, Puah SH. COVID-19 acute respiratory distress syndrome (ARDS): clinical features and differences from typical pre-COVID-19 ARDS. Med J Aust 2020;213(2):54–6.
149. Goligher EC, Ranieri VM, Slutsky AS. Is severe COVID-19 pneumonia a typical or atypical form of ARDS? And does it matter? Intens Care Med 2021;47;83–5.
150. Metlay JP, Waterer GW, Long AC, Anzueto A, Brozek J, Crothers K, et al. Diagnosis and treatment of adults with community-acquired pneumonia. An official clinical practice guideline of the American Thoracic Society and Infectious Diseases Society of America. Am J Respir Crit Care Med 2019;200(7):e45–67.
151. Australian Institute of Health and Welfare (AIHW). Australia's health. Australia's health series no. 15. Cat. no. AUS 199. Canberra: AIHW; 2016.
152. Osman M, Manosuthi W, Kaewkungwal J, Silachamroon U, Mansanguan C, Kamolratanakul S, et al. Etiology, clinical course, and outcomes of pneumonia in the elderly: a retrospective and prospective cohort study in Thailand. Am J Trop Med Hygiene 2021;104(6):2009–16.
153. Kline J, editor. Pulmonary embolism and deep vein thrombosis. 8th ed. Philadelphia: Elsevier Saunders; 2014.
154. Republished with permission of Thieme Verlag, from Wells PS, Anderson DR, Rodger M, Ginsberg JS, Kearon C, Gent M, et al. Derivation of a simple clinical model to categorize patients probability of pulmonary embolism: increasing the models utility with the SimpliRED D-dimer. Thromb Haemost 2000;83(3):416–20. Permission conveyed through Copyright Clearance Center, Inc.
155. Hargett C. Pulmonary vascular disease. In: Hess D, Macintyre NR, Galvin W, Mishoe SC, editors. Respiratory care. 3rd ed. USA: Jones & Bartlett Learning; 2016.
156. Singh B, Parsaik AK, Agarwal D, Surana A, Mascarenhas SS, Chandra S. Diagnostic accuracy of pulmonary embolism rule-out criteria: a systematic review and meta-analysis. Ann Emerg Med 2012;59(6):517–520.e1–4.
157. Bikdeli B, Wang Y, Minges KE, Desai NR, Kim N, Desai MM, et al. Vena caval filter utilization and outcomes in pulmonary embolism: medicare hospitalizations from 1999 to 2010. J Am Coll Cardiol 2016;67(9):1027–35.

158. Young T, Tang H, Hughes R. Vena caval filters for the prevention of pulmonary embolism. Cochrane Database Syst Rev 2010;(2):Cd006212.
159. Cameron P, Jelinek G, Kelly AM, Brown AF, Little M. Textbook of adult emergency medicine. 5th ed. Sydney: Churchill Livingstone; 2019.
160. Rose JJ, Wang L, Xu Q, McTiernan CF, Shiva S, Tejero J, et al. Carbon monoxide poisoning: pathogenesis, management, and future directions of therapy. Am J Respir Crit Care Med 2017;195(5):596-606.
161. Cruise DC. Carbon monoxide. In: Cameron P, Jelinek G, Kelly A, Brown A, Little M, editors. Textbook of adult emergency medicine. 5th ed. Edinburgh: Churchill Livingstone; 2019.
162. Oh S, Choi SC. Acute carbon monoxide poisoning and delayed neurological sequelae: a potential neuroprotection bundle therapy. Neural Regen Res 2015;10(1):36-8.
163. Studdert DM, Gurrin LC, Jatkar U, Pirkis J. Relationship between vehicle emissions laws and incidence of suicide by motor vehicle exhaust gas in Australia, 2001–06: an ecological analysis. PLoS Med 2010;7(1):e1000210.
164. Dorey A, Scheerlinck P, Nguyen H, Albertson T. Acute and chronic carbon monoxide toxicity from tobacco smoking. Mil Med 2020;185(1-2):e61–7.
165. Huang CC, Chung MH, Weng SF, Chien CC, Lin SJ, Lin HJ, et al. Long-term prognosis of patients with carbon monoxide poisoning: a nationwide cohort study. PLoS One 2014;9(8):e105503.
166. Lai CY, Chou MC, Lin CL, Kao CH. Increased risk of Parkinson disease in patients with carbon monoxide intoxication: a population-based cohort study. Medicine 2015;94(19):e869.
167. Lee FY, Chen WK, Lin CL, Kao CH. Carbon monoxide poisoning and subsequent cardiovascular disease risk: a nationwide population-based cohort study. Medicine 2015;94(10):e624.
168. Garg J, Krishnamoorthy P, Palaniswamy C, Khera S, Ahmad H, Jain D, et al. Cardiovascular abnormalities in carbon monoxide poisoning. Am J Ther 2018;25(3):e339-48.
169. Villalba N, Osborn ZT, Derickson PR, Manning CT, Herrington RR, Kaminsky DA, et al. Diagnostic performance of carbon monoxide testing by pulse oximetry in the emergency department. Respir Care 2019;64(11):1351-7.
170. Gozubuyuk AA, Dag H, Kaçar A, Karakurt Y, Arica V. Epidemiology, pathophysiology, clinical evaluation, and treatment of carbon monoxide poisoning in child, infant, and fetus. N Clin Istanbul 2017;4(1):100–7.
171. Wylie BJ, Kishashu Y, Matechi E, Zhou Z, Coull B, Abioye AI, et al. Maternal exposure to carbon monoxide and fine particulate matter during pregnancy in an urban Tanzanian cohort. Indoor Air 2017;27(1):136–46.
172. Weaver LK. Carbon monoxide poisoning. Undersea Hyperb Med 2020;47(1):151-69.
173. Rose JJ, Nouraie M, Gauthier MC, Pizon AF, Saul MI, Donahoe MP, et al. Clinical outcomes and mortality impact of hyperbaric oxygen therapy in patients with carbon monoxide poisoning. Crit Care Med 2018;46(7):e649.
174. Wang W, Cheng J, Zhang J, Wang K. Effect of hyperbaric oxygen on neurologic sequelae and all-cause mortality in patients with carbon monoxide poisoning: a meta-analysis of randomized controlled trials. Med Sci Monit 2019;25:768493.

CHAPTER 22
CARDIOVASCULAR EMERGENCIES

LESLEY FITZPATRICK, ALISON PARTYKA AND ZIAD NEHME

ESSENTIALS

- Cardiovascular disease (CVD) risk calculators are utilised to identify, stratify and optimise a patient's individual risk.
- The goal of the primary survey is the identification and simultaneous correction of life-threatening emergencies relating to the patient's airway, breathing, circulation and neurological assessment.
- Chest pain assessment is a time-critical, hierarchical diagnostic process based upon presentation, history, serial electrocardiograms, and cardiac biomarkers.
- A comprehensive history is of paramount importance in the assessment of the cardiac patient.
- A physical examination may reveal cardiac abnormalities on inspection (implanted device, raised jugular venous pressure), palpation (pitting oedema) and auscultation (adventitious lung sounds, heart sounds and murmurs).
- Acute coronary syndromes (ACS) encompass a range of conditions that includes unstable angina pectoris, ST-segment elevation (STEMI) and non-ST-segment elevation myocardial infarction (NSTEMI).
- Early and prompt recognition, assessment and treatment of acute coronary syndromes can reduce the extent of myocardial injury and prevent long-term adverse patient outcomes.
- Early identification and communication about STEMI with patients will enable timely reperfusion procedures to begin.
- Early assessment, time-critical intervention and ongoing monitoring could optimise revascularisation and improve patient outcomes.

INTRODUCTION

Globally, cardiovascular disease (CVD) is the leading cause of death with the majority of cases attributable to myocardial infarctions and cerebrovascular accidents.[1] CVD is an umbrella term for a range of conditions which affect the heart and blood vessels, and includes conditions such as coronary heart disease, chronic heart failure and cerebrovascular accidents. Across Australia, CVD is the second leading cause of death, affecting more than 1.2 million Australians and accounting for 591,000 hospitalisations.[2–4] CVD remains one of the most common causes for calls to the ambulance service, presentations to the emergency department (ED) and admissions to hospital.[2,3,5]

CVD is a largely preventable disease, with most Australians (64%) having three or more modifiable risk factors, including high blood glucose, tobacco use, smoking, hypertension, high blood cholesterol, physical inactivity, poor nutrition and obesity.[6] International and Australian guidelines recommend utilising CVD risk calculators to identify, prevent and manage a patient's individual risk of developing the disease.[7] The

Australian Heart Foundation recommends the National Vascular Disease Prevention Alliance (NVDPA) risk calculator[6] and the New Zealand Heart Foundation recommends PREDICT-T.[8] Aboriginal and Torres Strait Islander peoples experience CVD hospitalisation and death at twice the rate of non-Indigenous Australians,[7,9,10] and it is recommended that screening should commence at 18 years of age, while the NVDPA risk assessment should commence from 30 years of age.[9]

Across Australia and Aotearoa New Zealand, coronary heart disease (CHD) remains a leading cause of death in the community, with 25% of all deaths attributable to this condition.[4,11] There are over 161 acute coronary events per day, the highest demographic age group is over 75 years, and most events occur in males (> 57%).[11] CHD is commonly caused by a narrowing (stenosis) of one or more coronary artery vessels.[4] This vessel narrowing is usually the result of atherosclerotic plaques, which adhere to coronary artery walls. The narrowing leads to a reduction in blood flow and subsequent oxygen perfusion to the myocardium. Over time, atherosclerotic plaques (fatty plaques) lead to a chronic reduction in oxygen flow, resulting in symptoms of angina pectoris (chest pain), shortness of breath, arm pain or jaw pain.[12] As a result, during periods of exertion, the higher oxygen demand leads to the manifestation of the symptom angina. Alternatively, acute instability and/or rupture of atherosclerotic plaques can result in the life-threatening condition known as acute myocardial infarction.[12]

CHD can lead to congestive heart failure (CHF), a chronic disease that occurs when blood does not efficiently pump out of the left or right ventricle. Left-sided heart failure occurs when the left ventricle does not contract adequately or effectively to pump blood, which causes blood to build up in the pulmonary veins. Right-sided heart failure occurs when the right chamber is unable to pump effectively, which causes blood to build up in the veins.[12,13]

This chapter sets out the essential steps for emergency assessment in relation to diseases of the heart. In addition, serious CVD conditions are outlined, together with their paramedicine and nursing management.

ANATOMY AND PHYSIOLOGY

The heart is a four-chambered, fibromuscular, hollow organ which is about the size of the clenched fist of the individual. The heart is located within the thoracic cavity, with one-third to the right of the sternum and the remaining two-thirds to the left. The primary function of the heart and blood vessels is to transport oxygen, nutrients and cellular waste products around the body.[14] The upper portion of the heart is known as the *base*; this is comprised of the left atrium and a small part of the right atrium. The lower pointed section is known as the *apex (inferior)* and lies at the 5th left intercostal space at the midclavicular line.[15,16] The pumping function of the heart is achieved by two highly specific pump chambers (a left and a right), each with its own set of cardiac valves.[15–17]

CHAMBERS OF THE HEART

The human heart has four chambers—right and left atria, and right and left ventricles. The heart also contains two atrioventricular valves, the tricuspid and mitral valves, and two semilunar or cardiac valves, the pulmonary (or pulmonic) and aortic valves (Fig. 22.1).[16,17]

FIGURE 22.1 CROSS-SECTIONAL VIEW OF THE HEART. NOTE THE POSITION OF THE FOUR CARDIAC VALVES[18]

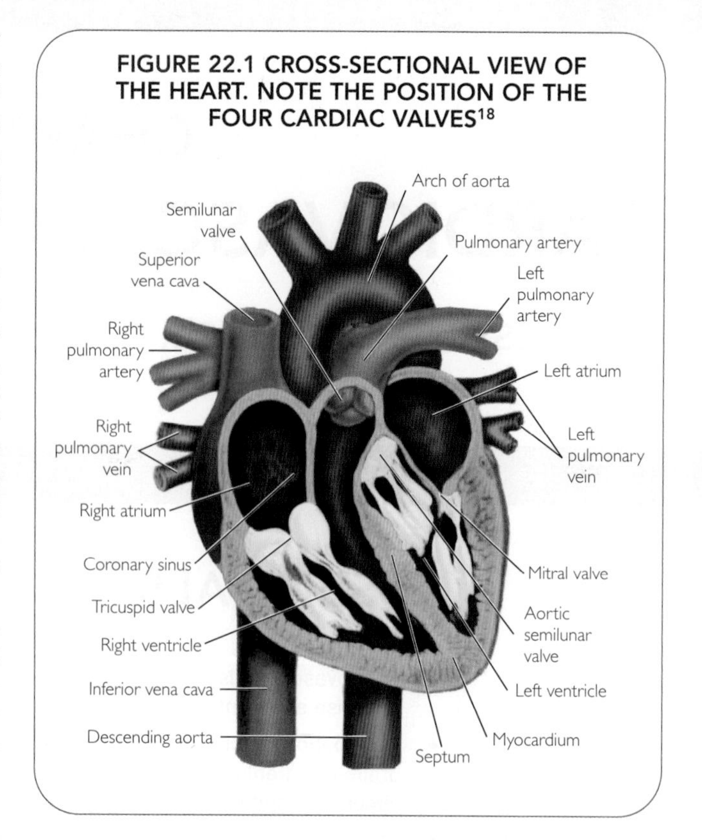

The annuli fibrosi is a fibrous skeleton within the heart that consists of rings of fibrous connective tissue. This tissue surrounds the cardiac valves and provides an internal supporting structure for the heart. The atria and the ventricles are divided by the fibrous skeleton, which also serves as an electrical insulator.[16,17] The atria are relatively thin-walled, as this chamber is a low-pressure environment, and are separated by a fibromuscular septum. The heart is filled passively: 70% occurs during diastole, and atrial contraction (known as atrial kick), and contributes approximately 25% to 30% to complete ventricular filling.[15,17]

The right ventricle is smaller than the left and has thinner walls, as it pumps blood into the low-pressure pulmonary circulation. The left ventricular wall is 2–3 times thicker than the right ventricular wall, as it pumps blood into the high-pressure systemic circulation.[16,17] The left ventricle must generate great force to eject blood into the aorta through the aortic valve, and it is for this reason that the left ventricle is the major pump of the heart. As a result, the anatomical thicknesses of the atrial and ventricular chamber walls differ (right atrium 2 mm; right ventricle 3–5 mm; left atrium 3 mm; left ventricle 13–15 mm).[16,17]

BLOOD FLOW THROUGH THE HEART

During passive cardiac relaxation (diastole), deoxygenated blood is returned to the right side of the heart from the body via the superior and inferior venae cavae. Blood enters the right atrium then flows through the tricuspid valve and into the right ventricle. From here it is forced through the pulmonary valve during cardiac contraction and into the pulmonary circulation, where it becomes oxygenated in the lungs. This is the pulmonary circuit.[15–17]

During cardiac contraction (systole), oxygenated blood is returned to the left side of the heart from the lungs through the pulmonary veins. Blood enters the left atrium then flows through the mitral valve and into the left ventricle. From here, blood is forced through the aortic valve during systole and into the circulation, which supplies blood to the body. This is referred to as the *systemic circuit*.[2,26,27]

VALVES OF THE HEART

The chambers of the heart are each separated by the *atrioventricular valves*, which include the tricuspid valve (right atrium and ventricle) and the mitral valve (left atrium and ventricle). The tricuspid valve consists of three cusps or leaflets, while the mitral (bicuspid) valve consists of only two cusps or leaflets. Both *atrioventricular valve* leaflets are composed of fibrous tissue covered by endothelium.[16,17] The *atrioventricular valve* leaflets attach to the fibrous skeleton of the heart and are anchored by fibrous cords called chordae tendineae. These cords attach the ends of the valve to papillary muscle and the ventricular wall. The opening and closing of these valves is passive and dependent on pressure gradients. The structure of the valves and the attachment of the leaflets to the ventricle walls allow for only one-directional blood flow.[16,17,19]

The semilunar valves are the pulmonary valve and the aortic valve. Both semilunar valves consist of three cusps, all about equal size, which are attached to the fibrous skeleton. The leaflets of the semilunar valves are comprised of fibrous connective tissue covered by endothelium. These valves separate the ventricles from their outflow arteries.[16,17] The aortic valve is the strongest of all the heart's valves as it is exposed to the greatest pressures during the cardiac cycle. The leaflets of the aortic valve are attached to the annuli fibrosi, which forms part of the Sinus of Valsalva; the coronary arteries open near the upper part of this sinus (Fig. 22.2). The names of the three cusps of the aortic valve correspond to the coronary arteries that lie behind each semilunar cusp: the right coronary aortic cusp, the left coronary artery aortic cusp and the non-coronary aortic cusp.[15–17]

LAYERS OF THE HEART

The heart is comprised of three tissue layers. The *pericardium* (parietal pericardium) is the outermost layer of the heart; it stabilises the heart in its fixed position and provides a physical barrier against infection. The *epicardium*, or visceral pericardium, completely encloses the external surface of the heart. Together, the pericardium and the epicardium form a sac around

FIGURE 22.2 PROXIMITY OF RIGHT AND LEFT ARTERIES TO AORTIC VALVE AND SINUS OF VALSALVA[15]

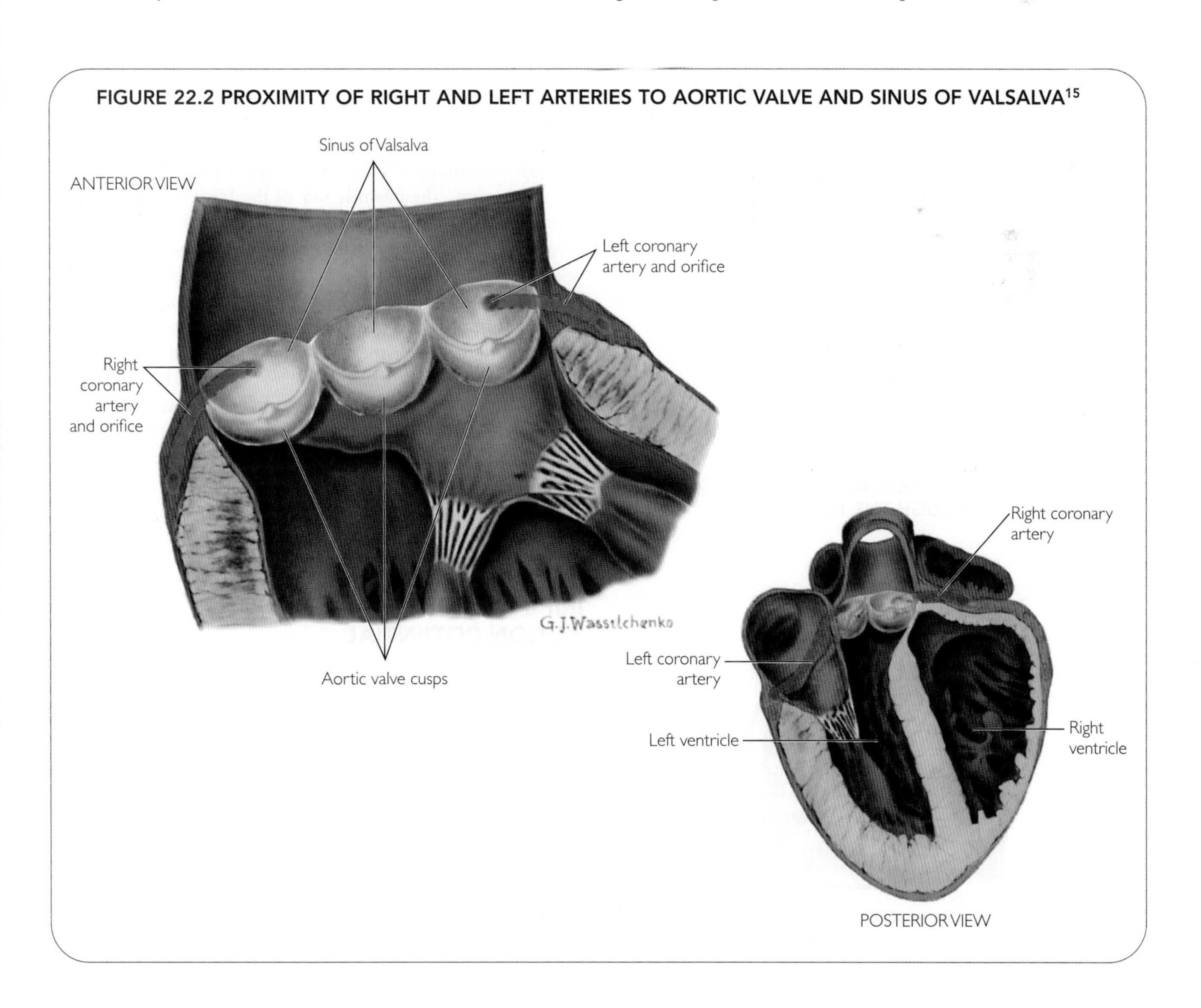

the heart. This sac normally contains 10–30 mL of serous fluid, which lubricates the moving surface of the heart.[15,17,19]

The thickest layer of the heart is known as the *myocardium* and is the muscle damaged during a myocardial infarction. The myocardium is a thick middle muscular layer that forms the bulk of the heart muscle. The myocardium is further divided into the subendocardium and the subepicardium (the outermost layer just below the epicardium).[19] The *endocardium* is the innermost heart layer and is comprised of endothelial cells, which are continuous with the internal lining of adjoining blood vessels—the tunica intima.[19]

THE CORONARY CIRCULATION

The coronary circulation consists of the blood vessels that supply oxygenated blood to the heart muscle (*coronary arteries*) and those that return deoxygenated blood to the circulation (*coronary veins*). Coronary arteries originate at the base of the aorta in the region of the sinus of Valsalva (Fig. 22.3). Coronary arteries extend over the epicardial surface of the heart and branch many times. Two coronary arteries originate at the aorta: the left coronary artery (LCA) and the right coronary artery (RCA). Coronary arteries are supplied with blood during diastole (heart relaxation) and as the aortic valve closes, blood flows down the coronary arteries to perfuse the myocardium and enable ventricular filling to occur.[16,19]

The left main coronary artery is a short vessel that divides into the left anterior descending branch (LAD) and the circumflex branch. In most people the right coronary artery (RCA) supplies the right atrium and right ventricle. It also supplies the sinoatrial (SA) node and the atrioventricular (AV) node. The LAD supplies the anterior surface of the left ventricle and the interventricular septum. The circumflex branch supplies the lateral aspect and part of the posterior aspect of the left ventricle (Fig. 22.4 and Box 22.1).[16] There is considerable variation in the normal anatomy of the coronary circulation. In approximately 90% of people, the RCA is the origin of the posterior descending artery (PDA); in the remaining cases, the PDA arises from the left circumflex artery. The RCA also supplies the SA nodal artery in 60% of people, the left circumflex artery in the remaining 40%.[19]

FIGURE 22.3 CIRCULATION OF BLOOD THROUGH THE HEART[20]

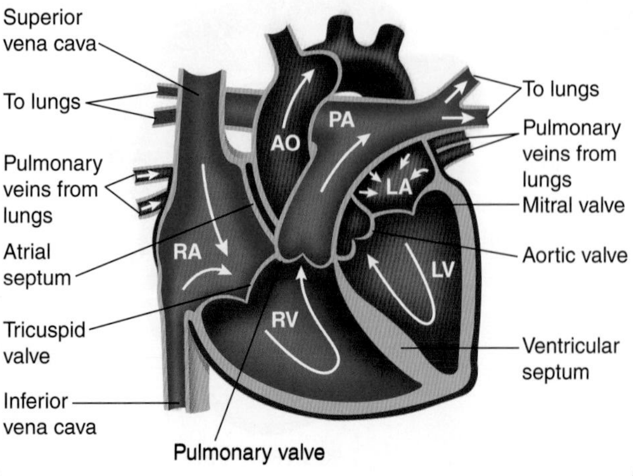

THE CONDUCTION SYSTEM

The specialised conductive system that controls and propagates cardiac contraction is known as the conduction pathway. The conduction pathway consists of three main areas of impulse generation: the sinoatrial (SA) node, the atrioventricular (AV) node and the bundle of His and Purkinje system.[16,17,19]

The *SA node* is referred to as the pacemaker of the heart, as it has the highest degree of automaticity or intrinsic rate: 60–100 times per minute. The SA node initiates each cardiac cycle. It is located on the posterior surface of the right atrium near the superior vena cava. Its anatomical position ensures that the atria are depolarised before the ventricles. Cells within the SA node initiate a wave of electrical depolarisation and the cardiac impulse spreads from the SA node to the AV node by myocardial cell-to-cell conduction.[15,17]

The *AV node* also possesses pacemaker cells that depolarise at an intrinsic rate that is less than that of the SA node—about 40–60 times per minute. The AV node is located on the right, posterior side of the interatrial septum. Non-conductive tissue separates the atria and the ventricles, and as the depolarisation arrives at the AV node from the SA node there is a slight delay. This delay allows optimal time for ventricular filling to occur and ensures that the ventricles do not respond to excessively rapid atrial depolarisation rates.[17,19]

The bundle of His conducts the electrical depolarisation from the AV node to the ventricles. The impulse is conducted rapidly through the bundle of His into the upper part of the interventricular septum. The intrinsic rate of the His/Purkinje system is approximately 15–40 times per minute. This delay is a result of the complex local circuitry and relatively small size of AV nodal cells.[17,19] Approximately 10–12 mm away from the AV node, the bundle of His divides into the right and left bundle branches. The right bundle branch consists of one fascicle, which continues down the right side of the interventricular septum and radiates towards the right ventricular apex.[16,17,19] The left bundle branch consists of two sets of fibres, referred to as the anterior and posterior fascicles. The anterior fascicle travels over the left ventricular wall to the papillary muscle. The left posterior fascicle travels inferiorly and posteriorly across the left ventricular outflow tract. When one of the left bundle branches is blocked or damaged, and non-conducting, it is referred to as a hemi-block or fascicular block.[15–17,19]

IMPULSE FORMATION AND THE ACTION POTENTIAL

Many cells in the human body can generate an electromechanical gradient between their intracellular and extracellular environment. The voltage difference across a cell's membrane is referred to as the 'membrane potential', and is controlled by a series of pumps and channels which work efficiently to shift ions; for example, sodium, potassium and calcium, across the cell membrane, and against their concentration gradients.[23] The movement of these ions across cell membranes in the heart is responsible for the electrical activation of heart tissue, commonly referred to as the 'action potential'. An action potential propagates along the membranes of excitable cells in the heart, generating an electrochemical wave that causes heart tissue to

FIGURE 22.4 ANTERIOR AND POSTERIOR VIEWS OF THE CORONARY ARTERY CIRCULATION AND MAJOR VESSELS[15]

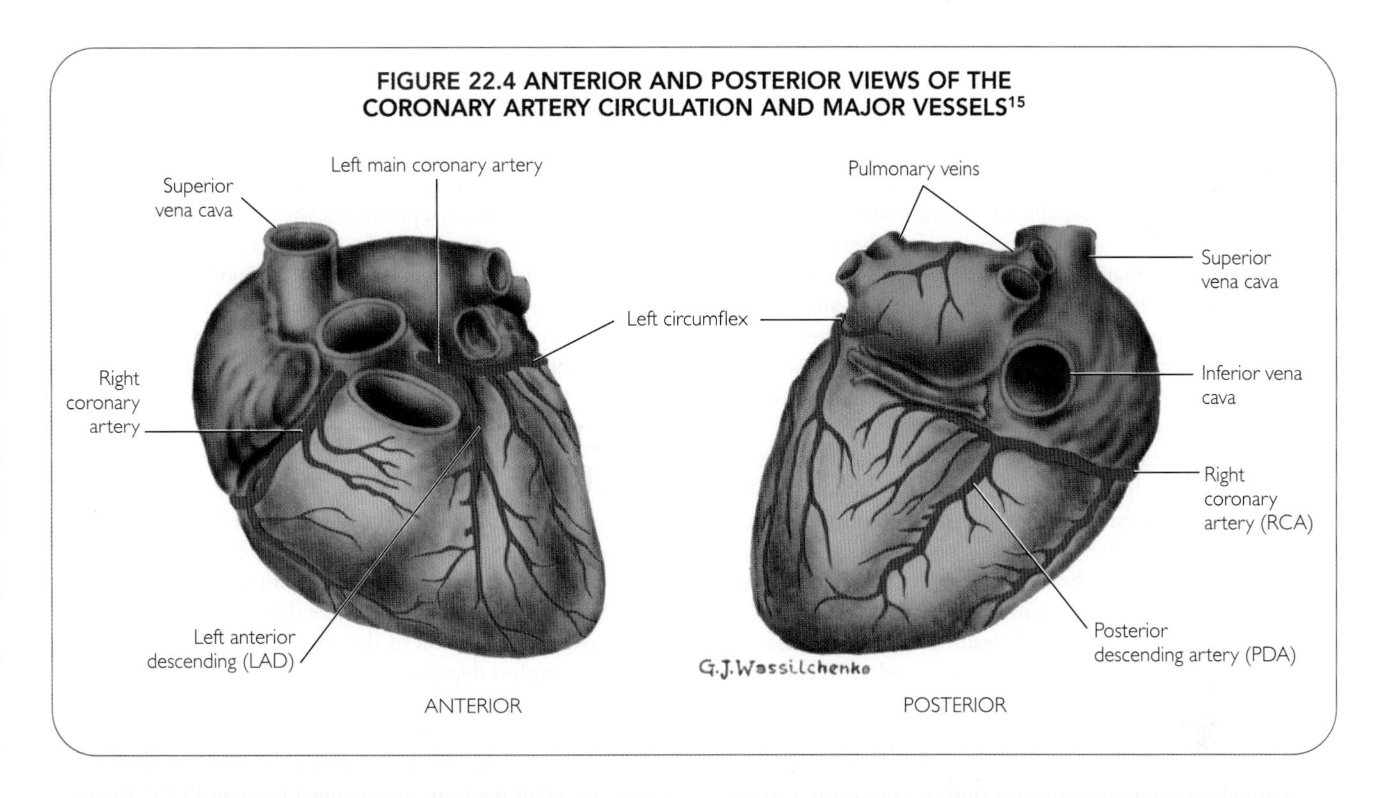

BOX 22.1 CORONARY ARTERIES IN MYOCARDIAL INFARCTION[22]

RIGHT CORONARY ARTERY

Supplies the following:

- right atrium
- right ventricle
- inferior/diaphragmatic surface of left ventricle
- sinoatrial node (55%)
- atrioventricular node (90%)
- bundle of His

Blockage causes the following:

- infarction of posterior or inferior wall of left ventricle
- right ventricle infarction
- in inferior myocardial infarction (leads II, III, aV_F), anticipate second-degree heart block or Mobitz type I block (Wenckebach)

LEFT CORONARY ARTERY

Left circumflex branch

Supplies the following:

- left atrium
- lateral wall of left ventricle
- sinoatrial node (45%)
- atrioventricular node (10%)
- posterior/inferior division of left bundle

Blockage causes the following:

- lateral wall infarction
- posterior wall infarction (near base)
- in lateral wall myocardial infarction, electrocardiogram changes seen in leads I, AVL, and V_5 and V_6

Left anterior descending branch

Supplies the following:

- anterior wall of left ventricle
- interventricular septum
- bundle of His
- right bundle
- posterior/inferior division of left bundle
- apex of left ventricle

Blockage causes the following:

- infarction of anterior wall of left ventricle
- effect on papillary muscle (which attaches to mitral valve)
- in anterior myocardial infarction (leads V_2, V_3, V_4), anticipate second-degree heart block, Mobitz type II block or third-degree block

contract and relax almost uniformly.[23] The speed and efficiency of this process is attributed to a network of intercalated discs which interconnect neighbouring heart cells and allow the rapid propagation of the action potential across the heart (known as 'the cardiac syncytium').

'Depolarisation' and 'repolarisation' are terms that are commonly used to describe key changes in the membrane potential of heart cells.[23] Depolarisation describes the contraction phase of heart tissue, and the inward influx of positively charged sodium and calcium ions inside cardiac cells. Repolarisation describes the relaxation phase and the return to resting membrane potential, caused by the outward shift of potassium ions. The electrical properties of cardiac cells can be divided into two types: pacemaker and non-pacemaker cells.[24] Pacemaker cells are found in the SA and AV nodes and some parts of the bundle of His and Purkinje system. Non-pacemaker cells, also known as 'worker cells', make up the bulk of the myocardium and represent the contractile cells of the atria and ventricles. Unlike non-pacemaker cells, pacemaker cells have smaller unstable resting membrane potentials and are capable of spontaneously depolarising, generating the intrinsic electrical activity of the heart – a process referred to as 'automaticity'.[24] In comparison, non-pacemaker cells have a large stable resting membrane potential and display a prolonged action potential with a plateau phase. Although non-pacemaker cells are unable to generate their own action potential, they are critically important in propagating the action potential through the cardiac syncytium.

The cardiac action potential of non-pacemaker cells has five phases which are helpful in understanding the pathophysiology and treatment of dysrhythmias, and have important clinical implications (Fig. 22.5).[25]

1. During phase 0, membrane permeability to potassium decreases and fast sodium channels open, causing an inward influx of sodium into the cell, leading to its depolarisation. Depolarisation gives rise to the P wave and QRS complex of the electrocardiogram.
2. During phase 1, there is partial (early) repolarisation as sodium channels begin to close and open potassium channels promote the outward shift of potassium, causing the membrane potential to fall.
3. During phase 2 (the plateau phase), membrane permeability to calcium increases maintaining a steady inward influx of positive ions across the cell's membrane. This phase helps to prolong depolarisation and the life of the action potential.
4. Phase 3 signals the start of rapid (final) repolarisation that helps to restore the resting membrane potential and is characterised by the closing of calcium channels and the outward shift of potassium.
5. Phase 4 is the resting member potential and is stable at approximately –90 millivolts.

The cardiac action potential lasts approximately 300 milliseconds in non-pacemaker cells. For the vast majority of this time, the cell is refractory to activation from other action potentials. In fact, once a cell has reached phase 1 of the action potential it remains refractory to other action potentials until it approaches approximately the halfway mark of phase 3, a period known as the absolute refractory period.[24] The action potentials of pacemaker cells in the SA and AV nodes are significantly different from those of non-pacemaker cells. The membrane potential at the onset of phase 4 is more depolarised (−50 to −65 mV) and undergoes a slow depolarisation with the influx of sodium ions, and gradually merges into phase 0.

ELECTROCARDIOGRAM INTERPRETATION

The electrocardiogram (ECG) records the electrical conduction system of the heart. The ECG represents electrical activity of the heart's depolarisation and repolarisation during the cardiac cycle. The ECG is divided into three distinct waveforms:

- P wave: depolarisation of the atria
- QRS complex: depolarisation of the ventricles
- T wave: repolarisation of the ventricles.

The 12-lead ECG is an important diagnostic tool and consists of six limb leads (standard leads) and six chest or praecordial leads. Twelve 'views' of the heart are obtained from an ECG. The limb leads (Fig. 22.6) should be positioned on each wrist and ankle; however, modification depending on the patient; for example, amputee or breast tissue, and context, such as trauma, may be required. The six chest leads are positioned in specific places on the chest wall around the praecordium, as shown in Fig. 22.7:

- V_1: fourth intercostal space, right sternal border
- V_2: fourth intercostal space, left sternal border
- V_3: midway between V_2 and V_4
- V_4: fifth intercostal space, midclavicular line
- V_5: anterior axillary line, same level with V_4
- V_6: midaxillary line, same level with V_4 and V_5.

FIGURE 22.5 THE FIVE PHASES OF THE CARDIAC ACTION POTENTIAL[21]

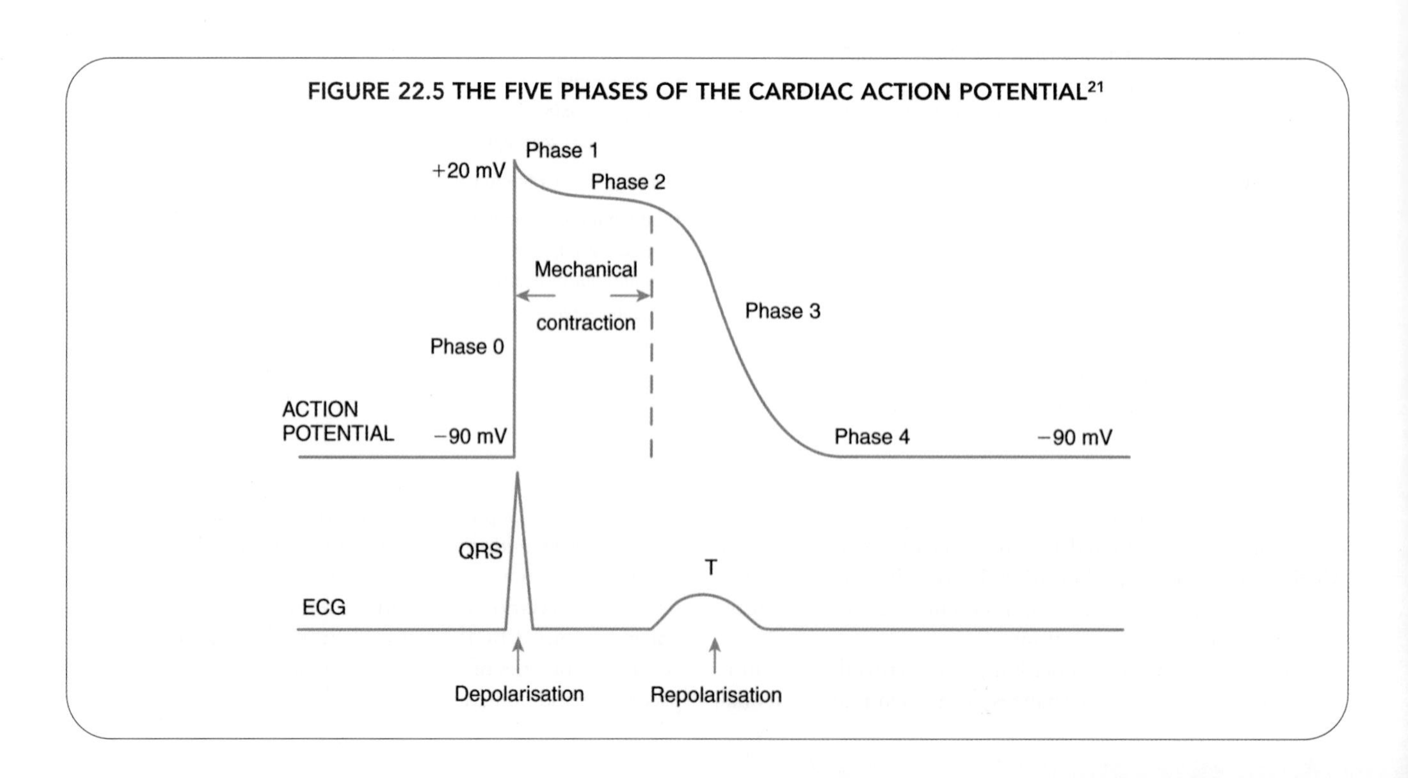

FIGURE 22.6 SIX LIMB LEAD (LEADS I, II, III, aV_R, aV_L AND aV_F) NORMALLY APPEAR AS SHOWN[26]

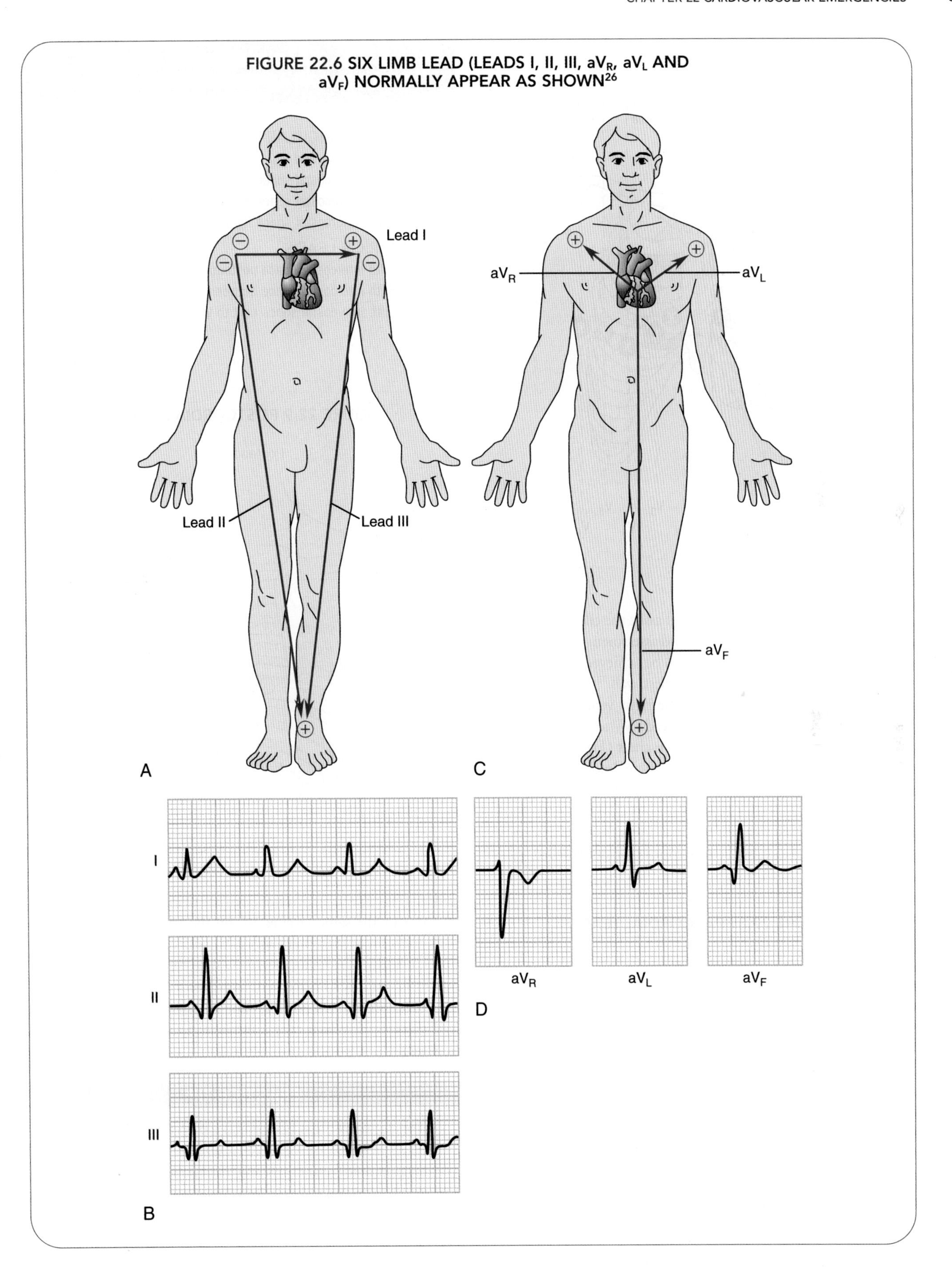

FIGURE 22.7 CHEST LEADS (V_{1-6})[26]

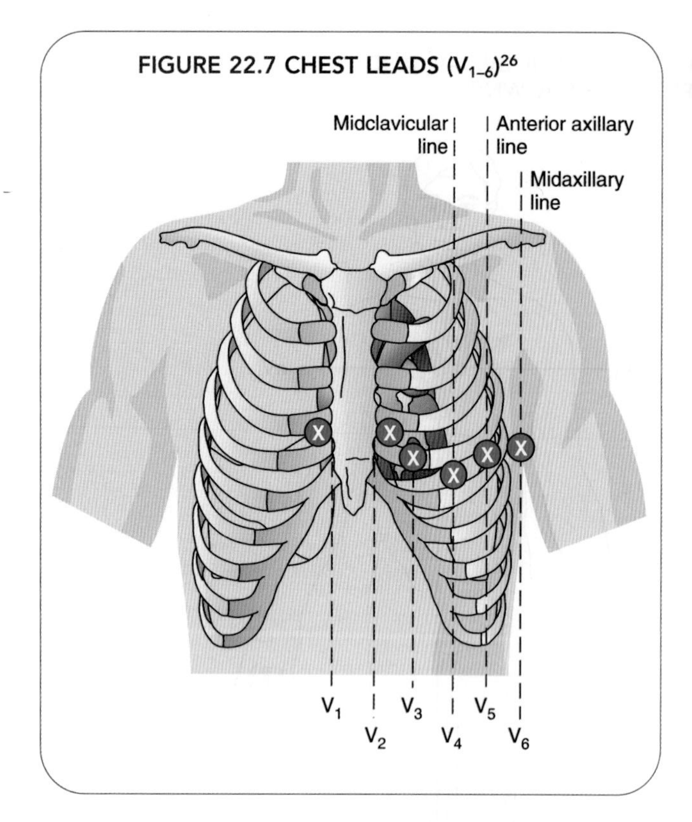

Twelve-lead ECG chest leads (V_1–V_6) assist the clinician to evaluate the left ventricle. The diagnosis and assessment of the posterior wall or right ventricle of the heart can be achieved by positioning the leads in different places on the chest wall.[12,27,28] When right ventricular infarction is suspected, the right ventricle can be assessed by swapping the position of leads V_3 to V_6 to a mirror-image position on the right side of the chest (Fig. 22.8). Should right-ventricular damage be present, these leads may show an injury pattern on the ECG. These leads should be clearly labelled on the ECG as V_{3R}, V_{4R}, V_{5R} and V_{6R} (Box 22.2).[12,27,29] Posterior leads can also be used to assess the heart's posterior wall. Leads V_4, V_5 and V_6 are replaced by the posterior leads and labelled V_7, V_8 and V_9 (Fig. 22.9).[29] Posterior leads are placed at the 5th intercostal space or the same level as V6 on the left side of the patient's back and mirror placement of V_4, V_5 and V_6 (Box 22.2).[19,29] Prehospital and in-hospital emergency care clinicians need to be expert in 12-lead ECG placement as the recording of electrical activity (direction and amplitude) can be affected by inappropriate lead placement, which may contribute to suboptimal treatment decisions.

FIGURE 22.8 PRAECORDIAL LEADS

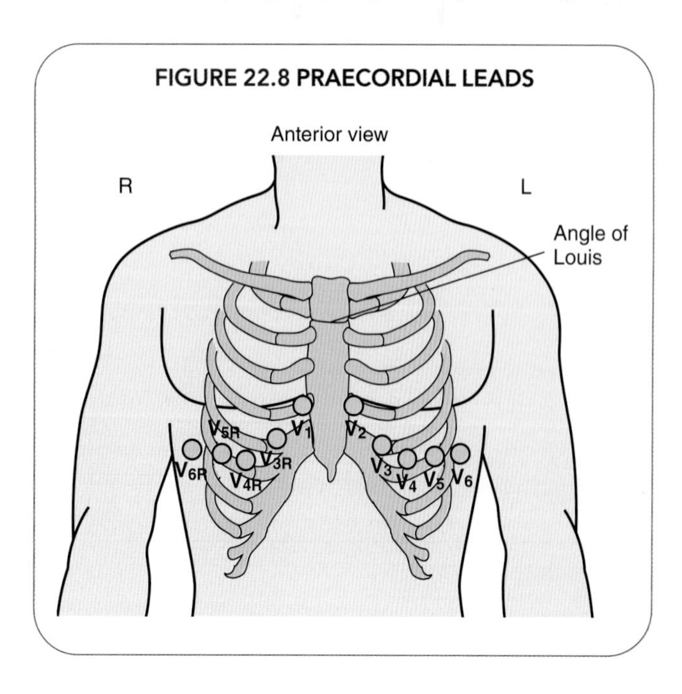

BOX 22.2 LEAD PLACEMENT FOR RIGHT VENTRICULAR AND POSTERIOR LEADS[12,27]

RIGHT VENTRICULAR LEADS

V_{3R} = Between V_1 and V_{4R}

V_{4R} = Fifth intercostal space right midclavicular line

V_{5R} = Fifth intercostal space right anterior axillary line

V_{6R} = Fifth intercostal space right midaxillary line

POSTERIOR LEADS

V_7 = Fifth intercostal space posterior axillary line

V_8 = Fifth intercostal space between V_7 and V_9

V_9 = Fifth intercostal space next to vertebral column

FIGURE 22.9 POSTCORDIAL LEADS

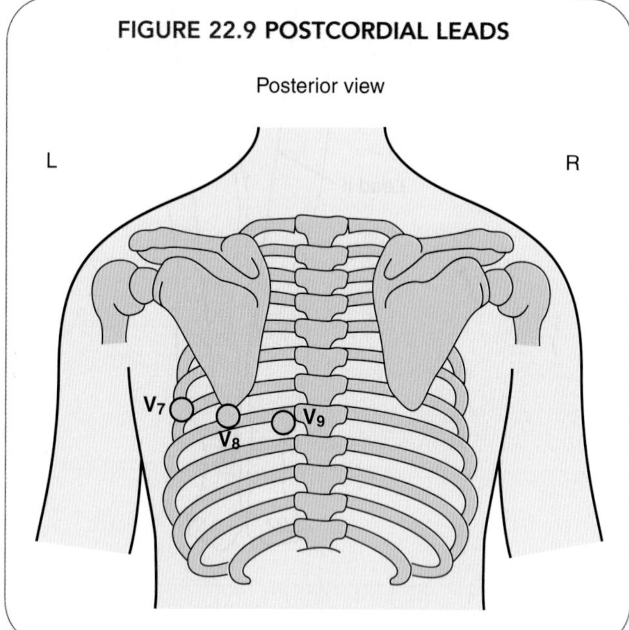

PRACTICE TIP

The placement of the 12-lead ECG is critical to maximising the quality of the tracing and assisting with interpretation, diagnosis and treatment. Some modification may be necessary for different diagnostic groups, clinical situations such as trauma and patient physiological constraints, for example amputee or breast tissue. Breast tissue has a negligible effect on ECG amplitudes, and in women with large breast tissue, the placement of chest leads over the breast rather than under the breast may help facilitate their placement in the correct anatomical location.[30]

CARDIAC AXIS

The QRS cardiac axis is the mean (overall) direction of a wave of ventricular depolarisation. The mean vector (electrical activity) travels downwards and towards the left due to the increased muscle mass of the left ventricle towards lead II. The mean vector can be plotted on a graph known as the hexaxial reference system (Fig. 22.10).[15] Lead I is the zero-reference point. The normal range of cardiac axis is –30° to +110°. An axis lying > –30° is referred to as a left-axis deviation and an axis > +110° is referred to as a right-axis deviation. Right-axis deviation may be a normal variant in newborns, infants and young adults. Axis deviation can be caused by hypertrophy of the ventricle, bundle branch blocks, Wolff-Parkinson-White syndrome, fascicular blocks or MI.[12,15,16]

Accurate assessment of cardiac axis can be achieved by examining all six limb leads. The hexaxial reference system shows that the flow of depolarisation towards a lead results in a positive deflection on the QRS complex, while a depolarisation away from a lead results in a negative deflection on the QRS. A depolarisation at 90° to a lead results in an equiphasic (equal amounts of positive and negative deflection) QRS complex (refer to Figs 22.10 and 22.11).[15,16,31]

The steps to assess the cardiac vector are:

1. Choose the lead that has the smallest or most equiphasic QRS complex. The axis lies approximately 90° to the right or left of this lead.
2. Using the hexaxial reference system, find the lead that is perpendicular (at a right-angle) to the lead chosen in step 1.
3. If the deflection of the lead you are now looking at is positive, then the axis is in this direction. If the deflection of the lead is negative, then it is the opposite pole, i.e. the direction of the axis.[15,16,31]

FIGURE 22.10 HEXAXIAL REFERENCE SYSTEM[15]

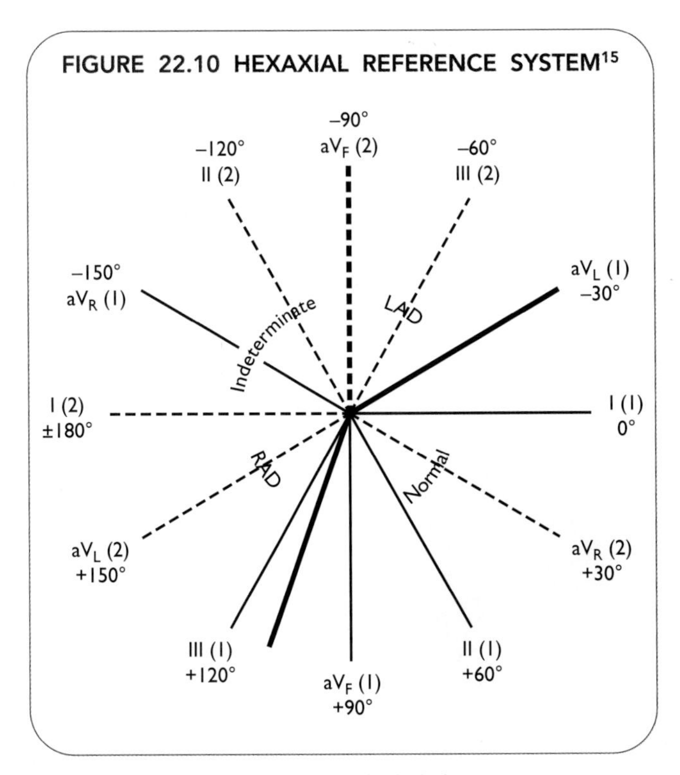

LAD: left-axis deviation; RAD: right-axis deviation.

CARDIAC DYSRHYTHMIAS

Sinus rhythm is the normal rhythm of the heart originating from the SA node, the natural cardiac pacemaker. The rate is between 60 and 100 beats/minute, the rhythm is regular, P waves are present and precede every QRS complex, all intervals are within normal limits and the conduction is through the typical pathway. Figure 22.12 illustrates the conduction in sinus rhythm. Table 22.1 lists the ECG criteria for sinus rhythm.

Cardiac dysrhythmia is a term used to indicate abnormal electrical activity in the heart (Box 22.3). Dysrhythmia may occur at any time in the cardiac cycle and originate anywhere in the cardiac conduction pathway: SA node, atria, AV node or junction and ventricles. A dysrhythmia may be a sign of the failure of the SA node to initiate an impulse, a delay or blockage in the conduction pathway, activation of aberrant conduction pathways and other foci initiating impulses causing ectopy (Table 22.2).[13,15,27,32,33]

Heart rate and stroke volume determine cardiac output and subsequent blood pressure; therefore, when a patient presents with symptoms including dizziness, syncope, chest pain, breathlessness and palpitations, assessment of the underlying cardiac rhythm is essential to avoid serious complications associated with low cardiac output.[16,19]

The presence of cardiac dysrhythmia requires continuous ECG monitoring to obtain a real-time electrical interpretation of the patient's cardiac rhythm in both pre-hospital and in-hospital settings.[27,29,31] For the ECG to be of diagnostic and/or therapeutic benefit, the clinician must be able to recognise and manage any abnormalities.[16,32]

SINUS BRADYCARDIA

Sinus bradycardia occurs when the SA node takes longer to depolarise than normal because of increased vagal (parasympathetic) stimulation. This produces a heart rate slower than 60 beats per minute, but fulfils all the other criteria for sinus rhythm.[13,16] Diastole is longer in sinus bradycardia, so that ventricular filling and coronary artery perfusion may not be reduced, but the heart rate may be insufficient to meet oxygen demands. Sinus bradycardia may then lead to reduced cardiac output that may not be tolerated well in patients with underlying heart disease.[12,15,16,27]

Sinus bradycardia can be caused by several factors, including physiological stimulation of the vagus nerve (vasovagal syncope, vomiting or straining of the bowel), hypoxia, ACS, raised intracranial or systemic blood pressure, hypothermia or hypothyroidism. Sinus bradycardia can also be produced by medications such as beta-blockers and digoxin.[13] Sinus bradycardia may also be physiological (i.e. not causing any perfusion problems) in athletes or during sleep (Fig. 22.13 and Table 22.3).[13,27,34]

Physiological bradycardia usually does not require treatment. Treatment options for symptomatic bradycardia should aim to address the underlying cause. Adjusting regular medications that affect heart rate and/or blood pressure in consultation with the patient's doctor or cardiologist should be considered. Severe symptoms and/or haemodynamic instability can be treated with intravenous adrenaline, atropine or temporary transvenous or external cardiac pacing.[16,27,33] If the cause is an ACS or heart failure, revascularisation with a stent or coronary artery bypass may be required. Patients with sinus node dysfunction and structural heart defects may also require a pacemaker.

FIGURE 22.11 PATTERNS OF AXIS DEVIATION AND ASSOCIATED CONDITIONS

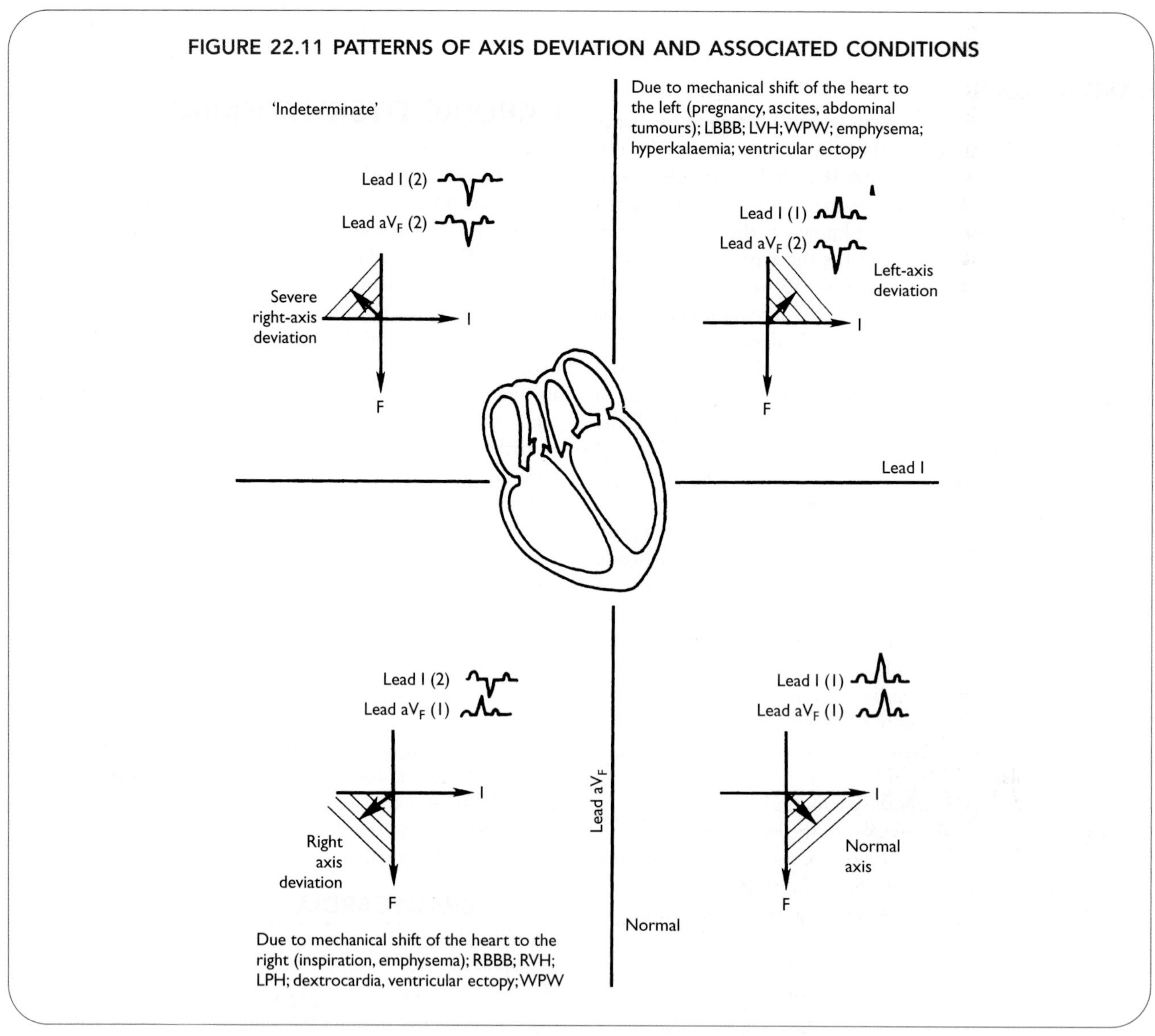

LBBB: left bundle branch block; LPH: left posterior hemiblock; LVH: left ventricular hypertrophy; RBBB: right bundle branch block; RVH: right ventricular hypertrophy; WPW: Wolff-Parkinson-White syndrome.

FIGURE 22.12

A. Normal sinus rhythm. **B.** Conduction pathway for normal sinus rhythm.

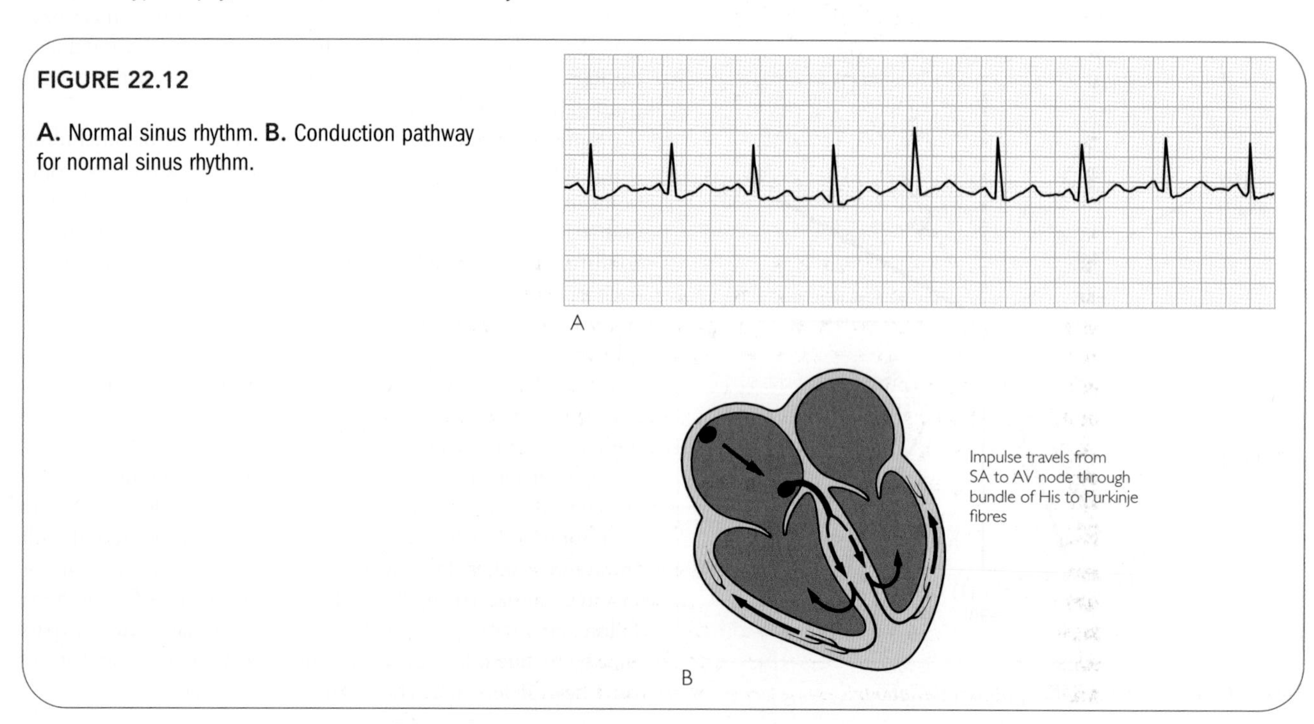

SA: sinoatrial; AV: atrioventricular.

TABLE 22.1 SINUS RHYTHM

Rate	60 to 100 beats/minute
Rhythm	Regular
P waves	Present
QRS complex	Present; normal duration 0.04–0.11 second
P/QRS relationship	P wave precedes each QRS complex
PR interval	Normal 0.12–0.20 seconds

BOX 22.3 SYSTEMATIC EVALUATION OF CARDIAC RHYTHMS

RATE

Bradycardia: < 60 beats/minute
Normal rate: 60 to 100 beats/minute
Tachycardia: > 100 beats/minute

RHYTHM

Is the rhythm regular or irregular?

P WAVES

Are P waves present?
Does one P wave appear before each QRS?
Is P wave deflection normal?

QRS COMPLEX

Normal is 0.06–0.11 second. Are the QRS complexes normal shape and configuration?
Does QRS complex follow every P wave?

PR INTERVAL

Normal is 0.12–0.2 second. Is the interval prolonged? Shortened?

TABLE 22.2 CARDIAC RHYTHMS BY POINT OF ORIGIN[22]

ORIGIN	RHYTHM
Sinus node	Normal sinus rhythm Sinus tachycardia Sinus bradycardia Sinus dysrhythmia
Atria	Premature atrial complexes Atrial flutter Atrial fibrillation Wandering atrial pacemaker Multifocal atrial tachycardia
Atrioventricular junction	Supraventricular tachycardia Premature junctional complexes Junctional escape rhythm Accelerated junctional rhythm Junctional tachycardia
Atrioventricular blocks	First-degree atrioventricular block Second-degree atrioventricular block, type I Second-degree atrioventricular block, type II Third-degree atrioventricular block
Ventricles	Premature ventricular complexes Ventricular tachycardia Ventricular fibrillation Idioventricular rhythm Accelerated idioventricular rhythm
Other	Pulseless electrical activity Asystole

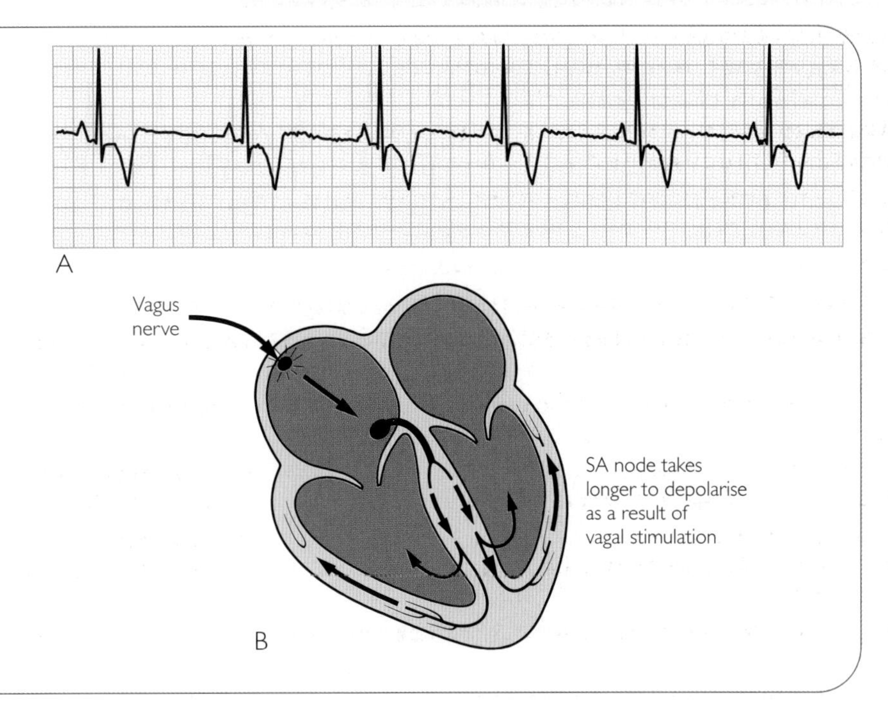
A
Vagus nerve
SA node takes longer to depolarise as a result of vagal stimulation
B

FIGURE 22.13

A. Sinus bradycardia. **B.** Conduction pathway for sinus bradycardia.

SA: sinoatrial.

TABLE 22.3 SINUS BRADYCARDIA[22]

Rate	Fewer than 60 beats/minute (age-dependent)
Rhythm	Regular
P waves	Present
QRS complexes	Present; normal duration
P/QRS relationship	P wave precedes each QRS complex
PR interval	Normal

SINUS TACHYCARDIA

Sinus tachycardia occurs when the SA node depolarises more quickly than normal. This results in a heart rate faster than 100 beats/minute and again fulfils all the other criteria for a sinus rhythm.[13,16] Diastole is shorter in sinus tachycardia, which means ventricular filling and coronary artery perfusion are reduced. Sinus tachycardia may lead to a reduction in cardiac output, which may not be tolerated in patients with underlying heart disease.[12,13,16,27]

Primary causes include stimulation of the sympathetic nervous system as a result of pain, anxiety, stress, exercise, hyperthyroidism, or a physiological response to hypotension and hypovolaemia. Sinus tachycardia may also be associated with the use of prescribed medications or stimulants (Fig. 22.14 and Table 22.4).[13,27,32]

Treatment of sinus tachycardia is usually conservative and should address the underlying cause. Treatment of hypovolaemia with intravenous fluids, blood or definitive operative management may be required. A beta-blocker may also be considered to reduce rate and myocardial oxygen demand where sinus tachycardia is secondary to ACS or stimulant use.[16,27,33]

SINUS DYSRHYTHMIA

Sinus dysrhythmia occurs when there is cyclic variation in a sinus rhythm. During respiration, intermittent stimulation of the vagus nerve results in beat-to-beat variations in the resting heart rate. As a result, the SA node speeds slightly at the end of inspiration and then slows down at the end of expiration. Sinus dysrhythmia is usually a sign of cardiovascular health and may be seen more often in young adults and paediatrics. If not related to respiration, sinus dysrhythmia may indicate SA node pathology or inferior MI (Table 22.5).[16,27,33] Sinus dysrhythmia is typically an incidental finding and is rarely associated with complications.

PREMATURE ATRIAL COMPLEXES

Premature atrial complexes (PACs) result from irritable atrial cells and increase the long-term risk of developing atrial fibrillation.[39] The pathway is abnormal as it does not originate from the SA node and results in an abnormal, premature P wave followed by a normal QRS complex. PACs may be singular or have multiple ectopic foci and often (re)occur in repeating patterns. PACs are generally a normal electrophysiological phenomenon not usually requiring treatment, with

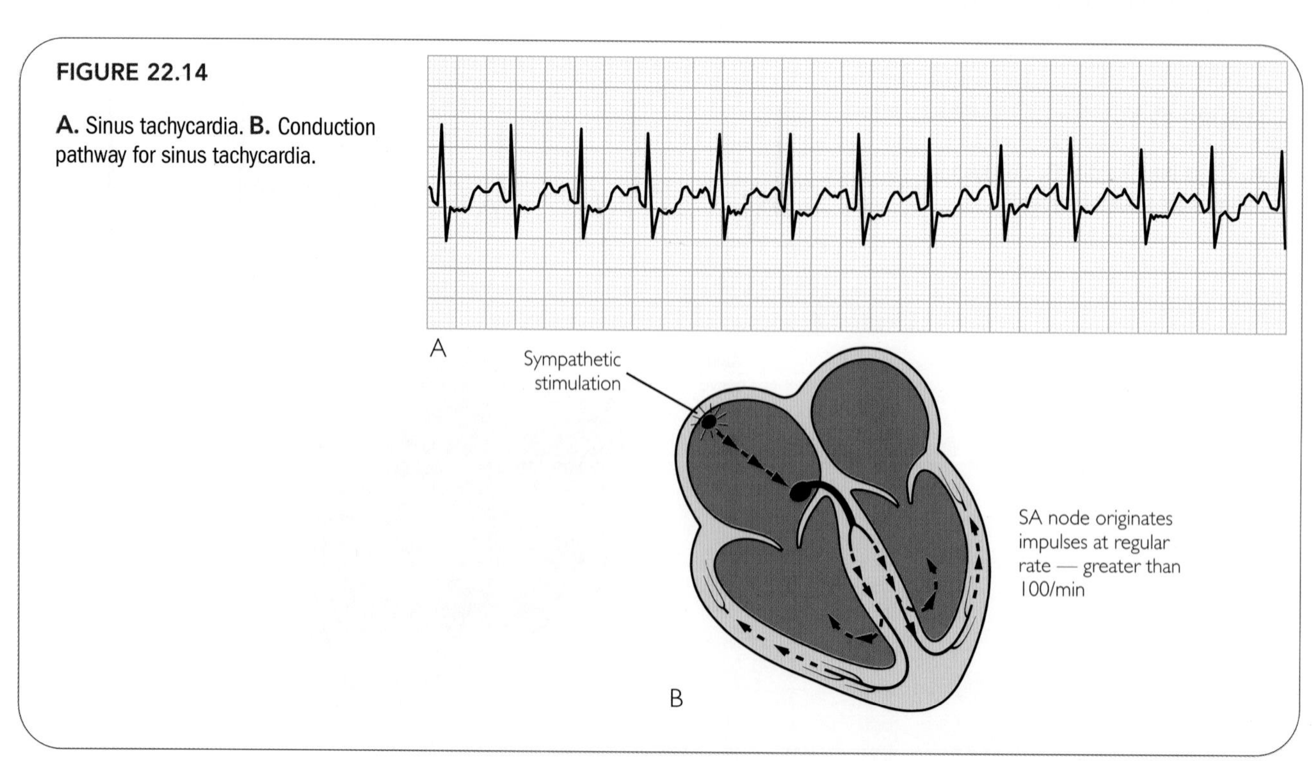
A
Sympathetic stimulation
SA node originates impulses at regular rate — greater than 100/min
B

FIGURE 22.14

A. Sinus tachycardia. **B.** Conduction pathway for sinus tachycardia.

SA: sinoatrial.

TABLE 22.4 SINUS TACHYCARDIA[22]

Rate	100 to 180 beats/minute (age-dependent)
Rhythm	Regular
P waves	Present, may merge with T waves
QRS complexes	Present; normal duration (width)
P/QRS relationship	P wave precedes each QRS complex
PR interval	Normal

TABLE 22.5 SINUS DYSRHYTHMIA[22]

Rate	60–100 beats/minute; may increase with inspiration and decrease with expiration
Rhythm	Slightly irregular; may be obvious on a rhythm strip but undetectable by palpation
P waves	Present
QRS complexes	Present; normal duration
P/QRS relationship	P wave precedes each QRS complex
PR interval	Normal

causes including fatigue, anxiety, alcohol and stimulants (Fig. 22.15 and Table 22.6).[16,27,33]

ATRIAL FIBRILLATION

Atrial fibrillation (AF) is the most recognised arrythmia and occurs frequently in older people. AF is characterised by rapid, irregular atrial contractions which produce a variable ventricular rate and absent P waves.[13,16] The ventricular rate is determined by the AV node, which is normally irregular, but conduction follows the usual intrinsic pathway producing a normal QRS complex.[13]

AF occurs when multiple atrial foci fire erratically, causing the atria to quiver or *fibrillate*, but with no effective atrial contraction. As a result, cardiac output may be affected with up to 25% loss due to atrial contraction flow impairment referred to as 'atrial kick'. The causes of AF are commonly cardiovascular in origin and include complete heart block, ischaemia, hypertensive heart disease, mitral valve disease and congestive heart failure (Fig. 22.16 and Table 22.7).[16,27,33] Non-cardiac causes of AF include hypoxia and pulmonary embolus.[16] In the long term, AF is a risk factor for stroke, heart failure and early death. In the short term, uncontrolled AF can reduce cardiac output and result in symptoms such as chest pain, shortness of breath, lightheadedness or syncope. AF may be either paroxysmal (short-term, intermittent, and usually terminating spontaneously),

TABLE 22.6 PREMATURE ATRIAL COMPLEXES[22]

Rate	60–100 beats/minute
Rhythm	Irregular because of early beats
P waves	Present, but (because they do not originate in the sinoatrial node) premature P waves have a different morphology
QRS complexes	Present; normal duration; noncompensatory pause
P/QRS relationship	A P wave precedes each QRS complex. If an ectopic P wave appears early in the cardiac cycle, a QRS complex may not follow (non-conducted premature atrial complex)
PR interval	Normal or prolonged

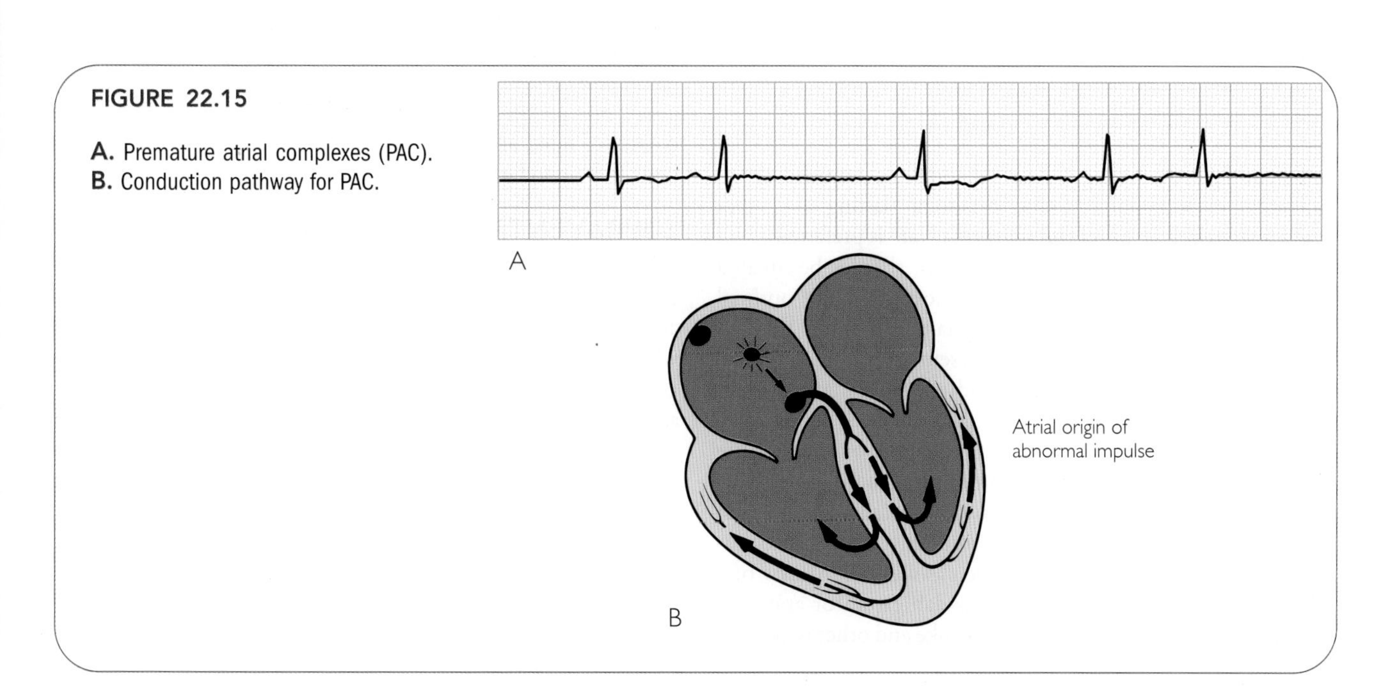

FIGURE 22.15

A. Premature atrial complexes (PAC).
B. Conduction pathway for PAC.

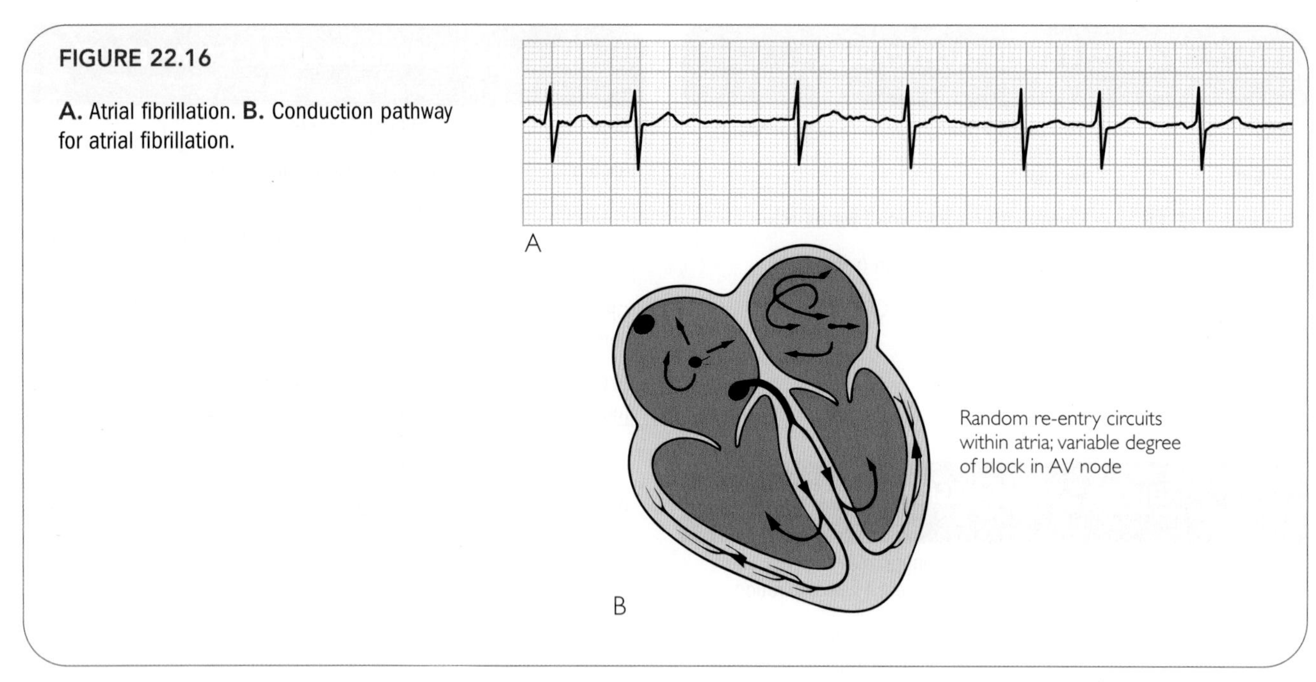

FIGURE 22.16

A. Atrial fibrillation. **B.** Conduction pathway for atrial fibrillation.

AV: atrioventricular.

TABLE 22.7 ATRIAL FIBRILLATION[22]

Rate	Atrial rate 400 beats/minute or more; ventricular rate varies
Rhythm	The ventricular rhythm is always irregular
P waves	No identifiable P waves
QRS complexes	Present, normal duration
P/QRS relationship	None identified; irregular ventricular response
PR interval	Not applicable

persistent (episodes lasting >7 days that do not terminate spontaneously) or long-standing and persistent (lasting ≥ 1 year where a strategy to control the ventricular rate is preferred).[36]

Haemodynamically unstable patients should be treated with urgent synchronised electrical cardioversion. The optimal pharmacological therapy for haemodynamically stable patients differs depending on whether the presentation is paroxysmal, persistent or long-standing. Beta-adrenoceptor antagonists, such as metoprolol, and some calcium channel antagonists; for example, verapamil, diltiazem, amiodarone or digoxin, are the preferred medications for controlling a rapid ventricular response.[36] Flecainide and amiodarone may also be used for chemical cardioversion (to restore a sinus rhythm). Anticoagulation with vitamin K antagonists such as warfarin or new oral non-vitamin K anticoagulants such as dabigatran or apixaban may also be used to reduce the risk of stroke and other ischaemic events in some AF patients.[36]

ATRIAL FLUTTER

A re-entry circuit within the right atria is thought to be responsible for atrial flutter. The atrial focus depolarises at a rapid rate of around 300 beats per minute, but most impulses are blocked by the AV node, usually to a regular, slower rate.[13,16] The AV node will allow every second, third or fourth flutter wave to reach the ventricles; consequently, there may be four flutter waves to every ventricular beat (4:1) or three or two flutter waves to every ventricular beat (3:1 and 2:1, respectively). Atrial flutter may be regular or irregular and although the atria do not contract well and thrombus formation may occur, it is less common than in atrial fibrillation.[13,16,27] Primary causes of atrial flutter include heart disease, right heart enlargement, chronic pulmonary disease, heart failure and thyrotoxicosis (Fig. 22.17 and Table 22.8).[13,16,27] Emergency management includes electrical cardioversion or chemical control of rapid atrial response rate with antiarrhythmic medications (e.g. amiodarone).[36]

SUPRAVENTRICULAR TACHYCARDIA

Supraventricular tachycardia (SVT) is a narrow complex tachycardia originating at the site of a rapid re-entry circuit in the atria or in the AV junction.[13,16] SVT is considered paroxysmal when it begins and ends abruptly and the rate may be as high as 280 beats per minute. Usually, the P wave is not clear or absent, although the QRS complex is normal (Fig. 22.18 and Table 22.9).[13,16,27,37] In some circumstances there may be two accessory pathways within the AV node and an electrical circuit or loop may be formed, which can continuously stimulate the ventricles to depolarise; thus called a re-entrant tachycardia. With such a rapid tachycardia, cardiac output may be compromised. Primary causes of SVT include: consumption of alcohol/stimulants, nicotine and caffeine and stress, although there may be no cause.[16,27,33]

FIGURE 22.17

A. Atrial flutter. **B.** Conduction pathway for atrial flutter.

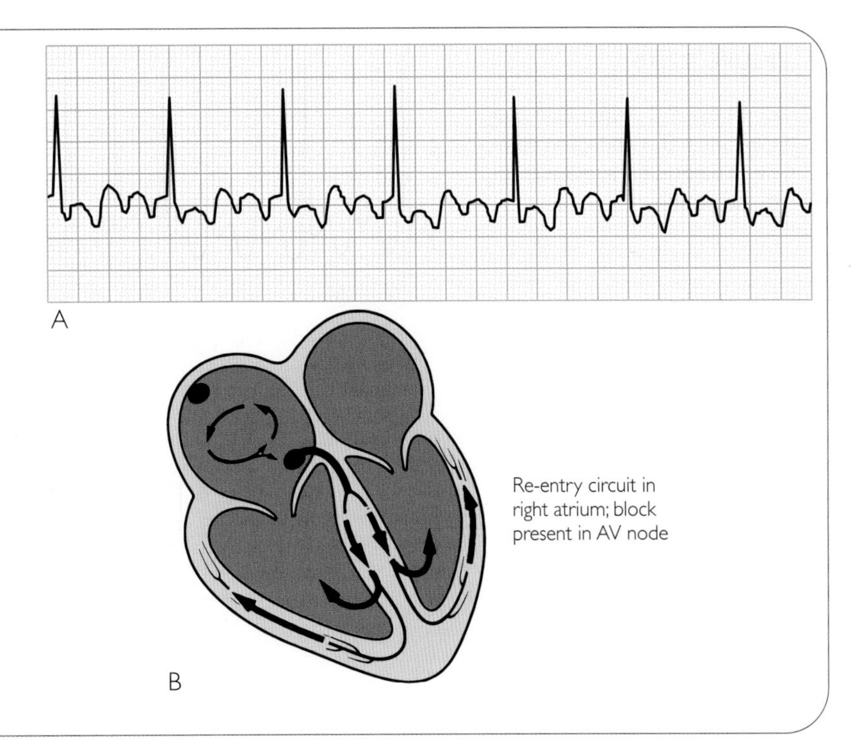

AV: atrioventricular.

TABLE 22.8 ATRIAL FLUTTER[22]

Rate	Atrial rate of 230 to 350 beats/minute; ventricular rate varies from normal to rapid
Rhythm	Regular if there is a fixed conduction ratio (a constant number of F waves to QRS complexes); irregular if there is a variable conduction ratio
P waves	A saw-toothed pattern of flutter waves (F waves)
QRS complexes	Present; normal duration
P/QRS relationship	Because of the rapid atrial rate, there will be two or more flutter waves for every QRS; the rhythm may be regular or irregular
PR interval	Not applicable

SVT is often self-limiting and can be easily terminated with vagal manoeuvres such as coughing or bearing down. For haemodynamically unstable patients, synchronised electrical cardioversion is the preferred treatment for SVT. For haemodynamically stable patients, treatment with vagal manoeuvres or adenosine is preferred.[34] The Valsalva manoeuvre is the most commonly used vagal manoeuvre in the out-of-hospital and ED setting and involves placing the patient in a semi-recumbent position and asking them to strain by blowing forcefully into a 10mL syringe for 15 seconds. Immediately following the strain, patients are laid flat and with their legs raised to 45 degrees for 15 seconds. The 'lying down with leg lift Valsalva' has success rates of over 40% after two attempts.[32]

FIRST-DEGREE ATRIOVENTRICULAR BLOCK

A first-degree AV block exists when the impulse is delayed in the AV node longer than normal, resulting in a prolonged PR interval. There is a P wave for every QRS. This is frequently an asymptomatic dysrhythmia, but may precede a more severe heart block (Fig. 22.19 and Table 22.10).[16,33,37] Emergency treatment is usually not required.

SECOND-DEGREE ATRIOVENTRICULAR BLOCK, TYPE I

Second-degree AV block, type I, is also known as Mobitz type I or Wenckebach. It is caused by delayed conduction through the AV node which progressively worsens over each consecutive beat. The PR interval gradually lengthens with each beat until it results in a non-conducted P wave and a resultant 'dropped' QRS complex; then the cycle begins again. It is as if the P wave is 'walking back' from its QRS complex (Fig. 22.20 and Table 22.11).[13,16,27] Emergency treatment should focus on identifying and treating the underlying cause; for example, digoxin toxicity. Although most cases are not associated with haemodynamic compromise, paramedics and emergency nurses should closely monitor the 12-lead ECG for progression into second-degree type II or third-degree block.

SECOND-DEGREE ATRIOVENTRICULAR BLOCK, TYPE II

Second-degree AV block, type II, is also known as Mobitz type II and exists when there is a regularly occurring block of the atrial impulse by the AV node. It may occur on a background of a normal or increased PR interval.[13,37] The block may occur in a pattern of conducted to non-conducted atrial impulses; for example, 2:1, 3:1 etc. Progression to complete

FIGURE 22.18

A. Paroxysmal supraventricular tachycardia. **B.** Conduction pathway for paroxysmal supraventricular tachycardia.

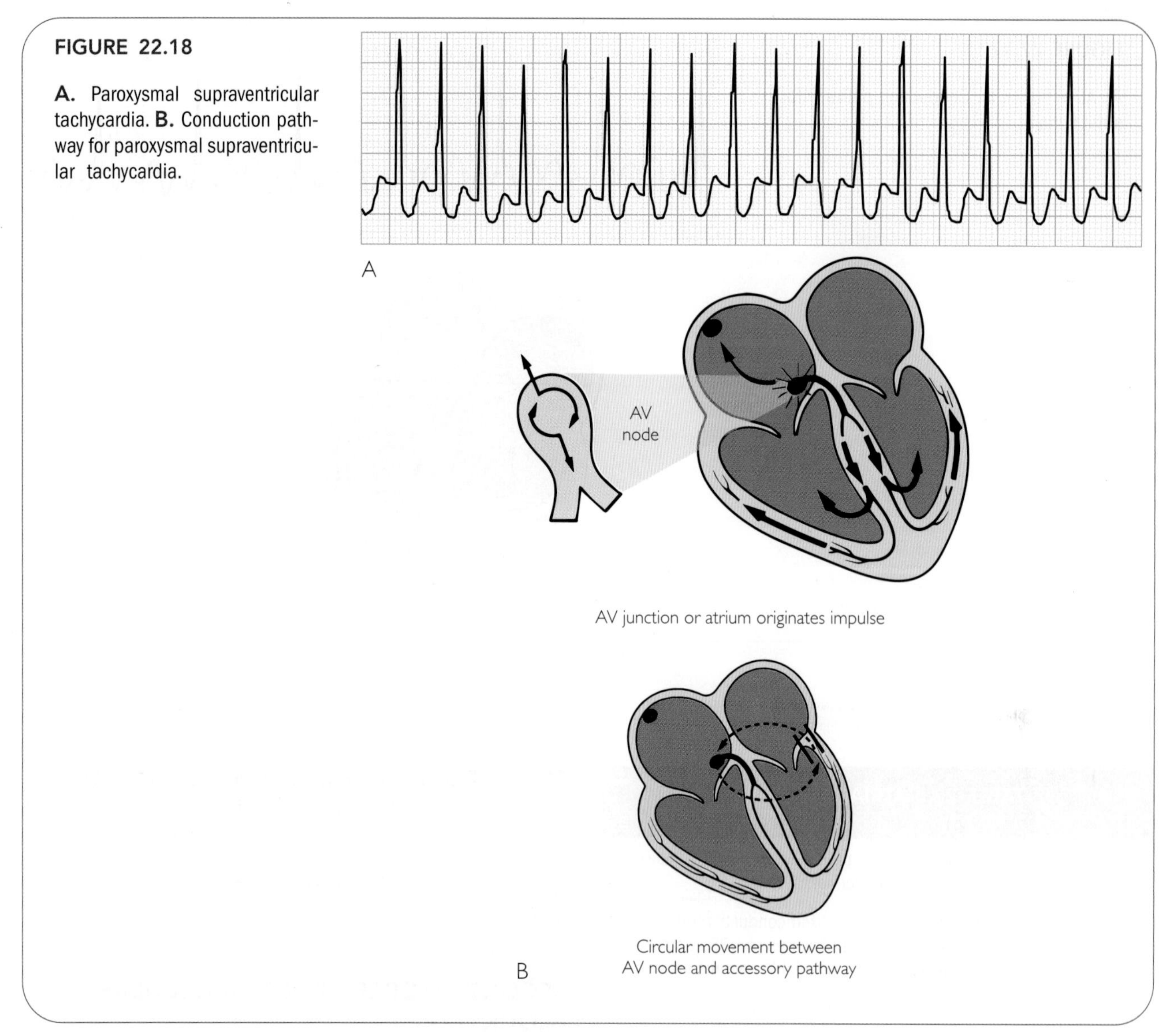

AV: atrioventricular.

TABLE 22.9 PAROXYSMAL SUPRAVENTRICULAR TACHYCARDIA[22]

Rate	100 to 280 beats/minute
Rhythm	Regular; sudden start and stop
P wave	May occur before the QRS; often distorted or buried within the QRS complex
QRS complexes	Present; duration is usually normal though the QRS may be wide
P/QRS relationship	A P wave for each QRS or none seen (buried in QRS complex)
PR interval	Short or none

heart block is not uncommon with this rhythm, and it is considered a high-risk presentation for deterioration (Fig. 22.21 and Table 22.12).[27,33] Where appropriate, emergency clinicians should identify and treat the underlying cause. The most common causes include ACS, thyroid disease, congenital heart defects, infective or inflammatory conditions of the heart and medication misuse; for example, beta-blockers, amiodarone, digoxin.[38] If symptomatic, intravenous atropine, a beta-adrenergic agonist (e.g. adrenaline or isoprenaline) or external cardiac pacing should be considered.[38]

THIRD-DEGREE AV BLOCK (COMPLETE AV BLOCK)

Third-degree heart block is also known as complete AV disassociation and exists when there is no conduction of the atrial

FIGURE 22.19

A. First-degree AV block. **B.** Conduction pathway for first-degree AV block.

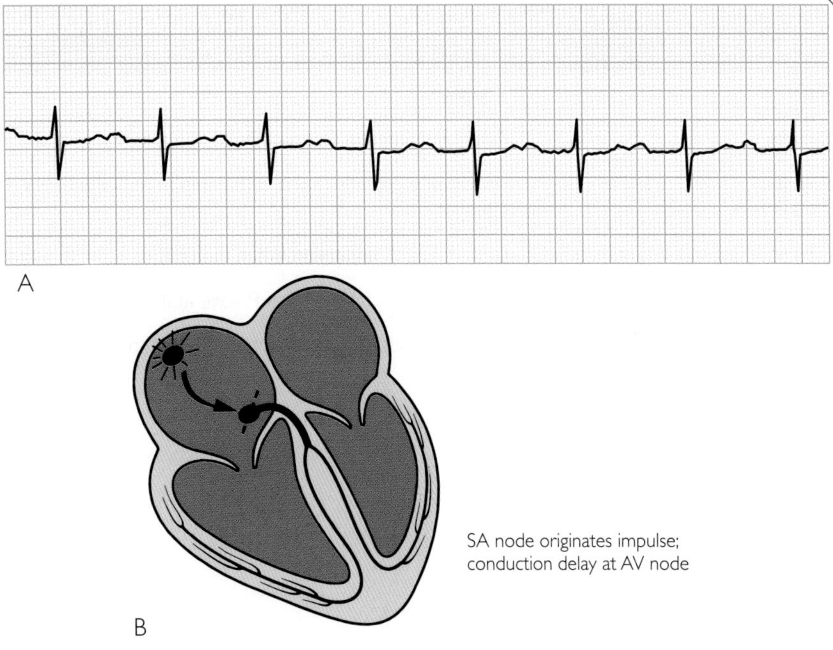

A

SA node originates impulse; conduction delay at AV node

B

SA: sinoatrial; AV: atrioventricular.

TABLE 22.10 FIRST-DEGREE ATRIOVENTRICULAR BLOCK[22]	
Rate	Usually 60 to 100 beats/minute
Rhythm	Regular
P waves	Present
QRS complexes	Present; normal duration
P/QRS relationship	A P wave precedes each QRS complex
PR interval	Prolonged (> 0.20 second) but consistent

impulse through the AV node to the ventricles. In response to the complete block by the AV node, a junctional or ventricular pacemaker will take over ventricular depolarisation.[16,27] As a result, the atria and the ventricles work completely independently (asynchronously) of each other. The atrial rate is around 60 beats/minute as it is initiated by the SA node, and the ventricular rate can be between 20 and 40 beats/minute depending on the site of the ventricular pacemaker. If the impulse originates within the ventricle, the QRS complex will be wide (> 0.12 sec).[16,33]

Cardiac output falls because of loss of atrial filling and bradycardia. If the heart block occurs gradually, as with conditions such as fibrosis associated with the ageing process, compensatory mechanisms will help maintain homeostasis. However,

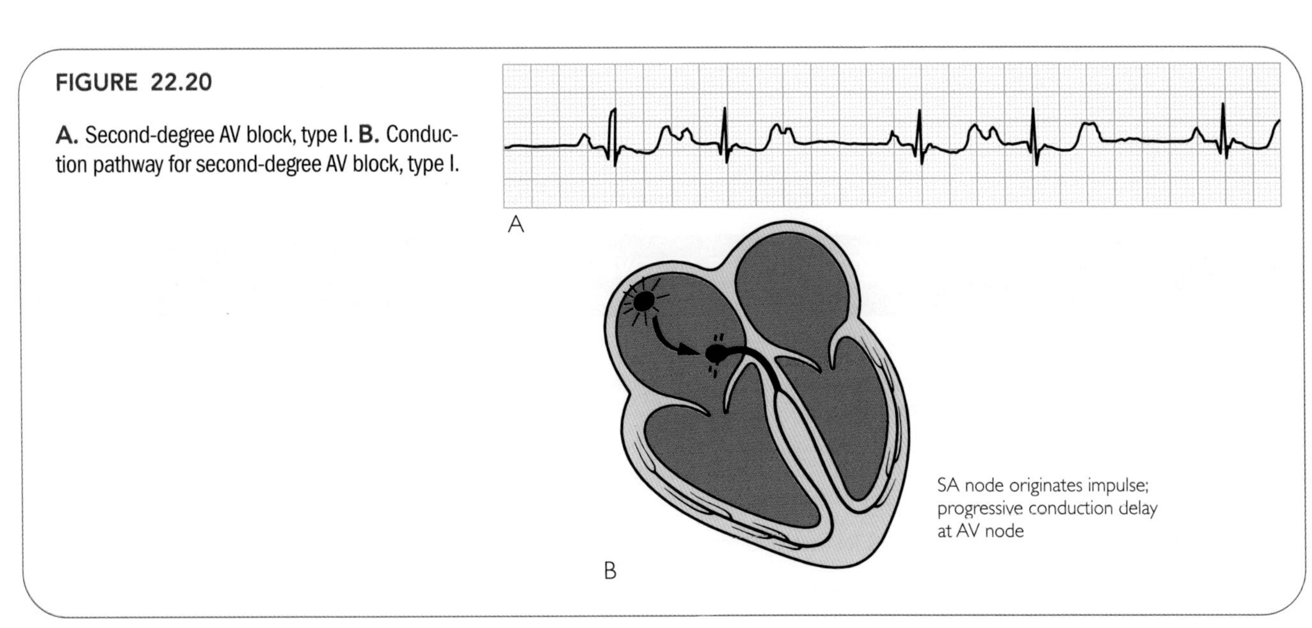

FIGURE 22.20

A. Second-degree AV block, type I. **B.** Conduction pathway for second-degree AV block, type I.

SA: sinoatrial; AV: atrioventricular.

TABLE 22.11 SECOND-DEGREE ATRIOVENTRICULAR BLOCK, TYPE I[22]	
Rate	Normal
Rhythm	Atrial beats are regular; ventricular beats are irregular
P waves	One P wave precedes each QRS complex until the QRS is dropped. This pattern recurs at regular intervals
QRS complexes	Cyclic missed conduction; when the QRS complex is present, it is of normal duration
P/QRS relationship	A QRS complex follows each P wave and then is dropped (absent) at patterned intervals
PR interval	Lengthens with each cycle until a QRS complex is dropped, and then the pattern repeats

FIGURE 22.21

A. Second-degree AV block, type II, with 2:1 conduction. **B.** Conduction pathway for second-degree AV block, type II.

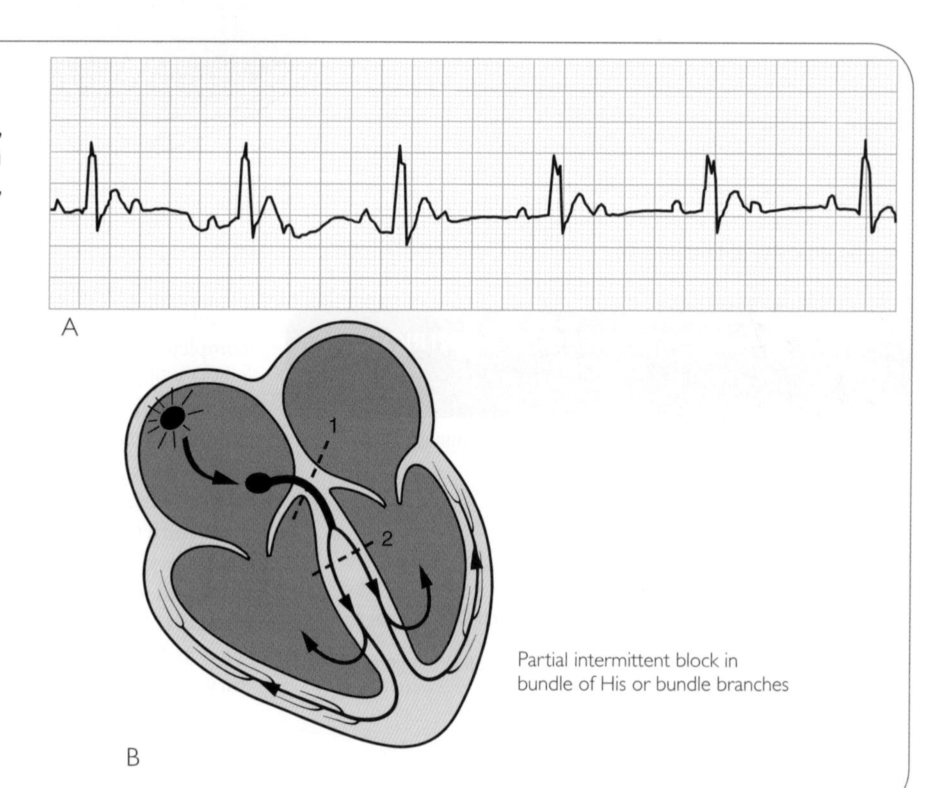

TABLE 22.12 SECOND-DEGREE ATRIOVENTRICULAR BLOCK, TYPE II[22]	
Rate	Atrial rate of 60 to 100 beats/minute; ventricular rate is often slow
Rhythm	Atrial rhythm is regular; ventricular rhythm is regular with a consistent conduction pattern but is irregular if conduction pattern is variable
P waves	One or more for every QRS complex
QRS complexes	When present, normal or prolonged duration
P/QRS relationship	One or more P waves for each QRS complex
PR interval	Normal or delayed for the P wave that conducts the QRS complex

FIGURE 22.22

A. Third-degree heart block. **B.** Conduction pathway for third-degree heart block.

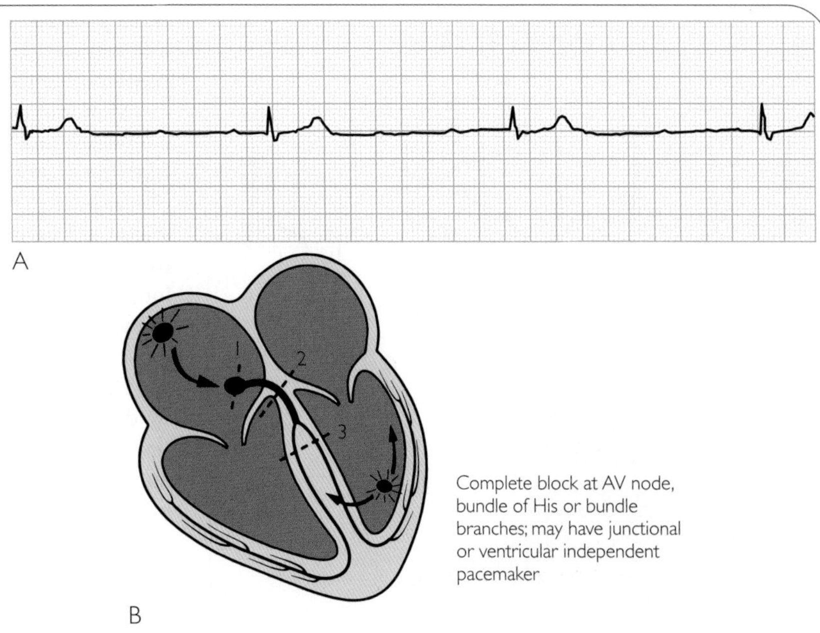

AV: atrioventricular.

TABLE 22.13 THIRD-DEGREE HEART BLOCK[22]

Rate	Atrial rate of 60 to 100 beats/minute; ventricular rate usually less than 60 beats/minute
Rhythm	Regular
P waves	Occurring regularly
QRS complexes	Slow; narrow if the QRS is a junctional escape beat, wide (0.12 second) if it is a ventricular escape beat
P/QRS relationship	The P wave and QRS complex are completely independent of each other
PR interval	Inconsistent

when cardiac output is compromised or the heart block occurs suddenly (as with ACS), rapid treatment may be required (Fig. 22.22 and Table 22.13).[16,27,37]

Causes of complete AV blocks include infarction of the conduction pathway; for example, anterior or inferior MI and reversible ischaemia of the AV node, aortic valve disease (degenerative), medications; for example, digoxin, beta-blockers, antiarrhythmics, carbamazepine, acute rheumatic fever, atrial septal defect, dilated cardiomyopathy and connective tissue disorders.[15,33]

Emergency clinicians should be prepared to provide basic and advanced life support as necessary (see Chapter 14 for Resuscitation). If symptomatic, intravenous atropine, a beta-adrenergic agonist; for example, adrenaline or isoprenaline, or external cardiac pacing, should be considered.

PREMATURE VENTRICULAR COMPLEXES

Premature ventricular complexes (PVCs) are extremely common abnormal impulses that are initiated from an ectopic focus within the ventricles.[16,27] When a single focus of the ventricle initiates an impulse, the complex will have the same configuration and is therefore said to be unifocal.[27] When multiple foci are involved in initiating ventricular impulses, the complexes present in a variety of configurations and are said to be multifocal (refer to Fig. 22.23 and Table 22.14).[16,27,33] A pair of PVCs is known as a couplet and three consecutive PVCs are known as a triplet. Three or more PVCs constitute a run of non-sustained ventricular tachycardia.

Increasing age, a taller height, a higher blood pressure, a history of heart disease, low physical activity, and smoking predict a greater frequency of PVCs in the general population.[39] Increased PVC frequency may also be caused by myocardial ischaemia, anxiety, stimulants, excess caffeine, electrolyte disturbances and digoxin toxicity. PVCs are a normal electrophysiological phenomenon and are typically benign. If the patient is symptomatic and the PVC frequency is high, acute management with a beta-adrenoceptor antagonist, or a nondihydropyridine calcium channel blocker should be considered.[39]

PRACTICE TIP

Bigeminy is a repetitive pattern of PVCs which occurs on every second beat; and in trigeminy, PVC occurs every third beat. Although typically a benign finding, emergency clinicians should monitor the patient closely for the development of symptoms; for example, palpitations, chest pain, shortness of breath or dizziness and haemodynamic compromise. In patients with underlying long-QT syndromes or ACS, frequent PVCs may increase the risk of developing lethal ventricular dysrhythmias; for example, ventricular tachycardia.

FIGURE 22.23

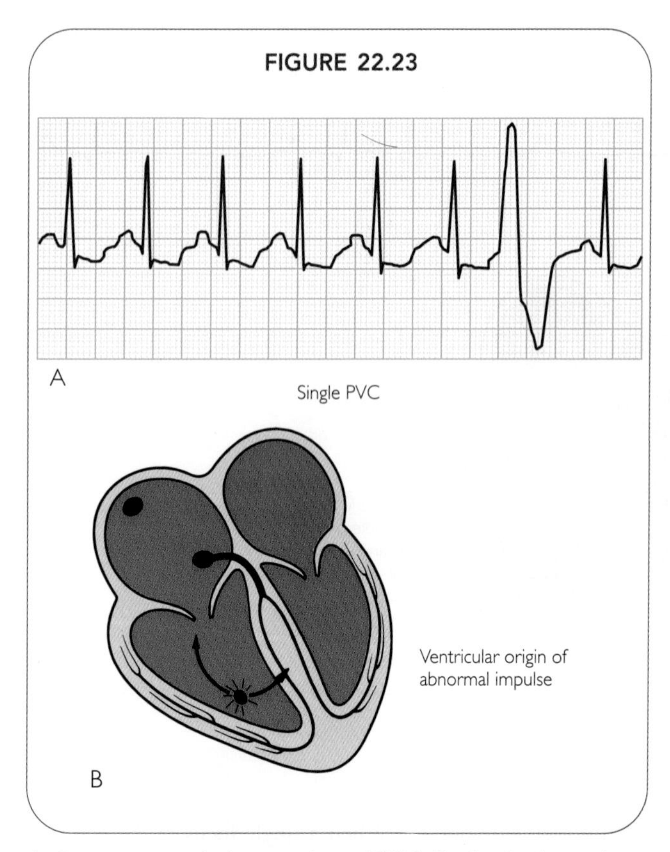

A. Premature ventricular complexes (PVCs). **B.** Conduction pathway for PVC.

TABLE 22.14 PREMATURE VENTRICULAR COMPLEXES (PVCs)

Rate	Varies with underlying rhythm
Rhythm	Irregular because of early beats
P waves	Present with each sinus beat; P waves do not precede premature ventricular complexes (PVCs)
QRS complexes	Sinus-initiated QRS complexes are normal; the QRS complexes of PVCs are wide (> 0.12 second) and bizarre and usually have a T wave of opposite polarity. Look for a full compensatory pause
P/QRS relationship	A P wave precedes each QRS complex in the normal sinus beats; no P wave precedes PVCs
PR interval	Normal in sinus beats; none in PVCs

VENTRICULAR TACHYCARDIA

Ventricular tachycardia (VT) is a rhythm frequently observed in patients with underlying heart disease. The regular, broad complex QRS originates within the ventricle and is considered to be a life-threatening dysrhythmia.[16,40] A patient with VT may present with a range of symptoms, from mild symptoms; for example, palpitations, dizziness, to severe haemodynamic compromise (unconscious with no or little perfusion). The following criteria support VT diagnosis: QRS complex > 0.12 second; rate > 100 beats per minute; > 3 consecutive beats; usually regular, dissociated P waves. If the diagnosis is in doubt, any wide-complex tachycardia should be considered VT until proven otherwise.

Monomorphic VT is characterised by symmetrical QRS complexes and is usually associated with left ventricular dysfunction and coronary heart disease. Polymorphic VT is a form of ventricular tachycardia characterised by non-symmetrical wide QRS complexes. A common type of polymorphic VT is torsades de pointes normally caused by medications that prolong the Q–T interval, such as amiodarone, or by toxicity due to medications such as tricyclic antidepressants (Fig. 22.24 and Table 22.15).[16,27,33]

The term paroxysmal (non-sustained) VT is usually defined by duration (less than 30 seconds), in contrast to episodes of sustained VT (lasting greater than 30 seconds). The VT rate and duration will usually determine the severity of symptoms, which may be exacerbated by pre-existing heart disease. The faster the rate, the more likely that cardiac output will be compromised. Haemodynamically stable patients with VT can be treated with antiarrhythmic drugs such as procainamide, amiodarone or sotalol.[41] For conscious patients, who are haemodynamically unstable, treatment with immediate synchronised electrical cardioversion is the optimal therapy. Cardiac arrest should be treated with immediate defibrillation, basic and advanced life support interventions (see Chapter 14 on Resuscitation). In patients presenting with torsades de pointes, correction of electrolyte disturbances and treatment with intravenous magnesium are the preferred treatment interventions.[41]

PRACTICE TIP

Polymorphic VT treatments include stopping all medications that prolong the QT interval, correction of electrolytes and the administration of intravenous magnesium sulfate. Avoid the administration of procainamide, amiodarone and sotalol as these medications may further prolong the QT interval, promoting the development of torsades de pointes.[15,27,41]

VENTRICULAR FIBRILLATION

Ventricular fibrillation (VF) exists when there is a rapid firing of ventricular ectopic sites at the same time, causing a fibrillatory waveform that originates in the ventricles.[16,27,40] This rhythm produces no effective ventricular contraction and therefore no cardiac output. Without immediate intervention it becomes a fatal dysrhythmia—the risk of death increases significantly with every minute delay to basic life support interventions (Fig. 22.25 and Table 22.16). Across all health settings, clinicians should be educated and trained in basic life support. However, paramedics and emergency nurses need to be skilled in providing advanced life support, given the complexity and acuity of patients and the likelihood of being involved in a cardiac arrest event. Refer to Chapter 14 for a detailed approach to basic and advanced life support techniques.

ASYSTOLE

Asystole is the complete absence of any electrical activity associated with ventricular depolarisation. Atrial impulses may or may not be present. This rhythm usually implies that the

FIGURE 22.24

A. Ventricular tachycardia (VT).
B. Conduction pathway for VT.

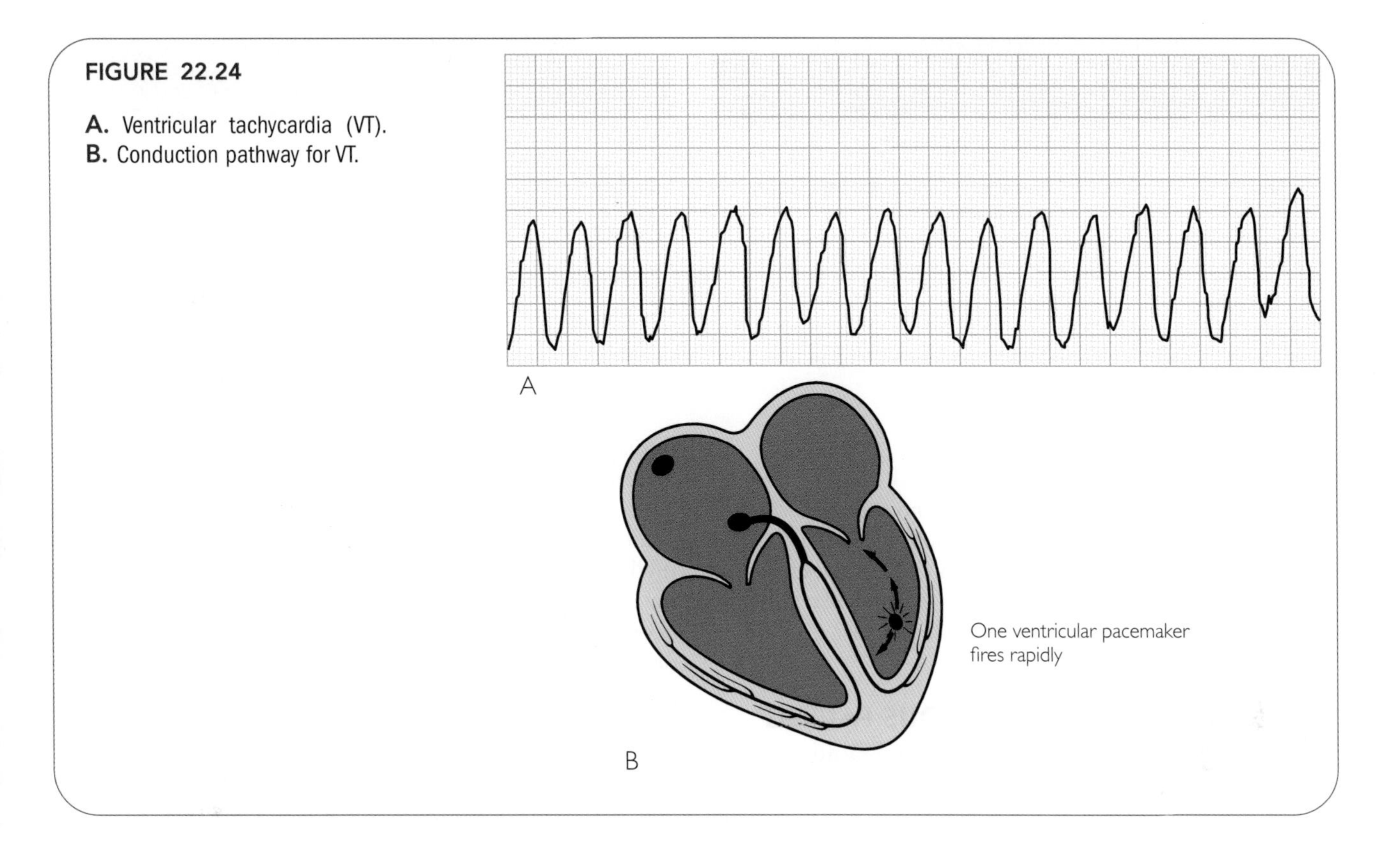

TABLE 22.15 VENTRICULAR TACHYCARDIA[22]	
Rate	100 to 250 beats/minute
Rhythm	Regular
P waves	Not seen
QRS complexes	Wide, regular, monomorphic
P/QRS relationship	None

patient has been in cardiac arrest for a prolonged time and is associated with a high mortality rate.[46] If atrial impulses are present (P waves) on the 12-lead ECG in the absence of the QRS complex, this is often termed ventricular standstill; a rhythm that carries a similar prognosis to asystole. The aim is to treat or correct the underlying cause (Fig. 22.26 and Table 22.17). Refer to Chapter 14 for basic and advanced life support approaches to resuscitation.

PULSELESS ELECTRICAL ACTIVITY

Pulseless electrical activity (PEA) is defined as organised electrical activity, with no detectable cardiac output (pulse). Patients who exhibit PEA generally have a poor prognosis unless the underlying reversible cause is identified and treated rapidly. Common causes of PEA include hypovolaemia, hypoxia, hypo- or hyperkalaemia, hypo- or hyperthermia, tension pneumothorax, cardiac tamponade, thrombosis (coronary or pulmonary), and poisoning.[42] Refer to Chapter 14 for basic and advanced life support approaches to resuscitation.

FIGURE 22.25

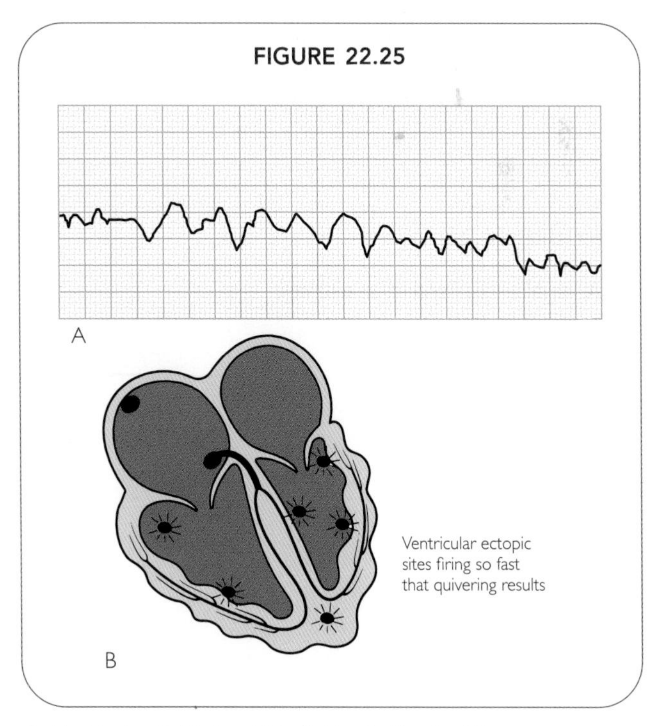

A. Ventricular fibrillation (VF). **B.** Conduction for VF.

CARDIAC PACING

Temporary cardiac pacing is used to provide emergency support of bradydysrhythmias. Cardiac pacing delivers an electrical current through the heart to increase heart rate, cardiac output and mean arterial pressure. The most common methods used to

TABLE 22.16 VENTRICULAR FIBRILLATION[22]

Rate	Rapid, disorganised
Rhythm	Irregular amplitude and wavelength (polymorphic)
P waves	Not seen
QRS complexes	None
P/QRS relationship	None
PR interval	None

TABLE 22.17 ASYSTOLE[22]

Rate	None
Rhythm	None
P waves	May or may not appear
P/QRS relationship	None
PR interval	None

enable cardiac pacing include the transvenous or transcutaneous approach. However, in the acute hospital setting cardiac pacing can be achieved by the insertion of epicardial pacing wires post-cardiothoracic surgery, and transthoracic where a myocardial pacing electrode is inserted via a cardiac needle into the right ventricle.[16,43,44]

TEMPORARY TRANSCUTANEOUS PACING

Temporary transcutaneous pacing is a straightforward and non-invasive procedure that can be delivered through most modern cardiac monitors/defibrillators. Pre-procedure, obtain patient consent, select appropriate analgesia and sedation, and apply standard chest leads. Apply defibrillator pads; place one anteriorly on the chest over the cardiac apex at the V_3 position and the other posteriorly and level with the inferior aspect of the left scapula, avoiding medication patches, implanted devices and injured areas (see Chapter 16 for information on applying cardiac pacing).[16,17] Select the appropriate mode; non-demand mode will deliver electrical impulses at the rate selected irrespective of the patient's intrinsic rhythm; or demand mode (preferred), which will identify the patient's intrinsic rhythm and provide necessary electrical impulses according to the rate selected.[17] The rate and energy level can be adjusted to maintain adequate capture, cardiac output and optimise patient comfort.[27,37,43,44] This is a relatively simple procedure for paramedics and emergency nurses, and should be part of routine resuscitation education and training.

TEMPORARY TRANSVENOUS PACING

This is a common procedure in coronary care units and is performed when the patient is haemodynamically compromised. The method involves inserting a pacing electrode into the right ventricle via the subclavian or external jugular venous route, under fluoroscopy or with a flotation-pacing catheter under guidance by the ECG. The electrodes are connected to a pulse generator where the output can be selected in milliamps along with the rate.[27,37]

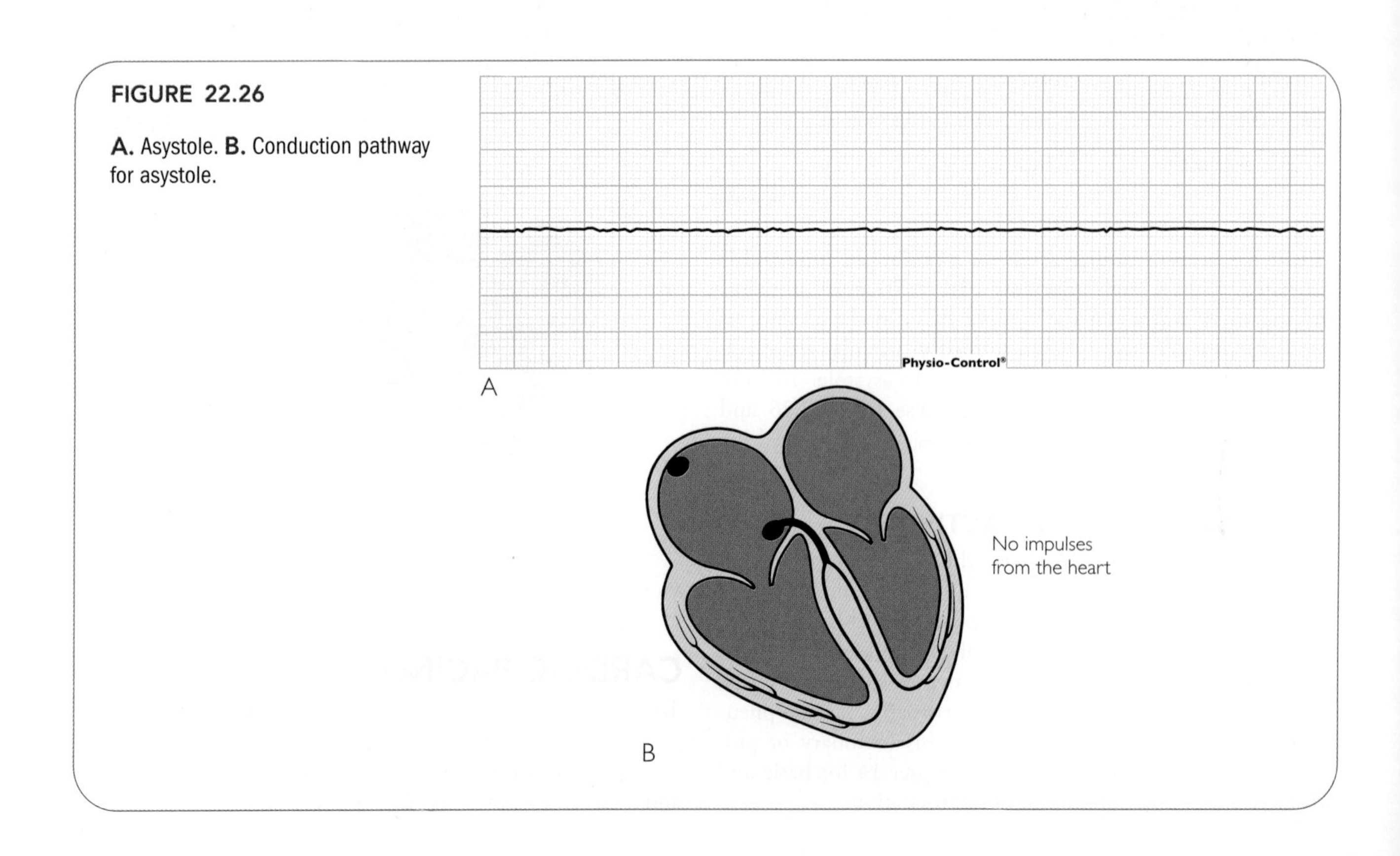

FIGURE 22.26

A. Asystole. **B.** Conduction pathway for asystole.

Either type of pacemaker can be at a fixed-rate mode or demand mode. Fixed rate is rarely used as it can have potential complications by delivering an impulse on the T wave and precipitating VF. Demand mode senses the patient's own QRS complexes and only generates an impulse when the heart does not produce its own intrinsic QRS complex.[16,17] Temporary cardiac pacing is indicated in symptomatic sinus bradycardia, sick sinus syndrome, heart blocks and ventricular standstill.[16,17]

EXTERNAL DEFIBRILLATORS

External defibrillators deliver an electrical counter-shock that interrupts the chaotic heart rhythm by depolarising a critical mass of myocardium at one time, thus stopping aberrant electrical and mechanical heart activity. The temporary halting of electrical activity within the heart allows for the heart's intrinsic pacemaker to regain its normal electrical activity. Chapter 14 provides a detailed overview of defibrillation, including pad placement.

IMPLANTABLE CARDIOVERTER DEFIBRILLATORS

Implantable internal cardioverter defibrillators (ICD) are effective in preventing sudden cardiac deaths from ventricular dysrhythmias[41] in patients with recognised heart disease, low ejection fraction conditions, heart failure, cardiomyopathy and cardiac channelopathies.[44,45] The ICD is inserted in the same way as a permanent pacemaker—the generator is implanted under the skin and subcutaneous tissue and the wires are directly inserted into the atria, ventricles, or both.

The ICD has the ability to perform defibrillation and synchronised cardioversion in order to treat ventricular fibrillation and tachycardia.[46–48] The ICD can also provide bradycardia pacing (to increase ventricular rate), and anti-tachycardia pacing, which has the ability to cardiovert tachydysrhythmias without the need for a painful shock. Anti-tachycardia pacing works by interrupting the re-entry circuit of ventricular and supraventricular tachycardias with a series of appropriately timed pacing stimuli delivered into the excitable gap of the re-entrant circuit. Once capture occurs, the ICD reduces the pacing rate considerably, slowing the ventricular rate.[44,47,48]

CARDIAC ASSESSMENT

A systematic and structured approach is required by clinicians to assess and treat patients with a cardiovascular emergency (Table 22.18). The goal of the primary survey is the identification and simultaneous correction of life-threatening emergencies relating to the patient's airway (A), breathing (B), circulation (C) and neurological assessment (D).[28]

A cardiac assessment involves obtaining details about the presenting problem, past medical history, current medications and a physical examination. This information will assist in identifying the differential diagnosis of the underlying condition. Cardiac-related symptoms often include chest pain, dyspnoea, palpitations, nausea, vomiting and syncope. Relevant risk factors for ACS include ischaemic heart disease, hypertension, dyslipidaemia, heart failure, respiratory disease, diabetes mellitus, renal disease or a past history cardiac surgery/intervention. A physical examination may reveal cardiac abnormalities on inspection (implanted device, raised jugular venous pressure), palpation (pitting oedema) and auscultation (adventitious lung sounds, heart sounds and murmurs).[49]

TABLE 22.18 CHEST PAIN MNEMONIC FOR CHEST PAIN ASSESSMENT[22]

LETTER	TRIGGER WORDS	ASSESSMENT
C	Commenced when?	When did the pain start? Was onset associated with anything specific? Exertion? Activity? Emotional upset?
H	History/risk factors	Do you have a history of heart disease? Is there a primary relative (parent/sibling) with early onset and/or early death related to heart disease? Do you have other risk factors, e.g. diabetes, smoking, hypertension or obesity?
E	Extra symptoms?	What else are you feeling with the pain? Are you nervous? Sweating? Is your heart racing? Are you short of breath? Do you feel nauseated? Dizzy? Weak?
S	Stays/radiates	Does the pain stay in one place? Does it radiate or go anywhere else in the body? Where?
T	Timing	How long does the pain last? How long has this episode lasted? How many minutes? Is the pain continuous or does it come and go? When did it become continuous?
P	Place	Where is your pain? Check for point tenderness with palpation.
A	Alleviates Aggravates	What makes the pain better? Rest? Changing position? Deep breathing? What makes the pain worse? Exercise? Deep breathing? Changing position?
I	Intensity	How intense is the pain? Rate the pain from 0 to 10.
N	Nature	Describe the pain. (Listen for descriptors such as sharp, stabbing, crushing, dull, burning, elephant sitting on my chest.) Do not suggest descriptors.

The secondary assessment includes a detailed pain assessment and various mnemonics exist to assist with a structured systematic assessment. PQRST (**P**rovokes/palliates, **Q**uality, **R**adiates, **S**everity, **T**ime) is a commonly used mnemonic for assessing pain.[50] Clinicians must be mindful that many patients experiencing an ACS may not report chest pain, instead they present with 'atypical' symptoms, including gastrointestinal pain, back pain, shoulder pain or simply a vague feeling of being 'unwell' or fatigued.[22] Importantly, women often present with a varying range of symptoms to men,[51] instead often describing signs and symptoms such as fatigue, sleep disturbances, shortness of breath, nausea and vomiting, and back or jaw pain.[52] Clinicians should not trivialise these symptoms in women or perceive that they have a lower risk of ACS than men, otherwise the diagnosis may be missed or undertreated.[53,54]

ACUTE CHEST PAIN

Chest pain can result from several cardiac and non-cardiac origins. Despite having non-specific findings on the ECG and negative biomarkers, approximately one-third of patients presenting with chest pain who have known cardiac disease will have an adverse cardiac event. The priority is to rapidly identify if the chest pain is related to an acute coronary event such as ACS. Favourable patient outcomes are dependent on early recognition, quantification of risk and appropriate management.[13]

It can be challenging to differentiate between a diagnosis of ACS and other causes of chest pain. Chest pain differential diagnoses must be considered, and you can refer to Table 22.19 for further detail.[22,55] Differential diagnoses can include aortic aneurysm, pericarditis/myocarditis, pneumothorax, and pulmonary embolus. Clinicians should have a high index of suspicion of ACS for patients who present with musculoskeletal or gastrointestinal complaints. It is not possible to exclude ACS accurately and safely in the pre-hospital setting, and even in the hospital setting a diagnosis may be missed. The severity of chest pain is not an indicator of the severity of myocardial damage.

Assessment

Chest pain assessment is a time-critical, hierarchical diagnostic process based upon presentation, history, serial ECGs and cardiac biomarkers.[13,46] A systematic patient assessment should include a primary and secondary cardiac assessment, including a focused history, physical examination and a pain assessment. Cardiac monitoring and vital signs need to be monitored regularly including blood pressure, mentation and pallor.

A 12-lead ECG should be obtained as soon as practicable, and the paramedic should transmit it to the receiving hospital or communicate the results according to local or state protocols if there is evidence of STEMI.[56] Early communication will ensure prompt and accurate identification of patients with STEMI and enable timely reperfusion procedures to begin, either by paramedics or emergency clinicians.

For patients presenting to an ED with chest pain, the Australasian Triage Scale recommends a Triage Category 2 (to be assessed within 10 minutes of presentation).[13,57] A 12-lead ECG must ideally be obtained and reviewed by an expert ED clinician within 10 minutes of presentation,[27,56,58] as this allows for early identification of a life-threatening cardiac diagnosis.

Investigations

Laboratory tests include electrolytes, full blood count, renal function, coagulation profile, blood glucose level and lipid screen. The preferred cardiac biomarker to detect myocardial injury (necrosis) is troponin-I and troponin-T. The determination of single or serial troponin measurements should be utilised in conjunction with risk calculators such as NVDPA, PREDICT-1 or HEART (History, Electrocardiogram, Age, Risk Factors and Troponin).[6,8,59,60] The Heart Foundation[61] assessment protocol recommends an initial troponin-I on arrival and the serial troponin-T can be repeated at 3 hours (highly sensitive assay) or 6 hours (sensitive assay), depending on risk stratification criteria. Emerging evidence recommends that a single negative troponin in conjunction with a low-risk HEART score can be safely used to rule out ACS so the patient can be discharged home from ED.[60] Creatine kinase-MB also detects myocardial necrosis, but may be elevated in non-cardiac causes. B-type natriuretic peptide (BNP) will aid in the diagnosis of heart failure and D-dimer can assist to exclude pulmonary embolism (PE). Serial measurements of cardiac biomarkers are often performed, as the time in which a biomarker peaks then returns to baseline provides essential information to identify and manage patients who are potentially suitable for early reperfusion therapy.[46,56] Table 22.20 provides the pattern for specific cardiac biomarkers.[15–17]

Medical imaging, in the form of a chest x-ray, may be required to enable identification of cardiac enlargement, aortic arch diameter changes and identification of non-coronary causes of chest pain.[24] A cardiac echo uses ultrasound to identify wall motion abnormalities (pericarditis), heart failure or complications of an MI. Computed tomography (CT) angiography will detect obstructive coronary disease (pericardial effusion, aortic dissection and PE), and a cardiac MRI will assess structures, functions and vasculature of the chest.[49]

Management

Initial pharmacotherapy for chest pain where ACS is the most likely diagnosis includes aspirin, nitroglycerin (GTN), and opioid analgesia; for example, titrated fentanyl or morphine. To assist with the assessment of chest pain, there are recognised protocols and pathways, such as HEART score, which have been validated in both retrospective and prospective trials.[59,62,63] These pathways are used to guide assessment, reduce unnecessary investigations, minimise delay in treatment and can facilitate early decision-making and disposition.[13] If an initial assessment has ruled out a STEMI, the patient can then be risk stratified into three categories: 1) high, 2) intermediate or 3) low risk. Further investigations and treatment are then subsequently based on the category and each facility will have its own management pathway.[58]

ACUTE CORONARY SYNDROMES (ACS)

ACSs encompass a range of conditions where there is a suspicion or confirmation of a myocardial ischemia or infarction. ACS conditions include ST-segment elevation myocardial infarction (STEMI), a non-ST-elevation myocardial infarction (NSTEMI) and unstable angina. NSTEMI and unstable angina are collectively described as 'NSTEACS',

TABLE 22.19 DIFFERENTIAL DIAGNOSIS OF CHEST PAIN[14,22]

CAUSE	ONSET OF PAIN	CHARACTERISTICS OF PAIN	LOCATION OF PAIN	HISTORY	PAIN WORSENED BY	PAIN RELIEVED BY	OTHER
Acute myocardial infarction	Sudden onset; lasts more than 30 minutes to 1 hour	Pressure, burning, aching, tightness, choking	Across chest; may radiate to jaws and neck and down arms and back	Age 40–70 years; may or may not have history of angina		Nothing; not movement, stillness, position, or breath holding; only relieved by medication (morphine sulfate)	Shortness of breath, diaphoresis, weakness, anxiety
Angina	Sudden onset; lasts only a few minutes	Ache, squeezing, choking, heaviness, burning	Substernal; may radiate to jaw and neck and down arms and back	May have history of angina; precipitating circumstances; pain characteristic; response to glyceryl trinitrate	Lying down, eating, effort, cold weather, smoking, stress, anger, worry, hunger	Rest, glyceryl trinitrate	Unstable angina occurs even at rest
Dissecting aortic aneurysm	Sudden onset	Excruciating, tearing	Centre of chest; radiates into back; may radiate to abdomen	Nothing specific, except that pain is usually worse at onset		Nothing	Blood pressure difference between right and left arms, murmur of aortic regurgitation
Pericarditis	Sudden onset or may be variable	Sharp, knifelike	Retrosternal; may radiate up neck and down left arm	Short history of upper respiratory infection or fever	Deep breathing, trunk movement, maybe swallowing	Sitting up, leaning forward	Friction rub, paradoxic pulse over 10 mmHg
Pneumothorax	Sudden onset	Tearing, pleuritic	Lateral side of chest	None	Breathing	Nothing	Dyspnoea, increased pulse, decreased breath sounds, deviated trachea
Pulmonary embolus	Sudden onset	Crushing (but not always)	Lateral side of chest	Sometimes phlebitis Deep vein thrombosis Recent surgery	Breathing	Not breathing	Cyanosis, dyspnoea, profound anxiety, hypoxaemia, cough with haemoptysis
Hiatus hernia	Sudden onset	Sharp, severe	Lower chest; upper abdomen	May have none	Heavy meal, bending, lying down	Bland diet, walking, antacids, semi-Fowler position	
Gastrointestinal disturbance or cholecystitis	Sudden onset	Gripping, burning	Lower substernal area, upper abdomen	May have none	Eating, lying down	Antacids	
Degenerative disk (cervical or thoracic spine) disease	Sudden onset	Sharp, severe	Substernal; may radiate to neck, jaw, arms and shoulders	May have none	Movement of the neck or spine, lifting, straining	Rest, decreased movement	Pain usually on outer aspect of arm, thumb or index finger
Degenerative or inflammatory lesions of shoulder, ribs, scalenus anterior	Sudden onset	Sharp, severe	Substernal; radiates to shoulder	May have none	Movement of arm or shoulder	Elevation of arm, support to shoulder, postural exercises	
Hyperventilation	Sudden onset	Vague	Vague	Hyperventilation, anxiety, stress, emotional upset	Increased respiratory rate	Slowing of respiratory rate	Be sure hyperventilation is from non-medical cause

TABLE 22.20 CARDIAC BIOMARKERS FOR ACUTE MYOCARDIAL INFARCTION[37,47]

CARDIAC MARKER	INITIAL ELEVATION AFTER ACUTE MYOCARDIAL INFARCTION (H)	MEAN PEAK TIME (H)	TIME TO RETURN TO BASELINE
Myoglobin	1-4	6-7	18–24 hours
Troponin-I (cTn 1) (cardiac-specific)	3-12	10–24	3-7 days
Troponin-T (cTn T) (cardiac-specific)	3-12	12–48	10–14 days
Creatine kinase-MB (CK-MB)	4-12	10–24	48-72 hours
CK-MB subforms: MB1 and MB2	1-6	18	Unknown
Lactate dehydrogenase (LDH)	8-12	24-48	10-14 days

Note: an LDH-1/LDH-2 ratio > 0.76 is significantly associated with acute myocardial infarction.

FIGURE 22.27 ATHEROSCLEROTIC PLAQUE FORMATION IMPEDES BLOOD FLOW

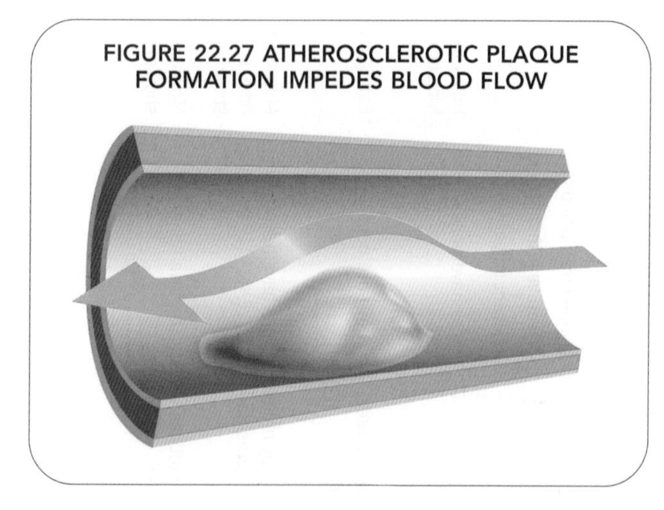

non-ST elevation acute coronary syndromes. ACS disease refers to a number of processes:

- unstable angina pectoris (UAP): history of cardiac disease with no ECG evidence of myocardial infarction and a negative troponin
- non-ST-segment elevation MI (NSTEMI): elevated serum troponin levels in the absence of ST elevation with partial thickness myocardial wall damage
- ST-segment elevation MI (STEMI): ST elevation on ECG or new left bundle branch block (LBBB) with full-thickness myocardial wall damage.[34,56]

ACSs are challenging to differentiate, but all are the result of cellular hypoxia, due to the partial or total coronary artery occlusion caused by one or multiple atherosclerotic plaques. Arteriosclerosis is abnormal thickening, hardening and loss of arterial elasticity of the arterial wall, which results in decreased blood flow to the myocardium (Fig. 22.27). Atherosclerosis is an inflammatory disease, which begins with endothelial injury, and then later as the disease progresses, accumulation of fatty, cholesterol and calcium deposits result in the development of a complicated plaque lesion.[32]

Management

The primary diagnostic goal in the early management of suspected ACS is to determine whether the patient is suffering a STEMI or NSTEACS. Early identification is critical to enable rapid reperfusion and to limit or halt the progression of the MI.[55] Clinical management of a suspected ACS includes:

- obtaining a comprehensive history to assist in identification of the underlying conditions
- a physical assessment to identify associated symptoms, including dyspnoea, nausea, vomiting, diaphoresis and raised JVP
- additionally, assessing and monitoring heart rate, blood pressure, respiratory rate, oxygen saturation, work of breathing, central and peripheral perfusion, and neurological status. Auscultate the chest, noting abnormal heart and valve sounds and adventitious lung sounds.[15,27,37]
  Oxygen therapy can be initiated if the patient has an oxygen saturation of < 93%, has increased work of breathing or shows signs of shock.[37,64]

Pharmacological treatment

- Administration of aspirin 300 mg if there are no contraindications.[13,17]
- Administration of a nitroglycerin tablet or spray (maximum three doses every 5 minutes) should be considered. Do not administer nitroglycerin tablet or spray if there are contraindications, e.g. hypotension.[17]
- Ongoing chest discomfort requires administration of analgesia by titrating intravenous morphine or fentanyl.[17]

UNSTABLE ANGINA PECTORIS (UAP)

UAP is commonly associated with atherosclerotic lesion (plaque) instability and can signal an increased potential for plaque rupture and thrombus formation. UAP is considered a medical emergency as it may result in myocardial infarction.[15,32] UAP refers to a change in the pattern of the patient's usual or stable angina pectoris symptoms. Symptoms may become more intense, unpredictable, easily provoked by minimal exertion, develop at rest, last longer in duration and be more difficult to

TABLE 22.21 COMPARISON OF CHARACTERISTICS OF ANGINA[55,56]

CHARACTERISTIC	STABLE ANGINA	UNSTABLE ANGINA	PRINZMETAL ANGINA
Location of pain	Substernal; may radiate to the jaw, neck and down arms or back	Substernal; may radiate to the jaw, neck and down arms or back	Substernal; may radiate to the jaw, neck and down arms and back
Duration of pain	1–15 minutes	Occurs progressively more frequently with episodes lasting as long as 30 minutes	Occurs repeatedly at about the same time of day. Episodes tend to cluster between midnight and 8 am
Pain characteristics	Commonly referred to as an aching, squeezing, choking, heaving or burning discomfort	Same as stable angina, but more intense	Distinctly painful
Severity of pain	Generally severity is the same as previous episodes	The severity, duration or frequency of events increases over time	Extremely severe
Other symptoms	None for most patients	Diaphoresis, weakness, S3 or S4 heart sound, pulsus alternans, transient pulmonary crackles	Diaphoresis, weakness, S3 or S4 heart sound, pulsus alternans, transient pulmonary crackles
Pain worsened by	Exercise, activity, eating, cold weather, reclining	Exercise, activity, eating, cold weather, reclining	Occurs at rest
Pain relieved by	Rest, glyceryl trinitrate, isosorbide	Rest, glyceryl trinitrate and isosorbide may provide only partial relief	Glyceryl trinitrate may be helpful
Electrocardiogram findings	Transient ST segment depression that disappears with pain relief	Patients often have ST segment depression or T wave inversion but the electrocardiogram may be normal	Episodic ST-segment elevation with pain. ST segment returns to baseline when the pain subsides. Patients are prone to develop ventricular dysrhythmias
Additional characteristics	Most common in middle-aged and elderly males and postmenopausal females	Most common in middle-aged and elderly males and postmenopausal females; often referred to as preinfarction angina	Generally occurs in younger patients; thought to result from coronary artery spasm

relieve.[15,32] Another type of angina is a non-ACS disease process called stable angina (angina pectoris), which is intermittent in nature, provoked by exertion or stress and relieved by rest or sublingual nitrates. Prinzmetal angina (or variant angina) occurs as a result of transient coronary artery narrowing from arterial smooth muscle constriction. This occurs more often in young patients and women, and can be exacerbated by substance misuse; for example, cocaine or cigarette smoking.[15,32] Table 22.21 compares the characteristics of the three types of angina pectoris: stable angina, unstable angina and Prinzmetal angina.

With unstable angina, coronary blood flow and myocardial perfusion are usually restored quickly by the patient's endogenous thrombolytic processes, with minimal or no myocardial injury. Therefore, serum cardiac biomarkers are often negative and ECG changes may be non-diagnostic or show ST-segment depression.[28,34,65]

Assessment and management

UAP is diagnosed from the patient's history of cardiac disease and presenting signs and symptoms. In the pre-hospital setting, patients experiencing UAP should have an ECG performed, continuous cardiac monitoring and administration of appropriate analgesia, nitrates, aspirin and oxygen titrated to normoxia. Patients should be transported to the nearest, most appropriate hospital, recognising that NSTEACS have the potential to evolve into STEMI.[12,16,17] Patients may complain of pain to the upper part of the chest, neck, jaw, shoulder, sternum, epigastric and intrascapular. The pain may often radiate to neck, jaw and arms. Management for UAP aims to reduce oxygen demand and inhibit further thrombus formation. UAP priorities include rest, analgesia, anti-ischaemic therapies, such as nitrates, beta-blockers, calcium channel blockers, antiplatelet agents, such as aspirin or clopidogrel, and anticoagulants, such as heparin.[66]

MYOCARDIAL INFARCTION (MI)

Myocardial infarction is described as the presence or absence of significant ST elevation and commonly occurs as a result of a ruptured or occlusive atherosclerotic lesion, but may result from other causes, such as trauma.[12,13,34] MIs are subdivided into either ST-segment elevation (STEMI) or non-ST-segment elevation (NSTEMI), as defined by a 12-lead ECG. Myocardial cell necrosis starts approximately 20 minutes after coronary arterial occlusion and proceeds from the subendocardium to the epicardium.[2] The surrounding myocardium becomes hypoxic and zones of ischaemia and necrosis form in the heart muscle around the site of occlusion (Fig. 22.28).[16,17,19,32]

FIGURE 22.28 ZONE OF ISCHAEMIA, ZONE OF INJURY AND ZONE OF INFARCTION, SHOWN THROUGH ECG WAVEFORMS AND RECIPROCAL WAVEFORMS CORRESPONDING TO EACH ZONE

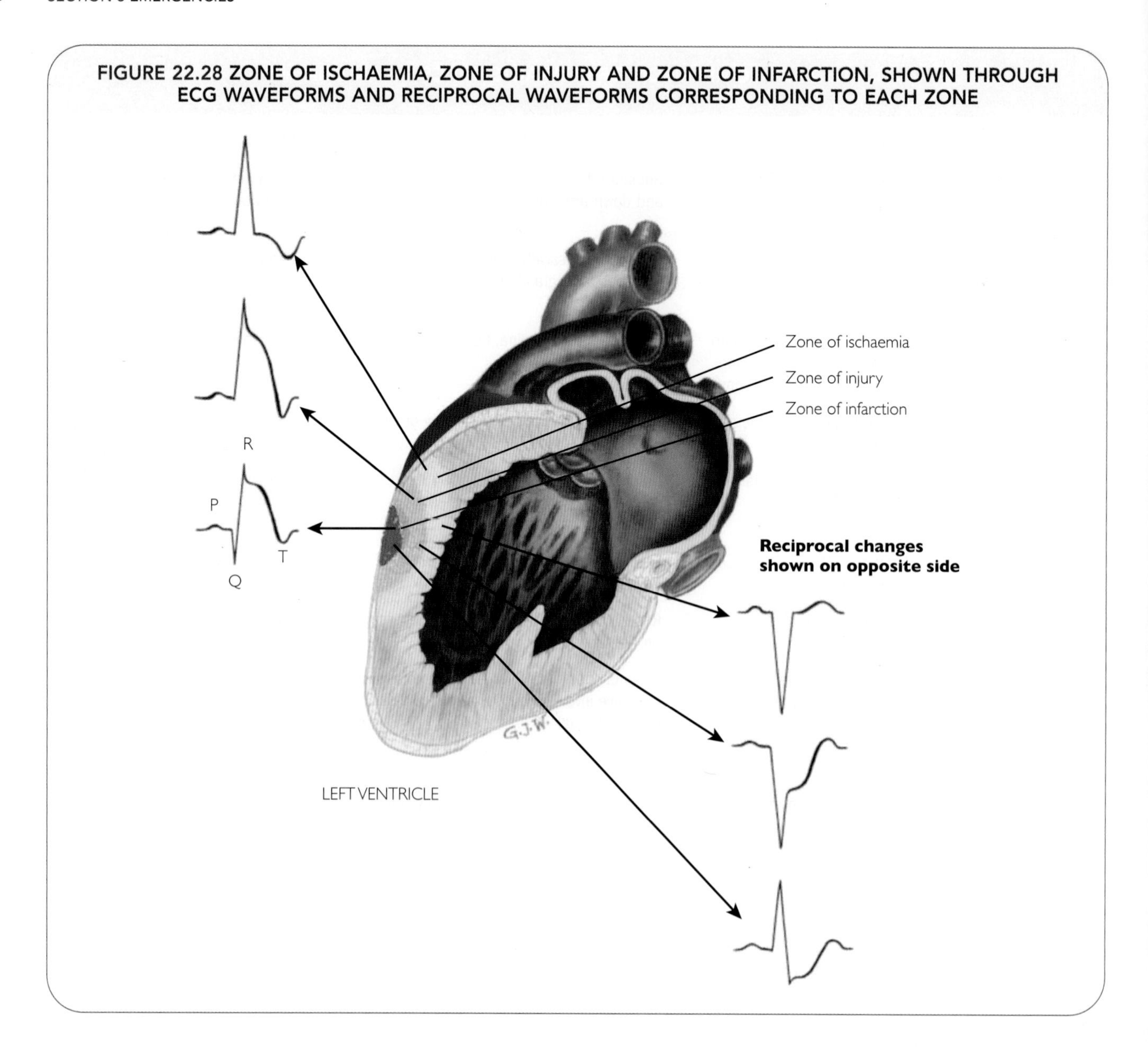

The areas of myocardial necrosis and cell death are called *zones of infarction*.

- The innermost zone, the zone of infarction, is comprised of necrotic or dead myocardium. ECG evidence of infarction is seen as new pathological Q waves. Q waves on the ECG are sometimes caused by lack of depolarisation in the area of infarction. When healed, the cells in the zone of infarction area are eventually replaced with scar tissue, which never fully function well. Q waves occur within 24 hours of irreversible myocardial necrosis.[15,27,32]
- The zone of injury surrounds the infarcted zone. This zone is still potentially viable if treated quickly. Repolarisation of cells in this area is affected as blood supply is decreased. This zone is characterised by ST-segment elevation on the ECG and is seen minutes after occlusion of the artery begins.[15,27,32]
- The outer region, known as the zone of ischaemia, is composed of viable cells. Repolarisation is temporarily impaired. This zone is evidenced on the ECG as T wave inversion and/or ST segment depression.[15,32]

Damage to the myocardium may lead to several complications related to contractility of the heart and electrical dysfunction. Haemodynamic changes occur as a result of an MI because myocardial contractility decreases and cardiac output is reduced with concomitant reductions in coronary artery perfusion. The reduced cardiac output leads to hypotension and activation of the sympathetic nervous system, resulting in widespread peripheral vasoconstriction. In addition, there is concomitant lung, kidney and gastrointestinal tract vasoconstriction.[16,19] Peripheral vasoconstriction redistributes blood flow to the heart and brain. In response to the reduced blood flow, hormonal compensation is activated within the renal system. Renin, angiotensin and aldosterone are released because of reduced renal blood flow. The increase in levels of aldosterone cause sodium and water retention, which increases circulating volume. If hypotension is not corrected, increased circulating volume may bring about an increase in cardiac workload for an already damaged and failing heart.[12,13,16,27]

NON-ST-ELEVATION MYOCARDIAL INFARCTION (NSTEMI)

NSTEMI occurs when an arteriosclerotic plaque ruptures, causing an intermittent or partial occlusive thrombus and resulting in distal myocyte necrosis of the region supplied by the affected coronary artery.[27,65] The occlusion causes minimal necrosis of myocardial tissue in the region supplied by the affected coronary artery.[27,32,65] An NSTEMI is associated with a rise in cardiac enzyme (troponin) levels without associated ST-segment elevation on the 12-lead ECG.[16,17] An NSTEMI may be defined on 12-lead ECG as ST-segment depression, T wave inversion or both, and represents up to 25% of acute MIs.[13,67] NSTEMI has a similar one-year mortality rate as STEMI.[13,67]

ST-SEGMENT ELEVATION MYOCARDIAL INFARCTION (STEMI)

STEMI occurs when an atherosclerotic plaque ruptures and causes a thrombus to fully occlude the coronary artery. Other causes of STEMI include coronary embolism, coronary dissection, and coronary artery spasm. A STEMI is defined as ST elevation on ECG or new LBBB with full-thickness myocardial wall damage.[34,56]

Emergency clinicians in the pre-hospital and in-hospital setting need to be familiar with ECG changes suggestive of ACS (Fig. 22.29). ECG changes (ST-segment elevation) can be noted within minutes of coronary artery occlusion and will often remain elevated for up to 24 hours. Within a few hours, T wave inversion occurs; the subsequent formation of Q waves develops at around 24 hours (Figs 22.30 and 22.31). Deep, wide Q waves may be representative of myocardial infarction if the Q wave amplitude is greater than or equal to 25% of the height of the succeeding R wave, or the duration of the Q wave is 0.04 seconds or more (Figs 22.31 and 22.32).[12,17,29] Myocardial necrosis is identified by the formation of a pathological Q wave.[12,15,16] When no electrical activity is recorded by any leads, the waveform tracing remains on the isoelectric line.[15,29] Twelve-lead ECG changes are not always evident during myocardial ischaemia or infarction (i.e. non-ST-segment elevation). The 12-lead ECG should be considered as one tool in the overall assessment of the patient and further diagnostic tests should be performed if there is suspicion of myocardial ischaemia, such as serum cardiac biomarkers and cardiac angiography.

FIGURE 22.29 ELECTROCARDIOGRAM CHANGES

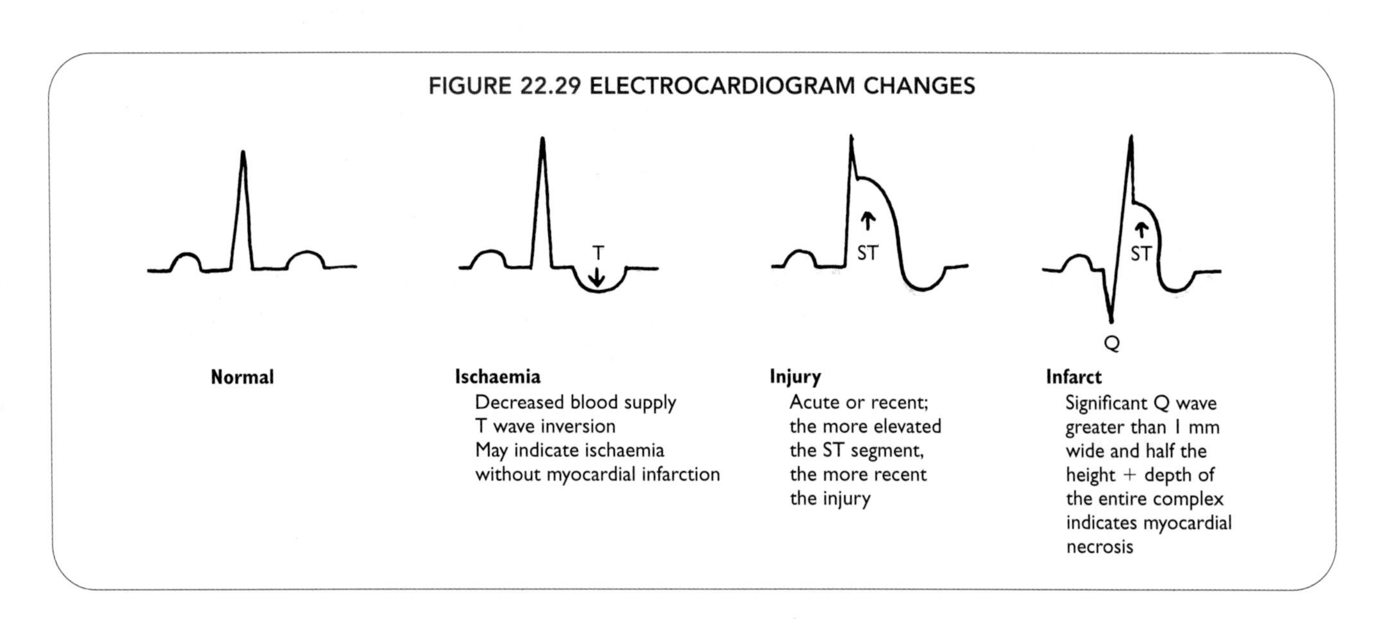

FIGURE 22.30 ANTERIOR MYOCARDIAL INFARCTION (V_2, V_3 AND V_4)

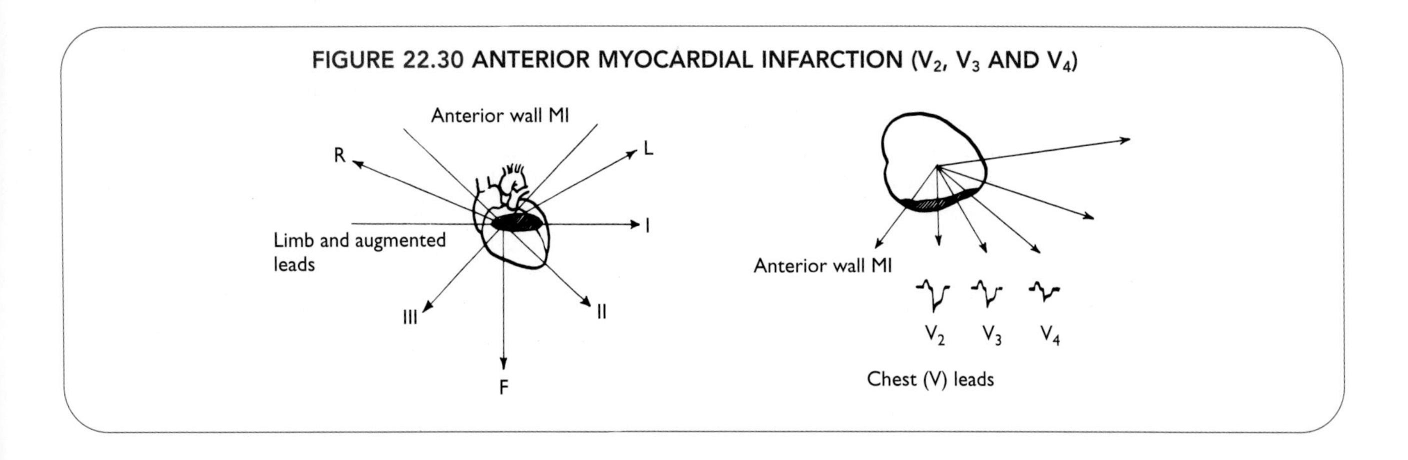

FIGURE 22.31 INFERIOR MYOCARDIAL INFARCTION (II, III AND aVF)

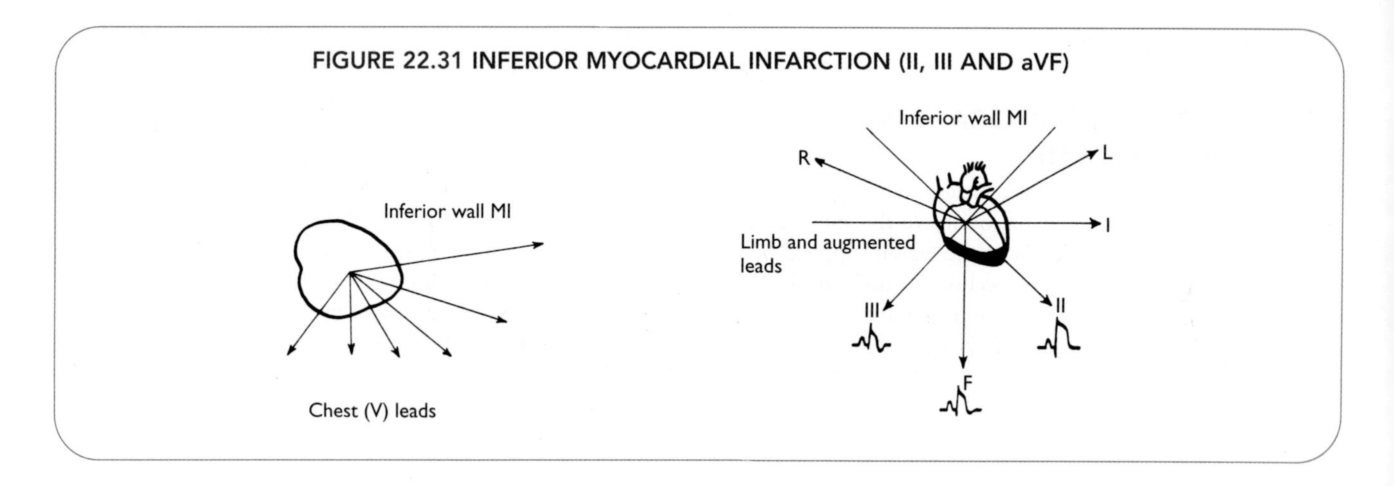

FIGURE 22.32 LATERAL MYOCARDIAL INFARCTION (I, aVL, V_5 AND V_6)

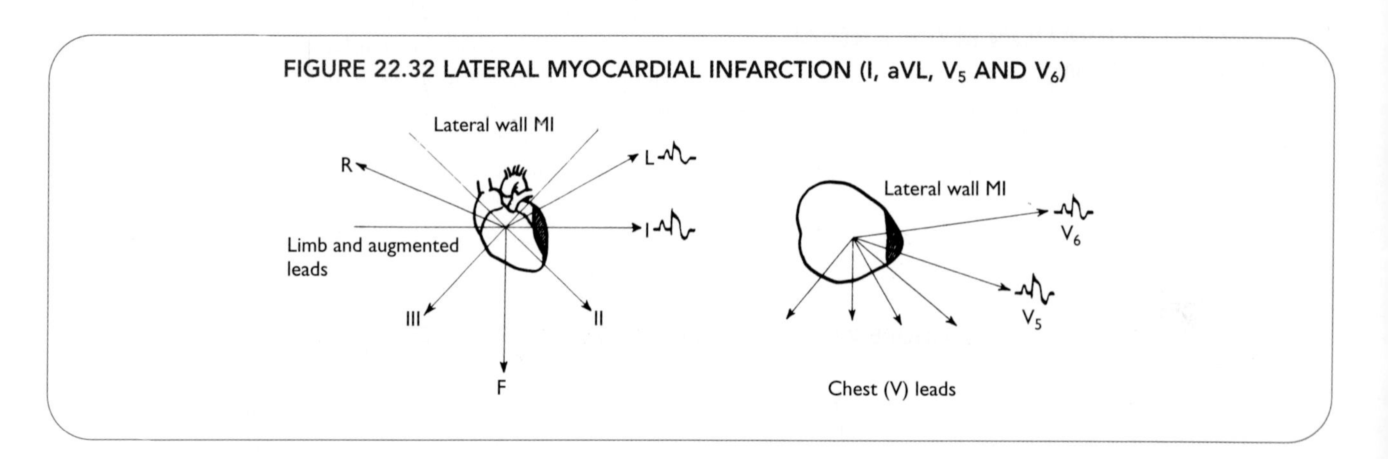

Diagnostic criteria for STEMI include:

- A clinical history of typical chest discomfort or pain ≥ 20 minutes duration and an ECG criterion with persistent ST-segment elevation (≥ 20 minutes) in ≥ 2 contiguous leads of:
  - Men under 40 years of age: 2.5 mm or more ST elevation in leads V_2–V_3 or
  - Men over 40 years of age: 2.0 mm or more ST elevation in leads V_2–V_3 or
  - In women: 1.5 mm or more ST elevation in V_2–V_3 or
    - 1.0 mm or more ST elevation in other leads or
    - development of new onset of LBBB.[13]

Assessment and management

Chest pain that is suggestive of an MI is usually central, crushing, retrosternal pain and described as more severe than angina pain. Associated symptoms may include shortness of breath, nausea, vomiting, diaphoresis, palpitations or a sense of impending doom. Atypical pain is more often reported by diabetic patients, elderly people, women and patients with renal disease.[12,15,27,46] The presentation is often different for women with an MI. Symptoms may be present from 2 weeks to 2 years prior to diagnosis of an MI. Women also more often present with bilateral basal lung crepitations because of existing heart failure, often the result of an unrecognised MI. Pain can occur at rest or exertion, lasts longer than 20 minutes and is unrelieved by nitrates. The pain can radiate to the neck, jaw or back, and can be associated with nausea, vomiting, diaphoresis, light-headedness and dyspnoea.[15,16,19,32]

The sympathetic nervous system response can cause tachycardia, hypertension, increased respiratory rate and elevated blood glucose. Infrequently, parasympathetic nervous response can cause bradycardia and hypotension to occur (inferior and posterior infarcts).[68] The priority management for STEMI is to restore myocardial perfusion and reduce the size of the infarct.

Prompt treatment to restore and maintain blood flow to the myocardium will reduce mortality and morbidity risk associated with an MI. Time to reperfusion is critical, as the longer the myocardium is without blood flow, the greater the chance of permanent damage.[54,69–71]

The evidence supporting improved patient outcomes associated with early reperfusion has meant that many Australian and international pre-hospital providers routinely perform 12-lead ECGs and are often capable of transmitting the results to the receiving hospital if there is a concern for a STEMI.[13,32,34,69,72] The transmission of the ECG to the receiving hospital enables confirmation of a STEMI pattern, allowing for prompt triage at an appropriate percutaneous coronary intervention (PCI) facility, with concurrent early activation of the catheterisation laboratory. In some situations the nearest hospital may be notified of the need for thrombolysis, or the paramedics may be advised to administer thrombolysis at the scene, in accordance with local clinical practice guidelines.[13,66,71] National guidelines recommend that patients should be advised to take aspirin while still at home or that paramedics should administer an initial dose of 150–300 mg aspirin while in transit to the receiving hospital.[15,73,74]

Management of NSTEMI is guided by a risk assessment that will guide pharmacological treatments and interventional procedures. Australian guidelines[13] recommend the following timing for invasive management of NSTEMI patients:

- Very high risk: patients with ongoing ischaemia, haemodynamic compromise, dysrhythmias, mechanical compromise, acute heart failure, recurrent dynamic or widespread ST-segment and/or T wave changes on ECG. Immediate angiogram or within 2 hours of admission.
- High risk: patients who experience within 24 hours of admission dynamic ST-segment and/or T wave changes on ECG or rise and/or fall in troponin, suggestive of an acute MI.
- Intermediate risk: recurrent symptoms or substantial inducible ischaemia on provocative testing, e.g. exercise stress test; perform an angiogram within 72 hours of admission.

Interventional procedures for NSTEMI include early coronary angiography and revascularisation.

Pharmacological management

Fibrinolytic therapy

Fibrinolytic agents are administered to dissolve coronary artery thrombus and restore vital blood flow to the myocardium. Fibrinolytic agents cause lysis by targeting elements of the clotting process to degrade the fibrin.[75] Fibrinolytic agents differ in action; Table 22.22 compares agents currently used in Australian hospitals. Indications for fibrinolytic therapy include acute chest pain less than 12 hours in duration with accompanying ST-segment elevation evident on the 12-lead ECG or a new left bundle branch block (STEMI). Fibrinolytic agents may be used cautiously in hypertension, trauma and recent surgery.[13,15–17,70] The major complications of fibrinolytic therapy are bleeding and haemorrhage. Clinical management should focus on hypotension, tachycardia, monitoring for reperfusion dysrhythmias and allergic reactions.[15,26,71,74] The administration of pre-hospital fibrinolysis minimises delays in patients receiving reperfusion therapy, and evidence to date has shown it to be safe and effective.[13]

There is an increasing role for paramedics to administer pre-hospital fibrinolysis specifically if primary PCI is unavailable at receiving hospitals. For paramedics, fibrinolysis should be considered as an appropriate treatment if there are transport delays due to geographical distance. A number of Australian emergency medical services provide pre-hospital thrombolysis models of care. These models of care have established protocols,

TABLE 22.22 COMPARISON OF FIBRINOLYTIC AGENTS[22]

AGENT	ACTION	DOSE	COMMENTS
Fibrin specific			
Tenecteplase	Activates clot-bound plasminogen to plasmin	IV: 30–50 mg bolus over 5 seconds Dosing based on patient weight*: < 60 kg $= 30$ mg 60 to < 70 kg $= 35$ mg 70 to < 80 kg $= 40$ mg 80 to < 90 kg $= 45$ mg 90 mg $= 50$ mg	More fibrin specificity and less incidence of bleeding than alteplase * In patients $\geq$75 years: administration of half the standard dose should be considered in reducing the risk of intercranial bleeding[3]
Alteplase	Proteolytic enzyme; direct activator of plasminogen; high degree of clot specificity	IV: Doses as per ECS[71] 15 mg bolus then 0.75 mg/kg (up to 50 mg) over 30 minutes then 0.5 mg/kg (up to 35 mg) over 60 minutes	Half-life in plasma is 5–7 minutes; may cause sudden hypotension; inline IV filters can remove as much as 47% of the drug
Reteplase	Activates the conversion of plasminogen to plasmin; high degree of clot specificity	IV: 10 units over 2 minutes; then repeat 10 units in 30 minutes after initiation of first bolus	Give normal saline fluid before and after administration of reteplase Reconstitute just before administration and use within 4 hours after reconstituting
NON			
Streptokinase	Exogenous plasminogen activator; not clot-specific	IV: 1.5 million units IV over 1 hr Intracoronary: 10,000 to 30,000 units; followed by maintenance infusion of 2000 to 4000 units/min until thrombolysis occurs (e.g. 150,000 to 500,000 units total)	Half-life in plasma is 18 minutes; has a prolonged effect on coagulation because of depletion of fibrinogen, which persists for 18–24 hours; antibodies to the drug may be present in persons who have been exposed to Streptococcus infection resulting in allergic reactions, e.g. rash, fever or chills; patients should not be re-treated with streptokinase for a period of 2 weeks to 1 year after initial administration because of secondary resistance to development of antibodies

IV: intravenous; TNKase: Tenecteplase.

comprehensive education and training and evaluation processes with medical oversight.[76,77]

Anticoagulation

Anticoagulants do not dissolve thrombi as do fibrinolytic agents, but they do inhibit any further formation of thrombin.[22,27] Anticoagulants are indicated for patients where ACS is suspected. Anticoagulants are used with fibrinolytic agents to prevent clot formation and subsequent re-occlusion of the affected vessel. The anticoagulant chosen is dependent on the type of ACS. Anticoagulants include subcutaneous injections of low-molecular-weight heparins, for example enoxaparin and unfractionated heparin. For patients with renal compromise, bivalirudin (direct thrombin inhibitor) should be considered for NSTEACS.

Advantages include simplified dosing, administration via subcutaneous injection and a reduction in the need to monitor the activated partial thromboplastin time (APTT); however, a disadvantage of low-molecular-weight heparin is its longer half-life, which may delay cardiac angiography.[13,15,17] Enoxaparin may be considered a safe and effective alternative to unfractionated heparin in the patient with STEMI. There have been recent studies challenging the routine use of glycoprotein IIb/IIIa inhibitor in patients with suspected STEMI or non-STEMI in the pre-hospital and ED setting, due to increased bleeding risks.[78] There may be a role for glycoprotein IIb/IIIa inhibitors in selected high-risk patients with NSTEACS, in whom a PCI is planned.[79]

Antiplatelet agents

Antiplatelet agents prevent platelet aggregation, which is essential in the early stages of thrombus formation. Antiplatelet aggregating agents have a primary role in the prevention of MI and ischaemic cerebrovascular accident. They are also effective in reducing the re-occlusion of arteries following stent insertion.[17,58] Early treatment should be initiated in patients, unless contraindicated for low- to high-risk NSTEACS. Aspirin is recommended in all ACS patients.

- *Aspirin* is the cornerstone of antiplatelet therapy. Activated platelets synthesise and release a powerful and potent vasoconstrictor thromboxane A2. Aspirin inhibits and thereby blocks thromboxane A2 synthesis in platelets. This reduces the aggregating properties of the platelet and, because the inhibition is irreversible, the effect lasts for the 7- to 10-day life span of the platelet. The initial dose of aspirin is 300 mg orally, followed by 100–150 mg daily.[13,27,80]
- *Clopidogrel* inhibits platelet aggregation by irreversibly binding to ADP platelet receptors ($P2Y_{12}$) and is the only antiplatelet agent recommended as post-fibrinolytic therapy.[24] The loading dose after fibrinolytic administration is 75 mg or 300 mg, depending on age and hospital/reperfusion protocol, followed by 75 mg daily. Dosage for pre-primary PCI or NSTEMI or unstable angina is 300–600 mg with a daily dose of 75 mg, dependent on age. Prasugrel and ticagrelor are both considered more effective in the setting of primary PCI.[13,71,81]
- *Prasugrel* has a more rapid onset of action and stronger inhibitory effect than clopidogrel and studies suggest that STEMI and diabetic patients may derive a greater benefit from more platelet inhibition with prasugrel, but older (age > 75 years) patients weighing < 60 kg and those with a history of stroke have a potential unfavourable bleeding risk.[16] The initial loading dose is 60 mg, then a 10 mg daily dose.[13]
- *Ticagrelor* is reversible, has a shorter half-life and requires twice-daily dosing. It acts in a dose-dependent manner with its antiplatelet effect having a rapid onset and offset. In the acute ACS setting, where surgery may be required and antiplatelet therapy ceased, ticagrelor is favoured.[15,16] For high-risk patients undergoing PCI, such as diabetics and stent thrombosis, prasugrel and ticagrelor should be considered as an alternative to clopidogrel. However, careful assessment of the bleeding risks should be undertaken prior to using these agents. Initial loading dose is 180 mg, then a 90 mg twice-daily dose.[13,82,83]
- *Glycoprotein inhibitors (GP IIb/IIIa)*—the GP IIb/IIIa complex is the most abundant receptor on the platelet surface. They block the final common pathway of platelet aggregation; however, GP IIb/IIIa antagonists do not prevent platelet adhesion, secretion of platelet products or thrombin activation.[13] GP IIb/IIIa inhibitors in combination with IV heparin are recommended at the time of PCI or for treating thrombotic complications among patients with ACS.[13]

Currently, there is no evidence of mortality benefit or harm with pre-hospital administration of ticagrelor or clopidogrel by paramedics. Further research is needed to explore pre-hospital administration of ADP receptor agonists if delays to PPCI are extensive.[67] It is important that in the pre-hospital setting antiplatelet agents should be undertaken within an appropriate model of care with close communication between paramedics, PCI facility cardiologists and emergency doctors. In addition, geographic, population, hospital resource factors and local systems of care should be accommodated within any new models of care.[45]

Beta-blocker therapy

Beta-blockers are effective in controlling hypertension and angina pain, and are considered essential treatment after AMI as secondary prophylaxis (Table 22.23). Beta-blockers block the beta-adrenoreceptors in the heart, bronchi and vascular smooth muscle. For haemodynamically stable patients, research evidence suggests that long-term oral beta-blockers should be administered within 24 hours post-STEMI, as a reduction in mortality rate has been noted.[70]

Beta-blockers are divided into two subtypes:

- beta-1 receptors: found in heart muscle (cardioselective)
- beta-2 receptors: found in bronchial and vascular smooth muscle (non-cardioselective).

Beta-blockers counteract the cardiac effects of adrenergic stimulation (fight or flight response). This stimulation increases myocardial oxygen demand by increasing heart rate, blood pressure and force of contraction. Bradycardic and negative inotropic effects of beta-blockers are relevant to the therapeutic effect in angina, as these changes reduce myocardial oxygen demand.[70,73,82,83]

Angiotensin-converting enzyme inhibitors

Angiotensin-converting enzyme (ACE) inhibitors are well supported by evidence for use in patients post-STEMI or with heart failure. ACE inhibitors act on the renin–angiotensin–aldosterone system by inhibiting the conversion of angiotensin

TABLE 22.23 BETA-BLOCKER THERAPY FOR THE PATIENT WITH MYOCARDIAL INFARCTION[84]

MEDICATION	DOSE
Esmolol	0.5 mg/kg bolus over 1 minute followed by a continuous infusion at 0.5 mg/kg/min. Maximum dose is 0.3 mg/kg/min. Titrate to effect. The half-life is short (2–9 minutes)
Metoprolol	5 mg slow intravenous (IV) push. Repeat as needed at 5-minute intervals to a total of 15 mg. Give 25–50 mg orally within 15 minutes of the last IV dose (unless contraindicated). Oral dose is 50 mg bid for 24 hours; then increase to 100 mg bid
Propranolol	0.1 mg/kg slow IV push, divided into three equal doses, at 2- to 3-minute intervals. Do not infuse faster than 1 mg/min. Repeat after 2 minutes if necessary
Atenolol	5 mg IV over 5 minutes, wait 10 minutes, and then give second 5 mg dose over 5 minutes. In 10 minutes (if tolerated well) start 50 mg orally and then 50 mg orally bid. Oral dose is 100 mg daily
Labetalol	10 mg IV push over 1–2 minutes. May repeat or double labetalol dose every 10 minutes to a maximum of 150 mg. Another option is to give the initial dose as a bolus and then start a labetalol infusion at 2–8 mg/min

I to angiotensin II, a powerful vasoconstrictor.[16,27,70,83] In patients post-MI, ACE inhibitors reduce mortality, improve left ventricular (LV) function, have a beneficial effect on the LV remodelling and delay the progression of heart failure. They are used in patients with signs and symptoms of heart failure or in patients with significant LV dysfunction, anterior wall infarctions and patients with LV ejection fraction less than 40%.[16]

Percutaneous coronary intervention (PCI)

Percutaneous coronary intervention (PCI) is a non-surgical coronary catheterisation procedure used to treat ACS such as UAP and STEMI. A patient's access to primary PCI is dependent on the availability of cardiac interventional services at the local or nearby hospitals. Primary PCI should be performed within 90 minutes of first medical contact.[85] First medical contact is defined as the time point when the patient is either initially assessed by a doctor, paramedic or nurse or other trained emergency service personnel who can obtain and interpret the ECG, and deliver initial interventions.[86,87] Timely PCI has benefits over fibrinolytic therapy, as thrombolysis does not have any effect on coronary artery stenosis; however, both will reperfuse the hypoxic myocardium.[70]

The choice of reperfusion therapy is usually between PCI or intravenous fibrinolysis. PCI is the most effective and definitive treatment when provided promptly by an appropriately qualified cardiologist at an appropriate facility. Cardiologists performing PCI should have expertise in both management of an AMI and coronary angioplasty. On-site surgical backup is not a requirement for primary PCI, and therefore the establishment of more centres providing these facilities is possible throughout rural Australia.[13,17,88]

A PCI procedure is performed in an acute hospital cardiac catheterisation laboratory. A catheter 'sheath' is inserted into the femoral artery or radial artery and a balloon-tipped catheter is inserted through the sheath and is guided through the arterial circulation, down the aorta and into the relevant coronary artery. The balloon is then positioned within the atherosclerotic lesion of the coronary artery and is intermittently inflated to expand the diameter of the vessel and push the atherosclerotic lesion back into the wall of the vessel.[16,17] A stent is a tubular metal scaffold which is then expanded into the atherosclerotic lesion of the vessel by the angioplasty balloon. Stents may comprise either bare metal or drug eluting compounds and are inserted to maintain the patency of the occluded vessel after balloon angioplasty, preventing coronary artery occlusion and promoting adequate blood flow (Fig. 22.33).

FIGURE 22.33 BALLOON COMPRESSION OF AN ATHEROSCLEROTIC LESION

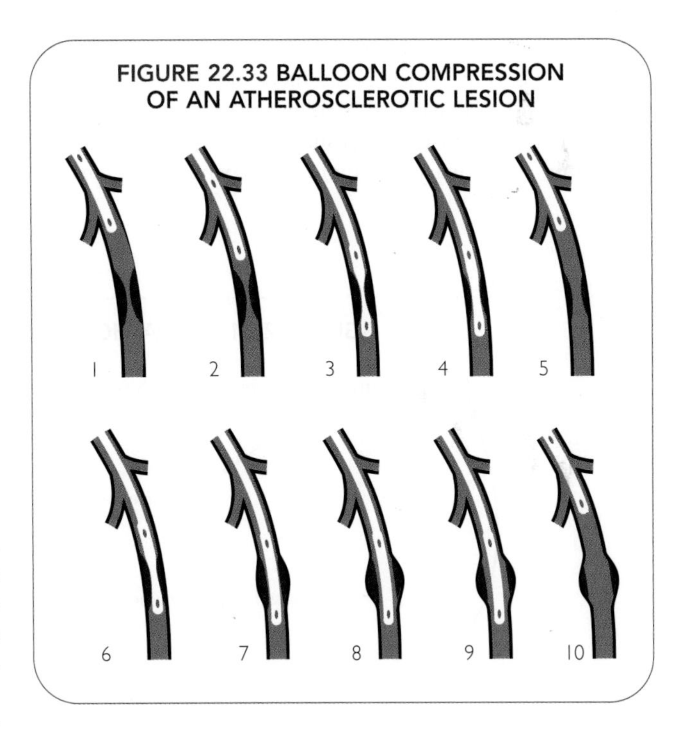

It is essential that pre-hospital clinicians are aware of the location of PCI cardiac catheterisation laboratory facilities, and the 24-hour availability of these services.[76,77] Maintaining a seamless patient-care continuum from pre-hospital to cardiac catheterisation laboratory is critical in order to minimise delays in patients receiving PCI. Reduction in door-to-balloon times for STEMI patients has been reported with the implementation of pre-hospital 12-lead ECG acquisition and transmission to cardiac interventional capable hospitals, including bypassing closer EDs.[63,88] Absolute contraindications to PCI include haemorrhagic stroke, internal bleeding or suspected aortic dissection.[89]

CARDIOGENIC SHOCK

Cardiogenic shock results from problems affecting the mechanical function of the heart, leading to diminished cardiac output, end-organ hypoperfusion, and tissue hypoxia (Box 22.3).[15,17,32,34,90] Development of cardiogenic shock due to MI is directly related to the extent of myocardial cell necrosis resulting in inadequate contractility of the heart muscle (pump failure). Cardiogenic shock is generally associated with extensive loss of myocardium (necrosis) and a loss of up to 40% of the left ventricle (Fig. 22.34).[15,16,19] Cardiogenic shock progresses in four stages: initial, compensatory, progressive and refractory.[15,19,91]

The *initial stage* of cardiogenic shock is associated with a reduction in blood flow leading to inadequate tissue perfusion.[17,19] Cardiac muscle fibres are not functioning and others are too weak to contract; consequently, the overall pumping ability of the affected ventricle is depressed and cardiac output is reduced.[17,19] The loss of contractility reduces stroke volume and cardiac output, which causes blood flow within the heart chambers to slow down. This results in a backflow of blood to the lungs, leading to increased lung tissue fluid or interstitial space fluid (pulmonary oedema) and impaired gas exchange. Hypoxaemia and the associated complications of hypoxia and acidosis complicate treatment efforts. Box 22.4 examines the clinical manifestations of cardiogenic shock.

Activation of the compensatory homeostatic mechanisms is known as the *compensatory stage* of shock.[16,17,19] As cardiac output falls, baroreceptors in the aorta and carotid artery junctions are activated to increase arterial blood pressure (neural compensation). Baroreceptors detect the decrease in blood pressure and inform the vasomotor centre in the medulla oblongata of the brainstem, resulting in peripheral arterial vasoconstriction. This sympathetic response redistributes blood flow to the heart and brain. Blood vessels in the skin, lungs, kidneys and gastrointestinal tract constrict in response to sympathetic activation. Vasoconstriction may achieve normotension, but this may be at the expense of peripheral tissue hypoperfusion and localised tissue hypoxia. Strong sympathetic stimulation also affects the heart by temporarily strengthening the functional muscle, increasing contractility and heart rate.[16,17,19] A reduction in blood flow to the peripheries and tissue perfusion often results in pallor and cold and clammy skin. Adrenaline, produced by a sympathetic response, stimulates diaphoresis, causing clamminess. Lactic acid is produced by anaerobic metabolism in poorly perfused tissue.[16,17,19]

In the renal circulation, hormonal compensation takes place when blood flow to the kidneys is reduced. The juxtaglomerular

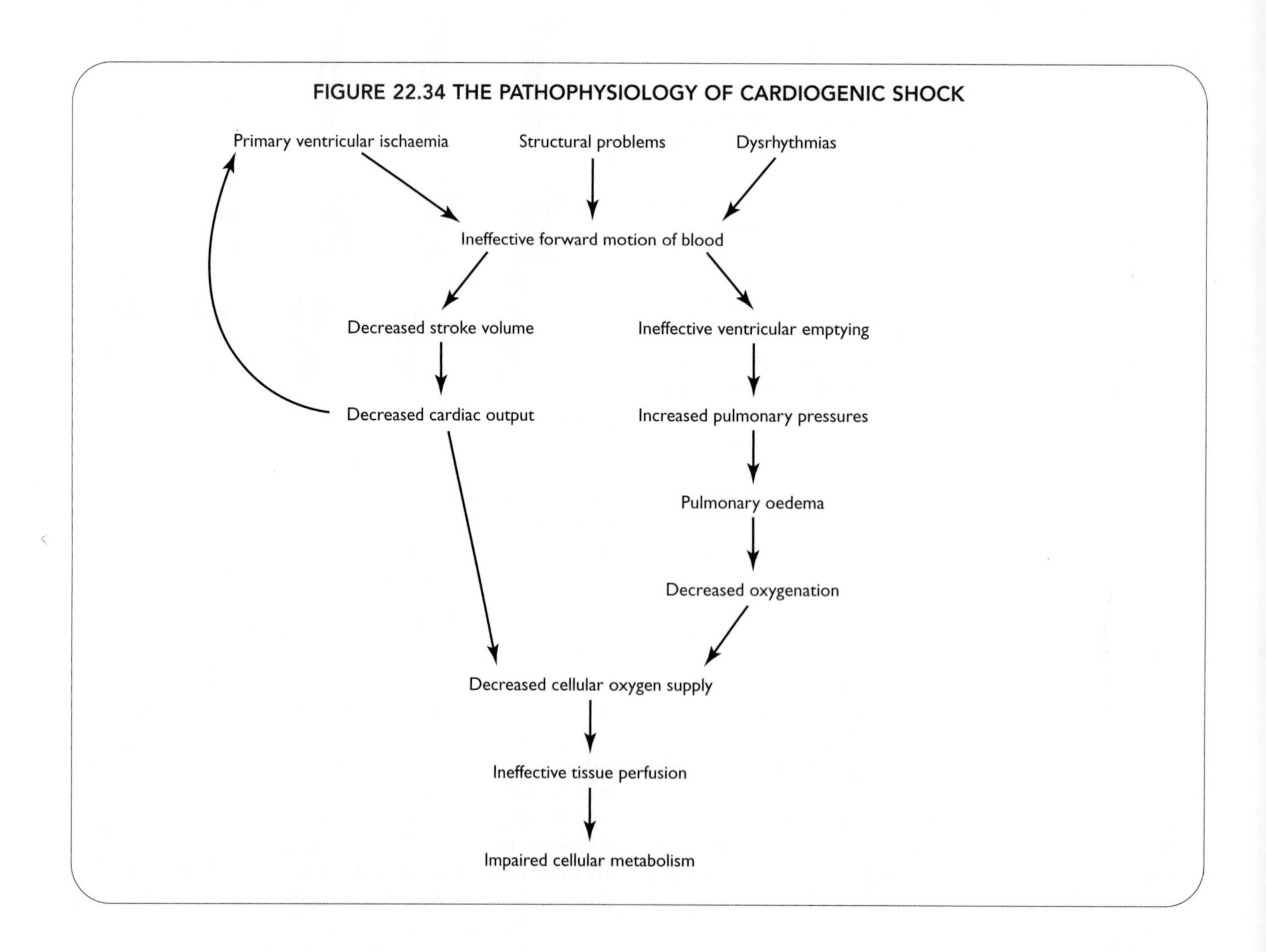

FIGURE 22.34 THE PATHOPHYSIOLOGY OF CARDIOGENIC SHOCK

BOX 22.4 CLINICAL MANIFESTATIONS OF CARDIOGENIC SHOCK[15]

Systolic blood pressure < 90 mmHg
Heart rate >100 beats/minute
Weak, thready pulse
Diminished heart sounds
Change in sensorium
Cool, pale, moist skin
Urine output < 30 mL/h
Chest pain
Dysrhythmias
Tachypnoea
Crackles
Decreased cardiac output
Cardiac index < 2.2 L/min/m^2
Increased pulmonary artery occlusion pressure
Increased right atrial pressure
Increased systemic vascular resistance

apparatus in the renal nephron produces renin. Renin released into the bloodstream activates the chemical angiotensinogen to produce angiotensin I. This circulates in the blood to the lungs, where it is converted to angiotensin II. This powerful vasoconstrictor aids in the maintenance of blood pressure. Angiotensin II also stimulates the adrenal gland to produce the hormone aldosterone. This stimulates the re-absorption of sodium ions. As blood levels of sodium increase, the pituitary gland in the brain releases antidiuretic hormone (ADH), which further reduces urine production (reabsorption of water) to increase circulatory volume.[16,17,19] The oedema leads to a ventilation/perfusion mismatch, resulting in impaired gas exchange and results in hypoxaemia.

The third, *progressive stage* of shock leads to multi-organ failure. Compensatory mechanisms eventually fail to maintain perfusion of the vital organs, which further reduces arterial blood pressure, which in turn reduces coronary artery and myocardial perfusion. An imbalance between myocardial oxygen supply and demand further decreases cardiac output and cardiac function. When renal blood flow or pressure is reduced to a critical point, arteriolar blood bypasses the nephron and flows back into the venule. Nephron necrosis as a result of hypoxia and acute tubular necrosis (ATN) develops.[16,17,19]

The fourth, *refractory stage* of shock leads to circulatory collapse, end-organ failure and death. Neurological insults diminish any capacity for a sympathetic response. Prolonged splanchnic vasoconstriction leads to gastrointestinal hypoxia and dysfunction. As a result of gastrointestinal hypoxia, endotoxin is released from dead intestinal bacteria. Endotoxin causes widespread vascular dilation and increases cellular metabolism. Further, cell deterioration occurs, and myocardial depressant factor is released as the pancreas becomes ischaemic. Myocardial depressant factor circulates in the blood and further depresses myocardial contractility. As a result, there is a decrease in heart rate and blood pressure resulting in circulatory collapse. This refractory stage of shock ultimately leads to end-organ failure and death.

Assessment and management

Not all patients who experience an ACS and hypotension will go on to develop cardiogenic shock. Other causes of hypotension should be considered, including narcotic or diuretic over-administration, or the effect of beta-blockers, calcium channel blockers or ACE inhibitors, or other causes for ischemia. Primary cardiac assessment will reveal dyspnoea, hypoxia, reduced cardiac output (pulse weak and rapid or severe bradycardia and hypotension) and tissue hypoperfusion (altered mental status, cool extremities). Other clinical signs include raised jugular venous pressure, peripheral oedema, and Cheyne-Stokes respiration. Laboratory tests include arterial blood gas, cardiac biomarkers, full blood count, electrolytes, renal function and coagulation profile. Diagnostic studies include ECG, chest x-ray, bedside ECG and possibly pulmonary artery catheterisation.[49] Cardiogenic therapy and management should focus on establishing immediate reperfusion using either thrombolysis or emergency angioplasty. Early treatment of cardiogenic shock should be aggressive to maximise patient outcomes. Early initiation of non-invasive ventilation and pharmacological therapy will often be the foundation of pre-hospital and ED treatment.

Non-invasive positive pressure ventilation (NIV)

There are two modes of NIV: continuous positive airway pressure (CPAP) and bi-level positive airway pressure (BiPAP). CPAP uses a single pressure that is applied during all phases of the respiratory cycle, whereas BPAP delivers two levels of pressure: inspiratory positive airway pressure and expiratory airway pressure.[90] CPAP is more useful to patients with hypoxic respiratory failure, while BiPAP is useful to patients with both hypercapnic and hypoxic respiratory failure. NIV has been shown to reduce in-hospital mortality and intubation rates as a result of improved oxygenation, improved pulmonary gas exchange and decreased work of breathing.[92] Patients in cardiogenic shock with acute respiratory failure are at risk of deterioration during pre-hospital transport. NIV can be initiated in the pre-hospital setting to provide ventilatory support as a bridge to hospital care.

Humidified high-flow nasal oxygen can be used as a bridge or prevent the need for NIV by using a humidified nasal cannula to deliver a predictable amount of fractured inspired oxygen (maximum FiO_2 1.0), with higher rates of gas flow (maximum 60 L/min). Humidified high-flow nasal oxygen has been increasingly employed for patients with hypoxic respiratory failure; for example, cardiogenic pulmonary oedema.[90,93] Refer to Chapter 21 for further discussion.

Intra-aortic balloon pump

Intra-aortic balloon pump (IABP) counterpulsation is commonly used in Australia in the setting of cardiogenic shock to improve cardiac output and subsequent tissue perfusion.[16,17,19] In a theatre or catheter laboratory, a helium-filled balloon approximately 10 cm long is inserted into the aorta via the femoral artery, just below the aortic arch. The purpose of IABP therapy is to reduce the workload of the heart; at the same time improving myocardial oxygen supply.[15–17,19]

Pharmacological therapy

The main aim of pharmacological therapy in cardiogenic shock is to decrease preload and afterload. Decreases in preload decreases myocardial wall tension with the end result being a decrease in myocardial oxygen demand. Decreasing afterload results in increased cardiac output and tissue perfusion by way of decreasing the left ventricle workload. In the ED the most common class of medications used to treat cardiogenic shock include:

- nitrates, namely nitroglycerin, which cause vasodilation at low doses and thereby reduce preload. At higher doses arterial dilation occurs, resulting in a reduction of afterload. In patients with persistent hypertension despite incremental increases in nitroglycerin dose, sodium nitroprusside may be considered.[90]
- diuretics, which should be administered in patients with significant signs of fluid overload.[90,95] Loop diuretics, such as furosemide, cause venous vasodilation and in turn decreases preload.[27]
- inotropic and vasopressor agents such as dobutamine, milrinone, epinephrine and norepinephrine, which can be used in the treatment of cardiogenic shock. Administration of these agents will increase myocardial contractility, heart rate and peripheral vascular tone, resulting in improved arterial pressure and cardiac output. However, inotropic and vasopressor agents have notable disadvantages, which can be deleterious for patients with myocardial ischaemia. Initial vasopressor therapy includes noradrenaline, a potent vasoconstrictor and inotropic stimulant that will increase contractility and heart rate.[16,17,19] Dobutamine increases cardiac contractility and is chronotropic and to a lesser degree causes peripheral vasodilation. Milrinone is a phosphodiesterase inhibitor which is considered to increase myocardial oxygen demand less than dobutamine. Evidence for its efficacy is equivocal; however, it is recommended in American Heart Association guidelines for the management of cardiac failure,[94,95] and is favoured by cardiologists. Current guidelines also recommend that inotropic medications are initiated only after optimising administration of nitrates and diuretics.[90]

CHRONIC HEART FAILURE

In Australia, the prevalence of chronic heart failure (CHF) is between 1% and 2% of the population with higher rates among elderly adults.[11,14,96] CHF is the most common reason for hospital admission and GP consultation in people aged 70 years and older, with 50–75% of patients dying within 5 years of CHF diagnosis.[90,94] Heart failure has several definitions and can be described as a systolic or diastolic dysfunction of the ventricles or both. There is an underlying structural abnormality or dysfunction impairing the filling or emptying ability of the ventricles. The poor contraction or relaxation of the heart muscle is characterised by haemodynamic, renal, neural and hormonal responses. CHF can be classified into four stages: Stage A occurs when the patient is at high risk due to a pre-existing condition; i.e. cardiomyopathy, hypertension, diabetes; Stage B occurs when the patient has developed left ventricular dysfunction; Stage C occurs when the patient has structural heart disease with ongoing symptoms; and Stage D occurs when the patient has advanced heart failure that is challenging to manage with standard treatment.[97] The common symptoms of CHF include shortness of breath, lethargy, bilateral pitting oedema, persistent coughing, exercise intolerance, or sudden weight gain.[27]

Assessment and management

Common causes of CHF are ischaemic heart disease, hypertension, dilated cardiomyopathy and diabetes (Table 22.24).[16,82,98,99] Systolic dysfunction of the left ventricle is the most common cause of heart disease in Western societies and although both systolic and diastolic CHF co-exist, distinguishing between the two is relevant to therapeutic management. Therefore, most CHF patients will have a diagnosis of left heart failure and some degree of right heart failure. Isolated right ventricular failure is rare. The term cor pulmonale is used to refer to right ventricular failure due to chronic pulmonary disease.[16,27,45] Some CHF patients may have asynchronous contraction of the left ventricle, especially if the duration of the QRS (0.12 sec) on the 12-lead ECG is prolonged. Evidence suggests clinical benefit from the use of biventricular pacing in heart failure, as this resynchronises cardiac contraction, improves ventricular performance and reduces frequency of hospitalisation.[90,92]

Signs and symptoms include: exertional dyspnoea, orthopnoea, dry and irritating cough, fatigue, dizziness, palpitations, which may indicate a dysrhythmia. Symptoms related to fluid retention such a pitting oedema may indicate a more advanced CHF.[16,27]

Patients with CHF experience symptoms that severely affect their quality of life, including shortness of breath, reduced exercise tolerance and lethargy. The Heart Foundation consumer resource focuses on patients learning how to manage their CHF to reduce symptoms and hospitalisation using self-management strategies, such as restricting fluid intake, adhering to a complex medication regimen and maintaining a low-sodium diet.

Implantable cardioverter defibrillators (ICDs) have a role in the prophylaxis of dysrhythmia management in patients with significant LV dysfunction from ischaemic heart disease and therefore CHF.[44] Prophylactic implantation of ICDs may be considered in patients with a low ejection fraction (< 35%); however, funding is a significant constraint to patients receiving therapy.[16,27,98]

Therapeutic interventions

- A structed primary survey and comprehensive history to assist in identification of the underlying condition.
- Vital signs need to be monitored regularly to assess cardiac and urine output, blood pressure, mentation and pallor.

TABLE 22.24 CAUSES OF HEART FAILURE[22]

TYPE	CAUSE
Left ventricular failure	Systemic hypertension, aortic stenosis, aortic regurgitation, mitral regurgitation, cardiomyopathy, bacterial endocarditis, myocardial infarction
Right ventricular failure	Mitral stenosis, pulmonary hypertension, bacterial endocarditis on the right side of the heart, right ventricular infarction
Biventricular failure	Left ventricular failure, cardiomyopathy, myocarditis, dysrhythmias, anaemia, thyrotoxicosis

- Titrated oxygen may be required, including the use of an NIV.
- Long term: lifestyle modifications may be required to improve diet and exercise.

Pharmacological therapy

- Diuretics can be used to maintain volume in patients with fluid overload.
- Beta-blockers are recommended, unless contraindicated.
- Angiotensin II receptor antagonists: used when patients are unable to tolerate ACE inhibitors.[81,84,100]

ACUTE PERICARDITIS

Acute pericarditis is inflammation of the pericardium, a sac containing serous fluid that surrounds the myocardium and maintains lubrication. Pericarditis occurs more often in adult males than in females and can be caused by infection, virus, MI, malignancy, medications, or it may be idiopathic (Table 22.25).[27,101–105]

Assessment and management

Chest pain, fever and a pericardial friction rub (one systolic and two diastolic heart sounds heard on auscultation) are common signs and symptoms. Chest pain usually occurs suddenly and is typically a persistent, sharp, stabbing pain aggravated by deep inspiration and coughing. Patients often experience relief when sitting upright and leaning forwards. A pericardial rub is produced by the movement of the inflamed pericardial layers moving against one another and is best heard with the patient sitting upright, forwards and on expiration.[31,74]

A severe complication of pericarditis is cardiac tamponade, which happens when a pericardial effusion occurs at a rapid rate. The rapid accumulation of fluid within the pericardial sac compresses the heart, preventing the ventricles from filling adequately to maintain stroke volume. The 12-lead ECG is a useful tool in diagnosing pericarditis; typical changes include ST-segment elevation in all leads except aV_R and V_1, although this is not to be misinterpreted as AMI when ST-segment elevation occurs in two or three leads with reciprocal changes in opposite leads.

Therapeutic interventions

- Primary survey, including medical imaging and pathology, is required.
- A comprehensive history is needed to assist in identification of the underlying causes.
- Vital signs need to be monitored regularly to assess cardiac and urine output, blood pressure, mentation and pallor.[27,101,103]

Pharmacological therapy

Pharmacological managements include pain relief with analgesia and/or non-steroidal anti-inflammatory medications.

AORTIC ANEURYSM

Aortic aneurysm is the localised weakness of the arterial wall that results in a bulge or alteration in the shape of the artery and therefore an alteration in blood flow. The weakness of the arterial wall may predispose the vessel to thrombus formation, embolisation or rupture.[12,27] Optimal cardiovascular risk management should focus on statin therapy, antihypertensive, antiplatelet and smoking cessation, as most cases of aortic aneurysm involve patients with a history of atherosclerosis.[106,107] The incidence of aneurysm is higher in men than in women and can occur anywhere along the aorta, but occurs more frequently in the abdominal region than the thoracic region.[103]

There are three types of aneurysm:

- a fusiform aneurysm, where the aneurysmal area radiates around the whole diameter of the vessel
- a sacculated aneurysm, which involves only one side of the vessel, usually the ascending aorta
- a pseudoaneurysm, which involves a dissection of the intimal layer of the vessel creating a false channel or lumen.[108]

TABLE 22.25 CAUSES OF PERICARDITIS

CATEGORY	DISCUSSION
Idiopathic	May follow a viral or febrile illness but the cause is often never established
Viral	Echovirus, coxsackievirus, adenovirus, varicella, Epstein-Barr, cytomegalovirus, hepatitis B, human immunodeficiency virus
Bacterial	Staphylococcus, Streptococcus, Haemophilus, Salmonella, Legionella, Mycobacterium tuberculosis
Fungal	Candida, Aspergillus, Histoplasma capsulatum, Coccidioides immitis
Parasitic	Entamoeba histolytica, Toxoplasma gondii, Echinococcus
Neoplasms	Lung, breast, lymphoma, leukaemia, melanoma, radiation therapy
Drugs	Procainamide, hydralazine, dantrolene, fibrinolytic agents
Connective tissue disease	Systemic lupus erythematosus, rheumatoid arthritis, scleroderma
Others	Uraemia, haemodialysis, myocardial infarction, chest trauma, aortic dissection, pancreatitis, irritable bowel syndrome

Assessment and management

Unruptured aortic aneurysm

Aortic aneurysms are often discovered incidentally during routine examination. The symptoms are usually vague and non-specific such as chronic back or abdominal pain.[108]

Ruptured aneurysm

An impending rupture of aortic aneurysm is frequently heralded by the sudden onset of pain in the flank or abdomen in a patient who is clinically shocked. There is also often the presence of a pulsatile abdominal mass.[108] The degree of shock and nature of pain varies according to the size and location of the aneurysm, as well as the time delay from initial rupture to presentation at hospital.

Therapeutic interventions

Rapid assessment and primary survey and then subsequent management are dependent on a variety of factors, including the patient's age, co-morbid state, the type of aneurysm, as well as its location and size, the risk of rupture, current medical management, and the patient's clinical condition.

Medical management

Medical management of aortic aneurysm generally involves cardiovascular risk reduction, including antiplatelet therapy, statin therapy and antihypertensive therapy.[109] Small aneurysms are often treated this way and continuously monitored as it is felt to be a safe approach with a risk/benefit approach to surgery. Unfortunately, medical management does not provide a definitive option.[109]

Surgical management

Previously surgical repair was the only option; however, advancements in the field have allowed for patients to be offered a stent/graft repair known as endovascular surgery at specialist cardiothoracic facilities.[110] Endovascular aneurysm repair, or EVAR, is performed by inserting graft components delivered via a sheath through the lumen inserted via the femoral artery. EVAR is associated with a notable reduction in mortality compared with open repair. This can be attributed to a reduction in aortic clamping and operative exposure of the aorta.[111]

AORTIC DISSECTION

Aortic dissection can occlude nearby vessels that branch off from the aorta, including the coronary arteries, carotid, spinal, mesenteric and renal arteries. There are two main subcategories of an aortic dissection based on their anatomical location. A dissection located in the ascending aorta or arch is referred to as type A and dissection isolated to the descending thoracic aorta is known as type B. There can be further classification based on the chronicity; for example, those present for fewer than or more than 14 days.[112]

Assessment and management

The most common initial presenting complaint in over 90% of acute aortic dissections is severe pain, often described as 'tearing', 'sharp' or 'ripping'. Differences in bilateral limb blood pressure should alert the clinician to the potential of aortic dissection. Reduced or absent carotid or femoral pulses usually indicate aortic dissection, and acute MI or ischaemia may involve occlusion of the coronary arteries.[12,103,113] A chest x-ray may assist in the diagnosis of an aortic aneurysm evidenced by a widened mediastinum. Pericardial involvement will be indicated by a pericardial rub, diminished heart sounds and cardiac tamponade, and its complications can result in sudden death. A focused bedside informal echo may be performed by an ED doctor to aid in early diagnosis.[114] Frequently, neurological deficits are also present, which may pose a challenge for clinicians.[114] Neurological deficits may include an altered level of consciousness and syncope or unilateral weakness or changes in sensation.

Therapeutic interventions

Immediate management should include a rapid primary survey with a focus on the control of hypertension and analgesia.

Medical management

An uncomplicated type B aortic dissection is, in most cases, managed with optimal medical management.[115] Medical management includes:

- antihypertensive therapy
- beta-blocking agents
- analgesia: pain is usually a significant issue for patients experiencing an aortic dissection. Opiate analgesics, such as morphine or fentanyl, will reduce chest pain and minimise anxiety. Clinical judgement should be used when administering narcotic analgesia in conjunction with antihypertensive therapy.[12,27,102]

Surgical management

Surgery should be anticipated based on the radiological findings, specifically type A dissection and the patient's clinical condition in order to prevent aortic rupture or cardiac tamponade.[12,27,102] Surgical advancements in endovascular aortic repair are currently occurring.

HYPERTENSIVE EMERGENCIES

Blood pressure is a result of both cardiac output and peripheral vascular resistance; in hypertension either one or both of these components are elevated.[116] Hypertensive emergencies are defined by a systolic blood pressure above 180 mmHg or a diastolic blood pressure above 120 mmHg and central nervous system compromise, altered level of consciousness and headache, cardiovascular compromise, chest pain, angina, STEMI, heart failure, haematuria, oliguria and renal failure. Common causes of hypertensive emergencies include non-compliance with medications, illegal drug usage, renal disease, pre-eclampsia and eclampsia.[117–119] Complications from uncontrolled hypertension include increased risk of stroke, heart disease and heart failure, renal disease and death.[12,27,118–120]

Malignant hypertension is defined as a sudden blood pressure increase whereby immediate intervention is required.[116] A hypertensive emergency develops rapidly over hours and involves a significant elevation in blood pressure that requires treatment within an hour to prevent end-organ damage. Hypertensive urgency develops over days and requires treatment within 24 hours of presentation.[12,118,120]

Therapeutic interventions

- Paramedic and emergency nursing management for the hypertensive patient should focus on identifying the causes while concurrently reducing the blood pressure without the introduction of adverse complications because of drug therapy.
- Regular observation, including neurological and cardiovascular assessment, will allow earlier interventions to be commenced if either is compromised.[37,55,116]

Pharmacological therapy

- Intravenous medications should be administered to reduce the mean arterial blood pressure (MAP) by 20–25% over a period of hours. Medications available include vasodilators such as GTN and sodium nitroprusside (SNP). GTN dilates both arteries and veins and has its greatest effect on the venous system. SNP infusion dilates both veins and arteries equally and reduces pre- and afterload with a minimal effect on cardiac output and is easily titratable. Beta-blockers and ACE inhibitors are also effective.[37,55,116]

SUMMARY

Cardiovascular emergencies are common pre-hospital and ED presentations. All clinicians require expert knowledge of anatomy and physiology and the pathophysiology of cardiovascular disease. This will enable the paramedic and emergency clinicians to critically assess, stratify and predict potential complications in patients presenting with a wide variety of cardiovascular emergencies. Careful assessment of a patient's condition and history can assist guidance of appropriate emergency care and optimise patient safety and outcome.

There is no doubt that cardiovascular emergencies are time-critical events and so paramedics and emergency clinicians need to be familiar with the latest treatments, diagnostic testing and therapeutic interventions. Early assessment and recognition are key to reducing adverse cardiac outcomes, improving patient safety, and enhancing quality of life. Early assessment, time-critical intervention and ongoing monitoring could optimise revascularisation and improve patient outcomes.

CASE STUDY

Mr Santos is a 65-year-old male whose wife has called for an ambulance, as he has had a 2-hour history of central, crushing chest pain and pain in his jaw. He has no known history of cardiac disease, and his wife says he takes medications for his high cholesterol. He is a smoker and is overweight. He has been unwell for the past few days with indigestion-type symptoms and has been feeling short of breath for the last few weeks.

Mr Santos is responded to by a paramedic who performs a 12-lead ECG (Fig. 22.35) and identifies an ST elevation myocardial infarction (STEMI). He is transported to the nearest facility with PCI capabilities. At the time his vital signs are recorded; blood pressure is 122/88 mmHg, pulse regular 83 beats/minute and respiratory rate 24 breaths/minute, and he is pale and diaphoretic. He is transported to the hospital and on arrival is triaged by an ED nurse.

QUESTIONS

1. Describe the initial assessment and treatment by the ambulance personnel on arrival at Mr Santos's home.
2. What other management options could be considered by the paramedics?
3. Describe the initial assessment at triage and then ongoing assessment of Mr Santos by the ED nurse on arrival to the ED.
4. What other treatment and investigations could be performed by the ED nurse?
5. Describe the changes shown on the ECG (Fig. 22.35).
6. Discuss the treatment options available for Mr Santos.

FIGURE 22.35 ST-ELEVATION MYOCARDIAL INFARCTION[121]

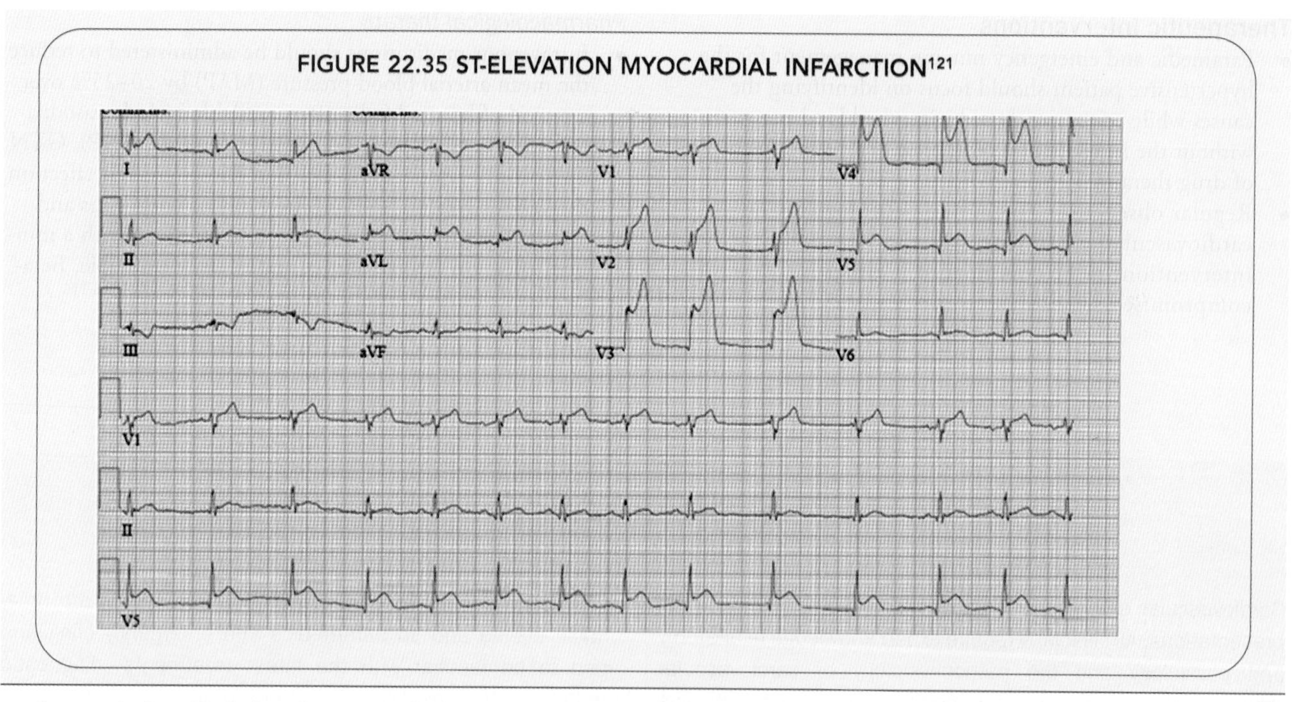

Answers to Case Study Questions can be found on evolve http://evolve.elsevier.com/AU/Curtis/emergency/ 

USEFUL WEBSITES

American Heart Association. Professional Heart Daily—resources for cardiovascular and stroke clinicians and scientists, professional.heart.org/professional/index.jsp.

Australian Heart Foundation. Resources on heart failure, www.heartfoundation.com.au.

Australian Institute of Health and Welfare. Contains the latest reports and statistics, www.aihw.gov.au/.

Cardiac Society of Australia and New Zealand. Contains position statements and practice guidelines, www.csanz.edu.au/for-professionals/position-statements-and-practice-guidelines/.

European Society of Cardiology. Evidence-based practice resources for emergency clinicians, www.escardio.org.

Heart Foundation—Heart failure tools and resources, www.heartfoundation.org.au/bundles/for-professionals/heart-failure-tools-and-resources.

Heart Foundation—Women and heart disease information, www.heartfoundation.org.au/bundles/your-heart/heart-conditions-in-women.

Heart Foundation—What is coronary heart disease? www.heartfoundation.org.au/bundles/your-heart/coronary-heart-disease.

Ministry of Health. Information on cardiovascular disease in New Zealand, www.health.govt.nz/our-work/diseases-and-conditions/cardiovascular-disease.

REFERENCES

1. World Health Organization (WHO). Cardiovascular diseases (CVDs). 2021. Online. Available from: www.who.int/news-room/fact-sheets/detail/cardiovascular-diseases-(cvds).
2. Australian Institute of Health and Welfare (AIHW). Australian health expenditure – demographics and diseases. Canberra: AIHW; 2017.
3. Australian Institute of Health and Welfare. Trends in cardiovascular deaths. Canberra: AIHW; 2017.
4. National Heart Foundation of Australia. Key statistics: coronary heart disease. Online. Available from: www.heartfoundation.org.au/activities-finding-or-opinion/coronary-heart-disease-key-stats.
5. Garofalo D, Grey C, Lee M, et al. Pre-hospital delay in acute coronary syndromes: PREDICT CVD-18. N Z Med J 2012;125(1348):1–22.
6. National Vascular Disease Prevention Alliance. Guidelines for the management of absolute cardiovascular disease risk. 2012. Online. Available from: https://informme.org.au/media/cuzjrcgz/absolutecvd_gl_webready.pdf.
7. Doust J, Bonner C, Bell K. Future directions in cardiovascular disease risk prediction. Aust J Gen Pract 2020;49:488–94.
8. Pylypchuk R, Wells S, Kerr A, et al. Cardiovascular disease risk prediction equations in 400 000 primary care patients in New Zealand: a derivation and validation study. Lancet 2018;391(10133):1897–907.

9. Agostino JW, Wong D, Paige E, et al. Cardiovascular disease risk assessment for Aboriginal and Torres Strait Islander adults aged under 35 years: a consensus statement. Med J Aust 2020;212(9):422–7.
10. Australian Institute of Health and Welfare (AIHW). Cardiovascular disease: Australian facts 2011. Canberra: AIHW; 2011.
11. Australian Institute of Health and Welfare (AIHW). Cardiovascular health compendium. Canberra: AIHW; 2022.
12. Foley A, Sweet V. Cardiovascular emergencies. In: Emergency Nurses Association, editor. Sheehy's emergency nursing: principles and practice. 7th ed. St. Louis: Mosby; 2019.
13. National Heart Foundation of Australia and Cardiac Society of Australia and New Zealand. Australian clinical guidelines for the management of acute coronary syndromes. Canberra: The Cardiac Society of Australia and New Zealand and Heart Foundation; 2016.
14. Herring N, Paterson DJ. Levick's introduction to cardiovascular physiology. 6th ed. London: Taylor & Francis; 2018.
15. Urden L, Stacy K, Lough M. Critical care nursing diagnosis and management. 9th ed. St. Louis: Elsevier; 2021.
16. Hatchett R, Thompson D. Cardiac nursing: a comprehensive guide. 2nd ed. Edinburgh: Churchill Livingstone; 2008.
17. Perpetua EM, Keegan P. Cardiac nursing. 7th ed. USA: Lippincott Williams & Wilkins; 2021.
18. Thompson JM, McFarland GK, Hirsch JE, Tucker SM. Mosby's clinical nursing. 5th ed. St. Louis: Mosby; 2002.
19. Tortora GJ, Derrickson BH, Burkett B, et al. Principles of anatomy and physiology. 3th ed. Australia: John Wiley & Sons; 2021.
20. Paediatric Heart Specialists. Normal heart anatomy and blood flow. 2022. Online. Available from: pediatricheartspecialists.com/heart-education/14-normal/152-normal-heart-anatomy-and-blood-flow.
21. Buckley T, Lin F. Cardiovascular assessment and monitoring. In: Aitken L, Marshall A, Chaboyer W, editors. ACCCN's critical care nursing. 3rd ed. Chatswood: Elsevier Australia; 2015.
22. Newberry L, Barnett GK, Ballard N. A new mnemonic for chest pain assessment. J Emerg Nurs 2005;31(1):84–5.
23. Katz AM. Cardiac ion channels. N Engl J Med 1993;328(17):1244–51.
24. Pinnell J, Turner S, Howell S. Cardiac muscle physiology. Contin Educ Anaesth Crit Care Pain 2007;7(3):85–8.
25. Grant AO. Cardiac ion channels. Circ Arrhythm Electrophysiol 2009;2(2):185–94.
26. Banasik JL. Cardiac function. In: Banasik JL, editor. Pathophysiology. 7th ed. St. Louis: Saunders; 2021.
27. Hammond B, Zimmermann P. Sheehy's manual of emergency care. 7th ed. Chicago: Mosby; 2012.
28. Tewelde S, Reynolds J. Cardiovascular emergencies: an issue of emergency medicine clinics of North America. St. Louis: Elsevier; 2015.
29. Wesley K. Huszar's ECG and 12-lead interpretation. 6th ed. US: Elsevier; 2021.
30. Rautaharju PM, Park L, Rautaharju FS, et al. A standardized procedure for locating and documenting ECG chest electrode positions: consideration of the effect of breast tissue on ECG amplitudes in women. J Electrocardiol 1998;31(1):17–29.
31. Sandau KE, Funk M, Auerbach A, et al. Update to practice standards for electrocardiographic monitoring in hospital settings: a scientific statement from the American Heart Association. Circulation 2017;136(19):e273–344.
32. Linton A. Introduction to medical-surgical nursing. 6th ed. St. Louis: Elsevier; 2015.
33. Cengiz P. Acute coronary syndrome. 2nd ed. Manchester: Lippincott Williams and Wilkins; 2015.
34. Lewis S, Bucher L, Heitkemper M, et al. Medical surgical nursing. St. Louis: Elsevier; 2017.
35. Prasitlumkum N, Rattanawong P, Limpruttidham N, et al. Frequent premature atrial complexes as a predictor of atrial fibrillation: systematic review and meta-analysis. J Electrocardiol 2018;51(5):760–7.
36. Brieger D, Amerena J, Attia JR, et al. National Heart Foundation of Australia and Cardiac Society of Australia and New Zealand: Australian clinical guidelines for the diagnosis and management of atrial fibrillation 2018. Med J Aust 2018;209(8):356–62.
37. Aitken L, Marshall A, Chaboyer W. ACCCN critical care nursing. 4th ed. Sydney: Elsevier; 2019.
38. Kusumoto FM, Schoenfeld MH, Barrett C, et al. 2018 ACC/AHA/HRS guideline on the evaluation and management of patients with bradycardia and cardiac conduction delay: a report of the American College of Cardiology/American Heart Association Task Force on Clinical Practice Guidelines and the Heart Rhythm Society. Circulation 2019;140(8):e382–482.
39. Marcus GM. Evaluation and management of premature ventricular complexes. Circulation 2020;141(17):1404–18.
40. Dresen WF, Ferguson JD. Ventricular arrhythmias. Cardiol Clin 2018;36(1):129–39.
41. Al-Khatib SM, Stevenson WG, Ackerman MJ, et al. 2017 AHA/ACC/HRS Guideline for management of patients with ventricular arrhythmias and the prevention of sudden cardiac death. Circulation 2018;138(13):e272–391.
42. Australian Resuscitation Council. ANZCOR Guideline 11.2: protocols for adult advanced life support. 2018. Online. Available from: www.resus.org.au.
43. Farzad A, Schussler JM. Acute myopericardial syndromes. Cardiol Clin 2018;36(1):103–14.
44. Mela T. Pacemakers and ICDs. Cardiol Clin 2014;32(2):xi–xii.
45. Australian Resuscitation Council. Electrical therapy for adult advanced life support. Melbourne: Australian Resuscitation Council; 2011.
46. Body R, Hendry C. Cardiac biomarkers in emergency care. Cardiol Clin 2018;36(1):27–36.
47. Angerstein RL, Thompson B, Rasmussen MJ. Preventing sudden cardiac death in post myocardial infarction patients with left ventricular dysfunction. J Cardiovasc Nurs 2005;20(6):397–404.

48. Gura MT. Implantable cardioverter defibrillator therapy. J Cardiovasc Nurs 2005;20(4):276–87.
49. Loscalzo J. Harrison's cardiovascular medicine. 3rd ed. Ohio: McGraw-Hill Education; 2017.
50. Stephens G. Using a structured clinical assessment to identify the cause of chest pain. Nurs Stand 2019;34:59–66.
51. Wenger NK. Juggling multiple guidelines: a woman's heart in the balance. J Womens Health 2016;25(3):213–21.
52. Australian Institute of Health and Welfare (AIHW). Cardiovascular disease in women. Canberra: AIHW; 2019.
53. Clerc Liaudat C, Vaucher P, De Francesco T, et al. Sex/gender bias in the management of chest pain in ambulatory care. Womens Health 2018;14:1745506518805641.
54. McDonnell LA, Turek M, Coutinho T, et al. Women's heart health: knowledge, beliefs, and practices of Canadian physicians. J Womens Health 2018;27(1):72–82.
55. Geller BJ, Abella BS. Evolving strategies in cardiac arrest management. Cardiol Clin 2018;36(1):73–84.
56. Chang AM, Fischman DL, Hollander JE. Evaluation of chest pain and acute coronary syndromes. Cardiol Clin 2018;36(1):1–12.
57. Australasian College for Emergency Medicine (ACEM). Guidelines for implementation of the Australasian Triage Scale in emergency departments. Melbourne: ACEM; 2016.
58. Moser D, Riegel B. Cardiac nursing: a companion to Braunwald's heart disease. St. Louis: Elsevier; 2008.
59. Backus BE, Six AJ, Kelder JC, et al. A prospective validation of the HEART score for chest pain patients at the emergency department. Int J Cardiol 2013;168(3):2153–8.
60. Wassie M, Lee M S, Sun BC, et al. Single vs serial measurements of cardiac troponin level in the evaluation of patients in the emergency department with suspected acute myocardial infarction. JAMA Netw Open 2021;4(2):e2037930.
61. National Heart Foundation of Australia. Assessment protocol for suspected ACS using a sensitive lab-based assay. 2016. Online. Available from: www.heartfoundation.org.au/getmedia/4618f6f4-12b6-45c5-a43b-b8675b96b6de/assessment_protocol_for_suspected_acs_using_a_sensitive_lab-based_assay-2016.pdf.
62. Brady W, de Souza K. The HEART score: a guide to its application in the emergency department. Turk J Emerg Med 2018;18(2):47–51.
63. Poldervaart JM, Langedijk M, Backus BE, et al. Comparison of the GRACE, HEART and TIMI score to predict major adverse cardiac events in chest pain patients at the emergency department. Int J Cardiol 2017;227:656–61.
64. Atherton JJ, Sindone A, De Pasquale CG, et al. National Heart Foundation of Australia and Cardiac Society of Australia and New Zealand: Guidelines for the prevention, detection, and management of heart failure in Australia 2018. Heart Lung Circ 2018;27(10):1123–208.
65. Hedayati T, Yadav N, Khanagavi J. Non-ST-segment acute coronary syndromes. Cardiol Clin 2018;36(1):37–52.
66. Emergency Nurses Association. Emergency nursing core curriculum. 7th ed. St. Louis: Elsevier; 2017.
67. Nikolaou NI, Welsford M, Beygui F, et al. Part 5: Acute coronary syndromes: 2015 international consensus on cardiopulmonary resuscitation and emergency cardiovascular care science with treatment recommendations. Resuscitation 2015;95:e121–46.
68. Humphreys M. Nursing the cardiac patient. Oxford: Wiley-Blackwell; 2011.
69. Hutchison AW, Malaiapan Y, Cameron JD, et al. Pre-hospital 12 lead ECG to triage ST elevation myocardial infarction and long-term improvements in door to balloon times: The first 1000 patients from the MonAMI project. Heart Lung Circ 2013;22(11):910–16.
70. Ibanez B, James S, Agewall S, et al. 2017 ESC Guidelines for the management of acute myocardial infarction in patients presenting with ST-segment elevation: the Task Force for the management of acute myocardial infarction in patients presenting with ST-segment elevation of the European Society of Cardiology (ESC). Euro Heart J 2018;39(2):119–77.
71. Savage ML, Poon KK, Johnston EM, et al. Pre-hospital ambulance notification and initiation of treatment of ST elevation myocardial infarction is associated with significant reduction in door-to-balloon time for primary PCI. Heart Lung Circ 2014;23(5):435–43.
72. Quinn T, Johnsen S, Gale CP, et al. Effects of prehospital 12-lead ECG on processes of care and mortality in acute coronary syndrome: a linked cohort study from the Myocardial Ischaemia National Audit Project. Heart 2014;100(12):944–50.
73. Ferri F. Ferri's clinical advisor 2018. St. Louis: Elsevier; 2018.
74. Sole ML, Klein DG, Moseley M. Introduction to critical care nursing. 8th ed. St. Louis: Elsevier; 2020.
75. Krittanawong C, Hahn J, Kayani W. Fibrinolytic therapy in patients with acute ST-elevation myocardial infarction. Interv Cardiol Clin 2021;10(3):381–90.
76. Saeedi M, Eslami M, Eslami P, et al. Effect of pre-hospital thrombolysis on mortality in patients with myocardial infarction: a systematic review and meta-analysis. J Maz Univ Med Sci 2018;28(164):170–8.
77. Davis P, Howie GJ, Dicker B, et al. Paramedic-delivered fibrinolysis in the treatment of ST-elevation myocardial infarction: comparison of a physician-authorized versus autonomous paramedic approach. Prehosp Emerg Care 2020;24(5):617–24.
78. Wang TY, White JA, Tricoci P, et al. Upstream clopidogrel use and the efficacy and safety of early eptifibatide treatment in patients with acute coronary syndrome: an analysis from the Early Glycoprotein IIb/IIIa Inhibition in Patients with Non-ST-Segment Elevation Acute Coronary Syndrome (EARLY ACS) trial. Circulation 2011;123(7):722–30.
79. Australian and New Zealand Committee on Resuscitation (ANZCOR). ANZCOR guideline 14.2: acute coronary syndromes: initial medical therapy. Emerg Med Australas 2016;23(3):308–11.
80. Phillips N, Hornacky A. Berry and Kohn's operating room technique. 14th ed. St. Louis: Elsevier; 2020.

81. Tiziani A. Havard's nursing guide to drugs. 11th ed. Sydney: Mosby Elsevier; 2021.
82. Roffi M, Patrono C, Collet JP, et al. 2015 ESC Guidelines for the management of acute coronary syndromes in patients presenting without persistent ST-segment elevation: task force for the management of acute coronary syndromes in patients presenting without persistent ST-segment elevation of the European Society of Cardiology (ESC). Euro Heart J 2016;37(3):267–315.
83. Nikolaou NI, Arntz HR, Bellou A, et al. European Resuscitation Council Guidelines for Resuscitation 2015 Section 8. Initial management of acute coronary syndromes. Resuscitation 2015;95:264–77.
84. Kizioe R, Hodgson K. Saunders nursing drug handbook 2018. St. Louis: Elsevier; 2018.
85. Bata I, Armstrong PW, Westerhout CM, et al. Time from first medical contact to reperfusion in ST elevation myocardial infarction: a Which Early ST Elevation Myocardial Infarction Therapy (WEST) substudy. Canad J Cardiol 2009;25(8):463–8.
86. Tewelde SZ, Liu SS, Winters ME. Cardiogenic shock. Cardiol Clin 2018;36(1):53–61.
87. Jentzer JC, Scutella M, Pike F, et al. Early coronary angiography and percutaneous coronary intervention are associated with improved outcomes after out of hospital cardiac arrest. Resuscitation 2018;123:15–21.
88. Theologou T, Field ML. Preoperative IABP in high risk patients undergoing CABG. HSR Proc Intensive Care Cardiovasc Anesth 2011;3(1):21–2.
89. Ahmad M, Mehta P, Reddivari AKR, et al. Percutaneous coronary intervention. In: StatPearls [Internet]. 2021.
90. Scott MC, Winters ME. Congestive heart failure. Emerg Med Clin N Am 2015;33(3):553–62.
91. Cecil R, Goldman L, Schafer A. Goldman's Cecil medicine. 25th ed. Philadelphia: Elsevier/Saunders; 2016.
92. Pang PS. Acute heart failure syndromes: initial management. Emerg Med Clin N Am 2011;29(4):675–88.
93. Bell N, Hutchinson CL, Green TC, et al. Randomised control trial of humidified high flow nasal cannulae versus standard oxygen in the emergency department. Emerg Med Australas 2015;27(6):537–41.
94. Yancy CW, Jessup M, Bozkurt B, et al. 2013 ACCF/AHA guideline for the management of heart failure: a report of the American College of Cardiology Foundation/American Heart Association Task Force on Practice Guidelines. J Amn Coll Cardiol 2013;62(16):e147–239.
95. Koster G, Bekema HJ, Wetterslev J, et al. Milrinone for cardiac dysfunction in critically ill adult patients: a systematic review of randomised clinical trials with meta-analysis and trial sequential analysis. Intensive Care Med 2016;42(9):1322–35.
96. Australian Institute of Health and Welfare (AIHW). Australia's health 2016. Canberra: AIHW; 2016.
97. Cleveland Clinic. Heart Failure (Congestive Heart Failure). 2022. Online. Available from: https://my.clevelandclinic.org/health/diseases/17069-heart-failure-understanding-heart-failure.
98. Eisenberg MJ, Gioia LC. Angiotensin II receptor blockers in congestive heart failure. Cardiol Rev 2006;14(1):26–34.
99. Turer AT, Rao SV. Device therapy in the management of congestive heart failure. Cardiol Rev 2005;13(3):130–8.
100. Krum H, Jelinek MV, Stewart S, et al. 2011 update to National Heart Foundation of Australia and Cardiac Society of Australia and New Zealand Guidelines for the prevention, detection and management of chronic heart failure in Australia, 2006. Med J Aust 2011;194(8):405–9.
101. Carter T, Brooks C. Pericarditis: inflammation or infarction? J Cardiovasc Nurs 2005;20(4):239–44.
102. Klein D. Thoracic aortic aneurysms. J Cardiovasc Nurs 2005;20(4):245–50.
103. Adler Y, Charron P, Imazio M, et al. 2015 ESC Guidelines for the diagnosis and management of pericardial diseases: the Task Force for the Diagnosis and Management of Pericardial Diseases of the European Society of Cardiology (ESC). Endorsed by: the European Association for Cardio-Thoracic Surgery (EACTS). Euro Heart J 2015;36(42):2921–64.
104. Imazio M, Gaita F. Acute and recurrent pericarditis. Cardiol Clin 2017;35(4):505–13.
105. Shabetai R, Oh JK. Pericardial effusion and compressive disorders of the heart: influence of new technology on unraveling its pathophysiology and hemodynamics. Cardiol Clin 2017;35(4):467–79.
106. Yoshimura K, Morikage N, Nishino-Fujimoto S, et al. Current status and perspectives on pharmacologic therapy for abdominal aortic aneurysm. Curr Drug Targets 2018;19(11):1265–75.
107. Soares Ferreira R, Gomes Oliveira N, Oliveira-Pinto J, et al. Review on management and outcomes of ruptured abdominal aortic aneurysm in women. J Cardiovasc Surg (Torino) 2018;59(2):195–200.
108. Mathur A, Mohan V, Ameta D, Gaurav B, Haranahalli P. Aortic aneurysm. J Transl Int Med 2016;4(1):35–41.
109. Chuen J, Theivendran M. Abdominal aortic aneurysm: an update. Aust J Gen Pract 2018;47:252–6.
110. Calero A, Illig KA. Overview of aortic aneurysm management in the endovascular era. Semin Vasc Surg 2016;29(1–2):3–17.
111. Chaer RA. Endovascular repair of abdominal aortic aneurysm. 2021. Online. Available from: www.uptodate.com/contents/endovascular-repair-of-abdominal-aortic-aneurysm.
112. Khayat M, Cooper KJ, Khaja MS, et al. Endovascular management of acute aortic dissection. Cardiovasc Diagn Ther 2018;8(Suppl. 1):S97–107.
113. Thrumurthy SG, Karthikesalingam A, Patterson BO, et al. The diagnosis and management of aortic dissection. BMJ 2012;344:d8290.
114. Taylor RA, Oliva I, Van Tonder R, et al. Point-of-care focused cardiac ultrasound for the assessment of thoracic aortic dimensions, dilation, and aneurysmal disease. Acad Emerg Med 2012;19(2):244–7.
115. Suzuki T, Eagle KA, Bossone E, et al. Medical management in type B aortic dissection. Ann Cardiothorac Surg 2014;3(4):413–17.
116. National Heart Foundation of Australia. Guide to management of hypertension in adults. Canberra: Heart Foundation of Australia; 2016.

117. Behan MW, Chew DP, Aylward PE. The role of antiplatelet therapy in the secondary prevention of coronary artery disease. Curr Opin Cardiol 2010;25(4):321–8.

118. Dimitriadis K, Tsioufis C, Tousoulis D. Modern management of hypertensive emergencies and urgencies: do we need more technology, paramedics, or physicians? J Clin Hypertens 2017;19(7):702–3.

119. Suneja M, Sanders ML. Hypertensive emergency. Med Clin N Am 2017;101(3):465–78.

120. Janke AT, McNaughton CD, Brody AM, et al. Trends in the incidence of hypertensive emergencies in US emergency departments from 2006 to 2013. J Am Heart Assoc 2016;5(12):e004511.

121. Peoples K, Kobe D, Campana C, et al. Hyperhomocysteinemia-induced myocardial infarction in a young male using anabolic steroid. Am J Emerg Med 2014;32(8):948.e1–e2.

CHAPTER 23

NEUROLOGICAL EMERGENCIES

JULIE CONSIDINE AND DAVID ANDERSON

ESSENTIALS

- Altered conscious state is a known predictor of poor patient outcomes and high mortality adverse events, such as cardiac arrest and unplanned intensive care unit (ICU) admissions.
- Adequate oxygenation and blood pressure are key priorities in the management of a patient with altered conscious state.
- Transient ischaemic attack (TIA) and stroke are a continuum: TIA is a major risk factor for stroke.
- Stroke is a medical emergency: early diagnosis and access to specialist services are pivotal to improved outcomes for stroke survivors.
- Physiological monitoring and maintenance of normal physiological parameters (oxygenation, blood glucose, temperature) are fundamental to optimal stroke management.
- Seizure management should be aimed at rapid seizure control, identifying precipitating factors and prevention of complications.
- Routine laboratory investigations and imaging are not warranted for patients with an uncomplicated first-time seizure and who make a complete recovery, and there is no evidence to currently support routine lumbar puncture in patients with seizure who are alert, afebrile and not immunocompromised.
- Head computed tomography is indicated in patients following seizure if the patient has focal neurological signs, does not recover fully or has a history of head trauma.
- Persistent or severe postictal confusion should not be presumed to be a consequence of the seizure and should be fully investigated.
- Severity of headache is an unreliable indicator of underlying pathology.
- Neuroimaging is recommended for patients with new headache and abnormal neurological assessment findings; new, sudden-onset severe headache; HIV-positive patients with new headache; and patients older than 50 years with new headache.

INTRODUCTION

Neurological emergencies relate to either illness or injury and can present as a minor discomfort or a severe life-threatening emergency requiring urgent medical and/or surgical intervention. Unresponsiveness with abnormal, ineffective breathing is the trigger to commence cardiopulmonary resuscitation,[1] and altered conscious state is both a marker of severity of both neurological and systemic illness, and a known predictor of out-of-hospital[2] and in-hospital adverse events.[3,4] It is imperative that emergency clinicians pay attention to subtle changes in conscious state and recognise behavioural disturbance, anxiety, restlessness and agitation as signs of clinical deterioration rather than dismissing these signs as disruptive behaviours or psychosomatic symptoms. The focus of this chapter is to provide a review of neuroanatomy and physiology, a guide to structured assessment of a patient with a neurological problem and an overview of the management of common neurological conditions. Trauma-related brain injuries are discussed in Chapter 43.

ANATOMY AND PHYSIOLOGY OF THE NERVOUS SYSTEM

MENINGES

The three membranes which cover the brain and spinal cord are the meninges (Fig. 23.1).[5,6] The outer layer is called the dura mater and is composed of fibrous connective tissue that supports and separates brain structures.[5,6] The arachnoid mater is a delicate layer of connective tissue membrane and the pia mater is the innermost layer of transparent fibrous membrane.[5,6] Two important folds in the dura mater that separate areas of the brain are the falx cerebri and the tentorium cerebelli.[5,6] The falx cerebri creates a longitudinal fissure that separates the two cerebral hemispheres and the tentorium cerebelli separates the hemispheres from and covers the cerebellum.[5,6] In between the meninges are spaces. The epidural space is the space between dura and skull and is more of a potential space, containing fat, connective tissue and blood vessels. The subdural space is the space between dura and arachnoid mater and contains serous fluid, and the subarachnoid space is the space between arachnoid and pia mater and contains circulating cerebrospinal fluid.[5,6]

FIGURE 23.1 CROSS-SECTION OF THE HEAD AND BRAIN[7]

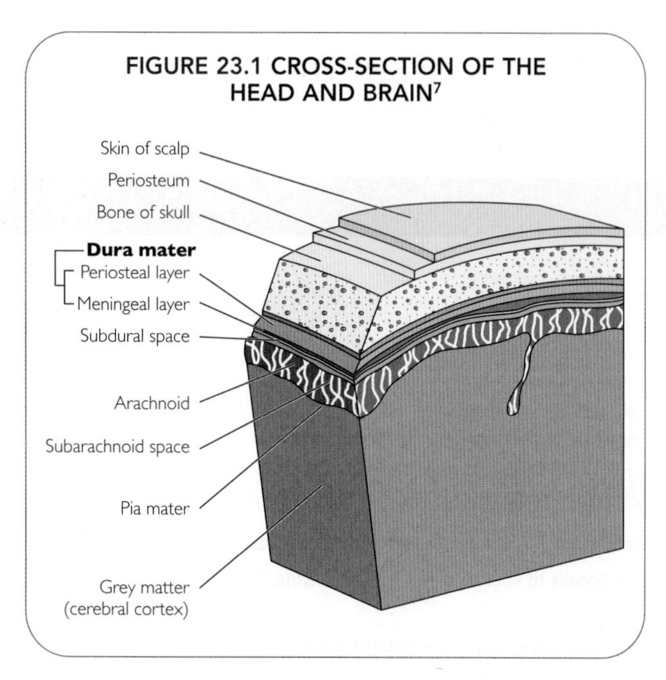

BRAIN

The adult brain is one of the largest organs of the body, weighing approximately 1300 g or 2% of total bodyweight. Structurally the brain is divided into three parts: the cerebrum, cerebellum and brainstem (Fig. 23.2).[5,6] The *cerebrum* accounts for about 80% of the total weight of the brain. The cerebrum is divided into the left and right cerebral hemispheres (Fig. 23.3).[5] Each hemisphere is made up of grey matter (nerve cell bodies and dendrites) and white matter (myelinated nerve fibres),[5,6] and the hemispheres are connected by a bundle of fibres called the corpus callosum. The corpus callosum relays information between the two hemispheres.[5,6] Each cerebral hemisphere has four lobes that are responsible for specific

FIGURE 23.2 MIDSAGITTAL SECTION OF THE BRAIN[8]

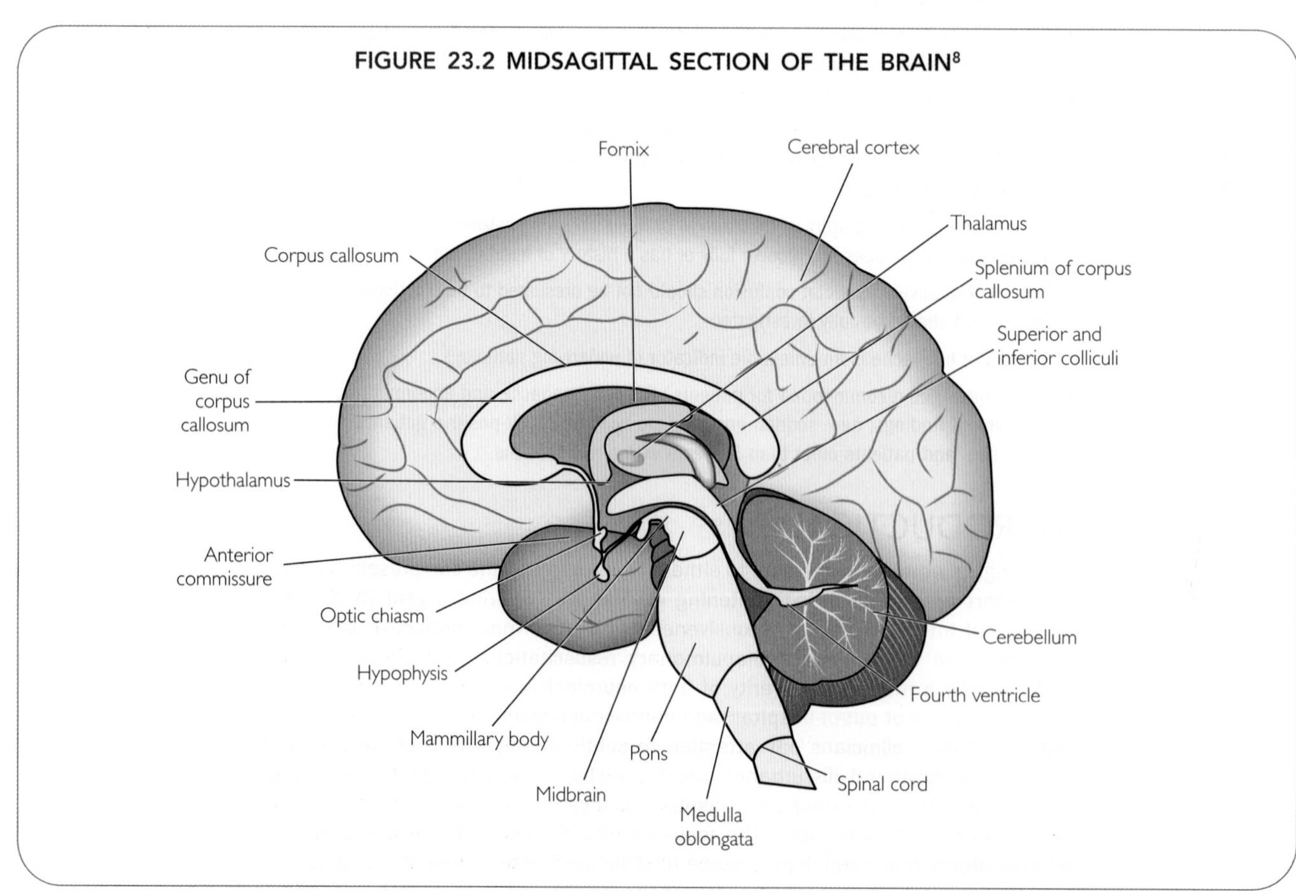

Note the relationships among the cerebral cortex, cerebellum, thalamus and brainstem and the location of various commissures.

FIGURE 23.3 LEFT HEMISPHERE OF CEREBRUM, LATERAL SURFACE, SHOWING MAJOR LOBES AND AREAS OF THE BRAIN[9]

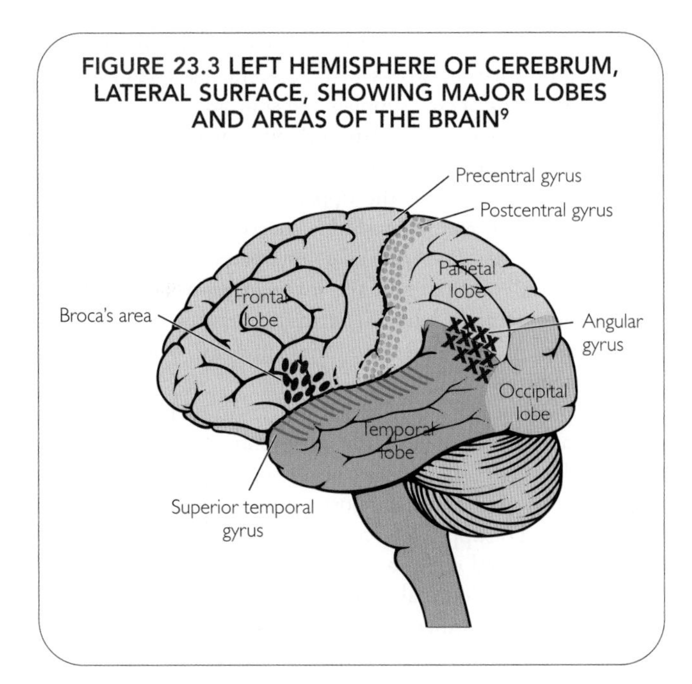

aspects of cerebral function (Table 23.1). The *cerebellum* is a butterfly-shaped structure located below the cerebrum.[5] The cerebellum controls subconscious skeletal muscle contractions required for coordination, posture and balance.[5]

The brainstem controls vital physiological functions and is composed of the medulla oblongata, the pons and the midbrain. The medulla is continuous with the upper spinal cord and forms part of the inferior brainstem. The medulla contains ascending and descending tracts that relay motor and sensory impulses between the brain and spinal cord.[5] Many tracts cross (or decussate) as they pass through the medulla,[5] which is why the right side of the brain controls the left side of the body and vice versa. Vital reflex centres are located in the medulla.[5] The cardiac centre controls heart rate and force of contraction, the medullary rhythmicity area controls respiratory pattern and the vasomotor area controls blood-vessel diameter.[5] The medulla also contains non-vital reflex centres such as those required for swallowing, vomiting, coughing and sneezing.[5] The pons lies directly above the medulla and relays impulses within the brain and between the brain and spinal cord.[5] The pons contains the pneumotaxic area and the apneustic area, both of which control

TABLE 23.1 LOCATION AND FUNCTION OF THE PARTS OF THE CEREBRUM[9]

PART	LOCATION	FUNCTION
Cortical areas		
Motor		
Primary	Precentral gyrus	Controls initiation of movement on opposite side of body
Supplementary	Anterior to precentral gyrus	Facilitates proximal muscle activity, including activity for stance and gait, and spontaneous movement and coordination
Sensory		
Somatic	Postcentral gyrus	Registers body sensations (e.g. temperature, touch, pressure, pain) from opposite side of body
Visual	Occipital lobe	Registers visual images
Auditory	Superior temporal gyrus	Registers auditory inputs
Association areas	Parietal lobe	Integrates somatic and special sensory inputs
	Posterior temporal lobe	Integrates visual and auditory inputs for language comprehension
	Anterior temporal lobe	Integrates past experiences
	Anterior frontal lobe	Controls higher-order processes (e.g. judgement, insight, reasoning, problem-solving, planning)
Other areas		
Language		
Comprehension	Wernicke's area	Integrates auditory language (understanding of spoken words)
Expression	Broca's area	Regulates verbal expression
Basal ganglia	Near lateral ventricles of both cerebral hemispheres	Controls and facilitates learnt and automatic movements
Thalamus	Below basal ganglia	Relays sensory and motor inputs to cortex and other parts of cerebrum
Hypothalamus	Below thalamus	Regulates endocrine and autonomic functions (e.g. feeding, sleeping, emotional and sexual responses)
Limbic system	Lateral to hypothalamus	Influences affective (emotional) behaviour and basic drives, such as feeding and sexual behaviour

respiration along with the medullary rhythmicity area.[5] The midbrain relays motor impulses from cerebral cortex to pons and spinal cord, and relays sensory impulses from spinal cord to thalamus.[5]

The thalamus and hypothalamus are situated on top of the brainstem. The thalamus surrounds the third ventricle and is an interpretation centre for sensory impulses (e.g. pain, temperature, touch and pressure).[5] The hypothalamus is located inferior to the thalamus[5] and controls vital functions (e.g. water balance, blood pressure, sleep, appetite and body temperature) and regulates the autonomic nervous system. The hypothalamus stimulates smooth muscle, controls heart rate and strength of contraction, controls gland secretions, receives and interprets sensory impulses from the viscera and is the main connection between the nervous system and the endocrine system.

SPINAL CORD

The spinal cord is located in the vertebral canal (cavity formed by the vertebral foramina) and like the brain, is also covered by the meninges. The spinal cord is continuous with the brainstem, beginning as a continuation of the medulla oblongata and terminating at the level of the second lumbar vertebra. The spinal cord is composed of H-shaped grey matter (nerve cell bodies) surrounded by white matter (nerve tracts and fibres). The spinal cord contains bundles of fibres called tracts: ascending tracts conduct impulses up the spinal cord (sensory) and descending tracts conduct impulses down the spinal cord (motor). These features are illustrated in Fig. 23.4. The spinal cord ends around the L1 lumbar vertebra. The *filum terminale* is a section of non-nervous fibrous tissue that extends inferiorly from below the lumbar enlargement to the coccyx, and the *cauda equina* is the tail-like collection of roots of spinal nerves at the inferior end of the spinal canal.

Spinal nerves

There are 31 pairs of spinal nerves, which are named and numbered according to the spinal cord region from which they emerge.[5] Each spinal nerve has two connections to the spinal cord: the *posterior* or *dorsal root* receives sensory input from sensory receptors and the *anterior* or *ventral root* contains a combination of efferent (motor) fibres.[5] Close to the spinal cord, spinal nerves divide into branches called *rami* and the anterior rami form networks with adjacent nerves called *plexuses*.[5] The *cervical plexus* supplies the skin and muscles of the head, neck and upper shoulders and innervates the diaphragm. The phrenic nerves also arise from the cervical plexus.[5] The *brachial plexus* innervates the upper extremities and shoulder region; the radial, median and ulnar nerves arise from the brachial plexus.[5] The *lumbar plexus* innervates the anterolateral abdominal wall and parts of the lower extremities, and is the origin of the femoral nerve. The sciatic nerve arises from the *sacral plexus*, which innervates the buttocks, perineum and lower extremities.[5]

The spinal nerves originating from T2 to T11 do not form plexuses and are known as the *intercostal nerves*5. Nerve T2 supplies the intercostal muscles of the second intercostal space, the skin of the axilla and the posteromedial aspect of the arm; nerves T3 to T6 supply intercostal muscles and the skin of the anterior and lateral chest; and nerves T7 to T11 supply intercostal muscles, abdominal muscles and overlying skin. The areas of skin that are innervated by specific spinal cord segments are called *dermatomes* (Fig. 23.5).

Cranial nerves

There are 12 pairs of cranial nerves, each with a name and numbered using Roman numerals.[5] The numbers indicate the order in which the nerves arise from the brain (front to back), and the name indicates the function of each nerve pair. Cranial nerve functions are not consciously controlled; therefore, assessment of cranial nerves provides an accurate picture of brainstem activity and neurological function.[5,6] Table 23.2 outlines the functions of each cranial nerve.

Cerebrospinal fluid

Cerebrospinal fluid (CSF) is produced in the cerebral ventricles by the choroid plexus and circulates through the cerebral ventricles and subarachnoid space.[5] CSF is a clear, colourless fluid containing oxygen, glucose, proteins, urea and salts.[5] Normally, the central nervous system contains 80–150 mL of CSF, and 20 mL of CSF is produced per hour.[5] CSF has protective and circulatory functions. It is a shock-absorbing medium for the brain and spinal cord and

FIGURE 23.4 CROSS-SECTION OF THE CERVICAL SPINAL CORD[10]

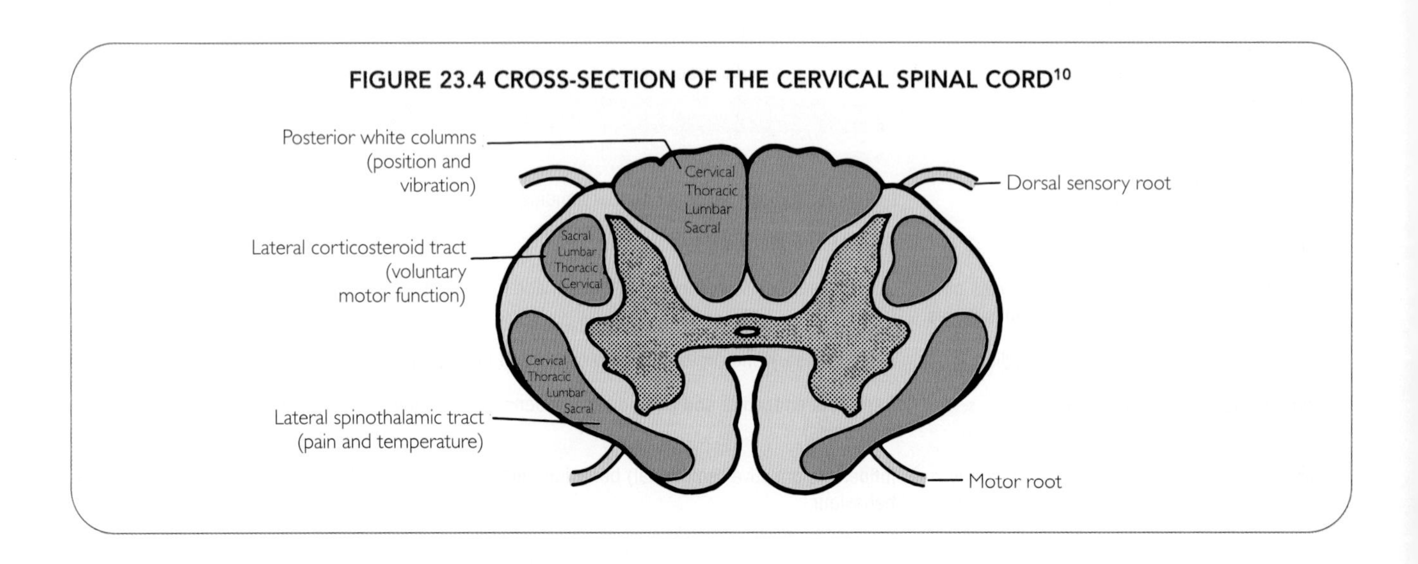

FIGURE 23.5 SENSORY DERMATOMES[10]

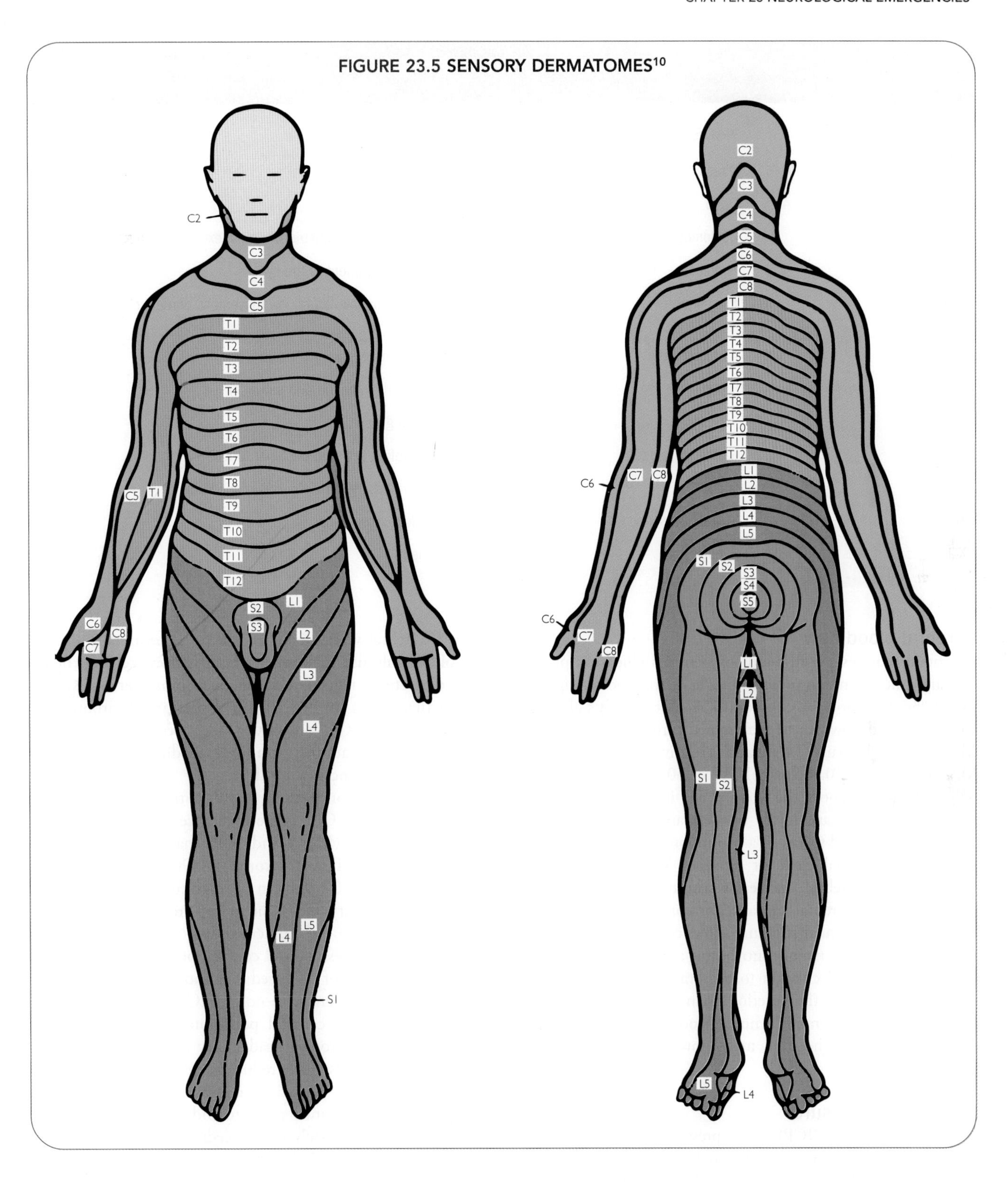

prevents the brain and spinal cord from crashing against bony structures. CSF also delivers nutrients filtered from the blood to the brain and spinal cord, and removes wastes produced by the brain and spinal-cord cells.[5] CSF also compensates for changes in intracranial pressure and volume.[5] The blood–CSF (or blood–brain) barrier is the interface between the peripheral circulation and the central nervous system and is made up of specialised endothelial cells.[11] The blood–brain barrier serves as a protective mechanism that prevents passage of certain substances from blood to CSF and then to the brain,[5] but also enables the maintenance of central nervous system homeostasis.[6] The blood–brain barrier has controlled reversible openings that are essential for normal cerebral physiological function.[6] Disruption to the blood–brain barrier from conditions such as stroke, head injury and cerebral inflammatory diseases often causes increased permeability, resulting in injurious substances causing further damage to the underlying brain[6].

TABLE 23.2 CRANIAL NERVES AND THEIR FUNCTIONS[9]

NUMBER	NAME	FUNCTION
I	Olfactory	Smell
II	Optic	Vision
III	Oculomotor	Elevate upper lid, pupillary constriction, most extraocular movements
IV	Trochlear	Downward, inward movement of the eye
V	Trigeminal	Chewing, clenching the jaw, lateral jaw movement, corneal reflexes, face sensation
VI	Abducens	Lateral eye deviation
VII	Facial	Facial motor, taste, lacrimation and salivation
VIII	Acoustic	Equilibrium, hearing
IX	Glossopharyngeal	Swallowing, gag reflex, taste on posterior tongue
X	Vagus	Swallowing, gag reflex, abdominal viscera, phonation
XI	Spinal accessory	Head and shoulder movement
XII	Hypoglossal	Tongue movement

Cerebral blood flow

The brain requires a continuous oxygen and glucose supply—although the brain comprises only 2% of total bodyweight, it uses 20% of the body's oxygen and 25% of the body's glucose.[5] Cerebral blood flow can be maintained across a wide range of Mean Arterial Pressure (MAP) and is relatively stable between a MAP of 60 and 150. Below a MAP of 50 cerebral blood flow will decrease and above the MAP it will increase, both potentially impacting on any injury to the brain. Adequate cerebral perfusion is required to ensure a continuous oxygen and glucose supply.[5] The arterial circle or circle of Willis is formed by the posterior cerebral, posterior communicating, internal carotid, anterior cerebral and anterior communicating arteries (Fig. 23.6). This circular structure allows compensation if blood flow from one of the major contributing arteries is reduced, and provides collateral circulation to the brain.[5,6] The internal carotid arteries supply the anterior brain and vertebral arteries supply the posterior brain.[5] Venous blood drains from the brain through sinuses in the dura mater into the internal jugular veins.[5]

Intracranial pressure

Intracranial pressure (ICP) is the pressure within the cranial cavity; normal ICP ranges from 5 to 15 mmHg.[13] The cranial cavity contains brain tissue (80%), blood (10%) and CSF (10%),[6] and increased ICP occurs when the volume of any of these components increases.[13] Small alterations in brain tissue, blood or CSF volume do not cause increased ICP because a small increase in volume of one component is compensated for by a decrease in the volume of the other components (Monro-Kellie doctrine).[11] CSF is the most easily displaced, and CSF volume is reduced via reabsorption.[11] If ICP remains elevated following CSF displacement, cerebral blood volume is reduced via vasoconstriction and compression of small intracranial veins.[14] Cerebral vessel diameter is a key determinant of cerebral blood volume. In normal circumstances, cerebral blood vessel diameter is regulated by the autonomic nervous system and fluctuations in the arterial partial pressure of carbon dioxide and oxygen ($PaCO_2$ and PaO_2). Increased $PaCO_2$ results in generalised vasodilation (including vasodilation of cerebral blood vessels) and increased ICP.[11]

Cerebral perfusion pressure (CPP) is the pressure required to perfuse the brain. CPP is the difference between mean arterial blood pressure (MAP) and ICP; that is, CPP = MAP – ICP.[11] Normal CPP ranges from 70 to 90 mmHg (but a narrower range of 50–70 will often be targeted in a patient with a traumatic brain injury (TBI) due to impaired autoregulation of cerebral blood flow).[11,13] Understanding the relationship between ICP, blood pressure and cerebral perfusion is important for the management of increased ICP and preservation of cerebral perfusion. A patient with normal ICP who is hypotensive will have inadequate cerebral perfusion. Similarly, a patient with increased ICP from a head injury or stroke and normal blood pressure will also have reduced cerebral perfusion. Cerebral perfusion will be especially compromised in the patient with increased intracranial pressure and concurrent hypotension. When ICP approaches or exceeds MAP, cellular hypoxia and death occur (Fig. 23.7).[11,14]

DIVISIONS OF THE NERVOUS SYSTEM

The major functions of the neurological system are to sense, interpret and respond to changes within the body and the outside environment.[5] The major divisions of the nervous system are the central and peripheral nervous systems. The *central nervous system* (CNS) is responsible for organising and coordinating all body system responses, including consciousness and

FIGURE 23.6

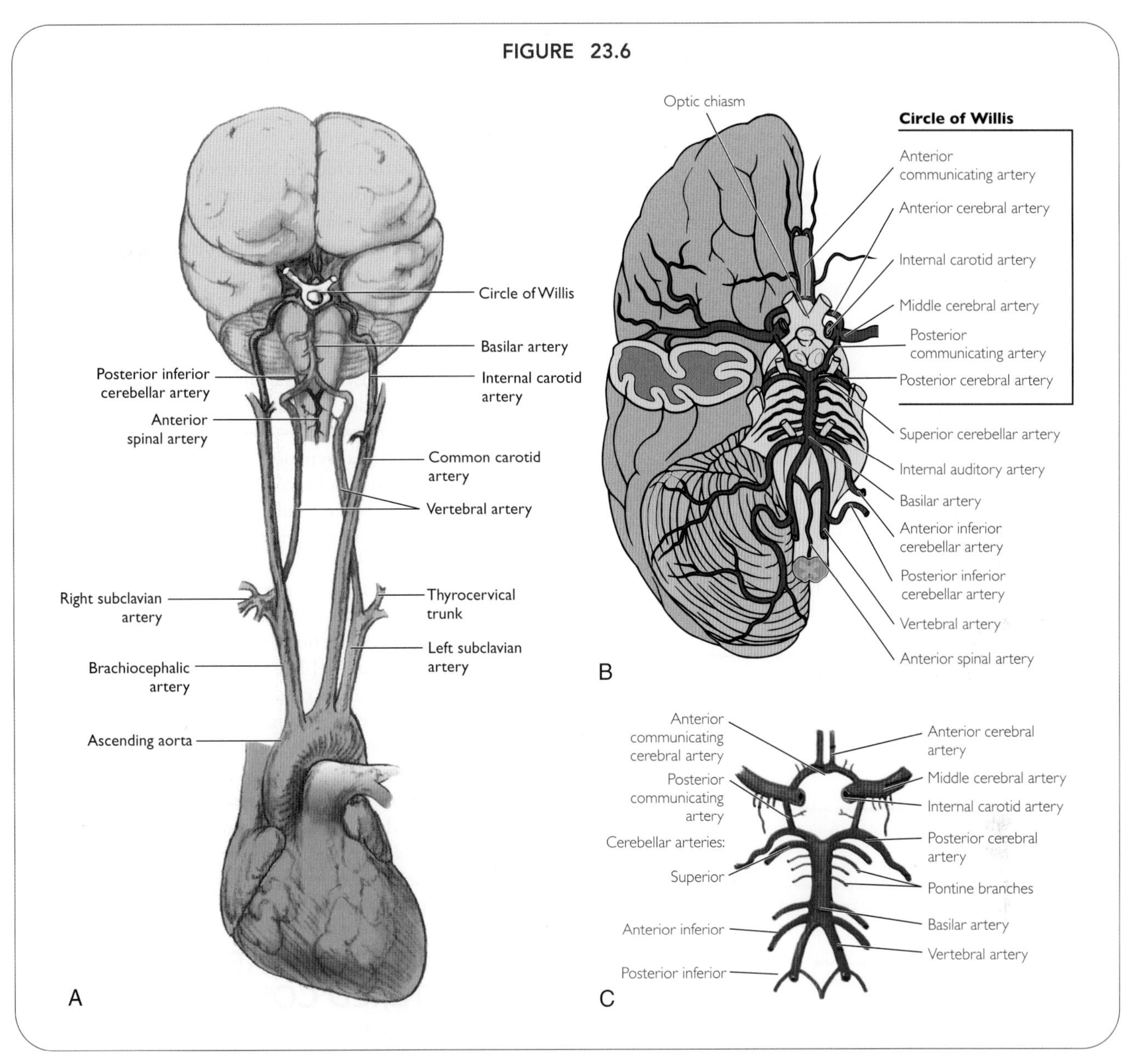

A. Origin and course of arterial supply to the brain.[12] **B.** Cerebral arteries and the circle of Willis. The tip of the temporal lobe has been removed to show the course of the middle cerebral artery.[12] **C.** Arteries at the base of the brain. The arteries that comprise the circle of Willis are the two anterior cerebral arteries joined to each other by the anterior communicating cerebral artery and to the posterior cerebral arteries by the posterior communicating arteries.[12]

cognition, while the *peripheral nervous system* (PNS) acts as the information pathway.[14]

CENTRAL NERVOUS SYSTEM

The CNS consists of the brain and the spinal cord.[5,6] Sensations are relayed from peripheral receptors to the CNS, then interpreted. The CNS is also responsible for the nerve impulses that stimulate the contraction of muscles and the excretion of glands.[5]

PERIPHERAL NERVOUS SYSTEM

The PNS is the processor that connects the brain with receptors, muscles and glands. It is divided into the *afferent (sensory)* system, which relays information from sensory receptors to the CNS, and the *efferent (motor)* system, which relays information from the CNS to muscles and glands.[5] The efferent nervous system is further divided into the *somatic nervous system*, which relays information from CNS to skeletal muscles, and the *autonomic nervous system* (ANS), which relays information from CNS to smooth muscle, cardiac muscles and glands.[5] The ANS is divided into the sympathetic nervous system and the parasympathetic nervous system.[5] These systems are discussed further in Chapter 10.

Autonomic nervous system

The ANS controls smooth muscle, cardiac muscle and gland function.[5] ANS activity is regulated by the centres in the cerebral cortex, hypothalamus and brainstem, and functions

FIGURE 23.7 PROGRESSION OF INCREASED INTRACRANIAL PRESSURE[16]

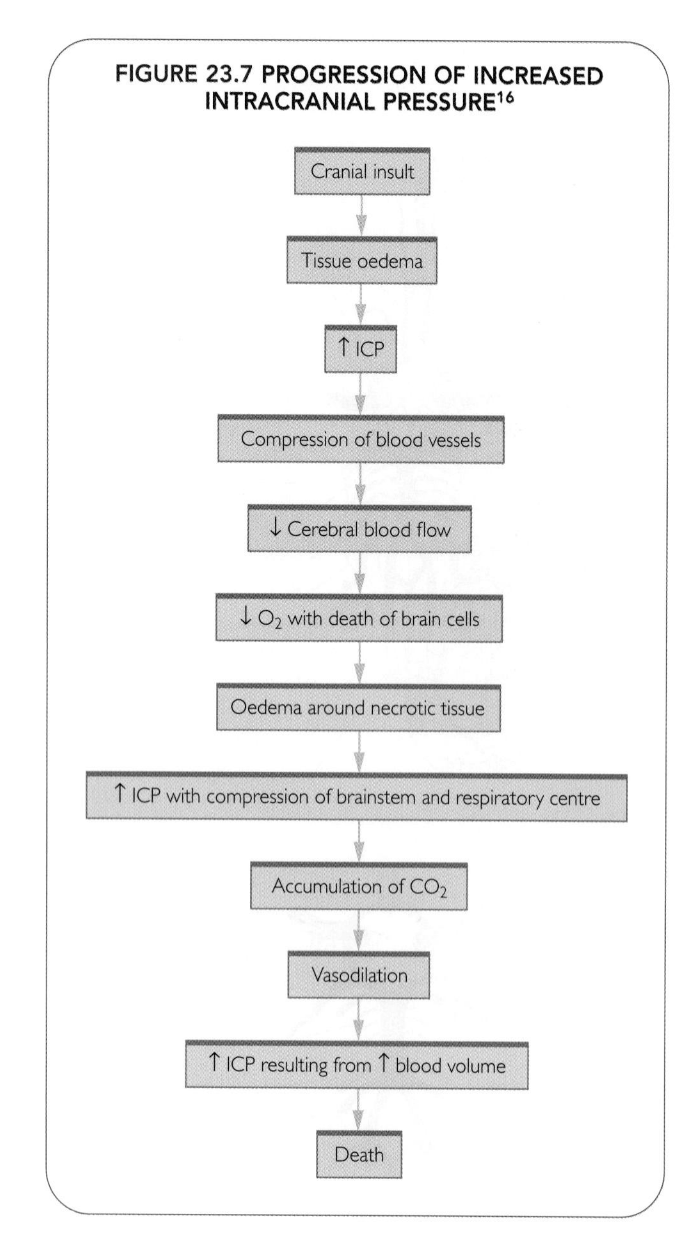

without conscious control or awareness.[5] The ANS is divided into the sympathetic and parasympathetic nervous systems.[5] Table 23.3 compares sympathetic and parasympathetic functions.

Sympathetic division

The sympathetic nervous system is responsible for the 'fight or flight' response and activates energy stores when required.[5,6] Sympathetic division domination occurs during fear, embarrassment, exercise, rage and emergency situations. It causes dilation of the pupils, increased heart rate and force of contraction, increased blood pressure, bronchodilation, decreased perfusion of gastrointestinal and genitourinary organs and increased glucose production and release.[5]

Parasympathetic division

The parasympathetic nervous system conserves and restores energy, resulting in effects that oppose sympathetic nervous system effects.[5,6] Parasympathetic stimulation results in decreased heart rate, bronchoconstriction and constriction of the pupils, and activities such as salivation, lacrimation, urination, defecation and digestion.[5]

NEURONS

Neurons are the structural and functional units of the nervous system. Neurons consist of three parts: a *cell body, dendrites* (or processes) that convey messages to the cell body and an *axon* (or nerve fibre) which carries impulses away from the cell body and towards another neuron, muscle fibre or gland cell (Fig. 23.8).[5] Propagation of impulses is known as the *action potential*. The junction between two neurons or a neuron and muscle or gland cell is called a *synapse*.[5,6] The synapse is the point at which impulses are transmitted between the axon of one neuron and the dendrite of another.

- *Nerve impulse transmission*—synapses may be electrical or chemical.[5] Electrical synapses are faster than chemical synapses and can synchronise large groups of neurons or muscle fibres.[5] As a result, electrical synapses are commonly found in visceral smooth muscle and cardiac muscle.[5]
- *Electrical transmission*—at electrical synapses, impulses are conducted directly between adjacent cells through gap junctions.[5] At gap junctions, ions flow from one cell to the next through tunnel-like structures called connexons, resulting in the transfer of action potential.[5]
- *Chemical transmission*—transmission of impulses between two neurons, a neuron and a muscle cell or a neuron and a glandular cell is controlled by neurotransmitters (Fig. 23.9).[5] Examples of neurotransmitters include acetylcholine, dopamine, noradrenaline, adrenaline and serotonin.[5,6] Neurotransmitters are partially responsible for pleasure, sexual desire, sadness, appetite, memory, anxiety and humour.

ASSESSMENT OF THE PATIENT WITH ALTERED CONSCIOUSNESS

A focused history and thorough physical assessment are fundamental to early identification and treatment of life-threatening neurological emergencies and are addressed in the following section.

HISTORY

Obtaining an accurate history in a patient with an altered level of consciousness can be difficult; therefore, family members or carers, police, paramedics, general practitioners (GPs) and bystanders are valuable sources of information. Causes of an altered level of consciousness are listed in Box 23.1.

The following information should be elicited:

- *History of presenting problem*—time and acuity of onset, history of trauma, including falls, consistency or fluctuation in symptoms, possibility of drug or alcohol use, environmental exposures (e.g. carbon monoxide exposure). Time of onset is particularly important in suspected stroke as reperfusion treatments may be administered or withheld based on time since the onset of symptoms.
- *Injury*—consider the need for cervical spine care if altered conscious state is associated with injury. Even a fall from standing height may result in a cervical spine injury. Have

TABLE 23.3 **EFFECT OF SYMPATHETIC AND PARASYMPATHETIC NERVOUS SYSTEMS**[17]

VISCERAL EFFECTOR	EFFECT OF SYMPATHETIC NERVOUS SYSTEM*	EFFECT OF PARASYMPATHETIC NERVOUS SYSTEM#
Heart	Increase in rate and strength of heartbeat (beta-receptors)	Decrease in rate and strength of heartbeat
Smooth muscle of blood vessels		
Skin blood vessels	Constriction (alpha-receptors)	No effect
Skeletal muscle blood vessels	Dilation (beta-receptors)	No effect
Coronary blood vessels	Dilation (beta-receptors), constriction (alpha-receptors)	Dilation
Abdominal blood vessels	Constriction (alpha-receptors)	No effect
Blood vessels of external genitals	Ejaculation (contraction of smooth muscle in male ducts (e.g. epididymis, ductus deferens))	Dilation of blood vessels causing erection in male
Smooth muscle of hollow organs and sphincters		
Bronchi	Dilation (beta-receptors)	Constriction
Digestive tract, except sphincters	Decrease in peristalsis (beta-receptors)	Increase in peristalsis
Sphincters of digestive tract	Contraction (alpha-receptors)	Relaxation
Urinary bladder	Relaxation (beta-receptors)	Contraction
Urinary sphincters	Contraction (alpha-receptors)	Relaxation
Eye		
Iris	Contraction of radial muscle, dilation of pupil	Contraction of circular muscle, constriction of pupil
Ciliary	Relaxation, accommodation for far vision	Contraction, accommodation for near vision
Hairs (pilomotor muscles)	Contraction producing 'goose bumps' or piloerection (alpha-receptors)	No effect
Glands		
Sweat	Increase in sweat (neurotransmitter, acetylcholine)	No effect
Digestive (e.g. salivary, gastric)	Decrease in secretion of saliva; not known for others	Increase in secretion of saliva and gastric hydrochloric acid
Pancreas, including islets	Decrease in secretion	Increase in secretion of pancreatic juice and insulin
Liver	Increase in glycogenolysis (beta-receptors), increase in blood glucose level	No effect
Adrenal medulla‡	Increase in adrenaline secretion	No effect

#Neurotransmitter is acetylcholine unless otherwise stated.

**Neurotransmitter is noradrenaline unless otherwise stated.*

‡Sympathetic preganglionic axons terminate in contact with secreting cells of the adrenal medulla. Thus, the adrenal medulla functions as a 'giant sympathetic postganglionic neuron'.

a very high index of suspicion for spinal injury in older people who have fallen.

- *Associated symptoms*—headache, seizures, nausea, vomiting, fevers, motor or sensory impairment, changes to speech, vision, memory, alterations to bladder and/or bowel function.
- *Past medical history*—similar episodes, past and concurrent medical and surgical history (particularly history of chronic neurological disorders or existing neurological deficits, headaches or migraines, seizure disorders, stroke/TIA (transient ischaemic attack), mental illness), results of previous investigations, allergies, medications (particularly anticoagulant or antiplatelet medications).
- *Social and employment history*—patterns of drug and alcohol use, environmental factors, stressors.

FIGURE 23.8 STRUCTURAL FEATURES OF NEURONS: DENDRITES, CELL BODY AND AXONS[9]

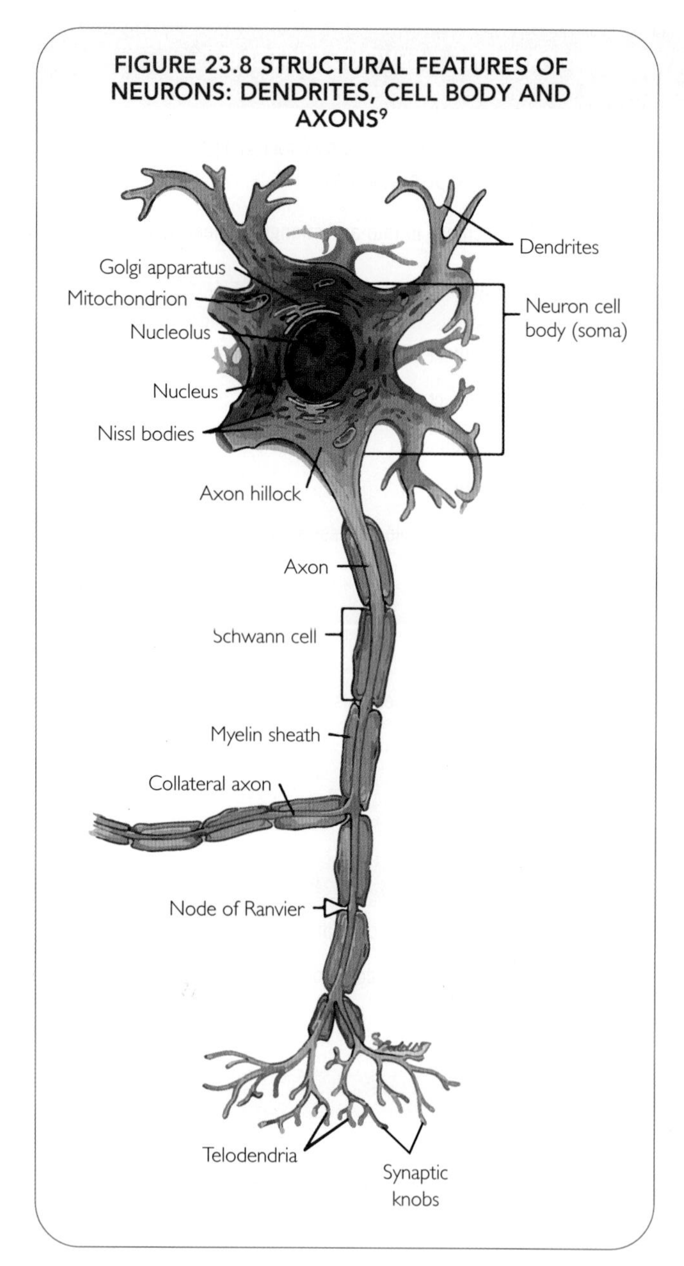

FIGURE 23.9 THE SYNAPSE IS LOCATED IN THE SPACE BETWEEN NEURON A AND NEURON B[9]

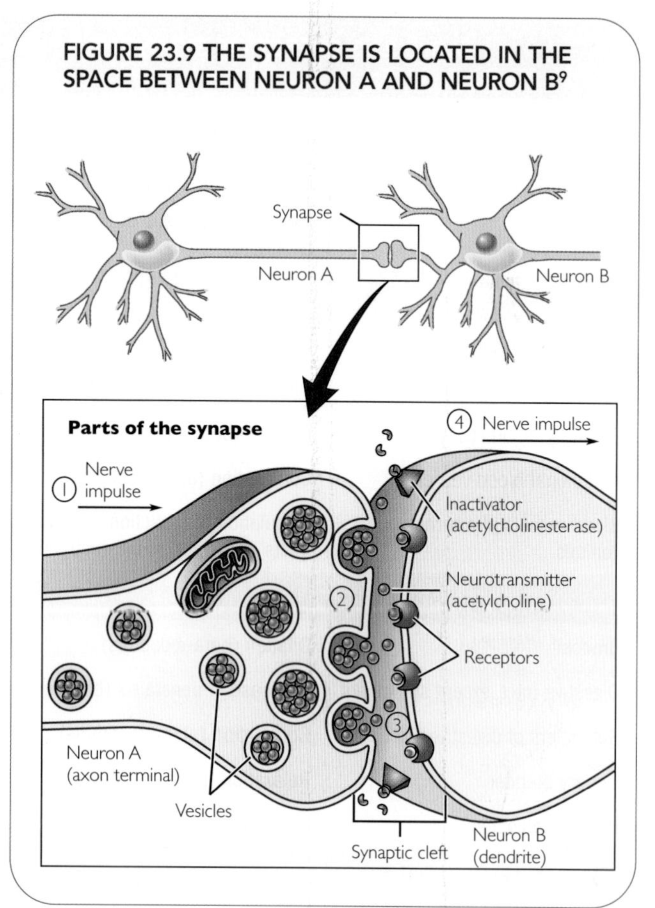

Parts of the synapse include the neurotransmitters, inactivators and receptors. The neurotransmitters are located in the vesicles of neuron A. The inactivators are located on the membrane of neuron B. The receptors are located on the membrane of neuron B.

- *Specific considerations for extremes of age*—developmental delay, intellectual disability, cognitive impairment, dementia, delirium (see Chapters 37 and 38).

Even when there is a history of illness that may easily explain an altered conscious state, all sudden deterioration should be treated as an acute event and thoroughly investigated.

PHYSICAL ASSESSMENT

As discussed earlier in this chapter, the brain is highly dependent on a continuous supply of oxygen and glucose.[5,6] Assessment priorities therefore include the identification and treatment (or exclusion and prevention) of hypoxia, hypotension and hypoglycaemia as causes of altered level of consciousness. The initial and ongoing assessment of patients with a neurological emergency is primarily aimed at identifying increasing ICP or evaluating the response to treatment for increased ICP. Frequent monitoring of vital signs (respiratory rate and pattern, heart rate and rhythm, blood pressure and oxygen saturation) provide important indicators of cerebral oxygenation and cerebral perfusion. Temperature should be measured to detect hypothermia, which, if extreme, may be a cause of altered level of consciousness (see Chapter 28). Conversely, an elevated temperature may suggest an infective cause or drug-related cause for an altered level of consciousness and, in severe cases, may cause altered level of consciousness.

As the brain is extremely sensitive to oxygen deprivation, a decreased level of consciousness is an early and reliable indicator of increased ICP.[11] Conscious state changes can be subtle (restlessness, agitation, anxiety, nausea or vomiting) or obvious (confusion, drowsiness and unconsciousness).[11] The Glasgow Coma Scale (GCS) assesses state of consciousness in adults, and in children the Paediatric Glasgow Coma Scale is used. The AVPU scale (Alert, responds to Voice, responds to Pain and Unresponsive) is useful as a rapid assessment tool, but should not replace formal assessment of GCS. Both of these scores assess eye opening, verbal response and motor response. The use of these scales in the emergency department (ED) is discussed in depth in Chapter 13.

Assessment of pupil size, equality and reactivity provides information regarding the presence and level of brainstem dysfunction.[11] Pressure on the oculomotor nerve (cranial nerve III) causes pupil dilation; however, this is a late sign of

BOX 23.1 CAUSES OF ALTERATION IN CONSCIOUS STATE[18]

STRUCTURAL INSULTS

Supratentorial

Haematoma
- Epidural
- Subdural

Cerebral tumour
Cerebral aneurysm
Haemorrhagic stroke

Infratentorial

Cerebellar arteriovenous malformation
Pontine haemorrhage
Brainstem tumour

METABOLIC INSULTS

Loss of substrate

Hypoxia
Hypoglycaemia
Global ischaemia
Shock
- Hypovolaemia
- Cardiogenic

Focal ischaemia
- Transient ischaemic attack/stroke
- Vasculitis

Derangement of normal physiology

Hypo- or hypernatraemia
Hyperglycaemia/hyperosmolarity
Hypercalcaemia
Hypermagnesaemia
Addisonian crisis
Seizures
- Status epilepticus
- Postictal

Post-concussive
Hypo- or hyperthyroidism
Cofactor deficiency
Metastatic malignancy
Psychiatric illness
Toxins
Drugs
- Alcohol
- Illicit
- Prescription

Endotoxins
- Subarachnoid blood
- Liver failure
- Renal failure

Sepsis
- Systemic

Focal
- Meningitis
- Encephalitis

Environmental
- Hypothermia/heat exhaustion
- Altitude illness/decompression
- Envenomations

increasing ICP. Patients with an altered conscious state should have a blood glucose test to exclude hypoglycaemia (see Chapter 26 for blood glucose sampling techniques). Hypoglycaemia is easily treated, quickly reversed and can present in many ways: agitation, confusion, restlessness, hemiplegia, slurred speech, fitting and unconsciousness. Hyperglycaemia may cause alterations in level of consciousness (see Chapter 26). Assessment of other symptoms such as pain, vomiting, fever, photophobia, urinary retention and under-sedation in the intubated patient should also be conducted, as they may further exacerbate increased ICP. Assessment of the unconscious patient is summarised in Box 23.2.

Herniation

If untreated, increased ICP will result in herniation of brain tissue—lateral (transtentorial), downward (central transtentorial) or medial (cingulate).[11,13]

- During lateral herniation, pressure on the oculomotor nerve results in sluggish, then fixed and dilated, pupils.[11]
- If herniation occurs laterally, pupillary changes will occur first in the ipsilateral pupil and then in the contralateral pupil.[11]
- During central herniation, pupils will be bilaterally small but reactive to light and then progress to bilateral fixed and dilated pupils.[11]
- If increased ICP continues, ischaemia of the vasomotor centre in the brainstem results in increased systemic blood pressure in an attempt to improve cerebral perfusion.[11]
- Cushing's reflex is a triad of the following signs: hypertension, widening pulse pressure and bradycardia; and is a late indicator of increased ICP indicating significant brainstem ischaemia.[11]
- Cheyne-Stokes respiration (deep, rapid breathing with periods of apnoea) and abnormal posturing may also be seen if brain herniation occurs.[11]

The structural changes that occur during herniation are shown in Figure 23.10.

INVESTIGATIONS

Investigations for the patient with neurological emergency may include routine blood tests, such as urea and electrolytes, full blood examination and coagulation profile. Specific tests that may be indicated, depending on the history and nature of presentation, may include drug levels, serum lactate, septic work-up and if envenoming is suspected, venom detection kits.[18] Routine drug screens are of limited clinical value.[18] A 12-lead electrocardiogram (ECG) should be performed to identify potential sources of cardiogenic emboli, cardiac dysrhythmias, specific rhythm changes related to hypokalaemia (J wave) and

BOX 23.2 **ASSESSMENT OF PATIENT WITH AN ALTERED CONSCIOUS STATE**[19]

PRIMARY SURVEY ASSESSMENT

Danger	Check for danger
Response	Check for patient responsiveness
Send for help	If the patient is unresponsive, send for help
Airway	Assess whether the patient is able to protect their airway If unable to protect airway, implement airway opening/protection manoeuvres
Cervical spine	Possible need for cervical spine care if neurological deficit is the cause or result of associated injury
Breathing	Respiratory rate Oxygen saturation–possible hypoxia Work of breathing
Circulation	Heart rate Blood pressure–possible hypo/hypertension Skin status 12-lead ECG–possible cardiac dysrhythmia, cardio-embolic event
Disability	AVPU GCS Assessment of pupils BSL–possible hypo/hyperglycaemia
Other	Temperature–possible sepsis

FOCUSED SYMPTOM ASSESSMENT USING THE PQRST MNEMONIC

Palliating/provoking factors	Known risk factors for: • headache, migraine • TIA/stroke/intracerebral haemorrhage • seizure disorders • dementia/delirium History of prescription medication/social or illicit drugs/alcohol use
Quality and quantity	Can the patient describe their symptoms? Are there other associated symptoms? • Fevers: possible CNS infection/sepsis • Rash: possible sepsis, allergy • Headache: possible migraine/headache syndromes/intracerebral haemorrhage • Tongue trauma/incontinence/soft-tissue injuries: possible seizure • Paralysis: unilateral = possible stroke; ascending = Guillain-Barré syndrome • Signs of head trauma: haematoma, soft-tissue injuries, Battle's sign, periorbital ecchymosis, rhinorrhoea, otorrhoea Do symptoms interrupt activities of daily living–sleeping, eating, bathing, walking?
Region/radiation	Headache? Do neurological symptoms affect other areas of the body–limbs, breathing?
Severity	How severe are the symptoms (pain/neurological deficits)? • 0 to 10 rating scale • Qualitative measures: mild, moderate, severe
Timing	How long does the symptom last? How often do symptoms occur? Are symptoms related to a particular time of day or a particular activity?

AVPU: Alert, Voice, Pain, Unresponsive; BSL: blood sugar level; CNS: central nervous system; GCS: Glasgow Coma Scale; ECG: electrocardiogram; TIA: transient ischaemic attack.

hypothermia (U wave) and myocardial ischaemia or infarction as potential sources of shock.[18]

LUMBAR PUNCTURE

Lumbar puncture (LP) examines the CSF, most commonly for CNS infections (meningitis, encephalitis), subarachnoid haemorrhage and cytological examination. ICP may also be estimated by LP, but dedicated ICP monitors are preferred.[18] Contraindications to LP include local infection at LP site, bleeding disorders and risk of CNS herniation.[20] Current recommendations suggest that adult patients with signs of increased intracranial pressure (e.g. papilloedema, altered mental status, focal neurological deficits, signs of meningeal irritation) should have CT imaging prior to lumbar puncture. In the

FIGURE 23.10 HERNIATION

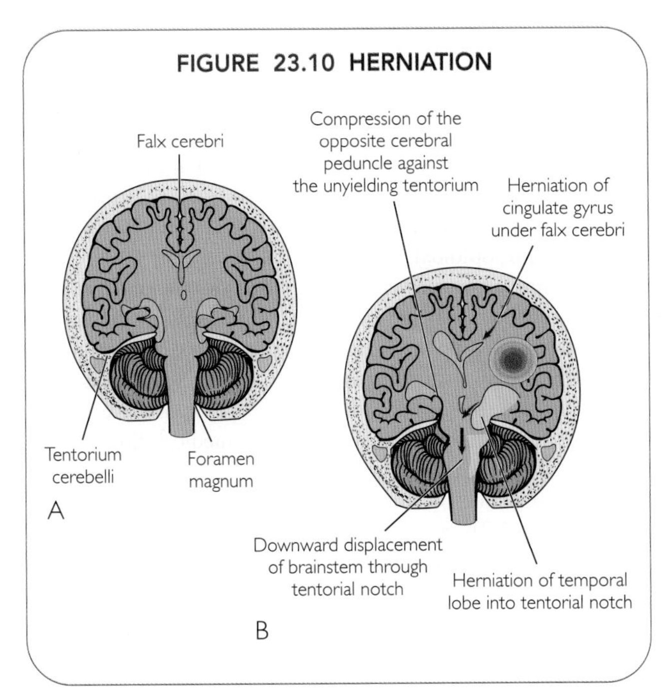

A. Normal relationship of intracranial structures.[16] **B.** Shift of intracranial structures.[16]

absence of signs of increased ICP, lumbar puncture can be performed without neuroimaging.[20] Intracranial imaging is most often performed using non-contrast CT brain scan and, depending on the nature of the presentation, a contrast-enhanced CT scan or MRI (magnetic resonance imaging) may also be performed.[18] All patients should have some form of local anaesthetic for lumbar puncture. Topical anaesthetic cream should be used (except where specimens are required urgently) and subcutaneous lidocaine should be used in addition to topical anaesthetic. Oral sucrose should be used for infants < 3 months, and sedation, including nitrous oxide, should be considered for those older than 6 months with normal conscious state.[21]

As an LP can be a stressful procedure, reassurance and explanation is vital. In children, the most important determinant of a successful lumbar puncture is a strong, calm, experienced assistant to hold the patient.[21] Patient position is critical. The patient should be positioned lying on their side with their back parallel to the edge of the bed. The patient's knees are flexed up to the chest with the chin touching the knees so that the back is arched. Alternatively, the patient may sit up leaning over a bed table. Ask the patient to slouch rather than bend from their hips.[20] Avoid over-flexing the neck, especially in infants, as this may cause respiratory compromise.[21] LP is a sterile procedure. Following preparation and draping of the site, vertebrae L3 and L4 are located and local anaesthetic is injected into the skin. The use of atraumatic needles reduces the risk of headache in adults; however, needle gauge has no effect on headache development.[20] Following the procedure, brief pressure and an occlusive dressing should be applied.

Post-lumbar puncture care

It is important to monitor for and be aware of potential complications related to LP. The most common LP-related complication is headache (sometimes called post-dural puncture headache, PDPH) and this affects as many as 85% of patients.[22] Onset of PDPH is usually 24–48 hours after LP, but can occur up to 12 days post-procedure. Headache is rarely present immediately following LP, so any headache present immediately post-procedure should be investigated to exclude increased ICP or displacement of intracranial structures. PDPHs are typically dull or throbbing, often start in frontal or occipital regions, but can become generalised, may radiate to the neck and shoulders and may be associated with lower back pain, nausea, vomiting, vertigo and tinnitus. The pathophysiology of PDPH is not well understood. Dural puncture does allow CSF to leak from the subarachnoid space, and it is thought that decreased CSF volume and pressure causes a downward pull on pain-sensitive structures resulting in a headache.[22] Another theory is that CSF loss may increase blood flow, resulting in PDPH from arterial and venous vasodilation.[22] The headache will continue until the hole heals and CSF pressure is restored; this headache typically lasts a few days and rarely more than 1 week. Factors that increase risk of PDPH are age less than 50 years, female gender, low body mass index, being postpartum, history of chronic headaches or previous PDPH.[22] Factors that do not increase risk of PDPH include patient position during LP, number of LP attempts, experience of clinician performing LP, volume of CSF removed and bed rest following LP.[22]

Most PDPHs (up to 85%) will resolve without any specific treatment,[20,22] and management, if required, is focused on symptom control. There is no strong evidence that bed rest prevents PDPH, but it may reduce headache intensity if PDPH occurs.[22] The evidence regarding use of additional oral or IV fluids to prevent or treat PDPH is inconclusive.[22] Gabapentin, hydrocortisone and theophylline have been shown to decrease pain severity scores in patients with PDPH.[20,22] Caffeine is a safe and effective option for PDPH as it causes vasoconstriction thereby decreasing cerebral blood flow and augments CFS production by activating sodium potassium pumps.[22] Caffeine is available as oral tablets; however, tea, coffee and cola drinks all contain sufficient caffeine to effectively treat PDPH and are often more practical to obtain. There is no evidence supporting the use of other medications, such as sumatriptan or adrenocorticotropic hormone.[22] The most common treatment for persistent PDPH is 'blood patch' which involves injecting 20–30 mL of the patient's blood into the epidural space so that the clot seals the dural perforation and prevents further CSF leak.[20] Blood patch is 70% to 98% effective if performed more than 24 hours post-LP.[20] Blood patch is contraindicated in patients with fever, local infection at the LP site and bleeding disorders.[22]

PATIENT MANAGEMENT

Management priorities for the pre-hospital and ED care of patients with an altered level of consciousness are preservation of airway, breathing and circulation, and optimisation of cerebral oxygenation and perfusion by ensuring adequate oxygenation and systemic blood pressure. Endotracheal intubation may be indicated for patients with a decreased level of consciousness if the patient is unable to maintain or protect his or her airway (see Chapter 16 for intubation procedures). A GCS score ≤ 8 is often used to indicate the need for endotracheal intubation, particularly in poisoned patients (see Chapter 30);

however, the GCS score on its own is a relatively poor predictor of the need for intubation and should be considered in the context of the overall patient presentation.[18] Supplemental oxygen or assisted ventilation may be warranted if hypoxia, hypercapnia or hypoventilation is present. Hypotension should be treated by fluid resuscitation and/or inotropes or vasopressors.[18] In the setting of increased ICP, hypercapnia and acidosis should be avoided and ventilatory settings should aim to achieve normocarbia and normoxia.[18]

The 'coma cocktail'—glucose, thiamine and naloxone—previously recommended for all unconscious patients, is no longer advocated,[23] although some agents may be useful, depending on the history and nature of the presentation. Point-of-care glucose testing can determine the need for glucose or dextrose supplementation (see Chapter 26 for blood glucose sampling procedure).[24] Administration of naloxone may be warranted if there is a history suggestive of opiate use and clinical signs such as pinpoint pupils and hypoventilation, and in this context naloxone may be both therapeutic and diagnostic.[23] Thiamine administration is recommended in patients in whom alcohol abuse or hepatic encephalopathy is suspected (see Chapter 40).[25] There is no evidence to support recommendations that thiamine should be administered prior to glucose administration and that correction of hypoglycaemia should occur prior to thiamine administration.[26] The routine use of flumazenil in patients with altered conscious state is not recommended.[24]

The management of altered conscious state in the context of traumatic brain injury is discussed in Chapter 43. Depending on the pathology, other medications may be considered: for example, steroids, anticonvulsants or antibiotics.

PRACTICE TIP

MANAGEMENT PRIORITIES IN THE PATIENT WITH ALTERED CONSCIOUS STATE

- Airway—position, endotracheal intubation if indicated
- Breathing—treat/prevent hypoxaemia, prevent hyperoxia, aim for normocarbia
- Circulation—ensure adequate blood pressure to increase cerebral perfusion pressure
- Disability—treat/prevent hypo/hyperglycaemia

DELIRIUM

Delirium is acute brain failure and commonly, but not always, affects older patients.[27] Delirium is rapid in onset (over hours to a few days), and key features are disturbed consciousness, inattention, impaired cognition and perception. Classically symptoms can fluctuate and periods of altered consciousness may alternate with relatively lucid periods.[27] Delirium can be classified as hypoactive (whereby the patient is quiet and withdrawn), hyperactive (whereby the patient is restless and agitated) or mixed.[27] When adjusted for age, delirium is associated with increased risk of death, length of hospital stay, falls risk, discharge to higher dependency of care and risk of developing dementia.[27] It is estimated that 10% to 18% of patients aged 65 years or older have delirium at the time of hospital admission, and 2% to 8% will develop delirium during their hospital stay.[27] A 2021 systematic review of 34 studies showed that the prevalence of ED delirium was 7% to 35%.[28] The factors strongly associated with ED delirium were residing in residential aged care, cognitive impairment, hearing impairment, history of stroke, ED length of stay of greater than 10 hours and severe pain (rather than the use of opioids).[28]

Delirium can be prevented and outcomes for patients with delirium can also be improved by early intervention. All patients should have screening for cognitive impairment using a validated tool, particularly if they are aged ≥ 65 years (≥ 45 years for Aboriginal and Torres Strait Islander peoples), or have known cognitive impairment or dementia, severe medical illness or hip fracture.[28] Patients and carers should also be asked whether the patient's behaviour or thinking has changed in the preceding hours or days.[28] There are a number of screening tools for cognitive impairment, delirium and dementia. The 4AT has been validated for use in EDs, acute care and subacute care settings and can also be used in patients with limited English proficiency or dementia.[29] There are also culturally sensitive screening tools such as the Rowland Universal Dementia Assessment Scale (RUDAS) and the Kimberley Indigenous Cognitive Assessment tools (KICA).[29] The Confusion Assessment Method (CAM) is one of the most widely used tools for assessing delirium, although there are concerns about variability in its application. The 3-Minute Diagnostic Assessment for Delirium (3D-CAM) is also used, but may underestimate delirium.[29]

Delirium may be prevented by reviewing medications, correcting states such as dehydration, malnutrition and constipation, enabling mobility, pain assessment and management, regular reorientation, including clocks, clear signage and, where possible, exposure to daylight via windows or skylights, activities for stimulating cognition, regular toileting and ensuring communication maintained through use of hearing and visual aids.[27] Non-pharmacological approaches to delirium, such as adequate lighting, psychosocial support, reorientation activities, and mobilisation, assist patients to interpret their surroundings correctly and are the standard of care.[24] The use of antipsychotic medicines for management of delirium should be minimised as they have a number of serious adverse effects for older people and can worsen delirium; however, they will occasionally be required to prevent immediate harm to the patient or carers.[27] There is no role for prophylactic antipsychotics in the prevention of delirium.[30] There are more details about acute confusional states and behavioural disturbance in Chapters 36, 37 and 38.

TRANSIENT ISCHAEMIC ATTACKS

Transient ischaemic attack (TIA) is defined as focal neurological symptoms due to focal ischaemia *that have fully resolved*.[31] Patients with ongoing or fluctuating symptoms should be treated as having an acute stroke.[31] The highest risk of stroke occurring following TIA is within the first 2 days; therefore, prevention of progression to stroke is a key focus of care of the patient with TIA.[31] Key aspects of the history that are useful to help identify TIA from other conditions are as follows:[31]

- *Age and other demographics:* is there a high probability of a cerebrovascular event from hypertension, ischaemic heart disease, diabetes, smoking, haematological disease?

- *Nature of the symptoms:* TIA involves the sudden onset of a focal neurological deficit: weakness, numbness (not paraesthesia in isolation), visual loss, speech disturbance
- *Duration:* the average duration is approximately 10 minutes, but all symptoms must be fully resolved within 24 hours.

ASSESSMENT

All patients with TIA should have an urgent and thorough clinical assessment, baseline blood tests, ECG and brain imaging.[31] It is essential that emergency clinicians obtain a thorough history in order to establish the risk of stroke. The highest risk of stroke occurring following TIA is within the first 2 days.[31] ABCD^2 is a risk-stratification tool that identifies **A**ge, **B**lood pressure, **C**linical characteristics, **D**uration and **D**iabetes risk factors for stroke after TIA.[31,32]

ABCD^2 can be used as an adjunct to clinical assessment but its use in isolation to determine clinical urgency is not recommended and may delay recognition of important risk factors such as atrial fibrillation and carotid stenosis.[31] The use of ABCD^2 has been called into question given the mixed results of ongoing validation studies,[33] thus, the ABCD^2 score has been modified to ABCD^3-I, which adds a history of ≥ two TIAs within the preceding week and imaging results (MRI and carotid imaging) to ABCD.^{2} The ABCD^3-I score has been shown to have superior performance as a risk-stratification tool for risk of early and 3-month ischemic stroke following TIA and minor stroke.[34]

Vital-sign monitoring in both pre-hospital and ED environments should aim to ensure adequate ventilation, oxygenation and cerebral perfusion, and frequent neurological observations should be performed to identify neurological deterioration or symptom progression. Blood glucose level should be measured to exclude hypoglycaemia as a cause for symptoms and to identify diabetes as a potential risk factor or TIA mimic (see Chapter 26 for blood glucose sampling procedure).[31,32] All patients with TIA should have a 12-lead ECG to exclude or confirm atrial fibrillation: a period of cardiac monitoring may also be indicated.[31,32] Brain imaging options include CT scan, MRI, ultrasonography (Doppler) and angiography;[31,32] all patients with TIA should have brain imaging to exclude stroke and intracerebral haemorrhage.[31,32] Carotid imaging should also preferably be performed during the initial assessment.[31]

MANAGEMENT

Management of TIA aims to identify and treat the cause and prevent progression to stroke.[31,32] The major treatment modalities for TIA are risk-factor modification, antiplatelet therapy and carotid endarterectomy.[31,32] Hypertension, diabetes, hyperlipidaemia, smoking and lack of exercise are all well-known risk factors for vascular disease, so patients with TIA should be referred to appropriate services for risk-factor reduction.[31,35]

Hypertension is a common feature in ED patients with TIA. If it is suspected that hypertension is causing neurological features, long-term oral antihypertensive therapy should be commenced; however, urgent blood pressure reduction in the ED is not indicated and may be harmful. Antiplatelet therapy is the most common treatment for TIA. One of the most commonly used antiplatelet agents in Australia is aspirin; however, other agents such as clopidogrel and dipyridamole may also be used in isolation or in combination with aspirin.[33]

Disposition and follow-up of patients with TIA will be dependent on institutional resources and patient risk factors. High-risk patients may warrant admission, whereas other patients may be discharged with antiplatelet therapy and neurology or primary-care follow-up. Irrespective of the source, early follow-up is important in patients who have suffered a TIA. TIA pathways involving primary care, EDs and stroke specialist teams are effective in ensuring that patients are managed as rapidly and comprehensively as possible. The 2020 National Stroke Audit of Acute Services, with data from 111 public and four private services, showed that 86% of hospitals had defined policies, processes of pathways for management of patients with TIA and 50% of hospitals had rapid TIA assessment clinics.[36]

PRACTICE TIP

TIA

Any patient with ongoing or fluctuating symptoms of TIA should be treated as if they are having an acute stroke.

VERTEBROBASILAR ATTACKS

Vertebrobasilar insufficiency is used to describe TIA syndromes of the posterior circulation.[32] Dizziness is the most common symptom of vertebrobasilar ischaemia; other symptoms include unilateral weakness, dysarthria, headache, nausea and vomiting.[37] Common clinical signs of vertebrobasilar ischaemia include unilateral limb weakness, ataxia, dysphagia, and visual disturbance.[37] Sensory deficits can be either contralateral or crossed (e.g. contralateral deficits involving the body suggest medial medullary infarct, and ipsilateral deficits involving the face suggest lateral medullary infarct).[37] Vertebrobasilar attacks may be a cause of collapse, syncopal episode or sudden loss of consciousness. Insufficiency may be provoked by position: turning the head partially can occlude the ipsilateral vertebral artery and invoke symptoms.[38] Very rarely, vertebrobasilar (basilar artery) occlusion from a thrombosis or embolism can result in 'locked in' syndrome.[37] Patients with 'locked in' syndrome appear unconscious and are paralysed and unable to speak, but have intact consciousness and understanding.[37] Investigations of symptoms include Doppler/ultrasound, CT or MRI angiography.[37] Treatment may include endovascular approaches, but is more commonly anti-platelet therapy, statins and blood pressure control.[38]

STROKE

Stroke is an acute neurological injury that is caused by interruption to the blood flow to an area of the brain.[32,33] Stroke is one of Australia's biggest killers and kills more women than breast cancer and more men than prostate cancer.[39] One Australian has a stroke every 19 minutes and stroke costs the Australian economy $6.1 billion per year.[40] Strokes can be classified as ischaemic or haemorrhagic.[32]

ISCHAEMIC STROKE

Approximately 80% of strokes are ischaemic, resulting from three major pathophysiological processes: thrombi, emboli and hypoperfusion.[32] The most common cause of stroke is thrombosis, or blood-vessel narrowing secondary to clot formation.[32,33] Atherosclerosis is the most common cause of thrombotic stroke; however, other causes include vasculitis, polycythaemia and infectious diseases. Embolic stroke occurs when a normal cerebral blood vessel is occluded by fragments from a clot arising from outside the brain, commonly the heart and major vessels.[32,33] Cardiogenic emboli most commonly results from atrial fibrillation; however, other cardiac causes such as AMI, valve disease resulting in vegetations and atrial or ventricular septal defects are recognised.[33] Less-common causes of embolic stroke are fat emboli, emboli arising from intravenous drug use or septic emboli.[33] Hypoperfusion is an uncommon cause of ischaemic stroke and occurs most often as a consequence of profound hypotension (such as may occur in septic or cardiogenic shock).[33] Hypoperfusion causes more diffuse injury than thrombotic or embolic strokes and typically causes infarcts in separate vascular territories.[33]

Cerebral injury from ischaemic stroke is directly related to lack of blood supply. As neurons are highly dependent on a continuous supply of oxygen and glucose, when blood flow is interrupted they die within a few minutes.[33] Even with complete occlusion of a cerebral blood vessel, collateral blood flow and local tissue pressure gradients preserve some perfusion to the ischaemic area[33]. Cell death occurs at the centre of the ischaemic area and this is surrounded by an area of potentially reversible injury (the penumbra).[33] The viability of cells in the penumbra is dependent on the severity and duration of the occlusion and the timing of re-perfusion.[33]

HAEMORRHAGIC STROKE

Approximately 20% of strokes are haemorrhagic and the commonest cause of haemorrhagic stroke is hypertension.[32] Other causes include haemorrhage from ruptured aneurysms, vascular malformations and tumours.[32,33] Cerebral injury occurs as a result of increased intracranial pressure, local compression and decreased perfusion.[33]

Subarachnoid haemorrhage

While typically presenting in a manner distinct to ischaemic or haemorrhagic stroke, subarachnoid haemorrhage (SAH) is classified as a kind of stroke. When a spontaneous SAH occurs, blood leaks into the subarachnoid space from a cerebral vessel.[33] In 85% of occurrences it is caused by a cerebral aneurysm rupture.[41] The incidence of subarachnoid haemorrhage is around 10 cases per 100,000 person-years and half of patients with SAH are aged less than 55 years.[41] A sudden onset of severe headache is a key feature of SAH: the headache is typically occipital and often described by patients as 'the worst headache of their life' which instantly peaks.[41,42] Associated symptoms (in addition to headache) that increase the likelihood of subarachnoid haemorrhage include exertional onset, syncope, nausea and vomiting, neck pain and seizure.[41,42] Patients are classified into clinical grades according to their conscious state and neurological deficit (Table 23.4).[41,42] Subarachnoid haemorrhage has a 40–60% mortality rate and as many as one-third of survivors of subarachnoid haemorrhage have a neurological deficit.[41]

TABLE 23.4 CLINICAL GRADING SCHEMES FOR PATIENTS WITH SAH[41,42]

GRADING SCHEME OF HUNT AND HESS

Grade	Symptoms
1	No symptoms or minimal headache, slight nuchal rigidity
2	Moderate to severe headache, no neurological deficit other than cranial nerve palsy
3	Drowsy, confused, mild focal deficit
4	Stupor, moderate to severe hemiparesis, vegetative posturing
5	Deep coma, decerebration, moribund

RISK FACTORS

Non-modifiable risk factors for stroke include age (stroke rate doubles for every 10 years after age 55), male gender and positive family history.[32] Hypertension is the single-most important risk factor that is amenable to change, and effective antihypertensive therapy has been shown to reduce the incidence of stroke. Risk of stroke is increased by risk factors for atherosclerosis (smoking, hyperlipidaemia, diabetes). Atrial fibrillation is the most significant cardiac risk factor; however, other cardiac risk factors include endocarditis, cardiac valve prostheses, recent AMI and mitral stenosis.[32] Carotid stenosis or a carotid bruit in asymptomatic patients is also a risk factor for stroke.[32]

SIGNS AND SYMPTOMS OF STROKE

The signs and symptoms of stroke are variable and clinical differentiation between an ischaemic and haemorrhagic stroke is unreliable.[32] As discussed earlier in this chapter, cerebral blood supply is divided into the anterior and posterior circulations. The signs and symptoms of ischaemic stroke depend on the brain area affected.

The anterior circulation supplies the optic nerve, retina and frontoparietal and temporal lobes.[32] Signs and symptoms associated with anterior circulation disruption are those classically associated with stroke such as unilateral weakness or paralysis, speech and comprehension difficulties (receptive and expressive aphasia) visual disturbance, motor and sensory facial deficits, difficulty writing and calculating numbers, unilateral neglect and difficulty dressing.[32] Less-common features are those associated with disruption to the supply from the anterior cerebral artery. These include sensory and motor changes commonly affecting the leg rather than the arm, subtle personality changes, conjugate gaze and urinary dysfunction.[32]

The posterior circulation supplies the cerebellum, brainstem, thalamus and temporal and occipital lobes.[32] Signs and symptoms associated with posterior circulation disruption include visual disturbance, motor and sensory deficits that may be unilateral or bilateral, cerebellar signs (ataxia, vertigo, nystagmus) and cranial nerve palsies resulting in dysarthria, vertigo and diplopia.[32] Brainstem strokes are characterised by ipsilateral cranial nerve or cerebellar signs.[32] Altered level of consciousness occurs when there is reticular-activating-system ischaemia.[32] Signs and symptoms associated with haemorrhagic stroke may include history of prolonged hypertension, sudden onset of symptoms, headache, vomiting, collapse and history of anticoagulant medications.[32]

ASSESSMENT

Stroke is a medical emergency and the triage of stroke patients should reflect the fact that early diagnosis, treatment and referral to specialist services is pivotal to improving patient outcomes and preventing complications.[31,43] Current guidelines recommend that ED clinicians use a validated stroke screening tool (such as ROSIER: Recognition of Stroke in the Emergency Room or NIHSS: National Institute of Health Stroke Scale).[31] Early assessment and management of acute stroke should focus on optimal triage decisions, physiological surveillance, fluid management, risk management and prevention of complications, and early referral to specialists.[31,43] Paramedics play a key role in prioritising transfer to hospital and early notification to EDs to facilitate efficient stroke management.[31,43] Triage decisions are a key determinant of care for patients with actual or potential acute stroke. The National Stroke Foundation 'FAST' test is useful for identifying patients with actual or potential stroke in both pre-hospital and ED environments.[43,45] 'FAST' stands for:[43,45]

- **F**ace: has the patient's mouth unilaterally drooped?
- **A**rms: can they lift both arms?
- **S**peech: is their speech slurred? Do they understand you?
- **T**ime: time is critical in patients with any of the above signs.

Patients with current or fluctuating symptoms should be treated as having a stroke and be immediately transported to an ED for stroke specialist assessment, investigations and consideration of reperfusion therapy.[31,43] Pre-notification should be provided to the receiving ED.[31,43] As thrombolysis or endovascular clot retrieval (ECR) are time-critical interventions in acute stroke, facilitation of rapid assessment and identification of patients who may be eligible for thrombolysis or ECR or transfer for thrombolysis should be a major priority for pre-hospital and ED triage personnel.[31,43]

In Australia, most patients with stroke arrive at hospital by ambulance (76%): 30% of patients arrive at hospital within 3 hours, and 37% arrive within 4.5 hours of stroke symptom onset.[36] In recent years, specialist stroke care has become available in the out-of-hospital environment via mobile stroke units (MSUs), which have onboard CT imaging, pathology testing capability and high-speed wireless data transmission.[47–50] A 2022 systematic review and meta-analysis of 14 studies (including three random clinical trials, three non-randomised trials and eight observational studies) found that, compared with usual care, patients managed by a MSU had a better neurological outcome at 90 days (OR of a Modified Rankin Score 0–1 was 1.64 (1.27–2.13)), an increased rate of thrombolysis (OR 1.83 (1.58–2.12)), and no increase in symptomatic intracranial haemorrhage.[51] There was no mortality difference noted; however, the analysis was not adequately powered to identify one.[51] Studies from Melbourne Australia show that compared to usual care, MSU care substantially reduced time to reperfusion therapies by a median time of 26 minutes ($p < 0.001$) for ambulance dispatch to hospital arrival, 15 minutes ($p < 0.001$) for hospital arrival to thrombolysis, and overall time-saving from ambulance dispatch to thrombolysis of 42.5 minutes.[50] For endovascular thrombectomy, the median time saving was 17 minutes ($p = 0.001$) for hospital arrival to arterial puncture.[50] In addition, MSU service was also cost effective in terms of disability-adjusted life years avoided.[49]

Although current stroke guidelines do not make clear recommendations about ED triage category allocation in actual or suspected stroke,[31] they do refer to stroke as a 'time-critical emergency'.[43] In Australia, these recommendations equate to Category 2 of the Australasian Triage Scale.[52] Like other groups of patients, such as trauma and acute coronary syndrome, patients with stroke benefit from organised systems of care that harness the skills of emergency clinicians and specialist stroke clinicians and 'Code Stroke' and stroke team activation from the ED is a common and important element of stroke care. All patients with suspected acute stroke, who have been pre-notified to the stroke or ED team, and who may be eligible for reperfusion therapy, should be met at arrival and assessed by the stroke team or other experienced personnel.[31]

History is an important factor in the diagnosis and management of stroke (see Case Study at the end of this chapter). Accurate information regarding onset of symptoms is vital to assist in deciding the treatment options available for patients. For example, current National Stroke Foundation Guidelines recommend that thrombolytics may be beneficial in selected patients with acute ischaemic stroke if administered up to 4.5 hours after symptom onset.[31] Issues related to thrombolysis administration in acute stroke are discussed later in this chapter.

PRACTICE TIP

INITIAL ASSESSMENT AND TRIAGE OF PATIENTS WITH STROKE

All patients with stroke should be managed as a time-critical emergency and be preferentially transported to a hospital capable of delivering reperfusion therapies and stroke unit care.

All patients who have current or fluctuating symptoms suggestive of acute stroke should be triaged to at least Australasian Triage Scale category 2.

INVESTIGATIONS

All patients with actual or suspected stroke should have a thorough examination, baseline blood tests, ECG and brain imaging.[31,44] Frequent neurological observations should be performed to identify neurological deterioration or progression of symptoms. ECG changes are not uncommon in patients with acute stroke.[53,54] Common ECG changes include prolonged QT interval, ST segment changes, and T wave abnormalities.[53,54] As many as 25% of patients have severe cardiac arrhythmias causing clinical symptoms or requiring urgent clinical evaluation within 72 hours of stroke, the most common of which is atrial fibrillation.[54] An ECG should be performed to identify sources of cardiogenic emboli, such as atrial fibrillation or recent AMI, and signs of pre-existing cardiac disease.[32] The duration and mode of cardiac monitoring should be guided by the patient's clinical status, but is recommended for at least the first 24 hours.[31]

Brain imaging

Urgent brain imaging in patients with acute stroke is needed to confirm cerebral ischaemia or intracerebral haemorrhage and exclude stroke mimics. MRI is more sensitive than non-contrast CT in the detection of ischaemia; however, delays in accessing MRI and limited availability in some settings means that CT remains a commonly used imaging modality for patients with stroke.[31] CT has good sensitivity for the diagnosis of haemorrhage. All patients with suspected stroke who are eligible for reperfusion therapies should undergo immediate brain imaging.[32] All other patients with suspected stroke should have urgent brain CT or MRI, preferably within 60 minutes.[32] Australian audit data from 2021 showed that 45% of patients had imaging performed within 1 hour of arrival to hospital, 73% of imaging was CT scans and the median time to brain imaging from ED arrival was 64 minutes.[36]

CT perfusion scanning may be used in addition to usual brain imaging. CT perfusion imaging involves repeated brain imaging with intravenous contrast bolus. Delayed blood flow may indicate an ischaemic stroke and regions with severely reduced blood flow are likely to be irreversibly injured: large regions with severely disrupted blood flow are associated with a worse prognosis whereas strokes with smaller areas of severely impaired perfusion and larger penumbras may respond better to reperfusion therapies.[31] Following initial brain imaging, imaging should be repeated if there is a change in the patient's clinical status, as there may be treatable or reversible evolving pathology.[31] Although it is likely the patient will not be in ED, brain imaging should be routinely repeated at 24 hours after reperfusion therapy to exclude the development of haemorrhagic complications that might alter subsequent antithrombotic management, and confirming infarct size, which also has treatment and prognostic implications.[31]

Vascular imaging

Patients who are potentially eligible for endovascular thrombectomy should have vascular imaging from aortic arch to cerebral vertex using CT or MRI angiography to determine whether there is a vascular occlusion that may be a target for thrombectomy and also to assess proximal vascular access.[31] Vascular imaging is not recommended for syncope or other non-focal neurological presentations.[31]

MANAGEMENT

The management priorities for a patient with stroke are dependent on the nature and site of the stroke, the underlying cause and assessment of treatment risks and benefits.[32]

Restoration of airway, breathing and circulation is the first priority for all patients, including patients with stroke.[32] For patients with stroke, adequate ventilation, oxygenation and cerebral perfusion are essential. Airway support by endotracheal intubation may be indicated in patients with decreased conscious state. Altered conscious state is uncommon in ischaemic stroke, but may occur with haemorrhagic stroke and is common in SAH (see Chapter 16 for intubation procedures). In a cluster randomised controlled trial of evidence-based nurse-led interventions for the management of fever, sugar and swallowing in stroke units resulted in a 16% reduction in 90-day death and disability.[55] Although a more recent cluster randomised controlled trial of the same interventions in EDs did not show an effect,[56] there is an evidence base to support the active management of fever, sugar and swallow.

Impaired swallowing is associated with increased mortality following stroke, so patients with acute stroke should have their swallowing screened within 4 hours of ED arrival and before being given any oral food, fluid or medication.[44] Swallow screening should be by a trained healthcare professional using a validated screening tool. Patients who fail swallow screening should have a swallowing assessment by a speech pathologist.[44] Mild hypoxia is common in stroke patients, affecting up to 63% of patients, and is associated with increased cerebral injury and neurological deterioration;[44] therefore, assessment of oxygen saturation is an important element of assessment in patients with stroke. Hyperoxia is also problematic for patients with stroke as it causes vasoconstriction and the formation of toxic free radicals that further damage the ischaemic brain.[44] The routine use of supplemental oxygen in patients with acute stroke who are not hypoxaemic is not recommended: supplemental oxygen should be given to patients who have an oxygen saturation of < 95%.[44] If supplemental oxygen is used, aiming for an oxygen saturation of 96–98% will avoid hyperoxia.

Hypertension can be a cause of stroke but also is often a physiological response to preserve cerebral perfusion pressure in the setting of cerebral ischaemia and increased intracranial pressure.[32] Hypertension occurs in as many as 75% of patients with acute stroke,[57] and as many as 70% of patients with stroke have a history of high blood pressure on admission.[44] Hypertension can be harmful in both acute ischaemic stroke and haemorrhagic stroke. In acute ischaemic stroke, hypertension is independently associated with poor outcomes (recurrent stroke, death and dependency).[57,58] In acute intracerebral haemorrhage, hypertension may be associated with increased bleeding and haematoma.[57,58] Current guidelines recommend that all patients with acute stroke should have their blood pressure closely monitored in the first 48 hours after stroke onset.[44]

Patients with acute ischaemic stroke eligible for treatment with intravenous thrombolysis should have their blood pressure reduced to below 185/110 mmHg before treatment and in the first 24 hours after treatment.[44] Patients with acute ischaemic stroke with blood pressure > 220/120 mmHg should have their blood pressure cautiously reduced (e.g. by no more than 20%) over the first 24 hours.[44] Other causes for hypertension, such as pain, vomiting or urinary retention, should be considered and, if present, treated appropriately. Patients with haemorrhagic stroke should ideally have their systolic blood pressure lowered to less than 160 mmHg. This will often require IV antihypertensives such as labetalol or sodium nitroprusside, invasive arterial blood pressure monitoring and ICU admission. However, there is some evidence that patients who present with initial SBP > 220 mmHg may do worse with aggressive blood pressure control.[59] All patients with haemorrhagic stroke require specialist neurology or neurosurgery input.

Hyperglycaemia after stroke is common and occurs in approximately one-third of patients, although reports in the literature vary between 8% and 83%, depending on the patient group and definition of hyperglycaemia.[44] Further, 16–24% of patients admitted with stroke have pre-existing but undiagnosed diabetes.[44] Hyperglycaemia fluctuates the most during the first 72 hours after acute stroke and this is the case irrespective of whether the patient has diabetes[44] and has been associated with poor neurological outcomes and increased infarct size.[44] All patients with acute stroke should have their blood glucose level monitored for the first 72 hours following admission, and hyperglycaemia (glucose levels greater than 10 mmol/L) should be actively treated, regardless of the patient's diabetic status:[44] glycaemic monitoring and management should commence in the ED. There is no evidence that tight glycaemic control (between 4.0 and 7.5 mmol/L) is of benefit, and in fact may be harmful so is not recommended.[44]

Hyperthermia in the early phase of acute stroke increases mortality and infarct size. Hyperthermia (temperature greater than 37.5°C) occurs in 20–50% of patients in the first few days of acute stroke.[44] Current guidelines recommend that all patients with acute stroke have their temperature monitored at least four times a day for 72 hours and that temperatures greater than 37.5°C should be treated with paracetamol.[44] Temperature monitoring and management should commence in the ED.

There are a number of pathways and guidelines for management of acute stroke, although in Australia, the National Stroke Foundation Guidelines would be considered a key source of evidence-based information.[31,43] The management of cerebral oedema and increased ICP is discussed in detail in Chapter 43.

Specialist referrals and interventions

One of the key principles of stroke care should be getting the patient to specialist expertise as soon as possible. There is good evidence that stroke unit care improves stroke outcomes, and getting the patient to a stroke unit in a timely manner is one of the single most important recommendations for improving stroke management.[44] Stroke units provide organised inpatient stroke unit care and improve a number of outcomes. For every 1000 stroke patients, stroke unit care results in 44 fewer deaths at 12 months; 64 fewer deaths or patients in institutional care at 12 months; and 54 fewer deaths or dependent patients at 12 months.[44] The evidence to date supports that stroke care must be delivered in the one area and mobile stroke teams are of little benefit[44]. While numbers of stroke units and stroke unit beds have increased between 2010 and 2016, the percentage of patients receiving stroke unit care has not increased.[44] Patient transfer from the ED to a stroke unit should be a high priority and ED clinicians should facilitate getting patients with acute stroke to definitive care. Based on current evidence, patients with stroke should be transferred directly to a stroke unit and not via assessment units or medical wards, irrespective of ED key performance indicators.[44]

Urinary and/or faecal incontinence can occur due to stroke-related impairments such as weakness, cognitive impairment and decreased mobility.[31,60] Incontinence is associated with stroke-related complications such as depression, and can precipitate other adverse events such as falls or can result in prolonged recovery.[31,60] Thorough assessment of continence may not occur in the ED, but it is important that use of indwelling catheters as initial management of urinary retention or incontinence should be avoided.[31,60] If catheterisation is required then intermittent catheterisation is preferable to the use of indwelling urinary catheters.[60]

ISCHAEMIC STROKE MANAGEMENT

There is high certainty evidence that shows aspirin significantly reduces death and dependency and recurrent stroke in patients with ischaemic stroke who are not receiving reperfusion therapy.[44] Therefore, patients with ischaemic stroke should receive aspirin within 48 hours.[44] Further, it is important that the patient can safely swallow if aspirin is to be administered orally. Reperfusion therapy may be intravenous thrombolysis or endovascular thrombectomy (clot retrieval).[44] Current National Stroke Foundation guidelines[44] recommend that thrombolysis (alteplase) should be given as early as possible in eligible patients, but may be used up to 4.5 hours after stroke onset.[44] Use of thrombolysis after 4.5 hours of symptom onset has not been shown to be of any benefit.[44] Clinicians should consult current National Stroke Foundation guidelines[44] and their organisational guidelines for the indications, contraindications and relative contraindications for thrombolysis in acute ischaemic stroke.[44] Decisions regarding the use of thrombolysis should be based on the patient's pre-morbid level of function rather than chronological age.[44] Thrombolysis rates in Australia and internationally remain low. The 2021 National Stroke Audit showed that 88% of Australian hospitals have thrombolysis capability.[36] In 2021 there was a reduction in delivery of thrombolysis within 60 minutes of hospital from 32% in 2019 to 27% in 2021.[36] Nationally, the median time from onset (patient awareness) of stroke symptoms to thrombolysis was 2 hours and 50 minutes which is also a significant decrease compared to previous audits.[36] Regional services with formal acute telehealth support have higher thrombolysis rates compared to regional services without telehealth.[36]

Endovascular thrombectomy (also called mechanical thrombectomy or endovascular clot retrieval) is a minimally invasive procedure performed via angiogram, most commonly via the femoral artery. Neuro-interventions are a rapidly emerging field and offer an alternative or an adjunct to thrombolysis which has a narrow time-window for administration, has a number of absolute and relative contraindications and limited efficacy in patients with proximal large arterial occlusions.[44] As with intravenous thrombolysis, the earlier the removal of the clot the more likely improved patient outcomes are, so time is of the essence.

Current recommendations are that for patients with ischaemic stroke caused by a large vessel occlusion in the internal carotid artery, proximal cerebral artery or with occlusion of both the cervical carotid and intracranial arteries, endovascular thrombectomy should be undertaken when the procedure can be commenced within 6 hours of stroke onset.[44] Eligible patients should receive intravenous thrombolysis while endovascular thrombectomy is being arranged: neither treatment should delay the other.[44] The 2021 National Stroke Audit data showed that 13% of participating hospitals had 24-hour per day endovascular thrombectomy capability; however, at the time of writing, endovascular thrombectomy was not available in the Northern Territory.[36] During 2021, there was a 15% increase in the number of endovascular thrombectomy procedures (1907 in 2019 versus 2194 in 2021).[36]

HAEMORRHAGIC STROKE MANAGEMENT

The management of intracerebral haemorrhage is dependent on the location, cause, neurological deficit and patient's clinical condition.[32] Cerebral oedema and increased ICP tend to occur more acutely in haemorrhagic strokes; however, ischaemic strokes can also have haemorrhagic complications that can occur spontaneously or as a result of anticoagulant or thrombolytic treatments.[32] Neurosurgical referral should occur early for patients with potential for surgical intervention[32] Management of SAH is directed at maintaining oxygenation, reducing hypertension and increased ICP[33] and surgical aneurysm clipping.[41] Re-bleeding and vasospasm are major complications of SAH.[33]. Re-bleeding is most likely to occur in the first 24 hours, and blood pressure control (mean arterial pressure of 110 mmHg) decreases the risk of re-bleeding and is associated with decreased mortality.[33] Cerebral ischaemia secondary to vasospasm can occur up to 3 weeks following aneurysm rupture. Oral nimodipine has been shown to decrease both the incidence and the severity of vasospasm in patients with SAH, and to improve patient outcome.[33] Other management strategies include anticonvulsant therapy if seizures occur, management of pain by administering analgesia, dimming lights and removing stimuli. Vomiting should be treated with antiemetics.[33] Surgical clipping of the neck of the aneurysm remains the definitive treatment of choice for ruptured cerebral aneurysm, as it prevents re-bleeding and removes the clot. It is essential that emergency nurses and paramedics monitor the patient's blood pressure and GCS frequently, and facilitate transfer to definitive care as soon as possible.

SEIZURES

A *seizure* is an 'episode of abnormal neurological function caused by abnormal discharge of brain neurons'.[61] A *convulsion* is an 'episode of excessive and abnormal motor activity'.[61] These definitions are important, as seizures can occur with or without convulsion.[61] A seizure can be an acute event or the result of a past neurological insult (e.g. stroke, head injury or hypoxic brain injury). A first-time seizure is a major event for patients and their families. Not only are there short-term health concerns, but concerns regarding long-term occupational, social and quality-of-life implications are also valid.[61]

The focus for seizure activity is a group of neuronal cells which have highly permeable plasma membranes and are therefore in a hypersensitive state.[13] Hyperexcited neurons fire impulses that increase in frequency and amplitude until impulses spread to adjacent normal neurons.[13] Excitation of the subcortical areas of the basal ganglia, thalamus and brainstem areas results in the *tonic phase* of seizure (muscle contraction with excessive tone), autonomic signs and symptoms, apnoea and loss of consciousness.[13] Hyperexcitation is interrupted by inhibitory neurons in the cortex, anterior thalamus and basal ganglia, resulting in the *clonic phase* of seizure (alternating muscular contraction and relaxation). During a seizure, energy demands are increased by 250%, there is a 60% increase in cerebral oxygen consumption and cerebral blood flow also increases by 250% in an attempt to keep up with cerebral oxygen and glucose demands.[13] Tonic–clonic seizures may be preceded by an aura or partial seizure that occurs immediately prior to a generalised tonic–clonic seizure. The patient may also experience prodromal symptoms in the hours or days preceding a seizure.[13] The International Classification of Epileptic Seizures classifies epileptic seizures as either partial or generalised, as discussed below.[61]

PARTIAL SEIZURES

Partial (or focal) epileptic seizures are classified as simple partial, complex partial or secondary generalised seizures, according to whether or not there is loss of consciousness.[61] Conscious state is not affected during a simple partial seizure; however, there is impaired consciousness in complex partial seizures and loss of consciousness in secondary generalised seizures.[13,61] Simple partial seizures can have the following local effects without impairment of conscious state: Focal motor signs that are usually clonic movements, and can occur with or without 'Jacksonian march' (Jacksonian marching is the spread of seizure activity in an organised manner to adjacent areas).[13] Somatic sensory symptoms can include altered sensation such as numbness, tingling, 'pins and needles' or visual, olfactory and auditory dysfunction. Autonomic signs and symptoms that are particularly characteristic of temporal lobe seizures may include lip-smacking, chewing, facial grimacing, patting or picking at clothing, psychic symptoms such as feelings of familiarity in an unfamiliar setting (*déjà vu*) or unfamiliarity in a familiar setting (*jamais vu*). During a complex partial seizure, consciousness is impaired and ability to respond to external stimuli is reduced.[13] Complex partial seizures may occur as a simple partial seizure followed by impaired conscious state, or conscious state may be impaired from the onset of seizure activity.[13] If impaired conscious state is delayed, symptoms as described above may occur. A secondary generalised seizure is thus a progression of a simple partial seizure that results in loss of consciousness.[13] During a simple partial seizure, the patient is conscious if the seizure is confined to one cerebral hemisphere. However, if seizure activity spreads to the other cerebral hemisphere and deeper brain structures, the patient will become unconscious.[13]

GENERALISED SEIZURES

Generalised epileptic seizures are further classified as:

- generalised tonic–clonic seizures (formerly referred to as grand mal seizures)
- non-convulsive seizures that include absence seizures (formerly referred to as petit mal seizures), myoclonic, tonic and atonic seizures.[61]

Tonic–clonic seizures are usually characterised by sudden loss of consciousness, falling to the ground, stiffening and extension of arms and legs and forceful closure of the jaw (often resulting in tongue-biting). A shrill cry may occur as air is forcibly exhaled through closed vocal cords and urinary and/or faecal incontinence may occur. During the tonic phase, the patient is apnoeic, may become cyanosed and the pupils are dilated and unresponsive to light. During the clonic phase, there is alternating muscular contraction and relaxation. Hyperventilation, eye-rolling, excessive salivation, profuse sweating and tachycardia also occur during the clonic phase.[13,62]

During the postictal period following a tonic–clonic seizure, the patient may have a decreased conscious state and[62] as conscious state improves, the patient may be confused, irritable and may complain of headache.[13,62] Fatigue and myalgia are also common following a generalised seizure.[13,62] Usually there is no recollection of the seizure.

Absence seizures occur in children aged older than 4 years and prior to the onset of puberty.[11] Absence seizures are characterised by abrupt cessation of activity with momentary loss of consciousness. A vacant stare or eye-rolling may occur and the lips may droop or twitch; however, the child will be responsive to verbal stimuli.[63] The duration of absence seizures is usually 5–10 seconds, after which the child usually resumes their previous activity.[63]

STATUS EPILEPTICUS

Status epilepticus is defined as two or more seizures without full recovery of consciousness between seizures or recurrent seizures for more than 30 minutes.[61] One of the major pathophysiological issues with status epilepticus is that compensatory mechanisms which usually occur during seizures begin to fail as the duration of seizure activity increases.[61] Prolonged seizure activity causes direct neuronal damage, and secondary neuronal injury occurs from hypoxia, hypoglycaemia, hyperpyrexia and acidosis.[61] There is also evidence to suggest that excitatory neurotransmitters such as glutamate and aspartate contribute to brain damage from prolonged status epilepticus.[61] The likelihood of permanent brain injury increases with the duration of status epilepticus: the mortality rate increases from 2.7% for seizures lasting less than 1 hour to 32% for seizures lasting longer than 1 hour.[61]

ASSESSMENT

Assessment of the patient with a seizure can be difficult, as many patients arrive in the ED after the seizure has resolved. History is an extremely important diagnostic factor in these patients.[61] It is important to attempt to distinguish seizure from cardiogenic syncope, although this may be difficult. Syncope is often associated with a brief tonic seizure and may also be associated with a head strike that results in a seizure. Typically, patients with syncope will recall all events leading up to the collapse and will recall waking up on the ground immediately following the collapse, whereas patients who have had a seizure will have a period of retrograde amnesia preceding the seizure and will not have any recall of events until sometime after regaining consciousness ('waking up in the ambulance'). Factors that should be considered include head trauma, drug and alcohol use and underlying or associated illnesses.[61] It is estimated that alcohol is a factor in 50% of ED presentations related to seizures and most alcohol-related seizures are due to withdrawal.[61] Acute drug and/or alcohol toxicity and alcohol withdrawal can also precipitate seizures, and seizures in the setting of acute drug overdose are associated with significant mortality and morbidity.[61] Pregnancy status should be ascertained in women of childbearing age because pregnancy will influence patient disposition and anticonvulsant drug therapy choices. In advanced pregnancy or the early postpartum period, eclampsia should be considered (see Chapter 34).

The signs and symptoms of seizures can vary, and seizures can affect motor, sensory and autonomic activity, level of consciousness, emotions, memory, cognition and behaviour. Tongue-biting, broken teeth and distal limb injuries commonly occur with generalised seizures.[61] If an altered conscious state is present, it should not be automatically attributed to a postictal state: thorough assessment and investigation is warranted.[61] When assessing the associated conditions and treatable causes of seizure, cause of seizures may be considered using the following categories:[61]

- acute symptomatic seizures that occur as a result of neurological insult during an acute illness or injury (e.g. hypoxia, hypoglycaemia, head injury, CNS infections, metabolic and electrolyte derangement, drug overdose, drug withdrawal, cerebral tumours or stroke)
- remote symptomatic seizures that occur in patients without a history of neurological insult
- progressive encephalopathy seizures that occur in association with a progressive neurological disease
- febrile seizures that occur almost exclusively in children
- idiopathic seizures (that are usually classified as epilepsy).

Routine laboratory investigations and imaging are not warranted for patients with an uncomplicated first-time seizure and who make a complete recovery.[61] However, glucose abnormalities and hyponatraemia are the most common laboratory abnormalities in patients with seizure disorder,[61] so blood glucose level is useful during initial patient assessment. Serum sodium may be indicated, depending on patient history and examination results.[61] There is no evidence to currently support routine lumbar puncture (LP) in patients with seizure who are alert, afebrile and not immunocompromised.[61] However, head CT scan and LP may be indicated in patients with an abnormal neurological examination and features of meningitis, encephalitis or subarachnoid haemorrhage.[61] Head CT is indicated in patients: (1) with focal neurological signs; (2) who do not recover fully; and (3) with a history of head trauma.[61] Less than 1% of patients with first-time seizure will have abnormalities on non-contrast CT scan.[61] Decisions about timing of CT scanning will depend on local resources: CT may be performed in the ED; however, outpatient neuroimaging is a safe alternative, provided there is reliable follow-up. Outpatient EEG may also be considered.[61]

MANAGEMENT

Key aims in general seizure management are highlighted in Box 23.3. Pharmacological agents that may be used in the treatment of status epilepticus include benzodiazepines and anticonvulsants. There are a number of benzodiazepines that may be used in this context (diazepam, midazolam, clonazepam,

BOX 23.3 AIMS OF SEIZURE MANAGEMENT

- **Airway protection and prevention of aspiration (lateral position, suction)**
- **Restoration and preservation of oxygenation (supplemental oxygen)**
- **Injury prevention (removing objects, use of pillows, bedrails)**
- **Cessation of seizure activity (intravenous access, drug therapy)**
- **Identify and treat precipitating factors**
- **Identify and treat complications**
- **Provide seizure prevention/management plan to optimise seizure control and quality of life**

lorazepam). Midazolam is used most commonly in the Australian setting; however, currently there is no evidence to suggest that one agent is superior to the others and all have advantages and disadvantages.[61] All benzodiazepines can cause respiratory depression and hypotension.[61] The IV route is preferred, but intramuscular or rectal administration are other options. Rectal administration of diazepam is highly effective in children, but the onset of action of rectal diazepam in adults can be slow and unpredictable.[61]

Seizures refractory to benzodiazepines should be treated with an IV anticonvulsant. Wherever possible the agent that the patient is usually on to control their seizures should be given IV for status epilepticus and phenytoin is now rarely used for baseline seizure control. Therefore, while phenytoin was classically used for termination of status epilepticus, agents such as levetiracetam or sodium valproate are now more commonly used. This practice is supported by a recent trial which randomised patients with status epilepticus to valproate, levetiracetam or phenytoin, and found no difference in efficacy with regards to seizure termination and no significant safety differences between the three drugs.[64] The clinical effects of phenytoin are not apparent until 40% of the dose has been given; therefore, phenytoin should be commenced early and given in conjunction with benzodiazepines.[61] A summary of medications used in seizure management is in Table 23.5. It is important that altered conscious state following a seizure is carefully assessed and not assumed to simply be due to a postictal state.[61] Other treatment issues for the patient suffering from status epilepticus are the management of secondary problems such as hypoxia, hypotension, hypoglycaemia, hyperpyrexia and cerebral oedema.[61] For specific issues related to seizures in children, please refer to Chapter 35.

PRACTICE TIP

PRIORITIES FOR THE MANAGEMENT OF A PATIENT HAVING A SEIZURE

- Maintain safety and prevent injury.
- Record the duration of the seizure.
- Once seizure activity stops: ensure airway patency, provide supplemental oxygen if hypoxaemic, assess vital signs and GCS, check blood glucose level, reassure the patient.

HEADACHE

Headaches are a common health problem. Although most headaches are innocuous, it is essential that emergency clinicians can rapidly identify life-threatening causes of headache. The management priorities for patients presenting with headache are pain relief and accurate diagnosis.

Headache, like many other painful symptoms, is not a disease state, but is the symptom of a pathological process.[65] The pathological processes that can result in headache are:[65]

- tension of neck and head muscles
- traction on intracranial structures
- vasodilation of cerebral blood vessels
- inflammation.

Intensity of pain or response to analgesia is an unreliable indicator of the seriousness or aetiology of headache.[65,66]

Headache may be classified as primary and secondary headache syndromes.[66] Primary headache syndromes include migraine headache, tension headache and cluster headaches (Table 23.6). Secondary headache syndromes may be considered in terms of extracranial or intracranial causes.[65,66] Intracranial causes may include cerebrovascular conditions, such as haemorrhage or temporal arteritis, CNS infections and CNS tumours. Extracranial causes of headache may include non-CNS infections such as systemic infection, herpes zoster or sinusitis, ophthalmic pathology, such as glaucoma, iritis and optic neuritis, referred pain from dental or optic conditions, and other conditions, such as nitrate administration, hypercapnia that results in vasodilation, carbon monoxide poisoning and hypertension. Causes of headache types are presented in Table 23.7.

ASSESSMENT AND MANAGEMENT

Baseline vital signs and neurological observations score should be recorded (see Chapter 13). When headache is a key feature, history is of paramount importance.[65] The PQRST mnemonic (see Box 23.2) provides a useful guide for focused symptom assessment. Specific aspects of past medical history that are important to note are hypertension and a history of neurological problems or seizure disorders. Specific considerations may include gender: migraine headaches are more common in women and may be influenced by hormonal factors.[14] In pregnant women, pre-eclampsia should be excluded as a cause of headache (see Chapter 33).

TABLE 23.5 MEDICATIONS USED IN SEIZURE MANAGEMENT[61]

AGENT	LOADING DOSE	POTENTIAL ADVERSE EFFECTS
Phenytoin	15–20 mg/kg slow IV push (no more than 50 mg/min)	Hypotension Arrhythmias Local pain at injection site
Sodium valproate	40 mg/kg (no more than 10 mg/kg/min) (max dose 3 g)	Hepatic toxicity Hyperammonaemia (may cause encephalopathy)
Levetiracetam	60 mg/kg over 15 mins (max dose 4.5 g)	None in acute setting

TABLE 23.6 COMPARISON OF TENSION-TYPE, MIGRAINE AND CLUSTER HEADACHES[67]

PATTERN	TENSION-TYPE HEADACHE	MIGRAINE HEADACHE	CLUSTER HEADACHE
Site	Bilateral, band-like pressure at base of skull, in face or in both	Unilateral (in 60%), may switch sides, commonly anterior	Unilateral, radiating up or down from one eye
Quality	Constant, squeezing tightness	Throbbing, synchronous with pulse	Severe, bone-crushing
Frequency	Cycles for several years	Periodic; cycles of several months to years	May have months or years between attacks; attacks occur in clusters: one to three times a day over a period of 4–8 weeks
Duration	Intermittent for months or years	Continuous for hours or days	30–90 minutes
Time and mode of onset	Not related to time	May be preceded by prodromal stage; onset after awakening; gets better with sleep	Nocturnal; commonly wakens patient from sleep
Associated symptoms	Palpable neck and shoulder muscles, stiff neck, tenderness	Nausea or vomiting, oedema, irritability, sweating, photophobia, phonophobia, prodrome of sensory, motor or psychic phenomena; family history (in 65%)	Vasomotor symptoms such as facial flushing or pallor, unilateral lacrimation, ptosis and rhinitis

The investigations that may be warranted in patients with headache include LP, CT scan or MRI.[65,66] In patients with acute headache, LP may be indicated. Concerns regarding herniation as a consequence of LP raises questions about head CT prior to LP. Currently there are no published randomised controlled trials answering the question of when it is safe to perform an LP. The current state of evidence suggests that it is safe to perform an LP without prior imaging in patients with normal neurological assessment, no focal neurologic deficit, and no history of immunosuppression.[66]

Neuroimaging should be considered in patients with high-risk features such as age over 50 years; sudden severe headache onset; fever; past history of immunocompromised state, malignancy, current or recent pregnancy or trauma; anticoagulant medications; substance misuse and family history that increases risk of aneurysm.[66] The aim of neuroimaging in these patients is to identify a treatable lesion (e.g. tumours, vascular malformations, aneurysms, subarachnoid haemorrhage, cerebral venous sinus thrombosis, subdural and epidural haematomas, infections, stroke, hydrocephalus, and others).

Sudden onset of new headache is a major risk factor for intracerebral haemorrhage, and patients with advanced HIV disease are at risk of CNS pathology, including infections and space-occupying lesions. The 'thunderclap headache' is often reported in the literature as a severe headache of sudden onset and almost instantaneous peak.[68] A 2022 international study of 4536 patients who attended ED with headache showed that 14% reported thunderclap headache.[68] Serious pathology was identified in 11% of patients with thunderclap headache compared with 6.6% of patients with a different headache onset ($p < 0.001$).[68] Subarachnoid haemorrhage occurred in 3.6% of patients with thunderclap headache versus 0.3% in patients with other headache types ($p < 0.001$).[68] The majority of patients (88%) with thunderclap headache did not have serious intracranial pathology.[68] Pregnant women are at increased risk of stroke that may involve headache as a symptom, and risk of subarachnoid haemorrhage is thought to be increased during pregnancy, delivery and the puerperium. For the majority of patients with migraine, investigations are not indicated. Investigations for suspected meningitis are discussed later in this chapter. CT scan or MRI may be indicated to exclude space-occupying lesion.

MIGRAINE

Migraine is a recurring headache disorder with gradual onset and lasting 4–72 hours, characterised by throbbing pain, a triggering event and manifestations associated with neurological and autonomous nervous system dysfunction which increases with physical activity.[14,65] Migraines are often accompanied by nausea, photophobia and phonophobia.[65,66] Many patients who suffer from migraine headaches are able to manage their symptoms without hospital care, so when patients call an ambulance or present to the ED it is often because self-medication has failed or symptoms are unusually prolonged or severe. Migraine headaches are more common in women and may be influenced by hormonal factors such as menstruation, use of oral contraceptives, pregnancy and menopause.[14]

The pathophysiology of migraine is unclear; however, it is thought interaction between the brain and cranial circulation in susceptible patients may contribute to migraine.[14] The phenomenon of aura is thought to be the result of 'cortical spreading depression', whereby there is a brief wave of depolarisation that moves across the cerebral cortex.[14] This state of excitability is followed by prolonged nerve-cell depression.[14] Some patients describe a preceding aura of symptoms, such as visual disturbance, diplopia, hemiparaesthesia, hemiparesis or speech difficulties that develop gradually and usually last less than 60 minutes.[14,65] If migraine aura is associated with neurological deficits (such as weakness, visual disturbance, sensory disturbance, speech impairments), symptoms should resolve prior to discharge from the ED. Emergency clinicians should have a high index of suspicion of significant pathology in patients

TABLE 23.7 CLASSIC CLINICAL COMPLEXES AND CAUSE OF HEADACHE[65,66]

SIGNS AND SYMPTOMS	CAUSE
Preceded by an aura Throbbing unilateral headache, nausea Family history	Migraine
Sudden onset Severe occipital headache; 'like a blow' Worst headache ever	Subarachnoid haemorrhage
Throbbing/constant frontal headache Worse with cough, leaning forward Recent URTI Pain on percussion of sinuses	Sinusitis
Paroxysmal, fleeting pain Distribution of a nerve Trigger manoeuvres cause pain Hyperalgesia of nerve distribution	Neuralgia
Unilateral with superimposed stabbing Claudication on chewing Associated malaise, myalgia Tender artery with reduced pulsation	Temporal arteritis
Persistent, deep-seated headache Increasing duration and intensity Worse in morning Aching in character	Tumour: primary or secondary
Acute, generalised headache Fever, nausea and vomiting Altered level of consciousness Neck stiffness ± rash	Meningitis
Unilateral, aching, related to eye Nausea and vomiting Raised intraocular pressure	Glaucoma
Aching, facial region Worse at night Tooth sensitive to heat, pressure	Dental cause

with 'migraine' that is notably different from their usual migraine headache.[65,66]

There are a number of pharmacological agents that can be used in the treatment of migraine, but current evidence suggests that phenothiazines (chlorpromazine and prochlorperazine) and selective serotonin receptor agonists (triptans) are the most effective agents. For mild-to-moderate migraine headache, aspirin in combination with metoclopramide has also been shown to be effective.[65]

TEMPORAL ARTERITIS

Temporal arteritis is a form of systemic vasculitis that commonly occurs in older patients (over 50 years of age) and is more common in women.[65,66] Headache is the most common symptom of temporal arteritis and occurs in 60–90% of patients.[65,66] The headache is usually severe and is often located in the temporal region.[65,66] The cardinal feature of headache in temporal arteritis is that it is new and often occurs in older patients with no history of headaches. Other classic signs and symptoms include jaw or tongue claudication, visual disturbance (usually diplopia or loss of vision), fever and polymyalgia rheumatica (pain and stiffness in shoulders, neck and hips that is worse in the mornings and improves throughout the day).[65,66] The signs and symptoms of temporal arteritis are due to local arterial inflammation causing endovascular damage, vessel stenosis and occlusion, resulting in tissue ischaemia or necrosis. The most devastating complication of temporal arteritis is irreversible blindness, usually due to ischaemic optic neuritis.[69] Blindness is rarely the first symptom of temporal arteritis, so there is always an opportunity to prevent permanent loss of vision.[69] Early identification, referral for temporal artery biopsy and treatment are therefore extremely important. Diagnostic criteria for temporal arteritis are:[66]

- age > 50 years
- new localised headache (onset or type)
- temporal artery tenderness or decreased pulse
- elevated erythrocyte sedimentation rate (ESR)
- abnormal temporal artery biopsy findings.

The aim of treatment of temporal arteritis is to prevent vision loss using corticosteroid therapy (usually prednisolone).[65,66]

CLUSTER HEADACHES

Cluster headaches are rare and usually self-limiting.[66] Unlike migraine headaches, cluster headaches are more common in men.[14,66] Cluster headaches are thought to be related to trigeminal nerve dysfunction and are characterised by severe unilateral, orbital, supraorbital or temporal pain that lasts from 15 minutes to several hours.[14,66] Cluster headaches are usually associated with at least one of the following symptoms that occur on the ipsilateral side: conjunctival infection, lacrimation, nasal congestion, rhinorrhoea, facial swelling, miosis or ptosis.[66] A distinguishing feature of cluster headache is that patients often pace, in contrast to patients with migraine, who often prefer limited movement and a quiet and dark room.[66]

Oxygen has been shown to be effective in the relief of cluster headaches, as has sumatriptan, intranasal lidocaine and inhaled dihydroergotamine.[14,66] Given the short duration of cluster headaches, oral agents are unlikely to be effective.

INFLAMMATORY BRAIN CONDITIONS

A comparison of inflammatory brain conditions is presented in Table 23.8.

MENINGITIS

Meningitis is an infection of the pia mater, arachnoid mater and subarachnoid space.[5,70] It is a neurological emergency and an infectious disease emergency. Meningitis can be caused by bacteria, viruses, fungi, parasites or toxins.[5,14,70]

TABLE 23.8 COMPARISON OF CEREBRAL INFLAMMATORY CONDITIONS[16]

	MENINGITIS	ENCEPHALITIS	BRAIN ABSCESS
Causative organisms	Bacteria (*Streptococcus pneumoniae, Neisseria meningitidis*, group B *Streptococcus*, viruses, fungi)	Bacteria, fungi, parasites, herpes simplex virus (HSV), other viruses (e.g. Murray Valley encephalitis)	Streptococci, staphylococci through bloodstream
CSF			
Pressure (normal: 60–150 mmH_2O)	Increased	Normal to slight increase	Increased
WBC count (normal: 0–8 × 10^6/L)	*Bacterial*: > 1000 × 10^6/L (mainly PMN) *Viral*: 25–500/mL (mainly lymphocytes)	< 5 × 10^6/L, PMN (early), lymphocytes (later)	0.25–3 × 10^6/L (PMN)
Protein (normal, 0.15–0.45 g/L)	*Bacterial*: > 5 g/L *Viral*: 0.5–5 g/L	Slight increase	Normal
Glucose (normal, 2.8–4.4 mmol/L)	*Bacterial*: decreased *Viral*: normal or low	Normal	Low or absent
Appearance of CSF	*Bacterial*: turbid, cloudy *Viral*: clear or cloudy	Clear	Clear
Diagnostic studies	Gram stain, smear, culture, PCR*	EEG, MRI, PET, PCR, IgM antibodies to virus in serum or CSF	CT scan, EEG, head x-ray
Treatment	Antibiotics, supportive care, prevention of ICP	Supportive care, prevention of ↑ ICP, aciclovir for HSV	Antibiotics, incision and drainage Supportive care

CSF: cerebrospinal fluid; CT: computed tomography; EEG: electroencephalogram; ICP: intracranial pressure; MRI: magnetic resonance imaging; PCR: polymerase chain reaction; PET: positron emission tomography; PMN: polymorphonuclear cells; WBC: white blood cell.

**PCR is used to detect viral RNA or DNA.*

BACTERIAL MENINGITIS

The most common bacterial agents causing meningitis vary with age group and location. In Australia, *Streptococcus pneumoniae* and *Neisseria meningitidis* are the common causes in adults.[70] The incidence of bacterial meningitis has decreased in recent years as a result of vaccines that cover a number of serotypes or strains and the largest reductions in meningitis have been in children.[70] Risk factors for meningitis include head trauma with basilar skull fractures, otitis media, sinusitis or mastoiditis, neurosurgery, systemic sepsis and immunocompromise.[5,70]

The classic symptoms of bacterial meningitis are fever, headache, stiff neck, and altered mental status.[71] Most patients have at least two of four of these symptoms, but their absence does not exclude meningitis.[71] Headache is the most common symptom and is seen in more than 85% of patients,[71] while fever is the second most common symptom.[71] Kernig's and Brudzinski's signs have been used in the clinical assessment of meningitis for many years, but their usefulness is doubtful as they are only present in approximately 50% of patients with bacterial meningitis.[70] Kernig's sign is resistance to leg extension when lying with hip flexed at a right-angle, and Brudzinski's sign is when neck flexion causes hip and knee flexion.[71] Kernig's and Brudzinski's signs are related to painful stretching of inflamed meninges from the lumbar region to the head.[5,71] Other symptoms of bacterial meningitis may include those associated with systemic infection, such as fevers, chills, tachycardia, petechial rash and generalised back, abdominal or limb pain. Neurological signs may include altered conscious state, photophobia, seizures, focal neurological deficits, nausea and vomiting.[14] Hydrocephalus and cranial nerve damage (particularly XIII cranial nerve resulting in deafness) can occur as a complication of bacterial meningitis, particularly in children.[14,70] Other signs and symptoms may be specific to the causative agent (e.g. petechial rash, a non-blanching rash with small purple or red dots on the skin surface or mucous membranes, is associated with meningococcal meningitis).[70]

Diagnosis of bacterial meningitis is made by history, physical examination and lumbar puncture.[70,71] LP findings are usually cloudy, purulent CSF that is under increased pressure.[70,71] CSF analysis shows increased white blood cells, increased protein content and decreased glucose.[70,71] Bacteria can also be seen on smear and culture.[70,71] Neuroimaging should be considered prior to LP in patients with signs of increased intracranial pressure or abnormal neurological findings; however, a normal head CT does not negate the risk of herniation.[70,71]

Early antibiotic administration (which may include pre-hospital administration) is important in preventing death or serious disability in patients with bacterial meningitis and antibiotic administration should not be delayed for investigations such as LP and head CT.[70,71] Agents that may be considered are third-generation cephalosporins and benzylpenicillin.[70,71] There is also some evidence to support the use of corticosteroids in conjunction with antibiotic therapy.[70,71] Supportive management includes preservation and monitoring of airway, breathing and circulation, and conscious state, analgesia, hydration and seizure management.[70]

VIRAL MENINGITIS

Viruses are the leading cause of meningitis.[70] Although viral meningitis most commonly affects children and young adults, older adults can also be affected.[70] Common viral agents include enterovirus, mumps virus, coxsackievirus, Epstein-Barr virus, herpes simplex virus 2 (HSV 2), varicella zoster virus, HIV and more recently SARS-CoV-2.[70] The clinical signs of viral meningitis are similar to those of bacterial meningitis, but are generally less severe[14] as the infection is limited to the meninges.[14] CSF analysis shows increased lymphocytes and moderate increase in protein and normal or mildly increased glucose content.[71] Acute viral meningitis is self-limiting and treatment is largely symptomatic, as described above.[14] Antiviral agents may be used in specific circumstances; for example, aciclovir, may be given for meningitis caused by HSV 2.[14]

GUILLAIN-BARRÉ SYNDROME

Guillain-Barré syndrome is an acquired inflammatory condition that causes demyelination of peripheral nerves.[72] One in three patients will require prolonged intensive care admission or mechanical ventilation.[72,73] Full recovery occurs in most patients, even in severe cases, but 20–30% of patients will have residual disability.[14,72] Guillain-Barré syndrome may be preceded by a mild infectious episode (typically respiratory, gastrointestinal or viral illness), surgical procedures or viral immunisations. *Campylobacter jejuni* is the causative organism in up to 40% of cases.[72] Zika virus and cytomegalovirus are also implicated as antecedents to Guillain-Barré syndrome.[14,72]

Signs and symptoms of Guillain-Barré syndrome include bilateral ascending paralysis, sensory symptoms, such as paraesthesia, pain and numbness, and decreased or absent deep tendon reflexes.[14,72] Severe back pain and distal limb paraesthesias with a 'tight band' feeling are common. Facial and oropharyngeal muscles are affected in 70% of patients, and weakness of these muscles may be the initial signs.[72,73] Progressive limb weakness, often with sensory and cranial nerve involvement, occurs 1–2 weeks post-infection and peaks in 2–4 weeks.[14,72] Diagnostically, Guillain-Barré syndrome is very distinctive because its symptoms are ascending in nature, are gradual in onset and are post-infectious.[72] Early diagnosis of Guillain-Barré syndrome is important: respiratory failure and complications secondary to ventilation are the major causes of morbidity and mortality. It is therefore important to thoroughly assess the respiratory function in patients with actual or suspected Guillain-Barré syndrome (see Chapter 16 for techniques on testing respiratory function). Cranial nerve weakness may result in facial weakness and difficulties swallowing, talking, chewing and coughing.[72] Autonomic dysfunction occurs in up to two-thirds of patients and causes heart rate and blood pressure changes and profuse or decreased sweating: severe changes in blood pressure and cardiac dysrhythmias can be fatal.[72] Diagnostic studies may include CSF studies, nerve conduction studies and electromyography (EMG). CSF findings in patients with Guillain-Barré syndrome include elevated protein levels.[72]

Emergency management of Guillain-Barré syndrome is aimed at preservation of oxygenation and circulation, and ongoing management involves supportive care for respiratory failure and management of autonomic dysfunction.[72] Depolarising neuromuscular blockers such as succinylcholine should be avoided in patients with Guillain-Barré syndrome due to the risk of a hyperkalemic response.[73] There is some evidence that intravenous immunoglobulins (IVIg) or plasma exchange is beneficial, particularly in patients with rapidly progressive weakness.[14,72]

SUMMARY

Preservation or restoration of airway, breathing and circulation are key priorities in the initial assessment and management of the patient with a neurological emergency. Neurological emergencies can have significant consequences for patients. Life-threatening conditions obviously carry a risk of mortality, but even non-life-threatening neurological conditions can have major effects on quality of life. Many neurological emergencies can have subtle or non-specific symptoms, making accurate symptom assessment and history important elements of patient assessment. Frequent monitoring of vital signs and level of consciousness and the correct and consistent application of assessment tools such as the GCS are vital to the early identification of deterioration. Emergency clinicians have a professional responsibility to ensure that their knowledge of assessment and management of neurological emergencies is current, based on the best available evidence and is regularly reviewed.

CASE STUDY

Joan is a 68-year-old woman who collapsed while out shopping with her wife. She suddenly grabbed her arm and said she felt dizzy, before becoming weak at the knees and slumping to the floor. Her wife says she helped her to the floor so she did not fall, but she was 'out to it' for a couple of minutes. When she woke, she was confused; she recognised her wife but did not know where she was, what day it was or what had happened. As she tried to stand up, she fell to the floor again as a result of a left hemiparesis. Her wife also states that her speech is slightly slurred.

QUESTIONS

1. What questions will you ask in this scenario to determine historical and clinical indicators of urgency and relevance?
2. Describe each aspect of your physical assessment and explain each step.
3. What investigations will you perform and why?
4. What ongoing monitoring will you provide?

Answers to Case Study Questions can be found on evolve **http://evolve.elsevier.com/AU/Curtis/emergency/**

USEFUL WEBSITES

Brain Foundation, nationally registered charity dedicated to funding world-class research Australia-wide into neurological disorders, brain disease and brain injuries, http://brainfoundation.org.au/disorders/stroke.

Heart and Stroke Foundation of Canada, is a source of information about stroke, heart disease, surgeries and treatments, www.heartandstroke.com.

National Stroke Foundation, Australia's authority on stroke and author of Australia's stroke guidelines, https://strokefoundation.org.au/.

REFERENCES

1. Australian Resuscitation Council. ANZCOR guideline 8: cardiopulmonary resuscitation. Melbourne: Australian Resuscitation Council; 2021. Available from: www.resus.org.au.
2. Clemency BM, Murk W, Moore A, Brown LH. The EMS Modified Early Warning Score (EMEWS): a simple count of vital signs as a predictor of out-of-hospital cardiac arrests. Prehosp Emerg Care 2022:26(3):391–9.
3. Smith RJ, Santamaria JD, Faraone EE, Holmes JA, Reid DA. Rapid response team diagnoses: frequencies and related hospital mortality. vol 1. College of Intensive Care Medicine; 2017.
4. Jones D, Mercer I, Heland M, Detering K, Radford S, Hart G, et al. In-hospital cardiac arrest epidemiology in a mature rapid response system. Br J Hosp Med 2017;78(3):137–42.
5. Tortora GJ, Derrickson BH. Principles of anatomy and physiology. 16th ed. New York, United States: John Wiley & Sons; 2020.
6. Butterfield RJ. Chapter 15: Structure and function of the neurological system. In: McCance K, Huether S, editors. Pathophysiology e-book the biological basis for disease in adults and children. 8th ed. St Louis: Elsevier; 2018.
7. Wedro B, MedicineNet. Head injury (brain injury). 2020. Available from: www.medicinenet.com/head_injury/article.htm.
8. Koeppen BM, Stanton BA. Chapter 4: The nervous system: introduction to cells and systems. In: Koeppen BM, Stanton BA, editors. Berne and Levy physiology. Elsevier; 2018.
9. Apapted from Brown D, Edwards H, Buckley T, Aitken RL, Lewis SL, Bucher L et al, editors. Lewis's medical-surgical nursing assessment and management of clinical problems. 5th ed. Chatswood: Elsevier Australia; 2020.
10. Rund DA, Barkin RM, Rosen P. Essentials of emergency medicine. 2nd ed. St Louis: Mosby; 1996.
11. Bautista C. Chapter 16: Disorders of brain function. In: Norris TL, editor. Porth's pathophysiology: concepts of altered health states. 10th ed. Philadelphia: Wolters Kluwer; 2019.
12. Davis JH, Drucker WR. Clinical surgery. vol 1. St Louis: Mosby; 1987.
13. Boss BJ, Huether SE. Chapter 17: Alterations in cognitive systems, cerebral hemodynamics, and motor function. In: McCance K, Huether S, editors. Pathophysiology e-book the biological basis for disease in adults and children. 8th ed. St Louis: Elsevier; 2018.
14. Boss BJ, Huether SE. Chapter 18: Disorders of the central and peripheral nervous systems and the neuromuscular junction. In: McCance K, Huether S, editors. Pathophysiology e-book the biological basis for disease in adults and children. 8th ed. St Louis: Elsevier; 2018.
15. Smith M. Cerebral perfusion pressure. Br J Anaesthes 2015;115(4):488–90.
16. Littlejohns L, Barr J, O'Brien EM. Chapter 55: Nursing management: acute intracranial problems. In: Brown D, Edwards H, Buckley T, Aitken RL, Plowman E, editors. Lewis's medical-surgical nursing assessment and management of clinical problems. 5th ed. Chatswood: Elsevier Australia; 2020.

17. Takahashi LK, McCance KL, Clayton MF. Chapter 11: Stress and disease. In: McCance K, Huether S, editors. Pathophysiology e-book the biological basis for disease in adults and children. 8th ed. St Louis: Elsevier; 2018.
18. Hew R. 8.4 Altered conscious state. In: Cameron P, Little M, Mitra B, Deasy C, editors. Adult textbook of emergency medicine. 5th ed. Sydney: Elsevier; 2020.
19. Munroe B, Hutchinson C. Chapter 13: Patient assessment and essentials of care. In: Curtis K, Ramsden C, Shaban RZ, Fry M, Considine J, editors. Emergency and trauma care: for nurses and paramedics. 3rd ed. Chatswood NSW: Elsevier Australia; 2019.
20. Engelborghs S, Niemantsverdriet E, Struyfs H, Blennow K, Brouns R, Comabella M, et al. Consensus guidelines for lumbar puncture in patients with neurological diseases. Alzheimer's Dement (Aust) 2017;8:111–26.
21. Royal Children's Hospital Melbourne. Lumbar puncture guideline. 2020. Available from: www.rch.org.au/clinicalguide/.
22. Patel R, Urits I, Orhurhu V, Orhurhu MS, Peck J, Ohuabunwa E, et al. A comprehensive update on the treatment and management of postdural puncture headache. Curr Pain Headache Rep 2020;24(6):24.
23. Srinivasan S, Bidkar PU. Approach to a patient with coma. In: Bidkar PU, Vanamoorthy P, editors. Acute neuro care focused approach to neuroemergencies. Singapore: Springer; 2020.
24. Mutter MK, Huff JS. Chapter 168: Altered mental status and coma. In: Tintinalli JE, Ma OJ, Yealy DM, Meckler GD, Stapczynski JS, Cline DM, editors. Tintinalli's emergency medicine: a comprehensive study guide. 9th ed. New York: McGraw-Hill Education; 2020.
25. Vlad I. 21.4 Alcohol-related illness. In: Cameron P, Little M, Mitra B, Deasy C, editors. Adult textbook of emergency medicine. 5th ed. Sydney: Elsevier; 2020.
26. Green S. Chapter 176: General management of poisoned patients. In: Tintinalli JE, Ma OJ, Yealy DM, Meckler GD, Stapczynski JS, Cline DM, editors. Tintinalli's emergency medicine: a comprehensive study guide. 9th ed. New York: McGraw-Hill Education; 2020.
27. Australian Commission on Safety and Quality in Health Care (ACSQHC). Delirium clinical care standard. Darlinghurst, NSW: ACSQHC; 2021. Available from: www.safetyandquality.gov.au/our-work/clinical-care-standards/delirium-clinical-care-standard.
28. Oliveira J, E Silva L, Berning MJ, Stanich JA, Gerberi DJ, Murad MH, et al. Risk factors for delirium in older adults in the emergency department: a systematic review and meta-analysis. Ann Emerg Med 2021;78(4):549–65.
29. Australian Commission on Safety and Quality in Health Care (ACSQHC). National Safety and Quality Health Service Standards User guide for health service organisations providing care for patients with cognitive impairment or at risk of delirium. Sydney: ACSQHC; 2019. Available from: www.safetyandquality.gov.au/sites/default/files/2019-06/sq19-027_acsqhc_cognitive_user_guide_accessible_pdf.
30. Oh ES, Needham DM, Nikooie R, Wilson LM, Zhang A, Robinson KA, et al. Antipsychotics for preventing delirium in hospitalized adults. Ann Intern Med 2019;171(7):474–84.
31. National Stroke Foundation. Clinical guidelines for stroke management. Chapter 2 of 8: Early assessment and diagnosis. Melbourne: National Stroke Foundation; 2021. Available from: informme.org.au/guidelines/clinical-guidelines-for-stroke-management#.
32. Aplin P, Morphett M. 8.2 Stroke and transient ischaemic attack. In: Cameron P, Little M, Mitra B, Deasy C, editors. Adult textbook of emergency medicine. 5th ed. Sydney: Elsevier; 2020.
33. Go S. Chapter 167: Stroke syndromes. In: Tintinalli JE, Ma OJ, Yealy DM, Meckler G, Stapczynski J, Cline D, editors. Tintinalli's emergency medicine: a comprehensive study guide. 9th ed. New York: McGraw-Hill Education; 2020.
34. Mayer L, Ferrari J, Krebs S, Boehme C, Toell T, Matosevic B, et al. ABCD3-I score and the risk of early or 3-month stroke recurrence in tissue- and time-based definitions of TIA and minor stroke. J Neurol 2018;265(3):530–4.
35. National Stroke Foundation. Chapter 4: Secondary prevention. Clinical Guidelines for Stroke Management. National Stroke Foundation; 2021. Available from: informme.org.au/guidelines/clinical-guidelines-for-stroke-management.
36. National Stroke Foundation. National stroke audit. Acute services report 2021. Melbourne; National Stroke Foundation; 2021. Available from: informme.org.au/stroke-data/Acute-audits.
37. Carvalho V, Cruz VT. Clinical presentation of vertebrobasilar stroke. Porto Biomed J 2020;5(6):e096.
38. Chandratheva A, Werring D, Kaski D. Vertebrobasilar insufficiency: an insufficient term that should be retired. BMJ Publishing Group Ltd; 2021.
39. National Stroke Foundation. Top 10 facts about stroke. 2022. Available from: strokefoundation.org.au/About-Stroke/Learn/facts-and-figures.
40. National Stroke Foundation. National Impact. Australia: National Stroke Foundation; 2022. Available from: strokefoundation.org.au/.
41. O'Sullivan Í. 8.3 Subarachnoid haemorrhage. In: Cameron P, Little M, Mitra B, Deasy C, editors. Adult textbook of emergency medicine. 5th ed. Sydney: Elsevier; 2020.
42. Marcolini E, Hine J. Approach to the diagnosis and management of subarachnoid hemorrhage. West J Emerg Med 2019;20(2):203–11.
43. National Stroke Foundation. Chapter 1: Pre-hospital care. In: Clinical guidelines for stroke management. Melbourne: National Stroke Foundation; 2021. Available from: informme.org.au/guidelines/clinical-guidelines-for-stroke-management.
44. National Stroke Foundation. Chapter 3: Acute medical and surgical management. In: Clinical guidelines for stroke management. Melbourne: 2021. Available from: https://informme.org.au/guidelines/clinical-guidelines-for-stroke-management#.
45. National Stroke Foundation. Stroke symptoms. 2022. Available from: strokefoundation.org.au/.
46. Singletary EM, Zideman DA, Bendall JC, Berry DA, Borra V, Carlson JN, et al. 2020 International consensus on first aid science with treatment recommendations. Resuscitation 2020;156:A240–A82.
47. Bil C, Walter S, Sauer J, Feldmann S. Towards an air mobile stroke unit for rapid medical response in rural Australia. ATDE: IOS Press; 2019.

48. Fatima N, Saqqur M, Hussain MS, Shuaib A. Mobile stroke unit versus standard medical care in the management of patients with acute stroke: a systematic review and meta-analysis. Int J Stroke 2020;15(6):595–608.
49. Kim J, Easton D, Zhao H, Coote S, Sookram G, Smith K, et al. Economic evaluation of the Melbourne Mobile Stroke Unit. Int J Stroke 2021;16(4):466–75.
50. Zhao H, Coote S, Easton D, Langenberg F, Stephenson M, Smith K, et al. Melbourne mobile stroke unit and reperfusion therapy. Stroke 2020;51(3):922–30.
51. Turc G, Hadziahmetovic M, Walter S, Churilov L, Larsen K, Grotta JC, et al. Comparison of mobile stroke unit with usual care for acute ischemic stroke management. JAMA Neurol 2022;79:281–90.
52. Australasian College for Emergency Medicine. Guidelines on the implementation of the Australasian Triage Scale in emergency departments. November 2000 (rev July 2016). Available from: https://acem.org.au/getmedia/51dc74f7-9ff0-42ce-872a-0437f3db640a/G24_04_Guidelines_on_Implementation_of_ATS_Jul-16.aspx.
53. Guo W, Liu L, Wen F, Shen Y. Analysis of neurogenic electrocardiographic changes in acute stroke patients. Int J Clin Experiment Med 2020;13(10):7787–93.
54. Scheitz JF, Nolte CH, Doehner W, Hachinski V, Endres M. Stroke–heart syndrome: clinical presentation and underlying mechanisms. Lancet Neurol 2018;17(12):1109–20.
55. Middleton S, McElduff P, Ward J, Grimshaw JM, Dale S, D'Este C, et al. Implementation of evidence-based treatment protocols to manage fever, hyperglycaemia, and swallowing dysfunction in acute stroke (QASC): a cluster randomised controlled trial. Lancet 2011;378(9804):1699–706.
56. Middleton S, Dale S, Cheung NW, Cadilhac DA, Grimshaw JM, Levi C, et al. Nurse-initiated acute stroke care in emergency departments: the T3 implementation cluster randomised controlled trial. Stroke 2019;50:1346–55.
57. Appleton JP, Sprigg N, Bath PM. Blood pressure management in acute stroke. BMJ 2016;1(2):72–82.
58. Bath PM, Appleton JP, Krishnan K, Sprigg N. Blood pressure in acute stroke. Stroke 2018;49(7):1784–90.
59. Qureshi AI, Huang W, Lobanova I, Barsan WG, Hanley DF, Hsu CY, et al. Outcomes of intensive systolic blood pressure reduction in patients with intracerebral hemorrhage and excessively high initial systolic blood pressure. JAMA Neurol 2020;77(11):1355–65.
60. National Stroke Foundation. Chapter 6: Managing complications. In: Clinical guidelines for stroke management. Melbourne: 2021. Available from: informme.org.au/guidelines/clinical-guidelines-for-stroke-management.
61. Wilkes G. 8.5 Seizures. In: Cameron P, Little M, Mitra B, Deasy C, editors. Adult textbook of emergency medicine. 5th ed. Sydney: Elsevier; 2020.
62. Kornegay J. Chapter 171: Seizures and status epilepticus in adults. In: Tintinalli JE, Ma OJ, Yealy DM, Meckler GD, Cline DM, Thomas SH, editors. Tintinalli's emergency medicine: a comprehensive study guide. 9th ed. New York: McGraw-Hill Education; 2020.
63. Butterfield RJ, Huether SE. Chapter 20: Alterations of neurologic function in children. In: McCance K, Huether S, editors. Pathophysiology e-book the biological basis for disease in adults and children. 8th ed. St Louis: Elsevier; 2018.
64. Kapur J, Elm J, Chamberlain JM, Barsan W, Cloyd J, Lowenstein D, et al. Randomized trial of three anticonvulsant medications for status epilepticus. NEJM 2019;381(22):2103–13.
65. Kelly A-M. 8.1 Headache. In: Cameron P, Little M, Mitra B, Deasy C, editors. Adult textbook of emergency medicine. 5th ed. Sydney: Elsevier; 2020.
66. Koyfman A, Long B. Chapter 165: Headache. In: Tintinalli JE, Ma OJ, Yealy DM, Meckler GD, Cline DM, Thomas SH, editors. Tintinalli's emergency medicine: a comprehensive study guide. 9th ed. New York: McGraw-Hill Education; 2020.
67. Roberts D, Plueger M, Matiuk S. Chapter 57: Nursing management: chronic neurological problems. In: Brown D, Edwards H, Buckley T, Aitken RL, Plowman E, editors. Lewis's medical-surgical nursing assessment and management of clinical problems. 5th ed. Chatswood: Elsevier Australia; 2020.
68. Roberts T, Horner DE, Chu K, Than M, Klim S, Kinnear F, et al. Thunderclap headache syndrome presenting to the emergency department: an international multicentre observational cohort study. Emerg Med J 2022;39(11):803–9.
69. Ling ML, Yosar J, Lee BW, Shah SA, Jiang IW, Finniss A, et al. The diagnosis and management of temporal arteritis. Clin Exp Optom 2020;103(5):572–82.
70. Singer A. 9.2 Meningitis. In: Cameron P, Little M, Mitra B, Deasy C, editors. Adult textbook of emergency medicine. 5th ed. Sydney: Elsevier; 2020.
71. Tanski ME, Ma OJ. Chapter 174: Central nervous system and spinal infections. In: Tintinalli JE, Ma OJ, Yealy DM, Meckler G, Cline D, Thomas S, editors. Tintinalli's emergency medicine: a comprehensive study guide. 9th ed. New York: McGraw-Hill Education; 2020.
72. Green T, Rogan EM. 8.7 Weakness. In: Cameron P, Little M, Mitra B, Deasy C, editors. Adult textbook of emergency medicine. 5th ed. Sydney: Elsevier; 2020.
73. Gupta N, Andrus P. Chapter 172: Acute peripheral neurologic disorders. In: Tintinalli JE, Ma OJ, Yealy DM, Meckler G, Cline D, Thomas S, editors. Tintinalli's emergency medicine: a comprehensive study guide. 9th ed. New York: McGraw-Hill Education; 2020.

CHAPTER 24
GASTROINTESTINAL EMERGENCIES

WAYNE F. VARNDELL AND LESLEY FITZPATRICK

ESSENTIALS

- Abdominal pain is a symptom of disease, not a diagnosis.
- Management of acute abdominal pathology involves a combination of systematic history-taking, physical examination and is aided by diagnostic studies.
- Examination always begins with a primary survey. The airway, breathing and circulatory status must be addressed to include airway patency; breathing pattern, including rate; pulse; blood pressure/capillary refill time and postural changes. The brain must be adequately perfused and the level of consciousness will provide a useful indicator.
- Fluid resuscitation must be considered immediately if derangements in circulation are evident.
- Complete assessment must include accurate fluid balance. Output must be maintained.
- Peritonism or abdominal rigidity is an abdominal emergency.
- Early consultation and referral are essential for all gastrointestinal bleeding, especially when there is haemodynamic instability.
- Be certain to consider pathology outside the abdomen.
- Repeat examination and assessments, including vital signs. The trend and changes are key to a deteriorating patient.

INTRODUCTION

Abdominal pain and diseases of the digestive system account for 5.4% of the 8 million Australians who present to emergency departments (ED) every year.[1] Although gastrointestinal (GI) conditions are a common reason for visits to the ED and calls to ambulance services, they must be approached in a serious manner. The complexity of GI conditions can make the assessment, diagnosis and management difficult, as the nature of presentations may constitute acute illness, chronic illness, or a combination of both. GI emergencies can vary from minor problems to more serious life-threatening conditions. Vigilance in assessment, observation and management aims to ensure that underlying abdominal pathophysiology is identified and treated promptly and appropriately.

A patient's condition may be variable. Changes in a condition may be related to clinical improvement, patient deterioration or a response to intervention. It is important to assess and elicit an understanding about the direction of clinical change. Pre-hospital assessment of patients with gastrointestinal emergencies includes a systematic history of the pain and identification of any high-risk symptoms, coupled with examination as part of an Airway, Breathing, Circulation, Disability and Exposure (ABCDE) approach to formulate ideas about the nature and cause of the pain and associated symptoms. In the pre-hospital setting, it can be difficult to differentiate between the many GI and non-GI causes of abdominal complaints. The chief aims of pre-hospital management consist of pain relief, early initiation of therapies, such as fluid resuscitation to stabilise the patient, and prompt transportation of patients with life-threatening injuries/symptoms to hospital. Where critically ill patients require prompt transportation to hospital, a pre-notification message through radio transmission will be sent to the receiving ED. Paramedics will provide a structured handover to the ED by using the mnemonic IMIST-AMBO (Identification, Mechanism/Medical complaint, Injuries/Information about complaint, Signs and Symptoms, Treatment, Allergies, Medications, Background history and Other).[2] Early communication of the patient's status enables the ED to prepare for the patient's arrival. On arrival to ED, patients are rapidly assessed by the triage nurse to establish the patient's level of clinical urgency. Triage of the patient is a dynamic process and provides a snapshot view of the progression of illness. Within the ED, the patient's triage assessment is categorised according to clinical acuity and is placed into one of the five Australasian Triage Scale categories (discussed in Chapter 11). Ongoing reassessment, professional communication and clinical handover at every stage of patient care is vital to the management of the patient.

Classic indications of dysfunction in the GI system include reflux, belching, nausea, vomiting, bloating, constipation, diarrhoea, chest pain, abdominal pain, back pain and bleeding.[3] This chapter focuses on conditions frequently seen in the ED. A brief overview of relevant anatomy and physiology is provided, followed by a discussion relating to patient assessment, physical examination and the relevant screening (e.g. urinalysis, blood sugar level) and diagnostic investigations (e.g. haematology, biochemistry) most often carried out. Treatment provided is based upon the history, assessment, investigation and findings. Pain relief is humane, and the most often prescribed initial treatment. Specific GI conditions will be covered and include: gastroenteritis, gastrointestinal bleeding, bowel obstruction, diverticulitis, gastro-oesophageal reflux disease (GORD), appendicitis, cholecystitis, pancreatitis and liver failure. Trauma to the GI system is discussed in Chapter 46.

FIGURE 24.1 ANATOMY OF THE GASTROINTESTINAL SYSTEM[4]

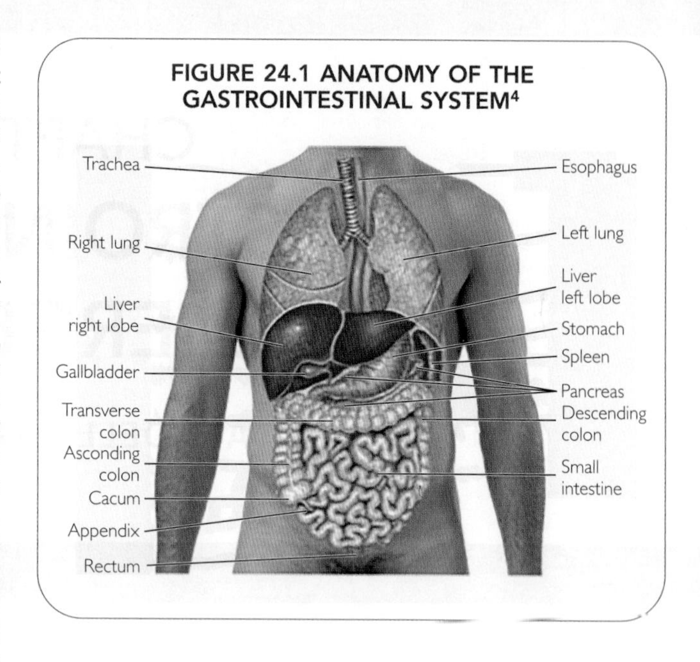

ANATOMY AND PHYSIOLOGY

Normal GI function requires ingestion of nutrients and fluids and is followed by elimination of waste products formed from metabolic activities. Major organs and structures of the GI system include the mouth, oesophagus, stomach, large and small intestines, liver, pancreas, gallbladder and peritoneum (Fig. 24.1).

MOUTH

The beginning of the digestive process starts normally in the mouth. The bite, movement of the tongue and pushing against the walls of the mouth begin the physical breakdown of food. Food is chewed and mixed with saliva, which begins one of many chemical interactions within the GI system. Saliva lubricates the tissues of the mouth and creates a semi-solid of the food being eaten. Salivary amylase, the enzyme of saliva, begins carbohydrate metabolism.

Pathology of the mouth includes trauma and dental and gum disease. Infection may occur in any part of the mouth, including the salivary glands or ducts: parotid, submandibular and sublingual. Further information on oral and dental emergencies can be found in Chapter 31 and on faciomaxillary trauma in Chapter 44.

OESOPHAGUS

The major function of the oesophagus concerns the movement of food. The oesophagus is a straight, collapsible fibromuscular tube of approximately 25 cm in length and up to 3 cm in diameter. The oesophagus extends from the pharynx to the stomach. Structurally, the oesophageal wall is composed of four layers: an inner mucosal layer; a supporting submucosa layer of connective tissue; muscularis propria, a thin layer of muscle; and adventitia, the outermost layer of connective tissue. Unlike the remainder of the GI tract, the oesophagus has no serous membrane. Secretions from mucous glands organised throughout the submucosa layer in longitudinal rows keep the inner lining moist and lubricated. The upper third of the oesophagus wall is skeletal-type striated muscle. As the oesophagus extends from the pharynx, the striated muscle fibres are gradually replaced by smooth muscle fibres, with the last third of the oesophagus wall being entirely smooth muscle. The upper and lower ends of the oesophagus function as sphincters. The upper oesophageal sphincter is at the proximal end of the oesophagus and is formed from thickened striated muscle that prevents air from entering during respiration. The lower oesophageal sphincter (also called the cardiac sphincter) is not identifiable anatomically and occurs at a point 1 to 2 cm from the distal junction of the oesophagus and stomach. The lower oesophageal sphincter prevents regurgitation from the stomach into the oesophagus. No absorption of nutrients takes place in the oesophagus until it transitions through the stomach and into the small intestines.

STOMACH

The stomach is a J-shaped, muscular, hollow organ situated below the diaphragm between the oesophagus and the small intestine. Stomach functions include food storage, combining food with gastric juices, limited absorption and moving food into the small intestine. The stomach is subdivided into four regions: the fundus, an expanded area curving up above the cardiac sphincter; the body or intermediate region that forms the central and largest portion of the stomach; the antrum, the lowermost, funnel-shaped region of the stomach; and the pylorus region, that narrows to join the duodenum (Fig. 24.2). The pyloric sphincter controls food movement from stomach to duodenum. Distinct layers of the stomach wall are outer serosa, muscular layer, submucosa and mucosa. The mucosal layer contains numerous folds called rugae that straighten as the stomach fills to accommodate more volume. Completely relaxed, the stomach holds up to 1.5 L.[6] Gastric juices containing pepsin, hydrochloric acid, mucus and intrinsic factor are secreted by glands in the thick mucosa membrane. These agents begin food breakdown. Acids in the stomach maintain the pH of gastric juices at 1.0. Absorption of some substances, including alcohol, actually begins in the stomach.[7]

INTESTINES

The intestines are vital organs in the GI tract of the digestive system, and consist of the small intestine, large intestine and rectum. The small intestine, or small bowel, is a tubular organ extending from the pyloric sphincter to the proximal large intestine, and has three distinct regions: the duodenum, the jejunum and the ileum. The duodenum attaches to the stomach at the pyloric sphincter in the retroperitoneal space and represents the only fixed portion of the small intestine. The duodenum is approximately 25 cm long and 5 cm in diameter. The jejunum and ileum are mobile and lie free in the peritoneal cavity.[6] The length of the small intestine is dependent upon the height of the person. On average, it is approximately 6 metres in length, but can vary greatly from 2.75 to 10.49 metres.[8] Secretions from the pancreas and liver complete digestion of nutrients in chyme, a semi-liquid mixture of food and gastric secretions that is passed from the stomach through to the small intestine. The small intestine absorbs nutrients and other products of digestion and transports residue to the large intestine.

Recognised regions of the large intestine are: the caecum, a pouch-like, dead-end passage that branches inferiorly from the end of the ileum and where the appendix is attached; the colon, the largest region of the large intestine; the rectum and anal canal where faeces are held until defecation occurs as the anal sphincter muscles of the anal canal relax. The large intestine is approximately 1.5 m long, beginning in the lower right side of the abdomen where the ileum joins the caecum. The colon is divided into ascending colon, transverse colon, descending colon and sigmoid colon (Figs 24.3A and B). Primary functions of the large intestine are absorption of water and electrolytes, formation of faeces and storage of faeces. Approximately 1500 mL of chyme pass through the ileocaecal valve each day.[6]

LIVER

The liver, the largest gland in the body, is a wedge-shaped organ located in the right upper quadrant (RUQ) of the abdomen and is divided into right and left lobes (Fig. 24.4). Functional units of the liver, called lobules, contain sinusoids and Kupffer cells. Each lobule is supplied by a hepatic artery, sublobular vein, bile duct and lymph channel (Fig. 24.5). The liver is extremely vascular; approximately 1450 mL of blood flows through the liver each minute, accounting for 29% of resting cardiac output.[6] Sinusoids in

FIGURE 24.2 PARTS OF THE STOMACH[5]

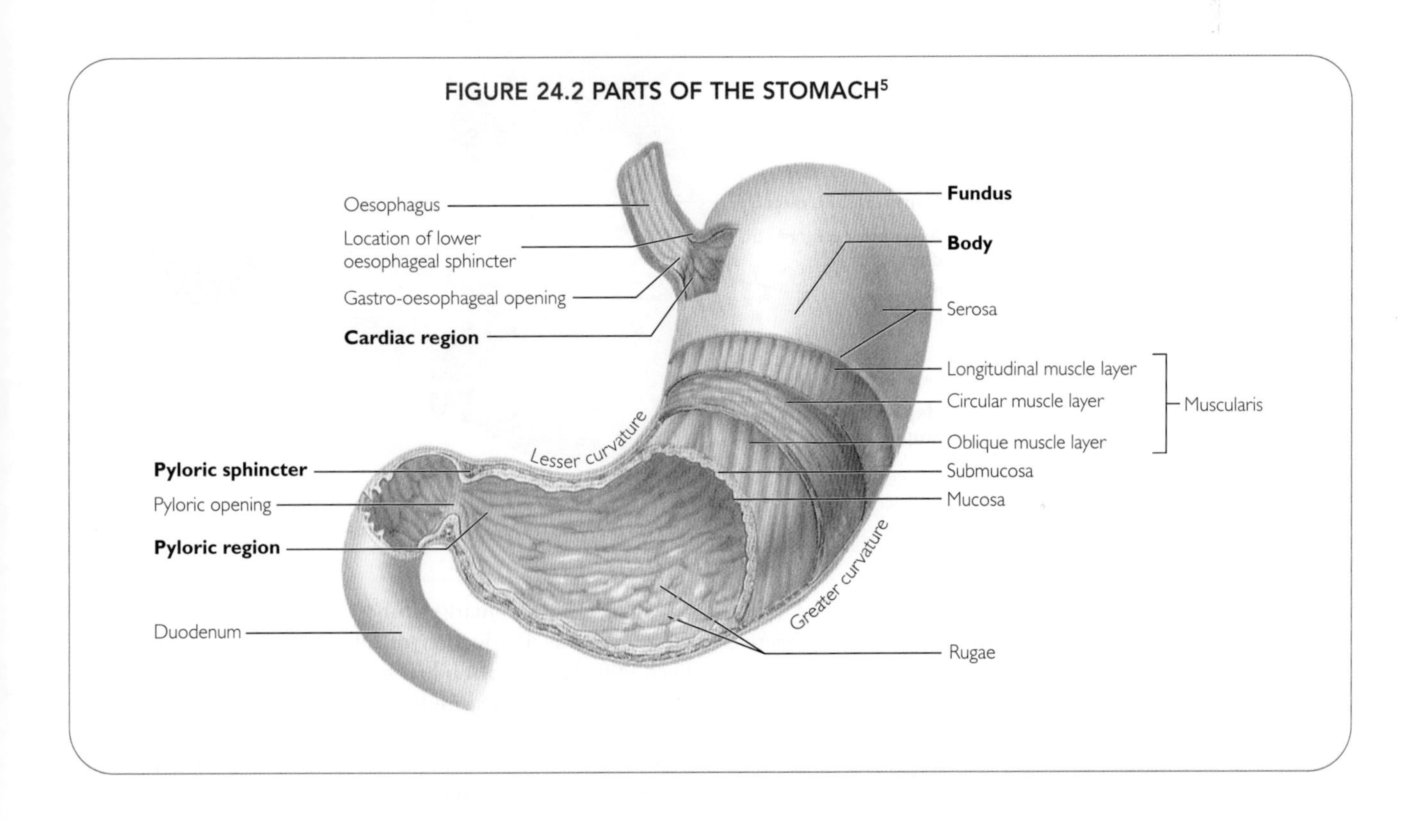

FIGURE 24.3 A, B. LARGE INTESTINE SHOWING THE ASCENDING COLON, TRANSVERSE COLON, DESCENDING COLON AND SIGMOID COLON[5]

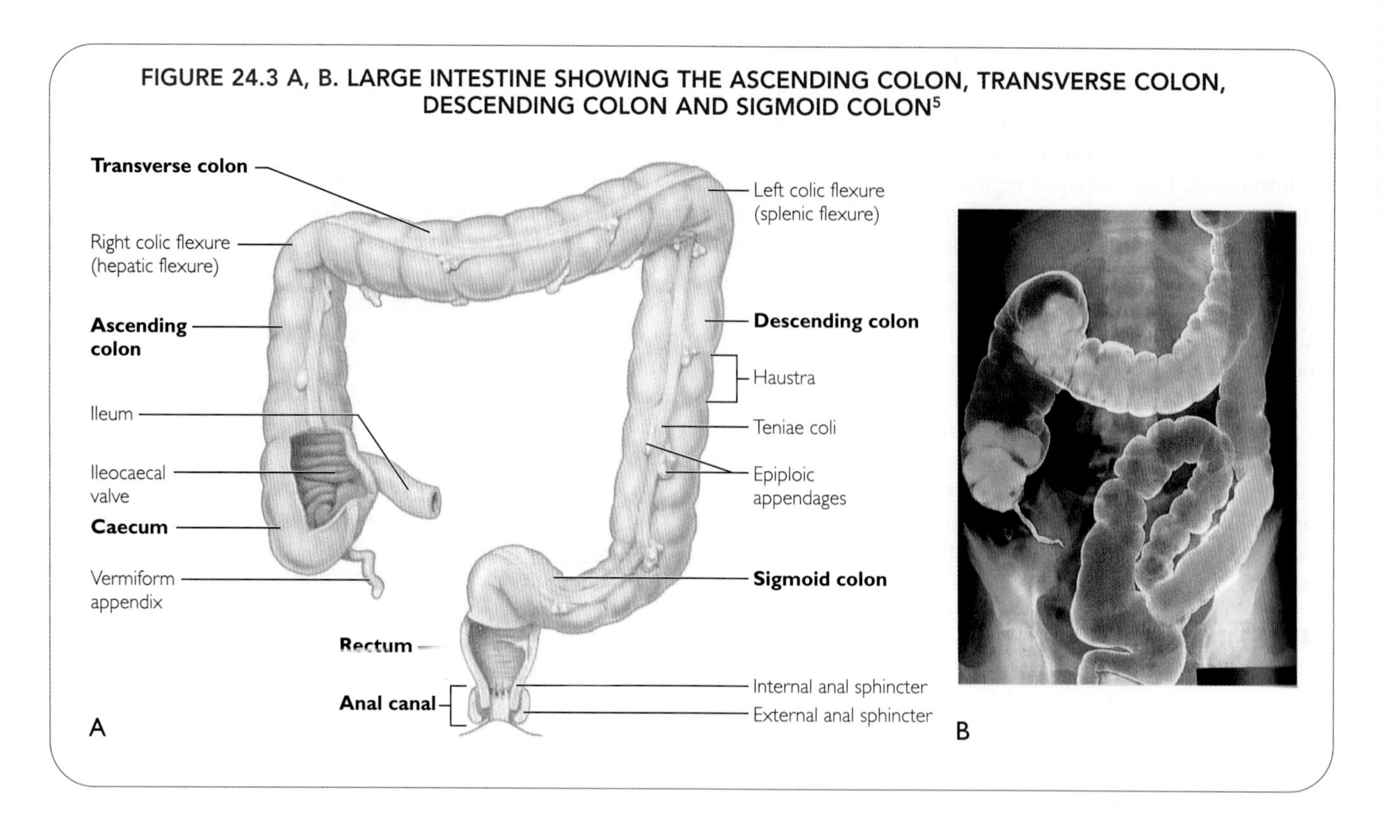

FIGURE 24.4 GROSS STRUCTURE OF THE LIVER, GALLBLADDER, PANCREAS, SPLEEN AND DUCT SYSTEM[5]

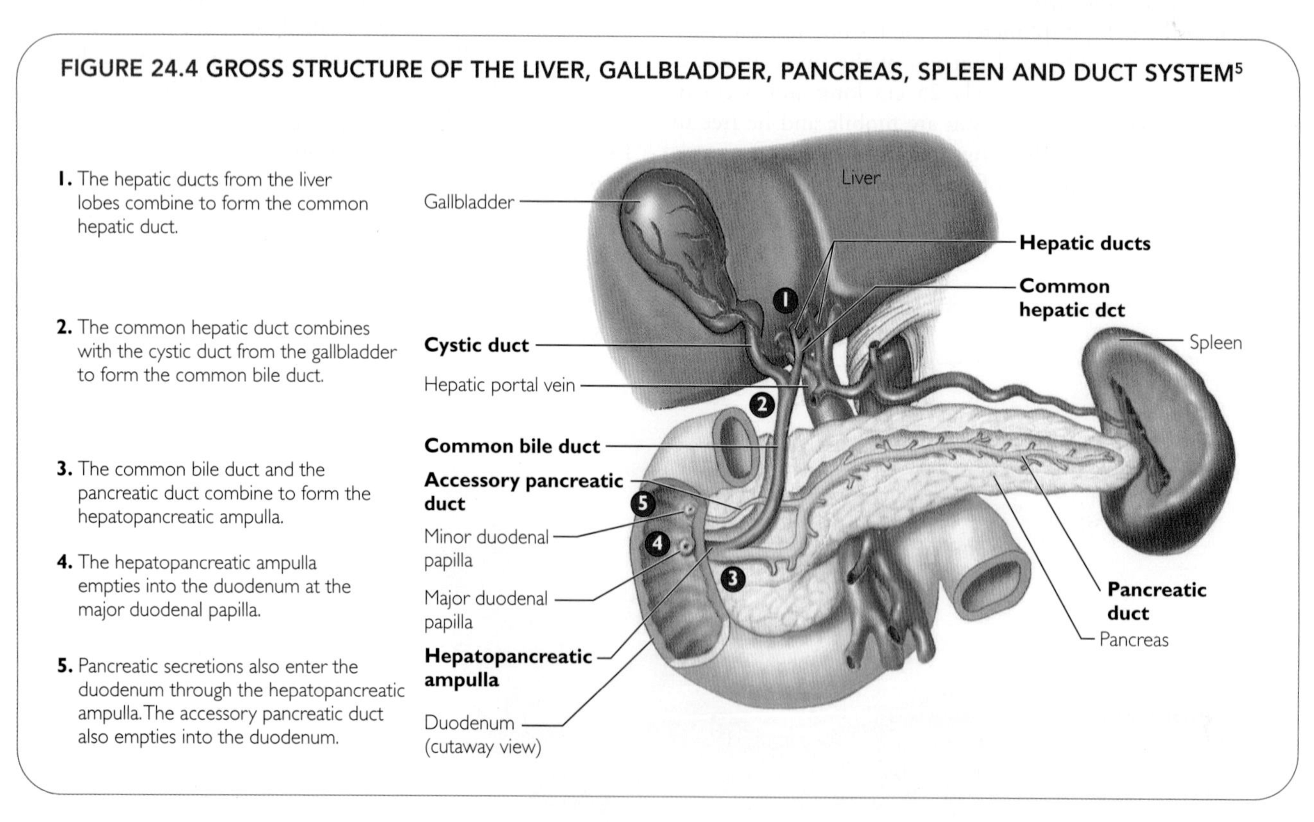

lobules act as a reservoir for overflow of blood and fluids from the right ventricle. A thick capsule of connective tissue, known as Glisson's capsule, covers the liver. The liver is involved in hundreds of metabolic functions, including metabolism of nutrients, gluconeogenesis, and produces biochemicals necessary for digestion and drug metabolism.

Table 24.1 summarises functions related to nutrition and waste removal. Production of bile is a major function of the liver: 600–1200 mL of bile is secreted each day. Bile is essential for digestion via the emulsification of lipids, and absorption and excretion of bilirubin and excess cholesterol. Bilirubin is an end-product of haemoglobin destruction. Fig. 24.6 illustrates processes involved in bilirubin conjugation.

FIGURE 24.5 MICROSCOPIC STRUCTURE OF THE LIVER LOBULE[5]

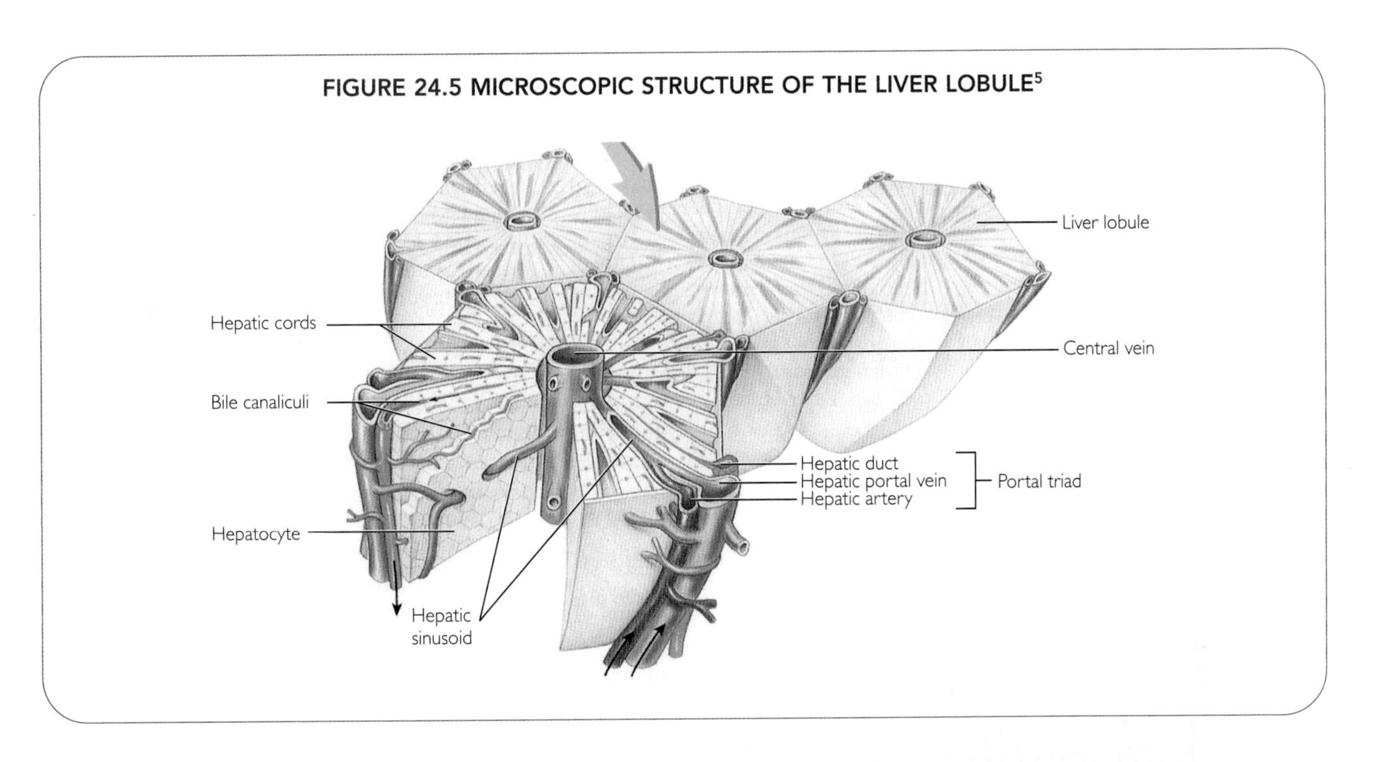

TABLE 24.1 MAJOR FUNCTIONS OF THE LIVER[9]

FUNCTION	DESCRIPTION
Metabolic functions	
Carbohydrate metabolism	Glycogenesis (conversion of glucose to glycogen), glycogenolysis (process of breaking down glycogen to glucose), gluconeogenesis (formation of glucose from amino acids and fatty acids)
Protein metabolism	Synthesis of non-essential amino acids, synthesis of plasma proteins (except gamma-globulin), synthesis of clotting factors, urea formation from NH3 (NH3 formed from deamination of amino acids and by action of bacteria on proteins in colon)
Fat metabolism	Synthesis of lipoproteins, breakdown of triglycerides into fatty acids and glycerol, formation of ketone bodies, synthesis of fatty acids from amino acids and glucose, synthesis and breakdown of cholesterol
Detoxification	Inactivation of drugs and harmful substances and excretion of their breakdown products
Steroid metabolism	Conjugation and excretion of gonadal and adrenal steroids
Bile synthesis	
Bile production	Formation of bile, containing bile salts, bile pigments (mainly bilirubin) and cholesterol
Bile excretion	Bile excretion by liver about 1 L/day
Storage	Glucose in form of glycogen; vitamins, including fat-soluble (A, D, E, K) and water-soluble (B_1, B_2, cobalamin and folic acid); fatty acids; minerals (iron and copper); amino acids in form of albumin and beta-globulins
Mononuclear phagocyte system	
Kupffer cells	Breakdown of old red blood cells, white blood cells, bacteria and other particles, breakdown of haemoglobin from old red blood cells to bilirubin and biliverdin

PANCREAS

The pancreas is a glandular organ approximately 20 cm long, lobulated, contains endocrine and exocrine cells, and lies deep in the abdomen behind the stomach.[6] The organ is divided into the head, body and a thin, narrow tail that extends towards the spleen (Fig. 24.7). The pancreas has an internal hormonal role (endocrine) and an external digestive role (exocrine). The endocrine role is conducted by hormonal tissue distributed along the pancreas in which the islets of Langerhans are situated. Cells in the islets of Langerhans secrete insulin and regulate

FIGURE 24.6 BILIRUBIN METABOLISM AND CONJUGATION[10]

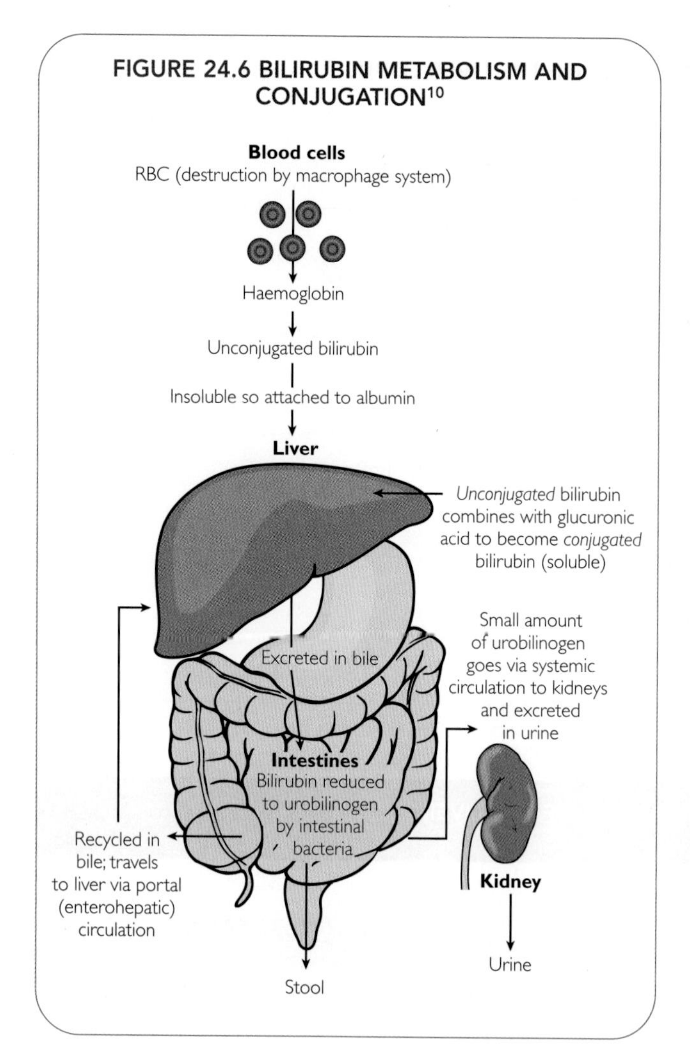
Blood cells
RBC (destruction by macrophage system)
Haemoglobin
Unconjugated bilirubin
Insoluble so attached to albumin
Liver
Unconjugated bilirubin combines with glucuronic acid to become conjugated bilirubin (soluble)
Small amount of urobilinogen goes via systemic circulation to kidneys and excreted in urine
Excreted in bile
Intestines
Bilirubin reduced to urobilinogen by intestinal bacteria
Recycled in bile; travels to liver via portal (enterohepatic) circulation
Kidney
Urine
Stool

glucose levels. The exocrine cells form 98% of the pancreatic tissue and consist of clusters of acini cells. These are responsible for secretion of enzymes required for the digestion of fats, carbohydrates, proteins and nucleic acids.[11] Pancreatic enzymes enter the intestines through the pancreatic duct at the same juncture as the bile duct from the liver and gallbladder. The pancreatic and bile ducts join at a short, dilated tube called the ampulla of Vater. A band of smooth muscles, called the sphincter of Oddi, surrounds this area and controls exit of pancreatic enzymes and bile. In a normally functioning pancreas, the enzymes are prevented from being activated until they reach the intestines.[11]

GALLBLADDER

The gallbladder is a pear-shaped hollow organ located in a shallow depression on the inferior surface of the right lobe of the liver. The gallbladder is approximately 7–10 cm in length. The organ's main functions are collection, concentration and storage of bile. Maximum volume is 30–60 mL; however, input from the liver can reach 450 mL over 12 hours. Concentration of bile in the gallbladder can be 5–20 times that of bile in the liver.[6] Bile is predominantly (80%) water, with the remaining volume comprised of bile acids (10%), phospholipid (4% to 5%) and cholesterol (1%).[12]

PERITONEUM

The peritoneum is a serous membrane covering the liver, spleen, stomach, and intestines, which acts as a semipermeable membrane; it contains pain receptors and provides proliferative cellular protection. The peritoneum is the largest serous membrane in the body and consists of two continuous layers: the parietal layer, which comes into contact with and is loosely attached to the abdominal wall, whereas the visceral peritoneum covers the viscera; the layers are separated by a thin layer of serous fluid called the peritoneal cavity. Many vital abdominal organs and structures are housed behind the peritoneum and therefore are retroperitoneal: adrenal glands, aorta and inferior vena cava, duodenum (except the proximal 2 cm, the duodenal cap), pancreas (except the tail), ureters, colon (ascending and descending sections), kidneys, oesophagus and rectum. However, the liver, spleen, stomach and intestines are suspended into the peritoneum and considered intraperitoneal organs.[12] Omenta are folds of peritoneum that surround the stomach and adjacent organs. The greater omentum extends from the stomach to cover the transverse colon and folds of the intestine. It is extremely mobile and spreads easily into areas of injury to seal off potential sources of infection. The lesser omentum extends between the transverse fissure of the liver and the lesser curvature of the stomach and covers parts of the stomach and proximal intestines but is not as movable as the greater omentum.

The peritoneum is permeable to fluid, electrolytes, urea and toxins. Somatic afferent nerves sensitise the peritoneum to all types of stimuli. In acute abdominal conditions, the peritoneum can localise an irritable focus by producing sharp pain and tenderness, voluntary or involuntary abdominal muscle rigidity and rebound tenderness.[12]

GENERAL ASSESSMENT

Assessment of a patient with a GI emergency should initially focus on airway (e.g. vomiting, obstruction), breathing pattern (rate, work of breathing) and circulation, including vital signs.[13] A completed primary assessment then allows a systematic and focused assessment. The patient's general appearance will provide an important first impression (pale, grey, jaundiced, flushed, diaphoretic). A patient who is calm and responding to questioning is initially easier to assess than one who is extremely agitated and distressed due to pain. An air of control and calm needs to be obtained, as a distressed patient coupled with a distressed clinician makes for difficult work.[14]

The initial assessment will provide a clue to recognition of an underlying GI-related disorder, such as severe dehydration, intense pain, shock, and metabolic and biochemical disturbances. The respiratory system may be activated to assist with maintaining normal blood pH (see Chapter 21). Abdominal pain may also affect breathing and lead to shallow respirations. Heart rate is often elevated as a result of a number of causative factors. Pain alone may increase heart rate; however, underlying pathology, such as fever, sepsis or shock, will also increase the heart rate and it is important to remain objective about physiological observations. Care must be taken not to assume that pain is the only factor to raise the heart rate. Blood pressure (BP) must be obtained to detect life-threatening hypotension, which may be associated with severe fluid shifts and poor perfusion. Temperature may be elevated when infection is an underlying causative factor. Time-critical abdominal emergencies for

FIGURE 24.7 ASSOCIATED STRUCTURES OF THE DUODENUM AND EXOCRINE PANCREAS[5]

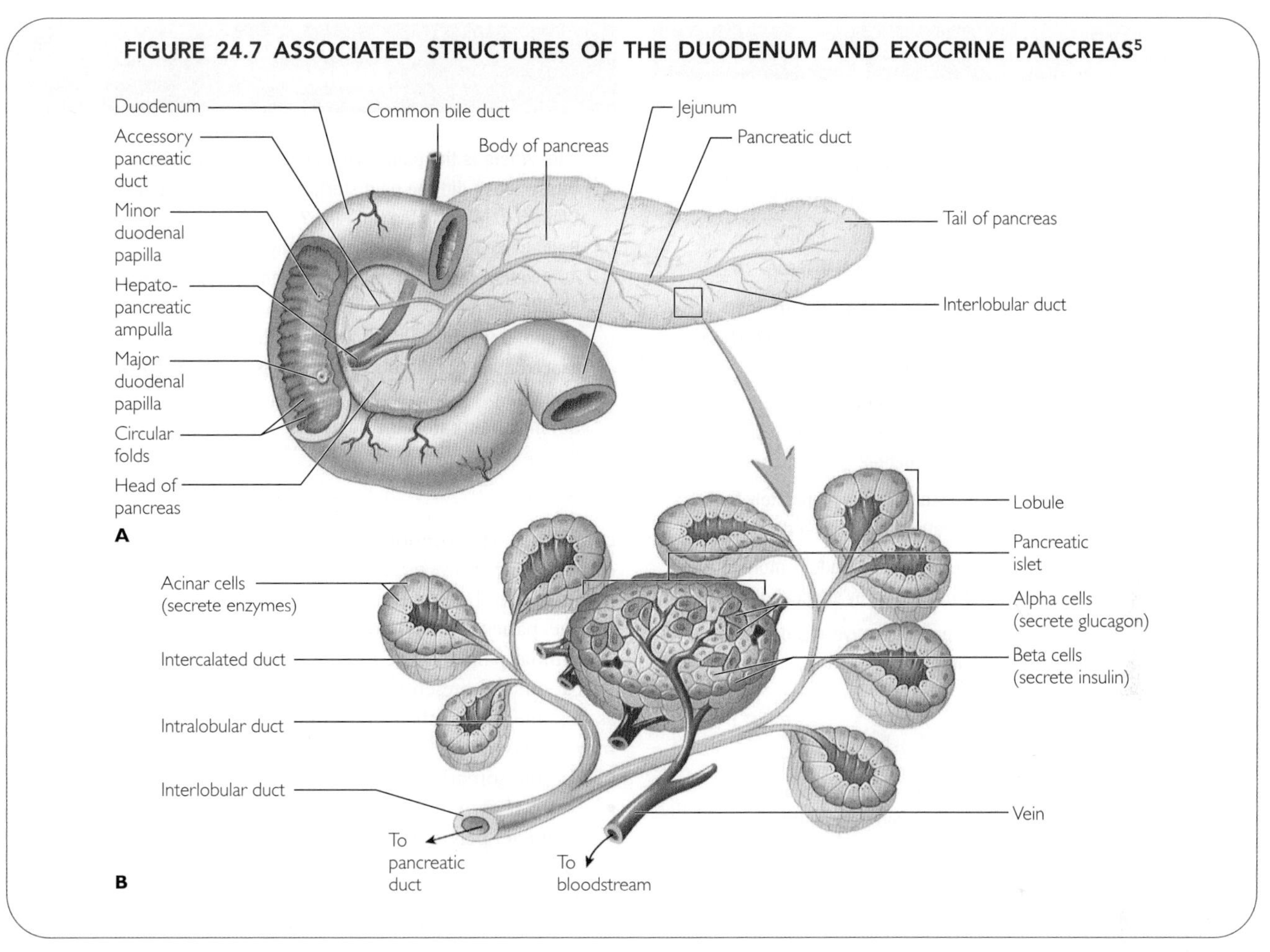

A. The head of the pancreas lies within the duodenum curvature, with the pancreatic duct emptying into the duodenum. **B.** Histology of the pancreas showing both the acinar cells and the pancreatic duct system.

paramedics include a ruptured abdominal aortic dissection (AAA), peritonitis, uncontrolled GI haemorrhage, acute bowel obstruction and acute pancreatitis.[15] Consideration must be given to the very young, older or immunosuppressed patient who may have a serious infection and not be able to mount a significant fever in response to infection.[16] Observe skin colour, diaphoresis, rashes, scars, wounds, abdominal-wall abnormalities and characteristics of any pain.

PATIENT HISTORY

Obtaining a complete focused patient history is the cornerstone of accurate symptom evaluation, appropriate test ordering and diagnosis. The history should be as complete as possible and include a description of the patient's pain and associated symptoms, and include past medical, surgical and social history, to aid in directing investigation and management plan decisions. Past medical history provides essential clinical information; however, maintain a view that this presentation may differ from that of previous presentations (see Chapter 13). Obtain a social history. Information may be gleaned from the patient, family members, friends, other healthcare professionals or old medical records.[14] Assessment should include questions related to respiratory, cardiovascular, gynaecological and genitourinary (GU) symptoms as they may also cause abdominal pain, nausea and vomiting. When appropriate, a complete assessment should also gain understanding about sexual contacts or sexual history, drug and alcohol use and any recent overseas travel. High-yield historical questions have been posited within the literature,[16,17] a summary of which is provided in Box 24.1.

PRACTICE TIP

Not all abdominal symptoms are caused by GI disease. Take a broad and detailed history.

PAIN

The nature and quality of abdominal pain provide key clues as to the potential cause and diagnosis; it is therefore important to undertake a detailed assessment. While the assessment of pain using the mnemonic PQRST (Provokes, Quality, Radiates, Severity, Time) (see Chapter 13) may provide for a systematic approach to assessing pain in general, it does not allow for a smooth patient interview regarding abdominal pain. An alternative pain assessment mnemonic SOCRATES (Site, Onset, Character, Radiation, Associations, Time, Exacerbating/relieving factors, Severity) may better suit the evaluation of abdominal pain and the patient interview (Box 24.2).[19] As part of assessing abdominal

BOX 24.1 HIGH-YIELD HISTORICAL QUESTIONS[18]

How old are you?	Advanced age is associated with increased hospitalisation, surgical intervention and mortality.
Which came first, pain or vomiting?	Pain that is worse before vomiting suggests surgical disease.
How long have you had the pain?	Pain lasting less than 48 hours is more likely to be caused by surgical disease.
Have you ever had abdominal surgery?	Previous abdominal surgery increases the risk of adhesions or obstruction.
Is the pain constant or intermittent?	Constant pain is more likely to be caused by surgical disease.
Have you ever had this before?	No previous episode is more likely to be caused by surgical disease.
Do you have a history of cancer, diverticulosis, pancreatitis, kidney failure, gallstones or inflammatory bowel disease?	All are suggestive of more serious pathology.
Are you immunocompromised (e.g. receiving chemotherapy, on immunosuppressant therapy)?	Consider occult infection of drug-related pancreatitis.
How much alcohol do you drink per day?	Consider pancreatitis, hepatitis or cirrhosis.
Are you pregnant?	Test for pregnancy; consider ectopic pregnancy.
Are you taking any antibiotics or steroids?	May potentially mask infection.
Did the pain start centrally and migrate to the right lower quadrant?	High specificity for appendicitis.
Do you have a history of vascular or heart disease, hypertension or atrial fibrillation?	Consider mesenteric ischaemia or abdominal aneurysm.

pain, the clinician must consider individual and cultural variations in expressions of pain. Each person reacts differently to pain. Older patients may not exhibit the same level of pain as younger patients;[16] men may hide pain because expression of pain is not considered masculine in many cultures. Conversely, dramatic expression of pain may be expected in some cultures. It is important to remember that pain is a symptom, not a diagnosis.[3] Interventions should focus on identification and treatment of the source of pain, as discussed in Chapter 13.

Location

Potential causes based on location of pain are listed in Table 24.2; Table 24.3 reviews pain descriptions associated with certain

BOX 24.2 SOCRATES PAIN ASSESSMENT MNEMONIC[20]

Site: Where is the pain? Where is the maximal site of pain?
Onset: When did the pain start, and was it sudden or gradual?
Character: What is the pain like?
Radiation: Does the pain radiate anywhere?
Associations: Are there any other signs or symptoms associated with the pain?
Tempo: Does the pain follow any pattern?
Exacerbating or relieving factors: Does anything change the pain?
Severity: How bad is the pain?

conditions. The location of pain may assist in localising the area of pathology; however, this may be misleading, especially if the pain is referred. Further, decreased perception of pain in advancing age, patients with diabetes, delirium/confusion or widespread abdominal pain may be unable to localise pain.[16,21] Obtain details about the presenting problem and dig for specifics as much as possible. Often the only symptom is abdominal pain, which may or may not be related to the GI tract. Abdominal pain may be visceral, somatic or referred.

- *Visceral pain* results from activation of nociceptors of the thoracic, pelvic or abdominal viscera. Visceral structures are highly sensitive to distension; the pain that arises is often described as cramping or a sensation of gas usually centred on the umbilicus or below the midline. Diffuse pain makes localisation of pain difficult, due to intraperitoneal organs being bilaterally innervated resulting in stimuli being perceived by both sides of the spinal cord. For example, stimuli from visceral fibres in the appendix enter the spinal cord at about T10, resulting in midline periumbilical pain. Other symptoms, such as diaphoresis, nausea, vomiting, hypotension, tachycardia and abdominal-wall spasms, may be present. Conditions associated with visceral pain are appendicitis, acute pancreatitis, cholecystitis, and intestinal obstruction.
- *Somatic pain* is the most common type of pain that occurs when pain receptors in tissues (skin, muscles, skeleton, joints, and connective tissues) are activated. Somatic pain is characterised as sharp and well localised to one area. Typically, a patient lies with legs flexed and knees pulled to the chest to prevent stimulation of the peritoneum and subsequent increase in pain. Associated findings include involuntary guarding and rebound tenderness.
- *Referred pain* occurs at a distance from the original source of the pain and is thought to be caused by development of nerve tracts during fetal growth and development. Biliary pain can be referred to the subscapular area, whereas a peptic ulcer and pancreatic disease can cause back pain (see Chapter 18). Referred pain to the shoulder tip (Kehr's sign) can be an important sign of diaphragmatic irritation, due to blood, fluid, or space occupying lesions (e.g. tumours) that accumulate from intra-abdominal pathology. This may be present following abdominal surgery, injury, trauma, or a spontaneous perforation.

TABLE 24.2 POTENTIAL SOURCES OF ABDOMINAL PAIN, BY LOCATION

LOCATION	POTENTIAL CAUSE	
Right upper quadrant	Cholecystitis	Pancreatic abscess
	Hepatic abscess	Duodenal ulcer perforation
	Hepatitis	Right lung pneumonia
	Hepatomegaly	Right renal pain
Left upper quadrant	Pancreatitis	Left renal pain
	Splenic rupture	Pericarditis
	Myocardial infarction	Left lung pneumonia
	Gastritis	
Right lower quadrant	Appendicitis	Ovarian cyst
	Cholecystitis	Pelvic inflammatory disease
	Perforated ulcer	Endometriosis
	Intestinal obstruction	Right ureteral calculi
	Meckel's diverticulum	Incarcerated hernia
	Abdominal aortic aneurysm, dissection or rupture	Gastric ulcer perforation
	Ruptured ectopic pregnancy	Colon perforation
	Twisted right ovary	Urinary tract infection
Left lower quadrant	Appendicitis	Left ureteral calculi
	Intestinal obstruction	Left renal pain
	Diverticulum of the sigmoid colon	Urinary tract infection
	Ruptured ectopic pregnancy	Incarcerated hernia
	Twisted left ovary	Perforated descending colon
	Ovarian cyst	Regional enteritis
	Endometriosis	

TABLE 24.3 DESCRIPTION OF PAIN ASSOCIATED WITH CERTAIN CLINICAL CONDITIONS

PAIN DESCRIPTION	ASSOCIATED CLINICAL CONDITIONS
Severe, sharp pain	Infarction or rupture
Severe pain controlled by medication	Pancreatitis, peritonitis, small bowel obstruction, renal colic, biliary colic
Dull pain	Inflammation, low-grade infection
Intermittent pain	Gastroenteritis, small bowel obstruction

PRACTICE TIP

- 'Abdominal pain' is a symptom, not a diagnosis.
- Abdominal pain with vomiting, no flatus or bowel movements and a midline abdominal scar suggests small bowel obstruction unless otherwise excluded.
- Constipation, gastroenteritis, irritable bowel syndrome and non-specific abdominal pain are diagnoses of exclusion.

PHYSICAL EXAMINATION

Although an essential component of all routine physical examinations, evaluating abdominal pain requires a systematic approach: observation, auscultation, percussion and palpation. Patient position should be noted because patients assume positions of comfort.[14] Prior to the examination, it is important to explain the procedure, expose only what needs to be seen and ensure patient privacy.

- *Observation* is often the first approach. Observe the patient's face (a central perspective) for facial expression, signs of discomfort, diaphoresis and skin colour (e.g. flushed, pale). Look at the abdomen for colour (e.g. pale, jaundiced, mottled); the abdominal wall for pulsations, movement, masses, symmetry or surgical scars.
- *Auscultation* should be done before palpation and percussion to prevent the creation of false bowel sounds by palpation. Auscultation can be difficult to perform in a noisy environment. Auscultate bowel sounds in all four quadrants, determining frequency, quality and pitch.
  - Normal bowel sounds are irregular, high-pitched gurgling sounds occurring 5–35 times per minute.
  - Decreased (hypoactive) or absent bowel sounds suggest peritonitis or paralytic ileus (also called functional bowel

obstruction), whereas increased (hyperactive) bowel sounds represent increased intestinal activity; in the context of nausea, vomiting and diarrhoea suggests gastroenteritis. When bowel sounds are not present, one should listen for a full 3 minutes before determining bowel sounds are absent.
  - Irritation of serosal surfaces may produce a sound (rub) as an organ moves against the serosal surface.
  - Frequent, high-pitched bowel sounds occur with bowel obstruction.
  - Vascular sounds such as venous hums or bruits are abnormal findings (see Chapter 18).
  - Due to low accuracy associated with interpreting bowel sounds, clinical decisions in patients with possible bowel obstruction should not solely be based upon auscultatory assessment of bowel sounds.[22]
- *Percussion* is performed in all four quadrants. Dull sounds occur over solid organs or tumours, whereas tympanic (hollow drum-like) sounds occur over air masses. Tympany is the normal sound heard when percussing the abdomen. Like performing auscultation, environmental noise can reduce the effectiveness and specificity of this assessment and thus the value of the findings.
- *Palpation* is important. Feeling the abdomen provides rapid and useful clinical information to underlying pathology. Initially, palpate away from areas of pain, noting areas of tenderness, guarding, rigidity or masses. Gently palpate towards the painful area last. Tenderness, guarding, rigidity and peritonism are all important clinical pointers to a patient suffering an acute abdominal event. Care is to be taken, as a soft and non-tender abdomen is not necessarily without pathology; it may be intermittent or transient and the patient as a whole must be considered with other clinical findings and history.
- *Specific abdominal signs* have been described within the literature as being associated with specific diagnosis (Table 24.4). Sensitivity and specificity vary between patient populations and pathologies. However, the sensitivity and specificity of all abdominal signs or assessment techniques is not known.

Nausea and vomiting are commonly encountered symptoms with a broad list of possible causes that accompany most GI emergencies. Specific treatment varies with the suspected underlying cause. Care must be taken to understand the causes of vomiting. Vomiting may be related to a condition of the GI system that directly initiates vomiting, for example, a toxin or virus. Alternatively, the vomiting may be secondary to a mechanical condition such as a bowel obstruction or a sign of raised intracranial pressure. If vomiting is present, observe or enquire if it contains blood or bile. Gain an understanding into the frequency; several times versus many or intractable. Table 24.5 lists various drugs that may be used for nausea and vomiting.

PRACTICE TIP

Patients unable to tolerate fluid without vomiting are not suitable for discharge.

TABLE 24.4 SPECIFIC SIGNS IN PATIENTS WITH ABDOMINAL PAIN

SIGN	DESCRIPTION	ASSOCIATION
Cough test	Post-tussive abdominal pain	Peritonitis (sensitivity 50–85%; specificity 38–79%)[23-28]
Cullen's sign	Periumbilical ecchymosis	Retroperitoneal haemorrhage, 37% increase in mortality rate[29]
Grey-Turner's sign	Flank ecchymosis	Retroperitoneal haemorrhage, 37% increase in mortality rate[29]
Heel-drop sign	Pain at RLQ on dropping heels to floor from standing on tiptoes, or from forcefully banging the patient's right heel with clinician's hand	Appendicitis (sensitivity 74–93%)[30]
Kehr's sign	Severe pain radiating to left shoulder tip, especially when the patient is supine	Intraperitoneal bleeding[31]
McBurney's sign	Tenderness located two-thirds distance from anterior iliac spine to umbilicus on right side[32]	Appendicitis (sensitivity 50–94%; specificity 75–86%)[25,33]
Murphy's sign	Exquisite pain is elicited by applying gentle pressure below the right sub-costal arch below the liver margin during deep inspiration[14]	Acute cholecystitis (sensitivity 48–97%; specificity 48–98%)[34,35]
Obturator's sign	The right hip and knee is flexed and then right hip is internally rotated	Appendicitis (sensitivity 8%; specificity 94%)[36]
Psoas sign	With the patient lying down on the left side, the right hip is then hyperextended. Painful hip extension is the positive response[37]	Appendicitis (sensitivity 13–42%; specificity 79–97%)[36]
Rovsing's sign	Pain at RLQ when palpating LLQ	Appendicitis (sensitivity 19–75%; specificity 58–93%)[38]

TABLE 24.5 DRUG THERAPY IN NAUSEA AND VOMITING[10,13]

CLASSIFICATION	DRUG
Antiemetic and antipsychotic	Chlorpromazine
	Haloperidol
	Perphenazine
	Prochlorperazine
	Trifluoperazine
Antihistamine	Dimenhydrinate
	Diphenhydramine
	Promethazine
Prokinetic	Domperidone
	Metoclopramide
Serotonin antagonist	Dolasetron
	Ondansetron
	Tropisetron
Antimuscarinic	Hyoscine
Other	Dexamethasone

Gain an understanding about the patient's dietary and fluid input (anorexia, increased thirst), as well as output in terms of urination (anuria, oliguria, polyuria, dysuria) and bowel motion activity (constipation/diarrhoea, consistency, colour). Information related to food and fluid intake and tolerance should also be noted.

Findings such as fever, malaise and chills are usually found with infective processes. Intractable vomiting or feculent vomiting (faeces in emesis) suggest bowel obstruction. Haematemesis (blood in emesis) occurs with gastritis, upper GI bleeding or mucosal tearing. Diarrhoea occurs with gastroenteritis; black, tarry stools suggest upper GI bleeding; and clay-coloured stools are found with biliary tract obstruction. Steatorrhoea, fatty, foul-smelling, frothy stools that float due to higher fat and gas content, commonly occurs with pancreatitis. Table 24.6 presents the factors that increase the probability of non-benign diarrhoea and Table 24.7 details causes of infectious diarrhoea.

INVESTIGATIONS

Abdominal complaints can represent a spectrum of conditions from benign and self-limited disease to surgical emergencies. Despite an in-depth history and physical examination, many patients may not present 'classically', therefore further diagnostors and physical examination, aid in determining the diagnosis.

Bedside

Urinalysis

Urinalysis is an important screening test for all patients presenting with any type of abdominal pain. Women of childbearing age (even if uncertain about pregnancy status) should have a screening urine pregnancy test, in the setting of abdominal pain. Pregnant women should undergo routine urine screening for the presence of protein, glucose or infection. The purpose for urine testing is to test pH (identifying acid–base disturbances), the presence of glucose (glycosuria, hyperglycaemic states), protein (proteinuria, renal damage), ketones (ketonuria, metabolic anomaly), blood (haematuria, renal damage, coagulopathy), bilirubin (liver and gallbladder states), specific gravity (indication of urine osmolarity), nitrates and leucocytes (markers of infection). The test is simple, quick, inexpensive and may uncover remarkable underlying causes or associated conditions related to the presentation. The test should not be limited to patients with abdominal pain, but extended to most patients who pass urine, and more so the unwell patient. Conditions such as diabetes or its complications, urinary tract infections, bleeding disorders, metabolic disturbances, dehydration, renal pathology and pregnancy are some of the important findings that can be revealed upon urinalysis.

PRACTICE TIP

There are many other abdominal causes of pyuria and microhaematuria that should be considered, such as appendicitis, pyelonephritis and renal abscess or tumour.

Electrocardiogram (ECG)

Patients experiencing acute coronary artery events may present with a variety of atypical symptoms, some of which manifest as abdominal conditions: epigastric pain, nausea, vomiting and indigestion.[41] Further, atypical acute coronary events may present more frequently in patients aged over 75 years, in women, and in patients with diabetes, chronic renal failure or dementia.[42] It is therefore important that an ECG be performed in cases where acute coronary syndrome (ACS) is suspected.

Capillary blood sugar

Patients with diabetic ketoacidosis may present with symptoms and signs imitating the acute abdomen: abdominal pain (especially in children due to gastric distension or stretching of the liver capsule), vomiting, polyuria, polydipsia and diarrhoea.[43]

Venous blood gas (VBG)

Critically unwell patients require immediate baseline exclusion of acidosis, alkalosis and compensated states. VBG has comparable results to an arterial blood gas (ABG) analysis (excluding evaluations of oxygenation) to guide initial management strategies and conduct serial analyses to determine response of treatment.[44] Early identification of anaemia and lactic acidosis is beneficial for the GI bleeding patient.[45] For a clinical estimation of renal function, the creatinine can be checked on the VBG to estimate the glomerular filtration rate (GFR) prior to contrast computerised tomography (CT) scan.[46]

LABORATORY TESTS

Diagnosing patients who present in the ED with acute abdominal pain is challenging. In addition to history-taking and physical examination, laboratory tests may be required to exclude diagnoses that can mimic acute abdominal pain. Appropriate laboratory test ordering will vary depending upon

TABLE 24.6 FACTORS INCREASING PROBABILITY OF NON-BENIGN DIARRHOEA[10,13,39]

FACTOR	SPECIFIC PATHOGEN(S)/OTHER CONSIDERATIONS
Presentation to a healthcare facility	Degree of illness overall greater in patients presenting for evaluation; increased probability of 'not norovirus' aetiology to 50%
Travel history	Especially foreign travel and to endemic areas of dysenteric disease
Recent hospitalisation	*Clostridium difficile* from antibiotic exposure
Day-care attendance	Rotavirus, *Shigella*, *Giardia*
Nursing-home residence	*C. difficile*, medication side-effects, tube feedings, ischaemic colitis, faecal impaction and overflow diarrhoea
Wilderness exposure	*Giardia* or *Cryptosporidium*
Antibiotic therapy	*C. difficile*, antibiotic side-effects
Raw shellfish, farm animals and show livestock, pet reptiles or amphibians, petting zoos	*Salmonella* spp., *Escherichia coli* O157:H7 and non-O157 Shiga-toxin-producing *E. coli*, *Vibrio* spp.
Epidemic of multiple patients with a short time of onset	Norovirus; less commonly, *Campylobacter jejuni*, *Salmonella* spp., *Cryptosporidium*
Acute vomiting and diarrhoea after suspected contaminated food	*Bacillus cereus*, *Clostridium botulinum*, *Staphylococcus aureus*
Epidemic of severe gastroenteritis traced to eggs, poultry, meat or dairy products	C. jejuni, *Salmonella* spp.
Oral–anal sexual practices (anilingus)	*Giardia lamblia*, *Entamoeba histolytica*
Abdominal pain	
Nausea, vomiting	
Bloody stool	
Fever	
Rectal pain	
Tenesmus	Severe bacterial infections: *Salmonella*, *Campylobacter*, *Shigella*, EPEC, *Yersinia* or *Vibrio* spp.
Also consider surgical abdomen, GI bleeding	
Inflammatory bowel disease	
Diarrhoea > 7–14 days' duration	Protozoa and microsporidia, *C. difficile*, *Campylobacter*, Shiga-toxin-producing *E. coli*
Haemolytic uraemic syndrome	*E. coli* O157:H7 or other species
Stool WBC count	Not reliable for diagnosis of bacterial aetiology
Colonic ulcerations	Inflammatory bowel disease
Proctitis	Bacterial aetiology highly probable
Pseudomembranes	Toxic megacolon, *C. difficile*
Chronic disease (e.g. cirrhosis, DM)	Complicated course expected with any form of diarrhoeal illness
Organ transplantation	Abnormally severe illness from rotavirus and adenovirus
Increased frequency of cytomegalovirus	
Severe illness from dysenteric diarrhoea	
Spore-forming protozoa and microsporidia	
HIV infection, other immunodeficiency disorders	Severe illness from common bacteria/spore-forming protozoa and microsporidia
Increased frequency of cytomegalovirus and *Mycobacterium avium* complex	

DM: diabetes mellitus; EPEC: enteropathogenic E. coli*; HIV: human immunodeficiency virus; WBC: white blood cell.*

TABLE 24.7 PATHOGEN-SPECIFIC SYNDROMES[40]

CAUSATIVE AGENT	INCUBATION PERIOD	DURATION OF ILLNESS	PREDOMINANT SYMPTOMS	FOODS COMMONLY IMPLICATED
Bacteria				
Campylobacter jejuni	3-5 days	2-5 days, occ. > 10 days	Sudden onset of diarrhoea, abdominal pain, nausea, vomiting	Raw or undercooked poultry, raw milk, meat, untreated water
Escherichia coli enteropathogenic, enterotoxigenic, enteroinvasive, enterohaemorrhagic	12–72 hours (enterotoxigenic); longer in others	3-14 days	Severe colicky abdominal pain, watery to profuse diarrhoea, sometimes bloody. May cause haemolytic uraemic syndrome	Many raw foods, unpasteurised milk, contaminated water, minced beef
Salmonella serovars	6-72 hours	3-5 days	Abdominal pain, diarrhoea, chills, fever, malaise	Meat, chicken, eggs and egg products
Shigella spp.	12-96 hours	4-7 days	Malaise, fever, vomiting, diarrhoea commonly with blood and/or mucus	Any contaminated food or water
Yersinia enterocolitica	3-7 days	1-21 days	Acute diarrhoea sometimes bloody, fever, vomiting	Raw meat and poultry, milk and milk products
Vibrio cholerae	Few hours to 5 days	3-4 days	Asymptomatic to profuse dehydrating diarrhoea	Raw seafood, contaminated water
Vibrio parahaemolyticus	12-24 hours	1-7 days	Abdominal pain, moderate diarrhoea/vomiting of moderate severity	Raw and cooked fish, shellfish, other seafoods
Viruses				
Small round structured viruses (SRSVs) such as astrovirus, adenovirus, calicivirus	24-48 hours	12–48 hours	Severe vomiting, diarrhoea	Oysters, clams, other food contaminated by human Norwalk virus, excreta
Rotaviruses	24-72 hours	3-7 days	Malaise, headache, fever, vomiting, diarrhoea	Contaminated water
Parasites				
Cryptosporidium	1-12 days	4-21 days	Profuse watery diarrhoea	Contaminated water and food
Giardia lamblia	1-3 weeks	1-2 weeks to months	Loose pale greasy stools, abdominal pain	Contaminated water, food contaminated by infected food-handlers
Entamoeba histolytica	2-4 weeks	Weeks–months	Colic, mucus or bloody diarrhoea	Contaminated water and food
Toxin-producing bacteria				
Bacillus cereus (toxin in food)	1-6 hours	< 24 hours	Nausea, vomiting, diarrhoea, cramps	Cereals, rice, meat products, soups, vegetables
Clostridium perfringens (toxin in gut)	8-20 hours	24 hours	Sudden-onset colic, diarrhoea	Meats, poultry, stews, gravies (often reheated)
Staphylococcus aureus (toxin in food)	30 mins–8 hours	24 hours	Acute vomiting, purging, may lead to collapse	Cold foods (much-handled during preparation), milk products, salted meats

the clinical presentation;[47] however, the clinical value of most laboratory tests ordered in differentiating surgical from non-surgical abdominal pain is limited. Commonly ordered laboratory tests in the evolution of acute abdominal pain are full blood count, C-reactive protein, amylase, lipase and liver function tests.

Inflammatory markers, such as white cell count (WCC) and C-reactive protein (CRP), are commonly part of the main battery of tests ordered in ED in the evaluation and differentiation of abdominal pain.[48,49] More recently, procalcitonin (PCT), the pro-hormone form of calcitonin secreted by the extra-thyroid immune cells, has also been promoted as a biomarker in the assessment and diagnosis of abdominal pain, with greater sensitivity and specificity for bacterial infection.[50,51] The role of WCC, CRP and PCT in differentiating abdominal pain, as exemplified in diagnosing appendicitis, is not perfect and in some instances misleading.[49,51–55] Earlier studies[56,57] examining raised WCC found that 10–60% of patients with surgically proven appendicitis had WCCs within the normal range. More recent studies examining the diagnostic value of WCC, CRP and PCT further demonstrated wide-ranging sensitivity and specificity.[58,59] In terms of accuracy, CRP has shown the greatest accuracy, followed by WCC and procalcitonin in diagnosing appendicitis.[59] Inflammatory biomarkers have been studied as an aid to differentiating between minor illness and more serious disease. Most of the studies have shown a moderate relationship between raised inflammatory biomarkers and the target condition, but conclude that if used in isolation are insufficient to rule in or out the condition safely.[60]

Serum lipase is the principal biomarker used for diagnosing acute pancreatitis, and has largely replaced amylase in terms of diagnostic value.[61] While both lipase and amylase are produced by the acinar cells of the pancreas, amylase is also produced by the salivary glands, small intestine mucosa, ovaries, placenta, liver and fallopian tubes, thus limiting its sensitivity and specificity in diagnosing pancreatitis.[62] In the setting of acute pancreatitis, both lipase and amylase become elevated at about the same time (4–8 hours), but lipase may rise to a greater extent and remain elevated much longer (7–10 days versus 12–72 hours respectively). The degrees to which serum lipase levels elevate are not proportional to the severity of the disease. Further, in some instances, both serum lipase and amylase levels may be normal in patients with recurrent pancreatitis or alcoholism.[63] These limitations notwithstanding, lipase is the most useful test in patients suspected of pancreatitis.

Liver function tests (LFT) consist of total bilirubin, conjugated bilirubin, alkaline phosphatase, alanine aminotransferase, aspartate aminotransferase, gamma-glutamyl transpeptidase, serum albumin and serum globulin. The term 'liver function test' is a misnomer as few of the tests actually assess liver function; the majority are based upon some property of the damaged hepatocyte (serum aminotransferases), biliary tract disorder (serum alkaline phosphatase, gamma-glutamyl transferase [GGT]) or synthetic function (serum albumin and prothrombin time/international normalised ratio). While abnormal liver-enzyme levels may signal liver damage or alternation in bile flow, abnormal results are frequently detected in patients who are asymptomatic.[64] Therefore, the decision to obtain LFTs should be determined in conjunction with information gathered from the history, identification of risk factors and physical examination of the patient.[65] Similarly, interpreting LFT results should be done with reference to this information as well as the pattern of LFT abnormality.[66] LFT abnormalities can often be grouped into one of three patterns: hepatocellular, cholestatic or isolated hyperbilirubinaemia.

Patients presenting with a hepatocellular process (e.g. alcoholic liver disease, hepatotoxicity) generally have a disproportionate elevation in serum aminotransferases compared with alkaline phosphatase (AP), while those with a cholestatic process (e.g. biliary flow obstruction) have the opposite findings. In the setting of cholestasis, whether extrahepatic or intrahepatic biliary obstruction, alkaline phosphatase is typically elevated to at least four times the upper limit of normal.[67] Differentiating between extra- and intrahepatic cholestasis is achieved through RUQ ultrasonography. The presence of biliary dilation on ultrasonography suggests extrahepatic cholestasis (e.g. gallstones, strictures or malignancy). The absence of dilation suggests intrahepatic cholestasis (e.g. primary biliary cirrhosis or viral hepatitis). Lesser degrees of alkaline phosphatase elevation are non-specific and may suggest several other types of liver disease. High serum GGT may also assist in confirming hepatobiliary disease; however, elevated levels can be attributed to a wide variety of other clinical conditions such as pancreatic disease, myocardial infarction (MI), renal failure, chronic obstructive pulmonary disease (COPD), diabetes, alcoholism and in patients taking phenytoin and barbiturates.[66]

PRACTICE TIP

Normal vital signs, laboratory results, history and physical examination findings are not reassuring in the older patient presenting with abdominal pain. Take the worst-first approach to ensure patient safety and prevent deterioration.

Rectal and pelvic examination

The inclusion of digital rectal examination (DRE) in all patients with abdominal pain has a longstanding history as a mainstay component in a complete physical examination, despite being unsupported by the literature.[68–71] Studies examining clinicians' use of DRE in the management of acute, undifferentiated abdominal pain in the ED concluded that it contributes no additional information that could not be obtained from history-taking and abdominal examination and, further, it has minimal predictive value.[39,70–73]

Pelvic examination is a key part of the evaluation of a woman presenting with abdominal pain or vaginal bleeding to the ED. Examining the pelvic organs may yield further information regarding the possible gynaecological or obstetric causes of abdominal pain in women. Pelvic examination begins with inspecting the external genitalia for discharge, erythaemia, ulceration, atrophy, masses and old scars. This is then followed by speculum examination of the cervix and bimanual palpation of the pelvic organs.[14] Consideration of testicular pathology in men presenting with lower abdominal pain is also important.

IMAGING

Plain x-rays

Abdominal radiography can be requested in ED, but contributes little to patient treatment while exposing patients to significant doses of unnecessary radiation.[74] Current indications for abdominal x-ray are few: suspected bowel obstruction, oesophageal foreign body (chest x-ray to be performed first) and suspected sharp/poisonous foreign body.[74–77] With the exception of these indications, abdominal radiography sensitivity and specificity is poor (23% and 38% respectively) in patients presenting with non-traumatic acute abdominal pain.[78,79] For patients requiring investigation beyond clinical history, physical examination and lab results, the clinician should be encouraged to request more definitive imaging such as ultrasound and CT.

Ultrasound

Ultrasound is a rapid, non-invasive examination that does not involve exposing the patient to ionising radiation. Most solid intra-abdominal organs (e.g. liver, spleen, gallbladder, pancreas and kidneys) can be imaged using ultrasound. Point of care ultrasound (POCUS) has contributed to the diagnosis and management of abdominal aortic aneurysm (> 3 cm), acute cholecystitis, ectopic pregnancy and, in the presence of free fluid, haemoperitoneum bleeding. It may be beneficial as an initial investigation to diagnose gastrointestinal perforation, small bowel obstruction and appendicitis.[80,81] Ultrasound sensitivity and specificity is largely operator-dependent; however, patient characteristics such as obesity, bowel gas and surgical emphysema can also reduce image quality. Within the context of the emergency care setting, bedside ultrasound is an appropriate first-line approach to assessing, monitoring and triaging abdominal pain;[82–84] however, further diagnostic modalities may be required, such as CT.

Computer tomography

Computer tomography (CT) imaging has been demonstrated to have a positive effect on the accuracy and certainty in the clinical diagnosis of patients with abdominal pain,[82,85–87] and direct decisions regarding patient management.[88] However, while CT imaging has been associated with improving timely diagnosis and treatment of patients presenting with abdominal pain, it is costly[89,90] and is a growing source of exposure to radiation in adults.[91,92] To minimise radiation exposure, a non-enhanced CT should be considered for all patients with non-traumatic acute abdominal pain.[93] Intuitional protocols, radiologist preference, patient's history and severity of condition are key factors in determining administration of contrast CT scans. The majority of abdominal contrast studies focus specifically on appendicitis and have concluded that non-enhanced CT is preferable.[94,95] If the patient requires contrast, electrolyte abnormalities and/or dehydration should be corrected, and electrolytes monitored for patients with severe diarrhoea.[96] The frequency of CT imaging and subsequent exposure to radiation in some instances could be reduced by initially screening abdominal pain patients using ultrasound.[82]

UPPER GASTROINTESTINAL EMERGENCIES

UPPER GASTROINTESTINAL BLEEDING

Bleeding is functionally categorised by location—upper or lower GI bleeding. Fig. 24.8 highlights various sites and causes of GI bleeding. Upper GI bleeding refers to blood loss

FIGURE 24.8 SITES AND CAUSES OF GASTROINTESTINAL BLEEDING[97]

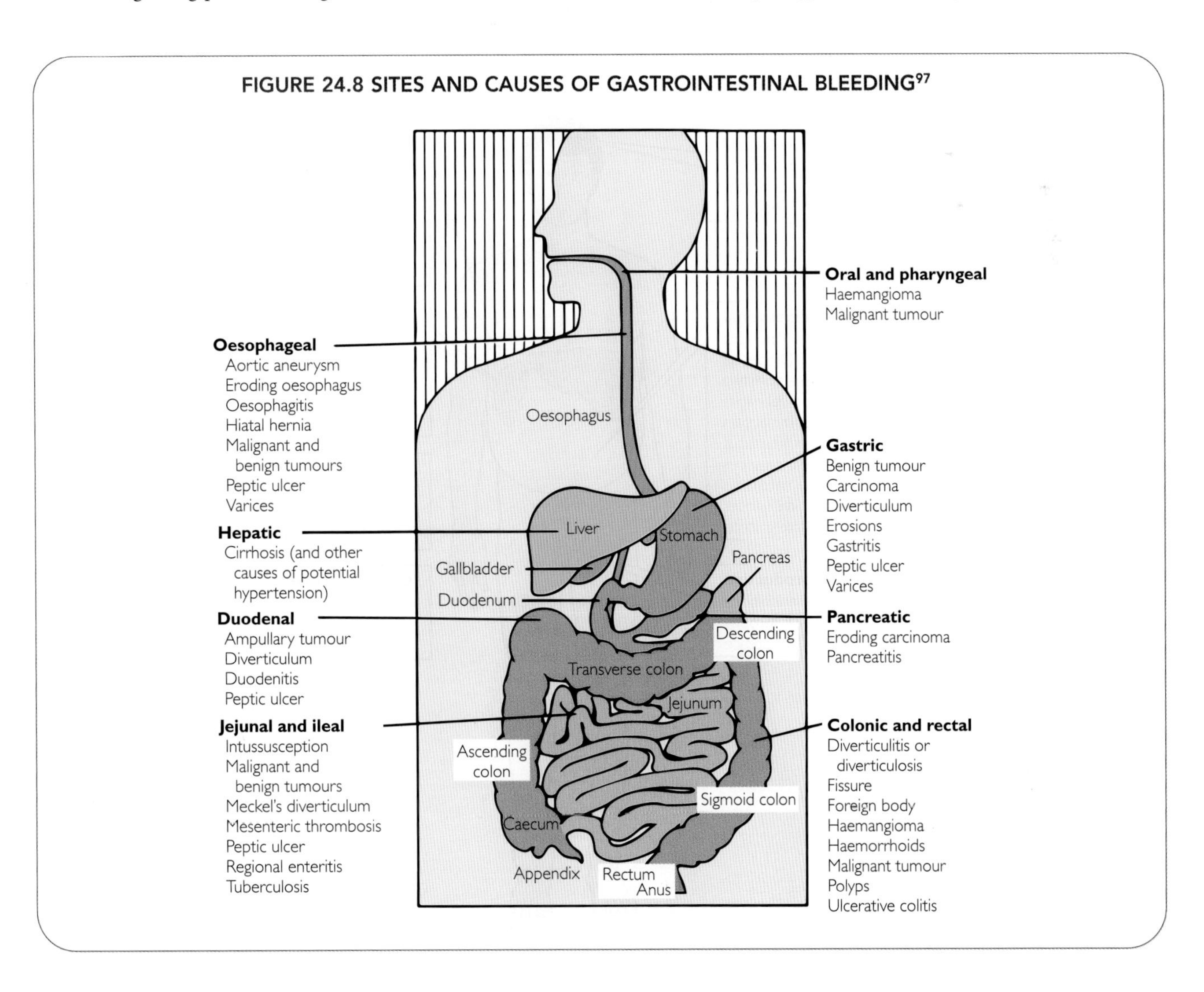

occurring between the upper oesophagus and duodenum at the ligament of Treitz. Bleeding is categorised as either variceal or non-variceal. Upper GI bleeding is more common in males.[98] The risk for death is greater with variceal bleeding because of the occurrence of haemorrhage in these patients.[99] Gastro-oesophageal varices are enlarged venous channels and are dilated by portal hypertension. As portal hypertension increases, varices continue to enlarge and eventually rupture, causing massive haemorrhage. Cirrhosis, mainly from alcohol and chronic viral hepatitis, is the most important cause of portal hypertension in the Western world, while schistosomiasis is the leading cause in developing countries.[100] Fig. 24.9 highlights systemic manifestations of cirrhosis. Bleeding from varices requires immediate intervention and close observation following initial control of bleeding, potentially including endotracheal intubation to protect airway patency. More than 40% of patients with variceal bleeds will re-bleed within 48–72 hours.[101] Non-variceal bleeding is due to erosion or ulceration of the oesophageal or gastroduodenal mucosa which extends into an underlying blood vessel.

Peptic ulcer disease is an infectious process caused by *Helicobacter pylori* and is the most common cause of upper GI bleeding in adults and children.[101] Gastric and duodenal ulcers are two types of peptic ulcers that account for half of major upper GI bleeding, with a mortality rate of 4%. Improvements in the prevention and management of ulcers are seeing a decline in bleeding complications from ulcers in certain parts of the world. This is perhaps due to control of *H. pylori*, safer use of non-steroidal anti-inflammatory drugs (NSAIDs) and prophylaxis with proton pump inhibitors.[98]

Other causes of upper GI bleeding include: drug-induced erosions (e.g. aspirin); retching and vomiting, which cause lacerations in the gastro-oesophageal mucosa (Mallory-Weiss syndrome); vascular anomalies; and gastritis.

Clinical signs and symptoms are variable and may be life threatening. They include pallor, dizziness, lethargy, abdominal pain, nausea, vomiting blood or dark 'coffee grounds' (haematemesis) and passing of dark or bright blood in the stool (malaena or haematochezia). Fluid volume status is important to assess, and signs of hypovolaemia such as tachycardia, postural hypotension, dizziness, confusion or syncope may also occur.

Assessment and management

Assessment and management begins with control of the ABCDEs, and a full assessment of the vital signs including heart rate, blood pressure, baseline mental status or Glasgow Coma Scale score (GCS) and capillary refill time (see Chapter 13). Pre-hospital management includes maintaining airway

FIGURE 24.9 SYSTEMIC CLINICAL MANIFESTATIONS OF LIVER CIRRHOSIS[9]

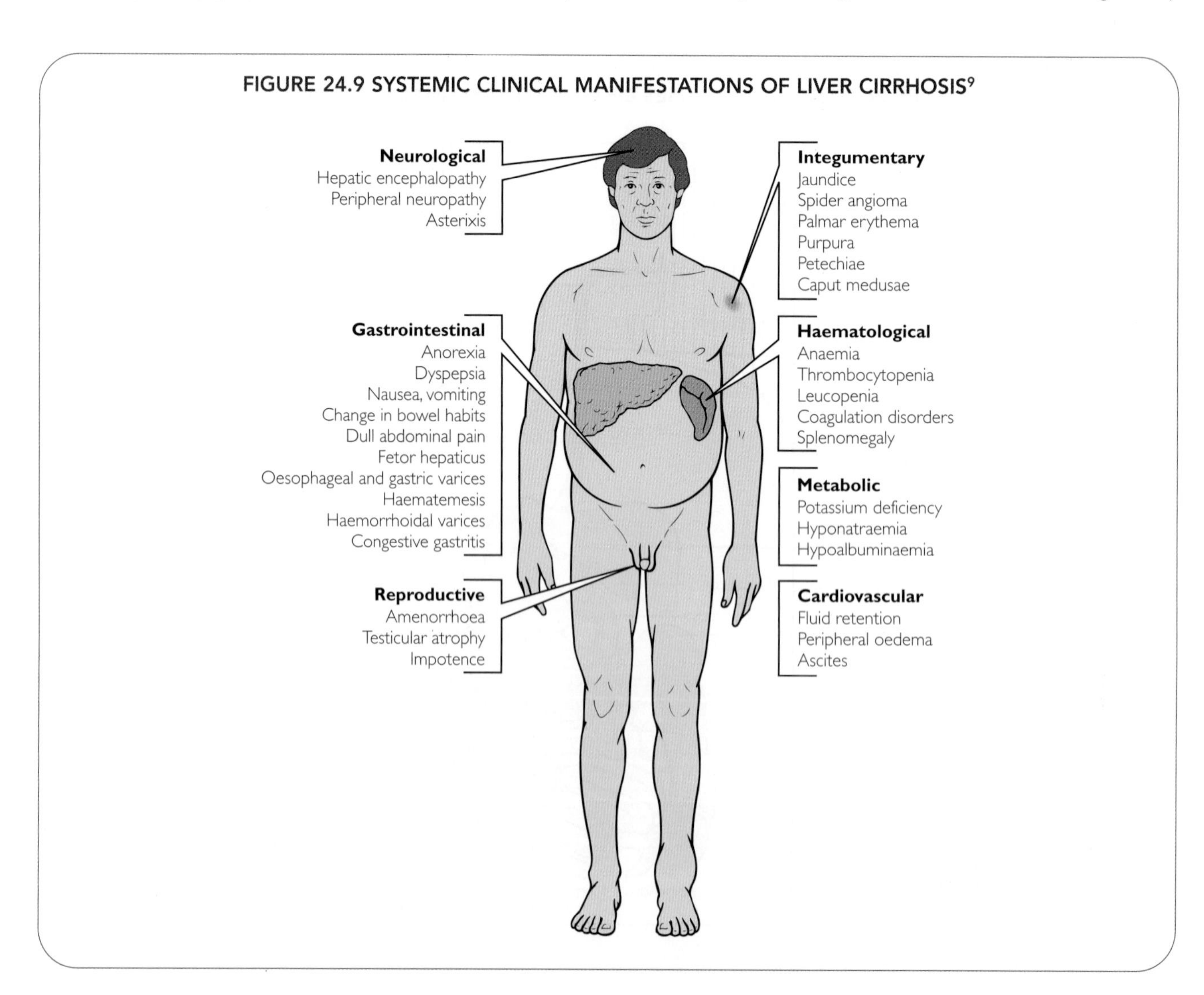

patency by positioning and suctioning of blood, inserting an advanced airway, high-flow oxygen via non-rebreather mask for decreased oxygen saturation, insertion of a large-bore cannula and maintaining perfusion of vital organs.[15] Fluid replacement begins with crystalloid or colloid solutions, followed by blood (packed red blood cells (PRBCs) or whole blood) replacement if the patient's condition does not improve. A restrictive transfusion strategy of a haemoglobin threshold of 70 g/L is recommended.[102,103]

The initial triage assessment must gain an understanding of clinical risk based on several factors. Patients at increased risk include age > 60 years, hypotension, tachycardia, the presence of comorbidities and evidence of blood in the vomit or stool. Bleeding can originate anywhere in the GI tract and can occur at any age.[97,104] The age group most often affected is individuals 50–80 years of age. Factors associated with high morbidity rates are haemodynamic instability, repeated haematemesis, haematochezia and a co-existent organ-system disease.[97] Further comorbidities include medication history, with particular attention to NSAIDs, antiplatelet agents and anticoagulants. New oral anticoagulants (e.g. rivaroxaban, apixaban, dabigatran, etc) may increase the risk of GI bleeding highest in patients with acute coronary syndrome and deep vein thrombosis or pulmonary embolus.[105]

Using a cardiac monitor and continuous measurement of heart and respiratory rate, blood pressure and pulse oximetry is recommended for patients with actual or potential significant blood loss. Be aware that patients with considerable blood loss have lost a large amount of red blood cells and thus oxygen-carrying ability, so are at risk of hypovolaemia and ischaemic conditions such as myocardial infarction. The older patient with poor compensatory mechanisms is further predisposed to ischaemic conditions and can deteriorate rapidly.

A nasogastric tube is recommended for patients with upper GI bleeding. Aspiration of blood or suspicious-coloured dark material confirms a source of bleeding. However, a non-bloodstained return may signify that bleeding is occurring outside the stomach; for example, the duodenum. Concerns that passage of a nasogastric tube may provoke bleeding are unwarranted.[97]

Monitoring of fluid balance is essential and may involve passing a urinary catheter to monitor output or if oliguria is present. A complete abdominal assessment should involve a rectal examination and testing for faecal occult blood.

Baseline laboratory studies include full blood count (FBC), 'group type and hold' or cross-match (for a minimum of two units) depending upon clinical picture, electrolytes, urea, creatinine and serum glucose. Normal creatinine with increased urea suggests bleeding with breakdown of blood in the gut, dehydration or diuretic therapy. Liver function and coagulation studies are also recommended to rule out coagulopathies or liver disease. Serial venous blood gases will show lactate clearance, a predictor of active bleeding and also determine success of resuscitation efforts.[106] An upright chest x-ray can provide valuable information if perforation is suspected; however, this is not feasible if significant haemodynamic compromise is present. An ECG should be obtained to assess for dysrhythmias or ischaemic changes related to blood loss.

Treatment modalities include endoscopy to identify the source of bleeding and control, if needed, medications and surgical interventions. Medical therapy for non-variceal bleeding includes administration of proton pump inhibitors, antacids and H_2 antagonists (Table 24.8). If a bleeding ulcer is detected on endoscopy, it is often managed by an adrenaline injection or cautery into the base of the lesion and a proton pump inhibitor.[97] Gastro-oesophageal variceal bleeding is treated with balloon tamponade (e.g. Sengstaken-Blakemore tube) or one of the variants to control bleeding. Peptic ulcer disease is treated endoscopically with thermal coagulation or injection therapy, whereas gastro-oesophageal varices are treated endoscopically with injection sclerotherapy or variceal band ligation. Endoscopic procedures may be done on a limited basis in EDs across the country. Surgical intervention may be necessary for variceal or non-variceal bleeding. Complications related to upper GI bleeding include aspiration, pneumonia, respiratory failure and hypovolaemic shock. Bleeding stops spontaneously in 80% of hospitalised patients.[107] In the initial stages of presentation to the ED, patients suspected of GI bleeding should be initially nil by mouth (NBM) and if the bleeding is significant a nasogastric tube should be passed.[108] This will rest the gut, reduce additional pressure in the stomach and reduce the likelihood of vomiting. If a patient is NBM, consideration must be made to the underlying fluid balance status with supplementation of intravenous (IV) fluids.

GASTRO-OESOPHAGEAL REFLUX DISEASE (GORD)

Transient gastro-oesophageal reflux is a normal physiological event that occurs at various intervals without causing disease or symptoms. Rosen suggests that it occurs daily in 7% of patients and at least monthly in 15%.[10] Regardless, those who experience an increased frequency of reflux will experience some type of symptoms. Reflux disease is common in Australia. Between 15% and 20% of adults experience heartburn and indigestion each week, and it is estimated that the prevalence of GP-diagnosed GORD in Australia is approximately 10% of patients attending GPs.[111] Conditions associated with GORD are decreased lower oesophageal sphincter (LOS) pressure, decreased oesophageal motility and increased gastric emptying time. Box 24.3 lists specific causes for each situation. It is of interest that acid secretion does not increase in patients with GORD.

Assessment and management

Chest pain or heartburn is the most common symptom associated with this condition. Patients experience a variance of pain or discomfort ranging from mild to quite severe. Relaxation of the LOS during pregnancy increases the occurrence of heartburn during pregnancy; at least 25% of pregnant women experience daily heartburn. Chest pain as the only symptom of GORD is reported in 10% of patients with the disease.[112] A key aspect of pain associated with GORD is that it radiates, usually to the neck, jaws, shoulders, arms and abdomen. Similarities to the clinical presentation of ischaemic heart disease require thoughtful consideration. It is often difficult to distinguish between these very different conditions in the ED. The healthcare professional should pay close attention to the appearance of the patient, the history, clinical assessment and changes in vital signs and clinical condition. Characteristics unique to GORD include worsening of symptoms with stooping, lying or leaning forward. Other symptoms associated with GORD are summarised in Box 24.4.

TABLE 24.8 DRUG THERAPY IN GASTROINTESTINAL (GI) BLEEDING[7,107,109,110]

DRUG	SOURCE OF GI BLEEDING	MECHANISM OF ACTION
Antacids	Duodenal ulcer, gastric ulcer, acute gastritis (corrosive, erosive and haemorrhagic)	Neutralises acid and maintains gastric pH above 5.5; elevated pH inhibits activation of pepsinogen
H_2-receptor antagonists Cimetidine Famotidine Nizatidine Ranitidine	Duodenal ulcer, gastric ulcer, oesophagitis, acute gastritis (especially haemorrhagic)	Inhibits action of histamine at H_2 receptors on parietal cells and decreases HCl secretion
Proton pump inhibitors Omeprazole Esomeprazole Lansoprazole Pantoprazole		Inhibits activity of proton pump and binds to hydrogen-potassium ATP at secretory surface of gastric parietal cell, blocking gastric acid production
Terlipressin	Oesophageal varices	Causes vasoconstriction and increases smooth muscle activity of the GI tract; reduces pressure in the portal circulation and arrests bleeding
Octreotide	Upper gastrointestinal bleeding, oesophageal varices	Somatostatin analogue that decreases splanchnic blood flow; decreases HCl secretion via decrease in release of gastrin

ATP: adenosine triphosphate; HCl: hydrochloric acid.

BOX 24.3 FACTORS AFFECTING LOWER OESOPHAGEAL SPHINCTER PRESSURE[9]

INCREASE PRESSURE

Bethanechol	Metoclopramide

DECREASE PRESSURE

Alcohol	Tea, coffee (caffeine)
Anticholinergics	Beta-adrenergic blockers
Chocolate (theobromine)	Calcium channel blockers
Fatty foods	Diazepam
Nicotine	Morphine sulfate
Peppermint, spearmint	Nitrates
Progesterone	Theophylline

BOX 24.4 CLINICAL SYMPTOMS OF GORD

TYPICAL	ATYPICAL
Chest pain	Non-cardiac chest pain
Heartburn	Asthma
Dysphagia	Persistent cough
Odynophagia	Hiccups
Regurgitation	Hoarseness
Water brash	Frequent throat clearing
Belching	Nocturnal choking
Early satiety	Sleep apnoea
Nausea	Recurrent pneumonia
Anorexia	Recurrent ENT infections
Weight loss	Loss of dental enamel
	Halitosis

ENT: ear–nose–throat; GORD: gastro-oesophageal reflux disease.

Consider the classic presentation for ischaemic heart disease and note the similarities and differences in presentation of patients who present with epigastric discomfort or chest pain of a GI origin. This is an important consideration, as both may have very similar presentations and symptoms, although one is immediately life threatening while the other is not. Therefore, management of GORD in the emergency sense begins with elimination of other conditions that are more lethal (e.g. myocardial infarction).[112] Vital signs must be obtained, with the regularity of observations dependent on the clinical picture. Patient assessment and studies such as ECG, chest radiograph and pathology investigations are primarily used to rule out other conditions. Additional imaging studies include endoscopy and barium studies. Specific treatment in the ED includes symptomatic relief through use of antacids, H_2 blockers and other medications.[112] Antacids are given with viscous lidocaine to increase effectiveness. Table 24.9 highlights specific medications and their actions.

TABLE 24.9 DRUG THERAPY FOR GORD[113]

MECHANISM OF ACTION	EXAMPLES
Increase LOS pressure	
Cholinergic	Bethanechol chloride
Dopamine antagonist	Metoclopramide
Serotonin antagonist	Cisapride
Neutralise acid	
Antacids	Alka-Seltzer: $NaHCO_3$ and/or $KHCO_3$ Andrews Antacid: $CaCO_3$, $MgCO_3$ Equate: $Al(OH)_3$ and $Mg(OH)_2$ Gaviscon: $Al(OH)_3$ Maalox (liquid): $Al(OH)_3$ and $Mg(OH)_2$ Maalox (tablet): $CaCO_3$ Milk of magnesia: $Mg(OH)_2$ Pepto Bismol: $C_7H_5BiO_4$ Pepto-Bismol Children's: $CaCO_3$ Rolaids: $CaCO_3$ and $Mg(OH)_2$ Tums: $CaCO_3$ Mylanta: contains $Al(OH)_3$ Eno Gelusil (tablet, syrup) Alusil MPS (tablet)
Antisecretory	
Histamine H_2-receptor antagonists	Ranitidine Cimetidine Famotidine Nizatidine
Proton pump inhibitors	Esomeprazole Omeprazole Lansoprazole Pantoprazole Rabeprazole
Cytoprotective	
Alginic acid antacid	Gaviscon: contains alginic acid and $NaHCO_3$
Antacids	Gelusil, Mylanta
Acid-protective	Sucralfate

LOS: lower oesophageal sphincter; $Al(OH)_3$: aluminium hydroxide; $C_7H_5BiO_4$: bismuth subsalicylate; $CaCO_3$: calcium carbonate; $KHCO_3$: potassium bicarbonate; $MgCO_3$: magnesium carbonate; $Mg(OH)_2$: magnesium hydroxide; $NaHCO_3$: sodium bicarbonate.

ACHALASIA (CARDIOSPASM)

In achalasia, peristalsis of the lower two-thirds (smooth muscle) of the oesophagus is absent. Pressure in the LOS is increased, along with incomplete relaxation of the sphincter. Obstruction of the oesophagus at or near the diaphragm occurs. Food and fluid accumulate in the lower oesophagus.[10] The result of the condition is dilation of the lower oesophagus (Fig. 24.10). The altered peristalsis is a result of impairment of the neurons that innervate the lower oesophagus. There is a selective loss of inhibitory neurons, resulting in unopposed excitation of the LOS. Achalasia affects all ages and both genders. The course of the disease is chronic. It is linked to increased incidence of carcinoma, possibly secondary to food stasis.

Assessment and management

Dysphagia (difficulty in swallowing) is the most common symptom and occurs with both liquids and solids.[114] Patients may report a globus sensation (a lump in the throat). Substernal chest pain (similar to the pain of angina) occurs during or immediately after a meal. Halitosis (foul-smelling breath) and the inability to eructate (belch) are other symptoms. Another common symptom is regurgitation of sour-tasting food and liquids, especially when the patient is in the horizontal position. Patients with achalasia may also report symptoms of GORD (e.g. heartburn).[112] Weight loss is typical.

Diagnosis is usually by radiological studies, manometric studies of the lower oesophagus and endoscopy. The exact cause of achalasia is not known, so treatment is focused on symptoms. Treatment consists of dilation surgery and the use of drugs. Drug therapy is used to manage early achalasia when there is no significant dilation. Drug therapy is used as a short-term measure and is considered as an alternative only in patients unfit to undergo surgery. Drugs used in management of achalasia include anticholinergics, calcium channel blockers

FIGURE 24.10 OESOPHAGEAL ACHALASIA[9]

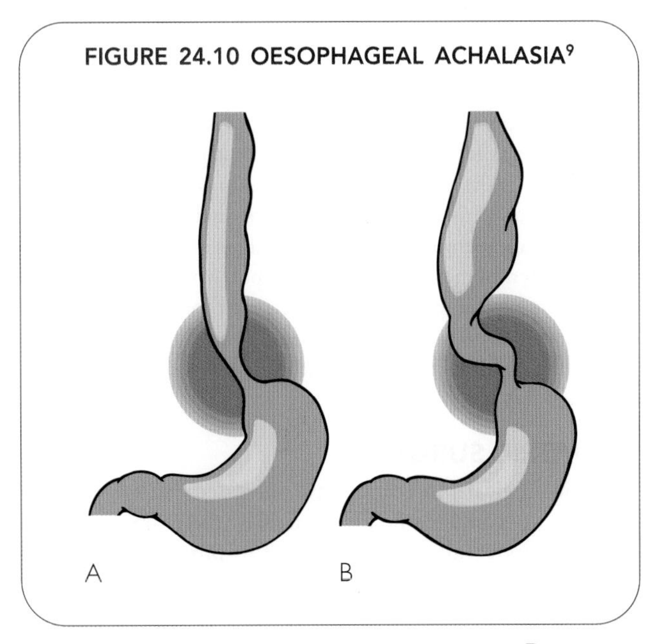

A. Early stage, showing tapering of lower oesophagus. **B.** Advanced stage, showing dilated, tortuous oesophagus.

(e.g. nifedipine) and long-acting nitrates, which act by relaxing the smooth muscle.[101]

GASTROENTERITIS

Gastroenteritis is inflammation of the gastrointestinal tract caused by viral, protozoal, bacterial or parasitic agents (see Table 24.7). Gastroenteritis is most commonly caused by viral infections resulting in vomiting and diarrhoea, of which norovirus, a highly infectious virus, is estimated to cause 677 million annual cases worldwide, resulting in 210,000 deaths, and is the leading cause of gastroenteritis in Australia. Viral gastroenteritis is generally self-limiting. Bacterial infection accounts for around 20% of acute diarrhoea disease,[3] of which *Campylobacter* is the most common cause of bacterial gastroenteritis in Australia (110.3 cases per 100,000 population);[115] it is frequently associated with eating contaminated poultry. Gastroenteritis may be caused by an imbalance of the normal flora (*E. coli*) resulting from the ingestion of contaminated food. Patients have nausea, vomiting, diarrhoea and abdominal cramps. Hyperactive bowel sounds, fever and headaches may also be present. Anal excoriation occurs with frequent episodes of diarrhoea. Diarrhoea accounts for 5 million to 10 million deaths annually in Asia, Africa and Latin America.[3]

Assessment and management

Appropriate diagnostic testing varies based on the clinical situation. Laboratory testing may include FBC, electrolytes measurement, stool for ova and parasites, and stool culture.[10] In the presence of dehydration in patients unable to tolerate oral hydration, obtain IV access for replacement of fluid and electrolytes. Administer antiemetics and analgesics as needed. Antibiotics are determined by patient history and presenting symptoms (Box 24.5). Successful treatment is based on identifying the causative agent and resting the intestinal tract.

In patients who are able to tolerate oral hydration, clear fluids should be encouraged. Suggested fluids should be dilute and gentle to the mucosa of the gastrointestinal tract and include various teas, ginger ale, broth and electrolyte replacement drinks or electrolyte ice blocks. Fluid replacement in children is critical to prevent dehydration. Electrolyte replacement substances such as ice blocks are an ideal first place to start. Oral rehydration is the preferred route to begin rehydration. Parenteral rehydration is reserved for patients unable to tolerate oral substances and demonstrating clinical signs of dehydration (dry mucous membranes, tachycardia, hypotension, lethargy and weakness). Rice, apple sauce, bananas and toast can be started as soon as diarrhoea subsides. Feeding should begin as soon as possible in children and adults, but only following an ability to tolerate fluids.

BOX 24.5 ANTIBIOTIC TREATMENT REGIMENS FOR GASTROENTERITIS[39,116]

GIARDIA LAMBLIA

Tinidazole 2 g orally as a single dose

OR

Metronidazole 400 mg orally, 8-hourly for 7 days

AMOEBIASIS

Metronidazole 600 mg orally, 6-hourly for 6–10 days

PLUS

Diloxanide furoate 500 mg orally 8-hourly for 10 days

SHIGELLOSIS

Norfloxacin 400 mg orally, 12-hourly for 7–10 days

OR

Ampicillin 1 g orally, 6-hourly for 7–10 days

OR

Co-trimoxazole (sulfamethoxazole and trimethoprim in ratio 1:5) 80 mg/400 mg orally, 12-hourly for 7–10 days

CAMPYLOBACTER

Erythromycin 500 mg orally, 6-hourly for 7–10 days

TRAVELLER'S DIARRHOEA

Norfloxacin 800 mg orally as a single dose or 400 mg orally 12-hourly for 3 days

OR

Co-trimoxazole (trimethoprim and sulfamethoxazole in ratio 1:5) 320/1600 mg orally, as a single dose or 160/800 mg orally, 12-hourly for 3 days

CLOSTRIDIUM DIFFICILE

Metronidazole 400 mg orally 8-hourly for 7–10 days. If unresponsive or severe disease: vancomycin 125 mg orally 6-hourly for 1–2 weeks

BARIATRIC SURGERY

Bariatric surgical procedures have increased exponentially in an effort to combat obesity. Currently there are two main forms of surgical therapy undertaken to promote weight loss and reduce patient morbidity and mortality; these are laparoscopic adjustable gastric banding and laparoscopic gastric bypass. Gastric bypass refers to any surgical procedure that first divides the stomach to leave a small pouch, which is then connected through rearranging the small intestine. In relation to Roux-en-Y gastric bypass surgery, this is commonly achieved laparoscopically. Similarly, in gastric banding an adjustable band is placed laparoscopically just below the gastro-oesophageal junction at a 45° angle towards the left shoulder, leaving a 50–80 mL size gastric pouch. Although the benefits and relative low mortality of bariatric surgery are clear,[117,118] postoperative abdominal pain is one of the most common and vexing problems increasingly presenting to ED. Clinical presentations are highly variable and evaluation may be complicated by the fact that obese patients feel abdominal symptoms more intensely compared to lean patients.[119] Therefore, a broad evaluation directed by history and clinical presentation is required. As a result, emergency clinicians have required increasing knowledge and expertise in managing patients presenting post-bariatric surgery with abdominal pain to the ED. It is imperative that ED clinicians remain vigilant in the evaluation and management of patients presenting following bariatric surgery, and seek surgical consultation as soon as possible. The assessment and management of both gastric banding and bypass surgery are discussed jointly below.

Assessment and management

Common emergencies occurring early (< 30 days) post-gastric bypass surgery include: anastomotic fistula formation leading to peritonitis (gastric bypass, 1–6%; sleeve gastrectomy, 3–7%);[120]

acute distension of the bypassed division of the stomach, typically developing in less than 7 days post-surgery; patients will present with nausea, dry-retching, left upper quadrant bloating, hiccups[121] and bleeding. Hepatobiliary complications in the form of gallstones occur most frequently (32%) postoperatively, due to rapid weight loss and resultant bile stasis with biliary sludge formation.[122] In open gastric bypass, incisional hernias occur much more frequently (15–20%)[123] compared to using a laparoscopic approach (6%).[124] Late gastric bypass surgical emergencies include stomal stenosis; small bowel obstruction may occur in the early or late postoperative period and has been described in up to 5% of Roux-en-Y gastric bypass operations. Aetiologies of small bowel obstruction post-gastric bypass surgery include adhesion, internal hernia and intussusception.[125]

A further potential complication post-bariatric surgery, whether by bypass or by banding, is pulmonary embolism secondary to deep vein thrombosis. Pulmonary embolism is the second-most common cause of death after bariatric surgery, with an incidence of 2% and a mortality of 20–30%.[118,126] Nutritional complications are more common with gastric bypass surgery than gastric banding, frequently resulting in iron-deficiency anaemia (20–49%) and B_{12} deficiencies (26–70%).[127] Similar complications have also been observed following laparoscopic gastric banding.

Superior mesenteric vein thrombosis after bariatric surgery is a diagnosis which should be considered in the presence of any postoperative abdominal pain. Initially a first aetiological assessment is performed (measurement of antithrombin III and of protein C and protein S, testing for activated protein C resistance).[120] Fistula after sleeve gastrectomy can develop even 3 months following surgery, and in the majority (90%) of cases, it is located at the upper level of the stapling (cardia).[128] Neurological complications occur in approximately 4% of patients after bariatric surgery and may develop 3–20 months after surgery, particularly in patients with repetitive vomiting.[127] They are characterised by neuropathy, myopathy and encephalopathy. Vitamin B_1 (thiamine) deficiency is usually the cause of these neurological problems.[129]

Laparoscopic adjustable gastric banding has gained popularity for treatment of morbid obesity worldwide, but has been associated with various complications. Pouch enlargement can occur in up to 12% of patients following gastric banding.[130] Pouch enlargement can frequently (77%) be resolved by deflating the band and conservative management (low calorie diet, re-enforcement of portion size control).[130] Band slippage can occur in up to 22% of patients, potentially leading to gastric perforation, necrosis, upper gastrointestinal bleeding and aspiration pneumonia.[131] Patients normally present complaining of dysphagia, vomiting, regurgitation and food intolerance,[132,133] and require surgical correction. Band erosion, whereby the band erodes through the stomach wall and into the gastric lumen, is uncommon ($< 1\%$).[131] However, despite its low incidence, ED clinicians should have a high index of suspicion as most patients present asymptomatically. When symptomatic, patients will complain of loss of restriction, vague epigastric pain, gastrointestinal bleeding, intra-abdominal abscesses or port site infection. Management involves the removal of the gastric band, which is made increasingly difficult by the extensive inflammatory response around the proximal stomach and left lobe of the liver.

Port-site infections, breakages and tubing malfunction can also occur. Port-site infections that manifest early following surgery are often present with the cardinal signs of erythaema, swelling and pain. Early infections with cellulitis alone can normally be managed with oral antibiotics, yet if the response is inadequate, intravenous antibiotic administration should be trialled. Should this fail, and the infection is limited to the port, then the port should be removed, and the tubing knotted and left inside the abdomen. Once the infection is resolved, a new port can be reconnected to the tubing. Late onset post-site infections are caused by delayed band erosion with ascending infection which manifests several months after surgery.[131,134] Late-onset port-site infections are normally unresponsive to antibiotic therapy. Left untreated, late port-site infections can develop into life-threatening intra-abdominal sepsis. Early gastroscopy and removal of the band is required. Damage to the port resulting in breakage typically presents as a slow-leak loss of injected fluid volume on aspiration. It is essential to only access ports with non-coring Huber needles to maintain port septum integrity. Any adjustment required of the gastric band must be undertaken using fluoroscopy. Similarly, assessing for tube leakage can be undertaken by injecting dilute non-ionic iodinated contrast into the port under fluoroscopy.[131,133]

ANALGESIA

Pain relief is a humane practice. The historical practices of withholding the administration of narcotic or other similar analgesia until a confirmed diagnosis is made or surgical consult obtained continues despite the overwhelming evidence that it does not lead to diagnostic error.[135,136] Evidence supports the early administration of analgesia to patients with abdominal pain, including children (see Chapters 18 and 35) and adults, finding that it enhances patient examination and facilitates diagnosis.[136] Education programs have also been established throughout Australian EDs to facilitate early narcotic and non-narcotic analgesia.[136,137]

For patients with severe ($\geq 7/10$) pain, pain management options include intravenous morphine sulfate or fentanyl depending on patient age and haemodynamic stability.[138] For patients with less severe pain, pain management includes paracetamol with the addition of oxycodone (immediate release) for those in moderate pain.[136]

LOWER GASTROINTESTINAL EMERGENCIES

LOWER GI BLEEDING

Lower GI bleeding is bleeding that occurs below the ligament of Treitz, and accounts for approximately 20–33% of episodes of GI haemorrhage.[139] Patients may have bright-red blood from mouth or rectum or black, tarry stools indicating bleeding from within the GI tract. Lower GI bleeding is seen more often in females.[104]

Common causes are haemorrhoids, diverticulitis (diverticular disease), colonic polyps, angiodysplasia, colon cancer or colitis. Diverticulitis and angiodysplasia are common causes of lower GI bleeding in the older patient, whereas haemorrhoids, anal fissures and inflammatory bowel disease occur most often in younger patients. Diverticulitis refers to pouch-like herniations on the colon (Fig. 24.11). What initially appears to be lower bleeding

FIGURE 24.11 DIVERTICULA ARE OUTPOUCHINGS OF THE COLON[9]

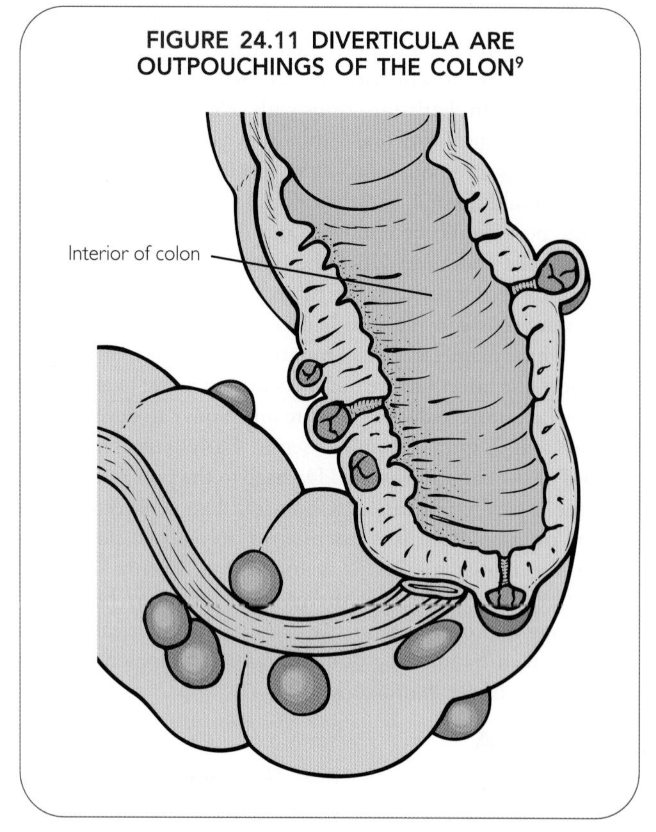

When they become inflamed, the condition is diverticulitis. The inflammatory process can spread to the surrounding area in the intestine.

FIGURE 24.12 ANATOMICAL STRUCTURES OF THE RECTUM AND ANUS WITH INTERNAL AND EXTERNAL HAEMORRHOIDS[9]

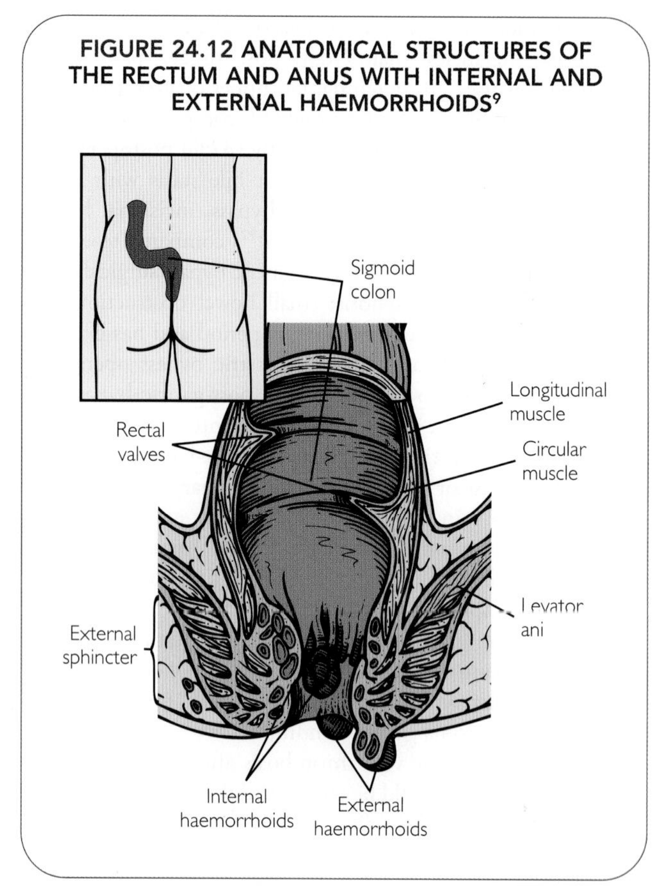

may in fact often be upper GI bleeding. Consideration should always be given to conditions of the upper GI tract when assessing patients with GI bleeding.

Haemorrhoids are the most common aetiology of lower GI bleeding.[104] Fig. 24.12 depicts internal and external haemorrhoidal veins, where haemorrhoids often erupt. Internal haemorrhoids are rarely associated with pain, whereas external haemorrhoids can cause significant discomfort.

Assessment and management

Approximately 11% of lower GI bleeding are secondary to brisk upper GI bleeding and are less severe in nature. Eighty-five per cent of patients with lower GI bleeding experience acute bleeds that are self-limiting and do not cause significant changes in haemodynamic status. Most patients with mild lower GI bleeding who are haemodynamically stable may be evaluated on an outpatient basis. Treatment includes identifying the source of bleeding with anoscopy, flexible sigmoidoscopy or barium enema. Patients with severe symptomatic lower GI bleeding require hospital admission for resuscitation, diagnosis and treatment. Colonoscopy may be performed to determine the source of bleeding after the patient is stabilised.[104]

The cardinal sign of lower GI bleeding is haematochezia. Patients may have bright blood or maroon stools, or there may be occult blood in the stool. Cramp-like abdominal pain may be present. Explosive diarrhoea with foul odour is frequently present. Painless bleeding also occurs. Pallor, diaphoresis and decreased capillary refill are present with significant bleeding. Postural changes in pulse or BP occur in many patients. Pedal oedema can occur with chronic bleeding because of protein depletion. The first priority is management of the ABCDEs and full assessment of the vital signs. Patients with signs or symptoms of hypovolaemia require immediate intervention, high-flow oxygen, ECG, BP and oxygen saturation monitoring, large-bore IV access and fluid resuscitation. Vigilant monitoring of fluid balance status is essential. Maintain NBM patients with attention to mouth care.

Baseline laboratory studies include FBC, platelet count, coagulation studies and 'group type and hold' or cross-match. Administration of PRBCs may be necessary in cases of significant blood loss. Determining the source of bleeding is a priority. Colonoscopy, bleeding scans or angiography may be performed, with surgical intervention required in some cases.

CHOLECYSTITIS

Inflammation of the gallbladder (cholecystitis) causes distension as the cystic duct becomes obstructed. Bacterial invasion, usually by *E. coli*, *Streptococcus* or *Salmonella*, also causes cholecystitis. The most common cause of biliary colic and cholecystitis is cholelithiasis (gallstones). Gallstones arise from the precipitation of cholesterol and calcium salts in saturated bile.[140] It is estimated that between 2% and 12% of patients suffering cholecystitis do not have gallstones.[10] Gallstones usually cause acute cholangitis, which is a potentially life-threatening bacterial infection of the biliary tree.[108] Gallbladder disease is a significant condition affecting Australians: over 70,000 people are hospitalised each year for illness relating to the gallbladder and biliary tree.[21] Cholecystitis usually affects obese, fair-skinned women of increasing age and parity. The female population is affected 3:1 with respect to males.[108]

Assessment and management

Symptoms include sudden-onset abdominal pain—usually after ingestion of fried or fatty foods.[114] Pain may radiate from the epigastrium to the RUQ or may be referred to the right supraclavicular area. Patients usually describe pain as colicky or intermittent in nature, waxing and waning in intensity. The symptoms are experienced when the gallbladder is contracting against an obstruction.[141] Eventual accumulation of fluid and bacterial proliferation may result, leading to empyema formation and possible perforation. Local and rebound tenderness may also be present. Marked tenderness and inspiratory limitation on deep palpation under the right subcostal margin (Murphy's sign) may also be present. A palpable gallbladder or fullness of the RUQ is present in 30–40% of cases. Low-grade fever, tachycardia, nausea, vomiting and flatulence are common findings.[10] Elderly patients (especially those with diabetes) may present with only vague symptoms. While localised tenderness may be present, historical and physical findings of pain and fever may be absent. If the common bile duct is obstructed, the patient may appear slightly jaundiced, with a history of pale stools. Untreated and progressive worsening of the condition may lead to deterioration, with a clinical picture of bacteraemia and sepsis. Elderly patients may deteriorate rapidly without warning. Acute cholangitis presents with the classic triad of symptoms of fever, RUQ pain and jaundice (Charcot's triad), which may lead to sepsis with symptoms of hypotension and decreased level of consciousness (Reynold's pentad).[108] Table 24.10 highlights clinical signs associated with obstructed bile flow.

Diagnostic tests include urinalysis, FBC, serum electrolytes, urea, creatinine, serum glucose and serum bilirubin levels; however, results may be non-specific. C-reactive protein is more accurate than white cell count to diagnose mild, moderate and severe cholecystitis.[142] Elevated amylase suggests pancreatitis rather than cholecystitis.[100] Leucocytosis may be mild to pronounced. POCUS is extremely useful in the emergency setting as it can detect a thickened gallbladder wall, gallstones, sonographic Murphy's sign and pericholecystic fluid.[143]

An ECG should be obtained to exclude the presentation with cardiac involvement. A cardiac cause should be considered, especially in patients with significant risk factors such as age, smoking, hyperlipidaemia, hypertension or previous cardiac pathology. Additional differentials include renal calculi, pancreatitis, gastritis and ulcer disease.[10]

Treatment of cholecystitis depends on the severity of the condition and the presence or absence of complications. Treatment may include the administration of IV crystalloid solution and medications for nausea and vomiting. A nasogastric tube may be necessary for gastric decompression. Monitor vital signs and intake and output. Broad-spectrum antibiotics are indicated if microbial infection is suspected. Narcotic analgesics are recommended for pain control. Definitive treatment for cholecystitis is surgery with traditional laparotomy or laparoscopic cholecystectomy.[140]

ACUTE PANCREATITIS

Acute pancreatitis results from inflammation of the pancreas.[144] Causes of acute pancreatitis are variable and include: bile or duodenal reflux due to gallstones, bacterial infection, pancreatic enzyme activation with autolysis and ductal hypertension. Some 70–80% of pancreatitis cases are due to biliary disease with probable obstruction of the common bile duct resulting in ductal hypertension and pancreatic enzyme activation.[10] Alcohol abuse causes toxic metabolites that injure the pancreas, leading to inflammation. Other causes include chronic hypercalcaemia, surgery, abdominal trauma, infections (mumps, cytomegalovirus infection), drugs, toxins (organophosphate insecticides) or endoscopic retrograde cholangio-pancreatography.[145] More than 85 drugs have been identified as causative agents for pancreatitis and together account for 2% of cases (Box 24.6).[10]

There exist both similarities and distinct differences between acute and chronic pancreatitis. Acute pancreatitis, with a mortality rate of $< 5\%$, may occur as isolated or recurring attacks where the gland is normal before the attack, returning to

TABLE 24.10 CLINICAL MANIFESTATIONS CAUSED BY OBSTRUCTED BILE FLOW[9]

CLINICAL MANIFESTATION	AETIOLOGY
Obstructive jaundice	No bile flow into duodenum
Dark amber urine, which foams when shaken	Soluble bilirubin in urine
No urobilinogen in urine	No bilirubin reaching small intestine to be converted to urobilinogen
Clay-coloured stools	No bilirubin reaching small intestine to be converted to urobilinogen
Pruritus	Deposition of bile salts in skin tissues
Intolerance for fatty foods (nausea, sensation of fullness, anorexia)	No bile in small intestine for fat digestion
Bleeding tendencies	Lack of or decreased absorption of vitamin K, resulting in decreased production of prothrombin
Steatorrhoea	No bile salts in duodenum, preventing fat emulsion and digestion

BOX 24.6 DRUG-INDUCED PANCREATITIS[9]

DEFINITE

Azathioprine	Tetracycline
Cisplatin	Thiazides
Furosemide	Sulfonamides
Colipase	

PROBABLE

Paracetamol	Mefenamic acid
Cimetidine	Opiates
Oestrogens	Sodium valproate
Indomethacin	

POSSIBLE

Bumetanide	Isoniazid
Carbamazepine	Isotretinoin
Chlorthalidone	Methyldopa
Clonidine	Metronidazole
Colchicine	Nitrofurantoin
Corticosteroids	Pentamidine
Cyclosporin	Piroxicam
Cytarabine	Procainamide
Enalapril	Rifampicin
Ergotamine	Salicylates
Ethacrynic acid	Sulindac

normal after the episode. In severe pancreatitis, there is pronounced inflammation, tissue necrosis and haemorrhaging of the gland, which gives rise to a systemic inflammatory response; the mortality rate is 10–50%.[45,146] After 5 to 7 days, necrotic pancreatic tissue can become infected by enteric bacteria. In contrast, chronic pancreatitis results in permanent structural changes to the pancreas, which impair the endocrine and exocrine functions of the gland.[11,145]

Regardless of mechanism, pancreatitis is characterised by acinar cell damage that leads to necrosis, oedema and inflammation. Acute pancreatitis affects 1.5 people per 100,000 population, but varies with the population.[33] Pancreatitis is the second-most frequent pancreatic emergency seen in the ED, a frequency exceeded only by diabetes (see also Chapter 26).[11,145]

Assessment and management

The cardinal symptom of acute pancreatitis is abdominal pain originating in the epigastric region and radiating to the back, which is characteristically dull, boring and steady. Usually, the pain is sudden in onset and gradually intensifies. Abdominal tenderness, rebound and guarding are usually present. Nausea, vomiting and abdominal distension may be present. Patients may be febrile with tachycardia, tachypnoea and hypotension. Decreased gastric motility causes hypoactive or absent bowel sounds. The presence of Cullen's sign (periumbilical bruising) or Grey Turner's sign (bruising of the flanks) is caused by retroperitoneal haemorrhage resulting from acute pancreatitis and is associated with a mortality estimate of nearly 40%.[29]

The initial diagnosis of acute pancreatitis is based on clinical presentation, although laboratory investigations, if required, can include CT, MRI or ultrasonography. Certain laboratory values can also aid in diagnosis of acute pancreatitis (Table 24.11). An elevated serum lipase level, and to some lesser degree, raised amylase levels, is pathognomonic for pancreatitis. Serum lipase is considered a more sensitive marker as it is only produced by the pancreas and persists after the onset of the attack. Lipase concentrations rise within 4–8 hours of the attack, peak at 24 hours and return to normal after 8–14 days.[11,145] Leucocytosis, decreased haematocrit, hyperglycaemia and glycosuria may also be present.[144] Continuing decreases in haematocrit suggest haemorrhagic pancreatitis. Persistent hypocalcaemia is associated with poor prognosis.[108] Serum amylase may be normal in patients with pancreatitis related to alcohol abuse or elevated triglycerides, or if testing is delayed. Amylase is a small molecule rapidly cleared by the kidneys; therefore, abnormally high levels in acute pancreatitis may be short-lived. Conversely, in patients with renal disease, a higher threshold of the upper normal values should be considered. A rapid urinary dipstick test trypsinogen-2 can be used as one of the diagnostic tools with comparable sensitivity and specificity of serum lipase and serum amylase.[147]

TABLE 24.11 DIAGNOSTIC STUDIES FOR ACUTE PANCREATITIS[108,144,147]

LABORATORY TEST	ABNORMAL FINDING	AETIOLOGY
Primary tests		
Serum amylase	Increased	Pancreatic cell injury
Serum lipase	Elevated	Pancreatic cell injury
Urinary amylase	Elevated	Pancreatic cell injury
Secondary tests		
Blood glucose	Hyperglycaemia	Impairment of carbohydrate metabolism resulting from beta-cell damage and release of glucagons
Serum calcium	Hypocalcaemia	Saponification of calcium by fatty acids in areas of fat necrosis
Serum triglycerides	Hyperlipidaemia	Release of free fatty acids by lipase

Radiographic studies are useful. A chest x-ray may reveal pleural effusions or pulmonary infiltrates, and the ileus may be detected on abdominal x-ray. Abdominal ultrasound can allow visualisation of dilated pancreatic ducts, ascites, or the presence of gallstones as an underlying cause. The optimal time for CT scan is at least 72–96 hours post onset of symptoms unless otherwise clinically indicated. Intravenous contrast may exacerbate pancreatitis, cause nephrotoxicity and allergic reactions.[148]

Management includes maintaining strict NBM status. Obtain IV access for fluid and electrolyte replacement with balanced salt solution to ensure renal perfusion. Antiemetics are administered for nausea and vomiting, and to minimise further fluid loss. Pain control is a high priority for the patient with pancreatitis. Table 24.12 highlights drugs used for management of acute and chronic pancreatitis.

Nasogastric suction helps alleviate nausea, vomiting and abdominal distension. Ongoing monitoring of respiratory, cardiovascular and renal functions and fluid balance is recommended.[150] The use of antimicrobial prophylaxis is not recommended in acute severe pancreatitis or sterile necrosis.[151]

Acute pancreatitis is a serious condition with significant mortality. Severe and life-threatening complications with acute pancreatitis are pleural effusion, fluid loss, abscess formation, jaundice, acute renal failure and adult respiratory distress syndrome. Respiratory complications can occur in 30–50% of patients.[10] Significant hypovolaemia can lead to hypovolaemic shock and ischaemia of lungs, heart and kidneys. Electrolyte imbalances such as hyperglycaemia and hypocalcaemia also occur. Septic complications include formation of pancreatic abscesses.[144]

APPENDICITIS

Obstruction of the appendiceal opening decreases blood supply and leads to bacterial invasion. Untreated, inflammation progresses so that the appendix becomes non-viable and gangrenous; at worst it may eventually lead to a rupture into the peritoneal space.[152] Appendicitis affects both sexes and all ages, and is most common in the 10- to 30-year age range. Approximately 6% of the population develops appendicitis in their lifetime. One in 2200 pregnant women develops appendicitis, making it the most common surgical procedure during pregnancy.[10]

Assessment and management

Variations in the position of the appendix, patient age and degree of inflammation make the clinical presentation of appendicitis challenging, with one in five cases misdiagnosed.[153] The archetypal presentation of anorexia, periumbilical pain followed by nausea, RLQ pain and vomiting occurs in only half of cases. Additional features may include patient reports of chills and fever. Abdominal pain may progress from diffuse to periumbilical to being intense and localised to the lower right quadrant. This pain migration pattern is the most discriminating feature, with a sensitivity and specificity of approximately 80%.[154] Classic pain associated with appendicitis is located in the right iliac fossa (inside the iliac crest at McBurney's point). Older patients are often afebrile and do not exhibit this classic pain. Pressure on the lower left abdomen intensifies pain in the RLQ (Rovsing's sign).[9] Pain may not always occur in this classic location because of normal variations in the location of the appendix. The position of comfort for most patients is supine with hips and knees flexed. Women may exhibit tenderness when the cervix is moved.[10]

If the appendix ruptures, peritoneal signs increase and involuntary guarding develops. Increased fever and rebound tenderness occur. Diagnosis is made by assessment of clinical signs and symptoms in tandem with physical examination. Diagnostic data may demonstrate an elevation of WBC count

TABLE 24.12 DRUG THERAPY IN ACUTE AND CHRONIC PANCREATITIS[108,144,149]

DRUG	MECHANISM OF ACTION
Acute pancreatitis	
Morphine, fentanyl	Relief of pain
Glyceryl trinitrate or papaverine	Relaxation of smooth muscles and relief of pain
Antispasmodics (e.g. propantheline bromide)	Decrease of vagal stimulation, motility, pancreatic outflow (inhibition of volume and concentration of bicarbonate and enzymatic secretion); contraindicated in paralytic ileus
Carbonic anhydrase inhibitor (acetazolamide)	Reduction in volume and bicarbonate concentration of pancreatic secretion
Antacids	Neutralisation of gastric HCl secretion and subsequent decrease in secretin, which stimulates production and secretion of pancreatic secretions
Proton pump inhibitors	Decrease in HCl secretion (HCl stimulates pancreatic activity)
Insulin	Treatment of hyperglycaemia
Chronic pancreatitis	
Pancreatin, pancrelipase	Replacement therapy for pancreatic enzymes
Insulin	Treatment for diabetes mellitus if it occurs or for hyperglycaemia

HCl: hydrochloric acid.

with increased neutrophils, although this is not invariable.[9] Ultrasound may occasionally demonstrate an enlarged appendix or collection of peri-appendiceal fluid, with 88–100% sensitivity and a specificity approaching 100%. Urinalysis should be performed to rule out genitourinary problems and pregnancy in women of childbearing age. CT has been used effectively in certain patients, but its broad use as a diagnostic tool for appendicitis has not been established.

Definitive therapy for appendicitis is surgical intervention, with laparoscopic surgery as the preferred method. In some situations, after consultation with surgeons, appendicitis can be managed with oral antibiotics. But most often, obtain IV access, administer prophylactic broad-spectrum antibiotic if clinically indicated, intravenous analgesia and instruct the patient to be NBM. Complications such as perforation, peritonitis and abscess formation can occur when treatment is delayed.

CROHN'S DISEASE

Crohn's disease is a chronic, non-specific inflammatory bowel disorder of unknown origin that can affect any part of the GI tract from the mouth to the anus. Crohn's disease may occur at any age, but occurs most often between the ages of 15 and 30 years. When it occurs in older adults, the morbidity and mortality rates are higher because of other chronic problems that may be present. Both genders are affected, with higher incidences in women. The incidence of Crohn's disease is slightly lower than that of ulcerative colitis.[9]

Crohn's disease is characterised by inflammation of segments of the GI tract. It can affect any part of the GI tract, but is most often seen in the terminal ileum, jejunum and colon. Involvement of the oesophagus, stomach and duodenum is rare. The inflammation involves all the layers of the bowel wall; the radiographic appearance in some patients with Crohn's disease is a section of normal bowel interspersed with segments of affected bowel (skip lesions).[10,152] Typically, ulcerations are deep and longitudinal, and penetrate between islands of inflamed oedematous mucosa, causing a classic cobblestone appearance. Thickening of the bowel wall occurs, as well as narrowing of the lumen with stricture development. The area of inflammation can extend through all the layers of the bowel wall. Abscesses or fistula tracts that communicate with other loops of bowel, skin, bladder, rectum or vagina may develop.[100]

The manifestation of the disease depends largely on the anatomical site of involvement, extent of the disease process and presence or absence of complications. The onset of Crohn's disease is usually insidious, with non-specific complaints, such as diarrhoea, fatigue, abdominal pain, weight loss and fever.

Assessment and management

Crohn's disease is a chronic disorder with unpredictable periods of recurrence and remission. Attacks are intermittent and subside spontaneously, usually recurring over a period of several weeks to months, with diarrhoea and abdominal pain which can be quite debilitating.[155] During a period of pain and inflammation, it is important to rest the GI tract and initially, in the acute phase, this may mean a short period of fasting or fluids only. During recovery, particular attention needs to be focused on a diet that is light and non-irritating.

Diagnosis of Crohn's disease can be made by means of a thorough history and physical assessment to establish clinical signs and symptoms. Barium studies will show characteristic inflammatory studies. Laboratory studies may determine electrolyte disturbance and presence of anaemia. C-reactive protein is an accurate biochemical marker to evaluate disease activity.[156] Treat symptoms while in the ED, arrange for appropriate follow-up, discharge information and resource access to modify lifestyle or dietary approach, should this be necessary. Drug therapy for Crohn's disease is presented in Table 24.13.

DIVERTICULITIS

Diverticulitis is defined as an inflammation of one or more diverticula, small pouches created by herniation of the mucosa into the wall of the large intestine (see Fig. 24.11). Diverticular disease accounts for over 51,000 hospitalisations per year in Australia;[159] it affects more women than men,[149] and 50% of the population aged 60 years and over.[157] Weakened areas that predispose the colon to herniation of inferior tissue layers in combination with a low-fibre diet lead to this primarily painless disorder.[152] Fewer than 10% of patients with diverticulosis experience pain. However, pain is the most-reported complaint when diverticula become inflamed, and diverticulitis develops. Inflammation develops when faecal material is trapped in the pouches, causing trauma to the intestinal lining, which ultimately leads to inflammation. Diverticular disease includes a spectrum of conditions that range from asymptomatic, symptomatic uncomplicated to complicated diverticular disease. Persistent pain associated with diverticulitis is localised in the left lower quadrant, as most diverticula occur in the sigmoid colon.[108,160] Fever, chills, nausea and vomiting are seen when infection is present; other symptoms include cramping and constipation. Older people, those on corticosteroids and patients who are immunosuppressed may have an unremarkable clinical examination, even in the presence of severe diverticulitis. Complications of diverticulitis include intestinal obstruction, haemorrhage, perforation, abscess, stricture, and fistula.[9,100]

Assessment and management

Diagnostic evaluation includes FBC and urinalysis. Results of the FBC show a left shift resulting from infection; an increase in the number of immature leucocytes in the peripheral blood due to consumption surpassing supply during bacterial infection, particularly neutrophil band cells.[161] The presence of WBCs and RBCs in urine is also a common finding. Blood cultures should be obtained in severely ill patients or in those with complicated disease. Given the typical location of LLQ pain, a pregnancy test must be performed in any female of childbearing age to exclude ectopic pregnancy, as well as prior to radiological studies. Graded compression ultrasound can be used as an initial diagnostic tool to detect abscesses, thickness of the bowel wall and pericolonic inflammation.[162] POCUS or x-ray can exclude perforations or bowel obstructions. Abdominal CT is the preferred diagnostic modality because it is more effective in identification of processes outside the colon's lumen (i.e. diverticulitis).[155] Barium enema and endoscopy may also be used.

Treatment of patients with diverticulitis includes rehydration with a saline solution, resting the bowel by making the patient NBM and inserting a gastric tube if persistent vomiting is present.[153] Anticholinergics are used to reduce colonic spasms, with opiates reserved for more-aggressive pain management. Oral or

TABLE 24.13 DRUG THERAPY IN INFLAMMATORY BOWEL DISEASE[157,158]

CATEGORY	ACTION	EXAMPLES
Antimicrobials	Prevent or treat secondary infection	Metronidazole
5-aminosalicylic acid (5-ASA)	Decrease GI inflammation*	Systemic Sulfasalazine Mesalazine Olsalazine Rectal suppository
Corticosteroids	Decrease inflammation	Systemic: corticosteroids (cortisone, prednisolone, budesonide) Enemas: prednisone Rectal suppository: prednisone
Anticholinergics	Decrease GI motility and secretions and relieve smooth-muscle spasms‡	Propantheline bromide
Sedatives	Reduce anxiety and restlessness	Diazepam
Antidiarrhoeals	Decrease GI motility‡	Diphenoxylate
Immunosuppressants	Suppress immune response	Azathioprine, cyclosporin
Immunomodulators	Inhibit the cytokine tumour necrosis factor-alpha (TNF-α) Block lymphocyte adhesion to blood vessel walls and subsequent migration into tissues	Infliximab
Haematinics and vitamins	Correct iron-deficiency anaemia and promote healing	Oral ferrous sulfate, ferrous gluconate; iron polymaltose injection Vitamin B_{12}, zinc

GI: gastrointestinal.

**Mechanism of action unknown, possibly antimicrobial, as well as anti-inflammatory.*

‡Used with caution during severe disease because of potential to produce toxic megacolon.

parenteral antibiotics may be given depending on clinical presentation. Emergency surgery is required when there is evidence of peritonitis.[33]

ULCERATIVE COLITIS

Ulcerative colitis is characterised by inflammation and ulceration of the colon and rectum. It may occur at any age, but peaks between the ages of 15 and 25 years. There is a second, smaller peak of onset between 60 and 80 years of age. Ulcerative colitis affects both genders equally.[9]

The inflammation of ulcerative colitis is diffuse and involves the mucosa and submucosa, with alternating periods of exacerbation and remission. The disease usually begins in the rectum and sigmoid colon and extends up the colon in a continuous pattern. The ulcerations also destroy the mucosal epithelium, causing bleeding and diarrhoea.[155] Loss of fluid and electrolytes occur because of the decreased mucosal surface area for absorption. Breakdown of cells results in protein loss through the stools. Areas of inflamed mucosa form pseudopolyps that have the appearance of tongue-like projections into the bowel lumen.[152] Granulation tissue develops and the mucosal musculature becomes thickened, shortening the colon. Although the precipitating factors involved in ulcerative colitis are poorly understood, it is clear that, once initiated, the inflammatory response is involved.

Assessment and management

Ulcerative colitis may appear as an acute fulminating crisis or, more commonly, as a chronic disorder with mild-to-severe acute exacerbations that occur at unpredictable intervals over many years.[152] The major symptoms of ulcerative colitis are bloody diarrhoea and abdominal pain. Pain may vary from mild lower abdominal cramping associated with diarrhoea to severe, constant abdominal pain that may be associated with perforations. In severe cases, diarrhoea is bloody, contains mucus and occurs 10–20 times per day. In addition, fever, weight loss, tachycardia and dehydration are present.[9]

Diagnostic studies include FBC, serum electrolyte levels and serum protein level. The FBC typically shows iron-deficiency anaemia from blood loss. An elevated WCC may indicate toxic megacolon or perforation. A decrease in serum electrolyte levels, such as sodium, potassium, chloride, bicarbonate and magnesium, are due to fluid and electrolyte losses from diarrhoea and vomiting.[104,108] Hypoalbuminaemia is present in severe cases and is due to protein loss from the bowel. The stool should be examined for blood and pus; a sample should be cultured to rule out an infectious cause of inflammation. Drug therapy is an extremely important aspect of treatment (see Table 24.15).

BOWEL OBSTRUCTION

Bowel obstruction occurs in either sex, at any age, and from a variety of causes.[11] The most common cause is adhesions from previous abdominal surgery, followed by incarcerated inguinal hernia.[6] Other causes include foreign bodies, volvulus, intussusception, strictures, tumours, congenital adhesive bands, faecal impaction, gallstones and haematomas (Fig. 24.13).

Bowel obstructions are classified as mechanical or non-mechanical.

- *Mechanical obstruction* results from a disorder outside the intestines or blockage inside the lumen of the intestines (Fig. 24.14A and B). Fig. 24.15 is a radiographic illustration of a small bowel obstruction.
- *Non-mechanical obstruction* results when muscle activity of the intestine decreases and movement of contents slows (i.e. paralytic ileus) (Fig. 24.16).

When obstruction occurs, bowel contents accumulate above the obstruction. This leads to rapid increase in anaerobic and aerobic bacteria, which causes an increase in methane and hydrogen production.[33] McQuaid indicates that 'the more proximal the obstruction, the greater the discomfort' and the shorter the time between symptom onset and presentation.[100] Peristalsis increases, so more secretions are released, which worsens distension, causes bowel oedema and increases capillary permeability. Plasma leaks into the peritoneal cavity with fluid trapped in the intestinal lumen, so absorption of fluid and electrolytes decreases.

Assessment and management

Clinical signs vary with the location of the obstruction. Table 24.14 compares clinical manifestations of obstructions in the large and small intestines. Symptoms include colic, cramping and intermittent and wavelike abdominal pain. At times, pain may be severe, and analgesia should be titrated accordingly. Abdominal distension may also be present. Patients may have diffuse abdominal tenderness, rigidity and constipation. Hyperactive bowel sounds or absent bowel sounds may be noted. The patient may also be febrile, tachycardic and hypotensive with nausea and vomiting. Emesis (secondary to reverse peristalsis) usually has an odour of faeces from proliferation of bacteria.[100]

Laboratory studies include FBC, urea, serum glucose, electrolytes, creatinine, amylase and arterial blood gas measurements. A WBC count greater than 20×10^{10}/L suggests bowel gangrene, whereas elevations greater than 40×10^{10}/L occur

FIGURE 24.13 BOWEL OBSTRUCTIONS[9]

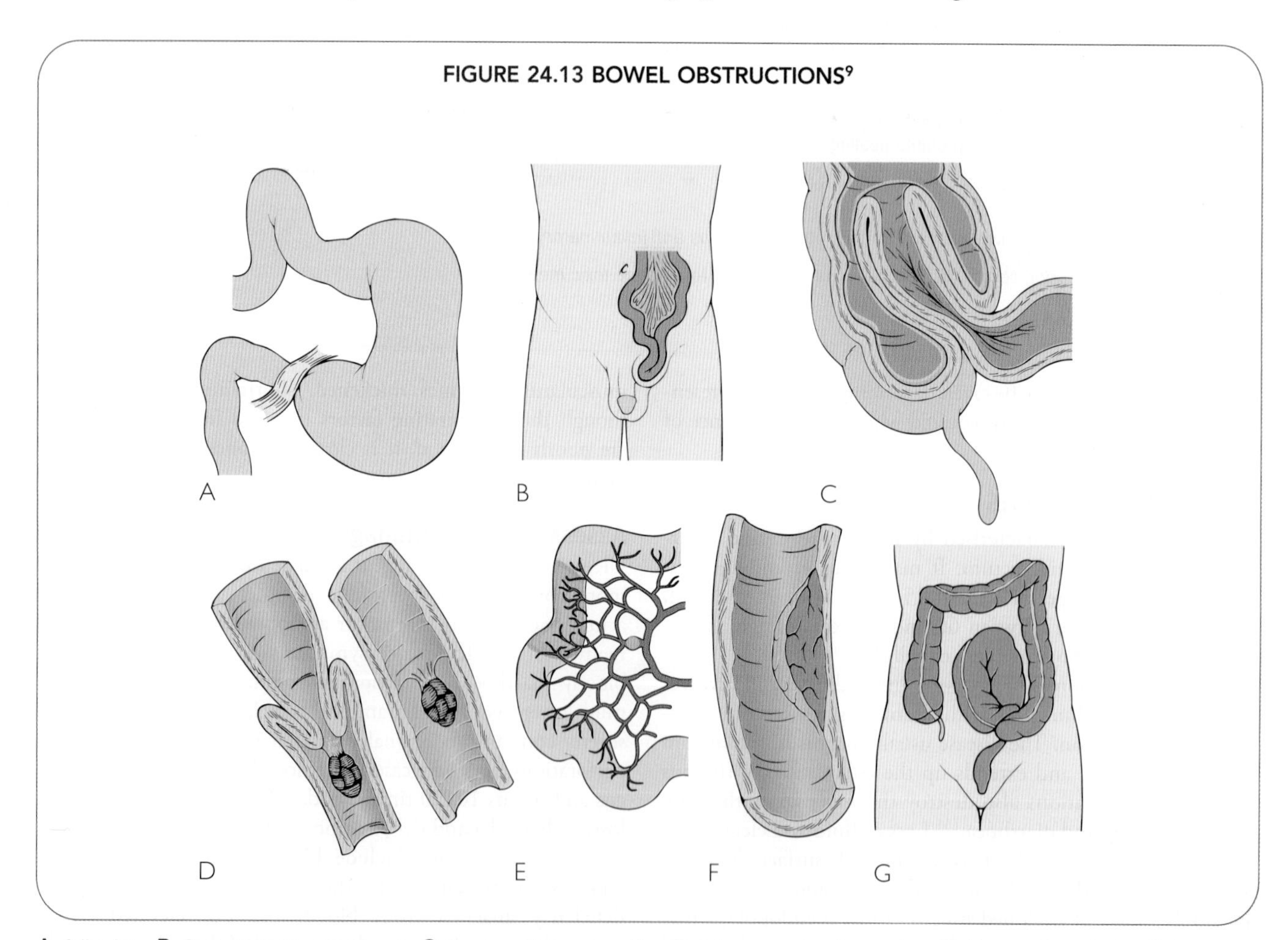

A. Adhesions. **B.** Strangulated inguinal hernia. **C.** Ileocaecal intussusception. **D.** Intussusception from polyps. **E.** Mesenteric occlusion. **F.** Neoplasm. **G.** Volvulus of the sigmoid colon.

FIGURE 24.14 MECHANICAL BOWEL OBSTRUCTION[163]

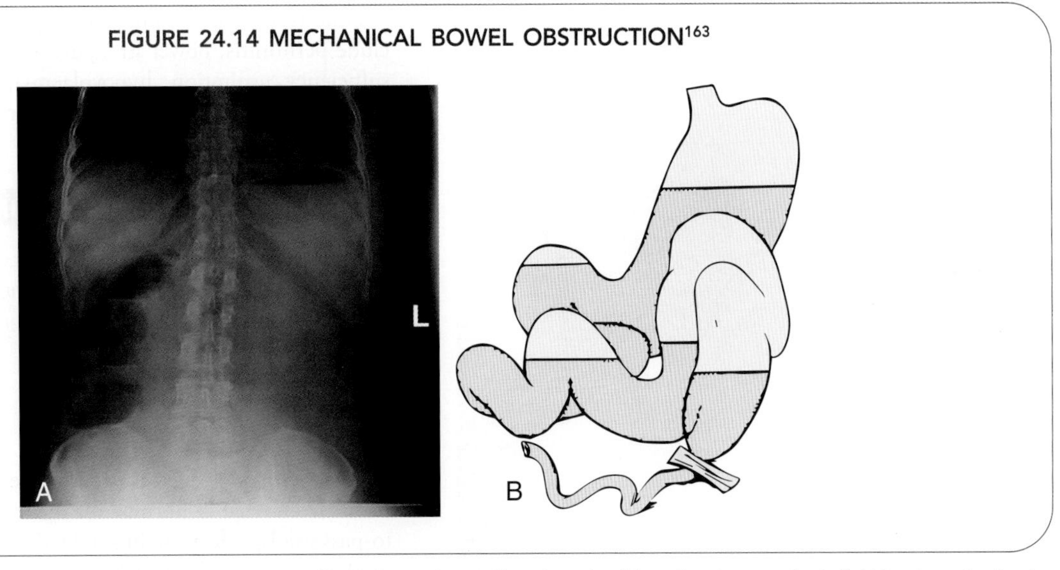

A. Localised air-fluid levels seen on upright film of abdomen. **B.** Diagram shows dilated proximal bowel and stomach air-fluid levels and adhesive band causing obstruction.

FIGURE 24.15 RADIOGRAPHIC ILLUSTRATION OF A SMALL BOWEL OBSTRUCTION

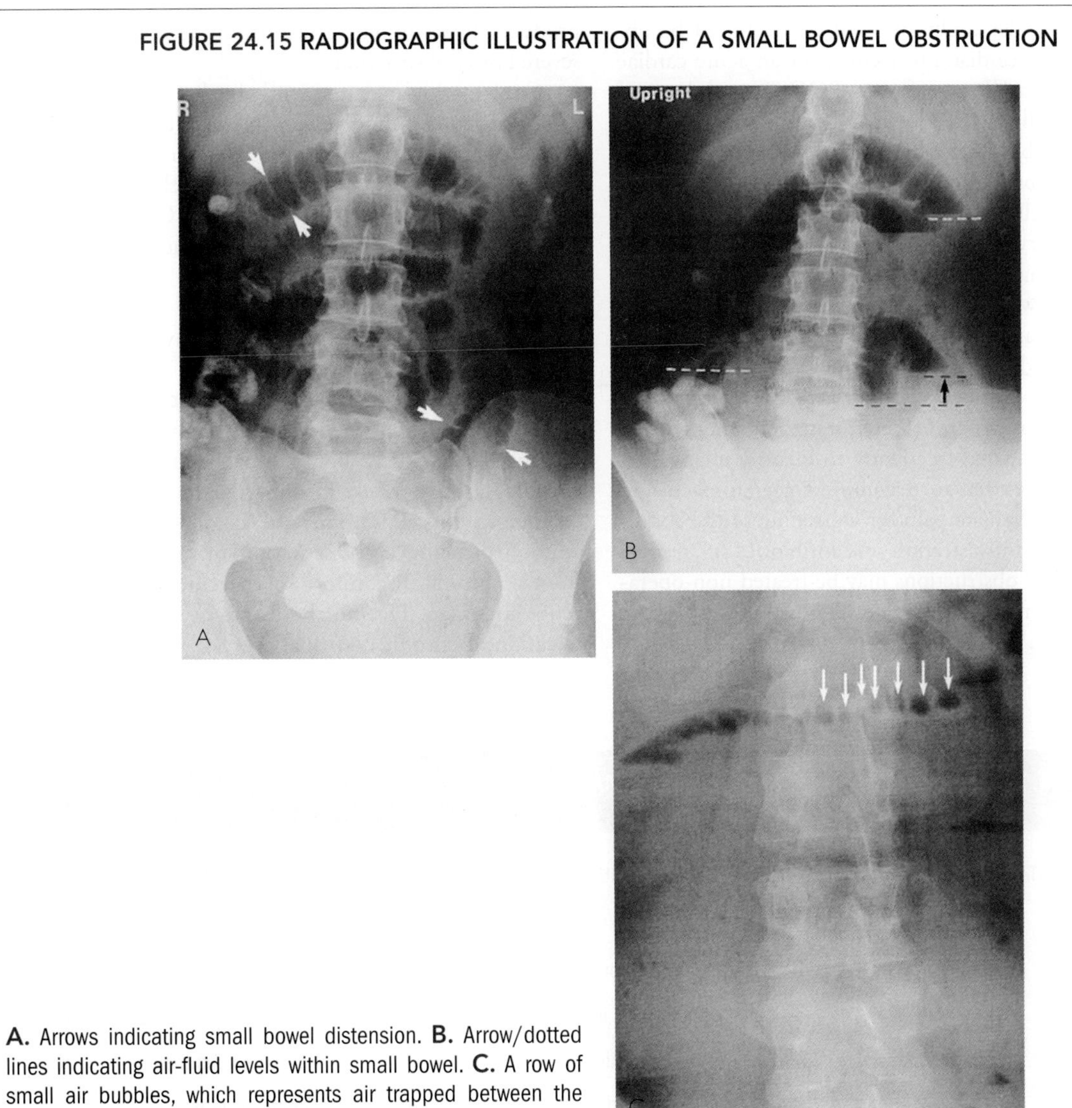

A. Arrows indicating small bowel distension. **B.** Arrow/dotted lines indicating air-fluid levels within small bowel. **C.** A row of small air bubbles, which represents air trapped between the valvulae conniventes, also known as the 'string of pearls' sign.

FIGURE 24.16 PARALYTIC ILEUS (FUNCTIONAL BOWEL OBSTRUCTION) ON ABDOMINAL X-RAY[164]

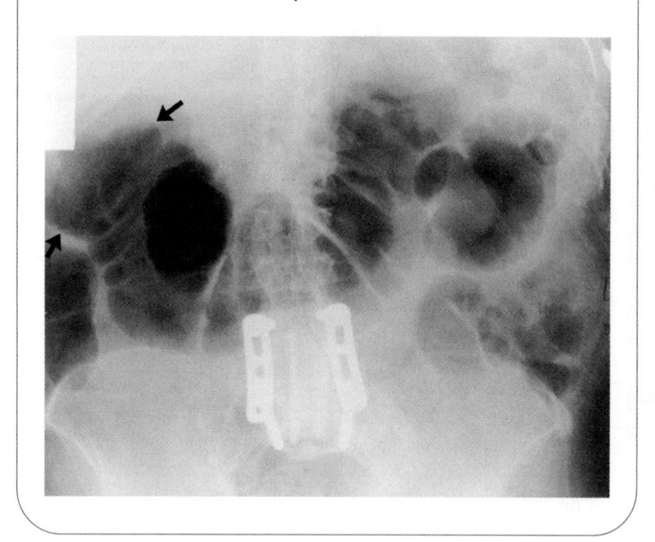

Note dilated loops of bowel.

with mesenteric vascular occlusion.[6] An ECG should be obtained to confirm no cardiac involvement or an acute cardiac event presenting like a GI presentation. POCUS or abdominal x-rays show dilated, fluid-filled loops of bowel with visible air-fluid levels.[165,166] Table 24.15 highlights radiographic differences with specific obstructions.

Management includes IV access for fluid and electrolyte replacement using crystalloid solution to maintain haemodynamic values and renal perfusion.[152] Fluid balance monitoring is important, along with an understanding of the balances of intake and output and patient response to therapy, which should be monitored. Early identification of reduced renal blood flow or hypovolaemia by recognising oliguria is vital to prevent an unwell patient from deteriorating further. Bowel sounds should be evaluated frequently to identify changes. A nasogastric tube is inserted to decompress the stomach and reduce vomiting.[107] Evaluate pain for worsening of the condition. Prophylactic administration of antibiotics is recommended. Small bowel obstructions may be treated non-operatively and most patients with large bowel obstructions require surgical intervention.[148]

Life-threatening complications of bowel obstruction include peritonitis, bowel strangulation or perforation, renal insufficiency, aspiration, hypovolaemia, intestinal ischaemia or infarction, and death. Untreated obstruction that progresses to shock has a 70% mortality rate.[6]

PRACTICE TIP

Mesenteric ischaemia can present covertly in the older patient. It is important to have a higher degree of suspicion when assessing an older person.

CONSTIPATION

Constipation is a decrease in the frequency of bowel movements from what is 'normal' for the individual. Hard, difficult-to-pass stools, a decrease in stool volume and retention of faeces in the rectum is the usual clinical pattern.[152] Normal bowel elimination may vary from 3 times a day to once every 3 days. Because of this, it is important for the clinician to ascertain the patient's normal pattern. It is important to remember that changes in bowel habits may also indicate bowel obstruction produced by a tumour. Constipation itself can become quite a severe bowel obstruction.

Constipation may frequently be due to insufficient dietary fibre, inadequate fluid intake, medications and lack of exercise. Constipation may also be due to environmental constraints, ignoring the urge to defecate, chronic laxative abuse and multiple organic causes (Box 24.7). Conditions that affect nerve function may also have an impact on bowel motility function.

Changes in diet, mealtime or daily routines are some of the few environmental factors that may cause constipation. Depression and stress can also result in constipation. For many patients, it is not possible to identify the underlying cause.[9] Some patients believe that they are constipated if they do not have a daily bowel movement. This can result in chronic laxative use and subsequent cathartic colon syndrome. In this condition, the colon becomes dilated and atonic. The clinical presentation of constipation may vary from a chronic discomfort to an acute event mimicking an acute abdomen. Haemorrhoids are the most common complication of chronic constipation.

TABLE 24.14 CLINICAL MANIFESTATIONS OF SMALL AND LARGE INTESTINAL OBSTRUCTIONS[9,10]

CLINICAL MANIFESTATION	SMALL INTESTINE	LARGE INTESTINE
Onset	Rapid	Gradual
Vomiting	Frequent and copious	Rare
Pain	Colicky, cramp-like, intermittent	Low-grade, cramping abdominal pain
Bowel movement	Faeces for a short time	Absolute constipation
Abdominal distension	Minimally increased	Greatly increased

TABLE 24.15 RADIOGRAPHIC AND CLINICAL EVIDENCE OF SPECIFIC BOWEL OBSTRUCTIONS[9]

TYPE	RADIOGRAPHIC FINDINGS	CLINICAL SIGNS AND SYMPTOMS
Bowel obstructions (general)	Air-fluid levels may appear as 'string of beads' and thus serve as an important diagnostic clue to mechanical obstructions. More than two air-fluid levels reflect mechanical obstruction, adynamic ileus, or both. Fluid-filled loops form a proximal impediment and are indicative of bowel obstruction Routine films or contrast studies show air-fluid levels, distortion, abscess formation, narrow lumens, mucosal destruction, distension and deformities at site of torsion	Pain, distension, vomiting, obstipation and constipation
Strangulation obstruction	'Coffee bean' sign appears on radiograph (dilated bowel loop bent on itself, assuming shape of coffee bean) Gas- and fluid-filled loops may have unchanging locations on multiple projection films Pseudotumour (closed-loop obstruction filled with water that looks like tumour) may be present	Abdominal tenderness, hyperactive bowel sounds, leucocytosis, rebound tenderness, fever
Gallstones	Air in gallbladder tree, distension of small bowel and visualisation of stone	
Hernia		Extra-abdominal or intra-abdominal hernia may be present: in men, most commonly inguinal; in women, right-sided femoral hernias
Volvulus		Torsion of mesenteric axis creating digestive disturbances
Intussusception	'Coiled spring' appearance seen on contrast radiograph	

Assessment and management

In the presence of constipation or faecal impaction secondary to constipation, especially in the older patient, colonic perforation may occur. Perforation of the colon, which is life-threatening, causes abdominal pain, nausea, vomiting, fever and an elevated WBC count. An abdominal x-ray or POCUS can show the presence of free air, which is diagnostic of perforation and bowel obstructions.[80,167]

A thorough history and physical assessment should be performed so that the underlying cause of constipation can be identified, and treatment started (see Table 24.16). Laxatives should always be used cautiously because with chronic overuse they may become a cause of constipation. See Table 24.17 for cathartic agents.

Patient and family education should emphasise the need for a high-fibre diet, ensuring adequate water intake, avoiding excess laxatives and a regular exercise regimen (Box 24.8).

LIVER FAILURE AND CIRRHOSIS

When damage to the liver parenchyma is so severe that metabolic functions are no longer possible, liver failure occurs. Irrespective of the cause of liver insult, the syndrome of acute liver failure (ALF) develops.[99] The clinical features are characterised by jaundice, ascites, coagulopathy, hepatic encephalopathy, haemodynamic changes, electrolyte disturbance and renal failure (hepatorenal syndrome [HRS]).[169–172] ALF is associated with multiple organ failure and a poor prognosis. Alcohol is the leading cause of liver failure; however, other aetiologies include chronic hepatitis B or C, biliary obstruction, haemochromatosis, chemical toxins, fatty liver disease and cirrhosis.[169]

Cirrhosis is often a 'silent' disease, with patients remaining asymptomatic until decompensation occurs.[170] Cirrhosis refers to a progressive, diffuse, fibrosing nodular condition that disrupts the entire normal architecture of the liver. The sequela of cirrhosis is liver failure. Risk factors for cirrhosis include alcohol as the major precipitant; others include hepatitis B or C, cystic fibrosis, biliary obstruction, haemochromatosis and autoimmune causes (see Chapter 40).[171]

The clinical features of cirrhosis include jaundice, organomegaly, ascites and encephalopathy. The following points summarise important considerations in the presentation and physical appearance of cirrhosis and liver failure.[170,173]

- Stigmata of chronic liver disease include spider naevi, palmar erythema, gynaecomastia, caput medusa.
- Oesophageal varices develop as a consequence of portal hypertension, and bleeding may initially present with small or significant haematemesis, malaena or rectal bleeding.
- Hepatorenal syndrome is a functional disorder whereby renal failure develops (elevated serum creatinine) in the context of liver failure, ascites and structurally normal kidneys.
- Jaundice is characterised by yellowish skin colour and whites of the eyes caused by an increase of bilirubin in the blood. Pre-hepatic jaundice is an increased rate of haemolysis, hepatocellular jaundice occurs when the liver is unable to metabolise or excrete bilirubin, and post-hepatic jaundice is caused by a biliary obstruction.[174]

BOX 24.7 CAUSES OF CONSTIPATION[152]

COLONIC DISORDERS	SYSTEMIC DISORDERS
Luminal or extraluminal obstructing lesions	**Metabolic/endocrine**
Inflammatory strictures	Diabetes mellitus
Volvulus	Hypothyroidism
Intussusception	Pregnancy
Irritable bowel syndrome	Hypercalcaemia/hyperparathyroidism
Diverticular disease	Phaeochromocytoma
Rectocoele	**Collagen vascular disease**
Drug induced	Systemic sclerosis (scleroderma)
Antacids (calcium and aluminium)	Amyloidosis
Antidepressants	**Neurological disorders**
Anticholinergics	Hirschsprung's megacolon
Antipsychotics	Neurofibromatosis
Antihypertensives	Autonomic neuropathy (secondary to diabetes mellitus)
Barium sulfate	Multiple sclerosis
Iron supplements	Parkinson's disease
Bismuth	Spinal cord lesions or injury
Calcium supplements	Stroke
Laxative abuse	

TABLE 24.16 NURSING ASSESSMENT IN CONSTIPATION[9]

SUBJECTIVE DATA	OBJECTIVE DATA
Important health information	**General**
Past health history—colorectal disease, neurological dysfunction, bowel obstruction, environmental changes, cancer, irritable bowel syndrome	Lethargy
Medications—use of aluminium and calcium antacids, anticholinergics, antidepressants, antihistamines, antipsychotics, diuretics, narcotics, iron, laxatives, enemas	**Integumentary** Anorectal fissures, haemorrhoids, abscesses
Functional health patterns	**Gastrointestinal**
Health perception/health management—chronic laxative or enema abuse; rigid beliefs regarding bowel function; malaise	Abdominal distension; hypoactive or absent bowel sounds; palpable abdominal mass; faecal impaction; small, hard, dry stool; stool with blood
Nutritional/metabolic—changes in diet or mealtime; inadequate fibre and fluid intake; anorexia, nausea	**Possible findings**
Elimination—change in usual elimination patterns; hard, difficult-to-pass stool, decrease in frequency and amount of stools; flatus, abdominal distension; tenesmus, rectal pressure; faecal incontinence (if impacted)	Positive faecal occult blood test (but should not do if patient is constipated); abdominal x-ray demonstrating stool in lower colon
Activity/exercise—change in daily activity routines; immobility; sedentary lifestyle	
Cognitive/perceptual—dizziness, headache, anorectal pain; abdominal pain on defecation	
Coping/stress tolerance—acute or chronic stress	

- Ascites is the pathological accumulation of fluid in the peritoneal cavity. Approximately 85% of patients with ascites have cirrhosis.
- Sepsis may occur due to the immunosuppressive nature of cirrhosis. The clinician should have a low threshold for severe infection in unwell patients who have cirrhosis. The classic febrile state may not always be seen in immunocompromised patients. Consider also other markers of sepsis and shock, such as tachycardia, hypotension and poor peripheral perfusion. Particular attention should be given to the possible development of spontaneous bacterial peritonitis (SBP), especially in patients with ascites. Empirical antibiotic therapy is recommended.
- Encephalopathy may be mild and be manifested only as low-grade confusion or sleep disturbances. Conversely, the encephalopathy may be severe and be associated with a

TABLE 24.17 DRUG THERAPY IN CATHARTIC AGENTS[109,168]

CATEGORY	MECHANISMS OF ACTION	EXAMPLE	ONSET OF ACTION	COMMENTS
Bulk-forming	Absorbs water; increases bulk, thereby stimulating peristalsis	Metamucil, Konsyl, Citrucel	Usually within 24 hours	Contraindicated in patients with abdominal pain, nausea and vomiting and in patients suspected of having appendicitis, biliary tract obstruction or acute hepatitis; must be taken with fluids
Stool softeners and lubricants	Lubricate intestinal tract and soften faeces, making hard stools easier to pass; do not affect peristalsis	Mineral oil, dioctyl sodium sulfosuccinate, Colace, Doxidan	Softeners up to 72 hours, lubricants up to 8 hours	Can block absorption of fat-soluble vitamins such as vitamin K, which may increase risk of bleeding in patients on anticoagulants
Saline and osmotic solutions	Cause retention of fluid in intestinal lumen caused by osmotic effect	Magnesium salts: magnesium citrate, milk of magnesia Sodium phosphates: Fleet enema, Phospho-Soda Lactulose Polyethylene glycol saline solutions	15 minutes to 3 hours	Magnesium-containing products may cause hypermagnesaemia in patients with renal insufficiency
Stimulants	Increase peristalsis by irritating colon wall and stimulating enteric nerves	Anthraquinone drugs: cascara sagrada, senna	Usually within 12 hours	Cause melanosis coli (brown or black pigmentation of colon); are most widely abused laxatives; should not be used in patients with impaction or obstipation

BOX 24.8 PATIENT AND FAMILY TEACHING GUIDE IN CONSTIPATION (ADULT)[6]

EAT DIETARY FIBRE

Eat 20–30 g of fibre per day. Gradually increase the amount of fibre eaten over 1–2 weeks. Fibre softens hard stools and adds bulk to stool, promoting evacuation.

Foods high in fibre: raw vegetables and fruits, beans, breakfast cereals (All Bran, oatmeal)

Fibre supplements: Metamucil, Mucilax

DRINK FLUIDS

Drink plenty of clear fluids, but not excessively and no more than 1 extra litre a day.

EXERCISE REGULARLY

Walk, swim or ride a bike at least three times per week. Contract and relax abdominal muscles when standing or by doing sit-ups to strengthen muscles and prevent straining. Exercise stimulates bowel motility and moves stool through the intestine.

ESTABLISH A REGULAR TIME TO DEFECATE

First thing in the morning or after the first meal of the day is a good time because people often have the urge to defecate at this time.

DO NOT DELAY DEFECATION

Respond to the urge to have a bowel movement as soon as possible. Delaying defecation results in hard stools and a decreased 'urge' to defecate. Water is absorbed from stool by the intestine over time. The intestine becomes less sensitive to the presence of stool in the rectum.

Record your bowel elimination pattern

Develop a habit of recording on your calendar when you have a bowel movement. Regular monitoring of bowel movement will assist in early identification of a problem.

AVOID LAXATIVES AND ENEMAS

Do not overuse laxatives and enemas because they can actually cause constipation. The normal motility of the bowel is interrupted and bowel movements slow or stop.

marked reduction in level of consciousness. Note that hepatic encephalopathy is a diagnosis of exclusion, and other possible causes to an altered mental state must be excluded.
- Jugular venous distension, a sign of right-side heart failure, suggests hepatic congestion.
- Abdominal examination should focus on the size and consistency of the liver and spleen, and the presence of ascites.

Assessment and management

Investigations into liver function can be assisted by laboratory evaluation, radiographic studies and biopsy. Utilising pathology is useful; however, the standard liver function assays do not reflect the function of the liver correctly. When interpreting the biochemistry along with the clinical picture, an impression of certain liver diseases may evolve.[171]

When liver disease is suspected, FBC with platelets; prothrombin time; enzymes aspartate transaminase (AST) and alanine transaminase (ALT); alkaline phosphatase; GGT; bilirubin; and albumin are useful.[172] Rather than a single measurement of a value, repeated testing over a period of time is warranted and may prove useful in assisting diagnosis. Imaging such as ultrasonography is a valuable first-line modality, as it provides information regarding the gross appearance of the liver and associated anatomy. It is relatively inexpensive, does not pose a radiation risk and does not require potentially toxic contrast. CT and MRI have limitations in detecting early changes with cirrhosis. They can accurately demonstrate nodularity, atrophy or hypertrophic changes, as well as ascites and varices in advanced disease. CT and MRI are valuable in follow-up studies.

The goals of treatment include resuscitation and stabilisation initially. Airway protection is vital and aspiration is a risk in any vomiting patient. Early pharmacology (vasoactive drugs, e.g. octreotide, to reduce portal pressures) and endoscopy improve outcomes for variceal haemorrhage. Sepsis is frequently a feature in liver failure; therefore, septic screening and use of antibiotics are recommended. Renal function needs to be closely monitored. Removal of hepatotoxic agents and liver insults is important to reduce the impact and effect of cirrhosis and liver failure. Eliminating alcohol, drugs and medications which are known to be toxic to the liver are vital to ensure what function is left is operating at maximum ability.[169,172]

PRACTICE TIP

Patients with alcoholism may have a combination of pancreatitis, hepatitis and gastritis. It is important to undertake a thorough history and examination to ensure patient safety.

SUMMARY

GI emergencies can be minor or life-threatening. Most GI emergencies present with similar clinical manifestations, so a detailed history and physical assessment play an important role in the management of these patients. The ability to differentiate conditions that require immediate attention is a requisite skill for the emergency healthcare professional (Fig. 24.17A–D).

FIGURE 24.17 COMMON CAUSES/DIAGNOSIS RELATING TO ABDOMINAL PAIN IN VARIOUS QUADRANTS

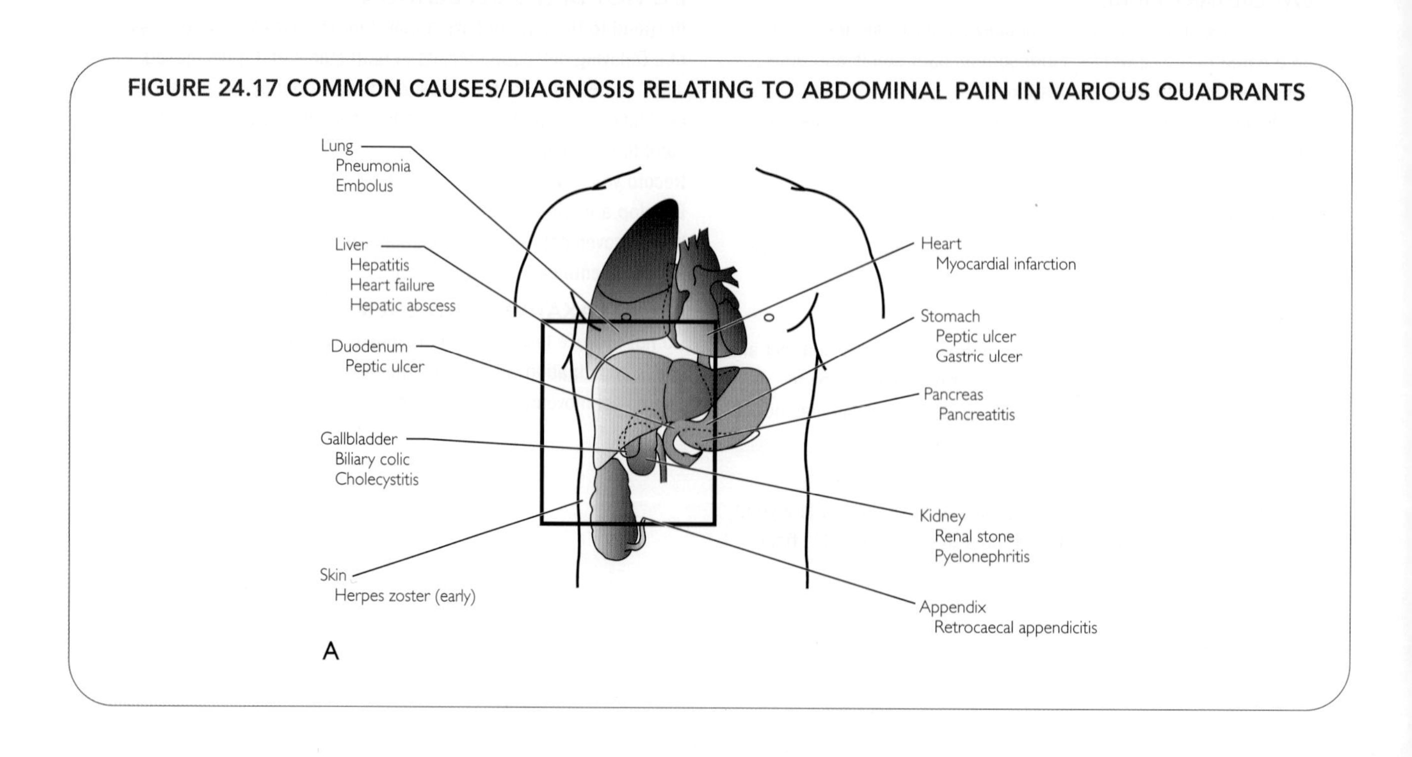

FIGURE 24.17 COMMON CAUSES/DIAGNOSIS RELATING TO ABDOMINAL PAIN IN VARIOUS QUADRANTS—cont'd

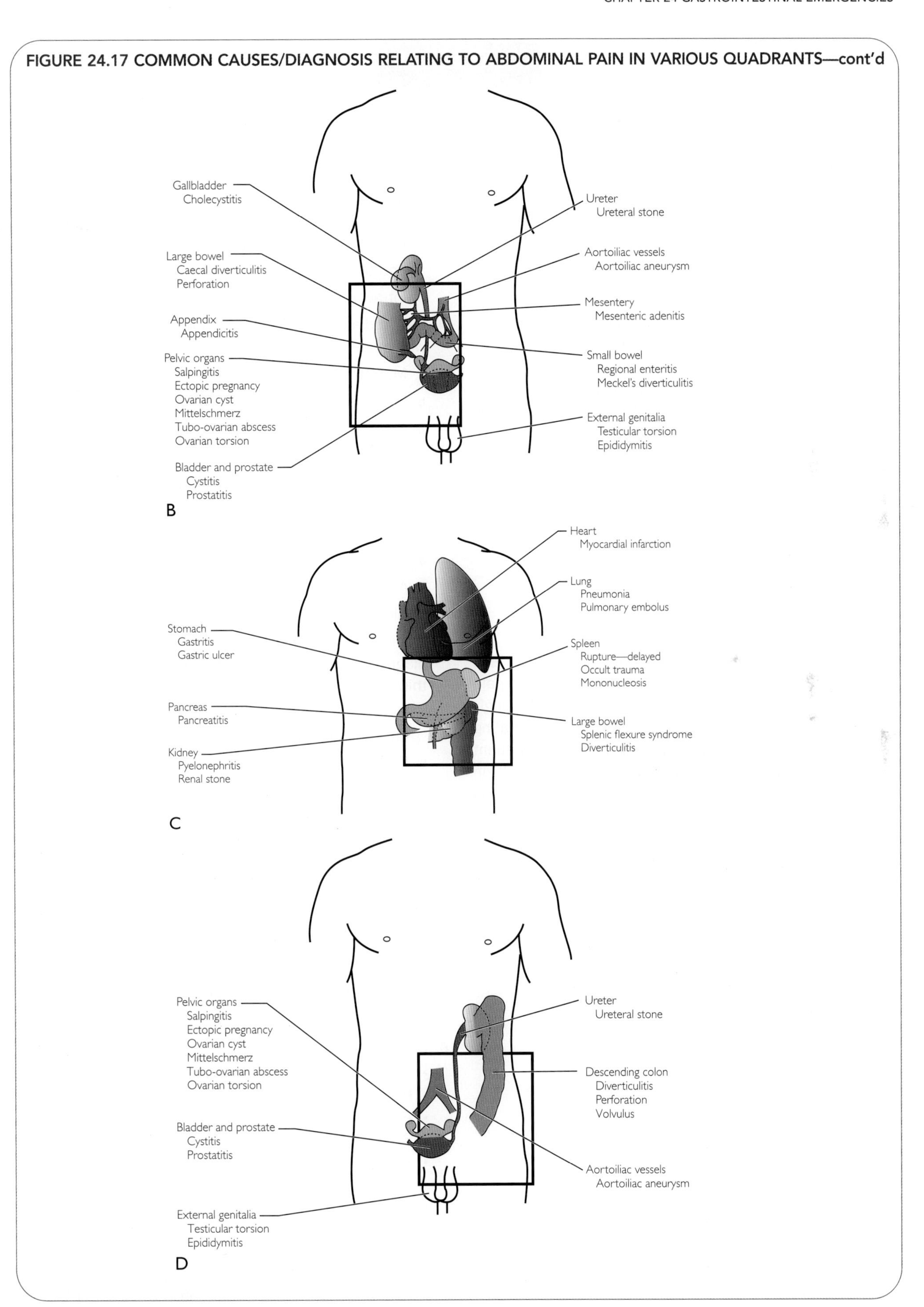
Gallbladder
Cholecystitis
Large bowel
Caecal diverticulitis
Perforation
Appendix
Appendicitis
Pelvic organs
Salpingitis
Ectopic pregnancy
Ovarian cyst
Mittelschmerz
Tubo-ovarian abscess
Ovarian torsion
Bladder and prostate
Cystitis
Prostatitis
Ureter
Ureteral stone
Aortoiliac vessels
Aortoiliac aneurysm
Mesentery
Mesenteric adenitis
Small bowel
Regional enteritis
Meckel's diverticulitis
External genitalia
Testicular torsion
Epididymitis
B
Heart
Myocardial infarction
Lung
Pneumonia
Pulmonary embolus
Stomach
Gastritis
Gastric ulcer
Spleen
Rupture—delayed
Occult trauma
Mononucleosis
Pancreas
Pancreatitis
Large bowel
Splenic flexure syndrome
Diverticulitis
Kidney
Pyelonephritis
Renal stone
C
Pelvic organs
Salpingitis
Ectopic pregnancy
Ovarian cyst
Mittelschmerz
Tubo-ovarian abscess
Ovarian torsion
Ureter
Ureteral stone
Descending colon
Diverticulitis
Perforation
Volvulus
Bladder and prostate
Cystitis
Prostatitis
Aortoiliac vessels
Aortoiliac aneurysm
External genitalia
Testicular torsion
Epididymitis
D

CASE STUDY

A 24-year-old man complains of increasing abdominal pain, with nausea and shortness of breath when sitting or lying down for the past 4 hours. In the course of your assessment you obtain information about the onset of his symptoms and past medical history. The previous evening following work, the patient had played rugby from 1830 hrs. During the match the patient was substituted off the field after being shoulder-charged in the abdomen and then vomiting. After the match ended, the patient went home, had a small dinner and took paracetamol (1 g) for 'stomach pain'. On exploring the patient's past medical history, the patient describes no significant medical history, denies smoking or recreational drug use. The patient works at the weekend as a bartender, and attends university during the week where he is studying for a law degree. His observations are:

- blood pressure 134/65 mmHg
- heart rate 122 beats/minute and regular
- temperature 36.8°C
- oxygen saturation 98% on room air
- respiratory rate 28 breaths/minute, breaths are short and staggered
- Glasgow Coma Scale score 15.

On asking the patient to describe the location and nature of the abdominal pain, he states that the pain is primarily over the upper left quadrant, increasingly intense when sitting or lying down, with pain radiating to the left shoulder tip when lying down. The patient rates the pain as 6/10 when standing and 10/10 on sitting or lying down. On examination, the patient finds it difficult to lie still as he finds it painful to straighten his body. On visual examination of the abdomen, there is no bruising or signs of injury. On light palpation, the patient is tender in the epigastric region and left upper quadrant. Deep palpation over the left upper quadrant elicits guarding. No tenderness noted elsewhere on palpating the abdomen; bowel sounds are normal.

QUESTIONS

1. Your immediate intervention on presentation following triage is to:
   a. Obtain a family history
   b. Provide pain relief
   c. Conduct a primary survey
   d. Obtain a blood sample to measure serum lactate.
2. The next clinical intervention is likely to be:
   a. Intravenous cannulation and blood sampling
   b. Arterial line insertion to monitor blood pressure
   c. Abdominal or girth measurement
   d. Urinalysis.
3. The best type of analgesia for this patient would be:
   a. Oral medication
   b. Nil at present; he needs to be assessed by a surgeon in case he has a surgical emergency requiring theatre
   c. Start with a non-steroidal anti-inflammatory drug and titrate response
   d. Intravenous narcotic analgesia.
4. Pain radiating to the left shoulder tip suggests which specific abdominal sign?
   a. Murphy's sign
   b. Kehr's sign
   c. Cullen's sign
   d. Grey-Turner's sign.
5. The best type of bedside diagnostic test for this patient would be:
   a. Urinalysis
   b. eFAST scan
   c. Abdominal x-ray
   d. Blood sugar level.
6. Ancillary tests are conducted to assist the diagnosis. The most useful initial blood tests for this patient would be:
   a. Full blood count; urea electrolytes and creatinine; amylase and lipase
   b. Full blood count; blood group and cross-match
   c. Lipase, troponin, full blood count
   d. Coagulation profile, liver and renal function tests, lipase and amylase.
7. Radiology will assist in diagnosis, and the inclusion or exclusion of other conditions. A useful initial investigation would be:
   a. Abdominal ultrasound
   b. Abdominal CT
   c. Abdominal magnetic resonance imaging
   d. Chest x-ray.
8. Blood tests reveal:
   - White blood cell count 13,000/mm^3
   - Haemoglobin 149 g/L
   - Packed cell volume 29%
   - Serum amylase 445 U/L
   - Serum lipase 65 U/L
   - Urea 5.4 mmol/L
   - Creatinine 7.9 microg/L
   - Sodium 141 mmol/L
   - Potassium 3.9 mmol/L
   - Chloride 104 mmol/L
   - Gamma GT (gamma-glutamyl transpeptidase) 41 U/L

- ALT (alanine amino transferase) 31 U/L
- AST (aspartate amino transferase) 21 U/L.

What are your findings?

a. Pancreatitis

b. Cholecystis

c. Splenic rupture

d. Myocardial infarction

9. If treated appropriately, most patients with acute pancreatitis will recover well. There are several complications associated with the disease of pancreatitis, and they include:

a. Liver failure

b. Coagulopathies and deep venous thrombosis

c. Pulmonary complications and effusions

d. Renal calculi.

Answers to Case Study Questions can be found on evolve **http://evolve.elsevier.com/AU/Curtis/emergency/** 

WEBSITES

The Gastroenterological Nurses College of Australia (GENCA). This is the professional nursing body representing gastroenterology and endoscopy nurses in Australia. GENCA promotes safe practice through the development of national standards and education courses and national and international representation, www.genca.org/.

Gastroenterology nursing courses. The Queensland University of Technology provides a range of academic courses specific to gastroenterology nursing to assist registered nurses to develop skills in professional practice, clinical care and collaborative practice, www.qut.edu.au.

REFERENCES

1. Australian Institute of Health and Welfare (AIHW). Emergency department care 2017–18: Australian hospital statistics. Health services series no.93. Cat. No.216. Canberra: AIHW; 2018.
2. Iedema R, Ball C, Daly B, Young J, Green T, Middleton PM, et al. Design and trial of a new ambulance-to-emergency department handover protocol: 'IMIST-AMBO'. BMJ Qual Safety 2012;21:627–33.
3. Makrauer F, Greenberger N. Acute abdominal pain: basic principles and current challenges. In: Greenberger N, Blumberg R, editors. Current diagnosis and treatment: gastroenterology, hepatology and endoscopy. 3rd ed. New York: McGraw-Hill; 2016.
4. Giddens JF, Wilson SF. Abdomen and gastrointestinal system. In: Health assessment for nursing practice, 7th ed. Philadelphia: Elsevier; 2022.
5. VanPutte C, Regan J, Russo AF, Seeley RR, editors. Anatomy and physiology. 12th ed. Boston: McGraw-Hill; 2019.
6. Gordon C, Craft J. The structure and function of the digestive system. In: Craft J, Gordon C, Huether S, McCance K, Brashers V, editors. Understanding pathophysiology. 3rd ed. Sydney: Elsevier; 2018.
7. Tortora G, Derrickson B. Principles of anatomy and physiology. 16th ed. New York: John Wiley and Sons; 2020.
8. Dibaise J, Parrish C, Thompson J. Short bowel syndrome: practical approach to management. New York: CRC Press; 2016.
9. Harding M, Kwong J, Roberts D, Hagler D, Reinisch C, editors. Lewis's medical-surgical nursing: assessment and management of clinical problems. 11th ed. St. Louis: Elsevier; 2019.
10. Walls R, Hockberger R, Marx J, editors. Rosen's emergency medicine—concepts and clinical practice. Philadelphia, PA: Elsevier; 2017.
11. Sargent S. Pathophysiology, diagnosis and management of acute pancreatitis. Br J Nurs 2006;15(18):999–1005.
12. Norris T, editor. Porth's pathophysiology: concepts of altered health states. Pennsylvania: Lippincott Williams & Wilkins; 2018.
13. Rossoll L. Abdominal emergencies. Emergency nursing core curriculum. 7th ed. Philadelphia: Elsevier; 2017.
14. Thomas J, Monaghan T. Oxford handbook of clinical examination and practical skills. 2nd ed. Oxford: Oxford University Press; 2014.
15. Service QA. Clinical practice guidelines: abdominal emergencies. State of Queensland; 2017. Available from: www.ambulance.qld.gov.au/docs/clinical/cpg/cpg_abdominal%20emergencies.pdf.
16. Laurell H, Hansson LE, Gunnarsson U. Acute abdominal pain among elderly patients. Gerontology 2006;52(6):339–44.
17. Lewis LM, Banet GA, Blanda M, Hustey FM, Meldon SW, Gerson LW. Etiology and clinical course of abdominal pain in senior patients: a prospective, multicenter study. J Gerontol Series A, Biol Sc Med Sci 2005;60(8):1071–6.
18. Penner R, Fishman M. Evaluation of the adult with abdominal pain. UpToDate; 2021. Available from: https://www.uptodate.com.acs.hcn.com.au/contents/evaluation-of-the-adult-with-abdominal-pain.
19. Gregory J. Use of pain scales and observational pain assessment tools in hospital settings. Nurs Stand 2019;34(9):70–4.
20. Clayton HA, Reschak GL, Gaynor SE, Creamer JL. A novel program to assess and manage pain. Medsurg Nurs 2000;9(6):318–21, 317.
21. Jones J, Sim TF, Hughes J. Pain assessment of elderly patients with cognitive impairment in the emergency department: implications for pain management-a narrative review of current practices. J Pharm Ed Pract 2017;5(2):30.
22. Breum BM, Rud B, Kirkegaard T, Nordentoft T. Accuracy of abdominal auscultation for bowel obstruction. World J Gastroenterol 2015;21(34):10018–24.

23. Bennett DH, Tambeur LJ, Campbell WB. Use of coughing test to diagnose peritonitis. BMJ (Clin Res Ed) 1994;308(6940):1336.
24. Fenyö G, Lindberg G, Blind P, Enochsson L, Oberg A. Diagnostic decision support in suspected acute appendicitis: validation of a simplified scoring system. Euro J Surg 1997;163(11):831–8.
25. Hajalioghli P, Mostafavi S, Mirza-Aghazadeh-Attari M. Ultrasonography in diagnosis of appendicitis and its complications in pediatric patients: a cross-sectional study. Ann Pediatr Surg 2020;16(1):12.
26. Hallan S, Asberg A, Edna TH. Estimating the probability of acute appendicitis using clinical criteria of a structured record sheet: the physician against the computer. Euro J Surg 1997;163(6):427–32.
27. Jahn H, Mathiesen FK, Neckelmann K, Hovendal CP, Bellstrøm T, Gottrup F. Comparison of clinical judgment and diagnostic ultrasonography in the diagnosis of acute appendicitis: experience with a score-aided diagnosis. Euro J Surg 1997;163(6):433–43.
28. Mahadevan M, Graff L. Prospective randomized study of analgesic use for ED patients with right lower quadrant abdominal pain. Am J Emerg Med 2000;18(7):753–6.
29. Barlotta KS, Stack LB, Knoop KJ. Grey turner sign and Cullen sign. In: Knoop KJ, Stack LB, Storrow AB, Thurman RJ, editors. The atlas of emergency medicine. 5th ed. New York, NY: McGraw-Hill; 2021.
30. Ahn S, Lee H, Choi W, Ahn R, Hong JS, Sohn CH, et al. Clinical importance of the heel drop test and a new clinical score for adult appendicitis. PLoS One 2016;11(10):e0164574.
31. Kendall JL, Moreira ME. Evaluation of the adult with abdominal pain in the emergency department. UpToDate; 2020. Available from: www.uptodate.com.
32. Marek V, Záhorec R, Durdík S. Acute appendicitis: clinical anatomy of the new palpation sign. Clin Anat 2021;34(2):218–23.
33. Andersson R, Swärd A, Tingstedt B, Akerberg D. Treatment of acute pancreatitis: focus on medical care. Drugs 2009;69(5):505–14.
34. Mills LD, Mills T, Foster B. Association of clinical and laboratory variables with ultrasound findings in right upper quadrant abdominal pain. South Med J 2005;98(2):155–61.
35. Navarro Fernández JA, Tárraga López PJ, Rodríguez Montes JA, López Cara MA. Validity of tests performed to diagnose acute abdominal pain in patients admitted at an emergency department. Rev Esp Enferm Dig 2009;101(9):610–8.
36. Rastogi V, Singh D, Tekiner H, Ye F, Mazza JJ, Yale SH. Abdominal physical signs and medical eponyms: movements and compression. Clin Med Res 2018;16(3–4):76–82.
37. Wagner JM, McKinney WP, Carpenter JL. Does this patient have appendicitis? JAMA 1996;276(19):1589–94.
38. Rastogi V, Singh D, Tekiner H, Ye F, Kirchenko N, Mazza JJ, et al. Abdominal physical signs and medical eponyms: physical examination of palpation part 1, 1876–1907. Clin Med Res 2018;16(3–4):83–91.
39. Werner JC, Zock M, Khalil PN, Hoffmann J, Kanz KG, Jauch KW. Evidence for the digital rectal examination in the emergency assessment of acute abdominal pain. Zentralbl Chir 2013;138(6):669–76.
40. Antibiotic Expert Groups. Therapeutic guidelines: antibiotics: acute gastroenteritis, Version 15. Melbourne: Therapeutic Guidelines Limited; 2021. Available from: https://tgldcdp.tg.org.au/etgcomplete.
41. Hamm CW, Bassand JP, Agewall S, Bax J, Boersma E, Bueno H, et al. ESC guidelines for the management of acute coronary syndromes in patients presenting without persistent ST-segment elevation: the task force for the management of acute coronary syndromes (ACS) in patients presenting without persistent ST-segment elevation of the European Society of Cardiology (ESC). Eur Heart J 2011;32(23):2999–3054.
42. Hammer Y, Eisen A, Hasdai D, Goldenberg I, Shlomo N, Cohen T, et al. Comparison of outcomes in patients with acute coronary syndrome presenting with typical versus atypical symptoms. Am J Cardiol 2019;124(12):1851–6.
43. Kitabchi AE, Umpierrez GE, Miles JM, Fisher JN. Hyperglycemic crises in adult patients with diabetes. Diabetes Care 2009;32(7):1335–43.
44. Byrne AL, Bennett M, Pace N, Thomas P. Peripheral venous blood gas analysis versus arterial blood gas analysis for the diagnosis of respiratory failure and metabolic disturbance in adults. Cochrane Database System Rev 2013;11:CD010841.
45. Benitez Cantero JM, Jurado Garcia J, Ruiz Cuesta P, González Galilea A, Muñoz García-Borruel M, García Sánchez V, et al. Early evaluation of anaemia in patients with acute gastrointestinal bleeding: venous blood gas analysis compared to conventional laboratory. Med Clin (Barc) 2013;141:332–7.
46. Levey AS, Stevens LA, Schmid CH, Zhang YL, Castro AF, Feldman HI, et al. A new equation to estimate glomerular filtration rate. Ann Intern Med 2009;150(9):604–12.
47. Australasia College for Emergency Medicine, RCPA. Guideline on pathology testing in the emergency department (G125). Melbourne: ACEM; 2018.
48. Macaluso CR, McNamara RM. Evaluation and management of acute abdominal pain in the emergency department. Int J Gen Med 2012;5:789–97.
49. Panagiotopoulou IG, Parashar D, Lin R, Antonowicz S, Wells AD, Bajwa FM, et al. The diagnostic value of white cell count, C-reactive protein and bilirubin in acute appendicitis and its complications. Ann Royal Coll Surg Eng 2013;95(3):215–21.
50. Bezmarevic M, Mirkovic D, Soldatovic I, Stamenkovic D, Mitrovic N, Perisic N, et al. Correlation between procalcitonin and intra-abdominal pressure and their role in prediction of the severity of acute pancreatitis. Pancreatology 2012;12(4):337–43.
51. Wu JY, Chen HC, Lee SH, Chan RC, Lee CC, Chang SS. Diagnostic role of procalcitonin in patients with suspected appendicitis. World J Surg 2012;36(8):1744–49.
52. Al-Gaithy ZK. Clinical value of total white blood cells and neutrophil counts in patients with suspected appendicitis: retrospective study. World J Emerg Surg 2012;7(1):32.
53. Jangjoo A, Varasteh AR, Bahar MM, Meibodi NT, Aliakbarian M, Hoseininejad M, et al. Is C-reactive protein helpful for early diagnosis of acute appendicitis? Acta Chir Belg 2011;111(4):219–22.

54. Meyer ZC, Schreinemakers JM, van der Laan L. The value of C-reactive protein and lactate in the acute abdomen in the emergency department. World J Emerg Surg 2012;7(1):22.
55. Schellekens DH, Hulsewé KW, van Acker BA, van Bijnen AA, de Jaegere TM, Sastrowijoto SH, et al. Evaluation of the diagnostic accuracy of plasma markers for early diagnosis in patients suspected for acute appendicitis. Ac Emerg Med 2013;20(7):703–10.
56. Lau WY, Ho YC, Chu KW, Yeung C. Leucocyte count and neutrophil percentage in appendicectomy for suspected appendicitis. ANZ J Surg 1989;59(5):395–8.
57. Lyons D, Waldron R, Ryan T, O'Malley E. An evaluation of the clinical value of the leucocyte count and sequential counts in suspected acute appendicitis. B J Clin Pract 1987;41(6):794–6.
58. Sushruth S, Vijayakumar C, Srinivasan K, Raj Kumar N, Balasubramaniyan G, Verma SK, et al. Role of C-reactive protein, white blood cell counts, bilirubin levels, and imaging in the diagnosis of acute appendicitis as a cause of right iliac fossa pain. Cureus 2018;10(1):e2070.
59. Yu CW, Juan LI, Wu MH, Shen CJ, Wu JY, Lee CC. Systematic review and meta-analysis of the diagnostic accuracy of procalcitonin, C-reactive protein and white blood cell count for suspected acute appendicitis. Br J Surg 2013;100(3):322–9.
60. van Ravesteijn H, van Dijk I, Darmon D, van de Laar F, Lucassen P, Olde Hartman T, et al. The reassuring value of diagnostic tests: a systematic review. Pat Ed Counsel 2012;86(1):3–8.
61. Yang RW, Shao ZX, Chen YY, Yin Z, Wang WJ. Lipase and pancreatic amylase activities in diagnosis of acute pancreatitis in patients with hyperamylasemia. Hepatobil Pancreat Dis Int 2005;4(4):600–3.
62. Prinzen L, Keulemans JC, Bekers O. The diagnostic benefits of lipase values in acute pancreatitis. NTvG 2013;157(38):A6432.
63. Sutton PA, Humes DJ, Purcell G, Smith JK, Whiting F, Wright T, et al. The role of routine assays of serum amylase and lipase for the diagnosis of acute abdominal pain. Ann Royal Coll Surg Eng 2009;91(5):381–4.
64. Malakouti M, Kataria A, Ali SK, Schenker S. Elevated liver enzymes in asymptomatic patients – what should I do? J Clin Transl Hepatol 2017;5(4):394–403.
65. Limdi JK, Hyde GM. Evaluation of abnormal liver function tests. Postgrad Med J 2003;79(932):307–12.
66. Gopal DV, Rosen HR. Abnormal findings on liver function tests. Interpreting results to narrow the diagnosis and establish a prognosis. Postgrad Med J 2000;107(2):100–2, 105–9, 113–4.
67. Pratt D. Liver chemistry and function tests. In: Feldman M, Friedman L, Sleisenger M, editors. Sleisenger and Fordtran's gastrointestinal and liver disease: pathophysiology, diagnosis and management. 10th ed. Philadelphia: Saunders; 2016.
68. Kessler C, Bauer SJ. Utility of the digital rectal examination in the emergency department: a review. J Emerg Med 2012;43(6):1196–204.
69. Manimaran N, Galland RB. Significance of routine digital rectal examination in adults presenting with abdominal pain. Ann Royal Coll Surg Eng 2004;86(4):292–5.
70. Quaas J, Lanigan M, Newman D, McOsker J, Babayev R, Mason C. Utility of the digital rectal examination in the evaluation of undifferentiated abdominal pain. Am J Emerg Med 2009;27(9):1125–9.
71. Bonello JC, Abrams J. The significance of a 'positive' rectal examination in acute appendicitis. Dis Colon Rectum 1979;22:97–101.
72. Dixon JM, Elton RA, Rainey JB, Macleod DA. Rectal examination in patients with pain in the right lower quadrant of the abdomen. BMJ (Clin Res Ed) 1991;302(6773):386–8.
73. Takada T, Nishiwaki H, Yamamoto Y, Noguchi Y, Fukuma S, Yamazaki S, et al. The role of digital rectal examination for diagnosis of acute appendicitis: a systematic review and meta-analysis. PLoS One 2015;10(9):e0136996.
74. Smith JE, Hall EJ. The use of plain abdominal x rays in the emergency department. Emerg Med J 2009;26(3):160–3.
75. Ahn SH, Mayo-Smith WW, Murphy BL, Reinert SE, Cronan JJ. Acute nontraumatic abdominal pain in adult patients: abdominal radiography compared with CT evaluation. Radiology 2002;225(1):159–64.
76. Maglinte DD, Reyes BL, Harmon BH, Kelvin FM, Turner WW, Hage JE, et al. Reliability and role of plain film radiography and CT in the diagnosis of small-bowel obstruction. Am J Roentgenol 1996;167(6):1451–5.
77. Suri S, Gupta S, Sudhakar PJ, Venkataramu NK, Sood B, Wig JD. Comparative evaluation of plain films, ultrasound and CT in the diagnosis of intestinal obstruction. Acta Radiol 1999;40(4):422–8.
78. Gans SL, Stoker J, Boermeester MA. Plain abdominal radiography in acute abdominal pain; past, present, and future. Int J Gen Med 2012;5:525–33.
79. MacKersie AB, Lane MJ, Gerhardt RT, Claypool HA, Keenan S, Katz DS, et al. Nontraumatic acute abdominal pain: unenhanced helical CT compared with three-view acute abdominal series. Radiology 2005;237(1):114–22.
80. Kameda T, Taniguchi N. Overview of point-of-care abdominal ultrasound in emergency and critical care. J Intens Care 2016;4:53.
81. Pourmand A, Dimbil U, Drake A, Shokoohi H. The accuracy of point-of-care ultrasound in detecting small bowel obstruction in emergency department. Emerg Med Int 2018;2018:3684081.
82. Laméris W, van Randen A, van Es HW, van Heesewijk JP, van Ramshorst B, Bouma WH, et al. Imaging strategies for detection of urgent conditions in patients with acute abdominal pain: diagnostic accuracy study. BMJ (Clin Res Ed) 2009;338:b2431.
83. van Randen A, Laméris W, van Es HW, van Heesewijk HP, van Ramshorst B, Ten Hove W, et al. A comparison of the accuracy of ultrasound and computed tomography in common diagnoses causing acute abdominal pain. Euro Radiol 2011;21(7):1535–45.
84. Varndell W, Topacio M, Hagness C, Lemon H, Tracy D. Nurse-performed focused ultrasound in the emergency department: a systematic review. Australas Emerg Care 2018;21:121–30.

85. Cartwright SL, Knudson MP. Diagnostic imaging of acute abdominal pain in adults. Am Fam Phys 2015;91(7):452–9.
86. Supreme Court Library Queensland. Donoghue v Stevenson [1932] AC 562. 2016. Available from: https://legalheritage.sclqld.org.au/donoghue-v-stevenson-1932-ac-562.
87. Sala E, Watson CJ, Beadsmoore C, Groot-Wassink T, Fanshawe TR, Smith JC, et al. A randomized, controlled trial of routine early abdominal computed tomography in patients presenting with non-specific acute abdominal pain. Clin Radiol 2007;62(10):961–9.
88. Esses D, Birnbaum A, Bijur P, Shah S, Gleyzer A, Gallagher EJ. Ability of CT to alter decision making in elderly patients with acute abdominal pain. Am J Emerg Med 2004;22(4):270–2.
89. Broder J, Warshauer DM. Increasing utilization of computed tomography in the adult emergency department, 2000–2005. Emerg Radiol 2006;13(1):25–30.
90. Mitka M. Costly surge in diagnostic imaging spurs debate. JAMA 2005;293(6):665–7.
91. Brenner DJ, Hall EJ. Computed tomography–an increasing source of radiation exposure. N Eng J Med 2007;357(22):2277–84.
92. Griffey RT, Sodickson A. Cumulative radiation exposure and cancer risk estimates in emergency department patients undergoing repeat or multiple CT. Am J Roentgenol 2009;192(4):887–92.
93. McQuown CM, Frey JA, Wilber ST. Noncontrast abdomen/pelvis computed tomographic scan in the evaluation of older adults. Am J Emerg Med 2016;34(11):2230–2.
94. Hlibczuk V, Dattaro JA, Jin Z, Falzon L, Brown MD. Diagnostic accuracy of noncontrast computed tomography for appendicitis in adults: a systematic review. Ann Emerg Med 2010;55(1):51–59.e1.
95. Kepner AM, Bacasnot JV, Stahlman BA. Intravenous contrast alone vs intravenous and oral contrast computed tomography for the diagnosis of appendicitis in adult ED patients. Am J Emerg Med 2012;30(9):1765–73.
96. The Royal Australian and New Zealand College of Radiologists. Iodinated contrast media guideline. 2018. Available from: www.ranzcr.com/college/document-library/ranzcr-iodinated-contrast-guidelines.
97. Society of Gastroenterology Nurses and Associates. Gastroenterology nursing: a core curriculum. 6th ed. Chicago: Society of Gastroenterology Nurses & Associates; 2019.
98. Ziebell C, Kitlowski A, Welch J, Friesen PA. Upper gastrointestinal bleeding. In: Tintinalli JE, Stapczynski JS, Ma O John et al., editors. Tintinalli's emergency medicine: a comprehensive study guide. 8th ed. Sydney: McGraw-Hill; 2015.
99. Roline C, Reardon R. Disorders of the small intestine. In: Marx J, Hockberger R, Walls R, editors. Rosen's emergency medicine—concepts and clinical practice. 9th ed. Philadelphia, PA: Saunders; 2017.
100. O'Grady J. Acute liver failure. In: Feldman M, Friedman L, Brandt L, editors. Sleisenger and Fordtran's gastrointestinal and liver disease pathphysiology, diagnosis and management. 11th ed. Philadelphia, PA: Saunders; 2020.
101. McQuaid K. Gastrointestinal disorders. In: McPhee S, Papadakis M, editors. New York: McGraw-Hill; 2017.
102. Odutayo A, Desborough MJ, Trivella M, Stanley AJ, Dorée C, Collins GS, et al. Restrictive versus liberal blood transfusion for gastrointestinal bleeding: a systematic review and meta-analysis of randomised controlled trials. Lancet Gastroenterol Hepatol 2017;2(5):354–60.
103. Villanueva C, Colomo A, Bosch A. Transfusion for acute upper gastrointestinal bleeding. N Eng J Med 2013;368(14):1362–3.
104. Lo B. Lower gastrointestinal bleeding. In: Tintinalli JE, Ma O. John, Yearly D, Meckler GD, Cline DM, Thomas SH, editors. Tintinalli's emergency medicine: a comprehensive study guide. 9th ed. Sydney: McGraw-Hill Education; 2019.
105. Holster IL, Valkhoff VE, Kuipers EJ, Tjwa ETTL. New oral anticoagulants increase risk for gastrointestinal bleeding: a systematic review and meta-analysis. Gastroenterology 2013;145(1):105–12.e15.
106. Wada T, Hagiwara A, Uemura T, Yahagi N, Kimura A. Early lactate clearance for predicting active bleeding in critically ill patients with acute upper gastrointestinal bleeding: a retrospective study. Intern Emerg Med 2016;11(5):737–43.
107. Meguerdichian D, Goralnick W. Gastrointestinal bleeding. In: Marx J, Hockberger R, Walls R, editors. Rosen's emergency medicine—concepts and clinical practice. 8th ed. Philadelphia, PA: Saunders; 2017.
108. Cydulka R. Pancreatitis and cholecystitis. Sydney: McGraw-Hill; 2017.
109. Therapeutic Guidelines. Functional gastrointestinal disorders. 2021. Available from: https://tgldcdp.tg.org.au/etgcomplete.
110. Therapeutic Guidelines. Gastric disorders. In: eTG complete Melbourne: Therapeutic Guidelines Limited; 2021. Available from: https://tgldcdp.tg.org.au/etgcomplete.
111. Knox SA, Harrison CM, Britt HC, Henderson JV. Estimating prevalence of common chronic morbidities in Australia. Med J Aust 2008;189(2):66–70.
112. Gastroenterological Society of Australia. Gastro-oesophageal reflux disease in adults. 2011. Available from: www.gesa.org.au/resources/clinical-guidelines-and-updates/gastro-oesophageal-reflux-disease/.
113. Therapeutic Guidelines. Disorders of the oesophagus. 2021. Available from: https://tgldcdp.tg.org.au/etgcomplete.
114. Wyatt J, Illingworth R, Graham C, Hogg K, Clancy MJ, Robertson CE, editors. Oxford handbook of emergency medicine. New York: Oxford University Press; 2012.
115. Department of Health. National notifiable diseases surveillance system. Canberra: Australian Government; 2017. Available from: www9.health.gov.au/cda/source/rpt_2.cfm.

116. Services VGDoHaH. The Blue Book: guidelines for the control of infectious diseases. Melbourne, Victoria: Victorian Government Department of Human Services; 2005.
117. Christou NV. Impact of obesity and bariatric surgery on survival. World J Surg 2009;33(10):2022–7.
118. Flum DR, Dellinger EP. Impact of gastric bypass operation on survival: a population-based analysis. J Am Coll Surg 2004;199(4):543–51.
119. Foster A, Richards WO, McDowell J, Laws HL, Clements RH. Gastrointestinal symptoms are more intense in morbidly obese patients. Surg Endoscop 2003;17(11):1766–8.
120. Kassir R, Debs T, Blanc P, Gugenheim J, Ben Amor I, Boutet C, et al. Complications of bariatric surgery: presentation and emergency management. Int J Surg 2016;27:77–81.
121. Gorecki P, Wise L, Brolin RE, Champion JK. Complications of combined gastric restrictive and malabsorptive procedures: Part 1. Curr Surg 2003;60(2):138–44.
122. Sugerman HJ, Brewer WH, Shiffman ML, Brolin RE, Fobi MA, Linner JH, et al. A multicenter, placebo-controlled, randomized, double-blind, prospective trial of prophylactic ursodiol for the prevention of gallstone formation following gastric-bypass-induced rapid weight loss. Am J Surg 1995;169(1):91–6; discussion 96–7.
123. Byrne TK. Complications of surgery for obesity. Surg Clin N Am 2001;81(5):1181–93, vii–viii.
124. Comeau E, Gagner M, Inabnet WB, Herron DM, Quinn TM, Pomp A. Symptomatic internal hernias after laparoscopic bariatric surgery. Surg Endoscop 2005;19(1):34–9.
125. Carucci LR, Turner MA. Radiologic evaluation following Roux-en-Y gastric bypass surgery for morbid obesity. Eur J Radiol 2005;53(3):353–65.
126. Belle SH, Berk PD, Courcoulas AP, Flum DR, Miles CW, Mitchell JE, et al. Safety and efficacy of bariatric surgery: longitudinal assessment of bariatric surgery. Surg Obesity Rel Dis 2007;3(2):116–26.
127. Podnos YD, Jimenez JC, Wilson SE, Stevens CM, Nguyen NT. Complications after laparoscopic gastric bypass: a review of 3464 cases. Arch Surg 2003;138(9):957–61.
128. Fuks D, Verhaeghe P, Brehant O, Sabbagh C, Dumont F, Riboulot M, et al. Results of laparoscopic sleeve gastrectomy: a prospective study in 135 patients with morbid obesity. Surgery 2009;145(1):106–13.
129. Yarandi SS, Griffith DP, Sharma R, Mohan A, Zhao VM, Ziegler TR. Optic neuropathy, myelopathy, anemia, and neutropenia caused by acquired copper deficiency after gastric bypass surgery. J Clin Gastroenterol 2014;48(10):862–5.
130. Moser F, Gorodner MV, Galvani CA, Baptista M, Chretien C, Horgan S. Pouch enlargement and band slippage: two different entities. Surg Endoscop 2006;20(7):1021–9.
131. Eid I, Birch DW, Sharma AM, Sherman V, Karmali S. Complications associated with adjustable gastric banding for morbid obesity: a surgeon's guides. Can J Surg 2011;54(1):61–6.
132. Suter M. Laparoscopic band repositioning for pouch dilatation/slippage after gastric banding: disappointing results. Obes Surg 2001;11(4): 507–12.
133. Tran D, Rhoden DH, Cacchione RN, Baldwin L, Allen JW. Techniques for repair of gastric prolapse after laparoscopic gastric banding. J Laparoendoscop Adv Surg Tech 2004;14(2):117–120.
134. Msika S. [Surgery for morbid obesity: 2. Complications. Results of a Technologic Evaluation by the ANAES]. J Chirurg (Paris) 2003;140(1):4–21.
135. Manterola C, Vial M, Moraga J, Astudillo P. Analgesia in patients with acute abdominal pain. Cochrane Database Syst Rev 2011(1):Cd005660.
136. Schug S, Palmer G, Scott D, Alcock M, Halliwell R, Mott JF, editors. Acute pain management: scientific evidence. 5th ed. Melbourne: ANZCA & FPM; 2020.
137. Varndell W, Fry M, Elliott D. Pain assessment and interventions by nurses in the emergency department: a national survey. J Clin Nurs 2020;29(13–14):2352–62.
138. Schug S, Palmer G, Scott D, Halliwell R, Trinca J. Acute pain management: scientific evidence. 4th ed. Melbourne: ANZCA & FPM; 2015.
139. Qayed E, Dagar G, Nanchal RS. Lower gastrointestinal hemorrhage. Crit Care Clin 2016;32(2):241–54.
140. Elwood DR. Cholecystitis. Surg Clin N Am 2008;88(6):1241–52, viii.
141. Craft J, Gordon C, Huether S, McCance K, Brashers V. Understanding pathophysiology. Sydney: Elsevier; 2014.
142. Beliaev AM, Marshall RJ, Booth M. C-reactive protein has a better discriminative power than white cell count in the diagnosis of acute cholecystitis. J Surg Res 2015;198(1):66–72.
143. Summers SM, Scruggs W, Menchine MD, Lahham S, Anderson C, Amr O, et al. A prospective evaluation of emergency department bedside ultrasonography for the detection of acute cholecystitis. Ann Emerg Med 2010;56(2):114–22.
144. Berkowitz R, Rose G. Acute pancreatitis. In: Marx J, Hockberger R, Walls R, editors. Rosen's emergency medicine: concepts and clinical practice. 9th ed. Philadelphia, PA: Saunders; 2017.
145. Amcrine E. Get optimum outcomes for acute pancreatitis patients. Nurse Pract 2007;32(6):44–8.
146. Freedman S. Pancreatitis. In: Porter R, Kaplan J, editors. The Merck manual of diagnosis and therapy. 19th ed. Whitehouse Station, NJ: Merck Sharp and Dohme Corp; 2011.
147. Rompianesi G, Hann A, Komolafe O, Pereira SP, Davidson BR, Gurusamy KS. Serum amylase and lipase and urinary trypsinogen and amylase for diagnosis of acute pancreatitis. Cochrane Database System Rev 2017;4(4):Cd012010.

148. Working Group IAP/APA. IAP/APA evidence-based guidelines for the management of acute pancreatitis. Pancreatology 2013;13(4 Suppl 2): e1–15.
149. Guidelines T. Chronic pancreatitis. 2021. Available from: https://tgldcdp.tg.org.au/etgcomplete.
150. Lewis S, Bucher L, Heitkemper M, Harding MM, Kwong J, Roberts D. Medical–surgical nursing: assessment and management of clinical problems. 10th ed. St. Louis: Mosby; 2016.
151. National Institute for Health and Care Excellence. Pancreatitis: diagnosis and management: guideline. London: NICE; 2018.
152. Peterson M. Disorders of the large intestine. In: Marx J, Hockberger R, Walls R, editors. Rosen's emergency medicine—concepts and clinical practice. 9th ed. Philadelphia, PA: Saunders; 2017.
153. Kryzauskas M, Danys D, Poskus T, Mikalauskas S, Poskus E, Jotautas V, et al. Is acute appendicitis still misdiagnosed? Open Med (Wars) 2016;11(1):231–6.
154. Yeh B. Evidence-based emergency medicine/rational clinical examination abstract. Does this adult patient have appendicitis? Ann Emerg Med 2008;52(3):301–3.
155. Cameron P, Little M, Mitra B, Deasy C, editors. Textbook of adult emergency medicine. 5th ed. London: Elsevier; 2019.
156. Chamouard P, Richert Z, Meyer N, Rahmi G, Baumann R. Diagnostic value of C-reactive protein for predicting activity level of Crohn's disease. Clin Gastroenterol Hepatol 2006;4(7):882–7.
157. Guidelines T. Inflammatory bowel disease. 2021. Available from: https://tgldcdp.tg.org.au/etgcomplete.
158. Marx J, Hockberger R, Walls R, editors. Rosen's emergency medicine: concepts and clinical practice. 9th ed. St. Louis: Mosby; 2017.
159. Australian Institute of Health and Welfare (AIHW). Separation statistics by principal diagnosis (ICD-10-AM 11th Edition) Australia 2019-20. AIHW; 2021. Available from: www.aihw.gov.au/reports/hospitals/principal-diagnosis-data-cubes/contents/data-cubes.
160. Baskin B. Acute abdominal pain. In: Fitch M, Joing S, Wang V, editors. Tintinalli's emergency medicine manual. 8th ed. Sydney: McGraw-Hill; 2017.
161. Honda T, Uehara T, Matsumoto G, Arai S, Sugano M. Neutrophil left shift and white blood cell count as markers of bacterial infection. Clin Chim Acta 2016;457:46–53.
162. Laméris W, van Randen A, Bipat S, Bossuyt PM, Boermeester MA, Stoker J. Graded compression ultrasonography and computed tomography in acute colonic diverticulitis: meta-analysis of test accuracy. Eur Radiol 2008;18(11):2498–511.
163. Tavakkoli A, Ashley SW, Zinner MJ. Small intestine. In: Brunicardi FC, Andersen DK, Billiar TR, Dunn DL, Kao LS, Hunter JG, et al., editors. Schwartz's principles of surgery, 11 ed. New York, NY: McGraw-Hill Education; 2019.
164. Chen MYM. Chapter 8. Plain film of the abdomen. In: Chen MYM, Pope TL, Ott DJ, editors. Basic radiology. 2nd ed. New York, NY: McGraw-Hill; 2011.
165. Clarke C, Dux A. Abdominal x-rays for medical students. West Sussex, England: Wiley-Blackwell; 2015.
166. Jang TB, Schindler D, Kaji AH. Bedside ultrasonography for the detection of small bowel obstruction in the emergency department. Emerg Med J 2011;28(8):676–8.
167. McDonald G, Wong C. Gastrointestinal emergencies. In: Fulde S, Fulde G, ediors. Emergency medicine. 7th ed. Sydney: Elsevier; 2020.
168. Wald A, Talley N, Grover S. Management of chronic constipation in adults. UpToDate; 2021. Available from: www.uptodate.com.acs.hcn.com.au/contents/management-of-chronic-constipation-in-adults.
169. Friedman S, Runyon B, Robson K. Clinical manifestations and diagnosis of alcohol-associated fatty liver disease and alcoholic cirrhosis. Waltham, MA: Wolters Kluwer; 2021. Available from: www.uptodate.com.acs.hcn.com.au/contents/clinical-manifestations-and-diagnosis-of-alcohol-associated-fatty-liver-disease-and-cirrhosis?search=alcoholic%20fatty%20liver&source=search_result&selectedTitle=1~34&usage_type=default&display_rank=1.
170. Heidelbaugh JJ, Bruderly M. Cirrhosis and chronic liver failure: part I. Diagnosis and evaluation. Am Fam Phys 2006;74(5):756–62.
171. Larson A. Diagnosis and management of acute liver failure. Curr Opin Gastroenterol 2010;26:214–21.
172. Friedman S, Chopra S, Grover S. Approach to the patient with abnormal liver biochemical and function tests. UpToDate; 2021. Available from: www.uptodate.com/contents/clinical-manifestations-and-diagnosis-of-alcohol-associated-fatty-liver-disease-and-cirrhosis.
173. Macnaughtan J, Thomas H. Liver failure at the front door. Clin Med (Lond) 2010;10(1):73–8.
174. Vizzutti F, Arena U, Laffi G. Acute on chronic liver failure: from pathophysiology to clinical management. Trends Anaesth Crit Care 2013;3:122–9.

CHAPTER 25
RENAL AND GENITOURINARY EMERGENCIES

ANN BONNER AND LEANNE BROWN

ESSENTIALS

- Urinalysis is an important, simple, quick and non-invasive assessment.
- Early and aggressive treatment of hypotension or hypovolaemia will prevent the development of acute kidney injury.
- Acute kidney injury can result from nephrotoxic agents such as contrast media.
- Infections are common causes of AKI.
- In remote locations, consider acute post-streptococcal glomerular nephritis as a cause of acute kidney injury.
- Chronic kidney disease should be considered likely in people with diabetes or hypertension, regardless of whether or not it is diagnosed.
- Arteriovenous fistulae should be regularly assessed for patency and should never be cannulated.
- Peritonitis is the most common complication associated with peritoneal dialysis.
- Urinary tract infections and pyelonephritis can be the cause of septicaemia, particularly in older people.
- The pain associated with renal calculi requires regular assessment and administration of appropriate analgesia.
- Scrotal pain needs urgent assessment and referral to preserve testicular function.

INTRODUCTION

Genitourinary (GU) problems are common in the community and often result in presentation to the emergency department (ED). Urinary tract infections (UTIs) are highly prevalent bacterial diseases, and up to 20% of women will experience at least one UTI in their lifetime. Uncomplicated UTIs are mostly managed by general practitioners and nurse practitioners. Nephrolithiasis (renal calculi) affects over one million Australians, and it is likely that the hot, dry climate causes more stone formation than in many other countries in the world. In Aotearoa New Zealand, 10–15% of the population may develop nephrolithiasis during their life. Acute kidney injury (AKI) is a common complication of any trauma. Hypovolaemia results in severe hypotension and this precipitates the development of acute tubular necrosis and subsequent AKI. The global incidence of chronic kidney disease (CKD) is rapidly rising in developed and developing nations. CKD is now classified into five grades, with those in grade 5 classified as being in kidney failure (formerly end-stage kidney disease [ESKD]).[1] It is estimated that one in three adults are at risk of developing CKD, and 10% of the Australian and Aotearoa New Zealand population has CKD. First Nation populations from both Australia and Aotearoa New Zealand (Aboriginal peoples,

Torres Strait Islander peoples, Māori and Pacific Islanders) are overrepresented in the number of people with all CKD grades.

Patients with compromised kidney function require the assistance of paramedics and many will present to the ED with life-threatening fluid and electrolyte imbalances. Specific GU emergencies discussed in this chapter are acute kidney injury, rhabdomyolysis, chronic kidney disease, UTIs, acute urinary retention, urinary calculi, testicular torsion, epididymitis and priapism. Refer to Chapter 33 for discussion of sexually transmitted infections (STIs) in women and to Chapter 46 for discussion of genitourinary trauma.

ANATOMY AND PHYSIOLOGY

The genitourinary tract consists of the kidneys, ureters, urinary bladder, urethra and external genitalia. The kidneys are responsible for regulation of fluid and electrolyte homeostasis. The kidneys also have a major role in acid–base balance, regulation of blood pressure, excretion of toxins (such as urea, creatinine and drugs), production of erythropoietin and synthesis of vitamin D.[2] Urine is transported by the ureters to the bladder for storage and then drained from the bladder by the urethra. Figure 25.1 shows structures of the GU system. Male external structures of the GU system have reproductive functions.

KIDNEYS

The kidneys are located behind the peritoneum on either side of the vertebral column in the abdomen. The kidney is shown in cross-section in Fig. 25.2. The *hilum*, medial aspect of the kidney, is where the renal artery and nerve enter and the renal vein and ureter exit. The hilum opens into the *renal pelvis*, an enlargement of the urinary channel. Renal calyces open into the renal pelvis. Each kidney contains 20 minor calyces that open into 2–3 major calyces. The kidney has an outer *cortex* and an inner layer or *medulla*. Cone- or triangular-shaped structures called *medullary pyramids* located in the renal medulla open into a minor calyx. The cortex surrounds the medulla and extends between pyramids in columns to the renal pelvis. The *renal artery* is a branch off the abdominal aorta that enters the kidney through the renal sinus to supply blood. The *renal vein* then empties blood into the abdominal inferior vena cava.

FIGURE 25.1 ORGANS OF THE URINARY SYSTEM[3]

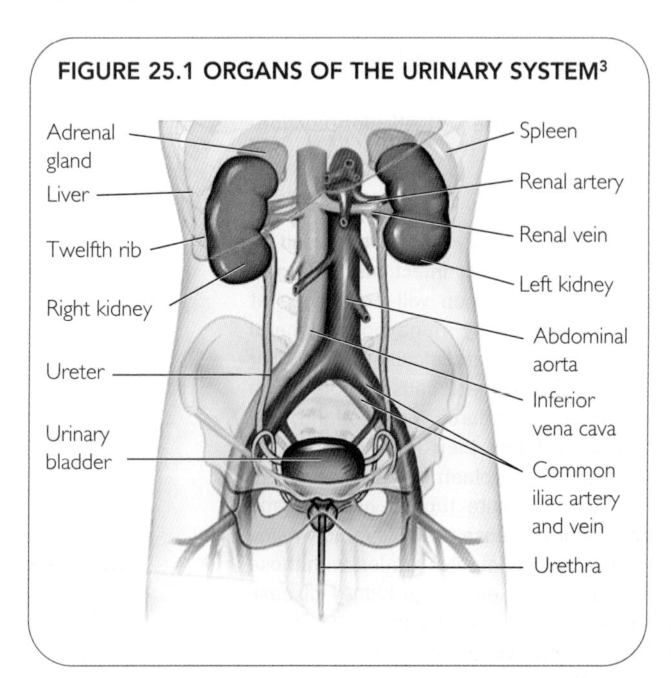

FIGURE 25.2 KIDNEY STRUCTURE[3]

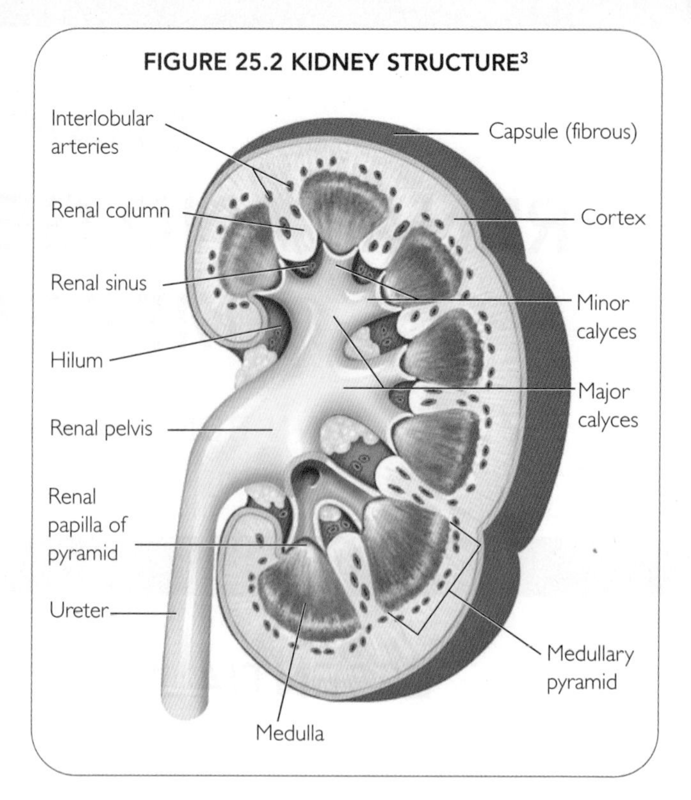

NEPHRON

The functional unit of the kidney is the *nephron*, and it comprises the renal corpuscle, proximal convoluted tubule, loop of Henle, distal convoluted tubule and collecting ducts (Fig. 25.3). There are an estimated 1,000,000 nephrons in each kidney, which are individually capable of producing urine through the processes of filtration, reabsorption, secretion and excretion. Nephrons cannot be reproduced once destroyed. The *glomerulus* is in the renal corpuscle and is a web of tightly convoluted capillaries. Surrounding and supporting the glomerulus is *Bowman's capsule*. Blood enters the glomerulus through the afferent arteriole and then out through the efferent arteriole. Each minute approximately 1–1.5 L of blood (25% of cardiac output) is passed through the glomeruli, where ultrafiltration takes place.[4,5]

In 15% of nephrons, at the point where the afferent arteriole enters the glomerulus there is a group of specialised cells called juxtaglomerular cells. Juxtaglomerular cells form a cuff and combine with the macula densa, a portion of the distal convoluted tubule that lies adjacent to the renal corpuscle between the afferent and efferent arterioles.[4,5] Together, the juxtaglomerular cells and the macula densa form the juxtaglomerular apparatus, which senses changes in either or both sodium concentration or blood pressure which then initiates the renin–angiotensin–aldosterone (RAA) system. Juxtaglomerular nephrons have a greater capacity to concentrate urine because they have longer loops of Henle, which extend into the medulla.

The first step in urine production involves filtration of plasma in the renal corpuscle. Pressure is generated as blood moves through the tight web of capillaries in the glomerulus,

FIGURE 25.3 COMPONENTS OF THE NEPHRON[3]

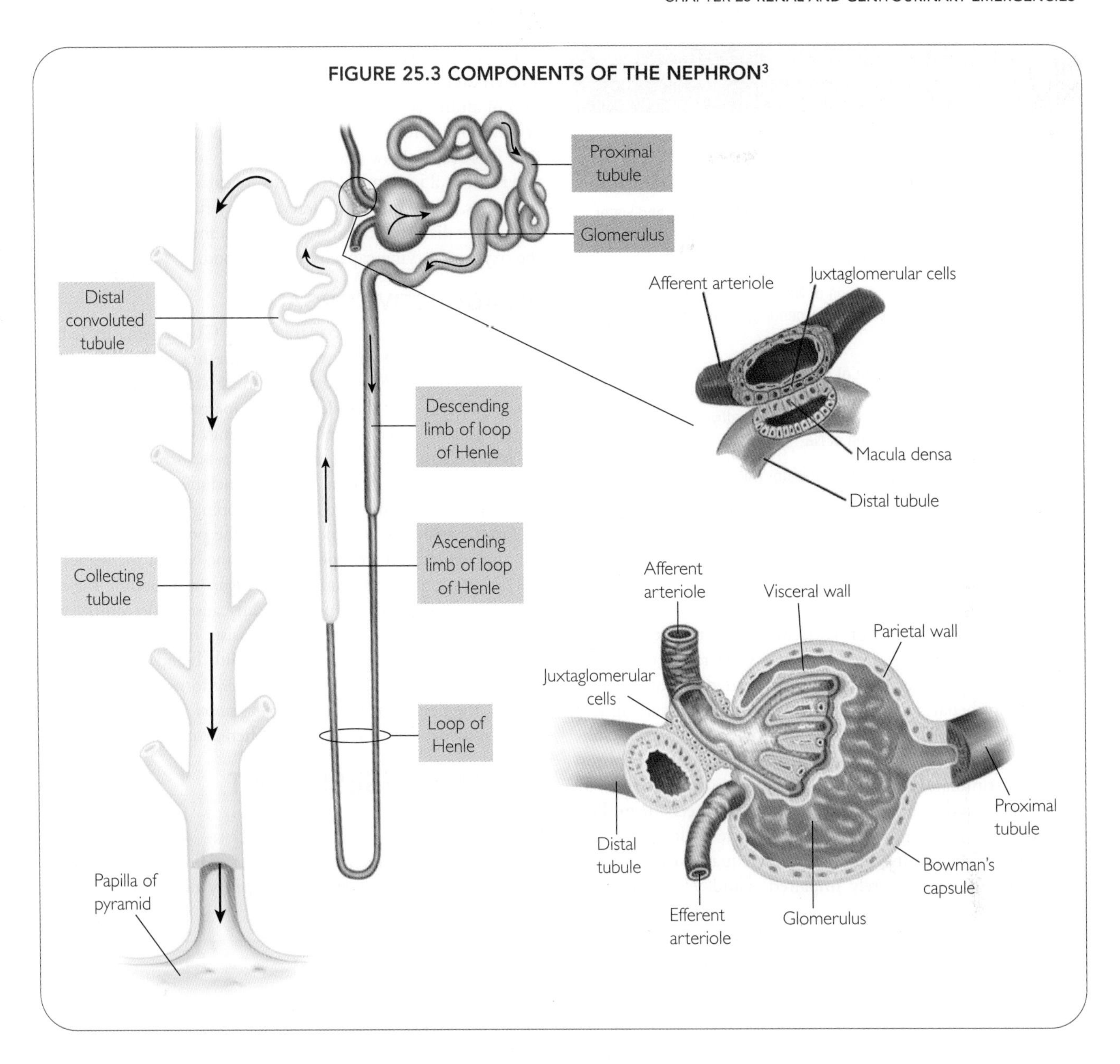

and oncotic pressure within the blood creates a greater pressure than the pressure exerted by Bowman's capsules. Thus the pressure enables plasma (termed filtrate) and small solutes to cross the semipermeable capillary lining. When the glomerulus is damaged, usually by ischaemia or inflammation, there is an increase in the permeability of the capillary membrane and this allows larger molecules (red blood cells [RBCs], epithelial casts, protein or white blood cells [WBCs]) to cross into the filtrate. Decreased oncotic pressure, often due to decreased serum albumin levels or decreased pressure within the glomerulus due to systemic hypotension, decreases glomerular filtration rate (GFR) and this in turn eventually lowers urine output. GFR in the average adult is 125 mL/min or 180 L/day.[4,5] The functions of the segments of the nephron are summarised in Table 25.1.

Tubules, loops of Henle and collecting ducts function to excrete waste products (e.g. urea, nitrogen, creatinine, drug metabolites), reabsorb water and solutes (potassium, sodium, chloride, hydrogen, glucose, amino acids) and secrete excess solutes the body doesn't need into filtrate.[4,5] Osmosis, diffusion and active transport occur between the nephron and surrounding capillaries. Hormonal control regulates reabsorption and secretion in the nephron. In comparison to nephrons, tubular cells have the capacity to regenerate following ischaemia (e.g. acute tubular necrosis).

RENIN–ANGIOTENSIN–ALDOSTERONE MECHANISM

Feedback loop systems in the body activate or switch off the renin–angiotensin–aldosterone system (RAA) (Fig. 25.4) and antidiuretic hormone (ADH) within the body, so that homeostasis is maintained. Increase in serum osmolarity causes stimulation of the hypothalamus, which releases ADH. Nephron permeability increases, so additional water is reabsorbed, causing serum osmolarity to return to normal, and then ADH release ceases.[4,5] A process of *autoregulation* controls pressure changes in the glomerulus through vasodilation and constriction of the afferent

TABLE 25.1 FUNCTIONS OF NEPHRON SEGMENTS[6]

COMPONENT	FUNCTION
Glomerulus	Selective filtration
Proximal tubule	Reabsorption of 80% of electrolytes and water, glucose, amino acids, HCO_3^-. Secretion of H^+ and creatinine
Loop of Henle	Reabsorption of Na^+ and Cl^- in ascending limb and water in descending loop. Concentration of filtrate
Distal tubule	Secretion of K^+, H^+, ammonia. Reabsorption of water (regulated by ADH) and HCO_3^-. Regulation of Ca_2^+ and PO_4^{3-} by parathyroid hormone. Regulation of Na^+ and K^+ by aldosterone
Collecting duct	Reabsorption of water (ADH required)

ADH: antidiuretic hormone; Ca^{2+} calcium; Cl^-: chloride; H^+: hydrogen; HCO_3^-: bicarbonate; K^+: potassium; Na^+: sodium; PO_4^{3-}: phosphate.

arteriole. This autoregulation is needed to protect renal blood flow and preserve GFR, even within a wide range of systolic blood pressures. When the range is exceeded, autoregulation fails and epithelial damage occurs, with eventual scarring and sclerosis, followed by decreased glomerulus permeability, resulting in lowered GFR and urine output. Inadequate nephron perfusion stimulates the reabsorption of sodium and water by the nephron under the influence of the RAA mechanism. Perfusion to the nephron increases and the cycle is altered.

Without functioning kidneys and adequate urine production, homeostasis is severely impaired. Fluid, electrolyte and acid–base imbalance, accumulation of urea and creatinine, decreased excretion of drug metabolites and inadequate reabsorption of amino acids and glucose occur. The kidneys also secrete erythropoietin for stimulation of red blood cell (RBC) production in bone marrow and help convert vitamin D into the active form (1,25-vitamin D_3) to ensure calcium absorption from intestines. Consequently, altered kidney function causes severe electrolyte disturbances and decreases bone mineralisation and the oxygen-carrying capacity of the blood.

REPRODUCTIVE ORGANS

External genitalia are also part of the GU system. In female genitalia, the space into which the urethra and vagina open comprises the *vestibule* and surrounding *labia minora* and *majora* (Fig. 25.5). The short length and anatomical location of the female urethra explains the high frequency of UTIs in females.

Male external genitalia include the *penis*, *scrotum* and *scrotal contents* (Fig. 25.6). Scrotal contents include the *testes*, tubules that secrete testosterone and carry developing sperm cells, and the *epididymis*, which is positioned along the posterior testes and is the final maturation area for sperm. At the base of the bladder is the *prostate*, a glandular and muscle organ surrounding the urethra. Enlargement of the prostate can cause outlet obstruction and urinary retention. The penis consists of three columns of erectile tissue that become engorged with blood, producing an erection (Fig. 25.7). The *corpora cavernosa* form the dorsum and sides of the penis and the *corpus spongiosum* forms the base and glans. In men, external genitalia are often involved in GU disease.

PATIENT ASSESSMENT

HISTORY

General health assessment of the GU system should determine history of diabetes, hypertension, history of renal calculi and

FIGURE 25.4 RENIN–ANGIOTENSIN–ALDOSTERONE SYSTEM[7]

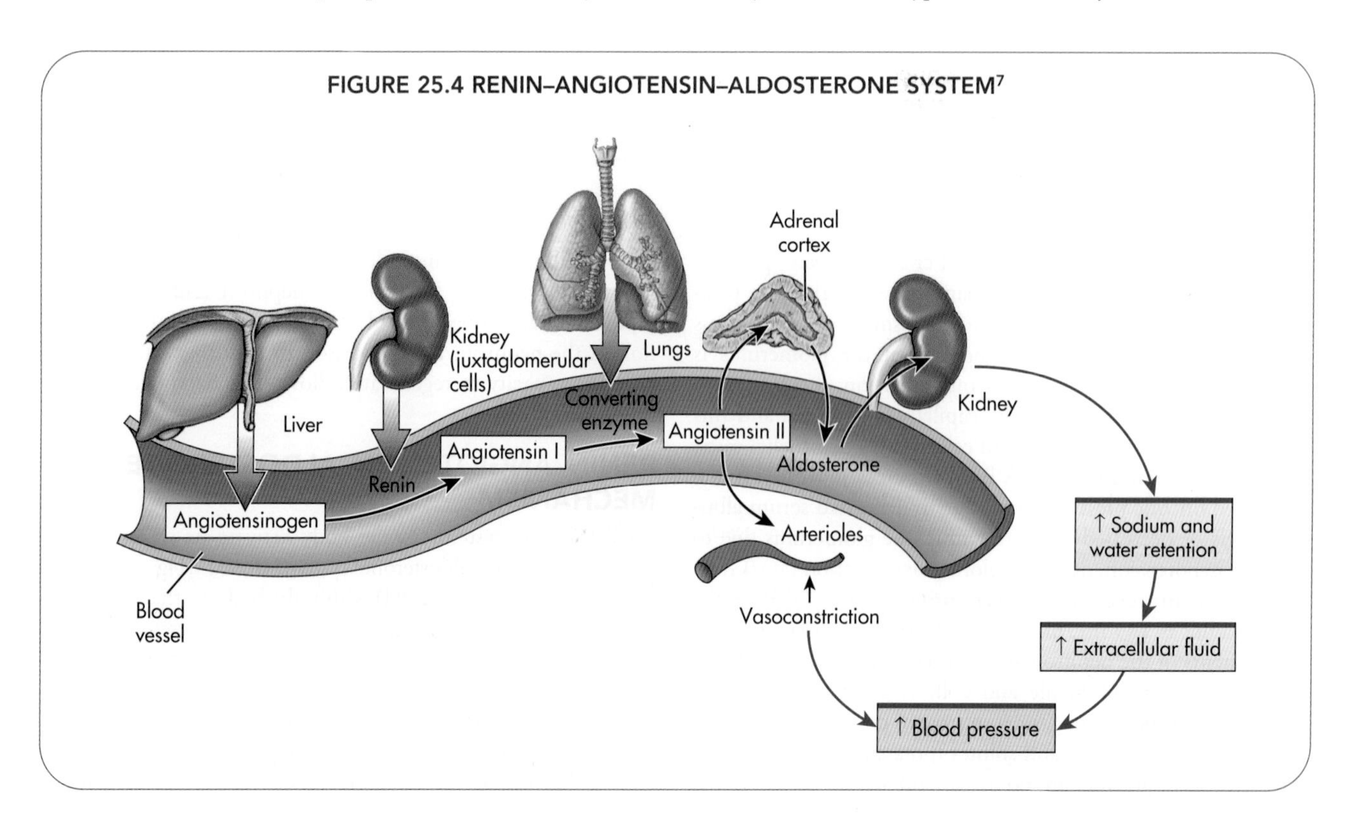

FIGURE 25.5 EXTERNAL FEMALE GENITALIA[8]

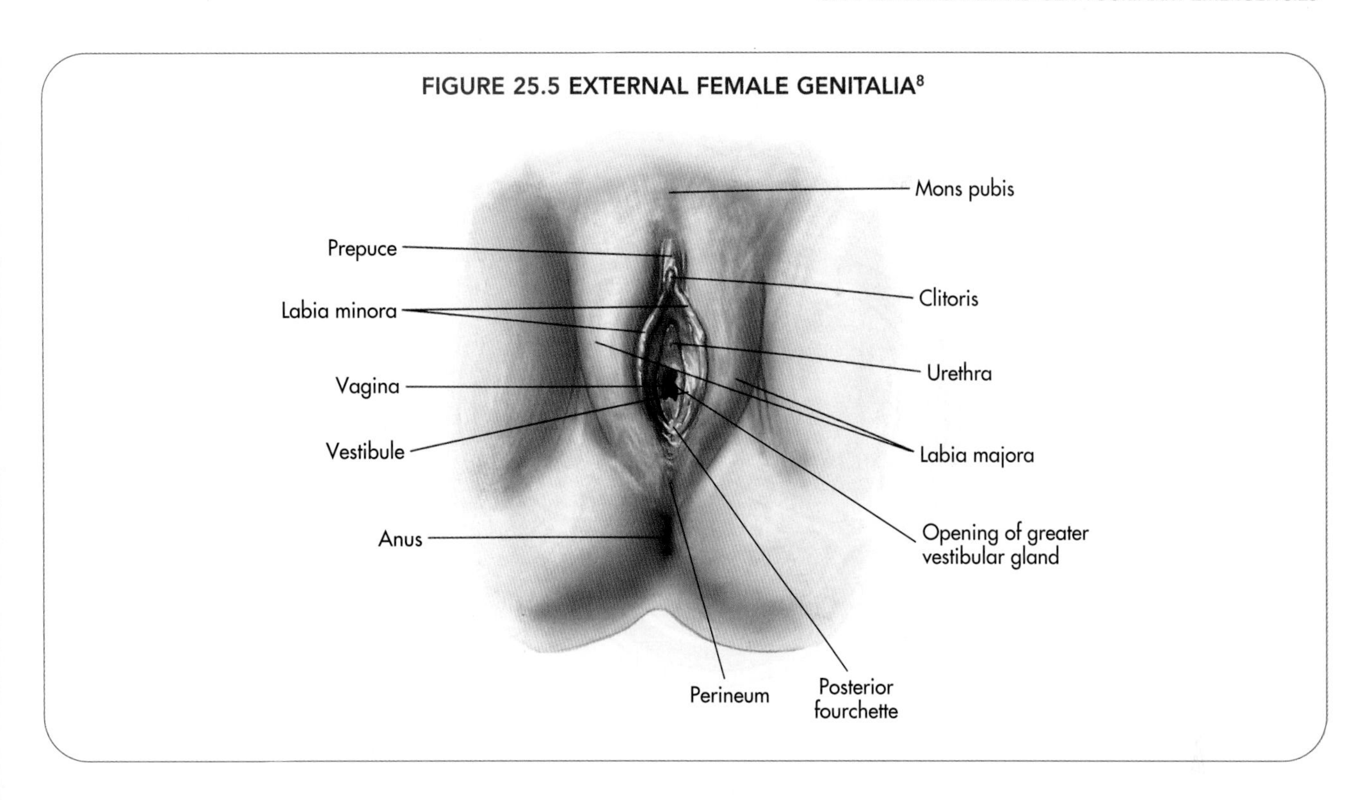

FIGURE 25.6 EXTERNAL AND INTERNAL MALE SEX ORGANS[9]

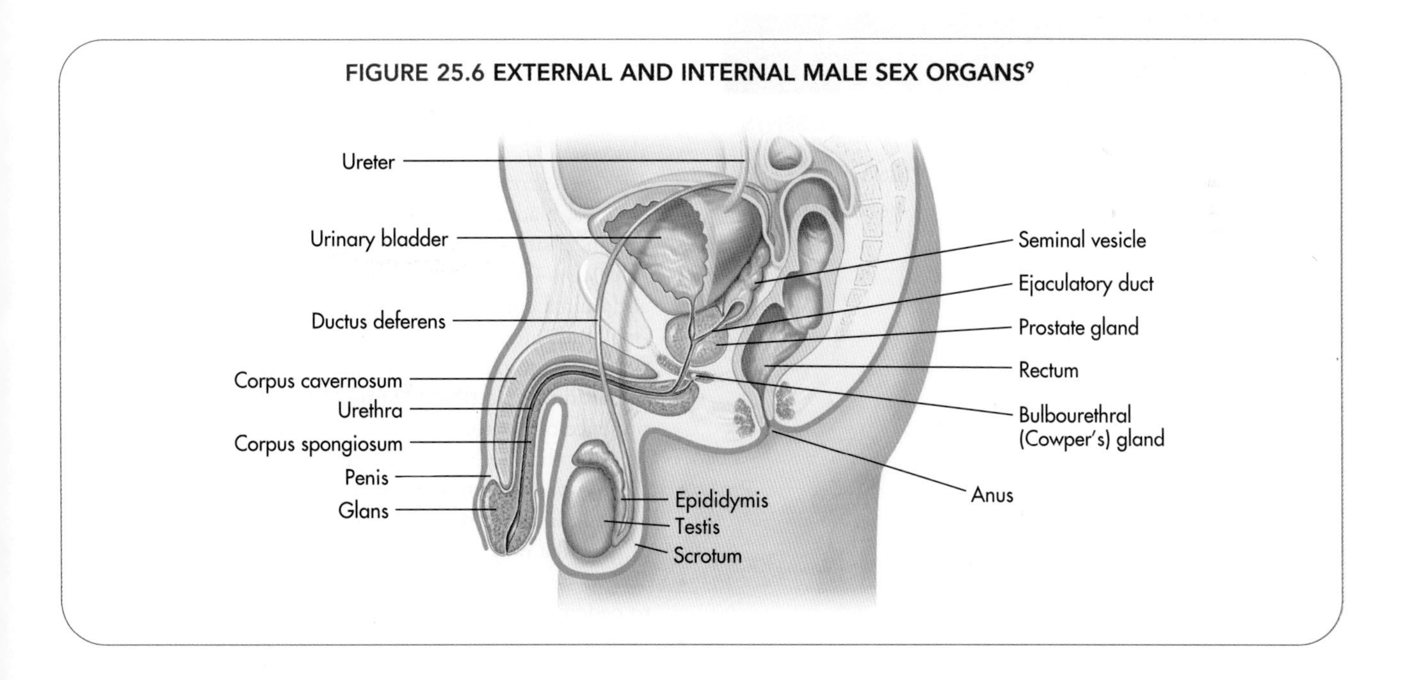

recurrent UTIs, prostatitis, urethritis, bladder or urethral damage during childbirth.[4,11] A comprehensive medication list, including prescription, over-the-counter (OTC) and illicit drugs, should be obtained. Recent medical and surgical history is also important, such as urethral instrumentation (catheterisation) or other urological procedures (e.g. transurethral resection of prostate [TURP], uterine prolapse repair [colpopexy]). Identification of any history of exposure to chemicals or toxins, including recent intravenous contrast media (e.g. for CT or angiography) or those encountered in the workplace, may identify contact with substances that could cause nephrotoxicity (Table 25.2). Sexual history should identify risk factors that can cause GU symptoms (e.g. use of contraceptive jellies or creams, multiple partners, abnormal penile or vaginal discharges, unsafe sexual practices, history of sexually transmitted infections [STIs]). Changes in urinary patterns, such as frequency, dysuria, urgency, dribbling, nocturia or incontinence may indicate GU problems. In a patient currently receiving kidney replacement therapy (i.e. haemodialysis, peritoneal dialysis or functioning kidney transplant), additional renal-specific history should be obtained.

FIGURE 25.7 CROSS-SECTION OF PENIS[10]

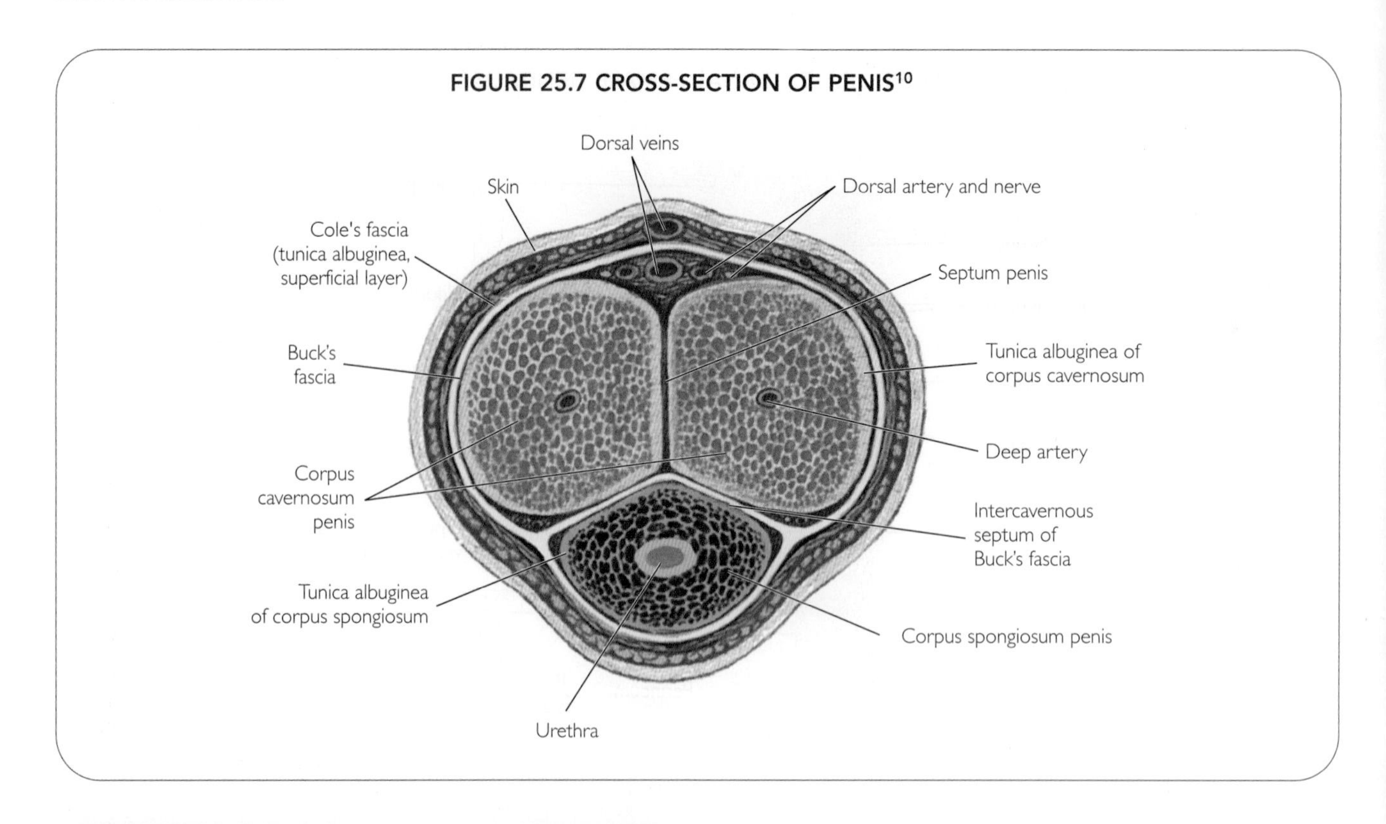

TABLE 25.2 POTENTIALLY NEPHROTOXIC AGENTS[6]

ANTIBIOTICS	OTHER DRUGS	OTHER AGENTS
Amphotericin B	Captopril	Gold
Cephalosporins	Cimetidine	Heavy metals
Gentamicin	Cisplatin	
Neomycin	Cocaine	
Polymyxin B	Cyclosporin	
Streptomycin	Ethylene glycol	
Sulfonamides	Heroin	
Tobramycin	Lithium	
Vancomycin	Methotrexate	
	Nitrosoureas (e.g. carmustine)	
	Non-steroidal anti-inflammatory drugs (e.g. ibuprofen, indomethacin)	
	Phenacetin	
	Quinine	
	Rifampicin	
	Salicylates (large quantities)	

PHYSICAL ASSESSMENT

INSPECTION

Inspection of the patient with renal or urological dysfunction may reveal characteristic changes.[4]

- *Skin*—pallor, yellow-grey, excoriations, changes in turgor, bruising (particularly thorax, abdomen and flank have the potential for injury to the renal and genitourinary system), texture (e.g. rough, dry skin), capillary refill time.
- *Mouth and throat*—stomatitis, ammonia breath odour, inflammation, state of dentition or presence of peritonsillar abscess.
- *Face and extremities*—generalised oedema, peripheral oedema, bladder distension, masses, enlarged kidneys, presence, site and type of vascular access for dialysis.
- *Abdomen*—skin changes described earlier, as well as striae, abdominal contour for midline mass in lower abdomen (may indicate urinary retention) or unilateral mass (occasionally seen in adult, indicating enlargement of one or both kidneys from large tumour or polycystic kidney), presence of peritoneal dialysis catheter exit site and whether the site is inflamed, leaking or encrusted.
- *Genitourinary*—presence of blood at the urinary meatus is a strong indication of trauma to the urethra; visualisation of genitalia may reveal injuries.
- *Weight*—current and ideal weight, weight gain secondary to oedema; weight loss and muscle wasting in renal failure.
- *General state of health*—fatigue, lethargy and diminished alertness.

PALPATION

As the kidneys are posterior organs protected by the abdominal organs, the ribs and the heavy back muscles, it is rare to palpate a normal-sized left kidney. Occasionally the lower pole of the right kidney is palpable. A landmark useful in locating the kidneys is the costovertebral angle (CVA) formed by the rib cage and the vertebral column.[5]

To palpate the right kidney, the examiner's left hand is placed behind and supports the patient's right side between the rib cage and the iliac crest (Fig. 25.8). The right flank is elevated with the left hand, and the right hand is used to palpate

FIGURE 25.8 PALPATING THE RIGHT KIDNEY[3]

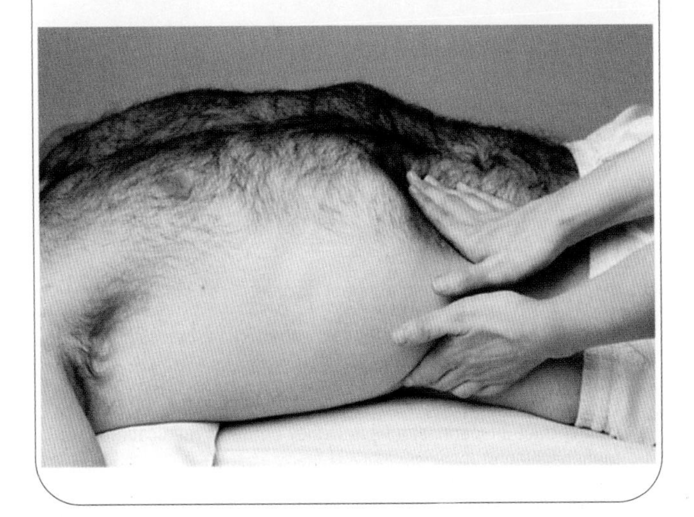

deeply for the right kidney. The lower pole of the right kidney may be felt as a smooth, rounded mass that descends on inspiration. If the kidney is palpable, its size, contour and tenderness should be noted. Kidney enlargement is suggestive of neoplasm or other serious renal pathological conditions. The urinary bladder is normally not palpable unless it is distended with urine. If the bladder is full, it may be felt as a smooth, round, firm organ and is sensitive to palpation.

PERCUSSION

Percussion is used to determine tenderness in the flank area. This technique is performed by striking the fist of one hand against the dorsal surface of the other hand (kidney punch), which is placed flat along the posterior CVA margin.[5] Normally a firm blow in the flank area should not elicit pain. If CVA tenderness and pain are present, it may indicate a kidney infection or polycystic kidney disease.

AUSCULTATION

The diaphragm of the stethoscope may be used to auscultate over both CVAs and in the upper abdominal quadrants. With this technique, the abdominal aorta and renal arteries are auscultated for a bruit (an abnormal murmur), which indicates impaired blood flow to the kidneys.[5] Arteriovenous fistula and grafts should also be auscultated with a stethoscope to determine the presence of a bruit which indicates the vascular access is patent. See Chapter 16 for further information and vascular access techniques. Bladder ultrasound, if available, can be used to verify urine volume and ability to empty bladder.

Table 25.3 presents clinical manifestations of disorders of the urinary system and Table 25.4 presents common assessment abnormalities.

URINALYSIS

In evaluating disorders of the urinary tract, one of the first studies done is a urinalysis (Table 25.5). This test may provide information about possible abnormalities, indicate what further studies need to be done and supply information on the progression of a diagnosed disorder. For a routine urinalysis, a specimen may be collected at any time of the day. The specimen should be examined within 1 hour of urinating. If it is not, bacteria multiply rapidly, RBCs haemolyse, casts (moulds of renal tubules) disintegrate and the urine becomes alkaline as a result of urea-splitting bacteria. If it is not possible to send the specimen to the laboratory immediately, it should be refrigerated. The results of a urinalysis usually include a description of the appearance, specific gravity (mass and density), pH, glucose, ketones, blood, protein and leucocytes in the urine and a microscopic examination of urine sediment for WBCs, RBCs, crystals and casts (Table 25.5). It is preferable to avoid an invasive procedure such as urinary catheterisation to collect a urine specimen for routine urinalysis.

If the urinalysis indicates a likelihood of infection, a reliable method to collect a mid-stream urine sample is required. In patients with severe cognitive impairments or non-toilet-trained children[5] insertion of a urethral catheter (e.g. in/out catheter) will enable a non-contaminated urine specimen to be collected.

TABLE 25.3 SIGNS AND SYMPTOMS OF URINARY SYSTEM DISORDERS[8]

GENERAL SIGNS AND SYMPTOMS	OEDEMA	PAIN	PATTERNS OF URINATION	URINE OUTPUT	URINE COMPOSITION
Fatigue	Facial (periorbital)	Dysuria	Frequency	Anuria	Concentrated
Headaches	Ankle	Flank or costovertebral angle	Urgency	Oliguria	Dilute
Blurred vision	Ascites	Groin	Hesitancy of stream	Polyuria	Haematuria
Elevated blood pressure	Anasarca	Suprapubic	Change in stream		Pyuria
Anorexia	Sacral		Retention		Colour (red, brown, yellowish green)
Nausea and vomiting			Dysuria		
Chills			Nocturia		
Itching			Incontinence		
Excessive thirst			Stress incontinence		
Change in bodyweight			Dribbling		
Cognitive changes					

TABLE 25.4 COMMON ASSESSMENT ABNORMALITIES OF THE URINARY SYSTEM[6]

FINDING	DESCRIPTION	POSSIBLE AETIOLOGY AND SIGNIFICANCE
Anuria	Technically no urination (24-hour urine output < 100 mL)	Acute kidney injury, kidney failure (end-stage kidney disease), bilateral ureteral obstruction
Burning on urination	Stinging pain in urethral area	Urethral irritation, urinary tract infection
Dysuria	Painful or difficult urination	Sign of urinary tract infection, interstitial cystitis, and wide variety of pathological conditions
Enuresis	Involuntary nocturnal urination	Symptomatic of lower urinary tract disorder
Frequency	Increased incidence of urination	Acutely inflamed bladder, retention with overflow, excess fluid intake, intake of bladder irritants
Haematuria	Blood in the urine	Cancer of genitourinary tract, blood dyscrasias, kidney disease, urinary tract infection, stones in kidney or ureter, medications (anticoagulants)
Hesitancy	Delay or difficulty in initiating urination	Partial urethral obstruction, benign prostatic hyperplasia
Incontinence	Inability to voluntarily control discharge of urine	Neurogenic bladder, bladder infection, injury to external sphincter
Nocturia	Frequency of urination at night	Kidney disease with impaired concentrating ability, bladder obstruction, heart failure, diabetes mellitus, finding after renal transplant, excessive evening and night-time fluid intake
Oliguria	Diminished amount of urine in a given time (24-hour urine output of 100–400 mL)	Severe dehydration, shock, transfusion reaction, kidney disease, kidney failure
Pain	Suprapubic pain (related to bladder), urethral pain (irritation of bladder neck), flank (CVA) pain	Infection, urinary retention, foreign body in urinary tract, urethritis, pyelonephritis, renal colic or stones
Pneumaturia	Passage of urine containing gas	Fistula connections between bowel and bladder, gas-forming urinary tract infections
Polyuria	Large volume of urine in a given time	Diabetes mellitus, diabetes insipidus, chronic kidney disease, diuretics, excess fluid intake, obstructive sleep apnoea
Retention	Inability to urinate even though bladder contains excessive amount of urine	Finding after pelvic surgery, childbirth, catheter removal, anaesthesia; urethral stricture or obstruction; neurogenic bladder
Stress incontinence	Involuntary urination with increased pressure (sneezing or coughing)	Weakness of sphincter control, lack of oestrogen, urinary retention

CVA: costovertebral angle.

HAEMATURIA

The presence of blood in the urine, haematuria, may be the primary problem or may be associated with other symptoms,[12] and is an indication of a serious underlying disease. Macroscopic haematuria is the hallmark of GU trauma and is also commonly associated with urological cancer, benign prostatic hypertrophy, glomerulonephritis, infection or renal calculi. Microscopic haematuria is found during urinalysis. Bleeding at the start of urination suggests urethral problems, haematuria during urination indicates upper GU tract bleeding, and bleeding at the end of the void suggests bladder neck or urethral bleeding. Most patients with haematuria will need to be admitted for further investigation. If the urine is discoloured, a detailed medication and diet history may uncover other causes. Box 25.1 highlights possible causes of red or dark-red urine.

Presence of gross blood at the urethral meatus strongly suggests urethral injury, generally associated with pelvic fractures (see Chapter 48 for further details). An indwelling urinary catheter (IDC) should not be inserted without first doing a retrograde urethrogram to ensure urethral integrity, or consulting with senior medical/urology clinicians.[13] If required, a suprapubic catheter will be inserted in the ED. In non-traumatic situations, patients with haematuria will need an IDC inserted. Where possible, determine from the patient the colour of the urine and the presence of clots.

PRACTICE TIP

Thick bloody urine with clots frequently requires a 22–28 F three-way IDC which enables the bladder to be continually washed and irrigated to prevent clot retention.

TABLE 25.5 URINALYSIS FINDINGS[6]

TEST	NORMAL	ABNORMAL FINDING	POSSIBLE AETIOLOGY AND SIGNIFICANCE
Colour	Amber yellow	Dark, smoky colour	Haematuria
		Yellow-brown to olive green	Excessive bilirubin
		Orange-red or orange-brown	Phenazopyridine
		Cloudiness of freshly voided urine	Infection
		Colourless urine	Excessive fluid intake, kidney disease or diabetes insipidus
Odour	Aromatic	Ammonia-like odour	Urine allowed to stand
		Unpleasant odour	Urinary tract infection
Protein	Random protein (dipstick): 0–trace	Persistent proteinuria	Characteristic of acute and chronic kidney disease, especially involving glomeruli. Heart failure
	24-hour protein (quantitative): < 150 mg/day		In absence of disease: high-protein diet, strenuous exercise, dehydration, fever, emotional stress, contamination by vaginal secretions
Glucose	None	Glycosuria	Diabetes mellitus, low renal threshold for glucose reabsorption (if blood glucose level is normal). Pituitary disorders
Ketones	None	Present	Altered carbohydrate and fat metabolism in diabetes mellitus and starvation; dehydration, vomiting, severe diarrhoea
Bilirubin	None	Present	Liver disorders May appear before jaundice is visible (see Chapter 24)
Specific gravity	1.003–1.030	Low	Dilute urine, excessive diuresis, diabetes insipidus
	Maximum concentrating ability of kidney in morning urine (1.025–1.030)	High	Dehydration, albuminuria, glycosuria
		Fixed at about 1.010	Renal inability to concentrate urine; end-stage kidney disease
Osmolality	300–1300 mOsm/kg (300–1300 mmol/kg)	< 300 mOsm/kg > 1300 mOsm/kg	Tubular dysfunction. Kidney lost ability to concentrate or dilute urine (not part of routine urinalysis)
pH	4.0–8.0 (average, 6.0)	> 8.0	UTI. Urine allowed to stand at room temperature (bacteria decompose urea to ammonia)
		< 4.0	Respiratory or metabolic acidosis
RBCs	0–4/hpf	> 4/hpf	Calculi, cystitis, neoplasm, glomerulonephritis, tuberculosis, kidney biopsy, trauma
WBCs	0–5/hpf	> 5/hpf	UTI or inflammation
Casts	None Occasional hyaline	Present	Moulds of the renal tubules that may contain protein, WBCs, RBCs or bacteria. Non-cellular casts (hyaline in appearance) occasionally found in normal urine
Culture for organisms	No organisms in bladder $< 10^4$ organisms/mL result of normal urethral flora	Bacteria counts $> 10^5$/mL	UTI; most common organisms are Escherichia coli, enterococci, Klebsiella, Proteus and streptococci

hpf: high-powered field; UTI: urinary tract infection.

PAIN

Pain should be assessed using the PQRST mnemonic—**P**rovocation, **Q**uality, **R**egion or radiation, **S**everity and **T**iming (see Chapter 18 for further details).

Renal colic caused by calculi (nephrolithiasis) causes the most severe pain associated with the GU system. Sudden, unbearable pain is due to an increased pressure and dilation of the kidney and upper urinary collecting system. The patient usually presents with restlessness and pallor, and complains of severe flank pain that often radiates to the abdomen and groin, often termed *loin-to-groin pain*.[14] If the stone is in the bladder, urinary frequency and urgency develop. Pain can cause

BOX 25.1 NON-HAEMATURIA CAUSES OF ABNORMAL COLOUR CHANGES IN URINE

FOOD	DRUGS	PATHOLOGICAL CONDITIONS
Beetroot (red)	Adriamycin (red)	Chyluria (white milky)
Rhubarb (red)	Aminosalicylic acid (red)	Jaundice (yellow to brown)
Blackberries (red)	Ibuprofen (red)	Myoglobinuria (red/brown/rust)
Food colouring (rhodamine B) (red)	Methyldopa (red)	Porphyrins (red to black)
Senna (yellow to brown, red)	Metronidazole (dark yellow)	Uric acid crystalluria (pink)
	Nitrofurantoin (brown)	
	Phenytoin (Dilantin) (red)	
	Rifampicin (red)	

tachypnoea, tachycardia and hypertension, although patients with these symptoms should not have other causes lightly excluded. Relief of renal colic requires substantial amounts of analgesia, as discussed later in the chapter.

OLIGURIA AND ANURIA

Presenting symptoms of urine output less than 400 mL in 24 hours is oliguria, or when urine output is less than 100 mL in 24 hours it is termed anuria.[15] Dehydration or obstruction are the usual causes of oliguria; anuria is more likely to be due to acute kidney injury or kidney failure. Serum biochemistries should be evaluated for elevated urea and creatinine (azotaemia), which indicates renal failure from prolonged urinary obstruction, leading to hydronephrosis or other causes. If the patient has a urinary catheter in situ, patency should be assessed. Acute urinary retention can be identified by palpating the bladder as a firm mass above the symphysis pubis, sometimes with an urge to void on palpation (more details later in this chapter).

SPECIFIC CONDITIONS

ACUTE KIDNEY INJURY

Acute kidney injury (AKI) is the rapid and sudden deterioration of kidney function resulting in impaired fluid and electrolyte balance, metabolic acidosis, and the retention of metabolic wastes (azotaemia).[15] It usually develops over hours or days and typically follows severe, prolonged hypotension or hypovolaemia or exposure to a nephrotoxic agent. In AKI there is an increase in serum creatinine and/or a reduction in urine output.[15] Unlike chronic kidney disease, AKI is potentially reversible if the precipitating factors can be removed or corrected before permanent kidney damage has occurred. Despite advances in kidney replacement therapies, AKI continues to have a mortality rate of approximately 80% in patients admitted to the intensive care unit.[15] The acronym RIFLE (**R**isk, **I**njury, **F**ailure, **L**oss and **E**nd-stage kidney disease) is used to classify the severity (R, I, F) and the outcome (L, E) (Table 25.6).[15] The causes

TABLE 25.6 RIFLE CRITERIA FOR STAGING ACUTE KIDNEY INJURY[8]

STAGE	GFR CRITERIA	URINE OUTPUT CRITERIA
Risk	Serum creatinine increased × 1.5 or GFR decreased by 25%	Urine output < 0.5 mL/kg/hr for 6 hr
Injury	Serum creatinine increased × 2 or GFR decreased by 50%	Urine output < 0.5 mL/kg/hr for 12 hr
Failure	Serum creatinine increased × 3 or GFR decreased by 75% or Serum creatinine > 4 mg/dL with acute rise ≥ 0.5 mg/dL	Urine output < 0.3 mL/kg/hr for 24 hr (oliguria) or Anuria for 12 hr
Loss	Persistent acute kidney failure; complete loss of kidney function > 4 wk	–
End-stage kidney disease	Complete loss of kidney function > 3 months	–

GFR: glomerular filtration rate; AKI: acute kidney injury.

**All serum creatinine references are based on changes from baseline.*

of AKI are commonly categorised as *prerenal* (55–60%), *intrarenal* (35–40%) and *postrenal* (< 5%).[15]

Prerenal

Prerenal causes are more commonly seen in the ED, as this form of AKI results from any external factors which cause a sudden and severe reduction in blood flow to the kidneys, and there is a subsequent reduction in glomerular perfusion and filtration rate.[16] The effective circulating volume of the blood can be lowered by hypovolaemia, decreased cardiac output, decreased peripheral vascular resistance and vascular obstruction. Oliguria occurs as the kidneys respond to the decreased blood flow by activating the RAA mechanism. This compensation by the kidneys results in sodium and water conservation. Decreased renal perfusion also decreases clearance of wastes (azotaemia). As decreased perfusion continues, the kidneys lose their ability to engage in compensatory mechanisms, and intrarenal damage to renal tissue occurs. The result is low urine output due to the kidneys' inability to excrete water, a rise in serum urea and creatinine proportional to each other (ratio of > 10 : 1), and the inability of the kidneys to conserve sodium (low spot urine sodium < 20 mmol/L). Prolonged hypotension and/or hypovolaemia will result in acute tubular necrosis (ATN). Causes of AKI, specific pathophysiology, general treatment, and diagnostic markers are listed in Box 25.2. Fig. 25.9 highlights clinical manifestations of AKI.

Intrarenal

Acute tubular necrosis (ATN) is a type of intrarenal AKI usually resulting from prolonged ischaemia, nephrotoxins (e.g. amino-glycoside antibiotics, contrast media—also called contrast-induced nephropathy [CIN]), haemoglobin released from haemolysed red blood cells (RBCs), myoglobin released from necrotic muscle cells or toxins released from severe sepsis.[11] Those at greatest risk of developing ATN include elderly people, patients who have diabetes or those with a history of CKD. Emergency clinicians should be alert to the potential for AKI in these patients, particularly if there has been recent exposure to contrast media or other nephrotoxins.[11] Ischaemic and nephrotoxic ATN are responsible for 90% of intrarenal AKI cases.[17] Primary renal diseases, such as acute glomerulonephritis and systemic lupus erythematosus, may also cause AKI.

ATN typically develops following prolonged ischaemia when perfusion to the kidney is considerably reduced, and in some patients ATN can eventuate after only a few hours of hypovolaemia or hypotension.[11] The renal protective mechanisms of autoregulation of renal blood vessels and activation of the RAA system are able to increase renal perfusion during the early stages of AKI. If, however, blood flow is reduced for longer than 1 hour, these protective mechanisms begin to weaken, triggering a variety of factors which result in the development of ATN.

BOX 25.2 COMMON CAUSES OF ACUTE KIDNEY INJURY[6]

PRE-RENAL	INTRA-RENAL	POST-RENAL
HYPOVOLAEMIA • Dehydration • Haemorrhage • GI losses (diarrhoea, vomiting) • Excessive diuresis • Hypoalbuminaemia • Burns **DECREASED CARDIAC OUTPUT** • Cardiac dysrhythmias • Cardiogenic shock • Heart failure • Myocardial infarction **DECREASED PERIPHERAL VASCULAR RESISTANCE** • Anaphylaxis • Neurological injury • Septic shock **DECREASED RENOVASCULAR BLOOD FLOW** • Bilateral renal vein thrombosis • Embolism • Hepatorenal syndrome • Renal artery thrombosis	**NEPHROTOXIC INJURY** • Drugs: aminoglycosides (gentamicin), amphotericin B • Contrast media • Haemolytic blood transfusion reaction • Severe crush injury • Chemical exposure: ethylene glycol, lead, arsenic, carbon tetrachloride **INTERSTITIAL NEPHRITIS** • Allergies: antibiotics (sulfonamides, rifampicin), non-steroidal anti-inflammatory drugs, ACE inhibitors • Infections: bacterial (acute pyelonephritis), viral (CMV), fungal (candidiasis) **OTHER CAUSES** • Prolonged pre-renal ischaemia • Acute glomerulonephritis • Thrombotic disorders • Toxaemia of pregnancy • Malignant hypertension • Systemic lupus erythematosus	Benign prostatic hyperplasia Bladder cancer Calculi formation Neuromuscular disorders Prostate cancer Spinal cord disease Strictures Trauma (back, pelvis, perineum)

ACE: angiotensin-converting enzyme; CMV: cytomegalovirus; GI: gastrointestinal.

FIGURE 25.9 MANIFESTIONS OF ACUTE KIDNEY INJURY[18]

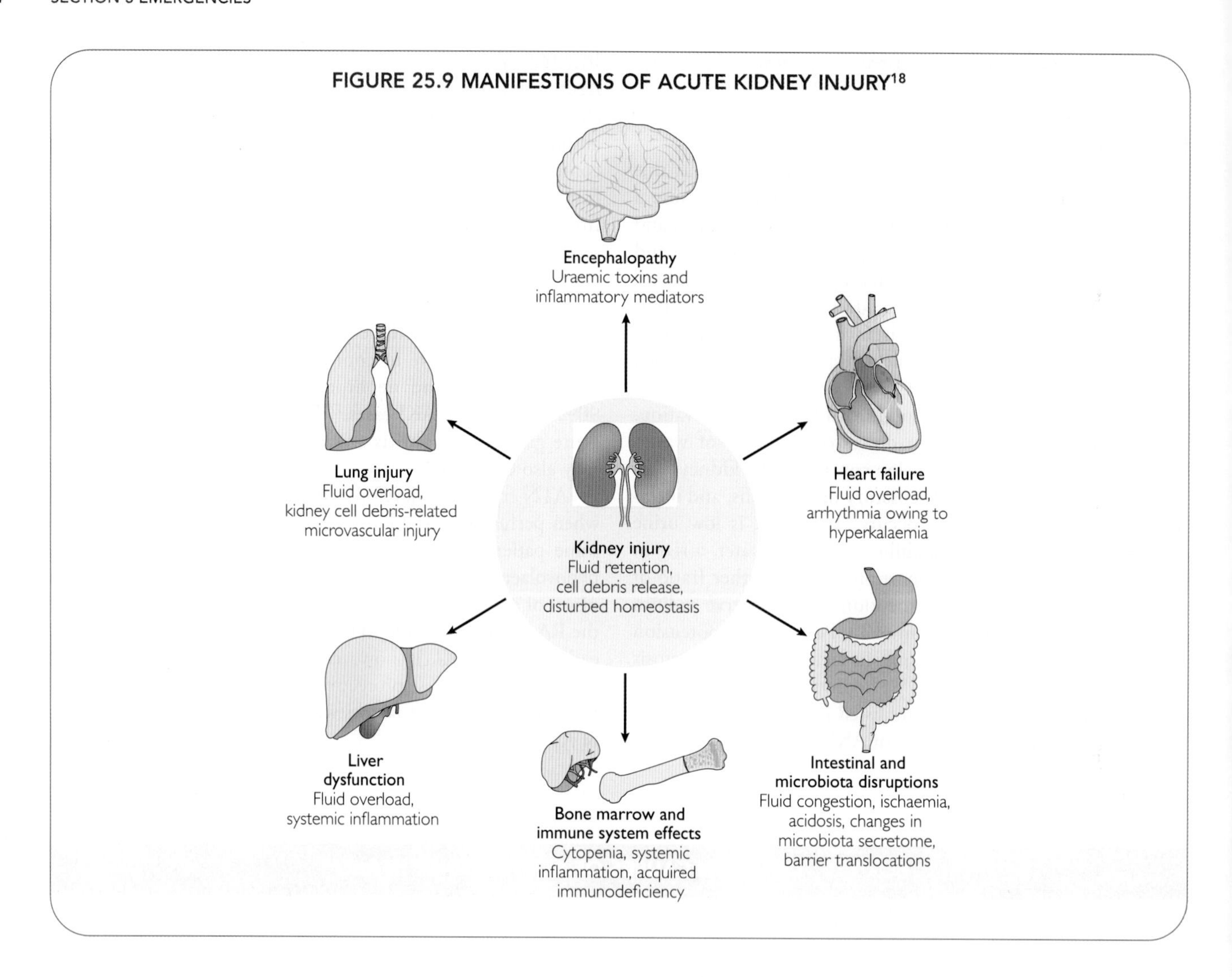

Postrenal

Postrenal AKI results from an obstruction of urine outflow from the kidneys. The obstruction can occur in the kidneys (e.g. renal cell carcinoma), ureter (e.g. renal calculi), bladder (e.g. cancer) or urethra (e.g. prostatic hypertrophy). Prostatic hypertrophy is the most common underlying problem. Urinary tract obstruction causes an increase in pressure proximal to the obstruction which often leads to dilation of the proximal collecting system (i.e. hydroureter and hydronephrosis). The elevated pressure in the collecting system is transmitted back into the tubular network and eventually stops glomerular filtration. Postrenal AKI is a urological emergency that requires immediate relief of the obstruction and decompression of the urinary system, otherwise permanent renal damage can occur.

Management of acute kidney injury

AKI is potentially reversible if the basement membrane of the glomerulus is not destroyed and the tubular epithelium regenerates. Prerenal and postrenal AKI resolve relatively easily when they are identified early and treatment is commenced quickly.[15] Intrarenal failure and ATN have a prolonged course of recovery because actual parenchymal damage has occurred. Clinically, AKI usually progresses through four phases: initiating, oliguric, diuretic and recovery. In some situations, the patient does not recover from AKI and chronic kidney disease results.

The primary goals of treatment are to eliminate the cause, manage the signs and symptoms and prevent complications while the kidneys recover.[15]

PRACTICE TIP

The first step is to determine if there is adequate intravascular volume and cardiac output to ensure adequate perfusion of the kidneys. Urine output may be decreased or increased. This can be assessed by bolus amounts of crystalloids. Diuretics (e.g. furosemide) are rarely used. It is crucial to monitor fluid status primarily through assessing jugular vein distension, vital signs (mean arterial pressure [MAP]) and urine output.

If AKI is already established, forcing fluids and/or administering intravenous diuretics will not be effective, and may in fact result in life-threatening fluid overload and pulmonary oedema. It is essential that paramedics accurately document and communicate fluids given, and the ED nurse commences and maintains an accurate fluid-balance chart, including fluids given pre-hospital.

Hyperkalaemia, hyponatraemia, hypocalcaemia, hyperphosphataemia, metabolic acidosis and hypervolaemia are the most common electrolyte and fluid imbalances resulting from loss of kidney function. Compromise of airway, breathing, circulation

BOX 25.3 TREATMENT ALTERNATIVES FOR ELEVATED POTASSIUM LEVELS[6]

REGULAR INSULIN IV

- Potassium moves into cells when insulin is given.
- IV glucose is given concurrently to prevent hypoglycaemia.
- When effects of insulin diminish, potassium shifts back out of cells.

SODIUM BICARBONATE

- Therapy can correct acidosis and cause a shift of potassium into cells.

CALCIUM GLUCONATE IV

- Generally used in advanced cardiac toxicity (with evidence of hyperkalaemia ECG changes).
- Calcium raises the threshold for excitation, resulting in dysrhythmias.

HAEMODIALYSIS

- Most effective therapy to remove potassium.
- Works within a short time.

SODIUM POLYSTYRENE SULFONATE

- Cation-exchange resin is administered by mouth or retention enema.
- When resin is in the bowel, potassium is exchanged for sodium.
- Therapy removes 1 mmol of potassium per gram of drug.
- It is mixed in water with sorbitol (or lactulose) to produce osmotic diarrhoea, allowing for evacuation of potassium-rich stool from body.

SALBUTAMOL

- Shifts potassium into the cells
- Administer via nebuliser

DIETARY RESTRICTION

- Potassium intake is limited to 40 mmol/day.
- Primarily used to prevent recurrent elevation; not used for acute elevation.

IV: intravenous.

and neurological function requires prompt intervention. Other symptoms may include nausea and vomiting, haematemesis, dysrhythmias, dyspnoea, short-term weight gain or loss, stupor or coma. Fever may be associated with infections or inflammatory events. Regular reassessment of vital signs is essential.

Hyperkalaemia is a medical emergency.[15] Tall peaked T waves, widened QRS and a prolonged P-R interval on ECG are secondary to hyperkalaemia. The various therapies used to treat elevated potassium levels are listed in Box 25.3. Both intravenous (IV) insulin and sodium bicarbonate shift potassium into the cells within 15–30 minutes, but it will eventually shift back out. IV calcium gluconate works within minutes by raising the action potential threshold at which dysrhythmias will occur, but of short duration, as evidenced by return of ECG changes. Nebulised salbutamol can be used as adjuvant therapy. Only sodium (or calcium) polystyrene sulfonate (e.g. Resonium) and dialysis actually remove potassium from the body. When administered rectally, sodium (or calcium) polystyrene sulfonate's onset of action is 60 minutes, with further delay in onset of action when administered orally (120 minutes).

After initial stabilisation, history and diagnostic testing focus on identifying the cause of AKI. Tests include serial blood chemistries, urinalysis with sodium and potassium concentrations, chest radiograph, renal ultrasounds and Doppler studies or computed tomography (CT) scan. Imaging procedures are usually done without contrast media because of toxic effects of the media on renal tubules. In patients with diabetes receiving metformin, there is a high risk of lactic acidosis if metformin has not been ceased for 48 hours. Acetylcysteine can also be used to prevent the nephrotoxic effects of contrast media in people at high risk of developing AKI, although this is controversial. If a patient requires the use of contrast media during imaging, adequate pre- and post-procedure hydration, particularly for those with diabetes and/or known chronic kidney disease, and close follow-up, are more effective in avoiding AKI.[19]

Emergency dialysis is required when stupor or coma (caused by rising serum urea), hypervolaemia and pulmonary oedema, dangerous hyperkalaemia and metabolic acidosis occur. Haemodialysis requires vascular access (usually via a temporary subclavian or femoral dual-lumen catheter) and an artificial kidney (dialyser) to act as a semipermeable membrane. The dialysate is on one side of the semipermeable membrane and blood is on the other; then the processes of diffusion and osmosis occur. A blood pump is required to move blood through the dialyser (Fig. 25.10). The ED nurse should be prepared to transfer the patient to the intensive care or dialysis unit, be familiar with transport equipment and have documented preceding events and communicated with the patient and their family.

Monitoring fluid volume status is the most important nursing and paramedic intervention of all patients at risk for the development of AKI or during the course of AKI.[15] Accurate measurements of blood pressure, pulse, bodyweight, urine output and jugular or central venous pressure, as well as assessment of lung fields, skin turgor, mucous membranes and presence of oedema, are all vital in determining the patient's fluid volume status. Monitoring the use, as well as careful administration, of potentially nephrotoxic agents is also an important clinician responsibility.

RHABDOMYOLYSIS

Rhabdomyolysis is due to destruction of skeletal muscle, which releases myoglobin into the circulatory system, and can then lead to AKI.[11] There are a number of different causes of rhabdomyolysis, including crush injuries, compartment syndrome, excessive physical exertion (e.g. long-distance running, working outdoors in the heat), muscle ischaemia (e.g. immobile or comatose person), drug or toxin ingestion, envenomation, infection, burns, temperature extremes or metabolic disturbances. Drugs, toxins and venoms are the largest causes of rhabdomyolysis. Those at risk of developing rhabdomyolysis due to excessive physical exertion can include military recruits and long-distance runners. See Chapter 48 for a detailed discussion of compartment syndrome and crush injuries.

When there is breakdown of muscle tissue and ensuing cell deterioration and death, there is a rapid release of myoglobin and potassium into the plasma circulation. Profound hypovolaemia is due to massive fluid shifts from the intravascular space into the interstitial space, and causes hypoperfusion of the kidneys, thereby decreasing the GFR. The electrolyte abnormalities seen in rhabdomyolysis include hyperkalaemia (which can be rapidly increasing), hypocalcaemia, hyperphosphataemia

FIGURE 25.10 COMPONENTS OF A HAEMODIALYSIS SYSTEM[6]

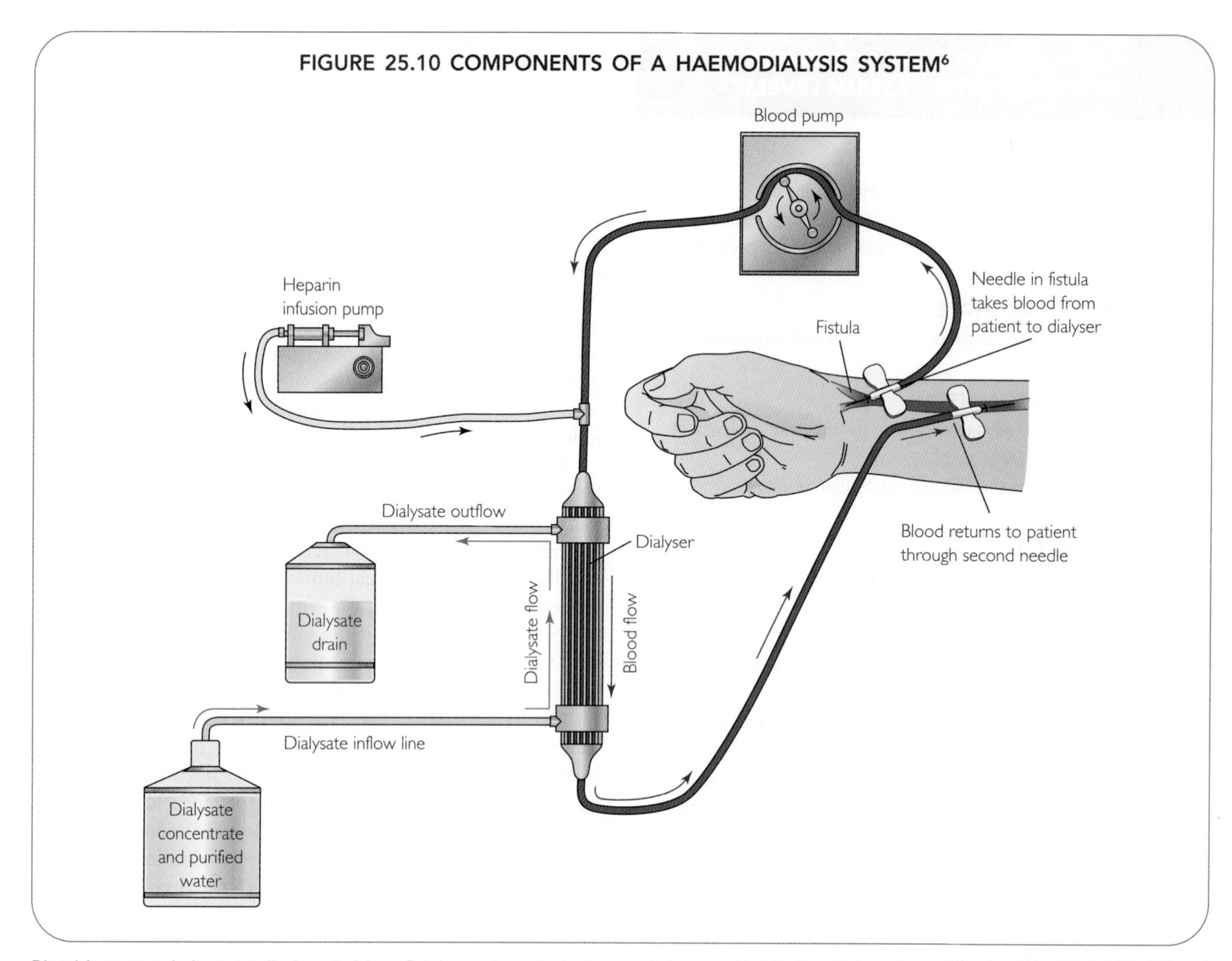

Blood is removed via a needle inserted in a fistula or via catheter lumen. It is propelled to the dialyser by a blood pump. Heparin is infused either as a bolus pre-dialysis or through a heparin pump continuously to prevent clotting. Dialysate is pumped in and flows in the opposite direction to the blood. The dialysed blood is returned to the patient through a second needle or catheter lumen. Old dialysate and ultrafiltrate are drained and discarded.

and hyperuricaemia. There is a massive increase in serum creatinine phosphokinase (CK) levels; anywhere from 10,000 to 200,000 U/L. The urine may have a characteristic reddish-brown colour ('tea-coloured'). Myoglobin reacts with the haemoglobin reagent on urine dipsticks causing a positive result; however, on microscopic examination, no RBCs are seen. Proteinuria is also noted on urinalysis. Muscle aches or acute muscle pain are often presenting symptoms, and general weakness, fever and muscle tenderness may also be present.

Early and aggressive fluid-volume replacement, monitoring and maintenance of electrolyte balance are essential treatment for rhabdomyolysis.[20] To help flush myoglobin through the kidneys, urine output should be increased. Sodium bicarbonate may be added to IV fluids to alkalinise the urine which decreases the precipitation of myoglobin. If sodium bicarbonate is used, urine pH and serum bicarbonate, calcium and potassium levels should be monitored, and if the urine pH does not rise after 4–6 hours of treatment or if symptomatic hypocalcaemia develops, alkalinisation should be discontinued and hydration continued with normal saline. If the patient progresses to AKI, management is the same as previously described.

CHRONIC KIDNEY DISEASE

One in three Australians is at risk of developing chronic kidney disease (CKD) due to the increasing number of people with risk factors such as diabetes, hypertension, obesity or smoking; 10% of Australians have CKD.[21] CKD is characterised by a progressive and irreversible destruction of kidney function that occurs over varying periods of time, ranging from a few months to decades. There are five grades of CKD, and the prognosis and course of CKD are highly variable, depending on the aetiology, patient's condition, age and adequacy of medical follow-up. Most individuals with CKD grades 2–3 live normal, active lives, whereas others may rapidly progress to stage 5 (ESKD). First Nations people from both Australia and New Zealand are overrepresented in the number of people with CKD. The major causes of CKD grade 5 in Australia are diabetes mellitus (38), glomerulonephritis (18%) and hypertension (12%).[22] Regardless of the stage of CKD, it is also possible to develop AKI, particularly due to the administration of nephrotoxic agents such as contrast media or antibiotics and the impact of untreated infections. Consequences of CKD are hypertension, elevated urea and creatinine levels, metabolic acidosis, mineral

FIGURE 25.11 SIGNS AND SYMPTOMS OF CHRONIC KIDNEY DISEASE[6]

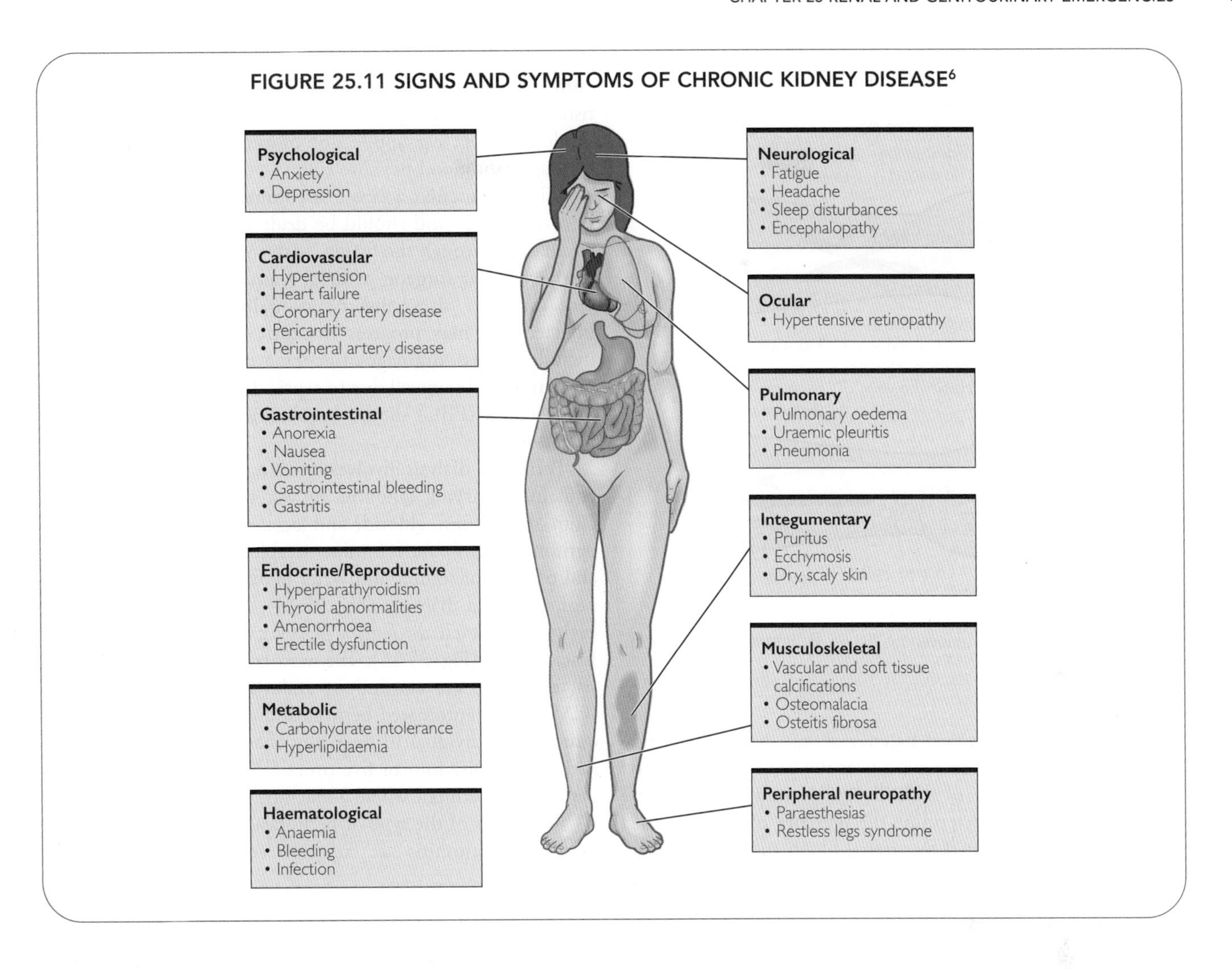

bone disorder and anaemia. In kidney failure (CKD grade 5), there are multisystem effects of uraemia, fluid overload and worsening effects of altered electrolytes (Fig. 25.11). When an individual has severely impaired kidney function (CKD grades 4 and 5), extra care should be taken with the rapid administration of intravenous fluids; in some patients, greater than 1000 mL in 8 hours can cause substantial fluid overload and/or pulmonary oedema can result quickly.

Dialysis complications

Kidney replacement therapy (KRT) is needed for people with kidney failure (CKD grade 5) to sustain life. KRT is commenced when $<$ 10% of kidney function remains and is provided by haemodialysis, peritoneal dialysis or a kidney transplant. Haemodialysis can be provided in a variety of locations. The most common location is in hospital ('in-centre'); it is also undertaken in satellite haemodialysis units that are often isolated from the main hospital or located in separate community facilities. These units are only staffed by nurses who in an emergency call the paramedic team. In addition, there are increasing numbers of patients who are performing haemodialysis at home—with or without a dialysis partner (e.g. spouse) in the home. Typically, a patient who is being managed with haemodialysis will receive a minimum of 4 hours of treatment on three occasions each week, although home haemodialysis patients may dialyse overnight or every second day. Peritoneal dialysis is exclusively performed at home.

Regardless of the reason for presentation to an ED, all patients with an arteriovenous (AV) fistula require special precautions to prevent infection and clotting of the vascular access. There are three main types of vascular access: AV native fistula, AV grafts and central lines. An AV fistula is a surgical connection of an existing artery (e.g. radial) with an existing vein (e.g. cephalic) in any extremity, but particularly the wrist, forearm and upper arm. See Chapter 16 for further information on types of vascular access and techniques. Alternatively, an AV fistula can be created with the use of material (e.g. Gortex) to form the AV connection (Fig. 25.12).

PRACTICE TIP

Regardless of the type of vascular access, it is crucial that paramedics and ED staff are aware of the presence of an AV fistula in a patient and that the access should be assessed (and preserved) at all times. For patients performing haemodialysis at home, emergency discontinuation involves stopping the blood pump, clamping all lines and leaving cannula in situ (flush with normal saline). If time permits and trained assistance is available (e.g. spouse), then blood in the circuit can be returned as it will increase circulating volume. If time does not permit, disconnect and discard the blood-filled circuit.

FIGURE 25.12 CIRCULATORY ACCESS FOR HAEMODIALYSIS[6]

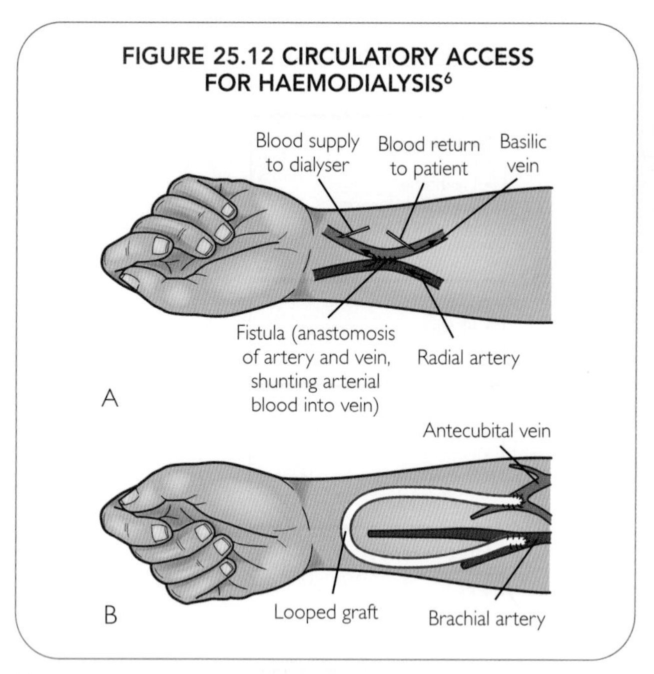

A. Internal (permanent) arteriovenous fistula. **B.** Internal (permanent) arteriovenous graft.

Assessment of AV access patency should be routine and involves two steps: first, palpation over the anastomosis site to determine the presence of a thrill; and second, auscultation with a stethoscope to determine the presence of a bruit. The bruit and thrill are created by arterial blood rushing into the vein. A limb with a fistula should never have a blood pressure cuff applied, insertion of IV lines or venepuncture. An AV fistula will clot during episodes of hypotension or constriction of blood vessels (e.g. application of tourniquet, circumferential bandaging or blood pressure cuffs).

Clotted vascular access is a common reason for presentation to the ED and should be dealt with urgently to restore circulation through the fistula, with the patient being referred to the vascular surgeon or renal team. Central venous catheters insertion sites and occasionally AV fistula become infected and may progress to septicaemia. Local symptoms include redness, drainage or oedema, although many patients present as quite unwell due to sepsis. Blood cultures and a full blood count (FBC) should be obtained to rule out systemic infection.

Peritoneal dialysis involves instilling 2–3 L of dialysate fluid containing varying amounts of water, glucose, sodium, calcium, magnesium, chloride and lactate into the abdomen. The peritoneal membrane is semipermeable and allows for diffusion and osmosis of solutes and water between the vascular peritoneal space and dialysate (Fig. 25.13). Access to the peritoneal cavity is achieved through a plastic catheter held in place by Dacron cuffs (Fig. 25.14). The most common peritoneal dialysis techniques are continuous ambulatory peritoneal dialysis (CAPD) and automated peritoneal dialysis (APD). CAPD requires the individual to manually change the dialysate in the peritoneal cavity four or five times each day. APD is normally performed overnight where a machine exchanges the dialysate.

Regardless of the type of peritoneal dialysis, exit-site infections and peritonitis are common complications and often

FIGURE 25.13 PERITONEAL DIALYSIS[6]

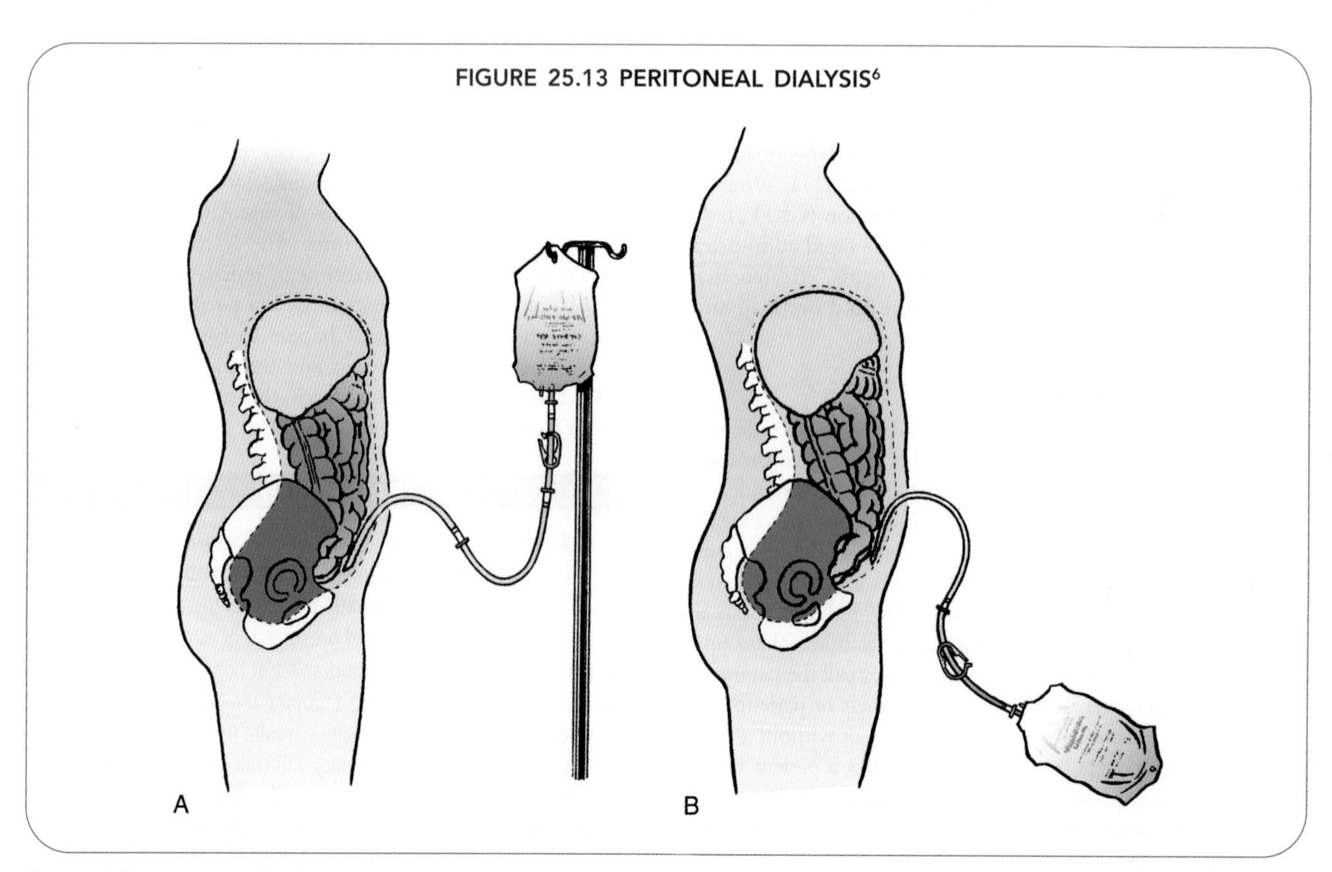

A. Inflow. **B.** Outflow (drains to gravity).

FIGURE 25.14 PERITONEAL CATHETER EXIT SITE[6]

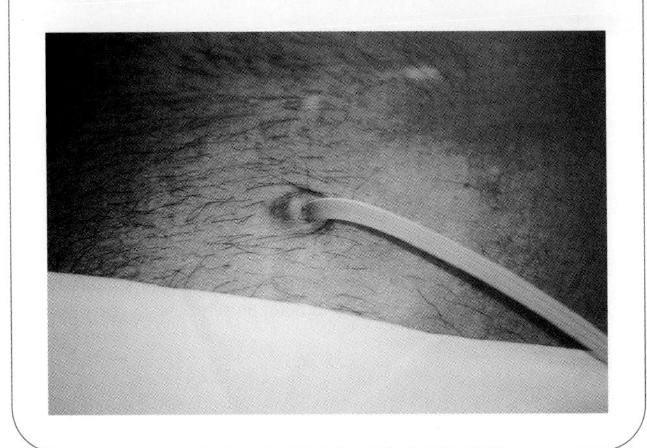

Courtesy of Mary Jo Holechek, Baltimore, MD.

bring the patient to the ED with complaints of abdominal pain, nausea and vomiting, fever and cloudy dialysate fluid.[23]

PRACTICE TIP

Patients undertaking peritoneal dialysis at home have been instructed by the renal unit to bring the most recent bag exchange (i.e. effluent) to the ED (providing it has been stored in the refrigerator); paramedics should ensure the patient is accompanied by the bag.

Peritonitis is a potentially life-threatening complication, so the patient needs to be assessed urgently, a sample of effluent sent to the microbiology department and the patient commenced on antibiotics, which are added to the dialysate (IP).[23] Most EDs have peritonitis protocols to inform practice. In some cases, catheter removal is needed and haemodialysis initiated until the peritonitis clears. The catheter can be surgically replaced and peritoneal dialysis reinitiated, although scarring may impair the permeability of the peritoneal membrane, necessitating permanent transfer to haemodialysis.

Kidney transplantation is also an option for most patients with kidney failure. The donor kidney is placed in the iliac fossa and native kidneys are not removed. Immunosuppression (e.g. prednisone, mycophenolate and tacrolimus or cyclosporin) is required to avoid rejection. Kidney transplant recipients commonly present to the ED with cardiovascular events or infections, particularly severe pyelonephritis.

URINARY TRACT INFECTIONS

Urinary tract infections are a frequent presenting problem to the ED, particularly for older adults[24] and young children.[25] It is the source of infection in 30% of patients presenting to Australian and New Zealand EDs. Symptoms include pyuria, haematuria, chills and fever, leucocytosis, nausea, vomiting and signs of bladder irritability, such as frequency, dysuria and urgency. Dull flank pain and costovertebral angle tenderness are associated with pyelonephritis. Older adults may not experience these symptoms and often experience non-localised abdominal discomfort. In addition, they are at risk of confusion or

FIGURE 25.15 SITES OF INFECTIOUS PROCESSES IN THE UPPER AND LOWER URINARY TRACTS[42]

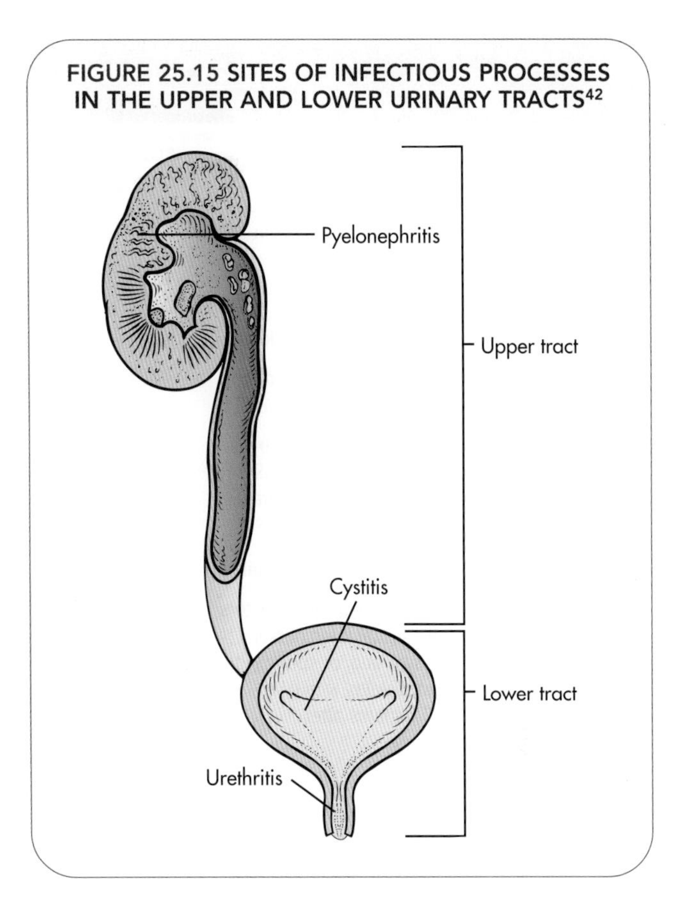

cognitive impairment and rapid progression to sepsis. UTI occurs in about 5–10% of children and should be considered in all febrile infants.

Fig. 25.15 illustrates infectious processes of the urinary system. Diagnosis is made by history, presenting signs, urinalysis, urine culture and sensitivity and FBC with differential. A KUB (kidneys–ureters–bladder) radiograph may show a hazy outline of the kidney secondary to oedema, although it is not always warranted. Kidney function is assessed via serum urea, creatinine and electrolyte results.

Approximately 80% of uncomplicated infections are caused by Gram-negative bacilli, such as *Escherichia coli*, *Klebsiella pneumoniae*, *Enterobacter*, *Proteus* and *Serratia*.[26] Table 25.7 compares common GU tract infections that present to the ED. Persistent microscopic or gross haematuria, symptoms of obstruction or presence of urea-splitting bacteria associated with staghorn renal calculi require work-up with renal ultrasound, cystogram or intravenous pyelogram. Negative cultures may indicate urethral infections due to *Chlamydia trachomatis* or *Neisseria gonorrhoea*.

In uncomplicated UTIs, commonly used antimicrobial therapy includes trimethoprim-sulfamethoxazole (TMP-SMX) and cephalexin.[26] Older patients, particularly from nursing homes, often have an infection that is resistant to TMP-SMX, so ciprofloxacin or cephalexin are used. Antimicrobial therapy is adjusted once culture and susceptibility are known. Collaborative interventions involve antibiotics, adequate fluid intake and urinary alkaliniser (Box 25.4). Intravenous rehydration may be needed in severe cases. Hot packs can relieve the discomfort associated with a UTI. Education about the risk

TABLE 25.7 COMMON GENITOURINARY INFECTIONS

TYPE	DESCRIPTION	ADDITIONAL SIGNS AND SYMPTOMS	INTERVENTIONS	COMPLICATIONS AND COMMENTS
Pyelonephritis	Involves renal parenchyma and pelvis Usually unilateral Kidneys enlarged by oedema More prevalent in women and diabetics Most commonly caused by ascending Escherichia coli infection from lower GU tract		Antibiotics specific to C&S Antipyretics and antiemetics Adequate hydration Monitor intake and output Bed rest	Complications uncommon but may include septicaemia Follow-up urine C&S to ensure effective antibiotic therapy Recurrence may require continuous antibiotic prophylactic suppression
Urethritis	More common in women; E. coli most common organism Associated behavioural factors include sexual intercourse, diaphragm and/or spermicide use, not voiding within 10–15 minutes after intercourse		Short-term antibiotics May need continuous antibiotic, prophylactic suppression or postcoital antibiotic	Associated behaviours UTIs Direction of wiping after defecation Tampon use Bubble bath Douche Tight clothing Carbonated beverages, coffee, alcohol Resisting urge to void Decreasing oral fluids Synthetic underwear
Epididymitis	Bacterial infection in older men Usually preceded by STI or urethritis in young men	P–lifting, sexual excitement, trauma Q–dull ache, sharp R–scrotum, lower abdomen S–increased with sex, decreased with elevation and support T–gradual onset Scrotum red, swollen and warm	Antibiotics Post-treatment culture Bed rest Scrotal support Avoid heavy lifting and straining	Teach safe sex and condom use, complete antibiotic regimen
Prostatitis	Expressed prostate secretions have more WBCs than urine	May have bladder outlet obstruction Low back pain Tender, boggy, hot prostate on manual exam	Antibiotics, urinalysis C&S and expressed prostate fluid C&S	
Non-specific urethritis	Causative agents: E. coli, Staphylococcus, Klebsiella, Pseudomonas	White discharge Urethral itching Perineal, suprapubic or testicular pain	Antibiotics as result of discharge C&S	

C&S: culture and sensitivity; GU: genitourinary; STI: sexually transmitted infection; UTIs: urinary tract infections; WBCs: white blood cells.

BOX 25.4 **COLLABORATIVE CARE IN URINARY TRACT INFECTION**[9]

DIAGNOSTIC STUDIES
- History and physical examination
- Urinalysis
- Urine for culture and sensitivity (if indicated)
- Imaging studies of urinary tract (e.g. IVP, cystoscopy) (if indicated)
- Collaborative therapy

UNCOMPLICATED UTI
- Antibiotic, 1- to 3-day treatment regimen: trimethoprim-sulfamethoxazole, nitrofurantoin
- Adequate fluid intake
- Urinary alkaliniser
- Counselling about risk of recurrence and reduction of risk factors

RECURRENT, UNCOMPLICATED UTI
- Repeat urinalysis and consideration of need for urine culture and sensitivity testing
- Antibiotic, 3- to 5-day treatment regimen: trimethoprim-sulfamethoxazole, nitrofurantoin
- Sensitivity-guided antibiotic (ampicillin, amoxycillin, first-generation cephalosporin, fluoroquinolone)
- Consider 3- to 6-month trial of suppressive antibiotics
- Adequate fluid intake
- Urinary alkaliniser
- Counselling about risk of recurrence and reduction of risk factors
- Imaging study of urinary tract in selected cases

IVP: intravenous pyelogram; UTI: urinary tract infection.

of recurrence and reduction of risk factors is important (Box 25.5). Cranberry juice or tablets can prevent UTIs in adults and children, although there is insufficient evidence in older adults.[27]

ACUTE PYELONEPHRITIS

Acute pyelonephritis is a dangerous infection involving the renal parenchyma and collecting system, usually caused by ascending organisms, that may result in septic shock and/or permanent renal damage.[28] Acute pyelonephritis occurs more frequently in women, who present with costovertebral angle pain and tenderness, often accompanied by fever greater than 38°C. Urinalysis and urine culture confirm the diagnosis of acute pyelonephritis, with *E. coli* responsible for more than 80% of cases. In severe illness, blood cultures may be collected.

Acute pyelonephritis can usually be managed with oral antimicrobial therapy such as trimethoprim-sulfamethoxazole or ciprofloxacin. Severe systemic symptoms of infection (high fever, haemodynamic instability and nausea or vomiting) warrant IV therapy and hospitalisation (see also septic shock in Chapter 27). An aminoglycoside, such as gentamicin, remains appropriate first-line therapy, although ceftriaxone, cefotaxime, piperacillin, ticarcillin, imipenem or meropenem can be used.[28] In older children, acute pyelonephritis can be treated with trimethoprim-sulfamethoxazole or cephalexin. Infants are usually hospitalised and receive IV therapy with ceftriaxone.

BOX 25.5 **RISK FACTORS FOR URINARY TRACT CALCULI**[6]

METABOLIC
Abnormalities that result in increased urine levels of calcium, oxaluric acid, uric acid or citric acid

CLIMATE
Hot climates that cause increased fluid loss, low urine volume and increased solute concentration in urine

DIET
Large intake of dietary proteins that increases uric acid excretion

Excessive amounts of tea or fruit juices that elevate urinary oxalate level

Large intake of calcium and oxalate

Low fluid intake, which increases urinary concentration

GENETIC FACTORS
Family history of stone formation, cystinuria, gout or renal acidosis

LIFESTYLE
Sedentary occupation, immobility

URINARY CALCULI

Calculi formation (urolithiasis) is more common in Australia due to the hotter and drier climate, affecting about 4–8% of the population who are mostly between 20 and 55 years of age.[29] Hypercalciuria is a primary risk factor for the development of renal calculi. UTI, gout, excessive ingestion of certain foods, family history, dehydration and pregnancy are also associated with calculi formation (Box 25.5). Calculi can recur in up to 50% of patients. Calculi are often asymptomatic until relocation along the urinary tract causes intermittent backache, urge to void, dysuria, renal colic and haematuria. The pain caused by either a partial or a complete obstruction to the flow of urine in the renal pelvis is referred to as *renal colic.*

Renal colic typically presents with flank pain that radiates to the groin and is often described as a constant, gnawing ache in the costovertebral region (the point on the back corresponding to the 12th rib and lateral border of sacrospinal muscle). The symptoms of renal colic can be so severe that patients find it impossible to be still, and writhe in agony. The pain can cause a sympathetic response of nausea, vomiting, pallor and cool, clammy skin. Proteinuria or bacteraemia may also be found on urinalysis. Diagnostic studies include FBC, serum urea, creatinine, electrolytes and uric acid, urinalysis with culture and sensitivity (C&S) and KUB (and rarely an IVP). Non-contrast helical CT scans are the primary diagnostic study when investigating an episode of acute renal colic.[30] Fig. 25.16 shows a calculus on a CT scan. Up to 90% of calculi are expelled spontaneously; however, if unpassed, removal may require laparoscopy, lithotripsy or surgical intervention.

Initial management includes insertion of an IV cannula, the commencement of IV fluids and administration of analgesia.

FIGURE 25.16 A 59-YEAR-OLD FEMALE WITH OBSTRUCTING URETERAL CALCULUS[31]

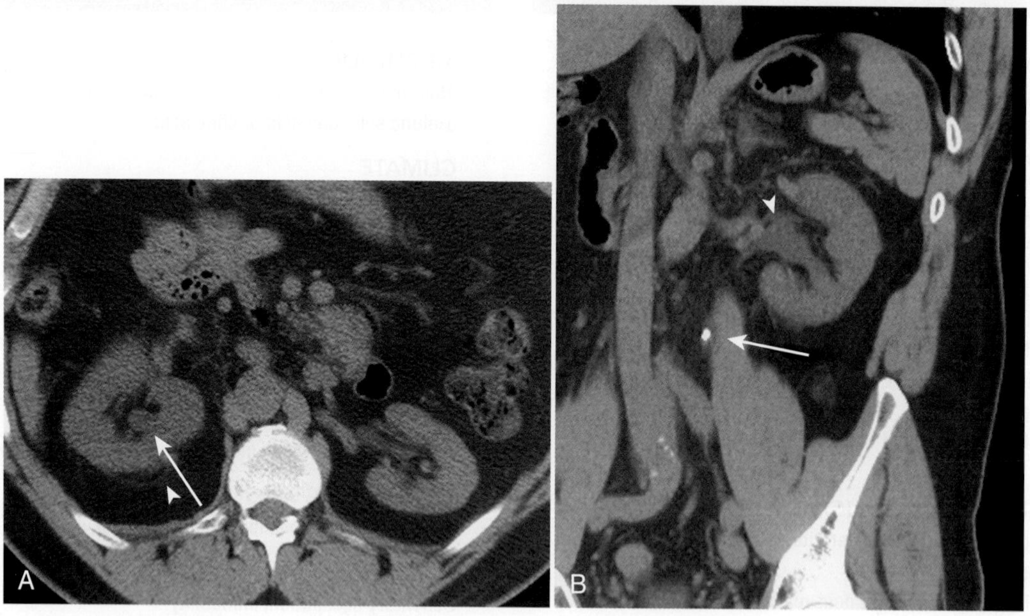

A. Axial unenhanced computed tomography (CT) image demonstrates mild, diffuse enlargement of the right kidney with hydronephrosis (arrow) and mild perinephric stranding (arrowhead). **B.** Coronal unenhanced CT image demonstrates hydronephrosis (arrowhead) and the ureteral stone (arrow).

Once in the ED, nursing interventions include ongoing analgesia, urinalysis, fluid balance monitoring and increased fluids. Current Australian recommendations are that all urine should be strained for 48 hours following an episode of ureteric colic and any calculi submitted for chemical analysis. It is crucial that regular pain assessment and management occurs in these patients because of the severity of their pain. Depending on the severity of the pain, either opioids (morphine sulfate or fentanyl via IV injection) or non-steroidal anti-inflammatory drugs (NSAIDs; ketorolac, naproxen) administered orally or rectally can be used; a combination of these is usually most effective.[32] In broad terms, patients receiving NSAIDs achieve greater reduction in pain scores and are less likely to require further analgesia in the short term. NSAIDs are contraindicated in patients at risk for gastrointestinal bleeding or CKD. Guidelines recommend NSAIDs and paracetamol and suggest they have better analgesic efficacy than opioids.[33] Intravenous paracetamol (1 g) can also be used as first-line analgesia in patients with renal colic.

Tamsulosin, an oral alpha-blocker (adrenergic alpha$_1$-receptor antagonist), more commonly used in the non-surgical treatment of benign prostatic hypertrophy, has been shown to be effective in increasing the expulsion rate of renal calculi and reducing analgesic requirements.[34] It can be used for a short period (2–4 weeks) and requires follow-up with a urologist.

Complications of renal calculi include altered elimination, UTI and rarely ischaemia at the obstructive site. Admission from ED occurs in about 10% of patients, and this is mostly due to the need for frequent doses of analgesia, large diameter stones, if the person has one kidney, paralytic ileus or severe infection. If the patient is discharged from the ED, information should be provided to them about returning if pain increases, excessive vomiting or fever and chills. Urological follow-up will be required. A high fluid intake (approximately 3 L per day) is recommended to produce a urine output of at least 2 L per day. High urine output prevents supersaturation of minerals (i.e. dilutes the concentration) and flushes them out before the minerals have a chance to precipitate and form a stone. Increasing the fluid intake is especially important for the patient who is active in sports, lives in a dry climate, performs physical exercise, has a family history of stone formation or works in an occupation that requires outdoor work or a great deal of physical activity that can lead to dehydration. Water is the preferred fluid, and consumption of colas, coffee and tea should be limited, because high intake of these beverages tends to increase rather than diminish the risk of recurring urinary calculi.

Dietary intervention may be important in the management of urinary calculi. In the past, calcium restriction was routinely implemented for the patient with kidney stones. However, more-recent research suggests that a high dietary calcium intake, which was previously thought to contribute to kidney stones, may lower the risk by reducing the urinary excretion of oxalate, a common factor in many stones.[35] Initial nutritional management should include limiting oxalate-rich foods and thereby reducing oxalate excretion.

ACUTE URINARY RETENTION

Acute urinary retention (AUR) is the sudden, painful inability to urinate spontaneously and is one of the most common GU emergencies.[36] It is characterised by lower abdominal pain, complete or partial urinary retention, overflow incontinence, bladder distension and irritative voiding. Elderly men are at the highest risk because of prostatic enlargement. History will reveal progressive lower urinary tract symptoms (LUTS), such as decreased urinary stream, hesitancy, nocturia and dribbling (often secondary to an enlarged prostate); rarely, AUR can occur following a transurethral resection of the prostate. Medications may also cause AUR, such as anticholinergics, antihistamines, decongestants, hypnotics, NSAIDs and narcotics. Neurological assessment is also required to rule out spinal cord injury or disease that can interfere with the micturition reflex. Assessment includes bladder palpation/ultrasonography and digital rectal examination of the prostate.

AUR requires prompt recognition and rapid and complete bladder decompression through indwelling urethral or suprapubic 2-way catheters is required. The catheter should be left in situ to ensure the bladder decompresses even if the volume is greater than 500 mL.[37] A Coudé catheter can be used in preference to a Foley's catheter in men with suspected prostatic hypertrophy as the cause of the AUR. This catheter is more rigid than other straight catheters and has a tapered, curved tip. Force should not be used to insert a catheter. A suprapubic catheter or assistance from a urologist may be necessary. If AUR is due to haematuria (i.e. clots), then a three-way catheter should be used so that continuous bladder irrigation can be established. The insertion technique is the same as a two-way catheter. Fig. 25.17 shows different urinary catheters.

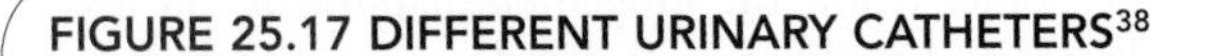

PRACTICE TIP

Use aseptic technique when catheterising. A Coudé catheter is inserted with tip pointing upwards. There is no evidence to support the clamping of urinary catheters as a strategy to avoid post-obstructive diuresis, hypotension and haematuria from rapid bladder decompression. Bladder irrigation for acute obstruction using a 60 mL syringe (either sterile water or normal saline) is recommended, but vigorous flushing/aspiration should be avoided due to the risk of damaging bladder mucosa.

FIGURE 25.17 DIFFERENT URINARY CATHETERS[38]

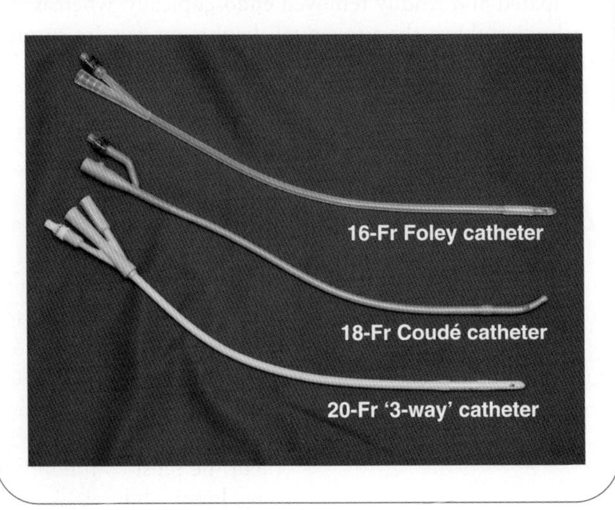

If sufficient oral hydration cannot be maintained during the diuresis phase or if marked polyuria (> 200 mL/h) occurs, then IV fluid replacement is required. Further diagnostic evaluation is needed if the target residual volume is minimal (< 100 mL) to identify the cause.

Patients with uncomplicated AUR are not admitted, but hospitalisation is indicated when there is kidney failure or urosepsis. Simple discharge instructions should be provided on the management of the catheter and drainage bags. Referral to the urologist and community nurse is also required.

TESTICULAR TORSION

Testicular torsion causes vascular compromise of the testes within 6–12 hours, which can lead to tissue infarction and loss of spermatogenesis. It is more common in adolescent males with about 50% occurring during sleep. Congenital abnormality of the tunica vaginalis, the canal from which the testes descend, is often an associated risk factor.[39] Recognition by paramedics and triage nurses can help in the immediate management of patients through referral pathways that will improve the long-term prognosis.

Clinical manifestations include upwardly retracted testes with redness and oedema to the site of the torsion, abdominal pain and nausea and vomiting. Fig. 25.18 compares normal testicular structures with testicular torsion. It can be difficult to differentiate between testicular torsion and epididymitis. Scrotal examination is urgently required in case there is torsion. Prehn's sign can be useful in differentiating testicular torsion from epididymitis.

PRACTICE TIP

To assess for Prehn's sign, the scrotum is gently elevated to the level of the symphysis. In testicular torsion, pain increases; however, in epididymitis, a decrease in pain is noted.[41] Colour Doppler ultrasound can be used to confirm the diagnosis and to determine blood flow to the testis.

FIGURE 25.18 TESTICULAR TORSION[40]

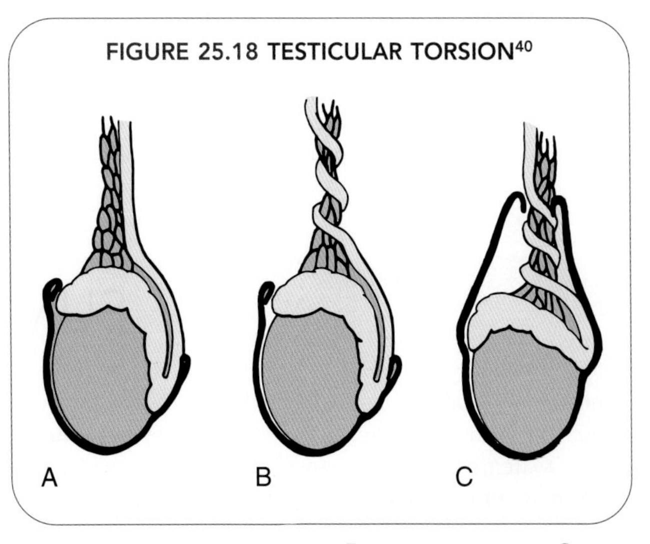

A. Normal tunica vaginalis insertion. **B.** Extravaginal torsion. **C.** Intravaginal torsion with abnormally high vaginalis insertion.

Analgesia should be administered as necessary and urological or paediatric consultation is urgently sought, as surgery must be performed within 6 hours or orchidectomy may be necessary. Manual detorsion may also be performed under local anaesthesia. Good communication skills are required as patients are often embarrassed young males.

EPIDIDYMITIS

Epididymitis, inflammation of the epididymis, is due to an infection (sexually or non-sexually transmitted), and is more common in sexually active males between 18 and 50 years of age. The causative organisms are often *C. trachomatis* or *N. gonorrhoeae*. Extreme physical strain or exertion can also cause epididymitis. Orchitis can also be a consequence; this is termed epididymo-orchitis.

Signs and symptoms of epididymitis include severe scrotal pain, which can radiate into the abdomen, tenderness along the spermatic cord, swelling, fever, pyuria and, occasionally, urethral discharge. A positive Prehn's sign may also be observed. An elevated WBC count will be present, and urinalysis will reveal bacteria.

Treatment of epididymitis includes administration of antibiotics (e.g. fluoroquinolones or doxycycline), antipyretics and analgesics. Supportive care includes scrotal support and elevation, ice packs to the affected area and sitz baths to alleviate pain. There should be an avoidance of physical strain and sexual activity.

PRIAPISM

Priapism is persistent, painful erection not associated with sexual desire. The corpora cavernosa are engorged but the corpus spongiosum and glans are not involved.[42] Venous drainage is obstructed causing a build-up of viscous deoxygenated blood, interstitial oedema and eventual fibrosis. Severity of pain increases with duration, and when there is urinary obstruction and bladder distension, pain can be prolonged for 24 hours or longer. Aetiologies include diabetes mellitus, spinal cord injury, multiple sclerosis, psychotropic drugs, prolonged sexual activity and marijuana or cocaine use. In addition, many common medications such as anticoagulants, corticosteroids and prazosin can result in priapism. Priapism from use of papaverine for impotence is occurring more frequently. Prolonged priapism is a medical emergency.

After a regional nerve block is administered, acute detumescence requires a large-bore needle is to be inserted into the corpus cavernosa. (Chapter 16 contains information on administering a regional nerve block.) Tissue removal may be necessary to relieve any obstruction or surgical venous anastomosis between glans and cavernosa may be needed. A urinary catheter to relieve bladder obstruction and distension is needed in about 50% of patients. Development of scar tissue or fibrosis in the cavernous spaces related to the duration of priapism and decompression can result in impotence. Paramedics and triage nurses need to be aware that men will often be embarrassed when calling for paramedic assistance or when presenting to the ED.

FOREIGN BODIES AND PIERCING

There are numerous case reports of various types of foreign bodies found in the urethra, bladder and genitalia. In adults, most foreign bodies are inserted for erotic stimulation. However, psychological disorders and drug ingestion are other frequent reasons for such activity. It is unusual for children to present with foreign bodies in the urethra. The most common reason for presentation is dysuria. Other complaints are suprapubic or perineal pain, urethral discharge, haematuria, difficulty urinating, swelling or abscess formation.

Complications of genital body piercing include local and systemic infections, poor cosmesis and foreign-body rejection. Piercing sites in men include the penile glans and urethra, foreskin and scrotum; sites in women include the clitoral prepuce or body, labia minora, labia majora and perineum.[43] Jewellery inserted through the glans penis often interrupts urinary flow. Paraphimosis (the inability to replace a retracted foreskin) has been associated with urethral and glans piercings in uncircumcised men. The foreskin may be reduced manually after a penile nerve block. Penile rings also can cause engorgement and priapism (i.e. persistent erection), requiring emergency treatment to preserve erectile function. Women with genital piercings can develop bleeding, infections, allergic reactions, keloids and scarring.

Clinical diagnosis is based on history and should always be considered in patients with chronic urinary tract infections. Radiographic studies, including plain x-rays, are usually helpful for radio-opaque objects. Xeroradiography is effective for detecting non-metallic foreign bodies traumatically or deliberately introduced into the genital tissues, including objects made of plastic, glass, rubber, cloth or wood. Foreign bodies below the urogenital diaphragm can usually be palpated and readily removed endoscopically, whereas foreign bodies above the urogenital diaphragm require surgical intervention.[44,45]

SUMMARY

Genitourinary emergencies, particularly AKI, require thorough evaluation of kidney function to identify any kidney involvement. The GU system maintains homeostasis, so disruption of kidney function interrupts almost all organ systems. In addition, emerging strains of resistant bacteria are challenging to prevent and manage. The roles of emergency clinicians are crucial in the detection and subsequent prevention of GU diseases.

CASE STUDY

Mr Perry is a 48-year-old man with type 2 diabetes (15 years) and grade 3A CKD (treated with Ryzodeg [70% insulin degludec, 30% insulin aspart] metformin, dapagliflozin, perindopril, amlodipine, furosemide). Other clinical history is cerebral palsy and hypertension. His carer called the ambulance to bring him in to ED due to general weakness and feeling dizzy. He has had nausea, vomiting and diarrhoea for last 3 days. On arrival the paramedic notes the following assessment:

- pulse 115 beats/minute
- respiratory rate 32 breaths/minute
- blood pressure 105/50 mmHg
- Mr Perry is conscious but somewhat confused as to the day and time.

His carer confirmed that Mr Perry had continued to take his medications during his illness and was not able to eat and drink normally; however, he may have missed a few doses of insulin. The paramedic undertook a BSL test, which was 10.5 mmol/L. Due to the appearance of dehydration, an intravenous cannula (IVC) is inserted and 1000 mL normal saline at 100 mL/h is commenced. Mr Perry is transported to the emergency department (ED) of the local hospital. On arrival his temperature is 36.3°C; other vital signs are the same as earlier. Urgent biochemistry reveals the following:

- sodium 133 mmol/L
- potassium 5.8 mmol/L
- urea 11.8 mmol/L
- creatinine 144 micromol/L
- C-reactive protein 8.4 mg/L
- urine analysis—glycosuria (1000 mg/dL), ketones (150 mg/dL), proteins (1 +), no infection
- Blood gases analysis showed severe metabolic acidosis with increased anion gap (pH 7.21, pCO_2 19.1 mmHg, HCO_3 7.6 mmol/L, anion gap 20 mmol/L) normal levels of lactate (9mg/dL)

QUESTIONS

1. What questions will you ask in this scenario to determine historical and clinical indicators of urgency and relevance?
2. What ongoing nursing assessment and monitoring will you provide? Why?
3. What does the clinical and pathology picture identify Mr Perry is experiencing?
4. What medication and clinical situation has probably caused euglycaemic ketoacidosis? Why?
5. The most important treatment for a patient with euDKA would be:
   a. fluid resuscitation (isotonic)
   b. treatment for nausea and vomiting
   c. ceasing medications (dapagliflozin, metformin, furosemide, perindopril)
   d. insulin infusion

Answers to Case Study Questions can be found on evolve http://evolve.elsevier.com/AU/Curtis/emergency/ 

USEFUL WEBSITES

Caring for Australasians with Renal Impairment, www.cariguidelines.org.

Kidney Health Australia, www.kidney.org.au.

Lions Australian Prostate Cancer Web Site, www.prostatehealth.org.au.

NSW Emergency Care Institute, urology emergencies and patient fact sheets, https://aci.health.nsw.gov.au/networks/eci/clinical/clinical-tools/urology.

New Zealand Kidney Foundation, www.kidneys.co.nz/.

Urological Society of Australia and New Zealand, www.usanz.org.au.

REFERENCES

1. Levey AS, Eckardt KU, Dorman NM, Christiansen SL, Hoorn EJ, Ingelfinger JR, et al. Nomenclature for kidney function and disease: report of a Kidney Disease: Improving Global Outcomes (KDIGO) consensus conference. Kid Int 2020;97(6):1117–29.
2. Hryciw D, Bonner A. Alterations of renal and urinary tract function across the lifespan. In: Craft J, Gordon C, Huether SE, editor. Understanding pathophysiology. 3rd ed. Sydney; Elsevier; 2018.
3. McCance KL, Huether SE, Brashers VL. Pathophysiology: the biologic basis for disease in adults and children. 8th ed. St. Louis, Missouri: Elsevier; 2019.
4. Powell K. Consultation and clinical assessment of the genitourinary system for advanced clinical practitioners. Brit J Nurs 2021;30(22):1288–94.

5. Reynard J, Brewster S, Biers S, Neal N. Oxford handbook of urology. 4th ed. Oxford: Oxford University Press; 2019.
6. Brown D, Edwards H, Buckley T, Aitken R, Plowman E. Lewis's medical–surgical nursing: assessment and management of clinical problems. Australia and New Zealand 5th edition. Chatswood, NSW: Elsevier Australia; 2020.
7. Herlihy BL. The human body in health and illness. 7th ed. St. Louis, Missouri: Elsevier Saunders; 2021.
8. Patton KT, Thibodeau GA, Patton KT. Anatomy & physiology. 10th ed. St. Louis, Missouri: Elsevier; 2019.
9. Patton KT, Thibodeau GA. The human body in health & disease. 7th ed. St. Louis, Missouri: Mosby; 2017.
10. Thompson JM. Mosby's clinical nursing. 5th ed. St. Louis, Missouri: Mosby; 2002.
11. Hooton T, Johnson RJ, Feehally J, Floege Jr. Comprehensive clinical nephrology. 6th ed. Edinburgh: Elsevier; 2019.
12. Ingelfinger, Julie R. Hematuria in adults. N Eng J Med 2021;385(2):153–63.
13. Battaloglu E, Figuero M, Moran C, Lecky F, Porter K. Urethral injury in major trauma. Injury 2019;50(5):1053–7.
14. Ranasinha N, Chandrasekera S. Symptoms, signs and basic investigations for urinary calculi. In: Ng ACF, Wong MY, Isotani S, editors. Practical management of urinary stone. Singapore: Springer; 2021. doi.org/10.1007/978-981-16-4193-0_1.
15. Ronco C, Bellomo R, Kellum JA. Acute kidney injury. Lancet 2019;394(10212):1949–64.
16. Sinert R, Peacock P. Acute kidney injury (renal failure). In: Emergency medicine: Medscape; 2019. Available from: https://emedicine.medscape.com/article/777845-overview?reg=1#a1.
17. Farrar A. Acute kidney injury. Nurs Clin North Am 2018;53(4):499–510.
18. Kellum JA, Romagnani P, Ashuntantang G et al. Acute kidney injury. Nat Rev Dis Primers 7(52) (2021):doi.org/10.1038/s41572-021-00284-z.
19. Davenport MS, Perazella MA, Yee J, Dillman JR, Fine D, McDonald RJ, et al. Use of intravenous iodinated contrast media in patients with kidney disease: consensus statements from the American College of Radiology and the National Kidney Foundation. Radiology 2020;294(3):660–8.
20. Sawhney JS, Kasotakis G, Goldenberg A, Abramson SB, Dodgion C, Patel N, et al. Management of rhabdomyolysis: a practice management guideline from the Eastern Association for the Surgery of Trauma. Am J Surg 2022;224:196–204.
21. Australian Institute of Health and Welfare (AIHW). Chronic kidney disease web report. Canberra: Commonwealth of Australia; 2020. Available from: www.aihw.gov.au/reports/chronic-kidney-disease/chronic-kidney-disease/contents/how-many-australians-have-chronic-kidney-disease.
22. Australia and New Zealand Dialysis and Transplant (ANZDATA). 44th Report, Chapter 1: Incidence of kidney failure with replacement therapy. ANZDATA, Adelaide: ANZDATA; 2021. Available from: www.anzdata.org.au.
23. Li PKT, Chow KM, Cho Y, Fan S, Harris T, Madero M, et al. ISPD peritonitis guideline recommendations: 2022 update on prevention and treatment. Perit Dial Int 2022;42(2):110–53.
24. Pinnell RAM, Ramsay T, Han W, Joo P. Urinary tract infection investigation and treatment in older adults presenting to the emergency department with confusion: a health record review of local practice patterns. Can Geriatr J 2021;24(4):341–50.
25. Tanaka Y, Oishi T, Ono S, Kono M, Kato A, Miyata I, et al. Epidemiology of urinary tract infections in children: causative bacteria and antimicrobial therapy. Pediatr Int 2021;63(10):1198–204.
26. Ahmed H, Farewell D, Jones H, Francis NA, Paranjothy S, Butler CC. Antibiotic prophylaxis and clinical outcomes among older adults with recurrent urinary tract infection: cohort study. Age Ageing 2019;48(2):228–34.
27. Duncan D. Alternative to antibiotics for managing asymptomatic and non-symptomatic bacteriuria in older persons: a review. Br J Community Nurs 2019;24(3):116–19.
28. Herness J, Buttolph A, Hammer NC. Acute pyelonephritis in adults: rapid evidence review. Am Fam Phys 2020;102(3):173–80.
29. Mami D, Alchinbayev M, Kazachenko A. Comparison of minimally invasive treatment methods for urinary stones: a retrospective analysis. Elect J Gen Med 2021;18(6):1-6.
30. Dai JC, Chang HC, Holt SK, Harper JD. National trends in CT utilization and estimated CT-related radiation exposure in the evaluation and follow-up of stone patients. Urology 2019;133:50–6.
31. Soto JA, Lucey BC. Emergency radiology: the requisites. 2nd ed. Philadelphia, Pennsylvania: Elsevier; 2017.
32. Minhaj FS, Hoang-Nguyen M, Tenney A, Bragg A, Zhang W, Foster J, et al. Evaluation of opioid requirements in the management of renal colic after guideline implementation in the emergency department. Am J Emerg Med 2020;38(12):2564–9.
33. European Association of Urology. EAU guidelines on urolithiasis. European Association of Urology; 2022. Available from: uroweb.org/guidelines/urolithiasis/chapter/guidelines.
34. Ze-Wei Y, Rui-Hong W, Chang-Cun Z, Gao JG. The efficacy and safety of alpha-adrenergic blockers for medical expulsion therapy in patients with ureteral calculi: a meta-analysis of placebo-controlled trials. Medicine 2021;100(37):e27272.
35. Goka SQ, Copelovitch L. Prevention of recurrent urinary stone disease. Curr Opin Pediatr 2020;32(2):295–9.
36. Mavrotas J, Gandhi A, Kalogianni V, Patel V, Batura D. Acute urinary retention. Brit J Hosp Med 2022;83(1):1–8.
37. Etafy MH, Saleh FH, Ortiz-Vanderdys C, Hamada A, Refaat AM, Aal MA, et al. Rapid versus gradual bladder decompression in acute urinary retention. Urol Ann 2017;9(4):339–42.
38. Roberts JR, Custalow CB, Thomsen TW. Roberts and Hedges' clinical procedures in emergency medicine and acute care. 7th ed. Philadelphia, PA: Elsevier; 2018.

39. Castle C, Beasley SW, Taghavi K. Access to emergency surgery for testicular torsion or intestinal volvulus in New Zealand a system perspective. J Paediatr Child Health 2022;58(1):146–51.

40. Price SA, Wilson LM. Pathophysiology: clinical concepts of disease processes. 5th ed. St Louis: Mosby; 1997.

41. Kumar V, Matai P, Prabhu SP, Sundeep PT. Testicular loss in children due to incorrect early diagnosis of torsion. Clin Pediatr 2020;59(4/5):436–8.

42. Muneer A, Alnajjar HM, Ralph D. Recent advances in the management of priapism. F1000Res 2018;7:37.

43. Schreiber ML. Tattoos and piercings: considerations for nursing practice. MedSurg Nurs 2019;28(2):130–4.

44. Maiers TJ. Management of genitourinary foreign bodies in a predominantly incarcerated population. Can J Urol 2020;27(6):10444–9.

45. He Y, Zhang W, Sun N, Feng G, Ni X, Song H. Experience of pediatric urogenital tract inserted objects: 10-year single-center study. J Pediatr Urol 2019;159(5):544e1–e8.

CHAPTER 26
ENDOCRINE EMERGENCIES

KELLI INNES AND MARGARET MURPHY

ESSENTIALS

- One of the key roles of the endocrine system is to maintain an optimal internal environment throughout the life span.
- Endocrine emergencies are rare and therefore constitute only a fraction of ED workload. The most frequent endocrine emergencies are related to diabetes.
- Diabetes is the fastest growing chronic condition in Australia.
- Clinicians should be aware of potential red flags for endocrine emergencies and not delay initiation of treatment while awaiting investigation results.
- It is also imperative that involvement of the endocrine team occur in a timely manner once endocrine involvement is suspected.
- Clinical assessment should follow the ABCD algorithm with interventions initiated if any of these parameters are compromised using rapid response systems.

INTRODUCTION

The endocrine system is comprised of glands capable of synthesising and releasing chemical messengers known as hormones. One of the key roles of the endocrine system is to maintain an optimal internal environment throughout the life span, and, in the context of acute or critical illness, to initiate adaptive responses when emergency demands occur. Endocrine emergencies constituted $<1\%$ of emergency department (ED) presentations in 2020–21,[1] and, as such, healthcare professionals working in out-of-hospital and emergency care may have limited experience in early detection and management of such emergencies. The most frequent endocrine emergencies are related to diabetes. With early detection and early interventions, diabetic emergencies may be successfully managed. In this chapter diabetic ketoacidosis, hyperglycaemic hyperosmolar syndrome and hypoglycaemia are discussed. Also discussed are less common endocrine emergencies related to the pituitary, thyroid and adrenal systems, as well as alcoholic ketoacidosis, with an emphasis on early assessment and initial management strategies.

ANATOMY AND PHYSIOLOGY

The endocrine system consists of the hypothalamus, pituitary, pineal gland, thyroid, parathyroid, adrenals, pancreas, testes (in males) and ovaries (in females) (Fig. 26.1). Hormone molecules are transported via blood to their target tissues, where each hormone exerts its characteristic regulatory function at a cellular and molecular level.[3] An overview of the major endocrine glands, hormones produced and functions is presented in Table 26.1.

Most hormones are proteins and are synthesised and produced in endocrine glands throughout the body. Hormone release occurs in response to altered cellular environment and is regulated by one or more of the following mechanisms:

- chemical factors
- endocrine factors
- neural control.[4]

The most important regulatory mechanism is the negative feedback system where the endocrine system is controlled through negative feedback loops. An example of negative feedback is where thyroid-stimulating hormone (TSH) released from the anterior pituitary stimulates the synthesis and secretion of thyroid hormones. TSH secretion is regulated by thyrotropin-releasing hormone primarily in the hypothalamus and is inhibited by the thyroid-secreted hormones thyroxine (T4) and, to a lesser extent, triiodothyronine (T3).

FIGURE 26.1 LOCATION OF THE MAJOR ENDOCRINE GLANDS[2]

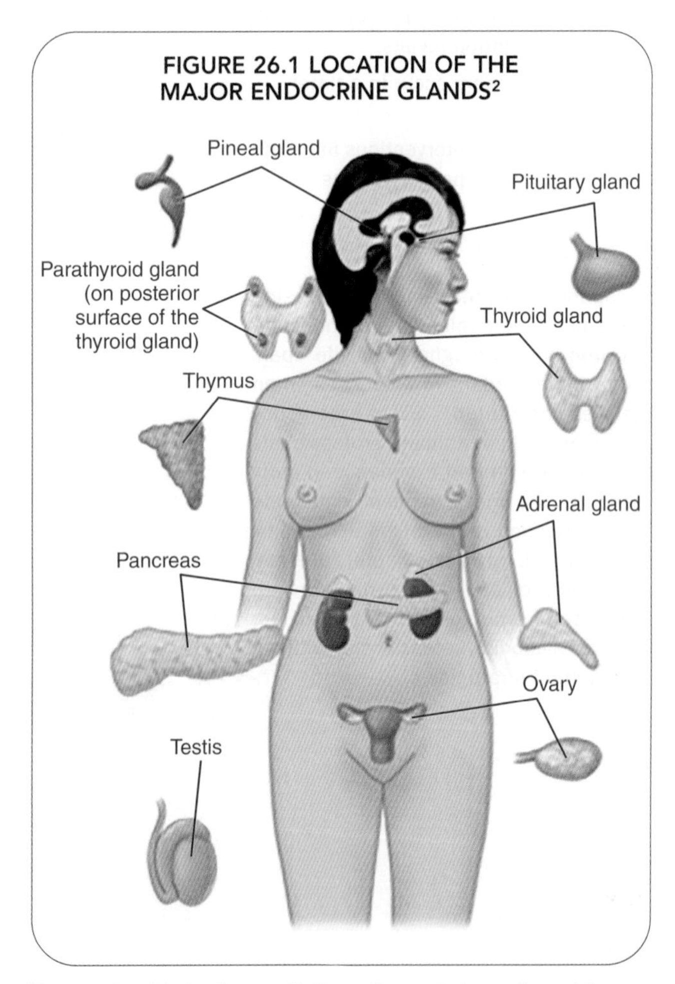

The parathyroid glands actually lie on the posterior surface of the thyroid gland.

Negative feedback systems maintain a delicate balance to ensure that hormone levels remain within physiological levels. Pathological conditions occur when there is a lack of negative-feedback inhibition, resulting in excessive hormonal levels. Alerted renal and liver function, and external factors, such as pain, fear and stress, all influence hormone release. Neural stimulation, for example, sympathetic activation during stress, results in increased levels of hormones, such as adrenaline and glucagon, which results in increasing heart rate, blood pressure and serum blood glucose levels (BGLs). When the stress reduces, adrenaline and glucagon levels decrease and symptoms subside. Intrinsic rhythms (e.g. circadian rhythms) vary from hours to weeks and provide another method of hormone control.[5]

Once secreted into the circulatory system, hormones may be either water soluble or lipid soluble or circulate in a free or active form. Water-soluble hormones usually have a short half-life (e.g. insulin with a half-life of 3–5 minutes), whereas lipid-soluble hormones (e.g. cortisol or thyroxine) have a considerably longer half-life of 60–90 minutes. Some hormones, such as cortisol, also have small amounts of unbound, free circulating cortisol, in addition to the bound form.[3,4]

HYPOTHALAMUS

The hypothalamus creates part of the walls and floor of the third ventricle of the brain and has central control of the automatic nervous centre (Fig. 26.2). Although the hypothalamus is small in size, centres in the anterior and posterior hypothalamus are responsible for performing numerous vital functions, most of which relate either directly or indirectly to the regulation of visceral activities (Table 26.2). The hypothalamus is responsible for limbic (emotional) regulation, as well as instinctual functions.[1,4]

The hypothalamus lies close to the pituitary gland and is linked to the brain by nerves and blood vessels. It produces neurosecretory chemicals that regulate anterior pituitary action through the stimulation or suppression of various hormones. These hormones are responsible for the regulation of other endocrine glands via the negative feedback loop. As the hypothalamus is one of the most vital structures of the body, dysfunction can have a serious effect on the autonomic, somatic or psychic functions of the body.[3,4]

PITUITARY

The pituitary is located on the inferior aspect of the brain in the region of the diencephalon, and lies within the sella turcica of the middle cranial fossa (Fig. 26.2). Pituitary secretions are controlled by the hypothalamus, as well as negative feedback from target glands. It is rounded and pea-shaped, measuring approximately 1 cm in diameter and is attached to the hypothalamus by the infundibular stalk.[3] The pituitary gland is structurally and functionally divided into the anterior and posterior regions. The anterior region contains secretory cells, and secretes trophic hormones—the term *trophic* meaning 'food'. The anterior pituitary hormones do not target food; rather, they result in hypertrophy of their targets when levels are high, and result in atrophy of target organs when levels are low. Hormones that are secreted by the anterior pituitary include growth hormone, adrenocorticotrophic hormone (ACTH), thyroid-stimulating hormone (TSH), prolactin, follicle-stimulating hormone and luteinising hormone.[3]

TABLE 26.1 PRIMARY ENDOCRINE GLANDS AND HORMONES[5]

HORMONES	TARGET TISSUE	FUNCTIONS
Anterior pituitary (adenohypophysis)		
Growth hormone (GH)	All body cells	Promotes protein anabolism (growth, tissue repair) and lipid mobilisation and catabolism
Thyroid-stimulating hormone (TSH)	Thyroid gland	Stimulates synthesis and release of thyroid hormones, growth and function of thyroid gland
Adrenocorticotrophic hormone (ACTH)	Adrenal cortex	Fosters growth of adrenal cortex; stimulates secretion of corticosteroids
Gonadotrophic hormones Follicle-stimulating hormone (FSH)-Luteinising hormone (LH)	Reproductive organs	Stimulate sex-hormone secretion, reproductive organ growth, reproductive processes
Melanocyte-stimulating hormone (MSH)	Melanocytes in skin	Increases melanin production in melanocytes to make skin darker in colour
Prolactin	Ovary and mammary glands in females	Stimulates milk production in lactating women; increases response of follicles to LH and FSH; has unclear function in men
Posterior pituitary (neurohypophysis)		
Oxytocin	Uterus; mammary glands	Stimulates milk secretion, uterine contractility
Antidiuretic hormone (ADH) or vasopressin	Renal tubules, vascular smooth muscle	Promotes reabsorption of water, vasoconstriction
Thyroid		
Thyroxine (T4)	All body tissues	Precursor to T3
Triiodothyronine (T3)	All body tissues	Regulates metabolic rate of all cells and processes of cell growth and tissue differentiation
Calcitonin	Bone tissue	Regulates calcium and phosphorus blood levels; decreases serum calcium levels
Parathyroids		
Parathyroid hormone (PTH)	Bone, intestine, kidneys	Regulates calcium and phosphorus blood levels; promotes bone demineralisation and increases intestinal absorption of calcium; increases serum calcium levels
Adrenal medulla		
Adrenaline	Sympathetic effectors	Response to stress; enhances and prolongs effects of sympathetic nervous system
Noradrenaline	Sympathetic effectors	Response to stress; enhances and prolongs effects of sympathetic nervous system
Adrenal cortex		
Corticosteroids (e.g. cortisol, hydrocortisone)	All body tissues	Promotes metabolism, response to stress
Androgens (e.g. testosterone, androsterone) and oestrogen	Reproductive organs	Promotes masculinisation in men, growth and sexual activity in women
Mineralocorticoids (e.g. aldosterone)	Kidney	Regulates sodium and potassium balance and thus water balance
Pancreas		
Islets of Langerhans		
Insulin (from beta cells)	General	Promotes movement of glucose out of blood and into cells
Glucagon (from alpha cells)	General	Promotes movement of glucose from glycogen (glycogenolysis) and into blood
Somatostatin	Pancreas	Inhibits insulin and glucagon secretion
Pancreatic polypeptide	General	Influences regulation of pancreatic exocrine function and metabolism of absorbed nutrients

Continued

TABLE 26.1 PRIMARY ENDOCRINE GLANDS AND HORMONES—cont'd

HORMONES	TARGET TISSUE	FUNCTIONS
Gonads		
Women: ovaries Oestrogen	Reproductive system, breasts	Stimulates development of secondary sex characteristics, preparation of uterus for fertilisation and fetal development; stimulates bone growth
Progesterone	Reproductive system	Maintains lining of uterus necessary for successful pregnancy
Men: testes Testosterone	Reproductive system	Stimulates development of secondary sex characteristics, spermatogenesis

FIGURE 26.2 ANATOMY OF THE HYPOTHALAMUS AND PITUITARY[6]

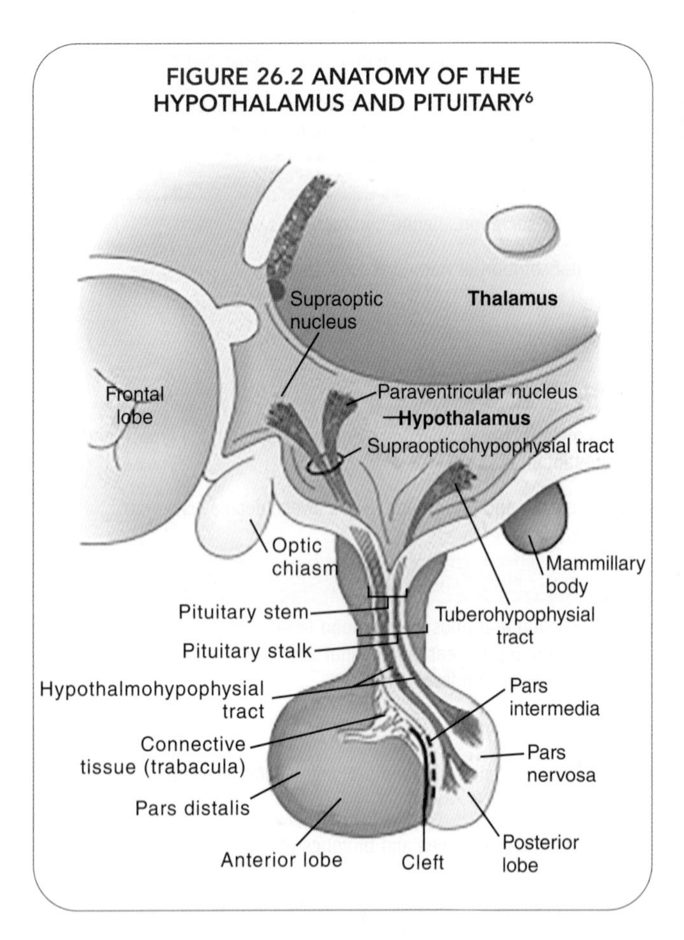

TABLE 26.2 CONTROL CENTRES OF THE HYPOTHALAMUS[7]

Control centre	Effect
POSTERIOR HYPOTHALAMUS	
Posterior hypothalamus	Increased blood pressure; pupillary dilation; shivering
Dorsomedial nucleus	Gastrointestinal stimulation
Perifornical nucleus	Hunger; increased blood pressure; rage
Ventromedial nucleus	Satiety; neuroendocrine control
Mammillary body	Feeding reflexes
Arcuate nucleus and periventricular zone	Neuroendocrine control
Lateral hypothalamic area	Thirst, hunger
ANTERIOR HYPOTHALAMUS	
Paraventricular nucleus	Oxytocin release; water conservation
Medical preoptic area	Bladder contraction; decreased heart rate; decreased blood pressure
Supraoptic nucleus	Vasopressin release
Posterior preoptic and anterior hypothalamic area	Temperature regulation; panting, sweating, thyroid-stimulating hormone

The posterior pituitary consists of neural cells that serve as a supporting structure for nerve fibres and nerve endings, and secretes two hormones into the circulation: antidiuretic hormone (ADH) and oxytocin. Both ADH and oxytocin are produced by the hypothalamus and stored in the pituitary's posterior lobe until required.[3]

THYROID

The thyroid is the largest of the endocrine glands. It is butterfly shaped and positioned just below the larynx, partially surrounding the trachea (Fig. 26.3). It consists of two lobes that lie on either side of the trachea which are connected anteriorly by a broad isthmus.[3] The initiating hormone is thyrotropin-releasing hormone (TRH), which is synthesised and stored in the hypothalamus and released into the hypothalamic–pituitary portal system, circulates to the pituitary and stimulates the release of TSH. TSH stimulates the thyroid gland to produce thyroid hormone, a process that requires iodide. Ninety per cent of thyroid hormone is in the form of thyroxine (T4), and the remainder, triiodothyronine (T3). These hormones are essential for proper growth and development, neurological function and the determination of basal metabolic rate (BMR).[3] Generally, thyroid hormones exert a number of permissive effects on many organs, but abnormally high or low levels can exert pronounced effects.

FIGURE 26.3 THYROID GLAND[8]

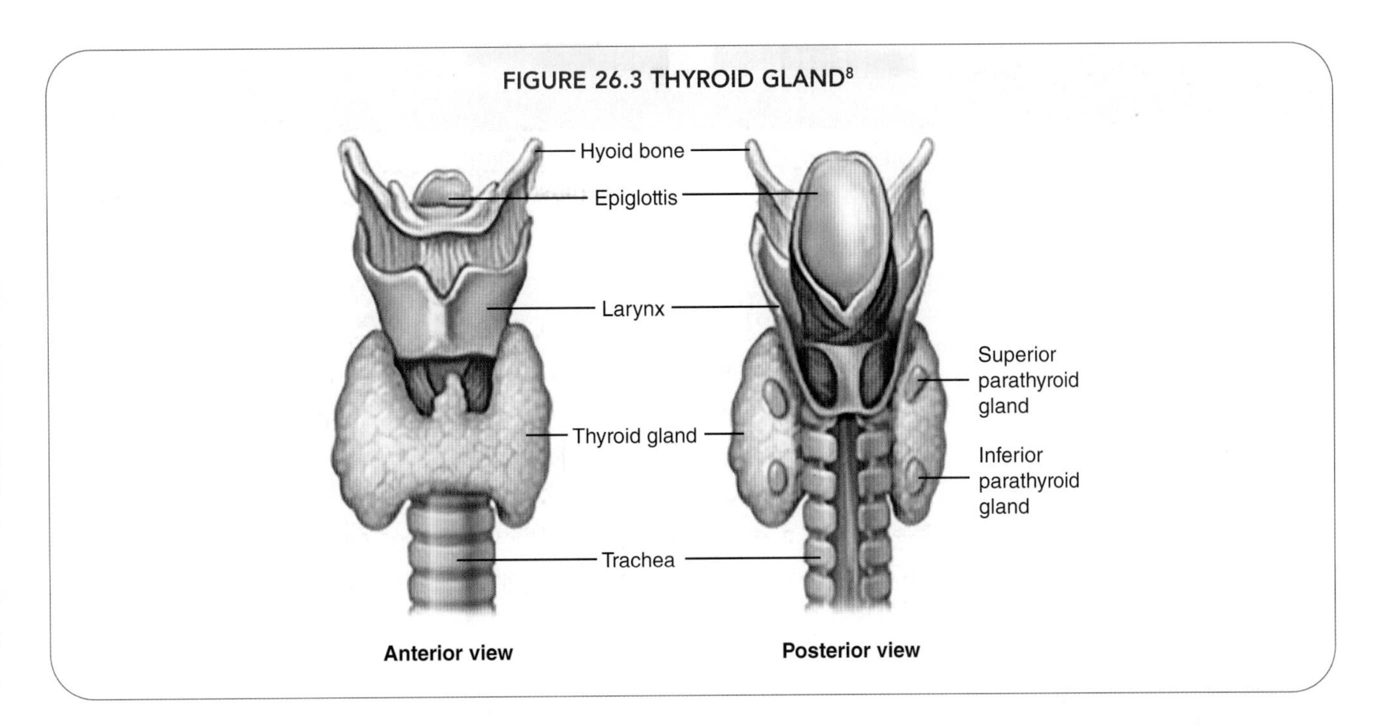

ADRENALS

The adrenal glands (also called the suprarenal glands) are paired organs located in the retroperitoneal area above the upper pole of each kidney and embedded against the muscles of the back in a protective layer of fat. The adrenal glands are generally pyramidal in appearance, measuring approximately 50 mm long, 30 mm wide and 10 mm deep. Like the pituitary, the adrenal glands have dual origins. Each gland consists of an outer cortical layer and an inner medullary layer. Functionally they are two different endocrine tissues, located in the same organ, and each secretes different hormones that are regulated by different control systems.[3]

The bulk of the gland is made up by the *adrenal cortex*, which is divided into three zones—outer zona glomerulosa, intermediate zona fasciculata and inner zona reticularis. The adrenal cortex secretes more than 50 steroid hormones, classified as glucocorticoids, mineralocorticoids and androgens.[3] Cortisol, the most abundant glucocorticoid, is necessary for the maintenance of life and protection from stress. With a half-life of approximately 90 minutes, cortisol increases BGLs through the promotion of hepatic gluconeogenesis by facilitating conversion of amino acids to glucose and inhibiting protein synthesis.[9] High levels of aldosterone have been associated with hypertension, atherosclerosis and heart failure.[10] Aldosterone is a potent mineralocorticoid that maintains extracellular fluid volume, regulated primarily by the renin–angiotensin–aldosterone system to alter serum sodium levels.

The *adrenal medulla* is composed of tightly packed clusters of cells, innervated by sympathetic neurons that are arranged around blood vessels. Impulses are initiated from the hypothalamus via the spinal cord when the sympathetic division of the autonomic nervous system (ANS) is stimulated. The cells of the medulla secrete the catecholamines adrenaline and noradrenaline in a ratio of approximately 4:1. Approximately 30% of adrenaline is secreted from the adrenal medulla; the remainder comes from nerve terminals. Adrenaline is up to ten times more potent than noradrenaline, although the latter has a longer duration of action.[3,4] Once released, catecholamines remain in the plasma for a very short duration, just several seconds, but result in increased cardiac output and heart rate, dilated coronary blood vessels, increased mental alertness, increased respiratory rate and elevated metabolic rate. Activation of the adrenal medulla, together with sympathetic division of the ANS, prepares the body for greater physical performance, the 'fight or flight' response.

Excessive stimulation of the adrenal medulla can result in depletion of the body's energy reserves and a high level of corticosteroid secretion from the adrenal cortex, which can significantly impair the immune system. The major functions of catecholamines are summarised in Table 26.3.

PANCREAS

The pancreas, a soft lobular gland, is situated behind the stomach and anterior to the first and second lumbar vertebrae, in the retroperitoneal space. The body of the pancreas extends horizontally across the abdominal wall, with the head in the curve of the abdomen and the tail touching the spleen. It is a soft, lobular gland (Fig. 26.4).[11,12] The pancreas has both endocrine and exocrine functions. Acini are exocrine cells that release amylase, lipase and other enzymes that aid digestion. The endocrine portion of the pancreas consists of scattered clusters of cells called the pancreatic islets, or islets of Langerhans. The islets account for less than 2% of the gland and consist of three types of hormone-secreting cells that produce hormones responsible for serum glucose regulation. Alpha cells produce and secrete glucagon, beta cells produce and secrete insulin and delta cells secrete somatostatin, which inhibits glucagon and insulin release.

Insulin, synthesised from the precursor proinsulin, is stimulated by increased serum glucose levels, amino acids arginine and lysine, serum free-fatty acids and parasympathetic stimulation.

TABLE 26.3 CATECHOLAMINE FUNCTIONS[7]

CLASS AND FUNCTION	ALPHA-ADRENERGIC	BETA-ADRENERGIC	DOPAMINERGIC
Agonist	Noradrenaline	Adrenaline	Dopamine
Antagonist	Phentolamine	Propranolol	Haloperidol
Actions			
Cardiac	Contracts	Inotropic and chronotropic	Inotropic
Smooth muscle		Relaxes	Mixed
Metabolic		Lipolysis Glycogenolysis Gluconeogenesis	
Molecular	Decreases cAMP	Increases cAMP	Increases cAMP

cAMP: cyclic adenosine monophosphate; this is a second messenger and regulates the effects of adrenaline and glucagon.

FIGURE 26.4 THE PANCREAS AND SURROUNDING STRUCTURES[11]

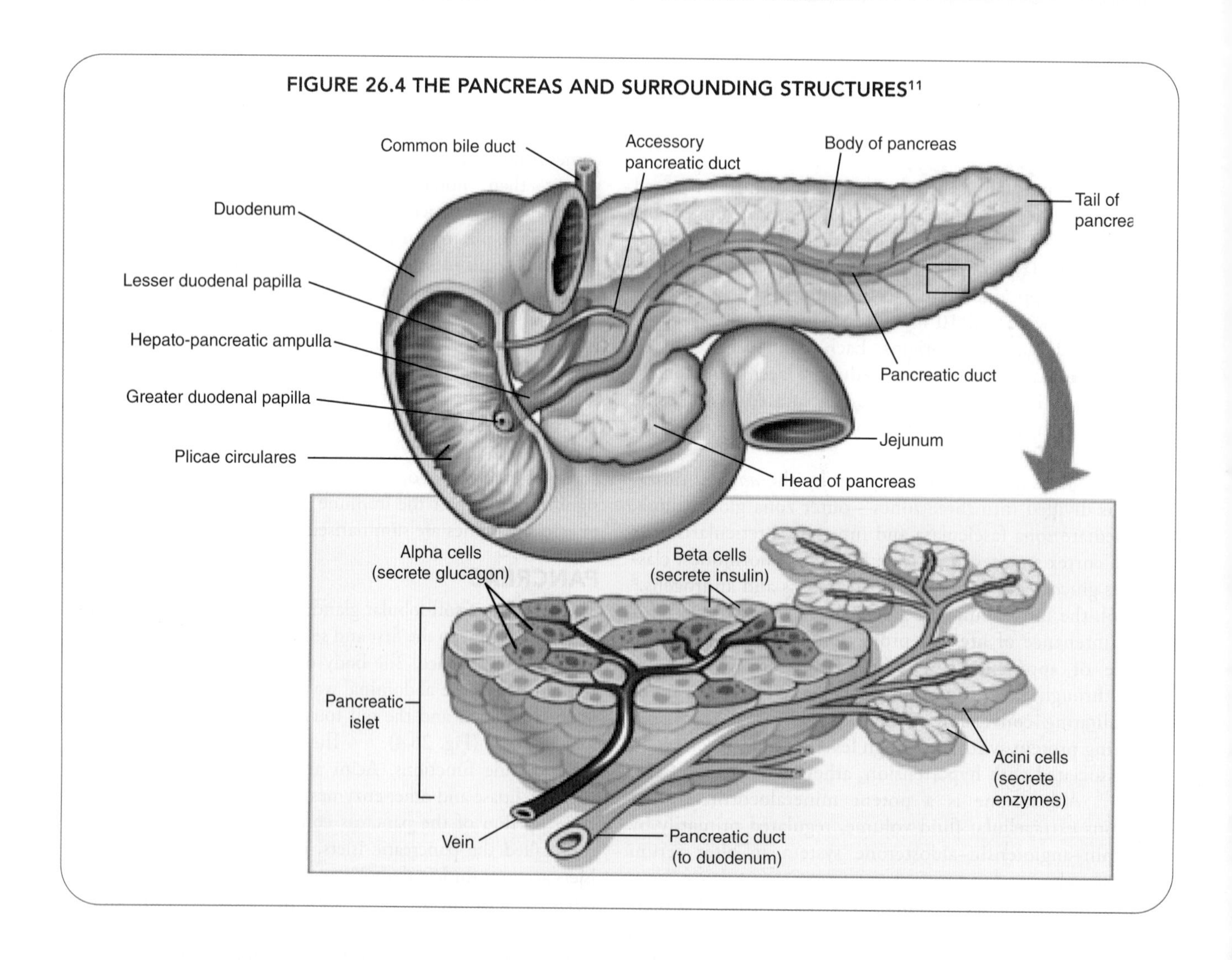

Conversely, insulin secretion reduces in response to low serum glucose, high levels of insulin through the beta-cell negative feedback system and sympathetic stimulation. An anabolic steroid, the primary role of insulin is to facilitate glucose uptake into cells, along with promoting synthesis of proteins, lipids and nucleic acids and resulting in increased metabolism (Table 26.4).[5,13]

Glucagon acts primarily on the liver, stimulating glycogenolysis and gluconeogenesis in response to hypoglycaemia, resulting in increased blood glucose.

TABLE 26.4 ACTION OF INSULIN[3]

ACTION	SITE OF INSULIN PROMOTED SYNTHESIS LIVER	ADIPOSE TISSUE	MUSCLE
Glucose uptake	Increased	Increased	Increased
Glycogenesis	Increased	-	Increased
Glycogenolysis	Decreased	-	Decreased
Glycolysis	Increased	Increased	Increased
Gluconeogenesis	Increased	-	-
Other	• Increased fatty acid synthesis • Decreased ketogenesis • Decreased urea cycle activity	• Increased fat esterification • Decreased lipolysis • Increased fat storage	• Increased amino acid uptake • Increased protein synthesis • Decreased proteolysis

DIABETES

Diabetes is a chronic disease caused by relative or absolute insulin insufficiency. Diabetes is the fastest growing chronic condition in Australia, with 280 people developing diabetes every day; that is, approximately 100,000 Australians developing diabetes every year. Almost 1.3 million Australians currently have diagnosed diabetes. This includes: type 1 diabetes (9% of all diabetes), type 2 diabetes (87% of all diabetes and rising), gestational diabetes (3%) and non-specific causes (<1%). Indigenous Australians are four times more likely to have type 2 diabetes compared with non-Indigenous Australians.[14] In 2017, 10% of all hospital admissions in Australia were associated with diabetes, and 1 in 10 deaths had diabetes as an underlying or associated cause of death.[10,14–18]

Diabetes is a group of chronic metabolic disorders resulting in elevated BGLs. This metabolic disorder disturbs the body's capacity to utilise glucose, fat and protein due to insulin deficiency or resistance. Diabetes occurs due to an absolute or relative lack of the hormone insulin. This is caused by the pancreas not producing enough insulin or cells of the body not responding to the insulin that is produced. There is currently no cure for diabetes and the condition requires lifelong management.[10,14–18]

Type 1 diabetes is characterised by destruction of insulin-producing beta cells caused by an autoimmune abnormality. Onset is usually rapid, although latent autoimmune diabetes (LADA) is a more slowly progressive autoimmune diabetes in adults. The exact cause of type 1 diabetes remains unknown and incidence has a strong family link. Type 2 diabetes is the most common form of diabetes in Australia.[13,14,16,17] Traditionally, type 2 diabetes has been associated with later adulthood, although the incidence is increasing in children. Type 2 diabetes may range from predominant insulin resistance to a predominant insulin secretory defect, with or without insulin resistance. Gestational diabetes refers to glucose intolerance with onset during pregnancy. Between 3% and 8% of pregnant women develop gestational diabetes around the 24th to 28th week of pregnancy. Women who develop gestational diabetes are at higher risk of developing type 2 diabetes.[14,17]

Other specific and less-common types of type 2 diabetes include:

- genetic defects of beta-cell function (e.g. MODY1–MODY6 sulfonylurea receptor (KCNJ11) genes)
- genetic defects in insulin action (e.g. type A insulin resistance and leprechaunism)
- diseases of the exocrine pancreas (e.g. pancreatitis, cystic fibrosis, haemochromatosis); endocrinopathies (e.g. Cushing's syndrome)
- drug-induced or chemical-induced diabetes (e.g. glucocorticoids)
- infections (e.g. congenital rubella, cytomegalovirus)
- uncommon but specific forms of immune-mediated diabetes (e.g. 'stiff-man' syndrome and anti-insulin-receptor antibodies)
- other genetic syndromes sometimes associated with diabetes (e.g. Down syndrome, Wolfram syndrome, Turner's syndrome and myotonic dystrophy).[5,19]

DIABETIC KETOACIDOSIS

Diabetic ketoacidosis (DKA) is an acute, life-threatening condition characterised by hyperglycaemia (blood glucose > 11 mmol/L) the presence of ketones in urine or blood (capillary ketones > 1.5) and acidosis (blood pH < 7.3 or HCO_3^- < 16). It has long been assumed that DKA is pathognomic of type 1 diabetes with most presentations occurring in individuals with type 1 disease. However, it is now recognised that it can also occur in type 2 diabetes, pregnancy and patients on certain oral glucose-lowering drugs, such as SGLT2 inhibitors (sodium-glucose co-transporter 2 inhibitors)[8,14,17,19] It occurs in 20–30% of all new-onset presentations of diabetes; therefore, acute presentation often results in a diagnosis of diabetes.[14,17] As a single episode, DKA is associated with a 5.2% risk of death within 4 years of follow-up, and for those with recurrent DKA admissions, the risk of death within 2 years is 23.4%.[18] Seventy per cent of diabetes-related deaths in children are attributed to DKA.

Hyperglycaemia is a result of severe insulin deficiency, either absolute or relative, which impairs peripheral glucose uptake and promotes fat breakdown. Relative glucagon excess promotes hepatic gluconeogenesis. Overall, metabolism in DKA shifts from the normal fed state characterised by carbohydrate metabolism to a fasting state characterised by fat metabolism (Fig. 26.5). Secondary consequences of the primary metabolic

FIGURE 26.5 PATHOPHYSIOLOGY OF DIABETES KETOACIDOSIS

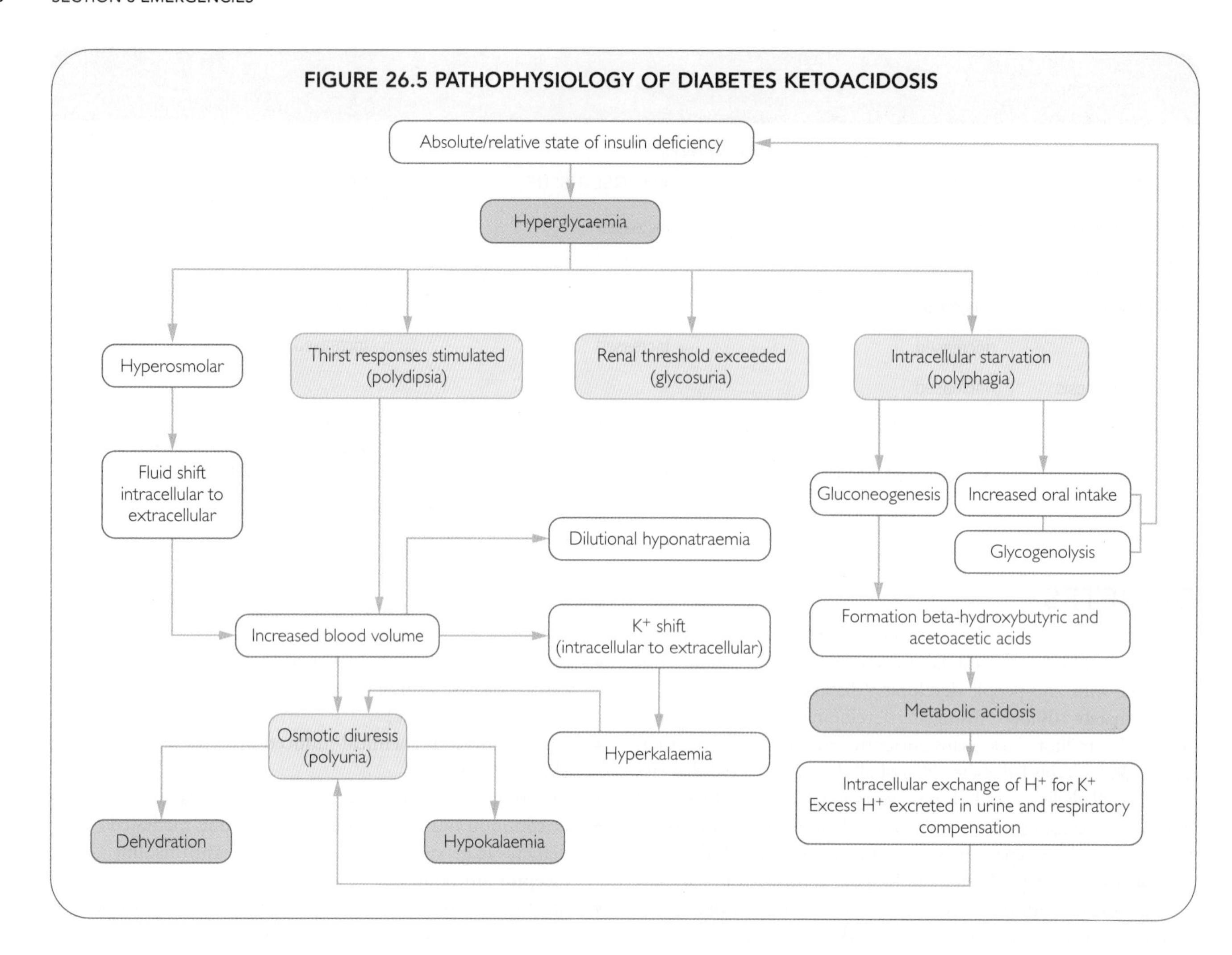

derangements include ketosis, caused by a switch to fat metabolism, leading to free fatty acid oxidation in the liver. As a result, the ketone bodies acetoacetic acid and 3-hydroxybutyric acid are formed. The dissociation of the ketone bodies (weak acids) results in acidosis due to depletion of extracellular and cellular buffers. Because of hyperglycaemic state, the renal threshold is surpassed and glucose is secreted in the urine, known as osmotic diuresis. This hyperglycaemia-induced osmotic diuresis depletes sodium, potassium, phosphates and water, as well as ketones and glucose, resulting in absolute dehydration and electrolyte depletion.

PRACTICE TIP

DIABETIC KETOACIDOSIS (DKA)

- DKA is a serious medical problem in patients with diabetes.
- Reducing the occurrence and severity of DKA depends on early detection of elevated serum blood ketones.
- All people with diabetes should test for ketones during acute illness, stress, when BGLs are consistently elevated, during pregnancy or when there are symptoms suggestive of ketoacidosis, e.g. nausea, vomiting, abdominal pain, excessive thirst, polyuria.
- The focus of management of DKA is glucose control.
- Treatment is directed at reducing ketones as the presence of ketones indicates an ongoing disturbance of glucose metabolism. Hence, an insulin infusion should be maintained until there is biochemical evidence that ketoacidosis has resolved.
- The most common mistake is to reduce the rate of insulin as the blood glucose falls before the acidosis is reversed.
- It can take up to 24 hours to reverse ketoacidosis. This is evidenced by normal pH, HCO_3^- and blood ketones < 0.5 mmol.
- Never cease insulin completely. The patient will be commenced on subcutaneous insulin and then the infusion ceased when ketoacidosis is reversed, plasma glucose levels are stable, and patient is tolerating oral fluids/diet.
- Identify, assess and manage precipitating factors, e.g. infection, acute coronary syndromes, non-adherence to insulin.

Clinical features

Diabetic ketoacidosis (DKA) tends to occur in young, type 1 diabetes patients and although symptoms may be present for several days, the presentation of DKA is usually rapid and

TABLE 26.5 CLINICAL MANIFESTATIONS OF DIABETIC KETOACIDOSIS (DKA) AND HYPERGLYCAEMIC HYPEROSMOLAR SYNDROME (HHS)[9,22,23]

SYSTEM	CLINICAL MANIFESTATIONS	
	DKA	HHS
Neurological	Lethargy, malaise and fatigue, gradually increasing restlessness and confusion; coma in extreme cases	Weakness, lethargy, drowsiness, delirium, visual changes, hemiparesis, sensory deficits, coma, seizures
Respiratory	Tachypnoea, Kussmaul's respirations, fruity acetone (ketone) breath, shortness of breath	
Cardiovascular	Tachycardia, hypotension, dysrhythmias, sunken eyes, weak pulse	Tachycardia, hypovolemia, dehydration (profound), hypotension, hypoperfusion
Integumentary	Flushed dry skin, dry mucous membranes, poor skin turgor,	Dry mucous membranes, poor skin turgor
Renal	Thirst, dry mouth, polyuria, ketonuria, glycosuria, polyuria, polydipsia	Polyuria, polydipsia
Gastrointestinal	Nausea, vomiting, anorexia, abdominal cramps or pain, polyphagia	Nausea, vomiting, abdominal pain (uncommon)
Other	Rapid weight loss, fever if infection, hypothermia (late)	Weight loss, fever if infection, hypothermia, muscle cramps

predictable. DKA may be precipitated by factors that result in increased circulating levels of stress hormones, such as adrenaline, growth hormone and cortisol, and the resulting increase in insulin resistance reduces the effectiveness of any residual insulin production or exogenous (injected) insulin. Examples of precipitating causes may include infection, acute coronary syndromes, cerebrovascular causes, influenza, surgical emergencies, cocaine use or stress.[20,21] These conditions often present with their own complex set of signs and symptoms, and therefore the possibility of DKA always needs to be considered in any diabetic patient presenting with any of the potential triggers listed above. Additionally, errors of insulin administration or manipulation with insulin treatment may be the precipitant of an acute DKA episode.[20,21]

After prolonged insulin deficiency, hyperglycaemia leads to thirst, polyuria, dehydration, electrolyte depletion and metabolic acidosis. Patients with DKA often complain of non-specific symptoms such as malaise and fatigue. Nausea, vomiting and abdominal pain are common and although it is not fully understood why these symptoms occur, it is thought to be the result of delayed gastric emptying, ileus, subacute pancreatitis, oesophagitis with ulceration or bowel ischemia.[21]

Physical signs include evidence of dehydration, such as tachycardia; hypotension may be the result of volume depletion, sepsis or both. Additionally, skin examination may reveal diminished skin turgor and dry mucous membranes due to dehydration. The most frequent cardiac rhythm is sinus tachycardia; however, dysrhythmias can occur secondary to electrolyte disturbances. Patients may also be tachypnoeic with Kussmaul's respirations and a fruity odour on their breath as a result of exhaled acetone.[18,20] The clinical features of DKA are summarised in Table 26.5.

Assessment and diagnosis

The first priority is to establish the severity of the presenting problem and hence the need for immediate intervention. The initial clinical examination, beginning with a primary survey, assesses the potential or actual threat to Airway, Breathing, Circulation and Disability. Interventions may need to be initiated if these parameters are compromised to ensure life-threatening conditions are identified first and treated. A focused secondary assessment then follows, usually directed by the presenting problem.

In determining the severity of the patient's illness and the need for intervention, it is important to determine the history of the presenting illness. Most patients presenting with DKA have a known history of diabetes, making differential diagnosis uncomplicated. However, as patients may also have signs and symptoms related to the precipitant factor, or trigger, of the DKA, laboratory tests will be needed to confirm DKA. The signs and symptoms may develop rapidly, but there is usually a history of being unwell for days, predominantly with gastrointestinal symptoms, such as vomiting, excessive thirst or urination and abdominal pain. In more advanced stages the patient may be confused or obtunded (lethargic). The patient's breathing pattern may be described as deep and rapid, referred to as Kussmaul's respirations with a distinctive 'sweet-smelling' odour. Dehydration, occasionally associated with hypotension, tachycardia and delayed capillary refill, may also be present. There may also be excessive urinary output resulting in significant weight loss (up to 5 kg/week).

In patients with the above presentation, bedside testing of capillary blood glucose and ketone (beta-hydroxybutyrate) levels using point-of-care testing will confirm the diagnosis of DKA (see Chapter 16 for information on blood glucose testing techniques). A diligent search for the precipitant is also essential. These causes may include infection, cessation of insulin, trauma or acute coronary syndromes (STEMI may be painless), to name a few. Other initial investigations that may assist diagnosis include urinalysis, electrocardiogram, point-of-care pathology and imaging (ultrasound).

Laboratory investigations

Laboratory tests should be obtained as early as possible. Diagnosis of DKA is confirmed in the presence of four clinical features:

1. Hyperglycaemia with serum glucose higher than 11 mmol/L
2. Ketones in urine or blood (capillary beta-hydroxybutyrate [blood ketones] > 1.5 mmol/L)
3. Metabolic acidosis with pH < 7.3 (or HCO_3^- <16)
4. Dehydration.[19,24]

Other possible laboratory findings are summarised in Table 26.6.

Patient management

While DKA generally requires specialist treatment, early assessment and initial treatments should commence as soon as possible in the pre-hospital setting. Once initial treatments have been commenced, endocrinology support and advice should be sought early. If a personal insulin pump is in situ, the pump must be stopped and disconnected before commencing treatment. Patients receiving intravenous insulin infusions need to be nursed in an intensive care or similar specialist unit as intravenous insulin infusions require intensive nursing resources and are potentially dangerous.

While most institutions have DKA management protocols to guide overall management, the generally agreed principles of DKA management are to:

- correct fluid depletion
- decrease BGL
- correct electrolyte imbalance; and
- treat the precipitating causes.[19,24,25]

To ensure efficacy and safety of treatments, patients with DKA will require close monitoring of clinical and metabolic status to monitor response to treatments and recognise changes to the patient's condition. For example, the onset of headaches or decreased level of consciousness may indicate the development of cerebral oedema and the need for more focused assessment and interventions in such patients.

Fluid depletion

Intravascular fluid depletion in adults with DKA can be significant. In the absence of heart failure, the fluid of choice in the resuscitation phase is sodium chloride 0.9%. If the patient is hypotensive (systolic blood pressure below 90 mmHg or heart rate > 120/minute), 1 L sodium chloride 0.9% is given intravenously while requesting senior medical review.[19] This rehydration therapy can be commenced by pre-hospital responders when treating adult patients. When the systolic blood pressure is above 90 mmHg, fluid replacement for people of average weight is 1000 mL within the first hour. Fluids should then be reduced to 1000 mL over 2 hours for 2 consecutive hours and, after that, titrated to maintain adequate blood pressure, pulse rate, urinary output and mental status. Correcting intravascular dehydration will reduce plasma osmolarity and BGLs. Care needs to be taken in cases of younger patients with DKA as rapid fluid infusion may result in cerebral oedema, which has a high mortality rate. For this reason, many pre-hospital guidelines do not advocate this therapy. As a guide, the aim should be to reduce serum osmolarity not more than 3 mOsm/L/hr or decrease sodium concentration by less than 1 mmol/hr to avoid potential cerebral oedema due to large fluid shifts. Additionally, if serum sodium rises above 155 mmol/L, switching to 0.45% sodium chloride may need to be considered, although the optimal time to use 0.45% sodium chloride remains uncertain.[26]

Many DKA protocols will recommend commencing glucose (5% dextrose) at 80–120 mL/h to prevent hypoglycaemia

TABLE 26.6 LABORATORY FINDINGS IN DIABETIC KETOACIDOSIS (DKA)[7]

LABORATORY ASSESSMENT	POSSIBLE FINDING	CLINICAL RELEVANCE
Sodium	For each 5.5 mmol/L increase in glucose from normal, serum sodium is lowered by 1.6 mmol/L	Increased sodium results from extravascular water movement to intervascular space due to the osmotic effect of hyperglycaemia.
Potassium	Initial serum potassium levels may be normal or slightly elevated	Potassium levels can rapidly decrease after commencement of insulin as potassium moves into the cells.
Beta-hydroxybutyrate	Levels greater than 0.5 mmol/L are considered abnormal, and levels of 3 mmol/L correlate with need for DKA treatment	Beta-hydroxybutyrate, the more common ketone body, is not detected by Ketostix. Serum or capillary beta-hydroxybutyrate can be used to follow response to treatment.
Osmolality	Blood levels may be increased due to intravascular dehydration	DKA patients who are comatose typically have values > 330 mOsm/kg. If the osmolality is less than this in a patient who is comatose, other causes of obtundation should be investigated.
Amylase	Hyperamylasaemia	Hyperamylasaemia may be seen even in absence of pancreatitis. It is not understood why this occurs, but it occurs in up to 75% of patients with DKA.
White cell count	Elevated white cell count > 15 × 10^9/L	Elevated white cell count may suggest underlying infection or response to stress.
Urea and creatinine	Elevated	Serum levels may be elevated due to dehydration.

when BGLs approach 15 mmol/L.[24] The glucose rate is adjusted to achieve a target BGL of 10–15 mmol/L in the first 12 hours. Thereafter glucose rate should be adjusted to achieve a BGL of 5–10 mmol/L. Occasionally 10% glucose may be needed. Normal saline will be continued if hydration status requires.

Blood glucose level (BGL)

Intravenous insulin will lower blood glucose concentration through increased glucose utilisation in peripheral tissues and a decrease in hepatic glucose production. Insulin will result in decreased ketone release, thereby correcting metabolic acidosis. Initial commencement of insulin infusion at a rate of approximately 5 units/hour (or 0.1 units/kg/h) is generally recommended to encourage a steady fall in BGLs. However, infusions may need to be increased if initial rates do not reduce BGLs after 2–3 hours. The treatment targets include the following; ketones decreasing by 0.5 mmol/L/hr, HCO_3 increasing by 3.0 mmol/L/hr and blood glucose decreasing by 3.0 mmol/L/hr. It is imperative that insulin therapy is continued until ketonaemia is resolved.[25]

BGLs should be monitored at least hourly, with the aim to prevent them falling below 10 mmol/L, and 5% dextrose should be added to the fluid replacement regimen once BGLs approach 12–15 mmol/L.[25] It is recommended that a mechanical pump or syringe driver is used to deliver the infusion. All intravenous tubing must be flushed with the prepared insulin solution prior to patient administration to ensure tubing is coated with insulin solution as insulin adheres to the tubing.[19]

The transition from intravenous insulin to subcutaneous injections is usually considered once glucose level is < 11 mmol/L, serum bicarbonate level > 18 mmol/L, venous pH > 7.30 and the patient has been eating and drinking for at least 24 hours. Normal diet should be resumed prior to ceasing the infusion. The subcutaneous insulin or oral hyperglycaemic medication is given with the next meal. An overlap time between the intravenous and subcutaneous insulin will be allowed depending on the type of insulin.

Electrolyte imbalance

Total body depletion of potassium can occur in DKA, despite initial normal or slightly elevated serum levels (Table 26.6). To prevent acute hypokalaemia with fluid and insulin therapy, potassium replacement should be considered once the patient's serum levels are known and adequate renal output established. No insulin infusions should be commenced until K^+ is > 3.5 mmol/L as insulin will lower the K^+. The aim is to maintain serum potassium levels between 4 and 5 mmol/L. Most DKA protocols will advocate commencing potassium replacement at a rate of 20 mmol/hr if potassium levels are < 3.5 mmol/L, adjusted in the succeeding hours to a replacement rate of 10 mmol/h to maintain a serum potassium level of 3.5–5.5 mmol/L.[19] The potassium infusion may be ceased when the patient's serum potassium is > 5.5 mmol/L.

While there are many slight variations on how to replace potassium, initial and 2-hourly monitoring of serum potassium and continuous cardiac monitoring is required during the resuscitation and treatment phases of DKA management. An example guide to potassium replacement is presented in Box 26.1.

BOX 26.1 POTASSIUM REPLACEMENT GUIDELINE

- **Serum potassium < 3 mmol/L, consider potassium 30–40 mmol/hour**
- **Serum potassium 3 to 4 mmol/L, consider potassium 20–30 mmol/hour**
- **Serum potassium 4 to 5 mmol/L, consider potassium 10 mmol/hour**
- **Serum potassium > 5 mmol/L, cease potassium infusion**

The clinical benefit of bicarbonate replacement in patients with initial metabolic acidosis remains controversial. However, in patients with severe acidosis (i.e. pH < 7), infusion of sodium bicarbonate may be considered, but only after consultation with an endocrinologist when pH is < 7.0 and the HCO_3^- is < 5.[21,25] An urgent referral to an endocrinologist is required before commencing a sodium bicarbonate infusion.

Although serum phosphate depletion is frequently observed in patients with DKA, replacement is not routinely recommended, with no clear benefit and a potential increased risk of hypocalcaemia and hypomagnesaemia. Serum phosphate level is often normal at presentation and may decrease with insulin therapy. Phosphate replacement may be considered necessary in patients with cardiac dysfunction, anaemia or respiratory depression if their serum phosphate level is less than 0.32 mmol/L. Replacement in such circumstances may consist of 20–30 mmol potassium dihydrogen phosphate in intravenous fluids over 4 hours.[25] In less urgent circumstances, if phosphate replacement is considered necessary, oral supplementation may be appropriate.

Paramedics may be confronted by patients in a poor conscious state presenting with hyperventilation to produce compensatory respiratory alkalosis. Some intensive care paramedic guidelines may allow for drug-facilitated intubation to assist with airway protection and ventilation maintenance. See Chapter 16 for intubation techniques. In such instances, the preservation of the compensatory alkalosis is imperative with end-tidal carbon dioxide values determined before any therapy is provided.

Investigate and treat precipitating cause

Identification of the precipitating cause is important both to prevent further occurrence and if appropriate to treat confounding illness. This will involve the following investigations:

- venous blood gases; arterial blood gases (if hypoxic) (see Chapter 16 for techniques)
- electrolytes (Ca, Mg, PO_4, urea, creatinine, osmolality)
- liver function tests, amylase, lipase
- lactate
- electrocardiograph (ECG) and troponin blood levels
- septic screen (blood cultures, CRP, chest x-ray, urine culture, wound swab)
- pregnancy test in females of childbearing age
- serum cortisol, if adrenal insufficiency is considered
- alcohol and drug screen, if drug use is suspected because acidosis will not resolve.

Co-existing illness, such as pelvic or rectal abscess, pneumonia and acute coronary syndrome should be excluded. Special concern exists in the pregnant woman presenting with DKA. The fetal mortality rate may be as high as 30% and up to 60% with ketoacidosis coma. Fetal death mainly occurs in women with overt diabetes, but may occur in gestational diabetes.[21]

PRACTICE TIP

MANAGEMENT OF DIABETIC KETOACIDOSIS

- Clinicians should be alert to altered mental status, especially in children with DKA, as this may indicate impending cerebral oedema.
- Keep the patient nil by mouth until ketonaemia has resolved.
- Insulin initially binds to plastic tubing. A priming and flushing procedure saturates the binding sites along the plastic tubing. To ensure the delivery of a stable insulin dose, prime the line with the insulin/intravenous solution. Leave for a minimum of 1 minute and then flush the solution from the tubing (4 mL), replacing it with fresh solution prior to commencing the infusion.
- Failure of the blood ketones to fall by 1 mmol/L, or BGL to fall by > 4 mmol/L after 2 hours of initial treatment with insulin therapy and fluids is a red flag. This may indicate that the insulin infusion line was not primed, or the patient is not responding to treatment correctly, and thus requires immediate medical assessment.
- Common errors in treatment include reducing the insulin infusion inappropriately, replacing potassium inadequately, failing to start glucose when BGL reaches 15 mmol/L, delay in identifying or treating the precipitating cause and too rapid a fall in glucose causing cerebral oedema.

HYPERGLYCAEMIC HYPEROSMOLAR SYNDROME

Hyperglycaemia hyperosmolar state (HHS) is a metabolic disorder that occurs in diabetes, sometimes as the initial presentation. It is characterised by hyperglycaemia, hyperosmolality and profound dehydration without significant ketoacidosis.

The HHS state occurs in type 2 diabetes and has a gradual onset occurring over several weeks, not days. Patients presenting with HHS typically have an underlying medical condition exacerbating often undiagnosed type 2 diabetes. Traditionally, patients presenting with HHS are middle-aged or elderly, but awareness of increased reports of type 2 diabetes in younger adults and children make presentations in these groups possible. Precipitating factors include infection (may be occult), acute coronary syndromes, pancreatitis, stroke or drugs (glucocorticoids, sympathomimetics, antipsychotics). A mixed picture of DKA and HHS may also occur.

It is associated with a 5–10% mortality rate, largely due to the age of the patient, their comorbidities, the precipitating illness and thromboembolic problems (Fig. 26.6). In the HHS state, BGLs rise slowly, and patients become progressively unwell. In most cases, sufficient insulin exists to prevent ketone formation and therefore metabolic acidosis is normally not present, except in extreme cases.[27]

CLINICAL FEATURES

Patients with HHS are dehydrated and clinically unwell, with marked hyperglycaemia (> 33 mmol/L) without significant hyperketonaemia (< 3.0 mmol/L) or acidosis (pH > 7.3, bicarbonate > 15 mmol/L). Serum osmolality levels are significantly elevated, in the region of 320 mOsm/kg or greater.

Differentiation between HHS and DKA may be difficult initially (Table 26.7). However, the treatment approach initially is similar to DKA, with a few modifications. When treating HHS, the emphasis is primarily on fluid replacement with supportive glucose control. The management of potassium and supportive treatments is the same as DKA.

For many presenting with HHS, this may be their first diagnosis with type 2 diabetes and therefore the diabetes team should be alerted early and involved in the patient's ongoing and future care.

Laboratory investigations

Important biochemical concepts need to be considered when interpreting laboratory results for patients with HSS. The first is the concept of sodium correction for hyperglycaemia. Sodium correction is required because sodium levels fall with hyperglycaemia and rise with lowering glucose due to osmotic shifts of water from the intravascular space. To calculate the 'true' sodium the following formula is used:

$$\text{Sodium (corrected)} = \text{Sodium (measured)} + (\text{blood glucose level}/4).$$

The second concept is that of calculated osmolality. The osmoregulatory mechanisms that adjust water balance are impaired in HSS due to hyperglycaemia. When hyperglycaemia occurs, the extracellular fluid osmolality rises because glucose entry into the cell is limited. Calculated osmolality is done using the following formula:

$$\text{Calculated osmolality} = 2 \times \text{sodium} + \text{urea} + \text{glucose (all measured in mmol/L)}$$

Diagnosis of HSS is confirmed in the presence of the following parameters:

1. Hyperglycaemia with serum glucose higher than 33 mmol/L without significant hyperketonaemia or acidosis
2. Bicarbonate greater than 15 mmol/L
3. Serum osmolality greater than 320 mOsm/kg.[19,24]

Other possible laboratory findings are summarised in Table 26.6.

Patient management

While most institutions have HHS management protocols, the generally agreed principles of management are to:

- normalise osmolarity
- restore euglycaemia
- prevent complications; and treat precipitants' causes.[19,24,25]

Patients with HSS require careful monitoring of clinical and metabolic status due to the age of the patients, their comorbidities, the precipitating illness and thromboembolic complications.

Fluid depletion

Patients with HHS require consideration of total body water deficit to guide fluid replacement. This is calculated using the formula: 0.6 × weight × (–140/serum sodium). Half of the predicted fluid deficit is replaced in the first 24 hours and the remainder over the next 12–36 hours. The clinical goal

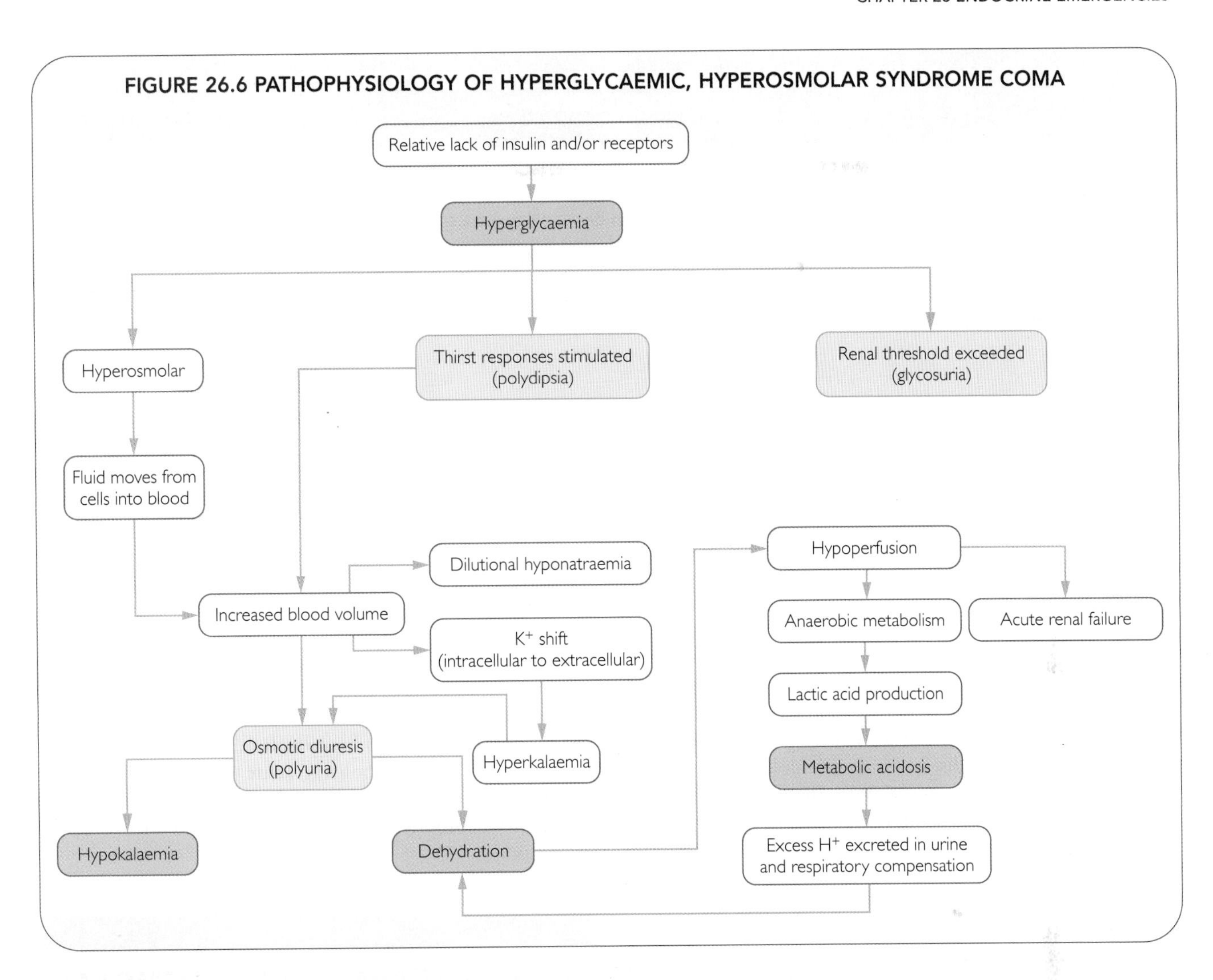

TABLE 26.7 COMPARISON OF HYPERGLYCAEMIC HYPEROSMOLAR SYNDROME (HHS) AND DIABETIC KETOACIDOSIS (DKA)[23]

CLINICAL PICTURE	HHS	DKA
General	Severe dehydrated, less acidotic	More acidotic and less dehydrated
	Frequently comatose	Rarely comatose
	No hyperventilation	Hyperventilation
Age frequency	Usually elderly	Younger patients
Type of diabetes mellitus	Type 2 or non-insulin-dependent	Type 1 or insulin-dependent
Previous history of diabetes mellitus	In only 50%	Almost always
Prodromes	Several days to weeks duration	Days duration
Neurological symptoms and signs	Very common	Rare
Underlying renal or cardiovascular disease	About 85%	About 15%
Laboratory findings		
Blood glucose	> 33 mmol/L	> 11 mmol/L
Capillary or serum ketones	< 3 mmol/L	> 1.5 mmol/L

Continued

TABLE 26.7 COMPARISON OF HYPERGLYCAEMIC HYPEROSMOLAR SYNDROME (HHS) AND DIABETIC KETOACIDOSIS (DKA)—cont'd

CLINICAL PICTURE	HHS	DKA
Serum sodium	Variable—usually low; can be normal or elevated	Usually low
Serum potassium	Normal or elevated (usual); can be decreased in severe cases	Variable—elevated (usual), normal or low
Serum bicarbonate	> 18 mmol/L	< 10 mmol/L
Anion gap	0-15 mEq/L	> 15 mEq/L
Blood pH	> 7.30	< 7.30
Osmolality (calculated)	High; usually ≥ 320 mmol/kg	Variable
Complications		
Thrombosis	Frequent	Very rare
Mortality	20-50%	1-10%
Diabetes treatment after recovery	Diet alone or oral agents (sometimes insulin)	Always insulin

should be to achieve a 2–3 L positive fluid balance by 6 hours. A central line is recommended for elderly patients and those with renal and cardiac disease to assist fluid and electrolyte management after initial resuscitation. The fluid of choice in the resuscitation phase is sodium chloride 0.9%. Hypotonic saline (0.45%) is only indicated if (calculated) serum osmolality is not declining despite adequate positive fluid balance.

Blood glucose levels (BGL)

BGLs must be reduced slowly to prevent extreme osmotic shifts. It will improve with rehydration. Insulin therapy is indicated if blood ketones are > 1 mmol/L. Commence insulin infusion (Actrapid®) at a rate of 0.05 units/kg/hr or if the BGL is not falling after initial rehydration. It is recommended to encourage a steady fall in BGL by no more than 4 mmol/L/hr. However, reduce insulin rate if BGL falls by > 4 mmol/hr or BGL reaches 15 mmol/L.

With the aim to prevent levels falling too rapidly, BGLs should be monitored at least hourly, and 5% dextrose should be added to the fluid replacement regimen once BGLs reach 14 mmol/L.[25] The glucose rate can be adjusted to maintain BGL between 10–15 mmol/L until the hyperosmolality is corrected.

Electrolyte management

Glucose, urea and electrolytes levels need to be monitored hourly and osmolality calculated and tabulated to guide resuscitation. The goals of resuscitation are a decrease in serum sodium by less than 10 mmol/L in 24 hours and osmolality by 3–8 mOsm/kg/hr. If osmolality falls rapidly, a reduction in the fluid replacement or insulin regimes may be indicated to prevent complication. Hypokalaemia is usually less significant than with DKA.

Identify 'red flags' and treat precipitants

Identification of precipitants is important. These are similar to DKA precipitants. Patients with HHS are also at high risk of developing arterial or venous thromboembolism and should be monitored for complications such as thrombosis and pulmonary embolism, acute coronary syndromes, cerebral oedema and fluid overload. All patients should receive DVT prophylaxis for the duration of their hospital admission.

PRACTICE TIP

HYPERGLYCAEMIC HYPEROSMOLAR SYNDROME (HHS)

- Traditionally, most patients with HHS are elderly and have an underlying medical condition.
- Suspect HHS based on history, physical assessment and medication review.
- Dehydration is usually significant, with fluid deficits of 10 L common in HSS.
- Fluid replacement is the priority of management. The choice of fluid used in the HHS state should consider age, sodium level (corrected for hyperglycaemia), degree of dehydration and patient's comorbidities.
- Treatment goals include normalising osmolarity, restoring euglycaemia, preventing complications and treating precipitants.
- Hypernatraemia is usual, but measured serum sodium may be spuriously low because of hyperglycaemia; it is important to calculate the 'corrected' sodium.
- Serious complications related to treatment for HHS include cerebral oedema (osmotic demyelination syndromes), respiratory failure, acute renal injury, fluid overload and thromboembolic events.

HYPOGLYCAEMIA

Hypoglycaemia most commonly occurs in type 1 diabetes, although it may also occur in type 2 diabetics.[16,28] Most episodes of hypoglycaemia are related to insulin treatment, although sulfonylurea drugs may also cause hypoglycaemic episodes.[29] Sulfonylurea medications act by binding to a high-affinity receptor on the surface of the pancreatic islet beta cells, potentiating normal glucose-stimulated insulin release in the presence of a pancreas with functioning beta cells.[18,29] An inevitable consequence of tight glycaemic control, most hypoglycaemic episodes are managed by the patients themselves, a family member or paramedics.

Hypoglycaemia should be considered in any unresponsive patient until proven otherwise, and insulin overdose considered in patients who present with hypoglycaemia that requires continuing doses of intravenous glucose to maintain blood glucose above 5 mmol/L. A lack of dietary intake, increased physical stress, liver disease, changes in insulin or oral medication regimens, pregnancy, pancreatitis, pituitary insufficiency, Addison's disease, alcohol ingestion and drugs such as non-steroidal anti-inflammatory drugs (NSAIDs), phenytoin, thyroid hormones and propranolol can all contribute to hypoglycaemia.[19] It is also worth noting that beta-blockers can mask the adrenergic warning symptoms, making symptoms sudden and unexpected in patients on such therapy.[19]

Definitions of hypoglycaemia

The normal BGL is 4.0–8.0 mmol/L. When the BGL is < 2.5 mmol/L, this is defined as severe hypoglycaemia. A blood glucose level of < 3.5 mmol/L is considered moderate hypoglycaemia.[19,30]

Additionally, hypoglycaemic symptoms may occur when a very high BGL falls too rapidly (e.g. a BGL of 16.7 mmol/L falling quickly to 10 mmol/L). This is especially true for patients with chronically elevated blood sugar levels.[31] Symptoms tend to be grouped as either:

- autonomic (i.e. sweating, warm sensation, anxiety, nausea, palpations and possibly hunger), or
- neurological (i.e. tiredness, visual disturbance, drowsiness, altered behaviour, confusion and, if untreated, seizures or coma).

Autonomic-related symptoms frequently occur with BGLs around 3.5 mmol/L, whereas neurological symptoms tend to be present with blood glucose levels closer to 2.5 mmol/L. A combination of sweating and reduced activity, along with depleted energy reserves, predisposes hypoglycaemic patients to hypothermia. Close attention to rewarming and protecting the patient from further heat loss is required during initial management.[30]

Treatment

Mild-to-moderate hypoglycaemia

If the patient is conscious and cooperative, a readily available and fast-acting glucose-containing food or drink (60–130 mL fruit juice, 75–150 mL lemonade, jelly beans, honey, 15 g of glucose in adults) may be considered, followed by a lower-glycaemic-load carbohydrate meal (sandwich, dried fruit).[19]

Severe hypoglycaemia

In episodes of severe hypoglycaemia, the person is likely to be unconscious or confused, requiring assistance. Treatment recommendations for hypoglycaemia in adults are glucose 10% or 50% given intravenously into a large vein, 0.5–2 mg intramuscular (IM) glucagon or subcutaneous (SC) glucagon 1 mg if the IV route is unavailable (treatment of choice for non-healthcare professionals), depending on availability and clinical setting.[19] The IM route has a quicker release rate and rectifies the BGLs more quickly, while the SC route is slower and more sustained. Response would be expected within 5–6 minutes of injection (either glucose or glucagon). However, prolonged hypoglycaemia associated with a seizure may take several hours for recovery of full consciousness and cognition. In the pre-hospital setting, use of glucose 50% is not advocated and glucose 10% by intravenous infusion (see below) or glucagon are preferred treatment choices.

Following successful reversal of hypoglycaemia, BGLs should be monitored every 1–2 hours initially, and then revert to the patient's usual testing regimen. Consultation with the diabetic specialist team is advisable to determine the cause of the hypoglycaemia; consider medication dose changes and commence education to prevent further episodes. Most patients are usually discharged home if the cause of the hypoglycaemic event can be identified unless they are on oral antihyperglycaemic medications that have a longer half-life.

PRACTICE TIP

HYPOGLYCAEMIA

If blood glucose level is < 2 mmol/L or severe symptoms of hypoglycaemia:

- administer 50% glucose 25-50 mL intravenously or glucagon 0.5-2 mg intramuscularly
- paramedics usually administer 10% glucose 150 mL intravenously for adults or 3 mL/kg intravenously for children. Can be followed by a further 100 mL or 2 mL/kg respectively if response is inadequate, or alternatively glucagon 0.5-2 mg intramuscularly if IV access unavailable
- consider hypothermia as a possible complication with the intent to maintain normothermia and protect from further heat loss.

If on insulin infusion:

- cease insulin
- bolus 100 mL, 5% glucose
- administer 50% glucose 25 mL (if asymptomatic) or 50% glucose 50 mL (if symptomatic) intravenously
- if pump is the patient's own insulin administration device, ask a carer or relative for assistance if unclear how to operate it. Recovery can still occur even if it is left operating.

In all cases, repeat BGL measurement every 15 minutes.

- Resume insulin at half the rate when BGL > 4.0 mmol/L if on insulin infusion.
- Where access to sugar-containing products is difficult, pre-hospital responders can use 15 g oral glucose paste as an alternative.
- Repeat BGL every 15 minutes.
- Give complex carbohydrate meal.

ALCOHOLIC KETOACIDOSIS

Alcoholic acidosis usually occurs in patients with chronic alcoholism in the setting of prolonged fasting, protracted vomiting and large alcohol ingestion.[30] The patient usually presents with severe hypoglycaemia, but will have concurrent accumulation of ketoacids and lactic acid. Insulin deficiency, depleted glycogen stores and volume depletion provide an appropriate milieu for the development of alcoholic ketoacidosis. Hypoglycaemia occurs, as gluconeogenesis is inhibited by ethanol and glycogenolysis is exhausted by a significant fasting state. If insulin levels are decreased, metabolism of glucose is altered, leading to the utilisation of fat and muscle tissue for energy. This results in ketosis, which, together with profound dehydration, continues the cycle of ketosis and acidosis.[32,33]

Management

The focus of treatment in the ED is rehydration with intravenous fluid and correction of hypoglycaemia with 5% dextrose. This treatment modality is usually enough to reverse the acidosis. Adjunctive therapy includes parental thiamine administration. Thiamine is often given before glucose administration to prevent precipitating Wernicke's encephalopathy, a neurological syndrome associated with ataxia (loss of muscle tone and balance), ophthalmoplegia and mental status changes.[24] Vital signs and neurological assessment are imperative to the nursing care of these patients, together with accurate monitoring of fluid, hydration and electrolyte status. Monitor also for signs of alcohol withdrawal.

ADRENAL INSUFFICIENCY

Adrenal insufficiency is a condition that occurs when glucocorticoid production is inadequate to meet metabolic requirements (Fig. 26.7).[34] It may be caused by structural or functional lesions of the adrenal cortex (*primary adrenal insufficiency*) or anterior pituitary gland/hypothalamus (*secondary adrenal insufficiency*).

FIGURE 26.7 PATHOPHYSIOLOGY OF ACUTE ADRENAL INSUFFICIENCY[5]

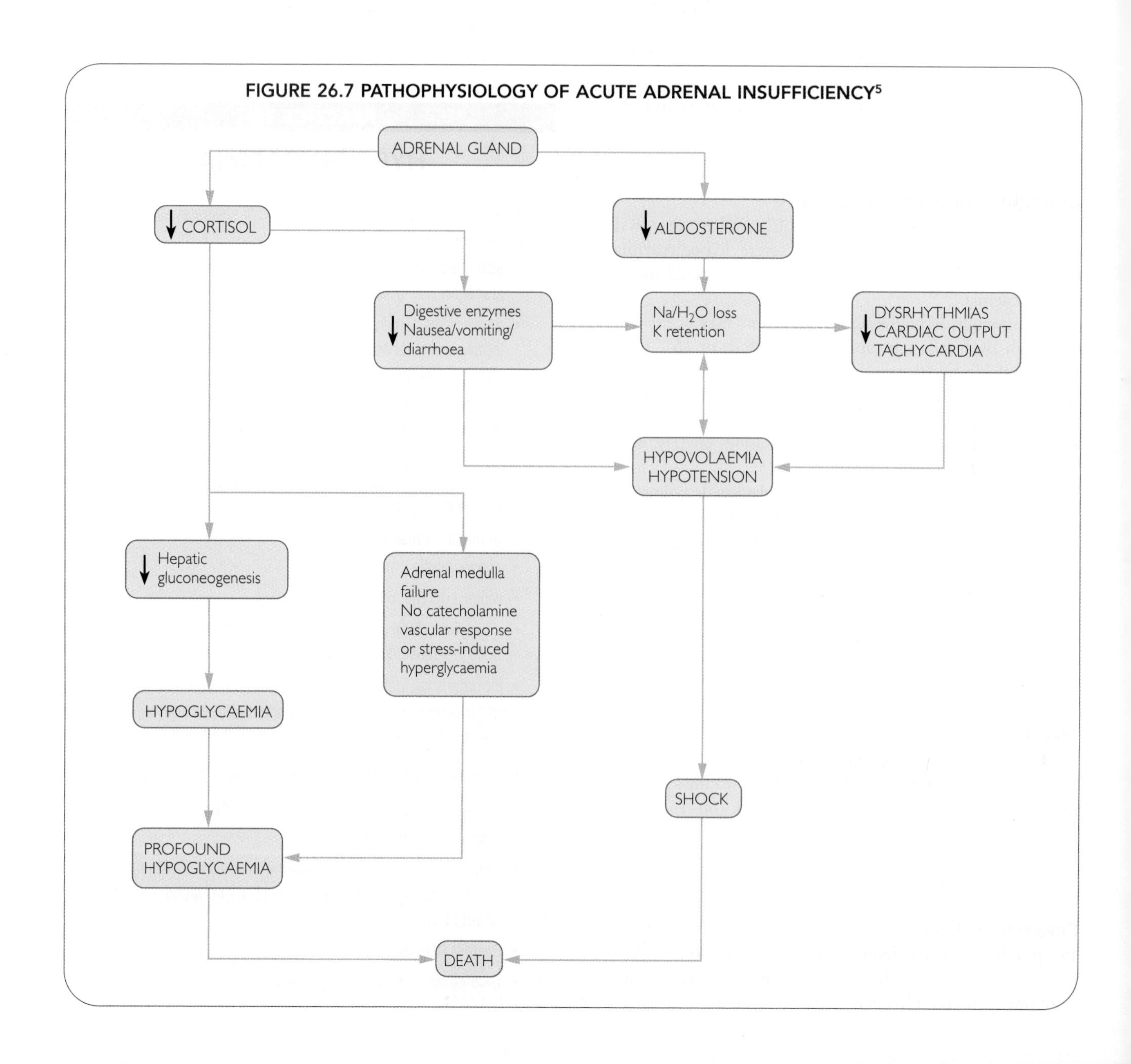

The presenting signs and symptoms can vary from non-specific clinical features, such as tiredness, nausea, anorexia, lethargy, mild hypotension, fever and abdominal pain, through to potentially life-threatening cardiovascular collapse. Historical indicators of the potential for adrenal insufficiency to occur include history of long-term glucocorticoid treatment and/or known adrenal failure.[30]

PRECIPITATING FACTORS AND AETIOLOGY

The aetiology of adrenal insufficiency is also diverse. It may result from abrupt withdrawal of glucocorticoid therapy or the onset of an acute illness or stressor, such as infection or trauma in steroid-dependent patients. Causes that are specific to the adrenal gland include autoimmune disorders, adrenal haemorrhage or infiltrates (carcinoma, sarcoidosis), bilateral adrenalectomy or drugs (ketoconazole). Pituitary and hypothalamic causes of adrenal insufficiency may be due to tumours, apoplexy or granulomatous disease.[34]

CLINICAL MANAGEMENT

As with all emergency presentations, the clinical assessment follows the ABCD mnemonic and interventions are initiated if a threat to any of these parameters is established. Establish intravenous access with a large gauge cannula. Obtain blood for electrolytes and glucose. Fluid resuscitation with intravenous fluids is usually required, titrated to the clinical response. Hydrocortisone 100 mg bolus is given immediately and continued every 6 hours for 24 hours.[19]

The initial assessment should be followed with a focused assessment to identify any precipitating event. Broad-spectrum antibiotic therapy may be indicated if infection is suspected. Having stabilised the patient, blood is sampled for random cortisol and adrenocorticotrophic hormone (ACTH) levels. This test is time-sensitive and needs to reach the laboratory within 30 minutes. The blood sample must be placed on ice for transport. Diagnosis is confirmed by performing a short ACTH stimulation (Synacthen) test.[34] Hydrocortisone therapy will be slowly reduced over the following 24–48 hours. The maintenance dose of glucocorticoid is usually hydrocortisone 10 mg twice per day.[19]

DISCHARGE ADVICE

A patient with adrenal insufficiency should be educated on the following key features of self-care on discharge. Patient education on glucocorticoid therapy is very important following an acute crisis. This education will include instructions to increase glucocorticoid dose at times of intercurrent illness. Wearing a 'medical alert' bracelet or necklace is advocated. Instructions on the use of an emergency injection pack (hydrocortisone), particularly when away from medical care, may also be included as part of the discharge advice. Above all, the early recognition of signs and symptoms suggestive of an adrenal crisis (nausea, vomiting, dehydration, feeling faint) are emphasised.

ACUTE PITUITARY APOPLEXY

This rare disorder is caused by infarction or haemorrhage of the pituitary gland associated with trauma, hypertension, anticoagulation, cardiac surgery and a large number of other conditions. Acute pituitary apoplexy is uncommon, affecting both males and females equally with an incidence of 0.6–9.1%.[19]

CLINICAL FEATURES

The clinical signs and symptoms are similar to those seen in raised intracranial pressure and include headache, vomiting, photophobia and altered level of consciousness. Neuro-ophthalmic signs, such as visual field defects and loss of vision, may also be present.[28]

TREATMENT

As with all emergency presentations, the clinical assessment follows the ABCD mnemonic and the initiation of interventions to support these systems. Hydrocortisone therapy is started immediately when signs of hypoadrenalism are absent by administering hydrocortisone 2–4 mg/h in an intravenous infusion.[19,35] Blood levels are taken prior to commencing steroid therapy. They include the following:

- cortisol
- prolactin
- follicle-stimulating hormone, luteinising hormone, oestradiol (women), testosterone (men)
- thyroid-stimulating hormone
- adrenocorticotrophic hormone.

Diagnosis is confirmed by urgent magnetic resonance imaging (MRI) or computed tomography (CT). A critical referral is then made for a neurosurgical consult, with operative management associated with improved outcomes especially in visual acuity.[35]

THYROID STORM

Thyroid emergencies are very rare but can be life threatening.[36] Abnormality, either hyperactivity or hypoactivity, can result in multisystem symptoms. Thyroid storm (hyperactivity or thyrotoxicosis) commonly occurs as a complication of Graves' disease, primarily in women aged between 30 and 40 years.[37] The hypothalamic–pituitary–thyroid counter-regulatory system is responsible for normal thyroid function.

PRECIPITATING FACTORS AND AETIOLOGY

Thyroid crisis occurs when any part of the circuit malfunctions. It is unusual for untreated hyperthyroidism to present as thyroid storm, as there are usually precipitating events. Hyperthyroidism can be divided into three categories: *true* (i.e. excessive thyroid hormones), *drug-induced* or *thyroid injury*. True hyperthyroidism is characterised by an overactive thyroid gland and excessive production of thyroid hormones. In Graves' disease, thyroid-stimulating immunoglobulins increase thyroid activity. Tumours and thyroid nodules also increase thyroid activity. A type of thyroid toxicosis occurs with increased circulating hormones without concurrent overactivity from the thyroid, as in thyroiditis or ingestion of thyroid hormones. Drugs such as iodine and iodine-containing agents, such as amiodarone and lithium, may potentially induce hyperthyroidism. Other thyroid-specific precipitation factors in thyroid storm may include thyroid injury such as palpation, infarction or an adenoma.[4,37]

CLINICAL FEATURES

An endocrine emergency, thyroid storm was first described in 1926 and remains a diagnostic and therapeutic challenge.[36] Thyroid storm occurs with rapid elevation in thyroid hormone levels and is a clinical diagnosis. General precipitating factors include: infection, non-thyroidal trauma or surgery, psychosis, parturition, myocardial infarction or other medical problems.[38] A concise medical history is imperative to the treatment of

TABLE 26.8 CLINICAL MANIFESTATIONS OF HYPERTHYROIDISM AND THYROID STORM[9]

SYSTEM	CLINICAL MANIFESTATIONS
Neurological	Nervousness, restlessness, tremors, confusion, agitation, delirium
Pulmonary	Tachycardia, dysrhythmias, hypertension
Respiratory	Shortness of breath, dyspnoea, rales, congestive heart failure
Gastrointestinal	Hyperactive bowel, abdominal pain, decreased appetite, weight loss, nausea, vomiting or diarrhoea, jaundice
Ocular	Exophthalmos, lid lag, staring gaze
Integumentary	Hyperthermia, flushed, diaphoresis, poor skin turgor

these patients, as it is unusual for untreated hyperthyroidism to present as thyroid storm. Assessment should include history of recent illnesses and medications. Red flags to observe for include recent weight loss despite increased appetite and increased caloric intake; abdominal pain is also a common complaint. The patient may be restless with a reduced attention span and prone to changing discussion topics frequently. Tremors and manic behaviours are also common. In the late stages, an alteration in mental status occurs, which can progress to coma. In extreme cases, hyperthermia can occur with temperatures reaching 40.5–41°C, as well as tachycardia, with heart rates of 200–300 beats/minute, which increases the risk of cardiac failure and arrest.[36] Rales secondary to cardiac failure may be heard. The skin can progress from warm and diaphoretic to hot and dry as dehydration worsens. Increased gastric motility can cause nausea, vomiting and diarrhoea. Hepatic tenderness, jaundice and thinning of the hair may also occur. Goitre, an enlarged thyroid gland, develops as the condition progresses. Eyes become protuberant, periorbital oedema develops and the patient has a staring gaze with heavy eyelids. The clinical manifestations of thyroid storm are summarised in Table 26.8.

TREATMENT

Treatment should be initiated promptly targeting all steps of thyroid hormone function, release and action. Thyroid hormone levels can help differentiate the causative factor; however, the hormone levels are frequently not readily available, making differentiation between thyroid storm and thyrotoxicosis difficult. If thyroid storm is suspected, therapy needs to be aggressive and rapid so that hormone levels are reduced and haemodynamic integrity is preserved. The treatment principles are to decrease the production and release of thyroid hormones, inhibit the peripheral effects of thyroid hormones using beta-blockers and identify and deal with the underlying precipitating factors.[36]

Beta-blocker medications (e.g. propranolol) can be given intravenously to reduce the heart rate. Younger patients and those in an acute crisis often require larger than normal doses. Propranolol acts to block the conversion of the T4 to T3. In cases where beta-blockers are contraindicated (e.g. in diabetes, pregnancy and asthma), digitalis may be used.[19]

Propylthiouracil, which inhibits thyroid hormone synthesis, and methimazole may be used to further block hormone synthesis. This can be given orally or through a gastric tube. Onset of action occurs within an hour; however, full potential is not reached for 3–6 weeks.[19] Iodine may be given 1 hour after antithyroid medications to slow the release of stored thyroid hormones from the thyroid gland. Iodine can be given orally or by intravenous infusion. Patients with Graves' disease and thyroid crisis metabolise and use cortisol faster than normal. Therefore, glucocorticosteroids, such as dexamethasone or hydrocortisone, may be prescribed as they prevent adrenal compromise and inhibit T4 and T3 conversion.[8]

Approaches to supportive therapy may include fluid resuscitation if required and reduction in core body temperature.

PRACTICE TIP

THYROID STORM

- Thyroid storm is very rare.
- In a patient with existing thyrotoxicosis, thyroid storm may be caused by intercurrent illness or by direct injury to the thyroid.
- Treatment includes the rapid inhibition of thyroid hormone synthesis with propylthiouracil, inhibition of the effects of excess thyroid hormone using beta-blockers and correction of the underlying cause.

MYXOEDEMA COMA

Myxoedema coma is a rare but potentially serious complication of untreated hypothyroidism.

PRECIPITATING FACTORS AND AETIOLOGY

The incidence of myxoedema coma is greater in men than in women. Precipitating causes include hypothermia, infection, myocardial infarction or congestive heart failure, cerebral vascular accidents, drug-induced respiratory depression (e.g. sedatives, anaesthetics or tranquillisers), trauma or gastrointestinal blood loss.[19] The disease usually progresses insidiously over months to years, with coma developing when the patient is subjected to stress. It is known to also affect elderly women who have longstanding hypothyroidism and those with undiagnosed hypothyroidism. The latter tends to occur in the winter months. Survival rates are increased when prompt hormone replacement with intense supportive care is received. In-hospital mortality rates have been reported recently at almost 30%.[39]

CLINICAL FEATURES

Thyroid hypoactivity results in reduced metabolic rate and activity. Pronounced fatigue, decreased activity tolerance, episodes of shortness of breath and weight gain may be displayed. Tongue swelling or macroglossia are common complaints. Patients may display elements of confusion and be slow to answer questions (Table 26.9). This alteration in mental

TABLE 26.9 CLINICAL MANIFESTATIONS OF HYPOTHYROIDISM AND MYXOEDEMA COMA[9]

SYSTEM	CLINICAL MANIFESTATIONS
Neurological	Confusion, lethargy, coma
Cardiology	Decreased stroke volume, decreased cardiac output, bradycardia, peripheral vasoconstriction, inverted T waves, prolonged QT interval
Respiratory	Macroglossia, obesity-related sleep apnoea, pneumonia, hypoventilation, hypercarbia
Gastrointestinal	Hypoglycaemia, constipation
Renal	Decreased renal blood flow, decreased sodium reabsorption, hyponatraemia

status can result in coma. Psychiatric symptoms such as hallucinations, paranoia, depression, combativeness and decreased concern for personal appearance may also be present, and are often referred to as 'myxoedema madness'.

Angio-oedema can result in airway occlusion in an unconscious or semiconscious patient. Weak respiratory effort with decreased respiratory drive results in alveolar hypoventilation and can predispose patients to infections. Alveolar hypoventilation also results in hypercarbia, which can cause alteration in mental status. Obesity-related sleep apnoea could further compromise the respiratory system (Table 26.9).

Cardiac changes include bradycardia, decreased stroke volume and decreased cardiac output. Widespread ST and T-wave changes may be evident, with prolonged QT intervals. Body temperature will be low and the skin pale and cool due to peripheral vasoconstriction. In myxoedema coma, the glomerular filtration rate and renal blood flow decreases. Generalised non-pitting oedema as a result of increased insulin sensitivity and decreased oral intake and constipation may also occur. Biochemical abnormalities may include hyponatraemia, increased creatine phosphokinase and lactate dehydrogenase, hypoglycaemia and normocytic or macrocytic anaemia. Thyroid-stimulating hormones may be modestly low in primary hypothyroidism or low in secondary hypothyroidism, but free thyroxine levels are usually low.[38,39]

TREATMENT

Even with prompt treatment, mortality can be as high as 30% in myxoedema coma. After the initial primary assessment and stabilisation, treatment focuses on hormone replacement which may take the form of intravenous T4 (levothyroxine). Large doses are used to saturate empty sites and replenish the circulating levels. T4 avoids adverse cardiac effects that might occur with a sudden increase in T3. Some treating clinicians may recommend a combination of both T3 and T4. As myxoedema coma is a rare condition, a lack of clinical trials to suggest best methods is lacking, and management is likely to be guided by an endocrinology specialist. ECG monitoring during careful titration of thyroid replacement is recommended.[19]

PRACTICE TIP

MYXOEDEMA COMA

- This condition carries a high mortality rate.
- The aim of treatment is prompt recognition, immediate thyroid replacement therapy, treatment of precipitating cause and supportive therapy including ventilation.

CUSHING'S SYNDROME

Cushing's syndrome is a rare endocrine disorder involving the hypothalamic–pituitary–adrenal glands, which results in excessive cortisol levels. Cortisol, a steroid hormone produced by the adrenal gland and normally produced in response to stress, can trigger physiological changes, resulting in a wide range of health problems, including hypertension, hyperglycaemia, muscle wastage and osteoporosis. Causes of Cushing's syndrome include:

- *iatrogenic factors*—prolonged administration of a glucocorticoid such as prednisone to treat conditions such as asthma or rheumatoid arthritis
- *ectopic factors*—production of cortisol by adrenal adenoma or carcinoma (e.g. lung cancer can produce ACTH which when added to the normal pituitary production of ACTH leads to excessive cortisol secretion)
- *problems in the hypothalamic–pituitary–adrenal axis*—resulting in excessive cortisol secretion from the adrenal glands due to overstimulation of the adrenal glands by ACTH.[40]

Features that best discriminate Cushing's syndrome from other common conditions include:

- *Skin*—easy bruising, facial plethora, purple striae
- *Musculoskeletal system*—proximal muscle weakness and/or myopathy; early osteoporosis with or without vertebral fractures or osteonecrosis of femoral or humeral head.

Other features of Cushing's syndrome include:

- *Skin and hair*—thin skin, poor wound healing, hirsutism or scalp thinning
- *Body habitus*—weight gain and central obesity; dorsocervical fat pad ('buffalo hump'), supraclavicular fat pads, facial fullness ('moon face')
- *Reproductive system*—menstrual irregularity, infertility
- *Psychiatric effects*—depression, psychosis, irritability, insomnia, fatigue
- *Metabolic effects*—diabetes
- *Cardiovascular effects*—congestive cardiac failure, hypertension, thrombosis (including deep vein thrombosis and myocardial infarction)
- *Immune system*—immunosuppression causing recurrent and atypical infection, including tuberculosis.[41]

ASSESSMENT AND INVESTIGATIONS

The diagnosis of Cushing's syndrome is generally based on laboratory investigations. Serum ACTH levels determine the aetiology of the excessive cortisol secretion. An elevated ACTH indicates ACTH-dependent disease, with further pituitary investigations required to identify the source. Normal ACTH levels identify the need for abdominal CT scanning to investigate the possibility of an adrenal tumour.

Other laboratory tests indicated include:

- serum glucose to establish if hyperglycaemia is present
- full blood count and white blood cell count—which may reveal elevated levels of both, but a decrease in lymphocytes
- electrolyte—particularly serum potassium which may be decreased
- 24-hour urine collection—may also be commenced to measure cortisol levels.[41]

TREATMENT

Treatment modalities are centred on removing the precipitating cause. Endogenous Cushing's syndrome requires surgical removal of the tumour causing the over-secretion of cortisol. Patients will require glucocorticoid replacement therapy for a period of time post-surgery due to adrenal insufficiency. Pharmacological blockade of cortisol production may be the treatment of choice in some patient populations, using metyrapone or mitotane. If the cause is iatrogenic due to long-term glucocorticoid therapy, the prescribed dose of steroids is gradually reduced.

Metyrapone

Metyrapone acts to reversibly inhibit the biosynthesis of cortisol, corticosterone and aldosterone in the adrenal cortex. Indications for use include:

- to establish the diagnosis of adrenocortical hyperfunction in Cushing's syndrome
- following pituitary surgery.

Standard dosage ranges between 500 and 1000 mg, orally three times a day. The key contraindication for metyrapone is adrenocortical insufficiency, and adverse reactions include nausea, vomiting, dizziness, light-headedness and abdominal pain.[19]

Mitotane

Mitotane is only available for restricted use in Australia via the Australian Therapeutic Goods Administration Special Access Scheme. Dosage is 500 mg orally initially, increasing up to 4–6 g daily.[19]

PRACTICE TIP

- Consider the diagnosis of Cushing's syndrome in patients who have discriminating signs (such as early osteoporosis, myopathy or easy bruising) or multiple features, especially if it is becoming progressively severe (such as refractory diabetes and hypertension associated with end-organ complications).
- Delayed diagnosis can cause life-threatening illness and irreversible organ damage and may compromise the management options of any underlying tumour.
- If endogenous Cushing's syndrome is suspected, refer to an endocrinologist; possible screening tests include urinary free cortisol, salivary cortisol and an overnight dexamethasone test.[40]

SUMMARY

Endocrine emergencies are rare, with hyperglycaemia and diabetic ketoacidosis being the most frequently encountered. Most institutions and health services have established protocols, which should be utilised when available. Clinicians should be aware of potential red flags for endocrine emergencies and not delay initiation of treatment while awaiting investigation results. It is also imperative that involvement of the endocrine team occur in a timely manner once endocrine involvement is suspected.

CASE STUDY

Thirty-two-year-old Dinesh Patel is attended by paramedics at 2 pm at his own residence. The 000 call was made by his wife for persistent vomiting, increasing abdominal pain and rapid breathing. During the assessment the paramedic obtains information on the onset of symptoms and past medical history. Mr Patel has been unwell for 2 days. He is unable to tolerate even clear fluids now. He does not report fever, coughs or dysuria. Patel is a type 1 diabetic, diagnosed at 10 years of age, who has recently immigrated from Sri Lanka. He was required to change insulin brands on arriving in Australia. He reports high readings using home blood glucose monitoring.

Paramedics find Mr Patel in bed, vomiting and feeling unwell. His vital signs are:

- blood pressure 95/60mmHg
- pulse rate 125 beats/minute
- temperature 37.6°C
- respiratory rate 40 breaths/minute
- oxygen saturation 97% on room air
- Glasgow Coma Scale (GCS) score 15
- BGL on glucometer was 'HI' and ketones are 7.2 mmol/L.

He is transported to the nearest emergency department (ED). The triage nurse assesses the patient and allocates a triage category 2. He is transferred to a resuscitation bay where an assessment is performed. The findings of the assessment are:

- Airway—patent, talking
- Breathing—increased work in breathing with a respiratory rate of 35 breaths/minute with Kussmaul's respirations and an acetone smell on his breath. He oxygenates well and has equal air entry bilaterally
- Circulation—warm to touch with a capillary refill of less than 2 seconds with dry mucous membranes. Monitored for sinus tachycardia, rate 134 beats per minute and his blood pressure is 85/45 mmHg.
- Disability—alert and orientated, although slightly drowsy. Temperature 36.5°C.
- BGL is reading 'HI' on bedside glucometer. Following the establishment of hyperglycaemia in this acutely ill patient, the next bedside test is serum ketone monitoring. The result is a serum ketone level of 7.1 mmol/L.
- Exposure—clothes are removed, and skin assessed for hydration status and integrity.

The priority is to establish the severity of Mr Patel's symptoms and hence the need for medical intervention. Circulatory support is established by inserting a large-bore cannula into his right arm, infusing 500 mL normal saline 0.9% to correct the hypotension. A venous blood gas is taken, confirming diabetic ketoacidosis (DKA) with pH 6.97, BGL 41.5 mmol/L and lactate 5.3 mmol/L.

Ketosis and hyperglycaemia are distinct metabolic problems. When these abnormal states occur together, diabetic ketoacidosis (DKA) may result. In determining the severity of Mr Patel's illness (DKA), it is necessary to consider a combination of clinical assessment findings, historical factors, diagnostic and laboratory testing and the outcome of interventions. A secondary assessment outlining these findings is given in Table 26.CS1.

With respect to the circulation and metabolic derangements that Mr Patel has suffered, the management goals are to:

- replace electrolyte and fluid losses
- stop lipolysis and inhibit glucose production with insulin
- identify and correct precipitant
- re-establish normal physiology.

TABLE 26.CS1 FOCUSED CLINICAL ASSESSMENT

	CLINICAL FINDING	FINDING/INTERVENTION
E	Exposure Expose patient to identify all injuries Recent overseas travel	Look for potential sites of infection Septic screening, including chest x-ray
F	Fluids • blood pressure 85/55 mmHg • heart rate 134 beats/minute • respiratory rate–Kussmaul's respirations • GCS 15 • pupils (equal and reacting to light) • SpO_2 98% • Temperature 37.6°C	Circulatory support was established Fluid resuscitation: 1 L NaCl 0.9% were infused stat followed by 1 L NaCl 0.9% over the next hour Indwelling catheter was inserted, which initially drained 650 mL dilute urine Hourly urinary measures were commenced to ensure a urinary output of 0.5 mL/kg/h ECG recorded–sinus tachycardia with no acute changes Haemodynamic monitoring was commenced via arterial line and continuous cardiac monitoring
G	Glucose	Formal blood sugar 41.5 mmol/L Serum ketones 7.1 mmol/L Commenced on insulin infusion therapy (50 units Actrapid in 50 mL NaCl infusing at 5 units/h)
H	History	Type 1 diabetic In the process of immigrating to Australia • In Australia 2 weeks

TABLE 26.CS1 FOCUSED CLINICAL ASSESSMENT—cont'd

	CLINICAL FINDING	FINDING/INTERVENTION
H	Head-to-toe assessment	
	Head/neck	Nil abnormalities detected
	Respiratory	Chest clear
		Kussmaul's respirations
		Acetone smell from breath
		ABG: severe acidosis
		pH: 6.95
		$PaCO_2$ 28.4 mmHg
		HCO_3^- 4.9 mmol/L
		BE -27.1 mmol/L
		Lactate: 5.39 mmol/L
	Cardiovascular	Warm peripheries
		Normal heart sounds
		CK $<$ 20 micromol/L (normal limits are: male 60–120 micromol/L, female 40–90 micromol/L)
		Troponin negative
		Excessive thirst
	Abdomen	Generalised abdominal pain scored 6/10
		Soft and non-tender to palpation
		Bowel sounds present
		LFTs normal
		Amylase and lipase normal
	Renal	Urinary output 120 m/hr
		Potassium 4.2 mmol/K (potassium replacement commenced at 10 mmol/h)
		Sodium 139 mmol/L; corrected sodium 153 mmol/L
		Anion gap 23 mmol/L

ABG: arterial blood gas; BE: base excess; CK: creatine kinase; GCS: Glasgow Coma Scale; HCO_3^-: bicarbonate level; LFT: liver function test; $PaCO_2$: arterial pressure of carbon dioxide; SpO_2: peripheral oxygen saturation.

The greatest dangers to Mr Patel are acidosis and electrolyte disturbances, especially hypokalaemia, not hyperglycaemia. The priority is fluid resuscitation to improve tissue perfusion and the tissue's response to insulin. Fluids also decrease the blood sugar levels by approximately 30%. Correcting Mr Patel's hypotension would also decrease the secretion of counter-regulatory hormones and improve acidosis.

As there is clear clinical evidence of ketoacidosis, the next priority is the commencement of an insulin infusion. The initial infusion rate is 5 units/h. The BGL progressively decreases from 28.4 mmol/L by 4.5–5.5 mmol/L over the next few hours. When Mr Patel's BGL drops to 14 mmol/L, a 5% dextrose infusion is commenced at 80 mL/h. This allows the BGL to be maintained until the acidosis is reversed by the insulin therapy and prevent hypoglycaemia developing.

The next most-critical management step is the recognition of the need to replace potassium. Potassium levels were 3.2 mmol/L. Potassium replacement is commenced at 10 mmol/h, and close monitoring is initiated in anticipation of a further fall in serum potassium due to the commencement of insulin therapy and the correction of the acidosis. Identification of the precipitating factor is the next vital step. This is identified as the change in the insulin brands from Sri Lanka to Australia. Mr Patel is transferred to the Level 1 intensive care unit. During his admission he is further resuscitated and stabilised. His acidosis and hyperglycaemia are corrected slowly. The endocrine team, diabetic educator and dietitian are consulted on his care. He is discharged 5 days later with a follow-up appointment in the diabetic clinic for ongoing management.

QUESTIONS

1. Describe the main characteristics of DKA.
2. Identify the key signs and symptoms reported by patients presenting to ED with DKA.
3. How would you prioritise your nursing management of DKA?
4. What are the overarching key principles of managing DKA?
5. What are common errors that occur when managing a patient with DKA?

Answers to Case Study Questions can be found on evolve **http://evolve.elsevier.com/AU/Curtis/emergency/**

USEFUL WEBSITES

American Thyroid Association: professional home for clinicians and researchers dedicated to thyroid health, www.thyroid.org/.

Diabetes Australia: resources for health professionals, educators, researchers and the community on awareness, prevention, detection, management and research, www.diabetesaustralia.com.au/.

Endocrine Society of Australia: national organisation of scientists and clinicians who conduct research and prastise in the field of endocrinology, www.endocrinesociety.org.au/position-statements.asp.

Endocrine Society: global community focused on improving patient care, shaping effective policy, and ensuring the future of our field, www.endocrine.org.

REFERENCES

1. Australian Institute of Health and Welfare (AIHW). Emergency department care. 2020–21. Available from: www.aihw.gov.au/reports-data/myhospitals/sectors/emergency-department-care.
2. Applegate E. The anatomy and physiology learning system. 4th ed. St. Louis: Saunders; 2011.
3. Guyton AC, Hall JE, editors. Textbook of medical physiology. Philadelphia: Saunders; 2020.
4. Kelly K. Endocrine system. In: Brown D, Edwards H, Buckley T, Aitken R, Plowman E, editors. Lewis's medical-surgical nursing. 5th ed. Sydney: Elsevier; 2017.
5. Brashers L, Huether S. Mechanisms of hormonal regulation. In: McCance KL, Huether SE, editors. Pathophysiology: the biological basis for disease in adults and children. St. Louis: Mosby; 2019.
6. Valentina LB, Karen CT. Mechanisms of hormonal regulation. In: Rogers JL, editor. McCance and Huether's pathophysiology: the biologic basis for disease in adults and children. 9th ed. St Louis: Mosby; 2024.
7. Buckely T, Murphy M. Endocrine emergencies. In: Curtis K, Ramsden C, Shaban R, Fry M, Considine J, editors. Emergency and trauma care for nurses and paramedics. Sydney: Elsevier; 2019.
8. Thibodeau GA, Patton KT. The human body in health and disease. 4th ed. St Louis: Mosby; 2005.
9. Brashers V, Jones R, Huether S. Alterations of hormonal regulation. In: McCance KL, Huether SE, editors. Pathophysiology: the biological basis for disease in adults and children. St Louis: Mosby; 2019.
10. Pedreanez A, Mosquera J, Munoz N, Robalino J, Tene D. Diabetes, heart damage, and angiotensin II. What is the relationship link between them? A minireview. Endocr Regul 2022;56(1):55–65.
11. Hoy A. The structure and function of the endocrine system. In: Rote NS, Huether SE, McCance KL, editors. Understanding pathophysiology. 2nd ed. Sydney: Elsevier Australia; 2015.
12. Craft J, Gordon C. The structure and function of the endocrine system. In: Craft J, Gordon C, editors. Understanding pathophysiology. Sydney: Elsevier; 2015.
13. Doumas M, Boutari C, Tsioufis C, Dimitriadis K, Triantafyllou A, Douma S. Clinical value of measuring the renin/aldosterone levels: optimising the management of uncontrolled/resistant hypertension. Curr Vasc Pharmacol 2017;16(1):10–14.
14. Mantzorus C, Serdy S. Insulin action. 2017. Available from: www.uptodate.com/contents/insulin-action.
15. Diabetes UK. Diabetes and the body. Available from: www.youtube.com/watch?v=X9ivR4y03DE&feature=youtu.be.
16. Australia Diabetes Association. Diabetes in Australia. 2019. Available from: www.diabetesaustralia.com.au/diabetes-in-australia.
17. Australian Institute of Health and Welfare. Diabetes. Available from: www.aihw.gov.au/reports/australias-health/diabetes.
18. Diabetes NSW & ACT. What is diabetes? Available from: www.diabetesnsw.com.au/useful-tools/audio-recordings/.
19. Tilenius H. Therapeutic guidelines: endocrinology. Version 5. Aust Prescrib 2015;38:19–20.

20. Brar P, Tell S, Mehta S, Franklin B. Hyperosmolar diabetic ketoscidosis – a review of literature and the shifting paradigm in evaluation and management. Diabetes Metab Syndr 2021;15(6):102313.
21. Westerberg DP. Diabetic ketoacidosis: evaluation and treatment. Am Fam Phys 2013;87(5):337–46.
22. Dickinson J. Diabetes mellitus. In: Brown D, Edwards H, Buckley T, Aitken R, Plowman E, editors. Lewis's medical-surgical nursing. 5th ed. Sydney: Elsevier; 2017.
23. Muneer M, Akbar I, Islam S. Acute metabolic emergencies in diabetes: DKA, HHS and EDKA. In: Islam M, editor. Diabetes from research to clinical practice. Advances in experimental medicine and biology. New York: Springer; 2021.
24. Little M. Endocrine emergencies. In: Cameron P, Little M, Mitra B, Deasy C, editors. Textbook of adult emergency medicine. Sydney: Elsevier; 2020.
25. Tran T, Pease A, Wood A, Zajac JD, Mårtensson J, Bellomo R, et al. Review of evidence for adult diabetic ketoacidosis management protocols. Nat Lib Med 2017;8:106.
26. Hirsch IB, Emmett M. Diabetic ketoacidosis and hyperosmolar hyperglycemic state in adults: Treatment. 2017. Available from: www.uptodate.com/contents/diabetic-ketoacidosis-and-hyperosmolar-hyperglycemic-state-in-adults-treatment?search=Diabetic+ketoacidosis&source=search_result&selectedTitle=1~150.
27. Avichal D, Blocher NC. Hyperosmolar hyperglycemic state. 2021. Available from: emedicine.medscape.com/article/1914705-overview.
28. Cryer P. Hypoglycaemia inadults with diabetes mellitus. 2021. Available from: www.uptodate.com/contents/hypoglycemia-in-adults-with-diabetes-mellitus.
29. Sola D, Rossi L Schianca G, Maffioli P, Bigliocca M, Mella R, et al. Sulfonylureas and their use in clinical practice. Arch Med Sci 2015;11(4): 840–8.
30. Heller SR. Glucose concentrations of less than 3.0 mmol/l (54 mg/dl) should be reported in clinical trials: a joint position statement of the American Diabetes Association and the European Association for the Study of Diabetes. Diabetes Care 2017;40:155–7.
31. Amiel S. The consequences of hypoglycaemia. Diabetologia 2021;64:963–70.
32. Long B, Lentz S, Gottlieb M. Alcoholic ketoacidosis: etiologies, evaluation and management. Clin Rev 2021;61(6):658–65.
33. Liu L, Li X, Wu J, Chen Y, Li H, Tian Z. Non-diabetic ketoacidosis: a case of alcoholic ketoacidosis accompanied by hyperglycaemia. Am J Emerg Med 2022;52:270.e5–e8. doi:10.1016/j.ajem.2021.08.063.
34. Nieman LK. Adrenal insufficiency overview. 2021. Available from: www.uptodate.com/contents/adrenal-insufficiency-addisons-disease-beyond-the-basics#H1.
35. Guijt M, Zamanipoor Najafabadi A, Notting I, Notting IC, Pereira AM, Verstegen MJT, et al. Towards a pituitary apoplexy classification based on clinical presentation and patient journey. Endocrine 2021;76:132–41.
36. Reyes-Castano J, Burman K. Thyrotoxic crisis: thyroid storm. In: Loriaux L, Vanek C, editors. Endocrine emergencies: recognition and treatment. New York: Springer; 2021.
37. Ross D. Thyroid storm. 2021. Available from: www.uptodate.com/contents/thyroid-storm#H1.
38. Field AG. Adrenal and pituitary disorders. In: Wolfson AB, Cloutier RL, Hendey GW, Ling LJ, Rosen CL, Schaider JJ, editors. Harwood-Nuss' clinical practice of emergency medicine. 6th ed. Philadelphia: Lippincott Williams & Wilkins; 2015.
39. Ono Y, Ono S, Yasunaga H, Matsui H, Fushimi K, Tanaka Y. Clinical characteristics and outcomes of myxedema coma: analysis of a national inpatient database in Japan. J Epidemiol 2017;27(3):117–22.
40. Ross D. Myxedema coma. 2021. Available from: www.uptodate.com/contents/myxedema-coma.
41. Fleseriu M, Auchus R, Bancos I, Ben-Shlomo A, Bertherat J, Geer EB, et al. Consensus on diagnosis and management of Cushing's disease: a guidance update. Lancet Diabetes Endocrinol 2021;9(12):847–75.

CHAPTER 27

HEALTHCARE-ASSOCIATED INFECTIONS AND INFECTIOUS DISEASES IN EMERGENCY CARE

RAMON Z. SHABAN, DEBOROUGH MACBETH, PHILIP L. RUSSO, BRETT G. MITCHELL, JAMES PEARCE AND CATHERINE VIENGKHAM

ESSENTIALS

The following Standard Precautions apply when providing emergency healthcare.[1]

HAND HYGIENE

- Hand hygiene must be performed in accordance with the Five Moments for Hand Hygiene. This includes before touching a patient, before a procedure, after a procedure or body-fluid-exposure risk, after touching a patient, and after touching a patient's surroundings.
- Alcohol-based hand rubs containing at least 70% v/v ethanol or equivalent should be used for all clinical situations in the healthcare environment where hands are visibly clean.
- Wash with soap and water when hands are visibly dirty or contaminated with proteinaceous material, or visibly soiled with blood or other body fluids, or if exposure to potential spore-forming organisms is strongly suspected or proven, or after using the bathroom.
- Hand hygiene must also be performed after removal of gloves.

PERSONAL PROTECTIVE EQUIPMENT

- Personal protective equipment (PPE) should be used appropriate to the task being undertaken to prevent exposure via established modes of transmission.
- Aprons or gowns should be worn for a single procedure or episode of patient care where there is a risk of exposure to blood and body substances, and removed in the area where the episode of care takes place.
- A surgical mask and eyewear must be worn during procedures or activities that are likely to result in splashes or sprays of blood, body fluids, secretions or excretions into the face and eyes.
- Gloves must be worn as a single-use item for each invasive procedure, contact with sterile sites and non-intact skin or mucous membranes; and for any activity that has been assessed as carrying a risk of exposure to blood, body fluids, secretions and excretions.
- Gloves must be changed between patients and after every episode of individual patient care.

- Sterile gloves must be used for aseptic procedures and contact with sterile sites.

HANDLING AND DISPOSAL OF SHARPS

- Sharps must not be passed directly from hand to hand and handling should be kept to a minimum.
- Needles must not be recapped, bent, broken or disassembled after use.
- The person who has used the sharp must be responsible for its immediate safe disposal.
- Used sharps must be discarded into an approved sharps container at the point-of-use. Do not fill above the mark that indicates the bin is three-quarters full.

ROUTINE ENVIRONMENTAL CLEANING

- Clean frequently touched surfaces with detergent solution at least daily, and when visibly soiled and after every known contamination.
- Clean general surfaces and fittings when visibly soiled and immediately after spillage.
- Clean shared clinical equipment between patient uses, with detergent solution.
- Use surface barriers to protect clinical surfaces (including equipment) that are touched frequently with gloved hands during the delivery of patient care, as these are likely to become contaminated with blood or body substances, or are difficult to clean (e.g. computer keyboards).
- Spills of blood or other potentially infectious materials should be promptly cleaned as follows: wear utility gloves and other PPE appropriate to the task; confine and contain spill, clean visible matter with disposable absorbent material and discard the used cleaning materials in the appropriate waste container; and clean the spill area with a cloth or paper towels using detergent solution.
- Use of chemical disinfectants should be based on assessment of risk of transmission of infectious agents from that spill.

Transmission-based Precautions are to be applied in addition to Standard Precautions in particular circumstances.

CONTACT PRECAUTIONS

- Implement contact precautions in the presence of known or suspected infectious agents that are spread by direct or indirect contact with the patient or the patient's environment.
- When working with patients who require contact precautions, perform hand hygiene, put on gloves and gown upon entry to the patient care area, ensure that clothing and skin do not contact potentially contaminated environmental surfaces and remove gown and gloves and perform hand hygiene before leaving the patient care area.
- To facilitate the mechanical removal of spores, meticulously wash hands with soap and water and pat dry with single-use towels.
- Use of alcohol-based hand rubs alone may not be sufficient to reduce transmission of spore-forming organisms.
- Use patient-dedicated equipment or single-use non-critical patient-care equipment (e.g. blood pressure cuffs).
- If common use of equipment for multiple patients is unavoidable, clean the equipment and allow it to dry before use on another patient.

DROPLET PRECAUTIONS

- Additional respiratory precautions are implemented for patients known or suspected to be infected with agents transmitted by respiratory droplets generated when a patient coughs, sneezes or speaks.
- The type of respiratory protection required will depend on a number of factors, most notably droplet size, which affects its distance of projection and time it spends suspended in the air.
- Respiratory precautions will typically involve donning a surgical mask or respirator when entering the patient-care environment.
- Patients who require respiratory precautions are placed in a single-patient room when available.

AIRBORNE PRECAUTIONS

- When respiratory droplets become increasingly small, it is likely for the infectious agent to be transmitted from person-to-person through the air.
- Wear a correctly fit-checked and fit-tested P2 (N95) respirator when entering the patient-care area when an airborne-transmissible infectious agent is known or suspected.
- Patients on airborne precautions should be placed in negative-pressure rooms or in a room from which the air does not circulate to other areas. Exceptions to this should be justified by risk assessment.

Implement transmission-based precautions for all patients colonised or infected with a multi-resistant organism, including:

- put on gloves and gowns before entering the patient-care area.
- use patient-dedicated or single-use non-critical patient-care equipment (e.g. blood pressure cuff, stethoscope).
- use a single-patient room or, if unavailable, cohort patients with the same strain of multi-resistant organism in designated patient-care areas; and ensure consistent cleaning and disinfection of surfaces near the patient and those likely to be touched by the patient and healthcare workers.

INTRODUCTION

As populations grow worldwide so do challenges for the control and prevention of infectious diseases and healthcare-associated infections (HAIs). Generally speaking, infectious diseases are diseases where the causative agent passes or is carried from one person or organism to another, albeit directly or indirectly. As a rule, HAIs are infections that are acquired in healthcare facilities ('nosocomial' infections) or are infections occurring as a result of healthcare interventions ('iatrogenic' infections), which may become evident after people leave the healthcare facility.[1,2] A variety of like and related definitions exist which are determined by, among other things, the setting or context in which they occur. Community-acquired infections are those acquired and detected within 48 hours of hospital admission in patients without previous contact with a healthcare facility.[3] A hospital-acquired infection is a localised or systemic condition resulting from an adverse reaction to the presence of an infectious agent(s) or its toxin(s), and was present 48 hours or more after hospital admission and not incubating at hospital admission time.[3–5] The clinical and epidemiological term HAIs are those infections detected within 48 hours of hospital admission in patients who had previous contact with a healthcare facility within 1 year.[4]

HOSPITAL-ASSOCIATED COMPLICATIONS

HAIs are one kind of 16 hospital-associated complications (HACs) identified by the Australian Commission on Safety and Quality in Health Care (ACSQHC).[6] The incidence of hospital-associated complications is high, with one in nine patients in Australian hospitals reported to experience a complication—an estimated 900,000 patients per year.[7] There are nine HAI types of HACs, namely: urinary tract infection, surgical site infection, pneumonia, bloodstream infection, infections or inflammatory complications associated with peripheral/central venous catheters, multi-resistant organism, infection associated with prosthetics/implantable devices, gastrointestinal infections, and other high-impact infections.[4,6]

The incidence of HAIs in acute healthcare facilities in Australia varies according to the data source. Early federal government data have shown less than 200,000 cases of HAIs each year,[8] whereas data described in the peer-reviewed literature from 2010 to 2016 revealed a yearly incidence of 83,096 HAIs.[9] Government reports of data from 2015 to 2016 showed a marked decrease in the incidence to 60,037 HAIs.[10] However, these findings must be interpreted with caution. Reports are limited by the lack of a national aggregated dataset and are mostly based on the best available evidence. For example, accounting for incomplete and missing data, a more likely incidence of HAIs from 2010 to 2016 is approximately 165,000 cases per year.[9] A 2018 cross-sectional study conducted across 19 Australian hospitals found that HAI prevalence rates ranged from 5.7% to 17% in acute adult inpatients and estimated over 170,000 annual cases and 7500 resulting deaths.[11,12] To increase the robustness and reliability of these data, researchers have called for a national consensus on definitions and reporting of surveillance methodology.[13] System-wide efforts to achieve the national mandate of eliminating preventable infections initially focused on financial penalties for specific events, such as bloodstream infections; subsequently, the government introduced system-wide financial penalties for hospital-associated complications from 2017.[14] Fundamentally, HAIs, cross-contamination and the spread of infection and infectious disease are risks in all healthcare settings.[15]

Effective management of HAIs is underpinned by timely administration of appropriate antimicrobials. An ongoing challenge is the development of antibiotic-resistant bacteria. For example, nationally in 2016, *Escherichia coli* (*E. coli*) caused 4108 of 11,163 cases (36.8%) of bloodstream infections; an issue was that *E. coli* was showing increased resistance to antibiotics, particularly fluoroquinolones, the 'last resort' group of antibiotics for infections not responding to other antibiotics.[16,17] Antimicrobial resistance is a leading worldwide threat to the wellbeing of patients, and the safety and quality of healthcare globally.[18,19] In Australia, effective antimicrobial stewardship for optimal use of antimicrobials and containment of antimicrobial resistance resulted in a 9% decrease in prescription of antimicrobials between 2010 and 2015,[17] and a further decrease of 14.8% between 2015 and 2019.[16] Effective antibiotic stewardship alone could potentially result in savings of $300 million for the Australian national healthcare budget.[15,18,19]

The human, financial and societal costs of HAIs are significant. Approximately one in 10 hospitalised patients will acquire an infection after admission, resulting in substantial economic cost.[4,11,18,19] The financial and health systems costs of HAIs are typically reflected by increasing length of stay, rates of readmission, increasing access block and bed block and additional diagnostic and therapeutic interventions. National data revealed patients who experienced a HAI have an average hospital length of stay 18.1 days longer in comparison to patients not burdened by an infection.[10] Nationally, surgical site infections are estimated to result in a total 206,527 excess bed days annually.[20] The human cost by way of unnecessary pain and suffering for patients and their families and prolonged hospital stays is difficult to quantify, but they are significant.[1] HAIs lead to substantial morbidity, and in some cases death.[10]

THE EMERGENCY SETTING

HAIs are, however, largely preventable adverse events rather than an unpredictable complication. It is possible to significantly reduce the rate of HAIs through effective infection control.[1] Effective infection prevention and control is thus a prerequisite to high-quality healthcare for patients and a safe working environment for those who work in healthcare settings. Successful approaches for preventing and reducing harm arising from HAIs involve applying a risk-management framework to manage 'human' and 'system' factors associated with the transmission of infectious agents. Understanding the modes of transmission of infectious organisms and knowing how and when to apply the basic principles of infection control is critical to the success of an infection-control program. This responsibility applies to everybody working and visiting a healthcare facility, including administrators, staff, patients and carers.[1]

Although the risk of infection and transmission of communicable diseases exists in all healthcare settings, some contexts present particular challenges.[21] The context of emergency nursing and paramedic practice are two such settings. The demand for emergency healthcare nationally and internationally is high.[22] Emergency nurses and paramedics provide clinical care to patients where there is a serious, unexpected or potentially dangerous situation requiring immediate action. The demands placed upon these healthcare professionals to render lifesaving care to the sick and injured are complex, time-pressured and high-stakes. Patients often present with complex, severe injuries and infections requiring rapid and aggressive intervention. The presentation of acute or chronic infections presents emergency nurses and paramedics with many challenges.

The ability to recognise infections and to determine their relative severity is critical to the practice of emergency nursing and paramedic practice. Severe or life-threatening infections, such as meningococcal septicaemia and sepsis,[23] require rapid identification and early intervention to ameliorate the high levels of morbidity and mortality.[24,25] If the care and interventions that emergency nurses and paramedics employ are to be effective and efficient, the strategies for infection prevention and control must be both high quality and safe. With increasing rates of presentations, increasing complexity of illness and disease, and a well-documented workforce shortage of skilled staff, healthcare professionals are expected to do more with less.[26,27] One of the consequences of this is that emergency nurses and paramedics are taking on new roles, extending their scope of practice, and consequently are more accountable for their clinical practice than ever before.[28] The rapid changes in the healthcare environment continue to precipitate challenges for healthcare professions regarding the sufficiency of professional practice standards, education and training, and clinical policy and procedures that ensure quality, safety and accountability in healthcare. As healthcare provided in primary and emergency care settings becomes more complex, so too do the complexities and risks of infection.

OVERVIEW OF INFECTION AND INFECTIOUS DISEASE

INFECTIONS AND OUTBREAKS

From time to time, new infections emerge to which individuals and populations around the world have little or no immunity. Infectious diseases account for approximately 25% of the 57 million deaths worldwide. Globally they are the leading cause of death for people under the age of 50 years.[29] The World Health Organization (WHO) estimates that new diseases are occurring at a rate of at least one per year. Occasionally, these outbreaks become pandemic. Historically, humankind has faced significant threats from infectious disease. The global 'Spanish flu' pandemic of 1918 caused an estimated 20–40 million deaths around the world. Influenza pandemics in 1957 and 1968 caused widespread morbidity and more than a million deaths worldwide, causing significant economic and social disruption.[30]

Australia has sustained relatively few outbreaks of infectious disease compared with the rest of the world. Although the demographic consequences have been minimal, the human and social impact on individuals and communities has been significant. The smallpox epidemics of 1881–82 and 1913–17 in Sydney, and the plague epidemic of 1900, led to the emergence of formal policies of isolation, quarantine, fumigation and cleansing and vaccination.[31] The most recent pandemic caused by SARS-CoV-2 (COVID-19) adversely affected every state and territory in the country, inducing strict mobility regulations, lockdowns, border closures and mask mandates. The outbreak of the novel virus placed an unparalleled strain on emergency healthcare workers, who were challenged by the need to constantly adapt to a rapidly changing situation, parse new and sometimes inconsistent information, handle surges in patient numbers, as well as mitigate the fear of contracting the disease and spreading it to family members.[32,33] Beyond this, there have been a few notable cases that captured public attention and were responsible for widespread fear and concern, which are listed in Table 27.1.[34]

Many of the infectious diseases that threatened public health and safety in the past continue to do so today. However, not all encounters with infectious agents lead to infection. For an infection to occur, a number of scientific conditions must be met. Understanding the science of infection and disease, including the modes of transmission of infectious organisms and knowing how and when to apply the basic principles of infection control, is critical to the success of an infection-control program.

Microorganisms are responsible for infectious disease. They are ubiquitous, and a necessary element of the environment. Not all of them, however, result in infection; not all are pathogenic all of the time. For microorganisms to cause infection, several criteria must be satisfied.

- There must be an agent that can cause disease.
- It must gain entry to the body of a susceptible host in sufficient numbers to overcome the body's defence mechanism.[35]
- The body must succumb to the infection, and for the spread to be sustained, it must leave the organism and spread to another.

This is referred to as the 'chain of infection' and is illustrated in Fig. 27.1.

For infection to occur, therefore, there must be a source of infection, a susceptible host and a means of transmission, and the *chain of infection* must be satisfied.

TABLE 27.1 NOTABLE INFECTIOUS DISEASE OUTBREAKS IN AUSTRALIA[34]

YEAR	DISEASE
1789-1790	Smallpox
1828	Smallpox
1857	Smallpox, influenza
1866/67	Measles
1875/76	Scarlet fever
1881/82	Smallpox
1894	Plague
1900/09	Plague
1913/17	Smallpox
1918/19	Spanish Influenza
1921	Plague
1937-1955	Polio
1940	Rubella
1957/58	Asian Influenza
1968/69	Hong Kong Influenza
1977/78	Russian Influenza
1997/1998	Cryptosporidiosis
1997	Hepatitis A
2000	Psittacosis
2009	Dengue fever (Queensland)
2009	H1N1 influenza
2020 - current	SARS-CoV-2 and COVID-19

THE CHAIN OF INFECTION

The chain of infection consists of six process points, each of which must occur concurrently for the spread of infection to be sustained.

1. Causative agent

First, there must be a causative agent. It may be caused by a variety of agents, such as a bacterium, virus, fungus or parasite. The property of an infectious agent that determines the extent to which overt disease is produced, or the power of an organism to produce disease, is called *pathogenicity*. Some agents are

FIGURE 27.1 THE CHAIN OF INFECTION

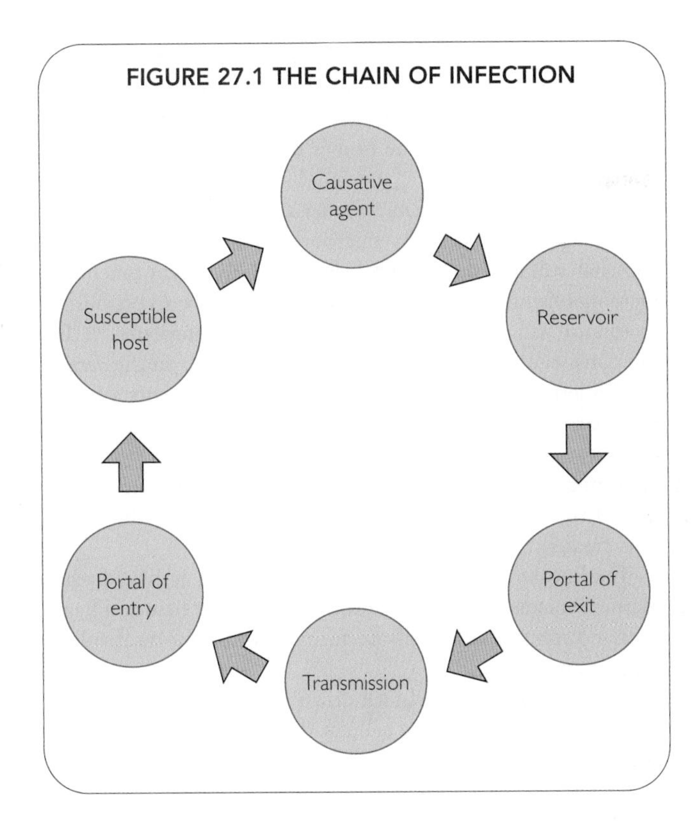

highly pathogenic and almost always produce disease, whereas others multiply without invasion and rarely cause disease.[36]

2. Reservoir

The causative agent that causes infection, such as bacteria, viruses, fungi, parasites and prions, can be involved in either colonisation or infection, depending on the susceptibility of the host.

- With *colonisation*, there is a sustained presence of replicating infectious agents on or in the body, without the production of an immune response or disease.
- With *infection*, invasion of infectious agents into the body results in an immune response, with or without symptomatic disease.[1]

Most microorganisms that cause disease in humans can only survive for limited periods outside the human body unless they are provided with an environment that will satisfy their requirements. Another animal or a non-living environment, such as soil or water, may provide an alternative environment or *reservoir* which will support the organism.

3. Susceptible host

To cause disease, the infectious agent must gain entry to a susceptible host. A susceptible host is one who lacks effective resistance to a pathogenic agent. Characteristics that influence susceptibility include age, sex, medical history, underlying pathology, lifestyle, nutrition, immunisation, medications and specific insult to the body, such as trauma.[36,37] The nature of the host response elicited by the pathogen often determines the pathology of a particular infection. The outcome of an infection depends on the balance between an effective host response that eliminates a pathogen, and an excessive inflammatory response that is associated with an inability to eliminate a pathogen and with resultant tissue damage that leads to disease.

In healthcare settings, the most common susceptible hosts are patients and healthcare workers. Patients may be exposed to infectious agents from themselves (endogenous infection) or from other people, instruments and equipment, or the environment (exogenous infection). The level of risk relates to the healthcare setting (specifically, the presence or absence of infectious agents), the type of healthcare procedures performed and the susceptibility of the patient. Healthcare workers may be exposed to infectious agents from infected or colonised patients, instruments and equipment, or the environment. The level of risk relates to the type of clinical contact healthcare workers have with potentially infected or colonised patient groups, instruments or environments, and the health status of the healthcare worker (e.g. immunised or immunocompromised).[1]

For some diseases, vaccination renders a potential host immune from infection, while for others it reduces the severity of disease and shedding of the microorganism if infected. It is the process whereby a person is deliberately exposed to an agent which is antigenic, but not pathogenic, to provide immunity to that specific antigen. Since the introduction of vaccination, the burden of many bacterial and viral diseases has been reduced. Healthcare workers have the potential to be exposed to many vaccine-preventable diseases. Vaccination against or proof of immunity to diphtheria, tetanus, pertussis, hepatitis B, varicella, measles, mumps, rubella, influenza and tuberculosis are recommended for healthcare workers throughout Australasia.[1]

4. Portal of entry

The major portals of entry are via the skin following trauma and via the mucous membranes lining the wall of the respiratory, gastrointestinal and genitourinary tracts. Pathogens may have a preferred portal of entry that gives access to an environment suitable for the establishment of growth. For example, *Bordetella pertussis*, which causes whooping cough, a disease of the respiratory system, enters via the mouth or nose.[38]

5. Transmission

There are five ways in which the causative agent may be transmitted: contact, inhalation, inoculation, ingestion and transplacenta, although in healthcare settings the main modes of transmission of infectious agents are contact (including bloodborne), droplet and airborne.[1]

The *contact route* consists of two subcategories: direct and indirect contact. The primary difference between the two is whether or not an environmental source is involved in disease transmission.

- With *direct contact*, there is no environmental source involved in disease transmission; the susceptible person comes into direct contact with an infected individual's contaminated body fluids.
- *Indirect contact* spread involves an intermediary contaminated environmental source between the infected person and the susceptible person.

In most situations, contact spread occurs when a healthcare worker's hands become contaminated with infectious particles and proper hand hygiene is not performed. Diseases such as scabies and methicillin-resistant *Staphylococcus aureus* (MRSA) are spread by contact transmission.[1]

The *droplet and airborne routes* are both forms of respiratory transmission, which involve the spread of infectious agents via respiratory droplets. Droplets can be projected from the respiratory tract via the nose or mouth when people sneeze, cough, talk or breathe—also known as aerosol-generating behaviours (AGBs). Furthermore, clinicians may also be involved in aerosol generating procedures, such as nebulising medications, performing CPR, RAT tests and the administration of inhaled analgesics that may cause a cough. These droplets contain millions of bacteria and viruses, and will vary in size, spread and air suspension. Larger respiratory droplets can infect healthcare workers within close proximity to the patient where they could inhale or come into contact with the infectious particles.

Increasingly small respiratory droplets may become airborne and be carried by air currents for long distances before settling onto the ground or a surface. They can remain suspended in the air for hours unless they are removed by ventilation or filtration systems and remain a risk to any nearby people who inhale the particles or touch contaminated surfaces. The person's respiratory tract (the mucous membranes of the nose, mouth or pharynx) then becomes the entry portal for pathogens to enter the body, either via direct inhalation or through contact with contaminated hands. Once the agent enters the body, it can replicate and cause an infection. Furthermore, direct contact with an infected person's respiratory secretions can also transmit infection. Infections such as influenzas and tuberculosis are examples of infectious diseases spread via respiratory droplets.[1]

Other modes of transmission also occur. *Trans-placental infections* are those that are transmitted vertically between mother and her embryo or fetus. Such infections are transmitted from the mother, who acts as the reservoir of infection. These infections include syphilis, rubella and viral hepatitis. Some infections are transmitted by *ingestion*, a form of contact, such as faecal–oral transmission for hepatitis A; and others via *inoculation*, such as hepatitis B and C. The modes of transmission vary by type of organism. In some cases the same organism may be transmitted by more than one route, such as influenza which can be transmitted by contact and droplet routes.[1]

6. Portal of exit

The agent may be transmitted in a variety of mediums, including blood, saliva, faeces, vomitus, discharge (wounds), urine and semen, or in other body tissues and/or fluids. The portal of exit is disease- and organism-specific. Some organisms present in one portal cannot be transmitted successfully in another. For example, hepatitis A exits the body via faeces, and hepatitis B and C by blood, and not vice versa.

WHEN INFECTION STRIKES: THE IMMUNE RESPONSE

The ability of the human body to resist infection depends on two major human defence mechanisms:[39] the *innate* or *non-specific* immune response and the *specific* immune response. These are outlined below.

Innate or non-specific immune response

The *innate* or *non-specific immunity* is the body's first line of defence. It relies on natural, mechanical and local barriers, does not discriminate one agent from another and acts in a similar way each time the same agent enters (or attempts to enter) the body. The function of the innate or non-specific immune response is to prevent the entry of pathogens into the tissues of the body, or to destroy them immediately if they do manage to enter. The skin and mucous membranes, certain cells, inflammation, various antimicrobial proteins and fever contribute to the body's non-specific response to a pathogen.[35]

The *skin* and *mucous membranes* are the body's first line of defence against invasion by microorganisms.[35] Intact skin and epithelial surfaces do not provide a friendly environment for microorganisms. The skin is dry, and mucosa have an established microflora and secretions with antimicrobial properties.[40] The skin consists of two distinct layers, the *epidermis* and the *dermis*. The epidermis is the tough outer layer and represents a formidable barrier to most organisms. The dermis contains sebaceous and sweat glands whose secretions inhibit the growth of some microorganisms. However, the bacteria that form the normal flora of the skin are tolerant and able to survive in the conditions created by the secretions.[35]

The human body's *cellular defence* system is activated when microorganisms or foreign substances enter the tissues. Phagocytes and natural killer cells perform a most important role in this system.

- *Phagocytes* ingest and break down foreign particles and dead tissue and remove cellular debris from the tissues; macrophages and neutrophils are the two major types of phagocytes. Macrophages, the largest of the phagocytic cells, are located in most tissues and organs of the body. Neutrophils, the most abundant of the white blood cells, are active in the bloodstream but also migrate into tissues in the early stages of infection and inflammation.
- *Natural killer cells* are large granular lymphocytes, which can destroy cancer cells and virus-infected cells. They do not recognise specific cells but attack a variety of targets.

Inflammation is the body's response to any injury or infection. The function of the acute inflammatory response is to prepare the injured area for the repair process by clearing the injured site of cellular debris and foreign material or pathogens. Once the injury has occurred, there is activation or release of a variety of chemicals, which cause dilation of the arterioles in the damaged area, increase the permeability of local capillaries and create an influx of phagocytic cells. This process creates the four main signs of acute inflammation: redness, heat, swelling and pain. *Chronic inflammation* occurs when the body is unable to clear the organisms or foreign particles from the damaged area.

Various *antimicrobial proteins*, the most important of which are the complement proteins, interferon and acute-phase proteins, also act non-specifically against foreign cells in the body. The complement system's major function is to enhance phagocytosis, produce inflammation and directly lyse foreign cells.

The hypothalamus (the body's thermostat) normally controls body temperature at around 37°C. *Fever*, a higher-than-normal body temperature, is the systemic response to invading microorganisms. Chemical substances called pyrogens that originate from within the body (endogenous) or outside the body (exogenous) produce fever. High fevers above 40°C may damage nerve cells and produce convulsions. However, a mild or moderate fever may be of benefit to the body, as temperatures above 37°C slow the rate of cell division of bacteria.

Specific immune response

Acquired or *specific immunity* is the body's second line of defence and is activated when microorganisms evade the non-specific defence mechanism. The specific and non-specific response systems overlap and interact with each other to protect the body.[35]

When a microbe evades the non-specific defences, the body reacts by producing an antigen-specific response. The specific immune response is tightly regulated and has unique properties: specificity for antigens, the ability to turn off the response once an exposure is cleared, and memory with augmentation, such that repeated exposure results in a more rapid and enhanced response.[40]

The specific or acquired immune system consists of a variety of cells, especially lymphocytes and macrophages, and various organs. There are two major populations of lymphocytes: the B lymphocytes (B cells) and the T lymphocytes (T cells). The B cells are mainly responsible for humoral immunity (immunity provided by antibodies), and the T cells provide cell-mediated immunity.[35]

Antibodies produced and secreted by plasma cells (derived from B cells) circulate in the blood and other body fluids. They bind to the invading microorganism and are most effective against bacteria and viruses before they enter host cells. An initial encounter with an antigen prompts a primary immune response, followed by a lag time during which there is activation and proliferation of B cells specific for the antigen. Specific serum antibody level will peak within several weeks and decline in weeks to months. If the body is exposed to the same microorganism a second time, then a secondary immune response occurs that is faster, stronger and longer-lasting. The response is prompt because of the priming of the immune system during the initial exposure when large numbers of memory B lymphocytes were produced.[35] This previously described process of antibody production is classified as *naturally-acquired active immunity*.

Immunity may also be acquired in other ways: *artificially-acquired active immunity* following vaccination; *artificially-acquired passive immunity* resulting from the transfer of premade antibodies from an immune person to a non-immune person; and *naturally-acquired passive immunity* when maternal antibodies pass across the placenta. Passive immunity provides only short-term protection against disease.

T-cells (cellular immunity) deal with intracellular pathogens by directly lysing the cells, or by releasing chemicals that enhance the inflammatory response and/or activate other defence cells to destroy the target cells. They are required for the proper functioning of both humoral and cell-mediated immunity. T-cell deficiency increases the susceptibility to viruses, intracellular bacteria and other intracellular parasites.[35]

BREAKING THE CHAIN—PREVENTING INFECTION

PRINCIPLES OF INFECTION PREVENTION AND CONTROL

The control and prevention of HAI and communicable diseases are high on the political and public agenda. The unacceptable burden of HAIs in economic and human terms is significant, with increasing patient length of hospital stay, re-admission, suffering, morbidity and mortality.[41–44] Ultimately, everyone pays the price for such infections.

The ACSQHC recognises the community concerns requiring urgent national consideration, and the role that infection prevention and control has on reducing hospital-acquired infections. The Commission's Healthcare Associated Infection Program[15] enables a national approach to reducing hospital-acquired infections by identifying and addressing systemic problems and gaps and ensuring that comprehensive actions are undertaken in a nationally coordinated way by leaders and decision-makers in both the public and the private health sectors.[45]

INFECTION PREVENTION PROGRAMS

The control and prevention of HAIs is a core function of all healthcare workers, including emergency nurses and paramedics. Infection prevention and control programs are formal structures and processes that together prevent, reduce and control transmission of HAI and the spread of infectious disease and enable the provision of safe and high-quality healthcare. Effective infection prevention guidelines and strategies for the control and prevention of hospital-acquired infections are required for all health contexts and settings, from large hospitals to emergency home and practice settings. Specific facilities require tailored programs and elements, but infection prevention principles remain the same across all healthcare settings. The success of infection prevention and control strategies relies on six key elements,[1] as shown in Fig. 27.2.

The *Australian Guidelines for the Prevention and Control of Infection in Healthcare* is the authoritative text for infection prevention and control across the range of healthcare establishments in Australia.[1] The recommendations for each setting

FIGURE 27.2 ELEMENTS OF SUCCESSFUL INFECTION PREVENTION PROGRAMS

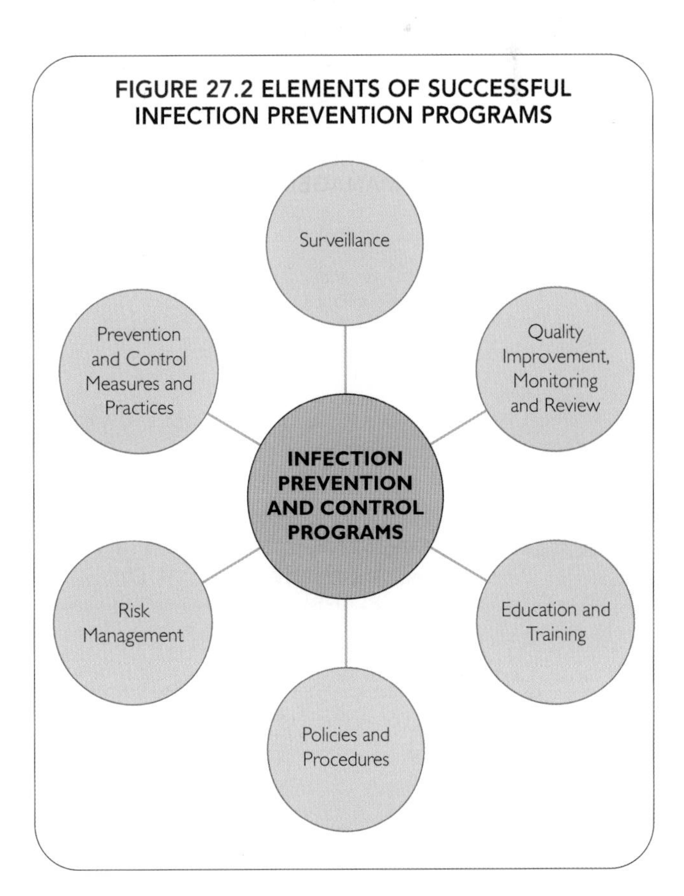

should be implemented in concert with state or territory legislative requirements that affect work practices at the local level. When using these guidelines, it is important to note that statutory requirements of the jurisdiction take precedence when difference exists. A range of resources and support materials are available for health professionals and agencies.[46]

INFECTION CONTROL MANAGEMENT PLANS

Work practices at the local level occur through the design, development and implementation of an infection-control management plan (ICMP), a formal and systematic clinical governance process that enables institutions to meet their infection prevention and control obligations within the broader corporate mission and goal.[1] They are designed to ensure that institutions and their people demonstrate accountability for quality in areas of infection prevention and control. Infection control management plans should risk-manage and reduce the incidence of preventable HAIs within organisational frameworks and systems that ensure quality and safety in healthcare.[47]

ICMPs should embrace, build and extend the organisational strategic plan, where they define the scope of an infection prevention program within the boundaries of areas such as client demographics, epidemiology of infection and restricted resources. The plan allows organisations to prioritise infection prevention activity in accordance with principles of risk management and to develop appropriate professional and program performance measures; thereby demonstrating professional and public accountability of the infection prevention program in terms of cost-effectiveness and/or cost–benefit.[47] Key elements of an infection-control program are outlined below (Fig 27.3).

An ICMP must incorporate all practice contexts, including the emergency care setting. The plan provides a strategic evidence base to guide work practices. The intentions documented in the strategic plan or activities outlined in the operational plan should form the basis of the infection control committee's (ICC) agenda, thereby assisting the ICC to steer activity.

Good infection control outcomes rely on clinicians and service providers complying with infection-control principles/standards and reporting various risk factors and/or situations that may lead to a risk of infection transmission. As such, leadership is required to obtain stakeholder buy-in at every level of the organisation. Key stakeholder input is required when setting policies/guidelines, targets and performance measures, as in most instances the performance being measured is that of the stakeholders. This fact needs to be clear for clinicians or service providers to be held accountable for their actions and outcomes.

In 2013, the ACSQHC released National Safety and Quality Health Service (NSQHS) Standards to improve the quality of health service provision in Australia. These Standards, revised in 2017 and updated in 2021, provide a nationally consistent statement of the level of care consumers should be able to expect from health service organisations.[2] There are currently eight NSQHS Standards focusing on areas that are essential to drive the implementation and use of safety and quality systems, including Preventing and Controlling Infections Standard.[48] This Standard aims to prevent patients acquiring preventable healthcare-associated infection and to effectively manage infections when they occur using evidence-based strategies.

For this to be successful, a variety of measures are required, as outlined in Box 27.1.[48,49] There must be formal governance and

FIGURE 27.3 CORE ELEMENTS OF AN INFECTION CONTROL MANAGEMENT PLAN

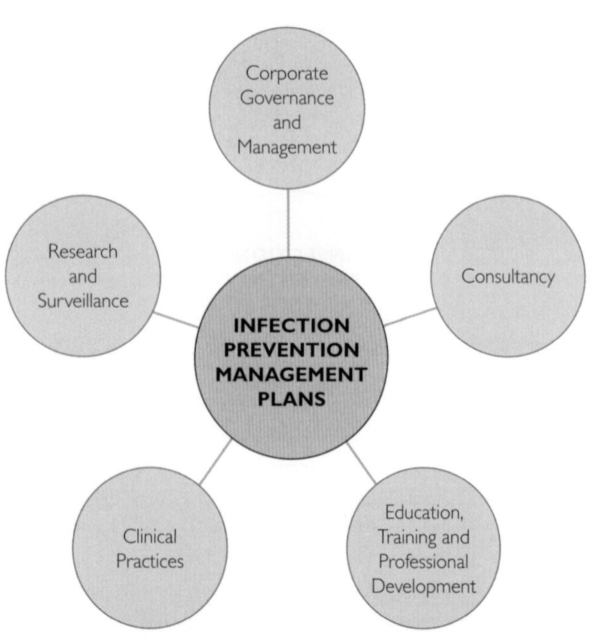

BOX 27.1 NATIONAL SAFETY AND QUALITY HEALTH SERVICE STANDARDS: PREVENTING AND CONTROLLING INFECTIONS STANDARD[48]

1. **Clinical governance and quality improvement to prevent and control healthcare-associated infections, and support antimicrobial stewardship**
   Systems are in place to support and promote prevention and control of healthcare-associated infections, and improve antimicrobial stewardship.
2. **Infection prevention and control systems**
   Evidence-based systems are used to prevent and control healthcare-associated infections. Patients presenting with, or with risk factors for, infection or colonisation with an organism of local, national or global significance are identified promptly, and receive the necessary management and treatment. The health service organisation is clean and hygienic.
3. **Reprocessing of reusable medical devices**
   Reprocessing of reusable equipment, instruments and devices is consistent with relevant current national standards, and meets current best practice.
4. **Antimicrobial stewardship**
   The health service organisation implements systems for the safe and appropriate prescribing and use of antimicrobials as part of an antimicrobial stewardship program.

Reproduced with permission from National Safety and Quality Health Service Standards (2nd ed), developed by the Australian Commission on Safety and Quality in Health Care (ACSQHC). Sydney: ACSQHC; 2021.

management systems for healthcare associated infections that operate systemically within quality assurance systems. Healthcare agencies and professionals must ensure strategies for the prevention and control of healthcare-associated infections are developed and implemented. Patients that present with or acquire an infection or colonisation during an episode or following episodes of care must be identified promptly and receive timely management and treatment, and they must be informed about their treatment and care. The healthcare environment must be clean and hygienic in accordance with best evidence and practice standards, in particular instrument and equipment reprocessing. Finally, safe and appropriate antimicrobial prescribing is a strategic goal of the clinical governance system. The Commission has developed tools and resources to assist emergency nurses, paramedics and other health professionals with the implementation of the Standards.[50]

BASIC MEASURES—STANDARD AND TRANSMISSION-BASED PRECAUTIONS

Central to the success of the implementation of NSQHS Preventing and Controlling Infections Standard is the implementation of systematic infection control practices. The emergency nurse and paramedic must adopt work practices that adhere to the two-tiered system of *Standard* and *Transmission-based* precautions.[48]

Standard Precautions

Standard Precautions are practices and procedures that are employed during the care of all patients to achieve a basic level of infection prevention and control. They are work practices that ensure that a basic level of infection control is applied to everyone, regardless of their perceived or confirmed infectious status. Implementing Standard Precautions as a first-line approach to infection control in the healthcare environment minimises the risk of transmission of infectious agents from person to person, even in high-risk situations.[1] The core elements of Standard Precautions include the following:

- Aseptic technique, including appropriate use of skin disinfectants.
- Personal hygiene practices, particularly handwashing and hand hygiene, and cough etiquette.
- Use of personal protective equipment.
- Appropriate handling and disposal of sharps and clinical waste.
- Appropriate reprocessing of reusable equipment and instruments, including appropriate use of disinfectants.
- Environmental controls, including design and maintenance of premises, cleaning and spills management.
- Appropriate provision of support services, such as laundry and food services.

In the clinical environment, transmission of an infectious agent to a susceptible host occurs by direct and indirect contact. Inappropriate hand hygiene is the most significant reason for hospital-acquired infections. In the absence of a true emergency, personnel should always perform hand hygiene in accordance with the Five Moments for Hand Hygiene (Fig. 27.4). Hand hygiene must be performed before and after every episode of patient contact. This includes before touching a patient, before a procedure, after a procedure or body-fluid-exposure

FIGURE 27.4 THE FIVE MOMENTS FOR HAND HYGIENE[51]

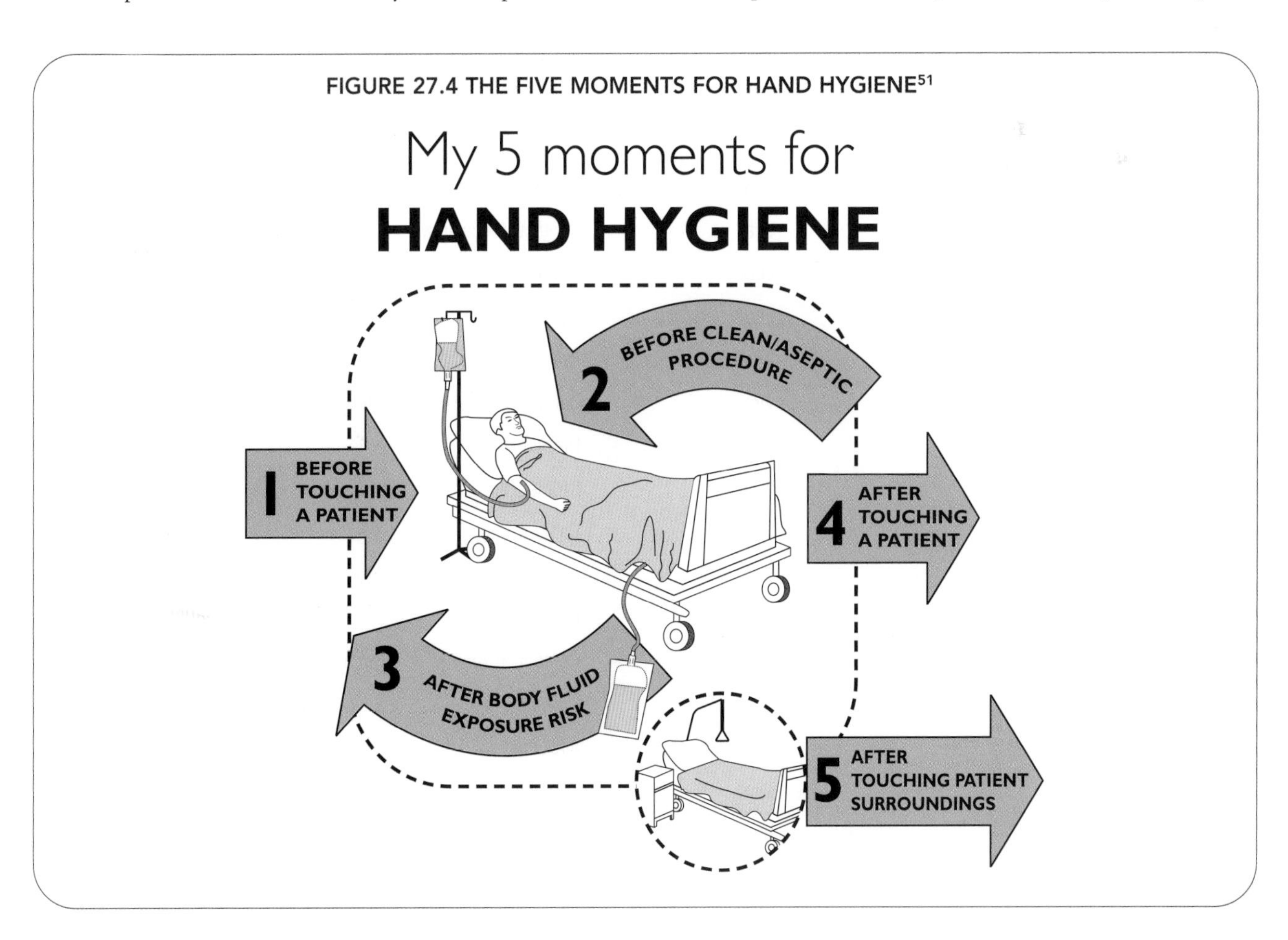

risk, after touching a patient and after touching a patient's surroundings. Hand hygiene must also be performed after removal of gloves. Alcohol-based hand rubs containing at least 70% v/v ethanol or equivalent should be used for all routine hand hygiene practices in the healthcare environment. Alcohol-based products may be used as an adjunct to traditional handwashing. However, visible soil must be removed by handwashing before using antiseptic products formulated for use without water.[1]

Transmission-based precautions

Transmission-based precautions are required in extra work-practice situations where Standard Precautions alone may be insufficient to prevent infection (e.g. for patients known or suspected to be infected or colonised with infectious agents that may not be contained with Standard Precautions alone. See Table 27.2).[1]

These precautions are tailored around specific infections or organisms, and may involve measures to prevent contact, airborne or droplet transmission (such as source isolation). Transmission-based precautions are also used in the event of an outbreak (e.g. gastroenteritis), to assist in containing the outbreak and preventing further infection, and must be tailored to the particular infectious agent involved and its mode of transmission.[1] This may involve a combination of the practices included in Box 27.2.

Transmission of infectious agents can occur in several ways. While these terminologies are used in current government documents, this area is subject to considerable debate and need for change. We present the modes of transmission as described currently in the literature, acknowledging there are limitations with this approach:

- *Indirect or direct contact transmission*, when a healthcare worker's hands or clothing become contaminated, patient-care devices are shared between patients, infectious patients have contact with other patients or environmental surfaces are not regularly decontaminated.
- *Droplet transmission*, when a healthcare worker's hands become contaminated with respiratory droplets and are transferred to susceptible mucosal surfaces, such as the eyes; when infectious respiratory droplets are expelled by coughing, sneezing or talking, and are either inhaled or come into contact with another's mucosa (eyes, nose or mouth), either directly into or via contaminated hands.
- *Airborne transmission*, when attending healthcare workers or others are exposed to small particles that contain infectious agents.[1]

TABLE 27.2 INFECTIONS WARRANTING TRANSMISSION-BASED PRECAUTIONS BEFORE LABORATORY CONFIRMATION OF INFECTION

INFECTION	TYPE	TRANSMISSION
Chicken pox and shingles (varicella zoster)	Viral	Airborne and contact (vesicular fluid)
Creutzfeldt-Jakob disease	Prion	Contact (CNS instruments)
Gastroenteritis	Bacterial	Contact (faecal-oral)
Gastroenteritis	Viral	Contact/droplet
Hepatitis A	Viral	Contact (faecal-oral)
Influenza (during outbreaks)	Viral	Droplet
Measles	Viral	Airborne
Meningococcal infection	Bacterial	Droplet
Norovirus	Viral	Contact/droplet (aerosolised vomitus)
Parvovirus B19	Viral	Droplet
Respiratory syncytial virus	Viral	Droplet (oral, fomites)
Rotavirus	Viral	Contact (faecal-oral)
Rubella	Viral	Droplet
Severe acute respiratory syndrome (SARS)	Viral	Droplet
SARS-CoV-2 (COVID-19)	Viral	Contact + droplet + airborne (for AGPs)
Staphylococcal infection	Bacterial	Droplet
Tuberculosis	Bacterial	Airborne
Viral haemorrhagic fevers	Viral	Contact
Whooping cough (pertussis)	Bacterial	Droplet

CNS: central nervous system.

BOX 27.2 TRANSMISSION-BASED PRECAUTIONS[1,8]

- Allocating a single room to an infected patient (isolation)
- Placing patients colonised or infected with the same infectious agent in a room together (cohorting)
- Personal protective equipment that is specific to the task being performed
- Using disinfectants effective against the specific infectious agent
- Providing a dedicated toilet
- Use of specific air-handling techniques
- Restricting movement of both patients and healthcare workers

For diseases that have multiple routes of transmission, more than one transmission-based precaution category is applied. Whether used singly or in combination, transmission-based precautions are always applied *in addition* to Standard Precautions, as outlined in Table 27.3. Transmission-based precautions remain in effect for limited periods of time until signs and symptoms of the infection have resolved or according to recommendations specific to the infectious agent as advised by infection-control practitioners.[1] Nurses and clinical staff should attend to signs on patient doors that indicate the level of PPE required prior to entering.

In Australia, a national system of surveillance operates to track the control and prevention of some organisms for which transmission-based precautions are used, referred to as 'notifiable diseases'. The National Notifiable Diseases Surveillance System was established in 1990 under the auspices of the Communicable Diseases Network Australia. It coordinates national surveillance of more than 50 communicable diseases or disease groups. Under this scheme, notifications are made to the state or territory health authority under the provisions of the public health legislation in their jurisdiction. Computerised, de-identified unit records of notifications are supplied to the Australian Government Department of Health and Ageing on a daily basis, for collation, analysis and publication on the internet and in the quarterly journal *Communicable Diseases Intelligence*.[1]

SPECIFIC CHALLENGES FOR INFECTION PREVENTION AND CONTROL IN EMERGENCY CARE

There are a variety of other special challenges in infection prevention and communicable diseases for emergency nurses and paramedics.

SARS-COV-2 AND COVID-19

The COVID-19 pandemic in Australia has resulted in cases and deaths recorded across every state and territory.[52] The early months of the pandemic saw a decline of 1.4% in the number of emergency department (ED) presentations compared to the previous year, most likely due to the mobility restrictions in place and public hesitation and fear of visiting hospitals.[53–56] Despite this, EDs still struggled, with ambulance services showing deteriorating response times, longer case times and hospital delays, probably as the result of ED crowding and limited capacity during lockdown.[57,58]

Healthcare and emergency care workers are at a significantly higher risk of infection compared to the general public,[33,59]

TABLE 27.3 APPLICATION OF STANDARD AND TRANSMISSION-BASED PRECAUTIONS[1,8]

	TYPE OF PRECAUTION			
	STANDARD	CONTACT	DROPLET	AIRBORNE
Examples of infectious agents	*Standard practices for all patients*	*Scabies, MRSA, VRE*	*Influenza, norovirus, pertussis*	*Pulmonary TB, varicella, measles*
Hand hygiene	✓	✓	✓	✓
Single room/cohort transport	×	✓	✓	✓ Negative pressure
Gloves	⊙	✓	✓	✓
Gown	⊙	✓	✓	✓
Mask	⊙	✓ Surgical mask if in sputum	✓ Surgical mask	✓ P2 (N95) respirator
Eye protection	⊙	⊙	⊙	✓
Equipment handling	⊙	Single use or reprocess	Single use or reprocess	Single use or reprocess
Visitors	×	⊙	Restrict number, and precautions as for staff	Restrict number, and precautions as for staff

MRSA: methicillin-resistant Staphylococcus aureus; *TB: tuberculosis; VRE: vancomycin-resistant* Enterococcus.

⊙ *As required—gloves to be worn whenever potential exposure to body fluids; gown if contamination with blood, body fluids, secretions or excretions likely; face and/or eye protection if splash likely (including during aerosol-generating procedures).*

particularly when PPE is inadequately donned or reused,[60] a practice further exacerbated by the fear of supply shortages during the beginning of the pandemic.[32,33,60] Outbreaks occurring among healthcare workers caused considerable issues with significant knock-on effects. The quarantining of positive workers and suspected contacts was the first line of defence in stopping the spread of the virus, but led to substantial limitations in hospital capacity and increased strain on the remaining providers.[53] The mental health toll on workers in response to a pandemic should also not be understated, with higher reports of depression, anxiety and distress,[61] emergency nurses and clinicians reporting greater workload and stress,[32] and a non-trivial proportion of the emergency nurses indicating an intention to leave the profession within the next 5 years.[62]

The situation improved gradually with greater understanding of the disease, access to more rapid testing, antiviral medications and greater observance of prophylactic measures, including the widespread dissemination and mandatory uptake of vaccinations.[63] Frontline workers and care staff were prioritised during the first national rollout of COVID-19 vaccines, which began in early 2021.[53] Furthermore, adoption of some clinical procedures can reduce the transmission of SARS-CoV-2 in the emergency setting, such as prioritising early insertion of supraglottic devices such as i-gel, rather than ventilating with a bag–valve–mask (BVM).

However, caution must continue to be exercised in response to the virus and its emerging variants, as well as changes in the protection offered by existing vaccinations over time.[64] ED presentations saw a resurgence in 2020–21, with numbers increasing by 6.9% despite continued, though sporadic, restrictions remaining in place across the country at the time.[54] Since the easing of restrictions upon meeting vaccination thresholds in late 2021, national case numbers and fatalities have rapidly increased.[65] The pandemic has highlighted the importance for a system-wide coordinated approach to managing patients and resources in EDs.[58]

INFECTIONS IN OLDER POPULATIONS

Older individuals are at an increased risk of morbidity and mortality from infection due to normal physiological changes, such as decreased mobility, impaired sight and hearing, and declining response to immunisations and medications. In addition, cognitive impairment and/or altered mental status changes put older people at risk from infection and make diagnosis more difficult. The frail elderly and those who live in institutionalised settings, such as long-term care or nursing homes and assisted living, tend to have limited mobility and comorbidities that put them at increased risk for infection.[21]

ED and emergency medical services personnel can expect to see infections frequently among older individuals and populations. Infection is the primary reason for hospital admissions among elderly individuals who reside in long-term care facilities such as nursing homes.[1] Infection may be difficult to diagnose in elderly people because most older individuals have a pulse/temperature dissociation that masks the signs of infection.[21] Diagnosis of infection may also be difficult because other normal signs of infection may be absent among older adults. Often, a change in behaviour or cognitive functioning, loss of appetite, or tachypnoea is the only symptom that indicates an infection is present in older individuals.[1]

The COVID-19 pandemic gravely elucidated the disproportionately adverse impact disease outbreaks have on older people, who were more likely to have additional comorbidities and experience greater severity of COVID-19 symptoms and mortality.[66] At the time of writing, the median age of COVID-19 deaths in Australia is 83.9, with the highest number of deaths occurring for those aged between 80 and 89, who have accounted for over one-third of total deaths.[67] The age groups with the second and third highest fatalities were those over 90 and those between 70 and 79 years of age, which accounted for 25.6% and 21.3% of total deaths respectively. This mortality rate is particularly critical when considering that Australians over 60 years of age comprise up to less than 10% of cases, yet account for over 90% of deaths.[65]

This trend has persisted since the beginning of the outbreak, where aged care residents were quickly identified as one of the most at-risk groups.[53] In addition to increased disease vulnerability, aged care residents live in close proximity to each other and in frequent contact with mobile care workers.[68] The first major outbreak in a residential aged care centre hit New South Wales in early 2020 and resulted in 61 confirmed cases across residents and staff, and 17 resident fatalities.[53,69] Several months later, a surge of outbreaks devastated Victoria, with active cases in over 200 aged care facilities and over 650 deaths by the end of the outbreak period.[70] During this time, written advice and guidelines for healthcare and emergency workers were available but inconsistent in execution amid the escalating situation.[71]

In particular, the decision for diagnosed residents to be removed from aged care facilities and transferred to hospitals was a contentious one. Initial recommendations based on WHO guidelines suggested immediate hospital transfer for any COVID-positive resident for the purpose of intensive care and separation from negative residents in the facility.[69] While this was practised by several facilities during the outbreak, the benefits of hospital care did not necessarily outweigh the complications associated with transfers and the ever-increasing burden on the healthcare system.[72] This recommendation was subsequently revised such that hospital admissions only occurred for those who required clinical care. Healthcare and emergency workers must be prepared to evaluate residents on a case-by-case basis with appropriate risk assessment that takes into consideration the health of the individual, the costs of transfer and the wellbeing of other residents within the aged care facility.[65]

INFECTIONS IN PAEDIATRIC POPULATIONS

Children are at increased risk from infection for a variety of reasons. First, very young children are dependent upon adult caregivers to ensure that proper hygiene needs are met. Secondly, children's immune systems are not as developed as adults, putting them at risk from infections that are generally not an issue in adults. In addition, young children tend to put objects into their mouths, which increases the risk of faecal–oral and contact transmission of infectious agents. Children also have a higher respiratory rate than adults and a disproportionate ratio of body surface area to weight, which puts them at risk from inhaling aerosolised infectious agents. Respiratory infectious diseases comprise a significant proportion of infectious diseases seen by emergency clinicians, particularly in seasonal patterns. Lastly, children are more at risk from vaccine-preventable diseases because they often have not yet developed full immunity to these agents. Similar to adults, children are at risk from hospital-acquired infections, multi-resistant organisms (MROs) and respiratory illnesses. Newborns and children with immunodeficiencies are at an increased risk from infection, especially during an infectious disease outbreak.

Emergency clinicians need to be prepared to address paediatric concerns in relation to infection prevention, including the need for special medical equipment/supplies that are specific to children. Examples of such equipment include different doses of medications (usually based on the child's weight), smaller endotracheal tubes, needles, intravenous kits, linen and other equipment.[1]

SEPSIS, WOUNDS, ANTIBIOTICS AND MULTI-DRUG RESISTANCE

Wounds, particularly chronic ones, present emergency nurses and paramedics with challenges. Wounds are often chronic and complex in nature, and emergency nurses and paramedics often manage them in resource-poor environments that may compound the complexity of wound care. Wound care is made more complex with multi-resistant organisms such as MRSA. The emergence and re-emergence of rapid-spread MROs is an ongoing international health priority.[16]

When *S. aureus* or another organism overcomes the body's defence mechanisms, as described earlier in the chapter, infection occurs. Local signs of infection include oedema, erythema and purulent exudate. If the infection becomes vascular, patients may deteriorate into sepsis or septic shock, a form of distributive shock with a higher risk of mortality.[73] In this event, fluid shift in the peripheral vasculature occurs, where extravascular spaces result in pooling of fluid, hypotension and poor tissue perfusion, as described in Chapter 14. In septic shock, patients present with systemic vasodilation, bounding pulse, tachycardia, bradycardia, hypoxia, altered mental state, alterations in core temperature and, in the late stages, a fall in blood pressure and oliguria. At the cellular level, there are alterations in microvascularity, vasodilation, poor perfusion, capillary endothelial leak and anaerobic respiration within the cell leading to the production of lactic acid.[25,74] Septic shock ultimately results in a cellular hypoxia, anaerobic metabolism and respiration and irreversible cell injury. Treating the infection is critical for resuscitation to be successful.

Identifying, treating and preventing wound infection, and sepsis, is a major challenge in emergency trauma and care, and there are well-established screening tools that should be deployed, such as qSOFA. In instances of sepsis and septic shock, patients require aggressive resuscitation and rapid, broad-spectrum antibiotic therapy until microbiological culture and sensitivities, and antibiograms, can be performed.[24,25] Box 27.3 summarises important principles of treatment for septic shock.

Historically, *S. aureus* has been a major cause of wound infections, septic shock and hospital-associated infection. It is the leading cause of healthcare-associated surgical-site infections, and the second leading cause of healthcare-associated bloodstream infections. It is responsible for infections such as osteomyelitis, septic arthritis, skin infections, endocarditis and meningitis.[76] MRSA continues to challenge the safety and quality of modern healthcare, and in some settings MRSA can constitute as many as 20% of all hospital-acquired infections. Endemic in most hospitals and epidemic in others, approximately 30% of all *S. aureus* infections present with some form of drug resistance.[77] First reported in 1961, MRSA is internationally endemic and one of the most challenging bacterial pathogens affecting clients in hospitals, including the ED. More recently, community-acquired MRSA (CA-MRSA) presents particular challenges. It occurs in otherwise healthy individuals with no risk factors for MRSA (such as recent hospitalisation, surgical procedure or antibiotic administration). The prevalence of CA-MRSA in EDs is increasing, especially in paediatric settings.[16]

The main route of MRSA transfer is from one client to another. Individuals transmit infection by failing to decontaminate their hands effectively before and after contact with individuals colonised or infected with MRSA. Attempts to eliminate endemic MRSA in hospitals have proven difficult, costly and have been largely unsuccessful. In some settings, identification of known carriers, prospective surveillance of clients and hospital workers and use of nasal mupirocin have helped control drug-resistant *S. aureus* infection rates.[77,78] Reported costs of a healthcare-acquired infection vary because of the wide range of study populations, sites of infection and methods used.[77]

Sometimes sepsis is due to MROs, making treatment even more challenging. Another organism that is significant, in that it results in increased morbidity, is *Clostridioides difficile*. *C. difficile* infections are on the rise in hospitals around the world, including Australia. Emergency clinicians are likely to encounter a patient with *C. difficile* infection; when this occurs, contact precautions should be utilised to prevent healthcare-associated spread.

Fundamentally, good hand hygiene is central to controlling and preventing the spread of infection.[1,8] Frequent and thorough hand hygiene and decontamination practices must be employed by emergency nurses and paramedics. Australian research suggests that nurses rely on facilities provided by the client for hand hygiene, and in the main nurses 'make do' when facilities, tools, inclination or time are inadequate.[79] In emergency nursing and paramedic practice settings, initiatives such as alcohol hand gels and rubs for use at 'point of care' are helpful. Emergency nurses and paramedics require an understanding of microbiology, and how and why microorganisms develop

BOX 27.3 PRINCIPLES OF TREATMENT FOR SEPTICAEMIA AND SEPTIC SHOCK

1. **Oxygen therapy (high-flow)**
2. **Fluid resuscitation**
3. **Urinalysis to ensure output of > 0.05 mL/kg/h**
4. **Blood and wound cultures**
5. **Broad-spectrum antibiotic therapy pending microbiological culture/sensitivity and antibiograms**
6. **Blood gas and haemodynamic monitoring, especially for lactic acidosis**
7. **Other interventions including glycaemic regulation, vasopressors (such as dopamine, adrenaline, noradrenaline and vasopressin), inotropic support (such as dobutamine), bicarbonate therapy (consideration for advanced acidosis), steroids.**[73,75]

resistance to antibiotics. This prepares them for preventing the spread of MROs, and equips them with the knowledge they need to teach clients and their families about infection control and antibiotic management.[80] Continued investment in comprehensive infection control programs that focus on sound hand hygiene practices, surveillance and rational and justified use of antibiotics are essential for emergency nursing and paramedic practice.

BACTERAEMIA ASSOCIATED WITH CANNULATION AND SEMI-CRITICAL DEVICES

Bacteraemias are life-threatening HAIs, and they are preventable. There are preventable and predictable risk factors for bacteraemia, typically the use of peripheral intravenous cannulas and other associated devices. Point-of-care ultrasound (PoCUS) percutaneous cannulation is increasingly used globally in emergency and critical care settings as routine practice and a core skill of practitioners. There is an ever-increasing body of evidence demonstrating its efficacy and safety as the preferred method for percutaneous cannulation for particular patient groups and presenting conditions.[81–83] The practice is, however, associated with significant risks to patients, in particular for healthcare-associated infections such as bloodstream infection and associated sepsis.[84] A recent study highlights this with an outbreak of *Burkholderia cenocepacia* bacteraemia and infection in 11 intensive and ED patients caused by contaminated sterile ultrasound gel used for central-line insertion and sterile procedures within four hospitals across Australia.[14] While the popularity of PoCUS percutaneous cannulation is ever-increasing, measures to protect patients from procedure-associated bacteraemia have not been as forthcoming. There are significant issues with a lack of systematic cleaning and decontamination of the equipment of this semi-critical device, related to both the high demand for its use in emergency care settings and a lack of recognition of the risks of healthcare-associated infection.[85,86] A lack of formal accreditation of practitioners in the use of PoCUS poses significant risks to patients. Formal training and certification of practitioners, including knowledge of and compliance with formal decontamination procedures, is required to ensure not only the efficacy of the procedure, but also its safety with respect to the significant risks of HAI.

INFLUENZA

Influenza is a contagious and acute viral infection that attacks the respiratory system. Influenza has evolved over hundreds of years, surviving the passing of time and the rising and falling of populations, to remain a significant global challenge. Over many years, multiple strains of influenza have been encountered globally. The 'Spanish flu' of 1918–19 was estimated to have killed 40–50 million people worldwide, including 11,500 in Australia—in an age before mass commercial air travel.[30] Outbreaks of avian influenza in bird flocks have affected many countries in Asia, the Middle East, Europe and Africa,[87,88] with as many as 15 different groups of avian influenza virus present in wild bird populations. The virus is largely asymptomatic in host populations. Humans appear to be accidental hosts of this infection, which is spread through bird faeces and contaminated water or dust. The pathogenicity of avian influenza changes as the virus mutates and spreads between host populations and can result in severe disease. Those strains with the highest mortality rates are referred to as 'highly pathogenic avian influenza' (HPAI) and are thought to have evolved from the 2003 strain (H5N1) found in Asia, which spread to most parts of the world through migratory birds and the poultry trade. Strict quarantine and infection-control measures successfully halted the spread of earlier infection; however, the current strain has moved across continents worldwide.[87]

Although H5N1 can cause severe and sometimes fatal infections in humans, the actual number of human cases around the world has been small relative to the levels of infection in host bird populations. Human cases have been in people who had close contact with infected poultry, usually from their own farms.[88] There is evidence that supports effective human-to-human spread of H5N1 infection.[88] An outbreak of H5N1, if significant, could have devastating economic and social impacts on Australia. Outbreaks of HPAI have occurred in Australia and around the world, and while outbreaks are quickly eradicated or are self-limiting, there is evidence and growing concern of contact between farmed poultry and wild waterfowl.[30]

Infection prevention for influenza is best aimed at reducing emergency risk and household transmission.[89] Personal hygiene, such as hand hygiene and cough etiquette, is an important infection-control measure in deterring household infection transmission, particularly for respiratory infections such as influenza.

EDs and emergency medical services are at the forefront of Australia's health disaster response, providing immediate patient care and system-wide patient facilitation. The H1N1 influenza 2009 demonstrated the diversity of roles of EDs in disease containment and management, but also provided an opportunity to describe the extended clinical impact of pandemic disease. Public awareness of H1N1 influenza 2009 led to a large number of patients presenting to both EDs and primary health services (including general practitioners). The H1N1 influenza 2009 outbreak had a significant impact on workload of EDs and ambulance services, with large numbers of patients presenting with flu-like illness. This impact occurred at a time when Australian and Aotearoa New Zealand emergency health services were confronting continual problems of overcrowding associated with access block and growing demand. EDs and ambulance services have responded to this demand and have adopted standard and transmission-based precautions to manage these patients, protect staff members and protect non-affected patients and visitors from potential cross-contamination. The response by EDs to the H1N1 influenza outbreak occurred during a period of evolving knowledge about the disease. Initial reports from Mexico raised serious concerns regarding the severity and mortality rate. Although the severity was subsequently shown to be less serious, the response by EDs and ambulance services was, and always will be, based on the information available at the time. Such events highlight the importance of pandemic planning by emergency health services.[90]

Recent research indicates that Australian and Aotearoa New Zealand hospitals have experienced significant increases in demand for service during peak periods of seasonal respiratory infections, in some states as high as a 10-fold increase, resulting in increased access block, ED overcrowding and ambulance ramping, all known to be associated with increased morbidity and mortality.[22,90] Other research indicates that many hospitals in Australia and around the world were unable to order sufficient supplies to care for H1N1 patients, including transport media for laboratory testing, masks, N95 respirators, disinfectant wipes, oseltamivir (e.g. Tamiflu) and other products needed for infection prevention.[91] While research demonstrates that prophylactic antiviral administration reduces time to first alleviation of symptoms, there are side-effects associated with its use. The evidence supporting clinically significant effects on complications from infection is limited. Moreover, the value and utility of stockpiling, particularly in economic terms, relative to potential benefits has been questioned.[92]

HIGH-CONSEQUENCE INFECTIOUS DISEASES INCLUDING SARS-CoV-1, MERS-CoV AND OTHER INFECTIONS

High consequence infectious diseases (HCIDs) are defined as a specific category of infectious diseases characterised by high case infectivity, communicability, mortality and that are difficult to prevent, contain and treat.[93] Public Health England further states that such diseases have been often difficult to detect rapidly and require significant system preparation and response to effectively manage.[94] While Australia does have nationally established guidelines for specific diseases that meet HCID criteria, it has not explicitly published an official list of HCIDs. Currently, international classifications from countries with similar demography and health systems are used instead. In the United Kingdom, Public Health England distinguishes two types of HCIDs: contact and airborne, which are listed in Table 27.4.[94] Contact HCIDs are spread through direct contact with the fluids or tissue of infected persons or via contaminated surfaces. Airborne HCIDs spread through respiratory droplets and aerosol transmission.

TABLE 27.4 PUBLIC HEALTH ENGLAND CLASSIFICATION OF CONTACT AND AIRBORNE HIGH-CONSEQUENCE INFECTIOUS DISEASES[94]

CONTACT HCIDs	AIRBORNE HCIDs
Argentine haemorrhagic fever (*Argentinian mammarenavirus*, formerly *Junin virus*)	Andes virus infection (hantavirus)
Bolivian haemorrhagic fever (*Machupo mammarenavirus*)	Avian influenza A H7N9 and H5N1
Crimean-Congo haemorrhagic fever (CCHF)	Avian influenza A H5N6 and H7N7
Ebola virus disease (EVD)	Middle East respiratory syndrome (MERS)
Lassa fever	Monkeypox virus
Lujo virus disease (*Lujo mammarenavirus*)	Nipah virus infection
Marburg virus disease (MVD)	Pneumonic plague (*Yersinia pestis*)
Severe fever with thrombocytopaenia syndrome (SFTS)	Severe acute respiratory syndrome (SARS)

Of particular concern are viral haemorrhagic fevers (VHF), a name given to a syndrome of acute and severe febrile illness caused by more than 30 viruses from four different taxonomic families, *Arenaviridae*, *Bunyaviridae*, *Flaviviridae* and *Filoviridae*.[95] These viruses do not occur naturally in Australia,[96] but are endemic to Africa, Asia, Eastern Europe and the Middle East.[1,97] Transmission of VHF is predominantly zoonotic, the ribonucleic acid (RNA) virus existing in nature in domestic animals and wildlife with the ability to transmit to humans, and subsequently spread by human-to-human contact.[95,98] There are four VHFs of primary concern: Lassa fever, Crimean-Congo haemorrhagic fever, Marburg virus haemorrhagic fever and Ebola virus disease (EVD).[1,97] The Arenaviruses include Lassa virus, causing Lassa fever, discovered in humans in Nigeria in 1969, and spread by rodent excreta.[99] The Bunyaviruses, *Nairovirus* genus, cause Crimean-Congo haemorrhagic fever, found in Crimea and subsequently isolated in the Congo in 1956, and spread by ticks.[100]

The more lethal Filoviruses, Marburg virus and Ebola virus, have been found in fruit bats in Africa and Asia.[98] The African strains of the Ebola virus have a reported high case mortality of 50–70%, contrasting with the Asian strain which does not cause disease in humans.[101] The Marburg virus was discovered in 1967 when laboratory workers in Marburg, Germany, and Yugoslavia developed VHF after working with tissue samples from green monkeys. A total of 31 cases were infected and seven (23%) died.[95,102] The Ebola virus was discovered in 1976, during simultaneous outbreaks in what is now Yambuku, Democratic Republic of Congo (near the Ebola River), and Nzara, South Sudan, with a mortality rate of 88% and 53%, respectively.[95,103] Pathogenicity of the African strain has been shown in approximately 30 EVD outbreaks since 1976, with the largest originating in West Africa from 2013–16, affecting over 28,000 cases with 11,308 deaths in Liberia, Guinea and Sierra Leone alone.[95,104] Spread of EVD to Europe and North America occurred with medical evacuations, and these cases had a reported lower mortality rate of 20%.[105] The second largest outbreak to date occurred between 2018 and 2020 in the Democratic Republic of Congo with a case fatality rate of 66%.[95,104]

In the early stages immediately following exposure, symptoms of viral haemorrhagic fevers are usually sudden, though non-specific, and are similar to many common illnesses, including fever, fatigue, myalgia and headache.[95] In EVD, the incubation period ranges from 2 to 21 days; inoculation resulting in a shorter incubation of 5–7 days, with an average of 9 days following contact via mucous membranes.[95] Within the first 4–6 days marked gastrointestinal symptoms begin, such as vomiting and diarrhoea with mild bleed in one-third of cases, as well as a sore throat and a transient maculopapular rash. Large fluid losses lead to electrolyte disturbances, acid–base imbalance, haemodynamic instability, acute kidney injury and liver dysfunction, with hypovolaemic and septic shock reported to be the most frequent cause of death. There is no cure for EVD and treatment is supportive with fluid resuscitation and symptom management. Large amounts of volume resuscitation require careful monitoring for the onset of multi-system organ dysfunction with hypoxaemia and acute lung injury. The provision of intensive care services with the addition of close monitoring of fluid and electrolyte replacement, vasopressors, renal replacement therapy, and ensuring adequate oxygenation with mechanical ventilation, undoubtedly contributed to the case mortality rate decreasing to 18.5% in resource-rich settings.[95,103]

Transmission of EVD human-to-human is via mucous membranes or non-intact skin directly contacting body fluids (e.g. blood, vomitus, faeces, urine, breast milk and semen) or organs of infected people, also materials and surfaces soiled with those fluids (e.g. clothing, bedding), and the cadaver.[103,106] During clinical management, inoculation through percutaneous injury is an efficient means of transmission, and aerosolisation could potentially occur when performing procedures such as bronchoscopies, endotracheal intubation and ventilation.[95] People become infectious when they experience symptoms and continue while the virus is present in their body fluids. A high Ebola viral load on admission to hospital is predictive of the likelihood of death, with infectivity peaking just before and after death. In convalescence, when the virus may not be detectable in the blood, it can persist in other sites, including vitreous humor, semen and cerebrospinal fluid; also the fetus, placenta and amniotic fluid of women infected while pregnant, and in breast milk, if infected when breastfeeding.[95,103] In a small proportion of survivors, the Ebola virus persisted in body fluids for longer than 9 months measured by a positive reverse transcriptase polymerase chain reaction (RT-PCR).[103]

Clinically, other infectious diseases, such as malaria, meningitis and typhoid fever, appear similar to EVD on presentation.[103] Confirmation of EVD is made using PCR in venous blood, and throat swabs or urine samples. Definitive testing for the Ebola virus includes: isolation of the virus and confirmation by the Centers for Disease Control, Atlanta; or detection of the virus by nucleic acid testing or antigen detection assay; or IgG seroconversion or a significant increase in antibody level, of a greater than or equal to fourfold rise in titres to the Ebola virus.[97]

In Australia, emergency nurses and paramedics are likely to be the first contact for people with suspected or confirmed EVD, including conducting risk assessments for probable and confirmed cases of EVD.[97] Paramedics could be involved in transporting a confirmed case to a specialist quarantine centre, particularly if the patient is critically ill. Healthcare workers who have followed the infection control recommendations, including wearing the appropriate PPE, are not considered to have exposure to EVD. Emergency nurses have expressed confidence in their preparation on a personal level and felt that organisations had planned an appropriate response if an outbreak should occur. However, some nurses expressed concern they might inadvertently put themselves at risk by breaching the protective equipment.[107] In these instances, healthcare organisations have recommended staff should continue working but monitor their temperature daily.[97]

Severe acute respiratory syndrome (SARS-CoV-1) emerged in the human population in 2002 in the Guangdong province of China, and avian influenza H5N1 re-emerged in Vietnam in 2003. SARS-CoV-1, caused by a coronavirus, is thought to have originated from contact with semi-domesticated animals such as the palm civet or the raccoon dog. Avian influenza, caused by a subtype of influenza A strain virus, occurs in the wild bird population and has spread to domestic poultry and humans in Asia, the Middle East, Africa and Europe. The virus was introduced to Hong Kong and then spread to 26 other countries around the world (including Australia), with an overall case fatality rate of approximately 11%. Avian influenza H5N1 does not yet demonstrate the ability for direct, sustained human-to-human transmission. It is thought that the droplet and contact routes may predominantly transmit both viruses, although during the SARS outbreak the airborne and possibly the faecal–oral routes may also have transmitted outbreaks of coronavirus. Healthcare workers in contact with SARS-CoV-1 or avian H5N1 influenza cases are advised to use Standard Precautions plus adhere to strict contact, droplet and airborne precautions.[108] Both diseases are notifiable by law, and must be notified in Australia to the Chief Medical Officer and in Aotearoa New Zealand to the local health authority.

Middle East Respiratory Syndrome Coronavirus (MERS-CoV) is a betacoronavirus that emerged in humans in 2012, identified as the causal organism for a fatal pneumonia in a patient in the Kingdom of Saudi Arabia. In March 2012, retrospective review of records identified MERS-CoV as causing previous infections in healthcare workers in Jordan.[109] The virus is thought to have originated in bats, spreading to humans via dromedary camels. The majority of cases to February 2022 have been confirmed in the Middle East, mainly in the Kingdom of Saudi Arabia ($n = 2184$), with spread occurring to 27 countries including Africa, Asia, Europe and the United States.[110,111] While it does not readily spread human to human, transmission is thought to be via multiple routes, with healthcare workers advised to use droplet and airborne precautions. Nosocomial spread among healthcare workers has been facilitated by inadequate infection control precautions, implicated in a multi-centre hospital outbreak ($n = 185$ cases) reported in the Republic of Korea in 2015.[111,112] During outbreaks in the Middle East, more than half of infected healthcare workers were nurses.[109] Worldwide, from September 2012 to February 2022 there have been 2585 confirmed cases with 890 case fatalities, an overall case fatality rate of 34.4%.[113] The WHO has identified MERS-CoV as an emergency.[114] To date no cases have been reported in Australia; as with SARS and H5N1 influenza, MERS-CoV is notifiable by law.

TUBERCULOSIS

Tuberculosis (TB) is one of the oldest diseases known to affect humans. Bacteria belonging to the *Mycobacterium tuberculosis* complex cause tuberculosis. The complex includes *M. tuberculosis, M. bovis, M. africanum, M. microti* and *M. canettii*.[115] In humans, the most frequent and important agent of disease is *M. tuberculosis*. The aetiological agent can be identified only by culture of the organisms. *M. tuberculosis* is a rod-shaped, non-spore-forming, aerobic bacterium which is often neutral on Gram-staining. However, once stained, the colour is not removed by acid alcohol, and therefore has the classification of acid-fast bacilli. *M. tuberculosis* grows very slowly compared with other bacteria.[38] Australia has one of the lowest rates of TB in the world, with an approximate incident rate of 5.8 cases per 100,000 population since the mid-1980s.[116] However, specific populations within Australia, such as Aboriginal and Torres Strait Islander people and people born overseas, exhibit four to five times as many cases compared to non-Indigenous Australian-born persons.[115,116]

The incubation period from infection to demonstrable primary lesion or significant tuberculin reaction is about

4–12 weeks.[37] The degree of communicability depends on the number of bacilli in the droplets, the virulence of the bacilli, adequacy of ventilation, exposure of bacilli to sun or ultraviolet light and opportunities for aerosolisation. Theoretically, as long as viable tubercle bacilli are discharged in the sputum, a person may be infectious.[37] Effective antimicrobial chemotherapy usually eliminates communicability within a few weeks.[117]

The disease usually affects the lungs, but it may affect any organ or tissue in the body. The sites of infection as a result of extrapulmonary TB include meninges, pleura, pericardium, kidneys, bones and joints, larynx, skin, intestines, peritoneum and eyes.[117,118] Extrapulmonary TB occurs more frequently among people infected with human immunodeficiency virus (HIV). Pulmonary tuberculosis can be categorised as primary or secondary.

- *Primary pulmonary tuberculosis* occurs when there is an initial infection with tubercle bacilli. The lesion formed in the lung at this time may not be detectable on chest x-ray, and in the majority of cases it will heal spontaneously.[115] In general, persons infected with tuberculosis have approximately a 10% risk for developing active TB during their lifetime. The risk is greatest during the first two years after infection.[37] In children and in immunocompromised people, primary tuberculosis may progress rapidly to clinical illness.
- *Secondary pulmonary tuberculosis* results from endogenous reactivation of latent infection, and is usually localised to the apical and posterior segments of the upper lobes.[115]

Diagnosis of TB is usually made by clinical signs and symptoms, or chest x-ray findings and results of tuberculin skin testing, also known as Mantoux test (see below). Confirmation of infection is demonstrated by the presence of acid-fast bacilli in sputum or tissue.[38] Primary TB is usually asymptomatic in immunocompetent people, and lesions in the lungs may not be detectable on chest x-ray. In symptomatic cases and/or secondary pulmonary TB, the signs and symptoms of disease may be non-specific and often insidious. Commonly there is fever and night sweats, weight loss, anorexia, general malaise and weakness. As the disease progresses, a cough develops, accompanied by the production of purulent sputum. The sputum often becomes blood-streaked because of erosion of a blood vessel. Chest x-ray may reveal infection, usually localised to the apical and posterior segments of the upper lobes. Eventually, because of extensive disease, there may be dyspnoea and adult respiratory distress syndrome.[115,119]

Directly observed treatments are recommended for TB infection. Australia has implemented this strategy with some modifications because of the low incidence of TB in the country. The treatment of TB may be protracted, particularly in cases of multi-drug resistance, where treatment may continue for many months. Drugs used to treat TB are classified into first-line and second-line agents. First-line agents are the most effective and are a necessity for any short-course therapeutic regimen. Contact tracing is an essential component of TB control. The TB prevention and control services or health department must always carry out contact tracing. The estimated risk of transmission of TB should guide the priority and rapidity of the contact management. The case should be categorised according to the likely degree of infectiousness (sputum smear result, and presence of symptoms), and the contacts according to risk of disease acquisition (i.e. the amount of time and type of contact they have had with the index case).

Patients diagnosed with pulmonary TB, or those where there exists a high index of suspicion, require transmission-based precautions for airborne transmission. The patient should be placed in a single, negative-pressure room with the door closed. People (healthcare workers and visitors) should wear a particulate filter mask when in the room. The patient should wear a surgical mask during transport. Receiving departments must be notified of the additional precautions required for patient management. Diagnosis of TB is notifiable by law, and must be notified to the TB prevention and control service and health department.[1,8]

The benefit of Bacille Calmette-Guérin (BCG) vaccine in adolescents and adults is not certain. BCG is recommended for the following: Aboriginal and Torres Strait Islander people, neonates living in regions of high incidence (Australia); neonates with one or both parents who identify as being Pacific people (Aotearoa New Zealand); neonates born to patients with leprosy or TB; children under the age of 5 years who will be travelling to live in countries of high TB prevalence for longer than three months; and children and adolescents aged less than 16 years (unable to be treated with antibiotics) who continue to be exposed to an individual with active pulmonary TB.[120]

HUMAN IMMUNODEFICIENCY VIRUS AND ACQUIRED IMMUNE DEFICIENCY SYNDROME

Human immunodeficiency virus is a retrovirus. Once inside the body, HIV replicates within white cells called CD4 cells. CD4 cells normally help coordinate the body's immune response; as the infection progresses, these cells are destroyed and the CD4 count gradually falls, reducing the ability of the immune system to ward off infections. As a result, HIV-infected people become susceptible to illnesses caused by the collapse of the body's immune system. Acquired immune deficiency syndrome (AIDS) is a severe, life-threatening consequence of HIV infection. This syndrome represents the late clinical stage of infection with HIV and is most often the result of progressive damage to the immune and other organ systems.

Within several weeks to months after infection with HIV, many individuals develop an acute, self-limited mononucleosis-like illness lasting for 1–2 weeks. Infected individuals may then be free of clinical signs or symptoms for months to years. Onset of clinical illness is usually insidious, with non-specific symptoms such as lymphadenopathy, anorexia, chronic diarrhoea, weight loss, fever and fatigue. Many opportunistic infections are considered AIDS-related illnesses, including several cancers, pulmonary and extrapulmonary tuberculosis, recurrent pneumonia, wasting syndrome, neurological disease (HIV dementia or sensory neuropathy) and invasive cervical cancer.[37]

HIV is transmitted by direct contact with blood or infected body fluids, through mucous membranes, non-intact skin or through percutaneous injury. The three significant routes of transmission for HIV are infected blood or blood products, infected sexual fluids and from infected mother to baby during pregnancy and delivery.[15] Antibodies to HIV usually develop within 2–8 weeks, typically within 12 weeks. However, most people do not feel unwell or develop symptoms of disease for years. All persons in the acute or chronic stage of infection who are HIV-antibody-positive are potentially infectious. The period of infectivity is believed to begin shortly after primary infection and to continue throughout life.[120] Epidemiological evidence suggests that infectivity increases with increasing immune deficiency, clinical symptoms and presence of other sexually transmitted infections.[37]

The most commonly used screening test for HIV, enzyme-linked immunoassay, is highly sensitive and specific. When this test is reactive, an additional test such as the Western blot or indirect immunofluorescence assay (IFA) should be obtained. Most individuals infected with HIV develop detectable antibodies within 1–3 months.

Susceptibility to HIV infection is universal. The risk of transmission of disease is dependent on the type of exposure and the concentration of HIV in the bloodstream of the source at the time of exposure. The risk of HIV transmission varies according to the type of exposure: 0.1% per act of unprotected sexual intercourse, 30% from mother to baby during pregnancy and delivery, and close to 100% if transfused with HIV-infected blood. The risk to healthcare workers of acquiring HIV from an occupational exposure is very small, with the average risk for HIV infection estimated to be 0.3% after percutaneous exposure (needlestick injury) and 0.09% following mucous membrane exposure.[120] However, any exposure to HIV must be managed in accordance with established protocols, including timely access to expert counselling and post-exposure prophylactic (PEP) treatments as required.

Patients with HIV are rarely treated in the ED, as it is a highly specialised field with the patient treated for the most part as an outpatient. However, the ED is often the first point of contact for these patients when they have an acute exacerbation of symptoms secondary to their disease, in the presence or absence of a diagnosis.

HEPATITIS

Hepatitis is injury and inflammation of the liver. Viruses are a major cause of hepatitis, but other microorganisms or non-infectious causes may also be responsible.[121,122] The non-viral causes include drugs and chemicals such as carbon tetrachloride, ethylene glycol, rifampicin, methotrexate, monoamine oxide inhibitors, chlorpromazine and paracetamol.[119,123] Table 27.5 outlines the characteristics of all viral hepatitis and the following discussion will address those most commonly encountered in Australia and Aotearoa New Zealand: A, B and C.

Inflammation of the liver caused by the hepatitis viruses may produce a variety of features. The common signs and symptoms of viral hepatitis include jaundice, fatigue, abdominal pain, arthralgia, anorexia, nausea and vomiting. During the acute phase, marked increases in the liver enzymes serum alanine aminotransferase (ALT) and serum aspartate aminotransferase (AST) can be detected. Liver failure or liver cancer may occur in more-severe manifestations of the disease.[122] Definitive diagnosis of the causative virus can only be made by laboratory testing.

Treatment of hepatitis differs depending on the virus type and the severity of infection. Acute presentations of hepatitis A, B and C require different kinds of treatment and management, but common to them all is rest, fluid intake and nutrition, and the avoidance of unnecessary medications.[125–127] Targeted treatment is necessary in instances where the disease becomes chronic. Antiviral medications are the most commonly used treatment to combat liver disease in patients with chronic hepatitis B and C.[126,127] Adoption of prophylactic measures is the ideal strategy for prevention of infection. Vaccinations do

TABLE 27.5 CHARACTERISTICS OF HEPATITIS VIRUSES[124]

CHARACTERISTIC	HEPATITIS A VIRUS	HEPATITIS B VIRUS	HEPATITIS C VIRUS	HEPATITIS D VIRUS	HEPATITIS E VIRUS
Nucleic acid	RNA	DNA	RNA	*	RNA
Serologic diagnosis	IgM anti-HAV	HBsAg	Anti-HCV	Anti-HDV	Anti-HEV
Major transmission	Faecal-oral	Blood	Blood	Needle	Water
Incubation period (days)	15–45	40–180	20–120	30–180	14–60
Epidemics	Yes	No	No	No	Yes
Chronicity	No	Yes	Yes	Yes	No
Liver cancer	No	Yes	Yes	Yes	No

*Incomplete RNA; requires presence of hepatitis B virus for replication.

Anti-HCV: antibody to hepatitis C virus; anti-HDV: antibody to hepatitis D virus; anti-HEV: antibody to hepatitis E virus; HBsAg: hepatitis B surface antigen; IgM anti-HAV: IgM antibody to hepatitis A virus.

exist to protect against some hepatitis viruses (A and B); however, immunisation against one disease does not extend to the types caused by different viruses.[125,126]

GASTROINTESTINAL DISEASES

Many microorganisms can produce symptoms of diarrhoeal disease. Gastrointestinal disease causes fluid loss and dehydration in people, regardless of the cause. Outbreaks of infectious diseases can occur sporadically and there are organisms that cause infections seasonally. Infections in healthcare may arise from staff, clients, visitors, air, food, water, sterile products, the environment and vermin. Most pathogens will enter the gastrointestinal tract via the faecal–oral route, from contaminated hands, food or fluids.[119] Diarrhoea may be caused by many viral, bacterial and parasitic pathogens, including (but not limited to) adenovirus, rotavirus, norovirus, *Campylobacter* spp., *Clostridioides difficile*, *Salmonella* spp., *Yersinia*, *Cryptosporidium* and *Giardia lamblia.*

Norovirus (formerly known as Norwalk-like viruses) is a common cause of non-bacterial gastroenteritis. Outbreaks have been reported in the ED, hospitals and aged care facilities. Norovirus commonly occurs in winter months, and is a syndrome of acute nausea, vomiting and explosive diarrhoea. Symptoms usually last between 24 and 48 hours, with an incubation period of the same; viral shedding continues for approximately 24 hours after the symptoms cease. The Norwalk-like viruses are small, structured ribonucleic acid (RNA) viruses classified as caliciviruses. This virus is transmitted via the faecal–oral route. Vomiting causes widespread aerosol dissemination of viral particles, resulting in environmental contamination and subsequent spread.

The general principles of infection prevention and control apply when providing care for clients in the emergency setting. Standard Precautions require strict hand hygiene after contact with clients who have signs and symptoms of gastrointestinal disease. Healthcare providers should encourage clients to practise good hand hygiene and toilet hygiene. Healthcare providers themselves should not attend work when symptomatic of gastrointestinal disease of unknown or infectious origin.

BIOTERRORISM

Bioterrorism has emerged as a key public health issue in the 21st century that presents unique challenges for emergency nurses and paramedics. Surprisingly, such challenges are not new. Numerous published papers, protocols and guidelines have focused for many years on the serious public health threat posed by the deliberate release of agents such as influenza, anthrax and smallpox.[128] As a phenomenon, bioterrorism comprises acts that are politically or religiously motivated and employ or threaten the use of biological agents/toxins to create deliberate harm or fear.[128] The threat of biological weapons and bioterrorism has been dramatically heightened since anthrax-tainted letters followed the terrorist attacks in the United States.[129] In September 2001, two mailed letters containing anthrax spores resulted in 22 cases of anthrax and five deaths. These incidents led to considerable emergency anxiety, confusion, mistrust and demand for chemoprophylaxis and increased overall demand on health service delivery. Similar events occurred in Australia in 2001 that received international attention, although no mortality or morbidity occurred.

Of all the infectious agents that pose challenges to humanity, few constitute significant threats in terms of their use in bioterrorism. Risk assessments are based on the severity and consequence of clinical disease, mode of transmission, potential for major public health impact and possible effects on public panic and social disruption. The most devastating potential bioterrorism threats are from high-consequence infectious diseases described earlier, including smallpox, anthrax, botulism, plague and viral haemorrhagic fevers such as Ebola, Marburg and Lassa fever.[96] Smallpox and anthrax are considered the greatest bioterrorism risk in Australia, although naturally-occurring smallpox was last seen globally in 1977.[128] Other important biological threats, such as plague and viral haemorrhagic fevers, are not endemic in Australia.[96]

Responding to bioterrorism, whether real or threatened, requires public health preparedness at an individual, emergency and societal level. Healthcare workers, particularly emergency-based individuals, lack adequate training, resources and opportunities for clinical education in bioterrorism preparedness.[128,129] An outbreak of avian influenza or another infectious disease spread via bioterrorism would have widespread social and economic impact on communities. Infections of pandemic magnitude have the potential to be catastrophic. Even with close collaboration between healthcare providers and the public health system, difficulties in early detection and diagnosis would compound the problems of containing the spread of disease and dealing with mass care, mass prophylaxis and mass fatality management.[130,131] Achieving the best health outcome in outbreaks depends on having a plan that will facilitate the rapid identification and treatment of affected and potentially exposed people, appropriate containment and robust communication mechanisms between clinical services, public health services and emergency services.[128] Adequate training and preparedness of clinicians in recognition and management of infection is vital for those working in emergency contexts. Swift and decisive responses and effective communication and collaboration between law enforcement officials, clinicians and public health officials are essential to contain outbreaks.[130,132]

Emergency nurses and paramedics should, in all instances, seek specialist assistance from local and state public health officials such as Australian Emergency Management, the Department of Health and the Communicable Diseases Network Australia. National emergency response and disaster management is coordinated by the Office of the Minister for Justice. Emergency nurses and paramedics must understand the specific nature of the various Commonwealth, state and local health threats and participate in preparing and testing comprehensive plans to manage the health threat within their facility.[128]

SUMMARY

In this chapter we have explored some contemporary challenges of healthcare-associated infection and communicable diseases and their control and prevention in emergency nursing and paramedic practice in the Australasian emergency care context. Recognition of the potential for disease transmission in emergency care is essential. Contacts between staff and patients are frequent and varied, allowing many opportunities for the transmission of infectious agents. All patients should be deemed a potential source of infection and Standard Precautions adopted to minimise the risk for disease transmission. The emergency nurse or paramedic should be aware of the modes of disease transmission and adopt the appropriate additional precautions when the airborne, droplet or contact routes transmit the infectious agent responsible for causing disease. Infection prevention and control is critical to providing high-quality, safe and timely emergency care. The practice environment of the emergency nurse and paramedic presents unique challenges requiring specialist knowledge and evidence.

CASE STUDY 1

You and your road partner are ambulance paramedics. You have been dispatched to a road traffic crash on a major highway 20 minutes from the station. It is reported to be a head-on collision between a passenger car and motorcyclist, with five patients, two of whom died instantly at the scene. On arrival, the mangled wreckage is off the side of the road in a shallow, muddy creek bed. There is mud and water everywhere. Of the three surviving patients, one patient (A) is trapped and unconscious, and the other two patients (B) and (C) self-extricated. Patient A has open head, chest and lower limb trauma. Patient B has a closed head injury and superficial grazes, and Patient C has an open fracture of the femur that has been contaminated by the mud from the creek. Both patients B and C are smoking cigarettes and were reported as consuming beer at the local hotel. The three surviving patients are transported to hospital, and all are admitted to the intensive care unit. Patient A develops a consolidated pneumonia two days post-admission.

QUESTIONS

1. What are the particular infection risks for each of the patients in this situation?
2. What prophylactic measures would be considered appropriate for each patient with respect to particular infectious diseases?
3. Would the pneumonia infection be classified as healthcare-associated? What factors would need to be considered for this assessment to be made?

Answers to Case Study Questions can be found on evolve **http://evolve.elsevier.com/AU/Curtis/emergency/** 

CASE STUDY 2

You are the triage nurse when Mrs V is brought in by ambulance to the emergency department. She is hypoxic, cyanotic and has a productive, purulent and unrelenting cough. She returned from an overseas holiday to Africa where she spent 3 months on safari. She is stabilised and admitted to a medical ward. The next day, microscopy of a sample of her sputum reveals acid-fast bacillus and active pulmonary tuberculosis.

QUESTIONS

1. What are the implications of this with respect to infection prevention and control?
2. What are the risks of the spread of infection to the paramedics and hospital staff, and what follow-up is required?
3. How should this incident be managed?

Answers to Case Study Questions can be found on evolve **http://evolve.elsevier.com/AU/Curtis/emergency/** 

REFERENCES

1. National Health and Medical Research Council. Australian guidelines for the prevention and control of infection in healthcare. Canberra, Australia: National Health and Medical Research Council; 2019.
2. Australian Commission on Safety and Quality in Health Care (ACSQHC). National safety and quality health service standards. 2nd ed. Sydney, Australia: ACSQHC; 2021.
3. Cardoso T, Almeida M, Friedman ND, Aragão I, Costa-Pereira A, Sarmento AE, et al. Classification of healthcare-associated infection: a systematic review 10 years after the first proposal. BMC Med 2014;12:40.
4. Shaban RZ, Mitchell BG, Russo PL, Macbeth D. Epidemiology of healthcare-associated infections in Australia. Australia: Elsevier Health Sciences; 2021.
5. Pop-Vicas AE, D'Agata EM. The rising influx of multidrug-resistant gramnegative bacilli into a tertiary care hospital. Clin Infect Dis 2005;40:1792–8.
6. Australian Commission on Safety and Quality in Health Care (ACSQHC). Hospital-acquired complications. 2018. Available from: www.safetyandquality.gov.au/our-work/indicators/hospital-acquired-complications/.
7. Shaban RZ. Tacking errors in healthcare: the rise of financial penalties for preventable hospital-acquired complications. Aust Hosp Healthcare Bull 2018;Spring:22–23.
8. National Health and Medical Research Council. Australian guidelines for the prevention and control of infection in healthcare. Canberra, Australia: National Health and Medical Research Council; 2010.
9. Mitchell BG, Shaban RZ, MacBeth D, Wood CJ, Russo PL. The burden of healthcare-associated infection in Australian hospitals: a systematic review of the literature. Infect Dis Health 2017;22(3):117–28.
10. Australian Commission on Safety and Quality in Health Care (ACSQHC). Healthcare-associated infection (detailed fact sheet). 2018. Available from: www.safetyandquality.gov.au/wp-content/uploads/2018/03/Healthcare-associated-infection-detailed-fact-sheet.pdf.
11. Russo PL, Stewardson AJ, Cheng AC, Bucknall T, Mitchell BG. The prevalence of healthcare associated infections among adult inpatients at nineteen large Australian acute-care public hospitals: a point prevalence survey. Antimicrob Resist Infect Cont 2019;8:114.
12. Lydeamore MJ, Mitchell BG, Bucknall T, Cheng AC, Russo PL, Stewardson AJ. Burden of five healthcare associated infections in Australia. Antimicrob Resist Infect Control. 2022;11(1):69.
13. Russo PL, Cheng AC, Mitchell BG, Hall L. Healthcare-associated infections in Australia: tackling the 'known unknowns'. Aust Health Rev 2018;42:178–80.
14. Shaban RZ, Maloney S, Gerrard J, Collignon P, Macbeth D, Cruickshank M, et al. Outbreak of health care-associated Burkholderia cenocepacia bacteremia and infection attributed to contaminated sterile gel used for central line insertion under ultrasound guidance and other procedures. Am J Infect Control 2017;45(9):954–8.
15. Australian Commission on Safety and Quality in Health Care (ACSQHC). Reducing harm to patients from healthcare associated infections: an Australian infection prevention and control model for acute hospitals. Canberra: Commonwealth of Australia; 2009.
16. Australian Commission on Safety and Quality in Health Care (ACSQHC). AURA 2021: Fourth Australian report on antimicrobial use and resistance in human health. Sydney, Australia: ACSQHC; 2021.
17. Australian Commission on Safety and Quality in Health Care (ACSQHC). AURA 2017: Second Australian report on antimicrobial use and resistance in human health. Sydney, Australia: ACSQHC; 2017.
18. Shaban RZ, Cruickshank M, Christiansen K, Antimicrobial Resistance Standing Committee. National surveillance and report of antimicrobial resistance and antibiotic usage for human health in Australia. Sydney: Antimicrobial Resistance Standing Committee; 2013.
19. Australian Commission on Safety and Quality in Health Care (ACSQHC). Windows into safety and quality in health care 2009. Sydney: ACSQHC; 2009.
20. Graves N, Halton K, Robertus L. Costs of healthcare associated infection. In: Cruickshank M, Ferguson J, editors. Reducing harm to patients from healthcare associated infection: the role of surveillance. Sydney: ACSQHC; 2008.
21. Johnson A, Roush RE, Howe JL, Palmisano BR, Perweiler EA, Roush RE, et al. Bioterrorism and emergency preparedness in aging (BTEPA). Gerontol Geriatr Educ 2008;26(4):63–86.
22. Lowthian JA, Curtis AJ, Jolley DJ, Stoelwinder JU, McNeil JJ, Cameron PA. Demand at the emergency department front door: 10-year trends in presentations. Med J Aust 2012;196(2):128–32.
23. Patocka C, Turner J, Xue X, Segal E. Evaluation of an emergency department triage screening tool for suspected severe sepsis and septic shock. J Healthc Qual 2014;36(1):52–61.
24. Burrell AR, McLaws ML, Fullick M, Sullivan RB, Sindhusake D. SEPSIS KILLS: early intervention saves lives. Med J Aust 2016;204(2):73.
25. Lelubre C, Vincent JL. Mechanisms and treatment of organ failure in sepsis. Nat Rev Nephrol 2018;14(7):417–27.
26. Fauchald SK, Smith D. Transdisciplinary research partnerships: making research happen! Nurs Econ 2005;23(3):131–5.
27. Shaban RZ. Scientific convenor's address. Balancing the art and the science. Seventh International Conference for Emergency Nurses. Gold Coast, 2009.
28. Shaban RZ. Paramedic knowledge of infection control principles and standards in an Australian emergency medical system (EMS). Aust Infect Control 2006;11(1):7.
29. World Health Organization (WHO). Primary health care: now more than ever. Geneva, Switzerland: WHO; 2008.

30. Brew N, Burton K. Critical, but stable: Australia's capacity to respond to an infectious disease outbreak. Canberra: Parliament of Australia; 2004.
31. Hess I, Curson P, Plant A. Bug breakfast in the Bulletin: outbreaks: the past, present and future. NSW Pub Health Bull 2005;16(6):2.
32. Li C, Sotomayor-Castillo C, Nahidi S, Kuznetsov S, Considine J, Curtis K, et al. Emergency clinicians' knowledge, preparedness and experiences of managing COVID-19 during the 2020 global pandemic in Australian healthcare settings. Australas Emerg Care 2021;24(3):186–96.
33. Chou R, Dana T, Buckley DI, Selph S, Fu R, Totten AM. Epidemiology of and risk factors for coronavirus infection in health care workers: a living rapid review. Ann Intern Med 2020;173(2):120–36.
34. Curson P. Epidemics and pandemics in Australia. Sydney: University of Sydney; 2010.
35. Lee G. The body's defence systems. In: Lee G, Bishop P, editors. Microbiology and infection control for health professionals. 4th ed. Sydney: Pearson Education Australia; 2010.
36. Bishop P. Epidemiology: how diseases are spread. In: Lee G, Bishop P, editors. Microbiology and infection control for health professionals. 4th ed. Sydney: Pearson Education Australia; 2010.
37. Newberry L. Sheehy's emergency nursing: principles and practice. 5th ed. St Louis: Mosby; 2003.
38. Lee G. Respiratory tract infections. In: Lee G, Bishop P, editors. Microbiology and infection control for health professionals. 4th ed. Sydney: Pearson Education Australia; 2010.
39. Doolan K. Infectious and communicable diseases. In: Curtis K, Ramsden C, Friendship J, editors. Emergency nursing and care. Sydney: Elsevier; 2008.
40. Borysiewicz LK. The host's response to infection. In: Warrell DA, Cox TM, Firth JD, editors. Oxford textbook of medicine. 4th ed. Oxford: Oxford University Press; 2003.
41. Lloyd-Smith P, Younger J, Lloyd-Smith E, Green H, Leung V, Romney MG. Economic analysis of vancomycin-resistant enterococci at a Canadian hospital: assessing attributable cost and length of stay. J Hosp Infect 2013;85(1):54–9.
42. Van Kleef E, Goldenberg SD, Robotham JV, Robotham JV, Cookson B, Jit M, et al. Excess length of stay and mortality due to Clostridium difficile infection: a multi-state modelling approach. J Hosp Infect 2014;88(4):213–17.
43. Mitchell BG, Ferguson J, Anderson M, Sear J, Barnett A. Length of stay and mortality associated with healthcare-associated urinary tract infections: a multi-state model. J Hosp Infect 2016;93(1):92–9.
44. Cassini A, Plachouras D, Eckmanns T, Abu Sin M, Blank HP, Ducomble T, et al. Burden of six healthcare-associated infections on European population health: estimating incidence-based disability-adjusted life years through a prevalence-based modelling study. PLoS Med 2016;13(10):e1002150. doi:10.1371/journal.pmed.1002150.
45. Australian Commission on Safety and Quality in Health Care (ACSQHC). Health care associated infection program. 2018. Available from: www.safetyandquality.gov.au/our-work/healthcare-associated-infection/.
46. Australian Commission on Safety and Quality in Health Care (ACSQHC). Tools and resources to implement the guidelines. 2010. Available from: www.safetyandquality.gov.au/our-work/healthcare-associated-infection/national-infection-control-guidelines.
47. Shaban RZ, Macbeth D, Vause N, Simon G. Documentation, composition and organisation of infection control progams and plans in Australian healthcare systems: a pilot study. Infect Dis Health 2016;21(2):51–61.
48. Australian Commission on Safety and Quality in Health Care (ACSQHC). Preventing and Controlling Infections Standard. In: National Safety and Quality Health Service Standards. Sydney, Australia: ACSQHC; 2021. Available from: www.safetyandquality.gov.au/publications-and-resources/resource-library/national-safety-and-quality-health-service-standards-second-edition.
49. Australian Commission on Safety and Quality in Health Care (ACSQHC). Standard 3 - Preventing and controlling healthcare-associated infection. In: National Safety and Quality Health Service Standards. 2nd ed. Sydney: ACSQHC; 2017. Available from: www.safetyandquality.gov.au/wp-content/uploads/2017/12/National-Safety-and-Quality-Health-Service-Standards-second-edition.pdf.
50. Australian Commission on Safety and Quality in Health Care (ACSQHC). Resources for NSQHS Standards. 2023. Available from: www.safetyandquality.gov.au/standards/nsqhs-standards/resources-nsqhs-standards.
51. World Health Organization (WHO). WHO Guidelines on hand hygiene in health care. Geneva, Switzerland: WHO; 2009.
52. Australian Government. Coronavirus (COVID-19) at a glance – 20 December 2020. In: Department of Health, editor. Canberra, Australia: Department of Health; 2020.
53. Australian Institute of Health and Welfare (AIHW). The first year of COVID-19 in Australia: direct and indirect health effects. Canberra, Australia: AIHW; 2021.
54. Australian Commission on Safety and Quality in Health Care (ACSQHC). Emergency department care. 2021. Available from: www.aihw.gov.au/reports-data/myhospitals/sectors/emergency-department-care.
55. Kam AW, Chaudhry SG, Gunasekaran N, White AJ, Vukasovic M, Fung AT. Fewer presentations to metropolitan emergency departments during the COVID-19 pandemic. Med J Aust 2020;213(8):370–1.
56. Jessup RL, Bramston C, Beauchamp A, Gust A, Cao Y, Haywood C, et al. Impact of COVID-19 on emergency department attendance in an Australian hospital: a parallel convergent mixed methods study. BMJ Open 2021;11(12):e049222.
57. Andrew E, Nehme Z, Stephenson M, Walker T, Smith K. The impact of the COVID-19 pandemic on demand for emergency ambulances in Victoria, Australia. Prehosp Emerg Care 2021:1–7. doi:10.1080/10903127.2021.1944409.
58. Dinh MM, Berendsen Russell S. Overcrowding kills: how COVID-19 could reshape emergency department patient flow in the new normal. Emerg Med Australas 2021;33(1):175–7.

59. Quigley AL, Stone H, Nguyen PY, Chughtai AA, MacIntyre CR. Estimating the burden of COVID-19 on the Australian healthcare workers and health system during the first six months of the pandemic. Int J Nurs Stud 2021;114:103811.
60. Nguyen LH, Drew DA, Graham MS, Joshi AD, Guo CG, Ma W, et al. Risk of COVID-19 among front-line health-care workers and the general community: a prospective cohort study. Lancet Pub Health 2020;5(9):e475–83.
61. Lai J, Ma S, Wang Y, Cai Z, Hu J, Wei N, et al. Factors associated with mental health outcomes among health care workers exposed to coronavirus disease 2019. JAMA Netw Open 2020;3(3):e203976.
62. Cornish S, Klim S, Kelly AM. Is COVID-19 the straw that broke the back of the emergency nursing workforce? Emerg Med Australas 2021;33(6):1095–9.
63. Communicable Diseases Network Australia. Coronavirus Disease 2019 (COVID-19): CDNA National Guidelines for Public Health Units. Canberra: Department of Health; 2021.
64. Tenforde MW, Self WH, Naioti EA, Ginde AA, Douin DJ, Olson SM, et al. Sustained effectiveness of Pfizer-BioNTech and Moderna vaccines against COVID-19 associated hospitalizations among adults—United States, March–July 2021. MMWR 2021;70(34):1156.
65. Australian Government Department of Health. Coronavirus (COVID-19) case numbers and statistics. 2022. Available from: www.health.gov.au/health-alerts/covid-19/case-numbers-and-statistics.
66. Shahid Z, Kalayanamitra R, McClafferty B, Kepko D, Ramgobin D, Patel R, et al. COVID-19 and older adults: what we know. J Am Geriatr Soc 2020;68(5):926–9.
67. Australian Bureau of Statistics (ABS). COVID-19 mortality in Australia. 2022. Available from: www.abs.gov.au/articles/australian-covid-19-mortality.
68. Communicable Diseases Network Australia. COVID-19 outbreaks in residential care: national guidelines for the prevention, control and public health management of COVID-19 outbreaks in residential care facilities. In: Department of Health, editor. Canberra, Australia: Commonwealth of Australia; 2020.
69. Royal Commission into Aged Care Quality and Safety. Aged care and COVID-19: a special report. Canberra, Australia: Commonwealth of Australia; 2020.
70. Australian Government Department of Health. COVID-19 outbreaks in Australia residential aged care facilities—9 October 2020. In: Department of Health, editor. Canberra, Australia: Australian Government; 2020.
71. Australian Government Department of Health. First 24 hours—managing COVID-19 in a residential aged care facility. In: Department of Health, editor. Canberra, Australia: Australian Government; 2020.
72. Dwyer R, Gabbe B, Stoelwinder JU, Lowthian J. A systematic review of outcomes following emergency transfer to hospital for residents of aged care facilities. Age Ageing 2014;43(6):759–66.
73. Rhodes A, Evans LE, Alhazzani W, Levy MM, Antonelli M, Ferrer R, et al. Surviving Sepsis Campaign: international guidelines for management of sepsis and septic shock: 2016. Intensive Care Med 2017;43(3):304–77.
74. Banasik JL. Shock. In: Banasik JL, Copstead LC, editors. Pathophysiology. St Louis, Missouri: WB Saunders; 2005.
75. Aitken LM, Williams G, Harvey M, Blot S, Kleinpell R, Labeau S, et al. Nursing considerations to complement the Surviving Sepsis Campaign guidelines. Crit Care Med 2011;39(7):1800–18.
76. Lee G. Cardiovascular and multisystem infections. In: Lee G, Bishop P, editors. Microbiology and infection control for health professionals. 4th ed. Sydney: Pearson Education Australia; 2010.
77. Rubin RJ, Harrington CA, Poon A, Dietrich K, Greene JA, Moiduddin A. The economic impact of Staphylococcus aureus infection in New York City hospitals. Emerg Infect Dis 1999;5(1):9–17.
78. Casewell MW. New threats to the control of methicillin-resistant *Staphylococcus aureus*. J Hosp Infect 1995;30(Suppl):465–71.
79. Praxis KB. Research and issues in community nursing: hand washing in the community setting. ACCNS J Comm Nurses 2002;7(2):3.
80. Kelly J. Addressing the problem of increased antibiotic resistance. J Prof Nurs 2001;17(1):4.
81. Simon EM, Summers SM. Vascular access complications: an emergency medicine approach. Emerg Med Clin North Am 2017;35(4):771–88.
82. Hoffman T, Du Plessis M, Prekupec MP, Gielecki J, Zurada A, Tubbs RS, et al. Ultrasound-guided central venous catheterization: a review of the relevant anatomy, technique, complications, and anatomical variations. Clin Anat 2017;30(2):237–50.
83. Sharma D, Farahbakhsh N, Tabatabaii SA. Role of ultrasound for central catheter tip localization in neonates: a review of the current evidence. J Matern Fetal Neonatal Med 2019;32(14):2429–37.
84. Spelman T, Pilcher DV, Cheng AC, Bull AL, Richards MJ, Worth LJ. Central line-associated bloodstream infections in Australian ICUs: evaluating modifiable and non-modifiable risks in Victorian healthcare facilities. Epidemiol Infect 2017;145(14):3047–55.
85. Shokoohi H, Armstrong P, Tansek R. Emergency department ultrasound probe infection control: challenges and solutions. Open Access Emerg Med 2015;7:1–9.
86. Rodriguez G, Quan D. Bacterial growth on ED ultrasound machines. Am J Emerg Med 2011;29(7):816–7.
87. World Health Organization (WHO). Epidemic and pandemic alert and response: avian influenza. Geneva: WHO; 2006.
88. Department of Health and Ageing. Avian influenza. In: Department of Health and Ageing, editor. Canberra: Australian Government; 2008.
89. Weber JT, Hughes JM. Beyond Semmelweis: moving infection control into the community. Ann Intern Med 2004;140(5):397–8.
90. Fitzgerald GJ, Shaban RZ, Arbon P. Emergency department impact and patient profile of H1N1 influenza 09 outbreak in Australia: a national study. H1N1 Influenza 09 Canberra. Canberra: Urgent Research Forum; 2009.

91. Rebmann T, Wagner W. Infection preventionists' experience during the first months of the 2009 novel H1N1 influenza a pandemic. Am J Infect Control 2009;37(10):e5–16.
92. Jefferson T, Jones M, Doshi P, Spencer EA, Onakpoya I, Heneghan CJ. Oseltamivir for influenza in adults and children: systematic review of clinical study reports and summary of regulatory comments. BMJ 2014;348:g2545.
93. Cieslak TJ, Herstein JJ, Kortepeter MG, Hewlett AL. A Methodology for determining which diseases warrant care in a high-level containment care unit. Viruses 2019;11(9):773. doi:10.3390/v11090773.
94. Public Health England. High consequence infectious diseases (HCID). 2018. Available from: www.gov.uk/guidance/high-consequence-infectious-diseases-hcid.
95. Leligdowicz A, Fischer WA II, Uyeki TM, Fletcher TE, Adhikari NK, Portella G, et al. Ebola virus disease and critical illness. Crit Care 2016;20(1):217.
96. Australian Government Department of Health. Overview of biological agents that could be used in a terrorist act. 2015. Available from: www.health.gov.au/internet/main/publishing.nsf/content/health-pubhlth-strateg-bio-agents.htm.
97. New South Wales Ministry of Health. Communicable diseases branch: NSW contingency plan for viral haemorrhagic fevers. 2016. Available from: www1.health.nsw.gov.au/pds/ActivePDSDocuments/GL2016_002.pdf.
98. CSIRO. Zoonotic disease threat. 2015. Available from: www.csiro.au/en/Research/BF/Areas/Protecting-Animal-and-Human-Health/Zoonotic-capability.
99. Centers for Disease Control and Prevention. Viral hemorrhagic fevers: Arenaviridae. 2013. Available from: www.cdc.gov/vhf/virus-families/arenaviridae.html.
100. Centers for Disease Control and Prevention. Viral hemorrhagic fevers: Bunyaviridae. 2013. Available from: www.cdc.gov/vhf/virus-families/bunyaviridae.html.
101. CSIRO. Case study Ebola virus research. 2015. Available from: www.csiro.au/en/Research/BF/Areas/Protecting-Animal-and-Human-Health/Zoonotic-capability/ebolavirus.
102. Centers for Disease Control and Prevention. Viral hemorrhagic fevers: Filoviridae. 2014. Available from: https://www.cdc.gov/vhf/virus-families/filoviridae.html.
103. World Health Organization. Ebola virus disease: fact sheet. 2018. Available from: www.who.int/en/news-room/fact-sheets/detail/ebola-virus-disease.
104. World Health Organization. Ebola virus disease. 2021. Available from: https://www.who.int/news-room/fact-sheets/detail/ebola-virus-disease.
105. Bell BP. Overview, control strategies, and lessons learned in the CDC response to the 2014–2016 Ebola epidemic. MMWR Suppl 2016;65(3):4–11.
106. New South Wales Health. Communicable diseases: Ebola virus disease control guideline. 2016. Available from: www.health.nsw.gov.au/Infectious/controlguideline/Pages/ebola-virus.aspx.
107. Pincha Baduge MS, Moss C, Morphet J. Emergency nurses' perceptions of emergency department preparedness for an ebola outbreak: a qualitative descriptive study. Australas Emerg Nurs J 2017;20(2):69–74.
108. Fauci AS. Emerging and re-emerging infectious diseases: the perpetual challenge. In: Robert H, editor. New York: Milbank Memorial Fund; 2005.
109. Suwantarat N, Apisarnthanarak A. Risks to healthcare workers with emerging diseases: lessons from MERS-CoV, Ebola, SARS, and avian flu. Curr Opin Infect Dis 2015;28(4):349–61.
110. Reperant LA, Osterhaus ADME. AIDS, Avian flu, SARS, MERS, Ebola, Zika... what next? Vaccine 2017;35(35, Part A):4470–4.
111. Food and Agriculture Organization of the United Nations. MERS-CoV situation update. 2018. Available from: www.fao.org/ag/againfo/programmes/en/empres/mers/situation_update.html.
112. New South Wales Health. Communicable diseases: Middle East respiratory syndrome coronavirus (MERS-CoV). 2017. Available from: www.health.nsw.gov.au/Infectious/alerts/Pages/MERS-Alerts.aspx.
113. World Health Organization (WHO). MERS situation update. February 2022. Available from: www.emro.who.int/health-topics/mers-cov/mers-outbreaks.html.
114. World Health Organization (WHO). Emergencies: Middle East respiratory syndrome coronavirus (MERS-CoV). 2018. Available from: www.who.int/emergencies/mers-cov/en/.
115. Communicable Diseases Network Australia. National strategic plan for TB control in Australia beyond 2000. Canberra: Commonwealth Department of Health and Ageing; 2002.
116. Bright A, Denholm JT, Coulter C, Waring J, Stapledon R. Tuberculosis notifications in Australia, 2015–2018. Canberra, Australia: National Tuberculosis Advisory Committee; 2020.
117. Tally NJ. Clinical gastroenterology: a practical problem based approach. Sydney: MacLennan & Petty; 1996.
118. Kasper DL, Braunwald E, Fauci AS. Section 7: infectious diseases. Harrison's manual of medicine. New York: McGraw-Hill; 2006.
119. van der Poel CL, Cuypers HT, Reesink HV. Hepatitis C virus six years on. Lancet 1994;334:1475–9.
120. Department of Health and Ageing. Infection control guidelines for the prevention of transmission of infectious diseases in the health care setting. Canberra: Biotext; 2004.
121. Wasley A, Miller JT, Finelli L, Centers for Disease Control and Prevention (CDC). Surveillance for acute viral hepatitis—United States 2005. MMWR Surveill Summ 2007;56(3):1–24.

122. Lee G, Bishop P. Gastrointestinal tract infections. In: Lee G, editor. Microbiology and infection control for health professionals. 4th ed. Sydney: Pearson Education Australia; 2010.
123. Moseley RH. Evaluation of abnormal liver function tests. Med Clin North Am 1996;80(5):10.
124. MSD. MSD manual. Professional version. 2023. New Jersey: Merck. Online. Available from: www.msdmanuals.com/professional/multimedia/table/characteristics-of-hepatitis-viruses.
125. World Health Organization (WHO). Hepatitis A. 2021. Available from: www.who.int/news-room/fact-sheets/detail/hepatitis-a.
126. World Health Organization (WHO). Hepatitis B. 2021 Available from: www.who.int/news-room/fact-sheets/detail/hepatitis-b.
127. World Health Organization (WHO). Hepatitis C. 2021. Available from: www.who.int/news-room/fact-sheets/detail/hepatitis-c.
128. McCall BJ, Looke D. The infection control practitioner and bioterrorism: threats, planning, preparedness. Aust Infect Control 2003;8(2):5.
129. Shadel BN, Rebmann T, Clements B, Chen JJ, Evans RG. Infection control practitioners' perceptions and educational needs regarding bioterrorism: results from a national needs assessment survey. Am J Infect Control 2003;31(3):129–34.
130. Flowers LK, Mothershead JL, Blackwell TH. Bioterrorism preparedness II: the community and emergency medical services systems. Emerg Med Clin North Am 2002;20(2):19.
131. Weant KA, Bailey AM, Fleishaker EL, Justice SB. Being prepared: bioterrorism and mass prophylaxis: part II. Adv Emerg Nurs J 2014;36(4):307–17.
132. Bratberg J, Deady K. Development and application of a bioterrorism emergency management plan. Prehosp Disaster Med 2012;20(Suppl. 3):158–9.

CHAPTER 28

ENVIRONMENTAL EMERGENCIES

IOANA VLAD AND BEN FISK

ESSENTIALS

- The severity of heat stress depends on physiological factors, the degree of heat, amount of humidity and length of exposure.
- Heat rash and heat oedema are compensated forms of heat stress that do not involve a rise in optimal core temperature.
- The lack of neurological sequelae is a significant difference between heat exhaustion and heat stroke.
- Treatment of heat stroke focuses both on rapid cooling of core temperature and life-supportive treatment.
- Gas exchange between the air and the human body is dependent upon the atmospheric pressure gradient between air at sea level and altitude. A reduced partial pressure of oxygen at altitude can lead to significant hypoxia.
- Hypoxaemia is at the maximum point during sleep. An increase of no more than 300 metres (1000 feet) in sleeping altitude per day is recommended.[1]
- Supplemental oxygen is essential for altitude sickness, although peripheral vasoconstriction may confound the use of oximetry as an indicator for oxygen administration. Acclimatisation can improve the body's ability to tolerate lower partial pressures of oxygen. A rapid reduction in altitude is critical following the onset of acute mountain sickness.[2]
- Snake bite is a rare but potentially lethal presentation in the emergency health setting. Once snake bite is considered a possibility, a standardised sequential approach to management is required, even in patients who are asymptomatic and have no obvious bite marks.
- Early, effective application of a pressure bandage with immobilisation (pressure immobilisation technique (PBI)) is a vital first-aid treatment for snake bite.
- Observation in the hospital and serial clinical and laboratory evaluation for at least 12 hours is required to exclude significant envenomation from a snake bite.
- Appropriate antivenom therapy should be given once the diagnosis of envenomation is made.
- In the event of cardiac arrest from a snake bite, early intravenous administration of undiluted antivenom is indicated. Call the Poisons Information Centre (13 11 26 in Australia or 0800 POISON/0800 764 766 in Aotearoa New Zealand).
- Redback spider bite is the most common medically significant arachnid envenomation syndrome in Australia. Funnel-web spider envenomation is much less common, but potentially lethal.
- Common marine envenomations are usually painful, and can be treated with hot-water immersion therapy and supportive care.
- Rarer marine envenomations (box jellyfish, Irukandji syndrome, blue-ringed octopus) can be lethal. Recognition of the clinical syndrome is essential, and advanced life support may be required.

INTRODUCTION

Interactions between humans and the natural environment create the potential for injury, illness and unpredictable emergency situations. Those working in pre-hospital emergency medical services, primary healthcare and emergency departments (EDs) should be aware of, and able to respond to, environmental emergencies. This chapter describes environmental emergencies resulting from a range of human-induced and natural events, including exposure to extremes of temperature, changes in atmospheric pressure, drowning and envenomations.

TEMPERATURE-RELATED EMERGENCIES

ANATOMY AND PHYSIOLOGY

Ambient temperature refers to the temperature around us and is a product of environmental temperature and humidity (the amount of moisture dissolved in the air). Increases in humidity will increase ambient temperature even when the environmental temperature remains constant. Optimal functioning of the human body and normal cellular function occur within a narrow temperature window between 36°C and 37.3°C. This temperature range is regulated by autonomic and endocrine feedback loops (Chapter 26). Metabolism of nutrients supports a range of biochemical functions, with endogenous heat being one by-product. The sum of all biochemical reactions is the basal metabolic rate (BMR), which, if unbalanced by cooling processes, would increase body temperature by 1.1°C per hour. Hyperthermia, defined by a core body temperature greater than 38°C, is less well tolerated than hypothermia.[3]

Temperature gain and loss are influenced by the properties of water and air. Heat transfer occurs via the processes of convection, evaporation, conduction and radiation. Water conducts heat at a rate greater than air, so is an ideal medium for both cooling and heating.[3] As indicated in Table 28.1, higher wind speed is associated with greater heat loss, and lack of wind will decrease the body's ability to reduce heat, especially in humid conditions. Wet clothing increases heat loss through conduction and evaporation, and can increase the risk of cold-related injury. The severity of heat or cold injury is related to the degree of temperature and length of exposure.

TABLE 28.1 WIND CHILL EFFECT[4]

WIND (km/h)	TEMPERATURE (°C)					
Calm	15	10	5	0	−5	−10
8	14	8	2	−4	−10	−17
16	11	6	1	−6	−12	-20
24	9	3	0	-7	−14	-22
32	6	0	−1	−8	−15	-23
40	2	−2	−4	−9	−16	-24

TABLE 28.2 BODY TEMPERATURE AND METABOLISM[5]

IF BODY TEMPERATURE RISES TO _°C	METABOLISM INCREASES BY _%
38	13
39	26
40	39
41	52
42	Insufficient oxygen to meet cellular needs

The significant effect of body temperature on metabolism, and thus oxygenation, is outlined in Table 28.2. As shown, for every 1°C rise in temperature, there is a correlating rise in oxygen consumption; and with each drop of 1°C in temperature below 36°C, there is a corresponding drop in both BMR and oxygen demand. Hyperthermia will produce a right shift in the oxygen–haemoglobin (O_2–Hb) dissociation curve, while hypothermia will produce a left shift (see Chapter 10). These responses are increased in non-acclimatised individuals. Acclimatisation is a process by which physiological adaptations occur in response to repeated exposures to heat or cold stress. Children and the elderly are at most risk of developing a temperature-related illness. Children have a greater body surface area by ratio to body mass and lose heat more easily (Chapter 35). Very young children have a reduced ability to shiver in response to cold and therefore cannot increase their body temperature in cold environments. Children are more reliant on others to avoid heat and to ensure an adequate fluid intake to prevent dehydration and associated heat stress. Those over the age of 50 have an increased risk of developing hyperthermia due to impaired thermoregulation, a reduced sweating response or comorbidities associated with the use of medications that inhibit thermoregulatory control (see Box 28.1).

HEAT-RELATED EMERGENCIES

By definition, hyperthermia is a core temperature above 38°C,[3,6] and the term 'thermal maximum' measures the magnitude and duration of heat that cells can encounter before damage occurs. In humans, this point is 42°C, beyond which further increases in temperature lead to rapid cellular damage, including progressive denaturing of a number of vital cellular proteins, failure of energy-producing functions and loss of cell membrane function. A right shift of the oxygen–haemoglobin (O_2–Hb) dissociation curve caused by hyperthermia means that Hb is less inclined to bind O_2, leading to more O_2 offloading and increased cellular oxygenation to meet increased metabolic demand. However, this means that a higher partial pressure of O_2 in the lungs is required to bind O_2 to Hb, and therefore good respiratory function is essential. At an organ system level, heat-influenced changes may manifest as rhabdomyolysis, acute pulmonary oedema (APO) (Chapter 21), disseminated intravascular coagulation (DIC) (Chapter 29), acute respiratory distress syndrome

BOX 28.1 RISK FACTORS FOR HEAT-RELATED EMERGENCIES[3,6]

AGE
Elderly
Infants

ENVIRONMENTAL CONDITIONS
Moderate to high environmental temperature
High relative humidity
Low wind speed
Lack of shade

ILLNESS
Cardiovascular disease
Chronic respiratory disease (e.g. cystic fibrosis, emphysema)
Diabetes
Obesity
Central nervous system disorders, e.g. prior stroke, dystonias
Skin disorders (e.g. large burn scars)
Infections

MEDICATIONS
Anticholinergics
Antihistamines
Antiparkinsonian drugs
Antispasmodics
Beta-adrenergic blockers

CALCIUM CHANNEL BLOCKERS
Diuretics
Phenothiazines
Salicylates
Tricyclic antidepressants

RECREATIONAL DRUGS
Stimulants, e.g. amphetamines, MDMA (ecstasy)
Hallucinogens, e.g. lysergic acid diethylamide (LSD), phencyclidine (PCP)

ALCOHOL

BEHAVIOURAL
Military personnel and manual workers
Athletes
Exertion
Inappropriate clothing or exposure (e.g. children in cars)

(ARDS), cardiovascular dysfunction, electrolyte disturbance, acute kidney injury, liver failure and neurological damage.

Heat illness will affect any individual who pushes their body past its ability to maintain thermal control and compensate for excessive heat production, either internally or externally. Heat illness may develop while exercising in ambient temperatures above 23°C. Because of the body's ability to lose heat, the capacity to maintain high levels of exercise without over-heating can be developed, although good physical condition does not preclude heat illness. Dehydration and intravascular volume depletion aggravate the risk in all age groups and fitness levels. Box 28.1 outlines the risk factors for heat-related illness. Heat waves are historically associated with significant morbidity and mortality. Rising baseline temperatures, especially at night, and longer periods of high daytime heat due to climate change are likely to worsen the incidence of heat-related emergencies. Heat oedema and heat cramps are mild heat-related conditions. Heat exhaustion and heat stroke are manifestations of decompensated heat-related stress. Differential diagnoses are listed in Box 28.2.

BOX 28.2 DIFFERENTIAL DIAGNOSES OF HEAT-RELATED EMERGENCIES

- Heat exhaustion
- Heat stroke
- Central nervous system injury
- Infection, e.g. meningitis, malaria
- Phaeochromocytoma
- Hyperthyroid storm
- Toxidromes: sympathomimetic, anticholinergic, serotonergic, neuroleptic malignant syndrome

Prevention of heat-related illness is essential, particularly as it exacerbates the risk of cardiac arrest in individuals with pre-existing co-morbidities. The community should be educated, both during pre-hospital encounters and prior to ED discharge, about the importance of changing behaviour to reduce the risk of heat-related illnesses. Health professionals should emphasise the critical importance of adapting behaviour to reduce ambient heat by choosing a cool environment, reducing activity to keep BMR low and maintaining hydration. Reliance on air-conditioning has reduced effective behaviours for staying cool on hot days, leaving many without options during power failures. Heat illness typically occurs with exercise during periods of high heat, when the elderly or ill are exposed to outside temperatures over 40°C, when housing is not optimised to reduce radiant heat, and when hydration and electrolyte balance are not maintained. It is also important to recognise that heat illness occurs more rapidly after the first exposure during any period of heat stress, and that rest for at least 12 hours afterwards is essential. For those who are required to work during periods of high temperature, heat–work–rest and water consumption tables (which incorporate thermal heat indexes) should be used. Workers should also be educated on how to recognise the symptoms of heat-related illnesses and what to do if they occur. See Useful websites section on Information on working in hot conditions.

Heat illness is generally associated with thermal regulation, and therefore sunburn is not a heat-related illness. Specific information on sunburn can be found in Chapter 49.

HEAT RASH AND OEDEMA

Heat rash is a fine, red, papular rash occurring on the torso, neck and in skin folds. The rash occurs when sweat ducts are obstructed and become inflamed, inhibiting sweat excretion. The rash usually occurs in warm weather, but has also been reported in cold weather as a result of excess clothing.

Heat oedema is characterised by swelling of the feet, ankles and fingers, and usually occurs in non-acclimatised individuals who exercise after prolonged periods of standing or sitting. The cause is believed to be cutaneous vasodilation and orthostatic pooling of interstitial fluid in gravity-dependent extremities following exposure to a hot environment. It is self-limiting and resolves in hours to days. Treatment includes heat, rest and elevation. While it is important to rule out other causes of peripheral oedema, especially in elderly people, overly vigorous diagnostic evaluation is unnecessary.

HEAT CRAMPS

Anatomy and physiology

Heat cramps are painful, involuntary muscle cramps (brief and intermittent), usually in the lower extremities, that develop suddenly after periods of exercise in a hot or humid environments in individuals who have perspired excessively. Heat cramps are presumed to be a result of both potassium wasting from persistent utilisation of aldosterone in order to maintain a euvolemic state and sodium loss through sweat and replacement of lost fluid with hypotonic solutions.[3]

Patient assessment and clinical interventions

Signs and symptoms may include weakness, nausea and tachycardia. As a form of compensated heat stress, the core temperature remains in the normal range as thermoregulation is not affected. Treatment includes removal from heat, rest and electrolyte replacement with oral or parenteral fluids.

PRACTICE TIP

Heat rash, oedema and cramps may be considered early warning signs and cues to implement prevention strategies to avoid more severe heat illness.

Discharge instructions are essential and should stress the importance of hydration and rest for at least 12 hours.

HEAT EXHAUSTION

Anatomy and physiology

Heat exhaustion occurs during periods of constant exercise in relatively high ambient heat when there is a failure to maintain fluid intake equal to losses experienced through perspiration and respiration. It is not uncommon to lose a litre or more of fluid per hour during periods of extreme heat stress. Cardiac output declines in response to a reduction in circulating fluid volume and poor venous return induced by vasodilation secondary to thermoregulatory demands. The subsequent response of the body to reduced cardiac output is peripheral vasoconstriction, thus preventing the usual mechanisms of heat loss to occur. Unable to cool itself, the body may heat up to a core temperature of 40°C.[3] In essence, heat exhaustion primarily involves significant volume depletion in the presence of an elevated temperature, following exposure to heat stress. The dehydration associated with heat exhaustion occurs in one of two forms: the first is *water depletion*, where the primary problem is a loss of water with subsequent reduced circulating volume. The second is *salt depletion*, with subsequent hyponatraemia and a milder degree of water depletion and associated hypovolaemia.

Patient assessment

Signs and symptoms include diaphoresis, pallor, hypotension, tachycardia, reduced urine output, nausea and vomiting, frontal headache, thirst, myalgia and syncope. The patient with heat exhaustion may be mildly confused, but does not demonstrate other mental-state changes or neurological sequelae. Because of the relatively ill-defined range of signs and symptoms, heat exhaustion is a diagnosis of exclusion.

Clinical interventions

Treatment is focused on active cooling, and fluid and electrolyte replacement. Cooling involves removing the patient from the source of heat, rest and removal of layers or tight clothing. When out of the heat the application of wet clothes will improve heat lost by evaporation, as will the use of a spray bottle and a fan to produce water mist. Where the core temperature is around 40°C, ice packs may be used in the armpit, groin and around the neck to enable rapid cooling. Fluid therapy is titrated to haemodynamic response and electrolyte replacement is based on serum electrolyte levels. Fluid and electrolyte replacement may be done orally if tolerated by the patient. All oral replacement is by commercially prepared oral rehydration solution (ORS). Where oral rehydration is not possible, intravenous therapy is used. If the patient is haemodynamically compromised and requires bolus fluid administration, the primary choice is 0.9% saline solution (normal saline). It is not uncommon for a fit young adult who has been exercising in the heat to receive up to 5–6 L of fluid replacement.

Core temperature should be monitored regularly during pre-hospital care, hourly in hospital, but preferably continuously if possible by using rectal or oesophageal probes (see Chapter 16). Active cooling should be ceased once core temperature decreases to 38°C, as shivering may occur and lead to a rise in core temperature. Admission should be considered for any patient who does not improve significantly within 3–4 hours of emergency treatment. Heat exhaustion is believed by some to be on the continuum to heat stroke, and therefore should be identified and treated early.

HEAT STROKE

Anatomy and physiology

Heat stroke is an uncommon but life-threatening form of heat-related illness. While difficult to define, heat stroke is always associated with altered mental status due to heat-induced encephalopathy in combination with a core temperature greater than 40.5°C.[3] As heat stroke is an interplay between the effects of heat and a range of inflammatory and coagulopathic responses, it has been argued that it should also be classified as a systemic inflammatory response syndrome (SIRS). However, unlike sepsis, the most familiar SIRS, heat stroke is commonly associated with rhabdomyolysis and guidelines for initial fluid resuscitation are less defined.[3]

Thermoregulatory failure will occur universally at ambient temperatures above 42°C and has a variable presentation at temperatures between 40°C and 42°C.[3] While a lack of perspiration is considered a key sign, perspiration may initially persist despite the presence of thermoregulatory failure. Therefore, dry skin and no sweating are not sensitive indicators. Mortality in heat stroke is dependent on the duration and intensity of hyperthermia. The more rapidly the condition is treated, the lower the incidence of both mortality and morbidity.

Heat stroke may be classified as non-exertional and exertional. Non-exertional heat stroke—also known as classic heat stroke—occurs as a result of prolonged exposure to sustained, high ambient temperatures and humidity. While anyone can be affected, the most susceptible are the elderly, children, the incapacitated, the chronically ill and those with mental health or substance-use disorders (suffering from disordered perception). This is in part due to the inability of these populations to initiate behavioural changes that will improve heat transfer, as well as the side-effects of some medications (see Box 28.1). These groups will have a diminished capacity to thermoregulate, adapt to hot climates and increase cardiac output. Paralysed and intoxicated patients are often unable to initiate autonomic responses to improve heat transfer. The elderly are more likely to suffer cardiac disease, which may limit their ability to increase cardiac output in response to heat stress, particularly in the presence of rate-controlling medications. In children, the younger the child, the greater their inability to thermoregulate and the more responsive they are to ambient temperature. Non-exertional heat stroke has been the cause of death in children locked in cars on warm to hot days, with inside temperatures rising rapidly in the first 10–20 minutes.

Exertional heat stroke is, by definition, the consequence of exercise or work. This type of heat stroke usually occurs in the presence of high ambient temperatures, where heat production exceeds the internal heat elimination mechanisms. It is most commonly seen in athletes, soldiers and manual labourers in hot environments. Individuals with one or more risk factors (Box 28.1) are at much greater risk for hyperthermia when exacerbating environmental conditions are present.[6,7] Heatwaves have significant potential to contribute to both non-exertional and exertional heat stroke and to exacerbate the risk of other adverse health events.

Patient assessment

Signs and symptoms of heat stroke are varied, and if not treated urgently can result in multi-organ failure. In 80% of cases, the onset of heat stroke is usually sudden. However, heat stroke may be preceded by a period of several hours during which heat illness presents as mild heat exhaustion. In the initial stages of heat stroke, central nervous system (CNS) dysfunction is observed. These are the first signs of thermoregulatory failure. Changes in the mental state include anxiety, confusion, hallucinations, ataxia (cerebellar dysfunction), combativeness and unconsciousness. Seizures occur most commonly during cooling. Direct thermal damage to cerebral tissue combined with decreased cerebral blood flow often produces cerebral oedema, further exacerbating CNS dysfunction. The cerebellum is particularly sensitive to thermal injury, and thus the range of neurological sequelae is broad.

PRACTICE TIP

The degree of neurological injury is directly related to the duration and magnitude of the increase in body temperature.

Initially, peripheral vascular beds dilate in an attempt to improve heat transfer, in turn producing a functional hypovolaemia, hypotension and tachycardia. Eventually, excessive sweating and inability to maintain adequate fluid intake in correlation with losses produce significant volume depletion[3,6] resulting in decreased renal blood flow and urine output. Hepatic damage is indicated by elevated serum aspartate aminotransferase (AST) and alanine aminotransferase (ALT) and is so common that its absence should raise doubts as to the diagnosis of heat stroke.[6] Coagulopathies are also common. While platelets may suffer heat damage, DIC is believed to occur secondary to a SIRS response.[3] Additional complications include rhabdomyolysis, multi-organ failure, hypoglycaemia, acid–base imbalance and ARDS. It is important to take into account pre-hospital care, as a patient may present to hospital with a normal temperature and still have demonstrated all the characteristics of heat stroke during initial care.

Clinical interventions

Early recognition and management is vital whether in the pre-hospital setting, in smaller medical facilities or tertiary centres. Early definitive airway intervention is important, as aspiration and seizures are common. Administer supplemental oxygen by the method most appropriate for the patient's level of consciousness and available resources. The use of non-depolarising agents to facilitate intubation and ventilation offers the advantage of decreasing heat production that might occur with fasciculations. The use of non-depolarising agents may also prevent the development of malignant hyperthermia. The choice of agents for initial and ongoing sedation should be considered carefully in the hyperthermic patient with suspected serotonin syndrome.

Pharmacological seizure control may be required in severely hyperthermic patients, with the understanding that concurrent active cooling is also essential.

Fluid replacement is essential, and correction of hypovolaemia with cool, crystalloid isotonic fluids will reduce temperature and support cardiac output. The volume delivered is titrated to response. As the body cools and thermoregulatory control is regained, the true extent of the fluid deficit will be easier to assess and treat. The use of isotonic fluid is important to avoid cerebral and pulmonary oedema. This most commonly involves normal saline or Hartmann's solution. Continuous monitoring should include haemodynamics, urine output, core body temperature, blood glucose level and oxygenation (see Chapter 16). It is important to observe for myoglobin in the urine, as rhabdomyolysis may occur secondary to heat damage of peripheral tissues. Regular assessment of serum liver enzymes and coagulation studies are useful in identifying complications.

Active cooling

Every minute the patient remains overheated, they are at increased risk of potential sequelae and mortality. Rapid cooling without producing over-cooling has demonstrated the best long-term outcomes. Cooling should occur simultaneously with primary survey intervention and should include removing the source of heat, appropriately removing clothing, immersion in cold water or ice pack application. While the practice may complicate the provision of other life-supporting measures, cold water immersion is recognised as the most effective strategy for rapid cooling. Nine minutes in a cool bath to a rectal temperature of 38.6°C is recommended.[6,8] Where it is not achievable, ice packs should be applied over and under the patient, especially over areas where large vessels are closer to the skin (i.e. neck, axillae, groins). Use of a fan is also effective, preferably in conjunction with ice or a cool water mist, as this technique will increase heat transfer away from the body. Other cooling methods, such as the use of cold IV fluids and a cooling blanket, can also be considered. If necessary, ice-water peritoneal or pleural lavage may be used to initiate rapid cooling.

Cooling should never produce shivering in the patient, as this will increase core temperature and oxygen consumption, although it is recognised that this may be challenging to regulate in the pre-hospital setting. Pharmacological agents, such as chlorpromazine, benzodiazepine and paralysing agents, may be considered to prevent shivering during the cooling process.[6,8]

PRACTICE TIP

Anti-inflammatories and paracetamol have not proved effective in reducing hyperthermia secondary to heat stroke. Regardless of the setting, the priorities are removal from the heat source, airway protection and rapid cooling.

COLD-RELATED EMERGENCIES

Compared to heat injuries, the body is better able to cope with cold exposure.[9,10] Cold-related emergencies occur following exposure to cold ambient temperatures or immersion in cold water, and severity depends on the extent and duration of the cold encountered. The effects of cold can be aggravated by the use of alcohol or other sedative agents, or pre-existing conditions, such as diabetes, renal failure and cardiac disease. Cold injuries can be classified as *localised* or *systemic*. Although uncommon, it is possible for localised and systemic cold injuries to occur concurrently. Localised injuries are almost uniquely peripheral, partly because human homeostasis places a priority on maintaining core temperature at the expense of peripheries. In humans adapted to cold, a reflex develops and cold-induced vasodilation occurs at regular intervals to provide peripheral protection against the hypoxic effects of vasoconstriction.[9] Thus, most localised cold injuries occur in poorly prepared, unadapted individuals who fail to protect their peripheries with adequate clothing. They can be categorised as *freezing* or *non-freezing* in nature. Frostbite is the primary localised freezing injury, while non-freezing injuries include chilblains, immersion and trench foot. Systemic effects of exposure to cold result in hypothermia which in severe cases can result in cardiac arrest.

IMMERSION AND TRENCH FOOT

Anatomy and physiology

Immersion and trench foot are the result of prolonged or constant exposure of a foot to both water and cold. The term 'trench foot' was coined in World War I—the era of trench warfare—when feet remained in the same boots, in subzero temperatures, deep in stagnant water for days. It is seen today among people who wear wet boots for long periods in temperate or cold, damp conditions. Immersion foot is a more severe form of trench foot and has been described in the past among sailors and downed pilots, who spent days in life rafts with their feet submerged in cold water. However, this is rarely seen nowadays with the use of EPIRBs, GPS and other rescue systems that decreased rescue times significantly. Soft tissue injury occurs with prolonged cooling of the foot and is accelerated by wet conditions. Primary injury is to peripheral nerves and vasculature.

Patient assessment and clinical interventions

Progression of the injury occurs over days. On assessment, the foot is cold, damp, pale, numb, pulseless and oedematous. The warming process produces vasodilation, erythema, intense burning and tingling, with perfusion returning to the foot over several days. In severe cases, anaesthesia may persist for many weeks after re-warming and may be permanent. Severe cases may also complicate with lymphangitis, cellulitis or liquefaction gangrene, requiring surgical intervention.

Treatment is focused on drying and warming the foot. Re-warming should occur gradually and is best achieved by exposing the area to warm air or soaking in warm water (37–39°C). The injury is reversible with timely treatment, a factor dependent on early presentation to care. Hospitalisation is only required in the presence of complications, which usually occur as the result of a delay in commencing treatment. Prevention is based on good-fitting boots, allowing feet exposure to air for at least 8 hours a day (during sleep if possible), changing into dry socks and allowing the footwear to dry. If trench or immersion foot is identified in the field, the focus should be on drying, warming and elevating the feet immediately.

FROSTBITE

Anatomy and physiology

Frostnip is the transient tingling and numbness after cold exposure, which resolves with warming and leaves no permanent damage. The lack of damage distinguishes frostnip from frostbite. Frostbite occurs with exposure to temperatures below freezing, with increased risk due to wind chill, prolonged inactivity, poor circulation, dehydration and wet peripheries (i.e. damp gloves or socks).[11] Cycles of warming and freezing are particularly damaging. As the temperature drops below 10°C, the cutaneous sensation is lost. Simultaneously, vasoconstriction reduces perfusion, blood viscosity increases and endothelial damage leads to interstitial leakage.

When skin temperature drops below freezing, ice crystals form initially in extracellular spaces. Crystal formation is increased if cold ambient temperatures occur in the presence of wind and moisture. Extracellular crystals prevent water movement in and out of cells, eventually resulting in cell dehydration and damage.[10] Intracellular crystal development enlarges and compresses cells, leading to membrane rupture, interruption of enzymatic activity, and alters intracellular metabolic processes. After thawing, in addition to the structural damage produced by crystal formation, sludging and microvascular collapse secondary to thrombosis occur. Reduced vascular flow is exacerbated by hyperviscosity and endothelial damage. Anaerobic metabolism eventually produces ischaemia and necrosis. Damage to the microvasculature ultimately determines the degree of permanent injury. The extent of frostbite is dependent on the degree and length of cold exposure, and estimation of the true extent of injury[7] may not be possible

TABLE 28.3 FROSTBITE CLASSIFICATIONS ACCORDING TO SEVERITY

CLASSIFICATION	DESCRIPTION	SYMPTOMS
Superficial		
First degree	Partial skin freezing Erythema, oedema, no blisters or necrosis	Transient stinging, burning Some throbbing pain ± hyperhidrosis
Second degree	Full-thickness skin freezing Erythema, significant oedema, vesicles Blisters which desquamate to form a black eschar	Numbness ± vasomotor disturbance
Deep		
Third degree	Full-thickness skin and subcutaneous freezing Haemorrhagic or violaceous blisters Skin necrosis, blue-grey discolouration	Anaesthesia Tissue 'feels like a block of wood' After re-warming–pain, burning, aching
Fourth degree	Full-thickness skin, subcutaneous, muscle, tendon and bone freezing Almost no oedema Initially mottled, deeply red or cyanotic Eventually dry, black and mummified	Anaesthesia Tissue 'feels like a block of wood' After re-warming–pain, burning, aching Possible joint discomfort

until several days post-injury. Table 28.3 summarises frostbite according to severity.

Patient assessment

All patients with frostbite will have some degree of sensory deficit. Areas at greatest risk are extremities: nose, digits, ears and penis. The most common symptoms include tingling, numbness or a burning sensation. Complete anaesthesia is the result of ischaemic nerve damage and should be considered an indicator of severe injury. The skin may appear white and waxy and frozen skin feels cold and stiff. After thawing the patient may feel a hot, stinging sensation or, more commonly, a dull continuous ache. Mottling and blisters may develop within hours to days of the injury (Fig. 28.1), progressing to gangrene if ischaemia is not resolved. Commonly, a dry black eschar will form over several weeks (Fig. 28.2). Oedema of the area is expected and in severe cases can persist for months.

Clinical interventions

In the pre-hospital environment, the focus of treatment is prevention of hypothermia, removal of constricting jewellery or material from the affected part with gentle handling and moderate elevation. Re-warming should be deferred if it is not possible to guarantee the part will not re-freeze.[7,10]

Preventing the onset of (or managing existing) hypothermia is essential in the pre-hospital setting, as hypothermia is life threatening and further aggravates frostbite. This can be achieved through temperature monitoring, judicious use of warm blankets, head coverings and warmed fluids. Hypothermia prevention and management should continue during hospitalisation.

FIGURE 28.1 BLISTER FORMATION 24 HOURS AFTER FROSTBITE[7]

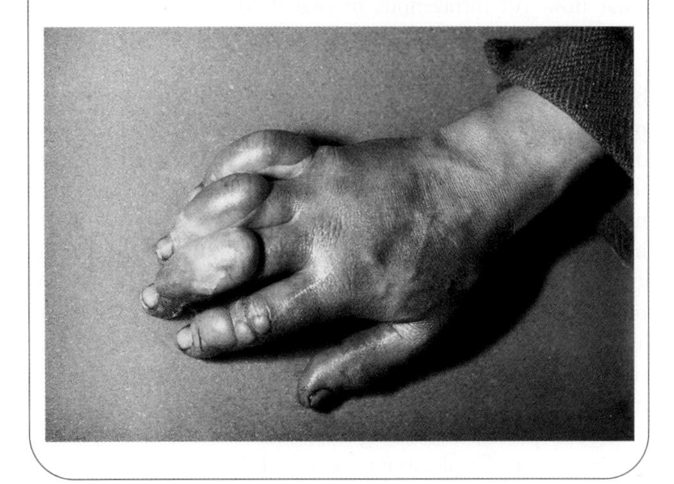

Scott Polar Research Institute/Science Photo Library.

If frostbite has occurred at altitude, supplemental oxygen may improve tissue oxygenation of the affected site since hypoxia causes vasoconstriction.[12]

If re-warming can be achieved without subsequent re-freezing, start by air drying and not rubbing the affected area, which is very fragile. If an extremity has been thawed, immobilise, protect with soft, thick dressings and elevate. This will continue in the ED. During the treatment phase, warm the room or vehicle in which the patient is kept. Rapid re-warming of the part under controlled conditions is the ideal for

FIGURE 28.2 GANGRENOUS NECROSIS 6 WEEKS AFTER FROSTBITE INJURY[7]

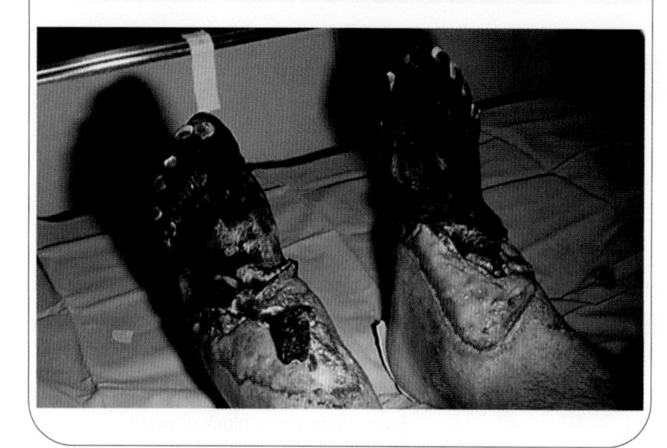

maintaining tissue viability. Thaw in a warm bath (40–42°C) for up to 30 minutes until the part is pliable and erythematous.[9,10] Alternatively, the application of warm wet dressings (at a similar temperature) and elevation provides gentle re-warming and improves vascular flow. This method is useful for areas such as the ears and face, although the dressings must be kept warm (changed as required). Avoid heavy dressings, blankets and clothes over the injured area, as it is fragile. Ensure hydration to reduce the effect of intravascular sludging on microvascular flow. All intravenous or oral fluids should be warmed prior to administration.

Wound management includes not debriding haemorrhagic blisters, tetanus prophylaxis, avoidance of vasoconstrictors, prohibition of weight-bearing on the affected part and fasciotomy for compartment syndrome. Antibiotics are only used for identified infections. Dress the thawed wound with dry, non-restrictive dressings and elevate the part. As the severity of injury usually takes a couple of weeks to months to determine, amputation is not considered during the early phase of treatment, although a surgical opinion is essential early. Eschars are allowed to develop as part of the demarcation process. Over time, viable tissue will reveal itself and wounds will be managed surgically.[9,10]

As the process of thawing frozen tissue is extremely painful, administration of analgesia is recommended. Intravenous narcotics are often required initially, and non-steroidal anti-inflammatory drugs (NSAIDs) are used for ongoing analgesia. Complications include secondary infections, tetanus, gangrene and ongoing paraesthesia.

HYPOTHERMIA

Anatomy and physiology

Hypothermia is defined as a core temperature below 35°C. It is considered mild if body temperature is 35–32°C, moderate 32–28°C and severe below 28°C.[5–9] Primary hypothermia is essentially caused by exposure to the environment, secondary hypothermia as a result of medical illness (e.g. any condition leading to a decreased BMR, including hypoglycaemia and CNS conditions interfering with thermoregulation or disrupting muscle movement and limiting the shiver response). Therapeutic hypothermia may be used in the post-resuscitation period for specific cases.

Primary hypothermia resulting from accidental exposure can be classified as *immersion-induced* or *non-immersion-induced*. Immersion hypothermia generally develops more rapidly due to the high rate of heat loss in water compared to air because water conducts heat much faster than air. Profound heat loss and rapid hypothermia can develop in water temperatures of 21°C or less. Non-immersion hypothermia occurs in cold environments that may be dry, damp or windy.

Common factors contributing to hypothermia are listed in Table 28.4. Behavioural patterns, including drug and alcohol use, and social situations such as homelessness, may alter a person's ability to prevent the onset of hypothermia. Elderly patients are more prone to hypothermia as a result of taking medications that alter body defences and the physiological decrease in basal metabolic rate, shivering response and sensory perception. Elderly patients are also more prone to falls at home or outside in domestic settings where they may not be found for hours or days.

Importantly, many patients and trauma patients in particular, are susceptible to hypothermia in the pre-hospital setting. Major trauma patients are susceptible to the systemic and physiological effects of hypothermia, coagulopathy, hypocalcaemia and acidosis. The processes of entrapment, extrication, assessment and resuscitation may all contribute to hypothermia due to continuous exposure, the presence of shock and the

TABLE 28.4 HYPOTHERMIA AETIOLOGIES[9]

Environmental	Cold, wet, windy ambient conditions
	Cold-water immersion
	Exhaustion
Trauma	Multitrauma (entrapment, resuscitation, head injury)
	Minor trauma and immobility (e.g. #NOF)
	Major burns
Drugs	Ethanol
	Sedatives (e.g. benzodiazepines) in overdose
	Phenothiazines (impaired shivering)
Neurological	CVA
	Paraplegia
	Parkinson's disease
Endocrine	Hypoglycaemia
	Hypothyroidism
	Hypoadrenalism
Systemic illness	Sepsis
	Malnutrition

CVA: cerebrovascular accident; #NOF: fractured neck of femur.

administration of cold fluids. It is essential to monitor temperature, keep the patient covered, re-warm the cold patient and administer warmed intravenous fluids or blood products as appropriate.

Patient assessment

The physiological effects of hypothermia produce symptoms and signs as indicated at the following core body temperatures:

- 35°C—cold, pale skin, poor muscle coordination, tachypnoea, piloerection and shivering, all designed to raise core temperature by retaining and generating heat.
- 35–32°C—decreased respiratory rate and carbon dioxide (CO_2) production,[7] resulting in lethargy, weakness, slurred speech, impaired reasoning, poor coordination and ataxia. Shivering may cease.
- 32–30°C—muscle rigidity, poor reflexes, dilated pupils, hypotension, bradycardia, coma.
- 30–28°C—flaccid muscles, fixed dilated pupils, dysrhythmias, cardiac arrest.
- A core temperature below 25.6°C is generally considered fatal.

The slowing of metabolic processes that occurs with hypothermia reduces cerebral oxygen requirements and is believed to provide some protection against hypoxic damage. A slowing of respiratory effort produces CO_2 retention, hypoxia and eventually acidosis. Oxygen delivery to the tissues is inhibited by a leftwards shift in the oxygen–haemoglobin dissociation curve, which represents an increased affinity of Hb for O_2. Consequently, Hb picks up O_2 more easily in the lungs, but is reluctant to offload it, leading to hypoxia at the tissue level. This is further aggravated by hypoperfusion due to peripheral shutdown. Cough and gag reflexes are depressed, increasing the risk of aspiration. While much has been said about the accuracy of arterial blood gases (ABGs) in hypothermic patients and the need to correct them prior to interpretation, it is recommended that ABGs be interpreted in their uncorrected form.[4]

Hypothermia produces bradycardia in proportion to the reduction in temperature, leading to reduced cardiac output and hypotension. Stroke volume is not affected. Concurrent hypovolaemia produced by dehydration will aggravate haemodynamic compromise. The cardiac conduction system is suppressed by hypothermia, resulting in QT prolongation and QRS widening on the electrocardiogram (ECG), and also the appearance of characteristic Osborne (J) waves (Fig. 28.3). An Osborne wave is a sharp, positive deflection at the end of the QRS complex, most prominent in leads II and V_3–V_6.[9,10]

Dysrhythmias, particularly ventricular fibrillation (VF), are a potential hazard once core temperature falls below 30°C. This is largely due to myocardial irritability, which can be aggravated by rough handling. Simply turning the patient can potentiate dysrhythmias. Therefore, gentle handling to avoid cardiac arrest is essential. The typical sequence for the progression of dysrhythmias is sinus bradycardia, atrial fibrillation with a slow ventricular response, VF and eventually asystole.[9,10] The temperature of 28°C is commonly considered the most likely point at which the patient will develop VF. Unfortunately, hypothermia increases transthoracic impedance and reduces the effectiveness of defibrillation below 30°C. As a rule, it is necessary to warm the patient before defibrillation can be effective. Anti-dysrhythmics have generally been shown to have little effect and may worsen the conduction disturbances.

Haemoconcentration, increased blood viscosity and reduced peripheral circulation have a tendency to produce thrombo-emboli, with subsequent complications. Platelet

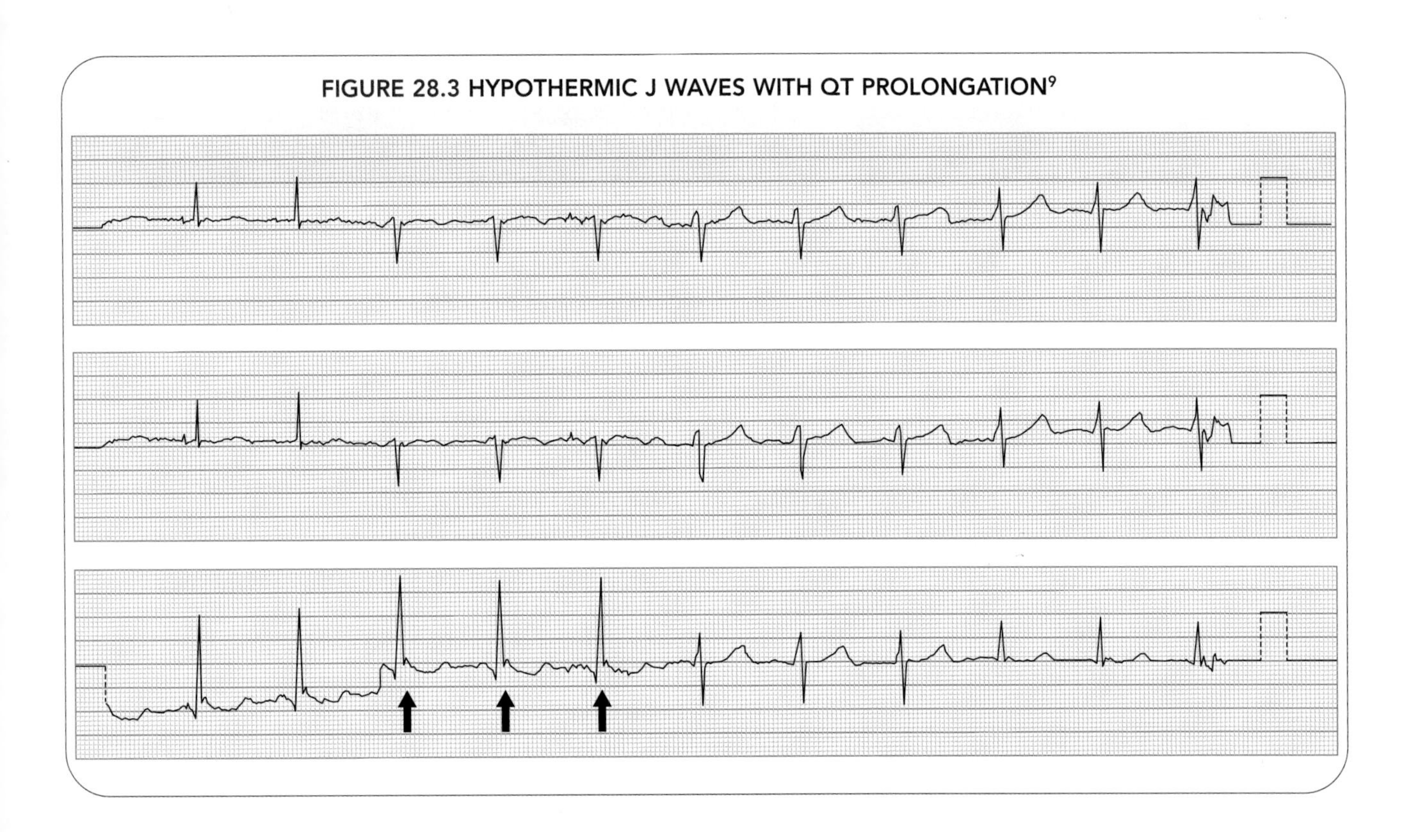

FIGURE 28.3 HYPOTHERMIC J WAVES WITH QT PROLONGATION[9]

function and the coagulation cascade are inhibited by cold, leading to a tendency to bleed (Chapter 30). As coagulation tests are performed at 37°C, cold-induced coagulopathies evident by clinical bleeding may not be confirmed in laboratory testing.[9,10]

The ability of the kidneys to concentrate urine is reduced in hypothermia, leading to a 'cold diuresis'. This results in volume losses, dehydration and a subsequent drop in urinary output. A failure of the kidney to concentrate urine makes the use of specific gravity and output poor indicators of haemodynamic status. In addition, the hypothermic patient who is immobile is at risk of rhabdomyolysis, myoglobinuria and renal failure.

Endocrine function is generally well preserved at low temperatures, with normal hormonal levels maintained. However, persistent shivering eventually uses glycogen stores, resulting in hypoglycaemia. In a percentage of patients, hyperglycaemia occurs secondary to reduced insulin release and decreased glucose use. A slowing in circulation reduces hepatic clearance. Thus medication half-lives are extended, and toxicity risks are increased. Below 30°C there will be inadequate circulation and no hepatic clearance.

PRACTICE TIP

The use of intravenous medications should be limited to those patients whose core temperature is greater than 30°C. Avoid the active management of bradycardia with output in severely hypothermic patients.

Clinical interventions

Treatment of hypothermia is focused on re-warming and life supportive interventions. If there is any detectable movement, pulse or cardiac rhythm capable of sustaining life, CPR should not be commenced due to the risk of precipitating VF.[7–10,13] However, where a cardiac arrest has already occurred, CPR is appropriate, and prolonged CPR in combination with rapid re-warming of patients in VF has resulted in neurologically intact survival. Re-warming procedures are active or passive, based on external warming or internal warming. The choice of warming technique is dependent upon the severity of hypothermia and the need to warm the patient in order to maximise the effectiveness of resuscitation. Table 28.5 outlines the options for re-warming.

The patient with mild hypothermia (32–35°C) requires simple external re-warming techniques to prevent further heat loss and to re-warm as rapidly as possible. Passive re-warming may at best increase the temperature 1–2°C per hour.[9] In the field, insulate the patient from the ground to prevent conductive heat loss; in windy conditions, use a windproof layer (e.g. tarps, sheets of plastic, reflective blankets) to prevent convective heat loss; and minimise further heat loss by removing wet clothing and covering the patient as effectively as possible.[13] Consider using a hypothermia wrap and be aware of the increased risk of a further drop in temperature if the patient remains immobile[11] but needs to be moved via stretcher carry. Once inside a warm ambulance or inside the ED, remove clothing if wet and provide dry clothes and warm blankets. Warming blankets, such as a Bair Hugger, and radiant heat lamps are all useful for more rapid and aggressive warming. All intravenous fluids should be warmed and in the hospital setting ideally include a percentage of glucose. Use hot, sweet drinks if the patient can tolerate fluids. Sugar is important as this produces heat through metabolism. Consider the use of humidified oxygen.

Be aware that re-warming will produce vasodilation, which in turn may precipitate hypotension as circulating volume redistributes into warmed peripheries. As the patient re-warms and renal flow improves, the urinary output will become a more predictive tool for haemodynamic status.

TABLE 28.5 OPTIONS FOR RE-WARMING PATIENTS

TEMPERATURE	WARMING OPTIONS	INTERVENTIONS
Core temperature 32 to 35°C	Passive external warming	Remove cold, wet clothing and dry the patient in warm environment
		Create improvised shelter if required to protect from wind, rain etc. Cover with warm blankets and/or hypothermia wrap
	Active external warming	Infrared radiant lamp (over bare skin)
		Heating blankets (e.g. Bair Hugger)
		Heating pads
Core temperature less than 32°C	Active core/internal warming	Warmed intravenous fluids at 39°C
		Warmed humidified oxygen at 42°C
		Gastric or bladder lavage with normal saline 20 mL/kg cycled 15 minutes at 42°C
		Peritoneal lavage with potassium-free dialysate 20 mL/kg cycled every 15 minutes at 42°C
		Pleural lavage
	Extracorporeal	Cardiopulmonary bypass

In the hypothermic patient with a core temperature below 32°C it is necessary to use both active external and internal (core) re-warming techniques. Active internal re-warming can include simple procedures such as heated inhalations via an endotracheal tube or warmed intravenous fluid, to more advanced procedures such as administration of warmed fluid via a peritoneal lavage, gastrointestinal or bladder irrigation. However, these procedures may not be effective for severe hypothermia with core temperatures less than 30°C and especially in cases of cardiac arrest, pleural lavage or extracorporeal re-warming via cardiopulmonary bypass may be required.[13]

Re-warming shock

Re-warming shock is a condition in which the core temperature continues to drop after re-warming is initiated. The improvement in blood flow with re-warming shifts cold, acidotic, potassium-rich peripheral blood to the central circulation, increasing ventricular irritability and leading to VF. This is compounded by peripheral vasodilation, which can precipitate hypotension and cardiovascular collapse. To this end, VF can occur on both the decline and the increase in temperature. This necessitates treating the patient very carefully and continuing warming methods until normal core temperature is reached. Active internal (core) warming may cease once the patient reaches 32°C, at which point re-warming continues via external methods. Active re-warming should discontinue when core temperature reaches 35°C, in order to prevent the onset of hyperthermia. Successful re-warming depends on the patient's age, general condition before the hypothermic event and length of exposure.[9,10]

Body temperature decreases 2°C in the first hour after death and 1.5°C for every hour thereafter. As a general rule, patients cannot be declared deceased secondary to hypothermia until they are warm and dead. One exception to this rule is a persistently declining temperature despite aggressive efforts to warm internally and externally, or a temperature that will not rise above 33°C despite aggressive actions. In this instance the patient can be declared deceased, despite a low body temperature.

DROWNING

Historically, drowning was defined as death within 24 hours from asphyxia associated with submersion in a fluid, with near-drowning defined as any degree of recovery with survival beyond 24 hours from the point of submersion.[7] In 2002, the International Liaison Committee On Resuscitation (ILCOR) established a more simple definition which does not discriminate between the two, where drowning is defined as a process of respiratory impairment resulting from immersion in a liquid regardless of the survival outcome. Drowning is one of the highest causes of death in childhood. In 2019–20 in Australia, 248 people died from unintentional drowning and there were 504 non-fatal drownings.[14] There is a downward trend, with 8% less deaths than the previous year. Most deaths occurred in the 25 to 34 years age group and after drowning in rivers or creeks. The number of deaths secondary to drowning in the 0–4 years age group has decreased significantly, probably due to improvements in public health promotion and laws mandating safety measures, such as pool fencing. However, the risk of drowning has increased in other areas due to drug and alcohol consumption and underlying medical conditions. The majority of drownings at beaches, in particular, is by people not familiar with the area, tourists and new arrivals in Australia, who are at particular risk due to lack of knowledge about the risks found at beaches.

Submersion events may be precipitated by trauma, risk-taking behaviour, hypothermia, syncope or seizures or disaster events such as flooding. Assessment for additional injury, intoxication or illness should be part of drowning management.

ANATOMY AND PHYSIOLOGY

Sudden immersion in cold water will elicit two separate physiological responses: the cold shock response and the diving reflex. The cold shock response is a sympathetic reaction characterised by gasping, hyperventilation, an increased heart rate and increased blood pressure.[15] The cold shock response may precipitate aspiration and drowning, and may induce arrhythmias in patients with cardiovascular compromise. Rapid cooling of the skin and peripheries may also induce muscle weakness and fatigue, and lead to rapid physical incapacitation.

The dive reflex (or mammalian dive reflex) is a parasympathetic response predominantly initiated by the combination of apnoea and immersion of the face in cold water. The dive reflex occurs due to stimulation of cold-sensitive neurons in the superficial epidermal layer of the skin and the trigeminal nerve. The dive reflex essentially acts to decrease oxygen demand and conserve oxygen supply during apnoea by decreasing heart rate and shunting the blood to the vital organs. The dive reflex is utilised by those who participate in the sport of freediving.

Following sudden immersion in cold water the cold shock response will predominate prior to the effects of the mammalian dive reflex coming into effect. Sudden immersion in rough and cold water in particular may quickly lead to aspiration and drowning.

Once thought to provide some protection against cerebral insult, it is now believed that the sympathetic stimulation associated with submersion of the head blunts the diving reflex in adults, although the diving reflex eventually predominates. However, submersion in cold water may provide protection due to rapid CNS cooling prior to the development of significant dysrhythmias.[16] Between the first 20 seconds and 5 minutes of immersion, a point is reached at which time the individual will breathe. This usually results in water entering the airway, producing laryngeal spasm and subsequent apnoea. Hypoxia, acidosis, convulsions and cardiac arrest follows.

There is a theoretical distinction between 'wet' and 'dry' drowning, separating those who aspirate and those in whom no obvious aspiration of fluid occurs and asphyxiation is secondary to laryngeal spasm.[16,17] Inhalation of fluid is usually broken up into occurrence in fresh or in salty water, although despite differences in the effects that each solution will have on the lungs, the type of water has no bearing on prognosis. Inhalation of salt water is believed to diffuse fluid from the pulmonary capillary network into the alveoli, resulting in pulmonary oedema, hypovolaemia and electrolyte disturbance. By contrast, freshwater exerts an osmotic force on the lungs that pushes water into the capillary network, potentially resulting in haemodilution and hypervolaemia. In reality, the amount of aspirated water is usually no greater than 3–4 mL/kg and the volumes are usually inadequate to have any significant effect on cardiovascular status.[15]

Patient assessment

Early basic life support is critical to increasing survival without neurological sequelae due to hypoxia. This should be complemented by rapid and aggressive management by paramedics, which may include advanced airway management, with urgent transfer to an ED for ongoing resuscitation and stabilisation. Without detracting from patient resuscitation, it is important to obtain a patient history. This should always include submersion time, medium, risk of water contaminants, temperature, level of consciousness (LOC) at the scene, first aid rendered and any other events that led to the incident.

It is possible for patients to present as relatively asymptomatic, although most will demonstrate respiratory distress ranging from shortness of breath to apnoea, pallor and a degree of cyanosis. Hypotension is common, secondary to bradycardia or other dysrhythmias. Profound bradycardia in combination with vasoconstriction may present as a pulseless patient from hypoxia, hypothermia or head injury. Peripheral vasoconstriction will produce pale, often mottled extremities, pupils will be dilated, and the patient will be extremely cold. The conscious patient may be vomiting and mildly confused. Evaluate the confusion as secondary to hypoxia early. Assess for signs of aspiration and other injury, particularly of the head and spine. An unconscious patient removed from the water should be managed as having a spinal injury until proven otherwise. Table 28.6 describes the association of presenting mental status post near-drowning with neurological outcome.

CLINICAL INTERVENTIONS

Early airway establishment with cervical spine control, if indicated, is critical. High-flow oxygen therapy administration for the conscious patient or intubation and ventilation for patients with a reduced GCS or persistent low arterial oxygen pressure (PaO_2) should occur.[15,18] See Chapter 16 for various airway management techniques, including intubation and positive end-expiratory pressure (PEEP), which is often used to improve the relationship of ventilation to perfusion and therefore gas exchange. Continuous cardiac, temperature and peripheral oxygen saturation (SpO_2) monitoring should be commenced, although SpO_2 monitoring may be impaired in the patient with hypothermia. Chapter 16 contains information on cardiac monitoring techniques.

A chest x-ray should be performed and is useful for evaluating the risk of aspiration or the presence of other trauma.[15,18] ABGs are useful for determining acid–base balance and gas exchange. An ECG should be performed, especially in the absence of a palpable pulse, as hypothermia is a significant cause of pulseless electrical activity (PEA). CPR is required in the pulseless patient and should continue until a palpable pulse is produced or the patient is warm. Fluid resuscitation is often required, although it should be administered judiciously, titrated to urine output, and the use of crystalloid fluids is recommended.[18] Inotropes may be required to support cardiac output and blood pressure. Gastric decompression will be required to remove gastric water and reduce the risk of aspiration. Gastric decompression should be performed early in children to minimise the effects of abdominal splinting on ventilation. Concurrent hypothermia is not uncommon and should be treated aggressively.[15]

There is a high incidence of injury associated with immersion, so a full secondary survey is essential (Chapter 42). Check glucose levels in all patients, particularly children and the hypothermic. Laboratory studies should include creatine kinase (CK) because of the reported risk of rhabdomyolysis. Blood alcohol level and urine drug screen should be considered where the cause of submersion is questioned. Depending on the events surrounding the submersion incident, haemoglobin (Hb), myoglobin and electrolyte levels may be useful investigations (Table 28.7).[6,7,15,18] Stroke, seizures, cardiac events, asthma and marine envenomation should be considered as precipitating events.

Primary complications are pulmonary, cerebral and cardiovascular, including pulmonary oedema, pneumonitis, ARDS, encephalopathy and cardiopulmonary arrest. Later complications are related to poor circulation and include cerebral oedema, DIC and renal failure.

Immersion pulmonary oedema (IPE) can complicate immersion and lead to drowning. IPE is known to occur in fit swimmers and divers and is believed to develop due to hydrostatic pressure contributing to an increased central blood volume. This in combination with cold-induced vasoconstriction, breathing against a negative pressure (snorkel or diving regulator) and exertion can lead to an increased pressure gradient between pulmonary capillaries and alveoli causing pulmonary oedema.[18] IPE is often of short duration, resolving within 24 to 48 hours after surfacing or exiting the water, but can also lead to hypoxia, unconsciousness and drowning.

TABLE 28.6 MODELL/CONN CLASSIFICATION OF MENTAL STATUS FOLLOWING DROWNING[18]

GRADE	DESCRIPTION OF MENTAL STATUS	EQUIVALENT GLASGOW COMA SCALE (GCS) SCORE	EXPECTED LIKELIHOOD OF GOOD OUTCOME (NEUROLOGICALLY INTACT) (%)
A	Awake/alert	14–15	100
B	Blunted	8–13	100
C	Comatose	6–7	> 90
C1	Decerebrate	5	> 90
C2	Decorticate	4	> 90
C3/4	Flaccid coma or arrest	3	< 20

TABLE 28.7 EMERGENCY MANAGEMENT OF SUBMERSION INJURIES[7]

AETIOLOGY	ASSESSMENT FINDINGS	INTERVENTIONS
Inability to swim or exhaustion while swimming	**Pulmonary** Ineffective breathing	**Initial** Manage and maintain ABCs
Entrapment or entanglement with objects in water	Dyspnoea	Assume cervical spine injury in all drowning victims and stabilise and/or immobilise cervical spine
Loss of ability to move secondary to trauma, stroke, hypothermia, acute myocardial infarction	Respiratory distress	Provide 100% oxygen via non-rebreather mask or BVM
Poor judgement due to alcohol or drugs	Crackles	Anticipate need for intubation
Seizure while in water	A cough with frothy pink sputum	Establish IV access with two large-bore cannulas for fluid resuscitation and cautiously infuse warmed fluids if appropriate (avoiding fluid overload)
	Cyanosis	Assess for other injuries
	Respiratory arrest	Remove wet clothing and cover patient with warm blankets
	Cardiac Tachycardia	Obtain temperature and begin re-warming if needed
	Bradycardia	Obtain chest x-ray and CT imaging (x-ray or CT)
	Dysrhythmia	Insert gastric tube
	Hypotension	**Ongoing monitoring** Monitor ABCs, vital signs, level of consciousness
	Cardiac arrest	Monitor oxygen saturation, cardiac rhythm
	Other Panic	Monitor temperature and maintain normothermia
	Exhaustion	Monitor for signs of acute respiratory failure
	Coma	
	Co-existing illness (e.g. acute MI) or injury (e.g. cervical spine injury)	
	Core temperature slightly elevated or below normal depending on water temperature and length of submersion	

ABCs: airway, breathing, circulation; BVM: bag–valve–mask; IV: intravenous.

ATMOSPHERIC-PRESSURE-RELATED EMERGENCIES

ANATOMY AND PHYSIOLOGY

Atmospheric pressure is the pressure of atmospheric gas and water, at any given altitude or depth. *Barometric pressure* is pressure (weight of air) exerted by the atmosphere against an object or human. At sea level, the human body is at zero on the atmospheric pressure scale and 760 mmHg barometric pressure.

Atmospheric pressure drops with the rise to a higher altitude, as the air becomes less dense and drier.[19] Conversely, with a descent to depth, pressure rises because the total pressure is a combination of both water and air. With every metre of descent, water exerts approximately 70 mmHg of pressure on the diver, which equates to exerting 1 atmosphere of pressure (700 mmHg) for every 10 m of descent.[20] The pressure changes on the diver are far greater and more significant with smaller distance changes than with altitude. For example, where a mountain climber needs to ascend to 5486 m (18,000 ft) to reduce atmospheric pressure by 50%, a diver needs to descend only 10 m (33 ft) to increase total pressure by 50%. Further, atmospheric pressure will vary with weather patterns and seasonal fluctuations.

Understanding the effects of pressure on the body requires an appreciation of several laws of physics and a few concepts. The human body and the environment are made of substances that are solid, liquid or gas. These substances are affected to varying degrees by pressure and temperature.

- Depending on its consistency, a solid experiences almost no change in the presence of either pressure or temperature.
- A liquid, while unaffected by pressure, will expand or contract with temperature. Pascal's law states that a pressure applied to a liquid will be transmitted equally throughout the liquid.
- Gas volumes experience the greatest changes in the presence of both pressure and temperature. As the majority of the human body is water, only the air-filled cavities demonstrate the effects of changes in pressure. Atmospheric pressure changes are greatest near sea level. A change of 1 atmosphere in water (10 m) will halve a gas volume on the descent and double a gas volume on the ascent.

PRACTICE TIP

The greatest changes in pressure and therefore the greatest risk for pressure-related trauma (barotrauma) occur during the last 10 m of ascent from depth. This is one of the most significant laws in respect to diving-related illness.

For example, if a diver with a residual volume of 1200 mL at the surface holds their breath and descends 10 m, they will end up with a residual volume of 600 mL. However, divers continually breathe compressed air, allowing their lungs to operate at normal volumes and thus maintaining normal lung capacity at all times. This works as long as they continuously breathe in and out during the dive. On ascent, a failure to exhale will result in a doubling of lung volume with every 10 m rise. If they start with a total lung capacity of 5000 mL at 30 m depth and rise without exhaling, they will have a total volume of 10,000 mL at 10 m and 20,000 mL at the surface. This will produce significant barotrauma and has been responsible for diver mortality.

The rate of change in the pressure–volume relationship described by Boyle (Chapter 15), relies on a constant temperature. However, temperature variations occur at both depth and altitude. For example, for every 300 m rise in altitude, the temperature drops 2°C. The effect of temperature on both the pressure and the volume of a gas is described by Charles's Law, which states that a change in temperature will result in a directly proportional change in volume and therefore gas pressure. Thus, as temperature rises, gas volume and, subsequently, pressure increase. The opposite is true with a drop in temperature. Equally, increasing a gas volume will result in an increase in temperature.

Every gas, based on its volume and consistency, will exert a pressure on the environment it is in. The pressure it exerts is known as *partial pressure*. Thus, as described by Dalton, the total pressure exerted by a mixture of gases is equal to the sum of the partial pressures of each gas in the mix. For example, atmospheric total pressure is 760 mmHg and is made up of approximately 21% oxygen (158 mmHg), 0.3% carbon dioxide (0.4 mmHg), 78% nitrogen (596 mmHg) and 0.7% water (5.7 mmHg). During an ascent to higher altitude, atmospheric pressure drops and thus the partial pressure of each gas in the mix drops. This means that while oxygen remains at 21% at higher altitudes, it has a lower partial pressure than at sea level.

Henry's Law refers to the dissolution of a gas in a liquid. At a given temperature, there is a directly proportional relationship between the partial pressure of a gas and how much of the gas will dissolve in a liquid. At higher pressures, more gas will dissolve in a liquid. This explains the accumulation of nitrogen in tissues and blood, increasing with depth and length of a dive. Ascent to lower atmospheric pressure will result in the gas dissolving out of the liquid. With a controlled, carefully timed ascent, this allows for dissolved gas to be exhaled via the lungs. However, if the ascent is rapid, nitrogen will expand in the blood or tissues forming bubbles and potentially block the microcirculation.

Moderate (intermediate) altitude is defined as between 1528 m and 2438 m (5000–8000 ft).[21] At these heights, exercise tolerance drops and minute ventilation rises. Part of the world's population live at high altitude (above 2438 m). Those populations are largely not at risk of altitude-related emergencies as they have adapted to their environment. Physiological adaptations (*acclimatisation*) to altitude include a relatively rapid increase in minute volume (MV) (hyperventilation), resulting in a decrease in $PaCO_2$ and a subsequent increase in PaO_2. Over days to months, changes occur with a reduction in total body water, bicarbonate concentration, haematocrit and haemoglobin. Cardiovascular compensation for maintaining near-normal oxygen delivery to the tissues includes initial tachycardia, elevated blood pressure and peripheral vasoconstriction; eventually returning to near-sea-level resting heart rate and blood pressure.[2,22] Extremely high altitudes occur above 5800 m (18,000 ft), and acclimatisation above this is not possible because of progressive physiological deterioration associated with chronic, profound hypoxia.

Rapid ascent has been enhanced by the advent of air and car travel and improved mountaineering equipment. Most significant altitude illness occurs above 3000 m (10,000 ft), with pathophysiological effects being noted once arterial oxygen saturation drops below 90%, causing hypoxia, hypoxaemia and subsequent pathophysiological changes such as oedema.[22] The shape of the oxygen–haemoglobin dissociation curve prevents significant desaturation until approximately 3658 m (12,000 ft), when desaturation occurs rapidly with small increases in altitude. The development of hypoxia is influenced by altitude, the rate of ascent, duration at altitude, individual tolerance and physical fitness, exercise at altitude, environmental temperatures and the use of medications or toxic substances.[2,22] Prevention of altitude illness focuses on controlling the rate of ascent, with the altitude at which someone is able to sleep (*sleeping altitude*) being the most important indicator of safe altitude. Altitude illness syndromes are a result of oedema formation initiated by the pathophysiological changes secondary to decreased PaO_2.

ALTITUDE EMERGENCIES

Acute mountain sickness

A relatively benign, self-limiting illness, acute mountain sickness (AMS) usually develops over several hours after ascent to critical altitude. *Critical altitude* is the point at which an individual can no longer maintain normal gas exchange, leading to hypoxia. In most people, this occurs around 2438 m (8000 ft). Underlying respiratory disease and anaemia will predispose a person to AMS. The primary signs and symptoms of AMS, as defined by the Lake Louise consensus criteria, are a headache and at least one of the following: anorexia, nausea, vomiting, fatigue, dizziness and insomnia in the setting of moderate-to-high altitude.[2,22]

PRACTICE TIP

Treatment for all cases of AMS is to cease ascent and reduce altitude if symptoms persist or worsen, or if there are pulmonary or cerebral signs. A descent of 500–1000 m is usually adequate to reverse symptoms.[2,22]

For mild cases, rest and increased fluid intake are usually adequate, allowing time for acclimatisation. Symptomatic treatment of headaches (anti-inflammatories, paracetamol) and nausea (antiemetics) is useful. For moderate or severe cases, acetazolamide is indicated,[2,22] as it aids the normal process of ventilatory acclimatisation by stimulating breathing, particularly during sleep when hypoxaemia is maximal; it helps to maintain cerebral blood flow despite hypocapnia and opposes fluid retention associated with AMS. Supplemental oxygen may be beneficial and immediate descent for severe or persistently moderate cases is required. Dexamethasone may have a benefit in severe cases, as it improves oxygen saturation and provides symptomatic relief.[2,22] Untreated and ignored, AMS can potentially lead to high-altitude cerebral oedema (HACE) or high-altitude pulmonary oedema (HAPE).

High-altitude cerebral oedema

High-altitude cerebral oedema (HACE) is a life-threatening condition developing over several days of exposure to critical altitude (usually above 3658 m (12,000 ft)) or following rapid ascent. As HACE is considered to be the end stage of AMS, clinically, the prevention and treatment for both are on a continuum.[2,22] HACE develops as hypoxaemia leads to cerebral hypoxia, increasing blood–brain barrier permeability, increasing cerebral blood flow, producing cerebral oedema and increasing intracranial pressure. Primary signs and symptoms may initially appear as severe AMS; however, severe headaches will remain unrelieved by analgesia.[2,22] Additional symptoms are likely to develop, with ataxia occurring early, followed by nausea and vomiting, altered mental state, seizures and unconsciousness.[2,22] Treatment for all cases is immediate descent, oxygen therapy, dexamethasone, rest, symptomatic treatment and, if available, hyperbaric therapy.

High-altitude pulmonary oedema

High-altitude pulmonary oedema (HAPE) is a life-threatening condition developing over several days of exposure to critical altitude or with very rapid ascent. Hypoxaemia leads to fluid retention, increased pulmonary blood volume, pulmonary artery hypertension and peripheral vasoconstriction secondary to cerebral hypoxia. The primary signs and symptoms are shortness of breath at rest, tachypnoea (worse at night), an initial dry cough which becomes moist, fatigue, rales and tachycardia.[2,22]

PRACTICE TIP

As with HACE, treatment for all cases of HAPE is to cease ascent and descend immediately and administer oxygen if available.

Mild cases of HAPE usually respond to rest, while moderate cases require supplemental oxygen. Oxygen provides excellent results in alleviating HAPE, although it may be required for more than 36 hours, so while it is recommended, oxygen is titrated to a SpO_2 of 90%; it is more critical in the field to conserve oxygen supplies for the duration of treatment.[1] Severe cases may require nifedipine, which lowers pulmonary artery pressure, assisting in the progressive clearing of alveolar oedema, and hyperbaric oxygen. The decision to administer nifedipine should take into account the risk of hypotension and concurrent HACE, as nifedipine may reduce cerebral perfusion and adversely impact cerebral oedema.

DIVING EMERGENCIES

The type of diving discussed in this section mainly refers to self-contained underwater breathing apparatus (SCUBA) diving, including the use of closed and open circuit systems which are used to deliver air, or other gas mixtures which allow divers to breathe at depth. Free-diving refers to breath-hold diving and, although some physiological effects are similar, it is important to distinguish between these two disciplines. SCUBA diving is pursued in a variety of aquatic environments, including caves, lakes, oceans and rivers.

Diving is central to tourism in many parts of Australia and Aotearoa New Zealand, to commercial fishing interests and military endeavours. An increase in the availability and affordability of diving equipment and training has increased the risk of diving-related accidents occurring. Accidents may occur due to a combination of human error, unexpected events and the increased risks associated with undertaking deep and technical dives. While the greatest physiological risk for divers is from changes in pressure (*dysbarism*), diving injuries are commonly associated with environmental exposure, aquatic hazards and interactions with marine wildlife. The diving-related injuries discussed in this section focus on those associated with pressure and gas exchange, including squeeze, barotrauma, nitrogen narcosis and decompression illness.

SQUEEZE

A 'squeeze' occurs during diving when the air is trapped on descent. The ears, sinuses, lungs, gastrointestinal tract, teeth and additional airspace, such as the face mask, are all potential areas for a squeeze to occur. During descent, external pressure exceeds the pressure inside air-filled cavities in the body. To avoid a squeeze, it is important that divers equalise their eustachian tubes and breathe slowly and regularly. Symptoms and signs include pain in the affected cavity, oedema, capillary rupture and bleeding. Treatment is to ascend until the pain is alleviated. A diver may then attempt to descend again or ascend completely for further treatment. Therapy is symptomatic and includes decongestants and NSAID analgesia. Antibiotics may be required in the presence of tympanic membrane (TM) rupture.[21] Prevention includes not diving with an upper respiratory tract infection, and it is not recommended to use decongestants prior to diving. A mask squeeze can be relieved by breathing out a small amount of air from the nose into the mask.

Barotrauma

Barotrauma refers to injuries produced as a result of volume increases in air-filled cavities expanding on ascent. Therefore, any gas-filled cavity susceptible to a squeeze is susceptible to barotrauma. Barotrauma is avoidable under normal diving conditions and occurs when trapped, expanding air or gas cannot equalise with the surrounding environment. To avoid pulmonary barotrauma, two fundamental rules of SCUBA diving are to ascend slowly and to breathe continually throughout ascent. If these rules are not adhered to, such as during an emergency ascent, severe barotrauma may occur as expanding air within the alveoli causes local tissue damage and rupture.[21] The most common causes of pulmonary barotrauma are panic, running out of air and buoyancy problems.

Patient assessment and clinical interventions

Barosinusitis is pain in the ethmoid, frontal or maxillary sinuses due to air entrapment during ascent or descent. It may be associated with epistaxis and is essentially self-limiting. Decongestants and antihistamines have proven useful, and antibiotics are only required if evidence of infection exists.[21] *Barodentalgia* is the pain associated with air trapped in a poorly filled dental cavity. The condition will self-limit and only requires analgesia until the pain subsides.

A failure to equalise the *middle ear* during ascent will produce the opposite of a squeeze. This usually only occurs when the diver has a pre-existing infection or inflammation of the middle ear or eustachian tubes. The initial symptom will be sudden acute pain, progressing to tympanic membrane (TM) rupture if the diver continues to ascend and fails to equalise. If the TM ruptures, the middle ear is exposed to cold water, producing a caloric response with subsequent nystagmus, vertigo, nausea and vomiting. Treatment is symptomatic.

Inner ear barotrauma involves injury to the cochleovestibular apparatus and, while less common than barotrauma of the middle ear, is associated with a greater level of morbidity. Initially, there is a failure to equalise, with increasing middle-ear pressure. The pressure is transferred via the ossicles to the oval window, where a pressure wave is created in the perilymph of the cochlea. This produces outward distension of the round window. If there is a sudden equalising of pressure or a harsh Valsalva, the round window may rupture. Clinically the patient will present with severe nystagmus, positional vertigo, ataxia and vomiting. The patient may have associated hearing loss or tinnitus. History and examination are primary in the initial diagnosis. Treatment is symptomatic, and referral to ENT is necessary.

Pulmonary barotrauma involves a number of conditions caused by expansion of gas on ascent, or occasionally by volume reduction on descent. The traditional term 'pulmonary over-pressurisation syndrome' (POPS) is now considered inadequate to describe the causes of pulmonary barotrauma. Pulmonary volume increases can be prevented as long as the diver exhales continuously on ascent to the surface. Respiratory illness predisposes to barotrauma. The clinical conditions associated with pulmonary barotrauma include pneumothorax, pneumomediastinum and arterial gas embolism (AGE). Pulmonary signs may include subcutaneous emphysema, mild substernal chest pain and shortness of breath. A chest x-ray will reveal a pneumothorax, pneumomediastinum or pneumopericardium.[21] Clinical assessment, signs and symptoms, mechanism of injury and dive profile should be used when in the field. Where any of these conditions are present, the patient should be assessed for neurological signs indicating AGE (discussed later). Interstitial emphysema without a pneumothorax will usually resolve without treatment. See Chapter 45 for assessment and management of pneumothorax. If non-invasive ventilation or intubation is required, the ventilation strategy and settings should be carefully considered. High pressures should be avoided as they may aggravate barotrauma.

NITROGEN NARCOSIS

In the words of Jacques Cousteau, nitrogen narcosis can be described as 'rapture of the deep', producing a euphoric state in which the diver becomes unaware of their condition and the need to surface. Nitrogen narcosis is the term describing the neurodepressant effect of high levels of nitrogen on the human body.[21] This effect varies in individuals, with some divers having a far greater tolerance to the effects of nitrogen. While nitrogen narcosis does not directly result in death, it can contribute significantly to death or diving injury by directly impairing a diver's judgement.

When SCUBA diving using compressed air, the gas inhaled is the same composition of atmospheric air and includes approximately 79% nitrogen. As depth increases during a dive, the volume of air within a dive tank decreases due to increased pressure, while the density and partial pressure of the air within the tank increases. The partial pressure of the individual components of air also increases, and therefore a diver at depth breathes and absorbs a greater concentration of nitrogen.

Symptoms and signs begin to appear at depths around 30 m (100 ft) or deeper and resolve with the ascent. Initially, the diver may feel euphoric and exhibit impaired judgement. Motor responses may slow, and proprioception may become lost. Below 60 m (200 ft) the diver may be unable to undertake fine and gross motor tasks, and unconsciousness can occur at approximately 90 m (300 ft). Prevention can be achieved by limiting dive depth and frequency over a given period and allowing adequate surface intervals between dives to enable off-gassing.

DECOMPRESSION ILLNESS

Injury mechanism

Decompression illness (DCI) is the current term that describes injury resulting from gas release and bubble formation as a result of diving using compressed gas.[20,21] Previously, diving incidents were divided into *decompression sickness* (DCS), a result of nitrogen bubbles, and *arterial gas embolism* (AGE), a result of pulmonary barotrauma releasing air into the circulation. The current understanding of DCI encompasses both DCS and AGE, recognising that while their aetiology differs, they are difficult to distinguish clinically and their initial management, prior to recompression, is identical.

Arterial gas embolism

Arterial gas embolism is second only to drowning as the cause of death among divers and has a mortality rate of 5% in divers who reach a compression chamber alive.[20,21] AGE occurs during ascent, due to gas expansion and increasing lung volume. If a diver fails to exhale during ascent, air is unable to escape the lungs, resulting in increased pressure and alveolar rupture. Micro-bubbles may then enter the circulatory system, migrating via the heart to the arterial system to produce AGE. Clinical signs of AGE are related to vascular obstruction by gas emboli. AGE most commonly appears within seconds to 10 minutes of ascent and alveolar rupture. Rarely, AGE can occur when a patent foramen ovale ruptures during diving, as a result of changes in the normal cardiac gradient from left to right.

PRACTICE TIP

Symptoms of arterial gas embolism (AGE) almost always begin within 10 minutes of surfacing and are primarily neurological in nature.

Cerebral emboli signs include vertigo, headache, visual changes, cranial nerve palsies, asymmetric multiplegia, confusion, seizures and loss of consciousness.[21] Coronary artery emboli may present as an acute myocardial infarction, dysrhythmia or cardiovascular collapse. Emboli may be widespread and cause shortness of breath or interruption to the vascular flow to the spinal cord, leading to spinal cord injury.

Decompression sickness

Known as 'the bends', and originally called *Caisson's disease*, the risk of developing decompression sickness (DCS) increases with the number, duration and depth of sequential dives. DCS occurs when the nitrogen absorbed into the body's tissues during a dive (as a result of pressure changes, Henry's Law) has inadequate time to slowly diffuse from the tissues back to the bloodstream and be eliminated by the lungs. During a rapid or uncontrolled ascent, gas expansion leads to the formation of nitrogen bubbles in the tissue, blood or lymphatic system. These nitrogen bubbles may then impair tissue perfusion and obstruct blood flow in the arterial system. Any organ in the body may be affected.

Symptoms of DCS usually begin within 6 hours of ascent and may be delayed for up to 36 hours.[21] Onset of symptoms within 10 minutes may suggest AGE; however, some individuals (30%) will exhibit symptoms before or on surfacing.[21] Obstruction of lymphatic tissue produces oedema, cellular distension and membrane rupture. Ischaemia in the pulmonary vasculature leads to dyspnoea, pleuritic chest pain, pulmonary oedema, cough or haemoptysis (the 'chokes'). Neurological symptoms include headache, fatigue, dizziness, paraesthesia, unconsciousness and seizures. Joint pain is a classic sign and, because of its tendency to reduce joint movement, gave rise to the name 'the bends'.

PRACTICE TIP

Joint pain can occur at depths less than 10 m (33 ft), and any joint pain within 24–48 hours of a dive should be treated as DCS.

The upper extremities are more susceptible than the legs, and signs, such as a rash, may occur due to the formation of cutaneous micro-bubbles. Spinal cord involvement occurs in up to 60% of DCS cases, often due to venous infarction of the cord, obstruction of the epidural vertebral venous plexus, inflammation or bubble emboli.[21] For this reason, back pain occurring within 24 hours of a dive should be evaluated for DCS. Diagnosis is primarily based on history and clinical findings, and it is important to recognise that DCS may exist simultaneously with AGE or barotrauma.

Patient assessment and clinical interventions

The diagnosis of DCI, encompassing DCS and AGE, is made on history and examination. The dive profile and history are particularly important, and the patient's dive computer will provide essential information about the number of dives, the depth, duration and surface interval between dives. Cold water, older age, fatigue, peripheral vascular disease, heavy work during or immediately after diving, multiple ascents, uncontrolled ascents and poor physical fitness aggravate the severity of DCI. Obesity lengthens the time during which the diver is at risk of DCI, as nitrogen is slowly absorbed and slowly released.[21] In addition to the physical fitness required to undertake diving, a degree of emotional and intellectual capacity is required to remain calm in a crisis, to understand and apply multiple rules and technological requirements associated with managing the risks associated with diving.

Full assessment should include vital signs, blood glucose levels, oxygen saturations and an ECG. One hundred per cent oxygen therapy should be applied to aid oxygenation and increase excretion of nitrogen by increasing the concentration gradient and rate of diffusion of nitrogen across the respiratory membrane. If intubation is required, the cuff should be inflated with saline rather than air, to avoid a change in volume on recompression. The patient should be left supine or in the left lateral position and should not be allowed to sit or stand, to prevent gas bubbles redistributing from the left ventricle to the brain[21]. A full blood count is useful, as intravascular fluid depletion is common and haemoconcentration may be affected. A chest x-ray is indicated if pulmonary barotrauma is suspected.

Intravenous crystalloids should be commenced and titrated in response to acute presentations. Importantly, note that fluid loading will affect microcirculation and may potentiate damage to the vascular endothelium, in combination with the effect of bubbles. Glucose-containing fluids may exacerbate CNS injury. Hypothermia should be corrected.

PRACTICE TIP

Definitive treatment for DCI is recompression and should be sought as soon as possible.[20] Patients retrieved by air should be flown in a pressurised aircraft (fixed-wing) and at the lowest safe altitude (rotary-wing). Awareness of changes in elevation, such as driving over mountainous terrain, is also important if retrieved by road.

Hyperbaric oxygen therapy reduces bubble size and aids diffusion of nitrogen. This then reduces obstruction and inflammation, and relieves ischaemia and hypoxia.[21] If air transport is the best option for timely patient transfer, every attempt should be made to avoid altitudes exceeding 100 m (300 ft). The higher the aircraft flies, the more the change in pressure will adversely affect the patient. Flying after diving can precipitate DCI. Even if there are no bubbles at the end of the dive, excess nitrogen will still be in the tissues waiting to be diffused and exhaled. Altitude can produce bubbles or enlarge existing asymptomatic ones. Current guidelines advise against flying for 12 hours after a single short dive, and 24 hours after multiple and decompression dives.[21] It is recommended that further diving is not done within 4 weeks of DCI symptom resolution. Twenty-four-hour assistance is available through the Divers Emergency Service 1800 088 200 (Australia), or 0800 4 DES 111 or 0800 4 337 111 (Aotearoa New Zealand).

ENVENOMATIONS

A standardised approach to envenomation, with appropriate first aid, clinical and laboratory evaluation, administration of antivenom and good supportive care, ensures a good outcome in most cases. Early discussion with a regional Poisons Information

Centre (Australia: phone 13 11 26 or Aotearoa New Zealand: 0800 POISON/0800 764 766) is beneficial. These centres provide expert advice in the management of envenomation syndromes. Venom is the poisonous secretion of an animal (snake, spider, scorpion or jellyfish), and is usually delivered by a bite or sting. The effects of toxins that are secreted by animals and cause poisoning once ingested (e.g. tetrodotoxin from puffer fish or bufotenine from cane toads) are managed in a similar manner to any toxic ingestions (see Chapter 30 Toxicology).

Venom is a complex, multicomponent substance containing various enzymes and toxins. Envenomation by terrestrial or marine animals in Australia can result in local and/or systemic effects:

1. Local effects
   Bites by brown, tiger, taipan or sea snakes have minimal or no symptoms at the bite site, while bites by black snake or death adder are associated with significant pain, tissue swelling and bruising (see Figs 28.4 and 28.5). Bites by Australian scorpions can be extremely painful, but rarely associated with systemic symptoms.
   Stepping on a stonefish often results in severe pain that can last for several hours, and spine fragments can also remain in the wound, causing ongoing foreign body reaction. Bluebottle and box jellyfish stings are associated with erythematous and painful welts (see Figs 28.6 and 28.7). Spider bites are usually painful. Redback spider bites can have delayed worsening of initial mild pain that can be distant to the bite site as well. Fang marks can often be seen after bites by funnel-web spiders.
2. Coagulopathy
   - Procoagulant agglutinins can cause a severe venom-induced consumptive coagulopathy (VICC), due to prothrombin activation and fibrinogen consumption (defibrination). This is a feature of the brown, taipan and tiger snake envenoming and is characterised by:
     - elevated activated partial thromboplastin time (aPTT) and international normalised ratio (INR) (usually unrecordable)
     - low fibrinogen (often undetectable)
     - elevated D-dimer (more than 10 times the upper limit of normal). Anticoagulant toxins cause a less severe coagulopathy, associated with mildly elevated aPTT and INR, but normal fibrinogen and D-dimer. In Australia, only black snakes cause anticoagulant coagulopathy.
3. Neurotoxicity
   - Australian snake venoms contain a mixture of presynaptic and postsynaptic neurotoxins. Presynaptic toxins inhibit

FIGURE 28.4 DEATH ADDER BITE[23]

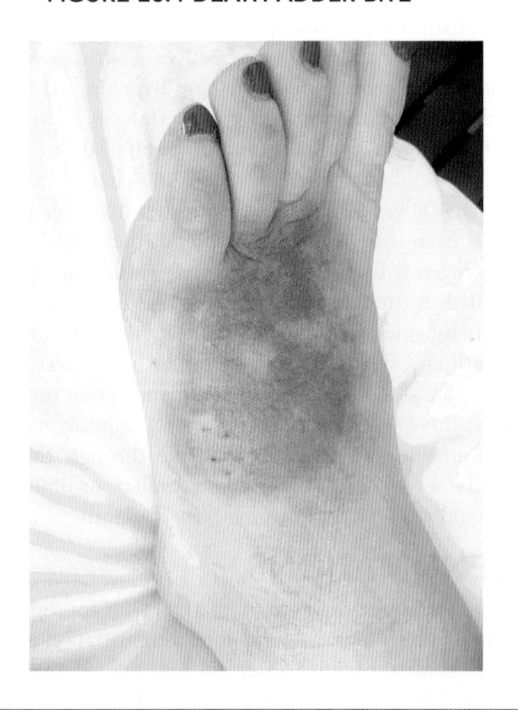

FIGURE 28.5 BLACK SNAKE BITE

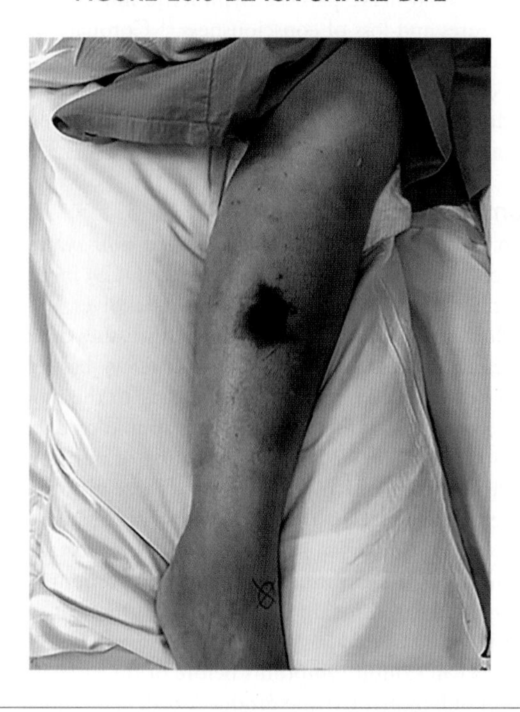

Dr Alan Gault

FIGURE 28.6 LINEAR WELTS CAUSED BY BLUEBOTTLE JELLYFISH STING[24]

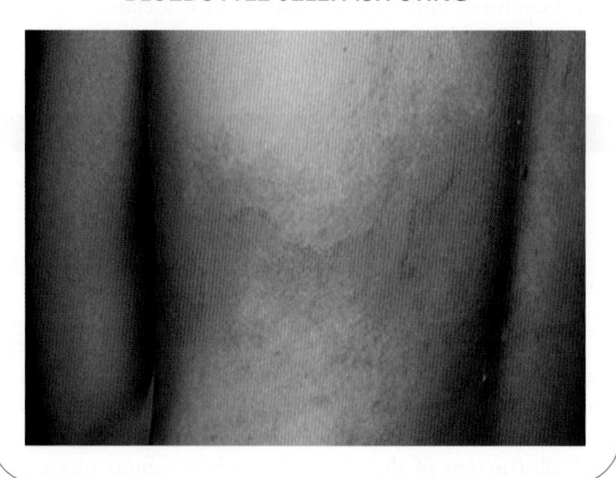

FIGURE 28.7

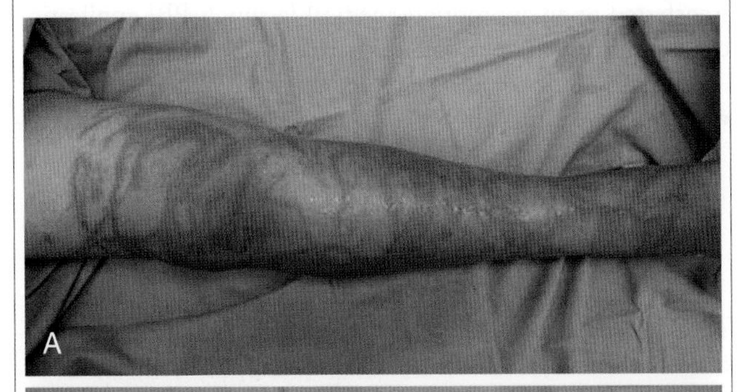

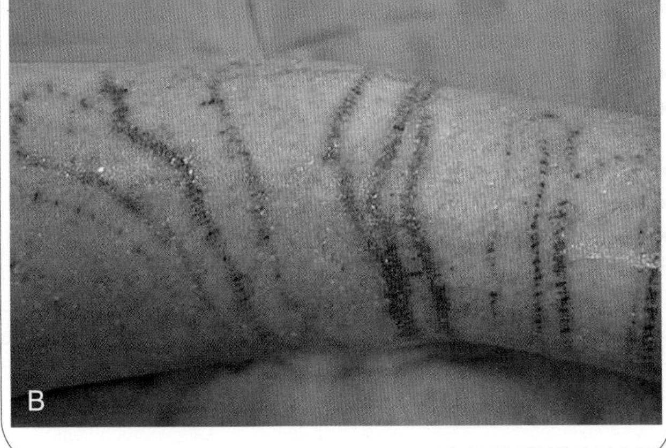

A. and **B.** Crosshatched linear welts caused by box jellyfish sting.[25]

acetylcholine release, while postsynaptic activity inhibits neuromuscular activation, resulting in a progressive, symmetrical, descending paralysis that can be seen with tiger, taipan, death adder and sea snake envenomations. The first signs of paralysis are usually evident in the small, ocular muscles (diplopia, ptosis, gaze palsies) and can progress to respiratory failure.
- Anosmia is a type of neurotoxicity that can occur after black snake envenomations.
- Tetrodotoxin is a neurotoxin that binds to sodium channels and inhibits the generation and propagation of action potentials resulting in a rapid, descending, symmetrical paralysis that can result in respiratory failure and hypoxic cardiac arrest. Paralysis secondary to tetrodotoxin may result from pufferfish ingestion or blue-ringed octopus envenoming. A similar type of paralysis can occur secondary to conotoxins from cone-shell envenomations.
- Presynaptic stimulation of catecholamine release due to envenoming by a funnel-web spider or Irukandji syndrome causes symptoms of sympathetic hyperstimulation, manifesting as hypertension, tachycardia or pulmonary oedema. Fasciculations, oral paraesthesia and muscle spasms can also occur.
- Redback spider venom stimulates acetylcholine and catecholamine release, resulting in a constellation of symptoms known as 'lactrodectism'.

4. Myopathy
   - Myotoxins are commonly found in Australian snake venom and cause significant muscle pain and rhabdomyolysis. Envenomations by all snake groups except brown (i.e. black, tiger, taipan, death adder, sea snakes) can cause rhabdomyolysis, which is often delayed in onset. It can be particularly severe following black snake envenomations.
5. Other effects related to venom are rare but can include:
   - cardiac arrest
   - collapse
   - seizures
   - non-specific symptoms, such as a headache, nausea and vomiting, haemolytic anaemia, thrombotic microangiopathy (TMA) and nephrotoxicity.

ANTIVENOM

Antivenoms are purified IgG antibodies against venom components which are produced by animals to injected venoms. A range of antivenoms for the treatment of snake, spider and marine envenomations are available.[26]

The decision to use antivenom is made once objective evidence of envenoming is obtained. All snake antivenom is administered intravenously, diluted in 500 mL of normal saline (20 mL/kg for children) and infused over 20 minutes. In cardiac arrest, antivenom may be given as undiluted intravenous (IV) bolus and may be lifesaving. Severe allergic reactions to these products are rare but can occur,[27] so they should always be given in an environment where full resuscitation facilities are available. Premedication with adrenaline, steroids or antihistamines to prevent anaphylactic reactions is not routinely indicated.

The dose of antivenom is the same in children as in adults (the amount of fluid for dilution differs) and it can be administered to pregnant women.[26,28]

SNAKE BITE

OVERVIEW

Definite or suspected snake bite is a common emergency presentation throughout Australia. Until envenoming is excluded, all suspected snake-bite patients should initially be assessed and managed in an area equipped for cardiorespiratory monitoring and resuscitation.[29] Snake bite is a time-critical emergency presentation, and a simple, standardised approach is required to diagnose envenomation and provide adequate treatment if it occurs (see Box 28.3, Table 28.8).

There are more than 70 venomous snake species in Australia, but the clinical envenomation syndromes can be grouped in six categories (tiger, brown, black, taipan, death adder and sea snake) and there are corresponding available antivenoms. See Table 28.9 for the clinical features of snake envenomation across the six categories. Early discussion with a regional Poisons Information Centre is extremely useful to aid in clinical management decisions. Although severe envenoming is rare, it is potentially lethal.[30] Any patient bitten by a snake, whether suspected or confirmed, should be considered for enrolment in the Australian Snakebite Project (see Useful websites at the end of the chapter).

FIRST AID

Most patients with a history of possible bite do not require immediate resuscitation. However, if resuscitation is required, it takes precedence over application of pressure bandage.

The use of a pressure bandage with immobilisation (PBI) is the standard first-aid treatment. It is indicated for bites by all

BOX 28.3 APPROACH TO SNAKE BITE

OUT-OF-HOSPITAL

1. First aid: pressure bandage with immobilisation
2. Consider taking antivenom to patient (in case they have a cardiac arrest) if responding to a remote location and if pre-hospital administration of antivenom is permitted (with medical advice). If antivenom is administered pre-hospital the paramedic(s) looking after the patient should watch for signs of and be prepared to treat anaphylaxis.
3. Transport: the patient should be transported as soon as possible to a hospital that meets all of the following criteria:
   a) doctor(s) able to manage snake bite
   b) laboratory capable of performing necessary investigations on a 24-hour basis
   c) adequate stock of antivenom to provide definitive treatment.

HOSPITAL

1. Resuscitation
2. Risk assessment: once snake bite is suspected, all patients should be considered potentially envenomed until proven otherwise. Serial regular assessment and observation over a period of at least 12 hours:
   a) history
   b) serial physical examination
   c) serial laboratory investigations.
3. If envenomation is confirmed, determine the type of monovalent antivenom required based on:
   a) geographical area (prevalent indigenous snakes)
   b) clinical and laboratory features.
4. Administer 1 ampoule of monovalent antivenom required to definitively treat the envenoming.
5. Provide adjuvant and supportive treatment.

Australian snake species, as well as bites from funnel-web spiders, blue-ringed octopuses and cone snails. It is not advocated for bites from other spiders or marine animals.

The PBI compresses the lymphatic vessels and inhibits limb muscle movement, thus retarding venom transport and preventing the venom from entering the systemic circulation.[31,32] It is not definitive medical treatment, but, when applied correctly, may prevent significant systemic symptoms while the patient is transferred to an appropriate medical facility.[32] PBI application can be difficult to optimise and is often performed poorly.

The principles of adequate PBI application are:

- Use a firm ~ 15 cm broad bandage (preferably elasticised—not crepe bandage) directly over the bite site and extend proximally to cover the whole of the affected limb. Then apply a further pressure bandage, commencing at the fingers or toes of the bitten limb and extending upwards covering as much of the limb as possible.

There are specific snake-bite bandages available, which have indicators indicating when correct tension is applied (see Fig. 28.8).

- Use firm pressure to occlude lymphatic flow but preserve blood flow—as for supporting a sprained ankle.
- Check for the distal pulses to ensure adequate blood flow.
- Include fingers and toes in the bandage to reduce limb movement.
- Splint the limb to further restrict movement.
- Immobilise the limb and the patient.
- Do not elevate the limb (as you might for a fracture).[31,32]

See Fig. 28.9 for a pictorial representation on applying PBI. Bites to body parts other than a limb pose a difficult problem as pressure dressings cannot be applied. Efforts should be made to completely immobilise the patient while transportation to a hospital is organised.

RESUSCITATION

Pre-hospital resuscitation should occur following standard BLS/ACLS algorithms. If the patient is in a setting where there is antivenom available, this should be administered as a rapid IV push as part of the resuscitation efforts.

Potential early life threats associated with Australian snake envenoming include:

- cardiac arrest
- syncope (brown snake, tiger snake, taipan)
- hypotension (brown snake, tiger snake, taipan)
- respiratory failure secondary to paralysis (taipan, tiger snake, death adder, sea snake)
- seizures (brown snake, tiger snake, taipan)
- severe coagulopathy with uncontrolled haemorrhage (brown snake, tiger snake, taipan).

TABLE 28.8 ASSESSMENT OF SNAKE BITE[28]

HISTORY	PHYSICAL EXAMINATION	LABORATORY INVESTIGATIONS
Geographical area where bite occurred	Vital signs	Full blood count (FBC)
Time of bite	Mental status	Renal function (U&Es)
Anatomical site of bite	Respiratory function (PEFR/FEV1)	Creatine kinase (CK)
Number of strikes	Aspect of bite site	Coagulation profile (aPTT, INR, fibrinogen, D-dimer)
Use of first aid (PBI)	Lymphadenopathy	Urinalysis for blood/myoglobin
Symptoms such as collapse, nausea, vomiting, bleeding and weakness	Abnormal bleeding (gums, IV cannula sites)	
	Descending symmetrical flaccid paralysis	

aPTT: activated partial thromboplastin time; FEV1: forced expiratory volume in one second; INR: international normalised ratio; PEFR: peak expiratory flow rate; PBI: pressure bandage with immobilisation.

TABLE 28.9 CLINICAL FEATURES OF SNAKE ENVENOMATION[28]

CATEGORY (GENUS)	VENOM INDUCED CONSUMPTIVE COAGULOPATHY (VICC)	ANTICOAGULANT COAGULOPATHY	NEUROTOXICITY	RHABDOMYOLYSIS	RENAL FAILURE	OTHER EFFECTS
Brown (Pseudonaja)	Present	Not present	Not present	Not present	Rare, can occur secondary to TMA	Thrombotic microangiopathy (TMA) and thrombocytopenia
Tiger (Notechis)	Present	Not present	Slow onset over hours	Onset over hours	Rare, can occur secondary to TMA and rhabdomyolysis	Thrombotic microangiopathy (TMA) and thrombocytopenia
Death adder (Acanthophis)	Not present	Not present	Present	Rare	Not present	Local bite site pain often present
Black (Pseudechis)	Not present	Present (can be very mild but it is used as indication to administer antivenom to prevent delayed rhabdomyolysis)	Not present	Slow onset over hours, can be severe	May occur secondary to rhabdomyolysis	Bite site pain may be significant Envenoming usually associated with nausea, vomiting, abdominal pain and headache Anosmia that can be irreversible
Taipan (Oxyuranus)	Present	Not present	May be rapid in onset	Onset over minutes/hours	Rare, can occur secondary to TMA and rhabdomyolysis	Thrombotic microangiopathy and thrombocytopenia
Sea snakes (Hydrophiidae)	Not present	Not present	May be rapid in onset	Onset over minutes/hours	May occur secondary to rhabdomyolysis	

aPTT: activated partial thromboplastin time

FIGURE 28.8 SNAKE-BITE BANDAGE[34]

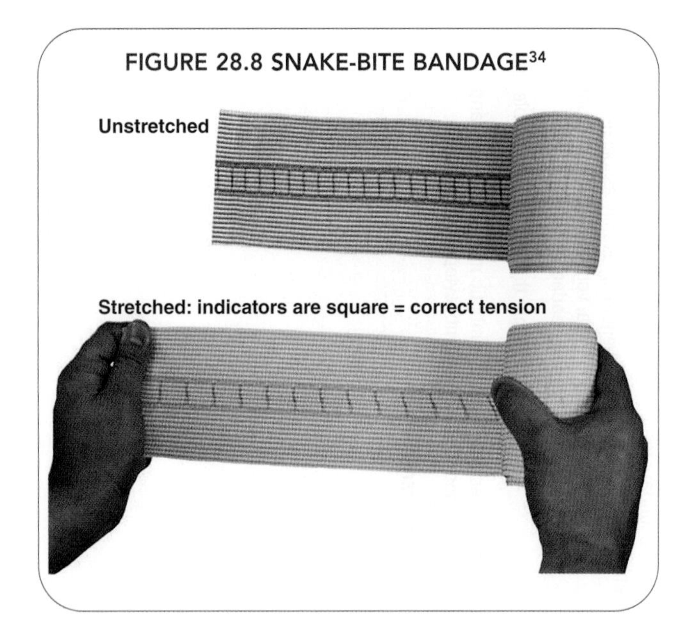

In cardiac arrest due to snake bite, undiluted antivenom administered as a rapid IV push may be lifesaving.

ASSESSMENT

Once snake bite is considered a possibility, systemic envenomation must be excluded. If envenomation is present, antivenom administration must be considered. These are vital steps in the management pathway and ensure that life-threatening cases are not missed.[28,30]

There is no risk stratification process that allows the clinician to identify patients who can be discharged early or without laboratory investigations. Patients with no obvious bite mark and no symptoms may still be envenomed. It is extremely unusual for a snake to be identified with sufficient reliability to preclude further observation or investigation.[26,28,30]

Patients do not necessarily have to be transferred to urban tertiary hospitals, but they need to be observed in a medical facility with:

- laboratory facilities on-site to perform serial blood tests
- antivenom available for the suspected snake genus
- a doctor who is able to deal with the life-threatening complications of snake bite or antivenom (respiratory failure secondary to neurotoxicity, bleeding, anaphylaxis).

Point-of-care devices that measure INR or D-dimer should not be used as there are reports of false negative results in patients who have VICC. Whole blood clotting tests should not be used either, as it is not reliable when assessing snake bites.[28,31,33]

DETERMINE IF THE PATIENT IS ENVENOMED

The aim of the hospital assessment is to seek objective evidence of envenoming based on history, physical examination and laboratory data. Serial physical examination (looking for signs of bleeding and neurotoxicity) and investigations (full blood count,

FIGURE 28.9 FITTING A PRESSURE BANDAGE WITH IMMOBILISATION (PBI)[35]

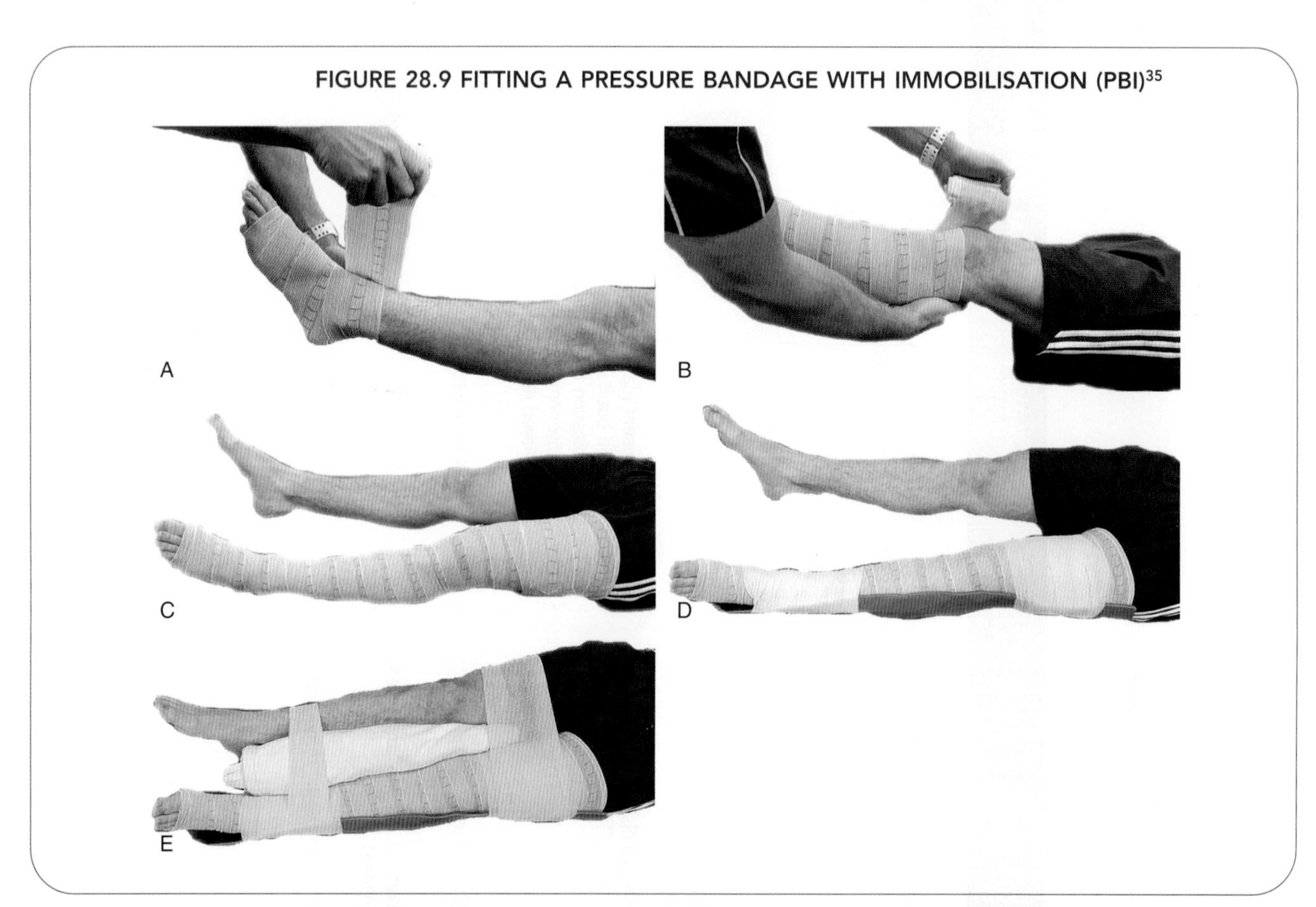

A and **B.** If bitten on a limb, apply a snake-bite bandage or broad elasticated pressure bandage (10–15 cm wide) over the bite. Then firmly apply an additional elasticised bandage, commencing at the distal end of the affected limb (i.e. fingers or toes) **C.** extending upwards, covering as much of the limb as possible. **D** and **E.** Splint the limb, keeping the patient and the limb completely at rest.

urea and electrolytes, creatine kinase and coagulation studies) are performed until envenoming is diagnosed *or* the patient is 12 hours post-removal of pressure bandage (see Table 28.9).

There are a number of non-specific symptoms related to a snake bite (nausea, vomiting, abdominal pain, malaise, mild headache) that *can* represent envenomation or significant underlying pathology (e.g. intracranial haemorrhage due to coagulopathy), so a thorough assessment is mandatory.

History of collapse, cardiac arrest, abnormalities of initial physical examination or laboratory studies consistent with snake envenoming prompt immediate antivenom therapy. However, if the patient is clinically well and initial laboratory studies are normal, then the PBI is removed. If there is a sudden clinical deterioration, the PBI is immediately reapplied, laboratory studies repeated and antivenom administered.

If there is no discernible deterioration following removal of the PBI, the patient is observed while physical examination and laboratory studies are repeated at 1, 6 and 12 hours. Twelve hours after removal of the PBI, the patient is reassessed and, if there is no evidence of envenoming, the patient may be discharged. Note that patients should not be discharged at night, as subtle, delayed neurotoxicity may not be detected.

In envenomed patients, snake venom detection kits have been used to determine what type of snake caused the envenomation. However, due to reports of false-negative and false-positive results, they have been removed from use in most states and are not recommended by current guidelines.[27]

ANTIVENOM ADMINISTRATION

All snake antivenom is derived from horse serum. Monovalent antivenom is preferred to polyvalent antivenom as it is safer (lower risk of allergic reactions) and cheaper. The choice of monovalent antivenom is based on:

- knowledge of snakes found in the area
- clinical presentation
- constellation of laboratory abnormalities.[28,30]

Antivenom dosages are based on consensus opinion and clinical experience, but there is minimal scientific data on the antivenom dose required to neutralise venom in vivo. Results from the Australian Snakebite Project suggest that for all snake bites 1 ampoule of antivenom is enough to ensure adequate treatment of envenoming syndromes.

Polyvalent antivenom contains the equivalent of 1 ampoule of each of the monovalent antivenoms for terrestrial snakes, and it does not contain sea snake antivenom. It includes a large protein load and thus has a higher probability of causing allergic reactions. Ideally, it should only be used in specific situations if it is not possible to use monovalent antivenom (Box 28.4).[28,30]

BOX 28.4 INDICATIONS FOR POLYVALENT ANTIVENOM[28,30]

1. Appropriate monovalent antivenoms not available.
2. The range of possible snakes requires the mixing of three or more monovalent antivenoms.
3. Exhausted monovalent antivenom stocks.

ADJUVANT THERAPY

In the rare case of anaphylaxis to antivenom, the infusion should be stopped immediately. Give oxygen, IV fluids and administer intramuscularly (IM) adrenaline 0.01 mg/kg (max 0.5 mg) to the lateral thigh and recommence the antivenom infusion cautiously once the clinical manifestations of anaphylaxis are controlled. Rarely, ongoing administration of adrenaline by titrated infusion may be necessary to complete antivenom administration. Adrenaline has to be carefully titrated to avoid hypertensive bursts in coagulopathic patients, as this could result in intracerebral haemorrhage.

Blood products, such as fresh frozen plasma (FFP) or cryoprecipitate, should be avoided unless there is an uncontrolled and life-threatening haemorrhage.[28,30] Recovery of clinically acceptable coagulation takes 12 to 18 hours.

The risk of infection or tetanus needs to be considered and standard wound care should be provided. Intramuscular tetanus toxoid should not be given to patients while coagulopathy is present due to a theoretical risk of developing an intramuscular haematoma.

Patients who receive antivenom should be counselled about the possibility of serum sickness, which can occur 4–21 days after antivenom administration. Symptoms include myalgias, fevers, malaise and arthralgias, and a palpable non-blanching rash. Treatment with oral steroids for 5 days may attenuate the severity of serum sickness, but not routinely prescribed as prophylaxis.[36]

SNAKE ENVENOMATION SYNDROMES

BROWN SNAKE

Clinical syndrome of brown snake envenomation can occur secondary to bites by the Eastern brown snake (*Pseudonaja textilis*), Western brown snake or *gwardar* (*P. nuchalis*), dugite (*P. affinis*) or other *Pseudonaja* species.

Brown snake envenoming is the most common cause of death from snake bite in Australia. These snakes are found in all parts of Australia, except Tasmania, Kangaroo Island in South Australia, and Carnac and Garden Islands in Western Australia.

Systemic envenoming may be heralded by collapse within a few minutes of the bite. The hallmark of brown snake envenoming is a severe defibrinating VICC. This may manifest clinically as bleeding gums, persistent haemorrhage at venesection or bite sites, haematuria, gastrointestinal bleeding or intracerebral haemorrhage.

Renal failure occurs in a small percentage of patients and is usually secondary to thrombotic microangiopathy (TMA), which is a rare complication. Oliguria may be present from the time of envenoming.

Rhabdomyolysis does not occur with brown snake envenomation, and neurotoxicity is very mild in the rare cases where it occurs.[37]

Management

Each ampoule of brown snake antivenom contains 1000 units and the dose required is 1 ampoule. Antivenom may treat other components of envenoming, but does not appear to hasten recovery from VICC.[38]

Recheck the coagulation profile 6 and 12 hours after the administration of antivenom. Marked improvements in aPTT and INR are better markers to assess recovery than fibrinogen levels,[37] and recovery is considered complete when INR < 2. Blood tests should also be performed up to 24 hours after envenomation to evaluate for less-common sequelae such as haemolysis or renal failure.

TIGER SNAKE

Bites by Common or Eastern tiger snake (*Notechis scutatus*), Western or Black tiger snake (*N. ater*), Copperhead (*Austrelaps* spp.), Broad-headed snake (*Hoplocephalus bungaroides*), Stephens' banded snake (*H. stephensii*), Pale-headed snake (*H. bitorquatus*) or Rough-scaled snake (*Tropidechis carinatus*) can cause tiger snake envenomation syndrome. These snakes are found along the coastal regions of the lower half of Australia, extending northwards into Queensland. They are the only terrestrial venomous snakes found in Tasmania and on Kangaroo, Carnac and Garden Islands.[26]

The features of tiger snake envenoming are VICC, progressive descending symmetrical flaccid paralysis and rhabdomyolysis.[39]

The initial stages of tiger and brown snake envenomation may be identical—the VICC is indistinguishable. However, patients with tiger snake envenoming are likely to develop rhabdomyolysis and progressive paralysis over the subsequent several hours. If there is a geographical risk of a bite from either snake and it is early in the clinical course, monovalent antivenom for both tiger *and* brown snakes is administered to ensure adequate treatment.[28]

The neurotoxic effects of the venom initially appear as diplopia or ptosis and can progress to diaphragmatic paralysis with respiratory failure. Antivenom does not reverse established weakness, but can prevent progression. Untreated, paralysis may persist for days before resolving. Regular assessments of peak expiratory flow rate (PEFR) or FEV_1 (forced expiratory volume) are useful objective markers of respiratory function.

Myotoxins in the venom can cause significant pain, muscle necrosis and rhabdomyolysis, and these symptoms can be notable features of envenomation.

Management

Each ampoule of tiger snake antivenom contains 3000 units. Initial dosage for envenomation is 1 ampoule. Recheck the coagulation profile 6 and 12 hours after the administration of antivenom. Marked improvements in aPTT and INR are better markers to assess recovery than fibrinogen levels, and recovery is considered complete when INR < 2.

BLACK SNAKE

Mulga or King brown snake (*Pseudechis australis*), Red-bellied (*P. porphyriacus*) or Blue-bellied (*P. guttatus*) can cause black snake envenomation syndromes after bites.

Black snakes are found throughout inland and northern Australia.[26,28] They are large and aggressive snakes that inflict a large and painful bite (see Fig. 28.5). Mulga is confusingly also known as the King brown snake, but it is not a brown snake and envenoming *will not* resolve with brown snake antivenom.

Black snake venom contains myotoxins, neurotoxins and anticoagulant toxins. Black snake envenomation causes an anticoagulant coagulopathy with isolated raise in aPTT, and normal fibrinogen and D-dimer levels. Bite by an Australian snake, associated with local pain, headache, nausea, vomiting and a mild anticoagulant coagulopathy (increased aPTT and normal fibrinogen and D-dimer), is highly suggestive of black snake envenoming.

Rhabdomyolysis secondary to black snake envenomation can be severe and delayed in onset.

Management

Each ampoule of black snake antivenom contains 18,000 units. Initial dosage for envenoming is 1 ampoule. Antivenom prevents progression of muscle injury, but does not reverse damage that has already occurred. Indications for antivenom administration are laboratory evidence of anticoagulant coagulopathy or CK that exceeds 1000 IU/L. Even mild elevations of aPTT should be considered an indication for black snake antivenom administration. A much lower threshold is used if the patient has significant pain from myonecrosis, or if non-specific features of abdominal pain, vomiting or a headache are severe and unresponsive to symptomatic treatment. CK is usually abnormal on arrival and may not become grossly elevated for many hours.

If the patient is envenomed and once antivenom is administered, CK should be checked 6-hourly in the symptomatic patient or 12-hourly in the asymptomatic patient until there is a definite improvement.

The red- and blue-bellied black snakes are black snakes, but can also be treated with tiger snake antivenom if necessary.[40,41]

DEATH ADDER

Death adders are found throughout most of mainland Australia, but bites and envenoming are uncommon as they are elusive and nocturnal snakes. A typical scenario is that the victim is bitten on the ankle after treading on the snake while walking outside with bare feet at dusk. The victim may feel little more than a sting and not see the snake.[42] Pain or stinging at the bite site is common; however, puncture wounds may not be apparent.

Prior to mechanical ventilation and antivenom availability, mortality was approximately 50%. The most significant venom toxin is a neurotoxin. Systemic envenoming is characterised by a progressive symmetrical descending flaccid paralysis, which usually manifests within 6 hours, but can be delayed. Early signs include ptosis, blurred vision, diplopia and difficulty swallowing. If left untreated, generalised paralysis, respiratory failure and secondary hypoxic cardiac arrest ensue. Regular assessments of PEFR or FEV_1 are useful objective markers of respiratory function.

With airway support, paralysis resolves spontaneously after 1–2 days. Neostigmine has been tried in the past to reverse the postsynaptic neurotoxic effects but not found to be beneficial. Coagulopathy and renal failure are not features of death adder envenoming. Mild rhabdomyolysis can rarely occur.

Management

Each ampoule of death adder antivenom contains 6000 units. Initial dosage for envenomation is 1 ampoule.

TAIPAN

Australian taipans are highly venomous snakes found in the northern part of Queensland, Northern Territory and Western Australia (coastal taipan), semi-arid Central East Australia and the Western Desert (inland taipan). Taipan snake envenoming is rare and is usually lethal without antivenom treatment. It is characterised by rapid onset of VICC, neurotoxicity and rhabdomyolysis due to potent pre- and postsynaptic neurotoxins, myotoxins and pro-coagulants. The coagulopathy is similar to that caused by brown or tiger snakes. Systemic envenoming may be heralded by collapse within a few minutes of the bite and paralysis is usually apparent within 1–2 hours. Seizures have been reported as an early manifestation of envenomation.[43]

Management

Each ampoule of taipan antivenom contains 12,000 units. Initial dosage for envenoming is 1 ampoule. Recheck the coagulation profile 6 and 12 hours after the administration of antivenom. Marked improvements in aPTT and INR are better markers to assess recovery than fibrinogen levels, and recovery is considered complete when INR < 2. Blood tests should also be performed up to 24 hours after envenomation to evaluate for less-common sequelae such as haemolysis or renal failure.

The antivenom halts the progression of paralysis, but does not reverse established neurotoxicity.[43]

SEA SNAKES

There are at least 30 species of sea snake found around the coast of northern Australia. They belong to the family Hydrophiidae and are closely related to the venomous Australian terrestrial snakes Elapidae. They are inquisitive but rarely aggressive, and bites always occur when they are handled—for example, when they are manually removed from fishing nets. Sea snakes have small fangs located in the rear of the mouth, so there is a lower risk of envenoming from a bite than with terrestrial snakes. However, it is essential to realise that a snake bite at sea, on the beach or in estuarine waters *may* be from a terrestrial snake as all snakes can swim.

Sea snake venom contains postsynaptic neurotoxins (paralysis) and myotoxins (rhabdomyolysis). Most bites are superficial, relatively painless and not associated with local swelling or lymphadenitis. Rhabdomyolysis manifests as myalgia and myoglobinuria and may progress to cause renal failure. Early signs of neurotoxicity include ptosis, blurred vision, diplopia and difficulty swallowing, progressing to symmetrical descending flaccid paralysis, which usually manifests within 6 hours. If left untreated, generalised paralysis can ensue, but this is rare.

Management

Each ampoule of sea snake antivenom contains 1000 units. Initial dosage for envenoming is 1 ampoule. Antivenom prevents progression of muscle injury but does not reverse injury that has already occurred. Antivenom is indicated if CK exceeds 1000 IU/L, or if there is evidence of neurotoxicity.

The polyvalent antivenom does not contain sea snake antivenom, so should not be administered when sea snake antivenom is not available.[28]

PRACTICE TIP

- PBI should be applied to all patients who sustain snake bites to the limbs.
- Snake identification is not required to appropriately manage snake-bite envenoming. Geographical location, clinical features and laboratory findings are more important in guiding snake-bite management.
- Once snake bite is suspected, all patients should be considered potentially envenomed until proven otherwise and have serial observations and blood tests to exclude envenomation.
- If there is a possibility of snake-bite envenoming, manage the patient as having a potentially life-threatening condition.
- Discuss envenoming cases with a clinical toxicologist at a Poisons Information Centre (phone 13 11 26 in Australia or 0800 POISON/0800 764 766 in Aotearoa New Zealand).

SPIDERS

OVERVIEW

Redback spider bite is the most common envenoming syndrome in Australia, with 2000 to 10,000 bites reported annually throughout Australia. Clinical features can be distressing and refractory to symptomatic treatment, but are not life threatening. Funnel-web spider distribution is limited to coastal New South Wales, Southern Queensland and a small area around Adelaide, and early recognition of this potentially lethal envenoming is vital.

FUNNEL-WEB SPIDER

The funnel-web spiders comprise 40 species in two genera (*Atrax* and *Hadronyche*) (Fig. 28.10). These potentially lethal spiders look very similar to other less dangerous, big black spiders, including the trapdoor spiders (families *Idiopidae* and *Nemesiidae*) and mouse spiders (*Actinopodidae* family). For this reason, it is important to have a clinical approach to a bite by a big black spider that occurs within the distribution area of the funnel-web species.

Both genera of funnel-web spider produce venom that contains potent neurotoxins. Robustoxin (*Atrax* spp.) and versutoxin (*Hadronyche* spp.) prevent inactivation of sodium channels, leading to a massive increase in autonomic activity and neuromuscular excitation. Patients usually give a history of a bite by a big black spider with large fangs. Not surprisingly, pain is severe, and fang marks are often visible. Severe systemic envenoming occurs rapidly, usually within 30 minutes and almost always within 2 hours.

Clinical features of funnel-web envenoming include:

- *general:* agitation, vomiting, headache, abdominal pain
- *autonomic:* sweating, salivation, piloerection, lacrimation
- *cardiovascular:* hypertension, tachycardia, hypotension, bradycardia, pulmonary oedema
- *neurological:* muscular fasciculations, oral paraesthesia, muscle spasm, coma

FIGURE 28.10

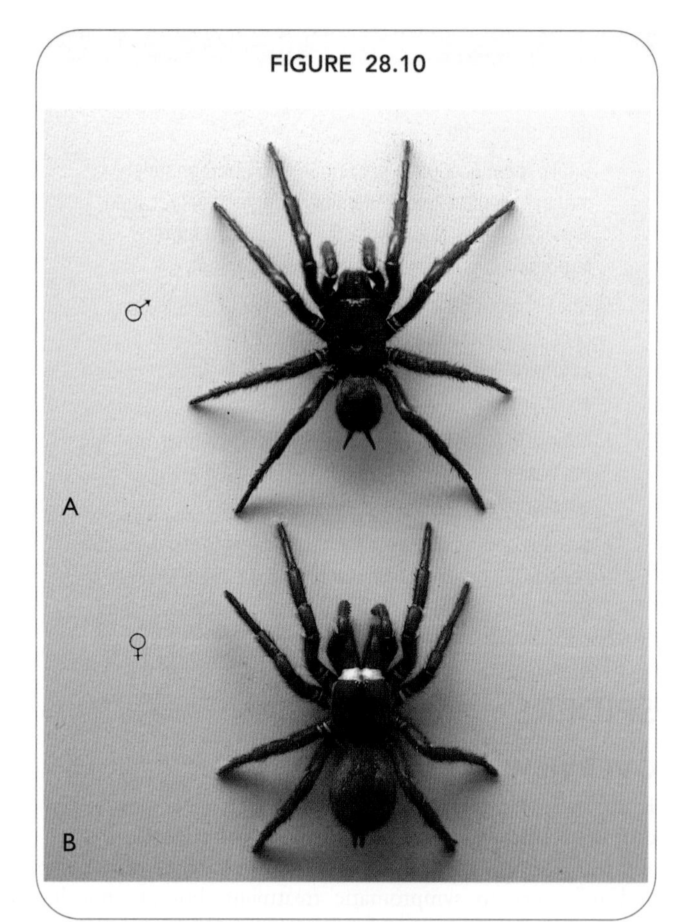

A. Male and **B.** female funnel-web. *Wikipedia/Sputniktilt/CC BY-SA 3.0*

FIGURE 28.11 REDBACK SPIDER

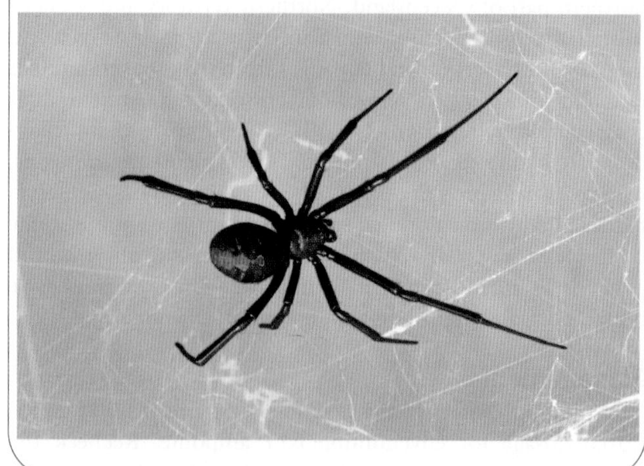

Shutterstock/Peter Waters

- *other:* in young children, the first indication of envenoming may be a sudden severe illness with inconsolable crying, salivation, vomiting or collapse.[44]

Bites by the other big black spiders (trapdoor and mouse spiders) may be associated with significant bite-site pain, but only mild systemic symptoms, such as nausea, headache, malaise or vomiting. Significant cardiovascular, autonomic or neurological symptoms do not occur.

Management

First aid is the same as for snake bite: apply direct pressure to the bite site, apply a PBI to the affected limb and transfer the patient to the nearest hospital capable of providing definitive care.

Funnel-web spider antivenom is derived from rabbit serum. Each ampoule of funnel-web spider antivenom contains 125 units. The freeze-dried antivenom is reconstituted in 10 mL of sterile water, and the initial dose is 2 ampoules diluted in 100 mL of normal saline (20 mL/kg in children) administered intravenously over 20 minutes.

Further doses can be considered for severely envenomed patients.

Redback spider

- Redback spider (Australia), *Latrodectus hasselti* (Fig. 28.11)
- Katipo spider (Aotearoa New Zealand), *L. katipo* (Fig. 28.12)

FIGURE 28.12 KATIPO SPIDER NURSING ITS EGG BALL

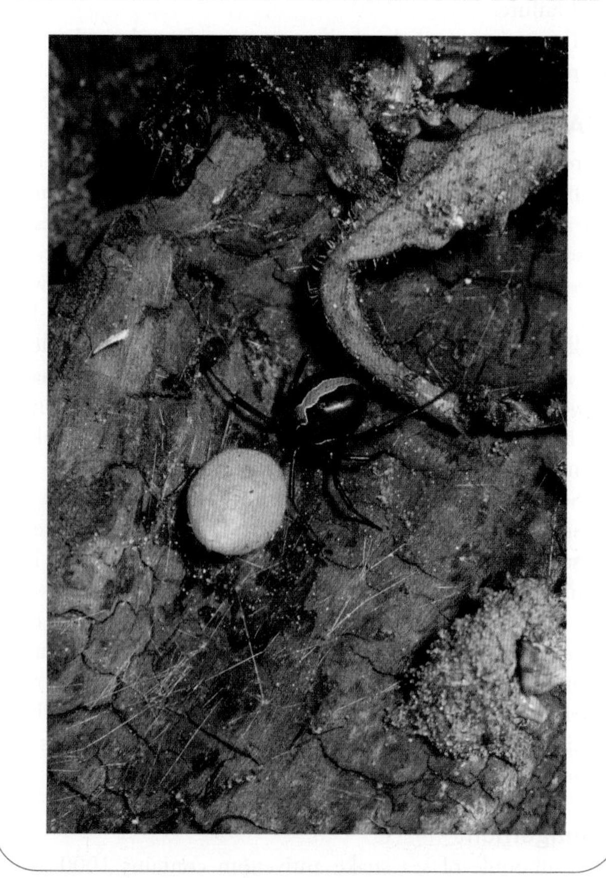

Richard Sharell. Gift of Mrs L. Sharell, 1987. © The Estate of Richard Sharell. Te Papa (CT.060847)

The redback and katipo spiders can both cause envenoming syndromes and are treated similarly. Whereas the redback lives in sheltered areas in close proximity to humans and bites are common, the katipo prefers grassy coastal regions and envenoming is rare and less likely to cause significant systemic features. The venom contains α-latrotoxin, which acts presynaptically to open cation channels (including calcium channels) and stimulate the release of neurotransmitters.[28,45]

Redback spider bites are not initially painful; however, local pain usually develops 5–10 minutes after the bite and is followed by localised sweating and piloerection within an hour. Puncture marks are not always evident and erythema, if present, is usually mild. The combination of pain, local piloerection and sweating are pathognomonic of redback spider bite.

Systemic envenoming (latrodectism) occurs in a minority of patients.[28,45] Pain typically radiates proximally from the bite site to become regional then general (e.g. pelvic, back, abdominal, chest or shoulder pain). Autonomic features include severe sweating, which may be regional (e.g. both legs) or generalised. Occasionally priapism may develop, especially in children. Latrodectism has been mistaken for conditions such as acute surgical abdomen, acute myocardial infarction and thoracic aortic dissection.

Non-specific features of envenoming include headache, nausea, vomiting and dysphoria.

If untreated, latrodectism may follow a fluctuating course lasting 1–4 days. Rarely, patients may feel unwell for up to a week. Very rarely, untreated patients report ongoing local symptoms that last weeks or months.

Management

Treatment with simple oral analgesia and ice applied to the bite site can be enough to treat mild to moderate envenoming. Severe envenoming can cause unremitting pain requiring parenteral opiate analgesia, and/or systemic toxicity (severe abdominal pain, generalised sweating).

Redback spider antivenom is derived from horse serum and has a low incidence of significant allergic reactions. It may be used for both redback and katipo spider envenoming. It is rarely recommended now after the RAVE study found that it provides minimally better pain relief than placebo. There is limited data about its efficacy for systemic effects.[28,46]

Each ampoule contains 500 units (1–1.5 mL), and initial treatment is 2 ampoules diluted in 100 mL normal saline (20 mL/kg in children) given intravenously over 30 minutes in a monitored area.

OTHER SPIDERS

The white-tailed spider (*Lampona cylindrata*) (Fig. 28.13) is ubiquitous throughout Australasia. The venom has been studied in detail, but no specific toxic components have been identified. Three local reactions to bites from *Lampona* species are reported:

- severe local pain of < 2 hours' duration
- local pain and a red mark lasting < 24 hours
- a persistent and painful red lesion that does not break down or ulcerate, and may continue for 5–12 days.

Mild, non-specific features may follow white-tailed spider bites, including nausea, vomiting, malaise and headache. Treatment with ice and simple analgesia such as paracetamol or anti-inflammatories is effective.

Bites from this spider were previously suspected to cause necrotic arachnidism, a syndrome of progressive cutaneous ulceration from spider venom. However, a study of 130 *Lampona* bites,[47] where the spider was caught and formally identified, showed that in every case other diagnoses (e.g. diabetic ulcers, infections) were responsible.

FIGURE 28.13 WHITE-TAILED SPIDER

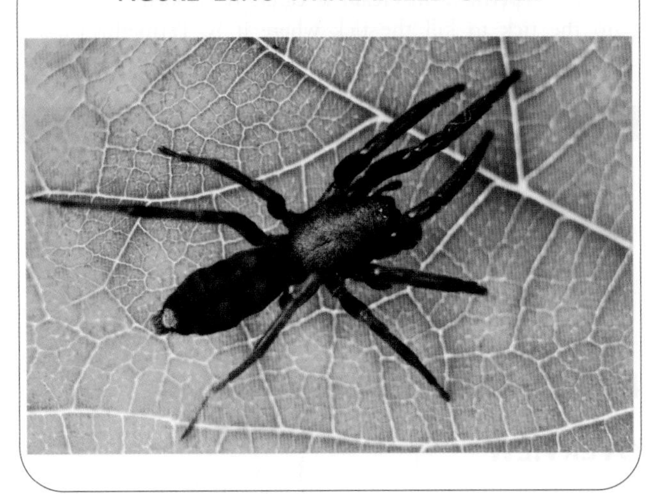

Shutterstock/ChameleonsEye

PRACTICE TIP

- Consider funnel-web or redback spider bite in children with inconsolable crying, acute abdominal pain or priapism.
- Administer antivenom in an environment staffed and equipped to manage anaphylaxis.
- Inform patients who receive antivenom of the potential for serum sickness in the weeks after administration.

OTHER TERRESTRIAL ENVENOMATIONS

There are a number of Australian scorpions that can cause painful stings, but there is limited knowledge about the components of the venom. They cause bite site pain, but not significant systemic effects. Pain relief with ice and simple analgesia is usually sufficient, and generalised symptoms are non-specific (nausea, headache and malaise) and self-limiting.

Anaphylaxis due to *Hymenoptera* spp. (honeybee and wasp stings) is a significant cause of morbidity and mortality related to envenomings. In southern Australia and Tasmania, bites from native ants (*Myrmecia* spp.) can also cause anaphylaxis.[27] Standard protocols for treatment of anaphylaxis, involving adrenaline, intravenous fluids and antihistamines, are the principles of management.

The Australian bush tick (*Ixodes cornuatus*, *I. hirsti* and *I. holocyclus*) can rarely cause a progressive descending flaccid paralysis in young children. Ticks can be hidden above the hairline or in skin folds, and a careful history and physical examination are required to confirm the diagnosis.[29] Attached adult ticks should be killed in situ by freezing them with ether-containing sprays to prevent allergic reactions to ticks. The dead tick should then be left to drop off. For ticks that can hardly be seen (nymph and larval ticks), it is recommended that a generous amount of permethrin cream is carefully dabbed or dropped onto the tick to kill the tick where it is. Permethrin-based creams and ether-containing spray are available from chemists.

CLINICAL PRACTICE TIP

For ticks you can see (adult ticks):
'Freeze it, don't squeeze it!'
For ticks you can hardly see (larval and nymph stage ticks):
'Dab it, don't grab'

MARINE ENVENOMATIONS

OVERVIEW

Encounters with marine animals are responsible for a broad spectrum of presentations to hospital in Australia. Envenoming from jellyfish can result in life-threatening reactions, and toxins from other creatures, such as the blue-ringed octopus or cone snails, can cause fatal paralysis. Traumatic injuries from stingrays or barbed fish require meticulous wound care to ensure good outcomes.

MAJOR BOX JELLYFISH

The box jellyfish (*Chironex fleckeri*) is found in tropical Australian waters, from Queensland around to the northern parts of Western Australia. Most stings occur between November and April, are benign and respond to supportive measures. Most stings are minor, but severe envenoming can happen, and it has been associated with at least 67 deaths in Australia.[25]

The venom components are thought to affect sodium and calcium channels, leading to abnormal membrane ion transport.

Stings usually occur in shallow water and are associated with immediate severe pain, typically lasting up to 8 hours. Linear welts characteristically occur in a cross-hatched pattern (see Fig. 28.7), and tentacles may remain adherent unless physically removed—gloves are required for this task to avoid secondary envenomation from undischarged nematocysts.

Systemic envenoming is heralded by collapse or sudden death within a few minutes of the sting. Cardiovascular effects include hypertension, hypotension, tachycardia or sudden cardiac arrest.[25]

Delayed hypersensitivity reactions occur in at least 50% of patients and manifest as pruritic erythema at the original sting site, 7–14 days after the sting.

Management

Cardiac arrest should be managed as per BLS/ACLS algorithms, and antivenom should be administered as a push during resuscitative measures.

For patients who do not require resuscitation, reassure them, wash off any remaining tentacles from the skin, then apply vinegar liberally followed by ice packs. The traditional recommendation, to apply generous volumes of vinegar (5% acetic acid) to all visible sting sites to inactivate all undischarged nematocysts (sting cells), has been challenged in a study where in vivo application of vinegar to already discharged nematocysts was shown to promote further discharge of venom.[48] However, the current recommendations remain that vinegar should be part of first aid. Do not apply a PBI as this can cause further nematocyst discharge, increased pain and may promote systemic envenoming.

Where appropriate and available, give simple oral analgesia such as paracetamol or anti-inflammatories prior to opioid analgesia, which is usually required. Patients with pain refractory to IV opioid analgesia should be administered 1 ampoule of box jellyfish antivenom diluted in 100 mL of normal saline (20 mL/kg in children) intravenously over 20 minutes. Further doses of 1 ampoule may be given, to a total of 3 ampoules, if pain persists.

If there is haemodynamic compromise, 3 ampoules diluted in 100 mL of normal saline (20 mL/kg in children) are recommended to be administered intravenously over 20 minutes, with repeat doses of 3 ampoules given until improvement is achieved.

Six ampoules may be given as a rapid IV push if the patient is in cardiac arrest.

Box jellyfish antivenom is derived from sheep serum. Each ampoule contains 20,000 units, and premedication with adrenaline is not required.

Magnesium can be tried in severe cases refractory to opioid analgesia and antivenom treatment.

IRUKANDJI SYNDROME

Irukandji syndrome is a painful sympathomimetic condition named after an Aboriginal tribe in North Queensland.[50] It is caused by envenoming by one of a number of different jellyfish species found in the coastal waters of tropical Northern Australia.[49,50] Best described is *C. barnesi*, a transparent thumbnail-sized carybdeid which can pass through stinger nets at patrolled beaches. It is one of a group of similar small jellyfish thought to cause the constellation of symptoms known as an Irukandji syndrome.[50] The mechanism of action of the venom has not been fully characterised, but is believed to cause massive catecholamine release.

The initial sting is usually minor, and there is a short delay in the onset of systemic symptoms. Local signs such as welts, dermal markings or tentacles can be minimal or absent.[49] Multiple systemic symptoms develop 30 to 120 minutes after contact with the jellyfish. These include a sense of impending doom, agitation, dysphoria, vomiting, generalised sweating and severe pain in the back, limbs or abdomen. Hypertension and tachycardia are common. Symptoms usually settle within 12 hours.

Severe envenoming manifests within 4 hours with ongoing significant opioid requirements. These patients are at risk of toxic cardiomyopathy, cardiogenic shock and pulmonary oedema and may require continuous positive airway pressure or intubation and mechanical ventilation. Fatal intracerebral haemorrhage has occurred in two patients, presumably due to uncontrolled hypertension.

Management

As in box jellyfish toxicity, PBI is not beneficial. Immersion in hot water may alleviate the pain. Parenteral opioids are usually required. Fentanyl in titrated doses is recommended, and intravenous magnesium is a commonly used but unproven adjunctive therapy. Antiemetics such as promethazine are also commonly used.

If significant cardiovascular toxicity develops, treatment with intravenous nitrate infusions will help with hypertension or pulmonary oedema. ICU management is warranted for patients with respiratory compromise. There is no antivenom available for the Irukandji syndrome, and box jellyfish antivenom is ineffective.

OTHER JELLYFISH

The bluebottle (*Physalia* spp., see Fig. 28.14) is a jellyfish-like hydrozoan responsible for thousands of stings on Australian beaches (and to a lesser extent in Aotearoa New Zealand) each year. Clinical features include intense local pain and dermal erythema. Unlike *Physalia* stings in other parts of the world, major systemic envenoming does not occur. Stings are mild, self-limiting and respond to first-aid measures.

Management

Hot-water immersion therapy is the most effective treatment for bluebottle stings (and most jellyfish stings apart from box jellyfish). Place the patient under a hot shower for 20 minutes (ideal temperature 45°C).[24] The shower should be hot but not scalding or uncomfortable. Administer simple oral analgesia such as paracetamol. Do not apply a PBI or vinegar, as these may worsen local symptoms. Transport to hospital is not usually required.

Bullous wounds from all jellyfish stings may be extensive enough to require dressings.

OTHER MARINE ENVENOMATIONS

The blue-ringed octopus (*Hapalochlaena* spp.) is a small brown octopus found in shallow waters around Australia. When handled or enraged, it changes colour and develops bright blue rings on its surface. The venom contains tetrodotoxin, a potent neurotoxin that the octopus delivers with a bite from the beak, not from the tentacles. The bite of the blue-ringed octopus is not necessarily painful, and there may be minimal local signs.[28]

Envenoming is characterised by a progressive descending flaccid paralysis, which develops rapidly over the course of minutes to hours and can lead to respiratory compromise requiring intubation and ventilation. Usually, symptoms are much less significant and are limited to mild perioral paraesthesia. A PBI is beneficial to limit systemic absorption of the toxin until the patient reaches hospital. There is no specific antidote, but with respiratory support, full recovery is expected over 24–48 hours.

A similar clinical presentation occurs after stings from the cone shell (*Conus* spp.), found in tropical waters around Australia. A barb from the end of the shell can deliver a sting containing conotoxins, which can also cause paralysis. There is no antidote, and supportive therapy is required if respiratory failure develops.

Stonefish (*Synanceia trachynis*) are found in the waters of Northern Australia. Their dorsal spines contain venom, which is injected into the skin when the animal is stood upon. Neurotoxins, stonustoxin and enzymes in the venom cause severe debilitating pain, and remnants of the spines may remain embedded in the limb, requiring surgical debridement.[28]

First-aid treatment for stonefish envenoming consists of hot-water immersion therapy and can be rapidly effective in providing analgesia. If pain does not resolve with this treatment, and the geographical location is stonefish habitat, antivenom can be considered.

Stonefish antivenom is derived from horse serum. Each ampoule contains 2000 units of antivenom, and 1 ampoule is administered diluted in 100 mL of normal saline (20 mL/kg in children) and given intravenously over 20 minutes.

A number of other barbed fish or stingrays can cause significant local tissue injury or pain. Hot-water immersion therapy is usually adequate analgesia for most marine toxins, although the mechanism is unclear. Regional anaesthesia is also useful, but if combined with hot-water immersion, the unaffected limb should also be placed in hot water to prevent inadvertent thermal injury if pain perception in the affected limb is impaired. Expert wound care (including removal of residual barbs or formal surgical debridement), tetanus prophylaxis and antibiotic therapy are all important considerations after such traumatic injuries.

Venomous sponges and corals are found throughout Australian coastal waters and if touched can cause local dermatitis characterised by localised itchiness, stinging, erythaema and occasional vesicles and swelling that can sometimes last a few weeks. Management is with simple analgesia, antihistamines and wound care.

FIGURE 28.14 BLUE BOTTLE JELLYFISH

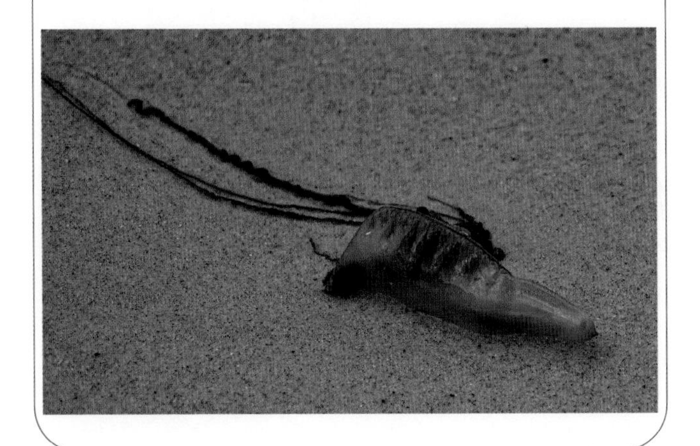

Shutterstock/Chris Andrews Fern Bay

PRACTICE TIP

Subtle neurological signs can be missed in potentially envenomed patients if they are discharged 'after hours', so discharge should occur in daylight hours accompanied by an adult.

- Consider envenomation in patients found unresponsive or collapsed around beaches.
- Hot-water immersion to treat stonefish envenomation can result in severe burns if used concomitantly with regional anaesthesia. Immerse a non-anaesthetised limb concurrently.
- Antivenom should not be withheld from children, pregnant or lactating patients.
- The dose of antivenom is the same for children and adults (the amount of fluid that it is diluted in varies).

SUMMARY

It is important to understand, recognise and effectively manage the effect of environmental impacts on the human body, such as temperature, submersion and environmental pressure. Onset may be insidious and difficult to identify, thus warranting a high index of suspicion when assessing and managing patients who have potentially been exposed to environmental hazards. Treatment should be timely and often based on clinical assessment, without the necessary benefit of diagnostic confirmation. Where appropriate, timely first aid and transfer to a facility capable of implementing required treatment is essential for best patient outcomes and reduced morbidity and mortality.

Early recognition of the patient with potential envenoming is essential for emergency clinicians. An understanding of the likely causes of envenoming based on clinical presentation and geographical possibilities is an important skill to develop. This enables appropriate triage categorisation for subsequent assessment and management.

Australia is home to many deadly snakes. There are few annual fatalities related to snake bite in Australia, and these usually occur pre-hospital. Antivenom availability, good supportive care and a standardised approach to managing snake-bite presentations are essential to ensure that this situation continues.

This chapter provides information on the major terrestrial and venomous marine creatures in Australasia and the management of envenoming syndromes. It should be used as a guide, in conjunction with information from services such as the Poisons Information Centres or other toxicology resources in Australia and Aotearoa New Zealand.

CASE STUDY

An ambulance is called to a 12-year-old boy who was bitten by a snake to the lateral border of the left foot 20 minutes previously. The patient is mildly nauseated, but is alert and feels otherwise well. There has been no first aid applied.

QUESTIONS

1. What is the most important initial intervention when arriving at scene?
2. What are the important examination findings that should be sought initially and on arrival to hospital?
3. What investigations should be performed in hospital?
4. What is the ongoing management plan for this patient?
5. What further treatment is required with this new information?

Answers to Case Study Questions can be found on evolve **http://evolve.elsevier.com/AU/Curtis/emergency/**

USEFUL WEBSITES

Information on working in hot conditions

Government of WA, Department of Mines, Industry Regulation and Safety. Working safely in hot conditions, www.commerce.wa.gov.au/worksafe/working-safely-hot-conditions

OHS representatives action plan:

Australia—working in heat: www.safeworkaustralia.gov.au/safety-topic/hazards/working-heat
www.safeworkaustralia.gov.au/resources-and-publications/guidance-materials/guide-managing-risks-working-heat
www.safeworkaustralia.gov.au/safety-topic/hazards/working-heat/checklist-managing-risks-heat-workplace

Information to manage envenomations

NSW Poisons Information Centre, www.poisonsinfo.nsw.gov.au/

Poison Information Centres 13 11 26 in Australia; 0800 POISON/0800 764 766 in Aotearoa New Zealand

Australian Snakebite Project research packs

www.newcastle.edu.au/research/centre/clinical-toxicology/research-study-packs

REFERENCES

1. Luks AM, Auerbach PS, Freer L, Grissom CK, Keyes LE, McIntosh SE, et al. Wilderness medical society clinical practice guidelines for the prevention and treatment of acute altitude illness: 2019 update. Wilderness Environ Med 2019;30(Suppl. 4):S3–18.
2. Rogers I. Altitude illness. In: Cameron P, Little M, Mitra B, Deasy C, editors. Textbook of adult emergency medicine. 5th ed. Amsterdam: Elsevier; 2020.
3. Santelli J, Sullivan JM, Czarnik A, Bedolla J. Heat illness in the emergency department: keeping your cool. Emerg Med Prac 2014;16(8):1–21.
4. NOAA's National Weather Service. NWS wind chill chart. Available from: www.weather.gov/safety/cold-wind-chill-chart.
5. Du Bois EF. The basal metabolism in fever. JAMA 1921;77(5):352–5.
6. Rogers I. Heat related illness. In: Cameron P, Little M, Mitra B, Deasy C, editors. Textbook of adult emergency medicine. 5th ed. Amsterdam: Elsevier; 2020.
7. Fong J, Bucher L. Emergency care situations. In: Brown D, editor. Lewis's medical-surgical nursing ANZ. 5th ed. Chatswood: Elsevier; 2019.
8. Rublee C, Dresser C, Giudice C, Lemery J, Sorensen C. Evidence-based heatstroke management in the emergency department. West J Emerg Med 2021;22(2):186–95.
9. Rogers I. Hypothermia. In: Cameron P, Little M, Mitra B, Deasy C, editors. Textbook of adult emergency medicine. 5th ed. Elsevier; 2020. p. 702–5.
10. Rischall ML, Rowland-Fisher A. Evidence-based management of accidental hypothermia in the emergency department. Emerg Med Pract 2016;18(1):1–18.
11. Dow J, Giesbrecht GG, Danzl DF, Brugger H, Sagalyn EB, Walpoth B, et al. Wilderness Medical Society clinical practice guidelines for the out-of-hospital evaluation and treatment of accidental hypothermia: 2019 update. Wilderness Environ Med 2019;30(Suppl. 4):S47–69.
12. McIntosh SE, Freer L, Grissom CK, Auerbach PS, Rodway GW, Cochran A, et al. Wilderness Medical Society clinical practice guidelines for the prevention and treatment of frostbite: 2019 update. Wilderness Environ Med 2019;30(Suppl. 4):S19–S32.
13. Dow J, Giesbrecht G, Danzl DF, Brugger H, Sagalyn EB, Walpoth B, et al. Clinical practice guidelines for the out-of-hospital evaluation and treatment of accidental hypothermia: 2019 update. Wilderness Environ Med 2019;30(Suppl. 4):S47–69.
14. Royal Lifesaving Society Australia 2020. 2021. Available from: www.royallifesaving.com.au/__data/assets/pdf_file/0003/33861/RLS_NationalDrowningReport2020LR-FINAL.pdf.
15. Schmidt AC, Sempsrott JR, Hawkins SC, Arastu AS, Cushing TA, Auerbach PS. Wilderness Medical Society clinical practice guidelines for the treatment and prevention of drowning: 2019 update. Wilderness Environ Med 2019;30(Suppl. 4):S70–86.
16. Datta A, Tipton M. Respiratory responses to cold water immersion: neural pathways, interactions, and clinical consequences awake and asleep. J App Physiol 2006;100(6):2057–64.
17. Gagnon DD, Pretorius T, McDonald G, Kenny GP, Giesbrecht GG. Cardiovascular and ventilatory responses to dorsal, facial, and whole-head water immersion in Eupnea. Aviat Space Environ Med 2013;84(6):573–83.
18. Mountain D. Drowning. In: Cameron P, Little M, Mitra B, Deasy C, editors. Textbook of adult emergency medicine. 5th ed. Amsterdam: Elsevier; 2020.
19. American Meteorological Society. The atmosphere aloft teachers guide. Project Atmosphere. 2012. Available from: www.ametsoc.org/ams/index.cfm/education-careers/education-program/k-12-teachers/project-atmosphere/training-opportunities/project-atmosphere-peer-led-training/project-atmosphere-peer-training-resources/atmosphere-aloft/.
20. Tetzlaff K, Thorsen E. Breathing at depth: physiologic and clinical aspects of diving while breathing compressed gas. Clin Chest Med 2005;26(3):355–80.
21. Smart D. Dysbarism. In: Cameron P, Little M, Mitra B, Deasy C, editors. Textbook of adult emergency medicine. 5th ed. Amsterdam: Elsevier; 2020.
22. Shroff NA, Balbin J, Shobitan O. High-altitude illness: updates in prevention, identification, and treatment. Emerg Med Prac 2021;23(9):1–18.
23. Johnston CI, O'Leary MA, Brown SGA, Currie BJ, Halkidis L, Whitaker R, et al. Death adder envenoming causes neurotoxicity not reversed by antivenom—Australian Snakebite Project (ASP-16). PLoS Negl Trop Dis 2012;6(9):e1841.
24. Loten C, Stokes B, Worsley D, Seymour JE, Jiang S, Isbister GK. A randomised controlled trial of hot water (45 degrees C) immersion versus ice packs for pain relief in bluebottle stings. Med J Aust 2006;184(7):329–33.
25. Currie BJ, Jacups SP. Prospective study of *Chironex fleckeri* and other box jellyfish stings in the 'Top End' of Australia's Northern Territory. Med J Aust 2005;183(11-12):631–6.
26. White J. A clinician's guide to Australian venomous bites and stings. Parkville, Melbourne, Victoria: CSL; 2013.
27. Johnston C, Ryan N, Page CB, Buckley N, Brown SG, O'Leary MA, et al. The Australian snakebite project, 2005–2015. Med J Aust 2017;207(3):119–25.
28. Murray L, Little M, Pascu O, Hoggett K. Toxicology handbook. 3rd ed. Sydney: Elsevier; 2015.
29. Miller MK. Massive tick (*Ixodes holocyclus*) infestation with delayed facial-nerve palsy. Med J Aust 2002;176(6):264–5.
30. Isbister GK, Brown SG, Page CB, McCoubrie DL, Greene SL, Buckley NA. Snakebite in Australia: a practical approach to diagnosis and treatment. Med J Aust 2013;199(11):763–8.
31. Australian Resuscitation Council[7]. Envenomation: pressure immobilisation technique. Guideline 9.4.8. Melbourne: ARC; 2011.

32. Canale E, Isbister GK, Currie BJ. Investigating pressure bandaging for snakebite in a simulated setting: bandage type, training and the effect of transport. Emerg Med Australas 2009;21(3):184–90.

33. Isbister GK, Maduwage K, Shahmy S, Mohamed F, Abeysinghe C, Karunathilake H, et al. Diagnostic 20-min whole blood clotting test in Russell's viper envenoming delays antivenom administration. QJM 2013;106(10):925–32.

34. St John Ambulance WA. Clinical resources: pressure immobilisation technique. 4 images technique. Available from: clinical.stjohnwa.com.au/clinical-skills/circulation/pressure-immobilisation-technique-(p.i.t).

35. St John Ambulance WA. Clinical resources: pressure immobilisation technique. 5 images technique. Available from: clinical.stjohnwa.com.au/clinical-skills/circulation/pressure-immobilisation-technique-(p.i.t).

36. Ryan NM, Kearney RT, Brown SG, Isbister GK. Incidence of serum sickness after the administration of Australian snake antivenom (ASP-22). Clin Toxicol (Phila) 2016;54(1):27–33.

37. Allen GE, Brown SGA, Buckley NA, O'Leary MA, Page CB, Currie BJ, et al. Clinical effects and antivenom dosing in Brown snake (*Pseudonaja* spp.) Envenoming–Australian Snakebite Project (ASP-14). PLoS One 2012;7(12):e53188.

38. Isbister GK, Williams V, Brown SGA, White J, Currie BJ. Clinically applicable laboratory endpoints for treating snakebite coagulopathy. Pathology 2006;38(6):568–72.

39. Isbister G, O'Leary M, Elliott M, Brown SG. Tigersnake (*Notechis* spp) envenoming: Australian Snakebite Project (ASP-13). Med J Aust 2012;197(3):173–7.

40. Churchman A, O'Leary MA, Buckley NA, Page CB, Tankel A, Gavaghan C, et al. Clinical effects of red-bellied black snake (*Pseudechis porphyriacus*) envenoming and correlation with venom concentrations: Australian Snakebite Project (ASP-11). Med J Aust 2010;193(11):696–700.

41. Johnston CI, Brown SGA, O'Leary MA, Currie BJ, Greenberg R, Taylor M, et al. Mulga snake (*Pseudechis australis*) envenoming: a spectrum of myotoxicity, anticoagulant coagulopathy, haemolysis and the role of early antivenom therapy - Australian Snakebite Project (ASP-19). Clin Toxicol 2013;51(5):417–24.

42. Johnston C, O'Leary M, Brown S, Currie BJ, Halkidis L, Whitaker R, et al. Death adder envenoming causes neurotoxicity not reversed by antivenom. Australian Snakebite Project (ASP16). PLoS Neglect Trop Dis 2012;6(9):e1841.

43. Johnston C, Ryan N, O'Leary M, Brown SG, Isbister GK. Australian taipan (*Oxyuranus* spp.) envenoming: clinical effects and potential benefits of early therapy-Australian Snakebite Project (ASP25). Clin Toxicol (Phila) 2017;55(2):115–22.

44. Isbister GK, Gray MR, Balit CR, Raven RJ, Stokes BJ, Porges K, et al. Funnel-web spider bite: a systematic review of recorded clinical cases. Med J Aust 2005;182(8):407–11.

45. Isbister GK, Gray MR. Latrodectism: a prospective cohort study of bites by formally identified redback spiders. Med J Aust 2003;179(2):88–91.

46. Isbister G, Page C, Buckley N, Fatovich DM, Pascu O, MacDonald SP, et al. Randomised controlled trial of intravenous antivenom versus placebo for lactrodectism: the second redback antivenom evaluation (RAVE II) study. Ann Emerg Med 2014;64:620–8.

47. Isbister GK, Gray MR. White-tail spider bite: a prospective study of 130 definite bites by Lampona species. Med J Aust 2003;179(4):199–202.

48. Welfare P, Little M, Pereira P, Seymour J. An in-vitro examination of the effect of vinegar on discharged nematocysts of *Chironex fleckeri*. Diving Hyperb Med 2014;44(1):30–4.

49. Nickson CP, Waugh EB, Jacups SP, Currie BT. Irukandji syndrome case series from Australia's Tropical Northern Territory. Ann Emerg Med 2009;54(3):395–403.

50. Little M, Pereira P, Carrette T, Seymour J. Jellyfish responsible for Irukandji syndrome. QJM 2006;99(6):425–7.

CHAPTER 29

ONCOLOGICAL AND HAEMATOLOGICAL EMERGENCIES

MEREDITH OATLEY AND JULIJA SIPAVICIUS

ESSENTIALS

- Recent advances in cancer care have resulted in a large outpatient population of cancer patients undergoing treatment that may present to emergency departments when they encounter treatment- or disease-related difficulties.
- Oncology and haematology patients may present with several life-threatening or highly debilitating syndromes, such as neutropenic sepsis, hyperviscosity, spinal cord compression, superior vena cava obstruction, hypercalcaemia, haemorrhage or disseminated intravascular coagulation.
- Early recognition, prompt intervention and appropriate emergency management reduces morbidity and mortality.
- Early recognition and intervention of neutropenic sepsis patients correlates highly with good patient outcomes.
- Administration of blood products, while commonplace in hospital, is hazardous.
- An understanding of the risks and of how to administer blood products safely is essential for emergency clinicians.

INTRODUCTION

In recent decades cancer treatments have become more effective, leading to a reduction in cancer incidence and mortality rates.[1] Advances in supportive care have allowed the use of more intensive treatment regimens, including chemotherapy, immunotherapy and targeted therapies and combinations of these treatments. Simultaneously, for both economic and quality-of-life reasons there has been a widespread trend away from hospitalisation and, where possible, treatments are administered in ambulatory care settings. Furthermore, for cases where a cure is not an achievable goal, long-term disease control has transformed some cancers into chronic diseases. Consequently, there are large numbers of people with cancer being cared for in the community and emergency clinicians are often the first to see, treat and manage such patients presenting with complications of their disease, treatment, or both.

CANCER INCIDENCE IN AUSTRALIA AND AOTEAROA NEW ZEALAND

CANCER INCIDENCE IN AUSTRALIA

Cancer is a major cause of illness in Australia and is responsible for 18% of the burden of ill health suffered by Australians. The Australian Institute of Health and Welfare (AIHW) estimated that in 2021 approximately 151,000 Australians would be diagnosed with cancer (413 per day) and 49,000 would die (135 per day).[1] Aboriginal and Torres Strait Islander peoples were 1.1 times more likely to be diagnosed with cancer than the non-Indigenous population. The number of new cases of cancer diagnosed in the non-Indigenous and Indigenous populations is estimated to increase to 185,000 in 2031. The survival rates for cancer have improved in recent decades with 70% of non-Indigenous people diagnosed with a cancer, excluding basal cell carcinoma (BCC) and squamous cell carcinoma (SCC), expected to survive at least 5 years from diagnosis. In the Indigenous population, the relative 5-year data is 50% of people expected to survive from diagnosis. These results demonstrate an improvement of 51% compared with data from 30 years ago.[1]

Cancer mortality rates continue to fall, with a sharper decline for males than for females. The age-standardised incidence rate of cancer is also decreasing. The most common cancers reported in Australia are breast, prostate, melanoma, colorectal, lung and lymphoma. Contributing factors in almost half of the cancer burden are attributable to personal and behavioural risk factors; including obesity and smoking. Improvements in public health programs raise awareness in the community about important risk factors and promote cancer screening. Patient participation in screening programs is important to facilitate early detection of cancers to enable early access to treatment and support better patient outcomes.[1]

CANCER INCIDENCE IN AOTEAROA NEW ZEALAND

Cancer is a leading cause of mortality in Aotearoa New Zealand.[2] Data from 2020 state that approximately 25,000 people are diagnosed with cancer each year, with nearly 3000 of those people being Māori. Each year approximately 9000 New Zealanders die from cancer. The most commonly diagnosed cancers are breast, lung, prostate and colorectal cancers. The patterns of incidence over time have shown decreases in stomach and lung cancers, and increases in liver and pancreatic cancers. Survival rates have been reported as improving significantly over the last 20 years with better access to screening and improvements in cancer treatment.

The leading causes of death in Aotearoa New Zealand are lung cancer and colorectal cancer (around 1700 and 1200 respectively). Cancer incidence has changed considerably over the past 20 years with both the Māori and non-Māori population reporting a gradual reduction in incidence since 1996. The Māori population is twice as likely to die from cancer as the non-Māori population. It is reported that up to 66% of all cancer patients will survive at least 5 years after diagnosis.[2]

CANCER PATHOPHYSIOLOGY

Cancer is a generic term for diseases in which abnormal cells divide without control and can invade nearby tissues. Cancer cells can also spread to other parts of the body through the blood and lymph systems.[3] Cancer is named based on the tissue that it arises from. For example, carcinomas refer to cancers that derive from the epithelial tissue; sarcomas are derived from the mesenchymal tissue; and haematologic malignancies, including lymphoma leukaemias and plasma cells dyscrasias, are derived from the haematopoietic tissue. Cancers nearly always arise from a genetic alteration within an original cell and are monoclonal in origin. Characteristically, most cancers have a broad heterogeneity in the cell population. This can lead to complications with treatment due to subsets of cells that will be resistant to therapy and continue to survive and proliferate.[4]

The process of carcinogenesis begins with a cellular genetic mutation that may be inherited or the result of damage to the chromosomal DNA (Table 29.1). Genetic mutations are common within cells and are generally fixed by normal cellular

TABLE 29.1 CARCINOGENS AND CANCER PROMOTERS

PROMOTERS/MUTAGEN/ CARCINOGEN	EXAMPLE	CANCER
Chemicals	***Aniline dyes***	***Bladder cancer***
	Asbestos	***Mesothelioma***
Smoking	Cigarettes and cigars, passive smoking	Lung, also thought to be linked with cancer of the oral cavity, larynx, oesophagus, kidney, pancreas, cervix, stomach and bladder
Ionising radiation	Nuclear radiation	Leukaemia and other cancers
Ultraviolet radiation	Sunlight	Skin cancers
Chronic inflammation	Inflammatory bowel disease	Bowel cancer
	Hepatitis	Liver cancer
Viruses	Epstein-Barr virus	Nasopharyngeal and some lymphomas
	Human papillomavirus	Anal and cervical cancer
Host immunosuppression	HIV	Lymphomas and other cancers
	Post-transplant immunosuppression	Skin and other cancers

repair mechanisms. However, where multiple genes are damaged over time—and particularly those whose function is to promote or inhibit cellular growth (proto-oncogenes or tumour suppressor genes respectively)—the first stage towards uncontrolled cellular division may occur. This is known as tumour initiation.[4]

Of all cancers, only 5–10% are inherited, germline cancers.[5] The remainder are the result of DNA damage through exposure to carcinogens that may be potentiated by individual host factors. Table 29.1 lists some of the currently known promoters/mutagens/carcinogens.[4]

Tumour promotion is the process whereby altered cellular division and gene expression occur in conjunction with immunosuppression, thus promoting tumour development.[6] This phase may take many years, which is why, although cancer is seen in children and in young people, it is predominantly a disease of ageing.[4,7] Cellular damage that occurs during this phase is still 'pre-malignant' and thought to be potentially reversible; for example, by removal of relevant cancer promoters.

The final stage in the development of the disease is cancer progression, whereby the malignant changes become irreversible and the collection of aberrant cells become a tumour with the capacity to spread not only locally, but also to distant sites (Fig. 29.1).[4]

FIGURE 29.1 SIMPLIFIED DIAGRAM OF THE MOLECULAR BASIS OF CANCER[6]

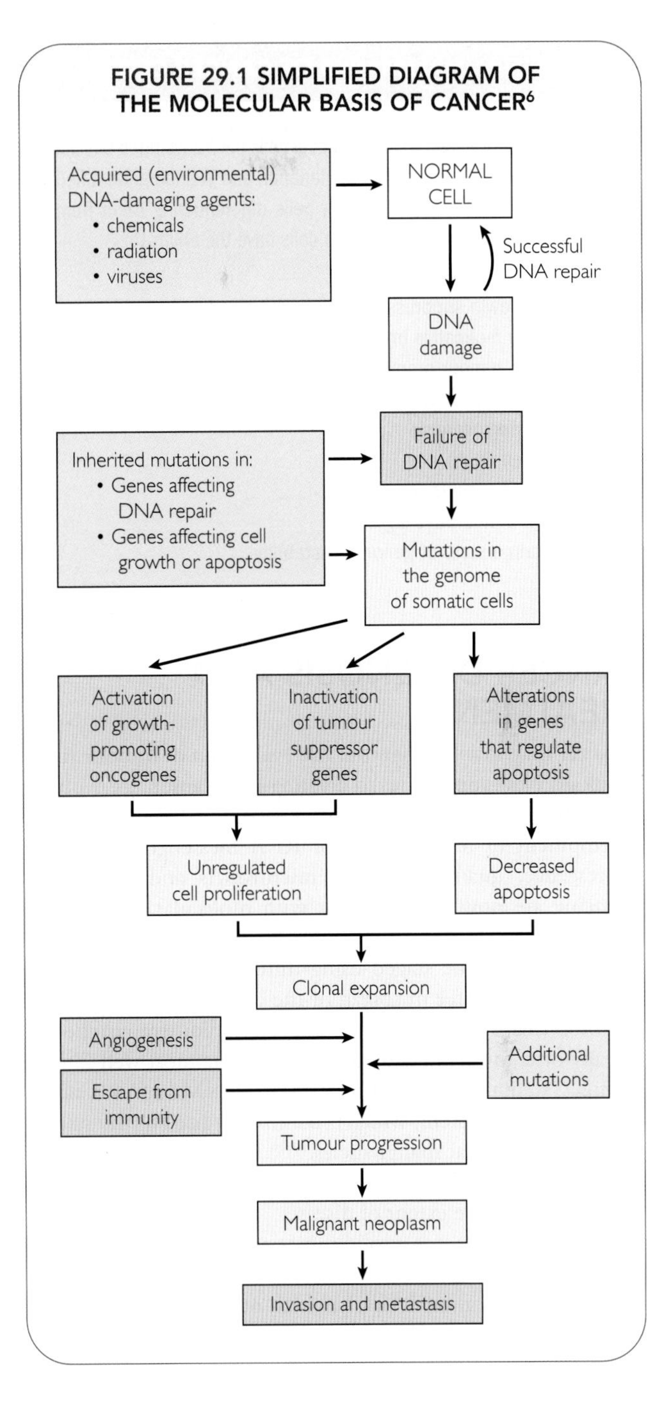

CANCER AND THE IMMUNE SYSTEM

Cancer cells are exquisitely refined to both manipulate their environment and evade immune detection (Box 29.1). To facilitate growth, the tumour surrounds itself with a supportive stroma providing nourishment and an inflammatory environment. It contains immunocompetent cells, such as T lymphocytes, macrophages, B cells and neutrophils, as well as cells normally associated with tissue repair—fibroblasts, endothelial cells and mesenchymal stem cells.[10] The regulatory mechanisms present in normal cellular growth and division break down in the malignant process, enabling tumour expansion. Healthy cells which usually cease replication when they come into contact with neighbouring tissue (*contact inhibition*) migrate into neighbouring tissues without boundaries.[11] Angiogenesis-promoting enzymes are released in order to supply the tumour with blood vessels to ensure adequate blood supply for expansion.[4]

The body has not evolved to be naive to this malignant cellular change. Specific lymphocytes are constantly circulating in order to detect cancer cells (immune surveillance). [7] Cancer cells display surface antigens, which under normal circumstances are recognised as 'non-self' by the immune system (tumour-associated antigens). Through a process of *immunological escape*, cancer cells are able to evade the immune system. [12] This is achieved by cancer cells:

- suppressing T cell stimulators
- expressing surface antigens weakly
- loss of antigenicity and/or loss of immunogenicity
- coordinating an immunosuppressive microenvironment
- blocking antibodies that bind to tumour-associated antigens
- inducing suppressor T cells. [7,12]

Immune checkpoints refer to a number of cellular pathways that are hard-wired into the immune system, whose normal function is to moderate the duration and amplitude of the body's immune responses in order to minimise damage to surrounding healthy tissue.[13] In short, checkpoints are the 'accelerator' or 'brake' pedals in immune responses, allowing them to be switched on or off. Activated T cells are important players in the immune response to foreign (or cancer) antigens, and express multiple checkpoint proteins. Two of note in oncology are cytotoxic T lymphocyte-associated 4 (CTLA-4) and programmed cell death protein 1 (PD-1).[14] Inhibition of CTLA-4 and PD-1 have been shown to enhance T-cell mediated immune responses. CTLA-4 and PD-1 are thus the targets for immunotherapy drugs, which have become very important in the treatment of a number of cancers. It is highly likely that drugs targeting specific parts of the immune pathway will become increasingly dominant in future cancer therapy.[14]

BOX 29.1 HALLMARKS OF CANCER CELLS[8,9]

In order to survive and to thrive, cancer cells have developed special characteristics. Seminal work by Hanahan and Weinberg identified a number of hallmarks of cancer cells differentiating them from normal cells.[10] Specifically, cancer cells have the ability to:

- avoid immune destruction
- evade growth suppressors
- maintain replicative immortality
- maintain tumour-promoting inflammation
- activate invasion and metastasis
- induce angiogenesis
- resist cell death
- deregulate cellular energetics
- sustain proliferative signalling
- maintain a state of genomic instability.

CANCER DIAGNOSIS AND TREATMENT

A cancer diagnosis is reliant on the evaluation of tumour tissue histology. New approaches to histologic evaluation are evolving and include immunohistochemistry analysis. Recent molecular development of identification of RNA messenger signatures, fluorescence, quantification of microRNAs and genetic sequencing are now used to assist with molecular diagnosis of many cancers.[4]

Tumours can be staged using different staging systems to determine the degree of spread of the cancer and to determine the best treatment approach (surgery, radiotherapy, chemotherapy or combinations of all of these). The most well-known staging system used internationally is the TNM (tumour, nodes and metastases) system, which is commonly used in the staging of solid oncological malignancies.[15,16] For haematological malignancies there are different staging systems that are used to grade and stage the extent of disease.

In simple terms, most solid tumour cancers can be staged in a four-step way:

- Stage 0: the cancer is 'in situ' with no spread at all.
- Stage 1: the cancer is small and has spread only a little into surrounding tissues and not at all into lymph nodes.
- Stage 2 and 3: the cancer is larger and has spread into nearby tissues or lymph nodes.
- Stage 4: the cancer has metastasised to distant sites of the body.

The traditional staging of cancer through histology, physical examination and imaging can have shortcomings. Considerable prognostic variation has been shown between patients of the same cancer stage using classification systems like the TNM.[15] The problem with this approach is that it focuses solely on the tumour and does not account for factors associated with host immune responses. As previously discussed, tumours are surrounded and infiltrated by large numbers of immune cells. Research in this area has demonstrated that the number, type and location of tumour-immune infiltrates in primary tumours are prognostic for response and overall survival.[15] Therefore, immunological 'scoring' is becoming an increasingly important part of the staging process.

Cancer staging has also changed considerably because of increasing commercial promotion of relatively affordable genome assays. This has meant that both tumour and host genomic profiles can be identified with the potential for 'precision' or 'personalised' medicine.[17] This can provide both prognostic and predictive information about, for example, the aggressiveness of the tumour and the likelihood of the patient responding to treatment. This, in turn, facilitates selection (or deselection) of appropriate targeted agent or treatment.[17,18] Excluding patients who are unlikely to respond to treatment spares them from toxicity symptoms and allows selection of more appropriate treatment.[19]

HAEMATOLOGICAL AND LYMPHOID MALIGNANCIES

Haematological and lymphoid tissue malignancies include a diverse group of diseases and include: lymphomas, leukaemias, myeloproliferative neoplasms, mast cell neoplasms, plasma cell neoplasms, histiocytic tumours and dendritic cell neoplasms. To classify these conditions, there are multiple classification schemes employed, Traditional classification systems use cytologic appearances of malignant cells. Immunophenotyping and cytogenetic and molecular genetic testing are used in more distinct entities to classify neoplasms.

The 2016 the World Health Organization (WHO) classified haematopoietic and lymphoid tumours into three categories:

1. Myeloid neoplasms—derived from bone marrow.
2. Lymphoid neoplasms—derived from B cell progenitors.
3. Histiocytic/dendritic neoplasms—derived from antigen presenting cells, i.e. dendritic cells.[20,21]

Leukaemia

Leukaemia is a malignant disorder of blood and blood-forming organs, characterised by excessive, abnormal growth of leucocyte precursors in the bone marrow. An uncontrolled increase in immature leucocytes decreases production and function of normal leucocytes (and other cell lineages).[21]

Different types of leukaemia peak at different ages, with acute myeloid leukaemia being most common in the over-60s and acute lymphoblastic leukaemia more common in children. Factors affecting the development of leukaemia are not clear, but may include a person's genetic history and exposure to intense radiation and certain chemicals, and viruses such as the human T-cell leukaemia virus.[21,22]

Leukaemia can affect either the granulocyte (myeloid) or lymphocyte (lymphocytic) lines, and may be either acute or chronic. Chronic leukaemias affect the blood cells when they are comparatively well differentiated. Acute leukaemia affects cells earlier in their maturation process, when they are closer to the undifferentiated stem cell (Fig. 29.2). There are four main leukaemias: acute myeloid leukaemia, chronic myeloid leukaemia, acute lymphoblastic leukaemia and chronic lymphoblastic leukaemia. Regardless of type, leukaemic cells have the capacity to invade the spleen, lymph nodes, liver and other vascular regions.[21,22]

Presentation with leukaemia may be subtle or more acute. Clinical manifestations include symptoms of fatigue, fever and weight loss. The patient may also complain of bone pain. Elevated uric acid levels, lymph node enlargement, hepatomegaly and splenomegaly are usually present. Neurological findings include headache, vomiting, papilloedema and blurred vision. Treatment

FIGURE 29.2 DEVELOPMENT OF BLOOD CELLS[23,24]

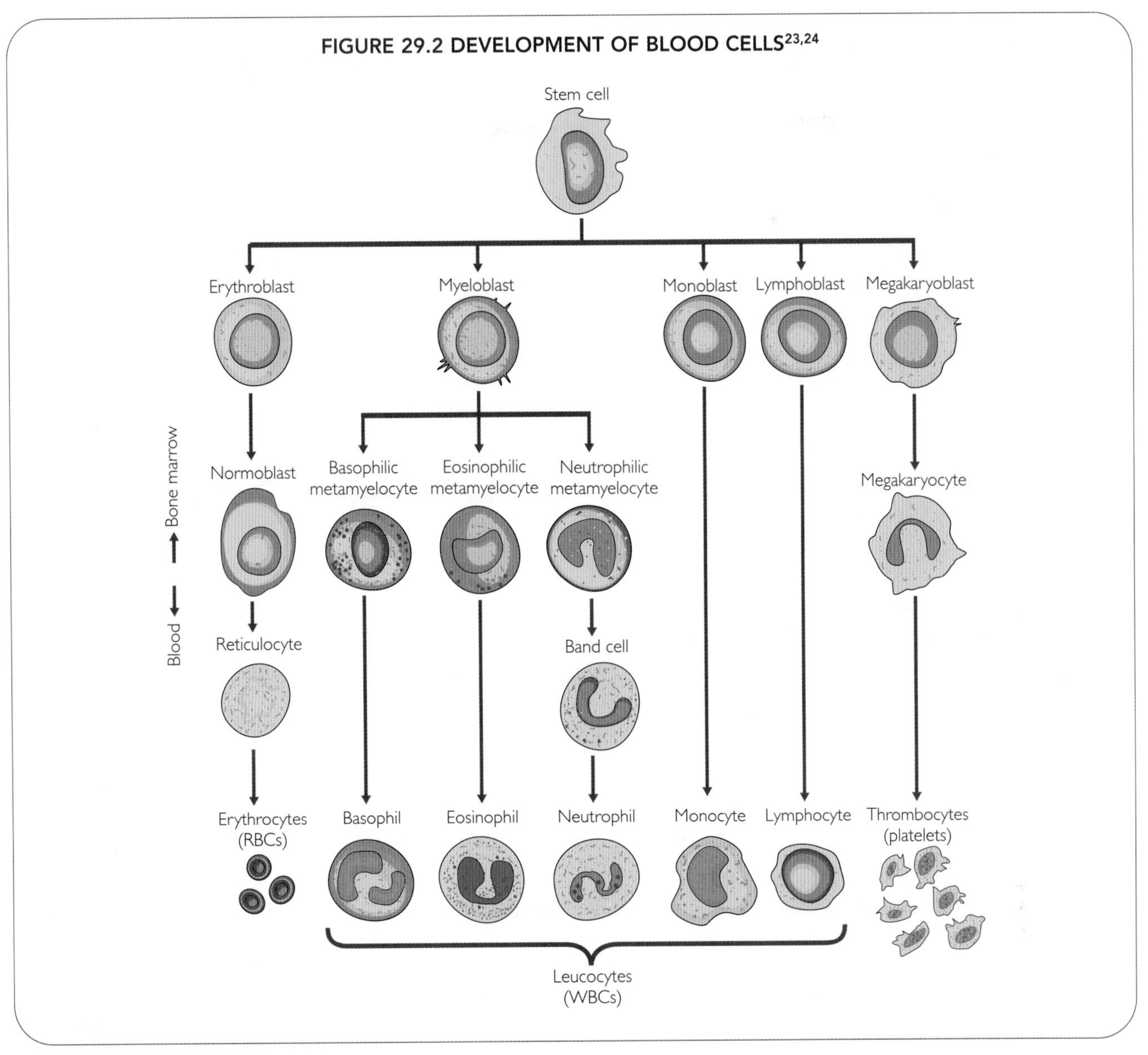

RBCs: red blood cells; WBCs: white blood cells.

for acute leukaemia generally begins within 24 hours of diagnosis and can include chemotherapy, radiotherapy, bone marrow or stem cell transplantation, or a combination of these.[21,22]

Lymphoma

Lymphomas are a diverse group of haematologic malignancies that derive from B cell, T cell or T/NK cell lineages or progenitor cells. They are a heterogeneous group of disorders caused by malignant lymphocytes that can accumulate in lymph nodes, leading to the characteristic clinical features of lymphadenopathy (Fig. 29.3). The clinical presentation can vary according to the histological subtype and the sites of involvement. Lymphoma may present as an oncological emergency as a new diagnosis or during the course of the disease and treatment. Burkett's lymphoma is a highly aggressive disease that requires prompt diagnosis and management as complications of the disease can be life threatening.[26,27]

Lymphomas are broadly divided into two distinct groups including Hodgkin lymphoma (HL) and non-Hodgkin lymphoma (NHL). The cause of lymphoma is not known; however, several key factors are thought to play a role in its development. These include infection with Epstein-Barr virus (EBV), genetic predisposition and exposure to occupational toxins such as herbicides, pesticides and benzene.[26–28]

Multiple myeloma

Multiple myeloma (MM) is a disease characterised by the malignant proliferation of plasma cells that produce a monoclonal immunoglobulin or paraprotein. Typically plasma cells proliferate and accumulate in the bone marrow leading to extensive skeletal destruction with lytic lesions, osteopenia and/or pathological fractures. Patients can present with symptoms related to this malignant process, including pain, increased serum protein, anaemia, hypercalcaemia or acute kidney failure.[29,30]

The cause of multiple myeloma is unknown, although exposure to radiation, organic chemicals (e.g. benzene), herbicides and insecticides may play a role, as may genetic factors and viral infection. The estimated number of new cases of MM in 2021

FIGURE 29.3 PALPABLE SUPERFICIAL LYMPH NODES[25]

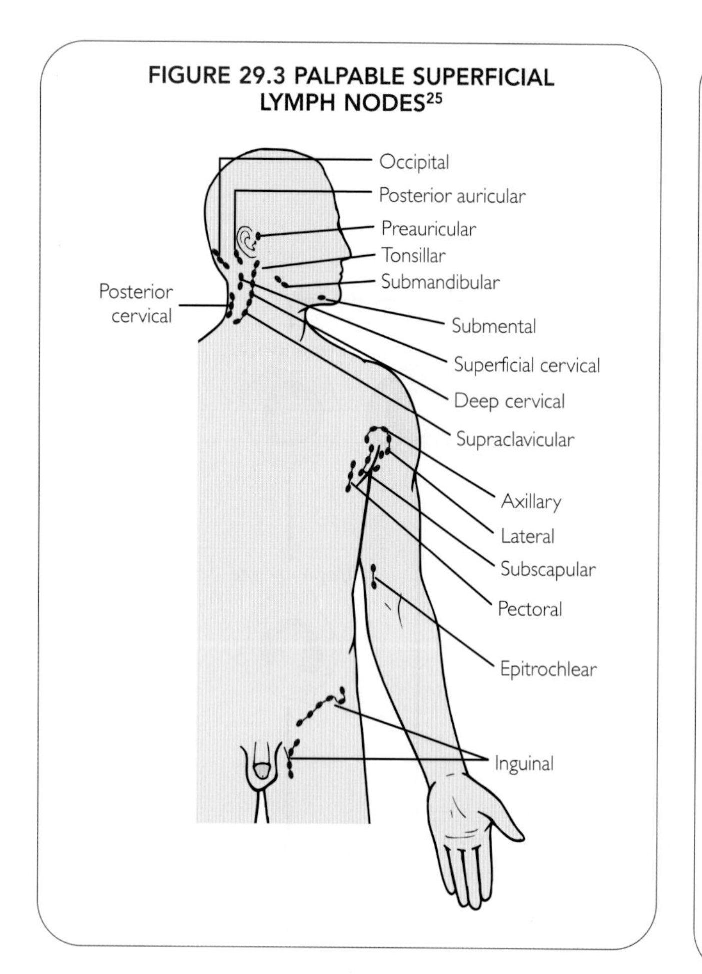

FIGURE 29.4 CELL CYCLE AND CANCER CHEMOTHERAPY[35]

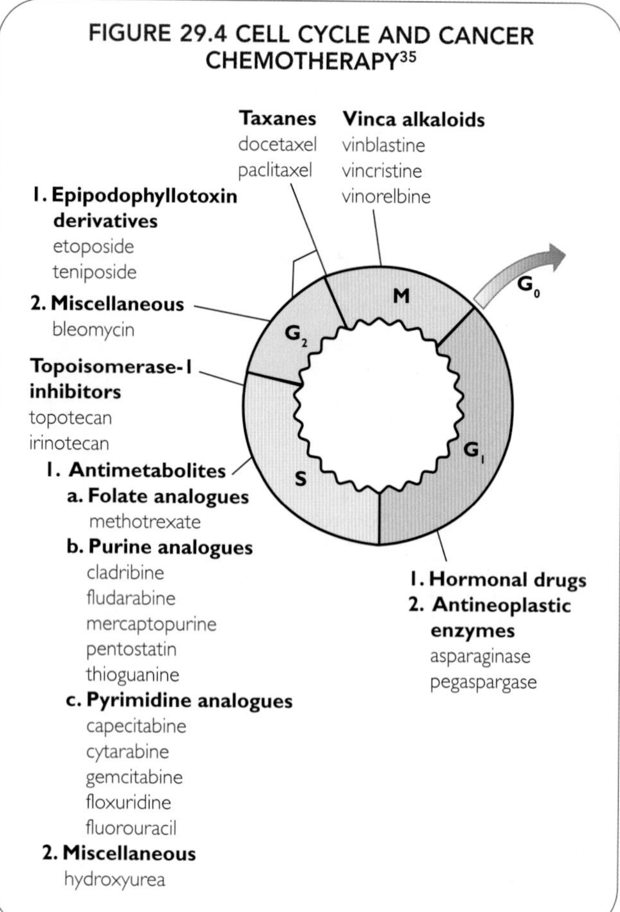

diagnosed in Australia was 2423.[31] Overall, MM is a rare disease, accounting for 1.6% of all cancers diagnosed in Australia.[31] MM is uncommon in people under 40 years of age, with almost 80% of all new cases diagnosed in people over the age of 60. It occurs more frequently in men than in women.[31]

CANCER THERAPY

Cancer treatments are wide ranging and are commonly managed by a range of specialties. Treatments are continually emerging and currently encompass one or a combination of: surgery, chemotherapy, radiotherapy, hormonal therapy, nuclear medicine, immunotherapy, CAR-T cell therapy and/or biological therapies.[32] Advances in the management of symptoms and improved supportive care interventions enable many patients receiving cancer treatment to be treated in outpatient clinics.[33]

Surgery

Surgery is an important treatment option for many cancers and is used to assist with the diagnosis and staging of the tumour. Surgery can constitute a complete cure without any further treatment (e.g. stage I or II tumours, in which complete resection is possible leaving negative tumour margins).[32,33] In other cases it can be used in combination with other therapies, including chemotherapy and radiotherapy, to assist with removing residual disease after completion of these treatments. In some circumstances surgery can be performed in the palliative setting to relieve symptoms caused from the tumour compressing or obstructing organs.[33]

Chemotherapy

Chemotherapy was first introduced into cancer therapy in the 1940s when the nitrogen mustards used in the First World War were recognised as having a cytotoxic effect.[7,32,34] Today there are many new chemotherapy drugs which are constantly being trialled, either on their own or in combination with other agents. The basic tenet of chemotherapy treatment is that it arrests the process of cell division during one of the phases of the cell cycle. The cell cycle is the process whereby the cell divides (Fig. 29.4). The diagram illustrates how different chemotherapy agents exert their effects at different stages of the cycle.

Chemotherapy is associated with a large range of acute and chronic adverse effects from mild to severe. The severity of adverse effects varies greatly between types of chemotherapy used and between individuals. Some side-effects are acute such as cytopenias, mucositis or diarrhoea, whereas other chemotherapy may cause long-term side-effects, such as nerve damage, infertility or heart and lung problems.

Acute toxicities include hypersensitivity reactions which may occur even after several exposures to a drug. Other side-effects are the result of chemotherapy's lack of specificity—chemotherapy targets *dividing* cells (not just *malignant dividing* cells). This means that chemotherapy drugs affect a number of body systems—particularly those which need rapid cell division to maintain their population, such as white blood cells. Neutropenia can be a major problem with some chemotherapy agents (see section on neutropenic sepsis).[36] Chemotherapy can also cause chronic organ damage, which may be exacerbated by other therapies such as radiotherapy or by infective episodes (e.g. pulmonary fibrosis, congestive heart failure). Table 29.2 lists how some common chemotherapy drugs can affect different organs. Below is a list of common side-effects from chemotherapy.

More common adverse effects of chemotherapy treatment

- *Nausea and vomiting*—can occur following treatment with chemotherapy. It can be acute, delayed, anticipatory, breakthrough or refractory to antiemetic therapy.[39]
- *Diarrhoea*—treatment-induced diarrhoea is the increased frequency and decreased consistency of bowel motions or ostomy output and can occur in response to chemotherapy. Patients may report abdominal pain, mucus or blood in the stool.

PRACTICE TIP

- Document the number of stools in 24 hours.
- Perform a stool specimen to eliminate an infective cause for the diarrhoea.

Note: some anticancer treatment can cause significant diarrhoea, so it is important to identify the treatment regimen.[40]

- *Constipation*—can occur as a result of chemotherapy agents, analgesia and antiemetics. There is an increased risk of constipation in patients diagnosed with gastrointestinal cancers, gynaecological malignancies and multiple myeloma.[41]

TABLE 29.2 SOME CYTOTOXIC AGENTS AND THEIR TOXICITIES[37,38]

TOXICITY	SYMPTOMS	SOME OF THE COMMON CHEMOTHERAPY AGENTS WHICH CAUSE THIS TOXICITY
Neurotoxicity	Cerebellar ataxia	Cytarabine
	Ototoxicity	Cisplatin, oxaliplatin
	Encephalopathy	Ifosfamide, cytarabine, 5-fluorouracil
	Peripheral neuropathies	Vincristine, vinblastine, paclitaxel, cisplatin, oxaliplatin
	Hemiparesis and facial palsy	Methotrexate
	Seizures	Busulphan, chlorambucil, procarbazine, temozolamide, vinblastine
Cardiovascular	Left ventricular dysfunction	Daunorubicin, doxyrubicin, epirubicin, high dose cyclophosphamide, cytarabine, mitoxantrone
	Dysrhythmias	Capecitabine, cisplatin, high-dose cyclophosphamide, daunorubicin, docetaxel, epirubicin, 5-fluorouracil
	Myocardial necrosis + myocarditis	Cyclophosphamide
	Pericarditis and pericardial effusion	Bleomycin, busulphan, cyclophosphamide, cytarabine, methotrexate
Pulmonary	Interstitial pneumonitis	Bleomycin, carmustine, chlorambucil, pacltitaxel, cyclophosphamide, etopiside, gemcitabine, irinotecan, mytomcin, mitoxantrone, methotrexate
	Non-cardiogenic pulmonary oedema	Cytarabine, docetaxel, gemcitabine
	Pulmonary fibrosis	Bleomycin, busulphan, carmustine, chlorambucil, cyclophosphamide, ifosphamide, melphalan, mercaptopurine, mitomycin C, oxaliplatin, procarbazine
Gastrointestinal	Oral mucositis	Methotrexate (can be severe and a sign of methotrexate toxicity), 5-fluorouracil
	Nausea and vomiting	Carmustine, cisplatin, cyclophosphamide, dacarbazine, temozolomide, chemotherapy combining more than one drug increases emetogenic potential to cause nausea & vomiting
	Diarrhoea	Irinotecan, 5-fluorouracil
Hepatic	Hepatic fibrosis	Methotrexate (chronic use)
	Hepatic necrosis	Dacarbazine, mercaptopurine
Renal/urological	Acute renal insufficiency	Carboplatin, irinotecan, oxaliplatin, carmustine
	Acute tubular necrosis	Cisplatin, iphosphamide, imatinib
	Chronic kidney disease	Cisplatin, gemcitabine, mitomycin C
	Haemorrhagic cystitis	Cyclophosphamide, ifosfamide

- *Pancytopenia*—neutropenia, thrombocytopenia and/or anaemia commonly occur after chemotherapy treatment and can lead to symptoms of infection, bleeding, anaemia and/or fatigue.[40]
- *Oral mucositis*—the erythematous ulceration of the mucous membranes of the oral mucosa and gastrointestinal tract, commonly occurring after chemotherapy and following radiotherapy treatment to the head, neck or oesophagus.
- *Peripheral neuropathy*—described as an altered sensation in the peripheries, including numbness, pain and weakness. It results from nerve damage related directly to some chemotherapy agents. Typically this is a symmetrical sensory neuropathy that can affect the fingers and toes, and can progress to the hands and feet. It occurs in response to some anticancer drugs, including taxanes, platinum-based compounds, vinca alkaloids and some drugs used to treat multiple myeloma.[39]

Table 29.2 lists how some common chemotherapy drugs can affect different organs.

Radiotherapy

Radiotherapy has been in clinical use since the beginning of the 20th century. It is an important primary adjuvant treatment option for many cancer types.[32] It is used as either a primary treatment or a combined treatment with systemic chemotherapy or surgery. Radiotherapy is also used in the management of patients in palliative care to manage difficult symptoms from advanced malignancy. Ionising radiation works by arresting cellular division and damaging cellular repair. Radiation treatment is associated with a number of toxicities, both localised (e.g. skin reactions) and systemic (fatigue).[41–43] The development of more targeted forms of radiotherapy (stereotactic radiotherapy) has facilitated *radiosurgery*, in which tumours that are difficult to access surgically can be treated with a high degree of accuracy using radiation with little damage to surrounding healthy tissues (e.g. prostate, brain tumours). Common side-effects from radiotherapy include:

- *radiation-induced cystitis*—occurs after acute radiation in the pelvic region and includes symptoms of cystitis, urinary frequency, urinary urgency, nocturia, bladder spasms and haematuria occurring in between 23–80% of patients.[40] Symptoms can be self-limiting and can last up to 3 months after treatment.
- *fatigue*—a common side-effect from radiation treatment, which can be pervasive and debilitating. Fatigue typically peaks towards the end of radiation treatment. Cancer-related fatigue is usually worst when the WBC counts are in the nadir 10–14 days following systemic treatment. Low haemoglobin levels also contribute to cancer-related fatigue symptoms.[40]
- *nausea and vomiting*—can occur when a patient receives radiation due to stimulation of the neurotransmitters that send impulses to the autonomic nervous system that induces nausea and stimulates the somatic and visceral system that leads to vomiting.[42]
- *skin reactions*—occur due to the damaging effects of ionising radiation in 95% of patients receiving radiation. Skin changes are visible within 2–3 weeks of treatment, including pruritus, erythema, dry or moist desquamation and can last for up to 2 weeks after treatment is completed.[40,43]
- *oral mucositis*—is the erythematous ulceration of the mucous membranes of the oral mucosa and gastrointestinal tract; commonly occurs after chemotherapy and following radiotherapy treatment to the head, neck or oesophagus.[40]

Immunotherapy

Immunotherapy drugs are monoclonal antibodies that target cytotoxic T lymphocyte-associated antigen 4 (CTLA4), and the programmed death-1 receptor (PD-1), and its ligand PD-L1 are becoming the standard of care for patients with certain types of cancer.[44] Traditional chemotherapy works by killing cancer cells through interfering with DNA synthesis, DNA replication and repair; in contrast, immunotherapy works by directly stimulating the immune system to enhance pre-existent anti-tumour immunity.[45,46]

Unlike traditional treatments, which often have acute and predictable toxicity, immune-related adverse events (irAEs) may occur at any time and involve any organ. The toxic effects from immunotherapy are caused by both on-target and off-target T cell toxicity against target antigens expressed in human tissue. This can lead to immune system enhancement, resulting in dermatological, gastrointestinal, hepatic, pulmonary, endocrine, neurological and other less common inflammatory processes. While most toxicities are mild, reversible and do not necessitate discontinuation of therapy, irAEs can be severe, such that early recognition and intervention are vital to reduce morbidity and mortality.[44] Clinicians need to be familiar and understand the individual drug toxicity profile to manage and mitigate the toxic effects to prevent adverse outcomes for patients.[47]

There are currently more patients receiving immunotherapy treatments due to government funding, clinical trials and wider indications for use. Therefore, irAEs related to treatment are presenting more commonly to outpatient cancer clinics and hospital EDs. It is important to know what type of immune checkpoint drug has been administered in order to determine the incidence and type of toxicity.[44] Furthermore, clinical trials combining two checkpoint inhibitors, nivolumab and ipilimumab, have demonstrated that irAEs were greater with combination therapy compared to when drugs were given individually.[48]

The most commonly occurring irAEs reported from immune checkpoint drugs can affect the skin, colon, endocrine organs, lungs and liver. Gastrointestinal (GI) toxicity is reported as a serious toxicity related to treatment with checkpoint inhibitors.[49] The most common symptom of GI toxicity is diarrhoea. It occurs frequently in 27–54% of patients treated with anti-CTLA4 checkpoint inhibitors. Severe diarrhoea can lead to a diagnosis of colitis, which if not managed carefully can progress to bowel obstruction, bowel perforation and possibly death. Rare and lethal toxicities, including hypophysitis, cardiac toxicity, rheumatologic, pancreatitis, neuropathies, diabetes, irdocyclitis, uveitis, nephritis and pneumonitis, have all been reported when using immune checkpoint inhibitors with varying degrees of severity.[44,49]

The incidence of irAEs can occur within weeks to 3 months after receiving treatment, but have also been reported up to 12 months following treatment and can be life threatening if not treated urgently. Treatment depends on the severity of symptoms presented and requires either temporarily or permanently withholding immunotherapy. Treatment with high-dose corticosteroids is the standard of care for grade 3–4 toxicities and patients require hospitalisation and specialist medical referral in accordance with the individual toxicity.[44,49]

Cytotoxic precautions

Prior chemotherapy administration should form part of the medical history for patients admitted to ED. This should include the agent/s used and the date of the last dose of chemotherapy administration (including tablets). This will be of significance in determining both cytotoxic status and in predicting blood count nadir. Patients undergoing chemotherapy will need to be managed using cytotoxic precautions if the last dose was administered within 7 days. (Box 29.2). Cytotoxic precautions require wearing a long-sleeved gown made from impermeable material, such as bonded polyethylene fibre, nitrile general purpose gloves, protective eyewear and a P2 (N95 mask) when handling patient body fluids.[50]

BOX 29.2 CYTOTOXIC PRECAUTIONS

Patients who are receiving infusional chemotherapy or have received chemotherapy within the last 48 hours may have cytotoxic residue in their blood, and therefore their body fluids should be treated as cytotoxic. This means avoiding handling body fluids (blood, urine, vomit, sputum) where possible. If contact is unavoidable, personal protective equipment (PPE) should be used—P2 mask, cytotoxic gloves, goggles and a cytotoxic gown (long-sleeved Tyvek gown).

- **Note that it is only necessary to wear protective clothing if handling body fluids—otherwise, contact with the patient should be completely normal.**
- **Disposal of cytotoxic waste should be in the designated cytotoxic bin.**

Radiation precautions

Patients are not radioactive when they receive external beam radiotherapy. Patients being treated for cervical, prostate or thyroid cancer may undergo brachytherapy, in which they have an implanted radioactive device that emits a low dose of radiation. This should not be hazardous to a normal healthy adult, but exposure to an infant, child or pregnant woman should be avoided.[40,51]

BIOLOGICAL THERAPIES

Advances in biological therapies that harness the immune system to identify and target cancer cells have led to an important new treatment modality for many cancer types. Biological therapies include haematopoietic growth factors, cytokines, erythropoietin, interferon, coagulation factors and monoclonal antibodies that target receptors on specific cancer cells.[52]

HAEMATOLOGICAL AND ONCOLOGICAL EMERGENCIES

The oncological and haematological emergencies that may present to the ED can result from an undiagnosed malignancy, symptoms related to anticancer treatment and/or the disease itself.

The different emergency scenarios described require prompt recognition and intervention in order to maximise best patient outcomes. Patients who present with advanced disease to the ED, and who are undergoing palliative care, should have advance care directives and resuscitation orders documented in their medical records so that clinicians can initiate the correct management for the patient.[53,54]

Cancer patients commonly present with pain to the ED.[55–58] For patients whose disease is incurable and whose treatment goals are palliative, correct management of these acute conditions can increase length and quality of life and minimise morbidity. In many cases, history and physical examination alone will be enough to alert the emergency clinician to one of the oncological or haematological emergencies discussed in this chapter.[55] On other occasions, however, it will be the blood count and coagulation screen that will be the key to diagnosis (Table 29.3).

TABLE 29.3 COAGULATION SCREEN

PARAMETER	NORMAL VALUE	WHAT IS BEING MEASURED	REASONS FOR ELEVATED VALUE
Prothrombin time (PT)—the international normalised ratio (INR) is calculated from the PT to take into account other coagulation variables	11-15 s	The time required for a fibrin clot to form via the extrinsic pathway	Liver disease, clotting factor deficiencies or patient on oral anticoagulants (where therapeutic goal is typically to maintain the value at 1.5-2.5 times the control value)
Partial thromboplastin time (PTT) or activated partial thromboplastin time (APTT)—APTT is a slightly more sensitive test	60-70 s; 25-38 s	The time required for a fibrin clot to form via the intrinsic pathway	Unfractionated heparin therapy, liver disease and clotting factor deficiencies (e.g. haemophilia), DIC, high-dose warfarin
Fibrinogen	200-400 mg/dL	Also known as factor I	Inflammatory response, acute infection, liver disease, DIC, menstruation, pregnancy, hyperthyroidism
D-dimer	400-500 ng/mL	D-dimer is a fibrin degradation product, indicating breakdown of the fibrin clot by plasmin	Pulmonary embolism, deep vein thrombosis, DIC, recent surgery, myocardial infarction/sepsis

In the next section we will look at emergencies related to an abnormal blood count or clotting screen, followed by a discussion of other cancer-related emergencies that may be encountered by emergency and paramedic staff that require expedited treatment and management.

HAEMATOLOGICAL EMERGENCIES

Emergencies in haematology patients can be classified broadly as conditions resulting from the cancer and/or resulting from complications related to the treatment directed against the malignancy itself. In addition to thorough physical assessment and comprehensive history, it is important to find out early during consultation what the patient has been told already. This is particularly important for those who have been newly referred from primary care with abnormal blood counts, as there may be significant anxiety and fear around a diagnosis of leukaemia or lymphoma.[54]

NEUTROPENIC SEPSIS IN HAEMATOLOGY AND ONCOLOGY PATIENTS

Neutropenic sepsis (also commonly referred to as febrile neutropenia) is one of the most common haemato-oncological emergencies. It is defined as an absolute neutrophil count (ANC) of $< 1.5 \times 10^9$/L (severe ANC < 0.5) in the presence of signs and symptoms of infection. In practice, the neutrophil count is often < 0.1.[59]

Immunosuppressed patients do not always show the signs and symptoms of infection, which can occur without fever, especially in the case of those patients taking corticosteroids.

Fever in this patient population is defined as a single oral temperature of greater than 38.3°C or a sustained temperature of greater than 38.0°C for more than 1 hour.[60] Further, neutropenic sepsis (FN) is defined as an oral temperature of $>$ 38.5°C or two consecutive readings of $>$ 38.0°C for 2 hours and an absolute neutrophil count (ANC) of $< 0.5 \times 10^9$/L, or expected to fall below 0.5×10^9/L.[34,60]

It is not usually the aim of outpatient chemotherapy regimens to render the patient severely neutropenic, but it is a potential toxicity, especially for patients with haematological malignancies. The neutrophil nadir can occur at any time from a few days to weeks post-chemotherapy administration, depending on the agents used.[34,60]

The depth and duration of neutropenia are the principal factors determining whether a patient will acquire an infection.[61] This risk is exacerbated by chemotherapy-induced mucosal damage, which allows the translocation of bacteria and fungi from the gut into the bloodstream.[54] Thus, in spite of all our attempts to manipulate the neutropenic patient's environment by reducing their contact with pathogens,[61] approximately 80% of neutropenic infections are believed to arise from the patient's own endogenous flora. In hospitalised patients, almost half of these infections are caused by organisms acquired during hospitalisation.[10,62]

Overall, the mortality rate from neutropenic sepsis is high, with reports in the literature of rates between 2% and 21%. Haematology patients are particularly at risk, with a mortality rate of 11% (compared with 1% for solid tumours).[34,60]

PRACTICE TIP

Questions to ask a patient with suspected neutropenic sepsis

- Is the patient post-stem cell transplant or do they have acute leukaemia?
- For a bone marrow/stem cell transplant patient, are they on immune suppression?
- When was the date of the last chemotherapy treatment given for acute leukaemia?

Note: Patients with acute leukaemia are at the highest risk of rapid onset neutropenic sepsis.

Management of neutropenic sepsis

Assessment

The absence of neutrophils in the neutropenic patient population can result in a lack of localising signs of infection and sometimes fever may be absent (more common in the elderly and patients taking steroids). For this reason, assessment must be thorough, observing for subtle signs, such as hypothermia, malaise or an isolated incidence of hypotension (Box 29.3).[60]

If neutropenic sepsis is suspected, the patient should undergo:

- comprehensive physical assessment
- FBC, EUC, CRP, LFT, CMP lactate, coagulation screen (DIC is a risk)
- blood cultures (peripheral and central lines), urinalysis and culture, sputum and stool microscopy
- swabbing of any skin lesions or wounds, including ostomies
- swabbing of central venous access catheters—including PICC lines, tunnelled catheters, power lines and implanted venous ports
- chest x-ray
- chemotherapy history (type, last dose).

Treatment

Any patient who is identified as febrile neutropenic must immediately commence empiric antibiotics to avoid progression to a sepsis syndrome. If not treated quickly, neutropenic sepsis can have a mortality rate of up to 50%.[60,64] International guidelines advocate that antibiotics should be commenced within 60 minutes.[64] One research paper reported that each hour of delay in antimicrobial treatment was associated with a 7.6% decrease in survival.[65] In practice, this means that it may not be possible to wait for all the microbiology samples to be obtained before beginning antibiotics.[34,60]

Ongoing management of the febrile neutropenic patient has been greatly assisted in recent years by the development of scales that allow stratification of patients according to risk, such as the MASCC (Multinational Association for Supportive Care in Cancer) scoring system.[66–68] High-risk patients will require close monitoring for signs of sepsis, admission for intravenous antibiotic and an aggressive approach to treatment. 'High risk' has been identified as a patient exhibiting one or more of the following risk factors:[60]

- ANC < 0.5 anticipated to last $>$ 7 days
- haemodynamic instability

BOX 29.3 **PRACTICE TIPS FOR THE FEBRILE NEUTROPENIC PATIENT**

ASSESSMENT

If neutropenic sepsis is suspected, the outcome is significantly improved by expedited action. Remember that a neutropenic patient may not necessarily have a temperature, but may still be septic; for example, paracetamol and corticosteroids can mask a temperature. Treat any abnormal signs with suspicion (e.g. confusion, decreased level of consciousness, hypotension, tachycardia, etc.). Also assess for symptoms or signs suggesting an infection focus, notably the presence of an indwelling venous catheter, infected central line and localised signs in the:

- respiratory system
- gastrointestinal tract
- skin
- perineal region/genitourinary discharges
- oropharynx
- central nervous system.[63]

INVESTIGATIONS

- Blood testing—full blood count; electrolytes, urea and creatinine (EUC); coagulation; C-reactive protein (CRP)
- Blood cultures (minimum two sets), including cultures from indwelling venous catheter
- Urinalysis and culture
- Sputum microscopy and culture
- Stool microscopy and culture (if diarrhoea present)
- Skin lesions/central lines (aspirate/biopsy/swab)
- Chest x-ray
- It may be helpful to also take a cross-match at this time.

On some occasions there may be a delay in obtaining some samples (e.g. stool, sometimes chest x-ray). If delay is unavoidable and likely to be protracted, antibiotics should be commenced immediately.

THERAPY

Intravenous hydration and if necessary oxygen therapy should be commenced immediately.

As soon as the septic screen is completed, intravenous antibiotics should be given. It is important to start these as soon as possible—do not wait, for example, for the next scheduled dose time.

Some institutions have programs that treat neutropenic patients with oral antibiotics on an outpatient basis. These patients will have to meet certain criteria in order to establish that they are 'low risk' and institutional guidelines should be followed.

- oral or gastrointestinal mucositis or severe diarrhoea
- neurological or mental status changes of new onset
- intravascular device infection
- new pulmonary infiltrates or hypoxaemia
- underlying lung disease
- uncontrolled or progressive cancer
- hepatic or renal dysfunction.

Today, prophylactic granulocyte stimulating factors are widely used to reduce the depth and duration of chemotherapy, especially among the higher-risk population. These growth factors include recombinant human granulocyte colony stimulating factor (g-CSF and pegylated G-CSF) and granulocyte-macrophage colony stimulating factor (GM-CSF). A number of consensus-based guidelines recommend the use of these agents when the anticipated incidence of neutropenic fever is 20% or higher.[67] Their use in the case of established fever and neutropenia is controversial. Despite their documented effects on neutropenia, prophylactic use of G-CSFs has not been shown to have an impact on survival in most clinical situations.[60]

Antibiotic regimens will vary between institutions and over time, dictated by trends in microbial prevalence. Interestingly, an infectious source is identified in only 20–30% of febrile neutropenic episodes.[61] Most commonly, however, the infective organisms are bacterial, although fungal infections may arise in higher risk populations. If a causative organism cannot be found and the patient remains febrile after 7 days of broad-spectrum antibiotics without a positive blood culture, it is recommended that the patient should be considered for antifungal cover.[60,69]

Low-risk patients, while still requiring expedited treatment, are less likely to develop sepsis and may be eligible for oral antibiotics and discharge home. 'Low risk' is defined as patients who are expected to be neutropenic for less than 7 days, who have no active comorbidities and no evidence of significant hepatic or renal dysfunction. Many cancer patients with solid tumours fall into this category.

PRACTICE TIP

Colony-stimulating factors administered to boost the neutrophil count are given as subcutaneous injections and are generally well tolerated. Toxicities include injection site reactions, arthralgias and myalgias, which are well managed with paracetamol.

SEPSIS

Unsuccessful emergency management or late presentation of the neutropenic patient will result in sepsis. A patient with sepsis[70] is around five times more likely to die than a patient who has suffered a heart attack or stroke.[70,71]

The global sepsis incidence is estimated to range from 22 to 240 per 100,000 people.[70] Fatality rates can reach up to 30% for sepsis, 50% for severe sepsis and 80% for septic shock.[70]

Sepsis is defined as a life-threatening dysfunction of the organs that is caused by an inappropriate regulation response by a patient to an infective event.[70] Sepsis is a continuum of states ranging from early sepsis (fever, bacteraemia) to septic shock ('sepsis that has circulatory, cellular and metabolic abnormalities that are associated with a greater mortality rate than sepsis alone').[70] The SOFA (sequential organ failure assessment) system has now been nominated to identify patients who are becoming septic—specifically the quick-SOFA (qSOFA) scale, a user-friendly tool with accurate prognostic value when used outside the ICU setting (Box 29.4).[70,71]

Those at high risk of developing sepsis are:[70,71]

- patients with cancer
- patients receiving treatment for cancer

BOX 29.4 QSOFA SCORING SYSTEMATIC[72]

QSOFA involves assessing three parameters:

- respiratory rate > 22 breaths/minute
- altered mentation
- systolic blood pressure < = 100 mmHg

Each scores 1 point and a score of > = 2 is associated with a poor outcome through sepsis.

- those who have had recent chemotherapy—administered last 7 days
- post-stem cell transplant recipients
- older adults.

The NSW Surviving Sepsis Campaign Guidelines for Management of Severe Sepsis and Septic Shock provides a framework for the management of the septic patient in the ED and inpatient areas.[73] The clinical picture of sepsis is similar to cardiovascular shock and/or respiratory failure including tachycardia, tachypnoea, hypotension, peripheral vasodilation, with or without fever >38°C.[70,71] Potential septic patients in ED should undergo urgent clinical assessment and management, including:

- administering oxygen
- venous access
- collecting bloods, including FBC/EUC/blood cultures/LFT/CMP/CRP lactate/coagulations screen/blood gas arterial
- commencing fluid resuscitation
- initiating septic screen (refer to local policies)
- administering empiric antibiotics within 30 minutes—DO NOT wait for blood results or septic screen
- consulting fluid balance chart—monitor urine output
- notifying intensive care/high dependency unit if indicated
- maintaining MAP > 65 mmHg and urine output > 0.5 mL/kg/hr
- if no improvement in MAP, administer vasopressors.[70]

Referral of the patient to appropriate retrieval or in-patient teams is essential for optimal care.

The Surviving Sepsis Campaign recently updated its guidelines providing an indication of the evidence base for each intervention.[70,71,73]

HYPER VISCOSITY

Hyper viscosity is defined as an increase in whole-blood viscosity as a result of an increase in either red blood cells, white blood cells or plasma components such as immunoglobulin. Excessive production of one protein or cell type may lead to hyper viscosity of the blood, which can cause leucostasis and inadequate organ perfusion—an emergency situation.[74,75]

Common haematology presentations associated with hyper viscosity are:

- Waldenström's macroglobulinaemia: involves over-production of immunoglobulin M (IgM)—a very large protein.[74]
- Multiple myeloma: where there is a proliferation of serum paraprotein.[29]
- Polycythaemia: the exponential rise in red blood cell volume—haematocrit of 0.5 or greater.[76]
- Acute leukaemias (AML, ALL): high blast cell count in peripheral blood at initial presentation.[22]

Hyper viscosity may be a presenting feature of a disease or may occur in its later stages.

Signs and symptoms

Signs and symptoms of hyper viscosity occur when plasma viscosity exceeds three times the normal value and are like those of leucostasis. Signs and symptoms may include dyspnoea and cough, mucosal bleeding (especially oronasal), visual disturbances, retinal haemorrhage and neurological symptoms, such as lassitude, confusion, dizziness and vertigo. Patients may also present with kidney failure due to congestion of the renal tubules. Hyper viscosity may be fatal if untreated and hence is classified as a haematological emergency.[75]

Management

If suspected, consult the apheresis unit immediately for prompt machine leukapheresis. If not available, venesection is recommended and replacement with isovolaemic fluid. Treatment is by therapeutic plasma exchange (TPE) in combination with chemotherapy. TPE involves the removal of a volume of diseased plasma and its replacement with healthy plasma or plasma substitute. The procedure uses the same apheresis machine that is used for leucostasis. Coagulation is checked pre- and post-procedure as replacement of clotting factors may be required.[75]

LEUCOSTASIS

Leucostasis is a condition in which there is an excessive number of circulating blast cells (abnormal immature white cells), usually in the capillaries, resulting in decreased tissue perfusion and subsequent organ damage. It is considered to be a medical emergency and is commonly seen in patients with acute myeloid leukaemia or chronic myeloid leukaemia in blast crisis.[77]

Common presentations of leucostasis are seen in:

- acute myeloid leukaemia, usually at diagnosis when there is a high circulating peripheral blast count.[77]
- chronic myeloid leukaemia in blast crisis (a stage of the disease in which there is a dramatic increase in circulating blast cells).

Patients presenting with leucostasis have a 20%–40% increased risk of death from severe pulmonary and neurological complications. Approximately 40% of these patients will also experience DIC and 10% will develop tumour lysis syndrome.[77]

Signs and symptoms

Leucostasis is a medical emergency. It is associated with the following symptoms:

- respiratory failure
- neurological symptoms (headache, tinnitus, confusion, potential spontaneous cranial haemorrhage)
- fever
- anaemia (although patients should not be transfused until the hyper viscosity has been rectified)
- visual (retinal haemorrhage, blurred vision)
- kidney failure
- severe metabolic abnormalities: hyperkalaemia, hyperphosphataemia, hyperuricaemia.[77]

Management

Urgent cytoreduction via leucapheresis is required for patients with marked leucostasis (> 50×10^9/L). Referral to the apheresis unit is indicated for urgent leucapheresis. Leucapheresis separates the blood into different blood components by either centrifugation or membrane filtration, and allows the removal of blasts and excess WBC.[77]

The role of apheresis in leucostasis has never been definitively proved in a randomised, controlled trial, and it has been argued that the procedure may not necessarily prevent death more efficiently than fluid therapy and the prompt initiation of chemotherapy.[78] AML patients with leucostasis have an increased mortality rate and reduced response rate to treatment when compared with leukaemia patients who do not have it.[77]

SICKLE CELL CRISIS IN ADULTS

Sickle cell disease (SCD) refers to one of the syndromes in which the sickle mutation is co-inherited—it includes sickle cell anaemia, sickle-beta thalassemia and haemoglobin SC disease. It is most prevalent in tropical Africa and parts of the Mediterranean, Middle East and India, occurring rarely in Caucasian people. While most serious acute complications of SCD occur during childhood, chronic symptoms are ongoing and worsen with age.[79,80]

SCD results from the production of abnormal haemoglobin which elongates into a sickle shape when it becomes deoxygenated. Subsequent re-oxygenation can reverse the process, but after repeated episodes the red cells become irreversibly sickled.[80] These sickled cells can result in the clinical manifestations of SCD—the major features being haemolytic anaemia and vaso-occulsion.[80]

Signs and symptoms

Clinical manifestations vary markedly between individuals and may be related to vascular obstruction and vaso-occlusion, severe anaemia or infection. Additionally, complications of long-term therapy can cause significant morbidity, particularly related to high iron burden secondary to chronic transfusion requirements and adverse effects related to opioid pain medication. Episodes of acute pain are one of the most common types of veno-occlusive events in SCD patients. They are responsible for a large number of emergency presentations and should be managed promptly.[80]

Assessment

Frequently patients will present to the ED with acute pain, although the nature and severity and duration varies significantly between people. Careful assessment of the sickle cell patient is required because episodes of pain can sometimes mask underlying pathology, such as acute chest syndrome, acute multi-organ failure, acute surgical abdomen (e.g. cholecystitis) or splenic sequestration.[80]

Management

Sickle cell crisis is an emergency. Seek urgent advice of senior haematology clinician.

Management includes:

- intravenous fluids and oxygen
- septic screening, including blood, urine and sputum cultures, chest x-ray
- commencing empirical antibiotic therapy if infection is suspected—do not await culture results
- analgesia as indicated—consider opiates in this patient group.[80]

OVERDOSAGE OF ANTI-THROMBOLYTIC THERAPIES

Anti-thrombolytic therapies are effectively used in a wide range of thromboembolic disorders for primary and secondary prevention and therapy. However, overdosage of any of the above listed agents can lead to life-threatening haemorrhage requiring emergency management. There are differences in how each class of agent is managed and monitored. Refer to local policies, national/international guidelines and seek senior haematology clinical advice.[81] Assess the severity of bleeding and the degree of anticoagulation through the patient's history and physical examination.

THROMBOLYTIC AGENTS

The risk of bleeding from anticoagulant therapy is a haemorrhagic complication from treatment. Signs of haemorrhage associated with anticoagulation include: bleeding or haematomas from venepuncture sites, bruising, surgical wounds, haematuria, epistaxis, headaches associated with possible intracranial haemorrhage.

Initial management of haemorrhage:

- consider allocating patient to the resuscitation area within ED
- discontinue anticoagulant medication
- discontinue any other anti-platelet agents
- apply local pressure to superficial bleeding sites
- administer intravenous volume replacement as required
- coagulation screening, including fibrinogen and continue monitoring
- FBC, LFT, EUC, CRP, blood transfusion group and hold
- cryoprecipitate, fresh frozen plasma and platelets may be required—seek haematology clinician advice.

Heparin

The mechanism of action of heparin is by directly binding to antithrombin lll and inactivate clotting factors lla (thrombin) and Xa. Heparin can cause severe thrombocytopenia and haemorrhage. Seek specialist haematology advice for management for reversal instructions.[81]

Warfarin

Warfarin is administered and monitored regularly (using INR) to maintain a therapeutic drug range. Haemorrhage secondary to warfarin overdosage may occur even in the setting of normal range INR. Treatment with intravenous vitamin K may be indicated to reverse the effect of warfarin within 24–48 hours for any bleeding. The use of fresh frozen plasma or prothrombin complex concentrate may be indicated in some cases for major bleeding caused by warfarin.[81]

Direct oral anticoagulants (DOACs)

DOACs reversibly inhibit coagulation factors and have a shorter half-life than wafarin.[82] The risk of major bleeding is low, but life-threatening haemorrhages have occurred.

Initial management:

- discontinue medication
- manage bleeding anatomically, pressure, surgery, gastroscopy
- administer blood products as required
- administer anticoagulant reversal agent. Refer to local and national guidelines specialist haematology advice.[83]

THROMBOCYTOPENIA EMERGENCIES

Thrombocytopenia results in a number of different clinical conditions and will not necessarily constitute an emergency. In certain conditions including chronic liver disease splenomegaly may be present leading to thrombocytopenia. Box 29.5 explains the workings of the spleen and its role in storing platelets. It also explains the causes of splenomegaly.

THROMBOTIC THROMBOCYTOPENIC PURPURA

TTP is always a medical emergency as without the prompt and appropriate treatment it is almost always fatal.[85,86] With appropriate treatment, survival rates of up to 90% are achieved.[85] In TTP, a deficiency in ADAMTS13 (an enzyme involved in clotting) brings about thrombotic microangiopathy (clotting in the capillaries), thrombocytopenia and haemolysis.[85]

TTP is a rare disorder that most commonly affects young adults, with the median age of diagnosis 41 years.[85] TTP can be acquired or hereditary, with approximately three cases of acquired TTP per one million adults per year. Hereditary TTP is extremely rare.[87]

Pregnancy and the postpartum state account for 12–25% of cases of TTP and the disorder is often associated with cancer. Other causes include toxins (e.g. from *Escherichia coli*), spider and bee venoms (see Chapter 30) or human immunodeficiency virus (HIV).

BOX 29.5 THE SPLEEN[84]

The spleen is an organ which is involved in the physiology of blood at various different stages.

1. **Erythropoietic: production of RBCs during fetal development.**
2. **Filtering: the spleen removes old and defective erythrocytes from the circulation.**
3. **Immunity: the spleen contains a rich supply of lymphocytes and monocytes. Splenectomy renders individuals at a very high risk of sepsis, and is discussed more fully below.**

Storage of platelets: an increase in spleen size (splenomegaly) results in an increase in the splenic platelet pool to the point that it might account for up to 90% of total body platelets. This leads to peripheral thrombocytopenia.

A large spleen results in abdominal pain and, depending on the cause, a splenectomy may be indicated. Splenomegaly may be caused by the following factors:[84]

- **haematological–lymphomas, leukaemias, haemolytic anaemias, haemoglobinopathies**
- **infectious–bacterial endocarditis, glandular fever, tuberculosis, malaria and a range of parasitic infections**
- **immunological–rheumatoid arthritis, systemic lupus erythematosus, sarcoidosis**
- **other–cysts, malignancies (rare), hyperthyroidism, portal hypertension–liver cirrhosis, right-sided heart failure.**

After splenectomy, IgM levels are reduced, and patients have a lifelong risk of infection, especially from organisms such as *Pneumococcus*, which is reduced by immunisation. Following splenectomy patients can present with overwhelming sepsis from encapsulated bacteria (*Pneumococcus, Neisseria meningitidis*). Such patients can deteriorate very quickly and require immediate treatment with intravenous antibiotics in the same way as febrile neutropenic patients (see Victorian Spleen Register in Useful resources).

Signs and symptoms

Immune TTP usually presents as severe microangiopathic haemolytic anaemia (MAHA) and thrombocytopenia (< 30) with or without symptoms in a previously healthy individual. Presenting symptoms can be subtle and nonspecific, including fatigue, dyspnoea, petechiae, dizziness, abdominal pain, and/or fever. In these patients the first indication of a possible TTP diagnosis is the full blood count that reveals severe thrombocytopenia and MAHA—the hallmarks of TTP.[85] Transient neurological defects are present with major neurological findings in 50% of patients. Kidney failure may occur late in the disease process.[85,87]

Management of TTP

Seek expert haematology advice and early involvement.

Initial treatment is to arrest any bleeding and provide supportive therapy.[88]

With presumptive diagnosis of TTP, several therapies are available:

- therapeutic plasma exchange—mainstay of treatment. Initiate as soon as possible
- glucocorticosteroids
- rituximab (monoclonal antibody).

Platelet transfusion is contraindicated unless there is active bleeding, but in some situations (when TPE cannot be instituted early enough), plasma infusions may be administered.[89]

HEPARIN-INDUCED THROMBOCYTOPENIA (HIT)

HIT is a severe prothrombotic adverse reaction following heparin administration, characterised by platelet-activating antibodies that recognise and bind to platelet factor 4 (PF4), heparin complexes PF4 activate platelets, causing arterial and venous thrombosis with a mortality rate as high as 20%.[90]

Suspect HIT in a patient receiving heparin who has a decrease in platelet count of more than 50% from baseline—even if maintained in the normal range. A higher risk of HIT has been observed among:

- women
- patients receiving unfractionated heparin rather than low molecular weight heparin
- surgical rather than medical patients
- older patients
- patients undergoing longer duration of therapy.[91]

The 4 Ts scoring system is recommended to assess for suspected HITS (Table 29.4). Unlike other forms of thrombocytopenia,

TABLE 29.4 THE 4 TS CLINICAL SCORING SYSTEM[92]

CATEGORY	2 POINTS	1 POINT	0 POINTS
Thrombocytopenia	Platelet count falls > 50% and platelet nadir $\geq 20 \times 10^9$/L	Platelet count falls 30–50% and platelet nadir 10–19 $\times 10^9$/L	Platelet count falls < 30% and platelet nadir < 10×10^9/L
Timing	Clear onset between 5 and 10 days or platelet fall $\leq$ 1 day (prior heparin exposure within 30 days)	Consistent with days 5–10 fall, but not clear (e.g. missing platelet counts), or onset after day 10, or fall $\leq$ 1 day (prior heparin exposure 30–100 days ago)	Platelet count fall < 4 days without recent heparin exposure
Thrombosis	New thrombosis (confirmed), or skin necrosis at heparin injection sites, or acute systemic reaction after intravenous heparin bolus	Progressive or recurrent thrombosis, or non-necrotising (erythematous) skin lesions, or suspected thrombosis (not proven)	None
Other causes of thrombocytopenia	Non-apparent	Possible	Definite

Probability of HIT: high, 6 to 8 points (21.4% to 100%); intermediate, 4 or 5 points (7.9% to 28.6%); low, 0 to 3 points (0% to 1.6%).

HIT: heparin-induced thrombocytopenia.

HIT is generally not associated with bleeding, instead with venous thromboembolism—the most common complication. Symptoms typically occur 4 to 10 days after the initiation of heparin therapy, although they may be seen later, even after discontinuation of heparin.

Complications include deep venous thrombosis, pulmonary embolism, myocardial infarction, occlusion to limb arteries, skin necrosis, and transient ischemic attack thrombosis, which may be venous (20–50%) or arterial (3–10%).[93]

Seek senior haematology clinical advice and refer to local policies.

Management of suspected or confirmed HITS

- Cease heparin and related products immediately.
- Initiate non-heparin anticoagulants.
- Warfarin (if used) should be postponed until platelet recovery is above 150×10^9/L.

Platelet transfusions are not recommended as they may increase the risk of thrombotic events unless the patient is actively bleeding or for prophylaxis prior to invasive or surgical procedures.[91,94]

THE PATIENT WHO IS BLEEDING

A patient who is bleeding in the absence of significant trauma or thrombocytopenia is likely to have a coagulopathy. Haemostasis refers to the processes that prevent blood loss after vascular damage (i.e. vascular spasm, platelet aggregation, coagulation and fibrinolysis). When injury occurs, the initial response is reflex vasoconstriction. Arterioles contract, reducing blood flow by decreasing vessel size and pressing endothelial surfaces together. Serotonin and histamine are released, also bringing about vasoconstriction and decreased blood flow to the injured area. Vasoconstriction is followed by platelet aggregation at the injury site, which prevents bleeding by sealing capillaries. This temporary measure may last for 20–30 minutes, allowing time for clotting factors to work. Clot formation requires activation of the coagulation cascade (Fig. 29.5). The coagulation cascade is a complex network of 12 different clotting factors (Table 29.5), and a defect of any clotting factor or an injury that overwhelms the entire system can cause its failure, leading to life-threatening haemorrhage. The coagulation cascade consists of two pathways: the intrinsic and the extrinsic. Physiologically, the two pathways work together, resulting in the stimulation of factor X, which (in the presence of factor V) activates the conversion of prothrombin to thrombin. The end result of the coagulation cascade is formation of a clot—a protein mesh made of fibrin strands.[90]

The process of haemostasis must also include clot resolution. The fibrinolytic system maintains the blood in a fluid state by removing clots that are no longer needed. Without this system, circulation to affected areas may be permanently lost because of obstructed blood vessels. In the clinical situation, blood coagulation is measured by performing a coagulation screen. The different elements of this screen are described in Table 29.3. There are a number of steps in the clotting cascade at which problems can occur and lead to an increased risk of bleeding. These are the result of clotting-factor abnormalities rather than platelet deficiency. Factor abnormalities may be either be inherited or acquired. Haemophilia is a hereditary clotting factor disorder of factor VIII. Acquired factor abnormalities include vitamin K deficiency, liver disease or disseminated intravascular coagulation (DIC).[90]

TREATMENT OF BLEEDING IN HAEMOPHILIA

Haemophilia A and B are X-linked coagulation factor disorders associated with bleeding of variable severity from life threatening to clinically silent.[95] The availability of factor replacement is essential in bleeding management, though patients do present to ED with acute bleeding symptoms requiring rapid intervention.

Haemophilia is an inherited, gender-linked disorder that occurs almost always in males. Currently there are approximately 2700 people in Australia with haemophilia and approximately

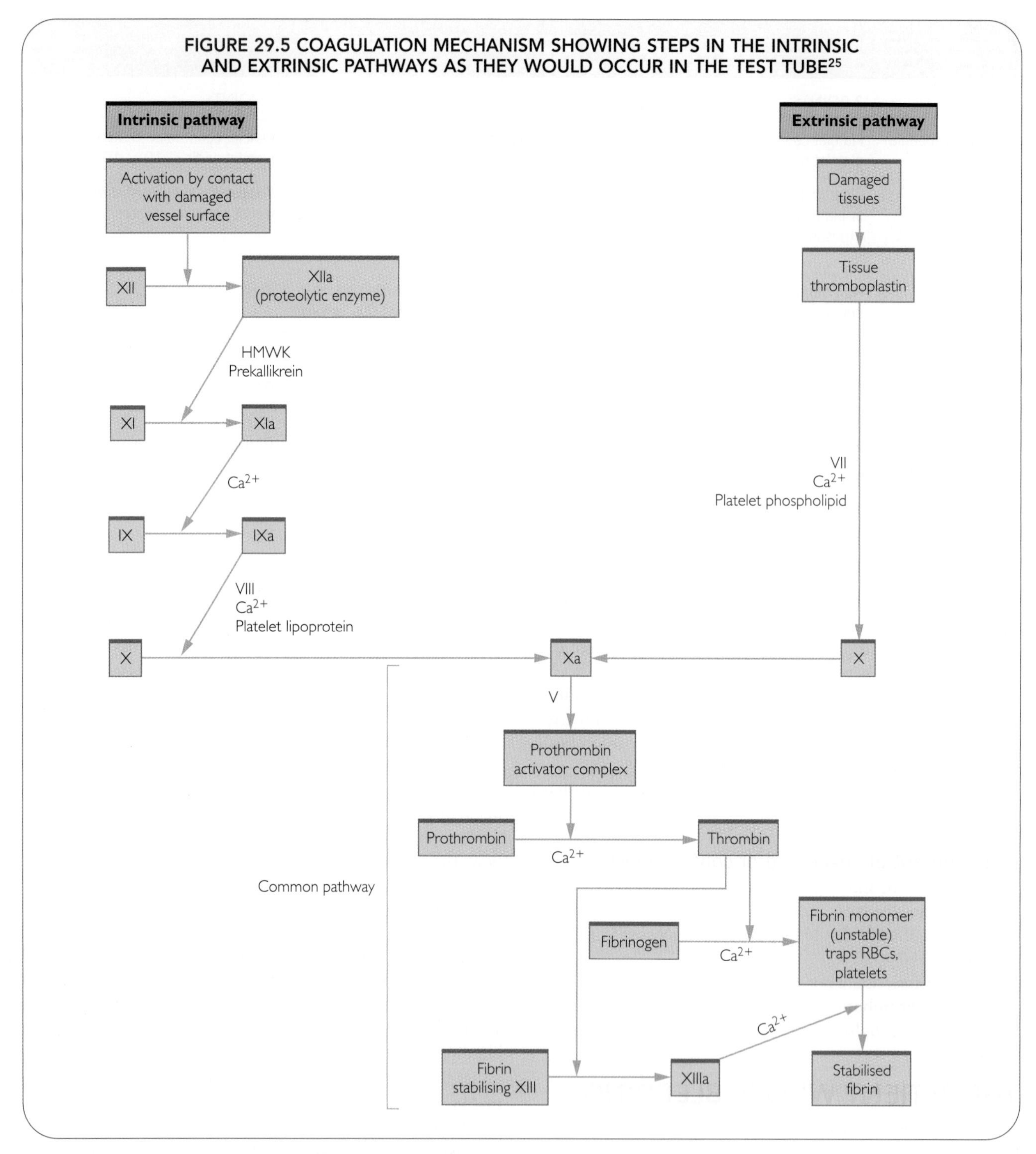

HWMK: high-molecular-weight kininogen; RBCs: red blood cells.

430 in Aotearoa New Zealand. Severity ranges from mild (6–60%) to severe (< 1%). The primary defect in haemophilia is absence or dysfunction of a specific clotting factor.[96]

Haemophilia A is due to a factor VIII disorder. In the majority of patients with haemophilia A, factor VIII is not missing; it may even be present in excess quantities. However, available factor VIII does not function adequately. Disease severity is directly related to the functional activity of factor VIII.[95]

Haemophilia B, or Christmas disease, occurs less often than haemophilia A. It is caused by the absence or functional deficiency of factor IX.[95]

Signs and symptoms

Haemophilia A and B have similar clinical presentations. Bleeding tends to be spontaneous or following trauma (including minimal trauma).[95,96]

TABLE 29.5 COAGULATION FACTORS

FACTOR	SYNONYMS	DESCRIPTION/FUNCTION
I	Fibrinogen	Fibrin precursor
II	Prothrombin	Is converted to thrombin in the presence of thromboplastin and calcium
III	Tissue thromboplastin	Thrombin precursor
IV	Calcium	Essential for prothrombin activation and fibrin formation
V	Labile factor, proaccelerin	Accelerates conversion of prothrombin to thrombin
VII	Prothrombin conversion accelerator	Accelerates conversion of prothrombin to thrombin
VIII	Antihaemophilic factor (AHF) A	Associated with factors IX, XI and XII; essential for thromboplastin formation
IX	Christmas factor, AHF-B	Associated with factors VIII, XI and XII; essential for thromboplastin formation
X	Thrombokinase factor, Stuart-Prower factor	Triggers prothrombin conversion; requires vitamin K
XI	Plasma thromboplastin antecedent, AHF-C	Formation of thromboplastin in association with factors VIII, IX and XII
XII	Contact factor, Hageman factor	Activates factor XI in thromboplastin formation
XIII	Fibrin-stabilising factor	Strengthens fibrin clot

Serious, life-threatening bleeding or head trauma is a medical emergency. It requires immediate replacement of factor to raise the level sufficiently to achieve haemostasis.

In the case of serious or life-threatening bleeding—DO NOT wait for blood results or imaging.

Sites of bleeding may include:

- ocular bleeding
- bleeding into the hip
- potential/suspected bleeding in central nervous system
- intra-abdominal bleeding
- bleeding affecting the airway
- deep muscle bleeding with neurovascular compromise
- prolonged bleeding not adequately responding to home-based therapy
- iliopsoas bleeding
- bleeding severe enough to cause anaemia requiring red cell transfusion
- significant injuries from MVA or falls from distance of several metres.

PRACTICE TIP

Do not wait for blood count results prior to patient management–facilitate urgent consult with haemophilia specialist physician. Often patients will carry haemophilia alert card with instructions on emergency management and treating centre contact details.

HAEMARTHROSES (BLEEDING INTO A JOINT)

Haemarthrosis involves primarily the knees, ankles and elbows. Patients often present to a healthcare facility with severe joint pain rather than active bleeding. Improperly managed haemarthrosis can lead to arthritis and ultimately joint destruction. Bleeding into tissue planes and tense haematomas in limbs can cause compartment syndromes.[95,96]

Bleeding into the neck or mouth may cause airway compromise. Central nervous system bleeding can be caused by minor head trauma, and patients will require hospital assessment and computed tomography (CT) scanning. If intracranial pathology is suspected, replacement therapy with appropriate clotting factors should be commenced prior to radiological investigation. Retroperitoneal bleeding should be considered if there is evidence of acute blood loss and the source cannot be found. Patients may also present with a complication of therapy, such as hepatitis or HIV as a result of exposure to viruses prior to the introduction of extensive screening of blood products. From the late 1970s to the mid '80s about half the people with haemophilia became infected with the HIV virus from using contaminated blood products. An estimated 90% of those with severe haemophilia were infected with HIV. Many developed AIDS and thousands died.[96] The risk of HIV transmission from blood products is low; however, the risk of contamination with other diseases is a real one and a consideration when deciding whether to use clotting factors prophylactically.

Management—refer to specialist centre

Acute management for bleeding/haemorrhage requires referral to a specialist centre.

The immediate goal is to replace factor activity to a sufficient level to achieve haemostasis. Replacement of deficient clotting factors is the primary means of support.[96]

For mild haemophilia A and certain subtypes of von Willebrand's disease, desmopressin acetate (DDAVP), a synthetic analogue of vasopressin, may be used to stimulate an increase in factor VIII and vWF, which subsequently binds with factor VIII, thus increasing its concentration. It can be administered intravenously, and the beneficial effects are seen within 30 minutes and last for more than 12 hours.[96]

Patients with moderate and severe haemophilia A will require factor VIII concentrate. Most haemophiliacs have personalised management plans and are able to manage minor incidents and administer factor VIII at home, but are aware that certain events—a large bleed, ongoing bleeding, severe pain, swelling of a muscle that restricts movement, head injury, swelling in the neck or mouth, haematuria, melaena and wounds in need of suturing—require medical attention. Acute interventions are related primarily to stopping the bleeding and are listed in Box 29.6.[96]

There is now considerable evidence that prophylactic factor administration results in a decreased incidence of haemorrhagic events and long-term complications of haemophilia. However, the costs are high in terms of the need for recurrent venous access (a central venous catheter may be required), time impact on family life and potential transmission of infection. Primary prophylaxis is for patients who have not had a bleeding episode, but are at high risk. Secondary prophylaxis is for those who have had more than one bleeding episode and intermittent prophylaxis is based on the patient's factor level.[96,97,99]

BOX 29.6 INTERVENTIONS FOR ACUTE HAEMOPHILIA PRESENTATIONS[97,98]

1. Stop topical bleeding as quickly as possible by applying direct pressure, ice, packing the area with Gelfoam or fibrin foam and applying topical haemostatic agents such as thrombin.
2. Administer the specific coagulation factor to raise the patient's level of the deficient coagulation factor.
3. When joint bleeding occurs, in addition to administering replacement factors, it is important to rest the injured joint totally until bleeding has stopped to prevent crippling deformities from haemarthrosis. The joint may be packed in ice. Analgesics are given to reduce pain, keeping in mind that those agents which affect clotting such as aspirin should never be used.
4. Monitor closely for life- and limb-threatening complications that may develop as a result of bleeding: airway obstruction from haemorrhage into the neck, decreased level of consciousness from acute head injury indicating cerebral bleeding, compartment syndrome developing from limb injuries.
5. Monitor for signs of ongoing blood loss such as hypovolemic shock: tachycardia, tachypnoea, altered level of consciousness, hypotension, pallor, diaphoresis, and decreased capillary refill.

In order to reduce the risks associated with repeated blood transfusion, it is recommended to rationalise and restrict blood transfusions if haemoglobin level is > 80 g/L, unless the patient reports symptoms of shortness of breath, excessive fatigue, or if they have a cardiac history.[43,97] Box 29.7 lists the steps that need to be taken in the event of a blood transfusion reaction.

BOX 29.7 BLOOD-PRODUCT TRANSFUSION[130]

- Haematopoietic stem cell transplant recipients require irradiated blood products
- Valid informed consent should be obtained from the patient and documented in their medical record. Blood products should be requested when the patient is ready, to avoid delays and wastage. Red blood cells taken out of storage for **less than 30 minutes** and unused can, on the discretion of the transfusion service provider, be accepted back into the blood bank. If out of storage for greater than 30 minutes then the transfusion should be completed within the next 4 hours
- 18 to 20 gauge venous access is recommended for adult non-emergency transfusion—a bigger gauge may be required in an emergency
- The standard blood-component-giving set should be used incorporating a 170–200 micron filter. It can be primed with blood component or normal saline—not dextrose which may cause the red cells to haemolyse.
- Giving set should be changed when transfusion complete or every 12 hours
- A RBC-giving set should never be used subsequently for platelets because the red cell debris in the filter could trap the platelets
- Blood-giving sets should never be 'piggy-backed' onto an infusion line
- Medications should never be given through a blood-component-giving set. When using multi-lumen central lines blood products and medications can be infused concurrently through different lumens but with caution if there is a history/high possibility of reactions to the medications
- Patients should be closely observed for the first 15–30 minutes of each new unit and regular visual observation is required throughout the transfusion
- The frequency of taking routine vital signs should be determined by institutional guidelines
- **At a minimum,** temperature, pulse, respiration rate and blood pressure should be recorded:
  - prior to the start of each blood component pack
  - 15 minutes after commencing each blood component pack, each hour
  - and on completion of each blood component pack
- Observations must be recorded in the patient's healthcare record.

Management strategies for haemolytic blood transfusions rest with prevention. Each hospital adopts its own policies, generally based on the guidelines set out by the Australian and New Zealand Society of Blood Transfusion (ANZSBT).[131] Box 29.8 lists the vascular access policies.

Exposure to transfused clotting factors may lead to the development of inhibitors—antibodies directed against the clotting proteins which are perceived by the body to be foreign. Factor VIII inhibitors are present in 25–30% of patients with severe haemophilia A.[96] A promising new monoclonal antibody, emicizumab, released in November 2017, is a subcutaneous medication for these patients.[95]

DISSEMINATED INTRAVASCULAR COAGULATION

Disseminated intravascular coagulation (DIC) is a secondary systemic process with the potential to cause simultaneous thrombosis and haemorrhage. It is usually the result of serious underlying disease, but may itself become life threatening.[100,101]

DIC is characterised by simultaneous activation of blood coagulation, consumption of clotting proteins, generation of thrombin, activation of platelets and secondary activation of the fibrinolytic system. Microclots form within the capillaries and deplete clotting factors in the circulating blood faster than the liver and bone marrow can replace them, resulting in haemorrhage. Intravascular clots obstruct the capillaries causing ischaemia in the tissues. The fibrinolytic system is activated to dissolve the clots and potent fibrin degradation products trigger further bleeding.

DIC can present as an acute, life-threatening emergency associated with a florid haemorrhagic/thrombotic syndrome or a chronic subclinical process, depending on the degree and tempo of the underlying cause.[100] DIC is a paradoxical condition characterised by both bleeding and thrombosis. It results from the release of pro-inflammatory cytokines, such as interleukins and tumour necrosis factor (TNF) as a response to one of the triggers listed in Box 29.3.[101]

- Sepsis: bacterial, (Gram negative and positive) viral, fungal and parasitic
- Malignancy: particularly acute promyelocytic leukaemia, pancreatic, gastric ovarian and brain tumours
- Immunological: anaphylaxis, heparin-associated thrombocytopenia, acute vasculitis
- Trauma: burns, trauma to central nervous system
- Obstetric complications: including eclampsia, dead fetus, uterine rupture
- Intravascular haemolysis: ABO red blood cell incompatible transfusion.

Diagnosis

In DIC all physiological anticoagulant pathways are functionally impaired. There is no single laboratory test with sufficient accuracy for the diagnosis of DIC. For the diagnosis of DIC a scoring system has been developed by Levy and Scully,[101] although DIC is a clinical and laboratory diagnosis.

Signs and symptoms

Signs and symptoms of DIC vary depending on the severity of the condition, and may include both bleeding and thrombotic events. Major bleeding is seen only in a minority of patients; more common is the occurrence of organ failure. Clinically, DIC in cancer has a less fulminant presentation than DIC seen in trauma or shock. Initial signs and symptoms are often subtle and may be overlooked until a catastrophic event occurs, such as a cerebrovascular accident, myocardial infarction, massive haemorrhage or acute kidney failure. For example, bleeding may be manifest only as generalised oozing from multiple intravenous catheter sites. Microvascular thrombosis may manifest itself as peripheral cyanosis. Neurological signs may include severe headache or altered behaviour, mood or level of consciousness. Patients may also exhibit haemodynamic instability (tachycardia and hypotension). Laboratory abnormalities are the most reliable way of diagnosing the disorder. Characteristically these will show:

- prolonged PT, TT (thrombin time) and APTT
- low platelet count
- low fibrinogen level
- elevated D-dimer
- reduced fibrinogen
- reduced protein C
- reduced antithrombin.[101]

PRACTICE TIP

DIC is often insidious in its presentation and small signs may alert the suspicions of the astute clinician. Be aware of bleeding from previous venepuncture sites, mucous membranes or the sclera and conjunctiva, particularly in the context of a clinically deteriorating patient. DIC should be considered in the management of any seriously ill patient, and suspected in an individual with generalised oozing from multiple sites or other signs of bleeding with an underlying condition associated with DIC such as malignancy.

Management

Treat the underlying cause in order to eliminate the stimulus for ongoing coagulation and thrombosis.[100]

Immediate goals for care will be dependent on the individual patient factors. They can include:

- haemodynamic and/or ventilatory support
- aggressive hydration for acute haemolytic transfusion reaction
- red blood cell transfusion for severe bleeding
- close monitoring for bleeding and thrombotic complications—treat as appropriate. The specific threshold for transfusion is individualised to the patient, including volume status and severity of bleeding, and the clinical setting.

Note: There is little evidence to support prophylactic anticoagulation or prophylactic administration of blood products.[102–105] The patient requires immediate transfer to a tertiary care hospital environment.

Prognosis

The mortality rate has been given as 40–80% in patients with severe trauma, sepsis and burns.[82] The median survival rate for cancer patients with DIC has been shown to be worse than that of cancer patients without DIC.[106]

METABOLIC EMERGENCIES

There are also a number of oncological and haematological emergencies that are unconnected to haemopoiesis. These are examined below.

TUMOUR LYSIS SYNDROME (TLS)

A small proportion of oncology and haematology patients will develop severe metabolic disturbances after commencing treatment for their disease in a condition known as tumour lysis syndrome (TLS). TLS is caused by the abrupt destruction of a large number of rapidly proliferating neoplastic cells.[107] The initiation of any cytotoxic therapy (chemotherapy, radiotherapy, immunotherapy) can cause TLS. In rare cases, TLS can be triggered following only steroid therapy. Patients are at risk of TLS in malignancies where there is a large tumour burden, with high proliferative rate and/or with high sensitivity to chemotherapy. Patients with malignancies such as Burkett's lymphoma and acute lymphoblastic leukaemia are at high risk for TLS.[107]

Pathophysiology

The breakdown of the malignant cells results in the release of intracellular contents into the circulation (potassium, phosphate, nucleic acids). Nucleic acid is catabolised into uric acid, which precipitates in the renal tubules inducing inflammation, oxidation and decreased blood flow, and resulting in acute kidney injury. The phosphate concentration of malignant cells is up to four times higher than that of normal cells, and so hypophosphatemia also occurs with secondary hypocalcaemia and also hyperkalemia.[107]

The emergence of effective targeted anticancer drugs in haematological oncology has led to an increase in the incidence and severity of TLS.[108] TLS occurrence in solid tumours is rare, but can occur in testicular or germ cell cancers, breast cancer, neuroblastoma and lung cancer.[108]

Signs, symptoms and management

Patients may present with metabolic abnormalities detectable from laboratory results but be otherwise asymptomatic. Initial symptoms may include nausea, vomiting, diarrhoea, anorexia, lethargy, dark urine, muscle cramps, which if left untreated may progress to cardiac dysrhythmias, heart failure, seizures, tetany, syncope and death. Effective management relies on identifying high-risk groups and instituting prophylactic therapy. Patients who are categorised as high risk will generally commence their treatment in hospital and will be closely monitored. TLS preventative treatment should be commenced prior to starting cytotoxic treatment. TLS prophylaxis includes:[107]

- aggressive fluid hydration (3000 mL/m^2 normal saline per day).[109] Close observation of fluid balance is necessary to monitor for signs of overload. Urinary alkalisation is no longer recommended.[109]
- *allopurinol*—decreases the formation of new uric acid crystals.
- *rasburicase*—an alternative to allopurinol, now considered to be superior in some cases, particularly for high-risk patients.[107]
- treatment of established TLS—patients with TLS who are likely to present to ED will be those for whom the syndrome was not predicted and effective prophylaxis was not implemented. Furthermore, TLS can occur spontaneously in some patients prior to the commencement of chemotherapy.

Intensive supportive care is required with continuous cardiac monitoring and measurements of electrolytes, creatinine and uric acid every 4 to 6 hours. Electrolyte replacement will be necessary in combination with vigorous hydration, attempting to flush uric acid crystals from the kidneys. Early involvement of a renal team is recommended.

HYPERCALCAEMIA

Hypercalcaemia is an elevated level of serum calcium which may result in life-threatening cardiac dysrhythmias, neurological symptoms and kidney failure. Its in-hospital mortality rate is 6.8% and is therefore considered to be an oncological emergency.[110]

The normal range for calcium varies between laboratories, but is generally between 2.2 and 2.5 mmol/L (8.5–10.2 mg/dL). As more than 50% of calcium binds to protein (principally albumin), albumin levels must also be taken into account when assessing calcium levels (Box 29.3). The BMJ Best Practice Guidelines classify hypercalcaemia into three categories using the adjusted serum calcium level:

- Mild: 2.6–2.9 mmol/L
- Moderate: 3.0–3.4 mmol/L
- Severe: 3.5 mmol/L or greater.[111]

Hypercalcaemia occurs in 10–30% of patients with cancer at some time during their disease and is reported consistently as being the most common metabolic disturbance in cancer patients.[69,112] It is unfortunately associated with a poor prognosis, with approximately 50% of patients with hypercalcaemia dying within 30 days.[62,113] It is more common among patients with bone metastases and patients with cancer of the breast and prostate, non-small cell lung cancer, lymphoma and multiple myeloma. Twenty per cent of MM patients are hypercalcaemic at diagnosis.[29,113]

Hypercalcaemia is caused by the inappropriate release of parathyroid hormone-related peptide (PTHrP) from tumour cells, resulting in a triad of processes: enhanced osteoclastic bone resorption, enhanced renal tubule reabsorption of calcium and enhanced intestinal absorption of calcium.[29]

Signs and symptoms

Signs and symptoms may be acute or gradual, but classically they include:

- fatigue—the most common symptom
- malaise
- joint, bone and muscle pain
- anorexia, nausea and vomiting
- constipation
- drowsiness, somnolence, confusion and hallucinations—a rapid rise in calcium is more likely to produce marked neurological symptoms than a gradual one, and these may be exacerbated by sedatives or narcotics
- cardiac dysrhythmias—an ECG reveals a shortened QT interval and the patient may develop dysrhythmias.[29]

Management

Prompt, effective therapy will minimise the severity of hypercalcaemia and reduce the possibility of renal failure. Management involves:

- *rehydration*—200–300 mL/hr dependent on renal and cardiac status
- *therapeutics medications*—principally bisphosphonates, such as pamidronate and zoledronic acid. These are generally well tolerated, but may be associated with flu-like symptoms, impaired renal function and rarely osteonecrosis of the jaw. Also withdraw medicine which may exacerbate hypercalcaemia, such as diuretics, vitamin D, antacids and lithium
- *dialysis*—may be used in severe cases and with patients who are likely to respond to cancer therapy[114]
- *calcitonin*—reduces calcium levels by inhibiting bone resorption and increasing renal excretion; however, resistance develops after repeated doses

- corticosteroids—sometimes helpful in haematological malignancies
- denosumab—for use in refractory hypercalcaemia. A monoclonal antibody which works by reducing the breakdown of bone by binding to a receptor activator.[29]

NON-METABOLIC ONCOLOGICAL EMERGENCIES

SPINAL CORD COMPRESSION (SCC)

Spinal cord compression results from either an intradural or, more commonly, an extradural metastasis pressing onto the spinal cord. It is seen in 5–10% of cancer patients. It occurs most commonly in multiple myeloma (15%), lymphoma (14%) and prostate cancer (6%).[115,116]

In 85% of cases, cord damage arises from extension of a vertebral body metastasis into the epidural space, but other mechanisms of damage include vertebral collapse (e.g. secondary to lytic lesions in myeloma), direct spread of tumour through the intervertebral foramen (as can be found with lymphoma) and interruption of the vascular supply.[117]

SCC is not immediately life threatening in itself, but can cause severe neurological morbidity.[118] Preservation of function is the primary goal of therapy, and this is why it is classified as an emergency: intervention needs to be timely in order to avoid irreparable spinal cord damage and paralysis. Unfortunately, the majority of SCC patients are not ambulatory at diagnosis.[115,119]

Cord compression may be associated with metastatic disease or may be the presenting feature of a new malignancy (sometimes lymphoma presents in this way). As a presenting feature it does not necessarily mean poor prognosis. In the metastatic setting it is generally indicative of a poor prognosis, with a median survival rate of approximately 4 months from diagnosis.[115,120,121]

Signs and symptoms

The most common presenting feature, noted by 83–95% of patients before diagnosis, is back pain. This may sometimes be associated with root irritation, creating a girdle or band of pain that tends to be worse on coughing, straining or lying down.[115,120] However, its significance is often missed. Presenting symptoms are put down to other factors, especially among children and in cases of advanced disease. In one British study,[122] the median delay in treatment for patients with spinal cord compression was 2 months from the onset of back pain and 14 days from the onset of symptoms of SCC. Increasing compression of the spinal cord is often—but not always—marked by improvement or resolution of the back pain.

Other neurological symptoms can vary enormously according to the rapidity of development of the lesion and its location. Leg weakness indicates progressive spinal damage and may initially be described as a feeling of stiffness rather than weakness, with tingling and numbness starting in both feet and ascending the legs. Pain generally pre-dates the onset of weakness by some weeks. Whereas the onset of pain may be gradual, the onset of weakness is generally sudden.[115]

Late neurological signs include urinary and bowel symptoms, such as hesitancy, retention or constipation. Both urinary and bowel symptoms are suggestive of extensive cord damage, except if the lesion is at the level of the cauda equina.[115,116]

Assessment and management

Expedited radiological imaging is required for thorough assessment. Ideally this is with CT or magnetic resonance imaging (MRI), although for patients unable to tolerate these, plain x-rays can provide some information if there are gross changes to the spinal cord. Physical assessment should consist of regular neurovascular observations, and at paramedical or nursing handover time these should be conducted with the receiving clinician to maintain consistency. Any alterations or deterioration should immediately be communicated with the treating medical team. It is not necessary to apply strict bed rest to these patients.[115,116]

Prompt diagnosis and appropriate intervention in cases of cord compression can have significant impact on quality of life. Neurological status at the start of treatment is the most important factor influencing outcome: if treatment is started within 24–48 hours of onset of symptoms, neurological damage may be reversible. After palliative radiotherapy, about one-third of patients who were not mobile *but not paraplegic* before treatment will regain the ability to walk, but only 2–6% of patients *who were already paraplegic* will regain this ability.[122]

High-dose glucocorticosteroid is the standard regimen for symptomatic SCC to reduce inflammation. Analgesia is also given for symptoms of acute pain associated with SCC. Patients who present with SCC are usually in pain that can impede the physical neurological examination. The dose of steroid and duration of therapy are individualised according to the radiological findings. Neural decompression, if indicated, is recommended within 24 hours to ensure the best outcome for the patient. There remains controversy about the role of radiation therapy versus surgery. In some studies it is reported that surgery followed by radiation can give better results, with higher ambulatory rates using this approach, while in other studies, radiation versus surgery showed no significant difference in patient outcomes.[121]

Conventional external beam radiation therapy may be indicated according to the degree of SCC in combination with high-dose corticosteroids. For some chemotherapy-sensitive tumours, such as Burkitt lymphoma, chemotherapy (and steroids) has a role in the management of acute SCC to reduce the size of the tumour.[115,123,124]

Fifteen per cent of patients with SCC develop a DVT due to blood stasis from paralysis of muscles and hyper coagulopathy. The evidence recommends that all patients should be anti-coagulated and wear compression stockings. Additionally, patients should be managed with nutritional support and laxative support. Bladder catheterisation may be indicated.[116]

PRACTICE TIP

For the triage nurse, if SCC is suspected urgent CT/MRI imaging is the most important radiological investigation for diagnosis. Initiate corticosteroids. Refer to radiation oncology/neurosurgery for decompression. If there are delays, permanent paraparesis may occur within hours.

SUPERIOR VENA CAVA SYNDROME

Superior vena cava syndrome (SVCS) refers to pressure on the superior vena cava that may arise from occlusion by extrinsic pressure, intraluminal thrombosis or direct invasion of the vessel wall. The result of this is reduced blood flow to the lungs and a backlog of blood in the venous circulation. The formation of venous collaterals occurs in an effort to compensate for the obstruction, resulting in an increase in venous pressure—particularly if the obstruction forms quickly, not giving enough time for adequate collateral development.[125–127]

The patient develops interstitial oedema in the tissues of the face and neck, and also nasal passage and larynx. The patient proceeds to become dyspnoeic and may develop hoarseness, cough and stridor. Cerebral oedema can develop leading to cerebral ischaemia and death, which is why it has traditionally been classified as an oncological emergency. Some argue against this, as the development of SVC obstruction is often over a number of weeks and the outcome is not related to duration of symptoms.[125] However, cases in which the individual presents with stridor due to central airway obstruction or severe laryngeal oedema, or coma from cerebral oedema, would generally be treated as an emergency situation.[125,127]

Most commonly, SVCS results from a tumour, although the increased prevalence of intravenous central lines has led to device-related SVC obstructions in recent years.[125,127] Intrathoracic malignancy causes 60–85% of SVC obstruction (SVCO), and in 60% of these cases the SVC obstruction is the presenting feature of a previously undiagnosed tumour. Up to 80% of patients who develop SVCS have right-sided lung lesions. Non-small cell lung cancer is the malignancy most commonly associated with SVCO, followed by diffuse large cell lymphoma. Together, these are responsible for 95% of the cases of SVCO caused by a tumour.[128,129]

Signs and symptoms

Most patients present after having developed symptoms over days to weeks. Symptoms include:

- neck swelling
- distended veins along the chest
- shortness of breath
- hoarse voice
- swelling in one or both arms
- tracheal oedema and shortness of breath
- cerebral oedema with headache, which becomes worse on stooping
- visual changes
- dizziness and syncope
- swelling of the face, particularly periorbital oedema
- tachypnoea
- cyanosis.[128]

Management

On arrival at hospital, initial management includes basic supportive measures, such as elevating the head and providing oxygen. The diagnosis of SVCS is made using radiological imaging, initially with chest x-ray and then CT chest or MRI. Mainstays of treatment include diuretics to reduce intravascular volume and at least a short course of parenteral steroids, followed by dexamethasone, 4 mg every 6 hours, to decrease oedema and tumour burden, although both these therapies remain unproven.[125,127,128]

Further management is dependent on diagnosis and will require histology if this is the first presentation of disease. For potentially curable diseases, such as lymphomas or germ cell tumours, chemotherapy and radiotherapy are often given. High-dose corticosteroids and surgical stenting of the superior vena cava are also treatment options.

BLOOD-PRODUCT ADMINISTRATION IN HAEMATOLOGY PATIENTS

Frequent blood transfusion may be required for patients with haematological diseases, either to correct anaemia related to disease status or as therapy to support treatment-related toxicities (see Boxes 29.7 and 29.8). In order to reduce the risks associated with repeated blood transfusion, it is recommended to rationalise and restrict blood transfusions if haemoglobin level is > 80 g/L, unless patient reports symptoms of shortness of breath, excessive fatigue, or if they have a cardiac history.[35,131]

HAEMOLYTIC BLOOD TRANSFUSION REACTIONS

Major ABO red blood cell incompatibility is infrequent,[35,132] though potentially fatal. It occurs as a result of intravascular haemolysis when the recipient has anti-A or anti-B antibodies that react with the transfused cells. Symptoms occur in minutes to hours. Close monitoring of vital signs is advised (Box 29.9).

Symptoms of reaction include:

- rapid temperature rise at start of transfusion—stop transfusion
- hypotension
- chills
- flushing
- restless
- lower back pain.

Nurses and clinicians should refer to Australian and New Zealand blood transfusion guidelines. Most major transfusion incompatibilities are the result of human error.[130] Management strategies for haemolytic blood transfusions rest with prevention.

BOX 29.8 VASCULAR ACCESS POLICIES[132,133]

- **Dressing the exit site of the line—all lines are dressed using an aseptic technique with a semipermeable membrane dressing and changed in accordance with institutional guidelines—usually every 7 days**
- **Infection-control practices in accessing the line—hand hygiene is required prior to using the line and the needleless capless valve should be decontaminated using alcohol solution prior to use[135]**
- **Flushing the central line is essential after access and blood taking—see institutional guidelines**
- **'Heparin locking'—some institutions 'lock' the line by injecting small volumes of low-dose heparin after flushing with normal saline when de-accessing—see institutional guidelines for management of central lines in your hospital/health service.**

BOX 29.9 STEPS TO BE TAKEN IN THE EVENT OF A BLOOD TRANSFUSION REACTION[130]

Acute transfusion reactions can present with a range of symptoms of varying severity. Signs of a mild transfusion reaction include rash, pruritus and a mild fever. A moderate or severe transfusion reaction may be accompanied by a greater temperature rise and inflammatory symptoms, as described below. Any temperature rise to $> 38°C$ or $> 1°C$ above baseline (if baseline $> 37°C$) should prompt the interruption of the transfusion and a clinical assessment of the patient.

If a mild transfusion reaction is suspected:

1. STOP the transfusion
2. Maintain IV access
3. Check vital signs: temperature, pulse, respirations and blood pressure
4. Check all documentation and patient identity including transfusion documentation
5. Contact medical staff immediately for further management and investigation.

If the temperature rise is $< 1.5°C$ above baseline or the patient has only localised rash or pruritus, the patient observations are stable and the patient is otherwise well, an antipyretic or antihistamines may be administered at the discretion of the doctor and the transfusion then continued with caution and close observation. If signs or symptoms persist, develop or deteriorate subsequently, STOP the transfusion and manage as for a severe transfusion reaction (following).

MODERATE-TO-SEVERE TRANSFUSION REACTIONS

Any of the following could be considered signs of a moderate-to-severe transfusion reaction:

- temperature 1.5°C above baseline
- hypotension/shock OR hypertension
- tachycardia
- tachypnoea, wheeze, stridor
- rigors or chills
- nausea, vomiting or pain (local, chest, back).

If a moderate or severe transfusion reaction is suspected, the following steps **MUST** be undertaken:

- **STOP the transfusion immediately and seek urgent medical advice;** Medical Emergency Team (MET) support may be required, depending on the specific clinical situation.
- Maintain venous access using a new administration set and 0.9% sodium chloride (normal saline), but do not discard the blood administration set and do not flush the original line.
- Repeat all clerical and identity checks of the patient and blood pack.
- Immediately report the reaction to the transfusion service provider, who will advise on returning the implicated product and administration set, and any further blood or urine samples required from the patient.
- Monitor and record the patient's temperature, pulse, respirations and blood pressure.
- Record the volume and colour of any urine passed (looking for evidence of haemoglobinuria).

Each hospital adopts its own policies, generally based on the guidelines set out by the Australian and New Zealand Society of Blood Transfusion (ANZSBT).[130]

PRACTICE TIP

The recommendations made by the ANZSBT are that vital signs are taken at the beginning of each unit and at the end of the transfusion episode.[130] The patient should be monitored closely for the first 15 minutes. The timing for taking vital signs after this is discretionary and should be guided by the clinical condition of the patient and institutional policy.

PRACTICE TIP

For all associated transfusion reactions and management refer to Australian and New Zealand policy/procedure/guidelines.

Severely immunosuppressed patients and recipients of haematopoietic stem cell transplantation are particularly vulnerable to GVHD, and thus (for life) receive irradiated blood products. The irradiation renders inactive any viable lymphocytes in the blood product.

SUMMARY

Particularly important areas for ED professionals include the management of neutropenic sepsis and the competent administration of blood products. Changes in haematological treatment strategies, coupled with a growing awareness of quality-of-life issues, is likely to further involve ED healthcare professionals in the management of oncology populations in the years to come.

CASE STUDY

John arrived home from work to find his partner Michael unwell with symptoms of fever, vomiting and confusion. He responded by calling 000 for urgent help. Michael is 66 years old with a new diagnosis of metastatic lung cancer, diagnosed two months earlier. Prior to the diagnosis Michael was well, with occasional asthma symptoms only, well controlled with salbutamol inhalers. Michael received his third cycle of the combined chemotherapy and immunotherapy protocol 5 days ago. To deliver this protocol an implantable venous access device was inserted (portacath), to facilitate the safe delivery of chemotherapy. To date, treatment had been uneventful with no complications.

Paramedics found Michael in bed, diaphoretic with a fever, vomiting, conscious but exhibiting signs of confusion.

On assessment they recorded his observations:

- Glasgow Coma Scale score 14
- JVP not visible
- temperature 38.6°C
- heart rate 120 beats/minute
- blood pressure 90/40 mmHg
- respiratory rate 30 breaths/minute
- oxygen saturation 92% RA.

Paramedics concluded that a possible differential diagnosis could be neutropenic sepsis given that he had recent chemotherapy. This was explained to Michael and his partner and they consented to him being transferred to the ED for urgent assessment. Oxygen was initiated and venous access gained. Fluid-resuscitation was commenced in response to hypotension.

On arrival at the ED, Michael was triaged by nursing staff and assigned a triage category 2. He was transferred to a resuscitation bay. Bloods were collected, including FBC EUC, CRP, LFTs, BSL; coagulation studies including d-dimer, lactate, cross-match and blood cultures were sent. Intravenous fluids continued and antibiotics commenced in accordance with the hospital protocol for the management of neutropenic sepsis. A COVID -19 multiplex PCR swab was collected in addition to a rapid antigen test.

Bloods results included:

- neutrophils 0.4×10^9/L
- haemoglobin 70×10^9/L
- CRP 230 mg/L
- lactate 2.5 mmol/L
- corrected calcium 2.83 mmol/L.

The results confirmed that the patient was neutropenic anaemic with an elevated CRP, lactate and a high calcium level. Bloods cultures results were not yet available. Access to the implanted venous port was obtained to enable more venous access to administer antibiotics and aggressive fluid replacement. He was also given antiemetics and IV paracetamol. A blood transfusion was commenced and IV bisphosphonate ordered.

Michael responded well to treatment and did not require transfer to a high dependency unit. Once hemodynamically stable, a bed was found for Michael on the oncology ward for continuation of antibiotics therapy and monitoring of his condition. No obvious source for the infection was found with blood cultures returning negative for pathogens. Michael was discharged home 5 days later when his blood counts had recovered. His next cycle of chemotherapy was delayed and dose-reduced.

QUESTIONS

1. What signs raised the paramedic's suspicion that Michael may be (a) neutropenic and (b) septic?
2. In addition to taking blood cultures, what other tests need to be performed if a cancer patient presents to the ED febrile and possibly neutropenic?
3. Michael was ordered intravenous fluids, a blood transfusion and intravenous antibiotics. In what order should these be given and why?
4. Hypercalcaemia of malignancy is a medical emergency. What signs did Michael present that indicated he may have this condition?
5. What is the international standard for time to antibiotics if a patient is suspected of having neutropenic sepsis?
6. Why was Michael anaemic? What questions would we need to ask when taking the patient's history in view of the acute anaemia?

Answers to Case Study Questions can be found on evolve http://evolve.elsevier.com/AU/Curtis/emergency/

USEFUL WEBSITES

Cancer incidence and prevalence

Cancer Australia, www.canceraustralia.gov.au/.

Cancer Council NSW, www.cancercouncil.com.au.

Cancer Society of New Zealand, www.cancernz.org.nz.

Global Cancer Map. Cancer's global footprint, www.globalcancermap.com.

Ministry of Health Manatū Hauora, Cancer, www.health.govt.nz/your-health/conditions-and-treatments/diseases-and-illnesses/cancer.

World Health Organization, www.who.int/cancer/en/.

Treatment

eviQ: A free resource of evidence-based, consensus-driven cancer treatment protocols and information for use at the point of care in the Australian context, www.eviq.org.au/.

Transfusion

Australian Red Cross Blood Service, www.lifeblood.com.au/health-professionals.

National Blood Authority Australia, www.blood.gov.au/pbm-guidelines.

Haematological disorders

Australasian Leukaemia and Lymphoma Group (ALLG), www.allg.org.au.

Haemophilia Foundation Australia, www.haemophilia.org.au.

Haemophilia Foundation of New Zealand, www.haemophilia.org.nz.

Leukaemia and Blood Cancer New Zealand, www.leukaemia.org.nz.

Lymphoma Australia, www.lymphoma.org.au/.

Spleen Australia, www.spleen.org.au.

Sepsis

NSW Government, NSW Health, Clinical Excellence Commission, www.cec.health.nsw.gov.au.

COVID-19

Communicable Diseases Network of Australia (CDNA). National Guidelines for the Prevention, Control and Public Health Management of Outbreaks of Acute Respiratory Infection (including COVID-19 and Influenza) in Residential Care Facilities, www.health.gov.au/resources/publications/national-guidelines-for-the-prevention-control-and-public-health-management-of-outbreaks-of-acute-respiratory-infection-including-covid-19-and-influenza-in-residential-care-facilities.

REFERENCES

1. Australian Institute of Health and Welfare (AIHW). Cancer in Australia, 2021. Canberra: Australian Government; 2021. 25 February, 2019. Online. Available from: www.aihw.gov.au/publication-detail/?id=60129558547.
2. Te Aho o Te Kahu, Cancer Control Agency. He Pūrongo Mate Pukupuku o Aotearoa 2020, The state of cancer in New Zealand 2020. Wellington: Cancer Control Agency; 2021.
3. National Cancer Institute. NCI Dictionary of cancer terms. Online. Available from: www.cancer.gov/publications/dictionaries/cancer-terms.
4. Clark JW, Longo DL. Cancer cell biology. In: Jameson JL, Fauci AS, Kasper DL, et al., editors. Harrison's principles of internal medicine. 20th ed. New York, NY: McGraw-Hill Education; 2018.
5. Polek C. Cancer. In: Lewis S, Bucherm L, Heitkemper M, et al., editors. Medical surgical nursing. 10th ed. Sydney: Elsevier; 2017.
6. Stephens M. Cancer. In: Craft J, Gordon C, Huether S, et al., editors. Understanding pathophysiology—ANZ adaptation. Sydney: Mosby; 2015.
7. Polek C. Cancer pathophysiology. In: Newton S, Hickey M, Brant J, editors. Mosby's oncology nursing advisor. 2nd ed. Sydney: Elsevier; 2017.
8. Polakowski T, Kerr M, Gregg Durand A. Caring for the continuum of patients with pancreatic cancer: the importance of survivorship care planning. Clin J Oncolog Nurs 2015;19(1):E21–4.
9. Hanahan D, Weinberg RA. Hallmarks of cancer: the next generation. Cell 2011;144(5):646–74.
10. Rote N, Virshup D. Biology of cancer. In: Huether SE, McCance KL, editors. Understanding pathophysiology. 6th ed. St. Louis: Elsevier; 2017.
11. Kumar V, editor. Robbins and Cotran pathologic basis of disease. 8th ed. Philadelphia: Saunders; 2009.
12. Beatty GL, Gladney WL. Immune escape mechanisms as a guide for cancer immunotherapy. Clin Cancer Res 2015;21(4):687–92.
13. Pardoll DM. The blockade of immune checkpoints in cancer immunotherapy. Nature Rev Cancer 2012;12(4):252–64.
14. Tsai H, Hsu P. Cancer immunotherapy by targeting immune checkpoints: mechanism of T cell dysfunction in cancer immunity and new therapeutic targets. J Biomed Sci 2017;24(1):35.

15. Amin MB, Greene FL, Edge SB, et al. The eighth edition AJCC cancer staging manual: continuing to build a bridge from a population-based to a more 'personalized' approach to cancer staging. CA Cancer J Clin 2017;67(2):93–9.
16. Bruni D, Angell HK, Galon J. The immune contexture and Immunoscore in cancer prognosis and therapeutic efficacy. Nat Rev Cancer 2020;20(11):662–80.
17. Roychowdhury S, Chinnaiyan A. Translating cancer genomes and transcriptomes for precision oncology. CA Cancer J Clin 2016;66(1):75–88.
18. Dizon D, Krilov L, Cohen E, et al. Clinical cancer advances 2016: annual report of progress against cancer from the American Society of Clinical Oncology. J Clin Oncol 2016;34(9):987–1011.
19. Salgado R, Moore H, Martens J, et al. Societal changes of precision medicine: bringing order to chaos. Euro J Cancer 2017;84:325–34.
20. Freedman AS, Friedberg JW, Aster JC, et al. Classification of the hematopoietic neoplasms. In: Lister A, Lowenberg B, editors. Haematological malignancies. USA: Wolters Kluwer; 2020.
21. Swerdlow SH, Campo E, Harris NL, et al., editors. WHO classification of tumours of haematopoietic and lymphoid tissues. Geneva, Switzerland: WHO Press; 2008.
22. Kolitz J. Overview of acute myeloid leukemia in adults. In: Larson R, editor. Leukemia. USA: Wolters Kluwer; 2022.
23. Shelton B, Rome S, Lewis S. Nursing assessment: haematological system. Sydney: Elsevier; 2008.
24. Patton K, Thibodeau G. Anatomy and physiology. 8th ed. Louis: Mosby; 2013.
25. Lewis S, Collier I. Medical surgical nursing: assessment and management of clinical problems. 7th ed. St. Louis: Mosby; 2007.
26. LaCasce A, Ng AK, Aster JC. Clinical presentation and diagnosis of classic Hodgkin lymphoma in adults. In: Freedman AS, editor. UpToDate. USA: Wolters Kluwer; 2022.
27. Freedman A, Friedberg JW, Aster JC. Clinical presentation and initial evaluation of non-Hodgkin lymphoma. In: Lister A, editor. UpToDate. USA: Wolters Kluwer; 2022.
28. Cancer Council. Types of cancer: lymphoma. 2022. Online. Available from: www.cancer.org.au/cancer-information/types-of-cancer/lymphoma.
29. Laubach J. Multiple myeloma: clinical features, laboratory manifestations, and diagnosis. In: Rajkumar SV, editor. UpToDate. USA: Wolters Kluwer; 2022.
30. Cowan AJ, Green DJ, Kwok M, et al. Diagnosis and management of multiple myeloma: a review. JAMA 2022;327(5):464–77.
31. Australian Government, Cancer Australia. Multiple myeloma in Australia statistics. Canberra: Australian Government; 2022. Online. Available from: www.canceraustralia.gov.au/cancer-types/myeloma/statistics.
32. Sausville EA, Longo DL. Principles of cancer treatment. In: Jameson JL, Fauci AS, Kasper DL, editors. Harrison's principles of internal medicine. 20th ed. New York, NY: McGraw-Hill Education; 2018.
33. Longo DL. Approach to the patient with cancer. In: Jameson JL, Fauci AS, Kasper DL, editors. Harrison's principles of internal medicine. 20th ed. New York, NY: McGraw-Hill Education; 2018.
34. Snyder J, Rainforth Collins S, Lilley L. Pharmacology and the nursing process. 9th ed. Elsevier; 2019.
35. Hillman R, Ault K, Leporrier M, et al. Haematology in clinical practice. 5th ed. New York: McGraw-Hill; 2010.
36. de Naurois J, Novitzky-Basso I, Gill MJ, et al. Management of neutropenic sepsis: ESMO clinical practice guidelines. Ann Oncol 2010;21(Suppl. 5): v252–6.
37. Young JS, Simmons JW. Chemotherapeutic medication and their emergency complications. Emerg Med Clin N Am 2014;32(3):563–78.
38. Livshits Z, Rao BR, Smith SW. An approach to chemotherapy-associated toxicity. Emerg Med Clin N Am 2014;32(1):167–203.
39. Cancer Institute New South Wales. Prevention of anti-cancer therapy induced nausea and vomiting (AINV). 2022. Online. Available from: www.eviq.org.au/clinical-resources/side-effect-and-toxicity-management/gastrointestinal/7-prevention-of-anti-cancer-therapy-induced-nausea.
40. Cancer Institute New South Wales. Side effect and toxicity management. 2022. Online. Available from: www.eviq.org.au/clinical-resources/side-effect-and-toxicity-management.
41. Davies A, Leach C, Caponero R, et al. MASCC recommendations on the management of constipation in patients with advanced cancer. Supp Care Cancer 2020;28(1):23–33.
42. McKenzie E, Zaki P, Raman S, et al. Radiation-induced nausea and vomiting: a comparison between MASCC/ESMO, ASCO, and NCCN antiemetic guidelines. Support Care Cancer 2019;27(3):783–91.
43. Lalla RV, Bowen J, Barasch A, et al. MASCC/ISOO clinical practice guidelines for the management of mucositis secondary to cancer therapy. Cancer 2014;120(10):1453–61.
44. Haanen J, Carbonnel F, Robert C, et al. Management of toxicities from immunotherapy: ESMO Clinical Practice Guidelines for diagnosis, treatment and follow-up. Ann Oncol 2017;28(Suppl. 4):119–42.
45. Kreamer KM. Immune checkpoint blockade: a new paradigm in treating advanced cancer. J Adv Pract Oncol 2014;5(6):418–31.
46. Weber JS. Challenging cases: management of immune-related toxicity. Am Soc Clin Oncol Ed Book 2018;38:179–83.
47. Gangadhar TC, Vonderheide RH. Mitigating the toxic effects of anticancer immunotherapy. Nature Rev Clin Oncol 2014;11(2):91–9.
48. Wolchok JD, Chiarion-Sileni V, Gonzalez R, et al. Overall survival with combined nivolumab and ipilimumab in advanced melanoma. N Engl J Med 2017;377(14):1345–56.
49. Cancer Institute New South Wales. Management of immune-related adverse events (irAEs). In: eviQ, editor. Sydney: Cancer Institute NSW; 2022.

50. Safework NSW. Cytotoxic drugs and related waste-risk management. Gosford NSW Government; 2017.
51. Cancer Council Australia. Facts and figures. 2018. Online. Available from: www.cancer.org.au/.
52. Shepard M, Lewis G, Thanos C, et al. Developments in therapy with monoclonal antibodies and related proteins. Clin Med 2017;17(3):220–32.
53. Klemencic S, Perkins J. Diagnosis and management of oncologic emergencies. West J Emerg Med 2019;20(2):316–622.
54. Halfdanarson TR, Hogan WJ, Madsen BE. Emergencies in hematology and oncology. Mayo Clin Proc 2017;92(4):609–41.
55. Alsharawneh A, Hasan AA. Cancer related emergencies with the chief complaint of pain: incidence, ED recognition, and quality of care. Int Emerg Nurs 2021;56:100981.
56. Koth J. Diagnosis and treatment of oncologic emergencies. Radiol Technol 2019;91(2):161–72.
57. Leikin JB. Foreword: an updated narrative review on the management of the most common oncological and hematological emergencies. Dis Mon 2022:101354.
58. Oatley M, Fry M, Mullen L. A cross-sectional study of the clinical characteristics of cancer patients presenting to one tertiary referral emergency department. Int Emerg Nurs 2016;24:35–8.
59. Bow EJ. Neutropenic fever syndromes in patients undergoing cytotoxic therapy for acute leukemia and myelodysplastic syndromes. Semin Hematol 2009;46(3):259–68.
60. Wingard J. Overview of neutropenic fever syndromes. 2022. Online. Available from: www.uptodate.com/contents/overview-of-neutropenic-fever-syndromes.
61. Bodey GP, Buckley M, Sathe YS, et al. Quantitative relationships between circulating leukocytes and infection in patients with acute leukemia. Ann Intern Med 1966;64(2):328–40.
62. Schimpff SC, Young VM, Greene WH, et al. Origin of infection in acute nonlymphocytic leukemia. Significance of hospital acquisition of potential pathogens. Ann Intern Med 1972;77(5):707–14.
63. Bone R, Balk R, Cerra F, et al. Definitions for sepsis and organ failure and guidelines for the use of innovative therapies in sepsis. The ACCP/SCCM Consensus Conference Committee. American College of Chest Physicians/Society of Critical Care Medicine. Chest 1992;101(6):1644–55.
64. Flowers CR, Seidenfeld J, Bow EJ, et al. Antimicrobial prophylaxis and outpatient management of fever and neutropenia in adults treated for malignancy: American Society of Clinical Oncology clinical practice guideline. J Clin Oncol 2013;31(6):794–810.
65. Legrand M, Max A, Peigne V, et al. Survival in neutropenic patients with severe sepsis or septic shock. Crit Care Med 2012;40(1):43–9.
66. Klastersky J, Raftopoulos H, Rapoport B. The MASCC Neutropenia, Infection and Myelosuppression Study Group evaluates recent new concepts for the use of granulocyte colony-stimulating factors for the prevention of neutropenic sepsis. Support Care Cancer 2013;21(6):1793–5.
67. Freifeld AG, Bow EJ, Sepkowitz KA, et al. Clinical practice guideline for the use of antimicrobial agents in neutropenic patients with cancer: 2010 Update by the Infectious Diseases Society of America. Clin Infect Dis 2011;52(4):427–31.
68. Penack O, Becker C, Buchheidt D, et al. Management of sepsis in neutropenic patients: 2014 updated guidelines from the Infectious Diseases Working Party of the German Society of Hematology and Medical Oncology (AGIHO). Ann Hematol 2014;93(7):1083–95.
69. Patel MJ, Connell BJ. Treatment of oncological emergencies. Hosp Med Clin 2017;6:283–94.
70. Evans L, Rhodes A, Alhazzani W, et al. Surviving Sepsis Campaign: international guidelines for management of sepsis and septic shock 2021. Intensive Care Med 2021;47(11):1181–247.
71. Gregory A, Schmidt MM. Evaluation and management of suspected sepsis and septic shock in adults. In: Parsons PE, Hockberger RS, editors. UpToDate. USA: Wolters Kluwer; 2022.
72. Singer M, Deutschman CS, Seymour CW, et al. The Third International Consensus Definitions for Sepsis and Septic Shock (Sepsis-3). JAMA 2016;315(8):801–10.
73. Burrell AR, McLaws ML, Fullick M, et al. SEPSIS KILLS: early intervention saves lives. Med J Aust 2016;204(2):73.
74. Ansell SM. Treatment and prognosis of Waldenström macroglobulinemia. In: UpToDate. USA: Wolters Kluwer; 2022.
75. Gertz MA. Acute hyperviscosity: syndromes and management. Blood 2018;132(13):1379–85.
76. Parnes A, Ravi A. Polycythemia and thrombocytosis. Prim Care 2016;43(4):589–605.
77. Schiffer C. Hyperleukocytosis and leukostasis in hematologic malignancies. UpToDate; 2017. Online. Available from: www.uptodate.com/contents/hyperleukocytosis-and-leukostasis-in-hematologic-malignancies.
78. Porcu P, Farag S, Marcucci G, et al. Leukocytoreduction for acute leukemia. Ther Apher 2002;6(1):15–23.
79. Teoh Y, Greenway A, Savola H, et al. Hospitalisations for sickle cell disease in Australian paediatric population. J Paediat Child Health 2013;49(1):68–71.
80. Vichinsky E. Overview of the clinical manifestations of sickle cell disease. In: UpToDate. USA: Wolters Kluwer; 2022.
81. Dhakal P, Rayamajhi S, Verma V, et al. Reversal of anticoagulation and management of bleeding in patients on anticoagulants. Clin Appl Thromb Hemost 2017;23(5):410–15.
82. Leung L. Direct oral anticoagulants (DOACs) and parenteral direct-acting anticoagulants: dosing and adverse effects. In: UpToDate. USA: Wolters Kluwer; 2022.
83. Levy JH, Ageno W, Chan NC, et al. When and how to use antidotes for the reversal of direct oral anticoagulants: guidance from the SSC of the ISTH. J Thromb Haemost 2016;14(3):623–7.

84. Kitchen G. Immunology and haematology. Edinburgh: Mosby; 2012.
85. George JN, Cuker A. Acquired TTP: clinical manifestations and diagnosis. 2018. Online. Available from: www.uptodate.com/contents/acquired-ttp-clinical-manifestations-and-diagnosis?source=search_result&search=TTP&selectedTitle=1~150.
86. Izak M, Bussel JB. Management of thrombocytopenia. F1000Prime Rep 2014;2(6):45.
87. Reese J, Muthurajah D. Children and adults with thrombotic thrombocytopenia purpura associated with severe acquired ADAMTS13 deficiency: comparison of incidence, demographic and clinical features. Pediatr Blood Cancer 2013;60(10):1676–82.
88. Michael M, Elliott E, Ridley GF, et al. Interventions for haemolytic uraemic syndrome and thrombotic thrombocytopenic purpura. Cochrane Database Syst Rev 2009;2009(1):CD003595.
89. Rathore B. Section 1: disease and disorders—thrombotic thrombocytopenic purpura. In: Ferri FF, editor. Ferri's clinical advisor. Philadelphia: Elsevier; 2018.
90. Crowther M. Clinical presentation and diagnosis of heparin-induced thrombocytopenia. In: Leung L, editor. UpToDate. USA: Wolters Kluwer; 2022.
91. Salter B, Weiner M. Heparin induced thrombocytopenia. J Am Coll Cardiol 2016;67(21):2519–32.
92. Lo GK, Juhl D, Warkentin TE, et al. Evaluation of pretest clinical score (4 Ts) for the diagnosis of heparin-induced thrombocytopenia in two clinical settings. J Thromb Haemost 2006;4:759–65.
93. Jevtic SD, Morris AM, Warkentin TE, Pai M. Heparin-induced thrombocytopenia. CMAJ 2021;193(20):E736.
94. Warkentin TE. Clinical picture of heparin-induced thrombocytopenia (HIT) and its differentiation from non-HIT thrombocytopenia. Thromb Haemost 2016;116(5):813–22.
95. Hoots WK, Shapiro AD. Hemophilia A and B: routine management including prophylaxis. 2018. Online. Available from: www.uptodate.com/contents/hemophilia-a-and-b-routine-management-including-prophylaxis?source=search_result&search=hemophilia&selectedTitle=1~150#H1521196374.
96. Haemophilia Foundation Australia. Fast facts about bleeding disorders. 2016. Online. Available from: www.haemophilia.org.au/about-bleeding-disorders/fast-facts.
97. Maclaren H. Anaemia. In: Cameron P, Jelinek G, Kelly AM, editors. Textbook of adult emergency medicine. Sydney: Elsevier; 2009.
98. Brack S. Nursing management of haematological problems. In: Lewis S, Collier I, Heitkemper M, editors. Medical surgical nursing: assessment and management of clinical problems. 7th ed. St. Louis: Mosby; 2007.
99. Bolton-Maggs P. Optimal haemophilia care versus the reality. Br J Haematol 2006;132(6):671–82.
100. Leung L. Clinical features, diagnosis, and treatment of disseminated intravascular coagulation in adults. 2017. Online. Available from: www.uptodate.com/contents/clinical-features-diagnosis-and-treatment-of-disseminated-intravascular-coagulation-in-adults.
101. Levi M, Scully M. How I treat disseminated intravascular coagulation. Blood 2018;131(8):845–54.
102. Iba T, Levy JH, Warkentin TE, et al. Diagnosis and management of sepsis-induced coagulopathy and disseminated intravascular coagulation. J Thromb Haemost 2019;17(11):1989–94.
103. Levi M, Toh CH, Thachil J, Watson HG. Guidelines for the diagnosis and management of disseminated intravascular coagulation. British Committee for Standards in Haematology. Br J Haematol 2009;145(1):24–33.
104. Squizzato A, Hunt BJ, Kinasewitz GT, et al. Supportive management strategies for disseminated intravascular coagulation. An international consensus. Thromb Haemost 2016;115(5):896–904.
105. Wada H, Thachil J, Di Nisio M, et al. Guidance for diagnosis and treatment of DIC from harmonization of the recommendations from three guidelines. J Thromb Haemost 2013. doi:10.1111/jth.12155.
106. Sallah S, Wan JY, Nguyen NP, et al. Disseminated intravascular coagulation in solid tumours: clinical and pathologic study. Thromb Haemost 2001;86(3):828–33.
107. Larson R, Pui C. Tumor lysis syndrome: prevention and treatment. UpToDate; 2018. Online. Available from: www.uptodate.com/contents/tumor-lysis-syndrome-prevention-and-treatment.
108. Howard S, Triffilo S, Gregory TK, et al. Tumor lysis syndrome in the era of novel and targeted agents in patients with hematological malignancies: a systematic review. Ann Hematol 2016;94(4):563–73.
109. Abu-Alfa A, Younes A. Tumor lysis syndrome and acute kidney injury: evaluation, prevention, and management. Am J Kidney Dis 2010;55(5 Suppl. 3): S1–13.
110. Wright J, Tergas A, Ananth C, et al. Quality and outcomes of treatment of hypercalcemia of malignancy. Cancer Invest 2015;33(8):331–9.
111. Shieh A, Martinez D. Hypercalcaemia of malignancy. BMJ Best Pract 2017.
112. Jameson J, Longo D. Precision medicine—personalized, problematic, and promising. N Engl J Med 2015;372:2229–34.
113. Zagouri F, Kastritis E, Zomas A, et al. Hypercalcaemia remains an adverse prognostic factor for newly diagnosed multiple myeloma patients in the era of novel antimyeloma therapies. Eur J Haematol 2017;99(5):409–14.
114. Stewart A. Hypercalcaemia associated with cancer. N Engl J Med 2005;352(4):373–9.
115. Laufer I, MBilsky M, Schiff D, Brown P. Treatment and prognosis of neoplastic epidural spinal cord compression. In: Wen P, editor. UpToDate. USA: Wolters Kluwer; 2021.
116. Casey K. Spinal cord compression. BMJ Best Pract 2017.

117. Skeoch G, Tobin MK, Khan S, et al. Corticosteroid treatment for metastatic spinal cord compression: a review. Global Spine J 2017;7(3):272–9.
118. Matsubara H, Watanabe K, Sakai H, et al. Rapid improvement of paraplegia caused by epidural involvements of Burkitt's lymphoma with chemotherapy. Spine 2004;29(1):E4–6.
119. Prasad D, Schiff D. Malignant spinal-cord compression. Lancet Oncol 2005;6(1):15–24.
120. Guo LY, Young B, Palmer LJ, et al. Prognostic factors for survival in metastatic spinal cord compression: a retrospective study in a rehabilitation setting. Am J Phys Med Rehab 2003;82(9):665–8.
121. Loblaw A, George KJ, Misra V. Surgical and radiotherapeutic management of malignant extradural spinal cord compression. Clin Oncol (R Coll Radiol) 2020;32(11):745–52.
122. Husband D. Malignant spinal cord compression: prospective study of delays in referral and treatment. BMJ 1998;317(7150):18–21.
123. Kovner F, Speigel S, Rider I, et al. Radiation therapy of metastatic spinal cord compression. Multidisciplinary team diagnosis and treatment. J Neurooncol 1999;42(1):85–92.
124. Glicksman RM, Tjong MC, Neves-Junior WFP, et al. Stereotactic ablative radiotherapy for the management of spinal metastases: a review. JAMA Oncol 2020;6(4):567–77.
125. Klein-Weigel PF, Elitok S, Ruttloff A, et al. Superior vena cava syndrome. Vasa 2020;49(6):437–48.
126. Cohen R, Mena D, Carbajal-Mendoza R, et al. Superior vena cava syndrome: a medical emergency. Int J Angiol 2008;17(1):43–6.
127. Drews R, Dimitry JR, Rabkin MD. Malignancy-related superior vena cava syndrome. 2017. Online. Available from: www.uptodate.com/contents/malignancy-related-superior-vena-cava-syndrome.
128. Prasad R, Kemnic T. Superior vena cava syndrome from extensive lung cancer. J Osteopath Med 2021;121(3):329–30.
129. Issani A. An updated narrative review on the management of the most common oncological and hematological emergencies. Dis Mon 2022: 101355.
130. Transfusion ANZSoB. ANZSBT guidelines for the administration of blood products. 2022. Online. Available from: anzsbt.org.au/guidelines-standards/anzsbt-guidelines/.
131. Hill S, Carless P, Henry D, et al. Transfusion thresholds and other strategies for guiding allogeneic red blood cell transfusion. Cochrane Database of Syst Rev 2002;(2):CD002042.
132. Böll B, Schalk E, Buchheidt D, et al. Central venous catheter-related infections in hematology and oncology: 2020 updated guidelines on diagnosis, management, and prevention by the Infectious Diseases Working Party (AGIHO) of the German Society of Hematology and Medical Oncology (DGHO). Ann Hematol 2021;100(1):239–59.
133. Schiffer CA, Mangu PB, Wade JC, et al. Central venous catheter care for the patient with cancer: American Society of Clinical Oncology clinical practice guideline. J Clin Oncol 2013;31(10):1357–70.
134. Toh C, Dennis M. Disseminated intravascular coagulation: old disease, new hope. BMJ 2003;327(7421):974–7.

CHAPTER 30
TOXICOLOGICAL EMERGENCIES

IOANA VLAD AND JAMES VINE

ESSENTIALS

- A standardised approach to the management of all poisonings allows the appropriate use of interventions in a timely, sequential manner.
- The risk assessment is of prime importance in guiding subsequent management decisions.
- Acute poisoning is a dynamic presentation, and deterioration can usually be predicted and managed effectively.
- Attention to airway, breathing and circulation will ensure the survival of most patients.
- Antidotal therapy is occasionally used in the resuscitation phase of acute poisoning, but more often is considered after immediate life threats have been treated.

INTRODUCTION

Clinical toxicology is a rapidly expanding area of core knowledge for paramedics and nurses working in emergency care. While virtually any agent ingested at sufficient dose is potentially toxic, so too all agents have a threshold dose below which they are relatively harmless; hence the need to have a thorough understanding of common agents and their particular toxic mechanisms.

DEMOGRAPHICS AND COMMON PRESENTATIONS

Poisonings may occur across the spectrum of the population. The most common scenarios in the adult population are deliberate self-harm or misadventure during recreational use. Chronic toxicity (as can occur with digoxin, lithium or lead) can occur secondary to accumulation of a prescribed medication or environmental toxin over time.

Iatrogenic poisonings can occur when patients are administered, dispensed or prescribed the wrong medication or wrong dose.

Accidental ingestions in children or patients with dementia or other disabilities are also possible. Accidental overdose may occur because of a confusional state or lack of information regarding the substance, leading to incorrect dosage, ingestion of substances that are contraindicated or resulting in significant drug interactions. Prescribed medications that have a narrow therapeutic range pose risks, if not monitored carefully, of a rise above the therapeutic dose to a toxic level. Misuse of regular medication, such as digoxin, lithium or warfarin, may lead to a toxicological presentation.

Most poisonings in children are accidental, either by incorrect dosage or because the inquisitive child gains access to a dangerous substance. However, within the adolescent age group, deliberate overdose is more common.[1]

BOX 30.1 RISK ASSESSMENT-BASED APPROACH TO POISONING[5]

RESUSCITATION

Airway
Breathing
Circulation
Control seizures
Correct hypoglycaemia
Correct hyperthermia/hypothermia
Consider resuscitation antidotes

RISK ASSESSMENT

(see Box 30.2)

SUPPORTIVE CARE AND MONITORING INVESTIGATIONS

Screening—12-lead ECG, paracetamol
Specific investigations
Decontamination
Enhanced elimination
Antidotes
Disposition

The history of poisoning is often unknown, unreliable or incomplete. The effective management of toxicology patients requires a systematic approach with initial resuscitation, followed by formulation of a risk assessment based on a worst-case scenario that should guide all further management decisions. A suggested approach to assessment and management is outlined in Box 30.1.

PRE-HOSPITAL MANAGEMENT OF THE POISONED PATIENT

With increased demands on global health services, the pre-hospital (000/999/112) system has increasingly become the first point of contact for a large proportion of patients presenting with drug ingestion, both accidental and intentional. Accounting for a significant percentage of total ambulance calls, these presentations are not confined to illicit drugs, as many prescription drugs can be misused, ingested or overdosed in an attempt to end patients' lives.

In a proportion of these presentations, this information will be volunteered, or it will be evident which substances have been taken, enabling paramedics to follow local or national guidelines, or utilise the support of the Poisons Information Centre (Australia 13 11 26 or Aotearoa New Zealand 0800 POISON/ 0800 764 766) early to ensure best outcomes.

The acute, emotive nature of these presentations, perceived legal implications or systemic effects of the ingestion, invariably make a standard approach to history-taking extremely challenging. This is where pre-hospital practitioners need to be diligent and have a high index of suspicion for poisoning as a differential for a wide variety of presentations, including reduced level of consciousness or agitation.

The information ascertained at the scene has the potential to significantly affect the acute management and clinical trajectory of the patient. Therefore, it is recommended that paramedics make the most of this opportunity, looking for any empty medicine packets or vessels in bins, dosette boxes, blister medicine packets, drug paraphernalia, wrappers, old prescriptions, or discharge letters, to take with the patient to hospital. This is also the opportunity to interview friends, family or other bystanders to ascertain past medical history, prescribed drugs/drug availability, potential timings and route. It is important to ascertain if the exposure was accidental or intentional, particularly if the amount is not known, since deliberate poisonings are often associated with higher doses, hence higher risk. This should not delay resuscitation, management or transportation to hospital. For certain poisonings or critically unwell patients, a pre-alert should be considered to afford the receiving emergency department (ED) time to collate further information from the patient's previous notes, and, if needed, to formulate a management plan in conjunction with the local Clinical Toxicology Service or Poisons Information Centre.

Poisoned patients might try to conceal the substance that they took or might be too unwell to accurately recall, so the history of substance ingested might be inaccurate. Also, it is not uncommon for patients to ingest or inject more than one substance and in this case their assessment and management can be extremely challenging. A comprehensive clinical assessment, utilising a systematic and disciplined approach, is imperative and, along with the physiological trends and clinical progression of symptoms, might indicate a certain toxidrome or group of drugs involved. In its simplest form it is about pattern recognition, but this has the potential to identify the time-critical nature/clinical progression of the ingestion, guide subsequent management, including antidote administration, and determine appropriate transport destinations.

Multiple acute non-toxicological conditions can present with altered level of consciousness or agitation, so the differential diagnosis should be kept broad, particularly if there is no clear history of drug exposure. Also, the potential for injuries should be considered in agitated or unconscious patients.

Scene safety is an important and integral concept that permeates all facets of both paramedic education and practice. It is made challenging by the unplanned, unpredictable nature and environments in which pre-hospital patients present and are managed, but is fundamental in the mitigation of both potential and actual risk to paramedics, patients and the public. The poisoning presentation poses its own unique challenges and specific safety considerations, but should still follow the same disciplined, methodical dynamic risk assessment that encompasses a high level of continued situational awareness. These considerations are:

- increased potential exposure to needles/sharps on scene or concealed on a patient.
- wearing normal personal protective equipment (PPE—gown, gloves and safety glasses) if transporting a patient whose skin or clothes are contaminated. Off-gassing secondary to vomit in a patient who has ingested phosphides could theoretically expose healthcare workers to toxic phosphine vapours.[2] These effects can be reduced by removing clothing, washing the skin and ensuring good ventilation.
- accidental exposure to toxic gases. This should be considered particularly when entering enclosed industrial or

agricultural spaces (e.g. phosphine in grain silos, ship hulls or clandestine methamphetamine laboratories).[3]

The Poisons Information Centre (Australia 13 11 26 or Aotearoa New Zealand 0800 POISON/0800 764 766) and fire and emergency services are also integral in ascertaining risk and the need for specialist decontamination procedures or specific protective equipment requirements. A multidisciplinary, interagency approach to establishing the potential risk is pertinent, but should not delay transport and patient care.

TRIAGE OF THE POISONED PATIENT

The triage of the poisoned patient is a vital part of the assessment and management. It should take into consideration any time-critical interventions, the risk of clinical deterioration and potential complications. Triaging the poisoned patient is often a complex task due to the subjective nature of triage and the confounding factors that often go along with deliberate self-harm, including psychiatric background, behavioural components and suicidality of the patient, attempts to conceal drug use, which can often make it difficult to take a history and confirm medication and doses taken. To effectively and competently triage a poisoned patient, the triage nurse needs to possess excellent history-taking skills, have a high index of suspicion and use resources available to them. Emergency medicine consultants, toxicologists, pharmacists and calling the Poisons Information Centre (Australia 13 11 26 or Aotearoa New Zealand 0800 POISON/0800 764 766) can all be of assistance.

High-risk triage pitfalls to be aware of include:

- cardiac medications (beta-blockers, calcium channel blockers, digoxin)
- metals (lithium, iron, potassium)
- oral hypoglycaemic agents, insulin
- organophosphates
- paraquat
- unusual chemicals
- sustained release preparations
- essential oils and hydrocarbons
- corrosive ingestions
- paediatric presentations.

GENERAL MANAGEMENT OF THE POISONED PATIENT

RESUSCITATION

Poisoning is a leading cause of death in patients under the age of 40 and is high in the differential diagnosis when cardiac arrest occurs in a young adult. Unlike cardiac arrest of other causes, resuscitation following acute poisoning may be associated with good neurological outcomes, even after prolonged periods (hours) of cardiopulmonary resuscitation (CPR). Thus, while poisoning is considered part of the differential diagnosis in a patient in cardiac arrest, resuscitation should continue until expert advice can be obtained.

Attempts at decontamination of the skin or gastrointestinal decontamination almost never take priority over resuscitation and institution of supportive care measures (except for paraquat poisoning). Therefore, clinicians should wear appropriate PPE, including gown, gloves, goggles and appropriate mask, at all times.

Some specific management issues for poisoned patients in cardiac arrest are:

- in cardiac arrest due to tachydysrhythmias post hydrocarbons abuse (e.g. glue sniffing), the pathophysiological mechanism is myocardial sensitisation to catecholamines, so adrenaline administration should be avoided. In hospital settings, beta-blockers are used in the treatment of these ventricular tachydysrhythmias.
- in patients who ingest paraquat, decontamination takes priority over resuscitation. Food or soil should be administered at the scene to decrease gastric absorption. Fuller's earth is traditionally recommended, but it is not readily available and has no advantage over activated charcoal. Oxygen should be avoided unless the oxygen saturation drops below 90%. If this occurs, oxygen administration is titrated to achieve saturation no greater than 91%.
- glucagon has no role in the management of hypoglycaemia secondary to poisoning. Dextrose should always be used to treat hypoglycaemia in the poisoned patient.

AIRWAY, BREATHING AND CIRCULATION

Acute poisoning is a dynamic medical illness and patients may deteriorate within minutes or hours of presentation. Altered level of consciousness, loss of airway protective reflexes or airway corrosive injury, arrhythmias and hypotension are common threats to life in the poisoned patient. As in all life-threatening emergencies, attention to airway, breathing and circulation is paramount and ensures the survival of the vast majority of patients.

Clinical scores, such as the Glasgow Coma Scale (GCS) or alert-verbal-pain-unresponsive (AVPU) system, although commonly used to describe a patient's mental status, have never been validated in poisonings. A patient's ability to guard their airway is not well correlated to the GCS and may change dramatically in a short space of time. An increased risk of aspiration has been noted with GCS scores of less than 12.[4]

Occasionally emergency antidotes are used during the resuscitation of a poisoned patient:

- Naloxone for opioid overdoses
- Sodium bicarbonate for tricyclic overdoses
- Atropine for organophosphate
- Calcium for hydrofluoric acid poisonings
- Dextrose for hypoglycaemia secondary to insulin overdoses.

CONTROL OF SEIZURES

Seizures of toxic cause are generalised, and can usually be controlled with intravenous benzodiazepines (e.g. midazolam, diazepam, clonazepam or lorazepam). Barbiturates are second-line therapy for refractory seizures in acute poisoning. Pyridoxine may be indicated in intractable seizures secondary to isoniazid. Phenytoin or other antiepileptic agents are not indicated in the management of seizures related to acute poisoning.

The presence of focal or partial seizures indicates a focal neurological disorder that is either a complication of poisoning (ischaemia or haemorrhage) or the result of a non-toxicological cause, and further investigations are required.

Venlafaxine, tramadol, amphetamines and synthetic cannabinoids are the most common causes of seizures in poisoned patients in Australia and Aotearoa New Zealand.

HYPOGLYCAEMIA

Hypoglycaemia is easily detectable and correctable to prevent significant neurological injury. Bedside serum glucose should be measured as soon as possible in all patients with altered mental status or seizures.

If the serum glucose is less than 4.0 mmol/L, boluses of 10% or 50% dextrose should be given intravenously in accordance with local protocols (usual recommendations are 50 mL of 50% dextrose or 200 mL of 10% dextrose in adults and 5 mL/kg of 10% dextrose in children) to urgently correct hypoglycaemia.

Insulin, sulfonylureas, beta-blockers, quinine, chloroquine/hydroxychloroquine, salicylates and valproic acid are the most common causes of hypoglycaemia in poisoned patients in Australasia.[5] Ethanol ingestion can cause hypoglycaemia in children.

HYPERTHERMIA

Hyperthermia can be associated with some life-threatening acute poisonings and is associated with poor outcome. A temperature > 38.5°C during the resuscitation phase of management is an indication for continuous core temperature monitoring. Temperature > 39.5°C is an emergency that requires immediate management to prevent multi-organ failure and neurological injury. Active cooling should be initiated immediately with ice packs or ice blankets and cold IV fluids. In severe cases, neuromuscular paralysis with intubation and ventilation is required as it leads to the cessation of muscle-generated heat production and a rapid reduction of temperature.

Paracetamol or non-steroidal anti-inflammatory agents have no role in hyperthermia secondary to acute poisoning as the most common cause is increased muscular activity.

ANTIDOTES

Administration of antidotes is sometimes indicated during the resuscitation phase of management. Examples include intravenous sodium bicarbonate ($NaHCO_3$) in tricyclic antidepressant poisoning, naloxone in severe opioid intoxication, digoxin-specific antibody fragments in severe digoxin toxicity, atropine for organophosphate poisoning and high-dose insulin euglycaemic therapy in severe calcium channel blocker poisoning.

RISK ASSESSMENT

Risk assessment should occur as soon as possible in the management of the poisoned patient. Resuscitation only takes a greater priority. It is the pivotal step in predicting the likely clinical course and potential complications.[6] The key components required to construct a risk assessment are listed in Box 30.2.

BOX 30.2 STEPS FOR CONSTRUCTION OF A RISK ASSESSMENT[5]

Takes into account:

1. **Agent(s) and formulation (liquid/immediate release/slow release)**
2. **Dose(s)**
3. **Time since ingestion**
4. **Clinical features and progress**
5. **Patient factors (weight and comorbidities)**

All subsequent management steps (supportive care and monitoring, investigations, decontamination, enhanced elimination, antidotes and disposition) are determined by the risk assessment. Patients with a normal mental status are usually able to give a good history from which an accurate risk assessment can be constructed. If altered mental status precludes obtaining a direct history, backup strategies are employed to gather necessary information. These include:

- asking the family to search for empty containers
- counting tablets to determine quantity missing
- checking medical records for previous prescriptions
- questioning relatives about agents potentially available to the patient
- any findings on clinical examination, such as the presence of track marks or transdermal patches, or other clinical findings suggestive of specific toxidromes (e.g. anticholinergic, serotonergic, cholinergic).

Under these circumstances, the risk assessment is less accurate and may, at least initially, be based on a 'worst-case scenario'. This is commonly the case with small children where ingestion is rarely witnessed. As the clinical course progresses, the risk assessment and management plan are refined.

In unknown ingestions, the patient's clinical status is correlated with knowledge of the agents commonly available in that geographical area. For example, the central nervous system (CNS) and respiratory depression associated with miotic pupils would indicate opioid intoxication in a young adult male in urban Australia, but is more likely to indicate organophosphate intoxication in India.

The agent, dose and time since ingestion should correlate with the patient's current clinical status. If they do not, the risk assessment needs to be revised. Acute poisoning is a dynamic process, and important decisions can often be made at particular time-points. For example, following deliberate self-poisoning with a tricyclic antidepressant, life-threatening events occur within 6 hours (and usually within the first 2 hours) of ingestion. Therefore, low-risk patients can be identified on clinical grounds at 6 hours post-ingestion. By contrast, following deliberate self-poisoning with sustained-release calcium channel blockers, patients may not exhibit clinical features of poisoning during the first few hours, and correct risk assessment anticipates the delayed onset of severe cardiovascular effects.

In most cases, risk assessment allows the early recognition of medically trivial poisonings, which reassures attending staff, family and patients, while preventing unnecessary investigations, interventions and observation. Supportive care may be instituted with early psychosocial assessment and discharge planning, resulting in a shortened hospital length of stay. Less commonly, but very importantly, risk assessment allows early identification of potentially serious poisoning and the implementation of a tailored proactive management plan. Balanced decisions about gastrointestinal decontamination can be made and appropriate investigations selected. If a specialised procedure or antidote might be required in the next few hours, early communication and disposition planning should begin.

RISK ASSESSMENT IN CHILDREN

Compared to adults, children usually ingest only one agent, usually small amounts (1–2 pills, a lick or a sip), as most medications and chemicals have a bitter taste. The risk for toxicity is

TABLE 30.1 POTENTIALLY LETHAL AGENTS IF 1–2 TABLETS OR A SIP ARE INGESTED BY A TODDLER WEIGHING 10 KG[5]

AGENT	SEVERE TOXICITY CHARACTERISTICS
Amphetamines (including ecstasy)	Confusion, agitation, hypertension and hyperthermia
Baclofen	Coma, respiratory depression
Calcium channel blockers (verapamil and diltiazem)	Rapid progression to hypotension, bradydysrhythmia, shock and cardiac collapse leading to cardiac arrest
Camphor/naphthalene	Seizures, haemolytic anaemia, methaemoglobinaemia
Carbamazepine	Coma
Chloroquine hydroxychloroquine	Coma and cardiac arrest
Clonidine	Coma, respiratory depression, bradycardia
Dextropropoxyphene	Seizure activity and cardiac toxicity leading to ventricular tachycardia; respiratory depression
Hydrocarbons (essential oil, e.g. eucalyptus oil), petrol	Seizures, coma, chemical pneumonitis
Opioids	Respiratory depression, cardiorespiratory arrest
Organophosphates and carbamate insecticides	Bradycardia, bronchospasm, bronchorrhoea, paralysis
Paraquat	Corrosive injury, pulmonary fibrosis, death
Propranolol	Hypoglycaemia, ventricular tachycardia, hypothermia, seizures and coma
Sulfonylureas	Hypoglycaemia which can be slow onset up to 8 hours post-ingestion
Theophylline	Vomiting, sinus tachycardia and central nervous system stimulation +/- seizures
Tricyclic antidepressants	Seizures and ventricular dysrhythmia
Venlafaxine	Seizures

also low as most agents found around the household are non-toxic, and children are usually brought to medical attention as soon as the ingestion is discovered.

The child presenting after ingesting an unknown tablet is a common and difficult clinical situation. All attempts should be made to determine what tablets were accessible to the child. Should this be impossible, the child should be observed for 12 hours, and never discharged overnight. There is no need to empirically administer activated charcoal unless definite ingestion of a potentially lethal poison has occurred, in which case a clinical toxicologist should be consulted for advice. There is a group of substances which, if ingested by a child, can be lethal with a one- or two-tablet dose or one sip (see Table 30.1), and management of a toddler who has ingested unidentified tablets must take this into consideration (see Box 30.3).

Some problems unique to poisoning in children include that the exact quantity and time of ingestion are often estimated (liquid spilt on clothes or the floor, a child left unsupervised for a period of time), or multiple children can be involved. In this case, the risk assessment should be constructed using a worst-case scenario: assume that everything that is missing has been ingested at the earliest possible time (except paracetamol) and that every child ingested the whole amount missing. If the tablets or substance cannot be identified, assume that it is potentially lethal until a period of observation has elapsed.

BOX 30.3 **MANAGEMENT OF A TODDLER WHO INGESTS ONE OR TWO UNIDENTIFIED TABLETS[5]**

1. Admit for a minimum 12-hour observation period.
2. Ensure healthcare facility has appropriate resources to observe, resuscitate and treat a patient if evidence of poisoning occurs.
3. IV access can be deferred until early evidence of toxicity is apparent.
4. Check bedside glucose level if child has symptoms suggestive of hypoglycaemia.
5. Brief staff regarding clinical features for which the patient is being observed (see Table 30.1).
6. Monitor level of consciousness, vital signs (pulse, blood pressure and respiratory rate) and for early clinical features of hypoglycaemia.
7. Cardiac monitoring may be instituted if there is any abnormality of conscious state or vital signs.
8. Discharge patients only during daylight hours.

Poisoning in children can also be a feature of non-accidental injury or neglect, and these should be considered if the child is under 12 months old/not walking or crawling yet, has unusually severe symptoms, the clinical features suggest large or repeated doses or multiple agents, or the history is inconsistent with clinical features. Other potential scenarios when poisoning can occur in children is if the pills are administered by older siblings, the incorrect dose is administered by mistake or lack of knowledge, or if there are substances of abuse in the house that children can be exposed to.

SUPPORTIVE CARE

Following resuscitation and risk assessment, supportive care and disposition planning can begin.

Poisoning morbidity and mortality usually result from the acute effects of the toxin on the cardiovascular, central nervous or respiratory systems. Support of these and other systems for the duration of the intoxication will ensure a good outcome in the vast majority of acute poisonings. Monitoring of the clinical status is essential to detect the progress of the intoxication and the timing of the institution, escalation and withdrawal of supportive care and other measures.

An initial period of close observation in the ED is usually appropriate. During this time the patient's clinical status is monitored closely to ensure that it correlates with the previous risk assessment. If early complications are expected (e.g. decreased level of consciousness requiring intubation in the following 2 hours), preparations can be made to secure the airway as soon as the intoxication declares itself, and before the patient is moved elsewhere. If unexpected deterioration occurs at any time, the clinician's priorities revert to resuscitation prior to revising the risk assessment. To ensure a comprehensive assessment is ongoing the patient should have:

- regular intervals of assessment of vital signs—the timeframe is determined by the severity of the presentation and the potential risks of the toxic substance
- cardiac monitoring until it is established that there is no further risk for cardiac complications
- neurological assessment/observation for seizures
- haemodynamic monitoring, including fluid input and urine output
- general physical assessment for signs such as diaphoresis, rashes or injuries caused by seizures or agitation
- psychological assessment to determine ongoing risks of self-harm or risks which may develop for psychotropic toxins.

If specific complications are anticipated, the correct in-patient clinical area must be identified to detect and manage them. Good practice includes the documentation of a comprehensive management plan, which informs the team looking after the patient of:

- expected clinical course
- potential complications according to the individual risk assessment
- the type of observation and monitoring required
- endpoints that must trigger notification of the treating doctor to review the patient
- management plans for agitation or delirium
- criteria for changing management
- psychosocial risk assessments with a contingency plan if the patient attempts to abscond prior to formal psychosocial assessment.

Patients who are admitted to hospital following an overdose or toxic exposure have the same risk of developing venous thromboembolism as any other patient, maybe even increased in certain groups (dehydration, comatose or delirious requiring bed rest). Thromboprophylaxis should be provided early in the clinical course. Patients with low GCS should have regular pressure care attended to.

Urinary retention is common, particularly if anticholinergic substances are ingested. It can be a significant cause for agitation, and it can result in overstretch injury and even acute renal failure, so prophylactic IDC insertion should be considered, or bladder scans regularly performed.

If available, the emergency observation unit is appropriate for the ongoing management of most acute poisonings, where general supportive measures and monitoring can be provided.

Criteria for admission to the intensive care unit (ICU) following acute poisoning include requirements for:

- airway control
- ventilation
- prolonged or invasive haemodynamic monitoring or support
- haemodialysis.

INVESTIGATIONS

Investigations in acute poisoning are employed either as screening tests or for specific purposes.

SCREENING TESTS

Screening refers to the performance of a medical evaluation and diagnostic test in asymptomatic persons in the hope that early diagnosis may lead to improved outcome. In the acutely poisoned patient, screening tests aim to identify occult toxic ingestions for which early specific treatment is indicated. The recommended screening tests for acute poisoning are 12-lead electrocardiogram (ECG) and serum paracetamol level.

The ECG is a readily available non-invasive tool that assists in the identification of potentially lethal electrical abnormalities, such as AV nodal blockade (PR prolongation), sodium channel blockade (QRS widening) or potassium channel blockade (QT prolongation).

Paracetamol is a ubiquitous analgesic sold under many commercial names in combination with various other medications and deliberate self-poisoning with paracetamol is common. Life-threatening paracetamol poisoning may be occult in the early stages and death can be prevented by timely administration of *N*-acetylcysteine. For this reason, it is advisable to screen for paracetamol in all cases of known or suspected deliberate self-poisoning. The screening paracetamol level may be performed at presentation and does not need to be delayed until 4 hours after ingestion. A non-detectable paracetamol level at more than 1 hour after ingestion excludes significant paracetamol ingestion and further paracetamol level tests are not required.

If paracetamol poisoning is suspected after the initial risk assessment, then a screening paracetamol level check is not required. Instead, a timed paracetamol level should be performed as soon as possible after 4 hours post-ingestion.

SPECIFIC INVESTIGATIONS

After appropriate risk assessment and the institution of supportive care, the patient may require no further investigations beyond the screening ECG and serum paracetamol measurement. Other investigations are ordered selectively as shown in Box 30.4.

BOX 30.4 **INDICATIONS FOR SPECIFIC INVESTIGATIONS**[5]

To:
- refine risk assessment or prognosis
- exclude or confirm an important differential diagnosis
- exclude or confirm an important specific poisoning
- exclude or confirm a complication that requires specific management
- establish an indication for antidote administration
- establish an indication for the institution of enhanced elimination
- monitor response to therapy or define an endpoint for therapeutic intervention.

TABLE 30.2 **GASTROINTESTINAL DECONTAMINATION**[5]

POTENTIAL BENEFITS	POTENTIAL RISKS
Improved clinical outcome (morbidity and mortality)	Pulmonary aspiration
More benign clinical course requiring lower level of supportive care	Distraction of staff from resuscitation and supportive care priorities
Reduced need for other potentially hazardous interventions or expensive antidotes	Gastrointestinal complications • bowel obstruction • perforation
Reduced hospital length of stay	Diversion of departmental resources for performance of procedure

Serum drug levels are indicated for only a few agents. These include lithium, salicylate, iron, theophylline, digoxin and CNS depressants such as sodium valproate, carbamazepine and barbiturates.

Qualitative urine screens for drugs of abuse (e.g. opioids, benzodiazepines, amphetamines, cocaine, barbiturates and cannabinoids) rarely alter the management of the acutely poisoned patient in the emergency department (ED).[7] They might be useful later on to the mental health team if a diagnosis of drug-induced psychosis is suspected, or in paediatric patients, particularly if non-accidental injury is suspected. Patients with acute intoxication with one or more of these agents may be managed according to their clinical presentation. A positive result from a patient without corresponding symptoms of intoxication rarely alters acute medical management. Electrolyte levels are a common assessment and are useful for identifying another underlying pathology; beta human chorionic gonadotrophin (beta-hCG) is useful for establishing pregnancy status, and urinalysis for assessing underlying pathology or the potential of rhabdomyolysis causing myoglobinuria associated with some toxic substances. Other pathology investigations will depend on the presentation and may include renal and liver function tests, full blood count (FBC) and venous blood gases. Chest x-ray might be needed to assess for complications such as aspiration pneumonia. Abdominal x-ray may be requested for evaluating radio-opaque substances such as iron, lithium, lead or arsenic (refer to Box 30.4).

GASTROINTESTINAL DECONTAMINATION

Historically, various methods have been employed in the reasonable expectation that by reducing the dose absorbed they will also reduce the subsequent severity and duration of toxicity. The Australian Poisons Information Centre and the New Zealand National Poisons Centre are available 24 hours a day and should be consulted for the most current treatment protocols for specific poisons.

These procedures do not provide significant benefit when applied to unselected deliberately self-poisoned patients and are no longer considered routine. The decision to decontaminate is one of clinical judgement, in which the potential benefits are weighed against the potential risks and the resources required to perform the procedure (see Table 30.2).

By employing this rationale, gastrointestinal decontamination is reserved for cases where the risk assessment predicts severe or life-threatening toxicity, and where supportive care or antidote treatment alone is insufficient to ensure a satisfactory outcome. Before proceeding, there should be reasonable grounds to believe that a significant amount of agent remains unabsorbed and is amenable to removal by the selected procedure. For certain poisonings that are associated with high mortality and have no antidotes available (e.g. colchicine, paraquat), decontamination should be considered even with delayed presentations. Gastrointestinal decontamination is never performed to the detriment of basic resuscitation or supportive care. To avoid pulmonary aspiration, the procedure is not performed without first securing the airway in a patient with a depressed level of consciousness or where the risk assessment indicates a potential for imminent seizures or decline in the level of consciousness.

INDUCED EMESIS

Emptying the stomach by inducing emesis is no longer advocated.

ASPIRATION OF GASTRIC CONTENT

If a naso- or orogastric tube is introduced, either because the patient is intubated or to facilitate administration of activated charcoal or whole-bowel irrigation, the stomach content should be aspirated and discarded in case it still contains toxic residues from the overdose.

SINGLE-DOSE ACTIVATED CHARCOAL

Oral activated charcoal consists of fine porous particles suspended in water or sorbitol. It reversibly adsorbs most ingested toxins and prevents them from being further absorbed from the gastrointestinal tract. However, it does not improve clinical outcome when applied to unselected patients with self-poisoning and should not be regarded as routine.[8]

Oral activated charcoal is indicated where it is likely that toxin remains in the gastrointestinal tract (within the first 2 hours for most agents and up to 4 hours for slow-release

TABLE 30.3 AGENTS POORLY BOUND TO ACTIVATED CHARCOAL[5]

HYDROCARBONS AND ALCOHOLS	METALS	CORROSIVES
Ethanol	Lithium	Acids
Isopropyl alcohol	Iron	Alkalis
Ethylene glycol	Potassium	
Methanol	Lead	
	Arsenic	
	Mercury	

preparations), and where the potential benefits outweigh the potential risks (see Table 30.2).

Activated charcoal is contraindicated if:

- the agent ingested is poorly adsorbed to charcoal (see Table 30.3)
- there is ingestion of corrosive agents with the risk of gastrointestinal perforation (except paraquat)
- there is a decreased level of consciousness, delirium or poor patient compliance (unless airway protected by endotracheal intubation) OR
- risk assessment suggests the potential for imminent onset of seizures or decreased level of consciousness
- risk assessment indicates non-toxic ingestion or that will have good outcome with supportive care and antidotal therapy alone.

The major risk is charcoal pulmonary aspiration due to loss of airway reflexes associated with the impaired level of consciousness or seizures.[9] Corneal abrasions have been described secondary to administration of activated charcoal. They can occur if charcoal is accidentally spilled on the patient's eyelids when administered via a nasogastric tube to an unconscious patient.

Due to its black colour, charcoal is often refused by young children. One way to overcome this is mixing it with ice-cream or juice to disguise the colour.

GASTRIC LAVAGE

Gastric lavage involves the sequential administration and aspiration of small volumes of fluid from the stomach via an orogastric tube to empty the stomach of toxic substances. This previously widely favoured method of gastrointestinal decontamination has now been all but abandoned, and few EDs remain experienced in its use.

The amount of toxin removed by gastric lavage is unreliable and negligible if performed after the first hour. Gastric lavage has also been associated with complications such as oesophageal rupture or aspiration pneumonia. There are few situations where the expected benefits of this procedure might be judged to exceed the risks involved and where administration of charcoal would not be expected to provide equal or greater efficacy of decontamination.

WHOLE-BOWEL IRRIGATION

This aggressive and labour-intensive form of gastrointestinal decontamination attempts to cleanse the entire bowel by administering large volumes of osmotically-balanced polyethylene glycol–electrolyte solution (PEG-ELS). It is rarely performed because risk-benefit analysis reserves this intervention for body packers or for life-threatening ingestions of sustained-release preparations or other agents, as outlined in Box 30.5.

BOX 30.5 CONDITIONS IN WHICH WHOLE-BOWEL IRRIGATION MAY BE POTENTIALLY USEFUL[5]

- **Iron overdose > 60 mg/kg**
- **Slow-release potassium chloride ingestion > 2.5 mmol/kg**
- **Life-threatening slow-release verapamil or diltiazem ingestions**
- **Symptomatic arsenic trioxide ingestion**
- **Lead ingestion**
- **Body packers**

PRACTICE TIPS

NURSING CARE OF WHOLE-BOWEL IRRIGATION

- 1:1 nursing care.
- Place nasogastric tube (NGT) and confirm placement.
- Give activated charcoal 50 g or 1 g/kg in children via NGT if it is an agent that binds to activated charcoal.
- Commence polyethene glycol electrolyte solution (PEG-ELS) at a rate of 2 litres per hour.
- Keep hydrated.
- Position patient on a bedside commode if possible as they will develop diarrhoea.
- Monitor until passing clear liquid stools (it may take several hours).

ENHANCED ELIMINATION

Techniques of enhanced elimination (Box 30.6) are employed to increase the rate of removal of an agent with the aim of reducing the severity and duration of clinical intoxication. These interventions are indicated if they reduce mortality, length of stay, complications or the need for other more invasive interventions. In practice, these techniques are useful only in the treatment of poisoning by a few agents that are characterised by:

- severe toxicity
- poor outcome despite good supportive care and antidote administration
- slow endogenous rates of elimination
- suitable pharmacokinetic properties.

Enhanced elimination is never carried out to the detriment of resuscitation and good supportive care, and once the decision is made to initiate a technique of enhanced elimination, it is essential to establish clinical or laboratory endpoints for therapy.

BOX 30.6 TECHNIQUES OF ENHANCED ELIMINATION AND AMENABLE AGENTS[5]

MULTIPLE-DOSE ACTIVATED CHARCOAL

- Carbamazepine
- Dapsone
- Phenobarbitone
- Theophylline
- Quinine
- *Amanita phalloides* mushroom

HAEMODIALYSIS AND HAEMOFILTRATION

- Lithium
- Metformin lactic acidosis
- Potassium
- Salicylate
- Theophylline
- Toxic alcohols
- Valproic acid

URINARY ALKALINISATION

- Phenobarbitone
- Salicylate
- MCPA (herbicide)

MULTIPLE-DOSE ACTIVATED CHARCOAL

Repeated administration of oral activated charcoal enhances the elimination of agents that enter the enterohepatic circulation and are excreted in the bile (Box 30.6).

Potential complications of administering multiple-dose activated charcoal include all those associated with single-dose activated charcoal, with the added risk of mechanical bowel obstruction.

URINARY ALKALINISATION

The production of an alkaline urine pH promotes the ionisation of highly acidic drugs and prevents their reabsorption across the renal tubular epithelium, thus promoting excretion in the urine. For this method to be effective, the drug must be filtered at the glomerulus, have a small volume of distribution and be a weak acid (e.g. salicylate overdose).

ANTIDOTES

Antidotes are medications that reverse the effects of certain poisonings. Contrary to popular belief, there is not an antidote for every poison. In fact, only a few exist and these are used for a limited number of poisonings, with many being used extremely rarely (e.g. chelating agents). Like all pharmaceuticals, antidotes have specific indications and contraindications, optimal administration methods, monitoring requirements, appropriate therapeutic endpoints and adverse effect profiles.

An antidote is administered when the potential therapeutic benefit is judged to exceed the potential adverse effects. While some antidotes, such as naloxone and benzodiazepines, are commonly used, many antidotes are rarely prescribed, expensive and not widely stocked. Planning for the stocking, storage, access, monitoring, training and protocol development are essential components of rational antidote use.[10] It is often appropriate for stocking to be coordinated on a regional basis in association with regional policies concerning the treatment of poisoned patients. It is frequently cheaper and safer to transport an antidote to a patient rather than vice versa. Commonly used antidotes are discussed with their specific target drugs in the following pages.

DISPOSITION

A period of observation is required for most patients who present with poisoning or potential exposure to a toxic substance. Those who have deliberately self-poisoned also require psychiatric and social review.

Patients must be admitted to an environment capable of providing an adequate level of monitoring and supportive care, and, if appropriate, where staff and resources are available to undertake resuscitation, decontamination, administration of antidotes or enhanced elimination techniques. Early risk assessment in the out-of-hospital setting, usually in consultation with Poisons Information Centre staff, often allows non-intentional exposures to be observed outside of the hospital environment. For those who present to the hospital, this can minimise the duration and intensity of monitoring. Frequently patients can be discharged directly from the ED immediately following assessment or after a few hours of monitoring. At other times, the risk assessment will indicate the need for ongoing observation, supportive care or the need for specific enhanced elimination techniques or antidote administration. In these circumstances, the patient must be admitted to an environment capable of providing a level of care appropriate for the anticipated clinical course. In many hospitals in Australia, this is now the emergency observation unit rather than the general medical ward. Patients requiring ongoing airway control, ventilation or advanced haemodynamic support are admitted to an ICU.

PRACTICE TIP

- Risk assessment, after resuscitation, is the most important step in the management of the poisoned patient as it determines subsequent management steps and patient disposition.
- Call the Poisons Information Centre (13 11 26 in Australia or 0800 POISON/0800 764 766 in Aotearoa New Zealand) when dealing with a time-critical toxicological emergency or for any toxicology advice.
- Meticulous supportive care and monitoring are sufficient to ensure a good outcome in most poisonings.
- Perform paracetamol levels and an ECG as screening tests in the poisoned patient.
- Gastrointestinal decontamination, enhanced elimination techniques and specific antidotes are rarely required, but in specific circumstances may be lifesaving.
- Most episodes of acute poisoning are an exacerbation of an underlying psychosocial disorder, which may determine the patient's final disposition.
- Administration of sodium bicarbonate prior to intubation may prevent deterioration from progressive acidosis in sodium channel blocker toxicity (e.g. tricyclic antidepressants).
- The absence of oral or lip burns does not exclude significant gastro-oesophageal injury following corrosive ingestions.
- Consider cyanide toxicity in the collapsed patient with severe lactic acidosis, especially following a house fire.

COMMONLY INGESTED AGENTS

ALCOHOL AND TOXIC ALCOHOLS

Ethanol

Ethanol ingestion causes rapid, dose-related CNS depression, with a high degree of inter-individual variability. The dose may be estimated if the number of standard drinks consumed is known. A standard drink contains approximately 10 g ethanol, which is equivalent to a 375 mL can of mid-strength beer (3.5%), a 100 mL glass of wine or a 30 mL shot of spirits.

Co-ingestion of other CNS depressants (e.g. sedative-hypnotic agents, opioids, antidepressants) increases the risk of CNS and respiratory depression. Other acute clinical effects include disinhibition, nystagmus, vomiting, tachycardia, seizures (in the setting of ethanol intoxication or withdrawal) and hypoglycaemia, particularly in children.

Ethanol is rapidly absorbed following oral administration and is distributed readily across the total body water. In the lungs, ethanol moves by passive diffusion from the capillaries into alveoli where it vaporises easily, being a volatile compound.

Investigations and management

Serum ethanol levels assist risk assessment in patients with CNS depression, but must not be assumed to be the sole contributor to CNS depression, and an appropriate evaluation for other causes, such as co-ingestants or trauma, is required. Measurement of breath ethanol concentration using a breathalyser can be used instead in cooperative patients as it provides a rapid, convenient bedside estimation of blood ethanol concentration, but the accuracy is influenced by multiple factors, including minute ventilation, body temperature and presence of vomit or blood in the mouth.

Management of ethanol intoxication is supportive and focuses on airway protection and adequate IV hydration. In alcoholic patients, this should also include administration of thiamine and the recognition that intoxication may be followed by alcohol withdrawal.

The major pitfalls are a failure to detect co-ingestants or co-existent injuries or medical conditions in intoxicated patients.

Toxic alcohols

Toxic alcohols include ethylene glycol, methanol and isopropyl alcohol. Ethylene glycol is usually found in antifreeze, window cleaners and brake fluids. Methanol can be found in home-made distilled alcoholic drinks or racing fuel. 'Methylated spirits' sold in Australia do not contain methanol, but do in Aotearoa New Zealand.

Ethylene glycol and methanol cause rapid-onset CNS effects similar to ethanol. Of note, both agents are metabolised by the alcohol dehydrogenase enzyme pathway to form acids, and the intentional ingestion of > 1 mL/kg ethylene glycol or 0.5 mL/kg methanol can result in potentially lethal metabolic acidosis.[11] Ethylene glycol also causes hypocalcaemia and acute renal failure, while methanol classically causes optic nerve injury and blindness. Small accidental ingestions of less than a mouthful are benign, but deliberate self-poisonings are assumed to be potentially lethal.

Isopropyl alcohol causes significant CNS depression. As little as 1 mL/kg of a 70% solution causes symptoms of inebriation. Ingestion of more than 4 mL/kg causes coma and respiratory depression.

Investigations and management

The diagnosis of both ethylene glycol and methanol toxicity can be made by a combination of history, clinical examination and biochemistry. Very few centres in Australia can perform ethylene glycol or methanol level measurements, and the results are not usually available within a clinically useful time-frame. However, serial measurements of serum osmolality (to calculate the osmolar gap), serum lactate, pH and bicarbonate are usually adequate to confirm or exclude the diagnosis. In the absence of ethanol, a raised osmolar gap (> 10 mmol/L), hyperlactataemia and a high anion-gap metabolic acidosis are suggestive of ethylene glycol or methanol poisoning. The presence of calcium oxalate crystals in the urine is pathognomonic for ethylene glycol intoxication. However, the absence of crystals does not exclude the diagnosis.

Significant ethylene glycol or methanol intoxication is initially treated with oral or intravenous (IV) ethanol. Ethanol competitively inhibits the formation of toxic metabolites by having a greater affinity for the enzyme alcohol dehydrogenase. Fomepizole is an alternative agent used to inhibit the action of alcohol dehydrogenase, but it is not widely available in Australia. Inhibition of toxic alcohol metabolism is, however, only a temporising measure and definitive treatment with haemodialysis must be arranged as soon as possible.

A common pitfall in management is not to recognise that co-ingestion of ethanol prior to the presentation will delay metabolism of the toxic alcohols and may mask their presence.

Isopropyl alcohol does not cause a metabolic acidosis but will cause an osmolar gap, which can be measured to confirm the diagnosis. Treatment is supportive, as for ethanol. Haemodialysis is effective at removing isopropyl alcohol, as it is with ethanol, but is rarely clinically indicated.

ANALGESICS

Aspirin (salicylates)

Salicylate toxicity occurs following irreversible inhibition of cyclooxygenase enzymes (COX-1 and COX-2), resulting in decreased prostaglandin synthesis and uncoupling of oxidative phosphorylation. This manifests initially as hyperventilation and respiratory alkalosis secondary to respiratory centre stimulation, followed by progressive metabolic acidosis as a result of oxidative phosphorylation uncoupling.[12]

Acute salicylate toxicity causes mild symptoms with ingested acetylsalicylate (aspirin) doses of < 150 mg/kg, but is potentially lethal with doses > 500 mg/kg. Methyl salicylate, found in numerous topical products such as oil of wintergreen, is more potent, with 1 g equivalent to 1.5 g of acetylsalicylate. Due to delayed absorption, symptoms may not occur for many hours post-ingestion.

Initial clinical features include profuse vomiting, tinnitus and diaphoresis (salicylism). Complicated acid–base disturbances occur in salicylate toxicity. The first of these is respiratory alkalosis due to hyperventilation (typically with increased tidal volumes rather than respiratory rate). This is caused by direct stimulation by salicylate of the medullary respiratory centre. Following this, metabolic acidosis occurs by inhibition of the Krebs cycle, causing an increase in lactic acid production. Also, lipid metabolism and protein catabolism are increased, leading to increased production of ketone bodies and amino acids respectively. The worsening acidosis enhances salicylate movement into the brain, resulting in cerebral oedema with coma and seizures. Hypoglycaemia can also develop, further complicating the management of these patients.

By contrast, chronic intoxication is more common in elderly people and usually presents with non-specific clinical features, such as dehydration, confusion, fever and acidosis. The diagnosis is frequently missed and, as a consequence, morbidity and mortality are greater in chronic intoxication.

Investigations and management

Specific investigations include venous blood gases and salicylate levels. Serial salicylate levels correlate poorly with actual toxicity, but are useful in determining treatment regimens and monitoring response to therapy.

Management consists of meticulous supportive care, decontamination and institution of enhanced elimination techniques.[11] Activated charcoal adsorbs salicylate very effectively and should be administered in patients with intact mental state, even many hours post-ingestion, as salicylates cause pylorospasm and may form pharmacobezoars, which result in ongoing delayed absorption.[12]

Renal elimination of salicylates is enhanced in alkaline urine, and this is achieved by administration of intravenous sodium bicarbonate bolus followed by infusion (target urine pH 7.5).[12]

Patients with confusion, acidaemia, renal failure or high salicylate levels should be referred for urgent haemodialysis. Deterioration in a conscious state is an ominous sign of salicylate poisoning and may require intubation while definitive therapy with haemodialysis is organised. Failure to maintain hyperventilation after intubation in patients with severe salicylate poisoning (to compensate for the metabolic acidosis) may lead to catastrophic deterioration from worsening acidosis.

Paracetamol

Paracetamol in acute overdose or with supratherapeutic administration has the potential to cause life-threatening hepatotoxicity. Hepatotoxicity is caused by the metabolism of paracetamol to *N*-acetyl-p-benzoquinone imine (NAPQI), which causes glutathione depletion and consequent hepatonecrosis. Other organ effects include nephrotoxicity, which may occur independently of hepatotoxicity, and coma, which is seen with massive ingestions.

Investigations and management

Paracetamol level testing at 4 hours or more post-ingestion should be performed in all patients who present after a deliberate overdose or after an accidental but potentially toxic overdose. Other tests such as hepatic transaminase levels, international normalised ratio (INR), FBC and renal function might be considered in some scenarios (delayed presentations, staggered ingestions etc.).

For single acute ingestions of immediate release paracetamol, the threshold for toxicity is considered to be > 200 mg/kg.[13] If the time of ingestion is known, a paracetamol level at 4–16 hours can be plotted on the paracetamol treatment nomogram for Australia and Aotearoa New Zealand.[13] If the level is above the treatment line, treatment with *N*-acetylcysteine is indicated. If the time of ingestion is not known, the decision to treat can be based on either a worst-case scenario (i.e. earliest possible time of ingestion), the presence of a raised paracetamol level or abnormal liver transaminases. The nomogram cannot be used for other scenarios of paracetamol poisonings, such as slow-release preparations, staggered overdoses or supratherapeutic ingestions.

Treatment with *N*-acetylcysteine, which replenishes glutathione, is close to 100% effective if started within 8 hours of acute ingestion. Every effort should be made to commence it within this time-frame if toxic ingestion is suspected or confirmed. Outside this period, if the risk assessment infers a potentially toxic dose, the safe management is to commence *N*-acetylcysteine before investigation results are available. The risk of anaphylactoid reaction with the infusion of *N*-acetylcysteine was reduced by the introduction of the 2-bag regimen. If an anaphylactoid reaction occurs, it is managed by slowing or ceasing the infusion, treating with an antihistamine such as promethazine and recommencing therapy at a lower rate.

Supratherapeutic administration of paracetamol is, in contrast to acute ingestions, a greater risk in children than adults. The decision to treat is based on abnormal hepatic transaminase levels (alanine aminotransferase [ALT] or aspartate aminotransferase [AST] > 50 IU/L) and/or raised paracetamol levels. These decisions should be made in consultation with a clinical toxicologist.

ANTICONVULSANTS

Carbamazepine

Carbamazepine inhibits inactivated sodium channels, blocks noradrenaline reuptake and is an antagonist at muscarinic and nicotinic receptors.

Intentional ingestion of carbamazepine causes CNS depression, anticholinergic symptoms and, in massive doses, dysrhythmias and haemodynamic instability. Clinical features are dose-dependent, but onset is dependent on the type of preparation ingested (immediate or controlled-release), and the patient may not become symptomatic for 8–12 hours.

Doses of 20–50 mg/kg predictably cause mild to moderate CNS effects, such as nystagmus, dysarthria, ataxia, sedation, delirium, mydriasis, ophthalmoplegia and myoclonus; and anticholinergic effects such as urinary retention, tachycardia and dry mouth. If > 50 mg/kg is ingested there is a risk of coma requiring intubation, hypotension and dysrhythmias.

Carbamazepine is slowly and erratically absorbed. Following large overdoses, ileus secondary to anticholinergic effects may result in ongoing absorption for several days.

Investigations and management

Carbamazepine levels are useful in comatose patients, but have little benefit in performing levels on patients who are awake and who can be monitored clinically.

Management is based on good supportive care and airway protection as required. In massive ingestions that result in ventricular dysrhythmias, sodium bicarbonate should be used. Carbamazepine is well adsorbed by activated charcoal and elimination is enhanced by the use of repeat-dose activated charcoal. In life-threatening cases, haemodialysis may be required. Avoidable pitfalls include failure to appreciate the potential for delayed onset of toxicity, failure to detect urinary retention or ileus from anticholinergic effects, and ongoing administration of multidose activated charcoal leading to bowel obstruction.

SODIUM VALPROATE

Valproate increases levels of gamma-aminobutyric acid (GABA), a central inhibitory neurotransmitter, and in large doses interferes with numerous mitochondrial metabolic pathways. It is usually well absorbed following oral administration, but absorption may be slow and erratic following overdose. Peak levels may be delayed up to 18 hours.

Most valproate overdoses result in various degrees of CNS depression that correlate with rising serum levels. Ingested doses < 200 mg/kg are asymptomatic, with the risk of coma developing at 400 mg/kg. With doses above this, patients are at risk of multi-organ toxicity with haemodynamic instability, cerebral oedema and bone marrow suppression. A dose of 1 g/kg is potentially fatal.

Investigations and management

Serial valproate levels can be used to confirm poisoning and guide therapy, particularly in the intubated patient. The valproate level on arrival can be normal even in a life-threatening overdose, so the level should be repeated if there is clinical deterioration or if the patient is comatose. Hypernatraemia, hypocalcaemia, hypoglycaemia, elevated lactate and hyperammonaemia are all associated with significant valproate toxicity.

Mainstays of treatment are good supportive care, airway protection and early dialysis, if indicated. Valproate is well adsorbed to activated charcoal, and this should be administered to the patient who has taken > 400 mg/kg. High serum levels, cardiovascular instability or development of lactic acidosis are the usual indications for haemodialysis, which can be lifesaving in the severely poisoned patient.

PREGABALIN

Pregabalin is a gamma-aminobutyric acid (GABA) analogue prescribed for neuropathic pain, epilepsy, fibromyalgia and anxiety. It has euphoric and dissociative effects and there is evidence of increasing recreational use worldwide.

Overdose results in various degrees of CNS depression ranging from drowsiness to coma.[14] Myoclonus can be a side-effect of normal therapeutic dosing and can occur in overdoses as well.

Pregabalin levels are not widely available. Management is largely supportive and seizures should be treated with benzodiazepines first-line, like other seizures of toxicological cause. Its elimination can be enhanced by haemodialysis.[14]

LAMOTRIGINE

Lamotrigine is an anticonvulsant also used in the treatment of bipolar mood disorders, enuropathic pain and migraine prophylaxis. It blocks voltage-gated sodium channels thus suppressing depolarisation, and decreases the release of excitatory neurotransmitters by blocking calcium channels.

Overdose most commonly results in CNS depression, which can range from drowsiness to coma depending on the amount ingested. Paradoxically there are reports of seizures and even status epilepticus in overdose. The most common cardiovascular manifestation is tachycardia, but QRS widening, wide complex tachycardias and cardiac arrest have been reported.[15]

Lamotrigine levels cannot be performed routinely. Activated charcoal should be considered for large overdoses, but it should only be administered after the airway is protected, due to the risk of CNS depression and seizures. Seizures should be treated with benzodiazepines first-line, like other seizures of toxicological cause. Sodium bicarbonate should be trialled to treat wide complex tachycardia; however, there are several reports of cases where it did not improve the conduction delay. Haemodialysis might have a role; however, there is very limited data about its use.[15]

ANTIDEPRESSANTS

Tricyclic antidepressants

Tricyclic antidepressant (TCA) poisoning remains a major cause of morbidity and mortality. Deliberate self-poisoning may lead to the rapid onset of CNS and cardiovascular toxicity. Prompt intubation, hyperventilation and sodium bicarbonate administration are lifesaving.

TCAs are noradrenaline and serotonin reuptake inhibitors, as well as GABA-A and muscarinic receptor blockers. However, their major toxic effect is through fast sodium channel blockade, which results in dysrhythmias, hypotension and seizures. TCAs are rapidly absorbed, highly protein-bound and have a large volume of distribution.

Ingestion of > 10 mg/kg is usually associated with major toxicity, which is manifest within 1–2 hours. Doses < 5 mg/kg cause minimal symptoms, and 5–10 mg/kg are associated with mild sedation and anticholinergic symptoms.

Investigations and management

The most useful investigation in TCA toxicity is the ECG. Sodium channel blockade causes prolongation of the QRS intervals, right axis deviation, and a prominent terminal 'R' wave in aVR (taller than 3 mm). A QRS width of > 110 ms is associated with an increased risk of seizures and > 160 ms with ventricular tachycardia.[16]

Severe toxicity is characterised by the rapid deterioration in clinical status within 1–2 hours of ingestion. Patients may present alert and orientated only to rapidly develop coma, seizures, hypotension and cardiac dysrhythmias. This clinical situation is managed by initial administration of 1 mEq/kg bolus of $NaHCO_3$ repeated every 3–5 minutes, as required, followed by endotracheal intubation and hyperventilation to a pH of 7.5–7.55. Adjunctive treatment measures include benzodiazepines for seizures and intravenous fluid boluses and vasopressors for hypotension.

Activated charcoal should only be administered once the airway has been secured.

Management of smaller ingestions is generally supportive, although anticholinergic symptoms may be problematic. Patients with a normal ECG and mental state at 6 hours may be removed from cardiac monitoring and referred for psychiatric assessment as appropriate.

Selective serotonin reuptake inhibitors

Deliberate self-poisoning with selective serotonin reuptake inhibitor (SSRI) antidepressants is common and usually follows a benign course if ingested as single agents. The SSRIs are rapidly absorbed following oral administration, are protein bound and have large volumes of distribution. They undergo hepatic metabolism to form less active and water-soluble metabolites, and elimination half-lives are approximately 24 hours. Clinically, most patients are asymptomatic or have mild symptoms, which resolve completely within 12 hours.

Ingestions may be associated with seizures or the development of symptoms of serotonin toxicity, particularly if co-ingested with other serotonergic agents such as monoamine oxidase inhibitors (MAOIs), two or more serotonin reuptake inhibitors (SSRIs), selective serotonin and noradrenaline reuptake inhibitors (SNRIs), TCAs, lithium, tramadol, pethidine, fentanyl, sympathomimetic recreational drugs (amphetamines or ecstasy) and herbal preparations (spirulina, St John's wort).

Serotonin toxicity manifests as agitation, tremor, tachycardia, mydriasis and hypertonia; when severe, it is associated with profound mental state changes, rigidity and hyperthermia that can be life threatening.[17] Two SSRI antidepressants, escitalopram and citalopram, apart from the risk of serotonin toxicity, can also cause dose-dependent QT prolongation and are more likely to cause seizures.

Investigations and management

A 12-lead ECG and serum paracetamol level are the only baseline investigations required following SSRI ingestion. Following citalopram overdose of > 600 mg or escitalopram 300 mg, all patients should have cardiac monitoring until 8 hours post-ingestion. A normal ECG at this time allows cardiac monitoring to cease.[17,18] If the ingested dose is > 1000 mg, or the QT interval is > 450 ms, cardiac monitoring is continued, and serial ECGs performed for at least 12 hours post-ingestion or until resolution occurs. Cases of torsade de pointes secondary to QT prolongation have been described in the context of citalopram and escitalopram overdoses; they should be managed with magnesium sulphate and overdrive pacing.

Patients with SSRI overdose other than citalopram who have a normal ECG do not require ongoing cardiac monitoring.

Seizures are usually short-lived and heralded by agitation and tachycardia, and are managed with benzodiazepines. Symptoms of serotonin toxicity are also well managed in almost all cases with benzodiazepines. Serotonin antagonists, such as cyproheptadine and olanzapine, can also be used in patients requiring large amounts of benzodiazepines. Life-threatening mental state changes, rigidity and hyperthermia require immediate intubation, paralysis and active cooling.[17,18]

Activated charcoal is rarely indicated as most ingestions are benign, and there is a risk of seizures in more significant ingestions. The exception to this are large citalopram ingestions (< 4 hours post-ingestion).

Monoamine oxidase inhibitors

Monoamine oxidase inhibitors (MAOIs) may be broadly classified into two groups:

- irreversible non-selective monoamine oxidase inhibitors, such as phenelzine and tranylcypromine, which are associated with potentially lethal serotonin toxicity in overdose and can cause significant adverse reactions, even with therapeutic dosing
- reversible and selective agents such as moclobemide are associated with a benign clinical course, but severe serotonin syndrome occurs when they are taken in combination with other serotonergic agents.[17,18]

MAOIs decrease the metabolism of sympathomimetic amines, in particular, dopamine, serotonin and noradrenaline. They are rapidly absorbed orally and metabolised prior to elimination.

Clinical features of significant ingestions include agitation, hypertonia, altered mental state, seizures, hyperthermia and cardiovascular instability with severe hyper- or hypotension. When symptoms occur, they are generally prolonged and may last for several days.

Investigations and management

There are no blood tests specific to these poisonings.

Management of severe toxicity is based on good supportive care and airway protection as required. Benzodiazepines, control of hyperthermia with paralysis if required and other antiserotonergic agents such as cyproheptadine or olanzapine may be indicated. Hypertensive crises are best treated with titratable, short-acting vasodilators (e.g. sodium nitroprusside, glyceryl trinitrate), as autonomic instability may result in profound hypotension and beta-blockers are contraindicated. Activated charcoal may be administered to intubated patients or if they present within 1 hour of overdose. Severely poisoned patients who require intubation and paralysis for hyperthermia may have prolonged ICU admissions.

ANTIPSYCHOTICS

Typical antipsychotic agents

Phenothiazines (e.g. chlorpromazine, pericyazine) and butyrophenones (e.g. haloperidol, droperidol) are therapeutic antagonists at central dopamine receptors. They are known as 'typical' antipsychotics because they were the initial agents used for psychotic disorders; however, they are rarely prescribed now for outpatient treatment. They have a number of adverse effects at $alpha_1$-adrenergic and cholinergic receptors, and in overdose, they cause CNS depression, orthostatic hypotension and anticholinergic effects. Cardiotoxicity is secondary to sodium and potassium channel-blocking effects. Extrapyramidal effects (dystonic reactions and akathisia) may occur after small ingestions, especially in children, and these may be delayed up to 5 days post-ingestion.

Investigations and management

The clinical features of intoxication occur within 2–4 hours of overdose. Sedation may occasionally require intubation for airway protection, and hypotension usually responds to volume resuscitation. Urinary retention is common, and anticholinergic delirium may complicate recovery from coma. Serial ECGs and cardiac monitoring are required if there are signs of toxicity (QRS widening and QT prolongation) and should be continued until these abnormalities resolve.

Atypical antipsychotics

This group includes quetiapine, olanzapine, asenapine, clozapine, risperidone, paliperidone, amisulpride, aripiprazole, ziprasidone and lurasidone. They are classified as atypical due to their decreased propensity to cause dystonia or extrapyramidal effects and have become an extremely common cause of drug-induced coma requiring intubation. Most of these agents have anticholinergic effects and the potential for mild hypotension.[19]

Following overdose, patients typically present with early-onset dose-related sedation, significant tachycardia, various degrees of QT prolongation and occasionally hypotension. Seizures are rare. Large ingestions of amisulpride and ziprasidone have been associated with QT prolongation, delayed broad-complex tachycardias and life-threatening cardiovascular collapse. Clozapine is associated with profuse salivation in overdose, and with agranulocytosis and cardiotoxicity with therapeutic use. Management of poisoning with these agents is, for the most part, supportive, although the management of torsade de pointes includes magnesium and overdrive pacing.

CARDIAC DRUGS

Beta-blockers

Beta-blockers are competitive antagonists at $beta_1$ and $beta_2$ receptors, leading to bradycardia and hypotension in overdose. Overdose involving the vast majority of beta-blockers is relatively benign and results in minimal toxicity only. However, large ingestions of propranolol or sotalol may be life threatening.[20]

Propranolol has sodium-channel blocking effects causing QRS widening and ventricular dysrhythmias, and crosses the blood–brain barrier reducing seizure threshold. Sotalol blocks cardiac potassium channels, disrupting cardiac repolarisation, and may lead to QT prolongation and, potentially, torsade de pointes.

The response to overdose is highly variable, but usually most significant in elderly patients with underlying heart or lung disease, or on concomitant treatment with calcium channel blockers or digoxin.

Investigations and management

Acute beta-blocker poisoning is a potentially life-threatening emergency that should be managed in an area equipped for cardiorespiratory monitoring and resuscitation. Bradycardia may be temporarily relieved with IV boluses of atropine 0.01–0.03 mg/kg, and in patients with significant concomitant hypotension, an infusion of adrenaline or isoprenaline should be considered.[21]

The threshold dose for severe toxicity from propranolol is approximately 1 g (15 mg/kg in children). Severe toxicity is characterised by the rapid deterioration in clinical status within 1–2 hours of ingestion. Patients may present as alert and orientated only to rapidly develop coma, seizures, hypotension and cardiac dysrhythmias. This clinical situation is similar to severe TCA toxicity except that the patients are usually bradycardic and asystolic cardiac arrest can occur. Patients are managed by administration of 1 mEq/kg bolus of $NaHCO_3$ repeated every 3–5 minutes, as required, endotracheal intubation and hyperventilation to a pH of 7.5–7.55. Bradycardia can be difficult to manage and is unlikely to respond to atropine. Adrenaline or isoprenaline infusion should be used and transcutaneous or temporary transvenous pacing attempted. The endpoints of successful treatment are an improvement in QRS duration or return of spontaneous circulation, and cessation of seizures.

Sotalol can cause QT prolongation in therapeutic dosing and in overdose. If torsade de pointes develops, treatment options include intravenous magnesium, overdrive pacing with isoprenaline or the insertion of a transvenous pacemaker.

Glucagon is no longer recommended for the treatment of beta-blocker poisoning as it offers no advantages over standard inotropic and chronotropic management. High-dose insulin euglycaemic therapy may have an emerging role in the management of severe and refractory beta-blocker toxicity.

Calcium channel blockers

Calcium channel blockers are well absorbed and following ingestion, peak levels and toxicity occur within 1–2 hours for standard preparations and 6–12 hours for SR preparations.

Verapamil and diltiazem cause potentially life-threatening cardiovascular collapse following an overdose, with the onset of symptoms delayed by several hours following ingestion of commonly prescribed slow-release (SR) preparations. In general, ingestion of 10 or more tablets causes significant haemodynamic symptoms in adults and the ingestion of 1–2 tablets of verapamil or diltiazem SR is potentially lethal in children. Advanced age and comorbidities, such as cardiac disease, increase the risk of significant toxicity.

Early signs of toxicity are bradycardia, first-degree heart block and hypotension. Hypotension results from severe peripheral vasodilation, bradycardia and decreased myocardial contractility, and typically is resistant to maximal doses of the usual inotropic agents.

Investigations and management

Early recognition of the potential for significant toxicity is vital. Ingestion of verapamil or diltiazem SR is an indication for decontamination with activated charcoal and consideration of whole-bowel irrigation. This can potentially be performed up to 4 hours after significant ingestion; however, the risk of aspiration needs to be considered if a patient becomes systemically unwell.

Significant or refractory hypotension is difficult to manage and requires a logical and methodical approach.

- Volume resuscitation with sodium chloride 0.9% or Hartmann's solution is first-line therapy.
- Intravenous calcium therapy aims to maintain ionised calcium level above 2.0 mEq/L.
- Vasopressor support with noradrenaline or vasopressin.
- High-dose insulin euglycaemic therapy should be started as soon as inotropic or vasopressor support is considered necessary. Calcium channel blockers block calcium channels in the pancreas as well, decreasing insulin release and thus creating a temporary hypoinsulinaemic/hyperglycaemic state. For this reason, the high insulin dose required to treat calcium channel blockers overdoses (1 units/kg bolus followed by infusion of up to 10 units/kg/hr) is usually well tolerated. Increasing dextrose requirements in this setting is usually a sign that poisoning is resolving.[5] High-dose insulin euglycaemic therapy takes 30–45 minutes to start working, so patience is required before deciding that it is either not effective or that the dose has to be increased.

Significant bradycardia can be difficult to manage. Atropine is unlikely to be effective, and it is often difficult to achieve electrical capture with ventricular pacing. Adrenaline infusion is occasionally effective. In isolated cases, extracorporeal membrane oxygenation (ECMO) and intra-aortic balloon pump have been successfully used as extraordinary manoeuvres.

Digoxin

Digoxin inhibits the membrane Na^+–K^+ ATPase pump and leads to an increase in intracellular calcium and extracellular potassium. Digitalis glycosides are also found in many poisonous plants (e.g. oleander, foxglove, rhododendron, desert rose) and animals (e.g. cane toads).

Acute digoxin toxicity occurs if more than 10 times the therapeutic dose is ingested. Ingestion of $>$ 10 mg in an adult or $>$ 4 mg in a child is potentially lethal and manifests as vomiting, hyperkalaemia and cardiovascular collapse refractory to conventional resuscitation measures.

Digoxin has a narrow therapeutic index, and elderly patients with multiple comorbidities are at risk to develop chronic toxicity. The clinical features of chronic digoxin toxicity are often non-specific and include cardiovascular (bradycardia, heart block, slow atrial fibrillation or ventricular ectopy), gastrointestinal (vomiting and abdominal pain) and neurological (confusion).

Investigations and management

Essential investigations include a serum digoxin level, urinalysis, electrolytes and serial 12-lead ECG. Serum digoxin levels of > 15 nmol/L (12 ng/mL) or serum potassium level > 5.5 mmol/L in the setting of acute overdose are potentially fatal.

The probability of digoxin toxicity increases with the number of clinical and ECG features observed, and the measured serum digoxin level.

Decontamination with activated charcoal is recommended if patients present in the first 2 hours post-overdose.

Prior to the availability of digoxin antibodies, overdoses were associated with significant mortality. Atropine and inotropes provide only temporary relief for haemodynamic instability. Hyperkalaemia should be treated using the usual measures (e.g. insulin + dextrose, sodium bicarbonate, salbutamol). There is a theoretical concern that calcium might worsen digoxin cardiotoxicity. However, there are several case reports published where it was used with no adverse incidents. Digoxin-specific antibodies (Fab) are available to treat both acute and chronic toxicity.

In acute overdose, the Fab dose is calculated on the presumption that one ampoule binds 0.5 mg of digoxin and taking account the clinical status of the patient. In case of cardiac arrest, 5 vials should be administered and attempts at resuscitation should continue for at least 60 minutes after the administration of digoxin immune Fab (e.g. Digifab®), as good outcomes have been reported. For patients who are not in cardiac arrest, 2 vials of digoxin immune Fab are recommended initially and then titration of further doses depending on clinical progression.

In chronic poisoning, empirical dosing starts with one ampoule. If the patient is in cardiac arrest the initial dose is 2 vials. It may take up to 6 hours to detect a clinical response. Digoxin bound to digoxin antibodies will be measured by the regular laboratory assays, so free digoxin levels should be requested to obtain an accurate measurement.

COLCHICINE

Colchicine is derived from the autumn crocus plant (*Colchicum autumnale*) and is used to treat gout. It binds to intracellular microtubules and prevents cell division. It has a narrow therapeutic window and is extremely toxic in overdose.

Severe gastrointestinal symptoms are the initial symptoms, and systemic features develop at doses of > 0.1 mg/kg. Ingestions of > 0.8 mg/kg are associated with multi-organ failure, cardiovascular collapse, hepatic failure and bone marrow suppression. Toxicity occurs at lower doses in patients with pre-existent renal or liver impairment or if co-ingested with certain drugs (cytochrome P-3A4 or P-glycoprotein inhibitors).

Investigations and management

Early recognition of the potential severity of colchicine overdose is vital. Because there is no antidote, the mainstays of treatment are early decontamination and good supportive care. Activated charcoal should be used as soon as possible, even in delayed presentation, as decreasing the absorption of even small amounts of colchicine may be lifesaving. Meticulous volume resuscitation and management in the intensive care unit is required in cases of significant poisoning.

LITHIUM CARBONATE

Lithium is a metal ion which modulates intracellular second messengers and is thought to affect neurotransmitter (including serotonin) production and release. It is available as both immediate- and slow-release preparations, and after absorption slowly redistributes to the CNS, where it is most toxic. It is almost completely renally excreted.

Lithium toxicity is classified into acute and chronic:

- *Significant acute* lithium overdose produces acute gastrointestinal symptoms, including nausea, vomiting, abdominal pain and diarrhoea. Provided adequate urinary lithium excretion is maintained, significant neurotoxicity should not occur with acute overdoses.
- *Chronic lithium toxicity* is most commonly diagnosed in patients with renal impairment on long-term lithium therapy; patients who have an intercurrent illness resulting in dehydration (e.g. gastroenteritis) or who are started on medications that interfere with lithium excretion (e.g. non-steroidal anti-inflammatory agents, ACE inhibitors). Patients usually present with signs of neurotoxicity, which can cause permanent neurological sequelae or death.

Clinical features of neurotoxicity include tremor, increased tone, hyperreflexia, confusion, myoclonic jerks, seizures and altered mental state. Nephrogenic diabetes insipidus and thyroid dysfunction can complicate therapeutic use and may contribute to chronic toxicity. Patients on long-term lithium therapy who have diabetes insipidus produce large amounts of urine, therefore requiring an increased water intake. Fluid restriction during their admission to hospital can precipitate lithium toxicity.

Investigations and management

Check urea and electrolytes following acute and chronic overdose to monitor renal function. Serum lithium levels > 5.0 micromole/L are not uncommon in acute ingestions, and with good management will not result in neurotoxicity. However, in chronic toxicity, clinical features of severe neurotoxicity may be present when the serum lithium level is only just above the normal range (i.e. > 1.0 micromole/L).

Management of acute poisoning depends on the dose ingested and renal function.[22] Doses < 25 g rarely cause significant toxicity in the setting of normal renal function. The routine use of whole-bowel irrigation is not indicated, but it can be considered in very large ingestions. Haemodialysis is reserved for those patients who, despite the implementation of conservative measures, exhibit renal impairment, significant neurotoxicity and deteriorating clinical status, or cannot tolerate the large amounts of IV fluids required to maintain adequate urine output.

Patients with chronic toxicity, which may be precipitated by renal failure or other drugs, such as NSAIDs and angiotensin-converting enzyme (ACE) inhibitors, usually present with established neurotoxicity and dehydration. They require fluid resuscitation and correction of renal impairment. If this fails, haemodialysis should be considered.

In patients with chronic lithium toxicity, signs of clinical improvement might take several days to a week post-treatment.

HERBICIDES

Glyphosate

Glyphosate, more commonly known by the tradename Roundup®, is a widely used herbicide. Intentional ingestion of large volumes of the concentrated solution can be life threatening. Ingested doses of < 50 mL of concentrated solution by an adult causes mild gastrointestinal symptoms, but doses of > 300 mL can cause refractory shock and death. Dilute over-the-counter preparations are normally benign, but can cause mild gastrointestinal irritation or pneumonitis secondary to pulmonary aspiration.

The toxicity is thought to be due to the surfactant that is combined with the glyphosate rather than the glyphosate itself, and involves uncoupling of mitochondrial oxidative phosphorylation.[23] Dermal exposure poses no risk of systemic toxicity.

Investigations and management

Specific investigations that may be useful in these patients include baseline renal and hepatic function, venous blood gases and a chest x-ray to assess for features of pneumonitis. Worsening acidosis and isolated elevations in potassium precede onset of refractory shock. Management is supportive. There is no role for enhanced elimination, although haemodialysis may be indicated as part of supportive care.

Paraquat

N, N'-dimethyl-4,4'-bipyridinium dichloride (commonly known as 'paraquat') is a herbicide that is potentially lethal with an ingested dose of as little as one mouthful. While small accidental ingestions may be salvageable with aggressive decontamination and early dialysis, intentional ingestions of large volumes are uniformly fatal.

Paraquat toxicity is due to the production of oxygen free radicals, which cause cellular injury and cell death. Paraquat is extremely corrosive to the gastrointestinal tract, resulting in severe upper airway and oesophageal burns. Following absorption, it accumulates predominantly in the lungs, and with large ingestions patients develop hypoxia, multi-organ failure and death occurs within days. Those patients who survive large ingestions are at risk of developing pulmonary fibrosis. Dermal exposure to intact skin poses no risk of systemic toxicity.

Investigations and management

Sodium dithionite is added to urine as a rapid qualitative test in cases of likely paraquat ingestion. Urine will turn blue in the presence of paraquat, and green in the presence of diquat, a related but less toxic agent.[4] Serum paraquat levels may be plotted on a nomogram to predict potential lethality following ingestions, but do not contribute to the acute management. Additional investigations include serial arterial blood gases, chest x-rays and endoscopy.

Management involves immediate aggressive decontamination—this even takes priority over initial resuscitation concerns. Activated charcoal adsorbs paraquat, but any ingested substance may limit absorption of paraquat—recommendations have even included eating soil if nothing else is immediately available. Excessive or routine supplemental oxygen should be avoided, as this worsens lung damage due to increased production of reactive oxygen species, but should not be withheld if significant hypoxia is present.

Following decontamination, the mainstays of treatment are haemodialysis (preferably within 2 hours of ingestion) and good supportive care.

Adjunctive treatments such as *N*-acetylcysteine, vitamin C, dexamethasone and sodium salicylate (or aspirin) are also recommended, although their role in management has not been validated in large studies.

INSECTICIDES

Organophosphates and carbamates

Intentional ingestion of organophosphates (OPs) or carbamates is potentially life threatening. They are used as insecticides and as 'nerve agents' in chemical warfare and are major problems in developing countries as a preferred mode of suicide. Cross-contamination between the patient and healthcare professional is possible, so contaminated clothing should be removed and exposed skin washed with water. Usual PPE is enough, and treatment should not be delayed by any further decontamination. There have been no documented cases of significant OP poisoning in healthcare professionals caring for poisoned patients.

Organophosphates and carbamates both act to inhibit acetylcholinesterase (AChE) enzymes and to increase acetylcholine (ACh) concentration at cholinergic receptors. Organophosphates, if left untreated, form a permanent bond with the AChE enzyme (known as ageing); whereas carbamates do not, and hence are self-limiting in their clinical effect.

Both groups of agents are well absorbed following ingestion, have large volumes of distribution and often accumulate in lipid stores. Carbamates have less CNS absorption than organophosphates and are associated with less significant neurotoxicity.

The timing of symptom onset is dependent on the agent, dose and route of exposure and may occur within minutes of ingestion or can be delayed many hours. Clinical features are classified according to the affected receptor.

- Muscarinic effects include diarrhoea, urination, miosis, bronchorrhoea, bronchospasm, bradycardia, emesis, lacrimation and salivation ('DUMBBBELS' mnemonic).
- Nicotinic effects include fasciculations and tremor, which can progress to respiratory muscle paralysis.
- Haemodynamic instability and CNS effects with seizures and coma may be seen. The most common cause of death in these patients is respiratory failure.
- An intermediate syndrome of muscle weakness may occur several days post-exposure, particularly in inadequately treated patients; some agents can cause organophosphate-induced delayed neuropathy (OPIDN), and chronic occupational exposure may result in neuropsychiatric sequelae.

Investigations and management

Red cell and plasma cholinesterase levels are used to confirm exposure and guide treatment after the acute resuscitation phase is completed.

Management of these poisonings requires aggressive early resuscitation, early intubation if indicated, and the use of antidotes.

- Atropine is the agent of choice for treating muscarinic symptoms. Dosage is commenced at 1.2 mg IV and doubled every 5 minutes until the patient is dry of secretions and has adequate air entry. Large doses may be required in severe cases until the desired clinical endpoints are attained.

- Pralidoxime reactivates the AChE enzyme that has been inhibited by being 'reversibly' bound to organophosphate molecules and is not effective if 'irreversible binding' (ageing) has occurred. Pralidoxime is not routinely used for organophosphate poisoning though due to suggestions of increased mortality.[24] It might be considered for certain patients after discussion with a clinical toxicologist.

A tragic but common impediment to adequate resuscitation is the concern that staff will be 'poisoned' following exposure to these patients. This has resulted in 'Hazmat' responses being instituted in the out-of-hospital setting with delays in transport to definitive care, and patients with life-threatening toxicity being refused entry into EDs. It is the vapours of the volatile hydrocarbon diluent and *not* the non-volatile organophosphate that may cause the treating staff to be aware of a strong odour and to produce mild symptoms such as a headache and dizziness if exposed for long periods, although this is not a significant threat to the health of staff. However, contact with body fluids should be avoided as per standard universal precautions, and staff should be rotated to reduce symptoms, but this should never take precedence over resuscitation of the patient.

CARBON MONOXIDE (CO)

Carbon monoxide poisoning occurs either secondary to deliberate self-poisonings with car exhaust fumes or accidentally, in domestic exposures to faulty gas heaters or when people try to warm themselves in winter by burning barbecue fuel inside the house. Exposure to house fires can result in both carbon monoxide and cyanide toxicity, as hydrogen cyanide is released from burning synthetic polymers used in building materials and furnishings.

Carbon monoxide has a higher affinity for haemoglobin than oxygen, making haemoglobin oxygen transport less effective and thus causing cellular hypoxia. In pregnant patients, the fetus is more susceptible to injury as carbon monoxide binds fetal haemoglobin more avidly.

Clinically poisoned patients present with headache, nausea, ataxia, confusion or poor concentration, symptoms that resolve with oxygen therapy. In more severe cases, they are found comatose, have ischaemic changes on the ECG and metabolic complications (lactic acidosis).

Deaths secondary to carbon monoxide poisoning usually occur out of hospital, and the large majority of patients who arrive at the hospital alive survive their poisoning but can have long-term neuropsychiatric sequelae.

Investigations and management

Carboxyhaemoglobin levels confirm the diagnosis but do not correlate with the symptoms. The presence of metabolic acidosis with raised lactate level on arterial or venous blood gases indicate more severe poisoning and can be a surrogate marker of toxicity. ECG and cardiac markers are done to look for myocardial ischaemia. All female patients of childbearing age should have a pregnancy test.

Management is along the usual lines of attention to airway, breathing and circulation, with the administration of high-flow oxygen as soon as possible, and continued until all symptoms resolve. Hyperbaric oxygen should be considered for all pregnant patients and those with severe toxicity and associated end-organ damage (collapse/coma/ongoing neurological signs, myocardial ischaemia).

IRON

Iron ingestions are particularly common in children. Iron has a direct corrosive effect on the gastric mucosa and, in large doses, acts as a direct cellular toxin on the heart, liver and central nervous system.

Toxicity is determined by the dose of elemental iron ingested. Ingested doses of > 20 mg/kg of elemental iron are associated with gastrointestinal irritation; > 60 mg/kg with systemic toxicity; and > 120 mg/kg may be lethal.

Clinically poisoned patients present with vomiting and diarrhoea, which then progresses to worsening acidosis, profound shock and multi-organ failure. Those patients who survive large ingestions are prone to long-term complications including fibrosis of the gastrointestinal tract and liver cirrhosis.

Investigations and management

An abdominal x-ray can be useful to confirm ingestion, particularly in children, as the tablets are radio-opaque. Iron levels are useful at 4–6 hours to help determine the need for chelation therapy. These may be repeated 6-hourly until they decline. In the absence of iron levels, serial serum bicarbonate and lactate levels may be used to detect developing systemic toxicity.

Management is based on decontamination, supportive care and the use of chelating agents. Iron is not adsorbed to activated charcoal, so this treatment is not indicated. For ingestions > 60 mg/kg, confirmed on x-ray, whole-bowel irrigation is the decontamination method of choice. Desferrioxamine chelation therapy is indicated where systemic toxicity (shock, metabolic acidosis, altered mental status) is present or predicted by a serum iron level > 90 micromol/L (500 microg/dL) at 4–6 hours post-ingestion.[5]

LOCAL ANAESTHETICS

Local anaesthetic toxicity is nearly always the result of a therapeutic error—either the inadvertent intravascular administration or incorrect dose. Topically administered local anaesthetic agents can be absorbed through skin or mucosa (teething gels, EMLA®, Co-Phenylcaine®) and there are case reports of paediatric fatalities after ingestion of lidocaine-containing topical anaesthetic preparations.

The local anaesthetic agents bind reversibly to sodium channels to inhibit the sodium flux necessary to initiate and propagate action potentials in peripheral nerves.

Clinical features of toxicity include tinnitus, dizziness, anxiety, confusion and perioral numbness, and in severe cases seizures, coma and cardiovascular effects (bradycardia, hypotension, atrial and ventricular dysrhythmias, cardiovascular collapse and asystole). Methaemoglobinaemia can also occur, but is not dose-related.

Investigations and management

Patients suspected of local anaesthetic toxicity should have serial ECGs, which might show evidence of Na channel blockade (QRS widening).

Ventricular dysrhythmias are treated with sodium bicarbonate 100 mEq (2 mEq/kg in children) IV repeated every 1–2 minutes until the restoration of perfusing rhythm. Intravenous lipid emulsion is indicated in severe cardiovascular toxicity or cardiac arrest refractory to standard resuscitation protocols. Hypotension should be treated with administration of intravenous crystalloid 20 mL/kg followed by inotropic support if necessary. Seizures are treated with benzodiazepines.

Methylene blue is the specific antidote for methaemoglobinaemia and is administered to symptomatic patients.

Local anaesthetic toxicity usually occurs in a hospital or clinic setting. The development of any neurological symptoms during or shortly after administration of a local anaesthetic should prompt close observation in an area equipped for cardiorespiratory monitoring and resuscitation. Once resuscitated, the patient should be managed in a high-dependency or intensive care setting until toxicity resolves.

HYPOGLYCAEMIC AGENTS

Insulin

Insulin stimulates the movement of glucose, potassium, magnesium and phosphate into cells. Profound refractory hypoglycaemia and clinically significant hypokalaemia may result.

Deliberate or accidental insulin overdose causes rapid onset of life-threatening hypoglycaemia. Large doses administered via subcutaneous injection create depots of insulin from which the drug is erratically released sometimes for several days.[25]

Clinical features of prolonged hypoglycaemia include seizures and depressed conscious state that, if left untreated, may lead to permanent neurological injury or death.

Investigations and management

Specific investigations include serial blood sugar levels and potassium levels. Blood sugar should be measured every 15–30 minutes for the first few hours, then 1- to 2-hourly when blood sugar levels have been stabilised. Potassium levels should be checked 2-hourly until stabilised.

Management is centred on the IV administration of dextrose for the duration of the poisoning. Initial hypoglycaemia is treated with boluses of IV dextrose (25–50 mL 50% in adults, and 5 mL/kg 10% in children), followed by dextrose infusion. Infusions are required for 24–48 hours, but may be longer with large overdoses. Potassium monitoring and replacement is also required. Protracted therapy with concentrated dextrose solutions must be given through a central line to prevent peripheral venous thrombophlebitis. Eight hours of euglycaemia off dextrose should be demonstrated prior to discharge and cessation of the dextrose infusion should not take place overnight.

Sulfonylureas

Sulfonylureas act by increasing the release of endogenous insulin from pancreatic beta islet cells and, if taken in excess, have the potential to cause life-threatening hypoglycaemia.[26] One tablet is enough to kill a child. Patients on therapeutic doses who develop renal failure are also at risk of toxicity. Due to the long half-lives of these agents the risk of hypoglycaemia can last several days with large ingestions.

Investigations and management

Serial blood sugar levels are the most useful investigations in these patients. As the onset of hypoglycaemia can be delayed by up to 8 hours following ingestion, patients often require overnight admission for observation and serial blood glucose measurements. During daylight hours, the conscious state can be used to guide the need for repeat blood glucose level testing, particularly for children who may find it traumatic.

Management is based on detection and treatment of hypoglycaemia (< 4.0 mmol/L in this setting). Activated charcoal may be considered < 2 hours following large intentional ingestion in patients with a normal mental state.

Initial hypoglycaemia is managed with IV dextrose (25–50 mL 50% in adults, 5 mL/kg 10% in children), but the definitive and specific antidote is octreotide. Octreotide inhibits endogenous insulin release and is so effective in this setting that patients rarely require further IV dextrose after its administration.[27] Patients must be normoglycaemic for at least 6 hours after cessation of octreotide infusion before being considered safe for discharge.

Metformin

Metformin is a biguanide that inhibits gluconeogenesis, reduces hepatic glucose output and stimulates glucose uptake in the peripheries. It is renally excreted.

Unlike sulfonylurea overdose, toxicity from metformin poisoning is secondary to lactic acidosis rather than hypoglycaemia, which is uncommon.

The greatest risk for metformin-induced lactic acidosis is in the setting of renal failure superimposed on therapeutic use, particularly in the elderly.[26] Acidosis with acute overdose is rare but potentially life threatening in patients who ingest more than 10 g or who have impaired renal function. Ingestion of less than 1700 mg in children is considered benign. Metformin increases production of lactate in the gut, so many patients will have raised lactate levels. High lactate levels become concerning if they are associated with worsening acidosis or if the patient has renal failure.

Investigations and management

Specific investigations include the renal function and serum lactate. Patients with serum lactate levels > 12 mmol/L are at risk of cardiovascular instability, and levels > 20 mmol/L are commonly fatal without immediate definitive care. Patients who are clinically well with normal serum lactate at 8 hours can be medically cleared.

Management is based on good supportive care with close attention to adequate hydration and urine output. Patients with refractory acidosis or rapidly rising lactate levels > 10 mmol/L will require haemodialysis.

CORROSIVE AGENTS

Chemicals with acid or alkaline pH can cause corrosive injury. Many household and farm products fall into this category:

- Alkalis: ammonia, potassium hydroxide, sodium hydroxide, sodium hypochlorite
- Acids: hydrochloric acid, sulfuric acid
- Other: glyphosate, paraquat, phenols, potassium permanganate, mercuric chloride, zinc chloride

Ingestion of corrosive agents can cause injury to the upper airway and gastrointestinal tract. The extent of the injury is dependent on pH, concentration and volume ingested. Upper airway injury is a life-threatening emergency and delay in management can cause significant airway oedema. Stridor, dyspnoea, dysphonia or throat pain after ingestion of a corrosive substance are highly concerning and should be a prompt for early airway management.

Significant gastro-oesophageal injury can also occur and can be complicated by perforation, infection or stricture formation. The absence of lip or oral burns does not exclude significant gastro-oesophageal injury.

Investigations and management

Symptomatic corrosive ingestion is a time-critical emergency managed in an area equipped for resuscitation. Early endotracheal intubation or surgical airway may be required.

The mouth may be rinsed with water as an immediate first aid measure, but do not induce vomiting, do not administer oral fluids or activated charcoal and do not attempt pH neutralisation. Do not insert a nasogastric tube and keep these patients nil by mouth until the extent of the injury is defined by endoscopy.

Patients who are asymptomatic and tolerating oral fluids at 4 hours post-ingestion do not require an endoscopy and can be discharged.

DRUGS OF ABUSE

Cannabinoids (marijuana)

Marijuana is the most widely used recreational illicit drug in Australia. It can cause unpleasant but not life-threatening symptoms in adults, but in children it leads to significant CNS depression.

Acute intoxication in adults is usually associated with mild sedation, disinhibition, mild disorientation and euphoria, and in higher doses with tachycardia, postural hypotension, CNS depression, anxiety, perceptual disturbances and even psychotic symptoms. Chronic use can lead to long-term neuropsychiatric sequelae. Treatment of acute intoxication is purely supportive.[5]

Heavy users can develop cannabinoid hyperemesis syndrome, which is characterised by cyclical severe vomiting, that can be resistant to usual antiemetics, and is characteristically relieved by hot showers. There are reports that haloperidol/droperidol and capsaicin cream might be effective therapies.[28]

Stimulants

Acute intoxication with amphetamines, cocaine, novel stimulant drugs, synthetic cannabinoid-receptor agonists, and novel hallucinogenic drugs result in sympathomimetic toxidrome.

Amphetamines are widely abused stimulant drugs that enhance catecholamine release and block their reuptake and also cause dopaminergic stimulation. Amphetamines are well absorbed following ingestion or inhalation/smoking.

Cocaine-intoxicated patients present very similar to amphetamines. Cocaine is also a sodium channel blocker and can cause QRS widening and ventricular tachydysrhythmias.[5]

Novel stimulant drugs, synthetic cannabinoid-receptor agonists, and novel hallucinogenic drugs are cheap, widely available and not detected by urine drug screens.

Novel stimulant drugs mimic established recreational stimulant drugs, such as methamphetamine. They are typically sold as powders or pills to be snorted or ingested, but can also be injected or smoked. Cathinones are the most common group and they are often sold under the street name of 'bath salts'. Other common street names are 'miaow-miaow' (4-methylmethcathinone), 'flakka' (alpha-pyrrolidinovalerophenone), 'ivory wave' (methylenedioxypyrovalerone) or 'bubbles' (methylenedioxymethcathinone).

Synthetic cannabinoid-receptor agonists are often termed 'synthetic marijuana' or 'synthetic cannabis', and are designed to mimic the effects of tetrahydrocannabinol (THC), the active ingredient in cannabis. There are hundreds of compounds in this group, usually sold as liquid formulations that are sprayed onto herbal mixtures, to be smoked. To disguise their intended use, they are often labelled as 'potpourri' or 'incense' with the disclaimer 'not for human consumption'. They are also used in e-cigarettes and vaporisers. The preparations have many names, depending on the specific formulation, including 'spice', 'K2', 'crazy monkey' or 'buddha blue'. Compared with cannabis use, seizures, paranoia and psychotic symptoms are more common and severe with synthetic cannabinoid-receptor agonists. Patients usually present in a hyperadrenergic state with agitation similar to stimulant drug poisoning. This is followed by CNS depression after 3 to 6 hours.

Novel hallucinogenic drugs are designed to mimic established hallucinogenic drugs, such as lysergic acid diethylamide (LSD) or ketamine. Their use often results in mental state and behavioural changes, serotonin toxicity and sympathomimetic toxidrome. Clinical features of sympathomimetic toxidrome include:

- CNS: anxiety, dysphoria, agitation and aggression, paranoid psychosis with visual and tactile hallucinations, rigidity and myoclonic movements, seizures
- hyperthermia
- cardiovascular: tachycardia, hypertension, dysrhythmias, acute coronary syndrome, acute cardiomyopathy, acute pulmonary oedema
- peripheral sympathomimetic: mydriasis, sweating and tremor
- rhabdomyolysis, dehydration and renal failure
- hyponatraemia (more common after ecstasy [MDMA] ingestion), due to temporary SIADH and increased water ingestion
- aortic and carotid artery dissection
- subarachnoid and intracerebral haemorrhage
- vasospasm (coronary, cerebral).

Investigations and management

Stimulant-intoxicated patients are often aggressive and difficult to manage initially. They might require physical and/or chemical restraint before performing any investigations.

All patients who present post-stimulant use should have an ECG looking for signs of cardiac ischaemia and dysrhythmias. Other investigations will be guided by the clinical scenario and the type of drug.

Tachycardia and hypertension are managed with benzodiazepines; in cases of severe refractory hypertension IV, GTN might be required temporarily. There are increasing case series reporting successful use of clonidine to control the blood pressure and heart rate. Seizures are managed with IV benzodiazepines.

Agitation is managed with benzodiazepines, but if psychotic features are significant an antipsychotic agent (e.g. droperidol, haloperidol, olanzapine) should be added early on.

Hyperthermia usually responds well to benzodiazepines and active cooling with ice packs and cold IV fluids; however, for temperatures > 39.5°C, early intubation and paralysis should be considered to facilitate cooling.

Other drugs of abuse

Gamma hydroxybutyrate (GHB) is a sedative drug that is abused in clubs and also used as a date-rape drug. Acutely intoxicated patients present with CNS and respiratory depression. Treatment is supportive.

Solvent abuse is a major public health problem in adolescents and Indigenous communities. The agent with the highest potential for abuse is toluene, found primarily in glues, spray paints and lacquers. Acute intoxication can lead to ventricular tachydysrhythmias, depressed GCS and seizures. Chronic toluene abuse can lead to renal tubular acidosis, ataxia, dementia and peripheral neuropathy. A fetal solvent syndrome, similar to fetal alcohol syndrome, has been described in children born to women who abused solvents during pregnancy.[5,29]

Another inhalant drug abused is nitrous oxide, which is often procured in the form of whipped cream cartridges (see Fig. 30.1). Long-term abuse of nitrous oxide can lead to inactivation of B_{12}-dependent enzymes. Patients can present with lower limb weakness, altered sensation and ataxia due to myelopathy involving the posterior columns of the spinal cord.[30]

PLANTS AND MARINE

There are many plants and marine organisms that can cause poisoning if ingested.[31] Cardiac glycosides can be found in oleander plants (Fig. 30.2), desert rose and foxglove. If ingested they can produce toxicity similar to digoxin, with gastrointestinal symptoms, hypokalaemia and various degrees of cardiac toxicity.

Rhododendron plants contain grayanotoxins which can cause paraesthesias, muscle weakness and brady or tachydysrhythmias.

Many mushrooms found in Australia can cause gastrointestinal symptoms (vomiting and diarrhoea), and some will also cause euphoria and hallucinations. Of concern is *Amanita phalloides* (Fig. 30.3) which is found in Adelaide Hills, Canberra and in some parts of Victoria.[5] It can cause hepatotoxicity, liver failure and death.

Castor bean plants (Fig. 30.4) are ubiquitously found in urban and rural Australia. All the parts of the plant contain ricin

FIGURE 30.1 WHIPPED CREAM CARTRIDGES (NITROUS OXIDE ABUSE)

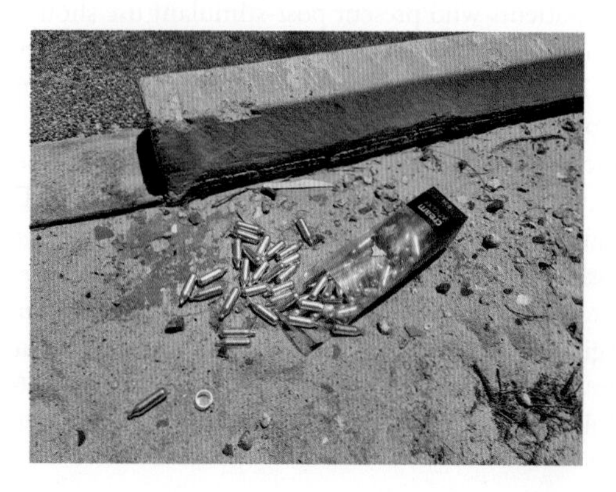

FIGURE 30.2 OLEANDER PLANT

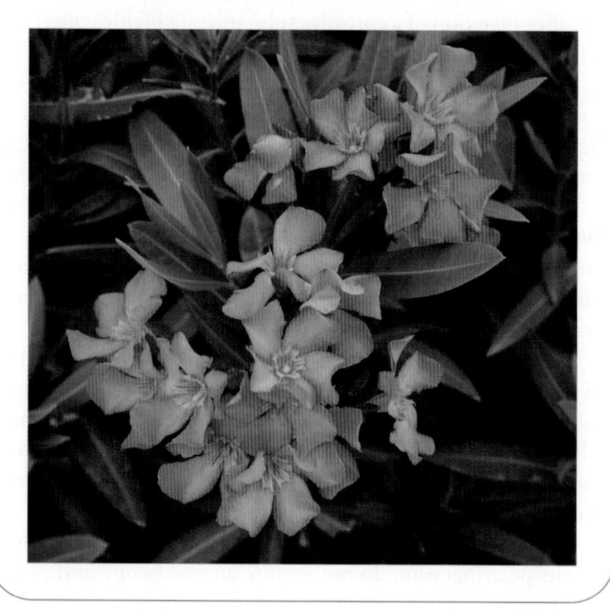

Shutterstock.com/Peter Maerky

FIGURE 30.3 *AMANITA PHALLOIDES* MUSHROOM

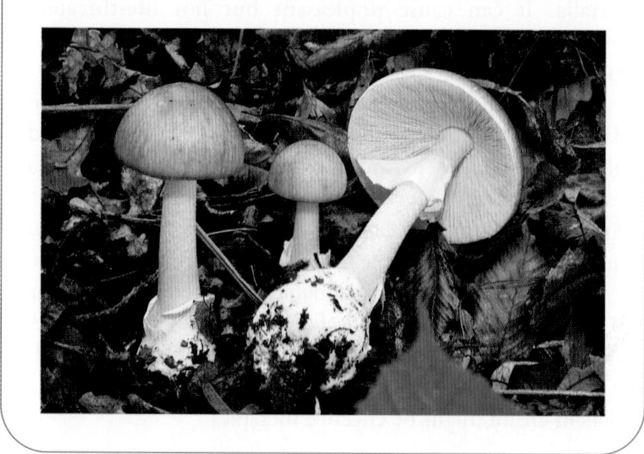

Shutterstock.com/el_cigarrito

FIGURE 30.4 CASTOR BEAN PLANT

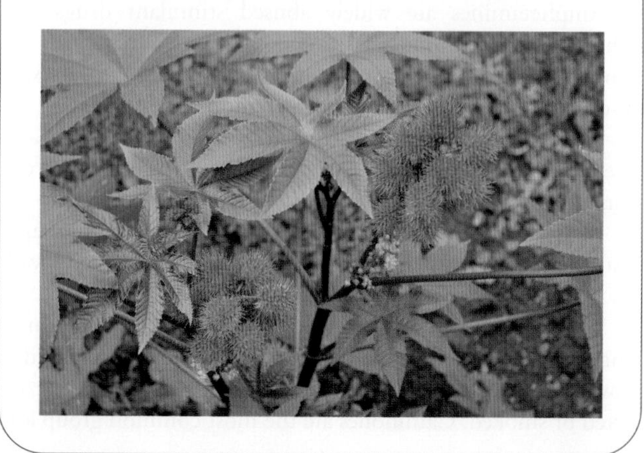

Shutterstock.com/Bubushonok

FIGURE 30.5 PUFFER OR BLOW FISH

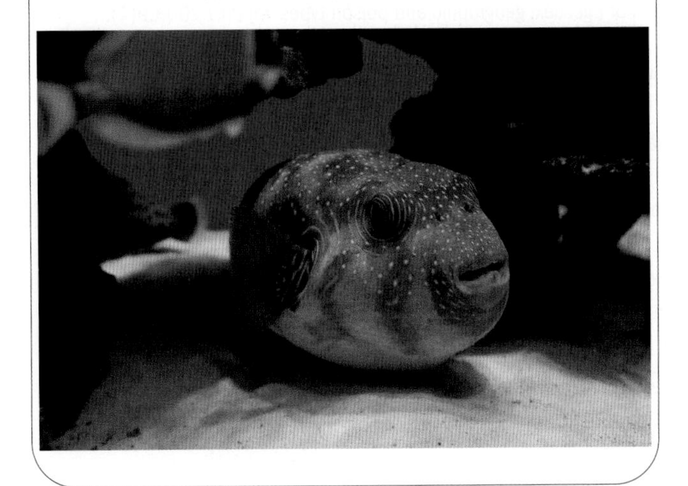

Shutterstock.com/Silk-stocking

and if enough is ingested can cause toxicity, initially manifested as gastrointestinal symptoms (vomiting and diarrhoea), and followed by multi-organ failure and death.

Puffer fish (Fig. 30.5) contain a potent neurotoxin, tetrodotoxin, which binds to sodium channels and inhibits the generation and propagation of action potentials, resulting in paralysis.

PRACTICE TIP

PITFALLS

- Inadequate airway management of the intoxicated patient with a decreased level of consciousness.
- Inappropriate decontamination of benign ingestions, the uncooperative patient or the patient at risk of aspiration.
- Failure to detect urinary retention in the agitated patient, particularly if there is evidence of anticholinergic toxicity.
- Failure to administer *N*-acetylcysteine within 8 hours of ingestion in the patient at risk of paracetamol toxicity.
- Stopping (without restarting) *N*-acetylcysteine infusions for paracetamol overdose because of an anaphylactoid reaction. These are common and usually benign: treat symptomatically and slow the infusion rate.
- Withholding high-dose insulin–euglycaemic therapy in severe calcium channel blocker toxicity due to fear of the large insulin doses required.
- Failure to recognise that sulfonylurea overdose can result in delayed and prolonged hypoglycaemia; should be treated with octreotide when hypoglycaemia first develops.
- Failure to recognise the high mortality rate of chronic digoxin toxicity.
- Compromising the care of patients with organophosphate poisoning due to unwarranted fears about nosocomial poisoning.

SUMMARY

Poisoning, whether accidental or deliberate, is an important ED presentation. The incidence differs between children and adults, with childhood presentations more likely to be accidental. Although the ingestion of pharmaceuticals is common in children, the rate of poisonings from household chemicals and plants is increasing. In most cases, children do not ingest significant amounts, and severe clinical symptoms are unlikely. However, the potential toxicity of some drugs, such as the agents described in this chapter, is high, and an accurate risk assessment and an appropriate period of observation are essential. Most importantly, one should treat the patient, not the poison. Meticulous supportive care is all that is required following most poisonings.

Adult poisonings are frequently deliberate. Self-harm attempts by drug overdose usually require hospital assessment and treatment. Emergency stabilisation and maintenance of airway, breathing and circulation are the priority. Following this, formulating a risk assessment guides all further care and management decisions.

CASE STUDY

The ambulance is called to a 72-year-old male farmer who ingested an unknown amount of paraquat 10 minutes ago.

QUESTIONS

1. What is the initial risk assessment?
2. What is the initial management of this patient?
3. What tests should be performed when he arrives in the emergency department?
4. What ongoing management is required for this patient?

Answers to Case Study Questions can be found on evolve http://evolve.elsevier.com/AU/Curtis/emergency/ 

REFERENCES

1. Lam LT. Childhood and adolescence poisoning in NSW, Australia: an analysis of age, sex, geographic and poison types. Inj Prev 2003;9(4): 338–42.
2. Shadnia S, Soltaninejad K. Fumigants. In: Nelson LS, Howland M, Lewin NA, Smith SW, Goldfrank LR, Hoffman RS, editors. Goldfrank's toxicologic emergencies. 11th ed. New York: McGraw Hill; 2019.
3. Little L, Murray L. Consensus statement: risk of nosocomial organophosphate poisoning in emergency departments. Emerg Med Australas EMA 2004;16:256–8.
4. Isbister GK, Downes F, Sibbritt D, Dawson AH, Whyte IM. Aspiration pneumonitis in an overdose population: frequency, predictors, and outcomes. Crit Care Med 2004;32(1):88–93.
5. Murray L, Little M, Pascu O, Hoggett K. Toxicology handbook. 3rd ed. Chatswood: Elsevier; 2015.
6. Daly FF, Little M, Murray L. A risk assessment based approach to the management of acute poisoning. Emerg Med J 2006;23(5):396–9.
7. Tenenbein M. Do you really need that emergency drug screen? Clin Toxicol (Phil, PA.) 2009;47(4):286–91.
8. Chyka PA, Seger D, Krenzelok EP, Vale JA. Position paper: single-dose activated charcoal. Clin Toxicol (Phil, PA) 2005;43(2):61–87.
9. Keller RE, Schwab RA, Krenzelok EP. Contribution of sorbitol combined with activated charcoal in prevention of salicylate absorption. Ann Emerg Med 1990;19(6):654–6.
10. Dart RC, Borron SW, Caravati EM, Cobaugh DJ, Curry SC, Falk JL, et al. Expert consensus guidelines for stocking of antidotes in hospitals that provide emergency care. Ann Emerg Med 2009;54(3):386–94.e1.
11. Megarbane B, Borron SW, Baud FJ. Current recommendations for treatment of severe toxic alcohol poisonings. Intensive Care Med 2005;31(2):189–95.
12. O'Malley GF. Emergency department management of the salicylate-poisoned patient. Emerg Med Clin North Am 2007;25(2):333–46, abstract viii.
13. Therapeutic Guidelines Limited. Paracetamol poisoning. In: Toxicology and Toxinology Group, editor. Therapeutic guidelines: oral and dental. Version 3. Melbourne: Therapeutic Guidelines Limited; 2020.
14. Wood DM, Berry DJ, Glover G, Eastwood J, Dargan PI. Significant pregabalin toxicity managed with supportive care alone. J Med Toxicol 2010;6:435–7.
15. Alyahya B, Friesen M, Nauche B, Laliberté M. Acute lamotrigine overdose: a systematic review of published adult and pediatric cases. Clin Toxicol 2018;56(2):81–9.
16. Bradberry SM, Thanacoody HK, Watt BE, Thomas SH, Vale JA. Management of the cardiovascular complications of tricyclic antidepressant poisoning: role of sodium bicarbonate. Toxicol Rev 2005;24(3):195–204.
17. Boyer EW, Shannon M. The serotonin syndrome. NEJM 2005;352(11):1112–20.
18. Therapeutic Guidelines Limited. Antidepressant drug poisoning. In: Toxicology and Toxinology Group, editor. Therapeutic guidelines: oral and dental. Version 3. Melbourne: Therapeutic Guidelines Limited; 2020.
19. Burns MJ. The pharmacology and toxicology of atypical antipsychotic agents. J Toxicol Clin Toxicol 2001;39(1):1–14.
20. Love JN, Howell JM, Litovitz TL, Klein-Schwartz W. Acute beta blocker overdose: factors associated with the development of cardiovascular morbidity. J Toxicol Clin Toxicol 2000;38(3):275–81.
21. Therapeutic Guidelines Limited. Beta-blocker poisoning. In: Toxicology and Toxinology Group, editor. Therapeutic guidelines: oral and dental. Version 3. Melbourne: Therapeutic Guidelines Limited; 2020.
22. Therapeutic Guidelines Limited. Lithium poisoning. In: Toxicology and Toxinology Group, editor. Therapeutic guidelines: oral and dental. Version 3. Melbourne: Therapeutic Guidelines Limited; 2020.
23. Lee HL, Chen KW, Chi CH, Huang JJ, Tsai LM. Clinical presentations and prognostic factors of a glyphosate-surfactant herbicide intoxication: a review of 131 cases. Acad Emerg Med 2000;7(8):906–10.
24. Eddleston M, Eyer P, Worek F, Juszczak E, Alder N, Mohamed F, et al. Pralidoxime in acute organophosphorus insecticide poisoning—a randomised controlled trial. PLoS Med 2009;6(6):e1000104.
25. Stapczynski JS, Haskell RJ. Duration of hypoglycemia and need for intravenous glucose following intentional overdoses of insulin. Ann Emerg Med 1984;13(7):505–11.
26. Harrigan RA, Nathan MS, Beattie P. Oral agents for the treatment of type 2 diabetes mellitus: pharmacology, toxicity, and treatment. Ann Emerg Med 2001;38(1):68–78.
27. McLaughlin SA, Crandall CS, McKinney PE. Octreotide: an antidote for sulfonylurea-induced hypoglycemia. Ann Emerg Med 2000;36(2):133–8.
28. Richards JR, Gordon BK, Danielson AR, Moulin AK. Pharmacologic treatment of cannabinoid hyperemesis syndrome: a systematic review. Pharmacotherapy 2017;37(6):725–34.
29. Bowen SE. Two serious and challenging medical complications associated with volatile substance misuse: sudden sniffing death and fetal solvent syndrome. Subst Use Misuse 2011;46(Suppl. 1):68–72.
30. Pema PJ, Horak HA, Wyatt RH. Myelopathy caused by nitrous oxide toxicity. AJNR Am J Neuroradiol 1998;19(5):894.
31. Barceloux DG. Frontmatter. Medical toxicology of natural substances: foods, fungi, medicinal herbs, plants, and venomous animals. Hoboken, N.J.: John Wiley & Sons; 2008.

CHAPTER 31
DENTAL, EAR, NOSE AND THROAT EMERGENCIES

TONY SKAPETIS AND JACQUELINE RYAN

ESSENTIALS

- Presentation is usually due to pain and discomfort, but serious airway compromise can occur.
- Dental emergencies are rarely life threatening. Treatment is usually stabilisation and referral to a dentist for definitive treatment.
- Appropriate initial diagnosis and treatment can reduce future dental expenses and improve patient outcomes.
- Earache can be debilitating and early analgesia is important.
- Taking a focused history will give clues to the diagnosis.
- The airway should be assessed and reassessed regularly as decline can be rapid.
- Patients presenting in the 'sniffing the air' position are already telling you their airway is compromised.
- Patients should never be forced to recline as this can immediately compromise their airway.
- Due to pain on swallowing, dehydration may be present. Intravenous cannulation should be attempted in an adult, but caution should be used in children as the added distress can further compromise their airway.
- Removal of a foreign body is generally most successful on the first attempt. It should not be rushed and only attempted in a controlled environment.

INTRODUCTION

With ear, nose, throat and dental emergencies, the initial presentation is usually because of pain and discomfort. Dental injuries usually occur as a result of trauma, such as a fall or an assault. Due to the close proximity of the structures in the facial area serious complications can arise, particularly if swelling of the airway is involved. Assessment of the patient's airway is a priority, along with providing adequate pain relief.

ANATOMY AND PHYSIOLOGY

MOUTH AND THROAT

The oral cavity is designed for articulation in speech and mastication of food, and also functions as an alternative airway.[1]

The mouth is sealed by the lips and they too are involved in articulation of speech. The oral cavity is lined by the buccal mucosa, which is rich in mucous glands. It consists of gums, alveolar bone, teeth, the hard and soft palates and the tongue. The floor of the mouth contains the openings of the submandibular and sublingual salivary glands (Fig. 31.1).

The gums are attached to the alveolar bone and are closely related to the teeth, whose roots lie within the alveolus.[2] Fig. 31.2 shows the structure of a tooth. Normal primary dentition begins erupting at 6 months of age, with 20 teeth by the age of 3 years. Permanent dentition begins at 6–7 years of age with eruption of the first molar, and is usually completed by age 16–18 to a total of 32 teeth.[3,4]

The throat, or pharynx, consists of the upper parts of the respiratory and digestive systems. It can be divided into three parts: the nasopharynx lies above the soft palate and behind the nasal cavities and contains adenoid tissue and the orifices of the eustachian tubes, the oropharynx extends from the inferior margin of the soft palate to the level of the hyoid bone, and the laryngopharynx extends from the hyoid bone to the opening of the larynx anteriorly and oesophagus posteriorly (see Fig. 31.3).[5] The larynx is made up of several muscles and cartilages. It functions autonomously in the

FIGURE 31.1 INTERIOR OF THE MOUTH AND THROAT[2]

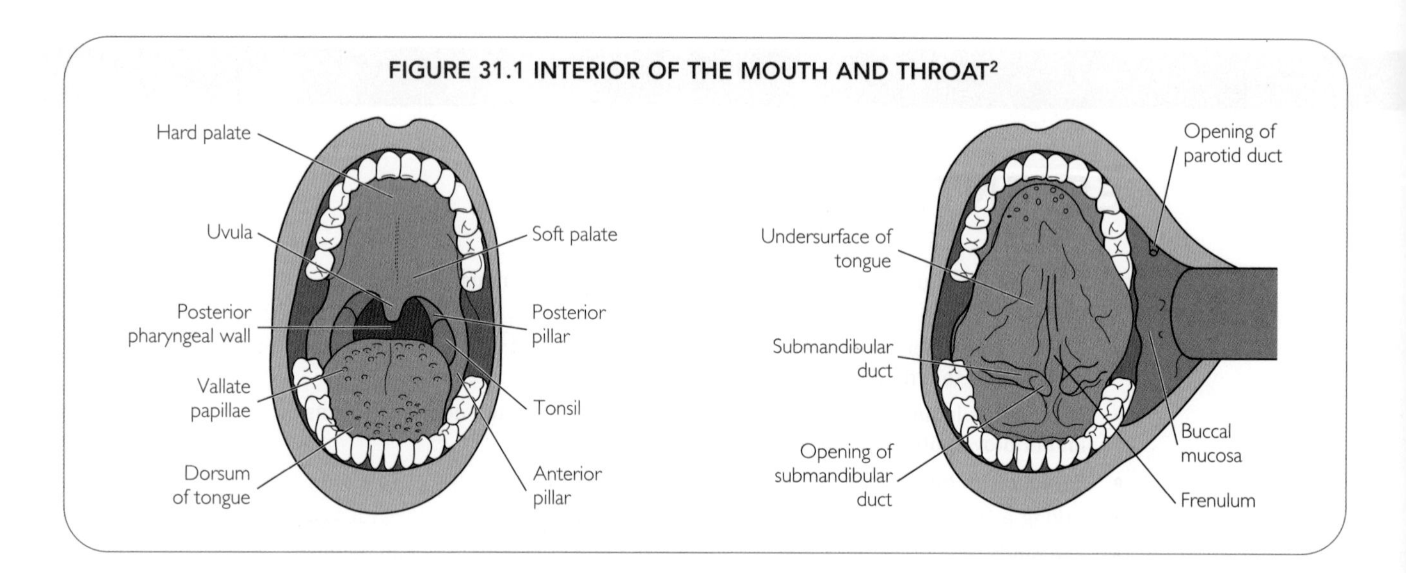

FIGURE 31.2 STRUCTURE OF THE TOOTH[3]

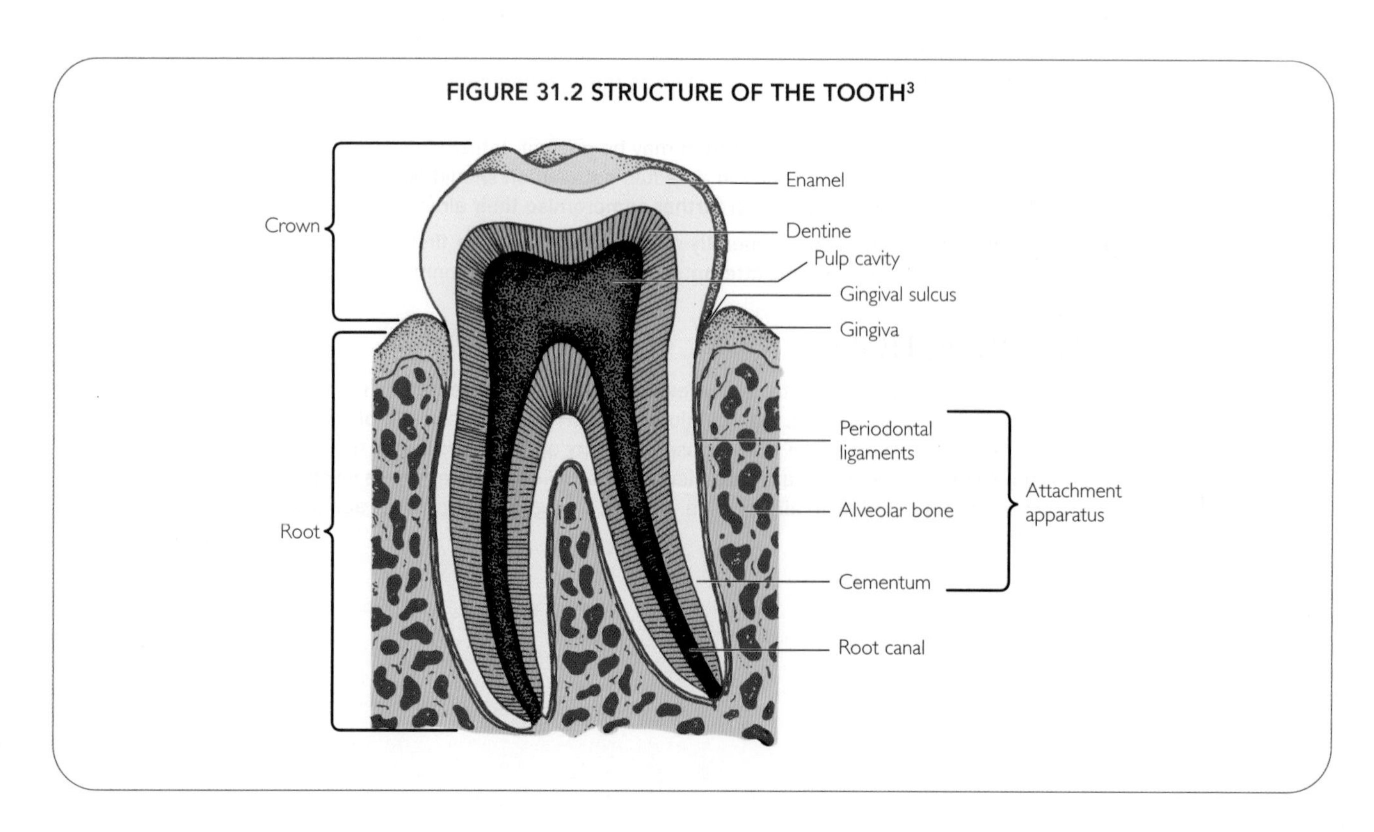

FIGURE 31.3 THE PHARYNX[6]

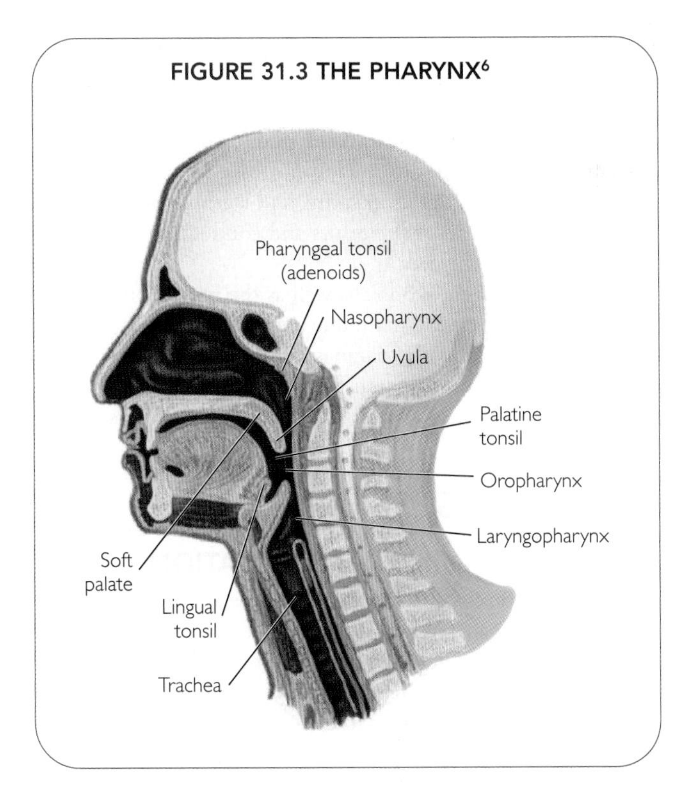

roles of respiration, airway protection, swallowing and phonation (producing sounds).[2,7]

EARS

The ear can be divided into three parts: the external, middle and inner ear (see Fig. 31.4). The external ear consists of the pinna, external auditory canal and the lateral surface of the tympanic membrane (eardrum). The external ear serves mainly to protect the tympanic membrane, but also collects

FIGURE 31.4 CROSS-SECTION OF THE OUTER, MIDDLE AND INNER EAR[2]

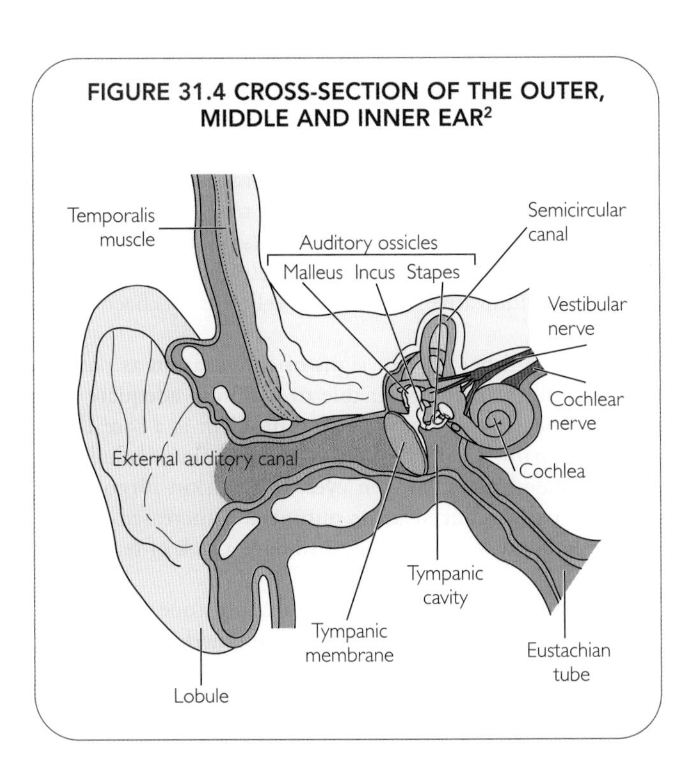

FIGURE 31.5 AUDITORY OSSICLES[2]

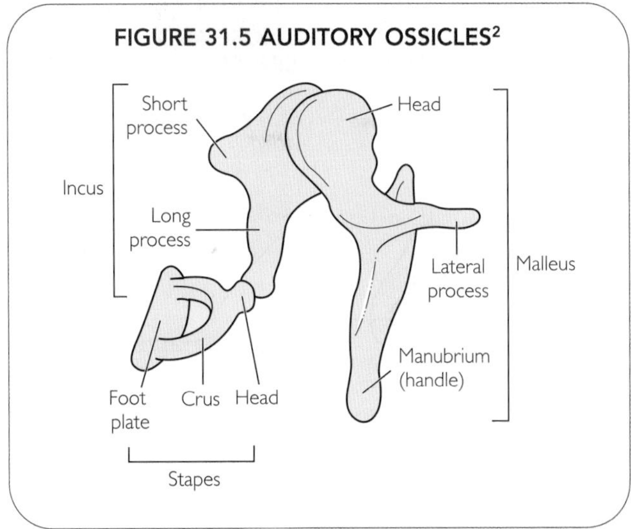

and directs sound waves.[1] Glands lining the canal secrete cerumen (earwax) to protect and lubricate the ear.

The middle ear is an air-containing space which communicates with the nasopharynx via the eustachian tube. It contains the three ossicles and is normally sealed laterally by the tympanic membrane. Its function is to transmit and amplify sound waves from the tympanic membrane to the stapes footplate, converting energy from an air medium to a fluid medium for the membranous labyrinth.[1] The relationship of the three ossicles is depicted in Fig. 31.5.

The inner ear or labyrinth communicates with the middle ear via the oval and round windows. The inner ear can be divided into two parts: the *cochlea* and the *vestibule*.[2] The cochlea converts sound waves into neural impulses with elaborate coding. The vestibule contains the utricle, the saccule and the semicircular canals which sense the position of the head and are important in maintaining the body's balance.

NOSE

The nose is responsible for the sense of smell, warming and saturating inspired air, removing bacteria and particulate debris as well as conserving heat and moisture from expired air.[1]

The nose consists of the *external nose* and the *nasal cavity*, which is divided into right and left halves by the midline nasal septum. Each half of the cavity has olfactory, vestibular and respiratory parts depending on the type of epithelial covering.[8]

The nose is mainly constructed from cartilage, apart from the upper third where the frontal and maxillary bones form the bony ridge. The nares are separated by a membranous columella anteriorly and by the nasal septum posteriorly. The nasal septum is both cartilaginous and bony (see Fig. 31.6). The lateral wall of each nasal cavity contains the inferior, middle and, sometimes, superior turbinates. These help to increase surface area and moderate air temperature.

The blood supply to the external nose is provided by the dorsal nasal artery (a terminal branch of the ophthalmic artery) and by the external nasal, lateral and septal branches of the facial artery. The main artery of the nasal cavity is the sphenopalatine. It supplies the mucosa over the turbinates and much of the septum. On the lower anterior part of the septum (Little's area), it anastomoses with the septal branch of the

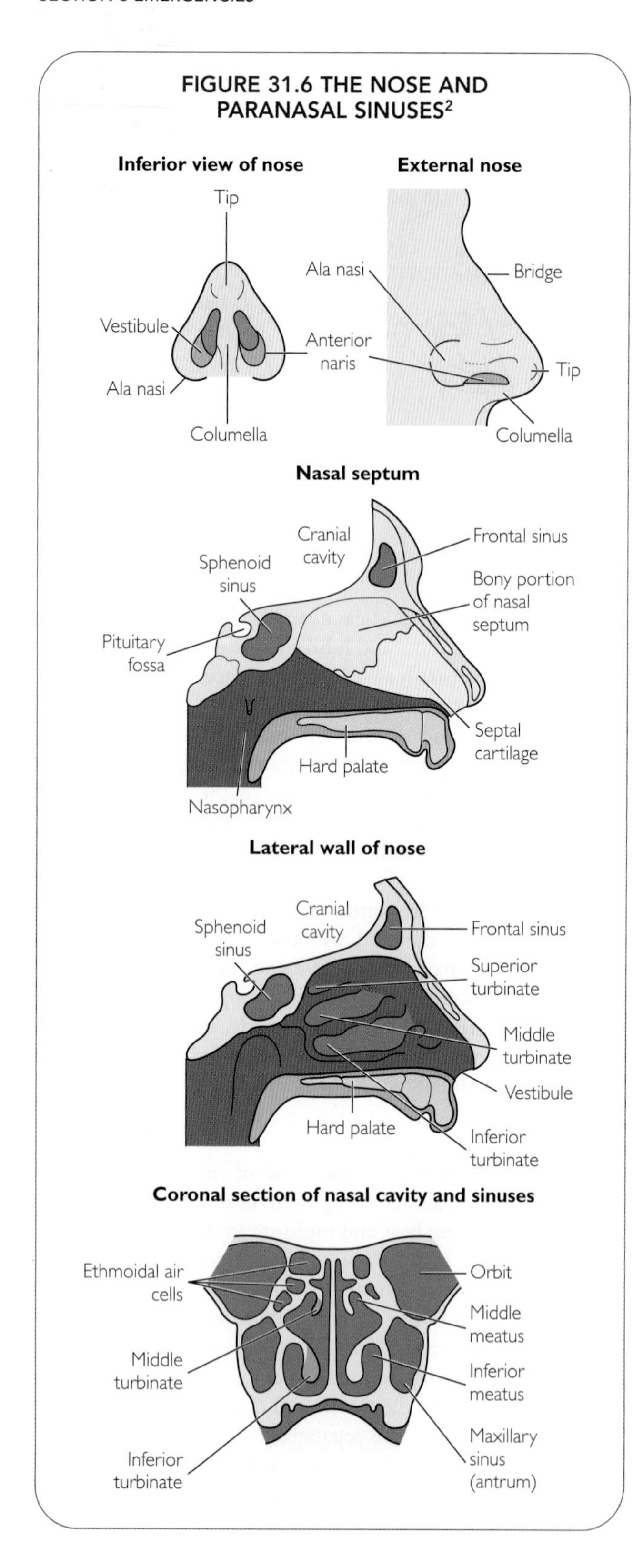

superior labial and the ascending branch of the greater palatine, so forming Kiesselbach's plexus, the common site for epistaxis (see Fig. 31.7).[8]

FACE

The face is the anterior part of the head bound between the eyebrow and chin vertically, and includes the ears laterally.[9] The facial skeleton is the front part of the skull, including the mandible.[8] Other important facial bones frequently injured include:

- the maxillae, which meet in the midline of the face and form the boundaries of the lower orbits
- the sphenoid, ethmoid, palatine and lacrimal bones, forming the basin of the orbits and conducting nerves and vessels to the eyes
- the zygoma or cheekbone as well as the temporomandibular joint between the mandible and base of skull.

The face also contains the paranasal sinuses (Fig. 31.8), which are air-filled sacs. They lighten the weight of the skull and add resonance to the voice, and are linked to the nasal passages for fluid drainage.

PATIENT ASSESSMENT

APPROACH TO INITIAL EVALUATION

Most presentations for a dental, ear, nose or throat problem will be due to pain. When assessing the patient, it is vital a DRSABCD approach (**D**anger, **R**esponse, **S**end for help, **A**irway, **B**reathing, **C**irculation and **D**isability) is taken due to the risk of potential complications, including airway obstruction and haemorrhage. These should be addressed before a history is taken from the patient, including relevant past medical history and medications.

PHYSICAL EXAMINATION

Physical examination will vary depending on the presenting problem and may include inspection and palpation or visualisation using an auroscope.

Identification and management of existing or impending airway obstruction takes precedence over other aspects of care.[11] A compromised patient is likely to have their head tilted back with their neck extended, and on reclining their symptoms may worsen due to airway impingement. Other signs to look for are a muffled voice, drooling due to swallowing difficulty, as well as trismus (limited mouth opening). These are signs that the airway is already compromised.

Inspection

The relevant external areas should be inspected. You should note asymmetry, asymmetry or swelling of the face. The opening and closing of the mouth should be smooth and complete with no limitations or hesitations. Erythema, warmth or drainage is indicative of abscess, cellulitis or haematoma formation.[5]

You should be alert for signs of dehydration as patients with significant pain are unable to maintain adequate fluid intake, especially if the presenting problem is a sore throat or dental pain. General signs of dehydration include dry mucous membranes, sunken eyes, loss of skin turgor, poor capillary refill, reduced urine output and increased drowsiness or lethargy. Children may also have a lack of tears when crying.

Ears should be examined with an auroscope if available, using the largest earpiece the ear can accommodate. The patient should sit with their head facing straight ahead. The pinna should be pulled gently upwards and backwards and slightly away from the head. Children are best seated on a parent's lap

FIGURE 31.7 ARTERIAL SUPPLY TO NASAL SEPTUM[3]

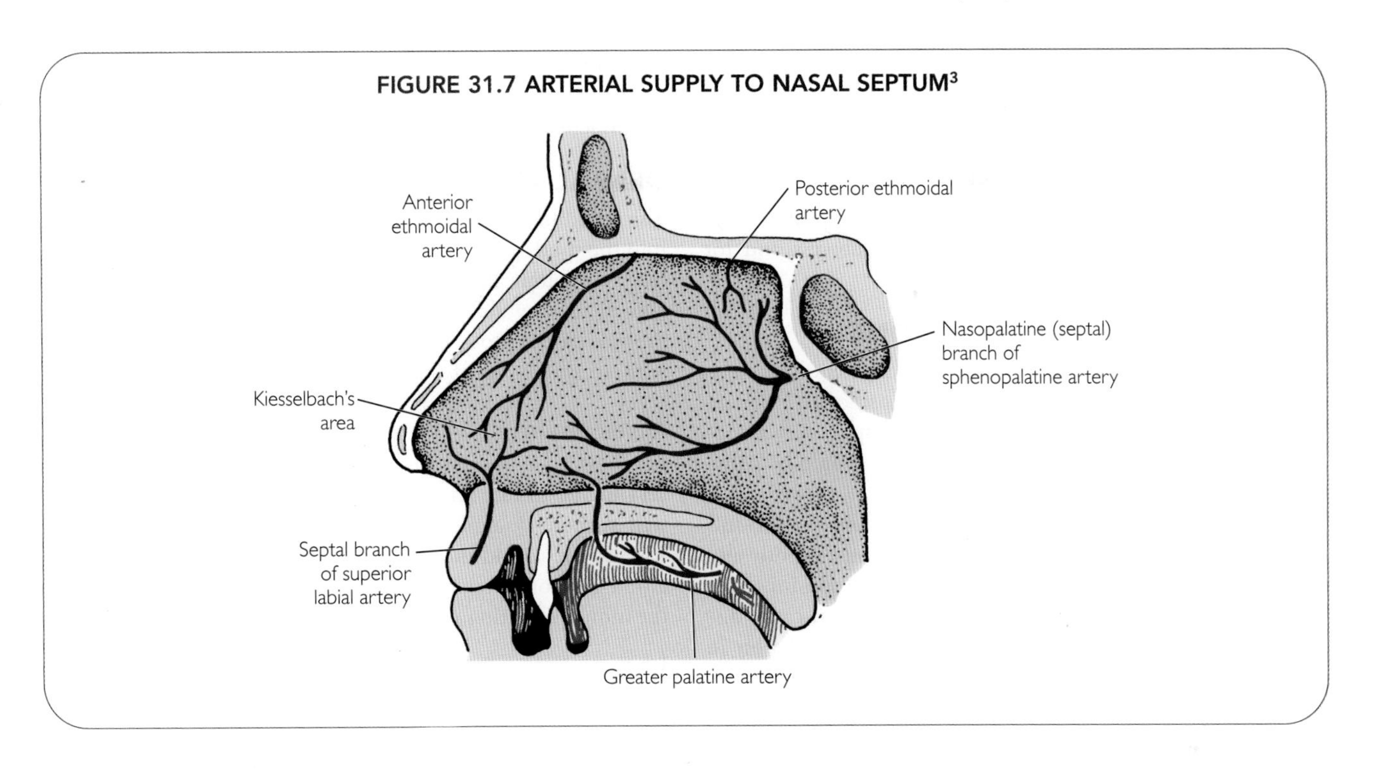

FIGURE 31.8 PARANASAL SINUSES[10]

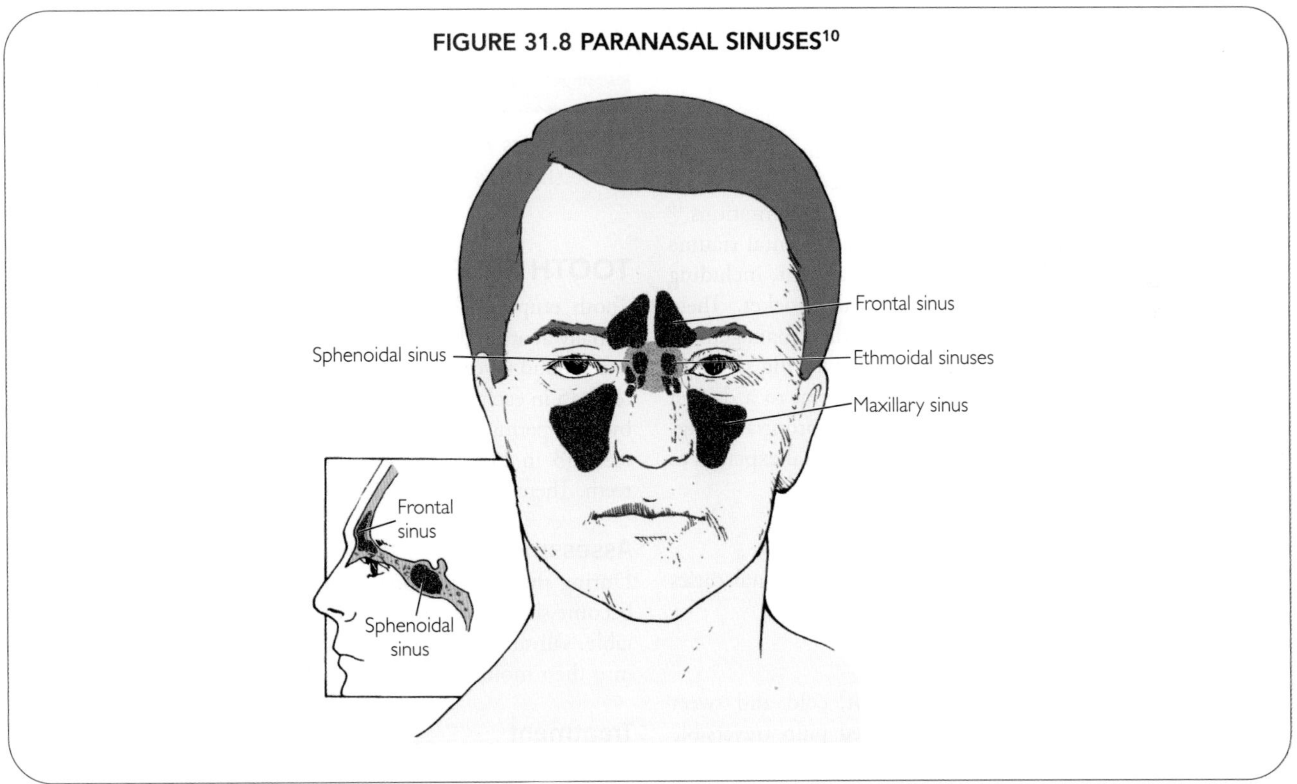

and held securely with their head resting on the parent's chest. In those younger than 3 years, the pinna should be pulled down to get a good view of the tympanic membrane.[12]

The throat should be examined for erythema, exudate and swelling, and uvula swelling or deviation should be noted.

Inspection of the mouth for dental injuries should take note of how many teeth are affected, their location and the whereabouts of any dental fragments in case they have been inhaled.

Palpation

The face and neck are palpated for tenderness, crepitus or step-offs (suggestive of bone fracture). Examination of the neck should also include palpating the lymph nodes. Enlarged tender nodes can be an indication of infection.

RADIOLOGY

For most ear, nose, throat and dental problems, radiology is not required. There are a few notable exceptions.

A chest x-ray is used to locate missing tooth fragments if aspiration is considered likely, or a facial x-ray if they are lodged in the lip or buccal mucosa. An orthopantomogram (OPG) is also useful to assess the extent of damage to the teeth and a PA of the skull is useful for mandibular fractures.

A computed tomography (CT) scan can be helpful in diagnosing mastoiditis, sinusitis, retropharyngeal abscess and for more severe dental infections.

INITIAL CLINICAL INTERVENTIONS

The patient should be encouraged to sit in a position of comfort. Often this is a seated or semi-erect position. Under no circumstances should a patient with signs of upper airway obstruction be forced to recline.[11] These patients should be delivered nasal high-flow oxygen.

Patients with upper airway obstruction commonly also suffer dysphagia (swallowing difficulty) and may consequently also be dehydrated. Intravenous (IV) fluids should be administered, but caution should be used in children so as to not cause distress and actually worsen their condition. IV cannulation in these cases should wait until arrival at hospital where airway management equipment is readily available.

A full set of vital signs should be recorded and repeated regularly, and analgesia should be given. Pre-hospital care is an important window during which pain should be assessed and treated.[12]

DENTAL EMERGENCIES

Dental emergencies are not uncommon presentations in the emergency department (ED).[13] They have been noted to account for between 1%[14,15] and 3.8% of ED presentations.[16] They include dental pain, dental infections and dental trauma as well as complications related to dental treatment, including haemorrhage from inside the mouth and dry socket. These presentations are rarely life threatening, and their management is usually of an empirical symptomatic basis involving stabilisation of acute conditions with appropriate referral to a dentist for more definitive treatment. Nevertheless, appropriate diagnosis and initial treatment can reduce future dental expenses as well as improve patient outcomes.

DENTAL PAIN

This type of pain can often be very acute, with dental caries being the principal cause.

Assessment

Initial symptoms include sensitivity to hot, cold and sweet stimuli, which are indicative of an inflamed pulp (reversible pulpitis).

Treatment

Symptoms are alleviated by avoiding any foods which provoke or exaggerate the pain, by covering any obvious tooth cavity using a temporary material such as Blu-Tack (is non-toxic) or a piece of chewing gum. Oral analgesics containing paracetamol are normally quite effective for such presentations.

Upon progression, the pulpitis may become irreversible with the pain intensifying and becoming more spontaneous. The addition of oral non-steroidal anti-inflammatory drugs (NSAIDs), or the combination of paracetamol and NSAIDs, is often indicated.[17,18] Irreversible pulpitis requires more extensive definitive dental treatment, such as root canal therapy or extraction.

DENTAL ABSCESS

This condition usually results through the ingress of bacteria into the tooth pulpal tissues resulting from dental decay or as a result of trauma and is more accurately described as a periapical abscess. It may also occur through bacteria progressing down the side of the tooth between the tooth root and surrounding gum, in which case it is referred to as a periodontal abscess.

Assessment

For both conditions the offending tooth or teeth become very tender to bite on, and may be associated with swelling, as well as more-systemic symptoms, including fever and malaise. Assessment should include consideration of any trismus (limitation in mouth opening), tongue swelling/hardness, floor of the mouth elevation or airway obstruction.

Treatment

Treatment is usually with antibiotics, but if trismus, tongue swelling or airway obstruction is present, then these would constitute a medical emergency and would require admission and likely surgical drainage.

PRACTICE TIP

Patients with suspected dental abscess involving swelling should be reassessed regularly for airway compromise.

TOOTH ERUPTION

Tooth eruption is a normal developmental process beginning initially at around 6 months of age for deciduous (primary) teeth and around 6 years of age for the permanent teeth. All deciduous teeth (5 in each quadrant and 20 in total) are eventually replaced by their permanent successors, with additional permanent molar teeth (3 in each quadrant) erupting behind all the deciduous teeth. There are 32 permanent teeth in total with 16 teeth per jaw.

Assessment

During the eruption phase, the gum overlying the tooth may become slightly red and swollen and children may become irritable, salivate excessively, and want to place fingers and objects into their mouth for relief or even tug on their ears at times.

Treatment

No treatment is usually necessary other than supportive care, with analgesia only indicated in more severe and persistent cases. Temporary use of such things as rusks and dummies may be of assistance.

PERICORONITIS

Pericoronitis refers to inflammation of gingival tissue overlying an erupting tooth and occurs when anaerobic bacteria and/or food debris penetrate from the mouth and infect the underlying tooth. It is commonly associated with erupting permanent third molars (commonly referred to as wisdom teeth) between the ages of 17 and 21 years.

Assessment

Pericoronitis may be of a mild nature consisting of only localised inflammation and intraoral swelling; at times it may be quite severe and include symptoms such as facial swelling, fever, malaise and trismus together with associated difficulty in eating.

Treatment

Treatment of mild cases involves oral analgesia as well as irrigating the site with 0.1–0.2% chlorhexidine solution (e.g. Savacol) using a 5–10 mL syringe and asking the patient to maintain good oral hygiene and rinse with the same solution twice a day for the next 5 days. In the more severe pericoronitis cases, appropriate antibiotics should be administered (targeting anaerobic bacteria), or even surgical drainage and/or extraction of the offending tooth following assessment by a dentist.

GINGIVITIS AND PERIODONTITIS

Gingivitis refers to inflammation of the gum and periodontitis to inflammation of the deeper supporting tissues of the tooth root. Both of these conditions are bacterial in origin and usually associated with poor oral hygiene habits. Gingivitis may be exaggerated during pregnancy due to hormonal changes. Varying degrees of gingivitis are common throughout most of the general population, while periodontitis with the associated periodontal disease is more prevalent in the adult population.

Assessment

Gingivitis causes the gum to become red and often bleed, with periodontitis also associated with the deepening of gum pockets surrounding the teeth, halitosis, loosening of the involved teeth due to surrounding bone loss (Figs 31.9–31.10) and even abscess formation.

Treatment

Symptoms for both conditions may be reduced through the use of a 0.1–0.2% chlorhexidine solution as a mouthwash twice a day for 1 week, together with improving oral hygiene especially through brushing. The use of analgesics may also be indicated in more-severe cases. Antibiotics are not usually indicated for either condition unless there is systemic involvement. Referral to a dentist is indicated for the longer term management of both conditions.

FIGURE 31.9 BONE LOSS FROM PERIODONTITIS

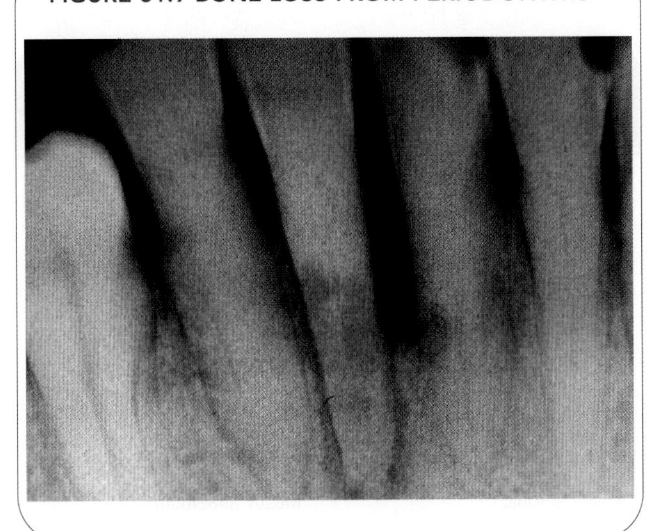

FIGURE 31.10 ADVANCED PERIODONTITIS CAUSING GINGIVAL OVERGROWTH AND LOSS OF TOOTH SUPPORT

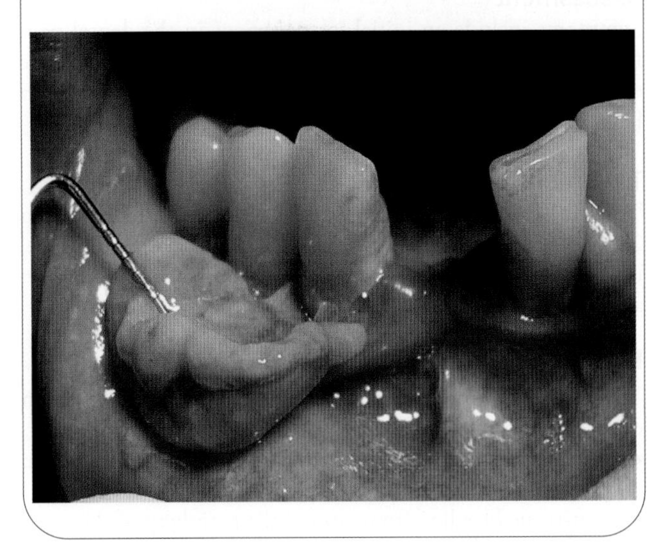

Note the plaque and calculus surrounding the teeth due to the poor oral hygiene.

MAXILLARY SINUSITIS

This condition refers to an infection involving the maxillary sinus. It is usually unilateral, but may also present bilaterally at times.

Assessment

It is common for the upper back teeth to ache in such presentations and become tender to biting. This is because the roots of maxillary premolars and molars often lie in close proximity to the maxillary sinus. Other symptoms include maxillary sinus palpation tenderness and pain worsening with changes in head position, when blowing the nose and exercising.

Treatment

Treatment involves sinus irrigation with saline, and use of antihistamines, analgesics and antibiotics.

PRACTICE TIP

If sinusitis is suspected, ask the patient to seal their mouth and pinch their nose between thumb and forefinger after which they should try and blow air out. In this way you increase intra-sinus pressure and the pain temporarily escalates.

ALVEOLAR OSTEITIS

This is commonly referred to as dry socket and is due to the breakdown in the granulation tissue process following a dental extraction. It occurs within a few days with a reported incidence varying greatly between less than 1% to greater than 20%[19] of extractions and is more commonly seen in smokers, difficult extractions and within the mandibular dental arch.[20]

Assessment

Symptoms include an initial improvement in the dental pain followed by a worsening of the pain several days after the extraction. Other symptoms include difficulty in chewing, with halitosis and a fetid odour commonly reported.

Treatment

This condition is self-limiting with symptoms subsiding within 2 weeks. Treatment involves flushing of the socket with saline, maintaining good oral hygiene and analgesics when necessary; antibiotics are not indicated.

POST-EXTRACTION HAEMORRHAGE

The causes of unexpected haemorrhage sometime after an extraction include:

- damage to small blood vessels within the bony walls of the extraction socket
- soft-tissue bleeding from around the periphery of the socket
- bleeding from residual granulation tissue
- disturbance of the blood clot due to the patient eating too soon, exercising, spitting, sucking, etc.
- presence of severe gingivitis or periodontal disease
- trauma or laceration bleeding from soft-tissue incisions performed during the course of the extraction
- dead-space haematoma arterial or venous bleeding from deeper parts of the wound.

PRACTICE TIP

Haemorrhage should be controlled during transportation by applying gauze which has been soaked in tranexamic acid if available using direct pressure to the bleeding site.

Treatment

Management of intraoral bleeds includes the use of one or more of the following:

- pressure applied with a rolled-up piece of gauze applied against the extraction site using bite pressure
- use of tranexamic acid 5% liquid solution (made up by crushing a 500 mg tranexamic acid tablet in 10 mL of saline) to soak the pressure gauze pack and promote coagulation
- packing the wound with oxidised cellulose (e.g. Surgicel), which acts as a resorbable clot matrix or alginate-based products such as Kaltostat
- use of a vasoconstrictor containing anaesthetic solution, which is injected around the bleeding socket
- suturing across the wound.

DENTAL INFECTIONS

Most odontogenic (of dental origin) infections are caused by a mix of aerobic and anaerobic bacteria with a large diversity of pathogens within the biofilm of the mouth. *Streptococcus viridans* is a common causative pathogen and 60% of infections also contain anaerobic rods. Aerobic pathogens typically initiate most of these infections followed by anaerobic pathogens, with a symbiosis between the two types of bacteria resulting in the more serious infections. Host factors such as age, tooth loss, diet, saliva and oral hygiene play an important role in regulating the composition and numbers of the oral flora. Dental infections will typically spread in the following ways:

- direct tissue spread
- vestibular spread with infections penetrating the dental alveolus into the vestibule (dental sulcus) of the mouth
- fascial spread with infections penetrating the dental alveolus and travelling along the tissue planes of the head and neck
- circulatory spread via blood vessels and lymphatics.

Maxillary infections typically spread to the buccal, canine and infratemporal spaces with mandibular infections spreading to buccal, submental, sublingual and submandibular spaces. Secondary spaces where odontogenic infections can spread include orbital, prevertebral, retropharyngeal, lateral pharyngeal, infratemporal, superficial and deep temporal, masseteric and pterygomandibular spaces. There is evidence that the frequency and severity of odontogenic infections requiring hospitalisation may be increasing in Australia.[21]

Assessment

Clinical features include local symptoms such as inflammation, swelling (intra-oral and/or extra-oral), suppuration, trismus, dysphagia and dysphonia with systemic symptoms, including fever, malaise, pallor and loss of function. Dental infections present as either a cellulitis or an abscess, or a mixture of both (Table 31.1).

Treatment

Management of odontogenic infections should include a determination of the severity of the infection using a complete medical and dental history, together with a physical examination and an evaluation of the patient's host defence mechanism. Use of antibiotics is often necessary where any of the following are present:

- fever and acute infection
- infection is not well localised and is spreading
- chronic infection despite drainage/debridement
- a diminished host response (immunocompromised patient)
- inadequate response to previous antibiotics
- osteomyelitis, sialadenitis, acute ulcerative gingivitis, localised juvenile periodontitis.

TABLE 31.1 SIGNS AND SYMPTOMS OF FACIAL CELLULITIS AND ABSCESS

CELLULITIS (SEE FIG. 31.11)	ABSCESS (SEE FIG. 31.12)
Acute duration	Chronic duration
Generalised pain	Localised pain
Large size	Smaller size
Diffuse borders	Well circumscribed
Indurated/doughy to palpation	Fluctuant
No pus	Pus present
Mostly aerobic	Mostly anaerobic

FIGURE 31.11 CELLULITIS

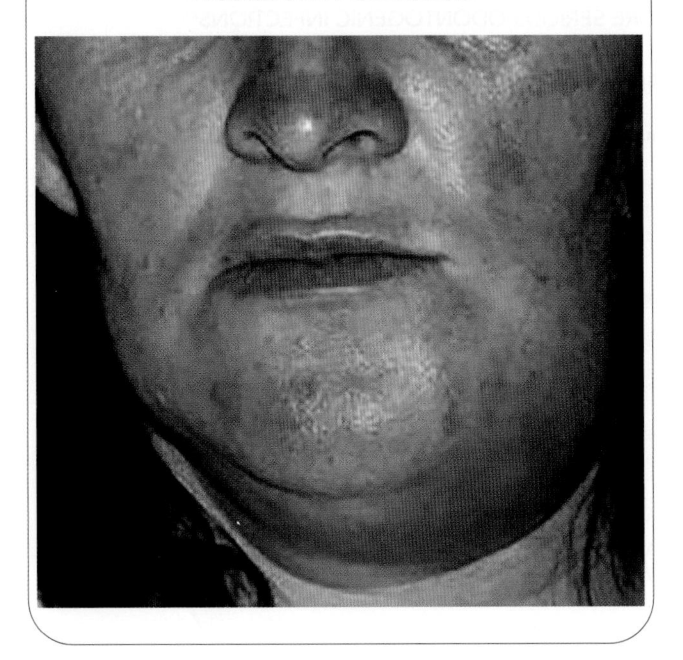

FIGURE 31.12 ABSCESS

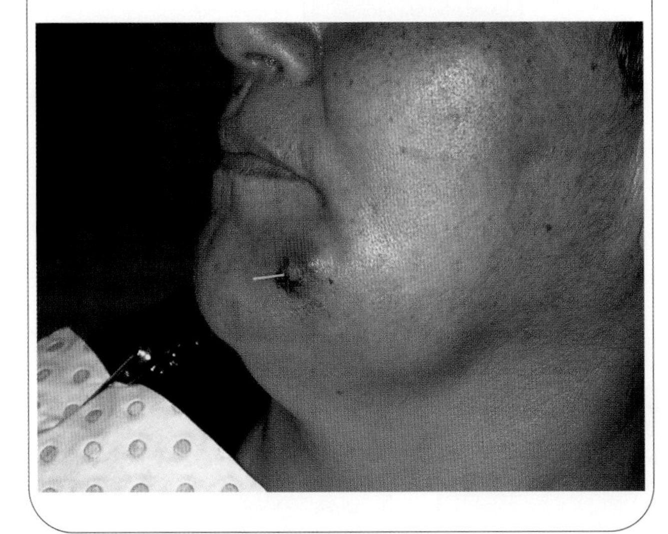

Fig. 31.13 summarises the appropriate management of dental infections in the ED; the darker shaded pathway represents the more serious odontogenic infections.[22]

DENTAL TRAUMA

Trauma to the teeth falls into two broad categories:[23]

- injuries to the hard dental tissues of the mouth, including both complicated and uncomplicated crown and crown–root fractures
- injuries to the periodontal or supporting tissues of the teeth, including tooth subluxation (loosening), luxation injuries where tooth displacement has been involved and tooth avulsion.

It has been estimated that more than one billion of the world population has suffered from a traumatic dental injury. The prevalence of these injuries is 23% in the primary dentition and 15% in the secondary dentition.[24] Acute morbidity from dental injury includes pain, swelling, bleeding and infection. Long-term morbidity arises from the need for cosmetic and functional tooth replacement which may cost the patient thousands of dollars.

Dental first aid is both simple and inexpensive and can dramatically improve future dental outcomes; however, it is rarely appropriately provided. It has been documented that emergency dental treatments provided by hospital doctors is often suboptimal and further training is warranted.[25–27] By simply covering and protecting an exposed pulp in a crown fracture or by the simple repositioning and splinting of a luxated or avulsed tooth, dental outcomes may be dramatically improved. In an effort to address the deficiency in dental trauma management dental kits have been distributed, at cost, by the NSW Rural Doctors Network in New South Wales and interstate to rural hospital EDs. These kits may be sourced at www.nswrdn.com.au/site/dental. The contents of the kit are listed in Box 31.1. These kits are to support dental education workshops (a collaboration between Western Sydney Local Health District Oral Health Network, NSW Rural Doctors Network and the University of Sydney, Sydney Dental School), which involve 4 hours of training in the management of dental emergencies and are being delivered across several Australian states to emergency medical personnel. The effectiveness of this education has been evaluated in several publications.[16,28] Furthermore, the emergency dental kit has been shown to be useful as a resource for providing emergency dental care, especially to rural and remote practice.[29] A more recent development by the Australian College of Rural and Remote Medicine has been the inclusion of the 'Introduction to Dental Emergencies and Odontogenic Infections' modules, delivered online and adapted for mobile devices.

UNCOMPLICATED CROWN FRACTURES

Crown fractures can be divided into two categories—uncomplicated and complicated. Uncomplicated crown fractures involve only the enamel, or the enamel in combination with the dentin.

Assessment

Patients who have damaged their dentin will complain of sensitivity to extremes of temperature, and on examination the yellow hue of the dentin will be noticed in contrast to the white of the peripheral enamel.

Treatment

If < 2 mm of tooth structure is broken, no intervention is often necessary; however, this type of injury may also be repaired.

BOX 31.1 EMERGENCY DENTAL KIT CONTENTS

- **GC Fuji IX pack (glass ionomer cement powder (GIC) + liquid + mixing pad)**
- **Dycal ($Ca(OH)_2$ base + catalyst)**
- **Microbrush applicators**
- **Emergency dental handbook for medical practitioners**

FIGURE 31.13 A SUMMARY OF THE APPROPRIATE MANAGEMENT OF DENTAL INFECTIONS IN THE ED; THE DARK BLUE PATHWAY REPRESENTS THE MORE SERIOUS ODONTOGENIC INFECTIONS[22]

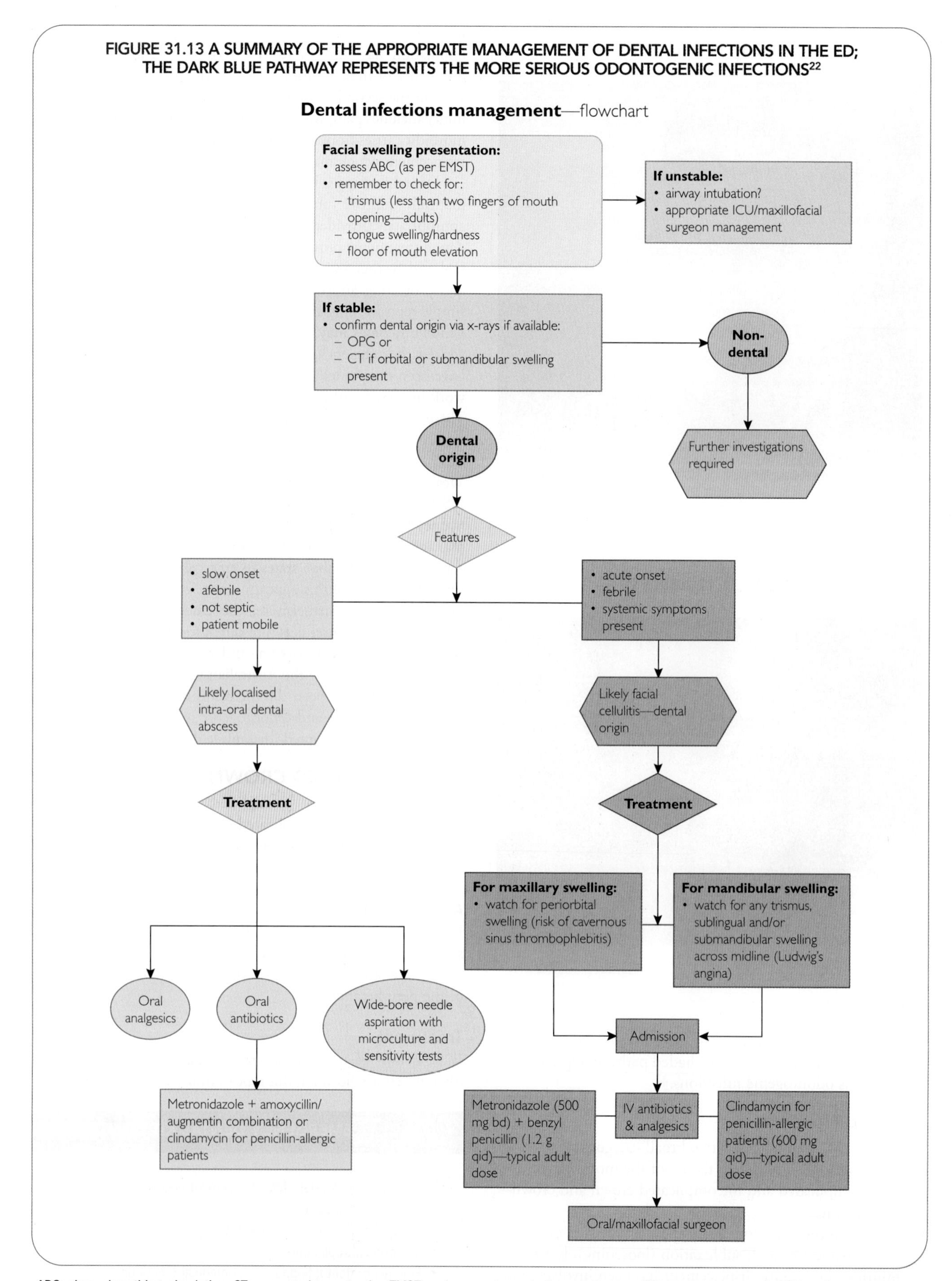
Dental infections management—flowchart
Facial swelling presentation:
• assess ABC (as per EMST)
• remember to check for:
– trismus (less than two fingers of mouth opening—adults)
– tongue swelling/hardness
– floor of mouth elevation
If unstable:
• airway intubation?
• appropriate ICU/maxillofacial surgeon management
If stable:
• confirm dental origin via x-rays if available:
– OPG or
– CT if orbital or submandibular swelling present
Non-dental
Further investigations required
Dental origin
Features
• slow onset
• afebrile
• not septic
• patient mobile
• acute onset
• febrile
• systemic symptoms present
Likely localised intra-oral dental abscess
Likely facial cellulitis—dental origin
Treatment
Treatment
For maxillary swelling:
• watch for periorbital swelling (risk of cavernous sinus thrombophlebitis)
For mandibular swelling:
• watch for any trismus, sublingual and/or submandibular swelling across midline (Ludwig's angina)
Oral analgesics
Oral antibiotics
Wide-bore needle aspiration with microculture and sensitivity tests
Admission
Metronidazole + amoxycillin/augmentin combination or clindamycin for penicillin-allergic patients
Metronidazole (500 mg bd) + benzyl penicillin (1.2 g qid)—typical adult dose
IV antibiotics & analgesics
Clindamycin for penicillin-allergic patients (600 mg qid)—typical adult dose
Oral/maxillofacial surgeon

ABC: airway, breathing, circulation; CT: computed tomography; EMST: early management of severe trauma; ICU: intensive care unit; OPG: orthopantomogram.

FIGURE 31.14 UNCOMPLICATED CROWN FRACTURE, COVERED

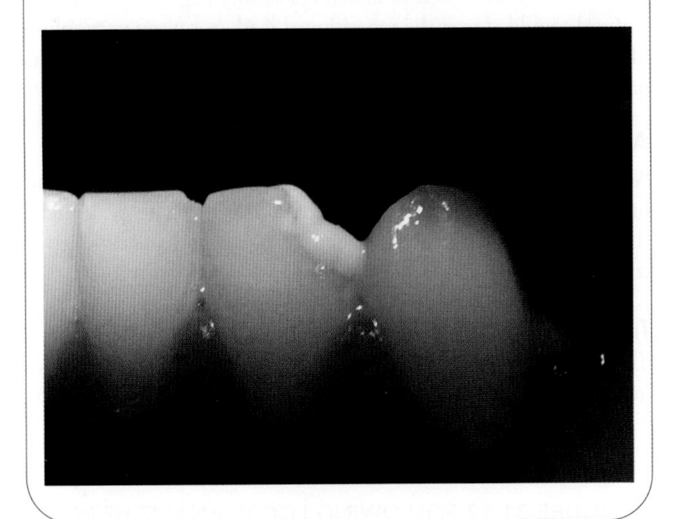

FIGURE 31.15 COMPLICATED CROWN FRACTURE WITH PULP EXPOSED

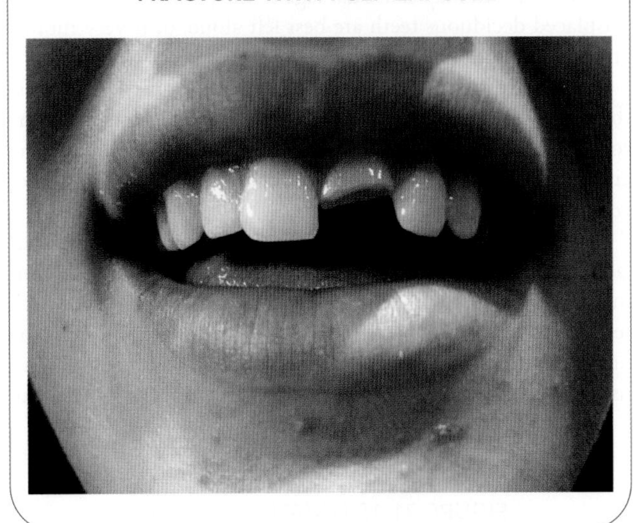

FIGURE 31.16 COMPLICATED CROWN FRACTURE WITH PULP EXPOSURE COVERED WITH CALCIUM HYDROXIDE

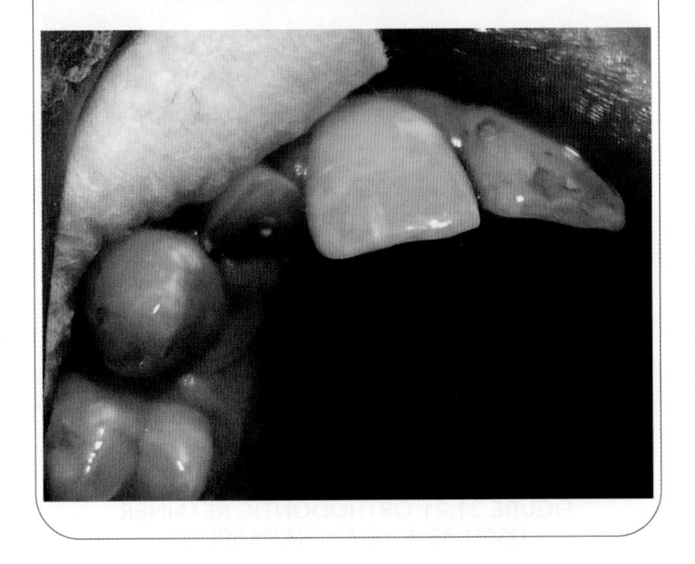

FIGURE 31.17 COMPLICATED CROWN FRACTURE COVERED WITH GIC (CEMENT) WITH CALCIUM HYDROXIDE BELOW

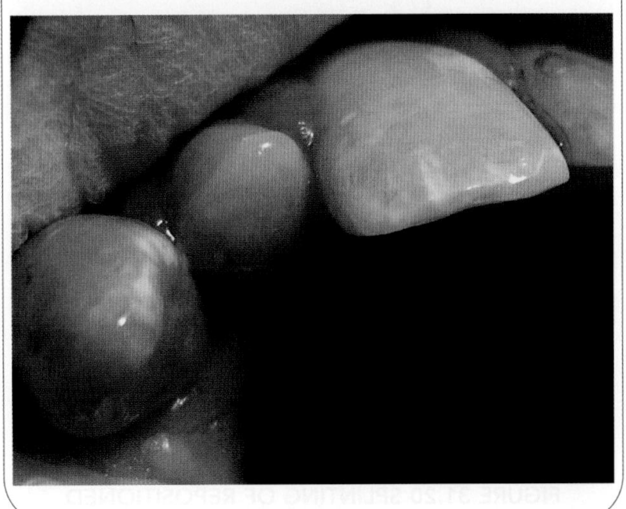

However, if > 2 mm of tooth structure is missing but no pulp (red centre) is exposed, either leave alone or cover with Blu-Tack as first aid or with GIC (cement) if available (Fig. 31.14).

COMPLICATED CROWN FRACTURES

Complicated crown fractures are where the pulp has been exposed (see Figs 31.15 and 31.16).

Assessment

If the fracture site is cleaned off with gauze, a pinkish blush or bleeding can be seen. Fractures through the pulp are usually extremely painful.

Treatment

The exposed pulp and fractured tooth is covered using Blu-Tack after drying. If available, calcium hydroxide ($Ca(OH)_2$), which has bactericidal and remineralising properties, may be placed first over the exposed pulp followed by GIC (Fig. 31.17).

LUXATION INJURIES

This is when the teeth are partially displaced from their sockets.

PRACTICE TIP

Loose or displaced teeth should not be manipulated unless airway intervention is required en route to the ED.

Treatment

Basic treatment principles include not repositioning deciduous teeth. Deciduous teeth are primary or baby teeth and will be replaced by their permanent counterparts which lie just below the deciduous tooth root. Repositioning or re-implanting a deciduous tooth may cause damage to the permanent successor. Displaced deciduous teeth are best left alone, or if very mobile and there is an inhalation risk, extract them.

When treating permanent-tooth injuries, give local anaesthesia when appropriate and reposition both teeth and surrounding bone (Figs 31.18 and 31.19). Splinting is done using either Blu-Tack with thick aluminium foil or with glass ionomer cement (GIC) if available.

The teeth should first be accurately repositioned, using the adjacent teeth positions as a guide. When completing the repositioning of the teeth, be sure that the patient can fully close their back teeth together and are able to chew properly. After repositioning the luxated teeth, they should be splinted against adjacent sound teeth using GIC alone or GIC and fine wire (Fig. 31.20). Other useful emergency splints include the use of the patient's orthodontic retainer or mouthguard if available (Fig. 31.21). Alternatively, a Stomahesive wafer (used to attach colostomy bags) may be cut to size and moulded over the repositioned teeth as a temporary splint. This wafer takes several hours to dissolve in the mouth, giving the patient time to access more definitive treatment.

AVULSION INJURIES

Avulsed teeth are a true dental emergency as the treatment and outcomes of these injuries is time critical.[30] The paramedic should attempt to locate the avulsed tooth and preserve it for transport as below.

Treatment

The most ideal treatment for an avulsed tooth is immediate re-implantation. Avulsed teeth (Figs 31.22 and 31.23) should be

FIGURE 31.18 LUXATION INJURY

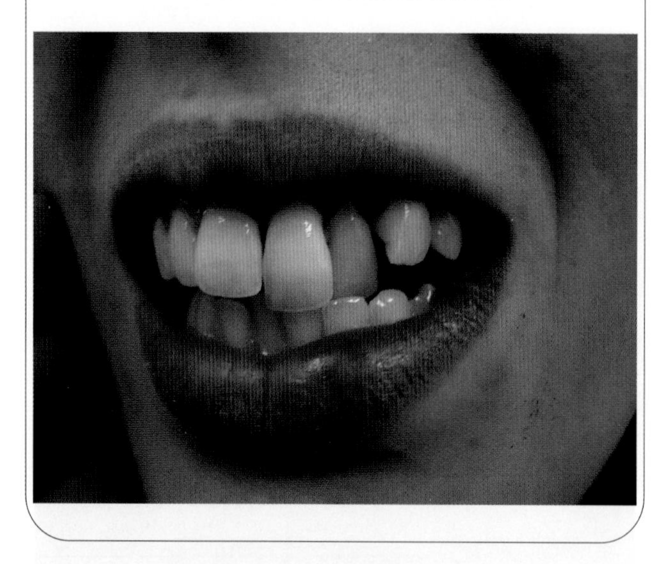

FIGURE 31.19 FOLLOWING LOCAL ANAESTHETIC, TEETH ARE REPOSITIONED WITH FIRM FINGER PRESSURE MAKING SURE BITE IS RE-ESTABLISHED

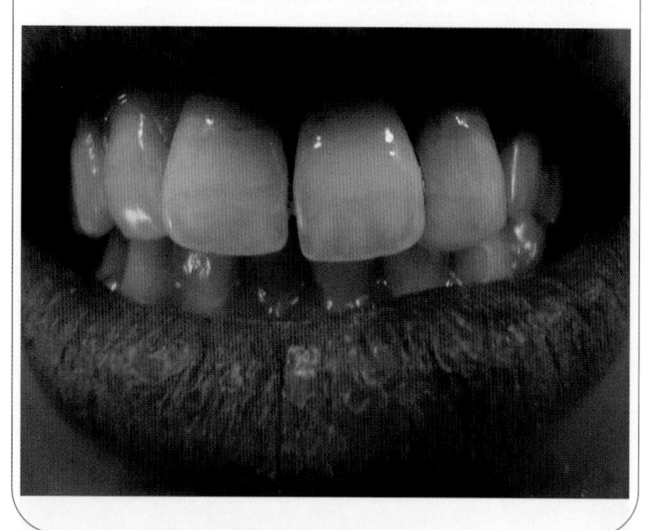

FIGURE 31.20 SPLINTING OF REPOSITIONED TEETH USING GIC TO RESTORE FUNCTION

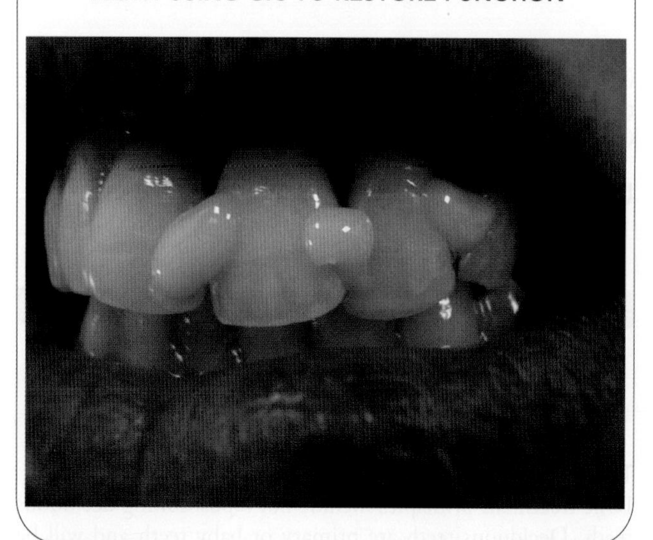

FIGURE 31.21 ORTHODONTIC RETAINER USED AS A TEMPORARY SPLINT

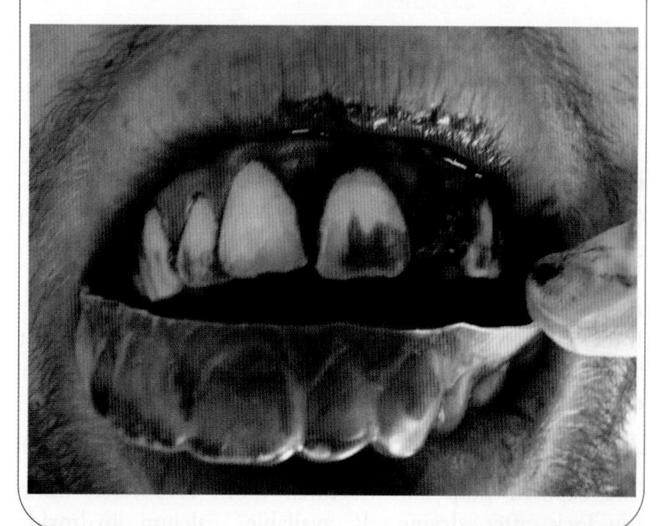

stored in cold milk during transport and re-implanted as soon as possible. Milk has an osmolality very similar to that of human blood, and therefore helps maintain the vitality of the periodontal ligament cells which line the root of the tooth, and which are critical for the tooth re-attaching back to the socket. Milk is in fact better than saliva as a transport medium as saliva carries a large bacterial load. Long-life, skim or soy milk are equally effective. Other suitable transport media include egg albumin and physiological saline, while tap water is unsuitable because of its osmolality. An avulsed tooth is not to be placed in the side of the cheek, as was suggested some years ago, since several children ended up swallowing these teeth.

If an avulsed tooth has been inappropriately stored dry for more than 1 hour, re-implantation may be attempted but success is limited. It is estimated that after 1 hour of dry storage, very few if any periodontal ligament cells are still viable on the root surface to allow the tooth to reattach. In addition, an avulsed deciduous (primary) tooth should never be re-implanted. This is because in trying to replace the deciduous tooth back into the socket there is the likelihood of damage to the developing permanent tooth which lies at the base of the socket just under the deciduous tooth.

The tooth socket should first be irrigated with saline to remove any residual clot which may inhibit replantation (Fig. 31.24). The avulsed tooth is handled only by the crown portion so as not to damage the periodontal ligament cells on the root surface which are essential for successful re-attachment (Fig. 31.25). The avulsed tooth is rinsed with saline for a few seconds to remove any gross debris, and then inserted back into

FIGURE 31.22 AVULSION INJURY

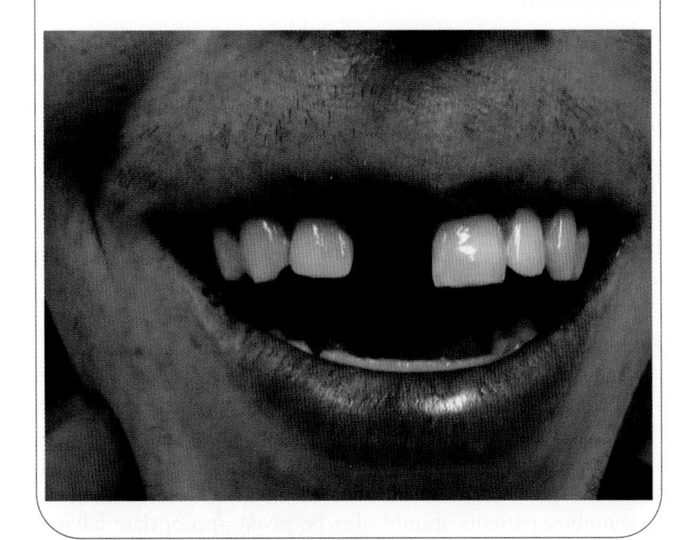

FIGURE 31.23 AVULSED TOOTH

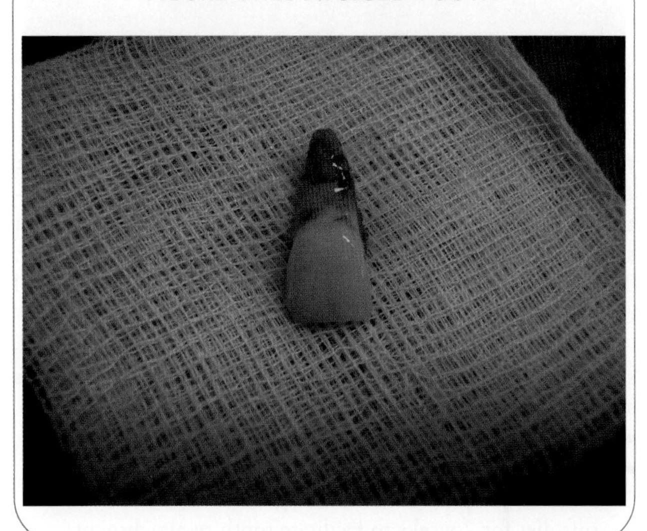

FIGURE 31.24 SOCKET IRRIGATED WITH SALINE TO REMOVE ANY CLOTS AND DEBRIS

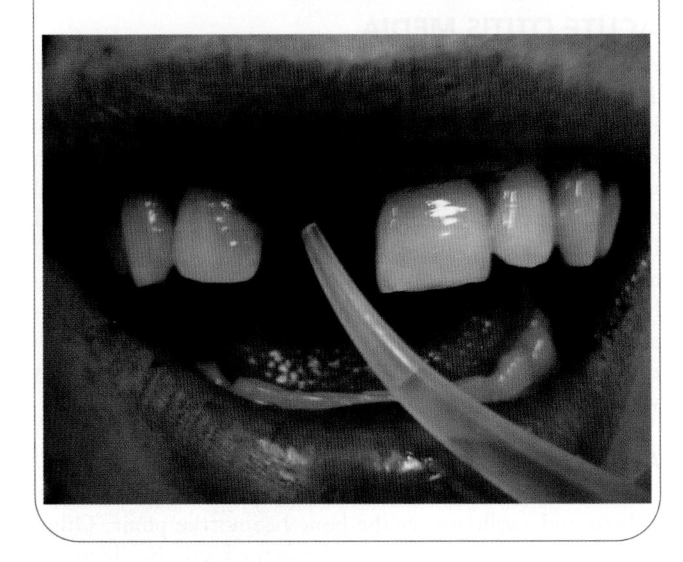

FIGURE 31.25 TOOTH HANDLED FROM CROWN AND NOT ROOT PORTION, THEREBY NOT DAMAGING PERIODONTAL MEMBRANE WHICH LINES THE ROOT SURFACE AND IS RESPONSIBLE FOR SUCCESSFUL RE-ATTACHMENT

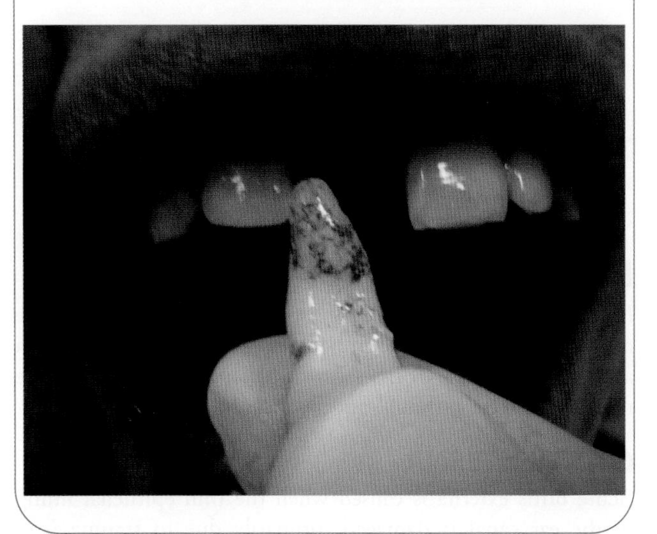

Note: The tooth is rinsed under running tap water for a few seconds prior to re-implantation.

FIGURE 31.26 TOOTH RE-IMPLANTED AND SPLINTED USING GIC

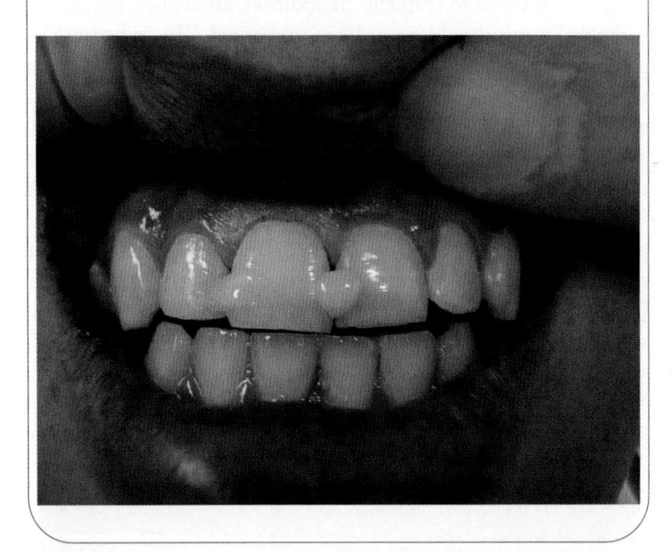

the socket (Fig. 31.26). It is important to avoid any aggressive cleaning as this may damage the vulnerable periodontal membrane cells. Once the tooth is correctly positioned the patient should be able to completely close their back teeth together. The tooth should then be splinted by using Blu-Tack with foil on top, or GIC if available (Figs. 31.26 and 31.27).

An assessment of the patient's tetanus immunisation status should be done, and post re-implantation treatment/instructions should include:

- amoxycillin or penicillin for 7 days[31]
- chlorhexidine (0.1–0.2%) mouthwash twice daily for 7 days to help maintain oral hygiene
- soft diet for 2 weeks to facilitate tooth re-attachment
- follow-up by dentist as soon as practical and ideally within 2 weeks.

PRACTICE TIPS

LUXATION INJURIES

- Hold avulsed tooth by the crown only.
- Transport in milk.
- Rinse the root briefly with saline before re-implanting.
- Secure the re-implanted tooth by splinting.

EAR EMERGENCIES

Most presentations to an emergency medical service are because of pain, infection or a foreign body lodged in the ear canal. Pain and earache are one of the most distressing symptoms and the need for pain relief should not be underestimated.[32]

OTITIS EXTERNA

Acute otitis externa is caused when the thin epithelial lining of the ear canal is damaged, primarily due to trauma (e.g. cleaning the ear with a cotton bud, or foreign-body insertion including hearing aids) or as a localised reaction to chemicals or excessive moisture. It is more common in the summer months and in humid conditions. It is also known as swimmer's ear. Patients with a pre-existing skin condition such as eczema or psoriasis may be predisposed.[33] Otitis externa may be bacterial or fungal in nature. Fungal infection is less common and usually follows a prolonged course of topical antibacterials and/or corticosteroids.[34]

PRACTICE TIP

Otitis externa is largely preventable, so patients should be educated not to put anything into their ear canal—including cotton buds.

Assessment

Patients present complaining of itchiness, ear pain, discharge or muffled hearing. The ear canal appears red and swollen and there may be a discharge in the ear canal. On examination, tenderness may be present on moving the pinna or opening the jaw.

Treatment

The ear should not be syringed with water, but debris and exudate should be removed. This can be done either by suctioning with direct visualisation or dry-mopping using cotton wool on a thin carrier. See Chapter 16 for a description of suctioning techniques. This should be followed with topical eardrops, which are a combination of a corticosteroid and an antibiotic, unless the patient is systemically unwell when oral antibiotics may be given.[35,36] Pain can usually be adequately controlled using paracetamol or ibuprofen.[35,37,38] Refer to Chapter 18 for pain management considerations. As otitis externa is largely preventable, patients should also be given appropriate advice about not inserting foreign objects into the ear (such as a cotton bud), keep the ear dry for 2 weeks while undergoing treatment and using eardrops to loosen cerumen.[32]

ACUTE OTITIS MEDIA

Acute otitis media (AOM) occurs mainly in children under 10 years, but can occur at any age. AOM is an infection or inflammation in the middle ear space (behind the tympanic membrane).[35] Pain is the major symptom; in young children unable to express the location of pain, irritability, crying and tugging at the earlobes may be the presenting symptoms. AOM is often preceded by upper respiratory tract infections (URTIs) and symptoms such as cough, dysphagia and sore throat may be found.[39] The infection can enter the middle ear via the Eustachian tube. Normally the middle ear is filled with air; however, after a cold or a URTI the space can be filled with mucus which can then become infected.[40]

Assessment

Patients will present with pain, which may be associated with redness and swelling over the bone behind the pinna. Other symptoms may include fever, tachycardia, headache, discharge and malaise. Diagnosis is confirmed by examining the eardrum with an auroscope. The tympanic membrane, which is usually pink, becomes a red or yellow colour and may have a lumpy

FIGURE 31.27

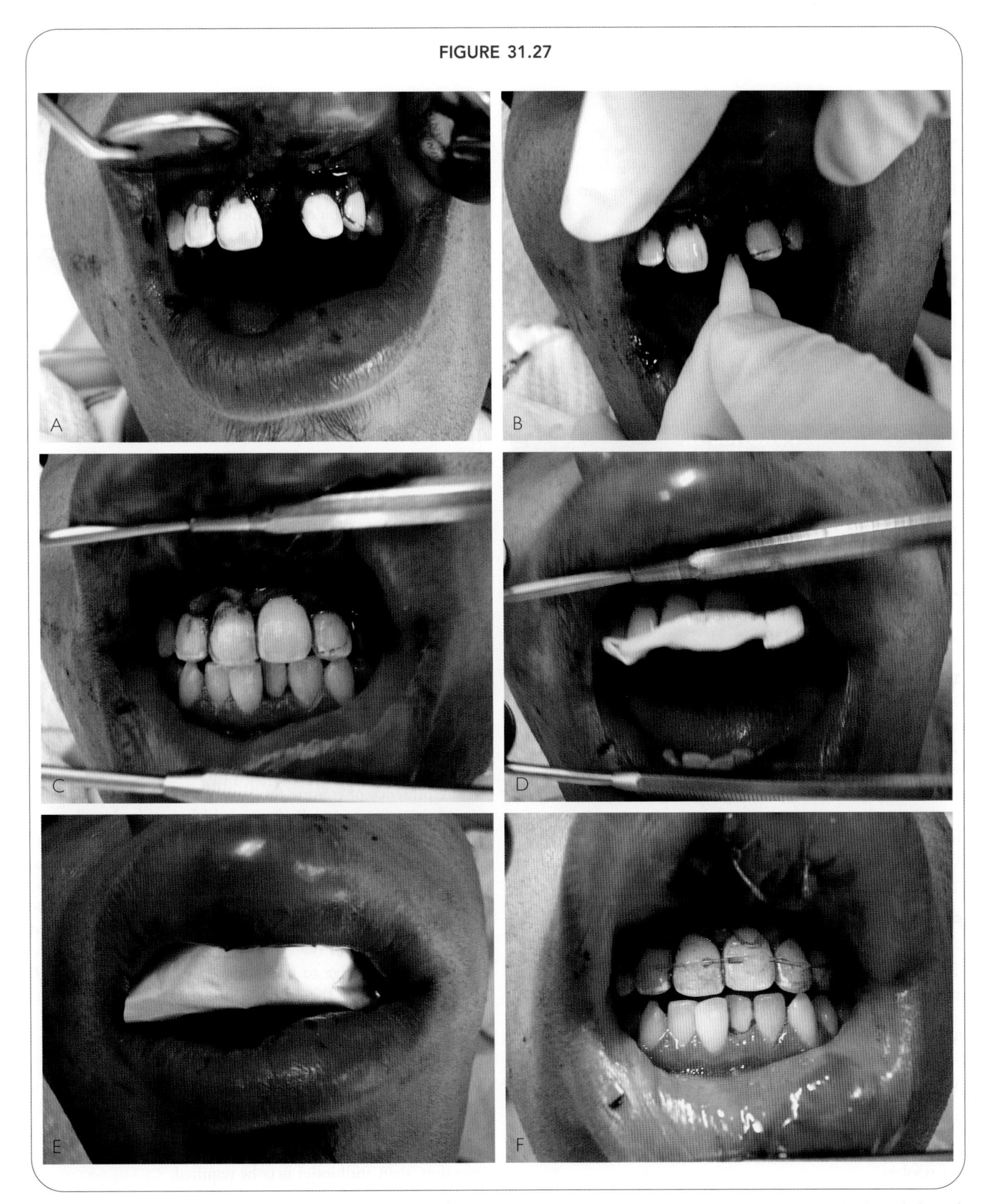

A. Tooth avulsion injury. **B.** Reinsertion of the avulsed tooth. **C.** Prior to splinting, the patient should be able to completely close their teeth together. **D.** Splinting with Yellow or Blu-tack. **E.** Covering the teeth with aluminium foiled paper (from a 'Jelonet' dressing package). **F.** The same patient splinted more definitively using GIC and some fishing line. *Courtesy Dr Tony Skapetis.*

appearance. It might also appear to bulge, with loss of normal landmarks. This is due to the pressure of mucus on the membrane.[40]

Treatment

Pain can usually be managed with either paracetamol or ibuprofen. Hot washcloths held over the ear can help by dilating the blood vessels and encouraging the reabsorption of fluid, and helping reduce swelling.

As most cases of AOM resolve spontaneously, antibiotics are not routinely required. However, if symptoms are not improving after 72 hours then a 5-day course of amoxicillin should be considered. Children between the ages of 6 months and 2 years should be followed up after 24 hours to see if further treatment is required. For children aged less than 6 months, Aboriginals and Torres Strait Islanders, treatment with antibiotics is recommended due to the risk of complications.[37]

PRACTICE TIP

A hot washcloth held over the affected ear can start to reduce pain while oral analgesics take effect. Ensure the temperature is not so hot as to cause a burn injury.

LABYRINTHITIS

Labyrinthitis is an infection of the inner ear and is thought to be associated with a viral illness.

Assessment

Sudden onset of symptoms include vertigo, nausea and vomiting, and loss of balance. Vertigo is more marked with movement of the head. Hearing loss may also be present on the affected side. Symptoms last from hours to weeks. However, vertigo can also be caused by intracranial pathology so this must be ruled out.

Treatment

Treatment includes bed rest, antiemetics and maintaining hydration (to counteract effects of vomiting).[5,41]

FURUNCULOSIS

Furunculosis is an abscess or furuncle in the ear canal. They can cause severe ear pain, which is made worse by moving the tragus or opening the jaw.[32]

Assessment

Furuncles usually present similarly to otitis externa, but the pain is much more severe.

Treatment

Treatment is with strong oral analgesia; the furuncle usually self-resolves.

MASTOIDITIS

The mastoid air-cell system is part of the middle ear cleft, so some degree of mastoid inflammation occurs whenever there is infection in the middle ear. In most cases this will not cause any problems, but in acute mastoiditis pus collects in the mastoid air cells and exerts pressure on the bony trabeculae, resulting in necrosis and formation of an abscess cavity.[42] Mastoiditis can be a complication of AOM; the symptoms usually become evident a few days after onset of AOM.

Assessment

Patients present with redness, swelling and tenderness over the mastoid process, and the pinna is displaced away from the side of the head.[33] The patient will be in severe pain and there may or may not be a discharge from the ear. Symptoms that indicate acute mastoiditis should be prioritised as urgent.[33]

PRACTICE TIP

Symptoms that indicate acute mastoiditis should be prioritised as urgent. Look for redness, swelling and tenderness over the mastoid process and a pinna which is displaced away from the side of the head.

Treatment

Mastoiditis can lead to a more serious intracranial infection, so treatment with IV antibiotics should begin as soon as possible and in some cases surgery is required for drainage of the abscess.

RUPTURED TYMPANIC MEMBRANE

A ruptured tympanic membrane (TM) can occur as a result of trauma or infection. Figs 31.28 and 31.29 show normal tympanic membranes. Types of trauma include penetrating trauma, such as inserting a cotton bud to clean the ear; altitude changes, such as in diving or flying; forcing air into the ear canal, such as being slapped over the ear or being in the vicinity of an explosion. Infection can cause the TM to rupture due to the pressure in the middle ear.

Assessment

In the presence of trauma the patient will present complaining of severe ear pain; discharge, which may be bloody; and hearing loss to the affected ear. In the case of infection the patient may state that the pain has gone; this may be due to the release of pressure caused by the rupture of the TM. In the case of a head injury associated with a ruptured TM, the patient may also have dislocated the ossicles and damaged the inner ear. Any of these injuries can result in hearing loss, dizziness and damage to the facial nerve as it passes through the temporal bone. The resulting injury can be either permanent or temporary.[2]

Treatment

Treatment for a ruptured TM usually consists of analgesia, and patient advice to keep water out of the ear canal. They usually spontaneously heal in a few months; however, ENT department follow-up may be advised. In the case of a rupture due to infection, then antibiotics may be required.[33]

FOREIGN BODY

Foreign bodies in the ear are a common presentation. The object can vary from an insect, beads and small toys to cotton buds. They prove problematic in their removal, as the area is sensitive and often the patient is a child. Removal should only be attempted by trained staff to avoid unnecessary trauma.[43] The first attempt at removal is likely to be the most successful,

FIGURE 31.28 NORMAL TYMPANIC MEMBRANE

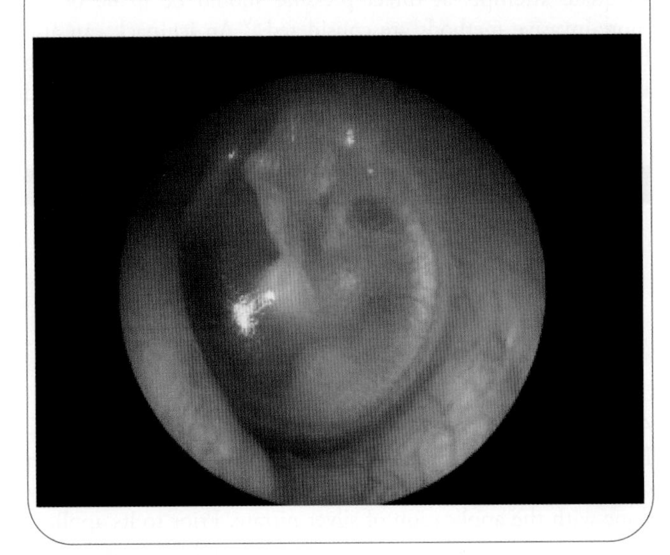

Courtesy Mr Simon A Hickey.

FIGURE 31.29 ANATOMY OF THE NORMAL TYMPANIC MEMBRANE[2]

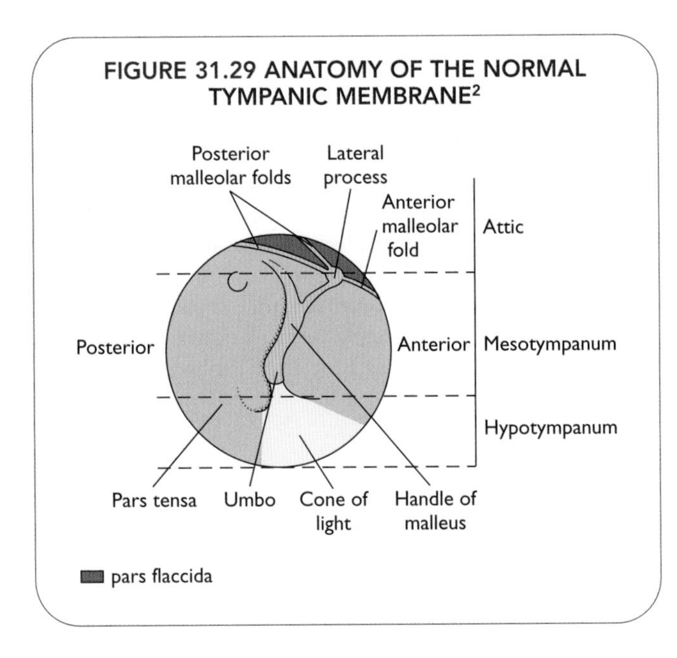

as repeated tries cause further swelling and bleeding and decrease patient cooperation.[44]

Assessment

An adult patient will usually be able to tell you what is stuck in the ear; however, children may be fearful of getting into trouble and may present due to secondary symptoms. Symptoms may include itching or discharge. If there is an insect in the ear, a buzzing may be heard or motion felt. The patient or parents/accompanying adult should always be asked about attempts to remove the object at home, as poorly executed attempts at foreign body removal may injure the ear canal, perforate the tympanic membrane or merely push the foreign body deeper into the canal.[45] Inspection of the ear canal should be performed using an auroscope. It is important to check that the tympanic membrane is intact.

PRACTICE TIP

After removing a foreign body, always re-examine the ear canal to make sure no further foreign body is present and to assess for any damage in removal of the original one.

Treatment

A patient presenting with an insect in the ear is usually very distressed due to the pain and noise associated with the insect. The first priority is to kill the insect. This can be done with olive oil, methylated spirits or lignocaine. Lignocaine has been reported to have an irritating effect that drives the insect out of the ear canal.[44] Once the insect is dead, the patient will be a lot calmer. The insect usually floats to the surface and can be easily retrieved.

Organic matter such as paper, vegetables and cottonwool cause an added problem as they swell in moist conditions, making it more difficult to retrieve them and making it difficult to flush them out. They may be grabbed onto using crocodile forceps, but the danger is that the object will be pushed further into the ear.

If the object is round and smooth, then forceps will not be able to grasp the item and other methods need to be considered. These include using gentle suction or a hook.

If the foreign body is successfully removed, then the ear canal should be inspected to ensure all matter is removed and no further damage has been caused by the removal.[33] If the object cannot be adequately visualised or retrieved, then referral to the appropriate ENT service is required and the patient should remain nil by mouth.

When approaching a child, a certain level of cooperation is required. It is helpful to gain their trust if possible by playing a few games before attempting to retrieve the object. However, if the first attempt is not successful then the chances of cooperation for subsequent attempts are reduced. Sedation may be an option if the resources are available.[43]

BLOCKED EARS

Cerumen or earwax, a naturally occurring substance in the ear, cleans, protects and lubricates the external ear canal. Blocked ears due to impacted wax are not something that can be dealt with in an ED. The patient should be advised to place wax-softening drops in the ear for a few days and then attend a general practitioner for syringing. The ED clinician should not perform ear syringing unless they have received formal training in the process. In the eyes of the law, you may be seen to be negligent if you do perform syringing and have not had the training or received a recent update of your skills.[45]

Trauma

A blunt force, such as a sporting injury or assault or a penetrative injury caused by a sharp object, are causes of trauma to the earlobe. An injury to the earlobe can result in a laceration to the pinna or a sub-perichondrial haematoma. Lacerations can involve the outer layer of skin or can be full-thickness involving the cartilage.

Assessment

A thorough inspection of the ear should be made and any bleeding stopped with direct pressure. The ear canal should also be inspected for injury using an auroscope. Clear fluid from the ear after trauma could be cerebrospinal fluid and brain injury should be suspected.

Treatment

Superficial lacerations can generally be treated by cleaning with normal saline and applying a non-pressure dressing. All foreign bodies should be removed to prevent tattooing or infection. Re-assessment of the wound should occur in 24 hours.[45] For lacerations involving the cartilage, referral to an ENT or a plastic surgeon is required. This is to ensure that the best cosmetic appearance is attained. A sub-perichondrial haematoma is a collection of blood between the cartilage and perichondrium. The blood exerts pressure on the cartilage, resulting in necrosis (leading to cauliflower ear if untreated). Treatment is evacuation of the blood followed by a pressure bandage to prevent re-accumulation.[33] See Chapter 16 for information on applying a bandage.

NASAL EMERGENCIES

Nasal problems can relate to trauma, infection or haemorrhage.

EPISTAXIS

Nosebleeds are a common occurrence with 60% of the population suffering a nosebleed at some time in their life.[46] Ninety per cent of nosebleeds stop spontaneously or with pinching of the soft tissue of the nose.[47] However, it can be life threatening in the elderly or those with comorbidities.[48] Epistaxis is more common in the winter months due to dry, cold air and subsequent drying of the nasal mucosa.[49] In the younger population, nosebleeds generally occur in the anterior area (Little's area or Kiesselbach's area), due to nose-picking or insertion of a foreign body, and account for 90% of incidences. In the elderly they tend to be posterior and account for the other 10%.[50]

Assessment

When a patient presents with active bleeding, it is not always easy to obtain a history straight away. After assessing airway, breathing and circulation and acting on any life-threatening findings, attempts should be made to stop the nosebleed. Once this has been done further history can be taken. A full set of vital signs needs to be obtained and repeated regularly to monitor haemodynamic stability. A nosebleed from only one nostril is usually anterior, whereas if the patient can feel the blood running down their throat it is more likely to be posterior.[49] The history should also include asking about bleeding disorders, medications including anticoagulants, trauma and estimated blood loss. Angina and chronic obstructive airways disease can be exacerbated due to hypovolaemia or anaemia, and presence of these conditions should be considered.[50] Hypertension is not generally a cause of nosebleeds but it can prolong the course of the nosebleed and is probably a stress response to the nosebleed.[2,50]

Treatment

Pressing on the nose beneath the nasal bone for 15 minutes without interruption can usually arrest bleeding. Patients should also be advised to sit up and tilt their head forward so as to allow blood to drain out of the mouth. Swallowing can cause pressure changes in the nose that dislodge recently formed clots, and swallowed blood irritates the stomach causing the patient to vomit and again dislodge the clot. At least two adequate attempts at direct pressure should be made before more-invasive methods are considered.[49] An ice pack can also be applied to the bridge of the nose.[47] In the pre-hospital setting if the bleed cannot be arrested, a large-bore cannula should be sited.

PRACTICE TIP

To stop epistaxis, press beneath the nasal bone (Little's area) with firm pressure for 15 minutes. Use a watch to time, as release before this time is unlikely to stop the bleeding. Consider applying an ice pack to the bridge of the nose.

Anterior management

If the bleeding site can be visualised then it may be possible to cauterise the vessel once haemostasis is achieved. This is usually done with the application of silver nitrate. Prior to its application it is important to protect the surrounding areas with a barrier cream to prevent injury to the unaffected areas. If bleeding continues then nasal packing will be required. This is usually as per department protocol and the type of packing available. Patients may be suitable for discharge if after initial treatment they maintain haemostasis. However, if bleeding reoccurs nasal repacking may be required. Patients may be considered for discharge with nasal packs in situ if they live close to the hospital and have a means to return, or have access to medical review within 24 hours. However, patients with risk factors for rebleeding (on anticoagulants, hypertensive and elderly people) are more safely observed in hospital.

A recent randomised controlled trial showed applying a topical application of injectable form of tranexamic acid was better than anterior nasal packing in the initial treatment of anterior epistaxis.[46]

Posterior management

If a bleeding site is not found or bleeding continues, then a posterior bleed is the likely cause. The use of a balloon catheter is usually required. The type will depend on departmental preference. The patient should be admitted to hospital for observation, as complications can arise. The pack can become dislodged and cause an airway obstruction. There is risk of infection, particularly sinusitis due to improper draining of the sinuses. It is a painful procedure, so adequate and ongoing analgesia should be given. Some patients can also experience difficulty in swallowing, so hydration needs to be monitored.[47,50,51]

FOREIGN BODY

Foreign bodies in noses generally occur in children aged 9 months and upwards following the development of the pincer grip and an inquisitive nature to explore their surroundings.

Assessment

The presence of a nasal foreign body should be suspected in patients with unilateral discharge and unexplained pain.[44]

Treatment

In an older child it is possible to try and get them to blow the object out of the affected nostril while occluding the unaffected one; however, there is a risk that the child will inhale instead and aspirate the object. Local anaesthetic spray can be applied to the nostril and then removal by forceps performed, but in an uncooperative child sedation may be required. Always re-examine the nose after removal of the object, as other foreign matter may also be in situ.[33,43]

Trauma

Trauma to the nose is usually a result of an accident or an assault. As with all trauma, the patient should be assessed for DRSABCD first and life-threatening injuries ruled out before treatment to the nose is commenced. Nosebleeds that follow head or facial trauma may indicate cerebrospinal fluid leak or an orbital blow-out fracture.[9]

Assessment

A history should be taken. Examination of the external surface of the nose should be conducted as well as examining the internal surfaces. A nasal speculum should be used for this.

Treatment

First-aid measures include applying ice and keeping the head elevated to reduce swelling.[50] If the patient has a nosebleed, then it should be stopped using the methods described above.

Any wounds to the nose should be cleaned and dressed as appropriate; tetanus status should be ascertained and a booster given if required.

Nasal injuries are often accompanied by soft-tissue swelling and so assessment of injury is difficult initially. The patient is usually followed up after 7–10 days, once the swelling has subsided. In children the fracture heals faster, so they should be seen within 5 days.[51] This is done in an ENT clinic if deformity is still present.

A septal haematoma should also be excluded where there is suspicion of a nasal fracture. Looking up the nose with a nasal speculum, it appears as a cherry pushing down. If left untreated it can become infected and lead to an abscess and necrosis of the nasal cartilage, leading to a cosmetic deformity. An ENT specialist usually performs an incision and drainage and referral should occur as soon as possible.[33]

SINUSITIS

Sinusitis is inflammation and swelling of the lining of the sinuses, causing the normal drainage mechanism of the sinus to become blocked. Acute sinusitis is diagnosed when symptoms are of less than 3 weeks duration. Viral upper respiratory tract infections and allergic rhinitis are the most common precipitants of acute sinusitis.[47] Chronic sinusitis occurs when symptoms persist for longer than 3 weeks.

Assessment

The patient will present with facial pain that increases with leaning forward, fever, yellow/green nasal discharge, nausea and headache. On palpation there may be tenderness over the sinus.

Treatment

For acute sinusitis with mild symptoms of less than 7 days' duration, symptomatic treatment is recommended. Paracetamol can be used for pain relief. Antibiotics should not be given unless symptoms persist for more than 7 days, or unless symptoms are severe.[47] Decongestants can also be used to reduce local oedema, promoting drainage and therefore helping to alleviate symptoms; but for no longer than 7 days due to rebound symptoms.[46] The patient should keep their head elevated, which can also relieve the stuffy feeling.

THROAT EMERGENCIES

Patients presenting with throat problems generally experience pain and may have difficulty breathing. There is little seasonal fluctuation in the incidence of sore throat, and about 10% of the Australian population will present to a primary healthcare service annually with an upper respiratory tract infection consisting predominantly of a sore throat.[52] A bacterial or viral infection, foreign body, trauma and irritation can cause sore throat from smoke, or seasonal allergy.[33,53]

PRACTICE TIP

Considerations for pre-hospital care for a child with a sore throat:

- Do not put anything in the mouth to visualise the pharynx.
- Do not site an intravenous line unless arrest is imminent.
- Allow the child to be transported in a position of comfort.
- Monitor heart rhythm for bradycardia.
- Transport rapidly to an emergency medical service.

There are two key issues that emergency medical personnel should focus on. First is being alert for signs of respiratory compromise. In these cases, high-flow oxygen should be given and the patient transported in the position that affords the most comfort. This is usually sitting upright or semi-erect. Under no circumstances should the patient be forced to recline. If complete airway obstruction occurs, then this should be managed with bag–mask ventilation, tracheal intubation or surgical airway, depending on the skill of the paramedic.

The second issue to consider is dehydration. Many patients with severe pharyngitis are unable to maintain adequate hydration. Intravenous fluids should be administered in these cases; however, caution should be exercised in children as emotional upset from having a cannula sited could worsen the airway obstruction.[52] Do not place anything in the mouth to visualise the pharynx in a child, as this could also exacerbate the potential airway obstruction. Rapid transfer to an emergency medical service should occur, with electrocardiograph monitoring as bradycardia can be a sign of impending arrest.[53] Epiglottitis is covered in Chapter 35.

PRACTICE TIP

Allow the patient to find a position which is the most comfortable for them. This may be seated or lying in a semi-recumbent position.

PHARYNGITIS

Pharyngitis is inflammation of the pharynx. Patients usually present complaining of a sore throat and difficulty swallowing. Pharyngitis tends to be viral, but a minority of cases are bacterial; clinically, it can be very difficult to differentiate the two. If the sore throat is accompanied by other cold-like symptoms such as a runny nose, cough and laryngitis (see below), the infection is most likely to be viral. Bacterial infection is much more likely in a patient presenting with only a sore throat. Group A beta-haemolytic *Streptococcus* (GABHS) is the most common bacteria found in bacterial pharyngitis. It can cause acute rheumatic fever and post-streptococcal glomerulonephritis; therefore, the patient may be treated with antibiotics if in a high-risk group such as a child with diabetes mellitus or immunodeficiency, a history of rheumatic heart disease or features of systemic illness due to the acute sore throat.[5,37,54,55]

Assessment

A history should be taken. Patients may complain of soreness on swallowing, general malaise, headache and fever. Past medical history should be taken and a history of rheumatic fever should be noted.[11] The patient's voice may be hoarse or sound muffled. A set of vital signs should be taken. The presence of fever is likely and tachycardia, tachypnoea and/or hypotension may mean the patient needs more immediate attention.

Examination can help reveal if the cause is viral or bacterial. In a viral infection, you would expect to find vesicular and petechial patterns on the soft palate and tonsils, and often associated with rhinorrhoea. In a bacterial infection, there is marked erythema of the tonsils and tonsillar pillars, tonsillar exudate; and when the neck is palpated, enlarged tender anterior cervical lymph nodes are found. Uvular oedema may also be seen.[56] Diagnosis of a GABHS is based on the Centor criteria, which state that the following four things must be present:

1. History of fever
2. Absence of cough
3. Tonsillar exudate
4. Enlarged tender anterior cervical nodes.[52]

PRACTICE TIPS

CENTOR CRITERIA

1. History of fever
2. Absence of cough
3. Tonsillar exudates
4. Enlarged tender anterior cervical nodes.

SCORING

- 4 Centor criteria = antibiotics
- 2-3 Centor criteria + positive throat swab = antibiotics
- < 2 Centor criteria and negative throat swab = no antibiotics

Treatment

For viral pharyngitis, treatment is conservative. Pain can be managed with over-the-counter analgesics like paracetamol and ibuprofen. Tablets that dissolve in water may be preferable, as they are easier to swallow.[54] Fluids should be encouraged to prevent dehydration.

For GABHS, treatment is based on how many positive Centor criteria signs are present. Those with Centor scores of 4 should be treated with antibiotics. Scores of 2–3 should have a throat swab, and antibiotics given only for those where the swab comes back positive. Those who score < 2 are treated symptomatically, as for viral pharyngitis.[52]

LARYNGITIS

Laryngitis is inflammation of the larynx and vocal cords due to viral or bacterial infection or irritation caused by allergens, chemicals or overuse. Episodes are usually self-limiting and can be influenced by weather conditions. The cords lose the ability to vibrate due to swelling and cause the voice to sound husky or to be lost altogether, breathing can be difficult and stridor may be heard. Obstruction of the airway can become serious and should be treated as soon as possible. See Chapter 35 for details on croup.

Assessment

Patients will give a history of a lowering of the normal pitch of the voice and hoarseness, which usually persists for from 3 to 8 days. They may also experience symptoms of a URTI, such as sore throat, rhinorrhoea, dyspnoea, post-nasal discharge and congestion. The diagnosis is often made on history alone.

Treatment

In the patient with loss of voice and sore throat, treatment consists of analgesia, steam inhalations and voice rest. Laryngitis is most often viral and antibiotics are not recommended.[54,56]

TONSILLITIS

The tonsils have many crevices that seem to harbour bacteria, but tonsillitis can be classified as either viral or bacterial and may occur in isolation or as part of a generalised pharyngitis.[57] It is more common in childhood. Rheumatic fever and acute glomerulonephritis are recognised complications of acute tonsillitis associated with GABHS. These diseases are rare in resource-rich countries, but do occasionally occur. They are still a common problem in certain populations, notably Aboriginal and Torres Strait Islander people, and may be effectively prevented in closed communities by the use of penicillin.[58]

Assessment

Patients with viral tonsillitis usually present complaining of a sore throat and may also have a blocked nose, cough and cold symptoms and general aches and pains. On examination, the tonsils will appear red, but may or may not have exudate on them. Bacterial tonsillitis tends to have more localised symptoms, such as sore throat, difficulty swallowing, referred ear pain, fever and malaise. A throat swab should be taken.

Treatment

Antibiotics are not recommended for tonsillitis; instead, the patient should rest, drink plenty of fluids and take regular analgesia for pain. However, if three or more of the Centor criteria are present or the patient has had a positive throat swab or appears systemically unwell, then antibiotics should be prescribed.

PERITONSILLAR ABSCESS

Peritonsillar abscess (quinsy) occurs when the bacterial infection of tonsillitis extends outside the tonsillar capsule and into surrounding tissue. The abscess is usually found in the potential space between the tonsillar capsule and the surrounding pharyngeal muscle bed. It is usually found in young adults who have a history of recurrent infections.

Assessment

The patient will usually present complaining of worsening pain, difficulty swallowing, trismus (spasm in jaw muscles causing pain on opening) and may be unable to swallow. Examination will reveal a grossly swollen tonsil deviating to the midline. Dehydration may be an issue in a patient who is unable to swallow and they should also be assessed for respiratory compromise.

Treatment

Intravenous antibiotics and fluids are commenced and referral is made to an ENT specialist who will perform an incision and drainage.

POST-TONSILLECTOMY BLEEDS

Post-tonsillectomy bleeding is an uncommon, but a potentially life-threatening event, estimated to occur in approximately 2–5% of patients undergoing tonsillectomy.[57] There are two types of bleeds; a primary bleed is considered to occur within the first 24 hours and those occurring after 24 hours (typically most frequently on days 5–9 and up to 28 days) are referred to as a secondary bleed. The majority of bleeds are usually minor and self-limiting; however, some require medical or surgical intervention. The main difficulties arising from bleeds are airway obstruction or hypovolemic shock.

Assessment

The patient will typically present with a history of bleeding or with current active bleeding from the tonsillar fossa. Examine the patient's throat to localise the source of bleeding, A full set of observations should be obtained to assess the haemodynamic stability of the patient. Children can tolerate blood loss to a certain point then will decompensate. Excessive swallowing may be an indicator of ongoing bleeding in younger children, as they swallow rather than spit out.

Treatment

Treatment is determined on the degree of bleeding and haemodynamic status of the patient. Cases of active bleeding and an unstable patient should be managed in the resuscitation room. Treat and manage airway, if obstructed (see Chapter 16), and manage hypovolaemic shock, if compromised (see Chapter 42). Early intravenous access should be obtained with large-bore cannula access; a second line should be considered when possible. The patient should be seated upright and leaning slightly forwards (to keep blood out of the airway) and encouraged to spit out blood if possible; suction should always be available. Keep the patient nil by mouth; obtain a VBG, full blood count for starting point of haemoglobin and platelets (this may not be representative of blood loss), coagulation profile (for unrecognised coagulopathy) and a Group and hold +/– crossmatch (depending on severity of symptoms). Co-phenylcaine spray to the oropharynx or adrenaline 1:10,000 via swab to the area of bleeding on tonsillar bed may be considered, but will require patient cooperation and a skilled hand. Administration of intravenous tranexamic acid may be required, and/or hydrogen peroxide 1% gargles. An ENT specialist should be contacted as soon as the condition is recognised to determine if surgical management and/or intravenous antibiotics are required.[57,58]

PARAPHARYNGEAL ABSCESS

Parapharyngeal abscesses can occur as a complication of bacterial tonsillitis or pharyngitis. Patients who present with severe symptoms of trismus, pain on swallowing, hot potato voice or muffled voice and shortness of breath should be carefully assessed to rule out this complication.

Assessment

Examination reveals asymmetric pharyngeal swelling, including the palate. Close observation of the airway is required, as it can be compromised by swelling into the neck.

Treatment

Treatment may require airway management and support if this is compromised. See Chapter 16 for airway management techniques. Surgical drainage of the abscess is usually required along with a course of intravenous antibiotics.[55,57]

FACIAL EMERGENCIES

Although the facial emergencies discussed here are not life threatening, they cause significant pain and distress to the sufferer. Facial fractures are discussed in Chapter 44.

TEMPOROMANDIBULAR JOINT DISLOCATION

The temporomandibular joint (TMJ) is a paired synovial joint capable of both sliding and hinge movements.[59] The TMJ articulates the mandibular condyle and the squamous portion of the temporal bone. The upper part of the joint allows for the sliding movement and this is separated from the lower joint by a fibrous meniscus. The lower part of the joint is responsible for the hinged movement. Young females tend to have laxer joints than males, and an unguarded yawn may take the condyle forwards and then a muscle spasm of the closing muscles holds it there.[60]

Assessment

Patients usually present with an open mouth. They may be quite distressed due to pain and anxiety.

Treatment

The dislocation can be reduced by manually pushing the mandible both backwards and downwards. Both hands are placed, with the thumbs outside the patient's teeth, on the lateral border of the mandible, which is then pushed downwards and backwards, placing the condyles back into the fossa. Gauze can be placed over the thumbs for protection. If the muscles are in spasm, then the patient may require a muscle relaxant such as diazepam. In more-severe cases a general anaesthetic may be required.[59] The patient may require anti-inflammatory medication for a few days for pain relief.

FACIAL CELLULITIS

Facial cellulitis usually occurs secondary to either odontogenic or auricular infections. Patients present with pain, swelling and redness over the affected area; treatment usually consists of antibiotics and analgesia, with no adverse outcomes. However,

Ludwig's angina is a submandibular space infection involving the suprahyoid region and floor of the mouth. It elevates the tongue and pushes it posteriorly. The spaces also communicate with the parapharyngeal space and so involvement of the epiglottis is not uncommon. Therefore the main risk for this patient group is airway obstruction.[3,5,61] Dental disease, particularly of the mandibular molars, is the most common predisposing factor.[9] Other precipitating factors include poor dental hygiene, recent dental work, local trauma, tongue piercing and immunocompromise.[9,61]

Assessment

A history should include exploration for any of the predisposing factors. Patients may present complaining of dental, mouth or neck pain. Trismus and/or drooling may also be present. A set of vital signs should be recorded, as fever, chills and tachycardia are common.

Treatment

Ludwig's angina can cause airway obstruction within hours, so constant monitoring of airway patency is essential. The swelling can make endotracheal intubation difficult and it has a high failure rate. Nasotracheal intubation is the preferred method, but an advanced airway kit should be kept close at hand and ready to use. If Ludwig's angina is suspected, then rapid transfer to an emergency medical service is required.

Definitive treatment is with surgical drainage of the abscess and IV antibiotics; however, dexamethasone reduces oedema and cellulitis and can improve the airway obstruction initially. Nebulised adrenaline can also help to reduce upper airway swelling.[61]

SUMMARY

This chapter has looked at common presentations to ED involving the ear, nose throat, face and teeth. Most presentations are precipitated by pain, but due to the intimate nature of structures, swelling and infection can spread to neighbouring areas. Therefore, all patients should be monitored closely for airway difficulties or symptoms of intracranial infection.

CASE STUDY 1

You are called to attend an 80-year-old woman. On arrival at the scene you find her sitting with her head over a bucket. She has had a large epistaxis, which is still actively bleeding. There is evidence of a large loss of blood. During transit the nosebleed is stopped using pressure but on arrival in the emergency department (ED) the epistaxis commences again. The site of bleeding cannot be visualised. She has a history of hypertension, atrial fibrillation and is warfarinised. Her blood pressure is 170/90 mmHg, pulse 110 beats/minute and respiratory rate 20 breaths/minute.

QUESTIONS

1. What is your first intervention?
   a. Lie the patient on her left side to prevent aspiration
   b. Obtain a full set of vital signs
   c. Insert a large-bore cannula
   d. Assess DRSABCD and apply firm pressure to the nostrils for 15 minutes.
2. What position should you get the patient into?
   a. Left lateral position
   b. Prone
   c. Semi-recumbent in a position of comfort
   d. Sitting up with head tilted forward
3. Which of the following treatment options would be most appropriate after your initial assessment?
   a. Give antihypertensive medication to reduce blood pressure
   b. Insert an appropriate nasal pack
   c. Organise crossmatch blood
   d. Reverse warfarin by administering vitamin K
4. What are the clinical red flags obtained during the history?

Answers to Case Study Questions can be found on evolve **http://evolve.elsevier.com/AU/Curtis/emergency/** 

USEFUL WEBSITES

American Academy of Otolaryngology head and neck surgery. This site provides clinical resources helpful for emergency clinicians, www.entnet.org/content/practice-management-resources-cerumen-removal.

Canadian Society of Otolaryngology head and neck surgery. This site provides clinical resources helpful for emergency clinicians, www.entcanada.org/education/medical-students/.

Ear, nose and throat: Emergency Care Institute, aci.health.nsw.gov.au/networks/eci/clinical/clinical-tools/ent.

Identifying high-quality medical education websites in Otolaryngology: a guide for medical students and residents. This site provides clinical resources helpful for emergency clinicians, www.ncbi.nlm.nih.gov/pmc/articles/PMC5445285/.

NSW Rural Doctors Network, Emergency dental kits, www.nswrdn.com.au/site/dental.

Statref.com. This is a suite of 3-D interactive models of human anatomy. Online ebook, www.merckmanuals.com/professional/index.html.

REFERENCES

1. Alford B. Core curriculum syllabus: review of anatomy—the larynx. Texas: Baylor College of Medicine; 2011.
2. Epstein O, Perkin GD, Cookson J, Watt IS, Rakhit R, Robins A, et al. Ear, nose and throat. Clinical examination. 5th ed. Sydney: Elsevier; 2019. p. 82–104.
3. Marx J, Hockberger RS, Wallia R. Rosen's emergency medicine. 8th ed. Philadelphia: Elsevier; 2014.
4. Berkovitz BKB, Holland GR, Moxham BJ. Oral anatomy, histology and embryology. 5th ed. London: Elsevier; 2017.
5. Association EN. Dental, ear, nose, throat and facial emergencies. In: Howard P, Steinmann R, Sheehy S, editors. Sheehy's emergency nursing: principles and practice. 7th ed. St Louis: Elsevier; 2012.
6. Wilson SF, Thompson JM. Respiratory disorders. St Louis: Mosby; 1990.
7. Hull JH, Backer V, Gibson PG, Fowler SJ. Laryngeal dysfunction: assessment and management for the clinician. Am J Respir Crit Care Med 2016;194(9):1062–72.
8. Sinnatamby C. Last's anatomy. 12th ed. Sydney: Elsevier; 2011.
9. Purcell D. Minor injuries: a clinical guide. 3rd ed. Sydney: Elsevier; 2016.
10. Barkauskas V, Pender N, Hayman L. Health and physical assessment. 2nd ed. St Louis: Mosby; 1998.
11. Benko K. Acute dental emergencies in emergency medicine. Emerg Med Pract 2003;5(5):1–24.
12. Curtis L, Morrell T. Pain management in the emergency department. Emerg Med Pract 2006;8(7):1–26.
13. Skapetis T, Curtis K. Emergency management of dental trauma. Australas Emerg Nurs J 2010;13(1):30–4.
14. Lewis C, Lynch H, Johnston B. Dental complaints in emergency departments: a national perspective. Ann Emerg Med 2003;42(1):93–9.
15. Gibson DE, Verono AA. Dentistry in the emergency department. J Emerg Med 1987;5(1):35.
16. Skapetis T, Gerzina T, Hu W. Managing dental emergencies: a descriptive study of the effects of a multimodal educational intervention for primary care providers at six months. BMC Med Ed 2012;12:103.
17. Moore PA, Ziegler KM, Lipman RD, Aminoshariae A, Carrasco-Labra A, Mariotti A. Benefits and harms associated with analgesic medications used in the management of acute dental pain: an overview of systematic reviews. J Am Dent Assoc 2018;149(4):256–65.
18. Laskarides C. Update on analgesic medication for adult and pediatric dental patients. Dent Clin North Am 2016;60(2):347–66.
19. Neugebauer J, Jozsa M, Kübler A. Die antimikrobielle photodynamische Therapie zur Prävention der alveolären Ostitis und des Dolor post extractionem. Mund Kiefer Gesichtschir 2004;8(6):350–5.
20. Tarakji B, Saleh LA, Umair A, Azzeghaiby SN, Hanouneh S. Systemic review of dry socket: aetiology, treatment, and prevention. J Clin Diagn Res 2015;9(4):ZE10–13.
21. Fu B, McGowan K, Sun J, Batstone M. Increasing frequency and severity of odontogenic infection requiring hospital admission and surgical management. Br J Oral Maxillofac Surg 2020;58(4):409–15.
22. Skapetis T, Naim A. Dental infections management flowchart. In: Skapetis T. Emergency dental: handbook for medical practitioners. 2nd ed. Sydney, NSW Rural Doctors Network; 2010.
23. World Health Organization (WHO). Application of the International Classification of Diseases to Dentistry and Stomatology (ICD-DA). 3rd ed. Geneva: WHO; 1994.
24. Petti S, Glendor U, Andersson L. World traumatic dental injury prevalence and incidence, a meta-analysis. One billion living people have had traumatic dental injuries. Dent Traumatol 2018;34(2):71–86.
25. Skapetis T, Gerzina T, Hu W. Review article: management of dental emergencies by medical practitioners: Recommendations for Australian education and training. Emerg Med Australas 2011;23(2):142–52.
26. Samaei H, Weiland TJ, Dilley S. Knowledge and confidence of a convenience sample of Australasian emergency doctors in managing dental emergencies: results of a survey. Emerg Med Int 2015;2015:148384.
27. Yeng T, Parashos P. An investigation into dentists' perceptions of barriers to providing care of dental trauma to permanent maxillary incisors in children in Victoria, Australia. Aust Dent J 2007;52(3):210–15.
28. Skapetis T, Gerzina T, Hu W. Can a four-hour interactive workshop on the management of dental emergencies be effective in improving self reported levels of clinician proficiency? Australas Emerg Nurs J 2012;15(1):14–22.
29. Skapetis T, Gerzina TM, Hu W, Cameron WI. Effectiveness of a brief educational workshop intervention among primary care providers at 6 months: uptake of dental emergency supporting resources. Rural Remote Health 2013;13(2):2286.
30. Kenny KP, Day PF, Sharif MO, Parashos P, Lauridsen E, Feldens CA, et al. What are the important outcomes in traumatic dental injuries? An international approach to the development of a core outcome set. Dent Traumatol 2018;34(1):4–11.

31. Fouad AF, Abbott PV, Tsilingaridis G, Cohenca N, Lauridsen E, Bourguignon C, et al. International Association of Dental Traumatology guidelines for the management of traumatic dental injuries: 2. Avulsion of permanent teeth. Dent Traumatol 2020;36(4):331–42.
32. Stevens D. Case book: earache. Pract Nurs 2008;19(4):193–6.
33. Reynolds T. Ear, nose and throat problems in Accident and Emergency. Nurs Stand 2004;18(26):47–53.
34. ACI. Earache agency for clinical innovation 2021. [updated 23 June 2021]. Available from: aci.health.nsw.gov.au/networks/eci/clinical/ndec/ndec-nmg/earache-nmg.
35. Leach A, Morris P, Castano R. Antibiotics for acute otitis media in children. (Protocol) Cochrane Database Syst Rev 2006(4):CD004401.
36. Ranakusuma RW, Pitoyo Y, Safitri ED, Safitri ED, Thorning S, Beller EM, et al. Systemic corticosteroids for acute otitis media in children. Cochrane Database Syst Rev 2018;3(3):CD12289.
37. Therapeutic Guidelines. Antibiotic version 16. West Melbourne, Therapeutic Guidelines; 2021.
38. Qureishi A, Lee Y, Belfield K, Birchall JP, Daniel M. Update on otitis media – prevention and treatment. Infect Drug Resist 2014;7:15–24.
39. Melbourne TRCsH. Acute otitis media. The Royal Children's Hospital Melbourne; 2021. [updated June 2021]. Available from: www.rch.org.au/clinicalguide/guideline_index/Acute_otitis_media/.
40. Peate I. Caring for the person with otitis media. Br J Healthc Assist 2009;3(4):167–70.
41. Ferri F. Labyrinthitis. Ferri's clinical advisor. Sydney: Elsevier; 2014.
42. Yates P. Otitis media. In: Lalwani A, editor. Current diagnosis and treatment in otolaryngology—head and neck surgery. New York: McGraw-Hill; 2017.
43. Mackle T, Conlon B. Foreign bodies of the nose and ears in children. Should these be managed in the accident and emergency setting? Int J Pediat Otorhinolaryngol 2006;70(3):425–8.
44. Grigg S, Grigg C. Removal of ear, nose and throat foreign bodies: a review. Aust J Gen Pract 2018;47(10):682–5.
45. Afolabi O. Foreign body in the ear: a review of methods of management. Savann J Med Res Prac 2019;8(1):1–7.
46. Zahed R, Moharamzadeh P, Alizadeharasi S, Ghasemi A, Saeedi M. A new and rapid method for epistaxis treatment using injectable form of tranexamic acid topically: a randomized controlled trial. Am J Emerg Med 2013;31(9):1389–92.
47. Waters T, Peacock IW. Nasal emergencies and sinusitis. In: Tintinalli J, Kelen G, Stapczynski J, editors. Emergency medicine: a comprehensive study guide. 8th ed. New York: McGraw-Hill; 2017.
48. Bertrand B, Eloy P, Rombaux P, Lamarque C, Watelet JB, Collet S. Guidelines to the management of epistaxis. B-ENT 2005;(Suppl. 1):27–41.
49. Bernius M, Perlin D. Pediatric ear, nose, and throat emergencies. Pediat Clin N Am 2006;53(2):195–214.
50. Pfenninger J, Fowler G. Management of epistaxis. Pfenninger and Fowler's procedures for primary care. 3rd ed. Sydney: Elsevier; 2011.
51. Pfaff J, Moore G. Otolaryngology. In: Marx J, Hockberger R, Walls R, editors. Rosen's emergency medicine: concepts and clinical practice. 8th ed. Sydney: Elsevier; 2014.
52. King B, Charles R. Pharyngitis in the ED: diagnostic challenges and management dilemmas. Emerg Med Pract 2004;6(5):1–24.
53. Sanders M. Mosby's paramedics textbook. 4th ed. Toronto: Elsevier Canada; 2011.
54. Shnayder Y, Lee K, Bernstein J. Management of adenotonsillar disease. In: Lalwani A, editor. Current diagnosis and treatment in otolaryngology—head and neck surgery. 4th ed. New York: McGraw-Hill; 2020.
55. Shores C. Infections and disorders of the neck and upper airway. In: Tintinalli J, Kelen G, Stapczynski J, editors. Emergency medicine: a comprehensive study guide. 7th ed. New York: McGraw-Hill; 2017.
56. Reveiz L, Cardona AF. Antibiotics for acute laryngitis in adults. Cochrane Database Syst Rev 2015;(5):CD004783.
57. Stallard T. Emergency disorders of the ear, nose, sinuses, oropharynx and mouth. In: Stone K, Humphries R, editors. Current diagnosis and treatment: emergency medicine. 8th ed. New York: McGraw-Hill; 2017.
58. Care TACoSaQiH. Chapter 15 – Antimicrobial stewardship in the Aboriginal and Torres Strait Islander population. Antimicrobial stewardship in Australian health care. Sydney: Australian Commission on Safety and Quality Health Care; 2018.
59. Goddard G. Temporomandibular disorders. In: Lalwani A, editor. Current diagnosis and treatment in otolaryngology: head and neck surgery. 4th ed. New York: McGraw-Hill; 2020. p. 405–12.
60. Juniper R. The temporomandibular joint. In: Yates C, editor. A manual of oral and maxillofacial surgery for nurses. Oxford: Blackwell; 2008. p. 189–212.
61. Buckley MF, O'Connor K. Ludwig's angina in a 76-year-old man. Emerg Med J 2009;26(9):679.

CHAPTER 32
OCULAR EMERGENCIES AND TRAUMA

JOANNA McCULLOCH

ESSENTIALS

- Never think of the eye in isolation; always compare the two eyes in assessment.
- A visual acuity of 6/6 does not necessarily exclude a serious eye injury, as both retinal detachments with the macula on and penetrating eye injuries can maintain good vision for a short period.
- No pressure should be applied to the globe if rupture or a penetrating injury is suspected. Apply a clear plastic shield to prevent pressure on the eye and loss of ocular contents.
- Do not try to open a swollen eyelid if there is a history of trauma, unless under the guidance of an ophthalmologist or senior medical officer, as a globe rupture may be present and ocular contents lost when lids are forced open.
- Slit-lamp assessment is essential if removing a corneal foreign body from the central cornea. It will provide the clinician with both depth and extent of the object. A risk of penetrating the cornea or corneal scarring can occur if the object is deeply imbedded in the cornea. This will result in vision loss.
- Do not apply ointment to a patient with a suspected penetrating eye injury.
- Chemical burns should be irrigated as soon as possible with any neutral fluid available (i.e. tap water), then irrigation continued until assessed as the cornea being clear, and no signs of limbal ischaemia.
- Do not prescribe ocular steroids unless directed by an ophthalmologist.

INTRODUCTION

Ocular-related presentations are common to the emergency department (ED). Paramedics will also be responsible for providing care for patients with ocular injuries. A relatively trivial traumatic presentation may mask a more serious underlying injury. Similarly, a relatively transient episode of visual loss with no abnormality found on examination may indicate potentially life-threatening cerebrovascular disease. All eye injuries presenting to paramedics and the ED should be carefully evaluated with the necessary equipment and skill.[1] In relation to trauma, it must always be remembered that life-threatening injuries are managed first. The ability to identify conditions that represent a threat to the patient's vision is essential to protecting the patient's vision. Concern about an eye condition is one of the biggest drivers to attend ED.[2] The goals of managing eye injury are to prevent further injury to the intact vision, then to assess the extent of the injury and refer the patient to ophthalmology for early management and/or intervention. This chapter provides the epidemiology of ocular trauma in Australia and Aotearoa New Zealand, as well as

a description of anatomy, ocular assessment, common ocular emergencies encountered in the ED and their management.

The availability of eye services varies widely in Australia and Aotearoa New Zealand. In urban centres the practitioner has greater access to ophthalmic services. In regional Australia, the practitioner may need to rely more on their own findings and experiences.[3] The Australian rural population has an increased prevalence of pterygium, lid lesions and ocular trauma in comparison to urban dwellers, and these people are more likely to have seen an optometrist, but less likely to have seen an ophthalmologist.

ANATOMY AND PHYSIOLOGY

OUTER EYE

The orbit is made up of 7 bones; the orbital floor and the medial wall are the thinnest points of the orbit. The volume of the orbit is 30 millilitres, its height 40 mm, width 35 mm and depth 40–50 mm (the average length of the eye is 23 mm). Beware of the close anatomical positioning of the sinuses to the lacrimal and orbital areas. Injuries that cause blow out fractures of the orbit, or orbital surgery, can encroach into the sinuses, risking subcutaneous emphysema or infection (preseptal/orbital cellulitis). The orbital structure has several openings, two key fissures being the superior orbital fissure and inferior orbital fissures, and the posterior optic canal.[4] These fissures and canal allow for cranial nerve pathways. Orbital fat cushions the posterior and lateral side of the eye (providing support, protection and facilitation of oxygen and nutrients via the blood vessels).

The eyelids and eyelashes are vital to protect the globe; the action of lids closing stops foreign bodies from entering the eye and reduces the force of blunt trauma. Blinking helps lubrication of the anterior aspect of the eye (spreading tears) (Figs 32.1 and 32.2). The upper lid is the larger lid; it crosses over the globe to protect it. By blinking, the tear film spreads across the anterior surface of the globe to lubricate it.

Lid movement

The space between the eyelids is termed the palpebral aperture or fissure. The *Orbicular oculi* muscle forms the eyelid in conjunction with the tarsal plate. Its circular orientation functions like a sphincter. It is comprised of broad, flat skeletal muscles with its innervation being from the facial nerve (cranial nerve VII). The orbicular oculi muscle is important for facial expression. The function of this muscle is to close the eyelids, and protect the anterior surface of the eye from injury by supporting tear film maintenance. The muscle helps pump lacrimal tears through the lacrimal system (punctum, canaliculi into the lacrimal sac). It is subdivided into three:

1. *Orbital*—closes the eyelid firmly and is controlled by a voluntary response. When the orbital portion of the orbicular oculi contracts, the eyes close tightly and areas surrounding the lids, forehead, temple and cheek are involved in this contraction.
2. *Palpebral*—which closes the eye gently, involuntary in nature (blinking refreshes precorneal tear film). The palpebral is further subdivided into pretarsal, preseptal and ciliary.
3. *Lacrimal*—via lacrimal sac receives tears and allows for tears to drain into the nasolacrimal duct.[6]

The primary function of the levator palpebrae superioris is to maintain normal lid position by opening the eyelids. It acts primarily on the upper lid. It has some tenuous fibres that act to retract the lower eyelid. This muscle is composed of both skeletal and smooth muscle fibres. The levator extends from the attachments at the orbital apex to attachments at the tarsal plate and skin (forming a skin crease). The skin of the lid is thin and loosely connected to underlying tissues; as a result, inflammation and haemorrhage can cause significant swelling and oedema. Eyelid position depends on the resting tone of the levator, and can be affected by a person's sense of arousal.[4] The lids are securely attached at either end to the bony orbital margin by the medial and lateral palpebral (or canthal) ligaments. Trauma to the medial ligament causes the lid to flop forwards

FIGURE 32.1 EYELIDS AND EYEBALL IN SAGITTAL SECTION[5]

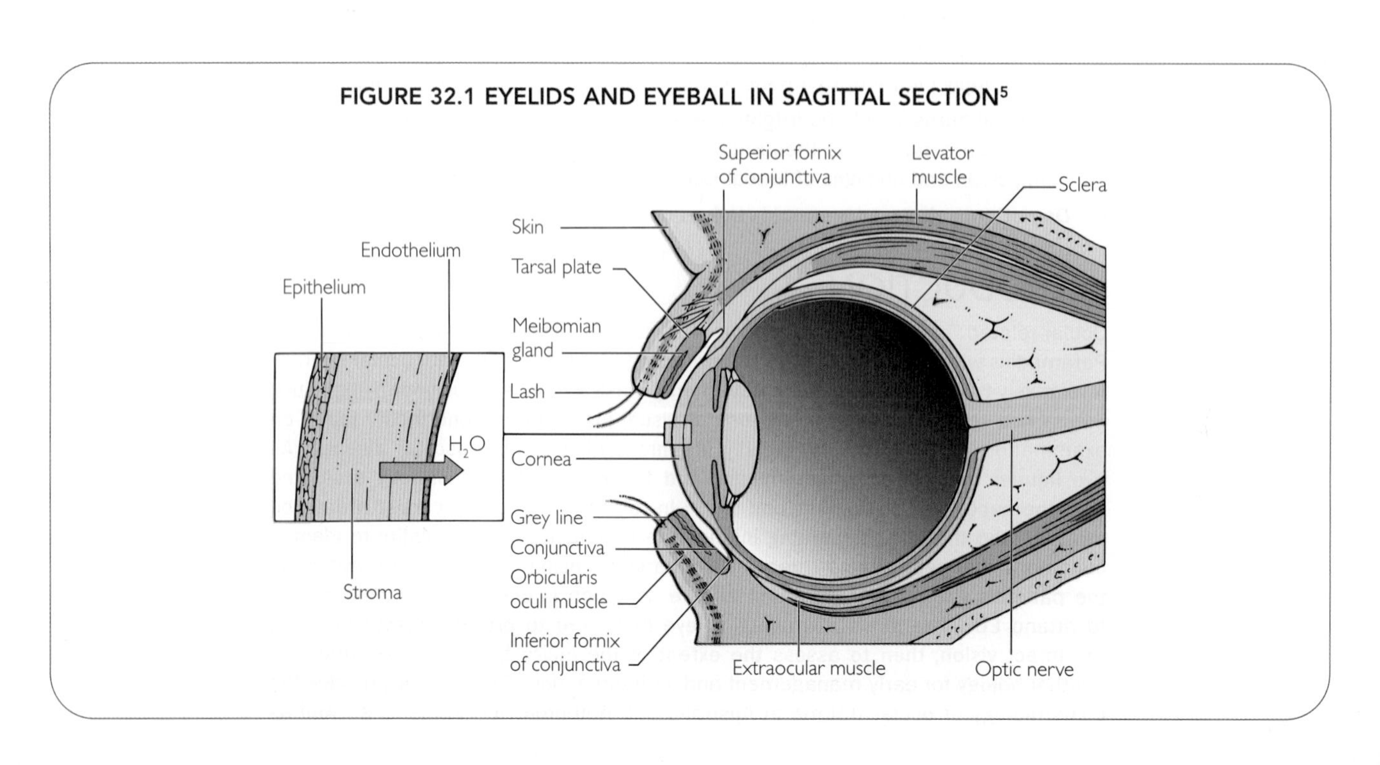

FIGURE 32.2 EYELID STRUCTURE ANTERIORLY (RIGHT EYE)[5]

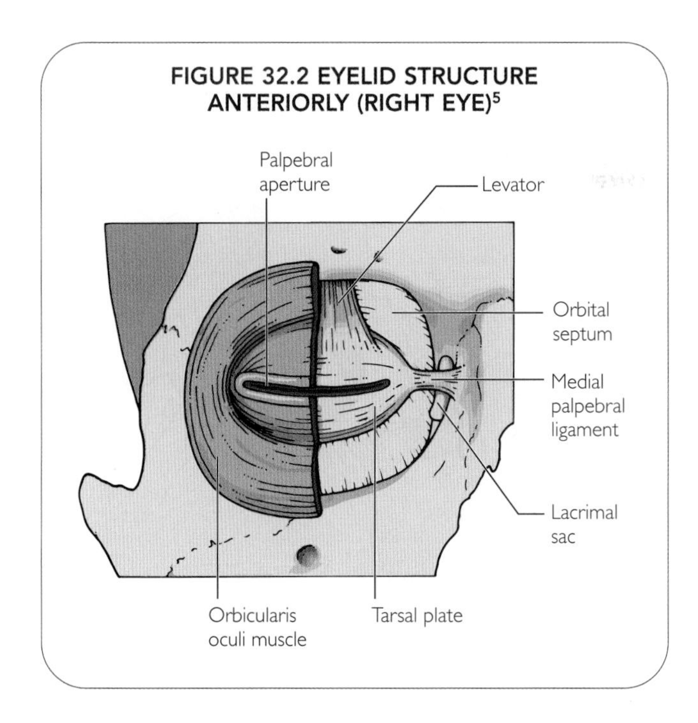

and laterally, impairing function and cosmesis. There is a brisk protective blink reflex: the afferent nerve is the optic (CNII), trigeminal (touch) (CNV) or auditory; the efferent nerve is the facial nerve (CNVII). The eyelashes are also protective.[5]

Skin and appendages

The semi-rigid tarsal plate lies behind the skin and orbicularis muscle and is lined posteriorly by conjunctiva. It contains the meibomian glands, which produce the oily lipid layer of tear film. There is a grey line (inter-marginal sulcus) as seen in Fig. 32.1, an important landmark in repairing lacerations of the lid margin, which is located between the eyelashes and the meibomian orifices.[5]

Innervation

Sensory innervation is from the trigeminal (fifth) cranial nerve, via the ophthalmic division (upper lid) and maxillary division (lower lid). The orbicularis oculi is innervated by the facial (seventh) nerve. Palsy causes an ectropion of the lower lid, but *not* ptosis. The levator muscle in the upper lid is supplied by the oculomotor (third) nerve. Palsy of the upper lid causes a ptosis. Note that all the nerves except the facial nerve reach the lids from the orbit.[5]

Blood supply and lymphatics

The eyelids are supplied by an extensive network of blood vessels, which form an anastomosis between branches derived from the external carotid artery via the face and from the internal carotid artery via the orbit. This accounts for excellent healing following trauma.

Lymphatic fluid drains into the preauricular and submandibular nodes. Preauricular lymphadenopathy is a useful sign of infective eyelid swelling (especially viral).[5]

Tear film

The tear film is the first defence against environmental harm to the surface of the eye. It also serves as the first refractive surface of the eye. Factors which influence the tear film include: blinking, eyelid position/functionality, lacrimal system, environment (temperature, humidity and airflow) and a person's emotions.

The globe

The eye, or globe, is described as almost spherical in shape and has two cavities with the crystalline lens dividing the two. Anterior to the lens is the anterior cavity (anterior segment) and posterior to the lens is the posterior cavity (posterior segment). The globe dimensions are on average 24 mm horizontally, 23 vertically and range from 22 to 25 mm in length (axial length). The total volume of the globe is 6.5 millilitres. The anterior segment comprises the cornea, anterior chamber, iris, posterior chamber and lens. The posterior segment involves the vitreous humour, retina, choroid and optic nerve/disc.[7]

The globe is just one part of the visual system; it must be remembered that it continues through the visual pathway to the visual cortex in the occipital lobe (lower, posterior part of cerebral cortex). The function of the occipital lobe is to process visual information from the eyes.[7]

Conjunctiva

The conjunctiva is a thin, transparent mucous membrane lining the eyelids and covering the anterior eyeball up to the edge of the cornea, where it ends at the limbus. The conjunctiva folds back onto itself forming two sacs, the superior and inferior fornices. These pockets are significant for presentations of foreign bodies and contact-lens loss. It is loosely connected to the globe, therefore inflammation can cause gross swelling of the fornices and bulbar conjunctiva. The conjunctiva comprises epithelium and an underlying stroma. Within the epithelium are goblet cells, which secrete the mucin component of the tear film.[5]

Cornea and sclera

The cornea and sclera form a spherical shell, which makes up the outer wall of the eyeball. Although the two are very similar in many ways, the corneal structure is uniquely modified to transmit and refract light.

The sclera is principally collagenous, avascular (apart from some vessels on its surface) and relatively acellular. It is tough despite being thin (the maximum thickness is 1 mm), and it gives attachment to the extraocular muscle, which at its thinnest point is 0.3 mm thick. It is perforated posteriorly by the optic nerve, and by the sensory and motor nerves and blood vessels to the eyeball. It has a protective function. The cornea and sclera merge at the corneal edge (the limbus).

The cornea is sensitive to touch (in contrast to the insensitive sclera) through nerve fibres from the ophthalmic division of the trigeminal nerve. The nerve endings lie under the epithelial layer. When the corneal epithelium is absent or abraded, this causes great pain.

The chief functions of the cornea are protection against invasion of microorganisms into the eye, and the transmission and focusing (refraction) of light. Refraction (bending of light rays) of light occurs because of the curved shape of the cornea and its greater refractive index compared with air. The cornea is transparent because of the specialised arrangement of the collagen fibrils within the stroma, which must be kept in a state of dehydration. This is achieved by an energy-dependent ion pump in the endothelium (direction of flow is from stroma to anterior chamber).

The cornea has five layers with the epithelium (surface layer) undergoing constant turnover with basal cells replicating, migrating to the surface and then being shed. The 'Bowman's layer', also known as the anterior limiting membrane, is not a membrane but a condensed layer of collagen; a tough layer that protects the corneal stroma. It does not regenerate when damaged. The stroma then makes up 90% of the corneal layer and is composed of parallel connective tissue. Descemet's membrane, or posterior limiting membrane, is a thin acellular layer that serves as the modified basement membrane of the corneal endothelium (the last layer). Descemet's membrane can regenerate when damaged. The endothelium is a simple squamous or low cuboidal monolayer of mitochondria-rich cells, responsible for regulating fluid and solute transport between the aqueous and the corneal stroma; in contrast to the epithelium, the cells of the endothelium do not divide. This is of great clinical significance, since there is sufficient pump activity to maintain corneal dehydration. In consequence, the cornea swells and loses its transparency; this is termed corneal decompensation or bullous keratopathy. Common causes of endothelial cell loss include normal ageing and intraocular surgery (including cataract surgery, retinal detachment surgery with either gas or oil).[5]

TEAR PRODUCTION AND DRAINAGE

Tears comprise water, mucus to bind the tear film to the corneal epithelium and an outer lipid layer to reduce evaporation of the water. Tears also contain some chemicals to protect against microorganisms.

The lacrimal gland secretes most of the aqueous component of the tear film. It lies in the supero-temporal part of the anterior orbit. Its anterior lobe can sometimes be seen in the upper conjunctival fornix; it is innervated by parasympathetic fibres carried by the facial nerve (Fig. 32.3).

Tears collect in a meniscus on the lower lid margin, are spread across the ocular surfaces by blinking, and drain into the superior and inferior puncta at the nasal end of the eyelids. Single canaliculi from the punctum unite in a common canaliculus, which ends in the lacrimal sac. This is in a bony fossa crossed anteriorly by the horizontally directed medial palpebral ligament. Finally, tears pass down the nasolacrimal duct and reach the nasopharyngeal cavity via the inferior meatus. This accounts for the unpleasant taste which follows administration of certain eye drops.

At birth, the nasolacrimal duct may not be fully developed, causing a watery eye. In most cases, full canalisation occurs within a year. Acquired obstruction of the nasolacrimal duct is a common cause of watery eye in adults. It may lead to an acute infection of the sac, which manifests as a cellulitic swelling just below the medial palpebral ligament.[5]

EXTRAOCULAR MUSCLES

There are six extraocular muscles which move the globe in all positions of gaze: four rectus and two oblique. The third cranial (oculomotor) nerve controls the superior, inferior and medial rectus, while the lateral rectus muscle is controlled by the abducent sixth cranial nerve and the superior oblique trochlear muscle is controlled by the fourth cranial nerve (Fig. 32.4).

FIGURE 32.3 EXTERNAL EYE AND LACRIMAL APPARATUS[8]

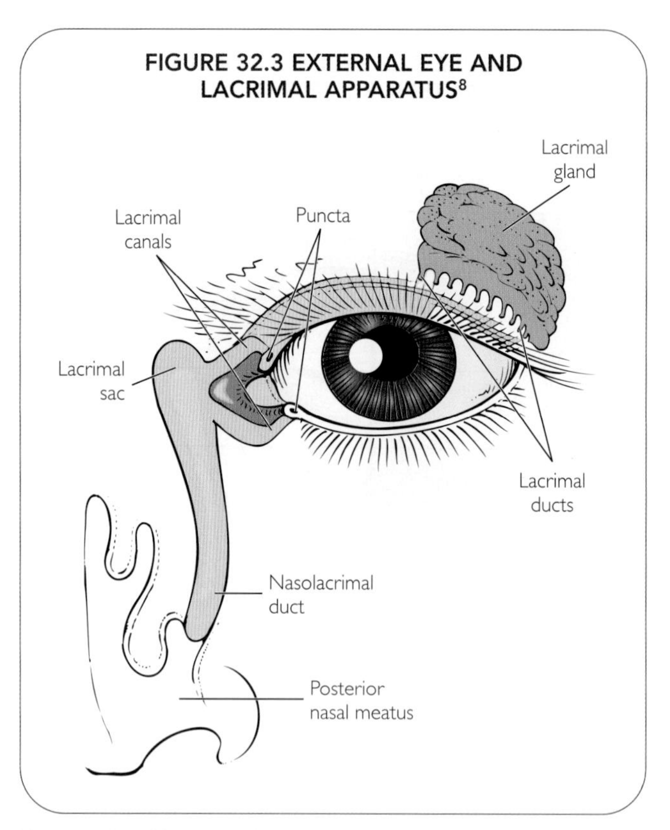

Tears produced in the lacrimal gland pass over the surface of the eye and enter the lacrimal canal. From there, the tears are carried through the nasolacrimal duct to the nasal cavity.

INNER EYE

The internal ocular structures function primarily to refine the image formed by the cornea, and to convert light energy into electrical energy for image formation by the brain. For light to reach the retina, it must pass through a number of structures: the cornea, aqueous humour, lens and vitreous humour (Fig. 32.5).

Uvea

The uvea comprises the iris and ciliary body anteriorly and choroid posteriorly.

Iris

The iris largely consists of connective tissue containing muscle fibres, blood vessels and pigment cells. A layer of pigment cells lines its posterior surface and at its centre is an aperture, the pupil. The chief functions of the iris are to control light entry to the retina and to reduce intraocular light scatter. Pupil dilation is caused by contraction of radial smooth muscle fibres innervated by the sympathetic nervous system (trigeminal nerve). Pupil constriction occurs when a ring of smooth muscle fibres (sphincter muscle) around the pupil contract. These are innervated by the parasympathetic nervous system (oculomotor nerve CN III).

Iris pigment (melanin) reduces intraocular light scatter. The amount of iris pigment determines eye 'colour': blue eyes have the least amount of pigment; brown eyes have the most. The amount of pigment can delay dilation and elongate the action of topical mydriatics.

FIGURE 32.4 EXTRINSIC MUSCLES OF THE EYE[9]

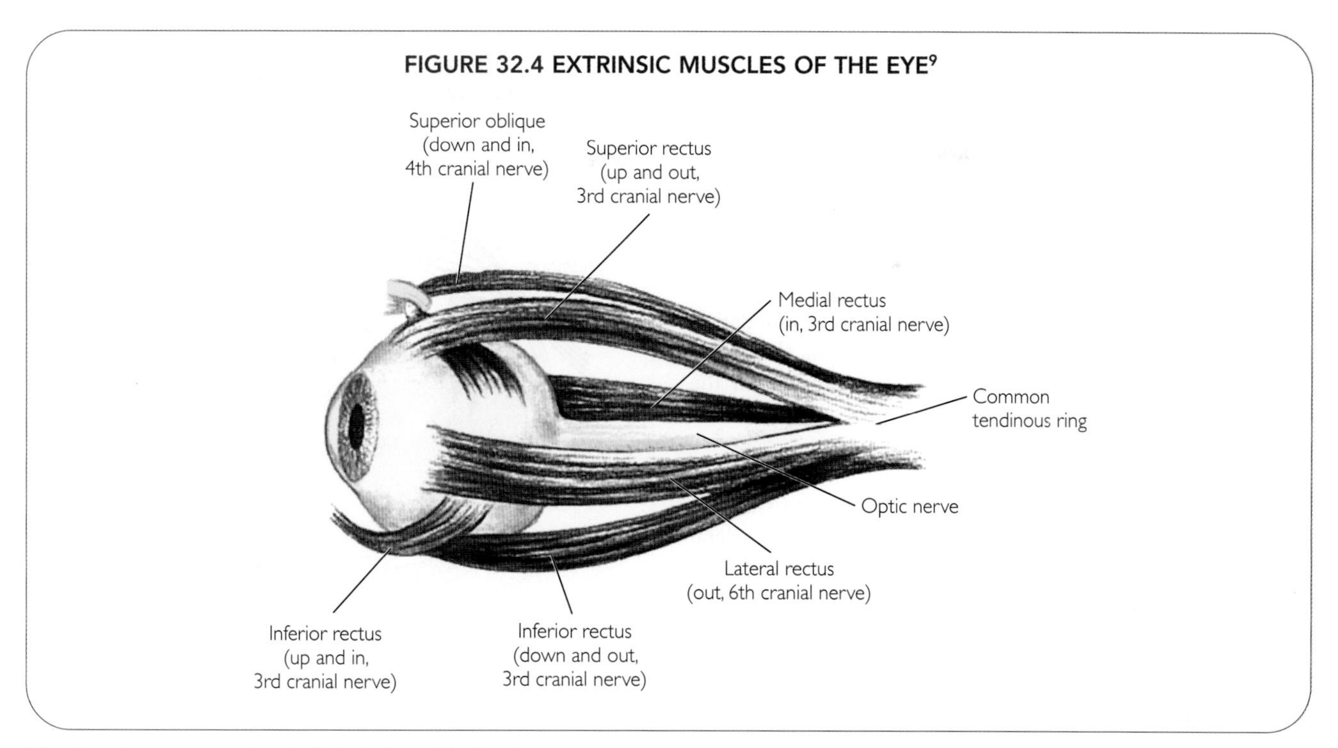

Direction of movement of eyeballs is indicated in brackets.

FIGURE 32.5 THE HUMAN EYE[8]

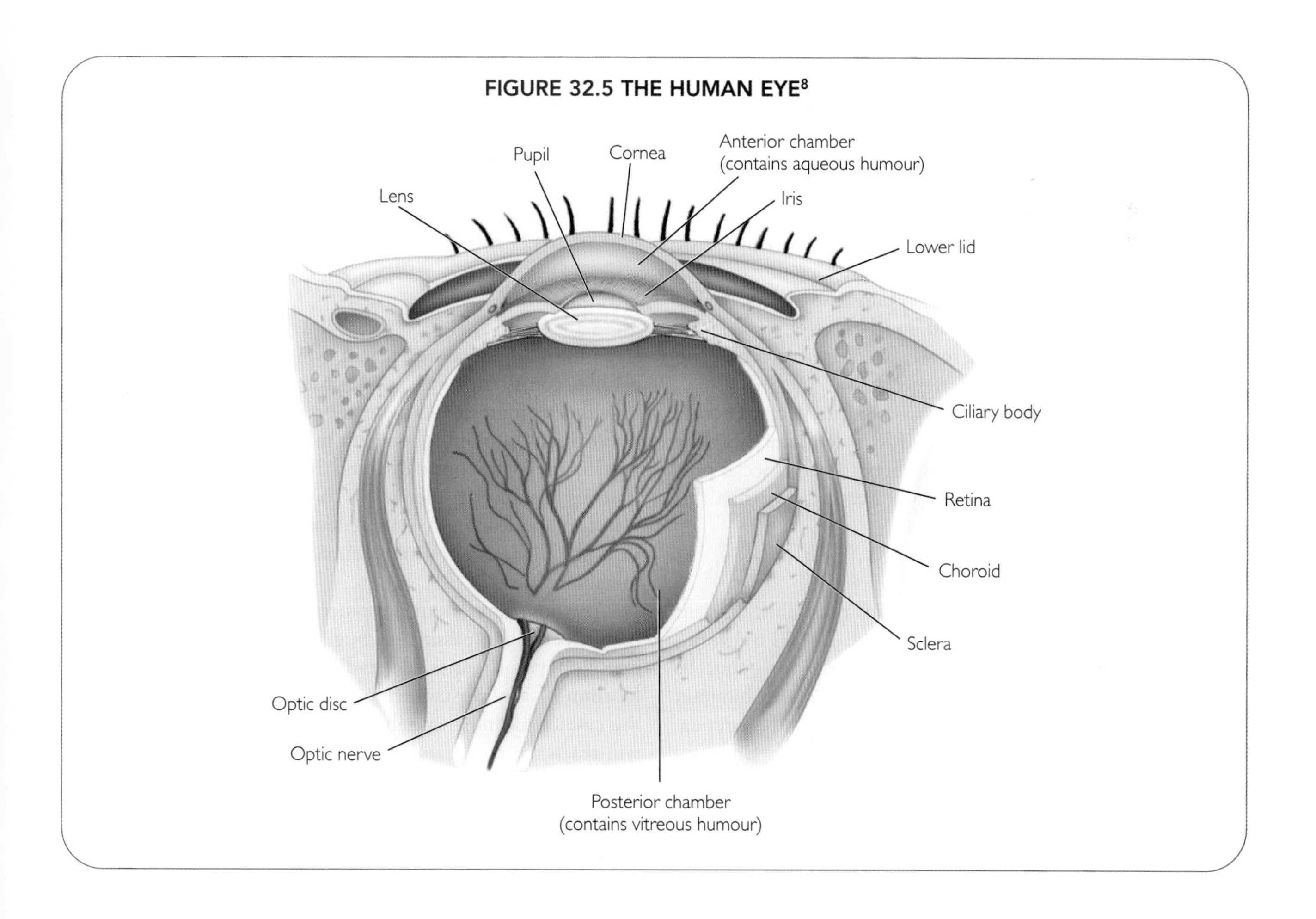

Ciliary body

The ciliary body is a specialised structure uniting the iris with the choroid. It makes aqueous humour and anchors the lens via zonules, through which it modulates lens convexity.

Anteriorly, the inner surface is folded into ciliary processes, which are the site of aqueous humour formation. Muscle fibres within the ciliary body contract, causing the inner circumference of the lens to reduce. This reduces the tension on the zonules, so that the natural elasticity of the lens causes it to become more convex to focus on near objects. This is called accommodation and is controlled by the parasympathetic system via the oculomotor nerve. Relaxation is passive, increasing tension on the zonules so that the lens is pulled flat for distance vision.[5]

Choroid

The choroid, consisting of blood vessels, connective tissue and pigment cells, is sandwiched between the retina and the sclera. It provides oxygen and nutrition to the outer retinal layers. There is a potential space between the choroid and the sclera, which can become filled with blood or serous fluid.[5]

The lens

The biconvex lens comprises a mass of long cells known as fibres. At the centre, these fibres are compacted into a hard nucleus surrounded by dense fibres, the cortex. The whole lens is enclosed within an elastic capsule and is deformable for accommodation. The ciliary muscle is a smooth muscle that alters the shape of the lens for near or far vision. It is controlled by the parasympathetic nerve signals transmitted to the eye through the third cranial nerve (oculomotor). Stimulation of the parasympathetic nerves contracts both sets of ciliary muscle fibres, which relaxes the lens ligaments, thus allowing the lens to become thicker and increase its refractive powers. With this increased refractive power, the eye can focus on objects that are nearer. Consequently, as a distant object moves towards the eye, the number of parasympathetic impulses impinging on the ciliary muscle must be progressively increased for the eye to keep the object constantly in focus. The sympathetic stimulation has an additional effect of relaxing the ciliary muscle, but this effect is so weak that it plays almost no role in the normal accommodation mechanism.[10]

Failure of accommodation with ageing (presbyopia) occurs through loss of capsule elasticity and lens deformability. The lens is relatively dehydrated and its fibres contain special proteins. This is why it is transparent. Cataract occurs when this organisation is disrupted.[8]

Intraocular fluid

The eye is filled with intraocular fluid, which maintains sufficient pressure in the eyeball to keep it distended. Fig. 32.6 demonstrates that this fluid can be divided into two portions—aqueous humour, which lies in front of the lens, and vitreous humour, which is between the posterior surface of the lens and the retina. The aqueous humour is a freely flowing fluid, whereas the vitreous humour, sometimes called the vitreous body, is a gelatinous mass held together by a fine fibrillar network composed primarily of greatly elongated proteoglycan molecules.[8]

Aqueous humour

The ciliary body forms aqueous humour by ultrafiltration and active secretion. Its composition is strictly regulated to exclude large proteins and cells, but it does contain glucose, oxygen and amino acids for the cornea and lens. Neural control is via the sympathetic autonomic nervous system (beta-receptors).[5]

FIGURE 32.6 FORMATION AND FLOW OF FLUIDS IN THE EYE[10]

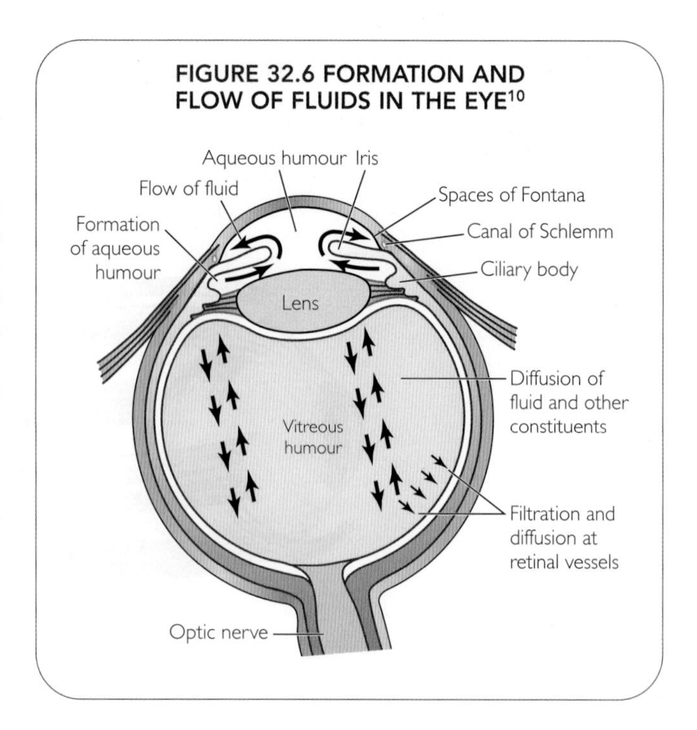

Aqueous humour circulates from the posterior to the anterior chamber through the pupil, leaving the eye through the trabecular meshwork, finally entering the canal of Schlemm, which empties into the intraocular veins.[8]

Aqueous production and drainage are balanced to maintain an appropriate intraocular pressure. Excess production or decreased outflow can elevate intraocular pressure above the normal 10–21 mmHg, a condition termed glaucoma.[11]

Vitreous body

The vitreous body is 99% water, but, vitally, also contains collagen fibrils and hyaluronic acid, which impart cohesion and a gel-like consistency. With increasing age, the vitreous body undergoes progressive degeneration and becomes more liquid. The vitreous humour is adherent to the retina at certain points, particularly at the optic disc and at the ora serrata. When the vitreous humour degenerates, it can pull on the retina, causing it to tear and leading to retinal detachment. The vitreous helps to cushion the eye during trauma and has a minor role as a metabolic sump.[5]

Any non-transparent substance within the vitreous humour may block light passing through the vitreous humour. The effect on vision varies, depending on the amount, type and location of the substance blocking the light. For example, in the case of haemorrhage into the vitreous humour, little light will reach the retina and vision will be severely compromised. However, cellular debris that accumulates from normal cell metabolism will cause only a relatively small shadow on the retina (a 'floater').[11]

Retina

The retina is the light-sensitive portion of the eye that contains the cones, which are responsible for colour vision, and the rods,

FIGURE 32.7 LAYERS OF THE RETINA[5]

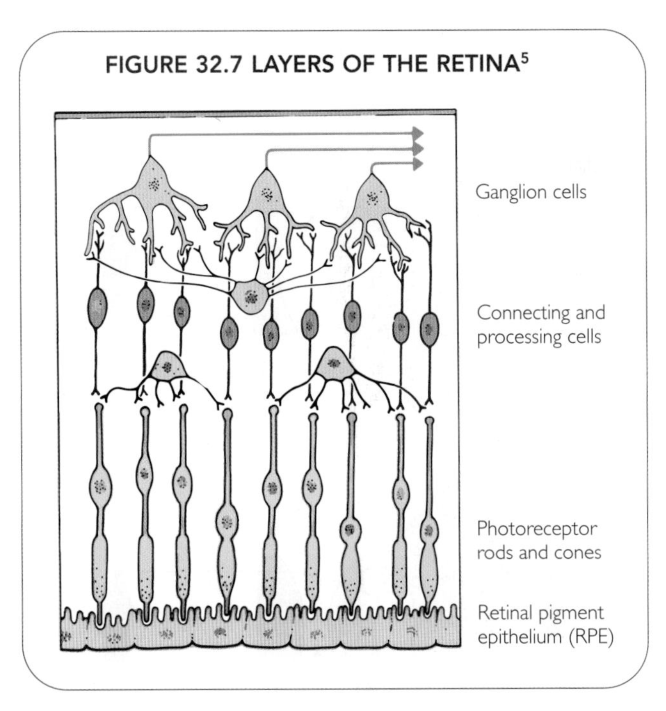

FIGURE 32.8 DIAGRAM OF THE RETINA (RIGHT EYE)[5]

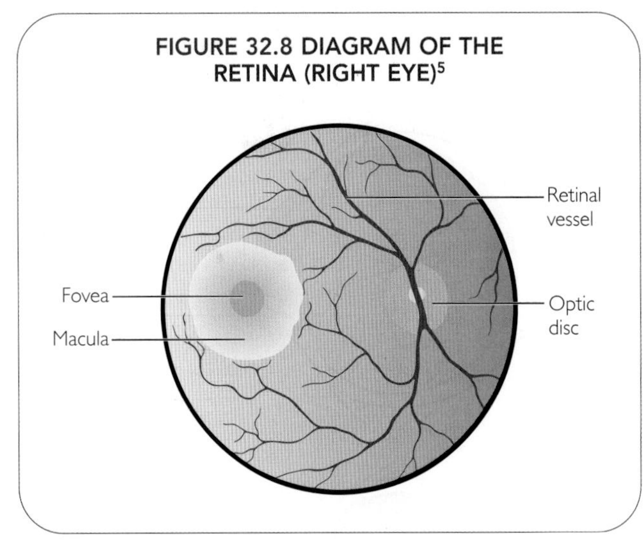

TABLE 32.1 PROPERTIES OF RODS AND CONES[5]

	RODS	CONES
Function	Vision in dim light, movement	Vision in bright light, colour, high resolution
Total number	> 100 million	6–7 million
Highest density	Peripheral retina	Fovea

which are mainly responsible for black-and-white vision (peripheral vision) and vision in the dark. When rods or cones are excited, signals are transmitted first through successive layers of neurons in the retina itself and finally into the optic nerve fibres and the cerebral cortex.[10]

The retina converts focused light images into nerve impulses (Fig. 32.7). It comprises the neurosensory retina and the retinal pigment epithelium (RPE). Light has to pass through the inner retina to reach photoreceptors, the rods and cones, which convert light energy into electrical energy (Table 32.1).[5] The inner retina is therefore transparent. Connector neurons modify and pass on the electrical signals to the ganglion cells. The axons run along the surface of the retina, then enter the optic nerve. An area called the macula provides for central vision. At its centre is a specialised area, the fovea, which is for high-quality vision. The rest of the retina is for peripheral vision (Fig. 32.8).

Cones concentrated at the macula are responsible for fine vision (acuity) and colour appreciation. Rods are for vision in low light levels and the detection of movement. They are distributed throughout the entire retina except the fovea. Photoreceptors contain visual pigments comprising retinol (vitamin A) linked to protein (opsin). Light absorption causes structural and then chemical change in visual pigments, which results in electrical hyperpolarisation of the photoreceptors.[5]

External to the neurosensory retina lies the RPE, a single layer of pigmented cells which is essential to the photoreceptor physiology. RPE cells recycle vitamin A for the formation of photopigments, transport water and metabolites, renew photoreceptors and help reduce damage by scattered light. Impairments of RPE function, which can occur with age and in many disease states, can lead to loss of retinal function and, therefore, sight.[5]

The principal blood supply of the retina is from the central retinal artery, a branch of the ophthalmic artery. The central retinal artery enters the retina at about the middle of the optic disc, an area where the optic nerve is attached and that contains no photoreceptor neurons (Fig. 32.8). After emerging through the disc, the central retina artery divides into superior and inferior branches, each of which subdivides into nasal and temporal branches. The central retinal vein drains blood from the retina through the optic disc.[12]

The blood–retinal barrier, consisting of tight junctions between the epithelial cells of the retinal vessels and between the RPE cells, isolates the retinal environment from the systemic circulation. Disruption of the barrier, as occurs in diabetic retinopathy, leads to retinal oedema and precipitation of lipid and protein, causing loss of retinal transparency and therefore loss of vision.[5]

Refraction errors

Refraction is the ability of the eye to bend light rays so that they fall on the retina. In the normal eye, parallel light rays are focused through the lens into a sharp image on the retina. This condition is termed emmetropia and means that light is focused exactly on the retina, not in front of it or behind it. When the light does not focus properly, it is called a *refractive error*.

- The individual with *myopia* can see near objects clearly (near-sightedness), but objects in the distance are blurred. A concave lens is used to correct the refraction (Fig. 32.9).
- The individual with *hyperopia* can see distant objects clearly (far-sightedness), but close objects are blurred. A convex lens is used to correct the refraction (Fig. 32.9).

FIGURE 32.9 REFRACTION DISORDERS[13]

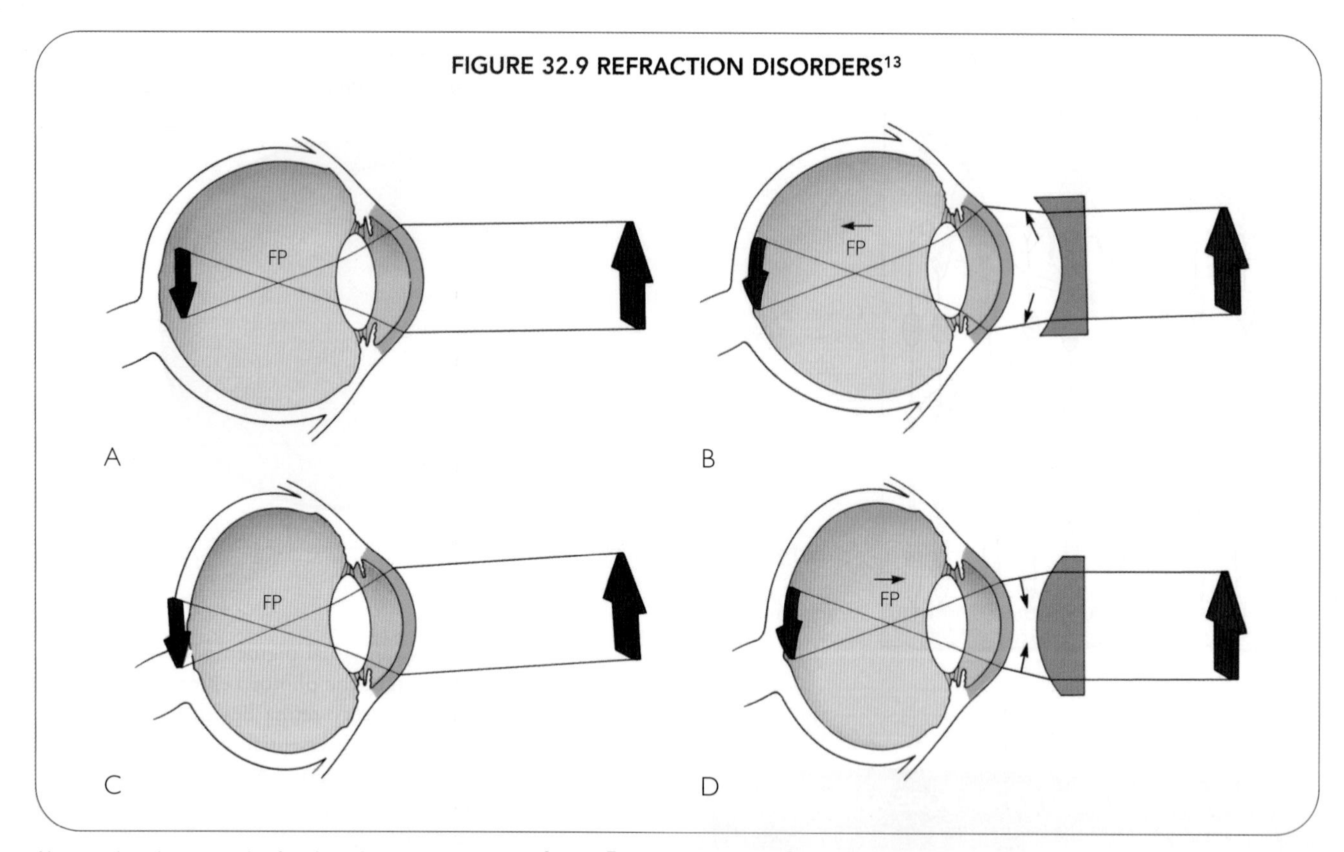

Abnormal and corrected refraction observed in myopia (**A** and **B**) and hyperopia (**C** and **D**). *FP: focal point.*

- *Presbyopia* is a form of hyperopia, or far-sightedness, that occurs as a normal process of ageing, usually around 40 years. As the lens ages and becomes less elastic, it loses refractive power and the eye can no longer accommodate for near vision.[11]
- *Astigmatism* is caused by unevenness in the corneal or lenticular curvature, causing horizontal and vertical rays to be focused at two different points on the retina, resulting in visual distortion. It can be myopic or hyperopic in nature in relation to where the image falls.

Optic nerve

The ganglion cell axons in the retinal nerve fibre layer make a right-angled turn into the optic disc, which has no photoreceptors and corresponds to the physiological blind spot. Most optic discs have a central cavity, the optic cup, which is pale in comparison with the redness of the surrounding nerve fibres. Loss of nerve fibres, as occurs in glaucoma, results in an increase in the volume of the cup.[5]

There are about 1,000,000 axons in the optic nerve. Behind the eyeball these axons become myelinated. Here the optic nerve is surrounded by cerebrospinal fluid in an anterior extension of the subarachnoid space and is protected by the same membranous layers as the brain.[5]

FIGURE 32.10 THE VISUAL PATHWAYS[8]

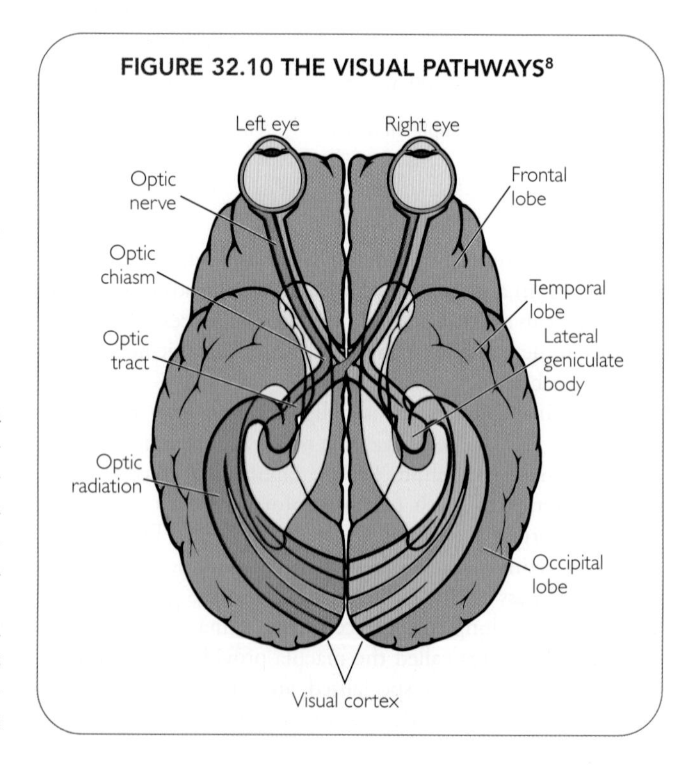

VISUAL PATHWAYS

Once the image travels through the refractive media, it is focused on the retina, inverted and reversed left to right (Fig. 32.10). From the retina, the impulses travel through the optic nerve to the optic chiasm where the nasal fibres of each eye cross over to the other side. Fibres from the left field of both eyes form the left optic tract and travel to the left occipital cortex. The fibres from the right field of both eyes form the right optic tract and travel to the right occipital cortex. This arrangement of the nerve fibres in the visual pathways allows determination of the anatomical location of abnormalities in those nerve fibres by interpretation of the specific visual field defect.[11]

PATIENT ASSESSMENT

The vast majority of ocular injuries are minor and involve the anterior segment only. It is important, however, to bear in mind the possibility of a more major trauma and not to rule it out without a comprehensive examination. If it is assumed that the eye injury is likely to be minor, sight-threatening injuries may easily be missed.[14] Visual outcomes depend on timely management and accurate assessment. The clinician needs to recognise and manage ocular trauma effectively. Chapter 16 contains information on some common eye emergencies and techniques on dealing with them.

The assessment of the patient with an ocular problem begins in the pre-hospital phase of care or at triage and continues into the treatment area. A potential threat to vision should be triaged as emergency, triage code 2 or 3 (Chapter 9), whereas a patient with a red eye and no potential loss of vision could be triaged as non-urgent if no other problems exist. The red eye is one of the most common complaints; differential diagnosis varies for a trivial complaint (conjunctivitis) to a patenting blinding (microbial keratitis).[15,16]

After assessment to ensure that the airway, breathing and circulation (ABCs) are stable, the patient is evaluated to identify any threats to vision, for example, globe penetrating, blunt trauma, vascular occlusion (sudden loss of vision), chemical burns and acute angle-closure glaucoma.

A focused assessment includes determination of precipitating events, duration of symptoms and identification of a worsening or improvement in signs and symptoms. Include information on the speed of onset of symptoms and when they were first noticed, and try to clarify some of the common symptoms; for example, discriminate between soreness, irritation and stinging versus pain, itching, burning or the sensation of something in the eye, and the degree and type of any reduction in vision. Was the vision loss gradual or sudden? partial or total? unilateral or bilateral? Have there been any recent changes to their medications (additions/ceased, especially those used in neurology, that can have retinal or visual field changes)?[17]

While assessing the patient, ensure a systematic approach is used to examine the eye, working from the outside of the eye (lids/orbit) inwards towards the anterior chamber (between the corneal and the iris). Commence with lids, conjunctiva/sclera and cornea; then the anterior chamber should be examined for the presence of blood (hyphaema) or pus (hypopyon), and the pupil size, shape, position and reaction to light should be checked (assess for a consensual response as well as direct pupil response). The iris should not look torn, and there should be depth evident between the cornea and the iris (A/C deep). Also check for any photophobia (sensitivity to light) and amount and type of discharge. Ask the patient if there has been any previous history of eye problems, or history and use of eye medication (prescribed or non-prescribed), if they have used corrective lenses, had past ocular surgery (including refractive) and have any diseases, such as diabetes. Document the assessment findings as per service or hospital policy. See Box 32.1.

The sudden presence of flashes (and explosion of floaters, web/veil-like substances in the field of vision) suggests a retinal tear or detachment.

If the patient has a history of trauma, determine when the injury occurred and the mechanism, velocity and timing of injury. Ask whether the patient was wearing protective eyewear, glasses or contact lenses at the time of the injury. Determine the patient's tetanus status. If the injury was a motor vehicle collision, did the airbag deploy? The force of airbag deployment can cause floaters or symptoms of blunt trauma, and the dust alkaline particles generated by the airbag contents can cause significant eye irritation and chemical burn.

OPHTHALMIC EXAMINATION

The primary elements of the ocular examination are visual acuity, external features, anterior segment and extraocular motility (Box 32.1). Fundamentally there are five vital signs or assessments for an effective eye examination: visual acuity, intraocular pressure (IOP), extraocular motility (EOM), pupil reactions and confrontational visual fields. Further examination includes a slit-lamp examination (viewing both the anterior and posterior segment of the eye with a 78- or 90-diopter lens) and direct ophthalmoscopy (posterior segment of the eye).

VISUAL ACUITY

Visual acuity should be tested on every patient presenting with a visual problem. A basic vision assessment should be undertaken by paramedics prior to transport to the hospital. It can be a simple test, such as holding up fingers to each eye separately. Avoid using the palm of the hand to cover the eye. Cup the hand, as the palm may press down on the globe causing pressure. Then ask the patient to identify the number of fingers seen. This will give valuable information around an intact visual system.[18] Assessment of visual acuity is the first priority and should be undertaken at triage; if possible, before any other investigation or treatment (except eye irrigation) is carried out. It is difficult to allocate an accurate triage category to a patient with an ocular problem without assessment of visual acuity.[14] Visual acuity results should be interpreted in context; optic nerve disease can affect colour vision before any changes in visual acuity. If visual acuity is not possible at triage, eye examination and history will

BOX 32.1 NORMAL PHYSICAL ASSESSMENT OF THE VISUAL SYSTEM[8]

- **Visual acuity 6/6 OU; no diplopia. Note a V/A of 6/6 does not exclude major ocular disruption**
- **External eye structures symmetrical without lesions or deformities**
- **Lacrimal apparatus non-tender without drainage**
- **Conjunctiva clear; sclera white**
- **Cornea clear**
- **Pupils equal, round, reactive to light and accommodation (PERRLA)**
- **Lens clear**
- **Vitreous clear**
- **Extraocular movements intact (EOMI)**
- **Disc margins sharp—no signs of cupping or swelling**
- **Retinal vessels normal with no haemorrhages or spots**

V/A: visual acuity.

indicate clinical urgency. Visual acuity is to be done at the earliest possible time.[19]

It is essential to understand the principles behind vision testing and be able to perform an accurate visual acuity test. Visual acuity is a measurement of central distance vision only: it assesses the pathway from cornea through to occipital cortex. Vision can be tested for both near (less than 30 cm) and distance (6 metres equivalent), but distance is the most common test.[10,20]

Normal distance vision (average vision) is normally defined as 6/6; it relies on the basis that both eyes are aligned (extra-ocular muscles functioning), cornea, lens, aqueous and vitreous humour are clear, the retina and other elements of the visual pathway are intact. The reasoning behind visual acuity is that it is one of the diagnostic tools that provides baseline data (similar to any baseline observations) and evaluates treatment while measuring the progress of any disease/condition. There may be legal implications after Workcover injuries, where a baseline vision is required.

There are numerous vision-testing tools. The Snellen chart is commonly used, and is designed to be read either at 6 or 3 metres (this is indicated on the chart). Vision charts are standardised for size and contrast and consequently are not to be photocopied or modified in any way (Fig. 32.11).

Visual acuity is a measure of best-corrected distance vision. Patients should be tested with either their distance glasses on or while wearing contact lenses. If the cause of their presentation is the contact lens, and they have removed the lens, test vision without correction and record accordingly. It is important to check that the glasses they are wearing were prescribed for that person, noting how old the script is, as well as whether the glasses are clean and scratch-free. Each eye needs to be tested separately; use an occluder or cupped hand to cover the eye that is not being tested. Avoid any pressure on the globe, especially if there is eye trauma. Ask the patient to read the chart until they cannot see the line clearly and make multiple mistakes. Encourage the patient to blink, as the eye will dry and vision will blur as it dries. If the patient does not reach the 6/6 line, use a pinhole to see if it improves vision. A pinhole can be created by putting a hole in a small square of cardboard or paper using a 19 g needle; the pinhole needs to be around 1.5 mm in size. If the pinhole improves vision, vision loss can be attributed in some part to a refractive error. This optical pinhole can correct up to 3 dioptres of astigmatism, myopia (short-sightedness) and hypermetropia (long-sightedness).[19]

Visual acuity is expressed as a ratio *x*/*y*; *x* is the testing distance in metres and *y* refers to the line containing the smallest letter the patient identifies. Record visual acuity for each eye and include vision of pinhole, if used (Fig. 32.12). Examples of recording of visual acuity are:

RVA (RIGHT VISUAL ACUITY)	LVA (LEFT VISUAL ACUITY)
6/9	6/6 with glasses
6/6 with pinhole	

- If the patient cannot see the top line of the Snellen/vision chart at 6 metres, walk them forward to 3 metres—record 6/60 at 3 metres.
- Ensure adequate lighting in the room when testing vision.

FIGURE 32.11 SNELLEN TEST TYPES SHOWN AT REDUCED SIZE

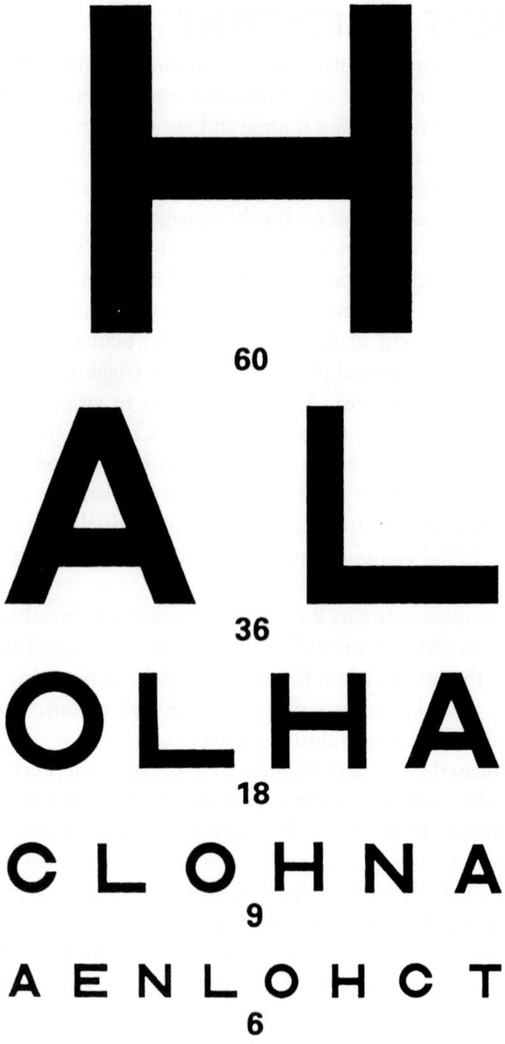

H
60
A L
36
O L H A
18
C L O H N A
9
A E N L O H C T
6

- If they are still unable to read the chart at 3 metres, hold your hand 1 metre away and ask the patient to count how many fingers, keeping your fingers still—record CF (count fingers) at 1 metre.
- If they cannot see fingers, move your hand slowly across the eye—record HM (hand movements) at 1 metre.
- If the patient cannot recognise hand movements, use a pen light to see if they have light perception (LP); record as NPL (no perception of light) if they are unable to see the torch going on and off.

PRACTICE TIP

VISUAL ACUITY

- Test each eye separately, using an occluder or cupped hand.
- Use distance correction if normally worn.
- Use a pinhole if the patient does not reach the 6/6 line.

FIGURE 32.12 VISUAL ACUITY MEASUREMENT[5]

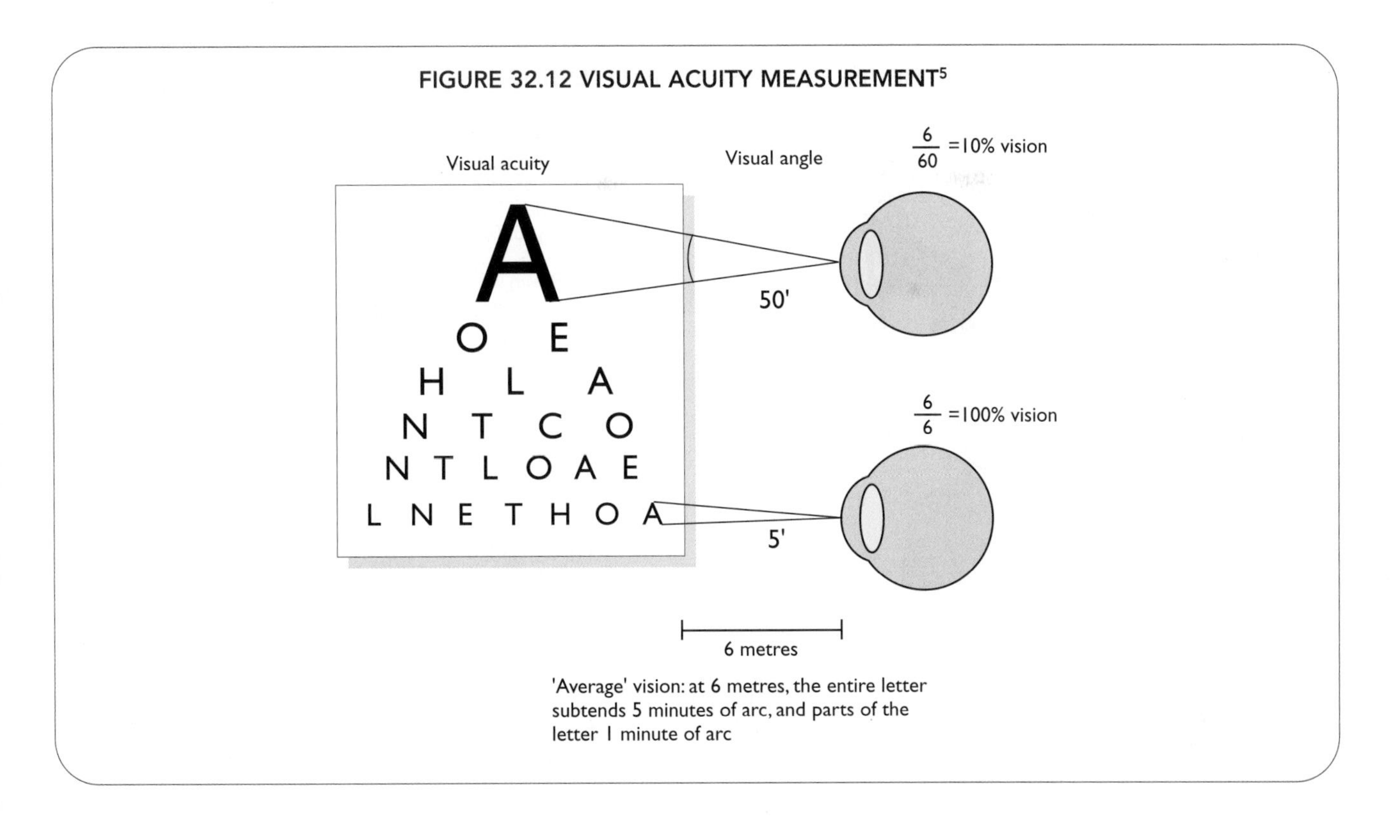

VISUAL FIELD

Using a simple confrontational technique easily identifies large, dense defects of the visual field. This test is quite straightforward. It is useful in detecting large visual field defects.[19] It should be noted that this is a quick gross visual field test; the test assumes that the clinician's visual field is normal, and the patient's visual field is checked against the clinician's.

Patients should not wear glasses when having their visual field assessed. The clinician should be at the same level and 1 metre away from the patient, who covers one eye. Use a pen, or 1–3 fingers, to test the four quadrants of the visual field. Do not bring the pen/fingers in at a vertical or horizontal position, as this will not be testing the visual field quadrants. Get the patient to look at a fixed point, such as the clinician's own eye, then slowly bring the pen in and ask the patient to say when they can see the pen tip. Repeat the test with the other eye. Document the findings.

EXTRAOCULAR MOTILITY (EOM)

When examining ocular movement, the first step is to look for asymmetry of the corneal light reflex with a pen torch, followed by observation of the movement of the eyes as they move onto the key nine positions of gaze (Fig. 32.13). Impaired ocular motility may occur with an entrapped muscle secondary to a blow-out fracture, muscular injury, orbital cellulitis or underlying central nervous system problem (CN III, IV, VI palsy).[1]

If the patient is complaining of pain on eye movement and diplopia (double vision), the full range of eye movements needs to be assessed. Have the patient look in the nine positions of gaze (Fig. 32.14): primary position (straight ahead), up, down, towards the nose (medial), towards the ear (lateral), up and then down towards the nose, and up and then down towards ear.[22] Ensure that the patient's eyes move freely with no pain. If the patient has mild pain when testing EOM, it is most unlikely to be optic nerve pain.[23] If the patient has restrictive eye movement due to cranial nerve palsy/trauma or muscle restriction, symptoms such as diplopia (seeing double) need to be assessed. Assessment includes whether it is binocular diplopia or monocular. Monocular is usually a form of refractive error in one eye. Typically, binocular diplopia will resolve when the patient closes one eye, whereas monocular will have no change.

EYE EXAMINATION

A pen torch provides adequate illumination for a systemic approach to eye examination starting with the eyelids, conjunctiva, cornea, pupil or iris for presence of any abnormality, including foreign body, discharge, loss of corneal clarity or corneal ulceration. Using the eyes to compare to each other provides additional information.

Fluorescein drops are a useful diagnostic aid. Fluorescein mixes into the tear film and adheres to areas of epithelial loss (ulcer or abrasion). It is best visualised using a blue light. It should be remembered that fluorescein can stain mucus, contact lenses, artificial eyes, cause allergic reactions and infection if poor technique is used. Too much dye may mask results (a wound leak—Seidel test).

PUPIL ASSESSMENT

Clinicians can only focus on size; older patients (≥ 73 years) typically have smaller pupils, and blue-eyed patients are prone to dilate (or it is more noticeable) in darker areas. Approximately 20% of patients have anisocoria (unequal pupil size), but pupil response should be as normal.[14] The most important aspects are differences between the sizes of the two pupils (direct response) and consensual responses (relative afferent

FIGURE 32.13 VISUAL FIELD TESTING[5]

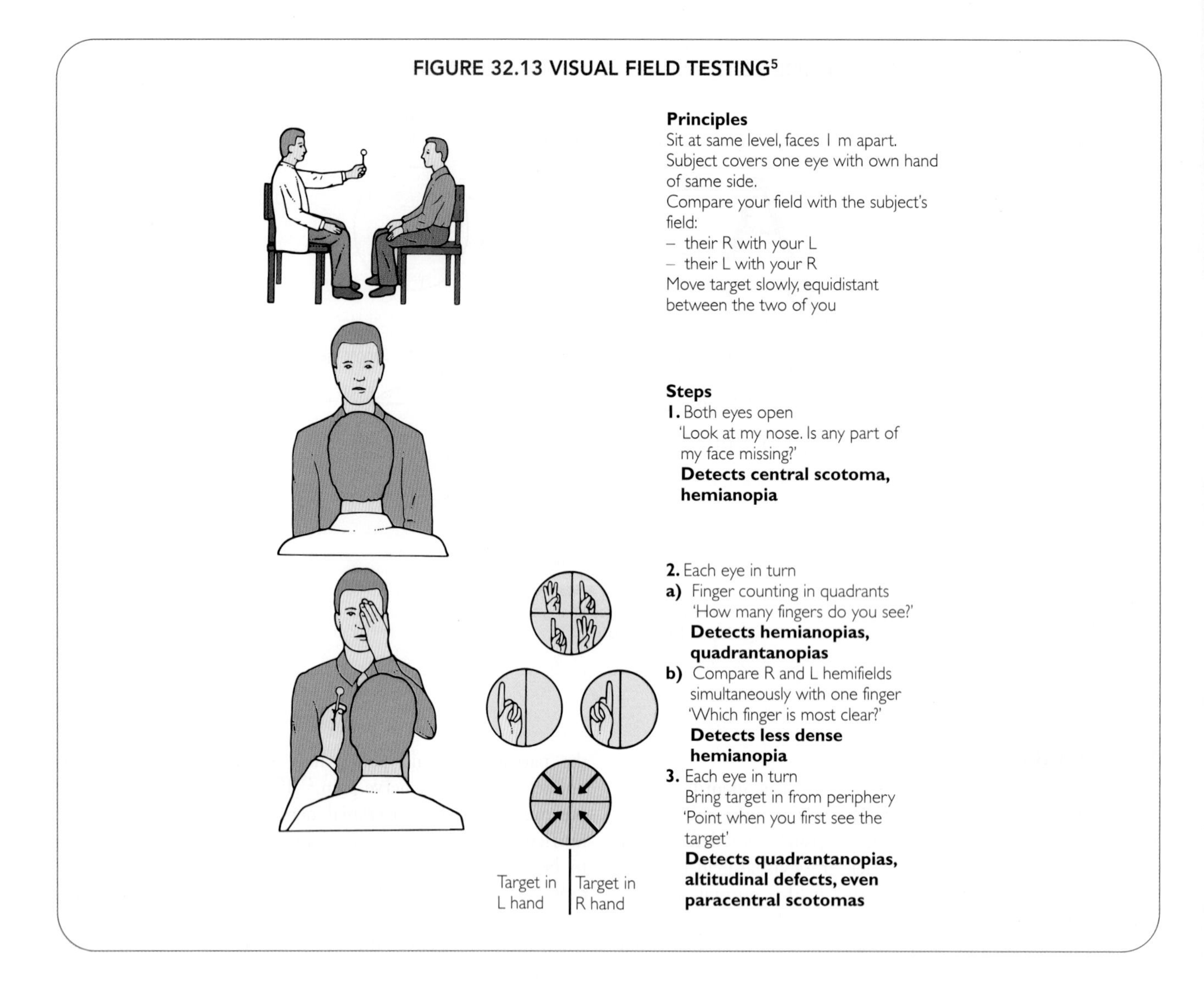
Principles
Sit at same level, faces 1 m apart.
Subject covers one eye with own hand of same side.
Compare your field with the subject's field:
– their R with your L
– their L with your R
Move target slowly, equidistant between the two of you
Steps
1. Both eyes open
'Look at my nose. Is any part of my face missing?'
Detects central scotoma, hemianopia
2. Each eye in turn
a) Finger counting in quadrants
'How many fingers do you see?'
Detects hemianopias, quadrantanopias
b) Compare R and L hemifields simultaneously with one finger
'Which finger is most clear?'
Detects less dense hemianopia
3. Each eye in turn
Bring target in from periphery
'Point when you first see the target'
Detects quadrantanopias, altitudinal defects, even paracentral scotomas
Target in L hand
Target in R hand

pupillary defect (RAPD). There are mild differences between pupils (anisocoria) in around 5% of the population. The pupils should respond in the correct manner to light. Use an ophthalmoscope or bright torch to test the reaction of the pupils to light and the red reflex. Checking should be carried out in a dim room, with the patient looking into the distance. The near response (looking at objects closely) makes the pupils constrict. Shine the light in one eye (for at least 3 seconds), then swing the light quickly to the other eye. If the response is for the pupil to dilate, then it is a positive relative pupillary afferent defect; the visual pathway is damaged at some point prior to midsection and there is less light being perceived by the visual cortex. There is a condition called hippus, where the pupil has spasms, making the pupil decrease and enlarge quickly. To tell the difference between RAPD and hippus, in RAPD the pupil will dilate immediately with the light, while with hippus, the pupil will constrict first then dilate. Visual acuity and RAPD do not necessarily correlate. Patients can have a RAPD and normal visual acuity (central distance vision). Often, extensive loss of peripheral vision correlates to RAPD (glaucoma).[19,23]

In an unresponsive patient, it should be recorded if the eyes are open or closed, and whether there is any resistance to opening an eyelid.

INNER EYE (FUNDUS)

Next examine the fundus (retina and optic disc) using an ophthalmoscope or a slit lamp with a 78- or 90-dioptre lens. For easier viewing, use mydriatic eye drops to dilate the pupil, so that the fundus can be viewed effectively. At the initial assessment and before instilling dilating topical medications, the pupil should be assessed for RAPD, as described above under Pupil assessment.[15]

SPECIAL INVESTIGATIONS

The slit lamp

The slit lamp provides a highly magnified and stereoscopic view. This provides high-quality assessment, especially when assessing depth and extent of penetrating eye injury or corneal foreign body. The pen torch can assess the extent of an injury, but not the depth—this is better calculated using a slit lamp.

FIGURE 32.14 NINE POSITIONS OF GAZE[21]

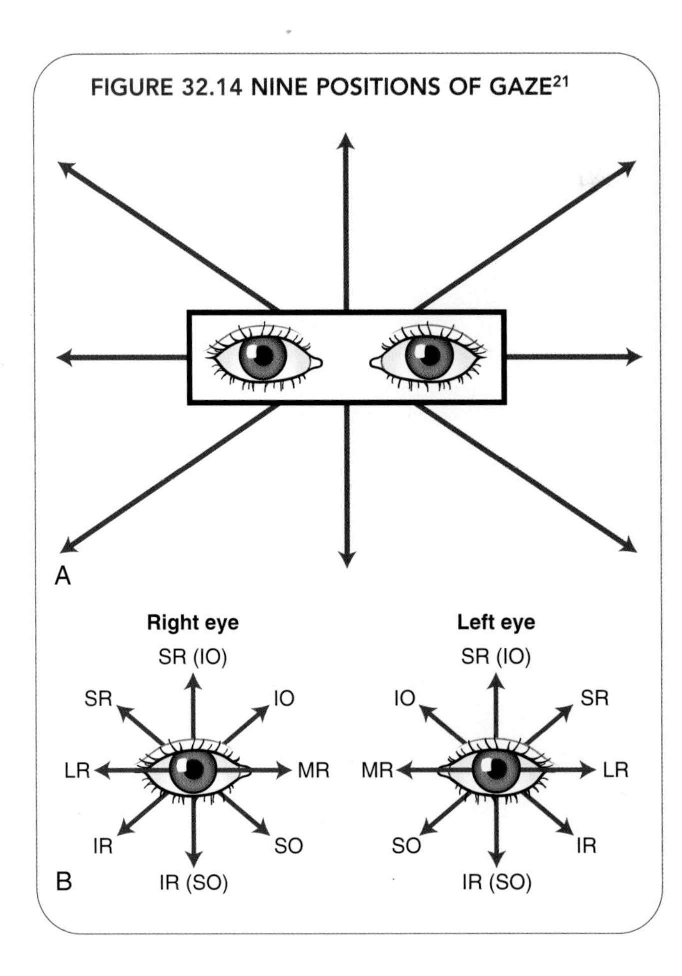

The basic apparatus enables only the anterior part of the eye, as far back as the lens, to be focused. A variety of supplemented lenses, both contact and non-contact, can be used to examine the inner eye (Fig. 32.15).

Intraocular pressure measurement (IOP)

Tonometry measures the intraocular pressure (IOP); normal pressures usually range from 10 to 21 mmHg. This can be performed with a device attached to the slit lamp (Goldman applanation tonometry) or by using a handheld electronic gauge (Tonopen). Both require contact with the cornea; topical anaesthetic is required to perform this measurement. There are now newer devices available that measure the IOP and require no topical anaesthetic drops; for example, ICare™ Tonometer. Eye pressures can be high (acute angle glaucoma) or low (ruptured globe) in many conditions. If using a device such as an IOP Tono Pen or ICare, ask the patient to avoid squeezing their eyelids as this will increase the pressure of their eyes. If there is high pressure in both eyes it may mean an incorrect technique is being used to test them. A simple way to check pressures is to palpate through closed eyelids. If there is high pressure the eye will feel hard, like a rock. Use the other eye as the control.[19]

PRACTICE TIP

If no device is available, ask the patient to close both eyes, and digitally touch both lids at the same time. If the intraocular pressure is very high (> 30), the eye will feel really hard, like a rock/stone and urgent review by an ophthalmologist is required.

EYE EMERGENCIES

Injury or disease may cause ocular emergencies. Situations encountered most often by the emergency clinician are discussed in this section (see also Chapter 16).

There are four basic principles for both the nurse and the paramedic to consider in the management of ocular trauma and other presenting ocular conditions: prevention of further injury, control of pain, control of nausea/vomiting and prevention of infection.

RED EYE

A unilateral red eye has a high suspicion rate, as there is a higher incidence of a more severe ocular condition (acute glaucoma, scleritis and penetrating (open) eye injury).

The ocular coat and tear film normally provide an excellent barrier to invasion of bacteria; however, if the conjunctiva or cornea is in some way compromised, bacteria may enter directly through these structures, causing a red appearance to the sclera/conjunctival area eye. In severe corneal infection, the cornea will appear cloudy or opaque, obscuring the view into the anterior chamber (A/C).[5]

PRACTICE TIP

When a patient presents with a red eye and complains of severe ocular pain not relieved by medication (i.e. paracetamol/NSAID), this is a red flag that increases triage weighting and urgency for review.

Subconjunctival haemorrhage

Subconjunctival haemorrhage (SCH) is often an isolated symptom, unilateral, and caused by minor trauma such as a sneeze, anticoagulant therapy, cough or the Valsalva manoeuvre; however, it can be an indicator of a more serious intraocular and orbital trauma.[16,18,26] Bungee jumping can cause a subconjunctival haemorrhage, but also can cause retinal detachments. The haemorrhage occurs when small blood vessels rupture and bleed, and it is painless (Fig. 32.16). Check the pain level; there should only be a dull ache and visual acuity. If it is reduced, suspect trauma. The typical presentation for trauma is that the haemorrhage spreads backwards, shows depth and has no clear borders. Blood pressure should also be assessed as a hypertensive patient can have spontaneous rupture of vessels.

Subconjunctival haemorrhage will spontaneously resolve within 2–4 weeks and the patient's visual acuity generally remains normal. Should healing be delayed, it is wise to check the patient's coagulation profile. There is rarely need for treatment.

PRACTICE TIP

The patient's history is important, assessing if the patient is hypertensive, on anticoagulants or has experienced recent eye trauma. Management by the general practitioner may be the more appropriate treatment option if the patient is hypertensive or a review of anticoagulant therapy is required.

FIGURE 32.15 THE SLIT LAMP[24]

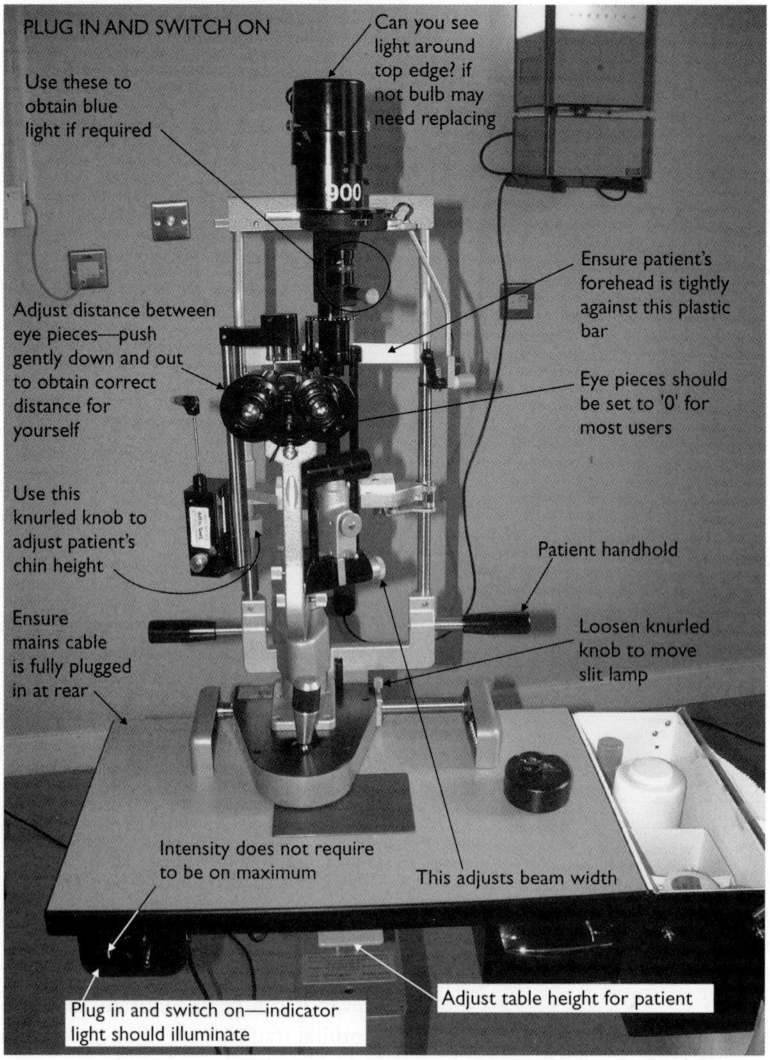

PLUG IN AND SWITCH ON

Can you see light around top edge? if not bulb may need replacing

Use these to obtain blue light if required

Ensure patient's forehead is tightly against this plastic bar

Adjust distance between eye pieces—push gently down and out to obtain correct distance for yourself

Eye pieces should be set to '0' for most users

Use this knurled knob to adjust patient's chin height

Patient handhold

Ensure mains cable is fully plugged in at rear

Loosen knurled knob to move slit lamp

Intensity does not require to be on maximum

This adjusts beam width

Adjust table height for patient

Plug in and switch on—indicator light should illuminate

FIGURE 32.16 SUBCONJUNCTIVAL HAEMORRHAGE[27]

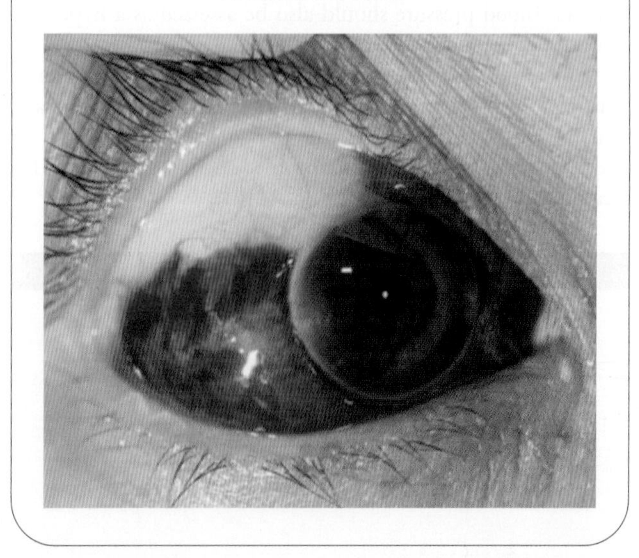

Conjunctivitis

Be aware of the diagnosis of unilateral conjunctivitis until all other more serious eye conditions are excluded.[28] Conjunctivitis is a common irritation or infection of the eye due to bacteria, viruses, chemicals or allergies.[16,29–33]

Discharge normally appears as a relatively clear mucous membrane on the surface of the eye and, if present, can cause the eyelids to stick together in the morning.[30] Multiple aetiological factors can cause swelling (chemosis) or dilation of the blood vessels in the conjunctiva (injection).[5,34] Repeated conjunctiva infections over a number of years causes conjunctival scarring and shortening of the upper eyelid, with the lashes turning inwards and rubbing the cornea, leading to corneal abrasion, ulcers or abscesses.[30]

Not all conjunctivitis is infectious: an accurate history and assessment will identify the cases that require appropriate precautions to prevent spread (Table 32.2). Differential diagnosis (Table 32.3) includes other, more serious, forms of 'red eye', such as keratitis, uveitis, scleritis and acute angle-closure glaucoma; typically these will see a reduced visual acuity and a

TABLE 32.2 COMPARISON OF TYPES OF CONJUNCTIVITIS[33]

CONDITION	AETIOLOGY	SIGNS AND SYMPTOMS	TREATMENT
Bacterial conjunctivitis	*Haemophilus influenzae* *Haemophilus aegyptius* *Streptococcus pneumoniae* *Staphylococcus aureus* *Moraxella catarrhalis*	Mucopurulent unilateral or bilateral discharge, normal vision, photophobia	Topical antibiotics, parenteral ceftriaxone for gonococcus, *H. influenzae*
Hyperacute bacterial conjunctivitis	*Neisseria gonorrhoeae* *Neisseria meningitides*	Conjunctival injection and oedema (chemosis); gritty sensation	
Viral conjunctivitis	Adenovirus, ECHO virus, coxsackievirus, herpes simplex virus	As above; may be haemorrhagic, unilateral	Self-limited
Neonatal conjunctivitis	*Chlamydia trachomatis* gonococcus, chemical (silver nitrate), *S. aureus*	Palpebral conjunctival follicle or papillae; as above	Ceftriaxone for gonococcus and erythromycin for *C. trachomatis*
Allergic conjunctivitis	Seasonal pollens or allergen exposure	Itching, incidence of bilateral chemosis (oedema) greater than that of erythema, tarsal papillae	Antihistamines, topical mast cell stabilisers or prostaglandin inhibitors, steroids
Keratitis	Herpes simplex virus, adenovirus *S. pneumoniae* *S. aureus, Pseudomonas Acanthamoeba*, chemicals	Severe pain, corneal swelling, clouding, limbus erythema, hypopyon, cataracts; contact lens history with amoebic infection	Specific antibiotics for bacterial/fungal infections; keratoplasty, aciclovir for herpes
Endophthalmitis	*S. aureus* *S. pneumoniae Candida albicans*, associated surgery or trauma	Acute onset, pain, loss of vision, swelling, chemosis, redness; hypopyon and vitreous haze	Antibiotics
Anterior uveitis (iridocyclitis)	JIA, post-infectious with arthritis and rash, sarcoidosis, Behçet disease, Kawasaki disease, inflammatory bowel disease	Unilateral/bilateral; erythema, ciliary flush, irregular pupil, iris adhesions; pain, photophobia, small pupil, poor vision	Topical steroids, plus therapy for primary disease
Posterior uveitis (choroiditis)	Toxoplasmosis, histoplasmosis, *Toxocara canis*	No signs of erythema, decreased vision	Specific therapy for pathogen
Episcleritis/scleritis	Idiopathic autoimmune disease (e.g. SLE, Henoch-Schönlein purpura)	Localised pain, intense erythema, unilateral; blood vessels bigger than in conjunctivitis; scleritis may cause globe perforation	Episcleritis is self-limiting; topical steroids for fast relief
Foreign body	Occupational exposure	Unilateral, red, gritty feeling; visible or microscopic size	Irrigation, removal; check for ulceration
Blepharitis	*S. aureus, Staphylococcus epidermidis*, seborrhoeic, blocked lacrimal duct; rarely molluscum contagiosum, *Phthirus pubis* *Pediculus capitis*	Bilateral, irritation, itching, hyperaemia, crusting, affecting lid margins	Topical antibiotics, warm compresses, lid hygiene
Dacryocystitis	Obstructed lacrimal sac: *S. aureus* *H. influenzae*, pneumococcus	Pain, tenderness, erythema, and exudates in area of lacrimal sac (inferomedial to inner canthus); tearing (epiphora); possible orbital cellulitis	Systemic, topical antibiotics; surgical drainage
Dacryoadenitis	*S. aureus, Streptococcus*, CMV, measles, EBV, enteroviruses; trauma, sarcoidosis, leukaemia	Pain, tenderness, oedema, erythema over gland area (upper temporal lid); fever, leucocytosis	Systemic antibiotics; drainage of orbital abscesses
Orbital cellulitis (post-septal cellulitis)	Paranasal sinusitis: *H. influenzae* *S. aureus* *S. pneumoniae*, streptococci Trauma: *S. aureus* Fungi: *Aspergillus*, *Mucor* spp. if immunodeficient	Rhinorrhoea, chemosis, vision loss, painful extraocular motion, proptosis, ophthalmoplegia, fever, lid oedema, leucocytosis	Systemic antibiotics, drainage of orbital abscesses
Periorbital cellulitis (preseptal cellulitis)	Trauma: *S. aureus*, streptococci Bacteraemia: pneumococcus, streptococci, *H. influenzae* *S. aureus*	Cutaneous erythema, warmth, normal vision, minimal involvement of orbit; fever, leucocytosis, toxic appearance	Systemic antibiotics

TABLE 32.3 DIFFERENTIAL DIAGNOSES OF EYE CONDITIONS

	CONJUNCTIVITIS	IRITIS	ACUTE GLAUCOMA	KERATITIS (FOREIGN-BODY ABRASION)
Discharge	Marked	None	None	Slight or none
Photophobia	None	Marked	Slight	Slight
Pain	None	Slight to marked	Marked	Marked
Visual acuity	Normal	Reduced	Reduced	Varies with site of the lesion
Pupil	Normal	Smaller or same	Large, oval and fixed	Same or smaller

painful red eye. During patient assessment it is important to check for abnormalities such as injury, foreign bodies, ulceration and cellulitis and refer as appropriate.

- *Allergic conjunctivitis* typically presents with an itchy, watery eye; everting the eyelid, view the conjunctival fornices, which will show papillary lesions. Treatment involves identifying and eliminating the allergic agent (if possible), cool compresses and lubricating drops without preservatives; frequently this is a self-limiting condition. Children presenting with repeated episodes of allergic conjunctivitis should be referred to a paediatric ophthalmologist for further investigation.
- *Viral conjunctivitis* frequently occurs and is concurrent with viral upper respiratory tract infection, and is very contagious. Presentation may involve red, watery eyes with a gritty feeling; it may begin in one eye and spread to the other within 2 days. Symptoms often get worse within 10 days. Both eyes are diffusely red, watery discharge can occur and visual acuity is normal. Viral conjunctivitis is frequently a self-limiting condition lasting about 10 days; treatment includes cold eye packs and lubricant drops.
- A particularly contagious viral conjunctivitis—*epidemic keratoconjunctivitis*—causes greater pain and redness, often with photophobia and eventual bilateral involvement. In contrast to other types of viral conjunctivitis, keratoconjunctivitis can last 3 weeks; treatment is supportive (Table 32.4).
- *Bacterial infection* may involve red eyes with a gritty feeling; it may begin in one eye and spread to the other, and presents as uniformly red because of widespread engorgement of the conjunctival vessels. Visual acuity is normal and purulent discharge can occur of varying colours (grey, yellow and green) and amounts. Typically, this is a self-limiting condition.[25] There is minimal to no pain or pre-auricular adenopathy.

  Antibiotic eye drops or ointment is the treatment of choice for bacterial infections (Table 32.4). Eyes should be swabbed for culture and sensitivity in high-risk populations, recurrent episodes and infants. The organism *Chlamydia trachomatis* causes repeated attacks of conjunctivitis in children, and is often transmitted from person to person, for example, by fingers, household cloths or by flies.[28] Large amounts of pus can indicate *Neisseria gonorrhoea.* If present, urgent treatment to prevent corneal ulceration and/or corneal melting is required and consists of intramuscular ceftriaxone plus frequent eye irrigation with saline. Topical antibiotics, such as erythromycin ointment, should also be prescribed. Referral to an outpatient ophthalmology service and sexual health service is required if the patient is photophobic or has reduced visual acuity or persistence of symptoms.[16,35,36]

The emergency nurse and paramedic should provide education, instructing the patient about hygiene—frequent washing of hands and not rubbing/touching eyes, non-sharing of towels, pillows or make-up to prevent cross-contamination. Ensure that patients and parents understand eye care and medication instructions prior to discharge and advise them to return if the patient develops pain or increased irritation.[30]

UVEITIS AND IRITIS

Uveitis is inflammation in the iris, ciliary body and choroid of the eye. Most commonly, anterior uveitis is seen, and this is known as iritis. This disorder may result from trauma, infections and autoimmune causes. Symptoms may include reduced vision, deep orbital aching, redness and consensual photophobia. An eye with anterior chamber cell inflammation will often feel pain when light is directed at the other eye because the light causes the ciliary body in both eyes to contract. The ciliary body is usually inflamed in persons with iritis, thus the contraction causes pain.[16] Synechiae (adhesions of the iris) may also be seen; dilating drops or heat should break this adhesion. Assess the pupil; with synechiae the pupil will be irregular due to the posterior iris sticking to the crystalline lens capsule or anterior iris to the cornea.[16]

Slit-lamp examination (slit lamp on maximum magnification) will identify flare and cells in the anterior chamber with suspended proteins causing fogginess of the slit-lamp beam.

Treatment consists of topical steroids and mydriatics/cycloplegics (Table 32.4); steroids should only be prescribed under the direction of an ophthalmologist. The patient should be referred to an ophthalmologist outpatient service as soon as possible if in an acute phase.[36]

TRAUMA

EPIDEMIOLOGY OF OCULAR TRAUMA

The workplace accounts for the majority of eye injuries, followed by the home. In Australia, the rate of hospital admissions as a result of work-related injury with eye trauma as the primary diagnosis is 3% of total admissions.[37] Eye injuries are a major cause of lost working days in Australia and Aotearoa New Zealand,

TABLE 32.4 SUMMARY OF DRUGS COMMONLY USED IN OPHTHALMOLOGY[8]

	EXAMPLES IN COMMON USE	MODE OF ADMINISTRATION	ACTION	SIDE-EFFECTS
Glaucoma treatment (note that different types of glaucoma may require different therapeutic approaches)	Beta-blockers; timolol, betaxolol, levobunolol	Topical	Reduce aqueous secretion by inhibitory action on beta-adrenoceptors in the ciliary body	Ocular: irritation Systemic: bronchospasm, bradycardia, exacerbation of heartblock with verapamil, nightmares
	Muscarinic (parasympathetic) stimulants: pilocarpine	Topical	Increase aqueous outflow via trabecular meshwork by ciliary muscle contraction	Ocular: miosis (reduced vision in presence of cataract, retinal examination impaired), spasm of accommodation, brow ache Systemic: sweating, bradycardia, gastrointestinal disturbance Long-term use leads to poor pupil dilation
	Alpha$_2$-stimulants: brimonidine, apraclonidine	Topical	Reduce aqueous secretion by selective stimulation of alpha$_2$-receptors and adrenoceptors in the ciliary body increase outflow by uveoscleral route	Ocular: allergy, mydriasis, eyelid retraction Systemic: dry mouth, hypotension, drowsiness, headache
	Prostaglandin derivatives: latanoprost, travoprost, bimatoprost	Topical	Increase aqueous outflow by the uveoscleral route	Ocular: iris darkening, conjunctival hyperaemia, eyelash growth
	Carbonic anhydrase inhibitors	Systemic (acetazolamide), topical (dorzolamide, brinzolamide)	Reduce aqueous secretion by the ciliary body	Ocular route: irritation, allergy Systemic (generally systemic use): malaise, paraesthesia, urea and electrolyte disturbance, aplastic anaemia
Mydriatics and cycloplegics (for retinal examination and objective refraction (retinoscopy))	Antimuscarinics: tropicamide, cyclopentolate, atropine	Topical	Inhibit muscarinic receptors of parasympathetic nervous system to paralyse pupillary sphincter and ciliary muscle	Ocular: blurred vision (especially for near), glare, angle-closure glaucoma Systemic: tachycardia, dry mouth, confusion, tremor
	Alpha-stimulant: phenylephrine	Topical	Stimulate dilator muscle of the pupil; no cycloplegic effect	Ocular: blurred vision, glare, angle-closure glaucoma, conjunctival blanching Systemic: hypertension (with use of 10%)
Lubricants A range of preparations is available for the treatment of dry eyes	Carbomers, hypromellose, polyvinyl alcohol, liquid paraffin	Topical	Exact mechanism depends on agent	Ocular: preservative allergy/toxicity, blurred vision (especially ointments)

Continued

TABLE 32.4 SUMMARY OF DRUGS COMMONLY USED IN OPHTHALMOLOGY—cont'd

	EXAMPLES IN COMMON USE	MODE OF ADMINISTRATION	ACTION	SIDE-EFFECTS
Anti-inflammatory agents Most important drugs in this category are corticosteroids; a variety of other agents is available, including systemic immunosuppressants	Corticosteroids: prednisolone forte (Prednisolone with Phenylephrine), dexamethasone fluorometholene	Topical, periocular injection, systemic	Suppression of broad spectrum of inflammatory processes	Ocular: glaucoma (especially with local administration), cataract (especially prolonged systemic use), exacerbation of some infections e.g. herpes simplex Systemic: negligible with topical use; common and varied with systemic administration
	Mast-cell stabilisers (cromoglycate, nedocromil, lodoxamide)	Topical	Stabilise mast cells	Ocular: irritation
	Antihistamines	Topical Ketotifen Olopatadine	Block histamine receptor (azelastine also stabilises mast cells)	Ocular route: irritation Systemic route: drowsiness
	Non-steroidal anti-inflammatory drugs: systemic help to control ocular pain and inflammation; topical increasingly used for pain of corneal abrasion, for inflammation after cataract surgery and to maintain pupil dilation during cataract surgery	Topical (ketorolac, diclofenac, flurbiprofen)	Modulate prostaglandin production	Systemic: peptic ulceration, asthma
Anti-infective agents Topically applied antibacterial and antiviral drugs are very commonly prescribed; the use of antifungal and antiparasitic agents is much less frequent	Antibacterials: chloramphenicol, gentamicin, Oflxacin	Topical, occasionally intraocular, systemic	Range of activities and specificities	Vary with agent Ocular: allergy; corneal toxicity common with intensive use Systemic: generally only with systemic use
	Antivirals: aciclovir	Topical, systemic, intravitreal	Inhibit herpes virus DNA synthesis	Ocular: blurred vision, corneal toxicity Systemic: rashes; kidney, liver and other effects may occur with systemic use
Local anaesthetics Major uses are to relieve pain and thereby assist with clinical examination, and the facilitation of surgical anaesthesia	Oxybuprocaine, proxymetacaine, tetracaine, lidocaine	Topical, periocular injection	Block conduction along nerve fibres	Ocular: irritation, corneal toxicity Systemic: generally iatrogenic intravascular or intrathecal (cerebrospinal fluid) injection during surgical anaesthesia: cardiac dysrhythmias, respiratory depression
Botulinum toxin Used in the management of certain ocular motility disorders and blepharospasm, and to induce ptosis for corneal protection		Injection at site of action	Prevent release of the neurotransmitter acetylcholine at neuromuscular junctions	Dependent on treatment site: e.g. unwanted ptosis or double vision

particularly in areas of production, such as manufacturing plants, construction sites, factories/warehouses, mines and farms in Australia. In Aotearoa New Zealand in 2020,[38] the incidence of eye injury is around 100/100,000. The most common mechanism of injury noted was being struck by an object, accounting for approximately 55% of cases. Injuries were more likely to occur at home, followed by industrial /commercial locations. Males 20–29 years of age incur the majority of the injuries.[37–41] In Australia and Aotearoa New Zealand, men living in rural areas are the most likely to experience eye injury.[38,42–44]

The injury profile for Aotearoa New Zealand (2020) is similar to Australia, with overall rates showing that males aged 20–29 represent the highest group.[38,44] European ethnicity account for around 74% of presentations.[38] Over 4000 cases of eye injuries are reported annually.[45]

Most eye injuries in industry are as a result of the eye being hit by moving parts. In Aotearoa New Zealand, 5% of all work-related injuries are caused by foreign bodies and 21% are lacerations (including the eyelid).[38,44] Tasks with the highest risk of eye injuries are grinding, welding and hammering. Other high-risk activities include cutting, drilling, spraying, smelting, sanding, chipping and chiselling.[38,40]

High-velocity ball and contact sports, such as tennis, golf or football, also account for a proportion of eye injuries and can result in permanent loss of visual acuity.[46] Behaviour modification and addressing attitudes towards wearing eye protection in some sports is occurring.[47] Less-frequent causes include farming incidents,[37,48] self-infliction,[49] stings[50] and animal-related injuries, such as falling off and being rolled on by a horse, which has resulted in several incidences of significant permanent loss of vision.[51]

Although injuries from airbag deployment do occur, in the vast majority of cases they protect rather than harm. The likelihood of sustaining an ocular injury increases significantly in cars in which the airbag did not deploy.[52–54]

Despite wearing approved and recommended eye protection and using screens, splatter burns from hot, moving particles and injury from flying metal particles continue to occur in the industrialised workplace and at home. This is partially because many models of approved protective eyewear, such as wide-vision spectacles, have gaps or fit poorly to the individual's face shape. Australian Standard/New Zealand Standard 1336:2014 states: 'wherever practicable, eye protectors should be fitted to the wearer by a person who[55] is competent to select the correct size and type'.[40] Injuries have occurred where the gap was as small as 5 mm and as large as 20 mm.[56] Research is continuing into improving design standards, and several eye injury prevention programs are in place.

INITIAL ASSESSMENT AND MANAGEMENT

The pre-hospital, initial or first-aid management of ocular trauma is presented in Box 32.2. The most important aspect is protection (Fig. 32.17). An accurate ophthalmic history includes previous eye conditions, ocular surgeries or use of eye medication, past or present. Vascular conditions such as diabetes or hypertension should be documented as they can affect the blood vessels of the retina (BRAO, CRAO, CRVO) or cause vitreous haemorrhages. If the eye patient is assessed inaccurately as a low priority it may lead to long-term effects, such as a major disability of vision impairment, which can also affect employment prospects. Any eye injury, whether it is a corneal abrasion or an orbital wound, should alert the clinician to the possibility of a ruptured globe.[21]

BOX 32.2 PRE-HOSPITAL MANAGEMENT OF OCULAR TRAUMA[57]

- **Control haemorrhage** around the eye or eyelids with direct pressure, but no direct pressure should be exerted on the eyeball itself.
- **Chemical burns** (caustic soda, lime, drain cleaners etc) If caustic powder present, remove particulate matter prior to irrigation with copious amounts of water or normal saline for 20 minutes. Do not allow the removal of particulate matter to delay irrigation. Continue irrigation for longer with more serious injuries, or if in doubt. Retract the lids to ensure thorough flushing of the eye. Remove contact lenses if in situ (before irrigation).
  - **Flash burns**—examine the eye to exclude chemical burn or foreign body, evert the upper eyelid to ensure no material in the conjunctiva. Remove any contact lens from the exposed eye. Pain management until seen in ED.
  - **Protect the eye** from pressure or rubbing with a shield or a modified polystyrene cup taped in place. The non-injured eye should not be padded as this causes needless disorientation to the patient.
  - **Beware of aggravating the injury**
  - Do not remove protruding or embedded bodies.
  - Do not replace an extruded eyeball. Support with a saline-moistened sterile dressing lightly taped in position.
  - Do not apply any pressure to penetrating injuries and situations with extrusion of ocular contents.
  - **Pain management**
  - **Antiemetic**—prevention of vomiting is very important in eye injuries.

PRACTICE TIP

- Airway and circulatory support take priority in patients with multiple injuries, but penetrating/perforated eye injuries or a globe rupture and preservation of sight warrant priority over conditions which are non-life threatening.
- If the patient has a suspected penetrating eye injury or ruptured globe do not instil any topical medications, as they are not compatible with ocular contents. If topical medications need to be used, e.g. fluorescein, to assess if there is a wound leak, use only single-use, preservative-free eye drops.
- When transporting patients, try to reduce conditions that induce vomiting; reduce eye movements and get the patient to close their eyes. If a hyphaema is present, patients should sit at a 45° angle to avoid corneal staining.
- Hypoxia will worsen an eye injury as the retina has a high oxygen demand.
- To avoid pressure on the globe, ensure face masks and oxygen masks do not place pressure on or near to the orbit.

FIGURE 32.17 APPLYING A DOUBLE EYE PATCH (A TO C). D, AN EYE SHIELD (USE INSTEAD OF A PATCH IN SUSPECTED PENETRATING EYE INJURY)[58]

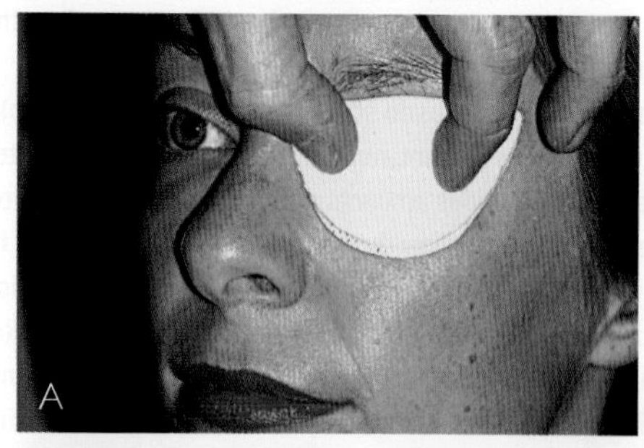

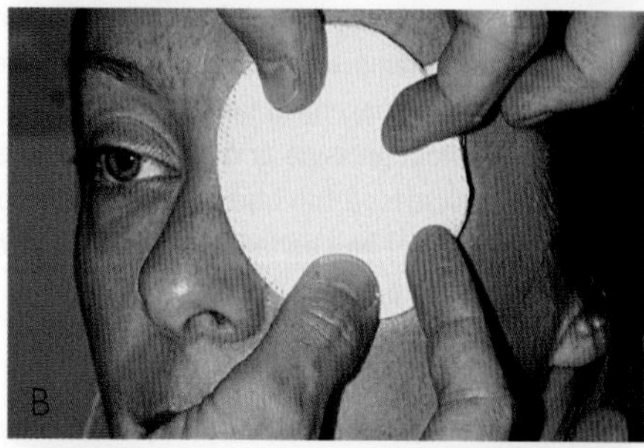

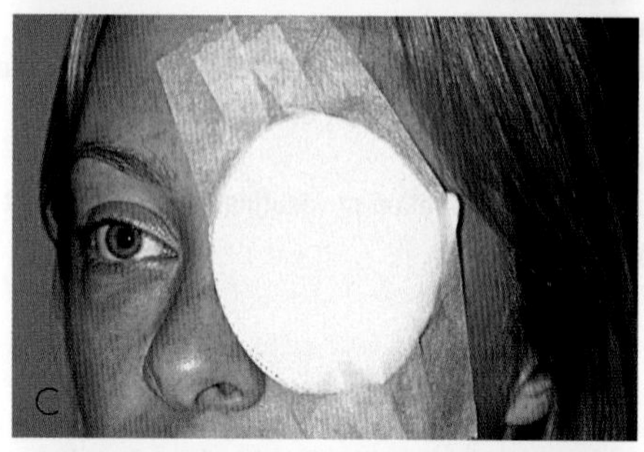

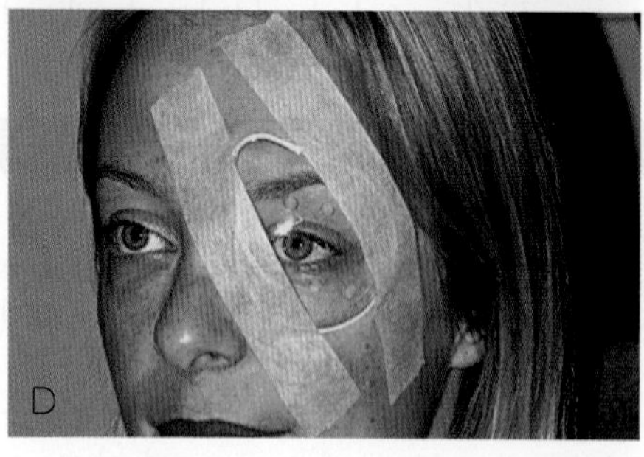

Clinicians should be aware there are two different classifications of eye trauma. The first is the Ocular Trauma Classification, where injuries are classified into open and closed globe injury.[55] An open globe injury is defined as a full thickness injury of the cornea and/or the sclera, while a closed globe injury presents as a contusion injury or lamellar (partial) laceration. Open globe injuries are further categorised into penetrating injury, ruptured globe, perforated injury and injury with retained intraocular foreign body (IOFB).

The second classification is the Birmingham Eye Trauma Terminology System (BETTS),[55] where closed globe injuries include cornea/sclera not totally perforated through contusions from blunt trauma and partial lamellar (partial) thickness wounds in cornea/sclera. An open globe injury is defined as a full thickness wound of the globe, ruptured globe, lacerations from sharp objects, penetrating and perforating injuries with a presence of an entrance wound and IOFBs.[59]

Eye assessment should occur as part of the secondary survey. Ocular injury often occurs in conjunction with head and facial trauma[56] (see Chapter 44); thus, the patient should be carefully evaluated for an associated eye injury.[60] Eye assessment should still be undertaken, even when periorbital oedema is present or the patient is comatose, uncooperative or combative, and it must be remembered that the extraocular appearance can be normal. Caution should be used when trying to open an eye with periorbital oedema when there is a history of severe trauma, as ocular contents may extrude if pressure is placed on the globe. A modified paper clip has been used as a tool to assist with the opening of the eyelid in the presence of periorbital oedema.[61] Obtain a history and assess the patient, as previously discussed. To ensure less pressure on the globe, use the orbital rim to support the clinician's fingers whilst gently opening the lids. This allows no pressure to be placed on the globe.

Check for contact lenses in the unconscious patient and remove them as soon as possible. As a result of trauma, contact lenses often become dislodged from the cornea and can be found in the superior or inferior ocular cul-de-sacs.[26] If no penetrating eye injury is present, topical fluorescein can be used to identify the contact lens position; the upper lid will need to be everted for access if contact lens is present.

Specific assessment and management for ocular injury as a result of blasts is discussed in depth in Chapter 42.

ORBITAL BLOW-OUT FRACTURE

The orbital contents may be forced through the orbital floor and into the maxillary sinus; this is known as a 'blow-out' fracture and is a common presentation to EDs. The medial aspect and orbital floor are common sites for fractures. The patient's history often includes recent blunt trauma. Patients may present with pain, especially with eye movements, diplopia (double vision), eyelid swelling and crepitus after blowing their nose. Vision may be reduced secondary to having a corneal abrasion, and there may be intraocular bleeding (hyphaema), retinal bruising or detachment.

The aim of pre-hospital management is to prevent further damage or assess level of ocular damage; initial action should be to inspect the eye area if possible. Do not try to open the eyelid if it is swollen shut, as ocular contents may be lost if there is a ruptured globe. If the eye is visible, check ocular movements and observe for signs of a trapped muscle or nerve.

Ice packs can be used to reduce swelling, but only if there is no evidence of a ruptured globe or a penetrating eye injury. Instruct patients not to sneeze or blow their nose.

Clinical features

These may include restricted eye movements, especially on upwards or lateral gaze, or both; subconjunctival haemorrhage; hyperaesthesia due to a trapped infraorbital nerve—affects cheeks and upper lip; enophthalmos (displacement of the globe backwards through the orbital fracture)—this can be masked by lid swelling.

Differential diagnoses that should be excluded are orbital oedema/haemorrhage without fracture, and cranial nerve palsy.[22]

Assessment and management

Assess extraocular muscle movement—ask the patient to look in all positions of gaze; compare both eyes looking for posterior globe displacement (enophthalmos). Primarily ask the patient to look up, down, left and right. To assess if there is nerve involvement, compare sensations between cheeks, top lip and front tooth. Palpate eyelids for crepitus (subconjunctival emphysema); educate patients not to blow their nose to avoid this from occurring.[5,14]

Evaluate globe patency—if there is no evidence of rupture, use a slit lamp to check for a hyphaema, traumatic iritis and retinal or choroidal damage. Further tests include an IOP check, testing for a relative afferent pupillary defect (RAPD). RAPD testing is a reliable way to implicate or rule out optic nerve disease. The usual response of healthy pupils to direct light is that both pupils contract equally, and if the light is moved quickly from one eye to the other, both pupils hold their level of contraction; if the light is moved too slowly (so that neither eye is 'dazzled'), the initial response from the first pupil is lost and both pupils dilate somewhat. With RAPD, shining the light in the good eye will cause both pupils to constrict; when the light is moved quickly to the bad eye *both* pupils will dilate. This is because a damaged optic nerve transmits light to a lesser degree, and more slowly than a healthy one; as a result, when the light is moved from the good to the bad eye, the brain interprets this as a decrease in the amount of light being shone. Colour vision testing will be performed in the ophthalmic clinic to rule out traumatic optic neuropathy. A simple test is to show a patient a red object and ask what colour it is. People with a colour deficit may say it is orange.

A computed tomography (CT) scan is recommended, especially if extraocular muscles are restricted, or periorbital oedema makes assessment of the eye patency difficult.

Treatment involves ice packs to reduce swelling for 24–48 hours to enable the clinician to view the eye, and nasal decongestants for 3 days. Broad-spectrum antibiotics should be prescribed for several days as a prophylaxis against periorbital cellulitis. A surgical repair is recommended within 24 hours if the CT shows a trapped muscle or enophthalmos. Other signs may also include diplopia, non-resolving bradycardia, heart block or nausea and vomiting. A neurological consultation is recommended if the orbital roof is fractured, as there is risk of intracranial haemorrhage.

Follow-up in an ophthalmic unit is 1–2 weeks after trauma, to evaluate whether there is persistent diplopia and enophthalmos after orbital oedema has reduced. Monitor also for secondary ocular trauma and advise patients accordingly for symptoms of orbital cellulitis and angle recession glaucoma (will present with high IOP). The patient should also be advised of the potential for retinal detachment, in which the retina peels away from its underlying layer of support tissue. Advise the patient to seek urgent medical attention if any of the following symptoms develop in the injured eye: very brief flashes of light in the extreme peripheral part of vision, a sudden and dramatic increase in floaters, a ring of floaters or hairs just to the temporal side of the central vision, a slight feeling of heaviness in the eye, a dense shadow starting in the peripheries and slowly moving to central vision, a sense of a veil or curtain being drawn over vision, straight lines that suddenly appear curved (positive Amsler grid test) or loss of central vision (signs of retinal detachment).

CORNEAL FOREIGN BODIES

Working with power tools, hammering or chiselling metal, explosions and gardening are common causes of corneal foreign bodies (Fig. 32.18).

The patient may complain of the sensation of a foreign body, mild irritation/pain and/or mild redness of eye. The use of fluorescein staining and anaesthetic drops can aid in the examination of the eye. Visual acuity is not affected unless the foreign body is lodged at the centre of the cornea. Subtarsal (evert the lid to view) or corneal foreign bodies can be removed with a moistened cotton bud after topical anaesthetic is instilled, using either a slit lamp or a pen torch, approaching the patient from the temporal aspect of the eye. Irrigation could also be tried to dislodge a foreign body.[62] As a precaution against fungal growth, patching should be avoided if the abrasive agent was a vegetative substance.[26] If the corneal foreign body cannot be removed within 24 hours, the patient should be referred to an ophthalmologist. If the foreign body is central and deep, do not try to remove it unless assessed by a skilled clinician, due to the risk of perforation and corneal scarring. If an intraocular foreign body is suspected, the patient should be referred to an ophthalmologist immediately. Only skilled clinicians should use the bevel of a 25-gauge needle to remove/flick out any foreign body.

Corneal rusting can occur as a complication following a metallic foreign body in the eye and may be loosened by the application of antibiotic ointment and padding for 24 hours, after which it is easily shelled out with the edge of a fine hypodermic needle. Use of a mechanical dental burr can result in large areas of epithelium removal.[1,26] Inflammation or ulceration can also occur as a complication. Short-acting cycloplegic eye drops (Cyclopentolate 1%) can be used for pain relief, and antibiotic drops or ointments are essential if the corneal epithelium has been disrupted. Patients need daily review until any ulceration is completely healed.

FIGURE 32.18 CORNEAL FOREIGN BODY[27]

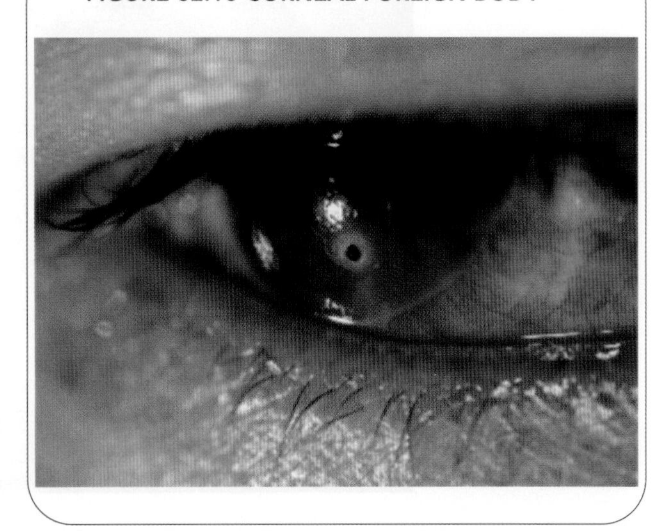

CORNEAL ABRASION

Corneal abrasions are defined as a defect in the superficial surface of the cornea (epithelium and Bowman's). Corneal abrasions become corneal ulcers when the injury penetrates further into the stroma. Corneal abrasion is a common injury that occurs in all age groups. Contact lens wearers are at most risk of injury. It is also the most common non-penetrating eye injury in children. Abrasion should be the differential diagnosis in infants and newborns with sudden onset of crying. Fingernail length and method of cutting nails are common issues in this group. Corneal abrasion can occur with dry eye in older people, corneal abrasion can occur with dry eye if it is not being affectively treated with lubricants (ointment/drops). Some patients can suffer from an abrasion post eye surgery—lid surgery. Epithelial cells adjacent to the injury site multiply (miosis) to enter and seal the defect; typically this takes 24–48 hours. If it reaches Bowman's level, scarring can occur. Ninety per cent of sharp pain/foreign body sensation will resolve with a topical local anaesthetic.[63]

Corneal abrasions can be caused by a foreign body, explosion, traumatic facial nerve damage (poor blink reflex), abnormal eyelid position (entropion, ectropion) and abnormal eyelashes (trichiasis) (Fig. 32.19). The patient may have a painful eye, photophobia, eye watering, blepharospasm (involuntary spasm of eyelid) and may be unable to open the eye for examination.

Wearing contact lenses can cause trauma and dry eye if not removed regularly. Symptoms may not occur immediately after injury, and patients may not be aware of the event that caused the injury. Reduced visual acuity may be suggestive of a more serious condition—keratitis, uveitis.

If the patient can open the eye, record visual acuity; instil local anaesthesia if necessary before trying to obtain a visual acuity. Treatment is the same as for corneal foreign bodies. Most corneal abrasions will heal within 24–48 hours and contact lenses can be worn 2 or 3 days after the abrasion has healed. Recurrence can occur at any time; repeated recurrent

FIGURE 32.19 CORNEAL ABRASION WITHOUT (A, B) AND WITH (C) WITH FLUORESCEIN STAINING[24]

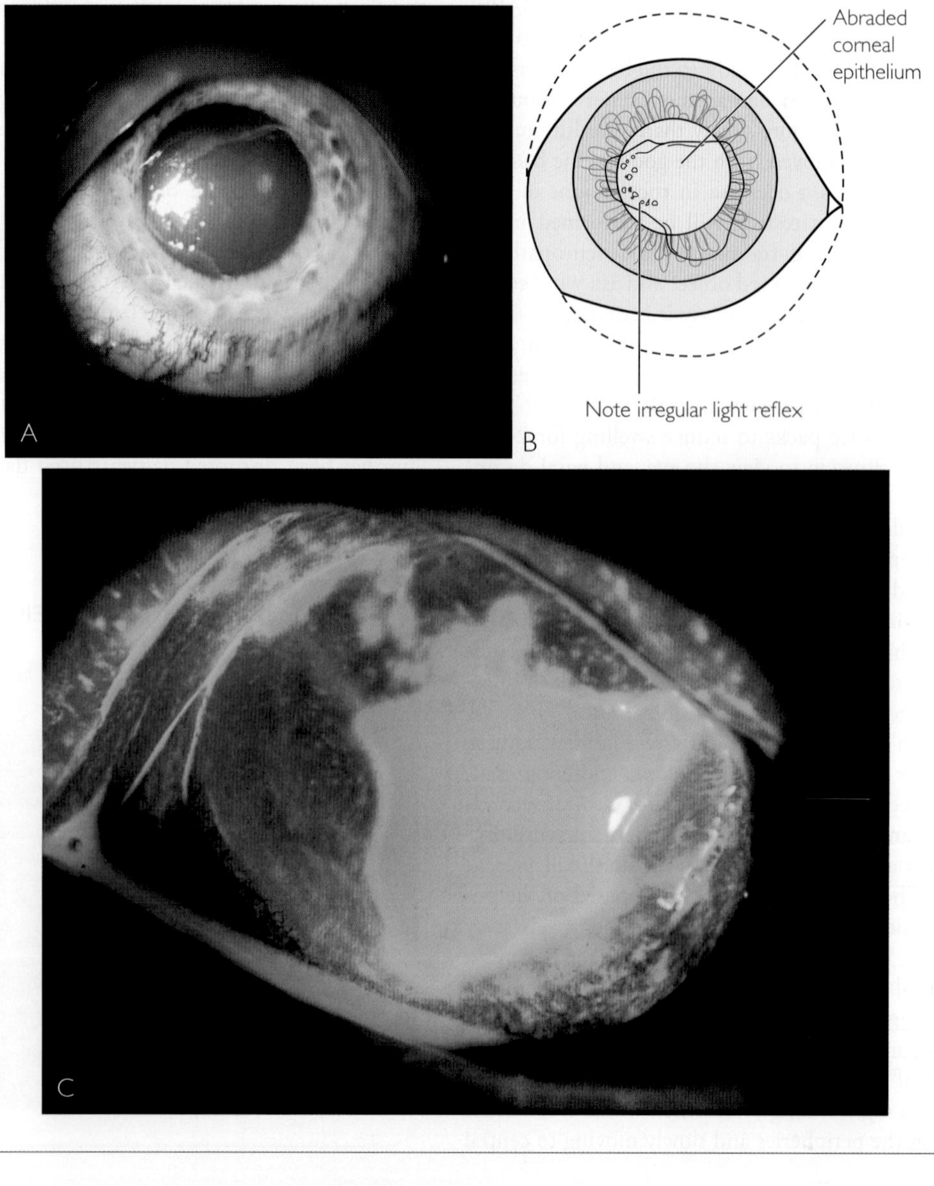

A

Abraded corneal epithelium

Note irregular light reflex

B

C

erosions should be referred to an ophthalmic outpatient department.

FLASH BURNS

Ocular trauma linked to flash burns has been declining over the last ten years. Exposure of the cornea to ultraviolet light from welding or devices such as photographer's lighting, halogen lamps, sun lamps, direct sunlight, reflection of light off water, fish tanks or snow at high elevations (snow blindness), and solar eclipse can cause radiation burns and abrasions/erosions of the cornea.[64,65]

Like most trauma statistics, the main demographic of those presenting to the ED are men, mainly between the ages of 10 and 49. Almost half of all ocular injuries due to welding were bilateral.

Three to 12 hours (average time is several hours) after exposure the patient begins to experience ocular symptoms; pain is mild to severe, red eyes (corneal injection), extreme light sensitivity/photophobia, foreign body sensation, tearing, blepharospasm (rapid blinking of eyelids) and blurred vision. If exposure occurs bilaterally, symptoms in the eye which was most exposed will be worse.

Metal Insert Gas (MIG) welding uses arc light, which is capable of burning the retina with anterior (front of eye) symptoms and visual changes only. It uses a longer wavelength and is not absorbed by the anterior segment (cornea to lens). Symptoms may be visual distortions and scotomas (blind spots in vision). In this case, referral to an ophthalmologist for further testing would be required.[4]

If the person wears contact lens, they should remove them immediately; wearing sunglasses will reduce glare/photophobia and reduce discomfort. Initial ocular assessment should be to exclude either chemical burns or corneal foreign bodies. Ensure you evert the lids to check there is no foreign material under the upper or lower eyelids. Welders have an elevated risk of a foreign body; questions around mechanism of injury will support clinical examination. Check for other flash burn injuries beyond the ocular surface.

For the clinician to accurately assess the eye, a drop of local topical anaesthetic in the affected eye is essential. The patient will not be able to open their eye without the use of local topical anaesthetic, which will also provide instant pain relief. Patients should not have topical anaesthesia to take home, as continued use will cause corneal toxicity. Oral analgesia (stronger than paracetamol) and ibuprofen are recommended to manage pain levels.

Vision can be slightly reduced, therefore assessing visual acuity is essential. When assessing the patient, consider examination with a slit lamp using fluorescein, which stains any corneal epithelial defects.

Treatment of the ocular flash burn involves a topical broad-spectrum antibiotic due to the corneal erosions/abrasions. Ointment form can be soothing for the patient, while a short-term mydriatic, such as Cyclopentolate 0.5%/1% twice daily for a few days, paralyses the ciliary muscle and stops painful spasms. Low preservative lubricants or artificial tears can improve the corneal surface.

HYPHAEMA

Hyphaema is blood in the anterior chamber of the eye (Fig. 32.20). It is caused by external compression, and secondary expansion of the angle with tearing of the iris root, ciliary body or pupillary margin causing blood to leak into the aqueous fluid of the anterior chamber.[66] Concurrent injuries are common, as a hyphaema is the result of severe ocular trauma. All hyphaemas need ophthalmology review. Micro hyphaema are not visible using a pen light or slit lamp; a form of magnification (such as Wood's eye examination lamp) is required to be able to view the anterior (A/C).

FIGURE 32.20 TRAUMATIC HYPHAEMA[67]

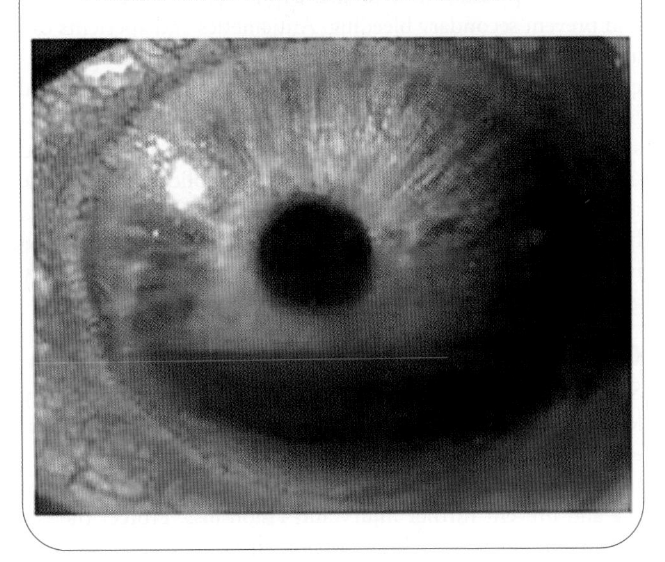

Hyphaema is graded as follows:

- grade 1: blood level < 1/3
- grade 2: blood level > 1/3 but < 2/3
- grade 3: blood level > 2/3 but < total
- grade 4: blood level fills up the anterior chamber totally.

Visual acuity may be greatly reduced and there may be a deep aching pain, reduced vision, photophobia and a red inflamed eye. Periorbital haematoma may be present.

Initial management should be to restrict the patient's movement; have them lie down at 45 degrees and place a protective eye shield over the eye until they are transported to hospital.

Management of a grade 1 hyphaema can be done at home if the patient is cooperative and able to return for regular check-ups. In general, all patients with hyphaema need to be examined daily for the first week to monitor intraocular pressure, corneal staining and to watch for re-bleeding. Re-bleeding, if it is going to occur, usually does so within 10 days of the initial injury, and can cause additional pathology.[26] Because of the risk of re-bleeding for high-grade hyphaema, strict bed rest is required for up to 5 days with elevation of the bed head—30–45° initially. An eye shield is used, not a patch. Fundal checks are required to ensure the retina is not detached or bruised. Management is variable and controversial, particularly in relation to activity, which ranges from quiet activity to strict bed rest.[68]

Pharmacological management includes:

- topical steroids to reduce inflammation
- mydriatic—to stop ciliary spasm and to avoid accommodation
- IOP management—topical alpha2-agonists, oral carbonic anhydrase inhibitor
- analgesia.

Medication, either topical or oral, can also be given to control intraocular pressure and to dilate the pupil, to rest the iris and prevent secondary bleeding. Antiemetics and aperients can also be used to prevent straining. Indications for surgery include raised intraocular pressure, unresolved clot or corneal bloodstaining. Anticoagulant therapy, salicylates and non-steroidal anti-inflammatory drugs (NSAIDs) should be avoided until reviewed by ophthalmology. Complications include the risk of re-bleeding, particularly 3–5 days after the injury, but may occur up to 14 days after the initial injury; increased intraocular pressure or corneal bloodstaining; and secondary glaucoma can occur acutely or months to years later.[66]

GLOBE INJURY

Severe closed globe injury involving the posterior segment may lead to permanent visual impairment and blindness through its effect on the lens, vitreous humour and retina.[69]

Initial management for any globe injury is to protect the eye and prevent further injury and vision loss. Protect the eye with a clear plastic shield if available; if not, cut down a polystyrene cup and secure. No pressure should be applied to the globe at any time. If there is bleeding around the site, irrigate with normal saline to assess the extent of the damage. If there is an obvious penetrating injury or ruptured globe (open globe injury), or a trauma history with a high suspicion of injury, cover the eye with a shield and provide pain management. If possible, transport the patient to the nearest hospital that has eye services, after trauma clearance.

Iris and lens trauma

Tears or holes may occur with trauma to the iris, which can result in pupillary irregularities and traumatic dilation. Blunt, non-perforating ocular trauma often results in acute iritis, an inflammatory reaction involving the iris and ciliary body. Symptoms include photophobia, tearing, pain; severe inflammation will cause an IOP increase and a decrease in vision. Treatment is topical cycloplegic drops plus a topical corticosteroid, unless there is an epithelial defect until healed; steroids will generally delay healing.[16,66]

Because of the crystalline nature of the lens, cataracts may develop rapidly or over weeks to months following trauma, and cause severe visual obscuration if the opacity is within the visual pathway.[70] Lens replacement (cataract surgery and intraocular lens implant) may be needed if sight is limited. If severe inflammation is associated with ocular injury, adhesions between the iris and the lens may develop (synechiae). The lens may subluxate/dislocate if sufficient force has been delivered, or as the result of a corneal laceration (Fig. 32.21); this may necessitate surgery for removal of the lens. Review the patient within 5–7 days, and within 1 month a check of the angle recession and fundus is recommended.

FIGURE 32.21 EXTRUSION OF LENS THROUGH CORNEAL LACERATION[26]

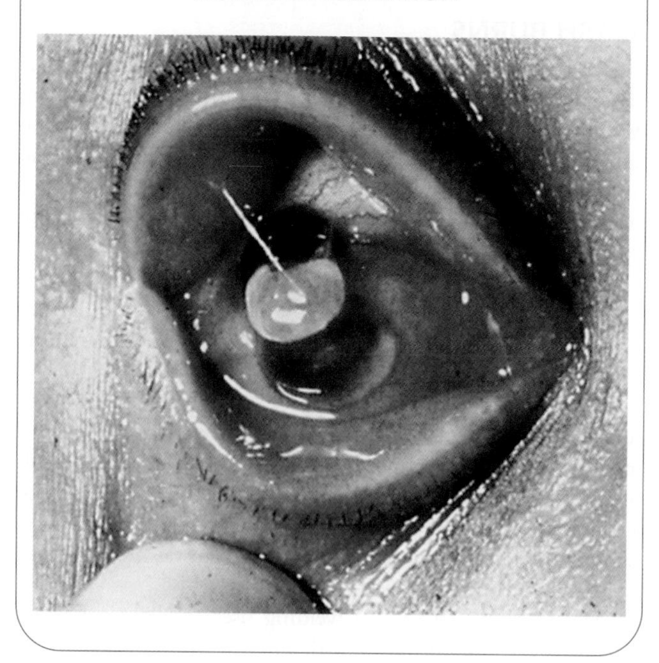

Retinal detachment

Retinal detachment is the separation of the sensory retina from the retinal pigment epithelium (RPE). It can occur following any globe injury (open and closed) where the retina breaks. Other possible causes of retinal detachment include myopia (short-sightedness) and systemic conditions like Marfan's syndrome and retinoschisis. In closed globe injuries, retinal detachments are known to result from enlargement in the equator region of the globe and tractions in the vitreous base that are caused by sudden compression of the eye in the anteroposterior direction.[71] These tears can take the form of small holes, horseshoe-shaped wide lesions with irregular borders, dialysis or giant tears. Retinal detachments occur immediately in 12% of patients and within 1 year after trauma in 80%.[72] The patient may have a painless loss of vision, described as a curtain or cobweb descending over vision; photopsia (flashes); or a sudden increase in floaters. If the macula is still on, the patient's vision will still be 6/6. If there is suspicion of a retinal detachment with a macula on, limit the patient's activity to lying flat on a bed until an urgent surgical repair can occur. Retinal detachments require surgical intervention. If the retinal detachment (macular off) is large, a RAPD is often found.

Patients may present with flashes and floaters; vitreous gel can undergo a change called syneresis (contraction of gel as part of the ageing process, accompanied by separating out of liquid), causing liquefaction and shrinkage of the vitreous diagnosed as posterior vitreous detachment. A high percentage (10–15%) of these progress to retinal breaks and detachments.

GLOBE RUPTURE (OPEN GLOBE INJURY)

A ruptured globe can be the result of either a blunt or a penetrating injury (Fig. 32.22), although rupture of an old, healed, large-incision cataract extraction wound is also a very common mechanism.[42] For a globe to rupture, the cornea and/or sclera must be perforated. There are anterior segment injuries, i.e. to the cornea, anterior chamber, iris and lens; and posterior segment injuries, i.e. to the sclera, retina and vitreous humour. Injuries of this nature usually occur with other severe injuries, in particular facial lacerations and fractures.

Signs of a globe rupture are:

- chemosis
- restricted eye movements

FIGURE 32.22 SEVERE EYELID LACERATION WITH ASSOCIATED PENETRATING TRAUMA TO GLOBE

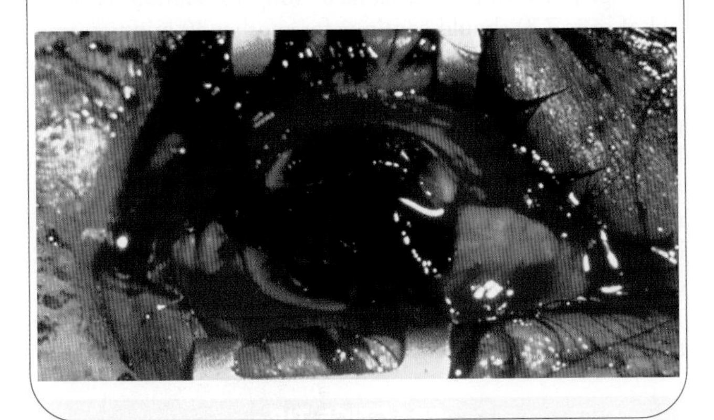

Reproduced, with permission, from Slide Scripts: Eye trauma and emergencies. San Francisco: AAO, 1985. © 2019 American Academy of Ophthalmology, www.aao.org

- pigment under the conjunctiva
- peaked pupil
- vitreous haemorrhage
- decreased IOP.

When a ruptured globe is suspected use an eye shield, or, if this is not available, a paper cup can be modified and taped over the eye to prevent any pressure being placed on the structures around the eye or on the globe itself. This should be done before the patient is moved. Do not attempt to remove a protruding foreign body from the globe. Relevant questioning at assessment includes when it happened, where the patient thinks the entry point was, duration of pain and whether there are any actions which make symptoms reduce or increase. Ophthalmology should be contacted and the orbit imaged on CT. The patient should be kept nil by mouth.

Specialised ophthalmic operating equipment is required to surgically repair penetrating or perforating injuries, and transfer to a specialist facility should be expedited once any other more serious injuries have been managed. Activities that cause an increase in intraocular pressure must be avoided. These include:

- coughing, gagging
- lying flat
- straining at bowel movements
- bending over
- lifting heavy objects.

Appropriate analgesia should be administered, such as NSAIDs. If opiates are required, consider concurrent antiemetic as vomiting increases intraocular pressure and may cause expulsion of ocular contents. Ondansetron should be used rather than agents that may precipitate dystonic reactions.[62] Sedation may be needed to prevent persistent coughing and vomiting, and aperients may be given to prevent straining during bowel elimination.

SYMPATHETIC OPHTHALMIA

Following repair of a globe which has been severely injured, the major concern is to prevent sympathetic ophthalmia. This is a rare condition characterised by a severe bilateral granulomatous uveitis. It may occur from day 5 to as late as years later. If untreated, the inflammatory response may result in loss of vision in the uninjured eye.[28] It is most probably an autoimmune response that needs aggressive treatment with systemic and topical corticosteroids. Enucleation (removal) of the injured eye may need to be performed, if there is no useful vision and disorganisation of ocular structures is severe, within 10 days to reduce risk of sympathetic ophthalmia. The patient will need psychological and emotional support.

SCLERAL RUPTURE AND VITREOUS HAEMORRHAGE

The most common cause of scleral rupture is penetrating and perforation injury. These injuries may occur in isolation or can be associated with severe facial injuries. Failure to aggressively manage lacerations of the sclera will result in visual loss.[3] In the presence of decreased or no light perception, and/or intraocular pressure of < 10 mmHg, hyphaema and/or chemosis, scleral rupture should be considered.[73] Management is as for a ruptured globe. The vitreous is normally a clear structure. If the retinal vessels or the underlying choroid have been torn by either penetrating or blunt trauma, the severity may vary from trivial to extremely severe haemorrhage. Symptoms include floaters and dark streaks that move with the eye.[74]

EYELID LACERATION

Any laceration other than superficial skin that is not involving the lid margin will need ophthalmic referral. Superficial signs may mask deeper lacerations; check for other injuries, especially in children, as they are poor historians. A full-thickness eyelid laceration is assumed to be a penetrating injury or ruptured globe until proven otherwise; consideration must be given to the possible need for tetanus prophylaxis.[28] X-rays and CT will assist in identifying foreign bodies (corneal, orbital or intraocular) and fractures. The laceration should be irrigated and debrided—do not debride if there is suspicion of penetrating eye injury (PEI)—sutured with 6/0 non-absorbable suture and the sutures removed in 3–5 days; however, repairs can be delayed 24–48 hours with excellent results. Treatment includes regular eye care, nursing in the semi-recumbent position at 30° head up, use of a cold pack to decrease swelling and application of chloramphenicol ointment.

LACERATION TO THE NASOLACRIMAL SYSTEM

Epiphora (tearing) from disruption of the tear drainage system occurs in:

- 0.2% of nasal fractures
- 3% to 4% of Le Fort II or III midfacial fractures and
- 17% to 21% of nasoethmoidal fractures.[75]

The diagnosis of the condition is made when there is a daily build-up of mucopurulent discharge, or epiphora since the injury. It may take several weeks to become apparent and the injury to the nasolacrimal system may have occurred during repair of other mid-facial injuries. Where there is conjunctival infection, give topical antibiotics. If the condition worsens, warm compresses, systemic antibiotics and systemic or topical nasal decongestants are required, and occasionally a needle aspiration. If lacrimal abscess occurs, incision and drainage may be needed.

OPTIC NERVE INJURY

Severe penetrating orbital injuries can result in optic nerve damage and sudden visual loss. Common causes are blunt orbital trauma (closed globe injury), objects severing the optic nerve and facial fractures.[24] The physical findings can include a pupil defect—the affected pupil is dilated and direct pupil reaction to light is absent; check relative afferent pupillary defect (RAPD) using the swing-torch test. Loss of vision can be caused by transaction, avulsion of the optic nerve, optic sheath haemorrhage, pressure on the optic nerve from bone fragments or orbital haemorrhage, direct contusion of the nerve or disruption of the blood supply to the nerve and globe. Often such injuries are irreversible; however, every effort must be made to restore vision. Fine-cut CT or MRI scans of the optic nerve and canal are important for evaluating the extent of injury. Surgical intervention and high-dose intravenous steroids are essential for managing optic nerve injuries. Steroids reduce inflammation and prevent further injury secondary to the inflammatory response.[26]

CHEMICAL BURNS

Initial management at the injury site is to irrigate with running tap water for at least 10 minutes, for example, under a shower with their eye open. Wash the patient's hands and face before commencing the irrigation. Ensure the patient's eyes are opening during the irrigation. Evert the eyelid and commence an irrigation using an intravenous giving set and normal saline on continuous flow. Remove contact lenses as the chemical can track behind the lens and continue to cause injury despite irrigation. Check with the patient what the chemical was, when did it occur? And did it enter both eyes? How much of the chemical entered the eye? If both eyes are affected, rotate the irrigation between them, or set up two intravenous giving sets and irrigate both eyes together. Irrigate the most affected eye first. The quicker the irrigation starts, the better the outcome for vision.[76,77]

- *Acid burns* (e.g. battery acids, sulfuric acid and hydrochloric acid) precipitate tissue proteins that set up barriers against deeper penetration. Damage is usually localised to the area of contact, with the exception of hydrofluoric acid and acids containing heavy metals, which tend to penetrate the cornea and anterior chamber.[34]
- *Alkali burns* (e.g. caustic soda, lime-plaster/cement and ammonia) penetrate the cornea rapidly because of their ability to lyse with the cell membranes. Damage is related to the alkalinity (pH) and permanent injury is determined by the nature and concentration of the chemical burn, as well as the time lapsed before commencement of irrigation.[34]
- *Alcohol and solvent burns* occur from splashes while painting and cleaning. Although the corneal epithelium is frequently burnt, it regenerates rapidly.[1]

The first principle of management is copious irrigation of the eyes with running water for at least 10 minutes. On arrival at the ED, these patients need to be fast-tracked to commence eye irrigation as soon as possible, or, if irrigation is commenced in the ambulance, continue the infusion for at least 30 minutes. The patient's history should include the type of chemical responsible and when it occurred. Note that acid or alkali burns have the same management, but the length of the irrigation may differ. Chemical burns are the only ocular condition where vision is not checked until after management. If the patient has been sprayed with pepper spray/oleoresin capsicum gas/capsicum spray, eye irrigation will reduce some of the effects of tearing and pain.

Irrigation with normal saline or Ringer's solution (closer to pH of tears 7.3) should continue for another 30 minutes; topical anaesthetic is required before commencing the irrigation. At some stage during the irrigation, whether done by ED staff or paramedics, the eyelid needs to be everted to irrigate under the lid. If the department uses a Morgan lens to irrigate, again a manual irrigation with an everted lid is required to remove trapped particles. Lime/cement on contact with the tears will harden and particles will be trapped under the upper lid, causing ongoing pain and a high pH.

Clinical appearance of the eye is a more accurate determination of how long the irrigation continues for.

PRACTICE TIP

Always wait 5-10 minutes after ceasing the irrigation to check pH, otherwise the test will be of the irrigation solution. Use Universal Indicator Paper, but do not use urine pH test strips to test tear pH, as these strips can cause more trauma to the eye. Insert small strips into both the lower lid fornices. Check the pH of both eyes, even if the chemical only entered one, as this provides a reference guide to what the person's normal pH is. Leave in until wet (eyes become quite dry after irrigation), then after 30 seconds read the test strip. Further irrigation will be required if pH is high (alkali burns).[27] The acceptable pH range is 6.5-8.5.[29]

Visual acuity can be checked after the 30-minute irrigation. Then the eye can be examined using a slit lamp to assess damage to the ocular surface and anterior chamber.

Assessment of the chemical burn should be done using topical anaesthetic drops and fluorescein staining to determine the area of surface injury (Fig. 32.23). If ischaemia is seen on limbus (if no ischaemia is present the junction of the cornea and sclera will be injected (red)), continue irrigating for another 30 minutes. Chemical burns where the epithelium is intact or minimally disturbed can wait 24 hours to be reviewed

FIGURE 32.23 FLUORESCEIN STAINING

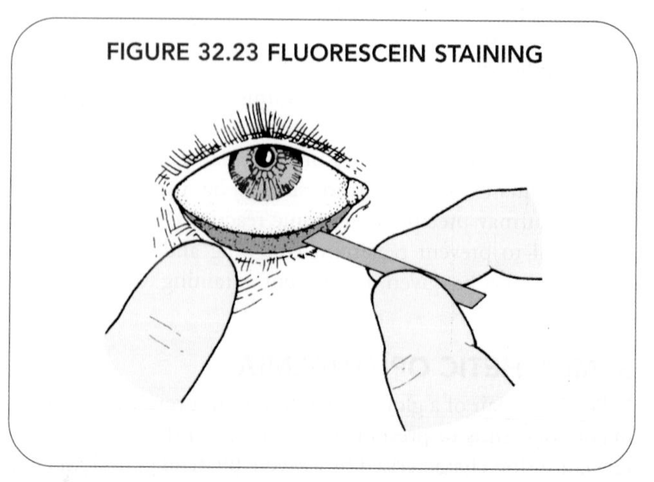

Touch moistened fluorescein strip to inner canthus of lower lid.

by an ophthalmologist. Burns involving more than one-third of the epithelium and the corneal edge, with any clouding of the cornea, are potentially more serious as there may be subsequent melting of the cornea and these should be referred immediately.

For more-serious alkaline burns, 10% citric and ascorbic drops 2-hourly for 48 hours over a week have shown significant outcomes, in combination with 1 g ascorbic acid daily. This regimen has an inhibitory effect on corneal melting. Topical antibiotics (chloramphenicol) and soluble steroids, such as prednisolone phosphate 0.5%, decrease inflammation.[1] A summary of nursing intervention for ocular trauma is provided in Table 32.5.

GLAUCOMA

The glaucomas are a mixed group of disorders that have some common features: optic disc cupping, visual field loss and, usually, raised intraocular pressure. Raised pressure without optic disc damage and visual field loss constitutes ocular hypertension: glaucoma in the absence of high pressure is known as normal, or low-tension, glaucoma.

ACUTE ANGLE-CLOSURE GLAUCOMA

Acute angle-closure glaucoma (AACG) is uncommon, resulting from the rapid and complete closure of the angle between the iris and trabecular meshwork of the anterior chamber. AACG (Fig. 32.24) is characterised by an acute impairment of the outflow of aqueous humour from the anterior chamber. This results in a rapid and severe elevation in the IOP. Pupil block due to synechiae may also lead to high IOP.

IOP rise is abrupt, causing pain, nausea, coloured halos or rainbows around light—physical signs of infection, opaque cornea, IOP > 30 shallow AC and mid dilated pupil. In AACG, the IOP can rise > 60 mmHg and above and damages the corneal endothelium, iris, optical nerve and retina (Fig. 32.25). Optic nerve damage and vision loss can result if untreated. This condition can occur suddenly from moving to a dark room with dim lighting (pupil naturally dilated and iris blocks angles). Topiramate and sulpha drugs can cause swelling of the ciliary body, which will push the iris forwards blocking the drainage angle. If there is ciliary body ischaemia, the use of aqueous humour suppression drugs will be ineffective.[16]

This manifests as severe pain, blurring of vision and redness. The pain can be severe enough to cause nausea and vomiting. Diagnosis is difficult because symptoms can mimic cardiovascular and gastrointestinal processes. Visual disturbances, including transition vision loss at night, can be preceded by halos around light, and in established cases is a result of corneal oedema. Relative hypoxia of the pupillary sphincter due to elevated pressure results in the pupil being oval and non-reactive to light stimulation. Acute angle-closure glaucoma is a true ocular emergency.

Treatment is aimed at lowering the IOP and allowing aqueous humour to flow from the posterior chamber to the anterior chamber. Acetazolamide 500 mg orally or IV may be effective in acutely lowering the IOP and thereby reducing pain, with alpha$_2$-agonists topically (iopidine, apraclonidine). Constriction of the pupil with 2% pilocarpine, a parasympathomimetic, 'breaks' the pupil block and re-establishes flow. The forward bowing of the iris is relieved and the angle opens to allow aqueous humour to leave the eye.[1,32,74] Re-check IOP 1 hour after initial therapy to assess effectiveness. Other

TABLE 32.5 NURSING AND PARAMEDIC INTERVENTION FOR OCULAR TRAUMA

All patients should leave the ED having had their visual acuity checked. For some patients (corneal abrasion), topical anaesthetic may be required before checking vision.

INJURY	NURSING MANAGEMENT
Subconjunctival haemorrhage	Check blood pressure
Vitreous haemorrhage	Slit-lamp assessment to assess if PEI
Hyphaema Ruptured globe Scleral rupture	Pain management Head up 45° or more Movement restriction depending on grade of hyphaema Protect eye with eye shield or modified plastic cup Antiemetics Aperients Caution with the use of anti-thrombolytics Educate patient about avoiding activities that cause an increase in intraocular pressure: • open mouth sneezing • straining during bowel elimination • bending over • lifting heavy objects Encourage deep breathing without persistent coughing
Iris trauma Lens trauma	Pain management Eye toilet Sunglasses to reduce glare
Lacerations, abrasions	Eye toilet–irrigate wound, remove any obvious debris If full-thickness laceration suspect PEI Head up 30° Corneal abrasion–instil local anaesthetic Apply ice/cold packs Chloramphenicol eye ointment may be ordered Eye pad only if strictly necessary due to risk of further corneal disruption
Laceration to nasolacrimal system	As above
Foreign bodies	Topical anaesthetic Remove foreign body Double-pad eye if large epithelial defect; only pad if necessary due to risk of further corneal abrasion Eye toilet if required

PEI: penetrating eye injury.

FIGURE 32.24 ACUTE ANGLE-CLOSURE GLAUCOMA: THE EYE IS RED, THE PUPIL IS OVAL. PART OF THE CORNEA IS HAZY[5]

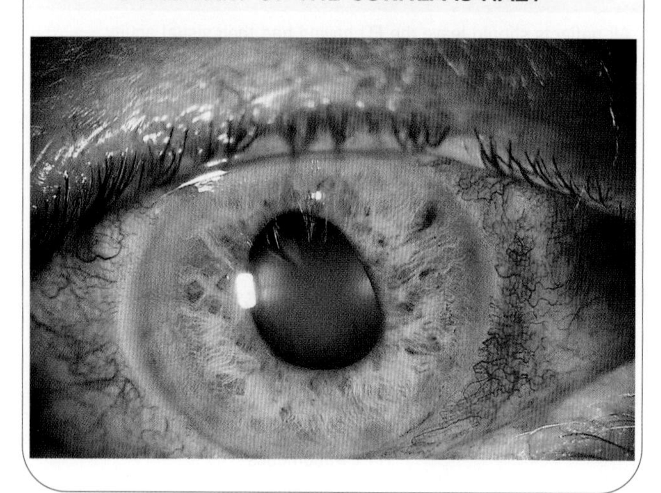

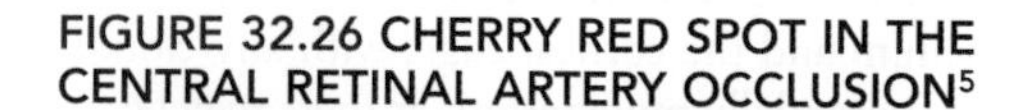

FIGURE 32.26 CHERRY RED SPOT IN THE CENTRAL RETINAL ARTERY OCCLUSION[5]

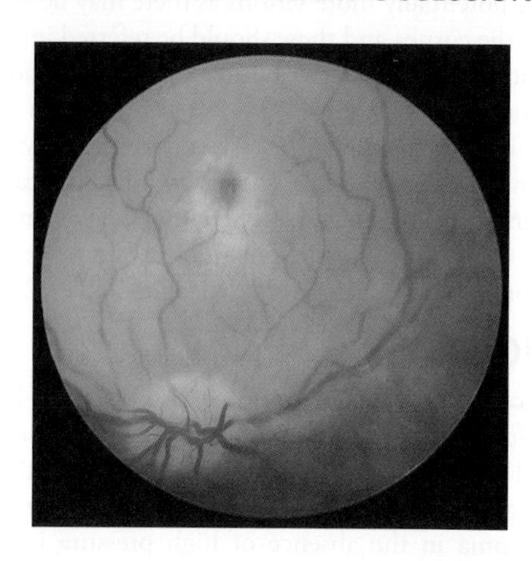

FIGURE 32.25 COMPARISON OF A, NORMAL ANGLE OF EYE WITH, B, CLOSED ANGLE IN ANGLE-CLOSURE GLAUCOMA

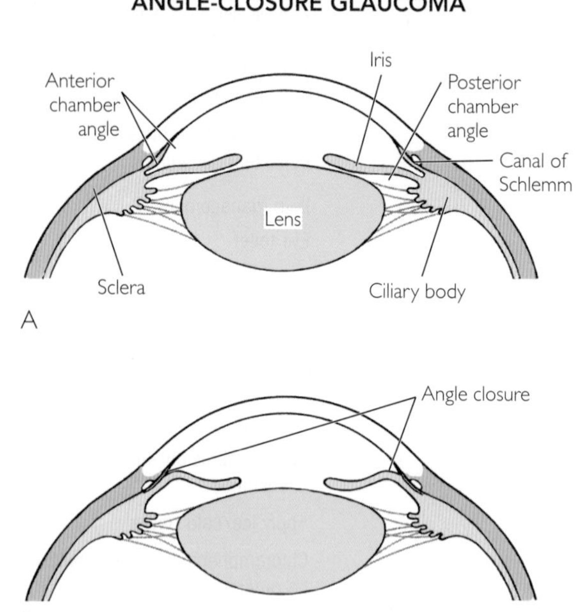

agents include a hyperosmotic (mannitol) if initial therapy is not successful.

After pressure reduction, admission under the care of an ophthalmologist is required for a peripheral iridotomy or a YAG laser iridotomy.

CENTRAL RETINAL ARTERY OCCLUSION

Central retinal artery occlusion (CRAO) produces sudden, painless blindness and is usually limited to one eye. This is a true ocular emergency. Retinal circulation must be re-established within 60–90 minutes to prevent permanent loss of vision. Occasionally, the patient may experience transient episodes of blindness, called amaurosis fugax, in the days prior to the occlusion. This can be equated to a transient ischaemic attack. The patient describes the episode as a shade coming down over the eye. Fundus examination shows creamy white retina oedema (cloudy swelling) with a central red fovea—the 'cherry red spot'—caused by the absence of oedema in the thinner retina at the fovea (Fig. 32.26). An embolus may be seen at any point along the retinal arterioles from the disc to the periphery.

Causes include embolus (carotid and cardiac), thrombosis, giant cell arteritis or a simple angiospasm (rare) associated with migraine or atrial fibrillation. To prevent permanent loss of vision and permanent damage, treatment includes pulsed ocular compression (ocular massage), IOP-lowering drugs, such as acetazolamide 500 mg, and vasodilation techniques, such as breathing into a paper bag. Full cardiac workup or stroke/assessment is required to exclude further embolus. No treatment has been proven effective in managing CRAO.

CENTRAL (BRANCH) RETINAL VEIN OCCLUSION

Central or branch retinal vein occlusion may present as a sudden painless loss of vision. Patients are usually in the older age group, often with systemic hypertension, diabetes mellitus and glaucoma. The characteristic fundus appearance is of extensive haemorrhage with a varied number of cottonwool spots. There may be disc oedema. There is no emergency management specific to vein occlusion. Giant cell arteritis needs to be excluded as a possible diagnosis before discharge from ED. The patient should be urgently referred to an ophthalmologist.

OCULAR PHARMACOLOGY

The effective administration of drugs to the eyes presents unique advantages and challenges. The eye is one of the few organs to which therapeutic agents can be administered directly by non-invasive methods.

Topical anaesthetics last approximately 20 minutes; instruct the patient not to rub their eye during this time. Never send patients home with topical anaesthetic, as its repeated use is toxic to the cornea.

Mydriatic and cycloplegic drops dilate the pupil and paralyse accommodation. The patient's near vision is therefore blurred for a period of time. Patients with darker irises (dark brown/black) who have multiple mydriatics can have dilated pupils for 1–5 days. Driving is not recommended until accommodation returns at 2–4 hours. The patient should be warned that if it is bright outside, they may find themselves dazzled by the sunlight and should wear sunglasses and take extreme care as depth perception can be impaired and falls results. The patient should be encouraged to have a relative take them home or to catch a taxi.[4]

Both patients and emergency nurses should be reminded about the importance of continuing topical medications for eye disease, as prescribed by the ophthalmologist. The emergency nurse should request that any already prescribed medication be brought into the ED on admission for the treating doctor to prescribe it, so that treatment can be continued. For information on commonly used drugs in ophthalmology refer to Table 32.4.

SUMMARY

Most ocular emergencies do not represent a threat to the patient's life; however, these conditions represent a great threat to the patient's wellbeing. Once lost, vision cannot be replaced. The paramedic and emergency nurse should assess patients who present with ocular problems and identify those with actual or potential threats to vision. Traumatic ocular injuries occur in many different circumstances, but must always be considered in any trauma involving the face. The primary survey has precedence no matter how severe the ocular injury. Early recognition of true ocular emergencies and preventing further damage is critical for the patient's optimal visual outcome.

CASE STUDY

Paramedics are sent to the home of a 26-year-old male at 1100. On arrival they find:

- mechanism—just 30 minutes ago the patient was applying chlorine powder in a swimming pool when a large volume of the substance flew up into his face. The patient washed his hands and face after the splash with tap water.
- injury—the patient is complaining of a high level of ocular pain and left eye chemical burn.
- signs—lids oedematous; it is hard to view the eye as the patient has difficulty opening it; heart beat 90 beats/minute, BP 130/80, respiratory rate 22 breaths/minute.

The patient is transported to hospital; paramedics have commenced irrigating the eye with normal saline using a giving set. On arrival at hospital at 1115, the patient is triaged as a category 2, and the irrigation continues by the fast-track nurse for another 30 minutes.

His vision was checked after completion of 2 L normal saline and found to be 6/12; pH was 8.

After examination of the eye by slit lamp, the patient is found to have no significant injury; he is treated for a corneal abrasion with Chloromycetin ointment, to be reviewed by his GP in 2 days.

QUESTIONS

1. If the patient had phoned the emergency department (ED), what initial aid advice could have been given to minimise damage to the ocular surface?
2. When a patient with a chemical eye injury arrives at the ED, what triage category could be assigned?
3. Outline your immediate eye emergency management and provide clinical rationale for each action.

Answers to Case Study Questions can be found on evolve http://evolve.elsevier.com/AU/Curtis/emergency/

REFERENCES

1. Kaufman D, Galbraith J, Walland M. Ocular emergencies. In: Cameron P, Jelinek G, Kelly A, editors. Textbook of adult emergency medicine. 2nd ed. Edinburgh: Churchill Livingstone; 2004.
2. Luk S, Stroman L, Kang S, Natkunarajah M, Duguid G. Patient perception and emotional disturbance in out-of-hour ophthalmic emergency care. Semin Ophthalmol 2017;32(5):559–63.
3. Manolopoulos J. Emergency primary eye care. Tips for diagnosis and acute management. Aust Fam Physician 2002;31(3):233–7.
4. ASORN. Essentials of ophthalmic nursing. 1st ed. San Francisco: American Society of Ophthamic Registered Nurses; 2013.
5. Batterbury M, Bowling B. Ophthalmology: an illustrated colour text. 2nd ed. Sydney: Elsevier; 2005.
6. Ahmad K, Wright M, Lueck CJ. Ptosis. Pract Neurol 2011;11(6):332–40.
7. Hildebrand GD, Fielder AR. Anatomy and physiology of the retina. In: Reynolds J, Olitsky S, editors. Pediatric retina. Heidelberg: Springer 2011.
8. Lewis S, Collier I, Heitkemper M. Medical–surgical nursing: assessment and management of clinical problems. 7th ed. St Louis: Mosby; 2007.
9. Rudy EB. Advanced neurological and neurosurgical nursing. St Louis: Mosby; 1984.
10. Guyton A, Hall J. Textbook of medical physiology. 11th ed. St Louis: WB Saunders; 2006.
11. Brown H, Edwards D, editors. Lewis's medical–surgical nursing: assessment and management of clinical problems. Sydney; Elsevier: 2005.
12. Tortora G, Anagnostakos N. Principles of anatomy and physiology. 6th ed. HarperCollins; 1990.
13. Lewis SM, Heitkemper MM, Dirksen S. Medical–surgical nursing: assessment and management of clinical problems. 6th ed. St Louis: Mosby; 2004.
14. Marsden J. Ophthalmic trauma in accident and emergency. Accid Emerg Nurs 1996;4(2):54–8.
15. Shah SM, Khanna CL. Ophthalmic emergencies for the clinician. Mayo Clin Proc 2020;95(5):1050–8.
16. Ossorio A. Red eye emergencies in primary care. Nurse Pract 2015;40(12):46–53.
17. Pane A. The neuro-ophthalmology survival guide. 2nd ed. London: Elsevier; 2017.
18. Vartsakis G, Fahy G. The profile of patients attending a triaged eye emergency service. Ir J Med Sci 2014;183(4):625–8.
19. Gorovoy IR. Pearls in ophthalmology for the emergency nurse. J Emerg Nurs 2015;41(1):19–22.
20. Madden AC, Simmons D, McCarty CA, Khan MA, Taylor HR. Eye health in rural Australia. Clin Exp Ophthalmol 2002;30(5):316–21.
21. Lavin PJM. Neuro-ophthalmology: ocular motor system. In: Janovic J, Mazziotta J, Pomerory S, editors. Bradley's neurology in clinical practice. 6th ed. London: Elsevier; 2016.
22. Dalpachitra SN, Rahmel BB. Orbital fractures in the emergency department: a review of early assessment and management. Emerg Med J 2016;33:727–31.
23. Huff JS, Austin EW. Neuro-ophthalmology in emergency medicine. Emerg Med Clin North Am 2016;34(4):967–86.
24. Webb LA. Manual of eye emergencies—diagnosis and management. 2nd ed. Edinburgh: Butterworth–Heinemann; 2004.
25. Kumar S, Yogesan K, Hudson B, Tay-Kearney ML, Constable IJ. Emergency eye care in rural Australia: role of internet. Eye 2006;20(12):1342–4.
26. Smith S. Ocular injuries. In: McQuillan K, Rueden K, Hartsock R, editors. Trauma nursing from resuscitation through rehabilitation. 3rd ed. Philadelphia: WB Saunders; 2002.
27. Beal C, Giordano B. Clinical evaluation of red eyes in pediatric patients. J Pediatr Health Care 2016;30(5):506–14.
28. Health NSW, S.O.S. Agency for Clinical Innovation (ACI). Eye emergency manual. Sydney: NSW Health; 2009.
29. Cronau H, Kankanala RR, Mauger T. Diagnosis and management of red eye in primary care. Am Fam Phys 2010;81(2):137–44.
30. Bannon A, Warrick B, McMurray P. Nurse practitioner clinical practice guidelines for the management of conjunctivitis. Sydney: Sydney West Area Health Service, NSW Department of Health; 2005.
31. Sheikh A, Hurwitz B, van Schayck CP, McLean S, Nurmatov U. Antibiotics versus placebo for acute bacterial conjunctivitis. Cochrane Database of System Rev. 2012;9.
32. Royal Flying Doctor Service of Australia (Queensland section). The primary clinical care manual. Brisbane: Queensland Health; 2003.
33. Olitsky SE. Disorders of the conjunctiva. In: Kliegman RM, Stanton BF, Geme JW, editors. Nelson textbook of pediatrics. Philadelphia Nelson; 2016.
34. Tintinalli J, Rothstein RJ, Krome RK. Emergency medicine: a comprehensive study guide. New York: McGraw-Hill; 1985.
35. Channa R, Zafar SN, Canner JK, Haring RS, Schneider EB, Friedman DS. Epidemiology of eye-related emergency department visits. JAMA Ophthalmol 2016;134(3):312–19.
36. Cline D, Ma O, Tintinalli J. Emergency medicine: a comprehensive study guide. Companion handbook. New York: McGraw Hill; 2000.
37. National Occupational Health and Safety Commission. Hospitalisation due to work-related injury in Australia 2000–01. Canberra: Commonwealth of Australia; 2004.
38. Wallace HB, Ferguson RA, Sung J, McKelvie. New Zealand adult ocular trauma study: a 10-year national review of 332,418 cases of ocular injury in adults aged 18 to 99 years. Clin Exp Ophthalmol 2020;48(2):158–68.
39. Victorian Injury Surveillance System (VISS). Injury surveillance and prevention in the Latrobe Valley. Melbourne: Monash University, Accident Research Centre; 1994.

40. WorkSafe Western Australia. Eye injuries. Perth: SafetyLine on the internet; 2006.
41. Shepherd M, Barker R, Scott D. Occupational eye injuries. Injury Bull 2006:2006(90).
42. Casson RJ, Walker JC, Newland HS. Four-year NHS. Review of open eye injuries at the Royal Adelaide Hospital. Clin Exp Ophthalmol 2002;30(1): 15–18.
43. McCarty CA, Fu CL, Taylor HR. Epidemiology of ocular trauma in Australia. Ophthalmology 1999;106(9):1847–52.
44. Archana P, Merriman M. Ocular trauma epidemiology: 10 year retrospective study. NZ Med J 2012;125(1348):61–9.
45. Save Sight Society NZ. Available from: www.savesightsociety.org.nz.
46. Jayasundera T, Vote B, Joondeph B. Golf-related ocular injuries. Clin Exp Ophthalmol 2003;31(2):110–13.
47. Eime R, McCarty C, Finch CF. Unprotected eyes in squash: not seeing the risk of injury. J Sci Med Sport 2005;8(1):92–100.
48. McAllum P, Barnes R, Dickson J. Ocular dangers of fencing wire. N Z Med J 2001;114(1136):332–3.
49. Spencer TJ, Clark B. Self-inflicted superglue injuries. Med J Aust 2004;181(6):341.
50. Winkel KD, Hawdon GM, Ashby K, Ozanne-Smith J. Eye injury after jellyfish sting in temperate Australia. Wilderness Environ Med 2002;13(3):203–5.
51. Fleming PR, Crompton JL, Simpson DA. Neuro-ophthalmological sequelae of horse-related accidents. Clin Exp Ophthalmol 2001;29(4):208–12.
52. Mohamed AA, Banerjee A. Patterns of injury associated with automobile airbag use. Postgrad Med J 1998;74(874):455–8.
53. Lehto KS, Sulander PO, Tervo TM. Do motor vehicle airbags increase risk of ocular injuries in adults? Ophthalmology 2003;110(6):1082–8.
54. Kenney KS, Fanciullo LM. Automobile air bags: friend or foe? A case of air bag-associated ocular trauma and a related literature review. Optometry 2005;76(7):382–6.
55. Kuhn F, Morris R, Witherspoon CD, Mester V. The Birmingham Eye Trauma Terminology system (BETT). J Fr Ophtalmol 2004;27(2):206–10.
56. Moller J, Bordeaux S. Eye injuries in the workplace occurring while wearing recommended and approved eye protection. Adelaide: Research Centre for Injury Studies, Flinders University; 2006.
57. Ambulance Service of New South Wales. Protocol eye injuries—T 13 Revised 2011. Available from: www.ambo.com.au/download/protocol_2011.pdf.
58. Payne A, Simcock P. Eye essentials for every doctor. Edinburgh: Elsevier; 2013.
59. Kadappu S, Silveira S, Martin F. Aetiology and outcome of open and closed globe eye injuries in children. Clin Exp Ophthalmol 2013;41(5):427–34.
60. Chang EL, Bernardino CR. Update on orbital trauma. Curr Opin Ophthalmol 2004;15(5):411–15.
61. Karssemakers LH, Forouzanfar T, Schulten EA, Karagozoglu KH. A simple tool for exposure of the eye in patients with periorbital edema. Am J Emerg Med 2013;31(9):1417.
62. Royal Children's Hospital Melbourne. Acute eye injury in children. Clinical practice guideline. Melbourne: Royal Children's Hospital; 2006.
63. Saccomano SJ, Ferrara LR. Managing corneal abrasions in primary care. Nurse Pract 2014;39(9):1–6.
64. Veugelen T, Coutteel C, Leys A. Flash photography-induced maculopathy. GMS Ophthalmol Cases 2011;1:Doc04.
65. Sehu W, Swamy B, Moore E, Grasso M. Eye emergency manual (EEM). 2nd ed. [online guide]. 2009. p. 56. Available from: https://aci.health.nsw.gov.au/networks/ophthalmology/eye-emergency-manual.
66. Wright K. Textbook of ophthalmology. Baltimore: Williams and Wilkins; 1997.
67. Harris P, Nagy S, Vardaxis N. Mosby's dictionary of medicine, nursing and health professions. Australian and New Zealand edition. Sydney: Elsevier; 2014.
68. Egging D. Ocular emergencies. 5th ed. St Louis: Mosby; 2004.
69. Matthews GP, Das A, Brown S. Visual outcome and ocular survival in patients with retinal detachments secondary to open- or closed-globe injuries. Ophthalmic Surg Lasers 1998;29(1):48–54.
70. Moore E, Feliciano D, Mattox K, editors. Trauma. 7th ed. New York: McGraw-Hill; 2004.
71. Ersanli D, Sonmez M, Unal M. Management of retinal detachment due to closed globe injury by pars plana vitrectomy with and without scleral buckling. Retina 2006;26(1):32–6.
72. Goffstein R, Burton TC. Differentiating traumatic from nontraumatic retinal detachment. Ophthalmology 1982;89(4):361–8.
73. Russell SR, Olsen KR, Folk JC. Predictors of scleral rupture and the role of vitrectomy in severe blunt ocular trauma. Am J Ophthalmol 1988;105(3):253–7.
74. Sherry E, Trieu L, Templeton J, editors. Trauma. Oxford: Oxford University Press; 2003.
75. Osguthorpe JD, Hoang G. Nasolacrimal injuries. Evaluation and management. Otolaryngol Clin North Am 1991;24(1):59–78.
76. Chau JPC, Lee DTF, Lo SHS. A systemic review of methods of eye irrigation for adults and children with ocular chemical burns. Worldviews Evid Based Nurs 2012;9(3):129–38.
77. Schrage N, Burgher F, Blomet J. Chemical ocular burns: new understanding and treatments. New York: Springer-Verlag; 2011.

CHAPTER 33
GYNAECOLOGICAL EMERGENCIES

DIANA WILLIAMSON, BELINDA FLANAGAN AND RACHAEL GRIST

ESSENTIALS

- Any woman of childbearing age presenting with abdominal or pelvic pain should be considered pregnant until proven otherwise.
- Life-threatening conditions, e.g. hypovolaemic shock secondary to blood loss and/or sepsis secondary to an underlying infection, should always be given a high index of suspicion, even in the healthy young patient.
- A detailed gynaecological and sexual health history must be undertaken for every woman presenting with pelvic and/or abdominal pain.
- Trust, rapport, sensitivity and privacy are essential when caring for women with gynaecological emergencies.
- Suspect ectopic pregnancy in women who present following a sudden onset of pain, with lateral pain relating to the tubes or ovaries and crampy midline pain, often uterine in nature.
- Differential diagnoses must always include ectopic pregnancy, appendicitis and peritonitis.
- Women who have been diagnosed with a sexually transmitted infection should also be counselled about referring their sexual partners for testing and treatment (known as 'contact tracing').
- Early referral to an infectious diseases doctor and/or sexual health nurse is paramount if a sexually transmitted infection is suspected or diagnosed.
- The diagnosis of a sexually transmitted infection and the need for emergency contraception can also be an opportunity for a conversation about safer sex practices.

INTRODUCTION

Women with gynaecological problems frequently present for both chronic and acute conditions. Knowledge of the normal reproductive system and functions are necessary to assess and manage women with these problems. Women may not seek care, or, despite seeking care, may not be forthcoming about all symptoms because of embarrassment or lack of knowledge. Cultural sensitivity and the need for privacy are fundamental to any discussion of problems related to the reproductive system.

This chapter focuses on gynaecological emergencies in the non-pregnant woman; obstetric trauma, obstetric emergencies and sexual assault are discussed in Chapters 34, 39 and 46. An overview of the anatomy and physiology of the female reproductive system is provided. Principles associated with assessment for women with gynaecological emergencies are discussed. The chapter addresses common conditions

seen in the emergency context, including vaginal bleeding, pelvic pain, infections, endometrial and ovarian emergencies and sexually transmitted infections (e.g. genital herpes, chlamydia, gonorrhoea, syphilis and genital warts).

ANATOMY AND PHYSIOLOGY

Gynaecological emergencies affect the non-pregnant woman's ovaries, fallopian tubes, uterus, cervix, vagina and external genitalia. External genitalia include the mons pubis, labia majora and minora, clitoris, vestibular glands, hymen, urethral opening and perineum (Fig. 33.1). The vestibule is located between the labia minora and contains the hymen, vaginal orifice, urethral orifice, ducts of the Bartholin's glands and Skene's ducts. Bartholin's glands secrete a mucus-like fluid during excitation. The perineum is a triangular-shaped area between the posterior portion of the vestibule and anus that supports portions of the urogenital and gastrointestinal tracts.[2]

The ovaries, fallopian tubes and uterus are located inside the peritoneal cavity. Ovaries are bilateral oval structures located between the uterus and lateral pelvic wall and diminish in size significantly after menopause. The number of ova present in the ovaries also decreases with age. Each month during ovulation one ovum is usually released by one of the ovaries, which is then transported down the fallopian tubes to the uterus. The fallopian tubes transport the ovum to the uterus through muscular contractions. These bilateral tubes are not contiguous with the ovaries, which means that ova can migrate into the peritoneal cavity. This is the basic mechanism which is thought to lead to endometriosis and ectopic pregnancy in the peritoneal space (Fig. 33.2).[2]

FIGURE 33.1 FEMALE PERINEUM[1]

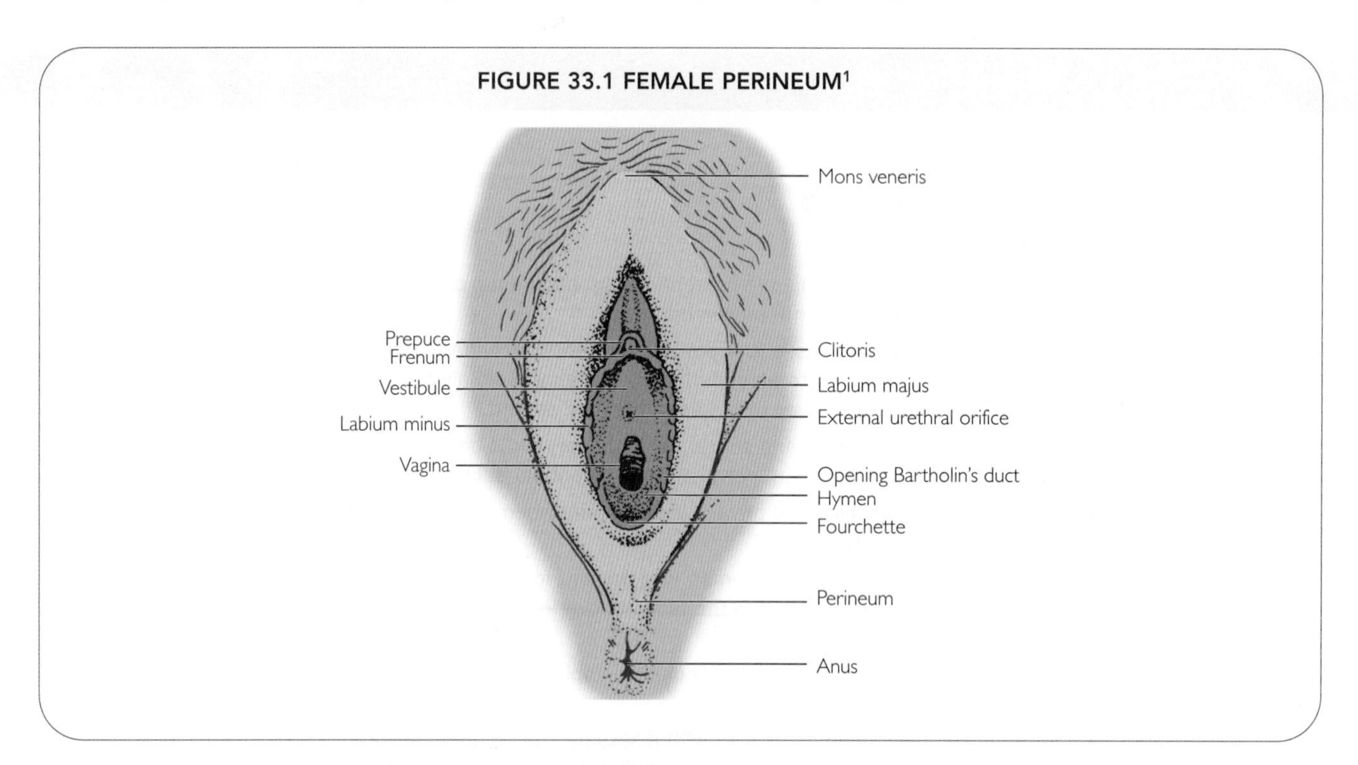

FIGURE 33.2 INTERNAL FEMALE REPRODUCTIVE ORGANS[1]

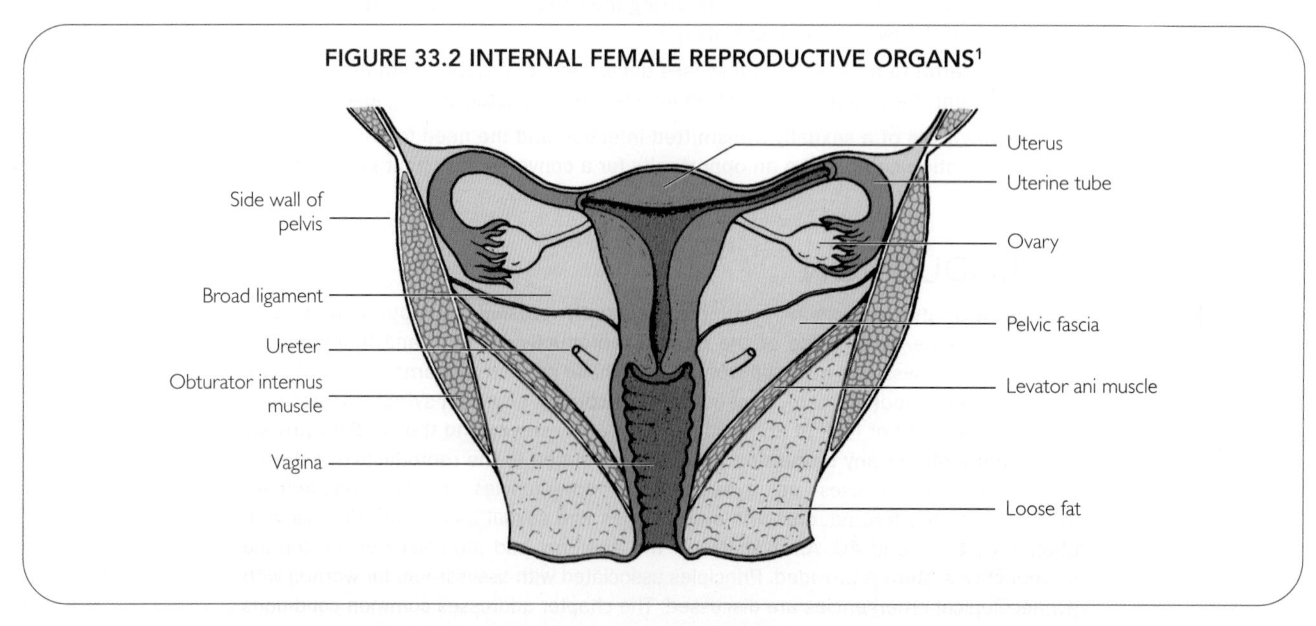

The uterus is a thick-walled organ shaped like an inverted pear. It is suspended in the anterior pelvis above the bladder and anterior to the rectum. A layer of peritoneum covers the superior portion of the uterus and forms the serous layer of the uterine wall. The middle layer of the uterine wall consists of smooth muscle with an inner mucous lining called the endometrium. The cervix provides entrance into the uterus. It is located in the vagina between the bladder on the anterior aspect and rectum posteriorly.[2]

The female sexual cycle consists of ovulation and menstruation, with each cycle regulated by hormones. Changes in hormonal levels prepare the endometrium for implantation of a fertilised ovum. If the ovum is not fertilised, the endometrium sheds the inner lining as menstrual flow. The length of each cycle ranges from 20 to 45 days, with an average of 28 days for most women. Menstrual flow lasts typically 3–7 days.[3]

PATIENT ASSESSMENT

PRE-HOSPITAL CARE

Women presenting with gynaecological issues are at times transported to the emergency department (ED) via ambulance. Pre-hospital care for all patients, including gynaecological presentations, is performed rapidly and efficiently by assessing the patient, employing a systematic patient assessment to identify any major problems and initiate relevant management and medical interventions with the implementation of appropriate protocols and pharmacology for the emerging situation.[4]

The most commonly presenting gynaecological emergency is non-specific pelvic pain, hypovolaemic shock secondary to blood loss and/or sepsis secondary to an underlying infection. It is important for the pre-hospital care provider to have an in-depth knowledge of normal female reproductive anatomy and physiology to identify and treat life-threatening disorders. Shock is discussed in further detail in Chapters 10 and 27.

THE PARAMEDIC

Paramedics may attend a woman with an acute gynaecological condition or an exacerbation of one. In addition to detecting and managing life threat, the paramedic role is to undertake a primary and secondary assessment while ensuring that their systematic approach includes focused questions relating to gynaecological symptoms/disease. These findings will determine the emergent need for transport and early transport to an appropriate facility. Assessment and management of pain and the need for haemostatic resuscitation are more likely presentations in the pre-hospital environment.

THE TRIAGE NURSE

The role of the triage nurse is to undertake a primary assessment to detect and/or recognise potential life-threatening conditions. Only after airway, breathing and circulation (ABC) have been assessed and considered stable should the focus move on to the woman's primary gynaecological complaint (Box 33.1). In this way, the triage nurse can determine within a few minutes the woman's clinical urgency, the need for the allocation of a bed and initiation of first aid or other interventions.[4] Assessment of pain and other symptoms should also be a key focus of the triage assessment. Refer to Chapter 13 for more details on a focused patient assessment.

BOX 33.1 TRIAGE INTERVIEW INFORMATION TO OBTAIN FOR GYNAECOLOGICAL CONDITIONS

- **Confirm the last menstrual period–whether normal, days lasted.**
- **If there is vaginal discharge, explore type, colour, consistency, odour and amount. Confirm if the vaginal discharge occurs around the time of normal period.**
- **Confirm the presence of local redness, swelling, itchiness or pain.**
- **If vaginal bleeding is present, determine the duration and volume.**
- **If bleeding is present, determine if it is associated with sexual intercourse.**
- **Confirm the presence or absence of other signs, such as fevers, vomiting and nausea.**

THE EMERGENCY NURSE

The emergency nurse needs to ensure that immediate interventions take place in the presence of life-threatening conditions. Airway, breathing and circulation must be stabilised, continuous haemodynamic monitoring and interventions such as fluid resuscitation should be commenced and pain should be assessed and managed (see Chapter 16 for haemodynamic monitoring procedures). The emergency nurse must assume that any woman of childbearing age presenting to the ED with abdominal or pelvic pain is pregnant until proven otherwise. This is important, as pregnancy expands the number of diagnoses that need to be considered, some of which are potentially life threatening; for example, ectopic pregnancy.[4]

HISTORY

A detailed gynaecological history must be undertaken for every woman presenting with pelvic or abdominal pain. The history should be undertaken in a private area and approached with sensitivity by a non-judgemental paramedic, nurse or doctor, and without other family members or friends being present, as many of the questions asked may be of a sensitive nature. The assessment of gynaecological conditions in the non-pregnant woman needs to include the presenting complaint with associated symptomology, including abnormal vaginal bleeding, discharge or fever, relevant medical and surgical history, including obstetric and menstrual history, sexual history (and contraception) and pain assessment.[5]

The investigation of pain assists in discriminating between urgent and non-urgent conditions. The differential diagnoses of pain are vast and symptoms are often non-specific. Gynaecological and non-gynaecological conditions can present with referred pain to the back, buttocks, perineum or legs. Recurrent episodes of acute pain may suggest conditions such as primary or secondary dysmenorrhoea. Pain history and assessment can also provide information on the most appropriate analgesic intervention, and for some women, parenteral analgesia will be required. The duration of the complaint may also be suggestive of slow leaking inflammatory mediators or an acute event, such as ischaemia or ruptured cyst.[6]

BOX 33.2 DETAILED HISTORY-TAKING OF PRESENTING PROBLEM[8]

- A description of the bleeding or vaginal discharge, including onset, precipitating factors, volume (number of pads used), colour, presence of clots and duration including abdominal pain, vaginal discharge.
- Pain history including any aggravating or relieving factors: does anything make it better or worse?
- Effects of passing urine, defecation, coughing on bleeding.
- Past medical, surgical, obstetric and gynaecological history: number of pregnancies; gravida/parity; contraception methods; and hormone replacement therapy.
- Menstrual cycle, including relationship of abnormal bleeding to menstrual periods, history of dysmenorrhoea, onset of menopause (if relevant).
- Sexual history, including dyspareunia, history of sexually transmitted infection (STI) and risk factors for infection: lower abdominal pain, pelvic pain, fever, chills, vaginal discharge.
- Experience of sexual assault, trauma or domestic violence.
- History of abnormal cervical screening tests.
- Any symptoms of weakness, syncope, anaemia (tiredness/lethargy) and/or coagulopathy (easy bruising, extensive bleeding).

The clinician should be wary of those women who present following a sudden onset of pain, with unilateral pain relating to the tubes or ovaries and crampy midline pain often uterine in nature as it may indicate a life-threatening ruptured ectopic pregnancy, indicating emergency surgery, especially in a haemodynamically unstable patient.[7]

Other important associated symptoms to elicit include the presence of fever (infection), nausea/vomiting (gastrointestinal), abdominal distension (obstruction), back pain or urinary symptoms (urinary tract infection, UTI). Further information that should be elicited in a detailed history for any woman presenting with a gynaecological emergency can be found in Box 33.2.[6]

PHYSICAL EXAMINATION

The physical examination should include an assessment of the general appearance of the woman and her vital signs, including signs of anaemia. The collection of vital signs (heart rate, blood pressure, respiratory rate, temperature and oxygen saturation) provides a useful reference point to discriminate between more or less urgent cases, including signs and symptoms of hypovolaemic and/or septic shock.[4]

The extent of physical assessment undertaken in the out-of-hospital setting or at triage may be limited because of the environment, but a full abdominal assessment is desirable. An abdominal examination should include inspection, auscultation and palpation of the abdominal and pelvic cavity, assessing for tenderness, guarding, rigidity and masses.[4] This may provide information on tumours and masses (e.g. ovarian cyst), tender areas (e.g. salpingitis) and signs of guarding suggestive of peritonitis (e.g. ruptured ovarian cyst).[4]

While pelvic examinations are not within a paramedic's scope of practice, for nurses a careful pelvic examination is essential. Ensure that privacy and a support person are provided. Inspection includes examination of the lower genital tract, both externally and, if indicated via speculum examination, looking for lacerations, foreign bodies, lesions/polyps, vaginal discharge, cervical os (open or closed) and bleeding from the cervical os. Bimanual pelvic examination is also generally indicated, looking for uterine and adnexal enlargement, masses, irregular contour and cervical motion tenderness (infection), masses (ovarian cyst, torsion or abscess) and to collect swabs. A rectal examination may be necessary to rule out masses, rectal bleeding and presence of haemorrhoids.[4,6]

This should be undertaken bearing in mind the possibility of past sexual abuse or domestic violence. Undertaking a vaginal examination in a woman who is already traumatised by sexual assault (either recently and/or in the past) may only exacerbate pain and trauma already experienced (see Chapter 39).[6]

CLINICAL INVESTIGATIONS

Following a complete history and gynaecological examination, pregnancy should always be excluded first in women of child-bearing age who present with vaginal bleeding. In paramedicine, considering a large-bore cannula, pain and fluid management as per service guidelines is appropriate. On admission to definitive care, insertion of a large-bore cannula and collection of blood samples for full blood count, group and cross-match are essentials. A quantitative beta-hCG (human chorionic gonadotrophin) test and pelvic ultrasound should be performed for confirmation of pregnancy, to exclude a miscarriage or ectopic pregnancy, and a urine specimen collected for evidence of infection, diabetes and/or haematuria.[9]

Other blood tests (endocrine, clotting function, iron studies) should only be undertaken if there is evidence of other underlying disease. In postmenopausal women, referrals should be made for further investigations including a Papanicolaou (Pap) smear, hysteroscopy and histological examination of tissue via a curettage, where clinically indicated.[10]

PSYCHOSOCIAL AND CULTURAL CONSIDERATIONS

Emergency clinicians must be sensitive when assessing a woman with a gynaecological condition. A public environment or even being in the presence of family and friends at home is not always conducive to private and sensitive discussions, and may prevent women from openly discussing problems.[6]

It is always preferable that the woman should be provided privacy while undertaking risk screening and assessment. A single room, for example, will ensure privacy, as the woman will require an abdominal palpation and, most likely, a vaginal examination. In the presence of a life-threatening event, however, the allocation of a single room may be inappropriate and unsafe. In addition, ensuring cultural safety must always be considered when discussing or assessing women.

As Australia and Aotearoa New Zealand are becoming increasingly multicultural, expected variations in care should be considered. In the context of gynaecological emergencies, certain cultural groups will need to see female clinicians only, health beliefs and health-seeking behaviours may be different and clinicians need to understand the influence of the caregiver's gender on the disclosure of sensitive information which may impact on the delivery of appropriate care.[11]

Female genital mutilation (FGM) is commonly performed in parts of Africa, with migrants from Somalia, Ethiopia, Sudan and Egypt, and sometimes the Middle East and Asia, comprising the majority of affected women seen in Australia. In Somalia and Sudan, more than 80% of women have undergone FGM, while the practice is banned in countries like Australia and Aotearoa New Zealand, meaning that presentations due to immediate complications is unlikely. Long-term gynaecological consequences of FGM include recurrent urinary tract infection (prolonged voiding time, difficulty obtaining a mid-stream urine specimen for analysis), recurrent vaginal infections, menstrual problems: haematocolpos, retained menstrual clots, as well as local scar complications (keloid, dermal cysts), local pain (chronic neuropathic pain), difficulty with even minor gynaecological procedures (e.g. Pap smear), as well as the psychological sequelae of post-traumatic stress disorder, anxiety and depression among these women.[11]

It is important to be culturally responsive and non-judgemental in these situations and to demonstrate knowledge and respect with appropriate referral for psychological support if required.[6]

PRACTICE TIP

Understand how gender, power and cultural differences can influence the dynamics of the relationship between the patient and healthcare provider and consequent effective communication. Be sensitive to history and examination processes and, if not sure, seek appropriate advice.

CLINICAL PRESENTATIONS

VAGINAL BLEEDING

There are several conditions that may cause vaginal bleeding. Such conditions may warrant a call to emergency services or presentation to an ED. Vaginal bleeding can occur in pregnant, non-pregnant and postmenopausal women, or female children. This section addresses vaginal bleeding in the non-pregnant woman. For bleeding in the pregnant woman, refer to Chapter 34.

TYPES AND CAUSES OF BLEEDING

Primary dysmenorrhagia is a common presenting problem for young women and is defined as pain and cramping during menstruation that interferes with normal activities. It is usually treated with non-steroidal anti-inflammatory drugs (NSAIDs) or the oral contraceptive pill (OCP). Some alternative therapies have also been shown to relieve or decrease pain in women suffering from primary dysmenorrhoea.[12]

PRACTICE TIP

In order to support the delivery of evidence-based clinical care the Australian Commission on Safety and Quality in Health Care (ACSQHC) has developed a Clinical Care Standard which addresses heavy menstrual bleeding.[13]

PRACTICE TIP

ALTERNATIVE THERAPIES FOR PRIMARY DYSMENORRHEA[14]

- Heating pads to the lower abdomen
- Exercise
- Massage
- Acupuncture
- Hypnosis
- Transcutaneous electrical stimulation (TENS)

Abnormal uterine bleeding refers to any bleeding that is outside of the normal menstrual cycle and can involve either too much or not enough bleeding. Dysfunctional uterine bleeding (DUB) is heavy and/or irregular bleeding that cannot be attributed to another cause.[15]

PRACTICE TIP

TERMS USED TO DESCRIBE ABNORMAL UTERINE BLEEDING[14]

- *Dysmenorrhoea*—the absence of a menstrual period in a woman of reproductive age
- *Oligomenorrhoea*—infrequent (or, in occasional usage, very light) menstruation > 35 days apart
- *Menorrhagia*—abnormally heavy and prolonged menstrual period at regular intervals
- *Metrorrhagia*—uterine bleeding at irregular intervals, particularly between the expected menstrual periods
- *Menometrorrhagia*—a condition in which prolonged or excessive uterine bleeding occurs irregularly and more frequently than normal.

DIAGNOSIS

The typical causes of abnormal vaginal bleeding include menorrhagia, intermenstrual bleeding, metrorrhagia and post-coital bleeding. The three most common causes of menometrorrhagia are uterine fibroids, adenomyosis and DUB. Other less common causes include endometrial polyps, endometrial carcinoma, presence of an intrauterine device (IUD), pelvic inflammatory disease (PID) and some coagulation disorders.

Typical pelvic findings for the most common causes of menorrhagia are:

- an abnormal-sized uterus
- an asymptomatically enlarged uterus (fibroids)
- a symmetrically enlarged uterus (adenomyosis).[16]

Abnormal vaginal bleeding in premenopausal women is bleeding occurring outside the regular cycle. Vaginal bleeding after menopause must always be investigated because of the increased risk of malignancy. Postmenopausal causes of vaginal bleeding include atrophic endometritis, vaginitis, endometrial cancer, cervical polyps, endometrial hyperplasia and exogenous oestrogens. Vaginal bleeding usually presents pain-free and is often considered as prolonged menorrhagia.[14,16]

Management

Most non-pregnant women presenting with abnormal vaginal bleeding do not require immediate interventions unless they prove to be haemodynamically unstable. The treatment regimens should be aimed at the specific underlying aetiology. There are four main treatment options for women with menorrhagia:

- pharmacotherapy
- medicated IUDs
- conservative surgical management
- hysterectomy.[14]

None of these options should be commenced in the ED due to the inability to follow up these women, and they should be referred to an appropriate gynaecological practitioner for decisions about treatment.

In postmenopausal women, prolonged bleeding (more than 12 months) after the last menstrual period has ceased should be investigated. This commonly occurs in the presence of atrophic endometriosis, and hormone replacement therapy will usually control symptoms. However, any postmenopausal bleeding should be considered abnormal and be investigated, given the increased risk of reproductive cancers in women in this age group. A referral to an appropriate gynaecological practitioner for a Pap smear, endometrial biopsy and/or ultrasound is necessary to definitively rule out malignancy and allow ongoing continuity of care.[14]

MISCARRIAGE

In Australia and Aotearoa New Zealand, miscarriage is generally defined as the loss of a pregnancy related to early pregnancy complications within the first 20 completed weeks of pregnancy or a birthweight less than 400 grams.[17] An estimated 10–20% of post-implantation pregnancies end in spontaneous miscarriage and 1.5–2% of pregnancies end due to an ectopic pregnancy.[18] Recent advances have led to earlier diagnosis and the adoption of more conservative treatment options. An ambulance response normally requires supportive care and transport to appropriate definitive care; however, many of these cases are managed on an outpatient or day-case basis to increase patient satisfaction and promote more efficient use of resources. Dedicated EPAS (Early Pregnancy Assessment Services) have been established across various locations in Australia, based on international models with recognised clinical benefits associated with the service.[9]

The terminology of miscarriage has changed over the last two decades in line with research and the significant psychological impact which women found distressing. The World Health Organization (WHO) classes miscarriage into the following categories:

- *Threatened miscarriage:* a threat of miscarriage with associated vaginal bleeding, with or without lower abdominal pain, which occurs in a pregnancy of < 22 weeks' gestation. The pregnancy may continue.
- *Inevitable miscarriage:* a miscarriage considered inevitable when specific clinical features indicate that a pregnancy is in the process of physiological expulsion. The pregnancy will not continue and will proceed to incomplete or complete miscarriage.
- *Incomplete miscarriage:* a miscarriage in which early products of pregnancy are partially expelled. Many incomplete miscarriages may be unrecognised missed miscarriages.
- *Complete miscarriage:* a miscarriage in which early products of pregnancy are completely expelled.[9]
- Other types of miscarriage:
  - *Missed miscarriage:* a miscarriage that is non-viable and confirmed on ultrasound, even in the absence of clinical features such as bleeding. Some women do recall a transient and/or brownish vaginal discharge, or a vague reduction in symptoms of early pregnancy.
  - *Recurrent miscarriage:* the spontaneous loss of ≥ 3 consecutive pregnancies before 22 completed weeks is regarded as recurrent miscarriage.[9]

Diagnosis

All women who present to the ED with a positive pregnancy test, abdominal and/or pelvic pain and bleeding require investigation for potential miscarriage. Blood is taken for a quantitative beta-hCG (beta-human chorionic gonadotrophin), which is used to confirm pregnancy and to assist the diagnosis of an ectopic pregnancy. During early pregnancy, hCG levels in the blood double every 2 to 3 days, but ectopic pregnancies normally have a longer doubling time.[19]

Blood grouping is also taken to determine Rhesus type. Rhesus disease is a condition where the antibodies in a pregnant woman's blood can destroy her baby's blood cells and occurs when the mother has rhesus-negative blood (RhD negative) and the baby in her womb has rhesus-positive blood (RhD positive). When a woman with RhD negative blood is exposed to RhD positive blood, sensitisation develops. This can occur during childbirth as their blood combines in the bloodstream, impacting all subsequent pregnancies. Rhesus disease is preventable by administering Rh(D) immunoglobulin (anti-D) within 72 hours of a sensitising event.[9,19]

An ultrasound is necessary to confirm the diagnosis of complete miscarriage and has a positive predictive value of 98%.[9]

Management

A thorough systematic clinical assessment is essential, especially if the patient is unwell. All vital observations, including an assessment of the vaginal blood loss, should be attended to. Paramedics are often the first to attend a woman who may have miscarried prior to or during an episode of care. If products of conception are visible, the fetal tissue or a noticeably developed baby should be retrieved and transported to hospital respectfully, ensuring that the parents can see and hold the baby, as it is an important part of the grieving process. In the emergency department (ED) the abdomen is examined for tenderness and a bimanual pelvic or speculum examination is considered if the woman is bleeding heavily or unwell. If products of conception are visible in the cervix they should be removed; consider taking swabs if signs of infection are evident. Any available products of conception should be sent to histology for processing.[20]

Appropriate psychological support should be offered, especially if the woman is alone, as this is usually an unexpected event with psychological sequelae associated with loss. The provision of information on miscarriage should be offered to each woman or couple to ensure that they are well informed of decisions that need to be made in relation to options, referrals and the sensitive issue relating to the disposal of fetal tissue.[20]

Appropriate referral and discharge processes are important to ensure the safety and quality of patient care. Women who are stable and suitable for discharge should be referred to the most appropriate follow-up care, for example, an obstetrician, general practitioner (GP) or appropriate service as available in their locality. Women requiring in-patient care, or where there is any question regarding best management, must be referred to the obstetric and gynaecological service.[20]

PRACTICE TIP

Presence of pain, hypotension, tachycardia and anaemia warrant exclusion of a life-threatening differential diagnosis, such as an ectopic pregnancy.

- The experience of a miscarriage is associated with a psychological impact of varying intensity in the short or long term, or both. All women should be offered counselling or psychological support.
- Anti-D is given within 72 hours of bleeding; it is the responsibility of any doctor or nurse who has seen the patient to ensure this occurs.

POSTPARTUM HAEMORRHAGE

Postpartum haemorrhage (PPH) is a growing concern, particularly as unplanned out-of-hospital birth rates increase and women are encouraged to partake in early postpartum hospital discharge programs. According to The Royal Australian and New Zealand College of Obstetricians and Gynaecologists, PPH within Australia and Aotearoa New Zealand remains a major cause of both maternal mortality and morbidity. It is common and in Australia the incidence is between 5 and 15%.[21] While most of these cases are minor, requiring little active management and causing minimal morbidity, it must be remembered that PPH remains a leading cause of maternal death, both globally and within the Australian and Aotearoa New Zealand context.[21]

PPH can be classified as early, which occurs within 24 hours of the birth and is usually caused by uterine atony or retained placenta. Late PPH, or secondary PPH, occurs from 24 hours to 6 weeks after delivery, and is generally due to retained placental tissue and/or infection; 99% of all PPH is classified as early.[21]

Diagnosis

PPH is the loss of 500 mL or more of blood during puerperium and severe PPH as loss of 1000 mL or more of blood.[22] The clinical diagnosis of PPH is characterised by heavy symptomatic vaginal bleeding post-birth that makes the patient symptomatic (e.g. pallor, light-headedness, weakness, palpitations, diaphoresis, restlessness, confusion, air hunger, syncope) and/or results in signs of hypovolaemia (e.g. hypotension, tachycardia, oliguria, oxygen saturation $< 95\%$).[21]

Pre-hospital management

Ambulance clinical practice guidelines (CPGs) determine initial treatment and management plans for women who are transported with a PPH. Common to all locally authorised CPGs are a primary assessment of the woman which includes the 4 Ts of primary PPH—Tone (uterine atony), Trauma (to the genital structures), Tissue (retention of placenta or membranes) and Thrombin (coagulopathy), as well as vital signs.[21]

Immediate interventions are commenced as appropriate—gentle massage of the uterine fundus if it is not firm, large-bore cannula, uterotonic medications, high-flow oxygen, fluid resuscitation, if indicated, bimanual compression and applying direct pressure to any visible lacerations. For any retained products, continuing to massage the fundus is encouraged while observing vaginal loss. In cases where an atonic uterus does not respond to uterotonic medications (now a standard in most services), and where the woman is haemodynamically compromised, external abdominal aortic compression and/or bimanual compression is indicated. Pain is managed as per the individual state or territory CPGs and urgent transport is necessitated. The continuing use of medications to induce uterine contractions should be referred to within authorised local CPGs.[21,23,24]

PRACTICE TIP

Minimal on-scene time is necessary to stabilise the mother and baby for transport to definitive care.

- The woman with a PPH should be treated like any other haemorrhaging patient and resuscitation measures should be commenced accordingly.

Management

On arrival at the ED, a primary assessment is undertaken to determine the woman's clinical urgency; she should be positioned flat and kept warm. Initial administration of high-flow oxygen is supported and wide-bore intravenous access should be established, with blood sent for full blood count, coagulation profile and cross-match. Blood cultures must be taken if the woman is febrile, or the vaginal blood/discharge is malodorous. Infusion of warmed fluids is ideal if fluids are indicated. The use of group-specific or group O RhD-negative blood should be given early to restore the woman's oxygen-carrying capacity and massive transfusion protocols administered where required. Facilities that provide obstetric care should adhere to a massive transfusion protocol and be familiar in its use.[21,23]

Early consultation with the obstetrics and gynaecology team is crucial to encourage good transition and communication from resuscitative to definitive care.[21]

A secondary survey and a more focused examination are necessary to assess the cause of the PPH, as previously described in pre-hospital care, which specifically refers to uterine atony, uterine rupture, trauma, retained placental tissue, uterine inversion and thrombosis.[24] Bedside ultrasonography (FAST) is used diagnostically to identify the cause and definitive care is undertaken based on these findings.[24]

PRACTICE TIP

The obstetrician/gynaecologist consultant should be contacted immediately as care for the patient is initiated to encourage good transition and communication from resuscitative care to definitive care.

PELVIC PAIN

Lower abdominal or pelvic pain is another common reason for a call to emergency services or presentation to an ED, particularly in young women. Pelvic pain can be acute, chronic or cyclic and will not always be pathological. A systematic approach will assist the diagnosis and management.[25]

Pelvic pain may originate from the genital tract, urinary tract or bowel, or may be referred from the musculoskeletal system. Physiological midcycle pelvic pain (Mittelschmerz) may be present at the time of ovulation in some women who are not taking the OCP.[26]

Pain may be psychosomatic, masking a psychological issue or concern. Underlying depression, anxiety state, sexual problem or history of domestic or sexual violence should always be kept in mind as a primary or secondary reason for pelvic pain.[27]

Differentiating urgent from non-urgent causes of pelvic pain is often the main challenge faced by emergency clinicians. Pelvic pain that lasts for > 6 months is considered chronic as opposed to sub-acute pain described as 3–6-month duration or acute pain which is < 3 months.[27,28] The common gynaecological and non-gynaecological causes of pelvic pain are summarised in the following sections.

Acute pelvic pain

The gynaecological causes of acute pelvic pain are outlined in Box 33.3. In the non-pregnant woman, the initial focus should be on differentiating abdominal pain causes from those that relate to gastrointestinal rather than pelvic causes. The non-gynaecological causes of acute pelvic pain are covered in other chapters in this text, and include:

- urological causes—cystitis, pyelonephritis, ureteric colic (see Chapter 25)
- gastrointestinal causes—acute appendicitis, diverticulitis, bowel obstruction (see Chapter 24)
- thrombotic causes—mesenteric thrombosis (see Chapter 46).

PRACTICE TIP[27]

- Nausea and vomiting more commonly occur with a gastrointestinal cause.
- Cervical motion tenderness suggests pain originating from the pelvic organs.

BOX 33.3 GYNAECOLOGICAL CAUSES OF ACUTE PELVIC PAIN[14]

- Threatened, incomplete or septic abortion (see Chapter 34)
- Ectopic pregnancy (see Chapter 34)
- Acute salpingitis
- Tubal or ovarian abscess
- Endometritis
- Pelvic peritonitis
- Complications of an ovarian cyst–rupture, haemorrhage into a cyst, torsion
- Ovulation pain
- Retrograde menstruation
- Primary dysmenorrhoea
- Trauma and/or sexual assault (see Chapters 39 and 40).

Chronic pelvic pain

Chronic pelvic pain is pain that is unrelated to pregnancy or the menstrual cycle and has been present for 6 months or more.[27,29] Common gynaecological causes of chronic pelvic pain are outlined in Box 33.4. The non-gynaecological causes of chronic pelvic pain are covered in other chapters in this text, and include:

- urological causes—bladder dysfunction, urinary tract calculi (see Chapter 25)
- gastrointestinal causes—appendiceal abscess, intra-abdominal adhesions, diverticulitis, irritable bowel syndrome, inflammatory bowel disease, Crohn's disease, malignancy of the large or small intestine (see Chapter 24)
- musculoskeletal causes—osteoarthritis, lumbar disc protrusion, pelvic nerve entrapment or other musculoskeletal or neurological disorders (see Chapter 48).

Diagnosis

An abdominal examination should assess for tenderness, guarding, rebound, abdominal distension or masses, and a vaginal examination (bimanual and speculum) may be indicated to assess for cervical motion tenderness, masses (ovarian cyst, torsion or abscess) and to collect swabs. Watch for diffuse peritoneal signs indicating a ruptured hollow viscus, pelvic inflammatory disease (PID) or an intra-abdominal haemorrhage (ectopic or ruptured ovarian cyst).[15]

Management

The management of pelvic pain will depend on the differential diagnoses that the history and examination suggest. It will also depend on the urgent nature of the problem; that is, how acutely unwell the woman is on presentation. It is essential that the clinician discuss the possible diagnoses with the woman and together plan the most appropriate management.[15,27]

Women who have long-standing chronic pelvic pain have often already seen many doctors and nurses, often with little relief. There may be hostility towards clinical staff, especially if the woman feels that her pain is being dismissed as 'psychological'. Studies have also shown that up to 60% of women with chronic pelvic pain have a history of sexual abuse with a significant association between physical abuse and chronic pelvic pain.[16,27]

It is essential to allow time to enable the woman to explore her feelings about her pain and her past care.[26] This may not always be feasible or possible in a busy ED; however, an effort should be made to ensure that the woman feels she is being listened to. Referral to a multi-disciplinary pain clinic or team may enable the multifaceted nature of chronic pelvic pain to be

BOX 33.4 COMMON GYNAECOLOGICAL CAUSES OF CHRONIC PELVIC PAIN[14]

- Chronic pelvic inflammatory disease
- Endometriosis
- Ovarian masses, both benign and malignant
- Complications of uterine fibroids
- Pelvic vascular congestion syndrome
- Response to past sexual abuse or domestic violence

addressed. If violence or abuse issues are disclosed, referral to the appropriate services is indicated.

PELVIC INFLAMMATORY DISEASE

Pelvic inflammatory disease (PID) refers to infections of the upper genital tract and includes endometritis, salpingitis, tubo-ovarian abscesses and pelvic peritonitis.[28,30]

The two most common causative organisms for PID are *Chlamydia trachomatis* and *Neisseria gonorrhoeae*.[28,30]

The major long-term consequences of unrecognised and untreated PID include scarring of the fallopian tubes leading to infertility (12%) and an increased risk of ectopic pregnancies.[28,30]

Diagnosis

The most frequent symptoms include acute pelvic pain, febrile illness, abdominal guarding and rebound tenderness, vaginal discharge and raised white cell count.[30] Postcoital or intermenstrual bleeding may also present as symptoms. During a vaginal examination the clinician should look for tenderness when moving the cervix laterally and/or adnexal or uterine tenderness.[28,30]

A high index of suspicion is required if the diagnosis of PID is not to be missed. The diagnosis is generally a clinical one based on signs and symptoms elicited during the examination, regardless of the results of the investigations.[28,30] Nonetheless, investigations should still be undertaken (Box 33.5).

Management

The management will depend on the causative organism. Common antibiotics include azithromycin, ceftriaxone, doxy-cycline and metronidazole. The most recent Therapeutic Guidelines: Antibiotics should guide management (see Useful websites for full details). In most cases, a patient with PID can be managed as an outpatient; however, clinicians should consider hospitalisation when the woman is pregnant or there is fever > 38.3°C, severe pain, tubo-ovarian abscess, concern for non-compliance and where outpatient therapy has failed.[30]

BOX 33.5 INVESTIGATIONS IN PELVIC INFLAMMATORY DISEASE[28,31]

- **Urine and/or serum hCG level to exclude pregnancy**
- **Full blood count and blood cultures**
- **Urine microscopy for culture**
- **Endocervical swab for chlamydia and gonorrhoea PCR and microscopy culture**
- **Pelvic ultrasound**
- **Screening for other STIs**
- **Investigation and treatment of the partner as required**

hCG: human chorionic gonadotrophin; PCR: polymerase chain reaction; STI: sexually transmitted infection.

OVARIAN EMERGENCIES

OVARIAN CYST

The development of an ovarian cyst, a small sac on the ovary, usually occurs as a result of hormonal level imbalance. An ovarian cyst is likely to develop from the following condition: if the developing Graafian follicle produces insufficient levels of oestrogen, then luteinising hormone (LH) levels may be inadequate to bring about ovulation. In this event the follicle-stimulating hormone (FSH) continues secretion resulting in follicle growth. Normally growth is restricted to about 2 cm. However, in this situation, growth is unrestricted and size may reach up to 8–10 cm.[15,16,32] Generally on presentation the woman reports significant pain usually unilaterally, delayed menstruation or menorrhagia. If the cyst has ruptured, life-threatening symptoms include acute pelvic or abdominal pain, peritonism and/or bleeding. For the most part, however, ovarian cysts are benign and asymptomatic and are often found incidentally.[33]

Diagnosis

The differential diagnosis must exclude ectopic pregnancy, appendicitis and peritonitis. The confirmation of hCG levels is important to rule out ectopic pregnancy. The ability to palpate the ovaries is usually suggestive of rupture of an ovarian cyst with localised haemorrhage. The definitive diagnostic test is a pelvic ultrasound which can guide monitoring and treatment options.[15,16,32]

Management

The main aim of emergency management includes pain control. NSAIDs are usually sufficient; however, for women with severe pain, narcotic analgesia may be necessary.[34] Close observation is necessary, with regular haematocrit and haemoglobin blood testing. Gynaecological referral is needed for potential operative management; however, surgical intervention is rarely required unless hypovolaemia is present.[34]

OVARIAN TORSION

In the presence of a tumour, such as a cystic teratoma, the fallopian tube or ovary can twist on itself to develop what is commonly referred to as torsion. These tumours are usually benign. Unilateral pain in the lower abdomen and possibly the flank is one of the most common presenting symptoms and fevers, dysuria and/or vomiting and nausea can be present.[35] The differential diagnosis of appendicitis must be excluded.

Diagnosis

While there may be an adnexal mass and tenderness, an ovarian torsion is notoriously difficult to diagnose.[16] Blood tests might confirm an elevated white cell count, although this can be a non-specific finding. The definitive test for torsion is a pelvic ultrasound with Doppler flow studies, but even this is often equivocal.[35]

Management

General management includes analgesia and appropriate resuscitation measures. If the torsion does not spontaneously resolve or the clinical diagnosis cannot be ruled out, then, despite an equivocal ultrasound, surgical intervention is necessary. If torsion is suspected, urgent gynaecological referral is needed for potential operative management.[16,35]

OVARIAN HYPERSTIMULATION SYNDROME

Ovarian hyperstimulation syndrome (OHSS) is a known complication of ovarian stimulation, occurring in 1–3% of patients during fertility treatment.[36] The aim of the treatment is to stimulate ovulation and produce multiple follicles without causing OHSS, which can be a potentially fatal condition. To stimulate ovulation, FSH injections (e.g. Gonal-F or Puregon) are administered, followed by a second injection of the antagonist (e.g. Cetrotide or Orgalutron) over a period of approximately 2 weeks.[36,37]

Careful monitoring of women is achieved using vaginal ultrasound and blood tests (serum oestradiol concentration) in order to determine the optimum number and size of developing follicles prior to egg collection. If untreated, OHSS can lead to life-threatening complications, including ascites, pleural and pericardial effusion, haemo-concentration, coagulopathy, adult respiratory distress syndrome, renal failure or even death.[36–38] OHSS has also been reported to have occurred spontaneously, unrelated to fertility treatments.[39]

Diagnosis

Abdominal swelling and fluid retention is a side-effect of fertility treatments, and in 1% of cases it can be severe, requiring hospital admission and treatment. If OHSS does occur, it is usually evident 2–8 days after egg collection and subsides 2–3 weeks later if a pregnancy does not occur. Where symptoms are associated with a pregnancy, then in up to 50% of cases the symptoms are more prolonged and severe.[36]

Symptoms requiring urgent medical attention include severe nausea and vomiting, increased abdominal pain, diarrhoea, shortness of breath, increasing thirst and decreased urine output.[36,37] On ultrasound the ovaries appear enlarged, sometimes greater than 10 cm, with multiple follicles and cysts; areas of haemorrhage within the ovary and free fluid may be seen surrounding the uterus or within the peritoneal cavity.[36]

Management

Mild symptoms are usually self-resolving and easily treated by rest, fluids (2–3 L per day) and mild pain relief. More severe symptoms, however, require hospitalisation with intravenous fluids, monitoring of renal function, anticoagulant therapy and sometimes drainage of fluid (ascites) from the abdominal cavity.[36]

INFECTIONS

TOXIC SHOCK SYNDROME

Toxic shock syndrome (TSS) was identified in the early 1980s and was associated largely with menses and tampon use (50–70%). The association between menses, tampon use and TSS has largely resolved in recent times with a declining annual incidence in Australia of 1–2 in 100,000 with an associated 3% case fatality[40] as a result of changes in the manufacturing of tampons. Today it is known that TSS is caused by *Staphylococcus aureus* and can occur in all age groups, and is associated with a range of conditions, for example, burns, surgery, trauma or childbirth. The incidence of non-menstrual TSS remains relatively constant with a 6% case fatality rate.[40,41]

Of greater concern and more prominent are streptococcal infections, which clinically mimic TSS. Similarly, these infections can result in severe systemic reactions, often presenting as a life-threatening event.[32,40,41] Streptococcal TSS is more clinically relevant for the emergency nurse as the incidence of this infection is more common and not isolated to gynaecological infections. Streptococcal infection may occur from either invasive or non-invasive infections.

Diagnosis

The clinical presentation usually involves a constellation of signs and symptoms associated with a septic presentation, and many could pose a life-threatening illness. Most commonly, fever (temperature > 38.9°C) is present and associated with hypotension and a diffuse macular erythematous rash. Scaling of the palms and hands (desquamation) is often present 1–2 weeks after the acute illness. Multisystem involvement, such as renal (elevated creatinine, urea nitrogen or the presence of a urinary tract infection), neurological (altered level of consciousness) and gastrointestinal (vomiting and/or diarrhoea), can also be evident.[32,41]

For suspected TSS in the febrile woman, a full septic work-up is necessary. This usually includes blood cultures, swabs, urinalysis, radiological investigations and a full blood count. It must be noted, however, that blood cultures are often negative as the exotoxin is absorbed through the vaginal mucosa.[40,41] Hospitalisation is likely when these investigations are indicated. A septic work-up may not be indicated if a recognised source for the sepsis is identified. For further information on the management of septic shock, refer to Chapters 10 and 27.

Management

Hospital admission with supportive and antibiotic therapy is required in most cases due to the significant mortality rate, 3–6%, of this disease. If a tampon is present, this must be removed.[40,41] For more severe cases where haemodynamic instability is evident, admission to an intensive care unit may be necessary. Supportive therapy usually involves airway management, fluids and drugs for refractory hypotension.[40,41]

The causative agent will determine antibiotic management. In addition, if a source for the infection can be identified then subsequent removal of this source is necessary, for example, drainage of an abscess. Antibiotics are the most common treatment. However, women may get worse before they recover, even with antibiotic treatment, because of release of exotoxins. The most recent Therapeutic Guidelines: Antibiotics should be consulted (see Useful websites). Usual antibiotic treatment involves a penicillin or first-generation cephalosporin. If the woman is unable to take penicillin because of allergic reactions, then clindamycin or vancomycin should be considered. Currently there is a lack of evidence to support steroid use.[41]

TUBO-OVARIAN ABSCESS

Tubo-ovarian abscess (TOA) can develop from acute salpingitis and/or persistent PID and can often result from a postpartum, post-termination or post-miscarriage infection. Left untreated, it can develop into a life-threatening condition (septic shock) because of rupture and contamination spilling into the peritoneal cavity.[6] This may occur as a complication of an untreated or undertreated PID. The woman may present with pelvic or lower abdominal pain, fever, tachycardia and offensive blood-stained lochia and signs of peritonitis.[5] For further information on the management of septic shock, refer to Chapters 10 and 27.

Diagnosis

The differential diagnosis of acute ruptured appendicitis must be excluded. It is important to obtain vaginal and endocervical swabs for identification and culture of organisms. Obtaining blood cultures during rigors will also assist in identification and culture of organisms. A pelvic ultrasound is usually the definitive diagnostic intervention, whereby fluid is usually identified in the pouch of Douglas. If fluid is present, signs of peritonism will usually be present on physical examination.[42]

Management

Immediate management involves correction of fluid, electrolytes and blood loss. Antibiotic management will depend on the causative organism, but urgent administration of broad-spectrum intravenous antibiotics is necessary. If the woman's condition deteriorates or fails to improve, surgical drainage of the abscess may be necessary. Urgent obstetric and gynaecological referral is needed for potential operative management.[42]

ENDOMETRITIS AND SALPINGITIS

Endometritis is the result of inflammation of endometrial tissue and is commonly associated with postpartum infections, including after termination or miscarriage. If this condition is allowed to spread, it can result in acute salpingitis (infection and inflammation in the fallopian tubes) and eventually widespread PID.[43,44]

Diagnosis

Common signs and symptoms associated with this condition include fever, tachycardia, abdominal tenderness, decreased bowel sounds, offensive-smelling lochia and an elevated white cell count (WCC). Vaginal swabs need to be obtained and examined for bacterial identification and antibiotic selection.[43,44]

Management

If this condition is left untreated, the woman can develop life-threatening complications, such as sepsis, abscess formation and disseminated intravascular coagulopathies (DICs), and it may also affect future fertility. General management includes pain and fever control and rehydration if required. The most common antibiotics include either clindamycin or gentamycin; however, management will depend on the causative organism.[43,44] Admission of women who are systemically unwell, intolerant to oral antibiotics or have evidence of a TOA is warranted.[43]

CANDIDIASIS

Candidiasis is caused by the organism *Candida albicans* and is commonly known as thrush. It is the most common vaginal infection in women and is not generally sexually transmitted. It is normal for women to have small numbers of the *C. albicans* yeast in the genital area, but a range of factors may cause it to overgrow and symptoms can develop.[45] Some of these factors include recent antibiotics, diabetes, pregnancy, soaps and detergents used in the genital area and tight clothing that promotes excessive sweating.[42]

Diagnosis

The signs and symptoms in women include an abnormal white or creamy yellow vaginal discharge (cottage cheese appearance), which is thick and has a slight yeasty odour. The skin around the vagina may become red, inflamed, itchy and may extend to around the anus.[45,46] Most cases of candidiasis can be diagnosed through clinical examination and history-taking for risk factors. A swab can be taken if necessary to confirm the diagnosis.[45,46]

Management

The infection, where uncomplicated, can be treated easily with antifungal topical treatments or a one-off dose of oral fluconazole. Follow-up should be recommended for those women who have symptoms that persist or if it recurs within 2 months of treatment.[45,46]

SEXUALLY TRANSMITTED INFECTIONS

Sexually transmitted infections (STIs) are very common, although often underestimated. They have been called the 'hidden epidemic' because their scope and consequences are often under-recognised by both the public and healthcare professionals. The rates of STIs are gradually increasing in most countries, including Australia and Aotearoa New Zealand. Rates of gonorrhoea are increasing, with an urban upswing in heterosexuals. There has also been a reappearance of syphilis in Northern Australia.[47,48]

Paramedics may attend females (and some males) presenting with symptoms of STIs. It is also important to acknowledge that the risk of STIs is high in adolescence post sexual assault.[49] Although the presence of STIs is not normally a reason for an emergency call to an ambulance service, as paramedics move into a more primary care role, the need to understand their pathophysiology, signs and symptoms, diagnosis and opportunities for referral is necessary. This may particularly be required in a rural or remote setting or industrial paramedics working in the resources sector with communal living arrangements. Consultation and/or referral to an infectious diseases doctor or sexual health nurse or doctor is important if an STI is suspected or diagnosed.[49]

Emergency nurses must work collaboratively with other healthcare providers to ensure that STIs are recognised and treated effectively. If one STI is diagnosed, it is often wise to recommend that the woman be tested for other STIs as well as the human immunodeficiency virus (HIV). These infections often occur concurrently as the modes of transmission are similar.

Consult the Therapeutic Guidelines: Antibiotics for specific information on the most appropriate antibiotic treatment for STIs (see Useful websites). Additional information and expanded topic advice is included based on general advice on common pathogens and contact tracing.

HISTORY-TAKING

Collecting a standard history from a woman who may have a risk of an STI or has presented with suggestive symptoms is no different from the standard history-taking process outlined earlier but should incorporate the detailed points in Box 33.6.

Effective communication skills are a key building block for effective professional relationships. Gathering a history from a woman in relation to an STI requires additional sensitivity and care. Non-verbal as well as verbal communication is particularly important when discussing these sensitive issues. Being non-judgemental, treating women and their families with respect and dignity[50] and being aware of the cultural component of communication will assist in ensuring that women feel comfortable to tell their story to the clinician. This is even more important for young women, including adolescents, who may be very reluctant to discuss these issues with someone they do not know.[50]

BOX 33.6 TAKING A SEXUAL HISTORY[50]

GENERAL POINTS:

- Ensure privacy and be non-judgemental and respectful.
- Avoid making assumptions about people, their sexual identity and their sexual practice.
- Make eye contact and have a relaxed body language.
- Provide a context for the questions that are to follow (e.g. 'I am going to ask you some questions about your sexual activity so that we can decide what tests to do.').

TERMINOLOGY:

- Generally use vernacular and colloquial expressions rather than more technical expressions, but use your judgement as this may make some women feel more uncomfortable.
- Adapt your language to the level of understanding of the woman.
- Use the language used by the woman, but be cautious as often people attempt to express issues in medical terms, but may get the meaning wrong.
- It may be helpful to check back with the woman that you have understood what has been said.

QUESTIONS:

- Questions should be open-ended (do not require a yes or no answer), clear and unambiguous.
- Ask 'how', 'what', 'where' type questions to explore behaviour.
- Avoid asking 'why' questions as they imply complex understanding of behaviour.
- Do not be afraid to be direct.
- Questions about sexual partners are important as they may be at risk of STIs because of their partner's sexual activity.
- Ask questions about risk-taking behaviours, e.g. What types of sexual activity do you engage in with your partner? vaginal/oral/anal?
- Ask about knowledge and use of condoms as this provides an opportunity for further information and education.
- Finish the interview with a general open-ended request for further information, for example: 'Is there anything else that concerns you or you would like to discuss?'

PRACTICE TIP

WHAT IS CONTACT TRACING?

The term is used to describe the process of finding and notifying sexual partners when a person has been diagnosed with a sexually transmitted infection.

- It can be very difficult, is a sensitive topic, and confidentiality is important.
- Further information can be accessed electronically through the Australasian Contact Tracing Guidelines and available at http://contacttracing.ashm.org.au/
- Causative agents, signs and symptoms, diagnosis and management of common STIs can be seen in Table 33.1.

PRACTICE TIP

HIGH-RISK GROUPS FOR STIS[53]

- Indigenous peoples
- Men who have sex with men
- People with HIV/AIDS
- Migrants from high-incidence countries
- Sex workers
- People who inject drugs
- Heterosexuals with recent partner change

PRACTICE TIP

FOLLOW-UP AFTER TREATMENT IN THE ED

Clinicians should always ask women diagnosed with an STI to follow up with their GP in 7–14 days so that the GP can:

- give the results of tests, so that the patient knows what STIs are present
- check that the response to initial treatment has been successful; in the case of ano-genital warts, usually further treatments will be necessary
- check adherence to medication (if necessary)
- check whether sexual contacts have been contacted and treated appropriately
- provide further information and education; essential in the case of both ano-genital herpes and syphilis, and often with HPV infection
- arrange further visits to check progress or to arrange further serology, e.g. syphilis (if necessary)
- arrange for a further STI screen in 3 months.

COMMON TYPES OF GENITAL TUMOUR

Many common benign genital tumours occur. Genital tumours that cause women to present to the ED include ovarian cysts, Bartholin's cyst or abscess, endometriosis of the pelvis or fibromyomata of the ovaries and/or uterus. Common malignant genital tumours include carcinoma of the cervix or endometrium, sarcoma of the uterus and serous cystadenocarcinomas of the ovary.

BARTHOLIN'S CYST OR ABSCESS

The Bartholin's gland is located within the vestibule and bilaterally at approximately 4 o'clock and 8 o'clock on the posterior lateral aspect of the vaginal orifice (Fig. 33.6).[14] The Bartholin's gland provides lubrication of the vestibule through secretion of a clear fluid. This adds to the normal vaginal secretions that result from vaginal transudate, cervical mucus, uterine secretions and the fallopian tube.[14,54]

TABLE 33.1 CAUSATIVE AGENTS, SIGNS AND SYMPTOMS, DIAGNOSIS AND MANAGEMENT OF COMMON STIS[51,52]

	GENITAL HERPES	CHLAMYDIA	GONORRHOEA	SYPHILIS	GENITAL WARTS	TRICHOMONAS
Causative agent	Herpes simplex virus type 2	*Chlamydia trachomatis*	*Neisseria gonorrhoeae*	*Treponema pallidum*	Human papilloma virus (HPV) types 6 or 11	*Trichomonas vaginalis*
Signs and symptoms	Blistering and ulceration of the directly affected areas (may include labia majora, labia minora, clitoris and urethra; see Fig. 33.3). These can be painful, tingling or itchy	In 70–90% of women, the infection is asymptomatic. When there are symptoms, these may include dysuria, abnormal vaginal discharge, abnormal vaginal bleeding, pelvic pain or pain during sex	In more than 60% of women the infection is asymptomatic. Where there are symptoms, these include cervicitis and a discoloured vaginal discharge	A primary chancre (painless sore) develops at the site (Fig. 33.4) after an incubation period of approximately 21 days. In the secondary stage, a rash on the palms of the hands or soles of the feet and on other parts of the body may be seen. Second stage symptoms, if they develop, usually occur from 7 to 10 weeks after infection	Present as small swellings and can appear as single or multiple fleshy lesions (Fig. 33.5). Others are flatter and harder to see	Frothy, green, offensive vaginal discharge
Diagnosis	A laboratory test (PCR test) is undertaken from a swab of the lesion	Detected from swabs collected from the cervix, urethra or anus or by a urine sample. PCR test or culture is undertaken	Detected by swabs collected from the cervix, urethra or anus and cultured for the organism	A sample of the chancre is taken for examination. Blood tests are used to diagnose primary and secondary syphilis	Direct examination. Confirmation by histological examination may be necessary	Detected from high vaginal swab
Management: refer to the eTG *Electronic Therapeutic Guidelines:* (2014) for specific information	Aciclovir in different doses and length of time depending on whether it is the first episode or a recurrence	Azithromycin, doxycycline or erythromycin are the commonly used drugs	Penicillin is most commonly used but ceftriaxone may also be prescribed. Follow-up cultures are recommended after completing treatment to ensure cultures are negative	Injections of penicillin are the most common treatment (e.g. doxycycline)	Treatment options include topical podophyllotoxin or imiquimod, cryotherapy, hyfrecation or surgery. The option depends on number and type of the warts	Metronidazole or tinidazole

FIGURE 33.3 GENITAL HERPES ON THE VULVA[1]

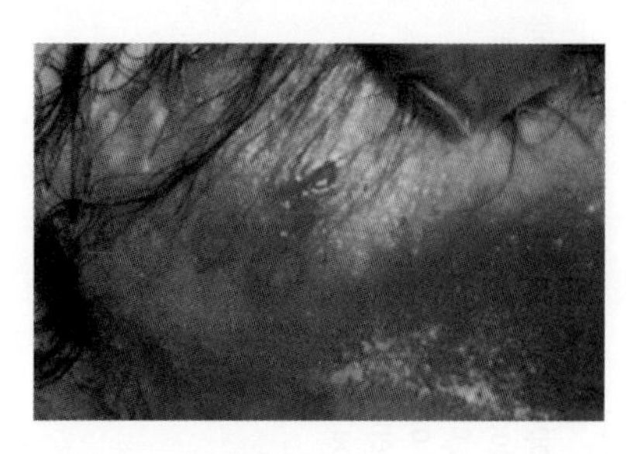

FIGURE 33.4 SYPHILIS, PRIMARY CHANCRE ON THE VULVA[1]

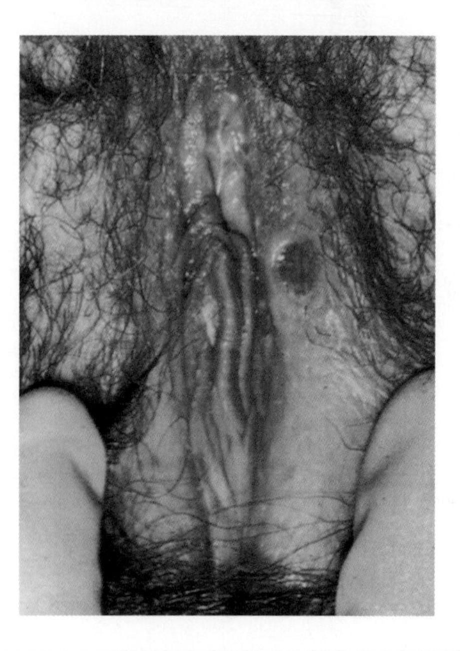

FIGURE 33.5 MASSIVE GENITAL WARTS IN PREGNANCY[1]

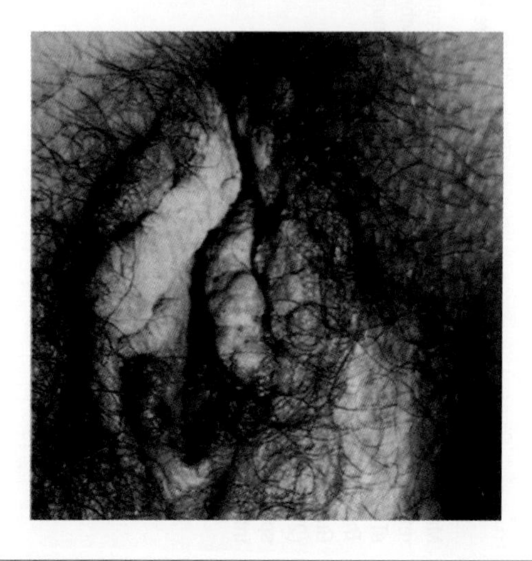

FIGURE 33.6 BARTHOLIN'S ABSCESS/CYST[55]

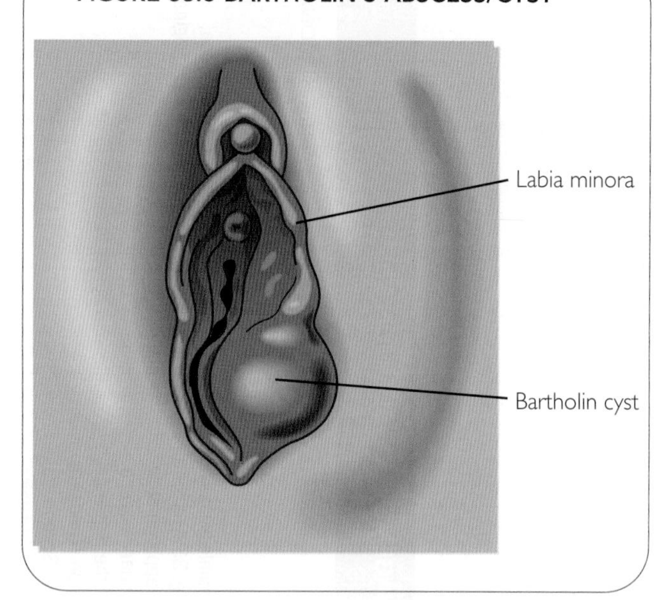

Diagnosis

When the Bartholin's gland is swollen (1–2 cm) the condition is usually benign and frequent sitz baths are usually sufficient treatment. A sitz bath is a warm-water bath taken in the sitting position that covers only the hips and buttocks.[54]

In the presence of infection, the Bartholin's gland can become obstructed, which often results in abscess formation. These abscesses can become quite large and are usually associated with severe pain and associated cellulitis. A Bartholin's abscess can develop over 2–3 days and any pressure against the vulva, induced by activities such as walking or sitting, can cause significant pain.[56]

Management

Immediate management of a Bartholin's abscess is appropriate analgesic administration. This condition is acutely painful and requires an analgesic such as an NSAID or a short-term narcotic agent. Given that this condition is more common in sexually active women, the possibility of associated STIs should be ruled out.[25] While spontaneous rupture can occur, the abscess usually benefits from surgical intervention. A Bartholin's abscess is unsuitable for drainage in the ED as there is a high incidence of re-collection if more definitive surgical treatment is not instituted. Antibiotics are not usually required if it is drained properly; however, it is recommended that the drainage is cultured for *N. gonorrhoeae* or *S. aureus*. For women experiencing recurrent Bartholin's abscesses, the surgical procedure 'marsupialisation' can be beneficial, whereby a permanent opening is constructed to assist gland drainage.[45]

ENDOMETRIOSIS

Endometriosis is a disease of the pelvic mesenchyme where endometrial glands and stroma are found outside the uterine cavity, thus altering the peritoneal environment. It has been estimated that about 10–15% of all women have endometriosis, with higher rates in infertile women (30–40%) and in women with chronic pelvic pain (20%).[14]

There are several theories on the aetiology of endometriosis. The main theories include retrograde menstruation, coelomic metaplasia (coelomic tissue makes up the peritoneal membrane of the pelvis) and an altered immune response to blood in the peritoneal cavity; or a combination of these. Oestrogen seems to be an important facilitator of endometriosis. The condition is not seen before adolescence and settles after menopause.[14]

DIAGNOSIS

The most common symptom is pelvic pain. This can be acute, but more frequently presents as a chronic problem. The pain is often worse 1 or 2 weeks before menses and peaks 1–2 days before the onset of menstruation. Other signs and symptoms can include dysmenorrhoea, menstrual irregularities, dyspareunia and infertility.[14]

Endometriosis is difficult to diagnose because the extent of the disease does not correlate with symptoms. The gold standard for diagnosis of endometriosis is through direct visualisation during a laparoscopy or laparotomy.[5] It is therefore essential that other causes of pelvic pain be excluded in the ED before referral for further investigation is undertaken.

MANAGEMENT

The overall management aim in the ED is to decrease pain, increase function, limit recurrence and maintain or ensure fertility. Acute management of endometriosis includes pain relief (NSAIDs), emotional support and appropriate gynaecological referral. Ongoing management options include medications such as oral contraceptive (progesterone), danazol and GnRH agonists and surgical diathermy or laser via laparoscopy.[14]

EMERGENCY CONTRACEPTION

Emergency contraception (EC), also known as postcoital contraception, is used to prevent pregnancy after an episode of unprotected sexual intercourse or in the case of contraceptive failure. Indications for EC are failure of a barrier method or contraceptive pill, unprotected intercourse, or sexual assault. The two types of EC available are emergency contraceptive pills (ECPs) or copper-releasing intrauterine contraceptive devices.[14]

EMERGENCY CONTRACEPTION PILLS

The most common method of EC is the ECP or 'morning-after pill', which must be taken as soon as possible, but within 72 hours, to be effective. ECP consists of two regimens: the progesterone-only (levonorgestrel) formulation or a course of high-dose oestrogen and progesterone combined pills. Women accessing ECP should be given information regarding timing, dosage, side-effects, follow-up and what to expect.[14]

Primary side-effects of the combined regimen include nausea, vomiting, headaches, dizziness and breast tenderness. These side-effects are considered less severe when the progesterone-only formulation is administered.[56] The progesterone-only (levonorgestrel) approach has been supported by research as the most appropriate method as it is better tolerated and more effective. Overall, if it is taken within 72 hours of unprotected intercourse ECP has a failure rate of 0.2%–3%. The sooner it is taken the more effective it is.[14] In Australia and Aotearoa New Zealand, the ECP is available over the counter from pharmacies without a prescription. It is also available from hospital EDs, GPs or sexual health clinics. Information regarding specific clinical therapeutic guidelines should be consulted before administration.

INTRAUTERINE CONTRACEPTIVE DEVICES

Copper-releasing intrauterine contraceptive devices (IUCDs) are also considered highly effective with a failure rate of $< 1\%$. It functions by eliciting a sterile inflammatory response within the uterus, making the environment unsuitable for fertilisation.[57] These may be used for those women where more than 72 hours has elapsed since unprotected intercourse. Copper IUCDs can be inserted within 5 days of unprotected intercourse and can be continued for long-term contraception once in situ, but has some other disadvantages, including the potential for rare complications such as infection.[5] An IUCD must be obtained from a GP and fitted by a trained professional. It is not suitable for women considered at high risk for STIs or for victims of sexual assault.[14]

In cases where women present to the ED with acute salpingitis or PID, the decision to remove the IUCD must be made urgently so the infection can clear. Appropriate antibiotic therapy should be commenced before the IUCD is removed. Persistent vaginal bleeding or pelvic pain related to an IUCD will require removal, but not as an emergency. The woman should be referred to the clinician who first inserted the device.[15]

PRACTICE TIP

- Where emergency contraception has not been administered within the recommended time-frames an unplanned pregnancy is likely; women should seek immediate medical consultation.
- ECP cannot be used for long-term contraception.
- The emergency contraception consultation is also an opportunity to discuss the possible risk of sexually transmitted infections, screening and unsafe sex practices.

SAFE SEX

Discussions around STIs and the need for emergency contraception in the ED can also be an opportunity for a conversation about safe sex. Regardless of whether the STI or pregnancy results are positive or negative, this can be an excellent time to talk about safe sex and ensure that women and their partners are aware of the risks associated with unsafe sex. Safe sex is the use of condoms and water-based lubricant during anal or vaginal intercourse. Safe sex can prevent HIV transmission, pregnancy and most STIs.[58]

PRACTICE TIP

More information on taking care of one's sexual health is available through most health department websites and specific organisations; for example, family planning organisations (www.fpnsw.org.au or www.familyplanning.org.nz).

SUMMARY

Women with life-threatening and non-life-threatening gynaecological emergencies regularly present for clinical care. A woman with a gynaecological emergency may have a problem that is directly related to her sexual practices or lifestyle and may feel embarrassed or uncomfortable discussing issues related to her problem. This presents challenging opportunities as the emergency clinician must focus on the woman in a caring, non-judgemental manner. Inability to do so can interfere with identification of potentially life-threatening gynaecological conditions and the recognition of non-life-threatening conditions. Recognition of potentially life-threatening conditions takes priority over other interventions. However, the emergency clinician must not lose sight of the long-range effect many gynaecological emergencies can have on women's fertility and sexuality.

An important part of the role of the emergency clinician is knowledge of the most appropriate referral points. In some cases, this will be a specialist gynaecologist; however, it may also be women's health or family planning clinic, pain services or counselling services.

CASE STUDY

An ambulance is called to a distressed 26-year-old woman with right-sided, lower abdominal pain and chills. The pain began 3 days ago and is associated with vaginal discharge. Her last menstrual period was 5 days ago. She uses an IUCD for contraception and had coitus 1 week ago, which she described as uncomfortable. There is no history of nausea, vomiting or diarrhoea. Her vital signs are blood pressure, 120/80 mmHg; pulse, 122 beats per minute; and temperature, 38°C. She is transported to a local emergency department (ED) for ongoing evaluation after pain management is administered.

QUESTIONS

1. In the pre-hospital setting, what red flags do you identify in the case study?
2. What questions will you ask in this scenario to determine historical and clinical indicators of urgency and relevance?
3. Describe each aspect of your physical assessment and explain each step.
4. What investigations will you perform, and why?
5. What ongoing monitoring will you provide?

Answers to Case Study Questions can be found on evolve **http://evolve.elsevier.com/AU/Curtis/emergency/** 

USEFUL WEBSITES

Australian Government Department of Health—provides information on the Department's policies, programs and services, www.health.gov.au.

Australian Indigenous HealthInfoNet—an excellent site for anyone interested in Indigenous health, www.healthinfonet.ecu.edu.au.

Australian Women's Health Network—good resources and excellent links to other resources covering a wide range of women's health issues. It can be found under the section Women's Health Information Links—Women's Health Issues, www.awhn.org.au.

eTG complete. Therapeutic Guidelines: Antibiotics. eTG complete is recognised as a leading source of accurate, independent and practical treatment to aid practitioners in making decisions to ensure their patients receive optimum treatment, https://tgldcdp.tg.org.au/etgcomplete.

Family Planning NSW—detailed information on safe sex and emergency contraception, www.fpnsw.org.au/.

Ministry of Health, New Zealand—access to publications, health education resources, data and statistics, guidelines, newsletters and online library catalogue, www.moh.govt.nz.

National Centre in HIV Epidemiology and Clinical Research—contains the Annual Surveillance Report for HIV/AIDS, viral hepatitis and STIs in Australia, https://researchdata.ands.org.au/national-centre-hiv-clinical-research/17070.

NSW Health Department—information about STIs, emergency contraception and safe sex for consumers as well as healthcare professionals, www.health.nsw.gov.au/Infectious/factsheets/Pages/default.aspx.

Royal Australian and New Zealand College of Obstetricians and Gynaecologists—provides access to publications, guidelines and other information pertaining to women's health and gynaecology, www.ranzcog.edu.au.

REFERENCES

1. Fraser D, Cooper M, editors. Myles' textbook for midwives. 15th ed. Edinburgh: Churchill Livingstone; 2009.
2. Patton K, Thibodeau G. Female reproductive system. Anatomy and physiology. 9th ed. St Louis: Elsevier; 2016.
3. Hall J. Female physiology before pregnancy and female hormones. In: Hall JE, editor. Guyton and Hall textbook of medical physiology. 13th ed. Philadelphia: Elsevier; 2016.
4. Steinmann R. Patient assessment. In: Howard PK, Steinmann RA, editors. Sheehy's emergency nursing: principles and practice. 6th ed. St Louis: Mosby; 2009.
5. Smith K. Abdominal pain. In: Walls RM, Hockenberger R, Gausche-Hill M, editors. Rosen's emergency medicine: concepts and clinical practice. 9th ed. St Louis: Elsevier; 2018.
6. Mendiratta VL, History G. Physical examination, and preventive health care. In: Lobo R, Gershenson D, Lentz G, editors. Comprehensive gynaecology. 7th ed. Philadelpia: Elsevier; 2017.
7. Ectopic pregnancy. ClinicalKey; 2017. Available from: www.clinicalkey.com.au.
8. Weston G, Vollenhoven B. Menstrual and other disorders. In: McDonald S, Thompson C, editors. Women's health: a handbook. Sydney: Elsevier; 2005.
9. Breeze C. Early pregnancy bleeding. Aust Fam Phys 2016;45(5):283–6.
10. The RACGP Curriculum for Australian General Practice women's health. 2011. Available from: http://curriculum.racgp.org.au/media/12308/womenshealth.pdf.
11. The Royal Australian and New Zealand College of Obstetricians and Gynaecologists. College Statement: Female Genital Mutilation; 2017. Available from: www.ranzcog.edu.au/RANZCOG_SITE/media/RANZCOG-MEDIA/Women%27s%20Health/Statement%20and%20guidelines/Clinical%20-%20Gynaecology/Female-Genital-Mutilation-(C-Gyn-1)-Nov17.pdf?ext=.pdf.
12. Kho KA, Shields JK. Diagnosis and management of primary dysmenorrhea. JAMA. 2020;323(3):268–9.
13. Care ACoSaQiH. Heavy menstrual bleeding. Clinical Care Standard. 2017. Available from: www.safetyandquality.gov.au/wp-content/uploads/2017/10/Heavy-Menstrual-Bleeding-Clinical-Care-Standard.pdf.
14. Callahan TL, Caughey A. Blueprints: obstetrics and gynaecology. 6th ed. Philadelphia: Lippincott, Williams and Wilkins; 2013.
15. Linda K. Gynecologic emergencies. In: Hammond BB, Zimmermann PG, Sheehy SB, editors. Sheehy's manual of emergency care. 7th ed. St Louis: Elsevier; 2013.
16. Collings JB, Baum NA. Gynecologic pain and vaginal bleeding. In: Adams JG, Barton ED, Collings JB, McBlieux P, Gisondi MA, Nadel ES, editors. Emergency medicine clinical essentials. 2nd ed. Philadelphia: Elsevier; 2013.
17. Parliament of Australia. Stillbirth statistics in Australia, Research paper series 2021–22. Canberra: Department of Parliamentary Services; 2022.
18. Queensland Health. Early pregnancy loss. Document number MN17.29-V5-R22. Queensland Government: Brisbane; 2018.
19. Murtaza UI, Ortmann MJ, Mando-Vandrick J, Lee AS. Management of first-trimester complications in the emergency department. Am J Health-Syst Pharm 2013;70(2):99–111.
20. NSW Health. Management of early pregnancy complications. 2012. Available from: www1.health.nsw.gov.au/PDS/pages/doc.aspx?dn=PD2012_022.
21. NSW Health. Guideline. Maternity–prevention, detection, escalation and management of postpartum haemorrhage (PPH). 2017. Available from: www1.health.nsw.gov.au/pds/ActivePDSDocuments/GL2017_018.pdf.
22. RANZCOG. Management of postpartum haemhorrage (PPH), Doc n.C-Obs-43. 2021. RANZCOG. Online. Available from: ranzcog.edu.au/statements-guidelines/obstetrics/postpartum-haemorrhage,-management-of-(c-obs-43).
23. Smith R. Postpartum hemorrhage treatment and management: medical therapy, management of obstetric hemorrhage, management of massive obstetric hemorrhage. 2017. Available from: https://emedicine.medscape.com/article/275038-treatment.
24. Yiadom MB. Postpartum hemorrhage in emergency medicine treatment and management: approach considerations, prehospital care, emergency department care. 2017. Available from: https://emedicine.medscape.com/article/796785-treatment.
25. Sanders JK. Gynecologic emergencies. In: Howard PK, Steinmann RA, editors. Sheehy's emergency nursing: principles and practice. 6th ed. St Louis: Mosby; 2009.
26. Trip D, Nickel C. Psychosocial aspects of chronic pelvic pain. IASP; 2013. Available from: www.iasp-pain.org/PublicationsNews/NewsletterIssue.aspx?ItemNumber=2063.
27. Polgar-Bailey P. Chronic pelvic pain. In: Buttaro TM, Trybulski J, Polgar-Bailey P, Trybulski J, editors. Primary care: a collaborative practice. 5th ed. St Louis: Elsevier; 2017.
28. Medina S. Pelvic inflammatory disease. In: Buttaro TM, Trybulski J, Polgar-Bailey P, Trybulski J, editors. Primary care: a collaborative practice. 5th ed. St Louis: Elsevier; 2017.
29. Royal College of Obstetricians and Gynaecologists (RCOG). RCOG release: treatment for women with chronic pelvic pain should consider the key role of the central nervous system, suggests a new scientific opinion paper. 2015. Available from: www.rcog.org.uk/en/news/rcog-release-treatment-for-women-with-chronic-pelvic-pain-should-consider-the-key-role-of-the-central-nervous-system-suggests-a-new-scientific-opinion-paper/.
30. Smith EM, Makai G. Pelvic inflammatory disease. In: Ferri F, editor. Ferri's clinical advisor. Philadelphia: Elsevier; 2018.

31. Cook K. Pelvic pain in females. In: Bourke S, editor. National management guidelines for sexually transmissible infections. Melbourne: SHSOV; 2008.
32. Frazier M, Drzymkowski J. Diseases and conditions of the reproductive system. In: Frazier M, Drzymkowski J, editors. Essentials of human diseases and conditions. 6th ed. St Louis: Elsevier; 2016.
33. Ross, E, Fortin C. Ovarian cysts, disease management. 2016. Available from: www.clevelandclinicmeded.com/medicalpubs/diseasemanagement/womens-health/ovarian-cysts/#top.
34. Muto M. Ovarian cysts. 2017. Available from: www.uptodate.com/contents/ovarian-cysts-beyond-the-basics.
35. Hopkins M, Patibandla J. Ovarian torsion 2017. BMJ Best Practice. Available from: http://bestpractice.bmj.com/topics/en-gb/792.
36. Yang-Kauh C. Complications of gynecologic procedures, abortion, and assisted reproductive technology. In: Adams JG, Barton ED, Collings JB, DeBlieux P, Gisondi MA, Nadel ES, editors. Emergency medicine clinical essentials. 2nd ed. Philadelphia: Elsevier; 2013.
37. Ovarian hyperstimulation syndrome. ClinicalKey; 2017. Available from: www.clinicalkey.com.au.
38. An assessment of emergency department visits for ovarian hyperstimulation syndrome (OHSS): have we improved? ClinicalKey; 2017. Available from: www.clinicalkey.com.au.
39. Mayo Clinic. Ovarian hyperstimulation syndrome. 2021. Available from: www.mayoclinic.org/diseases-conditions/ovarian-hyperstimulation-syndrome-ohss/symptoms-causes/syc-20354697.
40. Dye L. Toxic shock syndrome. ClinicalKey for Nursing; 2017. Available from: www.clinicalkey.com.au/nursing.
41. Fort G. Toxic shock syndrome. In: Ferri F, editor. Ferri's clinical advisor 2018. Philadelphia: Elsevier; 2018.
42. Soper D. Infections of the female pelvis. In: Mandell DB, editor. Principles and practice of infectious diseases. 8th ed. Cambridge: Saunders Elsevier; 2015.
43. Sciscione A. Endometritis. In: Ferri F, editor. Ferri's clinical advisor 2018. Philadelphia: Elsevier; 2018.
44. Dye L. Postpartum endometritis. ClinicalKey for Nursing; 2017. Available from: www.clinicalkey.com.au/nursing.
45. Bayram J, Malik M. Gynecologic infections. In: Adams JG, Barton ED, Collings JB, DeBlieux P, Gisondi MA, Nadel ES, editors. Emergency medicine clinical essentials. 2nd ed. Philadelphia: Elsevier; 2013.
46. Dye L. Candidiasis. ClinicalKey for Nursing; 2017. Available from: www.clinicalkey.com.au/nursing.
47. Institute of Environmental Science and Research. Surveillance Report: Sexually transmitted infections in New Zealand 2014; 2015. Available from: www.surv.esr.cri.nz.
48. Kirby Institute. HIV, viral hepatitis and sexually transmissible infections in Australia: annual surveillance report 2018. Sydney: Kirby Institute, UNSW Sydney; 2018. Available from: kirby.unsw.edu.au/sites/default/files/kirby/report/KI_Annual-Surveillance-Report-2018.pdf#page=134.
49. Bargad A. Sexually transmitted infections. In: Lewis SL, Bucher L, Heitkemper MM, Harding MM, Kwong J, Roberts D, editors. Medical surgical nursing. 10th ed. Sydney: Elsevier; 2017.
50. Altarum Institute. A sexual health and your patients. Providers guide. Washington, DC: Altarum Institute; 2016.
51. Donovan B, Bradford DL, Cameron S, Conway E, Coughlan L, Doyle F. The Australasian contact tracing manual. In: Australasian Society of HIV Medicine (ASHM). 3rd ed. Canberra: Commonwealth of Australia; 2006. Available from: www.ashm.org.au/images/publications/aust-contact-tracing.pdf.
52. Bradford D, Hoy J, Matthews G. HIV, viral hepatitis and STIs: a guide for primary care. Australasian Society for HIV Medicine (ASHM); 2008. Available from: www.ashm.org.au/images/publications/monographs/HIV_viral_hepatitis_and_STIs_a_ guide_for_primary_care/hiv_viral_hepatitis_and_stis_whole.pdf.
53. McAllister L, Street A. Talking with colleagues, patients, clients and carers. In: Higgs J, Sefton A, Street A, editors. Communicating in the health and social sciences. Melbourne: Oxford University; 2005.
54. Lentz GM, Lobo RA, Gershenson DM, Katz VL. Comprehensive gynaecology. Philadelphia: Elsevier Mosby; 2013.
55. Adams JG, Barton ED, Collings JL, DeBlieux PMC, Gisondi MA, Nadel S. Emergency medicine: Clinical essentials. 2nd ed. Philadelphia: Elsevier Saunders; 2013.
56. Bartholin cyst and abscess. ClinicalKey for Nursing, Elsevier; 2017. Available from: www.clinicalkey.com.au/nursing.
57. Bachman EA, Nothnagle MB. Emergency contraception. In: Ferri F, editor. Ferri's clinical advisor 2018. Providence: Elsevier; 2018.
58. Tilley D, Perks J. Understanding sexuality and sexual health. In: Crisp J, Douglas C, Rebeiro G, Waters D, editors. Potter and Perry's fundamentals of nursing. 5th ed. Elsevier; 2017.

CHAPTER 34
MATERNAL EMERGENCIES

NICOLE WATTS, BELINDA FLANAGAN AND JESSICA WOOD

ESSENTIALS

- Modifications to basic and advanced basic life support approaches are appropriate for the pregnant woman in cardiac arrest because of the physiological changes that are present in pregnancy and the early postpartum period. One important modification is the necessity to tilt or wedge a pregnant woman from a supine position into a left lateral position during ambulance transfer and cardiopulmonary resuscitation.
- Maternal collapse may be caused by thromboembolism, haemorrhage, amniotic fluid embolism, genital tract sepsis, drug overdose, anaphylaxis, eclampsia or pre-existing cardiac disease.
- Breathlessness and tachycardia are keys to the diagnosis of pulmonary embolism.
- Ectopic pregnancy should be considered in all women of childbearing age who are seen by paramedics or who present to the emergency department (ED) with abdominal pain.
- Women with a headache severe enough to seek medical advice or with new epigastric pain should have their blood pressure taken and urine checked for protein, as these are clinical indicators for pre-eclampsia.
- Sepsis is often insidious in onset with a fulminating course. The severity of illness should not be underestimated.
- Trauma in pregnancy can occur as a result of falls, vehicle collisions or domestic violence. Domestic violence has immediate and long-term effects on the woman and her baby.
- Amniotic fluid embolism is a rare emergency, but carries a high risk of mortality. The usual scenario is that the woman experiences acute respiratory distress, then collapses, often after pushing in the second stage of labour or immediately after the birth of the baby.
- A perimortem caesarean section can save the life of both the mother and baby if undertaken in the first 5 minutes after a cardiac arrest in the acute setting.
- The collapse and resuscitation of a pregnant woman is very stressful and difficult for the woman's family. They need accurate and timely information conveyed sensitively.
- Debriefing for all staff involved in maternal emergencies should occur as soon as possible.

INTRODUCTION

For most women, pregnancy is a normal life event and most babies are born healthy without complications. Maternal emergencies are fortunately rare; however, they can occur at home or in hospital settings. In hospital, most of these women will be in

maternity units (often a birthing unit); however, some women will present through the emergency department (ED) or be seen first by a paramedic. Knowledge of the normal reproductive system and functions is necessary to care for women who have a maternal emergency. This chapter will initially review the relevant anatomy and physiology in relation to the changes that occur during pregnancy and how these impact on emergency situations. This is followed by a description of the most acute of all maternal emergencies, that is, a maternal collapse or cardiac arrest requiring cardiopulmonary resuscitation (CPR). This includes a discussion of the modifications that need to be made to CPR in pregnant or newly postpartum women and the requirements for a perimortem caesarean section. Caring for the family and staff and investigating and learning from critical events such as these are also addressed. Integral to providing care is obtaining informed consent from the woman where possible and the next of kin where the woman is unconscious. A description of caring for a woman and baby where birth is imminent precedes a description of the major maternal emergencies that may be seen in women who are attended to by paramedics, present to EDs or who are admitted to intensive care units.

Maternal emergencies is a large topic and this chapter cannot cover them all in detail. Readers are advised to access other resources, including the midwifery textbook: *Midwifery: Preparation for Practice*, which has a chapter on life-threatening emergencies and covers a number of other maternal and neonatal emergencies in more depth.[1]

MATERNAL EMERGENCIES

The most recent UK Confidential Enquiry into Maternal Deaths[2] reported that early intervention by clinical staff to immediately recognise and act on the signs and symptoms of life-threatening conditions for pregnant women saves lives. A recommendation from the previous confidential enquiries into maternal deaths in the United Kingdom[3] is the use of a modified early obstetric warning system. Observation and response charts for deteriorating patients have been introduced in Australia, with some states and territories having modified the charts for pregnant women.[4]

The UK Confidential Enquiry into Maternal Deaths in 2011 found that 52 of the 350 women who died from direct, indirect or coincidental causes died in the ED.[3] The majority of these women had either collapsed in the community and were already undergoing CPR on arrival or collapsed shortly afterwards. Of the women whose care was assessed in relation to ED practice, the main causes were:

- pulmonary embolism
- ectopic pregnancy
- intracerebral bleed
- sepsis
- road traffic incidents.

The other significant maternal conditions that may be seen in the pre-hospital, ED or other critical care settings are newborn resuscitation, postpartum haemorrhage, eclampsia and amniotic fluid embolism.

As there are no similar data for Australian women who present through EDs, and many of the issues will be similar to the UK context, this information has been drawn upon throughout this chapter. In the most recent report on maternal deaths in Australia, there were 15 maternal deaths in 2018, with the most common causes being cardiovascular events, amniotic fluid embolism, sepsis and suicide.[5]

ANATOMY AND PHYSIOLOGY

From the onset of conception and throughout pregnancy, a woman's body undergoes many changes to allow her to accommodate and support her baby as it grows, and to prepare for birth and the postnatal period. These changes occur under the influences of the hormones of pregnancy and aim to maintain and develop the woman's pregnancy and the growing baby. These changes may also increase the risk factors for some women in emergency situations.

A brief description of the main changes is presented in the next section. The section is based on a number of textbooks and reference materials.[6,7] In addition, the textbook *Physiology in Childbearing*[8] provides a detailed description of the specific physiology and physiological changes.

INFLUENCE OF PREGNANCY HORMONES

Oestrogen, progesterone, human chorionic gonadotrophin (hCG), human placental lactogen and relaxin are the main hormones of pregnancy, and they produce significant physiological and anatomical changes during pregnancy. Progesterone and oestrogen, produced early in pregnancy by the corpus luteum, then by the placenta, work closely together for the maintenance of the pregnancy and adaptation of the mother's body in preparation for birth and breastfeeding.

Human chorionic gonadotrophin is produced early in pregnancy as the placenta is developing and the chorionic villi embed into the uterine wall. Its main function is to maintain the corpus luteum during early pregnancy, allowing for continued secretion of oestrogen and progesterone to maintain the pregnancy, and to prevent the shedding of the endometrium, as usually occurs during the menstrual cycle. Human chorionic gonadotrophin also suppresses the maternal lymphocyte response to prevent the maternal immune system from rejecting the placenta. The hCG levels present in either urine or blood are used as indicators of pregnancy.

The placenta produces human placental lactogen (also known as human chorionic somatomammotrophin). This hormone has the primary function of promoting fetal growth. It produces a degree of maternal insulin resistance, which then alters the maternal metabolism and use of protein, carbohydrate and fat. This process changes the availability of glucose, which may be metabolised by the growing baby.

Relaxin is produced by the corpus luteum and then the placenta. It has some effects—working with progesterone—in relaxing the uterus to inhibit uterine activity during pregnancy. It also aids in the relaxation of the ligaments within the woman's pelvis and softens the cervix during labour.

UTERUS

Under the influence of oestrogen and progesterone the woman's uterus relaxes and grows to accommodate the growing baby. The non-pregnant uterus weighs approximately 70 g and has a volume capacity of approximately 10 mL. As a result of growth of the muscle fibres and increased vascular supply, the uterus increases to a weight of 1000 g and a volume capacity of approximately 5000 mL by term.

The increase in the size of the uterus and the growth of the baby produces changes in the anatomical location of the uterus.

During early pregnancy, a woman's uterus is a pelvic organ; however, by the 12th week of pregnancy the uterus becomes an abdominal organ. At 20 weeks' gestation, the top of the uterus (fundus) is at the umbilical region, and by 36 to 40 weeks is at the level of the xiphisternum. The blood supply to the uterus is approximately 500 to 700 mL each minute at term, which is a significant contributing factor for haemorrhage being a leading cause of maternal death. The pregnant, or gravid, uterus poses the risk of compression of the inferior vena cava when the woman is lying supine. The inferior vena cava is compressed in the majority of pregnant women in the second trimester, and the compression may affect the uterine artery blood flow but not the fetal circulation.

As pregnancy progresses into the third trimester the uterus grows and develops an upper and lower segment. The upper segment is the ideal region for the placenta to be located as it has three layers of muscle fibres to anchor the placenta during pregnancy and to act as ligatures to the vessels of the placental site when the placenta separates at birth. The lower segment has two layers of muscle fibres. If the placenta embeds in the lower region of the uterus it may ultimately be anchored in the lower segment closer to the cervix. Low-lying placentas have a risk of premature separation leading to an antepartum haemorrhage. There is also a greater chance of a postpartum haemorrhage because of reduced ligature effects of the muscle layers of the lower segment.

CERVIX

Under the effects of oestrogen and progesterone, the cervix has increased vascularity and secretory effects. Early in pregnancy a mucus plug, called the operculum, develops in the cervix, which helps guard against ascending infection. Later in pregnancy there is a softening effect to allow for dilation and subsequent birth of the baby. There is a change to the cervical cells, which leads to a risk of bleeding directly from the cervix if the cells are disrupted, for example, during sexual intercourse or a vaginal examination.

VAGINA

Under the influence of oestrogen and progesterone, vaginal changes include increased vascularity, hypertrophy of the muscle and changes to the connective tissue, which allows for the passage of the baby at birth. Secretory changes create a more acidic environment as a protective mechanism against infection; this may also lead to a white discharge called leucorrhoea, which is a normal discharge during pregnancy.

BREASTS

During pregnancy, oestrogen and progesterone stimulate changes to the breasts by increasing blood supply and developing the glandular tissue and the duct system in preparation for lactation. The overall hormone effects cause enlargement of the breasts, up to 5 cm and 1400 g in weight by term.

RESPIRATORY

As the uterus enlarges and pushes up against the diaphragm and the unborn baby's need for oxygen supply and removal of carbon dioxide increases, respiratory changes occur to accommodate these demands. In addition, there is a slight flaring of the ribs to cater for the physical changes within the abdomen and thoracic cavity. The woman's residual volume decreases because of the enlarging uterus. There is decreased airway resistance, an increase in tidal volume, the arterial partial pressure of oxygen increases up to 105 mmHg and the maternal sensitivity to CO_2 is decreased to approximately 32 mmHg. The increased consumption of oxygen by the pregnant woman is necessary for the needs of the unborn baby.

CARDIOVASCULAR AND HAEMATOLOGICAL CHANGES

As pregnancy progresses, the vascular changes taking place within the uterus, cervix, vagina and breast tissue require an increase in circulating blood volume. Oestrogen and progesterone both have the effect of promoting fluid and electrolyte retention throughout pregnancy to meet these needs. Antidiuretic hormone and aldosterone also play a role in maintaining plasma volume.

Physiological effects include:

- an increase in plasma volume of approximately 45% by 32 weeks of pregnancy. The increase in blood volume predominantly supplies the uterus and helps to compensate for blood loss at birth through an auto-transfusion effect as uterine blood flow decreases and is shunted to the main circulation.
- vascular changes, which occur to allow for the increased blood volume. Metabolites of progesterone alter the response to the pressor action of angiotensin II, which leads to a vasodilatory effect and is evident in normal pregnancy by a drop in blood pressure. The peak effect is usually by 28 to 34 weeks of pregnancy.
- an increase in cardiac output by 30–40%. This is achieved through a slight increase in heart rate, an increase in stroke volume and a decrease in systemic vascular resistance. The heart muscle increases in size to meet the increasing workload and is also slightly displaced (turned to the left) as the uterus pushes up against the diaphragm. This may be represented by a left axis deviation on a 12-lead ECG. The woman's red blood cell count increases by approximately 25% to meet the increased metabolic demands; however, since the plasma volume increases at a greater rate the woman typically experiences a physiological anaemia.
- a decrease in anticoagulation components, and an increase in coagulation factors VII, VIII, IX and X; there is a slight increase in platelet numbers and an increased tendency for platelets to aggregate. The purpose is protective, to guard against haemorrhage; however, this does increase the risk of thromboembolism and pulmonary embolism, which is a leading cause of maternal mortality.

GASTROINTESTINAL TRACT

The gastrointestinal tract plays a role in maintaining intravascular fluid volume by decreasing motility and increasing absorption. This leads to a risk of constipation and the potential for mechanical obstruction. The woman's enlarging uterus also impinges on the gastrointestinal tract because her abdomen must accommodate the bowel and gravid uterus. The stomach is displaced, and emptying may be slowed due to increased intragastric pressures, which also increases the incidence of reflux. The growth of the uterus displaces the bowel and can affect how a physical assessment is performed.

HEPATIC SYSTEM

The increased metabolic demands of pregnancy increase the woman's hepatic workload. There is an increase in the viscosity of bile and the residual volume in the gallbladder, which increases the incidence of gallstone formation. The delayed bile flow can also result in mild jaundice and pruritus related to the deposits of bile salts in subcutaneous tissue—known as cholestasis of pregnancy.

RENAL SYSTEM

The increase in circulating volume leads to an increase in renal blood flow and glomerular filtration rate. The increase in glomerular filtration rate reduces the ability of the renal tubules to reabsorb substances such as glucose, amino acids, folic acid and some minerals.

ENDOCRINE SYSTEM

During pregnancy the woman enters into a mild hyperthyroid state which increases her basal metabolic rate to meet the increased demands of pregnancy. The increase in cardiac output and heart rate, combined with the effects of progesterone, causes vasodilation which accommodates the increased blood volume. The adrenal gland has some increase in function, in particular, increasing blood cortisol levels to meet the stressors of pregnancy and aldosterone to support the increased circulating volume. The pancreas increases the production of insulin; however, under the influence of human placental lactogen there is a decreased sensitivity to insulin, to allow for greater availability of glucose for the baby. The decreased sensitivity to insulin may also result in pregnancy-induced diabetes (gestational diabetes), which may pose risks to the woman and her unborn baby.

IMMUNE SYSTEM

During pregnancy there is a general depression of maternal immunity due to lymphocyte depressant factor and increased adrenal cortex activity. This is designed to prevent an immune response rejecting the baby which contains the father's 'foreign' DNA. Women who are Rhesus-negative and have a baby with Rhesus-positive blood are at risk of isoimmunisation, which occurs when fetal blood mixes with the maternal circulation and the mother develops antibodies to the positive Rhesus factor. Exposure may occur during miscarriage, amniotic fluid sampling and placental abruption, or at birth. Isoimmunisation is a complication for any subsequent pregnancies where the baby has a positive blood group as the mother's immune response is triggered to act against the fetal blood. Women who are Rhesus-negative should be given anti-D immunoglobulin within 72 hours of an actual or suspected exposure, to prevent isoimmunisation.

RECOGNITION OF THE SICK WOMAN

One of the core skills of being a clinician is the recognition of a patient who is unwell. This is not the same as making a diagnosis. In fact, the two skills are often independent of each other. Recognition of the seriously ill pregnant or postpartum woman relies on taking a complete history (listening to the cues given by her or her family) and measurement and understanding of vital signs such as heart rate, respiratory rate, temperature and pulse oximetry. It is important to reflect on the stages of shock in recognising a woman who is unwell, as these basic skills will provide valuable information. It is also important to remember that pregnant women who are sick often remain looking well for longer than they would if they were not pregnant due to the physiological compensatory changes of pregnancy.

Recognition of the sick woman does not depend on complex and time-consuming tests. Recognition of illness needs to be taught to all clinicians who attend to pregnant women on a regular basis. It is also important to make this teaching multidisciplinary.[9,10]

In recognising the sick woman, Hulbert,[9] an emergency doctor writing in the *UK Confidential Enquiry into Maternal Deaths*, stated that:

Tachycardia is without doubt the most significant clinical feature of an unwell patient and is regularly ignored or misunderstood. Measurements of respiratory rate and heart rate are infinitely more important than measurements of blood pressure. A normotensive patient may all too often be unwell and compensating. A tachycardic patient is hypovolaemic until proved otherwise. A patient with tachypnoea has a cardiorespiratory cause until proved otherwise. Attributing tachycardia and tachypnoea to anxiety is naïve and dangerous (p. 234).[9]

MATERNAL COLLAPSE

The cardiorespiratory collapse of a pregnant or postpartum woman (known as a maternal collapse) is the most dramatic of the maternal emergencies. Cardiac arrest complicates about one in 36,000 pregnancies, with a maternal survival rate of 58%.[11] There are a number of circumstances which could lead to a maternal collapse, including thromboembolism, haemorrhage, anaesthetic complications, amniotic fluid embolism, genital tract sepsis, drug overdose, anaphylaxis, eclampsia or pre-existing cardiac disease. Women are more likely to survive such an event if it happens in an acute care setting than in the community. All maternity care providers need to be adequately trained, with access to in-service education, such as emergency drill simulations to increase the survival rate for women suffering from maternal collapse.[12,13]

While maternal collapse and/or cardiac arrest are rare events, they have catastrophic consequences for mother and baby. Unfortunately, the early warning signs of impending maternal collapse often go unrecognised and the early detection of severe illness in pregnant women remains a challenge to all involved in their care. The relative rarity of such events, combined with the normal changes in physiology associated with pregnancy and childbirth, compounds the problem.[12]

PRACTICE TIP

The cardiovascular, respiratory and gastrointestinal changes that most affect resuscitation include:[6,7]

Increased:

- plasma volume by 40 to 50%
- erythrocyte volume by only 20%
- cardiac output by 40%
- heart rate by 15–20 bpm
- clotting factors
- sequestration of blood to the uterus—30% of cardiac output flows to the uterus
- oxygen consumption by 20%
- tidal volume (progesterone-mediated)
- laryngeal angle and pharyngeal oedema.

Decreased:
- arterial blood pressure by 10-15 mmHg
- systemic vascular resistance
- colloid oncotic pressure (COP) and pulmonary capillary wedge pressure
- functional residual capacity by 25%
- gastric peristalsis and motility
- effectiveness of the gastro-oesophageal (cardiac) sphincter of the stomach.

The physiological changes of pregnancy alter the resuscitation of women who have a maternal collapse. These alterations need to be considered whether maternal collapse occurs in or out of hospital. The main physiological changes to consider are related to the respiratory and cardiovascular systems.[14,15]

In the supine position the pregnant uterus compresses the descending aorta and the inferior vena cava, reducing cardiac output, blood pressure and venous return. This explains the rationale for tilting the woman towards her left side during resuscitation.

In pregnancy there is also a dilutional anaemia, which results in decreased oxygen-carrying capacity and increased CPR circulation demands. Pregnant women are also susceptible to thromboembolism. The respiratory changes mean that women are susceptible to a rapid decrease of PaO_2 with respiratory alkalosis and there are often difficulties with intubation related to laryngeal oedema which can occur in pregnancy. The gastrointestinal changes mean women have an increased risk of regurgitation and aspiration.

MODIFICATIONS OF BASIC LIFE SUPPORT IN MATERNAL COLLAPSE

Several modifications to basic life support (BLS) and advanced life support (ALS) approaches are appropriate for the pregnant woman in cardiac arrest because of the physiological changes that are present in pregnancy and the early postpartum period.[14–16] Fig. 34.1 describes the modifications required.

The primary assessment of a collapsed woman can be undertaken whether the woman is in hospital or in the community. Paramedics are often the front-line health professionals in these situations and need to consider the pregnancy related modifications required. It is essential that the pregnant woman is tilted using a wedge, pillow or IV fluid bag under her right hip during ambulance transfer and CPR.

Lifesaving surgery—caesarean section

A caesarean section is not only a last attempt to save the life of the baby, it is also an important intervention in the resuscitation of the woman in the acute care setting.[11,17,18] A caesarean section (known in this instance as a perimortem caesarean section) improves outcomes for both mother and baby where no possibility of survival would exist in a non-perfused uterus.[14] It is recommended that perimortem caesarean section be undertaken early in the resuscitation attempt (within 4 minutes of maternal collapse if there is no response to CPR), and that equipment to facilitate this should be available on the emergency trolleys, especially in labour wards and EDs (Box 34.1).[11,17,18]

PRACTICE TIP

Perimortem caesarean section is indicated when:
- personnel with appropriate skill and equipment to perform the procedure are available
- the woman fails to respond with a return of spontaneous circulation within 4 minutes
- the fundus is palpable above the umbilicus, as the main aim is maternal survival
- appropriate facilities and personnel are available to care for the woman and baby after the procedure.

It would be unusual for a perimortem caesarean section to be conducted in the community by paramedic staff, as it is unlikely that they would have the appropriate skill and/or equipment or have on hand the facilities and personnel to care for the woman and baby after the procedure.

Survival rates for the woman and her baby are improved when perimortem caesarean section is performed within 5 minutes of ineffective maternal circulation. It may still be worthwhile to undertake a caesarean section after this period as fetal mortality is 100% if no action is taken. Some infants have survived perimortem caesarean section up to 20 minutes after maternal death.[20] Perimortem caesarean section also increases the chance of the woman's survival. Maternal survival increases because removal of the baby results in an improvement in maternal circulation during CPR.[14]

CARING FOR THE FAMILY

The collapse and subsequent resuscitation of a pregnant woman is likely to be a very stressful and difficult time for the woman's family. Serious illness or death during pregnancy or early in the postnatal period is usually the furthest thing from any family's mind. They are likely to be shocked and express disbelief at what is happening. Particular attention needs to be paid to the woman's partner or support people who may be with her. It is likely that they will be very distressed with the situation and the resuscitation efforts that are occurring. One of the healthcare team needs to take responsibility to care for the partner and any other family or support people who are present. This may include staying with them in the room while the resuscitation takes place, but it may be that not being present is best. The partner and support people need accurate and timely information and this needs to be conveyed sensitively.

CARING FOR THE STAFF

A cardiac arrest or a major collapse of a pregnant woman can also be distressing for health professionals. Pregnancy is usually surrounded with positive feelings and happiness. The collapse of a pregnant woman, which may result in one or two deaths (mother and/or baby), is one of the hardest things that health staff will have to cope with.

Debriefing for all staff involved in the event should occur as soon as possible. Often a group discussion works well in these

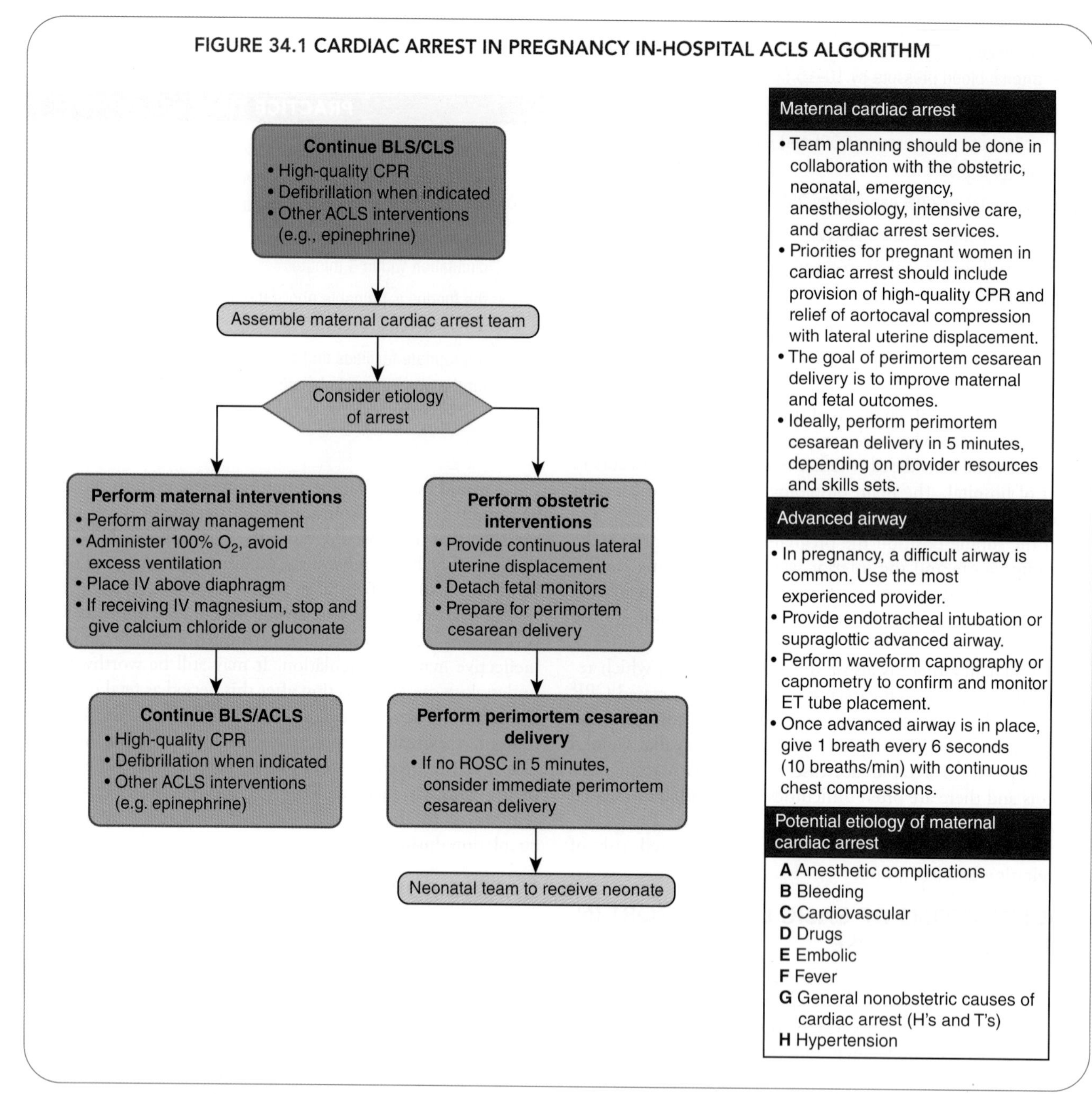

FIGURE 34.1 CARDIAC ARREST IN PREGNANCY IN-HOSPITAL ACLS ALGORITHM
Continue BLS/CLS
• High-quality CPR
• Defibrillation when indicated
• Other ACLS interventions (e.g., epinephrine)
Assemble maternal cardiac arrest team
Consider etiology of arrest
Perform maternal interventions
• Perform airway management
• Administer 100% O2, avoid excess ventilation
• Place IV above diaphragm
• If receiving IV magnesium, stop and give calcium chloride or gluconate
Perform obstetric interventions
• Provide continuous lateral uterine displacement
• Detach fetal monitors
• Prepare for perimortem cesarean delivery
Continue BLS/ACLS
• High-quality CPR
• Defibrillation when indicated
• Other ACLS interventions (e.g. epinephrine)
Perform perimortem cesarean delivery
• If no ROSC in 5 minutes, consider immediate perimortem cesarean delivery
Neonatal team to receive neonate
Maternal cardiac arrest
• Team planning should be done in collaboration with the obstetric, neonatal, emergency, anesthesiology, intensive care, and cardiac arrest services.
• Priorities for pregnant women in cardiac arrest should include provision of high-quality CPR and relief of aortocaval compression with lateral uterine displacement.
• The goal of perimortem cesarean delivery is to improve maternal and fetal outcomes.
• Ideally, perform perimortem cesarean delivery in 5 minutes, depending on provider resources and skills sets.
Advanced airway
• In pregnancy, a difficult airway is common. Use the most experienced provider.
• Provide endotracheal intubation or supraglottic advanced airway.
• Perform waveform capnography or capnometry to confirm and monitor ET tube placement.
• Once advanced airway is in place, give 1 breath every 6 seconds (10 breaths/min) with continuous chest compressions.
Potential etiology of maternal cardiac arrest
A Anesthetic complications
B Bleeding
C Cardiovascular
D Drugs
E Embolic
F Fever
G General nonobstetric causes of cardiac arrest (H's and T's)
H Hypertension

BOX 34.1 EQUIPMENT FOR PERIMORTEM CAESAREAN[19]

- Antiseptic solution
- Sterile gloves
- No. 10 scalpel blade
- Bandage (blunt end) scissors
- Absorbable suture
- Haemostats
- Cord clamps
- Towels
- Sterile sponges
- Laryngoscope with straight blades, no. 0 (preterm) and no. 1 (term)
- Suction catheters (5F to 14F)
- Neonatal endotracheal tubes (2.5 mm, 3.0 mm, 3.5 mm and 4.0 mm internal diameter)
- CO_2 detector
- Neonatal Ambu bag
- Newborn and premature-size face masks
- Oxygen source
- Neonatal incubator/warmer
- Cardiorespiratory monitor for mother and neonate, including pulse oximetry
- Delivery should be achieved within 5 minutes of collapse

situations where each person has a chance to talk about their experience. Often a person who was not directly involved in the event should facilitate such a group meeting as they will be more objective and can ensure the discussion and environment remains safe and supportive; elements of blame and recriminations are to be avoided. It is important to ensure that staff members are supported in their own shock and sadness and can reflect upon the event and the care provided. This is also an opportunity to reflect on the systems and assess which ones worked well and how things could be improved in the future if such an event happened again.

SUMMARY OF MANAGEMENT

A number of key points should be remembered when confronted with a pregnant woman who has a cardiorespiratory collapse and requires resuscitation. These are summarised in the box below. The immediate modifications to BLS are relevant to paramedic and hospital-based staff.

PRACTICE TIP

Key points if a pregnant woman has a cardiorespiratory collapse and requires resuscitation:

- Particular attention should be paid to minimising vascular compression caused by the pregnant uterus and to early advanced airway intervention.
- Early involvement of an obstetrician, midwife, neonatologist and neonatal nurse is crucial when dealing with a pregnant woman who collapses or has a cardiopulmonary arrest.
- Perimortem caesarean section may have to be undertaken early on (< 5 minutes) during the resuscitation attempt, while in the acute care setting with an experienced practitioner. Equipment should be immediately available.
- Contact with a retrieval service should be considered when appropriate staff, equipment or services are not available at the treating centre.

FIGURE 34.2 UPRIGHT POSITIONING FOR BIRTH

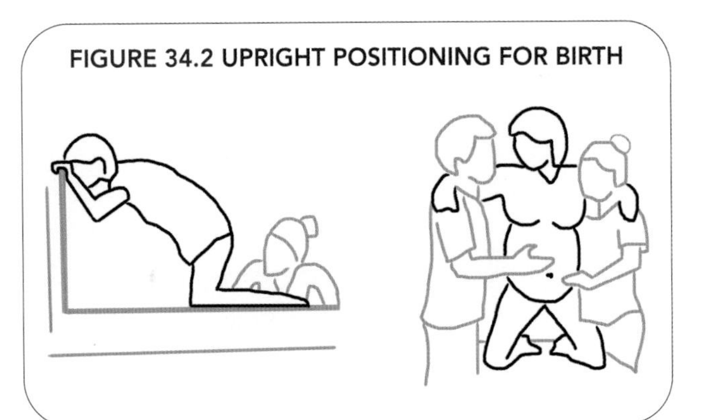

Courtesy of Amy McNicol

CLINICAL PRESENTATIONS

SUPPORTING A NORMAL BIRTH

This section provides an outline of how to support and attend a woman who unexpectedly presents to an ED in labour, or calls an ambulance in the community, and looks like she is progressing quickly to give birth. A normal vaginal birth is likely in this scenario. This section is based on clinical experience of the authors and midwifery texts.[7,19]

Most of the women presenting to an ED or who have called an ambulance, in advanced labour, will give birth to a baby who will present head-first (cephalic presentation). Sometimes, especially if the baby is premature (that is, the woman is less than 37 weeks pregnant), the baby may be born bottom-first, which is known as a breech presentation. The principles for both births in an emergency situation are essentially the same: call for help (hopefully a midwife is available in the maternity unit); ensure the woman is in a safe, private space; support the woman to be upright to give birth; and have a warm space for the baby and warm blankets and towels for both mother and baby. In the pre-hospital setting, it is wise to have a second crew dispatched to assist with the second patient, the baby.

Signs of an imminent birth include the woman having strong (usually painful), regular contractions. She will often describe a feeling of pressure in her vagina or rectum and an urge to push and will often be pushing involuntarily while making grunting noises. Call for assistance. Provide privacy for the woman and allow her to assume a comfortable position to give birth. Invite her support person to stay with her. Ask the woman or any support people she has with her for the baby's original due date as this will help determine if the baby will be premature and whether this is her first, second or subsequent baby (second and subsequent babies are usually born more quickly). It is important to keep calm and quiet and ensure that not too many people are in the room. Provide privacy and try not to disturb the woman unnecessarily.

Once the woman starts actively pushing, help her maintain a comfortable position. Being on hands and knees is the best position (Fig. 34.2). Try not to have her lying on her back at any time. With consent, assist her to remove her underwear. She may pass some blood-stained mucus from her vagina. She may also pass faeces or urine as the baby's head is descending; the area may be wiped if the woman consents, but it may be too sensitive. The membranes (the waters around the baby) usually rupture at this time and fluid will be observed draining from the woman's vagina. This is all very normal.

The woman may be very vocal, crying or quiet. It is important for the staff to keep quiet and calm and encourage the woman—tell her that she is doing well and the baby will be born soon. The baby's head will gradually come into view as the labia part. Talk calmly to the woman as you see the baby's head. Place a clean sheet under the woman and put on personal protective equipment, gloves, gown and eye protection. Open a maternity kit or birth pack if you have one (Fig. 34.3).

The woman will push involuntarily—just talk calmly to her. There is no need to tell the woman to push—she should be encouraged to push as she feels the urge. As the woman continues to push, the baby's head will slide over the perineum and be born. If the birth of the head seems fast, it is reasonable to apply two fingers to the baby's bony prominence and apply gentle counter pressure to slow the head down and limit perineal trauma. It is normal for the baby's face and head to appear bluish in colour. If faeces or meconium are present on the baby's

FIGURE 34.3 USUAL EQUIPMENT IN A BIRTH PACK

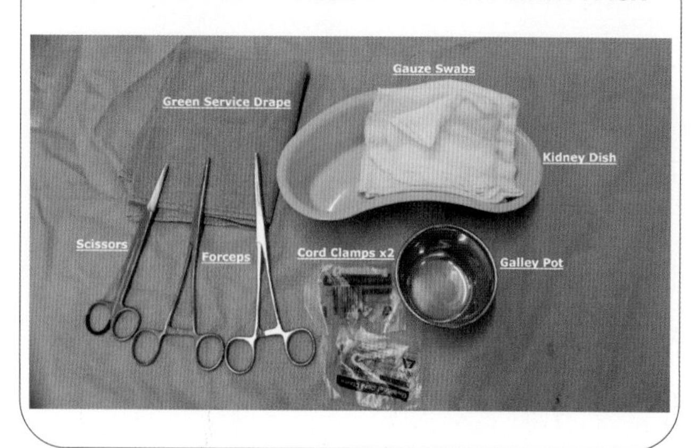

FIGURE 34.4 UPRIGHT BIRTH OF THE HEAD, RESTITUTION AND EXTERNAL ROTATION

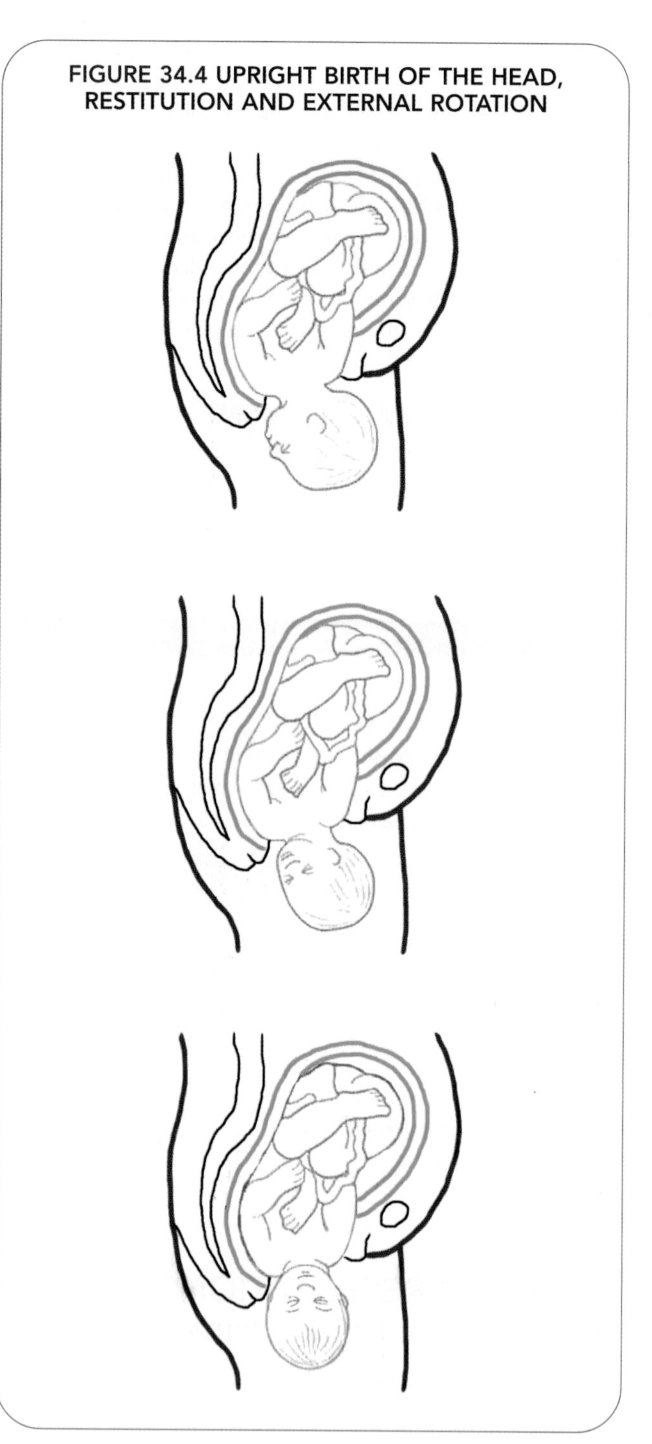

Courtesy of Amy McNicol

face, wipe it with a clean cloth. The birth of the head usually takes 30 to 60 seconds for a woman having her first baby, but can be just one or two contractions for a woman having her second or subsequent babies. There is no need to touch or pull on the baby; it will be born with the next contraction. At the time of the next contraction, usually 2–3 minutes later, the rest of the baby will be born. Initially the baby's head will rotate and the baby's shoulders will be born. If it seems to be taking a long time, ask her to change to a more upright position so that the shoulders will be eased out. Figs 34.4 and 34.5 show the anatomical positioning, restitution and rotation of the baby's head as it is being born. The pictures in each figure represent what will be seen in a woman who is birthing in the preferred upright position and in a woman who is supine.

It is not uncommon for the umbilical cord to be around the baby's neck; it can be unravelled when the baby is born. There is no immediate need to clamp and cut a tight nuchal cord prior to the birth of the shoulders. Manoeuvres, such as the Somersault manoeuvre, can be initiated if the cord seems to be preventing the baby from being birthed. A Somersault manoeuvre is achieved by holding the baby's head flexed and guiding it upwards or sideways towards the pubic bone or thigh, so the baby does a 'somersault', ending with the baby's feet toward the mother's knees and the head still at the perineum. If the membranes are still intact over the baby's face, wipe away the membrane with a clean cloth or gauze. Allow the baby to be born into the attendant's hands and immediately assist the woman to hold her baby. The attendant should always note the time the head was birthed and the time the baby was birthed, so prolonged birth of the shoulders can be calculated, and other interventions initiated promptly.

Assist the woman to place the baby on her chest and dry the baby with a warm towel while on the woman's chest. If the baby is well and crying, place the baby straight onto the woman's naked chest (skin-to-skin contact) and cover both of them in a warm blanket.

Immediately observe the baby's breathing, heart rate and colour. The baby may not cry, but you should be able to observe breathing patterns. The baby's colour will change from blue to pink within a minute or two. The hands and feet often remain bluish. Keep the baby on the woman in skin-to-skin contact and remove any wet or soiled linen and blankets. Perform an APGAR at 1 and 5 minutes, document. Place a name tag on the baby stating the mother's name and the date and time (if known) of the baby's birth. Leaving the baby on the woman's chest and initiating breastfeeding will assist delivery of the placenta and help to control bleeding.

If the baby is well and breathing, there is no rush to cut the umbilical cord. Evidence suggests that delayed cord clamping (at least 30–60 seconds) may benefit the neonate in reducing anaemia, and particularly the preterm neonate, by allowing time for transfusion of placental blood to the newborn infant, which can provide an additional blood volume and higher

FIGURE 34.5 RECLINING BIRTH OF THE HEAD, RESTITUTION AND EXTERNAL ROTATION

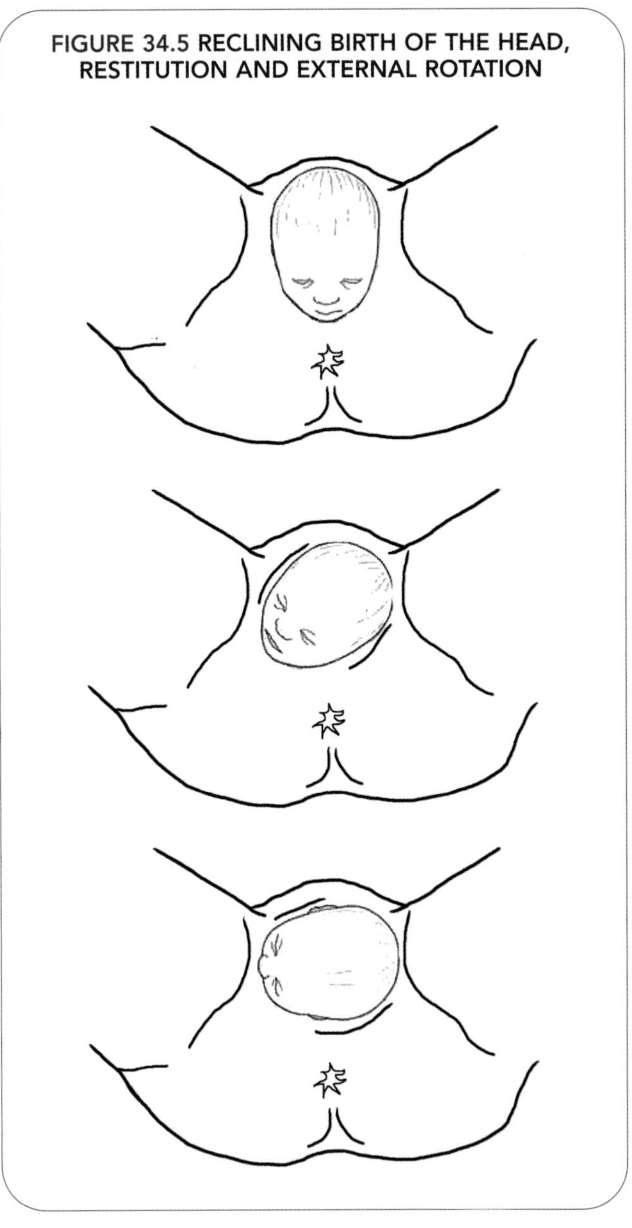

Courtesy of Amy McNicol

haemoglobin level.[21] In the ED, to cut the umbilical cord, place a cord clamp two finger breadths from the baby's abdomen on the umbilical cord and a clamp a few centimetres (cm) from the first cord clamp. Cut between the clamps to separate the baby from the placenta. In the pre-hospital environment it is recommended that clamps should be applied at 10 cm, 15 cm and 20 cm from the baby's abdomen, with cutting occurring between 15 and 20 cm. This provides extra cord length if a baby is compromised, and an umbilical vein catheter is required on admission to hospital.

The placenta and membranes are usually expelled spontaneously once the umbilical cord stops pulsating within the first hour of birth. There is no need to pull on the cord; the woman may express a feeling in her vagina that the placenta is coming, or it is visible at the vaginal introitus. Ensure a clean cloth is placed under the woman and have a kidney dish or a bowl available to collect the placenta in an attempt to measure the blood loss that is expelled at the time of the placenta being delivered.

Paramedics should manage third stage as per their practice guidelines, which may describe either modified active (to allow for delayed cord clamping) or expectant (physiological) management. If a midwife or experienced doctor is present, they may recommend active management of the third stage of labour to birth the placenta.[22] Active management of the third stage requires the use of the drug oxytocin given intramuscularly and controlled cord traction to deliver the placenta.

Keep the placenta for inspection by the midwife. Immediately after the placenta is delivered, rub the woman's fundus (this is the top of her uterus), which may now be at the level of her umbilicus. Rubbing of the fundus involves a circular massaging movement usually just above the woman's umbilicus. The uterus may initially feel soft (boggy), but usually will become contracted with the massage. It is important that the uterine fundus is firm (like a large tennis ball) and central as this will mean the bleeding is minimised. An atonic (boggy) uterus is the most common reason for a postpartum haemorrhage.

If the baby is vigorous, pink and breathing, dry thoroughly and remove the wet towel. Place the baby directly skin-to-skin on his or her mother and wrap both in a warm blanket. Skin-to-skin contact between a mother and her baby at birth promotes bonding and helps the mother to breastfeed successfully.[23] If the baby is not breathing, neonatal resuscitation will be required (see below).

Encourage the woman to breastfeed as this assists the uterus to stay contracted and reduces excessive blood loss. Measure the woman's vital signs and vaginal blood loss. Record the details of the birth in the woman's medical record. In the pre-hospital setting, maternal and neonatal observations should be recorded every 15 minutes for the first 2 hours. This should include vital signs and, in the mother, also vaginal blood loss and fundal tone. Offer the woman and her support person something to eat and drink. Congratulate everyone on a job well done.

Some newborns will need extra assessment and/or resuscitation and some mothers may experience a postpartum haemorrhage following birth. The next section describes in detail how to respond to both these events.

NEWBORN RESUSCITATION

The transition from fetus to extrauterine life is a normal physiological event and for most newborns this process requires minimal or no intervention. A very small amount (about 8%) of all babies will need positive pressure ventilation at birth to establish respirations and < 1% will need cardiac compression and ventilation.[24] With the first few breaths the fetal circulation undergoes unique changes that move amniotic fluid out of the lungs into the lymphatic system. This changes the lung environment from liquid-filled to air-filled. Fetal pulmonary and cardiac circulation also undergo changes to enable extrauterine life.[24] Most newborns, depending on gestation and risk factors, should be given the opportunity to do this for themselves.

About 10% of babies are born outside of a hospital or away from a planned home birth with a midwife. In these instances, frequently the first responder is a paramedic who will be the person to assist the woman to give birth. Two recent studies in Australia found that more than three-quarters of paramedic-attended births were uncomplicated births, if occurring at term; however, in these births the labour was often fast (precipitous).[25,26] These births were more than likely in women who had given birth before (multiparous). In about two-thirds of all obstetric-related callouts, however, the baby was born before the arrival of a paramedic.[25] In these instances the paramedic team arrived to attend two patients, the mother and the newborn. Nurses working in the ED should follow hospital protocol and the Australian and New Zealand Committee on Resuscitation (ANZCOR) guidelines for resuscitation of the newborn.[27]

The primary survey of the newborn, whether at the time of the birth or when a paramedic arrives, must include airway, breathing and circulation. A rapid assessment within the first minute of birth or on paramedic arrival should include:

- assessment of breathing, heart rate, muscle tone and reflexes
- stimulating and drying with a warm towel
- warmth, discard wet towelling and replace with dry towel or blanket.[24,28,29]

The newborn who has established respirations with stimulation and drying should be placed skin-to-skin on the mother's chest and left there with both covered in a warm dry towel or blanket. The mother's chest is the ideal heat source to regulate and maintain the newborn's temperature.[27]

Subsequent assessments of the newborn will be based on his/her breathing and heart rate, activity and colour. Respirations will be adequate if they maintain the newborn's heart rate > 100 beats per minute (bpm). If there is no respiratory effort or if the newborn is gasping, active resuscitation should be commenced. To determine heart rate, either auscultating the apical pulse or holding the base of the umbilical cord close to the baby's abdomen is most appropriate. A heart rate above 100 bpm is considered normal. The peripheral colour of the newborn is not a reliable indicator of wellness or need for oxygenation. It is normal for the newborn to have purple discoloured extremities (acrocyanosis) while adapting to extrauterine life. It can take several minutes of respirations for the newborn to register an oxygen saturation $> 90\%$.[29]

Newborn babies at any gestation are susceptible to hypothermia and this is reported as the biggest risk to infants born outside of the planned place and mode of birth.[24,28] Keeping the newborn warm immediately after birth will reduce cold stress and will reduce oxygen consumption. For premature newborns < 34 weeks gestation, covering in plastic wrap, and only drying the head will aid in reducing cold stress. A newborn that is cold-stressed will not respond to the efforts of resuscitation.[24,29]

The initial steps of newborn resuscitation are to maintain normal temperature of the infant, position the infant in a slightly extended 'sniffing' position, as depicted in Fig. 34.6,[28] to open the airway, clear secretions if needed, dry the newborn (unless premature and covered in plastic wrap), maintain normal temperature,[24] and to stimulate him/her to breathe. For the small percentage of newborns who do not establish spontaneous respiration or have laboured respiration and/or who have a heart rate persistently < 100 bpm, active resuscitation is paramount.

Place the newborn supine on a padded flat, firm surface (in the home this may be a table) and commence active resuscitation facing the newborn. ANZCOR have comprehensive guidelines for newborn life support when simple resuscitation is not adequate.[24–30] This algorithm is depicted in Fig. 34.7.[31] Follow this flowchart for advanced resuscitation.

1. Ventilation
   - For a baby with a heart rate between 60–100 bpm, commence bag-and-mask respirations at 40–60 breaths per minute. After 30 seconds, reassess breathing and heart rate.
   - If heart rate > 100 bpm and the newborn has spontaneous respirations, cease.
   - If heart rate 60–100 bpm, then continue positive pressure inflations.
   - If the heart rate is < 60 bpm, cardiac compressions must be commenced.
2. Cardiac compression
   - Place two thumbs just above the xiphisternum with the rest of the hands around the baby, as shown in Fig. 34.8.
   - Perform compressions at a ratio of 3 compressions to 1 breath 3 : 1.
   - Aim for 90 compressions each minute with a half second pause after each third compression for ventilation.[24,30]
   - Coordinate the compressions and ventilations to avoid giving a compression and the baby taking a breath at the same time. If the heart rate continues to be < 60 bpm, then escalation to administration of drugs as per individual paramedic or hospital protocol should begin.

FIGURE 34.6 POSITION OF THE NEWBORN HEAD FOR RESUSCITATION[19]

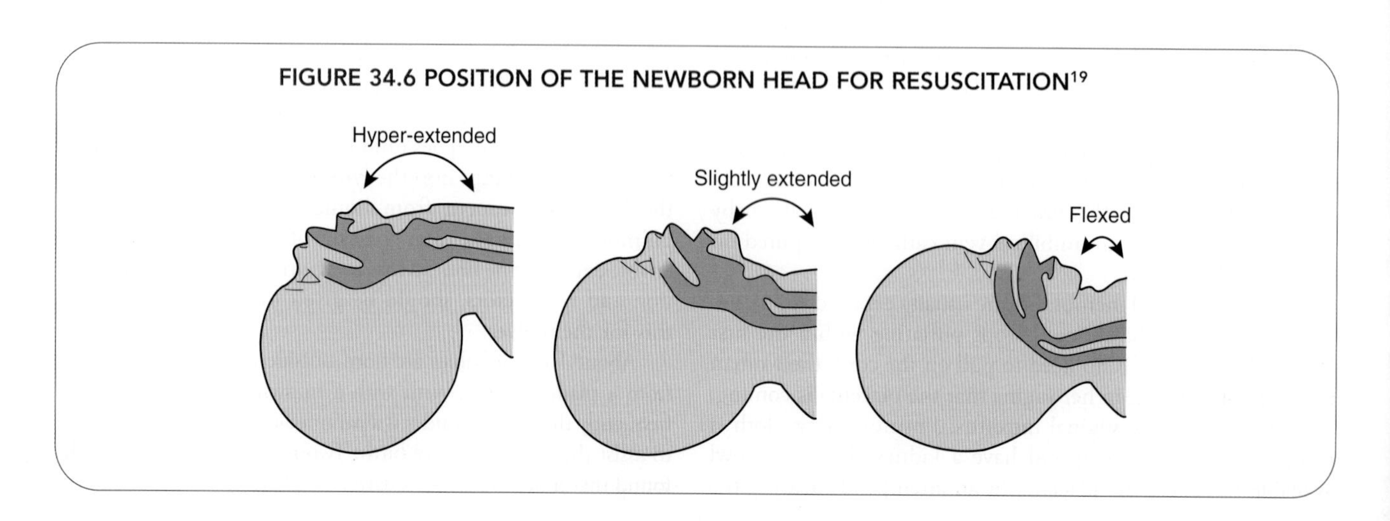

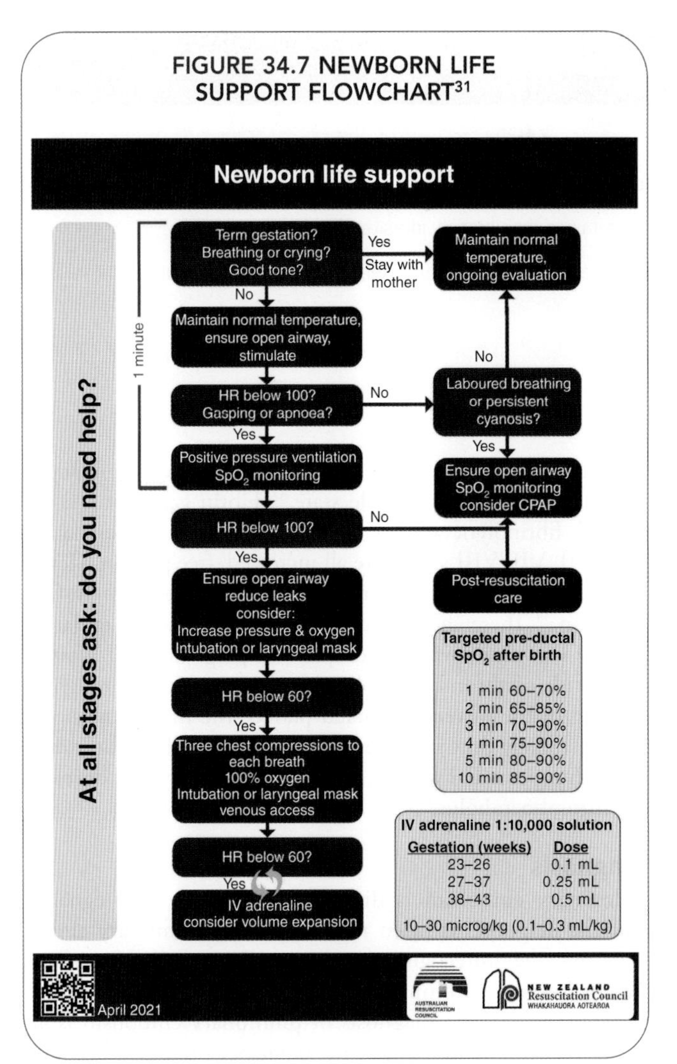

FIGURE 34.7 NEWBORN LIFE SUPPORT FLOWCHART[31]

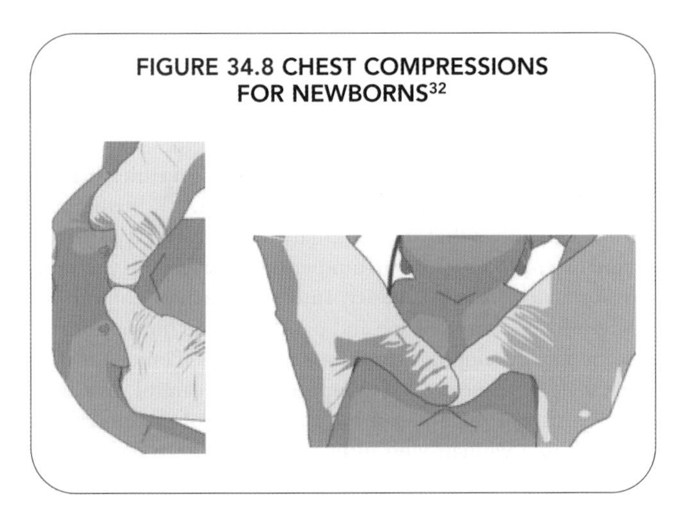

FIGURE 34.8 CHEST COMPRESSIONS FOR NEWBORNS[32]

POSTPARTUM HAEMORRHAGE

Globally, postpartum haemorrhage (PPH) is a major cause of maternal death and morbidity. Correct assessment and management of the third stage of labour is crucial. Australian data indicate that women whose births are attended by a paramedic have the same incidence of PPH as women having a planned birth in hospital.[26]

Primary PPH occurs within the first 24 hours of birth; secondary PPH from 24 hours post-birth until 6 weeks postpartum. It is well known that blood loss is often underestimated at birth and this can lead to under-recognition and treatment of PPH.[33] It can be difficult to visually estimate a woman's blood loss and quite often blood loss is underestimated. Misinterpretation of blood loss or maternal condition increases morbidity and the woman's risk of dying.[1,33]

The accepted definition of PPH in Australia and Aotearoa New Zealand for a primary PPH after a vaginal birth is a blood loss > 500 mL[33] or sufficient blood loss to cause deterioration in the woman's condition.[1]

The physiology of uterine and placental bed blood flow has been discussed earlier in this chapter. Given the large volume of blood flow, a woman can become critically hypovolaemic in just a few minutes from bleeding at the placental bed site after placental separation.[33] The most common cause of primary PPH is a relaxed uterus with poor tone (atonic) and the presentation is often dramatic with large blood loss in a short period of time. Close observation of blood loss and the woman's condition is essential for early recognition. Chapter 10 discusses hypovolaemic shock.

There are four factors to consider when assessing a woman who is bleeding heavily after birth. These are referred to in many settings as the 4 Ts and provide a logical sequence to follow when assessing the aetiology of the visible blood loss of the deterioration in the woman's condition. These are: tone, tissue, trauma and thrombin/thrombus. See Table 34.1 for a more detailed description of each.

The immediate and lifesaving management of PPH should be as follows:

- In the first instance, fundal massage should be attempted only after the placenta has been birthed. A well-contracted fundus should be about the level of the umbilicus, be centrally located and should feel firm, like a tennis ball. If the uterus feels boggy or is deviated to left or right, then begin fundal massage. Fundal massage is done with very firm pressure and will be painful for the woman, so a clear explanation of what you are doing to her and why is necessary. Cup your hand over the top of the fundus and pushing downwards, roll the hand around in a circular motion to stimulate the uterus to contract. This may need to be done for several minutes. Assist the woman to breastfeed if possible; this will help release the hormone oxytocin and help the uterus to contract.[34]
- With heavy blood loss, initiate the airway, breathing, circulation sequence as per life support protocols. Insert two 14–16-gauge cannulas and commence fluid resuscitation with a crystalloid. Begin oxygen therapy. If the equipment is available, insert a 16-gauge indwelling urinary catheter and give a uterotonic.[1] It is recommended for vaginal birth that Syntocinon 10 units or Syntometrine 1 mL should be given via intramuscular injection.[34] Of note, Syntometrine is contraindicated in women who have had any type of hypertension in pregnancy. If bleeding does not stop, consider bimanual compression, in which the uterus is compressed between a fist inserted into the vagina and pressure externally from the other hand.[34,35] This is demonstrated in Fig. 34.9. This is extremely painful for the woman and requires a clear explanation to the woman

TABLE 34.1 THE FOUR Ts—POTENTIAL CAUSES OF PPH[19]

FACTOR	INCIDENCE	CAUSE
Tone	80%	Atonic, not well-contracted uterus.
Tissue	10%	Retained placenta, retained membranes, invasive placenta
Trauma	9%	Vaginal or perineal lacerations, haematoma, uterine inversion, uterine rupture
Thrombin/Thromus	1%	Coagulopathies

FIGURE 34.9 BIMANUAL COMPRESSION[7]

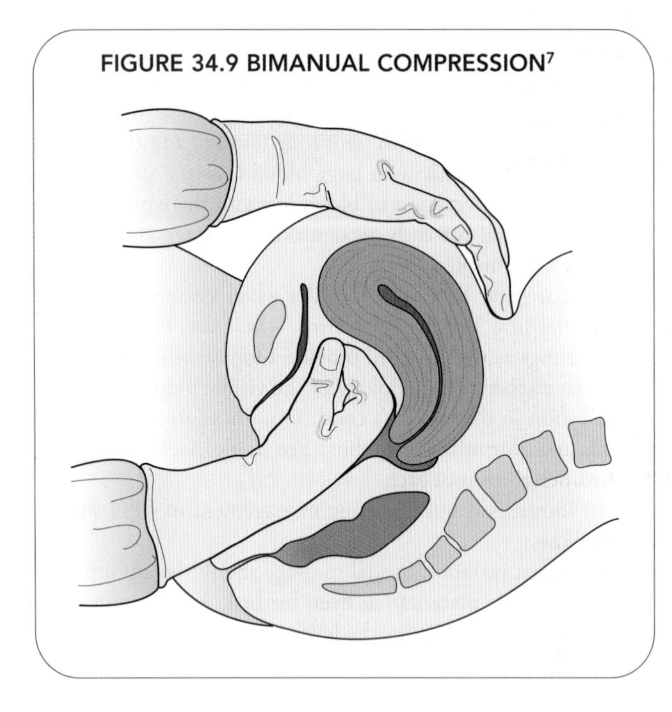

and continual dialogue while the procedure is being undertaken.

- If in the community, after this initial management, call for assistance and transfer to hospital for advanced management. If in the ED, an emergency call will bring help for advanced management of a PPH. Continual explanation of what is happening and why it is happening to the woman and any family members will keep her informed and included in the process. Women have reported symptoms of post-traumatic stress after a severe PPH.[36]

The next section of the chapter briefly outlines the major maternal emergencies that may be seen in women who call an ambulance, present to EDs or who are admitted to intensive care units. These are: pulmonary embolism; ectopic pregnancy; intracerebral bleed; eclampsia; sepsis; motor vehicle collisions; and amniotic fluid embolism.

PULMONARY EMBOLISM

Thrombosis and thromboembolism are the leading cause of direct maternal death in Australia.[5] Delayed diagnosis, delayed treatment and inadequate thromboprophylaxis account for many of the deaths because of venous thromboembolism (VT).[37]

Pregnant women are at risk of VT because pregnancy is considered a hypercoagulable state.[37] Fibrin generation is increased, fibrinolytic activity is decreased, levels of coagulation factors II, VII, VIII and X are all increased, free protein S levels are decreased and acquired resistance to activated protein C is common.[38] These changes mean there is increased coagulation activity in women with uncomplicated pregnancies.[39] Women are at risk of thromboembolism from conception through to the end of the 6-week postnatal period The third trimester is the most likely time in the pregnancy for thromboembolism to occur, but postnatal women are at the highest risk for developing thromboembolus.[40,41]

Diagnosis

Pulmonary embolism is difficult to diagnose in pregnancy and the diagnosis is often made too late. Pulmonary embolism may be unrecognised in a small number of women, mainly because pulmonary embolism is not always considered early enough.[42] The diagnosis of pulmonary embolism is already challenging in the non-pregnant person, but it becomes even more difficult during pregnancy.[37] The most common presentation of pulmonary embolism in pregnant women is dyspnoea and tachypnoea that may or may not be associated with chest pain.[43] Of those women who die from a potentially salvageable pulmonary embolism, many feel breathless prior to admission or presentation to hospital. Up to 75% of pregnant women will experience physiological breathlessness in pregnancy and this can start in any trimester.[44,45] It is important to remember that it is unusual to be breathless at rest in pregnancy or in the postpartum period, especially in the presence of tachycardia.[46] Obesity, smoking, medical comorbidities, advanced maternal age and parity > 3 are important risk factors for developing thromboembolism. Women at risk presenting with new chest symptoms need careful investigation.[45] It is not uncommon for a diagnosis of pneumonia to be made in a woman who ultimately is found to have a pulmonary embolism.

PRACTICE TIP

Breathlessness and tachycardia are keys to the diagnosis of pulmonary embolism. It is unusual to be breathless at rest in pregnancy or postnatally, especially in the presence of tachycardia. Careful measurement of vital signs in pregnant women is important.

Diagnosis requires the use of scanning using ionising radiation. There are concerns about the use of ionising radiation in pregnancy; however, the risk of missing the diagnosis of PE in pregnancy outweighs the exposure risks to the mother and baby.[47] A chest x-ray is useful to exclude diagnoses that mimic PE and to further triage patients to the most appropriate investigation. The D-dimer test is less useful in pregnancy; however, in women with a low probability of pulmonary embolism and a negative D-dimer, the diagnosis is excluded. Doppler ultrasound of both lower limbs has the benefit of being a radiation-free imaging modality. As venous thromboembolism is a continuous disease, the presence of a deep vein thrombosis can be used as a surrogate marker of PE and treatment commenced if present. The evidence to recommend either CT pulmonary angiogram or nuclear scintigraphy is complex. There are numerous issues to consider, including effects to the mother and fetus.[48] There is variation in scanning protocols between institutions and a decision as to the most appropriate test is best made after direct consultation with relevant specialists.

Management

The care of the pregnant woman with a pulmonary embolism requires a coordinated treatment strategy. Women who have a suspected or confirmed pulmonary embolism in late pregnancy should be treated with supplemental oxygen (to achieve an oxygen saturation of > 95%) and intravenous heparin and should be transferred to a hospital that has a maternal–fetal, neonatal and cardiothoracic unit for high-risk patients. As soon as the woman goes into active labour or a caesarean section is considered, the heparin should be stopped (and effect reversed with protamine if necessary). A caesarean section should not be performed while the woman is in a fully anticoagulated state; this can lead to uncontrolled bleeding and an increased risk of severe morbidity or mortality.[49]

ECTOPIC PREGNANCY

Many of the women who present with symptoms of ectopic pregnancy do not know or volunteer that they are pregnant and may not have a pregnancy test done as a routine test. Ectopic pregnancy should be considered in all women of childbearing age who present with these symptoms, regardless of contraceptive usage. Symptoms of an ectopic pregnancy include lower abdominal unilateral pain, light vaginal bleeding following a period of amenorrhoea, shoulder tip pain and, finally, shock.[50] Women may also present with less specific symptoms, including generalised abdominal pain and sometimes diarrhoea and vomiting. A negative pregnancy test can exclude ectopic pregnancy as a potential diagnosis in 99% of presentations; there have been reports of negative beta-hCG and ectopic pregnancy.[51]

Early and accurate diagnosis of ectopic pregnancy can be challenging, partly because cases present infrequently (1 in 100 pregnancies), but mainly because their presentation may not be classical. The triad of symptoms described in textbooks of emergency medicine are bleeding, abdominal pain and dysmenorrhoea, but many of the women who died, as well as some who survived, presented with non-specific symptoms and did not undergo a pregnancy test in the ED.[42]

Diagnosis

As explained above, women may present to paramedics or EDs with atypical signs of ectopic pregnancy. Ectopic pregnancy is occasionally associated with diarrhoea and vomiting and may mimic gastrointestinal disease. Fainting in early pregnancy may also indicate an ectopic pregnancy. There must be a low threshold for beta-hCG testing in women of reproductive age attending the ED with abdominal symptoms. A common practice in many departments is to undertake blood (serum) beta-hCG testing in all women of reproductive age who attend an ED with abdominal symptoms. In addition, it is recommended that pregnant women with abdominal pain should be reviewed by obstetrics and gynaecology staff, if available, or at least discussed with a specialist doctor by telephone.[42]

PRACTICE TIP

Ectopic pregnancy should be considered in all women of childbearing age who present with abdominal pain to paramedics or EDs. Undertake serum beta-hCG testing in all women of reproductive age who attend an ED with abdominal symptoms.

The diagnosis is made using beta-hCG measurements and transvaginal ultrasound.[52] Consultation and referral with an obstetrician and gynaecologist should occur as soon as possible to discuss ongoing management.

For women who are suspected of a ruptured ectopic, the following should occur:[53]

- IV access
- full blood count, blood type and Rhesus factor
- group and hold or crossmatch.

As best practice, women with a diagnosed ectopic or ruptured ectopic who are Rhesus-negative should be given anti-D immunoglobulin, to prevent isoimmunisation.[52,54]

MANAGEMENT

The most critical step in beginning the management is to have a high clinical suspicion for ectopic pregnancy (e.g. in any woman of childbearing age). After a positive blood pregnancy test, any necessary initial resuscitation and physical examination (including pelvic examination to rule out an open cervical os or completed miscarriage), a transabdominal pelvic ultrasonography, followed by a transvaginal ultrasonography if needed, should be performed to identify a definitive intrauterine pregnancy (yolk sac or fetal pole) or definitive ectopic pregnancy (extra-uterine yolk sac or fetal pole).[52,53]

Consultation with, and referral to, an obstetric specialist is essential in the effective management of women with a suspected ectopic pregnancy. Management options include surgical and medical approaches depending on the gestation of the pregnancy and the haemodynamic status of the woman. The current standard medical treatment of an unruptured ectopic pregnancy is methotrexate therapy.[44] Surgical management is via laparoscopy or open laparotomy and can involve complete removal of the fallopian tube (salpingectomy) or removal of the ectopic pregnancy and conservation of the tube (salpingostomy).[50] The decision for the type of management should be case-specific and should be made in conjunction with, if not by, a consulting obstetrician because there are a number of contraindications and cautions.[46]

> **PRACTICE TIP**
>
> A ruptured ectopic pregnancy is a medical emergency and needs to be managed urgently. Women may present with hypovolaemic shock secondary to blood loss and require urgent management to address their haemodynamic status. The insertion of two large-bore intravenous cannulas and vigorous fluid resuscitation is essential.

It is important to remember that women with an ectopic pregnancy are essentially losing their pregnancy, much like a miscarriage.[55] Losing a pregnancy may be seen as actually losing a baby, with all the hopes and dreams that come with this to the great majority of women, and it is likely that this will be accompanied by emotional shock, sadness and questions about this pregnancy and the future options. It is essential that the loss of this pregnancy is acknowledged, and women are cared for in a sensitive manner and provided with emotional support and the amount of information they feel ready to take in at the time. Private space and time and ensuring the woman can be with her partner are also important considerations and strategies. Ectopic pregnancy is also covered in Chapter 33.

INTRACEREBRAL HAEMORRHAGE

Intracerebral haemorrhage (also known as intracranial haemorrhage) in pregnancy is associated with pre-eclampsia and hypertension.[56] In the UK's 2019 report on maternal mortality,[57] intracerebral haemorrhage related to inadequate surveillance and failure of effective antihypertensive therapy were a common source of substandard care. In the report, 44 women died from intracerebral haemorrhage in the 20-year period from 1997–2017. In addition, it is recommended that all pregnant women presenting with new and potentially serious neurological symptoms be seen promptly by a specialist doctor. Neurological symptoms late in pregnancy mandate an urgent review and cerebral imaging.[57]

Diagnosis

Clinicians should be familiar with the means of diagnosis of an intracerebral haemorrhage and the subsequent management of people with this condition. Intracerebral haemorrhage is covered in Chapter 23. Paramedics may also see women with severe headaches in pregnancy or in the early postpartum period and may be the first healthcare professionals to be aware of possible diagnoses. It is important to remember that severe headaches in pregnancy or in the early postpartum period can be indicative of intracerebral bleeding, despite it being a rare event, and the timely diagnosis of intracerebral haemorrhage is vital for subsequent management and treatment.[56]

Management

Women with a headache severe enough to seek medical advice or with new epigastric pain should have their blood pressure taken and urine checked for protein as a minimum. For the most part, this will occur in the acute care setting.

Women with severe, incapacitating headaches described as the worst they have ever had should have an emergency neurological referral for brain imaging in the absence of other signs of pre-eclampsia. The threshold for same-day referral to an obstetrician is hypertension ≥ 140 mmHg systolic and/or ≥ 90 mmHg diastolic and/or proteinuria ≥ 1+ on dipstick. The systolic blood pressure is as significant as the diastolic. It is important to note that automated blood pressure machines can seriously underestimate blood pressure in pre-eclampsia. Blood pressure values should be compared with those obtained by manual auscultation.[58]

ECLAMPSIA

Eclampsia (seizures) complicates 0.1% of all births in Australia. Eclampsia is the endpoint of pre-eclampsia and presents as seizures. Eclampsia may occur antenatally, intrapartum or postnatally, usually within 24 hours of the birth of the baby, but occasionally later. Hypertension and proteinuria may be absent prior to the seizure, and not all women will have warning symptoms such as headache, visual disturbances or epigastric pain. There are no reliable clinical markers to predict eclampsia. In fact, the presence of neurological symptoms and/or signs is rarely associated with seizures.[2,58]

Pre-eclampsia is a multi-system disorder of pregnancy characterised by hypertension and involvement of one or more other organ systems and/or the unborn baby. Raised blood pressure is commonly, but not always, the first manifestation. Proteinuria is the most commonly recognised additional feature after hypertension, but should not be considered mandatory to make the clinical diagnosis.

> **PRACTICE TIP**
>
> Hypertension in pregnancy is defined as:[58]
> - systolic blood pressure greater than or equal to 140 mmHg, and/or
> - diastolic blood pressure greater than or equal to 90 mmHg (Korotkoff 5).
>
> These measurements should be confirmed by repeated readings over several hours in the acute care setting.
>
> Severe hypertension in pregnancy is defined as:
> - systolic blood pressure greater than or equal to 170 mmHg, and/or
> - diastolic blood pressure greater than or equal to 110 mmHg.[58]

A diagnosis of pre-eclampsia can be made when hypertension occurs after 20 weeks gestation and is accompanied by one or more of the following:

1. Renal involvement
   - Significant proteinuria—dipstick proteinuria subsequently confirmed by spot urine protein/creatinine ratio ≥ 30 mg/mmol
   - Serum or plasma creatinine > 90 micromol/L
   - Oliguria
2. Haematological involvement
   - Thrombocytopenia
   - Haemolysis
   - Disseminated intravascular coagulation
3. Liver involvement
   - Raised serum transaminases
   - Severe epigastric or right upper quadrant pain

4. Neurological involvement
   - Seizures (eclampsia)
   - Hyperreflexia with sustained clonus
   - Severe headache
   - Persistent visual disturbances (photopsia, scotomata, cortical blindness, retinal vasospasm)
   - Stroke
5. Pulmonary oedema
6. Fetal growth restriction
7. Placental abruption.[58]

The HELLP syndrome (Haemolysis, Elevated Liver enzymes and a Low Platelet count) represents a particular presentation of severe pre-eclampsia.

Diagnosis

The diagnosis of pre-eclampsia is made on the basis of the level of hypertension in pregnancy and the presence of the other factors outlined above. Most commonly, women present with hypertension and proteinuria, although other renal, haematological, hepatic or neurological manifestations may occur.

Diagnosing a seizure as eclampsia is often a process of exclusion of other diagnoses. The further from the birth of the baby that the seizure occurs, the more carefully other diagnoses should be considered. For example, cerebral venous thrombosis may occur in the first few days of the postpartum period and can present with seizure activity. It should be remembered that eclampsia is not the most common cause of seizures in pregnancy and the differential diagnosis includes epilepsy and other medical problems that must be considered carefully, particularly when typical features of severe pre-eclampsia are lacking.[58]

PRACTICE TIP

The differential diagnoses of seizures in pregnancy include:

- primary generalised epilepsy
- subarachnoid haemorrhage
- hypoglycaemia
- thrombotic thrombocytopenic purpura
- amniotic fluid embolism
- central venous sinus thrombosis
- water intoxication
- phaeochromocytoma
- local anaesthetic toxicity (e.g. epidural)
- overdose (e.g. tricyclic antidepressants).[57]

MANAGEMENT

Guidelines from SOMANZ[58] and the National Institute of Clinical Excellence (NICE)[59] provide comprehensive information to guide the management of women with hypertensive disorders of pregnancy. It is recommended that these are used to guide effective management and interventions. In particular, prompt treatment of severe hypertension (blood pressure of >/= 170 mmHg/110 mmHg) or seizures is mandatory. The presence of severe hypertension, headache, epigastric pain or nausea and vomiting are ominous signs which should lead to urgent admission and management,[58] as should any concern about fetal wellbeing.

The emergency management of eclampsia is outlined in Box 34.2. In the out-of-hospital setting the important management strategies include the first aid management of a seizure.[60] These include keeping the woman in a safe environment, removed from danger; avoiding restraining her; placing her in the left lateral position as soon as possible; and supporting her in the immediate postictal phase. Pharmacological management provided by paramedics may include an anticonvulsant such as midazolam and the administration of magnesium sulfate, both a loading and maintenance dose.[58] Most eclamptic seizures are self-limiting and once they are over the woman can be transported to an acute care setting.

SEPSIS

Sepsis is a major cause of morbidity and mortality in pregnant and postpartum women.[2,61] Severe sepsis with acute organ dysfunction has a 20–40% mortality rate.[62] Sepsis can occur in early and late pregnancy and is also commonly seen in the postpartum period. There have been reported deaths in early pregnancy often related to miscarriage or a termination of pregnancy and in later pregnancy related to the presence of a cervical suture. Infection should be suspected for women who present with pyrexia, persistent bleeding or abdominal pain, following recent miscarriage or termination of pregnancy.[3] An example of sepsis in early pregnancy in Box 34.3 is taken from the report into maternal deaths from the UK. This case has specific resonance for those who work in EDs.

Sepsis after the birth of the baby is often related to retained products of conception (fragments of placenta or membranes retained after the birth) or postoperative infection following caesarean section. As the caesarean section (CS) rate in many countries continues to rise (in 2015, the CS rate in Australia was 34%, with wide variations across states and territories and between public and private services, while in Aotearoa New Zealand it was 29%),[63,64] more women may potentially be at risk of infection post-caesarean section. In addition, as the hospital length of stay decreases in many places, more women will develop their infections outside of hospital and therefore present more readily to EDs. Genital tract sepsis related to pregnancy or childbirth can occur up to 6 weeks after the birth of the baby. Sepsis can result in septic shock, which is addressed in Chapter 27.

Pregnant women who present with a sore throat should have a throat swab collected as a common cause may be from community-acquired Streptococcal group A. Subsequently there should be a low threshold for using antibiotics.[3]

PRACTICE TIP

Other risk factors for sepsis include: obesity; impaired glucose tolerance/diabetes; impaired immunity; anaemia; vaginal discharge; history of pelvic infection; history of Group B Streptococcal infection; amniocentesis, and other invasive intrauterine procedures; insertion of a cervical suture; prolonged ruptured membranes; vaginal trauma during birth; caesarean section; wound haematoma; and retained products of conception, either after a miscarriage or after the birth.[61]

BOX 34.2 MANAGEMENT OF ECLAMPSIA[58]

Comprehensive protocols for the management of eclampsia (and severe hypertension) should be available in all appropriate areas.

There are four main aspects to care of the woman who sustains eclampsia.

1. RESUSCITATION

These seizures are usually self-limiting. Resuscitation requires assuring a patent airway, oxygen by mask and institution of intravenous access. Intravenous diazepam (2 mg/min to maximum of 10 mg) or clonazepam (1–2 mg over 2–5 minutes) may be given while the magnesium sulphate is being prepared if the seizure is prolonged.

2. PREVENTION OF FURTHER SEIZURES

Following appropriate resuscitation, treatment should be commenced with magnesium sulphate given as a 4 g loading dose (diluted in normal saline over 1–20 minutes), followed by an infusion of 1–2 g/hr, diluted in normal saline. Pre-diluted magnesium sulphate should be available in all appropriate areas for this purpose (4 g/ 100 mL normal saline). In the event of a further seizure, a further 2–4 g of magnesium sulphate is given IV over 10 minutes. Magnesium sulphate is usually given as an intravenous loading dose, although the intramuscular route is equally effective. Monitoring should include blood pressure, respiratory rate, urine output, oxygen saturation and deep tendon reflexes. Magnesium sulphate by infusion should continue for 24 hours after the last fit. Serum magnesium levels do not need to be measured routinely unless renal function is compromised.

Magnesium sulphate is excreted via the kidneys and extreme caution should be used in women with oliguria or renal impairment. Serum magnesium concentration should be closely monitored in this situation. Magnesium is not universally successful and the recurrence rate of seizures despite appropriate magnesium therapy is 10–15%.

3. CONTROL OF HYPERTENSION

Control of severe hypertension to levels below 160/100 mmHg is essential as the threshold for further seizures is lowered after eclampsia, likely in association with vasogenic brain edema. In addition, the danger of cerebral haemorrhage is real.

4. DELIVERY

Arrangements for delivery should be decided once the woman's condition is stable. In the meantime, close fetal monitoring should be maintained. There is no role, with currently available treatment, for continuation of pregnancy once eclampsia has occurred, even though many women may appear to be stable after control of the situation has been achieved.

PREVENTION OF ECLAMPSIA IN THE WOMAN WITH PRE-ECLAMPSIA

The drug of choice for the prevention of eclampsia is magnesium sulphate, given as a 4 g loading dose (diluted in normal saline), followed by an infusion of 1 g/hour. Although there is good evidence for the efficacy of this therapy, the case for its routine administration in women with pre-eclampsia in countries with low maternal and perinatal mortality rates is less than compelling. In some units, the presence of symptoms or signs, such as persistent headache, hyperreflexia with clonus, evidence of liver involvement or severe hypertension, are considered indications for prophylaxis with magnesium sulphate, although these symptoms have poor positive and negative predictability for eclampsia. It is appropriate for individual units to determine their own protocols and monitor outcomes.

BOX 34.3 A CASE OF A WOMAN WITH SEPSIS IN PREGNANCY WHO PRESENTED TO AN ED[3]

A woman in mid-pregnancy called an out-of-hours general practitioner (GP) as she was feverish, shivery and unwell and had a sore throat, but was diagnosed as having a probable viral infection. A few hours later the GP visited again as she had developed constant abdominal pain associated with vomiting, greenish black diarrhoea and reduced fetal movements, but no vaginal bleeding. The GP suspected placental abruption, and, although she was rapidly transferred to hospital, on admission she was critically ill with marked tachycardia, breathlessness, cyanosis and confusion. The correct diagnosis of septic shock was quickly recognised, fluid resuscitation was started, senior consultants were called, advice was sought from haematology and microbiology consultants and appropriate intravenous antibiotics were commenced immediately. Despite intensive life support she died a few hours after admission to hospital.

Diagnosis

Sepsis is often insidious in onset with a fulminating course. The severity of illness should not be underestimated.[63,64] Many pregnant women will maintain their haemodynamic status, often appearing deceptively well until they suddenly deteriorate and collapse. In later pregnancy, sepsis should be considered as a differential diagnosis when a woman presents with symptoms suggestive of placental abruption. Disseminated intravascular coagulation and uterine atony are common in genital tract sepsis and often cause life-threatening postpartum haemorrhage. Treatment, including facilitating the birth of the baby, should not be delayed once septicaemia has developed, because deterioration into septic shock can be extremely rapid.[61]

The most common pathogens found to cause severe maternal morbidity or mortality are Group A-beta-haemolytic *Streptococcus* (GAS) *pyogenes*, *Escherichia coli* and Group B streptococcus.[61]

The signs and symptoms of sepsis of genital tract origin are often non-specific and unless specifically considered in the differential diagnosis it may be missed until too late. The signs and symptoms are detailed in Box 34.4.

Management

In many cases of maternal mortality due to sepsis, there is a failure or delay in diagnosing, a failure to appreciate the severity of the woman's condition with resultant delays in referral to hospital, delays in administration of appropriate antibiotic treatment and late or no involvement of senior medical staff. It is essential that treatment is instigated promptly, as once septicaemia develops the woman's clinical condition may deteriorate very rapidly, resulting in her death.[63,64]

BOX 34.4 BACK TO BASICS—SEPSIS[43]

Associated red flag signs and symptoms that should prompt urgent referral for hospital assessment, and, if the woman appears seriously unwell, by emergency ambulance:

- **Pyrexia > 38°C**
- **Sustained tachycardia > 100 bpm**
- **Breathlessness (RR > 20; a serious symptom)**
- **Abdominal or chest pain**
- **Diarrhoea and/or vomiting**
- **Reduced or absent fetal movements, or absent fetal heartbeat**
- **Spontaneous rupture of membranes or significant vaginal discharge**
- **Uterine or renal angle pain and tenderness**
- **The woman is generally unwell or seems unduly anxious, distressed or panicky.**

A normal temperature does not exclude sepsis; paracetamol and other analgesics may mask pyrexia, and this should be taken into account when assessing women who are unwell.

Infection must also be suspected and actively ruled out when a woman who has recently given birth has persistent vaginal bleeding and abdominal pain. If there is any concern, the woman must be referred back to the maternity unit as soon as possible, certainly within 24 hours.

Women who present to out-of-hospital care clinicians with signs indicative of sepsis should be assessed and emergency management commenced before transfer to an acute care setting. Usual measures in the management of sepsis or septic shock should be commenced by paramedics, including intravenous cannulation, intravenous fluid replacement to maintain pulse and BP and transport to an appropriate centre.

Prompt early treatment with a combination of high-dose broad-spectrum intravenous antibiotics is required.[64] Time may be lost by waiting for microbiology results, although these results should be obtained as soon as possible. Fig. 34.10 details immediate management of a woman who presents with suspected sepsis; this can be enacted by both paramedics and nurses in the ED.

PRACTICE TIP

The expert advice of a consultant microbiologist and an obstetrician should be sought at an early stage. The source of sepsis should be sought and dealt with if possible and appropriate.

AMNIOTIC FLUID EMBOLISM

Amniotic fluid embolism (AFE) is a rare maternal emergency that carries a high risk of mortality, with reported mortality rates ranging from 11% to 44%.[65] The best available evidence for the overall mortality rate of women with an AFE is 1 in 5.[65] AFE is unpredictable, often occurring without warning and it is rapidly progressive. It occurs in about 1.9: 100,000 to 6.1:100,000 pregnancies.[66] Amniotic fluid embolism as the cause of maternal death has decreased over time. The reason for this is not clearly known, but the reduced mortality may be due to improved approaches in recognition and resuscitation when the collapse occurs.[3]

The pathophysiology and initiating event is often unclear. However, usually during labour or other procedures, amniotic fluid and debris, or some as yet unidentified substance, enters the maternal circulation. This seems to trigger either a massive anaphylactic reaction, or an activation of the complement system cascade, or both. Progression usually occurs in two phases. Initially, pulmonary artery vasospasm with pulmonary hypertension and elevated right ventricular pressure cause hypoxia. Hypoxia causes myocardial capillary damage and pulmonary capillary damage, left heart failure and acute respiratory distress syndrome. Women who survive these events may enter the next phase. This is a haemorrhagic phase characterised by massive haemorrhage with uterine atony and disseminated intravascular coagulation (DIC). In some cases, fatal consumptive coagulopathy may be the initial presentation. The usual clinical scenario is that the woman experiences acute respiratory distress, then collapses often after pushing or immediately after the birth of the baby.[67] Prodromal symptoms include breathlessness, chest pain, agitation, anxiety, confusion, seizures, chills and hypotension.[68] The presentation of amniotic fluid embolism can often be confused with other presentations; nevertheless, prompt effective resuscitation is essential despite the underlying cause.[2]

Diagnosis

Currently no definitive diagnostic test exists for AFE and often the diagnosis is only made at post-mortem examination. The diagnosis is often made by exclusion and any pregnant or newly postpartum woman who shows signs associated with pulmonary embolus, septic shock, acute myocardial infarction, cardiomyopathy, anaphylaxis, cardiorespiratory collapse or intractable haemorrhage must be systematically evaluated to exclude a diagnosis of amniotic fluid embolism.

The common features of AFE are:

1. acute hypotension, dysrhythmia or cardiac arrest
2. acute hypoxia and respiratory failure
3. coagulopathy or severe haemorrhage in the absence of other explanations
4. all of the above occurring during labour, caesarean section, dilation and evacuation of the uterus, or within 30 minutes postpartum with no other explanation of findings.[69]

PRACTICE TIP

The laboratory investigations to exclude amniotic fluid embolism in the acute care setting include:[1]

- full blood count with platelets
- coagulation parameters (prothrombin time, activated partial thromboplastin time, fibrinogen)
- arterial blood gases
- chest x-ray
- ECG
- echocardiogram.

Management

The management of a woman with suspected amniotic fluid embolism depends on her signs and symptoms. The

FIGURE 34.10 ASSESSMENT AND MANAGEMENT OF SEPSIS IN PREGNANCY[64]

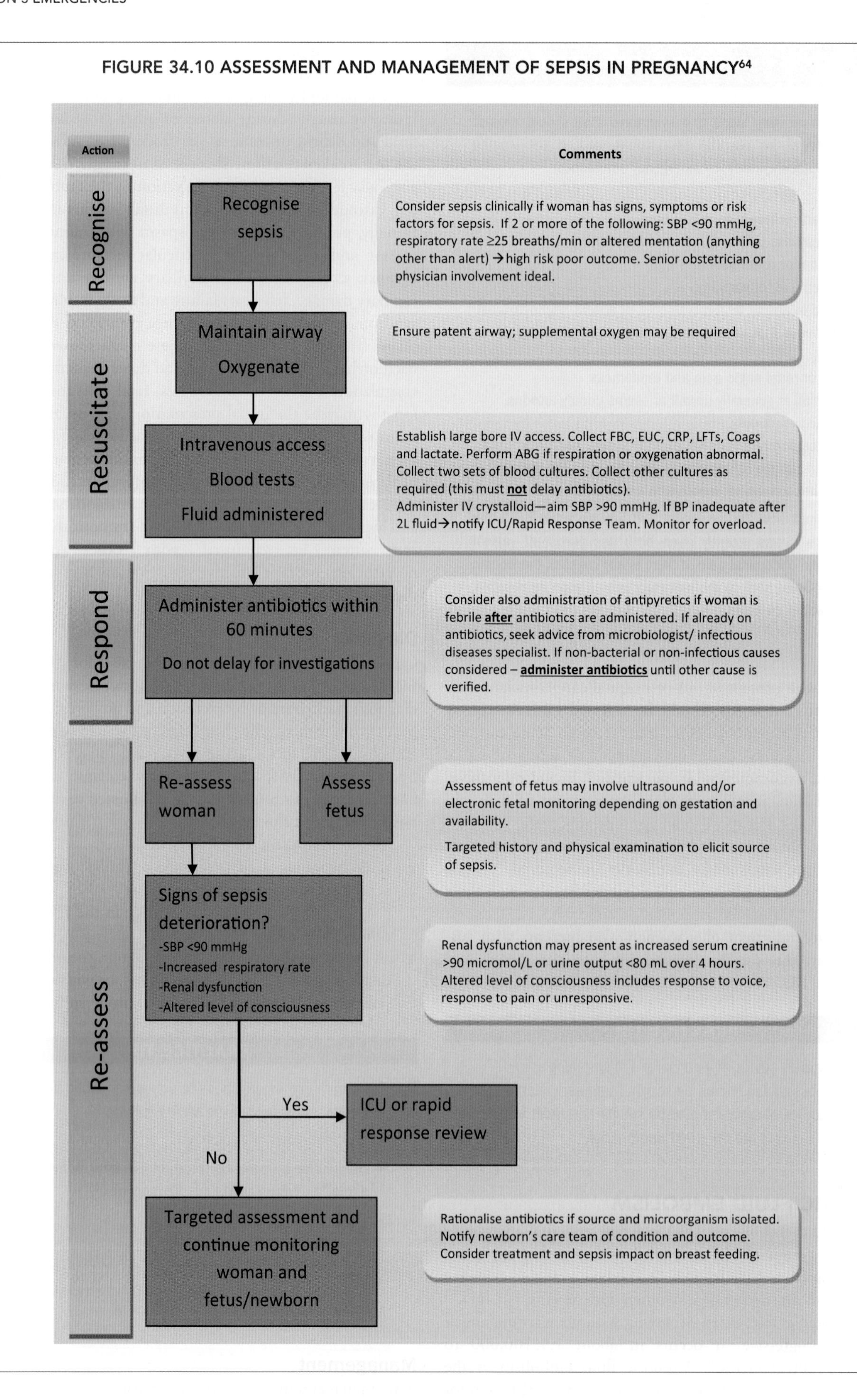

primary goals of management are to provide oxygen, maintain cardiac output and organ perfusion, correct coagulopathy and provide supportive therapies.[1] In the out-of-hospital setting, supportive management should occur, including oxygen therapy and intravenous fluids with urgent transport to hospital. The management in the acute care setting is essentially:

- administer oxygen to maintain normal saturation; intubate and ventilate if necessary.
- initiate CPR if the woman arrests. If she does not respond to resuscitation, perform a perimortem caesarean section.
- treat hypotension with crystalloid fluids, blood products and inotropes.
- consider pulmonary artery catheterisation in women who are haemodynamically unstable.
- continuously monitor the fetus.
- treat coagulopathy and thrombocytopenia using fresh frozen plasma, cryoprecipitate and platelet or whole-blood transfusion as appropriate.[69]

PLACENTAL ABRUPTION

Placental abruption is the partial or complete detachment of the placenta from the uterine wall at any time from 20 weeks gestation prior to the birth of the baby. Placental abruption complicates between 0.4% and 3.8% of all pregnancies[70] and is both a maternal and fetal emergency. It is a leading cause of maternal and fetal morbidity and mortality. Placental abruption can quickly lead to disseminated intravascular coagulation (DIC), uterine rupture, shock, and fetal demise if not correctly diagnosed and managed.[71] A placental abruption can either be partial or complete, the latter resulting in severe maternal and fetal morbidity and/or mortality if immediate management is delayed. Contributing factors include:

- blunt trauma (e.g. motor vehicle collision, physical violence)
- hypertension in pregnancy and pre-eclampsia
- history of caesarean section
- previous placental abruption
- cocaine, amphetamine or tobacco use
- multiparity
- advanced maternal age
- intrauterine infection.[71,72]

Diagnosis

Placental abruption typically presents with pain, tonic contractions of the uterus and/or changes in the fetal heart rate.[70] Vaginal bleeding is not a diagnostic feature of placental abruption because it may or may not be present. Often the bleeding is contained behind the area of detachment and not passed (concealed), or passed from the vagina (revealed).[73] Concealed placental abruption can lead to further detachment as blood fills and clots in the space between the uterine wall and the placenta (retroplacental clot).

Because of this, the degree of shock evident can seem at odds with the lack of blood visible.

A pregnant person who presents with localised or diffuse abdominal pain, uterine rigidity on palpation, contractions, signs of shock with or without bleeding must be considered for placental abruption.

PRACTICE TIP

Vaginal bleeding may not be present as a sign of placental abruption. A high level of suspicion for placental abruption should be taken for all presentations during pregnancy with abdominal pain, contractions and signs of shock. Prompt diagnosis and management can reduce maternal and fetal morbidity and mortality.

Management

When these symptoms present, early recognition and preventing hypotension and hypovolaemia can reduce the severity of shock in the person and the impact of hypoxia and compromise in the fetus.[74]

The priority is to replace circulating fluid volume and reduce shock. Insertion of two wide-bore cannulas and commencement of crystalloid IV fluids is the priority. The management of hypovolaemic shock is discussed in detail in Chapter 22 and Section 4.

Avoiding aortocaval compression by the weight of the fetus from 24 weeks gestation by positioning using a left tilt will aid in perfusion of the uterus and placental bed that remains attached to the uterine wall.[75] Using a wedge or rolled towel can facilitate this position.

Auscultation of the fetal heart via doppler or cardiotocograph (CTG) should be attended to to assess the condition of the fetus once in an ED or delivery suite.[75] The maternal and fetal condition and degree of placental abruption will determine the timing and mode of birth.

MAJOR TRAUMA FROM MOTOR VEHICLE CRASHES OR VIOLENCE

Although serious trauma during pregnancy is uncommon, it remains a major cause of maternal and fetal death and presents a variety of challenges because of the physiological changes due to pregnancy and because there are two people involved—mother and unborn baby.[76] Major trauma in pregnancy has the potential for significant maternal and fetal morbidity and mortality.[76,77] Trauma in pregnancy is the leading non-obstetric cause of maternal and fetal injury and death.[1,3,78] Unrestrained women were more likely to need non-obstetric surgery, suffer an abruption or fetal death.[79] Women should wear a three-point seatbelt, adjusted to fit well, with the lap strap placed beneath the pregnant abdomen and the diagonal strap above the abdomen and between the breasts.[3,80]

Unfortunately, Australian and Aotearoa New Zealand data on major trauma from MVC or violence during pregnancy is difficult to obtain. The most recent Australian Maternal Mortality Report (2010–19)[5] reported two deaths from MVC and 6 homicides. The deaths were classified as 'incidental' and, as such, were seen as being outside the scope of the report and not discussed further.

Trauma in pregnancy can also occur as a result of domestic violence. Domestic violence in pregnancy is a significant issue, as there are immediate and long-term effects on both the woman and her baby.[81,82] The prevalence of domestic violence varies depending on the context, population and measurement instruments. Reports vary regarding incidence, but the rates of women who experience domestic violence in pregnancy are generally reported as 3%–9%.[83,84] In Australia, in 2017–18, pregnant women made up 7.9% (292) of female assault hospitalisations by a spouse or domestic partner. Injuries directed at the torso (33%) were more common among pregnant females than among those who were not pregnant (12%).

Domestic violence in pregnancy can have catastrophic effects in relation to major trauma and death.[3,85] Studies report that women who sustained a physical assault during pregnancy experienced both immediate (placental abruption, increased fetal and maternal mortality) and long-term sequelae (prematurity and low birth-weight infants).[83,84] The Australian Bureau of Statistics[86] reports that 60% of women who had experienced violence were pregnant at some time during their relationship, 36% experienced it during their pregnancy and 17% experienced it for the first time when they were pregnant. Women are at risk of experiencing domestic violence with greater severity while they are pregnant.[87,88]

Major trauma in pregnancy, from whatever cause, has particular deleterious effects on the unborn baby. The unborn baby is more likely to die after traumatic injury than is the woman. Fetal and neonatal death is a significant outcome of trauma. It is reported that there is more than an eight-fold increase in fetal death and more than a six-fold increase in neonatal death for women who experience domestic violence.[84]

PRACTICE TIP

Major trauma in pregnancy can be as a result of a motor vehicle crash or from a physical assault, for example, in domestic violence. It is important to consider domestic violence as a cause when women present with trauma in pregnancy.

Diagnosis

The diagnosis of trauma in pregnancy is similar to that in non-pregnant women. The additional aspects are related to consideration of the effects of the trauma on the pregnancy, particularly on the baby. One of the major complicating factors is a placental abruption, where the placenta separates from the uterine wall. This is the most likely cause of preterm labour in a trauma patient.

The diagnosis of the cause of other trauma or domestic violence may be difficult. Pregnant women who have experienced an assault might be reluctant to talk about it. For example, a woman presenting with vaginal bleeding might not mention that it started after she had sustained a blow to the abdomen.[89] Sensitive and careful questioning in a private and safe space is important to enable women to tell their story.[87,90] It is important that women have time alone with a clinician, as often their partner will have accompanied her to the ED.

Paramedics will often be in an ideal position to assess a pregnant woman who has sustained trauma. Assessment will often take place outside the acute care setting and may be challenging in terms of determining the cause if family members are present. Sensitive questioning in a private environment in the home may be necessary to be able to fully understand the nature of the trauma and the possible cause.

PRACTICE TIP

Compression and displacement of the pelvic, abdominal and thoracic organs occur as pregnancy advances. This makes some injuries more likely and others harder to detect. The physiological changes due to pregnancy must be considered when assessing pregnant women with trauma.

Management

As with non-pregnant trauma patients, the focus of initial interventions remains the ABCs: airway, breathing and circulation.[76,91] Usual trauma care priorities do not change when the patient is pregnant; indeed, the baby's best chance for survival is effective resuscitation of the woman. An explanation of the physiological changes due to pregnancy and how these affect maternal resuscitation was discussed earlier in this chapter.

Identification that the woman is pregnant is the first step in effective resuscitation. In the primary survey by paramedics or assessment in the ED, every woman of childbearing age who presents with trauma should be asked when she last menstruated, whether she could be pregnant (if conscious) and a blood test performed for confirmation of pregnancy status.[91] Pregnant women with positive mechanism of injury according to time-critical guidelines should be transported to a major trauma centre. This applies even if the woman does not have evidence of physiological distress.

Early consultation with an obstetrician, midwife and neonatologist is essential in the case of these women. If the baby is likely to be born preterm, decisions need to be made about the most appropriate location for this to occur. Preterm babies are likely to require specialist care and it is generally easier to transfer the baby in utero rather than ex utero. This, of course, depends on the condition of the woman.

The unborn baby will be extremely sensitive to maternal hypovolaemia: fetal hypoxia and bradycardia can develop quickly. Fetal death can occur at any gestational age and usually results from fetal hypoxia. As highlighted earlier, the changes of pregnancy can mask the signs of decompensation normally present in patients going into shock. Pregnant women generally require two or more large-bore (14 to 16-gauge) intravenous catheters for potential fluid replacement,[76] as with most trauma patients. Resuscitation measures, including the volume of fluid replacement, should follow usual guidelines for patients who have experienced trauma (see Chapter 42 for more detailed information on resuscitation in trauma situations).

PRACTICE TIP

It is important to obtain an obstetric and general medical history from the woman and/or her partner. She may also have her antenatal record with her, which will contain relevant information. This will include the woman's estimated date of birth of her baby, the numbers of previous pregnancies and births and any complications of this or previous pregnancies. The admitting nurse should also establish whether she is currently experiencing contractions, vaginal bleeding or increased vaginal discharge (this could be amniotic fluid from around the baby), or backache or contractions, any of which could indicate that she is in preterm labour. Abdominal pain, contractions or vaginal bleeding might also indicate placental abruption where the placenta has separated from the uterine wall.[77]

Pregnant women who present with major trauma require the same diagnostic studies and interventions as non-pregnant patients. This is detailed in Chapter 46. This includes ultrasound in the first instance, all indicated on radiographic studies such as plain film x-ray, and computed tomography. The uterus should be shielded during radiographic procedures, except during abdominal or pelvic imaging.[76,92] As part of the primary physical assessment of an injured pregnant woman it is important to assess whether there is seatbelt bruising, as this will indicate whether the seatbelt was worn across or above the abdomen. Seatbelt bruising has been reported to significantly predict placental abruption after MVC in pregnant trauma patients. This warrants prompt stabilisation of the woman and fetal assessment.[93]

In addition, all Rhesus-negative women should receive full dose Rhesus immune globulin (more if indicated by Kleihauer-Betke test, the blood test used to measure the amount of fetal haemoglobin transferred from a fetus to the mother's bloodstream).

Fetal monitoring is an important aspect of the care of these women. Pregnant women who experience trauma beyond 23 weeks gestation should be monitored using an electronic fetal monitor continuously for a minimum of 4 hours.[94] Electronic fetal monitoring is usually available only in the labour ward setting, but a monitoring machine could be brought to the ED with a midwife to apply it and interpret the readings.

It is likely that women who experience trauma in pregnancy will be very anxious and concerned for the welfare of their baby. Their partner may also be present and will require support and information in a timely manner. It is important to provide as much information as possible in a caring and sensitive way. In some cases, the baby will have died before arriving at, or while in, the ED. A midwife can advise the staff about addressing this difficult and sad issue with the parents.

PRACTICE TIP

The anatomical and physiological changes of pregnancy can mask the signs of decompensation normally present in patients going into shock. Therefore, pregnant women with major trauma may not look like they are experiencing severe hypovolaemia until they collapse. Consider lower acceptable limits of vital signs as being significant in pregnant women.

CORD PROLAPSE

Umbilical cord prolapse is a true maternal emergency, with direct threat to the life of the neonate due to compression or occlusion of the cord between the fetal presenting part and pelvic brim or sidewall. The result can be asphyxia and mortality for the infant. The incidence of cord prolapse is low, with 0.1–0.6% occurring in vertex/cephalic presentations and approximately 1% in complete or frank breech presentations. Incidence in a footling breech presentation increases to approximately 10%.[95]

Cord prolapse is most common in situations where the presenting part of the fetus does not occlude the pelvic inlet well, such as in footling breech. Other contributing factors for cord prolapse include prematurity, high presenting part, polyhydramnios (excess amniotic fluid), and a long umbilical cord. Up to 50% of cord prolapse occurrences follow obstetric interventions, including rupturing the membranes with a high presenting part.[95]

DIAGNOSIS

Rapid identification and response to a cord prolapse may save the life of the baby.[96] Diagnosis is made by visual inspection or palpation on vaginal examination. The cord may be visibly extruding from the vagina, coiled inside the vagina, or wrapped across the presenting part. Where the cord is not observed extruding from the vagina, or felt upon vaginal examination, the only hint this emergency is occurring may be a sudden and severe variable deceleration or fetal bradycardia, particularly after membrane rupture.

Management

Following diagnosis, urgent management of the cord prolapse is required, aiming for birth as quickly as possible due to the risk of asphyxia and death. Management involves:

- rapid assessment of the baby's status through fetal heart rate monitoring or ultrasound.
- assessing the dilation and status of labour. In most cord prolapse situations, the safest mode of birth is through caesarean section; however, in the uncommon situation where a woman is fully dilated and able to birth vaginally, assistance via forceps or vacuum extraction may be performed.
- discontinuing the use of oxytocic medications (if in use).
- in preparing for caesarean section, elevate the presenting part out of the pelvis to minimise occlusion of the cord. This can be performed internally, using fingers to push the presenting part upwards. Alternatively, rapidly filling the bladder with 500 mL of saline solution and clamping the catheter has also seen some success in raising the presenting part. Women should be encouraged to adopt a deep knee-chest position while on all fours to further encourage the presenting part to move upwards. If being transported by ambulance, elevation of the presenting part should be continuously maintained until the commencement of the caesarean section.
- do not attempt to replace the cord back into the uterus.[95–97]

PRACTICE TIP

Prevention of cord prolapse may not always be possible, but risk can be minimised by identifying risk factors or by responding immediately to reduce cord compression and initiating urgent caesarean section. Women in the later stages of pregnancy who are at high risk of cord prolapse (e.g. polyhydramnios, footling breech) should be identified. Artificial rupturing of membranes should not occur when the baby's head is high in the pelvis. In situations where artificial rupture of membranes is essential to manage a difficult obstetric situation, access to operating theatres for caesarean section birth in the event of a cord prolapse is important.[97]

SUMMARY

This chapter has described the aspects of maternal physiology that affect maternal resuscitation and response to trauma during pregnancy and highlighted the modifications of BLS and ALS needed in pregnancy. Essentially, the anatomical and physiological changes of pregnancy can mask the signs of decompensation, and this has implications for resuscitation and the care of women who have maternal emergencies. The chapter also highlighted that effective resuscitation of the pregnant woman is an essential component of resuscitation of the unborn baby. This may include the undertaking of an emergency caesarean section. The chapter described the criteria for undertaking such a drastic procedure.

The diagnosis and management of pregnant or postpartum women who present to an ED with five maternal emergency situations was addressed. The most important considerations in relation to these emergencies are:

- recognition of the woman's pregnancy
- consideration of the physiological changes that will affect the diagnosis and management of the condition
- the psychological care of the woman and her family
- sensitive care around the possible death of the baby and the social and emotional impact on the parents
- sensitive care around the possible death of the woman and the social and emotional impact on the family
- consideration of the impact of a maternal emergency on the staff.

Maternal emergencies are unique in that there are two patients to consider and care for. Fortunately, for the most part, pregnancy is a normal life event and most babies are born healthy without complications.[7,98] Some women will experience acute maternal emergencies, and for those women the care discussed in this chapter is essential.

CASE STUDY

Lola Adams, a 34-year-old woman, presented to the ED on two occasions over a 48-hour period with a history of abdominal pain and diarrhoea. She was discharged on both occasions with a diagnosis of gastroenteritis, even though she had a history of collapse and measured heart rates of 130 and 144 beats per minute. At 10 pm that evening Lola's family called an ambulance with concerns as to her worsening condition. Lola was attended by a paramedic crew and transported to the nearest hospital.

QUESTIONS

1. With respect to your profession, what questions will you ask in this scenario to determine historical and clinical indicators of urgency and relevance?
2. Describe each aspect of your physical assessment and explain each step.
3. What investigations will you perform and why?
4. What ongoing monitoring will you provide?

This case study is a real story from the UK's *Saving Mothers Lives* report.[9] Lola (not her real name) arrested and died on this, her third, presentation. At post-mortem she was found to have had an ectopic pregnancy.

This case study highlights two important issues—the importance of tachycardia and the risk of overlooking an ectopic pregnancy. Tachycardia is, without doubt, the most significant clinical feature of an unwell patient and is regularly ignored or misunderstood. Measurements of respiratory rate and heart rate are more important than measurements of blood pressure. A normotensive patient may all too often be unwell and compensating. A tachycardic patient is hypovolaemic until proved otherwise.

Many of the women who call an ambulance or come into the ED with symptoms from ectopic pregnancy do not know or volunteer that they are pregnant. Performing a pregnancy test in the pre-hospital setting as a paramedic is unlikely; assumptions are generally made according to the history provided and presenting signs and symptoms. Occasionally these women on admission to an ED do not have a pregnancy test done as a routine. Without a pregnancy test it is hard to include ectopic pregnancy in the differential diagnosis.

Answers to Case Study Questions can be found on evolve http://evolve.elsevier.com/AU/Curtis/emergency/ 

USEFUL WEBSITES

Advanced Maternal and Reproductive Education (AMaRE), Australian registered not-for-profit organisation providing advanced education and training for maternity-related emergencies and situations, www.amare.org.au/

National Blood Authority Australia, blood management guidelines for obstetrics and maternity, www.blood.gov.au/pbm-module-5

PROMPT Maternity Foundation (PMF), UK. Not-for-profit organisation providing practical obstetric multi-professional training for maternal emergencies, www.promptmaternity.org

REFERENCES

1. Dixon L, Cooke H. Life-threatening emergencies. In: Pairman S, Tracey SK, Dahlen HG, Dixon L, editors. Midwifery: preparation for practice. 4th ed. Sydney: Elsevier Australia; 2019.
2. Knight M, Bunch K, Tuffnell D, Shakespeare J, Kotnis, R, Kenyon S, et al. Saving lives, improving mothers' care—lessons learned to inform maternity care from the UK and Ireland confidential enquiries into maternal deaths and morbidity 2015-2017. Oxford: National Perinatal Epidemiology Unit, University of Oxford; 2019.
3. Cantwell R, Clutton-Brock T, Cooper G, Dawson A, Drife J, Garrod D, et al. Saving mothers' lives: reviewing maternal deaths to make motherhood safer: 2006-2008. The Eighth Report of the Confidential Enquiries into Maternal Deaths in the United Kingdom. BJOG 2011;118(Suppl. 1):1-203.
4. Australian Commission on Safety and Quality in Health Care (ACSQHC). Observation charts for paediatric and maternity settings. Available from: www.safetyandquality.gov.au/our-work/recognising-and-responding-to-clinical-deterioration/observation-and-response-charts/observation-charts-for-paediatric-and-maternity-settings/.
5. Australian Institute of Health and Welfare (AIHW). Maternal deaths in Australia 2009-2018. Canberra: 2020. Available from: www.aihw.gov.au/reports/mothers-babies/maternal-deaths-in-australia/contents/maternal-deaths-in-australia.
6. Cunningham F, Leveno K, Bloom S, Dashe JS, Hoffman BL, Casey BM, et al. Williams obstetrics. 25th ed. New York: McGraw-Hill Medical; 2018.
7. Marshall J, Raynor M. Myles textbook for midwives. 17th ed. London: Elsevier; 2020.
8. Rankin J. Physiology in childbearing: with anatomy and related biosciences. Edinburgh: Elsevier; 2017.
9. Hulbert D. Specific recommendations for the management of pregnant women attending Emergency Departments (ED). In: Lewis G, editor. Saving mothers' lives: reviewing maternal deaths to make motherhood safer—2003-2005 The Seventh Report on Confidential Enquiries into Maternal Deaths in the United Kingdom. London: The Confidential Enquiry into Maternal and Child Health (CEMACH); 2007.
10. Ryan L. Recognition of the acutely unwell woman: maternal collapse and resuscitation. In: Marshall JE, Raynor MD, editors. Myles textbook for midwives. 17th ed. Edinburgh: Elsevier; 2020.
11. Pecher S, Williams E. Out-of-hospital cardiac arrest in pregnancy with good neurological outcome for mother and infant. Int J Obstet Anesth 2017;29:81-4.
12. Chu, J, Johnston TA, Geoghegan J. Maternal collapse in pregnancy and the puerperium. BJOG 2019;127(5):e14-52.
13. Hingston T. Maternal collapse. O&G Magazine 2017;19(2). Online. Available from: www.ogmagazine.org.au/19/2-19/maternal-collapse/.
14. Panchal, AR, Bartos JA, Cabañas JG, Donnino MW, Drennan IR, Hirsch KG, et al. Part 3: adult basic and advanced life support: 2020 American Heart Association guidelines for cardiopulmonary resuscitation and emergency cardiovascular care. Circulation 2020;142(16):S366-468.
15. Murphy NJ, Cullinan B. Maternal resuscitation and trauma (including amniotic fluid embolism). In: Leeman L, Quinlan JD, Dresang LT, Gregory DS, editors. Advanced life support in obstetrics provider manual. 8th ed. Kansas: American Academy of Family Physicians; 2017.
16. Australia and New Zealand Committee on Resuscitation (ANZCOR). Guideline 11.10 Resuscitation in special circumstances. 2014. 3 March 2022. Available from: https://resus.org.au/the-arc-guidelines/.
17. Martin-Gill C. Perimortem cesarean section. In: Cone DC, Brice JH, Delbridge TR, Myers JB, editors. Emergency medical services: clinical practice and systems oversight. 3rd ed. Oxford: John Wiley & Sons; 2021.
18. Beckett VA, Knight M, Sharpe P. The CAPS Study: incidence, management and outcomes of cardiac arrest in pregnancy in the UK: a prospective, descriptive study. BJOG 2017;124(9):1374-81.
19. Pairman S, Tracy SK, Dahlen HG, Dixon L. Midwifery: preparation for practice. 4th ed. Sydney: Elsevier Australia; 2019.
20. Tommila M, Pystynen M, Soukka H, Aydin F, Rantanen M. Two cases of low birth weight infant survival by prehospital emergency hysterotomy. Scand J Trauma, Resusc Emerg Med 2017;25:62.
21. Committee on Obstetric Practice, American College of Obstetricians and Gynecologists. Committee Opinion No.543: timing of umbilical cord clamping after birth. Obstet Gynecol 2012;120(6):1522-6.
22. Begley CM, Gyte GM, Devane D, McGuire W, Weeks A. Active versus expectant management for women in the third stage of labour. Cochrane Database Syst Rev 2011;(11):CD007412.
23. Moore E, Bergman N, Anderson G. Early skin-to-skin contact for mothers and their healthy newborn infants. Cochrane Database Syst Rev 2016;(11):CD003519.
24. Walker K, Dawson J. The compromised neonate. In: Pairman S, Tracy SK, Dahlen HG, Dixon L, editors. Midwifery: preparation for practice. 4th ed. Sydney: Elsevier Australia; 2019.
25. McLelland G, McKenna L, Morgans A, Smith K. Epidemiology of unplanned out-of-hospital births attended by paramedics. BMC Pregnancy Childbirth 2018;18:15.

26. Flanagan B, Lord B, Barnes M. Is unplanned out-of-hospital birth managed by paramedics 'infrequent', 'normal' and 'uncomplicated'? BMC Preg Childbirth 2017;17(1):436.
27. Australian and New Zealand Committee on Resuscitation (ANZCOR). ANZCOR Guideline 13.1—Introduction to resuscitation of the newborn. 2021. Available from: https://resus.org.au/the-arc-guidelines/.
28. Aziz K, Lee HC, Escobedo MB, Hoover AV, Kamath-Rayne BD, Kapadia VS, et al. Part 5: neonatal resuscitation. 2020 American Heart Association guidelines for cardiopulmonary resuscitation and emergency cardiovascular care. Circulation 2020;142(16 Suppl 2):S524–50.
29. Australian and New Zealand Committee on Resuscitation (ANZCOR). Guideline 13.3—Assessment of the newborn. 2021. Available from: https://resus.org.au/the-arc-guidelines/.
30. Australian and New Zealand Committee on Resuscitation (ANZCOR). ANZCOR Guideline 13.4—Airway management and mask ventilation of the newborn. 2021. Available from: https://resus.org.au/the-arc-guidelines/.
31. Australian and New Zealand Committee on Resuscitation (ANZCOR). ANZCOR neonatal flowchart. 2021. Available from: resus.org.au/flowcharts-3/.
32. Australian and New Zealand Committee on Resuscitation (ANZCOR). ANZCOR Guideline 13.6—Chest compressions during resuscitation of the newborn. 2021. Available from: https://resus.org.au/the-arc-guidelines/.
33. Hancock A, Weeks AD, Lavender DT. Is accurate and reliable blood loss estimation the 'crucial step' in early detection of postpartum haemorrhage: an integrative review of the literature. BMC Preg Childbirth 2015;15(1):230.
34. Evensen A, Anderson JM, Fontaine P. Postpartum hemorrhage: prevention and treatment. Am Fam Phys 2017;95(7):442–9.
35. Sentilhes L, Goffinet F, Vayssière C, Deneux-Tharaux C. Comparison of postpartum haemorrhage guidelines: discrepancies underline our lack of knowledge. Br J Obstet Gynaecol 2017;124(5):718–22.
36. Ricbourg A, Gosme C, Gayat E, Ventre C, Barranger E, Mebazaa A. Emotional impact of severe post-partum haemorrhage on women and their partners: an observational, case-matched, prospective, single-centre pilot study. Euro J Obstetrics Gynecol Reprod Biol 2015;193:140–3.
37. Khan F, Vaillancourt C, Bourjeily G. Diagnosis and management of deep vein thrombosis in pregnancy. BMJ 2017;357:j2344.
38. Costantine M. Physiologic and pharmacokinetic changes in pregnancy. Front Pharmacol 2014;5:65.
39. Macklon NS, Greer IA, Bowman AW. An ultrasound study of gestational and postural changes in the deep venous system of the leg in pregnancy. Br J Obstet Gynaecol 1997;104(2):191–7.
40. James AH. Thrombosis in pregnancy and maternal outcomes. Birth Defects Res Part C Embryo Today 2015;105(3):159–66.
41. Kamel H, Navi BB, Sriram N, Hovsepian DA, Devereux RB, Elkind MS. Risk of a thrombotic event after the 6-week postpartum period. N Eng J Med 2014;370(14):1307–15.
42. Tuffnell D, Mackillop K, Shakespeare J, et al. Lessons on caring for women with early pregnancy disorders. In: Knight M, Bunch K, Tuffnell D, Patel R, Shakespeare J, Kotnis, R, et al. Saving lives, improving mothers' care—lessons learned to inform maternity care from the UK and Ireland confidential enquiries into maternal deaths and morbidity 2015–2017. Oxford: National Perinatal Epidemiology Unit, University of Oxford; 2019.
43. Bhatia M, Mahtani KR, Rochman R, Collins SL. Primary care assessment and management of common physical symptoms in pregnancy. BMJ 2020;370:m2248. doi:10.1136/bmj.m2248.
44. Odejinmi F, Huff KO, Oliver R. Individualisation of intervention for tubal ectopic pregnancy: historical perspectives and the modern evidence based management of ectopic pregnancy. Euro J Obstet Gynecol Repro Biol 2017;210:69–75.
45. O'Shaughnessy, F, O'Reilly D, Ní Áinle F. Current opinion and emerging trends on the treatment, diagnosis, and prevention of pregnancy-associated venous thromboembolic disease: a review. Translat Rev 2020;225:20–32.
46. Singh S, Sandhu N, Singh S, Kumar P, Aziz A. Comparison between laparoscopy and laparotomy in the management of ectopic pregnancy: a retrospective study. Int J Repro Contra Obstet Gynecol 2020;9(2):705–9.
47. Cutts BA, Dasgupta D, Hunt BJ. New directions in the diagnosis and treatment of pulmonary embolism in pregnancy. Am J Obstet Gynecol 2013;208(2):102–8.
48. Tester J, Hammerschlag G, Irving L, Pascoe D, Rees M. Investigation and diagnostic imaging of suspected pulmonary embolism during pregnancy and the puerperium: a review of the literature. J Med Imag Radiat Oncol 2020;64:505–15.
49. Unger HW, Bhaskar S, Mahmood M. Venous thromboembolism in pregnancy. Obstet Gynaecol Repro Med 2018;28(11–12):360–5.
50. Deutchman M, Walker JE. First-trimester pregnancy complications. In: Leeman L, Quinlan JD, Dresang LT, Gregory DS, editors. Advanced life support in obstetrics provider manual. 8th ed. Kansas: American Academy of Family Physicians; 2017.
51. Hughes M, Lupo A, Browning A. Ruptured ectopic pregnancy with a negative urine pregnancy test. Proc (Bayl Univ Med Cent) 2017;30(1):97–8.
52. Lee R, Dupuis C, Chen B, Smith A, Kim YH. Diagnosing ectopic pregnancy in the emergency setting. Ultrasonography 2018;37(1):78–87.
53. Sepilian VP. Ectopic pregnancy differential diagnoses. Medscape; 2017. Available from: emedicine.medscape.com/article/2041923-differential.
54. Donaldson C. Challenges in pregnancy. In: Pairman S, Tracy SK, Dahlen HG, Dixon L, editors. Midwifery: preparation for practice. 4th ed. Sydney: Elsevier Australia; 2019.
55. Punches BE, Johnson KD, Gillespie GL, Acquavita SA, Felblinger DM. A review of the management of loss of pregnancy in the emergency department. J Emerg Nurs 2017;44(2):146–55.
56. Aoyama K, Ray JG. Pregnancy and risk of intracerebral hemorrhage. JAMA Netw Open 2020;3(4):e202844.
57. Tuffnell D, Bamber J, Banerjee A, et al. Messages for critical care In: Knight M, Bunch K, Tuffnell D, Shakespeare J, Kotnis R, Kenyon S, et al, editors. Saving lives, improving mothers' care–lessons learned to inform maternity care from the UK and Ireland confidential enquiries into maternal deaths and morbidity 2015–2017. Oxford: National Perinatal Epidemiology Unit, University of Oxford; 2019.

58. Lowe SA, Bowyer L, McMahon LP, Morton MR, North RA, Paech MJ, et al. Guideline for the management of hypertensive disorders of pregnancy. Society of Obstetric Medicine of Australia and New Zealand; 2014. Available from: www.somanz.org/content/uploads/2020/07/HTguidelineupdatedJune2015.pdf.
59. NICE. Hypertension in pregnancy: the management of hypertensive disorders during pregnancy. London: National Institute for Health and Clinical Excellence, RCOG Press; 2019. Available from: www.nice.org.uk/guidance/ng133.
60. ARCNZR, New Zealand Resuscitation Council. Guideline 9.2.4; first aid management of a seizure. 2014. Available from: www.revive2survive.com.au/wp-content/uploads/2016/09/guideline-9-2-4-nov-14.pdf.
61. Ambulance Victoria. Clinical practice guidelines for ambulance and MICA paramedics. 2018. Available from: www.ambulance.vic.gov.au/paramedics/clinical-practice-guidelines/.
62. Ali A, Lamont RF. Recent advances in the diagnosis and management of sepsis in pregnancy. F1000Res 2019;8:F1000 Faculty Rev-1546. doi:10.12688/f1000research.18736.1.
63. Mohamed-Ahmed O, Nair M, Acosta C, Kurinczuk JJ, Knight M. Progression from severe sepsis in pregnancy to death: a UK population-based case-control analysis. BJOG 2015;122(11):1506–15.
64. Bowyer L, Robinson HL, Barrett H, Crozier TM, Giles M, Idel I, et al. SOMANZ guidelines for the investigation and management sepsis in pregnancy. ANZJOG 2017;57(5):540–51.
65. Benson MD. Amniotic fluid embolism mortality rate. J Obstet Gynaecol Res 2017;43(11):1714–18.
66. Combs CA, Montgomery DM, Toner LE, Dildy GA. Society for maternal-fetal medicine special statement: checklist for initial management of amniotic fluid embolism. Am J Obstet Gynecol 2021;224(4):B29–32.
67. Guillaume A, Sananes N, Akladios CY, Boudier E, Diemunsch P, Averous G, et al. Amniotic fluid embolism: 10-year retrospective study in a level III maternity hospital. Euro J Obstet Gynecol Repro Biol 2013;169(2):189–92.
68. Ridhorkar A. Neurological emergencies during pregnancy. In: Gandhi A, Malhotra N, Malhotra J, Gupta N, Bora NM, et al, editors. Principles of critical care in obstetrics. New Delhi: Springer; 2016.
69. McDonnell NJ, Percival V, Paech MJ. Amniotic fluid embolism: a leading cause of maternal death yet still a medical conundrum. Int J Obstet Anesth 2013;22(4):329–36.
70. Downes KL, Grantz KL, Shenassa ED. Maternal, labor, delivery, and perinatal outcomes associated with placental abruption: a systematic review. Am J Perinatol 2017;34(10):935–57.
71. Eubank AA, Walzb S, Thiel LM. Maternal risk factors and neonatal outcomes in placental abruption among patients with equal access to health care. J Matern-Fetal Neonat Med 2021;34(13):2101–6.
72. Brennan K. Placental pathology: a review of placenta previa, placental abruption and placenta accrete. Update Anaesthesia 2019;39:51–5.
73. Donaldson C. Challenges in pregnancy. In: Pairman S, Tracy SK, Dahlen HG, Dixon L, editors. 4th ed. Midwifery preparation for practice. Chatswood; Elsevier; 2019.
74. Queensland Ambulance Service. Clinical practice guidelines: obstetrics/placental abruption. 2021. Available from: www.ambulance.qld.gov.au/docs/clinical/cpg/CPG_Placental%20abruption.pdf.
75. Page N, Roloff K, Modi AP, Dong F, Neeki MM. Management of placental abruption following blunt abdominal trauma. Cureus 2020;12(9):e10337.
76. Queensland Government. Queensland clinical guidelines: trauma in pregnancy. 2019. Available from: www.health.qld.gov.au/__data/assets/pdf_file/0013/140611/g-trauma.pdf.
77. Petrone P, Marini CP. Trauma in pregnant patients. Curr Prob Surg 2015;52(8):330–51.
78. Petrone P, Jiménez-Morillas P, Axelrad A, Marini CP. Traumatic injuries to the pregnant patient: a critical literature review. Eur J Trauma Emerg Surg 2017;45(3):383–92.
79. Acar B, Edwards A, Aldah M. Correct use of three-point seatbelt by pregnant occupants. Safety 2018;4(1):1.
80. Amezcua-Prieto C, Ross J, Rogozińska E, Mighiu P, Martínez-Ruiz V, Brohi K, et al. Maternal trauma due to motor vehicle crashes and pregnancy outcomes: a systematic review and meta-analysis. BMJ Open 2020;10(10):e035562.
81. Australian Institute of Health and Welfare (AIHW). Australia's mothers and babies 2019. Canberra: AIHW; 2019. Available from: www.aihw.gov.au/reports/mothers-babies/ncmi-data-visualisations/contents/labour-and-birth-indicators/caesarean-section.
82. Ministry of Health. Report on maternity 2021. Wellington: Ministry of Health; 2021.
83. Hill A, Pallitto C, McCleary-Sills J, Arcia-Moreno C. A systematic review and meta-analysis of intimate partner violence during pregnancy and selected birth outcomes. Int J Gynecol Obstet 2016;133(3):269–76.
84. Australian Institute of Health and Welfare (AIHW). Domestic and sexual violence. 2022. Available from: www.aihw.gov.au/reports/australias-health/health-impacts-family-domestic-and-sexual-violence.
85. Australian Institute of Health and Welfare (AIHW). Australia's mothers and babies: maternal deaths. 2021. Available from: www.aihw.gov.au/reports/mothers-babies/maternal-deaths-australia.
86. Australian Bureau of Statistics (ABS). Personal safety survey, Australia. 2012. Available from: www.abs.gov.au/ausstats/abs@.nsf/Lookup/4906.0Glossary12012.
87. Baird K, Saito AS, Eustace J, Creedy DK. Women's lived experience of intimate partner violence during pregnancy. Women Birth 2015;28:215–20.
88. James L, Brody D, Hamilton Z. Risk factors for domestic violence during pregnancy: a meta-analytic review. Violence Vict 2013;28(3):359–80.
89. Shneyderman Y, Kiely M. Intimate partner violence during pregnancy: victim or perpetrator? Does it make a difference? BJOG 2013;120(11):1375–85.

90. Salmon D, Baird KM, White P. Women's views and experiences of antenatal enquiry for domestic abuse during pregnancy. Health Expect 2015;18(5):867–78.
91. Jain V, Chari R, Maslovitz S, Bujold E, Gagnon R, Basso M, et al. Guidelines for the management of a pregnant trauma patient. J Obstet Gynaecol Can 2015;37(6):553–71.
92. Shakerian R, Thomson BN, Judson R, Skandarajah AR. Radiation fear: impact on compliance with trauma imaging guidelines in the pregnant patient. J Trauma Acute Care Surg 2015;78(1):88–93.
93. Tracy BM, O'Neal CM, Clayton E, MacNew H. Seat belt sign as a predictor of placental abruption. Am Surg 2017;83(11):452–4.
94. Gumm K, Kennedy M, Oats J, Lamb I, Harley N, Hogan C, et al. Pregnancy and trauma–trauma service guideline. Version 3.0 Melbourne: The Royal Melbourne Hospital; 2015.
95. Leeman L. Malpresentations, malpositions and multiple gestation. In: Leeman L, Quinlan JD, Dresang LT, Gregory DS, editors. Advanced life support in obstetrics provider manual. 8th ed. Kansas: American Academy of Family Physicians; 2017.
96. Sayed Ahmed WA, Hamdy MA. Optimal management of umbilical cord prolapse. Int J Women's Health 2018;10:459–65.
97. Chebsey CS, Fox R, Draycott TJ, Siassakos D, Winter C. Umbilical cord prolapse: green-top guideline no.50. Royal College of Obstetricians and Gynaecologists; 2014. Available from: www.rcog.org.uk/media/3wykswng/gtg-50-umbilicalcordprolapse-2014.pdf.
98. Department of Health. Clinical practice guidelines: pregnancy care. Canberra: Australian Government Department of Health; 2020.

CHAPTER 35

PAEDIATRIC EMERGENCIES

DIANNE CRELLIN, MICHELLE McCARTHY AND TOBY ST CLAIR

ESSENTIALS

- Accurately assessing and appropriately managing paediatric emergencies are contingent on having a good understanding of growth and development, and of the anatomical and physiological impact of immaturity and its effect on acute illness and injury across all systems.
- Effective collaborative healthcare is contingent on developing a therapeutic relationship with the patient and their family. Gaining the trust and cooperation of children requires an understanding of cognitive and emotional development and a flexible approach to assessment and management.
- The principles of assessment and management of children are the same as for adults, so this chapter should be read in conjunction with other chapters in the book addressing each topic.
- Acknowledging parental concern as an indicator of serious illness can identify early warning signs of subtle differences and can prevent deterioration and death.
- Tools are available to guide paediatric history-taking and examination to ensure that issues specific to children are not overlooked and that clinical findings are appropriately interpreted and prioritised. However, the principles of assessment, triage and management for children are the same as they are for adults presenting to the emergency department (ED).
- Children may rapidly deteriorate, and frequently exhibit few or non-specific signs and symptoms of significant illness due to immunological immaturity. For this reason, in addition to the attention given to the signs and symptoms of the illness, particular attention should be paid to feeding, urine output, activity levels and sleeping patterns.
- Respiratory illnesses are the most common illnesses occurring in children and account for 30–40% of acute admissions to hospital. As the aetiology is most frequently viral, treatment is focused on managing the symptoms of illness.
- Children react differently to shock and their compensatory mechanisms are effective only in the short term. Early recognition and aggressive treatment of physiological derangement is essential to avoid irreversible shock.
- Young children are also particularly susceptible to dehydration during episodes of illness, regardless of the type of illness, and hydration should be a focus of assessment and management of the unwell child.
- Changes in conscious state are also a feature of deterioration, regardless of the type of illness and should not be overlooked.
- Rashes can be grouped by appearance as vesicular, pustular, papular, eczematous, purpuric/vascular and erythematous, which will help determine the likely cause and therefore appropriate management.
- Injury is the major cause of mortality and morbidity in children and young people.

- The injuries children suffer and their response to trauma are affected by their size and their level of physical and cognitive development.
- Fever is a common symptom associated with illness in children and causes great concern in the community. However, treatment of fever in most circumstances is not recommended and management should be focused only on providing comfort. Furthermore, antipyretics are not recommended to prevent convulsions.
- Children are less likely to receive analgesics than adults in both the ED and pre-hospital settings, and infants and young children are less likely to receive analgesia than older children. Management should include adequate analgesia, regardless of the cause of the pain.
- Acute healthcare is the principal priority during the emergency presentation; however, it is also an opportunity for emergency clinicians to provide health education and address other health and lifestyle issues, such as immunisation, smoking cessation and weight management.

INTRODUCTION

Most children assessed and treated by emergency services are not seen by paediatric specialists but by paramedics and emergency clinicians, who require the skills to assess and manage both adults and children competently. Using a systematic approach to assessment and applying simple principles, it is possible to adequately assess and identify health-related problems in children presenting to emergency services and manage them effectively.

The aim of the chapter is to address the key differences that exist between infants, children and adults, and present some common and important paediatric presentations to emergency service providers. Where the presentation does not differ greatly from the adult and this is presented elsewhere in the book, these presentations have been omitted. For those that are presented in other chapters, but where the paediatric presentation differs, discussion in this chapter will chiefly focus on these differences. A list of useful websites and additional reading materials have also been included at the end of the chapter. Unless specified, the use of the term children in this chapter refers to both infants and children.

APPROACH TO PAEDIATRICS

ANATOMY AND PHYSIOLOGY

Accurately assessing and appropriately managing paediatric emergencies are contingent on having a good understanding of growth and development, and of the anatomical and physiological impact of immaturity and its effect on acute illness and injury across all systems. Children continue to grow in size and mature anatomically and physiologically until they reach adulthood. However, this is not uniform; for example, physiological maturity of many systems is achieved by the end of infancy, while skeletal maturity is not achieved until after puberty. This means that young children may have similar physiological responses to illness and require similar management to adults, while in other circumstances their responses and management may vary greatly.

These differences and their implications will be discussed throughout the chapter in relevant sections of the text. Table 35.1 supplements this discussion and should be consulted for a more comprehensive list of the anatomical and physiological differences that exist between adults, infants and children, and their clinical significance.

FAMILY-CENTRED CARE AND COMMUNICATION

In most circumstances, children present with a parent or caregiver who plays an integral role in maintaining the health and welfare of the child. Emergency care of children includes caring for the family unit, and this should be collaborative and based on a partnership. Parents and caregivers must be given the opportunity to negotiate their role in treatment decision-making and caring for their children and where children are sufficiently mature, they should be included in this collaboration. Please refer to Chapter 8 for a detailed discussion of patient-centred care and communication.

Paediatric emergency presentations require clinicians to rapidly develop rapport with adults and children, whose needs may be different, and the ways in which these needs can be met are also likely to be different. Parents experience a range of emotions when calling an ambulance or presenting with their children to the emergency department (ED); these may range from relief to great anxiety about the likely diagnosis and outcome, or guilt about the origins of the child's illness or injury. The parents may also have a range of concerns that they are reluctant to raise unless they feel comfortable.

Developing good rapport with parents and caregivers requires the clinician to listen carefully to the parents' concerns, ideally while seated, and not to interrupt. The circumstances of emergency care pre-hospital, at triage and during the diagnostic work-up and treatment phases of the emergency presentation can make this especially difficult to achieve. Simple strategies may help to overcome the limitations of the circumstances, such as using the parents' and child's names. Parents are often seeking information and reassurance, and this should be provided wherever possible. Acknowledging parental concern as an indicator of serious illness can identify early warning signs of subtle differences and can prevent deterioration and death. Parents most frequently complain that they were not listened to or taken seriously, or that they were not provided with sufficient information. Clinicians should be aware of their own body language, the language that they use and the messages that this may convey. For example, asking a question using 'why,' such as 'Why have you come today?', implies that they should have done something different.

Most children are discharged home where parents or family members will care for them, which makes it essential that they understand the information they were provided. Discharge education should provide families with sufficient detail to manage their child adequately and confidently at home. It should always include a comprehensive discussion of the criteria for re-presentation. Worsening of the symptoms of the viral illness or development of secondary infection may result in significant deterioration warranting review and treatment. On occasions, the diagnosis is difficult to make in the early stages of the illness and review may be necessary to identify the specific features of illness. Parents must be given the capacity to recognise signs of treatment failure and deterioration and the confidence to return to the ED for review.

Children are often frightened by clinicians and the healthcare setting. Gaining the child's confidence may improve

Text continued on p. 904

TABLE 35.1 THE ANATOMICAL AND PHYSIOLOGICAL DIFFERENCES BETWEEN INFANTS, CHILDREN AND ADULTS, AND THEIR CLINICAL SIGNIFICANCE

DIFFERENCE	DISCUSSION	CLINICAL IMPLICATIONS
Airway differences		
Airways –smaller –more airway soft tissue	Foreign matter such as blood, mucus, vomit and teeth easily obstruct small airways Small amounts of oedema may obstruct the airway, markedly increasing airway resistance	Visualisation and clearing of the airway more difficult Suctioning of airway may be required
Tongue–larger relative to the oropharynx	Airway may be obstructed by the tongue, where there is swelling or a decrease in conscious state	In the trauma patient, open the airway using the jaw-thrust manoeuvre Repositioning may be the only intervention needed to maintain a patent airway Oropharyngeal airways may be useful in the unresponsive child
Obligate nose breathers in early infancy (< 3 months of age)	Obstructed nasal passages can produce significant respiratory distress and/or feeding difficulty	Remove secretions using saline drops or suction
Trachea–shorter in length	Increased chance of bronchial intubation Changes in head position will cause movement in ETT Flexion of the neck displaces the tube further into the trachea Extension of the neck moves the tube further out of the trachea	Ensure air entry to both lung fields, confirm position on x-ray Secure tube carefully Record initial ETT position (centimetre mark at the gum) Maintain head in midline position and prevent extension or flexion of the neck Monitor ETT position regularly
Larynx–softer and more cartilaginous	More susceptible to compression with hyperextension or hypoextension of the neck	Maintain appropriate position to ensure airway patency Use jaw thrust in the trauma patient
Larynx–positioned more anteriorly and cephalad	Increased risk of aspiration Direct visualisation of the vocal cords is more difficult during intubation	Cricoid pressure may assist with visualisation of the vocal cords during intubation attempts
Epiglottis–shaped differently and relatively floppy	Epiglottis likely to 'flop' into airway obscuring view of cords during intubation	Ensure alternative laryngoscope blade (straight) available Lift epiglottis out of the way
Occiput–relatively large	Head pushed forward when lying supine, therefore neck not in neutral alignment; may result in airway compression	Place a small towel roll under the child's shoulders to maintain the appropriate airway position
Cervical spine differences		
Head–proportionately heavier Vertebral ligament–increased laxity Neck musculature–underdeveloped	Increases the risk that vertebrae may move, resulting in spinal cord injury in the absence of a fracture Pseudosubluxation of C2 on C3 Normal variant in up to 40% of children aged < 7 years and in < 20% of children aged < 16 years Secondary to ligamentous laxity Phenomenon called spinal cord injury without radiological abnormality (SCIWORA); seen predominantly in children	Normal cervical spine x-ray does not exclude cord injury Careful neurological examination needed CT scan and MRI may be useful adjuncts in the evaluation of possible spinal cord injuries Neurosurgical consultation should be obtained where extent of injury unclear

Continued

TABLE 35.1 THE ANATOMICAL AND PHYSIOLOGICAL DIFFERENCES BETWEEN INFANTS, CHILDREN AND ADULTS, AND THEIR CLINICAL SIGNIFICANCE—cont'd

DIFFERENCE	DISCUSSION	CLINICAL IMPLICATIONS
Fulcrum of flexion higher–C1–C2 in young children; C6–C7 in adults	Level of cervical spine injury occurs at fulcrum of flexion Affects outcome	Neurological deficits determined by level of injury
Growth centres in vertebrae	Increased susceptibility to shearing forces	Increases likelihood of cord injury
Ear–nose–throat		
Eustachian tubes–shorter and angle less acute	Reduced drainage of fluids	Increased number of ear infections
Respiratory differences		
Ribs –more cartilaginous –twice as compliant as those of an adult	Retractions are more common and reduce the infant's or small child's ability to maintain functional residual capacity or generate adequate tidal volume Ribs may not fracture under compression or with direct blow Provide less protection to underlying organs. Increased chest-wall compliance allows traumatic forces to be transmitted to underlying thoracic structures	Work of breathing the most useful indicator of level of respiratory distress Absence of rib fracture on x-ray does not exclude possibility of injury to underlying structures Suspect pneumothoraces and/or haemothoraces in the child who has significant chest trauma with or without rib fractures
Ribs–positioned more horizontally in infancy than the adults	Relatively fixed tidal volume	Dependent on rate to maintain minute volume
Mediastinum–more mobile	More likely to suffer damage due to shearing in an acceleration/deceleration injury	
Fatigue-resistant type I fibres–fewer in intercostal muscles	Become exhausted more quickly	Closely observe the child with continuous monitoring of heart rate, respiratory rate and effort, and pulse oximetry Treat respiratory distress Prevent increases to demand Allow parents to remain with child if their presence is comforting to the child Provide non-threatening environment and avoid noxious stimuli Treat pain
Diaphragm –performs most of the work of breathing –reduced role of intercostal muscles	Generation of tidal volume depends on diaphragmatic function Anything impeding diaphragm movement can lead to reduced tidal volume, e.g. distended stomach Diaphragmatic fatigue possible	Allow alert child to maintain own position of comfort to optimise respiratory effort If possible, maintain patient in upright position to support diaphragmatic function Avoid abdominal distension Smaller, more frequent feeds Nasogastric or orogastric tube insertion to decompress the stomach
Chest wall–relatively thin	Breath sounds are easily transmitted across the chest wall and over the abdomen Difficult to localise adventitious noises (including upper-airway-generated noises)	Breath sounds should be auscultated bilaterally over the anterior and posterior chest wall, and in the axillary areas, using a paediatric stethoscope Differences indicating pathology may be subtle Obtain chest x-ray films as necessary
Oxygen consumption–twice that of an adult	Higher minute volume to meet demand	Deliver highest possible concentration of oxygen to infants and children in respiratory distress

TABLE 35.1 THE ANATOMICAL AND PHYSIOLOGICAL DIFFERENCES BETWEEN INFANTS, CHILDREN AND ADULTS, AND THEIR CLINICAL SIGNIFICANCE—cont'd

DIFFERENCE	DISCUSSION	CLINICAL IMPLICATIONS
Respiratory muscles–greater oxygen and metabolite requirement	Work of breathing can account for up to 40% of the cardiac output, particularly in stressed conditions	Reduce work of breathing Mechanical ventilation to eliminate metabolic costs of work of breathing
Control of ventilation–immature	Responses to hypoxia are unpredictable	Monitor young infants closely for apnoea
Circulatory differences		
Myocardium –fewer actomyosin elements and mitochondria, therefore less capacity to increase contractility –less compliant	Greater reliance on increases in heart rate to increase cardiac output compared with the adult Higher atrial pressures at the same filling pressures Negative effect on preload Restricted capacity to increase stroke volume Relatively poor response to aggressive fluid resuscitation	Provide continuous cardiac monitoring with attention to trends in heart rate Larger volumes of fluid may be required to augment circulation
Compensation–better able to mount compensatory response by increasing peripheral vascular resistance	May remain normotensive until 25–40% of their blood volume is lost Hypotension is a late and often sudden sign of cardiovascular decompensation	Monitor other parameters, particularly heart rate, to detect hypovolaemia before hypotension apparent Aggressive resuscitation in response to earlier signs of hypovolaemia
Blood volume –larger volume per kg (child 80 mL/kg vs adult 70 mL/kg) –absolute volume much smaller	Smaller amounts of blood loss can cause volume depletion	Carefully estimate blood loss, including blood drawn for laboratory analysis Serial haemoglobin and haematocrit analysis should be obtained Consider blood replacement therapy after 40–60 mL/kg of isotonic crystalloids in the paediatric trauma patient with signs of shock or when acute blood loss totals 5–7% of the child's circulating blood volume
Vessels–smaller	Intravascular access more difficult	Cannula sizes will need to be adjusted Ensure most-competent clinician attempting access in time-critical situation Low threshold for using alternative access strategy, e.g. intra-osseous administration
Systemic vascular resistance–lower	BP lower	Ensure reference range for normal BP for varying age is available
Terminal rhythm differs –children: brady/asystole; adults: VF/VT	Bradycardia often result of hypoxia Bradycardia not well tolerated in children because it significantly reduces cardiac output	Provide adequate oxygenation and ventilation Treat symptomatic bradycardia
Fluid balance		
Percentage total body water Larger infants & children: 80%. adults: 65%	Infants and young children will lose larger amounts of water through evaporation than will the adult	Calculate maintenance fluids based on each child's weight in kilograms and clinical condition
Surface area/volume ratio–larger	Children have greater potential for dehydration Maintenance fluid requirements per kilogram of bodyweight are higher in children	Record all sources of fluid intake and fluid loss to calculate fluid balance and adjust fluid therapy accordingly

Continued

TABLE 35.1 THE ANATOMICAL AND PHYSIOLOGICAL DIFFERENCES BETWEEN INFANTS, CHILDREN AND ADULTS, AND THEIR CLINICAL SIGNIFICANCE—cont'd

DIFFERENCE	DISCUSSION	CLINICAL IMPLICATIONS
Renal blood flow and the glomerular filtration rate–lower	Less capacity to concentrate the urine infants 2 mL/kg children 1 mL/kg adults 0.5 mL/kg	Relatively higher volumes of urine are required to indicate adequate renal perfusion
Renal system–immature	Less able to acidify urine and therefore more susceptible to hyperchloraemic acidosis with aggressive resuscitation with normal saline	Avoid large volume resuscitation with normal saline without close monitoring of electrolytes
Neurological differences		
Head–proportionately larger and heavier	Higher centre of gravity acts as a missile If an infant or child falls or is thrown a significant distance, the initial impact more often will be to the head, which predisposes the child to head injury	Anticipate head injury in the traumatically injured child Suggest use of preventive measures, such as seatbelts, car seats and helmets, to patients and family members
Skull–thinner	Provides less protection for the brain	As above
Cranial sutures –do not fuse until approximately age 16–18 months –fontanelles are junction between sutures	Fullness of fontanelle is influenced by acute changes in intracranial volume –full = intracerebral infection, haemorrhage etc. –low = hypovolaemia Allow for growth of the skull and intracranial contents May allow for gradual increases in intracranial volume, i.e. hydrocephalus	Assess fontanelles for size and tension in the infant age 16–18 months or younger Measure head circumference with neurological examinations in the child up to age 16–18 months at risk for increasing intracranial pressure
Cognitive development–varies with age	Assessment of cognitive function influenced by level of development Cooperation influenced by development	Use modified GCS for neurological assessment Use age-appropriate assessment techniques Use age-appropriate management strategies
Metabolic and thermoregulatory differences		
Immune system–immature	Increased susceptibility to infection Response to infection differs; often poorly localised resulting in different constellation of symptoms	Assume serious illness in babies with generalised symptoms until focus found
Surface area to body mass ratio–higher Subcutaneous fat stores–lower	Increased heat loss through radiation and evaporation, especially from the child's proportionally large head Hypothermia can cause metabolic acidosis, hypoglycaemia, coagulopathies, CNS depression, respiratory depression and myocardial irritability, making resuscitation more difficult Less well-insulated by fat, adding to heat loss	Prevent heat loss Cover children with warm blankets or place them under warming lights if they cannot be covered Reduce draughts in clinical area Use warmed intravenous fluids or blood for volume resuscitation Warm and humidify supplemental oxygen if possible Consider placing small infants in isolettes with overbed warmers Monitor temperature in young babies in isolette with skin probe to avoid underheating or overheating and thermal injury
Heat production –infants aged < 3 months unable to rely on shivering –rely on fat stores	Increased risk of hypothermia in the small infant The burning of fat increases oxygen consumption, which can lead to hypoxia	As above

TABLE 35.1 THE ANATOMICAL AND PHYSIOLOGICAL DIFFERENCES BETWEEN INFANTS, CHILDREN AND ADULTS, AND THEIR CLINICAL SIGNIFICANCE—cont'd

DIFFERENCE	DISCUSSION	CLINICAL IMPLICATIONS
Glycogen stores—lower	Increased risk for developing hypoglycaemia	Monitor glucose frequently during and after resuscitation Administer glucose as ordered
Metabolic rate—higher	Increased oxygen and glucose consumption Increased demands associated with illness may not be met due to poor stores Results in higher nutritional needs per kilogram of bodyweight than in an adult	As above Provide supplemental oxygen to all seriously ill or injured children Consult with doctor and dietitian to provide early, adequate nutritional support to the compromised child
Abdominal differences		
Diaphragm—flattened	Pushes the spleen and liver down into the abdominal cavity Unprotected by the rib cage, increasing their exposure to injury Spleen and liver are the most commonly injured abdominal organs in children	Abdominal assessment for presence of injury vital in children involved in trauma Obtain early surgical consultation as necessary Monitor serial haemoglobin and haematocrit analysis for signs of haemorrhage Abdominal girth measurements may assist assessment
Abdominal wall—less musculature and less subcutaneous tissue	Provides less protection to underlying organs	As above
Bladder position—intra-abdominal organ until approximately 2 years of age	Increased risk of bladder trauma where there is injury to the abdomen	Urine specimens can be taken suprapubically in infants and young toddlers
Musculoskeletal differences		
Bones —incomplete bone calcification —more cartilaginous —more flexible and plastic	Afford less protection to underlying structures than the stronger, more rigid bones of the adult Can absorb larger amounts of force without bone injury, transferring force to underlying structures Change the injury profile as increased cartilage weakens the bone Weakest part of the musculoskeletal system (tendon/muscle/ligament/bone) Result in plastic deformation (bowing fractures, greenstick and torus fractures) in response to trauma	Index of suspicion for organ damage should be high even in the absence of fractures where the force was significant Obtain early surgical consultation as necessary Monitor for signs of internal haemorrhage Low threshold for x-ray of limb injuries even in the absence of obvious signs of fracture as plastic deformation, torus and buckle fractures less clinically apparent
Bones growing—physeal plate and secondary ossification centres present	Physeal plate is a point of vulnerability (2–5 times weaker than other parts of the bone) Increased blood flow to physeal areas of the bone increases likelihood of vascular deposition of bacteria, e.g. osteomyelitis	Presence of secondary ossification centres and physeal plates influence interpretation of radiological images Gain paediatric orthopaedic opinion if there is any doubt about images Index of suspicion for infection should be high
Bones growing—metabolic activity higher	Healing times are substantially shorter Growing bones allow for remodelling of the bony deformity particularly in the arc of movement	

BP: blood pressure; CNS: central nervous system; CT: computed tomography; ETT: endotracheal tube; GCS: Glasgow Coma Scale; MRI: magnetic resonance imaging; VF: ventricular fibrillation; VT: ventricular tachycardia.

the child's cooperation with history-taking and with the examination and help to reassure the parents. The strategies used to gain the confidence of the child will depend on their age and rely on showing creativity and an understanding of the cognitive development of the child and their likely fears.

Infants and young children will look to their parents for support, and they should not be separated unless absolutely necessary. Age-appropriate games and toys may be used to distract and help gain the child's confidence. These strategies serve as a way of relaxing the child, but are also an excellent aid to examination. For example, an infant watching and reaching for bubbles demonstrates normal cognition. Where possible, examination should be delayed until the child has become more comfortable with the clinician. The best results are generally achieved when the child is examined in a parent's arms or on their lap, with the clinician sitting on a low stool or on the ground rather than standing over the top of the child. The sequence of examination should see the more invasive and distressing techniques left until last.

As children get older, involving them as much as possible and explaining your intentions is likely to increase the child's confidence. Great care should be taken with the language used, as school-aged children can be very frightened by particular words and can take expressions quite literally. Magical thinking can exacerbate this, but is also an excellent foundation for age-appropriate games aimed at gaining their cooperation. It may be possible to make a game out of parts of the examination: for example, explaining that you think you saw a tiger in their ear, but you need to use a light to have a proper look to see if there really is one there. Reading stories and watching videos can also serve to distract the child.

Once children reach adolescence, they are usually striving for much more independence and are likely to look for this when seeking healthcare. Adolescents are also likely to demand greater privacy and may also wish to discuss their health concerns without the presence of their parents. However, this should not be assumed, and clinicians may need to negotiate everyone's roles during the presentation.

PRACTICE TIPS

- It is essential to rapidly gain the trust of the parents and the child to assess and manage the child in the ED.
- Parents and/or caregivers must be given the opportunity to negotiate their role in clinical decision-making and caring for their children.

ASSESSMENT

The physical, cognitive and developmental differences between infants, children and adults will influence the approach to assessment and interpretation of the findings. Using a systematic approach to assessment, such as HIRAID, is essential.[1] The following sections describe an approach to paediatric health assessment and highlight how the differences between adults, children and infants affect assessment.

HISTORY

There are some unique features to paediatric history-taking as it relies on building a rapport with both patient (child) and parent, and often relies on information provided by primary carers. However, it is important not to ignore the contribution made by quite young children. They are often capable of providing important details not known by the parent or primary carer. For example, a child with an arm injury may be able to confirm that the injury occurred once another child helped pull them up onto the play equipment and not from the fall as may have been assumed by the carer, supporting a diagnosis of 'pulled elbow' rather than 'fracture'. Additionally, siblings may also provide valuable information, particularly descriptions of the mechanism of injury responsible for the child's presentation.

Presenting complaint

This is a detailed account of the onset of the illness or the mechanism of injury, the range and extent of signs and symptoms, the precipitating and alleviating factors, and the treatment provided to date. There are some clinical and age-related factors that should be considered as they may alert the clinician to the presence of significant illness or injury.

Infants may rapidly deteriorate, and frequently exhibit few or non-specific signs and symptoms of significant illness due to immunological immaturity. For this reason, in addition to the attention given to the signs and symptoms of the illness, attention should be paid to feeding, urine output, activity levels and sleeping patterns. Research has shown that changes to any of these increases the likelihood that the infant or young child has a serious illness, and with the addition of a urine screen most infants with serious illness can be detected by reviewing these simple parameters.[2,3] Poor feeding may result from shortness of breath, lethargy or general malaise, and is associated with a range of illnesses, which include serious infection, moderate to severe respiratory illness and gastrointestinal disorders. The relationship between other symptoms and feeding should also be explored. In neonates and young babies, sweating and dusky skin colour during feeding suggests cardiac disease, while projectile vomiting soon after feeding suggests pyloric stenosis. Comparison with the feeding pattern of the child or infant when well is generally the best method for determining the adequacy of feeding and this information can be provided by the carer. However, it is useful to know the average volumes consumed by infants and children at varying ages, and these can be found in Table 35.2. Similarly, changes in urine output are best estimated by comparing current output with output when well. In infants this is determined indirectly via the number of wet nappies in a day. It is generally accepted that infants will have approximately six wet nappies per day.

TABLE 35.2 AVERAGE ORAL INTAKE FOR NEONATES, INFANTS AND CHILDREN

AGE	VOLUME
Infant	150 mL/kg/day
Small child	50 mL/kg/day
Older child	20 mL/kg/day

Serious illness in infants can be associated with irritability and disturbed sleep, or decreased activity and drowsiness, where the infant fails to wake for feeds. Sleep may also be disturbed by respiratory illness, shortness of breath, sleep apnoea caused by enlarged tonsils, pain, and a range of other circumstances.

Past history

A child's comorbidities and treatment and the potential effect on their acute condition should be considered. This should also include the infant's perinatal history, to identify health problems resulting from prematurity, the circumstances of the delivery or congenital abnormalities. For example, the infant with congenital lung disease resulting from prematurity is at risk of more significant respiratory dysfunction associated with an acute respiratory infection.

The history should determine whether the child is showing consistent weight gain and meeting normal growth and developmental milestones. Some illnesses and abnormalities become evident due to failure to thrive or arrested/delayed development[4] (refer to Table 35.3 for normal milestones in the first 2 years of life). Newborns in Australia and Aotearoa New Zealand are issued with an 'infant welfare' book (variously named in different jurisdictions) to document postnatal and maternal child health nurse examinations, including weight measurements and immunisations.

The immunisation schedule provides recommendations for the vaccination of children against a range of childhood diseases. The Australian and Aotearoa New Zealand government-funded schedules can be found in the list of Useful websites found at the end of the chapter. The immunisation status of the child should be established, and details should be obtained when vaccinations were administered overseas, where the schedule may vary from the Australasian schedules. Although it is uncommon for children not to be immunised, many children fall behind the schedule, often due to illness at the time vaccinations were due. A small number of families will identify as conscientious objectors to immunisation or will indicate that they have had their child homeopathically immunised. This is addressed in more detail in a later section focusing on preventative health measures.

Family history and social history

The family history will help determine whether familial or genetic disorders, such as asthma, diabetes, haemophilia etc, are likely. Relationships between family members and the illnesses suffered can be documented on a family tree for clarity. In some circumstances it may also be important to note consanguinity between parents, as this increases the risk of genetic and familial disorders and is common in some communities.

The health of siblings should also be explored, as they may be a potential infectious contact or exhibit similar signs of familial or genetic disorders. Attendance at childcare also increases the child's exposure to infectious diseases and it is important to note whether there has been a recent epidemic at the patient's childcare facility. Furthermore, childcare workers may also be able to contribute to the history.

The child's living circumstances should be observed by the paramedics and outlined in handover for consideration, to identify other risks to health such as cigarette smoke exposure, which increases the risk of respiratory diseases, meningococcal

TABLE 35.3 NORMAL MILESTONES IN FIRST 2 YEARS OF LIFE[5]

AGE	ACHIEVEMENT—MOTOR	ACHIEVEMENT—LANGUAGE AND SOCIAL
Neonate	Lifts head Visually fixes for period	Turns to voice
6 weeks	Follows past midline	Smiles
2–4 months	Rolls over Head steady when sitting Follows object 180 degrees	Smiles Squeals with enjoyment
5–8 months	Sits without support Transfers objects between hands	Makes babbling noises Feeds self hand-held food
9–12 months	Stands holding on for support, crawls Able to use a pincer grip for small objects	Says 'mama' and 'dada' Exhibits stranger anxiety Indicates needs by gesturing
12–16 months	Walks unassisted Able to make a stack of two blocks	Says single words Drinks from a cup
17–21 months	Walks up steps Scribbles with large Texta/crayon	Says several words Points to one part of the body
2 years	Runs and jumps Can copy drawing straight line	Combines words Can remove clothing

disease, Perthes' disease, sudden infant death syndrome (SIDS), etc.[6] In some circumstances, recent travel may be relevant to the current presentation.

A complete history should identify who acts as the primary carer and whether there are others who play a significant role as carer. Where a second person cares for the child for significant periods of time, this person may be able to add substantially to the history. Additionally, consideration should be given to providing this person with similar healthcare information as is provided to the parents to ensure that they are well placed to care for the child's health.

Child at risk

Mandatory reporting legislation in all jurisdictions in Australia demands that healthcare professionals report suspicions that a child has suffered physical, emotional or sexual abuse to the statutory child protection authority in that jurisdiction. A summary of the legislative duties can be found on the Australian Institute of Family Studies website.[7] Healthcare professionals responsible for the care of children must consider the possibility and respond appropriately where their suspicions have been aroused. Clinicians should also be alert to signs of family violence as this has profound effects on the wellbeing of the child. A detailed discussion of violence, abuse and assault is presented in Chapter 39.

The most common concern identified by paramedics and ED clinicians relates to injuries where the cause is thought to be non-accidental. Suspicion should be aroused when there are inconsistencies in the history provided, the version of events changes over time, it is reported differently by each of the parents, or the mechanism does not adequately explain the presenting injuries. Less commonly, the presentation may be for an unrelated health problem and evidence of injury or potential abuse is uncovered, or the parent alludes to their concern for their child's welfare while in their care or the care of someone else. Care of the child where abuse is suspected should involve a senior clinician. However, this does not abrogate responsibility for ensuring appropriate reporting occurs.

Alternatively, the carer may acknowledge that there has been family services involvement with the family, or this may be noted in the child's history. It is important to determine what responsibilities this places on the examining clinician; for example, reporting all injuries to state authorities, gaining consent from a state-appointed custodian, etc.

PRACTICE TIPS

HISTORY

- Parents, siblings and the patient may provide key historical data.
- Serious illness may be associated with non-specific signs and symptoms in infants, such as poor feeding, lethargy, irritability and poor sleeping.
- The perinatal history, immunisation status, infectious contact history, sibling and family history and childcare attendance frequently provide additional clues to the nature of the illness.

EXAMINATION

Physical examination of infants and young children and interpretation of the findings can be more difficult, as they frequently become distressed and are uncooperative when touched. Examination techniques may require significant adaptation and clinicians will need to rely more heavily on careful observation to elicit reliable examination data. Delaying the examination while you develop a rapport with first the parents and then the child is ideal.

Allowing infants to remain in their parent's arms during the examination, making a game out of parts of the examination for toddlers and providing clear explanations to older children of what is intended are examples of strategies that may help increase a child's confidence. Table 35.4 details some practical techniques for approaching infants and children of different ages.

The following sections will address the primary survey and the collection of vital signs, highlighting the significance of immaturity. This discussion is supplemented by the details in Table 35.1.

TABLE 35.4 AGE-SPECIFIC APPROACHES TO PHYSICAL EXAMINATION DURING CHILDHOOD[8]

POSITION	SEQUENCE	PREPARATION
Infant		
Best positioned on a parent's lap, particularly for sections of the examination that are likely to be distressing	If quiet, auscultate heart, lungs, abdomen first Palpate and percuss same areas Undress only when required to prevent babies getting cold Proceed in usual head-to-toe direction Perform traumatic procedures last (eyes, ears, mouth [while crying])	Clinician should sit on low chair in view of infant but out of reach while taking history, to allow infant to become more comfortable with clinician (older infant) Gain cooperation with distraction, bright objects, rattles, talking Smile at infant; use soft, gentle voice Pacify with feeding Enlist parent's aid for restraining to examine ears, mouth Avoid abrupt, jerky movements

TABLE 35.4 AGE-SPECIFIC APPROACHES TO PHYSICAL EXAMINATION DURING CHILDHOOD—cont'd

POSITION	SEQUENCE	PREPARATION
Toddler		
Best positioned on parent's lap, particularly for sections of the examination that are likely to be distressing	Take history first, while observing infant and allowing them to watch Use minimum physical contact initially Inspect body area through play: 'count fingers', 'tickle toes' Introduce equipment slowly Auscultate, percuss, palpate whenever quiet Examine injured limb last; start with the unaffected limb. Repeat to determine whether tenderness is reproducible Perform traumatic procedures last (same as for infant)	Clinician should sit on low chair in view of child but out of reach while taking history, to allow child to become more comfortable with clinician Ask parent to undress child well before examination is attempted, to allow child to settle before attempting to examine Allow child to inspect equipment; demonstrating use of equipment is usually ineffective If uncooperative, perform procedures quickly Use restraint when appropriate; request parent's assistance Talk about examination if cooperative; use short phrases Praise for cooperative behaviour
Preschool child		
Allow child to determine where they would like to sit—on parent's lap or on the trolley Ensure parents are close	If cooperative, proceed in head-to-toe direction If uncooperative, proceed as with toddler	Request self-undressing Allow to wear underpants if shy Offer equipment for inspection; briefly demonstrate use Make up story about procedure (e.g. 'I'm seeing how strong your muscles are' [blood pressure]) Give choices when possible Expect cooperation; use positive statements (e.g. 'Open your mouth')
School-age child		
Cooperative in most positions Younger child prefers parent's presence Older child may prefer privacy	Proceed in head-to-toe direction May examine genitalia last in older child	Respect need for privacy. Expose only area to be examined Request self-undressing Explain purpose of equipment and significance of procedure, such as otoscope to see eardrum, which is necessary for hearing Teach about body function and care Use simple language for explanations as they are easily frightened by misunderstood language
Adolescent		
Same as for school-age child Offer option of parent's presence	Same as older school-age child Leave intrusive/embarrassing examinations until last	Allow to undress in private and provide gown Expose only area to be examined Respect need for privacy Explain findings during examination: 'Your muscles are firm and strong' Emphasise normalcy of anatomy and development, including genitals Examine genitalia as any other body part; may leave to end

Airway

Evaluation of the airway will concentrate on determining airway patency. A narrower airway and increased soft tissue place the infant and child at greater risk of airway obstruction, and stridor is a common paediatric presentation. Other upper respiratory tract noises, such as snore and stertor, are also common, and can be the result of issues such as nasal congestion secondary to viral illness, enlarged tonsils, etc. Assessment of work of breathing, which is described in the next section, should make it possible to evaluate the extent of the airway obstruction. The pitch or loudness of upper respiratory noises should not be relied upon to assess severity of airway obstruction.

Breathing

Children tolerate respiratory distress very poorly. It is the most common antecedent to deterioration and paediatric cardiopulmonary arrest.[9]

The primary focus of respiratory assessment is an assessment of the work of breathing. Increased work of breathing has been shown to be an indicator of significant or serious illness in infants.[2,10] Increased work of breathing is reliably recognised in infants and children by the presence of subcostal, suprasternal and intercostal recession (Fig. 35.1), the severity of which is defined as *mild*, *moderate* and *severe*.[11]

Other clinical findings, which will contribute to the assessment of the severity of respiratory dysfunction, are:

- respiratory rate
- oxygen saturations (SpO^2)
- the presence or absence of nasal flaring.

Increasing respiratory rate suggests significant illness and is a better predictor of deterioration than other vital signs.[9] Rates over 50 breaths/minute in infants less than 2 months are predictive of hypoxia.[12] However, as infants and children become more exhausted, a drop in respiratory rate may signal deterioration. It has also been shown that the respiratory rates of well infants under the age of 6 months vary considerably, from 20 to 80 breaths per minute.[13] For these reasons, respiratory rate should be interpreted cautiously and not in isolation. Oxygen saturations support assessment of the efficacy of breathing, and in infants and children values less than 97% should not be considered normal.[14]

Some evidence suggests that measurement of the SpO_2 on presentation of infants and children with respiratory illness may assist in the prediction of those likely to require admission for respiratory observation and management.[15,16]

Systemic signs, such as colour, heart rate and mentation, will also assist in determining respiratory adequacy. Hypoxia results in increasing pallor and, in extreme circumstances, cyanosis. Respiratory inadequacy results in an increasing heart rate, but infants are extremely susceptible to hypoxia and quickly respond with bradycardia. Similarly, increasing respiratory dysfunction results in deteriorating mental state and infants can progress from irritability to drowsiness very rapidly.

Infants and young children use grunting to increase airway pressure and improve functional residual capacity and therefore oxygenation in respiratory illness. This involves closing of the glottis against expiration, resulting in positive end-expiratory pressure, which helps to prevent alveolar collapse. This creates the same effect as pursed-lip breathing, often seen in older people with chronic lung disease. Grunting should alert the clinician to the presence of significant pathology that has the potential to impact on oxygenation.

Lung sounds contribute to diagnostic decision-making rather than an assessment of respiratory efficacy. Wheezes are an expiratory noise reflecting narrowing of the airways. They are heard in several common paediatric illnesses, such as asthma and bronchiolitis, and in less common disorders, such as anaphylaxis and foreign-body inhalation. Other noises heard on auscultation are crackles, which may be widespread or localised. The small size of the chest and the thin chest wall can result in transmission of sounds across the lung fields and even from the upper airways, making it more difficult to localise adventitious sounds.

The infant or child presenting with respiratory illness and significant distress should be monitored closely for signs of deterioration, evidenced by changes in effort and efficacy of breathing. Oxygen saturation and respiratory and heart rate monitoring are routinely used to provide continuous monitoring of these children.

FIGURE 35.1 SITES WHERE RECESSION MAY BE VISIBLE ON AN INFANT

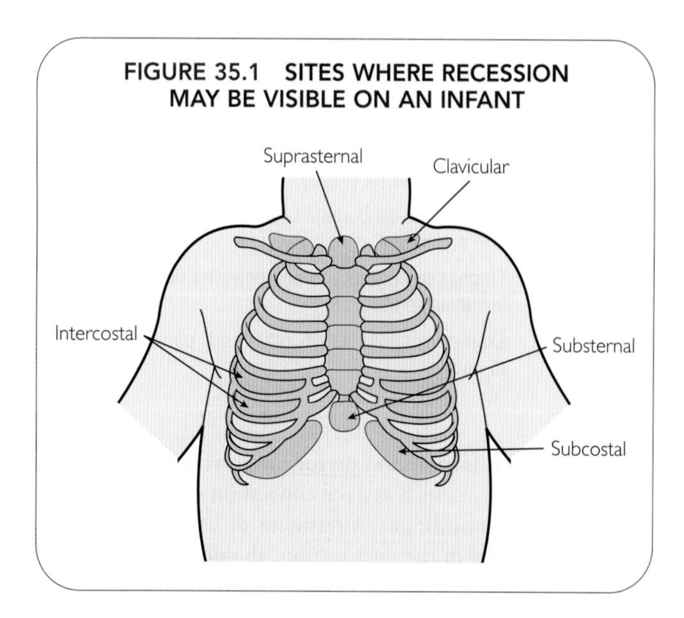

Circulation

Assessment of circulatory function should rely on clinical findings, which will detect dehydration and hypovolaemia in the early stages. Even in the early stages before dehydration is severe enough to result in hypovolaemia, there is considerable overlap in the signs of each of these states. Attempts have been made to identify the most sensitive and specific signs in children, with most studies focusing on dehydration.

Signs of vasoconstriction, such as skin pallor, mottling and delayed capillary refill time (CRT), are obvious signs of compensation aimed at improving cardiac output to secure adequate vital end-organ perfusion and are easily assessed pre-hospital and at triage without creating distress for the child. Sudden onset of pallor has been revealed by a series of studies as indicative of serious illness in infants.[2,17] Capillary refill time is considered an indicator of peripheral perfusion and therefore an indirect measure of cardiovascular function; 2 seconds is the accepted upper limit of normal.[18] However, clinicians are cautioned about relying exclusively on this parameter, as the evidence for its sensitivity for detecting shock in young children is not convincing, with no correlation shown between delayed CRT and bacterial infection,[19] and no correlation shown between capillary refill and invasive cardiovascular indices.[20] It should also be noted that ambient temperature and the technique and site of measurement are also likely to affect the sensitivity and specificity of the sign.[21,22] However, in the absence of more-suitable sensitive and specific non-invasive indices, CRT is still used for assessing peripheral perfusion and hydration for children pre-hospital and presenting to the ED.

TABLE 35.5 AVERAGE VITAL SIGNS BY AGE[18]

AGE GROUP	PULSE RATE (beats/minute)	RESPIRATION RATE (breaths/minute)	BLOOD PRESSURE (systolic, mmHg)
Neonate	120–180	40–60	60–80
Infant (1 month to 1 year)	110–160	30–40	70–90
Toddler (1–2 years)	100–150	25–35	80–95
Young child (2–7 years)	95–140	25–30	90–110
Older child (7–12 years)	80–120	20–25	100–120

Hypovolaemia is evidenced by signs of poor end-organ perfusion and compensatory efforts, such as tachycardia (see Table 35.5 for normal values for age).[23] As the child's condition worsens, the body initiates measures to overcome the derangements resulting from hypoperfusion; for example, tachypnoea to reduce acidosis. However, as the capacity to compensate deteriorates, evidence of inadequate perfusion, such as hypotension and deteriorating conscious state, become apparent.

Hypotension, defined in children as a systolic blood pressure (SBP) lower than the 5th percentile for age (see Table 35.5 for normal values),[24] occurs because of significant hypovolaemia. However, in children it is a late sign, which is not apparent until approximately 30% of circulating volume is lost. There are limited data to support these values and it may be slightly higher than the 5th percentile. As hypotension is an indicator of poor prognosis, blood pressure measurements should be recorded regularly for infants and children at risk of cardiac dysfunction and/or hypovolaemia. However, treatment decisions should not rest solely on this parameter.

Measuring a child's blood pressure provides practical challenges, which may affect the accuracy of the result. Young children are frequently uncooperative, are often anxious and distressed, and variation in their size affects cuff selection. There is also concern about the accuracy of ocillometric methods for estimating intra-arterial blood pressure.[25] A cuff most closely representing 40% of the circumference of the upper arm gives a measurement closest to invasive radial blood pressure values.[26] In some circumstances the cuff is applied around the calf. However, there are no data to determine the correlation between this measurement and arterial blood pressure measurements.

Reduced urine output is initially a mechanism to conserve fluid. However, as hypovolaemia progresses, renal perfusion deteriorates and urine output decreases further. The minimum permissible urine output for infants (2 mL/kg/h) and children (1 mL/kg/h) is much higher than the minimum volume accepted for adults (0.5 mL/kg/h).[18] Direct measurement of urine output in infants and children not yet toilet-trained is invasive and distressing to infants and children. To avoid catheterisation, which is common practice in adults to measure urine output, nappies are often weighed to provide an estimate of urine output. However, it has been shown that this is not an accurate measure and should not be used where the accuracy of the fluid balance assessment is critical.[27]

In summary, significant and potentially life-threatening hypovolaemia is characterised by a combination of signs, such as tachycardia, prolonged CRT, hypotension, tachypnoea, altered conscious state, decreased urine output and metabolic acidosis.

Disability

Conscious-state deterioration is a significant indicator of poor prognosis, and alteration in the level of activity has been shown to be an indicator of serious illness in children.[17] Decreased conscious state results from intracerebral pathology such as trauma and infection, but may also be an indication of inadequate oxygenation or circulation or other metabolic derangements. Children may manifest worrying changes in neurological status, such as lethargy, irritability, drowsiness, decreased activity and social interaction, including eye contact, and hypotonic posturing (extended limbs and abducted hips) with a broad array of illnesses. Clinicians should also be wary of the child who appears disproportionately miserable or lethargic with minor illness.

The variable developmental levels of children complicate neurological assessment and application of the Glasgow Coma Scale (GCS), a tool developed to standardise and quantify neurological assessment in adults. The GCS has been modified for use in children and is shown to compare favourably with the standard GCS for assessment of traumatic brain injury in older children.[28] The modified GCS is presented in Table 35.6.[29] The Advanced Paediatric Life Support course offers a simpler alternative as a crude way of defining conscious state in children, and this scale (AVPU) is presented in Box 35.1.[18] The AVPU scale describes four levels of consciousness from alert to unconscious. It is generally accepted that 'P' (responds to painful stimuli) equates to a GCS score of 8. Finally, parents are best placed to identify deviations from normal in their child's level of function.

A fontanelle is the intersection where three/four cranial bones met and create a small gap between the bones. The anterior and posterior fontanelles are palpable until, on average, 3 and 18 months of age respectively, at which time they generally close. The anterior fontanelle is the most described and palpated during an examination. Palpation of the tension of the fontanelle allows for a gross estimate of intracranial pressure (ICP; tense and bulging may indicate raised ICP) or hydration status (depressed/shrunken may indicate dehydration). There are limited data to support the sensitivity and specificity of these findings. In a study to determine the significance of a bulging fontanelle, 36% were associated with clinically significant

TABLE 35.6 THE MODIFIED GLASGOW COMA SCALE FOR CHILDREN[29–31]

AREA ASSESSED	INFANTS	CHILDREN	SCORE*
Eye opening	Open spontaneously	Open spontaneously	4
	Open in response to verbal stimuli	Open in response to verbal stimuli	3
	Open in response to pain only	Open in response to pain only	2
	No response	No response	1
Verbal response	Coos and babbles	Oriented, appropriate	5
	Irritable cries	Confused	4
	Cries in response to pain	Inappropriate words	3
	Moans in response to pain	Incomprehensible words or non-specific sounds	2
	No response	No response	1
Motor response	Moves spontaneously and purposefully	Obeys commands	6
	Withdraws to touch	Localises painful stimulus	5
	Withdraws in response to pain	Withdraws in response to pain	4
	Responds to pain with decorticate posturing (abnormal flexion)	Responds to pain with flexion	3
	Responds to pain with decerebrate posturing (abnormal extension)	Responds to pain with extension	2
	No response	No response	1

**A score is given in each category. The individual scores are then added to give a total score of 3 to 15. A score of < 8 is indicative of severe neurological injury.*

BOX 35.1 AVPU SCALE[18]

Alert
Responds to Voice
Responds to Pain only
Unresponsive

abnormalities.[32] Fontanelle assessment findings should be considered with findings and not in isolation. Pain assessment should also be included in neurological assessment, as pain may cloud capacity for accurate assessment and interpretation of other examination findings, particularly in children. Pain assessment is discussed in Chapter 18 and in the sections on pain management and procedural sedation in this chapter.

Vital signs

Vital signs (respiratory rate, heart rate, temperature, blood pressure and oxygen saturations) and other appropriately focused assessment parameters such as GCS, neurovascular observations, pain scores and blood glucose measurements should be recorded to provide a baseline (see Chapter 16 for information on blood glucose level sampling techniques). Normal values vary with age and are provided in Table 35.5. The regularity with which these parameters are then measured will depend on the nature and severity of the illness and the treatment implemented. However, establishing trend data via repeat measures is likely to be of greatest use, as single observations may be influenced by factors other than clinical deterioration or improvement, such as crying, sleeping, pain, etc.

Heart rate measurement in infants and young children should involve palpation of the pulse to provide other information in addition to the rate, such as strength and symmetry between right and left sides of the body. In infants where the carotid pulse may be difficult to locate due to their short neck, the brachial and femoral pulses provide a good alternative. Respiratory rate is most easily assessed during auscultation but may be affected by a change in respiratory pattern brought about by the child's awareness of being observed.

Infrared tympanic thermometers (ITTs) have become the standard tool for temperature measurement for adults and children in the ED and pre-hospital.

An oral temperature measurement, affected by hyperventilation, probe position and ingestion of hot or cold liquids, is also subject to inaccuracy and is not practical in infants and young children. Axillary temperature measurement has been advocated as a good alternative. However, studies have shown that this can be affected by ambient temperature and changes in skin perfusion;[33] measurements are on average likely to be from 0.4 (at low temperatures) to 1.0 degree (at temperatures over 39.0 degrees) lower than the oral or rectal temperature,[34] in contrast to tympanic and oral temperature measurements, which were shown not to be influenced by ambient temperature.[35]

The clinically rational approach is to avoid tympanic thermometers in young babies where the ear canal is not large enough to allow insertion of the probe, use the rectal route for measurement and to view a normal temperature reading in this age group with caution, regardless of the measurement technique. Furthermore, septic infants may present hypopyrexic rather than hyperpyrexic.[36]

Weight

In paediatric emergency care, the weight of the infant and child should be measured to provide important assessment data. Fluid loss is most accurately detected by repeat weight measurements, and infants and children with actual or potential for dehydration should be weighed naked 6-hourly during their hospital admission. Weight is also measured to guide medication dosing and fluid volume calculations.

For infants and children too unwell to weigh, this must be estimated. On average, newborns weigh approximately 3.5 kg and reach approximately 10 kg by 1 year of age, having gained an average of 200 g weekly for the first few months of life followed by 100 g per week. There is increasing evidence that traditional formulae such as (Age + 4) × 2 may underestimate the weight of many Australian children, and for this reason Advanced Paediatric Life Support Australasia has changed the method for calculating weight, which can be seen in Table 35.8.[18] Formulae are likely to underestimate the weight of overweight children. However, it is more appropriate to base medication doses on lean bodyweight, making this inaccuracy unlikely to be clinically concerning. This also means that on some occasions it may be more appropriate to use an estimated weight based on age and height, rather than measured weight for markedly overweight children to prevent significant overdose.

PRACTICE TIPS

EXAMINATION

- The severity of airway obstruction is determined by the severity of the respiratory distress.
- Work of breathing and mental state are the most useful indicators of the severity of respiratory distress.
- Hypotension is a very late sign of hypovolaemia in infants and children.
- Capillary refill measurement is a useful adjunct to assessment but should not be used as a single measure of peripheral perfusion.
- All infants and children with an actual or potential fluid and electrolyte imbalance should be weighed naked, as weight changes are the gold-standard measure for changes in fluid balance.
- A modified Glasgow Coma Scale score for infants and children is recommended for neurological assessments.
- A single set of vital signs may be difficult to interpret. Regular observations should be made to generate trend data.
- Age will influence the interpretation of diagnostic images and some pathology results.

DIAGNOSTIC TESTING

Diagnostic testing is employed to diagnose, exclude or identify the severity of disease, guide treatment options or determine the success of treatment. It is often invasive and distressing. Infants and children will require a combination of procedural sedation, local anaesthetic and analgesic, or in some cases a general anaesthetic for many diagnostic procedures, increasing the potential risks to the child. Therefore, it is important to be clear about what questions will be answered by the test results and whether answers to these questions are an important part of establishing a diagnosis or selecting management strategies.

The significance of age will also need to be considered when employing many sampling and imaging techniques and when interpreting test results.

Diagnostic imaging

Diagnostic images reveal anatomical differences that exist between infants, children and adults, and this influences interpretation of many images, including chest and skeletal plain film x-rays. For example, the shape of the ribs, the relative size and shape of the heart, the relatively flattened diaphragm and the presence in infants of a prominent thymus distorting the mediastinum will all impact on what constitutes a normal chest x-ray. Skeletal immaturity is evident on skeletal x-ray with the presence of secondary ossification centres and growth plates, and a higher proportion of cartilage in the bones of children, all of which influence interpretation.

Radiation safety is of concern for growing infants and children, and attempts should be made to reduce their exposure wherever possible. There are decision rules, such as the Ottawa ankle rules (see Chapter 17) and clinical decision rules for computed tomography (CT) in head injury,[37] validated for use in paediatrics to assist the clinician in determining whether diagnostic imaging is required.

Pathology

Diagnosis of illness in infants and children is less frequently dependent on pathology testing than it is for adults. Furthermore, paediatric presentations are less commonly complicated by comorbid disease, reducing the need for baseline evaluation of a range of measures of their underlying disease states.

The range of tests taken, methods for obtaining specimens and interpretation of the results are dependent on the presenting problem and the age of the patient. Smaller blood vessels and larger amounts of subcutaneous tissue make gaining intravascular access for blood sampling particularly difficult. Chapter 16 contains information on vascular access and catheter selection for all ages, and a section on paediatric considerations. It can also be difficult to aspirate large volumes of blood for testing, so laboratories capable of handling paediatric samples can perform these tests on much smaller samples collected in paediatric-sized blood tubes. It is important to confirm with the laboratory their capacity to test small samples before taking blood. Capillary samples from finger pricks are sometimes used as an alternative where intravenous access and larger volumes of blood are not required.

Urine specimens for microbiology and culture should be obtained from infants and young children not yet toilet-trained by urethral catheterisation or suprapubic aspirate. Urine bags applied to the skin to catch a urine specimen are not a satisfactory means to collect urine for this purpose as they are frequently contaminated.[38]

The reference ranges for some common pathology screening tests vary with age, and this must be considered when interpreting the results: haemoglobin, serum albumin, protein (CSF) base excess, serum creatinine, erythrocyte sedimentation rate (ESR), red blood cell (RBC) count, serum potassium, etc. Different laboratories use different testing methods and therefore report different ranges. Therefore, the reference ranges should be checked with the laboratory testing the samples.

TRIAGE

Paediatric triage assessment and decision-making, similar to adult triage practice, relies on recognising breaches to physiology which indicate the level of urgency (Chapter 11).

A brief history is taken to identify the chief complaint, along with past history, and family and social history risk factors for rapid deterioration in condition. The physiological approach to decision-making was developed by the Emergency Nurses Association, Victoria and was modified for paediatrics by the project team for the Department of Health Victoria-sponsored Consistency in Triage Project.[39] Although produced over 10 years ago it remains a useful tool to support decision-making and it is presented in Table 35.7.[39]

ASSESSMENT TOOLS

The value to paediatric assessment of evidence-based indicators of serious illness in infants and children has culminated in the development of several assessment tools.[17,40] Their role is to reinforce the features that should alert clinicians, including the triage nurse, to the increased likelihood of serious illness. The Paediatric Assessment Tool was designed to standardise the rapid assessment of infants and children by ED clinicians.[40] Clinicians are prompted to review the work of breathing, circulation to the skin and the appearance of the child to determine whether the child 'looks sick' or not, and to broadly identify whether this reflects cardiopulmonary, cerebral or metabolic derangement.

RESPIRATORY EMERGENCIES

RESPIRATORY FAILURE

Disorders of the respiratory tract are the most common illnesses in children. They account for up to 14% of hospital admissions and a quarter of ED presentations in Australia.[42] There are age-related factors that make infants and young children more susceptible to respiratory failure than older children and adults. Table 35.1 provides a comprehensive list of the respiratory differences between infants, young children and adults.

Oxygen consumption is much higher in infants and young children than it is in adults, which helps explain a significantly higher minute volume in this age group. Tidal volume (mL/kg) is relatively fixed, and increased alveolar ventilation is achieved by an increase in respiratory rate. However, the capacity to increase the respiratory rate to meet metabolic demands can be exhausted quickly in the sick or injured infant, predisposing them to respiratory failure. Therefore, a falling respiratory rate is not always a sign of improvement but may be a pre-terminal finding.

Infants and children also have a lower functional residual capacity (FRC), which is defined as the residual volume plus the expiratory reserve volume, which acts as a respiratory reserve. At FRC, the elastic recoil forces of the lungs and the chest wall are equal but opposite and there is no exertion by the diaphragm or other respiratory muscles. The smaller the FRC, the smaller the reserve and the greater the risk of hypoxia and respiratory failure. The situation is amplified in paediatric patients because of the chest-wall compliance, small thoracic cage and relatively large abdominal contents impinging on the diaphragm.[18,43]

The more compliant chest wall of the infant provides little support to the lungs. In addition to the effect that this has on FRC, increased chest-wall compliance makes it more difficult to maintain negative intrathoracic pressure, so the work of breathing is approximately three times that of an adult. However, the respiratory muscles of infants and young children are deficient in type I fatigue-resistant fibres and are therefore more susceptible to fatigue.[43]

Infants and young children have limited reserves to cope with respiratory illness and deteriorate rapidly once exhausted. Control of ventilation is immature in neonates and responses to hypoxic conditions are unpredictable and sometimes result in periods of apnoea.

Presentation

Infants and children in respiratory failure present with varying degrees of hypoxia and hypercarbia. The infant and young child with hypoxia will become increasingly restless and confused and will initially be tachycardic. Infants are particularly sensitive to hypoxia and rapidly become bradycardic if left untreated. Infants and young children suffering hypercarbia will become increasingly drowsy, have warm, flushed diaphoretic skin and are tachycardic. Neonates tolerate hypercarbia poorly and may suffer apnoea as a result.

Respiratory failure is a clinical diagnosis, which obviates the need for arterial blood gas (ABG) analysis to make the diagnosis and confirm the need for aggressive respiratory care. However, insertion of an arterial line for serial ABG analysis is justified in a child with severe respiratory illness receiving ventilatory support to monitor the effectiveness of treatments.

Management

Management of respiratory failure aims to improve ventilation, oxygenation or both. Furthermore, care should include strategies to minimise oxygen consumption such as keeping children as calm as possible, using the parents to reduce their distress and employing appropriate distraction techniques. Antipyretics may also play a role in reducing the metabolic costs associated with fever. Strategies to improve ventilation include bronchodilators, intubation and mechanical ventilation, while strategies to improve oxygenation include oxygen therapy, non-invasive ventilation to provide continuous positive airway pressure (CPAP), or bilevel positive airway pressure (BiPAP) and intubation and mechanical ventilation to provide positive end-expiratory pressure (PEEP). Oxygen therapy and mechanical ventilation will be discussed here.

Oxygen therapy

Oxygen therapy is the mainstay of respiratory management, and yet data detailing the effectiveness of therapy, or the appropriateness of different delivery systems, are limited. A 2014 Cochrane

TABLE 35.7 PAEDIATRIC PHYSIOLOGICAL DISCRIMINATORS DEVELOPED FOR THE AUSTRALASIAN (NATIONAL) TRIAGE SCALE[39]

	CATEGORY 1	CATEGORY 2	CATEGORY 3	CATEGORY 4	CATEGORY 5
Airway	Obstructed	Patent	Patent	Patent	Patent
	Partially obstructed with severe respiratory distress	Partially obstructed with moderate respiratory distress	Partially obstructed with mild respiratory distress		
Breathing	Absent respiration or hypoventilation	Respiration present	Respiration present	Respiration present	Respiration present
	Severe respiratory distress, e.g. severe use of accessory muscles, severe retraction, acute cyanosis	Moderate respiratory distress, e.g. moderate use of accessory muscles, moderate retraction, skin pale	Mild respiratory distress, e.g. mild use of accessory muscles, mild retraction, skin pink	No respiratory distress: no use of accessory muscles no retraction	No respiratory distress: no use of accessory muscles, no retraction
Circulation	Absent circulation Significant bradycardia, e.g. HR < 60 bpm in an infant	Circulation present	Circulation present	Circulation present	Circulation present
S/S dehydration: ↓ LOC/activity Capillary refill < 2 s Dry oral mucosa Sunken eyes ↓ tissue turgor Absent tears Deep respirations Thready/weak pulse	Severe haemodynamic compromise, e.g. absent peripheral pulses, skin pale, cold, moist, mottled, significant tachycardia capillary refill > 4 s	Moderate haemodynamic compromise, e.g. weak/thready brachial pulse, skin pale, cool, moderate tachycardia, capillary refill 2–4 s	Mild haemodynamic compromise, e.g.palpable peripheral pulses skin pale, warm, mild tachycardia	No haemodynamic compromise, e.g. palpable peripheral pulses, skin pink, warm, dry	No haemodynamic compromise, e.g. palpable peripheral pulses skin pink, warm, dry
Tachycardia ↓ urine output	Uncontrolled haemorrhage	> 6 S/S dehydration	3–6 S/S dehydration	< 3 S/S dehydration	No S/S dehydration
Mental health emergencies[40] (used with permission from South-eastern Sydney Area Health Service)	Definite danger to life (self or others), e.g. violent behaviour, possession of a weapon, self-destruction	Probable danger to life (self or others), e.g. attempt/threat of self-harm, threat of harm to others Severe behavioural disturbance, e.g. extreme agitation/restlessness, physically/verbally aggressive, confused/unable to cooperate Requires restraint	Possible danger to life, e.g. suicidal ideation Severe distress Moderate behavioural disturbance, e.g. agitated/restless intrusive behaviour, bizarre/disordered behaviour withdrawn, ambivalence re treatment Psychotic symptoms, e.g. hallucinations, delusions, paranoid ideas Affective disturbance, e.g. symptoms of depression, anxiety, elevated or irritable mood	Moderate distress, e.g. no agitation/restlessness, irritable, not aggressive, cooperative, gives coherent history, symptoms, of anxiety or depression without suicidal ideation	No danger to self or others No behavioural disturbance No acute distress, e.g. cooperative, communicative, compliant with instructions, known patients with chronic symptoms, request for medication, minor adverse effect of medication, financial/social/accommodation/relationship problem

Continued

TABLE 35.7 PAEDIATRIC PHYSIOLOGICAL DISCRIMINATORS DEVELOPED FOR THE AUSTRALASIAN (NATIONAL) TRIAGE SCALE—cont'd

	CATEGORY 1	CATEGORY 2	CATEGORY 3	CATEGORY 4	CATEGORY 5
Ophthalmic emergencies		Penetrating eye injury Chemical injury Sudden loss of vision with or without injury Sudden-onset severe eye pain	Sudden abnormal vision with or without injury Moderate eye pain, e.g. blunt eye injury, flash burns, foreign body	Normal vision Mild eye pain, e.g. blunt eye injury, flash burns, foreign body	Normal vision No eye pain
Risk factors for serious illness or injury should be considered in the light of history of events and physiological data. Multiple risk factors = increased risk of serious injury Presence of one or more risk factors may result in allocation of triage category of higher acuity.					
Mechanism of injury, e.g. penetrating injury fall > 2 × height MVC > 60 kph MBC/cyclist > 30 kph pedestrian ejection/rollover prolonged extrication (> 30 minutes) death of same-car occupant explosion	***Comorbidities,*** e.g. history of prematurity respiratory disease cardiovascular disease renal disease carcinoma diabetes substance abuse immunocompromise congenital disease complex medical Hx	***Age < 1 month and:*** febrile acute change to feeding pattern acute change to sleeping pattern ***Victim of violence,*** e.g. child at risk sexual assault neglect	***Historical variables,*** e.g. events preceding presentation to ED: apnoeic/cyanotic episode seizure activity decreased intake decreased output redcurrant-jelly stool bile-stained vomiting ***Parental concern***	***Other,*** e.g. rash actual/potential effects of drugs/alcohol chemical exposure envenomation immersion alteration in body temperature	

bpm: beats/minute; HR: heart rate; LOC: loss of consciousness; MBC: motorbike collision; MVC: motor vehicle collision; S/S: signs and symptoms.

FIGURE 35.2 NASAL PRONGS ON AN INFANT[45]

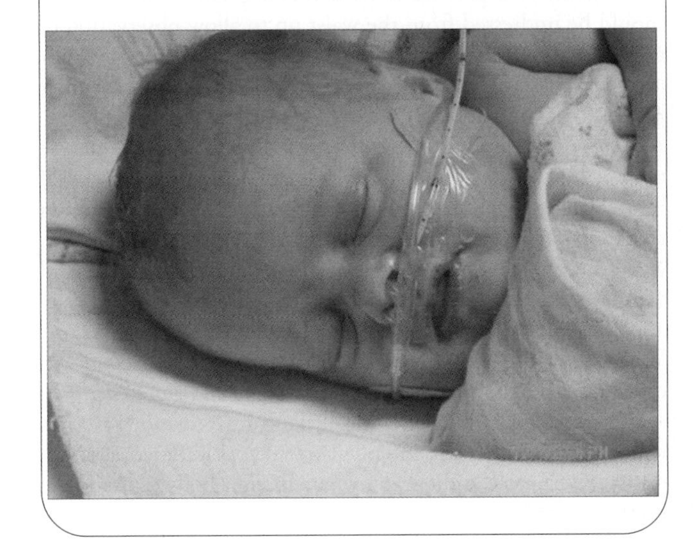

TABLE 35.8 FORMULAE FOR PAEDIATRIC EMERGENCIES[18]

PARAMETER	FORMULA
Weight	0–12 months (0.5 × age in months) + 4 1–5 years (2 × age in years) + 8 6–12 years (3 × age in years) + 7
Endotracheal tube diameter	Age/4 + 4
Endotracheal tube insertion depth (at the lip)	Age/2 + 12
Endotracheal tube insertion depth (at the nose)	Age/2 + 15
Adrenaline (bolus) 1 in 10,000	0.1 mL/kg
Defibrillation energy	4 J/kg

review, which aimed to determine the effectiveness of oxygen therapy and delivery methods in children, found no studies comparing oxygen with no oxygen, and only four randomised controlled trials evaluating delivery devices.[44] Nasal prongs or nasal cannulae, nasal catheters, oxygen tents and hoods and face masks are the methods used to deliver oxygen to spontaneously breathing infants and children. The choice of device is influenced by the age of the child, the oxygen flow required and the advantages and disadvantages of the available delivery systems. Ideally, oxygen is humidified. However, during pre-hospital transport and initial evaluation and resuscitation in the ED, this may not be possible and should not be a priority.

Nasal prongs, alternatively called nasal cannulae, in smaller sizes, are the preferred mode for oxygen delivery in young children and infants (Fig. 35.2). They can be taped to the cheeks in the same way as a nasogastric tube and are well tolerated. They allow the infant to feed and are not as restrictive as an oxygen mask.

A common practice among emergency clinicians is the use of a self-inflating resuscitation device to deliver oxygen to a spontaneously breathing patient. A mask is held over the patient's face, but the bag is not squeezed. In the spontaneously breathing patient this practice should be avoided; as sufficient negative inspiratory pressure is required to overcome the patient inspiratory valve, this may lead to entrained room air rather than oxygen resulting in highly variable FiO_2 delivery.[46]

Finally, in the absence of a well-tolerated oxygen delivery device, clinicians have used indirect means of delivery. Using a high-flow oxygen source, a stream of oxygen is aimed at the child's face. Although this practice is also not recommended, it is noteworthy that it has been shown that 30% oxygen can potentially be delivered if a face mask is held near but not against the face.[47] To achieve the best results, a non-rebreather mask or the tubing with a flow rate of 15 L/min should be on the child's chest directed up towards the face.

High-flow nasal cannula oxygen is gaining support as this therapy is well tolerated. In addition, evidence suggests that this therapy provides mild positive airway pressure and lung volume recruitment.[49] It should be used after a trial of low-flow nasal prong oxygen, or in the severely distressed child. Non-invasive ventilation is used increasingly in paediatrics to manage infants and children with lung disease to prevent the need for invasive ventilation.[48]

Invasive ventilation is indicated when other measures to secure adequate ventilation and oxygenation have been unsuccessful, including non-invasive ventilation (NIV) and medical management of respiratory conditions. The differences in anatomy and physiology of the airway and their impact on intubation, the equipment required, and the techniques used are described in the section on examination and are given in Table 35.1. The size of the equipment used is determined by the size of the child. Table 35.8[18] provides some useful formulae for calculation of tube size and insertion depth. There is increasing evidence that cuffed endotracheal tubes provide superior airway protection and improve ventilation, with no associated increase in adverse events supporting their use in children.[49] Appropriate initial ranges for the adjustable parameters and alarm limits for basic ventilation are presented in Table 35.9.

PRACTICE TIPS

RESPIRATORY EMERGENCIES

- Infants and young children are more susceptible to respiratory failure than adults.
- Tidal volume is relatively fixed in infants; however, because of higher respiratory rates minute volume is much higher.
- Infants are extremely sensitive to hypoxia and rapidly develop bradycardia.
- Hypercapnia in young infants may be responsible for apnoea.
- Nasal prongs/cannulae are the most effective way of delivering oxygen to infants in the ED. Older children may tolerate a mask.

TABLE 35.9 APPROPRIATE INITIAL SETTINGS FOR MECHANICAL VENTILATION[50]

PARAMETER	VALUE
Peak inspiratory pressure	20 cmH_2O
Tidal volume	6–7 mL/kg
Peak end-expiratory pressure	3–5 cmH_2O
Respiratory rate	Age-appropriate
Inspiratory time	0.8–1 second (to maintain I:E ratio of 1:3)
Peak inspiratory pressure (alarm)	30 cmH_2O
Low inspiratory pressure (alarm)	15 cmH_2O
Low minute volume (alarm)	75% of minute volume

I:E ratio: inspiratory–expiratory ratio.

Croup (laryngotracheobronchitis)

Croup is the most common cause of acute upper airway obstruction in children and accounts for approximately 15% of respiratory illness in children.[51] It is a clinical syndrome characterised by an abrupt onset of barking cough, hoarse voice and inspiratory stridor. It usually occurs in children from 6 months to 3 years of age, but may occur in children and adolescents. Croup is a seasonal disease and peaks in the winter when respiratory viruses are most prevalent.[51] Droplets and direct contact spread the illness and parainfluenza virus is responsible for approximately two-thirds of cases.[52] Other viruses, such as influenza type A, respiratory syncytial virus (RSV), rhinovirus, adenovirus and enterovirus, are also known to cause croup.

Croup causes inflammation of the upper airway, the larynx, trachea and bronchi. The swelling results in narrowing of the airway, including the subglottic area, which is the narrowest section of the paediatric airway, and this is responsible for increasing difficulty in breathing as the airway lumen narrows. Increased swelling to the larynx results in a hoarse voice and a barking cough. Worsening obstruction results in stridor.[51] Increased mucus production and the generation of negative pressure on inspiration obstruct the airway further. The size of the larynx, increased loose submucosal tissues and the tight fit of the cricoid ring around the subglottic region of the trachea in the younger child are responsible for more-pronounced signs of airway obstruction.

Presentation and diagnosis

Children with croup will generally present having had a prodrome featuring coryzal symptoms, a fever and a cough. The symptoms of barking cough and hoarse voice usually appear after 1–2 days and in 80% of children remain mild, and mortality rates are low.[16] Symptoms are generally worse at night and exacerbated by distress; patients with croup most commonly present to the ED between 10 pm and 4 am.[53] Moderate and more-severe croup presents with inspiratory stridor and increased work of breathing.

Children should be allowed to adopt a position of comfort and remain in a parent's arms if this alleviates distress. They should be undressed from the waist up to allow observation of respiratory effort and respiratory rate and limit the need for intrusive examination. They should also be observed for their level of activity, skin colour and the presence of stridor.

Croup severity should be assessed by evaluating the degree to which respiratory effort has increased. Saturations are of limited value in the assessment of croup. Increasing obstruction to the airway affects the capacity to ventilate, and oxygenation will only fall once the airway is significantly obstructed and ventilation is markedly impeded. This should become clinically apparent well before a decrease in oxygen saturations occurs. With increasing airway obstruction, a child will become increasingly tachypnoeic, tachycardic, restless and agitated.

The diagnosis is made clinically, and investigations are not required unless they are intended to rule out differential diagnosis; for example, radiograph where foreign-body aspiration is suspected.[51] Other differential diagnoses should be considered, in particular epiglottitis. Now rare since the introduction of the *Haemophilus influenzae* type B vaccine to the immunisation schedule, epiglottitis is a life-threatening infection which can result in complete occlusion of the airway by a swollen epiglottis. It manifests with abrupt onset of fever, pallor, signs of sepsis, drooling and a soft snore. As clinicians have less and less experience with this illness, they are at greater risk of confusing it with croup. Children with epiglottitis should be managed with great care—airway examination should *not* be undertaken to confirm diagnosis until a clinician with paediatric airway experience is prepared to intubate the airway and the resources to manage a difficult airway are available. Other presentations that may mimic croup include angio-oedema secondary to allergy, tracheitis or inhaled foreign body (FB).

Management

The mainstay of management for croup is steroids. However, children with only a cough do not require treatment with steroids.[54] Use of either 1 mg/kg of oral prednisolone or 0.15 mg/kg of oral dexamethasone is supported by the evidence for mild to moderate croup.[55] Studies comparing the two steroids have used a range of dosing regimens and evidence suggests that a single low dose of oral dexamethasone and prednisolone is non-inferior to dexamethasone 0.6 mg/kg dose.[56] Preference is given to dexamethasone due to its longer half-life and it has been demonstrated to be more palatable.[57] There is limited evidence to suggest that parenteral administration is superior to oral ingestion in a child who is not vomiting.[58]

Children with mild croup—no stridor at rest and minimal increase in respiratory effort—may be discharged from the ED following a dose of steroids. Children with moderate croup, characterised by an increase in respiratory effort and stridor at rest, should be observed in the ED and if they show adequate signs of improvement within several hours they may usually be safely discharged home.[59] In addition to improvement in condition, the decision to discharge a child with croup is influenced by factors such as their proximity to emergency services, the time of day (croup will typically deteriorate overnight) and parental concern. Children with more-severe croup, manifested by more-severe signs of respiratory distress, will need close monitoring, and may require nebulised adrenaline to alleviate significant obstruction. Nebulised adrenaline relieves symptoms by temporarily reducing bronchial and tracheal secretions and airway-wall oedema. Improvements occur within 30 minutes, with a duration of effect between 90 and 120 minutes, after which the symptoms return to baseline severity.[60] Most children treated with nebulised adrenaline will require hospital admission and may need a second dose of adrenaline. A standard volume for treatment, rather than weight-based dosing, is used most consistently in Australian EDs. This is most commonly 5 mg administered as 5 mL of 1 in 1000 (equivalent to 0.1% solution) solution or 0.5 mL of racemic adrenaline (1% solution) diluted with saline to a total of 2–4 mL and delivered by nebuliser mask.

Supplemental oxygen should be administered to a hypoxic child with croup. However, this should serve as a stimulus to seek expert airway assistance and prepare for intubation. This should also be considered for children requiring repeated doses of adrenaline with no improvement and those with signs of exhaustion.

Traditionally, steam and inhalational therapy have been used to manage croup and are still frequently recommended for home use despite no convincing evidence of their efficacy.

PRACTICE TIPS

CROUP

- Characterised by fever, barking cough, hoarse voice with or without stridor.
- Diagnostic tests are not required to confirm the diagnosis of croup.
- Changes in work of breathing are the most sensitive indicators of the severity of the airway obstruction.
- Corticosteroids, such as prednisolone or dexamethasone, are recommended for all infants and children suffering croup.
- Infants and children with severe croup may require nebulised adrenaline to relieve the symptoms of airway obstruction.

ASTHMA

Asthma is a chronic inflammatory disorder of the lower airways where smooth muscle contraction and swelling of the airway results in airway obstruction. This section should be read in conjunction with Chapter 21; it is not intended to be a comprehensive review of asthma, but will serve to highlight the ways in which paediatric asthma differs from adult asthma.

The prevalence of asthma in Australian children is estimated at 10% and is twice as high among children with a disability.[61] It is as high as one in six in Aotearoa New Zealand children,[62] which is higher than in adults and significantly higher than in other parts of the world.[63] The Indigenous populations of both countries have even higher rates of asthma prevalence. It is generally accepted that children older than 12 months may present with the features of asthma.

Presentation and diagnosis

The diagnosis of asthma in children is clinical and can be made based on a history of recurrent or persistent wheeze in the absence of other causes. The wheeze is associated with viral respiratory infection, exercise or exposure to allergens, such as grasses, animals and pollens. Children presenting with asthma will usually have a history or family history of atopy. Conditions such as eczema, allergic rhinitis or allergy are risk factors for persistent asthma beyond the age of 6 years. However, not all children with atopy develop asthma.[64] There is a greater prevalence in those children living in households with smokers.[65]

On examination, the child with asthma will have widespread expiratory wheeze, cough, increased respiratory effort and prolonged expiration. Asymmetry on auscultation may occur as a result of mucus plugging, but FB inhalation should be considered. Cough is frequently misdiagnosed as asthma in the absence of other features of asthma. Although a common feature of asthma, it is rare for it to be the only symptom experienced in asthma.[66] Persistent and recurrent non-specific cough frequently follows a viral respiratory infection and may not resolve for weeks to months. The cough is dry, exacerbated by exercise, is worse in the morning and is not responsive to treatment.

Severity, defined as mild, moderate, severe and critical, is primarily determined by the increase in respiratory effort and the effect of respiratory compromise on mental status. Secondary parameters, which may assist in quantifying the severity, are oxygen saturation, the ability to talk and heart rate. Other less-useful indicators, which are frequently described in texts, are wheeze intensity, arterial blood gases, pulsus paradoxus, central cyanosis, spirometry and peak flow rates.

The diagnosis is often confirmed based on a response to inhaled bronchodilators as this indicates that airflow limitation is reversible. Generally, children under the age of 5 years cannot perform spirometry reliably. Chest x-rays are also not of diagnostic value and do not provide evidence of severity of disease. However, a chest x-ray should be performed for infants and children with critical asthma or where the diagnosis is unclear.

Other causes of acute wheezing in children include bronchiolitis, *Mycoplasma* pneumonia, aspiration, allergy or heart failure, and should be considered when taking a history and performing an examination on the child presenting with wheeze. Preschool children frequently experience wheeze associated with a viral infection that is not responsive to asthma therapy.

Management

The management of asthma in children is similar to that of adults, and where it differs this reflects the differences in the natural history and pattern of asthma in children, the effects of the medications used and the potential for side-effects in these two populations. Guidelines recommending management for acute exacerbations are available from a number of sources; one of the most frequently used of these is the Royal Children's Hospital Asthma Management Clinical Practice Guideline, adapted for state-wide use with the support of the Victorian Paediatric Clinical Network.[67] Treatment recommendations based on presentation severity are clearly laid out and readers are recommended to use this or other evidence-based guidelines to guide dosing and scheduling of therapies for acute asthma management (see Useful websites section at the end of this chapter). This section will not address chronic asthma management and preventative therapy.

The evidence for inhaled bronchodilators to relieve the symptoms of acute asthma is strong. Furthermore, it has been shown that salbutamol delivered via spacer is as effective as nebulised salbutamol administered to children presenting with acute asthma.[68] There are no data about this delivery method in children with critical asthma. However, data supporting the safety of continuous undiluted (0.5%) nebulised salbutamol[69] and intravenous infusion of salbutamol are available.[70] There is a lack of consensus on the appropriate dosage for IV salbutamol as it is associated with increased risk of tremor and hypokalaemia.[71] Anticholinergics in combination with short-acting bronchodilators have been shown to reduce admission rates, improve lung function and clinical scores, and reduce nausea and tremor.[72] Furthermore, there is a trend to improved efficacy for more severe asthma. Ipratropium bromide is advocated for use in severe and critical asthma in the first hour of management, but confers no benefit if used beyond this period.[73]

Corticosteroids have been shown repeatedly to result in clinical improvement in paediatric asthma,[74] and the route of administration (oral versus intravenous) appears to have minimal effect on their efficacy. Specifically, intravenous steroid administration does not result in greater efficacy. Conversely, there is insufficient evidence to suggest that inhaled steroids are an efficacious alternative to systemic steroids.[75] Recent evidence recommends avoiding systemic steroids in preschool children unless they have been admitted or have had previous ICU admits with bronchodilator responsive wheeze, as there is increasing evidence that it does not improve symptom severity or aid in symptom resolution.[76]

The use of aminophylline in critical asthma is controversial, as it carries significant risk of serious side-effects and the data to support its efficacy is not convincing, however is becoming more frequently used.[77]

Decreased oxygen saturations should not be used as an indication for the need for additional bronchodilation in the absence of other signs of bronchospasm. Ventilation–perfusion mismatch, often exacerbated by beta-agonist use, and mucus plugging are responsible for deteriorating saturations and supplemental oxygen therapy should be commenced once saturations have dropped below 92%, which is the generally accepted, although arbitrary, threshold.

There is some interest in the role of intravenous magnesium sulfate to provide additional bronchodilation, as it appears to be an effective treatment option in children and has shown to improve lung function and reduce the need for hospital admission, but there is limited evidence.[77]

Guidelines for admission are generally consensus-based, as there is limited evidence on which to base admission criteria. The following factors should be considered when making a decision to admit or discharge a patient from the ED:

- the severity of the attack
- the response to therapy
- the time of day
- the proximity to emergency services
- the expertise of the parents to manage at home.

Risk factors for rapid deterioration and death, such as previous near-fatal asthma, previous admissions in the last year, previous admission to paediatric ICU, heavy use of beta$_2$-agonists and repeat attendance at the ED, should also lower the threshold for admission. On discharge, the family should receive a detailed action plan and advice about re-presentation.

The decision to commence a preventer is best not made in the ED, but rather by a clinician who will see the child regularly and monitor their response to therapy. Referral to a paediatrician, respiratory doctor or suitable GP should be made if the child has recurrent episodes of asthma and would be likely to benefit from a preventer. This also provides an opportunity to review and update their action plan.

PRACTICE TIPS

ASTHMA

- **A clinical diagnosis made on the basis of recurrent wheeze in the absence of other causes.**
- **Responsiveness to bronchodilation may be used to confirm the diagnosis.**
- **Chest x-rays and other diagnostic tests are not required to confirm the diagnosis and are of limited value to assess severity or determine treatment.**
- **Bronchodilators are used to control bronchospasm and should be given when work of breathing increases.**
- **Decreased oxygen saturations in the absence of other signs of bronchospasm should not be treated with bronchodilators.**

BRONCHIOLITIS

In Australia and Aotearoa New Zealand, viral bronchiolitis occurs in infants less than 12–18 months of age, and is characterised by wheeze, cough and varying degrees of shortness of breath. It is the most common lower respiratory tract infection in infants, and approximately 3% of infants will be hospitalised with bronchiolitis in their first year of life. However, most episodes are mild and can be managed at home. The aetiology includes respiratory syncytial virus (RSV), parainfluenza and influenza virus, rhinovirus and adenovirus, and as these viruses are more prevalent in winter this illness peaks during the winter. Infection causes acute inflammation and oedema of the epithelial cells lining the bronchioles, increased mucus production and bronchospasm, all of which contribute to airway obstruction.

Infants with pre-existing lung disease, congenital heart disease and infants younger than 6 months, born prematurely or failing to thrive, are at greater risk of increased severity of disease and more serious sequelae as a result of bronchiolitis.

Presentation and diagnosis

Bronchiolitis presents with features of upper and lower airway tract infection. There is no evidence to support the specificity or sensitivity of the clinical features of bronchiolitis for the purposes of making the diagnosis or to categorise severity. Parents usually describe the classic constellation of symptoms: a prodrome of coryza, mild cough and fever lasting for 1–2 days before wheeze, crackles and increasing shortness of breath become apparent. Dyspnoea may interfere with feeding, the extent of which will be dependent on the level of respiratory distress.

Examination findings include tachypnoea, tachycardia, fever, increased respiratory effort, a prolonged expiratory phase, hyperinflation and crackles and wheeze on auscultation. Reduced oxygen saturations and dehydration may be apparent in some infants. In severe cases hypoxia and cyanosis may occur, and young infants may suffer apnoeas.

TABLE 35.10 BRONCHIOLITIS MANAGEMENT BY SEVERITY[78,79]

SEVERITY	CLINICAL FEATURES	MANAGEMENT
Mild	Alert, pink in air Feeding well O_2 saturation > 90% Mild tachypnoea only No to mild chest-wall retractions	Disposition–can be managed at home Discharge advice: advise parents of the expected course of the illness, and when to return if there are problems; give parent information leaflet smaller, more frequent feeds Follow-up–review by GP within 24 hours
Moderate	Any one of: decreased feeding lethargy moderate chest-wall retractions suprasternal retraction nasal flaring underlying cardiorespiratory disease O_2 saturation 90–92% age < 6 weeks	Disposition–admit (may be discharged after a period of observation) Oxygen to maintain adequate saturation OVER 90% High-flow nasal cannula O_2 only if nasal prong O_2 fails Fluid management: nasogastric fluids if not feeding at least 50% usual Monitoring–1-2-hourly observations
Severe	Reluctant or unable to feed Increasing lethargy or irritability Marked chest-wall retractions Marked suprasternal retraction Marked nasal flaring O_2 saturations less than 90% Frequent and/or prolonged apnoeas	Consultation–involve senior staff/paediatric intensivist Disposition–admit. May require transfer to more appropriate facility with PICU Oxygen to maintain adequate saturation OVER 90% Consider high-flow nasal cannula O_2 delivery or CPAP Fluid management: nasogastric fluids if not feeding at least 50% usual Monitoring–cardiorespiratory monitor and hourly observations (more frequent if unstable)

ADH: antidiuretic hormone; IV: intravenous.

The severity of bronchiolitis, categorised as mild, moderate and severe, is not consistently defined in the literature. However, in numerous studies a number of clinical indicators are associated with more-severe disease:

- low oxygen saturation at the time of presentation
- young age (< 10 weeks)
- prematurity
- cyanosis
- increased work of breathing (including individually and in various combinations: increased respiratory rate, accessory muscle use, chest-wall retraction, recessions, nasal flare and/or grunting).

Table 35.10[78] provides a consensus-based guide for defining bronchiolitis severity based on respiratory effort, oxygen saturation, feeding and the extent of dehydration.

Bronchiolitis is a clinical diagnosis, obviating the need for investigation. Chest x-ray is of no diagnostic value unless considering an alternative diagnosis such as congestive cardiac failure, which may mimic bronchiolitis, particularly if precipitated by respiratory infection. Furthermore, evidence indicates that there is no correlation between chest x-ray results and the severity of the disease.

Management

The clinical presentation of bronchiolitis is very similar to asthma, and it seems reasonable to assume that the treatment for asthma would be likely to be effective to treat bronchiolitis. However, this appears not to be the case. Studies summarised in a Cochrane review, which evaluated the efficacy of bronchodilators, including adrenaline, $beta_2$-agonists and ipratropium bromide, have not confirmed the benefit of these agents to infants with bronchiolitis and cannot be recommended.[80,81] Improvement in signs in response to a salbutamol trial is at odds with the diagnosis of bronchiolitis and suggests that the infant has asthma. Steroids, although useful in the treatment of asthma and croup, have been shown to have no role in bronchiolitis.[83] The evidence for other potential treatments, such as antibiotics, ribavirin, immunoglobulin, decongestants and antitussives, is not sufficiently convincing to support their inclusion in the treatment regimen for bronchiolitis.[84] Nebulised hypertonic saline use in moderate to severe bronchiolitis has been explored and found modest reduction in hospital length of stay.[82] However, there does not appear to be widespread acceptance of this data and treatment recommendations do not currently include hypertonic saline.

Infants with bronchiolitis are managed based on severity, as detailed in Table 35.10.[78] Mild bronchiolitis can be managed safely at home. Under some circumstances, infants with moderate bronchiolitis can also be managed as outpatients, providing that regular review can be provided, and admission is possible if they show signs of significant dehydration and/or hypoxia.

Infants with more-severe bronchiolitis should be admitted to hospital, and the need for tertiary paediatric care considered for those with severe bronchiolitis and infants with the previously described risk factors for more-severe disease.

Inpatient management of bronchiolitis is conservative and confined to providing close observation, the provision of oxygen therapy to maintain acceptable oxygenation, and fluid management. Monitoring of respiratory parameters will depend on the severity of disease but should occur hourly at a minimum and include continuous oxygen saturation monitoring. The threshold at which to start oxygen therapy and the saturation that should be maintained are not supported by data. The effect of oxygen saturation on time to discharge in infants with bronchiolitis has been previously reported.[85] Administration of oxygen was described in a previous section and there is increasing support for the role of high-flow intranasal oxygen to manage bronchiolitis with hypoxia in an inpatient setting.[86] Early initiation of high-flow nasal cannula may reduce the escalation of care but it does not decrease the length of hospitalisation, duration of oxygen or intubation.[87]

Decisions surrounding hydration management are largely consensus-based in the absence of adequate evidence to guide clinicians. However, a multicentred trial has recently compared nasogastric and intravenous fluid therapy for infants with bronchiolitis requiring rehydration and results support nasogastric tube rehydration as a suitable mode for fluid delivery.[88] Consensus rather than evidence supports administering 75% of maintenance fluid volumes. Fluid management is also described in more detail in a previous section.

Two studies have examined the duration of illness; the median duration of symptoms was 2 weeks, but 20% of infants had symptoms for as long as 3 weeks. This should be explained to parents to ensure that their expectations for recovery are realistic.

PRACTICE TIPS

BRONCHIOLITIS

- Presents in infants less than 12–18 months of age with features very similar to asthma.
- Infants who were born prematurely, suffer a cardiac condition or are less than 6 months of age are more likely to suffer more-severe disease.
- Hydration status and oxygen saturations should be assessed in all infants with bronchiolitis, as these parameters define severity and the need for admission.
- Infants with moderate and severe bronchiolitis will require inpatient management for monitoring and may require oxygen therapy and/or rehydration.
- Although presentation is similar to asthma, steroids and bronchodilators are not helpful.

PERTUSSIS (WHOOPING COUGH)

Pertussis is a highly infectious, acute respiratory infection caused by *Bordetella pertussis* and is traditionally diagnosed in infants and toddlers, although it may affect adults. Vaccination for pertussis is included in the immunisation schedule to protect infants and young children from what can potentially be a very serious illness. Babies do not gain reliable protection from maternal antibodies and immunity from vaccination is not conferred until at least the second dose, making babies susceptible to pertussis infection in the first few months of life. This is of particular importance as very young infants are at greatest risk of severe morbidity and mortality.[89] There has been a worldwide resurgence in pertussis over the last 20 years and reasons for this are postulated, which include waning immunity following immunisation and improved diagnosis. The infection is usually mild in adults, so revaccination has not been routinely recommended. As adult pertussis has been increasingly implicated as the source of infection for unimmunised babies, this recommendation has been challenged more recently.[90,91] Government initiatives target vaccination for pregnant women, new parents and grandparents and others who care for young babies.[92] This indirect method of prevention has been shown to reduce the risk to the infant of contracting pertussis by 51%.[92,93] Despite the availability of routine pertussis vaccination, significant numbers of infants and young children still contract the disease and die. In Australia and Aotearoa New Zealand, epidemics occur every 3–4 years. Pertussis is a notifiable disease in both countries. In Australia there were 20,106 notifications made in 2016 and in 2015–16 rates were highest among 1- to 14-year-old children.[94] Similarly, Aotearoa New Zealand data confirms 872 cases in 2010, 1996 cases in 2011 and 5902 in 2012.[95]

Presentation and diagnosis

The classic course of pertussis can be divided into three stages of illness: the *catarrheal*, *paroxysmal* and *convalescent* stages. Infants and children usually present during the paroxysmal phase. The first stage (catarrheal), lasting 1–2 weeks, is characterised by rhinorrhoea, conjunctivitis, low-grade fever (although this can be uncommon), a mild cough that gradually increases rather than wanes, and malaise that is frequently considered insignificant by parents and clinicians.[96] Unfortunately, it is at this stage that they are most infectious. The developing cough becomes paroxysmal, marking the second stage, which can last from 2 to 6 weeks.

Pertussis is commonly known as whooping cough because of the characteristic 'whoop' that occurs with inspiration at the end of a coughing paroxysm. However, this is misleading as the whoop is only present in some cases.[97] The increase in intrathoracic pressure during a paroxysm results in bulging neck veins and a reddened face, and the child may vomit. In severe cases, the infant may become hypoxic, cyanosed and bradycardic during the coughing paroxysm, and some may experience apnoeas. In fact, some infants present only with apnoea and few classic symptoms. Young babies quickly become exhausted, which impairs feeding, leading to dehydration and failure to thrive. The disease is generally milder in older children, making it more difficult to recognise. Available data provide the foundation for the recommendation that where there is parental report of turning blue/purple or cyanosis, age less than 2 months and the presence of cough and rhonchi on examination, these findings should be considered to correlate with a diagnosis of pertussis and the child should be isolated and further testing completed to confirm the diagnosis.[98]

The final stage of the illness is the convalescent phase, during which the number and intensity of coughing episodes decreases. This stage may continue for many weeks.

Laboratory confirmation of the clinical diagnosis of pertussis is required and polymerase chain reaction (PCR), serology and culture are commonly used for this purpose. Isolation of *B. pertussis* from nasopharyngeal secretions is the gold standard for diagnosis during the first few weeks of cough as DNA bacteria significantly decreases beyond 4 weeks.[99] However, samples are frequently contaminated if not collected correctly and handled appropriately, lowering sensitivity. Furthermore, it takes 7–10 days before the results of the culture can be confirmed, making this test less useful clinically. The use of PCR to confirm diagnosis is increasing as it is a more sensitive test, and the Communicable Diseases Center (CDC) and the World Health Organization (WHO) now recommend positive PCR as a diagnostic criterion for the diagnosis of pertussis infection. Pertussis infection can also be confirmed by serology and can be distinguished from a serological response to immunisation. However, this test may be less sensitive and of less use early in the illness.

Management

The treatment of pertussis is largely conservative and supportive care is the mainstay, as antibiotics must be commenced within a week of the onset of illness for them to be of clinical value.[100] Their role in most cases is to shorten the infectious period of the illness and reduce the risk of the spread of pertussis to vulnerable individuals. Traditionally, erythromycin has been used for 14 days; however, recent evidence supports a 7-day course with newer agents such as clarithromycin or azithromycin, which have fewer side-effects and are better tolerated.[101] An appropriate resource, such as the *Australian Medicines Handbook* or the Therapeutic Guidelines, should be consulted for doses and dosing schedules (see the Useful websites section at the end of the chapter). At this stage there is not enough evidence to support the effectiveness of cough treatments such as corticosteroids, $beta_2$-adrengeric agonists, pertussis-specific immunoglobulin or antihistamines.[102]

Infants less than 6 months of age should generally be admitted to a high-dependency area for close monitoring. These infants are likely to require oxygen and fluid management, and are at risk of apnoea and other potential complications of pertussis, most commonly pneumonia. Children will require admission if they are experiencing significant respiratory distress or hypoxia with paroxysms or apnoea, regardless of age. Children with suspected as well as confirmed pertussis should be isolated and infection control officers alerted to their admission. It is recommended that close contacts who are not fully vaccinated also require treatment, and exposed children should be excluded from school for 14 days or until they have received a minimum of 5 days of antibiotic treatment, although the benefits of contact prophylaxis are not clear.[100,103] Pertussis is a notifiable disease in Australia and Aotearoa New Zealand, so the treating clinician must inform state surveillance units of the diagnosis.

Prevention serves as one of the best management strategies for pertussis. Routine vaccination for infants includes pertussis; the immunisation schedule is discussed elsewhere in this chapter. Vaccination of adults in contact with young babies and identification and treatment of pertussis in older children and adults is vital to prevent the spread of the disease to young babies, who are at great risk of serious sequelae.

PRACTICE TIPS

PERTUSSIS

- Pertussis can be a very serious disease, particularly in young babies who are at greatest risk of contracting the disease as immunity is not conferred until following the second vaccination at 4 months of age.
- Coughing paroxysms are the defining feature of the illness.
- The classic 'whoop' heard at the end of the coughing paroxysm is not heard in all cases and should not be relied upon to make the diagnosis.
- The diagnosis should be suspected in children with persistent cough for over 4 weeks.
- PCR (polymerase chain reaction) is recommended to confirm the diagnosis.
- Young babies should be monitored carefully as the characteristic coughing paroxysms may result in exhaustion or apnoea.
- Antibiotics are only of clinical value if commenced in the first week of illness; however, all cases should be treated to prevent community spread of the illness.
- Adults caring for infants should be revaccinated for pertussis as immunisation is unlikely to confer lifelong immunity.

PNEUMONIA

Pneumonia is described in detail in Chapter 21; this discussion serves only to highlight the key differences between paediatric and adult pneumonia. Pneumonia is an inflammation of the lung tissue, the aetiology of which is to some extent age dependent. As the causative organism is not isolated in 20–60% of cases, it is hard to accurately document their incidence, but it is estimated that viruses account for 15–35% of infections and are the most common aetiology in infants and young children, with RSV the single most-common virus.[104] In neonates and older children, bacterial causes become a more dominant aetiology for pneumonia. Bacterial pathogens in the neonatal period include *Escherichia coli* and Group B *Streptococcus*; in infancy they include *Pneumococcus*, *Haemophilus*, although less common since vaccination was introduced into the childhood schedule, and infrequently *Staphylococcus*; as children get older, bacterial pathogens also include *Mycoplasma pneumoniae*.[105]

Each year the influenza virus is responsible for severe pneumonia and several paediatric deaths in Australia. In 2009 influenza A (H1N1) was responsible for an outbreak of severe pneumonia in Mexico, where significant numbers of people, including children, died.[106] This pandemic soon spread to other parts of the world and large numbers of people, including children, contracted this virus in Australia and Aotearoa New Zealand. However, mortality was substantially lower than in Mexico where it originated.

Presentation and diagnosis

Cough, fever, dyspnoea, chest pain, vomiting, abdominal pain and anorexia are common although not specific symptoms of pneumonia.[104] Children with pneumonia frequently look unwell and are described as lethargic. Examination findings for children with pneumonia include tachypnoea, increased respiratory effort, grunting, reduced oxygen saturations and, on auscultation, crackles and decreased breath sounds.[107] Fever, tachypnoea and cough have been shown to be two of the single most-sensitive and specific signs of pneumonia.[107]

The signs and symptoms of pneumonia may vary with age, with infants presenting with more non-specific symptoms. Aetiology also varies with age. However, there appears to be limited correlation between the presenting signs and symptoms and the aetiology of pneumonia.[104,107] A large review identified that hypoxia and increased work of breathing were most associated with a diagnosis of pneumonia.[104] Wheeze is not characteristically present in children with pneumonia, although it may accompany viral pneumonia, and alternative diagnoses should be sought in the absence of findings, such as fever, coryza and tachypnoea, which suggest the diagnosis of pneumonia.[104] *Mycoplasma* is commonly associated with a more indolent pattern of illness in an older child, characterised by persistent cough.[108] In children with *Mycoplasma*, chest x-ray findings correlate well with clinical features such as consolidative lesions.[109]

Chest x-ray (anteroposterior view) is used for confirmation of the diagnosis of pneumonia, but is not necessary in mild illness. However, the chest x-ray may be normal in the early stages of the illness. There is also no convincing evidence that viral and bacterial pneumonia can be differentiated on the basis of the x-ray findings,[110] and routine chest x-ray has not been shown to affect the clinical outcomes.[111] Pathology does not aid diagnosis and does not usually alter management strategies, and therefore routine tests are not recommended.[110] However, the syndrome of inappropriate antidiuretic hormone (SIADH) is linked with pneumonia, and in the severely unwell, urea and electrolytes should be measured.

Management

Management of pneumonia is dependent on the severity of the illness and the likely aetiology. Most children presenting with community-acquired pneumonia will be well enough to be managed as outpatients. Viruses are the most common cause, but where bacterial pneumonia is suspected, empiric antibiotics are started and amoxicillin is best supported by available data, with recent evidence suggesting a lower dose and shorter duration was non-inferior to standard treatment, although none of the participants were colonised for penicillin-resistant pneumococci.[112] Oral therapy may be used in all but those children with signs of severe disease, such as hypoxaemia and dehydration.[113] Additional robust studies evaluating the efficacy of antibiotics for the treatment of *Mycoplasma* in children are required.[114] However, in children older than 5 years, a macrolide such as roxithromycin may be commenced to cover suspected *Mycoplasma* pneumonia. Where viral aetiology is considered the most likely, infants and children are treated symptomatically, and antibiotics are not prescribed. Infants and children managed as outpatients should be referred to their GP for review. There is no evidence that over-the-counter cough medicines provide any benefit to cough related to pneumonia.[115]

Management of infants and children with signs of more-serious illness (hypoxaemia and/or dehydration) will include admission and focus on respiratory support and fluid management. High-flow oxygen may be required to support acceptable oxygen saturations, fluid therapy commenced to support hydration and, in a small number of cases, fluid resuscitation. Penicillin is commenced for infants and children admitted with pneumonia unless there is convincing evidence that the infection is viral. The doses and dosing schedules for all antibiotics used in the treatment of pneumonia are available from a range of sources and the agents used will be influenced by geographic resistance patterns. Paediatric tertiary hospital CPGs, prescribing resources such as the Therapeutic Guidelines website and local resistance data, should serve as treatment guides.

PRACTICE TIPS

PNEUMONIA

- Pneumonia should be suspected in children presenting with the following symptoms: cough, fever, dyspnoea, chest pain, vomiting, abdominal pain and anorexia.
- In addition to the classic features of pneumonia, it should be suspected in children with fever, tachypnoea and abdominal pain.
- Viral and bacterial causes cannot be reliably differentiated on clinical and x-ray findings in most cases.

OTITIS MEDIA

Acute otitis media (AOM) is the most common cause of otalgia (earache) in children and is the most diagnosed childhood disease. At least 90% of children will experience AOM by the age of 2 years.[116] As described earlier in the chapter, the underdeveloped immune system coupled with the age-related differences in the Eustachian tube anatomy make the infant and young child more susceptible to ear infection than other age groups. The aetiology in children is generally viral (2%), *Streptococcus* pneumonia (23%), non-typable *Haemophilus* influenza (29%).[117,118]

The introduction of the pneumococcal conjugate vaccine 7 and 13 has seen a relative reduction in the epidemiology, but not the risk factors.[119,120] Childcare attendance, older siblings, younger age, dummy use and cigarette smoke exposure have all been shown by researchers and meta-analysis to increase the incidence of AOM in children.[121] The protective effect of breastfeeding has been debated in the literature; a meta-analysis suggests that exclusive breastfeeding during the first 6 months of life protects against having AOM in the first 2 years of life (43% reduction).[122]

Presentation and diagnosis

Infants and children with AOM present with fever, distress, interrupted sleep, and complaints of earache, or have been observed pulling at one or both of their ears. They may also have had discharge from the ear. There have usually been symptoms of an upper respiratory tract infection (URTI) for several days prior to the onset of more-specific symptoms. Approximately 90% of children suffering AOM will have rhinitis.

Examination usually reveals signs of URTI, such as coryza and rhinitis. Examination of the tympanic membranes is crucial in the diagnosis and is the best discriminator of AOM from otitis media externa (OME).[121] The tympanic membrane (TM) shows signs of inflammation and will be red, yellow or cloudy, and is usually full or bulging with signs of effusion. Redness with a lack of bulging TM may be related to crying or fever.[123] Where the TM is perforated, this may be visible or the canal may be occluded by yellow mucus discharge.

Consideration should be given to potential complications of AOM (such as hearing loss, mastoiditis and intracranial infection) or alternative aetiology for presenting symptoms (such as sepsis), particularly where infants or children present looking systemically unwell.

Management

Pain is a significant feature of AOM, so appropriate analgesics are essential. Despite analgesic recommendations, there is insufficient evidence on the difference between ibuprofen and paracetamol in short-term ear pain associated with AOM.[124] Several drops of lidocaine 1% may be instilled into the ear to provide temporary (up to 30 minutes) relief for severe pain.[125] There is limited evidence beyond 30 minutes in older children with AOM.[126] It is important to note that First Nations children have the highest rates of AOM with perforation in the world and it is generally not a painful condition; therefore it easily goes undetected and untreated, leading to chronic suppurative otitis media.[127,128]

A Cochrane review of the literature reports that fewer children treated with antibiotics will experience pain at 2 to 7 days or tympanic membrane perforation compared with children receiving a placebo. However, 82% of children settle spontaneously by 2 days and 20 children must be treated with antibiotics to prevent one child from unnecessarily experiencing pain beyond 2 days. Furthermore, 1 in 14 children treated with antibiotics will experience an adverse event.[129] Children less likely to achieve resolution within several days were those under 2 years of age with bilateral AOM and those who presented systemically unwell. This supports current recommendations that infants over the age of 1 year who are systemically well only receive antibiotics if the symptoms of ear infection persist beyond 2–3 days. However, there is insufficient evidence to guide the use of antibiotics alone or combining analgesics such as paracetamol or ibuprofen.

Amoxycillin is the antibiotic of first choice for the management of AOM. Although there is some evidence to suggest that children less than 2 years of age gain temporary benefit from a 10-day course rather than the standard 5 days, it is not convincing enough to merit altering dosing schedules for age-related subgroups. There is also evidence to suggest that the dosing schedule once- or twice-daily doses is as effective as three to four daily doses and is more convenient.[130] Amoxycillin and clavulanic acid may be considered when resistance to amoxicillin is suspected, such as in children with persistent symptoms following 48 hours of treatment with amoxycillin.[131] Guidelines and appropriate pharmacopoeias should be used to guide the choice of agent and the dose and dosing schedule.

Persistent middle-ear effusion (OME) frequently follows an episode of AOM. These children will be largely symptom-free, although may complain of a 'blocked ear' or difficulty hearing. They should be referred to their local doctor for review in 8–12 weeks to confirm resolution of the effusion, although approximately 25% of children will have persistent effusion at 12 weeks.[132] Treatment with antibiotics during the initial infection or following development of the effusion will not alter the course, and antibiotics are not recommended.[133] There is also no evidence to support the use of antihistamines or decongestants for OME.[134] Recurrent AOM and chronic effusions, where there is hearing loss, delayed language development or failure to thrive, should be referred to ENT.

PRACTICE TIPS

OTITIS MEDIA

- Frequently associated with a viral URTI.
- Pain management is the most important focus of otitis media.
- Antibiotic treatment should be withheld for 2 days in children who are over the age of 1 year and systemically well, as pain will subside spontaneously in approximately 80% of these children.
- Antibiotic therapy will not reduce the incidence or aid in the management of middle-ear effusion, a common outcome of acute otitis media.

PHARYNGITIS

Sore throat in paediatric emergency presentations is most commonly caused by viral pharyngitis. However, the aetiology in about one-third of presentations in Australia and Aotearoa New Zealand will be Group A *Streptococcus* (GAS), the majority of which will occur in school-age children. The complications that may occur following GAS infection, such as rheumatic fever, serve as the incentive for antibiotic treatment of presentations with a likely GAS infection. However, there is some controversy about this practice in some populations, such as non-Indigenous Australians and New Zealanders, where complication post-GAS infection is rare.[17] Conversely, the incidence of rheumatic fever in the Australian Indigenous community in the Northern Territory is the highest in the world,[135] and this is mirrored in the Māori community in Aotearoa New Zealand. Treatment of GAS will reduce this risk by approximately two-thirds.[136]

Presentation and diagnosis

Infants and children with pharyngitis present with fever, sore throat and/or decreased oral intake and mild irritability. Those with a viral aetiology will also present with coryza, cough and conjunctivitis. Those with Epstein-Barr infection will present with general malaise, fever and generalised lymphadenopathy and splenomegaly. The features of GAS infection are fever, pharyngotonsillitis, exudate and tender tonsillar lymph nodes. There is, however, considerable overlap between presentations of differing aetiology, making accurate diagnosis difficult. For example, exudate is present in approximately 30% of cases of non-GAS pharyngitis.[137]

Throat swabs are widely used to confirm GAS with 90–95% sensitivity.[138] They are not routinely recommended with the exception of high-risk groups and prior to commencing antibiotic therapy.

Management

Non-Indigenous Australian and Aotearoa New Zealand children under 4 years of age and older children with viral symptoms or signs of Epstein-Barr infection and no signs of GAS should receive symptomatic management and no antibiotic therapy. These children should be given regular analgesia to ensure that they are comfortable enough to drink. Evidence shows that approximately 6 more people out of 100 who take antibiotics will be better after 3 days than those who don't take antibiotics. Conversely, as many people will have problems such as rash, vomiting and diarrhoea from taking antibiotics. Children older than 4 years who have features of GAS infection should be treated with oral penicillin, as it has proven efficacy in eradicating the organism and preventing rheumatic fever secondary to GAS, it is safe and cost-effective[139,140] and no penicillin-resistant isolates have been reported.[141] There should be a very low threshold for treating Indigenous Australians and New Zealanders of any age with antibiotics. Pathology review in 2–3 days will confirm the need to continue the antibiotics. They can be stopped if the throat swab is negative for GAS.

There is insufficient evidence to support the role of other agents, such as steroids, in the treatment of pharyngitis in children,[142] although it should be acknowledged that vaccination for influenza and *Pneumococcus* reduces the incidence of pharyngitis.

PRACTICE TIPS

PHARYNGITIS

- Most pharyngitis, particularly in children under 4 years of age, is caused by viral infection.
- Throat swabs can be used in at-risk groups to diagnose Group B *Streptococcus* infection and determine the need for antibiotics.
- Penicillin remains the antibiotic of choice.

CARDIOVASCULAR EMERGENCIES

SHOCK

Shock is a complex physiological syndrome, but can be most simply defined as a state where inadequate perfusion results in profound tissue hypoxia. Shock is frequently classified by pathway to shock: hypovolaemic, cardiogenic, obstructive or distributive; and may be further defined by the predominant physiological derangement: an abnormality of preload, an abnormality of contractility, an abnormality of afterload or an abnormality of vascular tone. However, there is likely to be overlap between the precipitants to and the derangements of shock, and that once shock is well established a self-perpetuating inflammatory cascade, which is largely independent of the original cause, is established and is increasingly difficult to manage.[143] Chapters 10 and 22 describe shock in greater detail; this section will briefly focus on paediatric physiology and shock in infants and young children.

Acute illness demands an increase in cardiac output to supply oxygen and glucose to the tissues and remove waste products. Cardiac output is determined by heart rate and stroke volume, which are variable and tightly controlled to ensure adequate organ perfusion. However, infants have a relatively fixed stroke volume (Table 35.1) and are more dependent on an increase in heart rate to increase cardiac output.[143] Rates as high as 220 beats/minute may be seen in hypovolaemic infants.

Infant myocardial compliance is also lower than in adults, and so for the same ventricular filling volume infants will experience higher atrial pressures. This has a negative effect on preload and also restricts capacity to increase stroke volume.[144] This also helps explain the infant's relatively poor response to aggressive fluid resuscitation. Data exists to indicate that infants and children with higher central venous pressure (CVP) have higher mortality rates than those with lower CVP (< 8–12 mmHg).[145]

Infants are particularly susceptible to shock, as compensatory mechanisms are easily overwhelmed; unless the physiological derangements of shock are reversed, infants rapidly demonstrate a bradycardic response to deterioration, in contrast to the increasing tachycardia seen in older children and adults. This is the result of the presence of fewer beta-receptors in infant myocardium than are found in adult myocardium.[144]

Hypovolaemic shock reflects a loss of circulating blood volume; the most common causes in children are fluid loss from dehydration and blood loss from trauma. Other, less common causes are burns, diabetic ketoacidosis, reduced intake, and other third-space losses. Distributive shock is most commonly caused by sepsis. Sepsis is a complex syndrome mediated by bacterial toxins and the chemical mediators of inflammation that causes vasodilation and capillary leak, myocardial depression, and inhibition of cellular metabolism. An explanation of the pathophysiology of sepsis is beyond the scope of this chapter. In developed countries the following organisms are most commonly implicated in severe infection and sepsis in infants and children: *E. coli*, *Staphylococcus*, *Streptococcus*, *Neisseria meningitides*, *Enterobacteriaceae* and other Gram-negative bacterial infections causing pneumonia, skin infections, UTIs, meningitis and bacteraemia. In high-income countries, 4% of children admitted to hospital have sepsis and approximately 8% of those admitted to paediatric ICUs.[146] Mortality is approximately 5–50% depending on severity of illness, risk factors (such as age and pre-existing illness) and geographical location.[146]

Presentation

Typically, intravascular volume loss results in tachycardia to increase cardiac output, tachypnoea to increase oxygen supply and vasoconstriction, with a resulting narrowing pulse pressure to increase perfusion pressure. Poor circulating blood volume results in the infant or child exhibiting pallor, mottled peripheries, delayed capillary refill and deteriorating consciousness level. Hypotension is a late sign of shock and has been repeatedly shown to be associated with higher rates of mortality.[147]

The stages of septic shock are defined by different clinical findings. *Compensated* (warm) septic shock is characterised by evidence of a hyperdynamic circulation: tachycardia, tachypnoea, flushed warm skin, full pulses and widening pulse pressure. Deterioration sees this progress to *uncompensated* (cold) shock, characterised by increasing tachycardia, tachypnoea, and signs more consistent with hypovolaemia, such as pallor, cool to cold and mottled peripheries, delayed capillary refill and decreased consciousness state.

Infants and children can present with either warm or cold shock or with a combination of vasodilation and poor cardiac output, in contrast to adults, who usually present in the early stages with vasodilation and high cardiac output.[148] Immune-system immaturity is also responsible for unpredictable responses to sepsis in infants, who may present with hypothermia rather than hyperthermia and a range of non-specific symptoms.

Invasive monitoring, such as arterial pressures and central venous pressures, can provide more-accurate figures for determining the extent of the cardiovascular dysfunction. However, insertion of invasive cannulae for this purpose should not be an early priority as sufficient clinical data to make an assessment, establish a treatment plan and measure its success during the resuscitation phase can be gained from non-invasive monitoring. Central access will become a greater priority if inotropes are required.

Biochemical markers can be used as an indirect measure of the adequacy of cardiac output and tissue oxygenation. Markers such as lactate may serve as one of the earliest predictors of mortality in sepsis.[146,149] Hence, biochemical markers may be used as an indicator of the success of earlier treatment and a guide to ongoing resuscitation. However, they have a limited role in identifying children at risk of sepsis or guiding immediate fluid resuscitation, given the urgency of restoring an adequate circulation in a hypovolaemic child and the potential delay in accessing laboratory results.

Initial workup where sepsis is suspected should include collection of blood for culture, but this should not delay treatment and antibiotic choice should be made on the basis of age, infection site, comorbidities and local patterns of infection.[146]

Management

Management of shock must include airway and respiratory assessment and support and rapid administration of antibiotics. Children in shock will at least require high-flow oxygen and are likely to benefit from intubation and mechanical ventilation, which has been discussed previously. Empiric antibiotic therapy should commence without delay (within 1 hour of recognition of potential sepsis) as outcomes are improved by early treatment.[146] The focus of this section is circulatory management.

The aim of treatment, regardless of cause, is to improve organ perfusion. Potential for survival is improved by early normalisation of blood pressure values.[146] Crystalloid fluids have gained increasing favour as the fluid of choice for circulatory resuscitation as they are widely available, inexpensive and likely to remain in circulation as long as colloid fluids; evidence indicates that outcomes are equal to those where colloids have been used.[151] However, overuse can result in hyperchloraemic acidosis. Hartmann's solution (contains lactate, which when converted to bicarbonate acts as a buffer), Ringer's lactate solution or Plasmalyte® can be considered as alternatives. Colloid fluids may be recommended in specific circumstances; for example, albumin is the colloid most frequently recommended for sepsis and packed cells in trauma following 40 mL/kg of crystalloid. However, albumin is expensive, no more effective than crystalloids and synthetic colloids in sepsis have been linked to increased rates of renal replacement and higher mortality rates.[152]

Guidelines for fluid resuscitation most commonly recommend fluid boluses of 20 mL/kg.[18] This volume is based on results from a study which demonstrated that the signs of hypovolaemic shock become apparent with a loss of approximately 30% of circulating blood volume, which is equivalent to about 20 mL/kg. Fluid is rapidly redistributed and repeat boluses are usually required to maintain an adequate circulating volume, particularly where there is a total body fluid deficit or large volume shifts, as in sepsis. Data have shown that rapid resuscitation of septic infants and children presenting to the ED with in excess of 40 mL/kg increases survival when compared with those receiving smaller volumes of fluid.[153] However, there is a small body of evidence that aggressive fluid resuscitation may be associated with higher mortality.[154] A recent systematic review highlighted how few data there are on which to base decisions about fluid volumes for children in septic shock.[155] It is anticipated that the results of the SQUEEZE trial will go some way to answering this question.[156] Where intensive care is available, current recommendations are for 10–20 mL/kg boluses of fluid up to 40–60 mL/kg over the first hour titrated to provide adequate circulation without signs of fluid overload.[146]

Intra-osseous (IO) access to the circulation for delivery of resuscitation drugs and fluids is recommended where intravenous (IV) access cannot be rapidly achieved. Insertion of an IO needle is easier than IV insertion and is made easier with the use of insertion aids such as bone drills, which have been demonstrated as both reliable and safe in both the pre-hospital system as well as the ED.[157,158] Therefore, clinicians should have a low threshold for abandoning further attempts to site an IV (one or two brief unsuccessful attempts) and attempting IO access.

The type of access achieved will influence the rate and methods of fluid administration. Fluids given via the IO route must be pumped under pressure as they will not run on a gravity drip set. Manual blood pump sets, syringes and pressure bags can be used for this purpose. Small-bore IV cannulae also limit the flow of fluids, and higher pressures will be needed to deliver a fluid bolus. Low-volume fluid boluses can be given by 'pushing' fluids with a 20 mL or 50 mL syringe connected to a three-way tap in the fluid line, while larger volumes will require the use of infusion pumps, pressure bags or pump sets.

Fluid resuscitation is rarely sufficient to correct haemodynamic derangements in septic shock and delays to inotropes and/or vasopressors are associated with increases in mortality.[146] There is insufficient evidence to make strong recommendations regarding first-line inotropic support for infants and children. Available evidence supports adrenaline and noradrenaline in preference to dopamine.[156] In practice, clinicians may select agents based on treatment goals. Infants and children presenting with signs of high cardiac output and vasodilation, clinically manifested by warm peripheries and bounding pulses, benefit from agents that stimulate vasoconstriction, such as noradrenaline.[159] Alternatively, for those presenting with evidence of 'cold' shock, which is associated with vasoconstriction and clinically manifested by cold and mottled peripheries, weak thready pulses and delayed capillary refill, inotropic agents to improve contractility such as adrenaline are used.[160] In many cases where there are features of both vasodilation and poor cardiac output, combination regimens are best suited to improving perfusion. Furthermore, the haemodynamic status of children may change rapidly, requiring changes to inotropic regimens. Table 35.11 provides a guide to the dosing schedule and preparation of common paediatric inotrope infusions and Fig. 35.3 provides a clinical algorithm to guide haemodynamic management in the ED of septic infants and children.[156,162]

TABLE 35.11 INOTROPE INFUSIONS COMMONLY USED FOR SEPSIS MANAGEMENT

AGENT	PREPARATION	DOSING SCHEDULE
Adrenaline	0.3 mg/kg in 50 mL normal saline	0.05–0.1 microgram/kg/min
	= 6 microgram/kg/mL	0.5–1.0 mL/h
	If low doses are required, 0.15 mg/kg*	0.01–0.05 microgram/kg/min
	= 3 microgram/kg/mL	0.2–1.0 mL/h
Noradrenaline	0.3 mg/kg in 50 mL normal saline	0.05–0.1 microgram/kg/min
	= 6 microgram/kg/mL	0.5–1.0 mL/h
	If low doses are required, 0.15 mg/kg*	0.01–0.05 microgram/kg/min
	= 3 microgram/kg/mL	0.2–1.0 mL/h
Dopamine	15 mg/kg in 50 mL normal saline	5–10 microgram/min
	= 300 microgram/kg/mL	1–2 mL/h
Dobutamine	15 mg/kg in 50 mL normal saline	5–10 microgram/min
	= 300 microgram/kg/mL	1–2 mL/h

**At very low doses, small increases in rate may generate significant changes in blood pressure*

PRACTICE TIPS

SHOCK

- Infants rely almost exclusively on increasing heart rate to increase their cardiac output. However, once this is exhausted, they rapidly deteriorate.
- Infants may present with a low temperature associated with septic shock rather than a fever.
- Once compensatory responses are overwhelmed, infants and children may demonstrate a bradycardic response to rapid deterioration rather than the classic tachycardic response expected.
- Hypotension is a late sign of shock and is associated with poor prognosis.
- Pathology test results play no part in directing the initial fluid resuscitation of infants and children in shock.
- The aim of treatment is to improve end-organ perfusion by normalising circulating blood volume and blood pressure.
- Intra-osseous access to the circulation is recommended where intravenous access cannot be rapidly achieved.
- Infants and children may require up to 80–100 mL/kg of isotonic crystalloid solutions such as normal saline, and Hartmann's solution in boluses of 20 mL/kg to restore circulating blood volume.
- Infants and children in septic shock will usually require inotropic support to maintain end-organ perfusion.

Adjuvant therapies to treat shock, in particular septic shock, and other shock-related organ dysfunction and physiological derangements (e.g. hyperglycaemia), have been explored with mixed results. The role of fever management is unclear and no specific recommendations to treat or withhold antipyretics have been made.[156] The use of insulin therapy to maintain blood glucose levels less than 7.8 mmol/L is not recommended in children and although there are no studies to support its use to lower blood glucose levels above 7.8 mmol/L, it may be clinically appropriate to do so.[156]

A Cochrane review concluded that there is sufficient evidence to support the use of low-dose, long-term (> 5 days) steroids to improve sepsis mortality.[163] Two Cochrane reviews summarised the evidence for the use of human recombinant protein C in neonates[164] and in children and adults,[165] and both concluded that there is no evidence for this theoretically promising therapy. Researchers are increasingly exploring the role of vitamin D deficiency in sepsis, but as yet data from trials to evaluate the efficacy of treatment with vitamin D are not available.[156]

DEHYDRATION

Dehydration, due to poor oral intake and increased losses secondary to acute illness, occurs more commonly in infants than in adults, which can be explained by the physiological differences between adults and children and their responses to illness. Total body water is about 80 mL/kg at birth and falls to approximately 60–65 mL/kg by about 6–12 months of age, where it remains constant until adulthood. The distribution of fluids across fluid compartments also differs, evidenced by the difference in blood volume between infants (70–80 mL/kg) and adults (60–70 mL/kg); and like total body water,

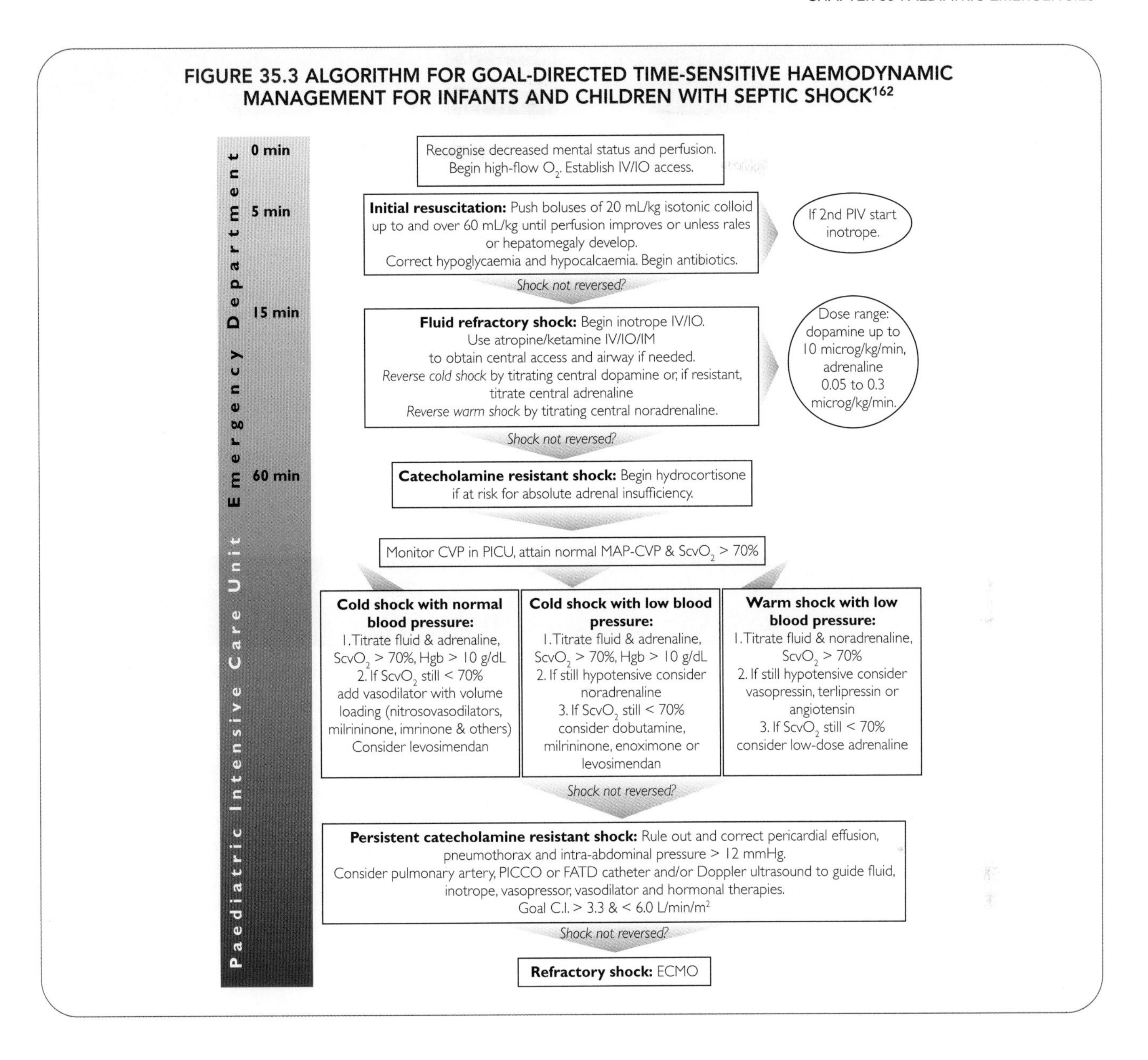

FIGURE 35.3 ALGORITHM FOR GOAL-DIRECTED TIME-SENSITIVE HAEMODYNAMIC MANAGEMENT FOR INFANTS AND CHILDREN WITH SEPTIC SHOCK[162]

fluid distribution resembles that of the adult by 6–12 months of age.[18]

Infant renal function differs from adult renal function, further reducing an infant's capacity to rapidly respond to hypovolaemia, dehydration and low cardiac output.[166] A lower glomerular filtration rate, renal blood flow and renal immaturity explain the differences in renal function between the infant and the adult. The infant kidney has less capacity to concentrate urine, excrete a solute load or acidify urine, and is more sensitive to hyperchloraemic acidosis resulting from large-volume resuscitation with normal saline than the adult kidney.[166]

Presentation

Changes in total bodyweight are considered the gold standard for assessment of dehydration. It has been shown that clinicians frequently overestimate dehydration severity, with one early Australian study revealing that this may be by as much as 3.2%.[167] This provides persuasive support for serial weight measurements for children presenting to the ED with the potential for fluid loss. All children with actual or potential fluid balance problems should have their bare weight measured as part of their initial assessment to provide a baseline for future assessments. However, accurate recent weight measurements are often not available to inform the initial hydration assessment, and clinicians are obliged to rely on clinical features to detect dehydration and determine the severity of the fluid loss.

Identifying clinical signs and symptoms, which are sensitive and specific for dehydration and its severity, has received significant attention from researchers. Traditionally, dehydration has been linked to a history of fluid loss (diarrhoea and vomiting), poor fluid intake and low urine output. However, data do not confirm this link, showing that these symptoms have low predictive value for moderate dehydration. Conversely, parental report of normal urine output positively predicts normal hydration.[168,169] The evidence to support signs to predict dehydration is variable and it is unlikely that any single sign can be used to identify dehydration or its severity.

TABLE 35.12 CLINICAL DEHYDRATION SCALE (CDS)[171]

CHARACTERISTIC	0	1	2
General appearance	Normal	Thirsty, restless or lethargic but irritable when touched	Drowsy, limp, cold, sweaty ± comatose
Eyes	Normal	Slightly sunken	Very sunken
Mucous membranes (tongue)	Moist	'Sticky'	Dry
Tears	Tears present	Decreased tears	Absent tears
Scoring			
0 = no dehydration			
1-4 = some dehydration			
5-8 = moderate-severe dehydration			

TABLE 35.13 ELECTROLYTE COMPOSITION OF FLUIDS COMMONLY OFFERED TO CHILDREN WITH DIARRHOEA AND VOMITING[180,181]

SOLUTION	SODIUM (mmol/L)	POTASSIUM (mmol/L)	CARBOHYDRATE (mmol/L)	OSMOLARITY (mOsm)
WHO recommendation	90	20	111	310
Reduced osmolarity solution	75	20	75	245
Hydralyte	55	20	80	230
Soft drink	2	0	700	750
Apple juice	3	32	690	730
Broth	250	8	0	500
Sports drink	20	3	255	340
Tea	0	0	0	5

WHO: World Health Organization.

Results demonstrate that dehydration assessment tools comprised of several signs have greater predictive value than individual signs. For this reason an approximation of the severity of dehydration should be based on the number of signs of dehydration identified, rather than the presence of specific individual signs and symptoms. Several tools using this approach have been developed and the Clinical Dehydration Scale (CDS) has recently been shown to be more accurate than other tools.[170] This scale is comprised of four items (appearance, eyes, mucous membranes and tears), each scored to generate a total ranging from 0 to 8. The scale and scoring system are shown in Table 35.12.[171]

The sensitivity of laboratory tests to detect dehydration and estimate the severity is not sufficiently high to support recommendations for routine laboratory tests for hydration assessment. Of those tests that are considered likely to be predictive of the severity of dehydration, bicarbonate has shown to be the most sensitive,[167,172–175] while parameters such as specific gravity of urine, the presence of ketones and urine output during rehydration show low predictive value.[173,176] Ultrasound has been tested as a means to identify severe dehydration with some success and as the use of bedside ultrasound grows there may be a role for ultrasound in the detection of dehydration.[177,178]

Management

Enteral fluid therapy is the most widely recommended approach to rehydration for children with dehydration in the absence of signs of hypovolaemia. Enteral fluid replacement is likely to avoid the potential fluid, electrolyte and acid–base imbalances that can occur with intravenous fluid management,[179] and has been shown to be potentially safer than IV rehydration, and at least as effective.[179] The composition of the optimal solution for oral rehydration (ORS) in developed countries is a reduced osmolarity solution based on WHO recommendations, which can be seen in Table 35.13,[180] alongside the composition of a number of other fluids commonly used for oral rehydration. Fruit juices and soft drinks

TABLE 35.14 ORAL AND ENTERAL REHYDRATION FLUID MANAGEMENT FOR THE FIRST 6 HOURS: AN EXAMPLE CALCULATION

REPLACEMENT CALCULATION	MAINTENANCE VOLUME CALCULATION	VOLUME / HOUR
15 kg child estimated as 6% dehydrated	4 mL/hr/kg up to 10 kg	= 150 + 50
6% of 15 kg = 900 g	2 mL/hr/kg for each kg between 10 and 20 kg	= 200 mL/hr
Therefore:	1 mL/hr/kg for each kg over 20 kg	
Deficit	Therefore:	
= 900 mL over 6 hours	(4 × 10) + (2 × 5)	
= 150 mL/hr replacement	= 50 mL/hr maintenance	

require considerable dilution (1 part to 4 parts water), if they are used as an alternative to ORSs for children refusing to drink ORSs, but their use in children with mild dehydration has been shown to result in fewer treatment failures than when ORS is used.[182]

Children with only mild dehydration can usually be encouraged to drink enough fluid to maintain adequate hydration. Frozen ORS prepared as an icy pole can be a good way of providing rehydration fluids, with results from a small study showing that children were more likely to tolerate frozen ORS than standard ORS.[183]

Many children will refuse to drink sufficient volumes of fluid or will not tolerate oral fluids. In the absence of signs of hypovolaemia, these children can in most circumstances still be rehydrated enterally via a nasogastric (NG) tube. Australian and Aotearoa New Zealand guidelines for rehydration strongly advocate for this route, claiming that it is effective and likely to be safer than IV rehydration. However, the evidence for this contention is not overwhelming and in many countries this practice is not so common.

The decision to rehydrate using an NG tube or intravenous (IV) access is complicated by the degree of procedural difficulty associated with NG tube and IV cannula insertion. Nasogastric tube insertion can be safely and quickly achieved in the ED to provide a route for fluid replacement,[184] and may prove to be easier than cannula placement in infants and young children with dehydration. However, although easier, NG tube insertion is considered one of the most painful procedures performed in the ED, and yet practice recommendations rarely advocate the use of analgesics or local anaesthetics. Although evidence is not available to support these practices in children, it is convincing in adults so clinicians should consider the use of agents such as lidocaine spray and nebulised lidocaine prior to NG tube insertion to alleviate the discomfort associated with this procedure.

As the need for NG rehydration is most likely to be necessary in infants and young children who are rarely cooperative, restraint is usually required to allow for insertion and to prevent them pulling out the tube. However, the least restraint necessary for the procedure should be used and removed as soon as possible. Delivery of fluids-only means that a fine-bore tube (size 8 French gauge) may be used to allow appropriate flow rates. Continuous administration of fluid by feeding pump or manual drip set will be better tolerated than regular boluses.

Where there is concern about the impact of rapid rehydration on fluid and electrolyte balance, it is recommended that replacement of losses occurs over 6 hours. The volume of fluid administered hourly is the sum of the estimated loss divided by 6, added to the hourly maintenance volume required. Table 35.14 provides an example of this calculation. Tables providing the volume of fluid administered by weight for children with moderate and severe dehydration are available, and can be found in the Australian Paediatric Improvement Collaborative (PIC) gastroenteritis clinical practice guidelines.[185] When electrolyte imbalance is not a concern, rapid rehydration regimens advocating 25 mL/kg/h to replace fluid losses over 3–4 hours may be used for rehydration.[186]

PRACTICE TIPS

DEHYDRATION

- All infants and children with actual or potential dehydration should be weighed, as short-term changes in bodyweight are the most sensitive indicator of fluid loss.
- Pathology tests to detect and determine the severity of dehydration are not sensitive enough to be of clinical value.
- Infants and children with dehydration (in the absence of signs of hypovolaemia) can be rehydrated enterally (orally or via a nasogastric tube) in most cases.
- Rapid enteral rehydration via nasogastric tube using 25 mL/kg/h over 3–4 hours may be used where electrolyte imbalance is not a concern.

Maintenance fluid management

Infants and children with acute illness often have higher losses of fluid (insensible, vomiting and diarrhoea) and drink poorly, impacting on their fluid and electrolyte balance. To overcome this, maintenance fluids are commenced as a means of providing sufficient water and electrolytes to maintain normal urine output at a similar osmolality to extracellular fluid.

Traditional maintenance fluid recommendations for hypotonic fluids were based on the needs of well children and have been shown to increase the risk of hyponatraemia and subsequent mortality and morbidity. Support for isotonic fluids was confirmed in a large RCT and echoed in a recent systematic review comparing isotonic and hypotonic fluids for maintenance fluid therapy in children.[187,188]

Infants and children suffering fever associated with infection have been shown to secrete higher levels of antidiuretic hormone (ADH) than well children. This prompts retention of water and higher rates of sodium excretion, potentially causing hyponatraemia and water overload. This is defined as the syndrome of inappropriate ADH secretion (SIADH), and is linked with illnesses such as meningitis, pneumonia, bronchiolitis and gastroenteritis. Although there is some concern that SIADH is over-diagnosed, this underpins the rationale for restricting the volume of fluids for some children to approximately two-thirds normal volumes where rates are calculated using bodyweight.

Maintenance fluids for infants and children should also contain glucose, as illness will increase their glucose consumption and infants have very limited stores of glycogen. Addition of 5% glucose to the IV fluids will prevent hypoglycaemia in most circumstances, but will only provide about 20% of daily required calories.

PRACTICE TIPS

MAINTENANCE FLUID THERAPY

- Isotonic fluids which contain glucose are recommended for maintenance fluid management for unwell children.
- Two-thirds of maintenance volumes are recommended for children suffering illnesses where water retention is possible, such as meningitis, pneumonia and bronchiolitis.

ABNORMAL PULSE RATE OR RHYTHM

Infants and children present to EDs with a range of cardiac dysrhythmias. Cardiac arrest rhythms are discussed elsewhere (Chapters 14 and 22), and these chapters provide considerable detail about a range of dysrhythmias common to both adults and children. This section will make brief reference to those common to infants and children and highlight the specific implications of these rhythms for infants and children. These dysrhythmias may also occur in neonates and the principles of management will be similar. However, it is beyond the scope of this text to discuss the needs of this population specifically and clinicians are encouraged to seek expert advice early if faced with a neonate with a dysrhythmia.

Bradydysrhythmias

Sinus bradycardia is the antecedent to most paediatric cardiopulmonary arrests and can usually be attributed to increased parasympathetic stimulus, as occurs during intubation, metabolic derangements such as hypoxia, raised intracranial pressure caused most commonly in children by head trauma and poisoning with agents such as beta-blockers. Infants and children are particularly sensitive to these precipitants and bradycardia is poorly tolerated, as cardiac output in infants is largely rate dependent. Infants and children quickly show signs of circulatory inadequacy, and if not treated promptly this is likely to progress to signs of circulatory collapse. Treatment should include addressing reversible causes such as hypoxia and, if the dysrhythmia is life threatening, basic life support including compressions is the priority (see Chapter 14).

Tachydysrhythmias

Sinus tachycardia is a physiological response to a range of stimuli, and as infants rely heavily on increasing their heart rate to increase cardiac output, the extent of the tachycardia in infants and young children is proportionately much greater than in adults in similar circumstances. Tachycardia in sick infants may be as high as 220 beats/minute and in young children 180 beats/minute.

Supraventricular tachycardia (SVT) is the most common tachydysrhythmia in children, occurring in 1 in 250–1000 children.[189] The pathophysiology is described in Chapter 22; in children the most common cause is atrioventricular re-entry, which involves an accessory conduction pathway between the atrium and the ventricles; and atrioventricular node re-entry, which involves a re-entry pathway within the atrioventricular node. It is usually paroxysmal, lasts on average 10 minutes and recurs.[189]

Older children present similarly to adults with SVT. However, infants will present with non-specific symptoms, such as restlessness, poor feeding and lethargy. These symptoms mimic many other presentations, and, therefore, recognition of SVT in infants can be delayed. With a longer duration of SVT, infants begin to show signs of respiratory distress, diaphoresis, pallor and mottling, and if prolonged for 24–48 hours, signs of congestive heart failure may become apparent.[189]

Supraventricular tachycardia is usually better tolerated in infants and children than adults. However, the need for resuscitation should be considered and unstable patients will need cardioversion (see Chapter 22). Stable patients with adequate perfusion should have oxygen therapy and cardiac monitoring commenced and a 12-lead ECG taken prior to attempts to revert the rhythm (Chapter 16 contains information on cardiac monitoring techniques). Vagal manoeuvres are usually attempted before pharmacological interventions. Young children may be asked to blow into a straw or blow with their thumb in their mouth. As an alternative, placing a bag containing cold water and ice across the forehead, eyes and bridge of the nose can stimulate the dive reflex. However, the success rates for these methods is unknown.[190] Where vagal manoeuvres have been unsuccessful, adenosine is the first-line treatment for SVT in infants and children and it is given as a bolus every few minutes until they return to sinus rhythm, starting with 0.1 mg/kg and increasing by 0.05 mg/kg increments each time to a maximum of 0.3 mg/kg (see Chapter 22 for further details). Cardioversion is used where adenosine fails to result in reversion.[189,190]

PRACTICE TIPS

ABNORMAL PULSE RATE OR RHYTHM

- Bradycardia is a pre-terminal rhythm and management should focus on correcting the cause (e.g. improve oxygenation) and maintaining the adequacy of the circulation.
- Infants suffering from supraventricular tachycardia often present with non-specific symptoms, such as restlessness, poor feeding and lethargy.

HEART FAILURE

Heart failure in neonates, infants and children occurs most commonly as a result of a congenital heart defect.[191] It is beyond the scope of this section to detail these anomalies or the pathophysiological syndrome of heart failure. It is generally accepted as a progressive clinical and physiological syndrome caused by cardiac and non-cardiac abnormalities that result in ventricular dysfunction, pressure overload or both and a characteristic constellation of signs and symptoms.[192] Congenital defects can be grouped as those that cause a left-to-right shunt with increased pulmonary blood flow (e.g. ventricular septal defect [VSD]) and atrial septal defect (ASD), those that cause acute obstruction (e.g. aortic or pulmonary stenosis, coarctation of the aorta) and complex anomalies, such as hypoplastic left heart syndrome, which cause a range of functional problems. In a small number of children, heart failure is precipitated by primary myocardial dysfunction (e.g. myocarditis), anaemia, metabolic derangements, toxins or dysrhythmias which result in a low output cardiac failure.[191,193]

Presentation and diagnosis

The age at which infants and children present with heart failure will depend on the cause. Congenital heart defects will result in heart failure in the days to months following birth, depending on the type of defect. Duct-dependent lesions will present within days to a few weeks of birth and defects causing left to right shunt after 1 month of age. Other causes for heart failure may present at any age.

Neonates and infants presenting with cardiac failure may have quite non-specific symptoms and early heart failure is often missed. Early signs most commonly include lethargy, reduced feeding, sweating and tachypnoea during feeding and failure to thrive.[194] Heart failure may be precipitated by a mild respiratory infection, so signs of URTI are often present. On examination, neonates and infants are usually tachypnoeic, tachycardic and show evidence of failure to thrive. A difference of at least 10 mmHg between blood pressures measured in right upper and lower limbs, hepatomegaly, a gallop rhythm, and circulatory dysfunction, which once failure is more progressed may include signs of shock may be detected.[195] A murmur may also be present, but may be difficult to hear on auscultation due to the heart rate. Neonates and infants with many congenital heart defects are unresponsive to oxygen and hence this diagnosis should be considered in an infant with respiratory and circulatory dysfunction with refractory hypoxia.

Cardiomegaly is confirmed on chest x-ray and evidence of fluid overload may also be present. Evaluation should also include an ECG, but interpretation will need to account for the normal age-related variations in the ECG. Electrical abnormalities may be present, but it may also be normal. Older children present with more-specific signs and symptoms consistent with those found in adults.

Management

Fluid resuscitation and oxygen therapy are used to resuscitate the shocked infant, regardless of the circumstances. However, in neonates and infants with a large right-to-left shunt, high-flow oxygen may worsen oxygenation. Furthermore, fluids are quickly restricted, and diuretics prescribed to control preload in neonates, infants and children suffering cardiac failure. Newborns who are only days old with duct-dependent circulation will require prostaglandin to prevent duct closure and worsening of their condition, but careful monitoring is essential as side-effects include apnoea and hypotension.[195] Digoxin and angiotensin-converting enzyme (ACE) inhibitors remain the mainstay of heart failure treatment in neonates, infants and children.[193,194,196]

Management is complex, and advice from a specialist paediatric centre to guide treatment should be sought early and arrangements made to transfer patients to a tertiary paediatric cardiac or intensive care unit. In the interim, the neonate or infant should be cardiac-monitored, and a 12-lead ECG should be taken.

PRACTICE TIPS

HEART FAILURE

- Heart failure is often precipitated by mild respiratory infections.
- It is frequently associated with non-specific symptoms, such as lethargy, decreased feeding, and failure to thrive.
- Fluid resuscitation and oxygen therapy should be used to resuscitate the shocked infant.
- Treatment of heart failure is complex, and expertise should be sought early.

MYOCARDITIS

As in adults, cardiomyopathy is caused by infections, inflammatory diseases and toxins. It has been linked to COVID infection and, since its widespread introduction in 2021, an increase in myocarditis has been reported in children and young adults worldwide following messenger RNA COVID-19 vaccinations.[197]

Presentation and diagnosis

Most children with myocarditis experience only mild symptoms and hence it probably goes unrecognised in many children.[198] The symptoms include chest pain, palpitations, shortness of breath and general malaise. Some children present with gastrointestinal symptoms, such as generalised pain, nausea and loss of appetite. There may be no abnormal examination findings or only mild tachycardia. Severe myocarditis may present with the signs of heart failure. Nearly all children with myocarditis will have ECG abnormalities and a cardiac troponin may also be useful in the initial workup where myocarditis is suspected. A guideline developed by the Australian Technical Advisory Group on Immunisation (ATAGI) has been released to assist clinicians to identify myocarditis following vaccination.[197]

Management

Management will depend on the severity of disease and is extrapolated from adults as there are limited studies evaluating therapies in children. The mainstay of treatment has been immune modulation ranging from non-steroidal anti-inflammatories in mild cases to intravenous immunoglobulins (IVIG) in more severe cases.[198] Treatment to improve myocardial function may also be needed and in extreme cases heart transplantation may be the only option. Early consultation and referral to a paediatric cardiologist is essential.

PRACTICE TIPS

MYOCARDITIS

- Most children experience only mild symptoms, but myocarditis may result in cardiac failure in small numbers of children.
- The mRNA COVID-19 vaccinations are associated with increased risk of myocarditis.
- Treatment planning should involve a paediatric cardiologist.

NEUROLOGICAL EMERGENCIES

SEIZURES

Seizure is a common paediatric presentation to the ED; approximately 4–10% of children will suffer a seizure during childhood and status epilepticus has a mortality of 2 to 4%.[199] A seizure occurs where there are excessive hypersynchronous discharges from neurons, resulting in a transient, involuntary alteration of consciousness, behaviour, motor activity, sensation or autonomic function. Seizure activity prompts an increase in cerebral metabolic rate, resulting in an increase in oxygen and glucose consumption and carbon dioxide and lactic acid production. Cerebral blood flow and systolic blood pressure increases. Once metabolic demands have exceeded the supply, cerebral ischaemia, lactic acidosis, rhabdomyolysis, hyperkalaemia, hypoglycaemia, hypoxia and hyperthermia occur, all of which may lead to irreversible brain damage. Data show that this is likely to happen within 45–60 minutes of continuous seizure activity.[200]

Seizures are broadly classified as *generalised*, which involves the whole brain, or *partial*, which involves a region of the brain and there are many subtypes within each category. Most commonly children suffer generalised tonic–clonic seizures.[200] Seizures may result from fever, metabolic derangements such as hypoglycaemia, hyponatraemia or hypoxia, poisoning with agents such as tricyclic antidepressants, vascular or traumatic lesions, local infection, such as meningitis and encephalitis; or alternatively they may be idiopathic. Seizures associated with fever are the most common seizure in infants and children. A febrile convulsion is a benign, usually self-limiting convulsion which occurs in infants and young children in association with fever but without signs of neurological disease, infection or injury, other pathology likely to cause seizure or a history of afebrile convulsions.[201] Febrile convulsions are discussed in the next section.

Epilepsy describes a condition where seizures are recurrent, and convulsive status epilepticus is defined as a continuous seizure or recurrent seizure without restoration of conscious state, lasting 30 minutes or more.[200] The majority of children experiencing status epilepticus in Australia are children with a previous history of seizures.[202]

Presentation

Infants and children may present during the seizure or in the post-ictal phase following a seizure. Subtle seizure activity can be difficult to detect, particularly in children with neurological deficits. Typical jerking movements may be absent and seizure activity may only result in stiffening of a limb, deviation of the eyes or an alteration in consciousness. For this reason, parents may not recognise the significance of the episode and children may occasionally present well after the seizure. Once a seizure has been identified, assessment of the infant or child should aim to determine the likely cause of the seizure.

Management

The priority for managing children with current seizure activity is to secure their airway, ensure adequate ventilation and perfusion, control the seizure, and identify and treat, where possible, the underlying cause of the seizure. Blood sugar levels should be checked at the bedside and hypoglycaemia treated promptly, as this may account for a small number of seizures in infants and children. Furthermore, children are more susceptible to developing hypoglycaemia with prolonged seizure.

Pharmacological control of the seizure is advocated if the seizure does not spontaneously terminate within 5 minutes and is best achieved using a benzodiazepine.[203] This may be repeated within 5 minutes if seizure activity continues. Second-line agents commonly used in Australia include phenytoin and phenobarbitone, which have recently been shown to be of equal efficacy.[204]

Prolonged seizure correlates with the need for airway management and ventilatory support, and this is likely in some cases to be related to respiratory depression as well as the need to control seizure activity. The evidence to support the selection of one particular anticonvulsant over another is not strong.[203] There is interest in the role of newer anticonvulsant agents for managing status. However, there is insufficient evidence to support any of these agents for first-line treatment in preference to the more traditional benzodiazepines. Fig. 35.4[205] details a commonly accepted algorithm for paediatric seizure management.

Post-seizure management will be determined by the underlying cause of the seizure, and some children will need aggressive management of these conditions. Where the likelihood of recurrence is high, anticonvulsant infusions should also be commenced. Intravenous fluids should contain glucose to prevent hypoglycaemia. Well-looking children who have recovered from an afebrile seizure and children who have recovered from a febrile convulsion where the focus of the fever has been identified can be managed as outpatients. Parents will require considerable support, as witnessing a seizure is frightening. First aid should be discussed prior to discharge and clinicians should be sensitive to parental concern about their capacity to manage another seizure at home. There should be a low threshold for admission for first-time seizure if the parents are not comfortable taking their child home.

PRACTICE TIPS

SEIZURES

- Focal seizure activity may go unrecognised.
- Benzodiazepines are the first-line treatment of seizure activity.
- Treatment should also include identifying and treating the underlying cause of the seizure.
- Check and correct hypoglycaemia, as this is a potential cause and a likely result of seizure activity in children.
- Where recurrent seizures are possible, an anticonvulsant infusion should be commenced.
- Seizures are frightening for parents, and they should receive considerable support once the child is stabilised.

FIGURE 35.4 ACTIVE SEIZURE FLOWCHART[205]

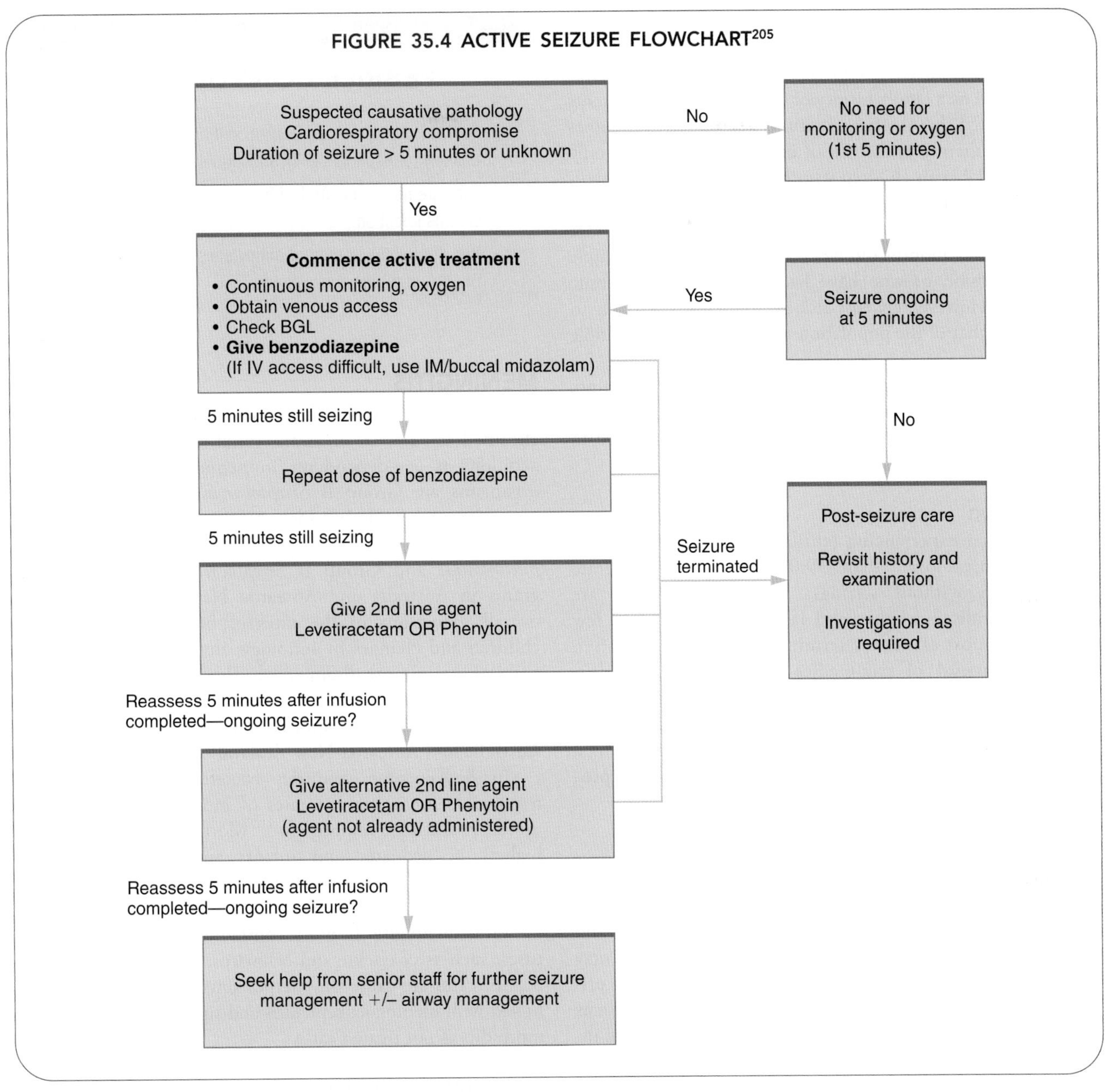

ABC: airway, breathing and circulation; BSL: blood sugar level.

FEBRILE CONVULSIONS

Febrile convulsions warrant specific attention given their frequency (2–4% of children worldwide), and the concern that they generate in the community. A febrile convulsion is defined as a seizure occurring in a child aged from 6 months to 5 years, in the setting of current or recent history of fever and no signs of neurological disease or CNS infection and no history of neurological disease or previous febrile seizure.[201] The illness causing the fever is most often mild, and there is no increase in the incidence of serious bacterial infection among children who have had a febrile convulsion.[206] They are classified as simple or complex, as follows.

- A simple febrile convulsion lasts no more than 15 minutes, is generalised, and occurs only once in 24 hours.
- Complex febrile seizures are either longer than 15 minutes, have focal features or occur more than once in 24 hours.

It has been suggested that the rapid rise in the temperature, rather than the height of the temperature, is responsible for febrile convulsions. However, there have been other theories postulated. Viral illnesses are usually associated with febrile convulsions and data from a number of studies have prompted a theory based on a viral aetiology (specifically human herpes virus 6B) for febrile convulsions.[207] An association between increased risk of febrile convulsion and measles, mumps and rubella (MMR) vaccine has been shown.[208,209] Furthermore, data has established a link between febrile convulsions and genetic factors.[210] Despite increasing awareness of these risk factors, the aetiology of febrile convulsions is still not known; it is likely to be complex and the result of multiple factors.

The rate of recurrence is 25–30%, and in 25–40% of children there will be a family history of febrile convulsion. Parents can be reassured that the risk of serious neurological outcomes is rare.[211] Furthermore, the risk of developing epilepsy is only fractionally higher in children who have had a febrile convulsion when compared with the rest of the population (increased risk 1%).[212] This risk is increased to 2.4% in children who were younger than 12 months old when they had their first simple febrile convulsion or who have had multiple simple febrile convulsions. However, epilepsy risk in children rises sharply to 30–50 times that of the population if the seizures are multiple and complex.[212]

Febrile convulsions are considered benign, self-limiting, and unlikely to result in significant sequelae. There are no deaths documented in the literature that can be attributed to febrile convulsions.

Presentation

Many children experiencing febrile convulsions will do so at temperatures lower than 39.0°C (and many tolerate higher fevers without seizing). Febrile convulsions are usually generalised seizures and last no longer than a few minutes. In most cases they terminate spontaneously, often before the arrival of paramedics or before the child is brought to the ED. However, a small number will seize for longer and a very small number will experience complex febrile seizures. Children usually recover quickly following a febrile convulsion and do not usually experience a pronounced post-ictal phase.

Management

Children in a convulsive state, regardless of aetiology, should be managed similarly. Basic life support and termination of the seizure are the first priorities of emergency service providers and ED clinicians. A small number in the post-ictal phase may briefly require simple airway management. In the ED, the priorities for management then become identification of the focus of the fever and parent education. Although the associated illness is usually mild, a potentially serious infection should be considered.

Simple febrile convulsions are not a reason for admission. If they are otherwise well enough, these children may be discharged home. Studies summarised in a recent systematic review continue to demonstrate that antipyretic therapy is not effective at reducing the risk of febrile seizure in children.[212,213] The use of antiepileptic agents during a febrile illness for children who are at risk of febrile convulsion, is also not supported as the adverse side-effects of these medications are substantial and outweigh any short-term benefit that may be gained from their use.[214] Management should concentrate on parent education and should include first aid for seizures and information about the likely aetiology and implications of febrile convulsions and advice about fever management and febrile convulsion prevention. Parents are likely to require a great deal of education and support to give them confidence to manage at home.

PRACTICE TIPS

FEBRILE CONVULSIONS

- Febrile convulsions are benign, self-limiting, and very unlikely to result in significant sequelae.
- They are not associated with an increased risk of more-serious infection.
- Regular administration of antipyretics does not reduce the risk of febrile convulsions.

MENINGITIS

Meningitis is an acute inflammation of the meninges and is classified as *bacterial* or *aseptic* (viral, fungal, etc.). Bacterial aetiology is age-dependent; in neonates the predominant organisms are Group B *Streptococcus*, *E. coli* and *Listeria monocytogenes*, while in older children (and adults) the predominant organisms are *Neisseria meningitides*, *Streptococcus pneumoniae* and Group B *Streptococcus*. Vaccination programs in Australia and Aotearoa New Zealand have seen overall reductions in the rates of bacterial meningitis in children and changes in aetiology: invasive *H. influenzae* in children has almost disappeared. The incidence of pneumococcal meningitis has decreased significantly, and serotype B is now responsible for approximately 85% of infections in Australia and Aotearoa New Zealand.[215]

In high-income countries bacterial meningitis is still responsible for significant rates of mortality and morbidity; up to 5% and 20% respectively.[216] Mortality and morbidity are highest in neonates and infants and are influenced by the organism, with rates highest for those infected with *S. pneumoniae*.[216]

Viral meningitis is most commonly caused by enteroviruses, such as coxsackie and echovirus. However, small numbers of cases are caused by herpes simplex 1 and 2, which is linked with meningoencephalitis and significant mortality and morbidity if not treated early.

Presentation and diagnosis

Older children may present with the classic features of meningitis, such as fever, headache, photophobia and neck stiffness, discussed in Chapter 23. However, infants and young children present with more non-specific signs and symptoms. Parents usually describe increased lethargy, irritability, poor feeding, fever and, in some cases, vomiting. On examination, these children generally look miserable and unwell, but may show few classic features of meningitis. The presence of photophobia, a positive Kernig's sign (inability to flex the knee when the leg is flexed at the hip) and a positive Brudzinski sign (flexing the head forwards resulting in flexing of the legs) are considered suggestive of meningitis, but the sensitivity and specificity for each of these tests is not high and hence cannot be relied upon exclusively to make the diagnosis.[217] Meningeal irritation may be manifested in infants and young children by increased irritability, particularly when handled. A bulging fontanelle is often described as a feature of meningitis in infants; however, the diagnosis should not be excluded if the fontanelle is found to be normal. The absence of meningeal signs and an abnormal cry reduce the likelihood of meningitis, but do not exclude it.

A provisional diagnosis of meningitis should be made, and treatment commenced based on clinical signs. Clinicians should approach the child who has commenced antibiotic treatment in the days prior to presentation with caution. The features of serious illness, including meningitis, are likely to be subtler and easily overlooked. The diagnosis is generally confirmed by cerebrospinal fluid examination. The presence of cells suggests meningitis, and an increase in protein and reduction in glucose implies a bacterial organism. Gram stain will usually identify the organism, providing antibiotics have not been administered well before specimen collection (CSF sterilisation may occur within 2–4 hours following a dose of ceftriaxone 50 mg/kg, depending on the organism). The contraindication to lumbar puncture is raised intracranial pressure, which may be evidenced by altered conscious state, focal neurology, abnormal posturing, seizure activity or papillo-oedema. Computed tomography (CT) is not a useful guide to the risks associated with lumbar puncture and is not routinely recommended.[218] Blood should also be collected for a full blood count, C-reactive protein, urea and electrolytes, glucose and culture.

Management

Resuscitation is the first priority. However, early treatment with antibiotics is also essential to improve outcomes. The antibiotic regimen will depend on the age of the infant and local resistance patterns. *N. meningitides* is showing some decrease in susceptibility to penicillin and resistance among pneumococci is also appearing in Australia and Aotearoa New Zealand; however, this is not yet clinically significant.[215,219] Antiviral agents, such as acyclovir, should be included if viral meningoencephalitis is suspected. Appropriate resources to guide choice of antimicrobials and the dose and schedule should be consulted to guide treatment. The tertiary paediatric hospitals across Australia and Aotearoa New Zealand offer CPGs which clearly define appropriate treatment choices.

Children with meningitis should be closely monitored, which should include neurological observations. Careful management of fluid and electrolyte balance is also an important component of meningitis management. The syndrome of inappropriate antidiuretic hormone (SIADH), which can result in hyponatraemia, can occur in children with meningitis. This serves as the rationale for current recommendations to restrict fluids to approximately 75% of maintenance, although evidence for this practice is not convincing and it is clear that under- or over-hydrating is linked to poor outcomes.[220]

The results from a Cochrane meta-analysis show that corticosteroids reduce the incidence of hearing loss but have not been proven to improve survival.[221] These findings support the current recommendation that children with meningitis receive steroids. However, steroids should not be administered to infants less than 2 months of age due to concerns about their impact on neurocognitive development.

PRACTICE TIPS

MENINGITIS

- Infants and young children usually present with non-specific signs of meningitis.
- The diagnosis cannot be excluded based on negative Kernig's and Brudzinski signs or a normal fontanelle.
- The symptoms of meningitis may be more subtle in children who have commenced antibiotic treatment in the few days prior to presentation.
- Lumbar puncture should not be attempted where there are signs of raised intracranial pressure, such as altered conscious state, focal neurology, abnormal posturing, seizure activity or papillo-oedema.
- Following resuscitation, fluid volumes should be reduced to approximately 75% of maintenance levels.
- Steroids should be given to infants and children over 2 months of age to reduce the risk of hearing impairment secondary to the infection.

ABDOMINAL EMERGENCIES

INFECTIOUS GASTROENTERITIS

Although death from acute gastroenteritis is relatively uncommon in developed countries, the yearly hospital admission rate for infectious gastroenteritis is second only to respiratory illness in Australia and Aotearoa New Zealand, at 10–12 per 1000 children,[222] and Australian data show that children younger than 3 years of age average 0.75 to 2.5 episodes per year (depending on how gastroenteritis is defined).[223,224] Viruses such as rotavirus, adenovirus and norovirus cause the majority of infections, although rotavirus rates have fallen since the introduction of the rotavirus vaccine to the Australia and Aotearoa New Zealand immunisation schedules. The common bacterial pathogens include *Campylobacter*, *Shigella* and *Salmonella* species; these are all communicable diseases and state health authorities should be notified of confirmed cases. Infrequently, gastroenteritis is caused by parasitic infection.

It is generally accepted that childcare attendance increases the risk of contracting infectious gastroenteritis.[225] It is also suggested that age (e.g. less than 6 months) and aetiology, specifically rotavirus, are risk factors for more-significant dehydration.[225] Finally, breastfeeding has been shown to reduce the incidence of diarrhoeal illness, but not the severity of the illness. The evidence for the value of breastfeeding is strongest in developing countries.[226]

Presentation and diagnosis

The defining feature of gastroenteritis is acute diarrhoea (defined most commonly as three or more loose stools per day), which may be accompanied by fever, general malaise and vomiting.[223] Infants and children may be intermittently irritable as a result of colicky abdominal pain. It is important to determine the extent of the child's symptoms: the number of vomits, the frequency of stools and an estimate of volume, their willingness to drink, the type of fluids offered, and the volume taken. This will assist in making the diagnosis, estimating fluid loss, predicting future losses, and planning treatment.

Gastroenteritis presents with few specific signs. Children with gastroenteritis may look unwell and exhibit the signs of dehydration. There will be no signs of peritonism on examination and no specific tenderness. However, they may show signs of colicky abdominal pain.

Stool cultures are not usually of clinical value.[226] In a significant proportion of samples sent for culture (estimated to be as high as 50%), the infecting organism is not isolated. The evidence for signs or symptoms or combination that can reliably distinguish between viral and bacterial aetiology is also poor. However, as management does not alter, identification of the agent is usually only of interest to public health programs monitoring the spread of communicable diseases.

Management

Gastroenteritis is managed symptomatically in all but a few cases, and the mainstay of treatment for gastroenteritis is fluid management. Intravenous fluid resuscitation is indicated for children with severe dehydration and evidence of hypovolaemia. However, data shows that there is no difference in hydration outcomes for infants and children treated with intravenous fluids and enteral fluids. The WHO and the American Academy of Pediatrics advocate oral rehydration for children who exhibit signs of mild to moderate dehydration. The section addressing management of dehydration provides more specific details regarding hydration management.

Most children presenting to the ED do not require resuscitation and hydration can be managed with oral fluids. Departments are advised to develop guidelines for commencing oral rehydration in the waiting room, as it has been shown to reduce the use of IV rehydration and admission for children with gastroenteritis.[227,228] Where oral rehydration is not feasible, children with moderate and moderate to severe dehydration without signs of hypovolaemia can be managed with enteral fluids (e.g. via an NG tube).

Oral rehydration solution is the fluid of choice during the rehydration phase; the recommended fluid regimens were described in an earlier section and an example is provided in Table 35.14. The evidence for the value of breastfeeding in reducing the risk of gastroenteritis is strongest in developing countries, because it reduces the risk of infection acquired via contaminated water. Reintroduction of diet is also recommended, although the evidence to support this is limited by the number and quality of the studies.[226] The only foods to be avoided are those high in sugar. There is some evidence, although of low quality, that a lactose-free diet for infants not predominantly breastfed may reduce the duration of the diarrhoea and reduce the risk of treatment failure.[229]

A 2020 meta-analysis confirms that ondansetron reduces the need for IV hydration in children who are unable to tolerate fluids due to vomiting,[230] and is now widely recommended in these circumstances.

Antibiotics are only used in the following circumstances: confirmed *Shigella* infection, confirmed *Salmonella* infection in infants less than 3 months of age, patients with immunodeficiency or who are systemically unwell, and for those who are unwell with signs of severe invasive diarrhoea.[226] No other pharmacological agents have proven to be of benefit in the treatment of gastroenteritis, although there is increasing interest in the potential role for probiotics and zinc.

Children with mild gastroenteritis and those with moderate dehydration who have tolerated rapid rehydration, evidenced by weight gain, may be discharged home from the ED. Parents must receive advice about the amount and type of fluid that should be offered prior to discharge and the indicators for representation. Gastroenteritis is highly contagious, and infection control practices should be discussed with parents and the need for rigorous standards of hygiene reinforced. In many circumstances, review with the GP or in the ED the following day should be recommended.

PRACTICE TIPS

GASTROENTERITIS

- Breastfed babies may be less likely to contract gastroenteritis, but for those who do contract it the illness is no less severe.
- Gastroenteritis is characterised by diarrhoea, so an alternative diagnosis should be sought for vomiting in the absence of diarrhoea.
- Stool cultures are not routinely recommended as the infecting agent is not isolated in as many as 50% of stool cultures and the aetiology of the infection does not usually affect treatment.
- Infants and children not showing evidence of hypovolaemia can generally be rehydrated enterally; an oral rehydration solution is the fluid of choice.
- Breastfeeding should be maintained throughout the illness.
- Solids should not be withheld other than during the rehydration phase of treatment. However, foods high in sugar should be avoided.
- Ondansetron may be of some use in infants and children with significant vomiting to support enteral rehydration.
- Antibiotics are only of use in patients with confirmed *Shigella* infection, confirmed *Salmonella* infection who are less than 3 months of age or who are systemically unwell, or patients who are unwell with signs of severe invasive infection.

CONSTIPATION

Constipation is a common problem among children and functional constipation has a prevalence of approximately 12%, occurring most commonly at the time of toilet training.[231] It is described as difficulty or a delay in the passage of stools and functional constipation is diagnosed when two or more criteria are meet for a minimum of 1 month.[231] There is considerable variation between individuals in bowel habits and stool frequency, particularly in breastfed infants, who may pass a stool following each feed or not for many days. Furthermore, straining while passing a stool (dyschezia) is normal in infants.

Parents are frequently concerned that constipation is a symptom of a serious physical problem, which should be excluded. However, the most common cause of constipation in infants and children is functional and occurs in the absence of a pathological condition. Infants and children will most commonly develop withholding behaviours following painful bowel movements or other trauma that is associated with bowel habits. Fluid is reabsorbed, and the stool becomes larger and harder as it is retained in the colon, increasing the child's reluctance to defecate.

Presentation and diagnosis

Parents will describe large, hard stools, infrequent stools or straining and distress with attempts to pass a stool. They may also observe the child becoming restless, clenching their buttocks, and wriggling to avoid passing the stool. These children tighten their anal sphincter in response to the sensation of a full rectum rather than relaxing it, making it impossible to pass a stool. Some children may also experience faecal soiling.[231]

A history of stool-withholding behaviour reduces the likelihood of organic disease.[231] An alternative aetiology should be sought if the presentation includes fever, weight loss or failure to gain weight, delayed passage of meconium, nausea, vomiting, abdominal distension, significant anorexia, or bloody stools in the absence of a fissure.

The examination is largely normal, although a faecal mass may be palpable in the abdomen and anal fissures may be visible in children with functional constipation. It is clinical and investigations (including abdominal x-ray) are used only to exclude alternative diagnoses or identify organic causes of constipation such as coeliac disease, hypothyroidism etc.

Management

There will often have been attempts to manage a child's constipation prior to ED presentation. However, they are often insufficient to restore regular bowel habits. Most commonly, treatments have not been used regularly or long enough. A regimen aimed at re-establishing a more suitable bowel pattern should be established. To achieve this, a stool-softener such as paraffin oil should be commenced with doses incrementally increased to achieve the desired outcome,[232] which is passage of a soft stool regularly (e.g. daily). If this does not result in a normal bowel pattern within several weeks or there are signs of faecal impaction, polyethylene glycol-based preparations have been shown to be most effective for disimpaction.[232] In the absence to support dosing regimens, clinical practice guidelines provide pragmatic guidance regarding treatment regimens (see Useful websites).

There is no data to suggest that increasing fluid will resolve constipation and little evidence to suggest that increasing fibre will have this effect.[232] Suppositories and enemas should only be used as a last resort, where evacuation of the rectum is needed as their use may reinforce withholding behaviours.[232]

Appropriate treatment may be commenced in the ED and should also include parent education regarding the treatment regimen. However, infants and children with constipation will require referral to a general paediatrician for ongoing management and families should be counselled that this is likely to continue for at least 6 months. Evidence for other interventions such as probiotics is weak and there is no role for ED clinicians to implement interventions other than laxatives.

PRACTICE TIPS

CONSTIPATION

- The most common cause of constipation in infants and children is withholding behaviours and not pathological.
- Abdominal x-rays should not be used to confirm the diagnosis.
- The focus of ED treatment should be a stool-softener to establish regular soft stools
- Disimpaction with a polyethylene glycol-based preparation may be needed before a maintenance regimen can be commenced.

ABDOMINAL PAIN

Abdominal pain is an extremely common non-specific symptom in children, which is associated with an extensive list of conditions, some of which are presented in this chapter or in Chapter 24. Table 35.15 provides a list of likely causes of acute

TABLE 35.15 COMMON CAUSES OF ABDOMINAL PAIN IN INFANTS AND CHILDREN[233]

COMMON	UNCOMMON	RARE
Non-specific	Volvulus secondary to malrotation	Sickle cell anaemic crisis
Appendicitis	Meckel diverticulitis	Henoch-Schönlein purpura
Mesenteric adenitis	Renal colic	Pancreatitis
Constipation	Pyelonephritis	Cholecystitis
Intussusception	Acute glomerulonephritis	Acute hepatitis
Urinary tract infection	Glandular fever	Diabetes mellitus
Torsion of the testis	Drug ingestion	Haemolytic-uraemic syndrome
Gastroenteritis	Peptic ulceration	Inflammatory bowel disease
Strangulated inguinal hernia		
Pneumonia		

abdominal pain.[234] Aetiology is influenced by age and gender, and in most cases the problem is not surgical and is associated with viral infection and constipation. In a recent study, a diagnosis of non-specific abdominal pain was the most frequently made diagnosis for children presenting to the ED with abdominal pain.[234]

Presentation and diagnosis

Clues to diagnosis can be gained from the age of the child, the infant's or child's history, the pattern and characteristics of the pain and other associated symptoms. In older girls, menstrual and sexual history should also be included, and diagnoses such as ovarian torsion should be considered in the setting of severe sudden onset pain. Examination should be similarly comprehensive and include other systems to identify or exclude the signs of important differential diagnoses for abdominal pain; in boys this should include the testicles. Older children will exhibit more specific signs associated with surgical conditions than younger children and infants, consistent with those of an adult.

The diagnosis of non-specific abdominal pain is one of exclusion, and it can be a diagnostic challenge to differentiate non-specific abdominal pain from more-significant pathology such as appendicitis. Diagnostic testing, including abdominal x-rays, should only be used to confirm or exclude specific diagnoses and should not be conducted for screening purposes.

Management

A small number of infants and children presenting with abdominal pain will require fluid resuscitation while larger numbers will require analgesics. As noted in Chapter 18, the rationale for withholding analgesics to enable diagnosis is fallacious and children should receive appropriate and timely analgesia consistent with the intensity of their pain. The diagnosis determines the definitive management of abdominal pain, which will be surgery in only a very small number of cases. Children with non-specific abdominal pain may be admitted for observation, but most can be discharged, and parents provided with criteria to guide the need for review. Children with recurrent non-specific abdominal pain can be referred to a general paediatrician for management strategies.

PRACTICE TIPS

ABDOMINAL PAIN

- The cause of most abdominal pain in children is not surgical. It is most commonly associated with viral infections, constipation or is non-specific.
- Abdominal x-rays should not be routinely ordered for screening purposes.
- Resuscitation, stabilisation and pain management may be required for children presenting with abdominal pain.
- Definitive management will depend on the aetiology of the pain and infrequently involves surgery.

INTUSSUSCEPTION

Intussusception is the invagination of a proximal segment of bowel into the distal bowel lumen. This results in compression of the perfusing vessels of this section of bowel, initially causing venous congestion and bowel wall oedema. If the intussusception continues, ischaemia and finally necrosis will result.

Intussusception is the most common cause of bowel obstruction in children aged between 3 months and 6 years, with a peak incidence at 5–9 months.[235] However, it may occur at any age. The aetiology of intussusception is not well understood and in 90% of cases it is thought to be idiopathic. However, there is a reported association with viral illness reinforced by reductions in the incidence of intussusception where there are corresponding reductions in infectious disease, such has been seen during public health directives to reduce social contact that have occurred during the COVID-19 pandemic.[236] A rise in the incidence of intussusception was also linked to the introduction of the original rotavirus vaccine, which points to an immunological or inflammatory link. A similar association between intussusception and the replacement vaccine has not been established.[237]

Presentation and diagnosis

The classic presentation for intussusception includes recent viral illness, intermittent abdominal pain demonstrated by pulling their legs up to their abdomen, redcurrant-jelly (bloodstained mucus) stool and a palpable abdominal mass. However, this constellation is not typical, with only 7.5–40% of presentations featuring these signs and symptoms and, when present, redcurrant stool is a late sign.[238] Vomiting is the most common feature in infants, but many will also present with unexplained distress and increasing lethargy. There may be some diarrhoea and as the illness progresses this may contain bloodstained mucus (redcurrant jelly), suggesting mucosal sloughing secondary to ischaemia. Many children are pain-free, some children will present with non-specific symptoms and there is considerable overlap between the presentation associated with intussusception and other abdominal conditions in infants and children.

The most useful physical sign is a palpable sausage-shaped mass. The remainder of the abdominal examination may be normal. As these infants become more unwell secondary to intestinal ischaemia and necrosis, they may begin to exhibit signs of hypovolaemia.

The most sensitive (~98%) and specific (88–98%) diagnostic tool currently available for the diagnosis of intussusception is ultrasound.[239] However, abdominal x-rays are frequently the imaging of first choice in the ED due to limited access to ultrasonography. As they may be normal (up to 25%), and results are only moderately sensitive (62%) to intussusceptions, they are not used for diagnosis but to exclude perforation and/or obstruction.[239]

Management

Management will depend on the condition of the infant. Fluid therapy and, in some instances, aggressive resuscitation may be needed and paediatric surgical review should be requested early. Limited evidence supports air enema as the most effective first-line approach to reduction of the intussusception.[240] There is some evidence to suggest that the addition of dexamethasone may improve air enema success.[240] However, this is not current practice in Australia and Aotearoa New Zealand. Where non-operative management has been unsuccessful, or there are signs of perforation or necrosis, these infants will require surgical reduction of the intussusception.

PRACTICE TIPS

INTUSSUSCEPTION

- Most infants and children presenting with intussusception do not present with the classic constellation of signs and symptoms, which includes 'redcurrant-jelly stools' and drawing up of the legs towards their abdomen.
- Ultrasound is the imaging modality recommended for detecting intussusception.
- Most intussusceptions can be managed non-surgically with an air enema.

PYLORIC STENOSIS

Pyloric stenosis occurs almost exclusively in young infants and is one of the most common causes of surgical emergency in this age group. The pyloric sphincter is hypertrophic and hyperplastic, causing narrowing of the pylorus and gastric outlet obstruction. The cause is unknown. Pyloric stenosis affects approximately 0.1–0.3% of infants, but recent figures show that there has been a decline over the last decade in the rates of pyloric stenosis in Aotearoa New Zealand.[241] It is more common in Caucasian infants, males (4 : 1), first-born and those born via caesarean section or preterm.[241,242]

Presentation and diagnosis

Classically, the infant presenting with pyloric stenosis is 3–6 weeks of age, but may present at between 2 and 8 weeks, is male, has a history of projectile vomiting soon after feeding and appears hungry and undernourished. Examination may reveal visible peristaltic waves and a palpable olive-shaped mass.[243] However, the pylorus can be difficult to palpate, particularly if the stomach is full. The infant is also likely to show signs of dehydration, the severity of which will depend on the extent of the vomiting and the delay to presentation.[243]

Identification of the enlarged pylorus on examination is a highly specific finding.[244] However, ultrasound is highly accurate (sensitivity ~98% and specificity ~100%) and the most commonly used technique to establish the diagnosis.[245] Blood should be collected to measure urea and electrolytes and a capillary blood gas sample sent for analysis to assess the impact of persistent vomiting and to guide treatment. Loss of stomach contents leads to loss of potassium, chloride and hydrogen ions resulting in the classic, but often late, findings of hypokalaemic, hypochloraemic and metabolic alkalosis.[246]

PRACTICE TIPS

PYLORIC STENOSIS

- The classic presentation is of a male infant aged between 2 and 8 weeks, with a history of projectile vomiting soon after feeding, who looks hungry and poorly nourished.
- These infants are likely to be dehydrated and may have electrolyte and acid-base imbalances.
- Fluid resuscitation and correction of metabolic derangements are the focus of emergency management.

Management

Fluid resuscitation and correction of the metabolic derangements resulting from vomiting is the focus of emergency management.[246] As metabolic alkalosis can impact on respiratory drive, infants should be monitored for apnoea with this risk increasing in younger infants. Surgical consultation will guide decisions regarding the need for additional diagnostic tests and operative management, and this should be sought early. In many centres a nasogastric tube to empty the stomach will be placed prior to anaesthetic.

HERNIAE

Herniae occur in all age groups, but are particularly common in infants. Inguinal herniae occur in approximately 1–4.5% of infants, and umbilical herniae in up to 18% of infants under 6 months of age.[247] Inguinal herniae are more common in premature neonates, boys and twins, and umbilical hernias are also more prevalent in premature neonates and more common in infants of Afro-Caribbean background. Both hernia types can be explained by the embryological development of intra- and extra-abdominal structures, which is beyond the scope of this text, but explains their prevalence in infants.

Presentation and diagnosis

Infants and neonates with an inguinal hernia will have a swelling in the inguinal region, and in some infants the swelling may extend into the scrotum or the labia majora. The swelling may only be evident when the infant is crying or straining or may be constantly present. Where the hernia is sustained, infants will become increasingly distressed.

Umbilical herniae present with a large swelling protruding through the umbilical ring and are symptom-free.

Management

Applying gentle pressure to the mass may reduce inguinal herniae that have not reduced spontaneously. In a small number, an inguinal hernia does not spontaneously reduce and cannot be reduced by a clinician. This is a surgical emergency, as prolonged hernia increases the risk of ischaemia and necrosis. Surgical consultation at the time of the presentation should also occur for a reducible hernia if it has been appearing with increasing frequency, the infant has experienced distress with the hernia or the infant is young (< 3 months). Most infants and young children with an inguinal hernia do not require urgent treatment and can be referred to a surgeon as outpatients, but all will require surgical repair.[248]

Conversely, umbilical herniae are rarely irreducible and rarely require surgical repair unless they have not closed spontaneously by 3 to 5 years.[249]

PRACTICE TIPS

HERNIAE

- Irreducible inguinal herniae are a surgical emergency.
- Umbilical herniae are benign and are unlikely to require correction.

RASHES AND SOFT-TISSUE INFECTIONS

Most rashes are not evidence of serious illness, and many do not require ED management. However, the presence of a rash frequently alarms parents and prompts them to seek medical assessment for their child. A diagnosis, some simple management strategies or a referral to a specialist will usually address their concerns. Rashes are extremely common presentations to the ED and are too numerous to attempt to describe them all in this chapter. The intent of this section is to discuss some principles when assessing paediatric rashes. They can be grouped into categories based on appearance, which will help narrow the likely cause.

A careful history detailing the development of the rash (location, appearance, spread, etc.), associated symptoms (e.g. itch, pain), the treatments used to control the rash and prodromal and concurrent systemic symptoms (e.g. fever, malaise) will provide vital information to assist in identifying the rash.

Rashes can be grouped by appearance as *vesicular*, *pustular*, *papular*, *eczematous*, *purpuric/vascular* and *erythematous*.[250] Furthermore, rashes can be *localised* or *widespread*. A number of terms used to describe rashes are listed in Box 35.2, and common diagnoses for each morphological category are provided in Table 35.16.[250]

Vesicles are small, monomorphic blisters on the skin filled with clear fluid, and when ruptured they leave a small round

BOX 35.2 TERMS USED TO DESCRIBE RASHES

Annular: Lesions found in a circular arrangement
Bulla: A raised, clear-fluid-filled lesion that is greater than 1 cm in diameter
Confluent: Lesions running together
Crusting: Dried exudate of plasma combined with blister roof which sits on the surface of the skin after acute dermatitis
Cyst: A raised lesion that contains a palpable sac containing solid material
Desquamation: Peeling of sheets of scale after acute skin injury
Discrete: Distinct and discretely separated from each other
Erosion: Moist, circumscribed, slightly depressed area, e.g. base of a blister
Eruption or rash: More-widespread skin involvement, comprised of multiple lesions
Excoriation: Oval or linear depression in the skin with complete removal of the epidermis exposing red dermis
Fissures: Linear, wedge-shaped cracks in the epidermis extending down to the dermis
Grouped: Lesions found closely adjacent to each other
Lesion: Describes an area of skin disease—generally small
Linear: Lesions found in a straight line
Macule: Flat area of skin with colour change
Nodule: Raised, solid lesion with indistinct borders and a deeper portion. May be intradermal or subcutaneous. A larger nodule is called a tumour.
Papule: Solid raised area of skin with distinct borders less than 1 cm in diameter
Plaque: Solid, raised, flat-topped lesion with distinct borders and an epidermal change larger than 1 cm in diameter
Pustule: A raised fluid-exudate-filled lesion that appears yellow
Scaling: Whitish plates on the skin surface
Vesicle: A raised, clear-fluid-filled lesion that is less than 1 cm in diameter
Wheal: An area of tense oedema in the upper dermis resulting in a raised, flat-topped lesion

TABLE 35.16 DIFFERENTIAL DIAGNOSIS OF RASHES OF VARYING MORPHOLOGY[250]

RASH MORPHOLOGY	DIFFERENTIAL DIAGNOSIS		
Vesicles	Varicella zoster	Herpes simplex	Herpes zoster
	Coxsackie virus	Contact dermatitis	Impetigo
Pustular	Impetigo	Acne	Varicella
	Scalded skin syndrome	Furuncles and boils	
Papular	Moluscum contagiosum	Insect bites	Scabies
	Urticaria	Acne	Warts
	Papular acrodermatitis		
Erythematous	Urticaria	Tinea	Streptococcal perianal disease
	Viral exanthema	Intertrigo	
	Cellulitis		
Eczematous (red and scaly)	Eczema	Psoriasis	Tinea
	Dermatitis–contact	Dermatitis–seborrhoeic	
Petechial	Meningococcal disease	Idiopathic thrombocytopenia	Viral infection
	Mechanical		

erosion. Larger blisters are called bullae. They are most commonly caused by infection or contact dermatitis. Varicella zoster (chicken pox), herpes simplex, coxsackie (hand, foot and mouth) and herpes zoster viruses are the common viral causes of vesicular rashes. However, the frequency of varicella is declining since the introduction of routine vaccination. Bullous rashes are generally bacterial. Pustular rashes look similar to vesicular rashes. However, the raised blister-like lesions are pus-filled, and the aetiology is bacterial. Pyoderma will be discussed in the next section.

The likely aetiology of papular rashes is wide and includes scabies, urticaria, molluscum, warts, acne, serum sickness and papular acrodermatitis. Papules can be red (e.g. acne) or skin-coloured (e.g. molluscum) and may be itchy (e.g. scabies); raised red rings are likely to occur with urticaria and bruising and/or purpura may suggest an associated vasculitis (e.g. Henoch-Schönlein purpura and urticarial vasculitis). Papular acrodermatitis is classically seen in children between 1 and 3 years of age, and is a reaction to a range of infectious illnesses or vaccination. Scabies infestation results in a secondary reaction to the scabies antigen, manifested by a papular rash. Molluscum lesions result from a viral infection and are characterised by pearly papules localised to areas such as the face and anogenital region, although they may appear anywhere.

Red scaly rashes include atopic dermatitis (eczema), seborrhoeic dermatitis (infants), contact dermatitis, psoriasis, tinea corporis and pityriasis rosea and versicolor. Redness indicates inflammation of the skin, and the scale indicates epidermal involvement. These rashes can present very similarly, and although common can be misdiagnosed or poorly managed. Eczematous rashes are characterised by itch, erythema, and disruption to the epidermis, and will be discussed in more detail in a following section.

Erythematous rashes are red, blanching rashes with lesions varying from small macules to large confluent areas of erythema. The most common erythematous rash is the one that accompanies a febrile illness, which is most often caused by a virus. Several of these presentations have specific features, such as measles and roseola infantum, while the majority are non-specific. Kawasaki's disease is a vasculitis, which presents with a non-specific erythematous rash in the setting of fever of over 5 days' duration, conjunctival injection, mucosal involvement, and erythema of the palms of the hands and soles of the feet. It is the leading cause of acquired coronary artery disease in children, and where the diagnosis is suspected, this should prompt referral to a specialist centre for further investigation (e.g. echocardiogram) and management.

Purpuric and petechial rashes should raise concern as they are linked with serious life-threatening illness. Infection with *N. meningitides*, *S. pneumoniae* and *H. influenzae* may present with fever and a non-blanching rash. Conversely, relatively benign viruses are also responsible for this type of rash. These children will be relatively well, unlike those with bacterial infections. Petechiae above the nipple-line may be the result of forceful coughing or vomiting, which may be associated with a febrile illness, making the presentation more difficult to differentiate from a child with a serious bacterial infection. Henoch-Schönlein purpura (HSP) may also present with a petechial rash. The classic triad of symptoms associated with HSP are rash, abdominal pain and swollen joints. It should be assumed that serious bacterial infection is the cause of a petechial rash until proven otherwise. Other significant conditions that should be considered in the setting of a non-blanching petechial rash include coagulation disorders, thrombocytopenia secondary to leukaemia and idiopathic thrombocytopenia. Always consider that intentional trauma patterns of bruising can be suggestive of non-accidental injury.

PYODERMA AND CELLULITIS

Pyoderma is a broad term used to describe a range of bacterial skin conditions, such as impetigo, folliculitis, furuncle and carbuncle, and they are one of the most common childhood skin diseases. The incidence is even higher in Indigenous children and children living in disadvantaged circumstances. It is highly contagious and spreads quickly through households and childcare centres. The most common causative organisms are Group A *Streptococcus* (GAS) *pyogenes* and *Staphylococcus aureus*; community methicillin-resistant *S. aureus* (MRSA) is appearing in increasing numbers, particularly in the Indigenous community.[251] Pyoderma frequently occurs secondarily to an existing skin disease such as eczema, scabies and molluscum. Post-streptococcal glomerulonephritis is rare in the non-Indigenous population, but a significant risk for Indigenous Australians and New Zealanders.

Cellulitis occurs in the subcutaneous fat layer and mainly involves the dermis, unlike impetigo, which is confined to the epidermal layers of the skin. Cellulitis may also spread to deeper layers, such as the muscle, and other associated structures with serious implications, such as periorbital cellulitis with spread to the structures of the eye. Cellulitis may result from a breach in the skin, which allows bacteria to colonise the wound; or alternatively it may occur with no apparent tissue injury. Cellulitis is caused by the same profile of organisms as pyoderma.

Presentation and diagnosis

Pyoderma generally presents with thick-crusted lesions, bullous lesions or the superficial ulcerations left by ruptured bullae. There is usually surrounding erythema and the lesions may be tender or itchy. Pyoderma may be associated with fever and malaise, although this is likely to be mild.[255] Where the child appears more unwell, a more significant infection such as cellulitis should be considered.

Cellulitis manifests with an area of significant erythema, oedema, warmth and marked tenderness. The margins of the infection may be identified by the extent of the erythema but are not palpable. Associated red streaking visible in the skin proximal to the area of cellulitis is characteristic of ascending lymphangitis. Regional lymphadenopathy and fever usually accompany cellulitis. On occasions, the macular erythema of cellulitis co-exists with areas of ulceration and frank abscess formation.

Cellulitis is frequently diagnosed in the setting of insect bite and a local allergic reaction is mistaken for cellulitis. The two can often be distinguished by their presenting features, although there is considerable overlap. An allergic reaction similarly presents with erythema, oedema and in most circumstances an itch rather than pain. In those circumstances, where the child complains of pain, it is probably secondary to swelling, and the degree of tenderness is disproportionately low given the extent of the reaction. Cellulitis is usually tender, and the child may exhibit signs of systemic illness.

Isolation of the causative organism is not always necessary in uncomplicated pyoderma and rarely possible in cellulitis. Furthermore, skin swabs do not reliably differentiate between infection and colonisation.[252] However, it is generally accepted that where there are crusted or moist skin lesions, a swab for microbiology and culture should be taken. This is particularly important for impetiginous rashes secondary to chronic skin disorders, where atypical and resistant bacteria may colonise and infect the skin.

Management

Pyoderma and cellulitis are treated empirically and in most cases as an outpatient with antibiotics. Topical antiseptics have not shown to be of benefit to treat pyoderma. However, data summarised in a Cochrane review and a separate systematic review support the use of topical antibiotics such as mupirocin for uncomplicated localised lesions.[253] However, the growing resistance to mupirocin should be considered when selecting an appropriate treatment. Extensive pyoderma and cellulitis should be treated with oral antibiotics to target *S. aureus* and *S. pyogenes*.[252] Penicillin is an effective treatment for GAS, but may be inadequate for *S. aureus*, so the antibiotic of choice is flucloxacillin or cephalexin. The frequency of dosing and the duration of therapy are not well supported by data and there may be some differences between CPG and pharmacopoeia recommendations. Hence, treatment choice should be based on local recommendations that are likely to have considered local organisms and resistance patterns.

Admission and IV antibiotics should be used for periorbital cellulitis, cellulitis with associated systemic symptoms or where oral treatment has failed. The parenteral antibiotics of choice are either flucloxacillin or a first-generation cephalosporin. Intravenous ceftriaxone at home (support by a local hospital program) has proven to be a safe option versus IV flucloxacillin in hospital.[254] Where there is a collection of pus, this must be drained to ensure treatment success, regardless of whether inpatient or outpatient management is proposed.

Rest, elevation and ice should be used where the cellulitis involves a limb to reduce the swelling and promote comfort. Children with extensive pyoderma or cellulitis may require regular analgesia to manage the discomfort and pain associated with infection.

Prevention of pyoderma in the developing world and among Indigenous communities has been given some attention, and improved sanitation and hygiene has been identified as an important prevention strategy.[255] Parent education should include the risk of spread and infection control practices to prevent the spread of infection to other members of the family.

PRACTICE TIPS

PYODERMA AND CELLULITIS

- Superficial bacterial skin rashes, such as impetigo, are highly infectious.
- Impetigo is characterised by crusts that must be regularly washed off for antibiotic treatment to be effective.
- Cellulitis involves the dermis and may spread to surrounding structures, making it potentially more serious.
- Local allergic reactions are frequently misdiagnosed as cellulitis. Although similar, allergy is usually associated with itch and cellulitis with pain.
- Drainage is required if there is an associated collection of pus.

ATOPIC ECZEMA (DERMATITIS)

Atopic eczema is a chronic inflammatory disease of the skin with complex pathogenesis, which includes genetic factors, immune dysregulation, and skin-barrier defects. In Australia and Aotearoa New Zealand, the incidence is higher than anywhere else in the world, and 30% of children will experience eczema. It generally improves with age and many children grow out of it. However, there is no cure for eczema and most infants and young children experience recurrent episodes of varying severity. Eczema can be difficult to control and, in some cases, may be a debilitating illness that has substantial psychosocial burden on children and their families.[256]

Presentation and diagnosis

Eczema is characterised by dry, inflamed and itchy skin and generally develops before the age of 2 years. Classically the rash distribution is age-dependent and first appears on the cheeks of infants, then spreads to include the chin, folds of the neck, torso and limbs, usually sparing the nappy area. In older children, eczema typically appears around the ankles and wrists and in flexures. Eczema variant, called discoid eczema, presents with round, well-demarcated eczematous lesions on the limbs or trunk; there is generally a history of dry skin and either a personal or a family history of atopy. More-severe eczema will be associated with excoriation and lichenification (skin thickening), particularly where it has been poorly controlled. Eczema may be secondarily infected and show impetiginous signs suggestive of bacterial infection or vesicles, suggestive of herpes simplex infection.

Eczema is very itchy, and the itch can be one of the most difficult symptoms to manage.[257] The itch frequently interferes with normal sleep patterns, with significant implications; for example, older children lose significant amounts of time at school. Infants with eczema become increasingly irritable and may begin to show signs of failure to thrive.

Assessment of severity is best achieved using the validated Scoring Atopic Dermatitis (SCORAD) tool developed by the European Task Force on Atopic Dermatitis.[258] The tool generates a composite score based on the extent of the following: inflammation, dryness, excoriation, crusting, lichenification, itch and the impact on sleep.

Eczema is a clinical diagnosis, and there are no diagnostic tests available to confirm the diagnosis. However, in certain circumstances children should be referred for allergy testing to determine the impact of allergy on their eczema. Eczema can often be mistaken for allergic or irritant dermatitis, psoriasis or scabies.

Management

Eczema treatment is comprised of daily skin care and management of exacerbations. Daily skin care should include avoidance of aggravating factors such as soaps, perfumes, woollen clothing, chlorines and other chemicals. Clothes should be rinsed a second time to remove detergents, moisturisers should be applied before swimming and the skin rinsed immediately afterwards, and products used on the skin, such as sunscreens, should be hypoallergenic. Moisturisers should be applied at least once a day following a bath or shower,[259] in which a cleansing agent with minimal defatting activity and neutral pH is used instead of soap; and if the skin is particularly dry, moisturisers should be applied twice a day. Committed used of moisturisers will reduce the need for steroid treatment. Furthermore, regular bleach baths have been recommended to reduce the incidence of infection. However, the data to support this to date is equivocal.[260]

Treatment of exacerbations will include steroids of variable potency, depending on the severity of the symptoms and the area of the body affected. As a principle, the steroid with the lowest potency possible should be selected. However, this should be balanced against the likelihood that it will adequately treat the eczema. A mild-potency steroid may be commenced on affected areas of the face, axilla and groin, and a mid-potency steroid on other affected areas of the body. High-potency steroids may occasionally be necessary to treat resistant eczema, but they should not be commenced without assessing the possibility of infection and ensuring that early specialist follow-up to ensure monitoring of response is available. Concerns about the side-effects of steroids are a common reason for prescription of suboptimal treatment and parental non-compliance with treatment regimens.[261] However, evidence suggests that treatment twice daily for 4 weeks with a mild- to moderate-potency steroid is safe.[261,262] Treatment must weigh the likely side-effects of steroid treatment against the likely outcome if treatment is withheld or is insufficient to address the problem.

As an alternative to steroids, topical calcineurin inhibitors, such as tacrolimus ointment (e.g. protopic) 0.03% and pimecrolimus cream (e.g. Elidel) 1%, have been shown to be effective.[263] The anti-inflammatory mechanism is different to steroids and the side-effect profile does not include skin atrophy, making them ideally suited for the face. During an exacerbation, moisturiser use should be increased, and, in some centres, wet dressings are recommended to increase moisture in the skin and provide cooling.[264] They may be a useful strategy to manage moderate to severe eczema, but their effect should be monitored carefully. Cool compresses may be used as an alternative to help reduce the itch. The use of non-sedating antihistamines has not shown to be of benefit for treating itch, but consideration can be given to sedating antihistamines to support sleep.[265]

Data suggests that there is a relationship (causation is unproven) between atopic dermatitis and immunoglobulin-E-mediated (IgE-mediated) food allergy, and that the strength of the association increases with the severity of the skin disease. Infants with moderate to severe eczema and infants and children with poorly controlled eczema, despite adequate treatment regimens, should be referred for allergy testing. Diet restrictions or other changes in lifestyle should not be implemented without allergy testing.

Many families will have sought care from several clinicians and will have had varying advice about the management of their child's eczema. Despite multiple consultations, the child's eczema frequently remains a problem. The concern that this causes, and the commitment required by families to manage their child's eczema, should not be underestimated. These families require support and understanding.

PRACTICE TIPS

ATOPIC DERMATITIS

- The incidence of eczema in Australia and Aotearoa New Zealand (approximately 30% of children) is higher than anywhere else in the world.
- It is characterised by dry, inflamed and itchy skin, which can be difficult to manage.
- Families presenting to the ED are often frustrated because their child's eczema is poorly controlled, despite having received advice and management from a number of professionals prior to presenting to the ED.
- Sudden increases in severity and/or crusting are likely signs of secondary infection and should be treated with antibiotics.
- Eczema management is comprised of daily skin care and management of exacerbations.
- As commitment to management plans is essential to control eczema, families should be provided with appropriate education prior to discharge from the ED.

Education is the mainstay of treatment; treatment failures can be attributed, among other things, to poor compliance, which is usually the result of inadequate education. Infants and children presenting to the ED should either be admitted for education regarding the management of the child's condition or be provided with preliminary education in the ED with rapid referral for review and eczema education. Educational interventions have shown benefit to severity of disease and improvements to quality of life.[266] Several resources are available to support emergency clinicians who need to provide education about the application of topical treatments and the use of wet dressings. Families should be provided with a written management plan to ensure adherence to the prescribed treatment regimen. The importance of maintaining daily skin care in the prevention of significant exacerbations should be stressed to parents.

URTICARIA

Urticaria is typically an itchy rash characterised by wheals, which may be clinically classified as ordinary urticaria (acute, chronic and episodic), physical urticaria (reproducibly induced by the same physical stimulus), angio-oedema without wheals, contact urticaria (induced by biological or chemical skin contact) and urticarial vasculitis (defined on skin biopsy).[267] This discussion will focus only on uncomplicated acute urticaria, which is defined as urticarial activity for up to 6 weeks and is not accompanied by vasculitis or angio-oedema, and is not precipitated by local contact. Uncomplicated urticaria is more common in children than adults.

Urticaria is commonly thought to be an IgE-mediated allergic reaction. However, there are likely to be a number of pathways and multiple causes for urticaria.

Activation of mast cells located in the skin results in rapid release of histamine, leukotriene, C4 and prostaglandin D_2, which causes vasodilation and leakage of plasma into the dermal tissues and hence the characteristic signs of urticaria. The delayed (4–8 hours) secretion of inflammatory cytokines is responsible for inflammatory infiltrate and longer-lasting lesions.

Presentation and diagnosis

Acute urticaria has a distinct and easily identified presentation. Parents will report the sudden appearance of a red blotchy rash, which may settle within 1–24 hours, only for new lesions to appear elsewhere. It may be described as itchy but is not usually associated with other symptoms.

The classic urticarial rash includes papules and larger wheals, which are usually surrounded by a reflex erythema. Urticaria may be associated with angio-oedema, which involves significant swelling of the lower dermis and subcutaneous tissues and may involve the mucous membranes. Infants and children should be assessed for the presence of airway obstruction and wheeze as evidence of angio-oedema. Infrequently, urticaria with associated angio-oedema may progress to anaphylaxis.[267]

Acute urticaria is a clinical diagnosis and investigations in the ED are not indicated. Where a possible precipitant has been identified, referral for allergy testing may be indicated.

Management

In the absence of angio-oedema affecting the airway or signs of anaphylaxis, acute urticaria can be managed simply with antihistamines and patient education. The evidence is weak for the role of antihistamines in the management of urticaria; loratadine and cetirizine both come in syrup preparations and are appropriate for children.[267] Conversely, the role of corticosteroids, which hold theoretical value, is debated. There are no paediatric-specific data available, but small-scale adult studies suggest that oral steroids may reduce the itch and the duration of the rash.[267] For this reason some clinicians may consider a 3-day course of oral steroids in severe or prolonged urticaria. Discharge education should include the signs and symptoms of airway involvement and anaphylaxis. Parents should also be provided with a realistic understanding of the potential prognosis (recurrent flares of rash over days to weeks).

PRACTICE TIPS

URTICARIA

- Urticaria is characterised by the appearance of itchy wheals of varying size which settle within 1–24 hours, often with new lesions appearing elsewhere.
- Urticaria is thought to be an allergic reaction, which may be associated with angio-oedema.
- Antihistamines are used to manage acute urticaria. Steroids are only recommended in severe or prolonged urticaria.

NEONATAL PRESENTATIONS

Neonates (babies aged less than 4 weeks of age) are a small cohort presenting to the ED. However, as the conditions likely to affect babies of this age can be different, their presentations very non-specific and they can deteriorate rapidly, they should be assessed and managed with this in mind, and their age treated as a substantial risk factor for serious illness. They should be treated with higher levels of urgency than older babies and young children for seemingly similar or simple problems. As they are such a unique population it is beyond the scope of this text to discuss health concerns related to prematurity and congenital abnormalities. In this section excessive crying and jaundice will be discussed. A specialist text should be relied upon for more comprehensive details regarding the management of neonatal presentations. This will also describe symptoms found alarming by parents which may be benign, such as minor swelling of the breast buds in female neonates.

THE CRYING BABY

Infant crying generally begins in the neonatal period at 2 weeks of age, peaks at 5–6 weeks, at which they average 126 minutes per day, and then settles at 3–4 months.[268] It may be a signal that the baby is hungry, tired, requires a nappy change or is seeking comfort. Colic is a syndrome of excessive crying. Although a universally agreed definition does not exist, the most accepted definition (ROME IV criteria) clinically defines colic as behavioural phenomenon in infants less than 5 months of age, characterised by prolonged crying, fussing or irritability in the absence of illness or failure to thrive.[231]

Crying frequently causes great concern among parents and is one of the most frequently reported problems in young babies. However, it is reported that fewer than 5% of infants have a significant organic cause for crying.[269] The range of possible causes is extensive, as it is a highly non-specific symptom.

Presentation and diagnosis

Parents present to the ED concerned about the wellbeing of their baby. There is either a sudden increase in crying or parents have become exhausted and are confused by the varying advice that they have received from family, friends and healthcare professionals about their baby's crying. An extensive history and examination should be undertaken to identify signs and symptoms of organic illness. This should always include urine analysis, as infants with urinary tract infections (UTIs) frequently present with non-specific symptoms and, of those babies presenting with excessive crying, a substantial number will have a UTI, despite the absence of a fever.[269] Feeding patterns, activity levels, weight gain and development should be explored to help determine the source of the crying.

Other causes of crying common to this age group which should be considered are cow's milk protein allergy, gastrointestinal reflux, raised intracranial pressure, hair tourniquet, surgical abdomen, irreducible hernia, corneal abrasion, injury and infection, to name a few. Although not common, clinicians should be alert to risk factors for abuse. Previous presentation to a healthcare professional is a risk factor for abuse in infants.[269,270] Parents may be attempting to seek assistance via an ED visit for non-specific symptoms. The history and examination will guide the need for further investigation. However, it is beyond the scope of this text to explore all causes in detail.

Management

The priority for emergency clinicians is to determine whether the crying is associated with organic pathology. The diagnosis of colic is one of exclusion. Colic mixtures containing simethicone are of no proven benefit; while anticholinergic medications do reduce crying, they have significant side-effects and are not recommended. Having made a diagnosis of excessive crying, management centres on education, reassurance and referral for strategies to manage excessive crying.[271] Referrals should be directed to clinicians such as maternal child health nurses, paediatricians and social workers with interest and expertise in crying babies. Emergency clinicians should also be aware of the enormous stress experienced by parents of crying babies and give consideration to the potential implications of this stress. In a large study, 6% of parents with crying babies admitted to physically abusive behaviours towards their babies.[272]

PRACTICE TIPS

CRYING BABY

- Crying is a normal behaviour in young babies; however, an increase in crying may be associated with significant illness or injury. Therefore, a detailed history should be taken, and the baby examined carefully to detect a potential pathological cause of the crying.
- Parents presenting with a crying baby are usually very concerned about their baby and will require advice and support to manage the crying if it is determined not to be pathological.

JAUNDICE

Jaundice occurs in approximately 60% of newborns, but few require treatment.[273] It is most commonly physiological jaundice, breastmilk jaundice or to a lesser extent secondary to sepsis. Infrequently, it is a symptom of liver disease, related congenital abnormalities such as biliary atresia, hypothyroidism, and a range of other uncommon causes. In most infants it is benign. However, unconjugated bilirubin toxicity, with neurological sequelae (kernicterus), may occur in a small number with more severe hyperbilirubinaemia.[273]

Bilirubin is produced by the catabolism of haemoglobin. Compared with older children and adults, newborns have a high rate of haemoglobin catabolism and bilirubin production because of their elevated haematocrit and red blood cell volume per bodyweight and the shorter life span of red blood cells in the infant (70–90 days). In contrast, conjugation and clearance of bilirubin can be slow. Immaturity of hepatic glucuronosyltransferase and inadequate milk intake can cause delayed clearance of bilirubin. Initially the breakdown of haemoglobin reveals lipid-soluble unconjugated bilirubin, which binds to albumin until binding sites are saturated. Free unconjugated bilirubin crosses the blood–brain barrier and is neurotoxic. Once in the liver, it is conjugated by glucuronosyltransferase to water-soluble conjugated bilirubin, which is easily excreted by the liver and biliary tract. Some bilirubin may be reabsorbed in the intestine and converted back to its unconjugated form.

Physiological jaundice in neonates results from the breakdown of foetal red blood cells and the resulting increase in haemoglobin and is more common in breastfed babies. Breastmilk jaundice is thought to be caused by a substance in breast milk that inhibits glucuronosyltransferase. In contrast, breastfeeding jaundice occurs when newborns do not receive sufficient breast milk and as a result bilirubin is reabsorbed from the intestine.

Presentation and diagnosis

Babies with jaundice may present with no associated symptoms or with lethargy and poor feeding. More-severe jaundice, if left untreated, results in opisthotonus, seizures and eventually kernicterus, which is the permanent neurological outcome of severe untreated hyperbilirubinaemia and is characterised by cerebral palsy, hearing loss and intellectual impairment.[273]

Clinicians should have a low threshold for considering full septic screening in a jaundiced neonate as the signs and symptoms of sepsis and those associated with jaundice, such as lethargy and poor feeding, are similar. Alternative less common causes should also be considered.

Investigation of the infant with jaundice should include a full blood count to look for anaemia, a smear for haemolysis, a reticulocyte count, total serum bilirubin and conjugated bilirubin levels, a direct antiglobulin (Coombs) test and an elution test to detect anti-A or anti-B antibodies on the baby's red cells (which is more sensitive than the Coombs test). Babies with physiological breastmilk jaundice or jaundice secondary to sepsis have increased serum concentrations of unconjugated bilirubin, whereas conjugated bilirubin is raised in jaundice secondary to most forms of liver disease.[274]

Management

Identification of the likely cause is paramount to neonatal jaundice management. Septic neonates should be managed accordingly and referred to a neonatal unit. Babies with increased conjugated bilirubin should be discussed with a specialist paediatric centre.

Management of babies with increased unconjugated bilirubin will depend on the bilirubin levels, the likelihood that it will continue to rise and the associated symptoms, such as lethargy and poor feeding. Most babies can be managed as outpatients with regular (daily in many cases) monitoring of bilirubin levels. Frequent feeding should be encouraged as this may reduce enterohepatic circulation of bilirubin. However, babies requiring admission for phototherapy, or where doubt exists about the cause or the severity, should be discussed with a neonatologist. In severe cases infants may need exchange transfusion. Thresholds and recommendations for treatment have been developed by the National Institute for Health and Clinical Excellence (NICE).[275]

PRACTICE TIPS

JAUNDICE

- Neonates presenting with jaundice should be screened for sepsis and liver disease, which, although uncommon, are a serious cause of jaundice in this age group.
- Neonates with lethargy and poor feeding, associated with increased unconjugated bilirubin, will require admission.

FEVER

Fever is a symptom associated with many paediatric illnesses and is of great concern to large numbers of parents. Considerable confusion still exists in the community and among healthcare professionals about what constitutes a fever, how and when a fever should be treated and the potential consequences of fever.[276–278]

Fever is an elevated core temperature, which is usually a component of the immune response of the host to a pathogen or foreign stimuli, the most common of which is infection. Immune cells release pyrogenic cytokines, cyclo-oxygenase-2 (COX-2) is induced, the arachidonic acid cascade is activated and biosynthesis of prostaglandin E_2 (PGE_2) is increased. These complex, immune-mediated reactions trigger a range of physiological events, including a rise in the hypothalamic temperature 'set point'. The physiological outcomes of these processes are increased metabolic rate resulting in increased cardiac output, which helps mobilise white cells; increased white cell activity; activation of T-lymphocytes; and stimulation of interferon production, to name a few. Moderate fever is considered to improve immune system function and potentiates the effects of antibiotics. There are few data to support the contention that fever associated with infection is harmful and increasing evidence to suggest that it may be of physiological benefit during infection.

In response to an increase in hypothalamic temperature set point, the body will mount a response to increase heat production and reduce heat loss to raise the body temperature. This is achieved by responses such as shivering and vasoconstriction. A drop in the set point will result in a reversal of these responses and vasodilation and diaphoresis will occur.

Presentation

Fever in children is defined as a temperature, measured tympanically or rectally, above 38.0°C. Infections are the most common reason for fever in children, the majority of which will be mild. However, a small number of children will have more-serious illness; in a large analysis of over 50,00 blood cultures in a UK hospital over 8 years, 2.5% were positive, of which 25% grew pathogens linked to clinically significant infections.[279] Despite these small numbers, as outcomes can be improved by early treatment it is crucial to identify these children early.

There is no convincing evidence to suggest that response to antipyretics is predictive of the severity of the illness.[280] Therefore, clinical decisions should not be delayed while waiting to assess response to antipyretics. There is also conflicting and limited evidence about whether the height or duration of the fever correlates with the severity of the infection, but it seems likely that infants less than 3 months of age with high temperatures are at increased risk of serious bacterial infection, and temperatures in children over 40.5°C are associated with serious bacterial infection.[281–283]

Management

Historically, it has been the practice to treat all fevers with antipyretics and a range of non-pharmacological measures, based on the assumption that fever is harmful, and that treating fever will eliminate its deleterious effects. However, limited evidence supports the benefits of fever to the host during infection and, conversely, has not been able to demonstrate that fever is harmful. The decision to treat fever must weigh the benefits of fever reduction against the benefits of fever. Animal data demonstrate that treatment with paracetamol increases viral shedding and reduces immune system activity. Human data is limited and conflicting: several studies indirectly infer that antipyretic therapy may impact negatively on mortality in severe infection and on morbidity in mild infection.[284] The potential adverse effects of antipyretics should also be considered when weighing the decision to treat fever.

It is now generally accepted that the focus should be on providing comfort to the febrile child and that this may include the use of antipyretics. Antipyretic therapy is not recommended for children who remain comfortable despite their fever, and it would be reasonable to recommend that subsequent doses are not given when the first was not considered to have conferred benefit to the child.

Once the decision to treat is made, a choice must be made about the methods used to treat. Authors of a recent systematic review conclude that paracetamol and ibuprofen are both effective and equally safe when used to treat fever and pain.[285] A Cochrane review comparing alternating with combined or monotherapy regimens concluded that the use of both in either a combined or an alternating regimen is likely to be more effective.[286] It should be noted that the use of combined or alternating regimens may increase the risk of dosing error and should only be recommended with caution.[287]

Non-pharmacological measures to treat fever, such as sponging, aim to overwhelm the capacity of the body to generate enough heat to maintain the febrile state. Findings from small studies support an initial reduction in fever following sponging; however, this is not sustained after 2 hours and is associated with increased discomfort.[288,289] Furthermore, the body will vigorously defend the higher 'set point', potentially at considerable metabolic cost. There are no studies evaluating the risk–benefit ratio for non-pharmacological measures to treat fever. However, as fever is likely to be of benefit and unlikely to come at significant cost, unlike cooling measures, non-pharmacological measures are not recommended.

The priority of ED management of fever is to determine the source of the infection. Septic work-up in infants and children, where an obvious focus of infection has not been identified on examination, is indicated to detect serious bacterial infections such as UTI, meningitis and bacteraemia. The extent of the work-up will be determined by the symptoms at presentation, the severity of the illness and the age of the child. Guidelines from various specialist paediatric centres are available to guide clinicians as to the appropriate diagnostic tests for febrile children of varying ages.[290]

Parents exhibit great concern about fever, but limited knowledge about its effect and management. Studies have shown that parents treating their children with over-the-counter medications, including antipyretics, are not always clear about the indications for and dosing of these medications.[291] Accurate information should be provided to ensure that parents can make appropriately informed decisions about the care of their febrile child, including when to seek medical advice.

PRACTICE TIPS

FEVER

- Fever improves immune responses to illness and there is no evidence that it is harmful.
- The height of the fever should not be used as an indicator of the severity of the infection.
- The response to antipyretics is also not predictive of the severity of the illness.
- The focus of fever management should be to provide comfort and not to treat the temperature.
- Antipyretics, such as paracetamol and ibuprofen, are the only therapies shown to be effective at reducing fever.

TRAUMA

Trauma is a major cause of mortality and morbidity in infants, children and adolescents. The size of the child should also be considered when predicting the likely pattern of injuries; for example, a young child hit by a car may suffer pelvic fractures, not femoral fractures like a taller adult hit by the same car. Furthermore, the proportions of the younger child increase the likelihood that they will suffer trauma to the relatively larger head.

Infants develop increasing mobility over their first year of life and injury occur when carers underestimate the extent to which they are able to move; for example, rolling off surfaces and falling. As they become toddlers their mobility improves, but they remain clumsy and typically fall an average of four times a day—usually sustaining no injury, but on occasions suffering minor trauma. As toddlers get older, parents and carers commonly provide increasingly less supervision. However, despite their improved coordination and capacity to understand simple rules, children of this age may not recognise the dangers associated with their activities, which increases their risk for injury. Injuries associated with bikes, skateboards and swimming pools are not uncommon. Teenagers may engage in risk-taking behaviours, such as experimenting with drugs and alcohol, sexual activity, and adventurous physical activities. Many young people are involved in a range of sporting activities that also increase their risk of injury.

Minor trauma is an extremely common reason for children to present to the ED. Children sustain fractures, sprains, strains, and other soft-tissue injuries, burns and lacerations. However, only major trauma, fractures, pulled elbows and foreign bodies will be considered in this section.

MAJOR TRAUMA

Major trauma is a significant source of mortality and morbidity in children aged 1–14 years. Although presentations are much lower than for the adult population, the small size of children results in transmission of force over a larger area of the body, making it more likely that they sustain multiple injuries.

The priority for trauma management and the sequence of assessment and management are the same for adults and children. The differences in approach relate to the specifics of assessment and management and are a result of different injury mechanisms and differences in anatomy and physiology between adults and children. Therefore, this section should be read in conjunction with Chapter 42, particularly the section on assessment, and Table 35.1. It is not intended to be a comprehensive review of major trauma management in children; the intent is to highlight some key areas of difference in paediatric trauma management.

Airway and circulation

Inadequate management of the obstructed airway and hypovolaemia are the main contributors to avoidable deaths in children following trauma. The sections in this chapter on respiratory failure and shock detail airway management, oxygenation and fluid resuscitation in children, and these principles can be applied to the child suffering major trauma requiring airway management, oxygenation and fluid resuscitation. Chapter 16 also contains further information on airway management techniques for paediatric patients.[292]

Cervical spine injury

Spinal injury is relatively rare in children, with the average overall annual hospitalisation rate of 9.43 (95% CI: 9.15–9.72) per 100,000 population from 2002 to 2012.[293] A number of injury patterns occur in children: fractures, fracture and subluxation or dislocation, subluxation or dislocation without fracture, and soft-tissue injury. Those under 8 years of age display different patterns to older children due to their unique anatomical differences, which makes them more likely to sustain a significant injury without bony fractures.[294] Subluxations and dislocations are more common in younger children, and cervical spine injuries in younger children usually involve occiput-C2 lesions as a result of the anatomical differences that exist between young children and adults. See Table 35.1 for full details. C1 dislocation is the most common specific injury in young children.[294]

Current practice for the management of the potentially injured cervical spine is to prevent further damage, and the likelihood of this occurring is small with the evidence building for the use of minimal or no cervical spine immobilisation.[295] Cervical spine protection presents a clinical challenge in the uncooperative child and for toddlers and infants, where available, immobilisation devices don't always fit well and may cause more harm than benefit. The Australian and New Zealand Resuscitation Council (ANZCOR) recommends initial management using manual alignment of the head and avoiding semi-rigid collars.[296] The optimal method of immobilisation is that which best secures the spine, and this will be determined by the circumstances. There is good evidence that rigid collars can have significant complications and it is now common practice in Australia and Aotearoa New Zealand to apply a foam cervical or no collar as part of the pre-hospital management. The soft collar is a visual flag and improves compliance and patient comfort. However, alternatives may be required for some children. For example, an infant held in its mother's arms with a rolled towel tucked around their neck may be better immobilised than one lying on a trolley in a poorly fitting collar. A child may be best extricated while still strapped in their car seat or capsule.[296] In children less than 8 years old it is recommended they be placed on foam padding called a thoracic elevation device to maintain neutral vertebral column alignment and prevent hyperflexion when lying supine.

There are also limited data to support criteria for clearing the cervical spine in children as many of the 'rules' were developed for adults.[297] The NEXUS criteria were based on a largely adult population and did not include sufficient numbers of children younger than 9 years of age to confidently apply these criteria to young children. Several studies have attempted to evaluate the capacity of cervical spine clearance protocols to detect injuries and reduce the need for imaging. However, the numbers of children in these studies with injuries is small, making it difficult to accept the results as evidence of the diagnostic accuracy of these tools. However, in the absence of evidence-based criteria specifically for children, the NEXUS criteria in conjunction with the Canadian C-Spine Rule[298] and clinical judgement serve as a reasonable basis for clearing the cervical spine in the conscious child. Plain radiographic imaging is recommended as first-line investigation for conscious children with risk factors for injury. To reduce radiation exposure, CT for children under 10 years of age is recommended only if the results of the plain films are unclear (review by a paediatric radiologist is advised) or there is a high suspicion of injury.[299] An observational study from a large tertiary paediatric centre reported two-thirds of children with potential cervical spine injuries undergo radiological evaluation; however, actual injuries are rare at $< 4\%$.[300] Recommendations vary widely and local decision-making algorithms should be referred to, many of these largely based on best practice consensus.

PRACTICE TIPS

CERVICAL SPINE INJURY

- Infants and children may sustain spinal cord injury without radiographic abnormalities (previously referred to as SCIWORA).
- Alternatives to the cervical collar should be sought.
- A pad should be placed under the infant's shoulders to ensure that the head does not flex forward if the infant requires a spine board.
- CT to detect injury should only be used if plain films are equivocal.

Head injury

The most common single-organ-system injury contributing to mortality in children is head injury. Anatomical differences render them more susceptible to head trauma (see Table 35.1). Varying levels of cognitive development have an impact on assessment and a modified version of the Glasgow Coma Scale (GCS) has been developed, but has not been adequately validated. The modified GCS may have overcome the limitations of the original GCS for younger children, and Holmes and colleagues demonstrated that it compares favourably with the original GCS for assessment of traumatic brain injury in older children.[28] However, it is generally accepted that the GCS is the most appropriate way of classifying the severity of traumatic brain injury and that trend data will be of most use. Many clinicians will also advocate for the modified GCS to account for the differences in potential verbal and motor responses in different age groups.

A number of rules to guide the decision to use CT for children with minor head injuries have been developed. The PREDICT Australian and New Zealand Guideline for Mild to Moderate Head Injuries in Children shows the highest levels of sensitivity and specificity of the available rules.[301] However, adherence to this rule may see a considerable rise in the number of CTs performed in Australasian hospitals, where practice is more conservative than in the US and Canada, with fewer scans requested without higher rates of missed injury. Skull x-rays have a very limited role in paediatric trauma.

Head injury management adopts the same principles in paediatric patients as in adults, with few exceptions, and much of the data to support these practices are extrapolated from adult data.[302]

Concussion

Concussion is a mild traumatic brain injury as a result from a direct or indirect force/blow to the head or body resulting in a range of symptoms.[303] Large numbers of children present to EDs straight from their sport games after having sustained a head injury with a suspected concussion. There has been much attention in the media and from sporting codes to develop stricter guidelines to assess for and manage concussion. Extensive research has shown males regardless of age and those in contact sports are more likely to sustain a sports-related concussion (SRC) and there is a strong association of risk of SRCs in those that have a history of prior SRCs.[304] Digital health technology has helped with on-field/sideline assessment of concussion with the evidence-based HeadCheck app, as it was recognised that those providing support in the community have limited knowledge about concussion.[305] The HeadCheck app is an accessible platform for disseminating best practice evidence and also provides monitoring and guidance for parents to help their children return to school and sport. Consensus remains that athletes/players have a cognitive and physical rest for approximately 24–48 hrs until symptom-free and then adopt a gradual and progressively active return.[304] Research for detecting biomarkers as more objective measure and prognostics biomarkers is currently being undertaken.

PRACTICE TIPS

HEAD INJURY

- Parents and the modified GCS should be used when assessing the infant or child's neurological state.
- CT is recommended for children with persistent vomiting, who suffer a seizure more than 20 minutes after the injury, have a history of loss of consciousness of greater than 1 minute and post-traumatic amnesia.
- Skull x-rays are rarely useful.
- Guide parents to avoid screen-use post-concussion for 24–48 hours, as there is evidence that 'screen time' lengthens recovery time from concussion.

Intra-abdominal trauma

Paediatric abdominal trauma typically occurs from a blunt injury; for example, seatbelts, and the spleen is the most common organ injured. Focused abdominal sonography for trauma (FAST) has increasingly become the standard for detecting blood in the peritoneum in adults and its use is widespread in adults in the ED. However, this technique remains controversial in paediatrics. A meta-analysis showed a pooled sensitivity of 35% and specificity of 96%.[306] The sensitivity and specificity of this tool in paediatrics is not comparable with use in adults. However, there is some evidence that a positive e-FAST indicates that intra-abdominal injury is likely and that a negative FAST following low-risk blunt trauma in a haemodynamically stable child may result in fewer children undergoing CT scans.[307] It may be a useful adjunct to the examination provided the FAST is performed by a trained clinician and the results are interpreted cautiously. It is also important to note that detection of free fluid is not sufficient to guide treatment in children where most injuries are managed conservatively, providing that the child is haemodynamically stable. In children, more than 90% of solid-organ injuries, including hepatic and splenic injuries, are safely managed non-operatively.[308–310]

PRACTICE TIPS

INTRA-ABDOMINAL TRAUMA

- Focused abdominal sonography for trauma (FAST) is of limited value for infants and children.
- Abdominal injuries are frequently managed non-operatively in infants and children.

FRACTURES

Fractures are a common paediatric injury and account for over 20% of all injuries in children. Fracture is more common than other types of musculoskeletal injury as a result of skeletal immaturity. To understand fractures in children it is essential that the anatomy of the paediatric bone is well understood; the sections of the growing bone are shown in Fig. 35.5. The differences between adult and paediatric bones are highlighted in Table 35.1, and this explains their impact on the types of injuries experienced by children and the differences in assessment and management. This section serves to highlight some of the key issues in paediatric fractures but does not detail assessment and management of specific common paediatric fractures.

Fractures in children can be categorised as either *physeal* (growth plate) or *non-physeal*. Injuries involving the physis can be further described using the Salter-Harris classification system, which is shown in Fig. 35.6. Salter-Harris type II injuries are the most common of these injuries. The type of fracture can also be used to describe fractures. Torus (periosteum intact) and greenstick (periosteum intact on one side) fractures are unique to growing bones, and reflect the softer, more malleable quality of children's bones compared with those of an adult. Fracture location is also influenced by age, with some fractures specific to paediatrics, such as supracondylar fractures, and others unlikely, such as scaphoid fractures in children < 10 years of age.

FIGURE 35.5 THE GROWING LONG BONE

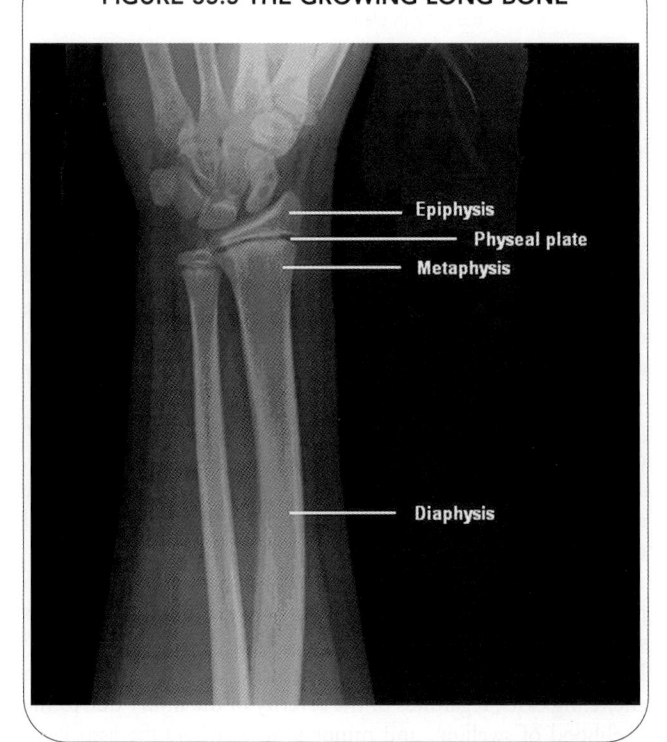

Presentation and diagnosis

Diagnosis of fracture in children can be more difficult than in adults. The history may be unclear in young children, particularly where the incident has been unwitnessed. Older children may be reluctant to provide details for fear that they may get into trouble. As children are more susceptible to fracture than adults, relatively insignificant mechanisms should not be overlooked as a possible mechanism for fracture.

Young children are often uncooperative, making examination more difficult. It can be hard to identify specific tenderness in a child distressed by examination. However, with careful palpation while watching the face of the child, it is often possible to detect subtle changes suggesting specific tenderness that are reproducible each time the area is examined. Swelling can also be difficult to detect in subtle injuries, particularly in toddlers, who have more subcutaneous tissue. If swelling is not visible, it may be evidenced by a slight fullness or firmness of the injured limb, which can be detected by feeling the injured and unaffected limb at the same time.

Consistent with practice in adults, neurovascular assessment should be included in injury assessment. Neurovascular injury is always a risk but is closely linked with specific injuries such as a supracondylar fracture due to the anatomy of the elbow and the potential distraction of neurovascular structures caused by fracture displacement and angulation. The features of neurovascular injury and compartment syndrome are detailed in Chapter 48 and will not be repeated here.

The avoidance of unnecessary radiation is a high priority in paediatric emergency care and identifying criteria to differentiate between children who require x-ray from those who do not has been attempted. The ankle and knee rules, adapted from the adult Ottawa rules (Chapter 17) and validated for use in paediatrics, are effective decision tools to guide the decision to x-ray in children over 5 years of age.[311] However, there are no data to support the predictive value of specific clinical signs and symptoms for fractures in general. In light of this and the often-subtle fractures sustained by children, it is reasonable to have a low index of suspicion for fracture and therefore a low threshold to x-ray.

Interpretation of plain films is greatly influenced by skeletal maturity and the presence of secondary ossification centres complicates interpretation. In some areas, such as the elbow, these ossification centres are numerous and appear at different stages of growth, further complicating interpretation. It is also important to recognise that some subtle fractures are not always visible on x-ray, requiring the clinician to review the x-ray for the presence of other indirect indicators of fracture, such as elbow joint effusion in the setting of occult supracondylar fracture. Ideally, a clinician with paediatric expertise should review x-rays. Ultrasound is also increasingly being used to diagnose fractures in children.[312]

Management

First-aid management of fractures is no different to first-aid management in adult injury and involves urgent reduction of the fracture if there is vascular compromise, immobilisation of the

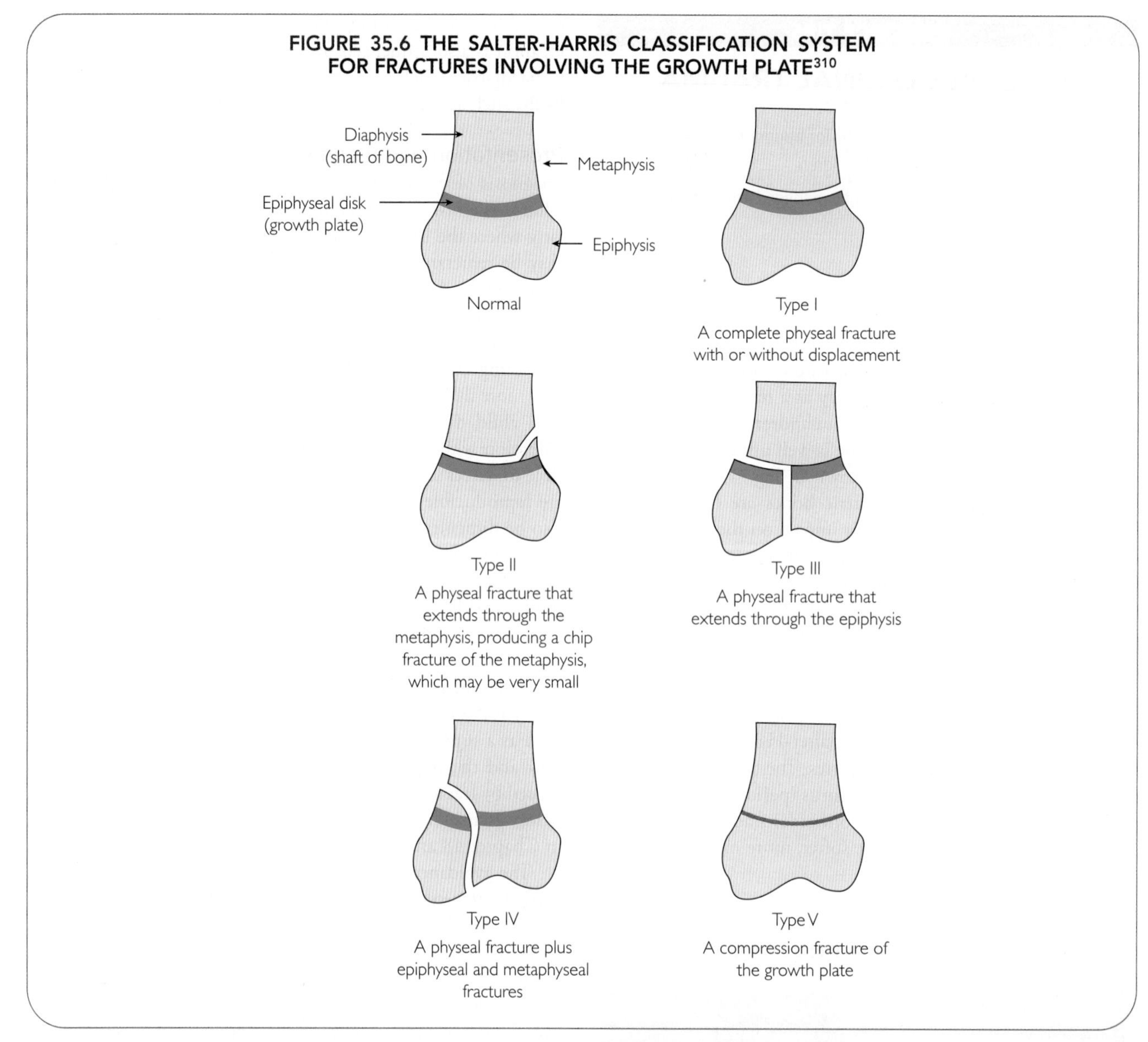
FIGURE 35.6 THE SALTER-HARRIS CLASSIFICATION SYSTEM FOR FRACTURES INVOLVING THE GROWTH PLATE[310]
Diaphysis
(shaft of bone)
Metaphysis
Epiphyseal disk
(growth plate)
Epiphysis
Normal
Type I
A complete physeal fracture with or without displacement
Type II
A physeal fracture that extends through the metaphysis, producing a chip fracture of the metaphysis, which may be very small
Type III
A physeal fracture that extends through the epiphysis
Type IV
A physeal fracture plus epiphyseal and metaphyseal fractures
Type V
A compression fracture of the growth plate

From the MSD Manual Professional Version (Known as the Merck Manual in the US and Canada and the MSD Manual in the rest of the world), edited by Sandy Falk. Copyright © 2023 Merck & Co., Inc., Rahway, NJ, USA and its affiliates. All rights reserved. Available at www.msdmanuals.com/professional.

injury and analgesics. Appropriate analgesic options for children with musculoskeletal injury are discussed later in the chapter.

Specific fracture management in children does differ from management of adult injuries and will depend on the type of injury and the age of the child. Paediatric fractures are frequently managed more conservatively than fractures of adults. Closed reduction is used more frequently, and more-significant displacement and angulation is tolerated as growth provides for significant remodelling of the injured bone with more-acceptable cosmetic and functional outcomes. There are no universal criteria for what degree of displacement of non-physeal injuries requires reduction; the need for reduction depends on the bone, the direction of the angulation/displacement (e.g. along the axis of movement), and the age of the child (e.g. remodelling time).[313] As a rule of thumb, injuries of long bones that look bent should be straightened regardless of the age of the child and the likelihood that it will remodel over time.

Displaced physeal and articular injuries require reduction (open or closed) and, in some instances, fixation. Improved function and a reduction of the risk of osteoarthritis are the reasons for reduction of these injuries. Concern often centres on the possibility of growth disturbance; however, this is unlikely and can be treated if it occurs. The advice of a paediatric orthopaedic surgeon should be sought if there is any doubt about the need for reduction. Some fractures are likely to be unstable, such as lateral epicondylar fractures of the humerus, and are therefore likely to require surgical management for fixation and referral should be made to a paediatric orthopaedic service.

Back-slabs, rather than encircling casts, are frequently used to provide analgesia and protection from further injury for injuries such as torus (buckle) fractures of the distal radial metaphysis.[314] Injuries of the elbow are also managed in back-slabs rather than encircling casts, regardless of the severity of the injury due to the likelihood of swelling, and minor injuries where the associated pain is only mild can often be managed in a simple collar-and-cuff sling.[315] The outcome for some injuries, such as ankle injuries, is improved by early mobilisation and full casts are not recommended for minor ankle injuries.

Paediatric fractures heal more rapidly, so where reduction is required, this may need to occur more urgently. This is significant for injuries where management is delayed while swelling resolves, for example, metacarpal fractures, nasal bone fractures. More-rapid recovery also means that young children are immobilised for shorter periods of time than adults with similar injuries. The Victorian Paediatric Orthopaedic Network provide detailed clinical guidelines to assist clinicians treating paediatric fractures in the ED, which can be accessed from their website (see Useful websites).

PRACTICE TIPS

FRACTURES

- Clinicians should have a high level of suspicion for fracture in infants and children presenting with musculoskeletal injury resulting from even minor trauma.
- Growing children have open physes (growth plates), which are a potential site of bony injury.
- Torus (buckle) and greenstick fractures are unique to growing bones and are frequently overlooked as they may present with only subtle signs.
- The Ottawa ankle and knee rules may be used in children to determine the need for ankle and knee x-rays.
- Skeletal maturity and the presence of secondary ossification centres will greatly affect interpretation of plain films.
- Management of specific fractures often differs from management of similar fractures in adults. In many cases, management is more conservative and immobilisation times shorter.

PULLED ELBOW

A radial head subluxation, commonly known as a pulled elbow or (in US literature) a nursemaid's elbow, is an injury that typically occurs in children aged 1–5 years. The characteristic mechanism is a 'pull' on the arm. However, in up to 50% of cases there is no history of a pull on the arm—either the mechanism was unwitnessed, or the parent describes a low-velocity fall.[316]

It is thought that under traction the annular ligament, which anchors the radial head to the capitellum, slips over the head of the radius and becomes trapped in the joint space. Movement pinches the ligament and causes pain. However, at rest the injury is painless, explaining the characteristic presentation.

Presentation

Children present with the affected arm hanging at their side, slightly flexed, and pronated, and they refuse to use the arm. There is usually no swelling or bony tenderness, and no distress provided the elbow is not moved. The child can move the shoulder and the wrist freely, but movement of the elbow, particularly supination, causes considerable distress. Radiographs are usually unnecessary. However, they may be used to rule out a fracture where the diagnosis is not clear or there have been two or three unsuccessful attempts at reduction.

Treatment

Treatment of a pulled elbow consists of manipulating the arm to reduce the subluxation. Two techniques have been described: forced pronation without flexion, and supination with flexion. For both techniques, the clinician places their hand under the elbow with their thumb on the radial head while the other hand holds the forearm. The forearm is either supinated and then flexed at the elbow, or while in extension the forearm is pronated. The authors of a Cochrane review[317] concluded that although the studies are of low quality, the pronation technique is likely to be more effective and less painful, making this the preferred technique for initial attempts, and supination–flexion as an alternative if forced pronation is unsuccessful. A 'click' is usually felt with successful reduction, which has a positive predictive value of more than 90%.[317] The child will usually resume normal movement of the arm within 15–30 minutes of reduction and may be discharged home. However, this may take longer where the child is older than 2 years and treatment has been delayed. Analgesia should be given prior to attempts to reduce the pulled elbow and to increase the likelihood that the child uses their arm quickly after reduction. Attempts to relocate the radial head should be limited to two or three, at which point if the clinician remains confident about the diagnosis, the child's arm can be placed in a sling, and they may be discharged home for review in 24–48 hours.

PRACTICE TIPS

PULLED ELBOW

- Approximately 50% of pulled elbows occur where there is no history of a pull on the arm.
- The characteristic features are refusal to use the affected arm, which hangs by their side, no swelling or bony tenderness and pain on movement of the elbow.
- Radiographs are only required to rule out an alternative diagnosis, as they are normal where there is a pulled elbow.
- Forced pronation with the arm extended should be the first technique used to resolve a pulled elbow.
- Where the 'click' is not felt and the child is still not using their arm 30 minutes following manipulation, it should be assumed that the pulled elbow has not been corrected.
- There should be no more than three attempts made to manipulate the elbow.

Spontaneous reduction will occur in some of these children prior to review, and the remainder will be reduced on re-presentation. Recurrence rates are about 20–25% and discharge should include education of the parents to avoid likely mechanisms for pulled elbow.

LIMP/REFUSAL TO WALK

A limp or refusal to walk in a young child is usually considered to be the result of trauma, and parents will frequently identify an event thought to be the cause of the limp. However, injury, transient synovitis of the hip, osteomyelitis, septic arthritis, Perthes' disease, discitis and neuromuscular disorders are among the potential causes of limp in this age group. Older children are generally able to be more specific about the onset of the limp and the precipitant. However, in this age group the limp associated with orthopaedic conditions, such as Perthes' disease and slipped upper femoral epiphysis, can be confused with limp associated with chronic injury and overuse. Furthermore, hip pain can be referred to the knee and therefore hip pathology can be overlooked.

The focus of this section is on the preschool-aged child with a limp/refusal to walk. Two of the most common reasons for limp or refusal to walk in this age group are toddler's fracture and transient synovitis. The cause of transient synovitis is not clear; however, it is considered a reactive arthritis of the hip, which may be provoked by recent viral infection. A toddler's fracture was first described as a spiral fracture of the tibial shaft in a preschool-aged child, which may or may not be visible on x-ray.[318]

Presentation and diagnosis

Young children with limp/refusal to walk present to the ED with sudden onset of limp following witnessed trauma, sudden onset of limp with no witnessed trauma or an unclear onset of limp with or without identified trauma. Careful questioning is necessary to identify the relationship between the limp and the traumatic event. Due to the subtlety of the limp or the insidious onset of the limp, the parents may attribute the limp to an unrelated trauma, when in fact the child was limping prior to this event. Examination of a child, which should include gait assessment, will provide additional clues to the likely diagnosis. An antalgic gait sees the child shorten the time that the painful limb takes weight and is linked to acute and painful conditions and differs from the alteration in gait seen with neurological conditions.

Transient synovitis

Where there is no convincing history of trauma to explain the limp, other causes need to be excluded. Classically, transient synovitis presents with a non-specific history of limp in a child aged between 2 and 5 years, generally following viral symptoms in the previous week or two.[319] Commonly, parents report that the child was walking normally yesterday, but was limping or refusing to walk when they got up that morning. The child may have a fever, but most commonly the temperature is normal, and they appear well. The child generally presents with an antalgic gait, although a small number of children may refuse to walk at all. However, this should increase suspicion of an alternative explanation for the limp. On examination, there is some limitation to the range of motion of the hip with resistance to internal rotation. These signs are usually subtle, and no other abnormalities are found. Significant resistance to passive movement of the hip should also prompt suspicion about an alternative diagnosis. Septic arthritis usually presents more floridly, with fever, malaise and significant joint tenderness and restricted range of motion, but at the onset of this infection limp may be the only obvious feature.

Plain radiographs are not useful to confirm the diagnosis, and inflammatory markers are either normal or only mildly elevated. Evidence to support the use of biochemical markers to differentiate septic arthritis from benign causes such as transient synovitis is weak.[320] Diagnostic ultrasound is not routinely used to diagnose transient synovitis, but may be used to exclude other pathology. It is gaining favour as a bedside tool to exclude more serious aetiology and confirm the diagnosis.[321] Evidence of fluid in the hip joint consistent with inflammation is the only abnormal finding seen on ultrasound in children with transient synovitis.

Transient synovitis is a diagnosis of exclusion, and the diagnosis is best made based on a constellation of clinical signs and symptoms. However, alternative diagnoses, such as septic arthritis, which may present similarly in the early stages, must be excluded and this may be achieved using x-ray and pathology.

Management

Transient synovitis generally resolves spontaneously within 2–5 days and, according to a recent systematic review, most children's symptoms will resolve within 2 weeks.[322] Improvement will be hastened by regular treatment with a non-steroidal anti-inflammatory drug (NSAID) such as ibuprofen.[323] The longer the duration of the limp without improvement, the more likely that an alternative diagnosis is the cause of the limp. Children discharged with a diagnosis of transient synovitis should be reviewed within several days and parents should be given careful instructions to return if the child develops fever, malaise, reduced range of motion or there is no improvement in 2–3 days.

Toddler's fracture

Toddler's fracture is more easily diagnosed if there is a clear history of witnessed trauma followed by limp or refusal to walk, or alternatively it can be seen on x-ray. The mechanism of injury is usually an event which exerts rotational force on the lower leg; for example, catching the foot on the slide as the child descends. However, in a small number of cases the mechanism is unclear. In these circumstances it is important to confirm that there was at least a clear and sudden onset of limp. Children with a toddler's fracture will usually refuse to walk, but some may walk with a limp. Many children will resort to crawling. Point tenderness is a moderately sensitive and specific clinical finding for toddler's fracture. However, its absence is not negatively predictive.[324] Pain with dorsiflexion of the ankle has also been reported, but is only seen in a few cases.

Plain films are taken in the ED to ideally confirm the diagnosis and rule out other pathology. However, normal x-rays on presentation have been reported in up to 25% of cases where a toddler's fracture was later confirmed.[325] In these circumstances the diagnosis is made clinically. Bone scans can provide a more definitive result. This may be used if confirmation of a toddler's fracture will allay concern about the potential for an alternative diagnosis. Ultrasound and plain radiographs about a week after the injury may also reveal a toddler's fracture, but are not routinely used where the diagnosis is clear.

Management

Management of a tibial fracture usually involves application of a plaster of Paris long leg cast. However, back-slabs/leg splints are used to immobilise toddler's fractures and increasing numbers of paediatric emergency clinicians are only using immobilisation to manage discomfort and to provide protection for the particularly active child. Limited data suggests that the time to weight-bearing is similar in children who were not immobilised when compared with those that were.[325] In contrast, side-effects associated with immobilisation are frequent.

PRACTICE TIPS

LIMP/REFUSAL TO WALK

- Limp and refusal to walk may not always be the result of trauma, so it is essential to take a careful history to determine the relationship between limp/refusal to walk and a history of trauma.
- Transient synovitis is considered a reactive arthritis that follows a viral illness. It should be differentiated from the much more serious septic arthritis.
- Radiographs and blood results are not useful in making the diagnosis, but may assist to exclude other potential causes for the limp/refusal to walk.
- Toddler's fractures are another common cause of limp/ refusal to walk that are associated with minor trauma.
- The signs are subtle, and the fracture may not be visible on x-ray.
- Toddler's fractures may be managed with no immobilisation, or for pain management and protection the leg may be immobilised in a back-slab.

FOREIGN-BODY ASPIRATION

Aspiration of a foreign body (FB) occurs most commonly in infants and toddlers; the average age is between 2 and 3 years, with a mortality rate of approximately 5–7%.[326] It is also one of the most common causes of accidental death in children under 1 year of age. The FB is often a piece of food; nuts are the most commonly reported organic FB. As children at this age have a tendency to put things in their mouths, small parts on toys and other small objects also pose a risk. Furthermore, the increasing number of toys and devices that are powered with small button batteries should prompt the clinician to consider the potential for button battery aspiration, which should be treated as an emergency.

Presentation and diagnosis

The clinical presentation of infants and children following FB inhalation is highly variable, and ranges from those presenting with a clear history of inhalation and obvious examination findings to those presenting with a less-obvious history of inhalation and/or equivocal examination findings. Furthermore, the level of evidence that establishes the sensitivity and specificity of the signs and diagnostic tests considered most useful for diagnosing FB aspiration is low.[327]

FB inhalation should be strongly suspected where the history details sudden onset of choking, coughing, dyspnoea, laboured breathing, dysphagia and gagging. Observational studies suggest that anywhere from 40% to 70% of children presenting with a combination of these symptoms will have a confirmed FB on bronchoscopy.[326] Depending on the size of the FB, the signs and symptoms of inhalation may be mild to absent following the initial choking episode,[326] or may only become apparent after days to weeks as the child continues to cough and develops signs of pneumonia. A choking episode may not be reported as it may not have been witnessed or was not considered significant, particularly if it was days or weeks ago. Therefore, FB inhalation should also be suspected where there is unexplained chronic cough in an infant or young child.

Examination findings may include signs of obvious upper or lower airway obstruction, such as stridor and marked increased work of breathing, decreased lung sounds or wheeze. Other respiratory signs, such as decreased oxygen saturation, are not pathognomonic for FB inhalation, but should raise suspicion. Although most children with FB aspiration will have abnormal chest auscultation, as many as 5% will have normal examination findings. Therefore, normal breath sounds cannot be considered negatively predictive. Where the history and/or examination is strongly suggestive of FB aspiration or the diagnosis cannot be excluded, a chest radiograph is indicated. However, in 25–30% of cases, the chest x-ray may be normal (e.g. FB is radiolucent and no lung findings).[327] Therefore, chest x-ray alone cannot be used to discriminate between those who have aspirated an FB and those who have not. Where the x-ray is abnormal, there will be signs of hyperinflation, mediastinal shift, localised air trapping or a radio-opaque FB.

The signs and symptoms of FB inhalation are not sufficiently sensitive or specific to support a diagnostic decision rule. In over 50% of cases, the diagnostic triad of signs and symptoms (wheeze, cough and gagging) are absent.[327] However, FB inhalation is unlikely in those children who present asymptomatically and have normal examination and radiological findings. All others should be considered at risk of an FB inhalation when an alternative diagnosis has not been made.

Management

Complete airway obstruction is an emergency and basic life support should be commenced immediately. Initial treatment involves removal of the object (if visible and safe to do so), airway-opening manoeuvres, back blows or chest thrusts, depending on the age of the child (see Chapter 14 for full details). Infants may be placed in a head downwards position prior to delivering back blows, for example across the rescuer's lap.[328]

The infant or child showing signs of partial airway obstruction but able to ventilate should be allowed to adopt a position of comfort while the adequacy of ventilation is observed. Children showing signs of significant respiratory distress will require urgent bronchoscopy to remove the FB. They should be monitored closely. However, interaction should be kept to a minimum to prevent distressing the child and increasing the risk to their airway. Clinicians with paediatric airway expertise should be immediately available or the child should be transferred to a centre with the resources to expertly manage a paediatric airway. For children presenting with less-obvious symptoms, but where there is suspicion of an inhaled FB, there should be a low threshold for performing bronchoscopy.

PRACTICE TIPS

FOREIGN-BODY (FB) ASPIRATION

- Presentation is highly variable and may include children with a less-obvious history of inhalation and/or equivocal examination findings.
- FB aspiration should be suspected in young children with unexplained cough.
- Chest x-rays are normal in 25–30% of cases of FB aspiration.
- There should be a low threshold for referring infants and children to ENT with a potential FB aspiration.
- No attempts to remove the FB should be made in the ED unless there is complete airway obstruction, the FB is visible, and it can be removed safely.

FOREIGN-BODY INGESTION

Foreign-body (FB) ingestion and FB insertion into the nose or ear are common paediatric presentations to the ED—food, small plastic toys, coins (60% of all ingested foreign bodies) and other small household objects are the most common FBs.[329]

Diagnosis is often delayed as the event is frequently not witnessed and parents are only alerted to the FB when the child or an older sibling informs them, or alternatively when they seek health advice for non-specific symptoms resulting from the FB, such as an offensive unilateral nasal discharge, bad breath or reduced hearing. Examination of a child who has inserted an FB into an ear or nostril should include both ears and nostrils, as children frequently insert FBs into multiple places.

Button batteries can be difficult to distinguish from a coin and early x-ray is important and the 'halo' sign is indicative if a button battery.[330] They should be removed from the oesophagus, aural canal or nasal passages immediately as generation of external electrolytic current will result in liquefaction necrosis and severe burns can occur within 2–2.5 hours. Children require urgent referral to ENT to ensure that removal occurs urgently. Children must also be referred for urgent follow-up, even if the battery has been rapidly and successfully removed in the ED as injuries extend after removal.[330] In extreme cases, injuries can be life threatening or result in life-long disfigurement.

Parents should be warned about the likelihood that this may occur again and the need to supervise children when eating and playing with objects small enough to swallow or insert into their ears or nose and the dangers of button batteries.

Ingested foreign bodies

Children frequently swallow foreign objects such as coins, causing significant alarm to their parents. Most commonly they pass into the stomach and are then rarely of concern. Radiographs are frequently used to locate radio-opaque FBs and demonstrate that they have passed into the stomach. These children may be discharged, and parents advised that it is not necessary to confirm passage of the FB through the intestinal tract by identifying the FB in the faeces or using repeat radiographs. Many clinicians suggest that in an asymptomatic child an initial radiograph is not needed as oesophageal obstruction under these circumstances is extremely unlikely. Ingestion of magnets is a notable exception to this rule, unless there is complete confidence that the child could only have swallowed one magnet. Where there is a possibility that there may be two, these children should be referred to a surgeon as the two magnets may be attracted and pinch adjacent bowel loops resulting in necrosis.[331] Although radio-opaque, the magnets may sit one behind each other and therefore appear as one magnet. Vomiting and abdominal pain are the most common initial symptom and modern magnets made from neodymium, creating a high-powered magnet, increase the risk of complications such as perforation.[331,332] There should remain a high level of suspicion for ingested FB in young children presenting with non-specific abdominal pain and vomiting.

Less frequently, the FB becomes lodged in the pharynx or the oesophagus and this is potentially a medical emergency. Children with an FB lodged in their oesophagus may present with a history of refusal to eat, may complain of feeling that something is stuck, vomiting, less commonly gagging, drooling, choking and coughing; or alternatively they may be asymptomatic.[330] These children should be referred to a paediatric general surgeon for potential removal of the obstruction. Depending on the likelihood of the FB passing, a conservative approach may be adopted, and surgical removal only used if the FB does not pass naturally. As noted above, button batteries lodged in the oesophagus should be removed urgently regardless of the symptoms and predicted likelihood that it may pass naturally. Uncommonly, but importantly, an FB, in particular a coin, may lodge in the oesophagus and cause airway obstruction. Airway protection is of highest priority and children should be managed in the same way as children with an FB aspiration and referred immediately to have the FB removed. Radiographs may assist in localising a radio-opaque FB. Children with an FB lodged in the oesophagus should be referred to general surgery, and where there are signs of airway obstruction, urgent referral to ENT should be made.

PRACTICE TIPS

FOREIGN-BODY (FB) INGESTION

- Most ingested FBs pass into the stomach and therefore do not require intervention (except button batteries).
- It is not necessary to confirm passage of the object by repeat x-rays or screening of the faeces.
- An FB lodged in the oesophagus or pharynx is a potential medical emergency.

Intranasal foreign bodies

Most common nasal foreign bodies (FB) are organic seeds and plastic beads.[333] Many children present with unilateral nasal discharge and offensive odour as the first clue to an intranasal FB. Foreign bodies pushed into the nose most frequently lodge in the floor of the nasal passage below the inferior turbinate, or in the upper nasal fossa anterior to the middle turbinate and are usually visible. They can generally be successfully removed in the ED. Alternatively, where the FB is a small lolly that will dissolve, it may be reasonable not to attempt removal and allow it to dissolve over time.

Small, round lightweight objects that are completely occluding the nostril may be removed by generating positive pressure in the nasal passage behind the object. If the child is old enough, this can be achieved by asking the child to blow their nose while occluding the other nostril, and if not old enough by having the parent blow into the child's mouth while occluding the patent nostril, a technique often referred to as a 'mother's kiss'. This has been shown to be effective approximately 60% of the time.[334] Parents benefit from a demonstration of the force of the breath used for this technique. It should be a short puff of air like blowing dust off something. The child will reflexively close the glottis to protect the lungs, preventing damage. Despite this, a forceful, large-volume breath should not be delivered.

Prior to alternative attempts to remove the FB, phenylephrine to reduce oedema and lidocaine to provide local anaesthetic should be applied to the nasal mucosa.[335] Techniques for removal include using suction, alligator forceps to grasp the object or a wax curette (metal to allow bending to a slight curve) or curved hook to slide behind the object and pull it forward (see Chapter 16 for suctioning techniques). Most children will require sedation to achieve sufficient cooperation to make FB removal possible (see the section on procedural sedation). However, care should be taken to ensure that they remain able to gag and cough to protect their airway during attempts to remove an intranasal FB.

Referral to ENT should be made when the FB cannot be adequately visualised, the child is not sufficiently cooperative to attempt removal or attempts to remove the FB have been unsuccessful. It is also suggested that a plain radiograph should be taken where the FB is not visible and there is suspicion that it may be a button battery, to prompt more expeditious management.

Aural foreign bodies

Foreign bodies inserted into the ear are the most difficult to remove and 20–33% of children will require general anaesthetic to facilitate removal.[336] The external auditory canal is cartilaginous and bony, lined with only a thin layer of skin, which provides very little cushioning for the periosteum. Therefore, attempts to remove the FB, in addition to being frightening to the young child, can be very painful. On occasions, the FB may become impacted deep in the canal as it narrows, particularly where previous unsuccessful attempts have been made, making removal even more difficult. Canal lacerations, rupture of the tympanic membrane and disruption of the ossicles are documented complications of removal attempts.[336]

Removal in the ED should only be attempted if the child will hold sufficiently still (see the section on procedural sedation for details), the FB can be adequately visualised, appropriate instruments for removal are available and the clinician is sufficiently skilled to remove the FB. Removal attempts are less likely to be successful in younger children, where the object is smooth and difficult to grasp, has been in the ear for an extended period and previous unsuccessful attempts have been made. Furthermore, these factors will also increase the rate of complications resulting from removal attempts, which may be as high as 43%.[336] Referral to ENT without first attempting to remove the FB in ED should be strongly considered if the object is smooth and spherical or there have been previous unsuccessful attempts made by other clinicians.

The techniques most frequently used with success are water irrigation and/or suction for small, lightweight objects, or removal using small alligator forceps to grasp the object or a wax curette to lever it out from behind the object. Irrigation should not be used where the FB is likely to be a button battery as this may increase the likelihood of the contents leaking from the battery. Alcohol, shown to be the most effective, should be used to kill live insects (found more frequently in older children) before attempts are made to remove them. However, this should not be instilled where there is tympanic perforation. A light and magnification source will improve visualisation of the FB and therefore the likely success rate. Most children will require sedation to assist staff to make a removal attempt possible.

PRACTICE TIPS

FOREIGN BODY (FB)—INTRANASAL AND AURAL

- Most FBs in the nose are visible.
- A lightweight object which is occluding the nose may be removed using positive pressure behind the object, achieved by the child blowing the nose or by a parent blowing into their mouth while occluding the unaffected nostril.
- Most children will require sedation to make safe removal of the object possible.
- Removal of aural FBs can be difficult; therefore, clinicians should have a low threshold for referring to ENT.

PAIN MANAGEMENT AND PROCEDURAL SEDATION

Pain is a frequent symptom in adult and paediatric patients presenting to the ED, and recommendations and clinical practice guidelines consistently emphasise the importance of the adequate management of acute and procedural pain and distress.

Despite this, it is widely accepted that pain and distress is inadequately managed in EDs, and some studies even show an *increase* in pain intensity between admission and discharge for some patients. Several subpopulations, such as children and geriatrics, are considered particularly vulnerable to suboptimal treatment for painful conditions and may needlessly experience pain with illness or injury. Studies have shown that children are less likely to receive analgesia than adults in the ED setting, and that young children are less likely to receive analgesia than older children. Unfortunately, most of the data that informs us about the pain-related experience of children in EDs comes from studies conducted over 15 years ago.

A more comprehensive overview of pain and pain management strategies has been presented in Chapter 18. The following sections add to this discussion by addressing some issues specific to paediatric pain and distress management.

ASSESSMENT

Pain and distress assessment

Fundamental to adequate pain management is pain assessment, and in children this presents a significant clinical challenge to emergency service clinicians due to children's varying levels of cognitive development. Pain can be assessed in several ways, such as the character of the pain, the region of the body affected, radiation, the effect of pain on activity and the intensity of the pain. Assessment in emergency services usually focuses on the character and intensity of the pain. Quantifying the intensity of pain has provided a commonly accepted language to describe pain and a baseline from which to measure the impact of treatments on pain. Numerous pain assessment tools are available for this purpose. However, they require adaptation depending on the child's age, i.e. behavioural tools for pre-verbal children, faces scales for early-verbal children and visual analogue scales for older children.

Self-report is considered the ideal standard for pain assessment, and the Visual Analogue Scale (VAS) is a reliable instrument for quantifying acute pain in adults.[337] However, young children may have difficulty using the VAS. To overcome this, scales using faces representing varying levels of pain intensity have been developed for this age group. Children may prefer the Wong-Baker FACES® Pain Rating Scale (Fig. 35.7).[338] However, the Faces Pain Scale-revised is likely to provide a more realistic assessment of the child's pain as the smiling face in the Wong and Baker may skew the child's score.[339] There is also increasing evidence that children between 3 and 5 years, while able to self-report pain, are unable to use a traditional scale based on six faces and may provide more valid reports of pain using a simplified scale with three faces to signify mild, moderate and severe pain intensity.[340]

Children under the age of 3–4 years lack the cognitive development to use self-report scales, hence observer rating scales are used for this group. The VAS Observer (VAS_{Obs}) appears in the literature as a proxy for self-report, where clinicians or parents perform the rating. However, clinicians and parents may underestimate the child's pain and scores are often not reliable.

An alternative to the VAS_{Obs} is the Face Legs Activity Cry Consolability (FLACC) scale (Table 35.17), which is an observational scale[341] focusing on behaviours that research has shown are indicative of pain in infants and young children. To administer FLACC, an observer looks at a young child's facial expression, leg movements, activity, whether they are crying, and the extent to which they can be consoled. Each of these five behaviours is given a score of 0, 1 or 2, resulting in a total score ranging from 0 (no pain/distress) to 10 (maximum pain/distress). There is some evidence of the capacity of the FLACC scale to provide valid pain/distress scores in children undergoing painful procedures in the ED.[342] However, assessments should also include factors other

FIGURE 35.7 THE WONG-BAKER FACES® PAIN RATING SCALE[338]

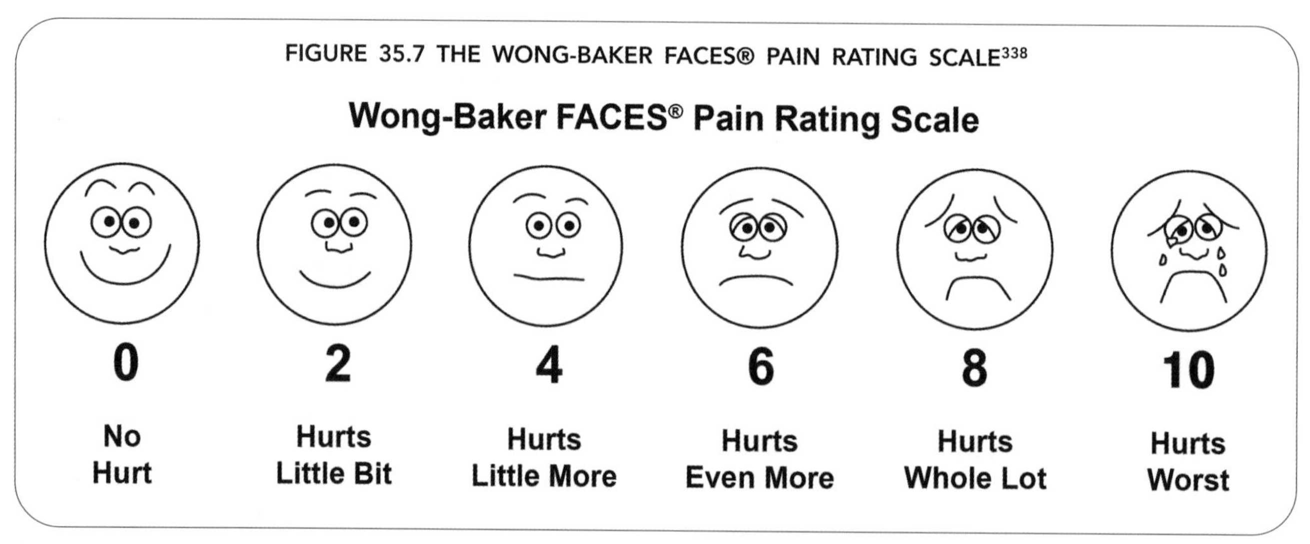

Wong-Baker FACES Foundation (2018). Wong-Baker FACES® Pain Rating Scale. *Retrieved 25/9/2018 with permission from www.WongBakerFACES.org.*

TABLE 35.17 THE FLACC (FACES LEGS ACTIVITY CRY AND CONSOLABILITY) SCALE[341]

	0	1	2
Face	No particular expression or smile	Occasional grimace or frown, withdrawn, disinterested	Frequent to constant frown, quivering chin, clenched jaw
Legs	Normal position or relaxed	Uneasy, restless, tense	Kicking or legs drawn up
Activity	Lying quietly, normal position, moves easily	Squirming, shifting back and forth, tense	Arched, rigid or jerking
Cry	No cry (awake or asleep)	Moans or whimpers; occasional complaints	Crying steadily, screams or sobs, frequent complaints
Consolability	Content, relaxed	Reassured by occasional touching, hugging, or 'talking to'; distractible	Difficult to console or comfort

BOX 35.3 UNIVERSITY OF MICHIGAN SEDATION SCALE[346]

- Awake/alert
- Minimally sedated–tired/sleepy, appropriate response to verbal conversation and/or sounds.
- Moderately sedated–somnolent/sleeping, easily aroused with light tactile stimulation
- Deeply sedated–deep sleep, rousable only with significant physical stimulation
- Unrousable

than the score, such as parent's perception of their child's pain, the circumstances etc., to guide management decisions.

Sedation assessment

Sedation scales have also been developed to quantify the level of sedation. The University of Michigan Sedation Scale (UMSS),[343] shown in Box 35.3,[343] is used in Australian and Aotearoa New Zealand EDs to score the level of sedation of children undergoing conscious sedation for a diagnostic or therapeutic procedure. Sedation is assessed on a 4-point scale, where scores of 1, 2 and 3 represent mild, moderate and deep sedation respectively, while a score of 4 is indicative of unconsciousness. The UMSS has been validated for children aged 6 months to 12 years of age,[343,344] and compares favourably with other scales.[344]

In addition to vital signs, a baseline sedation score should be recorded before administering sedation and then at regular intervals while the patient remains sedated. The level of sedation and the agent used will determine the frequency of assessment.

PRACTICE TIPS

ASSESSMENT OF PAIN AND SEDATION

- Children as young as 4 years of age can self-report pain but may require a simplified scale.
- The FLACC (Face Legs Activity Cry Consolability) scale is recommended for children younger than 4 years of age.
- The level of sedation achieved can be assessed using the University of Michigan Sedation Scale (UMSS) (see Box 35.3).[343]

ACUTE PAIN MANAGEMENT

Pain management has been described in some detail in Chapter 18, and many of the strategies described there are suitable for children. Pain relief is best achieved by using a range of strategies, both pharmacological and non-pharmacological. This section will discuss use of some of these strategies to optimally manage acute pain in children presenting to the ED.

The choice of pharmacological agent is based largely on the severity of the pain experienced by the child. However, the age of the child and their condition may play some role in influencing the agents chosen and the routes of administration. Table 35.18 provides a formulary of analgesic agents suitable for use in children with acute pain, which includes dosing regimens and the indications for use.

Mild pain is, in most circumstances, effectively managed with a non-opioid such as paracetamol or ibuprofen. There is low quality and limited evidence to suggest that ibuprofen may be more effective than paracetamol at relieving pain.[285] Although there is some concern about the role of prostaglandin in bone healing, there is no evidence from studies conducted in humans to confirm that NSAIDs have an effect on bone healing.[345] Short-term use in healthy children also places them at low risk for the other side-effects of NSAIDs,[285] making it reasonable to recommend their role in managing pain in children secondary to musculoskeletal injury.

Moderate and more-severe pain is most frequently controlled using opioids, such as fentanyl, morphine and oxycodone. Fentanyl administered intranasally is widely used pre-hospital and in the ED and has been shown to be effective as a first-line treatment for moderate to severe pain.[346] Oral oxycodone has replaced the use of oral codeine as it confers more reliable analgesic effect and is supported by a better safety profile than codeine.

Other agents used in adults or other clinical settings, such as tramadol and IV paracetamol, have not been widely studied in children and are not routinely recommended to treat acute pain in children.

Contemporary literature increasingly supports the use of multi-modal agents in the pre-hospital setting in managing acute onset severe pain. Optimal agents should be easy to administer, have predictable dose-response relationship and a short half-life. Combinations of medications such as either fentanyl or ketamine which can be delivered either via intranasal or intravenous route, along with inhalational methoxyflurane or intravenous paracetamol are becoming commonplace.[347–349]

PRACTICE TIPS

ACUTE PAIN MANAGEMENT

- Infants and children should be treated with an appropriate agent at an appropriate dose to manage their pain.
- Intranasal fentanyl is an effective way of administering opioid analgesia quickly and without the need to insert an intravenous cannula.
- Local anaesthetics can be used to manage condition-specific pain, such as otalgia associated with otitis media, oropharyngeal pain secondary to stomatitis and pain secondary to fracture.

Local anaesthetic agents are frequently used alongside analgesics to manage condition-specific pain. Some obvious examples are nerve blocks following long-bone fracture (see Chapter 18 for more details regarding their use). There are other occasions in paediatric emergency when these agents are used to manage pain and discomfort. However, data supporting their efficacy are limited. In one RCT, lidocaine used topically in the ear was shown to reduce earache in infants and children suffering otitis media.[126] Lidocaine in a viscous solution is often recommended for the pain and discomfort experienced by children with gingivostomatitis

TABLE 35.18 FORMULARY OF COMMONLY USED AGENTS FOR MANAGING ACUTE PAIN AND SEDATION IN CHILDREN

AGENT	DOSE	INDICATIONS	TIPS
Ibuprofen	5–10 mg/kg orally	Mild to moderate pain	May be more effective for some conditions than paracetamol, e.g. transient synovitis
Paracetamol	20 mg/kg orally (max 90 mg/kg/day)	Mild to moderate pain	Safe and effective Can be given in combination products, e.g. with codeine
Glucose	2 mL/procedure orally (max 5 mL/day)	Painful procedures in infants	Give several drops of glucose onto the tongue a minute or two before procedure commences and then at regular intervals throughout
Fentanyl	0.15 microg/kg intranasally	Moderate to severe pain	As effective as morphine given intranasally For larger volumes, dose can be divided, and half given into each nostril
Lidocaine	1% solution	Local anaesthetic for painful conditions	Instil several drops into painful ear
Lidocaine	0.5–2% solution Bier's block: 3 mg/kg Infiltration: 3 mg/kg	Local anaesthesia for painful procedures	Can be used to infiltrate wound Used for short-term nerve block, e.g. for LAMP
Ketamine	1–1.5 mg/kg	Procedural sedation	Better results if given intravenously Give as a slow bolus (2–3 minutes) to prevent respiratory distress
Ketamine	0.1–0.3 mg/kg IV; 0.5–1 mg/kg IM	Analgesics	At doses lower than sedation dosing, provides effective analgesia
Midazolam	0.5–1.0 mg/kg orally	Procedural sedation	Administer orally Intranasal administration is poorly tolerated, as it stings the nostril and runs down the back of the nose and is swallowed
Morphine	0.05–0.1 mg/kg	Moderate to severe pain	Can be titrated intravenously until analgesia is achieved
Oxycodone	0.1 mg/kg	Moderate to severe pain	More reliable analgesia than codeine
Nitrous oxide (NO_2)	30–70% inhaled	Analgesia and sedation for painful procedures	Establish sedation (at least 5 minutes of NO_2) before commencing the procedure

IV: intravenously; LAMP: local anaesthesia, manipulation and plaster.

and oral ulcers. However, an RCT conducted in an Australian tertiary paediatric ED has demonstrated that its use has no effect on oral intake.[350] However, its use to support fluid intake following discharge has not been tested and it may play a role in this context.

PROCEDURAL ANAESTHESIA, ANALGESIA AND SEDATION

Sedation is frequently used during procedures to reduce anxiety and improve cooperation[351–353] and in Australian and Aotearoa New Zealand EDs this is almost universally achieved using nitrous oxide or ketamine.[354] The specifics of dose, indication and administration are detailed in Table 35.18. Evidence from several large case series demonstrates that nitrous oxide is a safe and effective way to sedate infants and children in the ED sufficiently to undergo diagnostic and therapeutic procedures.[355–359] Vomiting and desaturation are the most frequent side-effects recorded and occur at rates of approximately 6–7% and less than 1%, respectively. Data from these case series do not record any serious adverse outcomes. Interestingly, in one series, longer fasting was linked to higher rates of vomiting, and deeper sedation with 70% nitrous oxide did not increase the number of adverse events. Furthermore, deep sedation occurred in only 3% of children in this series, placing only a small number at risk of aspiration. The success of nitrous oxide for procedural sedation can be improved by ensuring that the child is adequately sedated before commencing the procedure, which may take 3–5 minutes. It can be difficult to achieve a satisfactory outcome where the procedure is rushed, and the child becomes distressed before they have been adequately sedated.

Bone marrow toxicity and neurotoxicity are both reported with long-term use of nitrous oxide and neurotoxicity with short-term use, although rarely. There are no data to guide maximum exposure, but it is recommended that alternatives are sought for patients with metabolic diseases, such as methionine synthase deficiency, homocystinuria and methylmalonic acidaemia. Data are not available to determine the risk, but pregnant women should also avoid exposure.[337]

Ketamine, which produces a dissociated state of sedation conferring analgesia, amnesia, sedation and immobility with preservation of airway tone, is increasingly used in procedural sedation in the ED. It is ideally suited for procedures that require the child to be completely still, such as suturing of facial lacerations, or that are likely to be particularly painful and/or distressing, such as fracture manipulation. Data from numerous studies and RCTs confirm that ketamine can be used effectively for procedural sedation in the ED with a low rate of side-effects.[360]

The most common adverse events occurring in association with ketamine sedation are vomiting (12–17%), which occurs most frequently in the recovery phase, and hypersalivation (2–11%). Small numbers of children will require brief airway support, such as suctioning, due to hypersalivation; however, there are no reports of children requiring intubation resulting from ketamine sedation. Emergence reactions are acknowledged as a potential side-effect associated with ketamine sedation but rates are low (approx. 2%)[360] and recovery in a quiet environment with minimal stimulus reduces the rate of this phenomenon. In many departments, midazolam is no longer used routinely for procedural sedation as sedation results are less predictable and side-effects more common.

The prolonged recovery phase is one of the major limitations to ketamine sedation. A recent case series has demonstrated that intravenous administration of ketamine, rather than intramuscular, not only reduces the rate of some side-effects, but reduces the time to discharge following administration of ketamine by approximately 20 minutes.[361]

Sedation of children in the ED carries significant risk and measures should be employed to reduce the associated risks. EDs must be appropriately resourced (staffing and equipment) before attempting to sedate a patient. Staff providing sedation should be adequately trained to manage a sedated child and should have current basic and advanced life support skills. Furthermore, children undergoing conscious sedation should have continuous monitoring and a trained clinician should be dedicated to managing the sedation and to monitor for side-effects until the child has recovered.

With few exceptions, children undergoing painful procedures should receive analgesics and/or local anaesthetic in addition to sedation. Paracetamol, ibuprofen, oxycodone, intranasal fentanyl and intravenous morphine are appropriate analgesic options for painful procedures. Fentanyl and nitrous oxide are frequently used to manage procedural distress (pain and anxiety) with good effect and few side-effects.

Topical and infiltrated local anaesthetic agents can be given prior to procedures such as intravenous cannula insertion, lumbar puncture, urinary catheter insertion, wound closure, FB removal and eye irrigation. The results of a systematic review confirm that preparations containing amethocaine are more effective than emla®.[362]

Nebulised lidocaine has been shown to be safe and effective at reducing the pain related to NG tube insertion in adults,[363] which has been rated as the most painful procedure performed in the ED.[364] Theoretically it should be of similar value in infants and young children. However, the studies attempting to confirm this could not demonstrate similar results in young children and infants.[365,366] The authors question whether the considerable distress experienced by infants and children during NG tube insertion may have masked any alleviation of pain felt as a result of the lidocaine. Despite these results it is probably reasonable to consider topical anaesthetics for NGT insertion.

PRACTICE TIPS

PROCEDURAL ANALGESIA AND SEDATION

- Analgesia, local anaesthesia and sedation should be used in combination for procedures likely to be painful.
- Nitrous oxide is a safe and effective way to provide sedation for a range of diagnostic and therapeutic procedures.
- Ketamine may be used where deeper sedation is required. However, greater resources will be required to provide safe and effective sedation.
- Intravenous administration of ketamine is recommended as it reduces the rate of side-effects and the time to discharge.

NON-PHARMACOLOGICAL STRATEGIES

Non-pharmacological strategies to alleviate pain and distress should also be considered for children with pain related to illness or injury, and for those undergoing a painful and/or distressing procedure. There is a substantial volume of literature stressing the value of non-pharmacological measures, such as distraction and guided imagery in children with acute and chronic pain. Furthermore, there are several studies advocating for non-pharmacological techniques during painful procedures. However, the results from research evaluating its effectiveness are mixed. A Cochrane review concentrating on the effect of these techniques for needle-related procedural pain in children concluded that there is preliminary evidence to indicate benefit.[367] However, the quality of the studies included was not ideal and additional RCTs are needed. There is a scarcity of studies focusing on use of these techniques in the ED, and what literature is available focuses on their effect during painful and distressing procedures. A recent RCT shows that distraction, the most frequently used technique, has a positive effect on the level of pain and distress experienced by children of all ages.[368]

Some paediatric EDs may have the luxury of having play therapists available to assist with distraction. However, most children are seen in EDs which do not have these resources. Distraction can be provided by parents as well as staff, can be offered in the form of books, audio-visual aids, drawing and colouring-in, and should remain a priority despite limited resources. Bubble-blowing, games such as 'I-spy' and storytelling can be simple ways to provide distraction. Smartphones and other devices have increasingly replaced other tools for distraction and there have also been efforts made to explore the role of virtual reality for procedural and acute pain management.[369,370]

Techniques, such as immobilisation of injuries, dressing burns, hot packs, ice packs and other similar measures, are useful adjuncts to pharmacological treatment. However, infants and young children may tolerate some of these measures poorly. This requires some creativity on the part of the clinician to improve compliance. Using the child's imagination and playing games can be one way of overcoming a young child's reluctance to cooperate. Involving the parents, such as having them hold a heat or cold pack in place while cuddling a child or talking to them to distract them from or to persuade them to accept a treatment, can be another way to improve compliance. Pain management should be multimodal, and this may mean that pharmacological treatments are used to make non-pharmacological techniques possible; for example, providing nitrous oxide while a back-slab for support is applied.

Administration of small volumes (0.5–1 mL aliquots) of oral glucose solutions (25–35%) to newborns and very young infants moments before a painful procedure and at regular intervals throughout has been shown to reduce the pain experienced during the procedure.[371] This should be standard practice for infants having any painful procedure performed.

PRACTICE TIPS

NON-PHARMACOLOGICAL STRATEGIES TO MANAGE PAIN AND DISTRESS

- Employing non-pharmacological strategies to manage pain and distress should not be overlooked.
- Oral glucose (25-35%) solution should be given in small aliquots (0.5-1 mL) to neonates and infants having painful procedures.
- Distraction can be of great value to minimise the distress of procedures and improve cooperation.

HEALTH PROMOTION

Acute healthcare is the principal priority during an emergency contact; however, it is also an opportunity for emergency clinicians to provide health education and address other health and lifestyle issues, such as immunisation, smoking cessation and weight management. Clinicians should be aware of the various primary health and social services available to support families with children to provide recommendations where appropriate. In addition to providing clinical assessment, maternal and child healthcare nurses are often an excellent support and source of local community-based, health-related information for families of neonates, infants and young children.

OPPORTUNISTIC IMMUNISATION

The recommended schedule of immunisations is government-funded and is made available through local councils and other health services. The current Australian and Aotearoa New Zealand schedules can be found via the links in the list of Useful websites at the end of the chapter. However, for a number of reasons, significant numbers of children are inadequately vaccinated. In most circumstances, children fall behind for practical reasons, such as illness at the time that they are due for their next vaccination. It is reasonable to administer the scheduled vaccines which have become due or outstanding during the ED visit for most of these children. Guidance about contraindications and likely adverse reactions and parent information sheets can be accessed from the *Australian Immunisation Handbook* website (see Useful websites). Children who are well behind the schedule should be referred to their GP, an immunisation clinic, or a maternal child health nurse to have a 'catch-up' schedule planned. The *Australian Immunisation Handbook* also provides recommendations for scheduling catch-up vaccinations.

It is uncommon for parents to object to immunisation for their children. However, where this is the case, the majority cite the perceived risks associated with vaccination as the reason for their objection, despite scientific evidence demonstrating that the risks to health are greater from the disease than from the vaccination. These families should be referred to an immunisation or infectious diseases clinic to have an opportunity to discuss their concerns and explore the options.

WEIGHT MANAGEMENT

Obesity has become a major health concern in Australasia, and large numbers of children are now overweight. Excessive weight in childhood has wide-ranging impacts on health, contributing to poorer physical health, self-esteem and mental health, sleep, and lifelong weight-related health issues. Weight management is not the remit of the ED. However, ED clinicians have an opportunity to address this important health problem. The importance of healthy eating and exercise should be emphasised, and referrals made to dietitians and other experts to address weight-management issues.

SMOKING CESSATION

Passive smoking is a widely recognised risk to health, increasing the risk of a number of diseases; for example, respiratory illnesses, meningococcal disease, Perthes' disease and sudden infant death syndrome (SIDS). Efforts should be made to encourage parents to quit smoking and information provided to assist them. It has been shown that parents expect to be asked about smoking and advised to stop when consulting a healthcare professional about their child's health. Parents may be referred to their GP or Quit for smoking cessation advice, programs and support.

SUMMARY

The provision of emergency care to children requires that the clinician recognises the anatomical and physiological differences that exist between adults, children and infants, and understands the impact of immaturity on illness and injury, assessment and management. This chapter has provided a summary of these differences, a guide to recognition of serious illness and an overview of the presentation and management of many common paediatric presentations. This chapter should be read in conjunction with the many other chapters in this text that address presentations common in children.

CASE STUDY 1

A mother brings her 3-week-old infant to the emergency department (ED), stating that the baby has been crying more than usual for 2 days. The baby is alert and quiet, there are no signs of increased respiratory effort, and the baby is pink and warm.

QUESTIONS

1. Your triage assessment should identify which of the following?
   a. Airway—patent, Breathing—normal, Circulation—normal, Disability—normal, Risk factors—nil
   b. Airway—patent, Breathing—normal, Circulation—normal, Disability—normal, Risk factors—age
   c. Airway—patent, Breathing—normal, Circulation—normal, Disability—normal, Risk factors—age, increased crying
   d. Airway—patent, Breathing—normal, Circulation—normal, Disability—irritable, Risk factors—age, increased crying
2. Following more-extensive examination of the baby, it is also noted that the heart rate is 200 beats/minute. You note that:
   a. This is within normal limits for an infant of this age.
   b. This may be normal if the blood pressure is also normal.
   c. A rate this high is caused by a dysrhythmia such as supraventricular tachycardia.
   d. This is high for this age, which may reflect significant illness.
3. The temperature is also taken rectally and found to be 35.8°C. This may be for the following reason:
   a. The room is cool, and the baby is exposed.
   b. This is within the normal temperature range for young babies.
   c. The baby may be hypothermic secondary to infection.
   d. Rectal temperature measurement is unreliable.
4. If the baby begins to show signs of poor peripheral perfusion, treatment should include:
   a. An intravenous fluid bolus of 40 mL 4% dextrose and 1/5 normal saline
   b. An intravenous bolus of 80 mL normal saline
   c. An intravenous bolus of 80 mL 4% dextrose and 1/5 normal saline
   d. An intravenous bolus of 40 mL normal saline

For each of the following statements, state whether it is true or false:

5. Antibiotics should not be administered to treat suspected sepsis in neonates until microbiology results are available to confirm the diagnosis.
6. Neonates should receive maintenance fluids containing glucose (e.g. 10%) as they are at significant risk of hypoglycaemia.
7. Jaundice in neonates may be linked with sepsis.

Answers to Case Study Questions can be found on evolve http://evolve.elsevier.com/AU/Curtis/emergency/ 

CASE STUDY 2

A child aged 14 months with no past history has developed shortness of breath following a few days of cold symptoms. An ambulance is called by the parents and the child is transported to the ED of the local hospital.

QUESTIONS

1. As the first clinician to assess the child in the ED, your primary assessment of respiratory function should be:
   a. Work of breathing
   b. Oxygen saturations
   c. Respiratory rate
   d. Lung sounds
2. Wheeze is commonly associated with a number of conditions. Which of these sets includes one where wheeze is unlikely to be associated with this condition?
   a. Asthma, bronchiolitis, viral pneumonia
   b. Bronchiolitis, asthma, inhaled FB
   c. Asthma, croup, bronchiolitis
   d. Anaphylaxis, asthma, bronchiolitis

3. This child has moderate to severe increased work of breathing, widespread inspiratory and expiratory wheeze and his respiratory rate is 58. His oxygen SpO_2 is 96%. Therapy should commence with:
   a. A dose of adrenaline administered via nebuliser
   b. Oral steroids
   c. 5 mg salbutamol and 250 microg ipratropium bromide via nebuliser
   d. 6 puffs salbutamol and 4 puffs ipratropium via MDI and spacer
   e. 6 puffs salbutamol via MDI and spacer
4. This child's oxygen saturations when measured are now 86% in room air. The following is initially the most suitable delivery system and flow of oxygen:
   a. Nasal cannula at 6 L/min
   b. Nasal cannula at 2 L/min
   c. Face mask at 2 L/min
   d. Face mask at 6 L/min
5. Steroids are prescribed. They should be administered:
   a. Orally
   b. Intravenously
   c. Inhaled
   d. A or B—there is no significant difference in efficacy or onset
6. Children should be given a dose of salbutamol when:
   a. Wheeze can be heard (audibly or on auscultation)
   b. Wheeze can be heard and there is increased work of breathing
   c. There is a decrease in saturations and an increased respiratory rate
   d. Regularly to prevent deterioration
   e. B and C
7. There is evidence for the following agents to treat critical asthma:
   a. Aminophylline
   b. Magnesium sulphate
   c. Ketamine
   d. A and B
   e. A, B and C

For each of the following statements, state whether it is true or false:

8. All children admitted with asthma should have a chest x-ray.
9. It is unknown whether salbutamol administered via MDI and spacer is as effective as nebulised salbutamol to treat critical asthma.
10. Children under the age of 12 months should not be diagnosed with asthma.

Answers to Case Study Questions can be found on evolve **http://evolve.elsevier.com/AU/Curtis/emergency/** 

USEFUL WEBSITES

Advanced Paediatric Life Support (APLS), A not-for-profit training organisation providing multidisciplinary courses aimed at improving the early management of acutely ill and injured infants and children, www.apls.org.au/.

Australian Asthma Handbook. Australia's national guidelines for asthma management and National Asthma Council Australia's flagship publication, www.nationalasthma.org.au/health-professionals/australian-asthma-handbook.

Australian Immunisation Handbook provides clinical guidelines for healthcare professionals and others about the safest and most effective use of vaccines in their practice. These recommendations are developed by Australian Technical Advisory Group on Immunisation (ATAGI) and approved by the National Health and Medical Research Council (NHMRC), www.health.gov.au/resources/publications/the-australian-immunisation-handbook.

Department of Health Victoria, Disease Information and Advice. These guidelines for the control of infectious diseases provide detailed information about common and rare diseases that may pose public health concerns, www2.health.vic.gov.au/public-health/infectious-diseases/disease-information-advice.

DermNet NZ: A world renowned resource providing information about skin disease, https://dermnetnz.org/.

Don't Forget the Bubbles. This site provides a collection of paediatric-focused education and clinical resources created and collated by UK, Australian and New Zealand paediatric and emergency clinicians, https://dontforgetthebubbles.com/.

New Zealand Immunisation schedule. This site provides details about the NZ government recommended and funded immunisation schedule, www.health.govt.nz/our-work/preventative-health-wellness/immunisation/new-zealand-immunisation-schedule.

New Zealand Ministry of Health: Your Health A–Z. A source of paediatric health information and resources provided by the NZ Department of Health, www.health.govt.nz/your-health/full-a-z.

NSW Health. A source of paediatric health information for health professionals and families which includes policy directives and guidelines, parent information and other resources, www.health.nsw.gov.au/kidsfamilies/Pages/default.aspx.

Paediatric Research in Emergency Departments International Collaborative (PREDICT). This site details the work of PREDICT the paediatric research network for Australia and New Zealand. Links to their publications detailing the latest evidence for practice can be found on this site, www.predict.org.au/.

Pediatric Emergency Medicine Database. A web-based database cataloguing evidence addressing paediatric emergency practice. It is an independent not for profit site maintained by motivated health professionals, www.pemdatabase.org.

Royal Children's Hospital, Melbourne, Clinical Practice Guidelines (Including Statewide Guidelines). This site houses the clinical practice guidelines for acute paediatric care developed by the Royal Children's Hospital in collaboration with other paediatric experts in the State and used internationally, www.rch.org.au/clinicalguide/.

Royal Children's Hospital, Melbourne: Constipation, www.rch.org.au/clinicalguide/guideline_index/Constipation/.

Royal Children's Hospital, Melbourne: Kids Health Information. This site houses a range of parent Information/fact sheets for common paediatric health problems, www.rch.org.au/kidsinfo/.

Sydney Children's Hospital Network: Parent fact sheets. A similar repository of parent information sheets for common paediatric health problems, www.schn.health.nsw.gov.au/parents-and-carers/fact-sheets.

Therapeutic Guidelines: Antibiotics. The Therapeutic Guidelines are recognised as a leading source of accurate, independent and practical treatment advice for a wide range of clinical conditions, including infectious diseases, www.tg.org.au/.

Victorian Paediatric Orthopaedic Network, www2.health.vic.gov.au/hospitals-and-health-services/patient-care/specialist-clinics/specialist-clinics-program/vpon.

REFERENCES

1. Group HR. The implementation of an emergency nursing framework (HIRAID) reduces patient deterioration: a multi-centre quasi-experimental study. Int Emerg Nurs 2021;56:100976.
2. De S, Williams GJ, Hayen A. Accuracy of the 'traffic light' clinical decision rule for serious bacterial infections in young children with fever: a retrospective cohort study. BMJ 2013;346:f866.
3. Velasco R, Gomez B, Benito J, Mintegi S. Accuracy of PECARN rule for predicting serious bacterial infection in infants with fever without a source. Arch Dis Child 2021;106:143–8.
4. Davies K. Biological basis of child health 7: growth, development and the reproductive system. Nurs Child Young People 2020. doi:10.7748/ncyp.2020.e1308.
5. Starte D, Meldrum D. Developmental surveillance and assessment. In: Roberton MD, South M, editors. Practical paediatrics. Edinburgh: Churchill Livingstone; 2006.
6. Friedmann I, Dahdouh EM, Kugler P, Mimran G, Balayla J. Maternal and obstetrical predictors of sudden infant death syndrome (SIDS). J Matern Fetal Neonatal Med 2017;30:2315–23.
7. Mandatory reporting of child abuse and neglect 2013. 2019. Available from: https://aifs.gov.au/resources/resource-sheets/mandatory-reporting-child-abuse-and-neglect.
8. Hockenberry M, Wilson D. Wong's nursing care of infants and children. St Louis: Mosby; 2007.
9. Daw W, Kaur R, Delaney M, Elphick H. Respiratory rate is an early predictor of clinical deterioration in children. Pediat Pulmonol 2020;55:2041–9.
10. Nijman RG, Vergouwe Y, Thompson M. Clinical prediction model to aid emergency doctors managing febrile children at risk of serious bacterial infections: diagnostic study. BMJ 2013;346:f1706.
11. Clinical practice guideline: asthma acute. 2019. Available from: www.rch.org.au/clinicalguide/guideline_index/Asthma_acute/.
12. Rajesh VT, Singhi S, Kataria S. Tachypnoea is a good predictor of hypoxia in acutely ill infants under 2 months. Arch Dis Child 2000;82:46–9.
13. Fleming S, Thompson M, Stevens R, Heneghan C, Plüddemann A, Maconochie I, et al. Normal ranges of heart rate and respiratory rate in children from birth to 18 years of age: a systematic review of observational studies. Lancet 2011;377:1011–18.
14. Elder JW, Baraff SB, Gaschler WN, Baraff LJ. Pulse oxygen saturation values in a healthy school-aged population. Pediatr Emerg Care 2015;31:645–7.
15. Paniagua N, Elosegi A, Duo I. Initial asthma severity assessment tools as predictors of hospitalization. J Emerg Med 2017;53:10–17.
16. Bjornson CL, Johnson DW. Croup in children. CMAJ 2013;185(15):1317–23.
17. Hewson P, Poulakis Z, Jarman F, Kerr J, McMaster D, Goodge J, et al. Clinical markers of serious illness in young infants: a multicentre follow-up study. J Paediatr Child Health 2000;36:221–5.
18. Advanced Life Support Group. Advanced Paediatric Life Support: the practical approach. 6th ed. London: Wiley-Blackwell; 2017.
19. de Vos-Kerkhof E, Krecinic T, Vergouwe Y, Moll HA, Nijman RG, Oostenbrink R. Comparison of peripheral and central capillary refill time in febrile children presenting to a paediatric emergency department and its utility in identifying children with serious bacterial infection. Arch Dis Child 2017;102:17–21.
20. Otieno H, Were E, Ahmed I. Are bedside features of shock reproducible between different observers? Arch Dis Child 2004;89:977–9.
21. Raju NV, Maisels MJ, Kring E, Schwarz-Warner L. Capillary refill time in the hands and feet of normal newborn infants. Clin Pediatr (Phila) 1999;38:139–44.
22. Tibby SM, Hatherill M, Murdoch IA. Capillary refill and core-peripheral temperature gap as indicators of haemodynamic status in paediatric intensive care patients. Arch Dis Child 1999;80:163–6.
23. Fleming S, Gill P, Jones C, Taylor JA, Van den Bruel A, Heneghan C, et al. Validity and reliability of measurement of capillary refill time in children: a systematic review. Arch Dis Child 2015;100:239–49.

24. Haque IU, Zaritsky AL. Analysis of the evidence for the lower limit of systolic and mean arterial pressure in children. Pediatr Crit Care Med 2007;8:138–44.
25. Dionne JM, Bremner SA, Baygani SK, Batton B, Ergenekon E, Bhatt-Mehta V, et al. Method of blood pressure measurement in neonates and infants: a systematic review and analysis. J Pediatr 2020;221:23–31.e5.
26. Clark JA, Lieh-Lai MW, Sarnaik A. Discrepancies between direct and indirect blood pressure measurements using various recommendations for arm cuff selection. Pediatrics 2002;110:920–3.
27. Ledbetter L. Can they or can they not? Nurses' ability to quantify stool in superabsorbent diapers. J Pediat Nurs 2006;21:325–8.
28. Holmes JF, Palchak MJ, MacFarlane T, Kuppermann N. Performance of the pediatric Glasgow Coma Scale in children with blunt head trauma. Acad Emerg Med 2005;12:814–19.
29. Morray JP, Tyler DC, Jones TK. Coma scale for use in brain-injured children. Crit Care Med 1984;12:1018–20.
30. Davis RJ. Head and spinal cord injury. Baltimore: Williams & Wilkins; 1987.
31. James H, Anas N, Perkin RM. Brain insults in infants and children. New York: Grune & Stratton; 1985.
32. Tu YF, Chuang HY, Huang CC, Chuang CC, Wang SM, Tsai MC, et al. Frequency and prediction of abnormal findings on neuroimaging of infants with bulging anterior fontanelles. Acad Emerg Med 2005;12:1185–90.
33. Cusson RM, Madonia JA, Taekman JB. The effect of environment on body site temperatures in full-term neonates. Nurs Res 1997;46:202–7.
34. Falzon A, Grech V, Caruana B. How reliable is axillary temperature measurement? Acta Paediatrica 2003;92(3):309–13.
35. Chue AL, Moore RL, Cavey A. Comparability of tympanic and oral mercury thermometers at high ambient temperatures. BMC Res Notes 2012;5:356.
36. Goldstein B, Giroir B, Randolph A, International Consensus Conference on Pediatric S. International pediatric sepsis consensus conference: definitions for sepsis and organ dysfunction in pediatrics. Pediatr Crit Care Med 2005;6:2–8.
37. Babl FE, Borland ML, Phillips N, Kochar A, Dalton S, McCaskill M, et al. Accuracy of PECARN, CATCH, and CHALICE head injury decision rules in children: a prospective cohort study. Lancet 2017;389:2393–402.
38. Tosif S, Baker A, Oakley E, Donath S, Babl FE. Contamination rates of different urine collection methods for the diagnosis of urinary tract infections in young children: an observational cohort study. J Paediatr Child Health 2012;48:659–64.
39. Monash Institute of Health Services Research. Consistency of triage in Victoria's emergency departments: literature review. Clayton, Vic: Monash Institute of Health Services Research; 2001.
40. Dieckmann RA, Brownstein D, Gausche-Hill M. The pediatric assessment triangle: a novel approach for the rapid evaluation of children. Pediatr Emerg Care 2010;26:312–15.
41. Kelly J. The Paediatric Observation Priority Score (POPS); a useful tool to predict the likelihood of admissions from the emergency department. EMJ 2013;30:877–8.
42. Acworth J, Babl F, Borland M, Ngo P, Krieser D, Schutz J, et al. Patterns of presentation to the Australian and New Zealand Paediatric Emergency Research Network. Emerg Med Australas 2009;21:59–66.
43. Milner AD, Greenough A. Applied respiratory physiology. Curr Paediat 2006;16:406–12.
44. Rojas-Reyes MX, Granados Rugeles C, Charry-Anzola LP. Oxygen therapy for lower respiratory tract infections in children between 3 months and 15 years of age. Cochrane Database Syst Rev 2014;(12):CD005975.
45. Cambridge University Hospitals. Infant with nasal cannula [image]. Available from: www.cuh.org.uk/resources/images/rosie/neonatal/nicu/how_we_care/vital_needs/nasal_cannula_131008.jpg.
46. Grauman S, Johansson J, Drevhammar T. Large variations of oxygen delivery in self-inflating resuscitation bags used for preoxygenation—a mechanical simulation. SJTREM 2021;29(1):98.
47. Blake DF, Shih EM, Mateos P. The efficacy of oxygen wafting using different delivery devices, flow rates and device positioning. Australas Emerg Nurs J 2014;17:119–25.
48. Schibler A, Franklin D. Respiratory support for children in the emergency department. J Paediatr Child Health 2016;52:192–6.
49. Taylor C, Subaiya L, Corsino D. Pediatric cuffed endotracheal tubes: an evolution of care. Ochsner J 2011;11:52–6.
50. Henning R. Assisted ventilation. Edinburgh: Churchill Livingstone; 1999.
51. Leung AK, Kellner JD, Johnson DW. Viral croup: a current perspective. J Pediatr Health Care 2004;18:297–301.
52. Rihkanen H, Ronkko E, Nieminen T, Komsi KL, Räty R, Saxen H, et al. Respiratory viruses in laryngeal croup of young children. J Pediatr 2008;152:661–5.
53. Lee DR, Lee CH, Won YK, Suh DI, Roh EJ, Lee MH, et al. Clinical characteristics of children and adolescents with croup and epiglottitis who visited 146 emergency departments in Korea. Korean J Pediatr 2015;58:380–5.
54. Gates A, Johnson DW, Klassen TP. Glucocorticoids for croup in children. JAMA Pediatr 2019;173:595–6.
55. Gates A, Gates M, Vandermeer B, Johnson C, Hartling L, Johnson DW, et al. Glucocorticoids for croup in children. Cochrane Database Syst Rev 2018;8:CD001955.
56. Parker CM, Cooper MN. Prednisolone versus dexamethasone for croup: a randomized controlled trial. Pediatrics 2019;144:e20183772.
57. Fernandes RM, Wingert A, Vandermeer B, Featherstone R, Ali S, Plint AC, et al. Safety of corticosteroids in young children with acute respiratory conditions: a systematic review and meta-analysis. BMJ Open 2019;9:e028511.

58. Dobrovoljac M, Geelhoed GC. How fast does oral dexamethasone work in mild to moderately severe croup? A randomized double-blinded clinical trial. Emerg Med Australas 2012;24:79–85.
59. Parker R, Powell CV, Kelly AM. How long does stridor at rest persist in croup after the administration of oral prednisolone? Emerg Med Australas 2004;16:135–8.
60. Bjornson C, Russell K, Vandermeer B, Klassen TP, Johnson DW. Nebulized epinephrine for croup in children. Cochrane Database Syst Rev 2013;(10): CD006619.
61. Australian Centre for Asthma Monitoring. Asthma in Australia 2011: with a focus chapter on chronic obstructive pulmonary disease. Canberra: AIHW; 2011.
62. Health M. The Health of New Zealand children: key findings of the New Zealand Health Survey 2011/12. Wellington: Ministry of Health; 2012.
63. Lai CK, Beasley R, Crane J, Foliaki S, Shah J, Weiland S, et al. Global variation in the prevalence and severity of asthma symptoms: phase three of the International Study of Asthma and Allergies in Childhood (ISAAC). Thorax 2009;64:476–83.
64. Turner S. Gene-environment interactions—what can these tell us about the relationship between asthma and allergy? Front Pediatr 2017;5:118.
65. Campbell MA, Winnall WR, Ford C. Health effects of second hand smoke for infants and children. In: Greenhalgh E, Scollo M, Winstanley M, editors. Tobacco in Australia: facts and issues. Melbourne: Cancer Council Victoria; 2021.
66. Gibson PG, Chang AB, Glasgow NJ, Holmes PW, Katelaris P, Kemp AS, et al. CICADA: Cough in children and adults: diagnosis and assessment. Australian cough guidelines summary statement. Med J Aust 2010;192:265–71.
67. Asthma acute. 2020. Online. Available from: www.rch.org.au/clinicalguide/guideline_index/Acute_asthma/.
68. Cates CJ, Welsh EJ, Rowe BH. Holding chambers (spacers) versus nebulisers for beta-agonist treatment of acute asthma. Cochrane Database Syst Rev 2013;(9):CD000052.
69. Camargo Jr CA, Spooner CH, Rowe BH. Continuous versus intermittent beta-agonists in the treatment of acute asthma. Cochrane Database Syst Rev 2003:2003(4):CD001115.
70. Travers AH, Milan SJ, Jones AP. Addition of intravenous beta2-agonists to inhaled beta2-agonists for acute asthma. Cochrane Database Syst Rev 2012;12:CD010179.
71. Starkey ES, Mulla H, Sammons HM, Pandya HC. Intravenous salbutamol for childhood asthma: evidence-based medicine? Arch Dis Child 2014;99:873–37.
72. Griffiths B, Ducharme FM. Combined inhaled anticholinergics and short-acting beta2-agonists for initial treatment of acute asthma in children. Cochrane Database Syst Rev 2013;(8):CD000060.
73. Vezina K, Chauhan BF, Ducharme FM. Inhaled anticholinergics and short-acting beta(2)-agonists versus short-acting beta2-agonists alone for children with acute asthma in hospital. Cochrane Database Syst Rev 2014;(7):CD010283.
74. Rowe BH, Spooner C, Ducharme FM, Bretzlaff JA, Bota GW. Early emergency department treatment of acute asthma with systemic corticosteroids. Cochrane Database Syst Rev 2001;(1):CD002178.
75. Edmonds ML, Milan SJ, Camargo Jr CA, Pollack CV, Rowe BH. Early use of inhaled corticosteroids in the emergency department treatment of acute asthma. Cochrane Database Syst Rev 2012;12(12):CD002308.
76. Foster SJ, Cooper MN, Oosterhof S, Borland ML. Oral prednisolone in preschool children with virus-associated wheeze: a prospective, randomised, double-blind, placebo-controlled trial. Lancet Respir Med 2018;6:97–106.
77. Craig SS, Dalziel SR, Powell CV, Graudins A, Babl FE, Lunny C. Interventions for escalation of therapy for acute exacerbations of asthma in children: an overview of Cochrane Reviews. Cochrane Database Syst Rev 2020;8(8):CD012977.
78. The Royal Children's Hospital Melbourne. Clinical practice guideline: bronchiolitis guideline. 2017. Available from: www.rch.org.au/clinicalguide/guideline_index/Bronchiolitis/.
79. Fitzgerald DA, Kilham HA. Bronchiolitis: assessment and evidence-based management. Med J Aust 2004;180:399–404.
80. Gadomski AM, Scribani MB. Bronchodilators for bronchiolitis. Cochrane Database Syst Rev 2014;(6):CD001266.
81. Hartling L, Bialy LM, Vandermeer B, Tjosvold L, Johnson DW, Plint AC, et al. Epinephrine for bronchiolitis. Cochrane Database Syst Rev 2011;(6):CD003123.
82. Fernandes RM, Bialy LM, Vandermeer B, Tjosvold L, Plint AC, Patel H, et al. Glucocorticoids for acute viral bronchiolitis in infants and young children. Cochrane Database Syst Rev 2013;(6):CD004878.
83. Ralston SL, Lieberthal AS, Meissner HC, Alverson BK, Baley JE, et al. Clinical practice guideline: the diagnosis, management, and prevention of bronchiolitis. Pediatrics 2014;134:e1474–502.
84. Badgett RG, Vindhyal M, Stirnaman JT, Gibson CM, Halaby R. A living systematic review of nebulized hypertonic saline for acute bronchiolitis in infants. JAMA Pediatr 2015;169:788–9.
85. Cunningham S, McMurray A. Observational study of two oxygen saturation targets for discharge in bronchiolitis. Arch Dis Child 2012;97:361–3.
86. Moreel L, Proesmans M. High flow nasal cannula as respiratory support in treating infant bronchiolitis: a systematic review. Eur J Pediatr 2020;179:711–18.
87. Franklin D, Babl FE, Schlapbach LJ, Oakley E, Craig S, Neutze J, et al. A randomized trial of high-flow oxygen therapy in infants with bronchiolitis. N Engl J Med 2018;378:1121–31.
88. Oakley E, Borland M, Neutze J, Acworth J, Krieser D, Dalziel S, et al. Nasogastric hydration versus intravenous hydration for infants with bronchiolitis: a randomised trial. Lancet Respir Med 2013;1:113–20.

89. Chow MY, Khandaker G, McIntyre P. Global childhood deaths from pertussis: a historical review. Clin Infect Dis 2016;63(Suppl. 4):S134–41.
90. Leuridan E, Hens N, Peeters N, de Witte L, Van der Meeren O, Van Damme P. Effect of a prepregnancy pertussis booster dose on maternal antibody titers in young infants. Pediatr Infect Dis J 2011;30:608–10.
91. Amirthalingam G, Andrews N, Campbell H, Ribeiro S, Kara E, Donegan K, et al. Effectiveness of maternal pertussis vaccination in England: an observational study. Lancet 2014;384:1521–8.
92. Niewiesk S. Maternal antibodies: clinical significance, mechanism of interference with immune responses, and possible vaccination strategies. Front Immunol 2014;5:446.
93. Quinn HE, Snelling TL, Habig A, Chiu C, Spokes PJ, McIntyre PB. Parental Tdap boosters and infant pertussis: a case-control study. Pediatrics 2014;134:713–20.
94. National Notifiable Diseases Surveillance System Annual Report Writing Group. Australia's notifiable disease status, 2014: Annual report of the National Notifiable Diseases Surveillance System Part 1. Commun Dis Intell Q Rep 2016;40(1):E48–E145.
95. Ministry of Health (New Zealand). PHONZ: Public Health Observatory NZ. 2023. Online. Available from: https://www.ehinz.ac.nz/projects/public-health-observatory-of-nz/.
96. Marshall HS, Wood N. The potential for improved protection against pertussis. Lancet Infect Dis 2020;20:1220–2.
97. Chan MH, Ma L, Sidelinger D, Yen J, Inveiss A, Sawyer MH, et al. The California pertussis epidemic 2010: a review of 986 pediatric case reports from San Diego County. J Pediatr Infect Dis Soc 2012;1:47–54.
98. Mackey JE, Wojcik S, Long R, Callahan JM, Grant WD. Predicting pertussis in a pediatric emergency department population. Clin Pediatr (Phila) 2007;46:437–40.
99. Hale S, Quinn HE, Kesson A, Wood NJ, McIntyre PB. Changing patterns of pertussis in a children's hospital in the polymerase chain reaction diagnostic era. J Pediatr 2016;170:161–5.
100. Altunaiji S, Kukuruzovic R, Curtis N, Massie J. Antibiotics for whooping cough (pertussis). Cochrane Database Syst Rev 2007;(3):CD004404.
101. Centers for Disease Control and Prevention: Pertussis (whooping cough): postexposure antimicrobial prophylaxis. 2022. Online. Available from: www.cdc.gov/pertussis/pep.html.
102. Wang K, Bettiol S, Thompson MJ, Roberts NW, Perera R, Heneghan CJ, et al. Symptomatic treatment of the cough in whooping cough. Cochrane Database Syst Rev 2014;2014:CD003257.
103. Royal Children's Hospital Melbourne. Clinical practice guideline on whooping cough. Pertussis. 2019. Available from: www.rch.org.au/clinicalguide/guideline_index/whooping_cough_pertussis/.
104. Shah SN, Bachur RG, Simel DL. Does this child have pneumonia? The rational clinical examination systematic review. JAMA 2017;318:462–71.
105. Harris M, Clark J, Coote N, Fletcher P, Harnden A, McKean M, et al. British Thoracic Society guidelines for the management of community acquired pneumonia in children: update 2011. Thorax 2011;66(Suppl. 2):1–23.
106. Chowell G, Bertozzi SM, Colchero MA, Lopez-Gatell H, Alpuche-Aranda C, Hernandez M, et al. Severe respiratory disease concurrent with the circulation of H1N1 influenza. N Engl J Med 2009;361:674–9.
107. Korppi M, Don M, Valent F, Canciani M. The value of clinical features in differentiating between viral, pneumococcal and atypical bacterial pneumonia in children. Acta Paediatr 2008;97:943–7.
108. Wang K, Gill P, Perera R, Thomson A, Mant D, Harnden A. Clinical symptoms and signs for the diagnosis of Mycoplasma pneumoniae in children and adolescents with community-acquired pneumonia. Cochrane Database Syst Rev 2012;10(10):CD009175.
109. Cho YJ, Han MS, Kim WS, Choi EH, Choi YH, Yun KW, et al. Correlation between chest radiographic findings and clinical features in hospitalized children with Mycoplasma pneumoniae pneumonia. PLoS One 2019;14(8):e0219463.
110. Kumar P, McKean MC. Evidence based paediatrics: review of BTS guidelines for the management of community acquired pneumonia in children. J Infect 2004;48:134–8.
111. Cao AM, Choy JP, Mohanakrishnan LN, Bain RF, van Driel ML. Chest radiographs for acute lower respiratory tract infections. Cochrane Database Syst Rev 2013;(12):CD009119.
112. Bielicki JA, Stohr W, Barratt S, Dunn D, Naufal N, Roland D, et al. Effect of amoxicillin dose and treatment duration on the need for antibiotic re-treatment in children with community-acquired pneumonia: the CAP-IT randomized clinical trial. JAMA 2021;326:1713–14.
113. Rojas MX, Granados C. Oral antibiotics versus parenteral antibiotics for severe pneumonia in children. Cochrane Database Syst Rev 2006;(2):CD004979.
114. Biondi E, McCulloh R, Alverson B, Klein A, Dixon A, Ralston S. Treatment of mycoplasma pneumonia: a systematic review. Pediatrics 2014;133:1081–90.
115. Chang CC, Cheng AC, Chang AB. Over-the-counter (OTC) medications to reduce cough as an adjunct to antibiotics for acute pneumonia in children and adults. Cochrane Database Syst Rev 2014;2014;(3):CD006088.
116. Daly KA, Giebink GS. Clinical epidemiology of otitis media. Pediatr Infect Dis J 2000;19:S31–6.
117. Vadlamudi NK, Saatchi A, Patrick DM, Rose C, Sadatsafavi M, Marra F. Impact of the 13-valent pneumococcal conjugate vaccine on acute otitis media and acute sinusitis epidemiology in British Columbia, Canada. J Antimicrob Chemother 2021;76:2419–27.
118. Dyke M, Pirçon J, Cohen R, Madhi SA, Rosenblüt A, Macias Parra M, et al. Etiology of acute otitis media in children less than 5 years of age: a pooled analysis of 10 similarly designed observational studies. Pediatr Infect Dis J 2017;36:274–81.

119. de Sevaux JD, Venekamp RP, Lutje V, Hak E, Schilder AG, Sanders EA, et al. Pneumococcal conjugate vaccines for preventing acute otitis media in children. Cochrane Database Syst Rev 2020;11(11):CD001480.
120. Kaur R, Morris M, Pichichero ME. Epidemiology of acute otitis media in the postpneumococcal conjugate vaccine era. Pediatrics 2017;140(3): e20170181.
121. Shaikh N, Hoberman A, Rockette HE, Kurs-Lasky M. Development of an algorithm for the diagnosis of otitis media. Acad Pediatr 2012;12:214–18.
122. Bowatte G, Tham R, Allen KJ, Lau M, Dai X, Lodge CJ. Breastfeeding and childhood acute otitis media: a systematic review and meta-analysis. Acta Paediatr 2015;104:85–95.
123. Isaacson G. Acute otitis media and the crying child. Pediatr Infect Dis J 2016;35:e399–400.
124. Sjoukes A, Venekamp RP, van de Pol AC, Hay AD, Little P, Schilder AG, et al. Paracetamol (acetaminophen) or non-steroidal anti-inflammatory drugs, alone or combined, for pain relief in acute otitis media in children. Cochrane Database Syst Rev 2016;12(12):CD011534.
125. Bolt P, Barnett P, Babl FE, Sharwood LN. Topical lignocaine for pain relief in acute otitis media: results of a double-blind placebo-controlled randomised trial. Arch Dis Child 2008;93(1):40–4.
126. Foxlee R, Johansson A, Wejfalk J, Dawkins J, Dooley L, Del Mar C. Topical analgesia for acute otitis media. Cochrane Database Syst Rev 2006;(3):CD005657.
127. Taylor SL, Papanicolas LE, Richards A, Ababor F, Kang WX, Choo JM, et al. Ear microbiota and middle ear disease: a longitudinal pilot study of Aboriginal children in a remote South Australian setting. BMC Microbiol 2022;22(1):24.
128. Leach AJ, Morris PS, Coates HL, Nelson S, O'Leary SJ, Richmond PC, et al. Otitis media guidelines for Australian Aboriginal and Torres Strait Islander children: summary of recommendations. Med J Aust 2021;214(5):228–33.
129. Venekamp RP, Sanders SL, Glasziou PP, Del Mar CB, Rovers MM. Antibiotics for acute otitis media in children. Cochrane Database Syst Rev 2015;(6):CD000219.
130. Thanaviratananich S, Laopaiboon M, Vatanasapt P. Once or twice daily versus three times daily amoxicillin with or without clavulanate for the treatment of acute otitis media. Cochrane Database Syst Rev 2013;(12):CD004975.
131. Lieberthal AS, Carroll AE, Chonmaitree T, Ganiats TG, Hoberman A, Jackson MA, et al. The diagnosis and management of acute otitis media. Pediatrics 2013;131:e964–99.
132. Rosenfeld RM, Kay D. Natural history of untreated otitis media. Laryngoscope 2003;113:1645–57.
133. van Zon A, van der Heijden GJ, van Dongen TM, Burton MJ, Schilder AG. Antibiotics for otitis media with effusion in children. Cochrane Database Syst Rev 2012;(9):CD009163.
134. Griffin G, Flynn CA. Antihistamines and/or decongestants for otitis media with effusion (OME) in children. Cochrane Database Syst Rev 2011;2011(9):CD003423.
135. Katzenellenbogen JM, Bond-Smith D, Seth RJ, Dempsey K, Cannon J, Stacey I, et al. Contemporary incidence and prevalence of rheumatic fever and rheumatic heart disease in Australia using linked data: the case for policy change. J Am Heart Assoc 2020;9:e016851.
136. Spinks A, Glasziou PP, Del Mar CB. Antibiotics for treatment of sore throat in children and adults. Cochrane Database Syst Rev 2021;12(12):CD000023.
137. Danchin MH, Rogers S, Kelpie L. Burden of acute sore throat and group A streptococcal pharyngitis in school-aged children and their families in Australia. Pediatrics 2007;120:950–7.
138. Shulman ST, Bisno AL, Clegg HW. Clinical practice guideline for the diagnosis and management of Group A streptococcal pharyngitis: 2012 update by the Infectious Diseases Society of America. Clin Infect Dis 2012;55:1279–82.
139. Danchin MH, Curtis N, Nolan TM. Treatment of sore throat in light of the Cochrane verdict: is the jury still out? MJA 2002;177:512–15.
140. Bulloch B, Kabani A, Tenenbein M. Oral dexamethasone for the treatment of pain in children with acute pharyngitis: a randomized, double-blind, placebo-controlled trial. Ann Emerg Med 2003;41:601–8.
141. Lan AJ, Colford JM, Colford Jr JM. The impact of dosing frequency on the efficacy of 10-day penicillin or amoxicillin therapy for streptococcal tonsillopharyngitis: a meta-analysis. Pediatrics 2000;105:E19.
142. de Cassan S, Thompson MJ, Perera R. Corticosteroids as standalone or add-on treatment for sore throat. Cochrane Database Syst Rev 2020;5(5):CD008268.
143. Bronicki RA, Taylor M, Baden H. Critical heart failure and shock. Pediatr Crit Care Med 2016;17:S124–30.
144. Sivarajan VB, Schwartz SM. Structure and function of the heart. In: Fuhrman BP, Zimmerman JJ, Carcillo J, editors. Pediatric critical care. 5th ed. Philadelphia: Elsevier; 2016.
145. Choi SJ, Ha EJ, Jhang WK, Park SJ. Elevated central venous pressure is associated with increased mortality in pediatric septic shock patients. BMC Pediatrics 2018;18(1):58.
146. Weiss SL, Peters MJ, Alhazzani W, Agus MSD, Flori HR, Inwald DP, et al. Surviving Sepsis Campaign International guidelines for the management of septic shock and sepsis-associated organ dysfunction in children. Pediatr Crit Care Med 2020;21(2):e52–e106.
147. Alexander PMA, Checchia PA, Ryerson LM, Bohn D, Eckerle M, Gaies M, et al. Cardiovascular dysfunction criteria in critically ill children: the PODIUM Consensus Conference. Pediatrics 2022;149:S39–47.
148. Ceneviva G, Paschall JA, Maffei F, Carcillo JA. Hemodynamic support in fluid-refractory pediatric septic shock. Pediatrics 1998;102:e19.

149. Jasso-Contreras G, Gonzalez-Velazquez F, Bello-Aguilar L, García-Carrillo A, Muñoz-Rodríguez MR, Pereda-Torales L. Lactate levels as a predictor of mortality in patients with septic shock. Rev Med Instit Mex Seguro Soc 2015;53:316–21.
150. Kim YA, Ha EJ, Jhang WK. Early blood lactate area as a prognostic marker in pediatric septic shock. Int Care Med 2013;39:1818–23.
151. Medeiros DN, Ferranti JF, Delgado AF, e Carvalho WB. Colloids for the initial management of severe sepsis and septic shock in pediatric patients: a systematic review. Pediatr Emerg Care 2015;31:e11–16.
152. Long E, Duke T. Fluid resuscitation therapy for paediatric sepsis. J Paediatr Child Health 2016;52:141–6.
153. Carcillo JA, Davis AL, Zaritsky A. Role of early fluid resuscitation in pediatric septic shock. JAMA 1991;266:1242–5.
154. Maitland K, Kiguli S, Opoka RO, Engoru C, Olupot-Olupot P, Akech SO, et al. Mortality after fluid bolus in African children with severe infection. N Engl J Med 2011;364:2483–95.
155. Gelbart B, Glassford NJ, Bellomo R. fluid bolus therapy-based resuscitation for severe sepsis in hospitalized children: a systematic review. Pediatr Crit Care Med 2015;16:e297–307.
156. Parker MJ, Thabane L, Fox-Robichaud A. A trial to determine whether septic shock-reversal is quicker in pediatric patients randomized to an early goal-directed fluid-sparing strategy versus usual care (SQUEEZE): study protocol for a pilot randomized controlled trial. Trials 2016;17(1):556.
157. Szydlowski B, Nolte J, Vershilovsky E. Recent advances in intraosseous vascular access. Curr Emerg Hosp Med Rep 2021;9:82–8.
158. Ting A, Smith K, Wilson CL, Babl FE, Hopper SM. Pre-hospital intraosseous use in children: indications and success rate. Emerg Med Australas 2022;34:120–1.
159. Rizk MY, Lapointe A, Lefebvre F, Barrington KJ. Norepinephrine infusion improves haemodynamics in the preterm infants during septic shock. Acta Paediatr 2018;107:408–13.
160. Ramaswamy KN, Singhi S, Jayashree M, Bansal A, Nallasamy K. Double-blind randomized clinical trial comparing dopamine and epinephrine in pediatric fluid-refractory hypotensive septic shock. Pediatr Crit Care Med 2016;17:e502–12.
161. Dellinger RP, Schorr CA, Levy MM. A users' guide to the 2016 Surviving Sepsis Guidelines. Int Care Med 2017;43:299–303.
162. Brierley J, Carcillo JA, Choong K, Cornell T, Decaen A, Deymann A, et al. Clinical practice parameters for hemodynamic support of pediatric and neonatal septic shock: 2007 update from the American College of Critical Care Medicine. Crit Care Med 2009;37:666–88.
163. Annane D, Bellissant E, Bollaert PE, Briegel J, Keh D, Kupfer Y. Corticosteroids for treating sepsis. Cochrane Database Syst Rev 2015;(12):CD002243.
164. Kylat RI, Ohlsson A. Recombinant human activated protein C for severe sepsis in neonates. Cochrane Database Syst Rev 2006;(2):CD005385.
165. Marti-Carvajal A, Salanti G, Cardona AF. Human recombinant activated protein C for severe sepsis. Cochrane Database Syst Rev 2008;(1):CD004388.
166. Lynch R, Wood EG, Neumayer TM. Fluid and electrolyte issues in pediatric critical illness. In: Fuhrman BP, Zimmerman JJ, Carcillo J, editors. Pediatric critical care. 5th ed. Philadelphia: Elsevier; 2016.
167. Mackenzie A, Barnes G, Shann F. Clinical signs of dehydration in children. Lancet 1989;2:605–7.
168. Porter SC, Fleisher GR, Kohane IS, Mandl KD. The value of parental report for diagnosis and management of dehydration in the emergency department. Ann Emerg Med 2003;41:196–205.
169. Gorelick MH, Shaw KN, Murphy KO. Validity and reliability of clinical signs in the diagnosis of dehydration in children. Pediatrics 1997;99:E6.
170. Falszewska A, Szajewska H, Dziechciarz P. Diagnostic accuracy of three clinical dehydration scales: a systematic review. Arch Dis Child 2018;103:383–8.
171. Goldman RD, Friedman JN, Parkin PC. Validation of the clinical dehydration scale for children with acute gastroenteritis. Pediatrics 2008;122: 545–9.
172. Vega RM, Avner JR. A prospective study of the usefulness of clinical and laboratory parameters for predicting percentage of dehydration in children. Pediatr Emerg Care 1997;13:179–82.
173. English M, Waruiru C, Mwakesi R, Marsh K. Signs of dehydration in severe childhood malaria. Trop Doct 1997;27:235–6.
174. Teach SJ, Yates EW, Feld LG. Laboratory predictors of fluid deficit in acutely dehydrated children. Clin Pediatr (Phila) 1997;36:395–400.
175. Yilmaz K, Karabocuoglu M, Citak A, Uzel N. Evaluation of laboratory tests in dehydrated children with acute gastroenteritis. J Paediatr Child Health 2002;38:226–8.
176. Steiner MJ, Nager AL, Wang VJ. Urine specific gravity and other urinary indices: inaccurate tests for dehydration. Pediatr Emerg Care 2007;23: 298–303.
177. Chen L, Hsiao A, Langhan M. Use of bedside ultrasound to assess degree of dehydration in children with gastroenteritis. Ac Emerg Med 2010;17:1042–7.
178. Levine AC, Shah SP, Umulisa I, Munyaneza RB, Dushimiyimana JM, Stegmann K, et al. Ultrasound assessment of severe dehydration in children with diarrhea and vomiting. Acad Emerg Med 2010;17:1035–41.
179. Hartling L, Bellemare S, Wiebe N. Oral versus intravenous rehydration for treating dehydration due to gastroenteritis in children. Cochrane Database Syst Rev 2006;2006(3):CD004390.
180. Hahn S, Kim S, Garner P. Reduced osmolarity oral rehydration solution for treating dehydration caused by acute diarrhoea in children. Cochrane Database Syst Rev 2002;(1):CD002847.

181. Freedman SB, Willan AR, Boutis K, Schuh S. Effect of dilute apple juice and preferred fluids vs electrolyte maintenance solution on treatment failure among children with mild gastroenteritis: a randomized clinical trial. JAMA 2016;315:1966–74.
182. Gastanaduy AS, Begue RE. Acute gastroenteritis. Clin Pediatr (Phila) 1999;38:1–12.
183. Santucci KA, Anderson AC, Lewander WJ. Frozen oral hydration as an alternative to conventional enteral fluids. Arc Pediatr Adolesc Med 1998;152:142–6.
184. Stock A, Gilbertson H, Babl FE. Confirming nasogastric tube position in the emergency department: pH testing is reliable. Pediatr Emerg Care 2008;24:805–9.
185. Clinical Practice Guidelines. Gastroenteritis. 2020. Available from: www.rch.org.au/clinicalguide/guideline_index/Gastroenteritis/.
186. Powell CV, Priestley SJ, Young S, Heine RG. Randomized clinical trial of rapid versus 24-hour rehydration for children with acute gastroenteritis. Pediatrics 2011;128:e771–8.
187. McNab S, Duke T, South M, Babl FE, Lee KJ, Arnup SJ, et al. 140 mmol/L of sodium versus 77 mmol/L of sodium in maintenance intravenous fluid therapy for children in hospital (PIMS): a randomised controlled double-blind trial. Lancet 2015;385:1190–7.
188. McNab S, Ware RS, Neville KA, Choong K, Coulthard MG, Duke T, et al. Isotonic versus hypotonic solutions for maintenance intravenous fluid administration in children. Cochrane Database Syst Rev 2014;2014;(12):CD009457.
189. Manole MD, Saladino RA. Emergency department management of the pediatric patient with supraventricular tachycardia. Pediatr Emerg Care 2007;23:176–85.
190. Campbell M, Buitrago SR. BET 2: Ice water immersion, other vagal manoeuvres or adenosine for SVT in children. Emerg Med J 2017;34:58–60.
191. Shaddy RE, George AT, Jaecklin T, Lochlainn EN, Thakur L, Agrawal R, et al. Systematic literature review on the incidence and prevalence of heart failure in children and adolescents. Pediatr Cardiol 2018;39:415–36.
192. Kirk R, Dipchand AI, Rosenthal DN, Addonizio L, Burch M, Chrisant M, et al. The International Society for Heart and Lung Transplantation Guidelines for the management of pediatric heart failure: executive summary. J Heart Lung Transpl 2014;33:888–909.
193. Hinton RB, Ware SM. Heart failure in pediatric patients with congenital heart disease. Circ Res 2017;120:978–94.
194. Masarone D, Valente F, Rubino M, Vastarella R, Gravino R, Rea A, et al. Pediatric heart failure: a practical guide to diagnosis and management. Pediatr Neonatol 2017;58:303–12.
195. Strobel AM, Lu le N. The critically ill infant with congenital heart disease. Emerg Med Clin North Am 2015;33:501–8.
196. Watanabe K, Shih R. Update of pediatric heart failure. Pediatr Clin North Am 2020;67:889–901.
197. Immunisation ATAGI. Cardiac Society of Australia and New Zealand, Royal Australian College of General Practitioners, Australian College of Rural and Remote Medicine, Australasian College for Emergency Medicine, Paediatric Research in Emergency Departments International Collaborative. Guidance on myocarditis and pericarditis after mRNA COVID-19 vaccines. Canberra: Australian Government; 2021.
198. Putschoegl A, Auerbach S. Diagnosis, evaluation, and treatment of myocarditis in children. Pediatr Clin North Am 2020;67:855–74.
199. Barcia Aguilar C, Sanchez Fernandez I, Loddenkemper T. Status epilepticus—work-up and management in children. Semin Neurol 2020;40:661–74.
200. Riviello Jr JJ, Ashwal S, Hirtz D, Glauser T, Ballaban-Gil K, Kelley K, et al. Practice parameter: diagnostic assessment of the child with status epilepticus (an evidence-based review): Report of the Quality Standards Subcommittee of the American Academy of Neurology and the Practice Committee of the Child Neurology Society. Neurology 2006;67:1542–50.
201. American Academy of Pediatrics Febrile Seizures Subcommittee. Neurodiagnostic evaluation of the child with a simple febrile seizure. Pediatrics 2011;127:389–94.
202. Lewena S, Pennington V, Acworth J, Thornton S, Ngo P, McIntyre S, et al. Emergency management of pediatric convulsive status epilepticus: a multicenter study of 542 patients. Pediatr Emerg Care 2009;25:83–7.
203. McTague A, Martland T, Appleton R. Drug management for acute tonic-clonic convulsions including convulsive status epilepticus in children. Cochrane Database Syst Rev 2018;1:CD001905.
204. Dalziel SR, Borland ML, Furyk J, Bonisch M, Neutze J, Donath S, et al. Levetiracetam versus phenytoin for second-line treatment of convulsive status epilepticus in children (ConSEPT): an open-label, multicentre, randomised controlled trial. Lancet 2019;393:2135–45.
205. Royal Children's Hospital Melbourne. Clinical practice guidelines—afebrile seizures. Management flowchart for active seizures. 2022. Available from: www.rch.org.au/clinicalguide/guideline_index/Afebrile_seizures/.
206. Seltz LB, Cohen E, Weinstein M. Risk of bacterial or herpes simplex virus meningitis/encephalitis in children with complex febrile seizures. Pediatr Emerg Care 2009;25:494–7.
207. Epstein L, Nordli D, Hamidullah A, Pellock J, Frank M, Lewis D, et al. The role of primary human herpes virus 6, 7 (HHV-6, HHV-7) infection in febrile status epilepticus. Ann Neurol. 2005;58(suppl 9):S79–S80.
208. Gidengil C, Goetz MB, Newberry S, Larkin J, Maglione M, Hall O, et al. Safety of vaccines used for routine immunization in the United States: an updated systematic review and meta-analysis. Vaccine 2021;39:3696–716.
209. Feenstra B, Pasternak B, Geller F, Carstensen L, Wang T, Huang F, et al. Common variants associated with general and MMR vaccine-related febrile seizures. Nat Genet 2014;46:1274–82.
210. Seinfeld SA, Pellock JM, Kjeldsen MJ, Nakken KO, Corey LA. Epilepsy after febrile seizures: twins suggest genetic influence. Pediatr Neurol 2016;55:14–16.

211. Norgaard M, Ehrenstein V, Mahon BE, Nielsen GL, Rothman KJ, Sørensen HT. Febrile seizures and cognitive function in young adult life: a prevalence study in Danish conscripts. J Pediatr 2009;155:404–9.

212. Neligan A, Bell GS, Giavasi C, Johnson AL, Goodridge DM, Shorvon SD, et al. Long-term risk of developing epilepsy after febrile seizures: a prospective cohort study. Neurology 2012;78:1166–70.

213. Hashimoto R, Suto M, Tsuji M, Sasaki H, Takehara K, Ishiguro A, et al. Use of antipyretics for preventing febrile seizure recurrence in children: a systematic review and meta-analysis. Europ J Pediatr 2021;180:987–97.

214. Offringa M, Newton R, Nevitt SJ, Vraka K. Prophylactic drug management for febrile seizures in children. Cochrane Database Syst Rev 2021;6: CD003031.

215. Pennington K. Enhanced Invasive Pneumococcal Disease Surveillance Working Group, Communicable Diseases Network Australia. Invasive pneumococcal disease surveillance, 1 July to 30 September 2019. Commun Dis Intell 2020;44. doi:10.33321/cdi.2020.44.40.

216. Peltola H, Roine I, Kallio M, Pelkonen T. Outcome of childhood bacterial meningitis on three continents. Sci Rep 2021;11:21593.

217. Bilavsky E, Leibovitz E, Elkon-Tamir E. The diagnostic accuracy of the 'classic meningeal signs' in children with suspected bacterial meningitis. Eur J Emerg Med 2013;20:361–3.

218. April MD, Long B, Koyfman A. Emergency medicine myths: computed tomography of the head prior to lumbar puncture in adults with suspected bacterial meningitis - due diligence or antiquated practice? J Emerg Med 2017;53:313–21.

219. Lahra MM, Hogan TR. Australian Meningococcal Surveillance Programme annual report, 2019. Comm Dis Intell 2018;2020;44.

220. Maconochie IK, Bhaumik S. Fluid therapy for acute bacterial meningitis. Cochrane Database Syst Rev 2016;11:CD004786.

221. Brouwer MC, McIntyre P, Prasad K, van de Beek D. Corticosteroids for acute bacterial meningitis. Cochrane Database Syst Rev 2015;(9): CD004405.

222. Hall GV, Kirk MD, Ashbolt R, Stafford R, Lalor K. Frequency of infectious gastrointestinal illness in Australia, 2002: regional, seasonal and demographic variation. Epidemiol Infect 2006;134:111–18.

223. Mihala G, Grimwood K, Morley C, Lambert SB, Ware RS. Effect of definitions of acute gastroenteritis episodes using symptom diaries in paediatric cohorts: a systematic review. J Pediatr Gastroenterol Nutrit 2020;70(3):e54–8.

224. Mihala G, Grimwood K, Lambert SB, Ware RS. Community-level burden of acute diarrhoeal illness in the first 2 years of life in Brisbane, Australia: a birth cohort study. J Paediatr Child Health 2021;57(1):140–6.

225. Xie J, Nettel-Aguirre A, Lee BE, Chui L, Pang XL, Zhuo R, et al. Relationship between enteric pathogens and acute gastroenteritis disease severity: a prospective cohort study. Clin Microbiol Infect 2019;25:454–61.

226. Guarino A, Ashkenazi S, Gendrel D, Lo Vecchio A, Shamir R, Szajewska H, et al. European Society for Pediatric Gastroenterology, Hepatology, and Nutrition/European Society for Pediatric Infectious Diseases evidence-based guidelines for the management of acute gastroenteritis in children in Europe: update 2014. J Pediatr Gastroenterol Nutr 2014;59:132–52.

227. Carson RA, Mudd SS, Madati PJ. Evaluation of a nurse-initiated acute gastroenteritis pathway in the pediatric emergency department. J Emerg Nurs 2017;43:406–12.

228. Hendrickson MA, Zaremba J, Wey AR, Gaillard PR, Kharbanda AB. The use of a triage-based protocol for oral rehydration in a pediatric emergency department. Pediatr Emerg Care 2018;34:227–32.

229. MacGillivray S, Fahey T, McGuire W. Lactose avoidance for young children with acute diarrhoea. Cochrane Database Syst Rev 2013;(10):CD005433.

230. Nino-Serna LF, Acosta-Reyes J, Veroniki AA, Florez ID. Antiemetics in children with acute gastroenteritis: a meta-analysis. Pediatrics 2020;145(4):e20193260.

231. Hyams JS, Lorenzo C, Saps M, Shulman RJ, Staiano A, van Tilburg M. Childhood functional gastrointestinal disorders: child/adolescent. Gastroenterology 2016:S0016-5085(16)00181-5.

232. Southwell BR. Treatment of childhood constipation: a synthesis of systematic reviews and meta-analyses. Expert Rev Gastroenterol Hepatol 2020;14:163–74.

233. Magnúsdóttir MB, Róbertsson V, Þorgrímsson S, Rósmundsson Þ, Agnarsson Ú, Haraldsson Á. Abdominal pain is a common and recurring problem in paediatric emergency departments. Acta Paediatrica 2019;108:1905–10.

234. Beasley S. Abdominal pain and vomiting in children. In: Roberton DM, South M, editors. Practical paediatrics. Edinburgh: Churchill Livingstone; 2007.

235. Mandeville K, Chien M, Willyerd FA, Mandell G, Hostetler MA, Bulloch B. Intussusception: clinical presentations and imaging characteristics. Pediatr Emerg Care 2012;28:842–4.

236. Yoo IH, Kang HM, Jeong DC. Changes in the incidence of intussusception and infectious diseases after the COVID-19 pandemic in Korea. J Korean Med Sci 2022;37:e60.

237. Soares-Weiser K, Maclehose H, Bergman H. Vaccines for preventing rotavirus diarrhoea: vaccines in use. Cochrane Database Syst Rev 2012;11:CD008521.

238. Das MK, Arora NK, Mathai J, Sam CJ, Arunachalam P, Gupta B, et al. Profile and epidemiology of intussusception in children under-two years of age: a prospective surveillance. Indian J Pediatr 2021;88:1187–94.

239. Li XZ, Wang H, Song J, Liu Y, Lin YQ, Sun ZX. Ultrasonographic diagnosis of intussusception in children: a systematic review and meta-analysis. J Ultrasound Med 2021;40:1077–84.

240. Gluckman S, Karpelowsky J, Webster AC, McGee RG. Management for intussusception in children. Cochrane Database Syst Rev 2017;6:CD006476.
241. Yau A, Cha R, Jayaratnam S, Wilson T, Kukkady A, Evans SM, et al. Declining incidence of pyloric stenosis in New Zealand. ANZ J Surg 2019;89:1242–5.
242. Zhu J, Zhu T, Lin Z, Qu Y, Mu D. Perinatal risk factors for infantile hypertrophic pyloric stenosis: a meta-analysis. J Pediatr Surg 2017;52:1389–97.
243. Vinycomb TI, Laslett K, Gwini SM, Teague W, Nataraja RM. Presentation and outcomes in hypertrophic pyloric stenosis: an 11-year review. J Paediatr Child Health 2019;55:1183–7.
244. de Laffolie J, Turial S, Heckmann M. Decline in infantile hypertrophic pyloric stenosis in Germany in 2000–2008. Comp Stud 2012;129(4):e901–6.
245. MJPr HS. Pyloric stenosis: role of imaging. Pediatr Radiol 2009;39:134–9.
246. Dalton BG, Gonzalez KW, Boda SR, Thomas PG, Sherman AK, St Peter SD. Optimizing fluid resuscitation in hypertrophic pyloric stenosis. J Pediatr Surg 2016;51:1279–82.
247. Chang SJ, Chen JY, Hsu CK, Chuang FC, Yang SS. The incidence of inguinal hernia and associated risk factors of incarceration in pediatric inguinal hernia: a nation-wide longitudinal population-based study. Hernia 2016;20:559–63.
248. Olesen CS, Mortensen LQ, Oberg S, Rosenberg J. Risk of incarceration in children with inguinal hernia: a systematic review. Hernia 2019;23:245–54.
249. Zens T, Nichol PF, Cartmill R, Kohler JE. Management of asymptomatic pediatric umbilical hernias: a systematic review. J Pediatr Surg 2017;52:1723–31.
250. Phillips R, Orchard D, Starr M. Dermatology. In: Cameron P, Jelinlek G, Everitt I, editors. Textbook of paediatric emergency medicine. Edinburgh: Churchill Livingstone; 2012.
251. Abdalla T, Hendrick D, Fathima P, Walker R, Blyth CC, Carapetis JR, et al. Hospital admissions for skin infections among Western Australian children and adolescents from 1996 to 2012. PLoS One 2017;12(11):e0188803.
252. Raff AB, Kroshinsky D. Cellulitis: a review. JAMA 2016;316:325–37.
253. Koning S, van der Sande R, Verhagen AP, van Suijlekom-Smit LW, Morris AD, Butler CC, et al. Interventions for impetigo. Cochrane Database Syst Rev 2012;1:CD003261.
254. Ibrahim LF, Huang L, Hopper SM, Dalziel K, Babl FE, Bryant PA. Intravenous ceftriaxone at home versus intravenous flucloxacillin in hospital for children with cellulitis: a cost-effectiveness analysis. Lancet Infect Dis 2019;19:1101–8.
255. Romani L, Steer AC, Whitfeld MJ, Kaldor JM. Prevalence of scabies and impetigo worldwide: a systematic review. Lancet Infect Dis 2015;15:960–7.
256. Weidinger S, Novak N. Atopic dermatitis. Lancet 2016;387:1109–22.
257. von Kobyletzki LB, Thomas KS, Schmitt J, Chalmers JR, Deckert S, Aoki V, et al. What factors are important to patients when assessing treatment response: an international cross-sectional survey. Acta Derm Venereol 2017;97(1):86–90.
258. Schmitt J, Langan S, Deckert S, Svensson A, von Kobyletzki L, Thomas K, et al. Assessment of clinical signs of atopic dermatitis: a systematic review and recommendation. J Allergy Clin Immunol 2013;132:1337–47.
259. Cardona ID, Kempe E, Hatzenbeuhler JR, Antaya RJ, Cohen B, Jain N. Bathing frequency recommendations for children with atopic dermatitis: results of three observational pilot surveys. Pediatr Dermatol 2015;32:e194–6.
260. Chopra R, Vakharia PP, Sacotte R, Silverberg JI. Efficacy of bleach baths in reducing severity of atopic dermatitis: a systematic review and meta-analysis. Ann Allergy Asthma Immunol 2017;119:435–40.
261. Li AW, Yin ES, Antaya RJ. Topical corticosteroid phobia in atopic dermatitis: a systematic review. JAMA Dermatol 2017;153:1036–42.
262. Callen J, Chamlin S, Eichenfield LF, Ellis C, Girardi M, Goldfarb M, et al. A systematic review of the safety of topical therapies for atopic dermatitis. Br J Dermatol 2007;156:203–21.
263. Cury Martins J, Martins C, Aoki V, Gois AF, Ishii HA, da Silva EM. Topical tacrolimus for atopic dermatitis. Cochrane Database Syst Rev 2015;2015:CD009864.
264. Devillers AC, Oranje AP. Efficacy and safety of 'wet-wrap' dressings as an intervention treatment in children with severe and/or refractory atopic dermatitis: a critical review of the literature. Br J Dermatol 2006;154:579–85.
265. Matterne U, Böhmer MM, Weisshaar E, Jupiter A, Carter B, Apfelbacher CJ. Oral H1 antihistamines as 'add-on' therapy to topical treatment for eczema. Cochrane Database Syst Rev 2019;1(1):CD012167.
266. Moore EJ, Williams A, Manias E, Varigos G, Donath S. Eczema workshops reduce severity of childhood atopic eczema. Australas J Dermatol 2009;50:100–6.
267. Zuberbier T, Aberer W, Asero R, Abdul Latiff AH, Baker D, Ballmer-Weber B, et al. The EAACI/GA(2)LEN/EDF/WAO guideline for the definition, classification, diagnosis and management of urticaria. Allergy 2018;73:1393–414.
268. Vermillet AQ, Tølbøll K, Litsis Mizan S, Skewes J, Parsons CE. Crying in the first 12 months of life: a systematic review and meta-analysis of cross-country parent-reported data and modeling of the 'cry curve'. Child Dev 2022;93:1201–22.
269. Freedman SB, Al-Harthy N, Thull-Freedman J. The crying infant: diagnostic testing and frequency of serious underlying disease. Pediatrics 2009;123:841–8.
270. Reijneveld SA, van der Wal MF, Brugman E, Sing RA, Verloove-Vanhorick SP. Infant crying and abuse. Lancet 2004;364:1340–2.
271. Sung V. Infantile colic. Aust Prescr 2018;41:105–10.

272. Evanoo G. Infant crying: a clinical conundrum. J Pediatr Health Care 2007;21:333–8.
273. Olusanya BO, Kaplan M, Hansen TWR. Neonatal hyperbilirubinaemia: a global perspective. Lancet Child Adolesc Health 2018;2:610–20.
274. Khan A, Kim TY. Neonatal hyperbilirubinemia: recommendations for diagnosis and management in the emergency department. Pediatr Emerg Med Pract 2022;19:1–24.
275. Amos RC, Jacob H, Leith W. Jaundice in newborn babies under 28 days: NICE guideline 2016 (CG98). Archives of Disease in Childhood-Education and Practice. 2017;102(4):207–9.
276. Clericetti CM, Milani GP, Bianchetti MG, Simonetti GD, Fossali EF, Balestra AM, et al. Systematic review finds that fever phobia is a worldwide issue among caregivers and healthcare providers. Acta Paediatrica 2019;108:1393–7.
277. Gaffney GR, Bereznicki LR, Bereznicki BJ. Knowledge, beliefs and management of childhood fever among nurses and other health professionals: a cross-sectional survey. Nurse Educ Today 2021;97:104731.
278. MacMahon D, Brabyn C, Dalziel SR, McKinlay CJ, Tan E. Fever phobia in caregivers presenting to New Zealand emergency departments. Emerg Med Australas 2021;33:1074–81.
279. Theodosiou AA, Mashumba F, Flatt A. Excluding clinically significant bacteremia by 24 hours in otherwise well febrile children younger than 16 years: a study of more than 50,000 blood cultures. Pediatr Infect Dis J 2019;38(9):e203–8.
280. Gelernter R, Ophir N, Goldman M, Lazarovitch Z, Gamsu S, Oren-Amit A, et al. Fever response to ibuprofen in viral and bacterial childhood infections. Am J Emerg Med 2021;46:591–4.
281. Rosenfeld-Yehoshua N, Barkan S, Abu-Kishk I, Booch M, Suhami R, Kozer E. Hyperpyrexia and high fever as a predictor for serious bacterial infection (SBI) in children-a systematic review. Euro J Pediatr 2018;177:337–44.
282. Davis J, Lehman E. Fever characteristics and risk of serious bacterial infection in febrile infants. J Emerg Med 2019;57:306–13.
283. Gangoiti I, Zubizarreta A, Elgoibar B, Mintegi S. Occult bacteremia in young children with very high fever without a source: a multicenter study. Pediatr Infect Dis J 2020;39:e462–4.
284. Russell FM, Shann F, Curtis N. Evidence on the use of paracetamol in febrile children. Bull WHO 2003;81:367–72.
285. Tan E, Braithwaite I, McKinlay CJD, Dalziel S. Comparison of acetaminophen (paracetamol) with ibuprofen for treatment of fever or pain in children younger than 2 years: a systematic review and meta-analysis. JAMA Netw Open 2020;3(10):e2022398.
286. Wong T, Stang AS, Ganshorn H, Hartling L, Maconochie IK, Thomsen AM, et al. Combined and alternating paracetamol and ibuprofen therapy for febrile children. Cochrane Database Syst Rev 2013;2013(10):CD009572.
287. Sullivan JE, Farrar HC. Fever and antipyretic use in children. Pediatrics 2011;127:580–7.
288. Alves JG, Almeida ND, Almeida CD. Tepid sponging plus dipyrone versus dipyrone alone for reducing body temperature in febrile children. Sao Paulo Med J 2008;126:107–11.
289. Thomas S, Vijaykumar C, Naik R. Comparative effectiveness of tepid sponging and antipyretic drug versus only antipyretic drug in the management of fever among children: a randomized controlled trial. Ind Pediatr 2009;46:133–6.
290. Clinical Practice Guidelines: febrile child. 2022. Available from: www.rch.org.au/clinicalguide/guideline_index/Febrile_child/.
291. Dahmash DT, Shariff ZB, Kirby DJ, Terry D, Huynh C. Literature review of medication administration problems in paediatrics by parent/caregiver and the role of health literacy. BMJ Paediatr Open 2020;4(1):e000841.
292. Simon HK, Weinkle DA. Over-the-counter medications. Do parents give what they intend to give? Arch Pediatr Adolesc Med 1997;151:654–6.
293. Lystad RP, Curtis K, Soundappan SSV, Mitchell R. Trends of traumatic spinal injury-related hospitalizations in Australian children over a 10-year period: a nationwide population-based cohort study. Spine J 2020;20:896–904.
294. Leonard JC, Jaffe DM, Olsen CS, Kuppermann N. Age-related differences in factors associated with cervical spine injuries in children. Acad Emerg Med 2015;22:441–6.
295. Hood N, Considine J. Spinal immobilisation in pre-hospital and emergency care: a systematic review of the literature. Australas Emerg Nurs J 2015;18:118–37.
296. Australian and New Zealand Resuscitation Council. ANZCOR guideline 9.1.6 – management of suspected spinal injury. Melbourne: ANZCOR; 2016.
297. Slaar A, Fockens MM, Wang J, Maas M, Wilson DJ, Goslings JC, et al. Triage tools for detecting cervical spine injury in pediatric trauma patients. Cochrane Database Syst Rev 2017;12(12):CD011686.
298. Chung S, Mikrogianakis A, Wales PW, Dirks P, Shroff M, Singhal A, et al. Trauma association of Canada Pediatric Subcommittee National Pediatric Cervical Spine Evaluation Pathway: consensus guidelines. J Trauma 2011;70:873–84.
299. National Clinical Guideline Centre (UK). Spinal injury: assessment and initial management. London. National Institute for Health and Care Excellence (NICE); 2016.
300. Hopper SM, McKenna S, Williams A, Paediatric Research in Emergency Departments International Collaborative (PREDICT). Clinical clearance and imaging for possible cervical spine injury in children in the emergency department: a retrospective cohort study. Emerg Med Australas 2020;32:93–9.
301. Babl FE, Tavender E, Ballard DW, Borland ML, Oakley E, Cotterell E, et al. Australian and New Zealand guideline for mild to moderate head injuries in children. Emerg Med Australas 2021;33:214–31.
302. Lewis SR, Evans DJ, Butler AR, Schofield-Robinson OJ, Alderson P. Hypothermia for traumatic brain injury. Cochrane Database Syst Rev 2017;9(9):CD001048.

303. McCrory P, Meeuwisse W, Dvořák J, Aubry M, Bailes J, Broglio S, et al. Consensus statement on concussion in sport-the 5th international conference on concussion in sport held in 2016; Br J Sp Med 2017;51(11):838–47.

304. Rivara FP, Tennyson R, Mills B, Browd SR, Emery CA, Gioia G, et al. Consensus statement on sports-related concussions in youth sports using a modified Delphi approach. JAMA Pediatr 2020;174:79–85.

305. Davis GA, Thurairatnam S, Feleggakis P, Anderson V, Bressan S, Babl FE. HeadCheck: a concussion app. J Paediatr Child Health 2015;51:830–31.

306. Netherton S, Milenkovic V, Taylor M, Davis PJ. Diagnostic accuracy of eFAST in the trauma patient: a systematic review and meta-analysis. CJEM 2019;21:727-38.

307. Holmes JF, Kelley KM, Wootton-Gorges SL. Effect of abdominal ultrasound on clinical care, outcomes, and resource use among children with blunt torso trauma: a randomized clinical trial. JAMA 2017;317:2290–6.

308. Dodgion CM, Gosain A, Rogers A, St Peter SD, Nichol PF, Ostlie DJ. National trends in pediatric blunt spleen and liver injury management and potential benefits of an abbreviated bed rest protocol. J Pediatr Surg 2014;49:1004–8.

309. Notrica DM. Pediatric blunt abdominal trauma: current management. Curr Opin Crit Care 2015;21:531–7.

310. MSD Manual professional version. Copyright 2023. Merck & Co. Inc. Rahway, NJ, USA and its affiliates. All rights reserved. Online: Available from: www.msdmanuals.com/professional/injuries-poisoning/fractures/pediatric-physeal-growth-plate-fractures.

311. Dowling S, Spooner CH, Liang Y, Dryden DM, Friesen C, Klassen TP, et al. Accuracy of Ottawa Ankle Rules to exclude fractures of the ankle and midfoot in children: a meta-analysis. Acad Emerg Med 2009;16:277–87.

312. Lee SH, Yun SJ. Diagnostic performance of ultrasonography for detection of pediatric elbow fracture: a meta-analysis. Ann Emerg Med 2019;74:493–502.

313. Laine JC, Kaiser SP, Diab M. High-risk pediatric orthopedic pitfalls. Emerg Med Clin North Am 2010;28:85–102, viii.

314. Fitzgerald E, Mannion J, Boran S. Management of 'torus' or 'buckle' fractures of the distal radius: a systematic review. Ir J Med Sci 2021;22:1–8.

315. Oakley E, Barnett P, Babl FE. Backslab versus nonbackslab for immobilization of undisplaced supracondylar fractures: a randomized trial. Pediatr Emerg Care 2009;25:452–6.

316. Macias CG, Bothner J, Wiebe R. A comparison of supination/flexion to hyperpronation in the reduction of radial head subluxations. Pediatrics 1998;102:e10.

317. Krul M, van der Wouden JC, van Suijlekom-Smit LW, Koes BW. Manipulative interventions for reducing pulled elbow in young children. Cochrane Database Syst Rev 2012;1(1):CD007759.

318. Dunbar JS, Owen HF, Nogrady MB, Mcleese R. Obscure tibial fracture of infants—the toddler's fracture. J Can Assoc Radiol 1964;15:136–44.

319. Irfan A, Rose A, Roberts B, Foster S, Huntley JS. Epidemiology of irritable hip in western Scotland: a follow-up study. Cureus 2020;12:e10036.

320. Tu J, Gowdie P, Cassar J, Craig S. Test characteristics of history, examination and investigations in the evaluation for septic arthritis in the child presenting with acute non-traumatic limp. A systematic review. BMJ Open 2020;10:e038088.

321. Plumb J, Mallin M, Bolte RG. The role of ultrasound in the emergency department evaluation of the acutely painful pediatric hip. Pediatr Emerg Care 2015;31:54–58.

322. Asche SS, Rijn RM, Bessems JH. What is the clinical course of transient synovitis in children: a systematic review of the literature. Chiro Man Ther 2013;21(1):39.

323. Kermond S, Fink M, Graham K. A randomized clinical trial: should the child with transient synovitis of the hip be treated with nonsteroidal anti-inflammatory drugs? Ann Emerg Med 2002;40:294–9.

324. Halsey MF, Finzel KC, Carrion WV, Haralabatos SS, Gruber MA, Meinhard BP. Toddler's fracture: presumptive diagnosis and treatment. J Pediatr Orthop 2001;21:152–6.

325. Pelayo SL, Fernandez JR, Carbello, MTL Rubio Lorenzo M, García Alfaro MD, Arbona Jiménez C. Current diagnosis and management of toddler's fracture. Ann Pediatr 2020;92(5):262–7.

326. Foltran F, Ballali S, Passali FM, Kern E, Morra B, Passali GC, et al. Foreign bodies in the airways: a meta-analysis of published papers. Int J Pediatr Otorhinolaryngol 2012;76(Suppl. 1):S12–19.

327. Green SS. Ingested and aspirated foreign bodies. Pediatr Rev 2015;36:430–6.

328. Australian and New Zealand Resuscitation Council. ANZCOR guideline 4 – airway. Melbourne: ANZCOR; 2021.

329. Orsagh-Yentis D, McAdams RJ, Roberts KJ, McKenzie LB. Foreign-body ingestions of young children treated in US emergency departments: 1995–2015. Pediatrics 2019;143:e20181988.

330. Lee JH. Foreign body ingestion in children. Clin Endosc 2018;51:129–36.

331. Altokhais T. Magnet ingestion in children management guidelines and prevention. Front Pediatr 2021;9:727988.

332. Bauman B, McEachron K, Goldman D, Louiselle A, Zheng E, Mills D, et al. Emergency management of the ingested magnet: an algorithmic approach. Pediatr Emerg Care 2019;35:e141–4.

333. Sajid T, Shah MI, Qamar Naqvi SR. Pattern of presentation of nasal foreign bodies, an experience with 155 patients. J Ayub Med Coll Abbottabad 2018;30:548–50.

334. Handbook of Non Drug Intervention Project T, Glasziou P, Bennett J, Greenberg P, Green S, Gunn J, et al. Mother's kiss for nasal foreign bodies. Aust Fam Physician 2013;42:288–9.

335. Kalan A, Tariq M. Foreign bodies in the nasal cavities: a comprehensive review of the aetiology, diagnostic pointers, and therapeutic measures. Postgrad Med J 2000;76:484–7.

336. Prasad N, Harley E. The aural foreign body space: a review of pediatric ear foreign bodies and a management paradigm. Int J Pediatr Otorhinolaryngol 2020;132:109871.

337. Schug S, Palmer G, Scott D. Working Group of the Australian and New Zealand College of Anaesthetists and Faculty of Pain Medicine. Acute pain management: scientific evidence. 5th ed. Melbourne: ANZCA & FPM; 2020.

338. Wong-Baker FACES® Pain Rating Scale. 2018. Available from: www.WongBakerFACES.org.

339. Tomlinson D, von Baeyer CL, Stinson JN, Sung L. A systematic review of faces scales for the self-report of pain intensity in children. Pediatrics 2010;126:e1168–98.

340. von Baeyer CL, Chambers CT, Forsyth SJ, Eisen S, Parker JA. Developmental data supporting simplification of self-report pain scales for preschool-age children. J Pain 2013;14:1116–21.

341. Merkel SI, Voepel-Lewis T, Shayevitz JR, Malviya S. The FLACC: a behavioral scale for scoring postoperative pain in young children. Pediatr Nurs 1997;23:293–7.

342. Crellin DJ, Harrison D, Santamaria N, Huque H, Babl FE. The psychometric properties of the FLACC scale used to assess procedural pain. J Pain 2018;19:862–72.

343. Malviya S, Voepel-Lewis T, Tait AR, Merkel S, Tremper K, Naughton N. Depth of sedation in children undergoing computed tomography: validity and reliability of the University of Michigan Sedation Scale (UMSS). Br J Anaesth 2002;88:241–5.

344. Malviya S, Voepel-Lewis T, Tait AR. A comparison of observational and objective measures to differentiate depth of sedation in children from birth to 18 years of age. Anesth Analg 2006;102:389–94.

345. Herd D, Borland M. Intranasal fentanyl paediatric clinical practice guidelines. Emerg Med Australas 2009;21:335.

346. Setlur A, Friedland H. Treatment of pain with intranasal fentanyl in pediatric patients in an acute care setting: a systematic review. Pain Manag 2018;8:341–52.

347. Abebe Y, Hetmann F, Sumera K, Holland M, Staff T. The effectiveness and safety of paediatric prehospital pain management: a systematic review. Scand J Trauma Resusc Emerg Med 2021;29:170.

348. Murphy AP, Hughes M, McCoy S, Crispino G, Wakai A, O'Sullivan R. Intranasal fentanyl for the prehospital management of acute pain in children. Eur J Emerg Med 2017;24:450–4.

349. Whitley GA, Pilbery R. Pre-hospital intranasal analgesia for children suffering pain: a rapid evidence review. Br Paramed J 2019;4:24–34.

350. Hopper SM, Babl FE, McCarthy M, Tancharoen C, Lee KJ, Oakley E. A double blind, randomised placebo controlled trial of topical 2% viscous lidocaine in improving oral intake in children with painful infectious mouth conditions. BMC Pediatr 2011;11:106.

351. Hoeffe J, Doyon Trottier E, Bailey B, Shellshear D, Lagacé M, Sutter C, et al. Intranasal fentanyl and inhaled nitrous oxide for fracture reduction: the FAN observational study. Am J Emerg Med 2017;35:710–15.

352. Miguez MC, Ferrero C, Rivas A, Lorente J, Muñoz L, Marañón R. Retrospective comparison of intranasal fentanyl and inhaled nitrous oxide to intravenous ketamine and midazolam for painful orthopedic procedures in a pediatric emergency department. Pediatr Emerg Care 2021;37:e136–40.

353. Seiler M, Staubli G, Landolt MA. Combined nitrous oxide 70% with intranasal fentanyl for procedural analgosedation in children: a prospective, randomised, double-blind, placebo-controlled trial. Emerg Med J 2019;36:142–7.

354. Borland M, Esson A, Babl F, Krieser D. Procedural sedation in children in the emergency department: a PREDICT study. Emerg Med Australas 2009;21:71–9.

355. Annequin D, Carbajal R, Chauvin P, Gall O, Tourniaire B, Murat I. Fixed 50% nitrous oxide oxygen mixture for painful procedures: a French survey. Pediatrics 2000;105:E47.

356. Babl FE, Oakley E, Seaman C, Barnett P, Sharwood LN. High-concentration nitrous oxide for procedural sedation in children: adverse events and depth of sedation. Pediatrics 2008;121:e528–32.

357. Babl FE, Oakley E, Sharwood LN. The utility of nitrous oxide. Emerg Med J 2009;26:544–5.

358. Frampton A, Browne GJ, Lam LT. Nurse administered relative analgesia using high concentration nitrous oxide to facilitate minor procedures in children in an emergency department. Emerg Med J 2003;20:410–3.

359. Zier JL, Kvam KA, Kurachek SC. Sedation with nitrous oxide compared with no sedation during catheterization for urologic imaging in children. Pediatr Radiol 2007;37:678–84.

360. Jamal D, Powell C. Paediatric procedural sedation in the emergency department: is ketamine safe? Arch Dis Child Educ Pract Ed 2021;106:120–4.

361. Ramaswamy P, Babl FE, Deasy C, Sharwood LN. Pediatric procedural sedation with ketamine: time to discharge after intramuscular versus intravenous administration. Acad Emerg Med 2009;16:101–7.

362. Pywell A, Xyrichis A. Does topical Amethocaine cream increase first-time successful cannulation in children compared with a eutectic mixture of local anaesthetics (EMLA) cream? A systematic review and meta-analysis of randomised controlled trials. Emerg Med J 2015;32:733–7.

363. Lor YC, Shih PC, Chen HH, Liu SJ, Chao HC, Hwang LC, et al. The application of lidocaine to alleviate the discomfort of nasogastric tube insertion: a systematic review and meta-analysis. Medicine (Baltimore) 2018;97:e9746.

364. Babl FE, Mandrawa C, O'Sullivan R. Procedural pain and distress in young children as perceived by medical and nursing staff. Paediatr Anaesthes 2008;18:412–19.

365. Babl FE, Goldfinch C, Mandrawa C. Does nebulized lidocaine reduce the pain and distress of nasogastric tube insertion in young children? A randomized, double-blind, placebo-controlled trial. Pediatrics 2009;123:1548–55.

366. Craig SS, Seith RW, Cheek JA, Wilson K, Egerton-Warburton D, Paul E, et al. Lidocaine and phenylephrine versus saline placebo nasal spray for the pain and distress of nasogastric tube insertion in young children and infants: a randomised, double-blind, controlled trial. Lancet Child Adolesc Health 2019;3:391–7.

367. Uman LS, Chambers CT, McGrath PJ, Kisely S. Psychological interventions for needle-related procedural pain and distress in children and adolescents. Cochrane Database Syst Rev 2006;(4):CD005179.

368. Sinha M, Christopher NC, Fenn R, Reeves L. Evaluation of nonpharmacologic methods of pain and anxiety management for laceration repair in the pediatric emergency department. Pediatrics 2006;117:1162–8.

369. Arane K, Behboudi A, Goldman RD. Virtual reality for pain and anxiety management in children. Can Fam Physician 2017;63:932–4.

370. Garrett B, Taverner T, Masinde W. A rapid evidence assessment of immersive virtual reality as an adjunct therapy in acute pain management in clinical practice. Clin J Pain 2014;30:1089–8.

371. Stevens B, Yamada J, Ohlsson A, Haliburton S, Shorkey A. Sucrose for analgesia in newborn infants undergoing painful procedures. Cochrane Database Syst Rev 2016;7:CD001069.

CHAPTER 36
MENTAL HEALTH EMERGENCIES

MICHAEL A. ROCHE, TIM WAND, LISA CLEGG AND KATE EMOND

ESSENTIALS

- Incorporate the needs of individuals and their family/carers into clinically informed responses. People experiencing mental health concerns have better outcomes when clinical judgement is combined with the 'voice' of the individual and their family/carers.
- Seek help from specialist mental health/drug and alcohol workers to intervene early to prevent an escalation of crisis or recurrence of mental illness.
- Provide a positive, supportive response without further increasing the risk of stigmatising mental illness or enforcing excessive surveillance and scrutiny, which may increase distress and further alienate the individual.
- Undertake a thorough mental health assessment with all individuals experiencing mental health problems/mental illness. Active engagement with the individual, carers and other emergency personnel will help ensure that a comprehensive assessment is possible.
- Continue to conduct regular observations and communicate with the individual, ensuring that their concerns are listened to.
- Use an accredited interpreter whenever assessing a person who does not speak English. Non-accredited interpreters (such as family members and friends) should only be used in cases of extreme emergency.
- Be alert to the dangers of self-interest when working with a person who is acutely mentally unwell. Seek help and assistance and make decisions as a team. This is not the time to be a hero.

INTRODUCTION

This chapter aims to equip practitioners with information, practical strategies and suggestions for responding to people experiencing mental health challenges outside of hospital and on arrival at an emergency department (ED). The focus in this chapter is on common mental health presentations encountered by emergency staff, such as anxiety and panic, suicide and self-harm, depression, psychosis, toxicology and substance-related issues. Legal aspects are also addressed with consideration to mitigating restrictive practices in the context of promoting trauma responsive care. This chapter highlights the importance of interprofessional collaboration and the prevention of communication breakdown between individual practitioners and organisations.

BACKGROUND

Mental health is a growing national concern across Australia and Aotearoa New Zealand. Mental problems and substance use problems contributed 12% of Australia's total 'burden of disease' in 2015, making it the fourth highest group contributing to total burden. Of the total burden caused by mental conditions and substance use conditions, 98% was due to living with the effects of these conditions.[1] Mental and substance use challenges were the second highest group contributing to non-fatal burden (23%) after the first-ranked musculoskeletal conditions (25%).

The National Health Survey 2017–18[2] estimated that:

- 1 in 5 (20%, or 4.8 million) Australians reported that they had a mental health or behavioural condition during the collection period (July 2017 to June 2018)
- overall, 15–24-year-olds had the highest proportion of mental or behavioural conditions (26%) and 0–14-year-olds had the lowest (11%)
- of those participants who had a severe disability, 58% had a mental or behavioural condition compared with 14% of people with no disability or long-term restrictive health condition.[2]

The Australian Child and Adolescent Survey of Mental Health and Wellbeing 2013–14 (Young Minds Matter)[3] estimated that, in the 12 months before the survey:

- 560,000 children and adolescents aged 4–17 (14%) experienced a mental health condition
- Of the mental health conditions experienced by participants, the following were most prevalent: 'attention deficit hyperactivity disorder' (ADHD) (7.4%); anxiety (6.9%); depression (2.8%); and 'conduct disorder' (2.1%).[3]

The National Survey of People Living with Psychotic Illness 2010[4] estimated that:

- 64,000 people (or 4.5 cases per 1000 population) with a psychotic illness, who were aged 18–64, were in contact with public specialised mental health services in a 12-month period
- the prevalence of psychosis was higher for males than for females (5.4 and 3.5 cases per 1000 population, respectively). The age groups with the highest prevalence were 25–34 and 35–44 (5.6 cases per 1000 population for both age groups).[4]

There are similar concerns in Aotearoa New Zealand, particularly for young people. Results from the 2018 mental health monitor and the 2018–19 New Zealand Health Survey[5] found that mental distress is highest among young people (15–24-year-olds) and 1 in 5 New Zealanders aged 15 years and over are diagnosed with a mood and/or anxiety condition.

- There is a greater proportion of younger people in higher/more severe categories among anxiety and mental distress measures than older age groups (25–64 years old and 65+).
- 18–24-year-olds are more likely to report experiencing moderately severe or severe depression than older age groups.
- One-third (33%) of 15–17-year-olds and 25% of 18–24-year-olds reported difficulty doing everyday activities people their age can normally do caused by a long-term emotional, psychological or psychiatric condition.
- Young people in Aotearoa New Zealand have one of the highest suicide rates in the Organisation for Economic Co-operation and Development (OECD).[5]

Australian mental health policies[6,7] acknowledge that many of the determinants of good mental health, and of mental illness, are influenced by factors beyond the health system. The Fifth National Mental Health and Suicide Prevention Plan[7] stresses a commitment for governments across Australia to work together towards integrated planning and delivery of services, and ensuring that consumers and carers play a central role in the service planning, delivery and evaluation. It also emphasises the critical need to address social and emotional wellbeing across the nation, and to address the physical health needs of those experiencing mental illness. This is particularly important to paramedical and other health personnel working in the context of significant efforts being made to combine mental health services within the general health system and a community-based system of assessment, treatment and support. A whole-of-government, cross-sectorial approach is based upon principles of human rights and equity, and the belief that integrated mental health and community services could and should provide holistic care to individuals in a manner that contributes to the prevention of illness and the reduction of stigma.[8]

PRACTICE TIP

People who live with mental illness are also more at risk of physical health problems (e.g. cancer, cardiovascular illness or diabetes) and average life expectancy is shorter. Be equally alert to physical and mental health. Apply this knowledge to the person's assessment and treatment.

PREVALENCE OF MENTAL HEALTH PRESENTATIONS TO EDS

As indicated by the prevalence of mental health challenges in Australia and Aotearoa New Zealand, mental health in emergency situations is also a growing concern, with increasing numbers of distressed people presenting in mainstream hospital and community settings.[8,9] In 2019–20, 310,471 presentations to public Australian EDs were mental health-related, which was 3.8% of all presentations. This is a slightly higher proportion than in 2018–19 where mental health-related ED presentations comprised 3.6% of all presentations. Women aged 18–24 had the highest rate of mental health-related ED presentations (226.8 per 10,000 population), followed by men aged 35–44 years (202.0 per 10,000 population). The rate of mental health-related ED presentations was higher for males than for females (127.9 and 115.4 per 10,000 population respectively). Overall, those aged 18–24 years had the highest rate of mental health-related presentations (209.3 per 10,000 population); by contrast, people aged 85 years and older had the highest rate for all ED presentations (7850.9 per 10,000 population).

Aboriginal and Torres Strait Islander people, who represent about 3.3% of the Australian population, accounted for 12.0% of mental health-related ED presentations, compared with 7.5% of all ED presentations. The rate of mental health-related ED presentations for Indigenous Australians was more than four times that of non-Indigenous Australians (480.9 and 107.9 per 10,000 population respectively)

Certain mental health presentations are more common in EDs than others. In Australia, in 2019–20, for example, 28.1% of presentations were classified as 'Mental and behavioural disorders due to psychoactive substance use' and 27% were due to 'Neurotic, stress-related and somatoform disorders'.[10]

A report published by the Australasian College for Emergency Medicine[11] acknowledged a lack of national, publicly available data on people presenting to Aotearoa New Zealand EDs for mental health-related reasons. Data from two iterations of ACEM's Prevalence of Mental Health Access Block Study (POMAB), conducted over a 7-day period in December 2017 and in October 2018, were analysed for the participating Aotearoa New Zealand EDs. Six EDs participated in the 2017 iteration and five participated in the 2018 iteration. From these study sites the number and percentage of people presenting to Aotearoa New Zealand EDs for mental health-related reasons increased significantly between the 2017 and 2018 study periods, 3.7% of all presentations in 2017 to 7.4% in 2018. Moreover, people presenting in mental distress experienced a significant increase in ED waiting times between December 2017 and October 2018, and the proportion of mental health presentations who had an ED length of stay of 8 or more hours while waiting for an in-patient bed increased from 4.5% to 27.5%.[11]

PRINCIPLES OF RESPONDING TO PEOPLE IN MENTAL DISTRESS

Initial contact with an individual experiencing mental distress is particularly important, but it often occurs in less-than-ideal circumstances, such as on the street, in a busy ED, in the person's home or on the telephone. Regardless of the specific course of action required, it is critical that the individual is responded to with empathy and compassion by staff, as evidence indicates the quality of care a person receives in the ED can reduce anxiety, impact their future risk of suicide or self-harm, and help alleviate potentially volatile situations.[12,13]

Emergency assessment and treatment can be very challenging for people experiencing mental health issues and may trigger memories of previous traumatic events. People experiencing mental health issues therefore commonly consider ED presentation to be a negative event.[14,15] Despite the challenges of the emergency clinical environment, it is important to understand the potential link between previous traumatic experiences and the current presentation, to promote and protect the person's autonomy, and to remain aware that the patient needs to feel connected, valued and informed. A key aspect of responding to people experiencing mental distress is to communicate openly and honestly.[12,16]

SUPPORTING INDIVIDUALS IN THE OUT-OF-HOSPITAL ENVIRONMENT

As with all aspects of the assessment and management of patients, it is important to be able to review, synthesise and analyse the most recent literature and the various approaches to patient care in the out-of-hospital environment. A selection of international clinical practice guidelines and related literature have been examined and summarised here with respect to their approaches to the management of a person experiencing a mental health emergency.[17–33]

MENTAL HEALTH RESPONSE TEAMS

Guidelines for the management of an individual experiencing a mental health crisis in the out-of-hospital environment vary slightly across the states and territories of Australia and Aotearoa New Zealand, and in other jurisdictions around the world. In many areas, special co-responder teams exist, comprising a mental health professional, one or more police officers, or one or more paramedics, that respond to requests for the management of a person experiencing a mental health crisis. The focus of these teams is to provide a person-centred approach to assessment and intervention.[30,31,33] They can manage the person at the scene and, if required, facilitate transport to alternative destinations, such as a medical clinic or other type of mental health facility. The teams provide alternatives to management and transport by ambulance service paramedics, with the intent of reducing the burden on the ambulance services and hospital EDs.[32]

INTERVENTION BY PARAMEDICS

Prevalent across clinical practice guidelines is the importance of ensuring the personal safety of the patient, the paramedics and all others at the scene. If, upon initial contact, paramedics determine there is a potential for harm to themselves or others, then quickly exiting the scene to a place of safety is recommended. In addition, contact with police services is strongly advised to assist with management of the situation.

In most cases, an attempt to establish a rapport with the patient is recommended, along with the use of de-escalation techniques as an initial intervention. The primary focus of de-escalation is to enable the person to rapidly regain control of their own behaviour.[34] Supporting a person to shift from an agitated state to a calm state using a de-escalation technique should take between 5 and 10 minutes.[35] There is no universally accepted model of de-escalation,[36] but there are some commonly shared aspects of intervening with an aggressive or agitated person:

1. Respect personal space
2. Avoid provocation
3. Attentive listening
4. Display empathy
5. Calm, concise and clear verbal communication
6. Identification of the patient's needs, wants and feelings
7. Respect and dignity
8. Reassurance
9. Non-confrontational limit setting
10. Identify mutual goals
11. Offer choices
12. Remain optimistic.[36]

The normal rules of safety within a structure or outside area apply. These include:

- Ensure that you have clear access to an exit—never let the person or others get between you and that exit.
- Don't insist on performing clinical procedures like taking a BP or starting an IV. Focus on the issues at hand.
- Avoid verbal confrontations. Reassure the person that you are there to help.
- If you need to medicate the person, obtain their consent, whenever possible, and assure them that it will help them to calm down.[36]

PATHWAYS TO THE ED

People experiencing significant distress associated with their mental health can come to the attention of emergency mental health services in a number of ways. They may present to an ED via their own mode of transport, or that of a family member/carer. They may also be transported by a community mental health team, or by police officers. Alternatively, paramedics may transport the individual via ambulance. Whatever the pathway, the safety of the person in distress, the attending professionals, family members and bystanders are major priorities.

Guidelines for the transport of an individual to hospital via ambulance vary across the states and territories. The details here use current Victorian protocol[37] as an example (it is recommended that readers use this as a guide only, in conjunction with specific legislation and protocols within their state/territory). The Victorian protocol recognises the need to provide a person-focused approach, in which the individual, their family/carer and other health/mental health professionals are involved in the transport decision. Where a decision has been made that a person requires admission to an approved mental health service, a decision about the most appropriate form of transport should include assessing:

- the individual's physical and mental state
- the individual's immediate treatment needs
- the risk of harm the individual poses to themselves and others
- the likely effect on the individual of the proposed mode of transport
- expressed wishes of the individual and/or their carer(s), where practicable
- availability of the various modes of transport, including non-emergency patient transport vehicles
- the distance to be travelled
- the individual's need for support and supervision during the period of travel.

In certain circumstances, consideration should first be given to non-ambulance transport (other options include private vehicle, mental health professional agency vehicle, non-emergency patient transport vehicle). Transport via police vehicle should be regarded as a last resort (used only when absolutely necessary, such as when an individual is in police custody), due to the potential it can give the impression that the person is suspected of having committed a crime, which could cause unnecessary distress and anxiety, and perpetuate stigma. Where an individual is detained under the relevant Mental Health Act (see Chapter 4), police must maintain their custody and therefore will remain until the conclusion of the person's mental health assessment, even if the person is transported by ambulance to the ED.

If it is decided that an ambulance is the preferred mode of transport, the ambulance responses are categorised into the following three codes: emergency, urgent and routine (see Table 36.1). Generally, people experiencing a mental illness who may require transport to hospital need to be assessed by a health/mental health professional first, to determine whether hospitalisation is required, as well as what form of transport is needed. Sometimes, such as in cases of an overdose, an individual/family member/carer will need to contact ambulance services directly. In these instances, a judgement will be made by the ambulance service to categorise the request in accordance with Table 36.1. If, upon ambulance arrival, the person appears to have a mental illness but does not require hospitalisation, then the local mental health service triage must be contacted to

TABLE 36.1 CATEGORIES OF AMBULANCE RESPONSE[37]

AMBULANCE CATEGORY AND ACUITY	RESPONSE	DESCRIPTION
Code 1–emergency	Emergency response using lights and sirens, with person being transported to nearest appropriate ED for treatment/stabilisation.	There is an actual or potential risk that the person's life is immediately threatened (e.g. suicide attempt or overdose of harmful substance)
Code 2–urgent	A response (no lights and sirens) where the person is transported to the nearest ED or nearest appropriate mental health service.	The person: • exhibits evidence of acute mental illness, accompanied by agitation, distress, impulsivity, unpredictability and/or propensity to destructive acts • has attempted/threatened suicide but their life is not immediately threatened • is unable to be contained safely in a care or support situation in the community and has been sedated to enable safe transport • requires approved mechanical restraint for safe transport, or • is in crisis and has been apprehended by police under the Mental Health Act.
Code 3–routine	In some circumstances (e.g. in rural areas), a person will need to be transported to the nearest appropriate approved mental health service for admission (rather than the catchment area service the person should normally be admitted to). This may occur where either: • the person's wellbeing may be adversely affected by a long-distance transfer, or • a long-distance transfer at that time might adversely affect the provision of acute ambulance care in the rural community from which the ambulance would need to be dispatched.	Adequate care is currently being provided, but the person requires transport to an approved mental health service (e.g. inter-hospital transfers). Other forms of transport have been considered and deemed unsuitable by the mental health professional.

arrange appropriate management. If the person requires hospital treatment but refuses ambulance transport, the paramedics must contact the local area mental health service triage to organise a more urgent response.

OUT-OF-HOSPITAL ASSESSMENT AND MANAGEMENT

Responding to people experiencing mental health emergencies can be common for paramedics and therefore paramedics play a crucial role in out-of-hospital assessment, treatment and care, particularly in instances when assistance from mental health services is not present (e.g. when an ambulance has been requested by a member of the community, rather than by a community mental health team). Assessing the current status of the person's mental health can be accomplished by using one of several available assessment procedures.[19,26] A key component of this assessment is the requirement to eliminate all possible organic/medical causes for the person's behaviour, before initiating any interventions based on an assessment of mental illness. Such causes can include hypoglycaemia, hypoxia, sepsis, head injury, dementia and substance abuse.[23]

Paramedics are also well placed to undertake a screening mental state examination (mental health assessment) to determine if the person is at risk of self-harm or harm to others, is becoming aggressive and whether action is required to reduce this risk. A screening mental state examination involves enquiring about the individual's current circumstances and any recent changes in their life, as well as understanding their present thought processes and content, actions, emotions and feelings.[38] Consultation with any family and friends present can further assist with understanding the individual's current behaviour and experiences. Conducting screening risk and mental state assessments at first contact can also help build a clinical picture over time, documenting any significant change in behaviour, suicidal ideation or clinical presentation. An example of a mental state examination is provided in Table 36.2.

Once the assessment of the person's mental state has been completed, the paramedic must then decide which course of action is required. If a mental health assessment team is present, they can take responsibility for the person and determine if a referral is appropriate or if more definitive intervention is required.[33] If the team is not present, they can be requested to attend if the situation is deemed safe to do so. If a team is not available, then the paramedic must decide what course of action is in the best interest of the person.

Prior to transfer to the most appropriate place of care (and if time permits), paramedics are well placed to enquire about and document the immediate home or living environment and all collateral contacts, including any efforts to obtain collateral information from them. Other documentation to be completed by paramedics includes the use of mechanical devices or pharmacological agents for restraint and any adverse events that compromise safety to paramedics, the person being transported, family members or bystanders. In many instances, there will be no mental health professional present or available to

TABLE 36.2 MENTAL STATUS EXAMINATION[19]

PROCEDURE	MENTAL HEALTH ASSESSMENT GUIDE			
• Assess the patient appropriately to ascertain the cause of the presenting signs and symptoms • Exclude and/or manage causes of abnormal behaviour where possible • Using the guide to mental status examination, observe, question and note relevant information. This must be conducted in a highly respectful and empathetic manner. Judgemental attitudes, interrogatory questioning styles or other disrespectful stances will usually only serve to exacerbate a patient's condition. • Be mindful that different cultures hold different beliefs about mental illness. For some cultures, mental health is determined by physical and/or spiritual influences. For others, mental illness is a taboo subject and is not discussed openly.	Appearance	• grooming • posture • build • clothing • cleanliness	Thought form	• amount • rate • derailment • flight of ideas
	Behaviour	• eye contact • mannerisms • gait • activity level	Thought content	• disturbances • delusions • suicidal • obsessions
	Speech	• rate • volume • pitch • tone • flow • pressure	Perception	• illusions • thought insertion • broadcasting • hallucinations
	Mood	Emotion as described: • anxious • depressed • cheerful	Insight and judgement	• cognition • illness • understanding • cause and effect
	Affect	Emotion as observed: • restrictive • blunted • labile		

assess or assist with the person. In severe cases, paramedics may be required to administer pharmacological interventions, such as lorazepam or midazolam and provide physical restraints—sometimes without the need to consult a mental health practitioner.

PRACTICE TIP

Responding to a person experiencing mental health emergencies in the out-of-hospital environment requires an assessment of the person's current mental state, including an assessment of the person's presenting signs and symptoms, to eliminate alternative causes for their current presentation. A mental health assessment includes exploration of the person's appearance, behaviour, speech, mood, affect, thoughts, perception and judgement.

ED TRIAGE ASSESSMENT

Upon arrival at the ED, the first step in the care process is triage assessment. In mental health emergencies, the screening and classifying of distressed persons to determine priority needs and actions calls for sharp assessment skills and efficient use of human resources, equipment and other resources. If appropriate resources are not available for urgent cases, then steps should be taken to bring these to the individual as soon as possible. Table 36.3 presents an example of a mental health triage scale used in some New South Wales EDs[39] (again, it is important to ensure that readers also access protocols from their own state/territory, as these may vary). It outlines some key markers for determining mental health triage categories and the typical presentations observed or reported by secondary (non-consumer) sources. While these categories differ in their degree of risk, complexity and cross-cultural applicability, they do offer a consistent approach to decision-making following initial screening of all incoming referrals and admissions to the ED. It is worth noting that, similar to all ED presentations, 77% of mental health-related presentations in 2019–20 were classified as semi-urgent or urgent (individual to be seen within 60 minutes and 30 minutes respectively), around 16% were classified as emergencies, and approximately 1% required resuscitation.[10] For further information on triage practice see Chapter 11.

For each presentation the assessor should answer the following questions:

- Can I safely interview this person on my own, or do I need backup?
- Is the person going to be safe where they are?
- Can the person be left alone and/or with others safely?
- What degree of observation does the person need and can it be provided in the ED?
- Where is the most appropriate place to interview the person, given their level of arousal and agitation?

Answering these questions will help make the fullest and safest triage assessment possible, to benefit the person, their family/carers and the treatment team. The assessment must be recorded clearly and, if decisions are made, reasons given. In many instances the assessment will involve formulation of a differential diagnosis—most commonly for episodic referrals. It will be teamwork and interdisciplinary consultation, collaboration on the need for further investigations and active involvement of sub-specialties in clinical cases that will help determine an appropriate clinical pathway. The names of other colleagues who are consulted or involved in the decision must also appear in the clinical record.

AFTER TRIAGE

Once the triage assessment has been made, a brief mental state assessment will be conducted, usually by a general nurse and/or medical officer. As previously discussed, the purpose of the mental health assessment is to obtain information about specific aspects of the individual's mental health experiences and behaviour at the time of interview (see Table 36.2). If necessary, the individual will then be referred to the mental health team for a further interview, with an assessment conducted by a mental health liaison nurse consultant. Following this assessment, the mental health nurse, in consultation with the mental health team and the referring medical officer, will make a decision about the next course of action. In instances where immediate care is needed, the individual will then be admitted to hospital. Alternatively, if it is deemed safe and in the best interests of the individual to go home, the mental health nurse will provide them with information regarding support services in the community. These services should be as specific to the concerns experienced by the individual as possible. In instances where it is clear that additional community support is needed, the nurse will make a referral to a community mental health team. Refer to Chapter 11 for further discussion on triage.

REFERRAL AND CARE CONTINUITY

Crucial to the practice of effective mental health interventions is the way that an assessment is communicated, the way in which symptoms are described and the language used by both practitioners and the individual in this process. The formulation of a succinct summary of a person's history, current circumstances and main problems will help set the diagnosis in context.[39] It is particularly useful in conveying essential information upon discharge, when making a referral to a specialist mental health service or when referring for other specialist intervention. The time taken to communicate assessment findings will go a long way to help ensure continuity of information and, if more than one provider is involved, continuity of the therapeutic relationship and timely referral for additional assessment or care (Box 36.1).

THE ROLE OF ED MENTAL HEALTH LIAISON NURSES

In some Australian states and territories, general hospitals have employed mental health liaison nurses (MHLNs) to assist with clinical assessment and therapeutic care of people experiencing mental health problems/mental illness. The role is developed and defined by the needs of the hospital/health service. The main focus of the MHLN role is assessment and support for individuals with new or pre-existing mental health conditions (particularly self-harm and suicide), responding to the psychological complications of physical illness, and assisting in the response to behavioural disturbances typically due to intoxication with alcohol and drug use. High consumer and ED staff

TABLE 36.3 MENTAL HEALTH TRIAGE ASSESSMENT IN THE EMERGENCY DEPARTMENT[39]

TRIAGE CATEGORY AND TREATMENT ACUITY	DESCRIPTION	TYPICAL PRESENTATION OBSERVED AND/OR REPORTED
1 Immediate	Definite danger to self or others **Australasian Triage Scale states:** • Severe behavioural disorder with immediate threat of dangerous violence	Observed: • Violent behaviour • Possession of a weapon • Self-harm in ED • Displays extreme agitation/restlessness • Bizarre/disoriented behaviour Reported: • Verbal commands to do harm to self or others that the person is unable to resist (command hallucinations) • Recent violent behaviour
2 Emergency Within 10 minutes	Probable risk of danger to self or others AND/OR Client is physically restrained in ED AND/OR Severe behavioural disturbance **Australasian Triage Scale states:** Violent or aggressive: • Immediate threat to self or others • Requires or has required restraint • Severe agitation or aggression	Observed: • Extreme agitation/restlessness • Physically/verbally aggressive • Confused/unable to cooperate • Hallucinations/delusions/paranoia • Requires restraint/containment • High risk of absconding and not wanting treatment Reported: • Attempt/threat of self-harm • Threat of harm to others • Unable to wait safely
3 Urgent Within 30 minutes	Possible danger to self or others • Moderate behavioural disturbance • Severe distress **Australasian Triage Scale states:** • Very distressed, risk of self-harm • Acutely psychotic or thought-disordered • Situational crisis, deliberate self-harm • Agitated/withdrawn	Observed: • Agitated/restless • Intrusive behaviour • Confused • Ambivalence about treatment • Not likely to wait for treatment Reported: • Suicidal ideation • Situational crisis Presence of psychotic symptoms: • Hallucinations • Delusions • Paranoid ideas • Thought disordered • Bizarre/agitated behaviour Presence of mood disturbance: • Severe symptoms of depression • Withdrawn/uncommunicative • And/or anxiety • Elevated or irritable mood
4 Semi-urgent Within 60 minutes	Moderate distress **Australasian Triage Scale states:** • Semi-urgent mental health problem • Under observation and/or no immediate risk to self or others	Observed: • No agitation/restlessness • Irritable without aggression • Cooperative • Gives coherent history Reported: • Pre-existing mental health disorder • Symptoms of anxiety or depression without suicidal ideation • Willing to wait

Continued

TABLE 36.3 MENTAL HEALTH TRIAGE ASSESSMENT IN THE EMERGENCY DEPARTMENT—cont'd

TRIAGE CATEGORY AND TREATMENT ACUITY	DESCRIPTION	TYPICAL PRESENTATION OBSERVED AND/OR REPORTED
5 Non-urgent Within 120 minutes	No danger to self or others • No acute distress • No behavioural disturbance **Australasian Triage Scale states:** • Known patient with chronic symptoms • Social crisis, clinically well patient	Observed: • Cooperative • Communicative and able to engage in developing management plan • Able to discuss concerns • Compliant with instructions Reported: • Known patient with chronic psychotic symptoms • Pre-existing non-acute mental health disorder • Known patient with chronic unexplained somatic symptoms • Request for medication • Minor adverse effect of medication • Financial/social, accommodation or relationship problems

BOX 36.1 IMPORTANT ITEMS FOR REFERRAL TO ADDITIONAL SERVICES[39]

- **Description of the presenting complaint, its intensity and duration.**
- **Relevant current and past medical history and medication.**
- **A note of mental state examination results with key or contradictory findings highlighted.**
- **An estimate of degree of urgency in terms of risk to the consumer and others.**
- **Indication of referrer's expectations (assessment, advice, admission).**
- **The most urgent requests should be reinforced by telephone or email.**

satisfaction with the role has been found, particularly in terms of the service provided, information offered and improvements to consumer health outcomes.[40,41] Similarly, this role can play an important part in ED-based outpatient services, particularly regarding improved consumer access to specialised mental health care.[12,41,42]

PSYCHIATRIC EMERGENCY CARE CENTRES

A number of hospitals have Psychiatric Emergency Care Centres (PECCs), which are co-located with EDs. These centres serve to provide timely, specialist mental health assessment on-site in the ED.[43] Generally, these services offer 24-hour mental health staff presence. PECCs also provide high-level observation/immediate care for people requiring short-term mental health care (usually up to 48 hours). While the nature of work undertaken within a PECC may vary across jurisdictions, there is usually a protocol for fast-tracking mental health assessments of ED presentations. The PECC environment should be one that is constantly monitored, with the capacity to provide appropriate use of sedation and restraint only when necessary and in line with local policies and clinical protocols.

MENTAL HEALTH CONDITIONS

This section outlines various mental health conditions that may be seen in emergency situations. The symptoms and diagnostic characteristics described are based on the American Psychiatric Association's *Diagnostic and Statistical Manual of Mental Disorders*.[44] The WHO International Classification of Diseases[45] can also be used for diagnosis. It is critical to note that while these descriptions are important, each individual will experience mental health conditions differently, and so presentations of the same diagnosis might differ from person to person. Additionally, many individuals will experience comorbidity—that is, a diagnosis of more than one condition. At all times, care should be tailored to the individual as much as possible.

By their very nature, mental health conditions must be assessed holistically, taking account of psychosocial, cognitive, biological and interpersonal domains. Assessment therefore requires the practitioner to have an understanding and recognition of the symptoms of mental health conditions, and to be able to distinguish these from physical health diagnoses. Assessment is primarily made through talking to the individual and, where possible, their family/carers/friends and any other professionals involved in their care. Various assessment tools can be used for the different conditions, and typically these will be in a questionnaire-type format, addressing the experience of various symptoms. However, a richer and deeper understanding will come from listening to the individual sharing their story, as well as from observations of the individual's behaviour.

ANXIETY CONDITIONS

Anxiety is the most commonly experienced mental health condition, affecting approximately 11–15% of Australians and New Zealanders aged between 16 and 85 years, with a higher prevalence in women than men.[2,46] Some of the anxiety conditions include generalised anxiety, obsessive compulsive conditions, social phobia, panic condition, agoraphobia, specific phobia and post-traumatic stress. Common to all of these is excessive fear and anxiety, as well as related physical/behavioural symptoms; often this experience is so overwhelming that it can interfere with a person's day-to-day functioning.

While the causes of anxiety are not fully understood, it is likely that a particular anxiety condition is a result of several interacting factors and is affected by stressful life events and personality traits such as:[47]

- excessive or unrealistic worries (generalised anxiety condition)
- compulsions and obsessions which the individual cannot control (obsessive compulsive condition)
- intense excessive worry about social situations (social anxiety condition)
- panic attacks (panic condition)
- an intense, irrational fear of everyday objects and situations (phobia).

Symptoms and diagnostic criteria

The symptoms of anxiety involve excessive worry or concern about particular life domains, which is perceived to be difficult to control by the individual. Symptoms are both psychological and physical (see Box 36.2 for diagnostic criteria).

Management

Treatment can help people manage, reduce or eliminate anxiety symptoms. Diagnosis is generally made by a psychiatrist. Clinical psychologists, social workers or counsellors often manage ongoing treatment. Psychological treatments are the most effective way to treat most types of anxiety. These include cognitive behavioural therapy (CBT), exposure therapy or narrative therapy (among others), often supported by medication, community support and recovery programs.[47] During CBT, a person learns new and effective ways to cope with their symptoms. The skills of the nurse will include cognitive behavioural interventions, understanding the nature of the concern, offering reassurance and focusing on the positive abilities of the person to take control of the situation, to overcome the limitations of their thinking.

PANIC

Due to the associated physical symptoms of a panic attack, people experiencing this condition might present to the ED.[48] Panic condition has a high comorbidity with other anxiety and depressive conditions.[49]

Symptoms and diagnostic criteria

Panic condition is signified by recurrent, unexpected panic attacks. The acute panic attack usually begins with a sudden onset. Key diagnostic criteria are described in Box 36.3.

BOX 36.2 CRITERIA FOR RECOGNISING GENERALISED ANXIETY[44]

People who have been diagnosed with generalised anxiety describe excessive anxiety or worry for the majority of the week for at least 6 months. The person may be preoccupied about work and work relationships, performing well at school or at some other activity. Despite their best efforts, the person struggles to control or block out their worries and preoccupations. At the same time they may experience motor restlessness, irritability, difficulty in concentration, feeling highly strung and unable to process everyday information. The physical effects of generalised anxiety include tense and sore muscles and disturbed sleep.

BOX 36.3 CRITERIA FOR RECOGNISING A PANIC CONDITION[44]

People who have been diagnosed with a panic condition experience an overwhelming and abrupt surge of intense fear and discomfort that reaches a peak usually within a short time-frame (usually minutes). The person is visibly distressed, often sweating, with a rapid and thumping heartbeat. They may also be trembling and describe a sense of impending doom. Additional feelings and sensations include shortness of breath and a feeling that the person is not breathing in adequate amounts of air. The person may also feel as if they are suffocating or choking. The strength of emotions and feelings of dizziness and/or light-headedness may be accompanied by a fear of losing control or 'going crazy', or perhaps a fear of dying. The change in thought, feeling and behaviour is not attributable to the physiological effects of a substance or to another medical condition.

Management

The skills needed to manage panic are to be calm and reassuring and to reduce unnecessary or distressing stimulation. The practitioner should speak in a calm and controlled voice, asking the person to focus on their breathing, talking to them in such a way that they are helping to de-escalate the situation, letting the person know that they are in a safe and protective environment and that they are likely to feel better once they regain control of their situation. Actively helping the person to relax, and educating other practitioners to take a similar stance, will greatly enhance the person's ability to reduce the intensity of the panic. It may be necessary to have a relative, friend or carer sit with the person, working closely with the practitioner to reinforce that they are safe and that no one intends to make their situation worse or bring harm. Aspects of communication with a person in the acute phase of panic are discussed in Box 36.4.

BOX 36.4 ASPECTS OF COMMUNICATION WITH A PERSON IN THE ACUTE PHASE OF PANIC[48]

- ***Foster trust and confidence*—stay with the individual; ensure continuity of practitioners; reassure the individual that they are not dying, will not lose consciousness, that you are working with others to help resolve the situation and restore calm. This will help counter the feeling of being out of control, a fear of having a heart attack or of losing one's mind.**
- ***Model calmness and reassurance*—have the individual follow you in the taking of long, deep breaths. Breathing with the individual will help encourage teamwork and joint problem-solving. Slow, deep breathing can help reduce panic to a manageable level of anxiety. Individuals experiencing a panic state may take their physiological symptoms as an indication that they are going to die.**
- ***Self-monitor your own reactions to acute panic*—do some deep breathing, use quiet pauses and seek out support from colleagues to maintain self-confidence and clear thinking. Acute anxiety can be transmittable from one person to another and this can create a roller-coaster of emotions.**

PRACTICE TIP

Be alert to the contagion effects of anxiety and panic, and guard against them. Front-line workers working in high-stress environments must initiate self-care to reduce the impact of mental health presentations on their own health and wellbeing.

AFFECTIVE CONDITIONS

Affective conditions involve a change in affect or disturbance in mood. Affective conditions are experienced by women more than men (12% versus 9.5% in Australia; 9.5% versus 6.3% in Aotearoa New Zealand).[46,50] Affective conditions include major depression, bipolar affective disorder and postnatal depression.

MAJOR DEPRESSION

Depression affects the way someone feels, causing a persistent lowering of mood. In 2014–15 it was estimated that more than 2.5 million Australian adults experienced depression.[2,50] Globally, depression is a consistent leading contributor to the disease burden across all age groups.[51]

Recognising depression

Depression is often accompanied by a range of physical and emotional symptoms that can impede the way a person is able to function at home, at work and in their everyday life. Key criteria are outlined in Box 36.5.

Management

Management of depression can involve medication, individual therapy or community and social support programs—or a combination of all three. Medications assist the brain to restore its usual chemical balance, helping to control the symptoms of depression. Individual therapy involving a doctor, psychologist or other healthcare professional talking with the person about their symptoms, and discussing alternative ways of thinking about and coping with them, can be effective, particularly in building confidence and self-esteem. Similarly, community support programs are most helpful when they include information about the condition, accommodation support and options and help with finding suitable employment, training and education, psychosocial rehabilitation and mutual support groups. Understanding and acceptance by the community—including the therapeutic community in the ED—is also very important.

BOX 36.5 CRITERIA FOR RECOGNISING A MAJOR DEPRESSIVE CONDITION[44]

People who have been diagnosed with a major depressive condition often experience a feeling of depressed mood for most of the day, nearly every day for the week just past. There may be a markedly diminished interest or pleasure in most or a majority of activities. The marked diminished interest in pleasure is often indicated by a subjective account or observation from others (e.g. work colleagues or family members). At the same time there may be significant weight loss (when the person is not actively dieting) or weight gain, or a decrease in appetite nearly every day. They may have insomnia (either getting to sleep or staying asleep) or hypersomnia reported nearly every day. The subjective impression of the person is that they are 'not the same', with noticeable psychomotor agitation/retardation. An overwhelming feeling of fatigue and/or loss of energy may leave the person in a distressed and unsettled state of mind. There may also be impairment in family, social, employment or other important areas of daily functioning. The change in thought, mood and behaviour is not attributable to the physiological effects of a substance or to another medical condition.

POSTNATAL DEPRESSION

Postnatal depression is a significant clinical condition experienced by approximately 15% of women who give birth in Australia and Aotearoa New Zealand.[52,53] The risk factors for postnatal depression include a personal or family history of depression, severe 'baby blues', ambivalence towards or unwanted pregnancy and poor social and/or partner support. Postnatal depression is much less common than the postnatal blues, but if left untreated may become a chronic condition.

Symptoms

The clinical features of postnatal depression are similar to those of major depression, although during a mental state assessment there may be thought content that includes worries about going outside the home, and worries and concerns about the baby's health or the ability to cope adequately with the baby.

Management

Management of postnatal depression is largely supportive, educative and interactive between practitioner and consumer. Providing an explanation of the condition and education about treatment can provide a certain amount of relief. This can help women and their partners give meaning to their experience and prevent unhelpful worry that they are 'going crazy' or that their situation is one of personal failure because they are unfit to be a mother. Explaining what postnatal depression is, how it is not related to personal shortcomings and giving ample opportunity for the mother to talk openly and freely about such things as her relationship with her own mother, her partner, her disappointments, frustrations or stressors can generate trust and informed awareness of the situation. The emergency nurse can assist with organising help with childcare or respite, placing the woman in touch with support organisations and peer support workers, helping the woman recruit ongoing help and support from her GP, family and friends and referring the woman to professional mental health care.

DEPRESSION IN LATER LIFE

Global ageing estimates[54] predict that there will be approximately 8.8 million people aged 65 or over in Australia and Aotearoa New Zealand by 2050, and by the 2050s it is predicted that approximately 35% of those aged 65+ will be 80 years or older.[54] While many people can age well, growing older also presents certain challenges, including increased isolation and loneliness, deaths of partners and/or friends, as well as the development of medical conditions and cognitive decline,[55] all of which can contribute to feelings of alienation, hopelessness and lowered self-esteem.[56] Not surprisingly, depression is one of the most common mental health concerns in later life and can have severe effects on physical health and social relationships.

MANAGEMENT

Treating depression in older people requires flexibility and sensitivity, such as working at a slower pace, being prepared to repeat conversations if needed, and supporting the person's need to retain independence even if it takes time.[57] In addition, the use of pharmacological treatment needs to be considered with caution, as such treatments can place older people at increased risk of injury as a result of adverse effects.[58] The emergency nurse can support a person with depression in later life by promoting activities that improve nutrition, social interaction and social support and family relationships. While this might seem difficult to do in a busy ED, the promotion of supportive activities in the presence of family, for example, can go a long way to support messages that are being given by others (GPs, community nurses), who will also have contact with the consumer in the community.[55] Some consumers may have a negative view of themselves as people, of their contribution to family and society and of their future. Family members, social support networks and others important in the life of the consumer should be reminded that depression is not a weakness or a failure and that family education and social support and, in some instances, antidepressant medication can bring considerable benefit.

MANIC EPISODE

A manic episode is a period of unusually elevated mood and irritability which affects occupational and social functioning. Such an episode is typically experienced by individuals with a diagnosis of bipolar affective disorder.

Recognising a manic episode

A manic episode is primarily marked by symptoms of elevated mood and a tendency to engage in behaviour that could have serious social or financial consequences.[59] Key criteria are listed in Box 36.6.

BOX 36.6 CRITERIA FOR RECOGNISING A MANIC EPISODE[44]

At the time of a manic episode people experience a distinct period of abnormally and persistently elevated, expansive or irritable mood and out-of-character and persistently increasing goal-directed activity or energy. During the episode the person displays disturbed mood and increased energy or physical activity and there is a noticeable change from their usual behaviour, incorporating the following symptoms: a feeling of overstated self-esteem/grandiosity; a decreased need for rest or sleep; being extravagant and overly more talkative than usual, with a pressure to keep talking. There is a discernible rapid thinking—sometimes described as a 'flight of ideas'. The subjective experience at this time is that thoughts are racing and the person is easily distracted, giving rise to attention being too easily drawn to insignificant or immaterial external stimuli. Disturbance in mood causes marked impairment in functioning in social, family and work-related activity. The change in behaviour is not attributable to the physiological effects of a substance or to another medical condition.

Management

The specific management of a manic episode will include administration of medication (usually a benzodiazepine or antipsychotic in acute behaviour disturbance), keeping the environmental stimuli to a minimum, allowing the person to move yet remain under constant observation and providing physical supports as continuous motor activity, sleeplessness and overactivity may lead the patient to physically stop without much warning. The combined elements of this approach are designed to decrease the prospect of behaviour escalating and becoming out of control, and help restore calm at a time when the consumer does not have adequate internal control. This will also help promote physical safety for the person, staff and others present.

PSYCHOSIS

People in acute psychosis may present in a state of agitation or distress. Thought processes and communication can be fragmented and behaviour disorganised. Hypervigilance, a perception of threat, fear and paranoia associated with altered perceptions, unusual beliefs and delusions may also be evident. Voice hearing is also a common experience with psychosis, and visual hallucinations are mostly associated with substance-induced psychosis. Psychosis may be an acute short-term episodic experience or an enduring condition. People with long-term psychotic symptoms are typically given a psychiatric diagnosis of 'schizophrenia' or 'schizo-affective disorder'. They will be prescribed medication long term and may have a long association with in-patient and community mental health services. However, many individuals can also recover. With time and appropriate interventions, community support and acceptance, people can find a way to self-manage. Indeed, recovery principles have been enshrined in government mental health policy internationally, including Australia and Aotearoa New Zealand. Importantly, recovery does not mean 'cure' in the clinical sense, or a complete resolution of symptoms. It is a personal process of creating meaning and purpose in life beyond the constraints of diagnosis, and despite mental health challenges.

Family and social relationships may be strained or broken and, as a result of the episodic nature of psychosis, stigma, a reluctance to accept their condition, and other social factors, there may be an inability to maintain contact with individuals over prolonged periods. While the causes of psychosis are not fully understood, there is growing evidence that experiencing trauma, particularly in childhood, is a significant factor.[60,61] It is estimated that hearing voices in 77% of people diagnosed with 'schizophrenia' is related to traumatic experiences. The widely accepted contemporary view is that voice hearing is a normal human experience, that voices have meaning for individuals, and are parts of the self that should not be ignored. People are encouraged to accept voices and establish a dialogue with them.[62] In addition, drugs such as cannabis, LSD, cocaine and amphetamines can cause psychosis.

Management

When a person experiencing psychosis requires emergency mental health care, it is important to convey a message of safety, and to de-escalate their stress as much as possible. People experiencing psychosis can be challenging to establish rapport with, so it is important to use calming and reassuring verbal and non-verbal communication. Also be mindful that people who have had psychotic symptoms long term may have had negative experiences with emergency and mental health services previously and therefore are fearful of coercion. Responding to a person experiencing psychosis involves the following key features:[63]

- *Clarity and effective non-verbal communication*—ensure that communication is clear and not rushed, with short sentences and simple vocabulary. Be prepared to repeat statements as needed. Where possible use 'I' and 'you' rather than 'we' and 'us' to decrease the risk of misunderstanding. Non-verbal messages should be congruent with verbal statements, as some people may be very sensitive to whether the non-verbal supports the verbal message.
- *Model desired behaviours*—model expression of thought and feeling by interacting with other practitioners in the presence of the person in a calm and receptive fashion. Remain optimistic towards the person and provide suggestions rather than orders if you would like them to do something. Individuals with psychosis may take additional time to reach a level of trust where they can accept actions directed from healthcare professionals towards them.
- *Foster trust and relationship-building*—follow through on commitments made, inform the person when you will be talking to them, give careful explanations for treatments and medications and allow the person to control the amount of self-disclosure that takes place in the interaction. Such actions demonstrate trust by making the healthcare worker accessible to the person both physically and emotionally.

EATING CONDITIONS

An eating condition is characterised by persistent thoughts and disturbance regarding eating, eating-related behaviour and body weight. There is no single cause for eating conditions; a number of factors are involved to varying degrees in different people such as personal and psychological factors related to adolescence or family issues, and social factors such as media representation of body image. It is estimated that approximately 2 in every 100 people will develop some kind of eating condition at some time in their lives. More females than males tend to be affected, particularly young women. Typically, there is a high prevalence of comorbidity with other mental health conditions, particularly depression.[64,65]

Recognising eating conditions

Eating conditions can include limited food intake ('anorexia nervosa'), food intake followed by purging ('bulimia nervosa') or overeating ('compulsive overeating'); see also Box 36.7.[64] Anorexia nervosa is likely to be the greatest concern in emergency situations, due to the physical effects of extreme weight loss.

Management

Due to the physical manifestations associated with anorexia nervosa, management requires a multi-disciplinary approach involving endocrinologists, psychiatrists, dietitians, psychologists, nurses and others. In some instances, the associated medical implications will be severe, particularly when major organs are affected by prolonged reduced energy intake.[44,64] It is essential that these physical impairments are treated along with the psychological impacts. For example, initiating cardiovascular monitoring is important, considering the risk of profound bradycardia and electrolyte abnormalities associated with this condition (see Chapter 22 for cardiac monitoring techniques). Since many individuals will also experience depression or anxiety, and in some instances psychosis, this needs to be considered in the individual's management. Once the immediate physical implications are managed, some individuals may require admission to specialist eating condition wards for treatment.

BOX 36.7 RECOGNISING AN EATING CONDITION[44]

The overall clinical picture for people diagnosed with anorexia nervosa is marked by a restricted energy intake comparative to daily requirements, leading to a significantly lower body weight (defined as weight that is less than minimally normal/expected for age and gender, developmental stage and pre-existing physical condition). People experience an intense fear of gaining weight or express dogged behaviour that interferes with putting on weight, even though they are at a notably low weight. There are conspicuous changes in the way in which they describe and experience their body weight and shape, and this may be expressed in words or drawings. There is also a steadfast lack of personal recognition of the risk and potential seriousness of the current low body weight.

SEROTONIN SYNDROME

Serotonin syndrome is a relatively rare yet dangerous condition associated with the introduction of or increase in a serotonin agent (commonly selective serotonin reuptake inhibitors (SSRIs)).

Symptoms

Serotonin syndrome is characterised by altered mental state, racing thoughts and agitation, tremor, shivering, diarrhoea, hyperreflexia, myoclonus (spasm of a muscle or group of muscles), ataxia, hypertension and hyperthermia. It can occur as a result of overdose or drug combinations and, rarely, with therapeutic doses.[66] For example, serotonin syndrome may be precipitated by someone who is already taking an SSRI, then uses amphetamines, or starts taking another serotonergic agent such as St John's Wort. The onset is usually rapid and most acute cases resolve with appropriate treatment within 24 to 36 hours.

Management

First actions include making sure that offending agent(s) is/are ceased immediately. If the condition is due to over-dosage, activated charcoal should be considered (see Chapter 30). For the treatment of agitation, seizures and myoclonus, benzodiazepines may be considered. There is some evidence for the efficacy of the antihistamine cyproheptadine as a serotonin blocking agent.[67] Treatment for respiratory distress and dehydration should be accompanied by close monitoring of the consumer. If there is concern for dangerous medical complications, the consumer should be provided with close nursing supervision.

SUBSTANCE MISUSE AND DUAL DIAGNOSIS

Substance misuse conditions (dependency or harmful use of alcohol or other drugs) affect around 5% and 4% of Australian[68,69] and Aotearoa New Zealand adults[46] respectively. Between 30% and 40% of people who have a substance misuse condition also experience a mental health issue, often referred to as having a dual diagnosis.[69–71] Individuals with comorbid substance use and mental health issues often present as a diagnostic challenge as each condition may obfuscate the other, and treatment can be complicated as drug and alcohol and mental health services are often organisationally separate. Lack of early identification and treatment increases the cost for the individual, the family, healthcare systems and the community. Optimum treatment will involve an integrated multi-disciplinary approach that seeks to address both problems simultaneously rather than sequentially. As people with dual diagnosis are often seen in an emergency context, it is important to ensure coordination of different services for these individuals.

The outcome indicators of good clinical management include:

- collaboration between drug and alcohol services and the ED, bringing coordination of all matters pertaining to drug and alcohol issues, including prevention, treatment, health promotion, education and evaluation, into a coherent framework for action
- treating seriously ill individuals using an integrated model involving both psychiatric and drug and alcohol services.[70,72]

The combined effect of the above is improved connectedness with the person's preferences, stigma reduction and improved teamwork and collaboration across disciplines.[70,73] For more details regarding use of alcohol, tobacco and other drugs, and management of overdose, see Chapter 40.

SUICIDE AND SELF-HARM

Although suicide and self-harm are typically considered behaviours, not mental health conditions, those who are diagnosed with a mental health condition are more likely to experience suicide and/or self-harm ideation and behaviour.[74] Encountering individuals who experience suicidal and self-harming behaviours is common for emergency clinicians. Often, these behaviours will be experienced by individuals who present with dual diagnosis and who have recently experienced a situational crisis, such as relationship breakdown.

SUICIDE

The WHO defines suicide as 'the act of killing oneself … deliberately initiated and performed by the person concerned in the full knowledge, or expectation, of its fatal outcome'.[75] Across the globe in 2019, an estimated 703,000 people died by suicide, with suicide being the fourth leading cause of death for people aged 15–29 years.[75] Rates of suicide are thought to be under-reported, with 591 deaths by suspected suicide recorded in Aotearoa New Zealand,[76] and 3139 in Australia[77] in 2020, typically with higher rates among males and those living in rural areas.[76,77] The ED is central to any strategy for reducing the incidence and impact of suicide, particularly because a key predictor of death by suicide is a history of depression, a previous suicide attempt, experienced trauma and loneliness.[75,78–80] It is hoped that opportune intervention in the ED may prevent some suicides. Training specifically aimed at recognising, assessing and supporting individuals experiencing suicidal ideation and behaviour is needed.[7,81]

SUICIDE AND SELF-HARMING BEHAVIOUR

Many suicide attempts do not end in death and the incidence of suicidal behaviour and self-harm ('deliberate damage to the body without suicidal intent')[72] is much higher than that of suicide, occurring more frequently in females than males.[72] There were 10,736[82] reported incidents of intentional self-harm hospitalisations in Aotearoa New Zealand in 2020[82] and an estimated 28,600 in Australia during 2019–20.[77] Of those in Australia, 81.2% were accounted for by intentional self-poisoning and 12% by intentional self-harm by sharp object.[77] Other examples of non-fatal and self-harming behaviours include: jumping from heights, attempted hanging, deliberate high-speed motor vehicle crashes and use of firearms. While some people will only engage in these behaviours once, or for a short duration of time, others will continue for many years. There is a connection between suicide and self-harm, with previous attempts and expressions of self-harming behaviour being common among those who have died by suicide.[77,83,84]

IMMEDIATE CARE FOLLOWING SUICIDE AND SELF-HARMING BEHAVIOUR

Paramedics and ED nurses are often some of the first responders when a person has engaged in suicidal/self-harming behaviours, and therefore both play a crucial role in providing immediate care. Due to the nature of suicidal and self-harming behaviours, there is likely to be an immediate need to tend to the medical aspects of the behaviour (e.g. wound suturing).[85] Ensuring the safety of the individual and others present is also essential. This involves checking whether the individual is in possession of any items that could be used to cause further harm (e.g. sharp objects). Once these needs have been met, specific psychological care can begin.[86]

Following consultation with people with lived experience of suicide and clinical staff, as well as the international literature, the Black Dog Institute released a set of guidelines for providing care to people in EDs and other acute settings.[87] Readers are strongly encouraged to read this document, and consider it an adjunct to their state/territory and workplace recommendations. These guidelines suggest best practice for working with a person experiencing suicidal crisis, and aim to support those working in acute settings to provide the most supportive response to such individuals and their carers/family. At its core, the guidelines stress the importance of a collaborative person-centred approach.

SUICIDE ASSESSMENT AND MANAGEMENT

Central to supporting a person in suicide-related distress is gaining an understanding of their current experiences and recent life events. The best course of action when managing an individual experiencing a suicidal state is to directly raise the topic with the individual, with the view to understanding risk and protective factors for suicide. It is preferable to do so knowing something of the framework and/or system supports available to the practitioner if indeed suicide is a very real option for the individual. Warning signs are listed in Box 36.8.

BOX 36.8 WARNING SIGNS OF SUICIDAL INTENTIONS[13]

The majority of people give warning signs about their suicidal intentions. Some of these warning signs are:

- **expression of hopelessness or helplessness**
- **written or spoken notice of intention, saying goodbye**
- **dramatic change in personality or appearance**
- **irrational, bizarre behaviour**
- **overwhelming sense of guilt, shame or reflection**
- **changed eating or sleeping patterns**
- **severe drop in school or work performance**
- **giving away possessions or putting affairs in order**
- **lack of interest in the future**
- **self-harming actions, such as overdoses, which can be lethal to the person.**

While the approach taken must be non-threatening, open and confidential, confidentiality cannot always be unconditionally assured. A careful balance must be maintained between preserving confidentiality as a fundamental aspect of clinical practice and the need to breach it on rare occasions in order to promote the person's optimal interests and care, and/or the safety of others.[87,89] There will, however, be many professional situations that call for the sharing of information between practitioners. On occasions, individuals or relatives may be asked to provide a considerable amount of personal information, especially when consumers are first assessed or admitted. When this happens, it should be explained in a sensitive manner that other staff will have access to some of the information. Employees therefore have a duty of care to ensure that they are aware of the implications of any legislation relevant to their particular role, and follow the statutory requirements of legislation and the requirements of their employer.[87,88]

Empathy and a genuine interest in the inner life of the person involved must be apparent during the clinical interview. Establishing sound rapport can strengthen the motivation of the person to consider alternatives to suicide. An individual, biopsychosocial, narrative, approach is most appropriate, even within the time constraints of the ED. The person should be encouraged to share their story with the clinician, to facilitate a collaborative approach to identifying the needs of the individual.[89]

PRACTICE TIP

Be alert to behaviours that indicate a possible increased risk of suicide, such as giving away possessions, talking about suicide or the withdrawal from family, friends and normal activities. Document and communicate this knowledge to others as part of the consumer's assessment. Early recognition and communication of risk can improve outcomes and safety.

First contact: a positive, supportive response

Managing people experiencing suicidal thoughts and actions in crisis situations hinges upon ensuring safety for all concerned. This means scanning the environment for potential risks, speaking in a calm voice and favourably shifting risk as far as possible.[90] Many people in suicidal crisis are at high or imminent risk of suicide/self-harm, and require constant one-to-one monitoring and secure support. In the ED it is not always realistic or desirable for the primary support person to constantly be at the side of and interacting with someone while simultaneously recording observations. The important point here is for human contact with the distressed person, attending to any immediate health concerns following assessment. This is an opportunity for the clinician to generate trust with the person, maintaining support and facilitating appropriate expressions of emotions.

Clinical engagement with people who are experiencing suicidal crises can evoke mixed feelings in everyone and paramedics/ED staff are not immune to having thoughts and feelings which could be anti-therapeutic. It is important that the first response is not primarily defensive. It is critical to realise that not everybody has to take on the responsibility of treating those with suicidal thoughts/actions, but at the very least those who are in the situation where such persons may present should have the basic skills to provide a compassionate response and make a general assessment of suicidal persons (even though they should not feel obliged to continue management). Indeed, those involved should be aware of their limitations, and be willing to seek the assistance of colleagues with appropriate referral.

It is important to recognise that often people experiencing suicidal crises have recently perceived rejection, and a considerable degree of compassion and patience may be required in order to establish rapport. This can be achieved by communicating the wish to understand what is happening to that person and that time has been set aside to do so.

Having established a reasonable environment in which to assess the person, that person should be enabled to present their history in as full a manner as possible. When attempting to elicit information from individuals it should be remembered that challenging or direct questions that could be interpreted as critical will rarely help. Rather, open-ended and non-judgemental comments, such as: 'Things seem to be difficult for you right now' or 'You must have been feeling pretty upset about that', can encourage people to talk about their difficulties, and the open-ended question: 'Can you tell me more about it?' is often useful.

Some individuals may remain resistant, but by stressing that it is important to try to understand what is happening and by the therapeutic use of silence, which further indicates a willingness and openness to listen, most will respond and rapport can be achieved.

Assess the degree of suicidal intent

Recent best practice evidence indicates that although asking about suicide intent is critical and is not associated with an increased risk for suicide, evidence is still mounting to determine the best ways to ask about suicide.[91] Regardless, there is a general consensus that detailed questions should be asked in order to understand the extent of suicidal intent—including how, when, where and by what means the individual has considered ending their life, as well as the frequency, intensity and resistibility of these thoughts. It is also critical for paramedics and ED staff to recognise that, for many people, suicidal states fluctuate rapidly, indicating the need for ongoing and frequent assessment in order to best understand the individual's present experience.[92]

Assessment must recognise the basic human need for autonomy, as well as safety, and this means creating strategies to enable disclosure and trust wherever possible. More direct questions may be necessary in order to elucidate the degree of suicidal intent. Suicidal thoughts and behaviour usually revolve around interpersonal phenomena, and the role of persons of significance to the consumer should be sought. This may necessitate a systematic enquiry about the person's relationship with family members and friends. More specifically, suicidal intent can be determined on the basis of the degree of planning, knowledge of the lethality of the intended suicidal act, the degree of isolation of the person and also by asking open-ended questions, such as: 'What are your feelings—right now—about living and dying?' Such a question permits those with suicidal thoughts to express their feelings in a way that is not provided for by direct questions such as: 'Do you really want to kill yourself?', which may be too confronting and does not allow for the ambivalent feelings that are almost invariably present among people experiencing suicide-related distress.

PRACTICE TIP

Reassure people that no matter how challenging their situation is right now, the way forward is best achieved by working together. Where possible, use a conversational-style risk-assessment approach to create interactive dialogue and trust.

Commence initial management

The most important initial decision is based on assessment of the safety of the individual. It may be that the opportunity of ventilating thoughts and feelings to a concerned person has been sufficient for some people. In the absence of a mental condition, or if suicidal thoughts and actions have resulted in positive changes in personal relationships, further contact may be unnecessary, although the opportunity for further follow-up should be left open, particularly if there are inadequate social supports. Again, it is critical to remember that suicidal states fluctuate and that the presence or absence of suicide-related symptoms at one point in time is not indicative of future suicidal states for the individual.

For those who are profoundly suicidal with a severe mental illness, detention under the relevant Mental Health Act and hospitalisation may be necessary (see Chapter 4). Indeed, sometimes compulsory hospitalisation in order to reduce the likelihood of danger to the person or to others is required. If so, it must be emphasised to the individual and their relatives/carers/friends that it has been done in order to protect, not punish, the person. If this should happen, try to seek input from the relative, carer or friend in order to ensure that this is the best approach to the current situation.

Current evidence suggests that working with the individual to co-create a safety plan is an important suicide prevention strategy.[93] The safety planning intervention was initially developed in the United States for use in the ED, and involves working with the individual to develop a range of strategies to help keep them safe. A particular emphasis is placed on drawing on the person's internal resources and coping strategies, as well as involving supportive others and services. It should also include steps that the individual will take to remove/minimise lethal means from their environment. Each person's safety plan should be personalised to their experience, and should not be confused with a management plan. A safety plan can be commenced in the ED and then completed with external service providers. Various examples of safety planning templates exist, including the 'BeyondNow' application developed by beyondblue.[90]

SUICIDE AND SELF-HARM IN ABORIGINAL AND MĀORI COMMUNITIES

Despite the strength and resilience of Aboriginal people, the subject area of suicide and self-harm among Aboriginal Australians is one of persistent and overwhelming tragedy, marked by ongoing expressions of intergenerational pain, disconnection and despair. Based on data from New South Wales, Queensland, Western Australia, South Australia and the Northern Territory from 2016 to 2020, approximately one-quarter of deaths of Indigenous Australians aged under 24 were suicide.[77,94] Of note, suicide was the leading cause of death in Indigenous children 5–17.[94] Rates are typically higher for Indigenous men, particularly those in rural communities,[95,96] and often the death results from violent means, particularly hanging or firearms.[96] In contrast, self-harm is equally common among males and females.[77,95]

Several writers warn against a narrow focus on both suicidal and self-harming behaviour in the Aboriginal context.[97,98] All self-harming behaviour, they argue, should be seen as a drastic response to certain stressful experiences (risk factors) and violence in the broader social and emotional context of cultural meaning, cultural identity, historical and current socio-economic conditions.[97,98] Additionally, threats towards death by hanging may have significant historical messages of hurt, injustice, tyranny and domination for Aboriginal people.[99,100]

Rates of suicide and self-harm are also more prevalent among Māori peoples. In 2018, the suicide rate for Māori was 18.2 per 100,000 people, around 1.6 times greater than non-Māori (10.6 per 100,000). Rates were particularly high among males and youth.[76] These elevated rates can be attributed to higher rates of social deprivation and disadvantage, as well as acculturative stress, resulting from colonisation in the 1800s;[46] much like those factors faced by Aboriginal Australians.

It is critical for practitioners to be aware of the way that suicide is experienced in Aboriginal and Māori communities in order to ensure a culturally sensitive and competent approach to those experiencing suicide-related crises.

SUICIDE AND SELF-HARM AMONG PEOPLE SEEKING REFUGE AND PEOPLE SEEKING ASYLUM

Suicide and self-harm are common issues experienced by people seeking refuge and people seeking asylum, with suicide thought to be the leading cause of premature death for individuals in immigration detention in Australia.[101,102] A refugee is someone who, 'owing to a well-founded fear of being persecuted on account of race, religion, nationality, membership of a particular social group, or political opinion, is outside the country of their nationality, and is unable to or, owing to such fear, is unwilling to avail him/herself of the protection of that country'.[103] An asylum-seeker is someone who has left his or her country of origin in search of protection—whether or not their claim for refugee status has been determined.

Few studies have examined the ED use of immigration detainees in Australia, although some research has identified higher rates of use, and greater complexity in presentation.[104–109] The most common primary diagnosis of immigration detainee attendances to a Darwin ED in 2011 was psychiatric problems (24% of 770 total attendances), with many of these (138) being associated with self-harm, often among men.[107] Twenty of the total attendances were by children (9–17 years), of which 75% were related to self-harm.

Suicidal and self-harming behaviour among these populations may be associated with the considerable uncertainty for the individual, which can contribute to anxiety, mental distress and uncertainty for the future. Such factors are thought to be linked to depression, post-traumatic stress and other mental health concerns among these individuals.[109] Specifically, these behaviours might be associated with rejected visa applications and claims for permanent protection being refused, as well as being linked to past trauma and/or torture issues. Concerns are currently particularly high for those seeking asylum who have arrived in Australia by boat, with mental deterioration attributed to periods of prolonged uncertainty.[102,108]

The acts of suicide and self-harm by people seeking asylum are widely regarded by practitioners as among the most common and stressful emergency issues encountered by health and human service professionals. Emergency clinicians may feel overwhelmed and be left feeling unsure what to do by the complexity and the unusual depth of personal feeling they confront. For this reason, there is a real need for emergency clinicians to work together with advocate, migration, refugee and trauma services, so that all concerned can be supported in managing their own feelings and reactions while making themselves available to the individual. As with any individual engaging in these behaviours, it is important to ensure the safety of the person and to encourage them to feel listened to and validated.

OTHER CONSIDERATIONS WHEN PROVIDING EMERGENCY MENTAL HEALTH CARE

LEGAL CONSIDERATIONS

It is important to be reminded of the legal considerations when providing emergency mental health care. In particular, not all people come to the attention of emergency health services voluntarily. In some instances, a person may be treated without their consent or against their will. This situation arises when a person requires urgent treatment to save their life or to prevent serious harm to their health, or when the individual needs urgent treatment but is incapable of giving consent. Involuntary treatment orders can take the form of specific 'licence conditions', Community Treatment Orders (CTOs), or a legal order for care by an authorised officer for immediate detention under relevant legislation. For more detail and the Mental Health Acts for each state and territory, see Chapter 4.

In addition to involuntary detention, some Mental Health Acts also contain regulations for the administration of sedatives. For example, the New Zealand *Mental Health (Compulsory Assessment and Treatment) Act 1992* contains a provision that enables a medical practitioner, in certain circumstances, to administer an appropriate sedative to a person (Section 110A). If a medical practitioner administers urgent sedation, they must do so in accordance with relevant guidelines and standards of care and treatment issued by the Director-General of Health under section 130 of the Act.[109]

Occasionally, issues will arise when people with mental illnesses encounter the criminal justice system. There is much publicity of critical incidents involving 'mentally disturbed' people, which gives rise to the widely held belief that a high proportion of people with mental illness commit crimes. This is generally not the case. Most people with a mental illness, including those with major illnesses, do not commit crimes; but people with mental illness nevertheless are over-represented in the criminal justice system—rates up to 40% of prisoners in Australia reported having a previous diagnosis of mental illness.[110] Australian paramedics achieved national health professional registration in 2019, with the Paramedicine Board of Australia adopting professional capabilities for registered paramedics. While role activities may be governed by legislation that varies across health jurisdictions, all paramedics are required to meet Professional Competency Standards and Professional Capabilities for paramedics.[111] Paramedics must have a comprehensive understanding of their legislative obligations to comply with the various Mental Health Acts across the different geographical jurisdictions.

EARLY INTERVENTION IN AGGRESSION AND MITIGATION STRATEGIES TO PREVENT UNNECESSARY USE OF RESTRAINT AND/OR RESTRICTIVE PRACTICES

Not all people experiencing a mental health emergency display aggression and/or violence. Further, for many people displaying these behaviours, these are often unrelated to the individual's mental health. However, aggression and violence in healthcare is a growing concern, often leading staff to feel unsafe.[112–114] For example, a 2014 South Australian Ambulance Service report indicated a 74% increase in incidents of physical and verbal abuse directed at paramedics in the previous 2 years (from 57 incidents in 2012 to 99 incidents in 2013).[115] In addition to their role in dealing with the aftermath of out-of-hospital aggression and violence, EDs are also faced with occurrences of aggression and violence within the hospital setting.[112,113,116] ED nurses are frequently subjected to verbal abuse (e.g. swearing or obscenity, shouting and sarcasm) and physical abuse (e.g. pushing, hitting, use of a weapon and punching).[117] Risk factors associated with these incidences include a past history of violence, substance and alcohol misuse,[118] comorbid medical and mental health diagnoses,[119] long waiting times and time of day (with increased incidents in the evenings).[120] Some research indicates that those individuals who experience co-morbid psychoses and substance misuse are at a greater risk of violent behaviour;[121] others have found that this risk is no greater than for those individuals who have a substance use condition only.[122]

BOX 36.9 **DETECTION AND MANAGEMENT OF AGGRESSION**[120,123]

EARLY DETECTION OF THE POTENTIAL SIGNS OF AGGRESSION

- Being under the influence of alcohol or other drugs, particularly psychostimulants
- Having slurred speech, being sarcastic, abusive, threatening, using foul language
- Intruding personal space; defiant and uncooperative
- Hostile facial expression with prolonged eye contact and staring
- Bloodstained clothing, dishevelled appearance
- Possession of a weapon (actual or potential)
- Obvious motor restlessness, pacing, tapping feet (exclude akathisia), clenching of fists or jaws, twisting of neck.

OUT-OF-HOSPITAL AND ED MANAGEMENT GUIDELINES FOR AGGRESSION

- Consider personal safety at all times
- Avoid an argumentative, confrontational response
- Show you are listening–paraphrase back a summary of what is being said to you and communicate that you are trying to solve the problem
- Calm the person as much as possible, encouraging them to slow down prior to solving the problem
- Show concern through verbal and non-verbal responses. Avoid patronising their concerns
- Adopt a non-threatening body posture, voice tone and disposition more broadly
- Consider the safety of other consumers and their visitors at all times
- Avoid an audience or crowd forming around the consumer
- Place the person in a quiet and secure area and let staff know what is happening and why
- Never turn your back on the individual
- Don't walk ahead of the individual and ensure adequate personal space
- Avoid sudden movements or elevation of voice that may startle or be perceived as a threat, danger or attack
- Provide continuous observation and record behaviour changes in consumer notes
- Wear a personal duress alarm at all times
- Let the person talk
- Never block off exits and ensure you have a safe escape route.

Robust and assertive practice of early identification and early intervention of aggression and violence are the first steps in any de-escalation process. Where the prospect of violence is deemed to be real, staff must act in a defensive and anticipatory manner, at all times ready for the level of violence to escalate.[123] Early detection of the potential signs of aggression is the first step towards prevention and de-escalation. Some signs of potential aggression and general out-of-hospital and ED management guidelines are listed in Box 36.9. See also Chapter 11 for out-of-hospital triage assessment and management. The primary concern in the management of people displaying violent or aggressive behaviour (and of the impact of their behaviour on those present) is positive engagement and safety leading to de-escalation of the individual's behaviour in the least restrictive environment. This is not a time to be a hero. Rather, it is a time to ensure personal safety and for all involved to work using exemplary communication, teamwork and strategic use of medication and physical interventions.

PRACTICE TIP

Be alert to warning signs of aggression to prevent patient and staff harm. Aggressive behaviours that indicate an increased risk of aggression include intense staring, yelling, intoxication, threatening gestures. Use de-escalation techniques and seek support. This is not the time to be a hero.

MINIMISATION OF SECLUSION AND RESTRAINT

As discussed earlier in the chapter, certain situations (i.e. when an individual is behaving in ways that put them at risk to themselves or others) will require paramedics to implement processes of physical and/or chemical restraint in order to safely provide care and/or transport of the individual. For these same reasons, restraint is sometimes required in the ED. Each state, territory and emergency care provider has different legal regulations regarding seclusion and restraint (see Chapter 4), including which professionals (e.g. paramedics and nurses) are able to provide these responses. For example, in some states in Australia, paramedics have legislated powers of apprehension, treatment and transport to a medical facility.[124–126] Others require that the police detain the person under the Mental Health Act before an intervention can occur.[127] The least invasive means of restraint should always be used, with escalation to more intrusive means only when absolutely necessary. There must be legal justification for the use of restraint which is defined as self-defence, or the defence of others.[37]

In most cases, the use of verbal intervention skills, along with shared decision-making, can often resolve or de-escalate an incident. When the person is exhibiting signs of a condition such as severe anxiety, depending on the jurisdiction, a sedative agent, usually a benzodiazepine, can be administered once the person's capacity to consent to the intervention has been verified. If the person has been deemed to be competent, they maintain the right to refuse any treatment or transport. This is a major guiding principle in any interaction between a healthcare professional and a consumer of healthcare resources.

In instances where chemical restraint may be necessary, some of the more common agents used in this situation include diazepam, midazolam and haloperidol. While clinical observations after administration of intravenous medications will vary, depending upon local protocols, close monitoring after chemical restraint will involve recording vital signs every 15 minutes for the first hour, every 30 minutes for the second hour and then hourly for 4 hours (see Chapter 13, Patient assessment). If mechanical restraint (e.g. belts, harnesses, straps or handcuffs) is required, then the minimum type and amount of restraint should be used with caution. If a person has been mechanically restrained by paramedics, they should be transported, whenever possible, in the lateral position, avoiding the use of the prone position, which can restrict the person's ability to breathe and has been linked to restraint asphyxiation in patients.[128]

There are, however, some concerns about the use of these practices. For example, the primary concerns about ED seclusion rooms are three-fold. First, there is a danger that people *out of sight* are also *out of mind*, meaning that emergency clinicians may be less concerned with acts of self-harm, physical distress or injury. Second, such a setting may exacerbate mental distress by removing any capacity that the individual has to make decisions or take control of their situation. Removing personal control and freedom in this can have a traumatising and possibly re-traumatising effect.[14] Third, the person may perceive that being placed in a room against their will is the direct result of disclosing their distress and thoughts of self-harm to a health worker, resulting in the individual feeling punished for speaking honestly about their predicament. Each of these factors can hinder an individual's future encounters with the mental healthcare system.

Opposing this stance is the view that the person is unable to take control and it is the right of staff to have a safe, predictable and protected environment. Viewed this way, seclusion and restraint can, when used properly, be a lifesaving and injury-sparing measure designed to protect individuals in danger of harming themselves or others.[129] To be effective, seclusion and restraint must be supported by adequate policies and procedures which are periodically reviewed for determining when, why and how measures will be used and evaluated. Even in the most secure environments risk cannot be eliminated completely. Mental health support does not stop when a person is secluded. A clinically informed response means that staff continue to advocate for the individual. Staff must scrutinise the seclusion area so that it is, as far as possible, supportive and calming. It is imperative that the area is critically assessed so that it is free of hanging and other self-harm points.

CULTURAL CONSIDERATIONS WHEN PROVIDING AN EMERGENCY MENTAL HEALTH RESPONSE

As outlined in Chapter 5, Australia and Aotearoa New Zealand are increasingly becoming multicultural nations, and being aware of cultural nuances when providing mental health care is essential to good practice, regardless of the setting.

THE IMPORTANCE OF CULTURE

'Culture' gives meaning and context to the way people communicate thinking, action and events. Culture also allows people to make assumptions about social and emotional life, illness and death and how they should be understood within a particular context or setting. When individuals from one culture find themselves living in a different cultural context, there may be differences in the way that they communicate distress and suffering. In mental health emergencies it is important to look beyond taken-for-granted assumptions regarding the way that symptoms of mental distress are communicated and the personal meaning that people from culturally and linguistically diverse cultures give to diagnosis, treatments and outcomes. Consequently, people from culturally and linguistically diverse backgrounds remain a population group requiring special attention to their mental health status.[7] The challenges of a diverse population—of developing a culturally inclusive mental health assessment—remain.

CULTURAL AND LANGUAGE CONSIDERATIONS

Some of the cultural and language considerations relevant to the assessment of emergencies in mental health include:

- it is not uncommon for stress to increase the likelihood that a person from a culturally and linguistically diverse culture will revert to their language of origin
- if a person speaks a language other than English at home, it may be helpful to use an accredited interpreter service. Family members/friends should only be used in emergency situations
- be aware that a prior relationship between the individual and an interpreter can be a problem in small ethnic groups—in particular, new and emerging communities—where there tend to be fewer accredited interpreters and where individuals might have concerns about the confidentiality of involving an interpreter.

Cultural differences can result in markedly variable mental health presentations. Cultural differences can influence the way in which symptoms are presented, what is considered a good outcome, acceptance of prescription medication and help-seeking behaviour more generally.

PEOPLE SEEKING REFUGE AND ASYLUM

In recent years, there have been more people than ever affected by forced displacement. In 2020, over 135,000 refugees and people seeking asylum were in Australia and Aotearoa New Zealand.[130] The media pays heavy attention to the health and wellbeing of those in immigration detention, and it is not uncommon for these individuals to present to EDs. See Chapter 5 for further discussion of cultural considerations. Having an awareness and understanding of the ongoing impacts of uncertainty, isolation and trauma experienced by these individuals is essential to providing culturally appropriate, trauma-informed care.

Trauma-informed care acknowledges the significant prevalence of trauma among mental health consumers, many of whom have a lived experience of violence, abuse, neglect or other forms of trauma. The impact on individuals, family and the community often persists long after the trauma has ceased, and trauma survivors may present with multiple symptoms and behaviours. This emphasises the need for individual, flexible care, with a focus on the individual's physical and psychological safety, and an awareness of factors that may lead to re-traumatisation.[14]

PRACTICE TIP

Mental health assessment must be culturally competent to enhance the therapeutic relationship. Ask the person about how their situation would be understood and responded to by people from their own cultural group. This may mean asking about how their experiences would be expressed or explained in their cultural context.

COLLABORATION AND TEAMWORK BETWEEN MENTAL HEALTH PROFESSIONALS

Irrespective of practice setting, clinical conflict in mental health care is inevitable because of the episodic nature of mental illness, differing approaches to care and availability of resources. Consequently, service provision for individuals experiencing mental health problems can be hindered due to a breakdown of communication and deadlock between individual service providers, individuals and organisations. The solution to these problems is deadlock prevention and promotion of partnership. Also important is a commitment by managers, codified in formal policy, to deal with escalated conflict directly with their counterparts. It is acknowledged that a formal policy and process may seem cumbersome, especially when the issue (e.g. admission to hospital) is time-sensitive. But resolving the problem early in a collaborative, team-oriented manner, is ultimately more desirable in a health service, where many issues have significant implications for numerous parts of the service.[131,132]

When individuals and healthcare professionals collaborate more freely they are more likely to trust each other. When individuals trust healthcare organisations, they are more likely to give of themselves now in anticipation of future change and reward.

The benefits of creatively preventing and resolving conflict include:

- conflict resolution, which reduces individual and organisational ambiguity, and increases transparency and efficiency of healthcare
- new lines of communication and professional relationships, which facilitate timely access to appropriate mental health resources and supports
- a decrease in the number of problems that are pushed up the management chain.

SUMMARY

Paramedic and emergency health worker assessment and care of people experiencing mental health emergencies is dependent on a range of factors within the individual and the environment. The practitioner who takes a holistic approach to care will take account of social, psychological and medical interventions, which are essential if we are to address the many myths about the practice of mental health care. The 17th-century philosopher René Descartes conceptualised the distinction between the mind and the body when he viewed the 'mind' as completely separable from the 'body'. And, as we have seen in this chapter, mental health practitioners and advocates have been trying to put them back together. This separation between so-called 'mental' and 'physical' health has no real relevance to the scientific understanding of health in the 21st century, yet the myths and misinformation persist. It will be the skills of practitioners in their formulation of diagnosis and treatment of symptoms that can be bewildering to individuals and their relatives, the reassurance that they are working with others to improve quality of life and continuity of information about treatment that will help diffuse crisis and reduce suffering in some of the most vulnerable people in our society.

Mental health emergencies found out of hospital and in the ED are varied and challenging for both the individual and the emergency health worker. There is a range of factors that must be considered to make the fullest and most informed assessment possible, including the nature of the presenting problem, cultural considerations, quality of information available and interdisciplinary collaboration. Regardless of the presenting problem, it is important for the emergency practitioner to treat the person and their family with respect and empathy, while simultaneously operating within a human rights framework protecting the individual and others from harm.

CASE STUDY

Troy is a 19-year-old male who recently broke up with his girlfriend of 2 years. He was told by his former girlfriend that she had found someone new and 'wanted nothing more to do with him'. Troy's girlfriend had grown tired of Troy's mood changes and brooding. Some days he seemed fine, while at other times he was irritable and had ongoing difficulties at work and in his family.

Troy had been out drinking with his mates and had tried to call his former girlfriend several times by phone. She refused to take his calls. He wanted to see if he could get back together with her. When his calls went unanswered, Troy went to his former girlfriend's house by taxi. He tried to see her, to tell her 'he could not live without her' and that 'his life would soon be over'. His former girlfriend refused to come to the door. The police were called and Troy was removed from the property.

Troy returned home and continued drinking alone. He went out to his back shed, and with some rope strung a noose up across the central beam of the shed. He also bound his legs together with electrical tape. He then called his mate Phil and told him that he was 'going away for a while'. Troy was in an intoxicated state. He told Phil that he no longer needed his car and that Phil could now use it. Phil said that he would come over to see him, but Troy insisted that everything was now sorted and that he was fine and did not need any help. After the phone call, Phil drove to Troy's house. Troy was found hanging and barely alive. Phil grabbed Troy's legs to ease the strain of the rope. He also managed to attract a neighbour's attention. The neighbour came running to assist and with the aid of a ladder, both men removed the noose and lowered Troy's body to ground level. Police and ambulance were called.

QUESTIONS

1. What principles of mental health triage are important on arrival at Troy's house? Why are they important?
2. What mental health-related questions and observations might be useful at the first point of contact with Troy?

Troy arrives at the emergency department (ED).

3. What is the goal of initial contact and treatment for someone like Troy, and how might it be achieved?
4. What might be the purpose of a mental state assessment of Troy on arrival at the ED?

Answers to Case Study Questions can be found on evolve **http://evolve.elsevier.com/AU/Curtis/emergency/**

USEFUL WEBSITES

ABC 7.30 Report, Why are mentally-ill children tied up and tormented? Provides insight into child abuse, www.abc.net.au/news/2013-12-10/why-are-mentally-ill-children-tied-up-and-tormented/5148180.

Beyondblue. This site provides resources for support of mental health, www.beyondblue.org.au/.

Mental Health First Aid Australia. This site provides resources for support of mental health, https://mhfa.com.au/.

Mental Health Foundation of New Zealand. This site provides resources for support of mental health, www.mentalhealth.org.nz/.

National Eating Disorders Collaboration. This site provides resources for support of eating disorders, www.nedc.com.au/.

Refugee Council of Australia. This site provides resources for support of refugees, www.refugeecouncil.org.au/.

SANE Australia. This site provides resources for support of mental health, www.sane.org/.

Suicide and self-harm crisis interview. This site provides resources for support and understanding of suicide and self-harm, www.youtube.com/watch?v=fLXfDepZ-oO.

Suicide Prevention Australia. This site provides resources for suicide prevention, http://suicidepreventionaust.org/.

Teen suicide risk assessment. This site provides resources for support and understanding of teen suicide and self-harm, https://www.youtube.com/watch?v=WdC3nhxA66U.

REFERENCES

1. Australian Institute of Health and Welfare (AIHW). Australian burden of disease study: impact and causes of illness and death in Australia 2015. Canberra: AIHW; 2019.
2. Australian Bureau of Statistics. National health survey first results: Australia 2017–2018. Canberra, Australia: ABS; 2018.
3. Lawrence D, Johnson S, Hafekost J, de Haan KB, Sawyer M, Ainley J, et al. The mental health of children and adolescents: report on the second Australian child and adolescent survey of mental health and wellbeing. Canberra: Department of Health; 2015.
4. Morgan VA, Waterreus A, Jablensky A, Mackinnon A, McGrath JJ, Carr V, et al. People living with psychotic illness 2010. Report on the second Australian national survey. Canberra: Department of Health and Ageing; 2011.
5. Wilson A, Nicolson M. Mental health in Aotearoa: results from the 2018 mental health monitor and the 2018/19 New Zealand health survey. Wellington: Te Hiringa Hauora/Health Promotion Agency; 2020.
6. Council of Australian Governments. Roadmap for national mental health reform 2012–2022. 2013. Available from: www.health.gov.au/internet/main/publishing.nsf/content/mental-roadmap.
7. Australia Department of Health. The fifth national mental health and suicide prevention plan. Canberra: Department of Health; 2017.
8. Duggan M, Harris B, Chislett WK, Calder R. Nowhere else to go: why Australia's health system results in people with mental illness getting 'stuck' in emergency departments. Melbourne: Victoria University and Mitchell Institute; 2020.
9. Li X, Srasuebkul P, Reppermund S, Trollor J. Emergency department presentation and readmission after index psychiatric admission: a data linkage study. BMJ Open 2018;8(2):e018613.
10. Australian Institute of Health and Welfare (AIHW). Mental health services in Australia. 2021. Available from: www.aihw.gov.au/reports/mental-health-services/mental-health-services-in-australia.
11. Australasian College for Emergency Medicine. Mental health service use: a New Zealand context. West Melbourne: ACEM; 2019.
12. Wand T, D'Abrew N, Acret L, White K. Evaluating a new model of nurse-led emergency department mental health care in Australia; perspectives of key informants. Int Emerg Nurs 2016;24:16–21.
13. SANE Australia. How to help when someone is suicidal. Updated 10 September 2021. Available from: www.sane.org/mental-health-and-illness/facts-and-guides/sane-steps-how-to-help-when-someone-is-suicidal.

14. Molloy L, Fields L, Trostian B, Kinghorn G. Trauma-informed care for people presenting to the emergency department with mental health issues. Emerg Nurse 2020;28(2):30–5.
15. Hall A, McKenna B, Dearie V, Maguire T, Charleston R, Furness T. Educating emergency department nurses about trauma informed care for people presenting with mental health crisis: a pilot study. BMC Nurs 2016;15:21.
16. Muskett C. Trauma-informed care in inpatient mental health settings: a review of the literature. Int J Ment Health Nurs 2014;23(1):51–9.
17. St John Ambulance Western Australia. Clinical practice guidelines for ambulance care in Western Australia, disturbed and abnormal behaviour. Perth: St John Ambulance WA; 2017.
18. South Australia Ambulance Service. Clinical practice guidelines, acute behavioural emergencies. Adelaide: South Australia Government; 2017.
19. Queensland Ambulance Service. Clinical practice procedures: assessment/mental status. Brisbane: Queensland Government; 2017.
20. Queensland Ambulance Service. Clinical practice guidelines: behavioural disturbances/the physically restrained patient. Brisbane: Queensland Government; 2017.
21. Queensland Ambulance Service. Clinical practice guidelines: behavioural disturbances/the suicidal patient. Brisbane: Queensland Government; 2017.
22. Queensland Ambulance Service. Clinical practice guidelines: behavioural disturbances/acute behavioural disturbance. Brisbane: Queensland Government; 2017.
23. Pre-Hospital Emergency Care Council. PHECC clinical practice guidelines, mental health emergency. Osberstown, Ireland: Pre-Hospital Emergency Care Council; 2017.
24. New South Wales Ambulance Service. 2016 Protocol and pharmacology, mental health emergency. Sydney: New South Wales Ambulance Service; 2016.
25. National Association of Emergency Medical Services Officials. National Model EMS clinical guidelines, agitated or violent patient/behavioral emergency. Falls Church, Virginia: NASEMSO; 2016.
26. Ambulance Victoria. Clinical Practice Guidelines Ambulance and MICA Paramedics, Mental Status Assessment (Vol. CPG A0106). Melbourne: Ambulance Victoria; 2016.
27. Ambulance Victoria. Clinical Practice Guidelines Ambulance and MICA Paramedics Mental Health Conditions (Vol. CPG A0107). Melbourne: Ambulance Victoria; 2016.
28. Alberta Health Services. EMS medical control protocols, adult psychiatric non-combative – anxiety. Edmonton: Alberta Health Services; 2014.
29. Alberta Health Services. EMS medical control protocols, adult combative behaviour. Edmonton: Alberta Health Services; 2014.
30. Lamanna D, Shapiro GK, Kirst M, Matheson FI, Nakhost A, Stergiopoulos V. Co-responding police–mental health programmes: service user experiences and outcomes in a large urban centre. Int J Ment Health Nurs 2018;27(2):891–900.
31. Puntis S, Perfect D, Kirubarajan A, Bolton, S, Davies F, Hayes A, et al. A systematic review of co-responder models of police mental health 'street' triage. BMC Psychiatry 2018;18(1):256.
32. Molodynski A, Hollingsworth S, Penzenstadler L, Perfect D, Puntis S. An evaluation of the characteristics and outcomes of users of a street triage service: retrospective case note review. BJPsych Bull 2019;43(6):290–4.
33. Robertson J, Fitts MS, Petrucci J, McKay D, Hubble G, Clough AR. Cairns mental health co-responder project: essential elements and challenges to programme implementation. Int J Ment Health Nurs 2020;29(3):450–9.
34. Richmond JS, Berlin JS, Fishkind AB, Holloman Jr GH, Zeller SL, Wilson MP, et al. Verbal de-escalation of the agitated patient: consensus statement of the American Association for Emergency Psychiatry Project BETA De-escalation Workgroup. West J Emerg Med 2012;13(1):17–25.
35. Spencer S, Johnson P. Deescalation techniques for managing aggression. Cochrane Database Syst Rev 2016;(1):CD012034.
36. Patel MX, Sethi FN, Barnes TR, Dix R, Dratcu L, Fox B, et al. Joint BAP NAPICU evidence-based consensus guidelines for the clinical management of acute disturbance: de-escalation and rapid tranquillisation. J Psychiat Intens Care 2018;14(2):89–132.
37. Victoria Department of Health. Transport protocols for people with a mental illness. Victoria Department of Health; Updated 29 May 2015. Available from: www.health.vic.gov.au/practice-and-service-quality/transport-protocols-for-people-with-a-mental-illness.
38. Roberts L, Hains D. Mental health and mental illness in paramedic practice. Chatswood: Elsevier Health Sciences; 2021.
39. New South Wales Ministry of Health. Mental health for emergency departments—a reference guide. North Sydney: NSW Ministry of Health; 2009, amended 2015.
40. Wand T, Schaecken P. Consumer evaluation of a mental health liaison nurse service in the emergency department. Contemp Nurse 2006;21(1): 14–21.
41. Wand T, Collett G, Cutten A, Buchanan-Hagen S, Stack A, White K. Patient and staff experience with a new model of emergency department based mental health nursing care implemented in two rural settings. Int Emerg Nurs 2021;57:101013.
42. Wand T, White K, Patching J, Dixon J, Green T. Outcomes from the evaluation of an emergency department-based mental health nurse practitioner outpatient service in Australia. J Am Acad Nurse Pract 2012;24(3):149–59.
43. Huber JP, Wilhelm K, Landstra JM. Months of May: mental health presentations and the impact of a psychiatric emergency care centre on an inner-city emergency department. Emerg Med Australas 2021;33(4):691–6.
44. American Psychiatric Association. Diagnostic and statistical manual of mental disorders. 5th ed. Arlington, Virginia: APA; 2013.
45. World Health Organization (WHO). International statistical classification of diseases and related health problems (ICD). Available from: www.who.int/standards/classifications/classification-of-diseases.

46. New Zealand Ministry of Health. Te Rau Hinengaro: the New Zealand mental health survey: summary. Wellington: Ministry of Health; 2006.
47. Black Dog Institute. Anxiety causes. Black Dog Institute. Available from: www.blackdoginstitute.org.au/resources-support/anxiety/causes/.
48. Valdes B, Salani D, King B, de Oliveira GC. Recognition and treatment of psychiatric emergencies for health care providers in the emergency department: panic attack, panic disorder, and adverse drug reactions. J Emerg Nurs 2021;47(3):459–68.
49. Keefe JR, Chambless DL, Barber JP, Milrod BL. Treatment of anxiety and mood comorbidities in cognitive–behavioral and psychodynamic therapies for panic disorder. J Psychiat Res 2019;114:34–40.
50. Australian Bureau of Statistics (ABS). Mental health, 2017–18 financial year. ABS. Available from: www.abs.gov.au/statistics/health/mental-health/mental-health/2017-18#mental-and-behavioural-conditions.
51. Vos T, Lim SS, Abbafati C. Global burden of 369 diseases and injuries in 204 countries and territories, 1990–2019: a systematic analysis for the Global Burden of Disease Study 2019. Lancet 2020;396(10258):1204–22.
52. Health Promotion Agency. Postnatal depression in New Zealand: findings from the 2015 New Mothers' Mental Health Survey. Wellington: Health Promotion Agency; 2016.
53. Austin MP, Highet N, Expert Working Group. Mental health care in the perinatal period: Australian clinical practice guideline. 2017. Available from: www.cope.org.au/wp-content/uploads/2018/05/COPE-Perinatal-MH-Guideline_Final-2018.pdf.
54. United Nations. World Population Ageing 2020. Geneva: UN DESA; 2020.
55. Hamer HP, Lampshire D, Thomson S. Mental health of older people. In: Procter N, Hamer HP, McGarry D, editors. Mental health: a person-centred approach. 2nd ed. North Ryde: Cambridge University Press; 2017.
56. Olds T, Burton NW, Sprod J, Maher C, Ferrar K, Brown WJ, et al. One day you'll wake up and won't have to go to work: the impact of changes in time use on mental health following retirement. PLoS One 2018;13(6):e0199605.
57. Frost R, Nair P, Aw S, Gould RL, Kharicha K, Buszewicz M, Walters K. Supporting frail older people with depression and anxiety: a qualitative study. Aging Ment Health 2020;24(12):1977–84.
58. Wojt IR, Cairns R, Clough A, Tan EC. The prevalence and characteristics of psychotropic-related hospitalizations in older people: a systematic review and meta-analysis. J Am Med Dir Assoc 2021;22(6):1206–14.e5.
59. Semple D, Smyth R. Oxford handbook of psychiatry. 4th ed. Oxford: Oxford University Press; 2019.
60. Allsopp K, Read J, Corcoran R, Kinderman P. Heterogeneity in psychiatric diagnostic classification. Psychiatry Res 2019;279:15–22.
61. Huang ZH, Hou CL, Huang YH, He XY, Wang QW, Chen X, et al. Individuals at high risk for psychosis experience more childhood trauma, life events and social support deficit in comparison to healthy controls. Psychiatry Res 2019;273:296–302.
62. Mosquera D, Ross C. A psychotherapy approach to treating hostile voices. Psychosis 2017;9(2):167–75.
63. Bowers L. How expert nurses communicate with acutely psychotic patients. Ment Health Pract 2010;13(7):24–6.
64. Hay P, Mitchison D, Collado AEL, González-Chica DA, Stocks N, Touyz S. Burden and health-related quality of life of eating disorders, including Avoidant/Restrictive Food Intake Disorder (ARFID), in the Australian population. J Eat Disord 2017;5:21.
65. Drieberg H, McEvoy PM, Hoiles KJ, Shu CY, Egan SJ. An examination of direct, indirect and reciprocal relationships between perfectionism, eating disorder symptoms, anxiety, and depression in children and adolescents with eating disorders. Eat Behav 2019;32:53–9.
66. Scotton WJ, Hill LJ, Williams AC, Barnes NM. Serotonin syndrome: pathophysiology, clinical features, management, and potential future directions. Int J Tryptophan Res 2019;12:1178646919873925.
67. Jacobs ET, Akers KG, Vohra V, King AM. Cyproheptadine for serotonin toxicity: an updated systematic review and grading of evidence. Curr Emerg Hosp Med Rep 2020;8(4):151–9.
68. Australian Institute of Health and Welfare (AIHW). Alcohol and other drug treatment services in Australia annual report. 2021. Available from: www.aihw.gov.au/reports/alcohol-other-drug-treatment-services/alcohol-other-drug-treatment-services-australia.
69. Australian Institute of Health and Welfare (AIHW). Alcohol, tobacco and other drugs in Australia. 2021. Available from: www.aihw.gov.au/reports/alcohol/alcohol-tobacco-other-drugs-australia.
70. McDonough M, Baillie AJ, Clark PJ, Haber PS, Riordan BC, Winter DT, et al. Understanding and managing comorbidities for people with alcohol problems: polydrug use and dependence, co-occurring mental disorders, and physical comorbidities. MJA 2021;215(Suppl. 7):S3–32.
71. Australian Institute of Health and Welfare. National Drug Strategy Household Survey 2019: detailed findings. 2020. p. 104. Drug Statistics series. Available from: www.aihw.gov.au/getmedia/77dbea6e-f071-495c-b71e-3a632237269d/aihw-phe-270.pdf.aspx?inline=true.
72. Baker AL, Denham AMJ, Pohlman S. Treating comorbid substance use and psychosis. In: Badcock JC, Paulik G, editors. A clinical introduction to psychosis. Amsterdam: Academic Press; 2020. p. 511–36.
73. Barrett EL. Lived experiences of Australians with mental health and AOD comorbidity and their perspectives on integrated treatment. Aust J Psychosoc Rehab 2019: Summer 2018–19; 38–42.
74. Afzali MH, Sunderland M, Batterham PJ, Carragher N, Slade T. Trauma characteristics, post-traumatic symptoms, psychiatric disorders and suicidal behaviours: results from the 2007 Australian national survey of mental health and wellbeing. Aust N Z J Psychiatry 2017;51(11):1142–51.
75. World Health Organization (WHO). Suicide worldwide in 2019: global health estimates. Geneva: WHO; 2021.
76. New Zealand Ministry of Health. Office of the Chief Coroner: suicide web tool. New Zealand Ministry of Health; Updated 30 September 2021. Available from: minhealthnz.shinyapps.io/suicide-web-tool/.

77. Australian Institute of Health and Welfare (AIHW). Suicide and self-harm monitoring. AIHW; Updated 18 November 2021. Available from: www.aihw.gov.au/suicide-self-harm-monitoring/data/deaths-by-suicide-in-australia/suicide-deaths-over-time.
78. Shaw RJ, Cullen B, Graham N, Lyall DM, Mackay D, Okolie C, et al. Living alone, loneliness and lack of emotional support as predictors of suicide and self-harm: a nine-year follow up of the UK Biobank cohort. J Affect Disord 2021;279:316–23.
79. Roeder KM, Cole DA. Simultaneous longitudinal examination of hopelessness, thwarted belongingness, and perceived burdensomeness as predictors of suicide ideation. Suicide Life-Threat Behav 2019;49(4):1058–71.
80. Senior M, Burghart M, Yu R, Kormilitzin A, Liu Q, Vaci N, et al. Identifying predictors of suicide in severe mental illness: a feasibility study of a clinical prediction rule (Oxford Mental Illness and Suicide Tool or OxMIS). Front Psychiatry 2020;11:268.
81. Ferguson MS, Reis JA, Rabbetts L, McCracken T, Loughhead M, Rhodes K, et al. The effectiveness of suicide prevention education programs for nurses. Crisis 2018;39(2):96–109.
82. New Zealand Ministry of Health. National service framework library. MOH. Available from: nsfl.health.govt.nz/dhb-planning-package/system-level-measures-framework/data-support-system-level-measures/youth-slm—2.
83. Chan MK, Bhatti H, Meader N, Kaner E, Alderson H, Craig D, et al. Predicting suicide following self-harm: systematic review of risk factors and risk scales. Br J Psychiatry 2016;209(4):277–83.
84. Hawton K, Bergen H, Cooper J, Turnbull P, Waters K, Ness J, et al. Suicide following self-harm: findings from the multicentre study of self-harm in England, 2000–2012. J Affect Disord 2015;175:147–51.
85. Betz ME, Wintersteen M, Boudreaux ED, Brown G, Capoccia L, Currier G, et al. Reducing suicide risk: challenges and opportunities in the emergency department. Ann Emerg Med 2016;68(6):758–65.
86. Shand FL, Batterham P, Chan J, Pirkis J, Spittal MJ, Woodward A, et al. Experience of health care services after a suicide attempt: results from an online survey. Suicide Life-Threat Behav 2018;48(6):779–87.
87. Hill NTM, Halliday L, Reavley NJ. Guidelines for integrated suicide-related crisis and follow-up care in emergency departments and other acute settings. Sydney: Black Dog Institute; 2017.
88. Jones M, Ferguson M, Walsh S, Martinez L, Marsh M, Cronin K, et al. Perspectives of rural health and human service practitioners following suicide prevention training programme in Australia: a thematic analysis. Health Soc Care Community 2018;26(3):356–63.
89. Procter N, Baker A, Grocke K. Introduction to mental health and mental illness: human connectedness and the collaborative consumer narrative. In: Procter N, Hamer HP, McGarry D, editors. Mental health: a person-centred approach. 2nd ed. North Ryde: Cambridge University Press; 2017.
90. Beyond Blue. Information for health professionals. Beyond Blue. Available from: www.beyondblue.org.au/get-support/beyondnow-suicide-safety-planning/information-for-health-professionals.
91. Berman AL, Silverman MM. How to ask about suicide? A question in need of an empirical answer. Crisis 2017;38(4):213–16.
92. Kleiman EM, Turner BJ, Fedor S, Beale EE, Huffman JC, Nock MK. Examination of real-time fluctuations in suicidal ideation and its risk factors: results from two ecological momentary assessment studies. J Abnorm Psychol 2017;126(6):726–38.
93. Stanley B, Brown GK, Brenner LA, Galfalvy HC, Currier GW, Knox KL, et al. Comparison of the safety planning intervention with follow-up vs usual care of suicidal patients treated in the emergency department. JAMA Psychiatry 2018;75(9):894–900.
94. Australian Institute of Health and Welfare (AIHE). Suicide Prevention – AIHW Indigenous Mental Health & Suicide Prevention Clearinghouse. AIHW; Updated 6 December 2021. Available from: www.indigenousmhspc.gov.au/topics/suicide-prevention.
95. Pollock NJ, Naicker K, Loro A, Mulay S, Colman I. Global incidence of suicide among Indigenous peoples: a systematic review. BMC Med 2018;16(1):145.
96. Fitzpatrick SJ, Handley T, Powell N, Read D, Inder KJ, Perkins D, et al. Suicide in rural Australia: a retrospective study of mental health problems, health-seeking and service utilisation. PLoS One 2021;16(7):e0245271.
97. Dudgeon P, Bray A, Walker R. Self-determination and strengths-based Aboriginal and Torres Strait Islander suicide prevention: an emerging evidence-based approach. In: Page AC, Stritzke WGK, editors. Alternatives to suicide. Amsterdam: Academic Press; 2020.
98. Dudgeon P, Bray A, Ring I, McPhee R. Beyond evidence-deficit narratives in Indigenous suicide prevention. 2021. Available from: www.indigenousmhspc.gov.au/publications/evidence-deficit-narratives.
99. Hunter E, Reser J, Baird M, Reser P. An analysis of suicide in Indigenous communities of North Queensland: the historical, cultural and symbolic landscape. Canberra: Commonwealth Government Department of Health and Aged Care; 2001.
100. Rouen C, Clough AR, West C. Non-fatal deliberate self-harm in three remote Indigenous communities in Far North Queensland, Australia. Crisis 2019;40(6):422.
101. Procter N, Posselt M, Ferguson M, McIntyre H, Kenny MA, Curtis R, et al. An evaluation of suicide prevention education for people working with refugees and asylum seekers: improvements in competence, attitudes, and confidence. Crisis 2021;43(4):205–13.
102. Procter NG, Kenny MA, Eaton H, Grech C. Lethal hopelessness: understanding and responding to asylum seeker distress and mental deterioration. Int J Ment Health Nurs 2018;27(1):448–54.
103. United Nations High Commission for Refugees. Convention and protocol relating to the status of refugees. UNHCR. Available from: www.unhcr.org/en-au/3b66c2aa10.
104. Jessup RL, Bramston C, Beauchamp A, Gust A, Cao Y, Haywood C, et al. Impact of COVID-19 on emergency department attendance in an Australia hospital: a parallel convergent mixed methods study. BMJ Open 2021;11(12):e049222.

105. Hanes G, Chee J, Mutch R, Cherian S. Paediatric asylum seekers in Western Australia: identification of adversity and complex needs through comprehensive refugee health assessment. J Paediatr Child Health 2019;55(11):1367–73.

106. Banham D, Karnon J, Densley K, Lynch JW. How much emergency department use by vulnerable populations is potentially preventable? A period prevalence study of linked public hospital data in South Australia. BMJ Open 2019;9(1):e022845.

107. Deans AK, Boerma CJ, Fordyce J, De Souza M, Palmer DJ, Davis JS. Use of Royal Darwin Hospital emergency department by immigration detainees in 2011. Med J Aust 2013;199(11):776–8.

108. Procter N, Baker A, Kenny M, Ferguson M. Mental health of people of immigrant and refugee backgrounds. In: Procter N, Hamer H, McGarry D, editors. Mental health: a person-centred approach. 2nd ed. North Ryde: Cambridge University Press; 2017. p. 238–59.

109. New Zealand Ministry of Health. Guidelines For Medical Practitioners Using Sections 110 And 110a of the Mental Health (Compulsory Assessment And Treatment) Act 1992. New Zealand Ministry of Health. Available from: www.health.govt.nz/system/files/documents/publications/gmpmha.pdf.

110. Australian Institute of Health and Welfare (AIHW). The health of Australia's prisoners 2018. AIHW; 2019. Available from: www.aihw.gov.au/getmedia/2e92f007-453d-48a1-9c6b-4c9531cf0371/aihw-phe-246.pdf.aspx?inline=true.

111. Paramedicine Board of Australia. Professional capabilities for registered paramedics. AHPRA. Available from: www.paramedicineboard.gov.au/Professional-standards/Professional-capabilities-for-registered-paramedics.aspx.

112. Ayasreh IR, Hayajneh FA. Workplace violence against emergency nurses: a literature review. Crit Care Nurs Quart 2021;44(2):187–202.

113. Partridge B, Affleck J. Verbal abuse and physical assault in the emergency department: rates of violence, perceptions of safety, and attitudes towards security. Australas Emerg Nurs J 2017;20(3):139–45.

114. Egerton-Warburton D, Gosbell A, Wadsworth A, Moore K, Richardson DB, Fatovich DM. Perceptions of Australasian emergency department staff of the impact of alcohol-related presentations. MJA 2016;204(4):155.

115. Australian Broadcasting Corporation. SA Ambulance Service report shows attacks against paramedics on rise. Australian Broadcasting Corporation. Available from: www.abc.net.au/news/2014-07-18/sa-ambulance-violent-attacks-against-paramedics-are-on-rise/5606988?WT.ac=statenews_sa.

116. Maguire BJ. Violence against ambulance personnel: a retrospective cohort study of national data from Safe Work Australia. Public Health Res Pract 2018;28(1):e28011805.

117. Pich J, Roche MA. Violence on the job: the experiences of nurses and midwives with violence from patients and their friends and relatives. Healthcare (Basel) 2020;8(4):522. doi:10.3390/healthcare8040522.

118. Coomber K, Curtis A, Vandenberg B, Miller PG, Heilbronn C, Matthews S, et al. Aggression and violence at ambulance attendances where alcohol, illicit and/or pharmaceutical drugs were recorded: a 5-year study of ambulance records in Victoria, Australia. Drug Alcohol Depend 2019;205:107685.

119. Wu Y, Kang R, Yan Y, Gao K, Li Z, Jiang J, et al. Epidemiology of schizophrenia and risk factors of schizophrenia-associated aggression from 2011 to 2015. J Int Med Res 2018;46(10):4039–49.

120. Viottini E, Politano G, Fornero G, Pavanelli PL, Borelli P, Bonaudo M, et al. Determinants of aggression against all health care workers in a large-sized university hospital. BMC Health Serv Res 2020;20(1):215.

121. Černý M, Hodgins S, Kučíková R, Kážmér L, Lambertová A, Nawka A, et al. Violence in persons with and without psychosis in the Czech Republic: risk and protective factors. Neuropsychiatric Dis Treat 2018;14:2793–805.

122. Short T, Thomas S, Mullen P, Ogloff JR. Comparing violence in schizophrenia patients with and without comorbid substance-use disorders to community controls. Acta Psychiatrica Scand 2013;128(4):306–13.

123. Pitts E, Schaller DJ. Violent patients. Treasure Island, Florida: StatPearls Publishing; 2021.

124. Queensland. Mental Health Act 2016. Act No 5. Sydney: New South Wales Government; 2016.

125. New South Wales. Mental Health Act 2007. No 8. Sydney: New South Wales Government; 2007.

126. Australian Capital Territory. Mental Health Act 2015. A2015-38. Canberra: ACT Government; 2015.

127. Victoria. Mental Health Act 2014. Act Number 26/2014. Melbourne: Victorian Government; 2014.

128. Steinberg A. Prone restraint cardiac arrest: a comprehensive review of the scientific literature and an explanation of the physiology. Med Sci Law 2021;61(3):215–26.

129. Hall H, Smithard DG. A principlist justification of physical restraint in the emergency department. New Bioeth 2021;27(2):176–84.

130. United Nations High Commission for Refugees. Forced displacement in 2020. UNHCR. Available from: www.unhcr.org/flagship-reports/globaltrends/.

131. Wise S, Duffield C, Fry M, Roche M. Nurses' role in accomplishing interprofessional coordination. Lessons in 'almost managing' an emergency department team. J Nurs Manag 2022;30(1):198–204.

132. Wise S, Duffield C, Fry M, Roche MA. A team mental model approach to understanding team effectiveness in an emergency department: a qualitiative study. J Health Serv Res Policy 2022;27(1):14–21.

CHAPTER 37
PEOPLE WITH DISABILITIES

DAVID FOLEY

ESSENTIALS

- People with a disability are more likely to receive an incomplete assessment and inadequate care, because of diagnostic overshadowing and assumptions about their health.
- The number of people with an intellectual disability seeking both primary healthcare and emergency healthcare is increasing because of de-institutionalisation and longer life expectancy.
- Carers and personal support workers must be involved in the care of those with a disability.
- Family may be able to provide consent; however, personal support workers cannot act as the person responsible.
- The presence of pain is likely but difficult to assess, and it is better to assess distress based on prior observations of contentment and distress.
- The person with an intellectual disability may have difficulty expressing themselves, but are more likely to understand what is said to them.
- Use communication strategies from 'Communicating with People with Disabilities' developed by Advancing Care Excellence for People with Disabilities and recommended in Therapeutic Guidelines (2021).
- Check with the carer or personal support worker before touching the person with an intellectual disability.
- People with an intellectual disability are likely to have undiagnosed health problems.
- New presenting signs should not be assumed to be the result of an existing syndrome, but could be from a new undiagnosed pathology.
- Seizures are more likely in people with an intellectual disability.
- Anxiety is very disabling for most people with an intellectual disability and can adversely affect emergency care.
- Injury from falls is common.

INTRODUCTION

Definition of disability

Disability is a term that describes:

- impairment of bodily function or structure
- activity limitations, and
- participation restrictions.[1]

People's disabilities are categorised as intellectual, psychiatric, sensory, speech, physical and diverse. The term 'developmental disability' includes conditions that begin during development and affect intellectual functioning, social abilities or practical skills.[2] People with developmental disabilities, such as cerebral palsy or autism, may have no cognitive impairment. Intellectual disability is characterised by limitations in intellectual functioning and adaptive abilities that occur before the age of 18.[3] Fig. 37.1 shows the relationships between disability, developmental disability and intellectual disability.

In 2018, 17.7% of Australians[4] had a disability and 24% of New Zealanders[5] reported having a disability. Seventeen per cent of the world's population are estimated to have a developmental disability.[6] Disability used to be defined as a health condition; however, this medical approach placed 'the problem of disability' in the individual, and the answer to 'their problem' was to treat them. This fails to recognise how people fit into society. Disability is now acknowledged as a barrier that exists between a person and their social, legal and physical surroundings. Changing the environment overcomes these barriers. Instead of attempting to give someone back the ability to walk, the solution is to improve their mobility with easier access to public locations with ramps and lifts.

A person's activity limitations are categorised as:[1]

- *profound*—unable to perform the activity or always needs aid
- *severe*—sometimes needs help
- *moderate*—has difficulty but doesn't need assistance
- *mild*—uses equipment because of disability, but without difficulty.

More particularly, intellectual disability—the preferred Australian term—is defined as being present in a person when all three of the following criteria are met:

- Intelligence that is significantly below average, as measured with an intelligence quotient assessment.
- Considerable difficulties with the personal skills needed to live and work in the community.
- Limitations in intelligence and living skills that are evident before the person is 18 years old.[7]

HISTORICAL CONTEXT

It is important to review the history of how people with disabilities have been considered, as it reveals how beliefs about disability began, which subsequently determines how people act towards people with disability. It is important to understand this history in order to appreciate the present treatment of people with disabilities. (For further resources, see Useful websites at the end of this chapter.)

Aristotle supported the Greek practice of leaving 'deformed' babies to die of exposure. He is also supposed to have alleged that those 'born deaf become senseless and incapable of reason'.[8] This Greek custom continues to influence current thinking, that people with disabilities have a lesser value, and this may influence how healthcare professionals treat people with a disability.

During the medieval era, people with an intellectual disability (ID) were labelled generically as *natural fools* and *idiots*. They were cared for with others from the edges of society in charitable religious institutions, beginning the practice of institutional care, which continued and was developed during the Industrial Revolution with asylums.[9] Asylum institutionalisation shaped public opinion, so that people housed in asylums were believed to be 'unable, unworthy, or unfit to contribute to society and therefore best housed apart from society'.[9] During the 1970s and '80s the trend towards person-centred care and recognition of the rights of people with disabilities was recognised in

FIGURE 37.1 RELATIONSHIP BETWEEN DISABILITY, DEVELOPMENTAL DISABILITY AND INTELLECTUAL DISABILITY

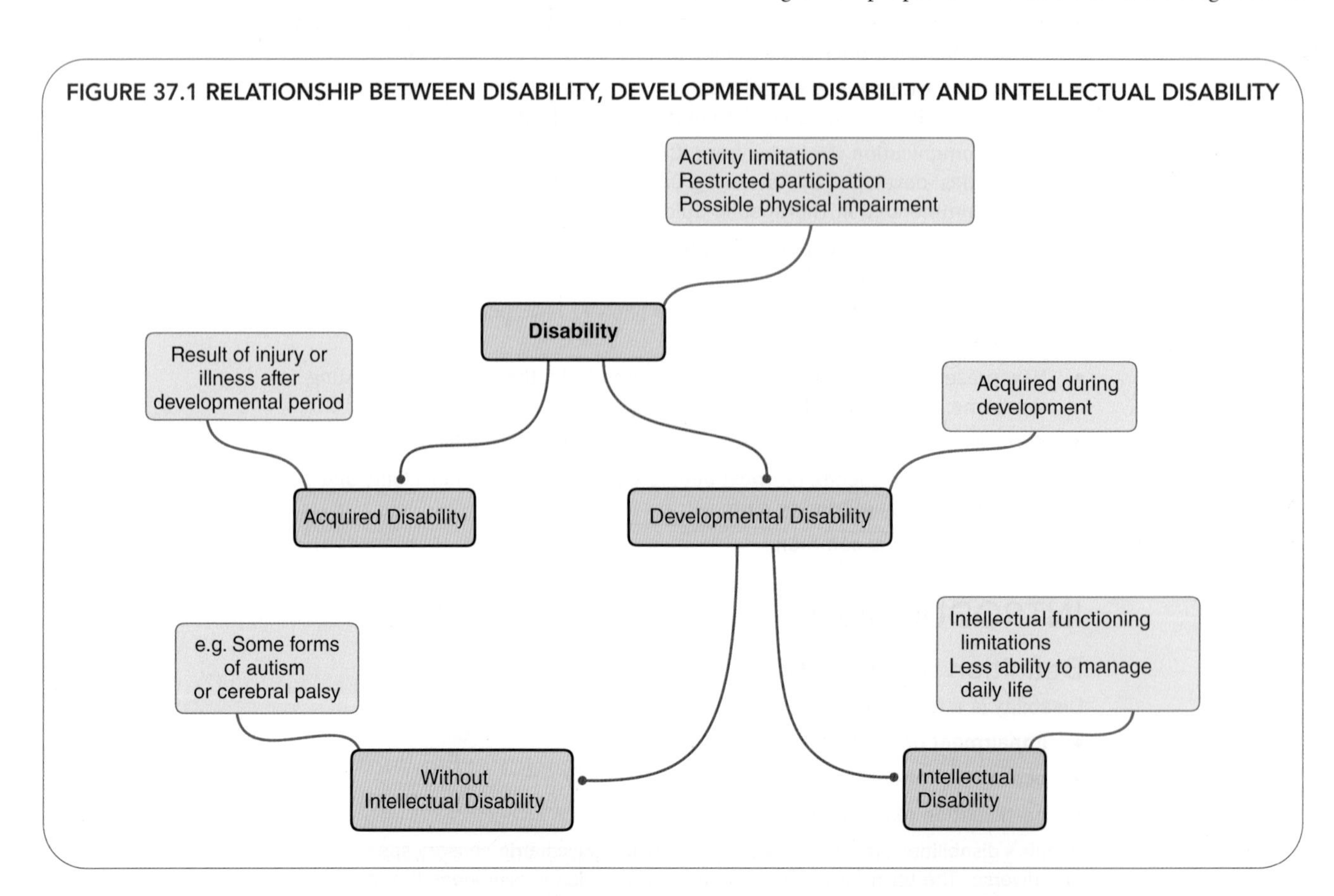

legislation, leading to de-institutionalisation. In Western countries, adults with intellectual disabilities now mostly live in community houses, supported independent living or in families that receive additional support. These improved living conditions, together with better medical care, mean that people with an intellectual disability are living longer. Not only are people living longer, but they are also using community health services rather than healthcare delivered within an institution. This means that the percentage of people with intellectual disabilities attending emergency departments (EDs) is increasing.

NATURE OF PROBLEM IN EMERGENCY CARE

In 2015, 26% of Australians with a disability had visited an ED.[10] The increasing number of people with disabilities who are using emergency services mean that difficulties with communication, management of pain, recognition of comorbid conditions and challenging behaviour are complicating emergency care. It is also difficult for emergency clinicians to determine what role carers and personal support workers should adopt when accompanying a person with a disability. When pain is not recognised or communication is impaired and carers are not involved, outcomes can be calamitous—as illustrated by the death of a young man from peritonitis caused by swallowing a plastic drink-bottle lid.[11] The purpose of this chapter is to address these issues and to suggest a strategy that includes carers in more effective emergency care.

NATIONAL DISABILITY INSURANCE SCHEME (NDIS) AND NEW ZEALAND DISABILITY STRATEGY

The Australian National Disability Insurance Scheme (NDIS) is designed to improve healthcare for people with disabilities by increasing individualised services that should reduce reliance on emergency services.[12] The aim of the NDIS is to fund the daily support that people with a disability need and to support their families and carers, consequently reducing unplanned ED visits through early intervention. The NDIS enables individuals who ask for financial assistance to be assessed using established criteria. People eligible for funding can then use this to purchase supports as part of an individualised plan.[13]

The New Zealand Disability Strategy is a 10-year (2016–26) plan that guides government agencies to build a 'non-disabling society'; it is guided by Te Tiriti o Waitangi (The Treaty of Waitangi) Convention on the Rights of Persons with Disabilities and involving people with disabilities in decision-making.[14] Outcome 3 of the strategy addresses health and wellbeing, to: 'Increase access to health services and improve health outcomes for disabled people with a specific focus on people with learning/intellectual disabilities' (see Useful websites).[14]

BROADER IMPLICATIONS

The predicament of people with an intellectual disability highlights issues that are common to many who seek emergency care. These include having:

- difficulty making themselves understood
- undiagnosed health problems
- pain that is difficult to assess
- threatening or frightening behaviour.

Better delivery of care to people with an intellectual disability will therefore lead to better ways to deliver emergency care to people who share these difficulties, and this could include people who are intoxicated, have dementia or delirium, or have a mental health problem.

PRACTICE TIP

Problems with communication, undiagnosed health problems, pain and confronting behaviour need to be considered and planned for when dealing with people who have an intellectual disability.

AETIOLOGY AND EPIDEMIOLOGY OF INTELLECTUAL DISABILITY

AETIOLOGY

Intellectual disability may be caused by genetic abnormalities, environmental factors or a combination of both. For disorders such as Down syndrome, the diagnosis may be made clinically at birth and confirmed with genetic testing. However, some diagnoses take years to establish, and some may never have a cause identified. There are up to 7000 genetic disorders known to be associated with cognitive disability.[15,16] For 50–70% of people who have an intellectual disability, the cause of their disability is not known. This is particularly so for people with a mild impairment. For people with a profound disability, the cause is usually genetic and identifiable.[17,18]

EPIDEMIOLOGY

Census data from 2012 identified that there were about 2.9% (n = 668,100) of Australians living with an intellectual disability.[19] In 2018, about 1 in 4 (23%), people with disability reported their main form of disability as mental or behavioural, with 6.5% of these describing this as intellectual and developmental.[20]

In Aotearoa New Zealand, it is estimated that about 2% of the population, or about 100,000 people, live with an intellectual disability.[5]

Most people with an intellectual disability have a mild disability and are aged between 5 and 64 years.[21,22] There are very few people over the age of 65 who have an intellectual disability; however, with better healthcare and accommodation, numbers in this group are expected to increase.

INTELLECTUAL DISABILITY MORBIDITY

People with an intellectual disability are likely to have poor health; they are at risk of abuse and neglect. Compared to the rest of the population they have more illness, and it is likely that they have additional medical problems associated with their syndrome.[23] Each intellectually disabled person may have between four and five medical conditions, half of which were undiagnosed at the time of the investigation.[24]

Epilepsy is the most common morbidity found in individuals with an intellectual disability; blindness, hearing loss, psychiatric illness, osteoporosis and obesity are also much more prevalent than in the general population.[25] As the presence of intellectual disability in people is associated with an increased morbidity, this group of people has an increased mortality, with death occurring 20 years earlier than the general population.[26]

DIAGNOSTIC OVERSHADOWING

When a person has an intellectual disability clinicians can be prone to attribute the presenting signs and symptoms to the intellectual disability or the syndrome that is associated with the intellectual disability rather than another disorder; this is *diagnostic overshadowing*.[27] For example, a loss of movement in someone with cerebral palsy may be assumed to have been present since birth as part of their condition and not recognised as a consequence of a new musculoskeletal, spinal or neurological injury.

PRACTICE TIP

Consider disability-linked health problems for all people with a disability who present for emergency care to avoid diagnostic overshadowing. Be careful to check for new problems.

PARTICULAR HEALTH PROBLEMS

Particular health problems occur with greater frequency in people with an intellectual disability. These include epilepsy and low-velocity injuries, such as occur with falls. These injuries are found more commonly when particular behavioural characteristics are present, often as a result of inadequate coping skills and an inability to understand consequences. In addition, diseases associated with particular syndromes, such as congenital heart disease and endocrine disorders associated with Down syndrome, should be expected. Furthermore, lifestyle diseases associated with a sedentary lifestyle occur with greater frequency.

More common health disparities experienced by people with an intellectual disability, summarised with relative risks calculated, are presented in Table 37.1.[28] It is also useful to recognise that there are medical conditions often associated with particular syndromes and these are summarised in Table 37.2.[30]

The most common health problems in people with an intellectual disability are:

- seizures, often intractable and difficult to manage
- chronic serous otitis media associated with anatomical alterations of the face and decreased immune function

TABLE 37.1 PREVALENCE OF HEALTH PROBLEMS IN PEOPLE WITH AN INTELLECTUAL DISABILITY[28]

HEALTH PROBLEM	PREVALENCE IN PEOPLE WITH AN ID (%)	PREVALENCE IN GENERAL POPULATION (%)	RELATIVE RISK INCREASE
Seizures	23.8	1.7	14.0
CNS conditions	24.9	5	5.0
Sensory loss	13.7	3.4	4.0
Hypothyroidism	5.7	3.2	1.8
Endocrine conditions	5.2	1.9	2.7
Chronic skin disease	17.2	7.1	2.4
Increased risk of fracture*	Low bone mass BUA: male: 52 ± 4 dB/MHz female: 34 ± 3 dB/MHz	Low bone mass BUA: male: 89 ± 2 dB/MHz female: 68 ± 2 dB/MHz	Approximately 4
Sleep problems	35.7	7.1	5.0
Hepatitis A (in institutionalised people)	54	22	2.5
Congenital disorders	5.0	0.4	12.5
Musculoskeletal impairment	6.0	0.5	12.0
Strabismus	5.3	1.1	4.8
Other disorders of the CNS	4.4	1.1	4.0
Deafness	6.3	2.3	2.7
Fracture of lower leg	5.0	1.9	2.6
Congenital anomalies, musculoskeletal system	3.1	1.3	2.4
STI (males)	2.6	0.4	6.5

BUA: broadband-ultrasound attenuation; CNS: central nervous system; ID: intellectual disability; STI: sexually transmitted infection.

**A fall of about 20 db/MHz is associated with a relative risk of fracture of 1.95 (95% CI 1.50–2.52, $p < 0.0001$)[29]*

TABLE 37.2 SYNDROME-ASSOCIATED CONDITIONS[28]

ID CAUSE	MEDICAL CONDITION	PREVALENCE BY CAUSE OF ID (%)
Cerebral palsy	Gastro-oesophageal reflux	8–10%
	Hearing loss	10%
	Hip dislocations, scoliosis, contractures, gait disorder	10%
	Seizures	33%
	Strabismus	50%
Down syndrome	Acquired hip dislocation	6%
	Atlanto-axial instability	14–22%
	Cataracts	15%
	Congenital heart disease	50%
	Deafness	75%
	Diabetes mellitus	1.4–10%
	Early Alzheimer's disease	near 100% > age 40 years
	Gastrointestinal atresias	12%
	Hirschsprung disease	1%
	Leukaemia	1%
	Psychiatric disorders	22%
	Seizure disorders	12–15%
	Severe refractive errors	50%
	Serous otitis media	50–70%
	Thyroid disease	15%
Fetal alcohol syndrome	Hearing loss	66%
	Heart defects	29–41%
	Recurrent serous otitis media	93%
	Renal hypoplasia, duplication of the kidney and collecting system, and bladder diverticula	10%
	Vision problems	94%
Fragile X syndrome	Autism	16%
	Mitral valve prolapse	22–77%
	Recurrent serous otitis media	60%
	Seizures	14–50%
	Strabismus	30–56%
Irradiation-induced intellectual disability	Microcephaly, leukaemia	2%
Trisomy 18	Congenital heart disease	99%

ID: intellectual disability.

- congenital heart disease
- viral myocarditis
- constipation and faecal impaction caused by medication and hypothyroidism
- gastro-oesophageal reflux disease (GORD); particularly in people with cerebral palsy
- chronic aspiration associated with GORD and dysphagia
- most musculoskeletal disorders occur in people with cerebral palsy and are usually a result of joint contractures, which result in limited mobility, osteoarthritis, pressure ulcers, discomfort, hip subluxation and scoliosis
- in about 20% of people with Down syndrome, the atlanto-axial joint of the spine is unstable due to lax ligaments and variations in bone morphology
- hypothyroidism, a particular problem in people with Down syndrome
- diabetes mellitus
- leukaemia, which has an increased incidence in people with Down syndrome
- dental disease.

PRACTICE TIP

Particular health problems should be considered when assessing people with known disability syndromes.

INJURY MECHANISM

The incidence of falls, burns, foreign-body aspiration, drowning and poisoning is higher in people with an intellectual disability.[31,32]

Falls are a particular issue for people with an intellectual disability; with up to 34% of people with intellectual disability experiencing a fall in the last 12 months,[33] with 30% visiting an ED.[34]

The incidence of injury for individuals with an intellectual disability is twice as high as for the general population and for people with autism spectrum disorder this increases by a further 54%.[34,35] Injury is the most common reason for a person with an intellectual disability to present to an ED.[36] Males with an intellectual disability are just as likely to be injured as females with an intellectual disability, a pattern quite different to the general population.[37] Thus, paramedics and emergency clinicians dealing with people who have an intellectual disability can expect to see just as many men as women, and to see proportionally more injuries as a result of falls, drowning, foreign-body aspiration and poisoning. Greater awareness of the likelihood of injury should raise the index of suspicion for these injuries when someone with an intellectual disability presents to the ED. Paramedics and emergency clinicians also need to be aware that this group of people has an increased chance of being moderately or severely injured. Consequently, they are more likely to be hospitalised, with admission rates from trauma almost double that of the general population.[37]

Of particular note is the risk of cervical nerve damage in people with Down syndrome, 3.8% of whom have atlanto-axial instability.[38] This is more of an issue in children with Down syndrome, as the instability resolves in many adults.

PRACTICE TIP

For people with intellectual disability, be suspicious that injury may be the result of foreign-body aspiration, drowning or poisoning.

MAJOR EMERGENCY CARE ISSUES FOR PEOPLE WITH AN INTELLECTUAL DISABILITY

Not only is the person with an intellectual disability at increased risk of injury and prone to particular health problems, but their treatment, including emergency care, is also more complex and yet neglected. Studies investigating the medical care of people with an intellectual disability have identified the following issues.[39–42]

- Hearing and visual loss are often not managed with corrective lenses or hearing aids. Consequently, a person with an intellectual disability may have an uncorrected sensory loss, threatening communication that is already difficult.
- Blood pressure measurement, Pap smears and prostate examinations are performed less frequently, and so easily detected problems remain undiagnosed.
- Health problems are under-investigated; consequently, more tests need to be conducted to establish the extent of the health problem.
- Known risk factors associated with intellectual disability syndromes are frequently neglected. For example, people with Down syndrome are more likely to have thyroid, cardiac and coeliac disease; therefore, people with Down syndrome presenting with vague symptoms need to be investigated for these diseases.
- Atypical behaviours are often expressed when a person is suffering a serious health disorder, and this can mask the problem. Irritability, inactivity, loss of appetite, disturbed sleep, speech which is more difficult to understand, self-injuring behaviour and loss of daily living abilities are all possible signs of a health problem.
- Not only might behaviours be atypical, but people with an intellectual disability who are usually able to communicate their needs also may not complain of discomfort or pain, and even people who know them well may not suspect that they are unwell.
- Significant health problems will be found in people who present with psychiatric problems or behavioural difficulties if they are carefully assessed.

In addition to these issues, there are extra barriers to the provision of quality emergency care that need to be overcome. Table 37.3 summarises these barriers.

ASSESSMENT OF PAIN

Most people with intellectual disability are able to express pain; however, their expression of pain may be idiosyncratic and difficult to interpret.[44,45] This can result in under-reporting a person's experience of pain, which is consistent for people who have an intellectual disability and who present for emergency care. These people with pain need to be carefully assessed as

TABLE 37.3 BARRIERS TO EFFECTIVE EMERGENCY CARE FOR PEOPLE WITH DISABILITY[43]

BARRIER ENVIRONMENT	BARRIER TO EFFECTIVE EMERGENCY CARE
Healthcare provider barriers leading to inadequate patient information	Knowledge, training and experience with people who have an ID
	Communicating with the person who has an ID
	Physical examination of the person with an ID
	Lack of time
	Consent for examination and treatment
Associated with patient and carer	Lack of understanding of the role and function of emergency services
	Explaining the problem
	Difficult past experiences with emergency care
	Unable to cooperate
	Atypical pain behaviour
Associated with the healthcare system	Long waiting exacerbates anxiety and consequent challenging behaviour
	Failure of preventative care, resulting in avoidable emergency visits
	Failure to recognise and account for issues associated with intellectual disability

ID: intellectual disability.

they are more likely to have pre-existing health problems that increase the likelihood of significant morbidity. It is also an imperative to reduce pain, and detect and treat its cause in all people. However, in many people who have an intellectual disability it is difficult to determine the presence of pain and often it is not possible to use self-reporting pain-scale tools; it is therefore important that other means of pain assessment are used.

People with mild or moderate communication impairments may be able to self-report pain.[46] However, they are less able to describe the location of the pain, take longer to respond to it and often do not demonstrate decipherable signs of pain.[47] For these patients, paramedics and emergency clinicians need to prudently assess the pain, consider its pathological cause and confirm observations with the person's carer.[48] This is important, as the patient's description is likely to be vague, poorly localised and possibly misleading.[47]

Before assessing pain, paramedics and emergency clinicians need to briefly assess cognitive and communication abilities, as people with profound intellectual disability are usually unable to indicate that they are in pain.[47,49] Pain assessment tools that rely on patients describing or grading their pain will not succeed. In people where communication is non-verbal, other methods of pain assessment need to be used and the best available form of pain assessment is skilled clinical assessment combined with a familiarity and understanding of the person. For emergency clinicians, paramedics and first responders, this is also unlikely to succeed as they probably do not know the patient. As communication with people who have profound communication impairment relies on the skill of carers to interpret behavioural, facial and verbal cues, carers become essential for pain assessment. In addition, each person will have an individual language of pain that cannot be generalised.[49]

Although carers and people who know the patient seem to intuitively identify signs of distress consistent with being in pain, they are usually unsure of their assessment. In response, a tool developed from palliative care, supplements and validates carer assessment. DisDAT (Disability Distress Assessment Tool) is a method that could be used by paramedics and emergency clinicians to assess distress in people with an intellectual disability. It is likely to be most effective if a carer who knows the patient has completed 'The Distress Passport' on the front page. However, the authors assert that anyone who cares for patients with severe communication difficulties will be able to use this tool to effectively detect distress.[50]

DisDAT is not a pain scale, as it does not score pain, but instead describes the context of distress and possible causes of distress.

In people with severe communication difficulties, there is no evidence that pain produces any specific or unique pain behaviours or signs. This has profound implications, since it means that pain cannot be an assessment goal in such patients. However, assessing distress can be, after which its cause must be determined.[50]

The goal of this tool is to reduce the signs of distress and associated behaviours as indicators that pain has been reduced.[50] The tool and its instructions for use are shown in Fig. 37.2.

PRACTICE TIP

It is often difficult to assess pain in a person with an intellectual disability, so consider using tools that measure distress, such as the DisDAT. This may assist emergency clinicians to treat signs of distress and associated behaviours, thereby reducing pain if present.

ASSESSMENT OF THE PERSON WITH AN INTELLECTUAL DISABILITY

FIRST ASSESSMENT CONSIDERATIONS FOR FIRST-RESPONDERS, PARAMEDICS AND EMERGENCY CLINICIANS

Emergency clinicians and first responders need to make a concerted effort to assess the patient in an area with as few distractions as possible, as many people with an intellectual disability are easily distracted, and anxiety is a common experience for people with an intellectual disability.[51]

Before beginning assessment, gather as much pertinent information as possible. Attempt to discover usual functional

FIGURE 37.2 DisDAT (DISABILITY DISTRESS ASSESSMENT TOOL)[50]

v19

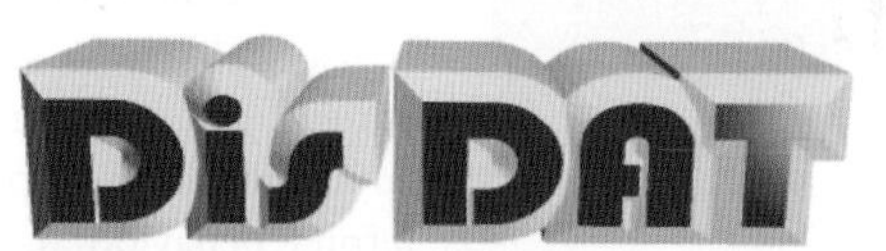

Disability Distress Assessment Tool

Individual's name:

DoB: **Gender:**

NHS No:

Your name:

Date completed:

Names of others who helped complete this form:

THE DISTRESS PASSPORT
Summary of signs and behaviours when content and when distressed

Appearance when CONTENT	**Appearance when DISTRESSED**
Face Eyes	Face Eyes
Tongue/jaw	Tongue/jaw
Skin	Skin

Vocal signs when CONTENT	**Vocal signs when DISTRESSED**
Sounds	Sounds
Speech	Speech

Habits and mannerisms when CONTENT	**Habits and mannerisms when DISTRESSED**
Habits	Habits
Mannerisms	Mannerisms
Comfortable distance	Comfortable distance

Posture & observations when CONTENT	**Posture & observations when DISTRESSED**
Posture	Posture
Observations	Observations

Known triggers of distress (write here any actions or situations that usually cause or worsen distress)

This tool relies on observed signs and behaviours to identify distress in people of any age with severe communication difficulties of any cause, and has features that help with monitoring and assessing the cause of the distress. A full-size version of the tool is available (see Useful websites).

FIGURE 37.2 DisDAT (DISABILITY DISTRESS ASSESSMENT TOOL)—cont'd

v19

Disability Distress Assessment Tool

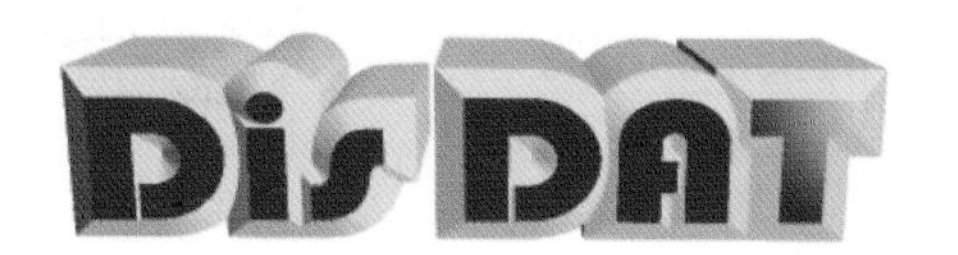

Please take some time to think about and observe the individual under your care, especially their appearance and behaviours when they are both content and distressed. Use these pages to document these.

We have listed words in each section to help you to describe the signs and behaviours. You can circle the word or words that best describe the signs and behaviours when they are content and when they are distressed.

Your descriptions will provide you with a clearer picture of their 'language' of distress.

COMMUNICATION LEVEL *

This individual is unable to show likes or dislikes	Level 0
This individual is able to show that they like or don't like something	Level 1
This individual is able to show that they want more, or have had enough of something	Level 2
This individual is able to show anticipation for their like or dislike of something	Level 3
This individual is able to communicate detail, qualify, specify and/or indicate opinions	Level 4

* This is adapted from the Kidderminster Curriculum for Children and Adults with Profound Multiple Learning Difficulty (Jones, 1994, National Portage Association).

FACIAL SIGNS

Appearance

Information / instructions	Appearance when content	Appearance when distressed
Ring the words that best describe the facial appearance	Passive Laugh Smile Frown Grimace Startled Frightened Other:	Passive Laugh Smile Frown Grimace Startled Frightened Other:

Jaw movement

Information / instructions	Movement when content	Movement when distressed
Ring the words that best describe the jaw movement	Relaxed Drooping Grinding Biting Rigid Other:	Relaxed Drooping Grinding Biting Rigid Other:

Appearance of eyes

Information / instructions	Appearance when content	Appearance when distressed
Ring the words that best describe the appearance	Good eye contact Little eye contact Avoiding eye contact Closed eyes Staring Sleepy eyes 'Smiling' Winking Vacant Tears Dilated pupils Other:	Good eye contact Little eye contact Avoiding eye contact Closed eyes Staring Sleepy eyes 'Smiling' Winking Vacant Tears Dilated pupils Other:

SKIN APPEARANCE

Information / instructions	Appearance when content	Appearance when distressed
Ring the words that best describe the appearance	Normal Pale Flushed Sweaty Clammy Other:	Normal Pale Flushed Sweaty Clammy Other:

FIGURE 37.2 DisDAT (DISABILITY DISTRESS ASSESSMENT TOOL)—cont'd

VOCAL SOUNDS (NB. The sounds that a person makes are not always linked to their feelings)

Information / instructions	Sounds when content	Sounds when distressed
Ring the words that best describe the sounds *Write down* commonly used sounds (write it as it sounds; 'tizz', 'eeiow', 'tetetetete'):	**Volume**: high medium low **Pitch**: high medium low **Duration**: short intermittent long **Description of sound / vocalisation**: Cry out Wail Scream Laugh Groan / moan Shout Gurgle Other:	**Volume:** high medium low **Pitch:** high medium low **Duration**: short intermittent long **Description of sound / vocalisation**: Cry out Wail Scream Laugh Groan / moan Shout Gurgle Other:

SPEECH

Information / instructions	Words when content	Words when distressed
Write down commonly used words and phrases. If no words are spoken, write NONE		
Ring the words which best describe the speech	Clear Stutters Slurred Unclear Muttering Fast Slow Loud Soft Whisper Other, e.g. swearing	Clear Stutters Slurred Unclear Muttering Fast Slow Loud Soft Whisper Other, e.g. swearing

HABITS & MANNERISMS

Information / instructions	Habits and mannerisms when content	Habits and mannerisms when distressed
Write down the habits or mannerisms, e.g. "Rocks when sitting"		
Write down any special comforters, possessions or toys this person prefers.		
Please Ring the statements which best describe how comfortable this person is with other people being physically close by	Close with strangers Close only if known No one allowed close Withdraws if touched	Close with strangers Close only if known No one allowed close Withdraws if touched

BODY POSTURE

Information / instructions	Posture when content	Posture when distressed
Ring the words that best describe how this person sits and stands.	Normal Rigid Floppy Jerky Slumped Restless Tense Still Able to adjust position Leans to side Poor head control Way of walking: Normal / Abnormal Other:	Normal Rigid Floppy Jerky Slumped Restless Tense Still Able to adjust position Leans to side Poor head control Way of walking: Normal / Abnormal Other:

BODY OBSERVATIONS

Information / instructions	Observations when content	Observations when distressed
Describe the pulse, breathing, sleep, appetite and usual eating pattern, e.g. eats very quickly, takes a long time with main course, eats puddings quickly, "picky".	Pulse: Breathing: Sleep: Appetite: Eating pattern:	Pulse: Breathing: Sleep: Appetite Eating pattern:

FIGURE 37.2 DisDAT (DISABILITY DISTRESS ASSESSMENT TOOL)—cont'd

Information and Instructions

DisDAT is

Intended to help identify distress cues in individuals who have severely limited communication.

Designed to describe an individual's usual content cues, thus enabling distress cues to be identified more clearly.

NOT a scoring tool. It documents what many carers have done instinctively for many years thus providing a record against which subtle changes can be compared.

Only the first step. Once distress has been identified the usual clinical decisions have to be made by professionals.

Meant to help you and the individual in your care. It gives you more confidence in the observation skills you already have, which in turn will give you more confidence when meeting other carers.

When to use DisDAT

When the team believes the individual is NOT distressed

The use of DisDAT is optional, but it can be used as a
– baseline assessment document
– transfer document for other teams

When the team believes the individual IS distressed

If DisDAT has already been completed it can be used to compare the present signs and behaviours with previous observations documented on DisDAT. It then serves as a baseline to monitor change.

If DisDAT has not been completed:

a) When the person is well known DisDAT can be used to document previous content signs and behaviours and compare these with the current observations

b) When the person is new to a carer, or the distress is new, DisDAT can be used to document the present signs and behaviours to act as a baseline to monitor change.

How to use DisDAT

1. **Observe the individual** when content and when distressed—document this on the inside pages. *Anyone* who cares for them can do this.
2. **Observe the context** in which distress is occurring.
3. **Use the clinical decision distress checklist** on this page to assess the possible cause.
4. **Treat or manage** the likeliest cause of the distress.
5. **The monitoring sheet** is a separate sheet, which may help if you want to see how the distress changes over time.
6. **The goal** is a reduction in the number or severity of distress signs and behaviours.

Remember

- Most information comes from several carers together.
- The assessment form need not be completed all at once and may take a period of time.
- Reassessment is essential as the needs may change due to improvement or deterioration.
- Distress can be emotional, physical or psychological. What is a minor issue for one person can be major to another.
- If signs are recognised early then suitable interventions can be put in place to avoid a crisis.

Clinical decision distress checklist

Use this to help decide the cause of the distress

Is the new sign or behaviour:

- Repeated rapidly?

Consider pleuritic pain (in time with breathing)
Consider colic (comes and goes every few minutes)
Consider: repetitive movement due to boredom or fear.

- Associated with breathing?

Consider: infection, COPD, pleural effusion, tumour

- Worsened or precipitated by movement?

Consider: movement-related pains

- Related to eating?

Consider: food refusal through illness, fear or depression
Consider: food refusal because of swallowing problems
Consider: upper GI problems (oral hygiene, peptic ulcer, dyspepsia) or abdominal problems.

- Related to a specific situation?

Consider: frightening or painful situations.

- Associated with vomiting?

Consider: causes of nausea and vomiting.

- Associated with elimination (urine or faecal)?

Consider: urinary problems (infection, retention)
Consider: GI problems (diarrhoea, constipation)

- Present in a normally comfortable position or situation?

Consider: anxiety, depression, pains at rest (e.g. colic, neuralgia), infection, nausea.

If you require any help or further information regarding DisDAT please contact:
Lynn Gibson 01670 394 260
Dorothy Matthews 01670 394 808
Dr. Claud Regnard 0191 285 0063 or e-mail on claudregnard@stoswaldsuk.org

For more information see
www.disdat.co.uk

Further reading

Regnard C, Matthews D, Gibson L, Clarke C, Watson B. Difficulties in identifying distress and its causes in people with severe communication problems. *International Journal of Palliative Nursing* 2003;9(3):173–6.

Regnard C, Reynolds J, Watson B, Matthews D, Gibson L, Clarke C. Understanding distress in people with severe communication difficulties: developing and assessing the Disability Distress Assessment Tool (DisDAT). *J Intellect Disability Res* 2007;**51(4)**:277–292.

Distress may be hidden, but it is never silent

abilities and communication strategies. It is also important to identify comorbid conditions, medical history medications and allergies.[52] The person from an institutional setting is likely to have a handheld health record (health diary or health passport) with them; this will describe much of this detail and is usually current.[53]

When first meeting the person with an intellectual disability, it is important that first responders, paramedics and emergency clinicians introduce themselves by name and role; this formality is frequently omitted, and distresses many emergency patients.[54] On introduction, it is imperative that emergency clinicians use more than visual appearance to assess the person's communication. Many people with significant communication difficulties do not have obvious physical deformities; alternatively, many people with obvious intellectual disability-associated syndromes have minimal communication difficulties. For example, a person with Down syndrome with obvious distinguishing features may be adept at understanding spoken language and may also have an extensive vocabulary. It is therefore important to attempt to gain a health history from the patient; this should then be confirmed with the carer or personal support worker. These accompanying people may be required to provide the history of the presenting complaint and relevant health information if the patient has severe communication impairment. The disclosure of health information with a carer (or responsible person) is permissible under the Privacy Act (Schedule 3 of the *Privacy Act 1988* amended 14 September 2006), but only under defined conditions; in particular: the person with a disability must be incapable of communicating, that this disclosure is necessary for care, is not contrary to the wishes of the person and is a limited disclosure. First responders, paramedics and emergency clinicians should familiarise themselves with the *Privacy Act 1988*.[55] The Office of the Australian Information Commissioner has produced a document with a poster that explains privacy principles.[56] In particular, sections 2.4 and 2.5 helpfully list when information can be shared and with whom. Privacy of health information in Aotearoa New Zealand is directed by the *Privacy Act 2020* (see Useful websites).

The occurrence of an acute illness or injury in the person with an intellectual disability can be accompanied by atypical responses. Any evidence of change in motor activity, irritability, refusal to eat, change in bowel habit, loss of weight or decrease in cognition should be investigated further.[39] There are numerous documented occurrences of behavioural change that are likely to be misleading. In an illustrative case, 'Ray' was 'cured' of his obsessive–compulsive behaviour when five ribs were found to be fractured.[57]

PRACTICE TIP

To most effectively assess the person with an intellectual disability and to preserve their dignity the following principles are recommended:

- Assume the person can understand what you are asking.
- Adapt your assessment communication style to the person's communication ability.
- If a carer accompanies a person, include them in your assessment.

PHYSICAL EXAMINATION

The physical examination is more important in this population of people, as a detailed history may be difficult to obtain, and as most disabilities are hidden, a careful clinical examination is required. It is also likely that the patient with an intellectual disability has other pre-existing, undiagnosed problems that complicate the presentation. It is important that health professionals consider that people with an intellectual disability are more likely to be injured and more likely to have chronic disease, and therefore need to be more carefully assessed. In addition to undiagnosed problems, people with a disability are more likely to have been prescribed one or more medications.[58] Consequently, the paramedic and emergency clinician need to identify what medication the person is receiving and to consider polypharmacy as a contributing factor.

In people with a disability, physical findings may be misleading or confusing; for example, a person with spastic quadriplegia is likely to have a stiff neck, which may be confused with significant CNS pathology. There are also documented cases of people with 'acute intestinal obstructions but few physical signs'.[57]

During the examination, a family member or personal care worker should be present; this will reduce anxiety in the patient and they may also be able to explain or interpret physical assessment findings.[54]

An explanation of what is going to be done in the physical examination with short, single-concept sentences using simple words must occur. The accompanying person must also receive an explanation; also check with this person for consent to perform the examination. They may be able to provide consent or indicate if the patient is able to consent.

It may also be appropriate to sedate the person for a thorough examination.

Ethical care and consent to medical treatment

When a person with a disability can understand the proposed treatment, the reason it is being given and how it will be administered, then that person is able to consent to the proposed treatment. If a person with a disability cannot give informed consent, then the person responsible will need to provide consent; however, this should not preclude paramedics and emergency clinicians from obtaining the permission of the person prior to any procedure, investigation or assessment. This is part of supported decision-making, which should be guided by the following principles, so that people with disability:[59,60]

- are notified and encouraged to exercise their fundamental human rights
- have the right to live free from neglect
- have the right to be respected for their worth, dignity, individuality and privacy
- have the right to access appropriate assistance and support that will enable them to maximise their capacity to exercise choice and control
- are allowed and encouraged to determine their own best interests, including the right to exercise informed choice and take calculated risks
- have procedures and investigations conducted unobtrusively, with the smallest infringements on the fewest rights
- are provided with services and support based on best evidence, best practice and with a strong focus on person-centred care.[61]

Inspection

- Observe the patient for signs of particular syndromes, for example, Down syndrome, fetal alcohol syndrome, fragile X, chromosome 22q11.2 deletion syndrome, and others that have particular facial characteristics. See Table 37.4 for a summary of the more prevalent syndromes and their physical features. Having some idea of the likely syndrome will help identify more-common risk factors.
- Observe for signs of distress as described in DisDAT (Fig. 37.2); also watch the part of the body that the person avoids touching or continually touches and rubs.
- Inspect teeth and gums, as more than half of all people with an intellectual disability have untreated dental caries.[63]
- Check for signs of dehydration, particularly dry mucosa.
- Obesity is prevalent in people with mild to moderate intellectual disability; however, lack of nourishment is more widespread in those with more-profound intellectual disability.
- Assess respiratory rate, breathing pattern, skin colour and oxygen saturation; this is particularly important as respiratory disease is the major cause of death.[64] This is because of reflux, aspiration pneumonia, poor thoracic expansion and frequent asthma.

Inspection is arguably the most important part of the assessment of a person with an intellectual disability, since a history may be difficult to obtain and the person may be unable to describe any symptoms. It is also possible that inspection is the only means available because touching the patient could be difficult, producing alarming behaviour. This is particularly so in people with autism spectrum disorder who may be averse to touch; it is also likely where anxiety is prominent. Before touching the patient, check with the carer for the best approach.

Auscultation

Using a stethoscope may be difficult if the patient does not like to be touched. Interpretation of breath sounds may also be difficult, as patients with an intellectual disability may not respond to requests to breathe deeply. Breathing may also be shallow. Despite these complexities, respiratory auscultation should be performed because of the high risk of respiratory problems.[64]

The assessment of indirect blood pressure measurement with a sphygmomanometer or electronic non-invasive blood pressure machine is often difficult. Many people with an intellectual disability do not like the sensation of increasing pressure as the bladder inflates. The assessment of indirect blood pressure may have to be omitted if it causes undue distress and is not vital for diagnostic considerations and/or treatment.

Palpation

As described previously, touch may be difficult because of behavioural responses; findings may also be misleading because of increased muscle tone that may mimic an acute abdomen. However, bowel obstruction, perforation and peritonitis are all causes of avoidable death in people with an intellectual disability.[65]

PARTICULAR CLINICAL PRESENTATIONS

SEIZURES AND EPILEPSY

Seizure activity in a person with an intellectual or physical disability such as cerebral palsy may be very difficult to recognise. Seizures may present as a behaviour change. Carers will usually be able to describe how a seizure might be recognised; however, there is a tendency for some carers to classify the seizure rather than describe it and this can lead to an inaccurate diagnosis.[66]

The cause of intellectual disability is often also the cause of epilepsy, and for some people this can mean that seizure activity contributes to cognitive decline. It is more prevalent in disorders such as tuberous sclerosis. A seizure in a person with Down syndrome may indicate the onset of Alzheimer's disease.[67]

Phenobarbitone and phenytoin, drugs often used in the general population, are to be avoided in people with an intellectual disability. Both agents can cause a decline in intellectual function, and phenytoin toxicity may result in enduring CNS injury. Furthermore, a small change in dose of phenytoin can produce a large alteration in the serum level (i.e. a narrow therapeutic range). The clinical manifestations of toxicity are subtle and are frequently overlooked, especially if the person is unable to describe any side-effects they may be experiencing.[68] For paramedics and emergency clinicians who encounter a person in an active seizure, the usual recommendation is to administer midazolam if the duration of seizure is greater than 5 minutes. For further information on the diagnosis and management of epilepsy, see Chapter 23.

NEUROLEPTIC MALIGNANT SYNDROME

Neuroleptic drugs are frequently prescribed for people with an intellectual disability, because of the severity of neuroleptic malignant syndrome (NMS) and the risk of death. It is important to assess for hyperthermia, muscle rigidity and hypertension. See Chapter 23 for management of this condition.

ALZHEIMER'S DISEASE

Almost all people with Down syndrome over the age of 40 years have the characteristic amyloid plaques of Alzheimer's disease, and this group of people is likely to develop dementia 20–30 years earlier than the general population.[69] The most important factor in the assessment of a person with Down syndrome who appears to have dementia is the exclusion of treatable or self-limiting health problems that produce a change in cognition.[69]

MUSCULOSKELETAL INJURY

Reduced weight-bearing, poor dietary intake of calcium, diminished vitamin D levels and the use of anticonvulsants all increase the risk of fractures in people with an intellectual disability.[70] As already indicated, many people with the disabilities described in this chapter are also prone to falls because of poor balance and risky behaviour. Furthermore, people with cerebral palsy are more likely to develop joint problems associated with contractures. It is therefore important that the presence of musculoskeletal injury should not be ruled out until properly assessed.[71]

ATLANTO-AXIAL INSTABILITY

The occiput, the atlas (C1) and the axis (C2) form a unit that is very mobile, allowing rotation of the head around the odontoid bone; however, the joint is not stabilised with bone: instead structures are kept in place with ligaments. This joint also allows flexion and extension, but this can be excessive in some individuals with Down syndrome who have lax ligaments. In

TABLE 37.4 SYNDROME FEATURES[62]

	CEREBRAL PALSY 1:500	DOWN SYNDROME 1:700	PRADER-WILLI SYNDROME 1: 10 000-25 000	FRAGILE X SYNDROME 1:6000	PHENYLKETONURIA 1:10 000-1:20000
AUDIOVISUAL	Visual Impairment Hearing Impairment	Visual impairment (multifactorial), cataracts Hearing impairment (multifactorial) (Annual assessments recommended)	Strabismus Myopia	Visual impairment (multifactorial) Hearing impairment Recurrent ear infections	
ENDOCRINE		Hypothyroidism (Annual TFT recommended)	Type 2 diabetes Hypogonadism Delayed puberty		
PSYCHIATRIC/ PSYCHOLOGICAL	Depression Variable intellectual capacity	Depression Alzheimer's type dementia—clinical onset uncommon before 40 yrs	Hyperphagia Impulse control difficulties Self-injury	Attention deficit/ hyperactivity Variable intellectual capacity Disabled in social functioning	Variable intellectual capacity Phobic anxiety Disabled in social functioning
CNS	Epilepsy	Epilepsy Usually clonic/tonic		Epilepsy—clonic/tonic, complex partial	Epilepsy Hyperactivity Tremor, pyramidal signs Extrapyramidal syndromes
CARDIOVASCULAR		Congenital heart defects (in 40 to 50%)		Aortic dilatation Mitral valve prolapse	
MUSCULAR/ SKELETAL and SKIN	Orthopaedic problems Neuromuscular problems	Atlantoaxial instability Skin disorders, alopecia, eczema	Scoliosis, Kyphosis Hypotonia Skin picking	Connective tissue dysplasia Scoliosis Congenital hip dislocation	
OTHER	Genito-urinary problems Incontinence Constipation Dental problems Recurrent aspiration Oesophagitis, gastroesophageal reflux +/- bleeding/anaemia Swallowing/eating difficulties	Blood dyscrasias childhood leukaemia Sleep apnoea Increased susceptibility to infections Coeliac disease	Infantile failure to thrive, then hyperphagia and severe obesity High tolerance to pain Decreased ability to vomit Sleep apnoea Osteoporosis Undescended testes Dental abnormalities	Herniae (CT related) Abnormalities of speech and language	Eczema
INHERITANCE		Most cases are sporadic; 4% due to translocation involving chromosome 21 or rarely parental mosaicism	Mostly sporadic; Microdeletion of 15q11 in 70%; rest—maternal disomy	X linked	Autosomal recessive

	ANGELMANN SYNDROME <1:10 000	WILLIAMS ?<1:20 000	RETT 1;14 000 FEMALES	NOONAN <1:10 000	TUBEROUS SCLEROSIS 1: 6000-17 000	NEUROFIBROMA-TOSIS 1:3000
AUDIOVISUAL	Glaucoma	Hyperacusis Strabismus	Refractory errors	Strabismus, refractive errors Vision/hearing impairments	Retinal tumours Eye rhabdomyomatas	Hearing impairment (Glioma affecting auditory nerve)
ENDOCRINE						Various endocrine abnormalities
PSYCHIATRIC/ PSYCHOLOGICAL	Easily excitable Hyperactive	Variable intellectual capacity Attention deficit problems in childhood	Severe intellectual disability	Mild intellectual disability	Variable intellectual capacity Behavioural difficulties Sleep problems	Variable intellectual capacity
CNS	Severe developmental delay Epilepsy	Perceptual and motor function reduced	Epilepsy Vasomotor instability	Epilepsy	Cerebral astrocytomas Epilepsy	Variable clinical phenomena depend-ing on site of the tumours Epilepsy
CARDIOVASCULAR		Cardiac abnormalities Hypertension CVAs Chronic hemiparesis	Prolonged QT interval	Pulmonary valvular stenosis ASD, VSD, PDA	Rhabdomyomatas Hypertension	
MUSCULAR/ SKELETAL/SKIN	Joint contractures and scoliosis (in adults)	Joint contractures Scoliosis Hypotonia	Osteopenia Fractures Scoliosis	Scoliosis Talipes equinovarus Pectus carinatum/ excavatum	Bone Rhabdomyomata	Skeletal abnormalities esp. kyphoscoliosis
OTHER	Speech impairment Movement and balance disorder Characteristic EEG changes	Renal abnormalities	Hyperventilation Apnoea Reflux Feeding difficulties Growth failure	Abnormal clotting factors, platelet dysfunction Undescended testes, deficient spermatogenesis Lymphoadenoma Hepatosplenomegaly Cubitus valgus, hand abnormalities	Kidney and lung hamartomata Polycystic kidneys Liver rhabdomyomata Dental abnormalities Skin lesions	Variable clinical phenomena depend-ing on the location of the neurofibroma Tumours are suscep-tible to malignant change Other varieties of tumours may be associated
INHERITANCE	Variety of genetic mechanisms on chromosome 15	Microdeletion on long arm of chromosome 7	Mainly sporadic	Autosomal dominant; may be sporadic	Autosomal dominant	Autosomal dominant

Reproduced with permission from Nick Lennox, Associate Professor and Former Director Queensland Centre for Intellectual and Developmental Disability, MRI/UQ, University of Queensland.

particular, laxity of the transverse atlantal ligament or possibly malformations of the odontoid bone lead to instability.[72]

Children with Down syndrome can be screened radiologically, although this is not recommended.[73,74] It is not usual to find atlanto-axial instability as a result of clinical symptoms; however, there have been rare fatalities as a result of this problem and so it needs to be considered.[75] It appears that this is mostly a problem in children with Down syndrome, with up to 20% affected;[76] in adulthood, the joint stabilises for most individuals. When there are clinical manifestations of spinal cord compression, they are rare with only about 1% affected and they usually occur slowly over weeks.[76]

The presence of the following signs and symptoms could be a result of spinal cord compression:

- neck stiffness or torticollis—an important sign
- unexplained behaviour change
- refusal to participate in usual activities
- changing hand preference
- neck pain
- ataxic gait
- increased reflexes
- clonus
- upgoing plantars
- urinary incontinence
- progressive spasticity in the legs.

PRACTICE TIP

Care should be exercised with procedures that involve hyperextension of the neck in people, particularly children with Down syndrome (such as intubation and instillation of eye drops), to prevent cervical injury due to lax ligaments.

COMMUNICATION WITH THE PERSON WITH AN INTELLECTUAL DISABILITY

Advice on communication with a person with an intellectual disability is given in Box 37.1.

BOX 37.1 COMMUNICATION WITH THE PERSON WHO HAS AN INTELLECTUAL DISABILITY[62]

Due to the high frequency of communication difficulties in people with intellectual disability, communication may take more time and the use of non-verbal communication may be necessary. The following are useful communication strategies to use with people with cognitive and/or communication difficulties.

- Always try to speak directly with the person with a disability, rather than a family member/carer or support worker. Find out if the person wishes the carer or support worker to stay for the consultation, and if they are happy for them to speak on their behalf.
- Be aware that while the person with a disability may have difficulty in speaking, he or she may be able to understand what is said to them.
- Find out how the person communicates, e.g. how do they indicate 'yes' or 'no', before asking questions.
- If a person uses a communication device, ask them to show you how to use it.
- Before you start, explain what will happen in the consultation, using brief, simple and direct sentences. Some people may be anxious, and not know what to expect or how to participate.
- Before examining the person, tell or show them what you are going to do and why you are doing it. Check they understand what you have said, and that they agree. Supplement verbal communication with pictures and gestures such as pointing to parts of the body.
- When giving advice or instructions, check that the person has understood by asking them to repeat what you have said in their own words. Let the person know you understand them. If you have trouble understanding, ask them to repeat. Don't pretend that you understand.
- Don't ask questions in a way that suggests an answer. Check responses to your question by asking again in a different way.
- Some people may take time to answer your questions. A good rule of thumb is to wait at least 10 seconds for a response.
- Some people may not be able to read letters, make appointments, tell the time or read instructions on medications. Family members, other carers or support workers can assist here.
- Understanding the concept of time may be difficult. Use examples from their daily routines, e.g. breakfast, lunch and dinner, rather than three times a day. Try to relate questions to familiar routines or events in their life.

OTHER CARE ISSUES

Intrathecal baclofen pumps

In order to reduce generalised hypertonia that occurs with cerebral palsy and spinal cord injuries, baclofen is inserted directly into the thecal sac surrounding the spinal cord and continuously infused using a pump.[77] If coma or signs of respiratory depression occur, overdose should be suspected and the pump should be stopped immediately. This requires a specialised device, and until it can be turned off or the reservoir emptied, airway, breathing and circulation need to be supported. If the pump fails or the infusing tube becomes blocked, then signs of withdrawal may become evident; these include tachycardia, blood pressure changes, hyperthermia, increased spasticity and rhabdomyolysis that may proceed to multi-system failure.[77]

VENTRICULOPERITONEAL SHUNTS

Ventriculoperitoneal (VP) shunts are catheters used to treat hydrocephalus; they are placed into the ventricles of the brain where they collect cerebrospinal fluid (CSF), which is then transported to the peritoneum. An obstruction in this drainage system causes a rise in intracranial pressure (ICP). Signs and symptoms are consistent with rising ICP and are likely to include irritability; headache; nausea and vomiting; reduced cognition; ataxia; changes in respirations, blood pressure and pulse; and a bulging fontanelle in infants. Emergency management should include elevating the person's head and managing their airway, breathing and circulation. If stable, the patient should have a computed tomography scan of the head and a neurosurgical consultation should be arranged for surgical shunt revision.[78]

If a child presents with signs of raised ICP and infection (fever, ill appearance, redness over the site, tenderness over the tubing, abdominal pain and tenderness), it may indicate that the shunt may be infected. In these circumstances a lumbar puncture with CSF collection for culture and sensitivity should occur, followed by appropriate broad-spectrum antibiotics.[78]

GASTROSTOMY TUBES

An increasing number of people with feeding difficulties are having enterostomy devices inserted. They are implemented to avoid aspiration and where nutritional intake is inadequate because of swallowing difficulties. These devices can be inserted via the nasogastric route or, for longer-term use, via a stoma.[79]

Percutaneous endoscopic gastrostomy tubes (PEGs or buttons) terminate in the stomach, whereas jejunostomy tubes (J tubes) terminate in the jejunum of the small bowel. PEGs are more routinely used for feeding, whereas J tubes are used for people with gastro-oesophageal reflux.

People with feeding tubes are likely to present for emergency care if the tube leaks gastric contents, becomes obstructed or is dislodged. The first assessment priority in all these circumstances is the person's level of hydration, as they may have a significantly reduced fluid intake. For the person who is unable to safely swallow fluids, intravenous hydration may be required to maintain fluid intake. Medication may also have been missed.[79]

PEG tubes that are blocked with food or medication can sometimes be cleared by flushing with warm water. This can be enhanced by using a push–pull technique and by rolling the tube while it is being flushed. A proteolytic enzyme solution may also be used; if this fails, replacement will be necessary.[80] Tubes that have come out need to be replaced quickly to prevent constriction and closure of the stoma; however, this should be attempted by an experienced and suitably trained person. Jejunostomy tubes need to be guided back into position under fluoroscopy. Attempts by inexperienced practitioners can result in false tracts being created.[81] If there is going to be some delay, an indwelling urinary catheter may be used to keep the stoma open.

When PEG tubes have been reinserted in the ED, their position needs to be confirmed radiologically. Patients should not be discharged until definitive tube placement has been achieved.[80]

CHALLENGING BEHAVIOUR AND ANXIETY

A change in behaviour is often a reason a person with an intellectual disability is brought to an ED. Often the abnormal behaviour is a result of distress, illness or pain.[82] Once a pathological cause has been ruled out or treated, only then can the behaviour be managed with a pharmacological, psychiatric or behavioural intervention.[83]

Two particularly difficult forms of challenging behaviour are 'stereotypical or self-stimulatory' and 'self-injurious'.[45] Stereotypical behaviour is characterised by repeated stimulation of a sense or senses. In the emergency setting it may be triggered by the unfamiliar and frightening surroundings that cause anxiety. As a result, the person may begin to rock, to tap or repeatedly taste things. If this behaviour is a result of anxiety, it may be managed with the help of the carer, who may effectively soothe the person; or a socially acceptable alternative could be provided, such as a piece of rubber to chew on. Self-injurious behaviour results in physical injury and may also be the result of anxiety; however, it may be more difficult to manage and be less socially acceptable, and so chemical or physical restraint may need to be used.[17] For all forms of behaviour the patient may have a healthcare plan that details the causes and describes management strategies and, in consultation with the accompanying carer, these strategies should be used.

Anxiety is a very common experience for people with an intellectual disability and this can be manifested as a diagnosable psychiatric disorder that may cause greater impairment than diminished cognitive abilities.[84] Carers and personal support workers must be involved in the prevention and management of anxiety in the emergency setting. Touching the patient to calm them is likely to exacerbate the problem. The person who knows the patient best should be the individual to use soothing techniques. However, once the patient becomes uncontrollably anxious there may be little that can be done apart from the administration of suitable pharmacological agents, restraint, or removal from the area.

THE ROLE OF CARERS, LEGAL GUARDIANS AND PERSONAL SUPPORT WORKERS

Carer is the term used for a person who lives with a person who has a disability; usually this will mean that they are a parent or sibling. Personal support workers (PSWs) are employed to perform this role. The term 'carer' is sometimes used for both roles. These people are integral to the delivery of effective care for the person with a disability. Some PSWs have known their clients for more than 20 years and may be more familiar with their health issues than many parents. It is therefore essential to involve carers and PSWs in the emergency care of patients with a disability.

Guardianship law in Australia is the principal mechanism for protecting the health of people with disabilities and each state and territory has its own guardianship legislation. There are, however, some general principles described by the Queensland Office of the Public Guardian. These principles stress that a person's guardian must respect their rights and presume that they have capacity and value.[85]

In Aotearoa New Zealand, guardians can be natural (parents), court appointed or testamentary (deceased parent names a person in their will) and the same principles apply.[86] Paramedics and emergency clinicians must therefore expect guardians to protect the person's best interests and guardians may provide consent on the person's behalf when the person does not have sufficient capacity.

Health professionals need to understand that local guardianship laws can vary across jurisdictions. Further, across Australia and Aotearoa New Zealand, citizen advocacy organisations are actively seeking to promote healthy and enduring relationships for people with disabilities and may play an active role in healthcare settings. These organisations strive to support, strengthen and improve the independent advocacy of people with disability.

PRACTICE TIP

Personal support workers and carers should be involved in the emergency care of patients with an intellectual disability. However, they cannot act as the 'person responsible' to provide consent unless they meet the jurisdictional principal requirements according to relevant guardianship laws.

SUMMARY

In Aotearoa New Zealand, 24%[5], and in Australia around 18%[1] of people, report having a disability; these people are more likely to present to an ED than people who do not have a disability. People with a disability are also likely to have hidden disabilities, undiagnosed health problems and they may have difficulty communicating their symptoms and history; paramedics and emergency clinicians therefore need to take extra care in their assessment of a person with a disability. People with an intellectual disability are a group in which these issues are amplified; they are at increased risk of disorders such as epilepsy and anxiety. People with an intellectual disability are most likely to die of a respiratory disorder. Having an intellectual disability predisposes the person to particular health conditions, many of which are related to the syndrome that caused their intellectual disability. Diagnostic overshadowing, a propensity by clinicians to attribute behaviour or clinical manifestations to a person's intellectual disability, can lead to inadequate or delayed treatment.

Depending on the communication ability of the person with a disability, assessing their emergency needs and level of pain or distress is difficult, and needs to be carefully performed with the assistance of the person who normally cares for them. Failure to acknowledge behavioural changes and signs of distress can result in inadequate assessment of serious pathologies. Generalisations cannot be applied when assessing pain, as people with disabilities may display their distress in idiosyncratic ways.

CASE STUDY

A 36-year-old intellectually disabled man is brought to the emergency department (ED) by ambulance. His personal support worker (PSW) accompanies him from his residential accommodation. He has been brought in because the staffing at his community house noticed that he was not his usual self and he had lost his appetite.

QUESTIONS

1. After introducing yourself to the patient and their PSW with your name and role, it is then important that you ask:
   a. the PSW to remain outside, so that the patient answers without fear of disclosing private details to the PSW.
   b. the PSW to remain with your patient and direct all questions to the PSW.
   c. the patient a simple question, such as 'Where does it hurt?' to determine their communication ability.
   d. the PSW what the patient's communication abilities are.
2. Your patient with an intellectual disability has a PSW at all times in his residential accommodation and a registered nurse visits when he needs assistance with his healthcare needs. How would you triage the patient?
   a. He needs to be urgently assessed and closely monitored.
   b. He can wait in the waiting room with his PSW.
   c. He should be moved to a quieter area.
   d. His triage priority should be determined on physiological parameters as for every other patient seeking emergency care.
3. You notice that your patient is slim, of short stature, has an extended face, enlarged ears and that he sits on the bed with widely abducted legs. These observations are important because:
   a. His elongated face and ears indicate that he may have Marfan's syndrome, indicating that he is at risk of aortic dissection and cardiac ischaemia.
   b. His facial features, short stature and mobile joints indicate that he may have Fragile X syndrome, indicating that he is more at risk of seizures and mitral regurgitation with congestive heart failure.
   c. His hypermobile hips indicate that he probably has Down syndrome, indicating an increased risk of thyroid disease, congenital heart disease and dislocated hips.
   d. These physical appearance findings, while informative, are unlikely to have much bearing on his emergency care.
4. You determine that your patient is unable to indicate that he has pain, as he has no language abilities. How will you best determine if he has any pain or discomfort?
   a. Ask his carer if he has pain.
   b. Use a tool to assess facial expression as an indicator of distress.
   c. If he appears in distress to you, he is likely to be in pain.
   d. Use information provided in his healthcare plan or from his carer to determine his appearance when content in comparison to when distressed.

Answers to Case Study Questions can be found on evolve **http://evolve.elsevier.com/AU/Curtis/emergency/** 

USEFUL WEBSITES

Australasian Society for Intellectual Disability, www.asid.asn.au.

Australian Citizen Advocacy, www.citizenadvocacytrust.com.au/what-is-citizen-advocacy/.

Australian Federation of Disability Organisations, www.afdo.org.au.

Australian Guardianship & Administration Council, www.agac.org.au/

Australian National Disability Insurance Scheme (NDIS), www.ndis.gov.au.

Australian Privacy Act, 1988, www.legislation.gov.au/Details/C2021C00452.

Centers for Disease Control and Prevention, Developmental disabilities, www.cdc.gov/ncbddd/developmentaldisabilities/index.html

Centre for Developmental Disability Health Victoria (CDDHV), www.cddh.monash.org.

Disability Advocacy Network Australia, www.dana.org.au.

Disability Service Australia, www.dsa.org.au.

Disability service standards, www.dsa.org.au/resources/disability-service-standards.

Disabled World towards tomorrow, www.disabled-world.com/disability/types/invisible/.

Distress and Discomfort Assessment Tool (DisDAT), www.stoswaldsuk.org/how-we-help/we-educate/education/resources/disability-distress-assessment-tool-disdat/

Donald Beasley Institute, www.donaldbeasley.org.nz.

Health Information Privacy Code 2020, www.privacy.org.nz/privacy-act-2020/codes-of-practice/hipc2020/

Historic England: a history of disability: from 1050 to the present day, https://historicengland.org.uk/research/inclusive-heritage/disability-history/

Inclusion Australia, www.inclusionaustralia.org.au/.

Intellectual disability mental health e-learning, www.idhealtheducation.edu.au.

National League for Nursing, Communicating with people with disabilities, www.nln.org/education/teaching-resources/professional-development-programsteaching-resourcesace-all/ace-d/additional-resources/communicating-with-people-with-disabilities-e030c45c-7836-6c70-9642-ff00005f0421

New Zealand Citizen Advocacy, www.caauckland.org.nz/

New Zealand Disability Strategy, www.odi.govt.nz/nz-disability-strategy/

New Zealand Guardianship Law, www.justice.govt.nz/family/care-of-children/guardians-and-guardianship/.

Office for Disability Issues Additional detail on the New Zealand Disability Strategy is available at: www.odi.govt.nz/nz-disability-strategy/.

Office for Disability Issues: Outcome 3—Health and wellbeing, www.odi.govt.nz/nz-disability-strategy/outcome-3-health-and-wellbeing/.

People with Disability, Australia, www.pwd.org.au.

Queensland Centre for Intellectual and Developmental Disability, qcidd.centre.uq.edu.au.

Understanding Intellectual Disability and Health, Changing Values, www.intellectualdisability.info/changing-values.

Understanding Intellectual Disability and Health, St George's, University of London, www.intellectualdisability.info.

REFERENCES

1. Australian Institute of Health and Welfare (AIHW). People with disability in Australia. Canberra: AIHW; 2020. Cat. no: DIS 72.
2. Sullivan WF, Diepstra H, Heng J, Ally S, Bradley E, Casson I, et al. Primary care of adults with intellectual and developmental disabilities: 2018 Canadian consensus guidelines. Can Fam Physician 2018;64(4):254–79.
3. Wen X. The definition and prevalence of intellectual disability in Australia. AIHW catalogue no DIS 2. Australian Government Publication. Canberra: AIHW; 1997.
4. Australian Institute of Health and Welfare (AIHW). People with disability in Australia. Canberra: AIHW; 2020.
5. Statistics New Zealand. 2013 New Zealand disability survey: Disability. Wellington: Ministry of Health; 2013. Online. Available from: www.health.govt.nz/our-work/populations/maori-health/tatau-kahukura-maori-health-statistics/nga-mana-hauora-tutohu-health-status-indicators/disability.
6. Olusanya BO, Davis AC, Wertlieb D. Developmental disabilities among children younger than 5 years in 195 countries and territories, 1990–2016: a systematic analysis for the Global Burden of Disease Study 2016. Lancet Glob Health 2018;6(10):e1100–21.
7. Disability Information Service. Intellectual disability: the facts. Fullerton SA: Disability SA, Department for Families and Communities; 2009.
8. Merriam G. Rehabilitating Aristotle: a virtue ethics approach to disability and human flourishing. In: Ralston DC, Ho J, editors. Philosophical reflections on disability. Dordrecht: Springer; 2010.
9. Brown I, Radford JP. Historical overview of intellectual and developmental disabilities. In: Brown I, Percy M, editors. A comprehensive guide to intellectual and developmental disabilities. 2nd ed. Baltimore: Paul H Brookes; 2007.
10. Australian Institute of Health and Welfare (AIHW). Access to health services by Australians with disability. Canberra: AIHW; 2017.

11. Chivell WC. An inquest taken on behalf of our Sovereign Lady the Queen at Adelaide in the state of South Australia, on the 2nd and 3rd and 17th of July 2001 and the 24th of August 2001, before Wayne Cromwell Chivell, a Coroner for the said State, concerning the death of Saverio Gadaleta. Adelaide: Coroners Court, South Australia; 2001.
12. Australian Institute of Health and Welfare (AIHW). Disability support services: services provided under the National Disability Agreement 2018–19. Canberra; AIHW; 2020.
13. NDIS. What is the NDIS? 2021. Online. Available from: www.ndis.gov.au/understanding/what-ndis.
14. Office for Disability Issues. New Zealand disability strategy. 2022. Online. Available from: www.odi.govt.nz/nz-disability-strategy/.
15. Karam SM, Riegel M, Segal SL, Félix TM, Barros AJ, Santos IS, et al. Genetic causes of intellectual disability in a birth cohort: a population-based study. Am J Med Genet A 2015;167(6):1204–14.
16. Percy M. Factors that cause or contribute to intellectual and developmental disabilities. In: Brown I, Percy M, editors. A comprehensive guide to intellectual and developmental disabilities. 2nd ed. Baltimore: Paul H Brookes; 2007.
17. Percy M, Brown I, Lewkis SZ. Abnormal behavior. In: Brown I, Percy M, editors. A comprehensive guide to intellectual and developmental disabilities. 2nd ed. Baltimore: Paul H Brookes; 2017.
18. Reichenberg A, Cederlöf M, McMillan A, Trzaskowski M, Kapra O, Fruchter E, et al. Discontinuity in the genetic and environmental causes of the intellectual disability spectrum. Proc Natl Acad Sci USA 2016;113(4):1098–103.
19. Australian Bureau of Statistics (ABS). 4433.0.55.003 – Intellectual disability, Australia. 2012. Online. Available from: www.abs.gov.au/statistics/health/disability/disability-ageing-and-carers-australia-summary-findings/2018.
20. Australian Bureau of Statistics (ABS). Disability, ageing and carers, Australia: summary of findings, ABS cat. no. 4430.0. Canberra: Australian Bureau of Statistics; 2019.
21. Bray A. Demographics and characteristics of people with an intellectual disability: review of the literature prepared for the National Advisory Committee on Health and Disability to inform its project on services for adults with an intellectual disability. Wellington: National Health Committee and Donald Beasley Institute; 2003.
22. Larson SA, Lakin KC, Anderson L, Kwak Lee N, Anderson D. Prevalence of mental retardation and developmental disabilities: estimates from the 1994/1995 national health interview survey disability supplements. Am J Ment Retard 2001;106(3):231–52.
23. Hall C, Amor D, Cohen J. Developmental disability. In: Therapeutic guidelines [Internet]. North Melbourne: Therapeutic Guidelines Ltd; 2021. Online. Available from: tgldcdp.tg.org.au/guideLine?guidelinePage=Developmental+Disability&frompage=etgcomplete.
24. Beange H, McElduff A, Baker W. Medical disorders of adults with mental retardation: a population study. Am J Ment Retard 1995;99(6):595–604.
25. Liao PA-O, Vajdic C, Trollor J, Reppermund S. Prevalence and incidence of physical health conditions in people with intellectual disability - a systematic review. PLoS One 2021;16(8):e0256294.
26. O'Leary L, Cooper SA, Hughes-McCormack L. Early death and causes of death of people with intellectual disabilities: a systematic review. J Appl Res Intellect Disabil 2018;31(3):325–42.
27. Kanne S. Diagnostic overshadowing. In: Volkmar FR, editor. Encyclopedia of autism spectrum disorders. New York, NY: Springer New York; 2013.
28. Jansen DE, Krol B, Groothoff JW, Post D. People with intellectual disability and their health problems: a review of comparative studies. J Intellect Disabil Res 2004;48(Pt 2):93–102.
29. Khaw KT, Reeve J, Luben R, Welch A, Wareham N, Oakes S, et al. Prediction of total and hip fracture risk in men and women by quantitative ultrasound of the calcaneus: EPIC-Norfolk prospective population study. Lancet 2004;363(9404):197–202.
30. Grossman SA, Richards CF, Anglin D, Hutson HR. Caring for the patient with mental retardation in the emergency department. Ann Emerg Med 2000;35(1):69–76.
31. Pal J, Hale L, Mirfin-Veitch B, Claydon C. Injuries and falls among adults with intellectual disability: a prospective New Zealand cohort study. J Intellect Develop Disabil 2014;39(1):35–44.
32. Petropoulou E, Finlayson J, Hay M, Spencer W, Park R, Tannock H, et al. Injuries reported and recorded for adults with intellectual disabilities who live with paid support in Scotland: a comparison with Scottish adults in the general population. J Appl Res Intellect Disabil 2016;30(2):408–15.
33. Pope J, Truesdale M, Brown M. Risk factors for falls among adults with intellectual disabilities: a narrative review. J Appl Res Intellect Disabil 2021;34(1):274–85.
34. Janicki MP, Davidson PW, Henderson CM, McCallion P, Taets JD, Force LT, et al. Health characteristics and health services utilization in older adults with intellectual disability living in community residences. J Intellect Disabil Res 2002;46(4):287–98.
35. Kalb LG, Vasa RA, Ballard ED, Woods S, Goldstein M, Wilcox HC. Epidemiology of injury-related emergency department visits in the US among youth with autism spectrum disorder. J Autism Dev Disord 2016;46(8):2756–63.
36. Lunsky Y, Balogh R, Khodaverdian A, Elliott D, Jaskulski C, Morris S. A comparison of medical and psychobehavioral emergency department visits made by adults with intellectual disabilities. Emerg Med Int 2012;2012:427407.
37. Sherrard J, Tonge BJ, Ozanne-Smith J. Injury risk in young people with intellectual disability. J Intellect Disabil Res 2002;46(Pt 1):6–16.
38. El-Khouri M, Mourao MA, Tobo A, Battistella LR, Herrero CF, Riberto M. Prevalence of atlanto-occipital and atlantoaxial instability in adults with Down syndrome. World Neurosurg 2014;82(1–2):215–18.
39. Anderson LL, Humphries K, McDermott S, Marks B, Sisirak J, Larson S. The state of the science of health and wellness for adults with intellectual and developmental disabilities. Intellect Dev Disabil 2013;51(5):385–98.

40. Carey IM, Shah SM, Hosking FJ, DeWilde S, Harris T, Beighton C, et al. Health characteristics and consultation patterns of people with intellectual disability: a cross-sectional database study in English general practice. Br J Gen Pract 2016;66(645):e264–70.
41. Daaleman TP. Primary care of adults with intellectual and developmental disabilities. South Med J 2016;109(1):12–16.
42. Morin D, Merineau-Cote J, Ouellette-Kuntz H, Tassé MJ, Kerr M. A comparison of the prevalence of chronic disease among people with and without intellectual disability. Am J Intellect Dev Disabil 2012;117(6):455–63.
43. Cheetham I, Lovering JS, Telch J, Percy M. Physical health. In: Brown I, Percy M, editors. A comprehensive guide to intellectual and developmental disabilities. 2nd ed. Baltimore: Paul H Brookes; 2007.
44. Doody O, Bailey ME. Understanding pain physiology and its application to person with intellectual disability. J Intellect Disabil 2019;23(1):5–18.
45. Huisman S, Mulder P, Kuijk J, Kerstholt M, van Eeghen A, Leenders A, et al. Self-injurious behavior. Neurosci Biobehav Rev 2018;84:483–91.
46. McKenzie K, Smith M, Purcell AM. The reported expression of pain and distress by people with an intellectual disability. J Clin Nurs 2013; 22(13–14):1833–42.
47. Amor-Salamanca A, Menchon JM. Pain underreporting associated with profound intellectual disability in emergency departments. J Intellect Disabil Res 2017;61(4):341–7.
48. Doody O, Bailey ME. Interventions in pain management for persons with an intellectual disability. J Intellect Disabil 2019;23(1):132–44.
49. Doody OE, Bailey M. Pain and pain assessment in people with intellectual disability: issues and challenges in practice. Br J Learn Disabil 2017;45(3):157–65.
50. Regnard C, Reynolds J, Watson B, Matthews D, Gibson L, Clarke C. Understanding distress in people with severe communication difficulties: developing and assessing the Disability Distress Assessment Tool (DisDAT). J Intellect Disabil Res 2007;51(Pt 4):277–92.
51. Jacinto M, Frontini R, Matos R, Antunes R. Effects of exercise programs on anxiety in individuals with disabilities: a systematic review with a meta-analysis. Healthcare (Basel) 2021;9(8):1047.
52. Anderson JS, Grossman SA. The intellectually disabled patient. In: Venkat A. editor. Challenging and emerging conditions in emergency medicine. Hoboken, NJ: Wiley-Blackwell; 2011.
53. Nguyen M, Lennox N, Ware R. Hand-held health records for individuals with intellectual disability: a systematic review. J Intellect Disabil Res 2014;58(12):1172–8.
54. Iacono T, Bigby C, Unsworth C, Douglas J, Fitzpatrick P. A systematic review of hospital experiences of people with intellectual disability. BMC Health Serv Res 2014;14(1):505.
55. Privacy Act 1988 No. 119, 1988, (2021).
56. Office of the Australian Information Commissioner. Australian privacy principles. Canberra: Australian Government; 2014.
57. Cheetham TC. Challenges in medical care for persons with developmental disabilities: an illustrative case: 'Ray'. Clin Bull Development Disabil Program 2001;12(3):1–9.
58. Haider SI, Ansari Z, Vaughan L, Matters H, Emerson E. Prevalence and factors associated with polypharmacy in Victorian adults with intellectual disability. Res Dev Disabil 2014;35(11):3071–80.
59. Bigby C, Whiteside M, Douglas J. Providing support for decision making to adults with intellectual disability: perspectives of family members and workers in disability support services. J Intellect Devel Disabil 2019;44(4):396–409.
60. Ellison C, Lante K. People living with disability: navigating support and health systems. In: Willis E, Reynolds L, Keleher H, editors. Understanding the Australian Health Care System. Chatswood: Elsevier Health Sciences; 2016.
61. Koutoukidis G. Health planning: an organisational approach to meeting the needs of individuals with a disability. Ageing and Disability Conference. Adelaide: National Disability Services; 2007.
62. Centre for Developmental Disability Studies. Health care in people with intellectual disability—guidelines for general practitioners. North Sydney: CDDS for NSW Health; 2006. CC BY 4.0 license.
63. Wilson NJ, Lin Z, Villarosa A, Lewis P, Philip P, Sumar B, et al. Countering the poor oral health of people with intellectual and developmental disability: a scoping literature review. BMC Public Health 2019;19(1):1530.
64. Trollor J, Srasuebkul P, Xu H, Howlett S. Cause of death and potentially avoidable deaths in Australian adults with intellectual disability using retrospective linked data. BMJ Open 2017;7:e013489.
65. Pilla M, Langlois NEI, Byard RW. Causes of death in a series of decedents with cerebral palsy in a medicolegal context. Aust J Forens Sci 2018; 50(4):428–34.
66. Kerr M, Linehan C, Thompson R, Mula M, Gil-Nagal A, Zuberi SM, et al. A White Paper on the medical and social needs of people with epilepsy and intellectual disability: the Task Force on Intellectual Disabilities and Epilepsy of the International League Against Epilepsy. Epilepsia 2014;55(12):1902–6.
67. Santoro JD, Pagarkar D, Chu DT, Rosso M, Paulsen KC, Levitt P, et al. Neurologic complications of Down syndrome: a systematic review. J Neurol 2021;268(12):4495–509.
68. Doran Z, Shankar R, Keezer MR, Dale C, McLean B, Kerr MP, et al. Managing anti-epileptic drug treatment in adult patients with intellectual disability: a serious conundrum. Euro J Neurol 2016;23(7):1152–7.
69. Hithersay R, Hamburg S, Knight B, Strydom A. Cognitive decline and dementia in Down syndrome. Curr Opin Psychiatry 2017;30(2):102–7.
70. Harper L. Optimal nutrition for bone health in people with a learning disability. Learn Disabil Prac 2017;20(1):31–5.

71. Novak I, Morgan C, Adde L, Blackman J, Boyd RN, Brunstrom-Hernandez J, et al. Early, accurate diagnosis and early intervention in cerebral palsy: advances in diagnosis and treatment. JAMA Pediatr 2017;171(9):897–907.

72. Talbot C, Alshryda S. Evidence-based treatment for musculoskeletal disorders in children with Down's syndrome. In: Alshryda S, Huntley, J, Banaszkiewicz P, editors. Paediatric orthopaedics: an evidence-based approach to clincal questions. Switzerland: Springer; 2017.

73. Capone G, Stephens M, Santoro S, Chicoine B, Bulova P, Peterson M, et al. Co-occurring medical conditions in adults with Down syndrome: a systematic review toward the development of health care guidelines. Part II. Am J Med Genet A 2020;182(7):1832–45.

74. Capone GT, Chicoine B, Bulova P, Stephens M, Hart S, Crissman B, et al. Co-occurring medical conditions in adults with Down syndrome: a systematic review toward the development of health care guidelines. Am J Med Genet A 2018;176(1):116–33.

75. Saad KF. A lethal case of atlantoaxial dislocation in a 56-year-old woman with Down's syndrome. J Intellect Disabil Res 1995;39(Pt 5):447–9.

76. Ali FE, Al-Bustan MA, Al-Busairi WA, Al-Mulla FA, Esbaita EY. Cervical spine abnormalities associated with Down syndrome. Int Orthop 2006;30(4): 284–9.

77. Woolf SM, Baum CR. Baclofen pumps: uses and complications. Pediat Emerg Care 2017;33(4):271–5.

78. Roepke C, Zada G, Pham M, Jhun P, Bright A, Herbert M. The lowdown on ventriculoperitoneal shunts. Ann Emerg Med 2016;67(3):414–6.

79. Molina Villalba C, Vázquez Rodríguez JA, Gallardo Sánchez F. Percutaneous endoscopic gastrostomy. Indications, care and complications. Med Clin (Barc) 2019;152(6):229–36.

80. Malhi H, Thompson R. PEG tubes: dealing with complications. Nurs Times 2014;110(45):18–21.

81. Lahham S, Assaf S, Fairley R. Mal-positioned gastrojejunostomy tube. West J Emerg Med 2015;16(7):1199–200.

82. Adirim TA, Rosenman ED. Evaluation of the developmentally or physically disabled patient. In: Marx J, Hockberger R, Walls R, editors. Rosen's emergency medicine: concepts and clinical practice. 8th ed. Philadelphia: Mosby; 2013.

83. Sheehan R, Hassiotis A, Walters K, Osborn D, Strydom A, Horsfall L. Mental illness, challenging behaviour, and psychotropic drug prescribing in people with intellectual disability: UK population based cohort study. BMJ 2015;351:h4326.

84. Reardon TC, Gray KM, Melvin GA. Anxiety disorders in children and adolescents with intellectual disability: prevalence and assessment. Res Develop Disabil 2015;36:175–90.

85. Queensland Public Guardian. The general principles. Brisbane: OPG; 2017. Online. Available from: www.publicguardian.qld.gov.au/__data/assets/pdf_file/0011/490556/opg-factsheet-general-principles.pdf.

86. Ministry of Justice. Powers to make decisions for others: what a welfare guardian does. Wellington: New Zealand Government; 2020. Online. Available from: www.justice.govt.nz/family/powers-to-make-decisions/welfare-guardians/what-a-welfare-guardian-does/.

CHAPTER 38
THE OLDER PERSON

GLENN ARENDTS, HELEN RAWSON AND TEGWYN McMANAMNY

ESSENTIALS

- Emergency ambulance and hospital presentations for older people are common and increasing.
- The ageing process affects human physiology.
- Emergency care must account for individual ageing processes particular to each person.
- The functional, cognitive and emotional status of the older person must be assessed and managed.
- Particular attention must be paid to the assessment and treatment of pain.
- Polypharmacy is such a significant cause of morbidity that it must be considered a contributing risk for all older people.
- It is helpful to bring patient medications to assist with patient assessment.
- Cognitive testing is an important part of assessment.
- Falls are the most common cause of injury.
- Malnutrition affects older people who seek emergency care.
- A serious infection can present with vague signs and symptoms.
- Carefully consider activities of daily living and function before discharge.
- Accurately and carefully complete standardised discharge or transitional care forms.
- It is particularly useful for paramedics to assess the living arrangements of older people to assist with discharge planning.

INTRODUCTION

What is an older person?

There is no standard definition of an 'older person' that encompasses all countries and population groups. The United Nations refers to older person as 60 years and over.[1] In Australia and Aotearoa New Zealand, and most developed countries, the chronological age of 65 years and over is the accepted definition of an 'older' person, historically based on the age when a person retired from the workforce.[2] For people 65 years and over, there are an additional three accepted phases of defining an older person: 'young-old' (65–74 years); 'middle-old' (75–84 years); and 'old-old' (85 years and over).[3] The definition of 'old age' for some population groups is earlier than 65 years. For Aboriginal and Torres Strait Islanders and Māori, the recognised age of an 'older person' is 50 years and over, due to the higher likelihood of developing serious medical conditions earlier in life, and the lower life expectancy in comparison to non-Indigenous groups.

DEMOGRAPHY

POPULATION DEMOGRAPHICS

The populations of Australia and Aotearoa New Zealand are ageing as a result of a large increase in the birth rate between 1946 and 1964 (demographic birth boom), improved healthcare and increasing life expectancy. Consequently, more people are entering older age than at any other time in history.[4] Between 1995 and 2020, Australia's population aged 65 years and over increased from 12% to 16% (representing 4.2 million people),[5] and this is projected to increase rapidly over the coming decades to between 21% and 23% of the total population by 2066.[6] The age profile among the older population is also projected to change. Currently over half of older Australians (56%) are aged 65–74 years, 31% are in the 75–84 years age group and those 85 years and over account for 13%. By 2066, the proportion of older people aged 65–74 years is projected to decrease to 45%, with projected increases among those 75–84 years (34%) and 85 years and over (21%).[6] The trend of women living longer than men is evident with increasing age. The male to female ratio is 95:100 for the 65–74 years age group; 85:100 in the 75–84 years age group, and decreases to 59 men for every 100 women in the 85 years and over age group.[7] A similar profile is observed for Aotearoa New Zealand's older population, where people 65 years and over represented 15.2% of the overall population in 2018, compared to 12.3% in 2006; this is projected to increase to 23.1% by 2048. In addition, the cohort aged 85 years and over is expected to more than triple from 1.8% of the total population in 2018 to 4.4% by 2043.[8]

The older populations of Australia and Aotearoa New Zealand are also culturally and linguistically diverse (CALD) with one in five older people in Australia born in a non-English speaking country.[9] Although 88% of Aotearoa New Zealand's older population identified themselves as European in 2013, this is projected to decrease to 77% by 2038. Among Aotearoa New Zealand's CALD older population in 2018, 5% were Asian, 6% Māori and 2% Pacific Islanders; these proportions are expected to increase to 13% Asian, 10% Māori and 4% Pacific Islanders by 2038.[10] Although older CALD populations are not homogenous and individual needs vary, overall people from CALD backgrounds have higher levels of disadvantage compared to Anglo-Australians, may experience substantial language barriers in accessing services, and may experience disadvantage as a consequence of having differing cultural practices and norms, which can result in a lack of understanding and barriers to service use.[11]

EMERGENCY CARE DEMOGRAPHICS

Older people presenting to the ED are more likely to arrive by ambulance, have higher acuity problems and take more time to evaluate.[12] The ageing population has meant a steady increase in the number and proportion of older people accessing emergency services. The fastest growth in the number of ED attendances is among persons 65 years and over, and they are more likely to be admitted to hospital or have repeated ED visits,[13] trends likely to continue in the future.[14] Currently 22% of ED attendances are for people 65 years and over.[15] While acute medical problems of older patients may be similar to those of younger adults, the presentation of older people is often different and the presence of comorbidities of ageing can complicate the presentation.[16] Compared to younger patients, older ED users and particularly frail older patients[17] can have chronic and complex conditions,[18] requiring multifaceted healthcare provision,[19,20] are more often acutely ill on presentation to the ED,[21,22] have longer lengths of stay in the ED[23] and have increased rates of adverse outcomes.[23]

EMERGENCY AMBULANCE USE

The rates at which older people use emergency ambulance services increase with age, with one study finding that while older adults comprised only 14% of the population in metropolitan Melbourne, they accounted for over 40% of the requests for emergency ambulance attendance.[24] In particular, there is a significantly higher ambulance attendance rate for older people who live in residential aged care (RAC) homes, with an average ambulance attendance rate of greater than 770 per 1000 people per year, in comparison to less than 210 per 1000 people per year for older people living independently within the community.[25] Increased demand is associated with increasing age, with the very old (those aged 85 years and over) eight times more likely to be transported by emergency ambulance compared to people aged 45–69 years.[26] With projected persistent growth in the older population, an impact on emergency ambulance use is likely. Falls, respiratory complaints and cardiac problems are the leading reasons for emergency ambulance requests for older patients.

ASSESSMENT OF NORMAL AGEING

The assessment of the older person requires an understanding of natural age-related changes. Without this understanding, normal ageing may be misinterpreted as pathology, and vice versa. Also, treatment of older people will not be tailored to the specific issues that ageing results in, leading to healthcare-induced harm. The ageing process is varied and dependent on genetics, nutritional status, level of fitness, lifestyle and presence of disease.[27] However, there are specific anatomical, physiological and immunological differences between older and younger adults.

ANATOMY

Skin and subcutaneous tissue

Structural changes of the skin occur with the epidermis flattening and losing papillae, leading to a decrease in adhesion between the layers of the skin. The outer layer of the skin is prone to peel off with shearing forces, leading to skin tears.[28] There is a loss of subcutaneous fat, with the characteristic wrinkled appearance of skin. Uneven colouring results from loss of melanocytes causing pallor, and capillary breakdown, causing bruising. There is a loss of sensory receptors and therefore a loss of light touch and temperature detection. Nails become thick, brittle and more prone to fungal infection.

Musculoskeletal

Muscle fibres decrease in number, being replaced by fibrous tissue. This atrophy of muscle results in decreased muscle strength and movement. Tendons shrink and harden. Cartilage atrophy and a reduction in bone mass result in increased kyphosis of the spine and loss of height, as well as increased risk of fracture with minor trauma.[29] Cartilage erosion in joints leads to osteoarthritis.

Chest and lungs

The trachea and rib cage become less flexible. A developing kyphosis increases the antero–posterior chest diameter. The muscles of inspiration become weaker. There is hypertrophy of mucous glands and loss of cilia, leading to an increase in the retention of respiratory secretions. Alveoli reduce in number, the lungs shrink and lose elasticity. Cumulatively, these changes impair lung function and put older people at increased risk of hypoxia.

Heart and blood vessels

Changes in the heart muscle are variable with ageing. Arteries typically lose elasticity and stiffen, with a resultant increase in peripheral resistance and, therefore, blood pressure. The extremities are often cold as flow is reduced through stiff peripheral arteries. Veins become engorged and varicosities are common. The heart valves become calcified and murmurs are common.

Kidneys and bladder

As people age there is a decrease in the number and size of nephrons, resulting in a 20% or more decrease in the size of the kidney by the age of 80.[30] Total renal blood flow also diminishes. This loss of nephrons and decrease in blood flow results in a decrease in the glomerular filtration rate (GFR), the key measure of renal function. The bladder wall loses smooth muscle and elastic recoil, resulting in incomplete emptying of the bladder and a risk of cystitis. The bladder sphincter weakens which can lead to incontinence.

Brain

The brain shrinks in size as neurons die off and the cortex atrophies. Blood flow to the brain decreases. As a result of these changes, many brain functions become less responsive, including reaction and response times. The blood–brain barrier becomes less effective, increasing the chance of meningitis and exaggerating responses to medications that cross this barrier, such as opiates.[31]

Sensory organs

The eye lens becomes less elastic and the muscles that help the lens adapt weaken. The middle ear bones degenerate, and inner ear hair cells are lost. Consequently, visual and hearing problems are very common. Other senses such as smell, taste and touch also tend to diminish with age.

PRACTICE TIP

Take particular care to avoid applying shearing forces to an older person's skin.

PHYSIOLOGY

Total body fluid and heat loss

With ageing, muscle mass decreases and adipose tissue increases, so that the proportion of total body fat increases.[29] As a result, total body fluid is diminished, which increases the risk of dehydration. Loss of subcutaneous fat results in poorer insulation and an increased risk of hypothermia.

Cardiovascular responses

The maximal achievable heart rate declines with age, so the heart is increasingly unable to mount a tachycardic response to a fall in cardiac output. Therefore, older patients with shock may not have the anticipated tachycardia, and clinicians should rely on other signs, such as poor skin perfusion and altered alertness, when assessing for shock. Postural hypotension is more common for multiple reasons, including reduced baroreceptor function. There is increased mismatch between myocardial oxygen supply and demand as the heart muscle stiffens. Heart failure may occur, even with a normal ejection fraction.

Kidney function

A decrease in GFR increases the chance of adverse drug reactions and drug-induced renal failure. The older person is less able to excrete excessive water.[32] Fluid overload is a real risk and fluid resuscitation must be titrated carefully; it is important to commence fluid balance charts and monitor vital signs, keeping in mind the potential for fluid overload.

PRACTICE TIP

- Always start a fluid balance chart.
- Dehydration is more likely.
- There is an increased risk of fluid overload with intravenous fluid administration.

Nervous system

There is a decline in cognitive functioning after the age of 20 years, which is usually evident in the performance of timed tests.[33] However, dementia is not part of normal ageing. The nervous system is also less able to effectively respond to changes in external temperature, predisposing the older person to hypothermia and hyperthermia. Balance and righting reflexes are impaired, contributing to falls risk. For bedridden patients, a decreased ability to detect or respond to the sensation of pressure increases the need for vigilance; turning older patients every 2 hours if they are immobile and using specialised mattresses reduces pressure injury.

SENSORY DEPRIVATION

The five senses—sight (vision), hearing (auditory), touch (tactile), smell (olfactory) and taste (gustatory)—enable communication and interaction with the world. There are two facets to normal sensory awareness: sensory reception—the ability to receive external information through various stimuli, and sensory perception—the ability to meaningfully organise and process the information. The ageing process can signal a decline in the senses, resulting in hearing loss, vision loss or diminished senses of taste, smell and touch. Consequently, age-related altered sensory function can impact older people's health-related quality-of-life outcomes.

Many of the chronic illnesses experienced by older people can also impair sensory functioning. Some medications also adversely affect sensory function in older people, and higher rates of polypharmacy in older patients places them at risk of medication-induced sensory impairment. Over 250 medications can affect taste or smell, and impairment of these senses has been linked to weight loss, mood change and functional decline in the older person.[34]

Sensory deprivation can significantly impact the health, wellbeing and safety of older people. While deprivation in one sensory system can result in problems, multi-system sensory deprivation, as a result of the decline in multiple senses, can occur. The National Health Interview Study found that combined vision and hearing loss significantly impacted older people's health and wellbeing.[35] They were three times more likely to have difficulty mobilising (i.e. walking, getting outside, getting into or out of bed or chair), managing medications and preparing meals. They were also significantly more likely to self-report a history of falling in the previous 12 months, as well as a history of hypertension, heart disease or stroke and limited participation in social activities.[35]

IMMUNE SYSTEM

Immunosenescence is the umbrella term given to the many immune changes with ageing that result in two main problems. Firstly, although levels of some white cells, such as neutrophils, are maintained with age, a reduction in T and B cell lymphocyte responses leads to reduced protection from acquiring viral or bacterial infection respectively.[36] Secondly, once the infection is acquired there is actually an exaggerated cytokine response to infection, with high levels of proinflammatory cytokines, leading to tissue damage. Therefore, older people are more likely than younger adults to become infected, and, once infected, develop more severe organ injury.

CONDITIONS OFTEN SEEN IN OLDER PEOPLE

There are certain conditions that, while occurring in all ages, are more prevalent in older people. When older people make contact with an ambulance service or ED, it is fairly rare for these problems to be the *sole reason* for their presentation. However, they are common background conditions that must be looked for in all older people because they critically influence holistic assessment and management. It is important to stress that even though these conditions are frequently present, they are not normal ageing conditions. In this section, the conditions are discussed in some detail, before screening and other assessment tools for paramedics and nurses are described.

CHRONIC DISEASE BURDEN

Chronic disease is the most significant burden on the health system today.[37] An ageing population has resulted in associated increases in disease burden and age-related disorders in older people (cardiovascular diseases, cancers, neurological and mental disorders, musculoskeletal diseases and chronic respiratory diseases),[38] with the overall burden increasing with age.[39] Three-quarters of Australians 65 years and over are reported to have at least one chronic condition that puts them at risk of serious complications and premature death.[37]

COGNITIVE IMPAIRMENT

Cognition refers to the mental processes involved in gaining knowledge and comprehension. These processes include thinking, knowing, remembering, judging and problem-solving. Cognition is important for older people to maintain functional independence, including understanding instructions and the ability to take medications accurately, and maintain effective communication, including processing and integrating sensory information and responding appropriately to others.[40] Changes in cognition occur as part of the ageing process and include decline in the ability to quickly process or transform information to make decisions.[40] Age-related diseases can accelerate cognitive decline, leading to cognitive impairments severe enough to impair everyday functional abilities.

The boundary between normal slowing of cognitive function with ageing and cognitive impairment is sometimes indistinct, but it is important to note that frank cognitive impairment is present in up to 40% of all people over the age of 70 who attend for emergency care.[41,42] Often this will never have been previously diagnosed, and so contact with emergency services represents an opportunity to screen for these conditions.

The most common cause of impaired cognition is dementia. In assessing and managing the older patient with impaired cognition, it is important to distinguish between delirium and dementia. Delirium is an acute state of confusion, whereas dementia is a permanent loss of memory and intellectual ability.[43]

Dementia is consistently listed as the number one disease people do not want in old age, higher than cancer or other illnesses. Older people therefore often do not seek help for dementia symptoms out of fear. But a diagnosis of cognitive impairment has many benefits for the patient, including possible treatments that can slow the disease and assist them with future life planning. With increases in the number of older adults 65 years and over, the increasing prevalence of age-associated neurodegenerative dementias, and the number and proportion of older people accessing emergency services, emergency clinicians will need to be aware of changes in cognition expected as part of the ageing process and changes that may indicate the onset of brain disease, such as dementia.

PRACTICE TIP

- Older people in emergency settings often have undiagnosed dementia or delirium.
- Routinely perform a cognitive screen.

FUNCTIONAL DECLINE

Functional decline is a loss of independence in self-care capabilities and is typically associated with deterioration in mobility and in the performance of activities of daily living (ADLs), such as dressing, toileting and bathing. The severity of the impact of this on an older person's life depends not only on the physical and/or cognitive problems causing their loss of ability, but on their home environment and the degree of support in place to compensate. It is particularly important to assess function at a point where decisions to not transport an older person to hospital by a paramedic, or to discharge a patient home from ED, are being contemplated.

MALNUTRITION AND FRAILTY

Frailty is defined as a state of heightened vulnerability to functional dependence or death in response to a stressor.[44] In other words, frail people who suffer injury or illness necessitating ED attendance have less reserve and so are not as likely to recover to their premorbid level, or survive, than the non-frail.[45] This is important to recognise as it may affect the treatment decisions; for example, we may be more likely to admit a frail

80-year-old with pneumonia than a fit 80-year-old with the same illness.

A hallmark of frailty is recent weight loss, and one of the possible treatments is high calorie and high protein diet. It is common for malnutrition and frailty to coincide, although why some older people are frail is far more complex than related to diet alone.

POLYPHARMACY AND OTHER MEDICATION ISSUES

Polypharmacy is typically defined as the use of six or more drugs together in the treatment of diseases. The definition also includes the prescribing of more medications than is clinically indicated, or at excessive dosages, or prescribed at too-frequent intervals.[46] It may be appropriate for older people with chronic conditions that require a range of medications to be on many different tablets. However, as the number of medications increases, the risk of drug interactions and redundant treatments also rises. It is estimated that one in five of all emergency presentations in older people are related in some way to medication misuse.[46,47] Confounding things for staff, less than one in four older patients can accurately detail all of their medications and doses, even when they have access to family members, medication lists and pill packages.[48]

Underlying medical problems, changing pharmacokinetics of ageing and treating side-effects of one drug with more medication exacerbate the problems of polypharmacy.[32] It is therefore important to assess for the presence of polypharmacy as a cause of or contributing factor in emergency presentations. Medications that are more likely to cause problems in the older patient include narcotics, sedative-hypnotics, antidepressants, diuretics, non-steroidal anti-inflammatory drugs (NSAIDs) and angiotensin-converting enzyme (ACE) inhibitors.[32] Narcotics and sedative hypnotics alter consciousness, increase the risk of falls and depress respiration. Electrolyte imbalances and dehydration may result from diuretics. Uraemia, hypertension, cardiac failure and sodium retention can all result from NSAID use, as well as the generally known problem of gastrointestinal bleeding.[32]

Polypharmacy implications extend beyond contributing to an emergency presentation; it may also complicate analgesia administration, as narcotics and NSAIDs are common and effective medications for controlling pain in the emergency health setting. When administering these agents, particularly narcotics, consider the effects by providing low doses slowly titrated. Box 38.1 describes common causes of medication errors made by older people.

PRACTICE TIP

Do not rely solely on an older person's memory for an accurate medication history–consult another source such as their pharmacist.

BOX 38.1 COMMON CAUSES OF MEDICATION ERRORS BY OLDER ADULTS[49]

- Forgetting to take medications
- Use of non-prescription over-the-counter drugs
- Use of medications prescribed for someone else
- Use of medications that are out of date (expired)
- Failure to understand instructions or the importance of drug treatment
- Taking an incorrect dose (lower or higher)
- Refusal to take medication because of undesirable side-effects, such as nausea and impotence
- Inappropriately combining the correct medication with food, drinks or other herbal substances

SOCIAL ISOLATION AND DEPRESSION

Although depression in older adults is actually less common than in younger adults, it is more often undiagnosed and undertreated in older people, leading to significant health consequences.[50] Depression is often associated with loneliness and insomnia, and it can be difficult to know what is cause and effect; however, enquiring about sleep patterns and social networks may help determine if further assessment for depression as a contributor to a person's ill-health is warranted. Older age may be accompanied by stressful life events, such as illness or death of a lifelong partner; relative immobility and more of the day spent being sedentary at home; disease states such as hypothyroidism; and other biological changes, such as neuronal loss and blood flow changes to the brain that can cause depression. Social isolation and loneliness are risk factors for poor ageing outcomes, and are linked to a range of physical and psychological conditions. Paramedics should assess the living situation of older people they care for in the pre-hospital environment, and ensure that relevant information is passed to the receiving ED at triage.

THE GERIATRIC ASSESSMENT IN THE EMERGENCY HEALTH SETTING

COMMUNICATION AND THE OLDER PERSON

Good communication between patients and healthcare professionals is important for safe and quality care delivery. The National Safety and Quality Health Service (NSQHS) Standards in Australia includes the Communicating for Safety Standard as recognition of the importance of effective communication for continuous, coordinated and safe patient care.[51] However, communication with older patients can be complex. Communication strategies adopted should differ according to the patient's needs and abilities. Impaired sensory function or cognition can impact on how the older person perceives or reports their health status.

As part of the usual ageing process, the older person may experience changes in their senses (sensory deprivation), speech, use of language and decline in memory, which can impact their ability to communicate effectively. The extent and severity of these changes will vary between individuals. In addition, changes in cognition, cultural and linguistic diversity and the debilitating nature of the patient's illness and condition can affect communication functioning in the older person. It is important for emergency clinicians to be aware of communication changes in older patients that are part of the normal ageing process and changes that may indicate a pathological condition.

PRACTICE TIP

When talking to an older person speak clearly, facing them, and make sure that hearing aids are in place and working. Also ensure that any glasses are worn, and reduce any background noise such as television or radio.

CULTURAL CONSIDERATIONS

All individuals are cultural beings embedded within the cultural and linguistic paradigms of their families, social groups, community, education and experiences.[52] Since older people from CALD backgrounds are a significant and growing proportion of Australia and Aotearoa New Zealand's older population, it is important for emergency care staff to be able to communicate effectively with this cohort of older people. Pivotal to successful communication is understanding that older people from CALD backgrounds are not a homogenous group and encounter different outcomes based on individual experiences and backgrounds.

Language is a key focus in communication with CALD older people. Government policies have focused on increasing language services as fundamental to improving health service quality and access for CALD groups, and higher levels of English language proficiency have been associated with better health, wellbeing and social inclusion outcomes.[11] Many healthcare organisations are focused on eliminating language barriers for patients through the use of interpreter services. In the ED, staff can access professional interpreters either remotely; for example, telehealth, or in person for consultations with CALD older patients. It is important to note that although using family members as interpreters is a regular occurrence in healthcare settings and may have some benefits, there are many disadvantages in using family members as interpreters.[53] In addition, while translated materials may seem an option to use with patients from CALD backgrounds, these materials may not be understood if the person has limited literacy in their first language.[11]

Communication, however, involves more than language proficiency and is one factor that emergency clinicians must consider when communicating with older people from CALD backgrounds. In addition to language, cultural practices and norms can impact on how some CALD groups manage health conditions and communicate with healthcare professionals.[11] Differences in cultural practices between healthcare professionals and CALD patients can lead to misdiagnoses, lack of understanding, medication mismanagement and barriers to service use. The use of traditional non-prescription medicines is the choice for the self-management of health conditions for some CALD groups,[54] and higher risk of medication mismanagement has been identified with some CALD groups compared to non-CALD populations.[55,56] Effective cross-cultural communication between CALD older patients and healthcare professionals must include cultural understanding and acknowledgement of traditional medicines, and clear instructions on taking medicines correctly.[57] It is important for emergency clinicians not to hold preconceived or stereotypical assumptions about care support for older CALD patients. While a preference for family members to provide care exists among older people from CALD backgrounds from some cultures, this should not be assumed as 'the norm' for all CALD groups.[58,59]

FAMILY AND CARERS

Families are generally considered to be the primary source of support for people with an illness,[60,61] and it is usually important to include them when communicating with older people. Encouraging patients and families to be involved in healthcare is increasingly recognised as important to improve efficiency of the healthcare system and to promote patient safety. The NSQHS Standard Partnering with Consumers promotes working with patients, families and carers to make decisions and plan care.[51] Family and carers can assist staff in communicating with older patients because of their knowledge of the person. They can provide emergency staff with information about the older person's physical condition, including reason for presenting to the ED or request for an emergency ambulance, changes in usual function, chronic illnesses and medication adherence; psychological condition, including cognitive function and sensory deprivation; and socialisation, including social engagement and cultural needs. Involving family members or carers can be beneficial in supporting older people with adhering to treatment and medication regimens.

Clinicians, however, must be aware that involving family or carers in communication with older patients should be at the agreement and inclusion of the older person whenever possible. Clinicians must seek the older person's consent to include a family member or carer in any communication. It is important not to ignore the older person when communicating with a family member or carer, and communication should always be between the patient, their family member or carer, and the clinician.

PRACTICE TIP

- Ensure that the patient's vision and hearing are intact as deficits could mislead to a conclusion of a cognitive impairment.
- Routinely assess cognitive function.
- Document cognition assessment undertaken and score achieved.

COGNITIVE SCREENING

Assessing the older person's cognition is important because an early and accurate assessment will provide a baseline understanding of the person's cognition and determine severity of impairment. This will aid early access to treatment and management, referrals, supportive care and ongoing information for patients, families and carers. An older person's cognition should be assessed if they, a family member or carer express concerns about changes in his or her memory or thinking. Emergency clinicians can also assess an older patient's cognition if they observe, or are concerned about, the person's memory, thinking or function. In general, it is difficult to determine a patient's cognitive function based on a routine, non-cognitive evaluation alone. Consequently, a number of tools have been developed that can be used to assess an individual's cognition. A selection of assessment tools are available which are relatively easy to administer by emergency staff and in the ED environment.[62–65] These tools are applicable to a broad range of older adults, including those from Indigenous and CALD groups. Clinicians must be aware of how to undertake these assessments and interpret the results. An example of a cognitive assessment is the 4AT.

The 4 'A's Test (4AT)

This is a brief tool, designed for rapid initial assessment of delirium and cognitive impairment, and is among the most widely-used clinical tests for delirium internationally (see Useful websites). The 4AT assessment takes approximately 2 minutes to complete and is designed to be used by any health professional at first contact with the patient, and at other times when delirium is suspected. This screening assesses a patient's alertness; response to questions on age, date of birth, place and current year; attention; and acute change in cognition.

PAIN ASSESSMENT

Untreated pain in older adults is associated with poorer outcomes, including significant physical and social consequences. Despite this, older people are often under-treated for pain due to misconceptions around pain and ageing: older people with cognitive impairment are the most severely affected by poor pain management.[66] Older people are less likely than their younger counterparts to receive pain management in the ED,[67,68] and there is some evidence that this disparity also occurs during pre-hospital care as well.[67] Effective pain management should begin with a patient self-report.[69] In patients who are unable to provide a self-report of pain, such as those with a cognitive impairment, communication disorders or lack of proficiency in the clinician's language, assessment should be based on validated observational pain scales. One such tool is the Pain Assessment in Advanced Dementia (PAINAD) tool, which measures pain in individuals with dementia using clinical observations.[70,71] The Geriatric Pain Web page (see Useful websites) provides access to these tools, as well as instructions for use.

If pain is detected it must be documented, treated and reassessed.[72] A combination of pharmacological and non-pharmacological means can be used to reduce pain and increase patient comfort. Prior to transfer, paramedics may need to consider splinting, cold/heat therapy and limb elevation as well as analgesia such as paracetamol, the administration of methoxyflurane, or intranasal fentanyl, morphine or ketamine depending on the treatment indication with the dose adjusted for age (taking into account the pharmacokinetics of older people).[73]

PRACTICE TIP

- It is essential that all older people be assessed for the presence of pain.
- A simple and effective tool to measure pain in individuals with dementia is Pain Assessment in Advanced Dementia (PAINAD) which measures pain using clinical observations.
- Treatment should include drug and non-drug therapies.
- In the ED, pain assessment should be repeated frequently to document efficacy of analgesia and trends in the patient's condition[72].

DISCHARGE RISK ASSESSMENT

Like most patients, older people prefer to be cared for in their own homes as much as possible. However, older patients discharged from the ED frequently experience adverse health outcomes,[45,74,75] and to be safe at home it is important that they have a risk assessment and receive comprehensive discharge planning that includes shared decision-making.[76–79] A variety of brief tools exist to highlight patients at high risk of adverse outcome after discharge (Table 38.1). The 'gold standard' risk assessment is a comprehensive geriatric assessment (CGA) (also termed a comprehensive health assessment), but this is usually too time-consuming to perform in the ED setting. The CGA is well recognised as being associated with improved outcomes for patients and is described as being significant to an older person's health, safety and quality of life outcomes.[80] It is a multidimensional and interdisciplinary information-gathering and decision-making process, designed to collect data on the medical, psychosocial and functional capabilities and limitations of older patients. It helps nurses and healthcare professionals to identify care needs and risks, and to make decisions about treatment and care options. The goal is to ensure that the often multifaceted problems experienced by older people are systematically identified, quantified and managed appropriately. The contribution of the interdisciplinary healthcare team is important in order to provide a detailed evaluation of the older person's overall health status.

TABLE 38.1 DISCHARGE RISK SCREENING TOOLS IN COMMON USE

TOOL	COMPONENTS
ISAR[81]	Six questions on memory, number of medications, need for home assistance before and since this illness, eyesight and recent hospitalisations
TRST[82]	Six questions on cognitive impairment, number of medications, living alone, falls, recent hospitalisations and staff concerns

PRACTICE TIP

- Discharging older patients back to a residential aged care facility needs to include a consideration of changes in functional and cognitive abilities.
- Residential aged care facilities are staffed and arranged to cater for different needs. It is important, therefore, that the older person's requirements for care are carefully assessed, documented and communicated to the relevant staff member in charge.
- Most residential aged care facilities have standardised hospital transfer forms, and these must be used and accurately completed.

FUTILITY CRITERIA

The concept of futility in healthcare is often subject to debate in relation to interpretation and moral dilemmas, yet futility in healthcare is still of immense concern in clinical practice.[83] Futility in healthcare refers to treatments, interventions or care that are unlikely to have any direct benefit for the patient.

Schneiderman[84] discusses that medical futility is '… unacceptable likelihood of achieving an effect that the patient has the capacity to appreciate as a benefit'. In emergency medicine, benefit to a patient is a vital part of decision-making.[85] Futility in medical care comprises a quantitative (the odds that a specific treatment will benefit the patient) and qualitative (the quality of benefit from treatment) component. It is important to note that futility refers to a specific intervention at a particular time for a specific person. For example, in an emergency situation, clinicians would have to decide whether resuscitation would be medically futile for the patient. Decisions on the futility of treatment in any given clinical situation should be undertaken in accordance with relevant institutional policies and procedures.

GERIATRIC EMERGENCIES

MAJOR TRAUMA AND FALLS

Diminished vision, hearing and touch expose older people to increased risk of injury. Loss of peripheral vision, decreased hearing and slowed reaction times increase the risk of older drivers being involved in vehicular trauma or pedestrians being struck by vehicles. Poorer vision in dim light, loss of proprioception and righting reflexes and muscle weakness are among many factors that predispose older people to falls in their home. These changes of ageing contribute to the increase in the rate of trauma in older people.

After adjusting for Injury Severity Score (ISS), geriatric trauma victims have twice the mortality of younger patients and significantly longer intensive care unit (ICU) and hospital stays.[86] Even one rib fracture results in significant morbidity and mortality. The principles of managing major trauma in older and younger adults are the same, but attention must be paid to:

- *under-triage*. An older person with the same ISS as a younger person is more likely to receive a lower priority triage in the field and on arrival to ED, and less likely to have a trauma team activation[87]
- *reduced cardiac and respiratory reserve*, and increased bone and skin fragility, that increase the risk of more severe injury
- *pain relief*. Attention must be paid to delayed and inadequate analgesia in trauma patients, which can impact morbidity and even mortality outcomes.

The process of resuscitation in the older trauma patient is conducted in the usual manner of prioritising care of the airway, breathing and circulation. It is vitally important that rapid, aggressive resuscitation is commenced in the unstable, older trauma patient and that careful informed and expedient assessment of the apparently stable patient occurs.[88]

Ground-level falls are the main cause for injury-related hospital separations (admissions or episodes of care) in people over 65 years of age.[89] In emergency settings, there are three key components of assessing patients that have fallen—what caused the fall; what injuries were sustained; and what mobility, functional and social circumstances need to be addressed for safe discharge.

Falls in older people are not necessarily a direct consequence of the ageing process, and it is important that the cause of the fall be investigated. The reason for the fall is likely to be complex and multifactorial, despite often being given a simple explanation by the patient, such as tripping. It is unlikely to occur without at least one precipitating risk factor.[90] Common disease risk factors include arthritis, neurological disorders such as stroke or Parkinson's disease, dementia, and cardiac problems causing syncope or postural hypotension.[45] Medications such as antihypertensives, benzodiazepines and opiates frequently contribute to falls risk.

In Australia in 2013, the estimated number of hospitalised injury cases due to falls in people aged 65 years and over was 98,704; an increase of over 24,000 falls in a 10-year period.[91] In Aotearoa New Zealand, falls are the leading cause of injury hospitalisation and one of the top three causes of injury-related deaths, with more than one-third of people over the age of 65 experiencing a fall every year,[92] and 10–20% of these falls result in injury, hospitalisation or death.[93] Falls in older people are a critical public health concern and a major issue for first responders, paramedics and emergency clinicians:

- Approximately 3–5% of falls cause fractures.[94]
- Mortality after a hip fracture remains significant, being 11–23% at 6 months and 22–29% at 1 year from injury.[95]
- 30% of older people entered in a trauma registry from falling suffered moderate-to-severe injuries.[96]
- Falls are a major cause of traumatic brain injury in older people.[97]

It is important that if no injury is found that requires hospitalisation following a fall, the older person should be referred to a multidisciplinary team that is able to provide suitable interventions in the home environment. Emergency medical services are beginning to develop and implement health screening programs[98] and falls assessment and referral programs for those patients who may not require immediate hospitalisation.[88] Where admission occurs, discharge planning must begin early with appropriate referral. Injury prevention activities are listed in Box 38.2.[99]

INFECTION

Sepsis and septic shock are most seen in older people, with two-thirds of cases occurring in people aged 60 or more. There are many factors that lead to infection in the older person.[100] The reasons that age contributes to an increase in susceptibility to infection are summarised in Box 38.3.

In addition to the increased susceptibility and mortality from infection, older people may present atypically, so that the expected signs of infection such as fever are absent. Older patients may present with weakness, fatigue and functional decline, perhaps combined with anorexia. These are not specific, making infection recognition difficult. Fever may be present in isolation or the older person with an infection may present with hypothermia. It is therefore important to suspect infection in the older person who presents with non-specific symptoms or signs.

DELIRIUM

Delirium is an acute deterioration in brain function that is characterised by acute onset, a fluctuating course over time and inattention.[101] Most older people with delirium are not agitated; they are quiet and withdrawn, which makes the diagnosis more difficult to spot and is the reason why

BOX 38.2 INJURY PREVENTION ACTIVITIES FOR THE OLDER PERSON

- Remove or tack down all scatter rugs.
- Check staircases for stability; install handrails whenever possible.
- Apply non-slip strips to stairways.
- Carpet areas that are prone to spills.
- Reduce clutter and open clear pathways through all rooms.
- Pad wooden or metal furniture edges.
- Install bright lights in hallways and entrances.
- Place non-slip mats in the bathtub and shower.
- Install grab bars near all bathrooms.
- Install smoke detectors, and check them at regular intervals.
- Obtain assistance with cooking, as needed. Extra care is required when using gas stoves.
- Do not wear loose-fitting garments while cooking.
- Use rear stove burners rather than front ones and avoid storing goods you may need over the stove.
- Reduce thermostat settings on water heaters and clearly label all hot water taps.
- Do not smoke, especially while resting.
- Keep easy-to-operate fire extinguishers readily accessible.
- Know how to access emergency help.
- Eliminate night driving if affected by night blindness.
- Wear seatbelts.
- Drive only in familiar locations, avoiding highly congested areas and roadways under construction.
- Contact vehicle licensing agency to enquire about an 'over-75 refresher course'.

BOX 38.3 AGE-RELATED INFECTION RISKS[43]

RISK FACTORS FOR ACQUIRING INFECTION

- Decreased pulmonary function and cough reflex
- Invasive devices (urinary catheters, nasogastric tubes)
- Thin, easily traumatised skin
- Immobility
- Inadequate nutrition and hydration
- Lack of immunisation
- Neurological diseases
- Close living proximity to others e.g. residential aged care

RISK FACTORS FOR INFECTION CAUSING ORGAN FAILURE AND DEATH

- Chronic diseases (diabetes, cardiac disease, renal disease, alcoholism)
- Exaggerated immune cytokine response causing organ injury
- Atherosclerosis and decreased capillary blood flow to organs
- Endocrine problems e.g. thyroid disease

screening tests outlined above are so important. Delirium is associated with a higher risk of falls, pressure injury and death in hospital.

It is vitally important that emergency clinicians are aware of, and institute, simple measures to either prevent or help manage delirium. Many cases of delirium are due to apparently simple factors—constipation; lack of access to food and hydration; restriction of patients to bed in an unfamiliar environment; and pain. In the busy ED environment it is sometimes easy to neglect these basic care needs that are so important in preventing delirium. Excellent guidelines exist to recommend simple care practices for people at risk of delirium, especially those with pre-existing dementia, and can be used in any environment.[102]

Identifying and treating the cause is the usual method for managing delirium. However, a few patients will be distressed and agitated and need their symptoms managed.[42] Physical restraints should be avoided as this increases agitation and is likely to worsen the delirium. Effective management may involve simple interventions, such as ensuring patients have their glasses and hearing aids, having familiar people beside them and turning off the lights to aid sleep.[102]

ELDER ABUSE

Elder abuse is any act occurring within a relationship where there is an implication of trust, which results in harm to an older person. Abuse may be physical, sexual, financial, psychological or neglect. Victims of abuse are at increased risk of many complications, yet it is estimated that only 5% of all cases are detected.[103] Most perpetrators are relatives or carers, which makes the situation complex, as the victim of abuse may be dependent on the perpetrator for their everyday support. The exception is abuse in aged care facilities, where the most common form of abuse is one resident with a dementing illness abusing another resident. Gentle enquiries regarding safety at home and threats made against them should be made of any older person with unexplained injury or who appears frightened or reluctant to provide full information in their history.

In Australia and Aotearoa New Zealand, there are specialised police units to investigate suspected cases of elder abuse, and hospital social workers also take referrals. There are also elder abuse helplines available (see Useful websites).

THE DYING PATIENT

There are three trajectories of dying (Fig. 38.1): sudden unexpected death in a previously well patient; rapid decline from a terminal illness such as cancer; or a slow dwindling decline and death from diseases such as heart failure or dementia. The first type of death occurs in older patients, but this is the minority. More older people experience death with a progressive decline.

Despite most people with inevitable decline expressing a wish to die at home, older people nearing death in such circumstances often call ambulances or come to ED. This may be because of new symptoms, poorly controlled chronic symptoms, or fear of death. Pre-hospital and ED staff should prioritise locating and referring to an advance health directive or advance care plan in these circumstances. Attention should be paid to supporting staff, relatives and carers that may become distressed in uncommon circumstances where a death is not congruent with the wishes of the older person.

FIGURE 38.1 DYING TRAJECTORIES

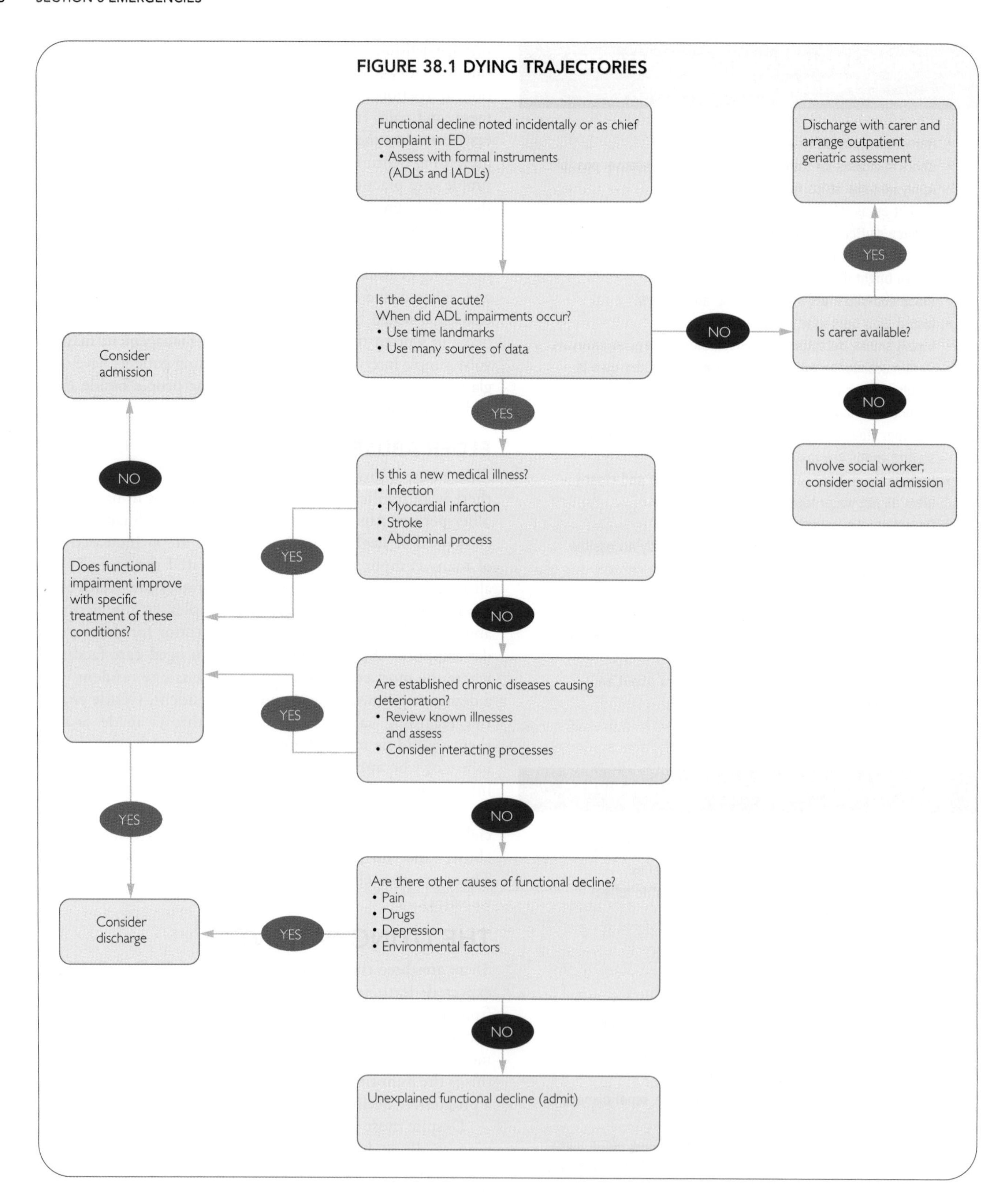

SUMMARY

To date, little attention has been paid to ED assessment and management of older people and the physiology affected by the ageing process. As the population age profile changes and older people use ambulances and attend our EDs more frequently, the knowledge required to effectively assess and manage the different diseases, comorbidities and psychosocial needs becomes fundamental to good clinical emergency practice. Optimal emergency care of older patients requires comprehensive care that can account for their individuality.

The majority of older people presenting to EDs do so with a symptom of pain. Pain is often poorly managed, especially in the cognitively impaired older person. Clinicians need to consider the use of validated pain assessment tools to improve detection and assessment of pain in the older person. Good communication is fundamental to the assessment, treatment and safe discharge of the older person. To assist in these processes, clinicians need to consider the functional, cognitive and emotional status of the older patient. It is therefore important that cognitive status testing occurs to help determine the need for further investigations, management and safe discharge.

CASE STUDY

Mrs Ioanna Demopoulos is a widowed 86-year-old Greek lady who recently moved to a residential aged care facility after living at home alone since her husband died 18 months ago. At 8.30 pm on Friday an emergency ambulance is called because staff are concerned about Mrs Demopoulos' poor food and fluid intake and distended abdomen. As the paramedic, you assess Mrs Demopoulos and she is unable to answer your questions. The staff inform you that Mrs Demopoulos only arrived at the facility 2 days ago and is unable to communicate in English. On your initial assessment, her radial pulse is 90 beats/minute, blood pressure is 150/90 mmHg and her respiratory rate is 18 breaths/minute. When you examine her abdomen, Mrs Demopoulos grimaces and grabs your hand. The staff also inform you that as a recent arrival to the aged care facility, Mrs Demopoulos is still waiting to be seen by a GP as her current GP will not be able to continue with her care.

QUESTIONS—PARAMEDICS

1. As the paramedic who receives the handover from the nurse in charge at the residential aged care facility, what will you need to consider before making an assessment of Mrs Demopoulos?
2. It is important to assess Mrs Demopoulos' condition, but in the absence of an interpreter how will you undertake this assessment?
3. Based on your assessment of Mrs Demopoulos, her medications and clinical symptoms, what illnesses and other factors would you consider for her?

Mrs Demopoulos is transferred to the nearest ED.

QUESTIONS—EMERGENCY NURSES

During the ambulance journey Mrs Demopoulos calls out at times, but is very quiet after her arrival in the ED. The paramedics hand over all the information they have on Mrs Demopoulos, including their initial assessment of her condition. On arrival in the ED her vital signs are assessed and have increased as follows: pulse rate is 100 beats/minute, blood pressure is 165/100 mmHg and respiration rate is 20 breaths/minute.

4. As the nurse in the ED, what do you think are the priorities for Mrs Demopoulos' nursing care needs?
5. What other nursing considerations should there be in preparation for Mrs Demopoulos' discharge from the ED, either to an inpatient ward or back to the residential aged care facility?

Answers to Case Study Questions can be found on evolve http://evolve.elsevier.com/AU/Curtis/emergency/ 

USEFUL WEBSITES

Acute Care Geriatric Nurse Network (ACGNN), www.acgnn.ca.

American College of Emergency Physicians, Geriatric emergency medicine guidelines, www.acep.org/by-medical-focus/geriatrics/geriatric-emergency-department-guidelines/#sm.00001hv1zjfnxcfn5zw2cnxbpxcl0.

Australasian College for Emergency Medicine Geriatric Section, https://acem.org.au/Content-Sources/Advancing-Emergency-Medicine/Geriatric-Emergency-Medicine.

Australian and New Zealand Society for Geriatric Medicine (ANZSGM), www.anzsgm.org.

Australian Institute of Family Studies, https://aifs.gov.au/elder-abuse-support-services.

Elder Abuse helpline NZ, www.healthpoint.co.nz/social-services/social/elder-abuse-helpline/.

4 'A's Test (4AT), www.the4AT.com.

Geriatric Pain Web page www.geriatricpain.org, A comprehensive health assessment of the older person template is available from the Department of Health, Victoria at https://www.health.vic.gov.au/residential-aged-care/comprehensive-health-assessment-of-the-older-person.

Geriatrics: a basic review for emergency health care providers, http://faculty.washington.edu/dgruen/table_of_contents.htm.

Royal Australian College of General Practitioners, Medical care of older persons in residential aged care facilities, www.racgp.org.au/your-practice/guidelines/silverbook/.

Urban Modified KICA tool (KICA Regional/Urban), for use in urban and regional settings, www.dementia.org.au/files/20130520_NAT_ATSI_KICADelphiQuestionnaireScoresAndComments.pdf.

REFERENCES

1. United Nations, Department of Economic and Social Affairs., Population Division. World population prospects: the 2017 revision, key findings and advance population tables. Working Paper No. ESA/P/WP/248. New York: United Nations; 2017.
2. Australian Institute of Health and Welfare (AIHW). Older Australians. 2021. Online: Available from: www.aihw.gov.au/reports/older-people/older-australia-at-a-glance/contents/summary.
3. Newson RS, Kemps EB. The influence of physical and cognitive activities on simple and complex cognitive tasks in older adults. Exp Aging Res 2006;32(3):341–62.
4. Khan HTA. Population ageing in a globalized world: risks and dilemmas? J Eval Clin Pract 2018;25(5):754–60.
5. Australian Institute of Health and Welfare. Older Australians at a glance. 2017. Online: Available from: www.aihw.gov.au/reports/older-people/older-australia-at-a-glance/contents/summary.
6. Australian Institute of Health and Welfare (AIHW). Older Australians at a glance. Australia's changing age and gender profile. 2017. Online: Available from: www.aihw.gov.au/reports/older-people/older-australia-at-a-glance/contents/demographics-of-older-australians/australia-s-changing-age-and-gender-profile.
7. Australian Bureau of Statistics (ABS). 2071.0 - Census of population and housing: reflecting Australia - Stories from the Census, 2016. 2021. Online: Available from: www.abs.gov.au/ausstats/abs@.nsf/Lookup/by%20Subject/2071.0~2016~Main%20Features~Ageing%20Population~14.
8. Statistics New Zealand. National Population Projections, by age and sex, 2016 (based)-2068 [data tables]. 2016. Online: Available from: http://nzdotstat.stats.govt.nz/wbos/Index.aspx?DataSetCode=TABLECODE7542#.
9. Australian Institute of Health and Welfare (AIHW). Older Australians at a glance: culturally and linguistically diverse older people. 2017. Online: Available from: www.aihw.gov.au/reports/older-people/older-australia-at-a-glance/contents/demographics-of-older-australians/culturally-linguistically-diverse-people.
10. Koopman-Boyden P. Older people – demographics of older people. 2018. Online: Available from: www.TeAra.govt.nz/en/older-people/page-1.
11. Federation of Ethnic Communities' Councils of Australia (FECCA). Review of Australian research on older people from culturally and linguistically diverse backgrounds. Canberra: Federation of Ethnic Communities' Councils of Australia; 2015.
12. Sweeny A, Keijzers G, O'Dwyer J, Arendts G, Crilly J. Predictors of a long length of stay in the emergency department for older people. Intern Med J 2020;50(5):572–81.
13. Covino M, Petruzziello C, Onder G, Migneco A, Simeoni B, Franceschi F, et al. A 12-year retrospective analysis of differences between elderly and oldest old patients referred to the emergency department of a large tertiary hospital. Maturitas 2019;120:7–11.
14. Arendts G, Lowthian J. Demography is destiny: an agenda for geriatric emergency medicine in Australasia. Emerg Med Australas 2013;25(3):271–8.
15. Australian Institute of Health and Welfare (AIHW). Older Australians: health service use. 2021. Online: Available from: www.aihw.gov.au/reports/older-people/older-australia-at-a-glance/contents/health-aged-care-service-use/health-care-gps-specialists/.
16. Lawson P, Richmond C. 13 emergency problems in older people. Emerg Med J 2005;22(5):370–4.
17. Ferguson C, Woodward J, Conroy S. Operationalising frailty definitions in the emergency department: a mapping exercise. J Nutrit, Health Aging 2009;13:266.
18. Driesen B, Merten H, Barendregt R, Bonjer HJ, Wagner C, Nanayakkara PWB. Root causes and preventability of emergency department presentations of older patients: a prospective observational study. BMJ Open 2021;11(8):e049543.
19. Considine J, Smith R, Hill K, Weiland TJ, Gannon J, Behm C, et al. Older people's experience of accessing emergency care. Australas Emerg Nurs J 2010;13:61–9.
20. Gallagher R, Gallagher P, Roche M, Fry M, Chenoweth L, Stein-Parbury J. Nurses' perspectives of the impact of the older person on nursing resources in the emergency department and their profile: a mixed methods study. Int Emerg Nurs 2015;23(4):312–16.
21. Leonard C, Bein KJ, Latt M, Muscatello D, Veillard AS, Dinh MM. Demand for emergency department services in the elderly: an 11 year analysis of the Greater Sydney Area. Emerg Med Australas 2014;26(4):356–60.
22. Lowthian J, Curtis A, Folley D, Stoelwinder JU, McNeil JJ, Cameron PA. Demand at the emergency department front door: 10-year trends in presentations. MJA 2012;196:128–32.

23. Gomes JCP, Dias RD, de Barros JV, Velasco IT, Jacob Filho W. The growing impact of older patients in the emergency department: a 5-year retrospective analysis in Brazil. BMC Emerg Med 2020;20(1):47.
24. Cantwell K, Morgans A, Smith K, Livingston M, Dietze P. Differences in emergency ambulance demand between older adults living in residential aged care facilities and those living in the community in Melbourne, Australia. Australas J Ageing 2017;36(3):212–21.
25. Dwyer R, Gabbe B, Tran TD, Smith K, Lowthian JA. Patterns of emergency ambulance use, 2009–13: a comparison of older people living in residential aged care facilities and the community. Age Ageing 2018;47(4):615–19.
26. Lowthian JA, Curtis AJ, Cameron PA, Stoelwinder JU, Cooke MW, McNeil JJ. Systematic review of trends in emergency department attendances: an Australian perspective. Emerg Nurs J 2011;28(5):373–7.
27. Herbert R. The biology of human ageing. In: Redfern S, Ross F, editors. Nursing older people. 4th ed. Edinburgh: Churchill Livingstone; 2005. p. 57–82.
28. Clothier A. Assessing and managing skin tears in older people. Nurse Prescribing 2014;12(6): 278–82.
29. Eliopoulos C. Gerontological nursing. 10th ed. Philadelphia: Lippincott Williams and Wilkins; 2021.
30. O'Sullivan ED, Hughes J, Ferenbach DA. Renal aging: causes and consequences. J Am Soc Nephrol 2017;28(2):407–20.
31. Kresevic D. Assessment of physical function. In: Boltz M, Capezuti E, Zwicker D, Fulmer TT, editors. Evidence-based geriatric nursing protocols for best practice. 6th ed. New York (NY): Springer Publishing Company; 2021.
32. Winterbottom F, Jenkins M. The older adult patient. In: Urden L, Stacy K, Lough M, editors. Critical care nursing: diagnosis and management. 9th ed. St Louis: Elsevier; 2022.
33. Jessen F, Amariglio RE, Buckley RF, van der Flier WM, Han Y, Molinuevo JL, et al. The characterisation of subjective cognitive decline. Lancet Neurol 2020;19(3):271–8.
34. Douglass R, Heckman G. Drug-related taste disturbance: a contributing factor in geriatric syndromes. Can Fam Phys 2010;56(11):1142–7.
35. Campbell V, Crews J, Moriarty D, Zack MM, Blackman DK. Surveillance for sensory impairment, activity limitation, and health-related quality of life among older adults, United States, 1993 and 1997. MMWR CDC Surveill Summ 1999;48:131–56.
36. De Gaudio AR, Rinaldi S, Chelazzi C, Borracci T. Pathophysiology of sepsis in the elderly: clinical impact and therapeutic considerations. Curr Drug Targets 2009;10(1):60–70.
37. Swerissen H, Duckett S, Wright J. Chronic failure in primary care. Carlton: Grattan Institute; 2016.
38. Prince MJ, Wu F, Guo Y, Gutierrez Robledo LM, O'Donnell M, Sullivan R, et al. The burden of disease in older people and implications for health policy and practice. Lancet 2015;385(9967):549–62.
39. Australian Institute of Health and Welfare (AIHW). Older Australians at a glance: burden of disease. 2017. Online: Available from: www.aihw.gov.au/reports/older-people/older-australia-at-a-glance/contents/health-and-functioning/burden-of-disease.
40. Murman DL. The impact of age on cognition. Semin Hear 2015;36(3):111–21.
41. Hustey FM, Meldon SW. The prevalence and documentation of impaired mental status in elderly emergency department patients. Ann Emerg Med 2002;39(3):248–53.
42. Wilber ST. Altered mental status in older emergency department patients. Emerg Med Clin N Am 2006;24(2):299–316, vi.
43. Sanders A, editor. Emergency care of the elder person. St. Louis: Beverly Cracom Publications; 1996.
44. Chen X, Mao G, Leng SX. Frailty syndrome: an overview. Clin Interv Aging 2014;9:433–41.
45. Crow RS, Lohman MC, Pidgeon D, Bruce ML, Bartels SJ, Batsis JA. Frailty versus stopping elderly accidents, deaths and injuries initiative fall risk score: ability to predict future falls. J Am Geriatr Soc 2018;66(3):577–83.
46. Pazan F, Wehling M. Polypharmacy in older adults: a narrative review of definitions, epidemiology and consequences. Eur Geriatr Med 2021;12(3):443–52.
47. Nickel CH, Ruedinger JM, Messmer AS, Maile S, Peng A, Bodmer M, et al. Drug-related emergency department visits by elderly patients presenting with non-specific complaints. Scand J Trauma Resusc Emerg Med 2013;21:15.
48. Goldberg EM, Marks SJ, Merchant RC, Nagy JL, Aquilante Jr JA, Beaudoin FL. How accurately do older adult emergency department patients recall their medications? Acad Emerg Med 2021;28(2):248–52.
49. Mira JJ. Medication errors in the older people population. Exp Rev Clin Pharmacol 2019;12(6):491–4.
50. Wei J, Hou R, Zhang X, Xu H, Xie L, Chandrasekar EK, et al. The association of late-life depression with all-cause and cardiovascular mortality among community-dwelling older adults: systematic review and meta-analysis. Br J Psychiatry 2019;215(2):449–55.
51. Australian Commission on Safety and Quality in Health Care (ACSQHC). National safety and quality health service standards. 2nd ed. Sydney, NSW: ACSQHC; 2021.
52. Commonwealth of Australia (Department of Social Services). National Ageing and Aged Care Strategy for People from Culturally and Linguistically Diverse (CALD) Backgrounds. Canberra: Federation of Ethnic Communities Councils of Australia; 2015.
53. Hilder J, Gray B, Dowell A, Macdonald L, Tester R, Stubbe M. 'It depends on the consultation': revisiting use of family members as interpreters for general practice consultations – when and why? Aust J Prim Health 2017;23(3):257–62.
54. Alhomoud F, Dhillon S, Aslanpour Z, Smith F. South Asian and Middle Eastern patients' perspectives on medicine-related problems in the United Kingdom. Int J Clin Pharm 2015;37(4):607–15.

55. Williams A, Manias E, Liew D, Gock H, Gorelik A. Working with CALD groups: testing the feasibility of an intervention to improve medication self-management in people with kidney disease, diabetes, and cardiovascular disease. Renal Soc Australas J 2012;8:62–9.
56. Chauhan A, Walton M, Manias E, Walpola RL, Seale H, Latanik M, et al. The safety of health care for ethnic minority patients: a systematic review. Int J Equity Health 2020;19(1):118.
57. O'Callaghan C, Quine S. How older Vietnamese Australian women manage their medicines. J Cross-cult Gerontol 2007;22(4):405–19.
58. Lo M, Russell C. Family care: an exploratory study of experience and expectations among older Chinese immigrants in Australia. Contemp Nurse 2007;25(1-2):3–8.
59. Walker R, Newman L, Tsianikas M, Panagiotopoulos G, Hurley C. The perspectives of older Greek-Australians toward changes in the nature of family support: implications for family care policies. J Aging Socl Pol 2013;25(4):320–34.
60. Benzein E, Johansson P, Arestedt KF, Saveman BI. Nurses' attitudes about the importance of families in nursing care: a survey of Swedish nurses. J Fam Nurs 2008;14(2):162–80.
61. Johnstone MJ, Hutchinson AM, Rawson H, Redley B. Nursing strategies for engaging families of older immigrants hospitalized for end-of-life care: an Australian study. J Pat Exp 2016;3(3):57–63.
62. Vertesi A, Lever JA, Molloy DW, Sanderson B, Tuttle I, Pokoradi L, et al. Standardized Mini-Mental State Examination. Use and interpretation. Can Fam Physician 2001;47:2018–23.
63. Hobson J. The Montreal Cognitive Assessment (MoCA). Occup Med (Lond) 2015;65(9):764–5.
64. Hsieh S, McGrory S, Leslie F, Dawson K, Ahmed S, Butler CR, et al. The Mini-Addenbrooke's Cognitive Examination: a new assessment tool for dementia. Dement Geriatr Cogn Disord 2015;39(1-2):1–11.
65. LoGiudice D, Smith K, Thomas J, Lautenschlager NT, Almeida OP, Atkinson D, et al. Kimberley Indigenous Cognitive Assessment tool (KICA): development of a cognitive assessment tool for older Indigenous Australians. Int Psychogeriatr 2006;18(2):269–80.
66. Cravello L, Di Santo S, Varrassi G, Benincasa D, Marchettini P, de Tommaso M, et al. Chronic pain in the elderly with cognitive decline: a narrative review. Pain Ther 2019;8(1):53–65.
67. Platts-Mills TF, Hunold KM, Weaver MA, Dickey RM, Fernandez AR, Fillingim RB, et al. Pain treatment for older adults during prehospital emergency care: variations by patient gender and pain severity. J Pain 2013;14(9):966–74.
68. Hwang U, Richardson LD, Harris B, Morrison RS. The quality of emergency department pain care for older adult patients. J Am Geriatr Soc 2010;58(11):2122–8.
69. Schofield P. The assessment of pain in older people: UK national guidelines. Age Ageing 2018;47(Suppl. 1):i1–i22.
70. Fry M, Chenoweth L, Arendts G. Can an observational pain assessment tool improve time to analgesia for cognitively impaired older persons? A cluster randomised controlled trial. Emerg Nurs J 2018;35(1):33–8.
71. Warden V, Hurley AC, Volicer L. Development and psychometric evaluation of the Pain Assessment in Advanced Dementia (PAINAD) scale. J Am Med Dir Assoc 2003;4(1):9–15.
72. Terrell KM, Hustey FM, Hwang U, Gerson LW, Wenger NS, Miller DK, et al. Quality indicators for geriatric emergency care. Acad Emerg Med 2009;16(5):441–9.
73. Thürmann PA. Pharmacodynamics and pharmacokinetics in older adults. Curr Opin Anesthesiol 2020;33(1):109–13.
74. McCabe JJ, Kennelly SP. Acute care of older patients in the emergency department: strategies to improve patient outcomes. Open Access Emerg Med 2015;7:45–54.
75. Westgård T, Ottenvall Hammar I, Holmgren E, Ehrenberg A, Wisten A, et al. Comprehensive geriatric assessment pilot of a randomized control study in a Swedish acute hospital: a feasibility study. Pilot Feasibil Stud 2018;4:41.
76. Ackermann S, Heierle A, Bingisser MB, Hertwig R, Padiyath R, Nickel CH, et al. Discharge communication in patients presenting to the emergency department with chest pain: defining the ideal content. Health Comm 2016;31(5):557–65.
77. Curran J, Bishop A, Plint A, MacPhee S, Zemek R, Chorney J, et al. Understanding discharge communication behaviours in a pediatric emergency care context: a mixed methods observation study protocol. BMC Health Serv Res 2017;17:276.
78. Hwang U, Shah MN, Han JH, Carpenter CR, Siu AL, Adams JG. Transforming emergency care for older adults. Health Affairs 2013;32(12):2116–21.
79. Lowthian JA, Straney LD, Brand CA, Barker A, Smit PV, Newnham H, et al. Predicting functional decline in older emergency patients—the Safe Elderly Emergency Discharge (SEED) project. Age Ageing 2017;46(2):219–25.
80. Health Victoria. Comprehensive health assessment of the older person. 2018. Online: Available from: www2.health.vic.gov.au/ageing-and-aged-care/residential-aged-care/safety-and-quality/improving-resident-care/comprehensive-health-assessment.
81. McCusker J, Bellavance F, Cardin S, Trépanier S, Verdon J, Ardman O. Detection of older people at increased risk of adverse health outcomes after an emergency visit: the ISAR screening tool. J Am Geriatr Soc 1999;47(10):1229–37.
82. Meldon SW, Mion LC, Palmer RM, Drew BL, Connor JT, Lewicki LJ, et al. A brief risk-stratification tool to predict repeat emergency department visits and hospitalizations in older patients discharged from the emergency department. Ac Emerg Med 2003;10(3):224–32.
83. Jox RJ, Schaider A, Marckmann G, Borasio GD. Medical futility at the end of life: the perspectives of intensive care and palliative care clinicians. J Med Ethic 2012;38(9):540–5.
84. Schneiderman LJ. Defining medical futility and improving medical care. J Bioeth Inq 2011;8(2):123–31.
85. Wang D, Creel-Bulos C. A systematic approach to comfort care transitions in the emergency department. J Emerg Med 2019;56(3):267–74.

86. Carpenter CR, Arendts G, Hullick C, Nagaraj G, Cooper Z, Burkett E. Major trauma in the older patient: evolving trauma care beyond management of bumps and bruises. Emerg Med Australas 2017;29(4):450–5.
87. The Trauma Audit and Research Network. Major trauma in older people – 2017 Report. Salford, UK: Trauma Audit and Research Network; 2017.
88. Snooks H, Cheung WY, Close J, Dale J, Gaze S, Humphreys I, et al. Support and Assessment for Fall Emergency Referrals (SAFER 1) trial protocol. Computerised on-scene decision support for emergency ambulance staff to assess and plan care for older people who have fallen: evaluation of costs and benefits using a pragmatic cluster randomised trial. BMC Emerg Med 2010;10:Art 2.
89. Australian Institute of Health and Welfare. Australian hospital statistics 2007–08. Canberra: AIHW; 2009.
90. Hammouda N, Carpenter CR, Hung WW, Lesser A, Nyamu S, Liu S, et al. Moving the needle on fall prevention: a Geriatric Emergency Care Applied Research (GEAR) Network scoping review and consensus statement. Acad Emerg Med 2021;28(11):1214–27.
91. Australian Institute of Health and Welfare (AIHW). Trends in hospitalisations due to falls by older people, Australia 2002–03 to 2012–13. Injury research and statistics series no. 106. Cat. no. INJCAT 182. 2017. Online: Available from: www.aihw.gov.au/getmedia/5f84eadd-6f25-4429-82fc-5e9072278335/aihw-injcat-182.pdf.aspx?inline=true.
92. Age Concern New Zealand. Falls prevention. 2021. Online: Available from: www.ageconcern.org.nz/Public/Public/Info/Health_Topics/_Falls_Prevention.aspx.
93. Safe Communities Foundation New Zealand. Falls injuries and prevention. 2016. Online: Available from: www.safecommunities.org.nz/application/files/3114/8115/6965/Fact_Sheet_8.pdf.
94. Wilkins K. Health care consequences of falls for seniors. Health Rep 1999;10:47–55(ENG), 47–57(FRE).
95. Haleem S, Lutchman L, Mayahi R, Grice JE, Parker MJ. Mortality following hip fracture: trends and geographical variations over the last 40 years. Injury 2008;39(10):1157–63.
96. Sterling DA, O'Connor JA, Bonadies J. Geriatric falls: injury severity is high and disproportionate to mechanism. J Trauma 2001;50(1):116–19.
97. Thomas KE, Stevens JA, Sarmiento K, Wald MM. Fall-related traumatic brain injury deaths and hospitalizations among older adults—United States, 2005. J Safe Res 2008;39(3):269–72.
98. Shah MN, Clarkson L, Lerner EB, Fairbanks RJ, McCann R, Schneider SM. An emergency medical services program to promote the health of older adults. J Am Geriatr Soc 2006;54(6):956–62.
99. Newberry L, Criddle L, editors. Sheehy's manual of emergency care. 6th ed. St Louis: Mosby; 2005.
100. Girard TD, Ely EW. Bacteremia and sepsis in older adults. Clin Geriatr Med 2007;23(3):633–47, viii.
101. Nagaraj G, Burkett E, Hullick C, Carpenter CR, Arendts G. Is delirium the medical emergency we know least about. Emerg Med Australas 2016;28(4):456–8.
102. Australian Commission on Safety and Quality in Health Care. Delirium clinical care standard. 2021. Online: Available from: www.safetyandquality.gov.au/our-work/clinical-care-standards/delirium-clinical-care-standard.
103. Hullick C, Carpenter CR, Critchlow R, Burkett E, Arendts G, Nagaraj G, et al. Abuse of the older person: is this the case you missed last shift? Emerg Med Australas 2017;29(2):223–8.

CHAPTER 39

VIOLENCE, ABUSE AND ASSAULT

AMBER PREECE, RUSSELL KRIEGER,
SAM MAALOUF AND SIMON SAWYER

ESSENTIALS

General

- Domestic and family violence significantly impacts the health and wellbeing of individuals and families. The physical and psychological impact of violence may span a lifetime and contributes to intergenerational cycles of disadvantage.
- While anyone can experience family violence, children and women experience domestic and family violence and abuse at far higher rates than males, and current evidence shows males perpetrate most of the most damaging violence and abuse.
- Individuals and families experiencing family violence may have a broad range of immediate and longer-term needs. It is recommended that services work collaboratively to provide a person-centred approach to care and support. This may include police, paramedics, nurses, doctors, social workers, counsellors and other specialist services.

Child abuse and neglect

- In Australia and Aotearoa New Zealand, any person who holds concerns about the physical or emotional safety of a child may make a report to the statutory child protection service; healthcare professionals are mandated to report suspected child abuse in several jurisdictions.
- Emergency clinicians and paramedics must be aware of the processes for responding to suspected child abuse and neglect, and understand the way in which organisational policies and procedures articulate with their legal responsibilities to report cases of suspected abuse and neglect.

Intimate partner violence (IPV) and sexual assault

- Intimate partner violence (IPV) is a pattern of behaviour that can include a range of different types of abuse, including physical, emotional, verbal, social, economic, psychological, technology facilitated, cultural and spiritual abuse, as well as other coercive controlling behaviours.
- The most common perpetrators of violence against women are male intimate partners or ex-partners. Though women can be violent in relationships with men, often in self-defence, men are far more likely to experience violent acts by strangers or acquaintances than by someone close to them.
- The role of the healthcare team is to provide a supportive and non-judgemental response to disclosures of abuse and/or assault, and to empower the individual to make decisions that will improve their personal safety and the safety of any dependent children.

- Traumatised people can often experience services, including health services, as unsafe, disempowering and invalidating. Trauma-informed practice emphasises physical, psychological and emotional safety and creates opportunities for victim-survivors to regain a sense of control and empowerment.
- The collection of evidence from victim-survivors of sexual assault must be performed by an experienced emergency doctor or nurse who has received specific training in the care of persons who have been sexually assaulted.

Elder abuse and neglect

- Elder abuse and neglect take different forms: the common feature is harm or potential harm to the health and wellbeing of an older person.
- Older people at risk of experiencing abuse should be provided with information about options, supported to make their own decisions and respected in their choice to accept or reject support if competent to make that decision.

INTRODUCTION

Violence is a major public health issue: for people in all age groups it is one of the leading causes of mortality and morbidity worldwide.[1]

In 2002, the World Health Organization's (WHO) report into violence and health sought to raise awareness among members of the general public about interpersonal violence and to highlight it as a problem that is amenable to preventative intervention. The important work of the WHO emphasises the crucial role that public health services have to play in helping society as a whole to address the causes and consequences of all types of violence.

Violence is currently defined by the WHO as:

The intentional use of physical force or power, threatened or actual, against oneself, another person, or against a group or community, that either results in, or has a high likelihood of resulting in, injury, death, psychological harm, maldevelopment or deprivation (p. 5).[2]

Box 39.1 contains definitions for different types of violence based on the key characteristics of the perpetrator.

Violence within families and intimate relationships is, by far, the most prevalent form of violence documented in developed countries. Research has demonstrated the adverse physical and mental health outcomes, in both the short and long term, resulting from domestic and family violence.[3-5] Healthcare systems and practitioners can play a critical role in terms of identification, assessment, treatment, crisis intervention, documentation, referral and follow-up with victim-survivors of domestic and family violence.[6]

To effectively identify, intervene and prevent violence and abuse, emergency practitioners must work collaboratively as part of a multidisciplinary and multi-professional team. In Australia and Aotearoa New Zealand, nurses, paramedics, doctors and police have professional obligations to report family violence involving child abuse or neglect.[7,8] Practitioners have a responsibility to be aware of the professional and legal obligations in their state and territory.[9]

BOX 39.1 DEFINITIONS FOR DIFFERENT TYPES OF VIOLENCE BASED ON THE CHARACTERISTICS OF THE PERPETRATOR

- Self-directed violence involves acts that are inflicted against oneself (suicide or deliberate self-harm).
- Interpersonal violence includes family and intimate partner violence, as well as community violence (violence between unrelated individuals).
- Collective violence involves social, political or economic violence perpetrated by larger groups, such as states or organised political groups.

THE CHILD AT RISK

Children and young people have the right to grow up safe, connected and supported in their family, community and culture. They have the right to grow up in an environment that enables them to reach their full potential.[10] Child abuse and neglect is a serious social and public health problem, as well as a children's rights issue worldwide. Abuse and neglect can lead to a wide range of adverse consequences for children and young people, impacting on short- and long-term physical and mental health, social development and functioning.[5,11] Research investigating the health effects of violence has identified behavioural, social, cognitive and emotional pathways by which exposures to adverse situations increase short- and long-term health risks.[12]

Data from the Australian Institute of Health and Welfare (AIHW)[7] show that:

- the number of children who are subject to a notification of child abuse or neglect, the number of children under care and protection orders and the number in out-of-home care are all on the rise in Australia
- Aboriginal and Torres Strait Islander children are over-represented in all of the above areas
- emotional abuse and neglect are the most common primary and co-occurring types of substantiated abuse and neglect.

Data analytics from Aotearoa Oranga Tamariki (New Zealand Ministry for Children)[13] show that:

- in the 12 months to June 2020, 12,861 children (around 1.1% of the population) had been found to be abused or neglected after an investigation or assessment was completed
- of all children in New Zealand, 0.7% had experienced emotional abuse, 0.3% physical abuse, 0.3% neglect, and 0.1% sexual abuse
- in 2018, 79,200 children (around 7.0% of the population) had been recognised as having a family violence notification.

Safe and Supported: the National Framework for Protecting Australia's Children 2021–2031 is Australia's framework to reduce child abuse and neglect and its intergenerational impacts. The shared goal of national, state and territory governments is to make significant and sustained progress in reducing the rate of child abuse and neglect and its intergenerational impacts. Under the National Framework, state and territory governments deliver family support, health, housing and education, mental health and therapy services and youth justice. They are responsible for child protection and areas of law, policies and services relating to child safety.[10]

Te Aorerekura: The Enduring Spirit of Affection[14] is Aotearoa New Zealand's national strategy to eliminate family violence and sexual violence. In Aotearoa, family violence includes intimate partner violence, elder abuse, child abuse, dating violence, stalking and violence towards another family or whānau member, including child-to-parent violence. This all-encompassing framework aims to eliminate family violence and sexual violence, to unify government action, public support and community. This wellbeing and strengths-based policy focuses on primary prevention, healing and the critical role of tangata whenua and community leadership for achieving intergenerational change. Te Aorerekura has been developed with Te Tiriti o Waitangi and Māori leadership at its heart.

NEGLECT

The AIHW defines neglect as:

> Any serious act or omissions by a person having the care of a child that, within the bounds of cultural tradition, constitutes a failure to provide conditions that are essential for the healthy physical and emotional development of a child (p.89).[7]

Neglect is the continued failure by a parent or caregiver to provide a child with the basic things needed for his or her proper growth and development, such as food, clothing, shelter, medical and dental care and adequate supervision. Neglect can have lasting mental and physical health implications throughout the child's lifetime. Neglect may be physically apparent in a child who is unkempt, left unattended, not dressed appropriately for the weather or malnourished.

Recognising neglect can be difficult in pre-hospital and emergency health settings. Practitioners should be alert for the signs and symptoms and develop skills in talking to patients about violence, abuse and neglect. Such knowledge and skills will support increased identification of neglect and provide opportunities for intervention to reduce overall harm.

FAILURE TO THRIVE

Although a consensus definition is lacking, failure to thrive is the condition in children whose growth persistently and significantly deviates from norms for age and sex based on national growth charts. Measurements for height, weight and head circumference are plotted against normal childhood growth patterns. Failure-to-thrive children show a trend downwards across centile growth charts representing a failure to gain weight, height or both.

The cause of failure to thrive may be organic, non-organic or mixed. Organic causes include medical conditions such as infection (e.g. gastrointestinal *Giardia* organism infection), autoimmune coeliac disease and other malabsorption states, acid reflux leading to food refusal and physical factors such as tongue-tie and cleft palate. Non-organic causes often represent caregiver issues, such as inability to produce breast milk. Psychosocial causes, however, are often linked to and reported as child neglect. Poor parenting practices, chronic family illnesses, parental depression and substance abuse among caregivers are often linked to failure to thrive.

The consequences of untreated failure to thrive include developmental and behavioural difficulties secondary to nutritional deprivation of the nervous system and other systems. Accordingly, a multidisciplinary approach to treating failure to thrive provides the best opportunity for success. Family assessment, nutritional counselling, medical intervention and family support are needed to address failure to thrive.

PRACTICE TIP

RECOGNISING FAILURE TO THRIVE

A review of the child's health record book containing past and present biometric data is an important part of evaluating and recognising failure to thrive. Parents should be encouraged to maintain this record with their routine health provider, keep it safe and present it for any medical encounter, so that it may be reviewed.

PHYSICAL ABUSE (NON-ACCIDENTAL INJURY)

The AIHW defines physical abuse as:

> Any non-accidental physical act inflicted upon a child by a person having the care of a child (p. 91).[7]

Physical abuse of a child typically entails a repeated pattern of behaviour, but may also include a single episode. Physical abuse involves an unreasonable level of force, and includes injury, torture and maiming. In Australasia, corporal punishment of children is also considered physical abuse. Vulnerability to child abuse is significantly influenced by age,[1] and fatal causes of physical abuse are largely found among young infants.[15]

Non-disclosure of physical abuse is common among children, who may harbour feelings of shame or confusion. In addition, children are often unaware that physical abuse is not only inappropriate but also unlawful. A further difficulty in identifying physical abuse is the number of conditions that may mimic abuse. For this reason, all possible physiological or pathological causes for any physical findings must be considered as part of the assessment of a child who presents to the ED with an injury.[16] Box 39.2 shows examples of some conditions that mimic physical abuse. It is important to rule out these conditions before attributing the presentation to abuse.

In addition to situations where physical signs may mimic abuse, two substantive patterns of physical abuse are particularly relevant to emergency presentations. These syndromes are abusive head trauma (including the term shaken baby syndrome) and factitious disorder imposed on another (previously known as Munchausen's syndrome by proxy). Please refer to Chapter 35 for more information about injury assessment in children.

ABUSIVE HEAD TRAUMA (NON-ACCIDENTAL HEAD INJURY, SHAKEN BABY SYNDROME)

Abusive head trauma includes injuries to the skull or intracranial contents of an infant or young child (under 5 years of age) due to inflicted blunt impact and/or violent shaking.[17] This definition, endorsed by the American Academy of Pediatrics in 2009, and now used widely throughout Australasia, broadens the aetiology of non-accidental head injury from shaking injuries to include direct trauma.

The mechanism underlying shaken baby syndrome (SBS) is acceleration–deceleration of the head, which can precipitate a number of injuries: subdural haemorrhage, retinal injury, an altered level of consciousness including coma and spinal cord injury. Importantly, there may be no external signs of trauma. Babies shaken into unconsciousness are often put to bed in the

BOX 39.2 SOME EXAMPLES OF CONDITIONS KNOWN TO MIMIC PHYSICAL ABUSE

- **Clotting disorders,** including haemophilia, thrombocytopenia and platelet dysfunction.
- **Mongolian spots** are birthmarks found predominantly in people with dark pigmentation. Mongolian spots do not change colouration or size over time and have a greyer appearance than bruises.
- **Multiple petechiae and purpura** of the face can occur when vigorous crying, retching or coughing increases vena cava pressure. Unlike intentional choking, there are no marks around the neck.
- **Bullous impetigo** may appear as an infected wound or burn. This condition may reflect neglect if caregivers are apathetic about care of lesions.
- **Cultural or ethnic practices,** such as coining or cupping, are used to treat pain, fever or poor appetite. *Coining*—rubbing a coin over bony prominences—causes a striated 'pseudoburn'. *Cupping* (warming a cup, spoon or shot glass in oil and then placing it on the neck, back or ribs) can result in a petechial or purpuric rash over the affected area.
- **Osteogenesis imperfecta** is an inherited disease that can result in multiple fractures with minimal trauma and causes a tendency to bleed easily.

hope that the injuries will resolve. In these cases, the window for therapeutic intervention is lost. The spectrum of symptoms arising from SBS vary; they may include vomiting and irritability in mild shakings and range to unconsciousness, convulsions (seizure) and even death in severe shakings.

If suspected, a fundoscopic examination of the pupils should be performed to look for retinal haemorrhages. Pupil dilation may be required in some patients. A computed tomography (CT) head scan may be obtained to identify brain haemorrhages, including subdural bleeds. Magnetic resonance imaging (MRI) can also evaluate these injuries without the associated radiation exposure of a CT scan, and may be more sensitive in evaluating subtle cortical brain injury not appreciated on CT. A skeletal x-ray survey can be obtained to evaluate the location and age of any bony fractures. Multiple fractures of differing ages and in unusual locations such as the ribs are suggestive of non-accidental injury.

FACTITIOUS DISORDER IMPOSED ON ANOTHER

Factitious disorder imposed on another (FDIA), previously referred to as Munchausen's syndrome by proxy, represents a complex multi-factorial form of abuse deliberately perpetrated against another. When perpetrated against a child, the caregiver's secondary gain is in the medical attention received and therefore may be encountered in the emergency setting. The outcomes for children involved are known to be poor, as the abuse is typically sustained and may go undetected for many years.[18] The *Diagnostic and Statistical Manual of Mental Disorders*, 5th edition (DSM-V)[18] specifies four key features of the syndrome:

1. Falsification of physical or psychological signs or symptoms or the induction of injury or disease in another associated with identified deception.
2. The individual presents another individual to others as ill, impaired or injured.
3. The deceptive behaviour is evident even in the absence of obvious external rewards.
4. The behaviour cannot be explained by another mental disorder.

In FDIA, the child is subjected to illnesses perpetuated by caregivers, who may administer drugs to induce symptoms, introduce pathogens or otherwise contribute to a child's illness. Caretakers may also falsify medical histories and symptoms. In this context, caregivers typically have little insight into their abusive patterns of behaviour. In extreme cases, caretakers have caused the death of a child.

In terms of management, the paramedic and nurse should attempt to project an objective, non-judgemental attitude. Despite their abusive behaviour, the parent has a right to nursing care that is provided respectfully and sympathetically. Communication with the parent is best focused on addressing initial concerns and the wellbeing of the child, rather than on confrontation about the behaviour or labelling. The treatment team should plan to communicate with the parent/caregiver in a unified manner, and communication around protection of the child must follow standardised procedures for mandatory reporting as per other types of abuse and neglect.[18]

EMOTIONAL AND PSYCHOLOGICAL ABUSE

Emotional abuse is defined as:

> Any act by a person having the care of a child that results in the child suffering any kind of significant emotional deprivation or trauma. Children affected by exposure to family violence are also included in this category (p. 86).[7]

Although emotional abuse is almost always found with every form of child maltreatment, this type of abuse is often very difficult to identify, as social and cultural factors appear to strongly influence the non-physical techniques that parents may choose to discipline their children.[2] Caregivers who use extreme measures of discipline, such as locking a child in a cupboard, or less-severe acts, such as habitual belittling, are sufficient to warrant notification to protective services.

SEXUAL ABUSE

Sexual abuse is defined as:

> Any act by a person having the care of the child which exposes a child to, or involves a child in, sexual processes beyond his or her understanding or contrary to accepted community standards (p. 93).[7]

Child sexual abuse is the involvement of children in sexual activities that violate social norms, usually with the intent of gratification or profit. Developmentally, children do not have the capacity to understand these acts of sexual abuse, so therefore are incapable of informed consent. Sexual abuse includes, but is not limited to: fondling, digital manipulation, exhibitionism, pornography and actual or attempted oral, vaginal or anal intercourse.

The legal and social systems that are intended to protect children from sexual abuse in Australasia are highly reliant on evidence from forensic examination. The integrity of evidence in sexual abuse cases is vital in the protection of children from further abuse and to prosecute the perpetrator(s). Emergency clinicians and paramedics must be able to recognise sexual abuse and ensure that children who have been sexually abused are cared for by personnel skilled in forensic examinations. All emergency departments (EDs) should have protocols for the screening, assessment and management of child sexual abuse.

CO-OCCURRENCE OF CHILD ABUSE AND INTIMATE PARTNER VIOLENCE

There is a high rate of co-occurrence between intimate partner violence and child abuse within the same families. Exposure to family violence or intimate partner violence is also a form of child abuse in itself. Children so exposed are more likely to have a range of health, development and social problems, both during childhood and later in life. In addition to this, these children are at a higher risk of perpetrating or being victims of violence themselves, making domestic violence a significant contributor to intergenerational cycles of disadvantage.[19] Children may be injured in the 'crossfire' of a violent assault or attack against an adult primary victim and can be used as 'weapons' by abusive (ex-)partners in the context of family or intimate partner violence.

PRACTICE TIP

VIOLENCE WITHIN FAMILIES

When there is suspected or confirmed child abuse or neglect, it is important to also assess the non-offending parent's safety. Joint safety planning and referral processes need to be implemented when both intimate partner violence and child abuse are identified.[20]

RESPONDING TO DISCLOSURES OF ABUSE

Healthcare provider response to disclosures of abuse are important in terms of maintaining rapport with the person, encouraging further disclosure and setting the foundation for further assessment. If a child or young person discloses any form of abuse, there are five good principles to follow. Let them know:

- you believe them.
- you are glad they told you.
- you are sorry it happened.
- it's not their fault.
- you will support them.

Ensure the child's immediate safety, trying not to alert the alleged abuser. It is important to listen and allow the child or young person to tell only as much as they want. False allegations are uncommon and it is far safer to act on the assumption that the child is telling the truth. A child old enough to disclose is probably old enough to be evidentially interviewed at a later date. It is therefore important not to interrogate the child, which may only cause distress and may confuse any subsequent evidential process. Keep questions to a minimum, keep them open-ended and document the conversation carefully in the clinical notes immediately afterwards.[20]

ASSESSMENT AND MANAGEMENT

Most acute care services have developed a streamlined and multidisciplinary approach to assessment and reporting.[10]

Regardless of the type of abuse that is suspected, the assessment priorities include:

- to diagnose, treat and document injuries to interpret the injury and/or behavioural patterns that have led to suspicion of abuse
- to notify the hospital social worker
- to comply with legislation governing the reporting of abuse
- to comply with organisational policies and procedures.

DIAGNOSE, TREAT AND DOCUMENT INJURIES

In all types of suspected abuse, assessment and treatment of urgent medical problems remain the priority. This should be done according to resuscitation principles.

Infants and children who are brought to the ED with an injury that is suspected to be of non-accidental origin require a full physical assessment. This needs to be carried out by an experienced medical officer. Care should be taken to collect any clothing that is removed during this process. A complete physical examination will contain height and weight measures—assessing failure to thrive—and a complete head-to-toe examination.

After the child's immediate care needs are met, further assessment can occur. A detailed history from the caregiver/s and child, with attention to the sequence of events, should be obtained. During the history-taking and assessment process, emergency care clinicians should recognise that the responsibility for investigation and prosecution of cases of child abuse rests with the police and protective services. It is important to establish the trust of the child and caregiver(s) and ensure that they know you are there as a carer and advocate. Giving children a degree of control by enabling choices can build a therapeutic relationship and a safe environment in which other concerns may be raised. Provide simple choices, such as: 'Which colour gown do you want—blue or red?' 'Is it okay if I listen to your heart, or do you want to listen to it first?' It is important to explain what you are doing and to be honest, particularly if something is going to cause discomfort or pain.

INTERPRET THE INJURY AND/OR BEHAVIOURAL PATTERN

In order to perform a physical examination and provide a report to protective services, consent is required from the child's parent or legal guardian. In an ED, the physical examination should be performed by an appropriately qualified and experienced medical practitioner and should only be performed once.

It is vital that the child is well prepared for medical or forensic examinations. A good time to explain the purpose of the examination is when the child is fully clothed, using a soft, calm and reassuring voice throughout the examination. Giving the child as many choices as possible will help them retain a sense of control, so it is useful to enable a child to choose who will be with them in the examination room, where they want to sit, if they want to be in a chair or on a bed. This will ensure that the child is always fully informed and will help to reduce anxiety. It is important to remind the child that they are in charge and give them control over what is happening: for example, if anything hurts, the child can ask the examiner at any time to stop and then together decisions will be made about what happens next or if there is an alternative way to do things. At the conclusion of the examination, the child should be given the opportunity to ask questions and be reassured.

Investigations should be undertaken as indicated and may include blood tests to exclude non-accidental injury mimics, such as a clotting profile and full blood count. X-rays are indicated if fractures are suspected. A bone scan or skeletal survey may be used to diagnose clinically unsuspected recent or old fracture sites.

In cases where sexual abuse is suspected, examination and the collection of evidence must be performed by appropriately trained and skilled medical practitioners. However, very limited inspections to determine the amount of bleeding or the extent of a rash are sometimes necessary and can be done with the cooperation of the child.

In the case of acute sexual assault, rapid evaluation is indicated and should occur within 72 hours of the assault. The primary responsibility of the emergency nurse in such circumstances is to notify the appropriate staff (medical and social worker), and to ensure that the child is comfortable and receiving the appropriate level of emotional support and privacy.

NOTIFY THE HOSPITAL SOCIAL WORKER

Contact with the nominated hospital social worker early in the presentation is recommended, and will assist with the overall evaluation and liaison with family and protective services.[21]

If a social worker is not available, practitioners should liaise directly with specialist child protection services. As resources vary between jurisdictions, each ED and ambulance service should ensure they are aware of the local and/or regional specialist child protection services.

COMPLY WITH LOCAL POLICY AND LEGISLATION GOVERNING THE REPORTING OF ABUSE

Health policies and clinical practice guidelines have been developed for medical and nursing staff to streamline assessment and management of suspected child abuse and neglect. Many state and territory ambulance services have developed local clinical practice guidelines to ensure a consistent approach to the management of situations of suspected abuse and neglect. Emergency clinicians and paramedics must be aware of these processes locally and understand the way in which organisational policies and procedures articulate with their legal responsibilities to report abuse and neglect.

Australia does not have a single child protection service, but rather eight separate child protection systems. The departments responsible for managing child protection across jurisdictions and the legislation under which each is governed also differ.[7] In Australia, any person who holds concerns about the physical or emotional safety of a child may make a report to the statutory child protection service. Nurses are specifically named as mandatory reporters in child protection legislation in a number of jurisdictions. The Australian Institute of Family Studies (AIFS) provides a helpful summary of mandatory reporting requirements by jurisdiction.[7] Currently, mandatory reporting does not exist in Aotearoa New Zealand. However, health workers are able to refer to police and/or Child Youth and Family Services where there is actual or suspected abuse and safety concerns warrant a statutory intervention.[21]

PRACTICE TIP

POLICY AND PRACTICE GUIDELINES

It is important that emergency clinicians familiarise themselves with the local policies, procedures and referral pathways for responding to child protection concerns.

INTIMATE PARTNER VIOLENCE

Intimate partner violence (IPV), often referred to as 'domestic violence' or 'domestic abuse', is a significant and complex problem in Australia and globally. The WHO defines intimate partner violence as:

> Behaviour by an intimate partner that causes physical, sexual or psychological harm, including acts of physical aggression, sexual coercion, psychological abuse and controlling behaviours (p. vii).[6]

This definition includes violence by both current and former partners and other intimate partners.

It is widely recognised that domestic abuse is a pattern of behaviour that includes one or many different types of abuse, including physical, emotional, verbal, social, economic, psychological, technology facilitated, cultural, spiritual abuse, as well as a range of other coercive controlling behaviours.[22–25] The tactics and methods of abuse employed by perpetrators are reflective of the characteristics of the individuals involved and their particular relationship. In each case, however, the fundamental and defining feature is one person exerting power and control over another.

IPV is primarily perpetrated by men against women and is understood to be independent of social, economic or religious factors. At every age in the life span, females are more likely to be sexually or physically assaulted by someone known to them than by a stranger or an anonymous assailant.[1] IPV has serious impacts for women's health, contributing to a range of negative health outcomes, including poor mental health, problems during pregnancy and birth, alcohol and illicit drug use, suicide, injuries and homicide.[23,26,27]

IPV contributes an estimated 5.1% to the disease burden in Australian women aged 18–44 years and 2.2% of the burden in women of all ages. Partner violence is ranked as the third leading risk factor for women aged 25–44, behind child abuse and neglect during childhood, and illicit drug use.[28] It is estimated to contribute five times more to the burden of disease among Indigenous women than non-Indigenous women, and is estimated to make a larger contribution than any other risk factor to the gap in the burden between Indigenous and non-Indigenous women aged 18–44 years.[23] IPV has serious consequences for the development and wellbeing of children living with violence, and is the single largest cause of homelessness for women.[29]

PREVALENCE

According to the WHO,[24] intimate partner violence is a globally pervasive public health problem—experienced by almost a third of all women worldwide. It is estimated that in Australia, 17% of women and 6% of men have experienced physical and/or sexual violence by a current or former partner. The prevalence of emotional abuse is even greater, with 23% of women and 16% of men experiencing emotional abuse by a current or former partner.[30] In Aotearoa New Zealand, one in three women have experienced physical and/or sexual violence by a male intimate partner in their lifetime and 18% of men have experienced IPV in their lifetime.[20] IPV and its health consequences occur among lesbian, gay, bisexual, transgender and queer (LGBTQ) individuals at rates equal to or higher than cisgender heterosexual individuals.[31] Further, LGBTIQ-identifying people are less likely to identify the experience as abuse, report violence to the police, or seek assistance from a domestic and family violence support organisation for fear of discrimination.[32]

The private nature of the relationships within which violence occurs and the fact that most incidents of domestic violence go unreported, suggests that it is impossible to measure the true extent of the problem.[33]

Historically, establishing prevalence rates of domestic violence in health services has been difficult because of discrepancies in definitions of domestic violence, lack of adequate reporting systems, the reluctance of victim-survivors to report violence as a reason for injury because of embarrassment, shame or fear and the failure of medical professionals to detect violence.[34] As a result, there is wide variance between prevalence estimates of IPV in healthcare contexts with estimates ranging between 2% and 37% of female ED visits being related to IPV.[35] However, we know that hospitalisations of women assaulted by a spouse or partner continue to rise.[28] Research has also shown that women who experience domestic violence have higher rates of healthcare service utilisation due to increased rates of physical and mental health issues that result directly and indirectly from the violence, with the highest figures for violence being identified in psychiatric, obstetrics and gynaecology and ED settings.[36] Aboriginal women experience significantly higher rates and severity of family violence than non-Indigenous women and are 32 times more likely to be hospitalised due to domestic violence-related assaults than other Australian females.[37]

DOMESTIC AND FAMILY VIOLENCE IN DIVERSE COMMUNITIES

Domestic and family violence (DFV) is prevalent across all of Australia's communities. It transcends cultural, social and economic boundaries. However, there are some people in diverse communities who are more vulnerable to DFV and experience violence more frequently and with more severity.[38] These population groups include Aboriginal and Torres Strait Islander people; people with a disability; lesbian, gay, bisexual, transgender and intersex people; people who are culturally and linguistically diverse, including migrants and refugees; people in regional, rural and remote (including isolated) communities; people experiencing mental illness; people who are or have been incarcerated; older people and younger people; and women who are pregnant or in early motherhood.[38] Healthcare workers need to be aware of these vulnerabilities, as well as the specific barriers to securing safety experienced by people from these diverse communities. Importantly, providers must also be aware that no matter which group or community they belong to, each survivor's experience of violence will be unique.[28,32,37,39–43]

PERPETRATORS

In the pre-hospital and ED setting, the stereotype of an abuser is the man who will not allow his partner to answer any questions, and will not allow her to be alone with the nurse. However, it is just as likely that the abuser will be very cooperative with nursing staff and appear compassionate towards his spouse, allowing her to interact normally. Importantly, control may be subtly communicated to the partner with very discrete gestures and expressions that only the victim can perceive.

While a great deal of work in the DFV field is with victim-survivors and children, it has been recognised that effective intervention with perpetrators is required to prevent violence and address this serious issue.[10] Interventions with perpetrators of family violence require specialist knowledge and skills, and there are specialist intervention services that provide this response. For further information go to https://mensline.org.au/health-professionals/.

RESPONDING TO DISCLOSURES OF INTIMATE PARTNER VIOLENCE

Research indicates that many people who experience abuse fear being blamed, judged or humiliated, and are reluctant to discuss their situation.[4] Victim-survivors have been interviewed regarding their experiences in the ED. Half of the women interviewed reported negative experiences in the ED, such as feeling humiliated, being blamed for their abuse, having abuse minimised and not being identified as victim-survivors of domestic violence.[44] On the other hand, survivors report that simple acknowledgement and a non-judgemental attitude helped them enormously in the emergency setting. The key principles for health worker responses to disclosures of IPV are to let them know:

- you believe them.
- you are glad they told you.
- you are sorry it happened.
- it is not their fault.
- you will support them.

Don't pressure the person to leave a violent relationship. A person needs to be well resourced and supported before this can be undertaken safely and effectively.[20]

ASSESSMENT AND MANAGEMENT

Healthcare workers, and in particular paramedics and ED workers, are in a unique position to create a safe and confidential environment for facilitating disclosure of abuse, while offering appropriate support and referral to other resources and services.[6] Identifying domestic violence and the provision of effective first-line responses in the pre-hospital or ED environment has the potential to be empowering, may contribute to enhanced health outcomes and are potentially lifesaving.[27]

In the pre-hosptial environment, paramedics have the capacity to witness signs of abuse that may be hidden from other healthcare workers, such as findings from the patient's home, or interactions with other family members. Paramedics should be mindful of scene findings which may indicate abuse, such as evidence of violence towards furniture (e.g. broken chairs, damaged walls), pets (fear responses or dishevelment), and fear responses from others on scene (e.g. children or relatives appearing withdrawn or unwilling to speak without approval of a controlling person in the scene).

The role of the emergency healthcare clinician in the management of people who have experienced domestic abuse must initially focus on ensuring that the physical and psychological needs of the individual are met. Patients who are experiencing IPV often have complex immediate and long-term needs. As with other forms of family violence, a multi-disciplinary and multi-professional approach is recommended to provide a supportive and non-judgemental response to disclosures of abuse, provide supportive counselling, information and/or referral to appropriate support services that will empower the individual to make decisions to improve their personal safety and the safety of any dependent children. Hospital social workers will often coordinate the healthcare response to IPV and can provide a great deal of information and/or support to other health workers.

SCREENING

There is clear evidence that screening by a skilled health worker directly asking questions increases the identification of women experiencing abuse,[45] and that screening has little or no adverse effect on women. Further, screening is supported by most women who have experienced abuse and can bring about benefits to women particularly when associated with referral to counselling.[26] Routine or universal screening involves routinely asking women about current or recent partner abuse using a standardised set of questions, regardless of the presenting issue. Although further research is required to establish the validity of screening tools, historically, three questions have been used to effectively identify victim-survivors of domestic violence.[46] These questions are listed in Box 39.3. Positive answers can be investigated further.

While there is currently no research evaluating the effectiveness of screening from the pre-hospital environment, the evidence does support women being open to non-judgemental and supportive enquiries about their relationship safety by healthcare professionals.[47] Provided this is performed by a trained practitioner, it would be reasonable to assume that screening for IPV in the pre-hospital environment would be safe.

Routine screening is distinguishable from case finding or targeted screening, which involves asking patients only in situations where there is a high index of suspicion due to the presence of physical, psychological, behavioural, social or other indicators of IPV.[48]

Privacy is essential for interviewing patients where IPV is suspected or confirmed. Questions should not be asked in a public place, such as a centrally located triage desk or waiting room, and the patient should never be questioned in the presence of a possible abuser. Where a concern about IPV has been identified, direct questioning is recommended. For example:

- Many women who have injuries like this have been deliberately hurt. Did someone hurt you?
- A lot of women we see are sometimes frightened of their partner. Have you ever been frightened of your partner?
- Do you feel safe to go home?
- Are you worried about your child's/children's safety?

Surveys of women in violent relationships and those not in violent relationships show that most are grateful to healthcare providers who enquire about violence and abuse in relationships and do not consider this line of enquiry offensive or intrusive.

DOCUMENTATION

Documentation in the medical record can be used as medico-legal evidence and can be very helpful for victim-survivors of abuse. The notes should be very specific. The clearer the information, the less likely the nurse will have to appear in court to explain them.

Documentation from paramedics should include descriptions of injuries or symptoms observed which may be associated with IPV, statements made or behaviours observed by the patient or others on scene, other scene findings that may be associated with IPV (such as damage to furniture or housing).[49] It is also useful to record the presence of children on scene, because in many countries allowing children to witness abuse can also be an offence.

Documentation from ED staff should include all standard nursing data, including time of arrival, preferred language, history of event, type and severity of injuries sustained (if any), and the nature of the examination that is conducted. In addition, the nurse should note whether the injuries are consistent with the history given, and if there have been previous episodes of domestic violence. If a patient denies abuse, the nurse should chart findings and document the suspicion that the findings do not fit the history and may indicate abuse.

Photographic evidence may be collected with the person's permission; alternatively, injuries can be recorded on a body map. The use of direct quotes from the victim-survivor can be powerful evidence. Direct quotes should be identifiable by the use of quotation marks. Ideally, the person's description of the incident and the name of the abuser should be asked and documented in direct quotation. Treatment provided, reports, referrals made, and the details of all agencies involved should also be noted in the medical record. Confidentiality of the medical record must be maintained. Practitioners should take care to ensure that they are not left available for the perpetrator of the abuse to read.

BOX 39.3 QUESTIONS TO ASK TO IDENTIFY VICTIM-SURVIVORS OF DOMESTIC VIOLENCE

1. Have you been hit, kicked, punched or otherwise hurt by someone within the past year? If so, by whom?
2. Do you feel safe in your current relationship?
3. Is there a partner from a previous relationship making you feel unsafe now?

PRACTICE TIP

DOCUMENTATION

Disclosures of domestic violence and documentation of injuries can constitute medico-legal evidence, which may be required in a range of legal proceedings. It is therefore imperative that documentation be accurate, thorough, timely and relevant.

REFERRALS

Providers need to be aware of, and knowledgeable about, resources available to refer women to when asking about intimate partner violence.[6] Resources vary between jurisdictions and each ED should become proactive by compiling and maintaining an up-to-date list of local refuges, and counselling and support services for people who have experienced domestic violence. Hospital social workers and/or local domestic violence services can assist with this process.

The network of community supports for victim-survivors of domestic violence includes telephone counselling and helplines, emergency shelters and accommodation, child protection agencies, police and legal services. The nurse may offer pamphlets or cards with phone numbers; however, the nurse should check first if it is safe for the patient to take home written material that deals with domestic violence. Ideally, ED clinicians will discuss possible referrals with the victim-survivor and establish an action plan in partnership with them.

REPORTING

While it is important to maintain privacy and confidentiality, clinicians must remember that, in certain situations, workers are unable to guarantee absolute confidentiality. For example, health workers may have to alert child protection services where there is significant risk of harm to a child as a result of IPV. Where mandatory reporting requirements exist, such reports MUST be made; the consent of the person involved is not required.

Any request by the victim-survivor to report to police should be facilitated immediately. Health policies in some jurisdictions require health workers to report to police where there is significant injury or risk of harm to the victim or the general public; for example, broken bones, gunshot wounds. In these situations, the consent of the victim-survivor is not required. However, best practice is to support and empower the victim in this process where possible. In all situations where health workers are *not* required to notify the police, the victim-survivor's right to pursue or not to pursue the crime with police and report the offence should be respected.

PSYCHOEDUCATION

While there is a growing recognition of non-physical forms of violence,[28] some victim-survivors are not aware that DFV includes a range of behaviours such as psychological, social and economic abuse, as well as coercive control. Supporting victims to identify or recognise their experience within a DFV framework is often a critical step in first-line responses to DFV.

Other options for education are posters and pamphlets. The best places to display posters and provide pamphlets on domestic violence are the treatment room and bathroom. The waiting room is too public, and the victim-survivor may have to walk in front of several people, including the perpetrator, to get the information. Treatment rooms and bathrooms provide the patient with a chance to read a pamphlet in private, even if he or she is not able to take it home.

RISK ASSESSMENT AND SAFETY PLANNING

All DFV should be considered a risk which requires a response. A risk assessment is a more comprehensive appraisal than asking routine questions. It involves gathering information to determine the level of risk, including any protective factors of the adult and child exposed to violence, as well as the likelihood and severity of future violence.[50] It is important that risk assessments are undertaken by workers who have the necessary skills, knowledge and training to conduct such assessments.

A central aspect of risk assessment and management is a focus on safety. Safety planning is aimed at decreasing the immediate and long-term risks to the safety of victim-survivors and children. It is vital that the nurse determines and documents the age, names and whereabouts of any children in the family, to ensure that they are in safe care. Thinking ahead and planning can increase the safety of victim-survivors and children, whether they are living in or leaving a violent relationship. Often, when victim-survivors manage to leave the abusive relationship, they will continue to experience abusive behaviours such as stalking, intimidation, harassment and systems abuse through family law proceedings, for example.[22,51,52] Further, separation or intent to separate has been identified as a key risk factor for intimate partner homicide.[53]

A safety plan is a personalised, detailed, action-oriented document that enables victims, with the support of professionals and services, to outline clear and specific help-seeking and escape strategies for themselves and their children, based on available resources. Multi-agency safety plans with clear and coordinated information sharing are particularly important in cases of high risk.[38]

For paramedics, safety planning is often best performed in the ED by trained ED staff, and the role of the paramedic is to ensure that scene findings are preserved and reported to facilitate this process. However, for instances where the patient won't be transported to ED, the paramedic should support the patient to consider their immediate safety needs, and that of their children. Providing advice and resources, such as when to contact the ambulance service or police, and other places to seek help can be useful, as well as providing referrals to services that can assist the patient with safety planning.

Safety planning needs to be done in consultation with the person who has experienced the abuse. This is important because they know the situation better than anyone else, and they are likely to have the clearest awareness of actions that might create further risk for them and their children. Plans for immediate safety may involve reporting the incident to the police and applications for police protection orders.

The emergency nurse can assist in this process by facilitating police contact. If the patient has decided not to go home, the nurse can help him or her explore resources. Is there availability of crisis accommodation? Does the patient have relatives or friends who they can stay with? Do they have financial and other material resources to meet immediate needs? Are there children still at home who must be protected?

When talking to patients about safety planning it is important to address immediate and future safety. Hospital social workers, local and national domestic and family violence services will have access to further resources to support safety planning.

SEXUAL ASSAULT

Sexual assault occurs in many contexts, both where the perpetrator is known to the victim-survivor (such as within families) and within the wider community where the perpetrator is unknown.

Sexual assault is a crime of power and control: sex is used as a way of controlling and humiliating the victim. It involves a wide range of behaviours with the common characteristic of unwanted sexual contact. Coercion encompasses a whole spectrum of degrees of force and may include psychological intimidation and threats.

TRAUMA-INFORMED CARE AND PRACTICE

There is increasing awareness in specialist sexual assault services of the need for, and value of, trauma-informed approaches to practice. Trauma-informed care and practice is a strengths-based framework that is grounded in an understanding of, and responsiveness to, the impact of trauma. Traumatised people can often experience services, including health services, as unsafe, disempowering and/or invalidating. To counteract this, trauma-informed practice emphasises physical, psychological and emotional safety for both providers and survivors and creates opportunities for survivors to regain a sense of control and empowerment. Trauma-informed practice incorporates the core principles of safety, trustworthiness, choice, collaboration and empowerment.[54]

ASSESSMENT AND MANAGEMENT

PRE-HOSPITAL MANAGEMENT

Paramedic management of survivors of sexual assault is detailed in practice guidelines developed by the Joint Royal Colleges Liaison Committee.[55] Although these inform practice in the United Kingdom, they are relevant to jurisdiction-based paramedic practice guidelines in Australia and Aotearoa New Zealand. Paramedics should be cautious about disturbing evidence, but this should not constrain the primary and secondary survey or management of significant threats to health. Paramedics may be called to respond to a recent sexual assault, or for physical, psychological or behavioural manifestations arising from previous sexual assault. In either situation, paramedics should be non-judgemental and should not elicit details about the alleged assault, other than information immediately relevant to the care of the individual. The sexual assault victim-survivor should be transported to an appropriate hospital and the hospital notified to assist in the early triage, so that triage does not occur in a public space.

INITIAL ED MANAGEMENT

The initial ED assessment and management of the sexual assault survivor requires careful planning, robust clinical governance in terms of specific policies and procedures, and staff who are well educated and skilled in meeting the needs of this vulnerable group. The goal of ED management is to provide sensitive, person-centred care in a manner that ensures legal and regulatory requirements are fulfilled. Attention in the first instance is given to the physiological needs of the survivor and the simultaneous preservation of evidence. Where possible, care of survivors of sexual assault should be managed in conjunction with appropriately skilled and resourced sexual assault teams.

Emergency medical care is always a priority. Following initial assessment by the triage nurse, the patient should be seen by a senior ED doctor, if injuries or medical condition warrant this. In the absence of an acute medical condition, the appropriate sexual assault service should be contacted and the patient should immediately be placed in an area of the ED that is safe and secure. It is never acceptable for a survivor of sexual assault to wait in the waiting room. An experienced emergency nurse should be allocated to care for the patient for the duration of their ED care to ensure reassurance and rapport, continuity of care and decrease the need for repetition. The patient should also have access to a support person, such as a family member, friend or clinician from a specialist support service.

DETAILED ASSESSMENT

The goal of ED care is to minimise additional stress for the sexual assault survivor. Patient consent should be confirmed before all interactions, and all interactions should occur with sensitivity and understanding. Emergency clinicians should ensure that patients have the opportunity to make informed choices about their care and the examination process.

Consent should also be obtained for evidentiary examination and photographs. It is important the patient understands that the evidence collected will be used in prosecution proceedings if a report is made. During ED care, many patients will not have contemplated the details of reporting their assault to police, or if they have made a report to police, they may not be fully aware of the process that will follow.

Examinations performed as soon as possible after the assault are more likely to yield evidence, especially in relation to bodily fluid forensic evidence collection; however, delayed presentation should not negate performing an examination. Emergency clinicians should minimise the use of jargon and, where possible, use simple, everyday language. Emergency clinicians need to be prepared to take their time when obtaining a history as this is likely to be a very challenging and emotional experience for survivors of sexual assault and patients' emotional responses to questioning can make it difficult to ascertain the information. ED documentation should be clear, legible and detailed, because if the case is called to court, emergency clinicians will be reliant on their documentation to answer questions about the case, which may occur months or even years after the episode of ED care.

Sexual assaults involving date-rape drugs (e.g. flunitrazepam [Rohypnol], gamma-hydroxybutyrate [GHB] and ketamine) and alcohol are referred to as drug-facilitated sexual assaults. The potential use of drugs to facilitate sexual assault should be assessed as part of history-taking and may assist in determining the need for drug screening.

COLLECTION OF EVIDENCE

In the pre-hospital environment, paramedics have a crucial role in collecting and preserving evidence. As discussed previously, documentation of scene findings is important. Additionally, transport of the patient along with evidence should be considered. Examples of this include advising the patient not to shower or wash any affected areas unless necessary for safety and collection of ripped or stained clothing to be transported with the patient. If possible, transport the patient on a stretcher and preserve the linen, as evidence may be collected here. It is important that paramedics explain each action they are taking and seek consent from the patient at each stage. Furthermore, paramedics should wear gloves at each stage to avoid evidence contamination.

Within the ED, the collection of evidence should be performed by an experienced emergency doctor, nurse practitioner, registered nurse or member of a sexual assault team who has received specific training in the care of people who have been sexually assaulted.

After urgent emergency care needs are attended to, laboratory tests, including a pregnancy test, should occur early in the ED episode of care. A negative pregnancy test is needed in order to administer emergency contraception. The patient's clothing should be collected and placed in paper rather than plastic bags and handed to police, adhering to the procedure to maintain the chain of evidence. Paper bags are preferred as plastic allows body fluids and other trace evidence to deteriorate more quickly.

The patient should be assessed using a head-to-toe approach, so that all injuries are identified. Documentation of injuries should include details such as the site, colour and size of bruises, abrasions, lacerations or avulsions. Semen on the patient's skin can be detected using a Wood's lamp or other ultraviolet light, which highlights semen as an orange or blue-green colour. When using Wood's lamp or similar lights, fluorescent areas should be swabbed with a moistened cotton-tipped applicator and the area adjacent to the fluorescent area should also be swabbed as a control. It is important to recognise that other materials such as lint also fluoresce when using Wood's lamps, so care should be taken when reporting Wood's lamp findings.

Oral swabs are taken for evidence of semen and as a reference sample. Reference samples include saliva, blood, semen, pubic hair and body hair, and are compared with specimens from potential suspects. For the female patient, the pelvic examination includes visual examination and photographs and magnified colposcopic photographs to detect and document genital trauma. Documentation should detail the site, size and appearance of injuries and whether the injury is apparent without use of the colposcope. Pubic hair is combed to look for foreign hairs. A representative number of the patient's pubic hairs are cut close to the skin for comparison. During the pelvic examination, swabs and slides are taken from the vaginal pool. Historically, baseline testing for chlamydia and gonorrhoea was undertaken, but some programs have stopped performing these tests because each patient is offered prophylactic antibiotic treatment. Rectal examination includes colposcopy, swabs, slides and baseline testing for sexually transmitted infections (STIs) (as indicated by local policy). The perianal area should be cleansed after taking vaginal/penile specimens to avoid contamination from vaginal or perianal drainage.

All swabs and slides must be labelled to identify the patient and the source, and placed in a drying box to prevent deterioration of evidence. All testing of swabs and slides occurs at a forensic laboratory, which also has the capability to undertake DNA linking of evidence to potential suspects. DNA testing methods allow detection of semen donor type as many as 5–6 days after a sexual assault. Evidence management is an important element of emergency care so emergency clinicians must prevent contamination of evidence collected, and ensure that all equipment that comes in contact with evidence is clean. Handling of evidence should be limited and emergency clinicians should wear gloves and not talk over evidence to avoid leaving their own DNA. To maintain validity of evidence collected and ensure that the chain of evidence is preserved, emergency clinicians must be able to verify the whereabouts of all evidence at all points in time. Any transfer of evidence to another person or agency, such as the police, must be carefully documented.

The patient should be offered a shower and clean clothing as soon as possible after the sexual assault examination. Options such as emergency contraception, prophylaxis for STIs and HIV should be discussed with the patient. Patients should be followed up within 2 weeks; if follow-up care is not part of the sexual assault program, referral to a gynaecologist or sexual health clinic is essential. Cultures for *Chlamydia* and *Neisseria gonorrhoeae* can be obtained and the details of HIV testing can be discussed during the follow-up appointment

ELDER ABUSE AND NEGLECT

The WHO currently defines elder abuse as:

> a single, or repeated act, or lack of appropriate action, occurring within any relationship where there is an expectation of trust which causes harm or distress to an older person (p. 3).[56]

Elder abuse can take various forms, including physical, psychological/emotional, sexual, financial and intentional or unintentional neglect. Elder abuse causes harm to an older person, usually deliberate harm such as assaulting an older person or stealing their money. It may also be harm caused by neglect, such as failing to feed or provide prescribed medications to an older person. Perpetrators of elder abuse may include, but are not limited to, family members, friends, health and social welfare professionals, and formal and informal carers. Elder abuse can occur in a range of settings, including community-based and institutional care settings.[57] An estimated 2–14% of older people in high- or middle-income countries are victims of abuse or neglect every year. Prevalence rates are likely to be much higher in institutional care settings than in community settings.[57] Elder abuse has a range of physical, psychological and financial consequences. It can result in pain, injury and even death, and is associated with higher levels of stress and depression and an increased risk of nursing home placement and hospitalisation.[58] The Australian Bureau of Statistics classifies older people as over 65 years. For Māori, Pasifika and Aboriginal and Torres Strait Islander peoples, all of whom are more likely to have age-related issues younger, a lower age of 45–50 years for those who are 'older' is considered appropriate.[57,59]

RISK FACTORS

There are different risk factors for different types of elder abuse. However, common overall risk factors identified include: when the older person has cognitive impairment or another disability, poor mental health, social isolation or a history of abuse, family violence or conflict.[60]

Several risk factors for the perpetration of elder abuse have been identified including: caregiver burden/stress, financial or emotional dependency on the older person, sense of entitlement, drug and alcohol abuse, history of family violence or conflict, and mental health difficulties.[58]

ELDER ABUSE IN DIVERSE COMMUNITIES

In the Aboriginal and Torres Strait Islander context, the terms 'elder' and 'abuse' have been considered problematic, as 'elder' has a specific meaning in Aboriginal communities, and 'abuse' may be considered inapt and confrontational.

There are not many studies in Aotearoa comparing elder abuse among cultures and ethnicities; however, one study found that Māori are more than twice as likely to be coerced, be verbally and emotionally abused, and feel uncomfortable with a member of their family than non-Māori.[61]

In culturally and linguistically diverse (CALD) communities, a number of factors can heighten vulnerability to abuse, including language difficulties for those whose primary language is not English, social dependence on family members for support and the potential conflict caused by cross-generational expectations in relation to care.[62]

IDENTIFYING ELDER ABUSE

As with other forms of abuse, paramedics are often able to witness signs in the patient's home environment, which can be recorded. As elder abuse is commonly associated with neglect, it is important for paramedics to be vigilant and document signs of neglect or control, such as poor hygiene, unclean bedding or living areas, inaccessible food, water, toileting or washing facilities or medications. Observe interactions with caregivers and document and report any concerns. Remember that neglect isn't always intentional, and many caregivers are simply unable to provide sufficient care, so it is important for paramedics to remember that caregivers may need support as well.

An ED visit provides a unique opportunity to identify elder abuse. Medical assessment for injury or illness may be the only time victimised older adults leave their home. Although extreme cases may be easy to identify, most cases are subtle and present with non-specific signs. Further, victims may be either unable or unwilling to report the problem. The same factors that are associated with vulnerability to elder abuse—social isolation and cognitive impairment—also present barriers to disclosure or identification and reporting.[63] The dynamics of dependence are also relevant, since an aged person may be reluctant to disclose abuse by someone on whom they depend for care, since disclosure may mean withdrawal of the care and potentially an unwanted change in living situation. When an older person has cognitive impairment, this may inhibit their capacity to disclose or mean they are not believed when they do disclose. Shame, embarrassment, fear of negative repercussions and/or a belief that disclosure and reporting may result in no consequences or negative consequences are also potential barriers to disclosure.[64]

In order to overcome the challenges in identifying elder abuse, a multi-disciplinary team-based approach is recommended, which incorporates the skills and perspectives of prehospital personnel, triage, nurses, doctors and social workers. Paramedics typically enter a patient's home when responding to a call. Examination of the home can provide important information about the overall safety of the environment and may also provide evidence of abuse. Once abuse is identified, paramedics should communicate with the ED care team about unusual family interactions; cleanliness and upkeep of the home; the availability of food, medications, heat and sanitation, and other safety issues. The triage nurses may be the only people to see and collect information from paramedics, family members or caregivers. It is important that information obtained at triage is accurately relayed to the ED care team. In the ED, nurses provide bedside care to patients and typically have significant face-to-face contact with patients, caregivers and other family and friends. Close observation by a nurse, with a focus on interactions and discordant information between the patient and caregivers, may identify red flags that require further investigation. Careful and complete examination of a patient during the provision of personal care may also uncover physical findings that provide evidence of abuse.[63]

INDICATORS OF ELDER ABUSE

Indicators of abuse are often subtle and can vary from person to person. Paramedics and emergency nurses should remain observant and aware of the abuse indicators, especially where there is no disclosure or witnessing of the abuse. Table 39.1 provides a summary of elder abuse indicators—behaviours and signs.

When screening for elder abuse, the patient and suspected abuser should be interviewed separately. A validated screening tool promoted by the Royal Australian College of General Practitioners is the Elder Abuse Suspicion Index (Box 39.4).

INTERVENTIONS

Older people at risk of experiencing abuse should be:

- provided with information about options
- supported to make their own decisions
- respected in their choice to accept or reject support if they are competent to make that decision.

Responses to abuse situations need to take into consideration whether the older person has capacity. Determining capacity requires a specialist legal test or medical assessment. An older person who has the mental capacity to make their own decisions may choose to stay in an abusive situation.

The overall aim of any intervention is to stop the abuse. Where this is not possible for any reason, the secondary objective becomes to prevent escalation of abuse; put protections and supports in place that maximise the older person's safety; and ensure the older person knows what information and resources are available to address the abusive situation.[66]

The needs of victims and abusers should be kept separate. However, the abuser's needs should be considered as this can sometimes be the key to stopping the abuse; for example, enhancing a stressed carer's skills and/or support.[66] When speaking with the abuser, it is important to avoid confrontation and to ensure that the older person will not be placed at further risk of harm as a result of the intervention.

Due to the complexity of elder abuse, intervention requires a multidisciplinary team approach. Such a team is able to assess aspects of the situation, such as physical injury, mental status, competency, financial irregularities, legality, treatment, assistance, protection or prosecution. Potential intervention strategies include referrals to community agencies for continual monitoring of the situation, support services to decrease caregiver stress, close healthcare follow-up to prevent switching to another healthcare provider, reports to adult protective services with removal of the individual from a harmful environment or use of 24-hour supervision through a home health agency. When there is a high degree of suspicion for elder abuse, or if you require support to determine appropriate intervention strategies, consult social services or the responsible agency in your area.

PRACTICE TIP

SUPPORT SERVICES

It is useful for clinicians to develop a resource that lists local support services that can assist in responding to violence within families and provide ongoing assessment and support.

TABLE 39.1 ELDER ABUSE TYPES—BEHAVIOURS AND SIGNS[57]

	FINANCIAL	PSYCHOLOGICAL	NEGLECT	PHYSICAL	SEXUAL
BEHAVIOURS	Threatening, coercing re: assets or wills; Taking control of the older person's finances against their wishes and denying access to their own money; Abusing Powers of Attorney; Stealing goods, e.g. jewellery, credit cards, cash, food, and other possessions; Unauthorised use of banking and financial documents; The recent addition of a signature on a bank account.	Pressuring, intimidating or bullying; Name calling, and verbal abuse; Treating an older person like a child; Threatening to harm the person, other people or pets; Engaging in emotional blackmail such as threatening to withdraw access to grandchildren, family, friends, services, telephone or placement in an aged care facility; Preventing contact with family and friends, or denying access to the phone or computer; Withholding mail; Preventing an older person from engaging in religious or cultural practices; Moving an older person far away from family or friends.	Failure to provide basic needs, i.e. food, adequate or clean clothing, heating, medicines; Under- or over-medication; Exposure to danger or lack of supervision, such as leaving the older person in an unsafe place or in isolation; An overly attentive carer in the company of others; Refusal to permit others to provide appropriate care.	Pushing, shoving, or rough handling; Kicking, hitting, punching, slapping, biting, and/or burning; Restraining: physical or medical; Locking the person in a room or home or tying to a chair or bed; Intentional injury with a weapon or object; Overuse or misuse of medications.	Non-consensual sexual contact, language or exploitative behaviour; Rape and sexual assault; Cleaning or treating the older person's genital area roughly or inappropriately; Enforced nudity of an older person.
SIGNS	Unexplained disappearance of belongings; Unexplained or inability to pay bills; Significant bank withdrawals and/or changes to wills; Inability of an older person to access bank accounts or statements; Stockpiling of unpaid bills or an empty fridge; Disparity between living conditions and money; No money to pay for essentials for the home including food, clothing and utilities.	Resignation, shame; Depression, tearfulness; Confusion, agitation; Feelings of helplessness; Unexplained paranoia or excessive fear; Disrupted appetite or sleep patterns, such as insomnia; Unusual passivity or anger; Sadness or grief at the loss of interactions with others; Withdrawal or listlessness due to people not visiting; Changes in levels of self-esteem; Worry or anxiety after a visit by specific person/ people; Social isolation.	Inadequate clothing, complaints of being cold or too hot; Poor personal hygiene, unkempt appearance; Lack of medical or dental care, or injuries that have not been properly cared for; Absence of required aids; Exposure to unsafe, unhealthy, and/or unsanitary conditions; Unexplained weight loss, dehydration, poor skin integrity, malnutrition.	Internal or external injuries (sprains, dislocations and fractures, pressure sores, unexplained bruises or marks on different areas of the body, pain on touching); Broken or healing bones; Lacerations to mouth, lips, gums, eyes or ears, missing teeth and/or eye injuries; Evidence of hitting, punching, shaking, pulling, i.e. bruises, lacerations, choke marks, hair loss or welts; Burns, i.e. rope, cigarettes, matches, iron, and/or hot water.	Unexplained STD or incontinence (bladder or bowel); Injury and trauma, e.g. scratches, bruises etc. to face, neck, chest, abdomen, thighs or buttocks; Trauma including bleeding around the genitals, chest, rectum or mouth; Torn or bloody underclothing or bedding; Human bite marks; and Anxiety around the perpetrator and other psychological symptoms.

REPORTING

Apart from limited obligations in relation to specific offences for Australian Commonwealth-funded care facilities, there are no statutory mandatory obligations on professionals to report abuse of older persons in Australia or Aotearoa New Zealand. However, you may have a duty of care or professional responsibility to report your suspicions of an incidence of elder abuse that has been disclosed to you or that you have witnessed. Check your workplace duty of care statement, policies and procedures for further details.[64]

ABUSE AND NEGLECT IN INSTITUTIONS

While this chapter has primarily outlined responses to abuse or neglect occurring within the community, emergency clinicians need to be aware and alert to incidences of abuse and neglect that may occur within institutional settings. As outlined in the

BOX 39.4 **ELDER ABUSE SUSPICION INDEX**[65]

THE ELDER ABUSE SUSPICION INDEX (EASI)

EASI Questions Q.1–Q.5 asked of patient; Q.6 answered by doctor.
While all six questions should be asked, a response of 'yes' on one or more of questions 2 to 6 may establish concern and warrant further investigation and assessment.
Within the last 12 months:

1	Have you relied on people for any of the following: bathing, dressing, shopping, banking or meals?	Yes	No	Did not answer
2	Has anyone prevented you from getting food, clothes, medication, glasses, hearing aids or medical care, or from being with people you wanted to be with?	Yes	No	Did not answer
3	Have you been upset because someone talked to you in a way that made you feel shamed or threatened?	Yes	No	Did not answer
4	Has anyone tried to force you to sign papers or to use your money against your will?	Yes	No	Did not answer
5	Has anyone made you afraid, touched you in ways that you did not want, or hurt you physically?	Yes	No	Did not answer
6	(to be answered by doctor) Elder abuse may be associated with findings such as: poor eye contact, withdrawn nature, malnourishment, hygiene issues, cuts, bruises, inappropriate clothing, or medication compliance issues. Did you notice any of these today or in the last 12 months?	Yes	No	Did not answer

final report of the Aged Care Royal Commission,[67] the abuse of older people in residential care is far from uncommon. The inquiry heard of physical and sexual abuse that occurred at the hands of staff members, and of situations in which residential aged care providers did not protect residents from abuse by other residents. The analysis of abuse also focused on restrictive practices and sub-standard care. The Aged Care Quality and Safety Commission can receive complaints of abuse or neglect of an older person living in an aged care facility or receiving a community-based aged care service subsidised by the Australian Government. In Aotearoa New Zealand, the Ministry of Social Development Elder Abuse Response Services (EARS) provide coordinated national services to those experiencing, or at risk of experiencing, abuse including institutional abuse.[59]

SUMMARY

Interpersonal violence is a pervasive, multi-factorial problem that affects the health and wellbeing of people in all countries and occurs across the life span. In every case of abuse, violence stems from the need to exert power and control over another person. The perpetrator of any form of violence transgresses the basic human rights of another for their own gain. Women and children are most often affected by violence, but men may also experience the various forms of interpersonal violence.

Paramedics have an important role in identifying cases of suspected abuse in individuals living in the community, and in referring these individuals to appropriate health agencies. As part of the multidisciplinary healthcare team, the emergency nurse is in a position to detect and manage the consequences of all types of interpersonal violence. In addition to their clinical role, emergency nurses have a responsibility to promote opportunistic self-disclosure of abuse among vulnerable populations when they are seeking emergency care for unrelated health problems.

Nurses and paramedics in many jurisdictions have statutory requirements to report child abuse and neglect in Australia, and it is vital that clinicians become familiar with the organisational and jurisdictional process for mandatory reporting of this type of abuse.

CASE STUDY

CHILD'S HISTORY

Charlie is an 18-month-old boy. He was found by a neighbour at approximately 1900 hours crawling in his front yard, wearing only a nappy and a light T-shirt. The neighbour could not find his mother inside the house or yard, so contacted the police. The police attended the home and in turn called an ambulance. Charlie was assessed for evidence of injury by paramedics, who comforted and warmed him before he was transported to the emergency department (ED) for further assessment and management.

On arrival in the ED, Charlie was found to be slightly dehydrated, cold and hungry. He was wrapped in a warm blanket and given a bottle, which he took well. At no time was he upset and was noted by the treating emergency doctor to be a happy and interactive child.

Charlie's medical records indicate that he was born via normal vaginal delivery at 32 weeks' gestation; he was of low birth weight and was substance-affected. He spent 3 months in the neonatal intensive care unit. Due to his prematurity, low birth weight and substance withdrawal, he had some initial feeding and attachment problems with his mother. Concerns of a mild developmental delay were raised by the maternal and child health nurse at 12 months and were to be followed up in the paediatric clinic of the outpatient department; however, Charlie's mother did not attend the scheduled appointment.

FAMILY HISTORY

Charlie is the youngest child in his family. He has two siblings (aged 3 and 4 years). His sister is currently living with his maternal grandmother; his brother is being cared for by his aunty. Charlie's mother Zoe is 20 years old and has a history of drug abuse, but has not used any illicit substances in the past 6 months.

Recently Zoe secured casual work and things were generally progressing very well for her and Charlie until she received a summons to attend court on the same day Charlie was taken to the ED. It was for this reason that Zoe needed to attend an urgent meeting with her solicitor and so left Charlie in the care of her boyfriend.

Charlie's father visits him one weekend per month. He currently lives approximately 2 hours away.

QUESTIONS

1. What are Charlie's actual and potential health problems?
2. Develop a care plan that addresses each of the problems you identify. In the plan include aims/goals, interventions and expected outcomes.
3. Outline the legal responsibilities of the nurse within your jurisdiction with regard to any protective concerns you have for Charlie.

Answers to Case Study Questions can be found on evolve http://evolve.elsevier.com/AU/Curtis/emergency/

USEFUL WEBSITES

Aged Care Quality and Safety Commission. Healthcare workers and consumers can access information on reporting serious incidents of elder abuse in residential aged care. https://www.agedcarequality.gov.au/

Australian Institute of Family Studies (AIFS) is the Australian Government's key research body in the area of family wellbeing. A number of research reports and factsheets about domestic and family violence and child abuse and protection are available, https://aifs.gov.au/.

Australia's National Research Organisation for Women's Safety (ANROWS), an independent, not-for-profit research organisation established to produce evidence to support the reduction of violence against women and their children, https://anrows.org.au/.

1800RESPECT National Sexual Assault, Domestic Family Violence Counselling Service. A confidential service available 24/7. Provides support for people experiencing, or at risk of experiencing, sexual assault, domestic or family violence. The website has useful resources and tools to support best practice, www.1800respect.org.au/.

Full Stop Australia, provides a range of counselling services for anyone who has experienced or is at risk of sexual violence, family or domestic violence and their non-offending supporters. The website has resources for professionals, and clinicians can contact the service for clinical consultation and/or debrief, (1800 385 578), https://fullstop.org.au/.

Men's Referral Service/No to Violence/, a men's family violence telephone counselling, information and referral service. It also provides support to professionals wishing to support a client who is using or experiencing family violence (1300 766 491), www.ntv.org.au/.

My Aged Care. The Australian Government's My Aged Care website and phone line provides assistance for older people, family members and professionals to access services and find information. My Aged Care website provides links to information, useful contacts and options for getting help for elder abuse in each state and territory, www.myagedcare.gov.au/legal-information/elder-abuse-concerns.

Secretariat of National Aboriginal and Islander Child Care (SNAICC), is the national non-government peak body for Aboriginal and Torres Strait Islander children. The website provides access to policy and research and a range of other resources, www.snaicc.org.au/.

REFERENCES

1. World Health Organization (WHO). World report on violence and health. Geneva: WHO; 2002.
2. World Health Organization (WHO). Global consultation on violence and health. Violence: a public health priority. Geneva: WHO; 1996.
3. Campbell J. Health consequences of intimate partner violence. Lancet 2002;359(9314):1331–6.
4. García-Moreno C, Hegarty K, d'Oliveira A, Koziol-McLain J, Colombini M, Feder G. The health-systems response to violence against women. Lancet 2015;385(9977):1567–79.
5. Felitti V, Anda R, Nordenberg D, Williamson DF, Spitz AM, Edwards V, et al. Relationship of childhood abuse and household dysfunction to many of the leading causes of death in adults: the Adverse Childhood Experiences (ACE) Study. Am J Prevent Med 1998;14(4):245–58.

6. World Health Organization (WHO). Responding to intimate partner violence and sexual violence against women: WHO clinical and policy guidelines. Geneva: WHO; 2013.
7. Australian Institue of Health and Welfare (AIHW). Child protection Australia 2019–20. Canberra: AIHW; 2021.
8. Australian Institute of Family Studies (AIFS). Mandatory reporting of child abuse and neglect CFCA Resource Sheet—September 2017. Canberra: AIFS; 2017.
9. Paramedicine Board Ahpra. Code of conduct (interim) for registered health practitioners. 2018. Online: Available from: www.paramedicineboard.gov.au/professional-standards/codes-guidelines-and-policies/code-of-conduct.aspx.
10. Australia Government, Department of Social Services. Safe and supported: the national framework for protecting Australia's children 2021–2031. Canberra: DOSS; 2021.
11. Moore S, Scott J, Ferrari A, Mills R, Dunne MP, Erskine HE, et al. Burden attributable to child maltreatment in Australia. Child Abuse Negl 2015;48:208–20.
12. Kendall-Tackett K. Treating the lifetime health effects of childhood victimization. Kingston, NJ: Civic Research Institute; 2013.
13. Oranga Tamariki – Ministry for Children. Prevalence of harm to children in New Zealand. Wellington: Oranga Tamariki—Ministry for Children; 2020.
14. New Zealand Government. Te Aorerekura: the enduring spirit of affection. The National Strategy to Eliminate Family Violence and Sexual Violence. Wellington: The Board for the Elimination of Family Violence and Sexual Violence Te Kāwanatanga o Aotearoa, New Zealand Government; 2021.
15. Reece R, Ludwig S, editors. Child abuse: medical diagnosis and management. 2nd ed. Philadelphia: Lippincott Williams and Wilkins; 2001.
16. Kirschner R, Wilson H. Pathology of fatal child abuse. 2nd ed. Philadelphia: Lippincott Williams and Wilkins; 2001.
17. Parks S, Annest J, Hill H, Karch DL. Pediatric abusive head trauma: recommended definitions for public health surveillance and research. Atlanta, Georgia: Centers for Disease Control and Prevention National Center for Injury Prevention and Control Division of Violence Prevention; 2012.
18. American Psychiatric Association. Diagnostic and statistical manual of mental disorders (DSM-V). 5th ed. Washington, DC: American Psychiatric Association; 2013.
19. Australia's National Research Organisation for Women's Safety (ANROWS). Examination of the health outcomes of intimate partner violence against women: state of knowledge paper. Sydney, Australia: ANROWS; 2016.
20. Fanslow J, Kelly P. Family violence assessment and intervention guideline: child abuse and intimate partner violence. 2nd ed. Wellington: Ministry of Health; 2016.
21. Royal Children's Hospital (RCH). Child abuse guideline. n.d. Online: Available from: www.rch.org.au/clinicalguide/guideline_index/Child_Abuse_Guideline/.
22. Stark E, Hester M. Coercive control: update and review. Violence Against Women 2019;25(1):81–104.
23. Webster K. A preventable burden: measuring and addressing the prevalence and health impacts of intimate partner violence in Australian women. Sydney: ANROWS; 2016.
24. World Health Organization (WHO). Violence against women prevalence estimates, 2018: global, regional and national prevalence estimates for intimate partner violence against women and global and regional prevalence estimates for non-partner sexual violence against women. Geneva: WHO; 2021.
25. Domestic Violence NSW. Good practice guidelines for the domestic and family violence sector in NSW. DVNSW; 2021.
26. Spangaro J, Ruane J. Health interventions for family and domestic violence: a literature review. Office of kids and families. Sydney: NSW Health; 2014.
27. State of Victoria. Royal Commission into Family Violence: summary and recommendations, Parl Paper No 132 (2014–16). Melbourne: State of Victoria; 2016.
28. Australian Institute of Health and Welfare (AIHW). Family, domestic and sexual violence in Australia: continuing the national story 2019. Canberra: AIHW; 2019.
29. Australian Institute of Health and Welfare (AIHW). Domestic and family violence and homelessness 2011–12 to 2013–14. Canberra: AIHW; 2016.
30. Australian Bureau of Statistics (ABS). Personal safety, Australia, 2016. Cat. no. 4906.0. Canberra: ABS; 2017.
31. Scheer J, Poteat V. Trauma-informed care and health among LGBTQ intimate partner violence survivors. J Interpers Violence 2021;36(13–14):6670–92.
32. Campo M, Tayton S. Intimate partner violence in lesbian, gay, bisexual, trans, intersex and queer communities: key issues. CFCA. Melbourne, VIC: Australian Institute of Family Studies; 2015.
33. Parliament of Australia. Domestic violence in Australia: an overview of the issues. Canberra: Parliament of Australia; 2011.
34. de Vries R, March L, Vinen J, Horner D, Roberts G. Prevalence of domestic violence among patients attending a hospital emergency department. ANZ J Pub Health 1996;20(4):364–8.
35. Btoush R, Campbell J, Gebbie K. Care provided in visits coded for intimate partner violence in a national survey of emergency departments. Women's Health Issues 2009;19(4):253–62.
36. Alhabib S, Nur U, Jones R. Domestic violence against women: systematic review of prevalence studies. J Fam Violence 2010;25(4):369–82.
37. Secretariat of National Aboriginal and Islander Child Care NFVPLS, & National Aboriginal and Torres Strait Islander Legal Services. Strong families, safe kids: family violence response and prevention for Aboriginal and Torres Strait Islander children and families (Policy Paper). Melbourne, Victoria: SNAICC; 2017.
38. Toivonen C, Backhouse C. National risk assessment principles for domestic and family violence. Sydney: ANROWS; 2018.

39. Campo MT. Domestic and family violence in regional, rural and remote communities: an overview of key issues. Melbourne: Australian Institute of Family Studies CFCA; 2015.
40. ANROWS. Improving family violence legal and support services for Aboriginal and Torres Strait Islander peoples: key findings and future directions (research to policy and practice). Sydney: ANROWS; 2020.
41. Frohmader C, Dowse L, Didi A. Preventing violence against women and girls with disabilities: integrating a human rights perspective. Melbourne: Women with Disabilities Australia; 2015.
42. Maher J, Spivakovsky C, McCulloch J. Women, disability and violence: barriers to accessing justice. Key findings and future directions. Sydney, NSW: ANROWS; 2018. Contract No. 2.
43. Vaughan C, Davis E, Murdolo A, Chen J, Murray L, Block K, et al. Promoting community-led responses to violence against immigrant and refugee women in metropolitan and regional Australia: The ASPIRE Project (State of knowledge paper 7). Sydney, NSW: ANROWS; 2015.
44. Hinsliff-Smith K, McGarry J. Understanding management and support for domestic violence and abuse within emergency departments: a systematic literature review from 2000–2015. J Clin Nurs 2017;26(23–24):4013–27.
45. O'Doherty L, Hegarty K, Ramsay J, Davidson LL, Feder G, Taft A. Screening women for intimate partner violence in healthcare settings. Cochrane Database of Syst Rev 2015:15(7):CD007007.
46. Ramsden C, Bonner M. An early identification and intervention model for domestic violence. Aust Emerg Nurs J 2002;5(1):15–20.
47. Feder G, Hutson M, Ramsay J, Taket AR. Women exposed to intimate partner violence: expectations and experiences when they encounter health care professionals: a meta-analysis of qualitative studies. Arch Intern Med 2006;166(1):22–37.
48. Ali P, McGarry J, Dhingra K. Identifying signs of intimate partner violence. Emerg Nurse 2016;23(9):25.
49. Sawyer S, Coles J, Williams A, Williams B. Paramedics as a new resource for women experiencing intimate partner violence. J Interpers Violence 2021;36(5-6):NP2999–3018.
50. Albuquerque M, Basinskaite B, Martins, Mira R, Pautasso E, et al. European manual of risk assessment. E-Maria. Göttingen: BUPNET; 2013.
51. Costello M, Backhouse C. Avoiding the 3 'M's: accurate use of violence, abuse and neglect statistics and research to avoid myths, mistakes and misinformation – a resource for NSW health workers. In: The NSW Health Education Centre Against Violence (ECAV) and Prevention and Response to Violence AaNPU, Ministry of Health. Sydney, NSW: The NSW Health Education Centre Against Violence (ECAV) and Prevention and Response to Violence, Abuse and Neglect (PARVAN) Unit, Ministry of Health; 2019.
52. Laing L, Humphreys C, Cavanagh K. Social work and domestic violence: developing critical and reflective practice. London: SAGE publications; 2013.
53. Team DVDR. NSW domestic violence death review team report 2017–2019. Sydney: Domestic Violence Death Review Team; 2020.
54. Kezelman C. Trauma-informed practice: how important is this for domestic violence services. Newsletter 2013:52.
55. Joint Royal Colleges Ambulance Liaison Committee (JRCALC). UK Ambulance Service clinical practice guidelines. Coventry: JRCALC; 2006.
56. World Health Organization (WHO). The Toronto declaration on the global prevention of elder abuse. Geneva: WHO; 2002.
57. Qu L, Kaspiew R, Carson R, De Maio J, Harvey J, Horsfall B. National elder abuse prevalence study: final report. Melbourne, VIC: Australian Institute of Family Studies; 2021.
58. World Health Organization (WHO). World report on ageing and health. Geneva: WHO; 2015.
59. Ministry of Social Development - Te Manatū Whakahiato Ora. Elder abuse in Aotearoa. The role and current state of MSD's Elder Abuse Response Services. Wellington: Ministry of Social Development—Te Manatū Whakahiato Ora; 2019.
60. Acierno R, Hernandez M, Amstadter A, Resnick HS, Steve K, Muzzy W, et al. Prevalence and correlates of emotional, physical, sexual, and financial abuse and potential neglect in the United States: the National Elder Mistreatment Study. Am J Pub Health 2010;100(2):292–7.
61. Waldegrave C. Measuring elder abuse in New Zealand: findings from the New Zealand Longitudinal Study of Ageing (NZLSA). Wellington: Family Centre Social Policy Research Unit; 2015.
62. Bagshaw D, Wendt S, Zannettino L. Preventing the abuse of older people by their family members. Sydney, Australia: Domestic Violence Clearing House; 2009.
63. Rosen T, Hargarten S, Flomenbaum N, Platts-Mills TF. Identifying elder abuse in the emergency department: toward a multidisciplinary team-based approach. Ann Emerg Med 2016;68(3):378–82.
64. Kaspiew R, Carson R, Rhoades H. Elder abuse: understanding issues, frameworks and responses. Melbourne: Australian Institute of Family Studies; 2016.
65. National Initiative for the Care of the Elderly (NICE). EASI: Elder Abuse Suspicion Index Canada. 2006. Online: Available from: www.nicenet.ca/tools-easi-elder-abuse-suspicion-index.
66. NSW Elder Abuse Helpline and Resource Unit. Responding to elder abuse. Sydney, NSW: NSW Elder Abuse Helpline and Resource Unit; n.d.
67. Royal Commission into Aged Care Quality and Safety. Royal Commission into Aged Care Quality and Safety Final Report: Care, Dignity and Respect Volume 1 Summary and recommendations. Canberra: Department of Health and Aged Care; 2021.

CHAPTER 40

ALCOHOL, TOBACCO AND OTHER DRUG USE

MICHAEL A. ROCHE AND ALAN EADE

ESSENTIALS

There are essential considerations regarding the safe care of people who may be affected by psychoactive substances such as alcohol, sedatives, opioids, psychostimulants or inhalants. These are:

- Never assume that the patient is merely affected by a psychoactive substance. All patients have the right to high-quality clinical assessment and treatment whether or not they are affected by psychoactive substances.
- A patient may present with an injury or other medical emergency and also be at risk of alcohol withdrawal, which can be life threatening.
- A patient who is intoxicated or similarly incapacitated and cannot safely manage their environment, thinking, problem-solving or physical functions adequately is at serious risk of injury, misjudging situations or other people's behaviour and communication, and is unlikely to be able to give informed consent.
- A patient who appears intoxicated may instead have (for example) head or other serious injury, acute infection, stroke, hypoglycaemia or other medical crises.
- A patient who is intoxicated can also have a serious injury or other medical condition (which may or may not be obvious).
- A patient who is intoxicated and has a concurrent mental health condition may present as a result of the intoxication, which may or may not exacerbate a concurrent mental health condition.
- A patient may present as moderately intoxicated, but still be at risk of imminent overdose due to the amount (dose) of a substance recently consumed still taking effect, e.g. excessive binge-drinking.
- A patient may be at imminent risk of toxicity or overdose due to recent consumption of more than one substance, such as alcohol and sedatives or opioids.
- A person may have ceased or significantly reduced their usual level (dose) of consumption of a substance before presentation and withdrawal.
- Alcohol withdrawal alone or in combination with withdrawal from other depressants can be life threatening.
- Always err on the side of caution until satisfied that the patient is medically safe to allow to leave.

INTRODUCTION

It is essential for the emergency clinician to have knowledge and understanding regarding alcohol, tobacco and other drug (ATOD)-related presentations. Developing

an understanding of the physiological and psychological effects of ATODs enables the anticipation, monitoring and early intervention and treatment of complications associated with ATOD use. Furthermore, developing an understanding of the clinical manifestations will assist you to provide care in a humane and compassionate manner.

This chapter provides an overview of common ATOD use and likely emergency presentations. Several case studies are referred to throughout to assist your learning. The common substances are summarised, the likely clinical features of each group are presented, and for a large number the specific care required for each overdose or withdrawal state is also presented.

An awareness and understanding of the physiological and psychological effects of ATOD is essential for all emergency clinicians. It enables clinicians to anticipate and monitor for potential complications and deterioration, commence assessment and treatment in the out-of-hospital setting and further assist with assessment, diagnosis and ongoing treatment in the ED environment. As point of first contact, emergency clinicians are uniquely placed to screen for ATOD use and detect risk factors and potential health problems. This provides an opportunity for early assessment and history, intervention and treatment.

OVERVIEW AND BACKGROUND

PSYCHOACTIVE SUBSTANCES: ALCOHOL, TOBACCO AND OTHER DRUGS (ATODS)

The term 'drugs' is often used in reference to illicit drugs; however, in this chapter we are referring to all psychoactive substances, whether they be legal or illegal. These include alcohol, tobacco (nicotine) and other drugs. They also include pharmaceuticals, alternative preparations and various substances. In Australia, fewer people overall use illicit drugs compared with legal drugs such as alcohol, caffeine and nicotine, and prescribed and over-the-counter (OTC) pharmaceuticals.[1,2]

ATODs have dose-related psychoactive effects on the central nervous system (CNS/brain), resulting in the person's altered physical function, mood and cognition. ATODs affect the CNS's (brain's) core body functions, such as respiration, temperature regulation, blood pressure, heart rate, consciousness and neural responses to external stimuli, including balance, movement, coordination and fine motor skills. ATODs can induce serious and often unpredictable adverse effects, including acute intoxication, overdose, toxicity and drug-induced psychosis. These effects can occur with first-time use, occasional use or regular dependent use. These are commonly used ATODs:[2–5]

- depressants, such as alcohol, sedatives, anaesthetics, ketamine, GHB, inhalants, opioids
- psychostimulants, such as nicotine, caffeine, ephedrine, pseudoephedrine, methamphetamine, amphetamines, cocaine, mephedrone and ecstasy (MDMA), which also has hallucinogenic effects
- hallucinogens, such as lysergic acid diethylamide (LSD), ecstasy, which also has psychostimulant effects, and magic mushrooms (psilocybin)
- THC (cannabis)—in a category of its own due to its multiple effects on mood and cognition including CNS depression, thought and perceptual distortion, mild paranoia and hallucinations.

Regular use of most psychoactive drugs develops tolerance due to the CNS adapting its functions so as to maintain homeostasis. Tolerance requires the person to use increasing amounts/doses to achieve the desired, original effect. Withdrawal can occur with cessation or rapid reduction in amount/dose of the ATOD use. The time of onset and length of the withdrawal symptoms depend on the type, action and half-life of the particular ATOD involved. *Note:* alcohol withdrawal can be life threatening.

ATOD-related problems are global. The World Health Organization (WHO) reports these to be within the top 10 risk factors for ill-health worldwide, with alcohol being the top risk factor for those aged between 15 and 49 years.[5] While harmful, ATOD consumption is preventable; risky use is associated with high rates of morbidity and mortality, representing a significant public and individual health and economic burden. More than 80% of Australians consume alcohol at some time, many from the age of 15 years, and many use prescribed and non-prescribed pharmaceuticals and 'alternative' medicine.[2] In Australia, the median age of illicit drug users has risen from 29 in 2001 to 34 in 2019, with recent drug use increasing for those in their 40s, 50s, 60s and older.[2]

The daily smoking rate has declined between 2016 and 2019, with a long-term decreasing trend in tobacco use.[2] There has been an increase in the use of 'roll-your-own' and e-cigarette use, as a proportion of those who smoke. According to the 2019 National Drug Strategy Household Survey of 22,274 Australians (over the age of 14) from households all across Australia:[2]

> ... since 1991, the proportion of daily smokers has more than halved while the proportion never taking up smoking has increased (from 49% in 1991 to 63% in 2019). The proportion of ex-smokers has remained fairly stable over this period and did not change between 2016 and 2019 (23%). In 2019, 11.0% of people aged 14 and over smoked daily (Table 2.1), declining from 12.2% in 2016. This equates to a reduction of about 100,000 daily smokers over the 3 years (from about 2.4 million to 2.3 million Australians).

Therefore, although tobacco use has declined over time, its longer-term health consequences are still impacting on continuing smokers, new smokers and those who have smoked.

The proportion of the population aged 14 or older who consumed alcohol at a level that puts their health at risk (see Box 40.1) shows a small decline between 2016 and 2019, continuing the trend of declining risky drinking since 2009:[2]

> In the case of lifetime risk, 17.2% of people in 2016, and 16.8% of people in 2019 drank more than 2 drinks per day on average, corresponding to 3.4 million people in 2016 and 3.5 million in 2019 ... The proportion of people drinking more than 4 drinks in 1 sitting at least monthly was about 1 in 4 in 2016 and 2019, representing around 5.1 million people in 2016 and 5.2 million in 2019.

According to the same 2019 survey, alcohol remains second to tobacco for morbidity and mortality, with 6355 deaths attributed. Drinking at risky levels has been stable over recent years, but approximately 1 in 6 drinkers have placed themselves or others at risk of harm while under the influence, typically by driving, and more than 1 in 5 people were victims of an alcohol-related incident (verbal or physical abuse) in 2019. Most (43%) alcohol consumption occurs on Fridays and Saturdays, with notable differences between males and females; males consuming more alcohol on average. There are also differences in age

BOX 40.1 GUIDELINES FOR RISKY DRINKING[6]

GUIDELINE 1: ADULTS

To reduce the risk of harm from alcohol-related disease or injury, healthy men and women should drink no more than 10 standard drinks a week and no more than 4 standard drinks on any one day.

GUIDELINE 2: CHILDREN AND PEOPLE UNDER 18 YEARS OF AGE

To reduce the risk of injury and other harms to health, children and people under 18 years of age should not drink alcohol.

GUIDELINE 3: WOMEN WHO ARE PREGNANT OR BREASTFEEDING

A. To prevent harm from alcohol to their unborn child, women who are pregnant or planning a pregnancy should not drink alcohol.

B. For women who are breastfeeding, not drinking alcohol is safest for their baby

groups, with those over 70 more likely to consume alcohol daily, and those in their 40s and 50s more likely to consume at risky levels.[2]

The risk of alcohol-related death or injury for healthy adult men and women is below 1 in 100 if they consume fewer than 10 standard drinks each week, i.e. up to two 10-gram beverages (10 to 20 grams of pure alcohol), and no more than 4 standard drinks on any one day.[6] There is no level of alcohol consumption that is without risk, but consumption above these levels significantly increases the risks of short- and longer-term alcohol-related injury, illness and death. This risk is greater for those 18–25 or over 60, or who have concurrent physical or mental health conditions.[6] Alcohol-related injury and illnesses greatly impact on ambulance, emergency units, hospitals and healthcare services.[7]

There has been a recent increase in the use of illicit drugs, alongside a decrease in non-medicinal use of pharmaceuticals (e.g. analgesics, opioids, anxiolytics), perhaps associated with the ban on OTC codeine in Australia. Legal and socially sanctioned drugs (e.g. tobacco and alcohol) are those most likely to cause serious injury, acute and chronic medical conditions, and death, to more people than those using illicit drugs (e.g. meth/amphetamines and heroin). They are also associated with more deaths and health problems overall.[2,6,8]

There are related, significant social and economic costs to individuals and the wider community from non-medical use of all psychoactive substances. It is estimated that the global burden is greater than 20 million years of 'healthy' life lost per annum;[1] approximately 300,000 in Australia.[9] Financial costs to the economies of Australia and Aotearoa New Zealand have been estimated at several billion dollars per annum.[9]

Harmful ATOD use seriously affects individuals, families, communities and healthcare systems. An Aotearoa New Zealand study[10] revealed that the average annual cost of harm per dependent user was $184,000 for meth/amphetamines and $9900 for cannabinoids in 2016, while for alcohol, 1 in 8 reported experiencing a harmful effect on their friendships, home life, finances, study, employment, capacity to learn, or had legal problems.[11,12]

Amphetamine use has fluctuated over the past decade, with present figures suggesting highest use among those in their 20s.[2] This is in the context of decreasing overall use of methamphetamines, but a high proportion of risky use with more frequent and injected use and availability of high purity crystal methamphetamine.[2,13,14] Clinicians at the 'frontline' report that they regularly encounter people acutely affected by methamphetamine and amphetamines:[3,14,15]

> the most common principal drug of concern in the middle age groups: almost 2 in 5 clients aged 30–39 (38%) and 3 in 10 clients aged 20–29 (31%) received treatment for amphetamines as a principal drug of concern.

This group was much more likely to report being diagnosed or treated for a mental illness than those who did not use illicit substances.[2,14,16] In 2021 the Australian Institute of Health and Welfare (AIHW) reported that tobacco, alcohol and illicit drug use accounted for 16.5% of the total burden of disease and injury in Australia in 2019.[3] The number of alcohol-related emergency department (ED) presentations in Australia has remained the same from 2016 to 2019 at approximately 1 in 8, while a decrease from 1 in 4 to 1 in 6 has been observed in Aotearoa New Zealand EDs.[14] Alcohol is a major contributor to premature death and hospitalisation, particularly for people in the lowest socio-economic group[8] and young people, who are more likely than older drinkers to undertake risky or anti-social behaviour consequent to alcohol use, and who may suffer adverse brain development leading to alcohol-related problems in later life. Alcohol-related presentations to the ED are more likely to be younger and male, to arrive by ambulance or police, and to require immediate treatment.[17]

UNDERSTANDING ATOD PROBLEMS

Humans have used psychoactive substances for thousands of years. It should be stated that ATOD use always serves a purpose, no matter how risky or harmful. For example, ATOD use may serve ceremonial, medicinal, social or personal purposes. Each person's ATOD experience, and any associated problems, is always influenced by the dynamic interrelationship between the:

- environment in which the use occurs
- type of drug and its effects; and
- the individual's physical and psychological characteristics, personal history, life experiences and cultural beliefs.

All staff involved in healthcare delivery need to have an understanding of how a particular patient's life context and history, mental health, physical health, family and socio-economic situation may influence their current pattern of ATOD use, and related health issues. For example, a person may have only used a particular drug once or they may use regularly. It should be considered whether a person has been living in an unsafe or violent family situation. Has the person been sexually or otherwise abused as a child or in their adult lives? Often, but not exclusively, people with substance-use issues have poor life opportunities and experiences.

TERMINOLOGY

As with any health condition, stigmatising language can impact the quality of care. Negative terms such as alcoholic or drug addict do not aid in treatment engagement and are therefore counterproductive. Professional language used to describe ATOD problems should therefore be framed in a health context that reflects the nature of the actual problem and related disorder or diagnosis.[18,19] It is important that all emergency clinicians, wherever they practise, use objective, accurate terms to describe a person's actual ATOD problem, and do not use stereotypical language or incorrect terms. Well-described conditions reliably convey a relevant diagnosis and related problems. For example, 'intoxication and short-term risk' and 'regular excessive use and long-term risk' are preferable to vague terms such as 'alcoholism'. It is important to refer to people as the 'person', 'client' or 'patient', which humanises them and their problem.[19] The terminology currently recommended in describing ATOD use is listed in Box 40.2.

SPECTRUM OF ATOD PROBLEMS

As well as understanding the dynamic interrelationship between the drug, the person and their environment, we must also understand that there is no 'one-size-fits-all' single ATOD-related problem.[19,21] Rather, there is a spectrum of varying health and social problems. For some, these problems may be a single episode and never repeated. For others, the problems may be sporadic and occur from time to time. For yet others, their issues may be complex and more enduring. A person may vary their pattern of use according to circumstance, and be at risk of different problems over their lifetime. They may move in and out of various patterns of use, or cease ATOD use at some stage.[22] A minority of people develop complex co-existing mental illness (comorbidity) involving ATOD dependence and mental illnesses. They can be stabilised if consistently offered integrated assessment and treatment and social support. Many, typically if untreated or undertreated, frequently relapse and have general and mental health complications requiring emergency care.[9,22] Comorbidity is a complex enduring condition.[23–25]

Take the case of a young person seriously injured while intoxicated with amphetamines (speed). He did not resume any amphetamine use once he had recovered. When he was older, in response to the grief of losing his best friend, he started binge-drinking, which quickly accelerated to daily drinking and dependence. His alcohol dependence was relatively short-lived, as he sought counselling and was assisted in working through his grief. He stopped drinking for 6 months as advised by his general practitioner. He did resume drinking later on, but within low-risk levels as a healthy adult male.

Fig. 40.1 illustrates how such problems may manifest, be interlinked, and can resolve. A useful way to conceptualise this is via Thorley's model, which describes three overlapping areas of drug use, discussed below.[26]

Depending on the nature and problems associated with a patient's ATOD use, and whether or not they want to have information or further assistance, an appropriate aftercare plan is required. This may include health information regarding ATOD use; information on access to local health and community services; and where to seek specialist services if needed. Offer the patient and/or their family up-to-date written material and phone numbers where they can get reliable ATOD information and advice.

BOX 40.2 TERMINOLOGY OF VARIOUS PATTERNS OF ATOD USE[19]

EXPERIMENTAL DRINKING OR DRUG USE

Drinking alcohol or another drug for the first time to experience the effects, or consuming unfamiliar types of alcoholic drinks or using other drugs. The person's experience of experimental drinking often determines whether or not they decide to drink again, or what type of alcohol they are likely to prefer. This pattern of drinking may be at low risk, or high risk to acute intoxication.

SOCIAL AND RECREATIONAL DRINKING OR DRUG USE

Drinking or using a drug to enhance personal pleasure in a social setting, and at levels which may or may not have harmful results. This term implies that the person is not dependent on the alcohol or other drug used.

INTOXICATION

Results from the acute pharmacological action of psychoactive drugs on the brain, in which the chemical (alcohol or other drug) changes brain function, perception and mood. The level of intoxication increases with *dose over time* (amount of drinks or drug consumed in a session), resulting in increasing levels of physical and behavioural changes and diminishing capacity.

RISKY DRINKING OR DRUG USE

Drinking or using a drug at a level and frequency that increases the short-term risk of harm to health and safety, for example, injuries or overdose from acute intoxication, such as can happen from experimental or occasional use; binge-drinking or binge drug use. If the person regularly drinks alcohol or uses drugs at a risky level, this is also referred to as *regular excessive use*.

HIGH-RISK DRINKING OR DRUG USE

Drinking or using a drug at a level and frequency that will cause harm to longer-term health, for example, physical (e.g. heart, liver or pancreatic disease) and mental health problems, such as suicidal thoughts, depression, anxiety and/or sleep disturbances. High-risk drinking or drug use often has serious adverse family and social consequences. Again, this pattern of drinking is also referred to as *regular excessive use*.

SYMPTOMATIC DRINKING OR DRUG USE

Drinking to change or reduce unpleasant feelings, pain, thoughts or experiences, or to avoid certain situations or responsibilities. The person may drink to get a feeling of emotional or physical numbness or temporary happiness.

TOLERANCE

Alcohol or other drug tolerance occurs after a person has regularly consumed a psychoactive substance such as alcohol, and higher amounts of alcohol are then required to produce the same feelings of intoxication. The National Health and Medical Research Council (NHMRC) explains this as:

> The immediate effects of alcohol on the brain are often less apparent in people who drink regularly, as they acquire a degree of tolerance. Tolerance occurs in part because the liver becomes more efficient at breaking down alcohol. The person learns to cope with, and compensate for, the deficits induced by alcohol.[6]

FIGURE 40.1 SPECTRUM AND RELATIONSHIP OF ATOD USE[20,26]

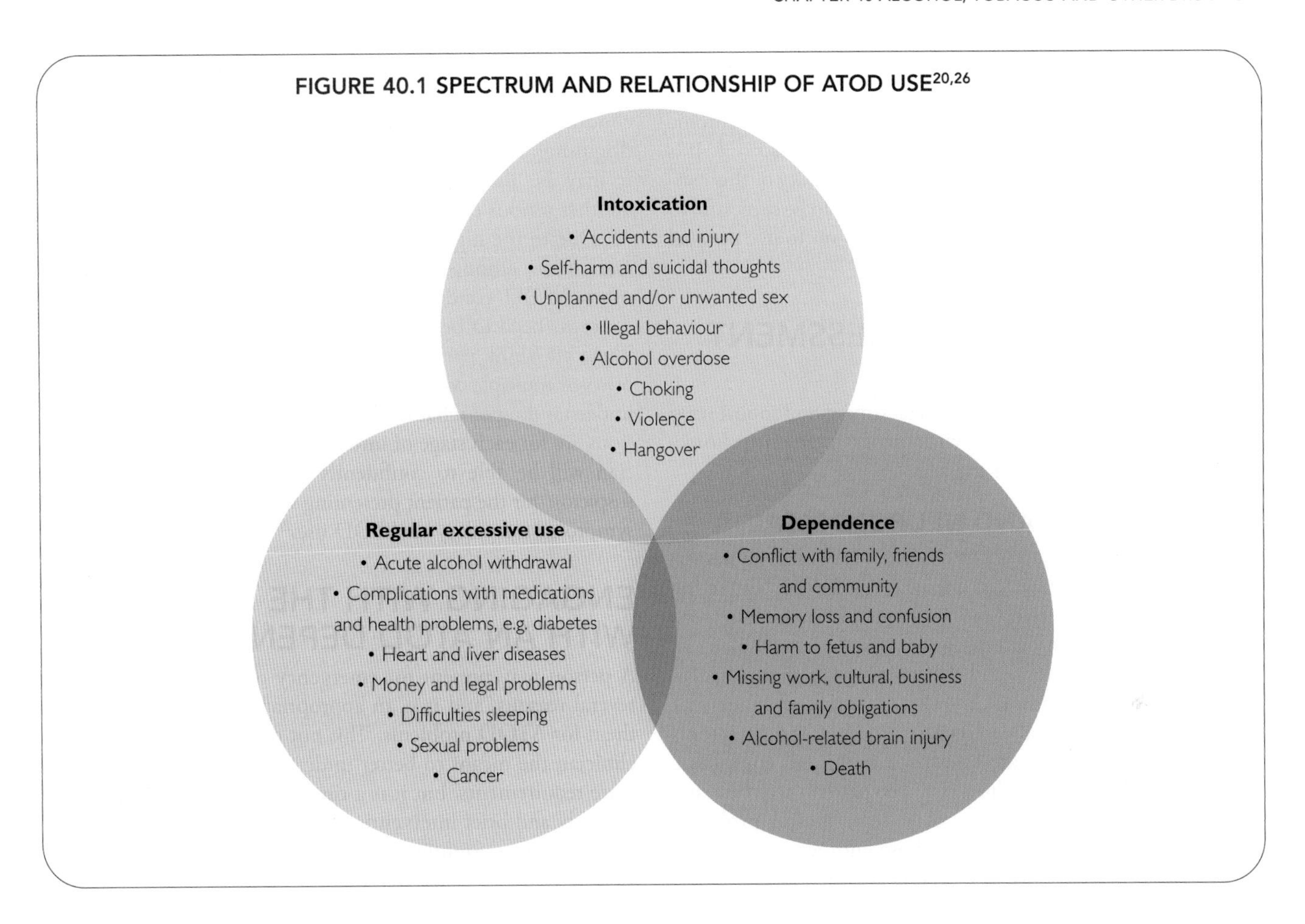

ATOD PRESENTATIONS

Intoxication

Intoxication is the acute action of psychoactive substances on the CNS (brain). The level of intoxication is according to dose and duration of continued consumption.[6,20,27] Intoxication may be a 'once-off' event, occasional or frequent. Intoxication can impact seriously on people's health, safety and social and personal situations. Importantly, the mood-altering effect and diminished cognitive capacity of an intoxicated person may place them at risk of self-harm, suicide or violence. Drug interactions may occur from concurrent use of other psychoactive drugs (poly-drug use). Accidental overdose may occur due to the ATOD itself.

Regular excessive use

Regular excessive use is the impact of regular excessive consumption of alcohol or another psychoactive substance such as a benzodiazepine or opioid; in other words, 'too much too often' but not at reliant levels (dependence). This has risks for both their short-term health and their longer-term health.[6,20,27] While the person will not be psychologically dependent, they may have become physically tolerant (neuro-adapted) to the drug or alcohol. They need to consume more to feel the original intoxicating effects.

Tolerance

Tolerance is the response of the brain (central nervous system, CNS) to ensure that all normal brain functions are maintained in the presence of regular effects of a psychoactive drug such as a depressant like alcohol. The brain adapts to the regular amount of alcohol or drug in the body. The person may experience social or health problems associated with their ATOD use, such as financial problems, family or work problems, hypertension, heart disease, pancreatic or liver disease, hepatitis C, memory and other cognitive problems, injury or cancer, and so on.[20,21,27]

Dependence

What we mean by *dependence* is when a person is physically tolerant to, and psychologically dependent on (addicted to), the ATOD they are using.[21] The following characteristics are common in people who are ATOD-dependent—the person:

- uses more of the drug than they intend to
- has made several unsuccessful attempts to cut down or control their use
- spends most of their time acquiring and using the drug—giving up or reducing time spent doing other important things (work, friends or family)
- continues to use despite knowing that there are associated medical, psychological or financial problems associated with using
- acquires physical tolerance (i.e. needs more of the drug to achieve the same effect)
- experiences psychological or physical withdrawal (often both) when they reduce or stop using the drug.

People who are dependent generally require medical, psychological and social support based on a comprehensive physical and mental health assessment, integrated comorbidity management as required and intensive multidisciplinary interventions. This approach is required to assist them in managing this chronic condition, and its social and emotional consequences.[20,21,27] It is important to understand that despite the complexity of this condition, many people experiencing dependence can be successful in overcoming their ATOD dependence and go on to live optimal lives.[28]

ATOD EMERGENCY ASSESSMENT AND SCREENING

Careful overall physical and ATOD assessment and monitoring are required, regardless of the environment, whether in a home, public place, in transit, or at the ED.

PHYSIOLOGICAL AND NEUROLOGICAL

Alcohol (or what seems to be) intoxication is commonly associated with trauma and serious medical conditions. Detecting whether alcohol is present, and subsequently measuring concentration, is critical in discerning the apparent effect. This can assist differential diagnosis and determining whether intoxication is the single condition, or if there is a risk of concurrent injury, toxicity or medical emergency.[29,30] Signs and symptoms related to ATOD effects are known to cause and complicate injuries and many serious illnesses.[27] The patient may be experiencing any one of a number of serious clinical problems associated with ATOD use, such as those outlined in Box 40.3.

The effects of frequently used ATOD are listed in Table 40.1. As with the assessment and management of any patients, first and foremost is safety of staff and patients, particularly regarding patients who exhibit challenging behaviours such as aggression. Useful strategies to minimise risk are outlined in Box 40.4.

ATOD screening and assessment are crucial to making an accurate diagnosis and deciding on and delivering safe and appropriate care.[32–35] It is very important for emergency clinicians to feel confident and competent in identifying and intervening effectively in these patients' acute ATOD problems according to the context of care delivery. Clinical manuals are often available and provide useful guidance.[35,36] Some diagnoses can be masked or confused by the presence of intoxication or withdrawal. This can lead to medical problems being wrongly diagnosed or overlooked. Examples of such problems are summarised in Box 40.5.

BOX 40.3 SERIOUS PROBLEMS ASSOCIATED WITH ATOD USE[9,20,23]

- Head or other serious injury
- Acute intoxication
- Complications from alcohol withdrawal
- Infection
- Overdose
- Psychosis
- Acute illness
- Unstable chronic illness
- Cognitive impairment

It is therefore very important to remember that what *may appear* to be an ATOD presentation *may not be.* It could be a condition that mimics intoxication or withdrawal and yet be disguising an acute injury or medical condition. Alternatively, it may be that intoxication or withdrawal is complicating another serious condition.[37]

Due to the high and frequent occurrence of serious injury and illness among people presenting with intoxication and other ATOD conditions to the emergency setting, two key concepts need to be kept in the forefront of clinicians' minds. These are 'think pathology first' and consider the possibility of other or multiple co-existing diagnoses. Through developing an understanding of what the behavioural and physical manifestations are for each stage of intoxication or withdrawal, the clinician will be able to confidently develop a clinical 'index of suspicion' for the patient presenting with behavioural or physical symptoms secondary to ATOD use.[20,21,27]

ENGAGING WITH THE PATIENT WITH AN ATOD DEPENDENCE

A person may present for emergency or unscheduled care for several reasons, and it is an appropriate opportunity to screen them for ATOD problems. This not only offers the emergency clinician the means to better understand their patient's immediate requirements, but it is a timely opportunity to provide:

- early and brief intervention
- access to community services
- referral to specialist treatment if needed.

This is as important for this patient as it is for a patient with any other serious health problem. All of these activities can be delivered quickly, with little difficulty and to good effect by emergency clinicians. These are not time-consuming and can be implemented while attending to the patient's general healthcare requirements. Importantly, they are known to be effective.[20,30,32,38]

Showing concern about how you may help the person will increase the likelihood of their engagement with the conversation about their recent ATOD intake and current concerns. It is of primary importance to be aware of your own beliefs about people's ATOD use, and to adopt a non-judgemental manner.[19] Patients need to be assured that this is usual practice for all patients, as ATOD use is a genuine health issue. Similarly, patients need to understand that in order to provide optimal care it is important to know what ATODs they use, and any problems related to this.[28,30]

Opening questions can be as simple as:

- 'Can you tell me if you currently use alcohol, tobacco or other drugs?'
- 'Can you tell me what you have been taking recently?'
- 'Was there anything different about what you chose to take today?'
- 'Can you tell me what you have taken today?'
- 'What time did you last take your alcohol, tobacco or other drug/s?'

It is essential that the questioning be empathetic in tone. Emergency clinicians want to help the patient by understanding the patient's circumstances and accurately assessing their needs. An interrogative tone by staff may result in the patient becoming defensive and evasive and in turn will give an inaccurate

TABLE 40.1 EFFECTS OF FREQUENTLY ABUSED SUBSTANCES[21,31]

SUBSTANCE	PHYSIOLOGICAL AND PSYCHOLOGICAL EFFECTS	EFFECTS OF OVERDOSE	WITHDRAWAL SYMPTOMS
Stimulants			
Nicotine	Increased arousal and alertness; performance enhancement; increased heart rate, cardiac output and blood pressure; cutaneous vasoconstriction; fine tremor, decreased appetite; antidiuretic effect; increased gastric motility	Rare: nausea, abdominal pain, diarrhoea, vomiting, dizziness, weakness, confusion, decreased respirations, seizures, death from respiratory failure	Craving, restlessness, depression, hyperirritability, headache, insomnia, decreased blood pressure and heart rate, increased appetite
Cocaine Amphetamines: amphetamine, chlorphentermine, dextroamphetamine, methamphetamine, methylphenidate	Euphoria, grandiosity, mood swings, hyperactivity, hyper-alertness, restlessness, anorexia, insomnia, hypertension, tachycardia, marked vasoconstriction, tremor, dysrhythmias, seizures, sexual arousal, dilated pupils, diaphoresis	Agitation; increased temperature, pulse, respiratory rate, blood pressure; cardiac dysrhythmias, myocardial infarction, hallucinations, seizures, possible death	Severe craving, severely depressed mood, exhaustion, prolonged sleep, apathy, irritability, disorientation
Caffeine	Mood elevation, increased alertness, nervousness, jitteriness, irritability, insomnia; increased respirations, heart rate and force of myocardial contraction; relaxation of smooth muscle, diuresis	Rare: hyperstimulation, nervousness, confusion, psychomotor agitation, anxiety, dizziness, tinnitus, muscle twitching, elevated blood pressure, tachycardia, extrasystoles, increased respiratory rate	Headache, irritability, drowsiness, fatigue
Depressants			
Alcohol Sedative-hypnotics: barbiturates: phenobarbitone, pentobarbitone benzodiazepines: diazepam, alprazolam non-barbiturates-non-benzodiazepines: chloral hydrate zolpidem zopiclone	Initial relaxation, emotional lability, decreased inhibitions, drowsiness, lack of coordination, impaired judgement, slurred speech, hypotension, bradycardia, bradypnoea, constricted pupils	Shallow respirations; cold, clammy skin; weak, rapid pulse; hyporeflexia, coma, possible death	Anxiety, agitation, insomnia, diaphoresis, tremors, delirium, seizures, possible death
Opioids			
Heroin Morphine Opium Codeine Fentanyl Hydromorphone Dextropropoxyphene Pentazocine Pethidine Oxycodone Methadone	Analgesia, euphoria, drowsiness, detachment from environment, relaxation, constricted pupils, constipation, nausea, decreased respiratory rate, slurred speech, impaired judgement, decreased sexual and aggressive drives	Slow, shallow respirations; clammy skin; constricted pupils; coma; possible death	Watery eyes, dilated pupils, runny nose, yawning, tremors, pain, chills, fever, diaphoresis, nausea, vomiting, diarrhoea, abdominal cramps

Continued

TABLE 40.1 EFFECTS OF FREQUENTLY ABUSED SUBSTANCES—cont'd

SUBSTANCE	PHYSIOLOGICAL AND PSYCHOLOGICAL EFFECTS	EFFECTS OF OVERDOSE	WITHDRAWAL SYMPTOMS
Cannabis			
Marijuana Hashish	Relaxation, euphoria, lack of motivation, slowed time sensation, sexual arousal, abrupt mood changes, impaired memory and attention, impaired judgement, reddened eyes, dry mouth, lack of coordination, tachycardia, increased appetite	Fatigue, paranoia, panic reactions, hallucinogen-like psychotic states	Mild, rare insomnia, hyperactivity
Hallucinogens			
Lysergic acid diethylamide (LSD) Psilocybin (mushrooms) Dimethyltryptamine (DMT) Diethyltryptamine (DET) 3,4-Methylenedioxy-methamphetamine (MDMA) Mescaline (peyote) Phencyclidine (PCP)	Perceptual distortions, hallucinations, delusions (PCP), depersonalisation, heightened sensory perception, euphoria, mood swings, suspiciousness, panic, impaired judgement, increased body temperature, hypertension, flushed face, tremor, dilated pupils, constricted pupils (PCP), nystagmus (PCP), violence (PCP)	Prolonged effects and episodes, anxiety, panic, confusion, blurred vision, increases in blood pressure and temperature	None
Inhalants			
Aerosol propellants Fluorinated hydrocarbons Nitrous oxide (in deodorants, hair spray, pesticide, whipped cream spray, spray paint, cookware coating products) Solvents (petrol, kerosene, nail polish remover, typewriter correction fluid, cleaning solutions, lighter fluid, paint, paint thinner, glue) Anaesthetic agents (nitrous oxide, chloroform) Nitrates (amyl nitrate, butyl nitrate)	Euphoria, decreased inhibitions, giddiness, slurred speech, illusions, drowsiness, clouded sensorium, tinnitus, nystagmus, dysrhythmias, cough, nausea, vomiting, diarrhoea, irritation to eyes, nose, mouth	Anxiety, respiratory depression, cardiac dysrhythmias, loss of consciousness, sudden death	None

history.[27] However, it should be recognised that the highly pressured and time-constrained out-of-hospital and ED environments might provide challenges to a consistently empathetic approach.

SCREENING FOR RISK

The first step to identifying the patient who is at risk from immediate or longer-term ATOD problems is to screen for patterns of use and risk of harm. To do this well, it is necessary to use valid, reliable screening instruments that are easy to use and not time-consuming. The result of a screening is an assessment of the patient's ATOD history and its impact on their current condition and overall health.[27,30,32,34] This forms the basis of a good diagnosis and informs which interventions may be required immediately, as well as longer-term strategies. While the emergency phase of care is usually very busy, it is necessary to remember the immediate and life-threatening risks a patient may present with. The screening process is not prolonged. However, the emergency clinician may feel they do not have enough time because of competing demands and may have difficulty maintaining patient focus. Nonetheless, screening is necessary for:

- duty of care of the patient
- making an accurate diagnosis of the current problem
- raising patients' awareness of risky practices
- longer-term benefits through referral and support mechanisms.

BOX 40.4 CLINICAL TIPS FOR THE ANGRY OR AGGRESSIVE INTOXICATED PATIENT[20]

Remember: your safety comes first. Try to:

- work in pairs
- stand slightly side-on, at least half an arm's length away, and with your feet slightly apart
- use space for self-protection—ensure that you have easy access to the open door
- give them space too—do not crowd them; keep furniture between yourself and them if feeling unsafe, etc
- speak in a calm, reassuring way
- avoid raising your voice. Keep your own emotions in check
- avoid challenging or threatening them by your tone of voice, eyes or body language
- let them air their feelings and acknowledge these
- determine the source of their anger and, if possible, alleviate it
- be flexible with their care, within reason
- be aware of workplace policies on preventing and managing aggression
- use available security measures or carry a personal duress alarm.

BOX 40.5 EXAMPLES OF MEDICAL CONDITIONS AT RISK OF BEING MISDIAGNOSED OR OVERLOOKED IN THE PRESENCE OF ATOD INTOXICATION OR WITHDRAWAL[20]

- Head injury
- Stroke
- Infection
- Hypoxia
- Hypoglycaemia
- Other metabolic imbalances
- Liver disease
- Impending overdose
- Adverse drug reaction
- Psychosis

Failure to adequately screen may have lethal consequences. A validated screening tool to identify alcohol, tobacco and other drug risk is the Alcohol, Smoking and Substance Involvement Screening Test (ASSIST).[32,39,40] ASSIST is designed for busy generalist clinicians. It is an easy-to-use questionnaire that takes between 5 and 8 minutes to administer, and from which the patient's score will indicate their level of risk. It screens for risky and high-risk use of alcohol, tobacco, cannabis, cocaine, amphetamines, sedatives, hallucinogens, inhalants and opiates. It also includes a guide for delivery of a brief intervention, which can be applied in any healthcare setting.[20,41]

If screening reveals there is risk due to the person's alcohol consumption or other drug use, they then need to be fully assessed. This involves taking the ATOD-use history in a safe, confidential place with sensitivity towards the patient (and their family). As always, respect for the patient's cultural identity and associated needs is paramount. Risky alcohol consumption may be best assessed using the three questions of the AUDIT-C.[17,42]

ASSESSMENT FOR DIAGNOSIS

Assessment should be carried out in a timely manner. The patient must not be intoxicated, acutely ill or incapacitated. During an unscheduled care episode it may be that their assessment is relatively brief, so as to determine the most pressing risk factors and how these may affect their condition. If time and the patient's condition allows, and depending on the resources available, a more extensive assessment can be undertaken by an emergency clinician, specialist ATOD liaison nurse or medical officer. Importantly, the findings from the ATOD assessment need to be communicated to all clinicians who participate in the patient's care throughout their care episode. This will form the basis of further diagnosis and the type of interventions required for the patient's particular condition. The wider multidisciplinary team may need to undertake more-detailed investigations and utilise specialist input as available.

Further assessment can be undertaken once the patient has been transferred to a ward or other relevant facility. Early referral within the health service or to a community service is important if the patient is likely to have an established or recurrent ATOD concern.

Dependence, with tolerance influencing risk of withdrawal, is a critical issue for ATOD assessment. Similarly, identification of any co-existing mental health or related physical concerns is crucial. Fig. 40.2 offers a systematic way of undertaking the ATOD assessment. If assessment has revealed concerns associated with the person's recent and longer-term ATOD use, then selections of key medical and psychological therapies need to be employed when appropriate.

Taking the ATOD history

When taking a patient's ATOD history, *show the patient you are concerned about their health and drug use without judging or rejecting them*—any substance use, including illicit drug use, is a legitimate health issue, not a moral issue. Again, it is about being aware of your own personal beliefs in order to ensure that you have strategies to combat these. Many patients feel embarrassed and ashamed, and have had bad experiences in the past with healthcare professionals who have refused help or been judgemental.[18,19] Offer high-quality health information about ATOD use for them to take home. Invite them to talk to a professional that you can refer them to. Alternatively, suggest they phone their local alcohol and drug information service (you can give them the phone number or even make the call for them at the time). If the patient is resistant or becomes anxious or angry, do not persist; rephrase the questions, leave the conversation to another time or desist altogether.[20,27] For general assessment guidance, see sources such as a clinical care manual[35] or Section 2.2 in *Alcohol, Tobacco and Other Drugs: Clinical Guidelines for Nurses and Midwives 2012.* For information about accessing validated assessment tools, see Section 4[20] or other examples.[36]

Some specific concerns

Mental health problems

It is important to recognise the need for mental health assessment and psychosocial support. If significant problems exist

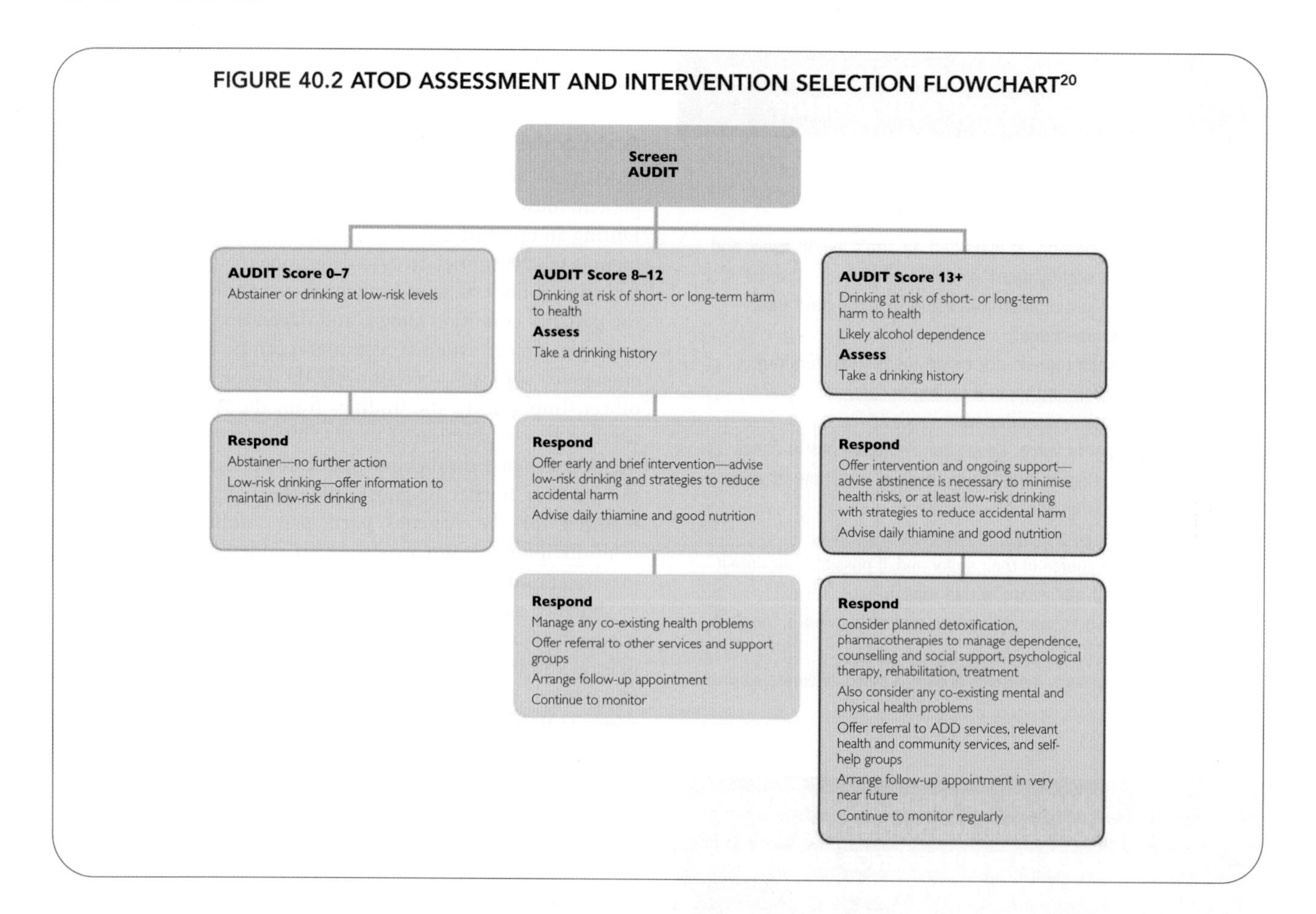

FIGURE 40.2 ATOD ASSESSMENT AND INTERVENTION SELECTION FLOWCHART[20]

at this time, ensure that a comprehensive mental health examination is undertaken once the patient is stable and able to be interviewed.

Transmission of blood-borne viruses

There may be a risk that serious medical complications are associated with the patient's injecting drug use; for example, if they have injected amphetamines or heroin and shared any of the injecting equipment, including needles, syringes, tourniquets, spoons and water when mixing the drug. Any of these items can spread bacterial infections causing septicaemia, cellulitis, endocarditis and pericarditis, and blood-borne viruses, such as human immunodeficiency virus (HIV) and hepatitis B and C. Other serious complications can occur from injecting drugs, including damage to blood vessels at injection sites, abscesses, thromboses, kidney or liver injury, electrolyte abnormalities and dysrhythmias.[20,27]

Physical signs of non-medical injecting drug use and thus risks of viral or bacterial infection include:[20,27]

- abnormal but even pupil size (uneven pupil sizes are associated with serious medical conditions) in association with:
  - puncture marks in cubital fossa, or other accessible veins
  - cellulitis associated with possible injection sites
  - phlebitis associated with possible injection sites.

Concealment of illicit drugs

The process of swallowing or inserting illegal packets of drugs for the purpose of evading detection can be fatal. Individuals engaged in such activities are frequently labelled in the media as 'body packers' or 'mules'. The most frequent cause of death among people concealing drugs is acute drug intoxication, overdose or toxicity from rupture of the package(s) within the gastrointestinal tract.[43,44] People who may have concealed drugs internally are often brought into the ED in the care of police and, less commonly, may seek care directly themselves, because the drugs they have concealed have begun to be absorbed, which is extremely dangerous and likely to cause rapid overdose or toxicity. Heroin, cocaine, methylenedioxymethylamphetamine (MDMA or ecstasy) are drugs known to be concealed during importation or entry to festivals, usually swallowed, or rectally or vaginally inserted in plastic bags, packets or condoms (Fig. 40.3).[2,11,43,45]

The perforation of a concealed package is life threatening. Each patient should be assessed immediately for signs of increasingly acute intoxication (discussed later in the chapter), treated accordingly, observed and monitored closely. Any patient that does not pass a primary survey (ABCD) at any time during their presentation must have the assessment halted and lifesaving measures implemented. These patients should all have an abdominal examination and, where available, a non-contrast abdominal computed tomography (CT) scan. No investigations can be undertaken without their consent. No CT should be performed on a woman who may be pregnant. If there is a possibility that she is pregnant, a beta-hCG (human chorionic gonadotrophin) test should be performed prior to CT to confirm whether or not she is pregnant. CT scans should be reported by an emergency or radiology registrar/consultant

FIGURE 40.3 COMPUTED TOMOGRAPHY SCAN DEMONSTRATING MULTIPLE RADIO-OPAQUE FOREIGN PACKAGES THROUGHOUT THE COLON, MEASURING APPROXIMATELY 1.7 CM × 1.0 CM AND CYLINDRICAL IN SHAPE. THE PATIENT HAD OVER 100 PACKAGES DETECTED

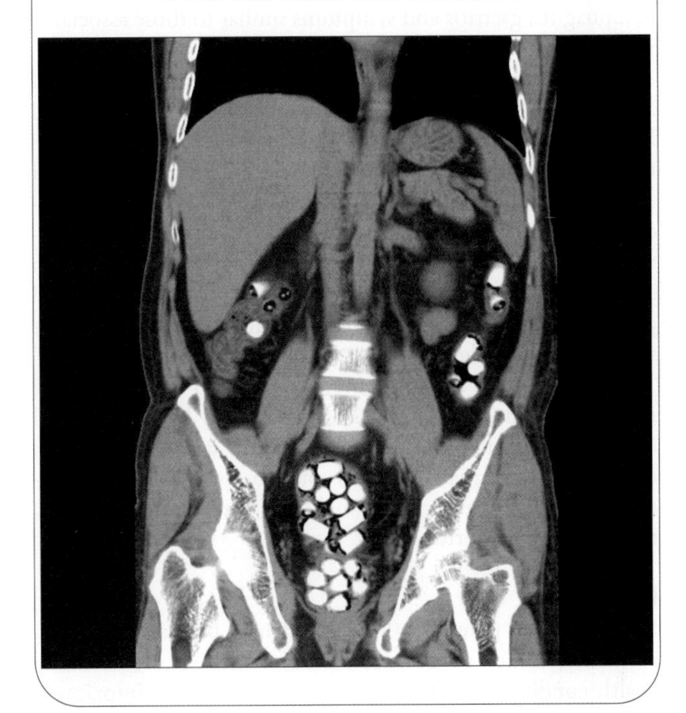

Courtesy Department of Radiology, St George Public Hospital, Sydney.

prior to discharging the patient. If there is a high clinical index of suspicion and the CT findings are equivocal, consent must be gained for an oral liquid bowel evacuation stimulant to be administered. The clinical staff and police (if the patient is in custody) must sight the resulting motions.

If concealment is confirmed, the patient should be observed closely and treated with privacy. Preparation of any applicable antidote or reversal agent for the concealed substance should occur for immediate administration. Continue to observe for signs of drug intoxication and any physical signs and symptoms of overdose. With consent from the patient, an oral liquid bowel preparation solution should be given to accelerate evacuation. Enemas and suppositories should not be used because of the risk of package perforation. If the patient refuses to take the preparation, they should be admitted and observed until all packages are passed. An estimate of the number of packages on initial CT should be made and a check CT carried out to confirm absence of further packages. The patient should remain in hospital until the repeat CT is clear and all packages are accounted for.

ATOD AND MENTAL ILLNESS (COMORBIDITY)

The term comorbidity refers to the co-existing issues of a psychiatric disorder and a substance-use disorder; patients with both are often described as having dual diagnosis.[24,25] Of all those using illicit drugs, around 30% have a co-existing mental health disorder; increasing to 42% in the case of methamphetamine users.[2] It is therefore recognised that people experiencing a serious ATOD problem, particularly dependence, are very likely to experience co-existing mental health conditions (comorbidity).[46] A significant number of these people present in crisis because they are seriously affected by their ATOD use and/or their mental health condition. Most commonly, these are anxiety disorders, particularly post-traumatic stress disorder or depression, and patients are at risk of self-harm or suicide. The less common disorders are psychotic conditions, such as bipolar disorder or schizophrenia. All of these patients require specialist assessment, monitoring and individualised treatment once their crisis is resolved (see Chapter 36, Mental health emergencies). Such patients will respond best if they are assessed and treated using an integrated, shared-care approach involving the medical team, nursing team, specialist ATOD and mental health teams. It is now well recognised that these patients can and will respond better to this combined approach to treatment being delivered simultaneously rather than sequentially, even though the latter still occurs in some areas. It is recognised that trying to treat one disorder before the other is far less effective, and also runs the serious risk of exacerbating relapse and worsening health overall.[20,21,24,25]

Drug-induced psychosis

The acute effects of some psychoactive drugs may induce acute psychosis, which is very likely to resolve, providing no further use of that drug occurs. These drugs are predominantly psychostimulants (e.g. amphetamine, methamphetamine, cocaine), THC (cannabis) and occasionally alcohol.[2,9] Which people are vulnerable to drug-induced psychosis is poorly understood. It may occur with 'once-off' or irregular use, or regular longer-term use. The patient needs to feel safe and protected from self-harm or endangering others. They may experience suicidal ideation.

Duration of drug-induced psychosis

The duration is variable due to the pharmacological properties of the drug and its action on the CNS and half-life. It is important to note that while psychostimulant-induced psychosis can resolve following cessation of psychostimulant use, this may take from days to weeks to fully resolve.[20,47]

Acute medical management

This patient requires pharmacological management typically involving a combination of benzodiazepines and antipsychotics.[27] Pharmacological interventions are usually necessary to adequately assess the patient for their mental health, ATOD and physical health condition/s. They may be detained under the appropriate Mental Health Act (Chapter 36), under which you must practise.

MAJOR ATOD GROUPS

To view the major categories and subgroups of commonly used ATODs within each group, see Section 3 in *Alcohol, Tobacco and Other Drugs: Clinical Guidelines for Nurses and Midwives 2012*[20] or the *Queensland Primary Clinical Care Manual.*[36]

DEPRESSANTS

ALCOHOL

Alcohol is absorbed rapidly across the wall of the small intestine and carried to the brain by the blood. It travels to every organ of the body, having a potentially toxic effect on all physiological systems.[6,20,30] While the rate of absorption is delayed slightly in the presence of food, especially proteins and fats, within only a short time (minutes), it is carried to the brain and intoxicates the person according to the amount consumed. Faster absorption occurs when alcohol is mixed with carbonated liquids. Metabolism of alcohol is predominantly by the liver, and occurs at a rate of about 1 standard drink (10 g of pure alcohol) per hour. This cannot be ameliorated by drinking water, juice, coffee or other means.

The concentration of alcohol in the body can be determined by assessing the breath or blood alcohol concentration (BAC). Alcohol may be measured in the blood within 15–20 minutes of ingestion, peaks in 60–90 minutes and is excreted in 12–24 hours. BAC is affected by the amount consumed, drinking rate, body size and composition, drink concentration, gender and hormones. For the healthy adult drinker who has not developed CNS tolerance, the BAC is generally predictive of the effects of alcohol. Importantly for the emergency clinician, a patient's BAC may still be rising for some time after presentation, depending on when they last drank.[48]

Updated Australian guidelines note that there is a risk of harm with *any* alcohol consumption, and that as consumption increases, so does the risk of negative consequences.[6] Each standard drink above the limits described in these guidelines (Box 4.1) increases the lifetime risk of alcohol-related disease or injury. These risks increase rapidly with greater consumption. Cancer, cardiovascular disease, stomach, pancreatic, liver and kidney disease, blood dyscrasias, osteoporosis, malnutrition, neurological and other serious conditions can all be caused or acutely and chronically exacerbated by alcohol.[6,30]

There is a high likelihood of comorbidity of mental health problems with alcohol dependence, particularly depression and anxiety disorders, as well as a range of serious physical illnesses.[3,9] Alcohol can interact with, or alter the effect of, many OTC and prescribed medications, as well as other drugs.[6,30]

Drugs that interact with alcohol in an additive or synergistic manner include opioids, sedatives, anti-hypertensive drugs, antibiotics, antihistamines, anti-anginal medications and salicylates (aspirin). Alcohol taken with aspirin may cause or exacerbate gastrointestinal (GI) bleeding. Alcohol taken with paracetamol can increase the risk of liver injury. Potentiation and cross-tolerance of alcohol with other CNS depressants is a serious risk when another CNS depressant is taken with alcohol, increasing the depressant effect and possibility of overdose; for example, benzodiazepines and opioids.

Effects

Alcohol has complex effects on the neurons in the brain. It increases the levels of dopamine, and depresses all areas and functions of the CNS. The effects of alcohol are related to the concentration of alcohol consumed (dose), how much is consumed over time and the person's age, gender, health status and individual susceptibility to the drug.[20,27]

High blood ethanol levels are associated with respiratory depression and an increased risk of vomiting and aspiration.[48] Aspiration is the most significant cause of death in non-injury ethanol-related deaths, due mainly to depression of the gag reflex. Ethanol is a vasodilator, especially of cutaneous vessels, partly due to a depressant effect on the central vasomotor centre, but also due to a direct effect on peripheral blood vessels.[27,49] This results in a small reduction in systolic blood pressure and stroke volume and a compensatory increase in heart rate and cardiac output. In addition, as ethanol directly irritates the lining of the oesophagus and stomach and induces vomiting, especially with large ingestion, a Mallory-Weiss tear causing haematemesis may result.[50] Minor effects include oesophagitis, gastritis and symptoms similar to those associated with gastro-oesophageal reflux disease.

The effects of ethanol on the elderly are often multi-factorial and additive. A combination of reduced lean body mass and liver enzyme function, together with decreased gastric motility, may lead to higher blood alcohol levels and an exacerbation of effects. In addition, because of altered pharmacokinetic parameters, especially metabolism and elimination, concurrent pharmacotherapy may be affected, particularly those drugs with a narrow therapeutic window such as digoxin, warfarin and potassium supplements and those relying on renal clearance such as opiate analgesics: for example, codeine.

It is important for emergency clinicians to be aware of the negative organic effects that can be caused by harmful alcohol use and how this may affect the patient's current condition, including differential diagnosis and co-morbidities, and increased risks of complications including toxicity, haemorrhage, thrombosis or hypertension.

Intoxication

Intoxication is potentially lethal and may be associated with accidental injury or overdose. It can also exacerbate many health conditions. When a patient presents in an intoxicated state, it is often not appropriate to try to educate or suggest to them that they stop drinking or offer them complex health information. They are unlikely to be able to understand or remember what you have said. What is important is not to assume they are 'just intoxicated'—*always assume* that there may be an underlying injury or serious medical condition.[6,20] Alcohol intoxication increases the likelihood of head injury, which is the predominant medical risk for intoxicated people and should always be the first consideration when assessing an intoxicated person or someone who appears intoxicated.

The acute effects of alcohol intoxication involve depressed respiration, diminished cough, diminished gag reflexes (potential for aspiration and asphyxiation) and cardiovascular dysfunction inducing various dysrhythmias. As with other depressant drugs, people are also at risk of accidental overdose from excessive alcohol, and there is a strong link between intoxication of alcohol and suicide.[6,30,51] Binge-drinking excessive amounts of alcohol over a brief period of time (hours not days) can lead to sudden cardiac dysrhythmias, shortness of breath, changes in blood pressure and sudden death. Older or frail people have an increased risk of falls and serious injury from drinking even small amounts. They may also experience serious drug interactions if they drink when taking medicines or other substances. Young people who drink to intoxication are often at greater risk because they lack experience and skills in managing drinking and can become very acutely intoxicated, leading to overdose.

Intoxication is evidenced with increasing BAC, increasingly diminished capacity of the person to manage their environment, their mood, behaviour and physical changes. Effects include an initial sense of relaxation, euphoria, loss of inhibitions; then

BOX 40.6 SIGNS OF ALCOHOL INTOXICATION[20,52]

- Positive blood alcohol concentration
- Flushing—dilation of peripheral blood vessels
- Altered cognition
- Inappropriate emotional responses
- Smell of alcohol
- Slurred or incoherent speech
- Mood swings
- Increasing sedation
- Ataxia
- Analgesic effect despite injury/illness
- Altered behaviour
- Decreasing consciousness

impaired judgement, poor concentration and mood swings. For example, a person may transition from elation to depression, possible aggression, irritability and emotional lability. Box 40.6 lists the common signs of alcohol intoxication.

The person who is alcohol-tolerant will have a higher BAC than expected from their observed behaviour, and an apparent lower level of intoxication. That is, they do not seem as intoxicated as one would expect looking at their clinical signs. This explains why some people who are tolerant to alcohol, as evidenced by high BAC (e.g. well over the legal driving limit for adults of 0.05% in Australia and 0.08% in Aotearoa New Zealand), genuinely believe that they are safe to drive or undertake other complex tasks. Also, be aware that an intoxicated person whose first language is not English may revert to their native tongue at this time and therefore have difficulty communicating or understanding instructions.

Fig. 40.4 illustrates the signs according to level of alcohol intoxication as detected by BAC in the non-alcohol-tolerant adult. This can be reliably obtained by blood or breath measurement.[32]

Out-of-hospital and ED management

As with all patients, management includes monitoring and responding appropriately to the patient's vital signs and level of consciousness. Guidelines for the level of observation and intervention for different levels of intoxication are outlined in Table 40.2. Like other depressants, alcohol can cause overdose if a person has consumed high doses over a short period of time. Alcohol-induced CNS depression leads to respiratory and circulatory failure manifested by depressed respirations, hypotension, hypothermia, decreasing level of consciousness and high BAC. This can occur with binge-drinking or drinking alcohol while taking other CNS depressants.

Priorities include maintenance of a patent airway and gas exchange (primary survey—ABCD). Interventions will be dependent on the individual clinician's scope of practice; in the out-of-hospital setting, this is usually achieved with appropriate

FIGURE 40.4 INCREASING BLOOD ALCOHOL CONCENTRATION (BAC) AND ASSOCIATED SIGNS AND SYMPTOMS IN THE NON-DEPENDENT DRINKER[53]

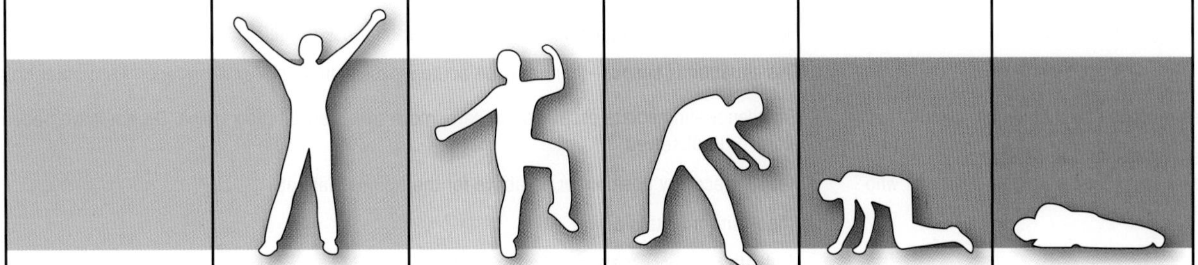

Stages	Feeling of wellbeing	Risky state	Dangerous state	Stupor	Death
Blood alcohol concentration	up to 0.05 g%	0.05–0.08 g%	0.08–0.15 g%	0.15–0.30 g%	over 0.30 g%
Likely effects	• talkative • relaxed • more confident	• attention impaired • judgement and movement impaired • inhibitions reduced	• speech slurred • balance and coordination impaired • reflexes slowed • visual attention impaired • unstable emotions • nausea, vomiting	• unable to walk without help • apathetic, sleepy • laboured breathing • loss of bladder control • possible loss of consciousness	• coma • death

Alcohol Treatment Guidelines for Indigenous Australians from Department of Health and Ageing, 2007.

TABLE 40.2 OBSERVATIONS AND ACTIONS REQUIRED TO CARE FOR THE INTOXICATED PATIENT[20,30]

PATIENT OBSERVATIONS/STATUS	ACTIONS REQUIRED
Opens eyes spontaneously Is orientated Makes appropriate verbal responses Obeys simple commands Stands without support BAC as expected in relation to observed intoxication	Conduct and record vital signs Conduct BAC test and record Conduct and record vital signs Observe hourly for first 3 hours, then 2-hourly if condition does not worsen Follow normal procedures for admission Ensure patient lies in recovery position on very low bed if not requiring spinal immobilisation. If so, have suction readily available and the patient in a very closely supervised area and be ready to log-roll the patient if they feel like or commence vomiting. An antiemetic should be administered prophylactically. Consider a high risk for falls—put bed rails up, assist with walking, follow health service guidelines for patients at high risk of falling Do not offer food or drink until patient has woken, is more sober and alert
Opens eyes spontaneously Is orientated Makes appropriate verbal responses Obeys simple commands Cannot stand without assistance Level of intoxication and BAC as expected	Conduct, monitor and record vital signs, including oxygen saturations and GCS score Conduct BAC test and record Observe no less than every 15 minutes Ensure patient can stand unaided at least 3 hours after admission Ensure patient lies in recovery position on very low bed, or as above for the trauma patient Do not shower or offer food or drink until fully alert and able to stand and walk unaided Follow health service guidelines for patients at high risk of falling Escalate care as appropriate
Opens eyes to simple stimuli (touch, voice) Obeys simple commands Not able to make appropriate answers Is disorientated or behaviour is of concern, particularly if not consistent with BAC	Conduct, monitor and record vital signs, including oxygen saturations and GCS score Conduct BAC test if possible Observe continually—if not possible, no less than every 5 minutes Keep patient in recovery position, or as above for the trauma patient Ensure immediate escalation in care Keep patient on at least half-hourly (30 minutes) observation until they are alert, are able to respond fully and can safely manage their environment Follow health service guidelines for patients at high risk of falling This situation is serious—there may be acute illness, injury and/or intoxication from other drugs
Does not open eyes to simple stimuli Does not respond to painful stimuli and/or is disorientated and unsure of who they are	Emergency—immediate escalation in care, move to a resuscitation space. Do not leave patient alone or unobserved Keep in recovery position, or as above for the trauma patient Check and maintain airway Ventilation as necessary, administer oxygen Commence CPR as necessary Ensure has patent IV cannula

BAC: blood alcohol concentration; CPR: cardiopulmonary resuscitation; GCS: Glasgow Coma Scale; IV: intravenous.

positioning but may include the insertion of supraglottic devices or the insertion of an endotracheal tube; emergency clinicians should be prepared for intubation if required and be proficient in the administration of oxygen. See Chapter 16 for airway management techniques. The establishment of intravenous (IV) access should be considered when possible, as hypotension can usually be corrected with IV fluids. Hypothermia can be corrected with either passive or active warming, dependent upon the available resources. It is essential to conduct a thorough health examination of the physical state, specifically assessing for any signs of injury. Exclude medical conditions other than alcohol intoxication (e.g. head injury, stroke, other drug overdose, hypoglycaemia, psychosis, severe liver disease), using blood tests, x-rays, scans and so on, as appropriate.

The management of the patient with an altered level of consciousness is discussed in Chapter 23. Because of the risk of vomiting and subsequent aspiration, offer ice chips rather than water. IV fluids are required to maintain hydration if the patient is not well enough to drink water safely after 12 hours. The administration of parenteral thiamine is required for those patients considered to be at risk of thiamine deficiency due to poor nutritional status (and this includes those who are regular drinkers). If the patient requires ongoing IV glucose in order to establish normal blood glucose levels, thiamine must be administered in order to prevent Wernicke's encephalopathy. Previously recommendations have been for administration of IV thiamine prior to administration of glucose in order to prevent Wernicke's encephalopathy. There are no clear guidelines in relation to this, and current literature suggests that a single dose of glucose is unlikely to cause this effect. The urgent treatment of hypoglycaemia with glucose should not be delayed in order for thiamine to be administered.[54,55]

Ascertain the patient's mental status (e.g. confusion, suicidal ideation, disorientation, panic, hallucinations, paranoia and psychosis). The intoxicated patient is at an extreme risk of falling: take all precautions to prevent this. For example, lower the bed, put padded bed rails up, do not ever leave them unaccompanied in the toilet, assist them to stand and walk if required and ensure the patient is closely observed. If the patient is to be admitted, emergency clinicians should ensure that regular vital signs are undertaken concurrently once commencement of monitoring with a validated withdrawal chart such as the CIWA-Ar has begun.[20]

It is important to have as accurate information as possible about the amount and frequency of drinking, and particularly *time of the last drink*. Document this clearly in the case notes and handover to team members in the ED and receiving ward. When taking a drinking history, do not accept or use phrases such as 'social drinker' or 'occasional drinker'. If the person cannot give exact amounts initially, ask in a non-judgemental manner questions such as:

- 'How many drinks have you had today?'
- 'What type of container was the alcohol in?'
- 'Is this how much you usually drink in a day?'
- 'How long have you been drinking like this?'

The intoxicated patient may present in various emotional states; Tables 40.2 and 40.3 show how the clinician can best respond and support them, taking into consideration possible risks.[20,27]

Thiamine deficiency: Wernicke's encephalopathy

Thiamine carries glucose across the brain barrier. Chronic alcohol consumption affects thiamine in the body in at least two ways: it decreases the absorption of thiamine from the GI tract and changes the structure of thiamine. The alteration of thiamine molecules prevents their utilisation in the cells. Insufficient thiamine leads to Wernicke's encephalopathy, which is an acute inflammatory haemorrhagic condition of the brain, and an acute medical crisis.

Thiamine (vitamin B_1) deficiency is common in people who are malnourished and/or regularly drink alcohol at high-risk levels. It is precipitated by the intake of glucose by the thiamine-deficient patient.[55,61] *If untreated*, it is likely to cause memory impairment and may lead to Korsakoff's syndrome, a form of amnesia characterised by permanent inability to learn, loss of short-term memory and dementia. In the clinical setting, if diagnosed quickly, accurately and treated appropriately, this condition can resolve. However, there may be some residual cognitive deficits in some patients.

Acute Wernicke's encephalopathy can occur in adult males who drink 80 grams or more of pure alcohol (8 standard drinks) daily or most days, and females or older/frail people who drink 60 grams or more of alcohol daily or most days.[20,61] This condition is largely preventable, requiring 100 mg thiamine daily throughout the person's drinking career.[62]

For acute management of thiamine deficiency and possible onset of encephalopathy, see Section 3 in *Alcohol, Tobacco and Other Drugs: Clinical Guidelines for Nurses and Midwives 2012*.[20]

All patients assessed as being at high risk of alcohol dependence should be examined for ocular abnormalities, including nystagmus (an involuntary eye movement), paralysis of the lateral rectus muscles (muscles of the eye), ataxia (abnormal gait) and a global confusion state. Signs and symptoms are summarised in Box 40.7.

Importantly, symptoms of Wernicke's encephalopathy can be difficult to distinguish from intoxication or withdrawal, and it is potentially reversible.[62]

Patients who drink at the levels cited above or who are withdrawing from alcohol may be hypoglycaemic from poor food intake, malabsorption or excessive vomiting, exacerbating thiamine deficiency.

Concerns related to the timing of thiamine and glucose administration focus on the potential for a glucose dose to utilise all thiamine, thereby precipitating Wernicke's encephalopathy. Recent evidence suggests timing is not as critical as once thought,[55] but, given the potential negative consequences, 100 mg IM or IV thiamine should be administered when considering ongoing glucose products administration.[55] Note that if IV thiamine is administered, there is a risk of anaphylaxis and resuscitation equipment should be available nearby. The person will require at least three 100–200 mg doses of thiamine three times a day for the first 3 days while acutely ill or withdrawing from alcohol, and should then continue with 100 mg oral thiamine daily (plus other essential vitamins and minerals) for the time they continue to drink alcohol.[20,27,55] It is critical to continue monitoring, assessment and intervention as needed until the patient is medically safe.

The patient should be reassured and re-orientated regularly. This patient group is particularly at risk of injury due to poor coordination and impaired judgement, and their safety must be a priority.[20,27]

Alcoholic hallucinosis

Alcohol hallucinosis is rare. It is a cluster of psychotic symptoms that appears during or following a period of heavy alcohol use, but is not due to acute intoxication alone and is not a symptom of the withdrawal syndrome. The disorder is characterised by hallucinations (typically auditory, but often involving other senses), perceptual distortions (usually visual, tactile or auditory), paranoid or other delusions, psychomotor

TABLE 40.3 BEHAVIOURAL STATES AND CARE OF THE INTOXICATED PATIENT[56–60]

PATIENT BEHAVIOUR	CARE
Anxious, agitated, panicky	Ensure close observation and supervision
	Approach them respectfully, calmly and confidently
	Move and speak in an unhurried way
	Ensure a simple, uncluttered environment
	Try to offer a quiet environment
	Provide frequent reassurance, e.g. 'It won't take much longer'
	Remain with them and calm them down
	Explain all interventions in simple, short sentences; repeat if needed
	Protect them from injury. Do not leave them unattended on a chair, in a bathroom or outside
	Consider whether you might need an interpreter
	Enable their family member or friend to sit with them, if possible
Confused or disorientated	Medical review is necessary
	Protect them from injury
	Settle them on a very low bed to prevent injury from falls
	Do not leave unattended
	Undertake frequent observation and close supervision
	Maintain an uncluttered environment; remove unnecessary equipment/furniture
	Do not disturb them unnecessarily once settled
	Provide well-lit surroundings to avoid strange/unusual perceptions
	Use a private area if possible
	Advise and explain to them what you need to do before touching them, when and why this is necessary
	Address them by their preferred name
	Help them to lie on their side in the recovery position
	Enable them to wear their own clothes if possible
	Regularly orientate—explain what is happening and where they are, who you are and your role, what day/time it is
	Use/display object(s) familiar to them such as their possessions they have with them
	Accompany them to any other place, e.g. bathroom
Altered perception and/or hallucinations	Medical review is necessary
	Ensure continual or very frequent observation and close supervision
	Explain perceptual errors; explain to them that they may be seeing things differently due to the acute effects of alcohol
	Continue to protect them from risk of injury
Angry, aggressive	Stand to the side of the patient, at least half an arm's length away
	Make sure you are not positioned in a corner or area that you cannot move from quickly
	Wherever possible, clear the area of other patients and staff not directly involved in the patient's care
	Speak calmly, reassure, use short sentences, be reasonably flexible with requests and actions
	Remind them that you want to help them and keep them safe. Keep your own emotions in check
	Do not challenge or threaten by tone of voice, eyes or posture
	Advise and explain to them before you touch them, when and why this is necessary
	Let them vent their feelings, and acknowledge their feelings
	Check what may be the possible source of anger, e.g. untreated pain, fear, psychosis
	Continue to protect them from injury, however possible
	If you *feel* unsafe, you are unsafe: get assistance and do not approach the patient unless there are skilled staff with you
	Call security

BOX 40.7 SIGNS AND SYMPTOMS OF WERNICKE'S ENCEPHALOPATHY*[21,63]

- Ophthalmoplegia (reduced eye movements or nystagmus)
- Ataxia—unsteady gait
- Acute disorientation
- Neuropathy—altered/lost sensation in extremities
- Confusion
- Poor concentration
- Impaired memory
- Labile mood.

** Wernicke's encephalopathy may co-exist with intoxication and withdrawal.*

disturbances and abnormal affect (ranging from intense fear to ecstasy). The sensorium is usually clear, although some degree of clouding of consciousness may be present. Supportive care and close supervision to prevent injury are the major focus of intervention. This includes withdrawal observations in order to identify and manage symptoms of the withdrawal syndrome that may also emerge.[6,20,27,30,64]

Alcohol withdrawal

Alcohol withdrawal can emerge in people who are physically dependent (tolerant) if they cease or drastically reduce their consumption level. This may have life-threatening effects. While people can experience uncomplicated withdrawal, a significant number will experience serious complications, particularly if injured or otherwise ill.[6,27,30,64] A patient may call for assistance or present for care after trying to 'detox' at home, and be 1 or 2 days into withdrawal with serious complications arising.

Withdrawal is due to the falling BAC and starts between 6 and 12 hours *after the last drink and before the BAC reaches zero*; for example, it may start at 0.1% BAC. This is due to CNS tolerance and neuro-adaptation. The severity of alcohol withdrawal ranges from mild through moderate to severe. It is unpredictable in terms of which person will experience complications, except when it is known that the person has a history of complications such as withdrawal seizures or hallucinations, in which case these are highly likely to recur.[6,27,65]

Signs and symptoms of alcohol withdrawal (Fig. 40.5) occur between 6 and 24 hours after the last drink. The usual course is 5 days, but can be up to 14 days. Further delays in onset may be caused by administration of other CNS depressants; for example, opioid analgesia or anaesthetics.[20,27,66] Symptoms range from mild (nausea, insomnia, mild sweating) to severe (hypertension, hallucinations, fevers, dehydration and electrolyte imbalances). Severe withdrawal may occur within 24 hours or may be delayed until 48 hours or more after the last drink. Alcohol withdrawal seizures account for 10–40% of all adult seizure presentations 6–48 hours after cessation of drinking and the peak is 12–24 hours. In elected or predicted alcohol withdrawal situations early intervention with benzodiazepines can prevent seizure activity.[56,65,67] The presence and severity of each of these symptoms varies with the level of severity of withdrawal. Presence of concomitant illness, infection, injury or other physical trauma and recent surgery increases the likelihood of complicated alcohol withdrawal.

See Box 40.8 for clinical index of suspicion of alcohol withdrawal and Table 40.4 for levels of severity.

Refer to Table 40.4 for the features of alcohol withdrawal; these are characterised as features of mild, moderate or severe withdrawal.

It is important to note that any seizure can be life threatening and all seizures should be investigated to establish a cause. Alcohol withdrawal seizures are preventable in people with a known history by use of prophylactic diazepam-loading regimens.

FIGURE 40.5 PROGRESS OF ALCOHOL WITHDRAWAL FROM TIME OF LAST DRINK[20]

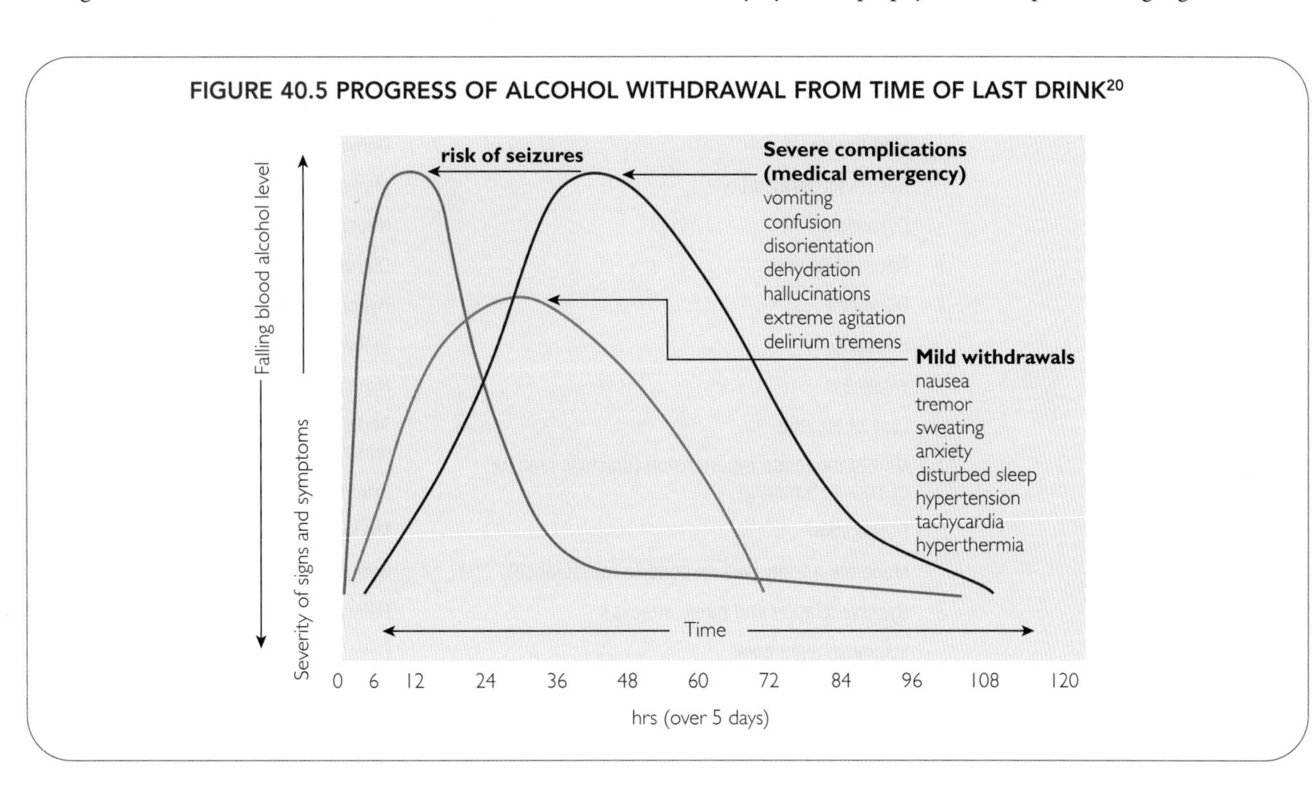

BOX 40.8 CLINICAL INDEX OF SUSPICION OF ALCOHOL WITHDRAWAL[20,56,65]

- History of adult male regularly drinking 80 grams or more (8 standard drinks) over several weeks or more.
- History of adult woman or older/frail person regularly drinking 60 grams (6 standard drinks) or more.
- The person is alcohol dependent.
- Symptoms occur less than 10 days since the last drink.
- Person is regularly drinking even smaller amounts of alcohol with other depressants, e.g. benzodiazepines or opioids.
- Previous episodes of alcohol withdrawal.
- Person has had alcohol withdrawal seizures or other serious symptoms before.
- The current presentation is alcohol related.
- Previous history of an alcohol-related condition (e.g. alcoholic hepatitis, alcoholic cardiomyopathy, pancreatitis, oesophageal varices, liver disease).
- Person's physical appearance indicates excessive drinking, e.g. facial vascularisation, reddened eyes, signs of liver disease (e.g. ascites, jaundice), muscle wasting, spider naevi, palmar erythema, previous injuries.
- Pathology results show raised serum gamma-glutamyl transpeptidase (GGT) and/or raised mean cell volume (MCV).
- Person is displaying or reporting symptoms such as hypertension, anxiety, sleep disturbance, agitation, tremor, sweatiness, nausea/vomiting or retching, possibly due to alcohol withdrawal.

Approximate time of onset of alcohol withdrawal complications after the last drink is:[56,66,67]

- seizures 6–48 hours
- disorientation 48 hours
- confusion 48 hours
- hallucinations 48 hours
- delirium tremens 2–6 days.

Alcohol withdrawal delirium

Alcohol withdrawal delirium (AWD), previously referred to as delirium tremens ('the DTs') is the most serious complication of alcohol withdrawal syndrome and is a *medical emergency*.[27] It usually develops 2–5 days after the last drink, but may occur earlier, or take 7 days to develop.[20,27,66] Dehydration, infection, dysrhythmias, hypotension and kidney failure can be precipitating factors of delirium tremens, which can lead to death in 20% of cases. If recognised and treated effectively, the mortality rate reduces to < 5%. Symptoms include exaggerated features of alcohol withdrawal; autonomic instability (e.g. fluctuations in blood pressure or pulse, may be hypertensive and tachycardic); disturbance of fluid balance and electrolytes; hyperthermia and sweating; extreme agitation, restlessness or disturbed behaviour—this may be to the extent where the person needs restraint or to be detained under the Mental Health Act for their protection; gross tremor; confusion and disorientation; paranoid ideation, typically of delusional intensity; and hallucinations affecting any of the senses, but typically visual (highly coloured, animal form).[65,68] The usual course is 3 days, but can be up to 14 days.

TABLE 40.4 FEATURES OF ALCOHOL WITHDRAWAL[20,27,56,66]

MILD WITHDRAWAL	MODERATE WITHDRAWAL	SEVERE WITHDRAWAL
Mild pyrexia, e.g. 37°C (no infection suspected)	Mild pyrexia, e.g. 37°C (no infection suspected)	Fever
Mild anxiety	Moderate sweating	Excessive sweating
Slight tremor	Mild tremor	Dehydration
Mild sweating	Restlessness/agitation	Marked tremor
Nausea	Dyspepsia	Nausea/vomiting
Vomiting	Nausea/vomiting	Diarrhoea
Mild dehydration	Diarrhoea	Hyperventilation and panic
Headaches	Headache	Tachycardia
Mild hypertension	Weakness	Hypersensitivity to stimulation
Tachycardia	Loss of appetite	Acute anxiety (may/may not respond to reassurance)
Dyspepsia	Mild-to-moderate hypertension (diastolic reading of 100–110 mmHg)	Extreme agitation
Malaise	Dehydration	Moderate/severe hypertension
	Moderate anxiety (will respond to reassurance)	Seizures (see note)
	Hyperventilation and panic attacks	Hallucinations (auditory, tactile, visual)
	Insomnia/nightmares	Disorientation/confusion (time, place)

Note: any seizure can be life threatening. All seizures should be investigated for cause. Alcohol withdrawal seizures are preventable in people with a known history by use of a prophylactic diazepam-loading regimen.

Clinical management of alcohol withdrawal

The most systematic and effective way to monitor and measure the severity of withdrawal is to use a validated and reliable withdrawal scale. A *withdrawal scale is not a diagnostic tool,* but merely guides in the identification and monitoring of symptoms indicative of the severity of the alcohol withdrawal syndrome. Used as a baseline, and then repeated regularly according to severity of symptoms, any changes in the patient's condition are measured and scored over time, assisting diagnosis and prescribing and administering medications—generally diazepam to prevent seizures. Other symptomatic medications may be required to reduce and contain alcohol withdrawal symptoms, and other complications.

The Clinical Institute Withdrawal Assessment for Alcohol—Revised Version (CIWA-Ar)[20,27,66] should be started as soon as the risk of withdrawal is suspected, either before or in the ED. It should be conducted hourly if scoring 8 or above (requires immediate medical examination), or 4-hourly if scoring less than 8. It is useful to include the Glasgow Coma Scale (GCS) score; temperature, pulse and respiration (TPR); and blood pressure assessment on the same case-note form as the CIWA-Ar to allow concurrent monitoring of health status, identifying other problems through objective clinical signs. The CIWA-Ar uses a 10-item scale for assessing and monitoring the clinical course of alcohol withdrawal. The scale allows a quantitative rating from 0 to 7—with a maximum possible score of 67—for withdrawal symptoms.

For more information on alcohol withdrawal management, see Section 3.1.1 in *Alcohol, Tobacco and Other Drugs: Clinical Guidelines for Nurses and Midwives 2012,* and for a CIWA-Ar alcohol withdrawal instrument see Section 4 Appendix 9.[20]

Withdrawal

The goal of treatment is to prevent any complications associated with alcohol withdrawal. Complications are more likely if there is co-existing injury, infection or serious illness. Monitoring, early recognition and effective management of the initial, milder stages of withdrawal are therefore crucial in preventing progression to severe, life-threatening stages. It is important to administer thiamine 100 mg parenterally as soon as possible during ongoing glucose/dextrose supplementation and then three times a day during acute illness and withdrawal. It is also essential to treat any concurrent conditions, and provide withdrawal symptom relief with medication, including antiemetics and analgesics. Hydration and electrolyte balance are critical and intravenous fluids are likely to be required.[20,27,66]

Pharmacological treatment may be required to prevent seizures and combat acute withdrawal symptoms. The most prescribed pharmacological treatment, known to be most effective for alcohol withdrawal, is diazepam. This is because it belongs to the only drug group that prevents alcohol withdrawal seizures, is long-acting and has cross-tolerance with alcohol.

Clinical specialist advice about alcohol withdrawal and recommended medication regimens may be available from specific drug and alcohol services in your area. Emergency clinicians should inform the treating team if dosing is inadequate to control withdrawal symptoms. Haloperidol may be required in addition to diazepam to control symptoms of alcohol withdrawal, especially when psychotic symptoms such as hallucinations or paranoid ideation are pronounced, particularly if they lead to the person exhibiting challenging behaviours such as aggression. Multivitamin and mineral preparations are also required. A daily fluid balance chart should be commenced, and fluids need to be encouraged, as dehydration from sweating, nausea, vomiting and diarrhoea may cause an exacerbation of the withdrawal syndrome. Electrolytes may be monitored as a component of medical management, including magnesium. To access advice on current best-practice alcohol withdrawal management, see relevant references and websites at the end of this chapter.

METHANOL

Methanol, sometimes referred to as wood alcohol, is a common ingredient in many solvents, including paint removers and window cleaners. It is sometimes used as a cheap alternative for alcohol and clusters of systematic substitution have been reported worldwide,[69] including in holiday locations frequented by Australians and New Zealanders.[70]

Effects

Methanol produces inebriation, but its metabolites are toxic with serious effects and high mortality.[69,71,72] Methanol-intoxicated patients often initially present with inebriation and gastritis. In the first few hours after ingestion acidosis is not usually present because of the slow production of the metabolites formaldehyde and formic acid by the enzyme alcohol dehydrogenase, which may take up to 30 hours to appear.[71,73,74] This period may extend if methanol has been consumed concurrently with alcohol, further delaying this metabolic process. After that period, severe metabolic acidosis will occur, with visual disturbances, blindness, seizures and death.

Management

Consistent with other instances of poisoning, the maintenance of airway and breathing are fundamental, with management of seizures or coma if they occur. If recent (30–60 minutes) ingestion can be clearly established, then aspiration of gastric contents may be appropriate. Charcoal or the induction of vomiting are not appropriate. Administration of alcohol (ethanol) will reduce or prevent the conversion of methanol to metabolites. It is a widely adopted initial treatment for cases of acute methanol poisoning as it has greater affinity for alcohol dehydrogenase, thereby blocking the conversion of methanol to formaldehyde.[69,72,73] Another effective antidote is fomepizole (4-methylpyrazole), although availability may be inconsistent.[72,75] Metabolic acidosis may be treated with intravenous sodium bicarbonate, with monitoring of arterial blood gases, and folic acid may also be administered to facilitate the conversion of formate to carbon dioxide and water. Haemodialysis should then proceed to enhance the elimination of both methanol and its metabolites from the system.[69,73]

BENZODIAZEPINES

The benzodiazepine group of sedative–hypnotics, and the similar non-benzodiazepines, known as Z-drugs[76] (collectively often referred to as minor tranquillisers) are commonly prescribed, and may be used problematically.[21,76] Benzodiazepines replaced barbiturates in the late 1980s for medical treatment of anxiety and poor sleep because they are far safer, having a wider therapeutic range than barbiturates, thus reducing the risk of overdose and causing less toxicity.[30,77]

Effects

Benzodiazepines have a general CNS-depressant effect that is dose dependent, and includes decreased anxiety, sedation and anticonvulsant effects. Even after taking therapeutic doses as prescribed, tolerance can develop quickly, even after only 2–3 weeks. Although there is a wide therapeutic margin of safety, rendering them relatively safe, benzodiazepines can have adverse reactions if tolerance has developed. These can include rebound anxiety and insomnia with short-acting benzodiazepines, and confusion and memory loss with longer acting drugs, causing the person to take increasing doses to get the original effect.[20,27,77]

Excessive doses cause initial euphoria; increasing intoxication; impaired cognition, judgement and fine motor coordination; slurred speech; loss of inhibitions and motor coordination; then progression from sedation to hypnosis and then stupor. Benzodiazepines can cause respiratory depression, but this effect is minimal unless other CNS depressants are used concurrently (e.g. alcohol and opioids), whereby a synergistic action may occur resulting in respiratory depression that can be life threatening. In rare cases there may be agitation, hostility and bizarre, uninhibited behaviour.[20,27,77]

These drugs are usually taken orally, but the capsule or tablet form may be injected intravenously, often causing serious vascular injury, cellulitis and tissue damage. Other complications from injecting these drugs include thrombosis, transmission of hepatitis B and C and HIV, and bacterial infections causing abscesses, necrosis, septicaemia and endocarditis.[20]

Overdose

Overdose of a major sedative–hypnotic such as a barbiturate can cause death from respiratory depression. This is far less likely with benzodiazepines than with barbiturates and opioids. Overdose of benzodiazepines is symptomatic and rarely treated with flumazenil, a specific benzodiazepine antagonist, although there is some risk of seizures and a panic-like response in some cases.[78] There are presently no known antagonists to counteract the effects of other sedative–hypnotic drugs. Emergency life-support measures must be taken in cases of overdose.[78] Table 40.5 presents emergency management of CNS depressants.

Withdrawal

If a therapeutic dose is prescribed, and continued for longer than 6 weeks, tolerance, physical dependence and withdrawal on cessation or rapid reduction will affect 15–50% of people. Common, less frequent, and uncommon symptoms of benzodiazepine withdrawal are listed in Box 40.9.

Acute withdrawal can last for up to 6 weeks, and longer-term use may result in withdrawal symptoms lasting from 6 months to 1 year, with intensity of symptoms gradually

TABLE 40.5 EMERGENCY MANAGEMENT OF OVERDOSE OF DEPRESSANT DRUG[30,73,78]

AETIOLOGY	ASSESSMENT FINDINGS	INTERVENTIONS
Ingestion, inhalation or injection of CNS depressants—accidental or intentional	Aggressive behaviour	**Initial**
	Agitation	Ensure patent airway
	Confusion	Anticipate intubation if respiratory distress evident
	Lethargy	Establish IV access
	Stupor	Obtain temperature and other vital signs
	Hallucinations	Obtain 12-lead ECG
	Depression	Obtain information about substance (name, route, when taken, amount)
	Slurred speech	Obtain specific drug levels or comprehensive toxicology screen
	Pinpoint pupils	Obtain a health history including drug use and allergies
	Nystagmus	Establish IV access
	Seizures	Administer antidotes as necessary
	Needle tracks	Perform gastric lavage if necessary
	Cold, clammy skin	Administer activated charcoal and cathartics as appropriate
	Rapid, weak pulse	**Ongoing**
	Slow or rapid shallow respirations	Monitor vital signs, temperature, level of consciousness, oxygen saturation, cardiac rhythm
	Decreased oxygen saturation	
	Hypotension	
	Dysrhythmia	
	ECG changes	
	Cardiac or respiratory arrest	

CNS: central nervous system; ECG: electrocardiogram; IV: intravenous.

BOX 40.9 BENZODIAZEPINE WITHDRAWAL SYMPTOMS[20,78]

COMMON WITHDRAWAL SYMPTOMS

- Anxiety
- Agitation
- Depression
- Insomnia
- Irritability
- Increased muscle tension
- Restlessness
- Poor concentration
- Sweating
- Headache
- Poor memory
- Muscle ache and twitching

LESS-FREQUENT SYMPTOMS

- Nightmares
- Panic attacks
- Decreased appetite
- Increased sensory perception (e.g. metallic taste)
- Gastric upset
- Agoraphobia
- Nausea
- Weight loss
- Palpitations
- Increased temperature
- Feelings of unreality
- Dry retching
- Sweating
- Tremor
- Ataxia
- Depersonalisation
- Light-headedness/dizziness
- Lethargy
- Blurred vision

UNCOMMON SYMPTOMS

- Delusions
- Seizures (more common with concurrent alcohol withdrawal)
- Paranoia
- Persistent tinnitus
- Hallucinations
- Confusion

diminishing. Not everyone will experience symptoms, and of those who do, the symptoms are not always disabling. Use of higher doses is more likely to produce a withdrawal syndrome with more severe symptoms. Withdrawal from short-acting benzodiazepines (e.g. oxazepam, temazepam, alprazolam and lorazepam) typically produces a faster and more severe onset of symptoms than withdrawal from long-acting benzodiazepines (e.g. diazepam and nitrazepam), and may be more difficult to endure.

People can experience withdrawal seizures and other serious complications, and so benzodiazepine use should never be ceased abruptly.[27,78]

Clinical management of benzodiazepine withdrawal

While emergency clinicians may not typically see benzodiazepine withdrawal, onset may occur in the presence of another acute condition if a patient has been ill and unable to access the benzodiazepine or have been trying to withdraw at home and presents with symptoms. If the patient presents for other reasons, their potential for withdrawal needs to be assessed and appropriate observation, monitoring and treatment implemented.

Pharmacological management of benzodiazepine withdrawal typically involves converting to longer-acting diazepam (maximum 80 mg per day) from the average daily dose of their particular benzodiazepine (e.g. a shorter-acting oxazepam). This is with the intent of implementing a gradual diazepam reduction regimen.[20,78] Diazepam is to be used with extreme caution or is contraindicated in certain conditions; for example, chronic airways disease, respiratory failure, liver disease. In such cases a shorter-acting benzodiazepine may be considered.[20,78] Other symptomatic medications can be used to prevent and reduce severity of withdrawal symptoms, providing this is safe in the presence of a current injury or illness.

Regular observations and monitoring are required to identify and effectively treat withdrawal symptoms, and prevent severe withdrawal. There is also the need to provide a safe, non-stimulating and non-judgemental therapeutic environment. Complementary therapies, such as warmth and massage for muscle tension, cramping and aching, can be helpful. The patient requires support and reassurance if they are experiencing any distortion of sensory stimuli.

OPIOIDS

Opioids are either naturally derived such as morphine, codeine and heroin,[57,77] or made synthetically. Opioids are CNS depressants that relieve strong pain.[77] Opioids *decrease spontaneous activity* of neurons in the CNS involving inhibition of adenyl cyclase activity and decrease in cellular concentrations of cyclic adenosine monophosphate (cAMP).[77] This produces the effects listed in Box 40.10.

Intravenous administration causes rapid absorption and CNS effects. Illicit morphine, codeine and heroin are consumed in Australia and Aotearoa New Zealand. As with any illicit drug, it is not possible to determine the dose or purity of heroin, although it is more possible to assess the doses used of

BOX 40.10 EFFECTS OF OPIOIDS[20,57,79]

- Analgesia
- Drowsiness
- Sense of tranquillity
- Sense of detachment from external environment
- Miosis (constriction of pupils)
- Slowed peristalsis
- Constipation
- Orthostatic hypotension
- Slurred speech
- Decreasing consciousness
- Respiratory depression
- In rare cases: delirium
- Respiratory arrest

BOX 40.11 ACUTE EFFECTS OF OPIOID INTOXICATION[20,57]

- Euphoria
- Orthostatic hypotension
- Constricted pupils (miosis)
- Respiratory depression
- Decreased level of consciousness
- In rare cases: delirium
- Constipation
- Appears tranquil

BOX 40.12 SIGNS OF AN OPIOID OVERDOSE[20,57,79,80]

- Increasing drowsiness (may be sudden)
- Decreasing level of consciousness
- Increasingly slowed respiration
- Cyanosis
- Subnormal temperature
- Miosis
- Weak pulse
- Bradycardia
- Pulmonary oedema

the non-medical (illicit) pharmaceutical opioids. In Australia and Aotearoa New Zealand, non-medical use of slow-release morphine and prescription codeine has recently reduced, consequent to the restrictions placed on codeine in 2018.[2] Over the past 20 years, use of illicit opioids has been consistently higher than that of heroin.[2]

Intoxication

The acute clinical manifestations of opioid intoxication are listed in Box 40.11. *Caution:* Opioid intoxication can rapidly progress to overdose, depending on the half-life and dose of opioid and the route of administration.[22,57] Additionally, the person may have also used another depressant, such as alcohol or benzodiazepine, which greatly increases risk.

Tolerance

Daily or almost-daily opioid use results in tolerance, neuroadaptation and lowering of pain threshold, within weeks or months.[79] The resultant hypersensitivity to even mild pain[80] can be problematic and increases the likelihood of continued use in greater doses as the person attempts self-medication. Where there is illness, surgery or injury, poorly assessed and managed pain can result in poor healing and extreme discomfort, and in frequent requests for pain relief, patient distress and possibly angry outbursts and premature self-discharge. This situation is often misinterpreted as drug-seeking behaviour rather than poorly relieved pain.

Pain in the opioid-tolerant patient therefore requires comprehensive assessment and additional pain relief, which may include larger doses of opioids, more-frequent or continuous administration of opioids and patient-controlled analgesia (PCA), possibly boosted by complementary analgesia such as non-steroidal anti-inflammatory medications, paracetamol, ketamine, and/or local block anaesthesia (Chapter 18).

Providing opioid analgesia and combinations of varying medications for analgesia will not make the patient relapse or become more drug dependent.[57,79] In fact, withholding opioids or under-dosing of opioid analgesia will more than likely exacerbate existing drug problems, precipitate relapse and inhibit optimal healing from their current medical condition.[80] Both ambulance paramedics and emergency nurses can play a significant role in ensuring patient comfort and therefore compliance by ensuring that adequate analgesia is administered and that their care is delivered in a non-judgemental manner.[20,81]

Overdose

Accidental overdose is not uncommon and may be associated with use of pharmaceutical opioids or 'street' heroin. It can occur with occasional use whereby tolerance is low or in dependent use and higher levels of tolerance. This is typically due to unknown doses or concurrent use of other depressants such as alcohol or benzodiazepines.[57,73]

Overdose is unpredictable due to unknown dose (potency) and purity of 'street' heroin. It can also be unpredictable when pharmaceutical opioids are used for medical or non-medical reasons. It is essential to try and view packaging or ask about what brand/type of opioids, and any other depressants, the person has taken—ideally identify trade name and dose.

Some additional overdose risks:

- Reduction in tolerance after period of abstinence (e.g. following release from prison, discharge from rehabilitation or hospital).
- Leakage and ingestion from packaged illicit heroin trafficking ('body stuffers'/'body packers').[43,44]

Signs of overdose are included in Box 40.12.

Clinical management of overdose

Overdose of opioids is a medical emergency. The patient's airway and oxygenation should be established immediately and a narcotic antagonist such as naloxone should be given as soon as life support is instituted. The patient should be monitored closely because narcotic antagonists have a shorter duration of action (half-life) than most opioids and may need to be re-administered. Because the longer plasma half-life of methadone is 24–48 hours compared with the much shorter half-life of heroin or morphine (2–3 hours), people who overdose from methadone and require emergency treatment with naloxone may seem to recover initially, but can lapse into respiratory depression and coma if not adequately monitored and treated.[20,73]

The effects of methadone or buprenorphine overdose can persist for up to 72 hours, even in cases where people have been resuscitated. Depending on the magnitude of the overdose, they should be closely observed for a period of up to 72 hours, and medical assessment will determine the need for additional naloxone administration.[20,57]

Pharmacological management of opioid overdose

Note that maintenance of airway and breathing are most important in depressant overdose management—follow CPR protocol. See Chapter 16 for a discussion of airway management techniques.

Naloxone (Narcan), an opioid antagonist, is used as a reversal agent and will reverse the effect of opioid overdoses. Following administration of naloxone, people who were previously sedated may become agitated, aggressive and difficult to manage due to sudden precipitated withdrawal syndrome. It is important to titrate the dose of naloxone to ensure the client improves their respiration but does not go into opioid withdrawal. The aim is a state of semi-consciousness with adequate respiration.

If the patient becomes fully conscious they may experience precipitated withdrawal and refuse further care. It is not uncommon practice to administer naloxone IM prior to giving the IV dose in case the patient does experience precipitated withdrawal syndrome and absconds after the IV dose. This strategy improves the wellbeing of the patient following emergency care, but does not guarantee it. The naloxone may still 'wear off', leading to decreased respiration and depressed conscious state due to the long-acting nature of the opioid.

Naloxone is a first-line treatment and should always be given in the case of respiratory depression.[57,73,79] A dose of naloxone may be administered in the community by the intranasal or intra-muscular route, or by an emergency clinician by these routes or the intravenous route. The aim is to use the lowest dose necessary to resolve the respiratory depression, as this is most likely to avoid the occurrence of acute withdrawal.[82,83] Doses vary by route of administration, but are usually 100 mcg IV, 400–800 mcg IM or SC, and 1.6–2 mg IN.[82,84] If respiratory function does not improve, other diagnostic options, such as other drug intoxication or other organic causes of loss of consciousness, including hypoglycaemia or traumatic brain injury, should be considered.[85] Naloxone is a short-acting drug. Therefore, repeated injections or IV infusion may be needed if a longer-acting opiate such as methadone or buprenorphine has been taken.[57,86] Following naloxone administration, patients may seem to recover initially. However, as a consequence of the long half-life of methadone or buprenorphine, patients may then lapse into respiratory depression. Naloxone can be given as a continuous intravenous infusion of 2 mg diluted in a 500 mL IV titrated at a rate determined by the clinical response.

The effects of methadone or buprenorphine overdose can persist for up to 72 hours, even in circumstances where people have been resuscitated. Depending on the magnitude of the overdose, they should be observed for a period of up to 72 hours. For high-dose intoxication, naloxone infusion should be considered.[57,79]

Withdrawal

Opioid withdrawal has a characteristic group of symptoms (syndrome) resulting from sudden cessation or reduction in daily prolonged use of an opioid drug (Box 40.10). People who use opioids regularly can experience a moderate-to-severe withdrawal, which, while distressing, is not life threatening.

Time of onset and intensity of withdrawal is associated with the half-life of the opioid used (Table 40.6).[57,79] Objective and subjective symptoms of opioid withdrawal can be seen in Box 40.13.[20]

Withdrawal from a shorter-acting opioid such as morphine or heroin can begin 4–12 hours after the last dose and last for between 4 and 10 days. Withdrawal from methadone, with its longer half-life, has a later onset, starting 24–48 hours after the last dose and lasting from 10 to 20 or more days. It is important for the clinician to know the half-life of each opioid drug, so as to more accurately predict likely time of onset of symptoms from the time of last dose, likely duration of withdrawal and identifying and effectively managing the withdrawal symptoms.[20,57,79]

Clinical management of withdrawal

Cessation or rapid reduction of opioids will precipitate withdrawal due to tolerance and neuro-adaptation. The opioid withdrawal syndrome has a characteristic group of symptoms ranging from moderate to severe, but these are not life threatening.

Providing a calm, non-stimulating, supportive and safe environment while undertaking adequate monitoring and assessment of withdrawal symptoms, and timely administration of medication and necessary treatments, can ensure the patient manages with fewer risks of complications. It is useful, if possible, to involve the patient in their own assessment, experience and management of severity of their withdrawal symptoms and pain. Considering and respecting the efficacy of their self-report of symptoms, and effectiveness (or not) of their current

TABLE 40.6 SIGNS OF OPIOID WITHDRAWAL[20,57,79]

TYPE OF OPIOID	TIME AFTER LAST DOSE SYMPTOMS APPEAR (HOURS)	DURATION OF WITHDRAWAL SYNDROME (DAYS)
Heroin/morphine	6-12 hours	5-7 days
Pethidine	3-4 hours	4-5 days
Methadone	24-48 hours	10-21 days
Morphine sulfate (e.g. Kapanol, Contin) (intravenously)	8-24 hours	7-10 days
Codeine (orally)	8-24 hours	5-10 days
Buprenorphine, naloxone	Variable, but generally around 48 hours	Can be prolonged, as with methadone, generally 10-14 days
Tramadol	12-20 hours	7 days or longer

BOX 40.13 OBJECTIVE AND SUBJECTIVE SYMPTOMS OF OPIOID WITHDRAWAL[20,57]

- Lacrimation
- Rhinorrhoea
- Yawning
- Sweating
- Piloerection
- Hot and cold flushes
- Mydriasis
- Tremor
- Restlessness
- Anxiety
- Muscle twitches
- Nausea/vomiting
- Abdominal cramps
- Muscle and joint aches
- Craving
- Hypertension

treatment, can greatly assist in reducing any anxiety they may have about being under-medicated or not believed.[20,27]

Buprenorphine is the preferred prescribed medication for a significant number of people experiencing opioid withdrawal symptoms (unless there is a risk of contraindications). It comes in sublingual tablets or film that dissolve under the tongue in about 5 minutes, and is absorbed directly through the lining of the mouth into the bloodstream. Crushing the tablets does not seem to have much impact on absorption. If it is swallowed whole, most of the drug will be metabolised by the liver before reaching the general circulation, and is therefore ineffective. The therapeutic effect lasts from 1 to 2 days.[57,79,80]

Symptomatic medications should be provided to relieve symptoms such as nausea, painful muscle cramps, diarrhoea, etc.

Naltrexone as well as opioid withdrawal

The possibility of naltrexone-precipitated withdrawal should be considered if a patient presents with signs of opioid withdrawal in conjunction with *delirium or intractable vomiting*. If the patient has a recent history of opioid dependence, they need to be carefully assessed, examined for signs of self-administered naltrexone or other drug use and questioned about the time of their last dose/use, particularly of opioids. An absence of track marks should not exclude this diagnosis.

The administration of an opioid agonist such as naltrexone is unhelpful, and patients should be warned that taking heroin or other opioids would not alleviate their symptoms. Antagonist-induced withdrawal is extremely traumatic, and the patient should be given appropriate nursing care and repeated assurance.

Treatment is therapeutically supportive based on symptoms.[57,79,80] The most important part of management is reassurance that symptoms, although severe, will be short-lived. There is a risk of delirium and agitation for approximately 4 hours with naltrexone-precipitated withdrawal. Symptomatic medications are likely to be required to relieve discomfort and anxiety.

Pharmacotherapy for opioid-dependent patients in a general hospital

If a patient is already receiving opioid-dependence treatment with prescribed methadone, buprenorphine or combined buprenorphine and naltrexone, their *usual prescribed dose must be continued* during their stay in the ED and if admitted to hospital. This is to maintain their pharmacotherapy regimen and ensure psychological and physical stability. This regimen will prevent withdrawal, *but will not* provide pain relief. It is important that the emergency clinician identify and communicate this to the medical team, especially as this patient will experience hypersensitivity to pain, particularly after-hours, so that arrangements can be made to obtain their usual pharmacotherapy medications, and that appropriate pain relief is also prescribed and administered. The continuation of the prescribed pharmacotherapy is essential to maintain the patient's regimen, prevent relapse and any other complications and ensure their maximum comfort and safety. Importantly, this will also influence effectiveness of pain management and healing.[57,80,81]

For more information on pain management for opioid-tolerant people, see Section 3.1.3 in *Alcohol, Tobacco and Other Drugs: Clinical Guidelines for Nurses and Midwives 2012*.[20]

SOLVENTS

Solvents (inhalants or volatile substances) include gases (e.g. nitrous oxide) and highly volatile compounds or mixtures of compounds; for example, petrol, paint, aerosols (anti-perspirants, flyspray, hydrocarbon-based adhesives and lighter fluid).[74,87,88] These products vaporise causing a 'high' feeling when inhaled. The commonly used term 'sniffing' relates to nasal or oral inhalation. It may be inhaled from a plastic bag or pre-soaked cloth or directly from a container; for example, a product container, soft drink can or drink bottle.[88,89]

How much has been used?

Quantification of solvent use is extremely difficult. Ask about and record the type of solvent used, and the frequency, quantity, date and time of last use. It may be possible to ask the patient why they are using this, any positives and negatives of use and if they intend to continue or stop use at this stage. Medical and social assessment should be undertaken, and health monitored to ensure physical and mental health is supported even if sniffing continues. There is a common perception that inhalant use is an exclusively 'Aboriginal' issue, which *is not the case*. Youths and adults of many cultural and socioeconomic backgrounds are known to have used inhalants.[90]

Effects

Solvent intoxication resembles alcohol intoxication. Onset of action is very quick, with CNS impairment generally clearing within a few hours of inhalation. High doses can cause coma and death. People may harm themselves (accidentally or intentionally) or become aggressive due to the intoxicating and hallucinating effects.[87–89]

While individual components of various compounds may differ, the overall effect of most solvents is CNS depression. People may experience acute problems associated with inhalant-induced malnutrition caused by the appetite-suppressant effects. Solvents induce respiratory depression and cardiac dysrhythmias, which can be fatal, with '*sudden sniffing death*' being recorded.[87-89] Sudden death can also result if the person is startled, such as when another person approaches and tries to remove the inhalant container from them.[88] Very high doses can result in convulsions and hallucinations and delusions can occur. Repeated use can result in, for example, rash and excoriation around the nose and mouth; weight loss and malnutrition due to lost appetite; respiratory problems; liver injury.[87] There can be serious injury to the nervous system, causing brain injury with cognitive and neurological disabilities. Some people may recover while others remain permanently disabled.[87] Self-harm may occur accidentally or intentionally.

Note: Removal of lead from all petrol has reduced the devastating impact from lead on short- and longer-term health; however, inhaling petrol is still dangerous. In some remote Australian communities, low aromatic fuel (LAF or OPAL) has replaced other petrol with success.[91,92] A story about this approach from the community perspective can be viewed on YouTube.[93]

For more information on the acute effects of solvent inhalants, see Section 3.5.2 in *Alcohol, Tobacco and Other Drugs: Clinical Guidelines for Nurses and Midwives 2012*.[20]

CANNABIS

Delta 9 tetra hydrocannabinol (THC) is the active ingredient that causes the psychoactive effects of cannabis. It is difficult to classify THC in cannabis due to its mixture of mood, cognitive, motor and perceptual effects. It therefore does not clearly belong to any particular class of drugs, and is presented here separately.[1,94]

THC effects include: perceptual changes, which can include frank hallucinations, psychomotor changes with slowed reaction time, distance judgement and impaired coordination, cognitive impairment with sedation, slowed thinking, difficulty concentrating and impaired memory. Toxicity, tolerance, withdrawal and psychosis can occur. Psychosis may co-exist or be triggered by cannabis (THC) use in some individuals.[95]

EFFECTS

At low-to-moderate doses, THC produces fewer immediate physiological and psychological effects than other classes of psychoactive drugs, including alcohol. Although its mechanism of action is uncertain and multi-faceted, THC affects dopamine and other neurotransmitter activity and a variety of receptors in the brain. When smoked, THC rapidly enters the bloodstream with plasma concentrations peaking within 30 minutes and effects lasting for up to 4 hours. If ingested, onset is about an hour and effects are milder, often experienced in waves.[95,96]

The psychoactive (intoxicating) effects of THC comprise a combination of stimulation and depression in low doses and, for some people, hallucinogenic and depressant effects in high doses. It can cause a slight increase in heart rate to about 20 beats/minute above baseline. Because it is stored in body fat, it is eliminated slowly, resulting in a half-life of 2–7 days. Its metabolites can be measured in blood or urine and are inactive, merely confirming that cannabis has been used at some time recently (e.g. in the last few weeks), and this does not confirm or refute intoxication.[96]

For more information on cannabis (THC) acute effects and withdrawal, see Section 3.2 in *Alcohol, Tobacco and Other Drugs: Clinical Guidelines for Nurses and Midwives 2012*.[20] See also Table 40.1 for the effects of frequently abused substances and a list of cannabis withdrawal symptoms.

PSYCHOSTIMULANTS

A range of symptoms and behaviours are associated with psychostimulant intoxication. These can vary in intensity according to people's individual differences and the actual drug consumed. Some useful tips for the clinician are given in Boxes 40.14 and 40.15. Psychostimulants are substances that increase CNS arousal and are typically sympathomimetics, acting like noradrenaline to increase cardiovascular tone and activity.[58] There are several types of psychostimulants: amphetamine-type stimulants; MDMA; cocaine; mephedrone and synthetic stimulants.[16,58,97,98] The clinical team should have a high degree of suspicion of acute intoxication from a psychostimulant in any patient who has dilated pupils, tachycardia, agitation, hyperactivity, fever and/or behavioural abnormalities. The possibility of cocaine or other psychostimulant use should be considered in a young person with unexplained myocardial ischaemia or infarction, dysrhythmias, myocarditis or dilated cardiomyopathy.[16,97,98]

BOX 40.14 CLINICAL TIPS FOR INTERACTING WITH THE PSYCHOSTIMULANT-INTOXICATED PATIENT[20]

GENERALLY

- Wherever possible, provide a quiet environment to reduce unnecessary CNS stimulation.
- Approach the patient in a quiet, calm and confident manner.
- Move and speak in an unhurried way.
- Introduce yourself and explain to them your role and what you are doing.
- Use their proper name when speaking to them.
- Remain with the person to calm them if anxious or frightened.
- Stand beside them rather than face to face.
- Control your body language so you do not appear aggressive or intrusive.
- Minimise how many clinicians are attending to them and minimise physical contact
- Reassure the person frequently (e.g. 'It won't take much longer', 'I am just going to do ... because ...').
- Explain any interventions needed, no matter how simple—such as moving the pillow, taking their TPR (explain what you mean by 'TPR').
- Protect them from injury, e.g. do not leave them unattended or on a bed without safeguards; lower the bed as close to the floor as possible.
- Brief and frequent attendances can reassure them that they are being cared for and prevent unnecessary agitation.

CONFUSION/DISORIENTATION

- Explain in simple terms what is happening.
- Provide frequent reality orientation.
- Reduce amount of unnecessary equipment and furniture nearby.
- Reduce amount of unnecessary noise.
- Display familiar objects for the person, e.g. personal belongings.
- Ensure frequent observation and close supervision.
- Accompany them to and from places (e.g. bathroom, lounge, x-ray).

ALTERED PERCEPTION AND HALLUCINATIONS

- Explain their perceptual errors; tell them that you understand what is happening but what is real (e.g. that the curtain does not have snakes on it).
- Provide care for them in well-lit surroundings to avoid perceptual ambiguities from poor light.

BOX 40.15 PHASES OF PSYCHOSTIMULANT CESSATION[20,21,59]

PHASE I—CRASH

The 'crash' (hangover) following cessation of psychostimulant use such as amphetamines begins about 9 hours after the last dose, and can last up to 2 days. This may be associated with a binge, and may or may not progress to the phase II withdrawal.

Crash symptoms include:

- extreme lethargy
- hunger
- formication
- headache
- anxiety
- insomnia
- irritability
- agitation
- aggression
- confusion
- mood lability.

PHASE II—WITHDRAWAL

If neuro-adaptation and dependence have developed, the crash will be followed by the second phase–withdrawal. This will be associated with a period of normal moods, little craving for the drug and normal sleep pattern for 1–4 days. However, dysphoria and craving for the drug then start to increase again, in conjunction with:

- flattened mood
- disturbed sleep
- agitation
- anxiety
- lack of energy.

Possible aggressive outbursts may return, and delusional (paranoid) thinking with hallucinations may occur. Craving for the drug can be intense.

PHASE III—EXTINCTION (PROLONGED WITHDRAWAL)

'Extinction' of withdrawal is characterised by gradual diminishing of the acute symptoms, and may last for weeks or several months. There can be episodic craving in response to environmental stimuli (cues) to use, and a feeling of anhedonia (inability to respond to pleasant events). The frequency of craving and the anhedonia does decrease over time, but likelihood of relapse is high.

For detailed information see Section 3 in *Alcohol, Tobacco and Other Drugs: Clinical Guidelines for Nurses and Midwives 2012*.[20]

COMMON PSYCHOSTIMULANTS

NICOTINE

Nicotine is a short-acting psychostimulant that results in rapid development of tolerance and physical dependence after a short period of use.[99] The CNS stimulation occurs for a short time, then reduces quickly, resulting in withdrawal and craving. Smoking one nicotine cigarette immediately raises blood pressure and heart rate, and decreases blood flow to body extremities and brain. It is important for the clinician to understand the acute physiological effects of nicotine and nicotine withdrawal, as they will alter the patient's physiological and psychological response to illness and create numerous risk factors for others. Note that nicotine consumption is measured by the strength in milligrams, and actual number of cigarettes smoked per day (not the number of packets).

Withdrawal management

A patient who is dependent on nicotine and requires long-distance retrieval or is in hospital will experience withdrawal symptoms because they have had to stop smoking. They will require clinical intervention and support during their retrieval or admission, and for in-patients this may be a time when they actually consider giving up, or, if they have relapsed, restarting their cessation program. Nicotine withdrawal starts 1–2 hours after the last cigarette and peaks at between 24 and 72 hours, due to the short half-life of nicotine. While not life threatening, it is characterised by distressing symptoms, including increased tension and agitation, disturbed sleep, muscle spasm, headache and loss of concentration (Table 40.1).

Acute nicotine withdrawal is associated with craving, which often leads to relapse.[99] The patient needs support and self-help information and should be put in touch with the Quitline free telephone support line as soon as they are able. They may wish to use nicotine replacement patches or gum as pharmacological assistance in managing their withdrawal while in acute care, and later for gradual cessation (if it is medically safe to administer). A combination of nicotine replacement therapies (NRTs) in the form of patches, spray or nicotine gum or lozenges decreases withdrawal symptoms more than any single NRT alone.[20,99] Emergency clinicians are ideally situated to help patients consider giving up smoking. Educating them about NRTs and how to use them (e.g. patches, gum and nasal spray), and how to contact the local QUIT service to get support, can boost their potential for success.[20,100]

It is *very important* to assess for immediate and longer-term harms associated with psychostimulants, including risk of withdrawal. People may present having been on a 3- or 4-day binge of any of these psychostimulants. If this occurs regularly, it is very likely that they have become tolerant and will experience withdrawal.

Onset and duration of acute effects

Amphetamine

- Onset of action when taken orally is about 30–60 minutes, with peak cardiovascular effect at 60 minutes and CNS effects at about 2 hours.[59,101]
- Duration of effect is about 4–6 hours. Intra-nasal intake (snorting) produces effects within a few minutes; smoking and intravenous use produces even faster effects.[59,101]

Ecstasy (MDMA) *also hallucinogenic*[97,102]

- Onset of action when taken orally is 30–60 minutes, with peak effect at 90 minutes.
- Duration of effect is about 4–6 hours.

Cocaine

- Cocaine is a powerful psychostimulant on the CNS derived from the coca plant. This action on the brain

BOX 40.16 SYMPTOMS OF COCAINE INTOXICATION[20,101]

- Pupils may be enlarged
- Increased BP and TPR
- Dry mouth
- Suppressed appetite
- Hyper-alertness and level of activity
- Pressured speech
- Increased self-confidence
- Euphoria
- Exhilaration
- Rapid mood swings
- Repetitious behaviour
- Panic
- Inability to sleep
- Paranoia
- Aggression
- Dysphoria and delirium.

BP: blood pressure; TPR: temperature, pulse and respiratory rate.

reward system magnifies pleasure and can quickly lead to tolerance and dependence.

- Cocaine increases levels of dopamine in the brain, producing euphoria and increasing energy and alertness.
- Onset of action when snorted is within minutes. When 'crack' is inhaled or cocaine is taken intravenously, action is within seconds.
- There is an immediate and marked 'rush' that is highly pleasurable with heightened cognitive awareness, energy and euphoria lasting for about 30 minutes.
- Rapidly diminished effects due to short half-life.
- There may be an interaction between alcohol and cocaine that extends the effect period of cocaine, albeit with lower potency.[59,101]
- Symptoms of cocaine intoxication are outlined in Box 40.16.

Withdrawal

Repeated binges over a time-frame of weeks can lead to marked tolerance, neuro-adaptation and physical dependence, and withdrawal on cessation or rapid reduction. In the first 9 hours to 14 days after the last cocaine use there is extreme exhaustion, hunger, a strong need to sleep, strong craving, marked agitation and mood swings, which may extend to serious depression and suicidal ideation. The three-phase pattern of cocaine withdrawal is very similar to amphetamine withdrawal.[59,103]

For more information on cocaine see Section 3.3.3 in *Alcohol, Tobacco and Other Drugs: Clinical Guidelines for Nurses and Midwives 2012*.[20]

AMPHETAMINES

Amphetamine is a synthetic psychoactive drug that stimulates the CNS, peripheral nervous systems and cardiovascular system. Peripherally, amphetamines stimulate the release of noradrenaline from stores in adrenergic nerve terminals, as well as directly stimulating adrenaline receptors. Centrally, amphetamines have a stimulating effect on several cortical centres including the cerebral cortex, medullary respiratory centre and reticular activating system. Amphetamines slow down catecholamine metabolism by inhibiting monoamine oxidase. The sum total of these effects can result in a clinical state of vasoconstriction, hypertension and tachycardia associated with hyperactivity and agitation.[14,101,104] There are medically prescribed psychostimulants for treatment of narcolepsy, attention deficit disorders and serious weight control, as well as illicit amphetamines.

Amphetamine (speed) and methamphetamine ('crystal', 'ice', and in Australia also referred to as 'speed'[105]) are illegal and are in increasing demand and availability worldwide.

Toxicity

Acute toxicity may be manifested by cardiac palpitations, tachycardia, increased respiratory rate and fever. At high levels of overdose, seizures, hypertension and dysrhythmias or myocardial ischaemia can occur. The patient experiences restlessness, paranoia, agitated delirium, confusion and repetitive stereotyped behaviours. Death is usually related to stroke, hyperthermia, fatal dysrhythmias or myocardial infarction.[59,101]

As with any illicit drug, the manufacture of illicit amphetamines lacks quality control, with unknown purity, dose and ingredients resulting in extreme variability in nature, quality and chemical composition of these drugs. These factors place people who use amphetamines at a very real risk of being exposed to lethal adulterants, unknown doses, unpredictable side-effects and toxicity.[59,106]

The acute toxic effects are due to increased stimulation and sympathomimetic activity of the CNS, possibly resulting in a drug-induced psychosis, paranoia, hyperthermia and seizures. The toxic effects are 'an extension of the pharmacological properties of the drug, being determined by dose, route of administration', as well as by the mental state of the person.[59] Without immediate medical intervention, death may occur from dysrhythmia, myocardial infarction, hyperthermia or cerebral haemorrhage (stroke). Any young person presenting with any of these conditions needs to be assessed for acute psychostimulant toxicity.[97]

People who use psychostimulants achieve a hyperarousal state and perceive the stimulus in their environment differently to those around them; they may experience persecutory delusions, feeling hostile and violent towards others, as a response to the intoxicated experience. Panic may result in irrational behaviour, causing harm to self or others.[97]

Amphetamine-induced psychosis may progress to perceptual disturbances, delirium, paranoid delusions and aggressive or violent behaviour, and may be difficult to differentiate from acute paranoid schizophrenia. Psychotic symptoms generally subside soon after the drug use ceases, although some people may experience persistent symptoms for weeks or months.[46]

Chronic toxicity can be manifested by depression, anxiety and panic attacks (suicidal ideation has been reported), nutritional deficits and weight loss. Neuropsychiatric complications include poor concentration and attention, memory impairment, sleep disturbances, hallucinations and flashbacks (vivid sense of reliving the past drug-use experience). Rhinorrhoea, nasal ulcers, epistaxis, sinusitis and perforation of the nasal septum often manifest chronic intranasal use.[59,101]

Complications of amphetamine use

Complications are directly related to the route of administration, rapidity with which the brain is affected, dose and the person's individual vulnerabilities. Chronic cocaine or amphetamine use may lead to impairment of concentration and memory, irritability, mood swings, paranoia and depression. With intranasal use, the nasal septum and mucosa may be damaged, and frequent sniffing and rhinitis are common signs of intranasal use. Smoking of methamphetamine is associated with oral injury, gum disease, tooth decay and poor dental hygiene. Injecting may result in thrombosis, cellulitis, bacterial infections, wound abscess, septicaemia, pericarditis, endocarditis and transmission of bacteria and blood-borne viruses—hepatitis B and C, and HIV.[20]

Psychostimulant-induced psychosis

A psychostimulant-induced psychosis can arise from once-off, occasional or regular use of psychostimulants. This form of psychosis is typically temporary. It generally progresses from paranoid delusions to visual hallucinations of 'snow lights', and tactile hallucinations of 'bugs' crawling under the skin. This drug-induced psychosis will settle with abstinence, usually within days or weeks. The acute phase is treated as for any other psychotic state. As well as good assessment and history-taking, skin excoriations from scratching and needle marks, and elevated blood pressure, heart rate and temperature may help differentiate a stimulant psychosis from other psychoses.[24,46]

When the person presents they may be very agitated, irritable and aggressive. Management involves careful 'first-line' assessment and treatment to ensure they can be safely treated. This may involve sedation or in some cases, physical restraint. Treatment is focused on 'safety first'. Consideration should also be given to whether an underlying pathology is a cause or is exacerbating the severe behavioural change, until excluded.[20,47,97,107]

Note: Physical restraint should be avoided if possible due to the risks of hyperthermia, rhabdomyolysis and renal failure.[24]

Psychostimulant withdrawal

People who are dependent on psychostimulants rarely use 7 days a week, but rather in 'runs' of 3–4 days, due to exhaustion. Nevertheless, tolerance soon develops, and withdrawal occurs with sudden cessation or reduction in amounts used.

Duration of acute withdrawal symptoms is associated with the type of psychostimulant drug used and its half-life, as well as duration of use, amount used and level of tolerance (e.g. 1–4 days for cocaine, up to about 3 weeks for amphetamines). Cessation results in what is often referred to as the immediate phase ('crash'), whereby the person experiences intense CNS-depressant-like symptoms, with a craving for sleep and feelings of exhaustion replacing the craving for the drug.[59,102] Withdrawal from psychostimulants is not life threatening, but severe depression can be a symptom of withdrawal and may lead to suicidal ideation, self-harm and possibly death. People also report subtle muscular aches and pains. Eventually mood can settle, but intense craving for the drug may remain for some time, similar to what happens with nicotine cessation. The three phases of withdrawal and cessation are outlined in Box 40.15.

Clinical management of withdrawal

To date there is little reliable evidence of which prescribed medication regimen is most effective for treating psychostimulant withdrawal. Tailored symptomatic treatment and good nursing care in a supportive and safe environment are essential. The following need to be attended to:

- Observe the person at least 4-hourly.
- Monitor stages of withdrawal and adapt care to changing needs.
- Monitor depressed mood to identify and prevent risk of self-harm.
- Ensure adequate food and fluid intake—expect variations, including hunger or poor appetite.
- Support during angry outbursts.
- Provide self-help information (e.g. *Getting through amphetamine withdrawal* from Turning Point in Victoria).
- Offer tips for coping with cravings, improving sleep, relaxation, coping with mood swings, aches and pains, nutrition and strange thoughts by focusing on the present.[20,59]

METHYLPHENIDATE

Methylphenidate (MPH, e.g. Ritalin) is a centrally acting sympathomimetic psychostimulant. It is prescribed to children and adolescents, and occasionally adults, diagnosed with attention deficit hyperactivity disorder (ADHD). This assists in reducing their overactive, impulsive behaviours and improves concentration. It is also prescribed for people with diagnosed narcolepsy. Some people use illicit MPH and ingest or inject crushed, diluted tablets which places them at risk of systemic toxicity.[73] Methylphenidate tablets are chalky in consistency, and if not filtered well prior to injecting can cause emboli in vessels of the eyes and lungs.

For more information on amphetamines see Section 3.3.2 in *Alcohol, Tobacco and Other Drugs: Clinical Guidelines for Nurses and Midwives 2012*.[20]

Ecstasy—hallucinogenic with psychostimulant effects

Ecstasy is 3,4-methylenedioxymethylamphetamine (MDMA). It is a psychostimulant with hallucinogenic properties that cause pleasant emotional effects, euphoria and increased energy. Illicit production of ecstasy has increased significantly in Australia.[2,3,97]

As with other psychostimulants, MDMA has created concern about the safety of its use because of large variations in quality, and frequent substitution of what is sold as MDMA by other highly toxic drugs. While the chemical process of production is not very complicated for those with the expertise, impurities and poor technical expertise often lead to highly toxic products being sold. Like amphetamine and methamphetamine, MDMA is smuggled in from South-East Asia and elsewhere, as well as produced locally in clandestine 'factories', resulting in large quantities being sold in both Australia and Aotearoa New Zealand.

Effects

As MDMA is related to mescaline and amphetamine, it has hallucinatory and stimulant properties. It induces pleasant emotional effects, euphoria and increased energy, although it is associated with potentially lethal complications such as hyperthermia.[59,97]

Autonomic effects:

- hypertension
- tachycardia
- poor temperature regulation—hyperthermia
- possible toxicity to serotonergic neurons.[63,73]

Quite common emergency MDMA presentations involve people with hyperthermia syndromes (see Chapter 28). MDMA appears to decrease heat loss through constriction of blood vessels near the skin, and possibly through increased heat production by muscles and the brain. These effects may be amplified by dehydration and a poor ability to cool by sweating. MDMA can mask the body's normal thirst and exhaustion responses, particularly if the person is dancing or otherwise physically active for long periods of time without hydration. Because of its effects, MDMA can temporarily reduce the body's ability to regulate core temperature. So in high-temperature surroundings (e.g. clubs) combined with physical exertion, hyperpyrexia can occur when the person cannot stay cool. Sustained hyperpyrexia can lead to rhabdomyolysis (muscle breakdown), which may rapidly progress to kidney failure and death.[59]

While dehydration is undesirable, people can experience water intoxication and hyponatraemia (dilution of the blood causing swelling of the brain) from drinking large amounts of water without salt replacement, causing water retention. There are also cases with no evidence of excessive water consumption, possibly due to MDMA-inducing release of anti-diuretic hormone (vasopressin) by the pituitary gland.[59,101,108]

The use of ecstasy can exacerbate depression and may produce temporary depression as an after-effect for some people. Some people may also experience unexpected mood swings 1 or 2 days after using MDMA. MDMA use can be very dangerous when combined with other drugs (particularly monoamine oxidase inhibitors [MAOIs] and antiretroviral drugs, in particular, ritonavir). Combining MDMA with MAOIs can precipitate a hypertensive crisis.[102]

Clinical management

The clinical management of acute MDMA (ecstasy) intoxication involves immediate treatment of symptoms and any complications as they emerge, as with other psychostimulants. There is some evidence that the drug dantrolene may be useful in the treatment of hyperthermia induced by the use of MDMA, but care needs to be taken in its use.[97,108,110] The clinical management of acute MDMA intoxication involves immediate treatment of symptoms and any complications as they emerge, as with other psychostimulants.

For more information on MDMA see Section 3.4.5 in *Alcohol, Tobacco and Other Drugs: Clinical Guidelines for Nurses and Midwives 2012*.[20]

SOME OTHER DRUGS

GAMMA-HYDROXYBUTYRATE (GHB)

GHB is a depressant neurotransmitter found naturally in the human CNS. GHB is not a true GABA agonist, but it is found naturally in the CNS, where it acts as an inhibitory neurotransmitter. Medical use of GHB as an IV anaesthetic agent in the mid- to late 1960s became unpopular due to its lack of analgesic effect, and risk of large doses causing seizures.[59,101,111]

GHB also has dopaminergic activity, increasing acetylcholine with endogenous opioids.[59,111] More recently, it has been used in the treatment of narcolepsy and alcohol dependence.

GHB is used as a 'street drug' with similar action to benzodiazepines, and known to be highly dose-dependent. It is mainly used for its euphoric effect. In high doses, profound sedation and seizures can occur; the short- and long-term effects of GHB can be seen in Box 40.17.

GHB, and similar agents (gamma-butyrolactone and -butanediol), have been known to be used illicitly. Street names include 'G', 'scoop', 'liquid x' and 'liquid E'. GHB can be masked when added to alcoholic beverages, causing drowsiness and eventual stupefaction at higher doses. It has been known to be used to 'spike' alcoholic drinks by perpetrators intent on sexual assault.[112] GHB is usually ingested as a liquid and is rapidly absorbed by the GI tract, with peak plasma levels occurring within 15–45 minutes. Most GHB is metabolised prior to excretion via the kidneys within 8–10 hours of ingestion.

Due to its rapid absorption and excretion (about 9 hours), it is difficult to gather laboratory evidence in cases of drug-facilitated sexual assault by the time a victim reports the crime.[112,113] It is strongly advised that for anyone presenting to ED with a report of unexplained memory loss and/or signs of sexual assault and alcohol consumption, a urine and/or blood drug screen test is taken as soon as possible (and other necessary forensic evidence) to assist with early diagnosis and medical management and investigation of this crime. The effects of

BOX 40.17 **GHB EFFECTS**[20,59]

LOW DOSE—SHORT-TERM EFFECTS

- A state of euphoria
- Feeling calm, relaxed or tranquil
- Dizziness
- Disinhibition
- Nausea
- Placidity
- Visual disturbance–usually blurred vision
- Hot/cold flushes
- Drowsiness
- Increasingly sociable
- Increased levels of confidence
- Talkative
- Diaphoresis

HIGH DOSE—SHORT-TERM EFFECTS

- Rapid onset drowsiness
- Impaired movement and speech
- Confusion/disorientation
- Vomiting and nausea
- Muscular stiffness
- Short episodes of unconsciousness
- Aggression when stimulated despite being near respiratory arrest
- Uncontrollable twitching (tics)
- Agitation
- Visual disturbances–hallucinations
- Seizures
- Respiratory depression, arrest
- Death

BOX 40.18 GHB OVERDOSE SYMPTOMS[20,73,111]

- Decreased level of consciousness/coma
- Acute delirium
- Severe respiratory depression
- Hypothermia
- Respiratory acidosis
- Vomiting
- Hypotension (occasionally)
- Bradycardia

GHB intoxication are associated with the dose of the substance, and are grouped together as short-term effects (low dose) and short-term effects (high dose) (Box 40.17).[20] The more serious effects are associated with higher doses of GHB.

Overdose

Concurrent use of alcohol or other CNS depressants is common in GHB overdose. Overdose should be considered in any case of unexplained sudden coma, i.e. without any evidence of head injury, intake of coma-inducing drugs or increasing intracranial pressure. People typically regain consciousness spontaneously within 2 hours of ingestion. GHB overdose symptoms are listed in Box 40.18.[59] Recovery from GHB toxicity is normally uneventful, although interim management of airway and respiration may be required. Close observation is always required, as ingestion of GHB can cause rapid onset of CNS and respiratory depression and, in severe cases, coma and death.[59,114,115] Management is supportive and based on symptoms. A recent study of 74 confirmed GHB-related deaths in Australia found a predominance of aspiration and pulmonary oedema, emphasising the priority of airway maintenance.[111]

For more information on GHB go to Section 3.1.5 in *Alcohol, Tobacco and Other Drugs: Clinical Guidelines for Nurses and Midwives 2012*.[20]

KETAMINE

Ketamine is a dissociative anaesthetic with stimulant properties when taken in low doses. Ketamine is mainly used non-medically for its euphoric effect. Ketamine may be swallowed, snorted, smoked or injected, and is often called 'K' or 'Special K'. It has multiple mechanisms of CNS action.[59,101,104]

Onset of action varies with route of administration, and ranges from 30 seconds (IV) to 10–20 minutes (oral). Typical duration of action is 1–3 hours, with a half-life of 3 hours. Potential dangers of ketamine use are drug-induced psychosis, violence, injury and marked psychomotor and cognitive impairment.[59,101,104]

It can produce a range of schizophrenia-like symptoms, including:

- flattened affect
- thought disorders
- depersonalisation
- catatonia.

BOX 40.19 FEATURES OF KETAMINE INTOXICATION[73,101]

- Initial rush
- Nausea and vomiting
- Slurred speech
- Blurred vision
- Numbness and ataxia
- Cardiovascular and respiratory stimulation
- Dissociative 'out-of-body' sensations (flying or floating), detachment from immediate environment
- Muscle rigidity
- Reduced response to pain
- Risk of respiratory collapse and failure
- Feelings of aggression
- Overstimulation
- Temporary paralysis
- Hallucinations
- Euphoria

Intoxication

Symptoms of ketamine intoxication are listed in Box 40.19. Ketamine overdose leads to:

- respiratory depression
- hyperthermia
- seizures—these can occur in people with known seizure disorders (ketamine use may induce or terminate seizures).[59]

For more information on ketamine, see Section 3.5.1 in *Alcohol, Tobacco and Other Drugs: Clinical Guidelines for Nurses and Midwives 2012*.[20]

HALLUCINOGENICS

Hallucinogens (psychedelics) include naturally occurring and synthetic substances. They distort thinking, mood and perception—typically inducing illusions or hallucinations. They are most commonly used 'once-off' or occasionally.

The acute effects of hallucinogens are due to the disrupted interaction between nerve cells and the neurotransmitter serotonin in the CNS. Distributed throughout the brain and spinal cord, the serotonin system is involved in the control of behavioural, perceptual and regulatory systems, including mood, hunger, body temperature, sexual behaviour, muscle control and sensory perception. Under the influence of hallucinogens, people can experience various forms of hallucinations, some of which produce rapid, intense mood swings from euphoria to paranoia and panic.[21,59]

Substances in this category include: lysergic acid diethylamide (LSD), phencyclidine (PCP), psilocybin and datura. These substances are not associated with a significant withdrawal syndrome, although some users report anhedonia and fatigue.[21,59]

Intoxication

Symptoms include:

- altered perception, thought, emotions
- unusual and vivid perception of shapes, colour, sounds
- blurred boundary between self and surroundings

- feeling of detachment
- dizziness
- weakness
- nausea.

For further information on hallucinogenics, see Section 3.4.1 in *Alcohol, Tobacco and Other Drugs: Clinical Guidelines for Nurses and Midwives 2012*.[20]

ANABOLIC ANDROGENIC STEROIDS (AAS)

In Australia and Aotearoa New Zealand AAS substances are available illegally through the 'black' market and on the internet, and are commonly veterinary preparations.[2] AASs can synthesise body tissue and increase muscle mass and promote development of male sexual characteristics.

AASs are synthetically modified derivatives of testosterone available in oral or parenteral form.

People commonly use AAS substances for increased physical stamina, sexual or sporting performance, muscle strength and definition and possibly 'health'.

AASs can be injected intramuscularly and those injecting may not consider that they can be at risk of contracting bacterial or viral infections including HIV and hepatitis B or C.[116]

People using AASs may also use other substances; for example, growth or reproductive hormones, diuretics, beta-2-AASs, thyroxin, insulin, creatinine monohydrate.[117] People seeking the effect of AAS usually prefer the high anabolic effects.

Examples of AAS

- Water-based. Stanazol is rapidly absorbed and more rapidly excreted than oil-based steroids, which may need to be administered twice a week. It is often injected with a 23-gauge or 21-gauge needle, as the powder in suspension can clog a narrower needle.
- Oil-based Deca 50 takes longer to absorb and take effect and has a longer effect than water-based steroids, e.g. between 2 and 3 weeks, although some people may use these more frequently. Oil-based steroids are usually injected with a 25-gauge needle.
- Anapolon 50 tablets are swallowed and the effects are short-acting. These tablets are taken twice a day.
- AAS tablets are associated with more-adverse side-effects due to the pharmacokinetics of the substance during its 'first pass' through the digestive system. This causes the substance to lose some of its potency and can cause liver injury. Some AAS tablets have a coating designed to prevent it from being destroyed by acids in the stomach, and are categorised as C-17 alpha alkylated, and the coating used is also toxic to the liver.[77]

Note: Anapolon may be more toxic than injectable steroids, but this remains unclear.

AAS use—serious risks[116,118,119]

- abscesses, cellulitis, endocarditis etc (blood-borne viruses, bacterial infections)
- tendon or ligament injury
- adenocarcinoma of prostate
- adenocarcinoma of colon
- Wilms tumour
- testicular atrophy
- gynaecomastia in men
- irregularities or cessation of menstruation
- hypokalaemic-induced dysrhythmia (due to concomitant diuretic use)
- hypertension
- oedema
- insulin resistance or impaired glucose tolerance
- diabetes
- increased low-density lipid proteins and decreased high-density lipid proteins
- salt and fluid retention
- cancer of liver, kidneys, prostate
- liver injury, e.g. jaundice, cirrhosis, tumours
- immunological changes
- sleeping difficulties
- acne
- loss of body hair
- aggression
- irritability
- labile mood
- depression
- mania
- psychosis.

AASs are often taken in combination with other substances and may potentiate or enhance the effects of other substances; therefore, it is important when assessing the patient who is using AAS to ensure a complete substance and medication history is gathered in order to anticipate and treat the more serious side-effects. Box 40.20 lists some of the clinical features likely to be noted and their association with other substances and medications.

BOX 40.20 CLINICAL MANIFESTATIONS OF ANABOLIC ANDROGENIC STEROID USE IN COMBINATION WITH OTHER SUBSTANCES[116,118]

AAS AND PSYCHOSTIMULANTS

- Increased body temperature
- Increased heart rate
- Increased blood pressure
- Masked pain
- Increased cardiac pressure resulting in convulsions and cardiac arrest
- Increased aggression
- Euphoria

AAS AND DEPRESSANTS, E.G. BENZODIAZEPINES, OPIATES, ALCOHOL

- Reduced responsiveness to pain

AAS AND DIURETICS

- Increased sodium levels causing fluid retention
- Altered sodium/potassium balance (kidney injury, muscle weakness, cardiac arrest)

AAS AND CLONIDINE

- Increased risk of kidney and liver disease

AAS AND INSULIN

- Risk of insulin-related death

SUMMARY

An awareness and understanding of the physiological and psychological effects of ATOD is essential for all emergency clinicians. It enables clinicians to anticipate and monitor potential complications and deterioration, commence assessment and treatment in the out-of-hospital setting and further assist with assessment, diagnosis and ongoing treatment in the emergency environment. Screening for ATOD use can detect risk factors and potential health problems, and is the first step towards assessment, early intervention and treatment.

High-quality care ensures that the health needs of individual patients are kept to the fore, and the patient is respected, well informed and provided with holistic care. Even in busy emergency environments or during assessment, stabilisation and transportation, clinical management needs to be focused on attending to this patient's immediate needs, and on empowering the person to better manage their own lives. Some people take longer than others to trust healthcare professionals and services, and to change their risky health behaviours, such as poor diet, smoking or risky drinking or drug use. If emergency clinicians can engage the patient and make them feel valued, they may consider taking up a suggestion for follow-up, return for treatment as required and move towards reducing or stopping harmful drinking or drug use.[20,27]

CASE STUDY 1—BRIAN

PART 1

You are a paramedic sent to the rear entrance of a local wine bar, to attend a man who has reportedly fallen and is unable to get up. It is 0200 on a cold winter Sunday morning. On your arrival, Mike, the manager of the wine bar, meets you, and he points you towards a man sitting upright against the fence, and tells you that this is Brian, his business partner. Brian is apparently asleep, with what looks like a handkerchief wrapped around his left hand. It is stained with blood. His shirt is vomit-stained, and he appears to have been incontinent. Brian rouses intermittently and becomes agitated and verbally aggressive. Mike says they finished work just before midnight, and had a 'few drinks' after closing for the night. Mike also tells you that Brian had been drinking steadily throughout the evening, and has probably consumed about 2–3 bottles of red wine. Brian was last seen taking a crate of empty bottles to the bin. Mike heard the sound of breaking bottles, and when he went to investigate found Brian lying among the broken glass. He had tried to stand, but was unable to get to his feet. Brian told Mike that he had slipped and fallen.

QUESTIONS

1. How will you ensure your safety and the safety of others while assessing Brian?
2. How will you assess Brian?
3. What do you think has happened? And why?
4. What would you do first?
5. What interventions and resources would you consider using?

PART 2

Brian allows you to examine him. While thankfully you find no other injuries, the hand laceration is deep. You bandage the wound, knowing that it will require suturing. You tell Brian that he needs to go to hospital. While Brian is not happy, with Mike's help he agrees to go in the ambulance to the hospital.

Brian arrives at the emergency department (ED). You are now the triage nurse. The paramedic gives you a detailed handover and describes his behaviour at the scene. The paramedic explains that once Brian had been loaded into the ambulance he seemed to settle down. The paramedic had also ascertained from Mike that when Brian drinks as he did tonight, he becomes aggressive. He has been drinking heavily for the last month and a half.

Brian appears to be asleep, and is snoring loudly with slow respirations. He is pale and his skin is cool. He has a weak radial pulse and is tachycardic. When you attempt to rouse him, he opens his eyes to painful stimuli only. He has a dressing on his left hand and smells strongly of alcohol. He rouses temporarily and tries to sit on the side of the wheeled hospital trolley bed.

6. What are treatment priorities of care for Brian?
7. Where is the most appropriate place for Brian to be nursed in the ED?
8. What interventions and resources might you anticipate using during Brian's stay in the ED?
9. Are there any other conditions that could mimic Brian's condition and behaviour? How would you assess for these?
10. What observations and interventions will Brian require?

11. Assuming that Brian is medically cleared and his hand sutured, what discharge advice could he be given?
12. What support services could be offered to Brian while he is in the ED, and for when he is ready to go home?

Answers to Case Study Questions can be found on evolve **http://evolve.elsevier.com/AU/Curtis/emergency/** 

CASE STUDY 2—OPIOID OVERDOSE

A 22-year-old female (Sue) was attended by paramedics at 4 pm outside an abandoned house. She was not breathing. Her friends said she had been to see her dealer, and was walking slowly on the footpath before she collapsed. Finding her unresponsive, and following the initial primary survey, the paramedic crew supported Sue's ventilation and administered an opioid antagonist (naloxone) from which she was roused. She appeared slightly intoxicated with alcohol, but otherwise alert. She was transported to the nearest emergency department (ED). Once in the ED she was medically examined and put in an observation area. About 20 minutes after her arrival a nurse walking past the cubicle saw that Sue was unconscious.

QUESTIONS

1. Why might this have happened?
2. How could this have been avoided?
3. What risks were there to her safety and wellbeing?
4. What advice would you give to other out-of-hospital emergency personnel, nurses and medical staff?

Answers to Case Study Questions can be found on evolve **http://evolve.elsevier.com/AU/Curtis/emergency/** 

CASE STUDY 3—NATALIE

PART 1

As a paramedic, you attend a 25-year-old woman (Natalie) who has been reported by a neighbour as behaving bizarrely.

When you arrive at the front door you hear shouting. You are met by a woman (Sandra) who says she called you because she is so worried about her friend. She tells you that Natalie was 'partying' 5 days ago and only came home about an hour ago. She has been behaving erratically ever since. When you try to enter the house, Natalie starts throwing plates at you and threatens you with a knife. She shouts that you are from the devil's army.

Natalie appears frightened and disorientated. She is unkempt, and while her clothes are intact they are dirty and very creased. Sandra tells you that it is common for Natalie to go out for a couple of days at a time, and take 'speed and ecstasy'. She does not know what Natalie has taken this time.

QUESTIONS

1. How can you ensure that you can safely assess Natalie?
2. What interventions and resources do you anticipate will be required?
3. What do you suspect has occurred? And why?

PART 2

The police are called and have arrived, and with Sandra's reassurance, Natalie allows you to assess her. She is still talking about the 'devil's army' in between incoherent, rambling speech. When asked, she tells you her name and date of birth, but does not know what day it is. Her attention span is brief, but she responds to instructions intermittently.

Her pupils are enlarged and react to light. She is tachypnoeic with a respiratory rate of 36 breaths/minute, and tachycardic at 140 beats/minute; her blood pressure is 90/60 mmHg. She has dry oral mucosa, and her skin is hot and dry to the touch. Sandra tells you that Natalie takes an injection for her diabetes, but doesn't know when she last injected. Natalie is unable to recall.

4. What assessments will you need to perform on Natalie?
5. What interventions will you initiate?
6. How will you ensure that Natalie can be safely transported to hospital?

PART 3

On arrival at the emergency department (ED), the paramedic provides you, the triage nurse, with a handover, which includes Natalie's condition, recent events, assessments and interventions undertaken prior to arriving at the ED. The police are also in attendance.

Continued

Natalie's airway is clear; she continues to be tachypnoeic and tachycardic with a weak pulse. The paramedic has established an intravenous line, and she is currently receiving normal saline. The paramedic also informs you of her known medical history and reports that a blood sugar level result reads 'high'. Natalie continues talking in rambling sentences, is agitated and intermittently verbally aggressive.

QUESTIONS (CONTINUED)

7. What is the safest environment in which to assess and treat Natalie?
8. What do you think has happened?
9. How does this explain her clinical signs and symptoms?
10. Once you are able to assess Natalie safely, what will be the priorities of her care?

Answers to Case Study Questions can be found on evolve **http://evolve.elsevier.com/AU/Curtis/emergency/** 

USEFUL WEBSITES

Alcohol, Smoking and Substance Involvement Screening Test (ASSIST), World Health Organization, www.who.int/publications/i/item/978924159938-2.

Drug and Alcohol Nurses of Australasia (DANA), www.danaonline.org/

New South Wales Ministry of Health. Handbook for Nurses and Midwives: Responding effectively to people who use alcohol and other drugs, www.health.nsw.gov.au/aod/professionals/Publications/handbook-nurses-aod.pdfAustralian Government. Drug and alcohol use information, www.australia.gov.au/information-and-services/health/drug-and-alcohol-use.

New Zealand Government Alcohol and Drug Abuse Information, www.health.govt.nz/your-health/healthy-living/addictions/alcohol-and-drug-abuse.

NSW Drug and Alcohol Withdrawal Clinical Practice Guidelines, https://www1.health.nsw.gov.au/pds/ActivePDSDocuments/GL2008_011.pdf.

Queensland Health Chronic Conditions Manual https://www.health.qld.gov.au/rrcsu/clinical-manuals/chronic-conditions-manual-ccm.

Queensland Health Primary Clinical Care Manual https://www.health.qld.gov.au/rrcsu/clinical-manuals/primary-clinical-care-manual-pccm.

Royal Australasian College of Physicians Addiction Medicine Resources, www.racp.edu.au/fellows/resources/addiction-medicine-resources.

South Australian Department of Health: Substance Misuse and Dependence. www.sahealth.sa.gov.au/wps/wcm/connect/public+content/sa+health+internet/clinical+resources/clinical+programs+and+practice+guidelines/substance+misuse+and+dependence/substance+misuse+and+dependence.

REFERENCES

1. United Nations Office on Drugs and Crime. World drug report 2021. Vienna: United Nations; 2021.
2. Australian Institute of Health and Welfare (AIHW). National drug strategy household survey 2019: detailed findings. Drug Statistics series. 2020. p. 104. Online: Available from: www.aihw.gov.au/getmedia/77dbea6e-f071-495c-b71e-3a632237269d/aihw-phe-270.pdf.aspx?inline=true.
3. Australian Institute of Health and Welfare (AIHW). Alcohol and other drug treatment services in Australia annual report. 2021. Online: Available from: www.aihw.gov.au/reports/alcohol-other-drug-treatment-services/alcohol-other-drug-treatment-services-australia/contents/about.
4. World Health Organization (WHO). Global status report on alcohol and health 2018. Geneva: WHO; 2018.
5. World Health Organization (WHO). World health statistics 2021: monitoring health for the SDGs, sustainable development goals. Geneva: WHO; 2021.
6. National Health and Medical Research Council, Australian Research Council, Universities Australia. Australian guidelines to reduce health risks from drinking alcohol. Canberra: Commonwealth of Australia; 2020.
7. Turning Point. AODStats. Eastern health. Online: Available from: https://aodstats.org.au/explore-data/.
8. Australian Institute of Health and Welfare (AIHW). Australian burden of disease study: impact and causes of illness and death in Australia 2018. 2021. Online: Available from: www.aihw.gov.au/reports/burden-of-disease/abds-impact-and-causes-of-illness-and-death-in-aus.
9. Australian Institute of Health and Welfare (AIHW). Impact of alcohol and illicit drug use on the burden of disease and injury in Australia: Australian Burden of Disease Study 2011. Canberra: AIHW; 2018.
10. McFadden M. The New Zealand drug harm index 2016. 2nd ed. Wellington: Ministry of Health; 2016.
11. Ministry of Health. Amphetamine use 2015/16: key findings of the New Zealand Health Survey. Wellington: Ministry of Health; 2016.
12. Ministry of Health. Annual update of key results 2017/18: New Zealand Health Survey. Ministry of Health. Updated 22 June 2021. Online: Available from: www.health.govt.nz/publication/annual-update-key-results-2017-18-new-zealand-health-survey.
13. Jones R, Woods C, Usher K. Rates and features of methamphetamine-related presentations to emergency departments: an integrative literature review. J Clin Nurs 2018;27(13-14):2569–82.
14. Australian College for Emergency Medicine. Alcohol and methamphetamine harm in emergency departments: findings from the 2019 Snapshot Survey. ACEM; 2019. Online: Available from: acem.org.au/getattachment/Content-Sources/Advancing-Emergency-Medicine/Better-Outcomes-for-Patients/Reducing-Alcohol-and-Drug-Harm-in-the-ED/Research/Alcohol-Snapshot-Report_R7.pdf?lang=en-AU.

15. NSW Ministry of Health. Methamphetamine use and related harms in NSW. Sydney: NSW Ministry of Health; 2017.
16. NSW Ministry of Health. Methamphetamine use and related harms in NSW: surveillance report to December 2018. St Leonards: NSW Ministry of Health; 2019.
17. Egerton-Warburton D, Gosbell A, Moore K, Moore K, Wadsworth A, Richardson D, et al. Alcohol-related harm in emergency departments: a prospective, multi-centre study. Addiction 2018;113(4):623–32.
18. Atayde AM, Hauc SC, Bessette LG, Danckers H, Saitz R. Changing the narrative: a call to end stigmatizing terminology related to substance use disorders. Addict Res Theory 2021;29(5):359–62.
19. Saitz R, Miller SC, Fiellin DA, Rosenthal RN. Recommended use of terminology in addiction medicine. J Addict Med 2021;15(1):3–7.
20. de Crespigny C, Talmet J, editors. Alcohol, tobacco and other drugs: clinical guidelines for nurses and midwives. 3rd ed. Adelaide: The University of Adelaide School of Nursing and Drug and Alcohol Services South Australia; 2012.
21. Saunders JB, Conigrave KM, Latt NC, Nutt DJ, Marshall EJ, Ling W, et al. Addiction medicine. Melbourne: Oxford University Press; 2016.
22. Ritter A, King T, Lee N. Drug use in Australian society. 2nd ed. Melbourne: Oxford University Press; 2017.
23. Marceau EM, Berry J, Lunn J, Kelly PJ, Solowij N. Cognitive remediation improves executive functions, self-regulation and quality of life in residents of a substance use disorder therapeutic community. Drug Alc Depend 2017;178:150–8.
24. Baker AL, Denham AMJ, Pohlman S. Treating comorbid substance use and psychosis. In: Badcock JC, Paulik G, editors. A clinical introduction to psychosis. London: Academic Press; 2020.
25. McDonough M, Baillie AJ, Clark PJ, Ritter A, Quinn C, Cunningham J, et al. Understanding and managing comorbidities for people with alcohol problems: polydrug use and dependence, co-occurring mental disorders, and physical comorbidities. MJA 2021;215(Suppl. 7):s28–s32.
26. Thorley A. The effects of alcohol. London: Junction Books; 1982. Drinking and problem drinking.
27. NSW Ministry of Health. Handbook for nurses and midwives: responding effectively to people who use alcohol and other drugs. St Leonards: NSW Ministry of Health; 2021.
28. Magill M, Martino S, Wampold BE. Goal setting and monitoring with alcohol and other drug use disorders: principles and practices. J Subst Abuse Treat 2022;132:108650.
29. Caputo F, Agabio R, Vignoli T, Patussi V, Fanucchi T, Cimarosti P, et al. Diagnosis and treatment of acute alcohol intoxication and alcohol withdrawal syndrome: position paper of the Italian Society on Alcohol. Intern Emerg Med 2019;14(1):143–60.
30. Haber PS, Riordan BC, Winter DT, Barrett L, Saunders J, Hides L, et al. New Australian guidelines for the treatment of alcohol problems: an overview of recommendations. MJA 2021;215(Suppl. 7):S3–S32.
31. Kizior RJ, Hodgson KJ. Drugs of abuse. In: Kizior RJ, Hodgson KJ, editors. Saunders nursing drug handbook 2018. St. Louis, Missouri: Elsevier; 2018. p. 1267–73.
32. Assanangkornchai S, Edwards JG. Clinical screening for illegal drug use, prescription drug misuse and tobacco use. In: Baldacchino AM, el-Guebaly N, Carrà G, Galanter M, editors. Textbook of addiction treatment. New York: Springer; 2021.
33. Bobes-Bascarán MT, Bascarán MT, García-Portilla MP. Clinical assessment of alcohol use disorders. In: Baldacchino AM, el-Guebaly N, Carrà G, Galanter M, editors. Textbook of addiction treatment. New York: Springer; 2021.
34. Saunders JB, Stjepanovic D, Connor JP. Screening and assessment for unhealthy alcohol use. MJA 2021;215:S6–S11.
35. Queensland Health. Primary clinical care manual 10th edition 2019. 10th ed. Brisbane: Queensland Health and the Royal Flying Doctor Service; 2021.
36. Queensland Health. Chronic conditions manual: prevention and management of chronic conditions in rural and remote Australia. 2nd ed. Brisbane: Queensland Health, the Royal Flying Doctor Service, and the Apunipima Cape York Health Council; 2020.
37. Secombe PJ, Stewart PC. The impact of alcohol-related admissions on resource use in critically ill patients from 2009 to 2015: an observational study. Anaesth Intens Care 2018;46(1):58–66.
38. Blow FC, Walton MA, Bohnert ASB, Ignacio RV, Chermack S, Cunningham RM, et al. A randomized controlled trial of brief interventions to reduce drug use among adults in a low-income urban emergency department: the HealthiER You study. Addiction 2017;112(8):1395–405.
39. Newcombe D, Tanielu-Stowers H, McDermott R, Stephen J, Nosa V. The validation of the Alcohol, Smoking and Substance Involvement Screening Test (ASSIST) amongst Pacific people in New Zealand. NZ J Psychol 2016;45(1):30–9.
40. World Health Organization (WHO). The Alcohol, Smoking and Substance Involvement Screening Test (ASSIST): manual for use in primary care. Geneva: WHO; 2010.
41. World Health Organization (WHO). The ASSIST-linked brief intervention for hazardous and harmful substance use: manual for use in primary care. Geneva: WHO; 2010.
42. Campbell CE, Maisto SA. Validity of the AUDIT-C screen for at-risk drinking among students utilizing university primary care. J Am Coll Health 2018;66(8):774–82.
43. Ghesglaghi F, Gomari M, Greene SL. A five-year report on body packing and body stuffing in Isfahan. Iran J Toxicol 2021;15(4):215–22.
44. Puntonet J, Gorgiard C, Soussy N, Soyer P, Dion E. Body packing, body stuffing and body pushing: characteristics and pitfalls on low-dose CT. Clin Imaging 2021;79:244–50.
45. Cappelletti S, Iaria A, Lombardo F, Vallone G, Vitale P, Ciallella C. Drug importation into Italy by body packing: an analysis of the UNODC individual drug seizures database. Med Leg J 2018;86(4):193–7.

46. Baldacchino AM, Sharma B. Substance-induced mental disorders. In: el-Guebaly N, Carrà G, Galanter M, Baldacchino AM, editors. Textbook of addiction treatment. Cham: Springer; 2021.
47. Cadet JL, Gold M. Methamphetamine-induced psychosis: who says all drug use is reversible? Treatment needs to take into account persistent cognitive impairment and comorbid disorders. Curr Psychiatry 2017;16(11):14.
48. Waring WS. Alcohols and glycols poisoning. Medicine 2020;48(3):185–8.
49. Varga ZV, Matyas C, Paloczi J, Pacher P. Alcohol misuse and kidney injury: epidemiological evidence and potential mechanisms. Alcohol Res Curr Rev 2017;38(2):283.
50. Marsano LS, Vatsalya V, Hassan A, McClain J. Clinical features, disease modifiers, and natural history of alcoholic liver disease. In: Chalasani N, Szabo G, editors. Alcoholic and non-alcoholic fatty liver disease. New York: Springer; 2016.
51. Chong D, Buckley N, Schumann JL, Chitty KM. Acute alcohol use in Australian coronial suicide cases, 2010–2015. Drug Alcohol Depend 2020;212:108066.
52. Kaestle CE, Droste N, Peacock A, Bruno R, Miller P. Perception of intoxication in a field study of the night-time economy: blood alcohol concentration, patron characteristics, and event-level predictors. Addict Behav 2018;76:195–200.
53. Department of Health and Ageing. Alcohol treatment guidelines for indigenous Australians. Canberra: Commonwealth of Australia; 2007.
54. Latt N, Dore G. Thiamine in the treatment of Wernicke encephalopathy in patients with alcohol use disorders. Intern Med J 2014;44(9):911–15.
55. Altman J, Ryan MF. Can Wernicke's encephalopathy be precipitated by administering glucose before thiamine in severely malnourished or alcoholic patients? Case Rep Clin Med 2019;8(9):245.
56. Sadacharan R, Wartenberg AA. Management of alcohol intoxication and withdrawal. In: Herron A, Brennan TK, editors. The ASAM essentials of addiction medicine. 3rd ed. New York: Lippincott Williams & Wilkins; 2020.
57. Morford KL, Tetrault JM. Management of opioid intoxication and withdrawal. In: Herron A, Brennan HK, editors. The ASAM essentials of addiction medicine. 3rd ed. New York: Lippincott Williams & Wilkins; 2020.
58. Herron A, Brennan TK. The ASAM essentials of addiction medicine. 3rd ed. New York: Lippincott Williams & Wilkins; 2020.
59. Wilkins JN, Danovitch I, Gorelick DA. Management of stimulant, hallucinogen, marijuana, phencyclidine, and club drug intoxication and withdrawal. In: Herron A, Brennan HK, editors. The ASAM essentials of addiction medicine. 3rd ed. New York: Lippincott Williams & Wilkins; 2020.
60. Wai JM. Management of sedative-hypnotic intoxication and withdrawal. In: Herron A, Brennan TK, editors. The ASAM essentials of addiction medicine. 3rd ed. New York: Lippincott Williams & Wilkins; 2020.
61. Teschke R. Alcoholic liver disease: alcohol metabolism, cascade of molecular mechanisms, cellular targets, and clinical aspects. Biomedicines 2018;6(4):106.
62. Shoaib S, Hyder M, May M. An atypical long-term thiamine treatment regimen for Wernicke encephalopathy. Fed Pract 2020;37(9):405.
63. Gallagher N, Edwards FJ. The diagnosis and management of toxic alcohol poisoning in the emergency department: a review article. Adv J Emerg Med 2019;3(3):e28.
64. Hides L, Riordan BC, Gullo M, Morley KC, Connor J, Quinn C, et al. Caring for and managing patients with alcohol problems: interventions, treatments, relapse prevention, aftercare, and long term follow-up. MJA 2021;215:S12–20.
65. Airagnes G, Ducoutumany G, Laffy-Beaufils B, Le Faou AL, Limosin F. Alcohol withdrawal syndrome management: is there anything new? Rev Med Interne 2019;40(6):373–9.
66. Duong T, Vytialingam R, O'Regan R. A brief guide to the management of alcohol and other drug withdrawal. Perth: Mental Health Commission 2018.
67. Maldonado JR. Novel algorithms for the prophylaxis and management of alcohol withdrawal syndromes–beyond benzodiazepines. Crit Care Clin 2017;33(3):559–99.
68. Grover S, Ghosh A. Delirium tremens: assessment and management. J Clin Experim Hepatol 2018;8(4):460–70.
69. Hassanian-Moghaddam H, Zamani N, Roberts DM, Brent J, McMartin K, Aaron C, et al. Consensus statements on the approach to patients in a methanol poisoning outbreak. Clin Toxicol 2019;57(12):1129–36.
70. Zacharov S. Challenges of mass methanol poisoning outbreaks: diagnosis, treatment and prognosis in long term health sequelae. Prague: Charles University in Prague, Karolinum Press; 2019.
71. Holt NR, Nickson CP. Severe methanol poisoning with neurological sequelae: implications for diagnosis and management. Intern Med J 2018;48(3):335–9.
72. Najari F, Baradaran I, Najari D. Methanol poisoning and its treatment. Int J Med Toxicol Forens Med 2020;10(1):26639.
73. Olson KR, Anderson IB, Benowitz NL, Blanc PD, Kim-Katz SY, et al. Poisoning and drug overdose. New York: McGraw-Hill Medical; 2017.
74. Yoshizawa T, Kamijo Y, Fujita Y, Suzuki Y, Hanazawa T, Usui K, et al. Mild manifestation of methanol poisoning half a day after massive ingestion of a fuel alcohol product containing 70% ethanol and 30% methanol: a case report. Acute Med Surg 2018;5(3):289–91.
75. Lao YE, Vartdal T, Froeyshov S, Latimer B, Kvaerner C, Mataric M, et al. Fomepizole dosing during continuous renal replacement therapy – an observational study. Clin Toxicol 2022:60(4):451–7.
76. Brandt J, Janzen D, Alessi-Severini S, Singer A, Chateau D, Enns M, et al. Risk of long-term benzodiazepine and Z-drug use following the first prescription among community-dwelling adults with anxiety/mood and sleep disorders: a retrospective cohort study. BMJ Open 2021;11(11):e046916.

77. Ritter J, Flower RJ, Henderson G, Loke YK, MacEwan D, Rang H. Rang and Dale's pharmacology. 9th ed. Edinburgh: Elsevier; 2019.
78. Baldwin DS. Clinical management of withdrawal from benzodiazepine anxiolytic and hypnotic medications. Addiction 2022;117(5):1472–80.
79. Torrens M, Fonseca F, Dinamarca F, Farré M. Opioid addiction and treatment. In: el-Guebaly N, Carrà G, Galanter M, Baldacchino AM, editors. Textbook of addiction treatment. New York: Springer; 2021.
80. Strayer RJ, Hawk K, Hayes BD, Herring AA, Ketcham E, LaPietra AM, et al. Management of opioid use disorder in the emergency department: a white paper prepared for the American Academy of Emergency Medicine. J Emerg Med 2020;58(3):522–46.
81. Macintyre PE, Roberts LJ, Huxtable CA. Management of opioid-tolerant patients with acute pain: approaching the challenges. Drugs 2020;80(1):9–21.
82. Rzasa Lynn R, Galinkin JL. Naloxone dosage for opioid reversal: current evidence and clinical implications. Ther Adv Drug Saf 2017;9(1):63–88.
83. Strang J, McDonald R, Campbell G, Degenhardt L, Nielsen S, Ritter A, et al. Take-home naloxone for the emergency interim management of opioid overdose: the public health application of an emergency medicine. Drugs 2019;79(13):1395–418.
84. Upfal J. Australian drug guide. 8th ed. Melbourne: Griffin Press; 2016.
85. Zhang X, Marchand C, Sullivan B, Klass EM, Wagner KD. Naloxone access for emergency medical technicians: an evaluation of a training program in rural communities. Addict Behav 2018;86:79–85.
86. Torrens M, Fonseca F, Galindo L, Farré M. Opioid addiction: short- and long-acting opioids. In: el-Guebaly N, Carrà G, Galanter M, editors. Textbook of addiction treatment: international perspectives. New York: Springer; 2015.
87. Balster RL. The pharmacology of inhalants. In: Herron A, Brennan HK, editors. The ASAM essentials of addiction medicine. 3rd ed. New York: Lippincott Williams & Wilkins; 2020.
88. Real T, Cruz SL, Medina-Mora ME. Inhalant addiction. In: el-Guebaly N, Carrà G, Galanter M, editors. Textbook of addiction treatment. New York: Springer; 2021.
89. Broussard L. Inhalants. In: Levine BS, Kerrigan S, editors. Principles of forensic toxicology. New York: Springer; 2020.
90. Crossin R, Cairney S, Lawrence AJ, Duncan JR. Adolescent inhalant abuse leads to other drug use and impaired growth; implications for diagnosis. ANZ J Pub Health 2017;41(1):99–104.
91. d'Abbs P, Shaw G, Field E. The impact of subsidized Low Aromatic Fuel (LAF) on petrol (gasoline) sniffing in remote Australian Indigenous communities. Subst Abuse Treat Prev Policy 2017;12(1):38.
92. Korff J. Petrol sniffing. Creative spirits. Updated 12 August 2020. Online: Available from: www.creativespirits.info/aboriginalculture/health/petrol-sniffing.
93. BP Australia. BP helps tackle petrol sniffing: the 10 year journey of Opal. 2015. Online: Available from: www.youtube.com/watch?v=9EjcA6tlFmE.
94. Bonnet U, Preuss UW. The cannabis withdrawal syndrome: current insights. Subst Abuse Rehabil 2017;8:9–37.
95. Connor JP, Stjepanović D, Le Foll B, Hoch E, Budney AJ, Hall WD. Cannabis use and cannabis use disorder. Nat Rev Dis Primers 2021;7(1):16.
96. Budney AJ, Sofis MJ. Cannabis use disorder and its treatment. In: el-Guebaly N, Carrà G, Galanter M, Baldacchino AM, editors. Textbook of addiction treatment. New York: Springer; 2021. p. 157–71.
97. Davies N, English W, Grundlingh J. MDMA toxicity: management of acute and life-threatening presentations. BJN 2018;27(11):616–22.
98. Gorelick DG, Baumann MH. The pharmacology of cocaine, amphetamines, and other stimulants. In: Ries RK, Miller SC, Saitz R, editors. The ASAM essentials of addiction medicine. 5th ed. New York: Lippincott Williams & Wilkins; 2015.
99. Sasiadek J, Durham N, George TP. Nicotine and tobacco. In: el-Guebaly N, Carrà G, Galanter M, Baldacchino AM, editors. Textbook of addiction treatment. New York: Springer; 2021. p. 197–214.
100. Gelberg L, Andersen RM, Afifi AA, Leake BD, Arangua L, Vahidi M, et al. Project QUIT (Quit Using Drugs Intervention Trial): a randomized controlled trial of a primary care-based multi-component brief intervention to reduce risky drug use. Addiction 2015;110(11):1777–90.
101. Gorelick DG, Baumann MH. The pharmacology of stimulants. In: Herron A, Brennan HK, editors. The ASAM essentials of addiction medicine. 3rd ed. New York: Lippincott Williams & Wilkins; 2020.
102. Miles LF, Austin K, Eade A, Anderson D, Graudins A, McGain F, et al. Characteristics, presentation and outcomes of music festival patrons with stimulant drug-induced serotonin toxicity. Emerg Med Australas 2021;33:992–1000.
103. Couch GA, White MP, de Gray LE. Central nervous system stimulants: basic pharmacology and relevance to anaesthesia and critical care. Anaesthes Intens Care Med 2020;21(10):503–11.
104. Docherty JR, Alsufyani HA. Pharmacology of drugs used as stimulants. J Clin Pharmacol 2021;61:S53–69.
105. The National Centre for Education and Training on Addiction. National alcohol & drug knowledg base glossary. Online: Available from: https://nadk.flinders.edu.au/glossary.
106. Solimini R, C Rotolo M, Pellegrini M, Minutillo A, Pacifici R, Busardò FP, et al. Adulteration practices of psychoactive illicit drugs: an updated review. Curr Pharm Biotechnol 2017;18(7):524–30.
107. McKetin R, Baker AL, Dawe S, Voce A, Minutillo A, Pacifici R, Busardò FP, et al. Differences in the symptom profile of methamphetamine-related psychosis and primary psychotic disorders. Psychiatry Res 2017;251:349–54.
108. Farkhondeh T, Roshanravan B, Shirazi FM, Mehrpour O. Can dantrolene be used in the treatment of cardioglycosides poisonings? Expert Opin Drug Metab Toxicol 2021;17(1):1–2.

109. Grunau BE, Wiens MO, Brubacher JR. Dantrolene in the treatment of MDMA-related hyperpyrexia: a systematic review. Can J Emerg Med 2010;12(5):435–42.
110. Nikoomanesh K, Choi J, Arabian S. Methylenedioxymethamphetamine (MDMA) overdose at rave parties, a case series. C42 Critical Care Case Reports: Toxicology And Poisonings 2. New York: American Thoracic Society; 2019. American Thoracic Society International Conference Abstracts.
111. Darke S, Peacock A, Duflou J, Farrell M, Lappin J. Characteristics and circumstances of death related to gamma hydroxybutyrate (GHB). Clin Toxicol 2020;58(11):1028–33.
112. Pettigrew M. Somnophilia and sexual abuse through the administration of GHB and GBL. J Forensic Sci 2019;64(1):302–3.
113. Madah-Amiri D, Myrmel L, Brattebø G. Intoxication with GHB/GBL: characteristics and trends from ambulance-attended overdoses. Scand J Trauma Resusc Emerg Med 2017;25(1):98.
114. Dutch MJ, Austin KB. Hospital in the field: prehospital management of GHB intoxication by medical assistance teams. Prehosp Disaster Med 2012;27(5):463–7.
115. Munir VL, Hutton JE, Harney JP, Buykx P, Weiland TJ, Dent AW. Gamma-hydroxybutyrate: a 30 month emergency department review. Emerg Med Australas 2008;20(6):521–30.
116. Pope Jr HG, Kanayama G. Neurobiology and treatment of anabolic-androgenic steroid-related disorders. In: Brady KT, Levin FR, Galanter MC, Kleber HD, editors. The American Psychiatric Association publishing textbook of substance use disorder treatment. Washington, DC: American Psychiatric Association; 2021. p. 315–31.
117. Moore D, Hart A, Fraser S, Seear K. Masculinities, practices and meanings: a critical analysis of recent literature on the use of performance-and image-enhancing drugs among men. Health (London) 2020;24(6):719–36.
118. Lehman D. The pharmacology of anabolic-androgenic steroids. In: Herron A, Brennan HK, editors. The ASAM essentials of addiction medicine. 3rd ed. New York: Lippincott Williams & Wilkins; 2020.
119. Liu JD, Wu YQ. Anabolic-androgenic steroids and cardiovascular risk. Chinese Med J 2019;132(18):2229.

SECTION FOUR
MAJOR TRAUMA

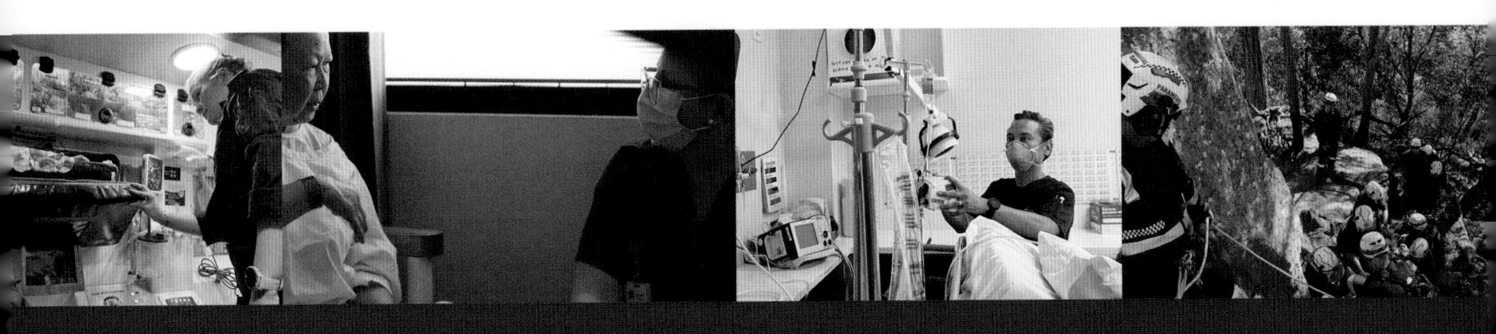

CHAPTER 41
EPIDEMIOLOGY OF INJURY

CAMERON PALMER AND TANEAL WISEMAN

ESSENTIALS

- Epidemiology is essential to understand trauma as both a clinical and a public health problem, because of its implications for clinical practice, social policy, public policy, legislation, injury prevention programs and as a source of data for trauma research.
- Injury is the third most common cause of death and disability worldwide; in Australia, it accounts for more years of lost life up to 75 years of age than cardiovascular disease and cancer combined. Male injury death rates are, on average, about twice those of females.
- Paediatric injury is a leading cause of hospitalisation and results in significant morbidity and mortality.
- Falls are the most commonly reported cause of admission for both males and females. Although fall rates are higher in older age groups, our understanding of contributing factors is limited by a lack of information about the nature of the falls.
- Suicide rates have increased in recent years. Men are three times more likely to commit suicide than women.
- Aboriginal and Torres Strait Islander suicide rates are nearly double the rate for other Australians, and the transport injury death rate almost three times as high.
- There is a relationship between alcohol and an increased risk of injury or death.
- The predominant cause of early death after trauma continues to be brain injury, followed by exsanguination.
- Australian and Aotearoa New Zealand firearm-related injuries are low in comparison with the rest of the world.
- The perception of injuries as preventable events rather than random, unexpected accidents is fundamental to the success of any injury prevention program.
- Each mechanism of injury generates specific biomechanical forces which act on the body. The type of force, duration and the surface area over which the force is applied determine the pattern of injury.
- The vast majority of trauma in Australia and Aotearoa New Zealand is blunt. The forces that result in blunt trauma are most commonly due to rapid deceleration or acceleration.
- Penetrating injury causes damage as it passes through the body or tissue, and with sufficient force may also affect surrounding tissues.
- Safety devices, such as restraints and airbags, have reduced injuries associated with some motor vehicle collisions. However, if these devices are faulty, or worn and/or installed incorrectly, preventable injuries may occur.
- Bombs and explosions can cause unique patterns of injury rarely seen outside combat areas.

INTRODUCTION

Although definitions of traumatic injury ('trauma') vary, all definitions involve the concept of energy transfer. This can include mechanical (kinetic, as in blunt or penetrating injury) or thermal energy, but also chemical energy (as in poisoning or corrosion) or energy deprivation (as in drowning or asphyxia). The effects of trauma can range from inconsequential to devastating; as well as significant mortality and short-term morbidity, trauma may result in long-term physical, mental and socio-economic impairment.

This chapter provides an overview of the epidemiology of trauma in Australia and Aotearoa New Zealand. Patterns of injury are examined, along with measures used to respond to trauma—injury prevention, the standardisation of clinical trauma management and the development of organised trauma systems. The chapter also explores mechanisms of injury, and the kinematics of trauma. Awareness of injury mechanisms can enhance clinical assessment by assisting in identifying common injury patterns within blunt, penetrating and blast trauma types.

Emergency clinicians should have a sound understanding of the mechanisms of injury, physiological responses to trauma, the determinants and extent of traumatic injury as a significant and burgeoning public health issue and organised approaches to trauma patient management. In this chapter, the epidemiology of trauma will be presented alongside the kinematics of specific injury mechanisms. An understanding of the role of trauma clinicians within these systems will promote optimal patient outcomes through the continuum of trauma care. The sources cited in this chapter are the most recent available at the time of publication; currency may vary across specific areas of injury.

THE BURDEN OF INJURY

Traumatic injury ('trauma') has many direct and indirect impacts on society, substantial costs to injured persons, their family and healthcare systems. These have been conceptualised in an injury List Of All Deficits (LOAD) framework, which describes the full range of deficits and adverse outcomes following injury and violence (Fig. 41.1).[1]

In 2019 it was estimated that 714 million people worldwide sustained injuries requiring healthcare interventions; of these, 4.3 million did not survive the injury.[2] The total number of deaths from trauma decreased only slightly between 2010 and 2019; however, death rates fell by 19.4%. Injury has remained the third highest cause of death globally since the coordinated Global Burden of Disease (GBD) project commenced in 1990.[2]

Disability-adjusted life-years (DALYs) are defined as years of healthy life lost. There are two summed components—the (weighted) number of years lived with disability (YLD) and the years of life lost (YLL). The DALY was developed and utilised by the GBD study as a powerful tool for priority setting, measuring disease burden from non-fatal as well as fatal conditions.

FIGURE 41.1 THE INJURY LIST OF ALL DEFICITS (LOAD) FRAMEWORK[1]

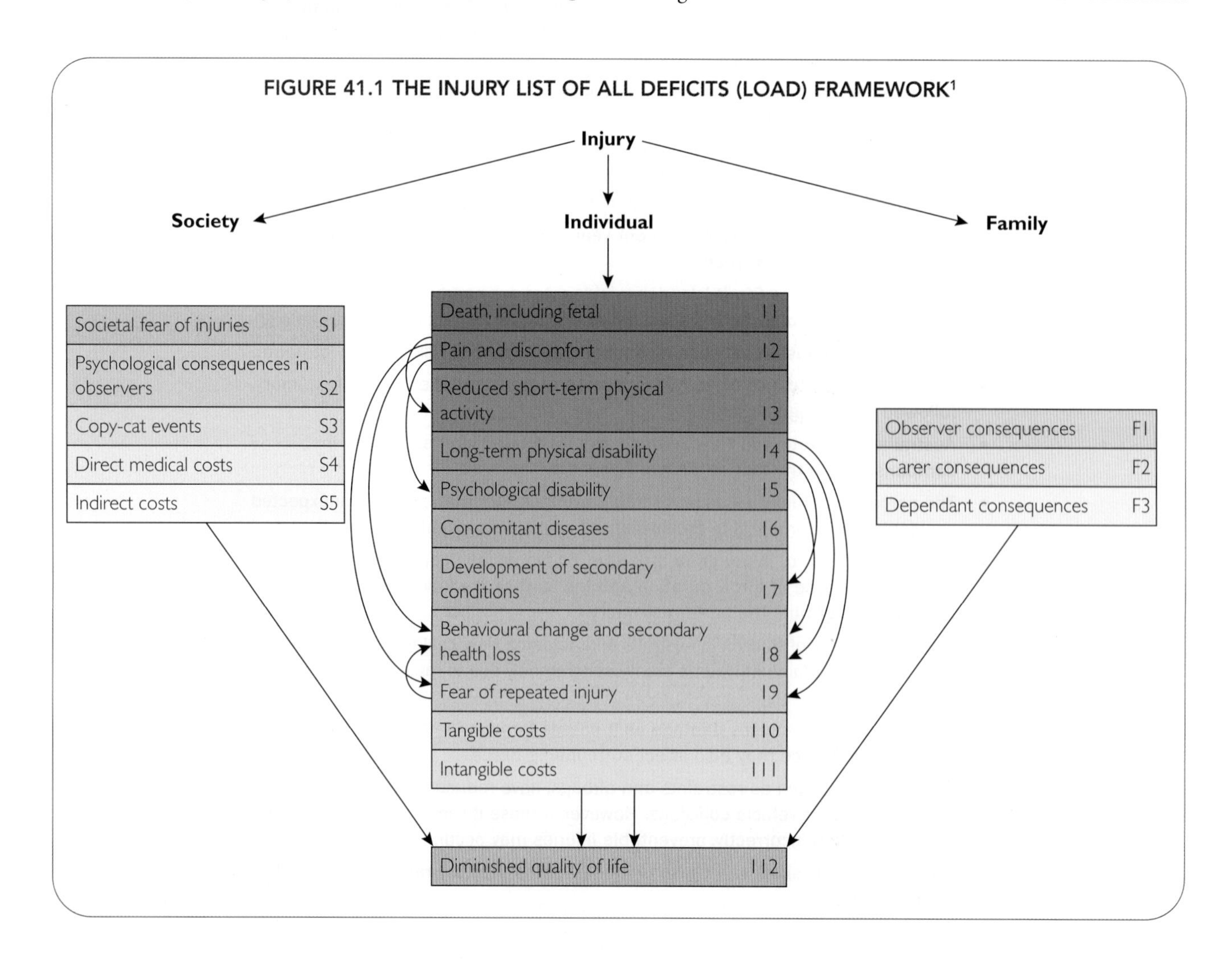

Despite reductions in injury over the previous decade, in 2019 it was estimated that injury resulted in 185 million YLLs and a further 63.9 million YLDs; as such, injury ranks third among global causes of YLD and YLL.[2] However, injury burdens, like all disease burdens, can be difficult to estimate.[3]

In Australia, injury is the leading cause of death in people aged 1–44 years.[4] The burden of trauma is immense, responsible for over 527,000 hospitalisations in 2019–20,[4] and accounting for 8.4% of the total disease burden in Australia in 2018.[5] In Aotearoa New Zealand, the total societal cost of injury has been estimated at more than $10 billion annually;[6] more recently, the cost of road trauma alone was estimated at $4.6 billion.[7] Injuries account for more potential years of life lost than cancer and heart disease combined;[8] in Australia, each fatal injury before the age of 75 years results in the loss of 32 years of potential life, compared with 9 years for cancer and 5 for cardiovascular disease.[9] In 2013 the social costs of road trauma alone in Aotearoa New Zealand were estimated to be $3.29 billion.[10]

Higher treatment costs are also associated with severity of injury, intensive care admission and traumatic brain injury. Once a patient has more than two body regions injured (i.e. polytrauma),[11] costs for medical care increase exponentially.[12] The complex nature of trauma patients does not allow for accurate funding prediction using the activity-based funding models currently employed in Australia; overall, trauma patients are underfunded for the care they require.[13] Strategies to decrease in-hospital cost and improve quality include multi-disciplinary rounds, case management and trauma coding strategies.[13] Compensation schemes in Australia and Aotearoa New Zealand vary between state, territory and country and may depend on injury mechanism (such as road transport).

Time-critical interventions can affect the outcome of severe trauma events.[14] Effective societal organisation and prompt, comprehensive medical care can reduce trauma-related mortality, improve outcomes and decrease the societal burden of trauma.[15] The role of the emergency clinician within such a system is crucial.

HISTORY

Morbidity and mortality resulting from injury have historically been a part of Australian and Aotearoa New Zealand societies, both in Indigenous populations and in the European colonisation of Australia and Aotearoa New Zealand. Traumatic injury was a common cause of death among convicts and settlers alike, and trauma was once considered an inevitable part of life in terms of both incidence and mortality risk.[16]

Contemporary understanding of patterns of injury and physiological responses to trauma were accelerated through periods of military conflict. An improved understanding of mechanisms of, and responses to, injury during World War II meant that many lives were saved through simple actions such as splinting and immobilising major fractures.[17] The Vietnam War saw significant improvements in understanding of the physiology of shock, and the importance of haemostasis and fluid resuscitation.[17] Improved survival rates of battlefield injuries have created awareness of the need for management of potentially permanent physical disabilities and post-traumatic stress. As a result, the expectations of trauma management and injury outcomes have changed significantly today.

In Australia, injury prevention has been recognised as a national health priority since at least 1986,[18] and the medical community in Australia and Aotearoa New Zealand has long recognised the need for improved, systematic care.[19] Since then, several national injury prevention plans have been developed in both countries, although as of late 2022, Australia's has been expired for several years.[8,20–23] Following many separate jurisdictional reports, trauma systems have also been progressively implemented in each Australian state and across Aotearoa New Zealand in the past 25 years. However, funding for injury research has consistently remained less than half that allocated for cancer research, and is less than diabetes, mental health, cardiovascular and obesity research.[24]

EPIDEMIOLOGY OF TRAUMA IN AUSTRALIA AND AOTEAROA NEW ZEALAND

This section serves to introduce broad concepts of trauma epidemiology. The overall societal effects of injury within Australia and Aotearoa New Zealand have already been discussed, and specific mechanisms are discussed in subsequent sections.

Injury admissions to hospital, and deaths from injury, are approximately two to three times as common for males than females up to 79 years. Blunt trauma accounts for 94% of severe injury presentations, with road trauma and falls making up around 80% of these statistics.[25] In Aotearoa New Zealand, the rate of major trauma is 51 per 100,000 people,[26] and injuries remain the fifth leading cause of health loss and the third leading cause of premature mortality.[27] Road trauma accounts for over 50% of severe injuries, with self-inflicted injuries and assaults being the leading causes of injury in young people, and falls a leading cause in those aged 65 years and older. Males account for nearly three-quarters of injury-related health loss. For adolescent males, injury is the leading cause of hospitalisation (43%), while for females it is the second leading cause of hospitalisation (10%), after complications of pregnancy and childbirth (43%).[28]

Aboriginal and Torres Strait Islanders and Māori are at greater risk of traumatic injury and resultant mortality than non-Indigenous and non-Māori populations. Other socio-economic factors, such as geographical location, can also affect injury risk. These will be discussed further below in the section on trauma determinants.

TRAUMA MORTALITY IN AUSTRALIA

Before 1991, the leading cause of death from external causes in Australia was motor vehicle collisions, although this is now dwarfed by suicide, falls and by drug and alcohol poisoning (Fig. 41.2).[29,30] Comparisons between the number of deaths obtained using the ABS mortality unit record data collection and the number of deaths obtained using data supplied by the National Coroners Information System (NCIS) has confirmed underestimation of road traffic injury and homicide.[31] Despite this, overall injury mortality in Australia has declined over recent years.[30]

As with all trauma, the mechanisms of injury resulting in death vary with age. For example, in Australia, infants are most likely to die of assault and suffocation, toddlers from drowning and teenagers through motor vehicle collisions.[32] There are approximately 250 child deaths due to injury each year in Australia.

Suicide

Suicide was acknowledged as a national public health concern in Australia during the 1990s, and continues to be a major

FIGURE 41.2 INTENT AND MECHANISM OF INJURY-RELATED MORTALITY IN AUSTRALIA, 2020[29]

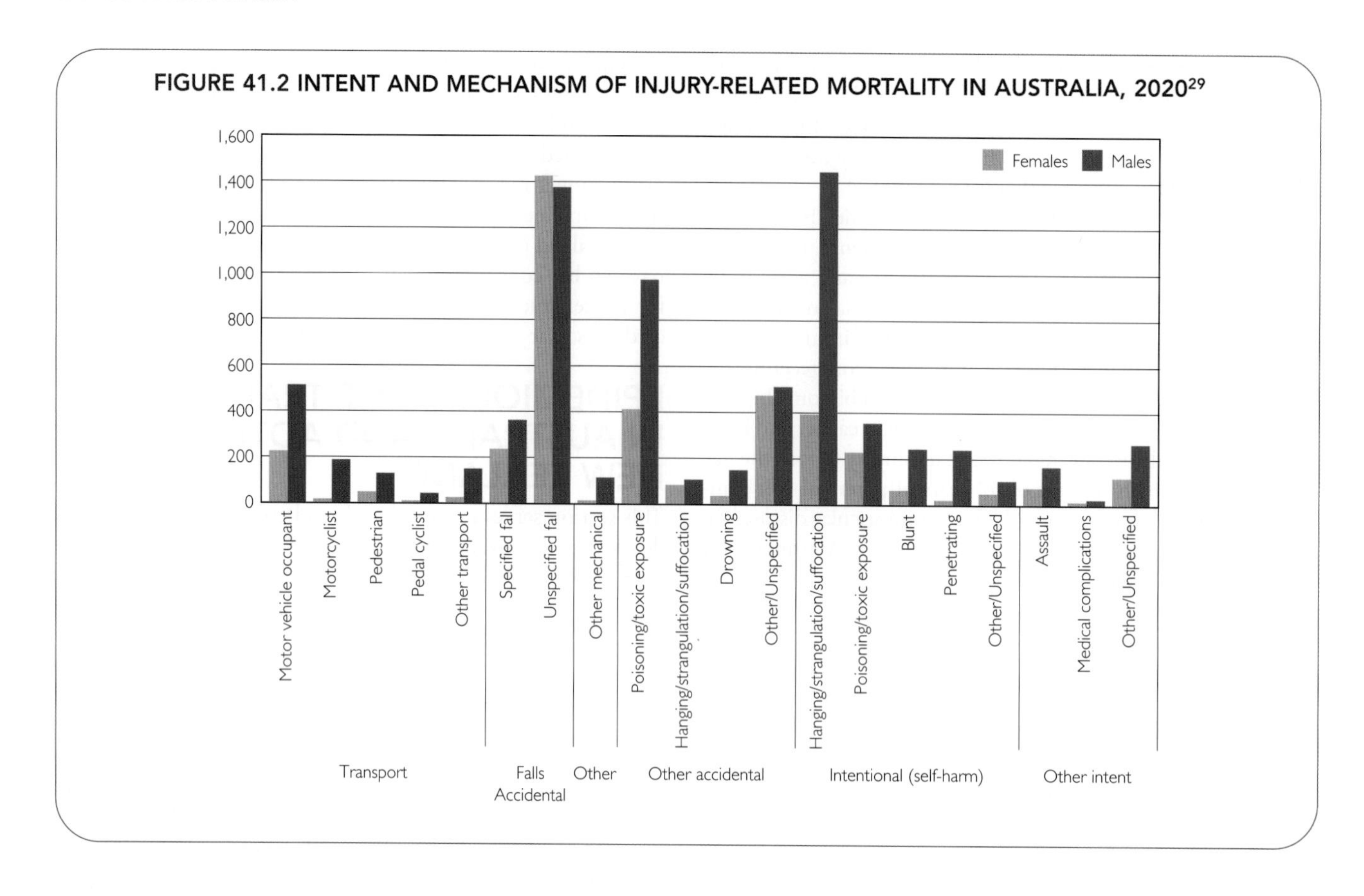

public health concern.[33] Suicide prevention strategies and investment in mental health services at both state and federal levels saw over $30 million invested into this cause between 2004 and 2014. However, between 2008 and 2020 there was a greater than 50% increase in the number of Australian suicide deaths, from 2191 to 3318.[30,33] In 2019, suicide was ranked as the 13th leading cause of all deaths. In 2012, three-quarters (75.0%) of people who died by suicide were male, primarily in the 20–24, 25–29 and 30–34-year age groups. Similarly, for females, suicide deaths comprise a higher proportion of total deaths in younger age groups compared with older age groups (32.6% of deaths of 15–19-year-olds and 25.2% of deaths of 20–24-year-olds).[32] Men remain three times more likely to commit suicide than women, regardless of age category.[30]

In 2012, the most frequent method of suicide was hanging, a method used in half (54%) of all suicide deaths. Poisoning was used in 23%, followed by firearms (6.8%). Other frequently used methods were jumping from a high place and contact with sharp objects (see also Fig. 41.2).[32]

Mortality data from the Australian Bureau of Statistics (ABS) are the main source of suicide statistics in Australia, although Coroners and the NCIS also contribute data in a complex process. Coding rules that form part of the International Classification of Diseases (ICD) can also affect the statistics.[31] It is believed that suicide data may be underestimated, and that observed changes over time are likely to have been affected by delays in Coroners finalising a cause. Undercounting of suicide cases could have more effect in some external-cause groups than in others; for example, suicide deaths from drowning can be difficult to distinguish from unintentional deaths by the same mechanism.[34]

Transport-related deaths

In 1970 there were 3798 deaths on Australian roads;[35] in 2021 there were 1123 road deaths.[36] This represents a decline in the rate of fatal crashes from 30 per 100,000 population to 4.4 per 100,000 in 50 years.[37] The largest proportion of motor vehicles involved in crashes were cars (94%).[36] Further details of transport-related injuries are provided later in the chapter.

Falls deaths

Fall rates are concentrated in the older age groups. Unlike other mechanisms of injury, males and females are injured in more equal numbers, as women make up a greater proportion of the elderly population. However, specific data about the nature of falls is absent in more than 80% of fall deaths (Fig. 41.2). As a result, our understanding of the factors which contribute to fall deaths is limited.

Even among older patients, residents of aged care facilities are significantly over-represented in hospital data.[37] To reduce the impact of fall-related injury among older people on the health system, significant resources are being directed towards the promotion of national level evidence-based falls prevention programs.[38] There is evidence to support injury prevention and fall reduction following the implementation of an exercise program, in particular, balance and strength exercises, tai chi and group exercise programs.[39]

Work-related fatalities

Between 2003 and 2020, 4136 workers were killed in work-related incidents, an average of nearly 20 per month.[40] There has been a gradual decrease in yearly deaths since a peak of 310 workers in 2007. In 2020, 194 workers (equal to 1.5 per

100,000 workers) were killed in work-related incidents; of these, 96% were male. The risk of workplace death increases with age; risks are highest for workers aged 65 years or over and workers aged 55–64 years are most common.[40]

Between 2016 and 2020, 65% of workplace deaths involved vehicles, with half of the vehicle-related incidents occurring on public roads, and the majority of deaths involving the occupant of a vehicle. More than 60% of workplace deaths occur within one of three industries: (1) transport, postal and warehousing; (2) agriculture, forestry and fishing; and (3) construction.

TRAUMA MORTALITY IN AOTEAROA NEW ZEALAND

As in Australia, injury is a leading cause of premature death and disability in Aotearoa New Zealand.[41] Suicide and motor vehicle collisions result in the greatest YLL.[42] In 2017, there were 50 reported fatalities across Aotearoa New Zealand resulting from workplace incidents, the most prevalent industries for workplace injuries being commercial fishing and forestry, mining and agriculture and manufacturing and construction.[43] Suicide is acknowledged as a public health concern in Aotearoa New Zealand; in 2018 it accounted for 623 deaths at a rate of 12.1 per 100,000 people. Similar to the Australian Indigenous peoples, the Māori population are over-represented in trauma volume, with incidence rates 1.5 times higher than the rest of the population.[26]

TRAUMA MORBIDITY

For every trauma patient who dies from their injuries, there are nearly six who survive to hospital discharge. This is exacerbated in children, where for every severely injured child, there are at least 13 children hospitalised with minor or moderate injuries. Childhood injury hospitalisation rates in Australia did not change in the 10 years to 2012.[44] Not all morbidities resulting from trauma are severe or result in long-term disability. Some may result in significant dysfunction, pain, cost or other sequelae, while many injuries—even serious injuries—can heal, leaving little or no physical residual dysfunction. In a significant proportion of patients with more serious injury, recovery is incomplete, and injury results in a degree of ongoing dysfunction or the onset of secondary conditions (such as osteoarthritis in injured joints). In addition, it has been suggested that minor trauma (such as 'whiplash' soft-tissue injuries) may account for a substantial proportion of population morbidity.[45]

Although there are specific risk factors (such as older age and compensability),[46] which are broadly predictive of worse outcomes, there is no reliable method for predicting which longer-term outcomes individual patients are likely to experience.[47] Also, although the link between major trauma and mental health sequelae is well recognised, it appears to be independent of the actual injuries sustained.[46] Early identification and intervention methods are areas of ongoing exploration.[48]

TRAUMA DETERMINANTS

Despite the nature of the injury and whether it was intended or not, most physical injuries can be prevented by identifying their causes and, where possible, eliminating or reducing them. Understanding some of the risk factors for injury may have a predictive value in anticipating patterns of trauma in certain populations and/or informing and evaluating injury prevention strategies. While examining all the trauma risk factors is beyond the scope of this text, determinants such as age, gender, Indigenous background, alcohol and other drugs, geography, temporal variations and the complex issue of driver distraction, may all contribute to injury risk and will be discussed below.

AGE

Age has a bimodal influence on risk of death from injury across the human life span. Among seriously injured patients who survive to hospital admission in Australia and Aotearoa New Zealand, the 20–29 and 45–59-year age groups are the most represented.[25,49] However, a comparison of the age-specific death rates for all injuries demonstrates that people aged 75 years and older have the highest death rates for all injuries; low falls, a common mechanism in older patients, have the highest mortality rate among hospital-admitted major trauma patients.[25,49]

Types of injury mechanism also vary with age. Falls and transport-related injuries are the most common mechanisms in all children admitted to hospital, although falls become less prevalent among older children and for other mechanisms.[44] In infants and children, the major causes of injury-related health loss vary depending on the age of the child or young person. Transport injuries are the predominant cause of health loss in children and young people, accounting for 45% of injury-related health loss. In infants, interpersonal violence accounts for over 40% of injury-related health loss. Drowning is an important cause of health loss in children under 9 years of age, with self-inflicted injury increasing from the age of 10.[27]

A second influence of age on morbidity and mortality risk relates to physiological responses to trauma. In children, the high ratio of body mass to surface area means that they are less able to absorb high-impact energies in trauma. Combined with their limited ability to physiologically compensate for traumatic injuries, this means that children are at high risk of death and permanent disability from a given mechanism of injury. At the other end of the chronological scale, trauma in older people is associated with increased severity and significant costs to health services, resulting in increasing recognition as a trauma subgroup.[50] People over the age of 55 years have a limited ability to compensate for physiological derangements induced by traumatic injury. Comorbidities and common medications taken in this age group, such as anticoagulants and antihypertensives, further complicate trauma resuscitation and rehabilitation. See Chapters 35 and 38 for detailed discussions of paediatric and elderly physiological differences.

GENDER

The difference in risk of injury between men and women is perhaps the most pervasive of all trauma risk factors. In Australia, male injury rates are, on average, about twice those of females.[51] This disparity between the genders is also reflected across most categories of injury death. In Australia, males are also three times more likely to commit suicide,[51] nine times more likely to be injured in a workplace incident[52] and have greater risk of being severely injured, regardless of mechanism.[25,49] Males are also over-represented in road trauma in both Australia and Aotearoa New Zealand. Despite females having an overall higher rate of hospital admissions due to falls, males require admission more frequently, with injuries from mechanical forces (e.g. sport) and assault.[51] The differences between males and females in the number of presentations, the type of injury mechanism and activities performed at the time of the injury illustrate gender differences found in many common social practices. Injury prevention messages need to take into account the complexity and interactive character of gender.[53]

INDIGENOUS POPULATIONS

Injury accounts for a higher proportion of disease burden among Indigenous Australians than non-Indigenous Australians. Injury accounts for 12% of disease burden, making it the second-highest contributor.[54] Aboriginal and Torres Strait Islander Australians are 1.2 times as likely as non-Indigenous Australians to be hospitalised after injury, and have a mortality rate from injury that is nearly double that of non-Indigenous Australians.[4] In 2021, leading mechanisms of injury resulting in hospitalisation were falls, assault and other mechanical forces;[54] assault was far more prevalent among Indigenous Australians, with 15 times the rate of hospitalisation.[4] Death and injury resulting from self-harm, assault, poisoning and traffic incidents all occurred at doubled rate (or more) in Indigenous Australians than non-Indigenous Australians.[4,22] Similar to all other age groups, the rate of injury in Indigenous children is significantly higher than for the remainder of the population.[55] As a result of higher rates of transport and intentional (assault or self-harm) injuries, the age profile of hospitalised Indigenous Australians is quite different to that of non-Indigenous Australians. Although the age-specific rate for injury hospitalisation peaks in the 65+ age group, among Indigenous Australians the highest rate is seen in the 25–44 years age group.[4] While rates of injury increase with geographic remoteness, death rates for Aboriginal and Torres Strait Islander people living in metropolitan cities remain about twice those of other residents.

In view of the high level of trauma morbidity and mortality risk among Indigenous Australians, a National Aboriginal and Torres Strait Islander Injury Prevention Plan has been developed through a consultative process. This plan is mindful of the sensitivities of Indigenous communities, and seeks to address the specific issues faced by the Aboriginal and Torres Strait Islander communities (see Chapter 5).[56]

In Aotearoa New Zealand, the incidence of injury in the Māori population was 69 per 100,000 head compared with 31 per 100,000 people in the non-Māori population.[41] Between 2017 and 2021, age-standardised incidence rates for severe trauma were 50% higher for Māori than non-Māori New Zealanders. Māori also experience twice the rate of injury-related health loss compared to non-Māori, with health loss from assault four times higher in the Māori population.[41]

ALCOHOL AND OTHER DRUGS

Alcohol and other drugs have been associated with many causes of traumatic injury. They impair cognitive function, attention span, judgement and reaction time, often well after they have been metabolised and excreted. The relationship between alcohol and an increased risk of injury or death has been demonstrated in many settings, including road trauma, violence and self-harm.[57] Similarly, a study in Aotearoa New Zealand demonstrated that more than 40% of alcohol-related crash injuries in Aotearoa New Zealand are suffered by people who have not been drinking; most innocent victims are car passengers, and this includes almost all children who are injured through drink-driving.[58]

The influence of other types of substance use on risk of injury has resulted in the introduction of legislation to support large-scale roadside saliva testing for substances other than alcohol across Australia. This will provide public health researchers with a unique opportunity to better assess the influence of substance use on injury risk. There is a dose-related increase in violent behaviour when an individual uses methamphetamine compared to when they do not. This risk of violent behaviour is also increased by psychotic symptoms and/or alcohol consumption.[59]

The collection of accurate data on drinking patterns of these patients would therefore be useful in determining whether ED can be used for these hard-to-reach population groups (see Chapter 40).[57]

GEOGRAPHY—THE TYRANNY OF DISTANCE AND TERRAIN

Both Australia and Aotearoa New Zealand have many communities in remote and rural regions. This means that there are large distances between medical facilities, and these are more likely to provide lower levels of medical care. Designated trauma centres are generally situated in metropolitan areas; rural trauma patients are consequently more likely to be assessed, stabilised or admitted to a non-trauma centre. For major trauma patients, distance from definitive care can have life-threatening consequences. Box 41.1 further illustrates some of the more practical issues around rural trauma.

In Australia, increasing geographic remoteness (as determined by the ABS) from major cities is associated with increasing rates of injury-related hospitalisation and death, for patients up to 64 years of age (Fig. 41.3).[4] Overall, people living in the most remote areas are 2.3 times as likely to be hospitalised, and 2.0 times as likely to die from injury. These risks are higher depending on age; children have an increased risk of dying as a result of their injury if they reside in a rural or remote area.[44] For young people aged 15–24 years, hospitalisation and mortality risks for those living in very remote areas increased by 3.3 times, and 4.1 times respectively. The greatest risk increase in mortality was seen in children aged 5–14 years; children in major cities have a death rate of 1.8 per 100,000 people compared with 23.1 per 100,000 in very remote areas (13 times higher). These

BOX 41.1 CHARACTERISTICS OF AND PROBLEMS ASSOCIATED WITH RURAL TRAUMA[60,61]

By comparison with metropolitan areas, in rural trauma there are:

- greater distances travelled
- higher speed of travel—more severe injuries
- poorer road quality
- older age and poorer condition of vehicles
- poor seatbelt compliance
- fatigue and alcohol issues
- delays in discovery times as a result of remoteness/longer transport times
- less well-equipped rural ambulances to deal with multiple trauma
- lower levels of rural practitioner trauma experience (less frequent)
- hospitals less well equipped to deal with major road crashes and multiple persons.

FIGURE 41.3 INJURY HOSPITALISATIONS AND DEATHS, BY REMOTENESS, BY AGE GROUP AND SEX, 2019–20[4]

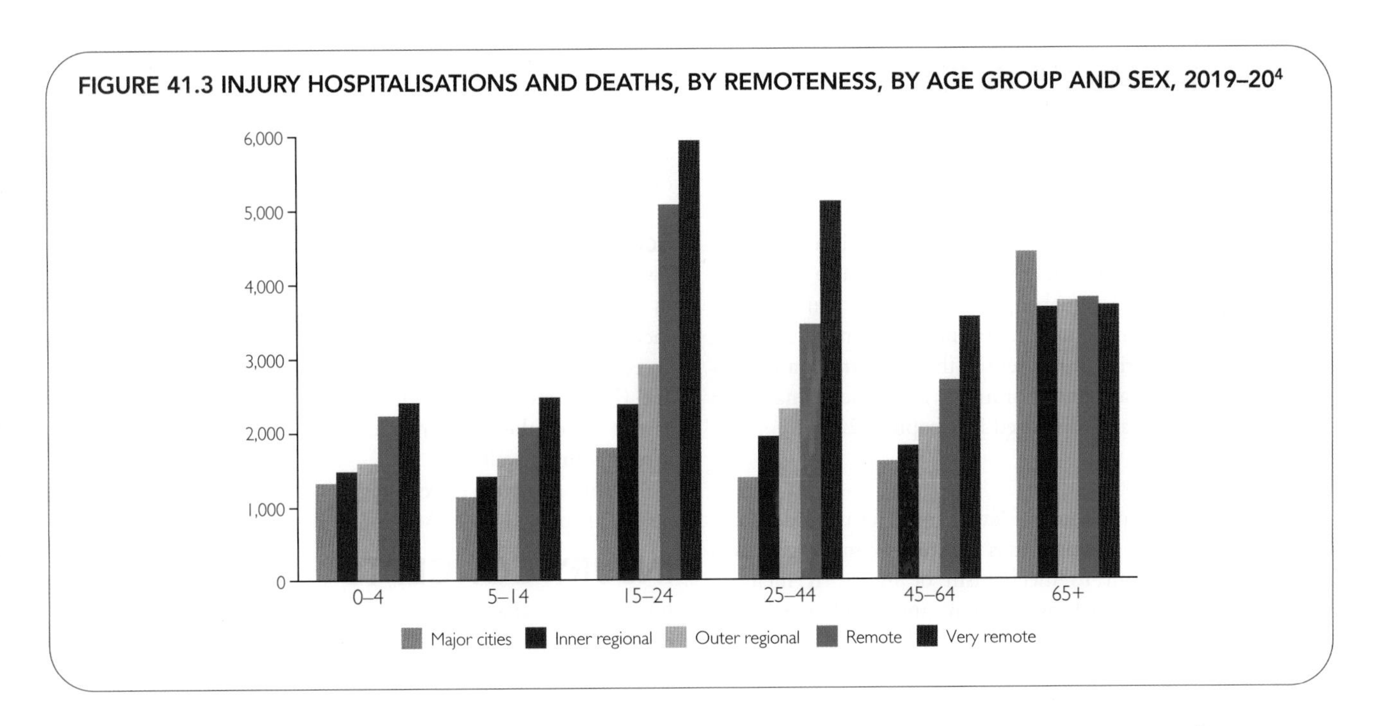

trends are seen for both males and females. In part, they may be attributed to the higher rates of injury among Indigenous Australians, who comprise a higher proportion of the population in more remote areas. Although all mechanisms of injury have higher rates (generally, 1.1 to 3 times higher) in regional and remote areas, rates of hospitalisation following assault are 18 times higher in very remote areas compared to in major cities.[4]

Overall trends towards higher rates of injury in rural areas are also seen in Aotearoa New Zealand.[26] Injury rates for hospitalised trauma are up to 81% higher in rural locations compared with major urban areas. It has also been reported that New Zealanders injured outside the vicinity of a major trauma hospital have a reduced chance of surviving their injuries.[41] As a result, Out-of-Hospital Destination Policies were launched in Aotearoa New Zealand in 2017 as a means of addressing the need for quicker, more efficient transfer to definitive care of injured patients. Emerging technologies in point-of-care testing, for example, venous blood gas, ultrasound and remote imaging, go some way to help guide early appropriate care.

DRIVER BEHAVIOURAL FACTORS

Behavioural factors continue to be implicated in many serious road crashes. At least 14% of all road trauma involves a distraction for the driver (either inside or outside of the vehicle); a significant portion of these result in road fatalities.[62]

Driver distractions may be visual (such as using an in-car navigation system) or auditory (e.g. when drivers focus on auditory signals such as conversation on a mobile phone). Biomechanical distraction involves the removal of one or both hands from the steering wheel to physically manipulate an object, resulting in difficulty steering or changing gears. Cognitive distraction includes any thoughts or cognitive processes that absorb a driver's attention to the point where they are unable to navigate safely through the road.[62]

External-to-vehicle driver distractions (such as billboard advertising) account for 30% of driver distractions in NSW alone; 36% of driver distractions are internal to the vehicle, such as other passengers and mobile phone use.[61] Speed, hand-held mobile phone usage and, for young people, having friends as passengers have been identified as contributing factors to road trauma.[63] Between 1% and 7% of drivers have been observed using mobile phones at any given moment during the day in Australia; this is more likely in younger drivers.[64] Reaction times are slower among drivers talking on a phone than among those talking to a passenger; however, this does not mean that a conversation with a passenger does not have distraction potential. Crash risk for young drivers is significantly increased by the presence of similarly-aged passengers in the vehicle,[62] particularly if they are having emotionally difficult conversations, which have been demonstrated to be more disruptive to driving with the passenger present than those conducted using a hands-free telephone.[65]

For pedestrians and drivers, more injuries are related to talking than texting, although for drivers, reaching for the phone accounts for the most injuries. These rates do not mean that texting is less distracting, but probably reflect a lower amount of texting while driving or walking.[66]

The full impact of driver distraction on the incidence of road crashes in Australia and Aotearoa New Zealand has yet to be systematically investigated and quantified. It is estimated that in Western Australia, speed is a contributor to 50% of road trauma deaths each year.[67] Similarly, in Aotearoa New Zealand, speed accounts for approximately 12% of fatal road incidents annually.[10]

The effects of fatigue on serious road casualties are difficult to quantify; however, it is estimated that 20–30% of all fatal crashes in Australia are due to fatigue. Fatigue is a contributing factor in crashes that involve long trips or trips when the driver has previously been deprived of sleep, placing shift workers particularly at risk. There is evidence that sleep deprivation can have similar hazardous effects to alcohol consumption. Studies have found that people driving after being awake for 17 to 19 hours perform more poorly than those with a blood alcohol concentration (BAC) of 0.05.[68]

MECHANISMS OF INJURY

Understanding the mechanism of injury is a vital part of trauma management. Knowing the mechanism of injury can assist in determining types of injury, and in identifying common injury patterns with mechanical (blunt and penetrating) and other types of trauma. It is essential that emergency clinicians develop sound knowledge and assessment skills in this area to accurately evaluate potential and actual injuries. However, while knowledge of injury patterns is useful, and raises the index of suspicion for certain injuries, it is essential that each trauma patient is assessed systematically and thoroughly using the primary and the secondary surveys, as discussed in Chapter 42.

KINEMATICS

It is important to appreciate the laws of physics to understand mechanism of injury. Kinematics is the study of moving objects and is highly relevant to mechanism of injury. It includes evaluation of aspects such as position, angle and speed, and how these affect the body in motion. A few laws relating to mechanism are discussed below.

1. *Newton's First Law of motion* (law of inertia) states that a body will remain at rest or in uniform motion unless acted on by an outside force.[69] Some examples of stationary objects set in motion by energy forces are pedestrians hit by a vehicle, and blast and gunshot victims. Moving objects interrupted or acted on to stop their motion include people falling from a height, vehicles hitting a stationary object or vehicles braking to a sudden stop.
2. *Newton's Second Law of motion* states that the force that an object exerts on another object is equal to the mass of the object multiplied by its acceleration ($F = ma$). This means that if either of these two variables increase, then the overall force applied to the object in question will also be increased.
3. *Newton's Third Law of motion* states that 'for every action there is an equal and opposite reaction'. This means for every action force, there is a reaction force in the opposite direction.
4. *The law of conservation of energy* states that energy is neither created nor destroyed, but changes form. As a car decelerates slowly, the energy of motion (acceleration) is converted to friction heat in braking (thermal energy) or sound.[70]
5. *The law of moving objects* states that kinetic energy (Ek) is the energy associated with motion, and reflects the connection between weight (mass) and speed (velocity).[71] The equation to calculate kinetic energy is $Ek = ½mv^2$, where m is mass and v is velocity.[72] Consequently, doubling the weight of the moving object doubles the impact, but doubling the speed *quadruples* the impact.

Scenario 1

A passenger travelling in a car will continue to travel at the same speed the car was travelling at when the car hits a wall, unless something (like a seatbelt) stops or alters this motion, demonstrating Newton's First Law. If the passenger was not wearing a seatbelt they would continue to travel at the speed they were travelling prior to impact, therefore being propelled from the car. Likewise, the passenger's internal organs are also travelling at the same speed and will be exerted to the same forces. The faster the car travels, the stronger the force will be (Second Law). Well-designed cars have a 'crumple zone', which absorbs the energy from the crash (law of conservation of energy).

Scenario 2

Two cars of the same mass travelling at 50 km/hr that collide in a head-on collision will apply the same amount of force onto each other (Second Law: $F = ma$). This force will then result in an equal reaction, resulting in both cars having the same damage (Newton's Third Law). The damage would be the same as the car of the same mass and travelling at the same speed hitting a brick wall.

If both cars were travelling at 100 km/hr, the damage would be quadrupled (Law of Moving Objects).

INJURY CONCEPTS

Injury occurs when an external source of energy dissipates more rapidly than the body's ability to tolerate it. A basic component in producing blunt injury is absorption of kinetic energy. Energy originates from several sources, including kinetic (motion or mechanical), chemical, electrical, thermal and radiation sources. An absence of heat or oxygen may also cause injury; for example, frostbite, drowning or suffocation.[73] Box 41.2 defines essential concepts for understanding mechanisms of injury.

Injuries can be classified by the type of forces applied into blunt, penetrating, blast, thermal, and other not as common mechanisms, such as drowning, inhalation injuries or hanging.

BLUNT TRAUMA

Blunt trauma can result from acceleration, deceleration, compression, shearing or direct forces. In both Australia and Aotearoa New Zealand, almost 95% of all major trauma is blunt.[25,49] The majority of major trauma is associated with transport-related injuries (44% in Australia and 50% in Aotearoa New Zealand), followed by falls (38% and 29% respectively); assault accounted for 5% of trauma in Australia and 8% in Aotearoa New Zealand.[25] Of all major trauma patients admitted to designated trauma centres across Australia and Aotearoa New Zealand, almost 40% have head injuries, either isolated or associated with other injuries. Patients with isolated head injuries alone have a higher mortality rate than other isolated body regions. Polytrauma patients, defined as patients with two or more significantly injured body regions,[11] have the highest mortality rate of all traumatic injuries and require an organised system to manage their care, commencing with pre-hospital management and on to surgical and critical care management.[11]

Acceleration injuries occur when a moving object strikes a stationary or slower-moving body (e.g. a blow from a blunt object). Deceleration injuries are the reverse and occur when a moving body hits a solid or slower-moving object. Compression injuries occur with a squeezing inward pressure applied to tissues. Shearing injuries occur when two oppositely directed parallel forces are applied to tissue. Shearing forces can cause organs such as the liver and heart to pull away or fold around muscles and ligaments that secure them in position.[74] This type of injury results in severe internal bleeding. Multiple injuries are common with blunt trauma. Lungs, bowel and other air-filled structures are subject to explosion injuries. Compression injuries to solid

BOX 41.2 ESSENTIAL CONCEPTS FOR MECHANISMS OF INJURY

- Acceleration–increase in velocity or speed of a moving object
- Acceleration/deceleration–increase in velocity or speed of object followed by decrease in velocity or speed
- Axial loading–injury occurs when force is applied upwards and downwards with no posterior or lateral bending of the neck
- Cavitation–creation of temporary cavity as tissues are stretched and compressed
- Compression–squeezing inward pressure
- Compressive strength–ability to resist squeezing forces or inward pressure
- Deceleration–decrease in velocity or speed of a moving object
- Distraction–separation of spinal column with resulting cord transection, seen in legal hangings
- Elasticity–ability to resume original shape and size after being stretched
- Force–physical factor that changes motion of body at rest or already in motion
- High velocity–missiles that compress and accelerate tissue away from the bullet, causing a cavity around the bullet and the entire tract
- Inertial resistance–ability of body to resist movement
- Injury–trauma or damage to some part of the body
- Kinematics–process of looking at a collision and determining what injuries might result
- Kinetic energy–energy that results from motion
- Low velocity–missiles that localise injury to a small radius from centre of the tract with little disruptive effect
- Muzzle blast–cloud of hot gas and burning powder at the muzzle of a gun
- Shearing–two oppositely directed parallel forces
- Stress–internal resistance to deformation, or internal force generated from application load
- Tensile strength–amount of tension tissue can withstand and ability to resist stretching forces
- Tumbling–forward rotation around the centre; somersault action of the missile can create massive injury
- Yaw–deviation of bullet nose in longitudinal axis from straight line of flight.

organs, such as the liver and spleen, may present with minimal external signs of injury. Hollow organs move out of the way more easily than solid organs; therefore, solid organs take the brunt of the force, resulting in contusions and tears. Blunt energy is transmitted in all directions, resulting in organs or tissues being susceptible to rupture if pressure is not released.[75]

ROAD TRAUMA

Road trauma makes up around half of the major trauma population in Australia and Aotearoa New Zealand.[25] In 2021, road deaths occurred from motor vehicle collisions (63%), pedestrians (12%), motorcycles (21%) and pedal cyclists (4%).[36,76] Pedestrians, motorcyclists and pedal cyclists are considered vulnerable road users as they have less protection from the kinetic energy involved in a road crash and are therefore more at risk.[77]

MOTOR VEHICLE COLLISIONS

With a motor vehicle collision, there are multiple phases that occur during deceleration.

1. Before a collision occurs, the occupant and vehicle are moving at the same speed. The first phase occurs when the vehicle impacts with another object—the motion of the vehicle continues until the kinetic energy is dissipated through damage to the vehicle or until the restraining force of the object is removed.
2. The next phase is deceleration of the occupant, which can result in compression or shearing trauma to the occupant. Injuries sustained will depend on the mass of the occupant and the protective devices within the vehicle. In addition, age impacts injuries sustained and children have greater skeletal compliance, which allows diffusion of energy, resulting in the reduced likelihood of fractures.[78]
3. The third phase occurs when internal structures continue to move until they collide with another internal structure, or vasculature, muscles or ligaments suddenly restrain them.

Determining the mechanism of injury in a motor vehicle collision is essential to avoid missed injury as different impact points result in different injury patterns.[79] Fig. 41.4 illustrates the three points of impact with sudden deceleration forces. The size of the occupant also deserves consideration. Due to the smaller size of children, any blunt-force impact will affect a larger portion of their body, potentially resulting in multisystem trauma.[78] Modern vehicles have been adapted with safety devices, such as seatbelts, airbags and crumple zones, which can dissipate the force of impact and reduce the severity of injuries that may occur; however, roll-over injuries are still associated with significant injuries.[79]

Paramedics should provide detailed information to emergency staff regarding the nature of the incident, as this will assist in determining possible injuries. Examples of questions to ask are outlined in Box 41.3.

MOTORCYCLE COLLISIONS

In 2021, there were 235 deaths of motorcyclists on Australian roads—the second highest cause of death after motor vehicle crashes; trends over the past decade have shown no change in the rate of motorcyclist deaths.[36] In Australian children over the age of 5, motorcycles are the second-most common transport-related reason for hospitalisation.[81]

The extent of injury from motorbike collisions is dependent on the amount and type of kinetic energy, the body part that sustains impact, and the safety gear used by the rider. However, motorcycle collisions have a high potential to cause severe injuries. Several factors impact the safety of motorcycle riders, including the effectiveness of the helmet and safety gear, the type and size of motorbike, motorcycle lane filtering laws and visibility of riders.[76] Indicators to the amount of force sustained during a collision include length of tyre skid marks, deformity of the motorbike, deformity of the helmet and stationary objects impacted. The condition of a motorbike driver is often like an occupant ejected from a vehicle.

Three types of motorbike impacts with predictable injuries are head-on impact, angular impact and ejection. During a head-on impact, the motorbike impacts an object that stops the bike's forward motion. The bike flips forwards, so the rider strikes or travels over the handlebars. As the rider strikes the

FIGURE 41.4 THE THREE PHASES OF A MOTOR VEHICLE COLLISION

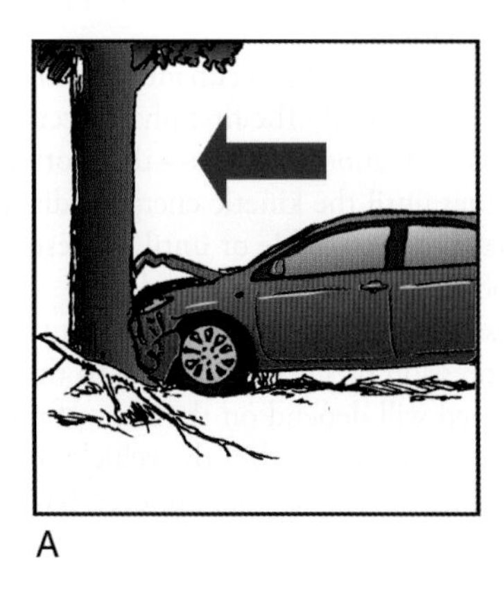

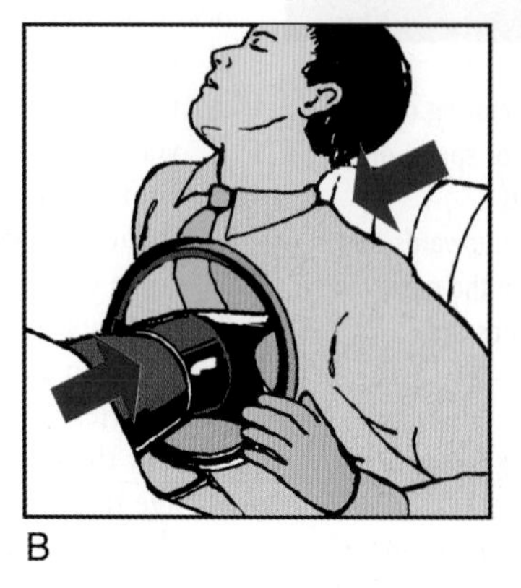

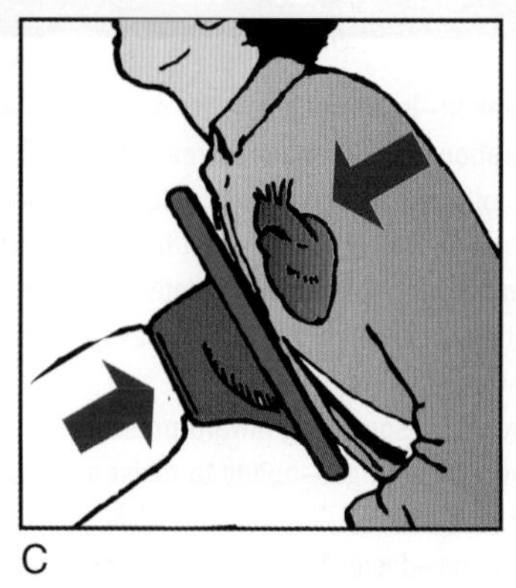

A. Car hits tree. **B.** Body hits steering wheel, causing fractured ribs and sternum. **C.** Heart strikes chest wall, causing myocardial contusion.

BOX 41.3 ADDITIONAL CONSIDERATIONS FOR BLUNT AND PENETRATING MECHANISM OF INJURY INFORMATION[80]

- What is the event type? (e.g. falls, motor vehicle collision)
- What was the estimated energy exchange?
- What protective devices were used? (e.g. seatbelt, helmet)
- What clues are evident from the scene?
- What are the obvious and potential injuries?
- Does the patient have any past medical history or take any medications that may affect their management?
- Is the patient under the influence of drugs and alcohol and what is the significance of this?
- What treatment has been initiated prior to hospital?
- How have they responded to any treatments given?

handlebars, abdominal, chest and pelvic injuries and shearing fractures of the tibia can occur. Bilateral femur fractures occur if the rider's feet are trapped at the time of impact. Neck injuries may occur as the helmet does not provide neck protection.

Angular impact may occur when the rider collides with signs, mirrors on cars or other such objects. When a motorbike is hit at an angle and collapses on the rider, the angular impact injures the side that is crushed between the rider and the ground. Injuries tend to occur in lower extremities, such as open fractures of the tibia or fibula, crushed legs, ankle dislocation and soft-tissue injuries. Abrasions and surface burns may occur if protective clothing such as boots, leather garments and helmets are not worn (Fig. 41.5).

When a rider is thrown or ejected off the motorbike, injuries occur to whatever body part is struck by another vehicle or object at the time of impact and at the point of impact when the body lands. The rest of the body absorbs energy from the impact. Helmet use in motorcycle riders is the most successful way to reduce risk of significant injury;[82] the same is seen in children (see Legislation section).[81]

FIGURE 41.5 EXTENSIVE DEGLOVING TO ABDOMEN AND LEFT THIGH FROM FRICTION SUSTAINED DURING A MOTORBIKE COLLISION

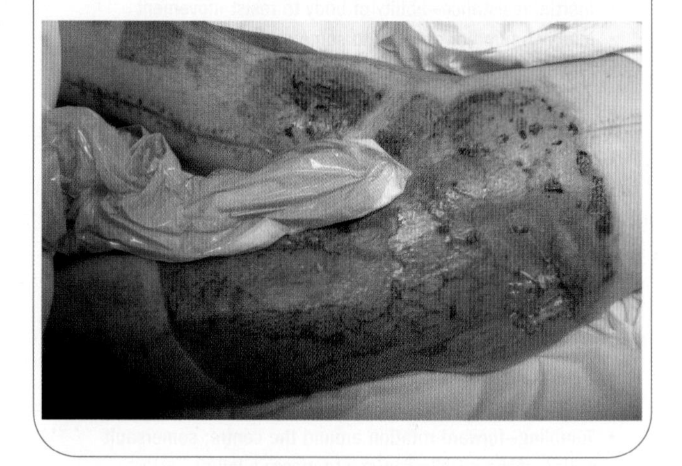

The patient was dragged along the road for 50 metres.

BICYCLE INJURIES

In Aotearoa New Zealand between 2015 and 2020, 58 cyclists died as a result of bicycle trauma, while 1022 were admitted to hospital with serious injury during the same time period.[83] Nearly a quarter of cyclists killed or injured in motor vehicle crashes are aged 10–19 years old and 74% of cyclists involved in police-reported crashes were male.[84] Similarly, in Australia, the majority of hospitalisations for pedal cyclists occurred in males. Cycle helmets are effective in reducing head and facial injuries, with those not wearing a helmet 5.5 times more likely to sustain a severe head injury, requiring three times higher treatment costs.[85,86] Mandatory helmet legislation has resulted in a sustained decline in bicycle-related head injuries in NSW, and cycling fatalities decreased by 2% per annum between 1991 and 2013.[87] Accurate data on cycling participation, use of injury prevention strategies and injury profiles will assist in reducing bicycle-related injury.

FIGURE 41.6 POTENTIAL PRIMARY INJURY SITES OF CHILD PEDESTRIAN[92]

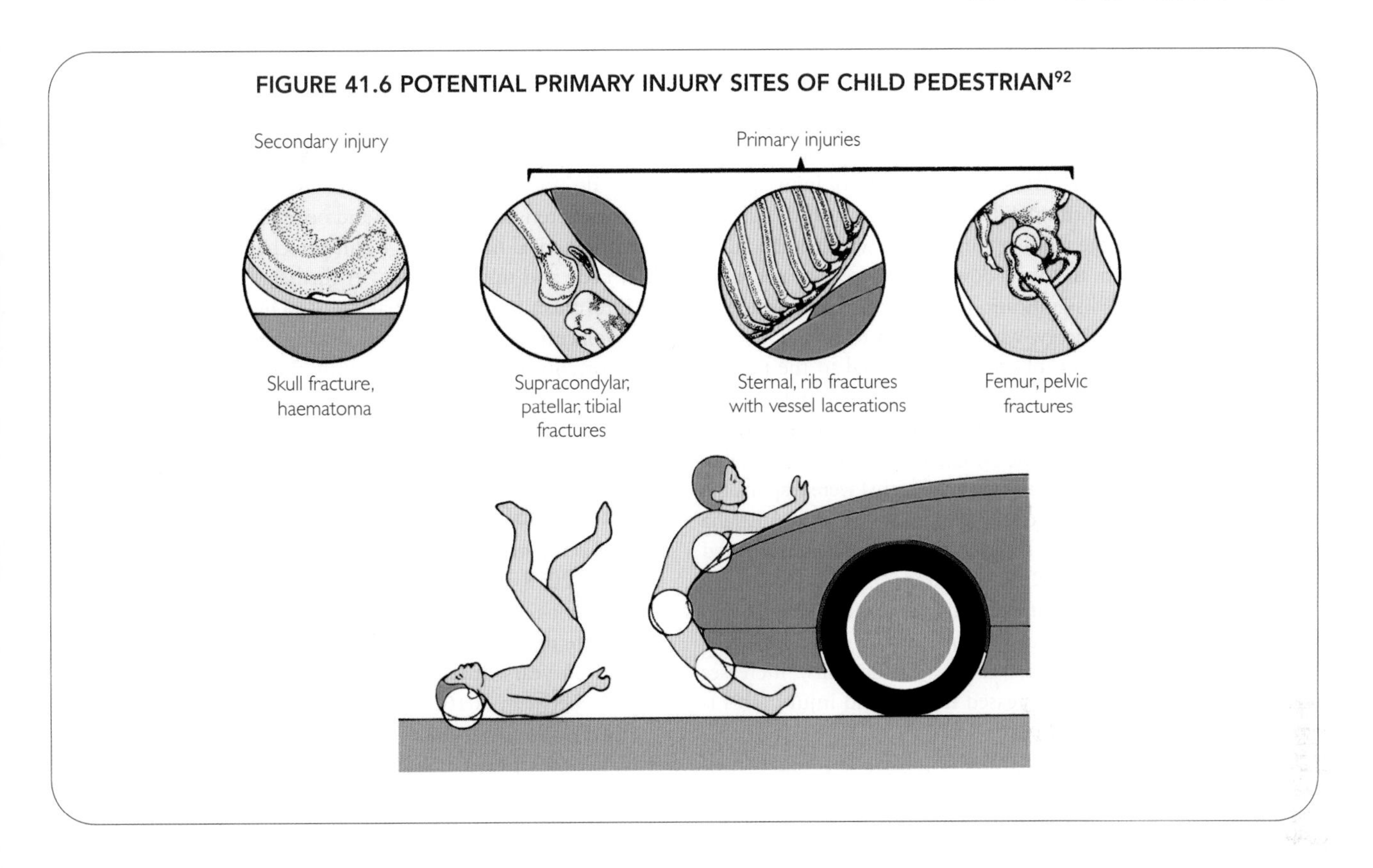

Common mechanisms of injury for bicycle injury are through falls and collisions with stationary or moving objects. The rider may fall as a result of losing control of the bicycle, which may be due to uneven ground surfaces, performing stunts, speeding or rider error.

The most common injuries in cyclists are lower limb, upper limb, head and facial.[88,89] Seat or straddle injuries can occur if there is impact with the middle bar or seat. This can lead to injuries such as vaginal tears, scrotal injuries and perineal contusions.

PEDESTRIAN TRAUMA

Pedestrians have higher mortality rates than other road users and are the most vulnerable. In Australia in 2021 there were 132 pedestrian road deaths.[36] In addition to the nature of the impact and vehicle size and speed, the height, posture and age of the pedestrian will have an effect on the type of injuries sustained.[90] Children tend to face the approaching vehicle; however, adults tend to protect themselves by turning sideways.[91] The mechanisms at play in pedestrian trauma are complex and injuries will vary with the height, mass and position of the pedestrian on impact as well as the vehicle speed, height and rotation.[90] There are three phases of injury in pedestrian trauma:

1. The initial impact occurs when the bumper of the vehicle impacts with the lower extremity of the pedestrian.
2. Following this, head, chest and abdominal injuries occur as the pedestrian hits the bonnet or windscreen.
3. The pedestrian may then fall to the ground, resulting in further head, chest and upper extremity injuries.[91]

Very small children are rarely thrown clear of the vehicle because of their low centre of gravity, size and weight. A child may be knocked down and under the vehicle, then run over. Multisystem trauma should be suspected in any child hit by a car. A combination of injuries, referred to as Waddell's triad, often occurs when a child is struck by a car (Fig. 41.6). Waddell's triad is characterised by injuries to the chest and abdomen, head and femoral shaft.[93] Musculoskeletal injuries are more common than head and neck injuries in the adult population; however, in the child population, head and neck injuries predominate, with musculoskeletal injuries being the second most prevalent.[94]

SERIOUS INJURY INVOLVING A RAILWAY TRAIN OR LEVEL-CROSSING INCIDENTS

In Australia in 2020, there were 65 fatalities involving a railway train or level crossing. In the period 2016–19, there were 137 seriously injured people involving a railway train or level crossing, with the majority of these the result of attempted and suspected suicide.[95] During 2020, most injuries were the result of car occupants or pedestrians on the track (66%) involved in a collision with a train. Other railway incidents included level-crossing events and derailments.[95]

Similarly in Aotearoa New Zealand, there were 13 deaths involving a railway train or level crossing in 2020. Nine people were seriously injured during the same time period.[96] During this time period, the majority of injuries were the result of car occupants (46.1%) and pedestrians (7.6%) involved in a collision with a train. Other railway incidents included level-crossing events and derailments.[96]

Major railway disasters are uncommon; however, they do occur. They often involve a number of fatalities and persons seriously injured and there have been a number of widely reported incidents in the media in both Aotearoa New Zealand and Australia.[97]

FALLS

Falls accounted for 29% of major trauma presentations in Aotearoa New Zealand in 2019 and 2020, and 38% in the same time period in Australia.[25] The mechanism of injury associated with falls is vertical deceleration. The severity and type of injury prevalence is often associated with the distance or height of the fall, the area of body impact, the landing surface and whether the fall is broken by objects on the way down.[73] Falls of greater than 3 metres are considered significant, as the person is subjected to gravitational potential energy, which converts to kinetic energy, resulting in a great amount of energy transferred to the person. In addition, it is important to consider the increasingly elderly population in Australasia: increased fragility and comorbidities lead to a greater risk associated with relatively minor falls (see Chapter 38).[98] Low falls (falls not from a height) were responsible for the greatest number of deaths (36%) in 2019–20 in Australia and Aotearoa New Zealand. This was ahead of transport-related deaths, which accounted for 29% of deaths.[25]

Children are of equal but different concern, as they have a relatively large head in comparison to body size and a less-well-developed neck musculature, which, during falls, increases momentum and results in increased risk of head injury. This is more prominent in infants.[78,99]

Head injuries may result from impulsive loading, which leads to movement of the brain within the skull; subsequent rotational movement may result in tearing of blood vessels, subdural bleeding and axonal injury. Impact loading may also occur, which may result in skull fracture or scalp lacerations. This force may create a pressure wave in the brain and skull, and cause brain contusions.[100]

If a person lands on their feet, they have the potential for Don Juan syndrome: a trio of injuries including bilateral calcaneus fractures, compression fractures of the vertebrae and bilateral Colles' fractures. The energy transferred from deceleration into the feet causes the calcaneus fractures. This energy then travels vertically upwards through the femurs, vertebral column and into the skull base, causing compression fractures in any of these areas.[74]

A fall that causes a person to place their hands out on impact will result in the transfer of energy up through the person's wrists, forearms and shoulders. This type of injury is common in falls from scooters or bicycles. Spinal injuries are another injury associated with falls. This is particularly common when the point of impact is the head, such as happens when diving head-first into water. With this impact, injuries occur because the weight and force of the torso, pelvis and legs bear down on the head and cervical spine. This type of injury is known as a compression injury or axial loading injury. Vertebral bodies are compressed and wedged, producing vertebral fragments that can pierce the spinal cord (see Chapter 47). However, it is important to remember that even simple falls, such as tripping, have the potential for people to hit their head, leading to significant head or spinal injury, or both.

CRUSH INJURIES

The most common mechanism of crush injury is blunt trauma, in which there is sudden or severe compression of the chest or upper abdomen; for example, on being wedged between a truck and a wall, or having a vehicle roll onto the individual and, most commonly, children being reversed over in the driveway. Other causes include natural disasters, such as earthquakes, and man-made disasters, such as terrorist attacks.[101]

A significant force can result in flail chest, head injury and traumatic asphyxia, and as many as 80% of patients with crush injury do not survive.[101] Traumatic asphyxia is a clinical condition characterised by cyanosis and oedema of the neck and face, subconjunctival haemorrhage and petechial haemorrhage of the face, neck and upper chest.[102] A further 10% of crush injuries go into crush syndrome, characterised by rhabdomyolysis and hypovolaemic shock, further increasing mortality.[101]

Mortality increases significantly with prolonged compression; therefore, it is important to consider the amount of force applied and the period of time it has been applied. Crush injury to limbs is discussed in Chapter 48.

INTERPERSONAL VIOLENCE

Assault is the most common form of violent crime in Australia. Between 2018 and 2019 there were 416 victims of homicide and violent-related offences in Australia. Over two-thirds of these were male (70%) and 25% of victims were aged between 25 and 34 years. Interpersonal violence increased in Australia by 10% between 2016 and 2019.[103]

Interpersonal violence occurs between individuals and is often divided into intimate partner, acquaintance and stranger violence, most commonly family and domestic related.[103] Patterns of assault injuries differ between communities due to cultural and social factors. Injuries resulting from assault will vary according to the force and object used. The most common injury sites are head, neck or face, and vary from minor abrasions to multisystem trauma. Bodily force or use of sharp or blunt objects are the most common methods used. Males are more likely to be injured by kicks, head butts or broken drinking glasses. Females are predominantly exposed to blunt violence. Defensive injuries are commonly found on the upper limbs, hands and back.[104] One type of interpersonal violence that is increasingly being reported in the media is the 'coward's punch' (previously known as 'king hit'). The coward's punch is generally characterised by a single blow to the head, causing the person to fall to the ground with a period of unconsciousness. The unconsciousness may result from the punch or as a result of the impact between the head and the ground. Shock waves from the rapid acceleration and deceleration involved in this mechanism are likely to cause tissue damage, swelling, inflammation, nerve disruption and skull fractures. Subarachnoid haemorrhage may also result from torsional injury to the vertebral artery due to rapid cranio-cervical rotation.[105] Interpersonal violence is particularly hard to assess because of the stigma connected to its reporting and the lack of non-healthcare epidemiological data available.

HANGING AND STRANGULATION

Self-inflicted strangulation is one of the most common successful suicide methods worldwide. The severity of injuries associated with hanging is dependent on the height of the fall, the type and position of the neck ligature used and whether the body is fully or partially suspended. The most common form of injuries are minor abrasions, bruising (with potential to increase swelling) and lacerations. More-serious associated injuries are hypoxic brain injury and/or spinal injuries, injuries to the larynx and trachea and vascular injuries.[106] Paramedics should consider these aspects at the scene and communicate to clinical staff during handover. Injuries can be significant due to the presence of the trachea, cervical spine and vital vessels.[107] The mechanisms of injury include venous obstruction leading to hypoxia and unconsciousness, arterial spasm due to carotid pressure, arterial dissection due to hyperextension of the neck and vagal collapse due to pressure on the carotid sinuses. Cervical spine and spinal cord injuries are rare, reported to occur in 0.6% of near hanging cases; however, these injuries should be considered, particularly if the drop height is greater than the height of the person.[108] It is important to remember that not all hanging incidents are self-inflicted; some may be unintentional, such as from window blind cords.

SPORTS- AND RECREATION-RELATED INJURIES

Sporting injury

Exercise is important in promoting health and wellbeing; however, sports may lead to injury. In Australia in 2019–20, 52,300 hospital admissions occurred as a result of a sports injury, were under 35 and the majority were men. The most common cause for sporting injury involved wheels, such as cycling and motor sports. Football-related injuries reduced during this period due to Covid restrictions.[109] In children, sporting injuries were most common in sports involving a ball, bat or stick, water sports or equestrian events.[44] Prevention approaches for sporting injuries in children may include skills education, use of protective gear including helmets, padding and mouthguards, particularly in sports involving a bat, ball and/or stick.[44]

In Aotearoa New Zealand between 2012 and 2016, rugby union was the most common cause of sporting injuries, followed by cricket, netball and rugby league. Moderate-to-severe concussion injuries were highest from each of these sports.[110]

The rate of major trauma, inclusive of deaths, due to participation in sport and active recreation, has increased over recent years; in Victoria, and likely across Australia, much of it can be attributed to cycling and off-road motor sports.[111]

Injuries associated with sports are generally caused by compressive forces or sudden deceleration. Twisting, hyperflexion or hyperextension can cause other injuries. Factors that affect injury include lack of protective equipment, lack of conditioning and inadequate training of the participant. Mechanisms associated with sports and recreational activities are similar to those involved in MVCs, motorcycle collisions and bicycle collisions. Potential mechanisms associated with individual sports are numerous; however, the general principles are the same as with falls and MVCs.

Damaged equipment, such as a broken or cracked helmet or buckled bicycle wheel, can help establish impact. Table 41.1 describes injuries associated with the common sporting and recreational activities in Australia and Aotearoa New Zealand.

TABLE 41.1 SPORTS- AND RECREATION-RELATED INJURIES[112–125]

SPORT/RECREATIONAL ACTIVITY	POTENTIAL INJURIES
Boxing	Concussion, cumulative brain damage, ocular injuries, facial lacerations, contusions, nasal fractures, hand fractures, carpometacarpal instability, boxer's knuckle
Cycling/bicycle riding	Head injuries, spinal cord injuries, abdominal injuries, vaginal tears, scrotal injuries, perineal contusions, facial lacerations, upper extremity injuries, lower extremity injuries
All-terrain vehicles	Head injuries, spine injuries, chest injuries involving rib and sternum, clavicle fractures, burns from exhaust
Gymnastics	Spinal cord injuries, shoulder injuries, ankle injuries
Football/rugby/soccer	Spinal cord injuries, head injuries, hamstring, hip, groin, knee, ankle, shoulder sprains/strains, fractures, lacerations, dislocations
Basketball/netball/hockey	Lower extremity sprains, strains, fractures, lacerations, contusions
Cricket	Head, neck injuries in batters. Upper and lower extremity sprains and strains in fielding and bowling
Skiing/snowboarding	Head injuries, upper and lower extremity fractures/sprains/strains, exposure to elements
Bungee jumping	Major impact-related injuries, intraocular haemorrhages, spinal cord injuries, perineal nerve injuries, soft-tissue injuries
Running	Lower extremity injuries, strains, sprains
Horse riding	Head injuries, thoracic injuries, spinal cord injuries, crush wounds, lower and upper extremity injuries
Skateboarding/scooter riding	Lower extremity injuries, upper extremity injuries, lacerations, head injuries, neck injuries, contusions, facial injuries, sprains, strains
Play equipment	Upper and lower extremity injuries, spinal cord injuries, head injuries
Body-boarding/surfing	Head injuries, lacerations, spinal cord injuries, abdominal injuries
Springboard and platform diving	Head injuries, spinal cord injuries, respiratory complications associated with near-drowning and drowning

All-terrain vehicles

All-terrain vehicles, also commonly known as 'quad bikes', were traditionally designed for use on unpaved off-road terrain such as farms. Between 2017 and 2021, there were 64 quad bike deaths in Australia, with the highest number[23] occurring in 2020; approximately 50% of these were work-related.[126] Capable of speeds up to 100 km per hour, these vehicles have low-pressure tyres and a high centre of gravity, making them more prone to rollover. More than half of the fatalities in Australia from quad bikes (2017–21) were as a result of rollover injuries.[126] Injuries associated with all-terrain vehicle recreational use were more likely to occur due to speed or loss of control; whereas the farm injuries were more likely to be related to rollovers or being pinned.[112,127]

Watercraft/boating

In Australia in 2017–18, 2670 people were hospitalised for a watercraft injury, with males being twice as likely to be injured as a result of a watercraft than females.[128]

Boating injuries can occur from colliding with another boat, explosions, capsizing, or an obstruction in the water. Occupants of boats are not routinely provided with restraint systems, and the boats are not built to absorb the energy associated with impacts. There is potential for drowning or hypothermia when occupants are thrown into the water and water temperatures are cold, in addition to severe injuries from motorised propellers. Other injuries may be similar to those seen in people ejected from a vehicle.

Personal watercraft, such as wave-runners and jet-skis, can also lead to injuries. Different styles allow the driver to sit, stand or kneel while operating the vehicle, with some vehicles allowing up to three passengers. Mechanisms of injury include collisions (with other watercraft, boats, swimmers or objects in the water), falls from the watercraft, handlebar straddle injuries, axial loading and hydrostatic injuries.[129] The potential for injury is very similar to the injury patterns seen with motorcycle collisions and all-terrain vehicles. Spinal fractures at the thoracolumbar region may occur from collisions or hard landing on the seat after the craft has been airborne.[130] Rectal, vaginal and perineal trauma may occur when passengers or drivers hit the water or seat at high speed and fractures occur in almost 50% of watercraft collisions.[128,131] Drowning is another complication associated with these types of incidents and is discussed in Chapter 28.

PENETRATING TRAUMA

Penetrating trauma refers to injuries caused by a foreign object piercing or entering the body, including firearm injuries, stabbing and impalement. The penetrating object creates energy that dissipates into the surrounding tissue. The extent of damage caused will be dependent on the object that is used to cause the injury, the amount of energy or force behind the object, the distance from the victim to the weapon and the type of tissue that is penetrated. Penetrating trauma may be divided into low- and high-velocity injuries. Low-velocity injuries most commonly include stab wounds and impalements, whereas high-velocity injuries refer to gunshot wounds.

Although penetrating injuries are a significant cause of severe injury and death in some other countries, deaths from stabbings and firearms constitute only a small proportion (4%) of trauma presentations in Australia and Aotearoa New Zealand.[25] However, in Australasia it is important to consider other objects, such as industrial and farming equipment, and those objects causing penetrating injuries due to secondary mechanisms, such as in MVCs or falls.

LOW-VELOCITY PENETRATING WOUNDS

Stab wounds

Stab wounds are categorised as low-velocity injuries as the energy exerted behind them is low.

When assessing patients with low-velocity penetrating trauma, it is beneficial to have insight into the object used and hence the size and length of the object. The position of the attacker and the victim will indicate the projected path of the object.[132] It is important to consider the victim's position at the time of penetration. If the victim is hunched over or leaning forwards in an attempt to ward off an attacker, the actual entrance point of the object when the patient is lying on a hospital bed may not correspond with the extent or location of the underlying tissue injury. In addition to this, the wound track may not be straight, making it difficult to determine the extent of the wound and where the wound track ends.[133]

Although stab wounds are considered low-velocity injuries, exerting minimal energy, a single stab wound can penetrate several body cavities with the potential to cause lethal injuries. For example, the object can enter both the chest and the abdominal cavity with one single penetration and may cause damage to more than one body organ.

PRACTICE TIP

Remember that small wounds may be deceptive: they may hide extensive internal damage caused by the attacker moving the object once penetration occurs.

IMPALEMENTS

Impalements are also generally classified as low-velocity injuries and can result from a multitude of factors, including falls, MVCs or secondary to flying or falling objects. While impalement injuries are rare, it is important to consider secondary mechanisms from industrial and farming equipment; for example, lawn mower-related projectiles resulting from debris thrown up from the mower.[134] Removal of impaled objects may result in extensive haemorrhage and hence an unstable patient.

PRACTICE TIP

Impaled objects should be secured in position until the patient is in a controlled environment where surgical support is immediately available.[70]

HIGH-VELOCITY PENETRATING WOUNDS

Gunshot wounds

Rates of injuries and deaths from gunshot wounds have been decreasing in both Australia and Aotearoa New Zealand over the past two decades, due primarily to gun legislation reform.[135,136] In 2013–14, there were 338 hospitalised cases and 209 deaths as a result of firearm-related injuries. Over 90% of each of these

FIGURE 41.7 POTENTIAL INJURY PATH OF HIGH- AND LOW-VELOCITY BULLETS[92]

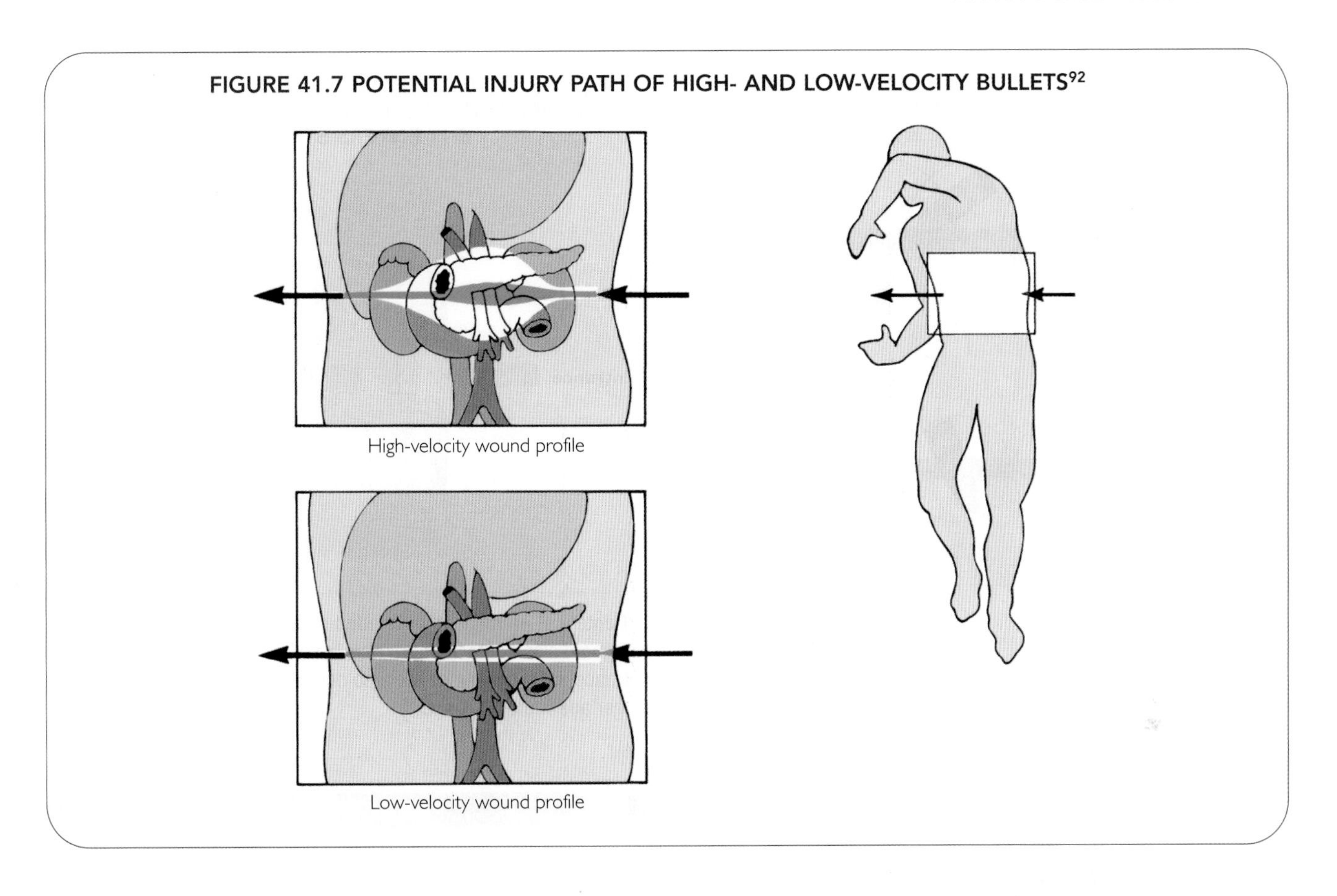

populations were male, with remote areas of Australia accounting for four times the amount of firearm-related injuries than urban areas. Of the 338 hospitalised cases or firearm-related injuries, 39% were caused by unintentional injury, 33% caused by assault, and in 19% of cases, the intent was undetermined. In contrast, 79% of deaths resulted from intentional self-harm (suicide) and 17% resulted from homicide.[137]

Experience in managing patients with gunshot injuries in Aotearoa New Zealand and Australia is limited in comparison to the United States and other countries where guns are more prevalent.

Ballistics is the study of the mechanics of flight, behaviour and effects of projectiles from guns. The type of weapon, type of bullet and type of tissue will all have an effect on the injury sustained. As in a MVC, due to the Law of Kinetic Energy if the velocity of the bullet is doubled, so will the energy.

Laceration or crushing may occur as the bullet passes through tissues, leading to shearing of tissues. If the kinetic energy is larger, the transfer of energy from a weapon may cause cavitation—where particles are moved out of position. Cavitation can be permanent or temporary depending on the amount of energy transferred and the elasticity of the object it hits.[138] Permanent cavitation causes a hole that remains after the energy has dissipated, whereas in temporary cavitation the tissue particles may return to their original location. Temporary cavitation may become permanent depending on the amount of energy transfer from the weapon to the tissue.[138] The size of permanent cavitation is affected by tissue elasticity. For example, cavitation through bone will result in greater permanent cavitation than that through more-elastic tissue.[139]

Low-velocity weapons include handguns and some short-barrel rifles. Bullets fired from these types of guns travel at 300 to 900 m/s, limiting the amount of tissue disruption to a temporary cavity of 3–6 times the diameter of the bullet. Low-velocity bullets cause tissue in the path of the bullet to be pushed aside, causing tissue damage to be relatively localised to the centre of the bullet tract.

High-velocity weapons include hunting and long-barrel assault rifles. Bullets travel at a speed > 900 m/s and, as a result, are responsible for greater tissue damage. High-velocity bullets can create a temporary cavitation of 30–40 times the diameter of the bullet. The high velocity of the bullet creates the cavity by compressing and displacing tissue around the bullet. Fig. 41.7 shows the cavitational differences between high-velocity and low-velocity bullets.

In addition to the velocity, bullet profile (and hence the shape of its nose) and the yaw, tumble and fragmentation of the bullet are important factors in determining the extent of damage. The yaw of the bullet refers to the deviation of the nose of the bullet from a straight path, causing it to hit the target at an angle. Tumbling refers to the change in rotation of the bullet as it hits the body, causing the bullet to somersault in a forward motion through the tissue and leading to extensive tissue destruction (Fig. 41.8).[74] Bullets such as hollow-point bullets are designed to mushroom or expand on impact, causing the bullet to tumble. This increases the frontal surface area, providing maximum energy transfer, reducing penetration with a hard target, but increasing the damage when it strikes a soft target.[140] Both yawing and tumbling increase the surface area of body tissue that the bullet comes into contact with, resulting in greater temporary and permanent cavities.

Some bullets, such as high-velocity jacketed and semi-jacketed bullets, are designed to fragment.[140] Fragmentation

FIGURE 41.8 EFFECT OF BULLET MOVEMENT ON WOUNDING POTENTIAL

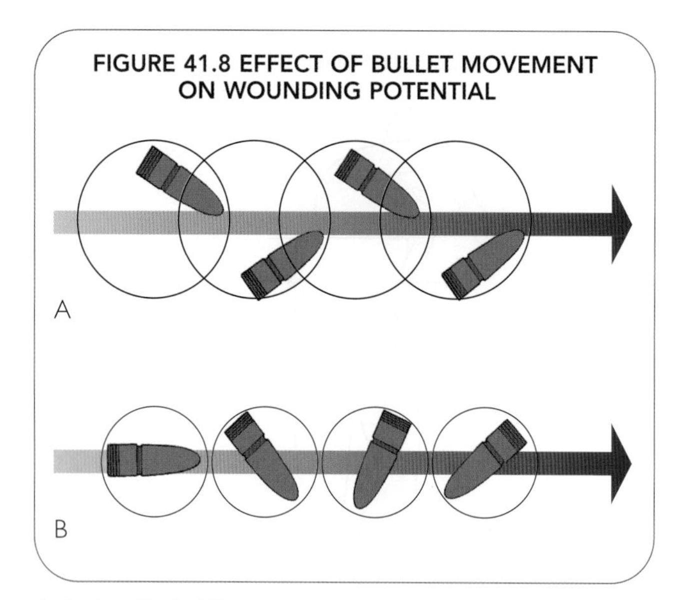

A. Yawing. **B.** Tumbling.

FIGURE 41.9 FRAGMENTATION

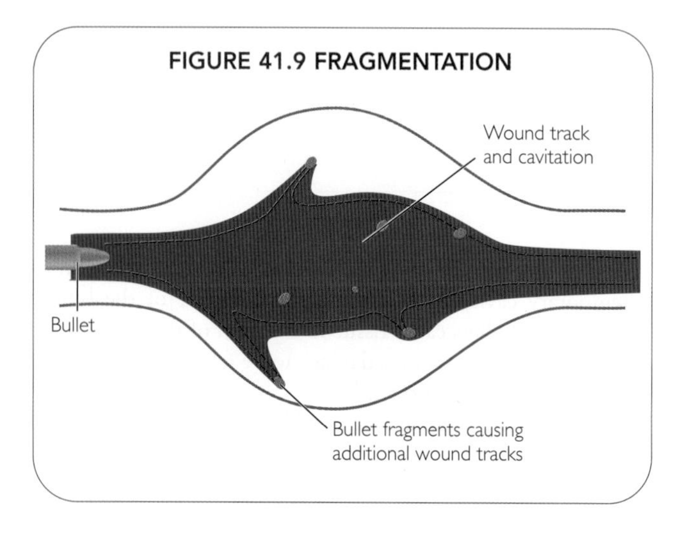

occurs when the bullet breaks apart on impact. This means that the bullet fragments will spread out over a wider area of tissue, causing damage to more areas (Fig. 41.9).

Identifying entry and exit wounds may help determine the pathway of the bullet and therefore indicate potential organs and bones the bullet may have come in contact with. Entrance wounds are usually round or oval in shape, whereas exit wounds are stellate or starburst in shape. Fig. 41.10 compares entrance and exit wounds.

If the gun has been fired within close range—less than 25 cm away—the entrance wound may also be accompanied by a graze or a small burning tattoo. The exit wound will not exhibit these features. Exit wounds may not always be found, as it is possible for the bullet to lodge itself within dense tissue or bone.

Secondary causes of death from firearm injuries are internal haemorrhage, wound infection and organ destruction.[141]

PRACTICE TIP

It is important not to wash around the patient's wound area or the patient's hands immediately as these may contain gunpowder traces essential for forensic investigations.[142]

FIGURE 41.10 A SPINNING MISSILE PRODUCES A 1–2 MM ABRADED EDGE ALONG THE WOUND IF IT ENTERS STRAIGHT

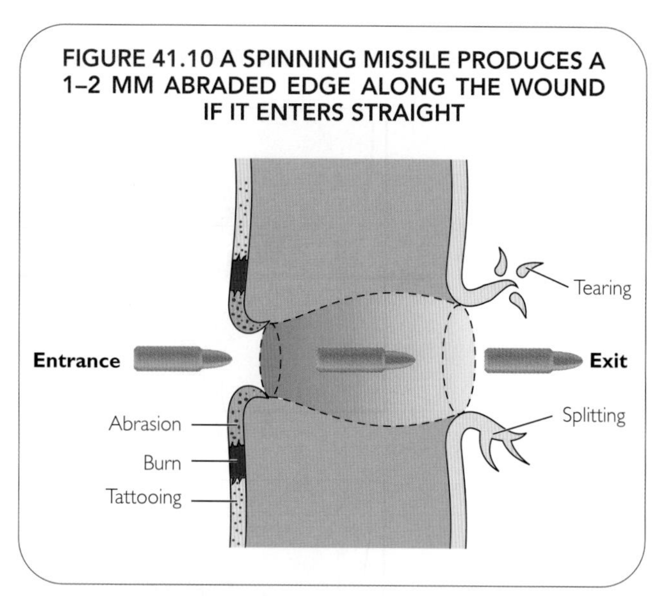

If it enters at an angle, the abraded side is on the bottom of missile, with more skin contact, and covers a much wider area. Differences in entrance and exit wounds are also depicted. Exit wounds are generally longer and more explosive.

PRACTICE TIP

When assessing a patient with a penetrating injury, it is useful to tape a metal object such as a paper clip to each wound prior to radiological imaging. This will assist with identifying trajectories.

BLAST INJURIES

Blast injuries are uncommon in Australasia; however, the potential exists, especially with hazardous explosions within industrial settings, such as oil refineries, mines, shipping docks and chemical plant sites. The potential for blast injuries has also heightened with increased terrorist activity globally and emergency clinicians working with the defence forces have recently had significant exposure to these injuries in conflict-ridden areas. An explosive refers to a high-energy substance with the ability to cause decomposition by the sudden release of a combination of thermal and kinetic energy.[143,144] Fig. 41.11 illustrates the types of injury from a blast.[140]

PRIMARY INJURIES

Primary injuries are associated with the effects of the pressure or blast waves associated with a high explosive substance. In essence, it is a form of barotrauma. The nature of expanding gas causes equal amounts of air to be displaced, known as a shock wave or 'overpressure'. The shock wave lasts several milliseconds and causes damage at the interface of tissues. The degree of damage is directly related to the power behind the blast and the duration of the shock wave. Following the shock wave, a vacuum is generated at the explosion site, which creates a negative pressure wave. It has a duration of up to three times that of the shock wave and is commonly associated with barotrauma injury. In addition, the point of impact and subsequent energy dispersal to underlying tissue of a pressure wave hitting an

FIGURE 41.11 EFFECTS OF AN EXPLOSIVE BLAST

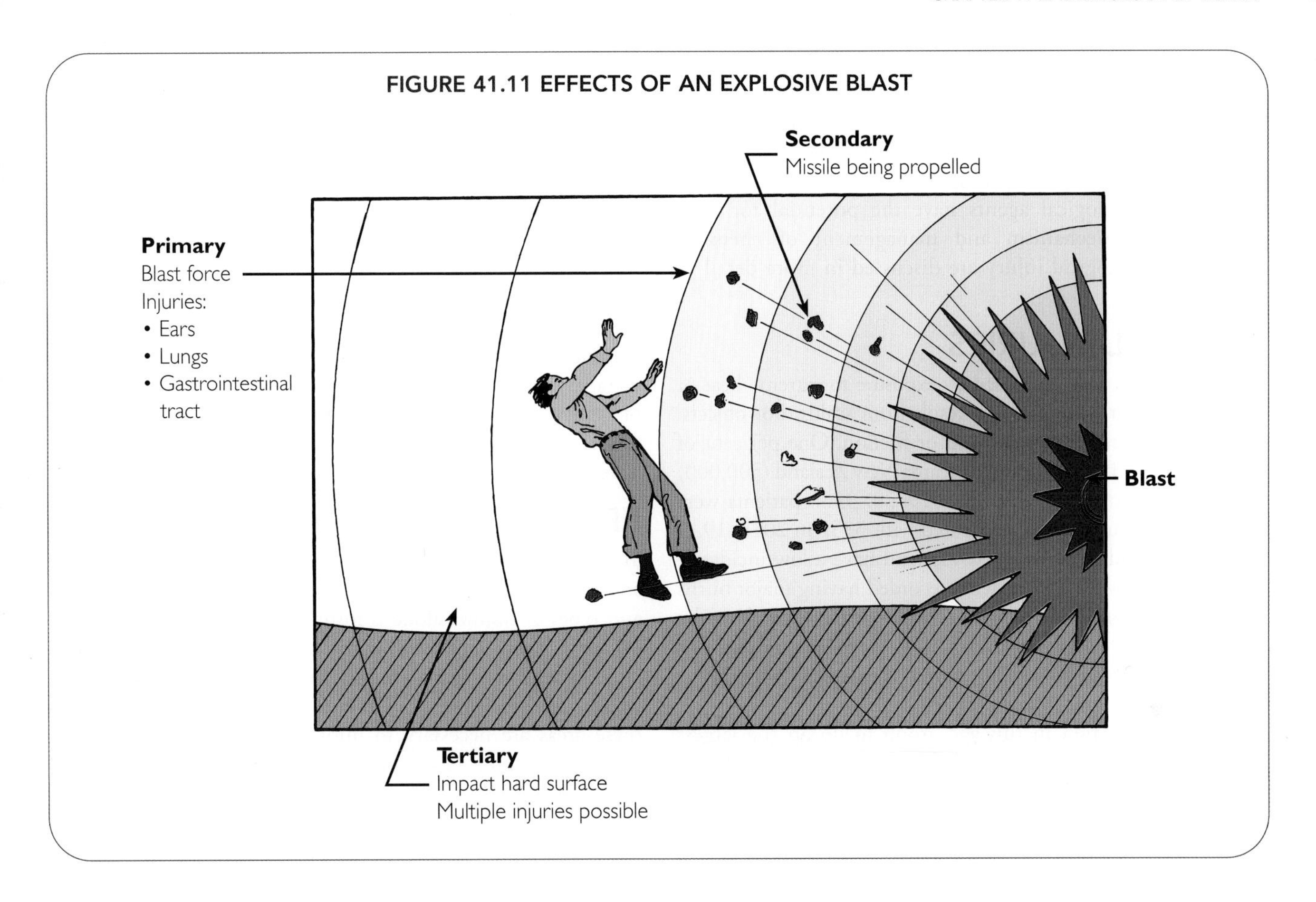

individual is affected by their position in relation to the wave. A wave passing over a person lying down is less likely to produce injury than one hitting the upright body.

Gas-containing organs, such as the lungs and bowel, are at greatest risk of primary blast injury.[144] Other injuries commonly associated with primary blasts include myocardial contusion, shearing of large cardiac vessels, detachment and tearing of the bowel, rupturing of the eardrum, pulmonary haemorrhage and rupture.[140]

SECONDARY INJURIES (BALLISTIC)

Secondary blast injuries involve the projection of bomb fragments and flying debris through the air, often at enormous speeds comparable to those of missiles. This occurs as a result of the blast wind that immediately follows the shock wave. Debris is any object between the blast epicentre and outer perimeter of the blast radius, and may include minutely small to large fragments, rocks, glass, dirt, human remains and structural items. The blast wave causes a mass displacement of air and is responsible for both penetrating and blunt injury.[144] Common injuries associated with secondary blast injury include penetrating injuries, lacerations, abrasions, lung contusions and ruptured bowel.[144]

TERTIARY INJURIES

Tertiary blast injuries result from the person being thrown into the air and displaced either onto the ground or into other objects. The displacement distance is an important question in the history process. The most common injuries are the same as for falls or ejection from a vehicle, with blunt head, spinal and pelvic injury, abrasions and contusions.[144] Impalement is less common. Children are particularly susceptible to tertiary blast injury, due to their smaller body mass.

QUATERNARY INJURIES

Miscellaneous injuries, also known as quaternary blast injuries, may result from, but are not limited to, building collapse leading to crush injuries, thermal injuries such as burn or hypothermia associated with prolonged extrication or toxic effects from chemicals, any pre-existing condition potentially aggravated by a blast, or psychological trauma and infection which occur after the explosion.[144]

QUINARY INJURIES

Quinary blast injury is a relatively recent term describing toxic absorption, either by inhalation or through wounds, producing an immunological response and unique early hyperinflammatory state.[145,146] This is associated with hyperinflammatory states manifested by hyperpyrexia, diaphoresis, low central venous pressure and a positive fluid balance.[140] This area requires further research for increased understanding of the mechanisms involved.

ADDITIONAL WEAPONS

The increasing terrorist activity around the world has not only heightened the interest in blast injuries, but also those of chemical, biological, radiological and nuclear (CBRN) weapons. Healthcare institutions need to be prepared with disaster plans as they require specialised equipment such as HAZMAT suits.[147] Chemical weapons contain chemicals with the potential to kill, injure or incapacitate humans. The health impact will be determined by the agent used, the concentration of the agent, the route, and rate of exposure and the spread of the agent and potential contamination of other people. Different routes of exposure are: inhalation, ingestion, irradiation, injection and skin exposure. The method of dispersing the agent will determine the depth of contamination.[148]

As such, biological agents have the potential for high lethality. The mechanism and management of chemical biological radiological injury are discussed in more detail in Chapter 12.

THERMAL INJURIES

Thermal injuries may be caused by exposure to extreme heat or lack of heat. Burns injuries can result from scalds, hot objects, chemicals, fire and flames and sun or friction. One per cent of the population of Australia and Aotearoa New Zealand (300,000) suffers from burns each year. In 2019–20, 3367 patients were admitted to a burns service compared with 3357 in 2018–19.

Australia and Aotearoa New Zealand have a low incidence of major burns, with 230 patients recorded having major burns in 2019–20, significantly lower than when compared to the United States.[149] However, over half of these burn admissions (57%) occurred in rural and remote areas with significant implications for transport and pre-hospital care.[150]

Burns in children in this age group made up the largest single group of burns victims, with 52% of paediatric burns resulting from a scald injury.[150] The vast majority occur at home (89%) and in the kitchen (47%). Trend estimates over the seven-year study period showed no evidence of decline (see Chapter 49).

Frostbite is a thermal injury caused by exposure to extreme cold. The injury is localised to the area of exposure and the tissues that are damaged. It typically occurs in people exposed to extremely cold climates; see Chapter 28.[151]

OTHER MECHANISMS

Less common mechanisms include inhalation or electrocution injuries, which account for less than 1% of severe trauma presentations.

INHALATION OR PULMONARY INJURY

Inhalation injury may be a result of three mechanisms: carbon monoxide poisoning, thermal injury and toxic chemicals such as chloring and cyanide. These may occur singularly or in combination, and can lead to the development of severe respiratory distress.[152] The three distinct categories of inhalation injury are carbon monoxide (CO) poisoning, upper airway injury and lower airway injury (Chapters 21 and 49).[153]

Carbon monoxide is a colourless, odourless and tasteless gas produced during combustion. When inhaled, it combines with haemoglobin, for which its affinity is more than 200 times greater than that of oxygen, reducing oxygen-carrying capacity. This results in hypoxia and asphyxiation.[154] Upper airway injury may be caused by direct heat or chemical damage of the structures of the upper airway leading to erythema, oedema and ulceration of the airway above the vocal cords. Lower airway injury refers to injury below the vocal cords, and usually results in death. All inhalation injuries require early airway management, ventilatory support and hard-line pulmonary hygiene.[152] Management of inhalation injury is discussed in more detail in Chapter 21.

DROWNING

Drowning is the submersion in a liquid above the airways, preventing the inhalation of air. The patient experiences breath holding, followed by laryngospasm, hypoxia and hypercarbia, swallowing of liquid, water inhalation, surfactant washout, hypoxia, loss of consciousness and then death if not removed to dry land.[155]

ELECTROCUTION

Electrocution injuries occur as a result of exposure to electric current. The severity of the injury may depend on the level of voltage. Electrocution injuries can include dysrhythmias, burns or asphyxiation due to tetany of muscles. Electricity will need to return to the ground to complete its circuit; therefore, victims will have an entry and exit wound, for example, the hand and foot.

EFFECTS OF INJURY ON SOCIETY

To understand the magnitude of trauma as a public health issue and its full burden on society, collecting data on the prevalence and types of trauma alone is insufficient. The impact of injury on acute health and rehabilitation services, the workforce and families and significant others needs to be monitored and understood. Ongoing measurements of the impact of trauma in these areas are necessary to inform public policy, legislation, funding, resource allocation and distribution. An understanding of the effects of injury on society is therefore essential for clinicians, from pre-hospital to rehabilitation.

In an effort to reduce trauma mortality, the focus of trauma management has been predominantly physiological. However, improved survival has resulted in a growing awareness of the psychological impact of traumatic injury. Two areas identified in the trauma literature include post-traumatic stress (PTSD) and the impact of trauma on cognitive function and personality.

POST-TRAUMATIC STRESS

As times of military conflict accelerated our understanding of physiological responses to traumatic injury, the problem of emotional sequelae stress reactions among trauma survivors has also emerged. After World War I, post-traumatic stress was called shell shock; during World War II, it was referred to as combat fatigue; following the Vietnam War, it was labelled the post-Vietnam syndrome; and after the Gulf War, Gulf War syndrome emerged, although its physiological and/or psychological origins remain a topic of intense debate.

According to the American Psychiatric Association,[156] PTSD is defined as an anxiety disorder that persists for a period of more than 1 month following a traumatic event involving actual or threatened death, and serious injury or threat to the physical integrity of oneself or others. It usually comprises the following symptoms, including disturbing and persistent memories of the trauma, avoidance of trauma-related factors, negative mood and social changes and self-destructive behaviours.[156]

Some studies have reported an incidence of up to 51% of patients who had sustained traumatic injuries meeting diagnostic criteria for PTSD,[48] yet psychological consequences such as PTSD are currently neglected in burden-of-injury calculations.[157]

According to the American Psychiatric Association's practice guidelines for the treatment of patients with acute stress disorder (ASD) and PTSD, ASD was added to the established list of psychiatric diagnoses in 1995 to distinguish individuals with PTSD-like symptoms that lasted for less than 1 month from persons who experienced milder or more-transient difficulties following a traumatic event. Further, trauma centres (while the patient is in hospital), outpatient clinics and general practitioners should screen patients for symptoms of depression, anxiety and stress to assist with early identification and intervention. Research continues to demonstrate that the majority of trauma patients experience high levels of anxiety and stress in hospital, and those with traumatic injury are likely to have ongoing mental health complications, including PTSD, depression, anxiety and stress.[158,159]

COGNITIVE/BEHAVIOURAL CHANGES

In addition to post-traumatic stress, there is a range of cognitive and behavioural changes that can result from traumatic brain injury, such as depression and PTSD. These changes vary according to the mechanism of injury and resultant focal or diffuse damage to cerebral tissue, but can have significant impacts on functional outcome and quality of life.[157] For example, in general, cognitive disorders result from disorders of attention, concentration and memory, problems with communication, difficulty with reasoning and judgement, and difficulties with planning and initiating daily activities. Behavioural sequelae may include impulsivity, irritability, agitation, aggression, depression and egocentrism in interpersonal relationships. Even in minor head injuries, these changes can have a significant impact on work performance and safety, subsequent workplace absence and on relationships with family and significant others. These effects represent an enormous hidden impact of trauma on individuals and their functioning in society.

As with other psychological sequelae of traumatic injury, clinicians have an important role to play in recognising symptoms of cognitive disorders and behavioural change in trauma patients and in initiating early/appropriate referrals; for example, by conducting the abbreviated post-traumatic amnesia score (AWPTAs) in minor head injury patients being discharged from the ED. For a more detailed examination of traumatic brain injury, see Chapter 43.

INJURY PREVENTION

In view of the impact of injury on the individual, family, health service and society, there has been an increasing emphasis on prevention strategies. For example, in Australia and Aotearoa New Zealand, legislative changes to improve road and workplace safety and Indigenous health have been implemented through multi-year, ongoing safety plans and strategies.[23,56,160,161]

Clinicians who care for trauma patients clearly recognise the need for prevention and control strategies to curb trauma mortality and morbidity. To initiate or participate in injury prevention programs, clinicians need to be aware of the principles that underlie injury prevention and understand accepted models of injury control. This responsibility is seen to be part of the role of the emergency physician and the trauma coordinator, and the presentation of a patient to hospital following injury often provides a teachable moment for future injury prevention. Trauma nurse coordinators, however, are often met with competing priorities and time restraints, making this aspect of their role difficult to fulfil.[162]

The perception of trauma as preventable events, rather than random, unexpected 'accidents', is fundamental to the success of any injury prevention program. There are a number of principles that underpin effective injury prevention and safety promotion—these are listed in Box 41.4.[20] Understanding these principles empowers clinicians to involve themselves in preventing injury rather than being limited to dealing with the physical, emotional and psychological sequelae of traumatic injury. Pre-hospital professionals such as paramedics are ideally placed to be significant contributors to injury prevention, as they see the actual scenes and potential contributing factors where people are injured and are equipped with skills to rapidly assess and control a trauma scene. One such injury prevention program is the 'Prevent Alcohol and Risk Related Trauma in Youth' (P.A.R.T.Y.) program, which is aimed at youth and has been shown to reduce alcohol-related offences, including effective decision-making regarding a sober driver, improving use of seatbelts and education of the risks of speeding.[163]

BOX 41.4 INJURIES WITH APPROPRIATE RESTRAINT SYSTEMS[20]

SPINAL

- Cervical vertebral fractures from flexion forces
- Neck sprains secondary to hyperextension
- Lumbar vertebral fractures secondary to flexion–distraction forces

THORACIC

- Soft-tissue injuries of the chest wall associated with belt placement
- Sternal fractures with or without myocardial contusion
- Fewer than three rib fractures if restrained; more than four if unrestrained
- Trauma to breast in females

ABDOMINAL

- Soft-tissue injuries (contusions, abrasions, ecchymosis)
- 'Seatbelt' friction burns or abrasion where seatbelt rests
- Injuries to small bowel secondary to crushing and deceleration
- Ruptured aorta secondary to longitudinal stretching of the vessel
- Injuries to the liver, pancreas, gallbladder and duodenum secondary to crushing forces

LEGISLATION

Seatbelts, child restraints

Seatbelt use, child restraints and wearing of helmets by motorcyclists and their passengers was made compulsory by legislation in all Australian states and territories by 1973.[164,165] This legislation led to a consistent decline in road trauma deaths over the following three decades. The use of seatbelts has shown a 51% reduction in fatalities globally, and a 67% reduction in fatalities when used in combination with airbags.[166] In addition to driver and passenger airbags, other safety features have been made mandatory on cars sold in Australia (and later Aotearoa New Zealand) over the past 20 years—specifically, antilock braking systems (ABS) and electronic stability control (ESC).

Legislation regarding child restraints was introduced in Australia in 2010. The Australian Transport Council (comprising transport ministers from across Australia) approved new laws which introduced a mandatory, size-appropriate restraint system for all children up to the age of 7 years in order to significantly improve the safety of children when travelling in vehicles. The introduction of mandatory child restraints significantly reduced the rate of serious injury and mortality in children involved in road crashes. Child restraints are effective as they distribute the force of the collision over the child's strongest body region and protect the child from hitting the interior of the vehicle. The main principle in reducing force involves restraining the child from moving downwards in a collision. The most common injuries of restrained children involved in motor vehicle collisions are head injuries, where their head collides with the internal structures of the vehicle.

Seating children from age 4 to under 7 years of age in an appropriate booster seat approved by Standards Australia[167] reduces their risk of injury in a crash by almost 60% when compared with a child sitting in an adult seatbelt without a booster seat. According to Australian and New Zealand Standard AS/NZS 1754 there are eight types of child restraints and children 7 years and younger must be seated in the rear of the vehicle when there are at least two rows of seats. If all the rear seats are occupied by children 7 years and younger, a child of 4 years of age or older may be secured by an age-appropriate device in the front seat. However, up to 79% of children are not always properly restrained or are placed in an ill-fitting seat. Injuries to the child occupant are substantially increased when child restraints are inappropriately used or fitted.[168] Some of the common forms of misuse include harness straps being poorly adjusted or incorrectly positioned, seatbelts being incorrectly routed or twisted, and incorrect fitting of locking clips.[169]

Speed limits, drink-driving laws, improved law enforcement technology

Reduced speed zoning has been used as a strategy to modify driver behaviour and reduce the risk of collisions in areas prone to motor vehicle crashes or pedestrian injury. By the end of 2001, the speed limit in all Australian streets was reduced from 60 kph to 50 kph (unless otherwise signed) and is linked to a 20% reduction in casualty crashes, with greater reductions for crashes involving serious injuries and fatalities. This has had particular benefits for pedestrians, who were at greatest risk of death following a collision with a motor vehicle in speed zones of 60 km/hr and greater.[170] Similarly, speed zoning near schools and places of high pedestrian activity has been reduced to 40 kph and 50 kph respectively during before and after school times, resulting in a 23% reduction in casualty crashes and a 24% reduction in all pedestrian and bicyclist crashes outside schools in Victoria.[171]

Random breath-testing for alcohol was initiated on a wide scale in Victoria in 1976. Speed and/or red-light cameras were first introduced in Victoria in 1983. The success of these law-enforcement initiatives led to their subsequent dissemination to other Australian states and territories. More recently, these technologies have further developed to include more-accurate laser-based speed-detection devices, digital imaging, red-light cameras and point-of-testing tools for the detection of other illicit substances.

It is estimated that following the introduction of random breath testing in Australia there has been a reduction of almost 50% in the number of fatal crashes across all states in Australia.[172]

Vehicle safety

'Design Rules for Motor Vehicle Safety' were introduced to Australian legislation through the *Motor Vehicles Standards Act* in 1989. This brought Australian vehicle design standards into line with many international standards. Design standards include improved tyres, windscreens, head restraints, lights, indicators and brakes; vehicle impact resistance in cars; increased occupant protection and rollover strength in buses; mandatory fitting of seatbelts in new passenger vehicles from 1970; the use of retractable belts and progressive extension of seatbelt requirements to other motor vehicles; mandatory use of anchorage points for child restraints; and installation of speed limiters in heavy vehicles.

Airbags

Airbags are not mandatory in all Australian or Aotearoa New Zealand vehicles; however, most recent-model cars are equipped with dual front, side and head impact airbags. Airbags are designed to protect occupants in frontal and lateral deceleration collisions by inflating on impact, cushioning the head and chest, then rapidly deflating. Further, in Victoria, since January 2011 new vehicles must be fitted with electronic stability control to be registered, and curtain airbags are mandatory in all new cars manufactured from 2012. The use of airbags in new vehicles is supported by the Australasian New Car Assessment Program (ANCAP), which in turn is supported by all Aotearoa New Zealand and Australian motoring clubs, the Aotearoa New Zealand Government, Australian state governments and the Fédération Internationale de l'Automobile (FIA).[173,174]

Airbags are a supplementary restraint and are most effective when used in conjunction with seatbelts. Australian airbags are triggered to deploy at higher-impact speeds compared with airbags in the United States; this reduces the likelihood of injury resulting from 'unnecessary' airbag deployment.

Injuries reported from airbag deployment include facial soft-tissue injury, facial and forearm bruising and corneal abrasions. Serious injuries have been seen in small drivers who adjust the seat closer to the steering wheel. Injuries to children from airbags have been reported in the United States; however, Australian and Aotearoa New Zealand standards for child restraints means that properly tethered restraints can only be mounted in the rear seats, where appropriate anchorage is provided.[175]

Helmets

Australia was the first country to make pedal cyclist helmets mandatory. Similarly, in Aotearoa New Zealand the wearing of helmets by pedal cyclists is mandatory. Helmet use has been shown to reduce the rate of serious and fatal head injuries and facial injuries in pedal cyclists. Motorcycle helmets manufactured in Australia and Aotearoa New Zealand must meet Australian/New Zealand Standard AS/NZS 1698:2006 Protective Helmets for Vehicle Users safety standards (refer to bicycle section above for further detail).

Motorcyclists and their passengers are also legally required to wear a helmet in Australia and Aotearoa New Zealand; however, this is not required to be a full-face helmet. Full-face helmets have been shown to reduce the risk of facial injury; however, they are suspected to be associated with an increased risk of skull base fractures. The incidence of significant head trauma has been shown to be higher in motorcyclists who were not wearing a helmet (63.81%) than in those who were wearing a helmet at the time of their injury (38.95%).[175]

Licensing restrictions for inexperienced drivers

Young people account for a significant portion of traumatic injuries and death, both globally and in Australia and Aotearoa New Zealand.[25,64] As a result, there is a significant focus on injury prevention for this cohort.

Graduated driver licensing (GDL) systems are regarded as the primary means of ensuring novice drivers (typically young drivers) are introduced to the use of motor vehicles in a safe, controlled and low-risk manner. Graduated driver licensing systems have been shown to reduce road trauma deaths in young drivers.[176]

The Australian approaches to GDL combine restrictions on young drivers with intensive training requirements, and add significant enforcement (zero tolerance with regard to speeding, driving while impaired by alcohol or other drugs and the use of mobile telephones by young drivers) and penalty components (particularly the suspension of a driver's licence for offences, the impoundment of motor vehicles and opportunities to attend traffic offender intervention programs as part of the penalty process). There is also a focus on restricting the number of passengers in the vehicle, resulting from research which showed that the risk of a road crash for a young driver increases where there are similar-aged passengers in the car and continues to increase where there are more passengers. The risk of injury increases further when there is more than one young passenger in the vehicle.[176]

Prior to the introduction of passenger restrictions in Victoria, carrying more than one passenger increased the fatal crash risk of first-year provisional-licence driver to four times the level of driving alone or with only one passenger. More than a quarter of these drivers involved in fatal crashes were carrying multiple passengers at the time of the crash.[164]

Workplace injury legislation

Stronger workplace legislation has been developed to enforce work safety standards in both Australia and Aotearoa New Zealand. In the 1980s, Australia followed the legislative trend of the United Kingdom after the recommendations of a parliamentary inquiry into occupational health and safety were mandated by law. In 2020, Australia reported a total of 194 workplace fatalities compared with 174 workplace fatalities in 2017.[177] Workplace fatalities have almost halved since the mid-1990s, with a significant decrease in the number of compensated claims in the same period.[177] The model Work Health and Safety (WHS) Regulations are made under the *Work Health and Safety Act* and outline a wide range of matters relating to work health and safety, including: managing risks to health and safety and general workplace management; hazardous work involving noise, hazardous manual tasks, confined spaces, falls, demolition work, electrical safety and energised electrical work; construction work; hazardous chemicals; mines and asbestos. They are model provisions only. To be legally binding they need to be enacted or passed by Parliament in each jurisdiction. In Aotearoa New Zealand, the *Health and Safety at Work Act 2015* and the *Hazardous Substances and New Organisms Amendment Act 2015* provide similar regulations.

TRACKING INJURY IN AUSTRALIA AND AOTEAROA NEW ZEALAND

Many trauma registries exist in Australia and Aotearoa New Zealand; most are based at single hospitals, but others collect data across organised systems of trauma management (such as regions or states). The Australia New Zealand Trauma Registry (ATR) collects data on major trauma patients (see below) admitted to one of 34 trauma centres across Australia and Aotearoa New Zealand, providing invaluable data on major injury. The ATR is being expanded each year to include regional hospitals that also collect trauma data; for example, Wollongong and Townsville.[25,178]

Across Australia and Aotearoa New Zealand, a Bi-National Trauma Minimum Dataset (BNTMDS) has been developed both to standardise the collection of data points across all trauma registries, and to serve as the data set collected by the ATR.[25,179] However, the exact data points collected at each local or regional registry will vary depending on resourcing (such as staffing, software and the availability of electronic data) and the audit, quality, research, education and injury prevention needs of those accessing the registry.

Trauma data is generally collected across several phases of care. This includes demographic data, injury event details, pre-hospital response, movement between hospitals, emergency department (ED) reception, post-ED management, injury coding and outcomes. Broadly, registries will focus on data capture at one of three ascending levels: injury surveillance (epidemiology); trauma system monitoring; and finally system performance and patient outcome monitoring.[178,180]

TRAUMA SCORES—MEASURING INJURY, ITS IMPACT AND OUTCOMES

Several trauma scores have been developed in an attempt to quantify injury severity and/or predict mortality likelihood. Many of these trauma scores were developed using data from the Major Trauma Outcome Study (MTOS), undertaken in North America in the early 1980s. The MTOS aimed to refine methods for injury severity scoring, establish national normative outcomes for trauma and provide trauma care institutions with objective evaluations of quality assurance and outcome.[181] They can be used for quality assurance and comparisons of outcome between or among hospitals or groups of patients.

Abbreviated Injury Scale

The most commonly used method of classifying injuries in Australian and Aotearoa New Zealand trauma registries is the Abbreviated Injury Scale (AIS).[182] The AIS is an anatomical injury classification which assigns individual injuries to a 6-point ordinal severity scale ranging from AIS 1 (minor) to AIS 6 (currently untreatable).[183] It is used as the basis of a number of commonly derived injury severity scores including the Injury Severity Score (ISS) and New Injury Severity Score (NISS), and forms a component of composite prediction and risk adjustment tools including the Trauma and Injury Severity Score (TRISS).

The AIS was first developed in the late 1960s to describe injuries from road crashes.[184] It has been revised several times since. Revisions have incorporated severities for different injury types (such as penetrating, burn and asphyxia injuries) and allowed for changes in injury diagnosis (such as the advent of CTs, and later MRIs) and management over time. In many cases, this has resulted in the severity levels assigned to particular injuries changing between AIS versions. The 2008 revision of the AIS is currently used across Australia and Aotearoa New Zealand, although a newer (2015) version is likely to be adopted from 2023.[183] Data coded using one AIS version cannot be directly compared to data coded using a different version, and mapping tools have been developed.[185] Current AIS versions each describe around 2000 different injuries.

Injury Severity Score

The Injury Severity Score (ISS)[186] is the most commonly used injury summary score. It is designed to reflect the overall severity of an injury event which may result in one or multiple separate anatomical injuries. To calculate the ISS, the body is divided into six regions. The ISS is the sum of the squares of the three highest AIS scores in the three most severely injured body regions.[186] ISS scores range from 1 to 75, and are ordinal—an ISS of 10 does not double the severity of an ISS of 5. Around the world, an ISS >15 was adopted as the definition of 'major trauma', equating to an increased risk of mortality, in the 1980s.[187] However, because AIS severities have changed over time, an ISS of > 12 is a more appropriate major trauma threshold for use with the 2008 AIS.[188] This threshold is used across Australia and Aotearoa New Zealand.

The ISS has many recognised mathematical, administrative and clinical limitations, and is outperformed in outcome prediction by a number of newer tools.[188] However, its simplicity and ubiquity have resulted in the ISS remaining the most widely used injury severity scoring system.

New Injury Severity Score

The New Injury Severity Score (NISS)[189] is a modification of the ISS.[186] Since its introduction in 1997, the NISS has been found to be more accurate than the ISS at predicting mortality and post-injury multiple-organ failure.[189] The NISS simplifies the process and allows more than one injury from the same region to count by taking the three highest AIS scores regardless of location. The NISS has been proposed as a better score for identifying major trauma patients,[190] but has not been widely adopted outside of Europe.

ICD-based severity scores

Since the 1970s, several prediction tools and severity indices have also been developed based on different iterations of the International Classification of Diseases (ICD) system, which is used for hospital discharge coding worldwide. The ICD Injury Severity Score (ICISS) is one such score, which, like the ISS, can be used to predict morbidity and mortality.[191] In a number of studies, the ICISS has outperformed the ISS in mortality prediction. However, the results of such studies can be dependent on the exact methodology used to generate severity estimates for the ICISS, as several variants have been developed.[192]

STANDARDISED CLINICAL TRAUMA MANAGEMENT

Since the introduction of the Advanced Trauma Life Support (ATLS) guidelines by the American College of Surgeons in 1978, many countries with organised systems of healthcare have attempted to standardise approaches to the clinical management of trauma.[193] In 1988, the Royal Australasian College of Surgeons introduced the Early Management of Severe Trauma (EMST) course in Australia and Aotearoa New Zealand, adapting the ATLS guidelines. EMST provides a common language and general approach to managing trauma for all emergency healthcare clinicians. Most errors in trauma management occur when the correct therapeutic and diagnostic measures are not performed at the right time, in the right amount or in the right order.[194]

A standardised trauma management environment holds the potential to ensure effective and coordinated trauma team response (trauma call), defined roles for trauma team members with clear leadership, shared goals and priorities in trauma management, evidence-based interventions, standard time-frames for trauma management (according to resource availability) and a systems approach to managing trauma that extends beyond primary and secondary survey. To meet the changing demands of resource variability, a principles approach to developing standardised trauma care is recommended.

PRINCIPLES OF STANDARDISING TRAUMA MANAGEMENT

Standardising trauma management is heavily dependent on local resources, the frequency and type of trauma received, the experience level of clinicians and the role of the facility in an organised trauma system. Similarly, standardising trauma management is also determined by the developed nature of the surrounding trauma system, including pre-hospital triage guidelines and systems for transferring patients to major trauma centres.

Pre-hospital trauma triage, using a series of protocols and guidelines, aims to get the right patient to the right hospital. With a common understanding and goals to work towards, all levels of trauma care within a system need to develop standardised approaches to managing trauma that meet and evolve with changing local resource constraints and demands for trauma services (Table 41.2).

Organised trauma systems in Australia and Aotearoa New Zealand

The aim of a trauma system is to facilitate timely treatment of the injured patient at the right hospital, resulting in optimal care for all trauma patients.[195] Across Australia and Aotearoa New Zealand, several state and regional trauma systems now exist; these encompass pre-hospital care, acute care in the hospital setting, recovery and rehabilitation (in both hospital and home settings) (Box 41.5). In Australia in 1993, the National Road Trauma Advisory Council (NRTAC)[196] published a report of the working party on trauma systems. This report formed the blueprint for the subsequent development of state-based, regionalised trauma systems in Australia. Being part of a trauma system requires hospitals to be 'designated' at a prescribed level of care. Having an inclusive trauma system, where all hospitals with 24-hour ED access are classified at different levels of trauma service (level 1 being the highest), facilitates these hospitals being included in ongoing aspects of trauma care, education and patient management. These hospitals are also supported by having well-defined triage and transfer protocols in place, in the event that trauma patients require treatment at a higher level of care within the system. The introduction of trauma systems across Australia has led to reductions in mortality.[195]

TABLE 41.2 PRINCIPLES OF STANDARDISING TRAUMA MANAGEMENT[20,194]

STANDARDISATION PRINCIPLE	RATIONALE
Use EMST guidelines as a beginning point	EMST guidelines offer a common language and understanding of the overall approach to trauma management and are therefore a good beginning point and overall structure for standardising trauma management.
Gather an evidence base	Knowledge and practice in trauma management is changing rapidly. To ensure best practice in trauma management, and therefore optimal trauma patient outcomes, it is important that standards of practice are based on current research and best practice in trauma management. Systematic approaches to reviewing literature and determining best practice in trauma management can seem like an overwhelming task for many hospitals already struggling with burgeoning clinical workloads. However, much of this sort of work is often undertaken by governmental bodies, such as NSW ITIM and major trauma services. The role of major trauma services and larger teaching hospitals that receive trauma patients is to share this sort of information. However, it is up to committed groups of clinicians at smaller hospitals to adapt this information for their own local resources.
Maintain a focus on the elements of care known to influence outcome	The multitude of tasks in trauma management demands that emergency clinicians prioritise what they do. It is therefore important that standardised approaches to trauma care maintain a clear focus on what improves patient outcome. For example, many sizeable hospitals in country regions have the resources available to perform CT scans on trauma patients. However, many of these facilities do not include an in-house or even on-call neurosurgeon. Trauma systems research suggests that trauma patients are more likely to survive the sooner they are transferred to a major trauma service. Clearly, the focus of smaller regional hospitals needs to be to stabilise the trauma patient and transfer them to the nearest major trauma facility as soon as possible. Delays incurred by unnecessary procedures such as CT scans (which are usually repeated at major trauma services) only threaten the trauma patient's chances of survival.
Develop a clear and transparent process for calling in a trauma team	Trauma management is clearly a team effort. Even in smaller country hospitals where resources are scarce, a clear and efficient means of calling in the additional resources required to manage trauma patients needs to be developed in institutions. Communications technology makes this easier, including long-range pagers and mobile phones, often already used by these smaller hospitals for other purposes.
Develop clinical practice guidelines, protocols and algorithm-based approaches to trauma management	Standardised approaches to trauma management require the development of clinical practice guidelines, trauma protocols or trauma algorithms to delineate team roles, ensure effective use of available resources, time-efficient management of the trauma patient and transfer to the appropriate level of care as soon as the trauma patient is sufficiently stable for transfer.
Develop clinical pathways for post-initial resuscitation, single-system-injured patients	Receiving trauma hospitals, both big and small, need to have clear clinical pathways to guide the post-initial resuscitation management of patients with isolated or single-system injuries.

BOX 41.5 EFFECTIVE INJURY PREVENTION PRINCIPLES[19]

- **The health sector needs to take a leadership role in injury prevention and safety promotion.**
- **Initiatives need to be evidence-based.**
- **Injury prevention programs and safety initiatives need appropriate resource levels to be effective.**
- **Prevention efforts need to be coordinated and integrated.**
- **There is need for an informed and capable injury prevention workforce.**
- **Access to high-quality data is required, including injury patterns, exposure to risks and population trends.**
- **Programs should reduce inequalities in injury outcomes, including cultural and economic barriers.**
- **Sustainable changes can be facilitated by supportive laws, policies and regulations operating at federal, state, local and community levels.**
- **Initiatives need to be well researched, monitored and evaluated.**
- **Injury prevention and safety promotion programs need to be sustainable, well networked and share resources and purpose with these networks.**

In NSW, all Ambulance Pre-Hospital Trauma Triage Protocol T1 mandates that major trauma patients who meet criteria should be transported directly to a major trauma centre if within 1 hour of transport from the scene.[197]

In 2011, the National Health Board established the Major Trauma National Clinical Network trauma system in Aotearoa New Zealand.[198] To facilitate revision of the NZ Optimal Care Guidelines, it encouraged the formation of trauma services in each hospital and described a major trauma minimum data set. In 2015, all trauma-receiving hospitals had an established process to collect the minimum data set on all major trauma admissions and submit that data to a National Trauma Registry. By describing a system of care, requiring the appointment of trauma clinicians and mandating the collection and submission of major trauma data, the quality of trauma care in Aotearoa New Zealand will be measurable and able to drive ongoing improvements in care.[41]

Trauma verification

The Australasian Trauma Verification Program is a multidisciplinary intercollegiate process, developed through the Royal Australasian College of Surgeons (RACS) to assist hospitals in analysing their system of care for the injured patient. The review covers the process of care from pre-hospital through to discharge from acute care, and identifies the strengths and weaknesses of the hospital's trauma service.[199] RACS verification defines four different levels of trauma centre. Part of the Trauma Verification process defines resource-level criteria and capabilities for each level. For example, a level 1 trauma centre must be capable of providing the full spectrum of care for the most critically injured patient, from initial reception and resuscitation through to discharge and rehabilitation. By contrast, a hospital designated level 4 is one where the major trauma patient is resuscitated and transferred out to definitive care as rapidly as possible. Trauma systems ensure that guidelines are in place to facilitate this process. Full criteria can be found on the RACS website (see Useful websites) (Box 41.6).[199] To date, Trauma Verification is voluntary and unmandated by government authorities, and significant resource and outcome variance exists between trauma centres.[200]

BOX 41.6 LEVELS OF TRAUMA CENTRES AND MODEL RESOURCE CRITERIA[199]

Level I—provides 24-hour full spectrum of care for the most critically injured patient, from initial reception and resuscitation through to discharge and rehabilitation, and, ideally, a surgical trauma admitting service (bed card). Also, research, education and fellowship training, quality improvement program, prevention and outreach programs and the principal hospital for reception of inter-hospital transfer of major trauma patients.

Level II—can be either metropolitan- or rural-based; provides comprehensive 24-hour clinical care identical to that of a Level I service without the additional leadership, research and education components.

Level III—provides prompt assessment, resuscitation, 24-hour on-call emergency general surgical and anaesthetic service, and stabilisation of a small number of seriously injured patients while arranging for their transfer to the responsible major trauma service. A Level III service can provide some definitive care for non-major-trauma patients according to patient needs and available resources.

Level IV—a resuscitating hospital where the major trauma patient is transferred out as soon as possible. A medical doctor needs to be in attendance within half an hour.

Level IV services are not intended to care for major trauma patients; however, they are recognised because they participate in the care of minor trauma, and because, on occasions, individual patients may self-present with major trauma, or in rural situations there may be an occasional need for resuscitation of a major trauma patient, with rapid transfer on. Guidelines should exist for this management and transfer process.

Level V—may be large, mature tertiary institutions, which are not designated for trauma care specifically. In the rural setting, these institutions will usually be very small and isolated hospitals or medical centres, with no immediately available medical practitioner.

Multidisciplinary approach

The increased percentage of injured patients arriving at hospital has resulted in the need for an effective, organised and timely approach to their management. As a result, trauma team training has become an important part of education for multidisciplinary staff and has been shown to be associated with a decrease in time from the ED to operating theatre and improves team communication.[201]

Within trauma centres, the multidisciplinary team is developed, led and evaluated by the trauma service. At a minimum, the trauma service that is responsible for coordinating the larger multidisciplinary team should consist of the trauma medical director, trauma coordinator, trauma data manager and administrative support. The trauma service may also include trauma fellows, trauma registrars and case managers. As the pre-hospital providers are an integral part of the trauma service, direct communication between pre-hospital and in-hospital care providers is of paramount importance and is facilitated when there is a dedicated ambulance liaison person. The trauma service is responsible for the education of the multidisciplinary team and the overall care rendered by the team (Fig. 41.12).

In Australia and Aotearoa New Zealand, the composition of trauma teams has a heavy reliance on subspecialty surgical care. The patient is generally admitted to a ward under the duty surgeon, and any specialty medical team as required (e.g. orthopaedics or neurosurgery). The bulk of operative management in severe trauma is performed by orthopaedic surgeons, followed by plastic and maxillofacial, and neurosurgery.[202] Due to the multi-specialty input, coordination and communication problems can arise in trauma patient

FIGURE 41.12 FUNCTION OF THE MAJOR TRAUMA CENTRE TRAUMA SERVICE

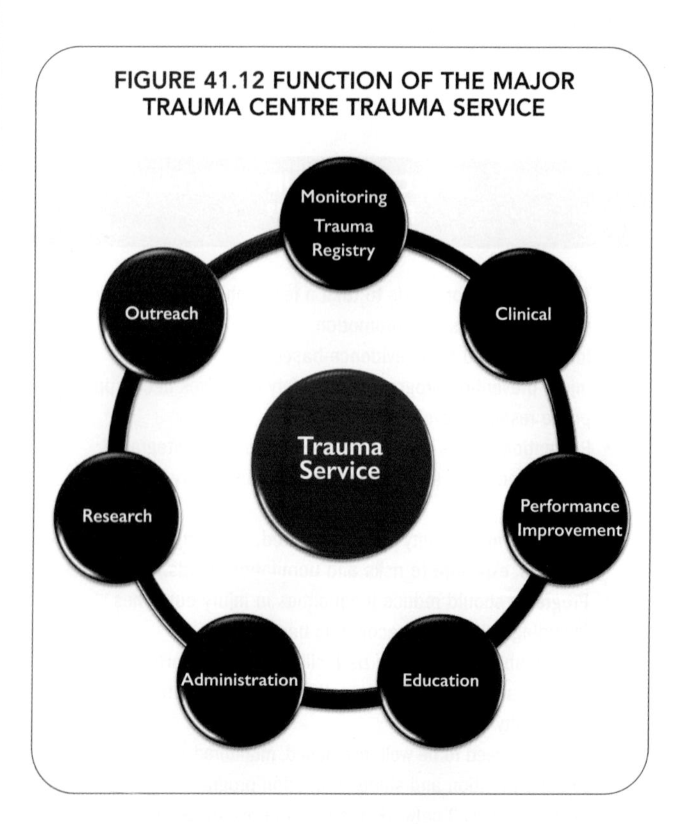

care, and using trauma case management or a dedicated trauma surgical team can alleviate these problems and improve patient outcomes.[203]

A multidisciplinary healthcare approach to the multiply injured patient may streamline post-injury rehabilitation, improve care and importantly reduce morbidity and mortality.[204]

TRAUMA SPECIALIST ROLES

The field of trauma encompasses a large variety of nursing and paramedic specialties. Nursing roles include injury prevention, emergency, perioperative, intensive care, high-dependency and ward surgical roles through to rehabilitation. However, the trauma case manager or trauma nurse specialist has additional knowledge and expertise in the complex care required of the traumatically injured patient throughout the whole span of trauma care. Trauma nurses work to ensure that all injured patients and their families are provided with complete physical and emotional care throughout the trajectory of their injury.

Trauma nursing was first established in wartime experiences, including those of Florence Nightingale in the Crimean War in 1854, and in the Korean and Vietnam Wars. These nurses established the first principles for nursing management of traumatic injuries, including triage, rapid evacuation, surgical intervention, stabilisation and early rehabilitation. In the United States in 1961, the civilian population recognised that an organised trauma system was essential, and the first trauma research nurse was employed in Maryland in 1961. Elizabeth Scanlan, Nursing Director of the Centre for the Study of Trauma when it opened in 1969, was visionary in her approach to developing a competent nursing staff specific to trauma and resuscitation. The first trauma nurse coordinator was appointed in Illinois, United States, in 1972.[205]

In Australia and Aotearoa New Zealand, the role of trauma nurse coordinator (TNC) has evolved since the 1980s, when two emergency nurses in large teaching hospitals in Sydney were appointed as trauma nurses. This was congruent with trauma system development in NSW and with progression of the concept of designated trauma centres. These nurses pioneered the specialty of trauma nursing in Australia. Along with their respective trauma medical directors, each was responsible for organising their institutions to receive and care for trauma patients.[206] There are two main roles for trauma nurse specialists. The first role is that of trauma coordinator or trauma program manager, which involves overseeing trauma care delivery alongside the medical directors. The role includes education, general trauma management, data collection, maintenance of a trauma database and evaluation and performance improvement of trauma care.

The second role is that of trauma case manager,[206] who is supervised by the trauma coordinator and is responsible for the day-to-day clinical coordination of trauma patient care and informal bedside staff education and patient advocacy. The case managers highlight any system problems or performance indicator violations and pass them on to the trauma coordinator for follow-up.

In 2010 in Canberra, ACT, the first trauma nurse practitioner position was introduced. Such roles have gradually been adopted across Australia and Aotearoa New Zealand. The roles of the trauma specialist are summarised in Table 41.3.[207]

Paramedics in Australia and Aotearoa New Zealand also have specialist roles for trauma, including the intensive care paramedic, rescue paramedic, special casualty access team paramedic and underwater medic. These paramedics need additional training and experience and respond to critical life-threatening emergencies including trauma. These roles are essential to pre-hospital trauma care as they need to be able to make quick, complex clinical judgements often unsupervised.[208] Refer to Chapter 2 for more information regarding the development of specialist paramedic roles.

TABLE 41.3 SPECIALIST TRAUMA NURSE ROLE RESPONSIBILITIES IDENTIFIED[207]

CLINICAL ACTIVITIES	EDUCATION	PERFORMANCE IMPROVEMENT	ADMINISTRATION	DATA COLLECTION	RESEARCH
• Direct patient care • Assessment and initial resuscitation • Ward rounds • Facilitation of medical team referrals • Allied health referrals • Multidisciplinary team reviews • Management of outpatient clinics • Advanced clinical skills	• Staff education and bedside teaching • Implementation of policy • Patient and family education • Maintenance of continued professional development • Presentation at conferences • Community outreach-injury prevention • Tertiary teaching	• Review of patient care for complications/adverse events • Audits • Policy/strategy development • Trauma committee meetings • Implementation of policy	• Management of staff • Rosters • Ordering stock • Attending meetings • Typing minutes • Budget preparation • Recruitment	• Trauma data collection • Maintenance of trauma registry • Report generation	• Initiating/participating in research programs • Implementation of research into practice

SUMMARY

Injury is a condition with a significant national and global burden, and demands the attention of healthcare providers on a daily basis, regardless of the care provided or the trauma systems in place. Clinicians must have a high level of understanding of the mechanism, incidence, prevalence and determinants of trauma in order to empower them to contribute to timely and effective trauma patient management and to contribute to the improvement of the trauma system in which they work.

Predominant patterns of injury mean that emergency clinicians in Australia and New Zealand are more expert in the management of blunt trauma. However, knowledge and skill in managing penetrating trauma and special patterns of injury need to be maintained if the trend towards increasing numbers of patients being injured by these mechanisms continues. The risk factors that help identify who is most likely to be injured can help clinicians comprehend and further develop their knowledge and skills bases in line with the diversity of injured patients they are likely to care for.

An in-depth knowledge of the nature, trajectory and outcomes of traumatic injury will assist in the facilitation of a multidisciplinary approach to the injured patient, and places emergency clinicians in a unique position to contribute to injury prevention and multidisciplinary trauma research. Standardising clinical trauma management holds the potential to reduce error and foster inter-organisational trauma research to improve trauma patient outcomes.

USEFUL WEBSITES

Australia New Zealand Trauma Registry https://atr.org.au/

Prevent Alcohol and Risk-Related Trauma in Youth partyprogram.com/. A program targeting injury prevention for youth, http://partyprogram.com/.

Royal Australasian College of Surgeons www.surgeons.org/.

The Institute for Health Metrics and Evaluation (IHME) is an independent global health research centre at the University of Washington that provides rigorous and comparable measurement of the world's most important health problems and evaluates the strategies used to address them. The Global Burden of Disease: Generating Evidence, Guiding Policy provides an overview of the reasons why the Global Burden of Disease (GBD) is an essential tool for evidence-based health policymaking. Data GBD Compare is new to IHME's line-up of visualisations and has countless options for exploring health data, www.healthdata.org/results/policy-reports.

The National Trauma Research Institute provides links to research, education, information and training opportunities for those working in trauma, https://ntri.org.au/.

REFERENCES

1. Lyons RA, Finch CF, McClure R, van Beeck E, Macey S. The injury list of all deficits (LOAD) framework—conceptualizing the full range of deficits and adverse outcomes following injury and violence. Int J Inj Cont Saf Promot 2010;17(3):145–59.
2. Institute for Health Metrics and Evaluation (IHME). GBD 2019 Cause and risk summary: Injuries - Level 1 cause. Seattle, USA: IHME, University of Washington; 2020.
3. Palmer CS. Commentary: epidemiological burden of minor, major and fatal trauma in a national injury pyramid. Br J Surg 2012;99(Suppl. 1):121.
4. Australian Institute of Health and Welfare (AIHW). Injury in Australia: all causes of injury. Canberra: AIHW; 2022. Report No. INJCAT 213.
5. Australian Institute of Health and Welfare (AIHW). Australian burden of disease study: impact and causes of illness and death in Australia, 2018. Canberra: AIHW; 2021.
6. O'ea D, Wren J. New Zealand estimates of the total social and economic cost of injuries. Inj Prevent 2012;18(Suppl. 1):A10.3–A1.
7. Ministry of Transport. Social cost of road crashes and injuries—June 2020 update. Wellington: Ministry of Transport; 2021.
8. Accident Compensation Corporation New Zealand Injury Prevention Strategy. Five-year evaluation—final report. Dunedin: ACC; 2010.
9. Australian Institute of Health and Welfare (AIHW). Hospital separations due to injury and poisoning, Australia 2004–05. Injury Research and Statistics Series no. 47. Cat. no. INJCAT 117. Adelaide: AIHW; 2008.
10. New Zealand Ministry of Transport. The social cost of road crashes and injuries 2013 update. Wellington: New Zealand Ministry of Transport; 2013.
11. Balogh ZJ. Polytrauma: it is a disease. Injury 2022;53:1727–9.
12. Curtis K, Lam M, Mitchell R, Black D, Taylor C, et al. Acute costs and predictors of higher treatment costs of trauma in New South Wales, Australia. Injury 2014;45(1):279–84.
13. Curtis K, Lam M, Mitchell R, Dickson C, McDonnell K. Major trauma: the unseen financial burden to trauma centres, a descriptive multicentre analysis. Aust Health Rev 2014;38(1):30–7.
14. Jurkovich GJ. Regionalized health care and the trauma system model. J Am Coll Surg 2012;215(1):1–11.

15. Gabbe BJ, Lyons RA, Fitzgerald MC, Judson R, Richardson J, Cameron PA. Reduced population burden of road transport-related major trauma after introduction of an inclusive trauma system. Ann Surg 2015;261(3):565–72.
16. Berndt RM, Berndt CH. The speaking land: myth and story in Aboriginal Australia. Vermont: Inner Traditions; 1994.
17. Kirkup J. Foundation lecture. Fracture care of friend and foe during World War I. ANZ J Surg 2003;73(6):453–9.
18. Better Health Commission. Looking forward to better health: volume 1. Final report. Canberra: Australian Government Publishing Service; 1986.
19. Royal Australasian College of Surgeons Trauma Committee, editor. Trauma care systems in the 90s. Melbourne: RACS; 1992.
20. National Public Health Partnership. The national injury prevention and safety promotion plan: 2004–2014. Canberra: NPHP; 2004.
21. National Public Health Partnership. The national falls prevention for older people plan: 2004 onwards. Canberra: NPHP; 2004.
22. National Public Health Partnership. The national Aboriginal and Torres Strait Islander safety promotion strategy. Canberra: NPHP; 2004.
23. Department of Health and Aged Care. National injury prevention strategy 2020–2030. Commonwealth of Australia; 2020. Online: Available from: www.health.gov.au/initiatives-and-programs/national-injury-prevention-strategy-2020-2030-0.
24. National Health and Medical Research Council. Funding facts 2014. Canberra: NHMRC; 2014.
25. McKie E. Australia New Zealand Trauma Registry, management of the severely injured, 1 July 2019 to 30 June 2020. Melbourne: Australia New Zealand Trauma Registry; 2021.
26. New Zealand Trauma Registry and National Trauma Network. Annual report 2020/21. Wellington: National Trauma Network; 2022.
27. Ministry of Health and Accident Compensation Corporation. Injury-related health loss: a report from the New Zealand burden of diseases, injuries and risk factors study 2006–2016. Wellington: New Zealand Ministry of Health; 2013.
28. Isles S, Christey G, Civil I, Hicks P. The New Zealand major trauma registry: the foundation for a data-driven approach in a contemporary trauma system. N Z Med J 2017;130(1463):19–27.
29. Australian Bureau of Statistics (ABS). 3303.0 – Causes of death, Australia, 2020. Canberra: ABS; 2021. Online: Available from: www.abs.gov.au/statistics/health/causes-death/causes-death-australia/2020/3303_1%20Underlying%20causes%20of%20death%20%28Australia%29.xlsx.
30. Australian Bureau of Statistics (ABS). Causes of death, Australia. Cat no. 3303.0. Belconnen: ABS; 2022. Online. Available from:www.abs.gov.au/statistics/health/causes-death/causes-death-australia/2020.
31. Henley G, Harrison J. Injury deaths, Australia 2004–05. Adelaide: AIHW; 2009.
32. Australian Bureau of Statistics (ABS). Causes of death, Australia. ABS; 2012. Online: Available from: www.abs.gov.au/ausstats/abs@.nsf/Lookup/by%20Subject/3303.0~2012~Main%20Features~Key%20Characteristics~10009.
33. Australian Bureau of Statistics (ABS). Causes of death, Australia, 2014. Cat. no. 3303.0. Belconnen: ACT; 2014. Online: Available from: www.abs.gov.au/ausstats/abs@.nsf/Lookup/by%20Subject/3303.0~2014~Main%20Features~Leading%20Causes%20of%20Death~10001.
34. Harrison J, Pointer S, Elnour A. A review of suicide statistics in Australia. Canberra: Australian Institute of Health and Welfare; 2009.
35. Bureau of Infrastructure Transport and Regional Economics (BITRE). Road deaths in Australia 1925–2008. Canberra: BITRE; 2010. Information sheet 38.
36. Bureau of Infrastructure and Transport Research Economics (BITRE). Road trauma Australia 2021 statistical summary. Canberra: BITRE; 2022.
37. Watson W, Clapperton A, Mitchell R. The incidence and cost of falls injury among older people in New South Wales 2006/07. Sydney: NSW Department of Health; 2010.
38. Public Health Association of Australia. Fall injury prevention in older people policy. Public Health Association of Australia; 2015. Online. Available from: www.phaa.net.au/documents/item/211.
39. Gillespie L, Robertson M, Gillespie W. Interventions for preventing falls in older people living in the community. Cochrane Database Syst Rev 2012;(9):CD007146.
40. Safe Work Australia. Work-related traumatic injury fatalities Australia 2020. Canberra: SWA; 2021.
41. New Zealand Major Trauma Registry, National Clinical Network. New Zealand Major Trauma Registry & National Clinical Network annual report 2016–2017. Wellington: Major Trauma National Clinical Network; 2018. Online: Available from: www.majortrauma.nz.
42. New Zealand Ministry of Health. Major causes of death. 2021. Online: Available from: www.health.govt.nz/our-work/populations/maori-health/tatau-kahukura-maori-health-statistics/nga-mana-hauora-tutohu-health-status-indicators/major-causes-death.
43. New Zealand Government. Workplace fatalities. New Zealand Government; 2018. Online: Available from: worksafe.govt.nz/data-and-research/ws-data/fatalities/workplace-fatalities-summary/2018.
44. Mitchell RJ, Curtis K, Foster K. A 10-year review of child injury hospitalisations, health outcomes and treatment costs in Australia. Inj Prev 2018;24:344–50.
45. Gustafsson M, Stigson H, Krafft M, Kullgren A. Risk of permanent medical impairment (RPMI) in car crashes correlated to age and gender. Traffic Inj Prev 2015;16(4):353–61.
46. Gabbe BJ, Simpson PM, Cameron PA, Ponsford J, Lyons RA, Collie A, et al. Long-term health status and trajectories of seriously injured patients: a population-based longitudinal study. PLoS Med 2017;14(7):e1002322.
47. Palmer CS, Cameron PA, Gabbe BJ. Comparison of revised Functional Capacity Index scores with Abbreviated Injury Scale 2008 scores in predicting 12-month severe trauma outcomes. Inj Prev 2020;26(2):138–46.
48. Wiseman T, Foster K, Curtis K. Mental health following traumatic physical injury: an integrative literature review. Injury 2013;44(11):1383–90.
49. Australian Trauma Quality Improvement (AusTQIP) Collaboration. Australia New Zealand Trauma Registry, management of the severely injured, 1 July 2019 to 30 June 2020. Melbourne, Victoria: Alfred Health; 2021.

50. Curtis K, Chan DL, Lam MK, Mitchell R, King K, Leonard L, et al. The injury profile and acute treatment costs of major trauma in older people in New South Wales. Australas J Ageing 2014;33(4):264–70.
51. Australian Institute of Health and Welfare, Pointer S. Trends in hospitalised injury, Australia 1999–2000 to 2010–11. Canberra: AIHW; 2013.
52. Safe Work Australia (SWA). Work-related traumatic injury fatalities. 2016. Online. Available from: www.safeworkaustralia.gov.au/resources_publications/.
53. Mitchell RJ, Curtis K, Fisher M. Understanding trauma as a men's health issue: sex differences in traumatic injury presentations at a level 1 trauma center in Australia. J Trauma Nurs 2012;19(2):80–8.
54. Australian Indigenous HealthInfoNet. Overview of Aboriginal and Torres Strait Islander health status 2021. Perth, WA: Australian Indigenous HealthInfoNet; 2022.
55. Henley G, Harrison J. Hospitalised farm injury, Australia, 2010–11 to 2014–15. Canberra: 2018. Online: Available from: www.aihw.gov.au/getmedia/279bb48f-d2fe-47b9-823c-63cdb2a1a3cf/aihw-injcat-189.pdf.aspx?inline=true.
56. Australian Government. National Aboriginal and Torres Strait Islander health plan 2013–2023. Canberra: Department of Health and Ageing; 2013.
57. Chikritzhs T, Evans M, Gardner C. Australian alcohol aetiologic fractions for injuries treated in emergency departments. Perth: National Drug Research Institute, Curtin University; 2011.
58. Connor J, Casswell S. The burden of road trauma due to other people's drinking. Accid Anal Prev 2009;41(5):1099–103.
59. McKetin R, Lubman DI, Najman JM, Dawe S, Butterworth P, Baker AL. Does methamphetamine use increase violent behaviour? Evidence from a prospective longitudinal study. Addiction (Abingdon, England) 2014;109(5):798–806.
60. Australian Transport Safety Bureau (ATSB). Road crash casualties and rates, Australia, 1925 to 2005. Canberra: ATSB; 2007.
61. Danne P. Trauma management in Australia and the tyranny of distance. World J Surg 2003;27(4):385–9.
62. Roads and Maritime Services. Driving distractions and crash risk. 2017. Online. Available from: www.rms.nsw.gov.au/roads/safety-rules/safe-driving/driving-distractions.html.
63. Scott-Parker B, Oviedo-Trespalacios O. Young driver risky behaviour and predictors of crash risk in Australia, New Zealand and Colombia: same but different? Accid Anal Prev 2017;99(Pt A):30–8.
64. World Health Organization (WHO). Mobile phone use: a growing problem of driver distraction. Geneva, Switzerland: WHO; 2011.
65. Lansdown TC, Stephens AN. Couples, contentious conversations, mobile telephone use and driving. Accid Anal Prev 2013;50:416–22.
66. Nasar JL, Troyer D. Pedestrian injuries due to mobile phone use in public places. Accid Anal Prev 2013;57:91–5.
67. Road Safety Commission. Government of Western Australia. 2014. Online. Available from: www.rsc.wa.gov.au/Statistics/Annual-Statistics.
68. Australian Transport Council (ATC). National Road Safety Strategy 2011–2020. Canberra: ATC; 2011.
69. Janik M, Straka L, Krajcovic J, Stuller F, Novomeský F, Hejna P, et al. All-terrain vehicle-related crashes among children and young adults. RJLM 2012;20(4):263–8.
70. Revere C. Mechanism of injury. St Louis: Mosby; 2003.
71. Venes D, editor. Taber's encyclopedic medical dictionary. Philadelphia: FA Davis; 2001.
72. Ionut RA, Corneliu C, Bogdan T. Mathematical model validated by a crash test for studying the occupant's kinematics and dynamics in a cars' frontal collision. Int J Auto Tech 2017;18(6):1017.
73. World Health Organization (WHO). Injury prevention and control: a guide to developing a multisectoral plan of action, surveillance and research. Cairo: WHO; 2006. Contract No.: WHO-EM/HLP/033/E.
74. Dickinson M. Understanding the mechanism of injury and kinetic forces involved in traumatic injuries. Emerg Nurse 2004;12(6):30.
75. McQuillan KA, Von Rueden KT, Hartsock RL, Flynn MB, Whalen E. Trauma nursing: from resuscitation through rehabilitation. 3rd ed. Philadelphia: WB Saunders; 2002.
76. NSW Government. Centre for road safety. Transport for NSW; 2022. Online. Available from: roadsafety.transport.nsw.gov.au/stayingsafe/motorcyclists/index.html.
77. Constant A, Lagarde E. Protecting vulnerable road users from injury. PLoS Med 2010;7(3):e1000228.
78. Moloney-Harmon PA, Czerwinski SJ. Nursing care of the paediatric trauma patient. St. Louis: Saunders; 2003.
79. Toney-Butler T, Varacallo M. Motor vehicle collisions. StatPearls [Internet]. Treasure Island (FL): StatPearls Publishing; 2021.
80. Cole E. Trauma care: initial assessment and management in the emergency department. Oxford: Blackwell; 2009.
81. Brown J, Schonstein L, Ivers R, Keay L. Children and motorcycles: a systematic review of risk factors and interventions. Inj Prev 2018;24(2):166–75.
82. Akbari M, Lankarani KB, Tabrizi R, Vali M, Heydari ST, Motevalian SA, et al. The effect of motorcycle safety campaign on helmet use: a systematic review and meta-analysis. IATSS Res 2021;45(4):513–20.
83. Te Manatu Waka Ministry of Transport. Enabling New Zealanders to flourish. Government NZ, editor. Wellington: Ministry of Transport; 2020.
84. New Zealand Ministry of Transport. Cyclists—crash statistics for the year ended 31 December 2012. Wellington: New Zealand Ministry of Transport; 2013.
85. Dinh MM, Curtis K, Ivers R. The effectiveness of helmets in reducing head injuries and hospital treatment costs: a multicentre study. MJA 2013;198(8):415.
86. Hwang MJ, Dillon JK, Dodson TB. Helmets decrease risk of bicyclist-related maxillofacial injuries but not severity. J Oral Maxillofac Surg 2019;77(10):2055–63.

87. Boufous S, Olivier J. Recent trends in cyclist fatalities in Australia. Inj Prev 2016;22(4):284–7.
88. Dinh MM, Kastelein C, Hopkins R, Royle TJ, Bein KJ, Chalkley DR, et al. Mechanisms, injuries and helmet use in cyclists presenting to an inner city emergency department. Emerg Med Australas 2015;27(4):323–7.
89. Mizuno K, Yamada H, Mizuguchi H, Ito D, Han Y, Hitosugi M. The influence of lower extremity postures on kinematics and injuries of cyclists in vehicle side collisions. Traffic Inj Prev 2016;17(6):618–24.
90. Pak W, Grindle D, Untaroiu C. The influence of gait stance and vehicle type on pedestrian kinematics and injury risk. J Biomech Eng 2021; 143(10):101007.
91. Hotz MG, Kennedy MA, Lutfi MK, Cohn SM. Preventing pediatric pedestrian injuries. J Trauma 2009;66(5):1492–9.
92. Neff JA, Kidd PS. Trauma nursing: the art and science. 2nd ed. St Louis: Mosby; 1993.
93. Paz MS, Mendez MD. Waddell Triad. StatPearls. Treasure Island (FL): StatPearls Publishing. © 2022. StatPearls Publishing LLC; 2022.
94. Chakravarthy B, Lotfipour S, Vaca FE. Pedestrian injuries: emergency care considerations. Calif J Emerg Med 2007;8(1):15–21.
95. Tracksafe Foundation. Suicide and attempted suicide on the Australian rail network. Adelaide: Office of the National Rail Safety Regulator; 2021.
96. Waka Kotahi NZ Transport Agency. Rail safety statistics through to the period ended 31 December 2021 report. 2022. Online: Available from: www.nzta.govt.nz/resources/rail-safety-statistics/.
97. Henley G, Harrison J. Serious injury due to transport accidents involving a railway train, Australia 2004–05 to 2008–09. Canberra: AIHW; 2012.
98. Cartagena LJ, Kang A, Munnangi S, Jordan A, Nweze IC, Sasthakonar V, et al. Risk factors associated with in-hospital mortality in elderly patients admitted to a regional trauma center after sustaining a fall. Aging Clin Exp Res 2017;29(3):427–33.
99. Mulligan CS, Adams S, Tzioumi D, Brown J. Injury from falls in infants under one year. J Paediat Child Health 2017;53(8):754–60.
100. Goldsmith W, Plunkett J. A biomechanical analysis of the causes of traumatic brain injury in infants and children. Am J Foren Med Pathol 2004;25(2):89–100.
101. Dimitriou N. Basics of trauma management: crush injuries. In: Pikoulis E, Doucet J, editors. Emergency medicine, trauma and disaster management: from prehospital to hospital care and beyond. Cham: Springer; 2021.
102. Richards CE, Wallis DN. Asphyxiation: a review. Trauma 2005;7(1):37–45.
103. Australian Bureau of Statistics (ABS). Recorded crime – victims. Australia. Canberra: ABS; 2020. Online. Available from: www.abs.gov.au/statistics/people/crime-and-justice/recorded-crime-victims/2019.
104. Shah Jainik P, Mangal HM, Vora Dipak H. Profile of defense injuries in homicidal deaths. Ind J Forens Med Pathol 2012;5(3):115–19.
105. Pilgrim JL, Gerostamoulos D, Drummer OH. King hit fatalities in Australia, 2000–2012: the role of alcohol and other drugs. Drug Alc Depend 2014;135:119–32.
106. Muralidhar N. Assessment of injury pattern and analysis of its outcome in patients presenting to emergency department after near hanging. Euro J Mol Clin Med 2021;8:1068.
107. Ursic C, Curtis K. Thoracic and neck trauma. Part four. Int Emerg Nurs 2010;18(4):177–80.
108. Nichols DS, McCarthy CM, Ekeh PA, Woods RJ, Walusimbi MS, Saxe JM. Outcome of cervical near-hanging injuries. J Trauma Inj Infect Crit Care 2009;66(1):174–8.
109. Australian Institute of Health and Welfare. Sports injury hospitalisations in Australia, 2019–20. Canberra: Australian Government; 2022.
110. King D, Hume P, A., Hardaker N, Cummins C, Gissane C, Clark T. Sports-related injuries in New Zealand: National Insurance (Accident Compensation Corporation) claims for five sporting codes from 2012–2016. Br J Sports Med 2019;53(16):1026–33.
111. Andrew NE, Gabbe BJ, Wolfe R, Cameron PA. Trends in sport and active recreation injuries resulting in major trauma or death in adults in Victoria, Australia, 2001–2007. Injury 2012;43(9):1527–33.
112. McIntosh AS, Patton DA, Rechnitzer G, Grzebieta R. Injury mechanisms in fatal Australian quad bike incidents. Traff Inj Prev 2016;17(4):386–90.
113. Olivier J, Walter SR, Grzebieta RH. Long term bicycle related head injury trends for New South Wales, Australia following mandatory helmet legislation. Accid Anal Prev 2013;50:1128–34.
114. Taylor JB, Ford KR, Nguyen AD, Terry LN, Hegedus EJ. Prevention of lower extremity injuries in basketball: a systematic review and meta-analysis. Sports Health 2015;7(5):392–8.
115. Loosemore M, Lightfoot J, Gatt I, Hayton M, Beardsley C. Hand and wrist injuries in elite boxing: a longitudinal prospective study (2005–2012) of the Great Britain Olympic boxing squad. Hand 2017;12(2):181–7.
116. Jayarao M, Chin LS, Cantu RC. Boxing-related head injuries. Phys Sportsmed 2010;38(3):18–26.
117. Siewe J, Rudat J, Zarghooni K, Sobottke R, Eysel P, Herren C, et al. Injuries in competitive boxing. A prospective study. Int J Sports Med 2015;36(3):249–53.
118. Bolling C, Leite M, Reis D. Junior gymnastic: incidence and injury profile. Br J Sports Med 2014;48(7):571.
119. Thorborg K, Krommes KK, Esteve E, Clausen MB, Bartels EM, Rathleff MS. Effect of specific exercise-based football injury prevention programmes on the overall injury rate in football: a systematic review and meta-analysis of the FIFA 11 and 11+ programmes. Br J Sports Med 2017;51(7):562.
120. Trojian TH, Cracco A, Hall M, Mascaro M, Aerni G, Ragle R. Basketball injuries: caring for a basketball team. Curr Sports Med Rep 2013;12(5):321–8.

121. Prakash A. Medical attention injuries in cricket: a systematic review of case reports. Ind J Orthopaed 2017;51(5):614–9.
122. Rust DA, Gilmore CJ, Treme G. Injury patterns at a large western United States ski resort with and without snowboarders: the Taos experience. Am J Sports Med 2013;41(3):652–6.
123. Sandiford N, Buckle C, Alao U, Davidson J, Ritchie J. Injuries associated with recreational horse riding and changes over the last 20 years: a review. JRSM Short Rep 2013;4(5):2042533313476688.
124. Keays G, Dumas A. Longboard and skateboard injuries. Injury 2014;45(8):1215–9.
125. Dimmick S, Gillett M, Sheehan P, Sutton C, Anderson SE. Acute injuries and chronic pathology of the head and face sustained while surf board riding. Trauma 2014;16(3):195–201.
126. Safe Work Australia. Quad bike fatalities. Canberra: SWA; 2022. Online. Available from: www.safeworkaustralia.gov.au/data-and-research/work-related-fatalities/quad-bike-fatalities#:~:text=As%20of%2016%20June%202022,were%2064%20quad%20bike%20death.
127. Mulligan CS, Brown J. 656 paediatric injury from motorcycles and off road vehicles. Inj Prev 2016;22(Suppl. 2):A235–6.
128. Pointer S, Harrison J. Boating and watercraft-related injury 2017–18. Injury research and statistics series no. 133. Canberra: AIHW; 2021.
129. Gill RS, Whitlock K, Jawanda AS, Gill SS, Karmali S. Epidemiology of personal watercraft injuries. J Trauma Treat 2012;1(2):112–15.
130. Lau SCP, Myhill NG, Ganeshalingam R, Quan GM. Cervical spinal cord injury at the Victorian Spinal Cord Injury Service: epidemiology of the last decade. Clin Med Insights Trauma Intens Med 2014;2014(5):1.
131. Culcu D, Ozban M, Aydin B, Aydin C. Colorectal injury in a personal watercraft (jet ski) passenger: a case report and review of the literature. Hong Kong J Emerg Med 2014;21(5):322–5.
132. Wong K, Petchell J. Severe trauma caused by stabbing and firearms in metropolitan Sydney, New South Wales, Australia. ANZ J Surg 2005;75(4):225–30.
133. Bird J, Faulkner M. Emergency care and management of patients with stab wounds. (learning zone: continuing professional development)(clinical report). Nurs Stand 2009;23(21):51.
134. Colville-Ebeling B, Lynnerup N, Banner J. Fatal lawn mower related projectile injury. Forensic Sci Med Pathol 2014;10(2):229–33.
135. McPhedran S, Baker J, Singh P. Firearm homicide in Australia, Canada, and New Zealand: what can we learn from long-term international comparisons? J Interpers Viol 2011;26(2):348–59.
136. Chapman S, Alpers P, Jones M. Association between gun law reforms and intentional firearm deaths in Australia, 1979–2013. JAMA 2016;316(3):291–9.
137. Australian Institute of Health and Welfare (AIHE). Firearm injuries and deaths fact sheet. Canberra: AIHW; 2017.
138. Rhee PM, Moore EE, Joseph B, Tang A, Pandit V, Vercruysse G. Gunshot wounds: a review of ballistics, bullets, weapons, and myths. J Trauma Acute Care Surg 2016;80(6):853–67.
139. Hunt J, Weintraub S, Marr A. Kinematics of trauma. In: Feliciano D, Mattox K, Moore E, editors. Trauma. 6th ed. New York: McGraw-Hill; 2008.
140. Wolf SJ, Bebarta VS, Bonnett CJ, Pons PT, Cantrill SV. Blast injuries. Lancet 2009;374(9687):405–15.
141. Shrestha R, Kanchan T, Krishan K. Gunshot wounds forensic pathology. Treasure Island (FL): StatPearls Publishing; 2021.
142. Taylor I. Emergency care of patients with gunshot wounds. Emerg Nurse 2009;17(4):32–9.
143. Venugopalan S. Demystifying explosives: concepts in high energy materials. London: Elsevier; 2015.
144. Moloney J, Welch M, Cardinal A. Applied pathophysiology of blast injuries. J High Threat Austere Med 2019;1(1):doi:10.33553/jhtam.v1i1.20.
145. Finlay SE, Earby M, Baker DJ, Murray VS. Explosions and human health: the long-term effects of blast injury. Prehosp Disaster Med 2012;27(4):385–91.
146. Mayo A, Kluger Y. Blast induced injury to air-containing organs. ADF Health 2006;7:40–4.
147. Olivieri C, Ingrassia PL, Della Corte F, Carenzo L, Sapori JM, Gabilly L, et al. Hospital preparedness and response in CBRN emergencies: TIER assessment tool. Euro J Emerg Med 2017;24(5):366–70.
148. Australian Government. Health CBRN Plan. Domestic health response plan for chemical, biological, radiological or nuclear incidents of national significance. Canberra: Australian Government, Department of Health; 2018.
149. Burns Registry of Australia and New Zealand (BRANZ). Annual report 2019/20. Melbourne: Monash University, Medicine DoEaP; 2021.
150. Bi-National Burns Registry Project Team. Bi-National Burns Registry annual report. Melbourne, Victoria: Australian and New Zealand Burn Association (ANZBA), Monash University Department of Epidemiology and Preventive Medicine; 2013.
151. Emet M, Ataç K, Çakmak MA, Saritemur M, Alğan S, Aslan S, et al. Frostbite. J Acad Emerg Med 2015;14(4):211.
152. Saeed O, Boyer NL, Pamplin JC, Driscoll IR, DellaVolpe J, Cannon J, et al. Inhalation injury and toxic industrial chemical exposure. Military Med 2018;183(Suppl. 2):130–2.
153. Urden LD, Stacy KM, Lough ME. Thelan's critical care nursing: diagnosis and management. 4th ed. St Louis: Mosby; 2002.
154. Schwartz S, Pantle H, McQuay N. Inhalation injuries. ICU Dir 2011;4(6):163–71.
155. Handley AJ. Drowning. BMJ (Clinical Research Ed) 2014;348:g1734.
156. American Psychiatric Association (APA). Diagnostic and statistical manual of mental disorders. Washington, DC: APA; 2013.
157. Haagsma JA, Polinder S, Toet H, Panneman M, Havelaar AH, Bonsel GJ, et al. Beyond the neglect of psychological consequences: post-traumatic stress disorder increases the non-fatal burden of injury by more than 50%. Inj Prev 2011;17(1):21–6.

158. Wiseman TA, Curtis K, Lam M, Foster K. Incidence of depression, anxiety and stress following traumatic injury: a longitudinal study. Scand J Trauma Resusc Emerg Med 2015;23:29.
159. Baecher K, Kangas M, Taylor A, O'Donnell ML, Bryant RA, Silove D, et al. The role of site and severity of injury as predictors of mental health outcomes following traumatic injury. Stress Health 2018;34(4):545–51.
160. New Zealand Government. Health and safety at work strategy 2018–2028. Wellington: New Zealand Government; 2018.
161. Infrastructure and Transport Ministers. National road safety strategy 2021–30. Canberra: Australian Government; 2021.
162. Curtis K, Leonard E. The trauma nurse coordinator in Australia and New Zealand: demographics, role, and professional development. J Trauma Nurs 2012;19(4):214–20.
163. Gunn A, McLeod J, Chapman R, Ball H, Fitzgerald M, Howard T, et al. Effect of the Prevent Alcohol and Risk-Related Trauma in Youth (P.A.R.T.Y.) program among senior school students. Emerg Med Australas 2018;30(2):209–13.
164. Koppel S, Charlton JL. Child restraint system misuse and/or inappropriate use in Australia. Traff Inj Prev 2009;10(3):302–7.
165. Conybeare J. Evaluation of automobile safety regulations: the case of compulsory seat belt legislation in Australia. Policy Sci 1980;12(1):27–39.
166. Fouda Mbarga N, Abubakari AR, Aminde LN, Morgan AR. Seatbelt use and risk of major injuries sustained by vehicle occupants during motor-vehicle crashes: a systematic review and meta-analysis of cohort studies. BMC Public Health 2018;18(1):1413.
167. Lennon AJ, Darvell M, Edmonston CJ, Biggs SE, Shaw L. Evaluation of the 2010 child restraint legislation in Queensland. Brisbane: Queensland University of Technology; 2011.
168. Bulger EM, Kaufman R, Mock C. Childhood crash injury patterns associated with restraint misuse: implications for field triage. Prehosp Disaster Med 2008;23(1):9–15.
169. Koppel S, Charlton JL, Rudin-Brown CM. The impact of new legislation on child restraint system (CRS) misuse and inappropriate use in Australia. Traff Inj Prev 2013;14(4):387–96.
170. Transport for NSW. Pedestrian Safety Action Plan 2014–2016. Sydney: NSW Government; 2014.
171. Pfeifer R, Tarkin IS, Rocos B, Pape HC. Patterns of mortality and causes of death in polytrauma patients–has anything changed? Injury 2009;40(9):907–11.
172. Ferris J, Mazerolle L. Random breath testing: impact on alcohol related crashes. Canberra: Australian Research Council; 2016.
173. Australasian College of Road Safety. Policies of the college. Mawson: ACT 2607; 2002.
174. Waka Kotahi New Zealand Transport Agency. Different types of airbags. 2022. Online. Available from: www.nzta.govt.nz/vehicles/choosing-the-right-vehicle/features-that-protect-you/airbags/.
175. Lastfogel J, Soleimani T, Flores R, Cohen A, Wooden WA, Munshi I, et al. Helmet use and injury patterns in motorcycle-related trauma. JAMA Surg 2016;151(1):88–90.
176. Centre for Road Safety. Australian graduated licensing scheme policy framework. NSW: Sydney: NSW Government, Transport for NSW; 2020.
177. Safe Work Australia. Work-related injury and disease: key WHS statistics Australia. Canberra: SWA; 2021.
178. Fitzgerald MC, Curtis K, Cameron PA, Ford JE, Howard TS, Crozier JA, et al. The Australian Trauma Registry. ANZ J Surg 2019;89(4):286–90.
179. Palmer CS, Davey TM, Mok MT, McClure RJ, Farrow NC, Gruen RL, et al. Standardising trauma monitoring: the development of a minimum dataset for trauma registries in Australia and New Zealand. Injury 2013;44(6):834–41.
180. Royal Australasian College of Surgeons Trauma Committee, editor. Establishing a minimum data set (M.D.S.) for Australasian trauma. RACS Data Collection Workshop. Albury–Wodonga: RACS; 1993.
181. Champion HR, Copes WS, Sacco WJ, Lawnick MM, Keast SL, Bain Jr LW, et al. The major trauma outcome study: establishing national norms for trauma care. J Trauma 1990;30(11):1356–65.
182. Gennarelli TA, Wodzin E, editors. Abbreviated Injury Scale 2005 – Update 2008. Barrington, IL: AAAM; 2008.
183. Association for the Advancement of Automotive Medicine, editor. The Abbreviated Injury Scale – 2015 Revision. Chicago, IL: AAAM; 2015.
184. States JD, editor. The abbreviated and the comprehensive research injury scales. 13th Stapp Car Crash Conf. Boston, MA: Society of Automotive Engineers; 1969.
185. Palmer CS, Tohira H. The Abbreviated Injury Scale is well described: a letter to the editor re: Loftis et al, 'Evolution of the Abbreviated Injury Scale: 1990–2015'. Traffic Inj Prev 2019;20(4):449–51.
186. Baker SP, O'Neill B, Haddon W, Long WB. The Injury Severity Score: a method for describing patients with multiple injuries and evaluating trauma care. J Trauma 1974;14(3):187–96.
187. Boyd CR, Tolson MA, Copes WS. Evaluating trauma care: the TRISS method. Trauma Score and the Injury Severity Score. J Trauma 1987;27(4):370–8.
188. Palmer CS, Gabbe BJ, Cameron PA. Defining major trauma using the 2008 Abbreviated Injury Scale. Injury 2016;47(1):109–15.
189. Osler T, Baker SP, Long W. A modification of the injury severity score that both improves accuracy and simplifies scoring. J Trauma 1997;43(6):922–5.
190. Ringdal KG, Lossius HM, Jones JM, Lauritsen JM, Coats TJ, Palmer CS, et al. Collecting core data in severely injured patients using a consensus trauma template: an international multicentre study. Crit Care 2011;15(5):R237.
191. Osler T, Rutledge R, Deis J, Bedrick E. ICISS: an international classification of disease-based injury severity score. J Trauma 1996;41(3):380–6.

192. Willis CD, Gabbe BJ, Jolley D, Harrison JE, Cameron PA. Predicting trauma patient mortality: ICD [or ICD-10-AM] versus AIS based approaches. ANZ J Surg 2010;80(11):802–6.
193. Carmont MR. The advanced trauma life support course: a history of its development and review of related literature. Postgrad Med J 2005;81(952):87–91.
194. Chua WC, D'Amours SK, Sugrue M, Caldwell E, Brown K. Performance and consistency of care in admitted trauma patients: our next great opportunity in trauma care? ANZ J Surg 2009;79(6):443–8.
195. Curtis KA, Mitchell RJ, Chong SS, Balogh ZJ, Reed DJ, Clark PT, et al. Injury trends and mortality in adult patients with major trauma in New South Wales. MJA 2012;197(4):233–7.
196. National Road Trauma Advisory Council. Report of the working party on trauma systems. Canberra: NRTAC, Commonwealth Department of Human Services and Health; 1993.
197. New South Wales Ambulance. Pre-hospital management of major trauma. Revised. Sydney: NSW Ambulance; 2018. Online. Available from: https://aci.health.nsw.gov.au/__data/assets/pdf_file/0005/243779/ASNSW-Protocol-T1-prehospital-management-major-trauma.pdf.
198. Royal Australasian College of Surgeons, Health Quality and Safety Commission New Zealand. Quality and Safety Challenge 2012 Final project report. Wellington: Health Quality and Safety Commission New Zealand; 2012.
199. Royal Australasian College of Surgeons. Australian and Aotearoa New Zealand Trauma Verification Program: model resource criteria for trauma services. Melbourne: RACS; 2022. Online. Available from: www.surgeons.org/-/media/Project/RACS/surgeons-org/files/trauma-verification/model-resource-criteria.pdf?rev=71ad3d4faf9049dcb542a38a18dd2e7e&hash=6757B62EFA5715EC752B85E35EC3FB45
200. Leonard E, Curtis K. Are Australian and New Zealand trauma service resources reflective of the Australasian trauma verification model resource criteria? ANZ J Surg 2014;84(7–8):523–7.
201. Murphy M, Curtis K, Lam MK, Palmer CS, Hsu J, McCloughen A. Simulation-based multidisciplinary team training decreases time to critical operations for trauma patients. Injury 2018;49(5):953–8.
202. Balogh Z. Traumatology in Australia: provision of clinical care and trauma system development. ANZ J Surg 2010;80(3):119–21.
203. Ursic C, Curtis K, Zou Y, Black D. Improved trauma patient outcomes after implementation of a dedicated trauma admitting service. Injury 2009;40(1):99–103.
204. Bach JA, Leskovan JJ, Scharschmidt T, Boulger C, Papadimos TJ, Russell S, et al. The right team at the right time – multidisciplinary approach to multi-trauma patient with orthopedic injuries. Int J Crit Ill Inj Sci 2017;7(1):32–7.
205. Beachley M. The evolution of trauma nursing and the society of trauma nurses: a noble history. J Trauma Nurs 2005;12(4):105–15.
206. Curtis K, Donoghue J. The trauma nurse coordinator in Australia and New Zealand: a progress survey of demographics, role function, and resources. J Trauma Nurs 2008;15(2):34–42.
207. Walter E, Curtis K. The role and impact of the specialist trauma nurse: an integrative review. J Trauma 2015;22(3):153–69.
208. Paramedics Australasia. Paramedicine role descriptors. Online. Available from: www.paramedics.org/paramedicine-role-descriptors/2016.

CHAPTER 42

MAJOR TRAUMA INITIAL ASSESSMENT AND MANAGEMENT

KELLIE GUMM AND BEN MEADLEY

ESSENTIALS

- Emphasis in the pre-hospital phase of care should be on the primary survey and include airway maintenance, control of external bleeding and shock, stabilisation and immediate transfer to the nearest highest level of care.
- Emphasis at the scene should be on obtaining and reporting information to the receiving hospital (time of injury, events and patient's history).
- Optimal patient outcomes require early trauma centre notification.
- Advance planning for the trauma patient's arrival is essential and the trauma team should be assembled and ready to treat the patient.
- The mechanism of injury and patient history form the fundamental information that help anticipate the care required for potential injuries and their severity.
- Primary and secondary surveys provide the standard sequence of priorities for the assessment of patients with multiple injuries.
- *Hypocalcaemia*, which is a key component of the coagulation cascade, plays an important role in coagulopathy and may change the trauma triad (hypothermia, hypotension and acidosis) to a diamond of death (hypothermia, hypotension, acidosis and hypocalcaemia).[1] The biggest impact of hypocalcaemia is on those pathways reliant upon calcium, such as platelet function, intrinsic and extrinsic haemostasis and cardiac contractility.[2] Calcium is lost in haemorrhagic shock and this loss is exacerbated by the blood products transfused, which contain citrate.
- Primary and/or secondary surveys should be repeated frequently to remain vigilant to deterioration and to identify any new treatments required.
- Tertiary survey > 24 hours to assist in identifying any missed injuries.

INTRODUCTION

Major trauma is a time-critical emergency and successful management results from prompt diagnosis of injuries, appropriate resuscitation and stabilisation and prevention of secondary injury. While trauma care is ideally provided in institutions that specialise in trauma,[3–6] the incidence of traumatic injury is not limited to

densely populated areas where there are short transport times and the majority of designated trauma centres are located. It is therefore incumbent on trauma clinicians to understand that, wherever they practise, essential clinical competencies and a sound knowledge base in trauma management is necessary to provide the highest-quality care to this fragile patient population. Although specialised trauma centres have designated trauma treatment areas and multidisciplinary staff allocated to trauma management inclusive of resuscitation through to rehabilitation, most emergency departments (EDs) must be able to provide trauma care while also dealing with innumerable other patients presenting with an assortment of ailments from sore throats to cardiac events.[7]

In the rural setting, trauma patient numbers may not be as great, but the seriousness of the situation faced by pre-hospital clinicians and emergency nurses, and their requisite knowledge, is similar. Importantly, for the 'occasional' trauma practitioner, getting the basics right (e.g. airway management and haemorrhage control) is paramount.

This chapter focuses primarily on trauma patient assessment, which is applicable in any clinical situation and the preparation for and management of the trauma patient during the resuscitative phase of the pre-hospital and ED care. Pre-hospital trauma management in the context of decision-making, equipment and extrication is discussed in Chapters 10 and 11.

PREPARATION

Trauma patients arrive in the ED in numerous ways. The amount of time taken from injury to arrival at the ED or trauma centre varies depending on location, length of time to report the injury, availability of emergency medical services (EMS), length of rescue and numerous other variables. Time has been a major influence on the development of world trauma systems and centres, especially the 'golden hour'.[5,8,9] This term was coined by R. Adams Cowley, who, using research from World War I, demonstrated that the mortality and morbidity of injured patients increased with the amount of time to resuscitation and definitive care: there was an increase of 10% with a 1-hour delay and an increase of 75% with a 10-hour delay. Thus, it was determined that the worst enemy of a trauma patient immediately after an injury was time.[10,11] However, in today's more-sophisticated trauma systems, the concept of the 'golden hour' can be interpreted as meaning the window of opportunity in which emergency clinicians can save a patient's life or limb. This could be a few minutes for some (threatened airway) or hours for others (vascular limb injury).[3,7,9,11] The golden hour may only be applicable to urban centres, whereas the 'silver day' is more appropriate and realistic for the remote areas of Australia and Aotearoa New Zealand. Increasingly, government health agencies are focusing on finding a balance between delivering effective pre-hospital medical services and retrieving appropriate patients in a timely fashion and ensuring their delivery to the highest level of care available, while balancing the unnecessary risks to EMS crews that are related to the rapid transport of patients.[7,12]

To decrease mortality and morbidity, a coordinated approach with EMS can assist in expediting care in the field and early notification, thus providing advance notice to ensure mobilisation of the trauma team and hospital set-up.[13] ED preparation is essential to maintain the principle of 'do no further harm', cited in the 2018 *Advanced Trauma Life Support Course Manual*,[5] and to expedite care. Preparation includes facility design for the trauma bay or resuscitation area cubicle, trauma team presence on patient arrival and necessary medications and equipment to handle potentially complicated injuries.

The first thing to consider is where the resuscitation will take place. Each ED has architectural strengths and weaknesses that require creative solutions for the maximum use of space and efficiency of personnel.

RESUSCITATION ROOM AND EQUIPMENT

The primary objective of a trauma resuscitation area is to facilitate rapid assessment of a severely injured patient, supported by adequate lighting, space and equipment. Consideration should be given to staff safety and welfare (i.e. personal protective equipment [PPE], room ventilation) in times of infectious diseases pandemic or cases of patient contamination. This will allow the identification and treatment of life-threatening injuries and seamless integration with the EMS staff into the department.[14,15]

PRACTICE TIP

Any immediate life-threatening haemorrhage should be managed concurrently with the airway and breathing assessment, then further stabilisation provided.

Most centres now have trauma guidelines to assist all practitioners in the identification, prioritisation and treatment of patient injuries. These guidelines should be readily available in various forms, such as applications for portable electronic devices, posters, laminated cards, desktop icons and/or online, to always ensure easy access. While Box 42.1 illustrates some of the essential equipment required, this is not an exhaustive list; however, it covers the essentials. Fig. 42.1A and B show the typical layout of a single patient trauma bay in a level 1 trauma centre purpose-built to resuscitate trauma patients.

STAFF TRAUMA EDUCATION

Managing today's complex pre-hospital and in-hospital environment requires skilled paramedical and nursing leaders, who understand and can manage the complex needs of high-acuity patients and the ward environment to ensure safe outcomes for patients and staff.

Gabbe,[4] Jashidimi,[18] Dans,[19] Copanitsanou[20] and Murphy[21] all demonstrated that patient outcomes improve with a good work environment, higher volume of patients, greater clinical experience, and nurses who have a higher education and more experience caring for the patient population.

The most sophisticated pre-hospital and in-hospital trauma systems are ineffective without a well-trained and organised trauma team; therefore, it is essential that, no matter the size of the facility, a multidisciplinary trauma team is available in the ED whenever needed.[5,22,23] All team members should have a minimum skill-set and knowledge base consisting of trauma patient triage, primary and secondary survey assessment, and adjuncts, including airway and spinal immobilisation, breathing, circulation and resuscitation skills. Roles can be interchangeable, with each role filled by the most experienced clinician present at the time.[24,25] This is especially relevant for the small rural urgent

BOX 42.1 **ESSENTIAL SUPPLIES, INSTRUMENTS AND TRAYS**[16]

AIRWAY
- Intubation supplies with various-sized blades, handles and tubes easily accessible
- Tracheostomy and cricothyroidotomy supplies
- Laryngeal mask various sizes

BREATHING
- Chest tube insertion trays with underwater-seal drains and chest tubes 28–32F
- Rapid-sequence induction medications
- Laerdal bag and various size masks
- Ventilator
- Oxygen

CIRCULATION
- Thoracotomy tray, including scalpel, black-handled scissors, rib spreaders (finochietto retractor), long retractors, dissecting scissors, vascular clamps, long-handled instruments, pledgets and cardiac sutures[17]
- Blood and fluid warmer (preferably high-volume devices)
- Venous access supplies for peripheral, intra-osseous and large-bore vascular access devices
- Defibrillator with paediatric and internal paddles

MISCELLANEOUS
- Resuscitation trolley containing ALS drugs
- Transport monitor with ECG, NIBP, pulse oximetry and end-tidal CO_2
- Dressings, suture supplies, splinting material
- Gastric tubes, urinary drainage system
- eFAST ultrasound machine
- Warming devices—convection blankets (e.g. Bair Hugger)

ALS: advanced life support; CO_2: carbon dioxide; ECG: electroencephalogram; FAST: focused abdominal sonography in trauma; NIBP: non-invasive blood pressure.

FIGURE 42.1A EMERGENCY DEPARTMENT TRAUMA RESUSCITATION BAY—CONFIGURATION

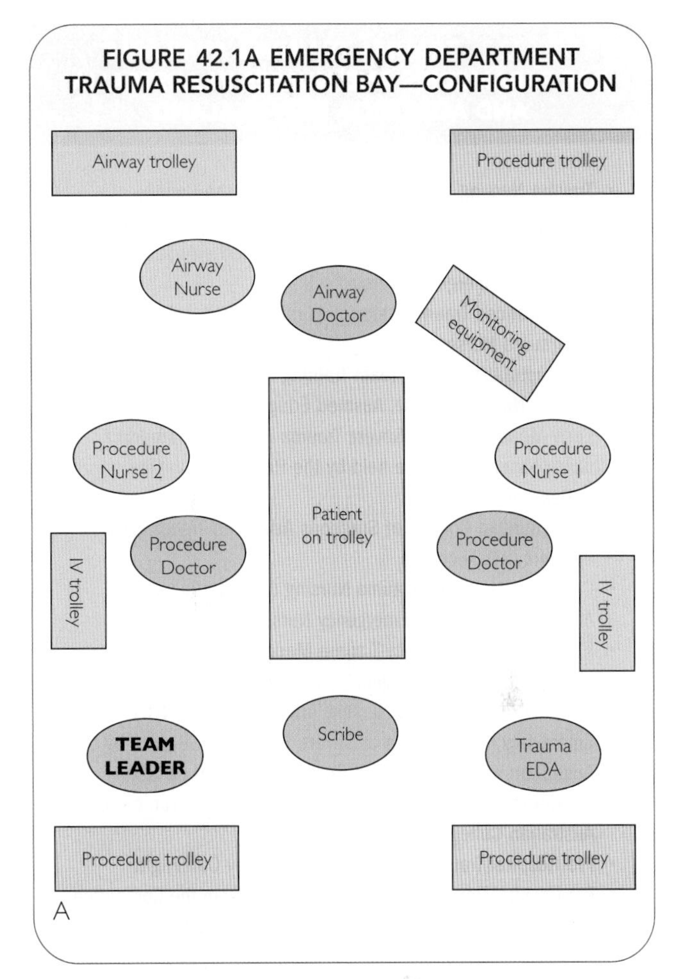

Based on diagram from The Royal Melbourne Hospital, Victoria.

FIGURE 42.1B EMERGENCY DEPARTMENT RESUSCITATION BAY

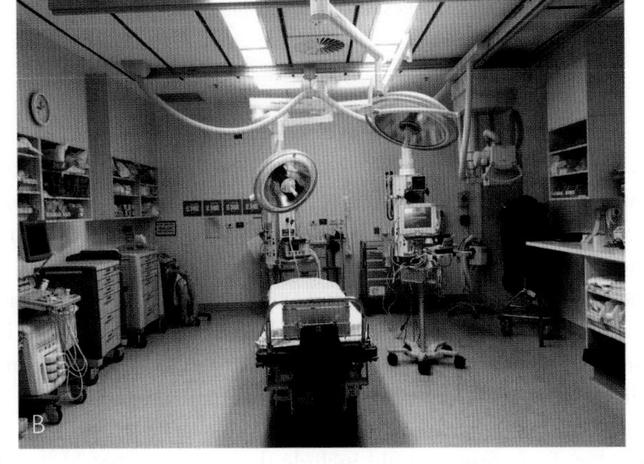

Courtesy of The Royal Melbourne Hospital, Melbourne, Victoria.

care centres where staff may have to rely on paramedics to fill roles out-of-hours.

Trauma education in many settings is evolving to include a wide range of learning modalities. These include online, low-fidelity (models) and high-fidelity (human patient simulators with heartbeats and constricting pupils) courses, making the simulation environment more realistic and hence improving the educational outcomes. Simulated trauma team training, practised as a standard part of routine ED education, can assist in team performance and is an effective way to achieve an advanced level of communication.[26,27]

See Box 42.2 for a list of a variety of trauma training available for paramedics and nurses in Australia and Aotearoa New Zealand. Further information on trauma courses and education can be provided by the trauma nurse coordinator at your nearest trauma centre.

THE TRAUMA TEAM

A trauma team (TT) is a group of health professionals with different skills, abilities and experience, aiming to successfully resuscitate an injured patient. Traditionally the TT would consist of medical and nursing staff; however, dependent on location and hospital resources, personnel may vary and the emergency clinician may be the most highly skilled staff member available. This will require them to have a more-developed

BOX 42.2 TRAUMA TRAINING AVAILABLE FOR PARAMEDICS AND NURSES IN AUSTRALIA AND AOTEAROA NEW ZEALAND

- Trauma Nursing Program (TNP) hosted by the College of Emergency Nursing Australasia
- Trauma Nursing Core Course (TNCC) from the Australian College of Emergency Nursing
- The Advanced Trauma Care for Nurses (ACTN), USA Society for Trauma Nurses
- The Australian Trauma Team Training update from ITEM
- Trauma Nursing Course, Ausmed Education Pty Ltd
- Early Management of Severe Trauma (EMST) paramedic/nurse observers course held by the Royal Australasian College of Surgeons
- The American College of Surgeons Advanced Trauma Life Support (ATLS) course
- Course in Advanced Trauma Nursing (CATN), run by the Australian College of Emergency Nurses
- ETM Course—Emergency Trauma Management Course—paramedic/nurse observers
- Definitive Perioperative Nursing Trauma Care (DPNTC)
- Emergency Management of Severe Burns (EMSB), run by the Australian and New Zealand Burns Association (ANZBA)
- International Trauma Life Support (ITLS) course, run by the Australian College of Emergency Nursing
- Pre-Hospital Trauma Course (PHTC), run by CareFlight
- Pre-Hospital Trauma Life Support (PHTLS), from the Committee of the National Association of Emergency Medical Technicians (NAEMT) in cooperation with the Committee on Trauma of the American College of Surgeons
- Managing Obstetric Emergencies and Trauma Course (MOET)
- Interactive web-based scenarios, learning modules, podcasts, videos, as well as information on upcoming trauma conferences and links to other web-based trauma resources such as trauma management guidelines, can be found on many state-based webpages, listed at the end of this chapter.

skill-set.[7,24] Table 42.1 illustrates the roles of the TT and the multidisciplinary team members who could fulfil each role. Team-member responsibilities are identified by the procedures they are required to conduct, such as establishing IV access or focusing on a specific anatomical area for assessment (e.g. head, left side of the patient's body). Responsibilities should be clearly defined, whether the trauma resuscitation is accomplished in a level 1 trauma centre or a small rural ED.[5,7,24]

A trauma team would consist of other staff in addition to this list. Such teams would include the core group of:[5,7,24]

- *team leader*: ED doctor on or the clinician with the highest level of trauma care skills; role is to control and manage the resuscitation, allocate roles, ensure preparation for patient reception, coordinate the resuscitation, discuss decision-making and debrief the team
- *airway*: nurse (airway competency if possible) and doctor (anaesthetists if available, someone experienced in airway management, i.e. ED clinical staff, GP, paramedic)
- *assessment*: doctor/nurse/paramedic conducts the primary survey, and the eFAST exam
- *procedure/circulation*: doctor (doctor/nurse/paramedic team) performs procedures required according to skill-set (i.e. IV/ IO insertion, indwelling catheters, fluid resuscitation, assists with log roll, secondary survey)
- *scribe*: preferably a senior nurse, able to take a leadership role while collating all information, keeps accurate record of all procedures and medications, provides a supporting role to the team, helping direct nursing care of less-experienced nurses in the procedure role[28,29]
- *emergency department assistant (EDA)/orderly/health care assistant*: trained aides who can help with removing clothes, applying warm blanket, log rolls, equipment, transport, blood delivery and collection, external cardiac massage
- *radiographer*: available to perform x-rays within 5 minutes
- *consultant surgeon and intensivist*: available in the hospital and within a short time of the patient arriving at the ED
- *surgical registrar*: undertakes secondary survey and examines the abdomen, can communicate with the surgical team and assist in decision-making.

In addition to the core TT, other medical and allied health personnel, who provide valuable background support, are also notified through a trauma paging system. Not all these need to be immediately present, but they can be notified of the arrival of the trauma patient by the trauma call page:

- blood bank
- biochemistry
- haematology
- operating theatre floor coordinator
- bed management trauma service.

There must be the capacity to directly communicate with other relevant specialists, such as neurosurgeons, orthopaedic surgeons, cardiothoracic surgeons, plastic surgeons and interventional radiologists, to assist in the ongoing management and definitive care of these patients.

It may be worthwhile to enlist the assistance of other personnel, such as social and/or pastoral care workers, to support the family from the time of the patient's admission.

Traumatic events experienced by trauma patients can often be psychologically traumatic for the trauma team caring for them. It is normal to need some extra support; a rapid trauma debrief can be very beneficial immediately after a trauma resuscitation. Almost every team member will be emotionally affected, and all will respond in a different way. Peer-support teams can provide any debriefing or peer support to staff involved in all trauma resuscitation, not just those perceived as 'distressing'.

PRACTICE TIP

To ensure ongoing quality and standards of care, evidence-based trauma protocols and guidelines should be followed throughout patient journey, from the incident scene through to discharge and rehabilitation.

TRAUMA TEAM NOTIFICATION

Trauma team activation criteria ensure early identification of a severely injured patient who requires specialised resources from

TABLE 42.1 CORE MULTIDISCIPLINARY TRAUMA TEAM[5,7,24]

ROLE	CORE COMPETENCIES/SKILLS
Team leader	**Competencies**
GP Surgeon (Registrar or Fellow) Anaesthetist Emergency doctor	Competent and experienced in assessment and management of the trauma patient according to EMST principles ***Skills*** *Supervision* of the team Appropriate *allocation* of team members Assessment of priorities and making team aware of these • listening to handover from EMS • overseeing of resuscitation Prioritising treatment and investigations Directing the performance of a range of invasive procedures, including: • endotracheal intubation and mechanical ventilation • prescription and administration of anaesthesia and analgesia • intercostal catheter insertion • intravenous cannulation and fluid resuscitation • venous blood gas sampling • environmental control (i.e. temperature/safety) Making appropriate referrals early in the treatment of the patient Ensuring that plans for *definitive management* are formulated at appropriate *pivotal points in resuscitation* Arranging for the transfer of patient to a place of definitive care
Airway nurse and doctor	**Competencies**
GP Anaesthetist MICA paramedic RN Paramedic	Competent and experienced in airway management ***Skills*** Maintenance of airway Application of O_2 Stabilisation and management of cervical spine (either in-line stabilisation or soft collar) Checking respiratory status and performing or assisting in endotracheal intubation and manual or mechanical ventilation Administration of anaesthesia and analgesia as necessary Insertion of nasogastric tube Assessment of GCS, checking pupil reaction, seeking information on next of kin Talking to patient, next of kin, relaying information to scribe
Procedure nurse and doctor	**Competencies**
GP Surgeon Surgical Fellow or Registrar ED doctor RN Paramedic	Competent and experienced in the invasive procedures to be performed or in assisting the set-up and assistance in insertion ***Skills*** Assistance with or performance of a range of invasive procedures, not limited to: • intercostal catheter insertion • intravenous cannulation and blood sampling • fluid resuscitation • arterial blood gas sampling/arterial line insertion • urinary catheterisation Attachment of monitoring equipment (ECG, NIBP, SaO_2, $EtCO_2$) Application of splints and dressings, performance of log-roll Performance of 12-lead ECG Performance of procedures as directed by the team leader
Scribe	**Skills**
Supervisor/RN Paramedic	Recording and documenting vital signs at frequent intervals Documenting the time of performance of procedures including the handover from EMS Documenting the time of administration of drugs Ensuring that procedures suggested by the team leader are carried out in a timely manner In conjunction with the team leader, controlling the access of personnel to resuscitation bay

ECG: electroencephalogram; EMS: emergency medical services; EMST: early management of severe trauma; MICA: mobile intensive-care ambulance; NIBP: non-invasive blood pressure; RN: registered nurse; SaO_2: oxygen saturation of arterial blood.

the hospital to form the TT. EMS[7,30] play a crucial role in the pre-notification by providing essential information about the patient's condition that will help in the decision to activate a TT or not. Notification of team members can be via overhead paging and/or a dedicated paging system. A degree of over-triage is required to ensure capture of all severely injured trauma patients.[31,32]

Designated trauma centres enhance communication to the team by establishing 'trauma call-out' criteria to notify the TT of a potentially major trauma patient's impending arrival. Trauma team activation was traditionally based on physiological criteria; specific high-risk injuries and mechanism of injury (see Box 42.3). The consensus that mechanism of injury alone is a criterion for TT activation is not predictive of severity of injury[35] or outcome and that physiological measurements are highly sensitive.

While it is necessary to mobilise the entire TT to manage multi-trauma patients with time-critical injuries, it is neither practical nor economical to mobilise them for every patient. Unnecessary activations divert resources away from other hospital activities, which could compromise patient care. Thus, most centres use a tiered response to enable them to differentiate between the severely injured patients who have a higher likelihood of increased mortality and those with a lower likelihood of mortality. Preventing under-triage is also important, as it can result in treatment delays. Serious injuries may not be diagnosed quickly enough, leaving the patient to clinically deteriorate and contributing to secondary complications.[3,36] Optimal triage systems can provide an appropriate balance of triage and resource allocation. Each hospital should have its own activation criteria based on its individual patient population to ensure that all major trauma patients and those with complex injuries receive adequate reception by the appropriately trained multidisciplinary team. While it may be difficult to minimise under- and over-triage rates, monitoring is essential to enable changes to be implemented as required.

Delayed trauma call based on clinician judgement and evolving patient condition in addition to pre-hospital TT activation should be available. For example, not all serious injuries meeting TT activation criteria may fall under one of the categories in Box 42.3. Thus, a senior clinician should be able to decide to activate the trauma team based on clinical judgement. And, if trauma criteria are not identified or evident on initial presentation, the TT should be activated immediately on recognition, regardless of time after presentation.

BOX 42.3 TRAUMA TEAM ACTIVATION CRITERIA[33,34]

VITAL SIGNS

- Systolic blood pressure < 90 mmHg
- Pulse rate < 60 or > 120 beats/minute
- Respiratory rate < 12 or > 24 breaths/minute
- Glasgow Coma Scale score ≤ 9
- Oxygen saturation < 90%

INJURIES

- All penetrating injuries to head, neck, torso or groin
- All blunt injuries to a single region or to two or more regions comprising head, neck, torso or groin

SPECIFIC INJURIES

- Suspected spinal cord injury
- Limb-threatening injuries and/or amputations
- Burns > 20% or suspected respiratory tract involvement
- Major compound fracture/open dislocation of limb
- Fractures of two or more of: humerus, femur, tibia
- Fractured pelvis

MECHANISM OF INJURY

- Ejection from vehicle
- Motor/cyclist impact > 30 kph
- Fall from height (> 3 m)
- Struck on head from objects falling > 3 m
- Explosion
- High-speed motor vehicle collision (60 kph or over)
- Pedestrian impact
- Prolonged extrication (> 30 minutes)

AND

- Pregnancy > 20 weeks with ruptured membranes/PV (per vaginal) bleeding/fetal heart rate < 100 beats/minute
- Age > 55 years
- Significant underlying medical condition

PRACTICE TIP

Trauma call, or upgraded trauma call, should be activated in the event of patient deterioration, or at the time it is recognised the patient meets the trauma call criteria—regardless of time after presentation.

PREPARATION

Preparation begins before the patient arrives; Box 42.4 gives a summary of preparation measures. Contemporary resuscitation planning may include concepts such as the 'zero point survey', optimising readiness for patient reception.[37] As stated previously, preparation includes an organised area within the scope of the facility's resources to accommodate resuscitation of a severely injured patient. The team notification should occur as soon as patient details become available with an expected time of arrival; once the team assembles, specific clinical details can be disseminated to all members in the moments available before the resuscitation begins, to enable prioritisation of tasks. This communication can clarify confusion about responsibilities, but also helps individual members focus as a team on anticipated injuries. The effectiveness of EDs and trauma centres depends on the entire team working together with a common vision of efficient, skilled and organised management.

In most instances, some prior notification by the ambulance service is provided. The person receiving the notification should elicit as much information as possible without compromising rapid transport of the patient. Knowing in advance the mechanism of injury, patient acuity and physiological status facilitates set-up of special equipment. Being aware, for example, that a patient in a vehicle rollover in winter was found in a paddock will help the TT anticipate and intervene early for hypothermia. Knowing that a patient has a penetrating abdominal injury and is hypotensive will enable activation of

BOX 42.4 PREPARATION FOR THE ARRIVAL OF A TRAUMA PATIENT

- Notification of trauma patient meeting the trauma call-out criteria
- Trauma call-out dispatched (on-call medical officers in rural areas notified)
- Standard room preparation—the trauma bay should be checked daily and then prior to patient arrival (ensuring all equipment is in working order and stock lists are adequate)
- Allocation of team roles, zero point survey can be used to prepare yourself, your team and your environment prior to resuscitations

EQUIPMENT

- Oxygen and suction
- Airway trolley, including preparation of intubation drugs
- Monitors, fixed and transport
- Defibrillator—ensure enough paper and battery is charged
- Procedure and IV trolleys
- Multipurpose packs and trays (1–2)
- Blood tubes for baseline blood and cross-match
- (ROTEM/TEG) if available
- Priming of fluid warming devices
- Turning on ultrasound machine
- Prepare equipment for assessment of clotting
- IV fluid bag and line primed ready to go
- Blood products and/or requesting massive transfusion packs if required (FFP, PLTS, Cryo & RBCs)

FORMS

- Pathology and x-ray
- Trauma flow sheet
- Wrist bands and labels

TRAUMA TEAM ARRIVAL

- Donning of lead gowns and standard precautions
- Allocation of staff roles and discussion of expected patient
- Notification of blood bank and pathology

massive transfusion protocols, early notification of the consultant surgeon, anaesthetist and operating suite. While it is not financially prudent to open a large number of supplies and trays before patient arrival, it is wise to secure necessary equipment ahead of time and have it readily accessible.

PRACTICE TIP

The 'zero point survey' precedes the primary survey, and allows for optimisation of the environment and team readiness prior to patient arrival. Ensuring a state of readiness prior to the first patient encounter sets the scene for expert team behaviours.

DOCUMENTATION

The ambulance patient care record should be filed in the inpatient paper or electronic medical record. It can assist in monitoring trends in the patient's condition, providing details of clinical events and describing the initial findings at the scene, which may not be evident to those who subsequently care for the patient. Accurate, succinct and timely documentation of the trauma resuscitation is essential to patient management, giving the scribe a pivotal role in the TT. The scribe's record captures the efforts of the paramedics at the scene to the first moments of a patient's arrival. It also provides data on the patient's physiological response to treatment and may be used as evidence in police investigations or the Coroner's Court (see Chapter 4). In addition, these records are used for case reviews and quality-assurance activities locally, nationally and internationally.

Accurate documentation is paramount for good trauma management. Documentation of vital-sign changes, blood loss, decreased urinary output and amounts and types of fluid administration quickly identify indicators that alert the astute clinician to physiological compromise in the patient's condition and allow regular updating of the TT leader. Tools used for documentation vary, but generally involve formatted paper or electronic trauma flow sheets, which can accommodate rapid documentation in the stressful atmosphere of trauma resuscitation. The flow sheet may also help guide the primary survey and ensure that all procedures are undertaken.

INITIAL RESUSCITATION

All trauma patients should have continuous assessment from the time of their injury through to hospital admission, using primary and secondary surveys. Life-threatening conditions are treated immediately before proceeding to the next phase of care.

Paramedics place emphasis on systematic assessment, airway maintenance, spinal immobilisation, haemorrhage control, fluid resuscitation (where indicated) and immediate transport, all while minimising scene time.[5,38–40] Once the primary survey is completed, patient assessment continues with the assessment of physiological status (i.e. vital signs survey) and is followed by the secondary survey, which includes anticipating plans for transport to a major trauma service or the closest most appropriate service. Pre-hospital triage guidelines enable identification of patients who should be immediately triaged to the highest level of trauma centre. The guidelines typically require assessment of physiological parameters, region or type of injury and mechanism of injury. The current time-critical guideline used by paramedics in Victoria is shown in Fig. 42.2. In the latest version, the timeframe has changed from 45 to 60 minutes.

Once the patient arrives at the ED or trauma centre, the process is repeated, beginning with the paramedic team handing over. Utilisation of the IMIST-AMBO mnemonic (see Box 42.5)[42] ensures that the most pertinent information is handed over in a timely manner. It is vital that the TT listens to the paramedic handover, as they were the first to conduct the

FIGURE 42.2 PRE-HOSPITAL MAJOR TRAUMA CRITERIA FOR VICTORIA[41]

Victorian State Trauma System

Pre-hospital Major Trauma Triage

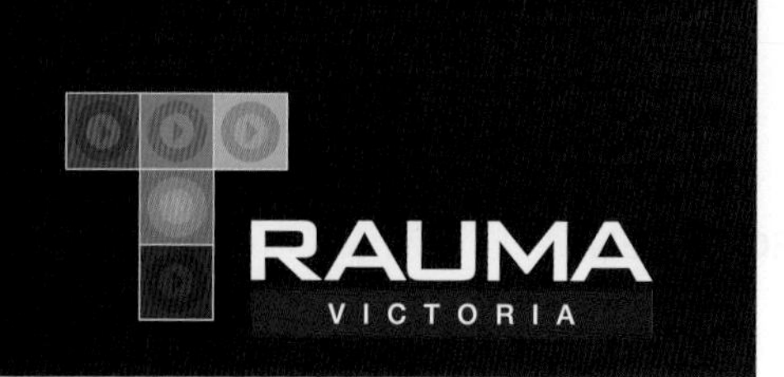
RAUMA
VICTORIA

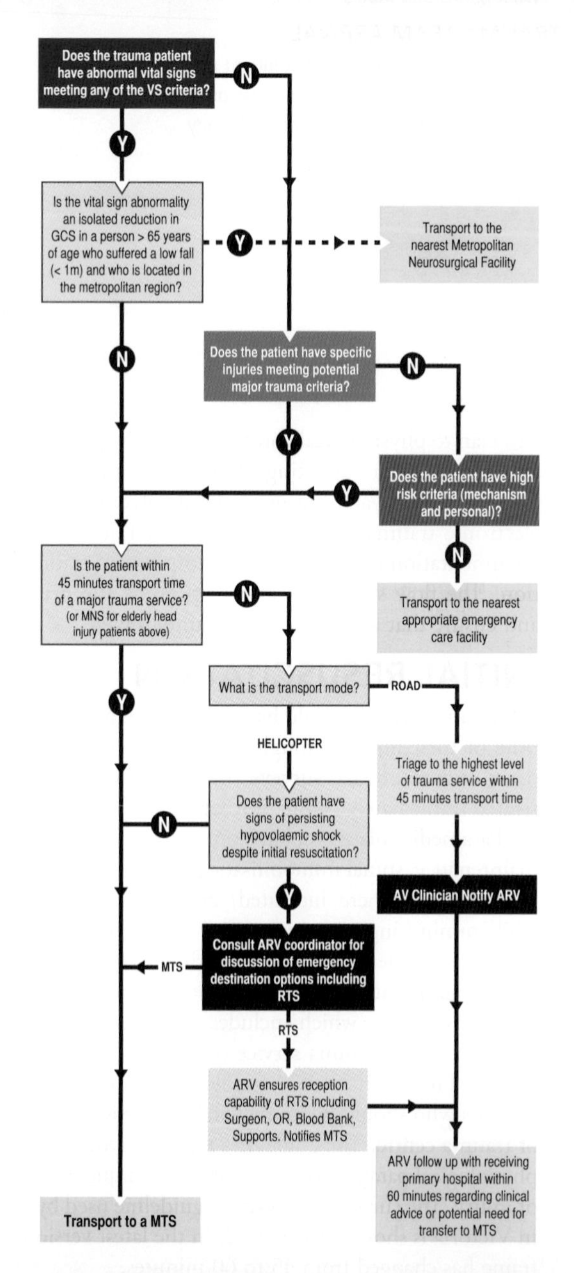
Does the trauma patient have abnormal vital signs meeting any of the VS criteria?
N
Y
Is the vital sign abnormality an isolated reduction in GCS in a person > 65 years of age who suffered a low fall (< 1m) and who is located in the metropolitan region?
Y
Transport to the nearest Metropolitan Neurosurgical Facility
N
Does the patient have specific injuries meeting potential major trauma criteria?
N
Y
Does the patient have high risk criteria (mechanism and personal)?
Y
N
Transport to the nearest appropriate emergency care facility
Is the patient within 45 minutes transport time of a major trauma service? (or MNS for elderly head injury patients above)
N
Y
What is the transport mode?
ROAD
HELICOPTER
Triage to the highest level of trauma service within 45 minutes transport time
Does the patient have signs of persisting hypovolaemic shock despite initial resuscitation?
N
Y
AV Clinician Notify ARV
Consult ARV coordinator for discussion of emergency destination options including RTS
MTS
RTS
ARV ensures reception capability of RTS including Surgeon, OR, Blood Bank, Supports. Notifies MTS
ARV follow up with receiving primary hospital within 60 minutes regarding clinical advice or potential need for transfer to MTS
Transport to a MTS

Pre-hospital Vitals Signs Major Trauma Criteria

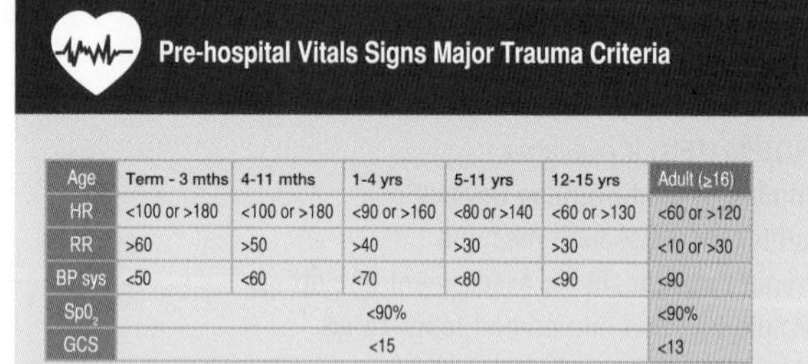

Age	Term - 3 mths	4-11 mths	1-4 yrs	5-11 yrs	12-15 yrs	Adult (≥16)
HR	<100 or >180	<100 or >180	<90 or >160	<80 or >140	<60 or >130	<60 or >120
RR	>60	>50	>40	>30	>30	<10 or >30
BP sys	<50	<60	<70	<80	<90	<90
SpO_2	<90%					<90%
GCS	<15					<13

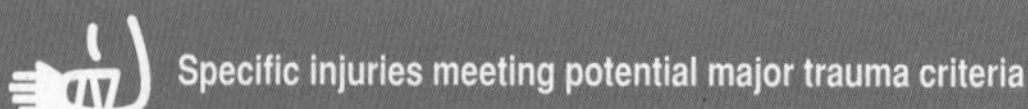

Specific injuries meeting potential major trauma criteria

All penetrating injuries (except isolated superficial limb injuries)

Blunt injuries:

- Serious injury to a single body region such that specialised care or intervention may be required, or such that life, limb or long term quality of life may be at risk.
- Significant Injuries involving more than one body region.

Specific Injuries:

- Limb amputation
- Suspected Spinal Cord Injury
- Burns > 20% BSA or suspected respiratory tract burns
- Serious crush injury
- Major compound fracture or open dislocation
- Fracture to two or more of: femur, tibia, humerus
- Fractured Pelvis
- Spinal Fracture

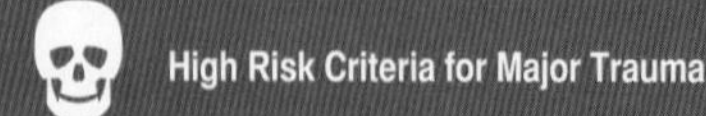

High Risk Criteria for Major Trauma

- Ejection from vehicle
- Motor / cyclist impact > 30 kph
- Fall from height > 3 m
- Struck on head by object falling > 3 m
- Explosion
- High speed MCA > 60 kph
- Pedestrian impact
- Prolonged extrication time

AND:

- Age <16 / >55
- OR Pregnant
- OR Significant comorbidity

ARV Adult Retrieval Victoria 1300 36 86 61 | PIPER Paediatric Infant Perinatal Emergency Retrieval 1300 13 76 50

AMBULANCE VICTORIA

28/07/2017 | Version 2.0 | Contact us: Trauma.Victoria@ambulance.vic.gov.au

BOX 42.5 **IMIST-AMBO—HANDOVER MNEMONIC**[42]

I	Identification of the patient
M	Mechanism of injury–time of the event, events related to the incident
I	Injuries–known or suspected injuries
S	Signs–vital signs (heart rate, blood pressure, conscious state, respiratory status)
T	Treatment–any treatment conducted at the scene or en route
A	Allergies
M	Medications (prescribed to the patient, if known, e.g. anticoagulants)
B	Background history (comorbidities, events leading up to the incident)
O	Other pertinent information (e.g. social status, relatives aware of incident)

primary survey in the pre-hospital environment and en route to the facility. This handover will provide valuable information on the mechanism of injury and the patient's injuries, treatment and vital signs.[5,40,42,43]

The IMIST-AMBO framework provides the structure necessary to ensure that the TT remains focused in a very distracting environment. It allows members of the TT to rapidly identify and treat immediate life-threatening injuries. A team member can then seek out the paramedic soon after for a more detailed history.

Once handover is complete, the initial resuscitation commences, with the TT conducting the primary survey, assessing and treating any life-threatening injuries. Once the primary survey is completed, patient assessment continues with the secondary survey, which includes anticipating plans for transfer or transport to another unit or trauma centre. The tertiary survey is the key third assessment of the patient. It is usually conducted 24–72 hours after admission and/or in addition to when a patient leaves the ICU and/or prior to patient transfer to assist in identifying missed or overlooked injuries.

PRIMARY SURVEY

Multi-trauma patients suffer from many and varied life-threatening injuries. If these injuries are not addressed in a clinically appropriate sequence, a potentially non-fatal threat can quickly escalate and become fatal.[7,9] It is essential that the initial systematic primary survey is prioritised and followed, in both the pre-hospital and the hospital phases of care.

The primary survey should be conducted in the following sequence (see below for trauma cardiac arrest [TCA], where addressing haemorrhage comes before airway; also when a trauma team is present ABCD can be addressed simultaneously and not sequentially):[5,7,44]

A. Airway maintenance with cervical spine control
B. Breathing and ventilation
C. Circulation with haemorrhage control
D. Disability: neurological status
E. Exposure and temperature control.

Most deaths due to trauma occur very early after the event and most are not preventable.[6] Patients in cardiac arrest due to trauma have different priorities of care than above and include haemorrhage control, restoration of circulating blood volume, airway management, relieving tension pneumothorax, all taking precedence over CPR. If traumatic cardiac arrest (TCA) is present on handover or during the primary survey, priorities of care should include immediate steps to identify and treat all reversible causes:[45]

- Stop the bleeding.
- Open the airway and assist with breathing.
- Decompress the chest (finger thoracostomy).[46]
- Establish adequate IV access and commence fluid/blood product resuscitation.
- Cardiac compressions are usually withheld until these procedures are complete.

In the next part of the chapter, the prioritised assessment and management will be discussed in sequence for the purposes of clarity; however, these steps are frequently accomplished simultaneously. Unless the patient is in TCA, as above, the primary survey is conducted using ABC; if in cardiac arrest, the CABC is utilised.

AIRWAY AND CERVICAL SPINE STABILISATION

Assessment of the trauma patient's airway and ventilatory status is the *top priority*. Patients at high risk of airway compromise include the unconscious, those with an altered level of consciousness, head injuries or blood loss, and those affected by alcohol and other drugs. Loss of airway could be lethal within 4 minutes.[7,44]

The goals of airway and ventilation assessment are to:

1. Secure a patent airway.
2. Ensure adequate oxygenation.
3. Provide adequate ventilation.
4. Monitor ongoing status of airway patency and ventilatory status.
5. Maintain in-line spinal immobilisation.

Airway, breathing and circulation assessment should be conducted using 'look, listen and feel' techniques.

The best way to assess the airway is to speak to the patient. If they are able to verbalise in a comprehensible orientated way, this is evidence that the airway is clear. If orientated, the patient's brain is being perfused and there is no immediate evidence of brain injury. On the other hand, no speech or incomprehensible or disorientated speech will reveal a compromised airway and/or potential traumatic brain injury.

Look for the presence of airway compromise: close examination of the patient may reveal obvious injuries that can cause airway obstructions, such as:

- foreign bodies (vomitus, blood, false teeth)
- evidence of airway burns (see Chapter 49)
- fractures or lacerations to the face, larynx, neck or maxillofacial region.

At this stage, pallor or cyanosis can help confirm the presence of an airway obstruction, with cyanosis being a late sign.

Listen for abnormal sounds, such as:

- snoring, gurgling
- stridor
- hoarseness
- inability to talk in sentences.

These sounds are all associated with a partial occlusion of the airway.

Feel for tracheal position and diminished air movement.

While assessing the airway, it is paramount that the cervical spine remains stabilised, no hyperflexion, hyperextension or rotation. The patient should be nursed in neutral position according to local guidelines, then manual in-line stabilisation is used for any manoeuvres. Emergency clinicians need to have a heightened awareness of the vulnerability of the spine, and all management must be aimed at preventing spinal cord injury or exacerbating a pre-existing injury.[47,48] See Chapter 47 for a discussion on cervical spine stabilisation techniques.

PRACTICE TIP

Be aware of the patient with maxillofacial trauma who refuses to lie down flat! This patient may have such severe injuries that they can only manage their secretions and maintain a patent airway while sitting up.[5] Let them sit up.

Table 42.2 illustrates life-threatening airway problems—which must be treated immediately—their signs and symptoms, and the interventions to manage these problems.

PRACTICE TIP

Treat all patients as if they are hypoxic until proven otherwise.

BREATHING AND VENTILATION ASSESSMENT

A breathing problem may have already been identified during the assessment of the airway. It is important to remember that adequate ventilation requires optimum functioning of the lungs, chest and diaphragm. During the initial assessment of the patient's breathing, each of these must be examined individually.[5,43,44,49]

Look closely and examine the patient's chest wall integrity for:

- fractures, lacerations and/or bruising, paradoxical chest movements, tachypnoea and/or abnormal respiratory rate and/or 'air hunger', use of accessory and/or abdominal muscles
- asymmetrical chest wall movement
- further assessment of patient colour.

Listen for absent or decreased breath sounds and unequal air entry.

Feel for:

- subcutaneous air
- chest wall instability and/or crepitus
- position of trachea
- dullness and/or hyperresonance.

If the patient is already intubated, confirm appropriate endotracheal tube (ETT) placement by assessing end-tidal carbon dioxide ($EtCO_2$) (see Chapter 16 for $EtCO_2$ monitoring techniques), visualising symmetrical chest rise and fall, auscultating over the stomach, then the lung field. These techniques should be performed after intubation and repeated whenever a patient is moved; for example, from trolley to CT table. Patients

TABLE 42.2 LIFE-THREATENING AIRWAY PROBLEMS[3,27,31]

PROBLEM	SIGNS AND SYMPTOMS	INTERVENTIONS
Airway obstruction (complete or partial)	Dyspnoea, laboured respirations Decreased or no air movement Presence of foreign body in airway Trauma to face or neck Breathlessness Agitation Combativeness Cyanosis Stridor Drooling	Airway opening manoeuvres: • jaw thrust • chin lift • foreign body/tongue removal • coughing/suction Airway adjuncts: • nasal airway • oral airway • laryngeal mask airway (LMA) • endotracheal tube Surgical airway: • cricothyroidotomy • tracheostomy
Inhalation injury	History of enclosed-space fire, unconsciousness or exposure to heavy smoke Dyspnoea Wheezing, creps, crackles Hoarseness Singed facial or nasal hair Carbonaceous sputum Burns to face or neck Blisters in the oral cavity	Provide high-flow oxygen (100%) via non-rebreather mask or bag-valve-mask device Prepare for endotracheal intubation as soon as possible

intubated prior to arrival at hospital may be moved several times, increasing the potential for ETT displacement. Where equipment in use by paramedics differs from hospital equipment, continue to use that of the paramedics until ready to change over in an orderly fashion. Once ETT placement is confirmed, further diagnostic studies should be obtained, such as chest x-ray, ongoing $EtCO_2$, oxygen saturation measurements and arterial blood gases (see Chapter 16 for information on collecting arterial blood gases).[5,43] The paramedic who intubated should state the reason for intubation, the technique used, a description of the patient prior to the procedure, what was used to secure the ETT, and include a description of the airway and any difficulties that were encountered. Note that pre-hospital airway procedures are governed by guidelines and protocols, and these may differ from what individual trauma hospital practitioners are used to.

PRACTICE TIP

An easy way to remember potential chest injuries is A–J:[50]

A Airway transection or tear
B Bronchial tear or rupture
C Cord (spinal) injury
D Diaphragmatic rupture
E Esophageal (oesophageal) injury
F Flail chest or rib fracture
G Gas in the chest or abdomen
H Haemothorax
I Infarction from AMI
J Jugular venous distension from cardiac tamponade.

Table 42.3 illustrates some of the life-threatening breathing problems a multi-trauma patient may be faced with, their signs and symptoms and interventions required.

CIRCULATION WITH HAEMORRHAGE CONTROL

Any immediate life-threatening haemorrhage should be managed concurrently with the airway and breathing assessment, then further stabilisation provided at this point. Haemorrhage is the principal cause of preventable death after traumatic injury.[51–53] It is essential that all hypotension in the setting of trauma is considered secondary to hypovolaemia until proven otherwise. Uncorrected haemorrhagic shock will lead to inadequate cellular perfusion, anaerobic metabolism and the production of lactic acid. This may lead to profound metabolic acidosis, which also interferes with blood-clotting mechanisms, and promotes coagulopathy and further blood loss. Hypothermia, acidosis and the consequences of massive blood transfusion contribute to the development of coagulopathy and mortality for these patients is three to four times higher than those without coagulopathy. Even if control of the primary site of bleeding is achievable, patients may continue to bleed from all lacerated surfaces. This leads to the worsening of haemorrhagic shock, and so to a worsening of hypothermia and acidosis, prolonging the vicious cycle.[52,54] For details on the physiology of shock, see Chapter 10.

The goals of circulation and haemorrhage control assessment are to:

- identify signs and sources of haemorrhage
- assess mental status
- assess pulses
- assess skin colour, temperature and moisture.

Key signs of significant blood loss are altered consciousness, poor perfusion, skin pallor, weakened or thready pulses and signs of external bleeding. When assessing a trauma patient, it is essential to consider that the shocked state may not be haemorrhagic and the patient could be suffering from other forms of shock (e.g. cardiogenic, neurogenic or anaphylactic shock). During the handover, the paramedic can provide a description of the amount of blood loss at the scene; this may help differentiate between the types of shock. However, clinician estimation of external blood loss has been shown to be unreliable.[55,56] Cardiogenic shock in the trauma patient may be due to a diaphragm injury, pericardial tamponade, blunt myocardial injury or tension pneumothorax. Pericardial tamponade should be suspected when there is hypotension unexplained by other findings, i.e. tension pneumothorax, haemothorax, abdominal or other haemorrhage.

PRACTICE TIP

The signs and symptoms of pericardial tamponade and tension pneumothorax are similar, thus careful assessment of the patient is paramount. For example, distended neck veins are a sign of cardiogenic shock and can be hidden by the cervical collar.[57]

Point-of-care ultrasound should be considered for confirmation or elimination of pericardial tamponade and pneumothorax.

Neurogenic shock results from spinal cord injury. This profound shock is due to loss of sympathetic tone and is characterised by hypotension with no tachycardia or vasoconstriction and a normal pulse pressure. Multi-trauma patients with suspected or confirmed spinal cord injury should always be treated initially as if hypovolaemic (see Chapter 47).

Assessment

Look for:

- level of consciousness
- obvious signs of external bleeding
- skin colour for pallor and/or cyanosis
- neck veins (collapsed or distended)
- abnormalities underneath a cervical collar.

Key changes in the patient's condition can indicate ongoing blood loss (see Table 42.4). Capillary refill time is a good measure of perfusion in children, but its usefulness decreases with patient age and diminishing health status, and is affected by ambient temperature, making this test less reliable in the field.

Listen for muffled heart sounds that indicate pericardial tamponade.

Begin basic and advanced life support measures for pulseless patients. Patients who are in TCA at the scene have an overall

TABLE 42.3 LIFE-THREATENING BREATHING PROBLEMS[5,25,30]

PROBLEM	SIGNS AND SYMPTOMS	INTERVENTIONS
Tension pneumothorax	Dyspnoea, laboured respirations Decreased or absent breath sounds on affected side Unilateral chest rise and fall Tracheal deviation away from affected side Cyanosis Jugular venous distension Tachycardia and hypotension History of chest trauma or mechanical ventilation Chest pain Decreased oxygen saturation Ultrasound: loss of lung sliding, 'Seashore' sign	Requires immediate intervention without radiological confirmation Provide high-flow oxygen (100%) via non-rebreather mask or bag–valve–mask device Perform rapid chest decompression by needle and/or finger thoracostomy on affected side Place chest tube on affected side
Pneumothorax	Dyspnoea, laboured respirations Decreased or absent breath sounds on affected side May have unilateral chest rise and fall May have visible wound to chest or back Bruising or abrasions on chest Pain May have decreased saturations History of chest trauma Ultrasound: loss of lung sliding, 'Seashore' sign	Provide high-flow oxygen (100%) via non-rebreather mask or bag–valve–mask device Chest decompression by needle and/or finger thoracostomy on affected side Place chest tube on affected side Place occlusive dressing over any open chest wound and secure on three sides with tape
Haemothorax	Dyspnoea, laboured respirations Decreased or absent breath sounds on affected side May have unilateral chest rise and fall May have visible wound to chest or back History of chest trauma (often penetrating) Tachycardia Bruising or abrasions on chest Pain May have decreased saturations	Provide high-flow oxygen (100%) via non-rebreather mask or bag–valve–mask device Consider autotransfusion Prepare for urgent transport to operating theatre for massive haemothorax-initially $>$ 1500 mL and/or $>$ 100 mL for 2–4 hrs
Sucking chest wound (open pneumothorax)	Dyspnoea, laboured respirations Decreased or absent breath sounds on affected side Visible, sucking wound to chest or back Chest pain May have decreased saturations	Provide high-flow oxygen (100%) via non-rebreather mask or bag–valve–mask device Cover wound with occlusive dressing and secure on three sides with tape Watch for signs of tension pneumothorax and remove dressing during exhalation if they are noted Place chest tube on affected side
Flail chest	Dyspnoea, laboured respirations Paradoxical chest wall movement Chest pain Tachycardia May have decreased saturations	Provide high-flow oxygen (100%) via non-rebreather mask or bag–valve–mask device Prepare for intubation and mechanical ventilation in compromised patients
Full-thickness circumferential burn of thorax	Dyspnoea, laboured respirations Shallow respirations Obvious circumferential burns to thorax	Provide high-flow oxygen (100%) via non-rebreather mask or bag–valve–mask device Prepare for immediate escharotomy

TABLE 42.4 LIFE-THREATENING CIRCULATION PROBLEMS, SIGNS AND INTERVENTIONS[3,58,59]

PROBLEM	SIGNS AND SYMPTOMS	INTERVENTIONS
External haemorrhage	Obvious bleeding site	Elevation where able Direct pressure Quick Clot Tourniquet
Shock	Tachycardia Weak, thready pulses Cool, pale, clammy skin Tachypnoea Altered mental state Delayed capillary refill Oliguria or anuria Abdominal free fluid on ultrasound	Provide high-flow oxygen (100%) via non-rebreather mask or bag-valve-mask device Place two large-bore IV lines and/or I/O cannula Infuse with warm isotonic crystalloid solution (Hartmann's or 0.9% NaCl) if needed to maintain systolic BP > 80 mmHg while awaiting early administration of blood components Consider fluid bolus (250 mL in adults or 5–10 mL/kg in children) Prepare to administer blood/products
Pericardial tamponade	Tachycardia Muffled heart sounds Distended neck veins Hypotension ECG showing pulseless electrical activity Signs of hypovolaemic shock Pericardial free fluid on ultrasound	Pericardiocentesis

ECG: electrocardiogram; IV: intravenous; NaCl: sodium chloride.

mortality rate of 95%, especially following blunt trauma (97%), with many deaths not being preventable, even with expert trauma care. The Australian Resuscitation Council (2016)[6,60] therefore suggests that unless injuries are obviously incompatible with life, attempted resuscitation of patients with cardiac arrest due to haemorrhage is not futile and should be attempted. There are caveats to this recommendation, as prolonged (> 10 minutes) cardiopulmonary resuscitation after reversible causes have been addressed is associated with poor outcomes.

TCA guidelines state:

- haemorrhage control: splinting, compression, tourniquet, direct pressure
- restoration of circulating blood volume: decompress tension pneumothoraces, insert appropriate IV or IO access, resuscitated with blood and blood products
- airway establishment: basic to advanced airway manoeuvres.

If these strategies fail to restore circulating volume, then the traditional ALS begins including CPR.

PRACTICE TIP

C comes before B in trauma cardiac arrest.

THINK OF THE 2H's AND 2T's:

- Hypoxia: open airway; oxygen
- Tension: bilateral finger thoracostomy
- Hypotension: 1:1:1:1 fluids
- Tamponade: EDT

BOX 42.6 ESTIMATING ADULT SYSTOLIC BLOOD PRESSURE (BP)

If the pulse is palpable, systolic BP is at least:

- **radial: 80 mmHg**
- **femoral: 70 mmHg**
- **carotid: 60 mmHg**

Feel:

- Assess skin for moisture and temperature.
- Palpate pulses for presence, quality, rate and rhythm.

Peripheral pulses may be absent following direct injury, hypothermia, hypovolaemia or vasoconstriction. For decreased systolic blood pressure, assess central pulses (femoral or carotid) bilaterally for quality, rate and regularity. Box 42.6 lists approximate minimal systolic blood pressures palpable in adults at various sites.

Consider that tachycardia often precedes hypotension and that patients may be on medications that regulate heart rate, thus tachycardia may not eventuate. Table 42.4 outlines the life-threatening circulatory problems, signs and interventions.

The extended focused abdominal sonography in trauma (eFAST) approach is a quick method to detect occult abdominal bleeding in shocked patients, and forms part of the primary survey if the patient is haemodynamically unstable and the

FIGURE 42.3 A AND B, SEATBELT SIGNS

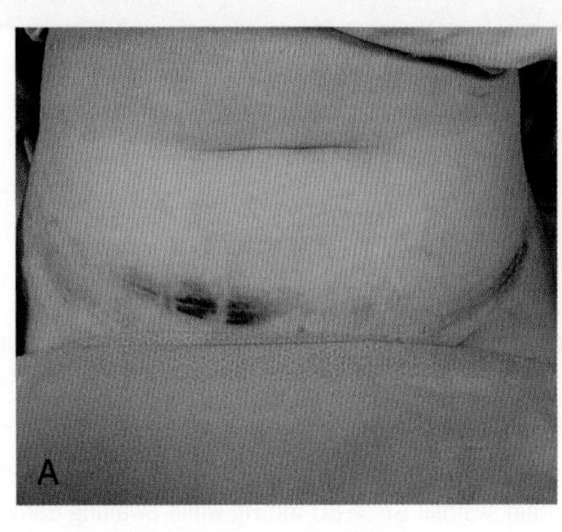

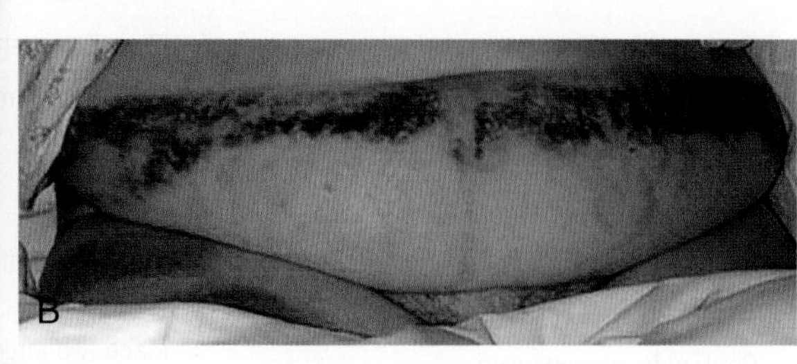

Courtesy of The Royal Melbourne Hospital, Victoria.

source of bleeding unknown; otherwise, this is an adjunct to the secondary survey. The indications for eFAST are altered sensorium, altered sensation, ambiguous physical examinations, those with a seatbelt sign (Fig. 42.3) and patients who will require prolonged sedation or anaesthesia (radiological investigations or operative procedures) and thus are unable to have a full abdominal examination.

eFAST is non-invasive, low-cost, safe, quick and accurate in the diagnosis of intraperitoneal bleeding, haemopneumothorax and pericardial tamponade, and is now universally accepted as an integral adjunct to the primary survey. eFAST scanning is now used in the pre-hospital environment by paramedic crews, with some studies finding that paramedics could achieve a high level of accuracy, with adequate training.[61,62] Performance of eFAST scanning in pre-hospital settings can be a challenge, as the paramedic has to deal with movement, combative patients, difficult access and short time-frames. NSW established the world's first eFAST course for nurses; its benefits include increased numbers of staff available to enable consistent, efficient and immediate care, which can be particularly advantageous to smaller centres without many medical resources. Many ultrasound machines are now more compact, easily usable and thus can be kept readily available. eFAST has the advantage of being able to be completed at the bedside in the trauma bay; it has the additional benefit of being easily repeatable. eFAST provides early, accurate information and has no side-effects, proving it to be a useful adjunct when considering management options. However, eFAST is very operator-dependent and requires training and practice; scans can be distorted by gas; and it is not sensitive to diaphragm, bowel and pancreatic injuries. It may also be unreliable in patients with ascites and subcutaneous air.[62]

DISABILITY (NEUROLOGICAL)

During the primary survey, a brief, focused neurological assessment is performed. This assessment is conducted at the end of the primary survey using the Glasgow Coma Scale (GCS) (see Chapter 13 for a detailed discussion) and the AEIOU mnemonic (Box 42.7). A decrease in the GCS is evidence of decreased cerebral perfusion and oxygenation; this could be due to hypovolaemia, hypoxia, brain injury or drug use. At this point, the oxygenation, ventilation and perfusion of the patient should be re-evaluated. The absence of spontaneous movement in the extremities and poor respiratory effort are early signs of spinal trauma.[5,47,63] If the patient is exhibiting motor posturing, or has gross pupillary dilation or asymmetry, consider mannitol, manoeuvres to maximise cerebral venous outflow, brief hyperventilation or emergent surgical intervention.

Any decreased level of consciousness or pupil abnormality will be investigated further during the secondary survey.[5,7,9,63] It is important to consider the patient's conscious state from the time of injury until the time of assessment; if the patient was brought in by ambulance, the paramedic will be able to provide information regarding the patient's conscious state, trends and changes during their management and any treatments provided that may have had some contributory impact.

BOX 42.7 AEIOU MNEMONIC[46]

A	Alcohol and drugs
E	Endocrine, encephalopathy
I	Insulin
O	Opiates and oxygen
U	Uraemia

If one of the above is not the primary cause of the decreased GCS score, it should be assumed as a traumatic cause until proven otherwise.

EXPOSURE AND TEMPERATURE CONTROL

Exposure of the trauma patient is the final step of the primary survey and prepares the patient for the secondary survey. Completely and rapidly remove the patient's clothing to assess for injuries, haemorrhage or other abnormalities; however, this step should not be completed until the patient reaches an environment where active warming can replace the patient's clothing, unless exposure is needed to diagnose or treat an injury.

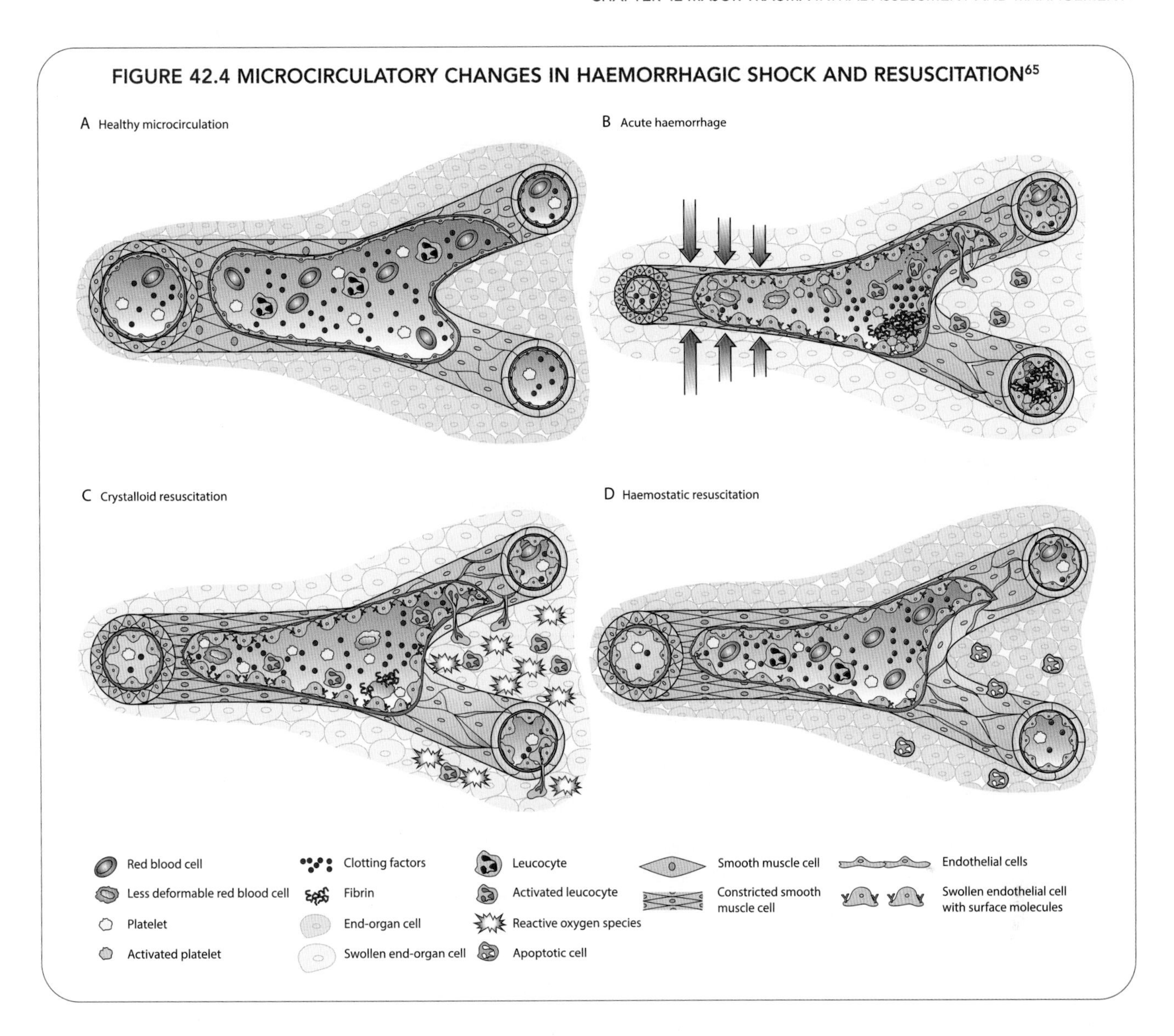

FIGURE 42.4 MICROCIRCULATORY CHANGES IN HAEMORRHAGIC SHOCK AND RESUSCITATION[65]

Observe the patient's overall general appearance, noting body appearance, asymmetry, guarding or the presence of odours such as alcohol, petrol and urine. The collection, securing and preserving of all patient clothing and belongings should be carried out.

TRAUMA-INDUCED COAGULOPATHY (TIC) AND THE DIAMOND OF DEATH

Acute traumatic coagulopathy (ATC) is an early endogenous coagulopathy that is characterised by systemic anticoagulation and fibrinolysis, exacerbated by hypothermia, acidosis and haemodilution, which contribute collectively to the established trauma-induced coagulopathy (TIC). TIC is defined as a hypercoagulable state that occurs after a traumatic injury and exacerbates blood loss. It is an imbalance of the dynamic equilibrium between procoagulant factors, anticoagulant factors, platelets, endothelium and fibrinolysis. *Coagulopathy* is present in up to a quarter of major trauma patients, and these patients are four times more likely to die than those who present with normal coagulation.[49,52,53,64]

Haemorrhage and resuscitation induce cellular changes that are characteristic of ischaemia and/or reperfusion injury (Fig. 42.4). This response is immune-inflammatory and compromises both intrinsic and adaptive immunity. When blood loss is severe a range of inflammatory mediators, cytokines and oxidants is almost immediately produced in large quantities and released. This dysregulation is the presumed cause of organ failure and death. The introduction of damage control resuscitation has been shown to improve haemostasis, achieve better haemorrhage control, limit haemodilution and hypothermia and improve outcomes of bleeding trauma patients. Patients who develop TIC have an increased likelihood of multi-organ failure (MOF), acute lung injury (ALI) infection, prolonged ventilation hours, ICU admission and increased early and late mortality. TIC can occur within minutes of an injury and is present in up to 25% of patients admitted to hospital. It is imperative that the paramedic and ED nurse mitigate progression of TIC as much as possible.

Hypothermia exacerbates TIC and is an indicator of severe injury. Hypothermia is associated with an increase in post-trauma

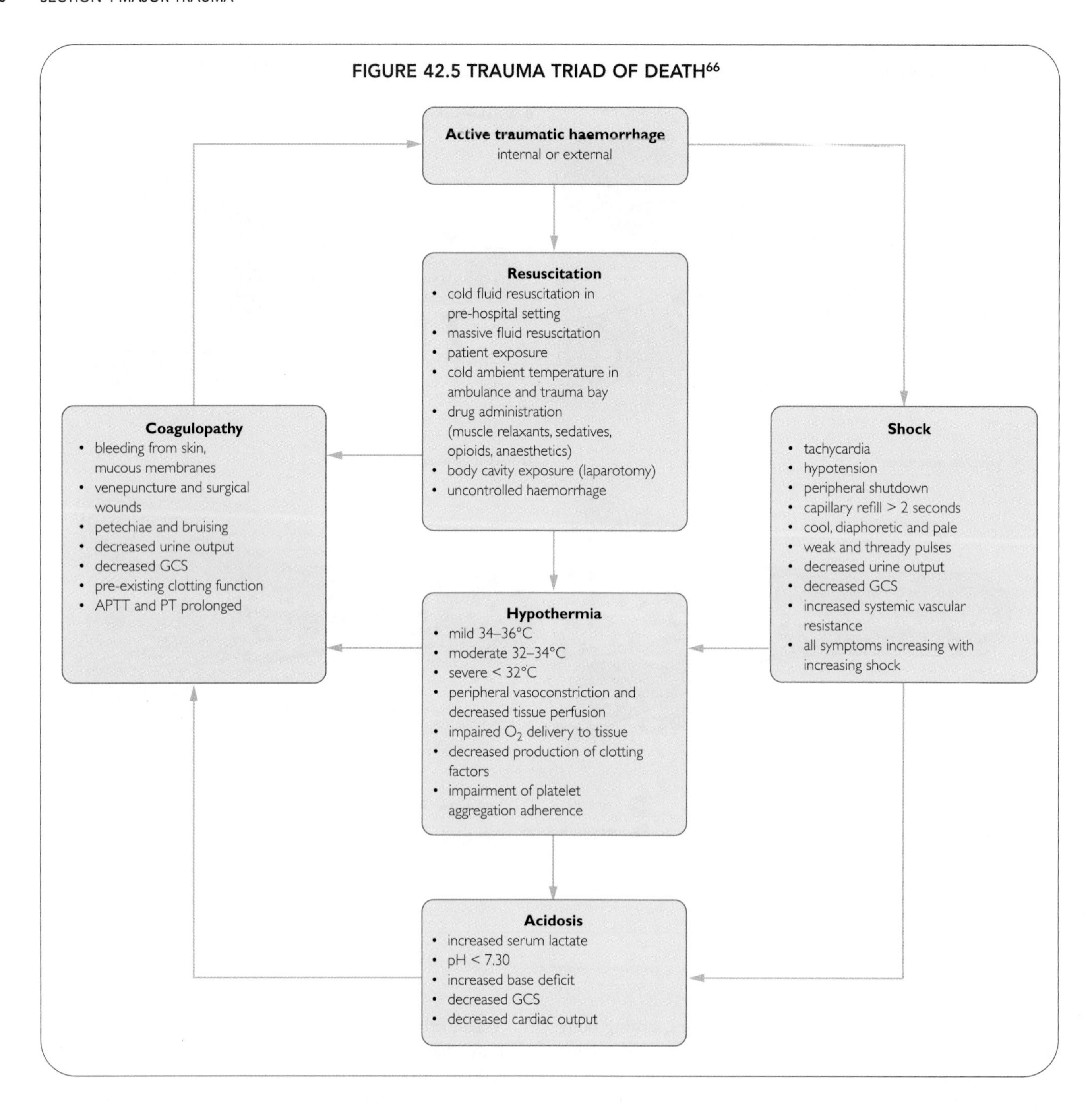

complications such as MOF, systemic inflammatory respiratory sepsis (SIRS) and sepsis. Most major trauma patients are hypothermic on arrival in the ED because of environmental conditions at the scene. Inadequate protection, intravenous fluid administration and ongoing blood loss worsens the hypothermic state. Haemorrhagic shock leads to decreased cellular perfusion and oxygenation, and inadequate heat production. Hypothermia has dramatic systemic effects on the body's functions, but most importantly in this context it exacerbates coagulopathy and interferes with blood homeostatic and platelet mechanisms. Hypothermia is defined as a temperature below 36.5°C, and can be classified as mild (34–36°C), moderate (32–34°C) and severe (< 32°C).[5,11,53]

Acidosis is caused by inadequate tissue perfusion, hypoxia and tissue injury and is another contributing factor that is worsened by the presence of hypothermia and coagulopathy. Acidosis has several negative effectors on haemostasis and includes platelet and coagulation dysfunction, especially in a pH < 7.2.[3] It can be an independent predictor of mortality and morbidity in major trauma; an increased base deficit increases transfusion requirements, causes multi-organ failure and increases major trauma patient mortality and morbidity. Fig. 42.5 illustrates some of the multifactorial conditions that contribute to the potentially lethal complication of hypothermia in a traumatic injury.

There is emerging evidence that *hypocalcaemia*, which is a key component of the coagulation cascade, plays an important role in coagulopathy and may change the trauma triad (hypothermia, hypotension and acidosis) to a diamond of death (hypothermia, hypotension, acidosis and hypocalcaemia).[1] The biggest impact of hypocalcaemia is on those pathways reliant

BOX 42.8 HYPOTHERMIA PREVENTION AND MANAGEMENT[5,7,16]

- Remove all wet, blood-soaked clothes, linen and covers
- Keep patient covered
- Apply blankets (external active rewarming temperature-regulated blankets)
- Warm all fluids and blood products before transfusion
- Increase room temperature
- Humidify inspired gases
- Control haemorrhage
- Reverse shock
- Be aware of causes of heat loss such as drugs, long operative events such as exploratory laparotomies, ongoing exposure.

upon calcium, such as platelet function, intrinsic and extrinsic haemostasis and cardiac contractility.[2] Calcium is lost in haemorrhagic shock and this loss is exacerbated by the blood products transfused, which contain citrate. In addition, shocked patients are unable to metabolise citrate due to the hypoperfusion and hypothermia affecting hepatic function. The presence of low calcium contributes to and exacerbates not only coagulation in the bleeding patient, but other outcomes, including increased inotrope use and ICU admissions, and sepsis and mortality.[1,2]

Once the patient enters the ED, all modalities of care should be implemented while trying to maintain or increase the patient's temperature (see Box 42.8).

During the primary survey, the five most important rules to remember are:[3,5,7,44]

1. Repeatedly reassess, particularly if clinical signs change.
2. Immediately address life-threatening conditions without delay.
3. Penetrating wounds and implements must be left for formal surgical exploration.
4. External bleeding should be stopped by using direct pressure.
5. Keep the patient warm.

PRIMARY SURVEY INTERVENTIONS

Primary survey interventions are implemented as they are identified in the clinical setting; they are outlined in this text according to priority.

Airway

Simple manoeuvres in the pre-hospital environment and ED can improve the patency of the patient's airway; interventions begin simply, then move to the more complex (see also Table 42.2). An experienced paramedic, ED or critical-care-trained nurse can implement many of the following simple manoeuvres.

1. Chin lift or jaw thrust.
   - Chin lift is performed by placing two fingers under the mandible and gently lifting it upwards, moving the chin anteriorly; caution should be exercised in patients with known or suspected spinal injuries.
   - Jaw thrust is useful to assist with maintaining a seal on a bag–valve–mask device if the patient requires ventilation assistance and for those with a potential spinal injury. The angles of the lower jaw are grasped with one hand each side and the jaw is displaced forwards.
2. Clear the airway.
   - This can be accomplished with a suction device or a manual scoop. If patients are required to be turned on their side to clear the airway, this should be done with a log-roll (see Chapter 47).
3. Insert nasopharyngeal or oropharyngeal airway.
   - The nasopharyngeal airway is passed into the posterior oropharynx by gently sliding it into one nostril. This airway may be better tolerated in the conscious patient, as it is less likely to induce gagging and vomiting.
   - Nasopharyngeal insertion is contraindicated in any significant maxillofacial injury or suspected basal skull fracture. In these cases an oropharyngeal airway should be used. The oropharyngeal airway is inserted into the mouth behind the tongue, and in adults it is best inserted upside down and turned 180° once it touches the soft palate. Caution needs to be exercised in the conscious patient (GCS ≥ 9) as oropharyngeal airways may cause gagging, vomiting and aspiration.[3,5,44]

PRACTICE TIP

Gagging in the neurological patient (trauma or otherwise) has a negative impact on intracranial pressure. Laryngoscopy and oropharyngeal airway insertion should be avoided, and the nasopharyngeal airway used only if no contraindications exist and hypoxia is present.

4. Definitive airway.
   - An endotracheal or nasotracheal (uncommon) airway is inserted if the above methods have failed to adequately maintain a patent airway. Other indications for a definitive airway in the trauma patient include patients with a GCS < 9, apnoeic patients, patients unable to protect their own airways from secretions or foreign matter or those with airway burns. The paramedic and ED nurse should anticipate the need for a cricothyroidotomy (Fig. 42.6). Indications include failure to intubate, airway swelling/burns and severe facial or neck trauma. Ensure that all equipment, including video and direct laryngoscopes, endotracheal tube cuff and pulse oximetry, has been thoroughly checked and is in working order prior to intubating the patient. A failure to secure an airway as a result of equipment failure can have a catastrophic conclusion.
5. Maintain cervical spine immobilisation.
   - Trauma patients should be treated as having a spinal injury until proven otherwise. Cervical spine immobilisation is achieved by keeping the spine in neutral alignment.[5,67] See Chapter 16 for cervical spine immobilisation techniques. Log-rolling a spinal immobilised patient requires the assistance of at least three people. In regional and rural areas, the paramedic and other support staff can assist with log-rolling should there not be enough nursing and medical staff available.
   - Airway management techniques can cause cervical spine movement. In particular, the chin lift/jaw thrust can

FIGURE 42.6 A. CRICOTHYROIDOTOMY TECHNIQUE[67] B. COMPLETED CRICOTHYROIDOTOMY

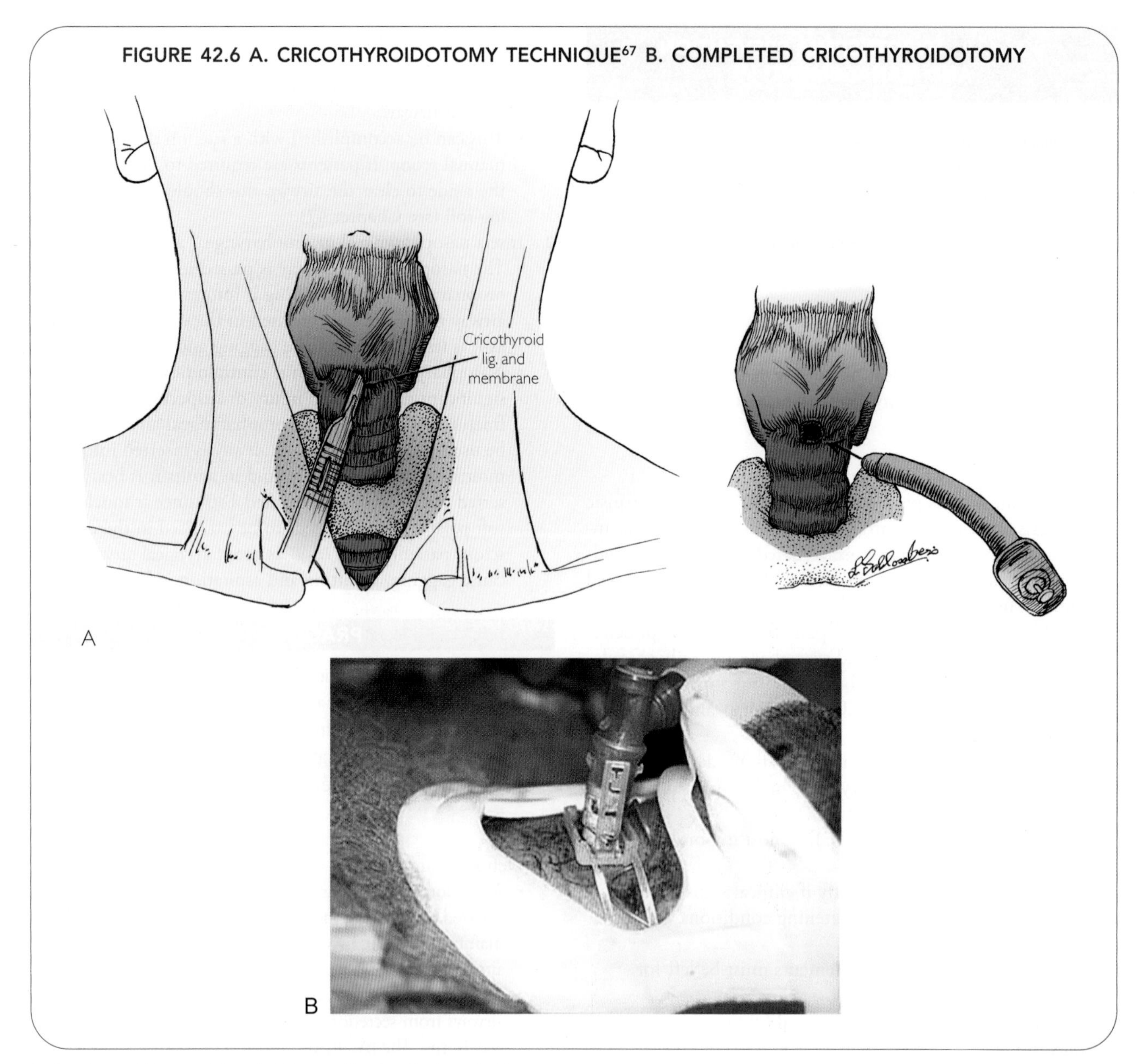

B. Courtesy of Liverpool Hospital Trauma Service, Sydney, NSW.

increase disc space by > 5 mm despite the presence of a collar. Likewise, oral endotracheal intubation produces a 3–4 mm increase in disc space. By contrast, oral/nasal airway insertion can be responsible for 2 mm posterior subluxation. Video laryngoscopes and bronchoscopes can reduce this even further. The spinal board should be removed on admission or at the first log-roll, to prevent pressure-related complications from prolonged spinal board use.[42]

- To maintain cervical spine alignment in children, a folded towel is placed under a child's shoulders as this prevents their relatively large head forcing their neck into flexion (Fig. 42.7).[68]

Breathing and ventilation

In the trauma patient, breathing and ventilation can be compromised for a variety of reasons, such as decreased GCS (caused by hypotension head injuries or drugs), mechanical failure (spinal injury), ventilation failure (generally caused by multiple rib fractures, flail segment, pulmonary contusion, tension pneumothorax or large haemothorax) or airway obstruction. A more detailed thoracic assessment is described in Chapter 45. However, the key interventions in breathing and ventilation are described below and are also listed in Table 42.3.

1. Oxygen administration.
   - All treatment should be aimed at correcting hypoxia—oxygen administration is the simplest intervention and should be titrated to the patient's needs.
   - Spontaneously breathing major trauma patients should have high-flow (15 L/min) oxygen delivered by a non-rebreather mask. If the patient requires some assistance or ventilation, then a bag–valve–mask device with a

FIGURE 42.7 YOUNG CHILD IMMOBILISED ON A STANDARD BACKBOARD.

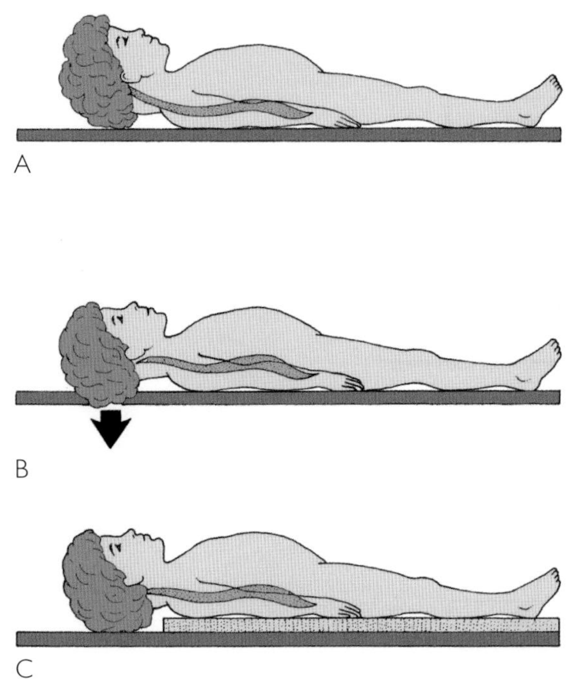

A

B

C

A. Note how the large head forces the neck into flexion. Backboards can be modified by an occiput cutout **B**, or a double mattress pad **C**, to raise the chest.[69]

reservoir can be used. If inadequate respiratory effort continues, the patient will likely require intubation.

- An oxygen saturation of > 95% is optimum (see Chapter 10). Oxygen saturation monitoring can be conducted by the ED nurse as an adjunct to the look, listen and feel techniques, using a SpO_2 device which estimates the peripheral arterial oxygen saturation. Be aware of SpO_2 inaccuracies in the presence of carboxyhaemoglobin, hypothermia, anaemia and hypovolaemia (mean arterial pressure [MAP] < 50 mmHg).
- Patients require continuous assessment to monitor for improvements and deterioration in their condition.

2. Chest decompression.
   - Chest decompression via needle or finger thoracostomy is indicated in patients with profound respiratory distress, unilateral breath sounds, subcutaneous emphysema, absence of lung sliding on ultrasound and any time that a tension pneumothorax is suspected. This should be conducted immediately without waiting for radiological confirmation (see Chapter 45 for technique).
   - The signs and symptoms of a tension pneumothorax include respiratory distress, neck vein distension, tachycardia, hypotension, trachea deviation and decreased breath sounds to the affected side. Assessment is more difficult in the intubated patient as some of these signs are altered due to the intubation, and the risk of tension pneumothorax is increased in those receiving positive-pressure ventilation.

PRACTICE TIP

Tension pneumothorax and pericardial tamponade signs and symptoms are very similar; therefore, care must be taken in patient assessment to differentiate between the two.

- *Tamponade*—distended neck veins, hypotension, muffled heart sounds, pulsus paradoxus, narrowing pulse pressure.
- *Tension pneumothorax*—respiratory distress, neck vein distension, tachycardia, hypotension, tracheal deviation, absent breath sounds on the affected side.

Needle or finger decompression converts a tension pneumothorax into a simple pneumothorax; the catheter should be left in place until an intercostal chest tube is in place.

3. Intubation.
   - Nasal/oral intubation or a surgical airway provides the ultimate definitive airway. The ED nurse or paramedic at the scene plays an important role in intubation, and must monitor the patient carefully throughout the procedure.
   - Rapid-sequence intubation (RSI) is a widely used and recommended airway technique (see Chapter 16: Clinical skills). The patient's breathing must then be maintained with manual bagging or, preferably, by attaching the patient to a ventilator. Ventilator observations which regularly assess air entry, ETT secretions, SaO_2 and ventilator settings should then be commenced, and ventilator settings adjusted accordingly.
   - If intubation fails, the paramedic and/or ED nurse should be ready to assist/manage the airway by anticipating the equipment needed and the procedure to be followed, given in the failed intubation algorithm shown in Fig. 42.8 (Chapters 13 and 16).
4. Sucking chest wounds.
   - Seal sucking chest wounds (open pneumothorax) with a three-sided occlusive dressing, followed by chest tube insertion. This creates a one-way valve; the dressing is sucked to the chest on inspiration, and then allows the air to escape on expiration.
   - If the dressing was to completely seal off and the air became trapped, a tension pneumothorax or further barotrauma is possible. If this occurs, the dressing should be removed and replaced after stabilisation.
5. Intercostal catheter insertion and management.
   - Indications for intercostal catheters (ICCs) in the trauma setting include both pneumothorax and haemothorax. If haemothorax is visualised on chest x-ray it should be treated with ICC. In addition, an ICC should be placed in all patients following needle decompression and should be considered in those even with small pneumothoraces requiring positive-pressure ventilation or transport in an air ambulance (helicopter or fixed-wing aircraft), as pressure changes can lead to tension pneumothorax. The ICC in a haemothorax evacuates blood and reduces the risk of clotted haemothorax; in pneumothorax the ICC facilitates removal of air and

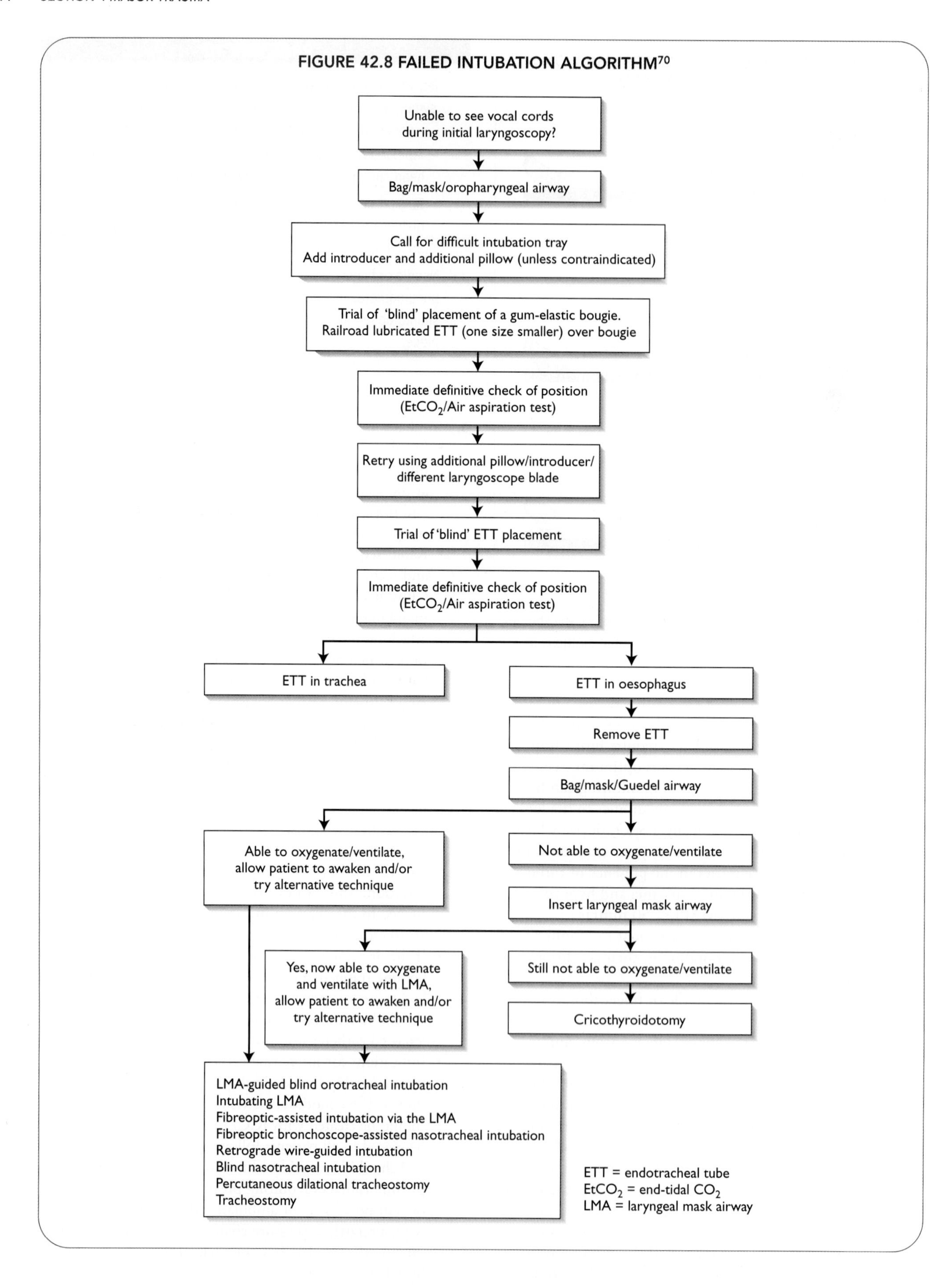
FIGURE 42.8 FAILED INTUBATION ALGORITHM[70]
Unable to see vocal cords during initial laryngoscopy?
Bag/mask/oropharyngeal airway
Call for difficult intubation tray
Add introducer and additional pillow (unless contraindicated)
Trial of 'blind' placement of a gum-elastic bougie.
Railroad lubricated ETT (one size smaller) over bougie
Immediate definitive check of position ($EtCO_2$/Air aspiration test)
Retry using additional pillow/introducer/ different laryngoscope blade
Trial of 'blind' ETT placement
Immediate definitive check of position ($EtCO_2$/Air aspiration test)
ETT in trachea
ETT in oesophagus
Remove ETT
Bag/mask/Guedel airway
Able to oxygenate/ventilate, allow patient to awaken and/or try alternative technique
Not able to oxygenate/ventilate
Insert laryngeal mask airway
Yes, now able to oxygenate and ventilate with LMA, allow patient to awaken and/or try alternative technique
Still not able to oxygenate/ventilate
Cricothyroidotomy
LMA-guided blind orotracheal intubation
Intubating LMA
Fibreoptic-assisted intubation via the LMA
Fibreoptic bronchoscope-assisted nasotracheal intubation
Retrograde wire-guided intubation
Blind nasotracheal intubation
Percutaneous dilational tracheostomy
Tracheostomy
ETT = endotracheal tube
$EtCO_2$ = end-tidal CO_2
LMA = laryngeal mask airway

fluid, allows expansion of the lung and prevents tension pneumothorax.

- The standard ICC should be a large 32-French gauge placed into the intercostal space above the 5th rib in the mid-axillary line. The nurse's role is not only to assist with set-up and insertion where necessary, but also to carefully monitor the ICC and underwater-seal drainage (UWSD) unit (see Chapter 16 for techniques on attaching a UWSD unit). An ICC is normally inserted in emergency conditions; however, an aseptic technique needs to be adhered to to reduce infection risks. The ICC should be sutured close to the skin and dressed with a secure, occlusive dressing to prevent any air leaving from the insertion site and any back-and-forth movement of the tube into the chest, which can increase the risk of infection.
- Drainage of 200 mL/h for 2 to 4 hours is an indication for exploratory thoracotomy. The patency of the tube is also important to monitor, as a tension pneumothorax can develop if the tube becomes blocked or kinked, removed or disconnected.[5,6] Patients with large blood loss may require early blood product transfusion.[5,52]

Circulation and haemorrhage control

The primary survey thus far has already provided clues to the sufficiency of the circulation, such as respiratory rate, skin pallor, level of consciousness and severe external bleeding. Progressive haemorrhage control is the next primary goal, followed by fluid resuscitation.

1. Haemorrhage control.
   - All signs of external haemorrhage must be identified and direct pressure applied to stop the bleeding. Fractures to the long bones and pelvis can result in large-volume blood loss and should be splinted in the pre-hospital environment. Most ambulances carry a range of splints suitable for the pelvis and the long bones; these should be applied at the scene without causing time delays, or on arrival at the ED.[71] There is also now a wide range of commercially available haemostatic agents that can be used as adjuncts. They are applied topically and include collagen, gelatine or cellulose products, fibrin and synthetic glues.[5,52]
   - Patients who are haemodynamically unstable with a pelvic fracture have a high mortality rate; thus, haemorrhage control should include early non-invasive pelvic stabilisation.[72–74] This can be achieved with a specially designed pelvic sling or with a sheet wrapped as tightly as possible at the level of the patient's greater trochanters and symphysis pubis. The sling should be tightened to 180 Newtons, which is equivalent to lifting an 18 kilo weight.[75] If a splint has not been applied prior to admission this can be done on arrival, either on transfer from the ambulance trolley or at the time of log-rolling (see Chapters 16 and 48 for an explanation of different splinting techniques). When applying splints, consider adequate analgesia. Splints and slings fitted in the pre-hospital stage should not be removed, even during the initial assessment, until the patient has been stabilised (Fig. 42.9).
   - Tourniquets can also be applied as an adjunct for life-threatening bleeding from open extremity injuries in the pre-hospital or hospital setting; complications of crush injury can occur if prolonged use is required > 2 hours.[58] Clinicians applying them must note time of application on the tourniquet.
   - eFAST should be conducted as part of the primary survey if the patient is shocked, as a means of identifying the source of blood loss. These tests are not organ-specific, but can identify free fluid in the peritoneum. The nurse needs to be aware that a positive result will mean that the patient will need to go to theatre, as ultimately haemorrhage control must be attended to in the operating suite. Therefore, the nurse should anticipate and prepare the patient for rapid transport to the operating or angiography suite.
2. IV access.
   - Insert two large-bore IV (16-gauge or larger) to allow for rapid fluid transfusion if required. The preferred site

FIGURE 42.9 PELVIC SLINGS

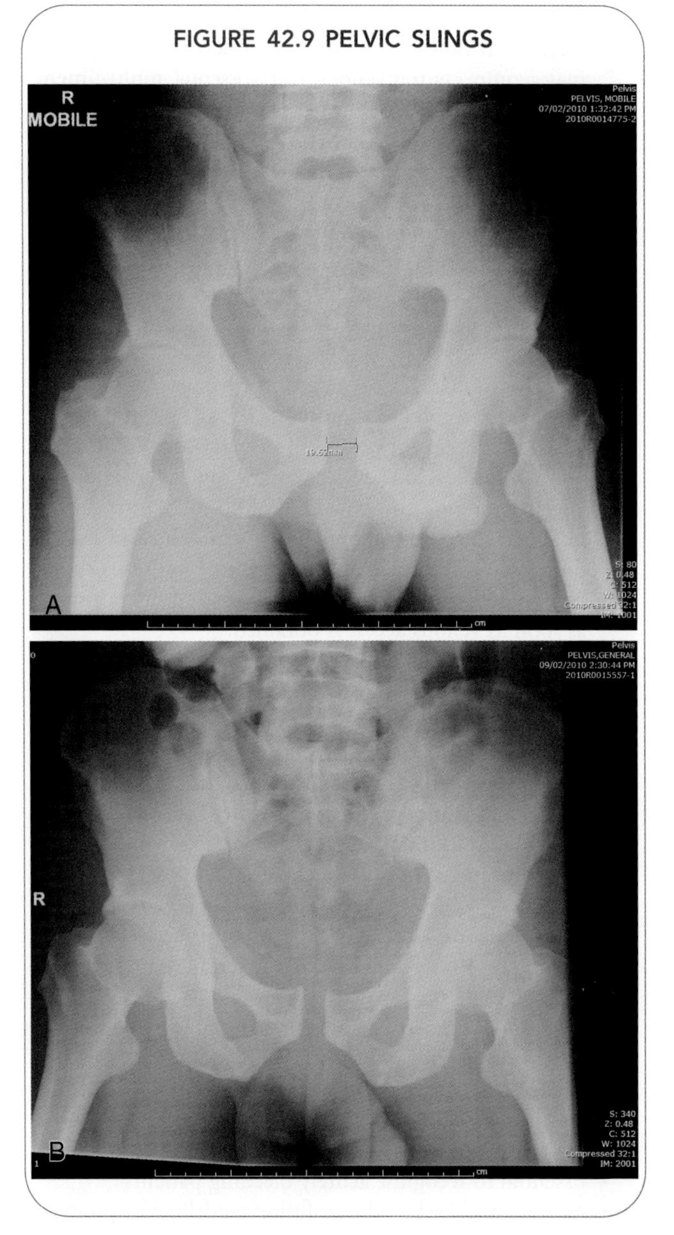

A. Separated sacroiliac joint prior to sling application: pubic symphysis diastases with widening up to 1.9 cm. **B.** SI joint reduction post application of sling, to 15 mm.

for these lines in the adult is the antecubital vein of the forearm. If cannula insertion is unsuccessful, the patient may require central venous, intra-osseous, multi-limen access catheter (MAC) or peripheral cutdown procedures to gain access.
- IV cannula placement in the field is often compromised by poor light, poor patient positioning, restlessness, pain or hypotension and inadequate skin cleaning prior to insertion. If IV access gained by paramedics is poorly sited or of a less desirable gauge, additional or alternative access should be sited at an appropriate time.
- Intraosseous (I/O) needles are an effective alternative for IV access and are appropriate for all ages when venous access is not possible or after two failed attempts. Intraosseous devices can be quickly inserted within 1 minute and flow rates of up to 125 mL/min obtained. Insertion sites include the proximal tibia, distal tibia and proximal humerus. I/O infusions should be limited to emergency resuscitation and discontinued as soon as venous access is obtained.[5]
- I/O infusions can be painful when fluid is infused—if this is the case, then lidocaine can be administered to assist with pain control. I/O must be closely monitored for other complications such as extravasation of fluids and medication, which could occur if not monitored closely and could lead to compartment syndrome. Other complications are fractures caused by insertion (with improper insertion technique) and osteomyelitis when I/O used for longer than indicated and/or is associated with either multiple attempts or aseptic technique. I/O is safe with ≤ 1% serious complication rate (Fig. 42.10).
- Ultrasound guided IV access is achievable by paramedics and nurses, and if trained staff and equipment are present, this method can be instituted rapidly and effectively.[76,77]

3. Fluid resuscitation.
   - Essential to recognise acutely bleeding patients
   - Activate massive blood transfusion guidelines or protocols early
   - Transfuse blood products in a 1:1:1 ratio, packed red blood cells (PRBC): fresh frozen plasma (FFP): platelets (Plts)
   - ROTEM or TEG are vivoelastic testing devices that assess the formation, strength and dissolution of a blood clot. These devices allow rapid identification of hypofibrinogenemia and trauma-induced coagulopathy, resulting in earlier targeted blood produce use.[7,78]

PRACTICE TIP

Lead with cryoprecipitate, platelets and fresh frozen plasma before the red blood cells in a bleeding patient or if able transfuse together. Consider early calcium replacement.

FIGURE 42.10 INTRA-OSSEOUS ACCESS[79,80]

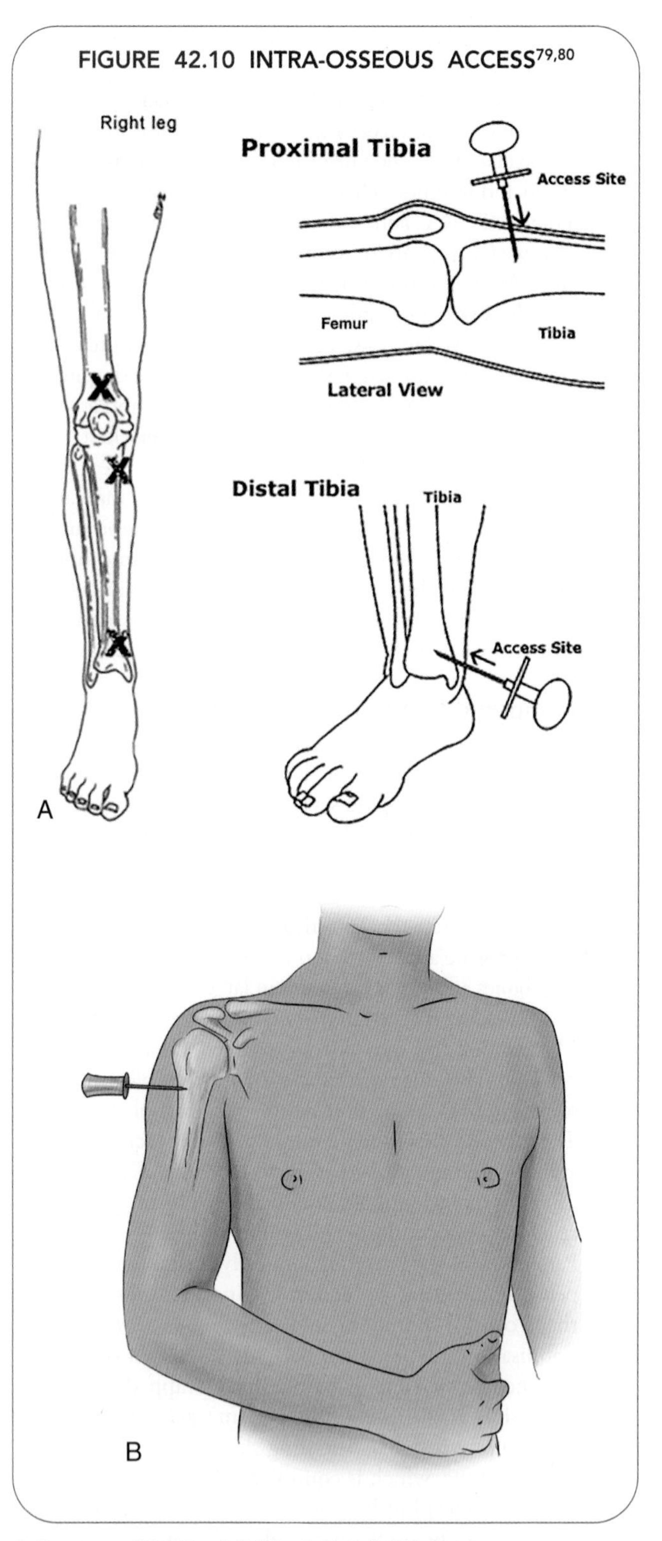

A. Courtesy of The Royal Children's Hospital Melbourne.

Damage control resuscitation

Damage control resuscitation (DCR) has resulted in a change in resuscitation practice over the last 10 years. This is a multi-pronged approach to resuscitation that aims to prevent and manage acidosis, hypothermia and TIC. The DCR strategies include active warming and heat-loss prevention, aggressive early blood product administration, aimed at preventing and reversing coagulopathy, restoring blood volume and hence oxygen delivery to the tissues. DCR typically is a temporising procedure and the patient will more than likely require lifesaving surgical or radiological intervention for ongoing management of these bleeding sources.[52]

- Permissive hypotension and minimum volume resuscitation is a concept of tolerating a lower blood pressure, which may prevent any clot that has formed at bleeding sites from being dislodged. Research on animals and in humans has shown that a systolic blood pressure of > 80 mmHg is enough to dislodge clots. This has contributed to the trend towards limiting fluid resuscitation until haemorrhage is controlled.[52,64] In the patient with a penetrating injury, limiting fluid resuscitation improves outcome due to platelet aggregation inhibition and dilution of clotting factors. An increase in blood pressure can cause a clot to be disrupted, reverse vasoconstriction and increase blood loss.[5,11]
- In the presence of uncontrolled haemorrhage in a patient with a known or suspected traumatic brain injury, one of the important goals is prevention of secondary brain injury from hypotension. Therefore, a systolic blood pressure (SBP) of at least 90 mmHg should be maintained, using fluid resuscitation and/or inotropic support,[7] while the optimal blood pressure in those without a traumatic brain injury with uncontrolled haemorrhage is an SBP of 80–90 mmHg.
- Treatment in the pre-hospital environment may differ from these guidelines; for example, Ambulance Victoria guidelines recommend fluid administration in blunt and penetrating cases in much smaller doses and to an SBP ≥ 70 mmHg (or 100 mmHg if a head injury is present), whereas in NSW fluid is administered to achieve a radial pulse.
- It is essential that paramedics and ED nurses monitor and titrate the amount and type of fluid being administered against the patient's response, and keep the treating medical staff constantly updated. In the pre-hospital and ED environment, keeping track of fluid resuscitation volumes can be challenging in stressful situations; keeping the empty fluid and blood bags aside can assist in keeping track of volumes administered. Fluid given in the pre-hospital environment should also be taken into consideration when blood products are administered.

PRACTICE TIP

PERMISSIVE HYPOTENSION AND MINIMUM VOLUME RESUSCITATION

- Transfuse to systolic blood pressure of 80–90 mmHg (be wary of head injury).
- Use small fluid boluses of 200 mL crystalloid initially.
- Early blood product administration, 1:1:1:1 packed red blood cells, fresh frozen plasma, platelets and cryoprecipitate, with a priority on fibrinogen replacement.
- Fluid and patient warming.

4. Blood administration.
   - Blood transfusion is fundamental to the care of the trauma patient. The main purpose of transfusing red blood cells is to restore the oxygen-carrying capacity of the intravascular volume. The circulating blood is often depleted of essential clotting products and the coagulation functions may also be affected. Essential blood products, such as platelets, fresh frozen plasma and cryoprecipitate, may need to be given, along with the red blood cells.
   - Early administration of clotting products and blood is intended to reduce coagulopathy and thrombocytopenia.[54,64] The estimated volume needed for transfusion is based on the percentage loss of circulating blood volume and the patient's ability to compensate. Estimated blood volume for an adult is 70 mL/kg.
   - Massive blood transfusion is defined as replacement of 50% of the patient's blood volume within 4 hours or more than 4 units administered within the first 4 hours of injury.[54,64]
   - When hypocalcaemic shocked patients arrive, calcium levels should be monitored throughout the trauma patient's resuscitation and maintained in a normal range [1.1–1.3 mmol/L] to assist in preventing worsening TIC and morbidity and mortality.[2,78] Complications of massive transfusion include thrombocytopaenia, coagulation factor depletion, hypocalcaemia, hyperkalaemia, acid–base disturbance, hypothermia, adult respiratory distress syndrome (ARDS) and multi-organ failure. The patient's clinical condition must be closely monitored, with early involvement of the blood bank for transfusion support.[3,52,64] A massive transfusion protocol should exist in each centre receiving trauma patients.
   - Since 2010, massive transfusion protocols/guidelines have begun to include tranexamic acid. In 2010, results were published of a study entitled CRASH-2, a large, multinational, randomised placebo-controlled trial which trialled the use of the antifibrinolytic tranexamic acid in trauma patients with or at risk of significant haemorrhage.[81] The study found that the administration of intravenous tranexamic acid in adult trauma patients with significant haemorrhage, within 8 hours of injury, can be used safely as an adjunctive therapy and may decrease bleeding and mortality. Further, tranexamic acid costs dramatically less than rFVIIa (less than one-tenth).
   - Currently, clinical trials are being conducted that look at the use of fibrinogen; low fibrinogen levels are associated with high transfusion requirements, so the studies are investigating if fibrinogen replacement can improve survival and reduce transfusion requirements and the associated morbidity; these studies are looking at both the use of factor concentrates cryoprecipitate or FFP.[56,82,83]
   - Many ambulance services have access to blood products. In the out-of-hospital environment, where transport times are short for hypotensive major trauma patients, there appears to be little benefit to blood product administration. However, for longer transport times and/or trapped patients, there may be some benefit.[83–85]

Emergency department thoracotomy

Rapid response times and improved EMS treatment at the scene and the increasing use of the TCA guidelines have seen improved survival rates for patients in TCA and extremis. Survival rates for those who require an emergency department thoracotomy (EDT) in penetrating trauma are 9–12% and up

TABLE 42.5 INDICATIONS FOR EMERGENCY DEPARTMENT THORACOTOMY (EDT)[3,87]

Penetrating trauma presenting to ED	
Extremis with signs of life—pupillary response to light, respiratory effort, response to pain, cardiac activity on ECG	Non-intubated patients: CPR < 5 minutes before admission Intubated patients: CPR < 10 minutes before admission
Witnessed cardiac arrest	
Persistent post-injury hypotension (systolic blood pressure < 60 mmHg) unresponsive to fluid resuscitation	
Refractory moderate post-injury hypotension (systolic blood pressure < 80 mmHg)	
Blunt trauma	
Witnessed cardiac arrest with vital signs present	

CPR: cardiopulmonary resuscitation; ECG: electrocardiogram.

to 38% where there are signs of life; as for blunt trauma, the rate is 1–2%, regardless of signs of life.[87–89]

The aim of an EDT is to evacuate haematomas, repair injuries and control haemorrhage, and in doing so prevent or treat air embolism.

The indications for EDT are listed in Table 42.5. Due to the very high mortality rates for EDT, it is usually undertaken in patients in extremis. ED nurses need to be familiar with the emergency thoracotomy instruments. It is also prudent to anticipate EDT in those patients receiving cardiopulmonary resuscitation or in TCA, as these patients usually require large volumes of fluid and urgent transfer to the operating theatre once haemorrhage control has been attained. Early notification to blood bank, haematology and theatre is essential.

The patient's pre-morbid state, age and comorbidities and the logistics of the procedure (available operating theatre, cardiothoracic surgeon, scrub staff) must be taken into consideration before going ahead with EDT.

ADJUNCTS TO THE PRIMARY SURVEY

All life-threatening injuries identified in the primary survey must be treated before progressing to the secondary survey. In the clinical setting with a full TT present, many of the following adjuncts can be completed in sequence with assessment and resuscitation. In a less-well-resourced setting, they should occur after life-threatening injuries have been addressed.

Monitoring

Monitoring should be applied in the pre-hospital environment and maintained until the patient's condition is considered stable. This includes continuous monitoring of the patient's vital signs, GCS and neurovascular status, which enables the paramedic at the scene and en route, and the TT, to identify the patient's injuries and titrate the patient's response to resuscitation. Cardiac and ventilatory monitoring leads, pulse oximetry, core body temperature monitoring and $EtCO_2$ should be commenced as soon as practical in the primary survey.[5]

Once the patient has arrived at the treating hospital and patency of the airway is established, venous (VBG) or arterial blood gases (ABG) should be taken to enable assessment of ventilation and to monitor the patient's transfusion state. Changes in pH and the base deficit can prompt not only ventilation changes but also transfusion requirements. Close monitoring of the $EtCO_2$ will assist in assessing the efficacy of ventilator settings and in confirming placement of the ETT at the time of intubation. Any deterioration should be immediately communicated with medical staff.

Urinary catheters and gastric tubes

An indwelling urinary catheter (IDC) is a vital adjunct, as urine output is a sensitive sign of the volume status in the patient and can give an indication of the patient's renal perfusion. Urethral injury is a contraindication for IDC insertion, and should be suspected in the presence of blood at the urethral meatus, perineal bruising, swelling, a high-riding prostate and in patients with a straddle or malaligned pelvic fracture. In females, additional signs, such as lower abdominal tenderness and macroscopic haematuria, are also contraindications. See Chapter 48 for urinary catheter insertion guidelines in pelvic trauma.

Gastric tubes are indicated to assist in stomach decompression, decreasing the risk of aspiration, especially in the patient who cannot protect their own airway, and to prevent obstruction of diaphragmatic motion in the paediatric patient. Patients with extensive faciomaxillary and/or suspected basal skull fractures should have their gastric tube placed orally. Orogastric tubes are not routinely placed in the pre-hospital setting, although orogastric tubes, particularly in children, may be placed in unconscious patients.

Laboratory tests

It is essential that, as an adjunct to the primary survey, baseline bloods are taken; this can be done at the time of peripheral or central line insertion. Blood tests should include group and hold, coagulation studies, full blood count and biochemistry. All female patients of childbearing age will require a beta-hCG (pregnancy) test; this can be done on a urine dipstick and confirmed with blood test. It is essential that the blood samples are correctly labelled and signed, as significant delays in obtaining cross-matched blood can occur with simple labelling errors. Table 42.6 lists the most common tests and their clinical implications. Massive transfusion protocols are moving towards goal-directed transfusion therapy, using viscoelastic haemostatic assays, such as ROTEM and TEG. These tools measure clot formation and breakdown in whole blood, enabling rapid and timely identification of coagulopathy and product replacement needs.

Primary survey x-rays

The 'trauma series' x-rays include lateral cervical spine, chest and pelvis. Diagnostic studies should not delay or interfere in any way with ongoing patient resuscitation. The chest and pelvic x-ray can quickly identify large sources of blood loss and help to guide resuscitation and early blood transfusion. The lateral cervical spine x-ray can identify a significant cervical spine fracture; however, if it is negative, this does not rule out cervical spine injury and spinal stabilisation must be maintained until formal assessment of the entire spine is conducted.

TABLE 42.6 COMMON LABORATORY TESTS[72,73]

LABORATORY TEST	CLINICAL IMPLICATIONS
Full blood count (FBC)	Haematocrit and haemoglobin may be normal or above normal despite acute haemorrhage; normal values do not exclude haemorrhagic shock
Electrolytes	Baseline data Creatinine to assess renal function Rule out electrolyte imbalance
Coagulation profile	Baseline data Rule out coagulopathies Include activated partial thromboplastin time (APTT) and international normalised ratio (INR) Fibrinogen
Amylase/ lipase levels	Baseline data Elevated value may indicate possible intraabdominal injury
Lipase	Baseline data Elevated value may indicate possible intraabdominal injury; has higher sensitivity for pancreatic injury
Lactate	Baseline data Elevated level correlates with acute haemorrhage, shock and increased anaerobic metabolism ROTEM/ TEG
Venous blood gas (VBG)	Assess ventilatory and respiratory status Acidosis, especially in the presence of normal or decreased $PaCO_2$ level, correlates with shock Base deficit of −6 or greater correlates with acute haemorrhage and shock Elevated $PaCO_2$ combined with low oxygen saturation (via pulse oximetry) may indicate an airway or breathing emergency This may correlate with $EtCO_2$, but if there is concurrent respiratory illness (e.g. COPD), the difference between $PaCO_2$ and $EtCO_2$ may be clinically significant
Liver function tests (LFTs)	Baseline data Elevated values may indicate liver damage
Type and cross-match	Prepare for administration of blood and blood products
Pregnancy	BHCG in female of childbearing age and to confirm gestation on patients with positive urine pregnancy test
Urinalysis	Dip for blood; gross haematuria suggests injury BHCG in females of childbearing age to rule out/ confirm pregnancy

$PaCO_2$: partial pressure of carbon dioxide in arterial gas; PaO_2: alveolar-arterial difference in partial pressure of oxygen; SaO_2: arterial oxygen saturation.

Depending on the size of the trauma centre primary screening of the cervical spine maybe with multidetector CT scanning in place of a lateral cervical spine x-ray.[5] See Chapter 47 for spinal clearance guidelines.

Do not avoid diagnostic tests in the pregnant patient. Radiation risk in pregnancy is related to the fetal radiation dose and the stage of pregnancy, being most significant during organogenesis (up to 9 weeks' gestation). Most diagnostic radiology procedures pose no substantial risk to the mother or fetus when compared with other risks throughout the pregnancy.[90] The pregnant woman presents two patients for care, but the principle of care is to provide trauma care to the mother. Optimal resuscitation of the mother will allow the optimal chance of fetal survival. Table 42.7 outlines the common radiology studies and their clinical implications.

UNIQUE PATIENT GROUPS

The paediatric, older adult, obstetric and bariatric patient should have the primary survey conducted systematically as for other patients; however, there exist special criteria in each group which need to be considered. Each of these groups also has increased psychosocial needs. Table 42.8 illustrates the differences in priorities for paediatric, pregnant, older adult and bariatric (obese) patients.

For paediatric patients, the quantities of blood, fluids and medications vary with the size of the child, as does the degree and rapidity of heat loss. Injury mechanisms and patterns are also different.[5] These are discussed in Chapter 35.

Older adult patients are over-represented in major trauma morbidity and mortality, and the frequency of cases is increasing.[91,92] The older adult patient will sustain more significant injury than will a younger patient from the same amount of force. The ED nurse should have a higher index of suspicion, as the older adult trauma patient has a significantly increased mortality and morbidity rate. For the older adult patient, special consideration needs to be given based on the physiological body changes of the older person, mechanisms of injury, pre-existing medical conditions and response to injury (see also Chapter 38).[93,94]

Pregnant trauma patient presentations are not frequent, but pregnancy must be considered in any female patient aged 10–50 years. The best treatment for the fetus is the provision of optimal treatment of the mother. It must be considered that the anatomical and physiological changes in pregnancy may modify the patient's response to the injury.[95] Early recognition of pregnancy by palpation of the abdomen for a gravid uterus, laboratory testing (beta-hCG), patient history of menstrual cycle and early fetal assessments and monitoring with early liaison with an obstetrician are important for maternal and fetal survival.

The pregnant or gravid uterus also poses the risk of compression of the inferior vena cava when the woman is lying supine. The inferior vena cava is compressed in the majority of pregnant women in the second trimester, and the compression may affect the uterine artery blood flow. To overcome this, manual manipulation of the uterus is required in emergency situations when clinicians are unable to place the pregnant female in the lateral position because of injury or treatment such as cardiopulmonary resuscitation. Manual manipulation is achieved by placing one hand on either side of the pregnant abdomen and lifting the uterus and fetus off the vena cava and

TABLE 42.7 PRIMARY SURVEY X-RAYS[3,12,25]

EXAMINATION	INDICATION	CLINICAL IMPLICATIONS
Chest x-ray	Blunt trauma Chest trauma or pain Shortness of breath Abnormal breath sounds	Should be taken immediately upon arrival if possible Anteroposterior examination with patient in supine position if immobilised Do not delay treatment of a suspected tension pneumothorax for a chest x-ray
Pelvic x-ray	Blunt trauma Pelvic pain or instability Blood at urethral meatus	Anteroposterior examination with patient in supine position Should be taken early in the resuscitation
Cervical spine x-ray	Blunt trauma Trauma above nipple line Neck tenderness Neurological deficit	Cross-table lateral film usually obtained early in resuscitation, with three views required to complete the series which include C1 to T1 Stabilisation should be maintained until spine is radiographically and clinically cleared

TABLE 42.8 PAEDIATRIC, OLDER ADULT, PREGNANT AND BARIATRIC PATIENT GROUP CONSIDERATIONS[3,58,93–96]

PAEDIATRIC (CH 35)	OLDER ADULT > 65 (CH 38)	PREGNANT (CH 34)	BARIATRIC
Special considerations			
Include the carer in emergency management Infants may rapidly deteriorate	Physiological effects of ageing Include the carer in in emergency management Ensure early cognitive assessment Will sustain a more significant injury than those younger with the same amount of force Higher index of suspicion Impact of pre-existing medical conditions	Consider pregnancy in all females 10–50 years of age Best treatment for the fetus is optimal care of the mother 12 weeks: uterus intrapelvic organ Uterus is thick-walled, of limited size and sits in bony pelvis 20 weeks: uterus at umbilicus Enlarged fetus is protected by amniotic fluid 34–36 weeks: uterus at costal margins If vertex presentation, fetal head is in the pelvis	Large size Significant increase in adipose tissue Oedematous limbs
Airway			
Be aware of anatomical differences Place padding beneath infant's and young child's shoulder to ensure neutral alignment of cervical spine Oropharyngeal airway not turned 180° Anticipate intubation	Require early intubation due to decrease in cardiopulmonary reserves Fragile tissues in oropharyngeal and nasopharyngeal airways Degenerative changes to laryngeal cartilage increases risk of fracture with neck trauma Arthritic changes to jaw and spine	Pregnant patients may have a normal $PaCO_2$ in respiratory failure due to changing tidal volume 8 times the risk of failed intubation due to mucosal oedema	Lack of landmarks and increased adipose tissue increase difficulty for intubation and cricothyroidotomy Be aware of airway obstruction when patient supine due to increase in adipose tissue Increased risk of aspiration caused by gastro-oesophageal reflux, hiatus hernia and increased abdominal pressure Regular O_2 mask too small Comorbidities of sleep apnoea V/Q mismatching due to reduced lung volumes

TABLE 42.8 PAEDIATRIC, OLDER ADULT, PREGNANT AND BARIATRIC PATIENT GROUP CONSIDERATIONS—cont'd

PAEDIATRIC (CH 35)	OLDER ADULT > 65 (CH 38)	PREGNANT (CH 34)	BARIATRIC
Breathing			
Difficult for children to increase tidal volume Children use abdominal muscles for respiration Signs of pneumothorax are less obvious in a child Ensure gastric tube in intubated patient Bradycardia a sign of hypoventilation	Decreased respiratory reserve and increase in chronic diseases (COPD) Caution with CO_2-retaining patients Decreased ability to increase work of breathing Pain control and physiotherapy essential Less tolerant of pulmonary injuries	BP falls by 5–15 mmHg in 2nd trimester Minute ventilation increases due to increased progesterone Decreased residual volume Beware of pregnant patient with $PaCO_2$ of 35–45 mmHg	Oxygen consumption and carbon dioxide production increases Breathing effort increases and efficiency of air exchange decreases Decreased functional residual capacity Decreased lung and chest wall compliance SpO_2 may not work on periphery due to increased adipose tissue Difficulty auscultating breath sounds
Circulation			
Heart rate assessed using brachial and femoral pulses Decreased BP ominous sign in a child Bradycardia a hallmark of impending cardiac arrest Small surface area makes children very prone to hypothermia	Decreased total blood volume Decreased cardiac function Predisposed to dysrhythmias More dependent on atrial filling to drive cardiac output Decreased glomerular filtration rate and renal blood flow Decreased creatinine clearance rates Beware of normal BP in an older adult patient Prone to anaemia Be cognisant of cardiac medications (beta-blockers)	Cardiac output increases 1.0–1.5 L/min by week 10 Beware that pregnant patient in supine position can compress vena cava and decrease cardiac output Heart rate increase 15 beats/minute 34 weeks: increase in plasma volume and decreased haematocrit Blood loss of 1200–1500 mL before signs of shock Increase in white blood cells Increase in clotting times Anaemia	Metabolic and cardiac demands increase Cardiac output, stroke volume increase Hypoxia and hypercarbia leads to pulmonary hypertension and right-sided heart failure Risk for venous thromboembolism Vascular access poor due to loss of landmarks, greater skin-to-blood vessels distance and short neck BP cuffs may not fit May need Dopplers for pulses due to oedematous limbs FAST scan useless Inability to CT scan or x-ray due to weight restrictions

BP: blood pressure; COPD: chronic obstructive pulmonary disease; CT: computed tomography; FAST: focused abdominal sonography in trauma; $PaCO_2$: partial arterial pressure of carbon dioxide; SpO_2: oxygen saturation; V/Q: ventilation–perfusion.

spine, and repositioning it to the lateral side of the abdomen. This relieves pressure on the vena cava, reinstating maternal circulation. A pillow can be placed under the left buttock, repositioning the pregnant female into the lateral position.[5] Placental abruption and other obstetric emergencies and physiology are discussed in Chapter 34.

Worldwide, obesity is rapidly becoming a significant public health issue. Globally in 2015 there were 107.7 million obese children and 603.7 million obese adults;[96] this is 5% of children and 12% of adults, equating to 23.2% of the world's population being overweight and 9.8% being obese. As in other developing countries, Australia is seeing a rapid increase in this population. It is estimated that worldwide by 2030 there will be 2.6 billion overweight individuals with 1.12 billion suffering from obesity.[96]

Obesity affects every body system and results in the patient being in a chronic inflammatory state. The patient's sheer physical size also increases the challenges involved in both the pre-hospital and the in-hospital environments, making every procedure more challenging. The mortality rate for the obese trauma patient is increased eight times when compared with a trauma patient in the normal weight range. Injury mechanisms also affect the obese patient differently. The increased adipose tissue means that there is an increased force when a traumatic mechanism is sustained; obese patients have an increased incidence of thoracic, pelvic and lower extremity injuries and a lower incidence of head injuries.[5,96] In the pre-hospital environment there are particular challenges in this group, mainly due to the physical size of the patient. Standard equipment carried in ambulances is often not suitable in managing the obese patient and there may be time delays in sourcing equipment such as spine boards or ambulance trolleys suitable for a weight over 230 kg. In some instances, alternative methods may need to be implemented for splinting and spinal immobilisation. Restrictions on air ambulances may also have impacts on triage and transfer decisions, potentially extending scene times and increasing transportation times. This could be fatal in a time-critical case. It is imperative that paramedics take a comprehensive history from the patient as early as possible so that the hospital can be prepared for the patient. This may be the only time that these details can be obtained.[5]

SECONDARY SURVEY

The secondary survey is not performed until the primary survey and its adjuncts have been completed. Many major trauma patients require transport to the operating suite for treatment of life-threatening injuries, such as damage control surgery/laparotomy (Chapter 46), and thus the secondary survey would need to be completed postoperatively.[3] The secondary survey is a complete physical examination using the 'head-to-toe' method. The aim is to identify all injuries and the interventions required. Table 42.9 outlines the secondary survey assessment guidelines and interventions, and Fig. 42.11 shows specific body region assessments.

TERTIARY SURVEY

Exit block exists in many hospitals and can result in considerable delays in transferring the trauma patient to the ward. If the patient has an extended length of stay in the ED, they require

TABLE 42.9 SECONDARY SURVEY INTERVENTIONS[3,5,78,97]

ASSESSMENT	INTERVENTIONS
F = Full set of vital signs/five interventions	In addition to obtaining a complete set of vital signs, consider the five interventions: Cardiac monitor Pulse oximeter (SpO_2) Urinary catheter if not contraindicated Gastric tube (oral or naso) Laboratory studies facilitate family presence
G = Give comfort measures	Verbal reassurance Touch Pain control
H = History Should include mechanism of injury (see Chapter 41). Can be obtained from family. AMPLE is a useful mnemonic to ensure all essential information is obtained: **A**llergies **M**edications currently used **P**ast illnesses/**P**regnancy **L**ast meal **E**vents leading up to incident	
H = Head-to-toe assessment	
Head, skull and face (see Chs 43 and 44)	
Look for lacerations, ecchymosis, deformities, contusions, bleeding, drainage from nose and ears, and check pupil size and reactivity, ocular bleeding, swelling, crepitus Feel for tenderness, note bony crepitus, deformity, bony step-offs and midface instability	Pain control Maintain airway patency Remove contact lenses Haemorrhage control
Cervical spine and neck (see Ch 47, Ch 16: Clinical Skills)	
For cervical spine examination, manual in-line stabilisation of the cervical spine should be used and the patient log-rolled to inspect and palpate the anterior surface and cervical spine. If the patient is wearing a collar this will need to be removed for the duration of the examination. Look for wounds, ecchymosis, deformities and distended neck veins Feel for tenderness; note bony crepitus, deformity, swelling, subcutaneous emphysema and tracheal position	Maintain spinal immobilisation with log-rolling and in-line manual stabilisation when moving the patient or removing the collar (if there is one in situ) Once complete ensure a correctly fitting appropriate cervical collar is reapplied (if clinically indicated). Use direct pressure if haemorrhage control required.

TABLE 42.9 SECONDARY SURVEY INTERVENTIONS—cont'd

ASSESSMENT	INTERVENTIONS
Chest (see Ch 45)	
Look for breathing rate and depth, wounds, deformities, ecchymosis, use of accessory muscles, paradoxical movement, expansion and symmetry	Prepare for decompression to relieve tension pneumothorax
Listen to breath and heart sounds	Prepare for chest tube insertion to follow decompression or for pneumothorax or haemothorax
Feel for tenderness; note bony crepitus, subcutaneous emphysema and deformity including clavicles and shoulders	Prepare for pericardiocentesis by needle for relief of pericardial tamponade
Abdomen and flanks (see Ch 46)	
Look for sounds, distension, ecchymosis or seatbelt signs and scars	Anticipate FAST
Listen for bowel sounds in each quadrant	Or
Feel four quadrants for tenderness, rigidity, guarding, masses and femoral pulses	Insert gastric tube and urinary catheter
	Anticipate transportation to CT scanner
	Maintain high index of suspicion of a lumbar spine fracture or hollow viscus injury if seatbelt sign present
Pelvis and perineum (see Chs 46 and 48)	
Look for wounds, deformities and lacerations; ecchymosis, priapism, blood at the urinary meatus or in the perineal area	Apply external pelvic immobilisation (i.e. pelvic sling or sheet) if not done already in patients with suspected pelvic fracture
	Assist with urethrogram if bladder trauma suspected
Extremities (see Ch 48)	
All four limbs and hands and feet should be examined	Check pulses in all limbs
Look for deformity, open wounds, ecchymosis and swelling, rotation, shortening	Apply splints to extremity fractures
Feel for ecchymosis, abnormal bony movement, joint instability wounds and deformities	Administer analgesia followed by pain assessment
	Assist with radiography studies
Assess motor and sensory deficits, circulation and capillary refill	Dress all open wounds with sterile dressings
Compartment syndrome pulses, pain, paralysis, paraesthesia, pallor	Administer antibiotics as required
Inspect posterior surfaces	Maintain spinal precautions
Maintain cervical spine stabilisation and support injured extremities while the patient is log-rolled	Control external haemorrhage
Look at posterior surface for wounds, deformities and ecchymosis	
Feel posterior surfaces for tenderness and deformities, pain, anal sphincter tone (if not performed previously)	

CT: computed tomography; FAST: focused assessment with sonography in trauma; SpO_2: oxygen saturation.

the performance of the tertiary survey in the ED rather than in the ward. The trauma tertiary survey, as defined by the American College of Surgeons,[5] is an evaluation that identifies and catalogues all injuries and operative interventions after the initial resuscitation. It encompasses a repeated primary and secondary survey, including a head-to-toe assessment. This should consist of a comprehensive review of the patient's medical records with emphasis on mechanism of injury and relevant co-morbidities, and examination of all blood tests, radiology and procedures.

The recommended time-frame for the tertiary survey is $\geq$ 24 hours, and once the patient regains consciousness post-injury.[98] The trauma tertiary survey is a vital part of the trauma patient's assessment: it provides continuity of care, promotes communication among the multidisciplinary trauma caregivers to meet the needs of the patient, strengthens the plan of care and maximises patient outcomes. Regular tertiary surveys have also been shown to decrease the mortality and morbidity in the multi-trauma patient and can be conducted by the ED nurse or medical staff members.

FIGURE 42.11 SECONDARY SURVEY ASSESSMENTS

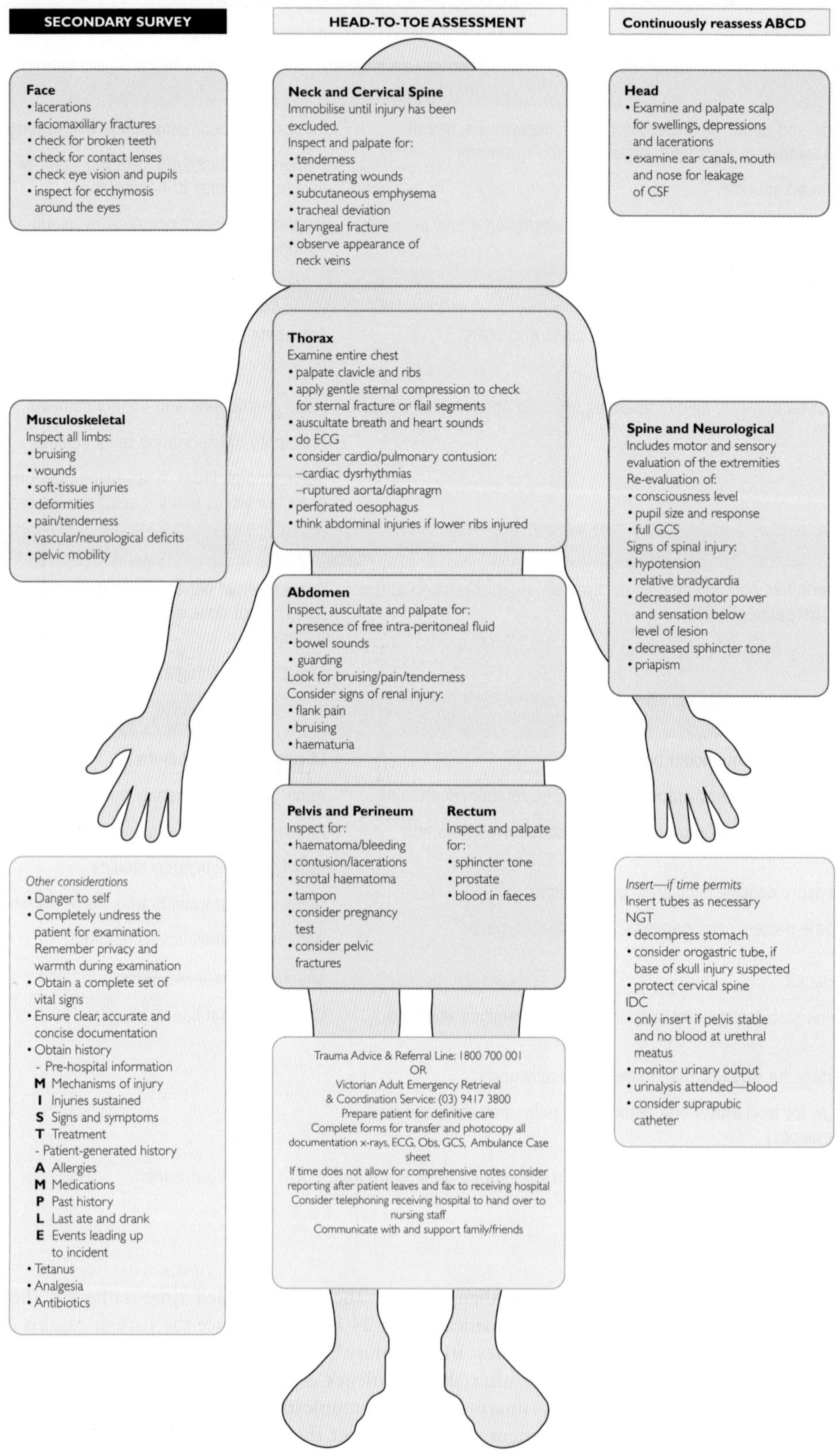

SECONDARY SURVEY

HEAD-TO-TOE ASSESSMENT

Continuously reassess ABCD

Face
- lacerations
- faciomaxillary fractures
- check for broken teeth
- check for contact lenses
- check eye vision and pupils
- inspect for ecchymosis around the eyes

Neck and Cervical Spine
Immobilise until injury has been excluded.
Inspect and palpate for:
- tenderness
- penetrating wounds
- subcutaneous emphysema
- tracheal deviation
- laryngeal fracture
- observe appearance of neck veins

Head
- Examine and palpate scalp for swellings, depressions and lacerations
- examine ear canals, mouth and nose for leakage of CSF

Thorax
Examine entire chest
- palpate clavicle and ribs
- apply gentle sternal compression to check for sternal fracture or flail segments
- auscultate breath and heart sounds
- do ECG
- consider cardio/pulmonary contusion:
  - –cardiac dysrhythmias
  - –ruptured aorta/diaphragm
- perforated oesophagus
- think abdominal injuries if lower ribs injured

Musculoskeletal
Inspect all limbs:
- bruising
- wounds
- soft-tissue injuries
- deformities
- pain/tenderness
- vascular/neurological deficits
- pelvic mobility

Spine and Neurological
Includes motor and sensory evaluation of the extremities
Re-evaluation of:
- consciousness level
- pupil size and response
- full GCS

Signs of spinal injury:
- hypotension
- relative bradycardia
- decreased motor power and sensation below level of lesion
- decreased sphincter tone
- priapism

Abdomen
Inspect, auscultate and palpate for:
- presence of free intra-peritoneal fluid
- bowel sounds
- guarding

Look for bruising/pain/tenderness
Consider signs of renal injury:
- flank pain
- bruising
- haematuria

Pelvis and Perineum
Inspect for:
- haematoma/bleeding
- contusion/lacerations
- scrotal haematoma
- tampon
- consider pregnancy test
- consider pelvic fractures

Rectum
Inspect and palpate for:
- sphincter tone
- prostate
- blood in faeces

Other considerations
- Danger to self
- Completely undress the patient for examination. Remember privacy and warmth during examination
- Obtain a complete set of vital signs
- Ensure clear, accurate and concise documentation
- Obtain history
  - Pre-hospital information
  - **M** Mechanisms of injury
  - **I** Injuries sustained
  - **S** Signs and symptoms
  - **T** Treatment
  - Patient-generated history
  - **A** Allergies
  - **M** Medications
  - **P** Past history
  - **L** Last ate and drank
  - **E** Events leading up to incident
- Tetanus
- Analgesia
- Antibiotics

Trauma Advice & Referral Line: 1800 700 001
OR
Victorian Adult Emergency Retrieval & Coordination Service: (03) 9417 3800
Prepare patient for definitive care
Complete forms for transfer and photocopy all documentation x-rays, ECG, Obs, GCS, Ambulance Case sheet
If time does not allow for comprehensive notes consider reporting after patient leaves and fax to receiving hospital
Consider telephoning receiving hospital to hand over to nursing staff
Communicate with and support family/friends

Insert—if time permits
Insert tubes as necessary
NGT
- decompress stomach
- consider orogastric tube, if base of skull injury suspected
- protect cervical spine

IDC
- only insert if pelvis stable and no blood at urethral meatus
- monitor urinary output
- urinalysis attended—blood
- consider suprapubic catheter

Adapted from Department of Health and Human Services, State Government of Victoria.

ONGOING NURSING CARE IN THE ED

After the initial resuscitation, patients not requiring urgent operative intervention may spend significant time in the ED. There are several key aspects of nursing care that will contribute to improved patient outcome and experience.

IV FLUIDS AND MEDICATION ADMINISTRATION

A fluid balance chart must be commenced or continued, ensuring that all fluids administered are recorded from the time of admission; this includes all fluid outputs, including estimations of blood and fluid loss. This is essential to assist in the monitoring not only of fluid resuscitation, but also to allow for monitoring of any signs of kidney injury post-contrast administration or from trauma. Ensure that there are adequate fluids prescribed for the ongoing care of the patient, and if the patient can eat and drink, ensure that this is documented and that the patient is commenced on diet and fluids as soon as they are able.

OBSERVATIONS AND PROGRESS NOTES

All essential details of patient admission should be documented, including any interventions and/or treatments, a list of valuables, next of kin details and any additional history.

Ensure that frequent observations are ordered and commenced, including vital signs, GCS, fluid balance chart, monitoring of ICCs and ventilation observations.

ANALGESIA

Ensure that the patient's pain score is recorded and measured, and that appropriate analgesia is prescribed and dosed according to the patient's response. If the patient is a child, record their weight for calculation of drug dosing. Paediatric patients present special challenges related to their age and development; it is key to all family/carers to be available to assist/nurse infants and toddlers during pain assessments for reassurance and assistance with assessment (see Chapter 35). If the patient has complex pain needs, referral to the acute pain service is appropriate. Injured patients are unprepared for the trauma pain experience and need education on what to expect during and after hospital discharge. Patients often experience intense and enduring injury pain at home, and clinicians should ensure the patient has adequate analgesia and information (communicated in a clear and simple way) to improve pain management, potentially preventing the long-term consequences of injury pain.[99]

VENOTHROMBOEMBOLISM PROPHYLAXIS

Early commencement of venothromboembolism (VTE) prophylaxis can prevent development of deep vein thrombosis (DVT) and/or pulmonary embolism (PE); this should be discussed with the treating team. Nurses should be aware of the contraindications for pharmacological prophylaxis and, if one of these exists, ensure that the patient has alternative VTE prophylaxis measures in place, such as compression stockings and/or electronic sequential calf compressors or foot pumps. Patient education regarding VTE prevention is also fundamental to the care of a trauma patient.

SPINAL CARE

If the patient requires spinal immobilisation for a suspected or confirmed spinal cord or column injury, ensure that regular 4-hourly log-rolling for pressure injury and collar care is attended to. This will enable visual inspection of the patient's skin surfaces, hygiene and assist in chest physiotherapy (see Chapter 13 for pressure-area and other essential nursing care).

CRITERIA FOR EARLY TRANSFER

All members of the TT must know their hospital's capabilities and limitations in caring for patients. The majority of patients will be easily cared for at a local level and will not require transfer; however, it is essential that those patients who do need to be transferred are referred early. The major trauma service has the resources to provide expert treatment throughout the span of trauma care. Each hospital should have established inter-hospital trauma transfer guidelines specific to their territory, region or state readily available to all staff. The ED nurse should be aware of these guidelines and aim to expedite transfer to definitive care if required within 30 minutes of arrival.[3] Table 42.10 defines major trauma patient characteristics, which indicate transfer is required to a major trauma service.

FAMILY PRESENCE

Family presence in trauma resuscitations is a highly controversial topic, with wide-ranging opinions offered.[100,101] Historically, both medical and nursing staff viewed family as guests rather than an integral part of the patient's illness, recovery and/or death. However, substantial research[101] has demonstrated that there are benefits for families in being present, such as allowing a shared experience between patient and family, helping to facilitate grieving if death occurs, assisting with closure and decreasing family fear and anxiety. Some researchers believe that these benefits far outweigh the risks, such as the effect that witnessing the resuscitation may have on the family, the increasing stress on the trauma team, interference from family, lack of support for the family during the resuscitation, as well as an increased risk of medico–legal action. In fact, many family members only recall the pain of the resuscitation and have no real memory of specific procedures and events. It should be remembered that 'family' not only pertains to those related by blood or marriage, but also to significant others who share an established relationship with the patient.

The success of the family presence depends on all TT members, particularly the nursing staff—who are usually responsible for preparing the family to enter the resuscitation—guiding and supporting them throughout and being able to answer their questions. Considerations for family presence are discussed further in Chapter 14. Most hospitals, especially trauma centres, will have as part of the TT a social worker or pastoral care worker who can be available to support the family throughout the resuscitation and throughout the patient's hospital stay in the case that a member of the TT team (medical or nursing) is not available to support families in this situation.[102–104]

POST-TRAUMATIC STRESS

Traumatic injury and mental health disorders are co-associated. Patients with traumatic injury report a substantial reduction in health-related quality of life compared to other patients, including long-term psychological and physical disability. The psychological impact of injury includes the development of acute and long-term mental health problems, such as post-traumatic stress disorder (PTSD), depression and anxiety. Acute stress disorder (ASD) occurs in up to 45% of injury

TABLE 42.10 CRITERIA FOR EARLY TRANSFER OF TRAUMA PATIENTS[25,100]

VITAL SIGNS (MAJOR TRAUMA IF ANY ONE OF THE FOLLOWING PRESENT)	ADULT > 15 YEARS	NEWBORN < 2 WEEKS	INFANT < 1 YEAR	CHILD 1–8 YEARS	LARGE CHILD 9–15 YEARS
Respiratory rate (breaths/minute)	< 10 or > 30	< 40 or > 60	< 20 or > 50	< 20 or > 35	< 15 or > 25
Cyanosis	Present	Cool/pale clammy	Cool/pale clammy	Cool/pale clammy	Cool/pale clammy
Hypotension (mmHg)	< 90	–	< 60	< 70	< 80
Glasgow Coma Scale	< 13	< 15	< 15	< 15	< 15
Injuries					

Serious or suspected serious penetrating injuries:
- to head/neck/chest/abdomen/pelvis/axilla/groin

Blunt injuries:
- patient with a significant injury to a single region: head/neck/chest/abdomen/pelvis/axilla/groin
- patient with injury to two or more of the above body regions

Specific injuries:
- limb amputations/limb-threatening injuries
- suspected spinal cord injury
- burns > 20% or suspected respiratory tract
- serious crush injury
- major compound fracture or open dislocation
- fracture to two or more of the following: femur/tibia/humerus
- fractured pelvis

survivors and, similar to PTSD, involves an anxiety response that includes re-experience of the traumatic event, intrusive memories, dreams and strong emotional distress on exposure to triggering events. Early identification of depression, anxiety and stress symptoms and associated prevention may reduce long-term symptoms and negative impacts. ICU admission and high levels of depression, anxiety and stress at 3 months post-injury are predictors for high levels of depression, anxiety and stress at 6 months.[105] Low levels of depression, anxiety and stress during hospital admission are correlated with low levels of depression, anxiety and stress at 3 and 6 months. It is recommended that a validated tool such as the DASS-21, which takes 2 minutes to complete, should be used as a screening tool in admitted trauma patients to identify patients at risk of long-term symptoms and facilitate preventive intervention.[105]

SUMMARY

The importance of thorough and accurate initial assessment and management of the trauma patient at all phases of care cannot be overstated. System, staff and departmental preparation minimises confusion and decreases the time to definitive care. A systematic approach to assessment and intervention improves patient outcomes through early recognition of potentially life-threatening injuries and intervention for identified problems. The paramedic and emergency nurse must advocate for trauma patient protection and prevent secondary insult as much as possible, while assisting with necessary lifesaving interventions. They should have solid trauma management knowledge and be able to assess the trauma patient, be aware of the patient's physiological status and treatment received and expedite the patient to definitive care.

CASE STUDY

PART 1—PRE-HOSPITAL

Mechanism

A 22-year-old male, the single occupant of a ute driven at high speed on a wet and cold night, crashes into a tree. He is trapped in the vehicle upside down by his legs for approximately 1 hour. He was drinking and using methamphetamine with his friends all afternoon, and there is a strong smell of alcohol on his breath. He is found by passers-by who call for an ambulance. He is transferred to hospital via helicopter. The scene is attended by the fire brigade who assist with the extrication.

Time-frame is:

- 2100 hours—ambulance called
- 2145 hours—paramedic arrival at scene
- 2230 hours—departure from scene
- 2310 hours—off stretcher.

Injuries

Altered conscious state, swollen and bruised left eye, seatbelt abrasion to chest and abdomen, complaining of pain to chest, abdomen and numbness and pain in lower legs. Spinal cord injury is suspected, obvious open lower leg fracture with large blood loss.

Signs—2150 hours

- Systolic blood pressure 90 mmHg
- Pulse rate 110 beats/minute
- Resp rate 22 breaths/minute
- Oxygen saturation unknown
- Glasgow Coma Scale (GCS) score 13 (eye 3, verbal 4, motor 6)
- Temperature 34°C.

Treatment

- Spinal stabilisation: head held in pouring rain, clothing removed from around neck and cervical foam collar applied.
- Extrication using spine board, patient initially upside down in vehicle held by seatbelt.
- Patient's wet clothing removed.
- Intravenous (IV) access 16G to right bicep, patient flailing around, very hard to cannulate and get blood pressure, SpO_2 not sensing as peripherally shut down.
- Oxygen applied 10 L/min via non-rebreather mask.
- Pelvis stabilised with a sheet or pelvic binder if available.
- Palpable surgical emphysema on the left chest wall, with decreased air entry, chest decompressed with finger thoracostomy, audible hiss.
- Splint to heavily bleeding lower leg and gauze pads applied.

QUESTIONS

1. What are the priorities of care by the paramedics?
2. Is the patient's treatment conducted according to the primary survey?
3. What alternatives to IV access could have been used in this case?
4. Why is the mechanism of injury important information in diagnosing injuries?

PART 2—EMERGENCY DEPARTMENT

The paramedic calls the MTS and provides handover to the receiving consultant. Based on this information, a trauma call is initiated and the patient is given a triage category 1.

- Mechanism—high-speed motor vehicle crash versus tree, then roll-over, entrapped possibly 60 minutes.
- Injuries—possible closed head injury, chest, abdomen and spine, open tibia fracture.
- Signs—heart rate 130 beats/minute, blood pressure 100 mmHg, respiratory rate 24 breaths/minute, oxygen saturation unknown, GCS 12 (eyes—3, verbal—4, motor—5) with loss of consciousness.
- Treatment—1 × IV cannula, IV fluids, oxygen, pelvic splint and ICC inserted.
- The trauma team assemble to meet the patient and primary and secondary surveys are performed.

Primary survey in ED

- Airway—patent, trachea midline, cervical spine collar in situ.
- Breathing—oxygen via non-rebreather 15 L/min, air entry, unequal, increased work of breathing, obvious chest deformity on right side, possible flail.
- Circulation—1 × IV cannula noted, unable to insert any others due to vasoconstriction and hypovolaemia, intra-osseous catheter inserted into left tibial plateau. Commence uncrossed O-negative red blood cell transfusion immediately and 1 unit fresh frozen plasma, 1 unit platelets.
- Disability—patient eye opening to voice, not obeying commands or verbalising, GCS 8 (eye 3, verbal 1, motor 4); patient's temperature was 34°C, hypothermia guideline was implemented, remaining wet clothes removed and warm fluids and blanket applied.

Signs—2310 hours

- Blood pressure 90/60 mmHg
- Pulse rate 110 beats/minute

- Respiratory rate 20 breaths/minute
- Oxygen saturation 92%
- Temperature 34°C
- GCS score 8
- Pupils PEARL 4+.

Treatment

A decision is made to intubate, $EtCO_2$ monitoring and equal entry confirm placement.

Adjuncts to primary survey

- Chest x-ray—confirmed ETT placement, multiple right-sided rib fractures, haemopneumothorax.
- Pelvis x-ray—open-book pelvic fracture.
- eFAST: negative.
- Oro.

Secondary survey

- HEENT—bruising and abrasions to left eye, external auditory canal NAD (no abnormalities detected), no crepitus or bony step-offs. Cervical collar in situ.
- Chest—seatbelt bruising, visible flail segment, reduced breath sounds to right side.
- Abdomen/pelvis—seatbelt abrasion to abdomen, pelvic sheet in place, abdomen soft, and pelvis not manipulated, blood at the external meatus.
- Extremities—NAD; obvious left leg tibial fracture?
- Neurological examination—patient sedated, unable to assess sensation and/or motor, was moving all limbs on arrival.
- Back/spine—nil bruising or deformity, step or abrasions, anal tone NAD.
- History—unable to attain past medical history as patient GCS 3 and intubated.

Adjuncts to secondary survey

- Trauma bloods—ethanol; full blood count; coagulation profile; urea, electrolytes, creatinine; liver function; cross-match.
- Insertion of arterial line.
- Venous blood gases: pH 7.30; PCO_2 45 mmHg, lactate 3.3 mmol/L.
- Computed tomography (CT) trauma series.
- X-ray right leg.
- Splint to open tibial fracture.

INITIAL TREATMENT PLAN

Patient has right side ICC inserted, which drains 200 mL of haemoserous fluid. An orogastric tube is inserted, which drains bile-stained fluid. Once stabilised, the sheet stabilising the patient's pelvis is replaced with a pelvic sling and he undergoes an emergency trauma urethrogram, which is normal and an IDC is inserted. He then has a CT trauma series (head, neck, chest, abdomen and pelvis) with CT angiography of chest. Emergency theatre is booked for open reduction internal fixation of his open tibial fracture and external fixation of his pelvis; spinal precautions are maintained.

The patient remains haemodynamically stable during transfer to CT, his blood pressure is maintained at 90–100 mmHg with blood products. He is commenced on morphine and midazolam infusions for sedation and analgesia. He remains intubated for the management of his chest injuries; he is admitted to the intensive care unit post-theatre for ongoing stabilisation, re-warming and resuscitation.

CT results

- Brain—closed head injury; isolated small frontal cerebral contusion.
- Cervical spine—NAD.
- Chest—fractured right ribs 1–9 with flail, pulmonary contusion and haemopneumothorax.
- Abdomen—grade 2 liver laceration.
- Pelvis: open-book pelvic fracture with 5 cm diastases of symphysis pubis and extremity fractures.
- Thoracolumbar spine—transverse processes of T5–9 level.
- Extremity—open, comminuted and displaced midshaft tibia and fibula fractures.

QUESTIONS (CONTINUED)

5. Does the patient meet trauma team activation criteria?
6. What would the indications for intubation be in this case?
7. What are the indications for activating a massive blood transfusion guideline?
8. What would impede the assessment of the patient's abdomen?
9. Outline the acute trauma coagulopathy and the steps in this case that may have prevented and/or worsened this condition.
10. How would a liberal transfusion strategy be managed in this case?
11. What steps would need to be taken to deem this patient's cervical spine injury-free?

Answers to Case Study Questions can be found on evolve http://evolve.elsevier.com/AU/Curtis/emergency/

USEFUL WEBSITES

Interactive web-based scenarios, learning modules, podcasts, videos, as well as information on upcoming trauma conferences and links to other web-based trauma resources, such as trauma management guidelines, care be found on many state and local trauma centre webpages.

Australian and New Zealand Burns Association, www.anzba.org.au.

Australian Emergency Nurses Association, www.acen.com.au.

CareFlight NSW, www.careflight.org.

Emergency Trauma Management, http://etmcourse.com/.

Institute of Trauma and Injury Management (ITIM), www.aci.health.nsw.gov.au/get-involved/institute-of-trauma-and injury-management.

NSW ACI clinical procedures app—short videos of 100 of the most common emergency procedures available online or as a free app, aci.health.nsw.gov.au/networks/eci/clinical/procedures.

Prehospital Trauma Life Support, www.sdc.qld.edu.au/phtls.htm.

Trauma Nursing Program (College of Emergency Nursing Australasia), www.tnp.net.au.

Trauma.org, www.trauma.org.

Trauma Victoria, http://trauma.reach.vic.gov.au/.

REFERENCES

1. Wray JP, Briwell RE, Schauer SG, Shackelford SA, Bebarta VS, Wright FL, et al. The diamond of death: hypocalcemia in trauma and resuscitation. Am J Emerg Med 2021;41:104–9.
2. Vasudeva M, Mathew JK, Groombridge C, Tee JW, Johnny CS, Maini A, et al. Hypocalcemia in trauma patients: a systematic review. J Trauma Acute Care Surg 2021;90(2):396–402.
3. Feliciano D, Mattox K, Moore EE. Trauma. 9th ed. New York: McGraw-Hill Medical; 2020.
4. Gabbe BJ, Simpson PM, Sutherland AM, Wolfe R, Fitzgerald MC, Judson R, et al. Improved functional outcomes for major trauma patients in a regionalized, inclusive trauma system. Ann Surg 2012;255(6):1009–15.
5. American College of Surgeons. ATLS®, Advanced trauma life support®. 10th ed. Chicago: American College of Surgeons; 2018.
6. ANZCOR. Management of cardiac arrest due to trauma: ANZCOR Guideline 11.10.1. Australian and New Zealand Council of Resuscitation; April 2016.
7. Cameron P, O'Reilly G. Trauma overview. In: Cameron P, Little M, Mitra B, Deasy C, editors. Textbook of adult emergency medicine. 4th ed. Sydney: Churchill Livingstone; 2015.
8. Cameron P, Gabbe B, Cooper D. A statewide system of trauma care in Victoria; effect on patient survival. MJA 2008;189(10):546–50.
9. Asensio J, Trunkey D. Trauma systems. In: Asensio JA, Trunkey DD, editors. Current therapy of trauma and surgical critical care. 2nd ed. Philadelphia: Elsevier; 2016.
10. Alarhayem A, Myers J, Dent D, Liao L, Muir M, Mueller D, et al. Time is the enemy: mortality in trauma patients with hemorrhage from torso injury occurs long before the 'golden hour'. Am J Surg 2016;212(6):1101–5.
11. Rossaint R, Bouillon B, Cerny V, Coats TJ, Duranteau J, Fernández-Mondéjar E, et al. The European guideline on management of major bleeding and coagulopathy following trauma: fourth edition. Crit Care 2016;20:100.
12. Rogers F, Rittenhouse K, Gross B. The golden hour in trauma: dogma or medical folklore? Injury 2014;46(4):525–7.
13. Fedor P, Burns B, Lauria M, Richmond C. Major trauma outside a trauma center: prehospital, emergency department, and retrieval considerations. Emerg Med Clin 2018;36(1):203–18.
14. ACEM. Emergency Department Design Layout. Australasian College of Emergency Medicine [Webpage]. Online. Available from: https://acem.org.au/Content-Sources/Advancing-Emergency-Medicine/COVID-19/Resources/Clinical-Guidelines/Emergency-Department-Design-Layout.
15. Frink M, Lechler P, Debus F, Ruchholtz S. Multiple trauma and emergency room management. Dtsch Arztebl Int 2017;114(29–30):497–503.
16. Emergency Nurses Association. Sheehy's emergency nursing: principles and practice. 7th ed. St Louis: Mosby; 2019.
17. Gumm K, Judson R, Thomson B, Antippa P, McCormick J, Shakerian R, et al. TRM04.02 Emergency Department Thoracotomy Guideline. Melbourne: The Royal Melbourne Hospital; 2018.
18. Jamshidi S, Parker J, Hashemi S. The effects of environmental factors on the patient outcomes in hospital environments: a review of literature. Front Architect Res 2020;9(2):249–63.
19. Dans M, Lundmark V. The effects of positive practice environments: leadership must-knows. Nurs Manag 2019;50(10):7–10.
20. Copanitsanou P, Fotos N, Brokalaki H. Effects of work environment on patient and nurse outcomes. Br J Nurs 2017;26(3):172–6.
21. Murphy M, Curtis K, Lam MK, Palmer CS, Hsu J, McCloughen A. Simulation-based multidisciplinary team training decreases time to critical operations for trauma patients. Injury 2018;49(5):953–8.
22. Clements A, Curtis K. What is the impact of nursing roles in hospital patient resuscitation? Australas Emerg Nurs J 2012;15(2):105–15.
23. Hughes KM, Benenson RS, Krichten AE, Clancy KD, Ryan JP, Hammond C. A crew resource management program tailored to trauma resuscitation improves team behavior and communication. J Am Coll Surg 2014;219(3):545–51.

24. Trauma Victoria Major trauma guidelines and education. Teamwork and communication. Trauma Victoria; Online. Available from: http://trauma.reach.vic.gov.au/sites/default/files/Teamwork%20and%20Communication_16102017.pdf.
25. ROTES. Review of trauma and emergency services. Melbourne: Department of Health Human Services; 1999.
26. Murphy M, McCloughen A, Curtis K. The impact of simulated multidisciplinary trauma team training on team performance: a qualitative study. Australas Emerg Care 2019;22(1):1–7.
27. Murphy M, Curtis K, McCloughen A. What is the impact of multidisciplinary team simulation training on team performance and efficiency of patient care? An integrative review. Australas Emerg Nurs J 2016;19(1):44–53.
28. Ford K, Menchine M, Burner E, Arora S, Inaba K, Demetriades D, et al. Leadership and teamwork in trauma and resuscitation. West J Emerg Med 2016;17(5):549–56.
29. Clements A, Curtis K, Horvat L, Shaban RZ. The effect of a nurse team leader on communication and leadership in major trauma resuscitations. Int Emerg Nurs 2015;23(1):3–7.
30. Trauma Victoria. Early trauma care guideline. Trauma Victoria. Online. Available from: https://trauma.reach.vic.gov.au/guidelines/early-trauma-care/introduction.
31. Moore LJ. Blood, balloons, and blades: state of the art trauma resuscitation. Am J Surg 2022;224:40–4.
32. Davis JW, Dirks RC, Sue LP, Kaups KL. Attempting to validate the overtriage/undertriage matrix at a Level I trauma center. J Trauma Acute Care Surg 2017;83(6):1173–8.
33. Cox S, Currell A, Harriss L, Barger B, Cameron P, Smith K. Evaluation of the Victorian state adult pre-hospital trauma triage criteria. Injury 2012; 43(5):573–81.
34. Gumm K, Read D, Putland D, Oppy A, Walsham N, Paspaliaris A, Shakerian R, et al. TRM08.05 Trauma Team Activation (Call and Alert). V. 6.0. Melbourne: The Royal Melbourne Hospital, The Trauma Services; June 2021.
35. Lerner EB, Shah MN, Cushman JT, Swor RA, Guse CE, Brasel K, et al. Does mechanism of injury predict trauma center need? Prehosp Emerg Care 2011;15(4):518–25.
36. Johnson G. Trauma triage and trauma system performance. West J Emerg Med 2016;17(3):331–2.
37. Reid C, Brindley P, Hicks C, Carley S, Richmond C, Lauria M, et al. Zero point survey: a multidisciplinary idea to STEP UP resuscitation effectiveness. Clin Exp Emerg Med 2018;5(3):139–43.
38. Heschl S, Andrew E, de Wit A, Bernard S, Kennedy M, Smith K, et al. Prehospital transfusion of red cell concentrates in a paramedic-staffed helicopter emergency medical service. Emerg Med Australas 2018;30(2):236–41.
39. Rosenbaum E, Cox S, Smith K, Fitzgerald M, Braitberg G, Carpenter A, et al. Ambulance management of patients with penetrating truncal trauma and hypotension in Melbourne, Australia. Emerg Med Australas 2020;32(2):336–43.
40. Brown J, Sajankila N, Claridge JA. Prehospital assessment of trauma. Surg Clin N Am 2017;97(5):961–83.
41. Trauma Victoria. Pre-hospital major trauma triage. Trauma Victoria [guideline]. 2017. Available from: https://trauma.reach.vic.gov.au/resources/trauma-victoria-posters.
42. Iedema R, Ball C, Daly B, Young J, Green T, Middleton PM, et al. Design and trial of a new ambulance-to-emergency department handover protocol: 'IMIST-AMBO'. BMJ Qual Saf 2012;21(8):627–33.
43. Trauma Victoria Early trauma care guideline trauma Victoria. 2017. Online. Available from: https://trauma.reach.vic.gov.au/guidelines/early-trauma-care/key-messages.
44. Genuit T, Rueda M. Initial assessment and resuscitation of the trauma patient. In: Cameron AM, Cameron JL, editors. Current surgical therapy. Philadelphia: Elsevier; 2020.
45. Camilleri D, Gumm K, Liersch K, Walsh M, Williams D, Morely P. TRM08.12 Traumatic cardiac arrest guideline. V. 2.0. Melbourne: The Royal Melbourne Hospital, The Trauma Services; 2018.
46. Emergency Care Institute New South Wales, Agency for Clinical Innovation. Emergency procedures. 2023. Online. Available from: https://aci.health.nsw.gov.au/networks/eci/clinical/procedures.
47. Kwan I, Bunn F, Roberts I. Spinal immobilisation for trauma patients. Cochrane Database Syst Rev 2001;2001(2):Cd002803.
48. Trauma Victoria. Spinal trauma guidelines. 2017. Online. Available from: https://trauma.reach.vic.gov.au/sites/default/files/Spinal%20Trauma%20Guideline_Ver%202.1_18122017.pdf.
49. NICE. Assessment and initial management. London: National Institute for Health and Care Excellence (NICE); 2016.
50. Cohen SS. Trauma nursing secrets: questions and answers reveal the secrets to safe and effective trauma nursing. Philadelphia: Hanley and Belfus; 2003.
51. Stephens CT, Gumbert S, Holcomb J. Trauma-associated bleeding: management of massive transfusion. Curr Opin Anaesthesiol 2016;29(2):250–5.
52. Spahn D, Bouillon B, Cerny V, Duranteau J, Filipescu D, Hunt BJ, et al. The European guideline on management of major bleeding and coagulopathy following trauma. 5th ed. Crit Care 2019;23(1):98.
53. Cohen M, Christie S. New understandings of post injury coagulation and resuscitation. Int J Surg 2016;33:242–5.
54. McQuilten ZK, Crighton G, Brunskill S, Morison JK, Richter TH, Waters N, et al. Optimal dose, timing and ratio of blood products in massive transfusion: results from a systematic review. Transfus Med Rev 2018;32(1):6–15.
55. Adkins AR, Lee D, Woody DJ, White Jr WA. Accuracy of blood loss estimations among anesthesia providers. Aana J 2014;82(4):300–6.

56. Harris W, Rotheram A, Pearson S, Lucas P, Edwards D, et al. Paramedic confidence in estimating external blood loss. Australas J Paramed 2017;14(3): https://doi.org/10.33151/ajp.14.3.535.
57. Netherton S, Milenkovic V, Taylor M, Davis PJ. Diagnostic accuracy of eFAST in the trauma patient: a systematic review and meta-analysis. CJEM 2019;21(6):727–38.
58. Victoria Ambulance. Haemorrhage control using combat application tourniquet (CAT) CWI/OPS/171. Victoria: Victoria Ambulance; 26 August 2016.
59. Taylor NB, Lamond DW. Stopping Haemorrhage by Application of Rope tourniquet or inguinal Compression (SHARC study). Emerg Med Australas 2021;33(5):803–7.
60. Kleber C, Giesecke M, Linder T, Haas NP, Buschmann CT. Requirement for structured algorithm in cardiac arrest following major trauma: epidemiology, management errors, and preventability of traumatic deaths in Berlin. Resuscitation 2014;85:405–10.
61. Meadley B, Olaussen A, Delorenzo A, Roder N, Martin C, St Clair T, et al. Educational standards for training paramedics in ultrasound: a scoping review. BMC Emerg Med 2017;17(1):18.
62. Delorenzo A, Meadley B. Point-of-care of ultrasound use in the pre-hospital setting. J Paramed Prac 2018;10(8):326–32.
63. Hawryluk GWJ, Rubiano AM, Totten AM, O'Reilly C, Ullman JS, Bratton SL, et al. Guidelines for the management of severe traumatic brain injury: 2020 update of the decompressive craniectomy recommendations. Neurosurgery 2020;87(3):427–34.
64. Cannon JW, Khan MA, Raja AS, Cohen MJ, Como JJ, Cotton BA, et al. Damage control resuscitation in patients with severe traumatic hemorrhage: a practice management guideline from the Eastern Association for the Surgery of Trauma. J Trauma Acute Care Surg 2017;82(3):605–17.
65. Gruen RL, Brohi K, Schreiber M, Balogh ZJ, Pitt V, Narayan M, et al. Haemorrhage control in severely injured patients. (author abstract). Lancet 2012;380(9847):1099–108.
66. Curtis K, Fraser M, Grant N. Adding insult to injury, hypothermia in the trauma patient: a trauma centre's experience in monitoring temperature. Arch Nurs 2004;6:30–5.
67. Zuidema GD, Rutherford R, Ballinger W, editors. The management of trauma. 4th ed. Philadelphia: WB Saunders; 1985.
68. Melbourne RCsH. Cervical spine assessment. Royal Children's Hospital Melbourne. 2020. Available from: www.rch.org.au/clinicalguide/guideline_index/Cervical_Spine_Assessment/. Accessed 22 March 2022.
69. Roberts J, Hodges J, editors. Clinical procedures in emergency medicine. Philadelphia: WB Saunders; 1998.
70. Jelinek G, Kelly AM, Brown A. Textbook of adult emergency medicine. 4th ed. Churchill Livingston; 2014.
71. Dawson J, Atassi O, Sun D, Sheth M. Emergency care of musculoskeletal injuries. In: Townsend CM, Beauchamp RD, Evers BM, Mattox KL, editors. Sabiston textbook of surgery. Missouri: Elsevier; 2022.
72. Tran T, Brasel K, Karmy-Jones RC, Rowell S, Schreiber MA, Shatz DV, et al. Western Trauma Association critical decisions in trauma: management of pelvic fracture with hemodynamic instability–2016 updates. J Acute Care Surg 2016;81(6):117–74.
73. Ruatti S, Guillot S, Brun J, Thony F, Bouzat P, Payen JF, et al. Which pelvic ring fractures are potentially lethal? Injury 2015;46(6):1059–63.
74. Gabbe BJ, de Steiger R, Esser M, Bucknill A, Russ MK, Cameron PA. Predictors of mortality following severe pelvic ring fracture: results of a population-based study. Injury 2011;42(10):985–91.
75. Liersch K, Gumm K, Judson R, Oppy D, McDonald D, McGurgan C, et al. TRM 06.02 pelvic binder guideline. Melbourne: The Royal Melbourne Hospital; 2019.
76. Feinsmith S, Huebinger R, Pitts M, Baran E, Haas S. Outcomes of a simplified ultrasound-guided intravenous training course for emergency nurses. J Emerg Nurs 2018;44(2):169–175.e2.
77. Stolz LA, Cappa AR, Minckler MR, Stolz U, Wyatt RG, Binger CW, et al. Prospective evaluation of the learning curve for ultrasound-guided peripheral intravenous catheter placement. J Vasc Access 2016;17(4):366–70.
78. Gumm K, Read D, Kelsey G, Haeusler M, Plunkett G, Williams D, The Advisory Commitee on Trauma and Melbourne Health Transfusion Committee. TRM08.01 Massvie blood transfusion in trauma. V. 4.4. Melbourne: The Royal Melbourne Hospital, Trauma Service; June 2021.
79. Royal Children's Hospital. Intraosseous access. 2018. Online. Available: www.rch.org.au/clinicalguide/guideline_index/Intraosseous_Access/.
80. Bardes J, Strumwasser A. Techniques of Intraosseous Access. In: Demetriades D, Inaba K, Lumb P, editors. Atlas of critical care procedures. New York: Springer; 2018.
81. Shakur H, Roberts I, Bautista R, Caballero J, Coats T, Dewan Y, et al. Effects of tranexamic acid on death, vascular occlusive events, and blood transfusion in trauma patients with significant haemorrhage (CRASH-2): a randomised, placebo-controlled trial. Lancet 2010;376(9734):23–32.
82. Curry N, Rourke C, Davenport R, Beer S, Pankhurst L, Deary A, et al. Early cryoprecipitate for major haemorrhage in trauma: a randomised controlled feasibility trial. Br J Anaesthes 2015;115(1):76–83.
83. Crombie N, Doughty HA, Bishop JRB, Desai A, Dixon EF, Hancox JM, et al. Resuscitation with blood products in patients with trauma-related haemorrhagic shock receiving prehospital care (RePHILL): a multicentre, open-label, randomised, controlled, phase 3 trial. Lancet Haematol 2022;9(4):e250–61.
84. Anto VP, Guyette FX, Brown J, Daley B, Miller R, Harbrecht B, et al. Severity of hemorrhage and the survival benefit associated with plasma: results from a randomized prehospital plasma trial. J Trauma Acute Care Surg 2020;88(1):141–7.
85. Shand S, Curtis K, Dinh M, Burns B. Prehospital blood transfusion in New South Wales, Australia: a retrospective cohort study. Prehosp Emerg Care 2021;25(3):404–11.
86. Hood N, Considine J. Spinal immobilisaton in pre-hospital and emergency care: a systematic review of the literature. Australas Emerg Nurs J 2015;18:118–37.

87. Seamon MJ, Haut ER, Van Arendonk K, Barbosa RR, Chiu WC, Dente CJ, et al. An evidence-based approach to patient selection for emergency department thoracotomy: a practice management guideline from the Eastern Association for the Surgery of Trauma. J Trauma Acute Care Surg 2015;79(1):159–73.
88. Menaker M, Scalea T. Trauma and emergency care: emergency department thoracotomy. In: Cameron D, Cameron A, editors. Current surgical therapy. 12th ed. Philadelphia: Elsevier; 2016.
89. Raja A. Thoracic trauma. In: Walls R, Hockberger R, Gausche-Hill M, editors. Rosen's emergency medicine; concepts and clinical practice. 9th ed. Philadelphia: Elsevier; 2018.
90. Mendez-Figueroa H, Dahlke JD, Vrees RA, Rouse DJ. Trauma in pregnancy: an updated systematic review. Am J Obstet Gynecol 2017;209(1):1–10.
91. Ferrah N, Dipnall J, Gabbe B, Cameron P, Ibrahim J, Beck B. Injury profiles and clinical management of older patients with major trauma. Australas J Ageing 2022;41(1):116–25.
92. Cox S, Morrison C, Cameron P, Smith K. Advancing age and trauma: triage destination compliance and mortality in Victoria, Australia. Injury 2014; 45(9):1312–19.
93. Trauma Victoria. Older person trauma. Trauma Victoria. Online. Available from: trauma.reach.vic.gov.au/guidelines/older-person-trauma/key-messages
94. System LMT London. Management systems: management of elderly trauma patients. London Major Trauma System; February 2017.
95. Gumm K, Lockie L, Shakein R, Woodward A, Plunkett G, Owen L, et al. TRM05.01 Pregnancy and trauma guideline. V. 4.4. Melbourne: The Royal Melbourne Hospital, Trauma Service; December 2019.
96. The GDB 2015 Obesity Collaborators. Health effects of overweight and obesity in 195 countries over 25 years. N Eng J Med 2017;377:13–27.
97. Trauma Victoria. Major trauma guidelines and education: Secondary survey. 2023. Online. Available at: trauma.reach.vic.gov.au/guidelines/early-trauma-care/secondary-survey.
98. Tammelin E, Handolin L, Söderlund T. Missed injuries in polytrauma patients after trauma tertiary survey in trauma intensive care unit. Scand J Surg 2016;105(4):241–7.
99. Goldsmith H, McCloughen A, Curtis K. Using the trauma patient experience and evaluation of hospital discharge practices to inform practice change: a mixed methods study. J Clin Nurs 2018;10(1):1589–98.
100. Trauma Victoria. Inter-hospital transfer guidelines. Trauma Victoria [PDF]. Online. Available from: trauma.reach.vic.gov.au/guidelines/inter-hospital-transfer/key-messages
101. Lederman Z. Family presence during cardiopulmonary resuscitation in the Covid-19 era. Resuscitation 2020;151:137–8.
102. Jabre P, Belpomme V, Azoulay E, Jacob L, Bertrand L, Lapostolle F, et al. Family presence during cardiopulmonary resuscitation. New Eng J Med 2013;368(268):1008–18.
103. O'Connell K, Fritzeen J, Guzzetta C, Clark AP, Lloyd C, Scott SH, et al. Family presence during trauma resuscitation: family members' attitudes, behaviors, and experiences. Am J Crit Care 2017;26(3):229–39.
104. Leske JS, McAndrew NS, Brasel KJ, Feetham S. Family presence during resuscitation after trauma. J Trauma Nurs 2017;24(2):85–96.
105. Wiseman T, Foster K, Curtis K. Mental health following traumatic physical injury: an integrative literature review. Injury-International Journal of the Care of the Injured 2013;44(11):1383–90.

CHAPTER 43
TRAUMATIC BRAIN INJURY

BEN FISK AND TAMSIN JONES

ESSENTIALS

- Traumatic brain injury is a significant cause of mortality and morbidity in our society. Injuries are described as occurring as a result of either a primary or a secondary cause.
- Primary injury occurs as a result of the direct effect of the initial insult and energy exchange with the central nervous system.
- Secondary injuries occur as an indirect result of the primary injury and the body's response to that injury. Hypoxia, hypotension and hypercapnia are potentially preventable contributors for the development of secondary brain injury. If these are not recognised and treated they have the potential to significantly worsen the initial primary injury.
- Close observation, monitoring and targeted interventions are paramount in order to lessen secondary insults.
- Guidelines for severe traumatic brain injury recommend the maintenance of systolic blood pressure ≥ 100 mmHg for patients aged 50–69 years or ≥ 110 mmHg for patients aged 15–49 or over 70 years of age. Intracranial pressure should ideally be < 20 mmHg,[1] cerebral perfusion pressure maintained between 60–70 mmHg[2] and jugular venous saturation > 50%.[2]
- Traumatic brain injuries are categorised as being mild, moderate or severe. A Glasgow Coma Scale score ≤ 8 may suggest a severe traumatic brain injury.
- Mechanism of injury and neurological findings can assist in guiding initial management, while computed tomography plays an important role in the diagnosis and management of traumatic brain injury.

INTRODUCTION

Traumatic brain injury (TBI) is defined as an alteration in brain function, or other evidence of brain pathology, caused by an external force.[2,3] The characteristics of the forces resulting in injury, along with the complexity of the brain's structures and functions, contribute to a broad range of TBI manifestations.[4]

Presentations range from mild TBI, with no apparent lasting effects, through to severe TBI, which can result in irreversible, permanent impairment. Such changes can adversely affect both family and interpersonal relationships, thus representing a significant social burden and cost. An important challenge in the clinical management of TBI patients is the prevention of injury progression.[5]

Post-injury complications, such as hypotension, hypoxia, seizures and other physiological events, have a profound impact on the degree of secondary injury sustained and ultimately the functional outcome of patients.[6] All clinicians involved in providing acute care play important roles in preventing or reducing these potential secondary injuries.

EPIDEMIOLOGY

TBI is considered to be the most significant traumatic injury pattern contributing to death and disability worldwide,[7] with the greatest burden of disease experienced in Southeast Asia and the Western Pacific regions.[7]

Despite significant advances in trauma system design, and the corresponding maturity of trauma registries and data capture, the incidence of TBI in Australia remains difficult to clearly quantify.[8] The incidence of mild TBI in particular is challenging to capture as patients may not seek medical care at the time of initial injury.[8] With similar population demographics between Australia and Aotearoa New Zealand, data extrapolation suggests that the national incidence of TBI in each country is between 790 cases per 100,000 person-years.[8] This number is inclusive of mild, moderate and severe TBI. Despite the lack of clarity regarding the true number of TBI cases in Australia and Aotearoa New Zealand, it is known that most deaths following TBI occur in the first 24 hours following injury,[9] and that less than 50% of severe TBI patients who survive the initial insult return to full pre-injury independence.[10]

Common causes of TBI in Australia and Aotearoa New Zealand are falls, transport-related events and sport-related activities.[11,12] Importantly, there is an over-representation of TBI in rural areas in both countries,[13] highlighting the importance of efficient transport to major trauma services able to provide definitive care and specialist rehabilitation.[14]

TBI has been predicted to be the leading cause of disability and death worldwide by 2030.[15] The high incidence, cost and loss of productive years associated with TBI reinforces the need to develop more-effective prevention strategies.[4]

This chapter begins with a brief review of TBI anatomy and physiology. It also provides an overview of assessment techniques for adult patients with TBI and current management strategies. Refer to Chapter 35 for discussion of paediatric trauma, Chapter 38 for trauma in the elderly and Chapter 34 for obstetric trauma.

INJURY MECHANISM

Traumatic brain injury is a complex mixture of two principal insults—primary brain injury and secondary brain injury. Primary brain injury is caused by the external forces on the skull and brain structures at the time of injury. Secondary brain injury is damage to the brain that results from both the evolution of the primary brain injury and from acute disorders of the respiratory and cardiovascular system that are associated with the direct TBI event and other trauma suffered.

Common examples of the evolution of primary brain injury include cerebral swelling, ischaemia and hypoxic damage, hydrocephalus, infection and the effects of raised intracranial pressure.[16] The consequences of other trauma may manifest as episodes of systemic hypoxia or hypotension. In both pre-hospital and hospital care, emphasis should be placed on avoiding hypotension and hypoxia in patients with TBI, with particular attention paid to preventing a combination of the two.[17]

ANATOMY

The hair, scalp, skull, meninges and cerebrospinal fluid (CSF) protect the brain from injury. The scalp consists of five layers of tissue: skin, subcutaneous tissue, epicranial aponeurosis, ligaments and periosteum. The skull is composed of many bones, including the frontal, parietal, temporal and occipital bones (Fig. 43.1).[18]

Cranial bones join with facial bones to form the cranial vault, a rigid cavity that can hold 1400–1500 mL of material. Internal bony structures of importance are depressions at the base of the skull called the anterior, middle and posterior fossa. The frontal lobe is located in the anterior fossa; parietal, temporal and occipital lobes in the middle fossa, while the brainstem and cerebellum are located in the posterior fossa.

Three layers of meninges surround the brain and provide additional protection. The outermost layer is the dura mater, which consists of two layers of tough fibrous tissue. The inner layer of the dura mater forms the falx cerebri and tentorium cerebelli. Potential spaces located above the dura mater (extradural/epidural) and below the dura mater (subdural) are at risk for haematoma formation as the middle meningeal artery lies in and above the dura, and veins are located within the subdural space. The middle layer is the arachnoid mater (meaning 'spiderlike'), a fine, elastic layer. Below the arachnoid mater, the subarachnoid space contains arachnoid villi, finger-like projections that form channels for CSF absorption. Adhering to the surface of the brain is the pia mater (Fig. 43.2).[18] More-detailed anatomy of the brain is presented in Chapter 23.

PHYSIOLOGY

Although the average brain accounts for only 2% of an adult's total bodyweight, it consumes approximately 20% of the body's resting oxygen consumption. It is a highly metabolic and active organ whose main energy source is oxygen and glucose. Cerebral blood flow, therefore, is vital to maintaining cerebral function.

Cerebral autoregulation is an important concept in healthy brain tissue, although its utility in pathological states such as TBI is unclear. Cerebral autoregulation may be defined as the intrinsic ability to maintain a constant cerebral blood flow over a range of blood pressures. Cerebral autoregulation maintains cerebral blood flow at an average of 50 mL/100 g brain tissue/minute between mean arterial blood pressures of 60–150 mmHg. This phenomenon protects the brain against ischaemia at low blood pressures, and against oedema and potential haemorrhage at very high blood pressures. Cerebral autoregulation is thought to be mediated through a combination of myogenic, neurogenic and metabolic mechanisms acting at the level of the vascular endothelium.[19]

In addition, oxygen, carbon dioxide and pH all exert an influence on cerebral blood flow. Hypoxia, hypercapnia and acidosis cause vasodilation that increases cerebral blood flow, cerebral volume and intracranial pressure (ICP). Hypocapnia causes vasoconstriction and lower cerebral blood volume. As such, brain tissue is very susceptible to hypoxia and hypoglycaemia.[16]

Secondary injuries limit the ability of the injured brain to adapt to minor variations in physiology and maintain adequate cerebral blood flow. Cerebral autoregulation is thought to be impaired after TBI, and cerebral blood flow may be pressure-dependent. Therefore, a decrease in cerebral perfusion pressure (CPP) may lead to ischaemia, while, conversely, increases in CPP can increase blood flow and raise ICP as a result (Fig. 43.3).[20]

Excitotoxic changes increase cerebral metabolism and may predispose ischaemia, even in the presence of normal or increased cerebral blood flow. The release of neurogenic factors

FIGURE 43.1 ANTERIOR VIEW OF THE SKULL[18]

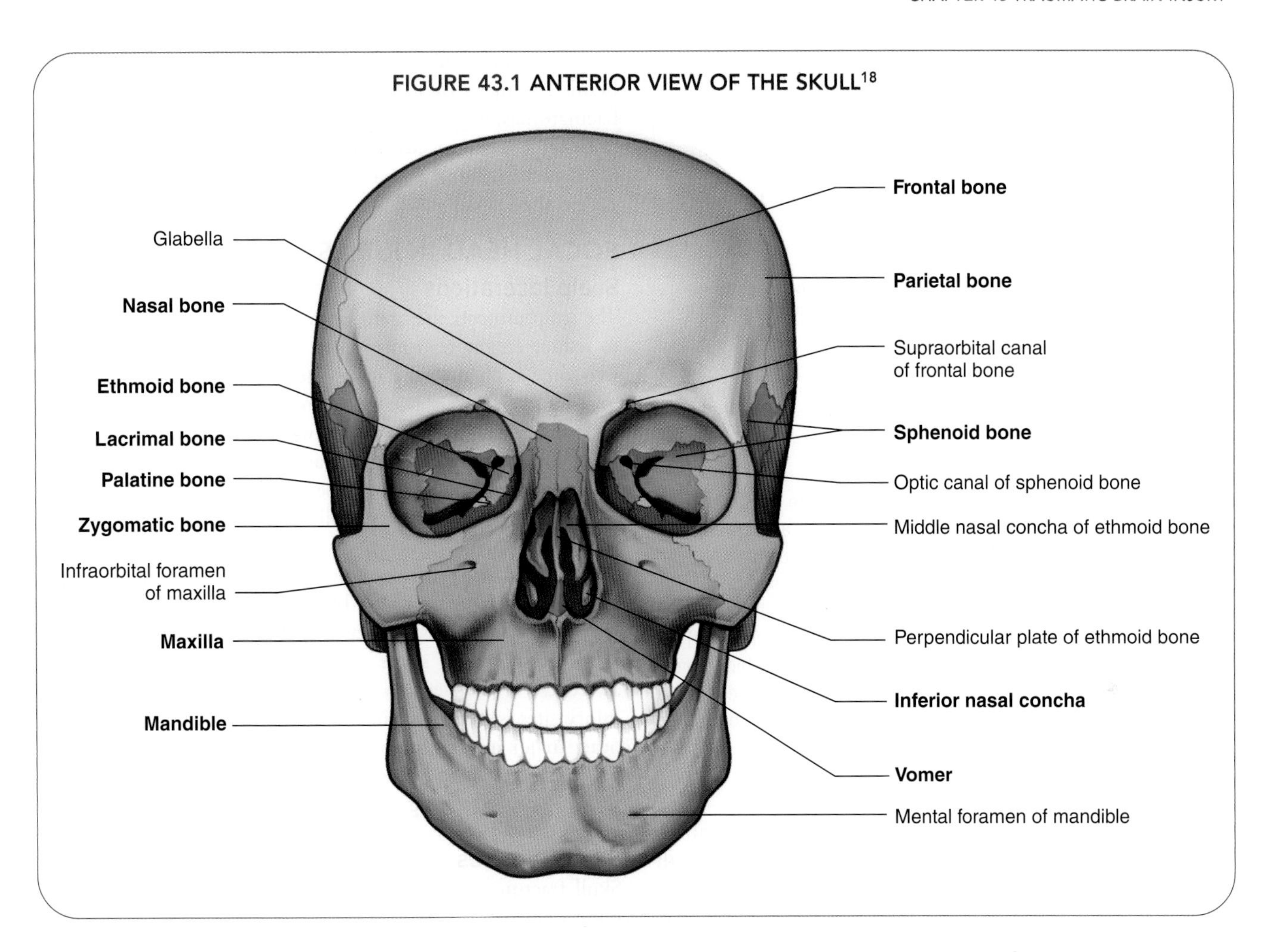

FIGURE 43.2 CORONAL (FRONTAL) SECTION OF THE SUPERIOR PORTION OF THE HEAD, AS VIEWED FROM THE FRONT. BOTH THE BONY AND THE MEMBRANOUS COVERINGS OF THE BRAIN CAN BE SEEN[18]

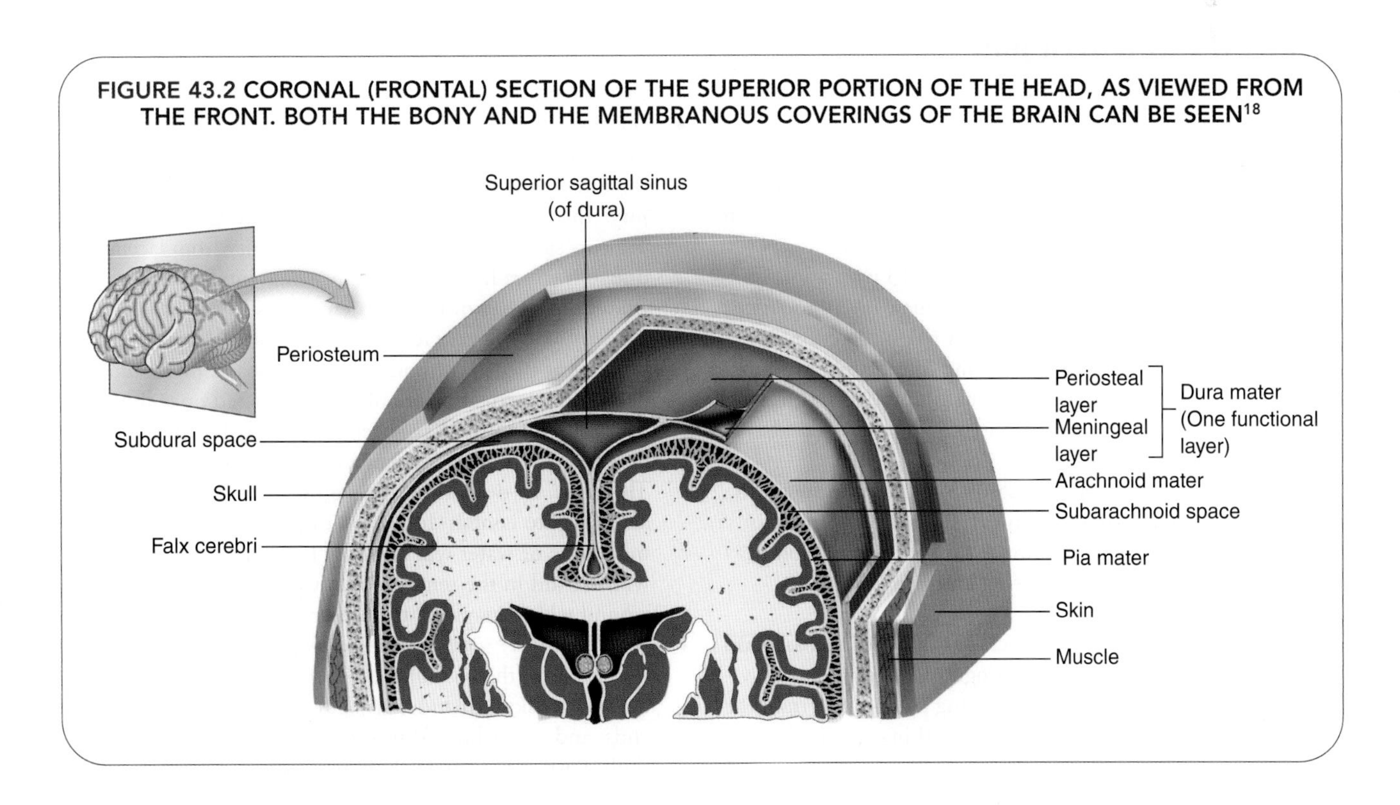

FIGURE 43.3 CEREBRAL AUTOREGULATION CURVE[20]

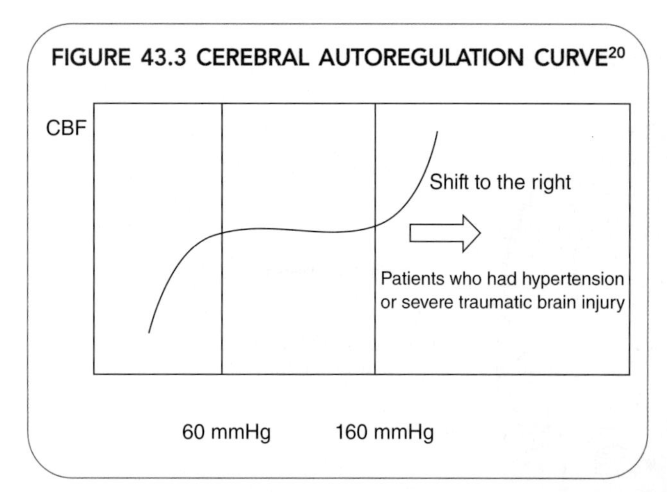

Cerebral blood flow (CBF) is constant when the mean arterial blood pressure (MAP) is tightly regulated between 60 and 160 mmHg. Vasoconstriction and/or vasodilation occurs as the cerebral vasculature changes to adjust to MAP. With hypertension or severe TBI, the autoregulation curve shifts to the right. Due to the rightwards shift (arrow), a MAP-dependent CBF reduction (brain ischaemia) or increase (hyperaemia) occurs, even for a small change in blood pressure. Note that the plateau range of CBF is presumably altered after TBI occurs. No clear data are available, however, on how this presumed alteration takes place. *CC BY 4.0 license.*

from damaged brain cells can also affect the cerebral vasculature. The resultant impact on the injured brain can be severe, with exacerbation of cerebral swelling, and in some cases coagulopathy will ensue.[16,21] As a result of these effects, clinicians may manipulate metabolic and physiological parameters in the management of patients with severe TBI.[16,21]

TBI CLASSIFICATIONS

TBI is commonly classified using the Glasgow Coma Scale (GCS) as mild, moderate or severe.

- *Mild TBI* is defined as a GCS score of 13–15 with a loss of consciousness up to 15 minutes. Patients with mild TBI do not generally require a hospital admission and are often discharged from the ED with close supervision.
- *Moderate TBI* is defined as a GCS of 9–13 with a loss of consciousness for up to 6 hours. Patients with a moderate TBI are hospitalised due to the high risk of deterioration from cerebral oedema and increasing intracranial pressure (ICP). Patients do not generally require ICP monitoring or ventilatory support unless systemic injuries make it necessary.
- *Severe TBI* is defined as a GCS of 3–8 after resuscitation, or patients that deteriorate to this level after 48 hours of admission. Patients require critical care admission, haemodynamic/ICP monitoring and ventilatory support.[21]

Numerous other scales for TBI classification exist based on severity, outcome, radiology and prognosis. A number of systematic investigations are currently taking place to ascertain the best classification system or systems for TBI in order to develop reliable individualised care.[4,20]

In this chapter, traumatic brain injury will be discussed as either a focal or a diffuse injury. *Focal injuries* have an identifiable area of involvement, whereas *diffuse injuries* involve the entire brain. Examples of focal injuries include skull fractures and haematomas, often occurring after a focal injury or fall; diffuse injuries generally occur as a result of rapid deceleration from high speeds (diffuse axonal injury) and movement of the brain within the cranial vault.

FOCAL HEAD INJURIES

Scalp lacerations

The scalp protects the brain from injury by acting as a cushion to reduce energy transmission to underlying structures. Excessive force applied to the scalp often causes a laceration, which may bleed profusely due to an extensive vascular supply with poor vasoconstrictive properties, which may lead to acute anaemia.[22] It is important to note that patients can exsanguinate via scalp lacerations, but most can be controlled with direct pressure to the affected area.[23] There will be cases where direct pressure is not able to be achieved or maintained,[24] especially where other urgent care is required, during transport or when fractures underlie the laceration.[23] If bleeding control is not achieved, scalp closure is necessary to assist in local pressure and to minimise the potential space for haematoma formation.[23,25] An awareness of the need to minimise bleeding from all external injury sites is important in the pre-hospital setting, even when other major injuries are present. The use of haemostatic dressings may assist with haemorrhage control from scalp injuries in the pre-hospital setting.

Skull fractures

Skull fractures occur when energy applied to the skull causes bone deformation. Clinical presentation of skull fractures is directly correlated to the type of fracture, area involved and the damage to underlying structures.

- A *linear skull fracture* is non-displaced and associated with minimal neurological deficit. Supportive care is usually all that is required.[21]
- A *depressed skull* fracture occurs as a result of bone deformation; the bone is depressed inwards (Fig. 43.4)[21] impacting the underlying brain tissue and resulting in a primary injury. This is usually the result of a high-energy impact and presents significant risk of secondary injury from laceration due to fracture fragments and increased intracranial pressure from haematoma or tissue oedema mass.
- An *open skull fracture* requires urgent neurosurgical referral because of the risk of underlying injury and infection. Appropriate irrigation should be conducted once life/limb threatening injuries have been addressed. Traumatic wounds almost always occur in a non-sterile environment. Therefore, by definition, the wounds will be contaminated and likely to contain foreign bodies. Irrigation with normal saline or water will not only facilitate assessment but will also aid in the removal of any contaminants from the wound which may lead to further injury.[21,26]
- A *basilar (base) skull fracture* develops when enough force is exerted on the base of the skull to cause deformity. The base of the skull includes any bony area where the skull ends, and is not limited to the posterior aspect of the skull. Portions of the facial bones comprise the base of the skull, such as the roof of the orbit. The occipital condyles are also part of the base of the skull, joining the occipital

FIGURE 43.4

A. Depressed skull fracture shows both brain tissue and bone injury. B. Bone window scan of the same depressed skull fracture shows the displaced fragments of bone.[21]

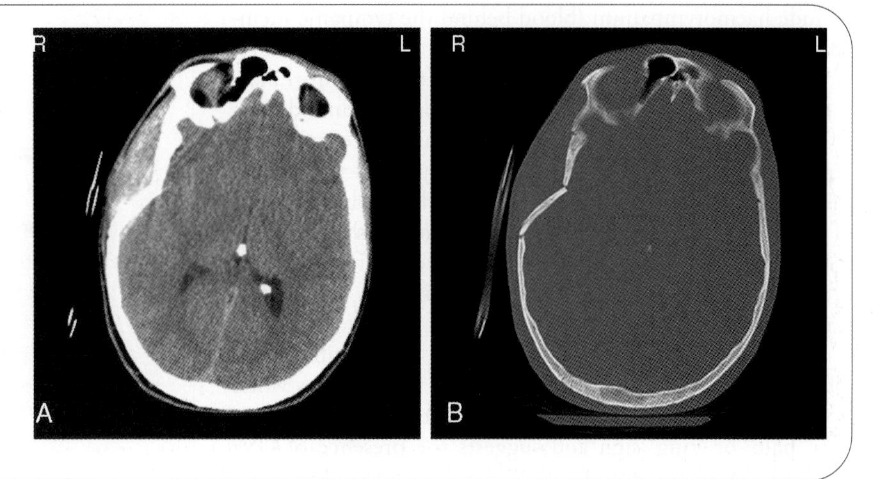

FIGURE 43.5 BASILAR SKULL FRACTURES THROUGH THE ANTERIOR SKULL BASE

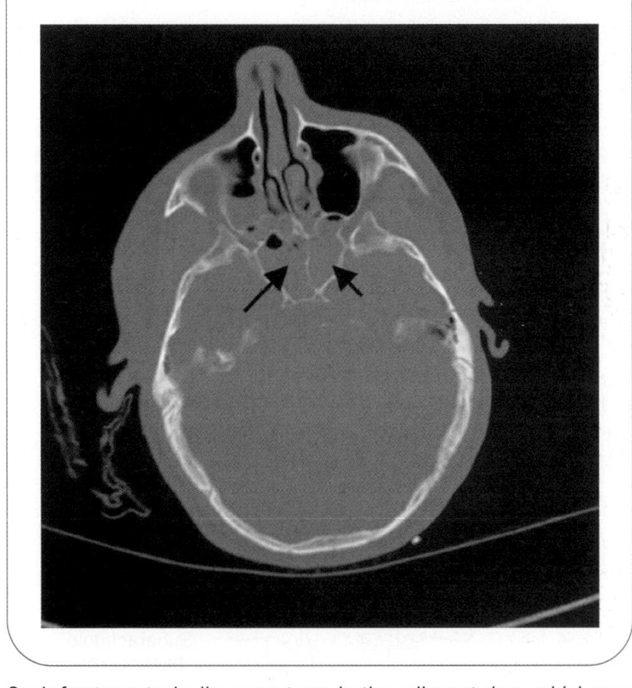

Such fractures typically cause tears in the adjacent dura, which may result in CSF rhinorrhoea. CT scans through the base of the skull may not show the fracture itself, but fluid in the sphenoid sinus (arrows) or the other paranasal sinuses is often seen (axial CT scan, bone window).[27]

FIGURE 43.6

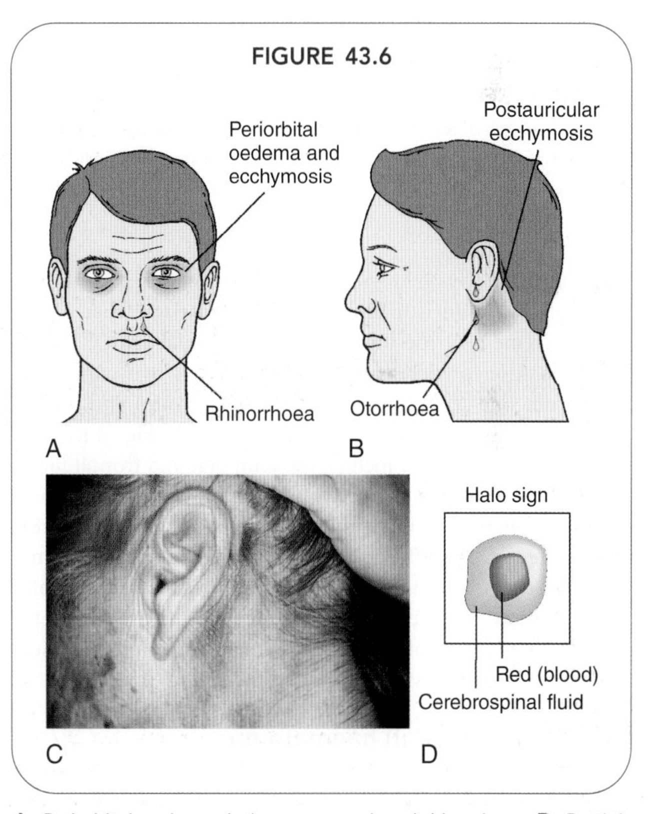

A. Periorbital ecchymosis (raccoon eyes) and rhinorrhoea. B. Battle's sign (postauricular ecchymosis) with otorrhoea. C. Battle's sign. D. Halo or ring sign.[28,29]

bone with the first cervical vertebra enabling the head to move relative to the cervical spine; fractures of these may increase the potential for cervical spine injury and thus must be considered.

A basilar skull fracture may be visualised on diagnostic imaging; however, this is not always true, and diagnosis may therefore also be made on the basis of clinical findings (Fig. 43.5).[27] Basilar skull fractures that overlay the middle meningeal artery are the cause of more than 75% of epidural haematomas. A basilar skull fracture may also cause intracerebral bleeding.

Clinical manifestations of basilar skull fractures may manifest 12–72 hours after the initial injury and include periorbital ecchymosis (Fig. 43.6A), which results from blood tracking into the periorbital tissue, and post-auricular ecchymosis, resulting from bruising over the mastoid process seen behind the ears (Fig. 43.6B and C).[28] Other clinical signs include haemotympanum (blood behind the tympanic membrane), caused by a fracture of the temporal bone, and CSF.

The most common injury sites that result in CSF rhinorrhoea involve fractures to the sphenoid, frontal, ethmoid sinus or the cribriform plate. CSF rhinorrhoea may also occur in the setting of a temporal bone fracture, if the tympanic membrane is intact and fluid drains through the eustachian tube. Fractures of the temporal bone that cause perforation to the tympanic membrane may result in CSF otorrhoea. However, the absence of visible CSF does not eliminate the possibility of a basilar skull fracture.

Suspected CSF fluid leak will form two distinct rings when the fluid drips onto filter paper or the patient's white bedsheet or pillow case. This is commonly referred to as a 'halo' or 'ring' sign and suggests the presence of CSF (Fig. 43.6D).[28] The fluid may be tested for glucose, as this is a normal finding in CSF; however, laboratory testing will provide more reliable confirmation. CSF rhinorrhoea or otorrhoea should be permitted to drain freely and not be obstructed. Nasal packing is not recommended for CSF rhinorrhoea, but may be required for haemorrhage control in the setting of complex facial fractures. To promote patient comfort, a nasal bolster is useful.

Clinical staff should exercise caution when considering a nasogastric tube, nasal endotracheal intubation or nasal temperature probe insertion due to a higher risk of these lodging intracranially.

Contusion

Cerebral contusion is a bruise of the brain tissue that occurs from movement of the brain within the cranial vault.[30] When an acceleration or deceleration injury occurs, two contusions may result: one at the initial site of impact (coup) and one on the opposite side of the impact (contrecoup) (Fig. 43.7).[29,31] Common areas affected include the temporal and frontal lobes.

On computed tomography (CT), contusions will appear as areas of hyperdensity within superficial grey matter. Areas of hypodensity from associated vasogenic oedema may often surround them.[32] The clinical presentation varies with size and location of the contusion. Commonly occurring symptoms include altered level of consciousness, nausea, vomiting, visual disturbances, weakness and speech difficulty.

Extradural (epidural) haematoma

Extradural haematoma (EDH) is bleeding between the inner surface of the skull and the dura mater. Commonly, a torn middle meningeal artery (caused by an accompanying skull fracture) leads to a rapidly forming haematoma; however, some patients may have no evidence of skull fracture (Figs 43.8 and 43.9). An acute EDH appears on CT as a well-defined, hyperdense, biconvex extra-axial collection. Mass effect, sulcal effacement, midline shifts and herniation are commonly seen.[34]

A rapidly expanding EDH is a neurosurgical emergency. Classical signs and symptoms include a brief period of unconsciousness followed by a lucid period, then another loss of consciousness. This brief lucid period is considered a hallmark of an EDH; however, it does not occur in all patients. If alert, the patient with an EDH will generally complain of a severe headache and may exhibit hemiparesis and an ipsilateral dilated pupil. Surgical intervention will be guided by the neurosurgeon.

FIGURE 43.7 WHIPLASH AND COUP–CONTRECOUP INTRACRANIAL FORCES.

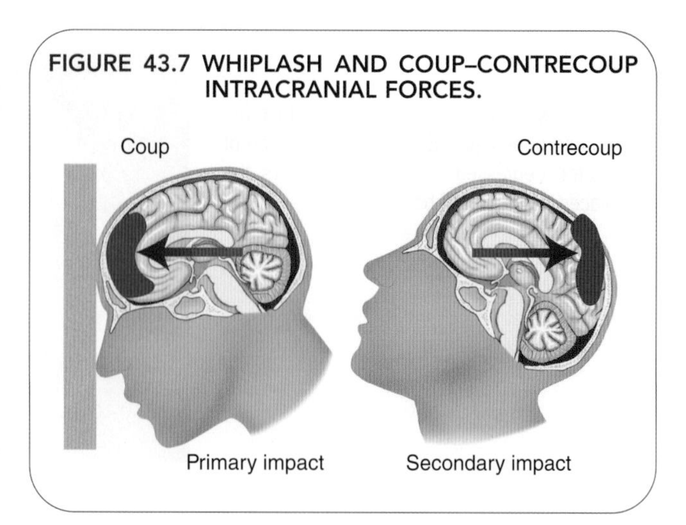

The primary site of injury results from the brain thrust against the frontal area from sudden whiplash and/or striking an object forcefully. The secondary site of injury results from the brain being thrust backward after impact in a recoil motion.[29]

FIGURE 43.8 LOCATIONS OF EPIDURAL, SUBDURAL AND SUBARACHNOID HAEMATOMAS[32]

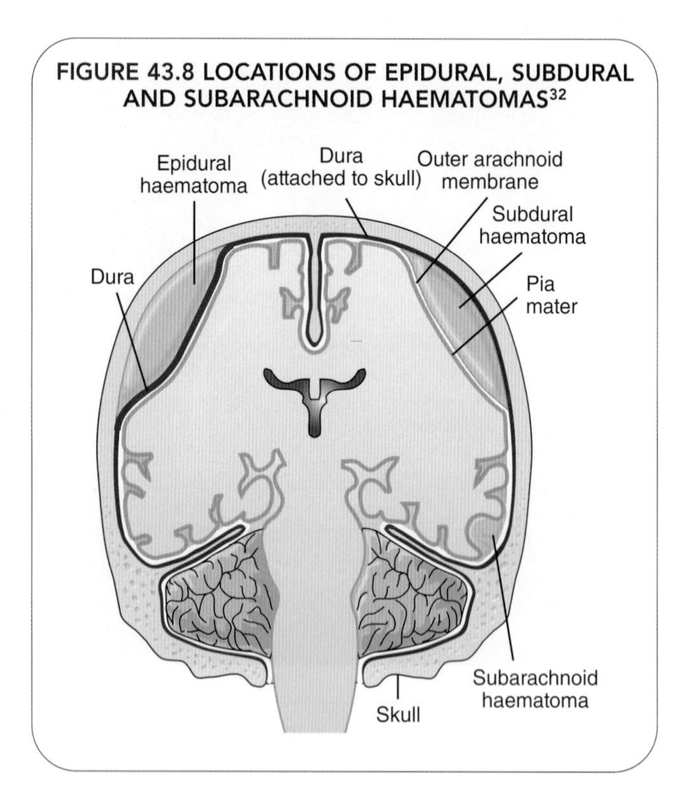

Subdural haematoma

A subdural haematoma (SDH) (Fig. 43.10) may be acute, subacute or chronic. Traumatic SDH usually results from shearing forces that rupture bridging cortical veins in the subdural space. This causes bleeding into the subdural space between the dura mater and arachnoid leading to the development of a haematoma. An acute SDH appears on CT as hyperdense, homogenous, crescent-shaped extra-axial collection.[27] SDHs are frequently associated with parenchymal injury and associated mass effect. Clinical features may include loss of consciousness, hemiparesis and fixed dilated pupils.

FIGURE 43.9 NON–CONTRAST-ENHANCED CT SCAN OF ACUTE EDH AT THE LEVEL OF RIGHT MIDCONVEXITY. THERE IS AN ASSOCIATED MASS EFFECT AND MODERATE MIDLINE SHIFT[33]

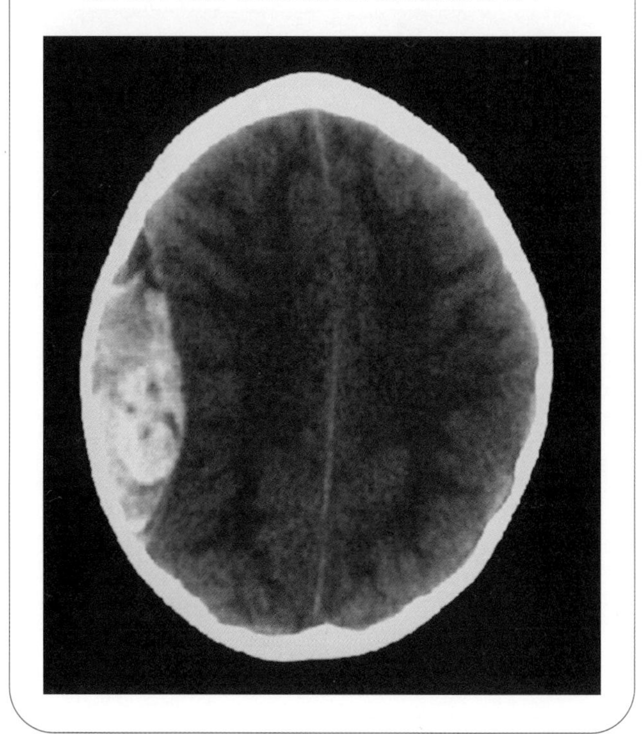

FIGURE 43.10 COMPUTED TOMOGRAPHY SCAN OF AN ACUTE SDH[35]

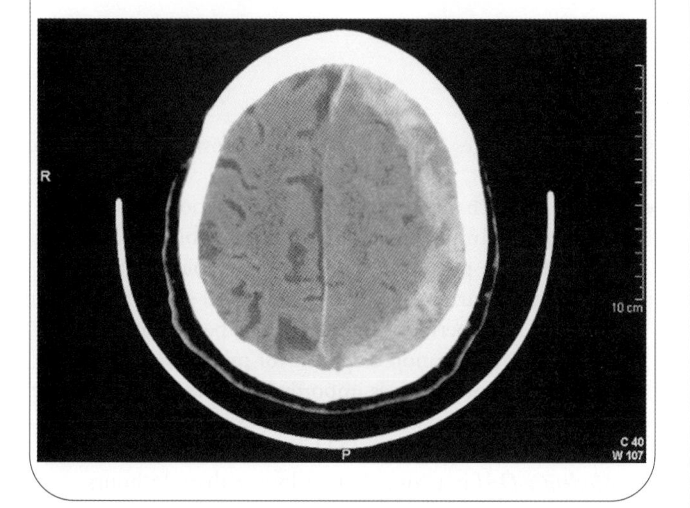

Subacute SDHs usually develop 48 hours to 2 weeks after injury. The clinical presentation is often seen as a progressive decline in level of consciousness as the haematoma slowly expands. The brain compensates as a result of slow blood collection over time, so decline in neurological function occurs gradually. After the SDH is drained, the patient may improve quickly with little or no lasting neurological deficit.

Chronic SDHs are frequently seen in elderly people and also progress slowly. Blood can collect over 2 weeks to several months. By the time a person is examined, the causative mechanism may have been forgotten. Chronic SDH is initially tolerated because of brain atrophy associated with ageing. As the brain decreases in size, the space within the cranial vault increases. A haematoma can collect over time without obvious changes in neurological status until its size is sufficient to produce a mass effect. SDH may be managed either surgically or conservatively, dependent on size, clinical presentation and the presence of other comorbidities.

Traumatic subarachnoid haemorrhage

Bleeding into the subarachnoid space is a common clinical finding in TBI patients. Traumatic subarachnoid haemorrhage (SAH) (Fig. 43.11)[16] can develop from the disruption of small pial vessels on the surface of the brain, or extravasation of contusion or haematoma into the subarachnoid space. An SAH is often seen occurring contralateral to site of impact (as seen in contrecoup injuries).

On CT, an acute SAH appears as linear, serpentine areas of high density conforming to cerebral sulci and cisterns. The major clinical associations with SAH are acute hydrocephalus and cerebral vasospasm.[36] Management is focused on minimising secondary brain injury.

Other focal injuries

Intraventricular haemorrhage (IVH) and intracerebral haemorrhage (ICH) (Fig. 43.12) are types of focal injuries. Management

FIGURE 43.11 COMPUTED TOMOGRAPHIC SCAN SHOWING A DIFFUSE, THICK SUBARACHNOID HAEMORRHAGE[37]

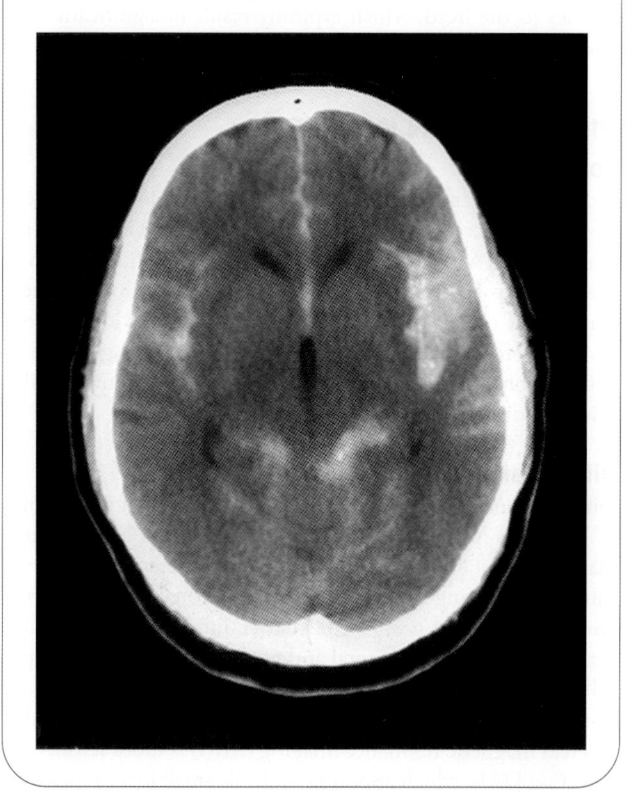

FIGURE 43.12 COMPUTED TOMOGRAPHY: LARGE INTRACEREBRAL HAEMATOMA[33]

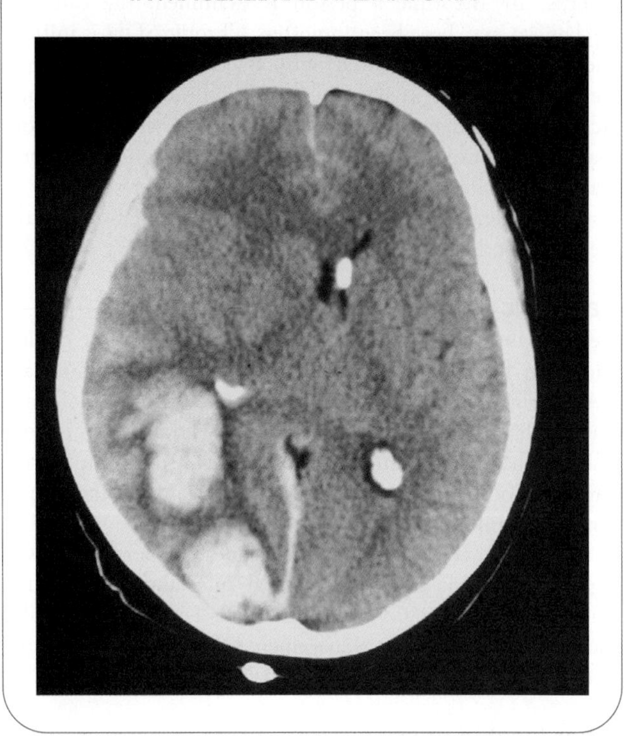

FIGURE 43.13 NON-CONTRAST-ENHANCED COMPUTED TOMOGRAPHIC VIEW OF A GUNSHOT WOUND TO THE HEAD

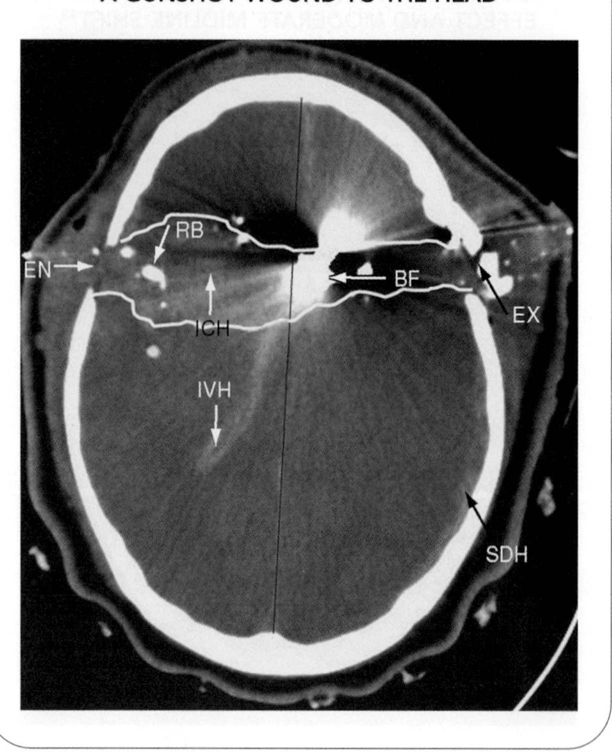

The wound crosses the sagittal plane, and is complicated by intracerebral and subdural haematomas and intraventricular haemorrhage. The permanent cavity is indicated by white lines.[37] *BF: bullet fragment; EN: entrance; EX: exit; ICH: intracerebral haematoma; IVH: intraventricular haemorrhage; RB: retained bone; SDH: subdural haematoma.*

depends on the size and source of bleeding. Surgical evacuation may be necessary in concert with medical management of increased ICP.

Firearms or other projectiles frequently cause penetrating injuries to the head, which typically result in significant focal injuries along the path of entry (Fig. 43.13).

DIFFUSE BRAIN INJURIES

Concussion

A concussion can occur as a result of a direct blow to the head or from an acceleration or deceleration injury in which the brain collides with the inside of the skull. Brief interruption of the reticular activating system may occur, causing transient amnesia. A classic concussion is characterised as loss of consciousness followed by transient neurological changes such as nausea, vomiting, temporary amnesia, headache and possible brief loss of vision.

Diffuse axonal injury

Diffuse axonal injury (DAI) is potentially the most severe form of TBI. This injury is almost always the result of blunt trauma that causes rotational acceleration and deceleration forces, resulting in shearing and disruption of neuronal structures, predominantly at the grey–white matter junction. DAI is most commonly seen in the frontal and temporal lobe (mild), corpus callosum (moderate) and midbrain (severe). On CT, DAI lesions appear as small petechial haemorrhages (Fig. 43.14A),[38] whereas magnetic resonance imaging (MRI) is more sensitive in detecting DAIs, which appear as multiple small foci of increased signal on T2 images (Fig. 43.14B).[38] Prognosis depends on the degree of injury.

- *Mild DAI* is characterised by loss of consciousness for 6–24 hours. Initially the patient may exhibit decerebrate or decorticate posturing, but improves rapidly within 24 hours. Return to baseline neurological status may occur over days, but periods of amnesia may be present.[35] Concussion is the common diagnosis for mild TBI with LOC < 6 hours; however, it is important to note that there have been reports that patients who have experienced an LOC of < 6 hours may have a DAI.[39]
- *Moderate DAI* is a coma lasting longer than 24 hours, possibly extending over a period of days. Brainstem dysfunction (decorticate/decerebrate) posturing is evident almost immediately and may continue until the patient begins to wake. Patients with moderate DAI usually recover, but rarely return to full pre-injury neurological functional capacity.[36]
- *Severe DAI* is characterised by brainstem impairment that does not resolve. Patients with severe DAI remain comatose for days to weeks. Autonomic dysfunction may also be present and overall prognosis is extremely poor.[36]

FIGURE 43.14

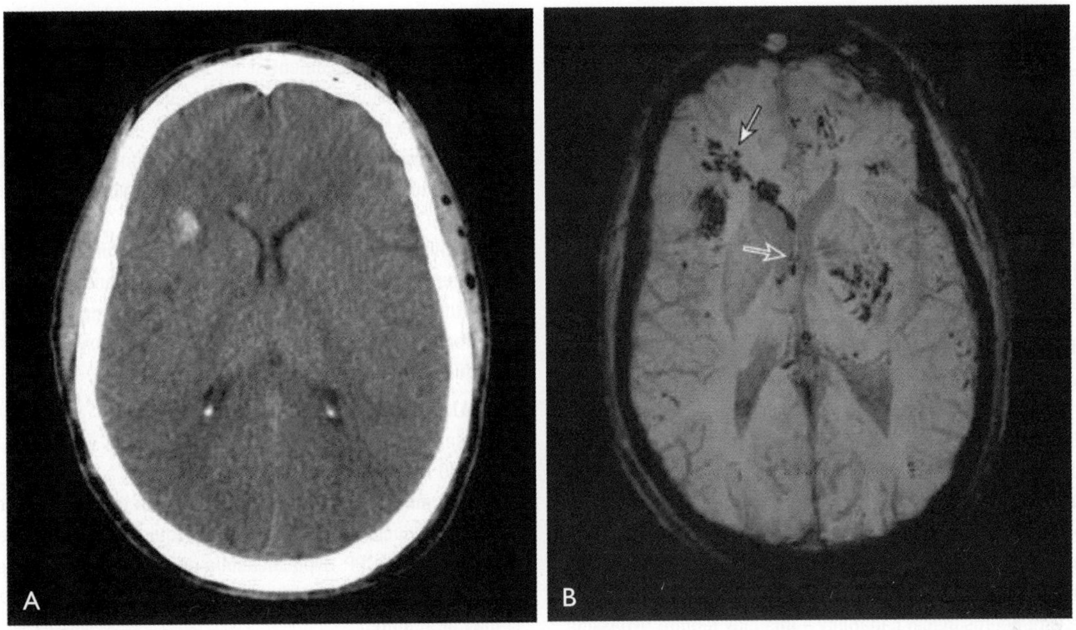

A. Several haemorrhagic lesions are seen at the corner of the right frontal horn in a 31-year-old with DAI following a motor vehicle collision. B. Much more extensive haemorrhagic lesions are apparent in the same region at the corner of the right frontal horn, also involving the genu of the corpus callosum. Lesions not apparent on CT are revealed in the left basal ganglia (solid arrow) and fornix (open arrow).[38]

PATIENT ASSESSMENT AND MANAGEMENT

The assessment of the patient with TBI follows the same systematic primary and secondary survey approach to trauma as discussed in Chapter 42.

PRE-HOSPITAL CONSIDERATIONS

The pre-hospital phase of care for the patient with TBI is an essential component of optimising subsequent recovery for patients.[21] The period that immediately follows a TBI is when cerebral tissue is at its highest risk for secondary injury due to cerebral oedema, disruption of cerebrovascular auto regulation and cerebral ischaemia. Fifty per cent of deaths from TBI occur within the first few hours of injury.[40]

Pre-hospital management should be directed towards prevention and/or limitation of the progression of secondary brain injury while facilitating rapid transport to an appropriate facility capable of providing neurocritical care evaluation and intervention.[17,21] Interventions in the pre-hospital setting should be directed towards maintaining adequate oxygenation, ventilation, blood pressure and monitoring oxygen saturations, end-tidal carbon dioxide ($EtCO_2$), neurological status and pupillary response. Emphasis is placed on regular, repeated observations and meticulous attention to basic supportive care in the field, as these areas have been shown to have the greatest impact on outcomes associated with TBI.[41] It is widely recognised that isolated episodes of hypotension (BP $<$ 90/systolic) or hypoxia (SpO_2 $<$ 90%) following TBI can significantly contribute to injury progression, and pre-hospital management should prioritise the avoidance and correction of these factors while commencing transport. This can be dramatically compounded in the setting of multi-trauma where significant external and internal injuries to other body areas may lead to compromised ventilation and hypo-perfusion. Recognition of the presence of TBI in multi-trauma will guide management towards neuroprotective strategies in preference to other principles of trauma management such as permissive hypotension.[41–45] Airway, breathing and ventilation management in TBI patients in the pre-hospital setting is likely to involve a spectrum of techniques, including manual airway manoeuvres, airway adjuncts and in some circumstances, drug-facilitated intubation using neuromuscular blocking agents.[43,46] Pre-hospital intubation may allow much more precision in ventilation and oxygenation, and allow tighter control of end-tidal CO_2. It is important to recognise that hyperventilation-induced hypocapnia contributes to cerebral vasoconstriction and hypoperfusion. Intubated patients are often inadvertently hyperventilated during resuscitations, causing a theoretical risk for ischaemic brain injury.[42,47] The decision to initiate advanced airway management in the pre-hospital setting needs to be guided by the severity of TBI, the presence of airway compromise and the need for oxygenation, and the transport time to a Major Trauma Centre.

Decompression of tension-pneumothorax and the provision of blood products may be required in the pre-hospital setting to further support oxygenation and perfusion. Severe TBI patients may require seizure control, but it must be recognised that common anti-seizure medication will have an adverse effect on perfusion.

BOX 43.1 **KEY CONCEPTS OF PRE-HOSPITAL TRAUMATIC BRAIN INJURY MANAGEMENT**[41,46]

ASSESSMENT

Primary survey

Correct life threats, ensure airway patency, optimise oxygenation, avoid hypotension and hypoxia

Secondary survey

Observations, including pulse oximetry, Glasgow Coma Scale (GCS)/ pupils, blood glucose level, and $EtCO_2$, invasive blood pressure monitoring and repeat ABGs to titrate ventilation (where pre-hospital scope of practice allows)

DECISION-MAKING

- Recognition of the presence of TBI, the severity of injury and the likely progression of injury
- Minimise out-of-hospital time, initiate early transport while commencing targeted management, provide notification to receiving Trauma Centre
- Remember - definitive care is provided at Major Trauma Centres, pre-hospital management needs to be efficient and expedient
- Direct transport to a Major Trauma Centre with neurosurgical centre with neurosurgical capability - this may require bypassing smaller hospitals
- Transport paediatric patients direct to a paediatric trauma centre (where possible)

AIRWAY

- Use airway adjuncts as required to maintain airway patency and keep $SpO_2 > 92\%$. In pre-hospital or retrieval services with specifically trained clinicians, this may include intubation using rapid sequence induction (RSI). The decision to initiate advanced airway management should be guided by the time and distance to a Major Trauma Centre
- Stabilise cervical spine as required—ensure it does not restrict venous return

BREATHING

- Provide supplemental oxygen, either via non-rebreather mask, bag-mask ventilation, or mechanical ventilation in conjunction with advanced airway management. With short transport times, basic airway management using 100% O_2 and bag-valve-mask ventilation, using an LMA in the absence of a gag reflex, can be just as effective as intubation
- Avoid hyperventilation (unless signs of imminent herniation). Utilise pulse-oximetry and ABGs (where scope of practice allows) to guide mechanical ventilation if utilised
- Recognise and manage major chest injuries in multi-trauma with suspected TBI. Pre-hospital ultrasound and eFAST can help identify tension-pneumothoraces. Chest decompression may be required, and may contribute to improved oxygenation and perfusion

CIRCULATION

Maintain SBP within recommended ranges

- $\geq$ 100 mmHg for patients aged 50–69
- $\geq$ 110 mmHg for patients aged 15–49 or over 70 years old
- Blood products (if carried) may be required to support perfusion and maintain CPP. Hypocalcaemia can result following the use of some blood products, the administration of calcium gluconate may be required
- Address all sources of external haemorrhage. Multiple sites of minor haemorrhage can contribute to cumulative blood loss and lead to hypotension
- Consider the presence of spinal cord injury in multi-trauma with TBI and the added challenges with perfusion management

DISABILITY

- Seizure management in severe TBI patients is rare but may be required
- Correct blood low blood sugar < 4.0 mmol/litre
- Elevate head of bed to 30 degrees where able
- Avoid heat loss - minimise exposure, utilise warming blankets and utilise heaters in ambulance vehicles or aircraft

Diagnosis of specific injuries is difficult in the pre-hospital environment despite the introduction of tools such as ultrasound. Consideration of the scene, mechanism, energy exchange, combined with a thorough assessment and a good understanding of neurological anatomy and physiology will enable the provider to prioritise and optimise care. Key concepts of pre-hospital TBI management are given in Box 43.1.[42–44,46] Chapter 16 contains information on $EtCO_2$ monitoring techniques.

PRIMARY SURVEY AND RESUSCITATION

In the primary survey, early cardiopulmonary stabilisation is essential for patients with severe TBI. Airway patency, maintenance of optimal oxygenation and tissue perfusion are vital, as the brain is adversely affected by secondary insults, particularly hypotension and hypoxia.[48,49] Patients with TBI need to be suspected of having sustained spinal injuries, therefore spinal precautions need to be maintained until cleared. Additionally, nasopharyngeal airways should be avoided in TBI patients until base of skull fractures can be ruled out. See Chapter 16 for airway management techniques.

While permissive hypotensive resuscitation is recommended for the bleeding hypovolaemic trauma patient, patients with head injuries will require slightly higher systolic blood pressure (SBP) until ICP and accurate MAP monitoring are available. While slight variation in systolic blood pressure targets in TBI may be identified in the literature,[42,44] it is recommended that a systolic blood pressure of > 110 mmHg be maintained for cerebral perfusion in adults.[50]

As level of consciousness is affected by both hypoxia and hypotension, any neurological assessments undertaken in the presence of these abnormalities should be well documented and repeated following correction. Consideration should also be given to the impact of alcohol and other drugs on neurological evaluation. Additionally, as noted in Chapters 13 and 16, it is important that an early blood glucose level (BGL) is established to eliminate BGL abnormalities as a potential cause of an altered conscious state and treated appropriately.

SECONDARY SURVEY AND ASSESSMENT

A formal secondary survey should only occur after completion of the primary survey, which includes the identification and treatment of lifesaving injuries. The assessing clinician should also consider the overall scene in order to appreciate the mechanism of injury and energy exchange. This can assist in identifying potential injuries and focus acute management strategies. For specifics regarding secondary survey and patient assessment refer to Chapters 42 and 13. While all aspects of secondary survey are required, it is essential that GCS, pupil examination and neurological assessment are always included for patients with TBI. If at any stage the patient deteriorates during the secondary survey, then the clinician needs to repeat a primary survey, communicate and escalate findings.

TIME TO DEFINITIVE CARE AND PATIENT DISPOSITION

All patients with TBI need careful consideration regarding their disposition. Ideal management of severe TBI patients begins with rapid transport to a tertiary facility with neurosurgical capability and early aggressive resuscitation, with meticulous airway and blood-pressure management.[43,48]

In Australia, patients can be vast distances and many hours from a major neurosurgical centre. Distance complicates the provision of emergency care for TBI.[51] In rural and remote settings an emphasis should be placed on airway protection, maintenance of adequate ventilation, and maintenance of sufficient circulation to achieve cerebral perfusion and brain tissue oxygenation while awaiting transfer/transport to a definitive centre.[51] Early consultation with the retrieval service and receiving facility specialists will assist in the coordination of patients' requirements and retrieval resources. Consider using Box 43.2 as a guide to ensure all relevant information is conveyed, and Box 43.3 as a guide to patient preparation for transfer.

BOX 43.2 TRAUMATIC BRAIN INJURY COMMUNICATION REGARDING ASSESSMENT AND REFERRAL[42]

COMMUNICATION

- **Patient age and mechanism of injury**
- **Pre-injury health, including regular medications**
- **Head CT findings (if available)**
- **Post resuscitation GCS with detailed neurological exam**
- **Completed interventions**
- **Focal motor findings**
- **Coagulation status and other pertinent laboratory findings**
- **Other injuries**
- **State of C-spine: cleared, not cleared, injury**
- **Current vital signs**

BOX 43.3 OTHER CLINICAL CARE PRIORITIES THAT WILL ASSIST BOTH PATIENT PREPAREDNESS FROM TRANSFER, AND OUTCOME

- **Scalp wounds are a source of significant blood loss**
  - **Where possible, these should be irrigated and closed prior to transfer**
  - **Any scalp wound left unsutured should be covered with a saline-soaked dressing**
- **Dressing and haemorrhage control for any other traumatic wounds**
- **Splinting and immobilisation of long bone fractures**
- **Ensure at least two points of intravenous access are secured**
- **Sites of suspected CSF leak should be covered with a bolster, do not pack**
- **Placement of an indwelling catheter**
- **Consider gastric tube insertion for protracted emesis and intubated patients.**

RADIOLOGY

Computed tomography (CT) remains the emergency neuroimaging modality of choice. Despite advances in magnetic resonance imaging (MRI) technology, CT acquisition is faster, is more reliable in identifying surgical lesions and is more practical for the critically injured patient.[2]

X-ray

Skull x-rays have limited application in the management of TBI.[36] Where CT scanning is unavailable, skull x-ray may be used as an adjunct to identify patients with skull fractures who are at greater risk of intracranial injury.[52] The presence of a skull fracture increases the probability of intracranial pathology and, therefore, increases the risk of deterioration.[53]

Computed tomography

CT scan remains the modality of choice for the initial assessment of acute head injury.

- CT is widely available in most urban centres and is a fast, highly accurate investigation for the detection of skull fractures and acute intracranial haemorrhage, and easily accommodates critical care support equipment.
- CT is recommended for all adult patients with moderate-to-severe TBI, and patients with open/depressed/skull base fractures, focal neurological deficit, or > 1 vomit post head injury.[54]
- CT angiography can be performed in addition when vascular injury or involvement is suspected. Traumatic vascular injuries are commonly associated with skull-base fractures.[55]

Magnetic resonance imaging

MRI is recommended for patients with acute TBI whose neurological findings are unexplained by CT. MRI is more sensitive for thin extra-axial smear collections, non-haemorrhagic lesions, brainstem injuries and SAH compared to conventional CT. The use of fluid-attenuated inversion recovery (FLAIR) imaging in

BOX 43.4 IMAGING OPTIONS FOR TRAUMATIC BRAIN INJURY (TBI)[53,56,57]

SKULL X-RAY
- as a screening tool in rural and remote settings, in absence of CT availability

COMPUTED TOMOGRAPHY (CT) IN ACUTE SETTING
- moderate and severe TBI; GCS < 13
- mild TBI with concurrent risks
- suspected skull fracture

MAGNETIC RESONANCE IMAGING IN ACUTE SETTINGS
- neurological findings unexplained on CT
- suspected DAI

ANGIOGRAPHY
- suspected vascular injury or infarction

conjunction with MRI improves the detection of focal cortical and white matter shearing injuries, such as DAI. Due to the magnetic field, limited critical-care support and equipment can be used on patients while in the MRI suite. A summary of imaging options for TBI is given in Box 43.4.[53,56]

ESSENTIAL CARE

The first priority for emergency and neurosurgical specialists caring for the head-injured patient is rapid resuscitation and stabilisation. It is important that clinicians identify and treat factors that may contribute to further brain injury, such as hypoxia, hypercapnia, hypotension, deranged BGLs and fever. Hypoxia and hypotension during the immediate post-injury period substantially increase the rate of morbidity and mortality.[58]

After initial stabilisation, consider other interventions that promote the return of optimal neurological function and reduce the risk of secondary brain injury. General guidelines for care of the patient with a head injury include ensuring a patent airway, ventilatory support to achieve oxygenation and carbon dioxide targets, ongoing neurological assessment, administration of pharmacological agents as needed (i.e. analgesia, anticonvulsants), optimal patient positioning, temperature management and other interventions based on patient condition.

Current recommendations for treatment of severe head injury specify that interventions to reduce ICP should be considered in the presence of clinical signs of cerebral herniation (Fig. 43.15). Signs include unilateral or bilateral pupillary dilation, asymmetric pupillary reactivity, motor posturing or continued neurological deterioration after physiological stability has been restored.[59]

Frequently, concomitant cervical spine trauma can be associated with TBI; therefore, cervical spine stabilisation should be maintained until adequate medical imaging examinations

FIGURE 43.15 CEREBRAL HERNIATION

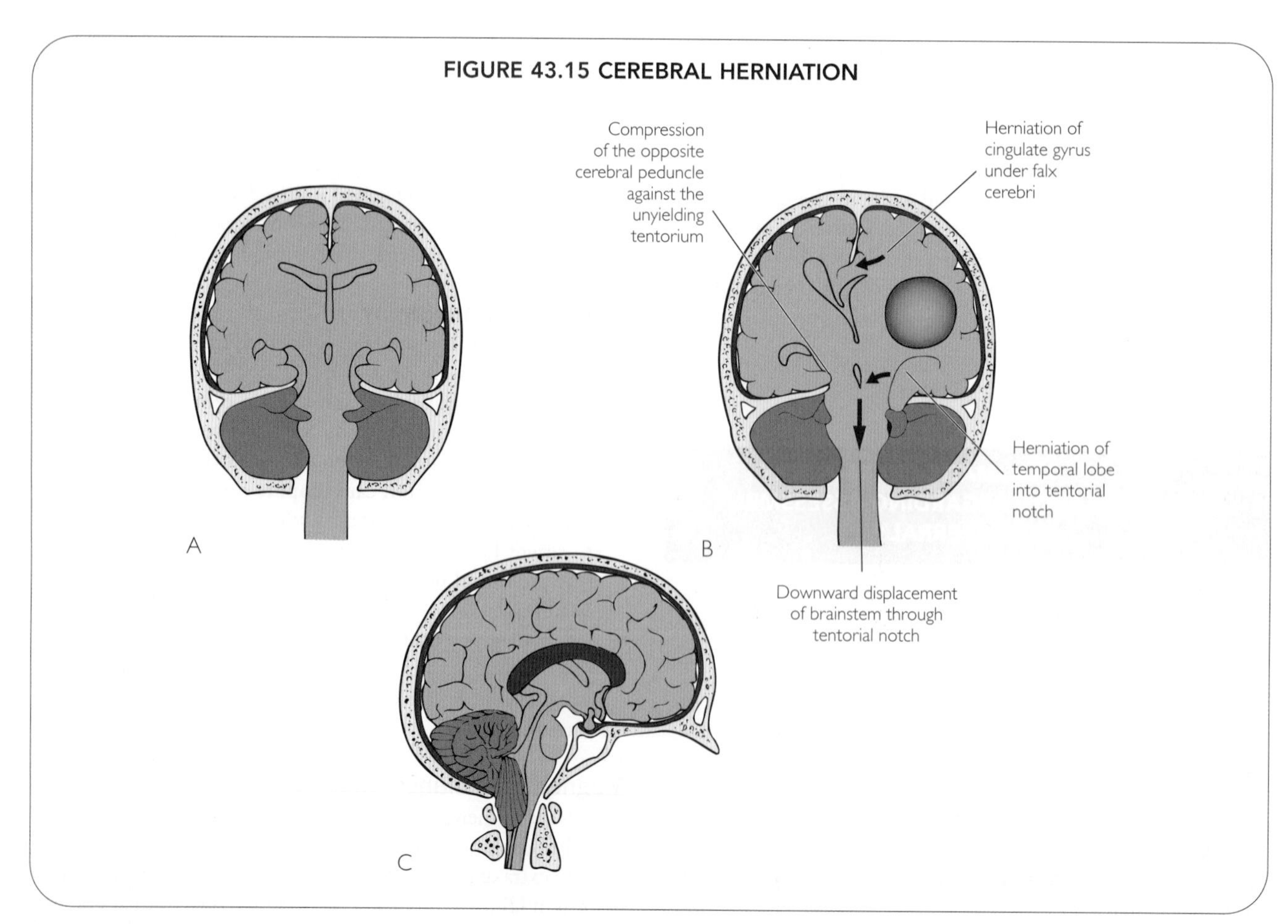

A. Normal relationship of intracranial structures. **B.** Shift of intracranial structures. **C.** Downward herniation of the cerebellar tonsils into the foramen magnum.

TABLE 43.1 ESSENTIAL NURSING CARE OF THE PATIENT WITH A TRAUMATIC BRAIN INJURY[21]

NURSING CARE ELEMENT	INTERVENTION	RATIONALE
GCS assessment	Half-hourly GCS monitoring for at least 4 hours after any TBI, then as ordered by the doctor	Enables early detection of deterioration in neurological status
	In a handover situation: the GCS should be done together with the nurse to whom the patient is being handed over, to ensure consistency in assessment and documentation	Inter-rater reliability in GCS assessments by nurses is problematic: this is a mitigation strategy
Head of bed elevation	30°–45° elevation	Promotes venous drainage of brain and reduces ICP
Cervical collar	Early clearance is key. Soft collars are recommended and may be removed in consultation with medical staff in intubated patients if sedation is adequate.	The neck can swell over the first 24 hours, and the collar can become constrictive and impair cranial venous return and cause a raised ICP Re-apply prior to all log rolls
Adequate analgesia and sedation	Careful patient monitoring for signs of pain and agitation; observe for tearing, tachycardia and ventilatory asynchrony in intubated patients Initial use of short-acting analgesia and sedation is preferred	Maintain normal ICP Reduce cerebral oxygen consumption and metabolism Optimise mechanical ventilation
Temperature monitoring; core temperature often rises in response to injury	Intubated patients should have continuous thermal monitoring—aim for normothermia	Avoid hyperthermia: as the core temperature rises, CO_2 production increases High $PaCO_2$ can cause raised ICP
Clustering of care	Group nursing interventions to provide a longer episode of rest, i.e. suctioning/washes/turns, mouth/eye care, etc.	Reduces noxious stimuli

exclude cervical spine trauma, or diagnosis and precautions are confirmed. Avoid compression of internal or external jugular veins with a tight cervical collar or tape fixation of the endotracheal tube as this can impede cerebral venous drainage and result in an increase in the ICP.[50] In patients with TBI, ensure the acute management plan clarifies options for collar release or removal. See Chapters 16 and 45 for discussion on cervical collars. Instigating a 'head-up bed tilt' while maintaining a neutral spine alignment, or if the patient condition permits elevating the head of the bed to 30°, may also facilitate venous drainage and ICP reduction.[50]

Table 43.1 outlines a number of key elements in the ongoing care of the patient with TBI, who require close observation and vigilance regarding early signs of deterioration.

An integral component of caring for head-injured patients is inclusion of the family or significant others in the plan of care. Head injuries can be overwhelming for the family; psychosocial support and education regarding the injury cannot be over-emphasised.

Following resuscitation and early CT imaging, it is the role of the emergency nurse to advocate for the patient to be transferred to an appropriate inpatient clinical setting for ongoing acute management. In many moderate and severe TBI cases this may be an intensive care or high dependency unit; in time-critical injuries such as symptomatic EDH, the patient is likely to go directly to theatre. Box 43.1 provides a succinct summary of key goals for initial TBI management with a particular focus on the pre-hospital setting. The application may differ in other settings such as remote clinics or regional hospitals, but the underlying principles and goals remain the same.

Oxygen and suction

To assist in the prevention of hypoxia, oxygen should be administered to all patients with signs and symptoms of TBI in the initial phase of care, especially in the multi-trauma patient. There are risks associated with both hypoxaemia and hyperoxaemia and, as such, oxygen should be considered as a drug that is prescribed and administered for specific indications, with a documented target oxygen saturation range, and with regular monitoring of the patient's response.[60] Hypoxia is generally accepted as an SpO_2 below 90%.[61] Variable targets enable wider clinical application and allow for inaccuracies in SpO_2 monitoring (these have been provided within the Australian and Aotearoa New Zealand context). ANZCOR and Trauma Victoria guidelines generally recommend SpO_2 of 94%–98%.[50,62]

As noted earlier in the chapter, a patent airway is required to provide appropriate oxygenation, with airway assistance options discussed in more detail in Chapter 16. The chosen option will depend upon the skill of the provider, patient requirement and resources available, with the preference to employ basic options first. Airway patency is essential and at times suctioning of the airway may be required; however, it is important to remember that suctioning of the airway in TBI can increase ICP[63] and removes oxygen from the airway, increasing the risk of hypoxia. Box 43.5 provides recommendations for safe suctioning on an endotracheal tube.

BOX 43.5 RECOMMENDATIONS FOR SAFE ENDOTRACHEAL SUCTIONING[64,65]

- Suctioning a patient with TBI is known to increase ICP
- Preoxygenate pre and post
- Suction only when necessary
- The suction catheter should occlude less than half the lumen of the endotracheal tube
- Use low suction pressure
- Avoid stimulation of the carina
- Avoid suctioning for longer than 15 seconds
- Avoid intermittent suctioning

Glasgow Coma Scale and pupil assessment

The GCS is a widely recognised and universal tool used for scoring consciousness and is explained in Chapter 13. Completing the GCS allows assignment of numerical values to clinical findings and assists in recognition of trends in neurological changes, facilitates prognostication and is a component to evaluating the severity of TBI.

PRACTICE TIP

- **GCS tips**
- Aim to acquire the highest level of response with the least stimulus.
- Watch for subtle changes in the level of consciousness. These are often early signs of deterioration in the patient with TBI.
- Where the GCS is < 15: Document by components, i.e.: E= / V= / M=

Interpretation of the GCS must be correlated with other clinical assessment findings. The presence of other physiological conditions, such as hypotension, hypothermia, abnormal blood glucose level, alcohol or intoxication, may artificially lower the total GCS score. Likewise, pre-injury impaired cognition, such as aphasia, will also artificially lower the GCS. In the absence of previously identified physiological conditions, a patient with a total GCS < 9 suggests a severe head injury. The motor response is a good indicator of overall nervous system function and integrity of cerebral cortex and spinal cord.[66]

The Paediatric GCS is an adapted version of the adult scale. Table 43.2 illustrates adult and age-appropriate paediatric responses. Paediatric GCS is described in Chapter 35.

Abnormal motor responses include inequality in movement from side to side, and posturing.

- Decorticate posturing is rigid flexion with arms flexed towards the core and lower extremities extended. This type of posturing is associated with lesions above the midbrain.
- Decerebrate posturing is rigid extension of the arms with wrist flexion and rigid extension of lower extremities. This type of posturing is associated with an insult to the brainstem.

TABLE 43.2 GLASGOW COMA SCALE: ADULT AND PAEDIATRIC[66]

ADULT		PAEDIATRIC
E: eye opening		
Spontaneous	**4**	Spontaneous
To speech	**3**	To speech
To pain	**2**	To pain
None	**1**	None
V: Verbal response—Best		
Orientated to time and place	**5**	Coos, babbles
Confused speech	**4**	Cries, but consolable
Inappropriate words	**3**	Persistently irritable
Incomprehensible sounds	**2**	Grunts to pain / restless
No response	**1**	No response
M: Motor response—Best		
Obeys command	**6**	Normal movements
Localises to pain	**5**	Localises to pain
Withdraws to pain	**4**	Withdraws to pain
Flexion (Decorticate)	**3**	Flexion (Decorticate)
Extension (Decerebrate)	**2**	Extension (Decerebrate)
No response	**1**	No response

The distinction between these two postures is important, as the decerebrate posture indicates a deeper level of coma. Fig. 43.16 illustrates decerebrate and decorticate posturing. If a patient's motor component of the GCS changes from decorticate to decerebrate, an immediate neurosurgical consult should be sought, as it may indicate rising ICP. Lateralisation occurs when patients with TBI have clinical signs of unilateral decorticate and decerebrate posturing. Posturing may be spontaneous or elicited by verbal or painful stimuli.

While not a component of the GCS, assessment of pupils is essential in patients with potential and confirmed TBI, as an abnormal pupillary response to light can indicate intracranial pathology. Normal pupillary response to direct light examination is constriction. Consensual reaction (constriction of the opposite pupil) should occur with direct light examination. Anisocoria, or unequal pupils, is a normal finding in 20–25% of the population, so assessment of reactivity in the dilated pupil is critical. Focal lesions, such as EDHs or SDHs, can cause pupil dilation as a result of compression of the third cranial nerve. Unequal pupils or bilaterally dilated pupils may suggest severe intracranial pathology and urgent neurosurgical intervention needs to be considered. Bilateral fixed and dilated pupils are indicative of impending cerebral herniation.[67]

Accurate GCS scoring and pupil assessment during the early management allows evaluation of neurological progress over time.

FIGURE 43.16 DECORTICATE AND DECEREBRATE POSTURING[28]

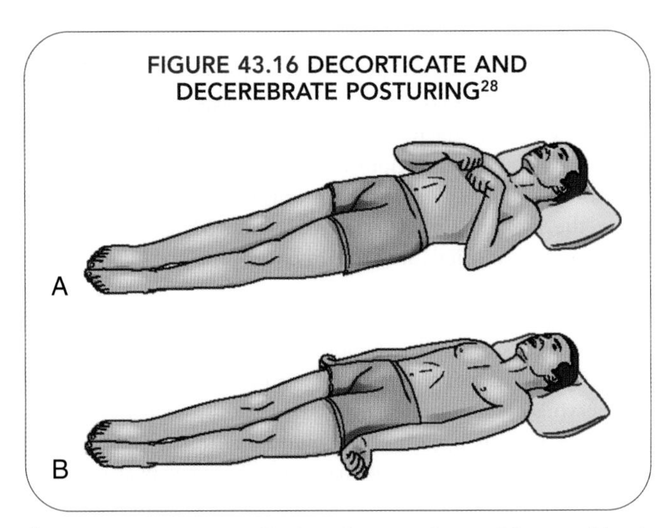

A. Decorticate response. Flexion of arms, wrists and fingers with adduction in upper extremities. Extension, internal rotation and plantar flexion in lower extremities. **B.** Decerebrate response. All four extremities in rigid extension, with hyperpronation of forearms and plantar flexion of feet.

PRACTICE TIP

GCS: Notify medical officer immediately if:

- ≥ 2 point reduction, at any time
- ≥ 1 point reduction in a GCS ≤ 9
- Always repeat the GCS assessment during handover to ensure both clinicians are clear and consistent on the interpretation of assessment findings

Note: Do not assume that anisocoria (unequal pupils) is pre-existing.

Intracranial pressure (ICP)

In the adult patient, the skull is a closed box containing the brain, CSF and blood. For ICP to remain within normal limits (0–15 mmHg), an increase in blood, CSF or brain mass must be accompanied by a reciprocal decrease of one of the other components. This is referred to as the Monro-Kellie doctrine.[1] Any condition that causes cerebral swelling, intracranial mass or reduces the flow of CSF or cerebral blood flow will affect ICP. In the acute phase of TBI, these are all likely. Sustained ICP > 20 mmHg is a neurosurgical emergency associated with increased mortality and morbidity.[1] Failure to reduce ICP may subsequently cause additional ischaemia and necrosis of brain tissue.

To measure ICP a monitoring device is inserted via a burr hole into the brain using an intraventricular, parenchymal or subdural catheter. ICP monitoring aids the detection of intracranial mass lesions, guides adjunctive therapies to control ICP and, with certain monitoring devices, such as an external ventricular drain, may facilitate a reduction in ICP by CSF drainage.[41] A further function of ICP monitoring is to allow a derived calculation of cerebral perfusion pressure.

Cerebral perfusion pressure

Cerebral perfusion pressure (CPP) is defined as the pressure gradient across the cerebral vascular bed, between blood inflow and outflow. Inflow pressure is taken as mean arterial pressure (MAP).[41] CPP is measured as the difference between the mean arterial pressure (MAP) and the ICP (CPP = MAP – ICP). To prevent cerebral ischaemia and secondary brain injury a target CPP of 60 to 70 mmHg is recommended.[2,41] Vasopressor agents, such as noradrenaline, can be used to augment MAP; however, care must be taken in the context of trauma to ensure that the underlying causative factor for hypotension is not hypovolaemia.[68]

A key factor in monitoring the CPP is accurate placement of the arterial pressure transducer. The arterial transducer should be level with and zeroed to the foramen of Monro. Failure to do this will result in either an under- or an over-estimation of CPP, which has the potential of being harmful to patients.[69]

PRACTICE TIP

- ICP zero point: external anatomical landmarks for the foramen of Munro
- Head elevated position: outer canthus of the eye
- Low Fowlers or supine position: the tragus, the top of the ear, or the external auditory canal

Glucose control

Hyperglycaemia is a common secondary insult in TBI, SAH and acute ischaemic stroke, and has repeatedly been associated with poor neurological outcome.[70] Ischaemia plays a major role in the pathology of injured brain and low cerebral glucose values are detected in ischaemia.[71] To date, the optimal glycaemic target range is uncertain and may not be uniform among TBI patients, varying between individuals at different time points during the clinical course. Future studies are needed to explore an optimal and safe glycaemic target range, to facilitate critical care of blood glucose control and to further research the relationship between brain cell metabolism and hyperglycaemia after severe TBI.[45,72] At present, avoidance of both hypo- and hyperglycaemia is appropriate.[71]

Coagulopathy and anticoagulation/antiplatelet awareness

The occurrence of coagulopathy in TBI patients, including those with isolated TBI, is high. Incidence approaches 40%–50% in severe TBI.[2] Any process that results in an increase in haemorrhage mass will affect ICP and should be addressed urgently. Identification of a pre-existing or rapidly acquired coagulopathy is important in the first critical hour and during the remainder of the hospital stay.[73]

Physiologically induced coagulopathy can be further compounded by the patient's past history, which may involve their prescription of anticoagulation or antiplatelet medications. It is important to promptly communicate any suspicion that the patient might be using any anticoagulation or antiplatelet medication to ensure relevant pathology is collected. Patients taking warfarin may be managed with prothrombin complex concentrate (PCC), fresh frozen plasma (FFP) and/or vitamin K, if identified as at risk of developing a warfarin-associated intracerebral haemorrhage.[74]

Tranexamic acid (TXA) should be considered for all trauma patients and ideally within 3 hours following injury. TXA inhibits the enzymatic breakdown of fibrin, therefore minimising excessive blood loss in surgical patients and the haemorrhage risk in patients with traumatic injuries.[48] While TXA has been shown to have significant benefit in reducing bleeding in trauma and surgery, further studies are required to determine the effectiveness in preventing progressive intracranial bleeding in patients with moderate–severe TBI.

Patients taking direct/novel oral anticoagulants (DOACs/NOACs) such as rivaroxaban, apixaban, dabigatran will need early input from haematology to guide effective reversal without thrombotic complications. Andexanet alfa is the antidote for apixaban and rivaroxaban; however, this is not yet approved for use in Australia. Idarucizumab is the reversal agent for dabigatran; however, its availability in Australia is often limited to major trauma hospitals. In addition to Vitamin K, TXA and PCC, recombinant activated factor VIIa (Novoseven) may be considered in life-threatening situations, but in consultation with a haemotologist.[50,75]

Osmotherapy

The use of intravenous solutions that exert an osmotic diuretic effect have been the mainstay of treatment for a critically elevated ICP. While there is insufficient clinical outcome evidence to support the use of specific agents,[42,48,75] mannitol 20% and hypertonic saline (> 1.5% saline) are the two most common agents used in Australia and Aotearoa New Zealand.

Mannitol 20% solution is an osmotic diuretic that reduces ICP by changing the osmotic gradient, causing fluid to leave cerebral extracellular tissues and move to intravascular beds. Movement of fluid reduces total brain mass, therefore decreasing ICP. A decision to utilise mannitol should be restricted to patients with signs of cerebral herniation or progressive neurological deterioration not attributable to extracranial causes.[43]

Prior to administration of mannitol the patient's overall volume status should be assessed. Ideally systolic blood pressure should be >110 mmHg prior to administration of bolus doses of 0.25–1.0 g/kg over 20 minutes.[2,58] The effect of mannitol is rapid, within 20–50 minutes, with a therapeutic duration of 2–8 hours.[76]

PRACTICE TIP

MANNITOL USE

Mannitol should be considered as a temporising therapy designed to provide time for confirmation of diagnosis or access to neurosurgical intervention.

- Administer only after neurosurgical consult or via established algorithmic pathways.

Hypertonic saline solutions of various concentrations are widely used for the interim treatment of raised ICP. Hypertonic saline has been shown to decrease cerebral water content and ICP with at least the same efficacy as mannitol. Hypertonic saline infusion causes plasma expansion via redistribution of fluid from the intravascular space and thus may be useful in patients who are hypotensive.[2] The resultant increase in MAP is achieved with less volume required than with isotonic fluids. Suggested doses of hypertonic saline to achieve effective reduction in ICP are 6–8 mL/kg of a 3% solution, or 4 mL/kg of 7.5% solution, given as a bolus or, alternatively, rapid infusion.[50] Higher concentrations of hypertonic saline solutions are available, such as 23.4%, and administered volumes are lower given the higher concentration of saline. Major trauma and neurosurgical hospitals are more likely to carry the higher saline concentrations.

There are a number of side-effects associated with the use of osmotic agents, including hypotension as a consequence of an induced diuresis and the accumulation of the agent in the central nervous system (which may paradoxically increase ICP) in the context of disruption of the blood–brain barrier. Inotropic support may be required to maintain SBP goal post osmotherapy.[42,43] It is important to remember that, as with hyperventilation, osmotic diuretics should be utilised only when signs of impending cerebral herniation are evident, as a temporising measure while neurosurgical intervention is considered.

OTHER THERAPIES AND CONSIDERATIONS

Seizure prophylaxis

Seizure activity can cloud the neurological evaluation in the acute phase, aggravate intracranial pathology and, in some patients, be the precipitating event that leads to herniation.[2] To minimise the risk of early seizure activity in patients with moderate and severe TBI, seizure prophylaxis should be administered. Levetiracetam and phenytoin are commonly administered seizure prophylaxis. Side-effects include complications related to prolonged sedation and acquired infections.

Prophylactic anti-convulsant therapy in closed head injury is usually not indicated beyond the first week. A neurosurgical consult is recommended if seizures occur and for general advice about prophylactic anticonvulsant therapy.

Infection prophylaxis

Intracranial infection may occur from any injury that enables contact of contaminants directly with cerebral tissue, for example, base of skull (BOS) fracture, compound skull fracture, CSF otorrhoea and rhinorrhoea. In these cases, the routine use of antibiotics is not recommended and neurosurgical consultation is advised.[77]

Severe TBI increases a patient's susceptibility to infection because of necessary intubation and mechanical ventilation to prevent airway obstruction, aspiration and consequential hypoxia, in addition to invasive monitoring. Infection risks, such as ventilator associated events (VAE) and central line associated bacteraemia, are increased in all critically ill patients.[42]

DVT prophylaxis

In addition to compression stockings, pharmacological prophylaxis may be considered if the brain injury is stable and the benefit is considered to outweigh the risk of increased intracranial haemorrhage.[42] Neurosurgical consultation should occur in order to determine the most appropriate medication and commencement.

Sedation

Patients who are intubated and mechanically ventilated commonly receive propofol for sedation. Propofol is widely used because its pharmacokinetic profile allows easy control of sedation and rapid wakening.[43] The use of propofol may directly correlate with the need for vasopressors, and caution is required as high dose propofol contributes to increased morbidity.[42] Patients with severe TBI will require deep sedation while in hospital until the neurosurgical team confirm the patient's ICP has been controlled. This is often achieved with a combination of fentanyl, midazolam and propofol. See Chapter 14 for post intubation/resuscitation care.

Sedation for non-intubated patients who are confused or agitated needs to be carefully considered and discussed with the neurosurgical team, as administration of sedation can impair neurological assessments.

Analgesia

Before prescribing analgesia, it is important to determine the cause of restlessness; for example, cerebral hypoxia from airway inadequacy, poor ventilation or poor perfusion, raised intracranial pressure, pain, alcohol intoxication or a full bladder. Medications other than paracetamol or codeine phosphate require neurosurgical consultation.

Multi-trauma patients with TBI requiring pain relief other than for headache may be given small incremental doses of a short-acting narcotic. Where CNS-depressant analgesics are used, such as those containing opiates, careful attention must be paid to monitoring the patient's neurological status. It is important to ensure that patients who have a TBI and are intubated receive sufficient analgesia, as pain contributes to increased ICP.

There are a number of non-pharmacological methods for treating pain, including reducing noxious stimuli by providing a quiet and dark environment, and allowing family to comfort the patient (providing they are not causing overstimulation). The intermittent use of cold packs can also provide an analgesic effect.

PRACTICE TIP

- **Non-pharmacological analgesia adjuncts**
- Reduce stimuli
- Aim for a quiet/dark environment: outside of the ED
- Position of comfort: preferably with head of bed elevated
- Consider cold packs
- Where possible, transfer to ward bed

FUTURE MONITORING

Hypothesis pertaining to monitoring and protocol-driven interventions for TBI management continue to be tested. Jugular venous oxygen saturation monitoring, brain-tissue oxygen monitoring, brain temperature monitoring and cerebral micro dialysis are all but a few of the current phenomena being researched. The near future will bring multimodal monitoring where multiple parameters can be successfully monitored via the one catheter.

At present, the only advanced monitoring modality supported by literature is that of jugular venous oxygen saturation. Current thinking recommends $< 50\%$ as the likely threshold to avoid in order to reduce mortality and improve outcomes.[42] Refer to the links at the end of this chapter for the most contemporary developments in TBI.

CONTROVERSIES IN CONTEMPORARY PRACTICE

Controlled or transient hyperventilation

Patients with severe TBI require definitive airway protection because they are at risk of pulmonary aspiration or compromised respiratory drive and function. Normal ventilation is currently the goal for severe TBI patients in the absence of cerebral herniation and normal partial pressure of carbon dioxide in arterial blood ($PaCO_2$) ranges from 35 to 45 mmHg, with the recommendation being to ventilate the patient to achieve the lower normal range ($PaCO_2$ 35–40 mmHg).[42]

The safety of hyperventilation is debatable,[47] and should be reserved as a temporising measure for those patients with unequivocal signs of raised ICP or impending cerebral herniation (witnessed neurological deterioration or lateralising signs or pupillary dilation) while neurosurgical intervention is considered.[43] In the instance where hyperventilation is required, physiological monitoring should be employed as changes in cerebral perfusion secondary to variations in $PaCO_2$ occur rapidly. Hypocapnia-induced cerebral vasoconstriction puts patients at risk for ischaemic brain injury and poorer functional outcomes.

For clinicians who lack cerebral oximetry monitoring, $EtCO_2 < 30$ mmHg has an effect on cerebral physiology, as $PaCO_2$ is a major determinant of cerebral vessel calibre and excessive hypocapnia may cause critical cerebral vasoconstriction and a reduction in cerebral blood flow (CBF).[43] Healthcare providers should be judicious with the use of hyperventilation/hypocapnia and should remain cognisant of the risks of inadvertent hyperventilation with the use of manual ventilation or bagging during resuscitation.[47]

PRACTICE TIP

Routine hyperventilation is not endorsed.[42]

It is reserved as a last-ditch 'rescue manoeuvre' when herniation is imminent and other means do not control high ICP.[43]

Thermoregulation

In the pre-hospital setting, hypothermia, when combined with acidosis, coagulopathy and hypocalcaemia, has been associated with poor long-term outcomes following major trauma.[78] Preventing hypothermia in this context is important, particularly when haemorrhage control is difficult to achieve. The use of fluid warmers when administering blood products and diligent patient packaging will help prevent further heat loss.

A rise in body temperature is common in the first few days of hospital admission after TBI as a result of the systemic inflammatory response to injury and direct damage to the hypothalamic control centres for thermoregulation. A rising core temperature can result in increased CO_2 production and may exacerbate injury via intracellular derangements and increased blood–brain permeability, which adds to cerebral oedema.[79]

Data from animal studies and observational case series in humans support the practice of avoiding fever and maintaining a normal body temperature; however, to date there have been no studies demonstrating that maintaining a normal temperature after TBI improves patient outcomes.

Induced hypothermia is a potential therapeutic strategy that remains controversial.[42] The hypothesis is that induced hypothermia may have neuroprotective properties, preventing or altering the biological cascade that causes secondary brain injury.

Steroids

Steroid use for reducing ICP in TBI patients in order to improve outcomes is not recommended. The use of high-dose methylprednisolone in severe TBI is contraindicated and associated with increased mortality.[42]

MILD TRAUMATIC BRAIN INJURY

Mild traumatic brain injury (mTBI) is a major public health concern, given the large number of patients affected each year. Approximately 80% of all TBI cases are categorised as mild head injuries, but this is believed to be conservative as it does not account for incidents of TBI in which the person does not seek medical care.[80]

Many patients admitted with an mTBI will exhibit subacute cognitive deficits, particularly in attention, memory, reasoning and thought-processing. In most cases recovery occurs within 3 months;[81] however, approximately 15%–25% of cases will experience ongoing symptoms, which can include headaches, dizziness, visual disturbance, memory difficulties, poor concentration, difficulty dividing attention, alcohol intolerance, fatigue, irritability, depression and anxiety.[82]

The difficulty associated with the assessment of these patients is that the cognitive deficits associated with mTBI are often too subtle to detect by routine examination.[82] Typically, symptoms subside naturally and recovery occurs within 3 months post injury. Some patients will experience at least one post-concussion symptom persisting beyond 3 months.[83]

ASSESSMENT OF MILD TRAUMATIC BRAIN INJURY

Deficits resulting from mTBI can cause a disruption in a person's ability to perform the activities of daily life. It is essential that all patients who present with mTBI have a thorough assessment, including both a cognitive and a functional assessment. The Abbreviated Westmead Post-traumatic Amnesia Scale (A-WPTAS) assesses PTA in patients with mild TBI.[84] Taking approximately 3 minutes to complete, the A-WPTAS is conducted within 24 hours of injury for patients with a GCS of 13–15. It includes the eye and motor response scales from the Glasgow Coma Scale (GCS), five orientation items and three novel memory items.[85] The A-WPTAS has been validated in adults[84] and facilitates detection of PTA in individuals with mTBI with normal levels of consciousness (GCS scores of 15).[86] A-WPTAS is reliable for use in children aged 7 years and older.[87] A patient is considered to be out of PTA the first time they attain a score of 18 out of 18.[86]

If the patient does not pass the A-WPTAS after 4 hours post-injury time, has a GCS of < 13 at the time of injury, or emerged from coma after 24 hours after injury, the full Westmead PTA scale should be commenced. For further information see the A-WPTAS education and screening tools webpage (see Useful websites).

SPORTS-RELATED mTBI (CONCUSSION)

The definition of concussion applied by both health and research staff is a point of conjecture with concerns that the term under-represents the potential severity.[87] Signs and symptoms that include headaches, dizziness, sleep disturbance and cognitive impairments, are all recognised as being associated with 'mild traumatic brain injury'.[87]

The Australian Institute of Sport states that, 'Concussion is a type of brain injury, induced by a force to the head or anywhere on the body, which transmits an impulsive force to the head'.[88] It commonly causes short-lived neurological impairment and the symptoms may evolve over the hours or days following the injury.[88] Symptoms may present directly after the traumatic force is applied or hours or even days later.

Sports-related concussion (SRC) is often defined as representing the immediate and transient symptoms of TBI.[89] At present, there is no perfect diagnostic test or marker that clinicians can rely on for an immediate diagnosis of SRC in the sporting environment. Because of evolving physiological processes, it is not possible to rule out SRC when an injury event occurs associated with a transient neurological symptom. In all suspected cases of SRC, the individual should be removed from the playing field and assessed by a licensed healthcare provider.[89]

An assessment of concussion/SRC must involve evaluation of the individual's cognitive function, assessing memory, attention/concentration, orientation and amnesia. An example of an assessment tool for health professional use is the Sports Concussion Assessment Tool (SCAT). The Concussion in Sport Group (CISG) released the SCAT5 (5th edn) following the Fifth International Consensus Conference on Concussion in Sport, Berlin in 2016.[90] The SCAT5 currently represents the most well-established and rigorously developed instrument available for sideline assessment by qualified staff[89] in the evaluation of individuals 13 years old or older who are suspected of having sustained an SRC.[90] The Child-SCAT5 is used to evaluate SRC in children 5–12 years old.[91]

As symptom presentations vary, treatment approaches should be tailored to the individual. Patient education and reassurance should be a primary intervention.[92] Individuals should be encouraged to rest in the acute phases; however, it has been demonstrated that prolonged rest can be detrimental to recovery and should not be extended past the first few weeks following injury.

Recently there has been a shift to better consider timelines for return to sport following TBI. Within the literature there exists a term of Second Impact Syndrome (SIS), which has garnered a lot of attention. SIS, or repetitive head injury syndrome, describes a condition in which the individual experiences a second head injury before complete recovery from an initial head injury.[93] There have been very few confirmed cases of SIS to date; therefore, the exact incidence, risk and pathophysiology of the condition are not well known.[94] While the literature remains divided on the occurrence of SIS, general consensus is for a period of cognitive and physical rest until the acute symptoms resolve, followed by a progressive return to activity according to a protocol of graded exertion.

'There is no good clinical evidence that currently available protective equipment will prevent concussion', according to Rosenfeld.[95] Australia's sporting authorities provide a clear message regarding head strikes and concussion in sport: 'If in doubt, sit them out'.[89] Education is required for parents/players about the importance of the return-to-play advice given to them.[96] Box 43.6 provides an overview of sports-related mTBI.

BOX 43.6 SPORTS-RELATED mTBI: OVERVIEW[89–92]

- In all suspected cases of concussion, the individual should be removed from the playing field as mTBI can evolve after several hours.
- If concussion is suspected, and a sideline healthcare provider is not present, refer directly to a medical facility.
- The patient should be assessed by an appropriate, licensed healthcare provider, and monitored for deterioration.
- age > 13: Sports Concussion Assessment Tool (SCAT5: 5th edition) 5-12: Child-SCAT5.
- If a child has a sport-related mTBI, ensure the school is aware of the injury.
- An initial rest period of 24–48 hours following injury may be of benefit.
- Review by a licensed healthcare provider prior to the resumption of sport.
- Graduated program for return to sport/work, as required.

POST-CONCUSSION SYNDROME (PCS)

It is important to understand that PCS is not a prolonged concussion, but rather a separate clinical entity. The International Statistical Classification of Diseases and Related Health Problems, 10th edition (ICD10)[97] recognises the code of post-concussion syndrome that occurs following head trauma (usually sufficiently severe to result in loss of consciousness) and includes a number of disparate symptoms such as headache, dizziness, fatigue, irritability, difficulty in concentration and performing mental tasks, impairment of memory, insomnia and reduced tolerance to stress, emotional excitement or alcohol.[29,98]

RESUMING FUNCTIONAL ACTIVITIES

Give verbal and printed discharge advice to patients with any degree of head injury who are discharged from an ED or observation ward.[57] After a brief period of rest during the acute phase (24–48 hours) after injury, patients can be encouraged to become gradually and progressively more active while staying below their cognitive and physical symptom-exacerbation thresholds (i.e. activity level should not bring on or worsen their symptoms).[89] Multiple variants of return to work/sport programs and guidelines now exist. The patient should be guided towards the most appropriate guidance, commensurate to their pre-injury level of functioning and lifestyle. Patient discharge advice is summarised in Box 43.7.

BOX 43.7 PATIENT ADVICE FOLLOWING HEAD INJURY[99]

Suggested written discharge advice card for patients aged over 16 years who have sustained a head injury

We think that it is alright for you to leave hospital now. We have checked your symptoms and you seem well on the road to recovery. When you get home it is very unlikely that you will have any further problems. But, if any of the following symptoms do return, we suggest you come back, or get someone to bring you back, to your nearest hospital emergency department as soon as possible:

- unconsciousness, or lack of full consciousness (for example, problems keeping eyes open)
- drowsiness (feeling sleepy) that goes on for longer than 1 hour when you would normally be wide awake
- problems understanding or speaking
- loss of balance or problems walking
- weakness in one or more arms or legs
- problems with your vision
- persistent headache
- vomiting (being sick)
- seizures (also known as convulsions or fits)
- clear fluid coming out of your ear or nose
- bleeding or discharge from one or both ears.

THINGS YOU SHOULDN'T WORRY ABOUT

You may feel some other symptoms over the next few days which should disappear in the next 2 weeks. These include: a mild headache, feeling sick (without vomiting), dizziness, irritability or bad temper, problems concentrating or problems with your memory, tiredness, lack of appetite or problems sleeping. If you feel very concerned about any of these symptoms in the first few days after discharge, you should go and see your own doctor to talk about them.

If these problems do not go away after 2 weeks, you should go and see your doctor. We would also recommend that you seek a doctor's opinion about your ability to drive a car or motorbike.

THINGS THAT WILL HELP YOU GET BETTER

If you follow this advice you should get better more quickly and it may help any symptoms you experience to go away:

- DO NOT stay at home alone for the first 24 hours after leaving hospital.
- DO make sure you stay within easy reach of a telephone and medical help.
- DO have plenty of rest and avoid stressful situations.
- DO NOT take any alcohol or drugs.
- DO NOT take sleeping pills, sedatives or tranquillisers unless they are given by a doctor.
- DO NOT play any contact sport (for example, rugby or football) for at least 3 weeks without talking to your doctor first.
- DO NOT return to your normal school, college or work activity until you feel you have completely recovered.
- DO NOT drive a car, motorbike or bicycle or operate machinery unless you feel you have completely recovered.

Telephone number to call at the hospital: ______________

LONG-TERM PROBLEMS

Most patients recover quickly and experience no long-term problems. However, some patients only develop problems after a few weeks or months. If you start to feel that things are not quite right (for example, memory problems, not feeling yourself), then please contact your doctor as soon as possible so that we can check to make sure you are recovering properly.

SUMMARY

Traumatic brain injuries are a major cause of traumatic deaths and cause significant long-term disability. Presentations to hospital for management of TBI are frequent, and this patient group will continue to confront emergency medical service providers and emergency nurses with multiple challenges. Recognition and prevention of secondary injuries related to ischaemia, increased ICP and hypoxia are essential for these challenging patients. Additionally, the increasing use of intoxicating illicit substances will continue to make the patient assessment and management process problematic. Preventing the injury from becoming worse, particularly from secondary brain injury, by having systems in place to recognise, report and action a deteriorating neurological state early, are the mainstays of clinical practice for this patient group.

CASE STUDY

A 28-year-old male patient presents with periorbital ecchymosis and confusion post assault, with a fluctuating level of consciousness.

QUESTIONS

1. Describe the immediate assessment.
2. What is his most likely injury, and why?
3. Differentiate between focal and diffuse traumatic brain injury.
4. Describe clinical strategies to minimise secondary brain injury.
5. Explain the rationale for the frequency of head injury observations.
6. Describe the rationale and transfer criteria for referral to a trauma centre with neurosurgical services.
7. Describe the rationale for maintenance of normal arterial blood gas values for the ventilated patient with signs of traumatic brain injury.
8. What is the earliest sign of deterioration in the patient with a head injury?
9. Explain the Monro-Kellie doctrine as it relates to raised intracranial pressure in the patient with traumatic brain injury.

Answers to Case Study Questions can be found on evolve **http://evolve.elsevier.com/AU/Curtis/emergency/** 

USEFUL WEBSITES

The following websites and links are provided as a guide to access further information.

Brain injury specific information

Brain Foundation, Australia. Good general information source. Good patient referral site, brainfoundation.org.au.

Brain Trauma Foundation, US. General information and guidelines with access to research links, braintrauma.org.

NSW-based agencies providing a range of resources, publications and links

Emergency Care Institute, NSW: aci.health.nsw.gov.au/networks/eci.

NSW Agency for Clinical Innovation: www.aci.health.nsw.gov.au/.

NSW Institute of Trauma Injury and Management: aci.health.nsw.gov.au/networks/itim.

Victorian-based agencies providing education and links

RACS Trauma Care Verification: www.surgeons.org/for-hospitals/trauma-verification/.

Trauma Victoria, major trauma guidelines and education, trauma.reach.vic.gov.au/.

Victorian State Trauma Outcomes Registry and Monitoring Group (VSTORM), www.monash.edu/medicine/sphpm/vstorm/home.

General information

Concussion in Sport Australia, www.concussioninsport.gov.au/.

World Health Organization, www.who.int/en/.

REFERENCES

1. Oropello JM, Kvetan V, Pastores SM. Lange critical care. McGraw Hill Professional; 2016.
2. Garvin R, Mangat HS. Emergency neurological life support: severe traumatic brain injury. Neurocritic Care 2017;27(1):159–69.
3. Menon DK, Schwab K, Wright DW, et al. Position statement: definition of traumatic brain injury. Arch Phys Med Rehabil 2010;91(11):1637–40.
4. Maas AI, Menon DK, Adelson PD, et al. Traumatic brain injury: integrated approaches to improve prevention, clinical care, and research. Lancet Neurol 2017;16(12):987–1048.
5. Stein DM, Feather CB, Napolitano LM. Traumatic brain injury advances. Crit Care Clin 2017;33(1):1–13.
6. Davanzo JR, Sieg EP, Timmons SD. Management of traumatic brain injury. Surg Clin N Am 2017;97(6):1237–53.
7. Dewan MC, Rattani A, Gupta S, et al. Estimating the global incidence of traumatic brain injury. J Neurosurg 2018;130(4):1080–97.
8. Fitzgerald M, Ponsford J, Lannin NA, et al. AUS-TBI Investigators, Gabbe B. AUS-TBI: The Australian Health Informatics Approach to predict outcomes and monitor intervention efficacy after moderate-to-severe traumatic brain injury. Neurotrauma Rep 2022;3(1):217–23.
9. Alexis RJ, Jagdish S, Sukumar S, et al. Clinical profile and autopsy findings in fatal head injuries. J Emerg Trauma Shock 2018;11(3):205.
10. Myburgh JA, Cooper DJ, Finfer SR, et al. Australasian Traumatic Brain Injury Study (ATBIS) Investigators for the Australian/New Zealand Intensive Care Society Clinical Trials Group. Epidemiology and 12-month outcomes from traumatic brain injury in Australia and New Zealand. J Trauma 2008;64(4):854–62.
11. Beck B, Bray JE, Cameron PA, et al. Trends in severe traumatic brain injury in Victoria, 2006–2014. Med J Aust 2016;204(11):407.
12. ACC. Traumatic brain injury strategy and action plan (2017–2021): improve the quality of life of New Zealanders by reducing the incidence, severity and impacts of traumatic brain injury. Wellington: 2017.
13. Heathcote K, Devlin A, McKie E, et al. Rural and urban patterns of severe injuries and hospital mortality in Australia: an analysis of the Australia New Zealand Trauma Registry: 2015–2019. Injury 2022;53(6):1893–903.
14. Kim HW, Yun J-H. Treatment experiences of traumatic brain injury patients using doctor-helicopter emergency medical service: early data in a regional trauma center. Korean J Neurotrauma 2020;16(2):157.
15. Hyder AA, Wunderlich CA, Puvanachandra P, et al. The impact of traumatic brain injuries: a global perspective. NeuroRehabilitation 2007;22(5):341–53.
16. Goldman L, Schafer AI. Goldman-Cecil medicine e-book. Elsevier Health Sciences; 2015.
17. Spaite DW, Hu C, Bobrow BJ, et al. The effect of combined out-of-hospital hypotension and hypoxia on mortality in major traumatic brain injury. Ann Emerg Med 2017;69(1):62–72.
18. Patton KT. Anatomy and physiology. 9th ed. Elsevier/Mosby; 2016.
19. Calviello L, Donnelly J, Zeiler F, Thelin E, Smielewski P, Czosnyka M. Cerebral autoregulation monitoring in acute traumatic brain injury: what's the evidence? Minerva Anestesiol 2017;83(8):844–57.
20. Kinoshita K. Traumatic brain injury: pathophysiology for neurocritical care. J Intensive Care 2016;4(1):1–10.
21. Urden LD, Stacy KM, Lough ME. Critical care nursing-e-book: diagnosis and management. Elsevier Health Sciences; 2017.
22. Basyuni S, Panayi A, Sharma V, Santhanam V. A missed scalp laceration causing avoidable sequelae. Int J Surgery Case Rep 2016;23:61–4.
23. US Department of Defense. Emergency war surgery. 4th US revision. Government Printing Office; 2014.
24. Holley J, Filips D. Hemorrhage control myth busters. 10 myths that need to be understood & addressed by emergency personnel. JEMS 2014;39(12):36–41.
25. Auerbach PS, Cushing TA, Harris NS. Auerbach's wilderness medicine. Elsevier Health Sciences; 2016.
26. Bryant R, Nix D. Traumatic wounds: bullets, blasts and vehicle crashes. In: Bryant R, Nix D, editors. Acute and chronic wounds. Elsevier; 2015.
27. Daroff RB, Jankovic J, Mazziotta JC, et al. Bradley's neurology in clinical practice E-Book. 7th ed. Clinical Key. Elsevier Health Sciences; 2015.
28. Lewis SL, Bucher L, Heitkemper MM, et al. Medical-surgical nursing e-book: assessment and management of clinical problems, single volume. 11th ed. Elsevier Health Sciences; 2019.
29. Lewis SL, Bucher L, Heitkemper MM, et al. Medical-surgical nursing: assessment and management of clinical problems. Philadelphia: Elsevier; 2011.
30. Ball JW, Dains JE, Flynn JA, Solomon BS, Stewart RW. Seidel's guide to physical examination-e-book. Elsevier Health Sciences; 2014.
31. Ferri FF. Clinical Advisor 2017: traumatic brain injuries. Philadelphia: Elsevier; 2016.
32. Copstead-Kirkhorn L-EC, Banasik JL. Pathophysiology—e-book. Elsevier Health Sciences; 2013.
33. Walls, R, Hockberger R, Gausche-Hill M. Rosen's emergency medicine: concepts and clinical practice. Philadelphia: Elsevier; 2017.
34. Servadei F, Picetti E. Traumatic subarachnoid hemorrhage. World Neurosurg 2014;82(5):e597–8.
35. Huff SJ, Wintermark M, Ghaemmaghami CA. Intracranial hemorrhages. Fig 103.3. Clinical Gate. Philadelphia: Elsevier; 2013.
36. Pervez M, Kitagawa RS, Chang TR. Definition of traumatic brain injury, neurosurgery, trauma orthopedics, neuroimaging, psychology, and psychiatry in mild traumatic brain injury. Neuroimaging Clin N Am 2018;28(1):1–13.
37. Winn HR. Youmans neurological surgery. Philadelphia, PA: Elsevier/Saunders; 2011.
38. Haaga JR. CT and MRI of the whole body. Fig 13 – 7A. Elsevier; 2016.

39. Jang SH. Diagnostic problems in diffuse axonal injury. Diagnostics 2020;10(2):117.
40. Taylor CA, Bell JM, Breiding MJ, Xu L. Traumatic brain injury-related emergency department visits, hospitalizations, and deaths—United States, 2007 and 2013. MMWR Surveill Summ 2017;66(9):1.
41. Dinsmore J. Traumatic brain injury: an evidence-based review of management. Contin Educ Anaesth Crit Care Pain 2013;13(6):189–95.
42. Carney N, Totten AM, O'Reilly C, et al. Guidelines for the management of severe traumatic brain injury. Neurosurgery 2017;80(1):6–15.
43. John R, Appleby I. Traumatic brain injury: initial resuscitation and transfer. Anaesth Intensive Care Med 2014;15(4):161–3.
44. Pélieu I, Kull C, Walder B. Prehospital and emergency care in adult patients with acute traumatic brain injury. Med Sci 2019;7(1):12.
45. Meyfroidt G, Bouzat P, Casaer MP, et al. Management of moderate to severe traumatic brain injury: an update for the intensivist. Intensive Care Med 2022;48(6):649–66.
46. Minardi J, Crocco TJ. Management of traumatic brain injury: first link in chain of survival. Mount Sinai J Med 2009;76(2):138–44.
47. Bagwell TA, Abramo TJ, Albert GW, et al. Cerebral oximetry with blood volume index and capnography in intubated and hyperventilated patients. Am J Emerg Med 2016;34(6):1102–7.
48. Wiles MD. Management of traumatic brain injury: a narrative review of current evidence. Anaesthesia 2022;77(1):102–12.
49. Sappenfield J, Galvagno SM, Blenko J. Initial treatment priorities for the physiological optimization of patients with severe traumatic brain injury. Open Access Emerg Med 2013;1(1).
50. Trauma Victoria. Traumatic brain injury guideline. 2017. Available from: https://trauma.reach.vic.gov.au/resources/trauma-victoria-guideline-pdf.
51. Gilligan J, Reilly P, Pearce A, Taylor D. Management of acute traumatic intracranial haematoma in rural and remote areas of Australia. ANZ J Surg 2017;87(1–2):80–5.
52. Currie S, Saleem N, Straiton JA, Macmullen-Price J, Warren DJ, Craven IJ. Imaging assessment of traumatic brain injury. Postgrad Med J 2016;92:41–50.
53. Reed D. Adult trauma clinical practice guidelines: initial management of closed head injury in adults. NSW Institute of Trauma and Injury Management; 2011. Online. Available from: https://static1.squarespace.com/static/52c9dd96e4b0268360dfa1f3/t/52c9eeede4b083e90ec350cf/1388965613934/Adult+Closed_Head_Injury_CPG_2nd_Ed_Summary_document.pdf.
54. Lamba I, Luthra A, Shinde V, et al. Using Canadian CT head rule in a developing nation: validation and comparing utilisation by emergency physicians and neurosurgeons. Am J Emerg Med 2021;45:112–16.
55. Dahlin BC, Waldau B. Surgical and nonsurgical treatment of vascular skull base trauma. J Neurol Surg B Skull Base 2016;77(5):396–403.
56. Zakharova N, Kornienko V, Potapov A, Pronin I. Neuroimaging of traumatic brain injury. New York: Springer International Publishing; 2014.
57. Hodgkinson S, Pollit V, Sharpin C, Lecky F. Early management of head injury: summary of updated NICE guidance. BMJ 2014;34–7.
58. Buttaro TM, Trybulski J, Polgar-Bailey P, et al. Primary care: a collaborative practice. St. Louis: Elsevier; 2016.
59. Bach L, Dries DJ. Management of traumatic intracranial hypertension: old questions with new answers. Air Med J 2017;36(4):156–9.
60. Beasley R, Chien J, Douglas J, et al. Thoracic Society of Australia and New Zealand oxygen guidelines for acute oxygen use in adults: 'Swimming between the flags'. Respirology 2015;20(8):1182–91.
61. Pakkanen T, Kämäräinen A, Huhtala H, et al. Physician-staffed helicopter emergency medical service has a beneficial impact on the incidence of prehospital hypoxia and secured airways on patients with severe traumatic brain injury. Scand J Trauma Resusc Emerg Med 2017;25(1):1–7.
62. ANZCOR. ANZCOR Guideline 11.6.1—Targeted oxygen therapy in adult advanced life support section 11—Adult advanced life support. ANZCOR; 2016.
63. Harrois A, Anstey JR, Deane AM, et al. Effects of routine position changes and tracheal suctioning on intracranial pressure in traumatic brain injury patients. J Neurotrauma 2020;37(20):2227–33.
64. Chowdhury T, Kowalski S, Arabi Y, et al. General intensive care for patients with traumatic brain injury: an update. Saudi J Anaesth 2014;8(2):256.
65. Pedersen CM, Rosendahl-Nielsen M, Hjermind J, Egerod I. Endotracheal suctioning of the adult intubated patient—what is the evidence? Intensive Crit Care Nurs 2009;25(1):21–30.
66. Mehta R, Chinthapalli K. Glasgow Coma Scale explained. BMJ 2019;365:l1296.
67. Heath Jeffery RC, Young B, Swann P, Lueck CJ. Unequal pupils: 'understanding the eye's aperture'. Aust J Gen Pract 2019;48(1/2):39–42.
68. Gupta B, Garg N, Ramachandran R. Vasopressors: do they have any role in hemorrhagic shock? J Anaesthesiol Clin Pharmacol 2017;33(1):3.
69. Abraham M, Singhal V. Intracranial pressure monitoring. J Neuroanaesth Crit Care 2015;2(3):193–203.
70. Alvis-Miranda HR, Navas-Marrugo SZ, Velasquez-Loperena RA, et al. Effects of glycemic level on outcome of patients with traumatic brain injury: a retrospective cohort study. Bull Emerg Trauma 2014;2(2):65.
71. Rostami E. Glucose and the injured brain-monitored in the neurointensive care unit. Front Neurol 2014;5:91.
72. Shi J, Dong B, Mao Y, et al. Traumatic brain injury and hyperglycemia, a potentially modifiable risk factor. Oncotarget 2016;7(43):71052.
73. Zehtabchi S, Baki SGA, Falzon L, et al. Tranexamic acid for traumatic brain injury: a systematic review and meta-analysis. Am J Emerg Med 2014;32(12):1503–9.
74. Tran HA, Chunilal SD, Tran H. An update of consensus guidelines for warfarin reversal. Med J Aust 2014;200(2):82.

75. Marehbian J, Muehlschlegel S, Edlow BL, et al. Medical management of the severe traumatic brain injury patient. Neurocrit Care 2017;27(3): 430–46.
76. Shawkat H, Westwood M-M, Mortimer A. Mannitol: a review of its clinical uses. Contin Educ Anaesth Crit Care Pain 2012;12(2):82–5.
77. Yellinek S, Cohen A, Merkin V, et al. Clinical significance of skull base fracture in patients after traumatic brain injury. J Clin Neurosci 2016; 25:111–15.
78. Wray JP, Bridwell RE, Schauer SG, et al. The diamond of death: hypocalcemia in trauma and resuscitation. Am J Emerg Med 2021;41:104–9.
79. Kirkman MA, Smith M. Therapeutic hypothermia and acute brain injury. Anaesth Intensive Care Med 2014;15(4):171–5.
80. Laskowski RA, Creed JA, Raghupathi R. Pathophysiology of mild TBI: implications for altered signaling pathways. Front Neuroeng 2015.
81. Rabinowitz AR, Li X, McCauley SR, et al. Prevalence and predictors of poor recovery from mild traumatic brain injury. J Neurotrauma 2015;32(19): 1488–96.
82. Ponsford J, Cameron P, Fitzgerald M, Grant M, Mikocka-Walus A, Schönberger M. Predictors of postconcussive symptoms 3 months after mild traumatic brain injury. Neuropsychology 2012;26(3):304.
83. Levin HS, Diaz-Arrastia RR. Diagnosis, prognosis, and clinical management of mild traumatic brain injury. Lancet Neurol 2015;14(5):506–17.
84. Meares S, Shores EA, Taylor AJ, et al. Validation of the Abbreviated Westmead Post-traumatic Amnesia Scale: a brief measure to identify acute cognitive impairment in mild traumatic brain injury. Brain Inj 2011;25(12):1198–205.
85. Tesson SA, Nogajski RR, Macey JA, et al. Reliability of the Abbreviated Westmead Post-traumatic Amnesia Scale in children: impact of age on test results. Emerg Med Australas 2016;28(1):73–7.
86. Meares S, Shores EA, Smyth T, et al. Identifying posttraumatic amnesia in individuals with a Glasgow coma scale of 15 after mild traumatic brain injury. Arch Phys Med Rehab 2015;96(5):956–9.
87. Sharp DJ, Jenkins PO. Concussion is confusing us all. Pract Neurol 2015;15(3):172–86.
88. Elkington LJ, Hughes DC. Australian Institute of Sport and Australian Medical Association position statement on concussion in sport. Med J Aust 2017;206(1):46–50.
89. McCrory P, Meeuwisse W, Dvorak J, et al. Consensus statement on concussion in sport—the 5th international conference on concussion in sport held in Berlin, October 2016. Br J Sports Med 2017;51(11):838–47.
90. Echemendia RJ, Meeuwisse W, McCrory P, et al. The Sport Concussion Assessment Tool 5th edition (SCAT5): background and rationale. Br J Sports Med 2017;51(11):848–50.
91. Davis GA, Purcell L, Schneider KJ, et al. The child sport concussion assessment tool 5th edition (child SCAT5): background and rationale. Br J Sports Med 2017;51(11):859–61.
92. Phillips MM, Reddy CC. Managing patients with prolonged recovery following concussion. Phys Med Rehab Clin 2016;27(2):455–74.
93. Stovitz SD, Weseman JD, Hooks MC, et al. What definition is used to describe second impact syndrome in sports? A systematic and critical review. Curr Sports Med Rep 2017;16(1):50–5.
94. Foris LA, May T, Donnally III CJ. Second impact syndrome. Treasure Island: Stat Pearls Publishing; 2017. Online. Available from: www.ncbi.nlm.nih.gov/pubmed/28846316.
95. Rosenfeld J. Practical management of head and neck injury. Elsevier Health Sciences; 2011.
96. Kemp JL, Newton JD, White PE, et al. Implementation of concussion guidelines in community Australian Football and Rugby League—the experiences and challenges faced by coaches and sports trainers. J Sci Med Sport 2016;19(4):305–10.
97. ACCD: Australian Consortium for Classification Development. The International Statistical Classification of Disease and Related Health Problems—Australian modification. 10th ed. Darlinghurst, NSW: Independent Hospital Pricing Authority (IHPA); 2017.
98. Crowe SF. The post concussional syndrome. The behavioural and emotional complications of traumatic brain injury. Taylor & Francis; 2012.
99. The Sydney Children's Hospital Network. Fact sheet: concussion and mild head injury. Elsevier; 2022.

CHAPTER 44
MAXILLOFACIAL TRAUMA

ROBERT J.W. KNIGHT AND TANEAL WISEMAN

ESSENTIALS

- Patients with maxillofacial injuries will be concerned about returning to normal function (eating, breathing and communicating) and appearance.
- Initial assessment and management must always follow basic trauma principles and the emergency clinician must not be distracted by injuries within the area of the face, which can often be very extreme, disfiguring and confronting.
- Airway problems commonly arise following maxillofacial injuries secondary to swelling. This can occur at any level of the airway and may result from fractures compressing the airway (extrinsic) or extensive soft-tissue haemorrhage or displacement leading to blood/tissue/vomitus within the airway (intrinsic). Intubate early if in doubt, especially in remote areas where deterioration may prove catastrophic to manage.
- While haemorrhage from maxillofacial trauma can be substantial, haemodynamic compromise may also be due to unidentified and internal bleeding, and a thorough assessment is always mandatory to exclude potential alternatives.
- Haemorrhage from maxillofacial trauma can usually be controlled through fracture reduction (forceps and/or traction) and packing. Uncontrolled bleeding may require angiographic embolisation.
- During repair of soft-tissue injuries to the face, the emergency clinician must ensure they are aware of the normal anatomy of the face and the potential structures that may have been injured (facial nerve branches, Stenson's duct, canthus, trochlea). A full assessment and exclusion of injuries is mandatory prior to repairing soft-tissue defects, which will otherwise have to be repaired in theatre with exploration under general anaesthetic.

INTRODUCTION

Trauma to the craniomaxillofacial (CMF) region can be alarming and confronting. This is largely due to the following; firstly, a person's face is the very first social impression they make and it also governs multiple other aspects of our psyche and emotional wellbeing. The stakes related to mismanagement are therefore high and this scares many people into inaction. Secondly, the proximity of the trauma to vital and unique anatomical structures makes anyone dealing with the area in question very nervous and reticent to touch any area for fear that they will make the issue worse. Lastly, and perhaps most importantly, the threat to a person's airway and the possible consequences of mismanagement will make most people anxious.

The principles that govern Advanced Trauma Life Support (ATLS) remain the same in the craniomaxillofacial region, with airway taking precedence. Pathology within this area often leads to significant bleeding and swelling, and special consideration needs to be given to timely management of the patient's airway. Consideration needs

to be given to how the injury will evolve over hours and whether delayed admission is safe.

Most acute craniomaxillofacial issues are related to either infection or trauma. Some of these presentations can be managed in the emergency department (ED), while others need to be referred for specialist care. This specialised care either can be delayed or will require immediate intervention by specialists in this area. In the case of paediatric patients, consideration should always be given to the possibility of non-accidental injury (NAI). Injury disproportionate to a child's abilities or mechanism should always prompt further investigation. All paediatric skull fractures acquired outside of the realms of motor vehicle collisions or similar high-velocity incidents should be investigated with caution.

ANATOMY AND PHYSIOLOGY

FACIAL SKELETON

The principal facial bones are the frontal, nasal, ethmoid, lacrimal, sphenoid, zygomatic and maxillary bones in the upper half, while the mandible comprises the lower jaw as it articulates with the temporal bone (Fig. 44.1).[1] Fig. 44.2 outlines the overlying facial contours. The inferior portion of the frontal bone articulates with the frontal process of the maxilla and nasal bone medially and with the zygoma laterally.[2] The orbit has a complex anatomy composed of the frontal and sphenoid bones superiorly, zygoma and sphenoid laterally, maxilla and palatine bones inferiorly and sphenoid, ethmoid and lacrimal bones medially. Paired nasal bones that form the bridge of the nose articulate with the frontal bone above and maxilla laterally (Fig. 44.3) forming the nasal bridge, which houses the nasal cavity that is divided by the nasal septum.[2] The zygoma forms the cheek prominence in conjunction with the greater wing of the sphenoid, the lateral wall and floor of the orbital cavity. Articulations with the maxilla, frontal bone and zygomatic process of the temporal bone form the zygomatic arch, which lends itself to the fullness across the posterior part of the cheek bone.

The maxilla forms the upper jaw, anterior hard palate, part of the lateral wall of the nasal cavity and part of the orbital floor. Below the orbit, the maxilla is perforated by the infraorbital foramen to allow passage of the infraorbital vessels and nerves. The inferior portion of the maxilla forms the alveolar process, which joins the left and right sides of the maxilla. The alveolar processes together form the alveolar arch, which houses the upper teeth.[3]

The mandible is a horizontal horseshoe-shaped body with two equal halves joined in the midline and each consisting of a body, angle and ramus, an anterior coronoid process and a posterior condylar process. The mandibular notch lies medial to the zygomatic arch and separates the two processes. The mandible articulates with the temporal bone to form the temporomandibular joint, while the superior border of the body of the mandible, called the alveolar ridge, contains the lower teeth. These in turn articulate with the upper teeth in a defined manner which has moulded over time and is directly proportionate to movements and habits of the individual.

FIGURE 44.1 FACIAL SKELETON[1]

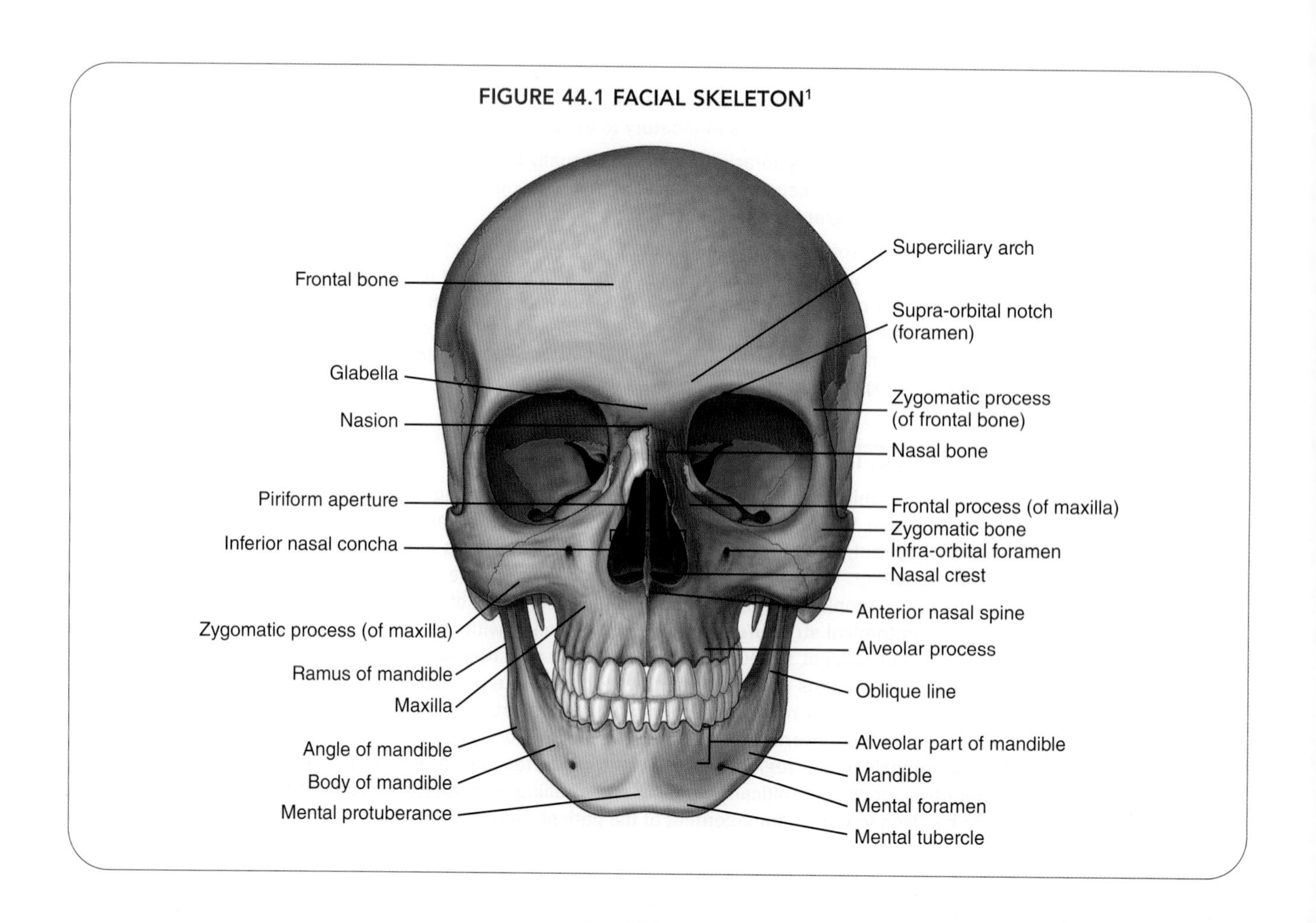

FIGURE 44.2 KEY SURFACE ANATOMY LANDMARKS OF THE HEAD AND NECK[2]

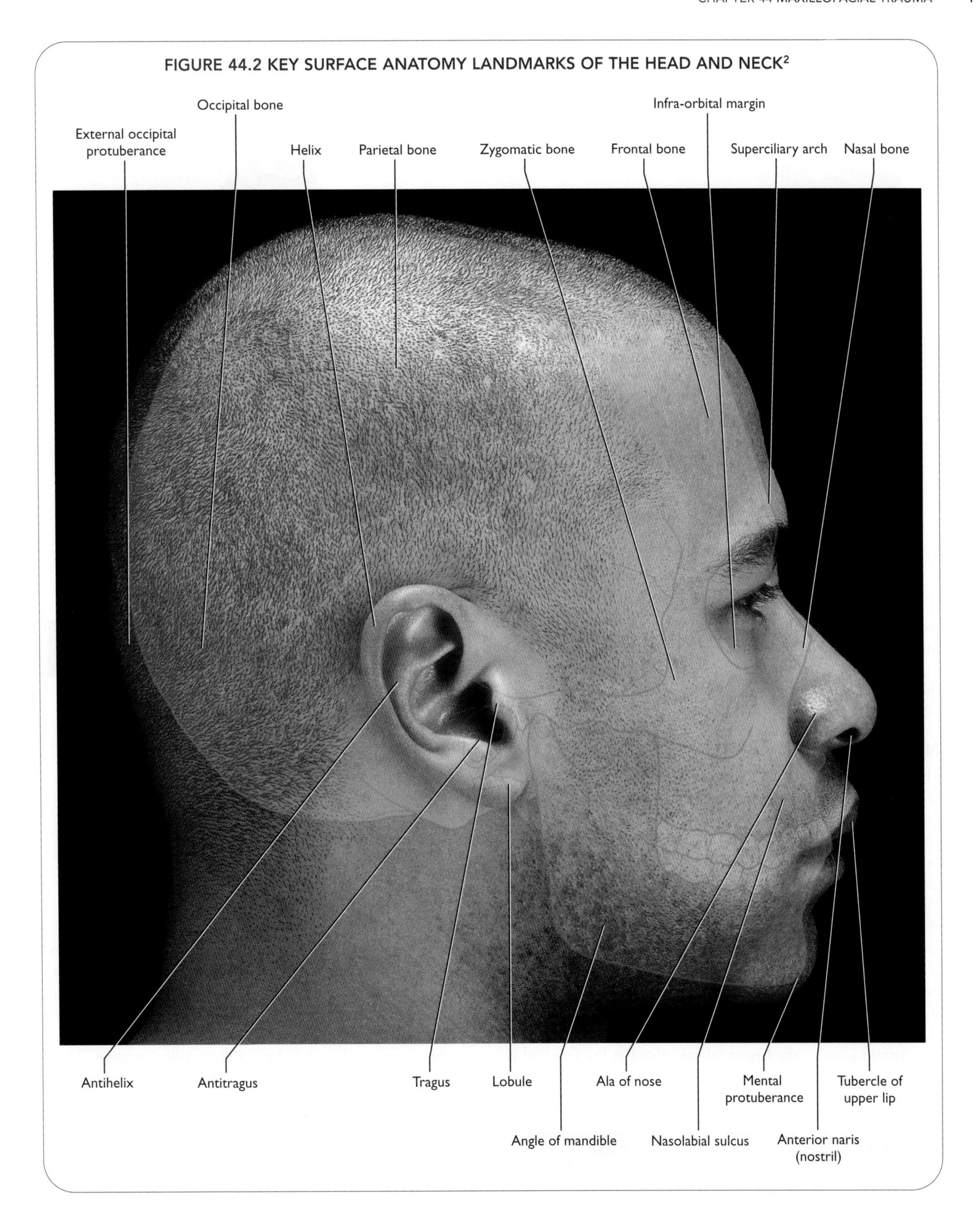

Sinus cavities are found within the maxilla (also referred to as the maxillary antrum), frontal bone and the ethmoid and sphenoid bones of the skull. The midface is a lattice of vertical and horizontal buttresses that resist functional forces, such as biting, and house the facial organs, such as the eyes, giving the face shape while preventing lateral crushing forces. Each buttress is consequently thickened to reflect its importance and loading force resistance characteristics. A common belief is that sinuses and the facial skeleton have evolved to provide a 'crumple zone' that protects the brain and eyes from injury while

FIGURE 44.3 NOSE (ANTEROLATERAL VIEW)[2]

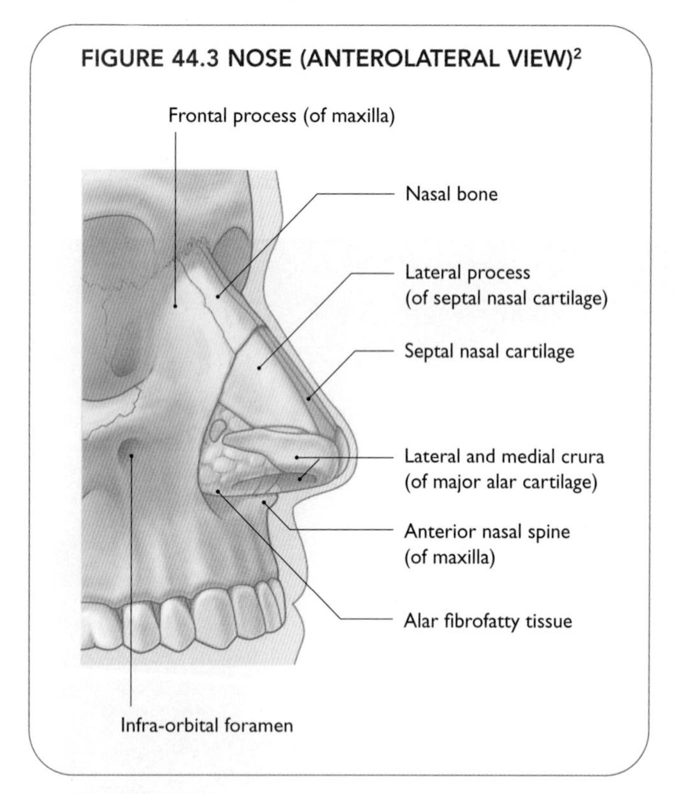

FIGURE 44.4 DISTRIBUTION OF FACIAL NERVE BRANCHES[5]

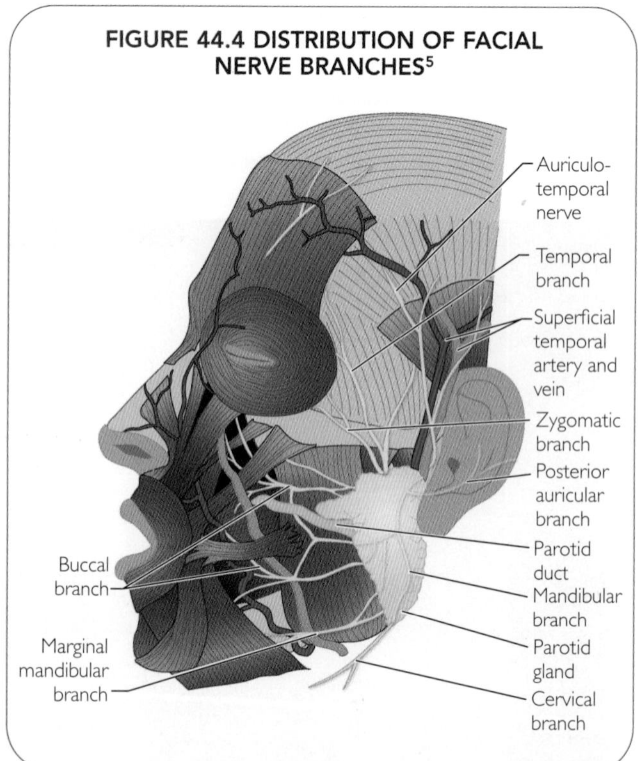

reducing cranial weight and enhancing the voice and humidifying one's breath.[3] It is worth noting that >10% of facial injuries have associated head injuries and therefore require a thorough consideration for intracranial pathology and should be assessed accordingly.[4]

NERVES, GLANDS AND BLOOD SUPPLY

The facial nerve (cranial nerve VII) provides motor, parasympathetic and sensory innervation to the face. Its origins are in the brainstem in the pontine region where it follows a tortuous course intimately related to the structures of the ear. It then exits the stylomastoid foramen inferiorly and medially deep to the external auditory canal. It then enters the deep surface of the parotid gland posterior to the ramus of the mandible where it divides into five main branches (Fig. 44.4).[5] Specific functions for each branch are listed in Table 44.1.

Other cranial nerves that may be affected by facial trauma are the oculomotor (cranial nerve III), trochlear (cranial nerve IV) and the three divisions of the trigeminal nerve (cranial nerve V). Function and testing for each nerve is described in Table 44.2.[6] The parotid gland is the largest salivary gland in the face and is located inferomedially to the anterior ear and drains into the oral cavity through the parotid duct (Stenson's duct) (Fig. 44.5).[7]

PRACTICE TIP

The airway should be constantly monitored for increasing oedema and haemorrhage, which may block the airway at a later stage. If there is any doubt that the airway may become compromised during transport, or that there may be issues related to clearance/suctioning of the airway, then endotracheal intubation should be guaranteed prior to transport and possible deterioration.

TABLE 44.1 FACIAL NERVE BRANCH FUNCTIONS

BRANCH	FUNCTION
Buccal	Wrinkle nose
Cervical	Wrinkle skin of neck
Mandibular	Purse and depress lips
Temporal	Raise eyebrows, wrinkle forehead
Zygomatic	Close eyelids

Blood supply to the face arises from both the internal and the external carotid arteries. They form a very rich network with multiple levels of communication that ensure both anterograde and retrograde flow as required. The larger vessels of note that supply the facial soft tissue include the facial, posterior auricular, superficial temporal, ophthalmic and maxillary arteries. Much of the bleeding encountered can occur in areas that are not accessible in order to apply pressure directly over the site of bleeding.[5] These include the sphenopalatine and pterygopalatine arteries that are situated behind the upper jaw (Fig. 44.6).

INJURY MECHANISM

History related to the injury is essential to allow context and is an important adjunct to a thorough clinical examination. It is also essential that the clinician bear in mind that greater than 50% of maxillofacial trauma is related to alcohol use.[4] This may assist with gaining accurate information regarding injury mechanism and possible injuries that are historically related to that specific mechanism.[8]

TABLE 44.2 TRIAGE GUIDELINES SPECIFIC TO MAXILLOFACIAL EMERGENCIES

PRIORITY CRITERIA	CRITERIA	EXAMPLES
IMMEDIATE REFERRAL		
	• Cervicofacial infections threatening airway or vision • Facial or neck soft-tissue injuries • Displaced facial fractures • Bleeding from the mouth, jaws or neck	Periocular erysipelas, fractured mandible
Priority 1		
Immediate referral to surgeon	• Any skull fracture—simple or compound • Panfacial trauma e.g. Le Fort type (I, II or III)/ zygomaticomalar fracture with mandibular fracture • Bilateral fracture of the mandible with an unstable and mobile segment • Any fracture of the face placing the airway at risk • Any periocular injury causing entrapment of the inferior rectus muscle of the eye or pressure on the optic nerve • Extensive soft-tissue injuries that involve major nerves, arteries or the parotid duct	Extensive fractures of both the upper and lower jaw simultaneously
Priority 2		
Urgent (< 24 hrs)	• Compound facial fractures • Orbital trauma without entrapment • Facial lacerations	Isolated fracture at risk
Priority 3		
Delayed (< 7 days)	• Isolated frontal sinus • Isolated naso-orbital ethmoid • Zygomatic arch fracture • Nasal bone fracture • Undisplaced/minimally displaced mandible fracture	Isolated fracture—no/low risk
DELAYED REFERRAL		
Category 1		
Appointment in 30 days—prefer 7–10 days Condition will require more complex or emergent care if assessment is delayed Condition will have a significant impact on the patient if not seen within 30 days	• Ulcer in mouth > 10 days • Facial skin cancers/lumps • Lichen planus • Facial growths affecting vision or oral intake • Any oral or oropharyngeal cancer • Acute unmanageable dental infection • Undisplaced fracture of the mandible, maxilla or orbit • Trismus—unexplained • Trigeminal neuralgia • Herpetic stomatitis • Complex immunocompromised patients that require complex care • Acutely infected hardware	• Malignancy of the face, neck or oral cavity • Uncontrolled pain of unknown source • Orofacial trauma that does not require immediate attention
Category 2		
Appointment within 90 days Condition will require more complex or emergency care if assessment is delayed more than 90 days Condition will have a significant impact on the patient if not seen within 90 days	• TMJ pain of dysfunction • Benign pathology of the face or jaws • Sinus pathology • Infected plates or screws—chronic • Benign salivary gland pathology • Salivary calculi	• Well-controlled pain • Facial or jaw cysts • Chronic infections • Pleomorphic adenomas
Category 3		
Appointment is not required within 90 days AND Will not deteriorate quickly AND Will not require more complex care if left for more than 365 days	• Aphthous ulceration • Branchial arch congenital anomalies e.g. tongue tie • Post-traumatic facial anomalies • Chronic TMJ issues • Hyperplastic tissue • Exostoses or hemihypertrophy	• Normal oral infections • Congenital anomalies • Craniofacial rehabilitation • Non-malignant growths

FIGURE 44.5 PAROTID GLAND AND DUCT (STENSEN'S) WITH THE SURROUNDING BRANCHES OF THE FACIAL NERVE.

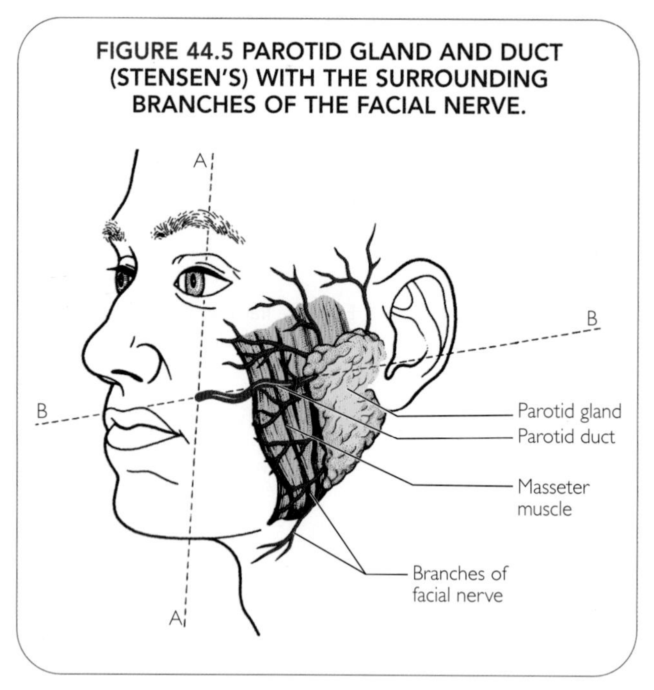

Line B approximates the course of the duct, which enters the mouth at the junction of lines A and B.[7]

FIGURE 44.6 ARTERIAL SUPPLY TO THE FACE AND SCALP[5]

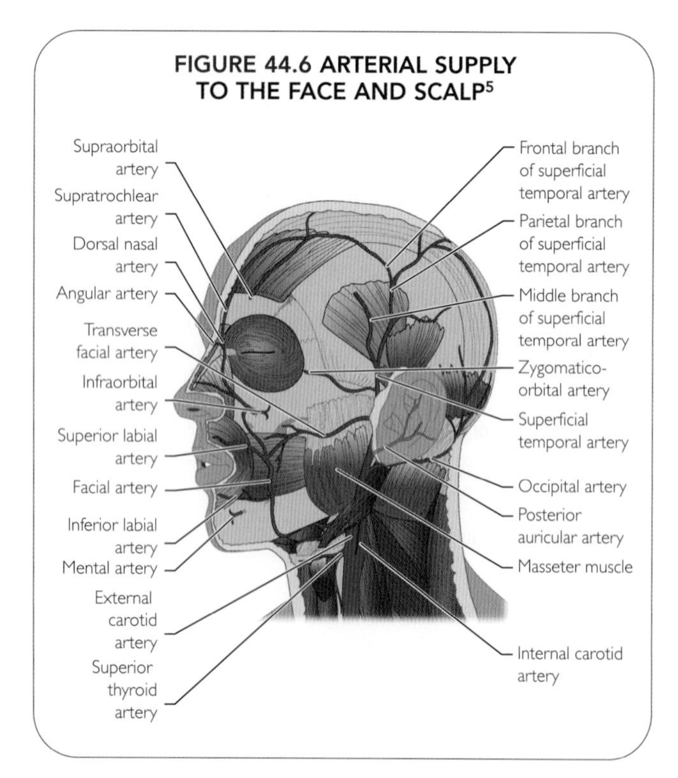

Most patterns of referral for assault to the ED are males aged 18 to 25 years. Unsurprisingly, 40% of many ED visits are related to assault. Within that cohort of assault victims, 30% will have a fracture of some sort and of that 30%, approximately 80% will have a craniomaxillofacial fracture. Motor vehicle-related facial injuries have reduced substantially since the onset of seatbelts and airbags, but increasingly, despite this well-documented decrease over the decades, we are now seeing a resurgence in facial trauma related to the craniomaxillofacial skeleton striking various parts of the vehicle.[9] Falls are becoming commonplace as our population ages, while sport injuries to this area are decreasing due to our understanding of concussion and its long-term effects.[10]

PATIENT ASSESSMENT

All trauma assessment should follow the ATLS method. This enables a structured patient assessment and ensures that life-threatening injuries are identified and managed in order to stabilise the patient prior to transfer and/or secondary survey.[11] Maxillofacial injuries that do not threaten the airway or cause life-threatening haemorrhage can be assessed as part of the secondary survey, no matter how disfiguring the injuries appear.[12]

INITIAL EVALUATION

Asphyxia due to upper airway obstruction is the major cause of death from facial trauma.[13] When performing a primary survey of the airway, the emergency clinician must maintain cervical spine precautions until cervical spine injury is excluded (see Chapter 42 for more detail on primary survey). On initial assessment, the patient's mouth should be observed for objects (e.g. dentures or avulsed teeth), which should be removed to prevent airway obstruction. Suctioning of any blood and vomitus is also essential.

Once the mouth and upper airway are clear, the clinician should assess for further airway compromise. The airway may be opened using chin lift or jaw thrust techniques if needed. If the mandible is displaced, the tongue loses anatomical support and occludes the airway, and may need to be manually held forward. In the pre-hospital setting it may be necessary to place the patient in the lateral position, or in life-threatening situations the patient is placed prone. In the ED, a towel clamp or heavy suture may be used to pull the tongue forward and provide stability to the tongue.[14] Altered mental status from alcohol, drugs or head injury can diminish the patient's gag reflex, increase the risk of vomiting and leave the airway unprotected. Severe fractures of the midface compromise the airway secondary to maxillary prolapse, haemorrhage, swelling and haematoma formation.[14] It may be necessary for the emergency clinician to place manual anterior traction on the maxilla to relieve obstruction from posteriorly displaced midface fractures.[15,16] Frequent suctioning of the oropharynx is required when bleeding or excessive secretions are present (see Chapter 16 for suctioning techniques), and anterior traction of fractured facial bones may increase haemorrhage.[16] If the patient is awake and talking, allow them to sit upright, or elevate the head of the bed or stretcher to promote drainage once the cervical spine has been cleared (Fig. 44.7).[17]

An oropharyngeal airway can be used in an unconscious patient to prevent obstruction from the tongue; however, nasopharyngeal airway use is not recommended in patients with maxillofacial trauma because of the risk of intracerebral malpositioning via the cribriform plate.[19] For the same reason, orotracheal intubation is preferred in patients with facial injuries. The success rate of emergency oral intubation in patients with oral swelling and haemorrhage can be as low as 80%, so a specific difficult airway algorithm and equipment is important.[20] If an airway cannot be maintained using the previously

FIGURE 44.7 PATIENT LEANING FORWARD TO CLEAR AND MAINTAIN OWN AIRWAY, ALLOWING FLOW OF SEVERE HAEMORRHAGE[18]

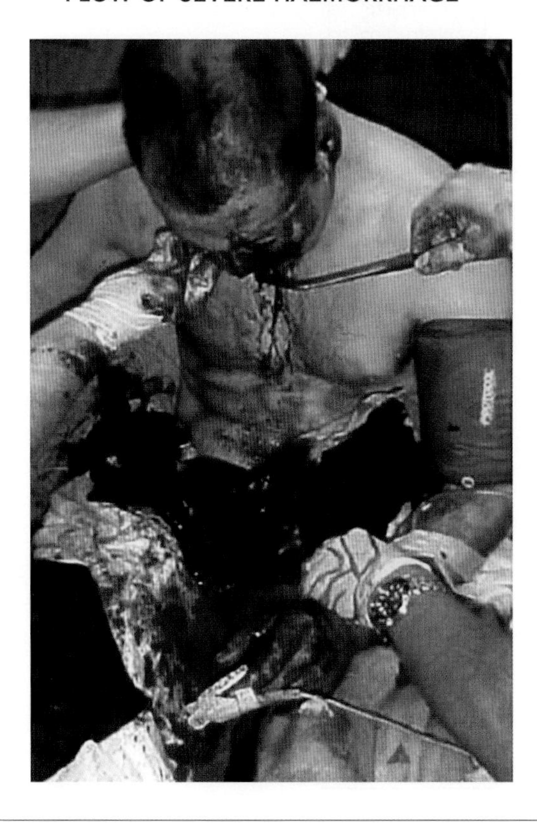

mentioned techniques, the paramedic qualified to do so will perform insertion of an endotracheal tube or a laryngeal mask airway (LMA) following local practice guidelines.[21] The LMA does not provide complete protection of the airway, so there is still the risk of aspiration (see Chapter 16 for LMA insertion techniques).[16]

In situations where intubation is not available, the airway should be managed using the safest patient position. Again, this may be the recovery/lateral position (or sitting up, leaning forward if the patient is alert) if haemorrhage and secretions are likely to block the airway or cause aspiration. If the patient is maintaining their oxygen saturation, an awake fibre-optic intubation in the operating theatre avoids potential airway emergencies.[21]

Rarely, intubation is required and cannot be accomplished due to excessive swelling or massive haemorrhage obscuring the vocal cords. In this situation a surgical airway such as a cricothyroidotomy needs to be performed.[21] Paramedics with sufficient training in the technique may perform this procedure following local practice guidelines. Cricothyroidotomy may also be performed in the ED (see Chapter 13). A needle cricothyroidotomy is recommended in children less than 12 years of age to prevent damage to the cricoid cartilage.[13] A tracheostomy will usually be required to provide a definitive airway once the patient is stabilised, if it is anticipated that they will require prolonged airway management and protection.[22] Due to the difficulties in airway management of the severely facially injured patient, a treatment algorithm will be useful (Fig. 44.8).[21]

Once a patent airway and satisfactory ventilation are established, the next priority is assessment of the cardiovascular function and intravenous access. In instances of massive haemorrhage with compromised blood pressure and cardiovascular stability, attention should be focused on the cause and management of haemorrhage. Massive blood loss causing haemorrhagic shock after facial bleeding is unusual, and the emergency clinician must search for alternative haemorrhage sites in the haemodynamically unstable patient (see Chapter 42 for haemorrhage assessment and management).[12,23,24] Alternative areas worth considering include retroperitoneal bleeds and long bone fractures, which are often covert and not as dramatic as open facial fractures that may bleed extensively. Rapid stabilisation and CT investigation of alternative sites may be required.

The dual nature of perfusion within the facial region from both the internal and the external carotid arteries can make haemostasis challenging. The substantial anastomotic network that allows anterograde and retrograde flow between the two systems often voids the proximal pressure principle to control bleeding. Haemorrhage therefore needs to be controlled in a timely manner with these principles in mind.[16] Blood transfusion may be required in cases of severe facial fractures with significant blood loss. Intravenous access is therefore mandatory in severe facial trauma, and also provides a means to administer analgesia, sedation and intubation drugs (see Chapter 42 for fluid management in major trauma).[25]

Most visible bleeding is often from the nose where the mucosa is most friable and where major anastomoses occur between the maxillary and ophthalmic systems.[23,24] In an attempt to stem the flow of blood and obtain haemostasis, blood clots should be removed from the nose and throat in an attempt to visualise the site of bleeding. When bleeding is anterior, a simple manoeuvre which may assist is pinching the nose between one's fingers and thumb while applying icepacks to the nose and forehead. Allow clots to run freely out of the patient's mouth and do not allow them to swallow the clots as this can lead to vomiting and elevation of blood pressure, which will lead to further bleeding. After pressure has been applied and if haemostasis has been achieved, pressure can be released and an attempt can be made to cauterise the area of concern, with either chemo-ablation or electrocautery. Adjunct manoeuvres include nasal tampons impregnated with vasoconstrictive drugs, such as lidocaine or tranexamic acid. Nasal balloons or foam rubber packs should always be checked to ensure that they are not causing pressure necrosis of the septum and established protocols should be employed when instituting pressure mechanisms within the nose (Fig. 44.9).[18,25]

If bleeding is posterior, nasopharyngeal packing secured to an external tether or a Foley catheter with traction or Epistat tube *with the balloon inflated within the nasopharynx* can be used to tamponade posterior bleeding.[13,23,24,26] PLEASE NOTE: intracranial insertion is a risk when inserting packing/pressure implements into the nose or nasopharynx in the context of a base of skull fracture. If a base of skull fracture is possible, a large-gauge catheter/bougie may be inserted by an experienced doctor.[27] All packing and instrumentation should be securely taped/sutured to the face to guarantee fixation and to

FIGURE 44.8 AN AIRWAY MANAGEMENT ALGORITHM FOR MAXILLOFACIAL TRAUMA[20]

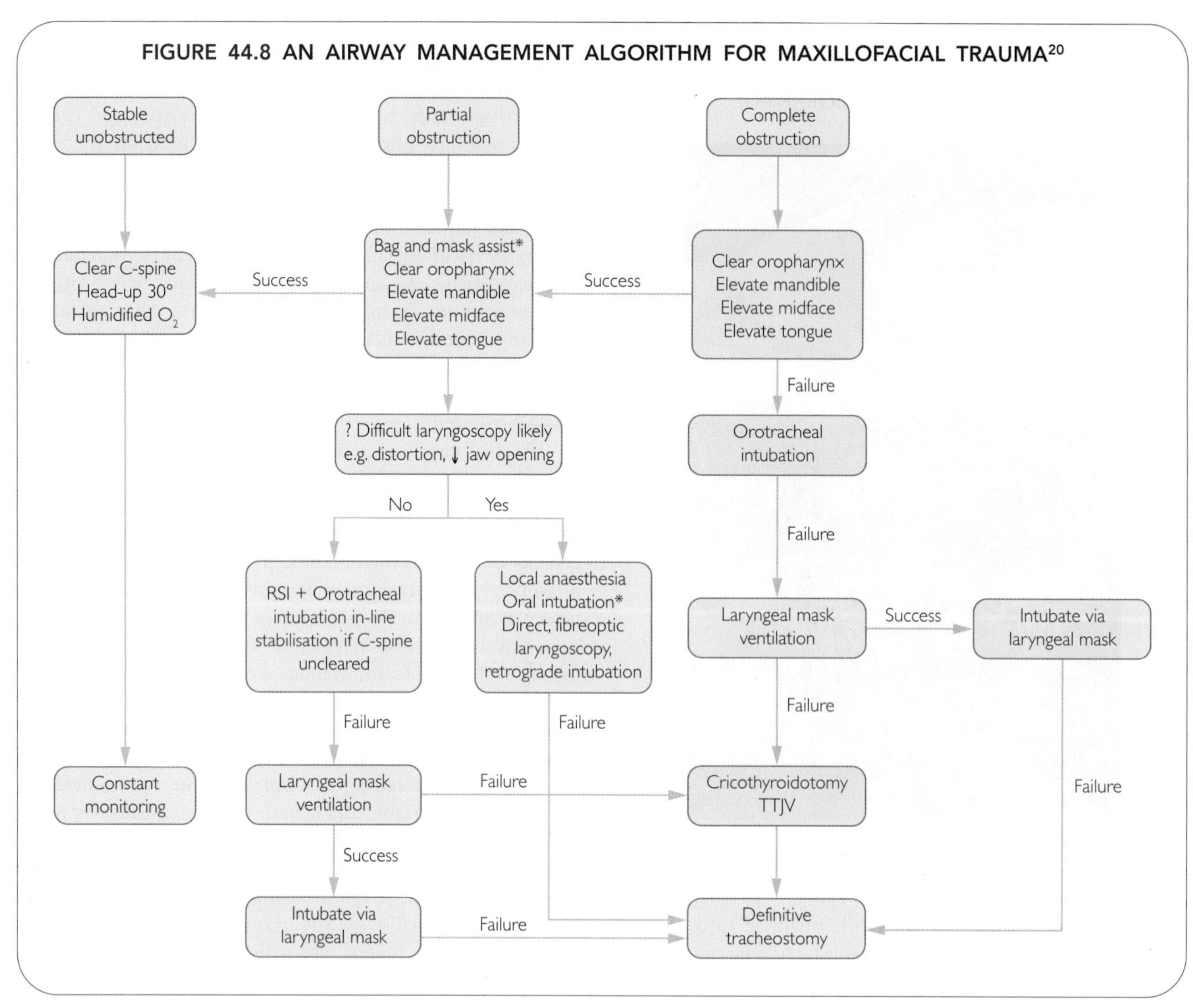

*C-spine = cervical spine; RSI = rapid sequence induction; TTJV = transtracheal jet ventilation. + Mask seal may be poor. *Nasotracheal route contraindicated in basilar skull fracture.*

FIGURE 44.9 PATIENT WITH MAJOR MAXILLOFACIAL INJURY WITH TRACHEOSTOMY, BITE BLOCKS, FOLEY CATHETERS AND PACKS (NOTE FACIAL SWELLING)[18]

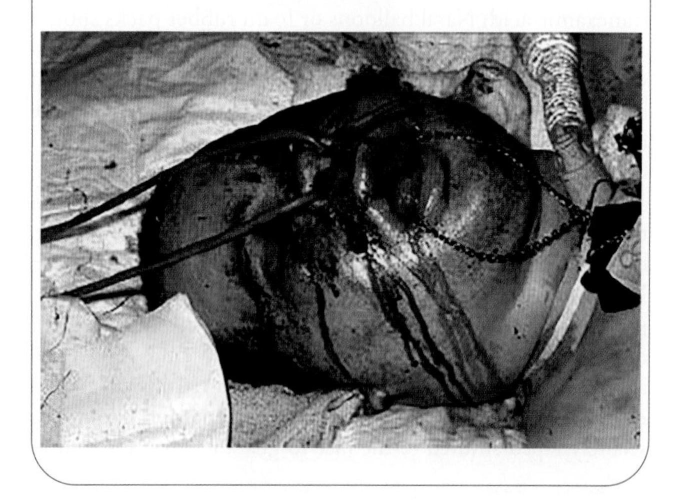

avoid aspiration. When fixation is tenuous, suture the tube/pack or implement to the face.

When simple manoeuvres have failed to ameliorate blood loss, severe haemorrhage from facial trauma may require manual reduction of the facial bones.[15] This can be performed by an experienced surgeon in the resuscitation bay while the patient is intubated, sedated and has been given adequate analgesia. If reduction fails to control the bleeding, then angiography and transcatheter arterial embolisation of bleeding vessels may be necessary,[23,24] and can also be performed prior to surgical fixation of fractures.[16] Ligation of arteries and veins may be necessary to control blood loss in institutions where angiography is not available or embolisation is unsuccessful. It is important for the emergency nurse to anticipate the need for the patient to be transferred for definitive care to a tertiary centre with angiography or operating suites and to expedite the process. Once haemorrhage is controlled, repair of fractures can be delayed while more urgent problems are managed.[16]

PRACTICE TIP

An ENT tray or trolley containing examination and packing equipment will expedite treatment of facial haemorrhage. Nurses can ensure adequate suction is available and if the patient is alert and orientated sucking on some ice may assist with vasoconstriction, decreasing swelling and provide some pain relief.

PRACTICE TIP

Blood loss may go unnoticed in the awake patient swallowing blood. Emergency clinicians need to encourage the patient to spit out blood and secretions to avoid nausea and vomiting. Suctioning is important and the patient may be given the opportunity to perform their own suction when possible.

Bleeding in the oral cavity can often be controlled by direct pressure. The emergency clinician can identify the bleeding source and ask the awake patient to apply direct pressure with gauze. If the patient is unconscious and intubated, the emergency clinician needs to pack the oral cavity laceration until the wounds can be sutured.

Prior to secondary survey the emergency clinician should assess the mental disability of the patient due to the significant association between maxillofacial trauma and head injuries.[4] A neurological examination is essential and will be discussed later in the chapter; however, a rudimentary assessment of pupil reactivity and posturing using the Glasgow Coma Scale (GCS) or the AVPU (Alert, Voice, Posturing, Unresponsive scale) is essential and needs to be documented. It is important that signs of raised intracranial pressure are not overlooked while focusing on an impressive facial fracture.

The patient's temperature is an essential consideration when dealing with trauma. There are very few circumstances other than anticoagulants that lead to catastrophic haemorrhaging. Euthermia is imperative to allow for the body's own coagulation cascade to function normally. Once the emergency clinician has control of the many variants that can alter outcome, a more detailed approach to the issues at hand is required through the secondary survey (see Chapter 42).

SECONDARY EVALUATION

Patient history

Patient history is important to gain insight into the context of their injury and to gain an understanding of the likelihood of different pathological processes. Without this insight, the examination that follows is most likely to be done at post-mortem. Every injury has context and identifies associated injuries that may be missed.

History of the injury must be documented and should include the following questions:

- Name of the person—indicates ethnicity, socio-economic background—allows family to be contacted.
- Age—indicative of physiological reserve.
- Occupation—work-related injury, considerations for recovery.
- Social—socio-economic background, access to care, health literacy, responsibilities, next of kin.
- Handedness—relates to brain injury and recovery milestones—handedness is important for rehabilitation.
- Time of injury—may indicate how much time the patient has left with regards to treatment response. May indicate why the clinical picture has changed and is inconsistent with the clinical findings.
- Who was present and was the injury witnessed—document their names and contact details.
- Perpetrator of the assault/incident/injury—specifics are important to determine mandatory reporting requirements, safety of patient.

The mechanism and location of the injury:

- What happened?
- Where was the patient struck?
- How hard was the patient struck?—speed of vehicle, the calibre of the rifle, the height of the roof
- How many times was the patient struck?—e.g. multiple strikes to the midface with a baseball bat
- What implement was used?

Associated results of the injury:

- Loss of consciousness—closed head injury occurs in 17% of facial fractures[9]
- Amnesia/concussive symptoms
- Bleeding—location and extent—nose, ears, mouth
- Vomiting
- Seizures
- Altered level of consciousness/confusion
- Altered vision/eye changes
- Altered occlusion—is their bite normal?
- Altered sensation on their face—region and distribution
- Loss or loosening of teeth—have all teeth been located?—teeth are an aspiration risk
- Does the patient have neck pain or altered sensation in their limbs?
- Is the patient continent?
- Are there any other areas of concern that require examination?
- Past medical history—loss of consciousness may be related to diabetes, previous self-harm/drug overdose
- Past surgical history—previous neurosurgery, trauma surgery, fractures
- Medications—may alter bleeding/level of consciousness/neurological function.

Clinical examination should always proceed in a top-down manner so as not to miss vital clues to the injury, and should be thoroughly documented. Assessment for deformity should occur as soon as possible, prior to swelling obstructing any bony deformities (Fig. 44.10). Assessment of vision-threatening injuries is also a priority. Observe for eyelid ecchymosis, assess for loss of vision, visual acuity, pupillary reactivity and symmetry, extraocular movements and diplopia. More detail on eye assessment is presented in Chapter 32, and on ear and dental assessment in Chapter 31.

- Fully expose the areas of concern to examine and look for swelling deformity and asymmetry.
- Palpate all areas for tenderness, fractures and subcutaneous emphysema.
- Vertex of scalp—examine the scalp extensively for swelling, haematomas, abscesses, previous scars.

FIGURE 44.10 PALPATION EXAMINATION TECHNIQUES FOR FACIAL INJURIES

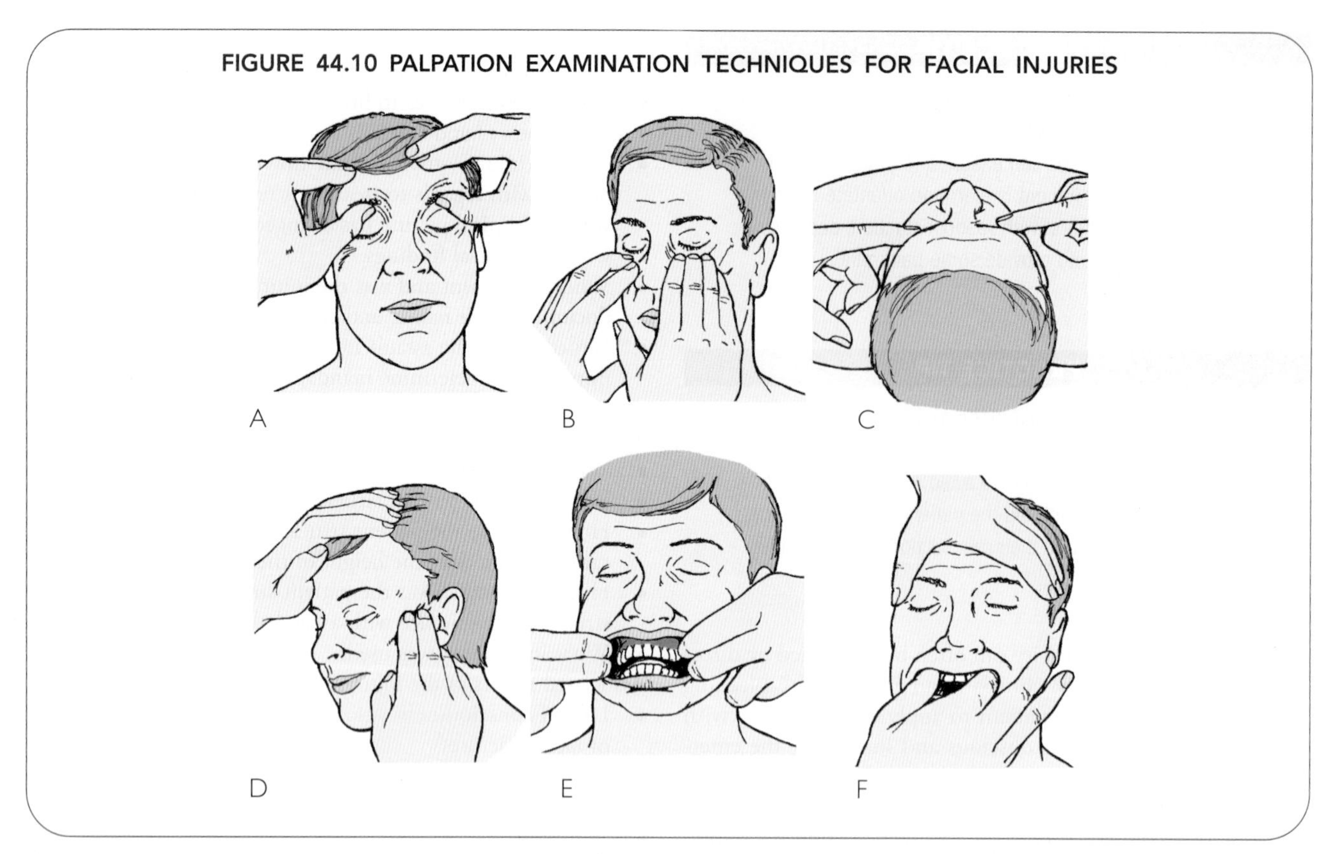

A. Palpation for irregularities of supraorbital ridge. **B.** Palpation for irregularities of infraorbital ridge and zygoma. **C.** Comparing height of malar eminences. **D.** Palpation for depression of zygomatic arch. **E.** Visualisation of gross dental occlusion. **F.** Manoeuvre to ascertain motion in maxilla.

TABLE 44.3 CRANIAL NERVES INVOLVED IN FACIAL TRAUMA

NERVE	NAME	FUNCTION	DESCRIPTION	ASSESSMENT
III	Oculomotor	Motor	Eyeball movement; supplies 5 of 7 ocular muscles	Pupil response; ocular movement to four quadrants
IV	Trochlear	Motor	Eyeball movement (superior oblique)	As above
V	Trigeminal	Motor and sensory	Facial sensation; jaw movement	Assessing pain, touch, hot and cold sensations, bite, opening mouth against resistance
VII	Facial	Motor and sensory	Facial expression; taste from anterior two-thirds of tongue	Zygomatic branch: have patient close eyes tightly
				Temporal branch: have patient elevate brows, wrinkle forehead
				Buccal branch: have patient elevate upper lip, wrinkle nose, whistle

- Paediatric patients should have their fontanelles examined.
- Ears—internal examination—bruising within the ear canal, bruising posteriorly—battle signs = base of skull fractures.
- Occipital areas and frontal areas—feel the contour of the aforementioned areas—step defects/pain, contour anomalies, altered sensation.
- Frontal bandeau—run your fingers along the brow and around the edges of the orbit looking for step deformities.
- Check the pupils—equal and reactive to light, subconjunctival haemorrhage, asymmetric gaze, diplopia, inability to track one's finger.
- Examine the cranial nerves in turn and systematically as these often allow for location of serious pathology especially if the signs change (Table 44.3).
- Place your thumbs over the maxillary sinuses and press posteriorly—assess sensation over the midface (Fig. 44.10).

FIGURE 44.11 EXAMINATION OF THE MIDFACE FOR INSTABILITY[28]

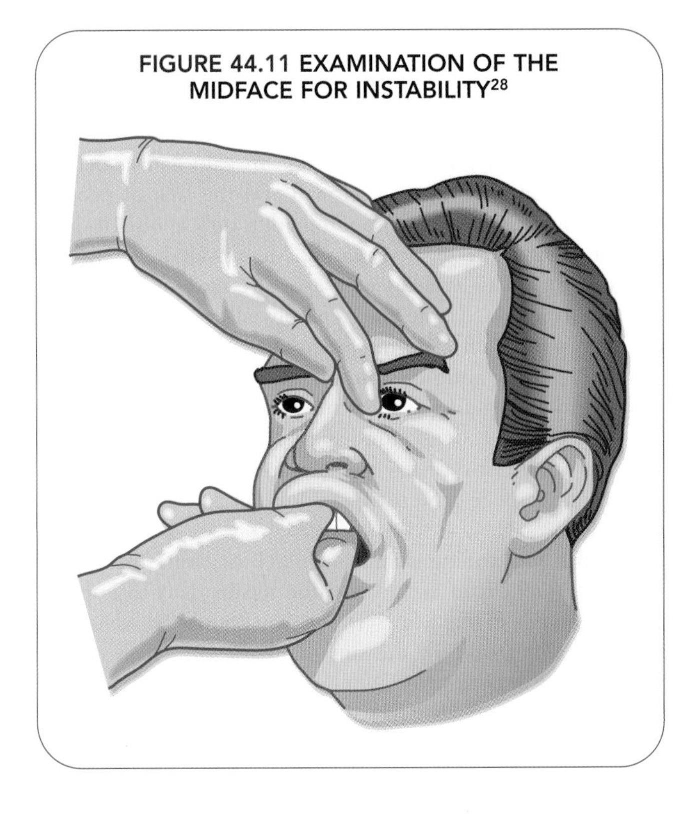

- Ask the patient to show you their teeth—check the dentition—false or native—good hygiene or poor dentition—note any swelling of the gums or floor of mouth.
- Hold the mandible with your thumb in the floor of the mouth and the forefinger under the chin and rock the mandible gently from side to side and open and close the mouth. This should be repeated in a similar fashion for the maxilla/midface. NOTE: Leave this until last as it may be very uncomfortable and the patient may not let you examine them again after this manoeuvre (Fig. 44.11).[28]
- Examine the C-spine if the patient is sitting upright (see Chapter 47 for cervical spine assessment and management). Approximately 20% of all C-spine injuries have an associated maxillofacial injury.[9] Remind yourself of the relevant anatomy while examining the facial skeleton (see Fig. 44.1).

Triage guidelines specific to maxillofacial emergencies can be found in Table 44.2.

CLINICAL INTERVENTIONS/CONSIDERATIONS

Lacerations

The treatment aim for soft-tissue trauma is complete closure of the wound to ensure functionality and cosmesis, and to enhance healing in sterile, vascularised conditions. Repair of facial lacerations should occur in a timely fashion, unless surgical repair to underlying structures is necessary.[29] If repair of underlying structures is required, then rudimentary closure often helps with transport, analgesia and temporary dressing, as long as there is a clear plan in place to explore the wound at a later date/time. Simple lacerations can be cleaned, debrided and sutured, primarily due to the sensitive aesthetic nature of the area involved. Given the unique dynamics of movement, careful consideration should be paid when considering how to repair the wound.

The question of whether specialist advice and treatment is required should also be considered whenever there is the possibility that there may be injury to underlying structures (e.g. glands, nerves, ducts, eye injuries). Avulsion injuries and trauma to functional aesthetic units such as noses, ears and eyelids deserve special consideration and probable specialist referral. While the main concern in repairing the structures is proper function, the aesthetic form and long-term result is what often determines patient satisfaction. If there is any doubt, refer the patient early to a specialist for tertiary care and management. Patients with multiple stab wounds to the face who do not receive early exploration and are not referred early for specialist care are at risk of significant facial nerve injury.[30] Deeper lacerations and those associated with compound fractures often require surgical exploration and sterile closure and should be referred to the treating specialist. Decontamination and reduction of bacterial load can often be performed by nursing and paramedic staff with pulse lavage. Pulse irrigation/lavage is best performed with normal saline solution,[31] and wounds consequently covered with saline-soaked gauze. Avulsed and degloved tissue in the facial region is often still viable tissue due to the rich vascular supply of the region. Excessive debridement and removal of tissue should therefore be avoided until definitively assessed.

Repair of facial lacerations in uncooperative patients is extremely difficult and often requires general anaesthetic for the safety and ease of treatment that a full theatre affords the surgeon. Delaying repair until the patient is more cooperative is therefore acceptable and any temporising measures by staff is acceptable in these circumstances. Use of povidone–iodine solution and hydrogen peroxide solutions should be avoided as they may delay tissue healing (see Chapter 16).[31,32]

Alignment of important aesthetic landmarks in eyebrows and eyelids is best achieved prior to excessive swelling. Every effort should be made to optimise the accurate alignment of the said landmarks given favourable circumstances. The eyebrows should never be shaved as this eliminates important landmarks.[31] When suturing the eyebrow, hairs are aligned so that they slant in a downward and outward direction. Vermilion–cutaneous and vermilion–mucosal margins are also important anatomical landmarks in the repair of lip lacerations. Ensure borders are perfectly aligned to prevent development of step deformities of the lip (Fig. 44.12).[31] Tissue loss from any anatomical structure that cannot be realigned with ease requires reconstruction by a plastic surgeon (Table 44.4).[24]

Intraoral injuries should be meticulously cleaned and irrigated. Superficial tongue, buccal mucosa and gingival lacerations do not need suturing as they often heal primarily within a few days.[31] Gaping intraoral and tongue lacerations should be sutured with minimal approximation, as should the gingiva overlying the mandibular and maxillary ridge.[31] The vascular supply of the mouth is so robust that even an amputated tongue is often able to be repaired with interrupted sutures.[33] The amputated tongue should be kept moist by wrapping it in saline-soaked gauze and the patient should present to emergency as soon as possible due to haemorrhaging and airway control as well as ease of surgery and haemostasis, which is preferentially performed in an operating theatre.

FIGURE 44.12 LIP LACERATION THROUGH THE VERMILION BORDER.

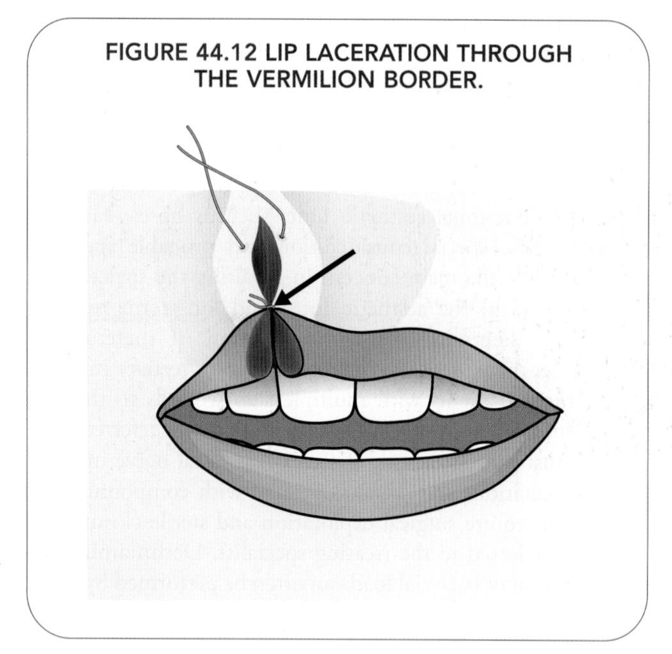

Closure requires proper alignment with the first suture placed at the vermilion-cutaneous border.

TABLE 44.4 RADIOGRAPHICAL EXAMINATION FOR MAXILLOFACIAL INJURY

TEST	DESCRIPTION
Water's view (posteroanterior)	Single most useful x-ray in maxillofacial injury Delineates orbital rim and floor Detects blood in maxillary sinus
Towne's view	Mandible condyles–subcondylar regions of orbital floor
Anterior, posterior and lateral	Skull Sinus, roof of orbit
Submental vertex (jug handle)	Zygomatic arch Details base of skull
AP and lateral oblique mandible	Condylar, coronoid, body and symphysis
Occlusal and apical	Palate, symphysis, roots of teeth
CT scan	Provides definitive diagnosis in cervical spine injury Standard for assessing soft-tissue injuries Standard for assessing complex facial fractures; should be ordered when concomitant brain and facial injuries are identified
MRI	Useful for identifying soft-tissue injuries in optic nerve Muscle herniation, infraocular and intraocular haematomas, entrapment

AP: anteroposterior; CT: computed tomography; MRI: magnetic resonance imaging.

Recovery is excellent and functionally the tongue has very few deficits.

Tissue adhesives, such as glue, can play a part in repair of low-tension facial lacerations in children and adults because of the speed of application, reduction in pain and anxiety of repair, resistance to bacterial growth and the lack of need to remove sutures.[34] Day-1 tensile strength is only about 10–15% of that of a suture-repaired wound. It cannot be used over joints or high activity areas with excessive movement, such as the mouth region. Tissue glue typically adheres for 7–14 days and then sloughs off with the epidermis. Petroleum-based ointments, including antibiotic ointments, should not be used on the wound after gluing as these substances can weaken the tissue glue.[35] Simple, small, non-gaping facial lacerations that are not over a joint or on hairy skin surfaces may also be repaired with wound tape (e.g. Steristrips) if it is not an area of excessive movement.[31]

Discharge planning should include instructing the patient to apply emollient to facial laceration repairs daily to improve the appearance of the scar.[35] The patient should be advised to avoid spending time in the sun or to use sunscreen on the wound for at least 2 years. Wounds to the oral cavity must be rinsed clean after meals.[31] The patient should be made aware of when sutures are to be removed, signs and symptoms of infection, pain relief strategies and wound care. Further information regarding wound care can be found in Chapter 16.

PRACTICE TIP

Discharge advice for facial wounds should include apply emollient to facial laceration repairs daily, avoid spending time in the sun or to use sunscreen on the wound for at least 2 years to improve appearance of the scar.

Bite wounds

Bite wounds include scratches, punctures, lacerations and avulsions. Initially, these wounds may look innocuous; however, they can lead to serious infections and complications. Lacerations/puncture wounds caused by animal or human bites are highly contaminated because of the bacteria and debris in the mouth. Facial bites, especially those in children, require meticulous management. Careful debridement, ample irrigation and cleansing and primary interrupted suture repair is important. Close follow-up is required for at least 5 days. Because subsequent plastic reconstruction may be needed, it may be useful to consult with a plastic surgeon at the time of initial repair. Extensive facial animal bites frequently require surgical exploration and repair, and in children may involve fractures to the face or skull.[36] Detailed discussion on the types of bacterial transmissions and management of bite wounds is found in Chapter 16.

Friction injuries

Bitumen rash and other friction injuries to the face present a unique problem because of potential tattooing or epidermal staining.[37] Gunpowder can cause permanent discolouration of skin and should be removed by using a local anaesthetic and scrubbing with a hard brush or hard-bristle toothbrush in the first hour, if possible, taking into consideration forensic implications. Early removal will also reduce the amount of burning from gunpowder to the epithelial and collagen layers of the skin. Moist wound healing is recommended for abrasions.[31] Visible glass fragments can be lifted with tape applied gently to the face. The aesthetic consequences of residual product are substantial, so if any doubt exists about residue, subsequent surgical debridement may be required and should be discussed with a surgeon.

INVESTIGATIONS

Each department has their own guidelines with respect to facial trauma investigations. While many departments still use x-rays as first-line treatment, they are often equivocal and will require further imaging. Furthermore, if any doubt exists or the history indicates that there is a high likelihood of a fracture that cannot be seen on x-ray, then due diligence would dictate that further imaging be performed (Table 44.5).

TABLE 44.5 FACIAL FRACTURES: CLINICAL AND RADIOGRAPHICAL FINDINGS, AND COMPLICATIONS FOR SPECIFIC FACIAL FRACTURES[38]

FRACTURE	CLINICAL PRESENTATION	RADIOGRAPHICAL FINDINGS	COMPLICATIONS
Naso-orbital	Symptoms: pain, visual abnormalities Signs: massive periorbital and upper facial oedema and ecchymosis, epistaxis, traumatic telecanthus, foreshortening of nose with telescoping; associated intracranial injuries	Views: CT scan Findings: disruption of interorbital space and comminution of nasal pyramid; frontal, zygomatic, orbital, maxillary fractures common	Residual upper midface deformity ('dish face'); telecanthus; frontal sinus-nasolacrimal system pathology with mucocoele, mucopyocoele, dacryocystitis
Zygoma			
Arch	Symptoms: pain in lateral cheek, inability to close jaw Signs: swelling, crepitus over arch, obvious asymmetry	Views: Water's submentovertex Findings: depression of arch, comminution	Contour irregularities of arch area, flattening of arch
Body 'tripod fracture'	Symptoms: pain, trismus, diplopia, numb upper lip, lower lid, bilateral nasal area Signs: swelling, ecchymosis of malar and periorbital areas; palpable infraorbital rim 'step-off'; entrapment of extraocular muscles with disconjugate gaze; scleral ecchymosis, displacement of lateral canthal ligament	Views: Water's submentovertex, CT scan Findings: clouding, air/fluid level maxillary sinus, separation of zygomaticomaxillary, zygomaticofrontal and zygomaticotemporal suture lines	Residual malar deformity, enophthalmos, diplopia, infraorbital nerve anaesthesia, chronic maxillary sinusitis
Orbital floor	Symptoms: diplopia, orbital pain Signs: periorbital oedema, ecchymosis, enophthalmos, extraocular muscle entrapment, disconjugate gaze; hyphaema, subluxation of lens, retinal detachment, rupture of globe with direct eye trauma	Views: Water's, CT scan, tomograms Findings: air/fluid level maxillary sinus, herniated adnexa and/or orbital floor fragments in maxillary sinus	Enophthalmos, diplopia; recurrent orbital cellulitis with implant (alloplastic) extrusion
Mandible			
Condyle	Symptoms: pain at fracture site, referred pain to ear Signs: crepitus, excessive salivation, swelling of condylar region, deviation of jaw towards fracture, cross-bite or open-bite deformity	Views: AP, oblique, Water's, OPG Findings: non-displaced, or displaced anteriorly and medially	Ankylosis of TMJ; chronic TMJ
Angle	Symptoms: pain at fracture site, inability to close mouth Signs: swelling at angle of jaw, ecchymosis, crepitus, malocclusion	Views: OPG, mandibular series Findings: non-displaced (favourable) or posterior fragment displaced upwards and medially (non-favourable)	Non-union, malunion, osteomyelitis
Body	Symptoms: pain at fracture site, limitation of movement Signs: swelling, ecchymosis, crepitus, malocclusion	Views: OPG, mandibular series Findings: non-displaced (favourable), or posterior fragment displaced upwards and medially, anterior fragments rotated lingually (non-favourable)	Osteomyelitis, infection (tooth in fracture line)

TABLE 44.5 FACIAL FRACTURES: CLINICAL AND RADIOGRAPHICAL FINDINGS, AND COMPLICATIONS FOR SPECIFIC FACIAL FRACTURES—cont'd

FRACTURE	CLINICAL PRESENTATION	RADIOGRAPHICAL FINDINGS	COMPLICATIONS
Symphysis	Symptoms: pain Signs: malocclusion, frequent association with soft-tissue wounds of lower lip, tongue	Views: mandibular series, submento-vertex Findings: non-displaced or lingual rotation or anterior fragments, may be associated with angle or condyle fractures	Residual malocclusion, loss of chin projection, asymmetry; osteomyelitis
Maxilla			
Le Fort I (transverse)	Symptoms: pain upper jaw, numb upper teeth Signs: midfacial oedema and ecchymosis, epistaxis, malocclusion, mobility of maxillary dentition	Views: Water's, OPG, CT scan Findings: opaque maxillary sinus, displacement of fragments of alveolus if comminuted; fracture through maxillary sinus and pterygoid plates	Loss of teeth, infection, malocclusion
Le Fort II (pyramidal)	Symptoms: pain midface, numb upper lip, lower lid, lateral nasal area Signs: midfacial oedema and ecchymosis, epistaxis, malocclusion, mobility of midface, nasal flattening, anaesthesia infraorbital nerve territory	Views: Water's, CT scan Findings: opaque maxillary sinuses, separation through frontal process, lacrimal bones, floor of orbits, zygomaticomaxillary suture line, lateral wall of maxillary sinus and pterygoid plates	Non-union, malunion lacrimal system obstruction, infraorbital nerve anaesthesia, diplopia, malocclusion
Le Fort III (craniofacial dysjunction)	Symptoms: pain face, difficulty breathing Signs: 'donkey-face' deformity, malocclusion, mobile face, marked facial oedema and ecchymosis, epistaxis, CSF rhinorrhoea	Views: Water's, CT scan Findings: separation of midthird of face at zygomaticofrontal, zygomaticotemporal and nasofrontal sutures, and across orbital floors; opaque maxillary sinuses	Non-union, malunion, malocclusion, lengthening of midface, lacrimal system obstruction

CT: Computed tomography; CSF: cerebrospinal fluid; AP: anteroposterior; TMJ: temporomandibular joint.

It is preferable to always scan the entire head and face in trauma situations. This avoids having images that are either inadequate or do not cover all the areas of concern. CT scan allows for evaluation of many areas simultaneously with negligible radiation exposure when considering the context of a person's entire life and radiation load. All patients with altered levels of consciousness should have a minimum of a CT scan.

Isolated nasal injuries do not require imaging. They serve no purpose and do not alter surgical management. Mandible fractures are also best viewed on CT scan, but can also be detected with an orthopantomogram (OPG). This is a scan that places the patient at the centre of a semicircle where they are required to place their chin in a holding frame and the beam then rotates around a central axis running through their head. This scan is very useful to determine a focal abscess at the base of a tooth and dental trauma. The emergency clinician should consider which imaging modalities would serve best in identifying pathology that marries up with the clinical picture and historical background. Repeat trips back to the scanner can be strenuous, stressful and dangerous for the unstable patient and should be avoided.

SPECIFIC FRACTURE MANAGEMENT

FRONTAL SINUS FRACTURES

Most facial frontal sinuses are designed to withstand at least 750 kg of force when struck directly. The initial design is to act as a shock absorber and to crumple to prevent coup and contra-coup injuries of the brain.

History of injury often involves a direct strike to the forehead region or indeed the forehead striking an immobile object. Clinical findings may be obvious with contour anomalies visible and associated swelling evident. Associated bruising, possible overlying lacerations and a CSF leak often direct the examiner to the area of concern. CSF leaks can be confirmed with a urine dipstick or beta transferring analysis of the liquid with a double ring sign often evident.

Management is largely based on well-devised algorithms concerning involvement of the frontal table alone or both the anterior and the posterior table with associated nasofrontal recess being affected or whether the fracture is compound or complex. Closed injuries with isolated table fractures often need to be assessed by a neurosurgical team to rule out any associated brain trauma, while the contour deformity can be managed as a delayed procedure. All CSF leaks must be assessed by a surgical team and preventive measures involving elevation of the head at 30 degrees to allow for drainage and swelling to subside. Antibiotic prophylaxis is recommended for any sinus exposure and any elevation of sinus pressure, such as blowing one's nose and flying, needs to be avoided for at least 2 weeks. If the brain is not exposed and there is no active CSF leak without a compound component, then the treatment can be delayed as long as the defect is not contributing to elevated intracranial pressure.

NASAL FRACTURES

These are one of the most common fractures seen in the ED. Overlooked nasal injury can lead to permanent deformity and airway obstruction from septal deviation and abnormal bone growth in children. The history usually relates to blunt trauma to the nasal region resulting in pain and swelling, as well as considerable bleeding in closed fractures. The bleeding is often from associated septal trauma to an area called Kiesselbach's plexus where multiple arteries coalesce to provide good blood supply to the nose. Tears elsewhere in the mucosa can also lead to bleeding and the amount of blood loss often leads to alarm. Careful examination of each naris can identify septal haematomas, lacerations and the ability of the patient to breathe through their nose. A septal haematoma appears as a bulging, tense bluish mass that feels doughy when palpated (Figs 44.13, 44.14).[39,40] Clinical findings include swelling, deformity, bleeding (epistaxis), contusion, periorbital bruising, pain and crepitus. Examination of an actively bleeding nose is fruitless and often distressing for both the patient and the staff. Palpation of the bridge of the nose also serves no purpose except to upset an already traumatised patient.

Attempts to try and stem the bleeding (epistaxis) include the following:[41,42]

- Calm and reassure the patient—elevated blood pressure leads to further bleeding.

FIGURE 44.13 NASAL FRACTURE WITH DISLOCATION OF NASAL BONES AND SEPTAL CARTILAGE[39]

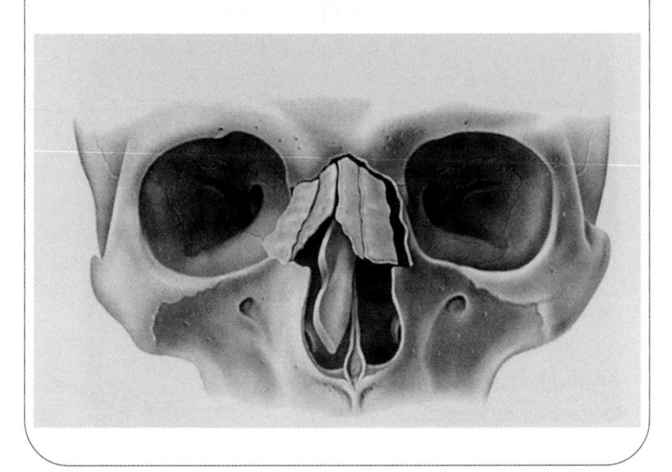

FIGURE 44.14 NASAL SEPTUM HAEMATOMA[40]

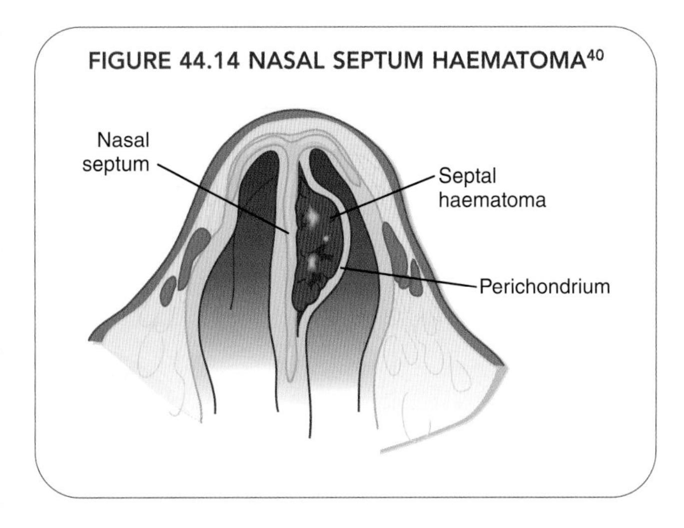

- Encourage the patient to allow the blood to flow outwards—swallowing of blood leads to nausea and vomiting and also masking of blood loss.
- Sucking ice or small sips of ice water helps to cool the collateral circulation and leads to vasoconstriction.
- Ice packs or ice water applied to the nose can also help stem the flow.
- Ask the patient to apply pressure to Kiesselbach's plexus—this requires the patient to pinch the nose, concentrating on the septum just inside the nose (Fig. 44.15). All of the above are important tips for the paramedic in the pre-hospital environment.
- If this does not help, then try to perform nasoendoscopy—look for areas of bleeding—if an area can be seen, attempt cautery—use either silver nitrate sticks or electrocautery.
- Packing often helps in these situations—Merocel® packs inserted horizontally and then inflated with ice water.
- If the bleeding stops—leave the packs in situ until the next day and then attempt removal.
- Septal haematomas observed need to be referred to ENT/plastic surgery specialists to drain (Fig. 44.14).
- If the bleeding continues but is mainly posterior, this can be dealt with directly with cautery.
- If the posterior bleed will not subside, then packing should be instituted and senior help should be sought to perform posterior endoscopy, Foley catheter traction pressure or sphenopalatine ligation.
- For most patients, epistaxis resolves with these manoeuvres and they can then be sent to their GP in 1 week for review. If their nose is deemed to be aesthetically displeasing they may be referred to a specialist. Fractures do not always lead to deformity and deformities are not always due to fractures—hence why pressing on the nasal bones is not helpful.
- Any correction of fractured nasal bones generally must occur with 2 weeks prior to bone healing.

Nasal bone fractures are usually managed either immediately (at the pitch side of the playing field) or more commonly expectantly and reviewed in 7–10 days. Symmetry and ease of breathing are then assessed and if the deformity warrants correction the patient has a general anaesthetic, at which time a closed reduction is performed with splinting.

FIGURE 44.15 VASCULAR ANATOMY OF NASAL SEPTAL BLOOD SUPPLY[40]

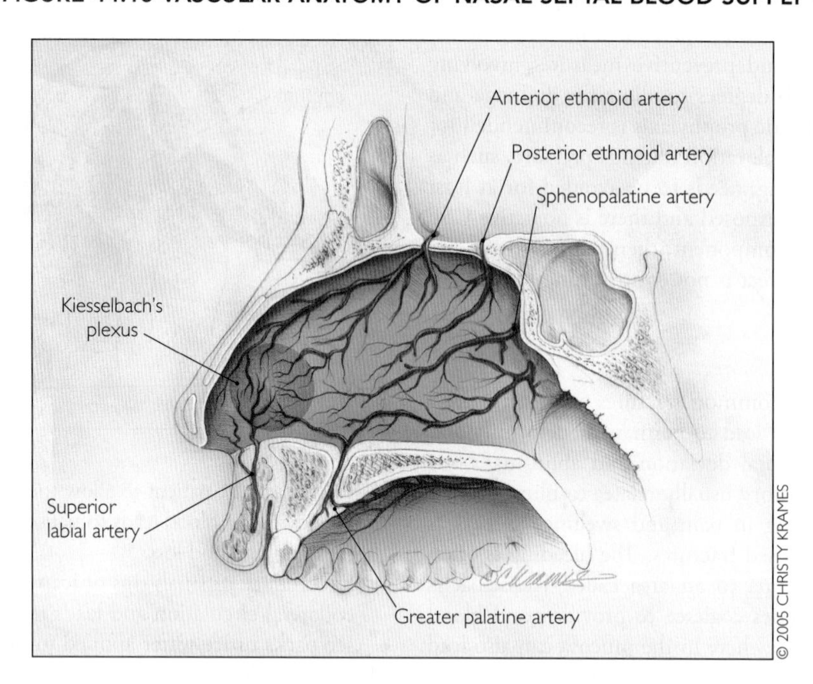

The emergency nurse should ensure that a definitive appointment exists for the patient to see an ENT or plastic surgeon within 7 days. Failure to do so will result in the patient missing a window of opportunity and having to undergo a rhinoplasty months later.

PRACTICE TIP

Pinching of the nose can be unreliable as it is tempting to intermittently check for bleeding. It also relies on the patient or caregivers to pinch the nose or hold the ice pack for extended periods. Using wooden tongue depressors as a nose clip for epistaxis is effective and simple.[43]

NASO-ORBITAL-ETHMOID FRACTURES

These fractures represent a more complex form of midface and nasal bone fracture in an area with minimal coverage and interspersed between three complexes. Patients often present with a history of trauma or the application of extreme force within the medial region of the eye socket or side of nose. This can be with a sharp implement or a blunt instrument.

Clinically, the most obvious deformity is telecanthus (patient's eyes appear too far apart). Loss of nasal bridge projection with peri-orbital oedema and orbital rim step deformities are obvious (Fig. 44.14). If the cribriform plate is affected and the dura torn, CSF rhinorrhoea occurs. CT scan is required to identify the extent of this complicated injury.

Imaging is preferably with CT scanning with fine cuts and zero degree gantry tilt. This allows a view of the canthal insertion both medially and laterally and for the anatomy of the nasolacrimal duct to be ascertained. Referral should be early as these patients often have exposed sinuses and associated orbital issues. Again 30 degrees of head tilt, antibiotics and restriction in sinus positive pressure should be employed.

ORBITAL FLOOR FRACTURES

These fractures are often called orbital blowout fractures. This is due to the proposed mechanism called the hydraulic hypothesis of the fracture, which exerts pressure on the globe from a punch, for instance, which then leads to a massive increase in intra-orbital pressure, leading to blowing out of the orbital floor. The second proposed mechanism is direct trauma to the inferior rim of the orbit leading to buckling and fracturing of the floor (Fig. 44.16).[28]

FIGURE 44.16 MECHANISM AND STRUCTURES INVOLVED IN AN ORBITAL BLOWOUT FRACTURE[28]

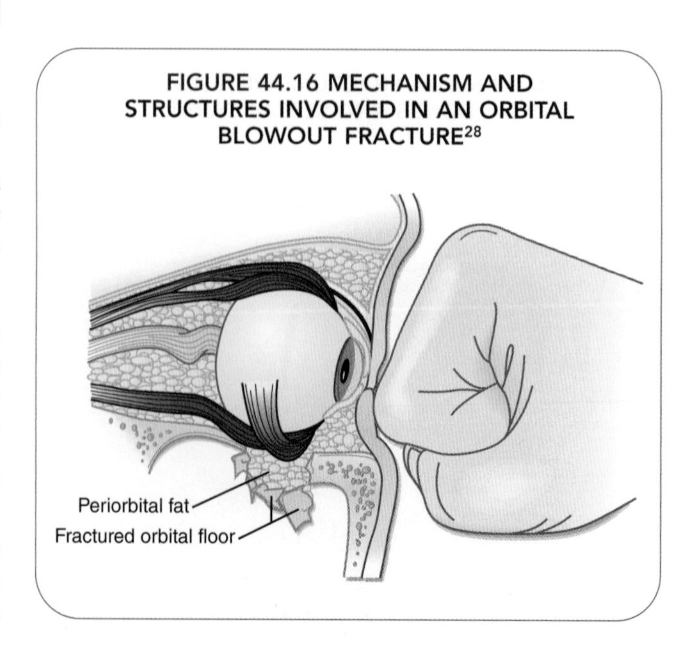

Clinical presentations include:

- diplopia, as the optical axis is disrupted through displacement, haematoma or herniation
  - binocular diplopia—visual axis has been affected and concordant gaze is disrupted
  - monocular diplopia—indicative of hyphaema, lens dislocation or globe disruption
- enophthalmos (retrusion of the globe into the socket), which often leads to a negative vector
- altered external eye movements, especially in children when the inferior rectus muscle is trapped
- dysaesthesia in the infraorbital nerve distribution. The fracture line often follows the contour of the natural orbital canals around the orbit which include the infraorbital canal.

Difficulty or pain in upward gaze within a child (usually below the age of 6 years) after trauma to the globe often indicates a trapped eye muscle.[44] Note: This is a surgical emergency and needs to go to theatre within 6 hours (see Chapter 32) (Fig. 44.17).

- Note: Injury to the globe can affect more than just the bones around the eye. The globe itself needs to be assessed. This includes everything from the cornea (abrasion) to the retina (bleeding). Any change in visual acuity needs to be assessed by an ophthalmic surgeon to determine the level of injury with a wide angle lens.
- Proptosis (bulging of the eye), epiphora (watering of the eye), nausea and vomiting accompanied by inconsolable pain are often preludes to retrobulbar haematomas (bleeding behind the globe). Note: This is a surgical emergency and if not corrected urgently will lead to irreversible loss of vision.
- Investigations for these fractures are with a CT scan—this allows for view of the natural axes of the globe, effacement of the periorbital musculature, assess the size of the defect of the floor and assess for subluxation of orbital contents.[45] It also allows assessment of medial orbital wall issues and provides a baseline if observation is deemed appropriate (Fig. 44.18).
- These patients will require oral antibiotics as the orbit is now exposed to the maxillary sinus and they should be encouraged to sleep with the head elevated at 30 degrees and to abstain from any nose-blowing for 2 weeks. While a fractured orbit does not preclude flight, equilibrating one's ears often is challenging when you are unable to blow your nose.
- Advise the patient not to smoke.
- While this fracture is not an emergency if the rectus muscle is not involved, it should be managed within 2 weeks.

ZYGOMATICO-MAXILLARY FRACTURES

This region of the face can be injured either in isolation (zygoma only) or as part of a complex that articulates with the rest of the face at multiple other suture lines. This area is often referred to as the cheekbone region and is injured through direct trauma. This area of injury has a high association with midface injuries and occlusal complaints and is erroneously called a 'tripod' fracture.[46] Isolated zygoma fractures need to be assessed by the treating surgical team to assess if it is to be managed conservatively or whether the contour anomaly/obstruction to the coronoid process of the mandible will be an issue later on (Fig. 44.19).

These patients usually present with a very swollen cheekbone that leads to closure of the ipsilateral eye. If the fracture is isolated there is no change in the occlusion of the teeth, but there will be altered sensation to the teeth. This is due to involvement of the inferior orbital rim and associated infraorbital nerve injury within its osseous canal. This fracture is also often associated with inferior orbital floor fractures, which may

FIGURE 44.17 AN ORBITAL FLOOR FRACTURE

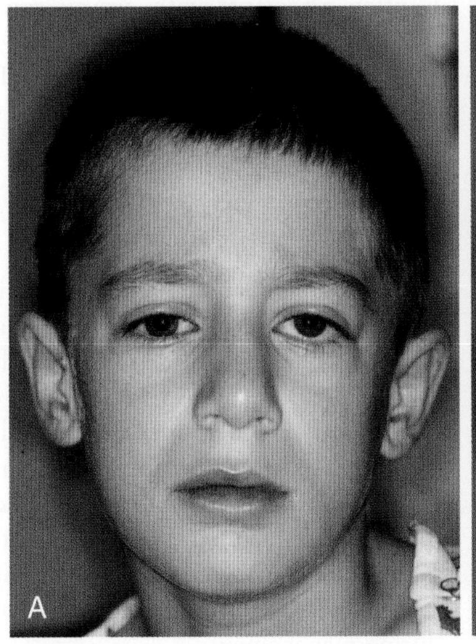

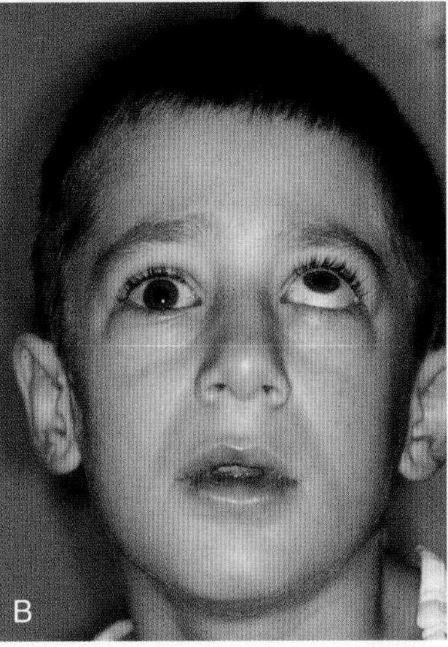

This injury represents a surgical emergency; the orbit must be explored and the muscle released expeditiously. **A.** Frontal gaze. **B.** Upward gaze.[44]

FIGURE 44.18 CORONIAL CT SHOWING A BLOW-OUT FRACTURE OF THE FLOOR OF THE RIGHT ORBIT[45]

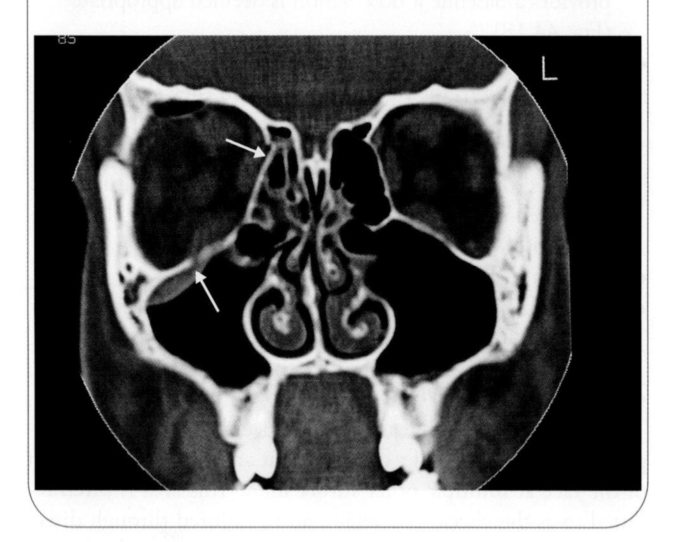

Fractures of the lamina papyracea (with blood within the ethmoid complex) and orbital floor (with herniation of orbital contents and air within orbital cavity) are indicated by arrows.

FIGURE 44.19 THREE-DIMENSIONAL RECONSTRUCTION DEMONSTRATING ZYGOMATICOMAXILLARY COMPLEX INVOLVEMENT AND DEGREE OF FRACTURE DISPLACEMENT[46]

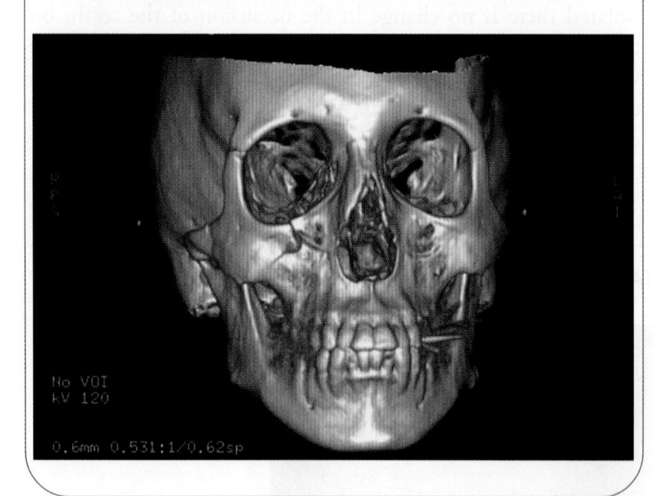

require fixation/correction. Depending on the length of time since presentation, the area may be visibly depressed with a contour anomaly. Again a high level of suspicion should accompany this pathology with regard to globe trauma. See other clinical associations (Box 44.1).

Investigations include examination of the oral cavity. Bruising may be evident in the upper buccogingival groove, and pain is often present in the retromolar area, as well as directly over the cheek projection. CT scanning is mandatory to determine the extent of the injury, as well as the possible associated orbital floor component (Fig. 44.19).

Again, oral antibiotics, head elevation and nose-blowing should be avoided due to communication of the maxillary sinus with the cheek region and the orbital floor. This fracture needs to be referred to the appropriate surgical management team for assessment.

BOX 44.1 TIDES MNEMONIC FOR ZYGOMATIC FRACTURES

T	**Trismus—tonic contracture of muscles of mastication**
I	**Infraorbital—hypoaesthesia or anaesthesia**
D	**Diplopia—double vision**
E	**Epistaxis—nosebleed**
S	**Symmetry absence—flatness or depression of cheek**

ALVEOLAR FRACTURES

These fractures are often very confronting as they involve the teeth. Consolation exists in that the teeth involved are often deciduous teeth and not the permanent equivalent in children. Adult presentations are just as distressing, but often have a good outcome as long as the alveolus is well aligned and allows for adequate bone stock for implant surgery to follow when trauma has settled.

Serious attention needs to be paid with regards to the teeth involved and their stability, both pre-hospital and during transport. Aspiration of dental matter can cause life-threatening pneumonia and every attempt should be made to clear a patient's airway and remove any debris, including teeth. Pieces of alveolus and teeth at a scene of the injury also need to be retrieved. Loose or threatened teeth need to be secured or removed. This can be done in the ED, either through a Fuji system where one tooth is welded onto another tooth using a splint for support or through removal manually. When in doubt, remove a tooth.

In unconscious patients the alveolus can often be re-approximated to a near-normal anatomical location. This fracture should be referred to a surgical team for stabilisation and reduction to optimise bone fixation and healing. This fracture is often associated with airway compromise and additional fractures of either jaw.

Investigations should include a CT scan and OPG to assess tooth viability and loss. A chest x-ray should be included in all work-ups related to this fracture.

MANDIBLE FRACTURES

These are fractures of the lower jaw. The pathophysiology of these fractures relates to extreme force being applied to this area. Such fractures are commonly isolated and related to punches to the face, but the fracture itself usually has two components. The area of direct impact is fractured, but often another area of the continuum is also injured.[47] Established fracture patterns are well described; for example, left paramedian and right angle of the mandible (Fig. 44.20). If only one part of the mandible is found to be fractured, the ipsilateral temporomandibular joint often bears the brunt of force distribution. Teeth are often collaterally damaged during the fracture and have to be considered during management.

Presentation is often pathognomonic. Patients are often intoxicated with evidence of trismus, malocclusion of their

FIGURE 44.20 FRACTURE SITES OF THE MANDIBLE[47]

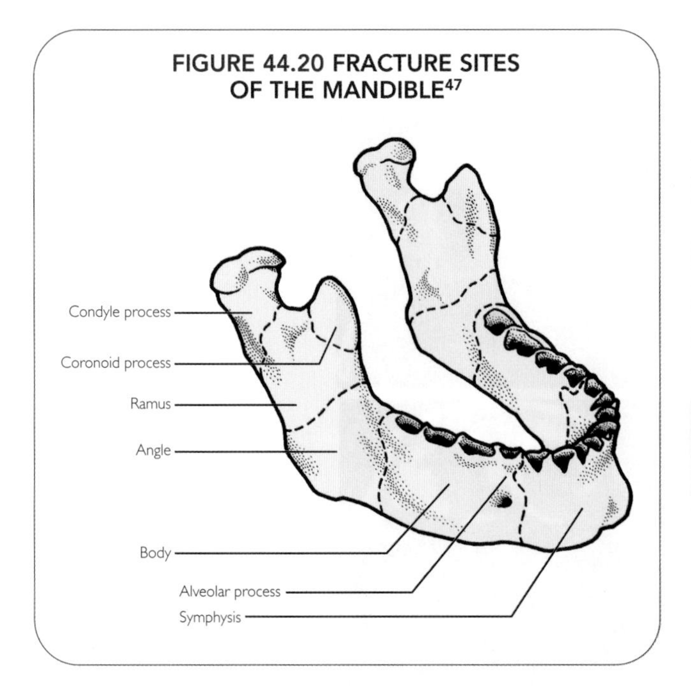

FIGURE 44.21 MALOCCLUSION CAUSED BY FRACTURE[48]

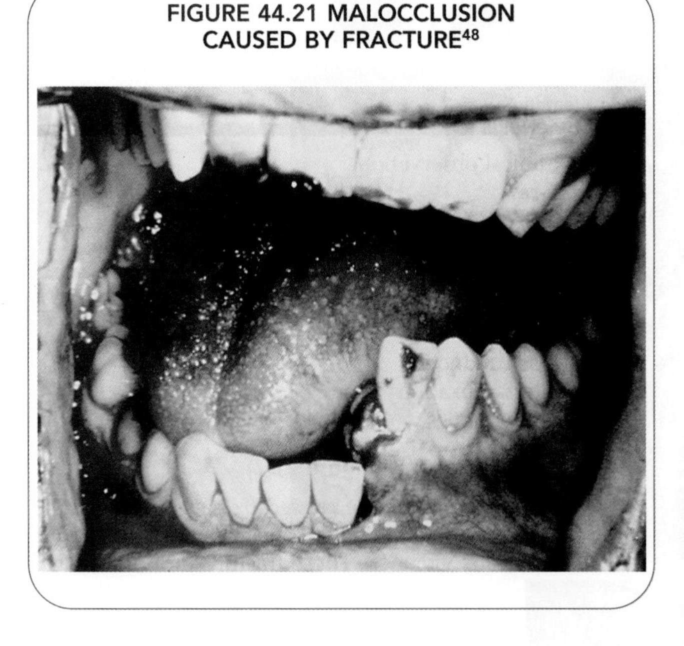

FIGURE 44.22 AN OPG OF A FRACTURED MANDIBLE

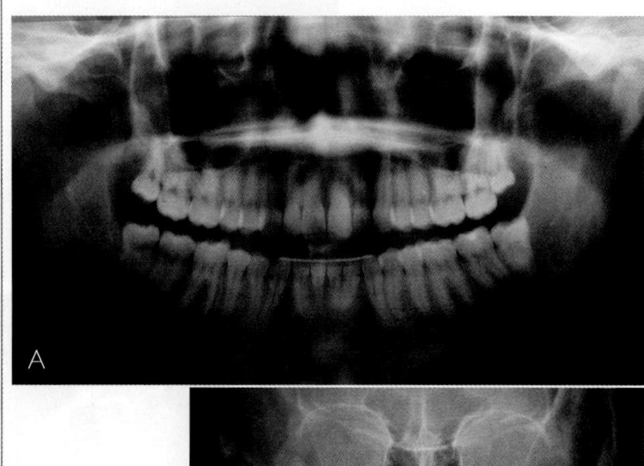

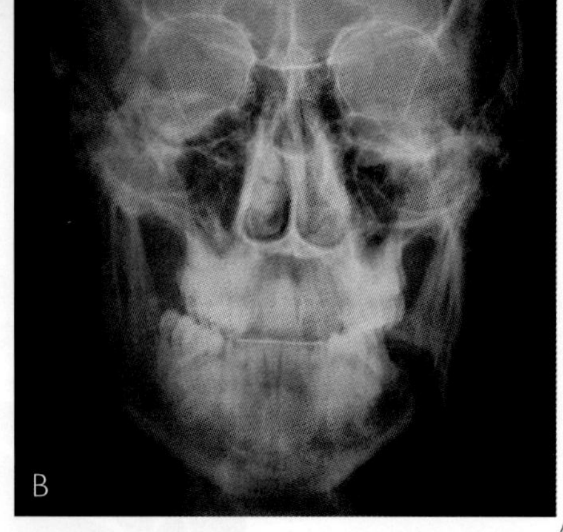

A. Panoramic radiograph demonstrating fracture at the left angle and right parasymphisis area. **B.** Posteroanterior radiograph of the skull showing severe displacement of the mandible angle on the left.[49]

FIGURE 44.23 THREE-DIMENSIONAL CT RECONSTRUCTIONS OF MINIMALLY DISPLACED MANDIBULAR FRACTURES[47]

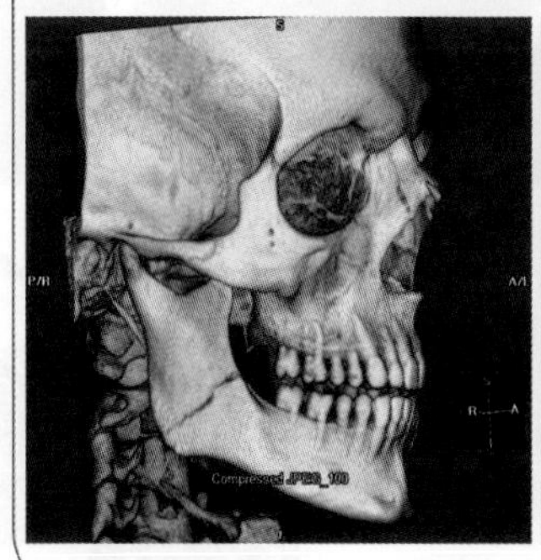

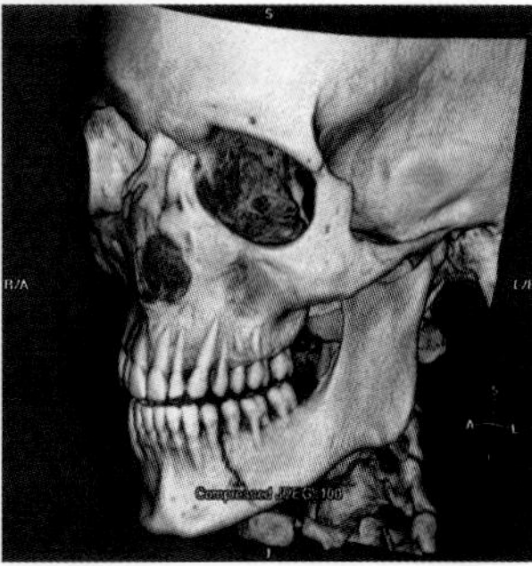

teeth, intra-oral bleeding and tenderness to various areas, as well as teeth (Fig. 44.21).[48] Clinical examination often yields areas of swelling, gingival bruising, teeth malalignment, drooling and obvious asymmetry of the mandible. Numbness of the chin and lower teeth is often present and palpation of the temporomandibular joint is often uncomfortable. Speech is often challenging and eating is a chore. Some patients are able to eat using the other side of the mandible while they may also complain of a blocked sensation within their ears due to swelling in the external auditory canal due to the proximity of a condyle fracture. The airway is rarely compromised in these patients unless associated with high collateral damage or force; for example, 0.44 Magnum shell.[49] Investigations include an OPG (Fig. 44.22) and CT scan (Fig. 44.23). These fractures need to be referred to the surgical management team early for assessment and pain management.

LE FORT FRACTURES—MIDFACE FRACTURES

These fractures involve various levels of disarticulation of parts of the upper face from the rest of the face or indeed the skull base (Fig. 44.24).[50] The fractures represent the very pinnacle of craniomaxillofacial trauma and the extreme end of the spectrum.

FIGURE 44.24 UNILATERAL LEFT-SIDED COMBINED LE FORT II & LE FORT III FACIAL FRACTURES (CASE 2):

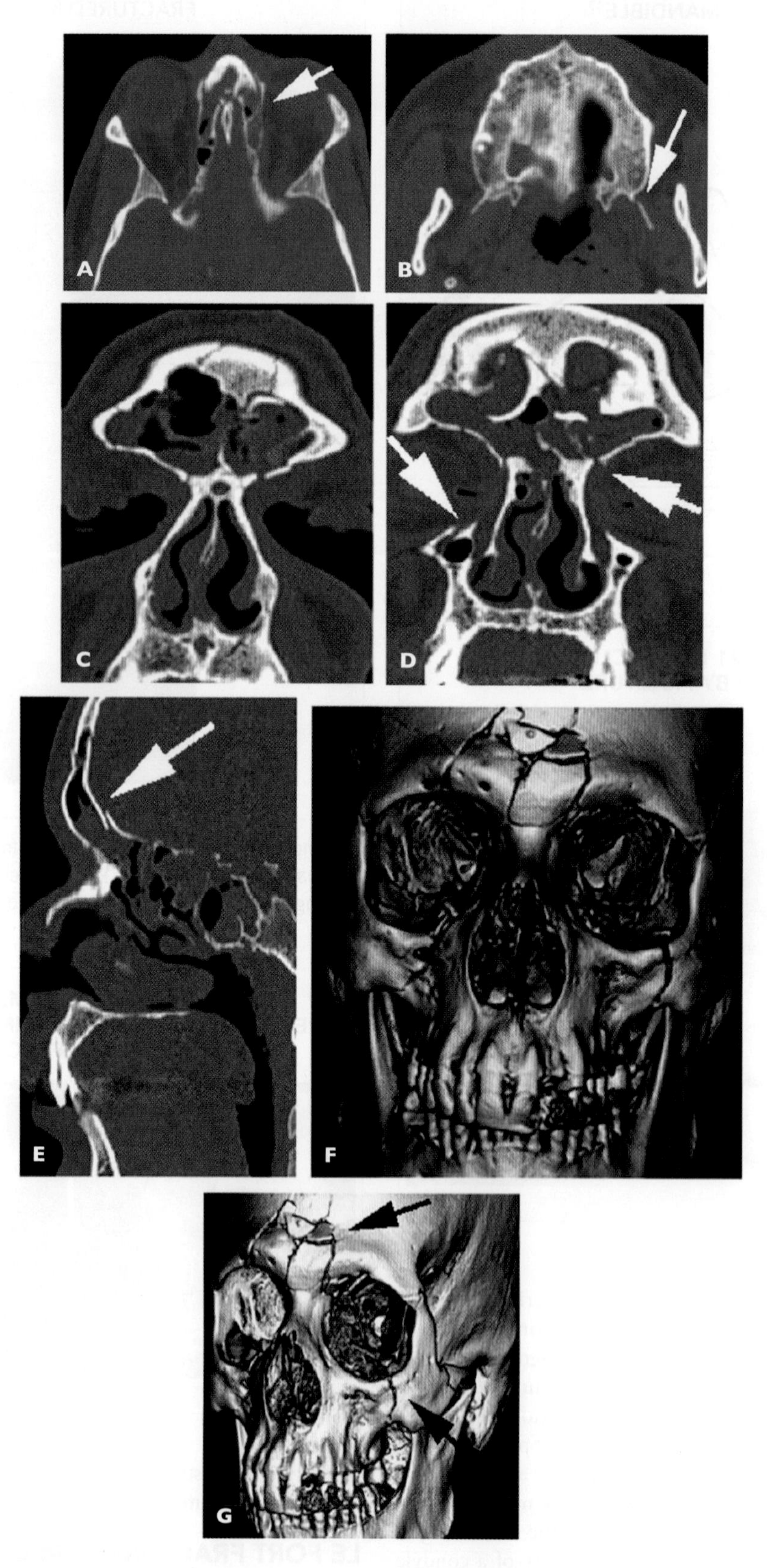

A and **B.** Non-enhanced axial CT images show fracture of the left pterygoid plate, both nasal bones and the lateral wall of left orbit. **C** and **D.** Coronal MPR images show the naso-frontal junction fracture, bilateral supra-orbital margin fractures and the frontal bone with frontal sinus opacification. **E.** Sagittal MPR image that displays the fracture of the nasal bone, the anterior and posterior walls of the frontal sinus. **F** and **G.** 3D VR images that demonstrate greatly the fractures involving frontal bone, both supra-orbital margins, the left inferior orbital wall, the left zygomatic arch, the left lateral orbital walls and the anterior wall of left maxillary sinuses.[50]

Considerable force is required to produce these fractures, which are extensive and often present with a considerable amount of bleeding. This bleeding is rapidly augmented with swelling and distortion and can lead to rapid airway compromise.

A history consistent with extreme trauma to the face, either through falling from a significant height or extreme force applied to the face, such as by a steering wheel or baseball bat, should make the emergency clinician concerned that this type of fracture may be present. Extreme bleeding from this injury can lead to hypovolaemic shock and even death while compromising the airway, as the patient has often lost consciousness. The fracture leads to extensive subcutaneous bleeding and swelling in retrofacial planes, with an unstable face that is prone to collapse with mask ventilation. Early intravenous access in multiple areas is mandatory, as well as early intubation to secure an airway that will often become unavailable. There is an extremely high association of this kind of injury with cervical spine trauma. All C-spine precautions should be employed until injury is definitively excluded by qualified personnel. Absent teeth need to be accounted for and x-ray of the neck, chest and/or abdomen need to exclude aspiration/ingestion. Le Fort fractures have three classifications:

- *Le Fort I fractures*—this fracture has led to separation of the upper dentition from the rest of the midface. There is a fracture line that crosses the face above the roots of the teeth on one side and extends backwards towards the base of the skull around the pterygoid plates leading to an independent segment that can collapse and no longer is attached by bone to the rest of the face. This occurs in impact to the lower half of the maxilla or inferior to the nose. This can be either unilateral or bilateral.
- *Le Fort II fractures*—this fracture involves separation of the midface from the base of the skull largely through the malar processes and extending down to the pterygoid plates. The orbits are generally preserved, but the relapse of the midface back into the nasopharynx as well as the associated bleeding often leads to considerable airway compromise.
- *Le Fort III fractures*—these resemble the Le Fort II fractures, except that they generally involve the orbits as well, and separation from the base of the skull has extended more rostrally and approached the cavernous sinus and optic nerve. There is no facial contour and orbits have not been spared with collapse of the face and even more extensive airway compromise.[51]

A summary of maxillofacial fractures, their clinical and radiographical findings, and complications can be found in Table 44.5.

SUMMARY

Craniomaxillofacial injuries are a common occurrence in the ED. Special attention should be given to clearing and maintaining a patent airway and controlling haemorrhage. Ongoing airway assessment is essential. The goal of treatment is to manage life-threatening airway problems and haemorrhage, return function and provide cosmetic repair.

CASE STUDY

Paramedics have been called to a patient allegedly assaulted with a baseball bat. The police are on-scene and report that the patient has been struck across the jaw and to the bridge of the nose. The patient is bleeding from the nose and mouth, and has a GCS of 13. The patient has significant swelling across the middle of their face and is drowsy but rousable. The patient appears to have difficulty opening their mouth and complains of severe pain across the bridge of their nose.

QUESTIONS

1. On arrival at the scene, what is your initial assessment of this patient?
2. What is your initial management plan?
3. On arrival at the ED, what is your initial assessment?
4. What is your initial management plan?
5. What is the likely definitive treatment for this patient?

Answers to Case Study Questions can be found on evolve **http://evolve.elsevier.com/AU/Curtis/emergency/** 

USEFUL WEBSITES

The AO Foundation online reference. This site has excellent interactive information about identifying and management bony injuries, www2.aofoundation.org/wps/portal/surgery?showPage=diagnosis&bone=CMF&segment=Overview.

REFERENCES

1. Drake RL, Vogl A, Mitchell A. Gray's basic anatomy. Philadelphia: Churchill Livingstone Elsevier; 2012.
2. Moses KP, Banks J, Nava P, Banks J, Petersen D. Atlas of clinical gross anatomy. 2nd ed. Philadelphia: Elsevier; 2013.
3. Kellman RM, Schmidt C. The paranasal sinuses as a protective crumple zone for the orbit. Laryngoscope 2009;119(9):1682–90.
4. Porto DE, Cavalcanti YW, Forte FDS. Maxillofacial trauma due to traffic accidents and falls: an exploratory study of associated factors. Med Oral Patol Oral Cir Bucal 2021;26(3):e349–e56.
5. Bogart BI, Ort V. Elsevier's integrated anatomy and embryology. St Louis: Mosby, Elsevier; 2007.
6. Dulak D, NIhwnnngb N. Neuroanatomy, Cranial Nerve 7 (Facial) StatPearls [Internet]. Treasure Island (FL): StatPearls Publishing; 2021. Online. Available from: www.ncbi.nlm.nih.gov/books/NBK526119/.
7. Mayersak R. Facial trauma. In: Marx JA HR, Walls RM, editors. Rosen's emergency medicine: concepts and clinical practice. 8th ed. Philadelphia: Philadelphia: Saunders Elsevier; 2014.
8. Joshi UM, Shashank R, Saujanya S, Patil S, Shah K. Brain injuries and facial fractures: a prospective study of incidence of head injury associated with maxillofacial trauma. J Maxillofac Oral Surg 2018;17(4):531–7.
9. Pietzka S, Kämmerer PW, Pietzka S, Schramm A, Lampl L, Lefering R, et al. Maxillofacial injuries in severely injured patients after road traffic accidents–a retrospective evaluation of the TraumaRegister DGU® 1993-2014. Clin Oral Investig 2020;24(1):503–13.
10. Ramisetty S, Gaddipati R, Vura N, Pokala S, Kapse S. Maxillofacial injuries in women: a retrospective study of 10 years. J Maxillofac Oral Surg 2017;16(4):438–44.
11. Esonu O, Sardesai MG. Initial assessment of the facial trauma patient. Semin Plast Surg 2021;35(4):225–8.
12. Tung TC, Tseng WS, Chen CT, Lai JP, Chen YR. Acute life-threatening injuries in facial fracture patients: a review of 1,025 patients. J Trauma 2000;49(3):420–4.
13. Ceallaigh PO, Ekanaykaee K, Beirne CJ, Patton DW. Diagnosis and management of common maxillofacial injuries in the emergency department. Part 1: Advanced trauma life support. Emerg Med J 2006;23(10):796–7.
14. Kellman RM, Losquadro WD. Comprehensive airway management of patients with maxillofacial trauma. Craniomaxillofac Trauma Reconstr 2008;1(1):39–47.
15. Perry M. Head, neck and dental emergencies. Oxford: New York: Oxford University Press; 2005.
16. Tuckett JW, Lynham A, Lee GA, Perry M, Harrington U. Maxillofacial trauma in the emergency department: a review. Surgeon 2014;12(2):106–14.
17. Perry M, Morris C. Advanced trauma life support (ATLS) and facial trauma: can one size fit all? Part 2: ATLS, maxillofacial injuries and airway management dilemmas. Int J Oral and Maxillofac Surg 2008;37(4):309–20.
18. Perry M, Dancey A, Mireskandari K, Oakley P, Davies S, Cameron M. Emergency care in facial trauma–a maxillofacial and ophthalmic perspective. Injury 2005;36(8):875–96.
19. Mithani SK, St-Hilaire H, Brooke BS, Smith IM, Bluebond-Langner R, Rodriguez ED. Predictable patterns of intracranial and cervical spine injury in craniomaxillofacial trauma: analysis of 4786 patients. Plast Reconstr Surg 2009;123(4):1293–301.
20. Edibam C, Robinson H. Faciomaxillary and upper-airway injuries. 7th ed. In: Berston A, Soni N, editors. Oh's intensive care manual. Sydney: Elsevier; 2014.
21. Barak M, Bahouth H, Leiser Y, Abu El-Naaj I. Airway management of the patient with maxillofacial trauma: review of the literature and suggested clinical approach. Biomed Res Int 2015;2015:724032.
22. Apfelbaum JL, Hagberg CA, Caplan RA, Blitt CD, Connis RT, Nickinovich DG, et al. Practice guidelines for management of the difficult airway: an updated report by the American Society of Anesthesiologists Task Force on Management of the Difficult Airway. Anesthesiology 2013;118(2):251–70.
23. Shimoyama T, Kaneko T, Horie N. Initial management of massive oral bleeding after midfacial fracture. J Trauma 2003;54(2):332–6; discussion 6.
24. Yang WG, Tsai TR, Hung CC, Tung TC. Life-threatening bleeding in a facial fracture. Ann Plast Surg 2001;46(2):159–62.
25. Cogbill TH, Cothren CC, Ahearn MK, Cullinane DC, Kaups KL, Scalea TM, et al. Management of maxillofacial injuries with severe oronasal hemorrhage: a multicenter perspective. J Trauma 2008;65(5):994–9.
26. Lynham AJ, Hirst JP, Cosson JA, Chapman PJ, McEniery P. Emergency department management of maxillofacial trauma. Emerg Med Australas 2004;16(1):7–12.
27. Veeravagu A, Joseph R, Jiang B, Lober RM, Ludwig C, Torres R, et al. Traumatic epistaxis: skull base defects, intracranial complications and neurosurgical considerations. Int J Surg Case Rep 2013;4(8):656–61.
28. Burton J. Facial trauma. In: Barton ED CK, DeBlieux PM, editors. James G. Adams emergency medicine. Saunders: Elsevier; 2013.
29. Ochs MW, Tucker M. Management of facial fractures. In: Ellis E, Hupp JR, Tucker MR, editors. Contemporary oral and maxillofacial surgery. 4th ed. St Louis: Mosby; 2003.
30. Singer AJ, Mach C, Thode Jr HC, Shrestha P, Allen R, Koos J, et al. Patient priorities with traumatic lacerations. Am J Emerg Med 2000;18(6):683–6.
31. Dulecki M, Pieper B. Irrigating simple acute traumatic wounds: a review of the current literature. J Emerg Nurs 2005;31(2):156–60.
32. Wilson JR, Mills JG, Prather ID, Dimitrijevich SD. A toxicity index of skin and wound cleansers used on in vitro fibroblasts and keratinocytes. Adv Skin Wound Care 2005;18(7):373–8.

33. Egozi E, Faulkner B, Lin KY. Successful revascularization following near-complete amputation of the tongue. Ann Plast Surg 2006;56(2):190–3.
34. Farion K, Osmond MH, Hartling L, Russell K, Klassen T, Crumley E, et al. Tissue adhesives for traumatic lacerations in children and adults. Cochrane Database Syst Rev 2002;2002(3):CD003326.
35. Brinker D, Hancox JD, Bernardon SO. Assessment and initial treatment of lacerations, mammalian bites, and insect stings. AACN Clin Issues 2003;14(4):401–10.
36. O'Brien DC, Andre TB, Robinson AD, Squires LD, Tollefson TT. Dog bites of the head and neck: an evaluation of a common pediatric trauma and associated treatment. Am J Otolaryngol 2015;36(1):32–8.
37. Ellis E. Soft tissue and dentoalveolar injuries. In: Ellis E, Hupp JR, Tucker MR, editors. Contemporary oral and maxillofacial surgery. 4th ed. St Louis: Mosby; 2003.
38. Ikeda A, Burke A. LeFort fractures. Semin Plast Surg 2021;35(4):250–5.
39. Reddy L. Nasal fractures. In: Fonseca R, editor. Oral and maxillofacial trauma. 4th ed. St Louis: Saunders, Elsevier, 2014.
40. Engelstad M. Naso-orbito-ethmoid fractures. In: Bagheri S BBR, Khan H, editors. Current therapy in oral and maxillofacial surgery. St Louis: Saunders, Elsevier; 2012.
41. Hall AC, Simons M, Pilgrim G, Theokli C, Roberts D, Hopkins C. Epistaxis management at Guy's Hospital, 2009–2011: full audit cycles. J Laryngol Otol 2014;128(1):82–5.
42. McClurg SW, Carrau R. Endoscopic management of posterior epistaxis: a review. Acta Otorhinolaryngol Ital 2014;34(1):1–8.
43. Offei OK, Osei-Ampofo M, Ekremet K, Antwi-Donkor K. Ujuzi (Practical Pearl/Perle Pratique). Af J Emerg Med 2015;5(2):96.
44. Bell RB, Al-Bustani S. Current therapy in oral and maxillofacial surgery. Philadelphia: Saunders, Elsevier; 2012.
45. Adam A, Dixon A. Grainger and Allison's diagnostic radiology. 5th ed. New York: Churchill Livingstone; 2008.
46. Papageorge MB, Oreadi D. Radiographic evaluation of facial injuries. In: Fonseca R, Walker RV, Barber HD, editors. Oral and maxillofacial surgery II. 4th ed. St Louis: Saunders Elsevier; 2013.
47. Marx J, Hockberger R, Walls R. Rosen's emergency medicine. 7th ed. St Louis: Mosby; 2010.
48. Sheehy SB, Jimmerson C. Manual of clinical trauma care. 2nd ed. St Louis: Mosby; 1994.
49. Steed MB, Bagheri DDS, Shahrokh C. Clinical review of oral and maxillofacial surgery: a case-based approach. London: Mosby, Elsevier; 2014.
50. Wahab MAKA, Ibraheim MA, Osman NM. The role of multi detector computerized tomography in evaluation of maxillofacial fractures. Egypt J Radiol Nuclear Med 2014;45(1):97–104.
51. Ikeda AK, Burke AB. LeFort Fractures. Semin Plast Surg 2021;35(4):250–5.

CHAPTER 45
THORACIC AND NECK TRAUMA

SARAH KOUROUCHE AND BENJAMIN CROOK

ESSENTIALS

- Simple manoeuvres, such as decompression of the chest, may be lifesaving.
- One of the earliest signs of clinical deterioration in patients with chest trauma is tachypnoea. If a patient cannot complete a sentence on one breath, this is a warning sign of impending respiratory failure.
- Early and effective analgesia is key.
- Do not delay definitive management in life-threatening chest trauma by waiting for a chest x-ray.
- Oxygen saturation is unreliable in determining the degree of hypoxaemia, but is useful for monitoring changes in a patient's condition.
- The presence of pain, chest wall tenderness and subcutaneous emphysema indicates underlying lung or airway injury, which may require intervention.
- Patients with blunt chest trauma will have lung contusions. Severe contusions evolve over time; may cause deterioration in respiratory status; require constant monitoring to detect deterioration.
- Multidisciplinary management involving physiotherapy, pain team, nursing and medical staff reduces morbidity and mortality in patients with blunt chest injury.
- Neck trauma presents challenges because of the concentration of critical structures in a confined space.
- CT angiography is the key to assessment of penetrating neck trauma.

INTRODUCTION

Injuries to the thorax and its contents encompass some of the most life-threatening situations in trauma care, and require rapid assessment and management. Thoracic injuries have the second highest mortality rate, second only to head injuries in severely injured patients in Australia.[1] They are one of the most common injuries, accounting for approximately 50% of all injuries in patients with severe trauma.[2]

Even in parts of the world with a relatively low prevalence of penetrating injuries, the most frequent regions affected are the thorax and abdomen,[3] with thoracic injuries having the highest mortality rate due to injury of the major thoracic vascular structures.[4] First responders need to know how to perform lifesaving interventions at the scene, since thoracic trauma resulting in such conditions as tension pneumothorax may be rapidly fatal unless managed appropriately. All staff caring for patients with major thoracic trauma must be familiar with the proper management of thoracic injuries to minimise potential mortality and morbidity.

The aim of this chapter is to review the anatomy of the thorax and neck, to consider mechanisms of injury as they relate to these structures, and to consider approaches to assessment and management of the most common injuries associated with trauma to the thorax and neck. The thorax and neck are presented separately.

THORACIC INJURIES

ANATOMY AND PHYSIOLOGY

The thorax extends from the supraclavicular fossae at the base of the neck inferiorly to the diaphragm, which is highly mobile. Diaphragmatic excursion may extend the limits of the thoracic cavity anteriorly down to and even slightly below the costal margins, and posteriorly to the 12th thoracic vertebra. As the diaphragm moves down, negative pressure is generated within the thoracic cavity, causing an influx of air via the nose or mouth, and expansion of the lungs.

The thoracic wall is comprised of the back and chest musculature, as well as the bony skeleton formed by the sternum, ribs and spine. It affords protection to the contents of the thoracic cavity. Within the thoracic cavity proper lie the thoracic viscera: the lungs and associated tracheobronchial tree, the oesophagus, the heart and major vascular structures (Fig. 45.1). Penetrating injuries of the torso, even beyond the defined anatomical boundaries of the thorax, may still damage intrathoracic structures.

The thoracic pleura cover both the inner aspect of the chest wall (parietal pleura) and the surface of the lungs (visceral pleura). These two layers fuse centrally at the pulmonary hilum to envelop the major vascular and bronchial structures. A thin film of clear pleural fluid separates and lubricates these two surfaces, keeping them in close apposition, so that the interpleural space, under normal circumstances, is only a 'potential space'. A mechanical breach of either pleural surface may result in influx into this space of air (pneumothorax), blood (haemothorax) or both (haemopneumothorax).

Injury mechanism

Mechanisms of thoracic injury fall into two main categories: blunt and penetrating. Other, less common mechanisms include burns (Chapter 49), drowning and blast (Chapter 41). Blunt trauma may be sustained following the sudden application of force over a broad surface area of the body, whether from a direct blow by moving solid objects (e.g. fists, cricket bats, falling rocks), sudden rapid deceleration (e.g. motor vehicle collisions, falls) or crushing (e.g. entrapment between wall and vehicle bumper). Penetrating injuries result from piercing or cutting of tissues from bullets, knives, shrapnel, glass shards or other implements. Mixed patterns of injury may be seen where combined mechanisms of energy transfer occur, such as blasts where blunt injury may result from the patient being thrown against a wall, penetrating injury occurs via the shrapnel generated by the blast and burns result from the direct thermal effects of the explosion.

Significant injury to most of the intrathoracic structures can be immediately life threatening. Death may occur secondary to exsanguination, severe respiratory failure with concomitant hypoxia, obstructive shock (tension pneumothorax) with resultant cardiac failure or direct cardiac injury. Oesophageal injuries can lead to significant morbidity and mortality from overwhelming mediastinal sepsis if missed, but the course is usually more protracted.

PATIENT ASSESSMENT

Approach to initial evaluation

Patients with thoracic injuries may present dramatically with profound shock or severe respiratory distress, but some may demonstrate only subtle physiological changes initially. An understanding of the history and mechanism of injury permits prediction of the likelihood of thoracic injury. Primary survey will assess and secure an airway, and should identify immediately life-threatening thoracic injuries, such as tension pneumothorax, massive haemothorax, or cardiac tamponade, which must be managed promptly before further assessment is undertaken. Noise in the environment may make it difficult for the clinician to hear breath sounds on auscultation; therefore, direct and continuous observation of the patient is paramount. Detailed secondary survey is essential to detect the presence of potentially life-threatening injuries, such as simple pneumothorax, simple haemothorax or pulmonary contusion.[5] Selective use of radiology, coupled with careful examination, should reveal even subtle thoracic injuries.

PRACTICE TIP

A rapid screening tool is to ask the patient their name and what happened. If the patient can answer, this indicates that their airway is clear. If they can complete the sentence in one breath it gives a rapid indication of respiratory status, and a lucid answer confirms adequate cerebral perfusion. Remember to repeat the exercise regularly since respiratory failure can occur progressively and rapidly in patients with significant thoracic trauma.

In the patient with thoracic trauma, assessment follows the sequence of inspection, palpation and auscultation. Measurement of vital signs, including pulse and respiratory rate, should be undertaken, and oxygen saturation should be recorded. In a cold, shocked patient, or one who is agitated or combative, pulse oximetry may not provide an accurate indirect measure of arterial blood oxygen, and should not be relied upon solely as an indicator of the physiological status of the patient. However, it is a useful gauge of any change in the patient's condition when considered in conjunction with the full assessment.

Tachypnoea or respiratory distress may indicate direct injury to the thoracic wall or underlying lungs, but can also be an early and sensitive indicator of severe circulatory shock.[6] Furthermore, severe brain injury can produce abnormalities of the respiratory system through impairment of brainstem function leading to hypoxic shock. Thus, any patient presenting in a confused or agitated state after sustaining a major mechanism of injury should first be presumed to be in either haemorrhagic shock or hypoxic shock (or both) until proven otherwise.

Inspection

Visual inspection of the chest should occur first, paying particular attention to less visible areas that could easily be ignored, such as the axillae. The patient should be fully exposed to facilitate thorough inspection and minimise the risk of missed injury, but hypothermia must be prevented, and the dignity of the patient preserved. When expedient, a log-roll must be performed to inspect the back, especially when there is a history of penetrating trauma. Relevant findings include ecchymosis (bruising), haematomas or abrasions that might indicate significant blunt force trauma. Discrete breaks in the

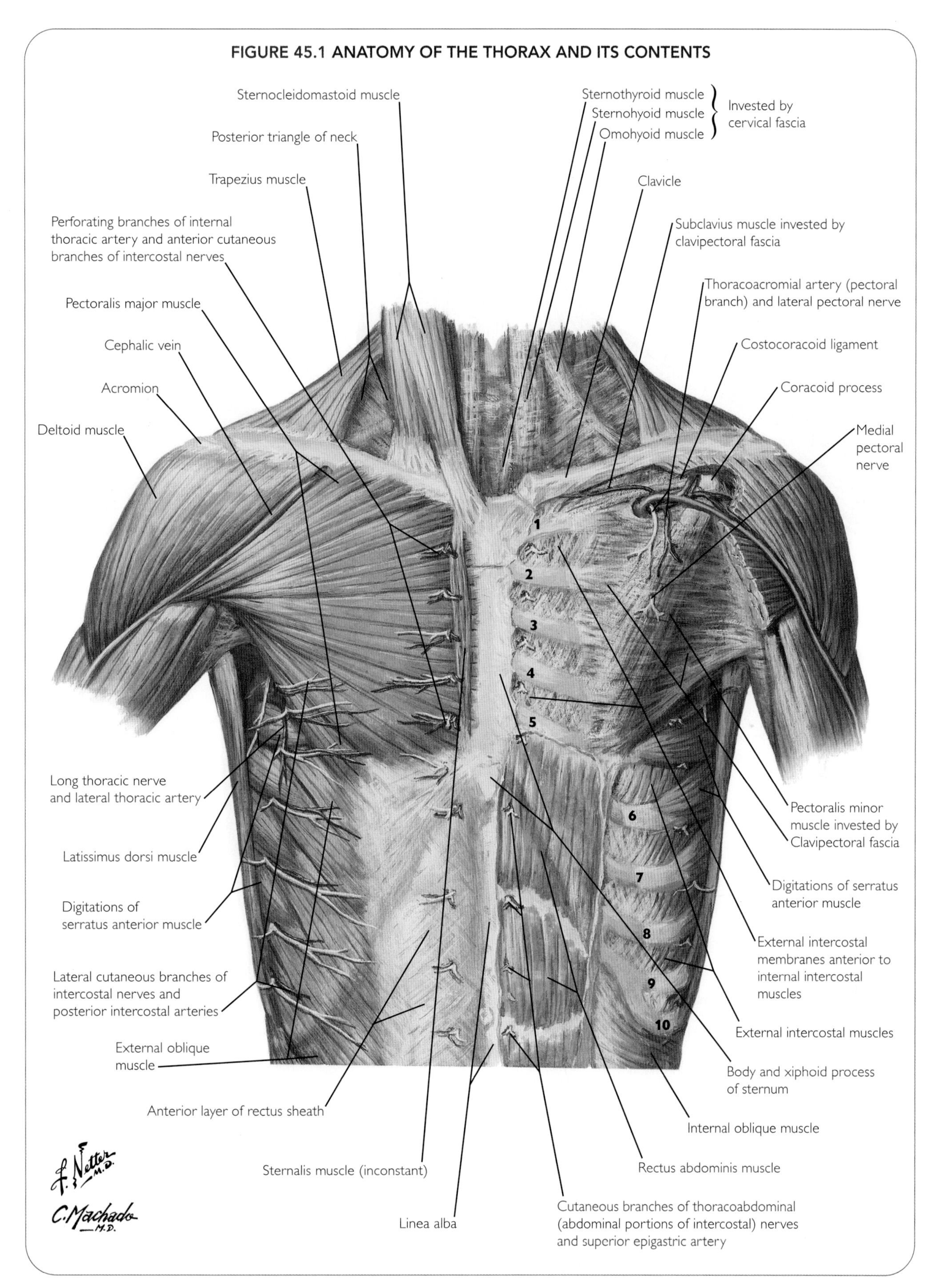
FIGURE 45.1 ANATOMY OF THE THORAX AND ITS CONTENTS
Sternocleidomastoid muscle
Posterior triangle of neck
Trapezius muscle
Perforating branches of internal thoracic artery and anterior cutaneous branches of intercostal nerves
Pectoralis major muscle
Cephalic vein
Acromion
Deltoid muscle
Sternothyroid muscle
Sternohyoid muscle
Omohyoid muscle
Invested by cervical fascia
Clavicle
Subclavius muscle invested by clavipectoral fascia
Thoracoacromial artery (pectoral branch) and lateral pectoral nerve
Costocoracoid ligament
Coracoid process
Medial pectoral nerve
1
2
3
4
5
6
7
8
9
10
Long thoracic nerve and lateral thoracic artery
Latissimus dorsi muscle
Digitations of serratus anterior muscle
Lateral cutaneous branches of intercostal nerves and posterior intercostal arteries
External oblique muscle
Anterior layer of rectus sheath
Sternalis muscle (inconstant)
Linea alba
Pectoralis minor muscle invested by Clavipectoral fascia
Digitations of serratus anterior muscle
External intercostal membranes anterior to internal intercostal muscles
External intercostal muscles
Body and xiphoid process of sternum
Internal oblique muscle
Rectus abdominis muscle
Cutaneous branches of thoracoabdominal (abdominal portions of intercostal) nerves and superior epigastric artery
F. Netter M.D.
C. Machado M.D.

Continued

FIGURE 45.1 ANATOMY OF THE THORAX AND ITS CONTENTS—cont'd

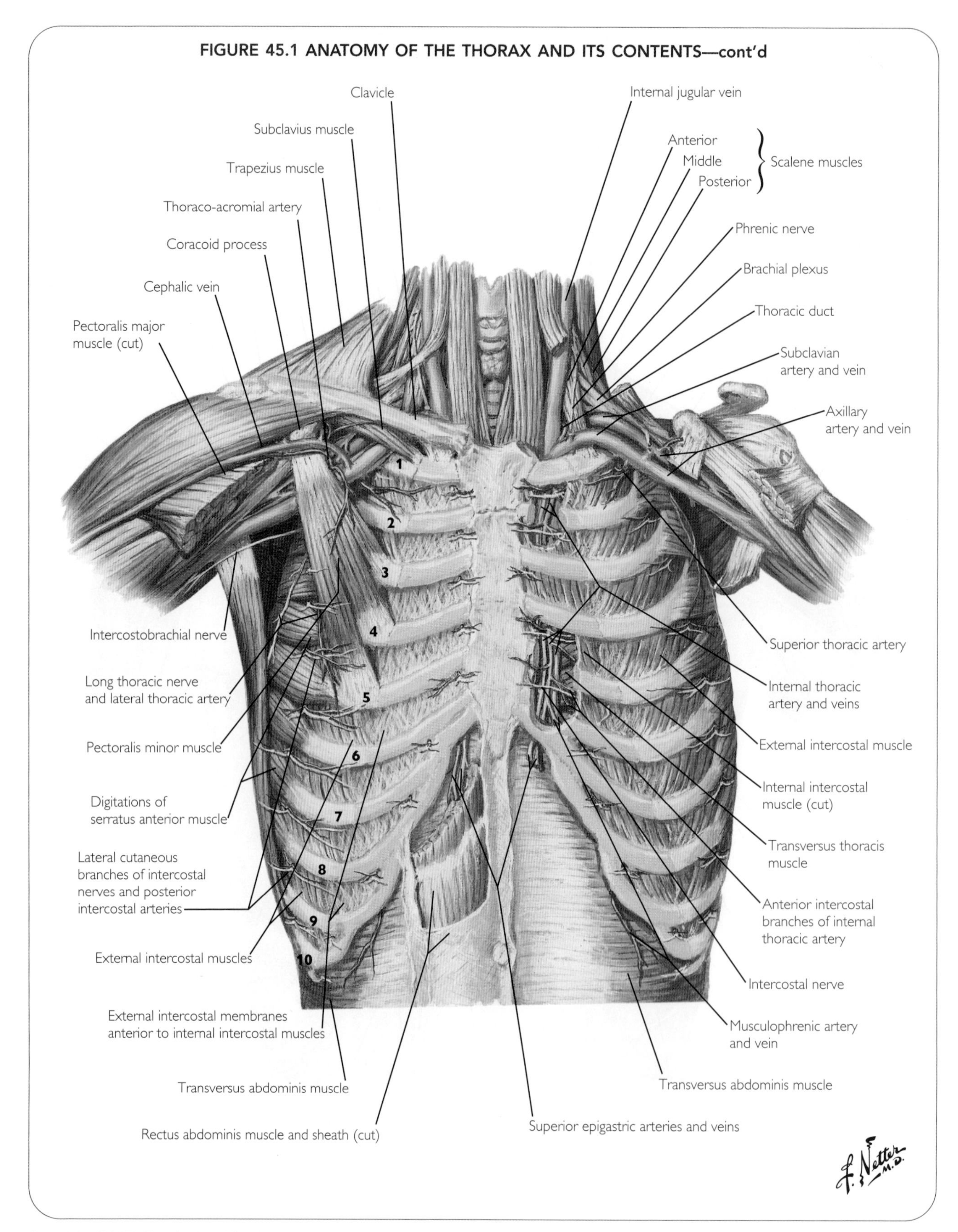
Clavicle
Subclavius muscle
Trapezius muscle
Thoraco-acromial artery
Coracoid process
Cephalic vein
Pectoralis major muscle (cut)
Internal jugular vein
Anterior
Middle
Posterior
Scalene muscles
Phrenic nerve
Brachial plexus
Thoracic duct
Subclavian artery and vein
Axillary artery and vein
1
2
3
4
5
6
7
8
9
10
Intercostobrachial nerve
Long thoracic nerve and lateral thoracic artery
Pectoralis minor muscle
Digitations of serratus anterior muscle
Lateral cutaneous branches of intercostal nerves and posterior intercostal arteries
External intercostal muscles
External intercostal membranes anterior to internal intercostal muscles
Transversus abdominis muscle
Rectus abdominis muscle and sheath (cut)
Superior thoracic artery
Internal thoracic artery and veins
External intercostal muscle
Internal intercostal muscle (cut)
Transversus thoracis muscle
Anterior intercostal branches of internal thoracic artery
Intercostal nerve
Musculophrenic artery and vein
Transversus abdominis muscle
Superior epigastric arteries and veins
F. Netter M.D.

skin, such as lacerations, incised wounds or punctures, are signs of penetrating injury. Do not overlook entry and exit wounds of projectiles. Where possible, haemorrhage should be controlled by direct pressure. Be aware that dried blood may hide underlying wounds; therefore, detailed inspection is essential. Photographs of wounds should be taken with an indicator of size (such as a tape measure), for forensic purposes. In some centres, digital photographs can be linked to the radiology system, allowing easy access.

Observation of the mechanics of breathing is essential. Segmental chest wall motion abnormalities may indicate rib fractures or a flail chest and highlight the presence of lung injury. Use of the accessory muscles of respiration, such as the intercostals and sternocleidomastoids, indicates increased work of respiration, which may rapidly lead to fatigue and respiratory failure. Respiratory rate and rhythm should be recorded since this may provide evidence of underlying physiological derangement.

Palpation

Palpation of the thorax and back will provide evidence, not only regarding the underlying integrity of the thoracic wall and rib cage, but also about the possibility of underlying lung injury, which has a high incidence of mortality.[7] Subcutaneous emphysema, typically felt as a fine crackling, indicates the presence of an air leak from either pneumothorax or tracheobronchial injury. Coarse crepitus felt over the ribs is caused by fractured rib ends grating against each other. In the awake, alert patient this will be associated with significant pain. Chest wall movement can be assessed by placing the hands on either side of the chest and noting their motion. Asymmetry indicates a major difference in air entry, suggesting the presence of pneumothorax, haemothorax or haemopneumothorax.

Auscultation

Although a detailed description of specific auscultatory findings is not really possible in the typically noisy pre-hospital or emergency department (ED) setting, auscultation of the chest walls laterally will confirm the presence or absence of breath sounds, and permit comparison of right and left sides.[8] Absence of breath sounds is a sinister sign indicating either tension pneumothorax or massive haemothorax, both of which may prove rapidly fatal unless urgent management is undertaken. The typical muffled heart sounds of pericardial tamponade may be difficult to distinguish due to ambient noise, and the diagnosis should be made based on associated clinical signs, which will be discussed below. Assessment of pain, especially on breathing and coughing, could indicate underlying injury to the chest wall and lung.

CLINICAL INTERVENTIONS

In the pre-hospital environment, the patient may exhibit severe respiratory distress coupled with worsening shock. It is essential to identify and treat life-threatening injuries to the chest quickly. Auscultation of the chest may reveal a unilateral absence of breath sounds. This is an emergency since these signs indicate a strong likelihood of tension pneumothorax, a condition that rapidly progresses to loss of consciousness and death if not treated by an urgent intervention to decompress the thoracic cavity. Finger thoracostomy involves an incision through subcutaneous tissue in the fifth intercostal space, midaxillary line.[9] Forceps are used to create a tract through the intercostal muscle and pleura, the finger is then inserted into the pleural space to sweep and assess for release of air or fluid. While this process increases the risk of fluid exposure, it allows a maximum release of air and fluid from the pleural space, as well as provision for further finger sweeps to assess for re-accumulation should the patient deteriorate. Alternatively, if the finger thoracostomy is not possible, needle thoracostomy is the placement of a large bore cannula in the second intercostal space, in the midclavicular line on the affected side. A hiss of air not only confirms the diagnosis, but also relieves the intrathoracic pressure. Needle or finger thoracostomy can be followed up with tube thoracostomy by a trained clinician. Tube thoracostomy may be performed in the field or in the ED prior to any radiological investigation.

The emergency clinician should ensure that oxygen is administered, preferably via face mask. In some trauma centres high-flow nasal prong (HFNP) oxygen is applied to patients with thoracic injury.[10] The benefits of HFNP include that the oxygen is warmed and moist, facilitating clearance of secretions, and a small amount of positive end-expiratory pressure (PEEP) is maintained, which is thought to diminish the work of breathing.[11] A full set of vital signs, including temperature, should be obtained and regularly repeated and, as above, pulse oximetry should be measured continuously to monitor changes in patient condition.

While the medical team are conducting the primary survey, a manual non-invasive blood pressure (NIBP) should be attended prior to the application of an automatic NIBP device, as automatic NIBP can be unreliable and take longer[12] in the acute trauma setting. The nurse should then place standard chest leads for continuous cardiac rhythm monitoring. Abnormalities on a full 12-lead electrocardiogram (ECG) may indicate either pre-existing cardiac disease or the presence of possible blunt cardiac injury. Subsequent ECG changes, including the development of dysrhythmias, may indicate either ischaemia or evolving cardiac injury. Venous blood should be taken for measurement of electrolytes, full blood count and coagulation studies. Remember, initial haemoglobin levels *do not* correlate with the extent of blood loss as it can take 8–12 hours before accurate blood levels are measurable once the interstitial fluids are redistributed into the blood plasma. Initial abnormal changes observed can be due to haemodilution from resuscitative efforts. Venous blood gas gives information about pH and lactate levels, which will indicate whether the patient is acidotic due to anaerobic metabolism (see Chapter 10). These parameters are also useful for monitoring response to resuscitation. Interpretation of venous blood oxygen content provides useful information about ventilation and perfusion. Where there is associated blunt abdominal trauma, measurement of liver enzymes and amylase and lipase may help reveal visceral injury.

Prompt, adequate analgesia in patients with significant blunt thoracic trauma may make the difference between survival and death, particularly in the elderly patient. Paramedics may be concerned about administering opioid analgesia in shocked trauma patients due to the vasodilatory response that may occur. If concerned then an agent such as ketamine or methoxyflurane (Penthrox) inhalational anaesthesia may be preferred options.[13] The use of ketamine is becoming more widespread in the paramedic practice setting.[14,15] The treating clinicians should ensure the patient receives pain relief in a timely manner. A patient whose pain is well controlled will more easily be able to cooperate with the remainder of the examination process. Furthermore, the psychological stress of major trauma may be diminished if pain is controlled early in the presentation.[16] Haemodynamically stable patients may receive parenteral opioids initially, but subsequently specialised pain team consultation should be obtained to determine the optimal analgesic regimen for the patient during the admission. Options include patient-controlled analgesia (PCA), with or without ketamine infusion, paravertebral or serratus plane blocks, or, in some patients, the placement of a thoracic epidural may be indicated.[17]

Clear documentation is essential, noting the initial assessment and management, plans for investigation or treatment and the times when observations or interventions are undertaken, including drug administration. Response to treatment should be recorded, including the time at which the observations are made. This allows trends in the patient's condition to be determined. Any deterioration in the patient's status, such as first notes of increasing shortness of breath or an inability to complete a sentence in one breath, should be documented and reported to the trauma team leader.

In a rural or regional centre, where the facilities may not be available to manage the patient with significant thoracic injury, transfer to a major trauma centre may be required. The emergency clinician will be responsible for expediting 'packaging' of the patient for safe transport. Preparation for transfer is discussed in detail in Chapter 15.

RADIOLOGY

Radiological studies are helpful in the initial evaluation of the patient with thoracic injuries. These tests vary not only in their availability, but also in their sensitivity and specificity for the diagnosis of particular injuries. The haemodynamic status of the patient must be considered when determining which radiological investigations to perform.[18] In the unstable patient not responding to resuscitation, treatment decisions must be made using clinical judgement without waiting for radiology or moving the patient out of the ED to obtain further investigations. Any transport of such a patient should only be to a location where definitive management of the underlying life-threatening injury can be performed, be this the operating theatre or the interventional radiology suite.

The chest x-ray

The single-view Anterior-Posterior (AP) chest x-ray (CXR) is a useful radiographic study that can be obtained during the initial evaluation of patients with suspected or confirmed chest injuries (Table 45.1). The bony structure of the chest wall and musculature are shown in Fig. 45.2. A portable, supine CXR is quite sensitive for diagnosing the most common life-threatening thoracic injuries. It may be sufficient to indicate the need for major therapeutic interventions, such as urgent thoracotomy in massive haemothorax, or be useful in planning management, such as the need for tube thoracostomy or chest computed tomography (CT).[19] Furthermore, plain CXR may provide evidence of injury to the mediastinal structures such as the thoracic aorta, which will be discussed further below. The importance of CXR in the initial evaluation of the patient with known or suspected thoracic injury is such that the radiographer should be a member of the multidisciplinary trauma team responding to all newly arrived major trauma patients.

TABLE 45.1 SUPINE CHEST X-RAY FINDINGS AND CORRELATING INTERVENTION

FINDING ON SUPINE PLAIN CHEST X-RAY	INTERVENTIONS
Large pneumothorax	Tube thoracostomy
Large haemothorax	Tube thoracostomy
Rib fractures	Analgesia; ensure physiotherapy; monitor for respiratory failure; suspect lung contusion or thoracic vascular injury
Elevated left diaphragm or viscera seen in lower left chest or nasogastric tube coiled in left lower chest	Suspect left diaphragm rupture
Pneumomediastinum	Suspect oesophageal injury
Widened/indistinct mediastinum	Search for thoracic aortic disruption

As an adjunct to primary survey, a normal initial CXR will rule out the thoracic cavity as a source of major occult haemorrhage in the patient presenting in shock. Conversely, lifesaving procedures should never be delayed until a CXR is obtained in patients with high clinical suspicion of major thoracic injury.[21] For example, a patient with respiratory distress, haemodynamic shock, tracheal deviation and unilateral absence/decrease of breath sounds has a tension pneumothorax and should undergo urgent chest decompression before a CXR is performed. In this situation any delay in definitive treatment may prove fatal.

Formal upright, two-view CXR (i.e. posterior–anterior and lateral projections), is now seldom used, due to the ease of access to CT and also the need to transfer the patient to the radiology department. This is important since thoracic wall injuries may be accompanied by bony spinal injuries, which would preclude the upright views.

In patients with penetrating injuries, all missile or knife entrance or exit wounds should be identified with a radio-opaque marker, such as an open paperclip, prior to CXR to facilitate determination of likely trajectories, and thus identify possible zones of major injury.

Ultrasound

Focused assessment sonography in trauma (FAST) was principally developed as an extension of normal ultrasound to determine the presence of free fluid in the abdominal cavity. FAST is used in EDs and pre-hospital settings as part of the primary survey. Extended FAST (eFAST) is now used to assess the thoracic cavity. A skilled operator can detect both fluid (haemothorax) and air (pneumothorax), and published reports indicate

FIGURE 45.2 FRONT AND BACK VIEW OF THE TRUNK SHOWING BONY AND SOFT TISSUE STRUCTURES

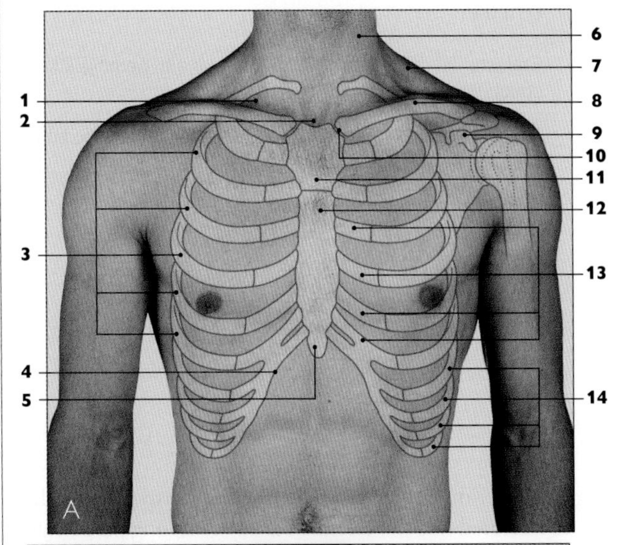

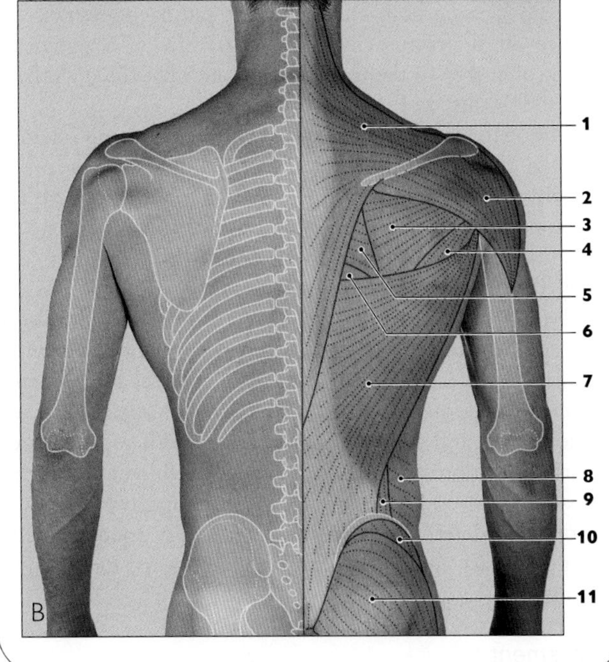

A. Frontal view. 1. Supraclavicular fossa. 2. Jugular notch. 3. True ribs. 4. Costal margin. 5. Xiphisternum. 6. Sternocleidomastoid. 7. Trapezius. 8. Clavicle. 9. Coracoid process. 10. Sternoclavicular joint. 11. Manubrium. 12. Body of sternum. 13. Costal cartilages. 14. False ribs. **B.** Posterior view. 1. Trapezius. 2. Deltoid. 3. Infraspinatus. 4. Teres major. 5. Rhomboid major. 6. Auscultatory triangle. 7. Latissimus dorsi. 8. External oblique. 9. Lumbar triangle. 10. Gluteus medius. 11. Gluteus maximus.[20]

high sensitivity.[22] In the pre-hospital setting it can indicate the need for chest decompression in the shocked polytrauma patient in whom the classic signs of tension pneumothorax (distended neck veins, absent breath sounds, tracheal deviation) may be difficult to elicit. The use of the eFAST has revolutionised the way trauma management occurs due to its ease of use, portability and advanced sensitivity.[23] Advanced care paramedics may also be trained in the use of the eFAST, especially as they are often the first point of contact.

Computed tomography (CT) scan

Compared to other imaging modalities, CT has a high degree of sensitivity and specificity for the detection of subtle injuries in the chest. While pneumothoraces or haemothoraces too small to be seen on plain CXR are readily detected by the CT, the clinical significance of such subtle findings remains unclear and comes with its own complications.[24]

Most Australian and Aotearoa New Zealand trauma centres do not have CT facilities co-located in the ED, thus requiring patients to be transported some distance away to get imaging. The dedicated trauma bay is a relatively controlled and safe environment for a seriously injured patient. During transport, transfer and time in the CT suite the ability of the trauma team to respond to acute deterioration in the patient's condition is limited by both space and resources. Multidetector computed tomography (MDCT) scanners are able to perform 'pan scans' in minutes; important information can be achieved in the metastable patient that may assist in planning the management course and appropriate interventions (Table 45.2).

In the assessment of thoracic aortic trauma, MDCT spiral technology with three-dimensional reconstruction has allowed CT scanning to catch up to angiography in terms of image quality; 64- or 256-slice scanners can image with submillimetre-section thicknesses and an image matrix rivalling digital subtraction angiography (DSA). A single intravenous administration of contrast material can be used for a combined vascular and non-vascular evaluation. MDCT scanning is the gold standard, especially in the detection of blunt thoracic aortic disruptions (Fig. 45.3). MDCT scanning has been shown not only to be faster, but also just as sensitive and specific as contrast aortography.[25,26]

Angiography

Historically, biplanar DSA has been considered the gold standard in the diagnosis of vascular injuries in stable patients and was for some time the only modality available to accurately delineate blunt and penetrating injuries to the thoracic aorta and its branches. However, as described above, significant improvements have occurred in CT technology over the last two decades, with MDCT scanners now producing superb images of the vascular tree in three dimensions and at sub-millimetre resolutions rivalling those derived from angiography. As MDCT resolution continues to improve, its non-invasive nature and ability to assess other injuries in the polytrauma patient are likely to convert those vascular surgeons who still routinely require angiography to confirm thoracic vascular injuries, and to decide between operative or endoluminal repair.

FRACTURES OF THE BONY THORAX

Managing patients with significant blunt chest wall trauma requires adequate and effective analgesia coupled with physiotherapy to permit clearance of secretions. Failure to combine these approaches increases the risk of the patient developing severe pulmonary dysfunction which may progress to pneumonia and respiratory failure. Adequate oxygen therapy, to prevent hypoxia, assists in reducing the work of breathing, thus minimising the risk of fatigue.[27]

TABLE 45.2 USE OF COMPUTED TOMOGRAPHY AS A DIAGNOSTIC TOOL IN THORACIC TRAUMA

MECHANISM	CLINICAL SCENARIO	UTILITY
Penetrating	Mediastinal missile traverse	Evaluate integrity of mediastinal vascular and aerodigestive structures
Blunt	'Abnormal' mediastinum on CXR	Indicate presence of mediastinal haematoma/thoracic aortic disruption
Blunt	Suspected diaphragmatic tear (elevated diaphragm or viscera overlying lower lungs fields on CXR)	Diagnose ruptured diaphragm
Blunt or penetrating	Persistent thoracic opacification on CXR	Differentiation between undrained/clotted haemothorax, lung contusion, atelectasis and lung consolidation

CXR: chest x-ray

FIGURE 45.3 THREE-DIMENSIONAL COMPUTED TOMOGRAPHY SCAN RECONSTRUCTION SHOWING TRAUMATIC PSEUDOANEURYSMS OF THE PROXIMAL DESCENDING AORTA (ARROW)

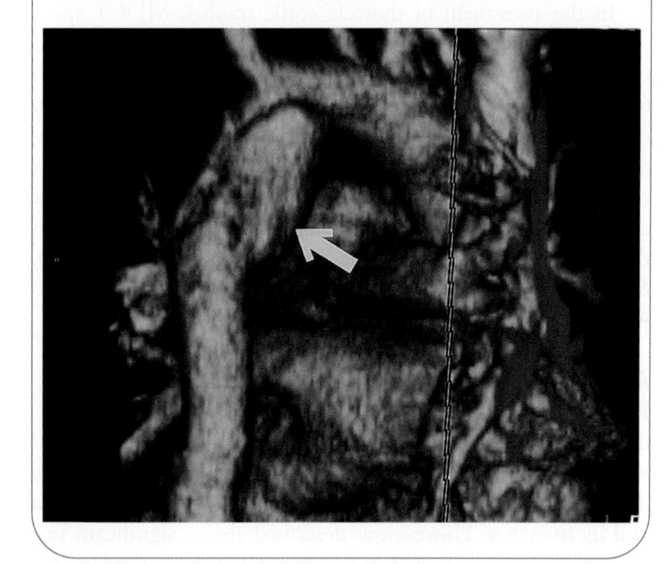

Courtesy Dr Caesar Ursic.

Rib fractures and pulmonary contusion

Rib fractures are the most common sequelae of blunt thoracic trauma, and may also follow some penetrating injuries. They cause severe pain, which results in decreased inspiratory effort and ineffective cough. Failure to clear respiratory secretions, with occlusion of small airways, contributes to a further decline in pulmonary function. If analgesia is inadequate, this can lead to alveolar collapse and consolidation. The presence of rib fracture in more than one anatomical region doubles the incidence of respiratory failure.[28] If the decline in pulmonary function is not reversed, then pneumonia and respiratory failure may ensue with the need for mechanical ventilation in severe cases. In patients with pre-existing pulmonary disease, or in the elderly, this may prove fatal.[28] Fractured ribs may result in haemothorax, most commonly as a result of damage to intercostal arteries which lie along the inferior border of each rib. Furthermore, the sharp edges of fractured ribs can lacerate the adjacent lung parenchyma, potentially causing both pneumothorax and haemothorax. The presence of rib fractures implies the transfer of a significant amount of energy to the thoracic cage, and that the underlying lung suffers injury as a result.

Pulmonary contusion associated with multiple rib fractures may lead to delayed-onset respiratory failure, and occurs in approximately one-fifth of patients with rib fractures.[29] The three components of pulmonary contusions are oedema, atelectasis and haemorrhage into the pulmonary interstitium and alveoli. The ensuing mismatch in pulmonary ventilation/perfusion leads to hypoxaemia (Fig. 45.4). Pulmonary contusions often do not manifest early on, so the presence of one or more rib fractures in a recently injured patient must lead to early prediction and management with adequate analgesia, chest physiotherapy and supplemental oxygen.[30] Where pulmonary contusions are present on initial scanning, this indicates that the patient has sustained severe thoracic trauma and they are at risk of rapid deterioration in their respiratory status. Patients with pulmonary contusions should be monitored for potential deterioration.

Assessment

Any patient complaining of pain and tenderness over one or more ribs after a blunt injury to the chest should be considered to have at least one fractured rib, regardless of x-ray finding. Within this context, the patient would be deemed to have a clinical rib fracture. Crepitus may be present, and if lung parenchymal or tracheobronchial tree injury has occurred, subcutaneous emphysema may be palpated. This results from entrapment in the muscles and subcutaneous tissues of air under pressure that has escaped from lacerated lung pleura.

It has been reported that screening CXRs miss rib fractures up to 20–30% of the time.[32] Treatment of the patient suspected of having fractured ribs should not be delayed pending radiological confirmation (Fig. 45.5). Dedicated rib views, i.e. x-rays taken at various oblique angles, are more sensitive in detecting fractured ribs, but they rarely change the management of the patient and are therefore unnecessary.[34] Finally, these fractures may be seen incidentally on chest CT scans, but CT performed

FIGURE 45.4 A 19-YEAR-OLD MALE PATIENT FOLLOWING A MOTOR VEHICLE CRASH

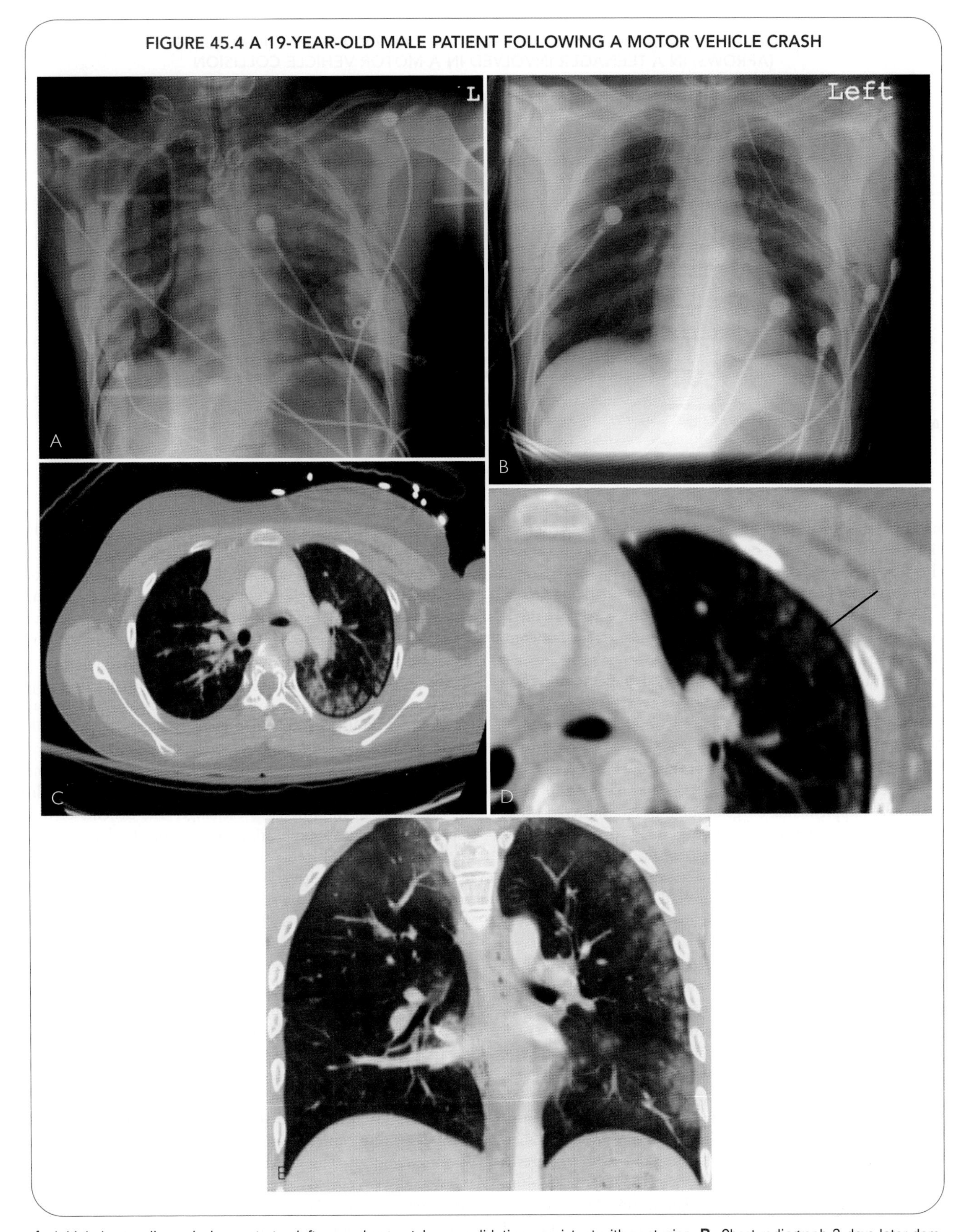

A. Initial chest radiograph demonstrates left upper lung patchy consolidation consistent with contusion. **B.** Chest radiograph 3 days later demonstrates rapid resolution of pulmonary contusion. **C.** Axial section through a CT scan demonstrates left-sided contusion affecting both the upper and the lower lobes, not confined to a single lobe. **D.** There is sparing of 1–2 mm of subpleural space (arrow). **E.** Coronal image demonstrates extent of lung contusion.[31]

FIGURE 45.5 HAEMOTHORAX (ASTERISK) AND ASSOCIATED RIB FRACTURES (ARROWS) IN A TEENAGER INVOLVED IN A MOTOR VEHICLE COLLISION

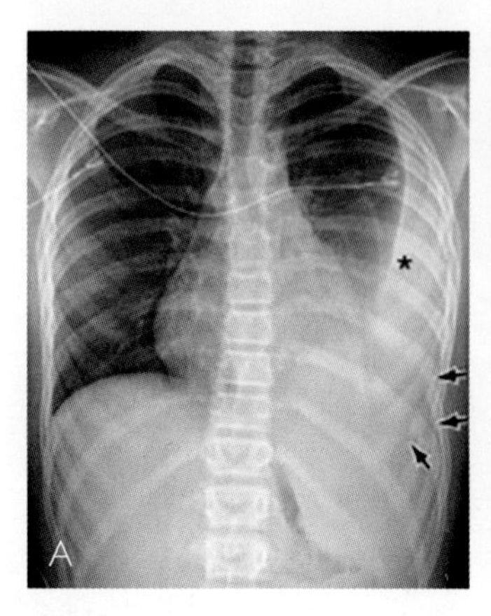

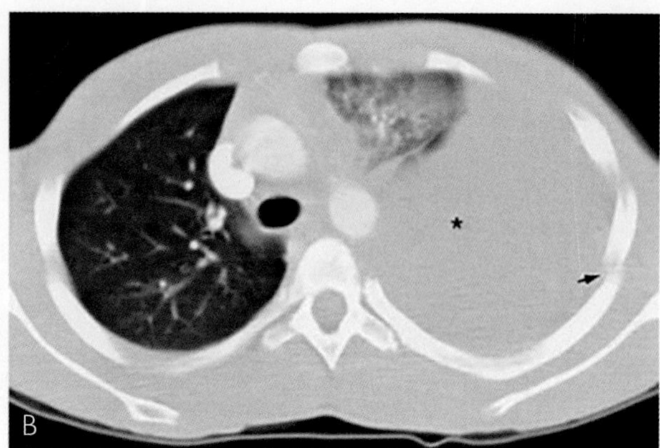

A. Chest radiograph. **B.** CT scan.[33]

purely to diagnose rib fractures in the absence of other indications is a costly and unnecessary investigation.[35] In most cases, the diagnosis of rib fractures should be a clinical one based on the history and physical examination of the patient. Should CXR reveal fracture of the first or second ribs, careful examination of the ipsilateral arm should include assessment of neurovascular status due to the close proximity of major neural and vascular structures, such as the brachial plexus, subclavian artery and vein.

Management

The mainstay of treatment for fractured ribs is early and adequate analgesia permitting effective inspiratory effort and coughing. Supplemental oxygen should be administered where required to maintain oxygen saturations above 94% (with the exception of patients with known lung disease). A chest injury bundle of care is recommended (Fig. 45.6) that incorporates early multidisciplinary notification and assessment, a coordinated pain management regimen, early physiotherapy intervention and patient education.[17] In patients with multiple rib fractures, and especially in the elderly, inpatient admission will be necessary to allow for administration of parenteral analgesia and close monitoring of respiratory function. Pain team review should be obtained since invasive techniques for analgesia delivery may be required. Regional analgesia can provide effective analgesia without the unwanted effects of systemic analgesia, and can be used in the out-of-hospital setting.[36] Thoracic epidurals have been shown to be superior to narcotic administration, but are time-consuming to establish and may be associated with complications.[37] If the location of the rib fractures is high in the thorax, the use of epidural anaesthesia can result in severe haemodynamic compromise. For unilateral rib fractures, paravertebral block may be useful using a catheter infusion of local anaesthetic.[38,39] Intercostal nerve blocks afford satisfactory analgesia, but the effect is short-lived, so that the procedure must be repeated frequently, making it impractical in most cases.[40] The advantage of analgesia using local anaesthetic is it is opioid sparing, which is particularly important in the elderly or patients with renal impairment.

Aggressive chest physiotherapy with encouragement of deep breathing and coughing is essential, and incentive spirometry provides a visual scale of respiratory effort and is useful for monitoring progress and improving lung function.[41] High-flow nasal prong (HFNP) delivery of humidified, high concentrations of oxygen is being used prophylactically in this group of patients,[10,42] though if not available venturi mask may be as effective.[43] HFNP has the added benefit of providing a small amount of positive end-expiratory pressure (PEEP), which not only prevents collapse by 'splinting' the alveoli (when the patient keeps their mouth closed), but may also recruit new alveoli, thus resulting in improved gas exchange. The benefits of this approach are that humidification of secretions facilitates clearance, the mechanical splinting of the alveoli reduces the work of breathing, thereby decreasing the risk of respiratory fatigue, and patient comfort is increased, since they are able to talk, thus increasing compliance. If respiratory fatigue occurs with progressive hypoxaemia or hypercarbia, then the use of non-invasive ventilatory assistance, such as continuous positive airway pressure (CPAP) or bi-level positive airway pressure (BiPAP), may prove beneficial in conjunction with adequate analgesia. Be aware of complications associated with BiPAP and CPAP use and monitor your patient carefully.

In certain cases of severe blunt thoracic trauma, especially when there are pulmonary contusions, the above multidisciplinary approach fails, and respiratory failure appears imminent. The nurse caring for these patients must be alert to the warning signs: worsening tachypnoea, use of accessory muscles and inability to complete a sentence in one breath. Do not wait for changes in oxygen saturation before calling for assistance as this is an unreliable indicator of hypoxaemia. These patients will require intubation (see Chapter 16) and mechanical ventilation until pulmonary contusions abate, respiratory mechanics improve, and pain control is optimised. Signs of pneumonia, such as fever, purulent sputum and progressive changes on

FIGURE 45.6 CHIP: EARLY NOTIFICATION CHEST INJURY PATHWAY

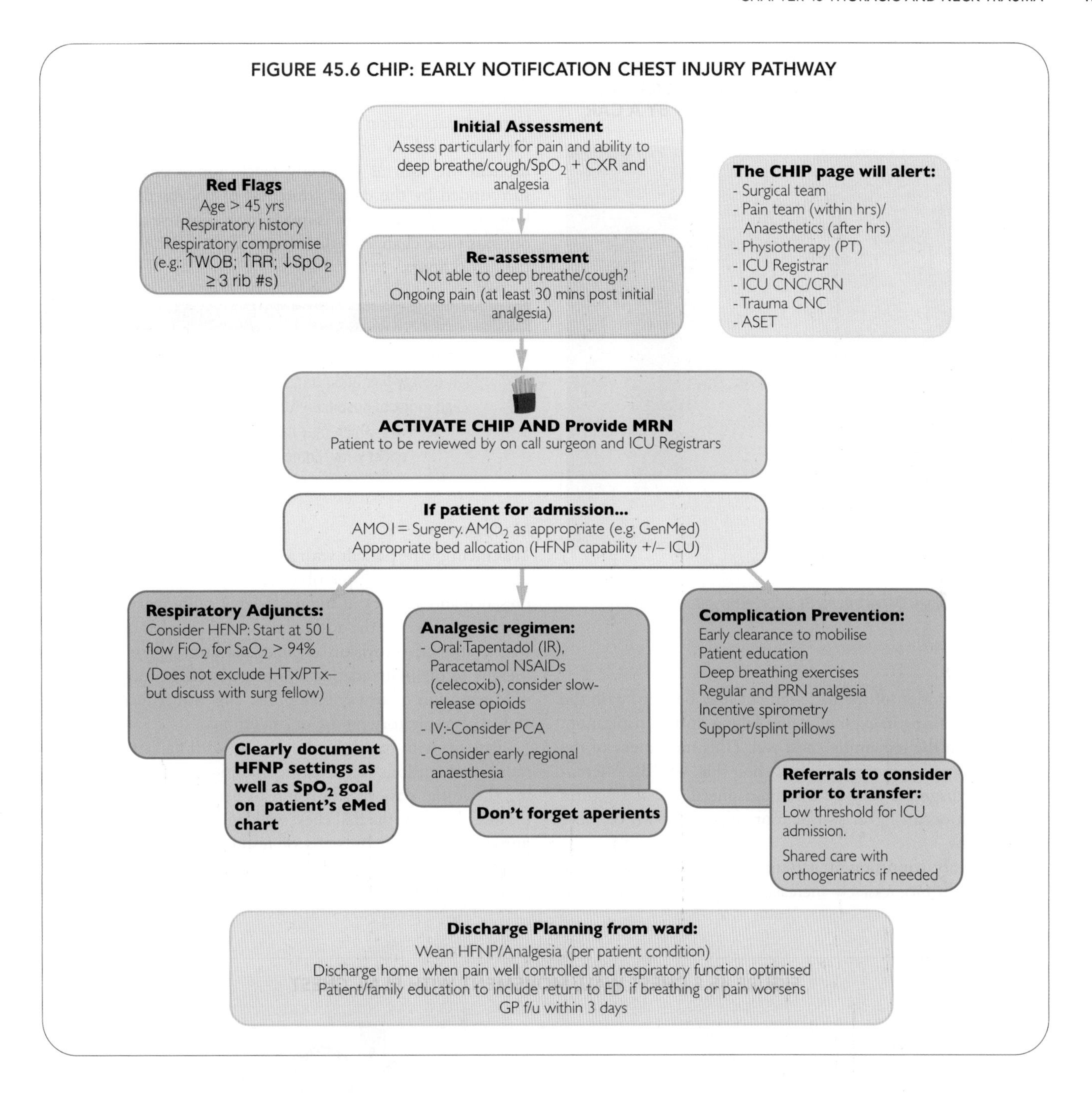

chest x-ray, should be treated with appropriate antibiotics. Finally, the patient should be cautioned that rib fractures can and do cause pain for many weeks, if not months. Patient compliance and education are imperative in their overall recovery.

Initial Assessment
Assess particularly for pain and ability to deep breathe/cough/SpO2 + CXR and analgesia
Red Flags
Age > 45 yrs
Respiratory history
Respiratory compromise
(e.g.: ↑WOB; ↑RR; ↓SpO2
≥ 3 rib #s)
The CHIP page will alert:
- Surgical team
- Pain team (within hrs)/ Anaesthetics (after hrs)
- Physiotherapy (PT)
- ICU Registrar
- ICU CNC/CRN
- Trauma CNC
- ASET
Re-assessment
Not able to deep breathe/cough?
Ongoing pain (at least 30 mins post initial analgesia)
ACTIVATE CHIP AND Provide MRN
Patient to be reviewed by on call surgeon and ICU Registrars
If patient for admission...
AMO1 = Surgery. AMO2 as appropriate (e.g. GenMed)
Appropriate bed allocation (HFNP capability +/– ICU)
Respiratory Adjuncts:
Consider HFNP: Start at 50 L flow FiO2 for SaO2 > 94%
(Does not exclude HTx/PTx– but discuss with surg fellow)
Clearly document HFNP settings as well as SpO2 goal on patient's eMed chart
Analgesic regimen:
- Oral: Tapentadol (IR), Paracetamol NSAIDs (celecoxib), consider slow-release opioids
- IV:-Consider PCA
- Consider early regional anaesthesia
Don't forget aperients
Complication Prevention:
Early clearance to mobilise
Patient education
Deep breathing exercises
Regular and PRN analgesia
Incentive spirometry
Support/splint pillows
Referrals to consider prior to transfer:
Low threshold for ICU admission.
Shared care with orthogeriatrics if needed
Discharge Planning from ward:
Wean HFNP/Analgesia (per patient condition)
Discharge home when pain well controlled and respiratory function optimised
Patient/family education to include return to ED if breathing or pain worsens
GP f/u within 3 days

PRACTICE TIP

To assess the effectiveness of analgesia in the patient with rib fractures, ask them to take a deep breath and cough. If unable to do so, titration of analgesic regimen is required.

Flail chest

The term 'flail chest' refers to a clinical condition resulting from the segmental fracture of two or more adjacent ribs in two or more places, with associated chest wall deformation (Fig. 45.7). Costochondral joint disruptions associated with rib fractures can also lead to a flail segment. Flail chest results from severe blunt chest trauma, and flail segment of chest wall (Fig. 45.8) is no longer mechanically attached to the relatively rigid surrounding bony rib cage. This segment is therefore uncoupled from the mechanical forces that move the chest wall during the breathing cycle. This is not itself dangerous, but is an indicator of severe underlying pulmonary contusion that is present as a result of the original trauma to the chest wall.[45]

As discussed above, the pain associated with the rib fractures contributes to poor inspiratory effort, and if an aggressive regimen of analgesia and physiotherapy is not instigated, significant deterioration in respiratory function may result, requiring intubation and mechanical ventilation.

FIGURE 45.7 X-RAY SHOWING A RIGHT-SIDED FLAIL CHEST WITH SIGNIFICANT DISPLACEMENT IN A 68-YEAR-OLD FEMALE PEDESTRIAN HIT BY A CAR

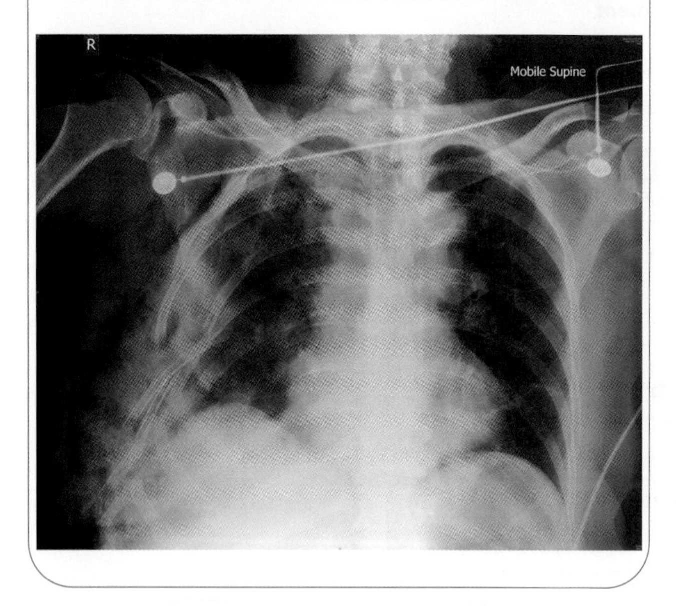

Courtesy Radiology Department, St George Hospital, Sydney.

Assessment

Paradoxical motion of the flail segment may be seen, with the rib segments rising in expiration and falling during inspiration, distinct from the remaining chest wall. This movement of the chest wall is pathognomonic of flail chest (Fig. 45.7B). Alternatively, the diagnosis may be a radiographical one if fractures can be seen occurring in two or more places on two or more adjacent ribs.

Pulmonary contusion after blunt chest wall injury can be deduced from progressively increasing respiratory distress and oxygen requirements in a patient with radiographical signs of lung opacification or consolidation. Although it may initially appear normal, the plain CXR soon shows areas of consolidation or opacification corresponding to the underlying contusion. So-called air bronchograms may be evident, where the bronchi are seen as distinctly black 'tubes' or cross-sections surrounded by the dense whiteness of collapsed/consolidated lung tissue. The CT scan is much more sensitive and will demonstrate these changes earlier than will the CXR, usually within the first 6 hours.

PRACTICE TIP

In the patient with multiple rib and scapula fractures, high energy has been transmitted to the thorax. Have a high index of suspicion for lung contusions in these patients, which may not be evident on initial chest x-ray/computed tomography.

Management

Treatment of the patient with a flail chest will be similar to that of a patient with multiple rib fractures, and will depend on the presence and severity of the underlying pulmonary contusion. Therapy consists of the administration of supplemental oxygen when required, provision of analgesia and aggressive physiotherapy to maintain adequate inspiratory effort and thus minimise retention of airway secretions. This will reduce the probability of respiratory failure or pneumonia.

Patients with multiple rib fractures with flail chest and pulmonary contusions may require endotracheal intubation during the initial days of admission to permit 'splinting' both of the alveoli and of the flail chest wall segment. In addition, if the nurse is concerned by signs of respiratory deterioration in a patient with multiple rib fractures, such as progressive tachypnoea and fatigue, then it is essential that medical review is

FIGURE 45.8 CHEST WALL MOVEMENT WITH FLAIL CHEST

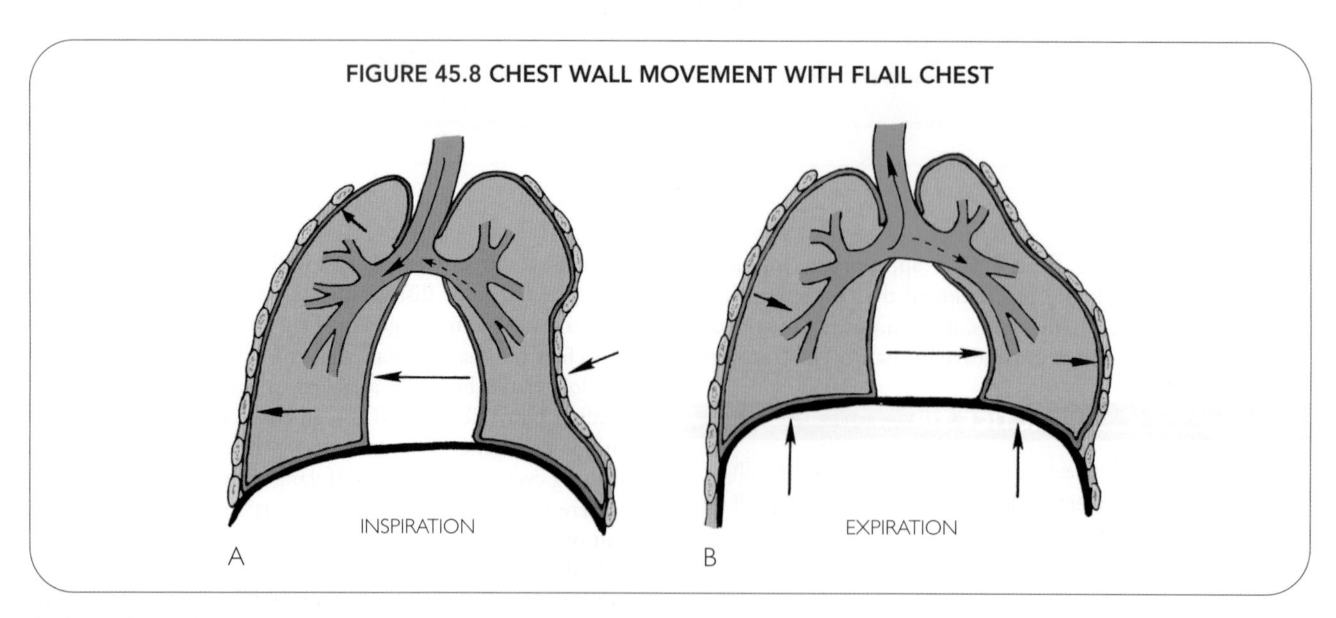

A. On inspiration flail section sinks in as chest expands, impairing ability to produce negative intrapleural pressure to draw in air. Mediastinum shifts to uninjured side. **B.** On expiration flail segment bulges outwards, impairing ability to exhale. Mediastinum shifts to injured side. Air may shift uselessly from side to side in severe flail chest (broken lines).[44]

FIGURE 45.9 INTRO-OPERATIVE RIB FRACTURE STABILISATION USING TITANIUM PLATES[46]

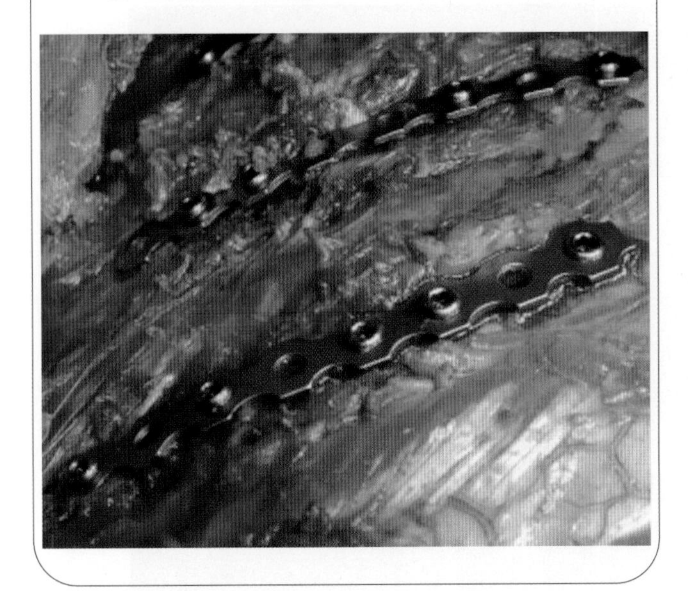

arranged in a timely manner, since these patients often require a period of mechanical ventilation as a prophylactic measure against the development of respiratory failure.

Antibiotics, steroids, diuretics and other anti-inflammatory agents have not been shown to alter the course of pulmonary contusions, which are generally self-limiting and usually resolve gradually over a period of days to weeks. In severe cases, surgical fixation of the segmented ribs has been performed with success, with reports that patients have improved long-term lung function (Fig. 45.9).[47]

Sternal fractures

Fractures of the sternum occur almost exclusively due to direct blows to the anterior chest. Some examples of this include injuries as a result of an MVC where the driver strikes the steering wheel when airbags are not employed, following a fall from height or as a result of interpersonal violence. Sternal fractures are among the most painful of the thoracic-wall injuries and in some cases are associated with multiple rib fractures and lung contusions. They may also be a predictor of blunt cardiac injury.[48] While they are not intrinsically life threatening, the painful nature of these fractures may lead to significant short-term disability with reduced respiratory effort. As with rib fractures, this in turn can soon progress to pulmonary atelectasis, bacterial pneumonia and respiratory failure, unless early and adequate analgesia is ensured.

Assessment

Patients with sternal fractures complain of severe pain and tenderness over the central chest wall. Palpation may reveal an irregularity of the fracture site if significant displacement and overlap of the bone ends has occurred, and crepitus may be felt on palpation and during deep inspiration and expiration. Displaced fractures may be visible on the anteroposterior (AP) CXR and fracture lines will be visible on chest CT scan. There is little need for a dedicated lateral sternal view since this will rarely influence management if a clinical suspicion of sternal fracture exists (Fig. 45.10). Electrocardiograph monitoring is essential and a 12-lead ECG should be performed on all patients with suspected sternal fractures.[49]

Management

Treatment of sternal fracture follows a similar pathway as that for rib fractures. The majority of isolated sternal fractures may be managed as outpatients. However, patients with polytrauma, associated blunt cardiac injury (discussed further below), or severe pain may need to be hospitalised.[49] Hospital admission may be required to establish an effective analgesic regimen and to ensure that the patient has adequate respiratory function prior to discharge. Weaning to oral analgesics or other regimens may proceed once pain control is deemed adequate and the patient is able to maintain adequate inspiratory effort and clear secretions. As above, monitoring for the early signs and symptoms of respiratory failure is essential to allow for timely intervention. In rare circumstances, the fracture segments will require surgical stabilisation if they fail to fuse over the ensuing months or if they override each other to such an extent that they produce significant cosmetic deformity.[50]

Clavicular fractures

Fractures of the clavicle are common after blunt thoracic trauma, including falls onto the shoulder, MVCs, and sport-related trauma. The usual site of injury is at the junction of the middle (shaft) and proximal third of this S-shaped bone. Although the fracture itself is neither life nor limb threatening, its presence should alert the clinician that a considerable amount of force has been applied to the chest and that underlying thoracic injuries may be present.

Assessment

Patients with fractured clavicles generally complain of localised pain and tenderness over the fracture site, which is aggravated by motion of the ipsilateral shoulder joint, and deformity or bruising of the soft tissues overlying the fracture may be noted. The standard AP CXR is very sensitive in demonstrating these fractures (Fig. 45.11), even though the diagnosis will be apparent clinically in patients who can cooperate with the physical examination.

A careful vascular examination of the arm is important to detect injury to vascular structures, since injury of the subclavian artery by the sharp bony ends of the clavicle may occur. Absent or diminished distal pulses may indicate vascular thrombosis or occlusion by an intimal flap; a pulsatile mass, palpable thrill or audible bruit in the supraclavicular fossa may signal an underlying traumatic arteriovenous fistula. Furthermore, neurological examination is essential to detect injury to the brachial plexus.

Management

The majority of clavicular fractures are treated non-operatively with oral analgesics. A sling to support the arm for a few weeks serves to decrease motion at the fracture site and can help diminish discomfort. Surgical fixation is generally required for the treatment of compound (open) fractures or more commonly for displaced fractures to avoid the complication of non-union and potential long-term pain.[51] Acute vascular injuries will also require urgent intervention when present.

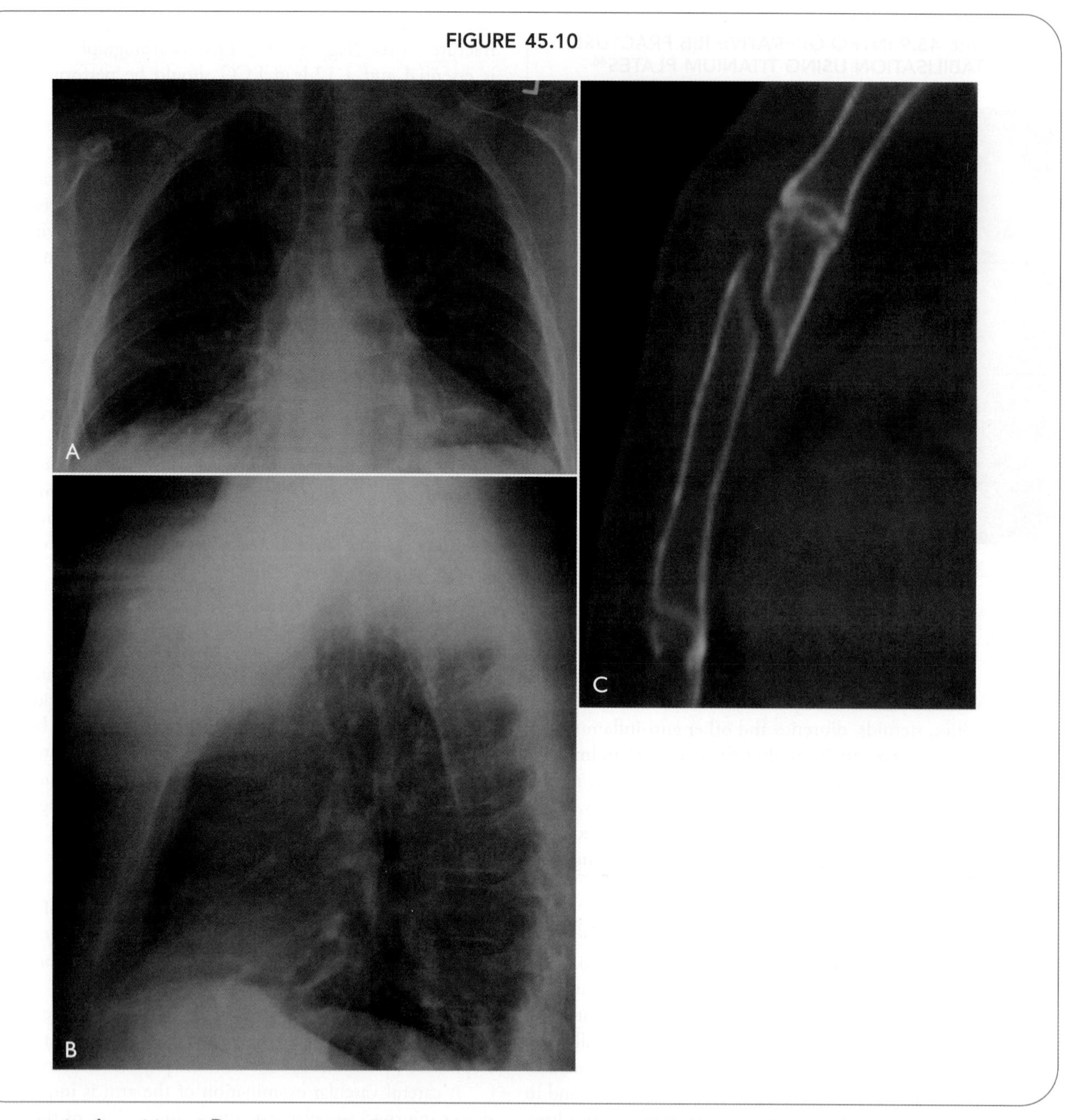

FIGURE 45.10

Anteroposterior **A**, and lateral **B**, radiographs of a 32-year-old male patient after an MVC. No sternal injury can be appreciated on these images. **C.** Sagittal reconstructed images through the sternum clearly show the minimally displaced sternal fracture that was not seen on plain radiographs.[31]

Scapular fractures

The scapula, one of the thickest bones of the human body, is not easily fractured. Rarely, scapulothoracic dissociation may result with severe and sometimes life-threatening consequences.

Assessment

These fractures manifest clinically with significant pain of the shoulder region, tenderness on palpation of the posterior shoulder, limited range of shoulder motion (due to pain) and occasional overlying soft-tissue haematomas and bruises. They are often visible on the plain CXR (Fig. 45.12A), but the full extent of the fracture, including any involvement of the glenohumeral joint, is best seen on CT scan (Fig. 45.12B). Distal radial and ulnar pulses should be documented. If a fracture has scapulothoracic dissociation, i.e. separation of the scapular articulation from the thoracic wall, this can be accompanied by frequent injury to the brachial plexus and the underlying axillary or proximal brachial artery.[52] These patients present with abnormal vascular, motor and sensory examinations of the involved extremity, and may have massive haemorrhage in and around the shoulder joint which can become life threatening. If scapulothoracic dissociation is suspected based on the clinical examination, an emergency arteriogram of the involved upper extremity is indicated to diagnose vascular injuries and stage their surgical repairs.

FIGURE 45.11 LEFT CLAVICULAR FRACTURE (ARROW) ON PLAIN CHEST X-RAY, SUSTAINED IN MVC

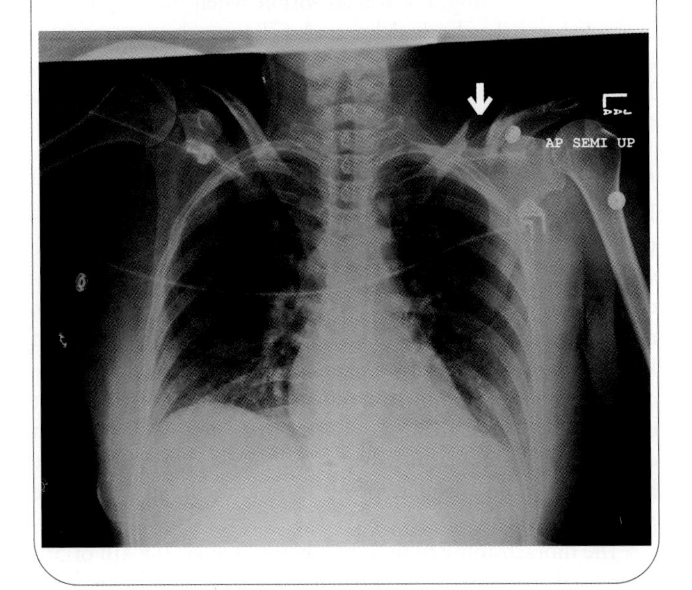

Courtesy Dr Caesar Ursic.

FIGURE 45.12 SCAPULA FRACTURE, PLAIN X-RAY AND CT SCAN

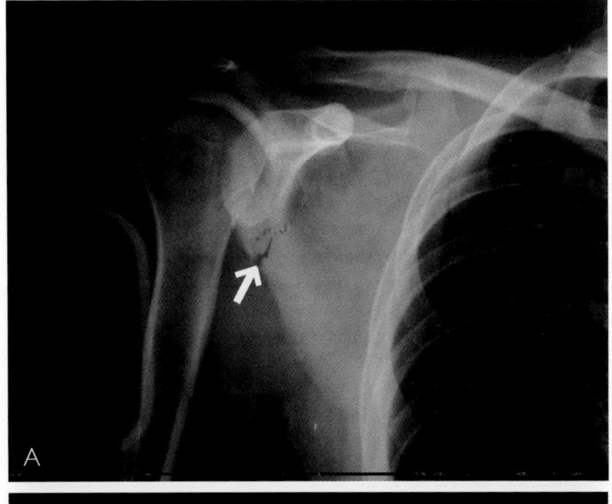

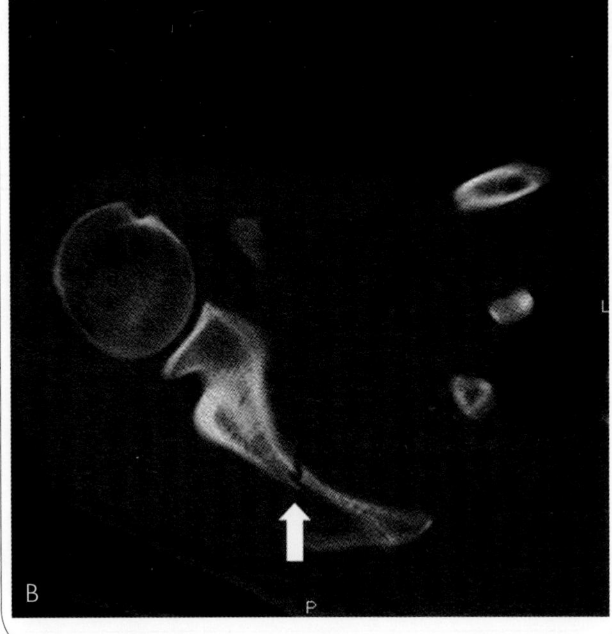

A. Scapular fracture, plain x-ray. **B.** Right scapular fracture, CT scan (glenoid joint is not involved). *Courtesy Dr Caesar Ursic.*

PRACTICE TIP

Scapular fractures indicate that great force has been transferred to the upper torso. Thus, a high index of suspicion should exist regarding the presence of underlying thoracic injury, notably pulmonary contusion.

Management

The majority of scapular fractures will not require operative intervention and can be treated with analgesics and temporary shoulder immobilisation with an arm sling to allow the fracture to stabilise. Only fractures involving the glenohumeral joint which are significantly displaced will benefit from open reduction and stabilisation, and this procedure may be delayed for several days until the patient's overall condition improves. Scapulothoracic dissociation, on the other hand, almost always requires some form of immediate surgical procedure; this usually being the repair of a torn or thrombosed axillary or brachial artery.

Pneumothoraces

When a mechanical breach to the pleural surface occurs after a penetrating or blunt injury, the pleural space may fill with air, blood or both; forming, respectively, a pneumothorax, haemothorax or haemopneumothorax.

Simple closed pneumothorax

Following blunt trauma, a pneumothorax may result from lacerations to the visceral pleura from the sharp edges of fractured ribs. Penetrating injuries may produce a pneumothorax due to direct pleural laceration, with air entering the thoracic cavity via the chest wall or the lacerated lung (Fig. 45.13). If air entry is self-limited, or if air can exit the thoracic space at the same rate at which it enters, this results in a simple pneumothorax.

Assessment

Acute, pleuritic chest pain, which may radiate to the opposite shoulder and/or dyspnoea may be indicative of simple pneumothorax. Simple pneumothorax may not produce significant respiratory or haemodynamic instability, especially when it is small or occult. In fact, the diagnosis may not be made until the initial CXR is reviewed. The chest wall should be inspected for evidence of blunt or penetrating trauma, which may be subtle. The history of the trauma will provide evidence on which to base the diagnosis; this may subsequently be confirmed on CXR (Fig. 45.14). Palpation may reveal not only the tenderness associated with rib fractures, but subcutaneous emphysema from air that has escaped via breaches in the pleura. The presence or absence of breath sounds should be noted on auscultation.

FIGURE 45.13 CLOSED PNEUMOTHORAX

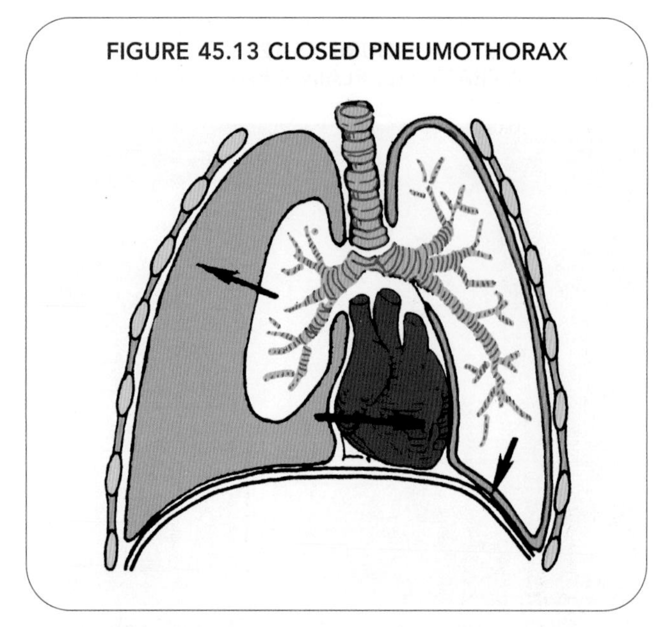

Simple pneumothorax is present in right lung with air in pleural cavity and collapse of right lung.[44,51]

Supine CXR will demonstrate the darker radiolucency of air between the chest wall and lung surface, which will be evident in the majority of clinically significant simple pneumothoraces. The edge of the lung, not usually visible when the lung is fully expanded, may be clearly delineated. CT is much more sensitive than CXR and can detect the smallest of pneumothoraces. Point-of-care ultrasound or eFAST is increasingly being used to identify pneumothorax during primary survey (Fig. 45.15).[22]

Management

In the presence of a simple pneumothorax and signs of respiratory distress, or in patients likely to require positive pressure ventilation, an intercostal catheter should be inserted. Previously assembled kits should be available in the trauma bay, along with several sizes of tube. The emergency clinician should know the location of these kits and how to assist with the procedure. There are various techniques for the proper placement of an intercostal catheter (ICC); all have several features in common as described in Table 45.3.[57] A checklist can also be helpful to ensure adequate preparation and completion of the procedure safely.

The thoracostomy tube is usually inserted via the 4th or 5th intercostal space at the mid-axillary line. An appropriate sized

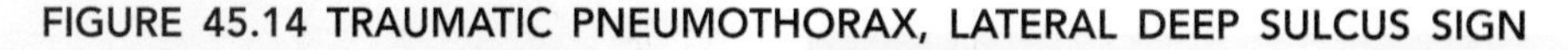

FIGURE 45.14 TRAUMATIC PNEUMOTHORAX, LATERAL DEEP SULCUS SIGN

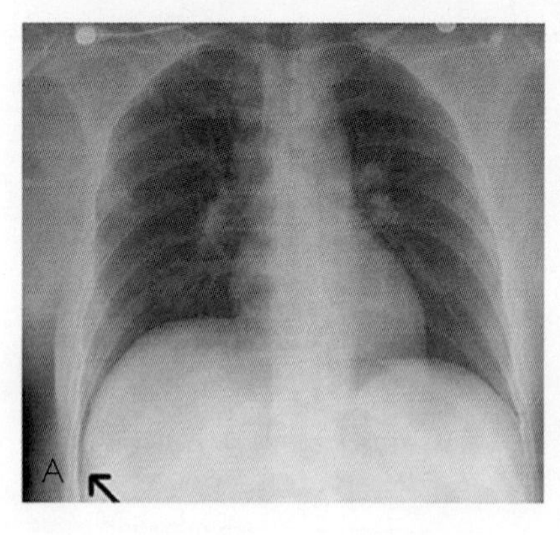

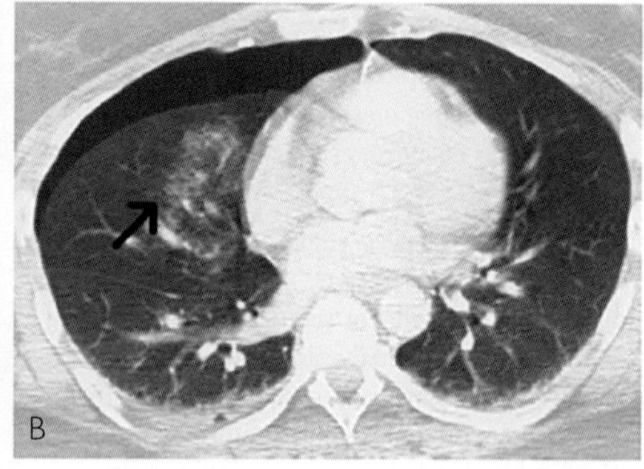

A. Anteroposterior chest radiograph in a 45-year-old female trauma victim shows right rib fracture and lucency extending deep into right lateral costophrenic angle (arrow). **B.** CT scan of chest confirms small anterior pneumothorax. Right middle lobe ground-glass opacities (arrow), consistent with pulmonary contusion, also are noted.[53,54]

FIGURE 45.15 ULTRASOUND
Transition between the barcode sign of a pneumothorax and the seashore sign of a normal lung.[55,56]

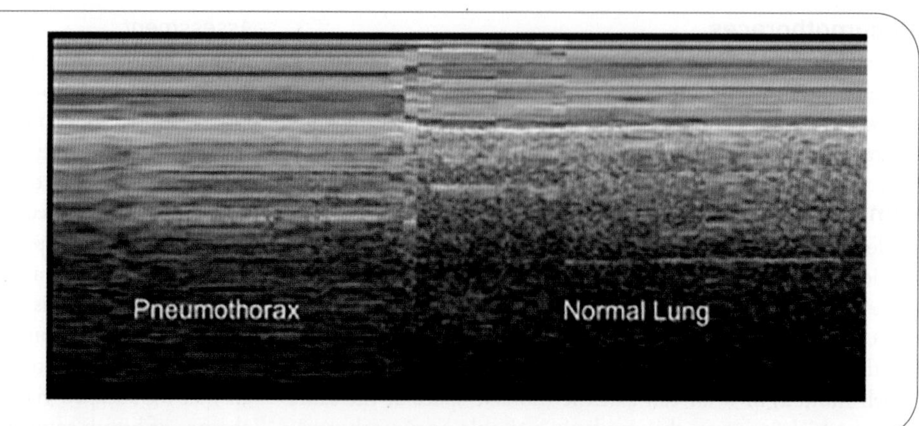

TABLE 45.3 PROCESS FOR INSERTION OF INTERCOSTAL CATHETER

PATIENT PREPARATION	Mechanical restraint of upper extremities (ipsilateral arm placed behind head whenever possible) Wide skin prepping and draping of chest wall with topical antibacterial solution and sterile towels/drapes Minimum of one large-bore intravenous cannula Continuous SpO_2, blood pressure and cardiac rhythm monitoring Time out
DRUGS	Supplemental oxygen 1% lidocaine for local anaesthesia Parenteral opioid analgesia and short-acting sedative
EQUIPMENT	Appropriately sized thoracostomy tube Low wall suction Closed thoracic drain reservoir device (pre-assembled with water) Tapes
RADIOLOGY	Confirmatory chest x-ray after procedure completed

SpO_2: partial oxygen saturation pressure.

tube should be inserted, with newer evidence suggesting that a smaller tube (such as a pigtail < 14 Fr) is adequate in most cases and better tolerated by the patient with fewer complications.[58] After connecting the tube to an underwater-seal collection bottle, a confirmatory CXR should be performed to document adequate tube placement within the chest. Some clinicians prefer that low continuous suction (3–4 kPa) is applied to the underwater-seal drain (UWSD), so nursing staff should discuss this with the admitting team. See Chapter 16 for information on applying a UWSD.

In the majority of patients with a simple pneumothorax, tube thoracostomy will be sufficient treatment, and can usually be removed in 1–2 days when the lung is fully inflated on follow-up CXR. A minority will continue to exhibit collapse of the lung on subsequent CXR or persistent air leak as demonstrated by continued bubbling in the drain. These patients will need placement of a second tube to fully re-expand the lung. An even smaller group of patients will require cardiothoracic surgical review for either a formal thoracostomy or a video-assisted thoracoscopic surgery (VATS) procedure to treat a persistent air leak or lung collapse.

Tension pneumothorax

A tension pneumothorax (Fig. 45.16) is a less common but much more dangerous variant of the simple pneumothorax, and occurs when air from a laceration in the lung tissue or via an open chest wall injury enters the interpleural space with each breath, but cannot escape. The progressive increase in volume of trapped air will compress the adjacent lung, limiting its expansion and leading initially to respiratory distress and hypoxaemia. As the intrathoracic pressure continues to increase, the mediastinal structures, including the venae cavae, the trachea and the heart, are also compressed, and displaced away from the affected side. This results in markedly decreased venous return to the heart with a drop in cardiac preload. The end result is severely compromised cardiac output, which may rapidly progress to cardiogenic shock and eventual cardiac arrest.

PRACTICE TIP

The diagnosis of a tension pneumothorax is a clinical one, not a radiographic one. A thorough clinical assessment is paramount.

Assessment

The hallmarks of the condition are the presence of shock and unilaterally absent breath sounds in a patient with clinical or historical evidence of thoracic trauma. The condition may be seen after both blunt and penetrating injury mechanisms, and the patient may present gasping for breath, and may be anxious or even combative due to hypoxia and early shock. A rapid primary survey usually discloses absent or diminished breath sounds on the affected side of the chest and may also reveal signs of chest wall injury, such as a penetrating wound, bruising and severe tenderness, subcutaneous emphysema or rib fractures. The trachea may be deviated away from the midline towards the uninjured side. However, this can be an unreliable clinical finding, which may only be noted on medical imaging. Distension of jugular veins in the neck may be observed because of increased intrathoracic pressures diminishing venous return, but this sign is also unreliable and may be absent in a patient with associated haemorrhagic shock from other injuries. In a patient with early tension pneumothorax without profound shock, where the radiographer responds rapidly to a trauma call, a CXR may in fact be taken which will show complete or almost complete collapse of the affected lung, and shift of the mediastinum away from the lung collapse, dragging the trachea towards the unaffected side.

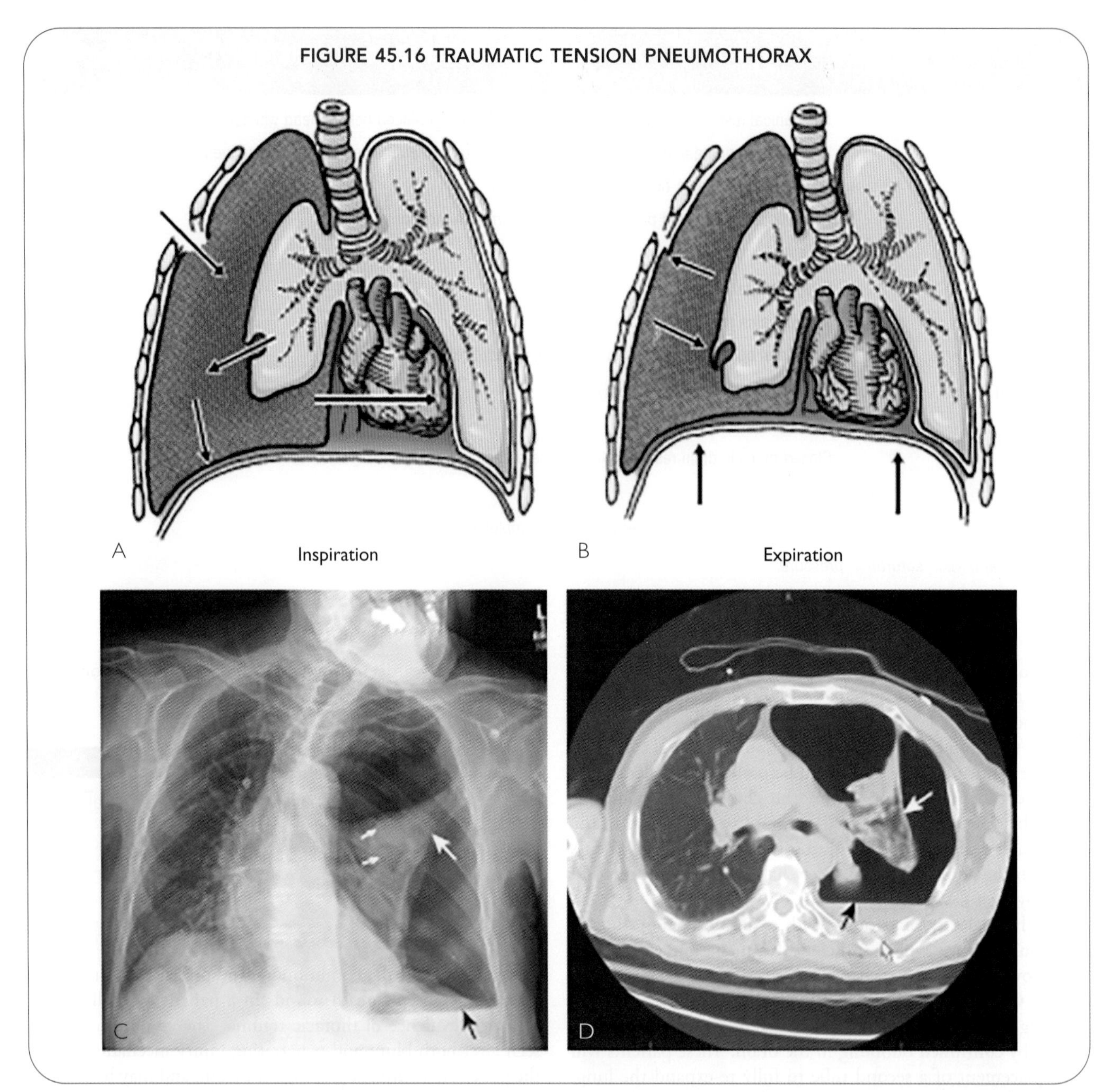

A and **B.** Pathophysiology of a tension pneumothorax. During inspiration, air enters the pleural space through a one-way valve either from the outside or from the lung itself. On expiration, the injury/valve closes and traps increasing amounts of air in the pleural space. Eventually, the mediastinum shifts and cardiac filling and ultimately cardiac output are compromised. **C.** This elderly patient sustained a tension haemopneumothorax after slipping and falling on ice. The left hemithorax is very dark (radiolucent) because of total collapse of the left lung (large white arrow). Note the dramatic shift of the mediastinum to the right, indicative of tension. Multiple posterior rib fractures are present but are difficult to appreciate on this film (small white arrows). The air-fluid level (black arrow) indicates the presence of fluid in the pleural cavity in addition to air. **D.** A computed tomography scan of the same patient redemonstrates the findings seen on the conventional radiograph.[59,60]

Management

Urgent decompression of the raised intrathoracic pressure is needed. In the ED or pre-hospital, in experienced hands, an emergency chest tube is the most appropriate measure, unless the patient is in established cardiogenic shock or near cardiac arrest, for which finger thoracostomy may be performed by trained personnel.

For finger thoracostomy, an incision is made through subcutaneous tissue between the 4th and 5th intercostal space, mid-axillary line on the affected side and is deepened through subcutaneous tissue down to muscle. Then using a blunt artery clip or a finger, the pleural cavity is entered. A hiss of air may confirm the position of the finger. The wound is left open and the trapped air leaking from the injured lung tissue escapes through the opening. This is a rapid procedure more suited to the confinement of a moving ambulance or retrieval aircraft than formal chest tube insertion. Once the patient arrives at the trauma centre an intercostal catheter is placed under sterile conditions, but not through the same wound. Bilateral finger thoracostomies may be lifesaving in the field for some patients with massive blunt chest injury.

An alternative approach is needle decompression, where a large-bore (14–16 gauge) cannula may be inserted into the chest via the second intercostal space in the midclavicular line on the affected side. An alternative site may be the 5th intercostal space anterior axillary line, which research suggests may have lower failure rates. Needle decompression will usually allow sufficient release of the trapped air to permit some increase in cardiac venous return and thereby improve cardiac output. Needle thoracostomy is only a temporary intervention to convert the tension pneumothorax into a simple pneumothorax or if there is a blockage in the ICC. The narrow diameter of the cannula imparts resistance to the outflow of the trapped air. The cannula length must be sufficient to penetrate all layers of the chest wall and enter the interpleural space. A cannula length of at least 4.5 cm is recommended especially in patients with a larger body habitus or where there is subcutaneous emphysema present.[61] As soon as practicable, or at the sign of any increase in respiratory distress or circulatory shock, a tube thoracostomy should be placed on the affected side. There is frequently an associated haemothorax, thus a tube of sufficient size should be placed (Fig. 45.17). In the pre-hospital setting, a patient with a tension pneumothorax may not respond to needle thoracostomy or may deteriorate en route to the trauma centre. Under these circumstances, check that the patient does not have bilateral pneumothoraces. Insert another large-bore cannula on the affected side, as the first may be blocked or dislodged. Should this manoeuvre fail then, for appropriately trained personnel, finger thoracostomies should be performed.

Occasionally, a patient presenting in extremis with a tension pneumothorax will fail to improve after insertion of one or more chest drains, remaining tachypnoeic, hypoxaemic and shocked. The chest radiograph will show a persistent lung collapse and there will be a large, continuous air leak. In these cases, serious consideration should be given to the presence of a major tracheobronchial injury (Fig. 45.18A and B).[40] This condition will require fibre-optic bronchoscopy for diagnosis and a prompt thoracotomy for direct surgical repair.

FIGURE 45.17 DEFINITIVE ASSESSMENT OF CHEST TUBE PLACEMENT IS WITH A CHEST RADIOGRAPH

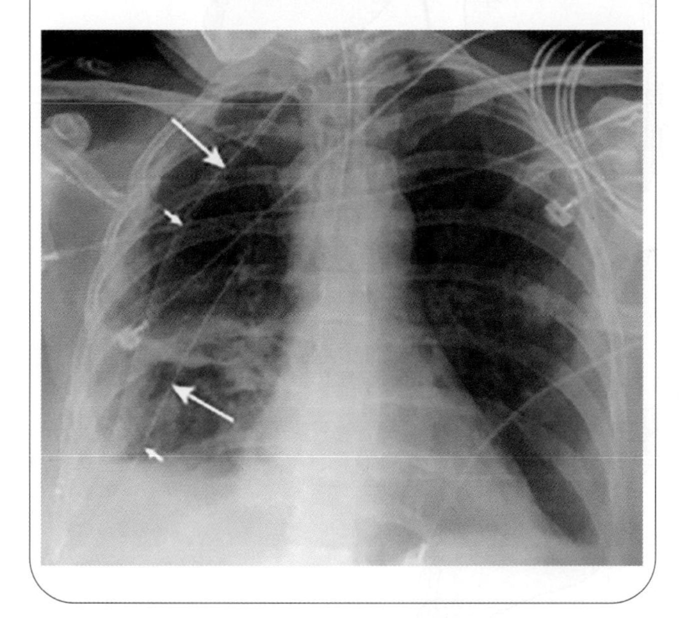

This patient has two chest tubes in place, and the radio-opaque marking lines on the tubes (large arrows) are readily visible. Chest tubes are manufactured so that these radio-opaque lines are interrupted at the level of the last drainage hole (small arrows). The gap in the line must be within the pleural cavity on the radiograph to ensure that the tube has been placed deep enough.[59,60]

Haemothorax

A collection of blood within the interpleural space is termed a haemothorax, and may arise from bleeding from the ends of fractured ribs, lacerated intercostal arteries or pulmonary parenchyma by sharp rib fragments or penetrating objects (knives, bullets, etc.), ruptured or lacerated intrathoracic blood vessels or (rarely) from haemorrhage from a cardiac chamber injury that is decompressing into the chest through a pericardial laceration. Fig. 45.19 demonstrates bleeding sources for a haemothorax.

Assessment

A haemothorax should be presumed present in any patient who has diminished or absent breath sounds on auscultation. If the patient is stable and time allows, a confirmatory CXR showing partial or complete opacification of the affected side is diagnostic showing a typical meniscus of layered blood within the chest. This will not be evident on a supine CXR, but the involved thorax will appear hazy. If the volume of blood within the chest is very large (massive haemothorax), complete opacification of the thorax will be noted in comparison to the unaffected side (Fig. 45.20). When the patient is in shock and the primary trauma survey does not clearly identify causes for the haemodynamic instability, treatment for haemothorax must proceed based on clinical signs alone without prior radiographical confirmation. The use of portable ultrasound (eFAST) for rapid bedside confirmation of haemothorax is now routine in many centres.[23]

Management

After blunt injury, small haemothoraces seen on CXR in asymptomatic patients may be managed without drainage, and the patient admitted for observation. Deterioration in respiratory status or repeat CXR after 24–48 hours showing an increase in size of the haemothorax will indicate the need for intercostal catheter placement. However, many of these small blood collections will not increase in size, but will be slowly reabsorbed by the pleura spontaneously without the need for drainage. Larger haemothoraces and those in patients who are hypoxaemic or complaining of shortness of breath require chest tube insertion. If large collections of blood are not drained, the result may be the formation of a 'fibrothorax', which results when fibrin deposition develops in an organised haemothorax and coats both the parietal and the visceral pleural surfaces, trapping the lung. The lung is fixed in position by this adhesive process and is unable to fully expand. Persistent atelectasis of portions of the lung and reduced pulmonary function then result. This then compromises respiratory

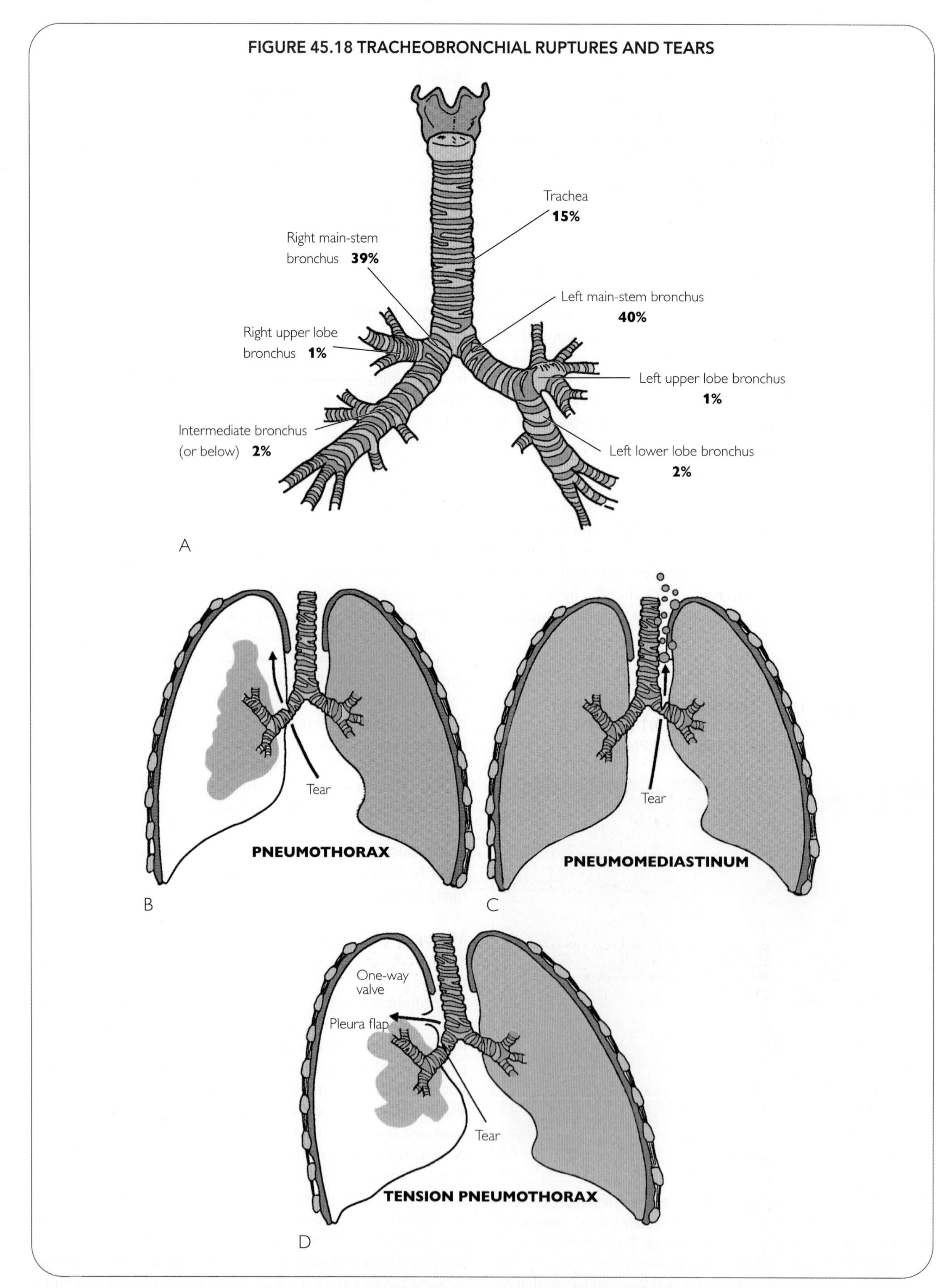

A. Tracheobronchial ruptures: general localisations based on literature review.[62,63] Complications of tracheobronchial tears. **B.** Pneumothorax.[64,65] **C.** Pneumomediastinum.[64,65] **D.** Progression of pneumothorax.[64,65]

FIGURE 45.19 SOURCE OF BLEEDING IN HAEMOTHORAX[62,63]

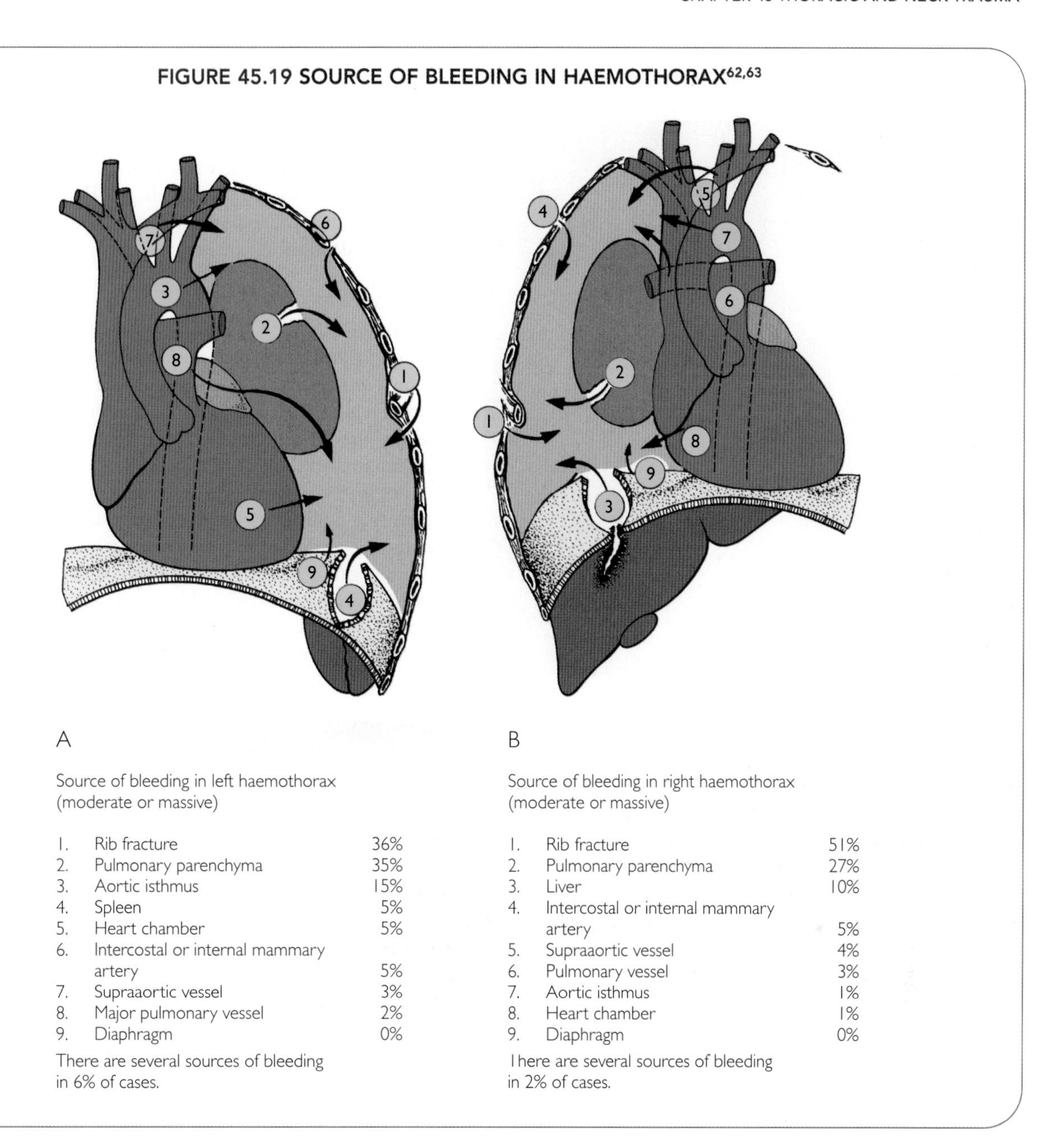

A

Source of bleeding in left haemothorax (moderate or massive)

1.	Rib fracture	36%
2.	Pulmonary parenchyma	35%
3.	Aortic isthmus	15%
4.	Spleen	5%
5.	Heart chamber	5%
6.	Intercostal or internal mammary artery	5%
7.	Supraaortic vessel	3%
8.	Major pulmonary vessel	2%
9.	Diaphragm	0%

There are several sources of bleeding in 6% of cases.

B

Source of bleeding in right haemothorax (moderate or massive)

1.	Rib fracture	51%
2.	Pulmonary parenchyma	27%
3.	Liver	10%
4.	Intercostal or internal mammary artery	5%
5.	Supraaortic vessel	4%
6.	Pulmonary vessel	3%
7.	Aortic isthmus	1%
8.	Heart chamber	1%
9.	Diaphragm	0%

There are several sources of bleeding in 2% of cases.

function, especially in individuals with pre-existing pulmonary disease, or in the elderly.[38] Observation of haemothoraces smaller than 300 mL and not observed on CXR (only CT) may be appropriately managed conservatively without chest tube insertion in patients not requiring mechanical ventilation.[68]

After penetrating injury, most haemothoraces large enough to be seen on CXR should also be drained, since the undrained thoracic blood in these cases has, by definition, been contaminated by external bacteria and the patient will be at increased risk for the development of an empyema. Most studies recommend only a single pre-procedure dose of an intravenous antibiotic with Gram-positive antimicrobial coverage (e.g. cephazolin), since continued antibiotic administration has not been shown to significantly reduce the incidence of wound infections or empyema in these patients.[69–71]

In approximately 85% of patients presenting with a haemothorax, no further intervention beyond the tube thoracostomy will be required.[57,72] However, in a minority, especially following penetrating injury, there will be persistent and ongoing bleeding that will require surgical intervention. The American College of Surgeons Committee on Trauma (ACSCOT) via its Advanced Trauma Life Support course (ATLS [EMST in Australia and Aotearoa New Zealand]) advises that initial drainage of 1500 mL of blood or more on insertion of a chest tube will usually dictate the need for surgery in that patient. The clinician assisting with chest tube placement should make note of this initial volume and communicate it to the medical team. Furthermore, even in the absence of an initial large volume of blood drainage, should the ongoing losses total more than 200 mL/hr over 4 or more hours, this is indicative of persistent haemorrhage which is likely to require surgical intervention to stop. It is crucial to monitor and record all output from the chest tube on a frequent and regular basis. The clinician must be mindful of blood replacement therapy, especially in the context of large haemothoraces causing altered haemodynamics.

FIGURE 45.20 HAEMOTHORAX

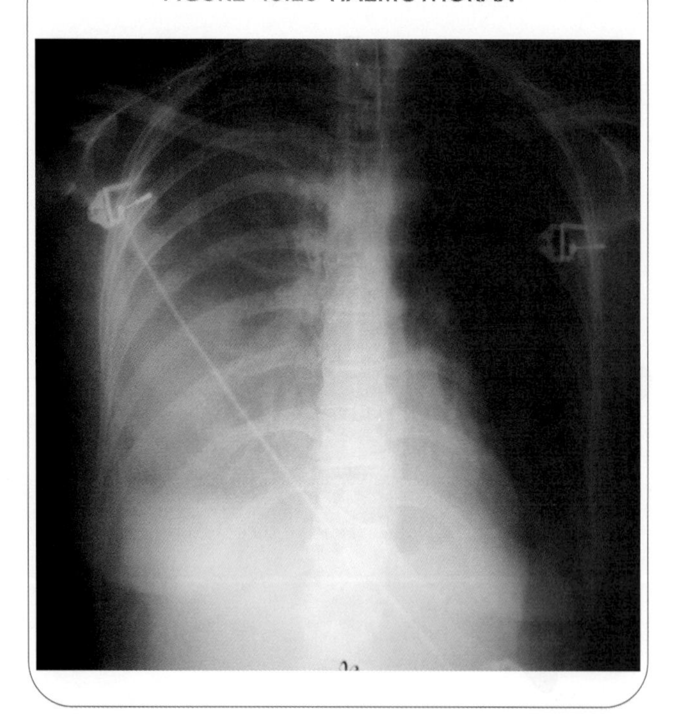

Chest radiograph of a 22-year-old female pedestrian hit by a bus. The hazy opacification within the right hemithorax is due to the presence of a large haemothorax caused by a ruptured intercostal artery.[66,67]

Open pneumothorax

Sometimes referred to as a 'sucking chest wound', this is an infrequent but dramatic injury which involves full-thickness loss of chest wall tissue leading to open and continuous external communication between outside atmospheric pressure and the thoracic cavity (Fig. 45.21). In civilian centres it may be seen after stabbings, shootings, or following wounding by large, rapidly moving sharp objects, such as watercraft propellers or industrial machinery. In the military setting, open chest wounds may result from blast injury or as a consequence of high-energy gunshot wounds. As a consequence of loss of the negative pressure within the thoracic cavity, the underlying lung completely collapses. If the lung itself has been lacerated there will be air leakage and associated haemorrhage. This leads to profound respiratory distress, hypoxaemia and shock, and may progress rapidly to death if not treated.

Management

The communication between the thoracic cavity and atmospheric pressure must be closed to restore negative pressure. In the prehospital setting this can be accomplished in a variety of ways: by placing a gloved hand over the hole in order to prevent any further passage of air into/out of the chest; taping an occlusive plastic dressing over the hole or using a dressing designed to allow egress but not ingress of air to prevent tension pneumothorax while also permitting drainage of any blood that accumulates in the chest cavity (Fig. 45.22). Eventually a chest tube will be required to restore negative intrathoracic pressure which will re-expand the lung and drain any associated haemothorax. This must be placed through uninjured chest wall and never through the injury itself. For large chest wall defects, surgical repair with musculocutaneous flaps may be required once the patient has stabilised.

PRACTICE TIP

If an occlusive taped dressing is used, it should only be taped on three sides to allow air to escape during expiration minimising the risk of raised intrathoracic pressure and tension pneumothorax.

OTHER THORACIC INJURIES

DIAPHRAGMATIC INJURY

The diaphragm is a thin yet complex sheet of muscle and tendon that separates the abdominal and thoracic cavities, and it

FIGURE 45.21 OPEN PNEUMOTHORAX

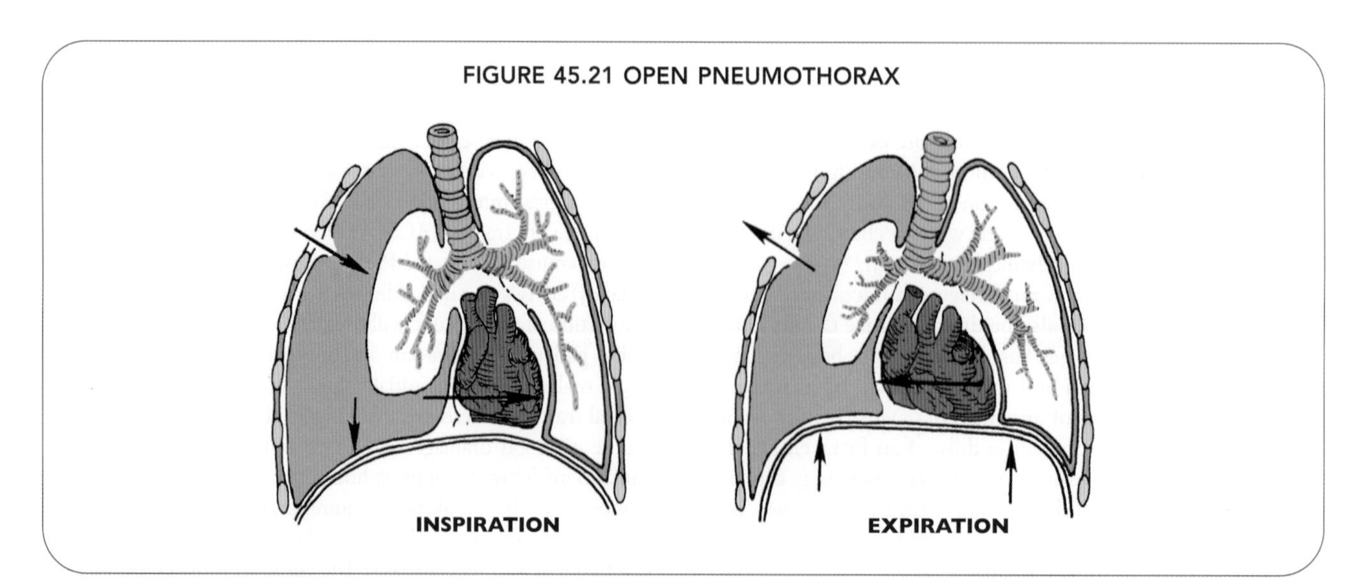

Collapse of right lung and air in pleural cavity occurs with communication to outside through defect in chest wall. In sucking chest wound, lung volume is greater with expiration.[44,51]

FIGURE 45.22 COMPARISON OF ASHERMAN vs BOLIN SEAL

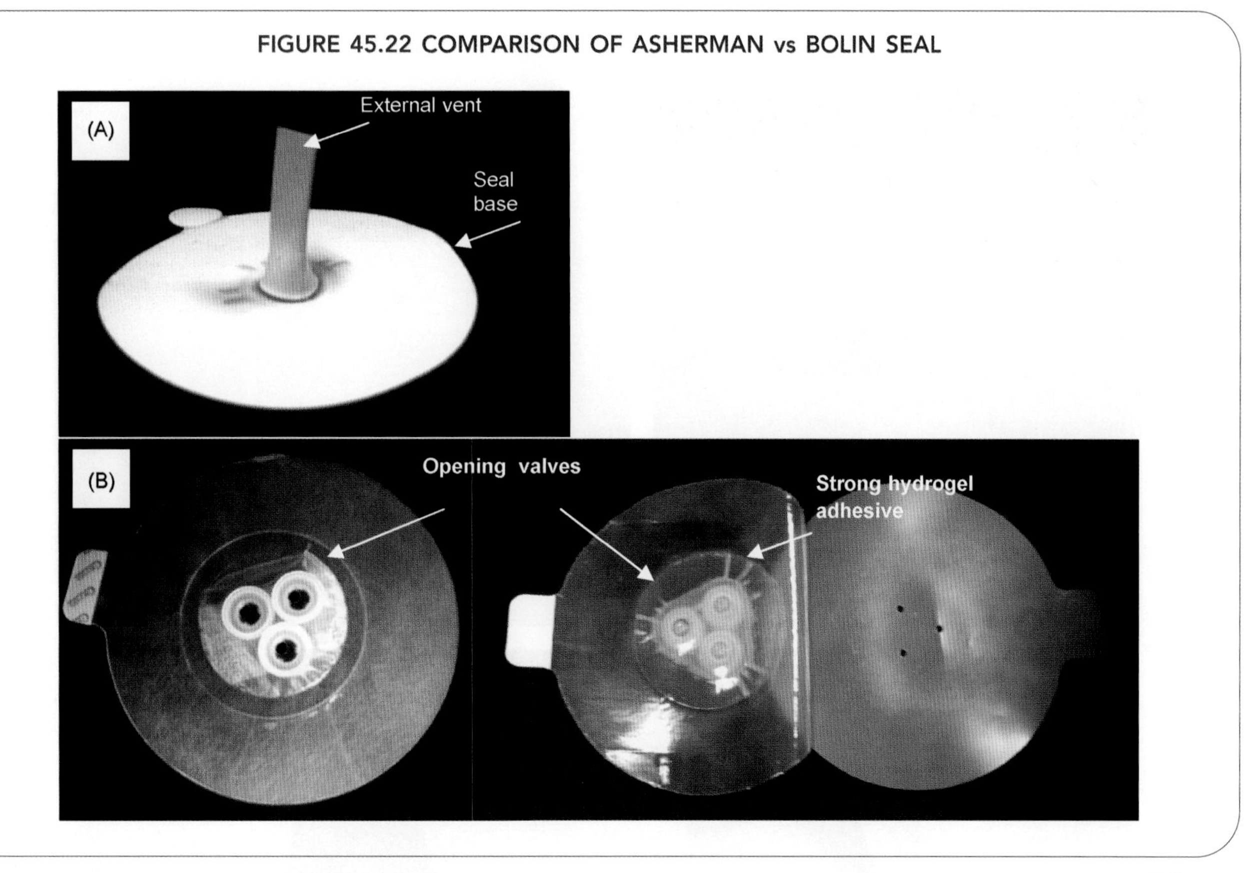

A. Asherman tube chest seal. **B.** Bolin 3-valve chest seal, both with a 15 cm diameter adhesive base—unopened and opened view.[73,74]

is critical to the mechanics of breathing. Its position varies with respect to respiration, rising as high as the 4th intercostal space on forced expiration, and moving as low as the inferior costal margins (T9) on deep inspiration. Diaphragmatic injury is very rare, less than 2% of the trauma population.[72]

Diaphragmatic rupture after blunt force trauma is more common on the left side because there is little or no liver in the left upper abdomen to absorb energy and thus protect the diaphragm from tearing. Penetrating diaphragmatic injuries occur at any point along the trajectory of the projectile or wounding weapon, and may result from penetration of the abdomen or thorax. Concomitant abdominal visceral injury is not uncommon, especially with gunshot wounds.[72] Injuries to the diaphragm, especially if the defect is small, may cause little clinical effect and may only be diagnosed if the patient needs laparotomy for intra-abdominal trauma.

Assessment

Patients may be asymptomatic, may complain of chest wall or abdominal pain due to the presence of associated rib fractures or may even be tachypnoeic and hypoxaemic if the amount of herniated viscera (stomach, colon, small bowel) in the thorax is large enough to compress the adjacent lung.[75] These patients may present in haemodynamic shock as a result of associated intra-abdominal injuries, but the effect of the herniated viscera in compressing the inferior vena cava and thus reducing cardiac preload must also be considered.

Blunt diaphragmatic injury may be suspected when the initial or subsequent CXR shows the presence of a high gastric bubble in the lower left chest (Fig. 45.23), suggesting that the stomach has herniated through the diaphragmatic defect. The pathognomonic radiographical sign is that of the nasogastric tube coiled in the left lower chest.[76] Occasionally, coils of small bowel or colon may be seen situated in the left thoracic cavity. If the injury is to the right diaphragm, assess the chest radiograph for an abnormal 'hump' in the lateral diaphragm, which is suggestive of a large laceration of the diaphragm with protrusion of the liver.

Modern CT scanners are sensitive enough to detect often subtle diaphragmatic ruptures after blunt trauma,[75] but even in the absence of CT findings, if the patient has suffered significant blunt force trauma to the thoraco-abdominal area a high index of suspicion must exist that a diaphragmatic injury may have occurred.

Injuries to the diaphragm may also be found at the time of exploratory laparotomy for penetrating trauma. Penetrating injury to the thoraco-abdominal region in an otherwise asymptomatic patient may best be assessed by diagnostic thoracoscopy or laparoscopy, at which time injury to the diaphragm can be detected and in some cases repaired.

Management

Diaphragmatic defects do not spontaneously close, regardless of the size, because of the negative pressure gradient between the thorax and the abdominal cavity caused by respirations. This tends to draw abdominal contents, such as omentum and/or viscera including bowel and stomach, through even small defects in the diaphragm, which subsequently enlarge. If undetected in the

FIGURE 45.23 DIAPHRAGMATIC RUPTURE

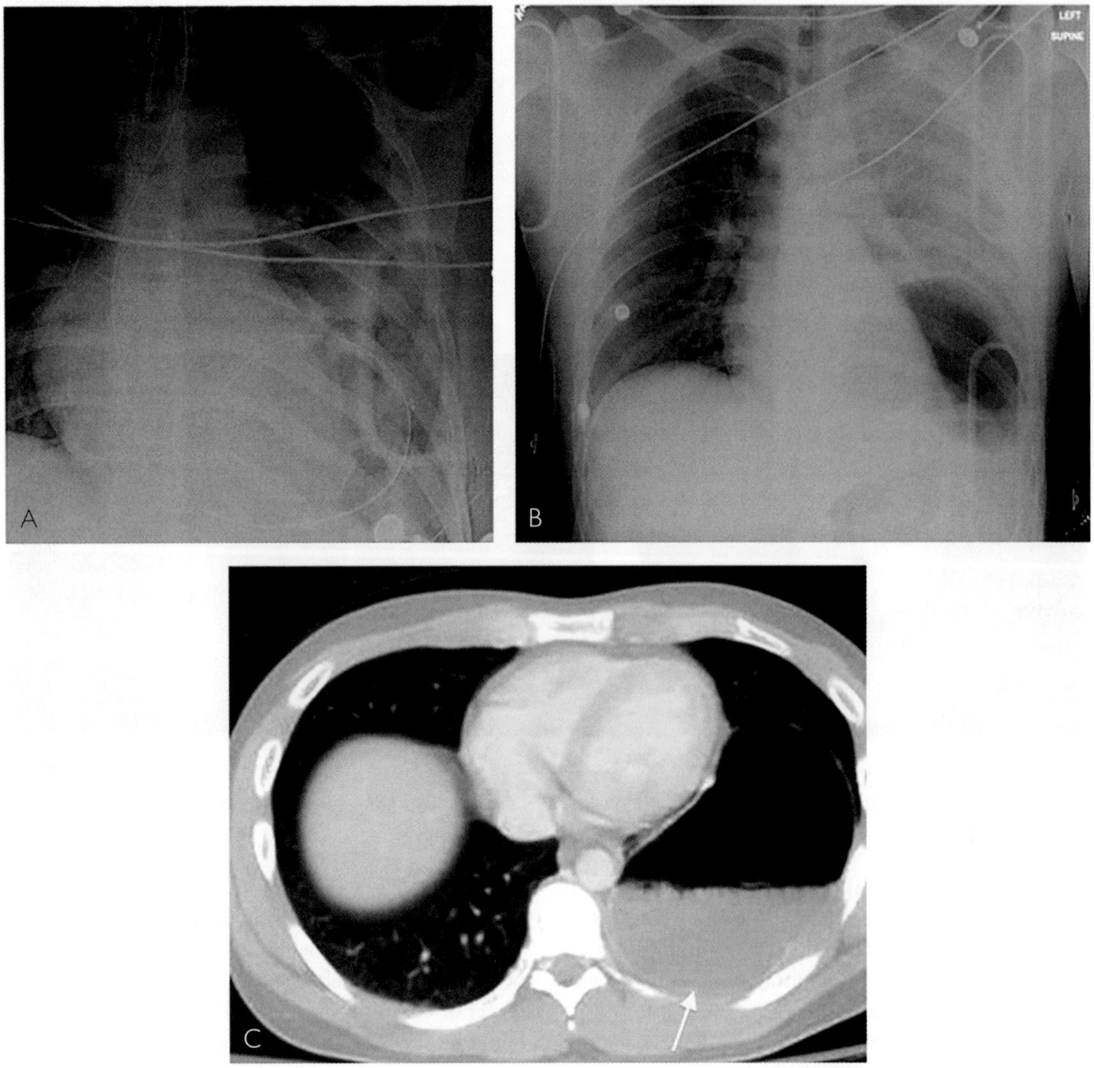

A. Chest radiograph shows the nasogastric tube coiled within an intrathoracic stomach (arrows), indicating diaphragmatic rupture in this trauma patient. B. In a different patient, chest radiograph shows an intrathoracic viscus in the left lower chest consistent with diaphragmatic rupture. The diffusely increased opacity on the left should also be noted, which suggests a haemothorax. C. CECT scan of the same patient demonstrates an intrathoracic stomach. Note that the stomach is in contact within the posterior chest wall, the 'dependent-viscera' sign (arrow). This is essentially diagnostic of diaphragmatic rupture.[66,67] *CECT: contrast-enhanced computed tomography.*

early period, non-specific abdominal complaints due to this intermittent herniation may be the subsequent presenting symptom, even well after discharge.[77] Visceral obstruction and incarceration may occur, and visceral ischaemia due to compression of vascular supply by the narrow hernial orifice can result with subsequent bowel necrosis. When patients who have suffered severe blunt thoraco-abdominal injury are intubated and sedated for other injuries, the possibility of such a missed injury or delay in diagnosis may result in serious life-threatening consequences.

As mentioned above, small defects detected at laparoscopy may be repaired at the time. Larger defects are approached via a laparotomy, where care is needed to return the abdominal contents to the peritoneal cavity without causing further injury to the vascular supply. The defect is repaired using heavy non-absorbable sutures. Where there is significant loss of tissue then repair using synthetic or biological mesh may be required. It is advisable that all diaphragmatic injuries are repaired at the time of their detection.

CARDIAC INJURY

Cardiac injury may occur following blunt or penetrating trauma. The literature shows a wide variance in incidence of cardiac injury in closed blunt chest trauma, anywhere between 2%[78] and 50%.[79] This wide range is mainly due to the variation in diagnostic criteria used, and the fact that there is no gold standard test for this diagnosis. In Australasia, blunt trauma is more commonly seen because of a lower incidence of gun-related injury. High-speed MVCs in which the patient impacts the steering wheel or pre-tensioned seatbelt account for the vast majority of cases, with pedestrians struck by vehicles, crush injuries and falls from great heights comprising the other groups of patients with blunt cardiac injury.[53] A slow but steady increase in interpersonal violence in Australasia has seen a parallel rise in the incidence of penetrating cardiac injuries presenting to EDs.

Cardiac injuries can be obvious and catastrophic to patient outcome, but in other cases the injury may be more subtle, making diagnosis challenging. Those who survive to reach the hospital may present in shock from acute pericardial tamponade, with severe heart failure from myocardial muscle, haemothorax compromising cardiac contractility, valve dysfunction or suffering a wide variety of potentially fatal cardiac dysrhythmias.[55]

Where cardiac damage is less obvious, the mechanism of injury, estimated energy transfer and clinical signs, such as bruising to the chest wall, must alert the treating team to the potential for cardiac injury.

BLUNT CARDIAC INJURY (BCI)

There is a wide spectrum of potential injuries to the heart after blunt chest trauma, including cardiac contusion, myocardial rupture, valvular disruptions and injury to the great vessels or the coronary arteries.

TABLE 45.4 BLUNT CARDIAC INJURY CLASSIFICATION AND MANIFESTATION

ANATOMY/PATHOPHYSIOLOGY OF BLUNT INJURY	CLINICAL MANIFESTATION
Free rupture of cardiac chamber into chest	Immediate death
Contained rupture (by intact pericardium) of cardiac chamber	Acute pericardial tamponade and cardiogenic shock
Rupture of cardiac valve leaflets or chordae tendineae	Acute or delayed valvular insufficiency
Tear of pericardium and cardiac herniation	Cardiogenic shock
Severe contusion of myocardium	Pump failure due to localised myocardial dyskinesis
Mild contusion of myocardium	Electrical conduction disturbances and possibly malignant dysrhythmias
Occlusion of coronary artery	Acute myocardial infarction

Myocardial contusion

Myocardial contusion is the most common injury to the heart after blunt trauma to the chest.[53] It is a well-defined entity with distinct pathological and biochemical abnormalities.[59] However, its manifestation varies widely, making diagnosis and quantification of incidence challenging.[80] The position of the right ventricle behind the sternum makes it particularly vulnerable to contusion. Myocardial contusions span a spectrum ranging from asymptomatic and transient elevations of various cardiac enzymes to patchy necrosis and haemorrhage, acute pericardial effusions, isolated tears to the pericardium with the potential for cardiac herniation, malignant dysrhythmias and immediately fatal cardiac chamber ruptures (Table 45.4).

Myocardial rupture

Most patients with uncontained myocardial rupture do not reach the ED alive. Of those who do, hypotension may reduce pressure on the injured myocardium, which may then worsen as fluid resuscitation restores blood pressure. Pericardial tamponade, usually rare following blunt cardiac injury, then develops. In the case of an intact pericardium with associated cardiac wall rupture, a pseudo-aneurysm may form, which buys time for detection and surgical intervention.[59] In a minority of patients, rapid diagnosis by echocardiography or CT scan and operative intervention can be lifesaving. Less severe injuries to the ventricular wall may lead to delayed necrosis and manifest as delayed rupture within several days of admission, therefore early identification is essential.

Valvular damage

Disruption of cardiac valves is rare and may present with a spectrum of disorders from new cardiac murmurs to fulminant cardiac failure.[81]

Dysrhythmia

Tachycardia in a trauma patient must always be presumed secondary to haemorrhage until proven otherwise. Only then in the setting of blunt chest trauma should persistent tachycardia, new bundle branch block or mild dysrhythmia raise suspicion of blunt cardiac injury.

Blunt cardiac injury typically occurs in severely injured patients who have associated significant thoracic trauma, such as multiple rib fractures, pulmonary contusions and haemopneumothorax.[81,82] Often none of the clinical features described above manifest until a complication occurs, which can be quite sudden. The injured area of myocardium may then become a focus for dysrhythmias, occasionally resulting in cardiac arrest from ventricular tachycardia or fibrillation. Injury to the conducting system can cause heart block. Injury to the myocardium can cause impaired heart contractility with reduced cardiac output, leading to cardiogenic shock and pulmonary oedema. As the pressure within the ventricles increases, a baroreceptor response is initiated to increase the heart rate and stroke volume in an attempt to increase cardiac output. Peripheral vasoconstriction shunts blood from the skin, gut and kidneys towards the brain, heart and lungs. The reduction in kidney blood flow precipitates water retention by way of antidiuretic hormone (ADH) and the renin–angiotensin–aldosterone system further increasing the load on the heart.

Assessment

Any patient whose history includes a known or potential major transfer of energy to the anterior chest should be considered at high risk for BCI. Examples include sudden decelerations onto a vehicle steering wheel or dashboard, and falls from heights > 3 m. Patients who have required CPR, chest drain placement, are unconscious or shocked pre-hospital should have a high suspicion for BCI.[83]

FIGURE 45.24 ELECTROCARDIOGRAM IN CARDIAC INJURY

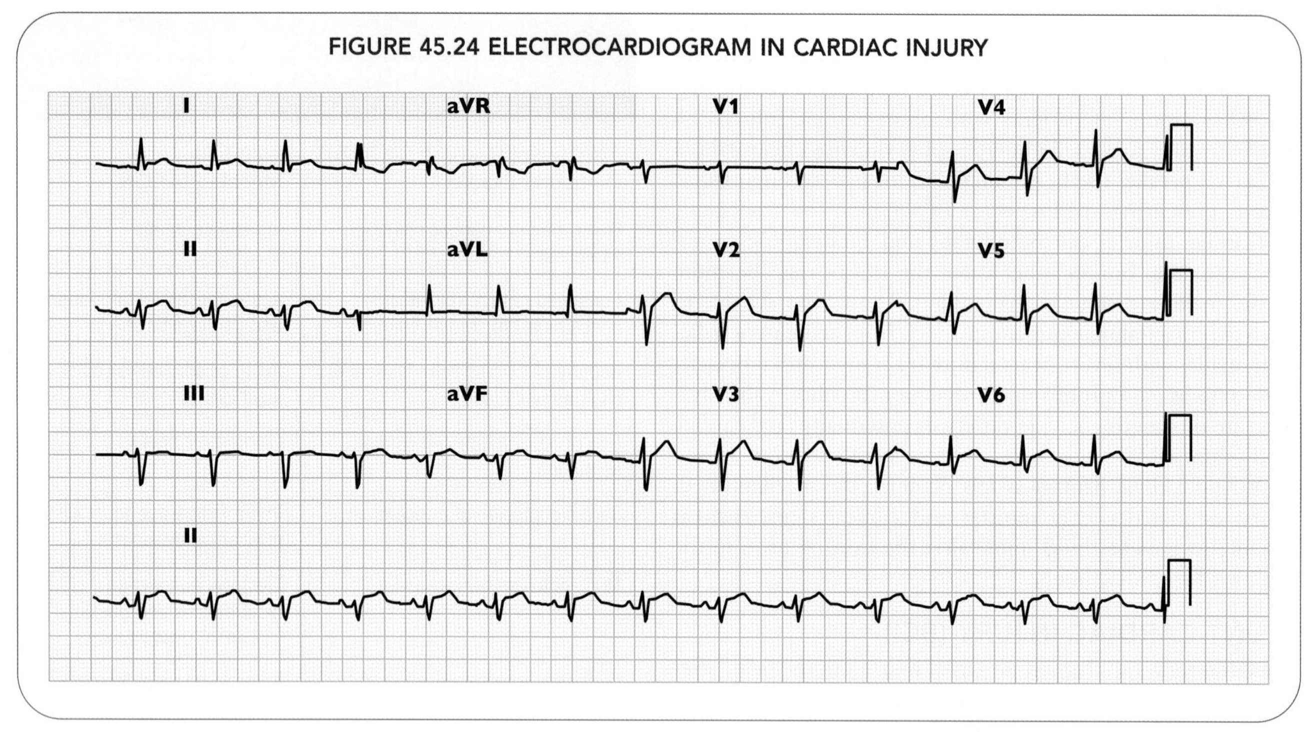

12-lead electrocardiogram demonstrating sinus rhythm with diffuse ST elevation across the anterior and inferior leads in a 37-year-old man with blunt cardiac injury following a motor vehicle collision.[62,84]

The most important assessment tool is the ECG. In haemodynamically stable patients, a normal ECG in the ED reliably identifies patients at low risk for cardiac complications who do not need any further cardiac investigations or ongoing cardiac monitoring (see Chapter 16).[83] Virtually any ECG abnormality may indicate cardiac contusion, such as sinus tachycardia, ectopic beats, ST segment deflections or T-wave changes.[62,83] All of these patients should be monitored and further investigated to differentiate BCI from myocardial infarction (Fig. 45.24). Where there is a clinical suspicion, FAST scan, now performed as an adjunct to primary survey, can assess the presence of haemopericardium.[64]

While elevation of serum troponin and wall motion abnormalities on echocardiography are also associated with adverse events, both of these tests lack adequate reliability for identifying patients who either need to be monitored for complications or can be safely left unmonitored. If malignant dysrhythmias arise, such as ventricular tachycardia, fibrillation or heart block, they will require prompt pharmacological intervention or electric cardioversion.

Abnormal movement of the heart in response to dysrhythmias can depress cardiac ejection fraction and significantly reduce cardiac output (see Table 45.4). In addition to the ECG, the echocardiogram is very useful in determining both the presence of cardiac dysfunction and the possible aetiology, and should be obtained as soon as the diagnosis is entertained.[70] The most frequent echocardiographic anomaly seen in unstable patients presenting with blunt cardiac injury is a localised or global dyskinesis of the heart chambers. Also seen are acute valvular insufficiencies due to tearing of the valve leaflets or adjacent supporting structures, ruptured interventricular septae and pericardial fluid collections indicating pericardial tamponade due to atrial or ventricular lacerations.

Management

Pre-hospital clinicians should manage any patient with potential blunt cardiac injury according to EMST guidelines with particular focus on airway, breathing and circulation. Rapid transport to the nearest major trauma centre should occur.

In the ED the emergency nurse should ensure that oxygen is applied and that cardiac monitoring leads are in place (see Chapter 16). Patients with cardiac dysrhythmias who are haemodynamically stable and have no evidence of depressed cardiac function will require no treatment beyond a 24-hour period of continuous ECG monitoring to ensure that there is no progression of their dysrhythmias to more malignant forms. Malignant dysrhythmias are treated according to their type and severity with pharmacological agents, electric cardioversion, or both. Nursing staff should be aware of clinical signs of deterioration which indicate hypoxaemia, including dysrhythmias, tachypnoea, decreased oxygen saturations, tachycardia, hypotension, decreased level of consciousness and increased temperature. The clinician should ensure that the patient is admitted to an appropriate acuity ward, that effective handover is given so that the receiving nurse is fully aware of the patient's injuries and any potential for deterioration, and that a plan is in place for multidisciplinary care, including effective analgesia.

Patients with structural heart injuries will generally require admission to an intensive care unit and may require inotropic support to maintain cardiac output.

PRACTICE TIP

The clinician should perform an ECG for the patient with suspected cardiac injury.

PENETRATING CARDIAC INJURY

Penetrating cardiac injury has an estimated pre-hospital mortality rate of over 80%.[71] Any penetrating mechanism to the left and central anterior chest, whether from a low-velocity piercing instrument such as a knife or a higher-velocity handgun missile, should be suspected of producing a cardiac injury until proven otherwise. Penetrating thoraco-abdominal injuries should also be suspected, with any penetrating chest injuries.[66] Entrance wounds located within the praecordial zone of injury, sometimes referred to as 'the box', should be assumed to have produced a cardiac injury and, in the stable patient, the full range of diagnostic measures described must be instigated to look for it. This zone is defined anatomically by an area encompassed superiorly by the clavicles, laterally by the right midclavicular line and the left midaxillary line, and inferiorly by the costal margins.

Assessment

The most widely available and sensitive means to non-invasively diagnose a cardiac injury remains the transthoracic echocardiogram.[85] This may be rapidly performed at the bedside by the trauma team as part of the initial FAST examination, or by a dedicated sonographer experienced in the technique of echocardiography if the patient is stable, but in whom there remains a high index of suspicion based on the location of the wound. Transoesophageal echocardiography is also a sensitive tool for this purpose, but is not readily available in most EDs.

Acute pericardial tamponade occurs following penetrating injury to the 'box'. It results when blood from injury to the cardiac chambers or coronary vessels accumulates between the heart and the rigid overlying fibrous pericardium, compressing the cardiac chambers and thus reducing cardiac output as a result of diminished ventricular filling during diastole (Fig. 45.25). Clinically, the patient will present with evidence of a diminishing cardiac output, which manifests initially by tachycardia, anxiety and agitation as cerebral perfusion decreases, but initially hypotension is rare. As the volume of blood within the pericardial space continues to increase and further compress the heart, the systolic blood pressure eventually drops, resulting in cardiac arrest and death due to compressive heart failure unless immediate action is taken to relieve the tamponade.

Cardiac tamponade is often characterised by a group of findings termed Beck's triad, which consists of hypotension, distant or diminished heart sounds on auscultation and elevated central venous pressure, as evidenced by distension of the neck veins.[73] In reality, the complete triad is rarely seen in patients with acute cardiac tamponade after trauma, so the diagnosis of tamponade should never depend on the patient exhibiting all three criteria. A patient exhibiting early to moderately advanced signs of tamponade (tachycardia and only small drops in systemic blood pressure) may be temporarily stabilised by administration of intravenous fluid boluses. This manoeuvre will delay the eventual and inevitable cardiac arrest by temporarily increasing ventricular filling pressures so as to overcome the extrinsic cardiac compression that is preventing normal cardiac output. However, early activation of MTP should be considered in all penetrating chest and abdominal injuries.

Management

Treatment of acute pericardial tamponade requires decompression of the pericardial space around the heart, as well as control and definitive repair of the cardiac injury from which the bleeding originated. This will require direct exposure of the injury via either a median sternotomy or an anterolateral thoracotomy incision. If a patient with a penetrating chest wound presents in pre-arrest or arrests on arrival in the ED, resuscitative thoracotomy (EDT) and decompression of a cardiac tamponade may be lifesaving. Otherwise, unstable patients with penetrating chest

FIGURE 45.25 ECHOCARDIOGRAM SHOWING PERICARDIAL EFFUSION CAUSING CARDIAC TAMPONADE

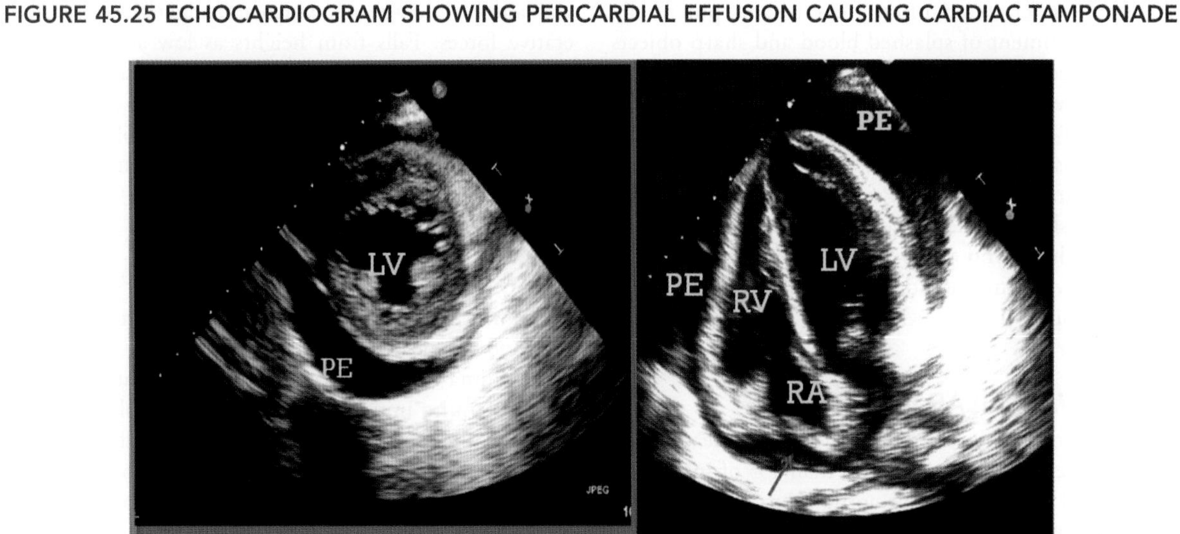

A subcostal view in early diastole shows a large circumferential pericardial effusion compressing the heart, with the right ventricle completely collapsed.[85,86] *Reprinted with permission from Priscilla Peters, Cooper University Hospital, Camden, NJ.*

wounds should be rapidly transported to the operating theatre for definitive management.[73]

Historically, needle pericardiocentesis (aspiration of blood from around the heart) has been performed in the emergency setting. However, this technique has been associated with iatrogenic cardiac and liver injury and is rarely effective since the blood is often clotted.[87] Subxiphoid pericardial window (SPW) is now the recommended, minimally invasive emergency intervention if the expertise to perform definitive EDT is not available. In the haemodynamically stable patient, the SPW can be both diagnostic and therapeutic, with the ability to identify major penetrating cardiac injury, and can be extended to a sternotomy if required.[88,89]

Any evidence of intra-pericardial fluid in a patient with a praecordial penetrating injury usually mandates immediate surgical exploration via either median sternotomy or thoracotomy to detect and repair the injured heart. In the stable patient, this is best done in the controlled environment of the operating theatre, where improved lighting, specialised anaesthesia and nursing support and greater instrument availability allow for a safer and definitive operation. However, patients with praecordial penetrating injuries who deteriorate rapidly in the ED or who suffer a cardiac arrest in the field, but have undergone less than 10 minutes of closed chest compression resuscitation, should undergo a prompt resuscitative ED thoracotomy if the surgical expertise is immediately available. This potentially lifesaving technique consists of rapidly opening the chest through a left anterolateral thoracotomy, cross-clamping the descending thoracic aorta, opening the left pericardial sac to evacuate the clot and relieve the compressive tamponade and digitally controlling the site of haemorrhage from the lacerated cardiac chamber while transporting the patient to the operating theatre for definitive repair under more-optimal surgical conditions.[71] Nursing personnel should anticipate transport and monitoring needs for these patients for, if the resuscitation is successful, the patient must be taken directly to the operating theatre if the chances for survival are to be optimised.

The ED resuscitative thoracotomy exposes all involved healthcare personnel to an often frenetic and potentially hazardous environment of splashed blood and sharp objects (instruments, needles, fractured rib ends, etc.) and should only be done when it is most likely to benefit the patient. The highest survival rates for ED thoracotomy are in those patients who sustain cardiac arrest after arrival to the ED from a stab wound to the heart. Patients who have sustained praecordial gunshot injuries have a much lower chance of survival, while those who arrest after a blunt mechanism of injury rarely survive and should not undergo an ED resuscitative thoracotomy (EDT).[71] Detail on the procedure is given in Chapter 42.

THORACIC VASCULAR INJURY

Blunt thoracic aortic injury is a major cause of death from blunt trauma. Despite representing less than 1% of injuries in patients involved in MVCs, blunt aortic injury is responsible for 16% of the deaths. The vast majority of patients die before arriving at the hospital.[90]

The thoracic aorta and its major branches, as well as the superior and inferior venae cavae and the azygous veins, carry very large blood flows and significant injury may lead to exsanguinating haemorrhage and death. Because of their relatively fixed position within the chest cavity, these large vessels (aorta, proximal innominate artery, proximal left subclavian and carotid arteries) are vulnerable to sudden decelerative forces after blunt trauma, which may result in the formation of traumatic pseudoaneurysms (i.e. contained partial ruptures of the vessel wall), partial or complete obstructions, lacerations or even total transections that cause massive haemothorax. High-speed MVCs are the most common blunt mechanism producing major intrathoracic vascular injury. Any occupant in the vehicle may sustain this type of injury, and it may occur even from laterally applied forces, such as the so-called left subclavian and carotid arteries, which are vulnerable to sudden decelerative forces. Falls from heights as low as 3 m can sustain this type of injury. Penetrating injuries, such as stab wounds and gunshot wounds, may disrupt the vascular tree at any point within the chest, producing uncontrolled haemorrhage and rapid death if not detected and treated expeditiously (Figs 45.26 and 45.27).

FIGURE 45.26 COMMON SITES OF AORTIC DISRUPTION

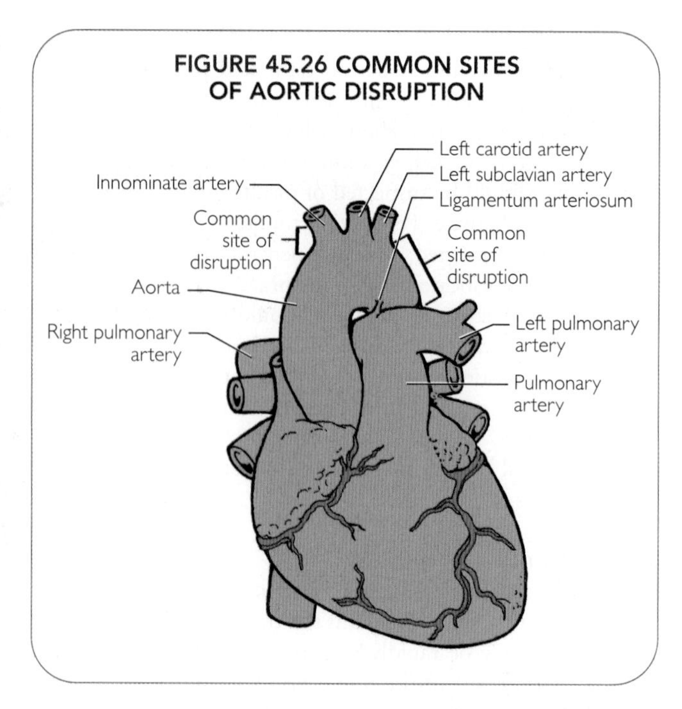

Assessment

The mechanism of injury and the patient's haemodynamic status will often provide evidence of thoracic vascular injury. Haemodynamically unstable patients with penetrating thoracic trauma who do not respond to resuscitative measures will usually require immediate surgery with a plain film CXR as the only preoperative radiological test. Stable patients with suspected intrathoracic vascular injuries should undergo further radiological evaluation to confirm and anatomically stage the injury. If the CXR demonstrates signs suggesting aortic injury then either CT angiography or digital subtraction angiography or both should be performed, a combined approach that allows for more-accurate preoperative localisation of the

FIGURE 45.27 RADIOGRAPHIC IMAGES OF THORACIC INJURIES

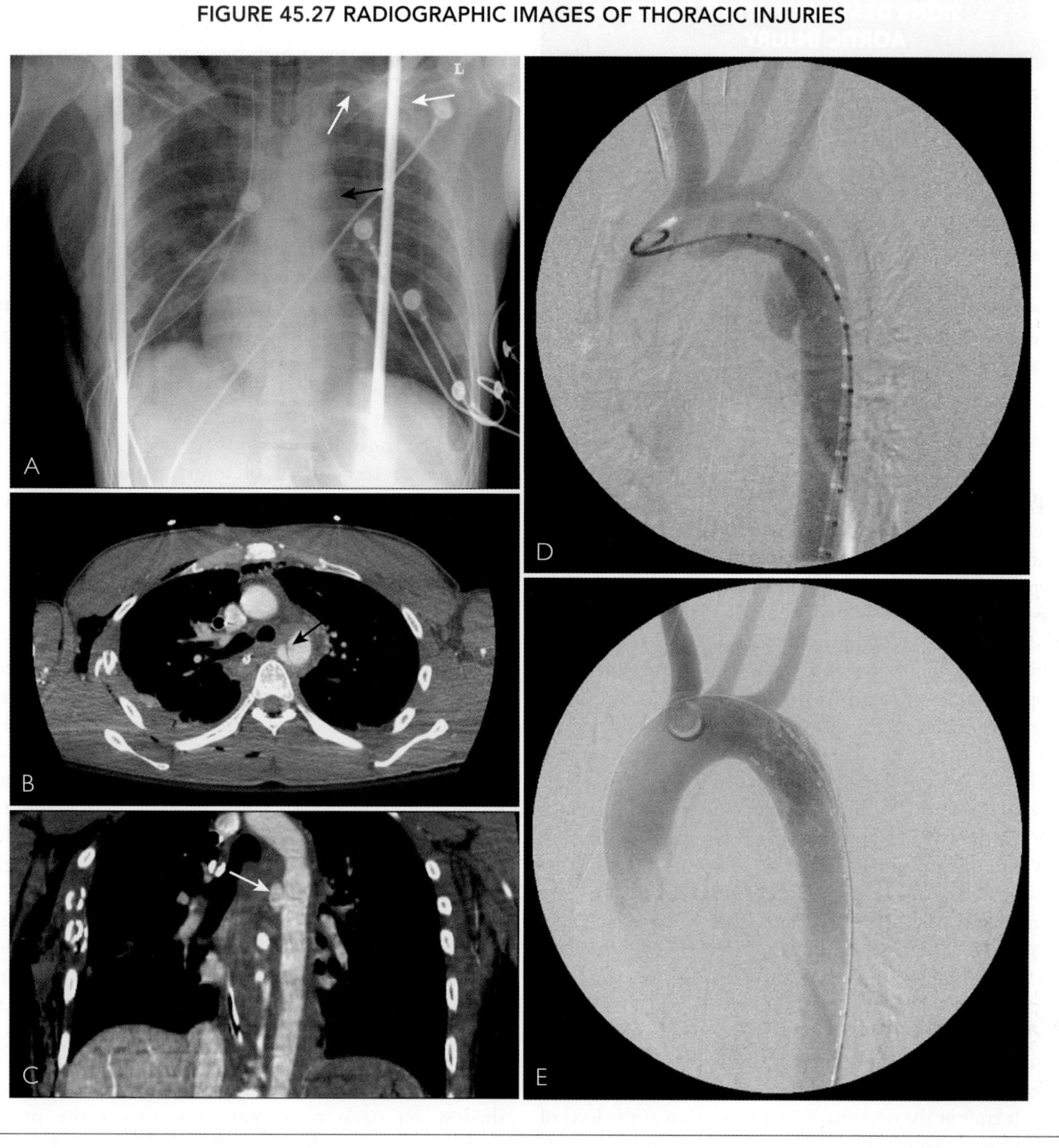

A. Portable chest radiograph shows an enlarged indistinct aortic arch (black arrow), a left apical pleural cap and upper rib fractures (white arrows). **B.** Axial computed tomography demonstrates mediastinal haematoma, intimal flap and pseudoaneurysm (arrow). **C.** Oblique coronal reformation shows the extent of pseudoaneurysm (arrow). **D, E.** Thoracic aortography before and after treatment with an aortic stent.[45,31]

injury and planning of the operation.[90] As mentioned above, improvements in CT technology and its ready availability have made CT angiography alone the investigation of choice in many centres. CXR signs suggestive of aortic injury are listed in Box 45.1.

Of these findings, the most important one, due to its high positive predictive value, is the 'funny looking mediastinum'. This admittedly imprecise term refers either to a superior mediastinum that appears on the CXR to be widened (more than the oft-quoted 8 cm maximum normal width at the aortic knob) or indistinct or poorly defined, especially along the superolateral border of the aortic knob and descending aorta (Fig. 45.27).

Contained aortic ruptures are prone to sudden rupture, which results in exsanguination into the thorax. Therefore, it is imperative that these injuries, when suspected, be diagnosed promptly. It should be remembered, however, that in a haemodynamically unstable patient with a widened mediastinum only, suggesting a contained bleed, other sites of haemorrhage such as the abdomen or the pelvis must be considered. A contained aortic transection will not cause hypovolaemic shock until it ruptures into the thoracic cavity.

BOX 45.1 SIGNS DEMONSTRATING POTENTIAL AORTIC INJURY

- 'Funny-looking mediastinum':
  - superior mediastinal width > 8 cm
  - indistinct or 'fuzzy' descending aortic margin
  - indistinct or 'fuzzy' aortic knob contour
- Fracture(s) of first or second rib(s)
- Fracture of scapula
- Depression of left mainstem bronchus
- Deviation of nasogastric tube to right
- Deviation of trachea to right
- Fractures(s) of upper thoracic vertebra(e)

Management

Treatment of major thoracic vascular injuries has traditionally been surgical repair via either a sternotomy or a thoracotomy. Pre-hospital clinicians should initiate damage control resuscitation protocols. Intravenous fluids should only be administered to maintain a systolic blood pressure around 80–90 mmHg, to avoid disrupting fresh clots and promoting further bleeding, coagulopathy and hypothermia. In the ED the nurse should alert the team leader to any change in haemodynamic parameters or in the conscious state of the patient. Heart rate and systolic blood pressure should be controlled with beta-blockers unless contraindicated.[91] This has been demonstrated to reduce mortality in the ED for those patients awaiting repair. Certain patients with thoracic aortic disruption following blunt trauma may now be suitable to undergo endovascular repair of the injury by percutaneous placement of a stent graft.[92] Where suitable, these injuries are often managed by the vascular surgeons rather than the cardiothoracic surgical team.

OESOPHAGEAL INJURY

The oesophagus is a long, muscular organ that begins at the pharyngo-oesophageal junction at the level of the 6th cervical vertebra. It ends at the oesophagogastric junction at the level of the 10th thoracic vertebra near the diaphragm. The surrounding organs and tissues provide protection from external force, therefore oesophageal injury is uncommon. In addition, the clinical symptoms and signs are non-specific, making the diagnosis difficult and often delayed. The risks of delayed diagnosis are high and include retropharyngeal abscess, mediastinitis, empyema, septic shock and death. A mediastinal crunch heard on auscultation is indicative of Hamman's sign, which should alert the clinician to underlying oesophageal pathology. Penetrating injuries of the oesophagus far outnumber blunt oesophageal injuries.[93]

Oesophageal injuries resulting from blunt trauma account for less than 1% of all oesophageal injuries. These injuries are most often located in the cervical oesophagus as the result of an anterior blow with the neck in a hyperextended position. Rarely an acute blow to a distended stomach may produce tears of the distal oesophagus due to a rapid increase in intraluminal pressure. In the same way, blast injury can result in oesophageal perforation.

Diagnosis

The rarity of oesophageal injuries means that even busy trauma centres that manage a high percentage of penetrating trauma may see very few. However, when encountered, penetrating oesophageal injuries pose a greater threat than blunt oesophageal trauma. Patients that suffer penetrating oesophageal trauma are more likely to have neck injuries, whereas blunt injuries are associated with spine injuries.[94]

These injuries do not occur in isolation and many penetrating wounds injure the aorta or heart, resulting in rapid death. Furthermore, since most penetrating injuries occur in the cervical oesophagus, injuries to adjacent structures are common, including the carotid arteries, jugular veins and trachea producing haemorrhage or airway issues that distract from investigation of oesophageal injury. Therefore, the keys to prevention of life-threatening complications related to delayed diagnosis is a high index of suspicion based on mechanism and a recognition of injury patterns associated with oesophageal injury. These injuries must be suspected in penetrating neck injuries that violate the platysma, in transmediastinal gunshot wounds, and significant chest trauma with associated tracheobronchial injuries.

Assessment

The clinical symptomatology is non-specific early after perforation. Studies have reported pain, located in the chest with cervical perforations and perhaps referred to the abdomen with thoracic perforations, as a frequent complaint by patients with oesophageal perforation, occurring in 70–90% of patients.[95] Other symptoms include dyspnoea in thoracic perforation and subcutaneous emphysema in cervical perforation. This pain may intensify with the swallowing of food (odynophagia), and be accompanied by dysphagia, vomiting, low-grade pyrexia and moderate leucocytosis. Tenderness to palpation and with passive motion, dyspnoea and/or hoarseness may be present. Expanding cervical haematoma is concerning, and the subsequent development of fever, cough and stridor may be the first signs of the massive inflammatory response, which can result from even minor perforations. Palpable subcutaneous emphysema or air within the soft tissues or a wide pre-vertebral shadow on neck x-ray may also suggest the presence of oesophageal injury, but radiological clues are subtle and may easily be missed. CT scan may detect even small amounts of subcutaneous emphysema in the neck or may demonstrate a pneumomediastinum.

The clinical findings associated with thoracic oesophageal injuries may initially be non-specific or even absent. In thoracic perforations dyspnoea is a common symptom. As mentioned above, pain may be referred to the abdomen and may be associated with abdominal tenderness and/or rigidity. Subcutaneous emphysema may track cranially from the mediastinum leading to cervical crepitus and Hamman's sign (mediastinal crunch on auscultation). Following penetrating thoracic trauma, the presence of pneumomediastinum and pleural effusion raise suspicion of oesophageal injury (Fig. 45.28).

While haemodynamically unstable patients with penetrating neck or thoracic trauma will require surgical exploration for associated wounds, the stable patient may present a diagnostic challenge.

FIGURE 45.28 OESOPHAGEAL INJURY X-RAY. STOMACH CONTENTS HAVE SPILLED INTO THE THORACIC CAVITY. POST-OESOPHAGEAL INJURY CAUSED BY A BULLET

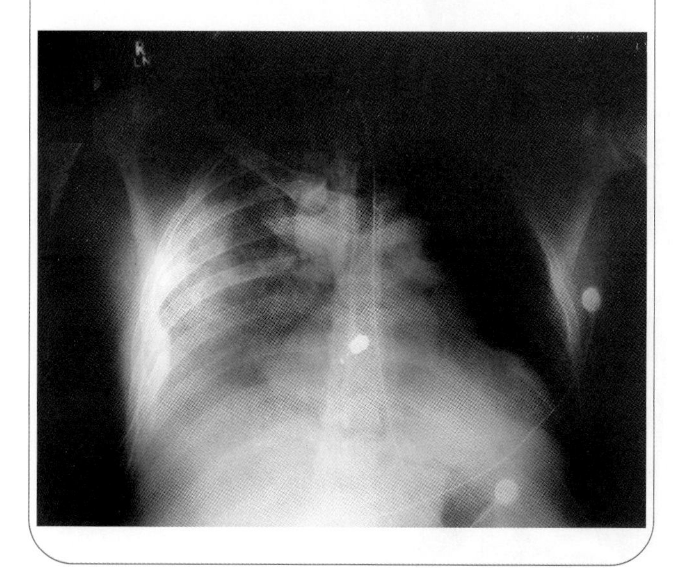

Courtesy Kate Curtis.

As will be discussed further below, in the past all penetrating neck wounds that breached the platysma underwent routine exploration. Since a more selective approach to the management of penetrating neck wounds is now accepted practice in most trauma centres, a diagnostic algorithm is required to exclude oesophageal perforation.

A water-soluble contrast oesophagram is the preferred first-line approach and can evaluate the entire oesophagus. It can be performed in intubated patients by withdrawing the nasogastric tube into the oesophagus and instilling contrast. If no leakage of contrast is seen, then dilute barium may be instilled as this adds a measure of safety in excluding injury. Coupling of oesophagoscopy with the oesophagram increases specificity to nearly 100%; however, given advances in endoscopic accuracy, recent literature recommends oesophagography only if endoscopic findings are equivocal.[96] The value of MDCT in assessing for possible oesophageal perforation is that it allows the tracts of missiles within the chest and mediastinum to be determined, thus potentially excluding oesophageal (as well as vascular) injuries with a high degree of certainty. In addition, when combined with oral contrast, MDCT may demonstrate pooling of contrast outside of the oesophageal lumen. Delayed images may be useful in detecting contrast extravasation.

Once an oesophageal injury has been diagnosed, the patient is kept fasted, a nasogastric tube is inserted, broad-spectrum antibiotics are initiated and resuscitation continues according to the patient's haemodynamic status.

Management

Since blunt trauma to the oesophagus is exceedingly rare, management is usually based on the approach to penetrating injuries.[97]

Operative fixation is the standard treatment for oesophageal injury. Some authors advocate for conservative management, showing no adverse outcome compared with surgical management in select cases, but the problem with these series is that they frequently encompass iatrogenic perforation, spontaneous rupture and chemically induced perforation.[96] Where operative exploration is undertaken, the approach is via a neck incision along the anterior border of the left sternocleidomastoid muscle for cervical perforations, and via left or right thoracotomy, depending on the proximal or distal location of thoracic oesophageal injury.

In the cervical oesophagus, primary suture repair and drainage is performed. If delayed diagnosis has led to late exploration, then the tissues may be markedly inflamed and friable. Under these circumstances drainage with a Penrose or soft silastic drain should be performed with the patient kept fasted and on broad-spectrum antibiotics. Oral intake can be commenced once healing is demonstrated on contrast swallow.

For injuries to the thoracic oesophagus, primary suture repair may be appropriate if the injury is diagnosed early before a massive inflammatory response and mediastinitis have made the tissues friable. The repair may be buttressed by a pleural or pericardial flap in the mid-oesophagus, or by fundoplication for the lower third. With penetrating trauma multiple injuries may be present and must be looked for.

Where severe mediastinitis and destructive inflammation are found at surgery the safest approach is debridement of the damaged tissue and tube drainage of the affected thorax, with a plan for delayed repair. Only rarely is oesophagectomy indicated.

NECK INJURIES

Few emergencies pose as great a challenge as neck trauma. Vital anatomical structures (e.g. airway, vascular, neurological, gastrointestinal) are in such close proximity that even a single penetrating wound is capable of causing multisystem injury. Furthermore, seemingly innocuous wounds may not manifest clear signs or symptoms, and potentially lethal injuries could be easily overlooked or discounted. Major neurovascular structures, including the carotid and vertebral arteries and the spinal cord, span the short gap between the head and the torso, and the trachea and oesophagus originate in the neck (Fig. 45.29). (Spinal injuries are discussed in Chapter 47, and oesophageal injuries are discussed above.)

Neck injuries are classified according to blunt or penetrating mechanism, in addition to the structures involved. The pattern of injury is often closely related to the mechanism of injury (mechanisms of injuries are discussed in Chapter 41). These injuries may result in exsanguinating haemorrhage or lead to airway occlusion, but often the signs of significant trauma may be far more subtle. Patients presenting with neck trauma should be assessed according to EMST principles to expeditiously identify life-threatening injuries and appropriately prioritise treatment.

Pre-hospital clinicians should be aware of the risk of airway compromise and unless the patient has sustained multiple injuries due to blunt force trauma, thus requiring spinal precautions, the patient should be allowed to sit forward to minimise the risk of aspiration of blood or secretions. In isolated penetrating trauma to the neck, the use of cervical spine protection is not indicated since the risk of cervical cord injury is very low.[99] Semi-rigid collars may also obscure expanding haematomas. Obvious haemorrhage should be controlled by

FIGURE 45.29 SUPERFICIAL VEINS AND CUTANEOUS NERVES OF NECK[98]

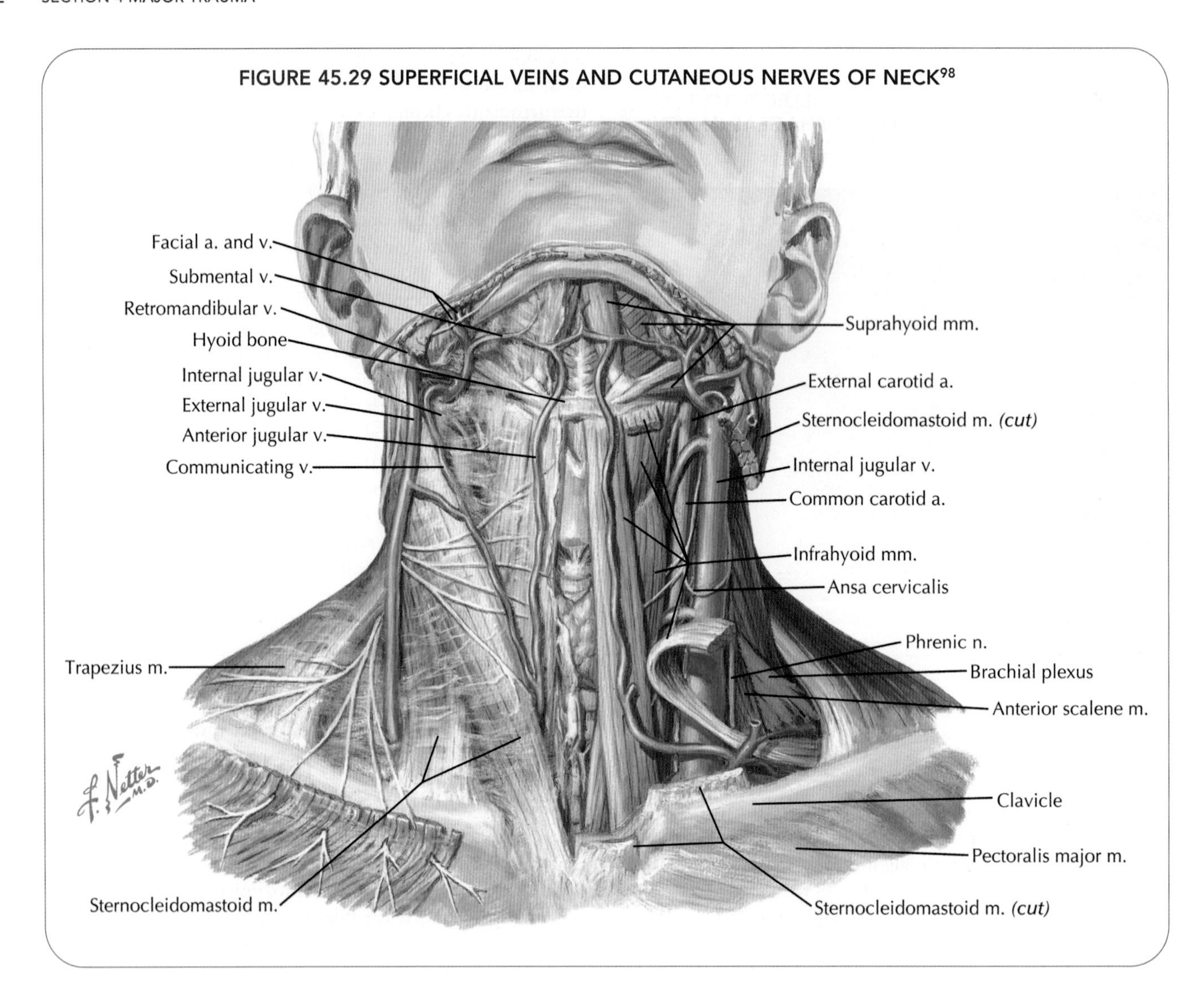

direct manual compression. Impaled objects should not be removed in the field. Intravenous access should be achieved in the extremity contralateral to the injured side in penetrating injury in case the ipsilateral venous system has been damaged, but fluid should only be given in accordance with damage control resuscitation principles (Chapter 42).

On arrival in the ED, the neck should be inspected after removal of any collars, articles of clothing and jewellery to allow for a complete, circumferential visual and manual examination. The posterior aspect of the neck is best examined during the log-roll.[99] Spinal alignment should be maintained by an assistant performing in-line stabilisation during the examination in any patient at risk of spinal column instability. As mentioned above, the use of cervical spine protection is not required in the ED in patients with isolated stab wounds who do not have neurological deficit at presentation. In the awake patient, refrain from oropharyngeal or nasal suction which may cause the patient to gag or cough, potentially dislodging blood clots and precipitating further haemorrhage. The patient may be given a sucker to use.

PENETRATING INJURIES

Assessment

Examination of the neck should look for evidence of underlying injury. A large or expanding haematoma usually indicates an injury to a major underlying vascular structure, typically the carotid arteries or one of their major branches. Tracheal deviation may be a late sign of an expanding haematoma; however, its absence does not exclude an underlying haematoma that may rapidly enlarge and occlude the airway. Gurgling or bubbling of air from the neck wound is diagnostic for a pharyngeal or tracheal injury. Signs of cranial nerve deficits may be present, such as tongue deviation caused by injury to the hypoglossal nerve. Haemoptysis is suggestive of injury to the pharynx or trachea, and odynophagia or dysphagia strongly suggests underlying oesophageal injury, as described previously.[100] Hoarseness indicates compression or direct injury to the larynx or recurrent laryngeal nerves. A loud 'machinery' bruit over the anterolateral neck is associated with traumatic arteriovenous fistulae between the carotid artery and jugular vein. Although most awake patients will exhibit tenderness over penetrating wounds, diffuse cervical tenderness should raise suspicions for underlying tracheo-oesophageal injury. Haemodynamically unstable patients with penetrating neck trauma or those with evidence of severe injury to the airway, vessels or digestive tract should have the airway secured immediately with an endotracheal tube or, if necessary, a surgical airway (described in Chapter 42).[84] Further evaluation and management should take place in the operating theatre, where emergency surgical exploration must be undertaken. Patients in this group include those with refractory shock, or who have expansile/pulsatile haematomas, or evidence of severe respiratory injury, the so-called 'hard signs' in neck injuries.[101]

Management

The surface anatomy of the neck has traditionally been divided into three discrete zones for the purpose of evaluating and treating penetrating neck wounds. More recently, based on the high specificity and sensitivity of MDCT and CT angiography to define critical neck structures and identify or exclude injury based on trajectory, the requirement to divide the neck into discrete zones has become outdated.[102] A 'no-zone' approach has been suggested as an alternative to limit unnecessary invasive neck exploration, especially due to the advancements in imaging technology. A no-zone approach treats the neck as a whole rather than three separate entities, as in the zone approach.[99]

Patients with any of the hard signs of vascular or aerodigestive tract injury should undergo surgical exploration.[101] The most common cause of death is exsanguination. Prophylactic antibiotics should be administered, usually a cephalosporin, and tetanus immunoglobulin should be given where there is any doubt about the tetanus status of the patient. Blood should be grouped and matched and the emergency clinician should notify the blood bank, should the team leader wish to activate the massive transfusion protocol.

Management of haemodynamically stable patients with neck trauma who have no clinical signs warranting immediate intervention has evolved over the last four decades.

Stable patients with no signs of injury should undergo CT angiography and can then be managed with observation only if no injury to vital structures is found. The focus should be primarily on physical examination regardless of the zone of injury.

BLUNT INJURIES OF THE NECK

Assessment

Assessment and maintenance of airway patency are the priority in blunt neck injury. The cervical airway, especially the larynx and associated structures, is vulnerable, and developing oedema or expansile haematoma from associated vascular injury can lead rapidly to airway occlusion. The paramedic or emergency nurse should prepare equipment for intubation and have the difficult airway kit available (see Chapter 16 for intubation techniques). Vascular structures, including the carotid and vertebral arteries, may be injured by direct trauma, by crushing against bony structures or by hyperextension and rotation of the neck causing intimal tearing.[103] Additionally, the cervical spine and spinal cord are frequently injured following blunt neck trauma and pre-hospital personnel should ensure that the neck is appropriately stabilised during both extrication and transport. Such immobilisation must be continued during all phases of evaluation and treatment of the status of the cervical spine stability can be definitively established (see Chapter 47).

The initial physical examination includes assessment of airway patency. Stridor or other changes in phonation are commonly associated with fracture of the larynx, which can promptly progress to localised oedema and complete upper airway obstruction. As stated above, a pulsatile or expansile haematoma places the airway at immediate risk. Patients with any of these findings require prompt intubation since delay may result in an obstructed airway and the need for surgical intervention.

Inspection of the neck may reveal skin bruising or soft-tissue haematomas, indicating possible underlying injuries. Subcutaneous emphysema of the cervical soft tissues may indicate an underlying tear to the distal pharynx or proximal trachea.

Investigations include lateral cervical spine x-ray, which may reveal air outside of the aerodigestive tract, but more commonly MDCT is the investigation of choice. Where a suggestion of vascular injury is visible, computed tomography angiography (CTA) is both sensitive and specific for diagnosis.

Blunt carotid and vertebral artery injuries, collectively termed blunt cerebrovascular injury (BCVI), are uncommon but potentially devastating events. The incidence of blunt cerebrovascular injury in patients sustaining blunt trauma is about 1%. Untreated blunt carotid injury is associated with mortality rates that range from 23–28%, with 48–58% of survivors suffering permanent severe neurological deficits.[86] Partial or complete occlusion of the vessel lumen pseudoaneurysm formation or complete transection of the carotid or vertebral arteries may result from sudden stretching or buckling of the artery, which leads to localised intimal tears and vascular dissections (Fig. 45.30).

Many of these injuries may be occult and initially the patient may be neurologically normal, only to suffer a sudden debilitating or even fatal ischaemic or embolic stroke hours to days later. Where the mechanism of injury or clinical examination raise suspicion of BCVI, it is imperative that appropriate investigations are undertaken. In most modern trauma centres, CTA is now the investigation of choice as it is more widely available and has comparable sensitivity and specificity to angiography, with angiography performed in any equivocal cases (Box 45.2).[104]

Management

Fractures of the larynx or trachea or ruptures of the oesophagus require surgical repair.[105] Where there is no contraindication, such as an intracerebral haemorrhage, small intimal tears of the carotid or vertebral arteries may be successfully treated with systemic anticoagulation, while larger pseudoaneurysms or occlusions are approached surgically and usually undergo resection and interposition of autologous venous grafts or artificial vascular prostheses. More recently, some of these injuries have been treated successfully by percutaneously-placed endoluminal stents, obviating the need for an open neck exploration. Postoperatively, many of these patients will return to the intensive care unit or ward with surgical drains in situ. Care should be taken to accurately record their outputs, keep their skin exit sites clean and avoid accidental dislodgement during patient turning and transport. Nurses should also be aware of any drain-output parameters that would mandate prompt notification of the surgical team.

FIGURE 45.30 LARGE RIGHT DISTAL INTERNAL CAROTID PSEUDOANEURYSM ASSOCIATED WITH DISSECTION AFTER BLUNT NECK TRAUMA[105]

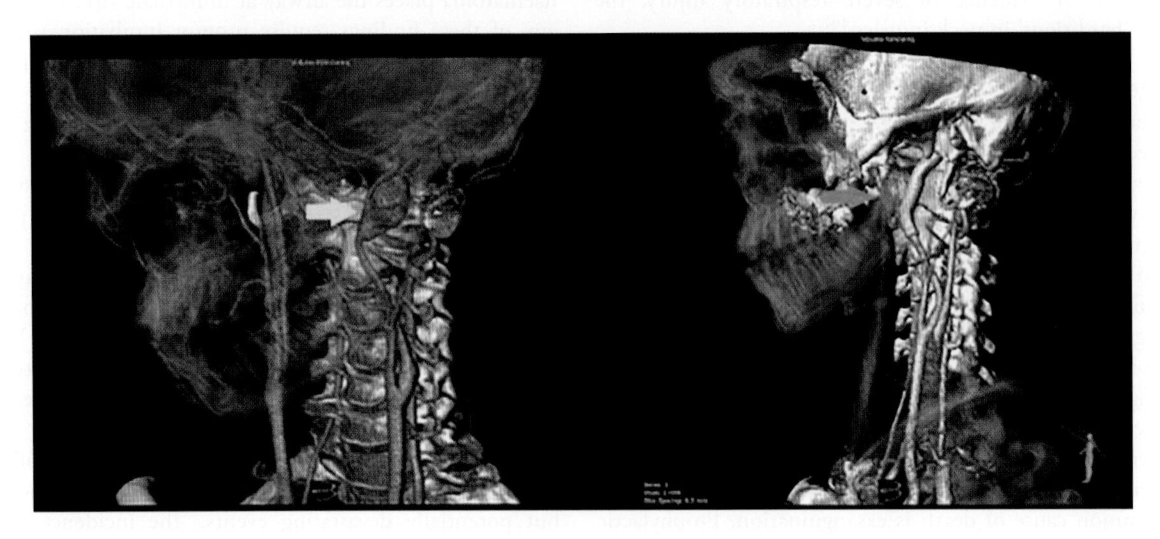

BOX 45.2 SIGNS AND SYMPTOMS ASSOCIATED WITH BLUNT CEREBROVASCULAR INJURY

- Unexplained neurological findings in the face of normal brain computed tomography scan
- Bruising of the lateral neck soft tissues—the 'seatbelt' sign of the neck
- Cervical spine fractures, dislocations or ligamentous injuries, especially those involving the first three vertebrae
- Severe maxillofacial fractures

SUMMARY

Trauma to the thorax or neck produces some of the most challenging and potentially life-threatening injuries. Injury to major vascular structures or airway compromise may produce death within minutes from shock or hypoxia if not promptly recognised and treated. The mechanism of injury should be determined as accurately as possible, since it often guides the diagnostic and therapeutic approach. As with any seriously injured patient, preservation of a patent airway and ensuring adequate oxygenation and ventilation are paramount in the evaluation and resuscitative phases of management.

The clinical examination of the chest as part of the primary survey includes inspection, palpation and auscultation and should provide sufficient information to allow for accurate diagnosis and treatment of immediately life-threatening problems, such as tension pneumothorax, pericardial tamponade or massive haemothorax. Chest decompression will often be the mainstay of management in thoracic injury since fewer than 10% of all patients with thoracic trauma will require operative intervention. The plain chest x-ray is performed as part of the trauma series. In many centres eFAST has become an adjunct to primary survey, but CT scanning is essential in blunt thoracic trauma as it allows assessment of the major vessels. CT angiography has a sensitivity similar to that of conventional angiography in the assessment of vascular injury. Adequate analgesia is paramount in thoracic trauma to prevent decreased respiratory effort secondary to pain, which can result in fatigue, atelectasis, hypoxia and subsequent respiratory failure. A multidisciplinary approach to the management of thoracic injuries improves outcomes.

Assessment of injuries to the neck should include examination of both the anterior and the posterior aspects with protection of the cervical spine by in-line stabilisation. CTA is an essential part of the assessment of neck trauma, replacing the need to consider the neck in discrete zones. Stable patients with no evidence of occult injury after serial examination or radiological evaluation will often require no operative intervention.

CASE STUDY

A 74-year-old man calls an ambulance after a fall from a ladder while putting up Christmas lights (approximately 4 metres). He is able to walk inside to the telephone and states that the left side of his chest hurts when he breathes.

QUESTIONS

1. What initial assessment would you perform for this patient on scene?
2. Pre-hospital his vital signs are:
   - Heart rate: 64 beats/minute
   - Respiratory rate: 26 breaths/minute, talking in full sentences
   - Blood pressure: 140/82 mmHg
   - Oxygen saturation (SaO_2): 94%
   - Glasgow Coma Scale (GCS) score: 15 (did not lose consciousness).

He has left chest wall tenderness, a small amount of subcutaneous emphysema and a scalp laceration.

   a. What treatment would you initiate? Why?
   b. If in an urban area, what type of hospital would you transport the patient to? Why?
   c. Given the patient's age, consider what comorbidities the patient may have that could affect his compensatory response or exacerbate his injury.

En route to the ED in the ambulance, you ascertain the patient's medical history—he has hypertension, takes warfarin for a mitral valve replacement and digoxin for atrial fibrillation. He stopped smoking 15 years ago.

3. a. What triage category would you give this patient? Why?
   b. Where would you place this patient in your department?

The patient arrives on your bed. You perform your initial assessment and find the following:

- heart rate: 64 beats/minute
- respiratory rate: 32 breaths/minute
- blood pressure: 150/84 mmHg
- SaO_2: 92%
- GCS score: 15.

The patient is in obvious discomfort despite 5 mg intravenous morphine. Air entry is decreased on the left.

4. a. What treatment do you initiate?
   b. What investigations should be performed? Why?
   c. What potential injuries does this patient have?
   d. What potential intervention will you prepare for?

The patient has an intercostal catheter inserted, which has drained 100 mL of blood and the underwater-seal drain is bubbling. His respiratory rate has reduced to 20 breaths/minute, and his SaO_2 increased to 98%. Nil other injuries have been detected at this stage. He has been admitted under the trauma team.

5. a. What type of ward should this patient go to?
   b. What referrals and communication (including medical charts and documentation) should you ensure have been completed prior to transfer?
   c. What potentially could go wrong with this patient, and why?

Answers to Case Study Questions can be found on evolve http://evolve.elsevier.com/AU/Curtis/emergency/ 

USEFUL WEBSITES

The following websites provide instruction, including video, on the insertion and management of chest drains and ED thoracotomy:

Emergency Care Institute procedure videos such as thorocostomy, https://aci.health.nsw.gov.au/networks/eci/clinical/procedures.

Emergency department thoracotomy procedure, www.trauma.org/index.php/main/article/361/.

Pleural Drains in Adults–A Consensus Guideline, NSW Agency for Clinical Innovation, www.aci.health.nsw.gov.au/resources/respiratory/pleural-drains/pleural-drains-in-adults.

Updated evidence-based clinical practice guidelines relating to trauma, www.east.org.

REFERENCES

1. Oliver M, Dinh MM, Curtis K, Paschkewitz R, Rigby O, Balogh ZJ. Trends in procedures at major trauma centres in New South Wales, Australia: an analysis of state-wide trauma data. World J Surg 2017;41(8):2000–5.
2. NSW Agency for Clinical Innovation. Major trauma in NSW: 2019–20. Sydney: ACI; 2020.
3. Curtis K, Caldwell E, Delprado A, Munroe B. Traumatic injury in Australia and New Zealand. Australas Emerg Nurs J 2012;15(1):45–54.

4. Friend J, Rao S, Sieunarine K, Woodroof P. Vascular trauma in Western Australia: a comparison of two study periods over 15 years. ANZ J Surg 2016;86(3):173–8.
5. Ludwig C, Koryllos A. Management of chest trauma. J Thorac Dis 2017;9(Suppl. 3):S172–7.
6. Wang IJ, Bae BK, Park SW, Cho YM, Lee DS, Min MK, et al. Pre-hospital modified shock index for prediction of massive transfusion and mortality in trauma patients. Am J Emerg Med 2020;38(2):187–90.
7. Elbaih A, Elshapowry I, Kalil N, El-Aouty H. Evaluation of thoracic trauma severity score in predicting the outcome of isolated blunt chest trauma patients. Int J Surg Med 2016;2(3):100–6.
8. Molaie M, Jafari S, Moradi M, Sprott JC. A chaotic viewpoint on noise reduction from respiratory sounds. Biomed Signal Process Control 2014;10:245–9.
9. Hannon L, St Clair T, Smith K, Fitzgerald M, Mitra B, Olaussen A, et al. Finger thoracostomy in patients with chest trauma performed by paramedics on a helicopter emergency medical service. Emerg Med Australas 2020;32(4):650–6.
10. Halub ME, Spilman SK, Gaunt KA, Lamb KD, Jackson JA, Oetting TW, et al. High-flow nasal cannula therapy for patients with blunt thoracic injury: a retrospective study. Can J Respirat Ther 2016;52(4):110–13.
11. Nishimura M. High-flow nasal cannula oxygen therapy in adults: physiological benefits, indication, clinical benefits, and adverse effects. Respir Care 2016;61(4):529–41.
12. Farner-Cordell C, Bitton A, Eeten K, Schmidt C, Brenden M. The need for manual skills in an automated world to obtain timely blood pressures in trauma patients. J Nurs Care Qual 2021;36(4):346–9.
13. Griffiths E. Efficacy and safety of methoxyflurane: managing trauma associated pain in UK SAR helicopter paramedic practice. J Paramed Prac 2017;9(3):108–20.
14. Bansal A, Miller M, Ferguson I, Burns B. Ketamine as a prehospital analgesic: a systematic review. Prehosp Disaster Med 2020;35(3):314–21.
15. Hollis GJ, Keene TM, Ardlie RM, Caldicott DG, Stapleton SG. Prehospital ketamine use by paramedics in the Australian Capital Territory: a 12-month retrospective analysis. Emerg Med Australas 2017;29(1):89–95.
16. Ahmadi A, Bazargan-Hejazi S, Heidari Zadie Z, Euasobhon P, Ketumarn P, Karbasfrushan A, et al. Pain management in trauma: a review study. J Inj Viol Res 2016;8(2):89–98.
17. Kourouche S, Buckley T, Munroe B, Curtis K. Development of a blunt chest injury care bundle: an integrative review. Injury 2018;49(6): 1008–23.
18. Ong D, Cheung M, Cuenca P, Schauer S. Clinical utility of routine chest x-rays during the initial stabilization of trauma patients. South Med J 2019;112(1):55–9.
19. Rodriguez RM, Langdorf MI, Nishijima D, Baumann BM, Hendey GW, Medak AJ, et al. Derivation and validation of two decision instruments for selective chest CT in blunt trauma: a multicenter prospective observational study (NEXUS Chest CT). PLoS Med 2015;12(10):e1001883.
20. Standring S. Thorax: overview and surface anatomy. In: Strandring, S. Gray's anatomy. The anatomical basis of clinical practice. 40th ed. Edinburgh: Elsevier; 2008.
21. Karmy-Jones R, Namias N, Coimbra R, Moore EE, Schreiber M, McIntyre Jr R, et al. Western Trauma Association critical decisions in trauma: penetrating chest trauma. J Trauma Acute Care Surg 2014;77(6):994–1002.
22. Staub LJ, Biscaro RRM, Kaszubowski E, Maurici R. Chest ultrasonography for the emergency diagnosis of traumatic pneumothorax and haemothorax: a systematic review and meta-analysis. Injury 2018;49(3):457–66.
23. Hamada S, Delhaye N, Kerever S. Integrating eFAST in the initial management of stable trauma patients: the end of plain film radiography. Ann Intens Care 2016;6(1):62.
24. Rodriguez RM, Hendey GW, Mower WR. Selective chest imaging for blunt trauma patients: the national emergency x-ray utilization studies (NEXUS-chest algorithm). Am J Emerg Med 2017;35(1):164–70.
25. Akgul Ozmen C, Onat S, Aycicek D. Radiologic findings of thoracic trauma. Therapeut Clin Risk Manage 2017;13:1085–9.
26. Schueller G, Scaglione M, Linsenmaier U, Schueller-Weidekamm C, Andreoli C, De Vargas Macciucca M, et al. The key role of the radiologist in the management of polytrauma patients: indications for MDCT imaging in emergency radiology. La Radiologia Medica 2015;120(7):641–54.
27. Brasel KJ, Moore EE, Albrecht RA, deMoya M, Schreiber M, Karmy-Jones R, et al. Western Trauma Association critical decisions in trauma: management of rib fractures. J Trauma Acute Care Surg 2017;82(1):200–3.
28. Witt CE, Bulger EM. Comprehensive approach to the management of the patient with multiple rib fractures: a review and introduction of a bundled rib fracture management protocol. Trauma Surg Acute Care Open 2017;2(1):e000064.
29. Miller C, Stolarski A, Ata A, Pfaff A, Nadendla P, Owens K, et al. Impact of blunt pulmonary contusion in polytrauma patients with rib fractures. Am J Surg 2019;218(1):51–5.
30. Martin TJ, Eltorai AS, Dunn R, Varone A, Joyce MF, Kheirbek T, et al. Clinical management of rib fractures and methods for prevention of pulmonary complications: a review. Injury 2019;50(6):1159–65.
31. Soto J, Lucey B. Emergency radiology: the requisites. Philadelphia: Mosby; 2009.
32. Macri F, Greffier J, Khasanova E, Claret PG, Bastide S, Larbi A, et al. Minor blunt thoracic trauma in the emergency department: sensitivity and specificity of chest ultralow-dose computed tomography compared with conventional radiography. Ann Emerg Med 2019;73(6):665–70.
33. Winnie G, Lossef S. Hemothorax. In: Kliegman R, Stanton B, Gemel J, Schor N, editors. Nelson textbook of pediatrics. 20th ed. Philadelphia: Elsevier; 2016.

34. Joseph A, Harris R, Dimmick S. Radiology in major trauma. In: Cameron P, Jelinek G, Kelly A-M, Brown A, Little M, editors. Textbook of adult emergency medicine. 4th ed. Edinburgh: Elsevier; 2014.
35. Singleton JM, Bilello LA, Canham LS, Levenson RB, Lopez GJ, Tadiri SP, et al. Chest computed tomography imaging utility for radiographically occult rib fractures in elderly fall-injured patients. J Trauma Acute Care Surg 2019;86(5):838–43.
36. Ibbotson WJ, Greenberg R, Brendt P. Erector spinae block for chest trauma in aeromedical prehospital and retrieval medicine. Prehosp Disaster Med 2020;35(4):454–6.
37. Britt T, Sturm R, Ricardi R, Labond V. Comparative evaluation of continuous intercostal nerve block or epidural analgesia on the rate of respiratory complications, intensive care unit, and hospital stay following traumatic rib fractures: a retrospective review. Local Reg Anesthes 2015;8:79–84.
38. Singh S, Jacob M, Hasnain S, Krishnakumar M. Comparison between continuous thoracic epidural block and continuous thoracic paravertebral block in the management of thoracic trauma. Med J Arm Force India 2017;73(2):146–51.
39. Galvagno SM, Jr., Smith CE, Varon AJ, Hasenboehler EA, Sultan S, Shaefer G, et al. Pain management for blunt thoracic trauma: a joint practice management guideline from the Eastern Association for the Surgery of Trauma and Trauma Anesthesiology Society. J Trauma Acute Care Surg 2016;81(5):936–51.
40. Hwang E, Lee Y. Effectiveness of intercostal nerve block for management of pain in rib fracture patients. J Ex Rehab 2014;10(4):241.
41. Sum SK, Peng YC, Yin SY, Huang PF, Wang YC, Chen TP, et al. Using an incentive spirometer reduces pulmonary complications in patients with traumatic rib fractures: a randomized controlled trial. Trials 2019;20(1):797.
42. Mu GH, Li X, Lu ZQ, Hu S, Hu S, Chen PF, et al. High-flow nasal cannula therapy for acute respiratory failure in patients with chest trauma: a single-center retrospective study. Injury 2020;51(11):2507–11.
43. Hsu JM, Clark PT, Connell LE, Welfare M. Efficacy of high-flow nasal prong therapy in trauma patients with rib fractures and high-risk features for respiratory deterioration: a randomized controlled trial. Trauma Surg Acute Care Open 2020;5(1):e000460.
44. Rosen P, Barkin R. Rosen's emergency medicine: concepts and clinical practice. 4th ed. St Louis: Mosby; 1998.
45. Phillips B, Murray E, Holzmer S. Bilateral flail chest: a review. J Trauma Orthopaed Surg 2017;12(2):2–7.
46. de Moya M, Mayberry J. Rib fracture management: a practical manual. Switzerland: Springer International; 2018.
47. Cataneo AJ, Cataneo DC, de Oliveira FH, Arruda KA, El Dib R, de Oliveira Carvalho PE. Surgical versus nonsurgical interventions for flail chest. Cochrane Database of System Rev 2015;(7):Cd009919.
48. Kralj E, Podbregar M, Kejžar N, Balažic J. Frequency and number of resuscitation related rib and sternum fractures are higher than generally considered. Resuscitation 2015;93:136–41.
49. Doyle JE, Diaz-Gutierrez I. Traumatic sternal fractures: a narrative review. Mediastinum 2021;5:34.
50. Ferree S, Hietbrink F, van der Meijden OAJ, Verleisdonk EJMM, Leenen LPH, Houwert RM. Comparing fracture healing disorders and long-term functional outcome of polytrauma patients and patients with an isolated displaced midshaft clavicle fracture. J Shoulder Elbow Surg 2017;26(1):42–8.
51. Frima H, van Heijl M, Michelitsch C, van der Meijden O, Beeres FJP, Houwert RM, et al. Clavicle fractures in adults; current concepts. Euro J Trauma Emerg Surg 2020;46(3):519–29.
52. Benns MV, Egger ME, Harbrecht BG, Franklin GA, Smith JW, Miller KR, et al. Does chest tube location matter? An analysis of chest tube position and the need for secondary interventions. J Trauma Acute Care Surg 2015;78(2):386–90.
53. Baldwin D, Chow KL, Mashbari H, Omi E, Lee JK. Case reports of atrial and pericardial rupture from blunt cardiac trauma. J Cardiothorac Surg 2018;13(1):71.
54. Horner P, Primack S. Chest radiography in the intensive care unit. In: Muller N, Silva C, editors. Imaging of the chest. Philadelphia: Saunders; 2008.
55. Grigorian A, Milliken J, Livingston JK, Spencer D, Gabriel V, Schubl SD, et al. National risk factors for blunt cardiac injury: hemopneumothorax is the strongest predictor. Am J Surg 2019;217(4):639–42.
56. Wu T. The CORE scan. Crit Care Clin 2014;30(1):151–75.
57. Anderson M, Fitzgerald M, Martin K, Santamaria M, Arendse S, O'Reilly G, et al. A procedural check list for pleural decompression and intercostal catheter insertion for adult major trauma. Injury 2015;46(1):42–54.
58. Tran J, Haussner W, Shah K. Traumatic pneumothorax: a review of current diagnostic practices and evolving management. J Emerg Med 2021;61(5):517–28.
59. Eghbalzadeh K, Sabashnikov A, Zeriouh M, Choi YH, Bunck AC, Mader N, et al. Blunt chest trauma: a clinical chameleon. Heart 2018;104(9):719–24.
60. Kirsch T, Sax J. Tube thoracostomy. In: Roberts J, editor. Roberts and Hedges' clinical procedures in emergency medicine. 6th ed. Philadelphia: Saunders; 2014.
61. Hohenberger GM, Schwarz A, Hohenberger F, Wickham S, Petermann JS. Evaluation of Monaldi's approach with regard to needle decompression of the tension pneumothorax–a cadaver study. Injury 2017;48(9):1888–94.
62. Curtis K, Asha S. Blunt cardiac injury as a result of a motor vehicle collision: a case study. Australas Emerg Nurs J 2010;13(4):124–9.
63. Besson A, Saegesser F. The color atlas of chest trauma and associated injuries. vol 1. Oradell: Medical Economics Books; 1983.
64. Edgecombe L, Sigmon DF, Galuska MA, Angus LD. Thoracic trauma. Treasure Island (FL): StatPearls Publishing; 2021.

65. Brenner B. Comprehensive management of respiratory emergencies. Rockville: Aspen Systems; 1985.
66. Lee TH, Ouellet JF, Cook M, Schreiber MA, Kortbeek JB. Pericardiocentesis in trauma: a systematic review. J Trauma Acute Care Surg 2013;75(4):543–9.
67. Adam A, Dixon A. Grainger and Allison's diagnostic radiology. 5th ed. New York: Churchill Livingstone; 2008.
68. Gilbert RW, Fontebasso AM, Park L, Tran A, Lampron J. The management of occult hemothorax in adults with thoracic trauma: a systematic review and meta-analysis. J Trauma Acute Care Surg 2020;89(6):1225–32.
69. Yuan K, Huang H. Antimicrobial prophylaxis in patients with major trauma. Curr Trauma Rep 2017;3(4):292–9.
70. Shoar S, Hosseini FS, Naderan M, Khavandi S, Tabibzadeh E, Khavandi S, et al. Cardiac injury following blunt chest trauma: diagnosis, management, and uncertainty. Int J Burns Trauma 2021;11(2):80–9.
71. Joseph B, Khan M, Jehan F, Latifi R, Rhee P. Improving survival after an emergency resuscitative thoracotomy: a 5-year review of the Trauma Quality Improvement Program. Trauma Surg Acute Care Open 2018;3(1):e000201.
72. Furák J, Athanassiadi K. Diaphragm and transdiaphragmatic injuries. J Thorac Dis 2019;11(Suppl. 2):S152–7.
73. Johnny CS, Vasudeva M, Gooi J, Waldron B, Ban EJ, Durbridge N, et al. Right atrial appendage rupture and cardiac tamponade secondary to blunt trauma. Trauma Case Rep 2022;38:100620.
74. Arnaud F, Tomori T, Teranishi K, Yun J, McCarron R, Mahon R. Evaluation of chest seal performance in a swine model: comparison of Asherman vs. Bolin seal. Injury 2008;39(9):1082–8.
75. Hammer MM, Raptis DA, Mellnick VM, Bhalla S, Raptis CA. Traumatic injuries of the diaphragm: overview of imaging findings and diagnosis. Abdom Radiol 2017;42(4):1020–7.
76. Kloth C, Vogele D, Brunner H, Beer M, Schmidt SA. Pathognomonic imaging signs in abdominal radiology. Abdom Radiol (NY) 2020;45(2):576–86.
77. Cocco AM, Ratnaraj V, Loveday BP, Gumm K, Antippa P, McCormick JJ, et al. Predictors of blunt diaphragm injury in Australia. Trauma 2021;0(0): 14604086211041857.
78. Turk EE, Tsang YW, Champaneri A, Pueschel K, Byard RW. Cardiac injuries in car occupants in fatal motor vehicle collisions—an autopsy-based study. J Forens Legal Med 2010;17(6):339–43.
79. El-Andari R, O'Brien D, Bozso SJ, Nagendran J. Blunt cardiac trauma: a narrative review. Mediastinum 2021;5:28.
80. Clancy K, Velopulos C, Bilaniuk JW, Collier B, Crowley W, Kurek S, et al. Screening for blunt cardiac injury: an Eastern Association for the surgery of trauma practice management guideline. J Trauma Acute Care Surg 2012;73(5 Suppl 4):S301–6.
81. Hill GED, Thorsen TN, Goelz AP, Miller RE, Almassi GH, Pagel PS. A rare consequence of remote blunt chest trauma. J Cardiothorac Vasc Anesth 2019;33(10):2875–81.
82. Kim M, Moore JE. Chest trauma: current recommendations for rib fractures, pneumothorax, and other injuries. Curr Anesthesiol Rep 2020;10(1): 61–8.
83. Huis In 't Veld MA, Craft CA, Hood RE. Blunt cardiac trauma review. Cardiol Clin 2018;36(1):183–91.
84. Simpson C, Tucker H, Hudson A. Pre-hospital management of penetrating neck injuries: a scoping review of current evidence and guidance. Scand J Trauma Resusc Emerg Med 2021;29(1):137.
85. Parrillo J, Dellinger P. Critical care medicine: principles of diagnosis and management in the adult: 5th ed. Netherlands: Elsevier; 2019.
86. Morales-Uribe C, Ramírez A, Suarez-Poveda T, Ortiz M, Sanabria A. Diagnostic performance of CT angiography in neck vessel trauma: systematic review and meta-analysis. Emerg Radiol 2016;23(5):421–31.
87. Eke OF, Selame L, Gullikson J, Deng H, Dutta S, Shokoohi H. Timing of pericardiocentesis and clinical outcomes: is earlier pericardiocentesis better? Am J Emerg Med 2022;54:202–7.
88. Dayama A, Sugano D, Spielman D, Stone Jr ME, Kaban J, Mahmoud A, et al. Basic data underlying clinical decision-making and outcomes in emergency department thoracotomy: tabular review. ANZ J Surg 2016;86(1–2):21–6.
89. Pang D, Hildebrand D, Bachoo P. Thoracic endovascular repair (TEVAR) versus open surgery for blunt traumatic thoracic aortic injury. Cochrane Database Syst Rev 2019;2(2):Cd006642.
90. Tran HV, Charles M, Garrett RC, Kempe PW, Howard CA, Khorgami Z. Ten-year trends in traumatic cardiac injury and outcomes: a trauma registry analysis. Ann Thoracic Surg 2020;110(3):844–8.
91. Tigkiropoulos K, Sigala F, Tsilimigras DI, Moris D, Filis K, Melas N, et al. Endovascular repair of blunt thoracic aortic trauma: is postimplant hypertension an incidental finding? Ann Vasc Surg 2018;50:160–6.e1.
92. Kou HW, Liao CH, Huang JF, Hsu CP, Wang SY, Ou Yang CH, et al. Eighteen years' experience of traumatic subclavian vascular injury in a tertiary referral trauma center. Eur J Trauma Emerg Surg 2019;45(6):973–8.
93. Sudarshan M, Cassivi SD. Management of traumatic esophageal injuries. J Thorac Dis 2019;11(Suppl. 2):S172–6.
94. Wahed S, Dent B, Jones R, Griffin SM. Spectrum of oesophageal perforations and their influence on management. Br J Surg 2014;101(1): e156–62.
95. Kuppusamy MK, Hubka M, Felisky CD, Carrott P, Kline EM, Koehler RP, et al. Evolving management strategies in esophageal perforation: surgeons using nonoperative techniques to improve outcomes. J Am Coll Surg 2011;213(1):164–71; discussion 171–2.

96. Ivatury RR, Moore FA, Biffl W, Leppeniemi A, Ansaloni L, Catena F, et al. Oesophageal injuries: position paper, WSES, 2013. World J Emerg Surg 2014;9(1):9.
97. Oteir AO, Smith K, Stoelwinder JU, Middleton J, Jennings PA. Should suspected cervical spinal cord injury be immobilised? A systematic review. Injury 2015;46(4):528–35.
98. Netter FH. Superficial veins and cutaneous nerves of neck. In: Netter F, editor. Netter's atlas of human anatomy. Philadelphia: Elsevier; 2011.
99. Nowicki JL, Stew B, Ooi E. Penetrating neck injuries: a guide to evaluation and management. Ann R Coll Surg Engl 2018;100(1):6–11.
100. Isaza-Restrepo A, Quintero-Contreras JA, Escobar-DiazGranados J, Ruiz-Sternberg ÁM. Value of clinical examination in the assessment of penetrating neck injuries: a retrospective study of diagnostic accuracy test. BMC Emerg Med 2020;20(1):17.
101. Tessler RA, Nguyen H, Newton C, Betts J. Pediatric penetrating neck trauma: hard signs of injury and selective neck exploration. J Trauma Acute Care Surg 2017;82(6):989–94.
102. Ko JW, Gong SC, Kim MJ, Chung JS, Choi YU, Lee JH, et al. The efficacy of the 'no zone' approach for the assessment of traumatic neck injury: a case-control study. Ann Surg Treat Res 2020;99(6):352–61.
103. George E, Khandelwal A, Potter C, Sodickson A, Mukundan S, Nunez D, et al. Blunt traumatic vascular injuries of the head and neck in the ED. Emerg Radiol 2019;26(1):75–85.
104. Spanos K, Karathanos C, Stamoulis K, Giannoukas AD. Endovascular treatment of traumatic internal carotid artery pseudoaneurysm. Injury 2016;47(2):307–12.
105. Moonsamy P, Sachdeva UM, Morse CR. Management of laryngotracheal trauma. Ann Cardiothorac Surg 2018;7(2):210–16.

CHAPTER 46

ABDOMINAL AND GENITOURINARY TRAUMA

KATE KING AND DEBRA McDOUGALL

ESSENTIALS

- Identify immediate life-threatening abdominal injuries during the primary survey and delayed life-threatening abdominal injuries in the secondary survey.
- Blunt abdominal trauma is the most common form of injury in Australia and Aotearoa New Zealand and is often treated with non-operative management. Penetrating injuries frequently require operative investigation.
- The organs most injured are the spleen, liver and bowel.
- The most common mechanism of injury for abdominal injuries is road trauma, falls, assaults and sporting injuries.
- Delayed recognition or diagnosis of intra-abdominal injuries can lead to death.
- Have a high index of suspicion for genitourinary trauma when abdominal trauma is identified.
- Follow local algorithms for the management of both blunt and penetrating abdominal injuries with early consultation with the surgeon.
- Consider early transfer to a tertiary hospital.

INTRODUCTION

Abdominal injury is a common result of trauma and, if undetected or inappropriately evaluated, can lead to significant morbidity and mortality. Abdominal injury frequently arises as part of multisystem injury following high-energy, blunt force trauma, including road trauma, high falls, sporting injuries, assaults and, much less frequently in Australia and Aotearoa New Zealand, penetrating injury. Accurate assessment, timely resuscitation and appropriate investigations are required to manage patients with abdominal trauma. The investigation and management of abdominal trauma continues to evolve. Strong team leadership ensures the appropriate triage, examination and prioritisation of care in the patient with multiple injuries. In patients where the abdomen is the compelling source of haemorrhage, the priority of the trauma team is to get the patient to the operating room or the interventional radiology suite for definitive treatment as soon as possible.

EPIDEMIOLOGY

Abdominal trauma can be divided in two main mechanisms: blunt and penetrating. The majority, 94% of hospital admissions in Australia and Aotearoa New Zealand, are as a result of blunt trauma.[1]

Approximately one-third of polytrauma patients have an abdominal injury, and up to 10% of these patients will have some form of genitourinary (GU) trauma, with renal trauma occurring in 1–5% of all traumas. Bladder, urethral, ureter, penile and scrotal trauma make up the remainder of GU trauma. GU trauma is also common in children, but rarely requires surgical management.[1,2] The kidneys of children have less peritoneal fat, are large in comparison with the abdomen as a whole and have a thinner capsule for protection.[3] Children also have a weaker abdominal musculature and a less ossified rib cage, which offers less kidney protection. Blunt urological injury, the most common form of trauma, accounts for 70–80% of all urological injuries.[4]

Of patients who survive major trauma and are transported to hospital, there are two significant mortality peaks in abdominal trauma patients.

- The first peak occurs early in the emergency department (ED) or operating room (OR) and is the result of significant damage to either abdominal vascular structures or gross injury to vital organ systems. The majority of haemodynamically unstable patients diagnosed with abdominal haemorrhage require emergency abdominal surgery to control bleeding; a small proportion of this population may benefit from interventional radiology treatments such as angioembolisation. It may be necessary to consider damage-control surgery or definitive surgery in these patients, which is discussed later in the chapter.
- The second mortality peak is for patients who survive the initial phase of resuscitation and management, but remain susceptible to the sequelae of major trauma. These patients are at risk of developing systemic inflammatory response syndrome (SIRS). SIRS is defined when two or more of the following criteria is met without evidence of infection, a temperature < 36 °C or > 38 °C, a heart rate > 90 beats/ minute, a respiratory rate > 20/minute or $PaCO_2$ < 32 mmHg and/or a white cell count < 4 $\times 10^9$/L, >12 $\times$ 10^9/L or ≥ 10% bands.[5] Regardless of infection, SIRS can progress to multi-organ dysfunction syndrome (MODS), which is associated with both high morbidity and high mortality. Although MODS is by definition multifactorial, abdominal complications, including anastomotic leaks, peritoneal contamination, abdominal compartment syndrome and haemorrhage are all significant contributing factors.[5–7]

ANATOMY

The abdomen extends from the thoracic diaphragm to the pelvic brim. Organs in the abdominal cavity include the liver, spleen, gallbladder, stomach, pancreas, kidneys, bladder, lower oesophagus and large and small intestines. The spleen, liver and kidneys are solid organs. The stomach and intestines are hollow organs. Solid organs fracture when injured; hollow organs collapse or rupture. The major vascular structures in the abdominal cavity include the aorta, vena cava, hepatic vein, iliac artery and the iliac vein. Most of these structures are found in the peritoneal space, and for the purposes of physical assessment are divided into four quadrants (Fig. 46.1). Functions of gastrointestinal (GI) and GU system organs are presented in Chapters 24 and 25, and are discussed below in relation to trauma.

PERITONEUM

Contained within the peritoneal cavity are most abdominal organs, including the liver, spleen, stomach, small bowel, parts of the duodenum and parts of the large bowel. The peritoneum is the largest serous membrane in the body, having a surface area about equal to that of the skin, and it is composed of a thin layer of squamous cells resting on a layer of connective tissue. It is made up of the parietal peritoneum, visceral peritoneum,

FIGURE 46.1 GASTROINTESTINAL STRUCTURES[4]

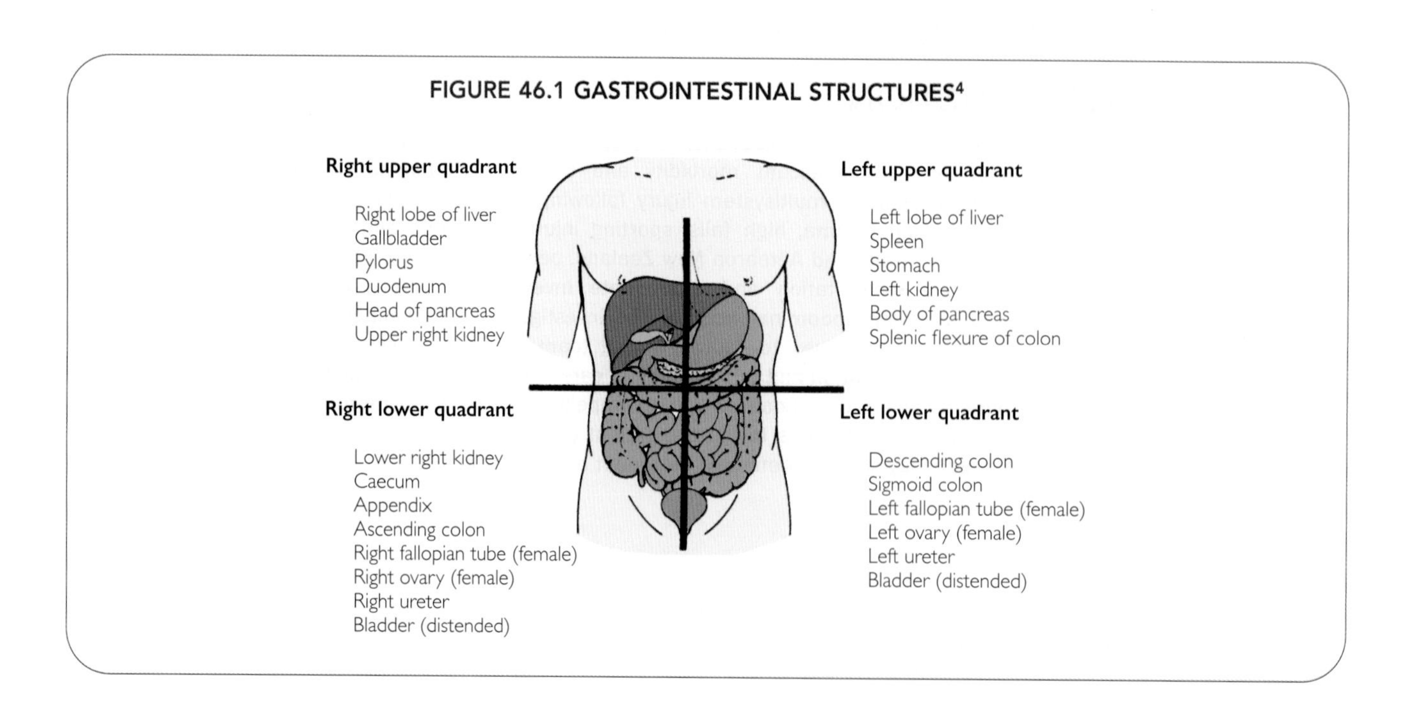

the peritoneal cavity, the retroperitoneal space and the mesentery. The parietal peritoneum lines the abdominal wall. The visceral peritoneum covers the abdominal organs. In females, the peritoneal cavity is continuous with the external environment via the fallopian tubes, the uterus and the vagina. The peritoneal cavity is closed in males.

The retroperitoneal space is the area posterior to the peritoneum. It contains the kidneys, major blood vessels and the reproductive organs in females. The mesentery consists of a double layer of peritoneum. This layer encloses organs and connects them to the abdominal wall. Folds of the mesentery are known as the greater and lesser omentum.

VASCULAR STRUCTURES

The arterial blood supply for the abdominal cavity is the aorta. The abdominal aorta sits to the left of the midline in the abdominal cavity. It bifurcates into the iliac arteries at the pelvic brim. The iliac arteries supply blood to the lower extremities. The abdominal organs are supplied by three arteries originating from the abdominal aorta—the coeliac trunk (which branches into the hepatic, left gastric and splenic arteries), the superior mesentery artery and the inferior mesentery artery (Fig. 46.2). The inferior vena cava, formed by the union of the two common iliac veins, is the major vein in the abdomen. Venous drainage is more complex than the arterial supply. Blood is drained from the small intestines, stomach, spleen and pancreas through the superior mesenteric and splenic veins and their tributaries, which join to form the portal vein, ultimately emptying into the hepatic veins and vena cava (Fig. 46.3).

GENITOURINARY SYSTEM

The GU system consists of the kidneys, ureters, bladder and urethra (Chapter 25). Kidneys are retroperitoneal organs that lie high on the posterior abdominal wall. The right kidney, 1–2 cm lower than the left, lies inferior and posterior to the liver and posterior to the ascending colon and duodenum. The left kidney lies posterior to the descending colon and is associated with the tail of the pancreas medially and the spleen superiorly. Ureters are small muscular tubes that are flexible and mobile and drain urine from the kidneys to the bladder. The ureters are rarely injured in blunt abdominal trauma because of their deep location in the retroperitoneal space and added protection from abdominal contents, spine and surrounding muscles. The bladder is an extraperitoneal hollow organ located in

FIGURE 46.2 ABDOMINAL AORTA AND BRANCHES[5]

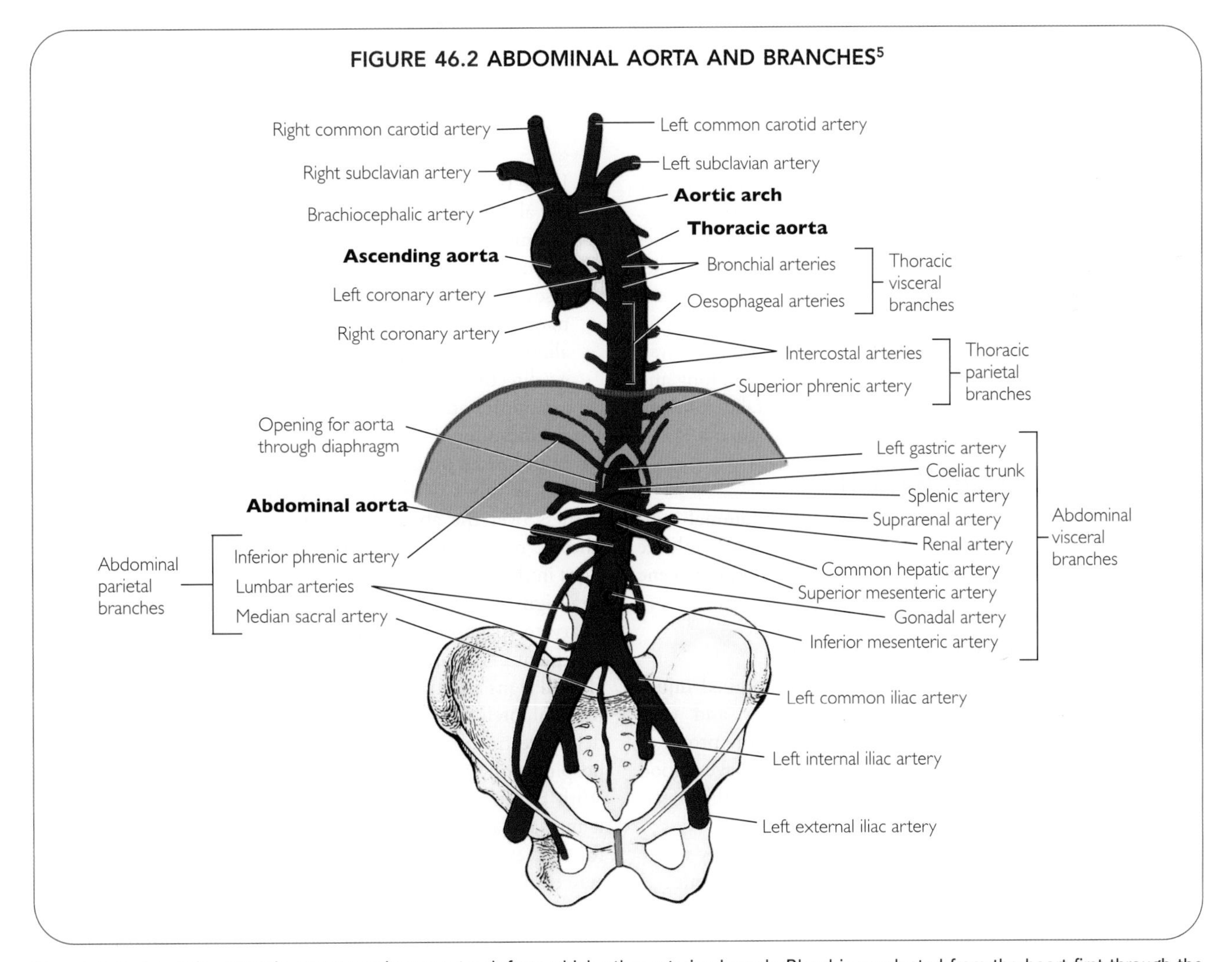

The aorta is the main systemic artery, serving as a trunk from which other arteries branch. Blood is conducted from the heart first through the ascending aorta, then the arch of the aorta, then through the thoracic and abdominal segments of the descending aorta.

FIGURE 46.3 INFERIOR VENA CAVA AND ABDOMINAL BLOOD SUPPLY[6]

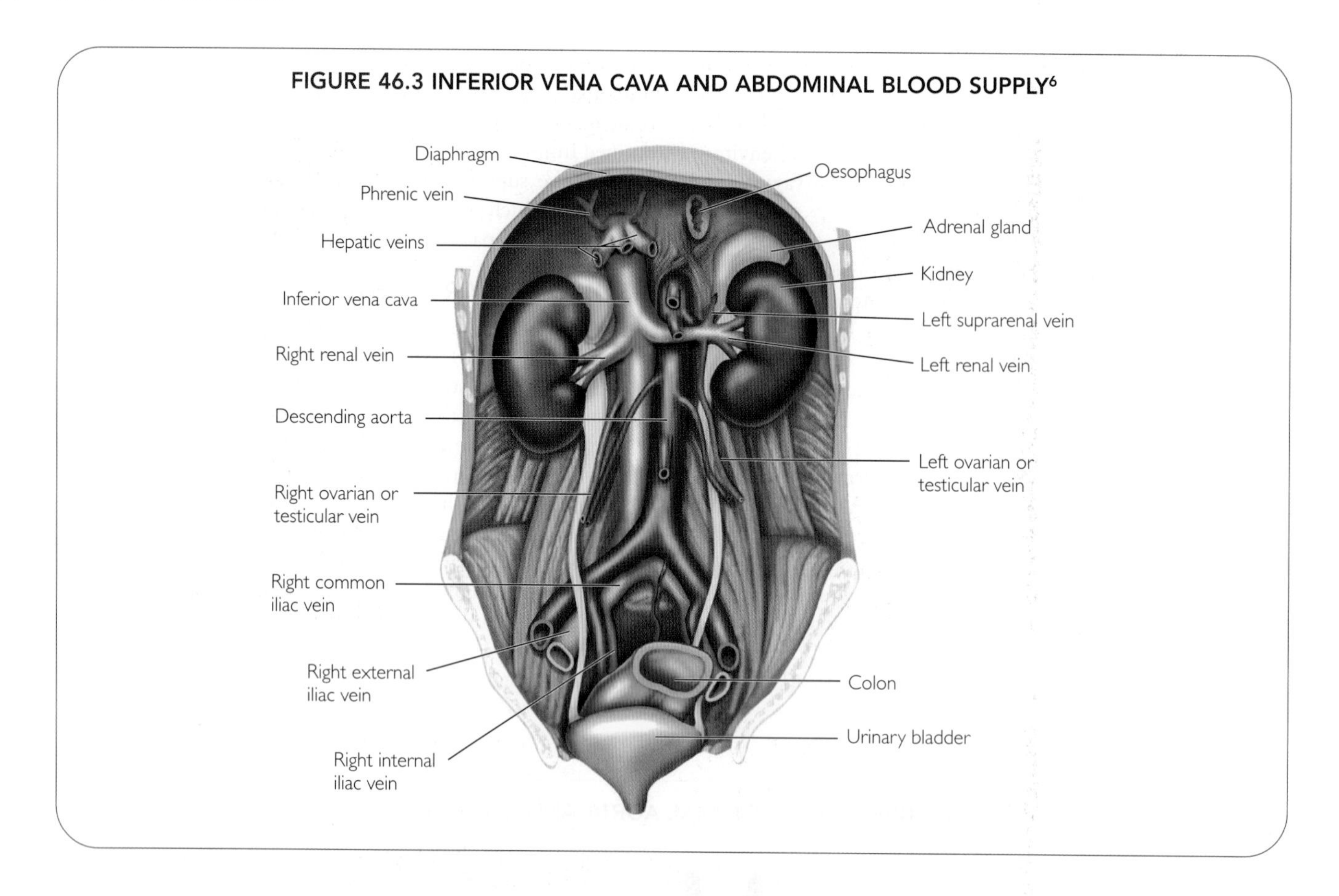

the pelvis that is well protected by pelvic bones laterally, the urogenital diaphragm inferiorly and the rectum posteriorly. Blood supply is abundant and mainly derived from branches of the internal iliac artery. In the male the prostate gland lies adjacent to the inferior margin and is fixed to the pubis anteriorly by ligaments and inferiorly by the urogenital diaphragm. The female urethra is short and well protected by the symphysis pubis. In the male the urethra is approximately 20 cm long and lies predominantly outside the body. The urogenital diaphragm divides the urethra into posterior and anterior segments.

MECHANISM OF INJURY

The most common mechanisms of injury for abdominal injuries are motor vehicle collisions (MVCs), interpersonal violence and falls.[8] Information provided from the pre-hospital scene can assist the emergency nurse in predicting injury patterns.

PRE-HOSPITAL CONSIDERATIONS

The priority of care for the patient with an abdominal injury remains the same: undertake a primary survey and treat any abnormalities according to local protocols before progressing to a secondary survey. The paramedic needs to have a good understanding of the anatomy of the abdomen and the effects of injury.

- If the patient has a solid organ injury, they are likely to bleed and therefore demonstrate signs of hypovolaemic shock.
- If the patient has a hollow organ injury, they are likely to display signs of peritonism, although this is a later sign, so may not be present in the pre-hospital setting.[9]
- If the patient has injured any of the major vessels of the abdomen, they will bleed heavily and are at risk of exsanguination.
- Some patients will have access to pre-hospital focused assessment sonography in trauma (FAST) scans, which may trigger protocols such as a Code Crimson,[10] which allows haemodynamically unstable abdominal injuries to go directly to the operating theatre or interventional suite, as appropriate, to increase survivability.[11]

Paramedics should have a high index of suspicion for abdominal injury based on mechanism, obvious external trauma to the abdomen, shock with no other identifiable cause, diffuse tenderness over the abdomen or signs of referred pain, such as phrenic nerve pain felt in the shoulder tip. The most reliable signs in the field for abdominal injury are pain and/or deranged vital signs. A rigid abdomen is an unreliable sign. It is not necessary to diagnose the exact injury, as there is no change in treatment in the pre-hospital setting. It is important to treat the clinical signs and transport the patient to the most appropriate hospital, preferably to a trauma centre so the patient can receive definitive treatment. Early communication with the receiving hospital will improve hospital trauma team response times. With penetrating injuries, if the object is still impaled, leave it in place and secure for transport and consider securing for forensic evidence. If the patient has an open abdomen with evisceration, do not attempt to put the contents back in; just cover with a wet dressing or cling wrap and transport the patient. As with all trauma patients, basic pre-hospital care for those with abdominal injuries should involve maintenance of airway, breathing and circulation (ABC), oxygenation, cannulation and timely transport according to local transport protocols.

PRACTICE TIP

- Use the MIST mnemonic for a clear and concise handover from pre-hospital to hospital setting. Also communicate estimated time of arrival and any clinical concerns to allow assembly of the most appropriate trauma team members.
- Limit pre-hospital fluids to avoid over-resuscitation sequelae, such as coagulopathy and abdominal compartment syndrome.

INITIAL ASSESSMENT AND MANAGEMENT

All trauma patients are assessed using the primary survey, and those fulfilling trauma call criteria should receive trauma team activation (Chapter 42). Patients with abdominal injury suspected from the mechanism of injury, the physical signs or associated injuries, should be triaged with a high priority and assessed and treated in the resuscitation room. The trauma team must maintain a high index of suspicion for abdominal injury in all trauma patients and have a low threshold for transfer to a trauma centre for investigation and referral to general/trauma surgeons.

ABDOMINAL ASSESSMENT

Although a full abdominal assessment is not part of the primary survey, evaluation of the abdomen as a source of bleeding is an integral part of the circulation aspect for the primary survey. The purpose of the initial clinical assessment in the unstable patient is to confirm or exclude the abdomen as a source of concealed bleeding that requires immediate surgery; the use of FAST as an adjunct to the primary survey will assist in destination decisions by senior clinicians. FAST in some practice environments is also being used in the pre-hospital setting.[11,12] During the secondary survey, the abdominal assessment is systematic and should be repeated throughout all phases of care, preferably by the same clinician, to provide the consistency necessary to evaluate changes. A missed abdominal injury is associated with high morbidity and mortality.[3] FAST scans should also be repeated as indicated and results should be clearly documented.[12,13]

Complaint of abdominal pain from an alert patient is indicative of abdominal injury, although many patients have an altered level of consciousness or distracting injury, and may be unable to provide reliable information. The usual four-step abdominal assessment, including inspection, auscultation, percussion and palpation, is not always practical in resuscitation, but all patients should have inspection and palpation performed. During the inspection phase look for abrasions, bruising, seatbelt signs, Morel-Lavallee lesions (closed soft-tissue degloving injury), and retroperitoneal haemorrhage signs, such as Cullen's sign or Grey Turner's sign. The initial clinical examination of the abdomen can often be misleading for the unwary. Blood may cause little peritoneal irritation initially; and drugs, alcohol, head injury or other distracting injuries can act to mask abdominal signs. If an abdominal injury is suspected, serial abdominal examinations by one practitioner can assist in early detection of deterioration, especially if radiology capabilities are limited.

IMMEDIATE RESUSCITATION CONSIDERATIONS

Several evidence-based algorithms guiding the clinician on penetrating and blunt abdominal trauma management have been developed over recent years (Figs 46.4 and 46.5). In the haemodynamically unstable patient with identified abdominal haemorrhage, following the stabilisation of airway and breathing, the priority of the trauma team is to expedite the patient's movement to the operating room for surgery. In some rare cases the patient may go to the interventional suite; this is a decision to be made by the treating surgeon. An organised and coordinated team approach is vital to achieve timely and safe transfer. Other patients with less-catastrophic injuries may respond rapidly to the initial fluid resuscitation and allow time for more-detailed investigation; however, subsequent cardiovascular deterioration in light of suspected abdominal injuries requires definitive treatment such as surgery. It is important for the ED nurse to be aware of the indications for trauma laparotomy (Box 46.1) to facilitate rapid transfer to definitive care.

Most institutions follow damage control resuscitation principles (Chapter 42), which includes limiting fluid administration, particularly crystalloid solutions, to the amount sufficient to maintain perfusion of the vital organs. Robust data on this approach—permissive hypotension in the context of damage control resuscitation (systolic blood pressure 80–90 mmHg)—is limited, although some research in penetrating trauma suggests that it confers a survival advantage. There is a theoretical basis for applying this principle to all trauma victims (with the exception of head injuries and blast injuries where it may have a detrimental effect) and resuscitating patients to a blood pressure sufficient to maintain perfusion of vital organs.[17] Minimum volume resuscitation is most likely to benefit those patients who have developed tamponade of their bleeding source. However, the priority in these patients remains rapid transfer of the patient to the operating room for surgical haemorrhage control (Chapter 42).

PRACTICE TIP

A senior clinician, such as a trauma surgeon, needs to make a destination decision for the haemodynamically unstable trauma patient within minutes of their arrival. Algorithms may assist in the decision-making processes.

HISTORY

Careful history-taking can provide valuable information that increases the clinician's index of suspicion for abdominal injury, even when it is not apparent in the first instance. The mechanism of injury (Chapter 41) is important as it provides guidance on the likely forces involved and potential injuries. In addition, patient signs and symptoms and response to treatment must be obtained from pre-hospital personnel. Unconscious patients, or those with obvious injuries above and below the abdomen, have an abdominal injury until proven otherwise.

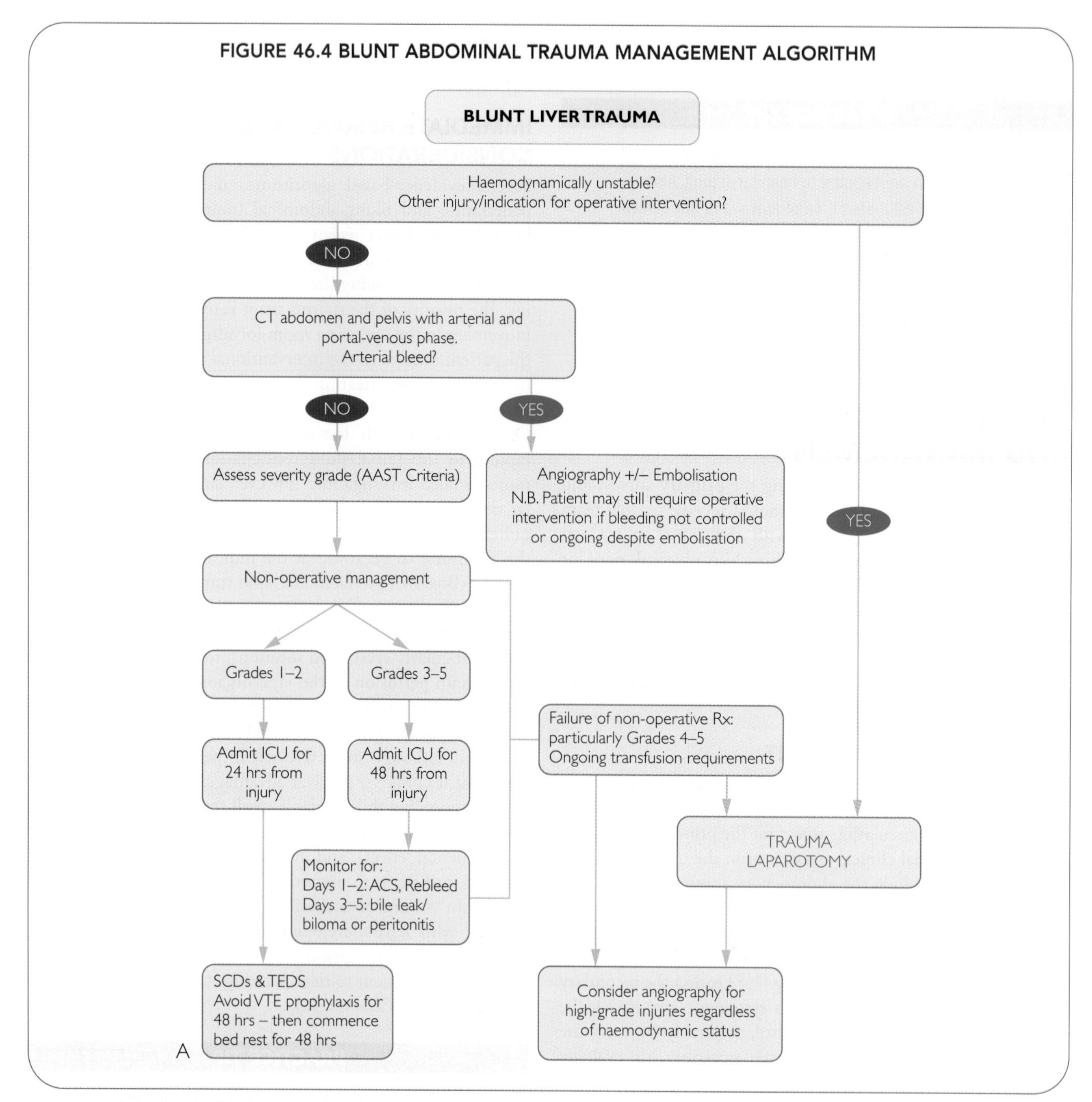

A. Blunt liver trauma.

ICU: intensive care unit; SCD: sequential compression device; TEDS: thrombo-embolus deterrent stockings; VTE: venous thromboembolism.

FIGURE 46.4 BLUNT ABDOMINAL TRAUMA MANAGEMENT ALGORITHM—cont'd

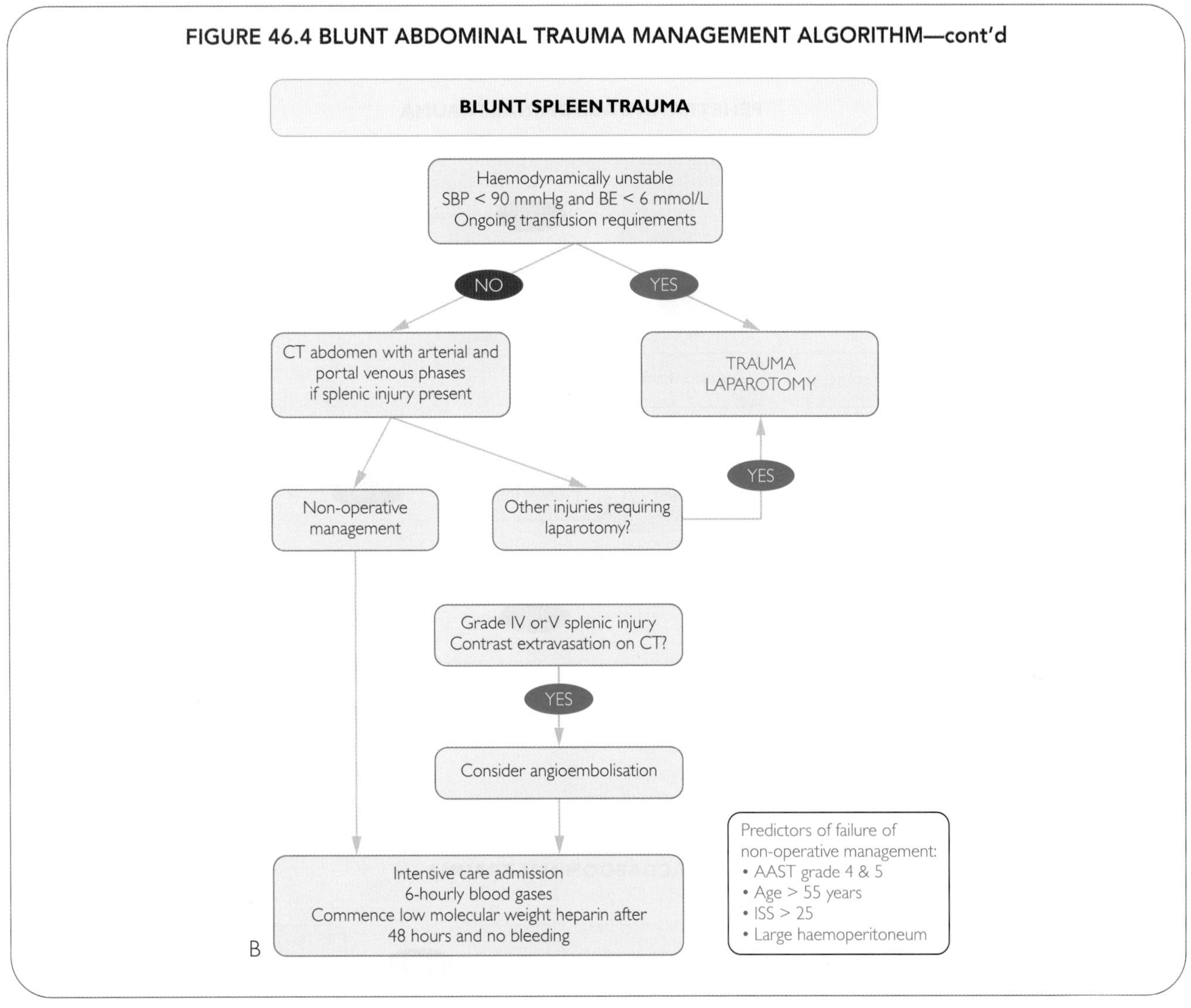

B. Blunt spleen trauma.
AAST: American Association for the Surgery of Trauma; ACS: abdominal compartment syndrome; BE: base excess; CT: computed tomography; ICU: intensive care unit; ISS injury severity score. Courtesy John Hunter Hospital Trauma Service.

Blunt or penetrating lower chest trauma can result in an abdominal injury, and should therefore be suspected, even in circumstances where the mechanism of injury does not appear to have directly affected the abdomen. The clinician's suspicions should be raised for splenic or liver injury if the patient has lower rib fractures. Seatbelt bruising, particularly if the bruising demonstrates an ill-fitting seatbelt, carries a high association with chance fractures of T12/L1 and bowel injury, although the appearance of bruising can be delayed.[18,19] Lumbar spine fractures from seatbelt acceleration/deceleration injury also have a high association with bowel perforation. The probability of abdominal injury increases significantly at velocities > 20 kph, age > 75 years, or the presence of head, leg or chest injuries, even at low velocities.[3,4] GU trauma is divided into upper urinary tract, lower urinary tract and genital injuries, and should be considered in patients with severe lower abdominal blunt trauma and pelvic fracture. Urinary tract injury should also be suspected for all patients with penetrating injuries to the abdomen, chest or flank until proven otherwise.

PRACTICE TIP

Using common mnemonics can assist with history—AT-MIST (Age, Time, Mechanism, Injuries, Signs and Symptoms and Treatment), and, if the patient is conscious, AMPLE (Allergies, Medications, Past medical history, Last time ate or drank and Environment surrounding the incident).

INSPECTION

Inspect the abdomen, flank, back and perineum for contusions, abrasions, lacerations, penetrating injuries, impaled foreign bodies, evisceration and pregnancy. This involves removal of all patient clothing, and, as with all trauma patients, conducting a log-roll to inspect posterior surfaces, keeping in mind the importance of re-covering the patient, preventing heat loss and maintaining patient dignity. Bruising that mirrors location of the seatbelt (seatbelt sign [SBS]) may be evident on admission to the ED, but usually does not occur for several hours after injury.

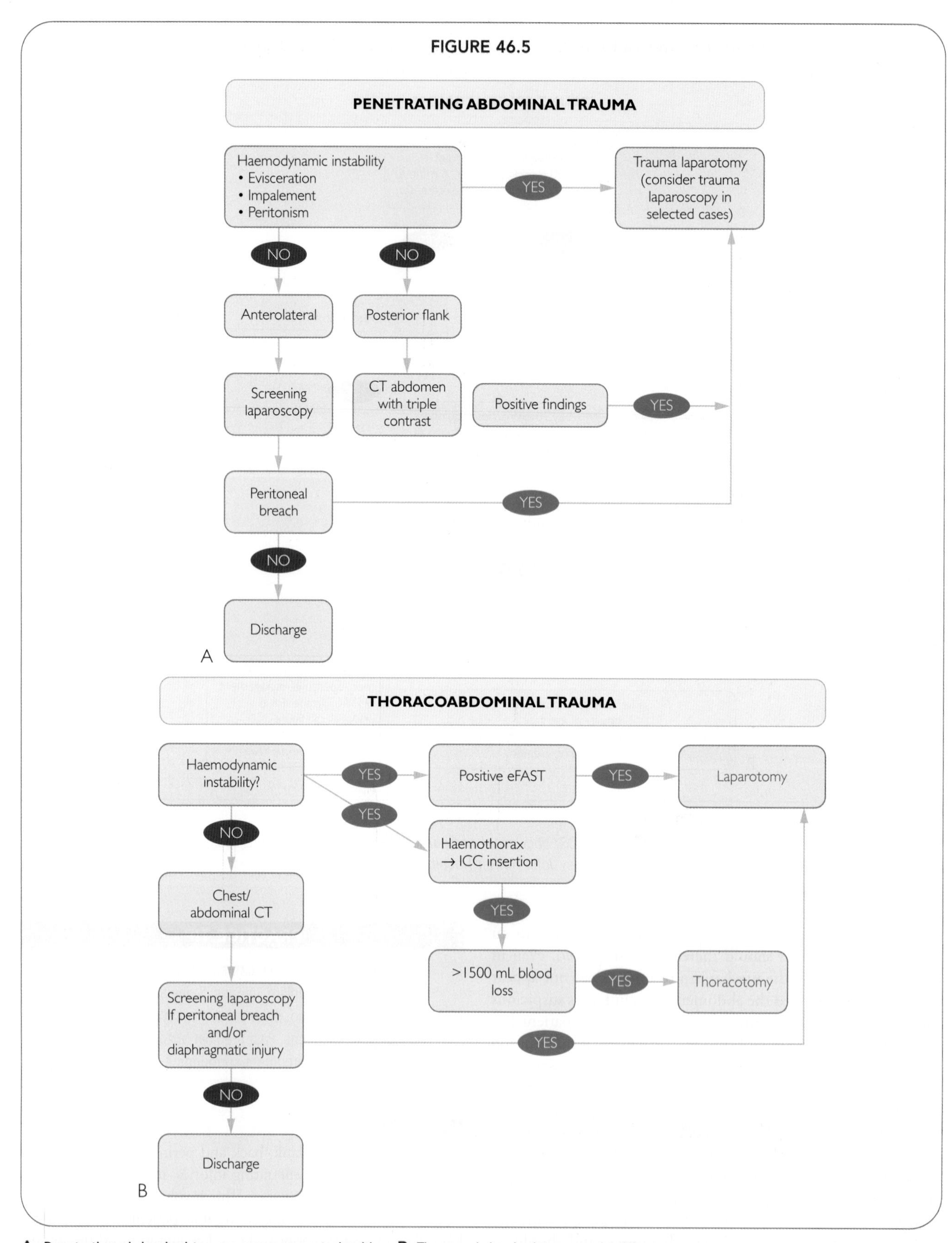

A. Penetrating abdominal trauma management algorithm. **B.** Thoracoabdominal trauma algorithm.
CT: computed tomography; eFAST: extended focused assessment sonography in trauma; ICC intercostal catheter. Courtesy John Hunter Hospital Trauma Service.

BOX 46.1 INDICATIONS FOR LAPAROTOMY[14–16]

- **Gross haemodynamic instability**
- **Evisceration**
- **Gunshot wound to abdomen/thorax**
- **Positive FAST with haemodynamic instability**
- **Stab wound with peritoneum breached**
- **Ongoing haemodynamic instability despite correction of estimated blood loss from extra-abdominal sites**
- **Frank peritonitis (initially or on repeat examination)**
- **Free gas on plain radiography**
- **Ruptured diaphragm**
- **Positive diagnostic peritoneal lavage**
- **Clinical deterioration during observation of suspected intra-abdominal injury**

FAST: Focused assessment with sonography for trauma.

There is some debate about the predictive nature of SBS and abdominal injuries, especially in the paediatric population.[19,20] A lap seatbelt contusion was associated with a 30% chance of a bowel injury; however, with improvements in car safety, including lap belts no longer being manufactured and airbags becoming standard, this incidence is decreasing.[21–23] Distension may be noted; however, it is not a reliable sign (2 L of intraperitoneal fluid increases abdominal girth by only 1.9 cm). Common signs of abdominal injury are listed in Table 46.1.

Consider old scars from previous abdominal surgery; this can provide information about past medical history, as well as providing a warning sign for internal scarring and adhesions.

PRACTICE TIP

A correctly fitted pelvic binder should not obstruct an abdominal examination.

AUSCULTATION

Auscultation of the abdomen can provide helpful information; however, it is usually difficult to hear percussion sounds in the middle of a trauma resuscitation. Auscultation can also provide helpful information about the presence or absence of bowel sounds. Absence of bowel sounds does not confirm intra-abdominal injury; the absence may be due to shock or to the presence of an ileus. Significantly decreased or absent bowel sounds have been reported in more than 50% of documented injuries. On the other hand, absent bowel sounds occur in a significant number (20%) of patients with no injuries at laparotomy.[9,25] Serial auscultation demonstrating a change in bowel sounds (i.e. diminishing or disappearing) is more diagnostic of abdominal trauma, peritonitis and/or ileus. Bowel sounds in the thorax may indicate a perforated diaphragm with herniation of the stomach or small bowel into the chest.[9,26]

PERCUSSION

Percussion of the abdomen is also of little practical value in the busy resuscitation room. The aim of percussion of the abdomen is to identify the presence of air, fluid or tissue. Tympanic sounds indicate air-filled spaces, such as stomach or gut, and a dull sound is present over organ structures.[27]

PALPATION

The abdomen is palpated carefully for pain, rigidity, tenderness and guarding, examining all four quadrants, progressing from light to deep palpation. Tenderness is the most frequent and reliable sign of abdominal injury of the corresponding underlying organs (Fig. 46.1). Palpation should commence on the side of no pain. Guarding and rebound tenderness are associated with peritoneal irritation, from either blood or bowel contents. However, even large amounts of blood can cause remarkably little peritoneal irritation and only very subtle signs on examination. The patient may experience referred pain, most commonly Kehr's sign, which is pain in the left shoulder tip secondary to diaphragmatic irritation caused by intra-abdominal blood, most commonly from splenic rupture (Table 46.1), although alterations in Glasgow Coma Scale (GCS) scores, distracting injury and drugs, can mask these subtle signs.

Rectal examination includes testing for gross blood and anterior tenderness, which can indicate active bleeding or peritoneal irritation. This is no longer common practice within the secondary assessment unless specifically indicated. A small group of patients will have an obviously distended or rigid abdomen; however, where the abdominal assessment is equivocal, special investigations must be used early and appropriately. A vaginal examination should be conducted if an injury is suspected.

Genitourinary trauma assessment

Rapid diagnosis and treatment of GU trauma can be very difficult because it seldom occurs in isolation and is often associated with abdominal injuries. The first rule of urological

TABLE 46.1 COMMON SIGNS OF ABDOMINAL INJURY[24]

SIGN	DESCRIPTION	SUSPECTED INJURY
Grey Turner's sign	Bluish discolouration of the lower abdomen and flanks 6–24 hours after onset of bleeding	Retroperitoneal haemorrhage
Kehr's sign	Left shoulder-tip pain caused by diaphragmatic irritation	Splenic injury, although can be associated with any intra-abdominal bleeding
Cullen's sign	Bluish discolouration around the umbilicus	Pancreatic injury, although can be associated with any peritoneal bleeding

trauma management is to actively seek and diagnose urological injury, because many of these injuries are not obvious at the onset. Pre-existing renal abnormalities can predispose the kidney to severe injury from even minor trauma, and previous injuries to the GU tract may have caused chronic urological infections and adhesions.

Certain mechanisms of injury carry a higher incidence of GU trauma, such as MVCs, assaults, high falls and, more recently, acts of terrorism or combat with the increased use of improvised explosive devices.[9,28,29] Several patterns of contusion and bruising are specific to GU injuries. Grey Turner's sign is bruising over the flank and lower back that occurs in retroperitoneal haematoma and is frequently present with pelvic fractures (Table 46.1). An oedematous and contused scrotum and perineal bruising may be seen with straddle injuries, pelvic fractures or dissecting retroperitoneal haematomas. Fractures of the 11th and 12th ribs have an increased potential for renal injury. The abdomen is gently palpated for presence of a distended bladder—an empty bladder is not palpable. It is important to note that a full bladder may indicate the inability to void. If the patient cannot urinate, the urinary meatus should be checked carefully for blood. Blood at the meatus is a cardinal sign for anterior urethral injury. A digital rectal examination provides information on condition of the prostate gland and posterior urethra, as well as spinal cord integrity. A high-riding prostate or boggy mass may indicate a posterior rupture of the urethra, but this is not always a reliable sign in young adult men.[30,31] Haematuria is the best indicator of GU trauma.[32,33] Radiological tests are discussed later in this chapter relative to specific injuries.

THE PREGNANT PATIENT WITH ABDOMINAL TRAUMA

In Australia and Aotearoa New Zealand, the incidence of abdominal trauma in the pregnant patient is rare,[34,35] and the vast majority suffer no obstetric complication. The exception to this is interpersonal violence, where pregnant women are one of the most vulnerable populations;[36] although worldwide, traumatic injury is the principal non-obstetric cause of maternal death and 7% of pregnant women suffer from trauma.[36,37] Blunt abdominal injury, even with seemingly minor mechanism of injury, can produce placental abruption and may cause uterine rupture.[38] Compared with other sites, abdominal trauma is associated more often with uterine contractions, premature labour and a positive Kleihauer–Betke (KB) test (used to detect transplacental haemorrhage enabling Rhesus-negative women to receive appropriate Rh(D) immunoglobulin [anti-D]). KB testing to predict placental abruption is controversial.[37,39]

Approximately 3–10% of pregnant patients injured sustain various degrees of damage to the uterus, placenta and fetus secondary to penetrating trauma,[39–41] with a maternal mortality rate less than 5%.[42,43] This low mortality rate is due to the protective effects of the gravid uterus, which can efficiently absorb projectile energy.[44–46] However, fetal mortality can be as high as 70%, as a result of direct missile injury or the effects of prematurity.[43] Penetrating wounds to the upper abdomen can produce complex injuries secondary to the displacement of the small bowel, because cephalad (movement of bowel towards the head) has been caused by the enlarged uterus. Depending on clinical status and the location of the wound and projectile, the pregnant penetrating trauma patient can be managed non-operatively.[41] However, when surgery is required, laparotomy alone is not an indication for delivery of the fetus, although delivery of the viable fetus by caesarean delivery should occur if the gravid uterus obstructs operative field exposure or evidence of fetal distress is noted. Delivery of a viable fetus within the first 5 minutes of cardiopulmonary resuscitation results in the highest infant survival rate without neurological dysfunction.[44,47]

Assessment and management

The pregnant trauma patient presents a major challenge to clinicians. The physiological changes that occur during pregnancy may significantly alter the clinical presentation of the patient (Chapter 34). Table 46.2 outlines some of the physiological changes that occur during pregnancy.[44] Pregnancy also distorts maternal anatomy. During the third trimester, the maternal blood volume increases significantly and the pregnant trauma patient may lose up to 35% (1.5–2 L) of their circulating blood volume without showing any overt signs of hypovolaemia.[46,47] Hence, the priority in the management of a pregnant patient who has sustained major trauma must always be maternal stabilisation. Fetal survival is best ensured with maternal resuscitation and adequate perfusion and oxygenation of the placenta; therefore, high-flow oxygen should be mandatory until all injuries have been identified.[43]

When the pregnant trauma patient is laid supine, the gravid uterus compresses the inferior vena cava impairing blood flow. To avoid this, the patient should be nursed with a 15-degree angle towards the left. If spinal injury is suspected, a wedge can be placed under the patient's right side without compromising spinal alignment.[46] Standard trauma radiological imaging for pregnant trauma patients is the same as for their non-pregnant counterparts. Shielding of the fetus during x-rays and consultation with a radiologist may be beneficial if multiple imaging is required.[37,41,49] Fig. 46.6 shows the algorithm for treating a pregnant trauma patient.

Fetal distress may occur subtly without overt clinical signs, and obstetric area monitoring should take place for a period of several hours. Patients with viable gestations require at least 6 hours of cardiotocographic monitoring (CTG) after even minor trauma. Pregnant trauma patients should be assessed simultaneously where possible by the trauma team and the obstetric team.[37,43,45,49,50]

TABLE 46.2 COMMON PHYSIOLOGICAL CHANGES DURING PREGNANCY[48]

Systolic blood pressure	Decreases by 5–15 mmHg
Diastolic blood pressure	Decreases by 5–15 mmHg
Heart rate	Increases by 10–15 beats/minute
Blood volume	Increases by 30–50%
Cardiac output	Increases by 30–50%
Oxygen consumption	Increases by 10%

FIGURE 46.6 ALGORITHM FOR THE MANAGEMENT OF ABDOMINAL INJURY IN THE PREGNANT PATIENT

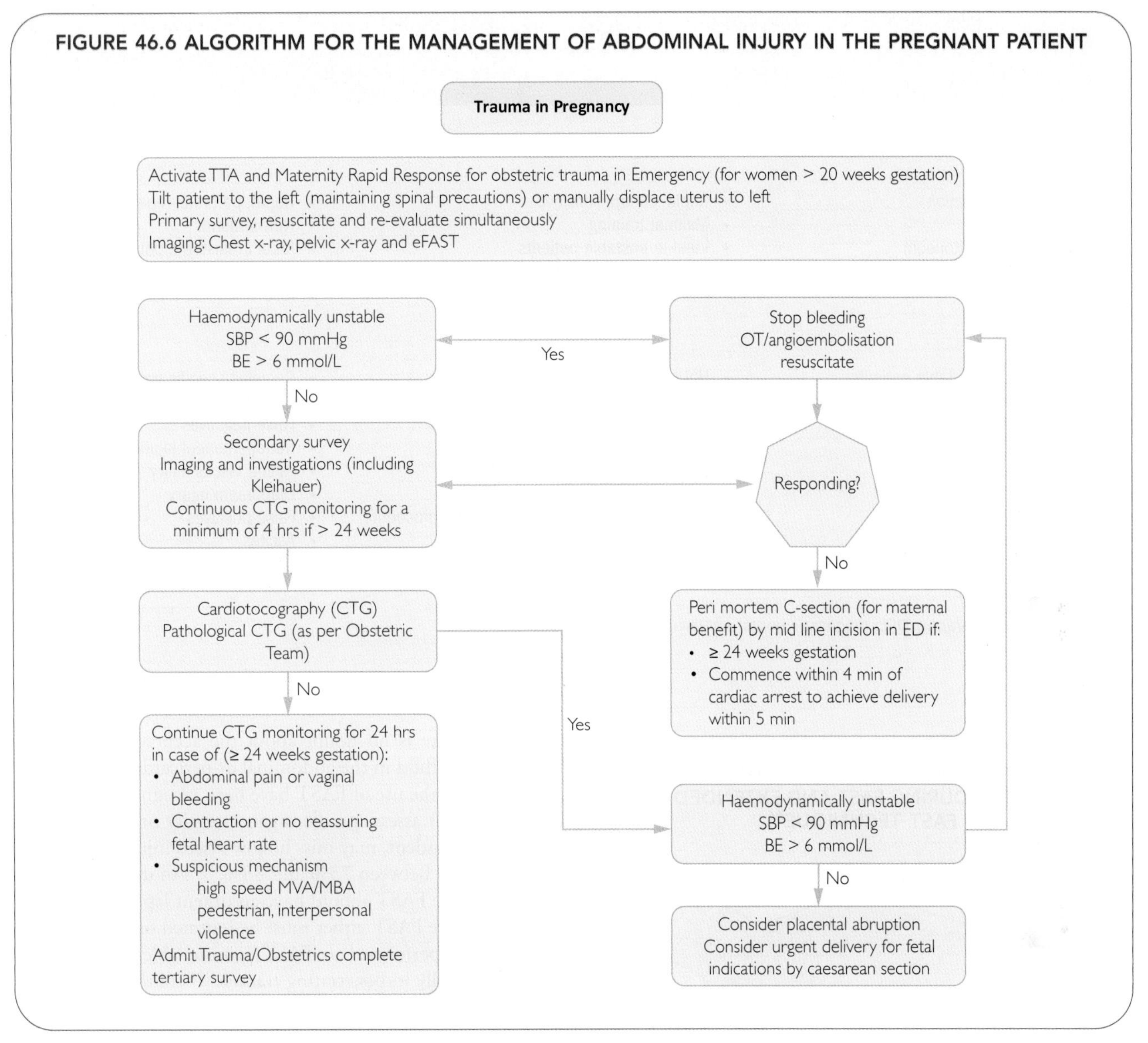

BE: base excess; CTG: cardiotocography; eFAST = extended focused assessment sonography in trauma; OT: operating theatre; TTA: trauma team. Courtesy John Hunter Hospital Trauma Service.

INVESTIGATIONS

The abdomen is a major source of missed injury and inadequate recognition of intra-abdominal bleeding.[51] Studies have highlighted the importance of rapid accurate abdominal investigation. The introduction of technology such as FAST and further sophistication of computed tomography (CT) in the assessment of the abdomen should allow rapid and accurate diagnosis of injury. The merits of these technologies are summarised in Table 46.3. However, these tools are generally not available in the rural setting, and the choice of investigation should be based on technical merit and individual patient circumstances.[52,53]

FOCUSED ASSESSMENT SONOGRAPHY IN TRAUMA (FAST)

FAST is a focused ultrasound examination to assess for free intra-abdominal or pericardial fluid, consisting of examination of four areas (Fig. 46.7). FAST is a rapid, reproducible, portable and non-invasive bedside test that may be performed simultaneously with ongoing resuscitation.[13,55] Research demonstrates that trained ED doctors, surgeons and nurses[56–58] can perform FAST accurately,[56,59,60] which has enabled FAST to become accepted as the bedside investigation of choice in abdominal trauma.[61,62] It is also being used by paramedics in the pre-hospital setting using small portable devices, and some large trauma centres are training their senior nursing staff to perform FAST.[56] It has also been shown to reduce CT and DPL rates in major trauma centres.[12,59] Modifications in the use of FAST to include assessment of the retroperitoneum and extremities[10] depend on the experience of the operator and have not yet been well evaluated in the literature. In recent years the introduction of the extended focused assessment sonography in trauma (eFAST) has allowed operators to assess the thorax for pneumothoraces and/or haemothoraces with greater sensitivity than plain radiographs (Chapter 47).

TABLE 46.3 COMPARISON OF ABDOMINAL CT, DPL AND ULTRASOUND FOR INVESTIGATION OF ABDOMINAL TRAUMA[44]

ABDOMINAL CT	DPL	ULTRASOUND
Advantages		
• Anatomical information • Non-invasive • Visualises retroperitoneum • Also views chest, pelvis	• Rapid, cheap, sensitive • Minimal training • Ideal in unstable patients • Can be done in resuscitation room	• Rapid, portable, repeatable • Non-invasive • Ideal in unstable patients • Can be done in resuscitation room • Also views heart, lungs, pelvis
Disadvantages		
• Not suitable for unstable patients • Requires transport from resuscitation room • Patient safety • Inaccessible while scanning • Time • Cost • False-negatives • Hollow viscus injuries • IV contrast reactions • Radiation exposure	• Not organ-specific • False-negatives • Retroperitoneal injuries • Hollow viscus injury • Diaphragm injury • Iatrogenic injury • Fluid and gas introduced during the procedure interfere with subsequent imaging	• Requires specific training • Operator-dependent • False-negatives • Retroperitoneal injuries • Hollow viscus injury • Diaphragm injury • False-positives • Ascites

CT: computed tomography; DPL: diagnostic peritoneal lavage; IV: intravenous.

FIGURE 46.7 PLACEMENT OF ULTRASOUND PROBES DURING FAST AND EXTENDED FAST TECHNIQUE[54]

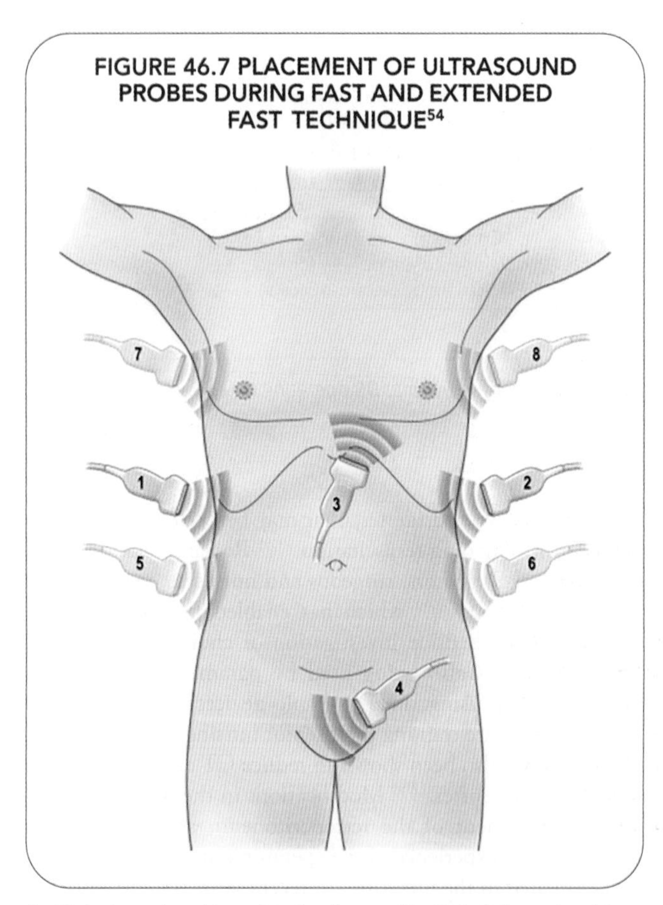

1. Right hypochondrium (Morison's pouch). **2.** Left hypochondrium. **3.** Pericardium. **4.** Pelvis (retrovesical space). **5.** Right renal fossa. **6.** Left renal fossa. **7.** Right chest base. **8.** Left chest base.

While there is no doubt about the accuracy of FAST in detecting free fluid in the abdominal or pericardial space,[57,63,64] limitations to the use of FAST have been recognised. The technique does not assess specific organ integrity or function; it is operator-dependent, may miss hollow viscus injury,[65] and has a low sensitivity between 73% and 88%.[9,25] An unstable patient with a positive FAST should have an urgent laparotomy; however, a negative FAST either must be repeated or an alternative investigation performed as FAST is unreliable in ruling out injury, especially in penetrating trauma where the sensitivity is only 50%.[66,67]

PRACTICE TIP

A negative eFAST scan does not exclude intra-abdominal injury. Repeat eFAST is warranted if there is a clinical deterioration.

ULTRASOUND/SONOGRAPHY

A formal ultrasound (different to a FAST scan) is another useful investigative modality for blunt abdominal trauma. Sonography is particularly helpful when trying to avoid radiation associated with CT scans in vulnerable trauma populations, most notably the paediatric and pregnant trauma populations. The use of ultrasound in these vulnerable populations is both reliable and sensitive in diagnosing blunt abdominal solid organ injury. Contrast enhanced ultrasounds are also gaining popularity in blunt abdominal injuries in the paediatric population.[2,68,69]

PLAIN RADIOGRAPH

While a plain abdominal film is of little use in trauma, an anteroposterior (AP) pelvic x-ray is recommended in the assessment of patients suspected of multisystem blunt trauma.[2,25,70–72] A pelvic x-ray should be conducted as an adjunct to the primary survey. If a pelvic fracture is identified, it alerts the clinician to have a higher index of suspicion for occult bleeding, particularly in the retroperitoneum. It is important to obtain a chest film, as thoracic injury is frequently associated with abdominal injury. In patients who have penetrating injuries and are haemodynamically stable, a plain abdominal film with metal markers at the entry and exit sites can provide information on the trajectory. Trauma patients requiring further abdominal assessment and potential surgery should be transferred to a trauma centre as soon as possible.

Initial radiographic evaluation of penetrating GU wounds consists of plain radiographs of the kidneys, ureters and bladder (KUB) to determine the path and appearance of the projectile. An abdominal x-ray may reveal loss of normal renal outline, loss of psoas muscle shadow on the affected side, scoliosis away from the kidney and a flank mass.[71–75] The KUB does not rule out renal trauma but does heighten the examiner's awareness of possible injury.[76,77] Intravenous pyelogram (IVP) is used in haemodynamically unstable patients with massive haemorrhaging and who require immediate laparotomy. Usually contrast is injected, then one radiograph is taken. However, an IVP has significant limitations in assessing associated intra-abdominal injuries and staging renal injuries. CT and CT angiogram are the imaging of choice in the haemodynamically stable patient.[3,55,68,78–82]

DIAGNOSTIC PERITONEAL ASPIRATION AND LAVAGE

Diagnostic peritoneal aspiration (DPA) refers to the insertion of a catheter in the peritoneal cavity and aspiration of any fluid. Diagnostic peritoneal lavage (DPL) involves infusion of normal saline, lavage of the cavity, and macroscopic and microscopic evaluation of the returned fluid.

- *DPL:* first developed in 1964 and historically performed to detect haemoperitoneum. While extremely sensitive (96% to 99%) and specific (98%), DPL is an invasive procedure with a complication rate of 1%. Currently, DPL has been largely replaced by FAST and CT.
- *DPA:* for rural and remote hospitals with limited access to radiology DPL or DPA may still be a viable option, remembering that most retrieval teams now carry portable FAST machines.[63,84–86]

SERIAL ABDOMINAL EXAMINATION

Serial abdominal examination (SAE), using the four-step approach, as previously described, is an alternative approach to assess for the development of abdominal signs and is used in those patients being admitted for observation for potential abdominal injury or non-operative management, particularly anterior abdominal penetrating wounds.[9,87] SAE is as safe and reliable as diagnostic laparoscopy for predicting the need for therapeutic laparotomy. It is not appropriate to include patients who will be unreliable with a clinical examination due to head or spinal injury or intoxication. There are several requirements for the patient who is admitted for serial clinical examination: the patient needs to be admitted for at least 24 hours, closely monitored from a haemodynamic point of view and have regular abdominal examinations looking for developing signs of peritonitis.[2,14] It is preferable that the same clinician does the examinations to avoid subjective components; if this is not feasible, then a clear handover should be done between the clinicians with the patient, so that there is agreement on signs and symptoms.

PRACTICE TIP

Serial examinations should be undertaken by one clinician to maintain objectivity and recognise early subtle changes. The exam assesses for distention, bowel sounds, tenderness, rebound tenderness, rigidity and guarding.

If the patient does develop any peritonism or haemodynamic instability, they will require a laparotomy. If the patient remains stable, they can start eating after the 24-hour mark. If they have persistent localised symptoms but not peritonitis, they require further investigation; for example, CT, laparoscopy or laparotomy.[14] The clinician should monitor and regularly assess the patient for increasing pain levels, rigidity, nausea, vomiting, increased heart and respiratory rates and temperature, which may indicate an acute abdomen, and ultimately a decreased blood pressure, indicative of septic or hypovolaemic shock, and should communicate any deterioration immediately to the treating medical team. There is no role for sequential girth measurements.

COMPUTED TOMOGRAPHY

Computed tomography (CT) is the investigation method of choice in haemodynamically stable trauma patients.[67] It provides accurate evaluation of the abdomen and retroperitoneum and is increasingly used in both blunt trauma patients and in penetrating ballistic trauma for the evaluation of trajectory and subsequent appropriate surgical approach if required.[70] Many institutions have developed CT protocols that encompass scans of the head, cervical spine, chest, abdomen and pelvis in patients with blunt multisystem injury known as a whole-body scan or a pan scan. Such an approach also allows evaluation of the thoracic and lumbar spine and re-formatting of the images for coronal and sagittal views. Whole-body CTs have been shown to improve survival in both haemodynamically stable and unstable patients,[78] although clinical assessment should guide the need for the considerable radiation exposure and risk of contrast induced neuropathy.[68,88]

PRACTICE TIP

Whole-body CT scans are often standard of care in the major poly blunt trauma, but should always be ordered after a clinical assessment and risks of harm have been weighed against benefit of a pan scan.

CT can demonstrate specific organ injury, allowing non-operative management protocols to be followed for low-grade injuries to the liver, spleen or kidney. CT is the best investigative modality to diagnose renal injury, particularly when used with intravenous (IV) contrast.[89] It also depicts the size and extent of retroperitoneal haematomas, urine extravasation and evaluates associated intra-abdominal injuries.[90,91] CT does, however, have varying degrees of sensitivity for hollow viscus injury because it is sometimes difficult to determine the significance of bowel-wall thickening or small pockets of free air.[74] Any patient with a high index of suspicion for abdominal injury with a negative initial CT scan should have serial abdominal clinical exams performed. Diagnostic sensitivity and accuracy may be related to the experience of the technician performing the scan and of the clinician interpreting the scan.[9,82,88] Very fast spiral CT provides shorter scanning time, but injury to the renal collecting system may be missed, so delayed scans are needed to rule out urinary extravasation.[73] CT cannot differentiate between various causes of traumatic vascular occlusion, such as thrombosis, vascular tears, avulsions, intimal tears and spasm.

CT is not appropriate for unstable patients, who may rapidly deteriorate while in the scanner. Although modern machines can complete scans in seconds, time is required to transport, load and unload the patient. It is essential that prior to transport, the ED nurse has and is familiar with appropriate, functioning monitoring and transport equipment. Heat loss and excess movement should be minimised. The use of oral contrast has not been demonstrated to increase the diagnostic accuracy of abdominal injury.[72,92,93] In addition, its administration delays CT scanning and puts the supine, immobilised patient at risk of aspiration.[2,9,68,78,94,95]

PRACTICE TIP

Oral contrast is rarely indicated for trauma CT scans.

CONTRAST STUDIES IN HOLLOW ORGAN INJURIES

Contrast studies can assist in the diagnosis of specific abdominal injuries if they are suspected. The timing of these studies should be decided by the appropriate specialty. The main studies used include urethrography, cystography, intravenous pyelography and gastrointestinal contrast studies. A retrograde urethrogram is essential before catheterising a patient who is suspected of having a urethral injury. Both CT cystography and conventional cystography are used to diagnose an intra-peritoneal or extra-peritoneal bladder rupture.[78,96,97] Intravenous pyelography (IVP) can be used to detect urinary system injuries if CT is not available. Injuries to retroperitoneal gastrointestinal structures (i.e. duodenum, colon, rectum, etc.) may best be imaged using specific GI contrast studies in conjunction with contrast CTs.[93]

TRAUMA LAPAROTOMY

While there are different techniques for trauma laparotomies, the objectives remain the same. Firstly, to control haemorrhage: this is usually done as a damage control procedure in conjunction with goal-directed haemostatic resuscitation. Other objectives include control contamination, repair vascular injuries, damaged or devascularised bowel and repair of retroperitoneal injuries and finally closure, if possible. Closure is dependent on several factors, including the amount of haemorrhage, volume of fluid resuscitation given, the degree of contamination and the patient's haemodynamic status.[98–101]

LAPAROSCOPY

Laparoscopy is slowly emerging as a useful tool in trauma patients with abdominal injuries. Traditionally laparoscopy was used as a diagnostic tool, but increasingly is being used for its therapeutic potential. The majority of the research into this area has involved penetrating injuries, specifically anterior abdominal stab wounds, but recently more evidence has emerged to support its use in blunt abdominal trauma.[102–104] Careful patient selection is vital. Patients that are haemodynamically stable and have a penetrating abdominal wound and suspected mesenteric injury may benefit. The use of laparoscopy has demonstrated decreases in hospital length of stay, infections and complications. Converting to laparotomy is less frequent as laparoscopy becomes more common; however, it is important to remember that, like any procedure, there are risks involved and there is still a chance of missed injury, such as bowel injury.[105]

LABORATORY TESTS

Blood samples should be collected as an adjunct to the primary survey when inserting large-bore cannulae. In the acute phase of trauma, the most relevant blood test is either an arterial or a venous blood gas (see Chapter 16 for information on interpreting test results). They are rapidly available serological markers of shock; lactate and base excess are highly sensitive in measuring tissue perfusion and demonstrating blood loss.[106] Standard blood tests are sent with each trauma patient, including a full blood count, urea and electrolytes, coagulation studies and cross-matching (Chapter 42), and while they may not always be of value in the initial resuscitation, they provide a baseline for ongoing assessment.[107]

Bloods relevant to abdominal trauma include lipase and amylase. Elevated amylase levels may indicate pancreatic or duodenal injury; however, some patients sustain injury to these organs without amylase elevation. The positive predictor of elevated amylase in pancreatic trauma is only 10%.[108] A serum lipase reading should be obtained if pancreatic injury is suspected, as it is an indicator of pancreatic function, and interpreted in conjunction with other investigative tools. In children, aspartate aminotransferase (AST) levels and physical assessment accurately predict intra-abdominal injury.[70,109] (AST is found in the liver, heart, lungs, muscle tissue, pancreas, spleen and kidneys and is released with damage, becoming elevated after 6–8 hours.)[106,110]

PRACTICE TIP

- Obtain a blood gas early. This allows for early assessment of microvascular perfusion and oxygen supply and can help goal-directed resuscitation for hypovolaemic shock.
- All women of childbearing age should have a quantitative beta-hCG (human chorionic gonadotrophin) level taken to determine pregnancy status.

ONGOING MANAGEMENT

Advances in resuscitation, assessment, new haemostatic agents and fundamental changes in the surgical management of the

BOX 46.2 ONGOING NURSING MANAGEMENT FOR ABDOMINAL TRAUMA

- Be aware of patient status, fluid balance, observations.
- Ensure warm fluid administration and prevent heat loss.
- Communicate all findings with the trauma team leader.
- Maintain documentation and anticipate requirements, such as preoperative checklist.
- Be familiar with and have appropriate equipment for monitoring for emergency transfer.
- Keep patient and family informed.
- Ensure nurse in charge is aware of progress.
- Facilitate ED discharge process to definitive care.
- Monitor for allergic reaction to radiological contrast.
- Regularly reassess the patient for signs of increased pain, blood loss and peritonism.
- When handing over, conduct an abdominal assessment with the new staff member to ensure consistency of interpretation.
- Ensure police have been notified of firearm injuries, as per legislation (Chapter 4).

most severely injured patients have evolved from an improved understanding of the physiological derangements associated with severe injury and may favourably affect the survival of patients with abdominal trauma.[2,9,87,111,112] Despite initial presentation, haemodynamically stable patients with penetrating abdominal trauma may have significant ongoing haemorrhage and major intra-abdominal injuries. Peritonitis should be a trigger for emergency operation regardless of vital signs, because haemodynamic 'stability' does not reliably exclude significant haemorrhage or soiling. Vascular injury, subsequent hypotension, blood transfusion and complicated postoperative course are common in this population.[95,113,114] The ED nurse should continue to monitor and assess the patient (Box 46.2).

Pre-hospital control of bleeding from the torso remains problematic and this is one area in trauma care that has seen developments in recent years. Limited evidence exists for the use of an Abdominal Aortic and Junctional Tourniquet (AAJT)[115–118] and Resuscitative Endovascular Balloon Occlusion of the Aorta (REBOA), which may temporise control of haemorrhage until definitive care at the trauma centre.[3,119,120]

- *AAJT*—initially designed for use in combat; a belt-like device used to apply external compression to major vascular structures and arrest blood flow in exsanguinating haemorrhage.
- *REBOA*—a procedure that involves placement of an endovascular balloon in the aorta to temporarily control non-compressible torso haemorrhage. Despite increased use of REBOA over the last decade and recent endovascular technology advancements, there is insufficient high-level evidence on its effectiveness for improving mortality in trauma.[115,116,118,121,122]

AAJT and REBOA are of interest in the initial management of major haemorrhage in both the pre-hospital and in-hospital arena; however, benefits in terms of overall reduction of trauma patient mortality are controversial. At present these are seen as a last-ditch effort to save life and are reserved for patient in extremis.[123]

MANAGEMENT TECHNIQUES

WOUNDS

All penetrating wounds of the abdomen need to be clearly documented in the patient record. Wounds, especially from ballistic injury, and even those apparently distant to the abdomen, need to be thoroughly evaluated for possible communication with the abdomen. Radio-opaque wound markers, such as a paperclip or cardiac monitoring dots, should identify entry and exit sites when plain x-rays are used to evaluate potential injuries. Protruding objects, such as a knife, should be left in situ and stabilised until operative removal, as they may be adjacent to or penetrating vascular structures. The sudden release of tamponade may result in catastrophic haemorrhage.[124–126]

PRACTICE TIP

Protruding foreign objects should be stabilised and protected until surgically removed.

EVALUATION OF PENETRATING ABDOMINAL INJURIES

Mandatory exploratory laparotomy of all patients who have sustained penetrating abdominal injuries will result in an extremely low incidence of delayed diagnoses or missed injuries, but an unacceptably high rate of negative abdominal explorations and potential surgery- and anaesthetic-related complications, especially in patients with low-velocity stab injuries.[111,127] Of course, laparotomy for penetrating abdominal injury is *always* indicated when the patient is unstable or in shock, thus all such patients should be transported promptly to the operating theatre without any further diagnostic interventions (Box 46.1). Most centres still advocate mandatory exploration for all patients sustaining gunshot wounds to the anterior abdomen irrespective of haemodynamic status, given the high probability of finding visceral (intestinal) injuries in these patients. Researchers from South Africa and the United States have advocated selective non-operative management of these patients with good results, but this practice has yet to spread to other major trauma centres worldwide.[2,111,128]

The stable patient with a stab wound to the anterior abdomen who presents without peritonitis, haematemesis, gross rectal bleeding or evisceration of abdominal contents through the wound may be initially managed non-operatively by performing wound exploration under local anaesthesia in the ED. The rationale for this approach is based on the fact that 15–30% of abdominal stab wounds do not actually violate the peritoneal cavity.[129,130] If the wound is followed through the tissue planes and found to end without violation of the peritoneal layer, then the patient may be discharged from the ED after wound irrigation and closure. The ED nurse should educate the patient on wound healing, maintenance and signs that indicate wound breakdown and the need for intervention. If, however, the wound is found to penetrate the abdominal cavity, or if its depth cannot be determined due to the patient's body habitus, four options exist:

1. Exploratory laparotomy without any further diagnostic interventions, which will reveal no intra-abdominal injuries in up to one-third of these stable patients.

BOX 46.3 DELAYED CLINICAL MANIFESTATIONS OF ABDOMINAL INJURY

INCREASING:	DECREASED:
• pain	• appetite
• rigidity	• bowel sounds
• bruising	• haemoglobin
• heart rate	• blood pressure
• respiratory rate	• urine output
• temperature	
• white cell count	
• nausea	
• vomiting	

2. Diagnostic laparoscopy under general anaesthesia, as previously discussed.
3. Admission for close observation, consisting of frequent (every 2–3 hours) serial abdominal examinations by an experienced clinician and repeated determinations of white blood cell (WBC) count. The nurse should monitor the patient for systemic signs of sepsis such as pyrexia, tachypnoea and tachycardia (Box 46.3),[131] which will lead to laparotomy and repair of injury. If, after 24 hours of observation, the patient does not show any signs of intra-abdominal injury, the likelihood of a missed injury is extremely low. The patient can be fed and, if oral intake is tolerated, discharged.
4. Performance of a diagnostic peritoneal lavage. Patients in whom the DPL is negative should be observed for a period of 24 hours, after which they may be released if no clinical signs of abdominal injury supervene.[12,85,132] Some have attempted to perform local wound exploration at the bedside using ultrasound rather than the traditional scalpel, with good results.[102,126,133,134]

Currently there is no clear evidence either way for the use of prophylactic antibiotics in penetrating abdominal trauma.[143]

SELECTIVE NON-OPERATIVE MANAGEMENT

Selective non-operative management (SNOM) of solid abdominal organ injury is a technique that was originally described in children, but has rapidly gained acceptance in the management of adult blunt and penetrating trauma. The improvement in critical care monitoring, CT scanning, as well as interventional radiology, assist SNOM.[135–137] A haemodynamically stable patient and accurate imaging by CT are prerequisites for this approach. Isolated injuries to the liver, spleen and kidneys are frequently self-limiting with minimal intra-abdominal blood loss.[138] These patients can be closely observed in a critical care area for any signs of deterioration or bleeding and the vast majority will avoid surgery—and require less blood transfusion and have fewer complications than surgical patients. Unstable patients and those who demonstrate evidence of ongoing bleeding require an urgent laparotomy and haemorrhage control.[9,98,111,128]

SNOM of liver and spleen injury is associated with a small incidence of missed bowel and pancreatic injury; therefore a high index of suspicion, especially with liver injury, should be maintained to detect this. It is thought that the greater amount and/or different vector of energy transfer needed to injure the liver versus the spleen accounts for the greater rate of associated injuries to the pancreas/small bowel.[9,139,140] Failure of SNOM is uncommon, typically occurs within the first 12 hours after injury and is associated with injury severity and multiplicity, as well as isolated pancreatic injuries.[141,142] The nurse should be aware of signs of deterioration and missed injury, as previously outlined in Box 46.3.

INTERVENTIONAL RADIOLOGY

Interventional radiology (IR) has a vital role to play in the management of abdominal trauma by providing therapeutic procedures alternative to surgery,[80,143,144] particularly in patients who are bleeding as a result of vascular injury.[66] IR has gained popularity as a management option for patients with isolated liver and spleen injuries,[145,146] and it can be used to gain an accurate diagnosis, and to evaluate for and control bleeding from pelvic and other vessels when clinically appropriate. Angiography is also a sensitive modality for staging renal injuries. In penetrating trauma, it can be used to identify pseudoaneurysms[83,123] and arteriovenous fistulas. The technique involves percutaneous access to the vessels, usually in the groin, and a catheter is then introduced under radiological screening. Contrast medium is injected while imaging continues, and extravasation of the contrast determines the site and degree of injury.

Various techniques can be attempted to control or stop the bleeding. Embolisation involves the deployment of multiple metallic coils through the catheter into the vessels supplying the injured organ. These act as scaffolding for clot formation, which then leads to occlusion of the damaged vessels. Embolisation can also be achieved by injecting topical haemostatic agents; these agents are absorbed into the body after about 5 days. Alternatively, balloon catheters can be passed either side of a bleeding point in a vessel and inflated to occlude flow to provide temporary control until surgical access is gained. Once again it is essential that the ED nurse has appropriate, functioning monitoring and transport equipment, as well as ensuring that communication with the patient and/or their family has occurred. The intravenous contrast that is administered as part of IR or CT may cause allergic reaction, so the nurse should monitor for signs of rash, hives, flushing of the skin or itching and contact the doctor immediately. Contrast can also impair renal function and so there is a need to monitor urine output and creatinine.

IR techniques may be employed in several situations. The presence of a contrast blush in the spleen on abdominal CT suggests ongoing bleeding. Arteriography and coil embolisation can be used to stop the bleeding and avoid surgery. Patients with significant liver injuries that require packing at surgery have a significant risk for ongoing bleeding. Arteriography can be used to define ongoing bleeding and to embolise bleeding vessels before planned return to the operating room. IR is also valuable in the diagnosis and control of pelvic bleeding in open-book pelvic fractures.[101,147–149]

PRACTICE TIP

IR suites are often very cold. Remember to continue to actively re-warm your patient with overhead heaters or a Bair-Hugger.

DAMAGE CONTROL SURGERY

It is well recognised that a combination of hypothermia, coagulopathy and metabolic acidosis is associated with a high level of mortality in trauma patients. The phrase encompassing these alterations, 'the triad of death', has been extended to the trauma diamond of death to incorporate hypocalcaemia (Chapter 42).[150] Damage control surgery (DCS), as a component of damage control resuscitation (Chapter 42), is a concept designed to minimise the time a patient is exposed to this diamond and expedite the patient to a higher care setting where further organ support can be instituted.[148,151,152] The aim of DCS is to prioritise the restoration of normal physiological parameters versus the normalisation of anatomy.[153–155] Indications for DCS are summarised in Box 46.4. Preparation is key, and the decision to perform DCS should be made in the ED or at the beginning of the operation. This allows a management strategy to be formulated, and communicated, with the anaesthetist, operating-room staff and critical care clinicians.

In short, the operating surgeon will initially deal with haemorrhage and contamination only, using a range of abbreviated techniques; the patient is then transferred to the intensive care unit (ICU) for correction of hypothermia, acidosis, hypocalcaemia and coagulopathy due to initial hypovolaemia/massive transfusion.[154,156] The aim is for the patient to return to the operating theatre for definitive surgery within 24–48 hours. This staged surgery allows the patient to be in a physiological state to normalise, giving the patient the best opportunity to recover.[157–159] The heterogeneous nature of the trauma patient needs to be considered when planning this staged approach. This applies equally to the timing of further investigations or radiological interventions; for example, CT scans. Premature return to theatre will convert what should be a definitive second operation into a second damage control procedure and result in further physiological insult for the patient. This should be balanced against undue delays, which may increase the risk of abdominal compartment syndrome, intra-abdominal sepsis and the progression of previously unrecognised injuries. The stages of DCS are outlined in Table 46.4.

BOX 46.4 CONSIDERATIONS FOR DAMAGE CONTROL SURGERY

- **Multiple penetrating injuries to the torso**
- **High-energy blunt trauma to the torso**
- **Multisystem trauma with competing operative/interventional priorities**
- **Profound haemorrhagic shock at presentation**
- **Evidence of worsening hypothermia, coagulopathy or metabolic acidosis on presentation or early in evaluation.**

PRACTICE TIP

Preventing or reversing the trauma diamond of death, hypothermia, hypocalcaemia, acidosis and coagulopathy, is one of the major goals in early trauma management.

SPECIFIC ORGAN INJURY

STOMACH

The location and relative mobility of the stomach generally protects it from blunt injury. Most trauma of the hollow, pouch-like stomach is penetrating, causing the release of digestive contents and hydrochloric acid into the peritoneal cavity. This may cause severe peritonitis, initially by chemical irritation

TABLE 46.4 STAGES OF DAMAGE CONTROL SURGERY

STAGE 1	Emergency department	Recognition—of the need for damage control surgery (DCS) during the initial evaluation	• Assess patient rapidly using ATLS protocol • Recognise anatomical and physiological patterns • Plan and prepare for DCS
STAGE 2	Operating room	Operative control—of life-threatening haemorrhage and gastrointestinal contamination	• Control haemorrhage by ligation, shunting or repair • Control contamination; do not perform stomas or anastomoses • Repair gastrointestinal discontinuity • Pack solid-organ and pelvic injuries • Consider IR procedures and mobilise early • Place temporary abdominal closure
STAGE 3	Intensive care unit	Resuscitation—in the surgical high-dependency or intensive care units, including correction of the diamond of death	• Assess resuscitation, set endpoints • Correct acidosis, hypocalcaemia, coagulopathy, hypothermia • Monitor for abdominal compartment syndrome • Consider adjunct procedures/studies: x-ray, IR, CT
STAGE 4	Operating room	Return—to operating room for further exploration and definitive management	• Identify and repair all injuries • Assess abdomen for fascial closure
STAGE 5	Operating room	Closure—of surgical and traumatic wounds	• Perform definitive wound closure

ATLS: advanced trauma life support; CT: computed tomography; IR: interventional radiology.

rather than bacterial.[65] Blunt injuries to the stomach are rare, with the incidence reported between 0.4% and 1.7% of all abdominal trauma; the mechanism is usually high-energy forces to the epigastrium with a full stomach.[3] The stomach has a rich blood supply from the splenic artery, gastroepiploic and short gastric arteries (Fig. 46.8).

Symptoms of gastric injury may include severe epigastric or abdominal pain, and signs of peritonitis. Blood loss is indicated by symptoms of hypovolaemia. Blood from a nasogastric tube and the presence of free air on abdominal x-ray may support the diagnosis.[82,128]

BOWEL INJURIES

Hollow-organ injuries from blunt trauma are rare, but associated with increased mortality and morbidity. While CT is the imaging modality of choice, its lack of sensitivity and specificity in diagnosing hollow-organ injuries is well reported in the literature. CT findings that are highly suggestive of bowel injury include bowel-wall discontinuity, extraluminal contrast and extraluminal air. However, the absence of these on CT does not completely rule out injury.[94,161] Regular serial clinical examination in the patient with significant seatbelt injury is vital. Symptoms usually develop slowly and include increased pain, guarding and distension and decreased bowel sounds.[161] Blunt injury to the bowel can be caused by direct blows, crushing the intestine between the external force and the spinal column and by shearing forces imposed by rapid deceleration. The presence of abdominal solid organ and lumbar spine injury are predictive of hollow viscus injury and thus the index of suspicion should be raised.[42,98,151,162] The small bowel (ileum and jejunum) has a neutral pH and harbours few bacteria, so clinical signs of injury may not be present on initial assessment. It is important for the ED nurse to be aware of the patient's mechanism of injury, the need for reassessment of the abdomen and signs of peritonitis.[18–20,71] The transverse colon (large bowel) crosses the upper half of the abdominal cavity from right to left, and then curves downwards beneath the lower end of the spleen to form the splenic flexure. The proximity of various parts of the colon to other organs that are injured should raise suspicion of potential colon injury. Trauma causing perforation of the large bowel is lethal if untreated, due to faecal contamination of the abdomen.[20,75,163]

Management

Early identification and management of bowel injury is essential to control for abdominal contamination and subsequent peritonitis and sepsis. Surgical management of a hollow viscus repair includes either resection or direct repair of the affected segment. Colonic injuries can be resected with primary anastomosis; however, in the face of shock, major blood loss, multiple organ injury, significant faecal contamination and a significant time delay prior to operative management, formation of a stoma may be required. This group of patients is likely to be physiologically challenged postoperatively, leading to poor splanchnic perfusion, increased acidosis and ultimately increased risk of anastomotic breakdown. The patient's physiological status should ultimately determine the extent of any surgical procedure. Complications such as wound infection are related to the extent of contamination and the site of the injury. In addition, other complications such as fistula formation, small bowel obstruction, ischaemic bowel and anastomotic breakdown have been reported.[94,161,162,164]

FIGURE 46.8 ARTERIAL SUPPLY TO THE STOMACH

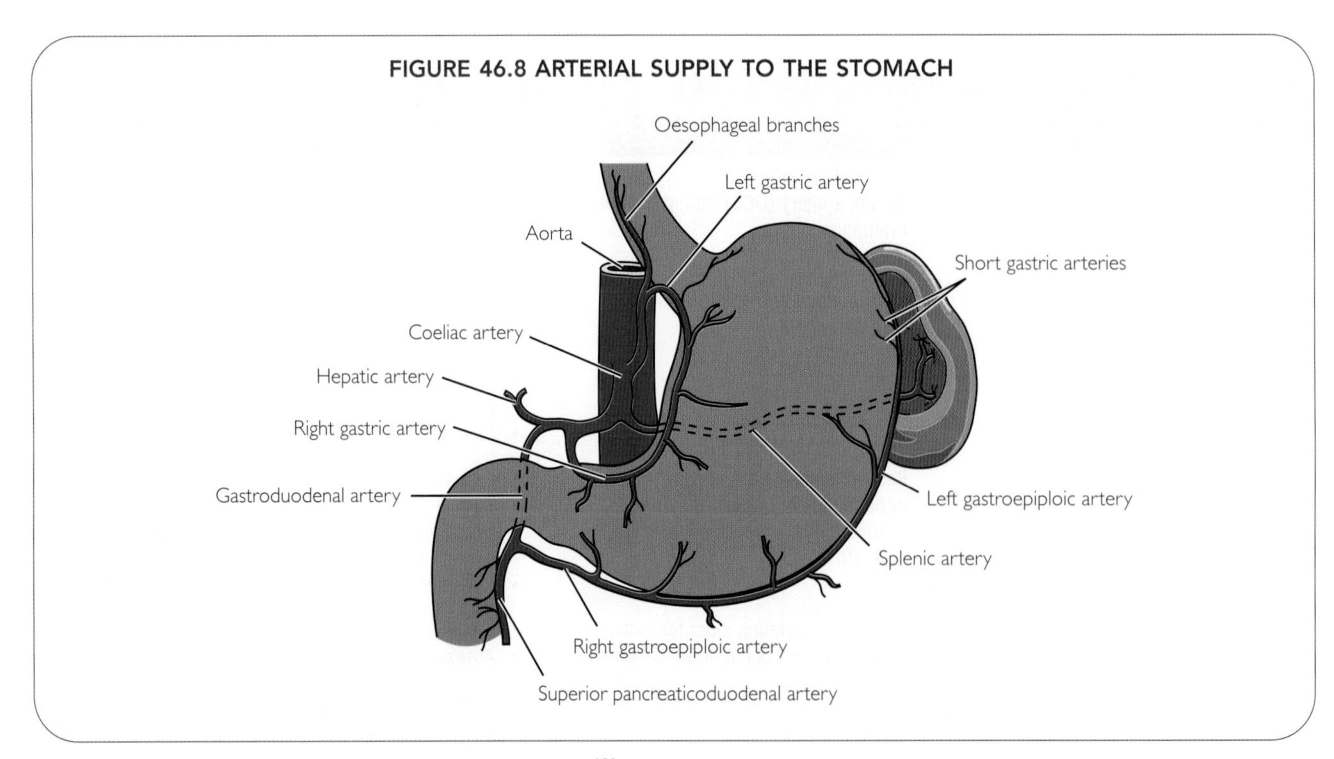

All the arteries are derived from branches of the coeliac artery.[160]

LIVER AND GALLBLADDER

The liver's large size and anterior location under the diaphragm and rib cage, occupying most of the right hypochondrium, makes it susceptible to injury and that is why it is the most commonly injured solid organ in the peritoneal cavity (Fig. 46.9). The most common mechanisms of liver injury are road trauma, falls and assaults. In penetrating or blunt trauma, hepatic injury should be suspected if there is right-sided chest-wall trauma.[128,137,138]

FIGURE 46.9 ANATOMICAL LOCATION OF THE LIVER[157]

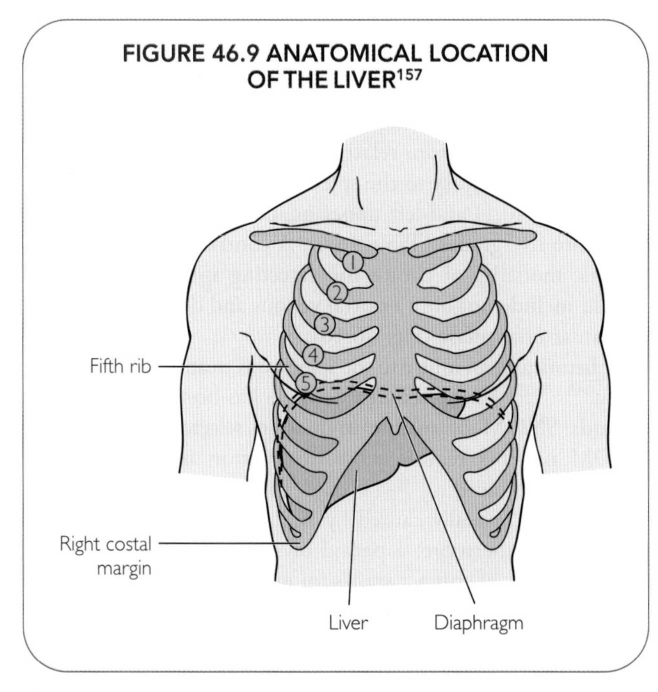

The upper border normally lies at the level of the 4th intercostal space or 5th rib, and the lower border does not normally extend more than 1-2 cm below the right costal margin.

Although only 15–20% of the liver is necessary to sustain life, death can occur in less than 12 hours after complete destruction of the liver. The liver has a dual blood supply from the hepatic artery and the portal vein. About 400 mL/min of blood enters the liver through the hepatic artery, and another 1000 mL/min enters through the valveless portal vein, making it vulnerable to injury and bleeding.[11,110,158,165,166]

CT is the imaging modality of choice to diagnose liver trauma in the stable patient. A delayed (venous phase) CT provides more detailed information about the extent of the injury and whether there is any active bleeding. In addition, and particularly in children, elevated blood aspartate aminotransferase (AST; children > 450 IU/L and adults > 360 IU/L) and alanine aminotransferase (ALT) levels are predictive of liver injury.[165–167]

Liver injury can be graded on a scale of I to VI (Table 46.5). Non-operative management of all grades of liver injury is now considered the standard of care if the patient is haemodynamically stable, and has been demonstrated to improve outcomes and decrease lengths of stay.[158] However, the higher the grade of liver injury, the higher the incidence of haemodynamic instability requiring OT and delayed complications causing an increase in morbidity, such as multiple organ dysfunction syndrome (MODS) and mortality.[112,169,170] If operative management is required, it is usually to control extensive venous haemorrhage. This is often achieved with packing. The operating surgeon will then decide whether a damage-control approach or a definitive repair should be carried out. Both management strategies will include ongoing resuscitation, and postoperatively the patient will require a critical care bed. Some patients may require angiography and embolisation after their initial surgery to assist with haemostasis[100,101,145,148,153,171]

The pear-shaped, hollow muscular gallbladder sac lies directly beneath the right lobe of the liver and stores from 20 to 50 mL of bile. Trauma to the gallbladder is rare, occurring in

TABLE 46.5 LIVER INJURIES[168]

GRADE	CATEGORY	DESCRIPTION
I	Haematoma	Non-expanding subcapsular haematoma less than 10% of liver surface
	Laceration	Non-bleeding capsular tear less than 1 cm deep
II	Haematoma	Non-expanding subcapsular haematoma covering 10–50% surface area; less than 2 cm deep
	Laceration	Less than 3 cm parenchymal penetration; less than 10 cm long
III	Haematoma	Subcapsular haematoma more than 50% surface area or one that is expanding; ruptured subcapsular haematoma with active bleeding; intraparenchymal haematoma more than 2 cm deep
	Laceration	More than 3 cm deep
IV	Haematoma	Ruptured central haematoma
	Laceration	15–25% hepatic lobe destroyed
V	Laceration	More than 75% hepatic lobe destroyed
	Vascular	Major hepatic veins injured
VI	Vascular	Avulsed liver

approximately 2% of all abdominal trauma cases, but when missed or improperly managed it may be associated with significant morbidity.[172–174] It is difficult to diagnose because of its vague symptoms and inconclusive test results and is most often found during laparotomy. In addition, it is often associated with liver, duodenal haematoma or perforation injury. The preferred management is cholecystectomy.[136,137,174]

PANCREAS AND DUODENUM

The pancreas, located behind the stomach, is in very close proximity to the duodenum. Blunt pancreatic and duodenal injuries[53,83,129] are rare, occurring in approximately 4% of all patients who sustain an abdominal injury. Major pancreatic injuries[83,141,142,175] are uncommon, but may result in considerable morbidity and mortality because of the magnitude of associated vascular and duodenal injuries or underestimation of the extent of the pancreatic injury. In addition, pancreatic injury has a high incidence of infectious complications.[170] Neglect of major pancreatic duct injury may lead to life-threatening complications, including pseudocysts, fistulas, pancreatitis, sepsis and secondary haemorrhage. Isolated pancreatic injury would be a relatively unusual finding due to its retroperitoneal[53] location and relative insulation by other organs.

Pancreatic and duodenal injuries are hard to identify on physical examination, but anyone complaining of epigastric pain following blunt or penetrating force to the area should be thoroughly investigated. Pancreatic damage is usually identified on CT scan (85% accurate) or at the time of surgery. Biochemical tests, such as amylase, are non-specific. Any breach of the retroperitoneum should instigate a thorough exploration for pancreatic injury. Debridement of devitalised tissue and drainage can be employed for most cases of pancreatic trauma. Most duodenal injuries can be managed with debridement and primary repair.[79,172] If there is significant ductal destruction of the body or tail of the pancreas, this damaged area can be resected and a good outcome expected. Destruction of the pancreatic head is often associated with duodenal injury. This may require a Whipple's procedure in the stable patient; the unstable patient may benefit from a damage-control procedure and delayed pancreaticoduodenectomy.

SPLEEN

This is a relatively large, very vascular organ found in the left upper quadrant behind and in close proximity to ribs 7 to 10, making it vulnerable to injury when those ribs are fractured and at equal risk of damage from both blunt and penetrating injuries to this area. It has a blood flow of 250 mL/min from the splenic artery and a normal volume of approximately 350 mL (Chapter 29). Splenic injuries are most commonly associated with blunt trauma. The spleen has a friable capsule leading to rupture from relatively minor trauma, for example, contact sports. Injury to the spleen may be indicated by Kehr's sign (Table 46.1) and left upper quadrant pain, and is categorised into five grades (Table 46.6). A contrast CT is the radiographic modality of choice for detecting splenic injuries and should include not only a portal venous and delayed phase, but also an arterial phase (Fig. 46.10).

Historically, an injury to the spleen was treated with a splenectomy.[146,177–179] In the last decade there has been a trend change towards SNOM of splenic injuries in selected patients.[168,179] SNOM patients require close observation in a critical care setting, as re-bleeding 7–14 days post-injury is a recognised complication, usually caused by rupture of a subcapsular haematoma. Furthermore, a period of self-imposed rest at home and avoidance of contact sports for a period of 2 months is also recommended following discharge from hospital. If a splenectomy is performed, the patient will require immunisation against encapsulated organisms, including *Pneumococcus* and *Haemophilus*, in an effort to prevent overwhelming post-splenectomy infections (OPSI). Although rare, OPSI can occur from 1 to 5 years after the operation. The illness presents with flu-like symptoms, such as nausea and vomiting, progressing

TABLE 46.6 SPLENIC INJURIES[168]

GRADE	CATEGORY	DESCRIPTION
I	Haematoma	Subcapsular; involves less than 10% surface area; haematoma does not expand
	Laceration	Non-bleeding capsular tear; less than 1 cm deep
II	Haematoma	Subcapsular haematoma covering 10–50% surface area Haematoma does not expand; intraparenchymal haematoma less than 2 cm wide
	Laceration	Capsular tear with active bleeding; intraparenchymal injury 1–3 cm deep
III	Haematoma	Subcapsular haematoma involving more than 50% surface area or one that is expanding; intraparenchymal haematoma less than 2 cm wide or expanding; ruptured subcapsular haematoma with active bleeding
	Laceration	More than 3 cm deep or involving intracellular vessels
IV	Haematoma	Ruptured intraparenchymal haematoma with active bleeding
	Laceration	Segmental laceration or one that involves hilar vessels Devascularisation of more than 25% of spleen
V	Laceration	Shattered spleen
	Vascular	Hilar vascular injury; spleen is devascularised

FIGURE 46.10 SPLENIC HAEMATOMA[177]

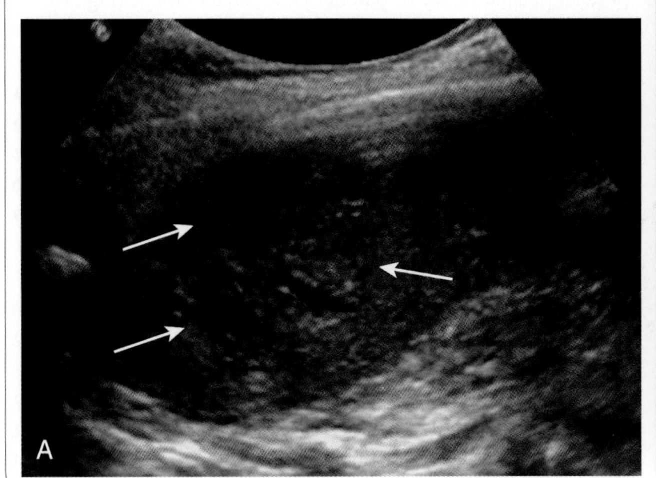

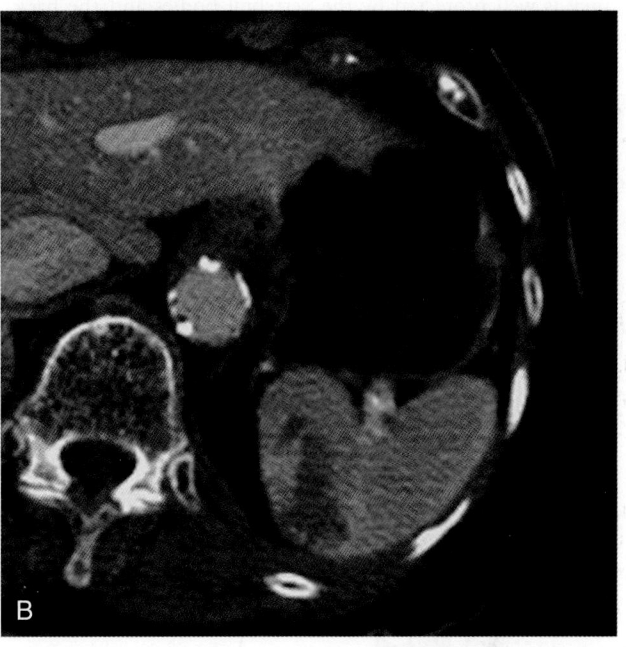

A. Focused ultrasound of the left upper quadrant demonstrates a focal region of heterogeneity in the spleen (arrows), suggestive of an acute splenic injury. **B.** Computed tomography performed following the initial ultrasound confirms the presence of an acute splenic haematoma.

rapidly to confusion, high fever and septic shock, leading to disseminated intravascular coagulation and death. Recent research has demonstrated a benefit in the use of spleen registries in reducing the mortality and morbidity associated with OPSI.[178,179]

VASCULAR INJURY

Major vascular injuries of the abdominal cavity or the retroperitoneum usually involve the aorta, vena cava, iliac arteries and their major branches, and are often associated with major pelvic fractures or sudden deceleration injuries. They manifest initially by severe or rapidly progressive haemorrhagic shock. The initial evaluation should be brief and directed towards ruling out haemorrhage, but it is often necessary to embark on an exploratory laparotomy without the benefit of full preoperative localisation of the source of bleeding. If operative facilities are not available, communication to transport the patient to definitive care must be of extremely high priority. The blood pressure should not be elevated above a systolic value of about 90 mmHg, in keeping with damage control resuscitation principles with permissive hypotension.[105,153,159]

Most decisions regarding the definitive control of these injuries are made intraoperatively by the surgeons once the actual anatomical injury is visualised. Nurses caring for such patients should ensure that high-flow oxygen is administered, any fluids given are warmed, an accurate record is kept of transfused fluid and vital signs, rapid transfer to the operating suite is facilitated by ensuring transport equipment and documentation are ready, the operating suite is aware of the patient and adequate amounts of blood products are available at all times by liaising with the blood bank. Activation of a massive transfusion protocol is very helpful in these situations (Chapter 42).

ABDOMINAL WALL HAEMATOMA/ RETROPERITONEAL HAEMATOMA

Occasionally, a penetrating abdominal injury will result in an abdominal-wall haematoma that requires full exposure under general anaesthesia to evaluate and control. If the haematoma is due to a stab wound or gunshot injury, it is usually explored, as there is a high likelihood of encountering and repairing a major vascular injury in these patients. It is dangerous to simply attempt to treat such injuries by applying local pressure or larger overlying masses of bandages in the hopes of tamponading the bleeding. It is rare that abdominal-wall haematomas due to blunt forces will require surgical intervention, as most resolve spontaneously with time and are self-limiting, although quite painful. The exceptions include internal degloving wounds such as a Morel-Lavallée lesion, where the skin separates from the underlying muscular fascia and forms a haemolymphatic mass, which may need to be drained.[180]

A general tenet of trauma surgery is that lateral and pelvic retroperitoneal haematomas due to blunt forces are usually left undisturbed (i.e. not surgically explored), unless the patient is unstable or in shock, while central haematomas are explored. If the haematoma is pulsatile or has visibly enlarged during the course of the laparotomy, then exploration is required.[181]

GENITOURINARY TRAUMA

RENAL TRAUMA

The kidneys are retroperitoneal organs that lie high on the posterior abdominal wall. They are enclosed by a strong fibrous capsule and lie within a fatty tissue layer. The perirenal space allows a large amount of blood to accumulate; however, the fascial layer can effectively tamponade renal bleeding in some cases. Normally, the kidneys are mobile within this area and can move up or down three vertebral spaces (Fig. 46.11). The kidney is well protected by the vertebral bodies and the back muscles posteriorly and the abdominal viscera anteriorly.

The kidney is the most commonly injured organ in the urinary tract. Renal trauma is difficult to assess and early recognition, management and referral is crucial.[77,112,182,183] Blunt trauma accounts for up to 90% of renal injuries, and penetrating trauma 5–10%.[184,185] Blunt injuries are most commonly caused by a MVC, assault, sports injuries or fall from a height. Injury from blunt trauma is due to three mechanisms—direct blow to the flank, laceration of renal parenchyma from a fractured rib or vertebrae or sudden deceleration that causes shearing which leads to renal pedicle injury or parenchymal renal damage (Fig. 46.12). Falls from heights are associated with ureteral avulsion at the ureteropelvic junction.

Between 4% and 25% of blunt injuries are classified as major lacerations or vascular injuries, compared with 27–68% of penetrating injuries.[3] Up to 60% of penetrating renal injuries are likely to have adjacent organ damage.[86,125,144,171,185] Damage to the kidney may be caused by a bullet, bullet fragment or blast effect. The majority of penetrating injuries require surgical intervention. In children, blunt abdominal trauma frequently results in renal injury due to their lack of perirenal fat, relatively larger size of the kidney in relation to other organs and decreased thoracic protection.[76,116,187,188]

Renal injuries have been classified by the American Organ Injury Scaling Committee from grade I (simple contusion) to grade V (complete vascular compromise). They are listed in Table 46.7 and illustrated in Fig. 46.13. These classifications have been demonstrated to be a reliable and predictable tool for clinical practice and are most commonly diagnosed through imaging.

The majority of renal pedicle injuries occur in children and young adults, with the left renal vein the most commonly injured vessel. Deceleration injury is the usual mechanism, through which the intimal layer of the renal artery is torn.[73,74,125,182] Renal vascular injuries include a vessel injury, renal artery thrombosis and disruption of the renal artery intimal layer resulting in an aneurysm or thrombosis. No signs or symptoms are specific for renal pedicle injury. Haematuria is absent in one-third of all cases.[172,193] Early diagnosis and surgical repair of pedicle injury is required to restore blood flow to the ischaemic kidney and salvage renal function. Total avulsion of the renal pedicle with

FIGURE 46.11 ANATOMICAL RELATIONSHIP BETWEEN THE KIDNEYS AND SPINE[182]

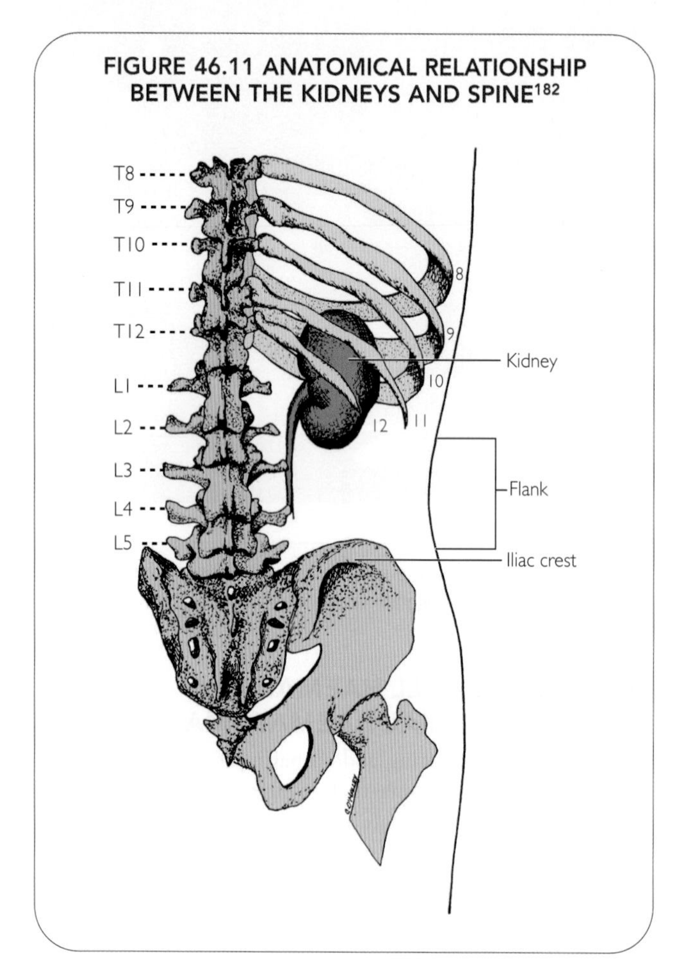

FIGURE 46.12 ACCELERATION/DECELERATION INJURY MAY PRODUCE A, DISRUPTION OF THE RENAL ARTERY AND B, THE UTEROPELVIC JUNCTION[186]

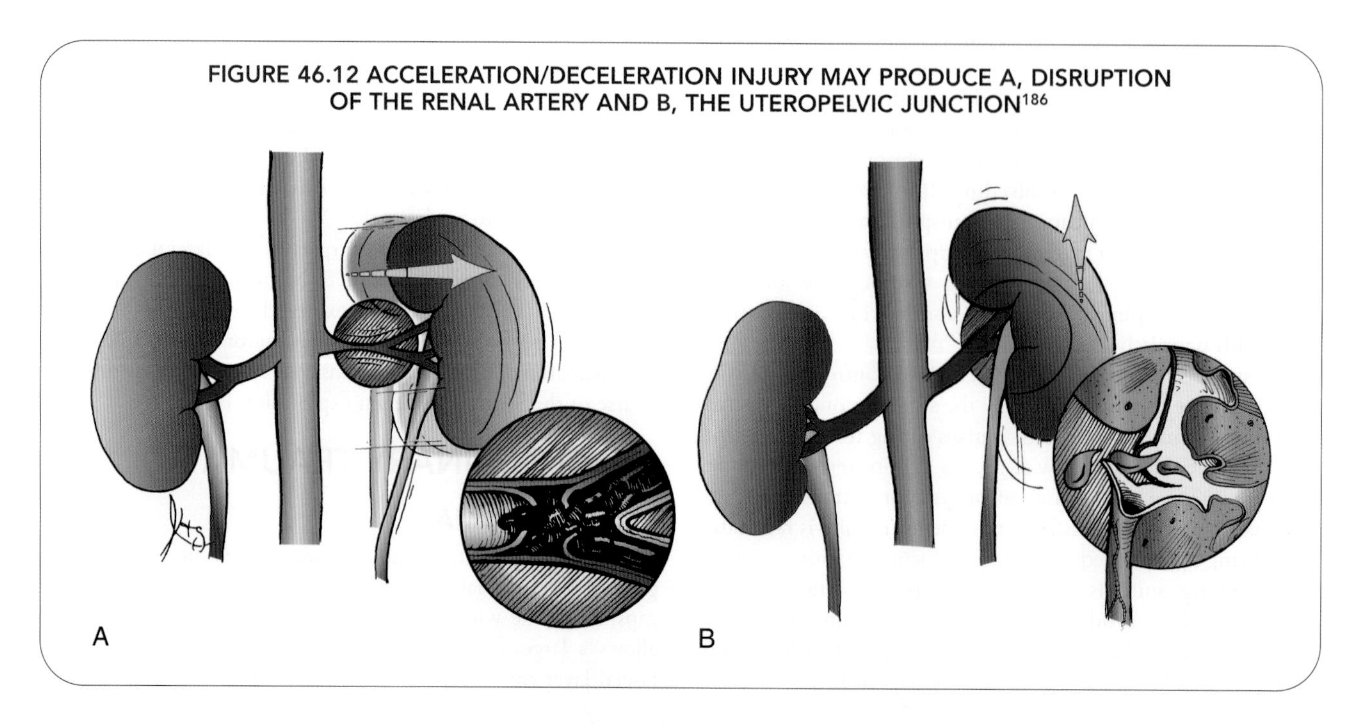

TABLE 46.7 CLASSIFICATION OF RENAL INJURIES[14,77,184,189]

GRADE	TYPE OF INJURY	DESCRIPTION OF INJURY
I	Contusion	Microscopic or gross haematuria, urological studies normal
	Haematoma	Subcapsular, non-expanding without parenchymal laceration
II	Haematoma	Non-expanding perirenal haematoma confined to renal retroperitoneum
	Laceration	$<$ 1.0 cm parenchymal depth of renal cortex without urinary extravasation
III	Laceration	$>$ 1.0 cm parenchymal depth of renal cortex without collecting-system involvement or urinary extravasation
IV	Laceration	Parenchymal laceration extending through renal cortex, medulla and collecting system
	Vascular	Main renal artery or vein injury with contained haemorrhage
V	Laceration	Completely shattered kidney
	Vascular	Avulsion of renal hilum which devascularises kidney

FIGURE 46.13 REVISED RENAL INJURY SCORING SYSTEM[77,192]

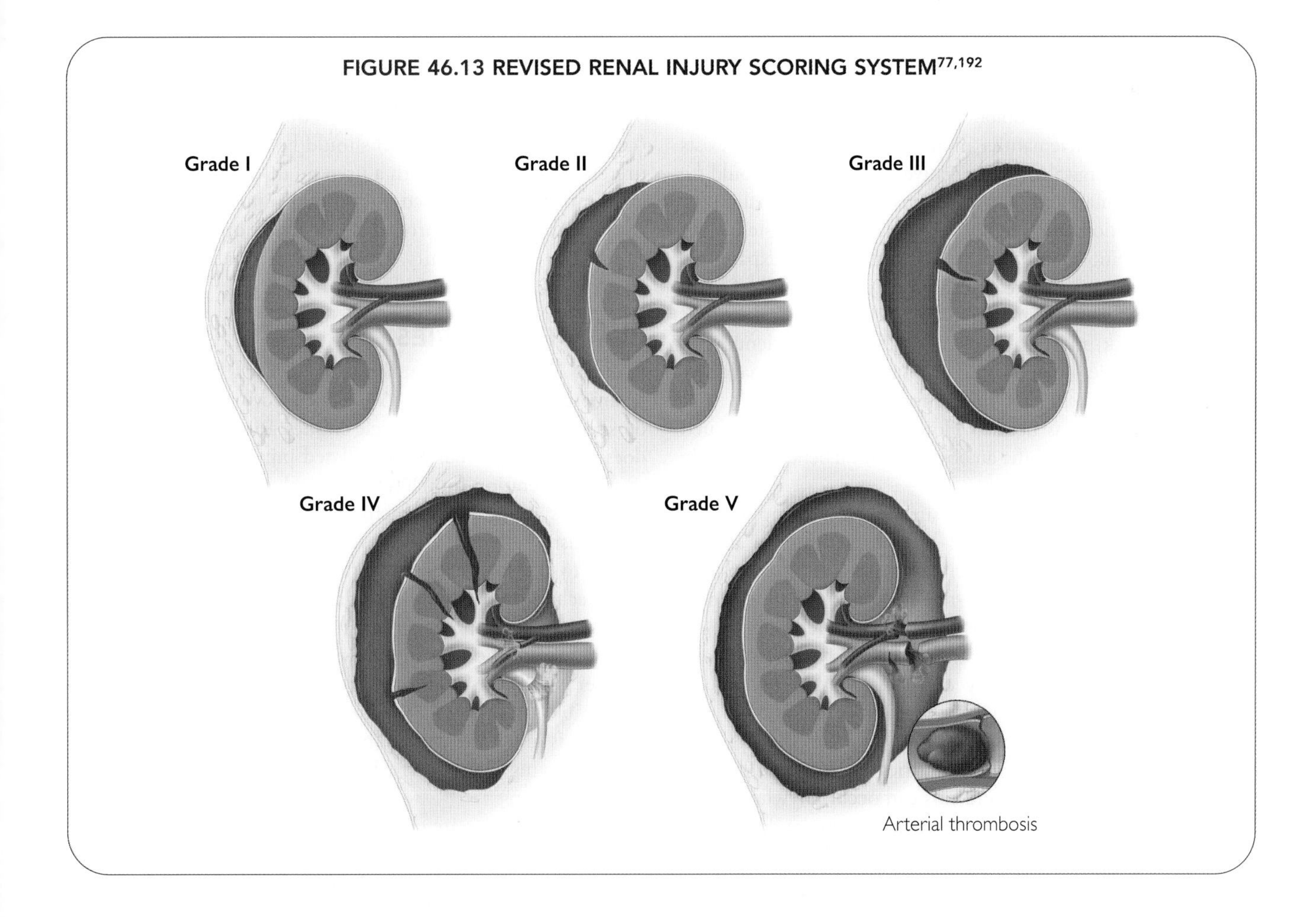

continuing intraoperative haemodynamic instability is often an indication for nephrectomy.[123,144] Postoperatively, an indwelling catheter is present and bed rest is maintained until gross haematuria clears.

Assessment and management

In addition to the assessment discussed earlier, clinical indicators of blunt renal injury include a history of a direct blow to the flank, lower thoracic or upper abdomen, and associated intra-abdominal injuries. Renal injury is often associated with costovertebral angle pain on palpation, lower rib fractures, fracture of the lumbar transverse processes, bruising of the body wall, flank mass and flank tenderness. Patients may develop microscopic or gross haematuria, with urine analysis the most important diagnostic investigation used to assess the patient with suspected renal injury. Haematuria is the best indicator of renal injury; however, the degree of haematuria does not always correlate with degree of injury.[27,92] The gold standard imaging modality to diagnose renal trauma is multi-slice CT with intravenous contrast.[144,192] To identify potential injuries to the collecting system excretory phase, CT is recommended. The primary role of imaging is to assess the severity and extent of injury and it also enables the clinician to evaluate for underlying disease and assess the function of the opposite kidney. Up to 36% of patients with major lacerations or vascular injury and 6–10% of patients with minor lacerations after penetrating trauma do not have haematuria.[102,111] Hypovolaemic shock secondary to a major renal laceration can occur.

Non-operative management for renal injuries has increased in popularity over the last 10 years and should be the first-line treatment option in paediatrics.[193,194] Surgical exploration is mandatory in patients with gunshot wounds, life-threatening haemodynamic instability, expanding/pulsatile perirenal haematoma and grade V vascular injury.[192] Management of stab wounds differs from management of gunshot wounds. Peripheral stab wounds, such as flank wounds posterior to the anterior axillary line, are more likely to injure non-vital structures.

Most blunt renal injuries, particularly grades I, II and III, can be treated non-operatively with hydration, frequent examinations, serial urinalyses, antibiotics and analgesics. Bed rest is required until gross haematuria resolves. Controversy still exists about whether surgical or conservative management should be used in haemodynamically stable patients with severe renal injury. Absolute indications for surgical exploration are persistent, life-threatening haemorrhage, renal pedicle avulsion and expanding, pulsatile or uncontained retroperitoneal haematoma.[195] Unless immediate exploratory laparotomy is indicated for associated injuries or shock, most haemodynamically stable patients with major renal injuries—penetrating or blunt—can be managed by non-surgical treatment and interventional radiology,[80,144] with delayed intervention as needed. However, salvaging the injured kidney does not seem to offer an obvious clinical benefit regarding postoperative renal function.[77]

The nurse should be aware of signs of early complications of renal injury, such as delayed bleeding, urinoma, abscess formation, renal insufficiency, urinary extravasation and fistula formation and renal failure post-nephrectomy.[183,196] Late complications include arteriovenous fistulas, hydronephrosis, stone formation, chronic pyelonephritis and pain. Hypertension can occur after renal artery injury or renal compression injury. Patients may become hypertensive within 24 hours of injury, or onset of hypertension can be delayed up to 10 years after injury. Patients with severe renal injuries are at risk of delayed or secondary haemorrhage, and this can occur anywhere from 2 to 38 days post-injury. These patients require long-term follow-up to identify hypertension, perinephric cysts, arteriovenous fistulas, stones, renal failure and retarded growth in the injured kidney.[197,198]

URETERAL INJURIES

Ureteral injuries are rare and account for only 1% of all GU trauma.[195] This is due to the protected location, small size and mobility of the ureters. Iatrogenic trauma, often following gynaecological surgery, is the leading cause of ureteral injuries, with penetrating trauma the next most-common mechanism.[114,132,190,199] Diagnosis of ureteral injury is difficult because early signs may not be evident on initial examination, with delayed diagnosis resulting in more significant complications. Blunt trauma usually causes avulsion of the ureteropelvic junction subsequent to major hyperextension of upper lumbar and lower thoracic areas. Penetrating injury can cause partial or complete ureteral transection. With penetrating lower abdominal injury, careful examination of the wound with the ureter in mind is essential.

Assessment and management

Physical findings of ureteral injury are non-specific and usually relate to an associated intra-abdominal injury. The clinician needs to have a high index of suspicion based on the mechanism of injury. Only when the ureter is obstructed and produces pain with classic radiation to the groin is diagnosis easy. Haematuria is an unreliable indicator of ureteral trauma, and is absent in 30–45% of cases.[200] Signs of urine leak, such as prolonged ileus, fever and persistent flank or abdominal pain, are indicators of missed ureteral injury.

Extravasation of contrast media is the hallmark sign of ureteral injury following either an IVP or retrograde ureteropyelography.[201] Delayed spiral CT scanning of the kidney 5–8 minutes or longer after injection of contrast medium (during the excretory phase) should be added to visualise the ureters. Most patients with a ureteral injury require operative exploration for associated abdominal injuries.[202] The type of reconstructive repair procedure depends on the nature and site of the ureteral injury. Untreated ureteral injury can lead to urinoma, abscess or stricture.

BLADDER INJURIES

Bladder injuries occur in less than 2% of blunt abdominal trauma cases, with up to 86% associated with ruptured bladders secondary to motor vehicle crashes. Rupture of the bladder does not usually occur as an isolated injury and is mostly due to direct laceration from a fractured pelvic bone, in particular a widened symphysis and sacroiliac joint fracture, or shearing mechanism.[73,191,203,204] The severity of the pelvic fracture correlates to the likelihood of both bladder and urethral injury. The mechanism of injury in bladder rupture varies with patient population, amount of urine in the bladder at the time of injury and location of injury within the bladder. When the bladder is full it rises into the lower abdomen, making it more susceptible to injury.[73] The incidence of bladder trauma in children is much lower than in adults, and is more common in boys following a pelvic crush injury and poorly fitting adult seatbelts.[29,175,202,205,206]

Bladder injuries are classified as contusions, extraperitoneal ruptures, intraperitoneal ruptures and combined injuries.[199,203] Twenty-five per cent are intraperitoneal and usually not associated with pelvic fracture; extraperitoneal bladder ruptures account for 54–56% of bladder trauma (Fig. 46.14), and are seen almost exclusively with pelvic fractures.[129] Injuries are usually caused by a suprapubic blow in the presence of a full bladder. The bladder tends to rupture at the weakest point (i.e. dome or posterior wall of the bladder). Intraperitoneal ruptures involve extravasation of blood and urine into the peritoneal cavity. Extraperitoneal bladder rupture involves perforation of

FIGURE 46.14 MECHANISM OF EXTRAPERITONEAL URINARY BLADDER RUPTURE

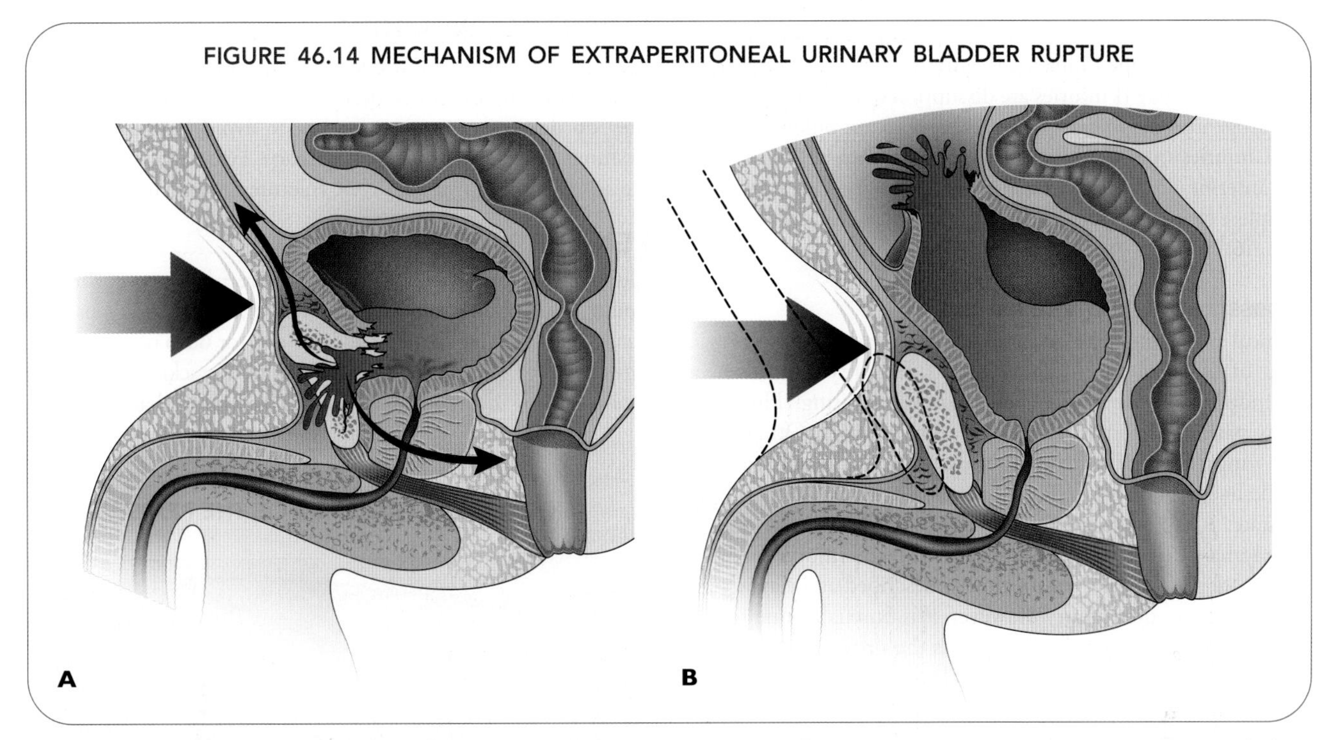

A. The public rami are fractured, and the bladder is perforated by a bony fragment. **B.** Mechanism of intraperitoneal vesical rupture. A sharp blow is delivered to the lower abdomen of a patient with a distended urinary bladder. The distensive force is exerted on all surfaces of the bladder, and it ruptures at its weakest point, usually the dome.[190]

the anterolateral bladder with extravasation of blood and urine into the retroperitoneal space. Combined intraperitoneal and extraperitoneal ruptures occur in up to 8% of cases, are associated with severe pelvic injury and are mainly diagnosed during surgery.[207]

Assessment and management

The classic combination of pelvic fracture and haematuria indicates immediate further investigation. Up to 95% of patients will have gross haematuria.[208] Often patients with bladder perforation are unable to void and have suprapubic pain. Haemodynamic instability is common because of extensive blood loss in the pelvis and associated injuries. Late signs and symptoms are abdominal distension, acute abdomen and increased blood urea nitrogen and serum creatinine levels.

Radiographic evaluation consists of retrograde urethrogram and cystogram in all male patients with pelvic fractures associated with gross haematuria, inability to urinate, blood at the meatus, perineal swelling or non-palpable prostate. Addressing haemodynamic instability should remain the priority and non-urgent investigations should be undertaken at an appropriate time. Insertion of an indwelling catheter prior to radiographic imaging remains controversial due to the potential for damage to the associated urethra.[209]

Female patients with a pelvic fracture should undergo careful visual inspection of the urethra. Extraperitoneal bladder rupture is managed conservatively with drainage (via either a Foley or a suprapubic catheter),[172,191,205] antibiotics and close clinical observation for sepsis. A repeat cystogram around day 10 often reveals a healed bladder, although approximately 15% of bladder ruptures may take up to 3 weeks to heal. Intraperitoneal ruptures do not close spontaneously and require surgical repair, which has been shown to significantly decrease associated morbidity.[136,153,159] Bladder injuries can lead to urinary ascites, abscess formation and urinary fistula formation and peritonitis.

URETHRAL INJURIES

A urethral injury should be suspected in any patient with a history of perineal or pelvic trauma (Chapter 48). Certain fracture locations are associated with increased risk for urethral injury; these are the sacroiliac joint, a widened symphysis and fracture of the inferior pubic ramus. Urethral trauma is much more common in men (75%) than women due to their longer urethra. Urethral injuries in females are rare and are usually associated with a significant pelvic fracture,[29,73,209,210] obstetric injury or anterior vaginal lacerations with labial oedema and haematuria present.[29,209] Proximal urethral injuries almost invariably occur in men secondary to a MVC (68–84%) or fall from height (6–25%). Iatrogenic injury to the urethra is not uncommon and can occur from traumatic catheter placement or transurethral procedures.

Traumatic urethral injuries are usually caused by shearing rather than direct laceration. If the injury is superior, the prostate can be forced upwards by a developing haematoma. In addition, 5–10% of patients with bladder rupture caused by pelvic trauma have a concomitant urethral injury.[29,197] Injuries to the anterior urethra can occur as a result of straddle injury, blunt trauma or sharp trauma to the penis caused by passage of a foreign body. Blunt trauma to the posterior urethra causes three general types of injuries, which may be incomplete or complete. With type I injuries, the urethra is stretched but does not rupture. Type II injuries are disruption of the urethra above the urogenital diaphragm; type III injuries are bulbomembranous injuries inferior to the urogenital diaphragm. Injuries to the anterior urethra are classified as contusions or partial or complete lacerations and frequently result from straddle injuries (Fig. 46.15).

Assessment and management

Clinical symptoms may be variable. Some patients have classic signs of blood at the urethral meatus, inability to urinate, a distended, palpable bladder and perineal bruising. However, many patients with partial urethral tears can void. Other signs and symptoms include pain on micturition; perineal, scrotal or penile haematoma or swelling; haematuria; and a 'high-riding' prostate. A digital rectal examination should be performed in all trauma patients to exclude associated rectal injury. Inability to palpate the prostate was previously described as a classic sign of posterior urethral injury; however, it is unreliable due to the significant haematoma that surrounds the prostate following a pelvic fracture, and only 34% of male patients will have a displaced prostate. A retrograde urethrogram is the study of choice for evaluation of urethral injuries.[29,32,73,199,210]

A urethral catheter should not be inserted if urethral injury is suspected. Such a procedure can convert a partial urethral disruption into a complete one, raise the risk of contamination and increase the risk of further haemorrhage. Absence of blood at the meatus and a palpable prostate on rectal examination are sufficient evidence to allow passage of a urethral catheter. Diagnostic investigation with a retrograde urethrogram is preferable prior to catheterisation. Postoperatively the patient is allowed to ambulate, but sitting is not advisable, requires intravenous antibiotics and erections are suppressed with diazepam. Impotence, urethral stricture and incontinence are the most severe complications of posterior urethral disruption. With anterior urethral injury, stricture formation is the most common complication. In females, urethral and bladder neck injury can cause significant sexual and lower urinary tract dysfunction.[207]

GENITAL INJURIES

Testicular and penile injuries are not common.[198,210–212] Injuries to the penis, testes and scrotum are rarely life threatening, but they do demand prompt attention to avoid long-term sexual dysfunction and psychological damage. Female genital injuries are associated with severe pelvic fractures and sexual assault.

PENILE TRAUMA

Blunt trauma to the erect penis via a direct hit can rupture the tunica albuginea surrounding the corpora cavernosa, causing a penile fracture (Fig. 46.16), and accounts for 60% of penile fractures.[198,212,214] The patient typically reports a 'cracking or popping sound' during intercourse, sexual play or masturbation, which

FIGURE 46.16 FRACTURE OF THE PENIS[213]

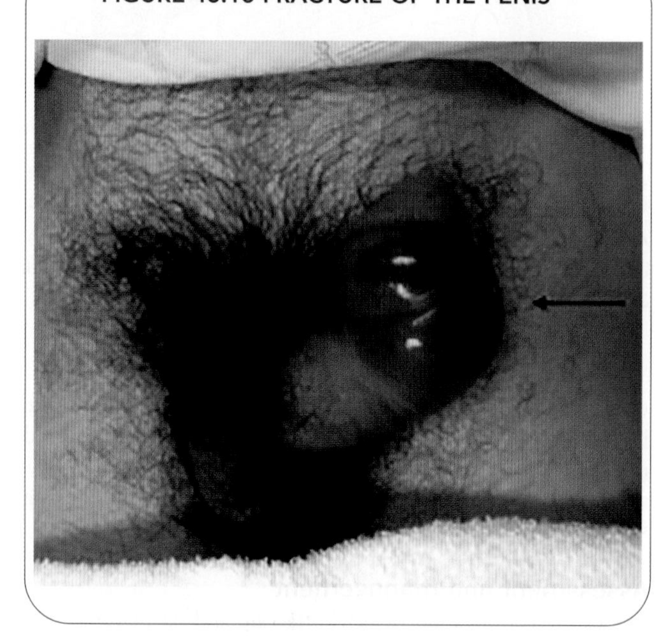

Traumatic rupture of the corpus cavernosum, usually associated with sexual activity, results in a profound penile haematoma most often requiring operative repair.

FIGURE 46.15 MECHANISM OF BLUNT ANTERIOR URETHRAL TRAUMA

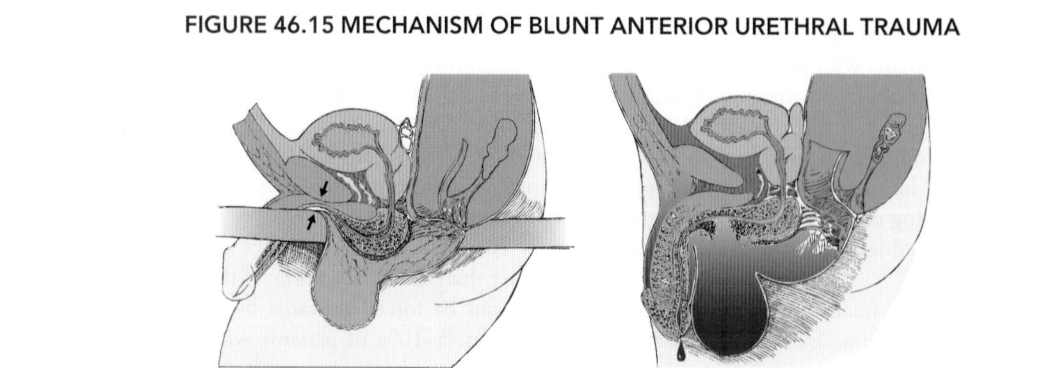

A. Straddle injury illustrating the bulbous urethra crushed against the pubic symphysis. **B.** Resulting urethral disruption with haemorrhage extending along the confines of Colles' fascia. Buck's fascia has been disrupted.[197]

results in severe pain and immediate detumescence. A haematoma with marked oedema develops in the penile shaft. Diagnosis is frequently made on clinical presentation. Most patients are able to void, but blood at the meatus and inability to void often indicates a lacerated urethra, so urethrography should be considered. Penetrating and degloving injuries of the penis can occur in the workplace. Penetrating injuries mandate exploration and reconstruction with liberal antibiotic coverage.[206]

Early surgical repair gives better outcomes of function and appearance, and is associated with a lower risk of adverse complications that have previously been associated with non-operative management, i.e. persistent penile angulation, longer hospital stay, missed urethral injury and more rapid functional return. Adequate analgesia is required until surgery commences.[185] Conservative treatment is only warranted in cases with minimal haematoma and no extravasation during a cavernosography. Treatment includes non-steroidal analgesia, ice packs and elevation of the penis. Sexually-related injuries involving strangulation or amputation of the penis have also been reported, and usually occur as a result of assault or self-inflicted wounds. Traumatic amputation requires preservation of the severed penis, as microsurgical reanastomosis is possible. Other penile injuries may be due to direct trauma from zippers, bites, machines or knives. Treatment is determined by the severity of the injury.

TESTICULAR TRAUMA

Traumatic injury to the testicles is an infrequent occurrence despite their exposed position in the male perineum. Injuries typically occur in young men, usually aged 15–40 years. Blunt trauma to the scrotum, such as from kicking and kneeing during rugby matches, accounts for approximately 85% of cases and can cause testicular rupture.[210,216,217] The patient with a scrotal injury may have acute pain, nausea, vomiting, syncope and urinary retention. Patients can have large scrotal haematomas that make examination difficult; therefore, scrotal ultrasound imaging with Doppler studies is the most sensitive and specific imaging modality to assess the vascularity and integrity of the testes.[216]

Minor cases are treated conservatively with scrotal support, non-steroidal analgesia, ice packs and bed rest for 24–48 hours.[27,182] Testicular rupture is best diagnosed on ultrasound and, if highly suspected or confirmed, should be repaired immediately as testicular salvage rates of 90% within the first 72 hours have been reported. All penetrating testicular injuries should be explored and repaired. Orchidectomy is necessary in some cases, but rarely indicated unless the entire testis is completely infarcted or shattered.

Avulsion injuries can cause loss of all or part of penile and scrotal skin (Fig. 46.17). Industrial or farming incidents are often responsible for such injuries. The penile shaft can be covered with skin grafts; return of function is expected. Partial scrotal skin loss is managed by primary closure. The scrotum regenerates to accommodate the testicles and spermatic cords. Total skin loss leaves the testicles unprotected, so the testicles are placed temporarily in thigh pouches when immediate grafting is not possible.

FIGURE 46.17 INJURIES INFLICTED BY A MANURE SPREADER[218]

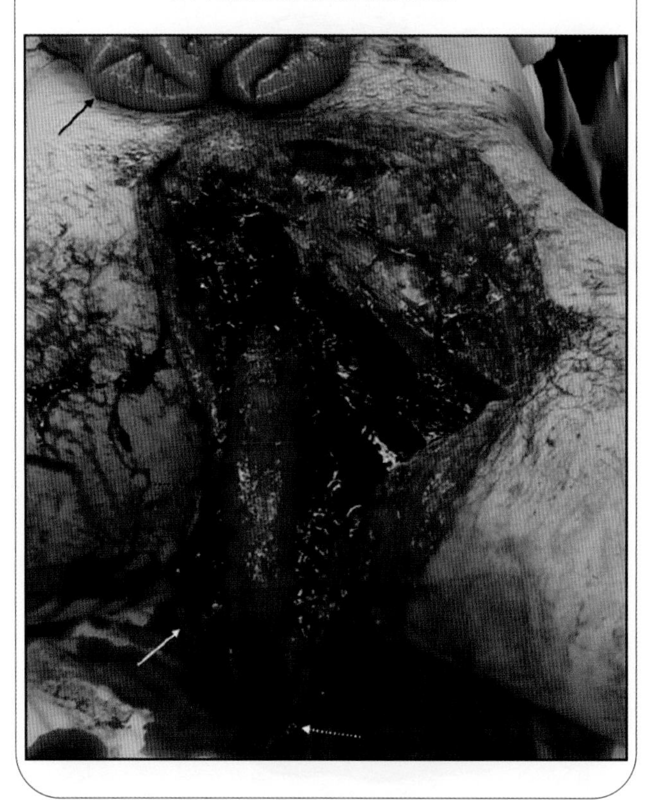

The groin laceration resulted in penis degloving (dashed black arrow), left lacerated spermatic cord (dashed white arrow), and right avulsed testicle (white arrow). The eviscerated bowel (black arrow) extrudes through an abdominal laceration (not shown).

STRADDLE INJURIES

Straddle injuries occur when a patient falls and takes the brunt of the fall on the perineum. The blow to the perineum compresses the perineal tissues and underlying urethra against the external object and the symphysis pubis.[219] These injuries commonly occur in young patients as they fall onto bicycle bars, motorcycles and fences, and can have a characteristic butterfly-shaped bruised area beneath the scrotum (Fig. 46.18). On examination of a female patient, a vulvovaginal laceration with extensive ecchymosis of the perineum may be evident. Straddle injuries in both sexes may result in blood at the meatus; and in men, many are unable to void. Associated urethral injuries and rectal tears should be ruled out. Insertion of urethral catheters should be avoided until after a retrograde urethrogram.[73]

Treatment of straddle injuries involves repair of the laceration with evacuation and drainage of haematomas. A supra-pubic and a urethral catheter are required postoperatively for 3–4 days. The urethral catheter is left in situ for 2–3 weeks. The most common complication in the immediate postoperative period is infection. Erectile dysfunction may also occur long term.

FEMALE GENITAL INJURIES

Female genital injuries are less common than male genital injuries; however, regardless of the mechanism of injury, all external genital injuries in females increase the suspicion of internal injuries and warrant further investigation. Vaginal bleeding is associated with pelvic fractures and urethral injuries, and requires a urethrogram. Female genital injuries occur in 20–53% of sexual assault victims,[215] and nursing support during physical

FIGURE 46.18

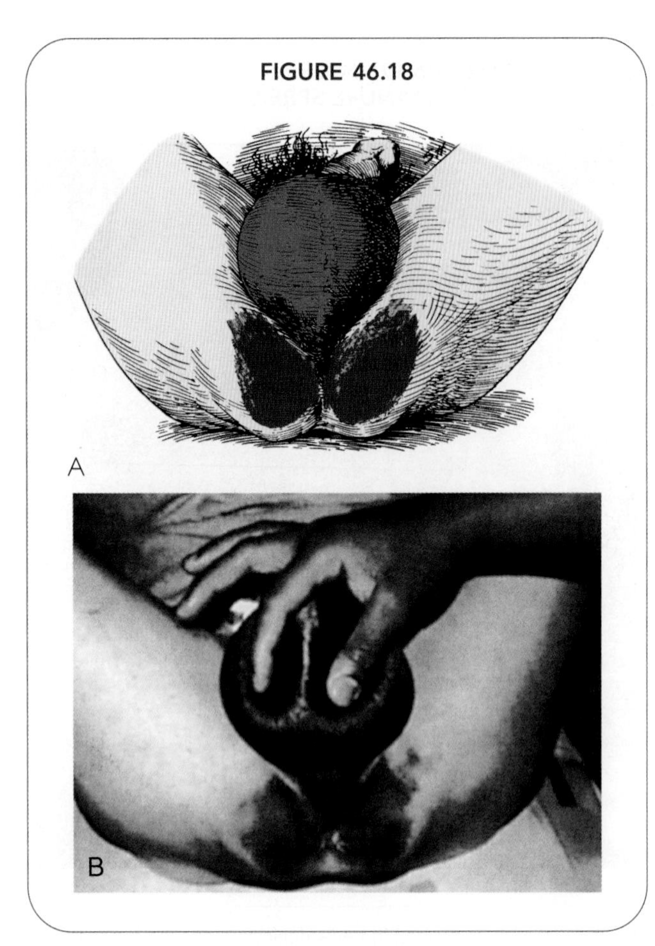

A. Diagram of a butterfly haematoma. **B.** Appearance of a patient with perineal butterfly haematoma.[190]

assessment and collection of specimens is required. Vulvar injuries, such as lacerations, can also be due to sports-related straddle-type injuries or from high-pressure water spray during water-based sports, and commonly present as haematomas. These injuries require non-steroidal analgesia and cold packs and, if the laceration or contusion is extensive, vulvar injuries require surgical intervention, drainage and repair and postoperative antibiotics. Internal lacerations may require speculum examinations under sedation to repair the laceration. Vaginal packing is used to establish haemostasis. Unrecognised genital injuries in females may result in abscess formation, vesicovaginal fistulae, sepsis and death.[220,221]

All clinicians should consider sexual abuse as a cause of both female and male genital trauma unless the mechanism is irrefutable.[73] Rarely seen in the Western world is injury from ritual genital surgery, which affects gynaecological, obstetric and sexual health. Given the large numbers of refugees and asylum seekers worldwide, such cases may increase slightly in the future.

RECTAL INJURIES

Rectal injury is rare, with a reported incidence of approximately 1 to 3% in civilian trauma centres,[33,222] but can lead to significant complications, and if missed are associated with an increased mortality rate. In blunt trauma, rectal injury is most commonly associated with complex pelvic fractures, particularly when the symphysis pubis is widened, and in penetrating trauma, with wounds, particularly gunshot, to the abdomen, thigh or buttock. During the secondary survey, findings of pelvic instability, blood at the urethral meatus, soft-tissue defect of the perineum, or penetrating injury near the pelvis should raise the index of suspicion for rectal trauma. Rectal examination, with the purpose of identifying blood, should be performed on all these patient groups, but diagnosis (or exclusion) of rectal injuries should not solely rely on the digital rectal examination which only has sensitivity of 33–52% for rectal injury. In the at-risk patient, a combination of diagnostics including a rectal examination, computed tomography (CT), contrast enema studies and endoscopy[223] may be used.[33,222]

OTHER CONSIDERATIONS

The volume and contents of drains should be recorded consistently throughout a 24-hour period. Abdominal dressings should be assessed daily for signs of infection (erythema, swelling, discharge, pain) and the dressing changed. Superficial wound infection can be managed by removing the skin sutures or clips. Deep wound infections or dehiscence of the wound requires a return to the operating room. Stomas should be monitored for viability and content of the stoma bag. An ischaemic or obviously necrotic stoma may necessitate a return to the operating room. Patients whose emergency laparotomy is delayed are at significantly higher risk of mortality and complication development.[224,225] Fascial dehiscence after trauma laparotomy is associated with technical failure, wound sepsis or intra-abdominal infection. Malnourishment and malignant obstructive jaundice predispose a patient to wound dehiscence by slowing the healing, and increasing the rate of wound infection.[224–226]

PRACTICE TIP

Triage and emergency nurses should have a high index of suspicion for missed abdominal injuries if patients re-present to ED with abdominal pain or other symptoms such as vomiting or haematuria and a recent history of abdominal trauma.

SUMMARY

Abdominal trauma is a significant cause of morbidity and mortality, and the patient can have life-threatening injuries with minimal evidence of injury or initially obvious clinical signs. This increases the importance of techniques such as FAST and CT in the thorough investigation of potential abdominal injury. The emergency nurse must assume that an injury is present until the possibility is ruled out. Consideration of how the patient was injured can highlight potential injuries and enhance patient assessment. GU trauma can be readily identified clinically and the extent of injury ascertained with radiographic imaging. An injured patient with potential urological injury has a host of general surgical concerns, particularly in conjunction with pelvic fractures; however, life-threatening concerns related to airway control, ventilation and haemodynamic status are still the priority. Decisions regarding urinary catheterisation are particularly important for these patients.

Ongoing assessment is critical for the patient with abdominal trauma; the patient's condition can change as the patient experiences continued blood loss or responds to bacterial contamination from a perforated intestine. Unstable patients who present with the lethal diamond of hypothermia, coagulopathy, hypocalcaemia and metabolic acidosis or show signs of deterioration may benefit from damage-control surgery. Operative management of these patients is often only the beginning of a long recovery phase, much of which is improved by attention to detail and continual reassessment of the patient. Success in returning abdominal trauma patients back to the community requires early recognition of injury and transfer to definitive care, coordination of a multidisciplinary trauma team and early involvement of healthcare professionals experienced in abdominal trauma.

CASE STUDY

It is 1130 hours when paramedics attend the scene of a motor vehicle collision. The following information is provided:

- *Mechanism:* A 25-year-old female restrained rear seat passenger in a high-speed MVC; hit telegraph pole driver's side. Self-extricated. The driver of the vehicle is deceased.
- *Injuries:* No LOC, c/o pain in neck, left shoulder and left upper quadrant pain. Seatbelt abrasion on neck, chest and abdomen.
- *Signs:* HR 74, BP 106/74, RR 20, SpO_2 98%, GCS 4,5,6, PEARTL, skin pale, radial pulse present.

QUESTIONS

1. What are your priorities as the paramedic assessing this patient?
2. In the emergency department (ED), you have received pre-hospital notification with a 15-minute estimated time of arrival of the patient. What will you do to prepare for the patient with the information provided by the paramedics?
3. What part of the MIST are you concerned about?

The patient arrives 15 minutes later. She is triaged as a category 1 and is offloaded into the resuscitation room where a full trauma team has assembled.

PRIMARY SURVEY

A: Patent, talking, cervical soft foam collar in situ

B: Spontaneous, good and equal air entry, trachea midline, SpO_2 98% on room air

C: HR 81, BP85/45, no external sites of bleeding

D: GCS 15, PEARTL, equal limb strength

E: T 35.3°C

4. What is your priority here?
5. What are the adjuncts to the primary survey you would like to see?
   - The patient receives an IDC and her βhCG is negative
   - FAST scan at 1155 hrs is positive
   - ABG
6. What does a positive FAST scan indicate?
7. Where are the possible sites of bleeding in the abdomen?
8. Where should this patient go and why?

TIME	TEMP. °C	PULSE BPM	BP mmHg	RR PER min	SpO_2	FiO_2
1154	35.3	82	85/45	12	98%	R/A
1155		75	85/45 manual BP	17	99%	
1200		85	75/45	26	100%	
1211		75	89/55	22	100%	

Observations in the ED

pH	7.26
CO_2	38
O_2	98
Hb	116
HCO_3	17
BE	-9.2
Lac	2.7

ABG on 15L PNRB

9. What does her ABG indicate?

   The patient receives 4 units of packed red blood cells and the first unit of FFP is commenced.

   A – Nil known

   M – Nil

   P – IVDU

   L – > 8 hours

   E – Refer to MIST handover

10. Where should the patient go now and why?

Answers to Case Study Questions can be found on evolve **http://evolve.elsevier.com/AU/Curtis/emergency/**

USEFUL WEBSITES

Eastern Association for the Surgery of Trauma, US site: The Eastern Association for the Surgery of Trauma (EAST) provides a forum for the exchange of knowledge to advance the care and rehabilitation of the injured patient. EAST places particular emphasis on interdisciplinary collaboration, scholarship, fellowship and developing leadership among young surgeons active in the care of the injured patient, www.east.org.

NSW ACI clinical procedures app–short videos of 100 of the most common emergency procedures available online or as a free app, https://aci.health.nsw.gov.au/networks/eci/clinical/procedures.

NSW Institute of Trauma and Injury Management (ITIM). Australian site: The NSW Institute of Trauma and Injury Management (ITIM), an institute within the Agency for Clinical Innovation (ACI), is the body responsible for overseeing, coordinating and supporting the NSW trauma system. It has some useful educational tools, including videos of talks by trauma clinicians throughout the state, www.aci.health.nsw.gov.au/networks/itim.

Trauma.org, UK site: trauma.org is an independent, non-profit organisation providing global education, information and communication resources for professionals in trauma and critical care, www.trauma.org.

Obstetric and gynaecological guidelines

Australian site that provides clear algorithms for the minimum standard of care for the pregnant trauma patient,

https://trauma.reach.vic.gov.au/guidelines/obstetric-trauma/rapid-reference-guideline.

A useful video demonstrating the technique for diagnostic peritoneal aspiration (DPL) can be found at https://youtu.be/O9BZamRIXVA.

ITIM app: For NSW health professionals this is a handy app to download which contains major trauma hospital protocols, guidelines and contact details, as well as other trauma-related information.

REFERENCES

1. Rasmussen TE, Tai NRM. Australia and New Zealand. In: Rasmussen TE, Tai NRM, editors. Rich's vascular trauma. 3rd ed. Philadelphia: Elsevier; 2016.
2. Arslan S, Okur MH, Arslan MS, Aydogdu B, Zeytun H, Basuguy E, et al. Management of gastrointestinal perforation from blunt and penetrating abdominal trauma in children: analysis of 96 patients. Pediatr Surg Int 2016;32(11):1067–173.
3. Brenner M, Hicks C. Major abdominal trauma: critical decisions and new frontiers in management. Emerg Med Clin North Am 2018;36(1):149–60.
4. Stillwell S. Mosby's critical care nursing reference. 4th ed. St Louis: Mosby; 2006.
5. Thibodeau GA, Patton KT. Anatomy and physiology. 7th ed. St Louis: Mosby; 2010.
6. Muckart DJ, Bhagwanjee S. American College of Chest Physicians/Society of Critical Care Medicine Consensus Conference definitions of the systemic inflammatory response syndrome and allied disorders in relation to critically injured patients. Crit Care Med 1997;25(11):1789–95.
7. Bone RC, Balk RA, Cerra FB, Dellinger RP, Fein AM, Knaus WA, et al. Definitions for sepsis and organ failure and guidelines for the use of innovative therapies in sepsis. The ACCP/SCCM Consensus Conference Committee. Chest 1992;101(6):1644–55.
8. McGeady JB, Breyer BN. Current epidemiology of genitourinary trauma. Urol Clin North Am 2013;40(3):323–34.
9. Bège T, Brunet C, Berdah SV. Hollow viscus injury due to blunt trauma: a review. J Visc Surg 2016;153(Suppl. 4):61–8.
10. ACI and ITIM. Trauma 'Code Crimson' pathway: streamlining access to definitive intervention in life-threatening haemorrhage. 31 January 2019. Available from: Trauma-Code-Crimson-Pathway-Final-20170919.pdf.
11. Oliver M, Dinh MM, Curtis K, Paschkewitz R, Rigby O, Balogh ZJ. Trends in procedures at major trauma centres in New South Wales, Australia: an analysis of state-wide trauma data. World J Surg 2017;41(8):2000–5.
12. Boutros SM, Nassef MA, Abdel-Ghany AF. Blunt abdominal trauma: the role of focused abdominal sonography in assessment of organ injury and reducing the need for CT. Alexand J Med 2016;52(1):35–41.

13. Akoglu H, Celik OF, Celik A, Ergelen R, Onur O, Denizbasi A. Diagnostic accuracy of the Extended Focused Abdominal Sonography for Trauma (E-FAST) performed by emergency physicians compared to computed tomography. Am J Emerg Med 2017;36(6):1014–17.
14. Brown CV, Velmahos GC, Neville AL, Rhee P, Salim A, Sangthong B, et al. Hemodynamically stable patients with peritonitis after penetrating abdominal trauma: identifying those who are bleeding. Arch Surg 2005;140(8):767–72.
15. Cameron P, Jelinek G, Kelly AM, Murray L, Brown AFT, Heyworth J, editors. Textbook of adult emergency medicine. 2nd ed. Edinburgh: Churchill Livingstone; 2004.
16. Ahmed N, Whelan J, Brownlee J, Chari V, Chung R. The contribution of laparoscopy in evaluation of penetrating abdominal wounds. J Am Coll Surg 2005;201(2):213–16.
17. Spahn DR, Bouillon B, Cerny V, Coats TJ, Duranteau J, Fernández-Mondéjar E, et al. Management of bleeding and coagulopathy following major trauma: an updated European guideline. Crit Care 2013;17(2):R76.
18. Masudi T, McMahon HC, Scott JL, Lockey AS. Seat belt-related injuries: a surgical perspective. J Emerg Trauma Shock 2017;10(2):70–3.
19. Onu DO, Hunn AW, Bohmer RD. Seat belt syndrome with unstable Chance fracture dislocation of the second lumbar vertebra without neurological deficits. BMJ Case Rep 2014;2014:bcr2013202412.
20. Vailas MG, Moris D, Orfanos S, Vergadis C, Papalampros A. Seatbelt sign in a case of blunt abdominal trauma; what lies beneath it? BMC Surg 2015;15:121.
21. Hayes C, Conway W, Walsh J, Coppage L, Gervin A. Seat belt injuries: radiologic findings and clinical correlation. Radiographics 1991;11(1):23–36.
22. Chandler CF, Lane JS, Waxman KS. Seatbelt sign following blunt trauma is associated with increased incidence of abdominal injury. Am Surg 1997;63(10):885–8.
23. Glover JM, Waychoff MF, Casmaer M, April MD, Hunter CJ, Trexler ST, et al. Association between seatbelt sign and internal injuries in the contemporary airbag era: a retrospective cohort study. Am J Emerg Med 2018;36(4):545–50.
24. Elliot D, Aitken L, Chaboyer W. ACCCN's critical care nursing. Sydney: Elsevier; 2006.
25. Coleman JJ, Zarzaur BL. Surgical management of abdominal trauma: hollow viscus injury. Surg Clin North Am 2017;97(5):1107–17.
26. Emery M, Flannigan M. How useful are clinical findings in patients with blunt abdominal trauma? Ann Emerg Med 2014;63(4):463–4.
27. Gondek S, Schroeder ME, Sarani B. Assessment and resuscitation in trauma management. Surg Clin North Am 2017;97(5):985–98.
28. Morey AF, Brandes S, Dugi DD, Armstrong JH, Breyer BN, Broghammer JA, et al. Urotrauma: AUA guideline. J Urol 2014;192(2):327–35.
29. Wardak SW, Nuttall MC. Genitourinary trauma. Surgery (Oxford) 2016;34(7):361–8.
30. Johnsen NV, Betzold RD, Guillamondegui OD, Dennis BM, Stassen NA, Bhullar I, et al. Surgical management of solid organ injuries. Surg Clin North Am 2017;97(5):1077–105.
31. Johnsen NV, Dmochowski RR, Young JB, Guillamondegui OD. Epidemiology of blunt lower urinary tract trauma with and without pelvic fracture. Urology 2017;102(Suppl. C):234–9.
32. Johnson MH, Chang A, Brandes SB. The value of digital rectal examination in assessing for pelvic fracture–associated urethral injury: what defines a high-riding or nonpalpable prostate? J Trauma Acute Care Surg 2013;75(5):913–15.
33. Jihun G, Min AL, Byungchul Y, Kang KC. Rectal injury associated with pelvic fracture. J Korean Soc Traumatol 2016;29(4):201–3.
34. Briggs C. An emerging trend in domestic violence: technology-facilitated abuse. Aust J Child Fam Health Nurs 2018;15(1):2.
35. Australian Institute of Health and Welfare (AIHW). New national statistical report sheds light on family violence. Canberra: Australian Government. 2018. Online. Available from: www.aihw.gov.au/news-media/media-releases/2018/february/new-national-statistical-report-sheds-light-on-fam.
36. Atkinson AL, Santolaya-Forgas J, Blitzer DN, Santolaya JL, Matta P, Canterino J, et al. Risk factors for perinatal mortality in patients admitted to the hospital with the diagnosis of placental abruption. J Matern Fetal Neonatal Med 2015;28(5):594–7.
37. Battaloglu E, McDonnell D, Chu J, Lecky F, Porter K. Epidemiology and outcomes of pregnancy and obstetric complications in trauma in the United Kingdom. Injury 2016;47(1):184–7.
38. Pearce C, Martin SR. Trauma and considerations unique to pregnancy. Obstet Gynecol Clin North Am 2016;43(4):791–808.
39. Jain V, Chari R, Maslovitz S, Farine D. Guidelines for the management of a pregnant trauma patient. J Obstet Gynaecol Can 2015;37(6):553–71.
40. Mendez-Figueroa H, Dahlke JD, Rouse DJ. Trauma in pregnancy: an updated systematic review. Am J Obstet Gynaecol 2013;209(1):1–10.
41. Sperry JL, Heller MT. The pregnant trauma patient. In: Falter F, Screaton NJ, editors. Imaging the ICU patient. London: Springer London; 2014.
42. Meisinger QC, Brown MA, Dehqanzada ZA, Doucet J, Coimbra R, Casola G. A 10-year restrospective evaluation of ultrasound in pregnant abdominal trauma patients. Emerg Radiol 2016;23(2):105–9.
43. Horstmann P, Larsen CF, Grønborg H. Adherence to protocol in pregnant trauma patients? A 12-year retrospective study. Euro J Trauma Emerg Surg 2014;40(5):561–6.
44. Hansen W, Moshiri M, Paladin A, Lamba R, Katz DS, Bhargava P. Evolving practice patterns in imaging pregnant patients with acute abdominal and pelvic conditions. Curr Prob Diagn Radiol 2017;46(1):10–16.
45. Raptis CA, Mellnick VM, Raptis DA, Kitchin D, Fowler KJ, Lubner M, et al. Imaging of trauma in the pregnant patient. Radiographics 2014;34(3):748–63.
46. Lucia A, Dantoni SE. Trauma management of the pregnant patient. Crit Care Clin 2016;32(1):109–17.
47. Petrone P, Jiménez-Morillas P, Axelrad A, Marini CP. Traumatic injuries to the pregnant patient: a critical literature review. Eur J Trauma Emerg Surg 2019;45(3):383–92.

48. Muench MV, Canterino JC. Trauma in pregnancy. Obstet Gynecol Clin North Am 2007;34(3):555–83.
49. van der Knoop BJ, Zonnenberg IA, Otten VM, van Weissenbruch MM, de Vries JIP. Trauma in pregnancy, obstetrical outcome in a tertiary centre in the Netherlands. J Matern Fetal Neonatal Med 2018;31(3):339–46.
50. Bouyou J, Gaujoux S, Marcellin L, Goffinet F, Chapron C, Dousset B. Abdominal emergencies during pregnancy. J Visc Surg 2015;152(Suppl. 6): S105–15.
51. Rostas J, Cason B, Simmons J, Frotan MA, Brevard SB, Gonzalez RP. The validity of abdominal examination in blunt trauma patients with distracting injuries. J Trauma Acute Care Surg 2015;78(6):1095–101.
52. Cameron P, Jelinek G, Kelly A, Murray L, Brown AF, Heyworth J, editors. Textbook of adult emergency medicine. 2nd ed. Edinburgh: Churchill Livingstone; 2004.
53. Lai CC, Huang HC, Chen RJ. Combined stomach and duodenal perforating injury following blunt abdominal trauma: a case report and literature review. BMC Surg 2020;20(1):217.
54. Catalano O. Abdominal trauma. In: Allan PL, Baxter GM, Weston MJ, editors. Clinical ultrasound. 3rd ed. United Kingdom: Elsevier Churchill Livingstone; 2011.
55. Carter JW, Falco MH, Chopko MS, Flynn Jr WJ, Wiles Iii CE, Guo WA. Do we really rely on fast for decision-making in the management of blunt abdominal trauma? Injury 2015;46(5):817-21.
56. Bowra J, Forrest-Horder S, Caldwell E, Cox M, D'Amours SK. Validation of nurse-performed FAST ultrasound. Injury 2010;41(5):484–7.
57. Frongillo E, Rea G, Tinti MG, Sperandeo M. Limitations of Focused Assessment with Sonography in Trauma (FAST) protocols in transthoracic US. Radiology 2017;285(2):693–4.
58. Hamada SR, Delhaye N, Kerever S, Harrois A, Duranteau J. Integrating eFAST in the initial management of stable trauma patients: the end of plain film radiography. Ann Intens Care 2016;6(1):62.
59. Talari H, Moussavi N, Abedzadeh-Kalahroudi M, Atoof F, Abedini A. Correlation between intra-abdominal free fluid and solid organ injury in blunt abdominal trauma. Arch Trauma Res 2015;4(3):e29184.
60. Gratton R, Olaussen A, Hassan M, Thaveenthrian P, Fitzgerald MC, Mitra B. Diagnostic performance of the cardiac FAST in a high-volume Australian trauma centre. J Emerg Med Trauma Acute Care 2017;2017(1):2.
61. Sue KMDC. The occasional ED ultrasound: focused assessment with sonography for trauma (FAST). Can J Rural Med 2015;20(1):33–9.
62. Montoya J, Stawicki SP, Evans DC, Bahner DP, Sparks S, Sharpe RP, et al. From FAST to E-FAST: an overview of the evolution of ultrasound-based traumatic injury assessment. Eur J Trauma Emerg Surg 2016;42(2):119–26.
63. Kumar S, Kumar A, Joshi MK, Rathi V. Comparison of diagnostic peritoneal lavage and focused assessment by sonography in trauma as an adjunct to primary survey in torso trauma: a prospective randomized clinical trial. Ulus Travma Acil Cerrahi Derg 2014;20(2):101–6.
64. Heidari K, Taghizadeh M, Mahmoudi S, Panahi H, Ghaffari Shad E, Asadollahi S. FAST for blunt abdominal trauma: correlation between positive findings and admission acid-base measurement. Am J Emerg Med 2017;35(6):823–9.
65. Aboobakar MR, Singh JP, Maharaj K, Mewa Kinoo S, Singh B. Gastric perforation following blunt abdominal trauma. Trauma Case Rep 2017; 10(Suppl. C):12–15.
66. Martin JG, Shah J, Robinson C, Dariushnia S. Evaluation and management of blunt solid organ trauma. Tech Vasc Interv Radiol 2017;20(4):230–6.
67. Shaider JJ, Barkin AZ, Barkin RM. Abdominal trauma, imaging. In: Schaider JJ, Barkin RM, Hayden SR, Wolfe RE, Barkin AZ, Shayne P, editors. Rosen & Barkin's 5-minute emergency medicine consult. Philadelphia: Lippincott Williams & Wilkins; 2015.
68. Armstrong LB, Mooney DP, Paltiel H, Barnewolt C, Dionigi B, Arbuthnot M, et al. Contrast enhanced ultrasound for the evaluation of blunt pediatric abdominal trauma. J Pediat Surg 2018;53(3):548–52.
69. Englum BR, Gulack BC, Rice HE, Scarborough JE, Adibe OO. Management of blunt pancreatic trauma in children: review of the National Trauma Data Bank. J Pediatr Surg 2016;51(9):1526–31.
70. Schaider JJ, Barkin AZ, Barkin RM, editors. Abdominal trauma imaging. Rosen and Barkin's 5-minute emergency medicine consult. Philadelphia: Lippincott Williams & Wilkins; 2015.
71. Johnson MC, Eastridge BJ. Redefining the abdominal seatbelt sign: enhanced CT imaging metrics improve injury prediction. Am J Surg 2017;214(6):1175–9.
72. Kim PK. Radiology for trauma and the general surgeon. Surg Clin North Am 2017;97(5):1175–83.
73. Dane B, Baxter AB, Bernstein MP. Imaging genitourinary trauma. Radiol Clin North Am 2017;55(2):321–35.
74. Gong J, Mei D, Yang M, Xu J, Zhou Y. Emergency CT of blunt abdominal trauma: experience from a large urban hospital in Southern China. Quantit Imag Med Surg 2017;7(4):461–8.
75. Kordzadeh A, Melchionda V, Rhodes KM, Fletcher EO, Panayiotopolous YP. Blunt abdominal trauma and mesenteric avulsion: a systematic review. Eur J Trauma Emerg Surg 2016;42(3):311–15.
76. Nerli RB, Patil A, Devaraju S, Hiremath MB. Renal pelvis injury in case of blunt trauma abdomen. Urol Case Rep 2015;3(4):109–10.
77. Buckley JC, McAninch JW. Revision of current American Association for the Surgery of Trauma renal injury grading system. J Trauma 2011;70:35–7.
78. Ali HI. Role of multislice computed tomography in assessment of non-solid organ injury in patients with blunt abdominal trauma. Egypt J Radiol Nuc Med 2016;47(3):749–56.
79. Alarhayem AQ, Myers JG, Dent D, Lamus D, Lopera J, Liao L, et al. 'Blush at First Sight': significance of computed tomographic and angiographic discrepancy in patients with blunt abdominal trauma. Am J Surg 2015;210:1004–111.

80. Johnson GE, Kogut MJ, Ingraham CR. The role of interventional radiology in trauma. J Radiol Nurs 2014;33(4):181–7.
81. Salcedo ES, Brown IE, Corwin MT, Galante JM. Angioembolization for solid organ injury: a brief review. Int J Surg 2016;33(Pt B):225–30.
82. Cinquantini F, Tugnoli G, Piccinini A, Coniglio C, Mannone S, Biscardi A, et al. Educational review of predictive value and findings of computed tomography scan in diagnosing bowel and mesenteric injuries after blunt trauma: correlation with trauma surgery findings in 163 patients. Can Assoc Radiol J 2017;68(3):276–85.
83. Krige JE, Kotze UK, Setshedi M, Nicol AJ, Navsaria PH. Surgical management and outcomes of combined pancreaticoduodenal injuries: analysis of 75 consecutive cases. J Am Coll Surg 2016;222(5):737–49.
84. Chereau N, Wagner M, Tresallet C, Lucidarme O, Raux M, Menegaux F. CT scan and diagnostic peritoneal lavage: towards a better diagnosis in the area of nonoperative management of blunt abdominal trauma. Injury 2016;47(9):2006–11.
85. Kuncir EJ, Velmahos GC. Diagnostic peritoneal aspiration—the foster child of DPL: a prospective observational study. Int J Surg 2007;5(3):167–71.
86. Kurtz MP, Eswara JR, Vetter JM, Nelson CP, Brandes SB. Blunt abdominal trauma from motor vehicle collisions from 2007 to 2011: renal injury probability and severity in children versus adults. J Urol 2017;197(3 Pt 2):906–10.
87. Adam N, Sorensen V, Skinner R. Not all intestinal traumatic injuries are the same: a comparison of surgically treated blunt vs. penetrating injuries. Injury 2015;46(1):115–18.
88. Benjamin E, Cho J, Recinos G, Dilektasli E, Lam L, Brunner J, et al. Negative CT can safely rule out clinically significant intra-abdominal injury in the asymptomatic patient after blunt trauma—prospective evaluation of 1193 patients. J Trauma Acute Care Surg 2018;84(1):128–32.
89. Brooke M, Victorino GP. Repeat computed tomography is highly sensitive in determining need for delayed exploration in blunt abdominal trauma. J Surg Res 2017;219:116–21.
90. Bates DDB, Wasserman M, Malek A, Gorantla V, Anderson SW, Soto JA, et al. Multidetector CT of surgically proven blunt bowel and mesenteric injury. Radiographics 2017;37(2):613–25.
91. LeBedis CA, Anderson SW, Bates DD, Khalil R, Matherly D, Wing H, et al. CT imaging signs of surgically proven bowel trauma. Emerg Radiol 2016;23(3):213–19.
92. Wilson CT, Clebone A. Initial assessment and management of the trauma patient. In: Scher CS, editor. Anesthesia for trauma: new evidence and new challenges. New York, NY: Springer New York; 2014.
93. Kong VY, Jeetoo D, Naidoo LC, Oosthuizen GV, Clarke DL. Isolated free intra-abdominal fluid on CT in blunt trauma: the continued diagnostic dilemma. Chin J Traumatol 2015;18(6):357–9.
94. Bates DDB, Wasserman M, Malek A, Gorantla V, Anderson SW, Soto JA, et al. Multidetector CT of surgically proven blunt bowel and mesenteric injury. Radiographics 2017;37(2):613–25.
95. Baygeldi S, Karakose O, Özcelik KC, Pülat H, Damar S, Eken H, et al. Factors affecting morbidity in solid organ injuries. Dis Markers 2016;2016:6954758.
96. Rahim S, Davidson J. Clinical approach to the trauma patient. J Radiol Nurs 2017;36(4):200–5.
97. Robinson JD, Sandstrom CK, Lehnert BE, Gross JA. Imaging of blunt abdominal solid organ trauma. Semin Roentgenol 2016;51(3):215–29.
98. Demetriades D, Velmahos G. Indication for and technique of laparotomy. In: Moore E, Feliciano D, Mattox K, editors. Trauma. New York: McGraw-Hill; 2006.
99. Dharap SB, Noronha J, Kumar V. Laparotomy for blunt abdominal trauma – some uncommon indications. J Emerg Trauma Shock 2016;9(1):32–6.
100. Parreira JG, Oliari CB, Malpaga JM, Fucs PMMB. Severity and treatment of 'occult' intra-abdominal injuries in blunt trauma victims. Injury 2016;47(1):89–93.
101. Chovanes J, Cannon JW, Nunez TC. The evolution of damage control surgery. Surg Clin North Am 2012;92(4):859–75.
102. Ahmed N, Whelan J, Brownlee J, Chari V, Chung R. The contribution of laparoscopy in evaluation of penetrating abdominal wounds. J Am Coll Surg 2005;201(2):213–16.
103. Chakravartty S, Sarma DR, Noor M, Panagiotopoulos S, Patel AG. Laparoscopy has a therapeutic role in the management of abdominal trauma: a matched-pair analysis. Int J Surg 2017;44(Suppl. C):21–5.
104. Chestovich PJ, Browder TD, Morrissey SL, Fraser DR, Ingalls NK, Fildes JJ. Minimally invasive is maximally effective: diagnostic and therapeutic laparoscopy for penetrating abdominal injuries. J Trauma Acute Care Surg 2015;78(6):1076–85.
105. French RL, Gilliam AD. Control of haemorrhage and damage control surgery. Surgery (Oxford) 2016;34(11):568–74.
106. Bloom BM, Grundlingh J, Bestwick JP, Harris T. The role of venous blood gas in the emergency department: a systematic review and meta-analysis. Eur J Emerg Med 2014;21(2):81–8.
107. Vohra T, Paxton J. Abnormal arterial blood gas and serum lactate levels do not alter disposition in adult blunt trauma patients after early computed tomography. West J Emerg Med 2013;14(3):212–17.
108. Williams KB, Christmas AB, Heniford BT, Sing RF, Messick J. Arterial vs venous blood gas differences during hemorrhagic shock. World J Crit Care Med 2014;3(2):55–60.
109. Parsikia A, Bones K, Kaplan M, Strain J, Leung PS, Ortiz J, et al. The predictive value of initial serum lactate in trauma patients. Shock 2014;42(3):199–204.
110. Zagory JA, Dossa A, Golden J, Jensen AR, Goodhue CJ, Upperman JS, et al. Re-evaluation of liver transaminase cutoff for CT after pediatric blunt abdominal trauma. Pediatr Surg Int 2017;33(3):311–16.

111. Biffl WL, Leppaniemi A. Management guidelines for penetrating abdominal trauma. World J Surg 2015;39(6):1373–80.
112. Bjurlin MA, Fantus RJ, Fantus RJ, Villines D. Comparison of nonoperative and surgical management of renal trauma: can we predict when nonoperative management fails? J Trauma Acute Care Surg 2017;82(2):356–61.
113. Boyd M, Keene DD. Management of shock in trauma. Anaesth Intens Care Med 2017;18(8):386–9.
114. Elliot D, Aitken L, Chaboyer W. ACCCN's critical care nursing. Sydney: Elsevier; 2006.
115. Hewitt CW, Pombo MA, Blough PE, Castaneda MG, Percival TJ, Rall JM. Effect of the abdominal aortic and junctional tourniquet on chest compressions in a swine model of ventricular fibrillation. Am J Emerg Med 2021;45:297–302.
116. Schechtman DW, Kauvar DS, De Guzman R, Polykratis IA, Prince MD, Kheirabadi BS, et al. Abdominal aortic and junctional tourniquet versus zone III resuscitative endovascular balloon occlusion of the aorta in a swine junctional hemorrhage model. J Trauma Acute Care Surg 2020;88(2):292–7.
117. Schwartz RB, Shiver SA, Reynolds BZ, Lowry J, Holsten SB, Akers TW, et al. The use of the abdominal aortic and junctional tourniquet versus combat gauze in a porcine hemicorporectomy model. J Spec Oper Med 2019;19(2):69–72.
118. Smith TN, Beaven A, Handford C, Sellon E, Parker PJ. Abdominal Aortic Junctional Tourniquet–Stabilized (AAJTS) can be applied both successfully and rapidly by Combat Medical Technicians (CMTs). BMJ Mil Health 2021:e001881.
119. Abid M, Neff LP, Russo RM, Hoareau G, Williams TK, Grayson JK, et al. Reperfusion repercussions: a review of the metabolic derangements following resuscitative endovascular balloon occlusion of the aorta. J Trauma Acute Care Surg 2020;89(2S Suppl. 2):S39–44.
120. Moore LJ, Rasmussen TE. A contemporary assessment of resuscitative endovascular balloon occlusion of the aorta (REBOA). J Trauma Acute Care Surg 2022;92(4):762–4.
121. Moore EE, Shackford SR, Pachter HL, McAninch JW, Browner BD, Champion HR, et al. Organ injury scaling: spleen, liver, and kidney. J Trauma 1989;29(12):1664–6.
122. Knapp J, Jakob DA, Haltmeier T, Lehmann B, Hautz WE. Resuscitative endovascular balloon occlusion of the aorta in severely injured patients in the emergency trauma room: a case series. Anaesthesist 2022;71:599–607.
123. Kokabi N, Shuaib W, Xing M, Harmouche E, Wilson K, Johnson JO, et al. Intra-abdominal solid organ injuries: an enhanced management algorithm. Can Assoc Radiol J 2014;65(4):301–9.
124. Barbois S, Abba J, Guigard S, Quesada JL, Pirvu A, Waroquet PA, et al. Management of penetrating abdominal and thoraco-abdominal wounds: a retrospective study of 186 patients. J Visc Surg 2016;153(Suppl. 4):69–78.
125. Fernández-Ibieta M. Renal trauma in pediatrics: a current review. Urology 2018;113:171–8.
126. Ferrada R, Birolini D. New concepts in the management of patients with penetrating abdominal wounds. Surg Clin North Am 1999;79(6): 1331–56.
127. Kuhajda I, Zarogoulidis K, Kougioumtzi I, Huang H, Li Q, Dryllis G, et al. Penetrating trauma. J Thorac Dis 2014;6(Suppl. 4):S461–5.
128. Coccolini F, Montori G, Catena F, Di Saverio S, Biffl W, Moore EE, et al. Liver trauma: WSES position paper. World J Emerg Surg 2015;10(1):39.
129. Phillips B, Turco L, McDonald D, Mause A, Walters RW. Penetrating injuries to the duodenum—an analysis of 879 patients from the National Trauma Data Bank, 2010 to 2014. J Trauma Acute Care Surg 2017;83(5):810–7.
130. Rezende-Neto JB, Vieira HMJ, Rodrigues Bde L, Rizoli S, Nascimento B, Fraga GP. Management of stab wounds to the anterior abdominal wall. Rev Col Bras Cir 2014;41(1):75–9.
131. John J. Algorithms for managing the common trauma patient. SAMJ 2015;105:502–7.
132. Aitken L, Niggemeyer L. Trauma management. In: Elliot D, Aitken L, Chaboyer W, editors. ACCCN's critical care nursing. Sydney: Elsevier; 2006.
133. Koto ZM, Mosai F, Matsevych OY. The use of laparoscopy in managing penetrating thoracoabdominal injuries in Africa: 83 cases reviewed. WJES 2017;12:27.
134. Matsevych O, Koto M, Balabyeki M, Aldous C. Trauma laparoscopy: when to start and when to convert? Surg Endoscop 2018;32(3):1344–52.
135. Alsikafi NF, Rosenstein DI. Staging, evaluation, and nonoperative management of renal injuries. Urol Clin North Am 2006;33(1):13–19.
136. Carrillo EH, Platz A, Miller FB, Richardson JD, Polk Jr HC. Non-operative management of blunt hepatic trauma. Br J Surg 1998;85(4):461–8.
137. Coimbra R, Hoyt DB, Engelhart S, Richardson JD, Polk Jr HC. Non-operative management reduces the overall mortality of Grade 3 and 4 of blunt liver injuries. Int Surg 2006;91(5):251–7.
138. Badger SA, Barclay R, Campbell P, Mole DJ, Diamond T. Management of liver trauma. World J Surg 2009;33(12):2522–37.
139. Goin G, Massalou D, Bege T, Contargyris C, Avaro JP, Pauleau G, et al. Feasibility of selective non-operative management for penetrating abdominal trauma in France. J Visc Surg 2017;154(3):167–74.
140. Hasanovic J, Agic M, Rifatbegovic Z, Mehmedovic Z, Jakubovic-Cickusic A. Pancreatic injury in blunt abdominal trauma. Med Arch 2015;69(2):130–2.
141. Negoi I, Paun S, Stoica B, Hostiuc S, Beuran M. High grade penetrating pancreatic trauma - case report and review of the literature. Chirurgia (Bucharest, Romania: 1990) 2015;110(6):554–8.
142. Siboni S, Kwon E, Benjamin E, Inaba K, Demetriades D. Isolated blunt pancreatic trauma: a benign injury? J Trauma Acute Care Surg 2016;81(5):855–9.
143. Carillo E, Spain D, Wohltmann CD, Schmieg RE, Boaz PW, Miller FB, et al. Interventional techniques are useful adjuncts in nonoperative management of hepatic injuries. J Trauma 1999;46(4):619–22.

144. Harper K, Shah KH. Renal trauma after blunt abdominal injury. J Emerg Med 2013;45(3):400–4.

145. Crichton JCI, Naidoo K, Yet B, Brundage SI, Perkins Z. The role of splenic angioembolization as an adjunct to nonoperative management of blunt splenic injuries: a systematic review and meta-analysis. J Trauma Acute Care Surg 2017;83(5):934–43.

146. Gaarder C, Gaski IA, Naess PA. Spleen and liver injuries—when to operate. Curr Opin Crit Care 2017;23(6):520–6.

147. Al-Hassani A, Jabbour G, El Labib M, Kanbar A, El-Menyar A, Al-Thani H. Delayed bile leak in a patient with grade IV blunt liver trauma: a case report and review of the literature. Int J Surg Case Rep 2015;14:156–9.

148. Lecky F, Bouamra O, Woodford M. Changing epidemiology of polytrauma. In: Pape HC, Peitzman AB, Rotondo MF, editors. Damage control management in the polytrauma patient. Cham: Springer International; 2017.

149. Smith JW, Nash N, Procter L, Benns M, Franklin GA, Miller K, et al. Not all abdomens are the same: a comparison of damage control surgery for intra-abdominal sepsis versus trauma. Am Surg 2016;82(5):427–32.

150. Wray JP, Bridwell RE, Schauer SG, Shackelford SA, Bebarta VS, Wright FL, et al. The diamond of death: hypocalcemia in trauma and resuscitation. Am J Emerg Med 2021;41:104–9.

151. Costantini TW, Coimbra R, Holcomb JB, Podbielski JM, Catalano R, Blackburn A, et al. Current management of hemorrhage from severe pelvic fractures: results of an American Association for the Surgery of Trauma multi-institutional trial. J Trauma Acute Care Surg 2016;80(5):717–25.

152. Matsumoto J, Lohman BD, Morimoto K, Ichinose Y, Hattori T, Taira Y. Damage control interventional radiology (DCIR) in prompt and rapid endovascular strategies in trauma occasions (PRESTO): a new paradigm. Diagn Interv Imaging 2015;96(7):687–91.

153. Malgras B, Prunet B, Lesaffre X, Boddaert G, Travers S, Cungi PJ, et al. Damage control: concept and implementation. J Visc Surg 2017;154(Suppl. 1): S19–29.

154. Roberts DJ, Ball CG, Feliciano DV, Moore EE, Ivatury RR, Lucas CE, et al. History of the innovation of damage control for management of trauma patients: 1902–2016. Ann Surg 2017;265(5):1034–44.

155. Harvin JA, Wray CJ, Steward J, Lawless RA, McNutt MK, Love JD, et al. Control the damage: morbidity and mortality after emergent trauma laparotomy. Am J Surg 2016;212(1):34–9.

156. Beal SL. Fatal hepatic hemorrhage: an unresolved problem in the management of complex liver injuries. J Trauma 1990;30(2):163–9.

157. Clochesy JM, Breu C, Cardin S, Rudy EB, Whittaker AA. Critical care nursing. 2nd ed. Philadelphia: WB Saunders; 1996.

158. Saverio S, Sibilio A, Coniglio C, Bianchi E, Biscardi A, Villani S, et al. A proposed algorithm for multimodal liver trauma management from a surgical trauma audit in a Western European Trauma Center. Minerva Anestesiol 2014;80(11):1205–16.

159. West N, Dawes R. Trauma resuscitation and the damage control approach. Surgery (Oxford) 2015;33(9):430–6.

160. Snell RS, Smith MS. Clinical anatomy for emergency medicine. St Louis: Mosby; 1993.

161. Khan I, Bew D, Elias DA, Lewis D, Meacock LM. Mechanisms of injury and CT findings in bowel and mesenteric trauma. Clin Radiol 2014;69(6):639–47.

162. Hamidian Jahromi A, Johnson L, Youssef AM. Delayed small bowel perforation following blunt abdominal trauma: a case report and review of the literature. Asian J Surg 2016;39(2):109–12.

163. Grünherz L, Startseva X, Kozomara-Hocke M, Barth BK, Simmen HP, Mica L, et al. Combined intra- and extraperitoneal urinary bladder rupture—a rare seat-belt injury: a case report. Int J Surg Case Rep 2017;38:119–21.

164. Pimenta de Castro J, Gomes G, Mateus N, Escrevente R, Pereira L, Jácome P. Small bowel perforation and mesentery injury after an unusual blunt abdominal trauma—case report. Int J Surg Case Rep 2015;7C:51–3.

165. Noyola-Villalobos HF, Loera-Torres MA, Jiménez-Chavarría E, Núñez-Cantú O, García-Núñez LM, Arcaute-Velázquez FF. Non-surgical management after blunt traumatic liver injuries: a review article. Cir Cir (English Ed.) 2016;84(3):263–6.

166. Richardson JD. Changes in the management of injuries to the liver and spleen. J Am Coll Surg 2005;200(5):648–69.

167. Notrica DM, Linnaus ME. Nonoperative management of blunt solid organ injury in pediatric surgery. Surg Clin North Am 2017;97(1):1–20.

168. Pearl WS, Todd KH. Ultrasonography for the initial evaluation of blunt abdominal trauma, a review in prospective trials. Ann Emerg Med 1996;27(3):353–61.

169. Safavi A, Skarsgard ED, Rhee P, Zangbar B, Kulvatunyou N, Tang A, et al. Trauma center variation in the management of pediatric patients with blunt abdominal solid organ injury: a national trauma data bank analysis. J Pediat Surg 2016;51(3):499–502.

170. van Wessem KJP, Hietbrink F, Leenen LPH. Attenuation of MODS-related and ARDS-related mortality makes infectious complications a remaining challenge in the severely injured. Trauma Surg Acute Care Open 2020;5(1):e000398.

171. Dantanarayana N, Ting F, Symons J, Evans D, Graham A. Isolated grade 5 renal trauma in a hemodynamically stable patient. Urol Case Rep 2016;4(Suppl. C):30–2.

172. Egawa N, Ueda J, Hiraki M, Ide T, Inoue S, Sakamoto Y, et al. Traumatic gallbladder rupture treated by laparoscopic cholecystectomy. Case Rep Gastroenterol 2016;10(2):212–17.

173. King K, Steggall M. Haematuria: from identification to treatment. Br J Nurs 2014;23(9):S28–32.

174. Ming Kwan BY, Plantinga P, Ross I. Isolated traumatic rupture of the gallbladder. Radiol Case Rep 2015;10(1):1029.

175. Bozdag Z, Kapan M, Ulger BV, Turkoglu A, Uslukaya O, Oğuz A, et al. Factors affecting morbidity and mortality in pancreatic injuries. Eur J Trauma Emerg Surg 2016;42(2):231–5.

176. Buzelé R, Barbier L, Sauvanet A, Fantin B. Medical complications following splenectomy. J Visc Surg 2016;153(4):277–86.

177. Soto JA, Lucey BC. Emergency radiology: the requisites. Philadelphia: Mosby; 2009.

178. Luoto TT, Pakarinen MP, Koivusalo A. Long-term outcomes after pediatric splenectomy. Surgery 2016;159(6):1583–90.

179. Navas-Cuéllar JA, Cañete-Gómez J, López-Bernal F, García-Rivera C, Pareja-Ciuró F, Padillo-Ruiz J. Spleen-preserving surgery after blunt abdominal trauma with splenic hilum involvement. Cir Cir (English Edition) 2015;83(6):516–21.

180. Greenhill D, Haydel C, Rehman S. Management of the Morel-Lavallée lesion. Orthoped Clin North Am 2016;47(1):115–25.

181. Breen KJ, O'Corragain E, Sweeney P. PD63-05 Blunt renal trauma: validation of a conservative follow-up imaging strategy. J Urol 2017;197(4):e1256.

182. Neff JA, Kidd PS, editors. Trauma nursing: the art and science. St Louis: Mosby; 1993.

183. Dagenais J, Leow JJ, Haider AH, Wang Y, Chung BI, Chang SL, et al. Contemporary trends in the management of renal trauma in the United States: a national community hospital population-based analysis. Urology 2016;97(Suppl. C):98–104.

184. Dixon MD, McAninch JW. American Urological Association update series, traumatic renal injuries, Part 1: assessment and management. Houston: The Association; 1991.

185. DuBose J, Inaba K, Teixeira PG, Pepe A, Dunham MB, McKenney M. Selective non-operative management of solid organ injury following abdominal gunshot wounds. Injury 2007;38(9):1084–90.

186. McQuillan KA, Von Rueden KT, Hartsock RL. Trauma nursing: from resuscitation through rehabilitation. 4th ed. Philadelphia: WB Saunders; 2008.

187. Lanchon C, Fiard G, Arnoux V, Descotes JL, Rambeaud JJ, Terrier N, et al. High grade blunt renal trauma: predictors of surgery and long-term outcomes of conservative management. A prospective single center study. J Urol 2016;195(1):106–11.

188. Maarouf AM, Ahmed AF, Shalaby E, Badran Y, Salem E, Zaiton F. Factors predicting the outcome of non-operative management of high-grade blunt renal trauma. Af J Urol 2015;21(1):44–51.

189. Kidney Injury Scale. The American Association for the Surgery of Trauma. Available from: www.aast.org/Library/TraumaTools/InjuryScoringScales.aspx.

190. Peters P, Sagalowsky A. Genitourinary trauma. In: Walsh P, Gittes R, Perlmutter A, editors. Campbell's urology. vol. 1. 8th ed. Philadelphia: WB Saunders; 2002.

191. Alfayez SM, Allimmia K, Alshammri A, Serro F, Almogbel R, Bin Dous A, et al. Urological injuries associated with pelvic fractures: a case report of a detached bone segment inside the bladder. Int J Surg Case Rep 2016;28(Suppl. C):188–91.

192. Hardee MJ, Lowrance W, Stevens MH, Nirula R, Brant WO, Morris SE, et al. Process improvement in trauma: compliance with recommended imaging evaluation in the diagnosis of high-grade renal injuries. J Trauma Acute Care Surg 2013;74(2):558–62.

193. Coccolini F, Catena F, Kluger Y, Sartelli M, Baiocchi G, Ansaloni L, et al. Abdominopelvic trauma: from anatomical to anatomo-physiological classification. World J Emerg Surg 2018;13(1):50.

194. Coccolini F, Moore EE, Kluger Y, Biffl W, Leppaniemi A, Matsumura Y, et al. Kidney and uro-trauma: WSES-AAST guidelines. World J Emerg Surg 2019;14(1):54.

195. Serafetinides E, Kitrey ND, Djakovic N, Kuehhas FE, Lumen N, Sharma DM, et al. Review of the current management of upper urinary tract injuries by the EAU Trauma Guidelines Panel. Eur Urol 2015;67(5):930–6.

196. Taken K, Oncü MR, Ergün M, Eryılmaz R, Güneş M. Isolated renal pelvis rupture secondary to blunt trauma: case report. Int J Surg Case Rep 2015;9:82–4.

197. Armenakas NA, McAninch JW. Acute anterior urethral injuries: diagnosis and initial management. In: McAninch JW, editor. Traumatic and reconstructive urology. Philadelphia: WB Saunders; 1996.

198. Sekyere EO. Trauma to the urogenital tract. In: David SS, editor. Clinical pathways in emergency medicine. vol. II. New Delhi: Springer India; 2016.

199. Lumen N, Kuehhas FE, Djakovic N, Kitrey ND, Serafetinidis E, Sharma DM, et al. Review of the current management of lower urinary tract injuries by the EAU Trauma Guidelines Panel. Eur Urol 2015;67(5):925–9.

200. Tausch TJ, Morey AF, Scott JF, Simhan J. Unintended negative consequences of primary endoscopic realignment for men with pelvic fracture urethral injuries. J Urol 2014;192(6):1720–4.

201. Zaid UB, Bayne DB, Harris CR, Alwaal A, McAninch JW, Breyer BN. Penetrating trauma to the ureter, bladder, and urethra. Curr Trauma Rep 2015;1(2):119–24.

202. Urry RJ, Clarke DL, Bruce JL, Laing G. The incidence, spectrum and outcomes of traumatic bladder injuries within the Pietermaritzburg Metropolitan Trauma Service. Injury 2016;47(5):1057–63.

203. Hsieh CH, Chen RJ, Fang JF, Lin BC, Hsu YP, Kao JL, et al. Diagnosis and management of bladder injury by trauma surgeons. Am J Surg 2002;184(2):143–7.

204. Johnsen NV, Young JB, Reynolds WS, Kaufman MR, Milam DF, Guillamondegui OD, et al. Evaluating the role of operative repair of extraperitoneal bladder rupture following blunt pelvic trauma. J Urol 2016;195(3):661–5.

205. Myers JB, Hotaling JM, Brant WO, Enniss TM. Management of a case of severe pelvic fracture related bladder trauma. Urol Case Rep 2015;3(2):32–4.

206. Zinman LN, Vanni AJ. Surgical management of urologic trauma and iatrogenic injuries. Surg Clin North Am 2016;96(3):425–39.

207. Johnsen NV, Kaufman MR, Dmochowski RR, Milam DF. Erectile dysfunction following pelvic fracture urethral injury. Sex Med Rev 2018;6(1):114–23.
208. Pereira BM, Reis LO, Calderan TR, de Campos CC, Fraga GP. Penetrating bladder trauma: a high risk factor for associated rectal injury. Adv Urol 2014;2014:386280.
209. Lückhoff C, Mitra B, Cameron PA, Fitzgerald M, Royce P. The diagnosis of acute urethral trauma. Injury 2011;42(9):913–16.
210. Hunter SR, Lishnak TS, Powers AM, Lisle DK. Male genital trauma in sports. Clin Sports Med 2013;32(2):247–54.
211. Dowlut-McElroy T, Higgins J, Williams KB, Strickland JL. Patterns of treatment of accidental genital trauma in girls. J Pediatr Adolesc Gynecol 2018;31(1):19–22.
212. Guerre D, Brehin C, Gurrera E, Pinnagoda K, Galinier P, Claudet I, et al. Management of unintentional pediatric female genital trauma. Arch Pediatr 2017;24(11):1083–7.
213. Minns AB, Sherry Y. Penile fracture in a patient presenting with groin pain. J Emerg Med 2011;40(4):441–2.
214. Terrier JE, Paparel P, Gadegbeku B, Ruffion A, Jenkins LC, N'Diaye A. Genitourinary injuries after traffic accidents: analysis of a registry of 162,690 victims. J Trauma Acute Care Surg 2017;82(6):1087–93.
215. Zilkens RR, Smith DA, Phillips MA, Mukhtar SA, Semmens JB, Kelly MC. Genital and anal injuries: a cross-sectional Australian study of 1266 women alleging recent sexual assault. Forens Sc Int 2017;275(Suppl C):195–202.
216. Bauer NJG. Case report: traumatic unilateral testicular rupture. Int J Surg Case Rep 2016;25(Suppl. C):89–90.
217. Nicola R, Carson N, Dogra V. Testicular trauma: role of sonography. Ultrasound Clin 2013;8(4):525–30.
218. Ward MA, Burgess PL, Williams DH, Herrforth CE, Bentz ML, Faucher LD. Threatened fertility and gonadal function after a polytraumatic, life-threatening injury. J Emerg Trauma Shock 2010;3(2):199–203.
219. Saxena AK, Steiner M, Hollwarth ME. Straddle injuries in female children and adolescents: 10-year accident and management analysis. In J Pediatr 2014;81(8):766–9.
220. Lo MK, Foley C, Healy C, Oliphant J, Kent S. A response to: macroscopically detected female genital injury after consensual and non-consensual vaginal penetration: a prospective comparison study. J Forensic Leg Med 2014;28:47–9.
221. Nelius T, Armstrong ML, Rinard K, Rinard K, Young C, Hogan L, et al. Genital piercings: diagnostic and therapeutic implications for urologists. Urology 2011;78(5):998–1007.
222. Clemens MS, Peace KM, Yi F. Rectal trauma: evidence-based practices. Clin Colon Rectal Surg 2018;31(1):17–23.
223. Parajuli P, Kumar S, Gupta A, Bansal VK, Sagar S, Mishra B, et al. Role of laparoscopy in patients with abdominal trauma at level-i trauma center. Surg Laparosc Endosc Percutan Tech 2018;28(1):20–5.
224. Leon M, Chavez L, Surani S. Abdominal compartment syndrome among surgical patients. World J Gastrointest Surg 2021;13(4):330–9.
225. Paduraru DN, Andronic O, Musat F, Bolocan A, Dumitraşcu MC, Ion D. Abdominal compartment syndrome—when is surgical decompression needed? Diagnostics (Basel) 2021;11(12):2294.
226. Cheatham ML, Safcsak K. Intra-abdominal hypertension and abdominal compartment syndrome in acute care surgery. In: Diaz JJ, Efron DT, editors. Complications in acute care surgery: the management of difficult clinical scenarios. Cham: Springer International; 2017.

CHAPTER 47
SPINAL TRAUMA

SARAH KOUROUCHE AND BELINDA KENNEDY

ESSENTIALS

Important considerations in the effective management of spinal trauma are the following:

- **Treat your patients with a high level of suspicion of spinal cord injury (SCI) until proven otherwise.**
- **Adequately maintain spinal alignment from the outset and throughout the course of treatment.**
- **Through adequate oxygenation and spinal alignment, avoid any progression of neurological deficits in the patient and enhance recovery if deficits exist.**
- **Through specialist intervention, provide the best opportunity for recovery for the SCI patient.**
- **If in doubt, always consult.**
- **Differentiate between neurogenic and hypovolaemic shock.**
- **Monitor respiratory function closely in high-level injuries.**
- **Provide regular pressure relief once the patient has been stabilised.**

INTRODUCTION

Trauma to the spinal column and the spinal cord can result in devastating injury. Spinal cord injury (SCI) is damage to the spinal cord that results in a loss of function such as mobility and/or sensation. The effects of SCI depend on the type and level of the injury. Before World War II, most people who sustained SCI died within weeks of their injury due to urinary dysfunction, respiratory infection or pressure injury. However, improved resuscitation and long-term management techniques and materials have meant that many people with SCI now approach the life span of the general population.

EPIDEMIOLOGY

Internationally, studies report between 5.5% and 9% of individuals with a spinal fracture had an associated SCI.[1,2] Each year traumatic SCI affects an estimated 180,000 new individuals, or 23 per million worldwide,[3] with considerable variance in estimates by region. In Australia, the incidence of SCI has been estimated to be between 21 and 32 people per million, based on population modelling.[4] The reported incidence of new SCI cases in Australia during 2017–18 was 187, or 8.6 per million population over 15 years, based on data from the Australian Spinal Cord Injury Register (ASCIR).[5] While trends show a steady decline over the last 20 years, the report underestimates the true incidence of SCI in Australia with the ASCIR data captured only from individuals treated at Australian spinal units who consent; this does not include data from paediatric facilities. A reduced number of cases were reported overall in 2017–18 to ASCIR, with factors such as COVID-19 and fewer consenting cited.[5]

The New Zealand Spinal Cord Injury Register (NZSCIR) was established in 2016, with data collected respectively to 2007 from the two spinal cord injury centres in Aotearoa New Zealand. Based on a retrospective review of data between 2007 and 2016, the mean annual incidence of SCI in Aotearoa New Zealand is 22 cases per million.[6]

In Australia, the main causative factors in traumatic SCI are land transport crash (n = 86, 46%) and falls (n = 67, 36%), with unprotected road users—motorcyclists, pedal cyclists and pedestrians—accounting for the largest proportion of land transport crash (n = 54, 29%). The incidence of SCI resulting from low falls was 14%, and from high falls 21% (Table 47.1).[5] This was inversely the case in Aotearoa New Zealand, where falls accounted for the highest percentage SCI (n = 66, 46%), followed by transport-related mechanisms (n = 36, 25%).[7]

The steady decline of motor vehicle collision (MVC)-related SCI can be partially attributed to injury prevention measures, such as speed-limit controls on freeways and open roads, stringent drink-driving legislation, improvements in vehicle safety and increased seatbelt usage.

ANATOMY AND PHYSIOLOGY

The vertebral column consists of a series of stacked bones which support the head and trunk, providing the bony case for the spinal cord. It consists of 33 vertebrae: 7 cervical, 12 thoracic, 5 lumbar, 5 fused sacral and usually 4 rudimentary coccyx vertebrae. The anterior column is held in alignment by the anterior and posterior longitudinal ligaments, and the posterior column by the nuchal ligament complex (supraspinous, interspinous and infraspinous ligaments), the capsular ligaments and the ligamentum flavum. Apart from the atlas/C1 and the axis/C2, all the vertebrae are anatomically similar, but differ in size and function (Figs 47.1 and 47.2). The spinal cord is a cylinder, flattened from front to back with the lower end tapering into a cone. Ventrally it possesses a deep midline groove, the anterior median sulcus, and dorsally it shows a shallow sulcus, from which a posterior median glial septum extends into the spinal cord. The posterior median septum within the spinal cord is attached to the incomplete posterior median septum of arachnoid in the subarachnoid space.

The spinal nerve roots, especially those of the lumbar and sacral segments, come to slope more and more steeply downwards as the body matures. The spinal cord is made up of two symmetrical enlargements (portions) supplying the upper and lower limbs (Fig. 47.3). The cervical enlargement supplies the upper limbs and the lumbar enlargement supplies the lower limbs. The spinal levels they occupy are C5 to T1 for the cervical and L2 to S3 for the lumbar enlargement. Both cervical and lumbar enlargements are due to the greatly increased mass of motor cells in the anterior columns of grey matter in these areas.

SPINAL NERVE ROOTS AND VASCULAR SUPPLY

Thirty-one pairs of spinal nerves originate from the spinal cord; these are discussed in Chapter 23. The distribution is 8 cervical, 12 thoracic, 5 lumbar, 5 sacral and 1 coccygeal pair of spinal nerves. Nerve roots and the muscles they innervate are shown in Fig. 47.4.

TABLE 47.1 MECHANISM OF INJURY OF ALL TRAUMATIC SCI AGED 15 AND OVER, BY SEX, 2017–18[5]

	MALES		FEMALES		TOTAL	
MECHANISM OF INJURY	NUMBER	%	NUMBER	%	NUMBER	%
Land transport crash						
Motor vehicle occupant	25	17	7	19	32	17
Unprotected land transport user	49	33	5	14	54	29
Fall						
Low fall (same level or < 1 metre)[a]	19	13	8	22	27	14
High fall (>1 metre)	28	19	12	33	40	21
Water-related	12	8	2	5	14	8
Heavy falling object	2	1	0	0	1	1
Horse-related	0	0	1	3	1	1
Football	2	1	0	0	2	1
Other and unspecified causes	13	9	2	5	15	8
Total[b]	150	100	37	100	187	100

a Includes falls from unspecified heights.
b Percentages may not equal 100, due to rounding.

FIGURE 47.1 THE VERTEBRAL COLUMN[3,8]

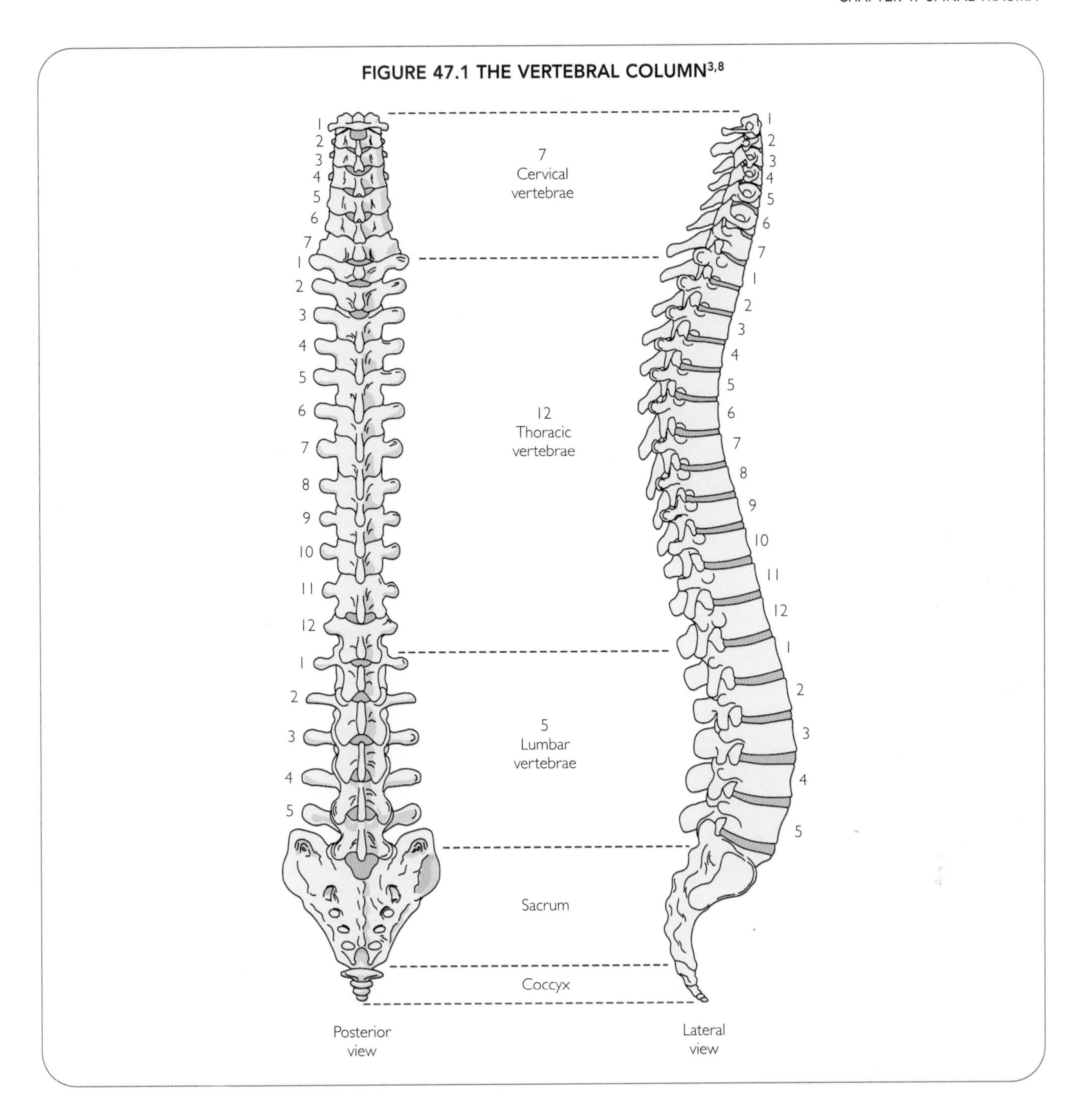

The vascular supply to the spinal cord originates from two main sources, namely the anterior and posterior spinal arteries, with a multitude of spinal rami that intercept the intervertebral foramina at successive levels. The anterior artery sits in the median fissure along the length of the spinal cord. The two posterior spinal arteries descend towards the emerging spinal roots. In effect, the anterior artery feeds the ventral two-thirds of the spinal cord, while the posterior arteries feed the remaining dorsal third.

If the vascular supply to the cord is damaged, the resulting effect is the deprivation of oxygen and essential nutrients, and ultimately necrosis of surrounding neural tissue. If the arterial supply is compromised, this may lead to ischaemia above the site where the injury has occurred—caused by proximal blood-flow loss. The spinal cord arteries are unable to compensate with collateral circulation to preserve neurological function if an injury occurs.

MECHANISMS AND ASSOCIATED INJURIES

The majority of injuries to the spine are closed. Energy causing injury can be transferred to the spine directly or indirectly, with common mechanisms including *flexion*, *extension*, *compression* and *rotation*.[10] The areas of the spinal column used specifically for mobility, the cervical and lumbar regions, are the areas where

FIGURE 47.2 TYPICAL VERTEBRAE[9]

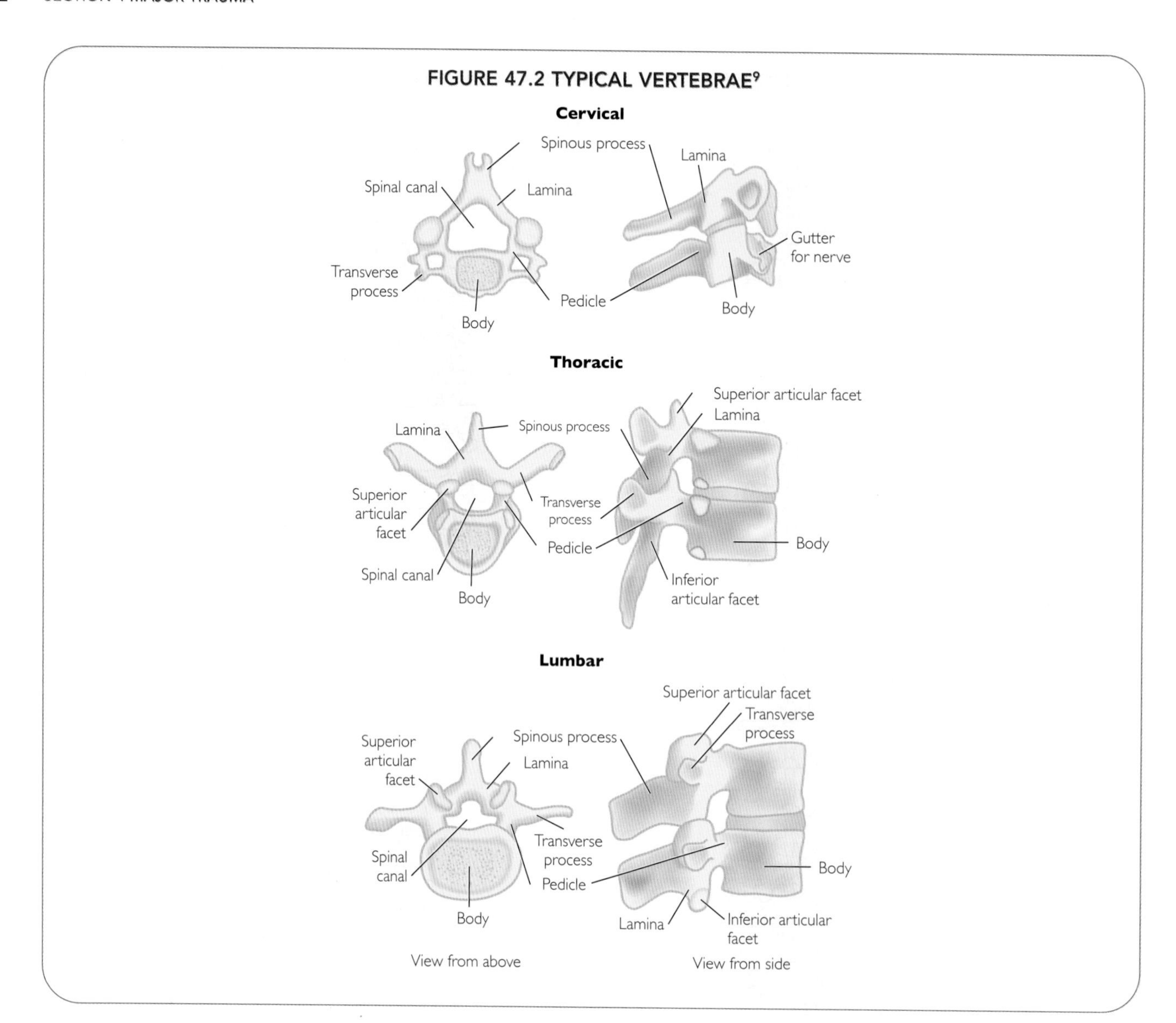

FIGURE 47.3 CROSS-SECTION OF SPINAL CORD

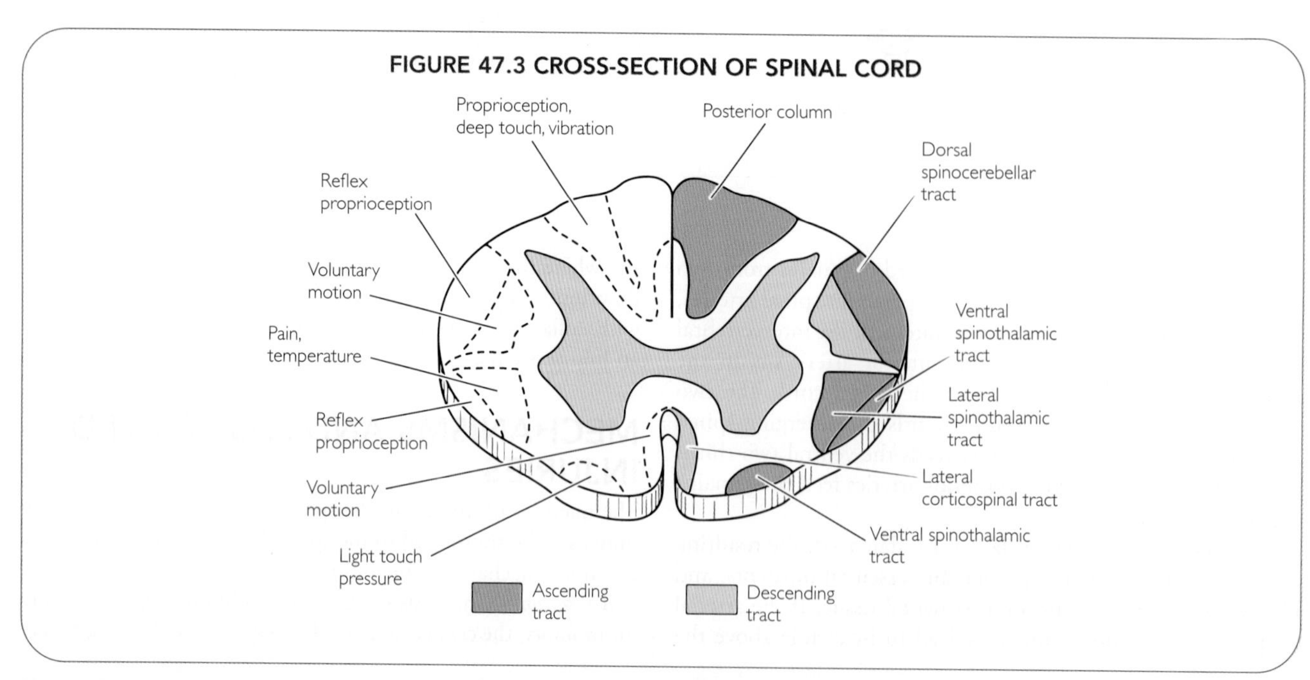

Marcus Cremonese, Medical Illustration Department, UNSW Faculty of Medicine.

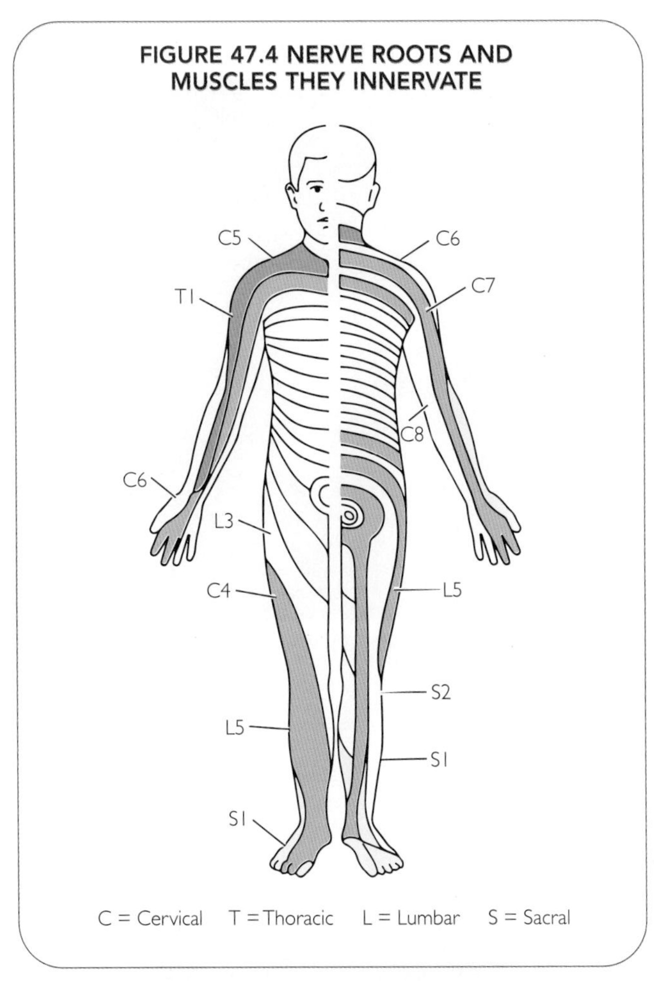

Marcus Cremonese, Medical Illustration Department, UNSW Faculty of Medicine.

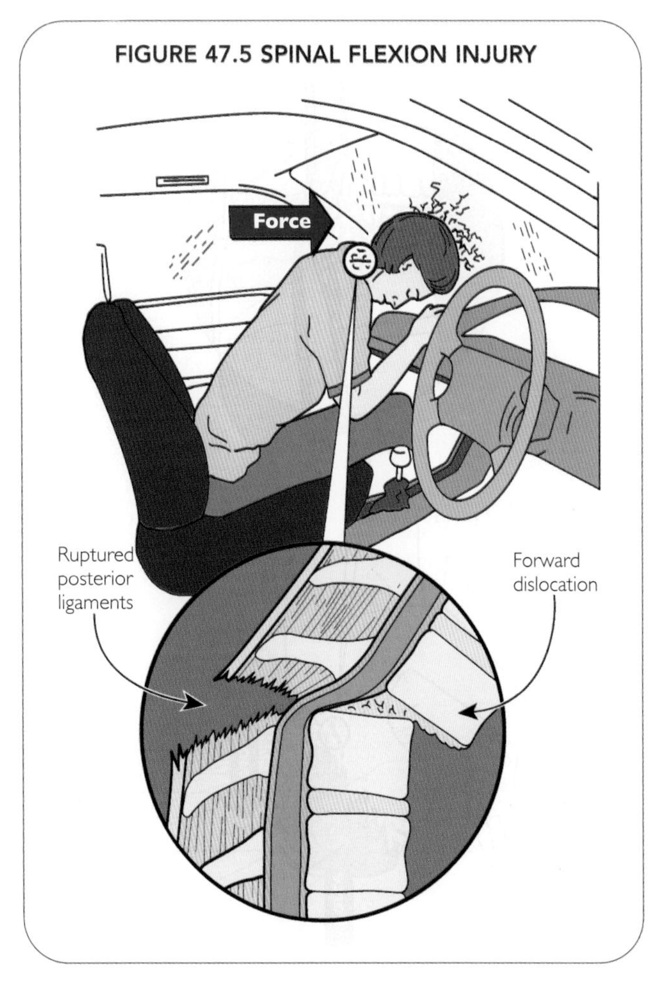

Marcus Cremonese, Medical Illustration Department, UNSW Faculty of Medicine.

most injuries occur. More significant force is required to produce a thoracic spinal injury compared to a cervical spine injury due to the rigidity of the column in this area and its immobility, largely due to the support from the rib cage and musculature. The greater the force, the greater the injury potential.

Hyperflexion injuries can cause rupture of tendons and ligaments, vertebral fractures and stretching of the spinal cord, which can result in tearing, swelling, bruising and impaired function (Fig. 47.5). Hyperflexion injuries in MVCs may occur in poorly restrained occupants where the patient has struck their head against the steering wheel or windscreen, forcing the spine into acute hyperflexion and throwing the chin forwards onto the chest. This may result in rupture of the posterior ligaments and dislocation of the spine, also known as an anterior subluxation.

Hyperextension injuries can also cause rupture of tendons and ligaments, vertebral fractures, and stretching of the spinal cord, which can result in tearing, swelling, bruising and impaired function (Fig. 47.6). Hyperextension injuries occur when the head and neck are forcibly extended backwards and are the most common way children injure their spinal cord. A common injury associated with hyperextension injuries is known as a hangman's fracture. In this instance, the anterior ligament is ruptured and the posterior elements of the vertebral body are fractured.

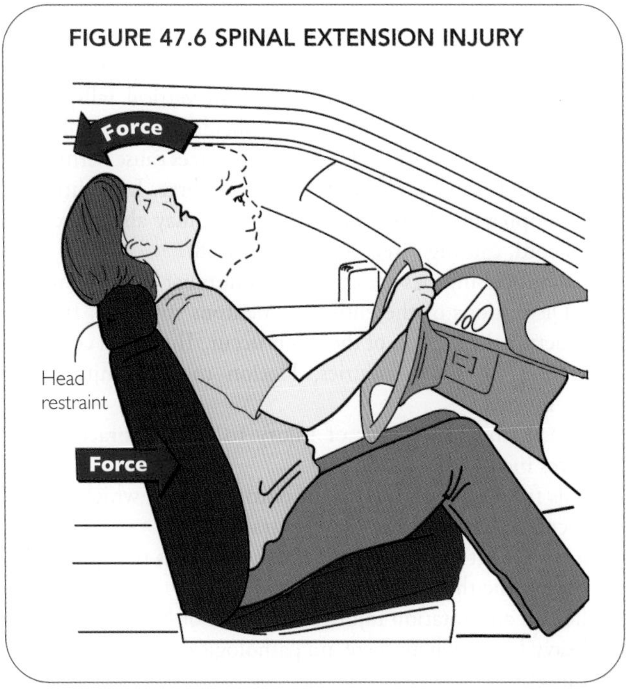

Marcus Cremonese, Medical Illustration Department, UNSW Faculty of Medicine.

FIGURE 47.7 SPINAL COMPRESSION INJURY

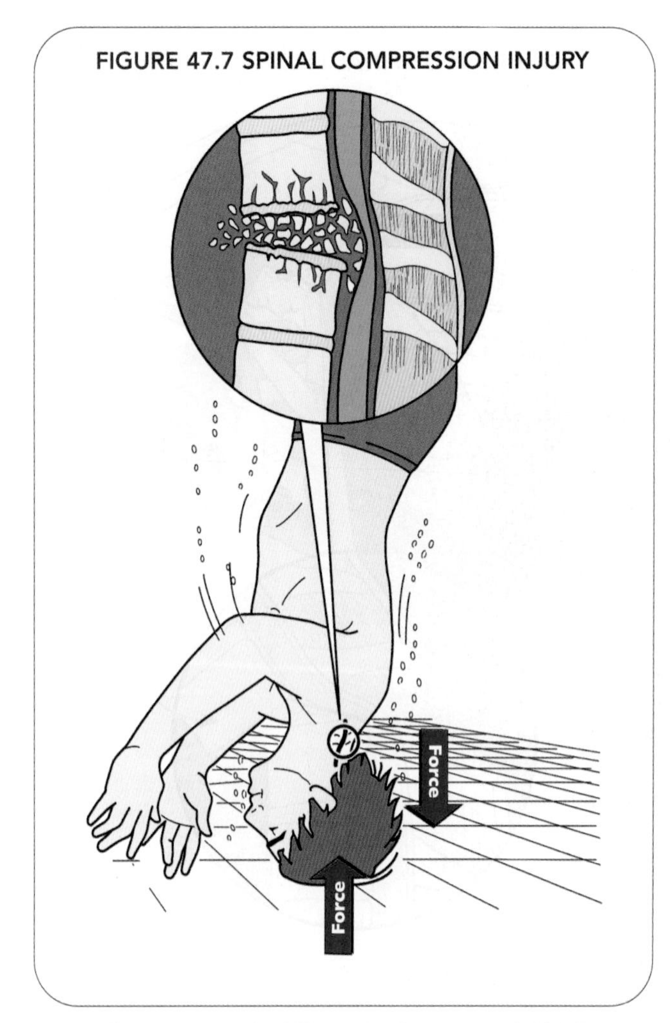

Marcus Cremonese, Medical Illustration Department, UNSW Faculty of Medicine.

FIGURE 47.8

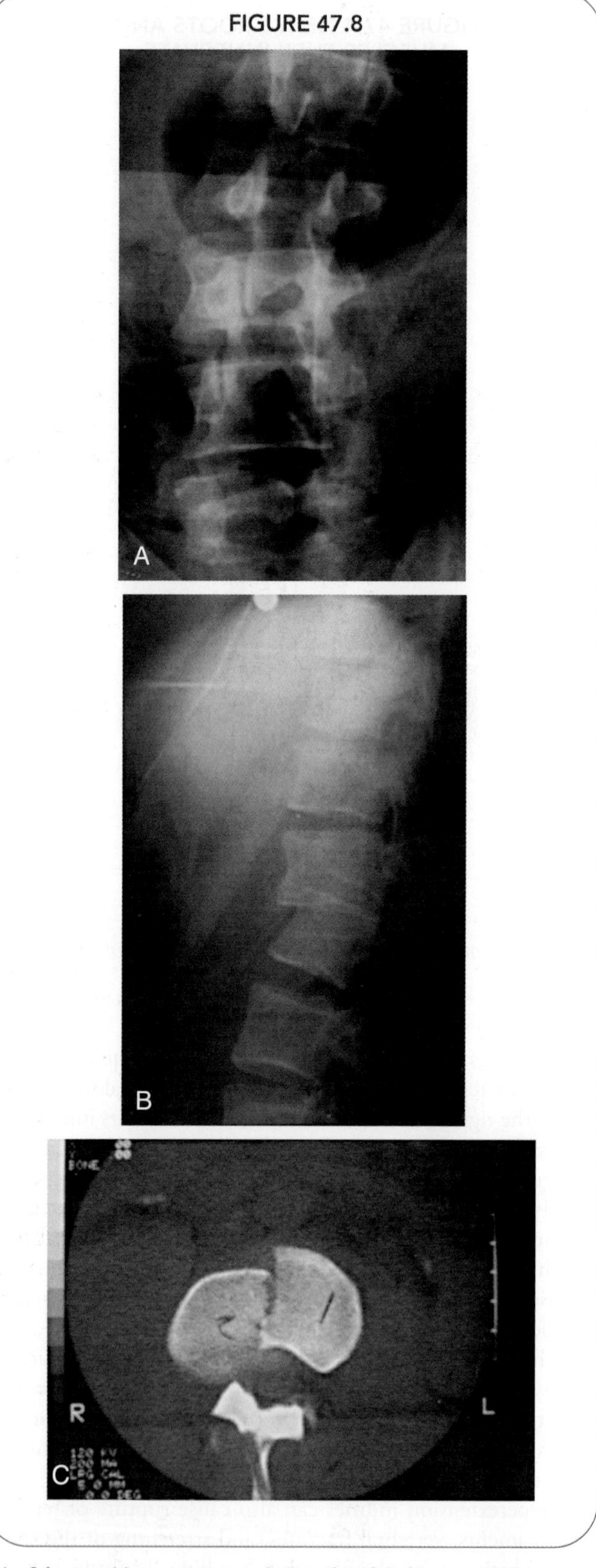

This 24-year-old man was a victim of a fall from a height, which resulted in a fracture-dislocation at L1–L2 and a complete spinal cord injury. **A.** An anteroposterior radiograph highlights the malalignment at L1–L2 with a significant rotatory component and lateral slip at this level. **B.** A lateral radiograph confirms the displacement with forward subluxation and overlap at L1–L2. **C.** A computed tomography scan through L1–L2 highlights the displacement and malalignment, resulting in significant canal compromise and spinal cord injury.[11,12]

Axial load injuries, also known as vertical compression injuries, are predominantly associated with vertical falls, either onto the head; for example, diving incidents, or a fall from height onto feet (Fig. 47.7). Compression forces cause herniation, rupture, and/or burst fractures of the vertebrae. In addition to cord compression, burst fracture segments may also pierce the spinal cord, causing direct injury (Fig. 47.8).

Rotational injuries are caused by a number of differing factors. Disruptions of the entire ligamentous structure, fracture and fracture dislocation of the facets occur. They are a common mechanism in sports injuries. Flexion rotation injuries are highly unstable.

The main mechanisms of injury to cause thoracolumbar fractures include:

- falls from a significant height onto the heels, which lead to increased anterior stress concentration
- a significant blow to the back, which causes the spine to bow at the thoracolumbar junction
- flexion and rotation injuries as a result of MVCs
- heavy lifting where there are pathological underlying causes.

Penetrating cord injuries occur when an object, most commonly a knife or bullet, penetrates the spinal cord. If the neural tissue is lacerated, a disruption of blood supply to the cord occurs. Gunshot wounds which have traversed the spinal column may produce incomplete, unstable injuries.

PRACTICE TIP

If there is one injury in the spine there may be additional non-contingent injuries. Examination to exclude other spinal injuries is required.

SPINAL COLUMN FRACTURES

Spinal fractures may or may not be associated with SCI. Fractures may be compression, burst or fracture-dislocation. The location of the fracture will determine the classification and severity. Vertebral fractures may be stable where the affected vertebra is still able to support spinal function and there are no neurological effects, or unstable where there may be associated neurological effects. Unstable fractures may deteriorate and cause further damage and worse outcomes, which is why spinal precautions are so important for the clinician to consider. Compression fractures require significant force and result in fracture of part of the vertebral body, usually associated with a loss of height secondary to the fracture. A burst fracture, a type of compression fracture, is the result of significant force causing multiple fractures within the one vertebrae.

PRIMARY AND SECONDARY SCI PATHOPHYSIOLOGY

SCI is divided into primary and secondary injury phases (Fig. 47.9). Primary injury results from the direct physical trauma to the spinal cord at the time of injury. This can be associated with cord compression, laceration, shear, contusion or stretch due to penetrating or blunt mechanisms. Secondary injury is a result of a progressive cascade of physiological, extracellular biomechanical and intracellular insults that commence from the time of injury and extend over the subsequent hours, days and weeks.

Mechanisms of secondary injury include ischaemia, hypoxia and oedema. Damage is caused by restricted blood flow, excitotoxicity, inflammation, oxidative cell damage, free-radical release and apoptosis, all of which contribute to ischaemia and ultimately cell death. Treatment should target neuroprotective strategies and therapies to help preserve functional tissue and limit the degree of secondary damage. Early management should be targeted at avoiding and ameliorating systemic insults while optimising provision of nutrients to the injured tissue. This includes prevention or correction of hypotension, shock, decreased arterial oxygen content, catecholamine release, hypercoagulability and hyperthermia.

SPINAL AND NEUROGENIC SHOCK

Neurogenic shock and spinal shock are sometimes confused; however, they are two different problems.[14]

Spinal shock refers to the symptoms associated with SCI. It occurs in cervical and upper thoracic injuries at the time of injury and has a duration lasting from days to weeks. It is defined as a sudden, complete loss of motor and sensory function below the level of SCI. Symptoms include loss of all spinal reflexes below the level of injury and flaccid paralysis, including the bladder and bowel. Sustained priapism may also be present.

FIGURE 47.9 PATHWAYS INVOLVED IN CELL DEATH AFTER SPINAL INJURY[13]

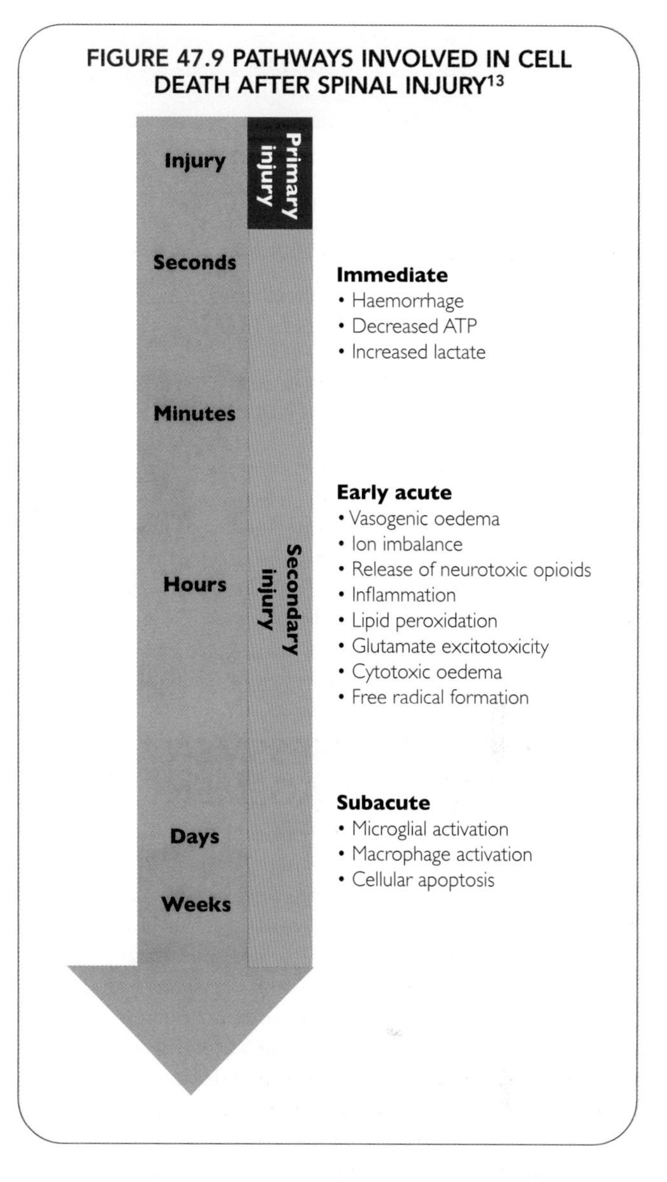

Resolution of spinal shock occurs when the reflex arcs below the level of injury begin to function again; the return of the bulbocavernosus reflex has traditionally been used to indicate the end of spinal shock. The severity of injury may not be fully appreciated until after spinal shock has resolved.

Neurogenic shock occurs as a result of interruption to the descending sympathetic tracts at or above T6, causing a loss in innervation to the heart and vasomotor tone. This results in profound vasodilation, and subsequently a decrease in venous return, cardiac output and tissue perfusion. Neurogenic shock is characterised by hypotension and bradycardia, and typified by warm extremities and preserved urine output. Thereby, often referred to as 'warm shock'. The early management of hypotension in these patients is of paramount importance to ensure optimal spinal cord perfusion.

PRACTICE TIP

It is important to differentiate between neurogenic and hypovolaemic shock, as they require very different treatment (see Chapters 10 and 42).

TABLE 47.2 DIFFERENCES BETWEEN NEUROGENIC AND HYPOVOLAEMIC SHOCK

NEUROGENIC SHOCK	HYPOVOLAEMIC SHOCK
Hypotension	Hypotension
Bradycardia	Tachycardia
Hypothermia	Hypothermia
Dry warm skin	Cool clammy skin
Related to nervous system injury	Related to massive blood or fluid loss

Neurogenic and hypovolaemic shock may co-exist in the multi-trauma patient and, in this instance, neurogenic shock exacerbates the effects of hypovolaemic shock by disabling the vasoconstrictive reflexes that ordinarily preserve blood flow to vital organs. Hypovolaemic and neurogenic shock differ in their presentation (Table 47.2).

PRE-HOSPITAL ASSESSMENT AND INITIAL MANAGEMENT

Pre-hospital clinicians play a significant role in influencing outcomes in the spinal injured patient. Early and accurate patient assessment, including the appropriate identification and management of potential spinal cord injuries, not only supports treatment and intervention decision-making, triage, transport requirements and destination decisions, but also aids in reducing inappropriate over-triage and unnecessary spinal immobilisation practices.[15,16]

The fundamental principles in the initial management of a trauma patient remain a thorough comprehensive primary and secondary survey (see Chapter 42). Early management strategies to optimise SCI outcome should be targeted at effective resuscitation, including the treatment of hypotension and prevention of hypoxia.[17] Early identification and treatment of immediate life-threatening injuries, such as the lost airway, is of the highest priority. It is important to protect the person's spine through all stages of assessment and intervention.

PRACTICE TIP

All unconscious trauma patients, or the awake patient complaining of spinal pain and/or neurological symptoms, should be presumed to have a SCI until proven otherwise.

PRIMARY SURVEY

Patients with known or suspected high SCI may require emergent airway protection manoeuvres/interventions, including intubation and ventilation, for airway protection, or to facilitate controlled mechanical ventilation. Although all airway interventions will cause some spinal movement, the clinical significance of this is still uncertain[18](see Chapter 16 for airway management techniques). Regardless of the means of securing the lost or compromised airway, limiting spinal movement during such procedures should be routinely practised. If emergent airway protection manoeuvres/interventions, including intubation and ventilation, for airway protection are required, the cervical collar should be removed, and manual in-line stabilisation applied (see images in Chapter 16).

The standard of care for spinal protection, in both the pre-hospital and acute care environment, has shifted away from rigid, blanket immobilisation strategies, to a more selective minimal handling strategy based on appropriate risk assessment.[19,20] If the patient is still wearing a helmet on arrival of paramedics, it should be removed as demonstrated in Fig. 16.17, p. 326 to facilitate assessment. Where there is immediate threat to life identified with initial assessment, all efforts to limit spinal movement without delay to treatment are required[21] (see Chapter 9 for extrication process). The efficacy of such devices as the Kendrick Extrication Device (KED) and long board use in pre-hospital extrication is under scrutiny.[22,23] Evidence suggests that self-extrication is reasonable and safe in many circumstances.[15,24] Expert consensus is that where casualties are conscious and have capacity to stand, professionally guided extrication independently or with minimal assistance should be the first consideration.[25] Spinal motion restriction, previously known as spinal immobilisation, is covered in more detail on the following page.

PRACTICE TIP

Self-extrication, guided by pre-hospital clinicians, should be the first consideration in the conscious patient with capacity to mobilise.

THE COMBATIVE PATIENT AND AIRWAY MANAGEMENT

Patients with known or suspected spinal injury may become agitated or restless due to shock, hypoxia, head injury, hypovolaemia or intoxication. As such, forced application of motion restriction strategies may exacerbate the risk of harm, and it is more beneficial to allow the patient to move unhindered. For those patients assessed as high risk, pharmacological agents may be necessary to ensure protection of both spine and airway.[26] Airway management in trauma patients with suspected or confirmed cervical spine injury requires expert clinical decision-making and technical execution. Significant airway assessment and management expertise are required to avoid adverse events.

PRACTICE TIP

In the pre-hospital setting where airway protection cannot be facilitated by on-scene clinicians, urgent assistance of critical care specialists should be requested, and if unavailable, transport to the nearest suitable facility should be prioritised.

Initial management strategies for the hypotensive trauma patient should remain targeted at treating a hypovolaemic cause (outlined in Chapter 42), until proven otherwise. Systemic hypotension in trauma patients with SCI, regardless of its cause, is associated with a worsened prognosis, higher mortality, and contributes to secondary SCI. Maintenance of MAP > 85–90 mmHg is the current recommended standard of care, to prevent hypoperfusion.[27] The evidence to support these recommendations is limited and it is recognised as an area requiring further research; however, consensus is that hypotension should be avoided post-SCI.[27,28] Neurogenic shock becomes a serious concern in lesions above T6, and characteristically consists of warm extremities, hypotension and bradycardia.[29] Neurogenic shock is an important consideration in all unstable trauma patients; however, it is relatively uncommon and is a diagnosis of exclusion after other forms of shock have been managed and/or excluded.

PAIN MANAGEMENT

In the acute phase, adequate pain management is crucial when providing care to trauma patients. It facilitates accurate patient assessment, controls post-injury stress responses, improves respiratory efficiency, patient experiences and outcomes, and is ethically moral. Adequate analgesia should be administered early in the care continuum, and titrated against the patient's pain score, physical dynamics and response (see Chapter 18). The choice of analgesic agent will be guided by pre-hospital protocols and clinician skill level. Adequate pain relief is essential to limit the effect of autonomic nervous dysfunction that can be triggered by pain.[27] Due to the risk of aspiration, prophylactic antiemetics should also be considered in patients prior to transport.

PRACTICE TIP

Early administration of appropriate analgesics facilitates accurate assessment, improves respiratory efficiency, controls post-injury stress responses and improves patient experiences and outcomes.

Hypothermia is common in trauma patients, and is associated with increased mortality and morbidity. Although there is growing evidence to support the role of therapeutic hypothermia in the treatment of trauma patients with acute traumatic spinal cord injury,[30] the priority in the pre-hospital setting, and emergency department (ED), remains with hypothermia prevention and management. This can be achieved through simple considerations and adjuncts, such as limiting exposure and scene time, avoiding excessive administration of cold intravenous fluid, applying warm blankets and removing all wet items of clothing (see Chapter 28).

SPINAL MOTION RESTRICTION/ STABILISATION

Application of spinal motion restriction continues to be a mainstay in both pre-hospital and acute trauma care for blunt trauma. There has been a shift away from rigid, blanket immobilisation strategies, to a selective minimal handling strategy based on appropriate risk assessment.[19] This shift is underpinned by the fact that the routine use of spinal motion restriction devices is often difficult, time-consuming, and in some cases counterproductive.[19,20,31] This selective approach should be complemented by the development and implementation of robust spinal triage tools, incorporating clinical decision rules and risk assessments that guide clinical practice. Spinal motion restriction is not recommended in isolated penetrating spinal trauma.[19]

Due to the risk of non-contiguous injury, where spinal motion restriction is indicated, restrictions are applied to the entire spine, until clinical and/or radiological examinations and clearance. Current recommendations advocate the use of vacuum mattresses and stretcher systems over hard surface systems for the transport of patients with suspected SCI.[32] Regardless of which devices/methods are used to assist in spinal motion restriction, there is consensus in the literature that a minimal handling strategy should be administered across all acute phases of care (Fig. 47.10).[19,33]

Cervical collars

There is evidence that cervical collars, particularly rigid collars, and prolonged spinal motion restrictions can lead to significant complications and morbidity.[19,31] Immobilisation of patients with significant degenerative deformity of the spine, including elderly patients with spondylosis, may result in abnormal positioning of the vertebral column and worsen fracture displacement or neurological injury.[34] There is a lack of evidence for the efficacy of cervical collars in the prevention of secondary SCI,[35,36] and although available devices may limit movement in the compliant patient within the cervical spine, no device has been shown to immobilise it completely.[15]

As such, most organisations have abandoned the use of rigid collars, and there is and greater acceptance and protocolisation of foam (soft) collars as the preferred, initial cervical collar of choice being implemented across pre-hospital and hospital settings.[37,38] While evidence is limited, an Australian retrospective review suggests the practice does not increase the risk of secondary SCI.[39] The application of a soft collar in this patient group provides both a visual and a physical cue to the patient, as well as staff, that the cervical spine has not been cleared, and to continue spinal motion restriction principles (log-roll with inline stabilisation) until formal assessment occurs. In the acute phases of care, occipital padding should be applied to optimise neutral alignment as required in adults (see Fig. 47.11A). Other common cervical collars used in the management of cervical spine injury include the Philadelphia, Aspen and Miami J collars. Measuring and application of collars is discussed in Chapter 16. Manual in-line stabilisation remains the best way to effectively limit the movement of the cervical spine at the lowest cost.

Positioning

Paediatric patients have several anatomical and physiological differences to adults, particularly in those younger than 8 years of age. These children have a prominent occiput and a larger head relative to body size than an adult. When supine, the neck becomes flexed, predisposing the airway to obstruction from the base of the tongue. As such, maintaining anatomical neck alignment and airway patency requires the patient to be positioned in the sniffing position. This is best obtained by placing a thoracic elevation device, such as a dedicated mat or

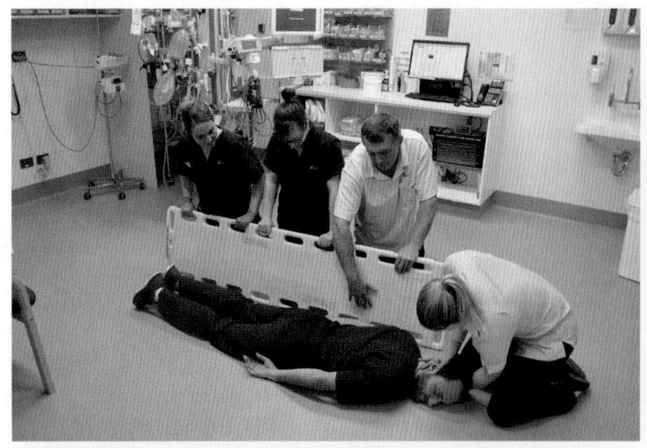

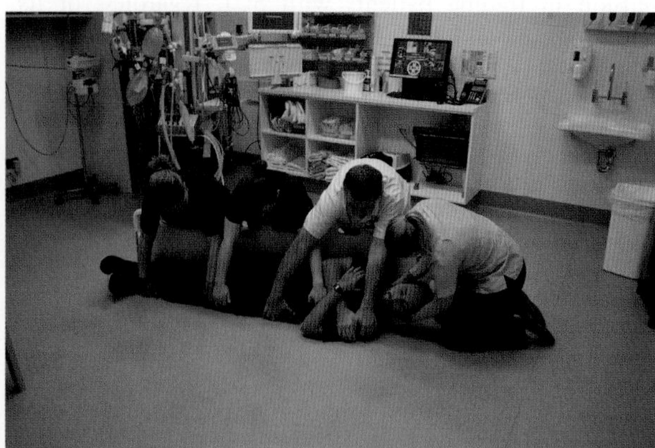

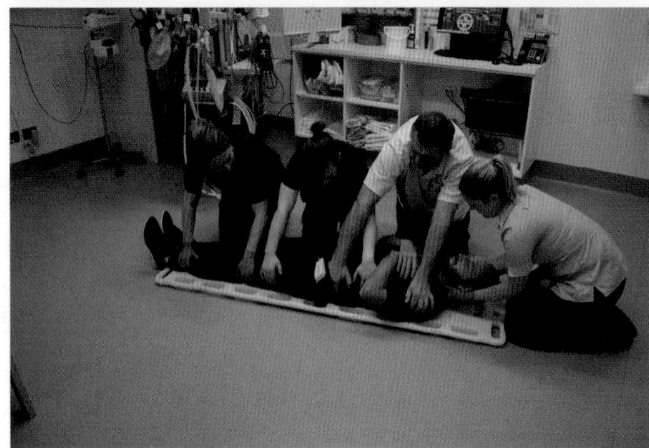

FIGURE 47.10 LOG-ROLLING THE PRONE PATIENT WITH A SUSPECTED SPINAL INJURY
Courtesy of Kate Curtis.

FIGURE 47.11A PADDING REQUIREMENTS FOR A, ADULT PATIENTS[40]

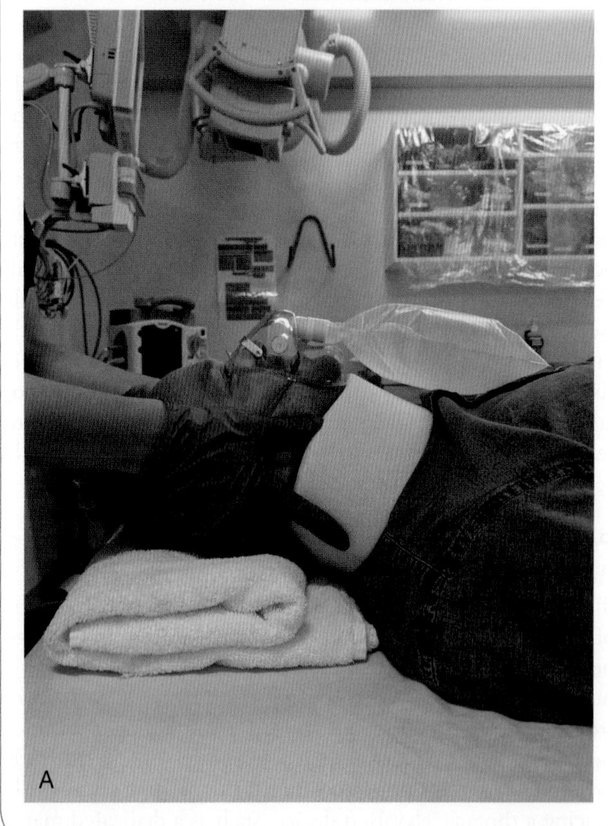

FIGURE 47.11B PADDING REQUIREMENTS FOR B, PAEDIATRIC PATIENTS

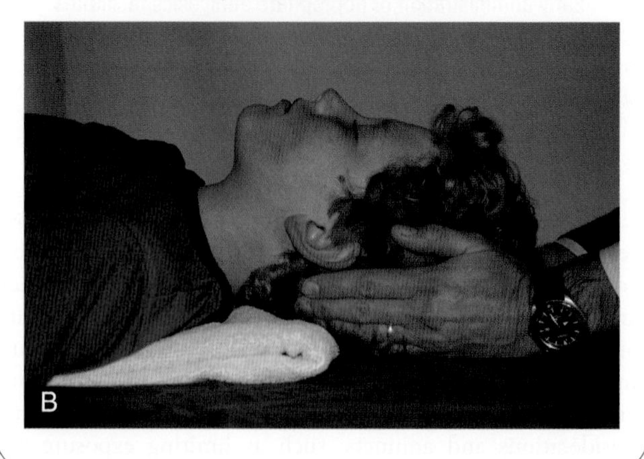

B: Courtesy of Kate Curtis.

folded towel, under the patient's torso to bring the cervical spine into the neutral position (Fig. 47.11B). Constant reassurance is advocated during this process to reduce anxiety and distress, especially in the uncooperative patient. In adults, occipital padding should be applied where necessary to promote neutral alignment. Conditions where the curvature of the spine is abnormal, such as kyphosis, require careful padding to maintain patient comfort as a 'neutral position' of the spine will not be possible.

PRACTICE TIP

A simple folded towel placed under the adult patient's head while using manual in-line stabilisation will generally improve patient comfort and be an effective measure to maintain neutral cervical spine alignment.

ONGOING ASSESSMENT

Once the airway has been assessed, deemed patent or secured, and spinal motion restrictions are in place, further examination of the patient can proceed. This should be conducted using the trauma primary survey principles outlined in Chapter 42.

As part of the primary survey, the multi-trauma patient requires a rapid examination of their entire body surface. This requires careful removal of the patient's clothing, while maintaining spinal motion restriction principles to prevent the flexion, extension and rotation of the neck. Often, the quickest and safest method of removing clothing is to cut the clothing off. Any clothing that remains under the patient can then be removed when the patient is log-rolled. It is important to assess and clear the entire spinal column, as secondary, concomitant, non-contiguous spinal fractures can occur in approximately 10% of cases.[41]

SECONDARY SURVEY AND LOG-ROLL

One of the key components of the secondary survey is to fully examine the patient's back. To enable this, a log-roll of the patient needs to be performed. While there have been no documented reports of sudden, movement-provoked neurological deterioration after blunt spinal trauma,[42] the possibility and amount of motion required to cause secondary injury is still unknown in the clinical setting. As such, the frequency of moving the trauma patient with suspected spinal injuries should be minimised, and where necessary, must be coordinated and designed to protect spinal integrity and alignment. The gold standard for trauma care requires a minimum of four members to safely execute a log-roll (Fig. 47.12).[41] The procedure is led by the most appropriately trained and qualified team member taking manual control of the cervical spine and head. This person will coordinate and remain in charge of the log-roll throughout the entire procedure until the point where the log-roll team is stood down. The remaining members of the team take responsibility of the thorax, abdomen, pelvis and lower extremities. The movement should be smooth and well coordinated to avoid any rotational movements of individual spinal segments. Due to the perceived risk of additional haemorrhage, if pelvic instability is suspected, it is recommended that a risk assessment be conducted before determining if and when to proceed with the log-roll.[43]

FIGURE 47.12 LOG-ROLLING THE TRAUMA PATIENT

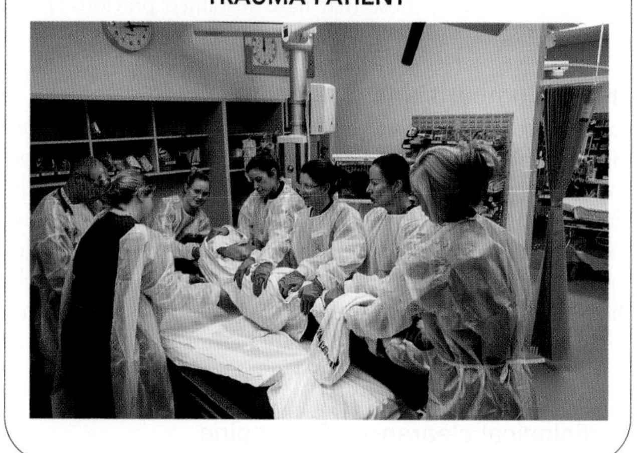

Courtesy of University of Sydney.

Palpation of the spine remains a fundamental component of the clinical examination process, and is useful in identifying areas of point tenderness and bony deformity.[41] This should be conducted during the log-roll, and only after all immediate and life-threatening injuries have been addressed. A comprehensive and thorough neurological examination of the patient's motor, sensory and reflex functions is of prime importance. Where SCI is suspected, or clinically indicated, assessment of rectal tone and sensation is required for complete neurological examination, and is necessary in classifying impairment as complete or incomplete.[44]

Examination of sensory responses to pinprick and light touch is completed by testing a key point in each of the 28 dermatomes on both sides of the body. A key element of assessment of the extent of injury is demonstrated by a display of a segmental pattern in the alteration of motor, sensory and reflex activity in the extremities. In the early acute management, repeat assessment is required, particularly once the patient is stabilised, to monitor for progression of any injury.[27]

SPINAL CLEARANCE

Spinal clearance should occur at the earliest, safest time to do so, and only when qualified clinicians have determined that no significant injury exists. This is only achievable after: 1) a risk assessment; 2) a comprehensive, and sometimes serial, physical examination; and 3) review of reported adjunctive radiological imaging where appropriate. Risk assessment and examination, through the application of validated clinical decision rules, inform either the clinical clearance of, or required radiological investigation of, patients with potential spinal injury. Delay in spinal clearance can significantly impact patient outcomes, with the greatest risk of mortality coming from associated complications, including pressure injury, and not the SCI itself.[45]

Clinical clearance of the cervical spine

Patients who are alert and cooperative are potential candidates for clinical clearance. There are two level 1 evidence-based clinical decision rules for cervical spine assessment: the Canadian C-Spine Rule (CCR) and the National Emergency X-radiography Utilisation Study (NEXUS). These validated rules are used to assist clinicians in distinguishing low-risk patients who do not require imaging of the cervical spine post blunt trauma, thereby reducing inappropriate use of diagnostic imaging, unnecessary spinal immobilisation, and waste.[46] Both clinical decision rules consistently yield high sensitivity[46] and can be safely and accurately applied by both emergency nurses[47,48] and paramedics[33] and are both used in Australia.[49]

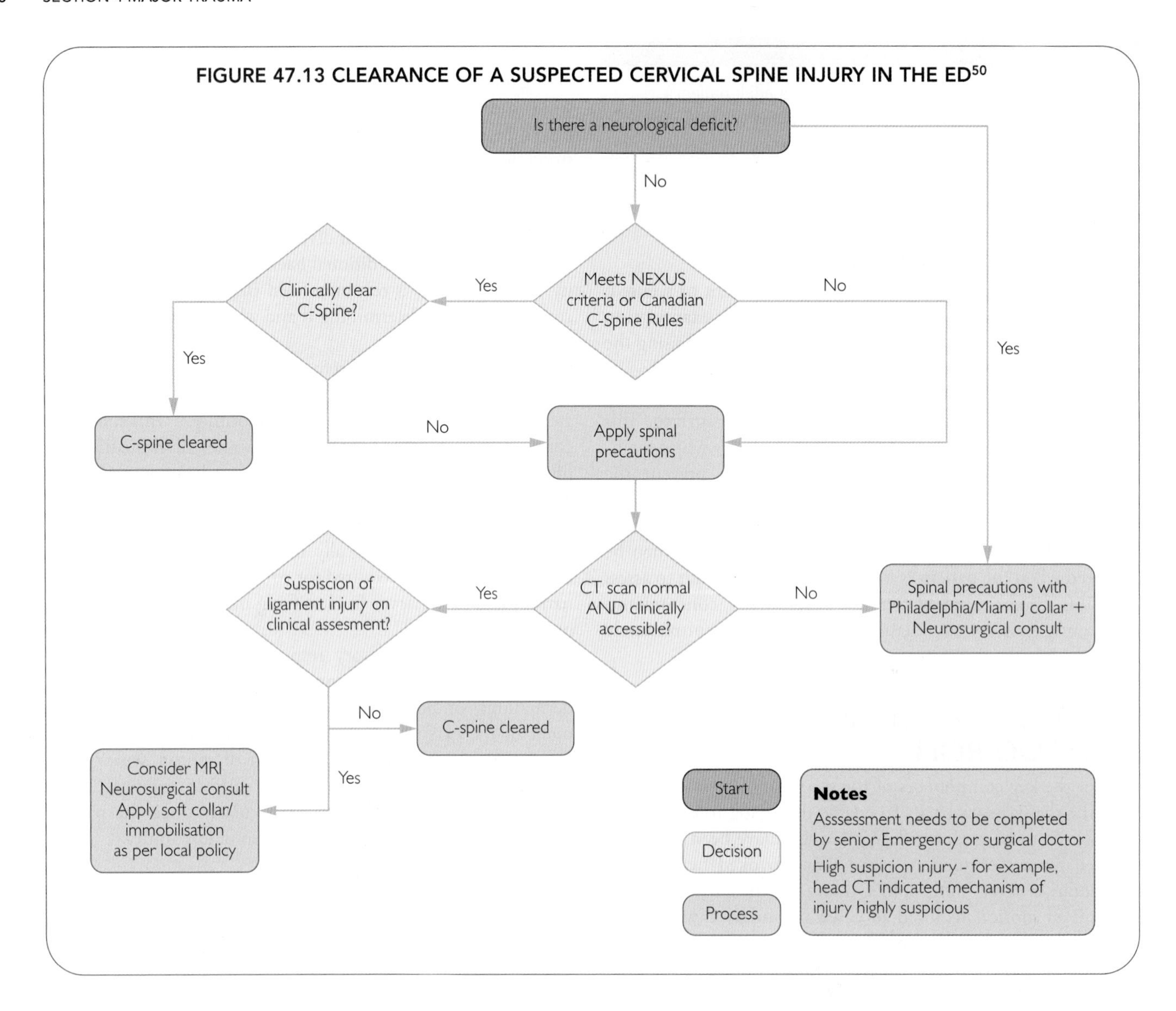

An example of the process to be followed for clearance of the cervical spine in the ED is illustrated in Fig. 47.13.

NEXUS low-risk criteria

The NEXUS low-risk criteria can be applied to all blunt trauma patients where there is a suspicion of cervical spine injury. It consists of five criteria (Fig. 47.14). If each of the five criteria are met, the cervical spine can be clinically cleared without the need for radiology. [45] Its sensitivity is reported between 0.83 and 1.00, and specificity ranged from 0.02–0.46.[51] The NEXUS criteria have been extrapolated and examined for use in the paediatric population.[52]

Canadian C-Spine Rule

The Canadian C-Spine Rule (CCR) adds an additional risk assessment, including mechanism of injury, age and a range of active neck motion tests to its criteria (Fig. 47.15).[53] If no high-risk criteria are met, then a single low-risk criterion allows for the safe assessment of active neck rotation. Providing the patient can actively rotate their neck 45° left and right, radiological evaluation of the cervical spine is not required, and clinical clearance can proceed. Its sensitivity has been reported between 0.90 to 1.00, and specificity ranged from 0.01 to 0.77.[50] Some limitations in its routine clinical application are its significant exclusion criteria, which consists of all pregnant patients, those with abnormal vital signs, those with pre-existing cervical spine abnormality, ankylosing spondylitis and/or rheumatoid disease, and those that have sustained previous spinal injuries.[54]

Thoracolumbar spine clearance

Patients who are alert and cooperative with a low-risk mechanism may be potential candidates for clinical clearance. Attempts have been made to develop clinical decision rules to support the clinical clearance of the thoracolumbar spine. However, these have not been validated or have not had significant results. Emerging evidence suggests that clinical examination alone lacks the sensitivity to safely clear the thoracolumbar spine, and that any decision-making algorithm should factor in such criteria as age, mechanism and other associated injuries.[55]

Radiological clearance of the spine

Radiological investigation is required for all patients with a suspected spinal injury that cannot be cleared clinically.

FIGURE 47.14 NEXUS LOW-RISK CRITERIA

According to the NEXUS Low-Risk Criteria, cervical spine radiography is indicated for trauma patients unless they exhibit ALL of the following criteria:

1. No posterior midline cervical spine tenderness
   and
2. No evidence of intoxication
   and
3. Normal level of alertness
   and
4. No focal neurological deficit
   and
5. No painful distracting injuries

Explanations:

These are for purposes of clarity only. There are not precise definitions for the individual NEXUS Criteria, which are subject to interpretation by individual doctors.

1. Midline posterior bony cervical spine tenderness is present if the patient complains of pain on palpation of the posterior midline neck from the nuchal ridge to the prominence of the first thoracic vertebra, or if the patient evinces pain with direct palpation of any cervical spinous process.

2. Patients should be considered intoxicated if they have either of the following: (a) a recent history by the patient or an observer of intoxication or intoxicating ingestion; or (b) evidence of intoxication on physical examination such as odour of alcohol, slurred speech, ataxia, dysmetria or other cerebellar findings, or any behaviour consistent with intoxication. Patients may also be considered to be intoxicated if tests of bodily secretions are positive for drugs (including but not limited to alcohol) that affect level of alertness.

3. An altered level of alertness can include any of the following: (a) Glasgow Coma Scale score of 14 or less; (b) disorientation to person, place, time or events; (c) inability to remember 3 objects at 5 minutes; (d) delayed or inappropriate response to external stimuli; or (e) other.

4. Any focal neurological complaint (by history) or finding (on motor or sensory examination).

5. No precise definition for distracting painful injury is possible. This includes any condition thought by the clinician to be producing pain sufficient to distract the patient from a second (neck) injury. Examples may include, but are not limited to: (a) any long bone fractures; (b) a visceral injury requiring surgical consultation; (c) a large laceration, degloving injury or crush injury; (d) large burns: or (e) any other injury producing acute functional impairment. Doctors may also classify any injury as distracting if it is thought to have the potential to impair the patient's ability to appreciate other injuries.

Adults

It has been demonstrated that plain film radiographs have low sensitivity in detecting cervical spinal injury with inadequate and repeat imaging required in between 37% and 72% of all cases.[56] As such, routine plain film radiography is not recommended and should be reserved for those institutions where multi detector computed tomography (MDCT) is unavailable.[56] MDCT provides volume data, which allows for reconstruction imaging and better visualisation, and will herein be referred to as CT.

CT is now considered the gold standard and first-line radiological investigation for spinal injury in adult trauma patients.[57] CT has been shown to have a sensitivity greater than 98% for cervical spine injuries,[56] and 97–100% for thoracolumbar spine injuries.[58] It has also been demonstrated to be a reliable and conclusive diagnostic tool for radiological clearance of the spine in the obtunded patient, with a best-case 0% cumulative literature incidence of unstable C-spine injuries after a negative initial imaging result with a cervical spine CT. Reformatted CT images of chest, abdomen and pelvis, as well as CT scout films, can be used for spinal assessment.

Routine adjunctive imaging, such as magnetic resonance imaging (MRI), after a negative CT scan increases the number of low-value diagnoses, places patients with multiple injuries at

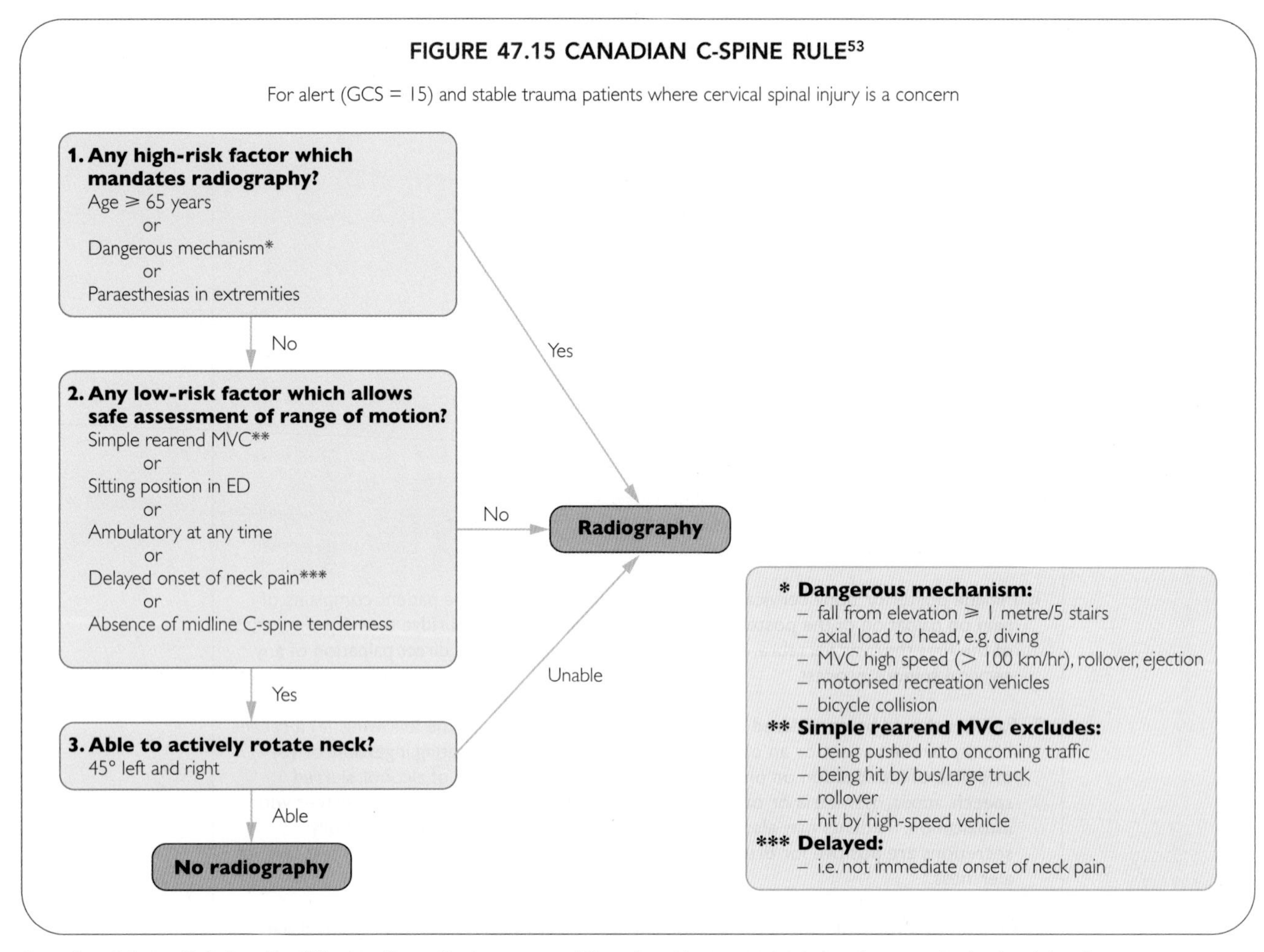

FIGURE 47.15 CANADIAN C-SPINE RULE53
For alert (GCS = 15) and stable trauma patients where cervical spinal injury is a concern
1. Any high-risk factor which mandates radiography?
Age ≥ 65 years
or
Dangerous mechanism*
or
Paraesthesias in extremities
No
Yes
2. Any low-risk factor which allows safe assessment of range of motion?
Simple rearend MVC**
or
Sitting position in ED
or
Ambulatory at any time
or
Delayed onset of neck pain***
or
Absence of midline C-spine tenderness
No
Radiography
Unable
Yes
3. Able to actively rotate neck?
45° left and right
Able
No radiography
* Dangerous mechanism:
– fall from elevation ≥ 1 metre/5 stairs
– axial load to head, e.g. diving
– MVC high speed (> 100 km/hr), rollover, ejection
– motorised recreation vehicles
– bicycle collision
** Simple rearend MVC excludes:
– being pushed into oncoming traffic
– being hit by bus/large truck
– rollover
– hit by high-speed vehicle
*** Delayed:
– i.e. not immediate onset of neck pain

Canadian C-Spine Rule for alert (Glasgow Coma Scale score = 15) and stable trauma patients where cervical spine injury is a concern

risk by additional movements outside of safe clinical spaces, is of high cost and, at best, results in the same clinical action of collar removal. However, MRI does have a role in the diagnosis, management and treatment of those patients with: 1) neurological deficit on examination; 2) moderate-to-severe spinal degenerative disease on CT; and 3) follow-up imaging to assess spinal cord injury related to a spinal fracture. MRI can also help evaluate soft-tissue injuries, though will not be an urgent investigation in the emergency department.[59]

Paediatrics

Anteroposterior and lateral plain film radiology continues to be the initial screening tool for assessment of spinal injuries in alert children without neurological deficit, with a sensitivity rate greater than 90%. Although CT is superior in sensitivity, at almost 100%, it is not routinely recommended in the paediatric setting due to the associated increase in radiation exposure and increased risk of malignancy. However, CT is superior to both plain radiographs and MRI in detecting bony injury, and specialised CT protocols are recommended to limit the radiation exposure in paediatric cervical spine imaging.[60,61] Additionally, some CT protocols will also recommend only imaging to the level of C3, due to most injuries of the paediatric cervical spine occurring at or above this level. MRI is a highly useful imaging modality in children as it reduces radiation exposure and has a high sensitivity to detect spinal cord and soft-tissue injuries.[62] MRI can play a fundamental role in clearing the cervical spine in the obtunded child, as well as in the evaluation of children with persistent symptoms and neurological deficit. There is the possibility of spinal cord injury without radiographic abnormality (SCIWORA) in children due to the underdeveloped spine. Imaging should be used to gather information and rule out other diagnoses.[63]

Table 47.3 outlines the various diagnostic procedures used to determine spinal column or cord injury.

PHARMACOLOGICAL MANAGEMENT

Currently, there are no pharmacological treatments available for SCI with proven, reproducible efficacy. Methylprednisolone, once the 'standard of care' in SCI management, and considered to be one of the few treatments to have demonstrated any clinical benefit, is no longer recommended in SCI treatment.[64,65] Other therapies are still in early phases of research and have not had demonstrated efficacy in human studies.[66]

ONGOING MANAGEMENT

Every system of the body is innervated by the spinal cord and during the emergency phase following SCI there are a number of interventions required to reduce the risk of secondary

TABLE 47.3 DIAGNOSTIC EVALUATION PROCEDURES FOR SPINAL CORD INJURY

PROCEDURE	COMMENTS
Radiography	Able to visualise the entire spine to delineate the exact site and specific nature of bony injuries
Anteroposterior (AP) and lateral views	Plain film radiography has a low sensitivity for cervical spine injuries in the adult population. However, plain film radiography, particularly AP and lateral films, continues to be the initial screening tool for assessment of spinal injuries in alert children without neurological deficit. Views should be examined for: • contour and alignment of vertebral bodies according to normal curvature of the spine • presence of cervical vertebrae • displacement of bone fragments into the spinal canal • fracture of the laminae, pedicles, spinous process to determine ligamentous stability • spinous process distances • degree of soft-tissue damage, especially important when no fracture is apparent (SCIWORA)
Computed tomography (CT) scanning	Thin-cut (2 mm) axial CT scanning of the spine is now considered the gold standard in those with suspected spinal injuries and is superior to both plain radiographs and MRI in detecting spinal column injuries. There is a reported best-case 0% cumulative literature incidence of unstable C-spine injuries after a negative initial imaging result with a cervical spine. The scan should include the entire vertebral body above and below the region of interest, as these must be undamaged for subsequent internal fixation. Widening, slippage or rotational abnormalities of the cervical vertebrae suggest soft-tissue injury. An absence of such signs appears to exclude significant instability. If there are abnormal findings on the CT scan, additional modalities, such as MRI, can be employed. Helical or multislice CT scanning from the occiput to T1 is performed at 2–3 mm collimation and 1.5 m pitch. Sagittal and coronal reconstructions must be closely examined for indications of ligamentous instability. Further, patients who undergo CT scan of the chest and abdomen can have spinal construction images created which can provide concise detail of the thoracolumbar spine.
Magnetic resonance imaging (MRI)	Non-invasive technique Uses radiofrequency radiation in presence of strong magnetic field to provide cross-sectional display of various anatomical structures, including soft tissues. MRI can play a useful role in the diagnosis, management and treatment strategies in those with spinal injury. It is considered an appropriate diagnostic tool in the paediatric population for its radiation sparing qualities, and can add valuable information in those patients with neurological deficits, abnormal CT findings or intervention planning. Difficult in intubated patient
Somatosensory evoked potential (SSEP)	Assists with establishing the extent of injury to the nervous system; often performed within 24–48 hours of admission Used to monitor intraoperative neural function during surgical reduction or instrumentation of the spine

complications, particularly to the respiratory, circulatory and the genitourinary systems.

RESPIRATORY

Respiratory complications after SCI are a major cause of morbidity and mortality. Patients with a SCI above the 12th thoracic (T12) spinal cord segment are at risk of respiratory complications and dysfunction. The higher the injury, the greater the likelihood dysfunction will occur.[67]

Patients with high SCI involving phrenic motor neurons above the fifth cervical (C5) spinal cord segment may develop diaphragmatic and expiratory muscle paralysis[67] or reduced respiratory effort due to spinal shock. These patients require immediate intubation and mechanical ventilation.[68]

At lower levels, cervical cord injury can lead to inspiratory and expiratory accessory muscle paralysis and the patient may also develop significant respiratory impairment due to diaphragmatic and accessory muscle weakness, impaired cough, increased secretion production and bronchospasm.[69] Refer to Table 47.4 for muscle innervation. These patients may benefit from non-invasive ventilation and assisted coughing techniques.[70]

Close respiratory monitoring of the patient's respiratory rate, depth and pattern is paramount in the early phases of care for all patients with suspected SCI. Impaired respiratory function may develop progressively, and serial observation for signs of fatigue, shallow or paradoxical breathing, increased accessory muscle use and hypoxia is essential to prevent deterioration.[71]

PRACTICE TIP

Recording baseline and ongoing respiratory function, including vital capacity (VC), forced expiratory volume (FEV_1), ABGs and oxygen saturation, can provide valuable indicators of respiratory compromise.[69]

TABLE 47.4 SPINAL NERVE MUSCLE INNERVATION AND PATIENT RESPONSE

NERVE LEVEL	MUSCLES INNERVATED	PATIENT RESPONSE
C4	Diaphragm	Ventilation
C5	Deltoid	Shrug shoulders
	Biceps	Flex elbows
	Brachioradialis	
C6	Wrist extensor	Extend wrist
	Extensor carpi radialis longus	
C7	Triceps	Extend elbow
	Extensor digitorum	Extend fingers
	Flexor carpi radialis	
C8	Flexor digitorum profundus	Flex fingers
T1	Hand intrinsic muscles	Spread fingers
T2 to L1	Intercostals	Vital capacity
	Abdominal	Abdominal reflexes
L2	Iliopsoas	Hip flexion
L3	Quadriceps	Knee extension
L4	Tibialis anterior	Ankle dorsiflexion
L5	Extension hallucis longus	Ankle eversion
S1	Gastrocnemius	Ankle plantar flexion
		Big toe extension
S2 to S5	Perineal sphincter	Sphincter control

Patients with SCI have a high likelihood of other injuries to the thorax. Pain and chest trauma, including rib fractures, pneumothorax and pulmonary contusions, can contribute to respiratory impairment, along with patient age and pre-existing conditions. Regular chest physiotherapy, incorporating deep breathing and coughing exercises, and the use of high-flow nasal prongs in patients that are not already intubated, can help prevent atelectasis and pneumonia. Assisted coughs can be provided manually or with an insufflation–exsufflation machine.

CIRCULATORY

Acute SCI results in interruption of sensorimotor and autonomic pathways and is associated with blood pressure and heart rate dysregulation and haemodynamic instability.[72] Cardiac dysrhythmias, particularly bradycardia, autonomic dysreflexia and orthostatic hypotension, are common cardiovascular complications following SCI, each having immediate and long-term negative effects on rehabilitation and quality of life.[72] To mitigate risks of hypoperfusion and secondary ischaemic cord injury, a goal of therapy is to maintain a mean arterial blood pressure of 85 mmHg or higher for 7 days.[27,28] This may be achieved through the use of vasopressors.[28] Clinician interventions such as turning the patient or suctioning may result in cardiovascular instability; the clinician should be aware of this risk.

Close monitoring of fluid status is important, as aggressive fluid resuscitation of a patient in neurogenic shock can result in pulmonary oedema. Cardiac, haemodynamic and respiratory monitoring will assist in early detection of potential complications and allow initiation of prompt treatment, which can lead to improved patient outcomes and reduced risk of complications.

All patients with SCI are at increased risk of venous thromboembolism due to reduced mobility and vascular contraction, loss of motor tone and reduced venous return. Mechanical prophylaxis, including compression stockings, sequential calf compression and regular position changes are not sufficient alone, but their use is recommended in conjunction with anticoagulant such as low molecular weight heparin.[73]

PRACTICE TIP

Where not contraindicated, prophylactic anticoagulant therapy, preferably low-molecular-weight heparin, should begin as soon as possible in conjunction with intermittent pneumatic compression device (calf compressors).

GASTROINTESTINAL AND GENITOURINARY

Gastrointestinal dysfunction is common after SCI. While the most common symptoms are obstruction, distension and abdominal pain,[74] it is reported that approximately half of all SCI patients will suffer from moderate-to-severe neurogenic bowel dysfunction (NBD).[75] NBD is colon dysfunction due to damage to the neuronal pathways that control gastrointestinal sensory and motor functions.[75] In the acute phases of care, the patient should be monitored for bowel sounds and abdominal distension at least every 4 hours.[70] A rectum examination should be performed to ensure the lower bowel is empty. The establishment of a multifaceted bowel regimen is considered the cornerstone in conservative management.[76] This regimen may include a regular diet, aperients, abdominal massage, digital rectal stimulation, manual extraction and the use of suppositories or enemas, depending on the level of injury and subsequent symptoms.[77] Electrical stimulation/neuromodulation is also a promising alternative intervention option in selected patients at the rehabilitation phase when paired with voluntary motor training.[78]

PRACTICE TIP

Insertion of an appropriate gastric tube is essential to relieve nausea and gastric distension, which can increase the risk of aspiration and further compromise respiratory function. Patient must remain nil by mouth until bowel sounds return and will require IV hydration until adequate oral intake can be tolerated. Abdominal injuries should be ruled out as may be more likely with a spinal injury.

Acute SCI, particularly cervical injuries, increases the risk of gastric ulcers; ideally, administration of intravenous prophylaxis should be started as soon as possible after injury.[79]

Genitourinary dysfunction is also common after SCI, with the loss of voluntary muscle control and reflexes causing either a neurogenic or an aneurogenic bladder. As such, during the acute phases of care, a urinary catheter must be placed to decompress the bladder and allow for strict urinary output measurement.

PRACTICE TIP

Insertion of an indwelling urinary catheter is required to facilitate drainage of urine and enable accurate monitoring of fluid balance.

OTHER SYSTEMS

Pain regulation

Sensory disturbances and the presence of acute and chronic neuropathic pain can be one of the most serious and debilitating consequences of SCI. In those with SCI, pathophysiological changes and activation of inflammatory mediators can influence and further heighten pain responses.[80] While an adequate treatment for neuropathic pain remains notoriously difficult to achieve and largely an unsolved problem,[81] the importance of appropriate and adequate pain relief in those with SCI is a fundamental requirement. Chronic neuropathic pain secondary to SCI is reported in up to 70% of all cases.[82] Common symptoms include pins and needles, burning, brush-evoked pain, electric shock/stabbing and tingling, and can manifest as regions of hypersensitivity with or without a stimulus.[83]

The pain relief chosen should not affect respiratory function and needs to take into account neuropathic pain requirements. Neuropathic pain does not respond well to many traditional analgesics, including opiates. Medications that have been found to provide effective pain relief include some anticonvulsant and antidepressant medications.[84] For further information on pain management, see Chapter 18.

PRACTICE TIP

It is essential to monitor and maintain normal body temperature of patients with spinal injuries at or above T6, as they lose the ability to autoregulate body temperature (poikilothermia), and will assume the temperature of their environment. This has significant implications for the haemorrhaging trauma patient.

Skin integrity

Pressure injuries are largely avoidable and prevention strategies should be implemented as part of the management of acute SCI. Patients with spinal cord injuries are at significant risk of pressure injury from decreased sensation and motor function, coupled with impaired circulation and use of hard support surfaces and cervical collars. Areas at highest risk are bony prominences below the level of injury and the occipital area for those wearing cervical collars.

Prolonged immobilisation should be avoided whenever possible, and pressure relief commenced once emergency medical conditions and spinal stabilisation permit. If a hard backboard has been used pre-hospital, it should be removed when the patient is transferred between stretchers. Ideally, assessment and documentation of the patient's skin condition would happen at this time, with reassessment occurring each time pressure relief is attended.

Use of pressure-relieving mattresses as appropriate to the patient's condition, along with regular turning or repositioning of individuals with acute spinal cord injury, should be attended every 2 hours if the medical condition allows. It is important to prevent shearing and friction and avoid stretching and folding of soft tissues, when moving and transferring patients. Box 47.1 summarises essential nursing care.

Thermoregulation

SCI results in reduced sensory input to temperature regulation centres and loss of sympathetic control of both temperature and sweat functions below the level of injury. The inability to maintain a core body temperature is referred to as poikilothermia, and results in passive dilation of dermal-level blood vessels. It is more common in high thoracic and cervical spinal cord injuries. As such, regular monitoring and maintenance of both core body and environmental temperature is important.

See Chapter 28 for the impact of hypothermia on the trauma patient.

DEFINITIVE CARE

All patients with SCI will need admission and specialist care. Once SCI is confirmed, the patient should have appropriate and timely transfer to the nearest spinal injury unit to ensure both best outcomes and resource utilisation.[85] As there are a small number of spinal injury units in Australia and Aotearoa New Zealand, many patients will be admitted to local and regional hospitals for their initial treatment. Depending on the level of injury and degree of neurological deficit, the patient may require admission to an intensive care unit or neurosurgical high dependency unit.

BOX 47.1 SUMMARY OF NURSING INTERVENTIONS FOR SCI

- Nasogastric tube
- Indwelling urinary catheter
- Intravenous fluids
- Cardiac monitoring
- Blood pressure monitoring
- Temperature
- Pulse
- Pulse oximetry
- Respiratory rate
- Pressure area care
- Analgesia
- Bowel regimen
- Deep vein thrombosis prophylaxis
- Gastric ulcer prophylaxis
- Arterial blood gases

PRACTICE TIP

Transfer to a dedicated spinal injury unit should not be delayed for unnecessary diagnostic procedures that will not alter management.

When transferring patients with spinal injuries, full spinal motion restrictions should be maintained, preferably using a vacuum mattress or split-scoop stretcher, or a lateral transfer board when moving the patient between flat surfaces.[86] Patients should never be left on a transfer device beyond the time taken to safely complete the designated task. Flat lifting scoop stretchers may be used in those patients with confirmed SCI; however, caution should be taken to avoid any disruption to skin integrity from application of the device.

TREATMENT OPTIONS

Treatment of spinal injuries can consist of surgical or conservative management, and will depend on the type of fracture, spinal cord involvement and patient condition. Early surgery for patients with a traumatic SCI is seen as the gold standard in acute management. Evidence suggests it not only reduces secondary damage, but also contributes to improved neurological recovery, reduced hospital stay, complications and costs.[87] Surgery is performed to reduce fractures and dislocations, decompress the spinal cord, stabilise injured segments, and restore optimal vertebral alignment. Surgery can be performed from an anterior or posterior approach; severe injuries may require both anterior and posterior surgery. Depending on the type of surgery performed, a number of internal fixation devices can be used to provide stability. Some factors that influence the surgical approach and type of internal stabilisation device used include the level and type of spinal column injury, the extent of spinal instability, the number of vertebrae requiring stabilisation, the extent of neurological impairment and the preference of the surgeon.

Non-operative management may be an option depending on patient condition and surgeon discretion. Therapeutic and complementary treatment options include the application and use of stabilisation devices, such as braces, casts, cervical collars and halo thoracic vests.

Conservative management is less common in SCI patients as it requires prolonged periods of bed rest and immobilisation strategies, and contributes to greater hospital lengths of stay and the risk of complications. However, conservative management strategies are still considered safe in selected patient groups.[88] Patients with spinal fractures without neurological involvement may be able to be managed conservatively without a brace with adequate analgesia and early ambulation.[89]

PSYCHOSOCIAL CARE

Those suffering with SCI will not only develop different levels of physical loss, but will often develop significant psychological difficulties and social limitations.[90] Immediately following SCI, it is common for the patient to struggle to comprehend what this means for them, their family and the rest of their life. Patients often ask questions regarding their long-term prospects, particularly whether they will be able to walk again. These questions are difficult to answer accurately, particularly until the acute phase of injury has passed and spinal shock has resolved. Reassurance, emotional support and honesty are valuable to patients and their family and friends at this time. Common feelings include anxiety, depression, shock, fear and helplessness. These psychosocial factors can have a significant impact on not only their physical rehabilitation, but also their ongoing quality of life.[91] Providing an explanation of all procedures and answering questions can help decrease the distress experienced due to feelings of loss of control in this unfamiliar environment.

CLASSIFICATION OF SPINAL CORD INJURIES

Injuries to the spine can be classified as complete or incomplete depending on the degree of sensory and/or motor deficits found on examination.[44] The American Spinal Injury Association Standards for Classification of Neurological Injury Scale form (Fig. 47.16) assists in the classification and documentation of spinal cord injury.

Classification of spinal cord injuries is determined using the American Spinal Injury Association (ASIA) scale.

- *Tetraplegia* is defined as 'impairment or loss of motor and/or sensory function in the cervical segments of the spinal cord as a result of damage to neural elements within the spinal canal'. Tetraplegia results in decreased function in the arms, trunk, legs and pelvic organs.
- *Paraplegia* is defined as 'impairment or loss of motor and/or sensory function in the thoracic, lumbar or sacral segments of the spinal cord, as a result of damage of neural elements within the spinal canal. Arm function remains intact, but trunk, legs and pelvic organs may be involved', depending on the level of injury. Injuries to the cauda equina and conus medullaris also fall into this category.
- The *neurological level of injury* may differ from the skeletal level of injury. The neurological level is defined as the lowest segment of the spinal cord with normal sensory and motor function on both sides of the body. Using the ASIA Impairment Scale, injuries are graded from A to E according to motor and sensory function, with A being a complete injury and E normal function (Box 47.2).

The sensory assessment consists of testing pinprick and light touch using 28 dermatomes. Each side is scored from 0 to 2, with 0 being absent sensation and 2 being normal. The motor assessment involves testing 10 myotomes on each side. Each muscle is graded from 0 to 5, with 0 representing total paralysis and 5 full strength. Dermatomes and myotomes unable to be tested are recorded as NT (not tested).

COMPLETE SPINAL CORD INJURY

Complete spinal cord injuries are those with an absence of sensory and motor function in the lowest sacral segment; S4–S5. This is tested by observing for voluntary anal contraction and presence of anal sensation. It is possible to have a zone of partial motor or sensory preservation in complete injuries which is recorded on the ASIA form, but there is very little opportunity for return of function in these injuries. Expected level of function in complete injuries can be predicted at an early stage (Table 47.5).

Diagnosis of complete or incomplete injury cannot be made until resolution of spinal shock.

FIGURE 47.16 INTERNATIONAL STANDARDS FOR NEUROLOGICAL CLASSIFICATION OF SCI (ISNCSCI) WORKSHEET[92]

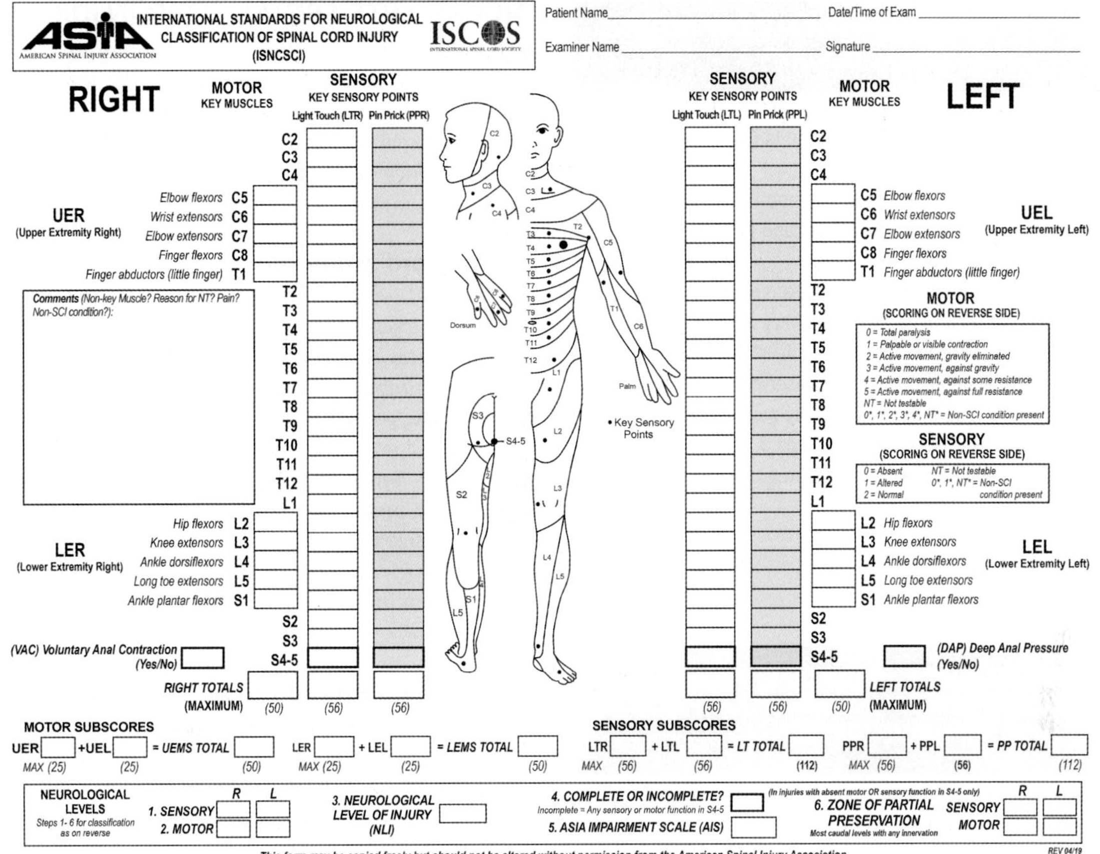
ASIA AMERICAN SPINAL INJURY ASSOCIATION
INTERNATIONAL STANDARDS FOR NEUROLOGICAL CLASSIFICATION OF SPINAL CORD INJURY (ISNCSCI)
ISCoS INTERNATIONAL SPINAL CORD SOCIETY

Patient Name ________ Date/Time of Exam ________
Examiner Name ________ Signature ________

RIGHT — MOTOR KEY MUSCLES — SENSORY KEY SENSORY POINTS: Light Touch (LTR) Pin Prick (PPR)
SENSORY KEY SENSORY POINTS: Light Touch (LTL) Pin Prick (PPL) — MOTOR KEY MUSCLES — LEFT

C2
C3
C4
UER (Upper Extremity Right) / UEL (Upper Extremity Left)
Elbow flexors C5
Wrist extensors C6
Elbow extensors C7
Finger flexors C8
Finger abductors (little finger) T1

Comments (Non-key Muscle? Reason for NT? Pain? Non-SCI condition?):

T2
T3
T4
T5
T6
T7
T8
T9
T10
T11
T12
L1

LER (Lower Extremity Right) / LEL (Lower Extremity Left)
Hip flexors L2
Knee extensors L3
Ankle dorsiflexors L4
Long toe extensors L5
Ankle plantar flexors S1

S2
S3
S4-5

(VAC) Voluntary Anal Contraction (Yes/No)
(DAP) Deep Anal Pressure (Yes/No)

RIGHT TOTALS (MAXIMUM) (50) (56) (56)
LEFT TOTALS (MAXIMUM) (56) (56) (50)

MOTOR
(SCORING ON REVERSE SIDE)
0 = Total paralysis
1 = Palpable or visible contraction
2 = Active movement, gravity eliminated
3 = Active movement, against gravity
4 = Active movement, against some resistance
5 = Active movement, against full resistance
NT = Not testable
0*, 1*, 2*, 3*, 4*, NT* = Non-SCI condition present

SENSORY
(SCORING ON REVERSE SIDE)
0 = Absent
1 = Altered
2 = Normal
NT = Not testable
0*, 1*, NT* = Non-SCI condition present

• Key Sensory Points
Dorsum
Palm
C2 C3 C4 C5 C6 C8 T1 T2 T3 T4 T5 T6 T7 T8 T9 T10 T11 T12 L1 L2 L3 L4 L5 S1 S2 S3 S4-5

MOTOR SUBSCORES
UER ___ + UEL ___ = UEMS TOTAL ___
MAX (25) (25) (50)
LER ___ + LEL ___ = LEMS TOTAL ___
MAX (25) (25) (50)

SENSORY SUBSCORES
LTR ___ + LTL ___ = LT TOTAL ___
MAX (56) (56) (112)
PPR ___ + PPL ___ = PP TOTAL ___
MAX (56) (56) (112)

NEUROLOGICAL LEVELS
Steps 1- 6 for classification as on reverse
R L
1. SENSORY
2. MOTOR
3. NEUROLOGICAL LEVEL OF INJURY (NLI)
4. COMPLETE OR INCOMPLETE?
Incomplete = Any sensory or motor function in S4-5
5. ASIA IMPAIRMENT SCALE (AIS)
(In injuries with absent motor OR sensory function in S4-5 only)
6. ZONE OF PARTIAL PRESERVATION
Most caudal levels with any innervation
R L
SENSORY
MOTOR

This form may be copied freely but should not be altered without permission from the American Spinal Injury Association.
REV 04/19

Muscle Function Grading

0 = Total paralysis

1 = Palpable or visible contraction

2 = Active movement, full range of motion (ROM) with gravity eliminated

3 = Active movement, full ROM against gravity

4 = Active movement, full ROM against gravity and moderate resistance in a muscle specific position

5 = (Normal) active movement, full ROM against gravity and full resistance in a functional muscle position expected from an otherwise unimpaired person

NT = Not testable (i.e. due to immobilization, severe pain such that the patient cannot be graded, amputation of limb, or contracture of > 50% of the normal ROM)

0*, 1*, 2*, 3*, 4*, NT* = Non-SCI condition present [a]

Sensory Grading

0 = Absent **1** = Altered, either decreased/impaired sensation or hypersensitivity

2 = Normal **NT** = Not testable

0*, 1*, NT* = Non-SCI condition present [a]

[a] Note: Abnormal motor and sensory scores should be tagged with a '*' to indicate an impairment due to a non-SCI condition. The non-SCI condition should be explained in the comments box together with information about how the score is rated for classification purposes (at least normal / not normal for classification).

When to Test Non-Key Muscles:

In a patient with an apparent AIS B classification, non-key muscle functions more than 3 levels below the motor level on each side should be tested to most accurately classify the injury (differentiate between AIS B and C).

Movement	Root level
Shoulder: Flexion, extension, adbuction, adduction, internal and external rotation **Elbow:** Supination	C5
Elbow: Pronation **Wrist:** Flexion	C6
Finger: Flexion at proximal joint, extension **Thumb:** Flexion, extension and abduction in plane of thumb	C7
Finger: Flexion at MCP joint **Thumb:** Opposition, adduction and abduction perpendicular to palm	C8
Finger: Abduction of the index finger	T1
Hip: Adduction	L2
Hip: External rotation	L3
Hip: Extension, abduction, internal rotation **Knee:** Flexion **Ankle:** Inversion and eversion **Toe:** MP and IP extension	L4
Hallux and Toe: DIP and PIP flexion and abduction	L5
Hallux: Adduction	S1

ASIA Impairment Scale (AIS)

A = Complete. No sensory or motor function is preserved in the sacral segments S4-5.

B = Sensory Incomplete. Sensory but not motor function is preserved below the neurological level and includes the sacral segments S4-5 (light touch or pin prick at S4-5 or deep anal pressure) AND no motor function is preserved more than three levels below the motor level on either side of the body.

C = Motor Incomplete. Motor function is preserved at the most caudal sacral segments for voluntary anal contraction (VAC) OR the patient meets the criteria for sensory incomplete status (sensory function preserved at the most caudal sacral segments S4-5 by LT, PP or DAP), and has some sparing of motor function more than three levels below the ipsilateral motor level on either side of the body.
(This includes key or non-key muscle functions to determine motor incomplete status.) For AIS C – less than half of key muscle functions below the single NLI have a muscle grade ≥ 3.

D = Motor Incomplete. Motor incomplete status as defined above, with at least half (half or more) of key muscle functions below the single NLI having a muscle grade ≥ 3.

E = Normal. If sensation and motor function as tested with the ISNCSCI are graded as normal in all segments, and the patient had prior deficits, then the AIS grade is E. Someone without an initial SCI does not receive an AIS grade.

Using ND: To document the sensory, motor and NLI levels, the ASIA Impairment Scale grade, and/or the zone of partial preservation (ZPP) when they are unable to be determined based on the examination results.

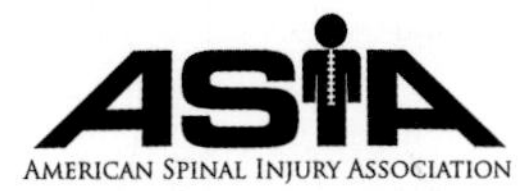

INTERNATIONAL STANDARDS FOR NEUROLOGICAL CLASSIFICATION OF SPINAL CORD INJURY

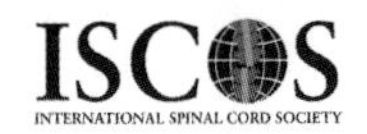

Steps in Classification

The following order is recommended for determining the classification of individuals with SCI.

1. Determine sensory levels for right and left sides.
The sensory level is the most caudal, intact dermatome for both pin prick and light touch sensation.

2. Determine motor levels for right and left sides.
Defined by the lowest key muscle function that has a grade of at least 3 (on supine testing), providing the key muscle functions represented by segments above that level are judged to be intact (graded as a 5).
Note: in regions where there is no myotome to test, the motor level is presumed to be the same as the sensory level, if testable motor function above that level is also normal.

3. Determine the neurological level of injury (NLI).
This refers to the most caudal segment of the cord with intact sensation and antigravity (3 or more) muscle function strength, provided that there is normal (intact) sensory and motor function rostrally respectively.
The NLI is the most cephalad of the sensory and motor levels determined in steps 1 and 2.

4. Determine whether the injury is Complete or Incomplete.
(i.e. absence or presence of sacral sparing)
*If voluntary anal contraction = **No** AND all S4-5 sensory scores = **0** AND deep anal pressure = **No**, then injury is **Complete**.*
*Otherwise, injury is **Incomplete**.*

5. Determine ASIA Impairment Scale (AIS) Grade.

Is injury Complete? If YES, AIS=A

NO ↓

Is injury Motor Complete? If YES, AIS=B

NO ↓ (No=voluntary anal contraction OR motor function more than three levels below the motor level on a given side, if the patient has sensory incomplete classification)

Are at least half (half or more) of the key muscles below the neurological level of injury graded 3 or better?

NO ↓ **AIS=C**

YES ↓ **AIS=D**

If sensation and motor function is normal in all segments, AIS=E
Note: AIS E is used in follow-up testing when an individual with a documented SCI has recovered normal function. If at initial testing no deficits are found, the individual is neurologically intact and the ASIA Impairment Scale does not apply.

6. Determine the zone of partial preservation (ZPP).
The ZPP is used only in injuries with absent motor (no VAC) OR sensory function (no DAP, no LT and no PP sensation) in the lowest sacral segments S4-5, and refers to those dermatomes and myotomes caudal to the sensory and motor levels that remain partially innervated. With sacral sparing of sensory function, the sensory ZPP is not applicable and therefore "NA" is recorded in the block of the worksheet. Accordingly, if VAC is present, the motor ZPP is not applicable and is noted as "NA".

BOX 47.2 ASIA IMPAIRMENT SCALE DEFINITIONS FOR SPINAL INJURY[92]

A. *Complete*—no motor or sensory function is preserved in the sacral segments S4-S5
B. *Sensory Incomplete*—sensory but not motor function is preserved below the neurological level and includes the sacral segments S4-S5
C. *Motor Incomplete*—motor function is preserved below the neurological level, and more than half of key muscles below the neurological level have a muscle grade < 3
D. *Motor Incomplete*—motor function is preserved below the neurological level, and at least half of key muscles below the neurological level have a muscle grade 3
E. *Normal*—motor and sensory function are normal

TABLE 47.5 GUIDELINES FOR EXPECTED FUNCTIONAL OUTCOMES FROM COMPLETE SPINAL INJURIES[52]

Level	Expected outcome
C1-C3	Loss of motor and sensory function below the neck Require permanent artificial ventilation Mobilise in mouth- or head-operated electric wheelchair
C4	Loss of motor and sensory function below the neck Some shoulder movement will remain intact Artificial ventilation may be required during the acute phase Mobilise in chin-operated electric wheelchair
C5	Loss of motor and sensory function below the neck Bicep function present Some shoulder movement will remain intact Mobilise in hand-operated electric wheelchair
C6	Presence of wrist extension Intact sensation extending down the outer arm to the thumb and forefinger Independence in most activities of daily living possible Mobilise in hand-operated electric or manual wheelchair
C7-T1	Intact tricep function Improved finger function Independent in all activities of daily living
T2-T12	Independent in all activities of daily living Sensation, balance and function increase with lower level injuries
L1-L5	Motor and sensory function in hips and upper leg increases with lower level injuries and walking with crutches or leg braces is possible
L2	Hip flexors
L3	Knee extensors
L4	Ankle dorsiflexors
S1-S5	Ankle plantar flexors intact Residual motor weakness in lower limbs but increased control of ankles and feet. May require leg braces to walk

INCOMPLETE SPINAL CORD INJURY

Incomplete injuries result in preservation of varying degrees of motor and/or sensory function below the level of injury, including the lowest sacral segment. This is determined by the presence of anal sensation and voluntary contraction of the anal sphincter. They can often be categorised into one of the following types of injury.

Central cord syndrome

Central cord syndrome occurs because of damage to the centrally lying tracts of the spinal cord and occurs predominantly in the cervical region (Fig. 47.17), and is the most common form of incomplete spinal cord syndrome. Hyperextension injuries are the primary cause of central cord syndrome and are particularly common in older people following falls. Degenerative changes and narrowing of the spinal canal, such as spinal stenosis, can predispose older people to this type of injury. It is possible to sustain central cord damage with no vertebral damage. Neurological loss in central cord syndrome is greater in the upper extremities, with variable bladder, bowel and sexual dysfunction.

Anterior cord syndrome

Anterior cord syndrome occurs due to injury to the anterior section of the spinal cord. This can be a result of decreased blood flow to the anterior spinal artery, which supplies the anterior two-thirds of the cord, resulting in infarction of anterior spinal cord. Other causes include contusion from bone fragments from the vertebral body, disc herniation and fracture dislocation from hyperflexion injuries. Anterior cord syndrome is characterised by variable loss of motor function, pain and temperature perception below the level of injury. Proprioception is maintained.

Brown-Séquard's syndrome

Brown-Séquard's syndrome occurs as a result of transection of half of the spinal cord, most commonly due to knife and bullet wounds or other penetrating injuries (Fig. 47.18). Less frequently, flexion and extension injuries cause Brown-Séquard's syndrome. It is characterised by ipsilateral (same side as lesion) motor paralysis with loss of proprioception and vibration sensation below the level of injury due to the severing of

FIGURE 47.17 CENTRAL CORD SYNDROME

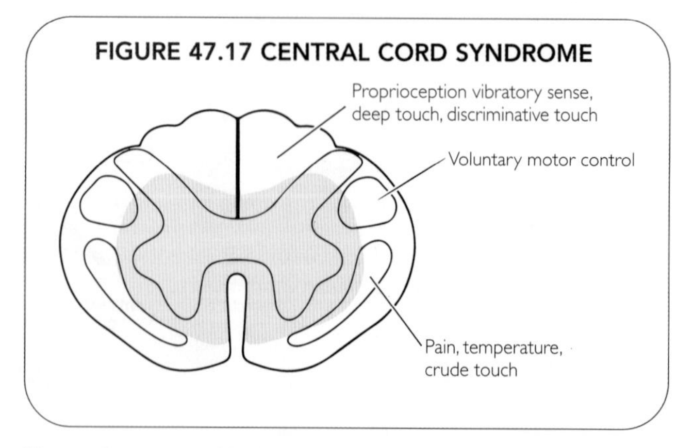

Marcus Cremonese, Medical Illustration Department, UNSW Faculty of Medicine.

FIGURE 47.18 BROWN-SÉQUARD'S SYNDROME

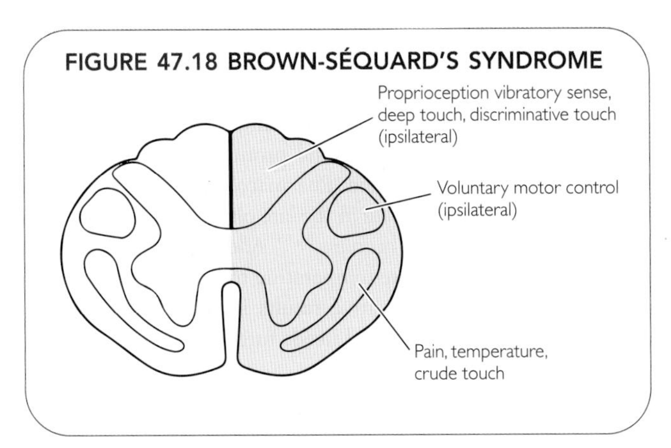

Marcus Cremonese, Medical Illustration Department, UNSW Faculty of Medicine.

corticospinal tracts. Pain and temperature sensation on this side remain intact as the spinothalamic tracts cross over soon after entering the cord. Contralateral (opposite side to lesion) loss of pain and temperature sensation occurs while motor function is retained. That is, poor motor function with good sensation on the same side as the injury and good motor function with poor sensation on the opposite side.

Nerve root injuries

The collection of nerve roots extending from the conus medullaris are referred to as the cauda equina. Lesions of the lumbosacral region may involve multiple roots of the cauda equina with a varying pattern of motor and sensory loss. These injuries are classified as lower motor neuron syndromes and result in an areflexic bladder and bowel, sexual dysfunction and flaccid lower limbs. Conus medullaris syndrome is defined by ASIA as an injury of the sacral cord (conus) and lumbar nerve roots within the spinal canal. Cauda equina syndrome is defined as an injury to the lumbosacral nerve roots within the vertebral canal (Fig. 47.19).

Penetrating injuries

Penetrating spinal cord injury is extremely rare in Australia. Penetrating injuries generally occur as a result of gunshot, blast and/or stab wounds to the spinal column. In most instances, there is no structural damage to the vertebrae and therefore no structural instability. Evidence for spinal stabilisation with collar or hard boards in a patient presenting with penetrating injuries is weak, and clinical context should be taken into account.[19] These injuries are unlikely to require surgery for stabilisation, but may require removal of foreign bodies or repair of vascular damage.

Spinal cord injury without radiographic abnormality (SCIWORA)

It is possible to sustain a spinal cord injury without any bony abnormality being visible on radiological tests. Although seen in all age groups, children are more susceptible to this type of injury, thought to be largely due to anatomical differences such as higher elasticity of spinal ligaments, immature osseous structures and higher head-to-body ratio causing greater deformation forces on the spinal cord. As a result, the spine is able to

FIGURE 47.19 MAGNETIC RESONANCE IMAGING SHOWING ACUTE L4 DISC HERNIATION WITH COMPRESSION OF THE CAUDA EQUINA[9]

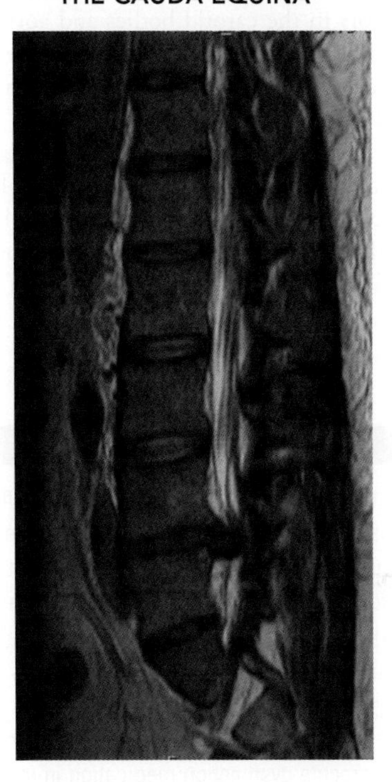

realign itself following a damaging displacement of the vertebrae which has resulted in cord damage. Patients with suspected SCIWORA should be assessed carefully and have MRI imaging to have their injuries assessed.[93]

AUTONOMIC DYSREFLEXIA/ HYPERREFLEXIA

PRACTICE TIP

Autonomic dysreflexia is a medical emergency which needs to be recognised and treated immediately.

Autonomic dysreflexia is a well-known complication of SCI, and is classically seen in those patients with neurological injuries at or above the sixth thoracic (T6) spinal cord segment. It is characterised by hypertension, pounding headache, bradycardia, flushing of skin and sweating above the level of lesion, nasal congestion, blurred vision, shortness of breath, anxiety, skin pallor and piloerection below the level of injury.[94] These symptoms may appear all together or in isolation. Autonomic dysreflexia is considered a medical emergency; without prompt treatment, the blood pressure can rise to dangerously high levels and result in seizures, cardiac dysrhythmia or intracranial haemorrhage. Stimuli below the level of spinal cord injury causes excessive, unmodulated reflex activity from the sympathetic nervous system. Overactivity of the sympathetic ganglia causes release of noradrenaline and dopamine, which cause severe vasoconstriction leading to a sudden rise in blood pressure, severe headache, skin pallor and piloerection. This activity is uncontrolled due to isolation from the normal regulatory response of the vasomotor centres of the brain. Parasympathetic activity occurs when the rise in blood pressure is detected by the baroreceptors in the carotid bodies and aortic arch. Compensatory bradycardia and vasodilation above the level of injury result but are unable to control the hypertension.[94]

The blood pressure of SCI patients needs to be considered in relation to their normal baseline reading. It is common for people with high paraplegia and tetraplegia to have a resting blood pressure of around 90–100/60 mmHg. A blood pressure of 20–40 mmHg above normal resting systolic pressure is considered significantly elevated for this group of people, with autonomic dysreflexia likely to occur within the normal blood pressure range for the general population.

PRACTICE TIP

The most common causes of autonomic dysreflexia are an overdistended bladder or bowel. Other causes include tight clothing, burns, kidney stones, urinary tract infection, haemorrhoids, bites, pressure ulcers, fractures and labour. The immediate treatment required is to identify and remove the cause if possible. Nitrates or captopril may be used according to local policy if the cause cannot be identified. Captopril is administered if there is a chance the patient has used erectile dysfunction medication in recent days.

THE FUTURE

NEUROPROTECTIVE THERAPY

Neuroprotective therapies focus on impeding or preventing secondary injury. Currently, several promising neuroprotective therapies are being investigated. Pharmacological agents, such as minocycline and Riluzole, are in the late phases of animal studies and undergoing trials in humans.[66,95] Additionally, therapeutic hypothermia, reducing core temperature to 32–34°C, is another emerging therapy with positive results in animal studies and small-scale human studies, and needs further research.[96]

RESTORATIVE THERAPY

Neuroregenerative therapies, such as Granulocyte colony-stimulating factor, focus on recovering neuronal circuitry functionality and regeneration, and have shown significant potential in promoting functional and sensory recovery in preclinical and clinical trials.[97] Currently, studies involve the use of various stem cell and cell-based therapies, including the use of glial cells, Schwann cells, bone marrow stromal cells, and even cellular reprograming.[98] Functional electrical stimulation therapy provides electrical currents to nerves and muscle to enhance activity and promote cardiovascular and respiratory conditioning. It has also been demonstrated to increase sensory feedback and muscle use and reduce atrophy.[78] Tissue-based bioengineered scaffolds and tissue grafts are also an emerging treatment in raising function recovery and outcomes in SCI patients, as is the use of nanotechnology materials.[99] However, the use of these technologies is still theoretical in humans.[99]

SUMMARY

While spinal cord injury is relatively rare, it is one of the most complex presentations of trauma that a paramedic, ED, intensive care or trauma ward nurse will face, as it impinges on every organ of the body. Highly developed skills of assessment are essential to differentiate between actual and potential problems. Also, a strong pathophysiology knowledge base is needed to cope with the interventions necessary in caring for the patient with an SCI. The goals of care in this setting are the immediate management of life-threatening conditions, stabilisation of the spine, treatment strategies to limit the degree of secondary injury, and early transfer to a specialist facility for definitive care, recovery, rehabilitation and reintegration back into the community.

CASE STUDY

Ian, an obese male motorbike rider, was out for a Sunday morning ride down the coast through the National Park. He was involved in a head-on collision at 60 kph with a car travelling at approximately 60 kph. He braked suddenly and was thrown over the car and hit the road behind. He was wearing protective gear.

QUESTIONS

1. What considerations need to be taken into account when paramedics first arrive on scene?
2. You receive pre-hospital notification of Ian's arrival. What nursing considerations are needed prior to the patient's arrival in the emergency department (ED)?

A trauma call is activated. On arrival at the ED, a primary survey and secondary survey takes place. The findings are below.

PRIMARY SURVEY

- Cervical spine stabilisation with soft collar, no midline tenderness.

- Effectiveness and rate: trachea centred, reduced breath sounds bilaterally.
- Skin temperature, pulse rate: tachycardic, blood pressure down to 90/40 mmHg. Cool peripherally. No active bleeding. FAST negative.
- Neurological deficit: GCS 14, PEARL. Unable to move legs bilaterally to T10.
- Temperature 34.8°C, clothes removed, blanket applied.

SECONDARY SURVEY

- Head: no obvious injury
- Neck: nil tenderness
- Abdomen: left upper quadrant tenderness. No blood at meatus. IDC inserted
- Lower limbs: 2 cm laceration to lower shin on right side
- Right ankle internally rotated/inverted
- Pinprick sensation lost from umbilicus
- Log-roll of Ian showed haematoma to mid thoracic back on left, very tender; anal tone absent

Plan for pan scan (head to pelvis) investigations and results showed:

- fracture T6 spinous process
- burst fracture T8/incomplete cord syndrome
- comminuted fracture T12
- cerebral oedema
- fractured scapula
- 2–9 fractures ribs/pulmonary contusion
- right haemopneumothorax.

3. Given the multiple body regions injured, and using a systematic approach, outline your monitoring and ongoing care needs for this patient.

FIGURE 47. CS1 BURST FRACTURE T8/T9

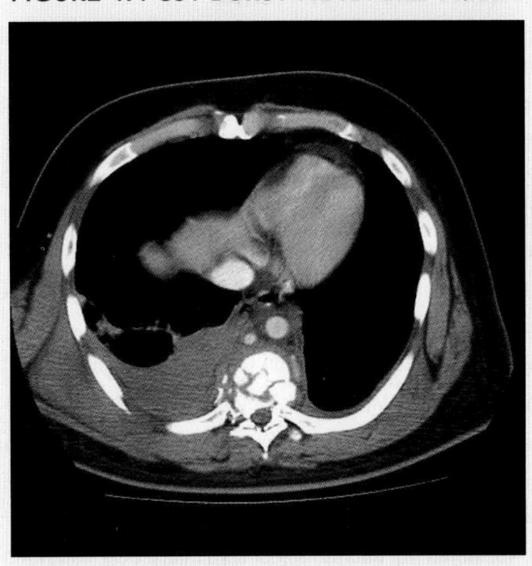

IAN'S JOURNEY

Ian spent 9 days in the intensive care unit, 5 of which were ventilated. He had an intracranial pressure monitor inserted for cerebral oedema. He then spent 7 days in the high-dependency unit and was transferred to a spinal rehabilitation unit for spinal fusion surgery. His ongoing rehabilitation was performed outside of the tertiary centre as Ian relocated to home in rural NSW. He is still having urinary issues, with recurrent urinary tract infections and a suprapubic catheter as intermittent catheterisation was difficult. Paraplegics with this level of injury are usually self-caring; unfortunately, due to Ian's large size, independent management of his activities of daily living has been impossible, with full-time care instituted. Ian has remained with his partner of 7 years and she is his main carer.

Answers to Case Study Questions can be found on evolve **http://evolve.elsevier.com/AU/Curtis/emergency/**

USEFUL WEBSITES

AO Spine Injury Classification Systems, www.aofoundation.org/spine/clinical-library-and-tools/aospine-classification-systems.

Em-docs. Cervical collars for C-Spine trauma: The facts, www.emdocs.net/cervical-collars-for-c-spine-trauma-the-facts/.

EM-RAP: A fib gets the royal treatment. Do we still need the C-collar? www.emrap.org/episode/feb2016emrap/dowestillneed.

JEMS: The Journal of Emergency Medical Services, Why EMS should limit the use of rigid cervical collars, www.jems.com/patient-care/why-ems-should-limit-use-rigid-cervical/.

Life in the Fast Lane: Acute traumatic spinal cord injury, https://litfl.com/acute-traumatic-spinal-cord-injury/.

Spinal Cord Injury Education and Resources Directory, https://aci.health.nsw.gov.au/networks/spinal-cord-injury/resources.

REFERENCES

1. Kristinsdóttir EA, Knútsdóttir S, Sigvaldason K, Jónsson Jr H, Ingvarsson PE. Epidemiology of spinal fractures and associated spinal cord injuries in Iceland. Spinal Cord Series Cases 2018;4(1):74.
2. Smits AJ, den Ouden L P, Deunk J, Bloemers FW. Incidence of traumatic spinal fractures in the Netherlands: analysis of a nationwide database. Spine 2020;45(23):1639–48.

3. Fitzharris M, Cripps R, Lee B. Estimating the global incidence of traumatic spinal cord injury. Spinal Cord 2014;52(2):117–22.
4. New PW, Baxter D, Farry A, Noonan VK. Estimating the incidence and prevalence of traumatic spinal cord injury in Australia. Arc Phys Med Rehab 2015;96(1):76–83.
5. AIHW, Harrison J, O'Brien D, Pointer S. Spinal cord injury, Australia 2017–18. Injury research and statistics series no. 136. Cat. no. INJCAT 219. Canberra: AIHW; 2021.
6. Mitchell J, Nunnerley J, Frampton C, Croot T, Patel A, Schouten R. Epidemiology of traumatic spinal cord injury in New Zealand (2007–2016). NZ Med J 2020;133(1509):47–57.
7. New Zealand Spinal Cord Injury Registry. New Zealand Spinal Cord Injury Registry Annual summary report 2020. 2021. Available from: nzspinaltrust.org.nz/wp-content/uploads/2022/10/NZSCIR-Annual-Report-2021-FINAL.pdf
8. Netter FH. Atlas of human anatomy E-Book. Philadelphia: Elsevier Health Sciences; 2014.
9. Marx J, Hockenberger R, Walls R, editors. Rosen's emergency medicine–concepts and clinical practice. 8th ed. St Louis: Mosby; 2014.
10. Flórez-Jiménez S, Bourassa-Moreau É, Mac-Thiong JM, Maurais G. Biomechanics and patterns of spine injuries associated with spinal cord injury. In: Rajendram R, Preedy VR, Martin CR, editors. Diagnosis and treatment of spinal cord injury. London: Academic Press; 2022.
11. Browner BD, Levine AM, Jupiter J, Trafton PG, Krettek C. Skeletal trauma. 4th ed. Philadelphia: WB Saunders; 2008.
12. van den Heuvel M, Jansz L, Xiong X, Singhal B. People with spinal cord injury in New Zealand. Am J Phys Med Rehab 2017;96(2 Suppl. 1):S96–8.
13. Hachem LD, Ahuja CS, Fehlings MG. Assessment and management of acute spinal cord injury: from point of injury to rehabilitation. J Spinal Cord Med 2017;40(6):665–75.
14. Eckert MJ, Martin MJ. Trauma: spinal cord injury. Surg Clin N Am 2017;97(5):1031–45.
15. Habibi Arejan R, Asgardoon MH, Shabany M, Ghodsi Z, Dehghan HR, Sohrabi Asl M, et al. Evaluating prehospital care of patients with potential traumatic spinal cord injury: scoping review. Eur Spine J 2022;31:1309–29.
16. Oteir AO, Smith K, Stoelwinder J, Middleton JW, Cox S, Sharwood LN, et al. Prehospital predictors of traumatic spinal cord injury in Victoria, Australia. Prehosp Emerg Care 2017;21(5):583–90.
17. Yue JK, Winkler EA Rick JW, Deng H, Partow CP, Upadhyayula PS, et al. Update on critical care for acute spinal cord injury in the setting of polytrauma. Neurosurg Focus 2017;43(5):E19.
18. Swain A, Sahu S, Swain BP. Cervical spine movement during intubation. J Neuroanaesthesiol Crit Care 2017;4(4):76.
19. Maschmann C, Jeppesen E, Rubin MA, Barfod C. New clinical guidelines on the spinal stabilisation of adult trauma patients–consensus and evidence based. Scand J Trauma Resusc Em Med 2019;27(1):77.
20. Tatum JM, Melo N, Ko A, Dhillon NK, Smith EJT, Yim DA, et al. Validation of a field spinal motion restriction protocol in a level I trauma center. J Surg Res 2017;211:223–7.
21. National Institute for Health and Care Excellence (NICE). Spinal injury: assessment and initial management. 2016. Available from: www.nice.org.uk/guidance/ng41.
22. Clemency BM, Natalzia P, Innes J, Guarino S, Welch JV, Haghdel A, et al. A change from a spinal immobilization to a spinal motion restriction protocol was not associated with an increase in disabling spinal cord injuries. Prehosp Disaster Med 2021;36(6):708–12.
23. Misasi A, Ward JG, Dong F, Ablah E, Maurer C, Haan JM. Prehospital extrication techniques: neurological outcomes associated with the rapid extrication method and the Kendrick extrication device. Am Surg 2018;84(2):248–53.
24. Häske D, Schier L, Weerts JO, Groß B, Rittmann A, Grützner PA, et al. An explorative, biomechanical analysis of spine motion during out-of-hospital extrication procedures. Injury 2020;51(2):185–92.
25. Nutbeam T, Fenwick R, Smith JE, Dayson M, Carlin B, Wilson M, et al. A Delphi study of rescue and clinical subject matter experts on the extrication of patients following a motor vehicle collision. Scand J Trauma Resusc Em Med 2022;30(1):41.
26. Braithwaite S, Stephens C, Remick K, Barrett W, Guyette FX, Levy M, et al. Prehospital trauma airway management: an NAEMSP Position Statement and Resource Document. Prehosp Emerg Care 2022;26(Suppl. 1):64–71.
27. American College of Surgeons Committee on Trauma. Best practice guidelines: spine injury. Chicago: American College of Surgeons; 2022.
28. Lee YS, Kim KT, Kwon BK. Hemodynamic management of acute spinal cord injury: a literature review. Neurospine 2021;18(1):7–14.
29. Taylor MP, Wrenn P, O'Donnell AD. Presentation of neurogenic shock within the emergency department. Emerg Med J 2017;34(3):157–62.
30. Martirosyan NL, Patel AA, Carotenuto A, Kalani MY, Bohl MA, Preul MC, et al. The role of therapeutic hypothermia in the management of acute spinal cord injury. Clin Neurol Neurosurg 2017;154:79–88.
31. Purvis TA, Carlin B, Driscoll P. The definite risks and questionable benefits of liberal pre-hospital spinal immobilisation. Am J Emerg Med 2017;35(6):860–6.
32. Fischer PE, Perina DG, Delbridge TR, Fallat ME, Salomone JP, Dodd J, et al. Spinal motion restriction in the trauma patient–a joint position statement. Prehosp Emerg Care 2018;22(6):659–61.
33. Kornhall DK, Jorgensen JJ, Brommeland T, Hyldmo PK, Asbjørnsen H, Dolven T, et al. The Norwegian guidelines for the prehospital management of adult trauma patients with potential spinal injury. Scand J Trauma Resusc Em Med 2017;25(1):2.
34. Peck GE, Shipway DJ, Tsang K, Fertleman M. Cervical spine immobilisation in the elderly: a literature review. Br J Neurosurg 2018;32(3):286–90.

35. Chen HA Hsu ST, Shin SD, Jamaluddin SF, Son DN, Hong KJ, et al. A multicenter cohort study on the association between prehospital immobilization and functional outcome of patients following spinal injury in Asia. Sci Rep 2022;12(1):3492.
36. Hawkridge K, Ahmed I, Ahmed Z. Evidence for the use of spinal collars in stabilising spinal injuries in the pre-hospital setting in trauma patients: a systematic review. Eur J Trauma Emerg Surg 2022;48(1):647–57.
37. Agency for Clinical Innovation. Use of foam collars for cervical spine immobilisation: initial management principles. Chatswood: NSW Institute of Injury and Trauma Mangement and Emergency Care Institute; 2018. Online. Available from: www.ambulance.qld.gov.au/clinical.html.
38. Queensland Ambulance Service (QAC). Clinical practice procedure: trauma/cervical collar. In: QAC. Digital clinical practice manual. Brisbane: Queensland Ambulance Service; 2021.
39. Asha SE, Curtis K, Healy G, Neuhaus L, Tzannes A, Wright K. Neurologic outcomes following the introduction of a policy for using soft cervical collars in suspected traumatic cervical spine injury: a retrospective chart review. Emerg Med Australas 2021;33(1):19–24.
40. Roberts JR. Prehospital immobilization. In: Roberts JR, editor. Roberts and Hedges' clinical procedures in emergency medicine. vol. 2. 7th ed. Philadelphia: Elsevier; 2019.
41. American College of Surgeons Committee on Trauma. Advanced trauma life support: student course manual. 10th ed. Chicago IL: American College of Surgeons; 2018.
42. Oto B, Corey DJ, 2nd, Oswald J, Sifford D, Walsh B. Early secondary neurologic deterioration after blunt spinal trauma: a review of the literature. Ac Emerg Med 2015;22(10):1200–12.
43. da Cunha Rodrigues IF. To log-roll or not to log-roll—that is the question! A review of the use of log-roll on patients with pelvic fractures. Int J Orthop Trauma Nurs 2017;27:36–40.
44. Kirshblum SC, Burns SP, Biering-Sorensen F, Donovan W, Graves DE, Jha A, et al. International standards for neurological classification of spinal cord injury (rev. 2011). J Spinal Cord Med 2011;34(6):535–46.
45. Stricsek G, Ghobrial, G, Wilson J, Theofanis T, Harrop JS. Complications in the management of patients with spine trauma. Neurosurg Clin 2017;28(1): 147–55.
46. Ala A, Shams Vahdati S, Ghaffarzad A, Mousavi H, Mirza-Aghazadeh-Attari M. National emergency X-radiography utilization study guidelines versus Canadian C-Spine guidelines on trauma patients, a prospective analytical study. PLoS One 2018;13(11):e0206283.
47. Fontaine G, Forgione M, Lusignan F, Mousavi H, Mirza-Aghazadeh-Attari M. Cervical spine collar removal by emergency room nurses: a quality improvement project. J Emerg Nurs 2018;44(3):228–35.
48. Smith N, Curtis K. Can emergency nurses safely and accurately remove cervical spine collars in low risk adult trauma patients: an integrative review. Australas Emerg Nurs J 2016;19(2):63–74.
49. Sharwood LN, Dhaliwal S, Ball J, Burns B, Flower O, Joseph A, et al. Emergency and acute care management of traumatic spinal cord injury: a survey of current practice among senior clinicians across Australia. BMC Emerg Med 2018;18(1):57.
50. Adapted from Asha SE, Curtis K, Healy G, Neuhaus L, Tzannes A, Wright K, Neurologic outcomes following the introduction of a policy for using soft cervical collars in suspected traumatic cervical spine injury: a retrospective chart review. Emerg Med Australas 2021;33:19–24.
51. Michaleff ZA, Maher CG, Verhagen AP, Rebbeck T, Lin CW. Accuracy of the Canadian C-spine rule and NEXUS to screen for clinically important cervical spine injury in patients following blunt trauma: a systematic review. CMAJ 2012;184(16):E867–76.
52. Lawner B, Parker B. The initial management and clearance of spinal injuries in emergency medical practice. Trauma Rep 2016;17(4):1–11.
53. Stiell IG, Wells GA, Vandemheen KL, Clement CM, Lesiuk H, De Maio VJ, et al. The Canadian C-spine rule for radiography in alert and stable trauma patients. JAMA 2001;286(15):1841–8.
54. Goergen S, Varma D, Ackland H, Michaleff Z, Rosenfeld JV, Malham G, et al. Education modules for appropriate imaging referrals: cinical decision rules. Adult Cervical Spine Trauma. Sydney: Royal Australian and New Zealand College of Radiologists; 2015.
55. Hercz D, Montrief TD, Kukielski CJ, Supino M. Thoracolumbar evaluation in the low-risk trauma patient: a pilot study towards development of a clinical decision rule to avoid unnecessary imaging in the emergency department. J Emerg Med 2019;57(3):279-89.
56. Vela JH, Wertz CI, Onstott KL, Wertz JR. Trauma imaging: a literature review. Radiol Technol 2017;88(3):263–76.
57. Odle TG. Computed tomography of thoracolumbar spine trauma. Radiol Technol 2017;88(3):299–319.
58. VandenBerg J, Cullison K, Fowler SA, Parsons MS, McAndrew CM, Carpenter CR. Blunt thoracolumbar-spine trauma evaluation in the emergency department: a meta-analysis of diagnostic accuracy for history, physical examination, and imaging. J Emerg Med 2019;56(2):153–65.
59. van Den Hauwe L, Sundgren PC, Flanders AE. Spinal trauma and spinal cord injury (SCI). Cham: IDKD Springer Series; 2020.
60. Arbuthnot M, Mooney DP. The sensitivity and negative predictive value of a pediatric cervical spine clearance algorithm that minimizes computerized tomography. J Pediatr Surg 2017;52(1):130–5.
61. Shah K, Tikoo A, Kothari MK, Nene A. Current concepts in pediatric cervical spine trauma. Open Orthopaed J 2017;11:346–52.
62. Srinivasan V, Jea A. Pediatric thoracolumbar spine trauma. Neurosurg Clin North Am 2017;28(1):103–14.
63. Kolcun JPG, Chang PY, Wang MY. C31389 Spinal cord injury: neurointensive care and surgical intervention. In: Kolcun JPG, Chang PY, Wang MY, editors. Neurotrauma: a comprehensive textbook on traumatic brain injury and spinal cord injury. New York: Oxford University Press; 2018.
64. Canseco JA, Karamian BA, Bowles DR, Markowitz MP, DiMaria SL, Semenza NC, et al. Updated review: the steroid controversy for management of spinal cord injury. World Neurosurg 2021;150:1–8.

65. Sultan I, Lamba N, Liew A, Doung P, Tewarie I, Amamoo JJ, et al. The safety and efficacy of steroid treatment for acute spinal cord injury: a systematic review and meta-analysis. Heliyon 2020;6(2):e03414.
66. Zhang Y, Al Mamun A, Yuan Y, Lu Q, Xiong J, Yang S, et al. Acute spinal cord injury: pathophysiology and pharmacological intervention (Review). Mol Med Rep 2021;23(6):417.
67. Gundogdu I, Ozturk EA, Umay E, Karaahmet OZ, Unlu E, Cakci A. Implementation of a respiratory rehabilitation protocol: weaning from the ventilator and tracheostomy in difficult-to-wean patients with spinal cord injury. Disabil Rehabil 2017;39(12):1162–70.
68. Schreiber AF, Garlasco J, Vieira F, Lau YH, Stavi D, Lightfoot D, et al. Separation from mechanical ventilation and survival after spinal cord injury: a systematic review and meta-analysis. Ann Intens Care 2021;11(1):149.
69. Berlowitz DJ, Wadsworth B, Ross J. Respiratory problems and management in people with spinal cord injury. Breathe (Sheff) 2016;12(4):328–40.
70. Bauman M, Russo-McCourt T. Caring for patients with spinal cord injuries. Am Nurse Today 2016;11(5):18–23.
71. Zakrasek EC, Nielson JL, Kosarchuk JJ, Crew JD, Ferguson AR, McKenna SL. Pulmonary outcomes following specialized respiratory management for acute cervical spinal cord injury: a retrospective analysis. Spinal Cord 2017;55(6):559–65.
72. Phillips AA, Krassioukov AV. Cardiovascular dysfunction following spinal cord injury. Neurological aspects of spinal cord injury. New York: Springer; 2017.
73. Weidner N, Müller OJ, Hach-Wunderle V, Schwerdtfeger K, Krauspe R, Pauschert R, et al. Prevention of thromboembolism in spinal cord injury—S1 guideline. Neurol Res Pract 2020;2:43.
74. Hagen EM. Acute complications of spinal cord injuries. World J Orthopaed 2015;6(1):17–23.
75. Sun X, Jones ZB Chen XM, Zhou L, So KF, Ren Y. Multiple organ dysfunction and systemic inflammation after spinal cord injury: a complex relationship. J Neuroinflamm 2016;13(1):260.
76. Martinez L, Neshatian L, Khavari R. Neurogenic bowel dysfunction in patients with neurogenic bladder. Curr Bladder Dysfunct Rep 2016;11(4): 334–40.
77. Bigford G, Nash MS. Nutritional health considerations for persons with spinal cord injury. Topics Spinal Cord Injury Rehab 2017;23(3):188–206.
78. Karamian BA, Siegel N, Nourie B, Serruya MD, Heary RF, Harrop JS, et al. The role of electrical stimulation for rehabilitation and regeneration after spinal cord injury. J Orthopaed Traumatol 2022;23(1):2.
79. Vermeijden HD, Leenen LPH, van Polen M, Dijkgraaf MGW, Hietbrink F. Analysis of two treatment modalities for the prevention of vomiting after trauma: orogastric tube or anti-emetics. Injury 2017;48(10):2106–11.
80. Hagen EM, Rekand T. Management of neuropathic pain associated with spinal cord injury. Pain Therapy 2015;4(1):51–65.
81. Kramer JL, Minhas NK, Jutzeler CR, Erskine EL, Liu LJ, Ramer MS. Neuropathic pain following traumatic spinal cord injury: models, measurement, and mechanisms. J Neurosci Res 2017;95(6):1295–306.
82. Agarwal N, Joshi M. Effectiveness of amitriptyline and lamotrigine in traumatic spinal cord injury-induced neuropathic pain: a randomized longitudinal comparative study. Spinal Cord 2017;55(2):126–30.
83. Soler MD, Moriña D, Rodríguez N, Saurí J, Vidal J, Navarro A, et al. Sensory symptom profiles of patients with neuropathic pain after spinal cord injury. Clin J Pain 2017;33(9):827–34.
84. Widerstrom-Noga E. Neuropathic pain and spinal cord injury: phenotypes and pharmacological management. Drugs 2017;77(9):967–84.
85. Satyarthee GD. Ways to improve outcomes of traumatic acute spinal cord injury: integrated approaches of improved prehospital care, the adoption of synergistic medical and surgical intervention, along with care for associated systemic injury and rehabilitation and social inclusion. World Neurosurg 2017;101:786–7.
86. Kreinest M, Ludes L, Turk A, Biglari B, Matschke S. Analysis of prehospital care and emergency room treatment of patients with acute traumatic spinal cord injury: a retrospective cohort study on the implementation of current guidelines. Spinal Cord 2017;55(1):16–9.
87. Qiu Y, Chen Y, Xie Y, Xie H, Dong J. Comparative analysis of the efficacy of early and late surgical intervention for acute spinal cord injury: a systematic review and meta-analysis based on 16 studies. Int J Surg 2021;94:106098.
88. El Masri W, Kumar N. Active physiological conservative management in traumatic spinal cord injuries–an evidence-based approach. Trauma 2017;19(1):1460408617698508.
89. Hoh DJ, Qureshi S, Anderson PA, Arnold PM, John HC, Dailey AT, et al. Congress of Neurological Surgeons systematic review and evidence-based guidelines on the evaluation and treatment of patients with thoracolumbar spine trauma: nonoperative care. Neurosurgery 2019;84(1):E46–9.
90. Tran J, Dorstyn DS, Burke AL. Psychosocial aspects of spinal cord injury pain: a meta-analysis. Spinal Cord 2016;54(9):640–8.
91. Lim SW, Shiue YL, Ho CH, Yu SC, Kao PH, Wang JJ, et al. Anxiety and depression in patients with traumatic spinal cord injury: a nationwide population-based cohort study. PLoS One 2017;12(1):e0169623.
92. American Spinal Injury Association (ASIA) & International Spinal Cord Society. International Standards for neurological classification of spinal cord injury. 2019. Available from: https://asia-spinalinjury.org/wp-content/uploads/2019/10/ASIA-ISCOS-Worksheet_10.2019_PRINT-Page-1-2.pdf.
93. Yaqoob Hakim S, Gamal Altawil L, Faidh Ramzee A, Asim M, Ahmed K, Awwad M, et al. Diagnosis, management and outcome of Spinal Cord Injury without Radiographic Abnormalities (SCIWORA) in adult patients with trauma: a case series. Qatar Med J 2021;2021(3):67.

94. Sharif H, Hou S. Autonomic dysreflexia: a cardiovascular disorder following spinal cord injury. Neural Regen Res 2017;12(9):1390–400.
95. Flack JA, Sharma KD, Xie JY. Delving into the recent advancements of spinal cord injury treatment: a review of recent progress. Neural Regen Res 2022;17(2):283–91.
96. Kafka J, Lukacova N, Sulla I, Maloveska M, Vikartovska Z, Cizkova D. Hypothermia in the course of acute traumatic spinal cord injury. Acta Neurobiol Exp (Wars) 2020;80(2):172–8.
97. Shah M, Peterson C, Yilmaz E, Halalmeh DR, Moisi M. Current advancements in the management of spinal cord injury: a comprehensive review of literature. Surg Neurol Int 2020;11:2.
98. Hejrati N, Fehlings MG. A review of emerging neuroprotective and neuroregenerative therapies in traumatic spinal cord injury. Curr Opin Pharmacol 2021;60:331–40.
99. Zimmermann R, Vieira Alves Y, Sperling LE, Pranke P. Nanotechnology for the treatment of spinal cord injury. Tissue Eng Part B Rev 2021;27(4):353–65.

CHAPTER 48

MAJOR ORTHOPAEDIC AND NEUROVASCULAR TRAUMA

JESSICA KEADY AND ANNA GRANT

ESSENTIALS

- History and understanding of the mechanism of injury is essential in predicting the pattern of fractures and underlying soft-tissue-structure damage; for example, a dislocated knee can tear the popliteal artery or rupture cruciate ligaments.
- Any variation of a neurovascular assessment requires closer observation and potential investigations.
- Splinting of the long bones is essential for reducing pain and attempting to restore anatomical alignment.
- All major trauma pelvic fractures should be splinted prior to moving the patient to decrease haemorrhage and further damage from bone ends.
- While pelvic binders are crucial in the acute phase, it is imperative that early plans for pelvic fracture are made to expedite the removal of the pelvic binder to minimise the risk of associated complications.
- A combination of pain treatment regimens should be considered to alleviate pain and reduce the effects of a stress response. These may include opioid analgesia, nerve blocks, ice, elevation, splinting. In severe circumstances, intubation may be required to give adequate analgesia and anaesthesia.
- Any amputated limb should be kept cool and dry.
- All open fractures should be splinted to prevent further breaching of the skin, and a sterile, saline-soaked dressing placed over the breach to prevent bone from drying out.
- Only those who are trained in application should apply skeletal or skin traction. Only the orthopaedic surgeon or registrar should prescribe traction weight.
- The basis for treatment of any patient with suspected fat embolism syndrome is supportive, such as prevention of hypovolaemia, the stress response and hypoxia, and stabilisation of fractures.
- All patients with significant soft-tissue trauma or fractures to the lower limbs are deemed to have a compartment syndrome until proven otherwise. Treatment remains to elevate the limb to heart level, ice, splint and monitor via neurovascular observations and visual examination, including a high index of suspicion and fasciotomy where necessary.
- Never elevate an injured limb above the level of the heart, as this will impede venous return and potentially lead to increased risk of compartment syndrome.

INTRODUCTION

This chapter outlines major musculoskeletal trauma incorporating injuries to the bone, muscle and vascular system. Subsequent physiological alterations to these systems are addressed. Extremity trauma itself is not usually life threatening, though major blood loss and vascular injury, if associated with these injuries, pose serious risks to life and limb. Musculoskeletal injuries that alter haemodynamic status significantly, such as massive pelvic injuries, amputations and major femur or multiple long bone fractures, require early identification and management. Fractures of the femur and pelvis can be associated with significant blood loss, contributing to hypovolaemic shock and haemodynamic instability, particularly in high-impact, blunt multi-trauma.

Assessment, resuscitation and therapeutic intervention are the basic principles of trauma care for life-threatening injuries. Patients who have multiple injuries will often have one or more skeletal injuries. Musculoskeletal injuries require timely recognition and management; however, this can only be done after management and stabilisation of catastrophic haemorrhage, airway, breathing, circulation and neurologic impairment, i.e. disability (CABCD), inclusive of damage control resuscitation to maximise patient stability.[1]

The musculoskeletal system is involved in approximately 66% of all injuries. Consequently, musculoskeletal injuries are widely seen in the healthcare setting, and are a major component of pre-hospital and emergency/trauma nursing care.[2]

Mechanism of injury is an important predictive tool and should raise one's index of suspicion of particular injury types when assessing musculoskeletal trauma, along with injury pattern and physiological symptoms. Fractures may occur as a result of either high- or low-energy forces, they may be blunt or penetrating injuries, and may occur from either twisting, bending or crushing forces.[3] The severity of fracture and damage to tissue, nerves, ligaments and muscles may be far greater in a fracture caused by a car travelling at high speed than a fracture caused by a low-energy fall.[2]

Extremity trauma can be complex and can result in long-term sequelae that are significantly disabling. Patients with major orthopaedic injuries, especially to the lower limb, are more likely to have long-term changes to their quality of life and functional outcomes. This chapter addresses the major aspects of extremity trauma, associated complications and recommendations for appropriate trauma assessment and management in the field and in the emergency department (ED).

ANATOMY AND PHYSIOLOGY

BONE

There are 206 bones in the human skeleton. These bones provide the architectural framework for the body (Fig. 48.1).[5]

Other structures, such as tendons, cartilage, ligaments, soft tissue and muscle, allow the bones to perform many functions, such as support, serving as a reservoir for minerals and haematopoietic function (production of red blood cells), shielding internal organs, and activities such as protection, work and play, which are coordinated by involuntary and voluntary muscle movement.[1]

Bone is dynamic and can adapt itself when forces are applied to it. Bones can be grouped based on shape, as flat (innominate—pelvis), cuboidal (vertebrae) or long (tibia). Furthermore, bones can be classified as cancellous (spongy or trabecular bone) or cortical (compact). Cortical bone is found where support matters most, in shafts of long bones and outer walls of other bones. Cancellous bone is 'honeycomb' in appearance and makes up the internal network of all bones.[1,5]

Periosteum surrounds bone and contains a substantial network of blood vessels that supply the bone with blood and nutrients. Inside the long bones is the medullary cavity containing yellow marrow (mostly fat) and red marrow (responsible for blood-cell production).[6] Therefore, when the long bone is fractured, blood loss occurs and fat can be released from the medullary cavity, potentially causing fat embolism.

Injuries to the soft tissue, which includes muscle, skin and subcutaneous fat, can occur in combination with fractures. Sometimes soft-tissue injuries are more significant and have more serious ramifications than the fracture itself. Appreciation of this is essential for preventing complications to fracture healing.[6] In understanding soft-tissue damage, it may help to try to envisage the mechanism of injury and the position of the limb at impact when the bone ends are separated. When the patient reaches the ED, soft tissues may have recoiled back to normal position. X-rays give little indication of the extent that soft tissue has been stretched.

Healing of an uncomplicated fracture may take from 6 weeks to 6 months. Vascular compromise, infection and other injuries may lengthen the healing process and, in some cases, non-union may occur.[6]

The five stages of fracture healing do not occur independently, but overlap as progression of the healing process occurs (Table 48.1 and Fig. 48.2).[10]

Strength and bone mass change considerably with age and may contribute to musculoskeletal trauma. During adolescence, bone mass increases rapidly, reaching a maximum level a decade after skeletal maturity; then it begins to decline. By the eighth or ninth decade, bone mass and strength has decreased to about half its maximum level. Menopause can cause a woman to undergo accelerated bone loss.[11] Age-related osteoporosis is accelerated around menopause. Menopause generally commences between the ages of 45 and 55 years. A sharp decline in oestrogen production leads to accelerated bone loss. Oestrogen, a hormone produced by the ovaries, has been revealed to have protective effects on bone by decreasing bone resorption with the reduction and activity of osteoclasts. During menopause, bone loss greatly surpasses that in men. Osteoporosis and osteopenia (low bone mass) occur when the rate of bone formation is markedly slower than bone resorption, resulting in thin, fragile bone and, consequently, fractures.[5,6]

MUSCULOSKELETAL TISSUE

There are two types of tissue in the musculoskeletal system: muscle and connective tissue. Connective tissue is specified as tendon, fascia, ligaments and cartilage. This will be addressed later in the chapter.[1]

Skeletal muscle

Skeletal muscle tissue is a voluntary muscle and has a unique ability to contract, therefore providing the body with the ability to move. Skeletal muscle has high metabolic demands and is provided with a rich blood supply by arteries and veins that

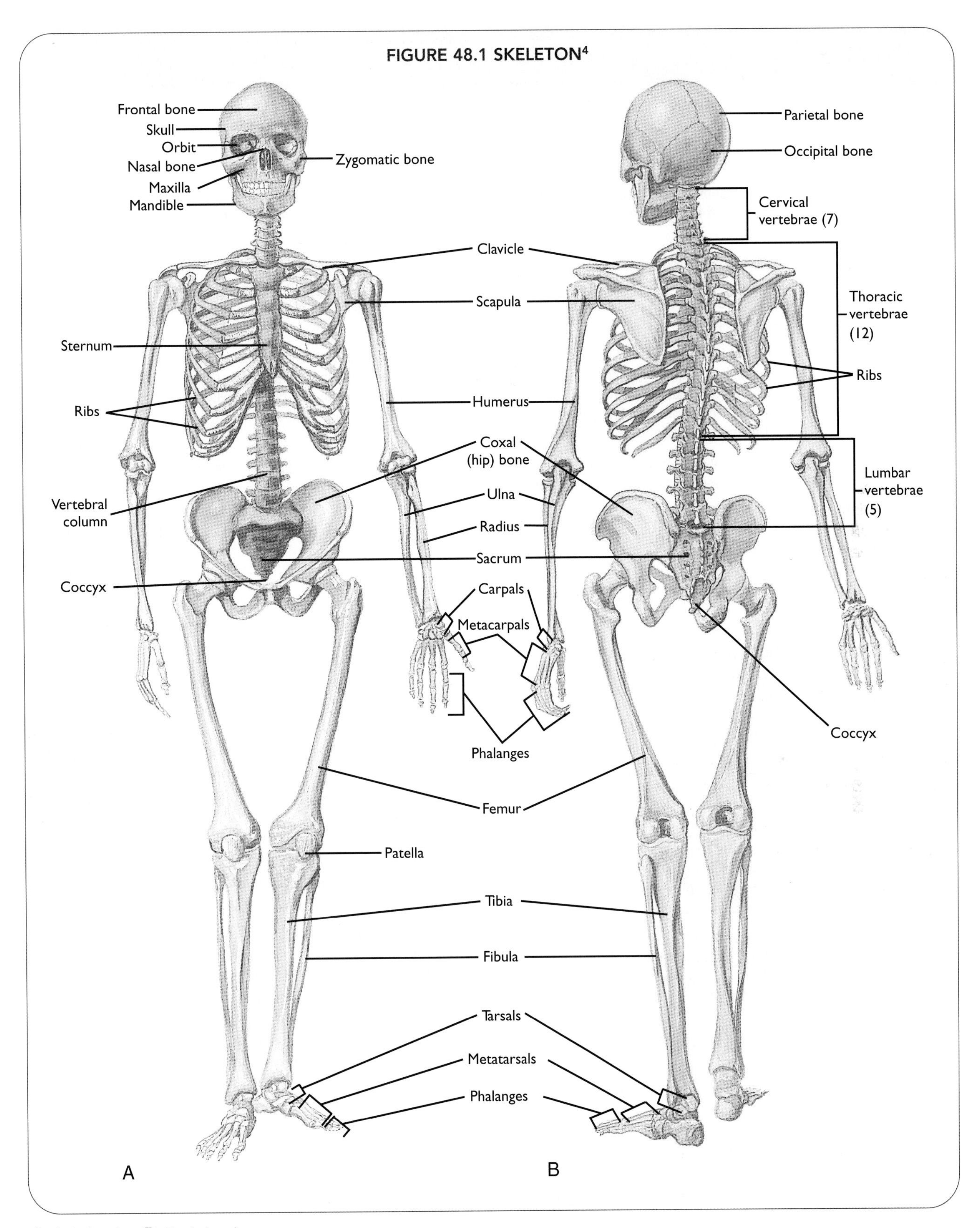

A. Anterior view. B. Posterior view.

TABLE 48.1 STAGES OF FRACTURE HEALING[7,8]

STAGE	DESCRIPTION	LENGTH
I–Haematoma formation	Immediately following fracture, bone ends rub together–called crepitus–causing pain. Amount of haematoma depends on the damage to bone, soft tissue and vessels around the fracture	48–72 hrs
II–Granulation	Granulation tissue forms after fibroblasts, osteoclasts and chondroblasts invade the haematoma as part of the inflammatory sequelae. Osteoclasts remove dead bone and osteoblasts produce bone	1–4 weeks
III–Callus formation	The fracture becomes 'sticky' due to plasma and white blood cells entering the granulation tissue. This material assists in keeping fragments of bone together. PTH increases and calcium is deposited. This is the most important stage; slowing or interruption at this stage means that the last two stages cannot progress, leading to delayed healing or non-union	2–6 weeks
IV–Ossification/ consolidation	Osteoblasts and connective tissue are prolific, bringing the bone ends together. Bridging callus envelops the fracture fragment ends and moves towards the other fragments. Medullary callus bridges the fracture fragments internally, thus creating a connection with the marrow cavity and cortices of the fracture fragment. Trabecular bone replaces callus along the stress lines. Unnecessary callus is absorbed. Bony union is thus achieved	3 weeks–6 months
V–Remodelling	Re-establishment of the medullary canal. Fragments of bone are united. Surplus cells are absorbed, bone is remodelled and healing is complete	6 weeks–1 year

PTH: parathyroid hormone.

FIGURE 48.2 BONE HEALING (SCHEMATIC REPRESENTATION)[9]

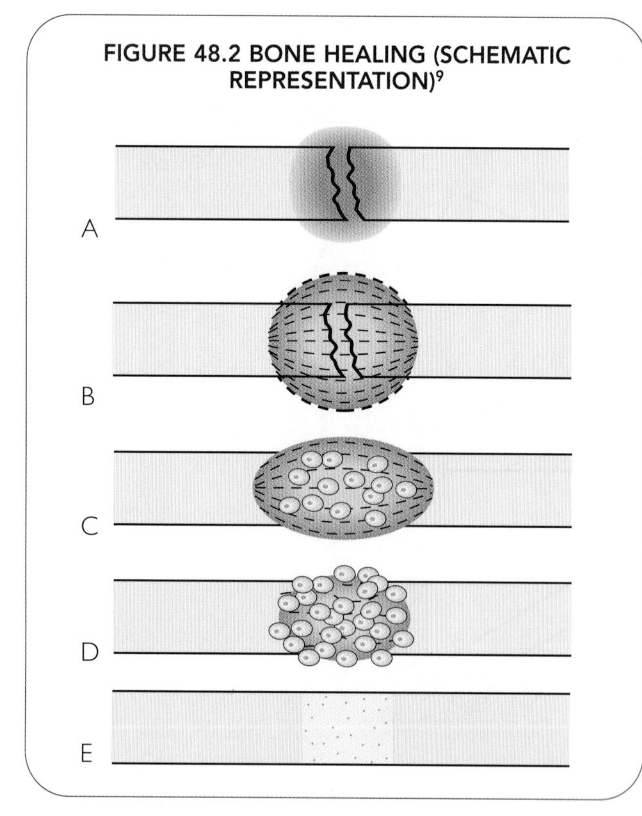

A. Bleeding at broken ends of the bone with subsequent haematoma formation. **B.** Organisation of haematoma into fibrous network. **C.** Invasion of osteoblasts, lengthening of collagen strands and deposition of calcium. **D.** Callus formation: new bone is built up as osteoclasts destroy dead bone. **E.** Remodelling accomplished as excess callus is reabsorbed and trabecular bone is laid down.

penetrate the epimysium (fascia), and are finally embedded in the innermost sheath, the endomysium.[12]

Muscles are enclosed within fascial compartments, which protect the muscle from damaged tissue swelling. Pressure within the compartment can increase so much that muscle ischaemia occurs, resulting in compartment syndrome, which is discussed later.[12]

Skeletal muscle declines with age because of decreases in the size and number of muscle cells. Commencing at the age of 25, skeletal muscle mass decreases by as much as 60%. This not only limits mobility, but increases the risk of falling, thus increasing the probability of injury.[11]

- *Nerve supply*—one or two nerves supply muscle. Each nerve includes efferent (motor) and afferent (sensory) fibres. Nerves provide movement and sensation. Sensory nerves carry impulses to the central nervous system (CNS). Motor nerves carry impulses away from the CNS. Traction, compression, ischaemia, laceration, oedema or burning can damage nerves, resulting in nerve deficit distal to the site of injury.[5]
- *Vascular supply*—the nutrient artery provides a rich blood supply to bone marrow and some cortex in adult long bones. The large ends of long bones are supplied by the circulus vasculosus (Fig. 48.3).[1]

Because of the close proximity of nerves and vessels to bony structures, any musculoskeletal injury can potentially cause vascular and/or neurological compromise (Table 48.2). This is a result of these systems being extremely sensitive to compression or stretch from the fracture, injury or haematoma and impaired circulation. If vascular supply is impaired, tissue perfusion is reduced and ultimately will lead to ischaemia. Irreversible damage to nerves, vascular structures and muscles

FIGURE 48.3 BLOOD SUPPLY OF A LONG BONE[7]

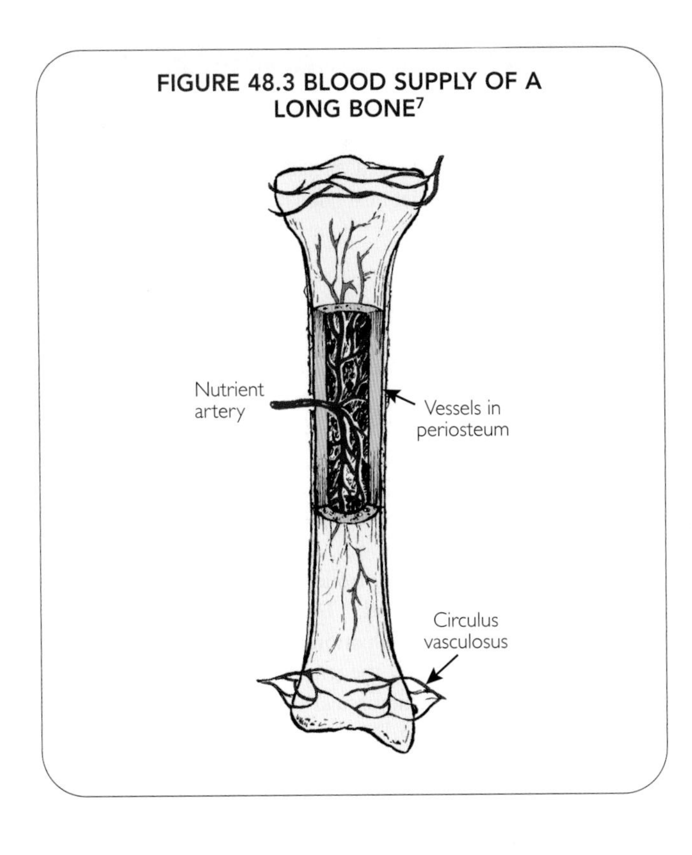

TABLE 48.2 JOINT FRACTURES AND DISLOCATIONS AND POTENTIAL NERVE/VESSEL INJURY[5,7,8,13]

SITE	NERVE/VESSEL INVOLVED
Hip and pelvis	Sciatic nerve
	Iliac arteries and veins and obturator vessels
Knee	Common peroneal or tibial nerve, popliteal artery/vein
Ankle	Posterior tibial nerve, tibial artery
Shoulder	Axillary nerve, brachial plexus, axillary artery
Humeral shaft	Radial nerve
Humeral supracondylar	Radial or median nerve, brachial artery
Elbow	Radial, median or ulnar nerve, brachial artery
Wrist	Median or ulnar nerve

can occur within 6–8 hours if progression from ischaemia to muscle necrosis occurs.[10] Poor arterial perfusion is evidenced by pallor, and cyanosis is suggestive of venous congestion.[6]

Improper handling of fractures can complicate further care of the patient and increase the degree of injury, as well as causing further bleeding, pain, increased incidence of fat embolism and further damage to soft tissue, nerves and vessels.[12]

PRACTICE TIP

When handling a fractured limb, always place one hand under the fracture site and the other hand distal to the fracture. This will prevent excessive movement at the fracture site.

PATIENT ASSESSMENT AND EARLY INTERVENTION

INSPECTION

Initially the patient's clothes should be cut away or removed, taking care not to overexpose the patient and contribute to hypothermia. Observe the patient during this procedure for grimacing or guarding when limbs are moved as this may suggest signs of injury; if possible, this should be confirmed with the patient. Observe for shortening, deformity/angulation or abnormal rotation.[10,14] Note impaired skin integrity, potentially due to open fractures, oedema/swelling and ecchymosis due to blood loss into the tissues and muscle spasm due to muscle contracting over the injured part. Observe extremity colour—dusky/cyanosed colour indicates venous congestion, and pallor is indicative of insufficient arterial blood supply.[10,14] Ensure important assessment findings are communicated through handover and documented in the patient's medical record, particularly for suspicion of open fracture and vascular injury, where time-critical intervention reduces risk of longer-term morbidity.

NEUROVASCULAR ASSESSMENT AND PALPATION

Extremity trauma is multifaceted; it remains a challenge as it can involve both skeletal and arterial injuries. Skeletal trauma accounts for 10–70% of all extremity arterial injuries. There is a substantially higher risk of limb morbidity and limb loss with combined arterial and skeletal trauma, particularly when diagnosis and revascularisation are delayed. Therefore, prompt diagnosis is essential with a high index of suspicion for arterial trauma in all injured extremities. Note whether hard signs of arterial damage are present, such as reduced or absent (late sign) distal pulses, bruit or thrill over wound, active haemorrhage, large, expanding or pulsatile haematoma and signs of distal ischaemia—the five Ps: **p**ain, **p**allor, **p**aralysis, **p**araesthesia, **p**olar (coolness). CT angiography has superseded angiography in most centres during the immediate diagnostic phase, and is mandatory in the presence of any of these hard signs. Additionally, disposition should be considered, with early transfer or retrieval to a trauma centre capable of damage control surgery, interventional radiology and/or vascular expertise to manage the threat to limb.

PRACTICE TIP

Distal pulses should be equal and bilateral. Always assess both pulses. For example, for dorsalis pedis, assess both feet.

If the injured limb has weak or absent pulses, this could be an indication of compromised circulation. Any deviation in pulses should be escalated immediately to the orthopaedic surgeon or the treating team, clearly documented and closely monitored.

TABLE 48.3 PARAMETERS FOR PERIPHERAL VASCULAR ASSESSMENT[13]

	INADEQUATE VENOUS RETURN	INADEQUATE ARTERIAL SUPPLY	NORMAL
Colour	Cyanotic (blue), mottled	White or pale	Pink
Capillary refill	Immediate	> 3 seconds	1-3 seconds
Temperature	Hot	Cool	Warm
Tissue turgor	Distended or tense	Prune-like or hollow	Full

Neurovascular assessment examines pain, vascular integrity and neurological integrity. Initial assessment should be thorough to establish a baseline against which further assessment can be compared (Table 48.3).[10]

Palpate each bone, observing any disturbance in integrity; this may be difficult as often the only signs of injury are pain, muscle spasm or crepitus. Essential components of palpation are:

- *pain*—bones are in essence insensate. Pain is generally caused by injury to periosteum, as periosteum has sensory innervation. Soft-tissue injury, swelling within fascial compartments and muscle spasm will also cause pain.[6,10]
- *muscle spasm*—caused by a continuous contraction of the muscle over the injured part.[6,10]
- *crepitus*—caused by fractured bone ends moving against each other; usually a grating sound can be heard and felt.[6,10]
- *capillary refill*—filling time of more than 2 seconds is abnormal and indicative of arterial injury.[6,10]
- *pulses*—presence, quality and absence over the full length of the extremity, rather than just distal to the apparent injury.
  - The upper extremity has three major pulses that should be palpated: radial, ulnar and brachial.
  - The lower extremity has four major pulses that should be palpated: femoral, popliteal, posterior tibial and dorsalis pedis. Note that 10% of the population will have a congenitally absent dorsalis pedis pulse, called peripheral occlusive arteriosclerosis. If pulse is absent or weak in one limb only, an ankle brachial index may be indicated, as this may be indicative of injury.[6,10,13]
- *Temperature*—feel if the skin is cold; this may indicate vascular compromise.
- *Sensation*—check for variation in sensation to stimuli. The conscious patient should be able to recognise numbness and tingling when normal pressure of your finger or slight pressure from your nail is applied. Do not use sharp implements that potentially break the skin integrity.
- *Movement*—do not test range of movement (ROM) on an injured limb, as this may cause further injury to ligaments, muscle and vessel. ROM testing may be passive, active or both.[10] The patient may be able to actively move the injured limb within pain limits.

PRACTICE TIP

Neurovascular status will vary, especially temperature and sensation, particularly if the patient has peripheral vascular disease or poor peripheral circulation. Always ask the patient what their normal status is.

PRE-HOSPITAL

In the pre-hospital environment, initial assessment and management of life-threatening injuries can occur concurrently and in accordance with PHTLS (Pre-Hospital Trauma Life Support)[15] and ITLS (International Trauma Life Support) principles. The priorities of CABCD take precedence over orthopaedic injuries, unless the orthopaedic injury is the cause of instability or haemorrhage (see Chapter 42). Any severe bleeding from an extremity that cannot be controlled with pressure or packing should have a tourniquet applied.[16] Tourniquet use will be discussed further within this section. Palpation and assessment of the pelvis and long bones (particularly the femur) should form part of the primary survey (C—cardiovascular assessment) for potential sources of internal bleeding.[16]

Extremity injuries are generally not the primary focus in the initial phase for multi-trauma and it is important for clinicians not to become distracted by non-critical extremity injuries, although they may appear painful and gruesome.[15] Further evaluation of extremities can occur during the secondary survey if patient stability allows, or en route to the trauma centre, if this can be done safely. If the paramedic suspects a fracture, then neurovascular observations should commence as soon as practicable.[10]

Urgent splinting and alignment

In general, major deformity requires straightening and realignment provisionally prior to splinting and immobilising. Formal reduction is generally delayed until the ED presentation; however, in some settings with critical care or advance paramedic practitioners, this reduction may be completed in the field (e.g. remote retrievals). In the case of neurovascular deficit, immediate realignment of the limb must be done by trained personnel. This should only occur after adequate analgesic administration and sedation where necessary, with neurovascular assessment pre- and post-intervention. Gross contamination of open fractures should be removed with saline solution and the wound or exposed bone covered with a saline-soaked sterile pad prior to realignment, splinting and packaging. Pre-hospital clinicians are unlikely to cause further injury by realigning severely deformed limbs in comparison with what was inflicted by the initial trauma, and there are negative impacts if a limb is left in a severely deformed position.[16]

Splints are adjuncts that can assist in further treatment of extremity injuries in the field and the ED. Splints can range from the simple cardboard splint and circumferential sheeting to commercially available traction splints or pelvic binders (see Chapter 16).[6] Suspected major pelvic and femoral fractures should have pelvic binder and traction splint applied for haemorrhage control in the pre-hospital phase of care.

The purpose of splinting is to reduce bleeding, pain, risk of fat embolism, and to reduce the risk of further damage to neurovascular structures, soft-tissue and skin injury or conversion to open injury due to movement of fracture fragments. The limb must be splinted above and below the fracture site.

Most commonly used by ambulance services are the CT-6 or Slishman femoral traction splints, which both provide skin traction. These devices allow for both immobilisation and traction of the affected limb, aligning the limb in a near-reduced position. The splinted limb must be continuously monitored for neurovascular compromise and increased pressure from the straps. Straps may need to be loosened and other areas may require further padding to prevent skin breakdown. The traction splint is a temporary measure and should be replaced by more definitive management once in the healthcare setting, such as skeletal or skin traction or internal fixation.[17]

Other removable splints include vacuum splints, which are conformable to a deformed limb, with air removed through a valve to provide rigid support. Caution must be used when applying vacuum splints as sharp objects may puncture the splint causing loss of vacuum and immobilisation. Box splints, cardboard splints and foam splints (SAM splint) are also used and are generally available in both long and short sizes. They are temporary and should be replaced as soon as practicable. They are useful for fractures of the forearm, wrist and ankle. In instances where prefabricated splints are unavailable, anything can be used as a temporary splint; for example, pillows, jumpers, cardboard, wood or towels. Patients with severe fractures should always be splinted to immobilise the limb and prevent further complications.[6] The application and use of casts and crutches is presented in Chapter 16.

Pelvic binders

Pelvic binders are a commercially available, non-invasive adjunct to unstable pelvic fracture management, also known as a pelvic circumferential compression device (PCCD). Unstable pelvic fractures require immediate attention and could be the cause of a patient's haemodynamic instability. Early application of the PCCD can be lifesaving, providing stabilisation and clot formation, preventing ongoing haemorrhage and trauma-induced coagulopathy. The mechanism is simple: 'close the book' and minimise bleeding by reducing pelvic volume, which reduces the amount of space for bleeding, realigning pelvic joints, stabilising bone ends, preventing clot disruption and compression of vasculature.

All patients with significant pelvic pain or tenderness, suspected pelvic fractures or instability, and who are haemodynamically unstable, should be placed in a PCCD during the pre-hospital phase of care. If the patient arrives to the ED without a PCCD and with haemodynamic instability, with clinical suspicion of pelvic fracture, or concerning mechanism of injury for pelvic fracture, a binder should be promptly applied. Ideally, the pelvic binder should be placed directly to skin. Commercially available devices include the Prometheus pelvic splint, SAM sling™ and T-pod®.

In 2002, Bottlang and colleagues[18] determined for the first time the amount of force required to reduce unstable pelvic fractures with a PCCD applied around the trochanters. More importantly, this study demonstrated the efficacy and absence of complications, such as over-compression, from a PCCD. Further studies have shown lower mortality and length of stay, haemorrhage control, reduced transfusion requirements, and improved analgesia.[19] PCCDs can be applied in the pre-hospital setting for early and effective stabilisation before and during transport. Correctly placed binders will not impede patient assessment and will aid in resuscitation.

For effective stabilisation, the PCCD should be placed directly over the greater trochanters and not the iliac crests. As such, anatomical landmarks mut be identified to correctly site the device. Misplacing the PCCD can reduce the amount of fracture reduction.[20] If a patient with multiple injuries requires both PCCD and femoral traction splint, the PCCD should be applied first.

Once an injury is discounted or identified, planning for the removal of the PCCD should commence. Most binders should be removed within a few hours, once pelvic ring disruption is excluded or surgical intervention with external pelvic fixation occurs.[21] The effectiveness of the PCCD depends on the classification of injury.[22] Anterior posterior compression (APC) type 1 and lateral compression (LC) type 1 fractures are considered stable fractures; therefore, in theory negate the need for a PCCD in all cases. For APC 2 and LC 2 injuries, it is reasonable to consider loosening the binder and repeating the AP pelvic x-ray to assess for any changes to the injury pattern that may have been masked by the PCCD before removing the binder completely.[23] When loosening/removing the PCCD, it is crucial to assess the patient for changes in haemodynamic status, increased pain or changes in neurovascular observations. If there is a change in haemodynamics or a reported significant increase in pain by the patient, the PCCD should be reapplied.

Soft-tissue and pressure injuries have occurred due to incorrect fitting of the PCCD, application over clothing, or a significantly long length of time left in the binder. While the PCCD is in place, the risk of pressure areas, especially over bony prominences, is of concern. It is important that the binder is only in place while necessary and if extended use is required, pressure area care should be attended every 2–3 hours, if haemodynamics allow, with the skin under the PCCD inspected every 12 hours as per manufacturer's guidelines.[24,25] Definitive management of the unstable pelvis should occur within 24 hours of application.[6,26] Pelvic binders should be removed where there is no confirmed pelvic fracture, it is an identified mechanically stable pelvic fracture, if the binder PCCD is not adding stability to the fracture, or there are no further bleeding or coagulation concerns.[26]

Tourniquet (life and limb threats)

Tourniquets are effective at controlling haemorrhage in severe extremity trauma and reducing blood product usage.[27] In the context of severe extremity trauma with uncontrollable blood loss, application of a widely commercially available tourniquet, such as the Combat Arterial Tourniquet™ (CAT), may be required. Tourniquets may be required in situations such as mangled limbs, blast or gunshot injuries, severe crush injuries (e.g. farming/industrial incidents) or deep penetrating injuries (e.g. shark bite). The tourniquet should be tightened until loss of the distal pulse or until bleeding stops. Important considerations are application time, with complication risk increasing with prolonged tourniquet time. Tourniquet application time should be recorded and clearly communicated with the accepting team on handover in the ED. Tourniquets can be used on arms and legs and should be applied proximally to the haemorrhage site (> 5 cm), as distal as possible, sparing joints and directly against skin if the situation allows.[28] If the tourniquet is ineffective after tightening, the provider may need to consider a second tourniquet placed proximal to the first.

There remains some controversy regarding tourniquet use due to potential adverse events, including permanent nerve and muscle injury, ischaemia, vascular injury or skin necrosis; however, recent studies have shown relatively low rates of complications in civilian settings if tourniquet time is kept to a minimum 60–100 minutes.[27–30] Preventing arterial flow to a limb will cause ischaemia and after 2 hours, tissue damage will ensue with nerve and muscle damage (rhabdomyolysis, compartment syndrome), vascular injury and skin necrosis. After 6 hours, muscle damage is significant with high risk of amputation. Therefore, there is some agreement that a tourniquet can be left on for up to 2 hours before complications occur.[31] There are no clear evidence-based guidelines on tourniquet use; however, the mantra 'save life over limb' is a pragmatic approach to their clinical use.

Tourniquet use is discussed further in Chapter 16.

PAIN MANAGEMENT

There is an enormous stress response produced after major trauma. Inadequate pain relief has been shown to amplify this stress response, with a resultant rise in morbidity. The adverse effects of trauma on ventilation, haemodynamic stability and renal and gastrointestinal function are said to be compounded when pain is untreated. Simple but important measures, such as splinting or immobilising an injured limb, should be instituted initially. These will help avoid further tissue damage and muscle spasm, and reduce pain. Elevating the limb promotes venous return, thus reducing venous congestion, and can aid in reducing discomfort. Cooling via ice packs can decrease swelling and oedema. There are numerous treatments for pain relief available; these include intravenous, oral, inhaled, local and regional anaesthetics.[2] Non-pharmacological methods, such as reassurance, distraction and stress management, may also have an important role in pain management for the trauma patient. See Chapters 16 and 18 for further information on pain management.

PRE-HOSPITAL PAIN MANAGEMENT

The prevalence of pain experienced by trauma patients in the pre-hospital setting is high with most experiencing moderate to severe pain.[32] Pre-hospital clinicians may have fewer pharmacological agents at their disposal, and choice may be limited by accessibility to the patient; for example, entrapment that complicates intravenous access.

Methoxyflurane is commonly used in the pre-hospital setting for trauma. It is delivered via a self-administered disposable inhaler to trauma patients with moderate-to-severe pain and has been found to be effective, well tolerated, and has a rapid onset of effective pain relief.[33] IV opioids (fentanyl, morphine) continue to be used with good analgesic effect in this setting, with fentanyl increasingly being delivered via the intranasal route if IV access presents challenges. Ketamine has become an important agent in the pre-hospital setting, particularly in the unstable trauma patient, for both its sedating and analgesic effects. Research has shown that ketamine is effective and safe when used alone for analgesic effects and is an acceptable alternative to opioids.[34] Ketamine is also increasingly being delivered by the intranasal route. Non-pharmacological methods such as immobilisation, ice and calming/distracting techniques, can also be effective in improving the pain experience.

ED assessment

In the ED, immediate attention should be given to assessment and resuscitation as part of the primary survey, in accordance with EMST/ITLS (Early Management of Severe Trauma/International Trauma Life Support) principles. The mantra 'find the bleeding, stop the bleeding' should be front of mind for clinicians in the early phase of care for unstable patients. Specific assessment of the extremities is left to the secondary survey in emergency, unless active haemorrhage requires controlling.

Detailed physical examination of the extremities should begin in the ED by gaining a comprehensive history with the patient, paramedic and/or family, regarding mechanism of injury, pattern of injury, and presenting symptoms, where appropriate. This may provide important clues to the type and severity of injury. The emergency clinician should then proceed to inspection and palpation.[10] Pain, deformity, crepitus, oedema, ecchymosis and reduced motion should raise suspicion for fracture with radiological investigation to diagnose or exclude a fracture. Prompt referral to the orthopaedic surgeon and/or trauma centre will ensure expedient management and expertise and in the case of major trauma, the orthopaedic surgeon may form part of the trauma team response.

Palpation for pulses, capillary refill examination and colour of the limb are included in the neurovascular assessment, which is essential when fractures are suspected or diagnosed (discussed on p. 1325). Frequency of neurovascular assessment is dependent on institutional protocols. Generally, in the first few hours after injury, neurovascular/extremity observations should be conducted half-hourly to hourly, or after interventions such as reduction of fractures/dislocations, application of splints/traction, application of plaster or inadvertent movement of the fractured limb. Neurovascular observations should continue at the frequency prescribed by the orthopaedic surgeon. These observations should then continue 4-hourly until definitive management occurs, such as internal fixation, then revert to hourly for the postoperative period.[10,35] When neurovascular status worsens, the orthopaedic surgeon should be notified immediately.

PRACTICE TIP

Use of a dedicated neurovascular observation chart, commenced in the ED, promotes consistency and the ability to view trends while monitoring an injured limb.

Peripheral neurological integrity is checked by assessing sensation and motion. The major nerves in the upper extremity are musculocutaneous, radial, ulnar and median, and in the lower extremity sciatic, peroneal and tibial nerves. Initially by touching an area innervated by a specific nerve, ask the patient what is felt, such as dull, sharp, numb or 'pins and needles'. To assess the motor function, ask the patient to move the affected limb. For the lower limb, ask the patient to dorsiflex and/or plantar-flex

FIGURE 48.4 NEUROVASCULAR ASSESSMENT OF THE UPPER AND LOWER EXTREMITIES[13]

Peroneal nerve

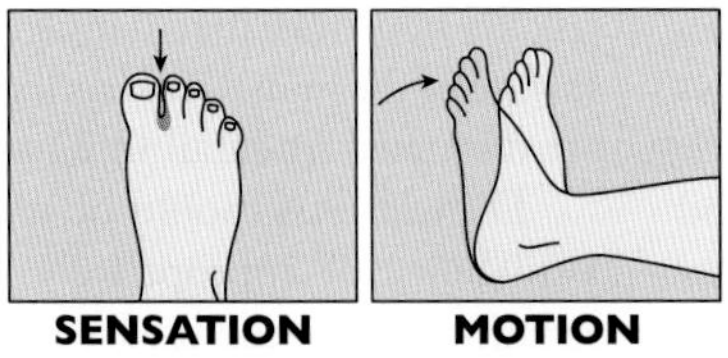

SENSATION MOTION

☐ **SENSATION**
Prick the web space between the great toe and second toe

☐ **MOTION**
Have patient dorsiflex ankle and extend toes at the metatarsal phalangeal joints

Tibial nerve

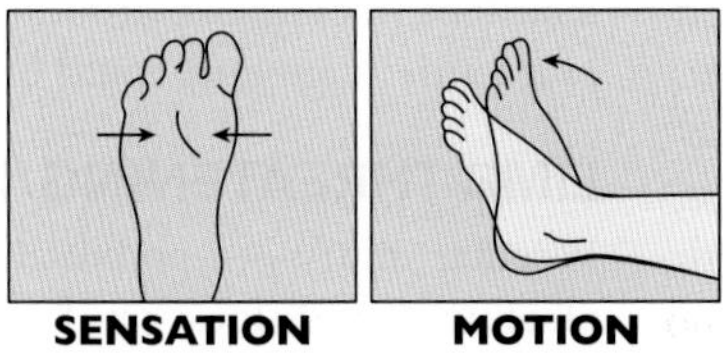

SENSATION MOTION

☐ **SENSATION**
Prick the medial and lateral surfaces of the sole of the foot

☐ **MOTION**
Have patient plantar flex ankle and toes

Radial nerve

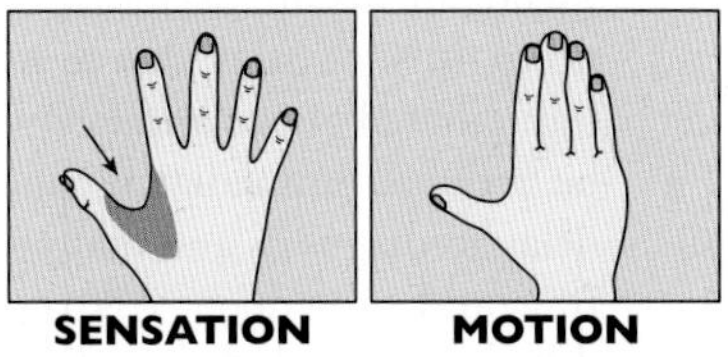

SENSATION MOTION

☐ **SENSATION**
Prick the web space between the thumb and index finger

☐ **MOTION**
Have patient hyperextend thumb then wrist and hyperextend the four fingers at the MCP joints

Ulnar nerve

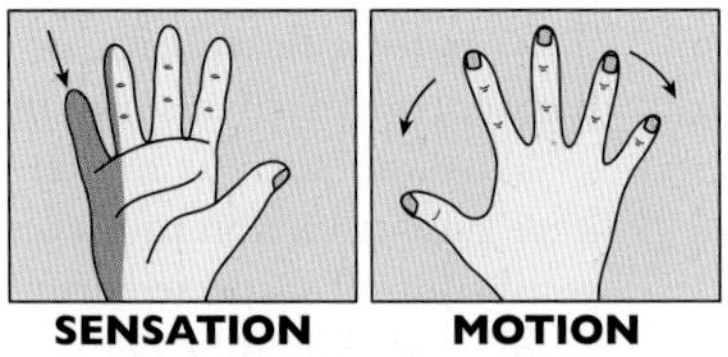

SENSATION MOTION

☐ **SENSATION**
Prick the distal fat pad of the small finger

☐ **MOTION**
Have patient abduct all fingers

Median nerve

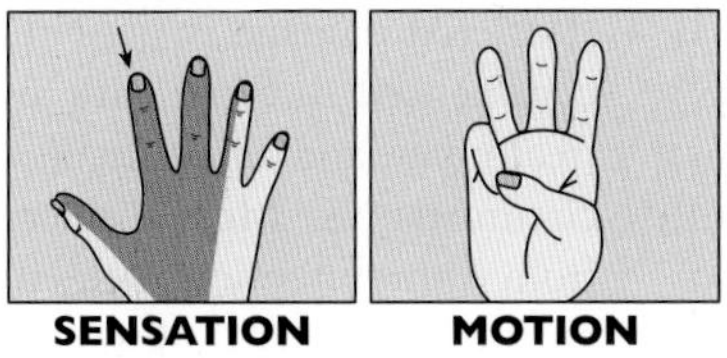

SENSATION MOTION

☐ **SENSATION**
Prick the distal surface of the index finger

☐ **MOTION**
Have patient oppose thumb and small finger; note whether patient can flex wrist

their foot. For the upper limb, the main motor test is flexion/extension of the wrist, and the strength and ability to flex and extend their fingers open and closed (Fig. 48.4).[11,35]

PRACTICE TIP

If distal pulses are difficult to digitally palpate, try using a hand-held Doppler and, once a pulse is located, the location should be marked on the patient's skin.

DIAGNOSIS

RADIOLOGY

X-ray

In all major trauma patients, an anteroposterior (AP) pelvis x-ray is recommended. Numerous other x-rays are performed to confirm or exclude musculoskeletal injuries. For standard plain films, there should be at least two views of the limb, AP and lateral, to detect displacement and degree of angulation. The exact zone of injury is often not fully appreciated; therefore x-rays of limbs must include areas distal and proximal to any suspected injury. For example, with a mid-shaft tibial fracture, x-rays of joints above and below the fracture are essential to rule out other fractures or dislocations. Pattern of injury and clinical examination will aid in determining what x-rays should be undertaken.

Significant force may cause more than one injury on more than one level; for example, with fractures of the calcaneus or femur, it is essential to also x-ray the pelvis and the spine.[14,36]

PRACTICE TIP

Always x-ray joints above and below a fracture.

Ultrasound

The use of ultrasound is becoming more widespread in EDs as more practitioners are accredited. The advantages of ultrasound over other imaging modalities are that it is portable, repeatable, dynamic, irradiation-free, cost-effective, and allows assessment of soft tissues and musculoskeletal body parts. Ultrasound is a dynamic process that is easily repeatable and provides real-time assessment; therefore, it can be a good alternative to MRI. It has a high resolution, enabling detection of nerve compression, foreign bodies, tendon and ligament injury and other soft-tissue injury. Ultrasound has been proven in studies to be accurate to rule extremity fractures in or out. It can also be used for therapeutic guidance, such as post-fracture reduction, drainage of collections, nerve blocks, etc. There is still conjecture regarding diagnosing fractures with ultrasound; it may not replace traditional radiography, but is helpful to rule a fracture in or out.

Computed tomography

Some x-rays may be inadequate in diagnosing fractures in the pelvis, knee and ankle; therefore, computed tomography (CT) scans are required to confirm minimally displaced or hidden fractures, and to evaluate the integrity of posterior pelvic structures, haematoma size and visceral injury, such as bladder rupture. Three-dimensional CT images are excellent in displaying fracture pattern and extent of injury, particularly in difficult sites such as the acetabulum, calcaneus and vertebral column.[5,37]

Magnetic resonance imaging

Soft-tissue, ligament and tendon injuries are not clearly identified radiologically; magnetic resonance imaging (MRI) should be performed if more-substantial damage is suspected. MRI is regarded as more sensitive than CT on soft-tissue structures.[38] MRI differentiates between muscle, ligaments and tendons, providing anatomical differentiation of structures of the joint. It is particularly useful in visualising anterior and posterior ligaments of the knee.[39]

Retrograde urethrogram/cystography

Evaluation of urethral injuries usually involves retrograde urethrogram. Commonly, fractures of the sacroiliac (SI) joint, symphysis pubis and sacrum are associated with bladder injuries. Fractures of the inferior rami, widened symphysis and SI joint are associated with urethral injuries. Bladder distension is directly related to bladder injury; a full bladder is more likely to be injured. Pelvic fractures in combination with blood at the meatus, inability to void, high-riding prostate, scrotal swelling and gross haematuria warrant immediate retrograde urethrogram/cystography to assess the lower urinary tract and bladder.[40]

FRACTURE CLASSIFICATIONS

DISLOCATIONS AND SUBLUXATIONS

A *dislocation* is when the articular (joint) surfaces are no longer in contact, and can be described as anterior/posterior or medial/lateral. A *subluxation* is partial displacement of the articular surfaces. Both injuries occur when the joint is forced beyond its anatomical range of motion. Symptoms of dislocations include loss of normal mobility, pain, change in contour of the joint and discrepancy in length of the extremity.[5,14] A dislocated joint is considered an orthopaedic emergency due to the risk of neurovascular damage and damage to the articulating surface of the joint.[3] Ankle, elbow, shoulder and patella dislocation are discussed in detail in Chapter 17.

Dislocations should be reduced as soon as practicable with availability of appropriately trained personnel, analgesia and sedation (if needed). If practicable, dislocations should be x-rayed before reduction to diagnose severity and rule out concomitant fractures. A dislocation may prove difficult to reduce as fracture fragments could be lodged in the joint.

LIMB-THREATENING/MAJOR DISLOCATIONS

Vascular injury is a potentially limb-threatening complication of acute knee dislocation. Knee dislocations frequently damage the nerves and the popliteal artery, including intimal tears, pseudoaneurysm, occlusion, avulsion, rupture or transection in up to 40% of cases, due to its location and constitution of being tethered above and below the knee. These injuries need to be reduced immediately, and arterial injury identified, with delay to diagnosis and management increasing warm ischaemic time and subsequent risk of above knee amputation.[40] Motor vehicle trauma is believed to be a key factor in the increased occurrence of traumatic knee dislocations, with dashboard injury against a flexed knee or the proximal tibia accounting for high-energy mechanism of injury.

A splint, such as a knee immobiliser, should support the knee post-reduction to prevent further dislocation. Further investigation of suspected arterial damage is required via angiography, and should be performed immediately, with contemporary convention favouring early diagnosis with CT angiography. If arterial damage is present, emergency treatment should be commenced directly, with surgical operation the mainstay of treatment, and endovascular treatment reserved for selected circumstances. Most dislocations post-reduction will benefit from immobilisation with either a sling or a splint, depending on the limb.[1,10,35,41]

Reduction can require intravenous sedation for muscle relaxation (see Chapter 16 for procedural sedation). Post-reduction x-rays are required to ensure alignment. Patients receiving intravenous sedation require one-on-one nursing for frequent observations such as respiratory, cardiovascular and neurovascular monitoring.[6]

Prior to reduction, a thorough neurovascular assessment should be completed to provide a baseline, as this will guide monitoring of the neurovascular status post-reduction for any changes and adverse effects post-reduction. Neurologic damage to the common peroneal nerve is reported in approximately 25% of cases of knee dislocation, potentially leading to foot drop and impaired gait.[42] While not limb threatening, this injury poses significant morbidity and early recognition is essential.

Common dislocations and management are listed in Table 48.4.

FRACTURES

Bone has some degree of elasticity. A fracture results from stress/force placed on the bone which it cannot absorb. It may be caused by direct or indirect trauma, stress or weakness of

TABLE 48.4 COMMON DISLOCATIONS[43]

BODY AREA	TYPICAL MECHANISM OF INJURY	CLINICAL FINDINGS	TREATMENT
Shoulder	Anterior fall on an outstretched arm, or a direct blow to the shoulder	Arm abducted, cannot bring the elbow down to the chest or touch the hand of the affected side to the opposite ear	Splint in a position of comfort; reduce as soon as possible
Posterior	Rare; strong blow to the front of the shoulder; violent convulsions or seizures	Arm held at the side, unable to externally rotate the arm	Same as for shoulder
Elbow: radius and ulna	Fall on an outstretched hand with the elbow in extension	Arm shortened; pain with motion; rapid swelling; nerve injury may occur	Same as for shoulder Surgical repair is required if the dislocation is associated with fracture of the radial head or olecranon
Radial head (children)	Sudden longitudinal pull, jerk or lift on a child's wrist or hand ('nursemaid's elbow')	Pain; patient refuses to use the arm; limited supination; can flex and extend at the elbow; may have no deformity	Reduce; place in a sling; advise parents that this may recur until the age of 5 years
Hip (usually posterior)	Blow to the knee while the hip is flexed and adducted (sitting with crossed knees); common in front-seat passengers in a motor vehicle collision	Hip flexed, adducted, internally rotated and shortened; may have an associated fracture of the femur; sciatic nerve injury (this nerve lies posterior to the femoral head)	Splint in a position of comfort; reduce as soon as possible
Patella	Spontaneous	The knee is flexed; the patella can be palpated lateral to the femoral condyle	Reduce dislocation (may occur spontaneously) or immobilise with a cast or splint
	Associated with other trauma	Excessive swelling, tenderness and a palpable soft-tissue defect	Surgical repair of soft-tissue injury or fractures is required
Knee (rare)	Severe direct blow to the upper leg or forced hyperextension of the knee	Ligamentous instability; inability to straighten the leg; peroneal nerve and popliteal artery injury are common; assess distal neurovascular function	Immediate neurovascular assessment is necessary; reduce dislocation
Ankle	The ankle is a complex joint, with multiple ligaments providing stability; dislocation is usually associated with other injuries such as fractures and soft-tissue trauma	Swelling, tenderness; loss of alignment and function	Splint ankle; ankle dislocation usually requires open reduction because the joint is complex and must be realigned accurately

the bone, or may be pathological in origin (Fig. 48.5).[11] The types of force used to cause fractures are direct violence, indirect (generally a twisting injury), pathological (generally a weak bone from tumour or osteoporotic bone) and fatigue (repeated stress on the bone, e.g. from military marches).

CLASSIFICATION

Fractures are classified as *stable* or *unstable*. Stable fractures are unlikely to be displaced, whereas unstable fractures are likely to be displaced and require reduction. Fractures are also classified as *open* (see open fractures for more detail) or *closed*. With closed fractures, there is no penetration of the skin by bone. Conversely, in open fractures the bone breaches the skin or one of the body cavities, or the force that caused the fracture penetrates the soft tissue.[5,6]

TYPE

- *Transverse fractures*—cross the bone at a 90° angle and are generally stable post-reduction.[6]
- *Oblique/spiral fractures*—are at a 45° angle to the axis, usually from a twisting force causing upward thrust. Most long-bone fractures are due to violent twisting motions, such as a sharp twist to the leg when the foot is stuck in a hole, producing a spiral fracture. They are difficult to maintain without internal fixation due to malrotation of the fracture.[6]
- *Comminuted fractures*—high-energy injuries where the bone is splintered in more than two fragments. These are generally associated with significant soft-tissue injury, and reduction and anatomical reconstruction is difficult (Fig. 48.6).[6]
- *Impacted fractures*—occur when one fragment is forced into another. The fracture line may be difficult to visualise.[6]
- *Crush fractures*—occur when cancellous bone is compressed or crushed. Reduction is difficult as there are no fragments to manipulate.[6]
- *Avulsion fractures*—occur when soft tissue and bone are torn away from the insertion site.[6]

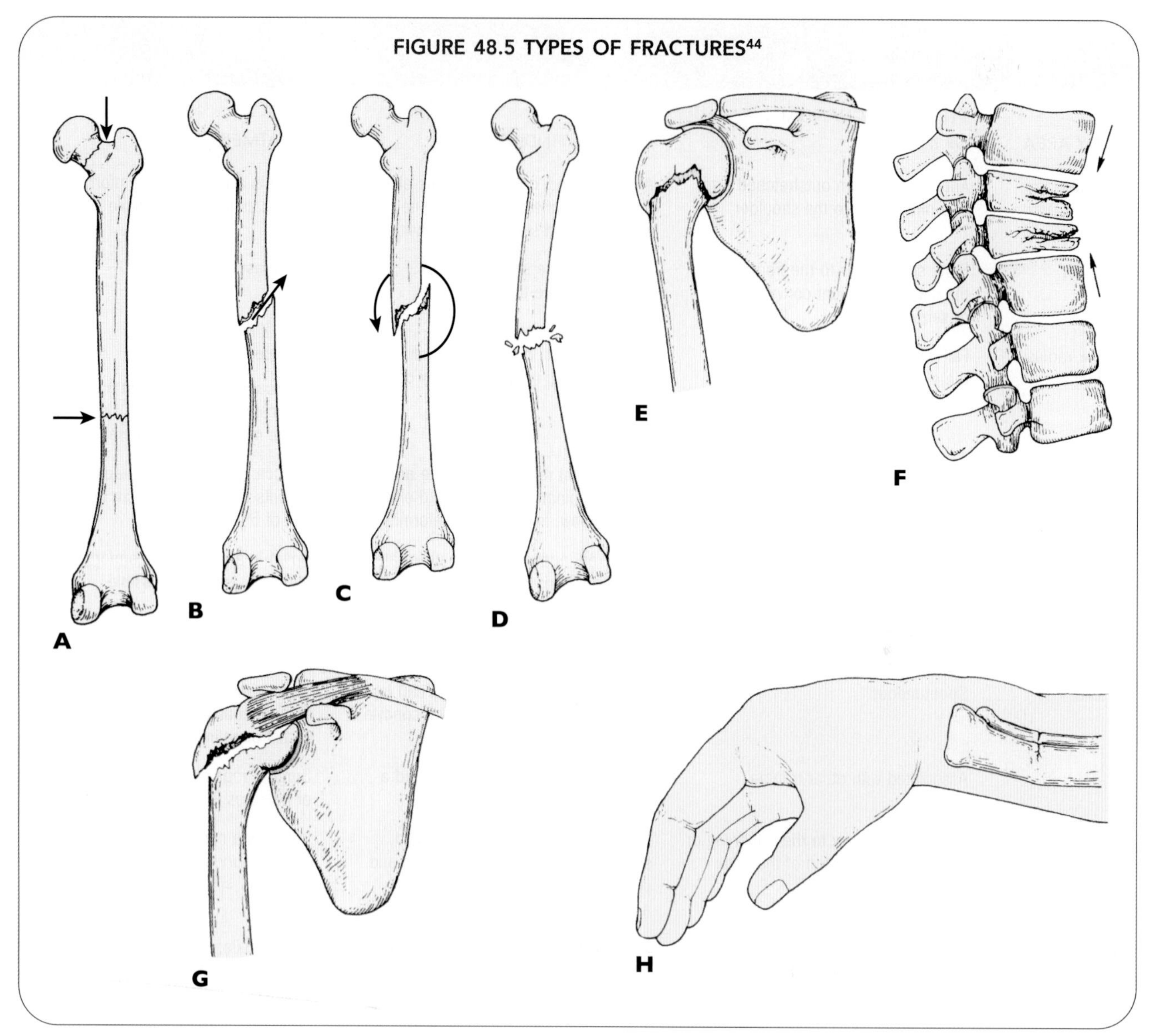

A. Transverse fracture. **B.** Oblique fracture. **C.** Spiral fracture. **D.** Comminuted fracture. **E.** Impacted fracture. **F.** Compression fracture. **G.** Avulsion fracture. **H.** Greenstick fracture.

- *Greenstick fractures*—occur when the compressed cortex bends/buckles. If the force persists, the cortex will fracture.[6] These are usually seen in children as their bones are much more porous and soft.
- *Epiphyseal or growth plate fractures* (Salter-type)—may affect future bone growth because of early closure of the epiphyseal plate and resultant limb shortening. Angulation may occur with partial growth plate fractures because bone growth continues in the non-injured area. Epiphyseal fractures require close orthopaedic follow-up for several months to monitor healing and identify growth abnormalities.

BLOOD LOSS FROM FRACTURES

Blood loss from long bones can be underestimated and is often not appreciated (Table 48.5). A patient with multiple fractures can experience significant blood loss. Third spacing occurs when blood accumulates in surrounding tissue causing fluid shifts into the interstitial space, increasing extremity size. Bleeding may be difficult to assess as it may be slow, as in the shoulder girdle. Blood loss can continue for up to 48 hours and is often greater than expected. Prompt reduction, immobilisation and gentle handling of fractures can limit bleeding. The amount of blood loss is dependent on the type of fracture and location, as well as previous medical history of the patient, such as if the patient is on anticoagulants.[45] See Chapter 42 for further reading on shock and fluid resuscitation.

Treatment

Box 48.1 outlines general guidelines for emergency fracture management.

CLOSED FRACTURES

Where skin integrity is not compromised, fractures are classified as closed. Emergency management includes regular neurovascular observations, pain relief, elevation and ice to reduce swelling, removal of jewellery—particularly in hand injuries (Fig. 48.7)—and splinting to reduce movement and prevent

FIGURE 48.6 COMMINUTED FEMUR FRACTURE[44]

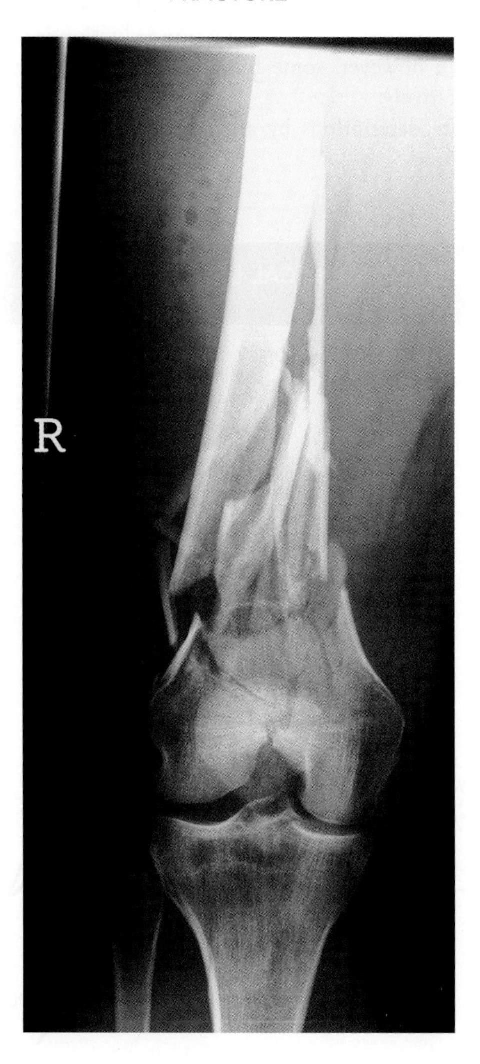

BOX 48.1 GENERAL GUIDELINES FOR FRACTURE MANAGEMENT[41]

- Perform primary survey and initiate appropriate interventions.
- Evaluate neurovascular status of each injured extremity.
- Secure any impaled objects.
- Manage pain.
- Remove rings, other jewellery and tight clothing/shoes from injured extremities.
- Immobilise extremities beyond the joints above and below the site of injury.
- Re-evaluate neurovascular status after repositioning or immobilisation.
- Cover open wounds with a sterile dressing.
- Apply ice packs to areas of swelling.
- Avoid putting cleaning solutions (i.e. hydrogen peroxide, povidone-iodine, chlorhexidine) directly on a wound.
- Elevate injured extremity.
- Obtain radiographs as indicated.
- Assess patient tetanus immunisation status and vaccinate as required.
- Ensure patient maintains nil by mouth status if emergency surgery is probable.
- Repeat radiographs after any manipulation.
- Obtain orthopaedic consultation.

TABLE 48.5 ESTIMATED BLOOD LOSS IN FRACTURES[4,10,13]

FRACTURE	BLOOD LOSS (mL)
Humerus	500–2500
Elbow	250–1500
Radius/ulna	250–1000
Pelvis	750–6000
Hip	1500–3000
Femur	500–3000
Knee	1000–2500
Tibia/fibula	250–2000
Ankle	250–1500
Spine/ribs	1000–3000

FIGURE 48.7 METACARPAL FRACTURE[48]

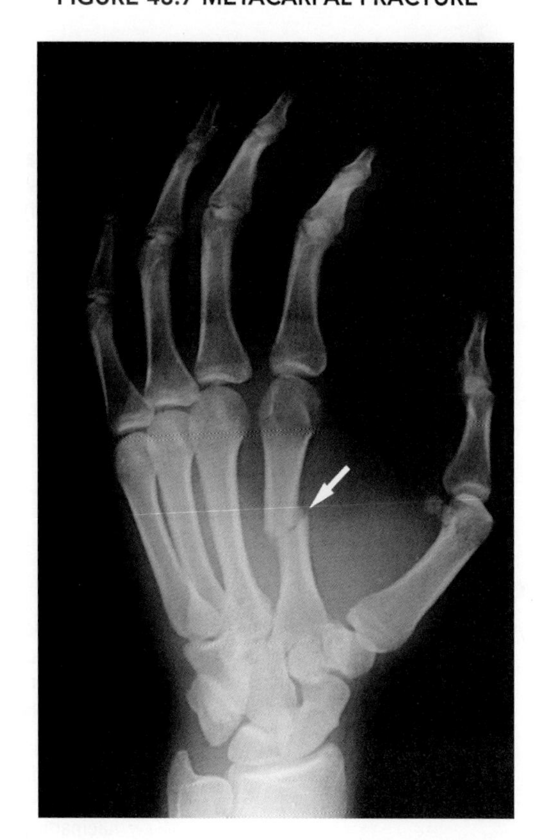

soft-tissue damage and pain, and lower the incidence of clinical fat embolism.[6,17]

Unstable, displaced fractures will require reduction to realign bony fragments, reduce damage to neurovascular structures and soft-tissue and tamponade bleeding. Reduction is painful and requires analgesia and generally procedural sedation. Post-reduction x-ray films are important in assessing successful anatomical realignment. Classification of fracture extent and type, and associated soft-tissue injuries, along with patient clinical status and assessment, will determine management planning and guide conservative versus operative approaches to care. Generally, fracture reduction is performed in the ED; however, some fractures will be openly reduced intra-operatively.

Fracture descriptions by anatomical location are listed in Table 48.6.

TABLE 48.6 FRACTURE NAMES AND DESCRIPTIONS BY ANATOMICAL LOCATION[15]

	DESCRIPTION	COMMON TREATMENT	ILLUSTRATION[46]
Humerus			
Anatomical neck	Two-part fracture of the true neck of the humeral metaphysis at the area of tendon attachment with angulatory or rotational deformity usually less than 45°	Sling and exercise program or collar/cuff and exercise program Operative—hemiarthroplasty[47]	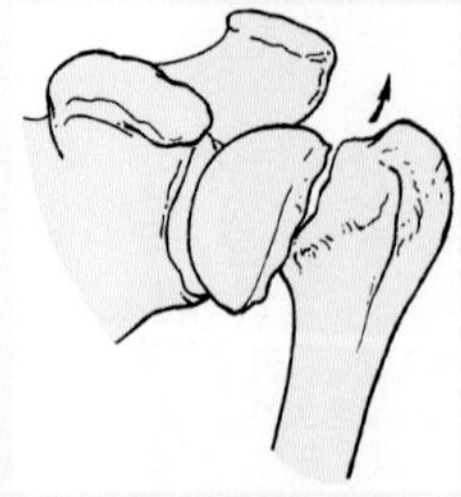
Surgical neck	Fracture occurring below the anatomical neck, usually angulated greater than 45 degrees or malrotated—may have associated non-displaced linear fracture extending into humeral head	Closed reduction with sling and swathe to maintain reduction Operative—ORIF, hemiarthroplasty, reverse total shoulder arthroplasty[47]	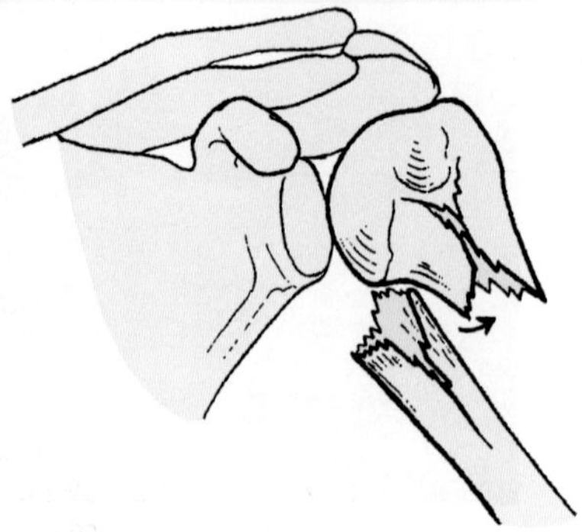
Diaphyseal	Fracture of the humeral shaft; middle third is most common site	Closed—hanging cast or coaptation splint (U-shaped plaster splint with collar/cuff) or sling and swathe Operative—compression plate and screws, intramedullary rods	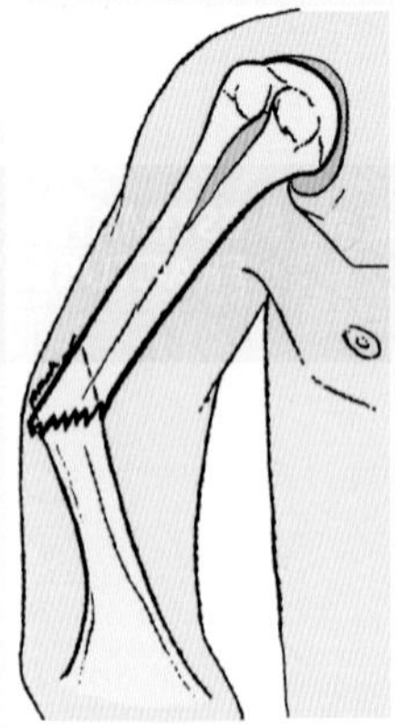
Elbow			
Condylar	Fracture of medial or lateral articular process of the distal humerus	Lateral: displaced (disrupts joint surface)—open reduction and internal fixation; undisplaced or minimally displaced—immobilisation Medial: displaced—open reduction and internal fixation or pin fixation; undisplaced—aspiration of haemarthrosis and posterior splint application	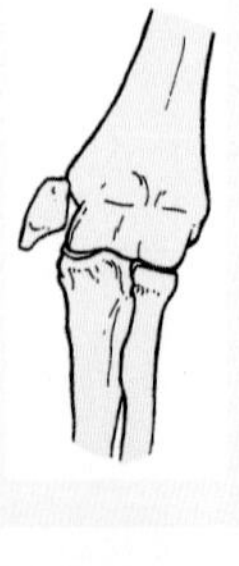

TABLE 48.6 FRACTURE NAMES AND DESCRIPTIONS BY ANATOMICAL LOCATION—cont'd

	DESCRIPTION	COMMON TREATMENT	ILLUSTRATION[46]
Epicondylar	Fracture through the medial or lateral epicondyle	Lateral–immobilisation until pain subsides, displaced over 2-3 cm requires open reduction and internal fixation Medial–open reduction and internal fixation and immobilisation	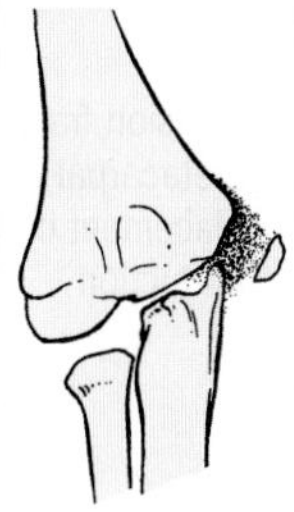
Supracondylar	Fracture of distal humeral shaft	Closed reduction under general anaesthesia and posterior splint, or percutaneous pinning Open reduction and internal fixation if reduction is unstable or fails Difficult to treat if displaced–watch for development of compartment syndrome	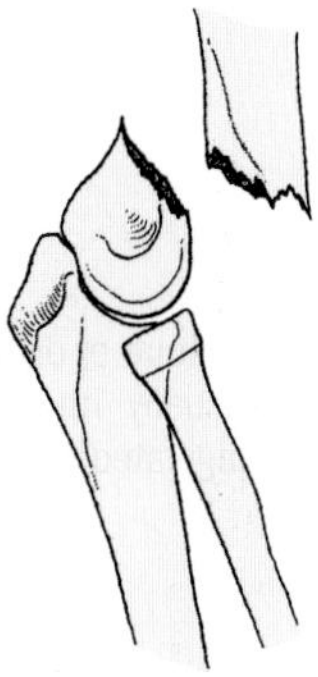
Olecranon	Fracture of the olecranon process of the ulna (prominent portion of ulna at the elbow)	Displaced–anatomical reduction and internal fixation or primary excision Undisplaced–long-arm cast with 45-90° elbow flexion	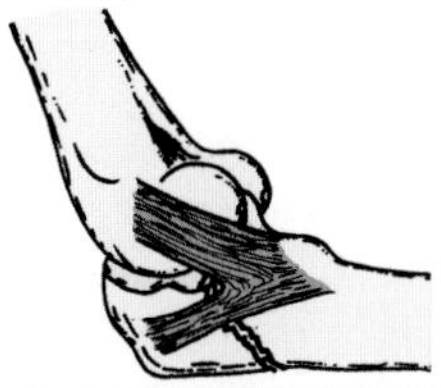
Forearm and wrist			
Colles'	Fracture through distal radial epiphysis within 13-19 mm of the articular surface with radial displacement and dorsal angulation of the distal fragment	Closed reduction and splint or cast Severely comminuted (uncommon)–external fixator	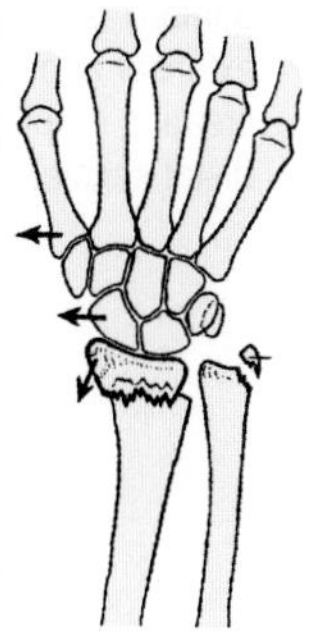
Radial head	Fracture of the most proximal part of the radius	Undisplaced–long-arm splint, sling or cast Displaced/single fracture line–open reduction and internal fixation Comminuted–excision with silastic implant	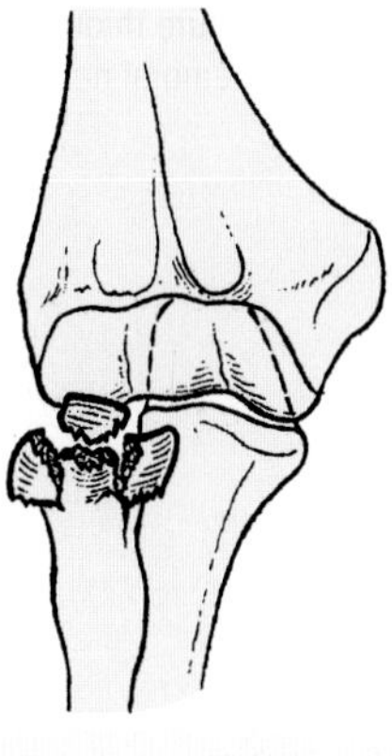

Continued

TABLE 48.6 FRACTURE NAMES AND DESCRIPTIONS BY ANATOMICAL LOCATION—cont'd

	DESCRIPTION	COMMON TREATMENT	ILLUSTRATION[46]
Hand			
Bennett's	Avulsion fracture of carpo-metacarpal joint with displacement caused by pull of abduction	Closed–reduction and immobilisation Operative–open reduction and internal fixation under direct visualisation or percutaneous pinning under image intensification	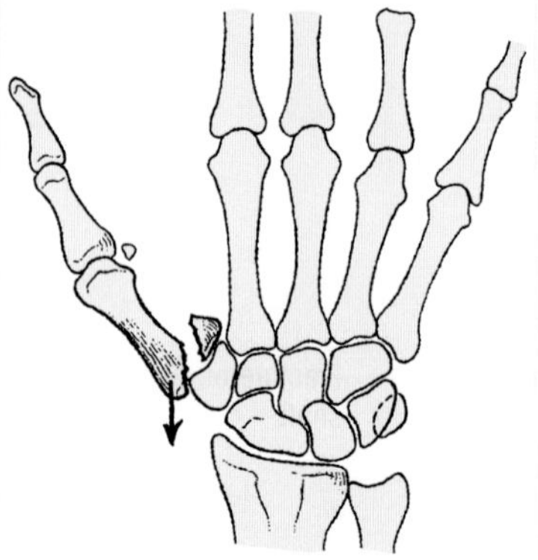
Boxer's	Fracture of distal metacarpal (usually 4th or 5th) angulated or impacted	Closed reduction and short-arm cast with finger splint; seldom requires open reduction with percutaneous pin fixation	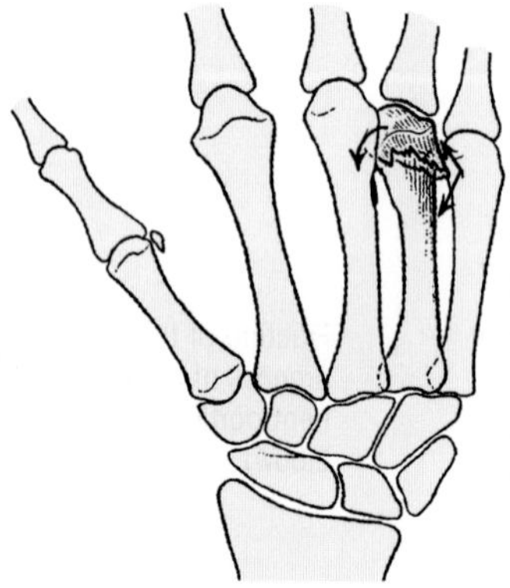
Mallet	Avulsion fracture of dorsal articular surface of distal phalanx of any digit involving extensor apparatus insertion, creating dropped flexion of distal segment	Closed reduction and dorsal splint, may require open reduction and internal fixation	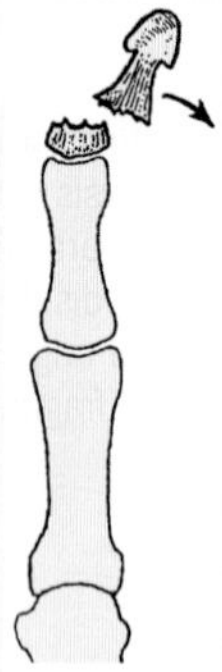
Proximal femur			
Femoral neck	Fracture through midportion of femoral neck	Anatomic reduction and stable internal fixation or prosthesis	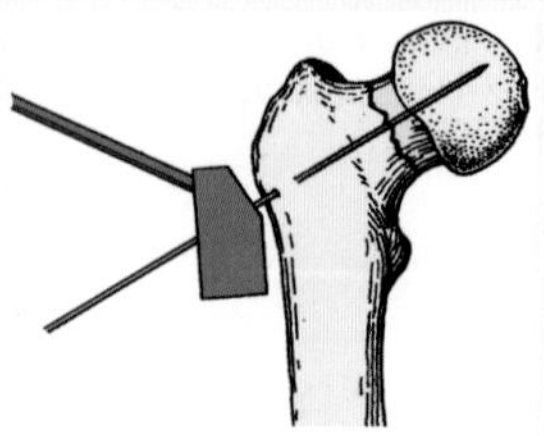

TABLE 48.6 FRACTURE NAMES AND DESCRIPTIONS BY ANATOMICAL LOCATION—cont'd

	DESCRIPTION	COMMON TREATMENT	ILLUSTRATION[46]
Greater trochanter	Avulsion fracture of greater trochanter	Slight displacement–protected weightbearing (as an isolated injury) Displaced–open reduction and internal fixation	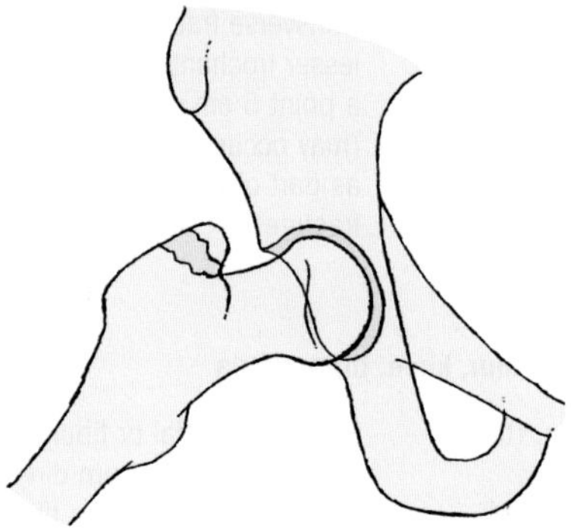
Intertrochanteric	Fracture along a line joining the greater and lesser trochanter	Reduction and internal fixation of proximal femur–fixed or sliding nail/plate device, intramedullary device	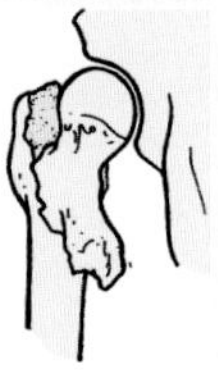
Lesser trochanter	Avulsion fracture of lesser trochanter	Bed rest 2–3 days with hip flexed, then protected ambulation (as an isolated injury)	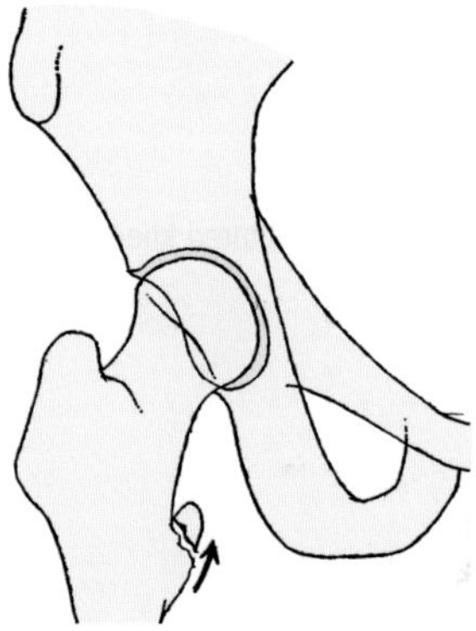
Shaft	Fracture between subtrochanteric and supracondylar area	Skeletal traction Cast brace External fixation Intramedullary fixation Closed medullary nailing Interlocking nail, plate and screws	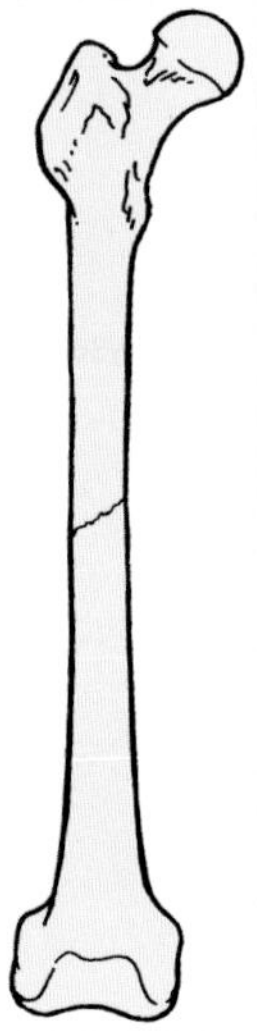

Continued

TABLE 48.6 FRACTURE NAMES AND DESCRIPTIONS BY ANATOMICAL LOCATION—cont'd

	DESCRIPTION	COMMON TREATMENT	ILLUSTRATION[46]
Subtrochanteric	Transverse fracture between lesser trochanter and a point 5 cm distally (may occur independently or as part of intertrochanteric fracture)	Open reduction and internal fixation Fixed-angle nail and plate AO blade plates Sliding compression hip screw Intramedullary devices	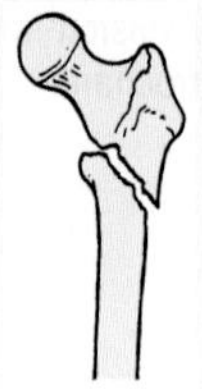
Distal femur, knee, tibia, fibula			
Bumper (tibial plateau)	Fracture of tibial or fibular condyle resulting from direct blow in the area of the tibial tuberosity	Displaced–open reduction and internal fixation or Undisplaced	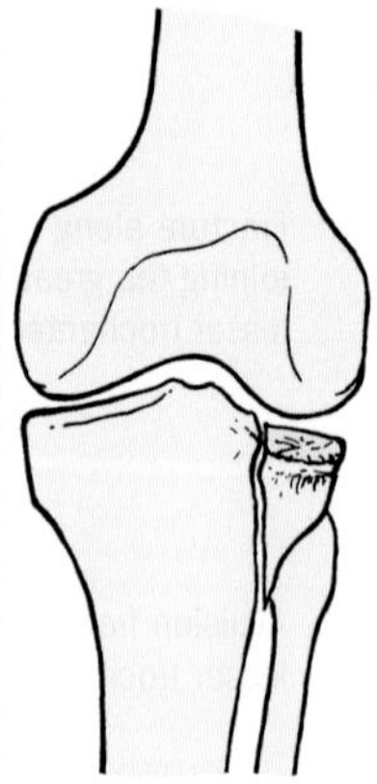
Patellar	Fractured kneecap	Undisplaced–cylinder cast Displaced or comminuted–operative fixation or excision	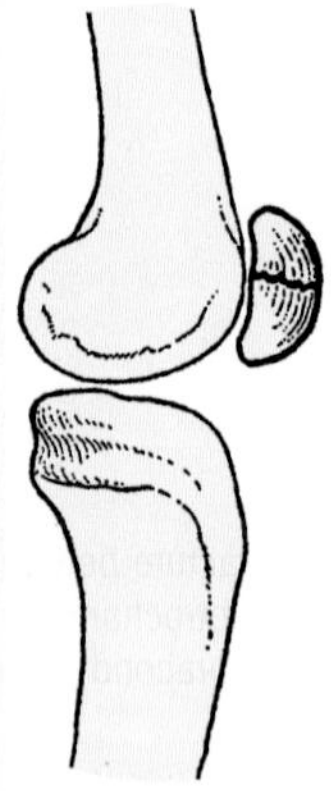
Shaft, fibula	Diaphyseal fracture of fibula	As single fracture–cast	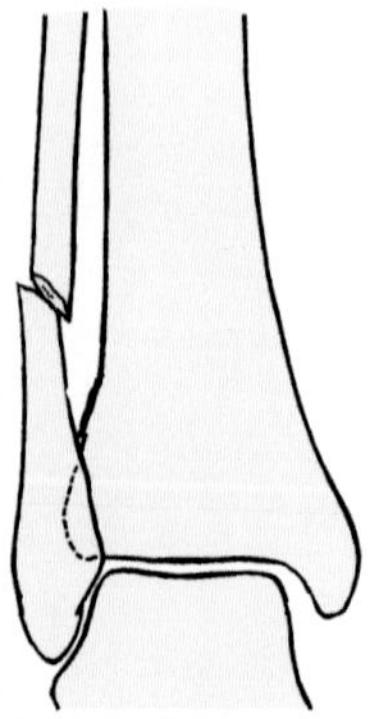

TABLE 48.6 FRACTURE NAMES AND DESCRIPTIONS BY ANATOMICAL LOCATION—cont'd

	DESCRIPTION	COMMON TREATMENT	ILLUSTRATION[46]
Shaft, tibia	Diaphyseal fracture of tibia	Closed reduction, long-leg cast, or pin/plaster or external fixation Open reduction–compression plating or plate and screws	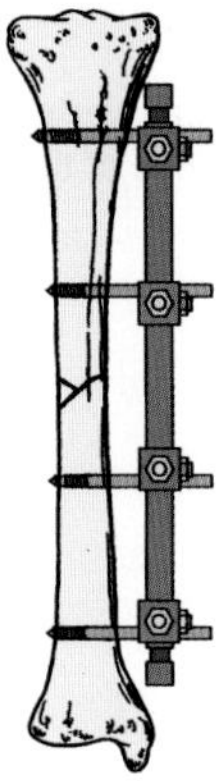
Supracondylar	Fracture of distal femoral condyle	Open reduction and internal fixation Medullary fixation Blade/plates Skeletal traction	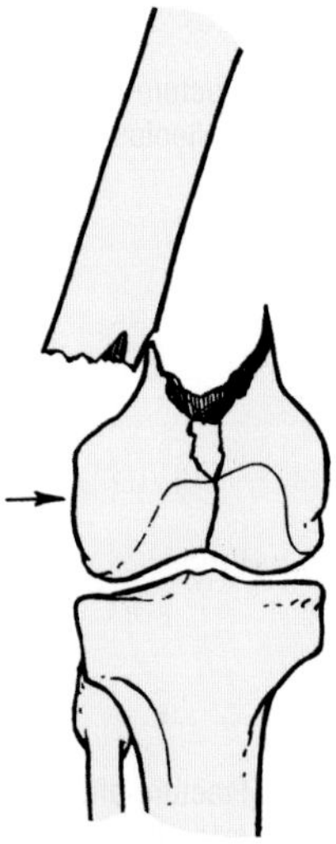
Tibial plateau	Fracture of proximal tibial articular surface	Soft dressing Cast Traction External fixation Closed or open reduction	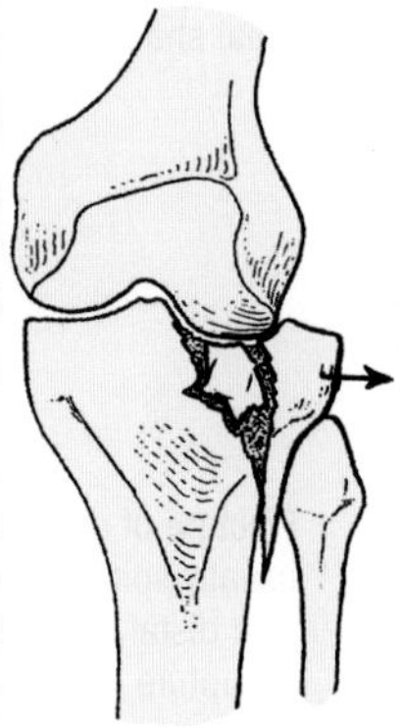
Tibial tubercle	Avulsion and proximal dislocation of tibial tubercle	Minimal or non-displaced–long-leg cast with full knee extension Displaced > 5-7 mm–open reduction and internal fixation	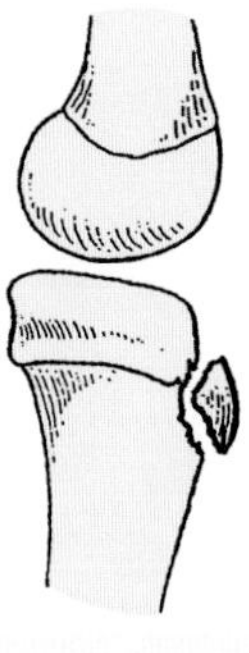

Continued

TABLE 48.6 FRACTURE NAMES AND DESCRIPTIONS BY ANATOMICAL LOCATION—cont'd

	DESCRIPTION	COMMON TREATMENT	ILLUSTRATION[46]
Ankle, foot			
Boot top	Transverse fracture of distal third of tibia	Stable–closed reduction if possible Unstable–intramedullary fixation	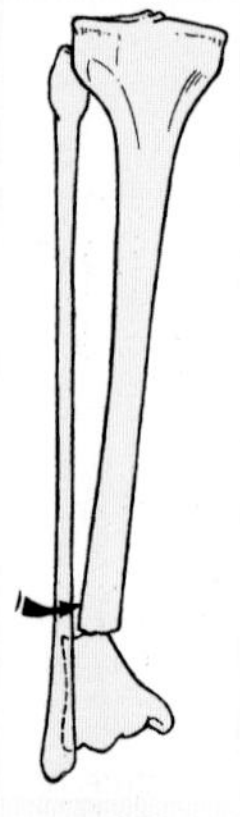
Paratrooper	Fracture distal tibial and malleolus	Open reduction and internal fixation	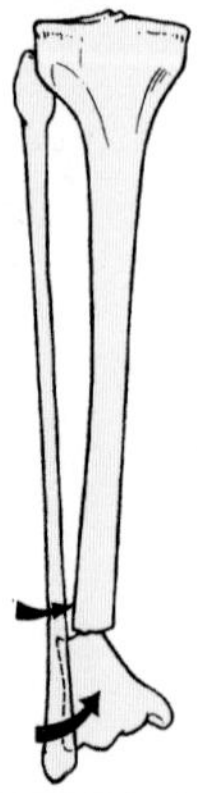
Plafond	Fracture of tibial plafond extending in a spiral or longitudinal fashion into tibial shaft	Open reduction and internal fixation	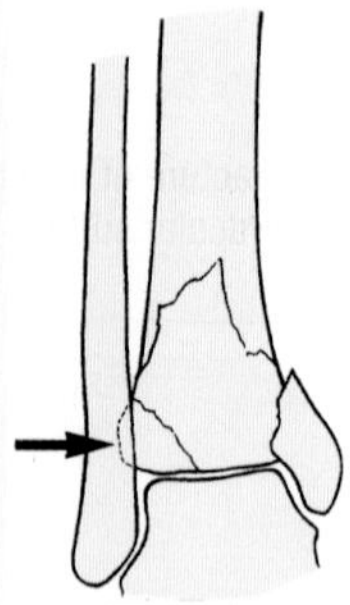
Pott's	Fracture of distal fibula, usually spiral/oblique, with distal tibial chipping or rupture of surrounding ligaments	Closed reduction or open reduction and internal fixation, followed by cast immobilisation	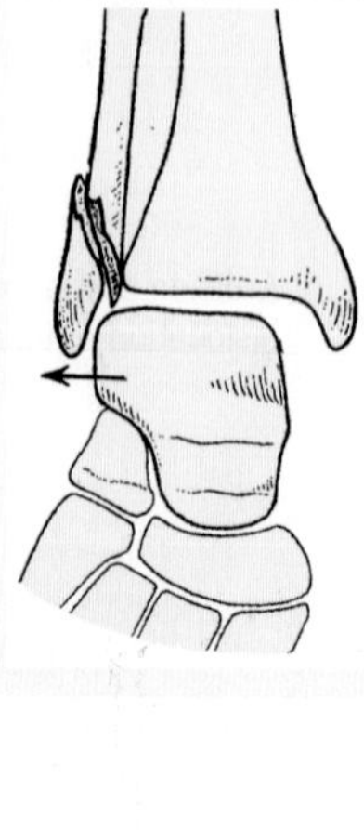

OPEN FRACTURES

An open fracture is where the bone has breached the skin or any of the body cavities, and may result from blunt or penetrating injury (Fig. 48.8).

Open fractures generally involve high-energy trauma. There can be significant soft-tissue stripping and devascularisation of bone and soft tissue.

The risk of compartment syndrome from an open fracture should not be underestimated, with regular patient and neurovascular assessment. Open fractures are largely associated with high infection risks. This is primarily due to the high risk of contamination by debris and foreign objects from the surrounding environment. Studies suggest early wound debridement and antibiotic administration is key in the reduction of infection, associated non-unions, and later osteomyelitis.

Assessment and management

Further x-rays of the limb are essential to establish the extent of bony injury. Broad-spectrum antibiotics should commence in the ED, if not given prior during the pre-hospital phase, with optimal timing $<$ 1 hour from injury to antibiotic administration. Tetanus prophylaxis needs to be considered if immunisation status is unknown, or greater than 5 years prior to presentation. Consider photographing wounds, prior to debridement, to prevent contamination from repeated removal of dressings by different clinicians assessing the injury. Ensure protocols cover the handling of photographic images for clinical decision-making. All open fractures should be examined, irrigated, debrided and stabilised in the operating suite.

Open fractures represent a limb-threatening and potentially life-threatening emergency. Wounds can be irrigated in the ED using copious amounts of sterile saline. This will only get gross contaminants out, such as grass and other debris. For optimal wound management, a pulse lavage (high pressure) system is used in the operating theatres. For many years the gold standard for open fracture management was rapid operative debridement to reduce infection. Recent studies have demonstrated that is not as vital as once believed. Current recommendations are for debridement to occur; immediately for grossly contaminated wounds; within 12 hours for high-energy open fractures (e.g. Gustillo-Anderson Type IIIa and IIIb) not grossly contaminated; and within 24 hours for all other open fractures.[26] Multiple studies have shown that early administration of prophylactic antibiotics has decreased the incidence of infection for open fractures. All grades of open fracture should be treated for Gram-positive bacteria, usually with intravenous Cefazolin.[3] Antibiotic prophylaxis administration should be given as soon as possible, ideally within 3 hours of injury with the total duration dependent on injury severity.[49] Initial surgical management includes extensive pulse lavage, thorough debridement, and often fracture fixation at another time. Despite these guidelines, in tertiary referral centres surgical delay is common due to patient transfers from other facilities and access/demand for emergency surgery.

FIGURE 48.8 GUNSHOT WOUND FRACTURE OF RADIUS AND ULNA WITH EXTENSIVE SOFT-TISSUE DAMAGE[48]

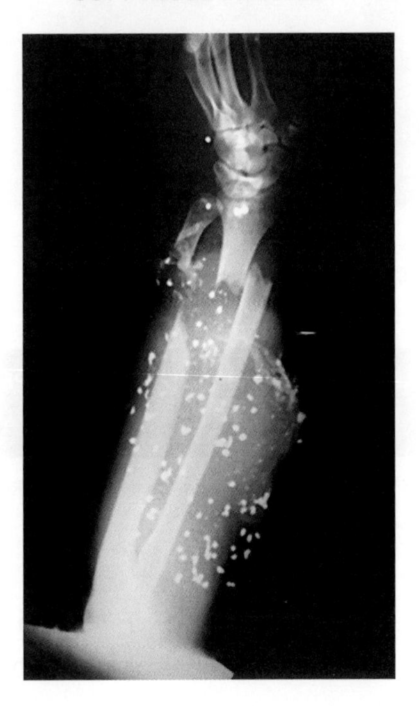

PRACTICE TIP

Always apply a sterile, saline-soaked dressing to open fracture wounds; this may assist in preventing the bone from dehydrating. Avoid gauze, as this can leave small fragments behind when removed.

PRACTICE TIP

Open fracture management basic principles: analgesia/sedation, fracture reduction, wound wash-out with copious amounts of sterile saline, sterile dressing, splinting and antibiotics.

CLASSIFICATION

The most widely cited classification of open fractures is Gustilo's. In 1976 Gustilo and Anderson divided open fractures into three categories: types I, II and III. Gustilo revised this classification in 1984, subdividing type III injuries into IIIA, IIIB and IIIC (see below).[50,51] There is collective agreement that open fractures require urgent surgical debridement and stabilisation.

Type I

There is minimal soft-tissue trauma due to a low-energy injury; type I is characterised by a small wound of less than 1 cm. Typically the bone 'spike' produces an inside-out puncture. There is minimal contamination. Fractures may be transverse or oblique and there is little comminution of the bone.[52]

Type II

This type represents variation of energy between type I (low energy) and type III (high energy). These fractures are associated with lacerations to soft tissue 1–10 cm long. There is moderate contamination, potentially minor periosteal stripping of bone fragments, and slight to moderate comminution/crush of the bone.[53]

Type III

This represents the most severe fracture patterns, divided into IIIA, IIIB and IIIC.

- IIIA—having adequate soft-tissue coverage, despite significant soft-tissue trauma. A reflection of the high energy is the presence of extensive flaps or lacerations. The bone may have a segmental fracture or severe comminution. Any open fracture is predisposed to extensive bacterial contamination.[53]
- IIIB—having significant soft-tissue damage, necessitating local or distant flap coverage due to areas of exposed bone. These are commonly associated with significant periosteal stripping, exposure of bone, massive contamination and severe comminution.[53]
- IIIC—an injury with related vascular trauma that requires surgical repair for limb survival regardless of extent of soft-tissue damage (Fig. 48.9).[53]

Infection rates of open fractures are listed in Table 48.7.

TRAUMATIC AMPUTATIONS

Traumatic amputations can be devastating injuries, whether they are a single digit or a limb. Fingertip amputations are common injuries that generally proceed to surgery for terminalisation. Finger amputations can be a clean transverse cut or contaminated crushing injuries. Management is aimed at producing a useful finger or joint. If the finger is insensate or is exquisitely tender, the patient will not use it. Therefore, it is better to have a useful stump than an ineffective finger. Traumatic amputation of the thumb is serious and disabling, as the thumb is an opposing digit and enables us to complete many tasks; it accounts for 40–50% of the hand's function.

Mechanism of injury is essential in determining the type of amputation.

- Cut- or guillotine-type amputations have wound edges that are well defined, and damage to nerves, tissue and vessels is localised.
- Crush-type amputations involve essentially more soft-tissue trauma, particularly to the vessels.
- Avulsion-type amputation is produced when stretching and tearing forces are exerted on the tissues, such as in blast injuries. Stress waves of sufficiently high intensity in blast injuries can produce limb avulsion. This is discussed in Chapter 41.

Traumatic amputations pose a challenge to the emergency clinician caring for the patient as well as the amputated part. Commonly, amputations are associated with industrial, farming or crush injuries (Fig. 48.10). Although salvage of the limb is important, other life-threatening injuries may need priority care, unless the amputation is the cause for gross haemodynamic instability.

Care of the amputated part includes keeping it dry and cool. Gently clean the amputated part, removing gross contamination, then place the part in a clean, sealed plastic bag and place the bag in iced water, or cold water if there is no ice. Care should be taken to ensure that the part does not become frozen, as freezing will result in irreparable tissue damage. The amputation

FIGURE 48.9 GRADE IIIC OPEN PROXIMAL TIBIA FRACTURE DISLOCATION FOLLOWING A MOTORBIKE CRASH

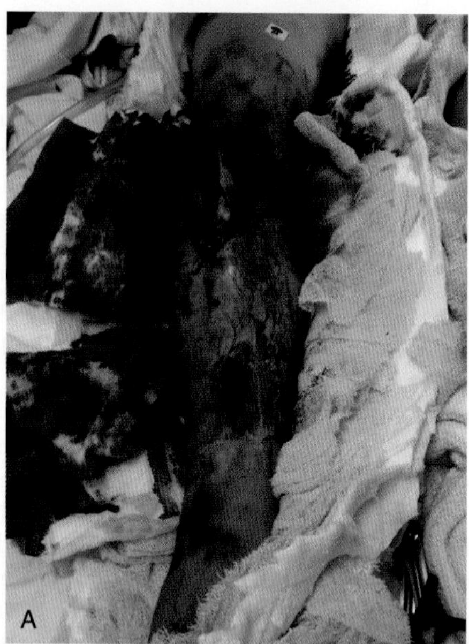

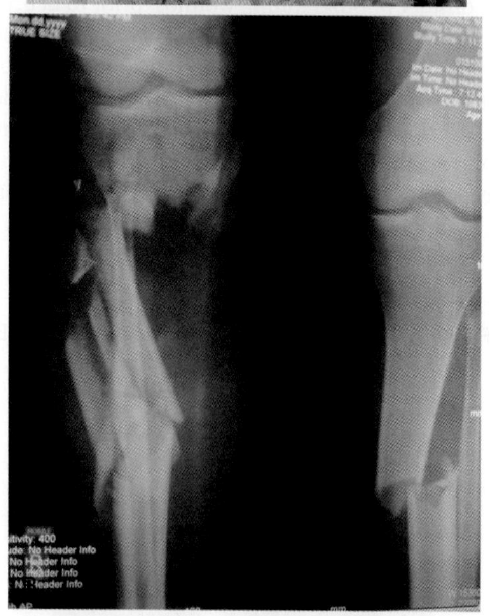

Courtesy of Celine Hill.

TABLE 48.7 INFECTION RATES OF OPEN FRACTURES[50]

FRACTURE TYPE	INFECTION RATES %
I	0-2
II	2-5
IIIA	5-10
IIIB	10-50
IIIC	25-50

FIGURE 48.10 A, B. RIGHT LEG CRUSH INJURY FROM A 100 KG STEEL GIRDER. C. 5 DAYS POST-CRUSH, PATIENT PROCEEDED TO OPERATING SUITE FOR BELOW-KNEE AMPUTATION.

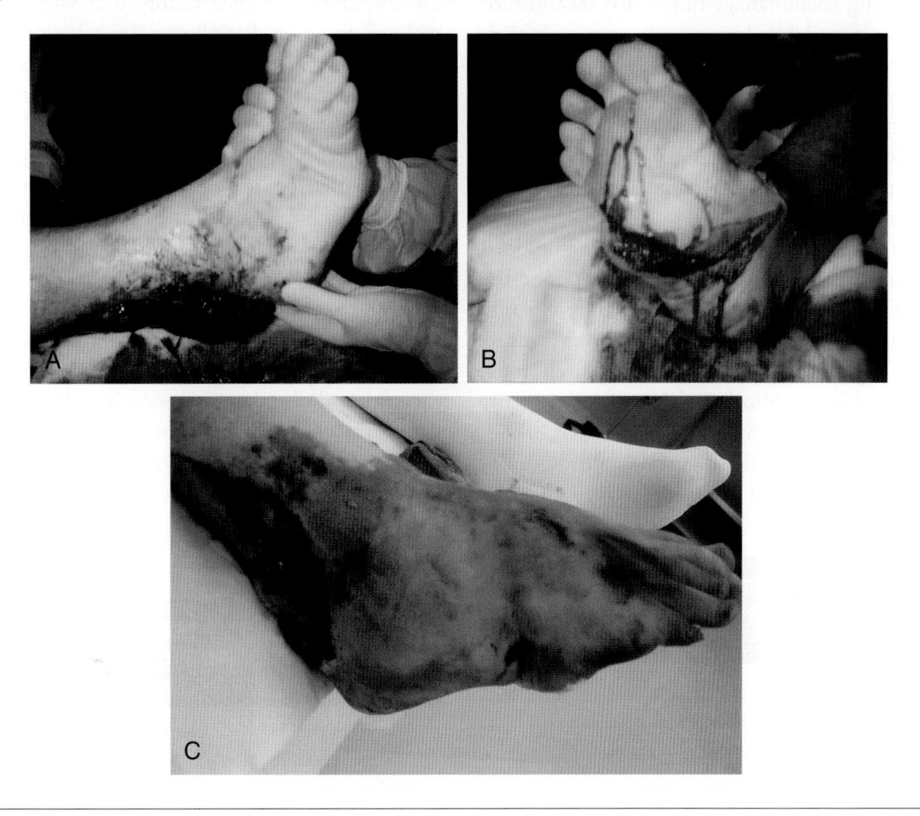

Courtesy of Celine Hill.

site should be cleaned with sterile saline and a moist saline dressing applied. Cooling the part slows metabolism, thus making it more resistant to ischaemia. It is extremely helpful for staff and patient in the postoperative phase if a photograph of the wound is placed in the medical record, as often the patient will have a better understanding of the operative management if they can visualise the extent of their injury.

The emergency nurse and medical officer should clearly document the time and type of amputation, level of amputation, completeness, warm and cold ischaemic time, amount of blood loss, sensation to the stump, previous injuries to the amputated limb and whether (part of) the dominant hand was amputated. Also document injuries to the same extremity at other levels (e.g. avulsion amputation of the humeral shaft can cause a shearing/tearing force on the brachial plexus, resulting in complete or incomplete loss of function and sensation of the arm) and degree of crush and contamination.

There is a high risk of infection due to contamination, and broad-spectrum antibiotics should be administered early. Administration of tetanus prophylaxis is required if the immunisation history is not up to date or is unknown. Re-implantation of amputated parts is based on the initial assessment, as stated above. Severely crushed tissue or devascularised tissue is not amenable to re-implantation. Soft tissue is very susceptible to ischaemia, so accurate time of warm ischaemia (without cooling) and cold ischaemia (with cooling) should be clearly documented.[54]

PRACTICE TIP

For amputated parts, clean gently, place in a sealed plastic bag and then in iced water or cold water. Never place them directly on ice as this destroys potentially viable tissue.

THE MANGLED LIMB

Management of severe lower limb injuries represents enormous challenges for clinicians. A mangled limb describes the most severe cases, where there are partially destroyed blood vessels, tissue, nerves, muscle and bone.[55] The definitive objective of reconstruction of a mangled lower extremity is salvaging a viable and functional limb, with the alternative of amputation. Patients who undergo salvage will endure more-complicated operations, have a longer length of stay and may suffer more complications than primary amputees. Sometimes these complications can be so significant and critical that secondary amputation is required.

Emergency management of the mangled limb is similar to that of open fractures. Immobilise the limb, administer pain relief, and ensure wounds are covered with a sterile, saline-soaked dressing, and in the ED administer antibiotics, tetanus inoculation and further pain relief. The use of tourniquets can be used to provide rapid haemorrhage control until operative control can be achieved.[56] For wounds that are unsuitable for tourniquet use, such as the groin or axilla, where tourniquet placement would be difficult to obtain or difficult to maintain pressure, consider a commercially available haemostatic dressing to control life-threatening haemorrhage in the first instance, or a junctional tourniquet if available. In some instances, a tourniquet, haemostatic dressing and application of direct pressure on the wound may be required to control life-threatening haemorrhage. Following damage control resuscitation, ongoing care will require orthopaedic, plastics and vascular surgical involvement and therefore patients with a mangled limb should be transferred to a tertiary facility.

A number of predictive scoring systems have been developed to assist in the decision of whether to salvage or amputate the mangled extremity. These are: the Mangled Extremity Severity Score (MESS); Predictive Salvage Index (PSI); Hannover Fracture Scale (HFS); Limb Salvage Index (LSI); Nerve injury, Ischaemia, Soft-tissue injury, Skeletal injury, Shock and Age of patient score (NISSSA); and Mangled Extremity Syndrome Index (MESI).

The MESS is the most commonly used today, although not as a sole predictor of management (Table 48.8).

These scoring systems lack sensitivity and specificity, they have limited clinical utility and should not be used as a sole criterion for amputation. Other factors that will help in the decision-making are multidisciplinary consultation, age-related factors, comorbidities, mechanism of injury, fracture pattern, soft-tissue injury, vascular injury, neurological injury, contamination, infection, haemorrhage and hypothermia.[57] The experience and judgement of a senior surgeon, patient consultation and the aforementioned factors will determine treatment choice. Treatment of the mangled limb is performed as a staged procedure and consists of seven stages described in Table 48.9.[55]

PELVIC FRACTURE

The pelvis is made up of two innominate bones and the sacrum, which in combination form a ring. The ring is held together by the strong iliolumbar and sacroiliac ligaments posteriorly and the weak symphysis joint anteriorly. The pelvis is rigid; therefore, a fracture in one point of the ring must be accompanied by a disruption at a second point, unless a direct blow causes an isolated fracture, for example, an acetabular floor fracture.[5]

TABLE 48.8 MANGLED EXTREMITY SEVERITY SCORE (MESS) SYSTEM[56]

CHARACTERISTIC	SCORE
A. Skeletal and soft-tissue injury	
Low energy (stabs, simple fracture, pistol, low-energy GSW)	1
Medium energy (open or multiple fractures, dislocations)	2
High energy (close range shotgun, high-energy GSW, crush injury)	3
Very high energy (gross contamination, tissue avulsion)	4
B. Limb ischaemia	
Pulse reduced or absent, perfusion normal	1*
Pulseless, paraesthesias, diminished capillary refill	2*
Cool, paralysed, insensate, numb	3*
C. Shock	
Systolic blood pressure always above 90 mmHg	0
Transient hypotension	1
Persistent hypotension	2
D. Age (years)	
0–30	0
30–50	1
50+	2
Result	
Score < 7 = salvageable extremity	
Score > 7 = non-salvageable extremity	

GSW: gunshot wound.
**Double score for ischaemia > 6 hours duration*

TABLE 48.9 MANAGEMENT OF THE MANGLED LIMB[55]

TREATMENT	DESCRIPTION
Irrigation and radical debridement	Gravity irrigation, debridement of devitalised tissue and vessels, antibiotic administration, tetanus inoculation, and bacterial wound culture swabs. Fasciotomy performed if indicated at this stage. Repeated debridements with 2nd and 3rd looks are often required (e.g. 24 and 48 hrs).
Skeletal stabilisation	Initially external fixation devices for anatomical alignment, converted to open fixation with rods or plates for definitive stabilisation.
Stabilisation and reduction of intra-articular fractures	Intra-articular fractures reduced and anatomically stabilised to allow joint mobility. Joint replacement or fusion of joints may be required in some complex cases.
Vascular reconstruction	Damaged arteries and veins are reconstructed using vein grafts
Tendon repair and tendomuscular reconstruction	Early primary tendon reconstruction ideal where possible. Tendon transfers can be performed at later stage.
Nerve reconstruction	Nerve exploration and repair (when possible) at initial stages of surgery. Better outcomes when performed early. Meticulous surgical techniques required, with non-surgical patient factors also affecting outcome. End-to-end epineural repair or primary nerve transfer.
Wound coverage	Timing and type of wound closure controversial. Negative wound pressure (e.g. VAC dressing) for less than 7 days. Closure with pedicle or free-flap muscle coverage.

Significant force is required to fracture a pelvis in young patients. Principal mechanisms of injury due to high-energy events include fall from height, road traffic collision (motorcycle, road cyclist, motor vehicle, pedestrian) or being pinned by a heavy force such as a vehicle.[58] Due to such high energies, the patients are often haemodynamically unstable and have concomitant injuries, such as urethral, bladder, vaginal and/or rectal injuries, torn iliac vessels and neurological deficits.[41] Other injuries which are potentially prone to haemorrhage due to high-energy trauma are the thorax and abdomen. Pelvic fractures can vary in severity. Mortality in the initial 24 hours post-injury is likely from an inability to control haemorrage.[59] Mortality in open pelvic fractures is three times that of closed fractures.[59] Pelvic fractures can be related to significant haemorrhage from iliac arterial branches, presacral venous plexus and cancellous bone. There are no rapid radiological studies that can swiftly confirm haemorrhage associated with disruption to the pelvic ring.[52,60] Early management decisions are based mainly on clinical condition and haemodynamic stability, rather than diagnostic pelvic ring classifications.

The patient can present with leg length discrepancy, groin, perineal, suprapubic and flank bruising.[61]

CLASSIFICATION

There are many pelvic fracture classifications in the literature. Tile classification is based on the integrity of the sacroiliac ligaments (Fig. 48.11). The most common one used is the Young–Burgess classification (Fig. 48.12). This is a system based on mechanism of injury.

- *Lateral compression (LC)*: graded from 1 (stable) to 3 (completely unstable)—caused by a blow/compression to the side of the pelvis, causing the ring to buckle and break. In road crashes or falls from a height, it is a side-on impact. On the side of the impact, the pelvis is rotated inwards. Posteriorly, there is significant sacroiliac strain, or a fracture of the ilium or sacrum. Anteriorly, the pubic rami can be fractured on one side, or both. Instability is due to considerable displacement of the sacroiliac joint. Treatment may include protected weight-bearing and early mobilisation for minor injuries. Major injuries may require open reduction and internal fixation, or bed rest for 6–8 weeks.[5,41,60,63]
- *Anterior posterior compression (APC):* graded from 1 (stable) to 3 (completely unstable)—caused by frontal impact to the pelvis. The innominate bones and symphysis pubis are sprung open and the sacroiliac ligaments are torn or the posterior part of the ilium is fractured. Separation of the symphysis pubis is stable when it is less than 2 cm, and unstable when it is greater than 2 cm separation. This disruption is often referred to as an 'open-book' pelvic injury. This injury can cause catastrophic haemorrhage from torn iliac vessels.[5,41,60,63]
- *Vertical shear*: caused typically by falls from a height with force being distributed upwards through the femur/s. One side of the pelvic ring, the hemipelvis, is sheared/displaced vertically, resulting in fractures to the pubic rami and disruption of the sacroiliac joint on the same side. The shearing injury can cause neurological injury and sacral plexus damage. Stabilisation of the pelvis is achieved by reduction of the hemipelvis. This may be achieved in the first instance with skeletal traction followed by external or internal fixation.[5,60,63]
- *Combined*: a combination of mechanisms may produce fracture patterns that do not fit the other categories. These injuries are a combination of ligamentous injuries and forces and are usually completely unstable.[5,60,63]

TREATMENT

Not all pelvic fractures are unstable, but for the purposes of this section treatment of unstable injuries will be addressed.

Initial management should follow the CABCs of trauma management. Attention is then given to stabilisation of the pelvis, initially by using a commercially available pelvic binder (or sheet in resource-poor environment) to achieve this rapidly at the scene or in the ED.

The theory behind the use of pelvic binders (see section above p. 1327), sheets and external fixation is to reduce the pelvic volume, which in turn reduces the potential space for bleeding, which may aid in the formation of blood clots. Aligning fracture surfaces may reduce bleeding from bones. Some patients may be suitable for early angiographic embolisation based on their injury pattern and clinical condition, or alternatively pre-peritoneal packing is indicated if this cannot be achieved due to time pressure, instability or requirement for other emergent operative interventions. External fixation should be considered early to allow for rapid restoration of pelvic and haemodynamic stability (Fig. 48.13).[60]

Care should be taken when log-rolling unstable pelvic fractures, particularly vertical shear fractures, as these fractures are vertically unstable and can continue to shift upwards when rolled. If not done correctly, log-rolling may cause clot dislodgement and further damage to muscle, vessels and other structures due to bone fragments shifting and causing a shearing/tearing force. In the unstable patient, turning the patient to facilitate pelvic splinting and scoop placement for packaging should be limited to 10–15 degrees.

Pelvic springing is controversial and not recommended. In addition to causing unnecessary pain to the patient, springing can dislodge clots that have tamponaded haemorrhage and cause further damage to muscle, vessels and other structures by bone fragments via a tearing/shearing force. An AP pelvic x-ray will almost always be attended to and will identify pelvic injuries without the need for pelvic springing. When reviewing an AP pelvic x-ray with a binder in place, consideration needs to be given to the masking of pelvic ring disruption due to the compression nature of the pelvic binder. On occasion, and in the presence of senior medical staff, binders may be loosened for x-ray if haemodynamics allow.

As discussed, pelvic fractures (namely APC 3, LC3 and Combined) have the potential for torrential haemorrhage. These cases will benefit from early angiographic embolisation, bearing in mind that angiography has its own morbidity and mortality risks.[63]

Emergency management includes frequent monitoring of haemodynamic status—patients can rapidly exsanguinate—and neurovascular status of both lower limbs. The emergency clinician should anticipate the need for blood transfusion and fluid resuscitation and ensure that a supply of blood and warm haemostatic products are available, and be prepared to urgently transfer the patient to definitive care.[63,65]

FIGURE 48.11 TILE CLASSIFICATION OF PELVIC FRACTURES.[62]

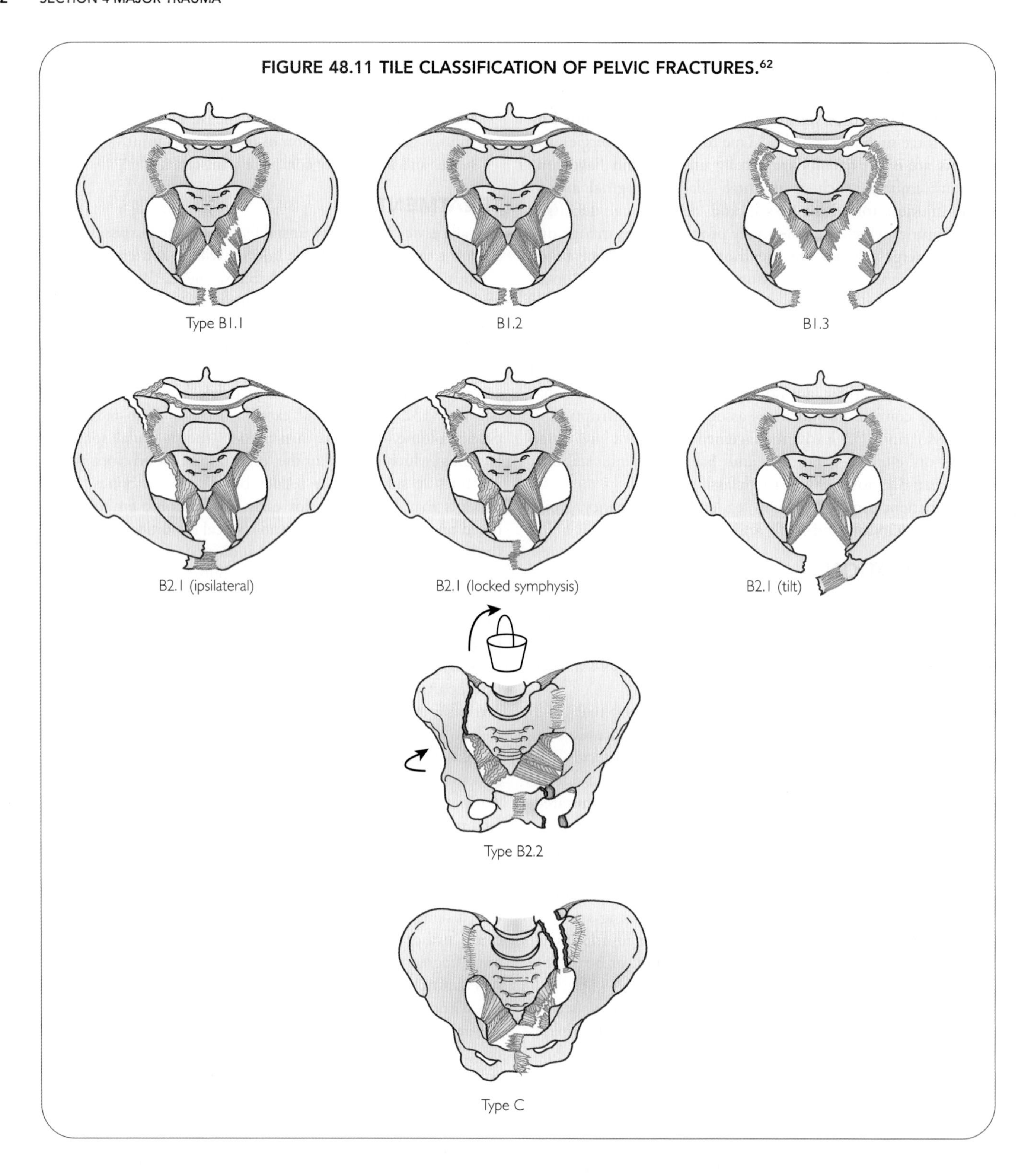

Damage to other structures, such as the rectum, vagina, urethra and bladder, can occur at the time of injury either due to the pelvic fracture, which may indicate an open fracture, or due to direct trauma. A rectal and/or vaginal examination must be performed if there is bleeding or suspicion of injury. Rectal and vaginal bleeding is indicative of tears to the walls of these structures. A rectal examination not only evaluates the rectum but also the urogenital tract, assessing for a high-riding prostate, which can indicate urethral disruption; although this is an unreliable finding in younger men. Blood at the urinary meatus is present in 37–93% of patients with urethral injuries, and this precludes urethral catheterisation until the urethra is adequately imaged. Additionally, pain on urination or inability to void with or without haematuria, or a palpable bladder suggests urethral trauma. If cystoscopy performed by a urologist for primary realignment over catheter fails initially, a suprapubic catheter is required and, depending on extent of urethral damage, various urological surgical options are available to repair the urethra.[66] Injuries to these systems have a high susceptibility to devastating infections, so early diagnosis and treatment is paramount.[63]

FIGURE 48.12 YOUNG AND BURGESS CLASSIFICATION OF PELVIC FRACTURES[62]

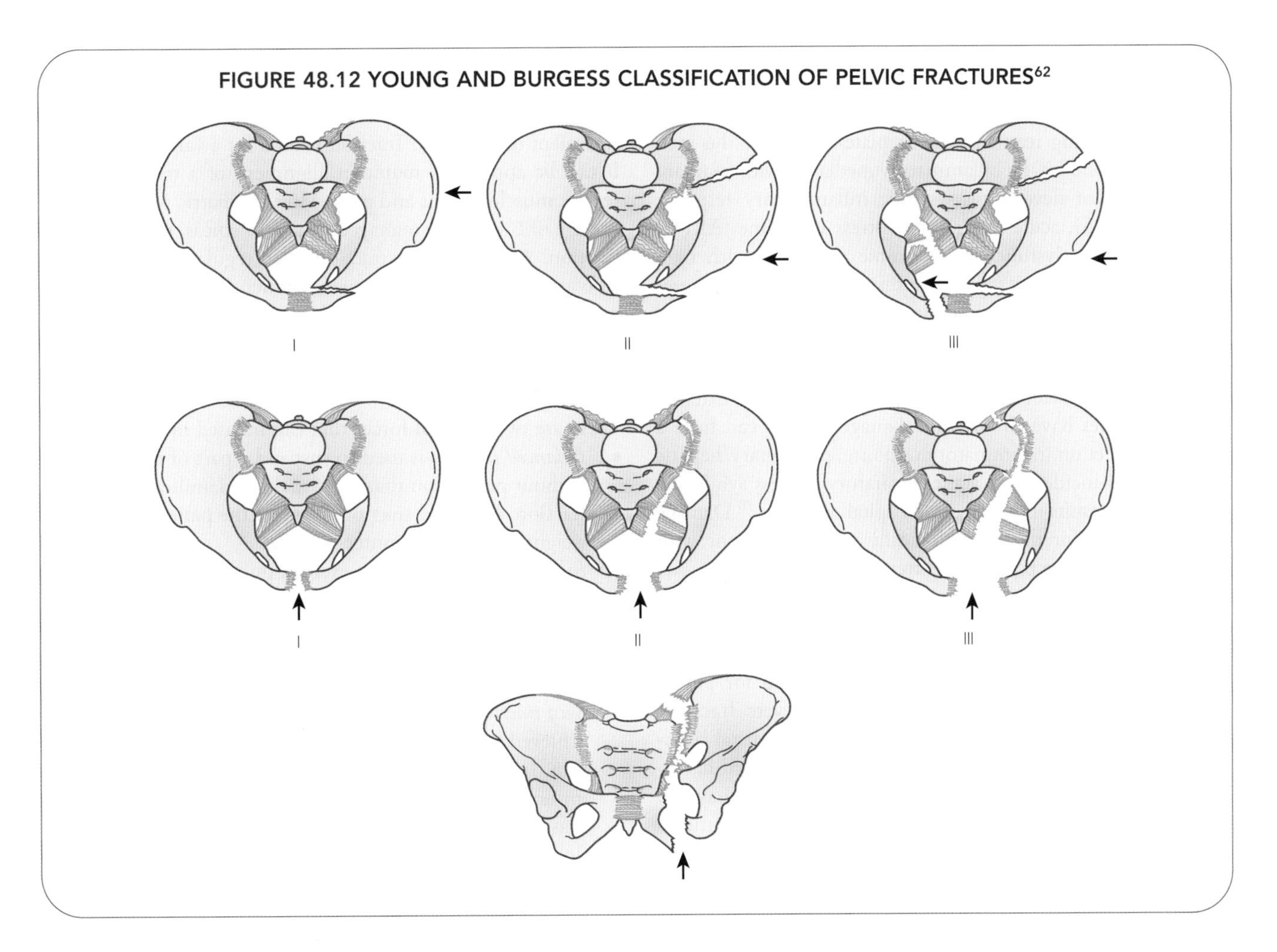

FIGURE 48.13 EXTERNAL FIXATOR: PELVIS[64]

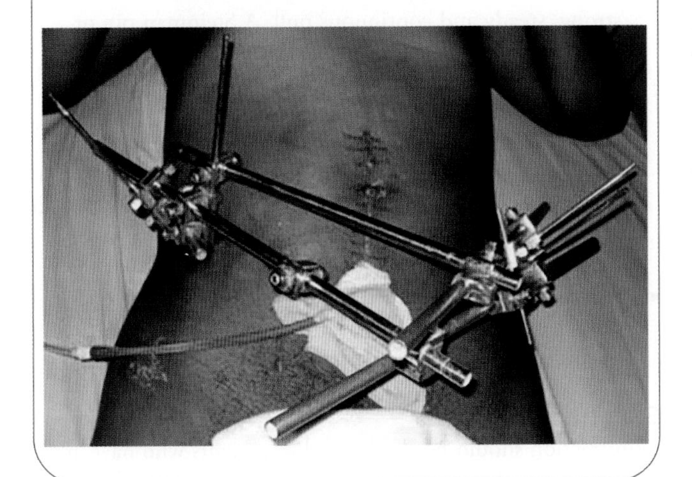

Neurological injury in pelvic fractures has been seen in up to 10–20% of patients.[66] The fracture pattern will determine the nature and risk of neurologic injury based on anatomical location of fracture fragments. Lumbosacral plexus or sciatic nerve damage can occur when there is a fracture of the sacrum or displacement of the sacroiliac joint. The sciatic nerve is responsible for dorsiflexion of the foot. Neurologic injuries can occur early or late and it is important they are not overlooked in the busy clinical setting. Bladder, bowel and sexual dysfunction are potentially devastating neurological consequences, and can be permanent.[67] Pelvic fractures, whether stable or unstable, require ongoing assessment and observation such as neurovascular observations, which should continue for days after the injury, daily blood tests (FBC, EUC), and review, as required, by orthopaedics, with any anomaly, however small, escalated and reviewed. Between 7% and 14% of stable pelvic fractures with retroperitoneal haemorrhage will require embolisation for haemostasis. Therefore, even if the patient's injury is classified as stable, pre-hospital and emergency staff need to remain vigilant for signs of haemodynamic instability.[68]

PRACTICE TIP

Pelvic springing is not recommended nor a reliable method of determining if the pelvic ring is intact. In cases where there is significant pelvic injury, springing the pelvis can cause significant pain and potentially worsen any underlying haemorrhage.

DAMAGE CONTROL ORTHOPAEDICS

Damage control orthopaedics are urgent techniques, such as external fixation, which are minimally invasive. Damage control focuses on controlling haemorrhage, managing soft-tissue injuries and provisional skeletal stabilisation, so that the overall condition of the patient is optimised. Damage control avoids additional insult to the patient. Performing major orthopaedic procedures in the initial stages of the unstable patient's surgical management, using reamed nails or plates, increases the incidence of a 'second hit' by inflammatory mediators with resultant increased risk of developing systemic inflammatory response syndrome (SIRS), acute respiratory distress syndrome (ARDS) and multi-organ dysfunction syndrome (MODs), with high morbidity and mortality.[69,70] Early surgical intervention increases blood loss, necessitating resuscitation and along with the 'second hit', may promote the 'diamond of death'—hypothermia, coagulopathy, hypocalcaemia and acidosis. The damage control concept promotes rapid skeletal stabilisation, generally with external fixation. Studies have shown that damage control can have a protective effect on inflammatory response, pulmonary/hepatic function, and incidence of acute respiratory distress syndrome (ARDS), and results in reduced in-hospital mortality.[70] Damage control is ideal for the physiologically unstable patient with severe injuries or the patient in extremis.[53]

ANGIOGRAPHY

Angiography can determine location of arterial occlusion or disruption. Angiographic embolisation is required for persistent haemorrhage from pelvic fractures and severe fracture/dislocations near the knee joint with compromised distal circulation. Pelvic fractures can be correlated with significant haemorrhage, largely from pelvic vasculature. Haemorrhage may also originate from abdominal visceral injury. Mortality in patients with haemorrhagic shock and unstable pelvic fracture pattern is higher than 52%; therefore, consideration should be given to angiography before laparotomy. Some facilities have the ability to perform 'on-table' interventional angiography in an operating suite. Fundamentally, early effective coordination between general surgeons, orthopaedic surgeons and the ED in prioritising definitive management is essential to prevent delay in diagnosis and haemostasis, as haemorrhage from unstable pelvic injuries is directly responsible for permanent disability for survivors or death from exsanguination.[71]

CLINICAL INTERVENTIONS

Any obvious or suspected musculoskeletal injury should be properly immobilised, and, if applicable, sterile, saline-soaked dressings applied to open wounds. Any immobilised areas should remain splinted (see Splints, p. 1326) to prevent further injury. Whenever turning or rolling the patient, one person should assume responsibility for maintaining alignment and immobilisation of the limb.[5,6]

Care should therefore be taken when applying plaster casts, bandages and traction over bony prominences, such as the head of the fibula, as compression of the common peroneal nerve can occur, leading to foot drop. With pressure on the radial nerve from humeral fractures or axillary crutches, wrist drop can occur.

PRACTICE TIP

Never elevate an injured limb above the level of the heart, as this will impede venous return and potentially lead to increased risk of compartment syndrome.

Traction

Overall, the use of traction—a pulling force on a part of the body—has been reduced due to the advances in orthopaedic treatment of fractures. Traction is used for a variety of reasons. It can be applied to maintain alignment of a fracture and to reduce muscle spasms and pain. Most paediatric patients under the age of 6 years are managed in plaster spicas, plaster casts or traction. All patients in traction need regular analgesia, pressure-area care, hydration, bowel regimen, deep venous thrombosis (DVT) prophylaxis and adequate documentation of fluid balance.[72]

Forces used in traction

There are two types of forces that can be used in traction:

- *Balanced traction* is used to suspend a part of the body without pulling on that part, such as Hamilton Russell traction. Balanced traction relies on the patient's bodyweight to provide counter-traction.[73]
- *Inline or running traction* exerts a pull on the axis of the long bone in one plane, such as Buck's skin traction.

Classifications of traction

There are three classifications of traction:

- *Skin traction*, being the most common type of traction, is achieved by the direct application of a pulling force on the skin. It is generally only a temporary measure to maintain immobilisation prior to surgery, and to reduce muscle spasm and therefore pain. Complications from skin traction are blisters, necrosis and compartment syndrome. Generally no more than 2.3–3.6 kg of weight should be applied to skin traction. Hamilton Russell traction has a 'block and tackle' effect; in other words, 2.3 kg of weight is applied, but the resultant traction pull is 4.5 kg.[74]
- *Skeletal traction* is applied directly to the bone and is a strong, steady and continuous pull. A Steinman pin or Kirschner wire (K-wire) is passed through the bone distal to the fracture (Fig. 48.14). It is useful in comminuted and complex fractures, as more weight can be applied in skeletal traction—4.5 kg or more. Skeletal traction can be the definitive treatment or can precede internal fixation. It is particularly useful in stabilising fractures in patients who are in extremis and too unstable to endure a lengthy orthopaedic procedure.[17]
- *Manual traction* is applied temporarily by the hands to immobilise an injured limb. Manual traction can be used during application of a plaster of Paris (POP) cast.[13]

Skin traction

Skin traction should not be applied to patients who have allergies to tape or have obvious circulatory or vascular disorders, such as varicose veins or ulcers. There is a variety of adhesive or non-adhesive skin traction kits on the market that come prepacked with skin strips, bandage and rope.

Application of the skin strips begins proximal to the malleolus, leaving the foot free for ROM exercises, and should end distal to the head of the fibula. These are areas of risk due to the common peroneal nerve being in close proximity (Fig. 48.15). Pressure on this nerve can produce foot drop. Leaving the foot free of bandaging also allows the nurse to assess the neurovascular status regularly. A bandage is provided in the kits and

FIGURE 48.14 K-WIRE

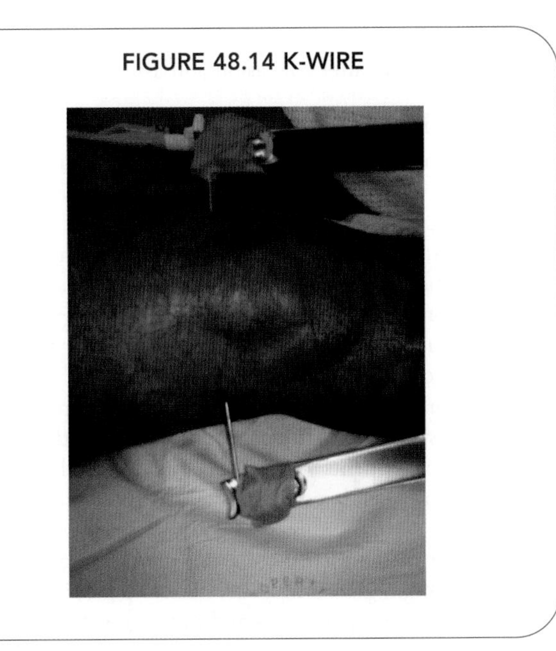

The K-wire is passed through the tibia to project equally medially and laterally. Points are protected with covers. *Courtesy of Celine Hill.*

FIGURE 48.15 COMMON, SUPERFICIAL AND DEEP PERONEAL NERVES[61]

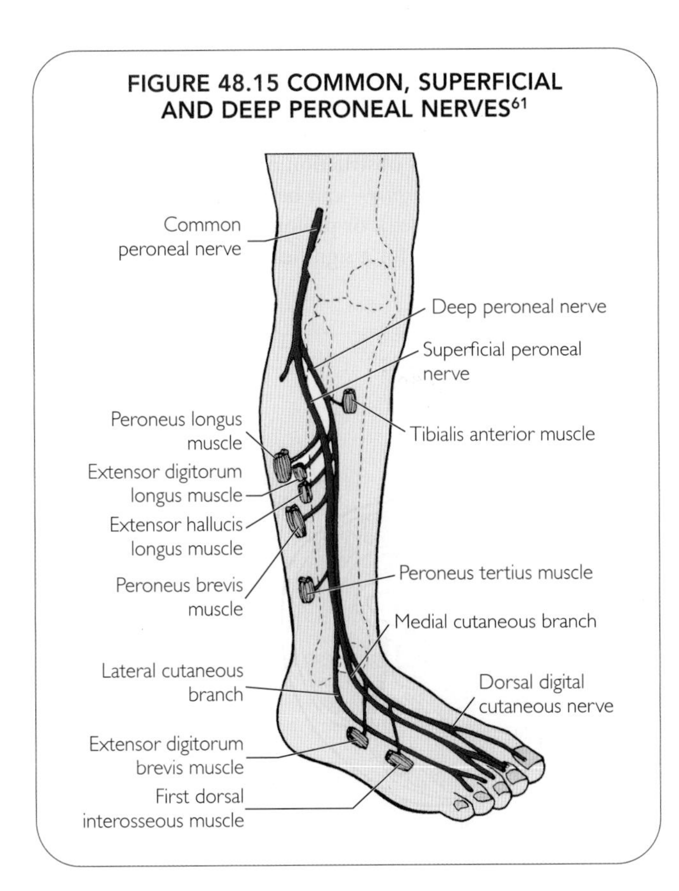

should be applied firmly and in one direction with no twists or creases (Fig. 48.16).

The rope is threaded through the pulley and the weight bag is applied. Neurovascular observations must be attended pre-application and at least hourly post-application.[75] Analgesia

FIGURE 48.16 SKIN TRACTION TO LOWER LEG

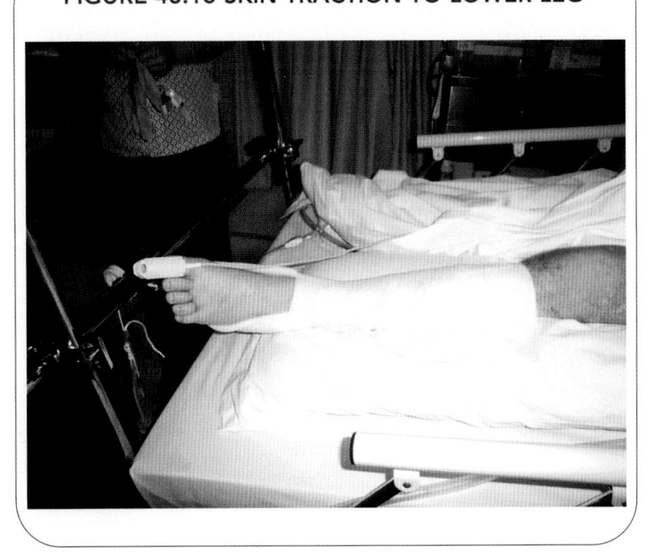

Courtesy of Celine Hill.

prior to traction application is essential. The use of opioids or femoral nerve blocks may assist in pain control.

PRACTICE TIP

Do not apply skin traction strips or bandage above the head of the fibula. This will cause compression of the common peroneal nerve which can potentially lead to foot drop.

Skeletal traction

Skeletal traction can be used for pelvic and femoral fractures. The rationale for traction is to reduce fractures, keep the limb out to length, for pain relief and to decrease haemorrhage. The type of pin used currently is Kirschner wire (K-wire). The k-wire is easily inserted while the patient is still in the ED. The K-wire should only be inserted by personnel who are trained to do so. Appropriate procedural sedation should be considered for the patient, as well as local anaesthetic to the periosteum. The K-wire is inserted from medial to lateral (to prevent vascular injury). Bend the wire at each end to capture the tensioning device. The K-wire is placed depending on the location of the fracture. Skeletal traction allows substantial weight to be applied directly to the bone.[73,76]

A simple traction set-up will consist of a rope attached to the tensioning device, passing through a pulley at the end of the bed, which is then attached to a hanging weight. The leg should be supported with pillows to reduce deformity and elevate the heel off the bed; 7–11 kg is generally enough to overcome muscle tension, restoring the femoral to length and reducing muscle spasm (Fig. 48.17).[76]

Pin-site care is often debated. A 2013 Cochrane review found no evidence for the best technique for pin-site care to minimise complications and infections.[77]

Complications

It is important to understand the complications associated with traction. Traction can cause inadequate alignment of fracture, neurovascular compromise, soft-tissue injury and skin

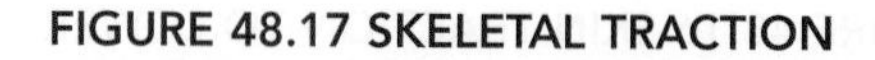
FIGURE 48.17 SKELETAL TRACTION

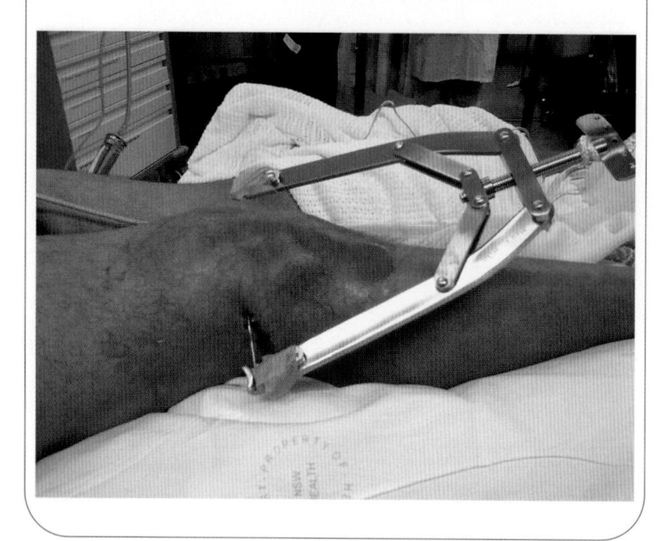

Courtesy of Celine Hill.

breakdown. Prevention of these problems includes neurovascular observations, regular pressure-area care and maintenance of traction. The application of traction requires a medical order. The order must include type of traction, weight to be applied and whether the traction can be removed for tests, such as CT or MRI.[13]

It is important that nurses are instructed by an experienced clinician on application of traction and the essential components of safety of application, assessment and monitoring. The advanced practice emergency nurse should be able to apply skin traction in the ED after education and assessment.

COMPARTMENT SYNDROME

Compartments are classified as closed spaces containing nerves, muscles and vascular structures that are enclosed within bone or fascia (Fig. 48.18).

Compartment syndrome is a complication that can occur with any patient who sustains a sprain or fracture, or as a complication from surgery. Compartment syndrome is defined as an increase in pressure within a restricted space. There are 46 anatomical compartments in the body, with 36 of these located in the extremities. In the extremities, muscle groups are covered by fascial tissue; fascia is tough and inelastic. In the lower leg, the four compartments most frequently involved in this syndrome are the lateral, posterior, deep posterior and anterior. The forearm contains three compartments: the dorsal, volar and mobile wad. Compartment syndrome can also occur in the upper arm, thigh, gluteal muscles, lumbar paraspinal, shoulder and extraocular compartments and in the foot.[4,79]

Aetiology

There are three categories of aetiology:

- *Decreased compartment size*—can be due to restrictive splints, casts or dressings, traction or early closure of fascia.[10,71]
- *Increased compartment content*—can be due to bleeding caused by a fracture, or vascular injury. Other aetiologies may include burns, overuse of muscles, envenomation, coagulopathy, venous obstruction or 'tissued' IV site.[71]
- *Externally applied pressure*—can be due to tight dressings (as previously discussed), or prolonged compression from lying in one position for a significant length of time.[71]

FIGURE 48.18 FASCIOTOMY OF THE THIGH[78]

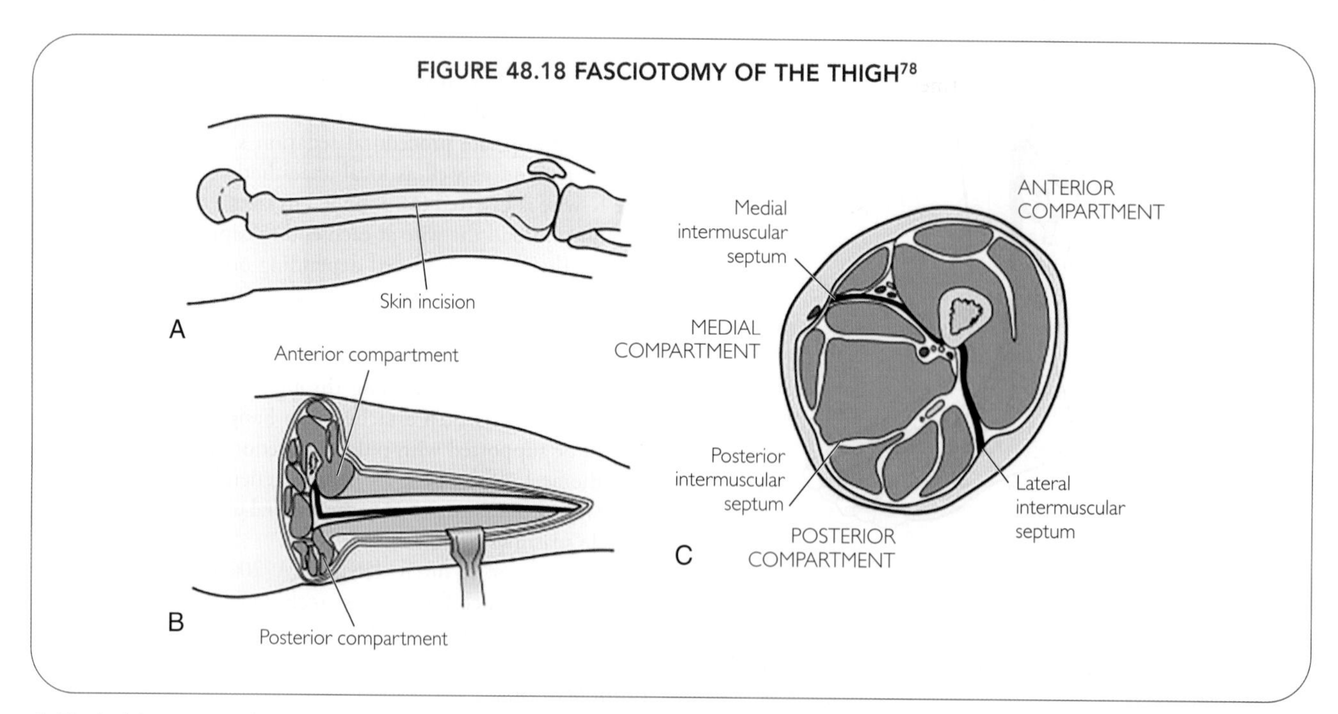

A. The incision extends from the intertrochanteric line to the lateral epicondyle. **B.** The anterior compartment is opened by incising the fascia lata. The vastus lateralis is retracted medially to expose the lateral intermuscular septum, which is incised to decompress the posterior compartment. **C.** Thigh compartments and appropriate incision.

Types

There are three types of compartment syndrome: acute, chronic and crush syndrome. For this section, we will only look at acute compartment syndrome.

Pathophysiology

Acute compartment syndrome (ACS) is the rise in interstitial pressure within the closed fascial compartment. This will result in microvascular compromise, neural dysfunction and tissue hypoxia. Local swelling and bleeding results in compressive damage to muscle groups. Due to the inelasticity of fascial compartments, swelling occurs inwards, causing compression and collapse of nerves, muscle cells and blood vessels. If hypoxia continues due to decreased circulation to muscle, the cells will become necrotic. The compartment affected may be distal to the injury, resulting in reduced blood flow, which, in turn, causes the capillaries to lose integrity. Oedema is exacerbated by colloid proteins escaping into soft tissue, pulling fluid with them.[71]

Elevated compartmental pressure is the most significant issue. As the pressure increases within the compartment, vessels begin to collapse as the soft-tissue pressure is greater than the intravascular pressure. Intracompartmental pressures of 30–40 mmHg are high enough to compromise muscle microcirculation. The decrease in blood outflow is directly linked to the collapse of venous structures, which eventually leads to obstructed outflow. If the pressure continues to increase, blood supply can be cut off, and the muscle will become necrotic. In the forearm, a pressure of 65 mmHg, and in the calf, one of 55 mmHg, can completely stop blood circulation in tissue in a normovolaemic patient. Normal compartment pressure is 8 mmHg or less. Total cessation of blood flow to the affected extremity is due to the imbalance in pressures between the outflow of venous blood and the inflow of arterial blood. Decreased capillary blood flow, due to tissue-fluid pressure and prolonged periods of microcirculatory ischaemia, will result in irreversible necrosis of intracompartmental tissues, which include nerve tissue and muscle.[79]

Signs and symptoms

The symptoms of increased compartment pressure are described in Box 48.2.

BOX 48.2 SIGNS OF INCREASED COMPARTMENT PRESSURE AND COMPARTMENT SYNDROME[8,80,81]

- *Pain*—a critical early sign. The patient may complain of diffuse pain not relieved by analgesia. Pain may be greater during passive motion, and may be out of proportion to the injury. Patients may describe the pain as throbbing, deep or burning: this is due to the ischaemic process of the syndrome.
- *Paraesthesia*—a subtle early sign. Patient may complain of tingling or burning as nerves are very sensitive to pressure. This can lead to numbness.
- *Pallor*—a late sign. Caused by pressure on the artery, it is a late and ominous sign. Skin may look pale, greyish or white. Patients will have a delayed capillary refill of greater than 3 seconds. Skin will feel cool to touch due to decreased capillary perfusion.
- *Paralysis*—a late symptom. Can be caused by either irreversible muscle damage or prolonged nerve compression.
- *Pulselessness*—a very late and ominous sign. The patient may have a very weak pulse or no palpable pulse. This is due to deficient arterial perfusion. This is an indication of tissue death. The pulse will be present until the very late stages.

Management

The emergency clinician can contribute to prevention of ACS by elevating the limb early and observing closely for early signs of swelling and increasing pain. Elevation above the level of the heart can actually impede venous return and further increase the risk. The emergency clinician must ensure that dressings are applied firmly but are not too tight. Consistent and regular neurovascular assessments are essential. There are a number of pressure monitors on the market that can be used to measure intracompartmental pressures. If the patient is unconscious or unresponsive, continuous monitoring can be used.[80]

If clinical signs and symptoms of compartment syndrome are present, the most important management is to relieve the pressure. This may begin with loosening casts or dressings or proceeding to the operating suite for a fasciotomy to decompress the compartment and halt the ischaemia cycle. Fasciotomies must be done early: within 6 hours and no later than 12 hours from onset of symptoms. Controversy exists regarding what upper pressure limits mandate a fasciotomy. Several protocols recommend compartment pressures of 30 mmHg or more as the determining level for mandatory fasciotomy.[79,82] If increased compartment pressure is suspected, the limb should not continue to be elevated as it further decreases venous flow. Post-fasciotomy the patient may have a vacuum-assisted wound-closure device, or return to the operating suite approximately every 2–3 days for dressing change and potentially further debridement until the wound is able to be surgically closed. If the fasciotomy is not able to be surgically closed, a split-skin graft (SSG) may be required.

PRACTICE TIP

If compartment syndrome is suspected, do not elevate the limb, as this will greatly reduce venous return in an already compromised limb.

PRACTICE TIP

If compartment syndrome is suspected the clinician should not delay escalation. ISBAR should be used when raising clinician concern with specific mention of the suspicion of compartment syndrome and/or threatened limb.

INFECTION

All patients are at risk of infection when there is a break in the skin. When a fracture is associated with skin trauma, a high risk of infection is possible and may lead to osteomyelitis.

This infection is most often attributed to *Staphylococcus aureus*. The emergency nurse's role in infection prevention is to try to prevent the onset. This includes ensuring aseptic technique is used in wound management, administering prophylactic antibiotics and determining requirements for tetanus prophylaxis.[83]

Osteomyelitis is a bone infection involving the bone marrow. Bacteria can invade via the blood; via direct introduction, such as in open fractures or penetrating wounds; or during surgery. Treatment includes antibiotic therapy, surgical debridement, irrigation and/or drainage.[5,83]

Necrotising fasciitis is an uncommon and rapidly accelerating infectious process. It primarily involves the fascia and subcutaneous tissue. It is a severe infection with toxin-secreting bacteria which leads to life-threatening soft-tissue destruction and necrosis. There are a variety of terms used to describe this condition: haemolytic streptococcal gangrene, Fournier gangrene and gas gangrene. Anaerobic bacteria in combination with Gram-negative organisms are most commonly found in necrotising fasciitis. They propagate in an environment of tissue hypoxia. Treatment should include administration of antibiotics, fluid replacement, thorough surgical debridement of necrotic fascia and decompression of compartments. Hyperbaric oxygen has been used to reduce the spread of gangrene, but its use remains controversial due to lack of level one data. The patient may rapidly decline due to toxaemia, which, if left untreated, causes coma and death. Necrotising fasciitis has a mortality rate of 15–50%.[5,84]

PRESSURE INJURIES

Patients with complex orthopaedic and/or neurovascular injuries are at risk of pressure injuries in both the acute and subacute phase of hospitalisation. Specifically, such patients may have splints, traction, fixation or post-operative movement restrictions that limit nursing staff attending to pressure-area care. See Chapter 13.

FAT EMBOLISM SYNDROME

Fat embolism syndrome (FES) results from long-bone fractures, intramedullary manipulation and blunt trauma. Classically, fractures can cause the release of lipid particles (fat emboli) from the bone marrow of fractured long bones, entering the venous circulation and lodging in vital organs.[6] It is a potentially serious, life-threatening complication. Fat embolism can produce embolic phenomena from fat within the circulation. FES has identifiable clinical signs and symptoms associated with fat in the circulation; it can also occur with massive soft-tissue injuries, especially adipose tissue, severe burns, severe infections and blunt trauma to fatty organs, particularly fatty livers,[79] culminating in embolisation of fat in the pulmonary and systemic systems, causing right ventricular failure and cardiovascular collapse.[6]

FES has been the subject of conjecture and controversy, as the syndrome is a series of signs and symptoms which can be common in other critical illnesses. FES is often diagnosed by excluding other injuries or illnesses.[85]

Signs of FES and recommended laboratory investigations for FES diagnosis are listed in Box 48.3. FES can be due to intramedullary reaming during fracture fixation; however, this theory remains controversial. Normal marrow pressure is 30–50 mmHg. During reaming this pressure can increase to up to 600 mmHg. The increase in marrow pressure can cause extravasation of fat emboli from the marrow of bones. The incidence of FES has been reported as 1–19%, while a much higher incidence (several times higher) has been noted in postmortem studies. Mortality can reach up to 10–50% in patients with marked respiratory failure and coma.[86]

BOX 48.3 SIGNS AND LABORATORY DIAGNOSIS FOR FAT EMBOLISM SYNDROME (FES)[6,12,85–87]

SIGNS OF FES MAY INCLUDE:

- petechial rash
- dyspnoea
- cyanosis
- hypoxaemia
- tachypnoea
- loss of consciousness with deepening coma
- fever
- anaemia.

LABORATORY TESTS FOR DIAGNOSIS OF FES

- *Measuring arterial blood gases (ABGs)*. This is an essential procedure that should be done early and frequently during the first 48 hours in all patients with significant bony injury.
- Platelet counts should be obtained daily for several days after injury. Platelet counts less than 150,000 per mL are indicative of thrombocytopenia and diagnostic of FES.
- Urine test for lipuria (the presence of fat in the urine). This test is too sensitive to be of clinical value, because about half of all patients with significant bony injury will have lipuria.
- Fat in the sputum is of no significance in the diagnosis of FES.
- Serum lipase testing is too sensitive to be of any clinical value, as elevation of serum lipase levels occurs in about half of all patients with fractures.
- Fat droplets in the circulating blood. This test is too sensitive to be of clinical value.

PRACTICE TIP

All other critical illnesses should be ruled out before FES is diagnosed.

Pathophysiology

Mechanical theory

Trauma disrupts fat cells in the marrow. With an increase in marrow pressure, fat droplets escape and are transported to the lung circulation and trapped as emboli. Smaller droplets may reach the kidney, brain, retina and skin. The release of fat is directly related to pressure and the duration of externally applied forces.[85–87]

Biochemical theory

Chylomicrons, lipid-containing particles, are released due to haemodynamic changes such as hypotension and various hormones. This mobilises fat stores, resulting in systemic fat droplet formation and deposition in end-organ vasculature. Free fatty acids are also mobilised due to an elevated concentration of catecholamines as a result of trauma. This chemical process results in aggregation of platelets and formation of fat globules, which leads to acute lung injury, pneumonitis and acute respiratory distress syndrome (ARDS).[79]

Signs and symptoms

FES is defined as a triad of hypoxia, petechiae and neurological impairment. Signs and symptoms usually occur between 12 and 60 hours, but can occur within a few hours.[79]

FES signs and symptoms have been divided into major and minor criteria.

Major

- *Petechial rash* can be transient and occurs in 50–60% of patients. The rash is usually distributed over the chest wall, axilla, conjunctiva and mucous membranes. The rash may be due to stasis, endothelial damage from free fatty acids, loss of clotting factors and platelets, all leading to the rupture of thin-walled capillaries.[79]
- *Respiratory and cardiac symptoms with diffuse pulmonary infiltrates on chest x-ray.* The lung responds to FES by secreting lipase, turning the fat into free fatty acid. This results in increased capillary bed permeability, destruction of the alveolar architecture and damage to lung surfactant, which results in immediate and serious impairment of oxygen transfer to haemoglobin (Hb). Hypoxia can be extreme and can result in death. The initial effect of pulmonary microembolism is an increase in perfusion pressure when vessels become engorged, rendering the lung more rigid. The work of breathing increases, which results in the right side of the heart attempting to increase output by dilation, which requires an increase in venous return. An ECG will demonstrate heart strain with prominent S waves, arrhythmias, right bundle branch block and T-wave inversion. The heart is now more susceptible to hypovolaemia with a decrease in central venous return. Death at this point is due to right-sided heart failure.[79]
- *Neurological changes* not explained by other medical conditions or trauma and hypoxaemia. Changes can be in the form of restlessness, irritability, headache, anxiety, disorientation, delirium, convulsions and constriction of pupils.[79]

Minor

- Tachycardia
- Fever $< 38°C$ due to the inflammatory response
- Decreased urine output or fat globules
- Decreasing haematocrit
- Fat globules in the sputum.

Diagnosis

FES is most likely to occur in patients with multiple long-bone fractures, poor fracture splinting, hypovolaemic shock and rough patient movement.

There is a variety of diagnostic tools that can be used in the diagnosis of FES. Transoesophageal echocardiography (TOE) can identify circulating embolic particles. It is argued that this has circumspect clinical significance. The best use of TOE is to identify cardiac defects from FES. Other scans such as MRI, CT, chest x-ray and ventilation–perfusion (V/Q) scan tend to be non-specific and have a decreased specificity to FES.[79] Laboratory tests that may diagnose FES are discussed in Box 48.2.

Treatment

Despite technological advances, the treatment of FES remains predominantly supportive—gentle handling and appropriate splinting of fractures, and the prevention and treatment of hypovolaemic shock. Clinicians must support the respiratory system by immediate administration of high-flow oxygen to all patients with significant fractures. In the patient who is intubated and mechanically ventilated, the clinician's main aim is to maintain reasonable ventilatory parameters. Continuous cardiac monitoring, regular arterial blood gas testing and regular analgesia should be performed. Early fixation of long-bone fractures remains controversial with regard to the type of fixation in the initial stages, i.e. intramedullary nailing versus external fixation. As discussed, early internal fixation may not be advantageous to patients, particularly patients with thoracic trauma.[87]

In summary, the basis of treatment is prevention of hypovolaemic shock, stress response and hypoxia, and then stabilisation of fractures operatively within 24 hours.

DELAYED COMPLICATIONS

Understanding how a fracture heals is essential in knowing how to treat it (Table 48.10). Factors such as immobilisation and/or internal fixation are important issues in facilitating the

TABLE 48.10 DELAYED COMPLICATIONS IN BONE HEALING

DELAYED COMPLICATION	DESCRIPTION[6,88–90]
Delayed union	When the fracture may take a substantial amount of time to heal, 3–12 months May be due to infection or fracture of the internal fixation device
Non-union	When the bone fails to complete bony union, usually greater than 6 months May be due to repetitive stress on the fracture site or insufficient blood supply, inadequate or improper immobilisation or infection
Malunion	When the bone heals in the standard amount of time, but in an unacceptable position with residual bony deformity May be due to unequal stress forces of muscle pull or improper reduction of the fracture
Angulation	When the fracture heals in an abnormal position
Pseudoarthrosis	A type of non-union which occurs at the fracture site where a false joint is formed
Refracture	When a new fracture occurs at the old/original fracture site
Myositis ossificans	A deposit of calcium in muscle tissue due to a blunt impact/trauma or repetitive muscle injury

healing process. In some cases, the normal healing process is hindered and bone fails to unite, causing delayed union, non-union and malunion. Causes of abnormal fracture healing can be severe damage to soft tissues (which makes union non-viable), abnormal bone, infection, movement at the fracture site and distraction and separation of fragments.[88]

Specific patient groups

- *The obese patient:* Due to the increasing epidemic of obesity, fracture management and treatment in the obese patients poses special challenges. Accurate reduction and fixation will require special considerations and equipment. Obese patients are at higher risk of significant complications, such as nerve injuries, compartment syndrome, medical complications and pressure ulcers. Obese patients may sustain severe fracture patterns from low-energy trauma. Due to the large soft-tissue covering, open femoral fractures are rare.[1]
- *The paediatric patient:* A child has thicker peristeoum compared to an adult; therefore, their fractures heal faster and are generally managed non-operatively. The epiphyseal, or growth plate, does not fuse until skeletal maturity is reached, after puberty. Fractures through the growth plate can severely affect future growth of the fractured bone or complete physeal arrest. Children's bones are more flexible due to being cartilaginous; therefore, greenstick fractures are common.[14]
- *The aged patient:* Generally after the age of 50 years we start to lose skeletal muscle mass. Around this time our bone remodelling is no longer in balance, whereby we resorb more bone than we can produce. This, along with poor calcium intake, will lead to osteoporosis, or 'brittle' bones. This will lead to an increased risk of fracture.[10]

PSYCHOSOCIAL ASPECTS

The paramedic or emergency nurse is frequently the first person the patient, family or friends have contact with to seek answers to their many questions. In the pre-hospital environment or a busy ED, there are often major pressures on the clinician's time. It is therefore essential that clinicians be acutely aware of the physiological and psychological impact of trauma, no matter how minor they perceive it to be. Some studies have looked at the psychological consequences of orthopaedic injury, and report that after 2 years at least 20% of patients who sustained a lower extremity injury report severe phobic anxiety and/or depression.[17] With this in mind, the paramedic and emergency nurse's perception of the injury will always be different from that of the patient, family and friends.

SUMMARY

For the paramedic and emergency trauma nurse, musculoskeletal trauma will continue to be challenging and demanding. Upwards of 70% of trauma patients will have fractures or injured limbs, and with improvements in treatment and surgical management, outcomes for these patients have improved. Research continues to improve options in assessment and management of musculoskeletal injuries. Early identification of patient deterioration or a limb at risk must be escalated promptly to facilitate senior clinician review/management with the aim of preventing mortality or further morbidity. Injury prevention remains a major focus for trauma.

CASE STUDY

PART 1—PRE-HOSPITAL

You are called to a 54-year-old male, who has fallen out of a tree approximately 4 metres high, landing on his back on a concrete driveway. The timing is as follows:

- 1026 hours—Ambulance call received
- 1039 hours—Paramedic arrival at scene
- 1051 hours—Depart scene
- 1055 hours—Triage
- 1058 hours—Off stretcher.

Using MIST, you note the following:

- Injury—lacerated occipital area. Alert but confused (GCS=14). Pupils 4 mm and reactive to light. Chest has decreased air entry on right side and decreased oxygen saturations. The patient is tachycardic and hypotensive. The abdomen is rigid, patient is moving all four limbs.
- Signs as in Table 48.CS1.

QUESTIONS

1. What potential injuries does this patient have?
2. What immediate treatment will you initiate?
3. What type of hospital will you transport the patient to?

PART 2—EMERGENCY DEPARTMENT

A trauma call is activated, and the patient given a Triage Category 1. A primary and secondary survey are

TABLE 48.CS1 VITAL SIGNS ON INITIAL ASSESSMENT

TIME	SBP	PR	RR	O_2 SATS	GCS	BREATH SOUNDS	AVPU	PUPILS
1018	89	145	40	90	13	D	V	+
1025	92	101	40	94	13	D	V	+
1041	92	108	36	96	13	D	V	+

AVPU: Alert, Voice, Pain, Unresponsive; GCS: Glasgow Coma Scale; O_2 sats: oxygen saturations; PR: pulse rate (beats/minute); RR: respiratory rate (breaths/minute); SBP: systolic blood pressure.

performed (see below). His medical history is further clarified as having hypertension. He has no known drug allergies.

Primary survey

- Airway: patent, trachea midline, cervical spine soft foam collar in situ
- Breathing: oxygen via non-rebreather, 15 L/min
- Circulation: IV normal saline 2 L (pre-hospital)
- Deficit: U GCS 13 (E3, V4, M6)
- Signs—see Table 48.CS2

Secondary survey

- Head: small occipital head laceration
- Face: NAD
- Neck: Patient noted to grimace during palpation of c-spine but unable to articulate specific location or whether pain is acute or longstanding
- Chest: decreased right side, focal tenderness around 4th, 5th and 6th rib laterally
- Abdomen: distended, upper quadrant guarding. Abrasions right upper quadrant
- Pelvis: binder in situ, complaining of pain (aching and constant in nature) right side which continues down his right leg
- Back: non-specific tenderness over thoracic and lumbar spine
- Upper limbs: no obvious deformity, pulses present
- Lower limbs: no obvious deformity, pulses present

TABLE 48.CS2 VITAL SIGNS AFTER ARRIVAL AT EMERGENCY DEPARTMENT

TIME	BP	PR	RR	O_2 SATS	GCS	TEMP	PUPILS
1059	99/68	100	20	88%	13	36.8	4+
1100	90/58	90		100%	13		4+
1150	122/70	105	25	100%	13		4+
1215	110/58	105			13	36.8	4+
1300	121/60	99	20	100%			
1340					13	36.9	4+

GCS: Glasgow Coma Scale; O_2 sats: oxygen saturations; PR: pulse rate (beats/minute); RR: respiratory rate (breaths/minute); SBP: systolic blood pressure; Temp: temperature (°C).

Adjuncts

- A full range of blood tests was performed, including cross-match.
- Veneous blood gas (VBG) results were: pH 7.15; partial carbon dioxide pressure (pCO_2) 54 mmHg, partial oxygen pressure (pO_2) 128 mmHg, bicarbonate 18.4 mmol/L, lactate 2.7 mmol/L, Base Excess – 4
- Chest x-ray: no pneumothorax, likely contusions right side with possible underlying fractures
- Pelvis x-ray: open-book fracture (Fig. 48.CS1)
- eFAST—pericardial view negative, perihepatic view negative, perisplenic view negative, pelvic view positive, thoracic view negative

QUESTIONS (CONTINUED)

4. Did the patient receive appropriate fluid management?
5. Discuss the concept of damage control resuscitation.
6. What is the relevance of the positive pelvic eFAST?

PART 3—MANAGEMENT

Initial treatment plan

The patient receives 1 U warmed packed red blood cells upon arrival. The patient is admitted under the trauma

FIGURE 48.CS1 PELVIS X-RAY

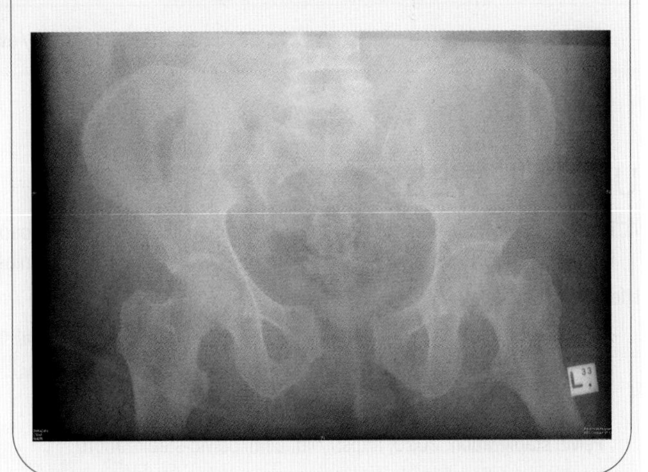

Courtesy Celine Hill.

team with his pelvic binder to remain on (Fig. 48.CS2). He undergoes computed tomography (CT) of head, abdomen/pelvis, cervical spine, chest. The patient remains haemodynamically stable during transfer to CT. He is given analgesia of fentanyl 25 microgram × 4.

CT scan results

- Brain: NAD
- Chest: rib fractures right 4, 5, 6 and 7
- Abdomen: NAD
- Fracture transverse process T11 and L1–5
- Pelvis: fracture through sacrum into sacroiliac joints bilaterally, left superior pubic ramus fracture, pubic symphysis diastasis. Open-book pelvic fracture
- Bilateral retroperitoneal haematoma extending into scrotum on right side

Orthopaedic surgery review

On review, the patient has palpable dorsalis pedis pulses. His L2 to S5 nerves are intact. A Kirschner wire (K-wire) is inserted into distal femur for skeletal traction (Fig. 48.CS2), and 10 kg of weight applied for pelvic fracture. He was transferred to the operating theatre at 1530.

Operating theatre (1535–2045)

Patient has an open reduction and internal fixation of pelvic fracture. In the operating theatre the patient receives a further 1 unit of packed red blood cells and 2 units of fresh frozen plasma.

Intensive care

The patient is transferred to the intensive care unit at 2050 hours intubated and ventilated. For the first 48 hours post-operation, he requires fluid resuscitation, blood products, correction of acidosis and hypocalcaemia and pain relief. Ventilation is weaned and the patient is extubated on day 4. The patient is transferred to the trauma high-dependency unit (HDU) on day 7. There is a delay in transfer to HDU due to bed availability. He remains in the trauma HDU for one day and is stable for transfer to the orthopaedic ward.

FIGURE 48.CS2 BINDER IN PLACE AND SKELETAL TRACTION (K-WIRE)

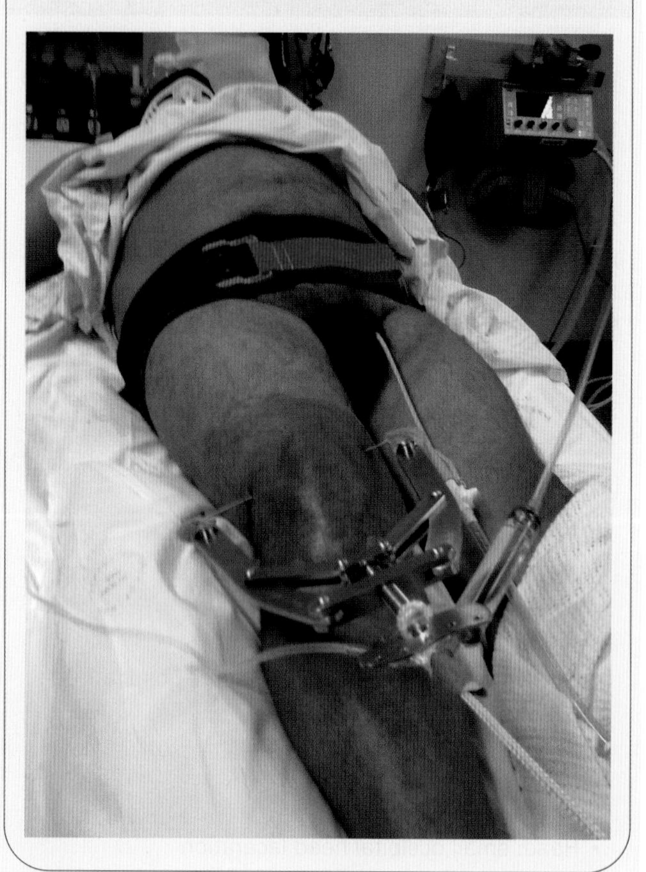

Courtesy Celine Hill.

QUESTIONS (CONTINUED)

7. Explain the complications and risks associated with an open-book pelvic fracture.

Answers to Case Study Questions can be found on evolve **http://evolve.elsevier.com/AU/Curtis/emergency/** 

USEFUL WEBSITES

ACT Health. Pelvic injury, identification, management and complications, broad overview and summary, www.health.act.gov.au/sites/default/files/2021-05/TORU%20-%20Pelvic%20Ring%20Fracture%20Classification%20Learning%20Package%202013%20v2.pdf.

Life in the Fast Lane:

Classification of pelvic fractures, 2020, https://litfl.com/classification-of-pelvic-fractures/.

Hip and pelvis injuries, 2020, https://litfl.com/hip-and-pelvis-injuries/.

Pelvic artery injury, 2020, https://litfl.com/pelvic-arterial-injury/.

Pelvic stabilization, 2020, https://litfl.com/pelvic-stabilization/.

MD+Calc, Mangled Extremity Severity Score (MESS) calculator, www.mdcalc.com/mangled-extremity-severity-score-mess-score.

NSW Institute of Trauma and Injury Mechanisms, Previous trauma events, www.aci.health.nsw.gov.au/networks/itim/events/previous-events#video-381818.

Pelvic fractures: ED presentations and management. emDOCS. 29 May 2017, www.emdocs.net/pelvic-fractures-ed-presentations-management/.

Trauma Victoria: Talking Trauma podcast: episodes, https://trauma.reach.vic.gov.au/podcasts:

- Interventional radiology in major trauma
- Pelvic trauma
- The role of ultrasound in trauma
- Traumatic limb injuries

REFERENCES

1. Walsh J, Vilaca T. Obesity, type 2 diabetes and bone in adults. Calcif Tissue Int 2017;100(5):528–35.
2. Stewart J, Allen T. Emergency and trauma care for nurses and paramedics. 2nd ed. Australia: Elsevier; 2016.
3. Dawson J, Atassi O, Sun D, Sheth M. Emergency care of musculoskeletal injuries. In: Townsand CM, editor. Sabiston textboook of surgery: the biological basis of modern surgical practice. St Louis: Elsevier; 2022.
4. Thibodeau GA, Patton KT. Anatomy and physiology. 6th ed. St Louis: Mosby; 2006.
5. Solomon L, Warwick D, Nayagam S. Apley's concise system of orthopaedics and fractures. 4th ed. London: Arnold; 2014.
6. Linton A. Introduction to medical surgical nursing. 6th ed. St Louis: Elsevier; 2016.
7. Dandy DJ, Edwards DJ. Essential orthopaedics and trauma. 5th ed. Edinburgh: Churchill Livingstone; 2009.
8. McQuillan KA, Makic MBF, Whalen E, editors. Trauma nursing: from resuscitation through rehabilitation. 4th ed. Philadelphia: WB Saunders; 2008.
9. Lewis S, Hagler D, Bucher L. Medical surgical nursing. 10th ed. St Louis: Elsevier; 2017.
10. Neff JA, Kidd PS. Trauma nursing: the art and science. St Louis: Mosby; 1993.
11. Ferri F. Osteoporosis. St Louis: Mosby; 2014.
12. Crowther-Radulewicz C, McCance K. Understanding pathophysiology. 6th ed. St Louis: Elsevier; 2017.
13. Maher AB, Salmond SW, Pellino TA. Orthopaedic nursing. 3rd ed. Philadelphia: WB Saunders; 2002.
14. Ball J, Dains J, Flynn J, Solomon BS, Stewart RW, editors. Seidel's guide to physical examination. 8th ed. St Louis: Mosby; 2015.
15. Moore EE, Feliciano DV, Mattox KL. Trauma. 8th ed. New York: McGraw-Hill; 2017.
16. National Association of Emergency Medical Technicians (NAEMT). PHTLS: Prehospital Trauma Life Support. 9th ed. Burlington, Mass: Jones and Bartlett; 2018.
17. Simon RR, Sherman SC, Koenigsknecht SJ. Emergency orthopedics: the extremities. 7th ed. New York: McGraw-Hill; 2014.
18. Bottlang M, Simpson T, Sigg J, Krieg JC, Madey SM, Long WB. Non-invasive reduction of open-book pelvic fractures by circumferential compression. J Orthopaed Trauma 2002;16(6):367–73.
19. Rice P, Rudolph, M. Pelvic fractures. Emerg Med Clin North Am 2007;25:795–802.
20. Bonner T, Eardley W, Newell N, Masouros S, Matthews JJ, Gibb I. Accurate placement of a pelvic binder improves reduction of unstable fractures of the pelvic ring. J Bone Joint Surg 2011;93(11):1524–28.
21. Kam C, Law P, Lau H, Ahmed R, Cheng M, Lee KB, et al. The 10 commandments of exsanguinating pelvic fracture management. Hong Kong J Emerg Med 2019;26(6):357–70.
22. Bakhshayesh P, Boutefnouchet T, Totterman A. Effectiveness of non-invasive external pelvic compression: a systematic review of the literature. Scand J Trauma Resusc Emerg Med 2016;24:73.
23. Jack C, Daurka D, Bircher M. Pelvic trauma. In: Dawson-Bowling S, Achan P, Briggs T, Ramachandran M, editors. Orthopaedic trauma–the Stanmore and Royal London guide. London UK: Taylor and Francis Group; 2015.
24. NSW Agency for Clinical Innovation (ACI). Pressure injury prevention for critically ill adults. 2014. Online. Available from: https://aci.health.nsw.gov.au/__data/assets/pdf_file/0014/240152/ACI14_PIP_1-1.pdf.
25. Q Medical Technologies. T-Pod FAQs: T-Pod pelvic stabilizer. 2018. Online. Available from: https://qmedical.co.uk/q-medical/t-pod-faqs/.
26. National Institute for Health and Care Excellence (NICE). Fractures (complex): assessment and management. 2017. Online. Available from: www.nice.org.uk/guidance/ng37.
27. McNickle A, Fraser D, Chestovich P, Kuhls DA, Fildes JJ. Effect of prehospital tourniquets on resuscitation in extremity arterial trauma. Surg Acute Care Open 2019;4(1):e000267.
28. Roman P, Rodriguez-Alvarez A, Bertini-Perez D, Ropero-Padilla C, Martin-Ibañez L, Rodriguez-Arrastia M. Torniquets as haemorrhage control measure in military and civilian care settings: an integrative review. J Clin Nurs 2020;31:3–4.
29. Wellme E, Mill V, Montain C. Evaluating tourniquet use in Swedish prehospital care for civilian extremity trauma. Eur J Emerg Surg 2021:47(6): 1861–6.
30. Benitez D, Ottolino P, Pereira B, Lima DS, Guemes A, Khan M, et al. Tourniquet use for civilian extremity haemorrhage: systemic review of the literature. Rev Col Bras Cir 2021;13(48):e20202783.

31. Lee C, Porter K, Hodgetts T. Tourniquet use in the civilian prehospital setting. Emerg Med J 2007;24(8):584–7.
32. Lourens A, Parker R, Hodkinson P. Prehospital acute traumatic pain assessment and management practices in the Western Cape, South Africa: a retrospective review. Int J Emerg Med 2020;13:21.
33. Porter K, Dayan A, Dickerson S, Middleton PM. The role of inhaled methoxyflurane in acute pain management. Open Access Emerg Med 2018;10: 149–64.
34. Yousfifard M, Askarian-Amiri S, Alavi S, Sadeghi M, Saberian P, Baratloo A, et al. The efficacy of ketamine administration in prehospital pain management of trauma patients; a systemic review and meta-analysis. Arch Ac Emerg Med 2020;8(1):e1
35. Jarvis C. Jarvis's physical examination and health assessment pocket companion. 2nd ed. Australia: Elsevier; 2016.
36. Lewis S, Hagler D, Bucher L. Medical surgical nursing. 10th ed. St Louis: Elsevier; 2017.
37. Beckmann N, Cai C. CT characteristics of traumatic sacral fractures in association with pelvic ring injuries: correlation using the Young-Burgess classification system. Emerg Radiol 2017;24(3):255–62.
38. Nacey NC, Geeslin MG, Miller GW, Pierce JL. Magnetic resonance imaging of the knee: an overview and update of conventional and state of the art imaging. J Magn Reson Imaging 2017;45(5):1257–75.
39. Alfayez SM, Allimmia K, Alshammri A. Urological injuries associated with pelvic fractures: a case report of a detached bone segment inside the bladder. Int J Surg Case Rep 2016;28:188–91.
40. Medina O, Arom GA, Yeranosian MG, Petrigliano FA, McAllister DR. Vascular and nerve injury after knee dislocation: a systemic review. Clin Orthopaed Rel Res 2014;472:2621–9.
41. Balbachesvsky D, Belloti JC, Doca DG, Jannarelli B, Junior JA, Fernandes HJ, et al. Treatment of pelvic fractures—a national survey. Injury 2014; 45(5):S46–51.
42. Karkos C, Koudounas G, Giagtzidis I, Mitka MA, Pliatsios I, Papazoglou KO. Traumatic knee dislocation and popliteal artery injury: a case series. Ann Vasc Surg 2018;50:298.
43. Kozin S, Berlet A. Pelvis and acetabulum. In: Kozin S, Berlet A, editors. Handbook of common orthopaedic fractures. 4th ed. Westchester: Medical Surveillance; 2000.
44. Cameron P, Jelinek G, Kelly A, Brown A, Little M, editors. Textbook of adult emergency medicine. 4th ed. Edinburgh: Churchill Livingstone; 2015.
45. Adams JG. Emergency medicine: clinical essentials. 2nd ed. Philadelphia: Saunders; 2013.
46. DePalma A, Connolly J, DePalma S. The management of fractures and dislocations. 3rd ed. Philadelphia: WB Saunders; 1981.
47. Cvetanovich G, Frank R, Chalmers P, Verma NN, Nicholson GP, Romeo AA. Surgical management of proximal humeral fractures: the emerging role of reverse total shoulder arthroplasty. Orthopedics 2016;39(3):465–73.
48. Frank ED, Long BW, Smith BJ. Merrill's atlas of radiographic positions and radiologic procedures. 12th ed. St Louis: Mosby; 2011.
49. Therapeutic Guidelines. Open fractures. 2021. Available from: https://tgldcdp.tg.org.au.acs.hcn.com.au/viewTopic?topicfile=open-fractures#toc_d1e233.
50. Gustilo RB, Anderson JT. Prevention of infection in the treatment of one thousand and twenty-five open fractures of long bones: retrospective and prospective analysis. J Bone Joint Surg 1976;58(4):453–8.
51. Gustilo RB, Mendoza RM, Williams DN. Problems in the management of type III (severe) open fractures: a new classification of type III open fractures. J Trauma 1984;24(8):742–6.
52. Marx J, Hockberger R, Walls R. Rosen's emergency medicine: concepts and clinical practice. 8th ed. Philadelphia: Saunders; 2014.
53. Kim P, Leopold S. Gustilo-Anderson classification. Clin Orthopaed Rel Res 2012;470(12):3624.
54. Engdahl R, Morrison N. Traumatic thumb amputation: case and review. Eplasty 2015;15:ic18.
55. Bumbasirevic M, Matic S, Palibrk T, Glišović Jovanović I, Mitković M, Lesić A. Mangled extremity – modern concepts in treatment. Injury 2021;52:3555–60.
56. Johansen K, Hansen S. MESS (Mangled Extremity Severity Score) 25 years on: time for a reboot? J Trauma Acute Care Surg 2015;79(3):495–6.
57. Stinner D, Edwards D. Surgical management of musculoskeletal trauma. Surg Clin North Am 2017;97(5):1119–31.
58. Coccolini F, Stahel P, Montori G, Biffl W, Horer TM, Catena F, et al. Pelvic trauma: WSES classification and guidelines. World J Emerg Surg 2017;12:5.
59. Burlew C, Moore E. Severe pelvic fracture in the adult trauma patient. (Internet). UpToDate; April 2020 (updated Jan 2022). Online. Available from: www.uptodate.com/contents/severe-pelvic-fracture-in-the-adult-trauma-patient.
60. Bolton P, Au J, Perriman D, Abbott L, Neeman T. AO pelvic fracture classification: can an educational package improve orthopaedic registrar performance. ANZ J Surg 2016;86(12):1019–23.
61. Jobe MT, Martinez SF. Peripheral nerve injuries. In: Canale ST, Beatty JH, editors. Campbell's operative orthopaedics. 12th ed. Philadelphia: Mosby; 2013.
62. Morrison W, Parvizi W, Weiss J. Pelvic and acetabular fractures. In: Miller MD, Sanders TG, editors. Presentation, imaging and treatment of common musculoskeletal conditions. Philadelphia: Saunders; 2012.
63. Wang H, Coppola P, Coppola M. Orthopaedic emergencies: a practical emergency department classficiation. Emerg Med Clin North Am 2015;33(2): 451–73.

64. Garden OJ, Parks RW. Principles and practice of surgery. 7th ed. Elsevier; 2018. All rights reserved. Fig. 27.27 'Damage control' by application of an external fixator in pelvis fractures can be life saving. Online. Available from: www.clinicalkey.com.au/#!/content/book/3-s2.0-B9780702068591000273?scrollTo=%233-s2.0-B9780702068591000273-f27-27-9780702068591.
65. Constantine TW, Coimbra R, Holcomb JB, Podbielski JM, Catalano RD, Blackburn A, et al. Pelvic fracture pattern predicts the need for haemorrhage control intervention—results of an AAST multi-institutional study. J Trauma Acute Care Surg 2017;82(6):1030–8.
66. Horiguchi A, Shinchi M, Ojima K, Masunaga A, Ito K, Asano T, et al. Evaluation of the effect of urethroplasty for anterior strictures by a validated disease - specific patient-reported outcome measure. World J Urol 2019;37(4):601–6.
67. Slater S, Barron D. Pelvic fractures - a guide to classification and management. Eur J Radiol 2010;74:16–23.
68. Bogden Y, Tornetta P, Jones C, Gilde AK, Schemitsch E, Vicente M, et al. Neurologic injury in operatively treated acetabular fractures. J Orthopaed Trauma 2015;29(10):475–8.
69. Volpin G, Pfeifer R, Saveski J, Hasani I, Cohen M, Pape HC. Damage control orthopaedics in polytraumatized patients - current concepts. J Clin Orthopaed Trauma 2021;12:72.
70. Yamamoto R, Udagawa K, Nishida Y, Ono S, Sasaki J. Damage control orthopaedics and decreased in-hospital mortality: a nationwide study. Injury 2019;50:2240–6.
71. Tesoriero RB, Bruns BR, Narayan M, Dubose J, Guliani SS, Brenner ML, et al. Angiographic embolization for haemorrhage following pelvic fracture: is it 'time' for a paradigm shift. J Trauma Acute Care Surg 2017;82(1):18–26.
72. Santy-Tomlinson J. Traction survival skills. Int J Orthopaed Trauma Nurs 2017;24:1–2.
73. Browner BD, Jupiter JB, Levine AM. Skeletal trauma: basic science, management and reconstruction. 5th ed. Philadelphia: WB Saunders; 2015.
74. Githens M, Alton T, Firoozabadi R, Bishop JA. Intraoperative distal femoral fine wire traction to facilitate intramedullary nailing of the femur. Orthopedics 2016;39(2):380–5.
75. Matullo K, Gangavlli A, Nivochuku C. Review of lower extremity traction incurrent orthopaedic trauma. J Am Acad Orthop Surg 2016;24(9):600–6.
76. Canale ST, Beatty JH, editors. Campbell's operative orthopaedics. 12th ed. Philadelphia: Mosby; 2013.
77. Roberts JR, Hedges JR. Clinical procedures in emergency medicine. 6th ed. Philadelphia: Saunders Elsevier; 2013.
78. Chung J, Modrall J. Compartment syndrome. In: Cronenwett JL, Johnston KW, editors. Rutherford's vascular surgery. 8th ed. Philadelphia: Saunders; 2014.
79. Stanley JC, Veith FJ, Wakefield TW. Current therapy in vascular and endovascular surgery. 5th ed. Philadelphia: Saunders; 2014.
80. Walls M. Compartment syndrome: an orthopaedic emergency. J Emerg Nurs 2017;43(4):303–7.
81. Prasarn M, Ovellette E. Acute compartment syndrome of the upper extremity. J Am Acad Orthopaed Surg 2011;19(1):49–58.
82. Lindsey RW, Harper A. Atypical acute compartment syndrome. J Bone and Joint Surg 2017;7(3):1–4.
83. Sagi C, Donohue D, Cooper S, Barei DP, Siebler J, Archdeacon MT, et al. Institutional and seasonal variations in the incidence and causative organisms for post traumatic infection following open fractures. J Orthopaed Trauma 2017;31(2):78–84.
84. Corona P, Erimeiku F, Reverté-Vinaixa MM, Soldado F, Amat C, Carrera L. Necrotising fasciitis of the extremities: implementation of new management technologies. Injury 2016;47(3):S66–71.
85. Hughes R. Fat embolism syndrome in long bone fractures. J Orthopaed Phys Assist 2016;4(2):5–9.
86. Miller A, Deal D, Green J, Houle T, Brown W, Thore C, et al. Use of the reamer/irrigator/aspirator decreases carotid and cranial embolic events in a canine model. J Bone Joint Surg 2016;98(8):658–64.
87. Zhou Y, Yuan Y, Huang C, Hu L, Cheng X. Pathogenesis, diagnosis and treatment of cerebral fat embolism. Chin J Traumatol 2015;18(2):120–3.
88. Elliott DS, Newman KJ, Forward DP, Hahn DM, Ollivere B, Kojima K, et al. A unified theory of bone healing and non union. Bone Joint J 2016;98(7):884–91.
89. Hildebrand F, Van Griensven M, Huber-Lang M, Flohe SB, Andruszkow H, Marzi I, et al. Is there an impact of concomitant injuries and timing of fixation of major fractures on fracture healing? A focused review of clinical and experimental evidence. J Orthopaed Trauma 2016;30(3):104–12.
90. Kulkami S, Kulkami G, Babhulkar S, Kulkarni MG, Kulkarni RM. Accuracy of valgus osteotomy using DHS. Injury 2017;48(2):S2–7.

CHAPTER 49
BURNS TRAUMA

ANDREW J.A. HOLLAND AND LINDA QUINN

ESSENTIALS

- Burns remain a common, potentially life-threatening injury for both adults and children.
- While visually dramatic, burns may occur in association with other forms of trauma.
- Appropriate first aid, which includes stopping the burning process and the application of at least 20 minutes of cold running water while avoiding hypothermia, may reduce the depth of the burn injury.
- Major burns (greater than 10% of total body surface area [TBSA] in children and 20% TBSA in adults), although appearing to involve only the skin, lead to a generalised increase in vascular permeability, in association with an intense and sustained metabolic response.
- All patients with major burns require supplementary oxygen, which should be warmed and humidified, together with intravenous fluids in proportion to the area of the burn. Children will also require maintenance fluids based on their weight.
- Oedema may result in rapid loss of the airway in the patient with facial, neck and inhalational burns, respiratory embarrassment in those with chest wall burns or distal ischaemia in those with limb burns. Early elective intubation must be considered, together with escharotomy, prior to transfer.
- Appropriate temporary burn wound dressings should be discussed with the receiving burns unit.
- Scarring and contracture formation remain important long-term sequelae in those patients with deep burns.

INTRODUCTION

'Burn' derives from the Old English word *baernan* for an injury as a result of heat, or a chemical, radiological or mechanical force simulating the action of heat. Despite improvements in prevention, either through legislation or education, or a combination of the two, a burn remains one of the most devastating forms of injury in all ages. Worldwide, it has been estimated that there are 180,000 deaths each year as a result of burn injury.[1] In the United States there were 450,000 patients in 2010 who required medical treatment for burn injuries and in 2008, 3400 deaths.[2] This comparatively high mortality rate reflects a combination of the systemic inflammatory consequences of major burn injury, the increased risks of sepsis, together with the impact of any associated inhalational injury. While the majority of burns occur in adults, children and older adults appear uniquely at risk as a result of a combination of their thin skin and different responses to burn injury. In Europe, a systematic literature review in 2010 identified an incidence of severe burns of between 0.2 and 2.9/10,000, with over 50% in the paediatric age group.[3] Worldwide, in 1997, burns caused the loss of 11.9 × 106 disability-adjusted life years (DALYs), resulting in a greater loss than that of diabetes, HIV and asthma.[4] Furthermore, these injuries are not evenly distributed geographically, with a much higher proportion occurring in low- to middle-income countries, especially South-East Asia.[4] Between 1990 and 2004, of the 505,276 children with burn injuries reported in the literature, 57% were located in Asia.[3]

From 1 July 2019 to 30 June 2020 there were 3367 people admitted to one of the 17 burns units in Australia and Aotearoa New Zealand; 230 with major burns in 2019–20 (a 20% increase from 2018–19).[5] Over half of these burn admissions (57%) occurred in rural and remote areas with significant implications for transport and pre-hospital care.[5] Further, the 2019–20 figure encompasses events that continue to have profound impacts on individuals and communities in Aotearoa New Zealand and Australia—the Whakaari/White Island volcano eruption and the bushfires in Australia. Nearly all people on the island who survived the eruption had severe burns, requiring many weeks and months of treatment in burn services in Aotearoa New Zealand and Australia. Then, over the ensuing summer, mega fires burned throughout South and Eastern Australia, directly killing 34 people and destroying homes, farms, and more than 20% of the nation's forests. Forty patients with severe burn injuries due to these bushfires were admitted to specialist burns services around Australia.[5]

For those clinicians dealing with burns patients, however, these numbers represent only part of the whole picture.[2] Increasing survival translates to a higher frequency of morbidity, with a very great burden on the patient, their family, clinicians and the healthcare system. Perhaps this feature, together with the need for excellent teamwork to achieve an optimal outcome, explains in part the *esprit de corps* that typically exists in burn units.[6] In addition, there is increasing evidence of long-term sequelae, both mental and physical, from burn injury. While these may be greater for those patients with major burn injury, even those patients with comparatively minor burns may suffer long-term health consequences of what should be considered a chronic disease.[7] Certainly, burn injury may represent one of the best examples of trauma care in which the provision of ideal pre-hospital treatment may directly affect the patient's final outcome, especially in relation to the depth of burn injury and the need for subsequent operative intervention.[8,9]

EPIDEMIOLOGY AND AETIOLOGY OF BURNS

Although there appears to be some conflicting data in the literature, several key facts remain. First, burns, like nearly all forms of trauma, generally affect males more commonly than females, with an average ratio of 1.6 : 1.[10] Second, while the overall incidence of burns requiring hospital admission has decreased over at least the last two decades in high-income countries, approximately 1% of the population in Australia and Aotearoa New Zealand will sustain some form of burn injury per annum.[10–12] In certain high-risk groups, such as children in South-East Asia and Australasia, the prevalence of burn injury may, in fact, be rising.[3,13,14] In part, these apparently conflicting data may reflect a failure to adequately account for differences between high-income and middle- to low-income countries.[3,15] A lack of agreement on age definitions and the increased use of ambulatory versus inpatient care in the management of burn injuries in many units make accurate comparison and analysis of trends difficult.[3,14,16]

The mechanism of burn injury also would seem both more complex and more dynamic than it might at first appear: historically, flame burns have accounted for the majority of burns in adults, followed by scalds and then contact burns.[11] In contrast, in children this order has been transposed, with scalds predominating, trailed by flame and then contact burns.[11] Depths of burn injuries are demonstrated in Fig. 49.1.

Some studies have suggested there is a rise in the proportion of scald burns in adults, perhaps in parallel with a greater proportion of the elderly being part of the adult population, although this may also reflect the inclusion of paediatric data.[17–19] In the paediatric age group, there appears to have been a rise in the number of contact burns, which has now replaced flame burns as the second most-common cause of burn injury in childhood after scalds.[20]

Knowledge of the likely aetiology of the burn injury remains important to paramedic, nursing and allied health personnel involved in the care of that patient, as it enables both

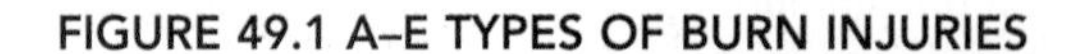

FIGURE 49.1 A–E TYPES OF BURN INJURIES

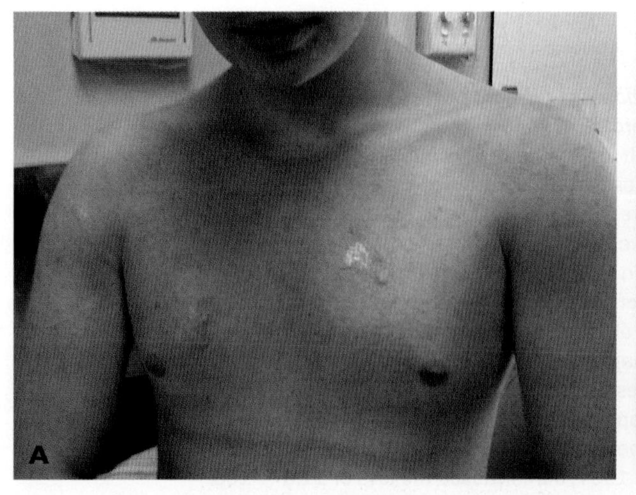

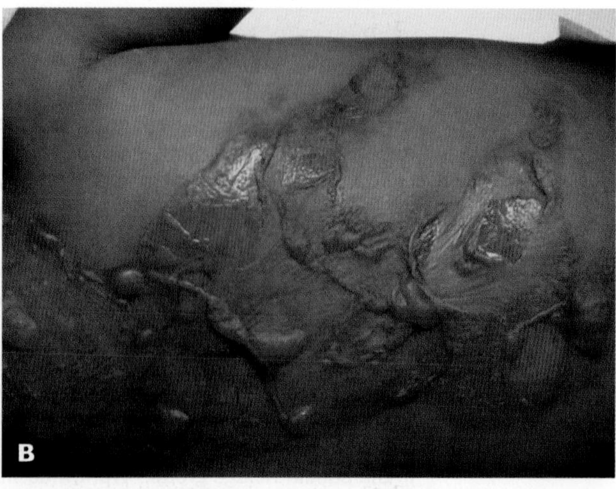

A. Epidermal burn. B. Superficial dermal burn.

FIGURE 49.1—cont'd

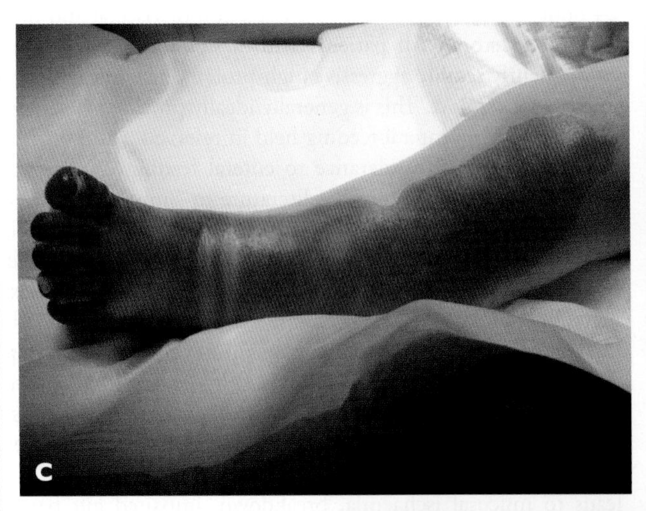

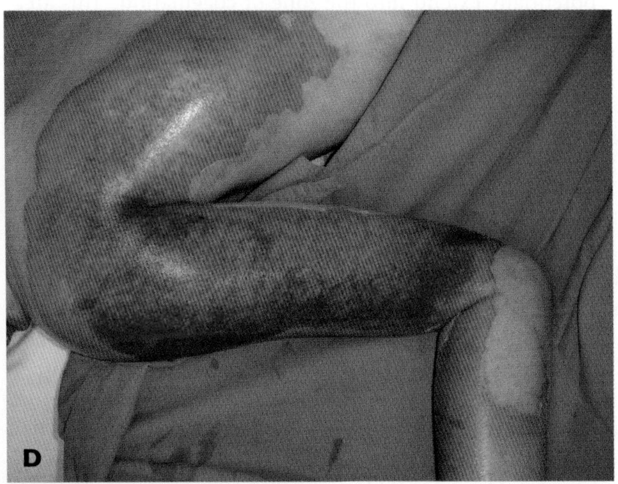

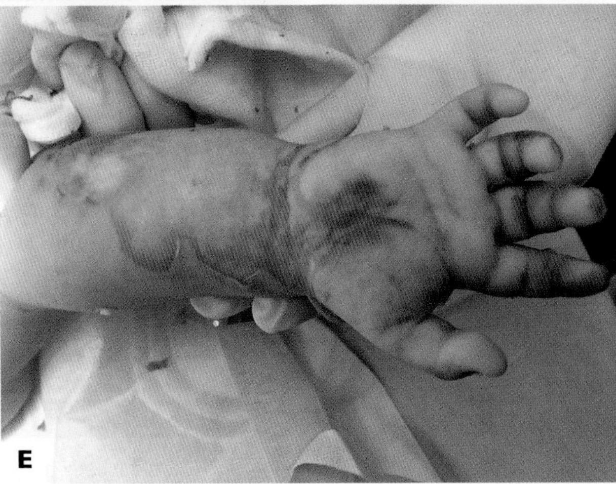

C. Mid dermal burn. D. Deep dermal burn. E. Full thickness burn. *SA Health, Government of South Australia. Women's and Children's Health Network; 2014.*

understanding and provision of optimal burns first aid treatment and provides an opportunity for advice on prevention.[8,14,21,22] Nearly a quarter (23%) of children with severe burns did not receive the recommended first aid treatment for burn injuries.[5]

PATHOPHYSIOLOGY

A burn injury has an effect on all of the five major functions of the skin:

- thermoregulation
- fluid and electrolyte imbalance
- immune response
- protection from bacterial invasion
- neurosensory interface.

LOCAL RESPONSE

To assist in understanding the pathophysiology of a burn, it is useful to look to Jackson's burn wound model (Fig. 49.2), first described in 1953.[4]

FIGURE 49.2 JACKSON'S BURN WOUND MODEL[4]

Zone of coagulation

Zone of stasis

Zone of hyperaemia

1. *Zone of coagulative necrosis*—this is the site of injury where the heat source is at its greatest, and rapid cell death occurs. This central zone of tissue death becomes deeper and wider as the heat intensifies and length of exposure increases. The damage in this zone is irreversible.
2. *Zone of stasis*—this area surrounds the zone of coagulation and the tissue damage is less severe; however, there

is damage to the microcirculation. Sluggish circulation makes this area susceptible to additional insult and may potentially extend into the zone of coagulation. This area is viable given appropriate fluid resuscitation and wound care, avoiding excessive oedema and infection.
3. *Zone of hyperaemia*—surrounding the zone of stasis is one of limited cellular damage, and complete recovery usually prevails. The inflammatory mediatory response causes widespread vasodilation and this increased blood flow brings necessary nutrients to support the zone of stasis.[12,23,24]

The final depth and area of the burn wound is dependent on the fate of the zone of stasis, and treatment is centred on facilitating the recovery of this area. The true extent of injury may take 3–5 days, as areas that acutely appear to be perfused often go on to show delayed healing. This is seen clinically as burn wound progression.

Recovery of the zone of stasis can be supported by:

- adequate burns first aid
- prevention of hypothermia
- good fluid resuscitation
- elevation of affected limbs
- prevention of infection
- covering of the burn wound
- analgesia.

SYSTEMIC RESPONSE

A burn injury induces changes in every organ system in the body, especially in those with injuries greater than 20% TBSA. These are caused by the release of inflammatory mediators and neural stimulation, with the most profound and immediate effect being on the circulation.[11] Vasodilation occurs, along with an increase in capillary permeability and a lowering of intercellular pressure. This causes mass movement of albumin out of the circulation and into the interstitial space, producing oedema. Changes in cell permeability result in an abnormal exchange of sodium. Sodium shifts into the cells in exchange for potassium, which results in further depletion of intravascular sodium. The decreased interstitial hydrostatic pressure is thought to be the predominant mechanism responsible for the initial rapid development of oedema. The generalised oedema seen in non-injured skin and organs of patients with injuries greater than 25% TBSA is due to the circulatory mediators.

Simple ways to assist with minimising oedema and increasing perfusion include:

- nursing with head of bed at 30°
- elevating limbs
- carefully observing for adequacy of fluid resuscitation
- active or passive range of motion exercises.

Hypermetabolic state and nutrition

As a result of a severe burn injury, stress hormones, such as cortisol, catecholamines and glucagon, are released, which in turn sets up a hypermetabolic state. The patient's metabolic rate can increase by as much as two to three times the normal rate; far in excess of that seen in any other disease state, including other major traumas.[25] The stress response causes the suppression of anabolic hormones (growth hormones, insulin and anabolic steroids), which results in considerable catabolism, including muscle protein breakdown.[7] We see these changes clinically as tachycardia, hyperthermia and protein wasting. This protein breakdown leads to the depletion of glycogen stores within 24 hours post-injury, along with depletion of visceral and muscle protein stores. All patients with a significant burn injury consequently require aggressive high-protein, high-carbohydrate nutritional support. This is generally ideally provided via enteral feeding, with parenteral feeding held in reserve for those with a prolonged ileus or intolerance to enteral feeding.[11,25] There is now a considerable volume of literature to support pharmacological modification of this hypermetabolic state, especially the use of propranolol, a non-selective β1 and β2 receptor blocker, to reduce the elevated resting heart rate, decrease the basal metabolic rate and reduce lipolysis.[7,26]

Depression of the immune mechanism causes immunosuppression; consequently, infection is still the leading cause of mortality in burn patients. The diffuse capillary leakage, hypovolaemia and release of vasoconstrictive agents following a severe burn injury cause a decrease in mesenteric blood flow.[27] This leads to mucosal ischaemia, breakdown, impaired gut barrier function, and an increase in bacterial translocation; another rationale for the early commencement of enteral feeds.[11,25]

The lungs commonly suffer from a post-burn systemic inflammatory response, resulting in acute respiratory distress syndrome (ARDS), even when not associated with an inhalation injury.

There are also widespread and long-term growth changes in the seriously burn-injured patient, which may never be restored. This may have special long-term consequences in children who sustain a major burn, particularly during their pubertal growth spurt.

PRACTICE TIP

Consider early passage of a gastric tube to both decompress the stomach and facilitate early enteral feeding.

PARAMEDIC AND FIRST AID TREATMENT

While burn injuries appear visually dramatic to patients, relatives and care providers, the general immediate care and management remains the same for any patient with trauma. It is vital that those tasked with the pre-hospital care of burns patients not allow themselves to be distracted by either the initial appearances of the injury or the apparent general wellbeing of the victim. Appropriate measures in relation to both provision of burns first aid treatment (BFAT) and application of general trauma care principles in relation to management of airway, ventilation and circulatory support, may have a profound impact on the patient's final outcome.

PRACTICE TIP

Remember that the burn patient is still a trauma patient. Always consider the possibility of blast, spinal or other traumatic injuries in the burn patient.

For all patients, it is crucial that the first responder/paramedic should initially ensure their own safety. It is certainly not uncommon that in providing first aid, the first responder will themselves sustain a burn injury, especially in the setting of flame, chemical, radiation or electrical burns, doubling the number of victims and therefore resources required for treatment. If the patient is still alight, the correct approach remains to 'stop, drop and roll'.[11] A blanket, towel or similar item may be used to smother the flames. In the case of an electrical burn, the first responder should exercise caution and ensure that the source of any current has been disconnected before approaching the patient, and use a non-conductor to separate the patient from the source.[28] Extensive chemical or radiological burns require the first responder to seek additional resources before providing effective care safely.

The second step in stopping the burning process is cooling the burn, while avoiding hypothermia.[29] Australian and New Zealand Burn Association (ANZBA) guidelines define this as the application of cool (but not iced) running tap water to the burn wound for at least 20 minutes within 3 hours of the burn injury.[11] Children and older adults would appear to be most at risk of hypothermia, especially with a greater than 20% TBSA burn cooled in a bath or shower. This may be avoided by warming the general environment and/or by the use of warm towels or a space blanket over that part of the patient that has not been burned.

In addition to the analgesic action of cool running water, there now exists considerable experimental and epidemiological evidence to support the efficacy of this regimen in reducing burn wound depth.[30–32] Based on experimental data from a scald burn wound model, not only does cool running water appear to be the most effective treatment when used for 20 minutes, but it also remains effective even when its use has been delayed for up to 1 hour post-injury.[31–34] Future studies may provide scientific evidence to support the efficacy of cool running water for up to 3 hours post-injury.

While apparently straightforward in the case of a contact burn involving a limb, the provision of optimal BFAT often proves challenging in the setting of more-extensive burns or outside the hospital environment. Several studies in both adults and children have identified the low number of patients provided with optimal BFAT.[14,35,36] While knowledge remains an issue, even among healthcare providers, there are often challenges in sourcing cool running water outside the domestic, industrial or hospital environments.[22] This has led to the development of a variety of commercial products based on a foam dressing combined with water and melaleuca oil. Their effectiveness in the provision of BFAT, however, remains unproven by independent trials and they are likely to be less effective than cool, running water.[32,37,38] Further, as with the use of cold running water, special care should be taken with these products to avoid the risk of hypothermia.

BFAT should be continued at the scene by paramedics while ensuring that management of the airway, breathing and circulation (ABCs) is not compromised.

PRACTICE TIP

Always check that the patient has had optimal burns first aid: cold running water for 20 minutes within 3 hours of the burn injury, avoiding hypothermia.

IMMEDIATE TREATMENT

A standard approach to the management of airway, breathing and circulation was given in Chapter 42 (see also Chapter 15). Several specific issues in relation to management of the burns patient require emphasis. First, any burn injury might be associated with other forms of trauma, including a cervical fracture or thoracic injury; the paramedic needs to recall this and avoid being distracted by the burn injury in isolation. Second, the airway may initially be readily maintained by the patient, but may be rapidly lost as a result of a combination of oedema secondary to the burn injury itself, compounded by the use of intravenous (IV) fluids. Particular caution is advised in the patient with an inhalational burn. Early indications of a potential airway burn include facial or neck burns, stridor, hoarse voice with a brassy cough and tachypnoea. While not necessarily requiring intubation at the scene, the airway requires careful monitoring to avoid a more complex, emergent intubation with the patient in transit. Supplementary oxygenation should always be given; preferably 100% humidified oxygen via a non-rebreathing Hudson mask.

In relation to breathing, a circumferential or near-circumferential burn of the chest and upper abdomen may restrict ventilation, acting as a cuirasse or tight 'binding'. This rarely occurs in the first 2–4 hours post-burn injury, but may develop insidiously, especially after the patient has been commenced on IV fluids. If combined with an inhalational burn, it may be rapidly fatal as a result of the combination of impaired chest-wall compliance, airway and pulmonary oedema, alveolar collapse and vessel shunting, and systemic toxicity from compounds such as carbon monoxide and cyanide.[11]

Finally, circulatory support in the form of resuscitation with IV fluids will be required for 'large' or major burns, defined as > 10% TBSA in children and > 15% TBSA in adults.[11] These fluids should be commenced as soon as practical by the paramedic, to help support the circulation, in addition to the benefits of helping reduce the potential depth of the burn as a result of prompt resuscitation. Monitoring resuscitation of the burn patient in the pre-hospital setting may prove problematic, as both blood pressure and pulse rate may be difficult to measure and inaccurate as a result of limb oedema. External monitoring of the heart rate, if available, may therefore be the most effective option.[39] Intravenous or intra-nasal opioids or ketamine should be given as required for analgesia.

It is often useful to document at this point the time and mechanism of injury, and what first aid (including its duration) and any other care has been provided. Often this information will otherwise be lost once the patient has been transferred to their definitive care location.

PRACTICE TIP

Optimal management of the patient's airway, breathing and circulation will assist in ensuring optimal management of the burn injury.

TRANSPORTATION AND TRANSFER

There appears to be clear evidence in the literature that, with the exception of a small minority of patients with life-threatening problems identified in the primary survey or those injured in a rural setting, optimal care for the major burns patient may be best

BOX 49.1 ANZBA REFERRAL CRITERIA

- Burn > 10% TBSA
- Full-thickness burn > 5% TBSA
- Burns of special areas:
  - face
  - hands
  - feet
  - genitalia and perineum
  - major joints
- Electrical burns
- Chemical burns
- Inhalational burn
- Circumferential burn of limb or torso
- Burns in children or the elderly
- Burns in patients with pre-existing illness
- Any burn with associated injuries

TBSA: total body surface area.

provided by direct transfer to a hospital with a burns unit.[40,41] ANZBA referral criteria are summarised in Box 49.1.

For patients with minor burns, initial consultation with the local burns unit may avoid an unnecessary transfer or, equally, an inappropriately delayed referral. Each emergency department (ED) should have their region's burns transfer protocols clearly displayed and readily available online. Despite increasing numbers of referrals to centres with a burns unit, there remain instances of stable patients having secondary transfers from hospitals without a burns unit.[42,43] As well as representing poor use of resources, this delays the provision of optimal, definitive care.

For those patients requiring transfer, careful consideration should be given in consultation with the receiving burns unit as to the ideal timing and mode of transfer.[11] During this consultation with the medical and nursing staff of the receiving burns unit, joint decisions over the current management of the patient can be made to assist in the patient receiving the best possible care prior to and during their transfer (Box 49.2).

Many centres now offer the option of submitting photographs of the patient's burn wound, so that a better-informed decision of the need and timing of transfer, or advice on immediate management, can be made. In addition to planning the transfer, advice can be given in relation to adequate BFAT, resuscitation, the need for escharotomies and use of dressings. Accurate determination of the TBSA of the burn remains crucial to assist in determining optimal resuscitation and fluid management, with both the more common overestimation and the less frequent underestimation equally deleterious to overall management of the patient and their burn wound.[42,44,45] For other principles relating to interhospital transfer of patients, such as communication and transport type, see Chapter 15.

PRACTICE TIPS

- If in doubt, always discuss referral with a burns unit.
- A digital photograph from a mobile phone or digital camera facilitates communication.

BOX 49.2 PREPARATION FOR TRANSFER

- Airway and breathing
- Secure airway
- 100% humidified oxygen
- Cervical spine protection if appropriate
- Circulation
- Two, secure large-bore intravenous cannulae
- Appropriate resuscitation fluids
- Monitor blood pressure, pulse and urine output
- Burn wound
- Cleaned chlorhexidine 0.1% or normal saline
- Appropriate dressing
- Review need for tetanus prophylaxis
- Nutrition and support
- Gastric tube
- Consider enteric feeding if > 10% TBSA in child or > 15% TBSA in adult
- Keep the patient warm
- Analgesia and documentation
  - Should be a narcotic, given intravenously
- Document management
- Copies of radiographs and other investigation results

TBSA: total body surface area.

BURNS SHOCK AND FLUID RESUSCITATION

Adequate fluid resuscitation is critical to the survival of a severely burn-injured patient. Prior to the understanding of the massive fluid shifts and vascular changes that occur during burn shock, the leading cause of death after burn injury was from hypovolaemic shock or shock-induced renal failure. Combined with the fluid loss from the exudating wound, there is insufficient blood flow throughout the body to maintain adequate tissue perfusion. Burn shock is both hypovolaemic shock and cellular shock, and is characterised by specific haemodynamic changes, including decreased cardiac output, extracellular fluid, plasma volume and oliguria. As in the treatment for other forms of shock, the primary goal is to restore and preserve tissue perfusion and ultimately avoid ischaemia. In burn shock, resuscitation is complicated by burn oedema and major fluid shifts. These fluid shifts are caused by the increase in capillary permeability and alteration in cell membranes, which in a severe burn can occur in areas that have not been heat-injured.[46] Correction of this hypovolaemia is a lifesaving task in the first hours following a major thermal injury,[17,46] with the aim to give the *least* amount of fluid necessary to maintain *adequate* organ perfusion.[47]

Estimating the fluid requirements is based on the extent of injury (TBSA), the patient's weight and by using a fluid resuscitation formula designed for the treatment of burns. The volume infused should be continually titrated so to avoid both under- and over-resuscitation.

PRACTICE TIPS

- The best measure of tissue perfusion in the major burns patient remains urine output.
- Over-resuscitation is more common and is as dangerous as under-resuscitation, especially in children and older people with major burns.

EXTENT OF INJURY

Burn assessment tends to be done poorly, even by those who are experts.[48] There are three commonly used methods to estimate burn size, and it is important that simple erythema is not included. This is a common error and can cause overestimation to occur and consequently fluid resuscitation to be overcalculated.

- *Palmar method:* the surface area of a patient's palm (including fingers) is approximately 1% of TBSA. Relatively small burns can be assessed this way, but it is inaccurate for more-significant burns.
- *Rule of nines:* the body is divided into areas of 9% (Fig. 49.3). This is a good, quick method to calculate adult burns. It is inaccurate for children because they have a different ratio of body-to-surface-area. Children have proportionately smaller hips and legs, and larger shoulders and heads than adults. This may seriously under- or overestimate the size of the burn if used.
- The *Lund and Browder chart* (Fig. 49.4) takes these considerations into account. If used correctly, it is the most accurate method. To make an accurate assessment, all of the burn must be exposed while keeping the environment warm. Pigmented skin can be difficult to assess, and if loose epidermal layers are not removed prior to estimation, the estimate will be undercalculated.[48]

FIGURE 49.3 THE 'RULE OF NINES'[39]

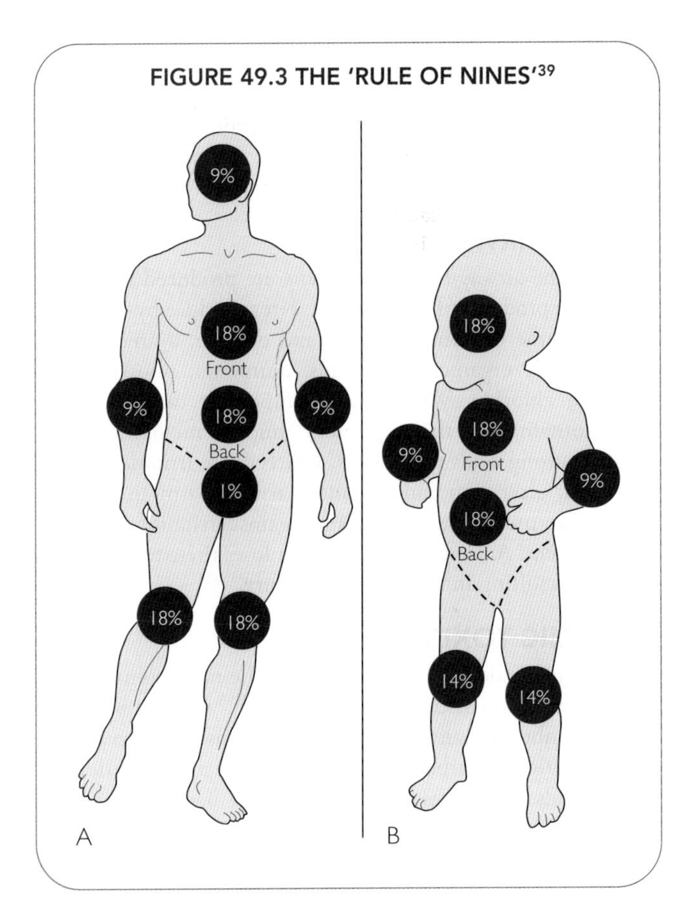

A. Adult. **B.** Child.

FIGURE 49.4 LUND AND BROWDER FORMULA (7.5 YEARS TO ADULT)[50]

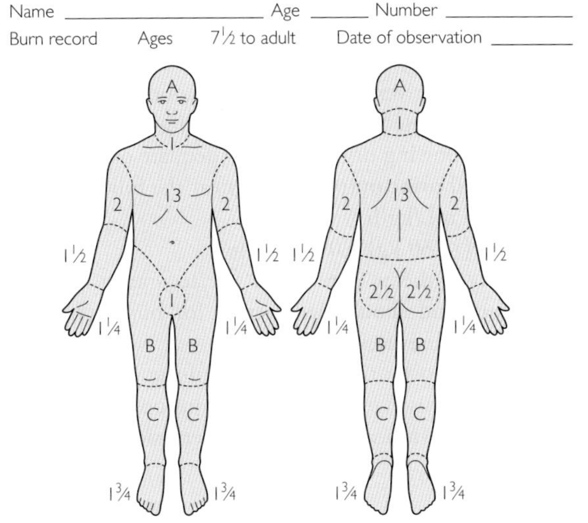

Relative percentages of areas affected by growth

Area	Age 10	15	Adult
A = ½ of head	5½	4½	3½
B = ½ of one thigh	4¼	4½	4¾
C = ½ of one leg	3	3¼	3½

% Burn by areas

Lund and Browder Chart
Estimation of extent of burn (7½ yrs–adult)

PRACTICE TIPS

- Study a burns chart before you meet your first burns patient.
- Consider a commercial application (such as uBurn) available for smartphones to assist with calculation of the area of the burn.[51]

Estimating fluid requirements

The commonly used formula as approved by ANZBA is the Parkland formula:

- 3 mL crystalloid (e.g. Hartmann's solution or normal saline)/kg bodyweight/percentage burn

These fluid requirements are required for children with burns > 10% TBSA and adults with burns > 15% TBSA. (See the section on burns in children for additional requirements.)

The calculation of fluid requirements commences from time of burn, not time of presentation. The calculated volume is that estimated for the first 24 hours. This is divided into two phases: half the calculated volume is given in the first 8 hours and the remaining half given over the succeeding 16 hours.[11,47]

Example: 70 kg man with a 40% burn

Parkland formula 4 × 70 × 40 = 11,200 for first 24 hours

Half this amount = 5,600 given from the time of burn, i.e. if 1 hour from injury, this is given over 7 hours = 800 mL/hour

Second half is given over the next 16 hours = 350 mL/hour

The most reliable method of monitoring fluid resuscitation is by closely following urine output. Adequate organ perfusion is maintained if urine output is kept near the following ranges:

- Adults 0.5 mL/kg/h
- Children (< 30 kg) 1.0 mL/kg/h

A urinary catheter is essential for accurately monitoring urine output, and should be inserted for burns that require intravenous fluid resuscitation.

Fluids need to be titrated, as large urine output indicates excessive fluid resuscitation with gratuitous oedema formation; low urine output indicates poor tissue perfusion.[11,47]

PAIN RELIEF

A burn injury is extremely painful and in all but the most minor cases the patient should be given narcotic analgesia intravenously. Taking into account any pre-existing disease or associated injury, IV morphine 0.1 mg/kg should be administered as soon as possible. Further doses are often required, but must be titrated against pain and sedation, followed by early commencement of narcotic infusion.

INHALATIONAL INJURY

Inhalation injuries, whether seen in conjunction with a cutaneous injury or in isolation, are one of the most critical injuries following a thermal injury and are strongly linked to an increase in mortality.[52,53] Inhalation injury requires early diagnosis and treatment and is classified according to the site of injury:

1. Airway injury above the larynx.
2. Airway injury below the larynx.
3. Systemic intoxication injury.

A patient may have one or more of the above types of injury. See Box 49.3 for clinical indicators of an inhalation injury and Fig. 49.5 for facial and inhalation injury.

BOX 49.3 CLINICAL INDICATORS OF AN INHALATION INJURY

- Burns to the mouth, nose and pharynx
- Sputum containing soot
- Change of voice
- Hoarse, brassy cough
- Inspiratory stridor
- Tracheal tug
- Singed nasal hairs
- Productive cough
- Respiratory distress
- Rib retraction
- Flaring of alae nasae
- Restlessness

FIGURE 49.5 FACIAL AND INHALATION INJURY[54]

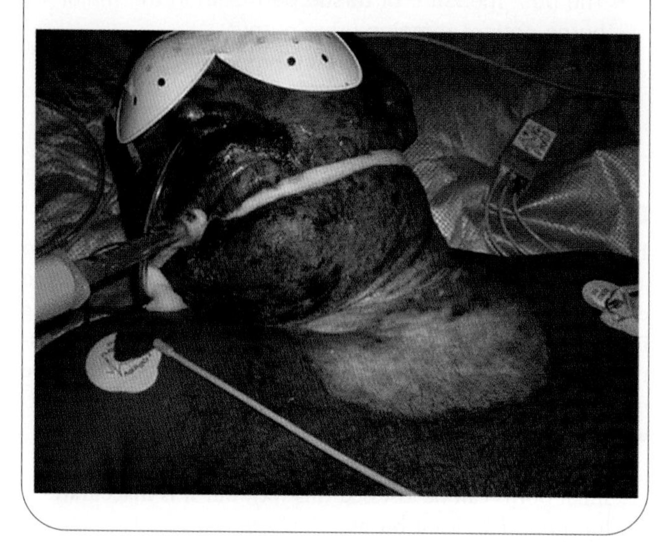

UPPER AIRWAY INJURIES

These are caused by the inhalation of hot gases and are most likely to occur in an enclosed space (if trapped in a fire) or with the inhalation of steam. As in thermal injury to skin, inhalation injuries above the larynx produce inflammatory mediators to cause oedema and loss of the protective functions of the mucosa. This leads to respiratory obstruction, which may not occur until 12–36 hours post-injury as the body responds to the injury, oedema progresses and fluid resuscitation fluid is given.

The upper respiratory tract has a tremendous ability to reflect heat; it is only after extreme heat exposure that pure heat damage to the lower respiratory tract occurs.[52,55,56]

LOWER AIRWAY INJURIES

Burns to the airway below the larynx are produced by inhalation of the products of combustion. Fires produce by-products, which include carbon monoxide and dioxide, cyanide, esters and complex organic compounds, ammonia, phosgene and hydrogen chloride. When these compounds dissolve in the water contained in the respiratory mucous membranes they produce strong acids and alkalis, which cause irritation, bronchospasm, ulceration and oedema. Laryngospasm and breath-holding are protective mechanisms against irritation in a conscious patient. An unconscious patient loses these mechanisms, however, resulting in a more severe injury.[55–57]

SYSTEMIC TOXINS

Carbon monoxide (CO) intoxication is the most common systemic intoxication associated with burns.[55,56] Oxygen is utilised during combustion and, in turn, CO is released due to incomplete oxidation of carbon. CO is a colourless and odourless gas which binds 200 times more readily with haemoglobin than oxygen, forming carboxyhaemoglobin (COHb). This reduces the oxygen-carrying capacity of the blood, and tissue anoxia occurs. CO can go on to bind with the intracellular cytochrome system, leading to further cell death.

Patients with CO intoxication are often misdiagnosed with alcohol intoxication as they often display similar symptoms. Therefore, CO intoxication must be ruled out prior to a diagnosis of alcohol intoxication.

Patients with an altered state of consciousness after a burn injury have CO intoxication unless proven otherwise. The majority of deaths occurring at the scene of a fire are due to CO intoxication; what we often hear reported as 'being overcome by the fumes'.

A thorough history is required, as burns in an enclosed space, such as a house, motor vehicle or aircraft, or burns with an associated explosion from petrol or gas fire or from a bomb, are likely to be associated with an inhalation injury. Symptoms of CO poisoning include cherry-red skin, tachypnoea, headache, dizziness and nausea, but commonly do not manifest until COHb levels are greater than 20% (Table 49.1).

ASSESSMENT AND TREATMENT

Maximum tissue oxygenation for all burn injuries during the initial assessment is facilitated by the administration of humidified oxygen at 10 L/min. This is especially imperative in those with a suspected inhalation injury. Intubation may be necessary in injuries above the larynx if increasing airway obstruction is detected, and without delay. In injuries below the larynx, intubation may be necessary to clear secretions, along with intermittent positive-pressure ventilation. (See Chapter 14 for details on intubation.)

The clinical indicators of an inhalation injury evolve over time, as with all traumas; therefore, repeat evaluation is critical. Constant observation of a change in these signs can detect the complications of an inhalation injury, which include airway obstruction, deteriorating consciousness, retained secretions, deteriorating oxygenation and respiratory failure. In assessing for an inhalation injury, one of the most useful tools is the fibre-optic bronchoscope, which allows for direct visualisation of the supraglottic airway and tracheobronchial tree.[56,57]

Treatment of systemic intoxication includes respiratory support, as described above, along with protection of the unconscious patient and allowing for the natural washout effect with time.[55,56,58] The use of inhaled beta-agonists, such as salbutamol, can assist in the severe bronchospasm resulting from the inhalation of irritants.[58] There has also been a reported benefit of using aerosolised heparin, which acts as a mucolytic to help prevent the build-up of secretions.[55,59] Fibre-optic bronchoscopy can also be effective in lavaging when physical therapy and pharmacological agents still fail to expectorate secretions.[55]

It must be noted that several studies have shown that the patient's fluid requirement is increased when an inhalation injury is present.[11,55]

TABLE 49.1 CARBON MONOXIDE INTOXICATION

CARBOXYHAEMOGLOBIN (COHb) %	SYMPTOMS
0-15	None (smokers, long-distance truck drivers)
15-20	Headache, confusion
20-40	Nausea, fatigue, disorientation, irritability
40-60	Hallucinations, ataxia, syncope, convulsions, coma
> 60	Death

PRACTICE TIPS

- Always consider the possibility of airway injury.
- Warmed, humidified, supplemental oxygen will benefit most patients, especially those with a major burn injury.

BURN WOUND ASSESSMENT AND MANAGEMENT

DEPTH

Burn depth is classified in Australia and Aotearoa New Zealand via the following system, depending on the depth of tissue damage:

- epidermal
- superficial dermal
- mid-dermal
- deep dermal
- full thickness.

It is important to remember, however, that all burns are a mixture of different depths. Refer to Table 49.2 and Fig. 49.6 for diagnosis of burn depth.

WOUND MANAGEMENT

The fundamental aim of all burn-care management is to achieve wound closure in a timely fashion with minimal complications. This is dependent on wound care, good nutrition, maintenance of function, oedema reduction, prevention of infection and adequate analgesia (see Chapter 16 for a discussion on types of wound management).

Wound care should promote spontaneous healing, prevent further tissue loss, prevent infection, provide optimal conditions for surgery if required and be as painless as possible.[62,63]

Debridement of the burn wound removes devitalised tissue from the wound and is an important measure in the promotion of wound healing. It reduces the wound's biological burden, clearing the debris that slows cellular movement necessary for healing and minimising infection.[62,63]

Warm and moist wound-healing principles are well supported; a burn dressing aims to protect the wound, provide patient comfort and function and reduce evaporative losses. There are many varieties of dressings available, including: silver dressings, foams, hydrofibres, calcium alginates, hydrocolloids, hydrogels, polyurethane-membrane-supported gels, film dressings and biological dressings. Different products seem to work in different centres, with contributing factors including patient demographics, local environment and product availability. The

TABLE 49.2 DIAGNOSIS OF BURN DEPTH[60]

DEPTH	COLOUR	BLISTERS	CAPILLARY REFILL	SENSATION	HEALING
Epidermal	Red	No	Present	Present	Yes
Superficial dermal	Pale pink	Small	Present	Painful	Yes
Mid-dermal	Dark pink	Present	Sluggish	±	Usual
Deep dermal	Blotchy red	±	Absent	Absent	No
Full thickness	White	No	Absent	Absent	No

±: may or may not be present.

FIGURE 49.6 BURNS OF VARYING TISSUE DEPTHS[61]

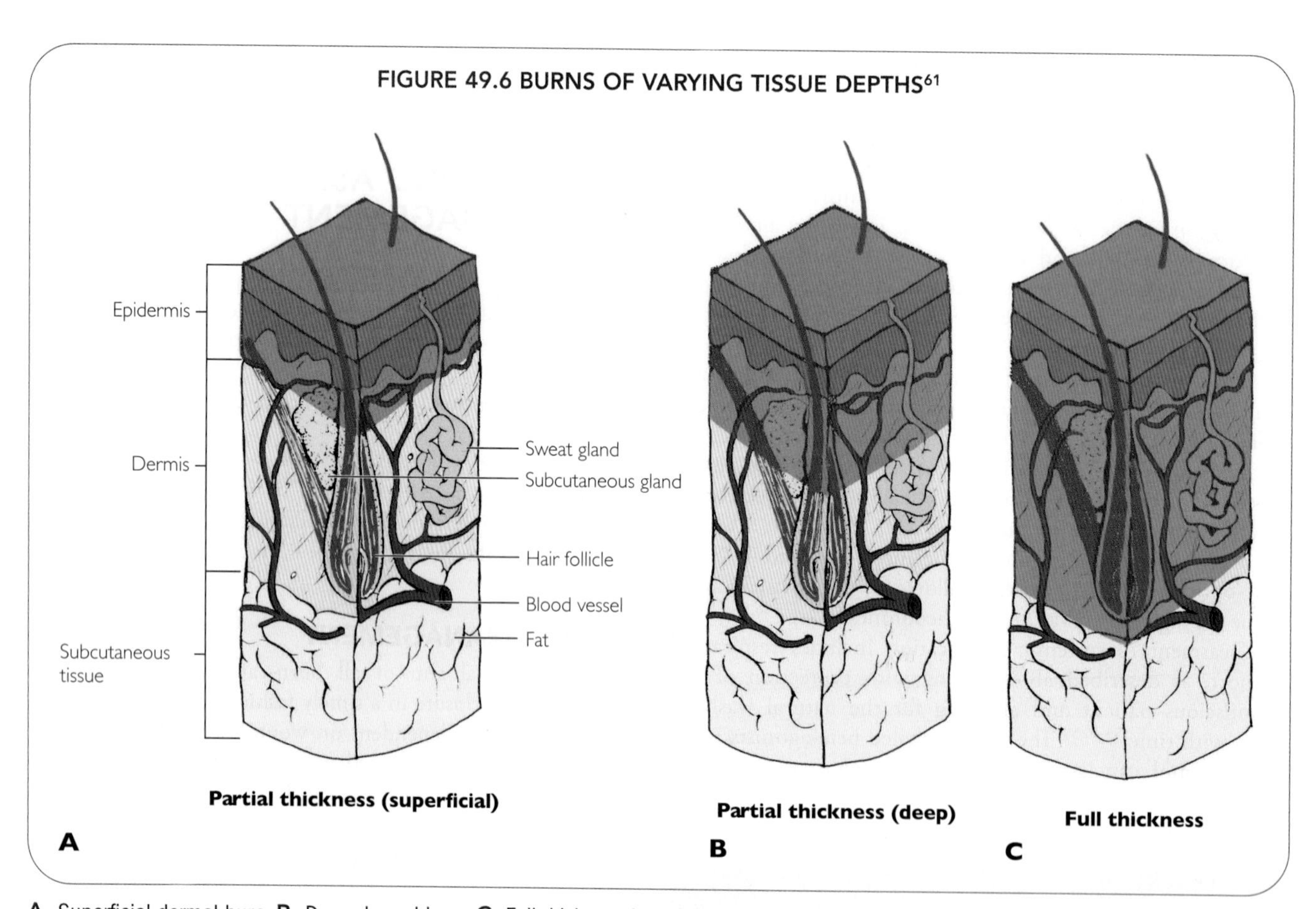

A. Superficial dermal burn. **B.** Deep dermal burn. **C.** Full-thickness burn injury.

important factors that need to be considered when selecting a suitable dressing are:

- depth of the burn (determines amount of exudate)
- site of the burn
- extent of the burn
- possibility of removing dressing without traumatising tissue
- type of burn first aid (e.g. cooling of burn in dirty river water may increase the risk of infection)
- cause of the burn (burns caused by flammable liquids or hot oil have a high risk of infection)
- whether it protects against mechanical trauma
- how functional and manageable it is by the patient (or caregiver), especially if managed in an ambulatory setting
- cost.

In the case of a patient who requires transfer to a burns unit, the wounds should be gently washed with chlorhexidine solution or normal saline and covered with cling wrap or a clean, dry sheet. Care must be taken not to wrap cling wrap around circumferential burns; lay it lengthways so as not to further restrict circulation. Advice on burn wound management will be discussed by consultation with the receiving burns unit, especially if transfer is going to be delayed. Advice on burn wound treatment for all burns can be gained through contact with your referral burns unit irrespective of the need for transfer.

SPECIFIC BURN MANAGEMENT

Epidermal/superficial dermal burns

The very superficial burn or epidermal burn that has no epidermal loss requires no dressing management. Sunburns or flash injuries typically fall into this category, and can be treated with a moisturising cream and pain relief as they are extremely painful.

Superficial dermal burns that involve skin loss can be treated with a variety of wound-care products that aim at encouraging re-epithelisation. These include hydrocolloids, foam dressings and calcium alginates.

An antimicrobial may need to be considered if infection is present or suspected.

PARTIAL-THICKNESS BURNS

Burns in this category include mid-dermal and deep dermal, depending on the extent of injury. After initial wound debridement—removing all devitalised skin, including blisters—these burns can be managed with products from the following groups:

- hydrocolloid
- foam dressings
- calcium alginates
- silver dressings.

Specialised burns units may also utilise temporary skin substitutes, such as Biobrane, for mid-to-deep dermal burns.

FULL-THICKNESS BURNS

Full-thickness burn injuries involve both the epidermal and the dermal layers, extending to the subcutaneous fat, and consequently require antibacterial dressings. The most common antibacterial dressings used in burn-care contain silver, and there are several varieties available. The choice of product is guided by the same principles as for any dressing. Full-thickness burn injuries require surgical intervention unless they are of limited size, and require referral to a specialised burns unit for ongoing treatment.

CIRCUMFERENTIAL BURNS

A deep dermal or full-thickness burn loses the ability to expand as oedema progresses. When the burn involves the whole of a limb or the chest, it may become necessary to release the burn wound surgically by incising the burned skin down to the subcutaneous fat. This procedure is known as an escharotomy (Fig. 49.7). If transfer to a burns unit is going to be delayed, this may have to be performed by the referral centre following consultation and advice.

Limbs

When a limb is burned circumferentially the rigid burned skin may interfere with circulation. Affected limbs must be elevated to limit swelling and closely observed for:

- deep pain at rest
- pain on passive movement of distal joints
- loss of distal circulation
- pallor
- decrease of capillary return
- coolness
- loss of palpable pulses
- numbness
- decrease in oxygen saturations.

FIGURE 49.7 PLACEMENT OF ESCHAROTOMIES

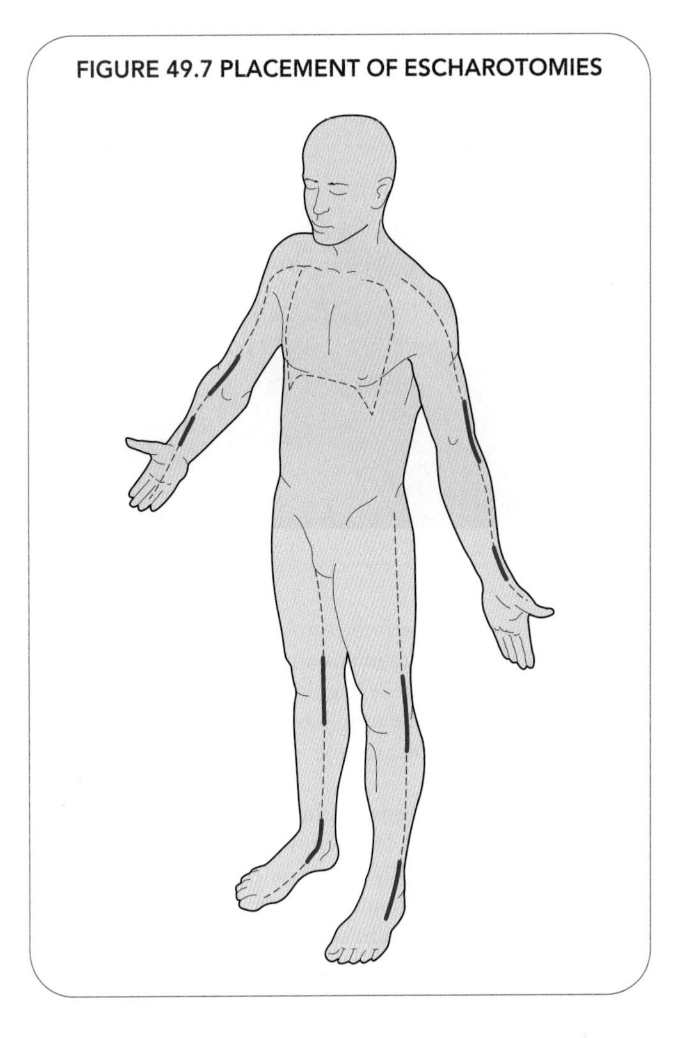

PRACTICE TIPS

- Initial appearances can be very deceiving: never reassure patients or relatives that the burn is 'just superficial and will heal in a few days'.
- Early escharotomy can be limb-saving.

ELECTRICAL BURNS

Electrical burns account for between 2% and 10% of all burn injuries.[64,65] As a result of occupational exposure, they remain more common in adults.[65,66] Traditionally, these burns have been classified by voltage, whether high (greater than 1000 V, including lightning burns) or low (less than 1000 V), although this may not necessarily reflect injury severity.[67] High-voltage injuries may be associated with cardiac or respiratory arrest at the scene.[11,65] In a number of cases, reported electrical burns may in fact represent a flash or flame burn as a result of a short-circuit in a high voltage supply.[68]

True electrical burns are characteristically full thickness and associated with an entry and exit site. A careful examination of

FIGURE 49.8 ELECTRICAL BURN INJURY[69]

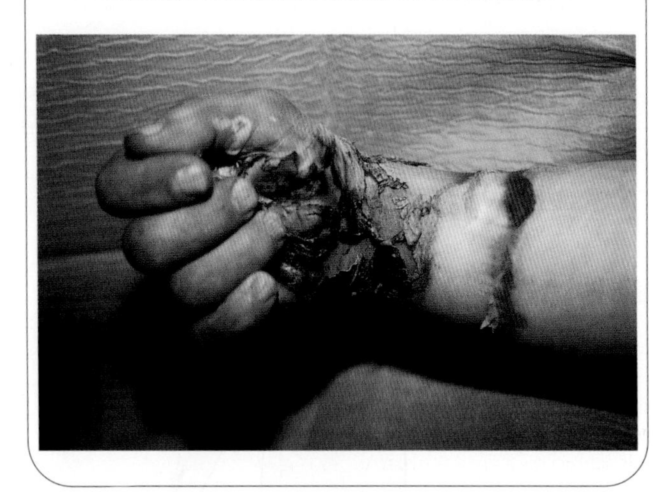

the patient should be performed to determine the location of both sites, as this provides important information on the likely path of the electrical current (Fig. 49.8). Those that have passed along a limb or across the torso have a greater risk of injury to deeper structures, compartment syndrome and myocardial dysrhythmias.[67,70]

While ECG monitoring has been generally recommended for 24 hours post-injury in patients with electrical burns, the risk of haemodynamically significant dysrhythmias would appear very low after 4 hours.[11,64,65] As a result of the greater heating effect of the electrical current on high-resistance structures such as bone, termed the Joule effect, apparently minor superficial electrical burns may be associated with extensive muscle oedema leading to compartment syndrome and, potentially, renal failure from secondary myoglobinuria.[11,65,67] As the risk of complications and associated injuries remains high, all patients with an electrical burn injury should be transferred to a burns unit.[11]

PRACTICE TIP

Ensure personal safety first in patients with electrical and chemical burns.

CHEMICAL BURNS

Chemical burns make up a small number of burn injuries seen, particularly in children.[71] Chemical burns, like all burn injuries, cause a denaturation of cell protein. The denaturation in burn injury may be due to heat, changes in pH or dissolution of lipids. Chemical burns can cause progressive damage until the chemical is inactivated. The severity of this type of burn depends on the type of chemical, strength of the agent, quantity, length of exposure, amount of tissue involved and the mechanism of action. Skin damage can range from erythema through to necrosis. There are three categories of chemical agents:

1. alkalis—producing liquefaction necrosis and loosening of tissue
2. acids—producing coagulative necrosis and precipitation of protein
3. organic compounds—causing chemical and systemic effects.[71,72]

Alkaline agents generally cause more tissue damage than acids, although paradoxically acid burns are at least initially more painful, with the destructive effects of alkali burns occurring more slowly over time. The first aid for chemical burns involves removing the agent from contact with the patient. It is important to ensure the protection of the first aid providers. Caution must be exercised so as not to cause damage to uninjured tissue by an inadvertent spread of the chemical agent. Dry powders should be brushed off before irrigation is commenced. Chemical burns require copious lavage, and irrigation may need to continue anywhere from 30 minutes to 2 hours, or until pain resulting from the chemical injury ceases. Alkali burns particularly require prolonged irrigation, generally for at least 1 hour.[11]

Hydrofluoric acid has several industrial applications such as metal cleaning, floor and wall cleaning and etching, etching silicon in semiconductor manufacture and glass etching. It is occasionally used in a domestic setting to clean alloy wheels and requires special mention because of its unique and rapid toxicity, even when only a very small TBSA has been involved.[73] The fluorine binds calcium ions, causing a profound hypocalcaemia, which leads to dysrhythmias and death. While irrigation with water should still be performed, calcium gluconate is a specific antidote, preferentially binding the free fluoride ions. It may be used topically as a gel, or given IV, with complete relief of pain the best indicator that adequate treatment has been provided.[11,73]

Interestingly, petrol may cause a chemical burn even when ignition has not occurred. While these burns are typically only partial-thickness, they may be readily avoided by prompt irrigation of all areas exposed.

Ingestion or aspiration of corrosive agents is really beyond the scope of this text, but fortunately has become much less frequent in Australasia as a result of improvements in prevention through the use of child-proof containers.[74] While such injuries remain more common in children, typically they now occur when an adult has elected to store a usually alkaline corrosive agent in a recycled drinks container. As with all alkaline burns, the severity of the injury will usually not initially be appreciated. All such patients should be carefully evaluated clinically and should have both chest and abdominal radiography performed to exclude free air from a perforation. Subsequent endoscopy to assess the pharynx, oesophagus and stomach should be performed, as the absence of intraoral burns does not necessarily exclude a clinically important injury of the aerodigestive tract. While IV steroids may be of benefit in reducing the inflammatory element of inhalational chemical burns, they appear to be of no proven benefit following caustic ingestion.[75]

BITUMEN AND FRICTION BURNS

Hot bitumen burns typically occur as an occupational injury. Immediate BFAT with cold running water should be applied, but no attempt made to physically remove the bitumen in the field, as this may cause further injury.[11] Subsequently, paraffin oil should be applied and the bitumen removed mechanically as part of a surgical debridement.

Friction burns may be seen in both adults and children, often as a result of falls from bicycles onto the road, pedestrian versus motor vehicle trauma or entrapment in a home treadmill.[76] With increasing use of exercise equipment at home, these injuries continue to occur despite prevention programs. The depth of these burns is often very difficult to appreciate initially and there may be underlying neurovascular or tendon involvement, especially in children. Wound management for these injuries is dependent on depth assessment and other considerations, as with all burn wounds.

EYES

Unless the mechanism of injury can rule out eye damage; for example, an isolated contact burn, all facial burns need to undergo an eye examination.[11] This is especially imperative in chemical injuries, which require copious irrigation with water for up to 3 hours.[71] Contact lenses, if worn, should be removed, as chemicals can track behind the lens and damage the cornea. Irrigation should continue after lens removal. Early eye examination using staining with fluorescein eye drops can detect any corneal damage before the resultant oedema makes it difficult and even impossible to perform.

BURNS IN CHILDREN

Burns in children remain distinct from those in adults as a result of physiological differences, psychological aspects in relation to the response to the injury, and important variations in aetiology and their impact on likely outcomes (see Chapter 35).[12,13] While the overall approach and management strategies remain the same, an understanding of the differences will facilitate improved outcomes in this important group of patients for whom the consequences of the injury may be lifelong.

AETIOLOGY AND PREVENTION OF BURNS IN CHILDREN

The predominance of scald injuries in children has been well documented, reflecting the propensity of toddlers exploring the home environment to sustain burn injuries while poorly supervised.[77,78] Approximately two-thirds of burn injuries in children will involve toddlers or preschool-age children with scald burns to the head, neck, upper torso and arms (Fig. 49.9).[21,29,77,78] Typically these burns will be mixed depth, with the child's relatively thin skin predisposing them to a proportionally deeper burn in relation to that suffered by an adult following exposure to the same hot liquid for the same time.[14] These same differences make accurate prediction of burn wound outcome problematic in children, stimulating the development of new technologies to determine the need for operative surgical intervention in deep burns.[79] Great caution should be exercised by first responders and all clinicians involved in the initial care of these patients regarding falsely reassuring parents or carers over the likely depth of the burn.

FIGURE 49.9 PAEDIATRIC SCALD BURN

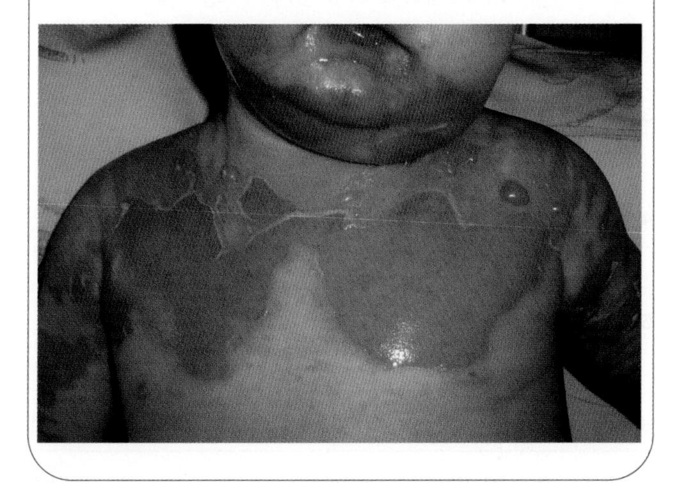

South Australia Health. Women's and Children's Health Network. 2014.

In addition to their propensity for scald burns, children remain at risk of several specific forms of burn injury infrequently seen in adults, including burns as a result of non-accidental injury. These include friction burns from home treadmills, hot noodle burns and those resulting from contact with inadequately insulated reflective oven doors, all recently identified as major sources of morbidity in the paediatric age group.[75,80–83] As with scald burns, prevention has been shown to be effective, but remains only sporadically applied and requiring constant re-enforcement.[76,83–86] Nursing, paramedic and allied health professionals remain uniquely positioned to influence the approach of parents and older children to this important issue.[23]

Health professionals need to show that they understand how difficult it is to watch a child constantly and how demanding it is to keep children safe.

It is not the task of health professionals to evaluate the probability of abuse and neglect. It is part of the burns assessment, however, to attempt to fully understand how the injury happened, so as to help reduce the risks of similar injuries to other children.

Any suspicion of neglect or an inflicted injury requires reporting to the appropriate mandatory body.

Indicators for a possible non-accidental burn

- Delay in seeking help.
- Different accounts of history of injury over time.
- Injury inconsistent with history or with the development capacity of the child.
- Past abuse or family violence.
- Inappropriate behaviour/interaction of child or caregivers.
- Obvious immersion patterns; for example, glove or sock patterns.
- Symmetrical burns of uniform depth.
- Restraint injuries on upper arms.
- Other signs of abuse or neglect such as numerous healed wounds.

RESPONSE TO BURN INJURY IN CHILDREN

The normal response in an adult would be to first avoid an obvious source of burn injury. Second, if suffering a burn, the adult would immediately withdraw and instinctively cool the burn. These three responses remain at best infrequent in children: in addition to unguarded exploration of their environment, preschool-age children will often simply cry out when sustaining a burn rather than withdraw from the painful stimulus. This predisposes them to a longer duration and therefore a deeper burn. These behavioural differences highlight the special importance of the first responder and paramedic in applying optimal BFAT for the paediatric burns patient.[8,14,35]

MANAGEMENT OF BURN INJURIES IN CHILDREN

As a result of their greater ratio of surface area to bodyweight, children have a proportionally greater metabolic rate and higher rates of water and heat loss than adults. A greater proportion of their total body water remains extracellular, further increasing fluid losses in burn injury. In addition, their compensatory mechanisms, such as shivering, are either reduced or much less effective, especially in the infant and toddler age groups. As a result, they are more likely to suffer hypothermia following a burn injury, and require resuscitation with IV fluids and nutritional support. Thus children with > 10% TBSA burns will require IV fluids and nutritional supplementation, usually initially via a gastric tube.[11] In addition to resuscitation fluids, children will require maintenance fluids with glucose to avoid hypoglycaemia (Box 49.4).[11,87] The predominantly diaphragmatic nature of breathing in children increases the likelihood of the need for an escharotomy of a chest or upper abdominal burn to permit adequate ventilation.

Just as there are differences in treatment, there are several differences in relation to monitoring the paediatric burn patient. Due to their usually normal cardiovascular system and enhanced reserves, but potentially rapid decline into shock, assessment of hypovolaemia requires a multimodal approach rather than a reliance on blood pressure and pulse alone.[11,39] In particular, skin colour, temperature and capillary refill should be frequently assessed in addition to urine output as a guide to the patient's status and response to resuscitation.[11,39]

BOX 49.4 IV FLUIDS IN PAEDIATRIC BURNS

- **Give resuscitation and maintenance fluids if the burn is > 10% TBSA**
- **Resuscitation fluids follow adult formula**
- **Maintenance fluids of 5% dextrose and 0.45% normal saline over the first 24 hours:**
  - **100 mL/kg up to 10 kg**
  - **plus 50 mL/kg from 10 to 20 kg**
  - **plus 20 mL/kg for each kg over 20 kg**
- **Monitor blood pressure, pulse and capillary refill**
- **Aim for urine output of 1.0 mL/kg/h**

TBSA: total body surface area.

SUMMARY

Burns represent a potentially devastating form of trauma with important long-term consequences. Optimal first aid and initial medical management, including securing the airway and ensuring appropriate fluid resuscitation, may make a significant positive impact in reducing the need for operative intervention and subsequent scarring. Just as a major burn may involve every organ system, so too will patients benefit from optimal management through the coordinated efforts of a multidisciplinary care team.

CASE STUDY 1

You have been called to the scene of a 20-year-old man weighing 80 kg after he sustained a flame burn. The injury occurred when his older brother threw petrol onto a camp fire, which ignited fuel vapour. He has burns to the front and backs of both legs and his abdomen.

QUESTIONS

1. Outline your initial examination of this patient.

SECONDARY SURVEY

2. Using the information below, calculate the total body surface (TBSA) area of this burn injury. You may want to use a body chart to assist you.

   Both legs: whole fronts of thigh and leg = 18%

   Backs of legs to mid-thigh = 18%

   Abdomen: below umbilicus to groin = 9%
3. Use your answer above to calculate the fluid requirements of this patient. How do you monitor the adequacy of the fluids?
4. During your examination you note circumferential burns to both legs. What does this indicate? What observations need to be carried out?
5. Your secondary survey reveals no further injury, and transfer to a burns unit is advised. Outline the reasons for transfer.
6. What wound care is required prior to transfer?

Answers to Case Study Questions can be found on evolve http://evolve.elsevier.com/AU/Curtis/emergency/ 

CASE STUDY 2

Using the Parkland formula, calculate the fluid resuscitation required for a 12 kg 17-month-old who sustained a 25% scald to her face, neck, chest, abdomen and thighs when she pulled a kettle of hot water onto herself this morning at 0930. You are called to the scene immediately. When you arrive the father is in the shower with the child.

QUESTIONS

1. Outline your initial response.
2. Calculate the fluid resuscitation using the Parkland formula.
3. Calculate the maintenance fluids with 5% dextrose and 0.45% normal saline.

Answers to Case Study Questions can be found on evolve http://evolve.elsevier.com/AU/Curtis/emergency/ 

USEFUL WEBSITES

Australian and New Zealand Burn Association (ANZBA), www.anzba.org.au/.

International Society for Burn Injuries (ISBI), www.worldburn.org/.

ANZBA and ISBI are both not-for-profit organisations for the body for health professionals responsible for the care of the burn injured. These websites provide information on available educational opportunities.

World Health Organization (WHO), www.who.int/.

REFERENCES

1. World Health Organization (WHO). Fact sheet: burns. Available from: www.who.int/en/news-room/fact-sheets/detail/burns.
2. Meyer AA. Death and disability from injury: a global challenge. J Trauma 1998;44(1):1–12.
3. Burd A, Yuen C. A global study of hospitalized paediatric burn patients. Burns 2005;31(4):432–8.
4. Jackson DM. The diagnosis of the depth of burning. Br J Surg 1953;40(64):588–96.
5. Burns Registry of Australia and New Zealand. Annual Report 2019–20. Department of Epidemiology and Preventive Medicine. Melbourne, Australia: Monash University; 2021.
6. D'Cruz R, Martin HC, Holland AJ. Medical management of paediatric burn injuries: best practice part 2. J Paediat Child Health 2013;49(9): E397–404.
7. Barrett LW, Fear VS, Waithman JC, Wood FM, Fear MW. Understanding acute burn injury as a chronic disease. Burns Trauma 2019;7:23.
8. Allison K. The UK pre-hospital management of burn patients: current practice and the need for a standard approach. Burns 2002;28(2):135–42.
9. Allison K, Porter K. Consensus on the pre-hospital approach to burns patient management. Injury 2004;35(8):734–8.
10. Pruitt BAJ, Goodwin CW, Mason Jr AD, editors. Epidemiological, demographic, and outcome characteristics of burn injury. London: Saunders; 2002.
11. Committee TE, editor. Emergency manual of severe burns course manual. 15th ed. Albany Creek: ANZBA; 2011.
12. Spinks A, Wasiak J, Cleland H, Beben N, Macpherson AK. Ten-year epidemiological study of pediatric burns in Canada. J Burn Care Res 2008; 29(3):482–8.
13. Tse T, Poon CH, Tse KH, Tsui TK, Ayyappan T, Burd A. Paediatric burn prevention: an epidemiological approach. Burns 2006;32(2):229–34.
14. Holland AJ. Pediatric burns: the forgotten trauma of childhood. Can J Surg 2006;49(4):272–7.
15. Forjuoh SN. Burns in low- and middle-income countries: a review of available literature on descriptive epidemiology, risk factors, treatment, and prevention. Burns 2006;32(5):529–37.
16. Foglia RP, Moushey R, Meadows L, Seigel J, Smith M. Evolving treatment in a decade of pediatric burn care. J Pediatr Surg 2004;39(6):957–60.
17. Forjuoh SN. The mechanisms, intensity of treatment, and outcomes of hospitalized burns: issues for prevention. J Burn Care Rehab 1998;19(5): 456–60.
18. den Hertog PC, Blankendaal FA, ten Hag SM. Burn injuries in The Netherlands. Accid Anal Prev 2000;32(3):355–64.
19. Hettiaratchy S, Dziewulski P. ABC of burns. Introduction. BMJ 2004;328(7452):1366–8.
20. Abeyasundara SL, Rajan V, Lam L, Harvey JG, Holland AJ. The changing pattern of pediatric burns. J Burn Care Res 2011;32(2):178–84.
21. Rea S, Kuthubutheen J, Fowler B, Wood F. Burn first aid in Western Australia–do healthcare workers have the knowledge? Burns 2005;31(8): 1029–34.
22. Burgess JD, Watt KA, Kimble RM, Cameron CM. Knowledge of childhood burn risks and burn first aid: Cool Runnings. Inj Prev 2019;25:301–6.

23. Rutan RL, editor. Physiological response to cutaneous burn injury. Missouri: Mosby; 1998.
24. Williams WG, editor. Pathophysiology of the burn wound. London: Saunders; 2002.
25. Norbury WB, Herndon DN, editors. Modulation of the hypermetabolic response after burn injury. Philadelphia: Saunders Elsevier; 2007.
26. Williams FN, Herndon DN, Kulp GA, Jeschke MG. Propranolol decreases cardiac work in a dose-dependent manner in severely burned children. Surgery 2011;149(2):231–9.
27. Beierle EA, Chung DH, editors. Surgical management of complications of burn injury. Philadelphia: Saunders Elsevier; 2007.
28. Mlcak RP, Buffalo MC, editors. Pre-hospital management, transportation, and emergency care. Philadelphia: Saunders Elsevier; 2007.
29. Kim LK, Martin HC, Holland AJ. Medical management of paediatric burn injuries: best practice. J Paediat Child Health 2012;48(4):290–5.
30. Nguyen NL, Gun RT, Sparnon AL, Ryan P. The importance of immediate cooling–a case series of childhood burns in Vietnam. Burns 2002;28(2):173–6.
31. Yuan J, Wu C, Holland AJ, Harvey JG, Martin HC, La Hei ER, et al. Assessment of cooling on an acute scald burn injury in a porcine model. J Burn Care Res 2007;28(3):514–20.
32. Cuttle L, Pearn J, McMillan JR, Kimble RM. A review of first aid treatments for burn injuries. Burns 2009;35(6):768–75.
33. Bartlett N, Yuan J, Holland AJ, Harvey JG, Martin HC, La Hei ER, et al. Optimal duration of cooling for an acute scald contact burn injury in a porcine model. J Burn Care Res 2008;29(5):828–34.
34. Rajan V, Bartlett N, Harvey JG, Martin HC, La Hei ER, Arbuckle S, et al. Delayed cooling of an acute scald contact burn injury in a porcine model: is it worthwhile? J Burn Care Res 2009;30(4):729–34.
35. McCormack RA, La Hei ER, Martin HC. First-aid management of minor burns in children: a prospective study of children presenting to the Children's Hospital at Westmead, Sydney. MJA 2003;178(1):31–3.
36. O'Neill AC, Purcell E, Jones D, Pasha N, McCann J, Regan P. Inadequacies in the first aid management of burns presenting to plastic surgery services. Irish Med J 2005;98(1):15–16.
37. Cuttle L, Kempf M, Kravchuk O, George N, Liu PY, Chang HE, et al. The efficacy of Aloe vera, tea tree oil and saliva as first aid treatment for partial thickness burn injuries. Burns 2008;34(8):1176–82.
38. Price J. Burnaid. Burns 1998;24(1):80–2.
39. DeBoer S, O'Connor A. Prehospital and emergency department burn care. Crit Care Nurs Clin North Am 2004;16(1):61–73.
40. Sanchez JL, Pereperez SB, Bastida JL, Martínez MM. Cost-utility analysis applied to the treatment of burn patients in a specialized center. Arch Surg (Chicago, Ill. 1960) 2007;142(1):50–7.
41. Wong K, Heath T, Maitz P, Kennedy P. Early in-hospital management of burn injuries in Australia. ANZ J Surg 2004;74(5):318–23.
42. Greenwood JE, Tee R, Jackson WL. Increasing numbers of admissions to the adult burns service at the Royal Adelaide Hospital 2001-2004. ANZ J Surg 2007;77(5):358–63.
43. Holland AJ, Jackson AM, Joseph AP. Paediatric trauma at an adult trauma centre. ANZ J Surg 2005;75(10):878–81.
44. Freiburg C, Igneri P, Sartorelli K, Rogers F. Effects of differences in percent total body surface area estimation on fluid resuscitation of transferred burn patients. J Burn Care Res 2007;28(1):42–8.
45. Chan QE, Barzi F, Cheney L, Harvey JG, Holland AJ. Burn size estimation in children: still a problem. Emerg Med Australas 2012;24(2):181–6.
46. Kramer GC, Lund T, Beckum OK, editors. Pathophysiology of burn shock and burn oedema. Philadelphia: Saunders Elsevier; 2007.
47. Perry V, Teague WJ. Same formula, different philosophy: more mindful use of the Modified Parkland Formula in severe burns. ANZ J Surg 2021; 91(4):490–2.
48. Hettiaratchy S, Papini R. Initial management of a major burn: II—assessment and resuscitation. Br Med J 2004;329(7457):101–3.
49. Elliot D, Aitken L, Chaboyer W, editors. ACCCN's critical care nursing. Sydney: Elsevier; 2006.
50. Hawley R, King J. Australian nurses' dictionary. 3rd ed. Sydney: Baillière Tindall; 2004.
51. Morris R, Javed M, Bodger O, Hemington Gorse S, Williams D. A comparison of two smartphone applications and the validation of smartphone applications as tools for fluid calculation for burns resuscitation. Burns 2014;40(5):826–34.
52. Woodson LC. Diagnosis and grading of inhalation injury. J Burn Care Res 2009;30(1):143–5.
53. Palmieri TL. Inhalation injury consensus conference: conclusions. J Burn Care Res 2009;30(1):209–10.
54. Medhat EH. Initial burn management. Austin J Surg 2014;1(2):1010. CC BY 4.0 License.
55. Toon MH, Maybauer MO, Greenwood JE, Maybauer DM, Fraser JF. Management of acute smoke inhalation injury. Crit Care Resusc 2010;12(1):53–61.
56. Fidkowski CW, Fuzaylov G, Sheridan RL, Coté CJ. Inhalation burn injury in children. Paediat Anaesth 2009;19(Suppl. 1):147–54.
57. Palmieri TL, Warner P, Mlcak RP, Sheridan R, Kagan RJ, Herndon DN, et al. Inhalation injury in children: a 10-year experience at Shriners Hospitals for Children. J Burn Care Res 2009;30(1):206–8.
58. Palmieri TL. Use of beta-agonists in inhalation injury. J Burn Care Res 2009;30(1):156–9.
59. Palmieri TL, Enkhbaatar P, Sheridan R, Traber DL, Greenhalgh DG. Studies of inhaled agents in inhalation injury. J Burn Care Res 2009;30(1):169–71.
60. Australia and New Zealand Burns Association. Emergency manual of severe burns: course manual (pamphlet). 10th ed. Albany Creek, Queensland: ANZBA; 2006.

61. Edlich R, Bailey T, Bill T, editors. Thermal burns. 5th ed. St. Louis: Mosby; 2002.
62. Kavanagh S, McRae S. Burns nursing study guides. Adelaide: University of Adelaide; 2005.
63. Alsbjorn B, Gilbert P, Hartmann B, Kaźmierski M, Monstrey S, Palao R, et al. Guidelines for the management of partial-thickness burns in a general hospital or community setting–recommendations of a European working party. Burns 2007;33(2):155-60.
64. Tomkins KL, Holland AJ. Electrical burn injuries in children. J Paediat Child Health 2008;44(12):727-30.
65. Rai J, Jeschke MG, Barrow RE, Herndon DN. Electrical injuries: a 30-year review. J Trauma 1999;46(5):933-6.
66. Arnoldo B, Klein M, Gibran NS. Practice guidelines for the management of electrical injuries. J Burn Care Res 2006;27(4):439-47.
67. Lee RC, editor. The pathophysiology and clinical management of electrical injury. Cambridge: Cambridge University Press; 1992.
68. Fordyce TA, Kelsh M, Lu ET, Sahl JD, Yager JW. Thermal burns and electrical injuries among electric utility workers, 1995–2004. Burns 2007;33: 209–20.
69. Barret JP, Herndon DN, editors. Color atlas of burn care. St Louis: WB Saunders; 2001.
70. Maghsoudi H, Adyani Y, Ahmadian N. Electrical and lightning injuries. J Burn Care Res 2007;28(2):255-61.
71. Nguyen AT, Chamberlain K, Holland AJ. Paediatric chemical burns: a clinical review. Eur J Pediatr 2021;180:1359-69.
72. Hardwicke J, Hunter T, Staruch R, Moiemen N. Chemical burns—an historical comparison and review of the literature. Burns 2012;38(3):383-7.
73. Wang X, Zhang Y, Ni L, You C, Ye C, Jiang R, et al. A review of treatment strategies for hydrofluoric acid burns: current status and future prospects. Burns 2014;40(8):1447-57.
74. Riffat F, Cheng A. Pediatric caustic ingestion: 50 consecutive cases and a review of the literature. Dis Esophagus 2009;22(1):89-94.
75. Fulton JA, Hoffman RS. Steroids in second degree caustic burns of the esophagus: a systematic pooled analysis of fifty years of human data: 1956–2006. Clin Toxicol (Philadelphia, Pa.) 2007;45(4):402–8.
76. Waltzman ML, Lee LK, Ozonoff A, Kupiec JK, Landschaft A, Kimia AA. Treadmill injuries in children. Am J Emerg Med 2021;46:495–8.
77. Eadie PA, Williams R, Dickson WA. Thirty-five years of paediatric scalds: are lessons being learned? Br J Plas Surg 1995;48(2):103–5.
78. Dewar DJ, Magson CL, Fraser JF, Crighton L, Kimble RM. Hot beverage scalds in Australian children. J Burn Care Rehab 2004;25(3):224–7.
79. Holland AJ, Martin HC, Cass DT. Laser Doppler imaging prediction of burn wound outcome in children. Burns 2002;28(1):11–17.
80. Jeremijenko L, Mott J, Wallis B, Kimble R. Paediatric treadmill friction injuries. J Paediat Child Health 2009;45(5):310–12.
81. Choo KL, Wallis B, Jain A, Ryan AB, Kimble RM. Too hot to handle: instant noodle burns in children. J Burn Care Res 2008;29(2):421–2.
82. Yen KL, Bank DE, O'Neill AM, Yurt RW. Household oven doors: a burn hazard in children. Arch Pediat Adolesc Med 2001;155(1):84–6.
83. Atiyeh BS, Costagliola M, Hayek SN. Burn prevention mechanisms and outcomes: pitfalls, failures and successes. Burns 2009;35(2):181–93.
84. Cagle KM, Davis JW, Dominic W, Gonzales W. Results of a focused scald-prevention program. J Burn Care Res 2006;27(6):859–63.
85. Spallek M, Nixon J, Bain C, Purdie DM, Spinks A, Scott D, et al. Scald prevention campaigns: do they work? J Burn Care Res 2007;28(2):328–33.
86. Durand MA, Green J, Edwards P, Milton S, Lutchmun S. Perceptions of tap water temperatures, scald risk and prevention among parents and older people in social housing: a qualitative study. Burns 2012;38(4):585–90.
87. Mlcak R, Cortiella J, Desai MH, Herndon DN. Emergency management of pediatric burn victims. Pediat Emerg Care 1998;14(1):51–4.

INDEX

A

C

D

E

F

I

Q

R

S